Fundamentals of Diagnostic Radiology

Second Edition

Fundamentals of Diagnostic Radiology
Second Edition

Edited by

William E. Brant, MD

Professor of Radiology
Department of Radiology
University of California, Davis
School of Medicine
Sacramento, California

Clyde A. Helms, MD

Professor of Radiology
Department of Radiology
Duke University Medical Center
Durham, North Carolina

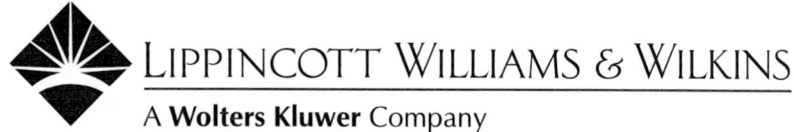
LIPPINCOTT WILLIAMS & WILKINS
A **Wolters Kluwer** Company
Philadelphia · Baltimore · New York · London
Buenos Aires · Hong Kong · Sydney · Tokyo

Editor: Charles W. Mitchell
Managing Editor: Grace E. Miller
Marketing Manager: Peter Darcy
Project Editor: Lisa J. Franko
Design Coordinator: Mario Fernandez

Copyright © 1999 Williams & Wilkins. Copyright is not claimed for Chapters 5, 56, 58, and 60-63, which were written by Federal Government employees. As such, these chapters are in the public domain and cannot be copyrighted. They may be reproduced without permission.

Portions of Section IX are borrowed from Helms: Fundamentals of Skeletal Radiology, 2nd ed., courtesy of W.B. Saunders.

351 West Camden Street
Baltimore, Maryland 21201-2436 USA

LIPPINCOTT WILLIAMS & WILKINS
530 Walnut St.
Philadelphia, PA 19106 USA
LWW.com

Printed in the United States of America

First Edition, 1994

Library of Congress Cataloging-in-Publication Data

Fundamentals of diagnostic radiology / (edited by) William E. Brant,
    Clyde A. Helms. -- 2nd ed.
        p.   cm.
    Includes bibliographical references and index.
    ISBN 0-683-30093-8
    1. Diagnosis, Radioscopic. 2. Diagnostc imaging. I. Brant,
    William E. II. Helms, Clyde A.
    (DNLM: 1. Diagnostic Imaging. WN 180 F981 1999)
    RC78.F86   1999
    616.07'57--dc21
    DNLM/DLC
    for Library of Congress   97-51178
                                                         CIP

The publishers have made every effort to trace the copyright holders for borrowed material. If they have inadvertently overlooked any, they will be pleased to make the necessary arrangements at the first opportunity.

This book is dedicated to my children, Dan, Ryan, Jon, and Rachel, who add so much to the joy of life, and to all residents and medical students whose quest for knowledge adds so much to the joy of teaching.

—WEB

To Nancy Marie Major, my beloved wife, and our son Austin Michael.

—CAH

Foreword to the Second Edition

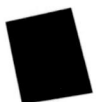

Creating a textbook that captures the essentials of diagnostic radiology and incorporates the broad range of technologic advances that have occurred during the past decade is a prodigious challenge. In their first edition, Drs. Brant and Helms sought to create "a comprehensive, succinct, and modern text" which could be used by beginning students of radiology. They intended it as the "beginning resident's first reader and the graduating resident's 'last reader.' " Clearly this was an ambitious goal but, as indicated by the broad acceptance of this text, one which the editors achieved admirably. The second edition of this text should continue to improve on the excellence of the first edition. All of the chapters have been updated to include the latest developments in diagnostic imaging. A new Section devoted to ultrasound, which was interspersed among many Sections in the first edition, has been created. The editors have retained most of the original authors from the first edition so that the style remains essentially the same. There is little doubt, given the success of the first edition, that this edition will continue to be extremely popular with radiology residents and indeed with any health professional desiring an overview of diagnostic radiology. This book admirably meets its editors goals and is well on its way to becoming a classic in the field.

Carl E. Ravin, MD

Foreword to the First Edition

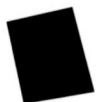

Radiologists are avid readers; the plethora of radiologic texts is a testimony to this fact. Despite the recent push to subspecialization, most of us who teach diagnostic radiology are still approached by residents and students with the request for a recommendation for a good single-volume text. It is expected that such a text would also deal with the new advances in our field such as computed tomography, magnetic resonance imaging, and ultrasound. Until Drs. Brant and Helms undertook this difficult task, there was no easy response to the query for there was no publication that could fulfill these criteria.

The authors have garnered contributions from an outstanding group of radiologists who represent the broad areas of subspecialization and who have presented succinctly the basic elements of their disciplines.

This work fulfills a requirement for those who are contemplating a career in radiology or who are new to the field and desire a broad overview. Drs. Brant and Helms are to be congratulated on recognizing the need and carrying it out in exemplary fashion.

Theodore E. Keats, MD

Preface to the Second Edition

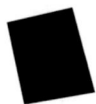

The feedback we have received from radiology residents from the across the country indicates that we have achieved, to a large degree, our goal of providing a useful text to serve as an introduction to learning of radiology as well as a review text for residents preparing for the American Board of Radiology examinations. We have been delighted to learn that a number of training programs recommend, and even provide, our text for their first-year residents. We are very gratified to learn of "Brant & Helms" clubs organized by residents to aid in their study of our exciting specialty. We greatly appreciate the enthusiastic endorsement of many residents and recent graduates of residency who have made many valuable suggestions and given us tremendous encouragement.

We have striven to make this second edition even better than the first. We have been very fortunate to retain nearly all of our outstanding authors who made gifted contributions to the first edition and have added a few new and talented authors for this work. A major change we made at the suggestion of many residents is to provide a separate Section for ultrasound. Thus, the current edition has Sections that correspond to the examination areas of the oral boards in diagnostic radiology. To maintain continuity, short descriptions of ultrasound findings of major lesions have been retained in chapters that review the appearance of lesions on the major imaging modalities. The ultrasound Section includes chapters on abdomen, genital, obstetric, vascular, chest, thyroid, parathyroid, and neonatal brain ultrasound. The chest Section has been reorganized and expanded into 9 chapters with many new illustrations and tables reflecting the exceptional teaching skills of Jeffrey Klein. In the cardiovascular Section, a new chapter on interventional radiology provides an introduction to rapidly maturing and expanding invasive techniques. The nuclear radiology Section has been extensively revised under the leadership of John Baumann working with Frederic Conte. The neuroradiology Section, under the guidance of Erik Gaensler, remains one of our favorites for its concise organization and discussion of complex topics. All the remaining Sections have been updated to reflect the rapid changes in radiology practice, new findings, and better understanding of previously described findings. Many new illustrations have been added and better examples substituted for some of the figures from the first edition.

We once again thank our friends at Williams & Wilkins for their always helpful advice, support, and their very professional guidance and encouragement. Williams & Wilkins provides a whole team of experts, but we specifically acknowledge the excellent work of Charles Mitchell, Grace Miller, and Lisa J. Franko.

William E. Brant
Clyde A. Helms

Preface to the First Edition

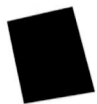

Diagnostic radiology is a captivating specialty with an exploding body of knowledge that overwhelms the neophyte resident, yet must be learned to practice effectively. A wide variety of excellent, and usually, multivolume texts are available for study of each subspecialty area of radiology. What is lacking is a comprehensive, succinct, and modern text that beginning students of radiology can use to achieve that basic framework of knowledge needed to initiate their learning of diagnostic imaging. We wrote this text to provide a complete, yet concise, beginning in radiology. Each Section of this book corresponds to a major subspecialty area on radiology, and deliberately, to categories for examination by the American Board of Radiology.

We visualize this monograph being used in two major fashions. We hope it will become the beginning resident's "first reader" and the graduating resident's "last reader." We provide an overview of the subject matter as residents begin their first rotations on chest or bone or gastrointestinal radiology. A few nights' study of the assigned Section provides a working knowledge of the fundamentals of that topic. Practical clinical experience in their residency will provide the cookbook details of performing each imaging study. Our text provides the basic approach toward interpretation of each study. Once students have mastered the framework of the body of knowledge, they can fill in the details by study of the subspecialty texts and studious attendance at teaching conferences and film reading sessions. By the final year of residency, with radiology board examinations looming, residents want a comprehensive review source that covers everything they "need to know" to pass boards. While there is no way a text of any kind can cover "everything needed to pass boards," we hope this text will resurrect the accumulated knowledge of the residency experience and help the residents to organize it in a memorable and usable fashion that will give them confidence taking the board examinations, and, more importantly, practicing excellent radiology.

To accomplish these lofty goals we have selected as contributors individuals with a proven ability to teach practical, important, patient care-oriented radiology. They know what it takes to be an effective radiologist and they know how to teach it to others. The text emphasizes differential diagnosis and supplements these differential considerations with numerous tables. The tables from all chapters are grouped in a list for easy reference. Each subspecialty of radiology is covered, including nuclear radiology, a topic not contained in most radiology texts.

Ultrasound, rather than being artificially sequestered as a separate Section, is integrated into the Sections identified by body system. This approach allows comparison of ultrasound to the other imaging modalities and more closely simulates the use of ultrasound in daily radiologic practice. Yet, all of the facets of ultrasound examination are covered including obstetrics, small parts, cardiac, and vascular sonography. Nuclear radiology is reviewed as a separate Section as well as being integrated into body system discussions.

We have provided copious illustrations for each chapter. Each figure is comprehensively labeled with an abundance of arrows and letters so the beginning student can readily identify the important findings and orient to the anatomy displayed. We utilize all of the imaging modalities and stress current concepts of their importance in solving each diagnostic problem. Anatomy, as the basis for all diagnostic imaging, is extensively reviewed in the appropriate Sections. While imaging modalities are developed and evolve with frightening speed, the basic principles of interpretation encompassing a firm understanding of anatomy and pathology change little. The latter is what is stressed in this book with examples of some of our best images. We emphasize the concept that a secure knowledge of anatomy and pathology can be applied to nuances of any existing or yet-to-be-developed imaging method to make a confident diagnosis. The student should avoid the concept of learning a check-list of findings for each disease on each imaging modality, but instead should stress understanding the disease process and the clinically applicable physics of each imaging method.

While obviously directed at the resident in diagnostic radiology, we hope that students and practitioners of other specialties will also find this book a useful reference and study guide as they use radiology in diagnosis.

We acknowledge the enthusiastic and professional assistance of personnel at Williams & Wilkins who provided us with constant encouragement and thoughtful suggestions. Tim Grayson, Will Passano, Editor-in-Chief, and Vicki Vaughn, Project Manager, were ardent driving forces promoting this book. Dr. Nancy Major, a resident in diagnostic radiology at the University of California, San Francisco, reviewed each chapter as it was written to provide us with invaluable resident perspective. Her insight resulted in numerous improvements and clarifications, and is deeply appreciated.

William E. Brant
Clyde A. Helms

Contributors

Jerome A. Barakos, MD
Section Chief
Department of Neuroradiology
California Pacific Medical Center
Assistant Clinical Professor
Department of Radiology, Neuroradiology Section
University of California, San Francisco
San Francisco, California

Robert M. Barr, MD
Neuroradiologist
Mecklenburg Radiology Associates
Presbyterian Hospital
Charlotte, North Carolina

John M. Bauman, MD
Chief, Department of Radiology
Madigan Army Medical Center
Tacoma, Washington
Clinical Associate Professor
Uniformed Services University of the Health Sciences
Bethesda, Maryland

Peter W. Blue, MD
Chief, Nuclear Medicine Service
Moncrief Army Community Hospital
Ft. Jackson, South Carolina
Professor of Radiology
University of South Carolina School of Medicine
Columbia, South Carolina

William E. Brant, MD
Professor of Radiology
Department of Radiology
University of California, Davis
School of Medicine
Sacramento, California

Jerrold T. Bushberg, PhD, DABMP
Clinical Associate Professor
Department of Radiology
University of California, Davis
School of Medicine
Sacramento, California

Frederic A. Conte, MD
Chairman, Department of Radiology
David Grant Medical Center
Travis Air Force Base, California

Marc G. Cote, DO, FACP
Chief, Nuclear Medicine Service
Department of Radiology
Madigan Army Medical Center
Tacoma, Washington

Peter Dietrich, MD
Professor of Diagnostic Radiology
University of Vermont School of Medicine
Burlington, Vermont

Raymond S. Dougherty, MD
Chief, Diagnostic Ultrasound
Department of Radiology
David Grant Medical Center
Travis Air Force Base, California

Erik H.L. Gaensler, MD
Bay Imaging Consultants Medical Group, Inc.
Assistant Clinical Professor of Radiology
University of California, San Francisco
San Francisco, California

Michael Galloway, MD
Assistant Clinical Professor
Department of Cardiovascular Medicine
University of California, Davis Medical Center
Sacramento, California

Alisa D. Gean, MD
Associate Professor of Radiology, Neurology and
   Neurosurgery
University of California, San Francisco
Chief of Neuroradiology
San Francisco General Hospital
San Francisco, California

Michael F. Hartshorne, MD
Professor and Vice-Chairman of Radiology
University of New Mexico School of Medicine
Chief, Joint Imaging Service
Veterans Administration Medical Center
Albuquerque, New Mexico

Anne S. Hayton, MD
Assistant Professor of Radiology
University of Vermont School of Medicine
Burlington, Vermont

Clyde A. Helms, MD
Professor of Radiology
Department of Radiology
Duke University Medical Center
Durham, North Carolina

Susan D. John MD
Associate Professor of Radiology and Pediatrics
Department of Radiology
The University of Texas Medical Branch
Galveston, Texas

Jeffrey S. Klein, MD
Associate Professor of Radiology
Chief of Thoracic Radiology
University of Vermont School of Medicine
Burlington, Vermont

Kelly K. Koeller, CDR, MC, USN
Chief, Neuroradiology Section
Department of Radiologic Pathology
Armed Forces Institute of Pathology
Washington, D.C.

Todd E. Lempert, MD
Staff Radiologist
Bay Imaging Consultants Medical Group, Inc.
Clinical Professor of Radiology
University of California, San Francisco
San Francisco, California

Karen K. Lindfors, MD
Professor of Radiology
Chief of Breast Imaging
University of California Davis School of Medicine
Sacramento, California

Mylon W. Marshall, MD
Vascular and Interventional Radiology
Radiological Associates of Sacramento
Sacramento, California

Mike McBiles, MD
Assistant Chief
Nuclear Medicine Service
Brooke Army Medical Center
Ft. Sam Houston, Texas
Assistant Professor of Radiology
University of Texas, San Antonio
San Antonio, Texas

Walter L. Olsen, MD
Radiologist, San Diego Diagnostic Radiology
Assistant Clinical Professor of Radiology
University of California, San Diego
San Diego, California

Todd Peebles, MD
Chief Resident in Radiology
University of Vermont School of Medicine
Burlington, Vermont

Howard A. Rowley, MD
Assistant Professor of Radiology and Neurology
Clinical Director of Biomagnetic Imaging Laboratory
University of California, San Francisco
San Francisco, California

David J. Seidenwurm, MD
Neuroradiologist
Radiological Associates of Sacramento
Sacramento, California
Assistant Professor of Clinical Radiology
University of California at San Francisco
San Francisco, California

David K. Shelton Jr., MD
Associate Professor of Radiology and Nuclear
  Medicine
Department of Radiology
University of California, Davis Medical Center
Sacramento, California

Leonard E. Swischuk, MD
Professor of Radiology and Pediatrics
Department of Radiology
The University of Texas Medical Branch
Children's Hospital
Galveston, Texas

Robert J. Telepak, MD
Associate Professor of Radiology
University of New Mexico School of Medicine
Albuquerque, New Mexico

James H. Timmons, MD, PhD
Chief, Computed Tomography Service
Department of Radiology
Madigan Army Medical Center
Tacoma, Washington

Austin Wand, MD
Clinical Assistant Professor of Radiology
Cornell University Medical College
New York, New York
Attending Radiologist
Coney Island Hospital
Brooklyn, New York

Philip W. Wiest, MD
Assistant Professor of Radiology
University of New Mexico School of Medicine
Albuquerque, New Mexico

John E. Williams, MD
Chief, Vascular and Interventional Radiology
Quantum Radiology, Northwest
Atlanta, Georgia

Rhonda A. Wyatt, MD
Chief, Nuclear Medicine
David Grant United States Air Force Medical Center
Travis Air Force Base, California

Contents

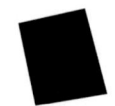

Section XI   **NUCLEAR RADIOLOGY**
Section Editors: John M. Bauman, Frederic A. Conte

List of Tables

xxii List of Tables

List of Universal Abbreviations

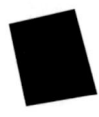

AIDS	Acquired immunodeficiency syndrome	LV	Left ventricle
ARDS	Adult respiratory distress syndrome	MR	Magnetic resonance imaging
CNS	Central nervous system	PA	Pulmonary artery
CT	Computed tomography	SPECT	Single-photon emission computed tomography
CSF	Cerebrospinal fluid		
GI	Gastrointestinal	RA	Right atrium
H	Hounsfield unit (applies to CT)	RV	Right ventricle
HIV	Human immunodeficiency virus	T1W1	T1-weighted image
HRCT	High resolution chest CT	T2W1	T2-weighted image
IV	Intravenous	US	Ultrasound
LA	Left atrium		

Section I BASIC PRINCIPLES

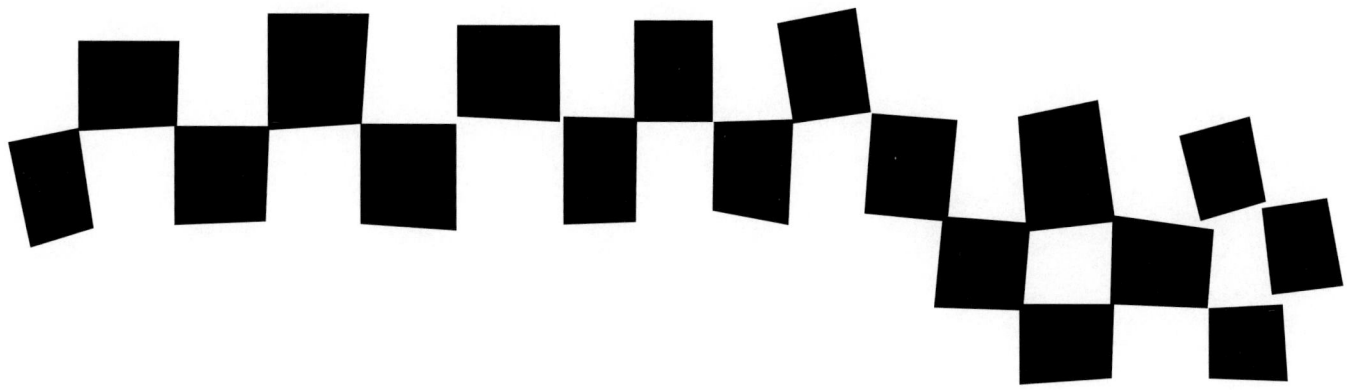

1 Diagnostic Imaging Methods
William E. Brant

1
Diagnostic Imaging Methods

William E. Brant

Diagnostic radiology is a dynamic specialty that has undergone rapid change with continuing advancements in technology. Not only has the number of imaging methods increased, but each one continues to undergo improvement and refinement of its use in medical diagnosis. This chapter reviews the basics of the major diagnostic imaging methods and provides the basic principles of image interpretation for each method. Contrast agents commonly used in diagnostic radiology are also discussed. The basics of nuclear radiology are discussed in chapters 53 and 54.

PLAIN FILM RADIOLOGY

Plain film examination of the human body dates back to the genesis of diagnostic radiology in 1895 and remains fundamental to its practice.

Image Generation. X-rays are a form of radiant energy similar in many ways to visible light (1,2). X-rays differ from visible light in that they have a very short wavelength and are able to penetrate many substances that are opaque to light. Plain film radiographs are produced by a photochemical interaction between x-rays and a screen coated with fluorescent particles inside a film cassette (Fig. 1.1). The fluorescent particles that are activated by x-rays emit light rays that expose photographic film within the cassette. As x-rays pass through the human body they are attenuated by interaction with body tissues (absorption and scatter), resulting in an image pattern recognizable as human anatomy (Fig. 1.2). The x-ray beam is produced by bombarding a tungsten target with an electron beam within an x-ray tube.

Naming Radiographic Views. Most radiographic views are named on the basis of the way that the x-ray beam passes through the patient. A posteroanterior (PA) chest radiograph is one in which the x-ray beam passes through the back of the patient and exits through the front of the patient to expose an x-ray film placed against the patient's chest. An anteroposterior (AP) chest film is exposed by an x-ray beam passing through the patient from front to back. A craniocaudad (CC) mammogram is produced by passing a beam through the breast in a vertical, cranial to caudad, direction. Views are additionally named by identifying the position of the patient. Erect, supine, or prone views may be specified. A right lateral decubitus view of the chest is exposed with the patient lying on his or her right side with a horizontal x-ray beam passing through the chest. Films taken during fluoroscopy are named on the basis of the patient's position relative to the fluoroscopic table because the x-ray tube is positioned beneath the table. A right posterior oblique (RPO) view is taken with the patient lying with the right side of his or her back against the table and the left side elevated away from the table. The x-ray beam generated by the x-ray tube located beneath the table passes through the patient to the film located above the patient.

Principles of Interpretation. Plain film radiographs demonstrate five basic radiographic densities: air, fat, soft tissue, bone, and metal (or x-ray contrast agents). Air attenuates very little of the x-ray beam, allowing nearly the full force of the beam to blacken the film. Bone, metal, and radiographic contrast agents attenuate a large proportion of the x-ray beam, allowing very little radiation through to blacken the film. Thus, bone, metallic objects, and structures opacified by x-ray contrast agents appear white on radiographs. Fat and soft tissues attenuate intermediate amounts of the x-ray beam, resulting in proportional degrees of film blackening (shades of gray). Thick structures attenuate more radiation than thin structures of the same composition. Anatomic structures are seen on radiographs when they are outlined in whole or in part by tissues of different x-ray attenuation. Air in the lung outlines pulmonary vascular structures, producing a detailed pattern of the lung parenchyma (Fig. 1.3). Fat within the abdomen outlines the margins of the liver, spleen, and kidneys, allowing their visualization (see Fig. 1.2B). The high density of bones enables visualization of their details through overlying soft tissues. Metallic objects such as surgical clips are usually clearly seen because they highly attenuate the x-ray beam. Radiographic contrast agents are suspensions of iodine and barium compounds that highly attenuate the x-ray beam and are used to outline anatomic structures. Disease states may obscure normally visualized anatomic structures by silhouetting their outline. Pneumonia in the right middle lobe of the lung replaces air in the alveoli with fluid and silhouettes the right heart border (Fig. 1.4). Squire and Novelline (3) provide an excellent text on the fundamentals of radiographic interpretation.

Conventional tomography provides radiographic images of slices of a living patient. This is done by simultaneously moving both the x-ray tube and the film about a pivot point centered in the patient in the

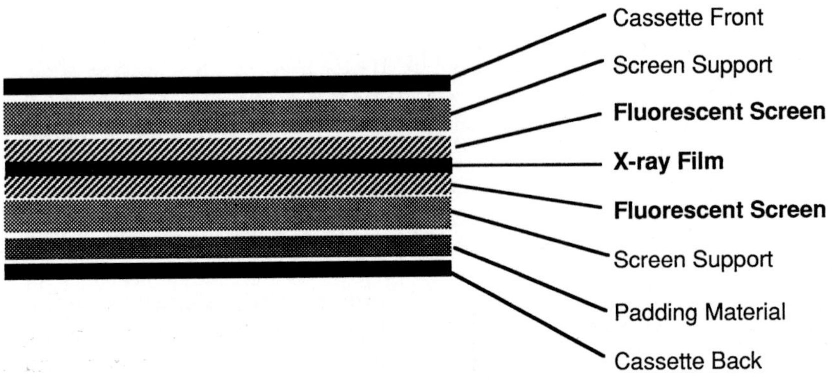

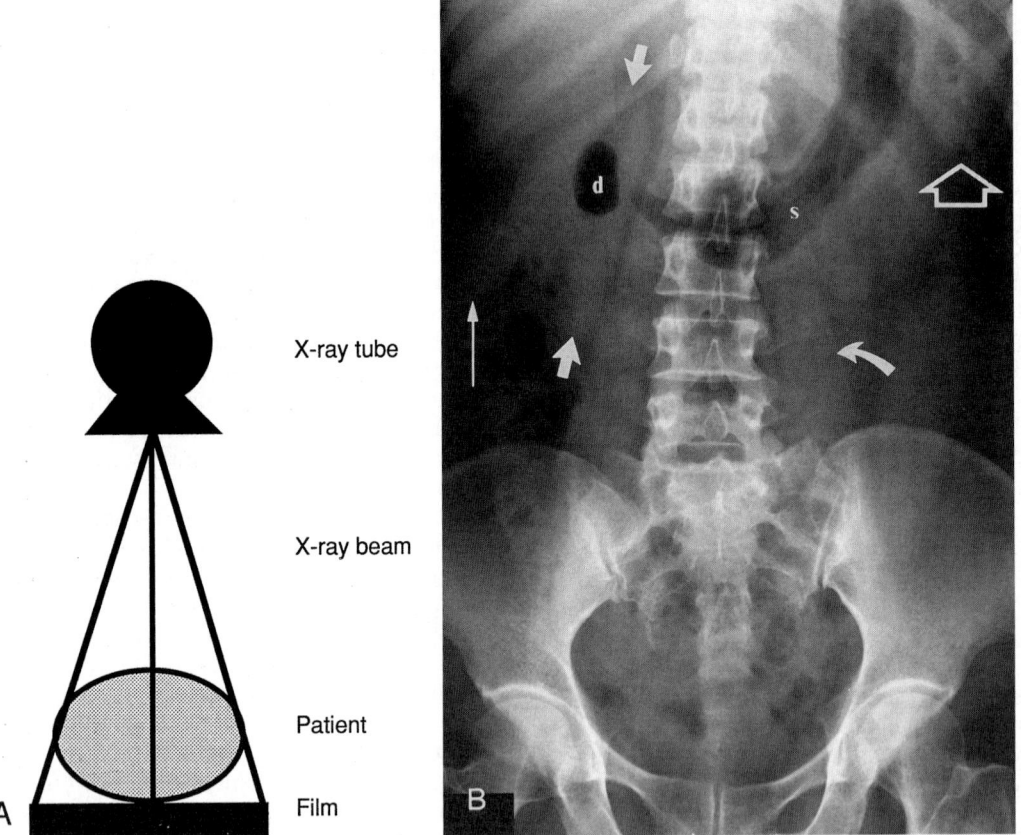

Figure 1.1. X-ray Film Cassette. Diagram demonstrates a sheet of x-ray film between two fluorescent screens within a light-proof cassette.

Figure 1.2. Plain Film Radiographs. A. Diagram of an x-ray tube producing x-rays that pass through the patient and expose the radiographic film. **B.** Supine AP radiograph of the abdomen reveals the patient's anatomy because anatomic structures differ in their capacity to attenuate x-rays that pass through the patient. The stomach (*s*) and duodenum (*d*) are visualized because air in the lumen is of different radiographic density than the soft tissues that surround the GI tract. The right kidney (*between short straight arrows*), edge of the liver (*long straight arrow*), edge of the spleen (*open arrow*), and the left psoas muscle (*curved arrow*) are visualized because fat outlines the soft-tissue density of these structures. The bones of the spine, pelvis, and hips are clearly seen through the soft tissues because of their high radiographic density.

plane of the anatomic structures to be studied (Fig. 1.5). Structures above and below the focal plane are blurred by the motion of the tube and film. Objects within the focal plane are visualized with improved detail as a result of the blurring of the overlying and underlying structures. Motion of the x-ray tube and

film may be linear, circular, elliptical, spiral, or hypocycloidal. Tomography is a useful adjunct to conventional radiographs in situations in which improved detail is needed for diagnosis.

Fluoroscopy enables real-time radiographic visualization of moving anatomic structures. A continuous x-ray beam passes through the patient and falls onto a fluorescing screen (Fig. 1.6). The faint light pattern emitted by the fluorescing screen is amplified electronically by an image intensifier, and the image is displayed on a television monitor. Fluoroscopy is extremely useful to evaluate motion such as GI peristalsis, movement of the diaphragm with respiration, and cardiac action. Fluoroscopy is also used to perform and monitor continuously radiographic procedures such as barium studies and catheter placements.

Angiography involves the opacification of blood vessels by intravascular injection of iodinated contrast agents. Conventional arteriography uses small flexible catheters that are placed in the arterial system usually via puncture of the femoral artery in the groin. With the use of fluoroscopy for guidance, catheters of various sizes and shapes can be manipulated selectively into virtually every major artery. Contrast injection is performed by hand or by mechanical injector and is accompanied by timed rapid-sequence filming or digital computer acquisition of the fluoroscopic image. The result is a timed series of images depicting contrast flow through the artery injected and the tissues that the artery supplies. Conventional venography is performed by contrast injection of veins via distal puncture or selective catheterization.

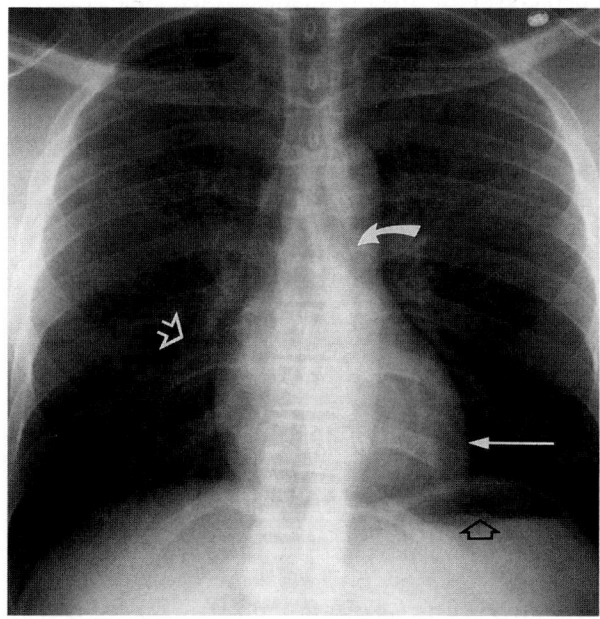

Figure 1.3. Erect PA Chest Radiograph. The pulmonary arteries (*white open arrow*) are seen in the lung because the vessels are outlined by air in alveoli. The left cardiac border (*long arrow*) is crisply defined by adjacent air-filled lung. The left main bronchus (*curved arrow*) is seen because its air-filled lumen is surrounded by soft tissue of the mediastinum. An air-fluid level (*open black arrow*) in the stomach confirms the erect position of the patient during exposure of the radiograph.

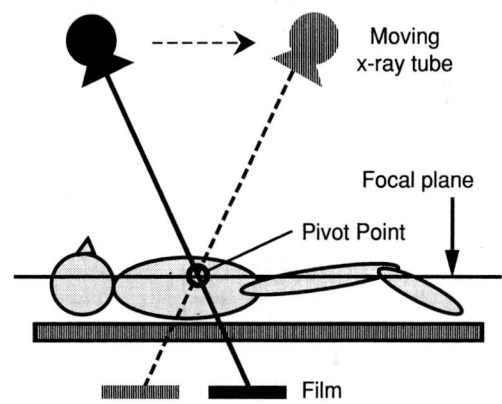

Figure 1.5. Conventional Tomography. In this technique, the x-ray tube and film simultaneously move about a pivot point at the level of the desired focal plane. Anatomic structures within the focal plane remain in sharp focus, whereas the structures above and below the focal plane are blurred by the motion of the tube and film.

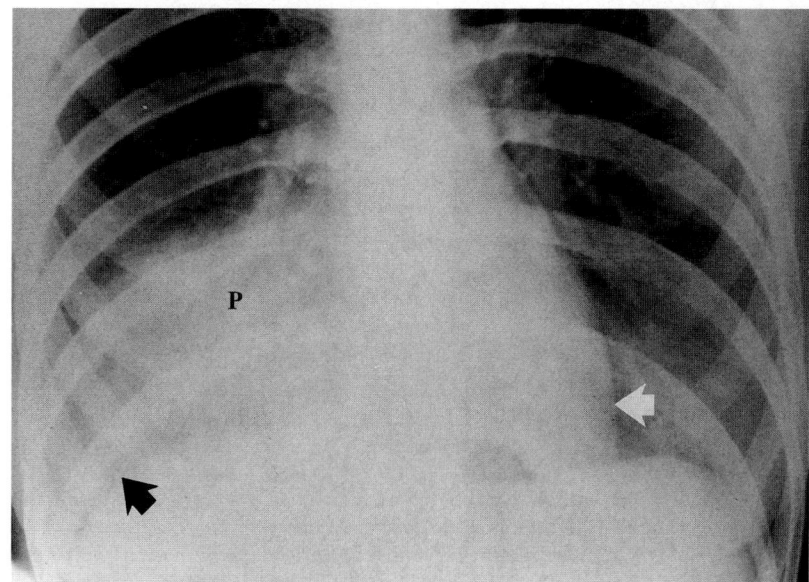

Figure 1.4. Right Middle Lobe and Left Lower Lobe Pneumonia. PA erect chest radiograph demonstrates pneumonia (*P*) in the right middle lobe replacing air density in the lung with soft-tissue density and silhouetting the right heart border. The dome of the right hemidiaphragm (*black arrow*) is defined by air in the normal right lower lobe and remains visible through the right middle lobe infiltrate. The left heart border (*white arrow*), defined by air in the lingula, remains well defined despite infiltrate in the left lower lobe.

CROSS-SECTIONAL IMAGING TECHNIQUES

CT, MR, and US are techniques that produce cross-sectional images of the body. All three interrogate a three-dimensional volume or slice of patient tissue to produce a two-dimensional image. The resulting image is made up of a matrix of picture elements (pixels), each of which represents a volume element (voxel) of patient tissue. The tissue composition of the voxel is averaged (vol-

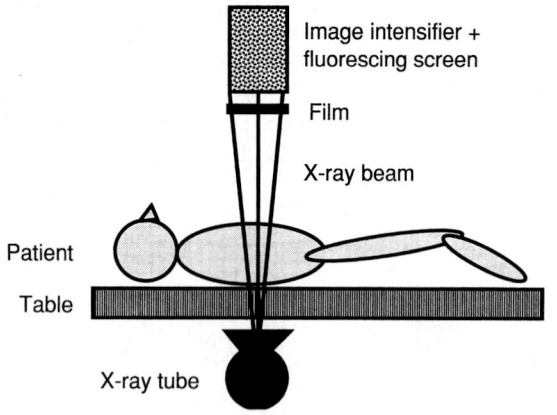

Figure 1.6. Fluoroscopy. Diagram of a fluoroscopic unit illustrates the x-ray tube located beneath the patient examination table and the fluorescing screen with the image intensifier positioned above the patient. Amplification of the faint fluorescing image by the image intensifier allows the radiation exposure to the patient to be kept at low levels during fluoroscopy. The real-time fluoroscopic images are viewed on a television monitor and may be recorded on videotape. Radiographs are obtained by placing a film cassette between the patient and the image intensifier and exposing the film with a brief pulse of radiation.

ume averaged) for display as a pixel. CT and MR assign a numerical value to each picture element in the matrix. The matrix of picture elements that make up each image is usually between 128 × 256 (32,768 pixels) and 560 × 560 (313,600 pixels), determined by the specified acquisition parameters (Fig. 1.7).

To produce an anatomic image, shades of gray are assigned to ranges of pixel values (Fig. 1.8). For example, 16 shades of gray may be divided over a *window width* of 320 pixel values. Groups of 20 pixel values are each assigned one of the 16 gray shades. The middle gray shade is assigned to the pixel values centered on a selected *window level*. Pixels with values greater than the upper limit of the window width are displayed white, and pixels with values less than the lower limit of the window width are displayed black. To analyze optimally all of the anatomic information of any particular slice, the image is photographed at different window-width and window-level settings optimized for bone, air-filled lung, soft tissue, and so forth (Fig. 1.9).

Computed Tomography

CT uses a computer to reconstruct mathematically a cross-sectional image of the body from measurements of x-ray transmission through thin slices of patient tissue (2). CT displays the imaged slice alone, without the superimposition of blurred structures that is seen with conventional tomography. A narrow, well-collimated beam of x-rays is generated on one side of the patient (Fig. 1.10). The x-ray beam is attenuated by absorption and scatter as it passes through the patient. Sensitive detectors on the opposite side of the patient measure x-ray transmission through the slice. These measurements are systematically repeated many times from dif-

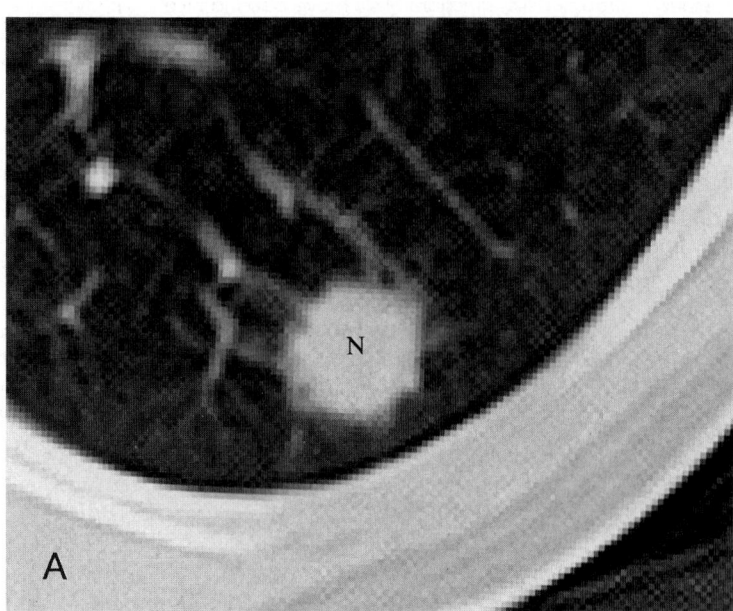

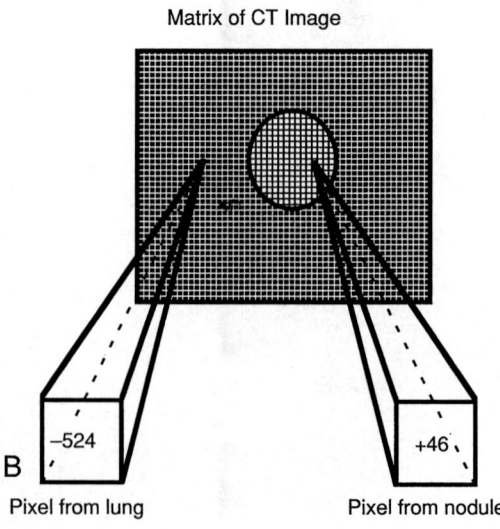

Figure 1.7. Image Matrix. A. Magnified CT image of a pulmonary nodule (*N*). The pixels that make up the image are evident as tiny squares within the image. The window width is set at 2000 H with a window level of −600 H to accentuate visualization of the white soft-tissue nodule on a background of gray, air-filled lung. **B.** Diagram of the matrix that constitutes the CT image. A pixel from air-filled lung with a calculated CT number of −524 H is gray, whereas a pixel from the soft-tissue nodule with a calculated CT number of +46 H is white.

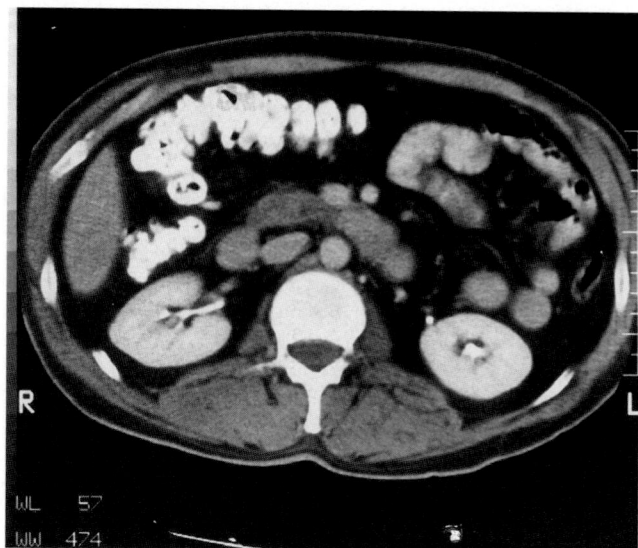

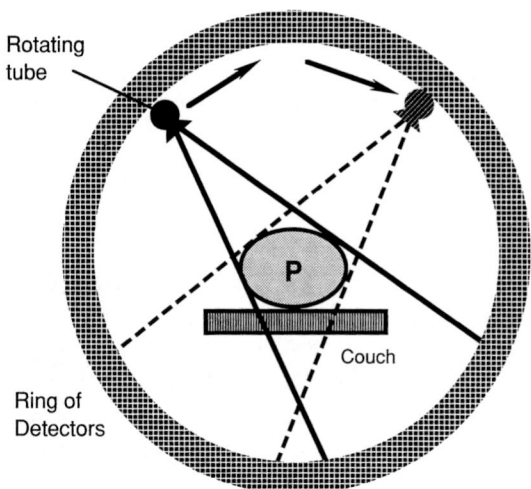

Figure 1.8. Gray Scale. A CT image of the abdomen includes a gray scale along its left edge. Each individual pixel in the CT image is assigned a shade of gray depending on its calculated CT number (H unit) and the window width and window level selected by the CT operator. This CT image is filmed at a window level **(WL) of 57** and a window width **(WW) of 474.** Along the right side of the CT image is a centimeter scale that can be used to measure the size of objects in the image. *R* indicates the patient's right side, and *L* indicates the patient's left side. Cross-sectional images in the transverse plane are routinely viewed from "below," as if standing at the patient's feet. This orientation allows easy correlation with plain film radiographs, which are routinely viewed as if facing the patient with the patient's right side to the viewer's left.

Figure 1.10. Computed Tomography. Diagram of a fourth-generation CT scanner. The patient (*P*) is placed on an examination couch within the core of the CT unit. An x-ray tube rotates 360° around the patient, producing pulses of radiation that pass through the patient. Transmitted x-rays are detected by a circumferential bank of radiation detectors. X-ray transmission data are sent to a computer, which uses an assigned algorithm to calculate the matrix of CT numbers used to produce the anatomic cross-sectional image. With helical CT scan technique, the patient couch moves the patient continuously through the rotating x-ray beam.

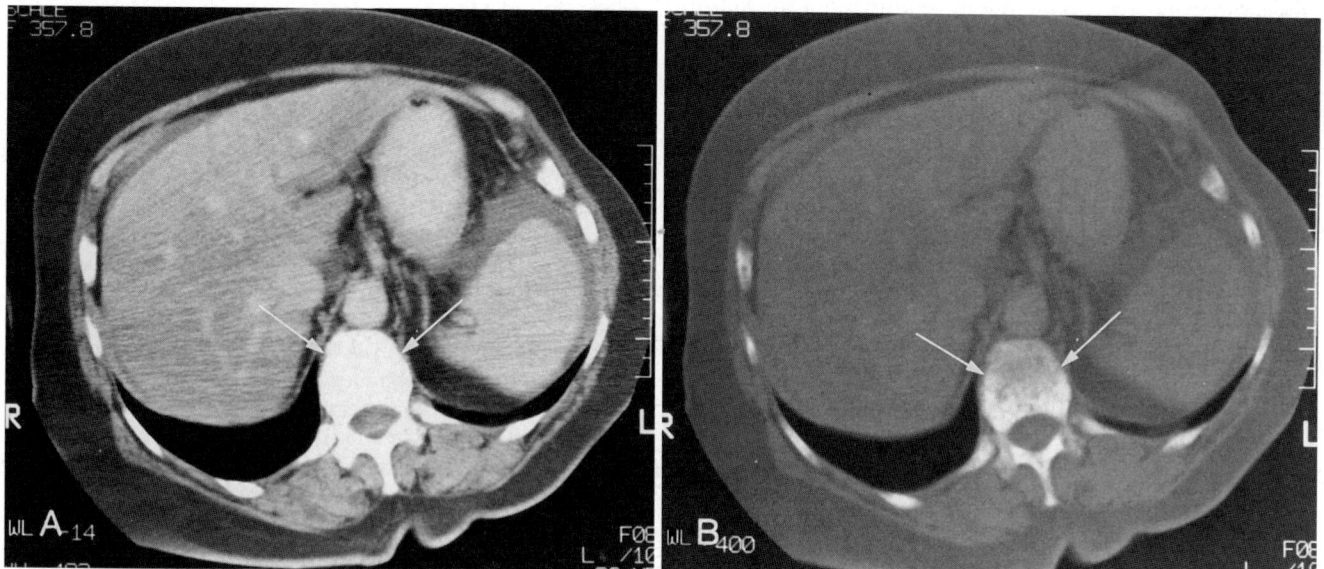

Figure 1.9. CT Windows. A. A CT image of the upper abdomen photographed with "soft tissue windows" **(window width = 482 H, window level = −14 H)** portrays a thoracic vertebra (*arrows*) entirely white with no bone detail. **B.** The same CT image rephotographed with "bone windows" **(window width = 2000 H, window level = 400 H)** demonstrates destructive changes in the vertebral body (*arrows*) owing to metastatic lung carcinoma.

Figure 1.11. CT Angiogram. A three-dimensional, shaded surface display, angiogram was created from a series of axial plane helical CT images obtained during rapid bolus IV contrast agent administration. Contrast enhancement greatly increases the CT numbers of the arteries and kidneys and allows removal of structures with lower CT density from the image by "thresholding." Only pixels with CT numbers higher than a specified threshold value are displayed. Computer algorithms create a "virtual" three-dimensional image from data provided by many overlapping axial slices. The three-dimensional image can be rotated and viewed from any desired angle. "Shading," simulating light cast from a remote light source, enhances the three-dimensional visual effect.

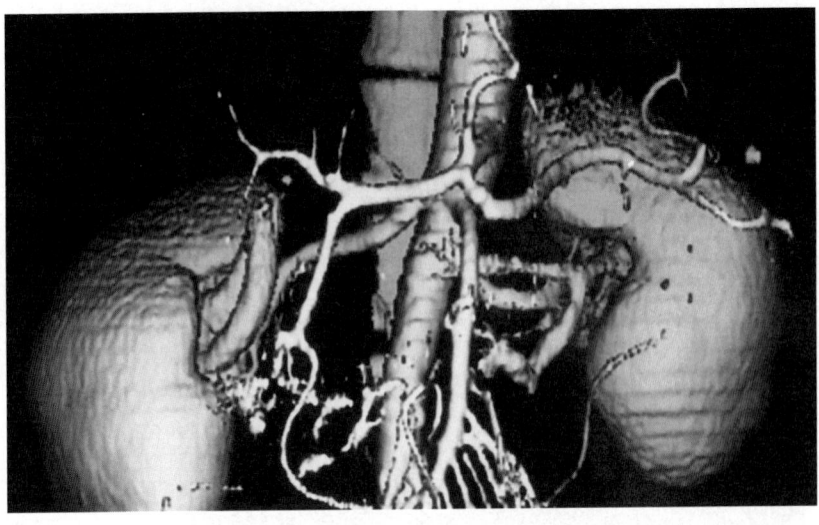

ferent directions while the x-ray tube is pulsed as it rotates around the patient. CT numbers are assigned to each pixel in the image by a computer algorithm that uses as data these measurements of transmitted x-rays (4). CT pixel numbers are proportional to the difference in average x-ray attenuation of the tissue within the voxel compared with that of water. A Hounsfield unit (H) scale, named for the inventor of CT, is used. Water is assigned a value of 0 H, with the scale extending from −1024 H for air to +3000–4000 H for very dense bone. H units are not absolute values but, rather, are relative values that may vary from one CT system to another.

Voxel dimensions are determined by the computer algorithm chosen for reconstruction and the thickness of the scanned slice. Most CT units allow slice thickness specifications between 1 and 10 mm. Data for an individual slice are routinely acquired in 1–3 seconds. Advantages of CT compared with MR include rapid scan acquisition, superior bone detail, and demonstration of calcifications. CT scanning is generally limited to the axial plane; however, images may be reformatted in sagittal, coronal, or oblique planes or as three-dimensional images (Fig. 1.11).

Conventional CT (nonhelical) obtains image data one slice at a time. The patient holds his or her breath, a slice is taken, the patient breathes, the table moves, and the sequence is repeated. This technique requires at least two to three times the total scanning time of helical CT for any given patient scan volume, making optimization of scanning during maximum contrast more difficult. Minor changes in lung volume with each breath-hold may make substantial changes in the chest and abdomen anatomy scanned, resulting in "skip" areas. More recent conventional scanners can simulate helical scanning by "cluster" technique. Several sequential scans are obtained during a single breath-hold..

Helical CT, also called spiral CT, is performed by moving the patient table at a constant speed through the CT gantry while scanning continuously with an x-ray tube rotating around the patient. A continuous volume of image data is acquired during a single breath-hold. This technique dramatically improves the speed of image acquisition, enables scanning during optimal contrast

opacification, and eliminates artifacts caused by misregistration and variations in patient breathing (5,6). The entire liver may be scanned in a single breath-hold; the entire abdomen and pelvis, in two to three breath-holds, all during the first 90 seconds of contrast administration. Volume acquisition enables retrospective reconstruction of multiple overlapping slices, improving visualization of small lesions and allowing high-detail three-dimensional CT angiography (Fig. 1.11) (7,8).

Some disadvantages of helical CT include vascular flow artifacts and increased volume averaging effects (9). When IV-administered contrast levels are at their peak in the arterial system, veins usually show no contrast opacification or show a confusing mixture of contrast with unopacified blood in the veins simulating thrombus. Delayed scans may be needed for optimal venous opacification.

CONTRAST ADMINISTRATION IN COMPUTED TOMOGRAPHY

IV contrast agents are administered in CT to enhance density differences between lesions and surrounding parenchyma, to demonstrate vascular anatomy and vessel patency, and to characterize lesions by their patterns of contrast enhancement (10). The normal blood–brain barrier of tight neural capillary endothelial junctions prevents access of contrast into the neural extravascular space. Defects in the blood–brain barrier associated with tumors, stroke, infection, and other lesions enable contrast accumulation within abnormal tissue, improving its visibility. In nonneural tissues, the capillary endothelium has loose junctions, enabling free access of contrast into the extravascular space. Contrast administration and timing of CT scanning must be carefully planned to optimize differences in enhancement patterns between lesions and normal tissues. For example, most liver tumors are predominantly supplied by the hepatic artery, whereas the liver parenchyma is predominantly supplied by the portal vein (≈70%), with a lesser contribution from the hepatic artery (≈30%). Contrast given by bolus injection in a peripheral arm vein will arrive earliest in the hepatic artery and enhance (that is, increase the CT density of) the tumor to a greater extent than the liver parenchyma (Fig. 1.12). Maximal enhancement of the liver parenchyma is delayed 1–2 minutes until the contrast has circulated through the intestinal tract and returned to the liver via the portal vein. Differentiation of tumor and parenchyma by contrast enhancement can thus be maximized by giving an IV bolus of contrast and by performing rapid CT scanning of the liver in the first 1–2 minutes following contrast administration. Helical CT is ideal for this early and rapid scanning of the liver. Oral or rectal contrast is generally required to opacify the bowel for CT scans of the abdomen and pelvis. Bowel without intraluminal contrast may be difficult to differentiate from tumors, lymph nodes, and hematomas.

COMPUTED TOMOGRAPHY ARTIFACTS

Artifacts refer to components of the image that do not faithfully reproduce actual anatomic structures because of distortion, addition, or deletion of information. Artifacts degrade the image and may cause errors in diagnosis (11).

Volume averaging is present in every CT image and must always be considered in image interpretation. The displayed two-dimensional image is created from data obtained and *averaged* from a three-dimensional volume of patient tissue. Slices above and below the image being interpreted must be examined for sources of volume averaging that may be misinterpreted as pathology.

Beam hardening artifact results from greater attenuation of low-energy x-ray photons than high-energy x-ray photons as they pass through tissue. The mean energy of the x-ray beam is increased (the beam is "hardened"), resulting in less attenuation at the end of the beam than at its beginning. Beam-hardening errors are seen as areas or streaks of low density extending from structures of high x-ray attenuation such as the petrous bones, shoulders, and hips (Fig. 1.13).

Motion artifact results when structures move to different positions during image acquisition. Motion is demonstrated in the image as prominent streaks from high- to low-density interfaces or as blurred or duplicated images.

Streak artifacts emanate from high-density sharp-edged objects such as vascular clips and dental fillings. Reconstruction algorithms cannot handle the extreme differences in x-ray attenuation between very dense objects and adjacent tissue (Fig. 1.14).

PRINCIPLES OF COMPUTED TOMOGRAPHY INTERPRETATION

Like all imaging analysis, CT interpretation is based on an organized and comprehensive approach. CT images are viewed in sequential anatomic order, examining each slice with reference to slices above and below. The radiologist must seek to develop a three-dimensional concept of the anatomy and pathology displayed. The study must be interpreted with reference to the scan parameters, slice thickness and spacing, administration of contrast, and artifacts. Optimal bone detail is viewed at "bone windows," generally a window width of 2000 H and a window level of 400–600 H (see Fig. 1.9). Lungs are viewed at "lung windows" with a window width of 1000–2000 H and window levels of −500 to −600 H. Soft tissues are examined at window width 400–500 H and window level 20–40 H. Narrow windows (width = 100–150 H, level = 70–80 H) increase image contrast and aid in the detection of subtle liver and spleen lesions.

Magnetic Resonance Imaging

MR is a technique that produces tomographic images by means of magnetic fields and radiowaves. Although CT evaluates only a single tissue parameter, x-ray attenuation, MR analyzes multiple tissue characteristics including hydrogen (proton) density, T1 and T2 relaxation times of tissue, and blood flow within tissue. The soft-tissue contrast provided by MR is substantially better than for any other imaging modality. Differences in the density of protons available to contribute to the MR signal discriminate one tissue from another. Most tissues can be differentiated by significant differences in their characteristic T1 and T2 relaxation times. T1 and T2 are features of the three-dimensional molecular environment

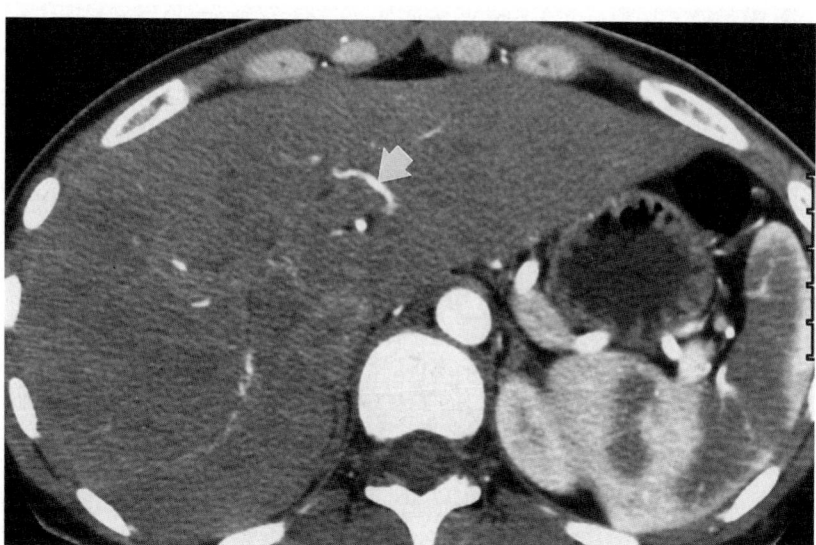

Figure 1.12. Early Contrast Enhancement. Helical CT image obtained during the early, arterial, phase of contrast enhancement shows normal early flow defects in the spleen and contrast enhancement of hepatic arteries (*arrow*) with negligible enhancement of the liver parenchyma. CT scans must be interpreted with recognition of the phase and pattern of contrast enhancement.

that surrounds each proton in the tissue imaged. T1 is a measure of a proton's ability to exchange energy with its surrounding chemical matrix. It is a measure of how quickly a tissue can become magnetized. T2 conveys how quickly a given tissue loses its magnetization. Blood flow has a complex effect on the MR signal that may decrease or increase its intensity.

The complicated physics of MR is beyond the scope of this book (2,12,13). In simplest terms, MR is based on the ability of a small number of protons within the body to absorb and emit radiowave energy when the body is placed within a strong magnetic field. Different tissues absorb and release radiowave energy at different, detectable, and characteristic rates. MR scans are obtained by placing the patient in a static magnetic field 0.02–4 T in strength, depending on the particular MR unit used.

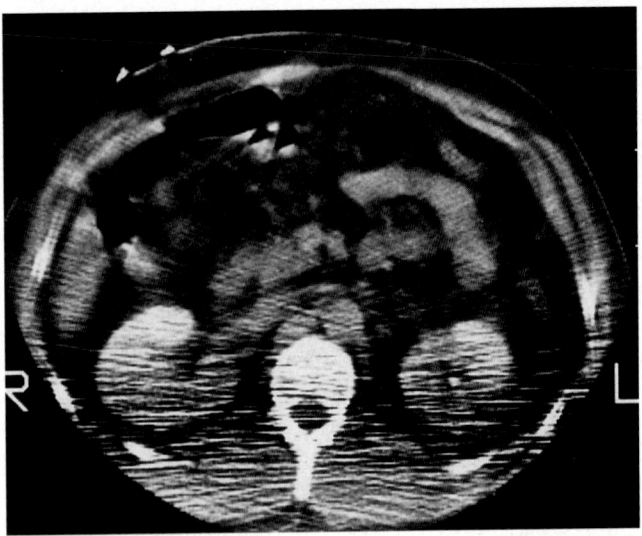

Figure 1.13. Beam Hardening Artifact. A CT image of the abdomen is severely degraded by beam hardening artifact that produces dark streaks across the lower half of the image. The artifact was caused by marked attenuation of the x-ray beam by the patient's arms, which were kept at his sides owing to injury.

Figure 1.14. Streak Artifact. Metallic surgical clips adjacent to the aorta produces dark and light streaks that obscure anatomy. The streak artifact is accentuated by motion of the pulsating aorta moving the metal clips.

Low–field strength systems (<0.1 T), midfield systems (0.1–1.0 T), and high-field systems (>1.0 T) each have their own advantages and disadvantages. The choice of unit for imaging is based on preference and local availability. A small number of tissue protons in the patient align with the main magnetic field and are subsequently displaced from their alignment by application of radiofrequency (RF) gradients. When the RF gradient is terminated, the displaced protons realign with the main magnetic field, releasing a small pulse of energy that is detected, localized, and then processed by a computer algorithm similar to that used in CT to produce a tomographic anatomic image. Slice location is determined by application of a slice selection gradient of gradually increasing intensity along the z-axis. The small energy pulses released by tissue protons are further localized by "frequency-encoding" in one direction (x-axis) and "phase-encoding" in the other direction (y-axis). Images can be obtained in any anatomic plane by adjusting the orientation of the x-axis, y-axis, and z-axis magnetic field gradients. Because the MR signal is very weak, prolonged imaging time is often required for optimal images. Standard spin-echo sequences produce a batch of images in approximately 10–20 minutes. Rather than obtaining data for each image one slice at a time, many MR sequences obtain data for all slices in the imaged tissue volume throughout the entire imaging time. Thus, motion caused by breathing and cardiac and vascular pulsation may degrade the image substantially. More recently available gradient recalled echo (GRE), fast spin-echo, and echo-planar techniques have significantly decreased imaging times, making breath-hold imaging practical (14). Continued rapid-paced technological improvements are making MR acquisition times comparable with those for CT.

Present MR technology relies on three major pulse sequence techniques, with many variations used by different MR manufacturers.

Spin-echo (SE) pulse sequences produce standard T1WI, T2WI, and proton density–weighted images. T1WI emphasize differences in the T1 relaxation times be-

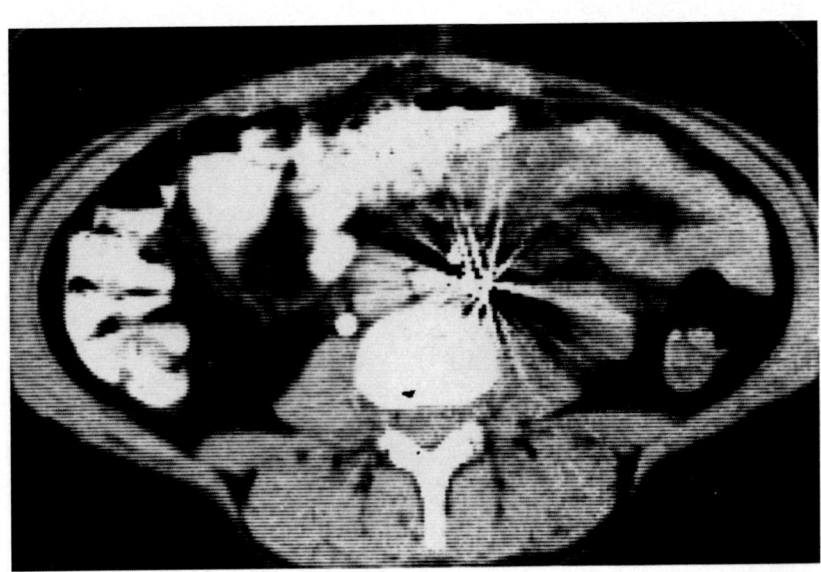

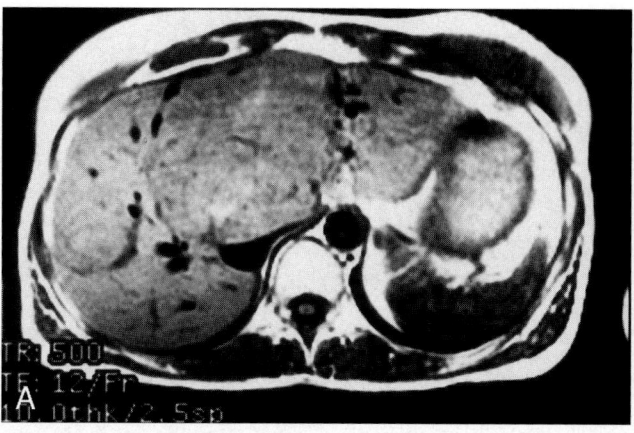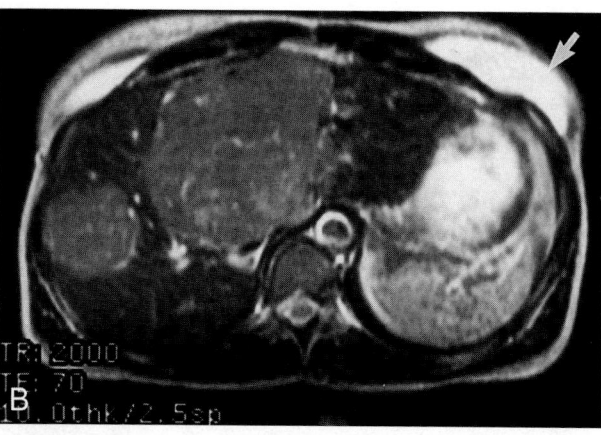

Figure 1.15. Spin-Echo MR. On the **left** is a T1WI (TR = 500, TE = 12) and on the **right** is a T2WI (TR = 2000, TE = 70). Note the substantially increased conspicuity of the mass lesions in the liver on the T2WI. The patient has silicone breast implants (*arrow*).

tween tissues. T1WI usually provide the best anatomic detail and are good for identifying fat and subacute hemorrhage. T2WI emphasize differences in the T2 relaxation times of tissues and usually provide the most sensitive detection of pathologic lesions. Proton density–weighted images accentuate proton density differences in tissues and are most useful in brain imaging.

Two major components of MR instrument settings selected by the operator for SE sequences are TR and TE. The time between administered RF pulses, or the time provided for protons to align with the main magnetic field, is TR (time of repetition). The time provided for absorbed radiowave energy to be released and detected is TE (time of echo). T1WI are obtained by selecting short TR (≤500 ms) and short TE (≤20 ms) settings for spin-echo sequences. T2WI use a long TR (≥2000 ms) and long TE (≥70 ms) (Fig. 1.15). Proton density–weighted images use a long TR (2000–3000 ms) and a short TE (25–30 ms) to minimize T1 and T2 effect and accentuate hydrogen-density differences in tissues.

Inversion recovery (IR) pulse sequences are used mainly to emphasize differences in T1 relaxation times of tissues. A delay time, TI (time of inversion) is added to the TE and TR instrument settings selected by the operator. Standard IR sequences, using a long TI, produce T1WI. Tissues with short T1 times yield a brighter signal. *Short TI inversion recovery* (STIR) sequences are the most commonly used. This sequence achieves additive T1-weighted, T2-weighted, and proton density–weighted contrast to increase lesion conspicuity (15). With STIR sequences, all tissues with short T1 relaxation times, including fat, are suppressed, whereas tissue with high water content, including many pathologic lesions, are accentuated, yielding a bright signal on a dark background of nulled short-T1 tissue (Fig. 1.16). STIR images more closely resemble strongly T2WI.

Gradient recalled echo pulse sequences are used to perform fast MR and MR angiography (16,17). Partial "flip angles" of less than 90° are used to decrease the time to signal recovery. Signal intensity arising from T2 relaxation characteristics of tissue is strongly affected by imperfections in the magnetic field on GRE images. Magnetization decay time with GRE imaging is termed

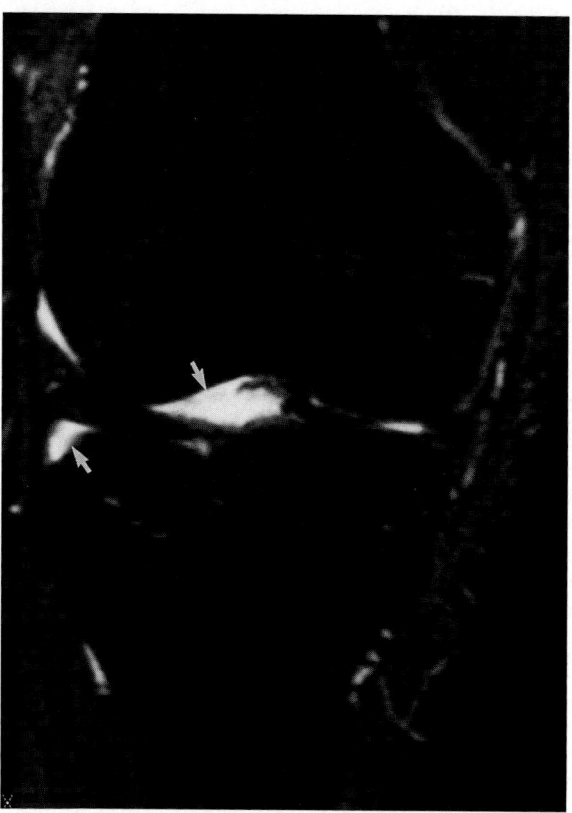

Figure 1.16. Inversion Recovery MR. A coronal plane inversion recovery (TR = 5000, TE = 54, TI = 140) MR of the knee in coronal plane demonstrates marked suppression of MR signal from all tissues except fluid in the joint space (*arrows*).

T2* ("T2 star") and is much shorter than the "true" T2 decay times seen with SE imaging. GRE images are characteristically low in image contrast, have prominent artifacts, and demonstrate flowing blood with bright signal (Fig. 1.17). T1-, T2-, T2*-, and proton density–image weighting is determined by the combination of flip angle, TR, and TE settings.

Echo-planar imaging is a fast MR technique that can produce single slice images in 20 milliseconds and mul-

Figure 1.17. Gradient Recalled Echo MR. Gradient recalled echo technique was used to create a "white blood" effect to demonstrate dissection of the descending thoracic aorta. The intimal flap is seen as a dark line extending across the lumen of the aorta separating the true lumen (*large arrow*) from the false lumen (*small arrow*).

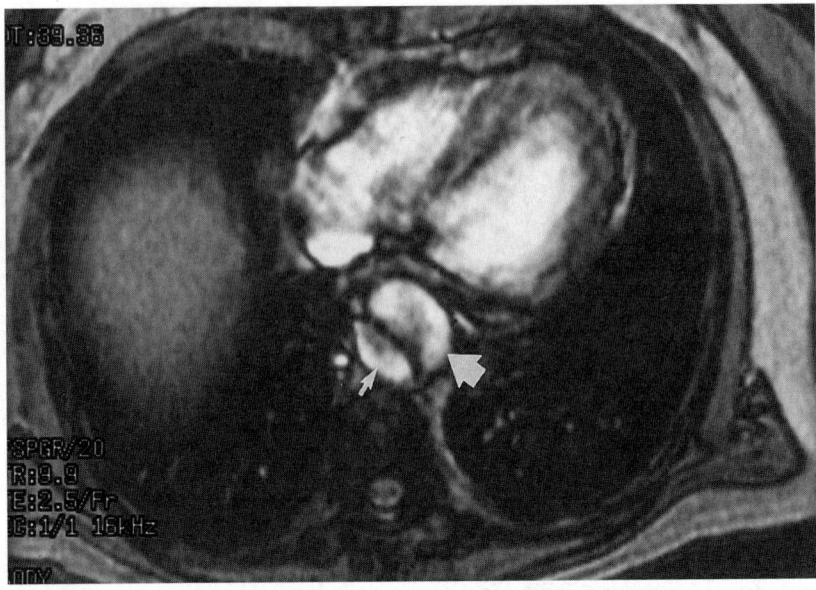

tislice studies in 20 seconds (18,19). All spatial encoding information is obtained after a single RF excitation, compared with the multiple RF excitations separated by TR intervals required for conventional MR. Motion artifact is reduced, and moving structures can be "freeze-frame" imaged. Special hardware is required for echoplanar imaging, but standard SE, GRE, and IR pulse sequences can be obtained. Echo-planar imaging overcomes many of the time and motion limitations of conventional MR and enables expansion of MR to new areas such as blood perfusion and cortical activation of the brain.

Advantages of MR include its outstanding soft-tissue contrast resolution, ability to provide images in any anatomic plane, and absence of ionizing radiation. MR is limited by its inability to demonstrate dense bone detail or calcifications, long imaging times for many pulse sequences, limited spatial resolution compared with CT, limited availability in many geographic areas, and expense. Because of the physically confining space for the patient within the magnet, a number of patients experience symptoms of claustrophobia and require sedation or are simply unable to tolerate MR scanning.

Safety Considerations. MR is contraindicated in patients who have electrically, magnetically, or mechanically activated implants including cardiac pacemakers, insulin pumps, cochlear implants, neurostimulators, bone-growth stimulators, and implantable drug infusion pumps (20,21). Patients with intracardiac pacing wires or Swan-Ganz catheters are at risk for RF current-induced cardiac fibrillation and burns. Ferromagnetic implants such as cerebral aneurysm clips, vascular clips, and skin staples are at risk for movement and dislodgment, burns, and induced electrical currents. Bullets, shrapnel, and metallic fragments may move and cause additional injury or become projectiles in the magnetic field. Metal workers and patients with a history of penetrating eye injuries should be screened with radiographs of the orbits to detect intraocular metallic foreign bodies

that may dislodge and cause blindness (22). A number of implants have been confirmed to be safe for MR, including nonferromagnetic vascular clips and staples, and orthopaedic devices composed of nonferromagnetic materials. Prosthetic heart valves with metal components and stainless steel Greenfield filters are considered safe because the in vivo forces affecting them are stronger than the deflecting forces of the electromagnetic field (23). No convincing body of evidence indicates that short-term exposure to the electromagnetic fields of MR harms the developing fetus, although it is not possible to prove that MR is absolutely safe in pregnancy (24). Pregnant patients can be scanned, provided the study is medically indicated (25).

MAGNETIC RESONANCE IMAGING ARTIFACTS

Artifacts are intrinsic to MR technique and must be recognized to avoid mistaking them for disease (26–28).

Ferromagnetic artifact is caused by focal distortions in the main magnetic field caused by the presence of ferromagnetic objects such as orthopaedic devices, surgical clips and wire, dentures, and metallic foreign bodies in the patient. The artifact is seen as areas of signal void at the location of the metal implant, often with a rim of increased intensity and a distortion of the image in the vicinity.

Motion artifact is common in MR because of prolonged image acquisition time. Random motion produces blurring of the image. Periodic motion, such as that caused by pulsating blood vessels, causes ghosts of the moving structures (Fig. 1.18). Motion artifacts are most visible along the phase-encoded direction. Swapping phase- and frequency-encoded directions may make the artifacts less bothersome.

Chemical shift misregistration occurs at interfaces between fat and water. Protons bound in lipid molecules experience a slightly lower magnetic influence than protons in water when exposed to an externally applied gradient magnetic field, resulting in misregistration of sig-

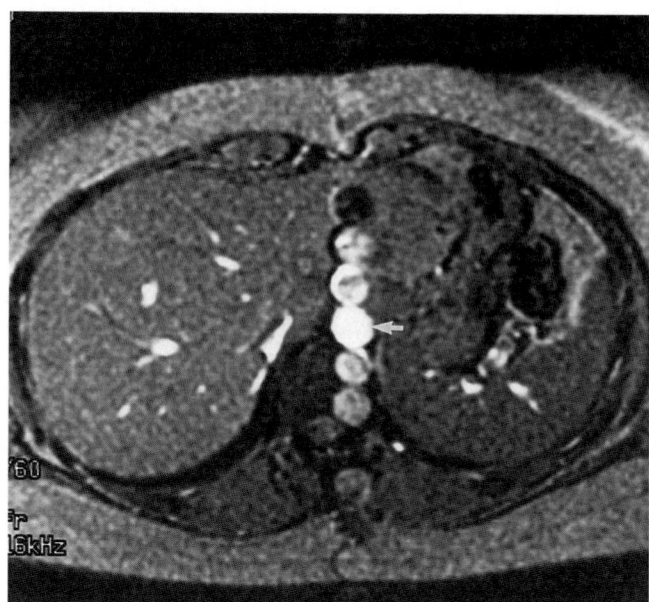

Figure 1.18. Motion Artifact. Pulsations of the aorta (*arrow*) produce numerous ghosts of the aorta in the phase-encoded direction. Swapping the phase-encoded direction with the frequency-encoded direction will enable evaluation of the left lobe of the liver.

nal location. The artifact is seen as a line of high-signal intensity on one side of the fat–water interface and a line of signal void at the opposite side of the fat–water interface (Fig. 1.19). Evaluation of the bladder wall and renal margins is difficult in the presence of this artifact.

Truncation error occurs adjacent to sharp boundaries between tissues of markedly different contrast. The artifact is attributable to inherent errors in the Fourier transform technique of image reconstruction. The artifact appears as regularly spaced alternating parallel bands of bright and dark signal. It may simulate a syrinx of the spinal cord or a meniscal tear in the knee.

Aliasing, or image wraparound, artifact occurs when anatomy outside the designated field of view but within the image plane is mismapped onto the opposite side of the image. For instance, on a midline sagittal brain MR, the patient's nose may be artifactually displayed over the area of the posterior fossa. Aliasing may be eliminated by increasing the field of view (at the expense of loss of image resolution) or by increasing the number of phase-encoding steps outside the field of view (oversampling).

PRINCIPLES OF MAGNETIC RESONANCE INTERPRETATION

Outstanding soft-tissue contrast is obtained in MR by designing imaging sequences that accentuate differences in T1 and T2 tissue relaxation times. Sequences that accentuate differences in proton density are fruitful in brain imaging but are generally less useful for extracranial soft-tissue imaging, in which proton density differences are small. Interpreting MR depends on a clear understanding of the biophysical basis of MR tissue contrast (29). Water is the major source of the MR signal in tissues other than fat. Mineral-rich structures such as bone and calculi, and collagenous tissues such

as ligaments, tendons, fibrocartilage, and tissue fibrosis, are low in water content and lack mobile protons to produce an MR signal. These tissues are low in signal intensity on all MR sequences. Water in tissue exists in at least two physical states: *free water* with unrestricted motion and *bound water* with restricted motion owing to hydrogen bonding with proteins. Free water is found mainly in extracellular fluid, whereas bound water is found mainly in intracellular fluid. Intracellular water is both bound and free and is in a condition of rapid exchange between the two states.

Free water has long T1 and T2 relaxation times, resulting in low signal intensity on T1WI and high signal intensity on T2WI (Table 1.1). Organs with abundant extracellular fluid, and therefore large amounts of free water, include kidney (urine); ovaries and thyroid (follicles); spleen and penis (stagnant blood); and prostate, testes, and seminal vesicles (fluid in tubules) (Table 1.2). Edema is an increase in extracellular fluid and tends to have the effect of prolonging T1 and T2 relaxation times in affected tissues. Most neoplastic tissues have an increase in extracellular fluid as well as an increase in the pro-

Table 1.1. Rules of MR Soft Tissue Contrast

T1-weighted Images		
Short T1	→	High Signal
Long T1	→	Low Signal
T2-weighted Images		
Short T2	→	Low Signal
Long T2	→	High Signal

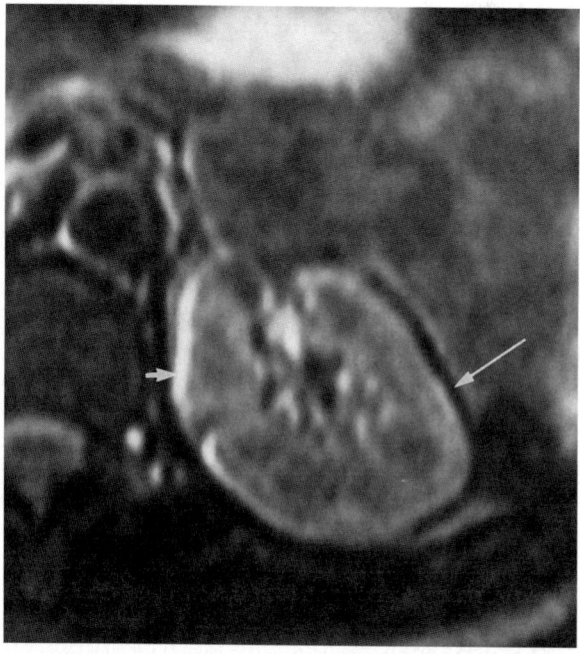

Figure 1.19. Chemical Shift Artifact. Chemical shift misregistration between fat and kidney tissue produces a high-density band (*short arrow*) on the medial aspect of the left kidney and a low-density band (*long arrow*) on its lateral aspect.

Table 1.2. MR of Tissues and Body Fluids

Tissue/Body Fluid	Examples	T1WI signal	T2WI signal
Gas	Air in lung Gas in bowel	Absent	Absent
Mineral rich tissue	Cortical Bone Calculi	Absent	Absent
Collagenous tissue	Ligaments Tendons Fibrocartilege Scar tissue	Low	Low
Fat	Adipose tissue Fatty bone marrow	High	Intermediate to High
High bound water tissue	Liver Pancreas Adrenal Muscle Hyaline cartilage	Low	Low to Intermediate
High free water tissue	Kidney Testes Prostate Seminal vesicles Ovary Thyroid Spleen Penis Simple cysts Bladder Gallbladder Edema Urine Bile Cerebrospinal fluid	Low	High
Proteinaceous fluid	Complicated cysts Abscess Synovial fluid Nucleus pulposis	Intermediate	High

Modified from Mitchell DG, Burk DL Jr, Vinitski S, Rifkin MD. The biophysical basis of tissue contrast in extracranial MR imaging. AJR AMJ Roentgenol 1987;149:831–837.

portion of intracellular free water, resulting in their visualization with bright signal intensity on T2WI. In organs, such as the kidney, that are also rich in extracellular or free water, neoplasms may appear isointense or hypointense compared with the bright normal parenchyma on T2WI. Neoplasms that are hypocellular or fibrotic appear dark on T2WI because fibrous tissue dominates their signal characteristics. Simple cysts, CSF, urine in the bladder, and bile in the gallbladder all reflect the signal characteristics of free water.

Proteinaceous Fluids. The addition of protein to free water has the effect of shortening the T1 relaxation time, thus brightening the signal on T1WI. T2 relaxation is also shortened, but the T1 shortening effect is dominant even on T2WI. Therefore, proteinaceous fluid collections remain bright on T2WI. Proteinaceous fluids include synovial fluid, complicated cysts, abscesses, many pathologic fluid collections, and necrotic areas within tumors.

Soft tissues with a predominance of intracellular bound water have shorter T1 and T2 times than do tissues with large amounts of extracellular water. These tissues, including the liver, pancreas, adrenal glands, and muscle, have intermediate signal intensities on both T1WI and T2WI. Intracellular protein synthesis shortens T1 even more; therefore, muscle, being less active in protein synthesis, is lower in signal intensity on T1WI than are organs with more active protein synthesis. Benign tumors with a predominance of normal cells, such as focal nodular hyperplasia in the liver, tend to remain isointense with their surrounding normal parenchyma on all imaging sequences. Hyaline cartilage has a predominance of extracellular water, but the water is extensively bound to a mucopolysaccharide matrix. Its signal characteristics resemble cellular soft tissues, and it is intermediate in strength on most imaging sequences.

Fat. Protons in fat are bound to hydrophobic intermediate-sized molecules and exchange energy efficiently within their chemical environment. T1 relaxation time is short, resulting in a bright signal on T1WI. T2 of fat is shorter than T2 of water, resulting in lower signal intensity for fat, relative to water, on strongly T2WI. On images with lesser degrees of T2 weighting, T1 effect predominates and fat appears isointense or slightly hyperintense compared with water. Specialized fat-saturation imaging sequences may be used to reduce the signal intensity of fat and enhance the visibility of pathologic processes within fat (30). STIR sequences suppress signals from all tissues with short T1 times, including fat (15).

Flowing Blood. The MR signal of slow-moving blood, such as in the spleen, venous plexuses, and cavernous hemangiomas, is dominated by the large amount of extracellular water present, resulting in low signal on T1WI and high signal on T2WI. Higher-velocity blood flow, however, alters the MR signal in complex ways depending on multiple factors. Protons may move out of the imaging plane between RF absorption and RF release, resulting in high-velocity signal loss. Alternatively, blood may be replaced by fully magnetized blood from outside of the image volume, resulting in flow-related enhancement. Flow-related enhancement predominates in GRE imaging, resulting in bright signal intensity ("white blood") for flowing blood (see Fig. 1.17), whereas high-velocity signal loss predominates in spin-echo imaging, resulting in signal void ("black blood") in areas of flowing blood.

Hemorrhage. MR of hemorrhage depends on the age of the hemorrhage, the physical and oxidative state of hemoglobin, the location of the hemorrhage, and whether the source of hemorrhage was arterial or venous (Table 1.3) (29,31). Hemorrhage in the first few hours (hyperacute) is high in free water and thus has low signal on T1WI and high signal on T2WI. Immediately following intraparenchymal arterial hemorrhage, red blood cells are saturated with oxygen and contain oxyhemoglobin, which is not paramagnetic and has little effect on the MR signal from surrounding water protons. Hemorrhage from a venous source contains deoxyhemoglobin, which is paramagnetic and does affect signal from surrounding water protons. Intracellular deoxyhemoglobin selectively shortens T2, reducing signal intensity on T2WI. Thus, acute hemorrhage from a venous source is not as bright on T2WI as is acute hemorrhage from an arterial source. Within a few hours, red blood cells, from either arterial or venous sources, desaturate and contain predominantly deoxyhemoglobin. The most hypoxic and desaturated portions of the hematoma have the lowest signal. The dark hematoma at this stage is of-

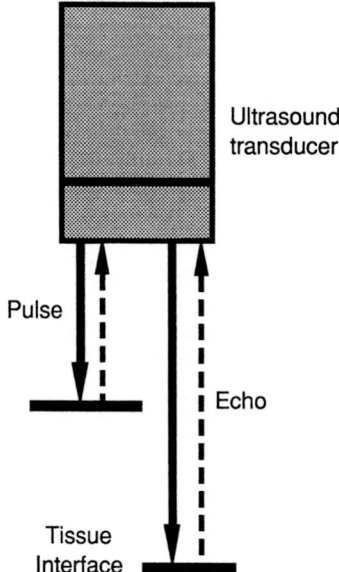

Figure 1.20. US Pulse-Echo Technique. The US transducer transmits a brief pulse of US energy into tissue. The transmitted US pulse encounters tissue interfaces that reflect a portion of the US beam back to the transducer. The depth of the tissue interface is determined by the round-trip time of flight for the transmitted pulse and the returning echo, assuming an average speed of 1540 m/s for sound transmission in human tissue.

ten surrounded by high intensity owing to encircling serum and edema. By approximately 1 week, intracellular deoxyhemoglobin is converted to intracellular methemoglobin beginning at the periphery of the clot. Intracellular methemoglobin is paramagnetic but has restricted motion and is heterogeneous in distribution, shortening T1 and selectively shortening T2, resulting in high signal on T1WI and low signal on T2WI. Lysis of red blood cells at 1 week to 1 month increases access of methemoglobin to water molecules, enhancing the T1 shortening effect. T1 shortening predominates over T2 shortening even on T2WI, resulting in high signal on both T1WI and T2WI. The more dilute the concentration of extracellular methemoglobin (the more water that is present), the higher the signal intensity on T2WI. Areas of low signal intensity on T2WI correspond to retracted clot with intact red cell membranes.

At approximately the same time as lysis of red blood cells is occurring centrally within the clot, releasing free methemoglobin, hemosiderin is being ingested by macrophages at the periphery of the clot. Hemosiderin is highly paramagnetic, but water insolubility precludes close interaction with water, thus restricting T1 shortening. Limited motion of hemosiderin in its intracellular location causes local inhomogeneous magnetic susceptibility and T2 shortening. The result is low signal on both T1WI and T2WI. Edema surrounding the hypointense band of hemosiderin produces a concentric outer rim of hyperintensity as long as edema is present. Hemosiderin-laden macrophages quickly enter the bloodstream, removing hemosiderin from hematoma in nonneural tissues and in areas of the brain where the blood–brain barrier is destroyed, such as in areas of

Table 1.3. MR of Hemorrhage

Age	Dominant Component	T1-weighted image signal	T2-weighted image signal
Hyperacute (<1 day) Arterial	Free water + Oxyhemoglobin	Low	High
Venous	Free water + Deoxyhemoglobin	Low	Less bright than arterial hemorrhage
Acute (1–6 days)	Deoxyhemoglobin	Low	Low
Chronic (>7 days) Intracellular	Methemoglobin	High	Low
Extracellular		High	High
Scar	Hemosiderin	Low	Low

Modified from Mitchell DG, Burk DL Jr, Vinitski S, Rifkin MD. The biophysical basis of tissue contrast in extracranial MR imaging. AJR Am J Roentgenol 1987;149:831–837.

hemorrhage into tumor. Where the blood–brain barrier is quickly repaired, the hemosiderin may remain in brain tissue for long periods and be seen as persisting low intensity. Differentiation of hematoma from other tissues generally requires at least two pulse sequences. Different areas of the hematoma may show signal intensity effects dominated by components in differing stages of evolution.

Ultrasonography

US imaging is performed by using the pulse-echo technique (Fig. 1.20). The US transducer converts electrical energy to a brief pulse of high-frequency sound energy that is transmitted into patient tissues. The US transducer then becomes a receiver, detecting echoes of sound energy reflected from tissue. The depth of any particular echo is determined by measuring the round-

trip time of flight for the transmitted pulse and the returning echo and by calculating the depth of the reflecting tissue interface by assuming an average speed of sound in tissue of 1540 m/s. The US instrument assumes that all returning echoes originate from along the line of sight of the transmitted pulse. The composite image is produced by interrogating tissue in the field of view with multiple closely spaced US pulses. The shape and appearance of the resulting image depend on the design of the particular transducer used (Fig. 1.21). Modern US units operate sufficiently quickly to produce nearly real-time images of moving patient tissue, enabling assessment of respiratory and cardiac movement, vascular pulsations, peristalsis, and the moving fetus. Most medical imaging is performed using US transducers that produce sound pulses in the frequency range of 1 to 10 MHz. Higher frequency transducers (5–10 MHz) yield the greatest spatial resolution but are restricted by

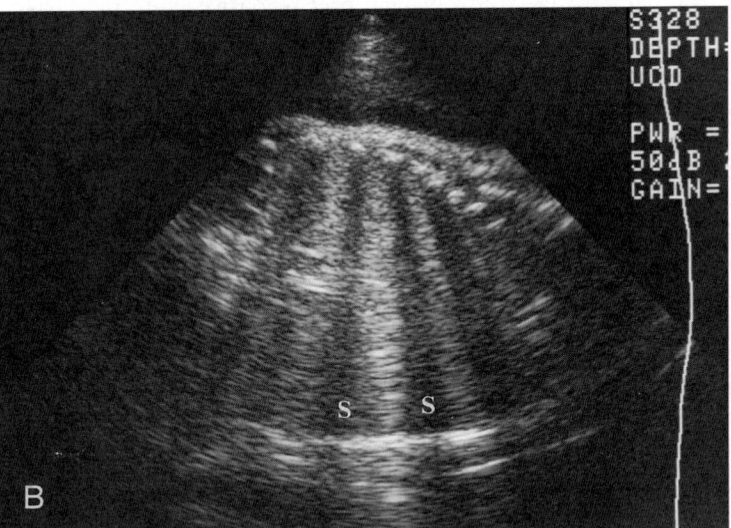

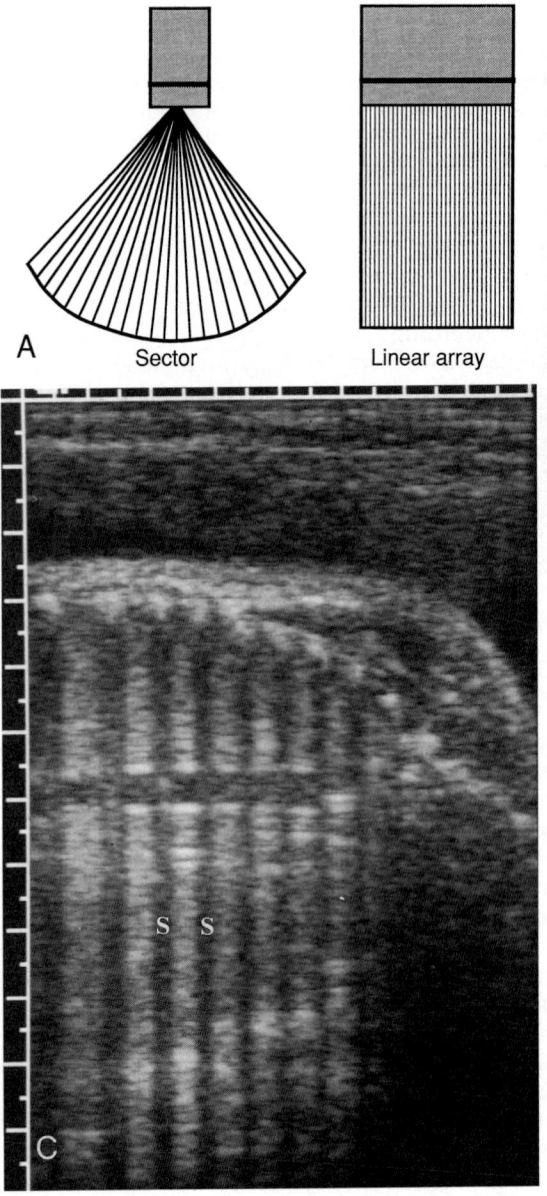

Figure 1.21. Sector Versus Linear Array US Transducers. A. Diagram of the diverging US beams transmitted by a sector transducer (left) and the parallel US beams transmitted by linear array transducer (right). Sector transducers have the advantage of wider field of view in the far field, whereas linear array transducers have a wider field of view in the near field. **B.** Sector transducer image of a fetus shows prominent shadowing (*S*) from the fetal ribs. Note how the width of the shadows expands with increasing depth because of the diverging US beams. **C.** Linear array transducer image of the same fetus shows parallel nonwidening shadows (*S*) from the fetal ribs. Note the improved visualization in the near field.

limited penetration. Lower frequency transducers (1–3.5 MHz) enable better penetration of tissues but at the cost of poorer resolution. High-frequency transducers are routinely used for endoluminal applications; examination of superficial structures such as thyroid, breast, and testes; and examination of infants, children, and small adults. Lower frequency transducers are used for most abdominal, pelvic, and obstetric applications.

US examinations are performed by applying the US transducer directly onto the patient's skin using a water-soluble gel as a coupling agent to ensure good contact and transmission of the US beam. Images may be produced in any anatomic plane by adjusting the orientation and angulation of the transducer and the position of the patient. The standard orthogonal planes—axial, sagittal, and coronal—provide the easiest recognition of anatomy but may not be optimal for demonstration of all anatomic structures. The quality of all US examinations depends heavily on the skill and diligence of the sonographer. US examinations generally provide the most diagnostic information when they are directed at solving a particular clinical problem.

Visualization of anatomic structures by US is severely limited by bone and by gas-containing structures such as bowel and lung. Sound energy is nearly completely absorbed at interfaces between soft tissue and bone, causing an acoustic shadow with limited visualization of structures deep to the bone surface. Soft tissue–gas interfaces cause nearly complete reflection of the sound beam, eliminating visualization of deeper structures. Optimal visualization of many organs is performed through "acoustic windows" that allow adequate sound transmission. The liver is imaged through the windows of the intercostal spaces. The pancreas is visualized through the window of the left lobe of the liver. Pelvic organs are examined through the urine-filled bladder, which displaces the gas-filled bowel out of the pelvis. US visualization of structures in the chest depends on finding windows between bone and air-filled lung. US examination may also be limited by surgical wounds, dressings, and skin lesions, which preclude firm transducer contact with the skin. Endoluminal techniques obviate many of the problems of surface scanning. Endovaginal transducers allow close and highly detailed visualization of the uterus and ovaries without intervening tissues. Endorectal transducers enable intimate examination of the prostate gland and rectum.

Doppler US is an important adjunct to real-time gray-scale imaging. The Doppler effect is a shift in the frequency of returning echoes, compared with the transmitted pulse, caused by reflection of the sound wave from a moving object. In medical imaging, the moving objects of interest are red blood cells in flowing blood (see Fig. 40.1). If blood flow is relatively away from the face of the transducer, the echo frequency is shifted lower. If blood flow is relatively toward the face of the transducer, the echo frequency is shifted higher. The amount of frequency shift is proportional to the relative velocity of the red blood cells.

Doppler US can detect not only the presence of blood flow but can also determine its direction and velocity.

The Doppler frequency shift is in the audible range, producing a sound of blood flow that has additional diagnostic value. *Pulsed Doppler* uses a Doppler sample volume that is time-gated to interrogate only a select volume of patient tissue for the Doppler shift. *Duplex Doppler* combines real-time gray-scale imaging with pulsed Doppler to enable accurate placement of the Doppler sample volume in visualized blood vessels or specific areas of interest (Figs. 40.2, 40.3). *Color Doppler US* combines gray scale and Doppler information in a single image (Fig. 40.9). Stationary tissue with echoes having no Doppler shift are displayed in shades of gray, whereas blood flow and moving tissue producing echoes having a detectable Doppler shift are displayed in color. Blood flow relatively toward the transducer face is usually displayed in shades of red, whereas blood flow relatively away from the transducer face is displayed in shades of blue. Lighter-color shades imply higher flow velocities. Doppler US is discussed in further detail in chapter 40.

ULTRASOUND ARTIFACTS

Artifacts are extremely common in US imaging and must be recognized to avoid diagnostic errors (32,33). Some artifacts, such as acoustic shadowing, are diagnostically useful.

Acoustic shadowing is produced by nearly complete absorption or reflection of the US beam, obscuring deeper tissue structures (Fig. 1.22). Acoustic shadows are produced by bone, metallic objects, gas bubbles, gallstones, and urinary tract stones. The presence of acoustic shadowing aids in the identification of all types of calculi.

Acoustic enhancement refers to the increased intensity of echoes deep to structures that transmit sound exceptionally well such as cysts, fluid-filled bladder, and gallbladder and some solid masses such as lymphoma-replaced lymph nodes. The presence of acoustic enhancement aids in the identification of cystic masses (Fig. 1.23).

Reverberation artifact is caused by repeated reflections between strong acoustic reflectors. Returning echoes are re-reflected into tissues, producing multiple echoes of the same structures that are portrayed on the image progressively deeper in tissue because of prolonged time of flight of echoes eventually returning to the transducer. Reverberation artifact is seen as repeating bands of echoes of progressively decreasing intensity at regularly spaced intervals.

Mirror image artifact is commonly evident when examining the upper abdomen and diaphragm. Multipath reflection from the strong sound reflection produced by the air-filled lung surface above the curving diaphragm results in depiction of liver or spleen tissue both below and above the diaphragm (Fig. 1.24).

Ring down, or comet tail, artifact is seen as a pattern of tapering bright echoes trailing from small bright reflectors such as air bubbles and cholesterol crystals. The artifact may result from vibrations of the reflector or multiple short-path reverberations.

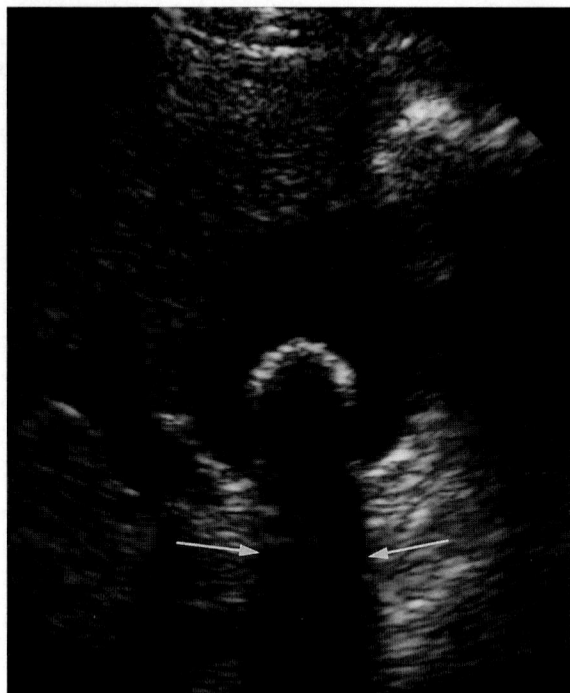

Figure 1.22. Acoustic Shadowing. A gallstone within the gallbladder produces a dark acoustic shadow (*arrows*) by absorption of the US beam. Demonstration of acoustic shadowing is important in the US detection of biliary and renal calculi.

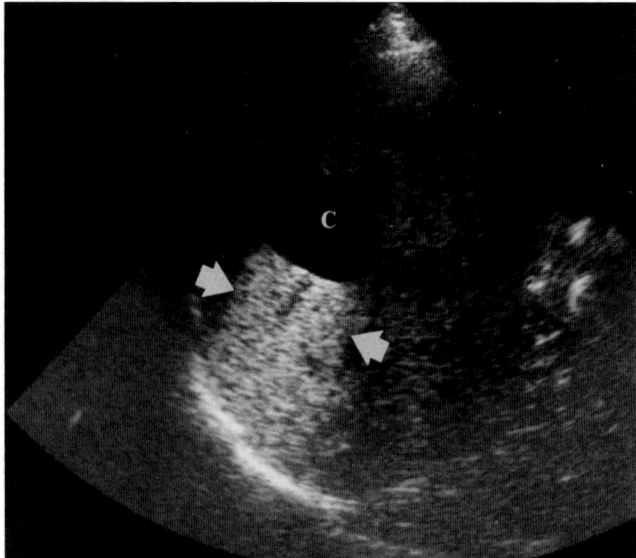

Figure 1.23. Acoustic Enhancement. US image of a cyst (*C*) in the liver demonstrates acoustic enhancement (*arrows*) as a band of bright echoes deep to the cyst.

PRINCIPLES OF ULTRASOUND INTERPRETATION

Interpretation of US examinations is best performed by the radiologist who has studied the images produced by the sonographer and who, with transducer in hand, has personally examined the patient. US in the hands of a skilled physician is a dynamic extension of physical examination. The examining physician has the opportunity to query the patient regarding current and past symptoms, previous surgery, and pertinent medical history. Suspected masses can be palpated as well as examined by US. Artifacts are more easily differentiated from true components of the image by real-time examination. Active examination enables rapid assessment of three-dimensional anatomic relationships. The real-time US examination yields thousands of images within a few minutes. The hard-copy recorded images serve only to document the dynamic real-time examination. All questions in interpretation should be answered by active sonographic examination.

Fluid-containing structures such as cysts, dilated calyces and ureters, and the distended bladder and gallbladder characteristically demonstrate well-defined walls, absence of internal echoes, and distal acoustic enhancement. Solid tissue demonstrates a speckled pattern of tissue texture with definable blood vessels. Fat is usually highly echogenic, whereas solid organs such as liver, pancreas, and kidney demonstrate lower degrees of echogenicity. Lesions within or arising from organs demonstrate mass effect with alteration of organ contour and displacement of blood vessels and with alteration in tissue texture. Lesions of lower echogenicity (lower intensity echoes) than surrounding parenchyma are termed *hypoechoic*, and lesions of greater echogenicity (higher intensity echoes) than surrounding parenchyma are called *hyperechoic*. The term *anechoic* refers to the complete absence of echoes, such as within simple cysts. Cystic structures containing echogenic fluid such as blood, pus, or mucin may cause confusion in the sonographic differentiation of cystic and solid lesions. Echogenic cystic structures demonstrate the absence of internal blood vessels, fluid–fluid layering, shifting con-

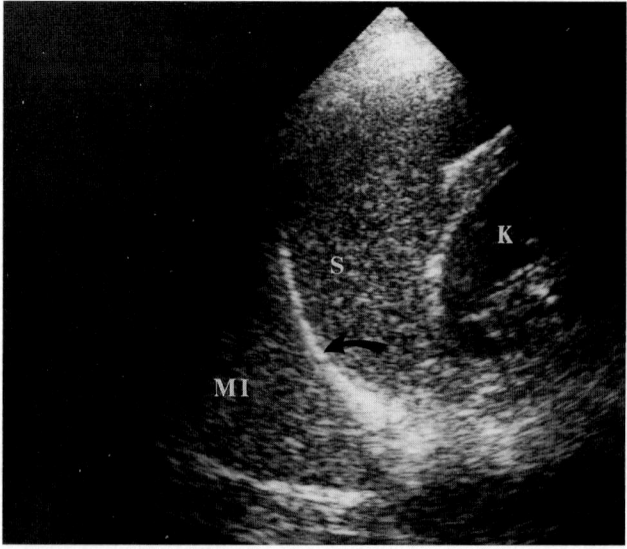

Figure 1.24. Mirror-Image Artifact. Longitudinal image of the left upper quadrant of the abdomen demonstrates the spleen (*S*), diaphragm (*arrow*), and artifactual mirror image (*MI*) of the spleen above the diaphragm. *K*, left kidney.

tents with transducer compression or change in patient position, and well-defined walls. Acoustic enhancement might or might not be present.

RADIOGRAPHIC CONTRAST AGENTS

Iodinated Contrast Agents

Water-soluble contrast agents, consisting of molecules containing atoms of iodine, are used extensively for intravascular applications in CT, urography, and angiography and for arthrography, cystography, fistulography, and GI opacification. Older, cheaper high-osmolar ionic agents are being replaced in many applications by newer but more expensive, low-osmolar agents because of safety considerations (34,35).

Ionic contrast agents (higher-osmolality contrast agents) have been considered safe and effective for more than 50 years. All iodinated contrast agents have a chemical structure based on a benzene ring containing three iodine atoms. Ionic media are acid salts that dissociate in water into a iodine-containing negatively charged anion (diatrizoate, iothalamate) and a positively charged cation, usually sodium or meglumine. To achieve a sufficient concentration of iodine for radiographic visualization, ionic agents are markedly hypertonic (approximately 6 times the osmolality of plasma). High osmolality and viscosity cause significant hemodynamic, cardiac, and subjective effects including vasodilatation, heat, pain, osmotic diuresis, and decreased myocardial contractility. Following IV injection, contrast media are distributed quickly into the extracellular space. Excretion is by renal glomerular filtration. Vicarious excretion through the liver, biliary system, and intestinal tract occurs when renal function is impaired.

Adverse reactions to IV contrast injection occur in approximately 5% of patients (36,37). Most (95%) of the reactions are mild or moderate; approximately 5% are severe. Death occurs as a result of contrast injection in approximately 1 in 40,000 patients. A feeling of warmth at the time of rapid ionic contrast injection is almost universal. Common reactions include nausea, vomiting, hives, and bronchospasm. More serious adverse effects include hypotension, bradycardia, vagal reactions, shock, seizures, and anaphylactoid reaction. Acute renal failure may also be precipitated by contrast injection. Extravasation of contrast media may rarely cause severe skin and subcutaneous tissue ulceration and necrosis (38). The patients at highest risk for contrast reactions include those with a history of previous contrast reaction, a history of allergies, the young (<1 year), the old (>60 years), and patients with heart disease, diabetes, or impaired renal function. An extended discussion of contrast media, adverse effects, and treatment is found in the *Manual on Iodinated Contrast Media* published by the American College of Radiology (39) and in several detailed reviews (40–45).

Lower-osmolality contrast agents (LOCAs) have an osmolality reduced to approximately three times that of blood, resulting in a significant decrease in the already low incidence of adverse reactions. Reduction in osmolality is achieved by making compounds that are non-ionic monomers (iopamidol, iohexol, ioversol), nonionic dimers (iotrol, iodixanol), or monoacidic dimers (ioxaglate). Iotrol and iodixanol are iso-osmolar with plasma. Reduced osmolality results in less hemodynamic alteration on contrast injection. A number of studies, none ideal in design, indicate at least a 50% reduction in the incidence of both minor and major adverse reactions. Because death is so uncommon, no study to date has included a sufficient number of patients to document a reduced incidence of fatal reactions. The cost ratio between LOCA and ionic media is as much as 13:1 in the United States, although the cost of LOCA has recently been decreasing. The decision to use LOCA or ionic media is heavily debated because of the cost implications. The decision to use LOCA in an individual patient must be based on analysis of medical benefit versus cost versus legal implications (35).

Magnetic Resonance Imaging Intravascular Contrast Agent

Gadopentetate dimeglumine, gadolinium-labeled diethylenetriamine penta-acetic acid (Gd-DTPA), is a U.S. Food and Drug Administration–approved contrast agent for MR. Gadopentetate is used, similar to the use of iodinated contrast agents in CT, to identify regions of disruption of the blood–brain barrier, to enhance organs to accentuate pathology, and to document patterns of lesion enhancement. Gadolinium is a rare-earth heavy metal ion with paramagnetic effect that shortens the T1 and T2 relaxation times of hydrogen nuclei within its local magnetic field. At recommended doses, Gd-DTPA shortens T1 to a much greater extent than it shortens T2. Increases in signal intensity resulting from T1 shortening resulting from concentrations of Gd-DTPA are best seen on T1WI. However, when very high tissue concentration is reached, such as in the renal collecting system, T2 shortening causes a significant loss of signal intensity that is best seen on T2WI. The Gd-DTPA is injected intravenously, diffuses rapidly into the extracellular fluid and blood pool spaces, and is excreted by glomerular filtration. Approximately 80% of the injected dose is excreted in 3 hours. Imaging is usually performed immediately after injection. Adverse reactions occur in 2–3% of patients and are similar in type to those encountered with iodinated contrast agents (46–48). They include nausea, vomiting, urticaria, bronchospasm, and anaphylactoid reactions. Only two contrast-related deaths have been reported. The osmolality of Gd-DTPA is 6.8 times that of serum. Extravasation of the contrast agent into the skin may cause ulceration and necrosis, but the risk is lower than for ionic iodinated media (38). Pregnancy, lactation, and renal failure are considered relative contraindications.

Gastrointestinal Contrast Agents

Barium sulfate is the standard opaque contrast agent for routine fluoroscopic contrast studies of the upper and lower GI tract. Modern formulations provide excellent coating of the GI mucosa. "Thin," more fluid, suspensions are used for single-contrast studies, whereas "thick," more viscous, suspensions coat the mucosa for double-contrast examinations. Barium preparations are remarkably well tolerated. Aspiration of barium rarely causes a clinical problem. Small amounts are cleared from the lungs within hours; however, huge amounts may result in pneumonia. Suspected allergic reactions including hives, respiratory arrest, and anaphylaxis have been rarely reported (49). Allergic reactions to latex used in enema balloons and rectal examination gloves are more common than reactions to the barium products themselves. The major risk from the use of barium sulfate is barium peritonitis resulting from the spill of barium into the peritoneal cavity as a result of perforations of the GI tract. Barium deposits act as foreign bodies, inducing fibrin deposition and massive ascites. Bacterial contamination from intestinal contents can lead to sepsis, shock, and death in up to 50% of patients.

Gas Agents. Air and carbon dioxide gas are effective and inexpensive contrast agents for both CT and fluoroscopic studies. A number of effervescent powders, granules, and tablets that release carbon dioxide on contact with water are routinely used. These preparations are excellent for distending the stomach for CT or barium studies. Air injected directly into the GI tract via a nasogastric or enema tube may be used to distend the stomach or colon.

Water-soluble iodinated contrast media opacify the bowel lumen by passive filling, rather than mucosal coating, and are considered by most radiologists to be inferior to barium agents for routine fluoroscopic GI studies. Because of the high mortality associated with barium peritonitis, however, water-soluble agents are indicated when GI tract perforation is suspected. Water-soluble agents are quickly reabsorbed through the peritoneal surface if perforation is present. Dilute solutions (2–5%) of ionic agents are routinely used in CT to opacify the GI tract. Ionic contrast agents stimulate intestinal peristalsis, which promotes faster opacification of the distal bowel on CT and may be useful in the postoperative patient with ileus. The major risk of oral water-soluble agents is aspiration, which causes chemical pneumonitis. Low-osmolar agents may be safer and are preferred when aspiration is deemed a risk. Large volumes of hypertonic water-soluble agents in the GI tract draw water into the gut and may result in hypovolemia, shock, and even death, especially in infants and debilitated adults.

References

1. Curry TS III, Dowdey JE, Murry RC Jr. Christensen's Introduction to the Physics of Diagnostic Radiology. 4th ed. Philadelphia: Lea & Febiger, 1990.
2. Bushberg JT, Seibert JA, Leidholdt EMJ, Boone JM. The Essential Physics of Medical Imaging. Baltimore: Williams & Wilkins, 1994.
3. Squire LF, Novelline RA. Fundamentals of Radiology. 4th ed. Cambridge: Harvard University Press, 1988.
4. Barnes JE. Characteristics and control of contrast in CT. Radiographics 1992;12:825–837.
5. Zeman RK, Zeiberg AS, Davros WJ, et al. Routine helical CT of the abdomen: image quality considerations. Radiology 1993;189:395–400.
6. Silverman PM, Cooper CJ, Weltman DI, et al. Helical CT: practical considerations and potential pitfalls. Radiographics 1995;15:25–36.
7. Bluemke DA, Chambers TP. Spiral CT angiography: an alternative to conventional angiography. Radiology 1995;195:317–319.
8. Zeman RK, Silverman PM, Vieco PT, et al. CT angiography. AJR Am J Roentgenol 1995;165:1079–1088.
9. Herts BR, Einstein DM, Paushter DM. Spiral CT of the abdomen: artifacts and potential pitfalls. AJR Am J Roentgenol 1993;161:1185–1190.
10. Baron RL. Understanding and optimizing use of contrast material for CT of the liver. AJR Am J Roentgenol 1994;163:323–331.
11. Brant WE. Computed tomography artifacts. In: Vogler JB, Helms CA, Callen PW, eds. Normal Variants and Pitfalls in Imaging. Philadelphia: WB Saunders, 1986:3–12.
12. Hendrick RE. Basic physics of MR imaging: an introduction. Radiographics 1994;14:829–846.
13. Saloner D. An introduction to MR angiography. Radiographics 1995;15:453–465.
14. Haacke EM, Tkach JA. Fast MR imaging: techniques and clinical applications. AJR Am J Roentgenol 1990;155:951–964.
15. Krinsky G, Rofsky NM, Weinreb JC. Nonspecificity of short inversion time inversion recovery (STIR) as a technique of fat suppression: pitfalls in image interpretation. AJR Am J Roentgenol 1996;166:523–526.
16. Elster AD. Gradient echo MR imaging: techniques and acronyms. Radiology 1993;186:1–8.
17. Price RR. Contrast mechanisms in gradient-echo imaging and an introduction to fast imaging. Radiographics 1995;15:165–178.
18. Edelman RR, Wielopolski P, Schmitt F. Echo-planar MR imaging. Radiology 1994;192:600–612.
19. DeLaPaz RL. Echo-planar imaging. Radiographics 1994;14:1045–1058.
20. Shellock FG, Morisoli S, Kanal E. MR procedures and biomedical implants, materials, and devices: 1993 update. Radiology 1993;189:587–599.
21. Shellock FG. MRI biologic effects and safety considerations. In: Higgins CB, Hricak H, Helms CA, eds. Magnetic Resonance Imaging of the Body. 2nd ed. New York: Raven Press, 1992:233–265.
22. Murphy KJ, Brunberg JA. Orbital plain films as a prerequisite for MR imaging: is a known history of injury a sufficient screening criterion? AJR Am J Roentgenol 1996;167:1053–1055.
23. Hartnell GG, Spence L, Hughes LA, et al. Safety of MR imaging in patients who have retained metallic materials after cardiac surgery. AJR Am J Roentgenol 1997;168:1157–1159.
24. Kanal E. Pregnancy and the safety of magnetic resonance imaging. MRI Clin North Am 1994;2:309–317.
25. Elster AD. Questions and Answers in Magnetic Resonance Imaging. St. Louis: Mosby, 1994:253–260.
26. Arena L, Morehouse HT, Safir J. MR imaging artifacts that simulate disease: how to recognize and eliminate them. Radiographics 1995;15:1373–1394.
27. Clark JA III, Kelly WM. Common artifacts encountered in magnetic resonance imaging. Radiol Clin North Am 1988;26:893–920.
28. Herrick RC, Hayman LA, Taber KH, et al. Artifacts and pitfalls in MR imaging of the orbits: a clinical review. Radiographics 1997;17:707–724.
29. Mitchell DG, Burk DL Jr, Vinitski S, et al. The biophysical basis of tissue contrast in extracranial MR imaging. AJR Am J Roentgenol 1987:831–837.

30. Semelka RC, Chew W, Hricak H, et al. Fat-saturation MR imaging of the upper abdomen. AJR Am J Roentgenol 1990; 155:1111–1116.

31. Granstrom P, Unger E. MR imaging of the retroperitoneum. MRI Clin North Am 1995;3:121–142.

32. Scanlan KA. Sonographic artifacts and their origins. AJR Am J Roentgenol 1991;156:1267–1272.

33. Kremkau FW, Taylor KJW. Artifacts in ultrasound imaging. J Ultrasound Med 1986;5:227–237.

34. Caro JJ, Trindade E, McGregor M. The cost effectiveness of replacing high osmolality with low osmolality contrast media. AJR Am J Roentgenol 1992;159:869–874.

35. Ellis JH, Cohan RH, Sonnad SS, et al. Selective use of radiographic low-osmolality contrast media in the 1990s. Radiology 1996;200:297–311.

36. Siegle RL. Rates of idiosyncratic reactions—ionic versus nonionic contrast media. Invest Radiol 1993;28:S95–S98.

37. McClennan BL. Adverse reactions to iodinated contrast media—recognition and response. Invest Radiol 1994;29: S46–S50.

38. Cohan RH, Ellis JH, Garner WL. Extravasation of radiographic contrast material: recognition, prevention, and treatment. Radiology 1996;200:593–604.

39. American College of Radiology. Manual on Iodinated Contrast Media. Reston, VA: American College of Radiology, 1991.

40. Katzberg RW, ed. The Contrast Media Manual. Baltimore: Williams & Wilkins, 1992.

41. Bettmann MA, Heeren T, Greenfield A, et al. Adverse events with radiographic contrast agents: results of the SCVIR contrast agent registry. Radiology 1997;203:611–620.

42. Bush WH, Swanson DP. Acute reactions to intravascular contrast media: types, risk factors, recognition, and specific treatment. AJR Am J Roentgenol 1991;157:1153–1161.

43. Lasser EC, Lyons SG, Berry CC. Reports on contrast media reactions: analysis of data from reports to the U.S. Food and Drug Administration. Radiology 1997;203:605–610.

44. Spring DB, Bettmann MA, Barkan HE. Deaths related to iodinated contrast media reported spontaneously to the U.S. Food and Drug Administration, 1978–1994: effect of availability of low-osmolality contrast media. Radiology 1997; 204:333–337.

45. Spring DB, Bettmann MA, Barkan HE. Nonfatal adverse reactions to iodinated contrast media: spontaneous reporting to the U.S. Food and Drug Administration, 1978–1994. Radiology 1997;204:325–332.

46. Nelson KL, Gifford LM, Lauber-Huber C, et al. Clinical safety of gadopentetate dimeglumine. Radiology 1995;196: 439–443.

47. Neindorf HP, Alhassan A, Geens VR, et al. Safety review of gadopentetate dimeglumine—extended clinical experience after more than five million applications. Invest Radiol 1994;29:S179–S182.

48. Murphy KJ, Brunberg JA, Cohan RH. Adverse reactions to gadolinium contrast media: a review of 36 cases. AJR Am J Roentgenol 1996;167:847–849.

49. Skucas J. Anaphylactoid reactions with gastrointestinal contrast media. AJR Am J Roentgenol 1997;168:962–964.

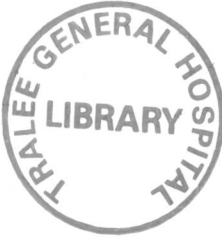

Section II NEURORADIOLOGY

Section Editor:
Erik H.L. Gaensler

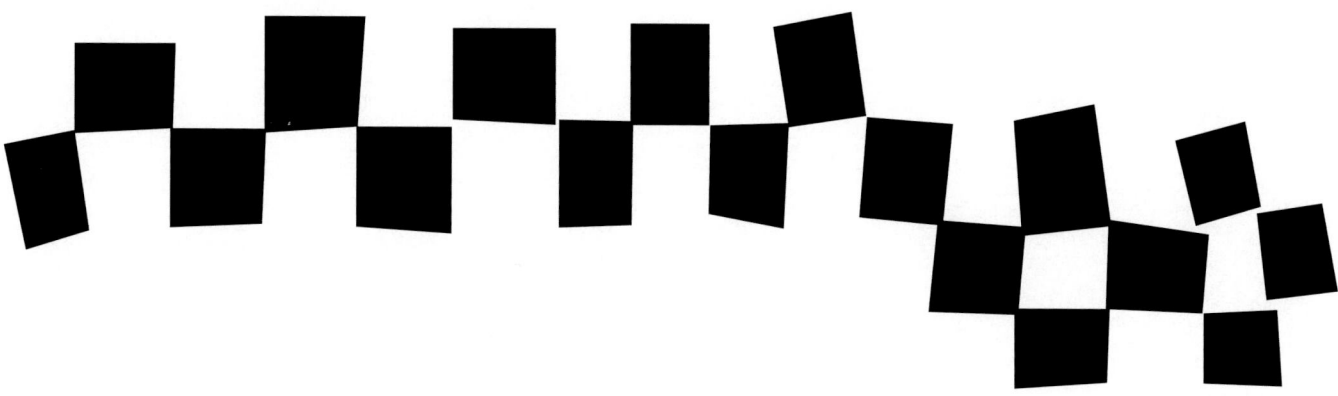

2
Introduction to Brain Imaging

David J. Seidenwurm

This chapter provides an atlas of neuroanatomy and a discussion of the principles of brain imaging and interpretation. Brain anatomy is shown on CT in axial plane (Figs. 2.1–2.4) and on MR in T2-weighted axial plane (Figs. 2.5–2.17) and T1-weighted coronal plane (Figs. 2.18–2.27) images. Figures 2.28–2.36 are examples of specialized high-resolution MR brain imaging.

LOOKING AT THE BRAIN

A few simple principles can be employed to ensure that no neurosurgical emergency is missed, even on a first cursory look at an emergency CT scan.

Midline. The middle of the patient's brain should be in the middle of the patient's head, and the two sides of the brain should look alike (Figs. 2.1–2.4). Although there are important functional asymmetries between the right and left hemispheres, the anatomic differences are subtle and play no role in clinical neuroradiology. Any shift of midline structures is presumed to represent a mass lesion on the side from which the midline is displaced. There are no "sucking" brain wounds that draw the midline toward them. If the interventricular septum and third ventricle are located in the midline, no subfalcine herniation is present (Fig. 2.1).

Symmetry of the brain is the key to radiologic evaluation. Only experience teaches how much asymmetry is within the range of normal variation. Generally, the sulcal pattern should be symmetric. The sulci on one side are the same size as the corresponding sulci on the other. The anterior interhemispheric fissure should be visualized (Figs. 2.1, 2.5). Loss of sulci may be attributable to compression resulting from mass or opacification of CSF owing to subarachnoid hemorrhage. The sulci extend to the inner table of the skull. In older patients, mild atrophy is normal. Significant medial displacement of the sulci may represent compressed brain caused by an extracerebral fluid collection such as a subdural or epidural hematoma. Because these may be bilateral and similar in density to brain, care needs to be taken in evaluating the periphery of the brain.

Basal Cisterns. More subtle, but more important, signs of intracranial mass include distortion of the CSF spaces of the posterior fossa and base of the brain. The

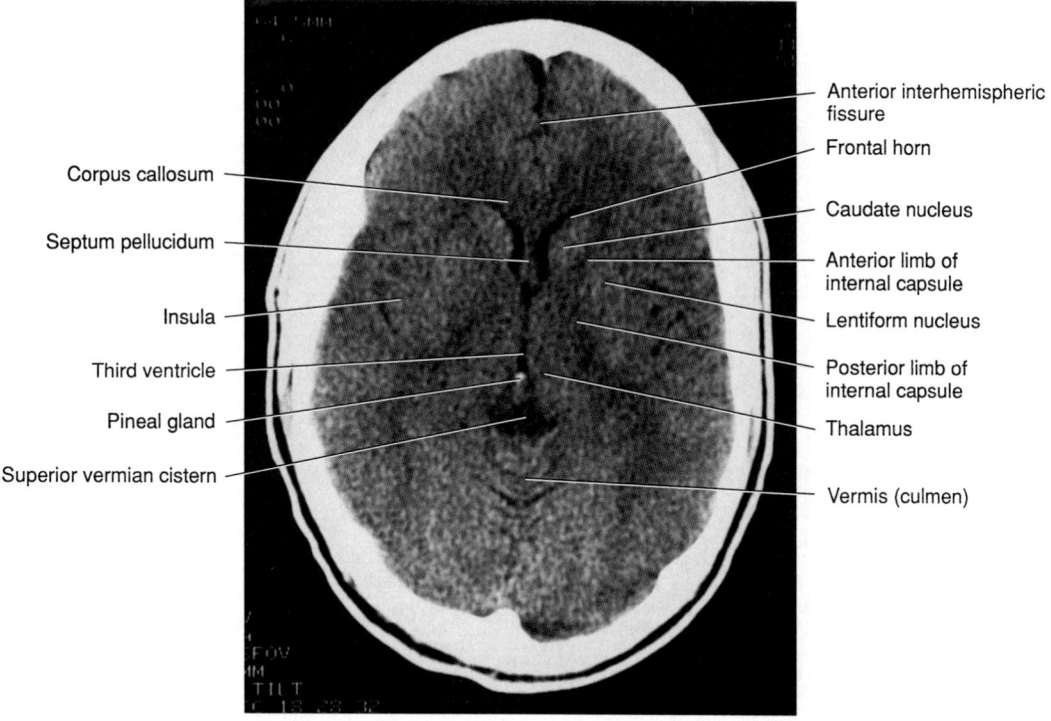

Corpus callosum

Septum pellucidum

Insula

Third ventricle

Pineal gland

Superior vermian cistern

Anterior interhemispheric fissure

Frontal horn

Caudate nucleus

Anterior limb of internal capsule

Lentiform nucleus

Posterior limb of internal capsule

Thalamus

Vermis (culmen)

Figure 2.1. Brain CT. Without IV contrast, axial plane through the third ventricle.

key structures here are the quadrigeminal plate cistern and the suprasellar cistern (Figs. 2.2–2.4; see Figs. 2.10,2.11,2.19). Because these CSF spaces are traversed by important neural structures, careful attention to these regions is essential. The quadrigeminal plate cistern in the axial plane has the appearance of a symmet-

ric smile (see Figs. 2.2,2.3). Any asymmetry must be suspect, and abnormality of this cistern may represent rotation of the brainstem from transtentorial herniation, effacement of the cistern resulting from cerebellar or brainstem mass, or opacification of the cistern as in subarachnoid hemorrhage.

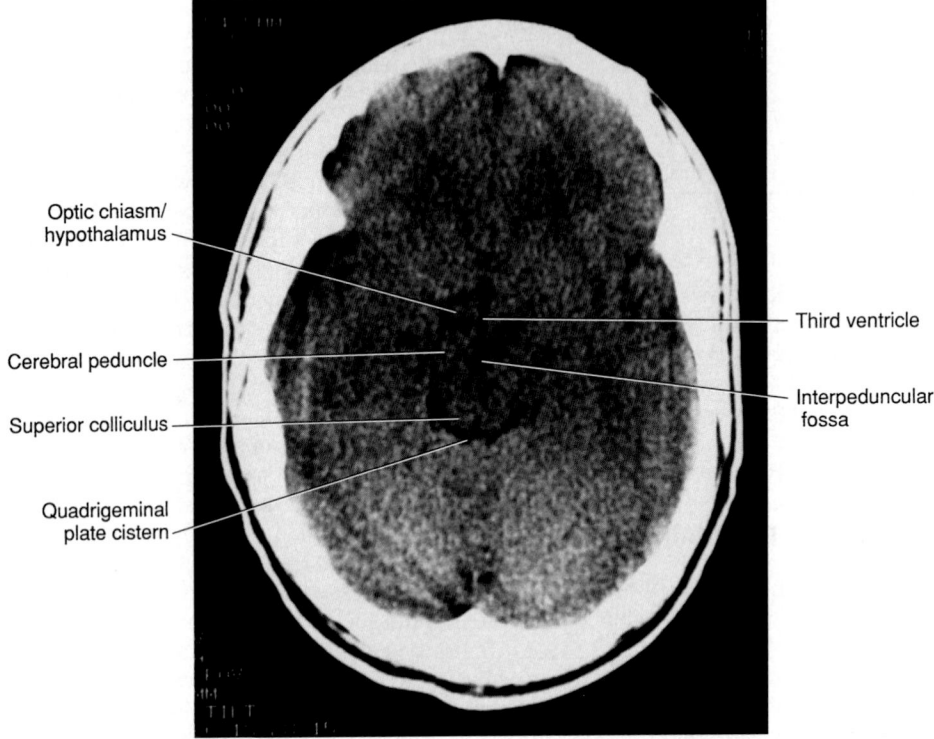

Figure 2.2. Brain CT. Without IV contrast, axial plane through the quadrigeminal plate cistern.

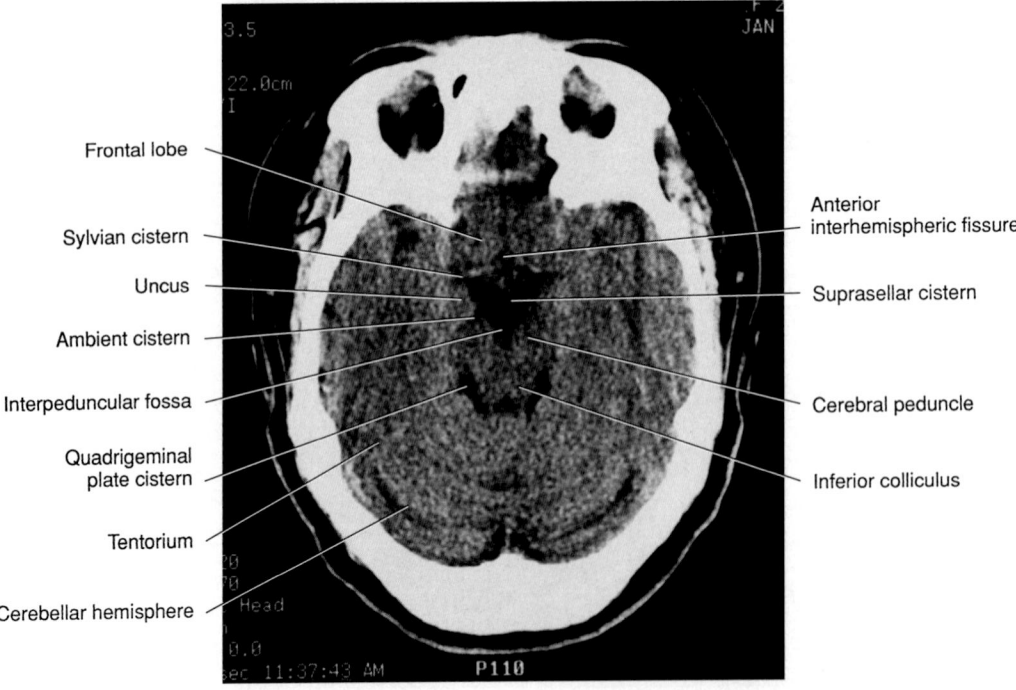

Figure 2.3. Brain CT. Without IV contrast, axial plane through the suprasellar cistern.

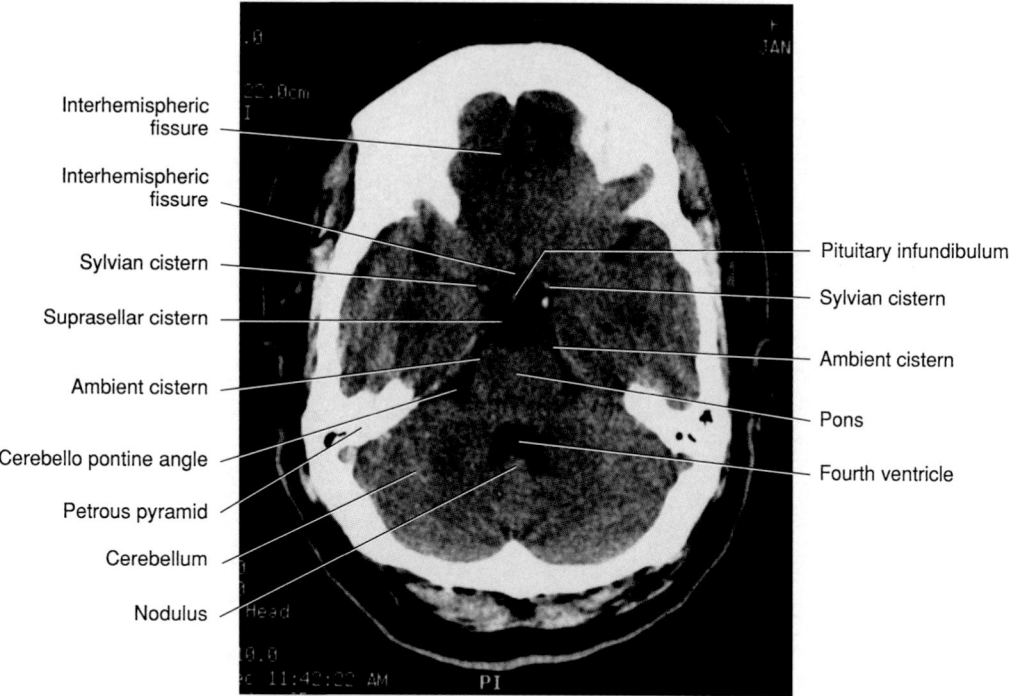

Interhemispheric fissure

Interhemispheric fissure

Sylvian cistern

Suprasellar cistern

Ambient cistern

Cerebello pontine angle

Petrous pyramid

Cerebellum

Nodulus

Pituitary infundibulum

Sylvian cistern

Ambient cistern

Pons

Fourth ventricle

Figure 2.4. Brain CT. Without IV contrast, axial plane through the pons and fourth ventricle.

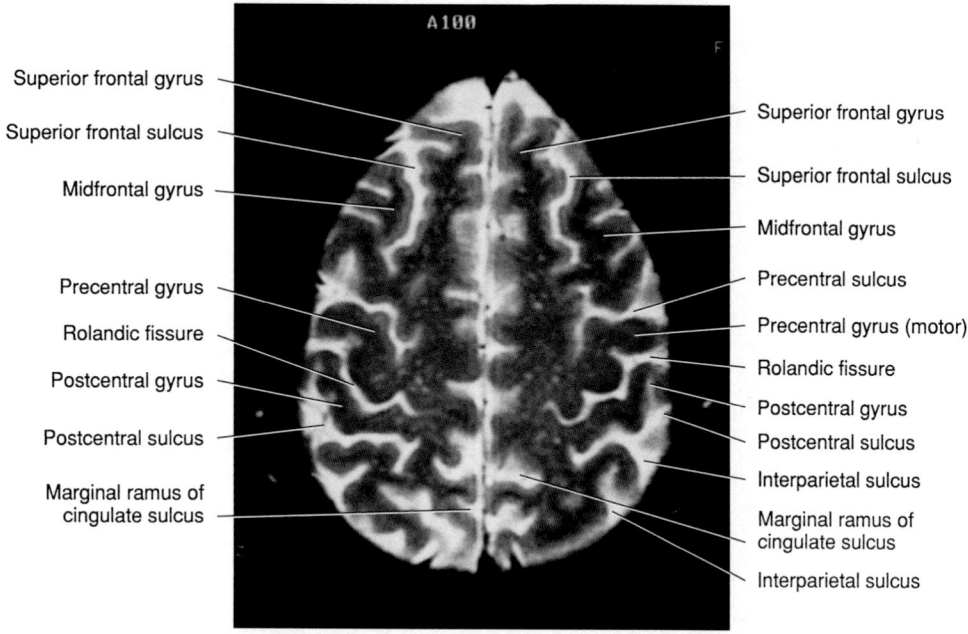

Superior frontal gyrus

Superior frontal sulcus

Midfrontal gyrus

Precentral gyrus

Rolandic fissure

Postcentral gyrus

Postcentral sulcus

Marginal ramus of cingulate sulcus

Superior frontal gyrus

Superior frontal sulcus

Midfrontal gyrus

Precentral sulcus

Precentral gyrus (motor)

Rolandic fissure

Postcentral gyrus

Postcentral sulcus

Interparietal sulcus

Marginal ramus of cingulate sulcus

Interparietal sulcus

Figure 2.5. Brain MR. T2-weighted, axial plane through the cerebral hemispheres.

The suprasellar cistern looks like a pentagon or the Star of David, depending on the angulation of the scan through it (see Figs. 2.3, 2.4, 2.10, 2.11). The five corners of the pentagon are the interhemispheric fissure anteriorly, the sylvian cisterns anterolaterally, and the ambient cisterns posterolaterally. The sixth point of the Star of David is in the interpeduncular fossa posteriorly. The cistern has the density of CSF, and the structure is symmetric. The anatomic continuations of the cistern are the same density as CSF. Significant asymmetry may be attributable to uncal herniation. Central mass may be because of sellar or suprasellar tumor. Opacification of the cistern may be the result of subarachnoid hemorrhage or meningitis.

Ventricles. The final structure that must be evaluated in a quick review of a brain scan is the ventricular system. It is best to start with the fourth ventricle in the posterior fossa because it is the hardest to see on CT scan-

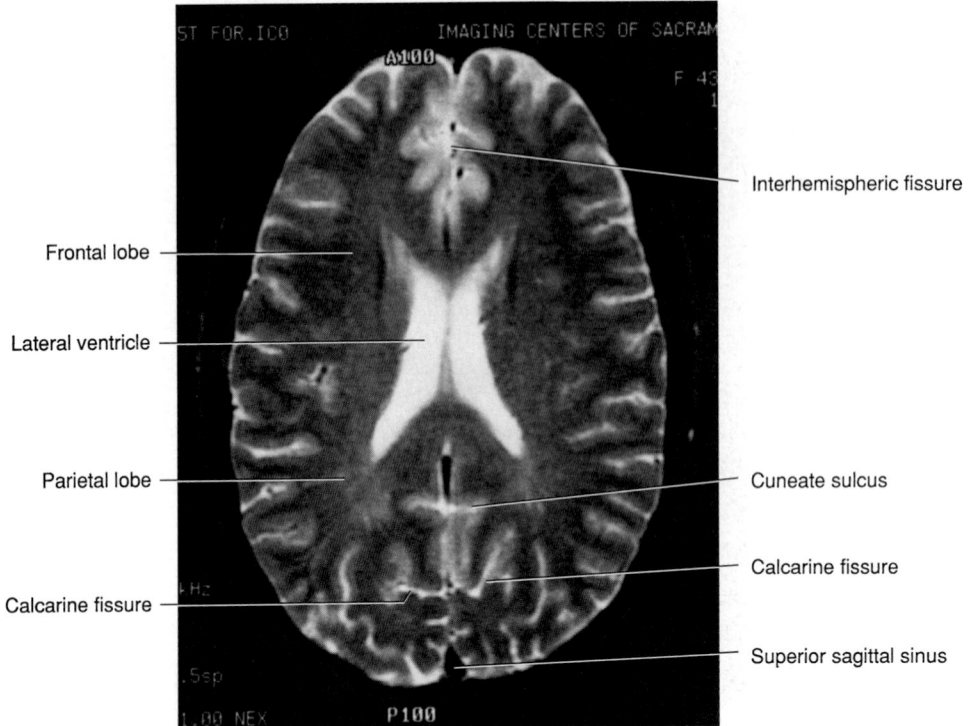

Frontal lobe

Lateral ventricle

Parietal lobe

Calcarine fissure

Interhemispheric fissure

Cuneate sulcus

Calcarine fissure

Superior sagittal sinus

Figure 2.6. Brain MR. T2-weighted, axial plane through the body of lateral ventricles.

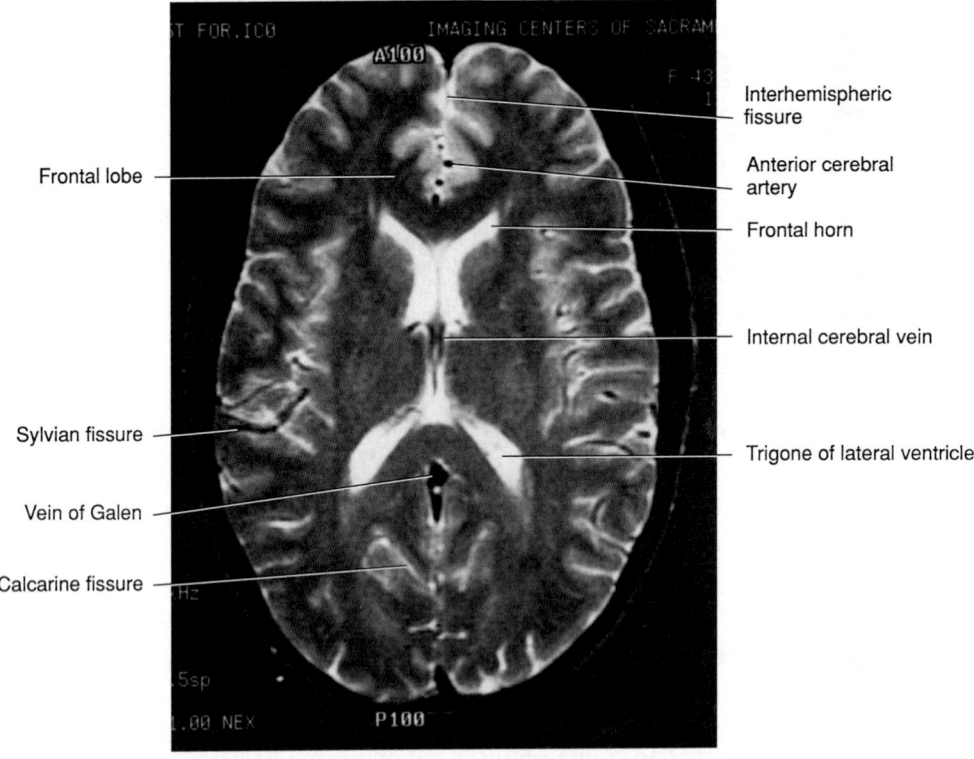

Frontal lobe

Sylvian fissure

Vein of Galen

Calcarine fissure

Interhemispheric fissure

Anterior cerebral artery

Frontal horn

Internal cerebral vein

Trigone of lateral ventricle

Figure 2.7. Brain MR. T2-weighted, axial plane through level of internal cerebral veins.

ning (Fig. 2.4). Subtle asymmetry of the fourth ventricle may be the only sign of significant intracranial masses.

The overall size of the ventricular system is assessed next (Figs. 2.1,2.2,2.4,2.6–2.16). Enlargement of the lateral ventricles and third ventricle in the setting of headache, or with signs of intracranial mass, may represent hydrocephalus, a potentially fatal yet easily treatable condition. Hydrocephalus is distinguished from enlargement of the ventricular system as a result of atrophy by a discrepancy in the degree of ventricular and

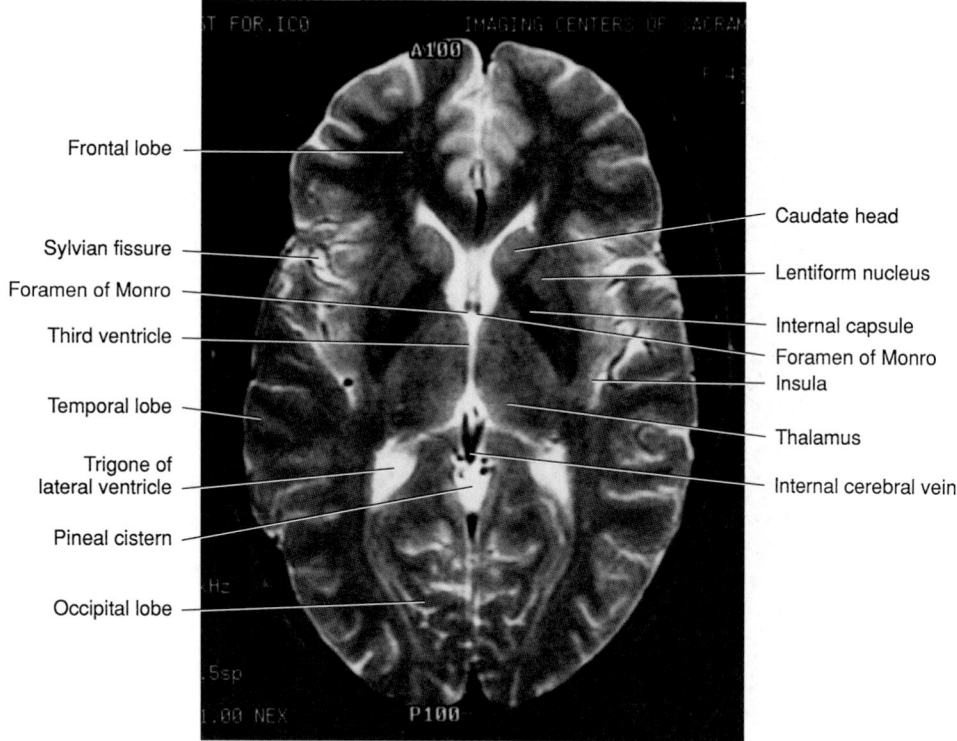

Frontal lobe

Sylvian fissure
Foramen of Monro
Third ventricle

Temporal lobe

Trigone of
lateral ventricle

Pineal cistern

Occipital lobe

Caudate head
Lentiform nucleus

Internal capsule
Foramen of Monro
Insula

Thalamus

Internal cerebral vein

Figure 2.8. Brain MR. T2-weighted, axial plane through foramina of Monro and third ventricle.

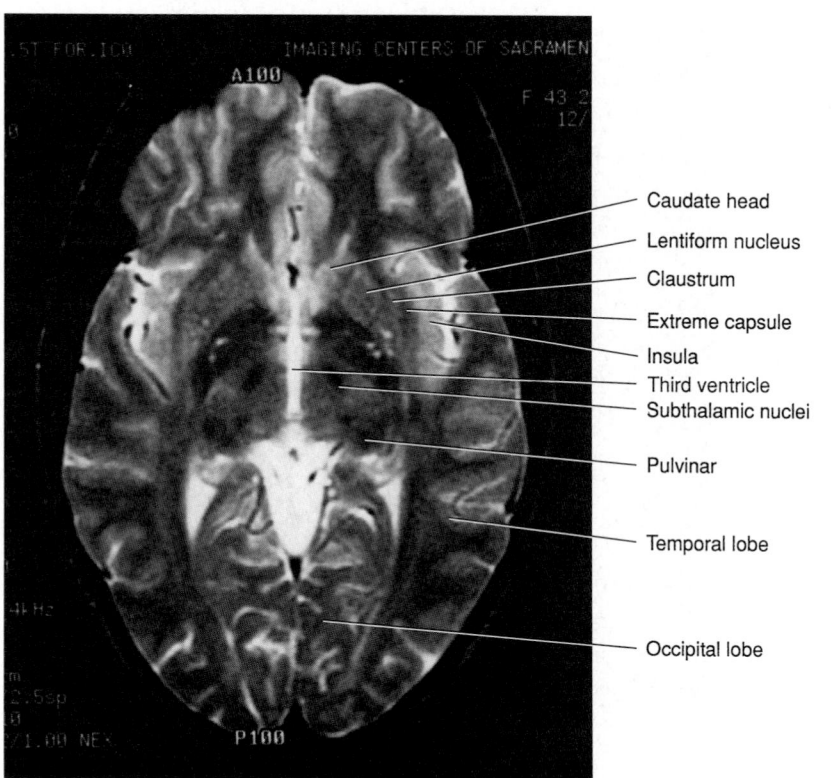

Caudate head
Lentiform nucleus
Claustrum
Extreme capsule
Insula
Third ventricle
Subthalamic nuclei

Pulvinar

Temporal lobe

Occipital lobe

Figure 2.9. Brain MR. T2-weighted, axial plane through third ventricle.

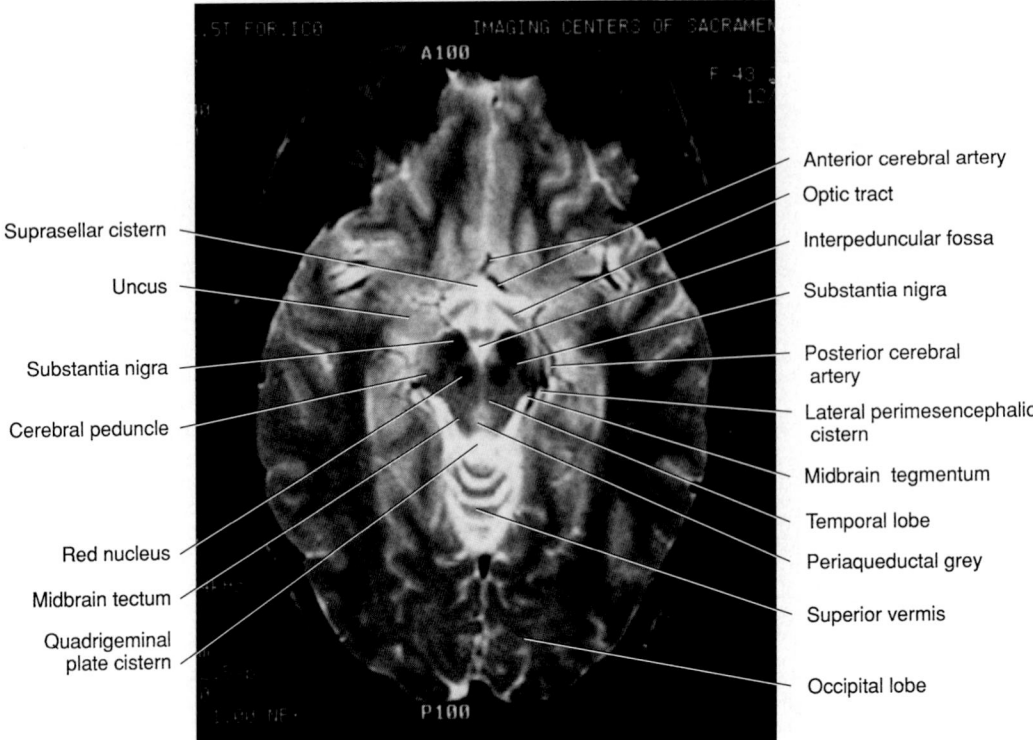

Suprasellar cistern

Uncus

Substantia nigra

Cerebral peduncle

Red nucleus

Midbrain tectum

Quadrigeminal plate cistern

Anterior cerebral artery

Optic tract

Interpeduncular fossa

Substantia nigra

Posterior cerebral artery

Lateral perimesencephalic cistern

Midbrain tegmentum

Temporal lobe

Periaqueductal grey

Superior vermis

Occipital lobe

Figure 2.10. Brain MR. T2-weighted, axial plane through midbrain and suprasellar cistern.

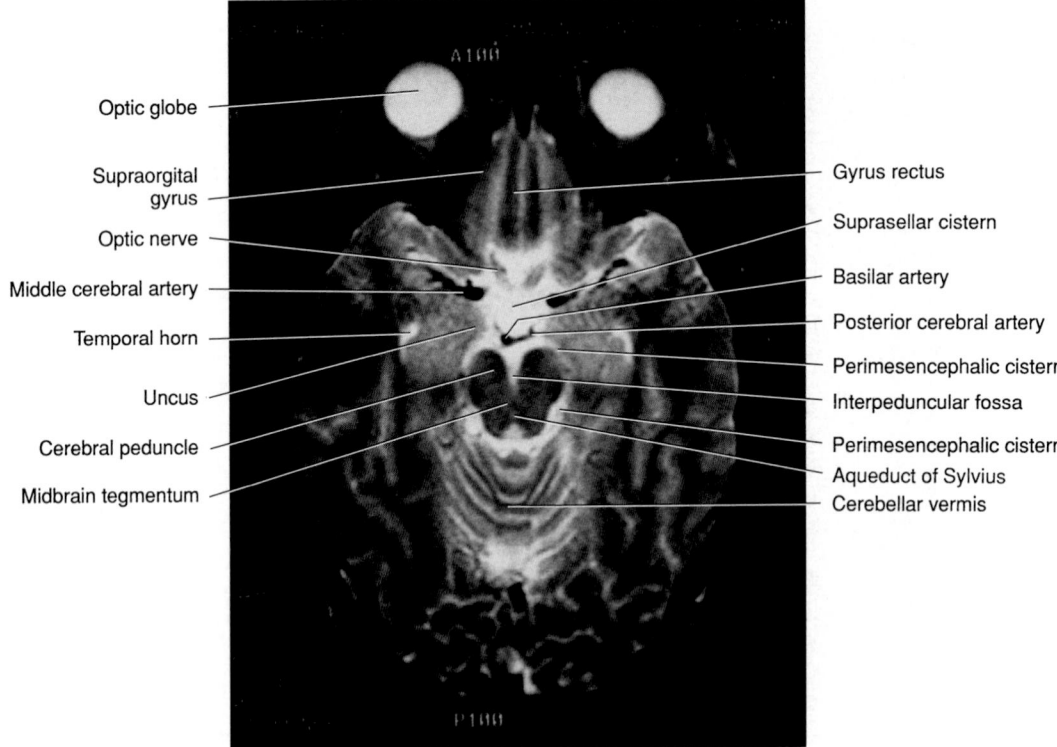

Optic globe

Supraorgital gyrus

Optic nerve

Middle cerebral artery

Temporal horn

Uncus

Cerebral peduncle

Midbrain tegmentum

Gyrus rectus

Suprasellar cistern

Basilar artery

Posterior cerebral artery

Perimesencephalic cistern

Interpeduncular fossa

Perimesencephalic cistern

Aqueduct of Sylvius

Cerebellar vermis

Figure 2.11. Brain MR. T2-weighted, axial plane through midbrain, vermis, and suprasellar cistern.

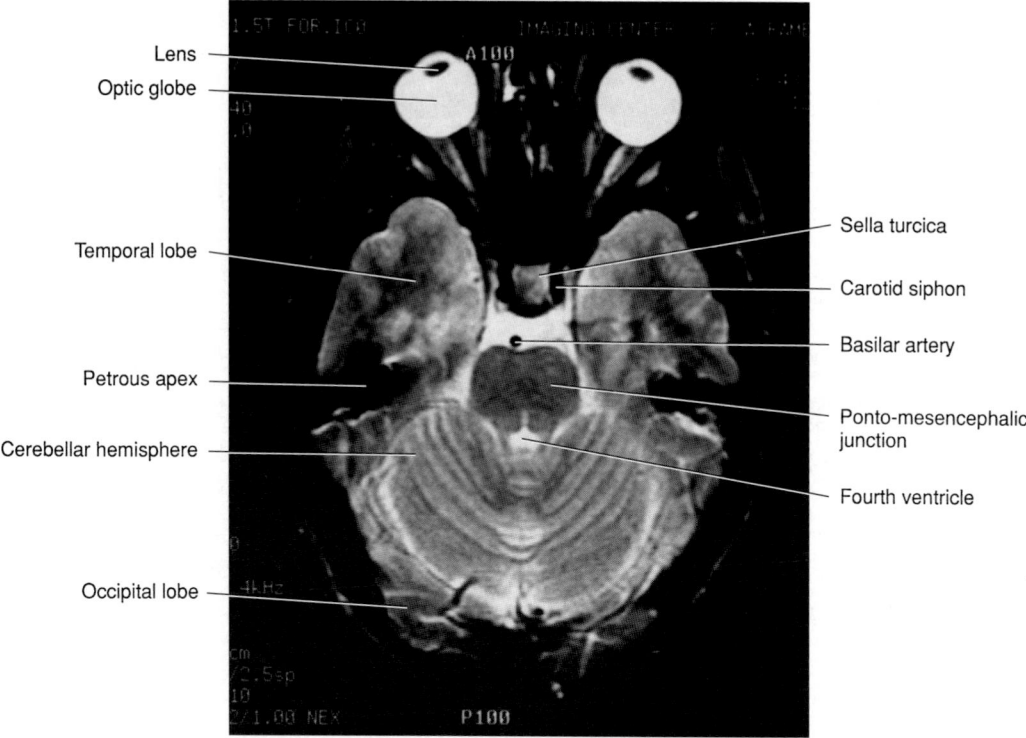

Figure 2.12. Brain MR. T2-weighted, axial plane through pontomesencephalic junction.

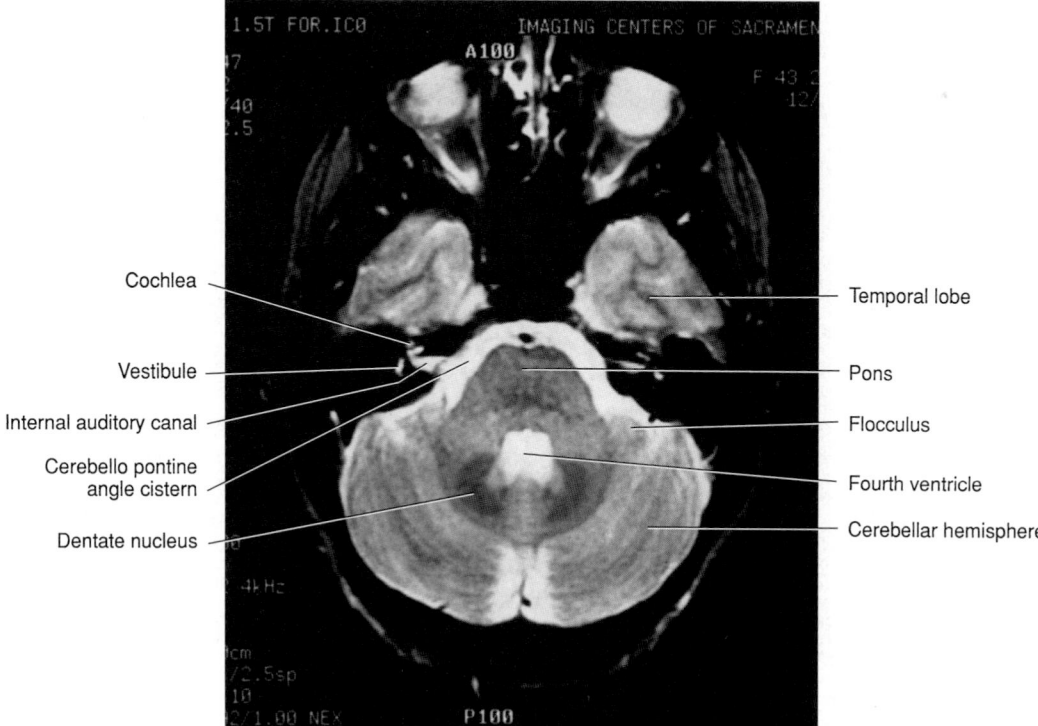

Figure 2.13. Brain MR. T2-weighted, axial plane through fourth ventricle.

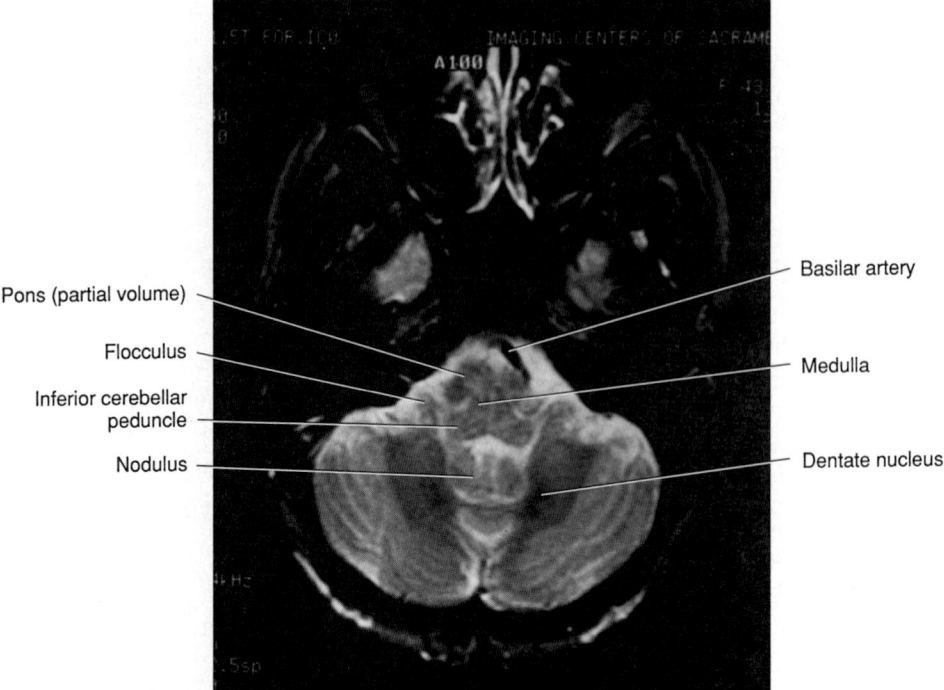

Pons (partial volume)

Flocculus

Inferior cerebellar
peduncle

Nodulus

Basilar artery

Medulla

Dentate nucleus

Figure 2.14. Brain MR. T2-weighted, axial plane through medulla.

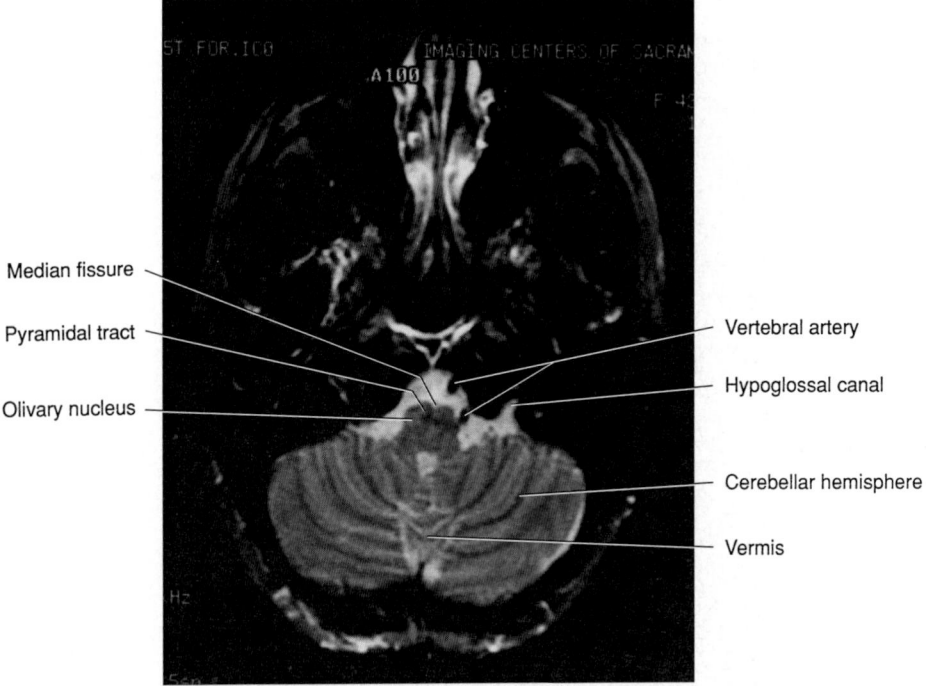

Median fissure

Pyramidal tract

Olivary nucleus

Vertebral artery

Hypoglossal canal

Cerebellar hemisphere

Vermis

Figure 2.15. Brain MR. T2-weighted, axial plane through the cerebellar vermis.

sulcal enlargement and by a characteristic pattern of frontal horn and temporal horn enlargement and a round appearance of the anterior portion of the third ventricle.

Emergency CT Checklist. When confronted with a CT scan under emergency conditions, ask yourself these five questions:

1. Is the middle of the brain in the middle of the head?
2. Do the two sides of the brain look alike?
3. Can you see the smile and the pentagon or Star of David?
4. Is the fourth ventricle in the midline and more or less symmetrical?
5. Are the lateral ventricles huge with effaced sulci?

If you can give the right answers to these five questions, there is no neurosurgical emergency. This approach leaves many important diagnoses unmade, but the diseases are untreatable or the treatment can safely be delayed several hours. Thrombolysis candidates, however, require close scrutiny of the basal ganglia and cortex for signs of early ischemia.

Midline Structures

The anatomy of the midline of the brain is extremely complex, and because the structures are not duplicated, principles of symmetry cannot be applied.

Suprasellar Region. The midline anatomy must be learned in detail. There are three prime locations to study. The first is the suprasellar and sellar region. During virtually every MR examination, it is possible to localize the sella turcica, the pituitary gland, pituitary infundibulum, optic chiasm, anterior third ventricle, mamillary bodies, and anterior interhemispheric fissure. Important vascular structures are also seen in this region. The tip of the basilar artery and the posterior cerebral arteries are seen posteriorly, and the anterior cerebral arteries are visualized anterior and superior to the sella (see Fig. 2.10). The anterior cerebral arteries travel in the interhemispheric fissure. Slightly off the midline, we see the "s"-shaped carotid siphons (see Fig. 2.10) and the posterior communicating arteries. Parallel to the course of the posterior communicating artery, we frequently see the third cranial nerve (see Fig. 2.29). In the parasagittal location, near the optic chiasm we see the optic nerve anteriorly and the optic tract posteriorly (see Figs. 2.10, 2.11, 2.29–2.31).

Pineal Region. The next important region to study in the midline is the pineal region (see Figs. 2.1, 2.8–2.11, 2.30, 2.31). It is crucial to identify the midbrain, the midbrain tegmentum (frequently with a small lucency representing the decussation of the superior cerebellar peduncle), the aqueduct of Sylvius, the midbrain tectum with superior and inferior colliculi, the pineal gland, and the superior cerebellar vermian lobules. If the precentral cerebellar vein can be seen in the superior vermian cistern, a mass here is unlikely.

Craniocervical Junction. Historically, the craniocervical junction (Fig. 2.17, 2.32) has been a relative blind spot to the neuroradiologist, so it is particularly important to study this region. The anterior arch of C-1, the odontoid process. and the cervical occipital ligaments are seen anteriorly. The sharp inferior edge of the clivus marks the anterior lip of the foramen magnum. The posterior lip is marked by the cortical margin of the occipital bone. The cerebellar tonsils should project no more than 3 mm below a line drawn between these two points.

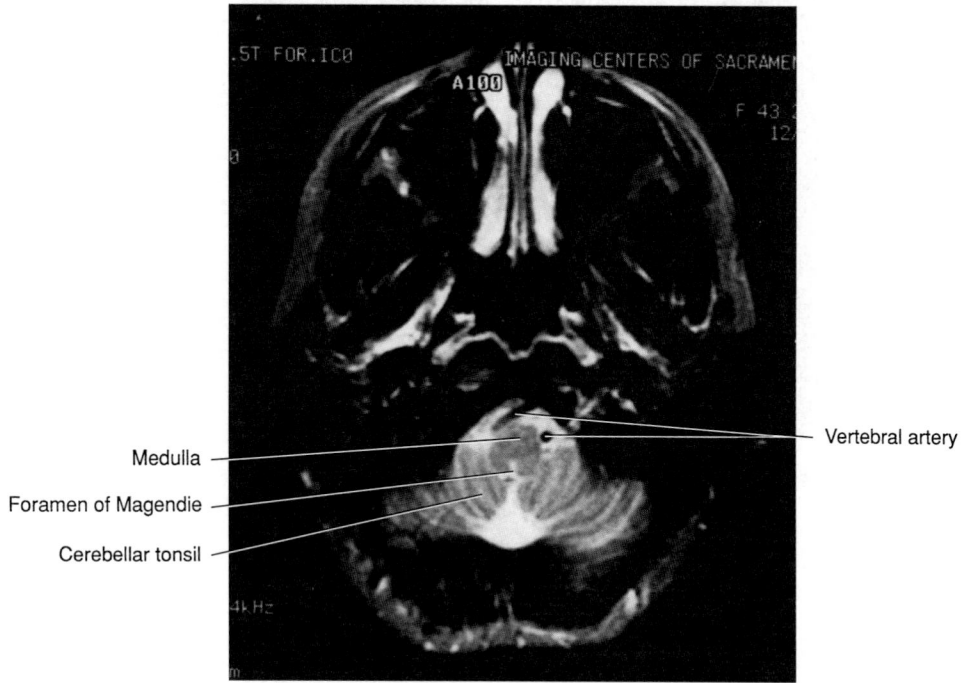

Figure 2.16. Brain MR. T2-weighted, axial plane through foramen of Magendie.

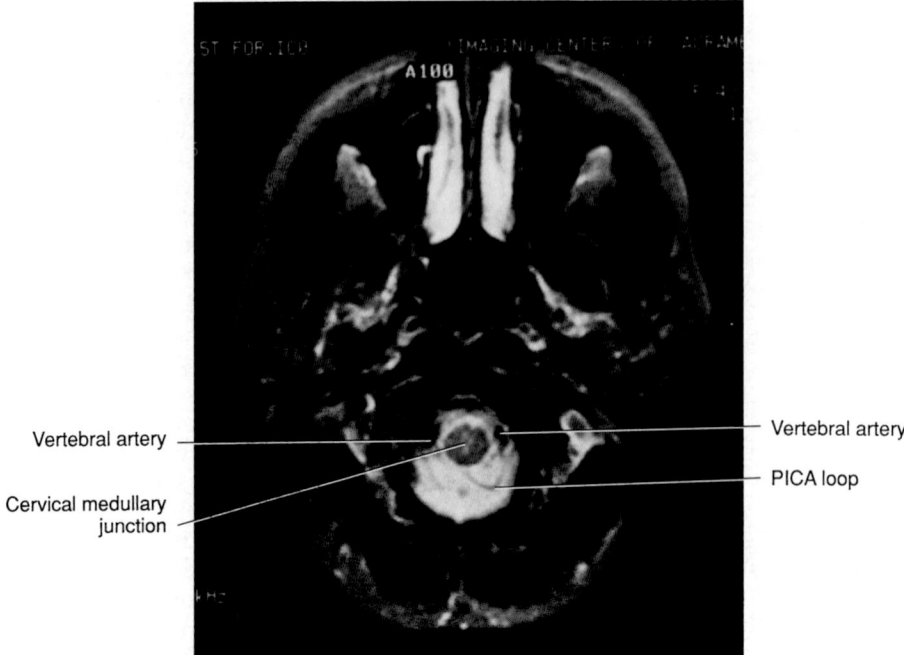

Vertebral artery

Cervical medullary
junction

Vertebral artery

PICA loop

Figure 2.17. Brain MR. T2-weighted, axial plane through cervical medullary junction.

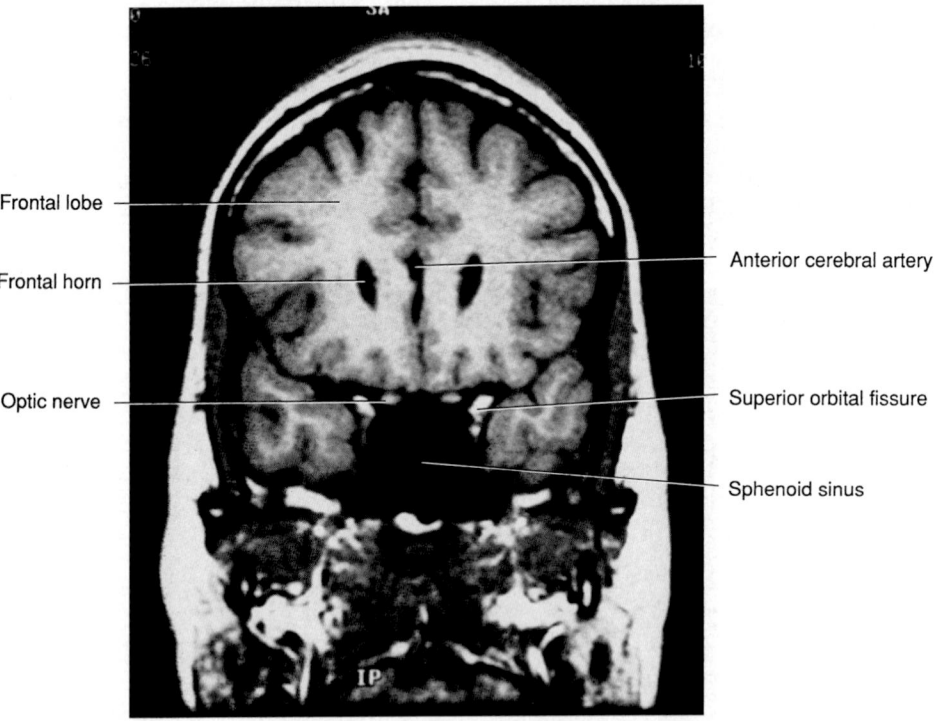

Frontal lobe

Frontal horn

Optic nerve

Anterior cerebral artery

Superior orbital fissure

Sphenoid sinus

Figure 2.18. Brain MR. T1-weighted, coronal plane through frontal lobes.

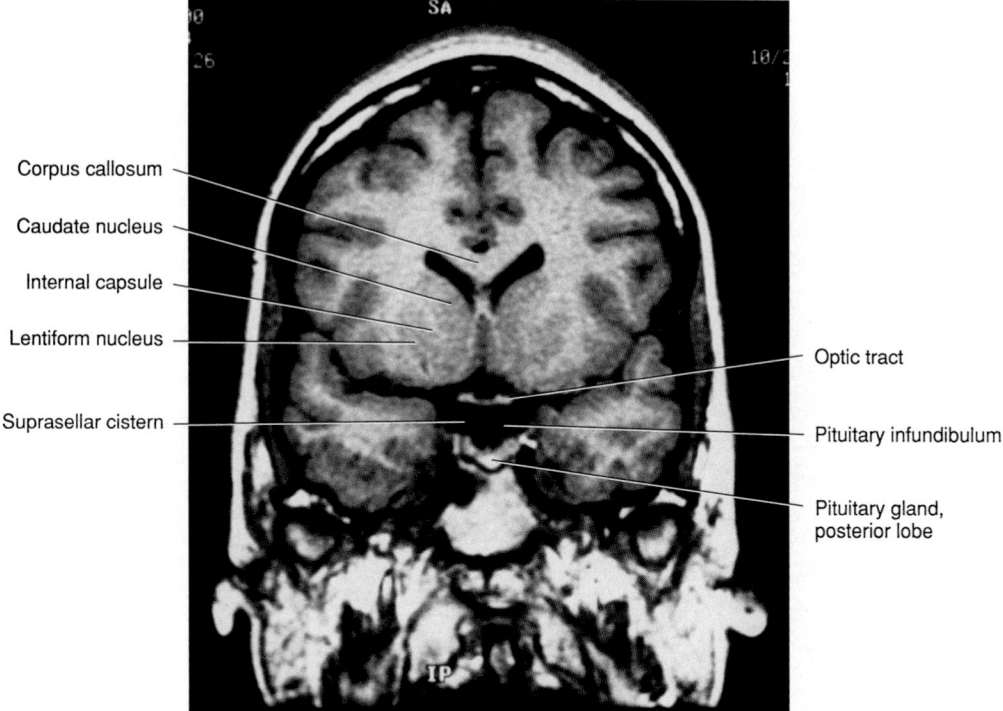

Figure 2.19. Brain MR. T1-weighted, coronal plane through pituitary infundibulum.

Corpus callosum

Caudate nucleus

Internal capsule

Lentiform nucleus

Suprasellar cistern

Optic tract

Pituitary infundibulum

Pituitary gland, posterior lobe

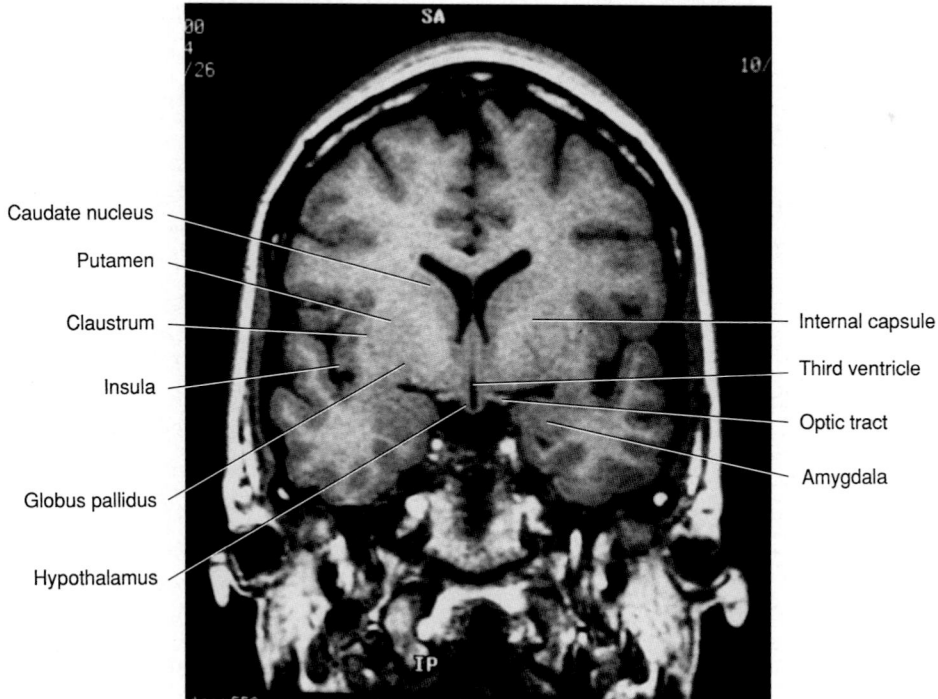

Figure 2.20. Brain MR. T1-weighted, coronal plane through optic tracts.

Caudate nucleus

Putamen

Claustrum

Insula

Globus pallidus

Hypothalamus

Internal capsule

Third ventricle

Optic tract

Amygdala

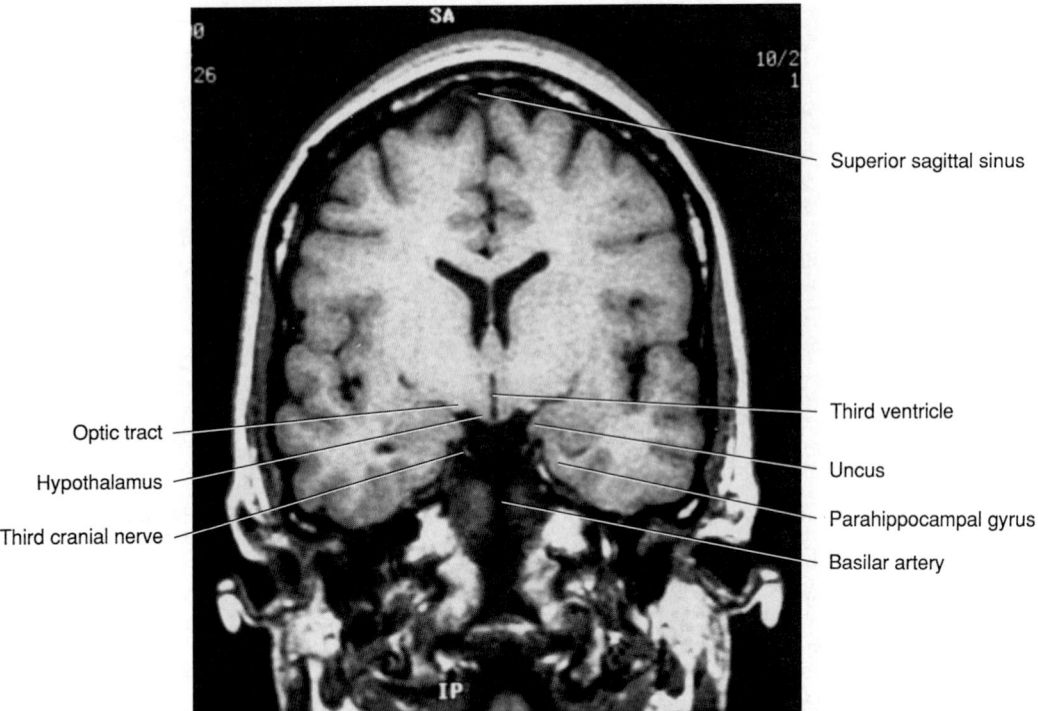

Figure 2.21. Brain MR. T1-weighted, coronal plane through uncus.

Superior sagittal sinus

Third ventricle

Uncus

Parahippocampal gyrus

Basilar artery

Optic tract

Hypothalamus

Third cranial nerve

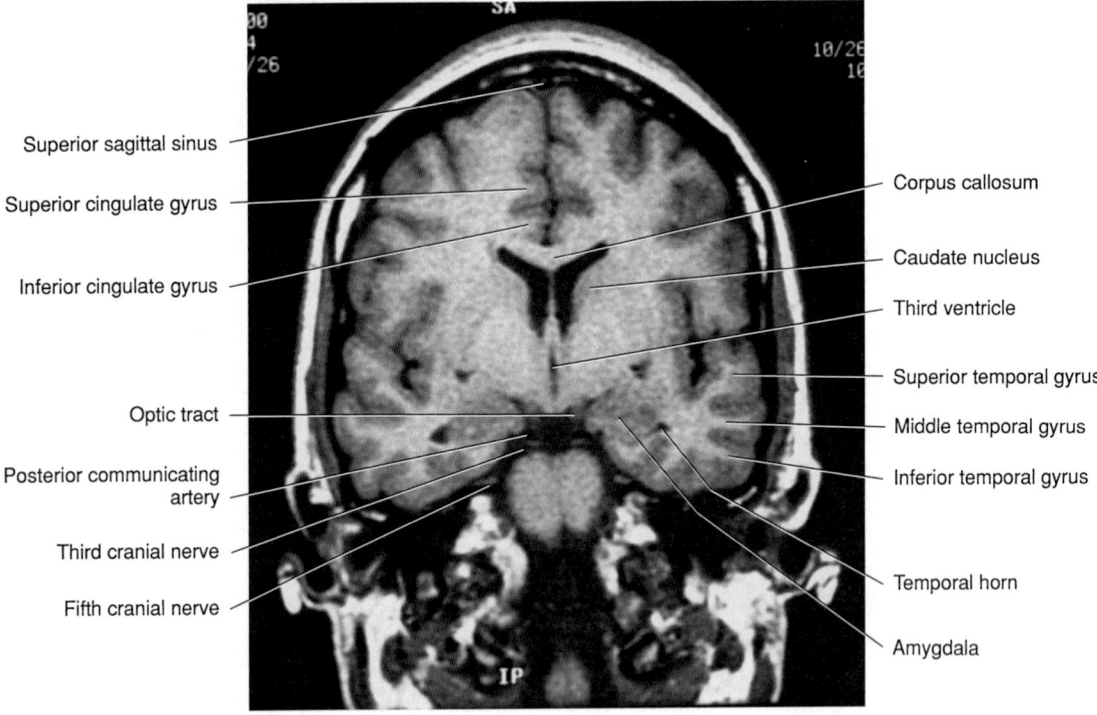

Figure 2.22. Brain MR. T1-weighted, coronal plane through anterior third ventricle.

Superior sagittal sinus

Superior cingulate gyrus

Inferior cingulate gyrus

Optic tract

Posterior communicating artery

Third cranial nerve

Fifth cranial nerve

Corpus callosum

Caudate nucleus

Third ventricle

Superior temporal gyrus

Middle temporal gyrus

Inferior temporal gyrus

Temporal horn

Amygdala

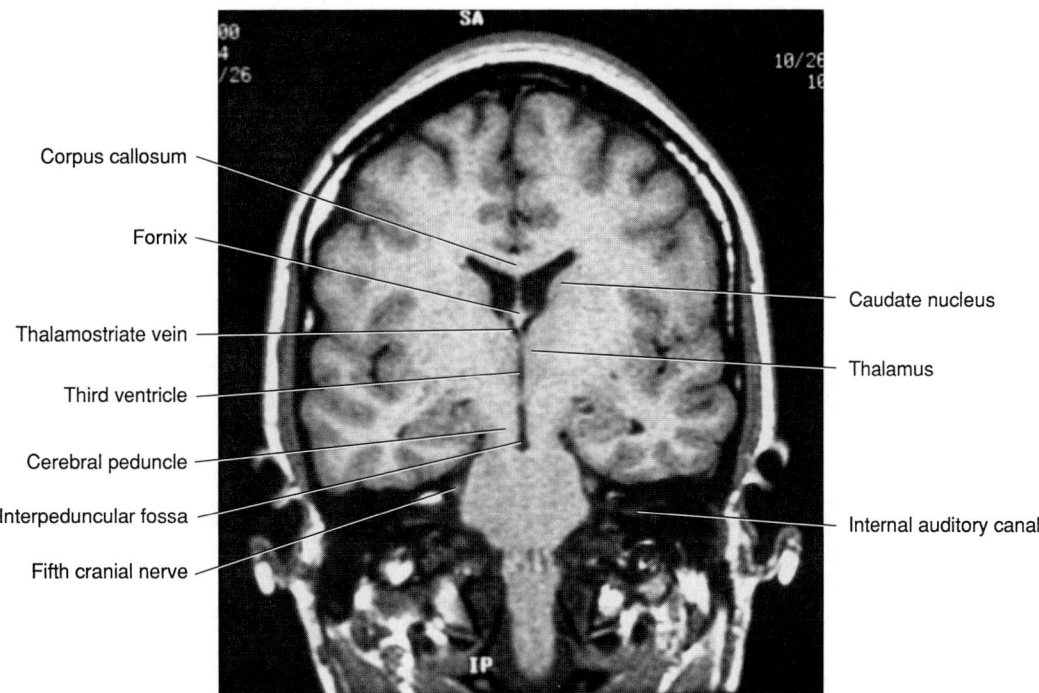

Figure 2.23. Brain MR. T1-weighted, coronal plane through third ventricle.

Corpus callosum

Fornix

Thalamostriate vein

Third ventricle

Cerebral peduncle

Interpeduncular fossa

Fifth cranial nerve

Caudate nucleus

Thalamus

Internal auditory canal

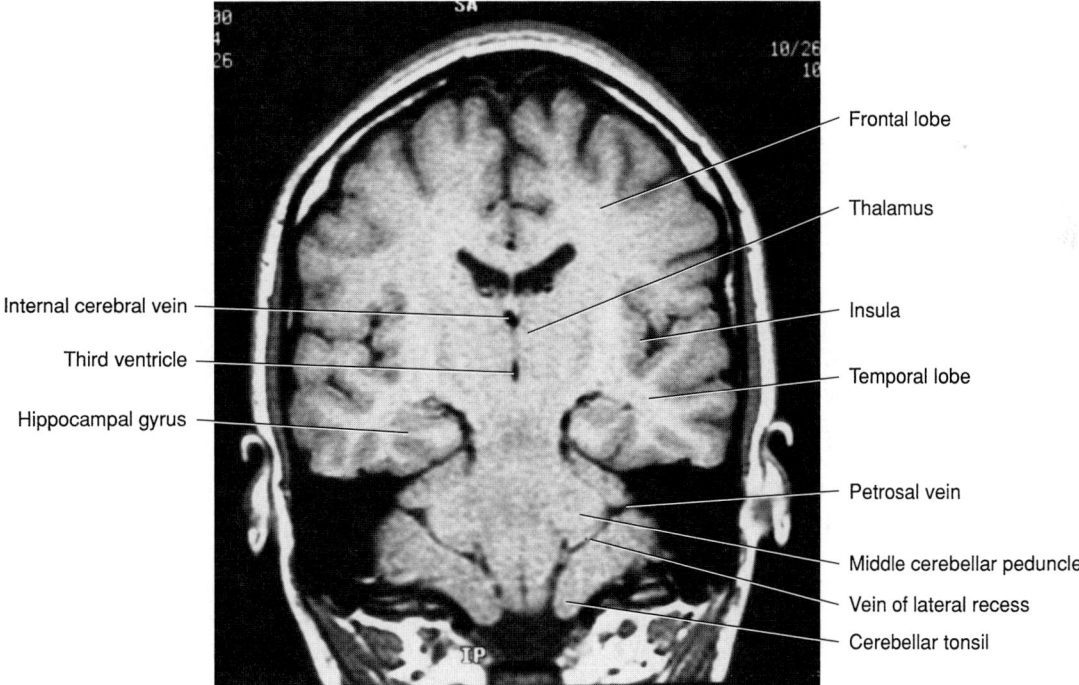

Figure 2.24. Brain MR. T1-weighted, coronal plane through middle cerebellar peduncle.

Internal cerebral vein

Third ventricle

Hippocampal gyrus

Frontal lobe

Thalamus

Insula

Temporal lobe

Petrosal vein

Middle cerebellar peduncle

Vein of lateral recess

Cerebellar tonsil

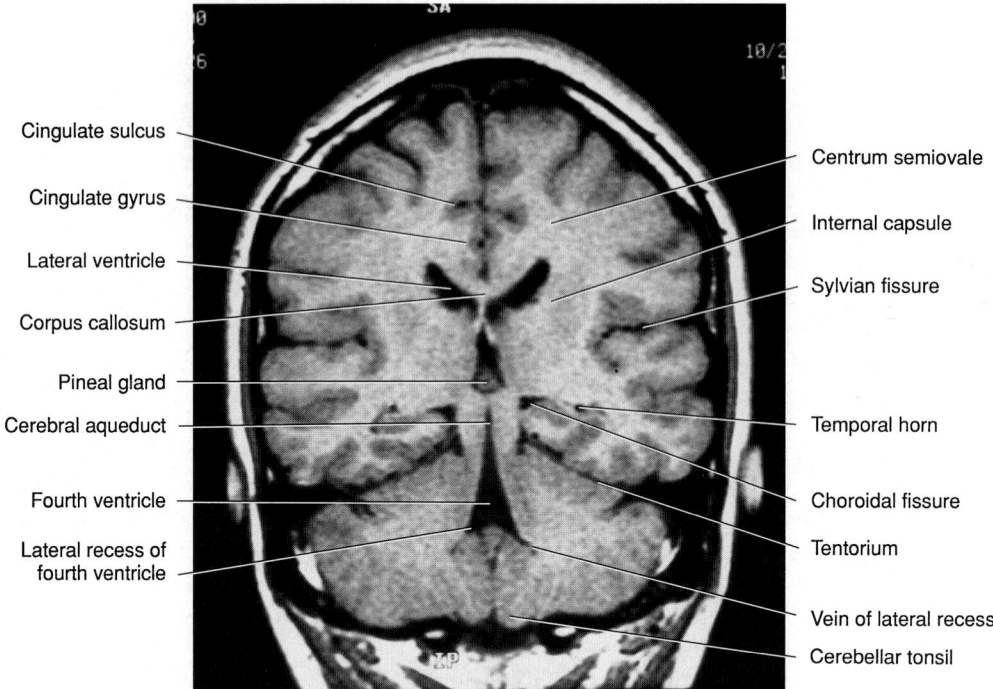

Cingulate sulcus
Cingulate gyrus
Lateral ventricle
Corpus callosum
Pineal gland
Cerebral aqueduct
Fourth ventricle
Lateral recess of fourth ventricle

Centrum semiovale
Internal capsule
Sylvian fissure
Temporal horn
Choroidal fissure
Tentorium
Vein of lateral recess
Cerebellar tonsil

Figure 2.25. Brain MR. T1-weighted, coronal plane through cerebral aqueduct.

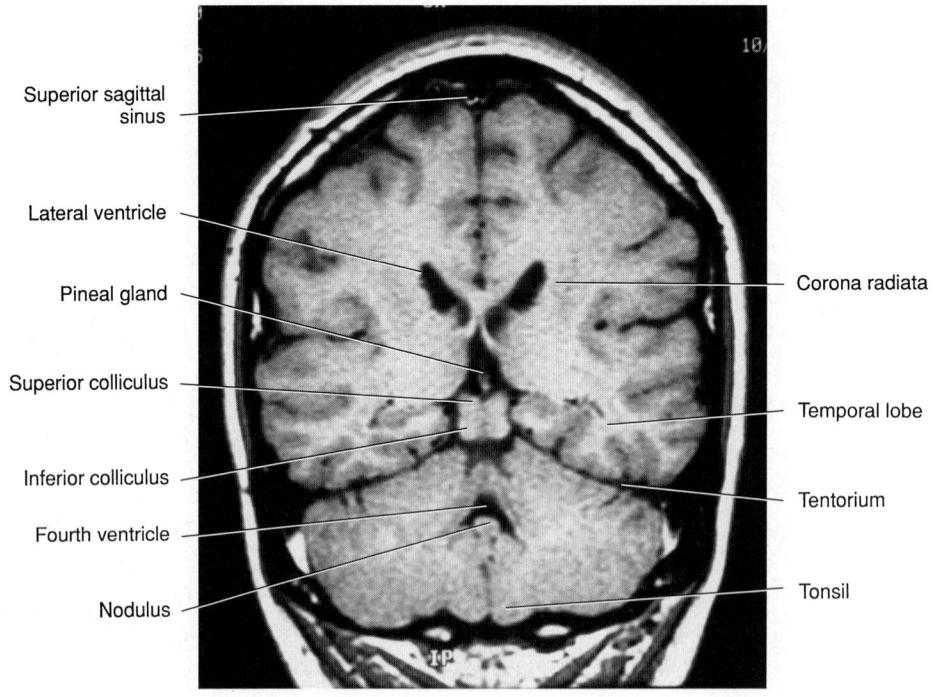

Superior sagittal sinus
Lateral ventricle
Pineal gland
Superior colliculus
Inferior colliculus
Fourth ventricle
Nodulus

Corona radiata
Temporal lobe
Tentorium
Tonsil

Figure 2.26. Brain MR. T1-weighted, coronal plane through fourth ventricle.

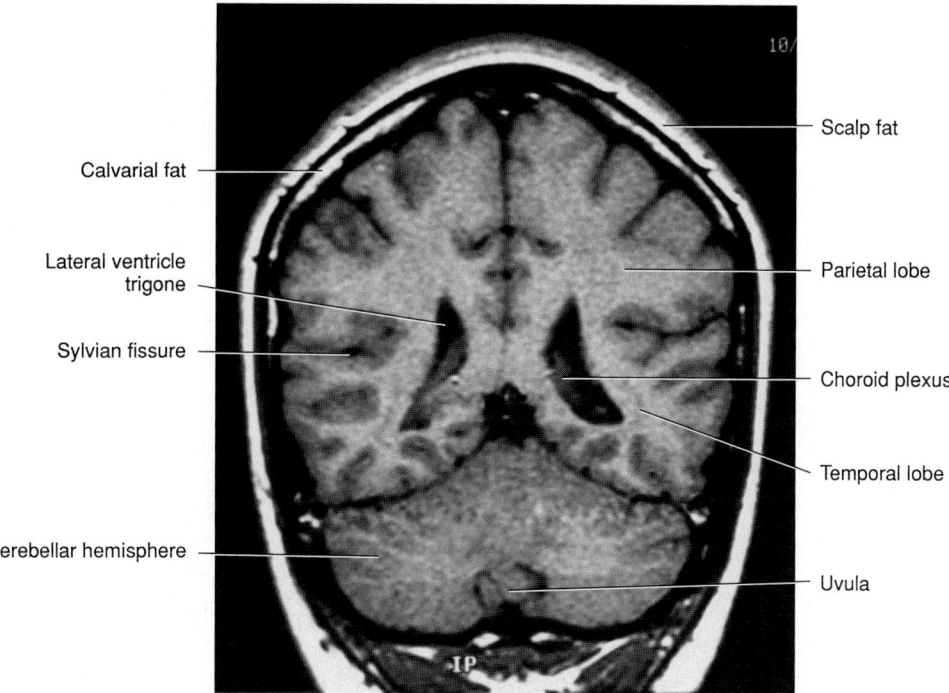

Figure 2.27. Brain MR. T1-weighted, coronal plane through trigones of lateral ventricles.

Calvarial fat

Lateral ventricle trigone

Sylvian fissure

Cerebellar hemisphere

Scalp fat

Parietal lobe

Choroid plexus

Temporal lobe

Uvula

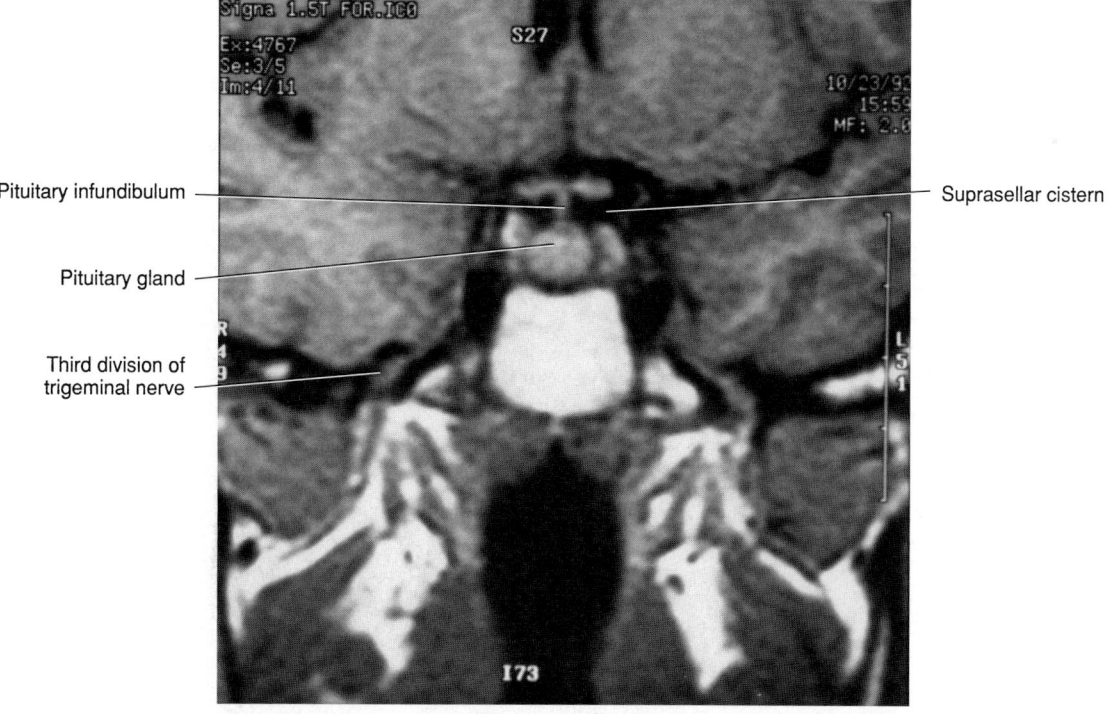

Figure 2.28. Brain MR. T1-weighted, coronal plane through pituitary gland.

Pituitary infundibulum

Pituitary gland

Third division of trigeminal nerve

Suprasellar cistern

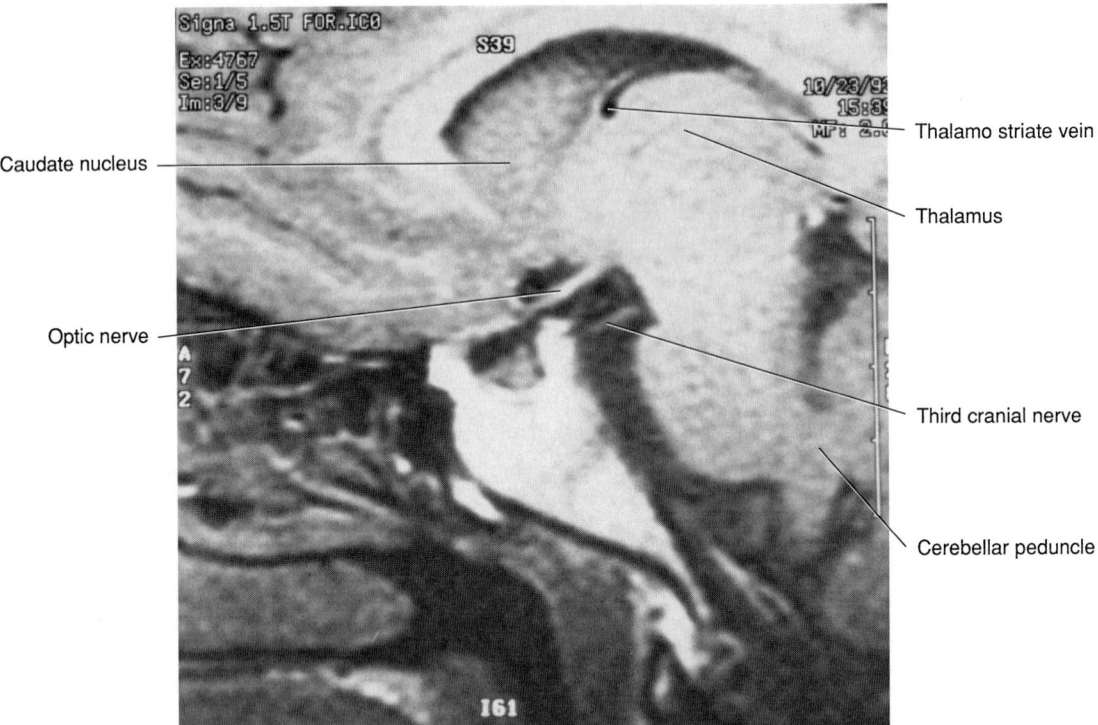

Caudate nucleus

Optic nerve

Thalamo striate vein

Thalamus

Third cranial nerve

Cerebellar peduncle

Figure 2.29. Brain MR. T1-weighted, sagittal plane through optic nerve.

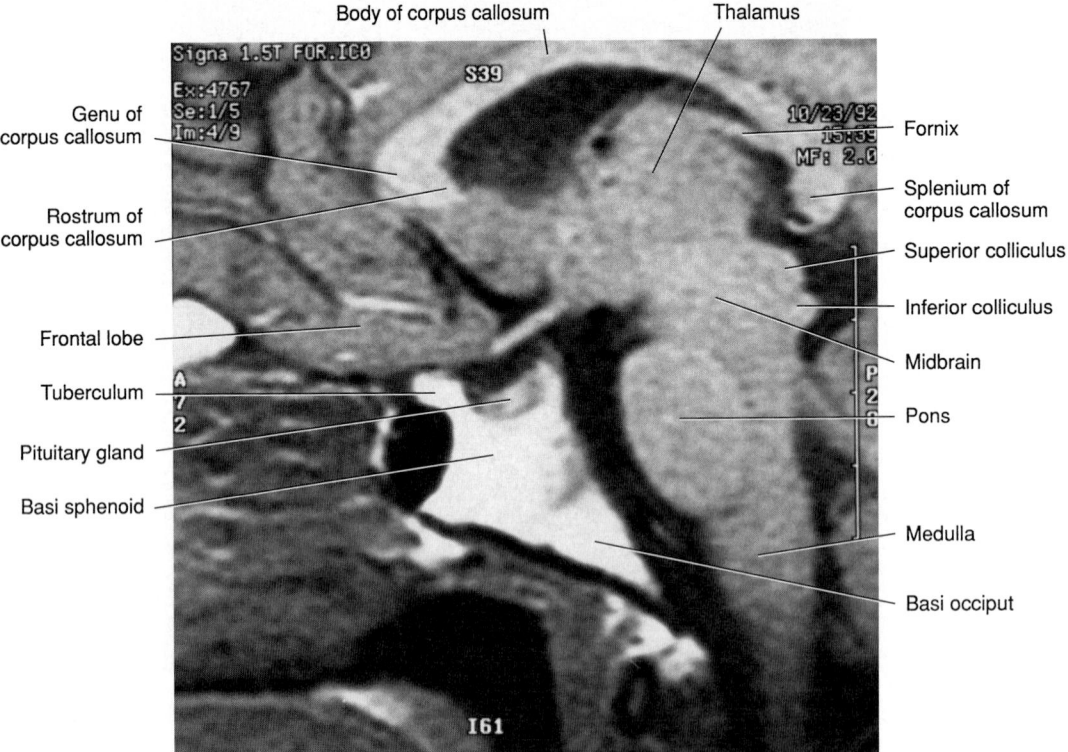

Body of corpus callosum

Thalamus

Genu of
corpus callosum

Rostrum of
corpus callosum

Frontal lobe

Tuberculum

Pituitary gland

Basi sphenoid

Fornix

Splenium of
corpus callosum

Superior colliculus

Inferior colliculus

Midbrain

Pons

Medulla

Basi occiput

Figure 2.30. Brain MR. T1-weighted, sagittal plane through parasellar region.

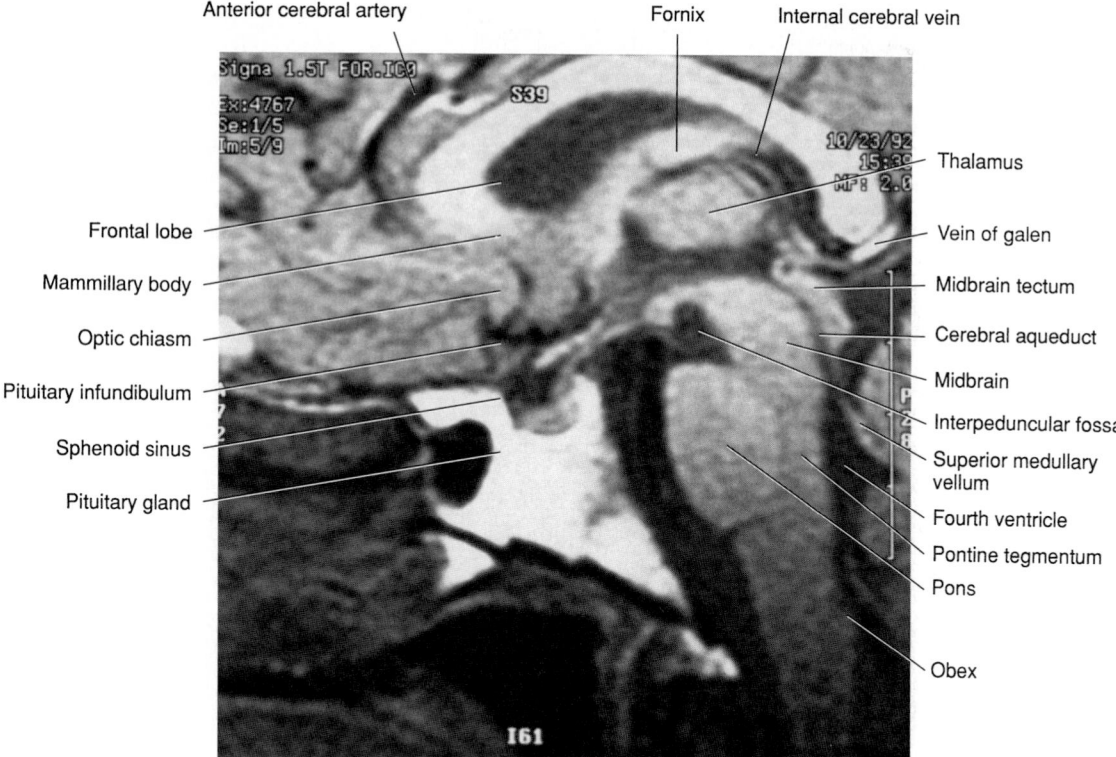

Anterior cerebral artery   Fornix   Internal cerebral vein

Frontal lobe

Mammillary body

Optic chiasm

Pituitary infundibulum

Sphenoid sinus

Pituitary gland

Thalamus

Vein of galen

Midbrain tectum

Cerebral aqueduct

Midbrain

Interpeduncular fossa

Superior medullary vellum

Fourth ventricle

Pontine tegmentum

Pons

Obex

Figure 2.31. Brain MR. T1-weighted, sagittal midline plane through pituitary infundibulum.

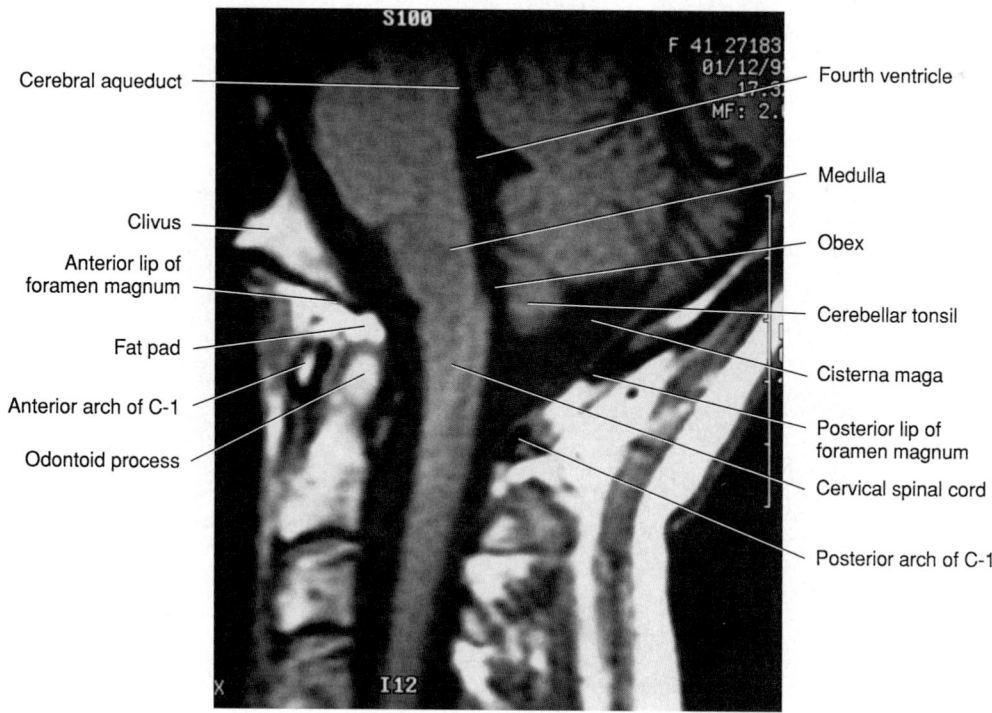

Cerebral aqueduct

Clivus

Anterior lip of foramen magnum

Fat pad

Anterior arch of C-1

Odontoid process

Fourth ventricle

Medulla

Obex

Cerebellar tonsil

Cisterna maga

Posterior lip of foramen magnum

Cervical spinal cord

Posterior arch of C-1

Figure 2.32. Brain MR. T1-weighted, sagittal plane through craniocervical junction.

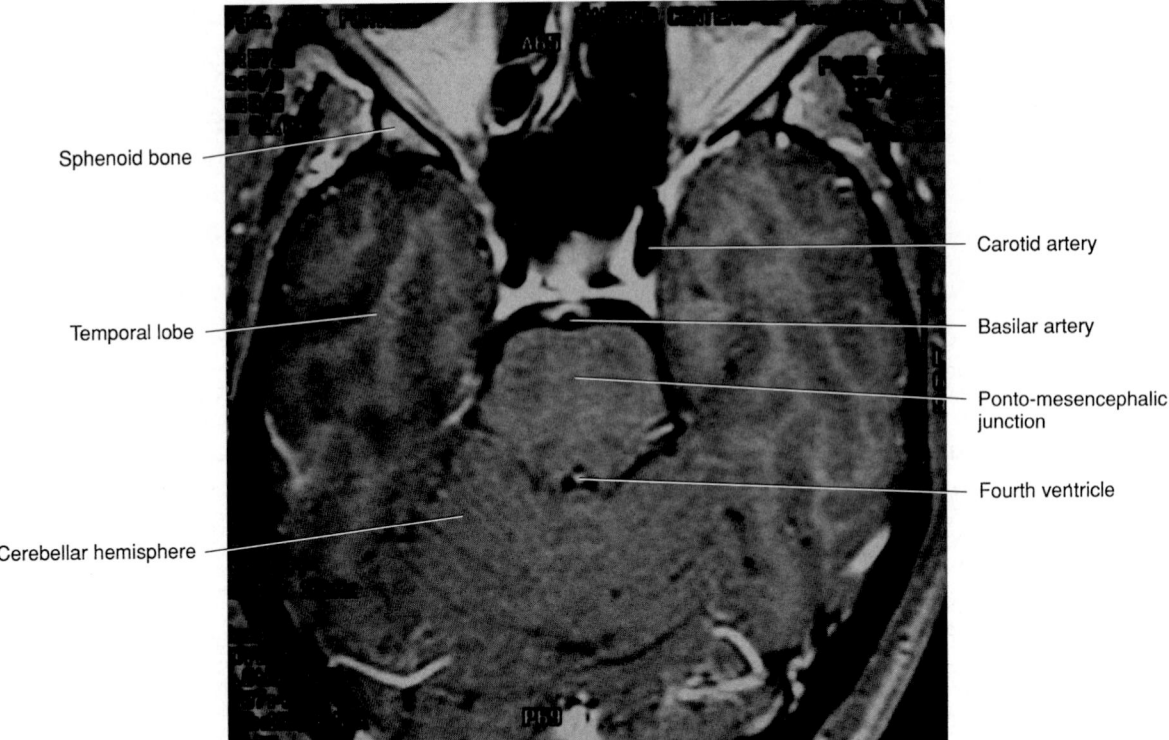

Sphenoid bone

Temporal lobe

Cerebellar hemisphere

Carotid artery

Basilar artery

Ponto-mesencephalic junction

Fourth ventricle

Figure 2.33. Brain MR. T1-weighted, gadolinium-enhanced, axial plane, through pontomesencephalic junction.

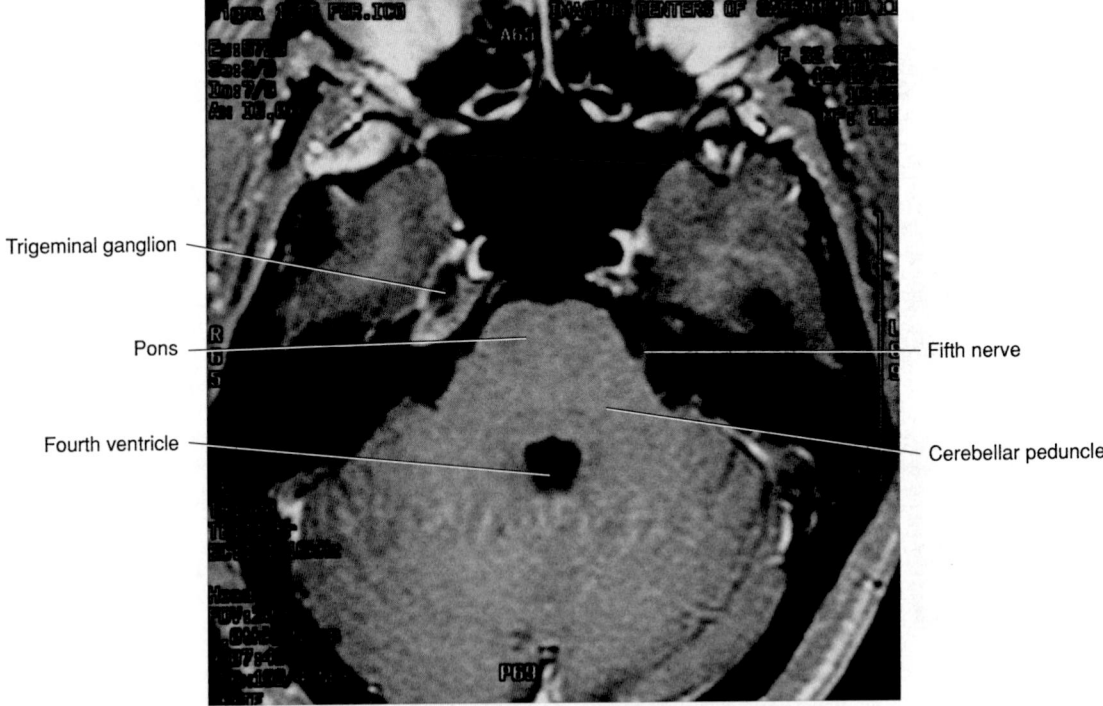

Trigeminal ganglion

Pons

Fourth ventricle

Fifth nerve

Cerebellar peduncle

Figure 2.34. Brain MR. T1-weighted, gadolinium-enhanced, axial plane, through fourth ventricle and fifth cranial nerve.

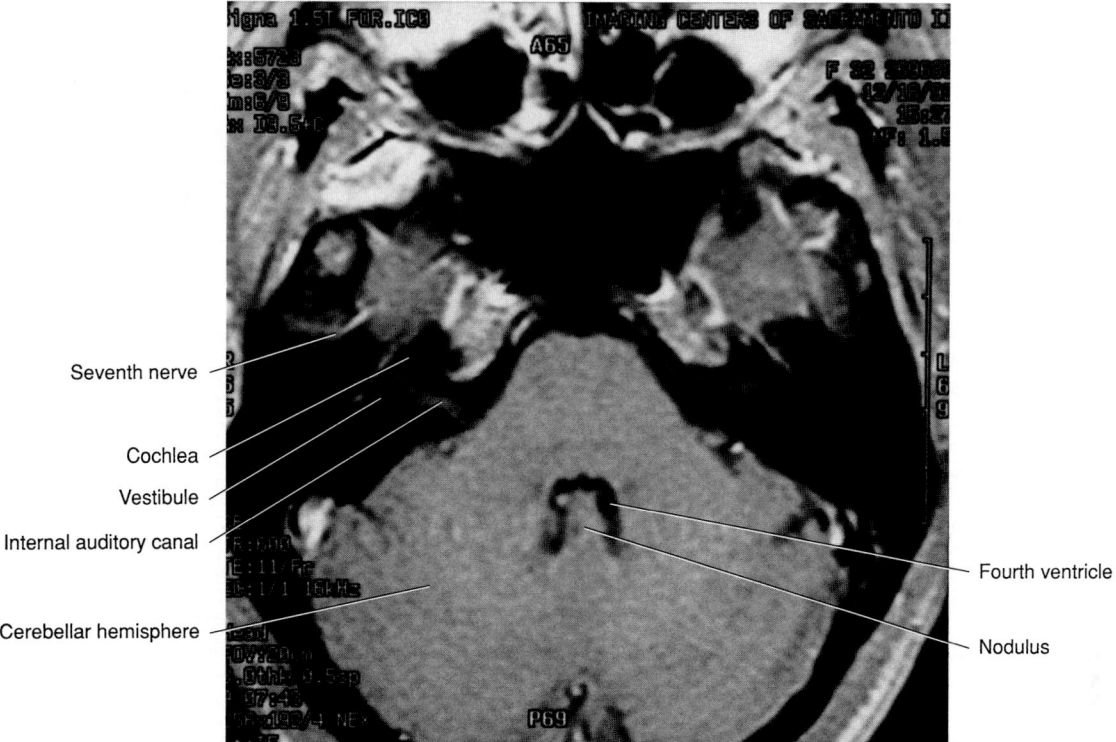

Figure 2.35. Brain MR. T1-weighted, axial plane through internal auditory canal.

Seventh nerve

Cochlea

Vestibule

Internal auditory canal

Cerebellar hemisphere

Fourth ventricle

Nodulus

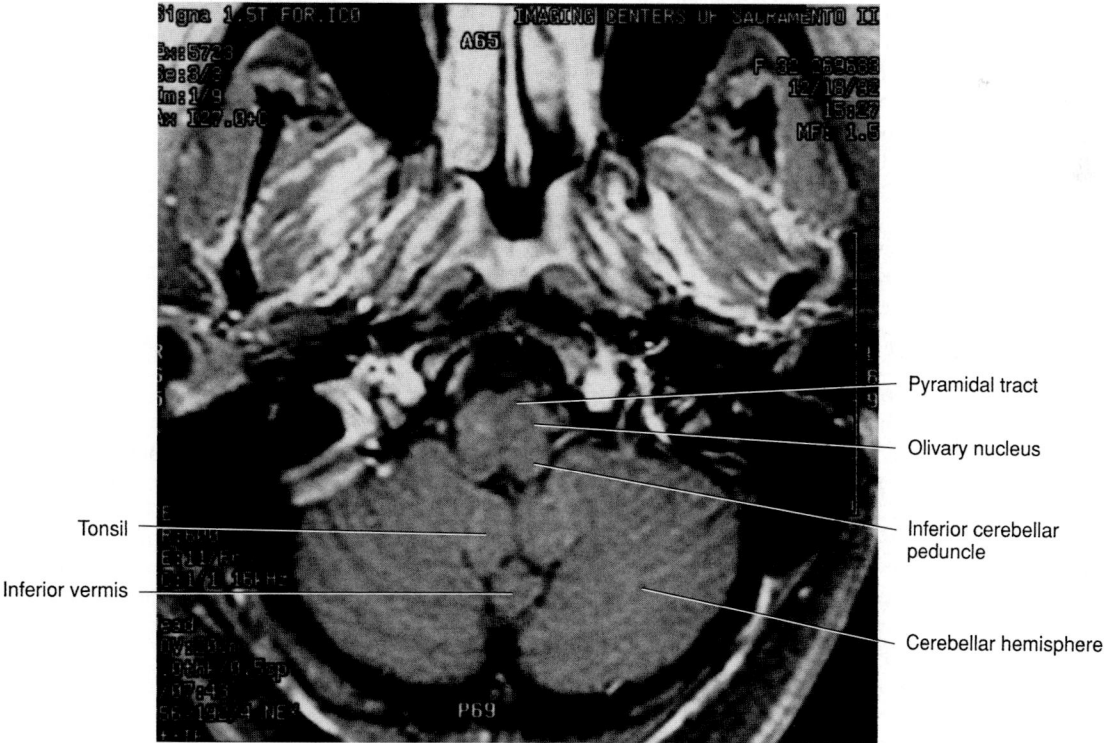

Figure 2.36. Brain MR. T1-weighted, axial plane through medulla.

Tonsil

Inferior vermis

Pyramidal tract

Olivary nucleus

Inferior cerebellar peduncle

Cerebellar hemisphere

The obex, the most posterior projection of the dorsal medulla, should lie above this imaginary line. The only structures visible at this level within the calvarium and spinal canal are the cervical medullary junction and a tiny bit of cerebellar tonsilar tissue. Any other soft tissue in this location is pathologic.

CHOOSING THE CORRECT STUDY

A bewildering array of examinations is available for imaging the brain. It is a difficult task to decide which of them is best for a given clinical situation. We can eliminate two from the start. Plain radiography is useless in patient management and is only of value in the documentation of fracture for medical or legal reasons. Nuclear medicine brain scans are only useful in certain very limited settings (see chapter 63). We still must decide between CT, MR, US, and angiography in the evaluation of the patient with acute neurologic complaints. We also need to decide whether to give IV contrast material. Angiography and US are used in the acute setting based on the appropriate combination of CT, MR, and clinical findings. The only contenders for the "first test" for the brain are MR and CT.

As a general rule in brain imaging, CT is performed for acute neurologic illness and MR for the more chronic and subacute cases. That is, if the onset of neurologic symptoms referable to the brain was within 48 hours, start with a CT. If the problem dates back more than 3 days, start with an MR. If the CT or MR suggests a primary vascular lesion, such as an arteriovenous malformation (AVM) or aneurysm, do a catheter angiogram or MR angiogram. If the CT or MR suggests tumor, give contrast. If the CT or MR fails to demonstrate an acute infarct and the symptoms suggest a transient ischemic attack or stroke, do a carotid Doppler US. Do not use IV iodinated contrast for CT in the acute setting unless brain abscess or tumor is a strong consideration. Give gadolinium for MR whenever there is a clinical finding that suggests a specific neurologic localization, a seizure, or a strong history of cancer or infectious disease. Exceptions to these general guidelines are few. Follow the rules and you will be doing the right thing in the majority of cases. Sometimes an MR will be required to clarify a questionable finding on CT. Also, remember that some patients are simply too sick to be studied easily with MR. These include patients with multisystem trauma or those who require assisted ventilation.

Although an almost infinite variety of clinical symptoms may related to the CNS, most patients can be divided into a limited number of categories (Table 2.1).

Acute Trauma. Patients with acute trauma have perhaps the most dramatic presentation. A noncontrast enhanced CT scan is preferred because CT can be obtained quickly and can be performed on virtually any patient. Furthermore, CT scanners are almost universally available in hospital emergency rooms. The most important abnormalities to be detected are extracerebral hematomas. These lesions produce devastating neurologic symptoms that can be completely reversed if treated early. Intracerebral contusions are of secondary interest because they are more difficult to treat surgi-

Table 2.1. Preferred Initial Imaging Study by Clinical Presentations

Clinical Presentation	CT Without Contrast	CT With Contrast	MR Without Contrast	MR With Contrast
Trauma	XX			
Stroke	XX			
Seizure	X	X	X	XX
Infection	X	X	X	XX
Cancer	X	X	X	XX
Acute Headache	XX			
Chronic Headache			XX	
Dementia			XX	
Coma	XX			

XX, best study; X, acceptable study (depends on circumstances).

cally and because the results of treatment are less encouraging.

Stroke. Noncontrast CT scan is the preferred initial imaging study. The majority of strokes are bland infarcts, and in the acute phase, the CT scan is normal or nearly normal. In these patients, we search for evidence of hemorrhage. A cerebral hematoma presenting as a stroke suggests hypertensive encephalopathy or amyloid angiopathy depending on the distribution of the lesion and the age of the patient. Subarachnoid hemorrhage requires further workup by MR or angiography or both to search for an aneurysm or AVM. If no hemorrhage is seen, a bland infarct is presumed to be present but currently occult to CT scanning. The absence of hemorrhage visible on CT enables the clinician to perform anticoagulation or thrombolytic therapy to prevent progression or even to reverse the neurologic deficit.

Prethrombolytic Evaluation. Recent developments in stroke therapy require further attention to the examination of patients considered for acute thrombolysis because hemorrhagic complications are more common when early signs of infarct are present on the initial CT. Loss of gray/white distinction, low attenuation in the basal ganglia, and poor definition of the insala may contraindicate thrombolytic therapy if correlated with clinical findings. Some consider mild sulcal effacement to be a contraindication as well.

Seizure. Patients suffering seizure present interesting problems for the radiologist. If it is the patient's first seizure, an intracranial tumor must be excluded. For this reason, contrast-enhanced MR or contrast-enhanced CT is the preferred approach. If the patient is in the immediate postictal state or if residual neurologic deficit is present at the time of imaging, a noncontrast CT scan should be obtained as the first study. If the seizure disorder is chronic, and particularly if it is refractory to medical therapy, then a detailed MR examination including high-resolution coronal images of the medial temporal lobes is performed. In pediatric patients, contrast enhancement is generally not required because congenital anomalies, rather than tumor, are the most common structural cause of seizures.

Infection and Cancer. In any patient in whom infectious disease or cancer is a strong consideration, contrast-enhanced MR is the preferred study. Parenchymal tumor or metastatic disease will be demonstrated with this study, and contrast-enhanced MR has the advantage of depicting meningeal disease much better than any other imaging modality. In some centers and under certain clinical conditions, contrast-enhanced CT is performed rather than MR. It is difficult to quantify the clinical impact of this choice of imaging strategy. It can be justified on grounds of economic cost and considerable clinical experience.

Headache is a frequent indication for imaging of the brain. Patients with severe acute headaches should undergo imaging with noncontrast head CT. Acute severe headaches may be attributable to subarachnoid hemorrhage, acute hydrocephalus, or an enlarging intracranial mass. The patient with chronic headache is generally evaluated by MR scanning. If the headache is not accompanied by focal neurologic symptoms, a noncontrast MR scan is usually sufficient. If the headache is associated with focal neurologic complaints, then gadolinium-enhanced MR scanning is indicated. When headache is the sole presenting complaint, the yield of imaging is low.

Coma. It is crucial to distinguish between a patient with an acute confusional state or coma and a patient who is chronically demented. The comatose or acutely confused patient undergoes imaging to detect an intracranial hemorrhage. These patients are studied urgently with noncontrast CT. The majority of patients who present in this manner will not have an acute structural lesion of the brain. Many will be comatose because of functional or physiologic abnormalities of the brain. An acute infarct may be present, but this may be invisible on CT.

Dementia. The patient suffering from chronic dementia is generally studied by noncontrast MR as a screening examination for large frontal masses, hydrocephalus, and other treatable abnormalities that may render a clinical picture indistinguishable from that of Alzheimer's disease. MR may also demonstrate small vessel ischemic changes in the cerebral white matter and small infarcts that also may clinically mimic Alzheimer's disease. If these findings are not present and the clinical picture is correct, the clinician may offer a diagnosis of Alzheimer's disease. Nuclear medicine studies may play a role in assessing prognosis.

ANALYSIS OF THE ABNORMALITY

When an abnormality is detected, the goal of the radiologist is to categorize the finding and, if possible, make a specific diagnosis. Given the large number and relatively infrequent specific findings of neurologic diseases, it is essential to adopt a systematic analytic method to narrow the range of differential diagnostic possibilities. Armed with an amalgam of basic clinical, anatomic, and pathologic knowledge, we can create such a system.

The central question in lesion analysis is the presence of mass or atrophy. Once the brain has completed its development, any injury resulting in tissue loss is permanent. Although functional recovery can occur, tissue loss is virtually never restored. Whenever focal or diffuse tissue loss is identified, a strong inference is drawn that the lesion is permanent and untreatable. On the other hand,

if the brain is expanded with normal structures displaced away from the lesion, the lesion is probably active and potentially treatable, and the urgency for specific diagnosis is greater.

Mass. The concept of mass effect is an essential starting point. A mass is recognized by displacement of normal structures away from the abnormality. The term *mass* is used in a sense that differs somewhat from our understanding of mass in physics, in which the central feature of mass is its gravitational affect. The term *mass* in neuroradiology is used in the sense of an object occupying space. Because two solid objects cannot coexist in the same space, the mass displaces normal cerebral structures away from it. The normal midline structures may be shifted contralateral to the mass. The sulci adjacent to the mass may be effaced, as the CSF in the sulci is displaced by the mass. Similarly, ipsilateral ventricular structures may be compressed by a mass, rendering the ipsilateral ventricle smaller than the contralateral ventricle. These specific points might be summarized by the question: Is there too much tissue within the skull?

Atrophy. Conversely, an atrophic lesion is recognized by widening of the ipsilateral sulci or enlargement of the ventricle adjacent to the lesion. We may ask the question: Is there too little brain? We have not listed shift of the midline toward the side of the lesion as a sign of atrophy. Shift ipsilateral to an atrophic lesion is very unusual. It is only seen commonly in congenital hemiatrophy. Even if a complete hemispherectomy is performed, shift of the midline toward the side of the hemispherectomy defect is almost always a sign of mass in the remaining cerebral hemisphere or of an extra axial mass compressing it.

When a pattern of diffuse cerebral atrophy is encountered, the first question we must ask is: What is the patient's age? If the patient is older than 65 years and has normal cognitive function, a diagnosis of age-appropriate cerebral atrophy can be made. Experience teaches us the range of normal to be expected for each age group. If the patient is demented, a diagnosis of Alzheimer's disease may be made on clinical grounds. It has been recently suggested that specific neuroradiologic features of Alzheimer's disease exist, such as focal atrophy of the hippocampal regions of the medial temporal lobe, but this has yet to be confirmed prospectively with sufficient reliability. If the patient is younger than 65 years of age, a large number of relatively rare conditions discussed in chapter 7 must be considered.

Reversible Atrophy. It is most important for the radiologist to consider the three common causes of cerebral atrophy. They are related to dehydration and starvation. Patients with Addison's disease or other causes of dehydration or abnormal fluid balance may occasionally present with a CT picture of atrophy. With treatment, a more normal appearance of the brain can be restored. Nutritional causes of reversible cerebral atrophy exist in anorexia nervosa and bulimia. The relative contribution of dehydration and starvation in these conditions is difficult to determine. Alcoholism may also occasionally result in reversible "cerebral atrophy." Although the neurotoxic effect of effects of alcohol are not reversible, it has been hypothesized that the accompanying nutritional deficiencies may be corrected restoring a more normal appearance to the brain on imaging studies.

Mass Lesion: Intra-axial or Extra-axial. Should a mass be identified, the first question we must ask is: Is the mass intra-axial, within the brain expanding it, or extra-axial, outside the brain compressing it? This distinction is usually obvious, but in some cases, it is very difficult to determine. Intra-axial masses are more dangerous to the patient and less easily treated than are extra-axial masses. We prefer to orient our approach to detect extra-axial masses reliably. Intra-axial masses are, most commonly, metastases, intracranial hemorrhages, primary intracranial tumors such as glioblastoma, and brain abscesses. Extra-axial masses are, most commonly, subdural or epidural hematomas, meningiomas, neuromas, and dermoid or epidermoid cysts.

To distinguish an intra-axial from an extra-axial mass, concentrate on the margins of the mass. Just as the beach is more interesting than the open sea, the interface between the mass and the surrounding brain is more interesting than the center of the mass. Extra-axial masses generally possess a broad dural surface. In contrast, intra-axial masses are surrounded completely by brain. In the posterior fossa, the most reliable sign of an extra-axial mass is widening of the ipsilateral subarachnoid space. The cerebellum and brainstem are displaced away from the bony margins of the calvarium by the mass. In contrast, intra-axial masses demonstrate a narrow ipsilateral subarachnoid space. In the supratentorial compartment, we evaluate a mass somewhat differently. With an intra-axial mass, the gyri become larger and the sulci become smaller and farther apart as we approach the center of the mass. The sulci adjacent to an extra-axial mass, on the other hand, become smaller as we approach the mass.

With the multiplanar capability of MR, we are frequently able to visualize direct displacement of the brain away from the dura by an extra-axial mass. When gadolinium is administered, extra-axial masses frequently show dural enhancement, whereas this is less common with intra-axial masses. Extra-axial masses tend to enhance homogeneously, for example, meningioma or neuroma, or not at all, for example, extracerebral hematomas and cysts. Intra-axial lesions tend to enhance in a ringlike or irregular fashion. In general, intra-axial masses have more surrounding edema than extra-axial masses of the same size.

Solitary or Multiple. Once a mass is identified and its location within or outside the brain is established, the next question we ask is: Is this a solitary lesion or multiple lesions? The implication is that a single lesion is more likely to be the result of isolated primary cerebral disease and that multiple lesions are more likely to be manifestations of widespread or systemic diseases. You should consider a single ring-enhancing lesion within the brain to be a glioblastoma. Multiple ring-enhancing lesions within the brain more likely represent metastases or abscesses. If a single infarct is identified, it is likely to be caused by a lesion within the carotid artery ipsilateral to the lesion. If multiple infarcts are seen, they may represent border-zone infarcts or may be attributable to a cardiac source of emboli.

Gray Matter or White Matter. If a lesion within the brain is primarily manifest by lucency on CT or increased signal on the T2-weighted MR, the most important question is whether the lesion involves gray matter, white matter, or both. Diseases primarily involving white matter without mass effect arise from a wide array of causes (see chapter 7). Lesions involving gray matter are usually the result of infarct, trauma, or encephalitis. If the lesion has mass effect, these conditions are likely acute. If the lesion is atrophic, it is likely chronic.

If the white matter is exclusively involved and the lesion is expansile, a pattern of edema is present. Usually, this will represent vasogenic edema caused by an intracerebral mass. The frondlike pattern of white matter extension and mass effect is typical. This form of edema results from disturbances in tight capillary junctions that occur in association with cerebral tumors, abscesses, or hematomas. This type of edema tends to progress relatively slowly and persist over time. If there is relatively more edema compared with the size of the lesion, a tumor or abscess is considered to be more likely than a hematoma.

If there is white matter expansion and increased T2 signal on MR or lucency on CT with gray matter involvement, cytotoxic edema is present. Cytotoxic edema is the result of increased tissue water content attributable to the neuropathologic response to cell death. In these cases, infarct, trauma, or encephalitis should be considered. This is called the gray matter pattern.

Lesion Distribution. When a gray matter pattern is identified, the distribution of the gray matter abnormality allows us to distinguish between infarct, trauma, and encephalitis. Infarcts are distributed according to vascular patterns described in chapter 4. For example, if a wedge-shaped lesion involves the opercula of the sylvian fissure and the underlying white matter and basal ganglia, a diagnosis of middle cerebral artery territory infarct is made. Similarly, if the medial aspect of the cerebral hemisphere anteriorly and over the convexity is involved, an anterior cerebral infarct is diagnosed. If the area of involvement falls between two major vascular territories, a border-zone or "watershed" infarct is likely. With multiple border-zone infarcts, global hypoperfusion from cardiac arrest must be suspected. If the deep gray matter structures bilaterally are involved, pure anoxia resulting from carbon monoxide poisoning or respiratory arrest should be considered.

Traumatic lesions are also distributed in a characteristic fashion (see chapter 3). Because of the transmission of forces through the brain and the relationship of the brain to the surrounding skull, traumatic lesions tend to occur at the orbital frontal and frontal polar regions, the temporal poles, and the occipital poles in acceleration or deceleration injuries. A direct blow produces injury beneath the site of blow and opposite the site. The lesion opposite the blow is called the contra-coup injury. Penetrating brain wounds are distributed according to the path of the missile or the location of the trauma.

Herpes simplex encephalitis is also distributed in a characteristic fashion. This disease spreads from the oral and nasal mucosa to the trigeminal and olfactory ganglion cells and then transdurally to the brain. The most common locations for involvement are the medial temporal lobes adjacent to the trigeminal ganglia, and the orbital frontal regions adjacent to the olfactory bulbs. Other forms of encephalitis are less common and are diagnosed by typical clinical presentation, characteristic CSF findings, cultures, and mixed gray and white matter pattern of involvement at other sites.

Contrast Enhancement. The next question we ask about a cerebral abnormality is whether it is associated with abnormal contrast enhancement. Enhancement of the brain parenchyma means that the blood–brain barrier has broken down and that the process is biologically active. In the astrocytoma tumor line, an increase in enhancement correlates with higher tumor grade; however, enhancement does not imply malignancy. Infarcts, hemorrhages, abscesses, and encephalitis all can demonstrate contrast enhancement. In these nonneoplastic processes, enhancement only appears in the acute phase and resolves with time.

Signal Intensity or Attenuation Pattern. Patterns of signal intensity are specific to the imaging modality or MR pulse sequence used and are the least generally applicable and to a great extent the least reliable radiologic findings. Knowledge of the physical basis for imaging with CT and MR is necessary to understand the pattern of signal intensities within the brain. As a starting point, one need only know that if an abnormality is white on CT or white on T1 MR or black on T2 MR, hemorrhage must be considered. This topic is discussed extensively elsewhere.

Suggested Readings

Atlas S. MR of Brain and Spine. Philadelphia: Lippincott-Raven, 1996.

Brodal A. Neurological Anatomy in Relation to Clinical Medicine. 3rd ed. New York: Oxford, 1981.

Burger PC, Scheithauer BW, Vogel FS. Surgical Pathology of the Nervous System and Its Coverings. New York: Churchill-Livingstone, 1991.

Davis RL, Robertson DM. Textbook of Neuropathology. 3rd ed. Baltimore: Williams & Wilkins, 1997.

DeGroot J. Correlative Neuroanatomy. 21st ed. Norwalk: Appleton & Lange, 1991.

Poirier J, Gray F, Escourolle R. Manual of Basic Neuropathology. 3rd ed. Philadelphia: WB Saunders, 1990.

Greenberg JO. Neuroimaging. New York: McGraw-Hill, 1995.

Grossman RI, Yousem DM. Neuroradiology. St. Louis: Mosby, 1994.

Hayman LA, Hinck VC. Clinical Brain Imaging. St. Louis: Mosby, 1992.

Osborn A. Diagnostic Neuroradiology. St. Louis: Mosby, 1994.

Plum F, Posner JB. The Diagnosis of Stupor and Coma. 3rd ed. Philadelphia: FA Davis, 1980.

Sox HC, Blatt MA, Higgins MC, et al. Medical Decision Making. Stoneham: Butterworth, 1988.

Von Kummer R, Bozzao L, Manalfe C. Early CT Diagnosis of Hemispheric Brain Infarction. Berlin: Springer, 1995.

Watson C. Basic Human Neuroanatomy. 4th ed. Boston: Little Brown, 1991.

Woodruff WW. Fundamentals of neuroimaging. Philadelphia: Saunders, 1993.

3
Craniofacial Trauma

Robert M. Barr
Alisa D. Gean

HEAD TRAUMA

Imaging Strategy

CT. Imaging of acute head trauma is performed to detect treatable lesions before secondary neurologic damage occurs. Currently, this is best performed by CT for several reasons: it is quick, widely available, and highly accurate in the detection of acute intra- and extra-axial hemorrhage, as well as skull, temporal bone, facial, and orbital fractures. Monitoring equipment is easily accommodated. CT images must be reviewed using multiple windows. A narrow window width is used to evaluate the brain, a slightly wider window width is used to exaggerate contrast between extra-axial collections and the adjacent skull, and a very wide window is used to evaluate the skull itself (see Figs. 3.1, 3.6). Contiguous 5-mm sections through the brain provide sufficient detail and can be obtained with modern scanners in less than 15 minutes. Thinner sections are used to evaluate the orbits, facial skeleton, and skull base. IV contrast media is not used in the acute setting because it may mimic or mask underlying hemorrhage.

When CT is performed in unconscious patients with severe head injury, it may be wise to include routine coverage of the craniocervical junction. A recent study by Link et al. (1) found that 18% of these patients had fractures of C-1, C-2, or the occipital condyles and that roughly half of all fractures were missed by plain radiographs.

MR imaging has traditionally been less desirable than CT in the acute setting because of the longer examination times, difficulty in managing life-support and other monitoring equipment, and inferior demonstration of bone detail. MR, however, has been shown to be comparable to CT in the detection of acute epidural and subdural hematomas and nonhemorrhagic brain injury (2,3). MR is also more sensitive to brainstem injury and both subacute and chronic hemorrhage. Newer imaging sequences, such as fluid-attenuated inversion recovery ("FLAIR") and diffusion-weighted imaging, may further improve detection of acute hemorrhage and early neuronal injury (4,5). In the majority of cases, MR is the modality of choice for patients with subacute and chronic head injury and is recommended for patients with acute head trauma when neurologic findings are unexplained by CT. MR is also more accurate in predicting long-term prognosis. With the development of faster sequences, improved monitoring equipment, and greater scanner availability, MR is likely to play an increasing role in the evaluation of acute head trauma.

Skull Films. Unfortunately, plain films continue to be used in evaluating patients with acute head trauma, despite abundant evidence that they are not helpful (6–8). Patients who are judged to be at low risk for intracranial injury on the basis of a careful history and physical examination should be observed, and patients at high risk should be imaged by CT. Plain films virtually never demonstrate significant findings in the low-risk group and are inadequate to characterize or exclude intracranial injury in the high-risk group. Further, the absence of skull fractures on plain films clearly does not exclude significant intracranial injury. In fact, in one large autosopy series of patients with fatal head injuries, only 75% had skull fractures (9). The decision to obtain a head CT in the setting of trauma must be based on clinical grounds. Skull films are poor predictors of significant intracranial pathology and should not be used either to prevent or encourage further diagnostic evaluation.

Scalp Injury

When interpreting CT scans for head trauma, it is helpful to begin by examining the extracranial structures for evidence of scalp injury or radiopaque foreign bodies. Scalp soft-tissue swelling is often the only reliable evidence of the site of impact. The subgaleal hematoma is the most common manifestation of scalp injury and can be recognized on CT or MR as focal soft-tissue swelling of the scalp located beneath the subcutaneous fibrofatty tissue and above the temporalis muscle and calvarium.

Skull Fractures

Nondisplaced linear fractures of the calvarium are the most common type of skull fracture. They may be difficult to detect on CT scans, especially when the fracture plane is parallel to the plane of section. Fortunately, isolated linear skull fractures do not require treatment. Surgical management is usually indicated for depressed and compound skull fractures, both of which are seen better on CT scans than on plain films (Fig. 3.1). Depressed fractures are frequently associated with an underlying contusion. Intracranial air ("pneumocephalus") may be seen with compound skull fractures or fractures involving the paranasal sinuses. Thin-section CT using a bone algorithm is the best method to evaluate fractures in critical areas, such as the skull base, orbit, or facial bones. Thin sections can also be helpful to evaluate the degree of comminution and depression of bone fragments.

Temporal Bone Fractures

Thin-section, high-resolution CT scanning has led to a dramatic improvement in the ability to detect and characterize temporal bone fractures. Patients with fractures of the temporal bone may present with deafness, facial nerve palsies, vertigo, dizziness, or nystagmus. Clinical symptoms are often masked in the presence of other se-

rious injuries. Physical signs of temporal bone fracture include hemotympanum, CSF otorrhea, and ecchymosis over the mastoid process ("Battle's sign"). Temporal bone fractures may be first suspected on standard head CT scans performed to exclude intracranial injury. Findings such as opacification of the mastoid air cells, fluid in the middle ear cavity, pneumocephalus, or occasionally, pneumolabyrinth, should raise the suspicion of a temporal bone fracture. Optimal evaluation of a suspected temporal bone fracture requires thin-section (1–1.5 mm) axial and direct coronal CT imaging using a bone algorithm.

Fractures of the temporal bone can be classified as longitudinal or transverse depending on their orientation relative to the long axis of the petrous bone. If the fracture parallels the long axis of the petrous pyramid, it is termed a "longitudinal" fracture; fractures perpendicular to the long axis of the petrous bone are termed "transverse" fractures. "Mixed" fracture types also occur.

The longitudinal temporal bone fracture represents 70–90% of temporal bone fractures (10). It results from a blow to the side of the head. Complications include conductive hearing loss, dislocation or fracture of the ossicles, and CSF otorhinorrhea. Facial nerve palsy may occur, but it is often delayed and incomplete. Sensorineural hearing loss is uncommon (Fig. 3.2).

The transverse temporal bone fracture usually results from a blow to the occiput or frontal region. Complications are usually more severe and include sensorineural hearing loss, severe vertigo, nystagmus, and perilymphatic fistula. Facial palsy is seen in 30–50% of these cases and is often complete (10). Transverse fractures may also involve the carotid canal or jugular foramen, causing injury to the carotid artery or jugular vein.

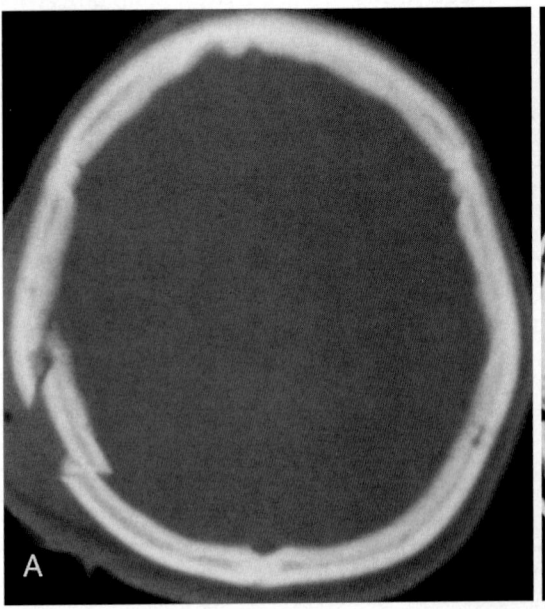
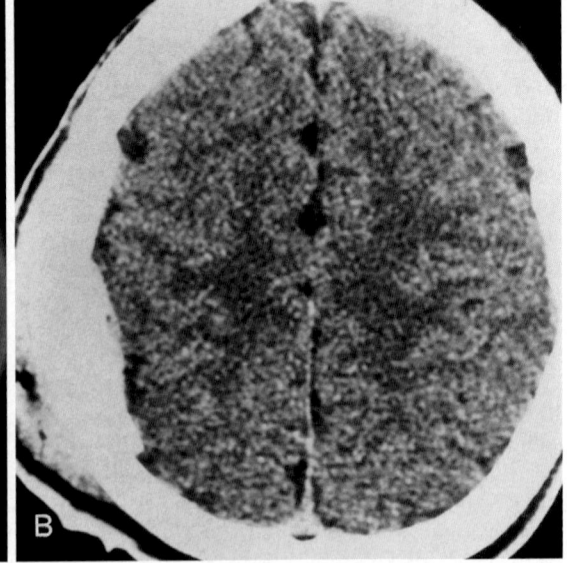

Figure 3.1. Depressed Skull Fracture. A. Axial CT scan demonstrates a right parietal depressed skull fracture with overlying soft-tissue swelling. The fracture is well seen using a wide window in order to enhance contrast between bone and soft tissue. **B.** The narrower window demonstrates excellent contrast between gray and white matter but fails to show the fracture. A small extra-axial hematoma is seen in the right parietal area.

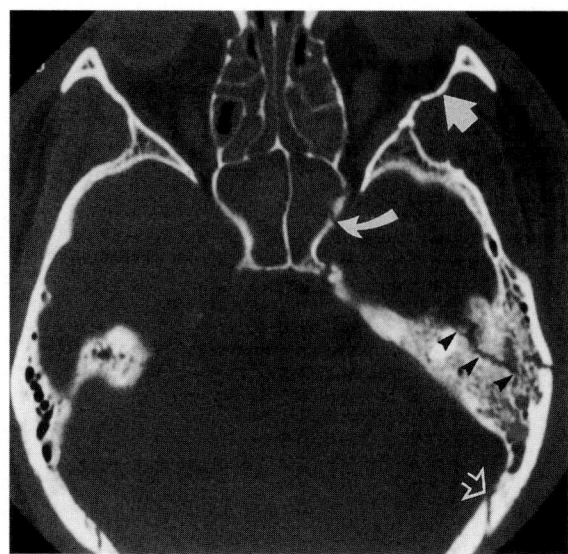

Figure 3.2. Longitudinal Temporal Bone Fracture. Axial CT scan shows a longitudinal left temporal bone fracture (*arrowheads*) with opacification of the mastoid air cells. Diastasis of the left lambdoid suture (*open arrow*) and fractures of the sphenoid sinus (*curved arrow*) and left lateral orbital wall (*arrow*) are also present. (Reprinted with permission from Gean AD. Imaging of Head Trauma. Philadelphia: Lippincott-Raven, 1994:63.)

Mixed or complex temporal bone fractures represent approximately 10% of temporal bone fractures. They involve a combination of fracture planes and generally follow severe crushing blows to the skull. Patients with mixed temporal bone fractures have a high incidence of associated intracranial injury.

CLASSIFICATION OF HEAD INJURY

Traumatic head injury can be divided into primary and secondary forms. Primary lesions are those that occur as a direct result of a blow to the head. Secondary lesions occur as a consequence of primary lesions, usually as a result of mass effect or vascular compromise. Secondary lesions are often preventable, whereas primary injuries, by definition, have already occurred by the time the patient arrives in the emergency department.

Primary lesions include epidural, subdural, subarachnoid, and intraventricular hemorrhage, as well as diffuse axonal injury (DAI), cortical contusions, intracerebral hematomas, and subcortical gray matter injury. Direct injury to the cerebral vasculature is another type of primary lesion.

Secondary lesions include cerebral swelling, brain herniation, hydrocephalus, ischemia or infarction, CSF leak, leptomeningeal cyst, and encephalomalacia. Brainstem injury, which is also divided into primary and secondary forms, is discussed later in this chapter.

Primary Head Injury

EXTRA-AXIAL INJURY

Epidural Hematomas are usually arterial in origin and often result from a skull fracture that disrupts the middle meningeal artery. The developing hematoma strips the dura from the inner table of the skull, forming an ovoid mass that displaces the adjacent brain. They may occur from stretching or tearing of meningeal arteries without an associated fracture, especially in children. Overall, skull fractures are seen in 85–95% of cases. In approximately a third of patients with an epidural hematoma, neurologic deterioration occurs after a lucid interval (11).

Most epidural hematomas are temporal or temporoparietal in location, though frontal and occipital hematomas can also occur. Venous epidural hematomas are less common and arterial epidurals and tend to occur at the vertex, posterior fossa, or anterior aspect of the middle cranial fossa. Venous epidural hematomas usually occur as a result of disrupted dural venous sinuses.

On CT, acute epidural hematomas appear as well-defined, high-attenuation lenticular or biconvex extra-axial collections (Fig. 3.3). Associated mass effect with sulcal effacement and midline shift is frequently seen. Bone windows usually demonstrate an overlying linear skull fracture. Because epidural hematomas exist in the potential space between the dura and inner table of the skull, they usually will not cross cranial sutures, where the periosteal layer of the dura is firmly attached (Fig. 3.4). Near the vertex, however, the periosteum forms the outer wall of the sagittal sinus and is less tightly adherent to the sagittal suture. Therefore, vertex epidurals, which are usually of venous origin from disruption of the sagittal sinus, can cross midline. Occasionally, an acute epidural hematoma will appear heterogeneous, contain-

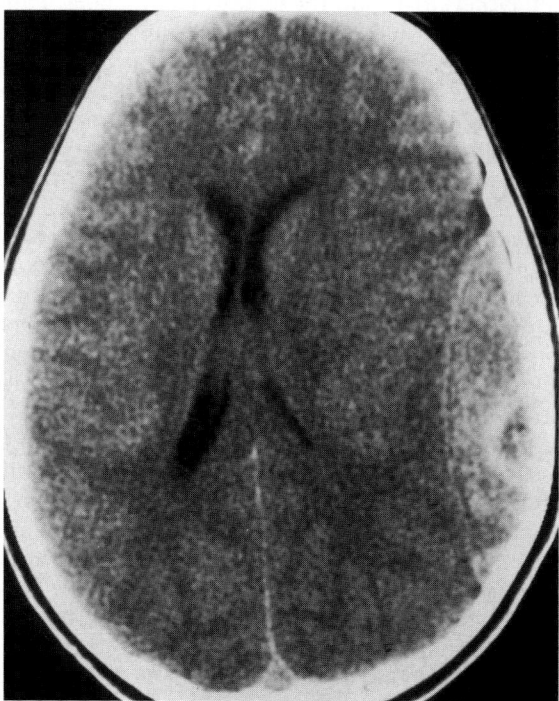

Figure 3.3. Epidural Hematoma. Axial CT scan demonstrates a biconvex high attenuation extra-axial collection causing mass effect on the left temporal lobe and mild midline shift (subfalcial herniation).

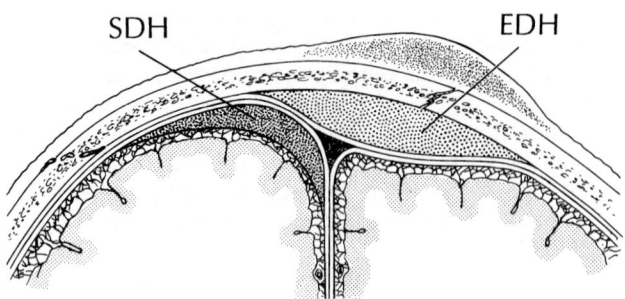

Figure 3.4. Epidural Versus Subdural Hematoma. Axial diagram of the brain surface in the frontal region demonstrates the characteristic locations of the epidural hematoma (*EDH*) compared with the subdural hematoma (*SDH*). Note how the EDH is located above the outer dural layer and the SDH is located beneath the inner dural layer. Only the EDH can cross the falx cerebri. (Reprinted with permission from Gean AD. Imaging of Head Trauma. Philadelphia: Lippincott-Raven, 1994:76.)

ing irregular areas of lower attenuation. This finding may indicate active extravasation of fresh unclotted blood into the collection and warrants immediate surgical attention.

Subdural Hematomas are usually venous in origin, resulting from stretching or tearing of cortical veins that traverse the subdural space en route to the dural sinuses. They may also result from disruption of penetrating branches of superficial cerebral arteries. Because the inner dural layer and arachnoid are not as firmly attached as the structures that make up the epidural space, the subdural hematoma typically extends over a much larger area than the epidural hematoma. Patients with a subdural hematoma commonly present after acute deceleration injury from a motor vehicle accident or fall. The same mechanism can cause cortical contusions and DAI, which are frequently seen in association with acute subdural hematomas.

On axial CT, acute subdural hematomas appear as crescent-shaped extra-axial collections of high attenuation (Fig. 3.5). Small subdural hematomas may be masked by adjacent cortical bone when viewed on a narrow window width but will be seen with an intermediate window width (Fig. 3.6). Most subdural hematomas are supratentorial, located along the convexity. They are also frequently seen along the falx and tentorium. Because dural reflections form the falx cerebri and tentorium, subdural collections will not cross these structures (see Fig. 3.4). Unlike epidural hematomas, subdural hematomas can cross sutural margins and, in fact, are frequently seen layering along the entire hemispheric convexity from the anterior falx to the posterior falx. Diffuse swelling of the underlying hemisphere is common with subdural hematomas. Because of this, there may be more mass effect than would be expected by the size of the collection and there may be little or no reduction in midline shift after evacuation of a hemispheric subdural hematoma.

The CT appearance of subdural hematomas changes with time. The density of an acute subdural hematoma initially increases because of clot retraction. By the time

most acute subdural hematomas are imaged, the collection is hyperdense, measuring 50–60 H, relative to normal brain, which measures 18–30 H. The density will then progressively decrease as protein degradation occurs within the hematoma. Occasionally, acute subdural blood may be isodense or hypodense in patients with severe anemia or active extravasation ("hyperacute" subdural hematoma). Rebleeding during evolution of a subdural hematoma causes a heterogeneous appearance from the mixture of fresh blood and partially liquefied hematoma (Fig. 3.7). A sediment level or "hematocrit effect" may be seen either from rebleeding or in patients with clotting disorders (Fig. 3.8). Chronic subdural hematomas have low attenuation values similar to CSF (Fig. 3.9). On noncontrast CT scans, it can be difficult to distinguish them from prominent subarachnoid space secondary to cerebral atrophy. Contrast enhancement can help by demonstrating an enhancing capsule or displaced cortical veins.

During the transition from acute to chronic subdural hematomas, an isodense phase occurs, usually between several days and 3 weeks after the acute event. Although the subdural hematoma itself is less conspicuous during this isodense phase, there are indirect signs on a noncontrast CT scan that should lead to the correct diagnosis. These include effacement of sulci, displacement of cortex with white matter "buckling," and midline shift (Fig. 3.10).

The MR appearance of subdural hematomas depends on the biochemical state of hemoglobin, which varies with the age of the hematoma (see chapter 4). Acute

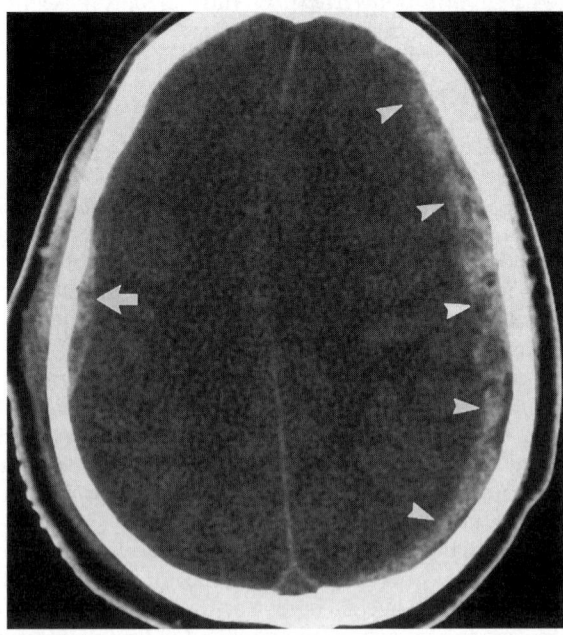

Figure 3.5. Left Subdural and Right Epidural Hematomas. Axial CT scan demonstrates a crescent-shaped high-attenuation collection extending along the entire left hemisphere consistent with a subdural hematoma (*arrowheads*). Compare the appearance with that of a small epidural hematoma seen on the **right** (*arrow*), where overlying scalp soft-tissue swelling is also present. (Reprinted with permission from Gean AD. Imaging of Head Trauma. Philadelphia: Lippincott-Raven, 1994:120.)

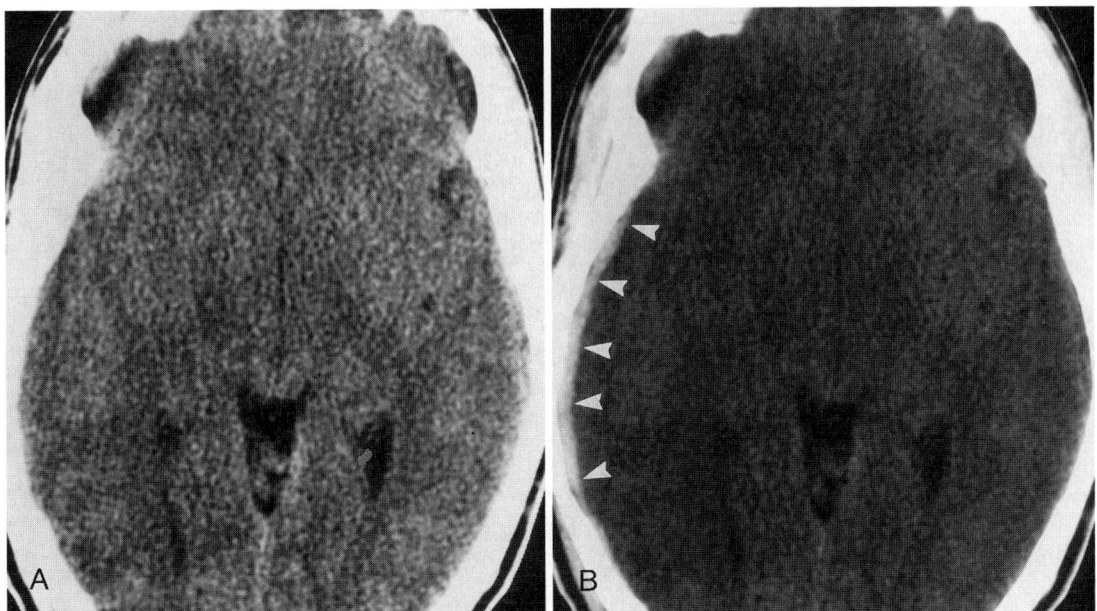

Figure 3.6. Subdural Hematoma Seen on Intermediate Window Only. A small right temporal subdural hematoma is masked on this CT using a narrow window **(A)** but is clearly seen **(B)** (*arrowheads*) with an intermediate (or subdural) window.

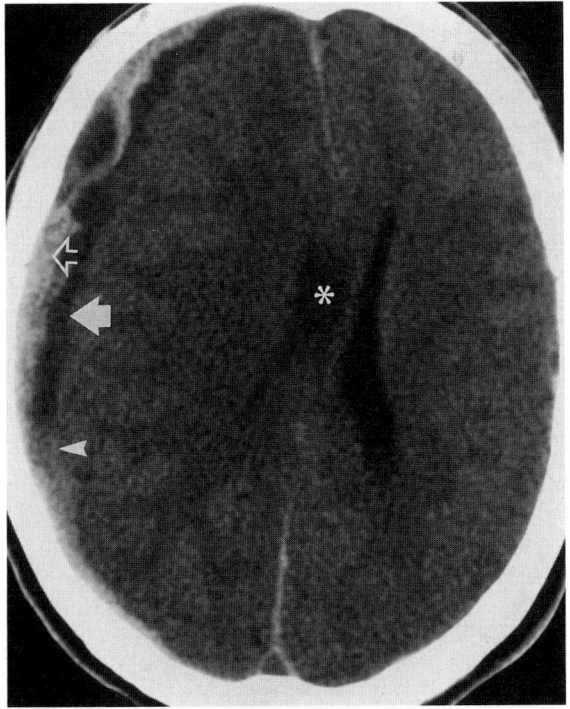

Figure 3.7. Acute and Chronic Subdural Hematoma. Axial CT scan demonstrates the heterogeneous appearance of superimposed acute and chronic subdural hematomas. The higher attenuation material (*open arrow*) represents fresh bleeding into a chronic, low-attenuation subdural hematoma (*closed arrow*). Layering of acute blood products is seen in the posterior aspect of the collection (*arrowhead*). Midline shift or "subfalcial herniation" is also present, evidenced by displacement of the right lateral ventricle (*asterisk*) across midline.

subdural hematomas are isointense to brain on T1WI and hypointense on T2WI. MR is particularly helpful during the subacute phase, when the subdural hematoma may be isodense or hypodense on CT scans. T1WI will demonstrate high signal intensity caused by the presence of methemoglobin in the subdural collection. This high signal clearly distinguishes subdural hematomas from most nonhemorrhagic fluid collections. MR also reveals that subacute subdural hematomas frequently have a lentiform or biconvex appearance when seen in the coronal plane, rather than the crescent-shaped appearance that is characteristic on axial CT scans (Fig. 3.11). The multiplanar capability of MR scanning is helpful in identifying small convexity and vertex hematomas that might not be detected on axial CT scans because of the similar attenuation of the adjacent bone.

Subarachnoid Hemorrhage is common in head injury but is rarely large enough to cause a significant mass effect. It results from the disruption of small subarachnoid vessels or direct extension into the subarachnoid space by a contusion or hematoma. On CT, subarachnoid hemorrhage appears as linear areas of high attenuation within the cisterns and sulci (Fig. 3.12). Subarachnoid collections along the convexity or tentorium can be differentiated from subdural hematomas by their extension into adjacent sulci. Occasionally, the only finding is apparent effacement of sulci when the sulci are filled with small amounts of blood. In patients who are found unconscious after an unwitnessed event, detection of subarachnoid hemorrhage may indicate a ruptured aneurysm, rather than trauma, as the prima-ry cause. In such cases, angiography needs to be considered.

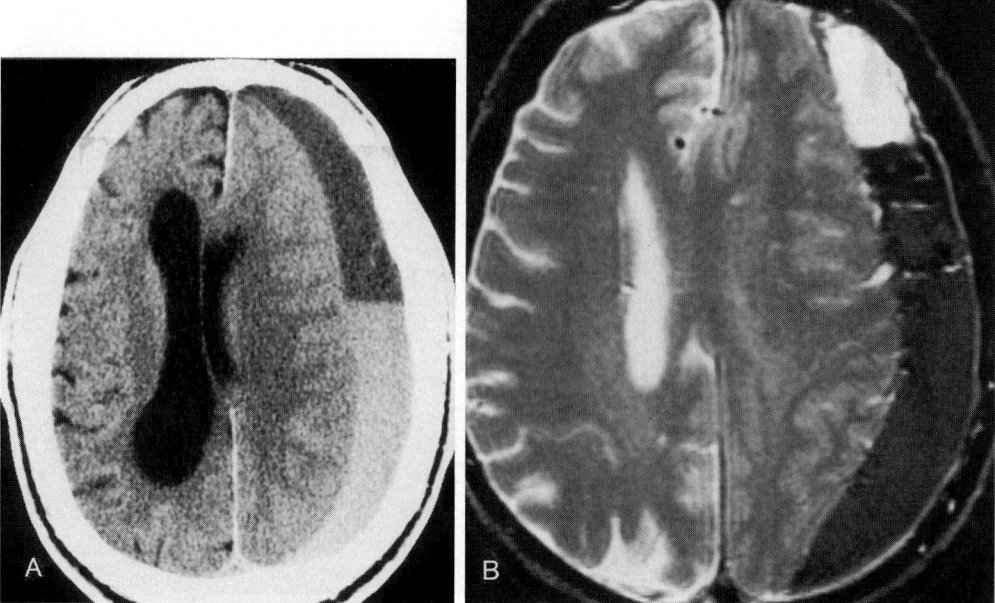

Figure 3.8. Subdural Hematomas with Hematocrit Effect. A CT scan **(A)** and T2-weighted MR scan **(B)** in two different patients show large left hemispheric subdural hematomas with fluid–fluid levels, known as the hematocrit effect. This appearance can be seen in patients with clotting disorders or in patients with rebleeding into an older subdural collection. (Reprinted with permission from Gean AD. Imaging of Head Trauma. Philadelphia: Lippincott-Raven, 1994: 89,95.)

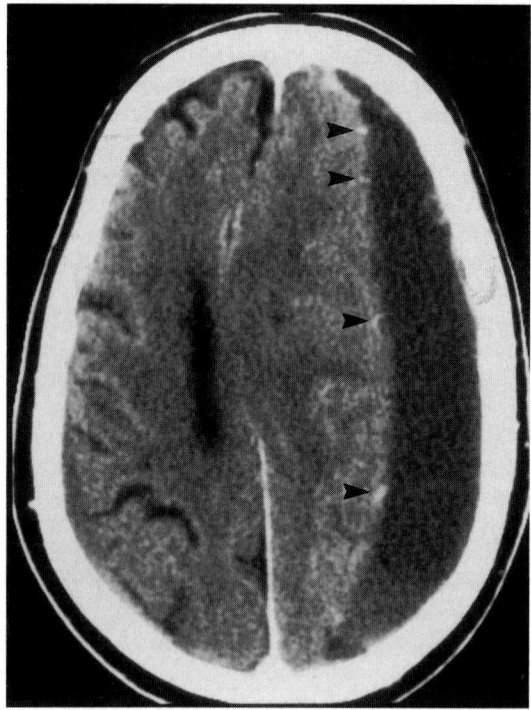

Figure 3.9. Chronic Subdural Hematoma. Contrast-enhanced CT scans shows a large water-density left subdural collection consistent with a chronic subdural hematoma. There is considerable mass effect with midline shift. Displaced cortical veins can be seen along the brain surface *(arrows)*. (Reprinted with permission from Gean AD. Imaging of Head Trauma. Philadelphia: Lippincott-Raven, 1994: 96.)

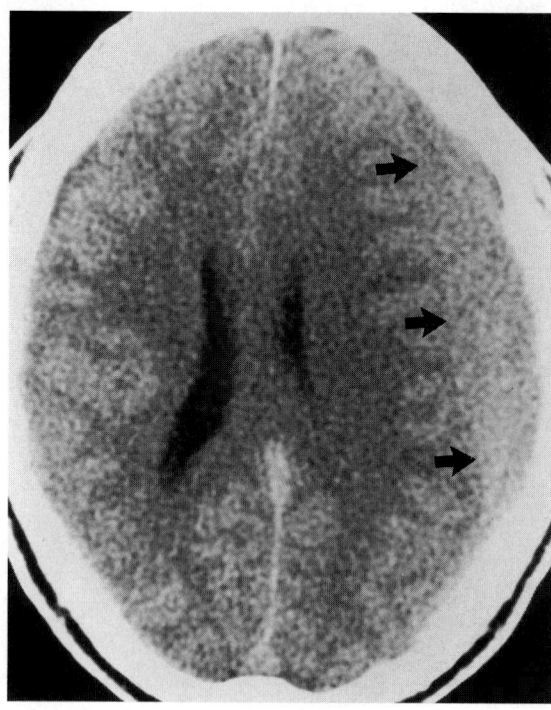

Figure 3.10. Subacute Subdural Hematoma on CT. Noncontrast CT scan shows an isodense left subdural hematoma with displacement of the underlying cortex *(arrows)*, compression of the lateral ventricle, and mild midline shift.

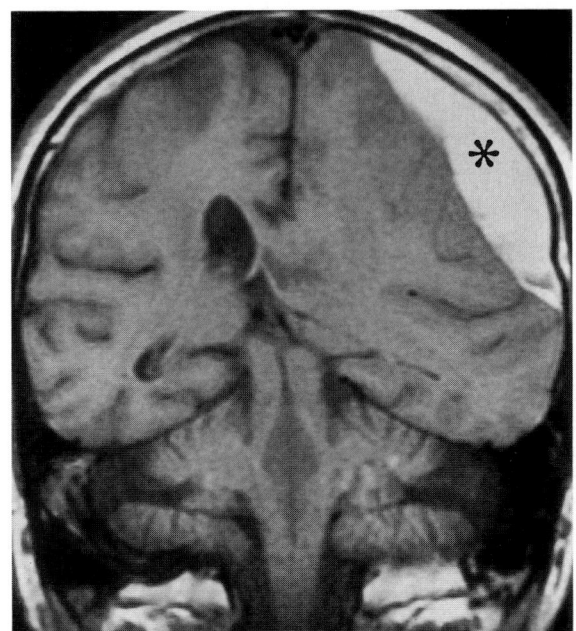

Figure 3.11. Subacute Subdural Hematoma on MR. Noncontrast coronal T1-weighted MR scan shows a well-defined, uniform, hyperintense extra-axial collection (*asterisk*) with associated mass effect on the left cerebral hemisphere. This represents a subacute subdural hematoma. The increased signal intensity on a T1-weighted sequence is attributable to methemoglobin. Subdural hematomas can appear crescent-shaped in the axial plane and biconvex in the coronal plane.

Acute subarachnoid hemorrhage is more difficult to detect on MR than it is on CT scans because it is isointense to brain parenchyma. Subacute subarachnoid hemorrhage may be better appreciated on MR because of its high signal intensity at a time when the blood is isointense to CSF on CT. Chronic hemorrhage on MR scans may show hemosiderin staining in the subarachnoid space, which appears as areas of markedly decreased signal intensity on T1- and T2-weighted sequences ("superficial hemosiderosis"). Subarachnoid hemorrhage may lead to subsequent hydrocephalus by impaired CSF resorption at the level of arachnoid villi.

Intraventricular Hemorrhage is commonly seen in patients with head injuries and can occur by several mechanisms. First, it can result from rotationally induced tearing of subependymal veins on the surface of the ventricles. Another mechanism is by direct extension of a parenchymal hematoma into the ventricular system. Third, intraventricular blood can result from retrograde flow of subarachnoid hemorrhage into the ventricular system through the fourth ventricular outflow foramina. Patients with intraventricular hemorrhage are at risk for subsequent hydrocephalus by obstruction either at the level of the aqueduct or arachnoid villi.

On CT, intraventricular hemorrhage appears as hyperdense material, layering dependently within the ventricular system. Tiny collections of increased density layering in the occipital horns may be the only clue to intraventricular hemorrhage.

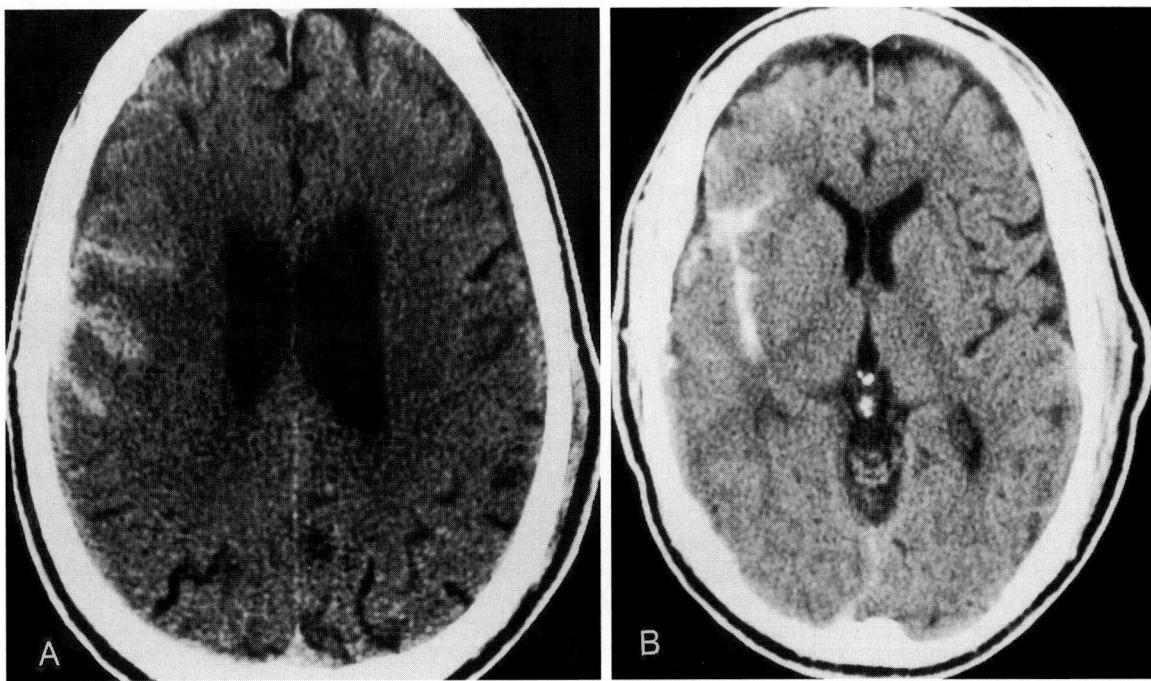

Figure 3.12. Subarachnoid Hemorrhage. Noncontrast axial CT scans in two different patients demonstrate high-attenuation material within the sulci **(A)** and right sylvian fissure **(B)** consistent with subarachnoid hemorrhage. (Reprinted with permission from Gean AD. Imaging of Head Trauma. Philadelphia: Lippincott-Raven, 1994: 130,131.)

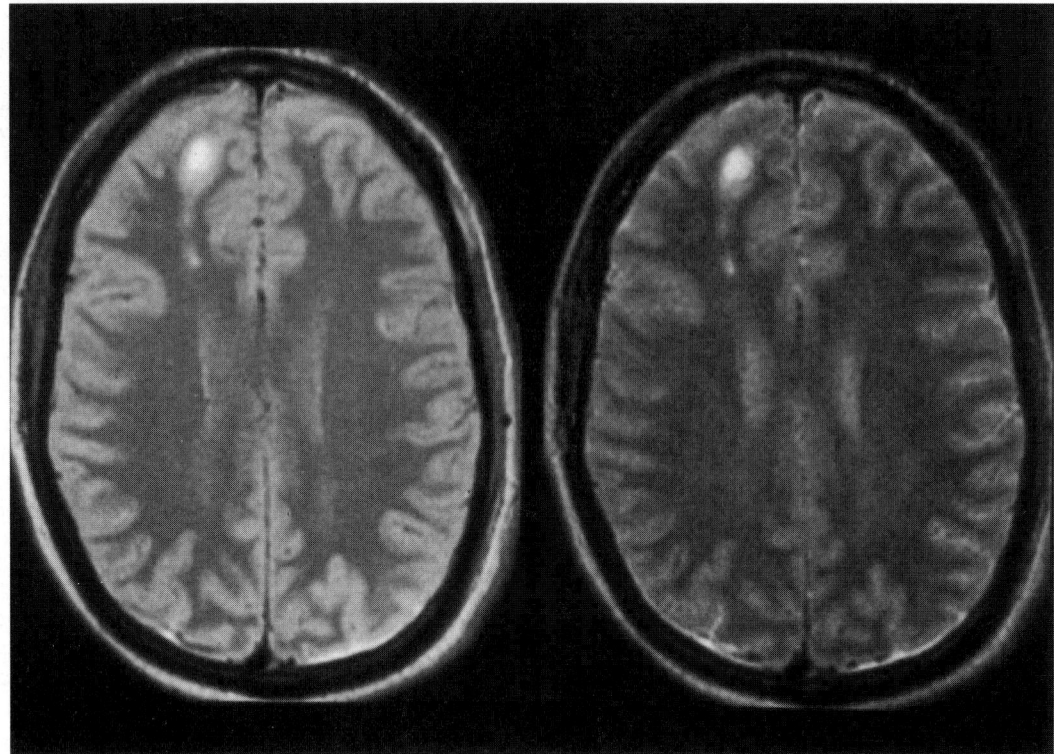

Figure 3.13. The MR Appearance of Acute DAI. Proton-density **(left)** and T2-weighted **(right)** MR images show several adjacent foci of high signal representing DAI in the right frontal parasagittal white matter. (Reprinted with permission from Gean AD. Imaging of Head Trauma. Philadelphia: Lippincott-Raven, 1994:225.)

INTRA-AXIAL INJURY

Diffuse Axonal Injury (DAI) is one of the most common types of primary neuronal injury in patients with severe head trauma. As the name implies, DAI is characterized by widespread disruption of axons that occurs at the time of an acceleration or deceleration injury. The affected areas of the brain may be distant from the site of direct impact; in fact, direct impact is not necessary to cause this type of injury.

The incidence of DAI was likely underestimated until recently because of the difficulty in visualizing these lesions on existing imaging studies as well as on histologic specimens. DAI is much better seen by MR than CT. This factor accounts to a large degree for the increased success of MR at explaining neurologic deficits after trauma and in predicting long-term outcome. Though MR has improved the detection of DAI in patients suffering head trauma, the incidence of this form of injury is probably still underestimated.

Patients with DAI are most commonly injured in high-speed motor vehicle accidents. These lesions have not been seen as a consequence of simple falls, such as when a patient falls from the standing position. Loss of consciousness typically starts immediately after the injury and is more severe than in patients with cortical contusions or hematomas.

On MR, nonhemorrhagic DAI lesions appear as small foci of increased signal on T2WI (T2 prolongation) within the white matter (Fig. 3.13). The lesions tend to be multiple, with as many as 15–20 lesions seen in patients with severe head injury. If seen on T1WI, they appear as subtle areas of decreased intensity. Petechial hemorrhage causes a central hypointensity on T2WI and hyperintensity on T1WI within a few days as a result of intracellular methemoglobin. The conspicuity of DAI on MR diminishes over weeks to months as the damaged axons degenerate and the edema resolves. Residual findings might include nonspecific atrophy or hemosiderin staining, which can persist for years and is especially obvious on gradient-echo sequences (Fig. 3.14).

DAI is seen in characteristic locations that correlate with the severity of the trauma. Patients with the mildest forms of injury have lesions confined to the frontal and temporal white matter, near the gray–white junction. The lesions typically involve the parasagittal regions of the frontal lobes and periventricular regions of the temporal lobes. Patients with more severe trauma have DAI involving lobar white matter as well as the corpus callosum, especially the posterior body and splenium. The corpus callosum accounts for approximately 20% of all DAI lesions (11). Initially thought to be caused by direct impact from the falx, experimental work shows (12) that injury to the corpus callosum is most commonly caused by rotational shear forces, like all forms of DAI. The corpus callosum may be particularly susceptible to DAI because the falx prevents displacement of the cerebral hemispheres. DAI of the corpus callosum is almost always seen in association with lesions in the lobar white matter. DAI in the most severe cases involves the dorsolateral aspect of the midbrain and upper pons in addition to the lobar white matter and corpus callosum (see Brainstem Injury).

CT findings in DAI can be subtle or absent. Only approximately 20% of lesions contain sufficient hemorrhage to be visible on CT scans, accounting for the low sensitivity of this modality. Most common is the finding of small, petechial hemorrhages at the gray–white junction of the cerebral hemispheres or corpus callosum (Fig. 3.15). Ill-defined areas of decreased attenuation on CT may occasionally be seen with nonhemorrhagic lesions.

Cortical Contusions are areas of focal brain injury primarily involving superficial gray matter. Patients with cortical contusions are much less likely to have loss of consciousness at the time of injury than are patients with DAI. Contusions are also associated with a better prognosis than DAI. They are very common in patients with severe head trauma and are usually well seen on CT scans. Contusions characteristically occur near bony protuberances of the skull and skull base. They tend to be multiple and bilateral and are more commonly hemorrhagic than DAI. Common sites are the temporal lobes above the petrous bone or posterior to the greater sphenoid wing, and the frontal lobes above the cribriform plate, planum sphenoidale, and lesser sphenoid wing (Fig. 3.16). Less than 10% of lesions involve the cerebellum (13). Contusions can also occur at the margins of depressed skull fractures.

The CT appearance of cortical contusions characteristically varies with the age of the lesion. Many nonhemorrhagic lesions are initially poorly seen but become more obvious during the first week because of associated edema. Hemorrhagic lesions are seen as foci of high attenuation within superficial gray matter (Fig. 3.17). These may be surrounded by larger areas of low attenuation secondary to surrounding edema. During the first week, the characteristic CT pattern of mixed areas of hypodensity and hyperdensity ("salt and pepper" pattern) becomes more apparent. Occasionally, surgical decompression of the contused brain is required to alleviate severe mass effect. Areas of prior contusion can often be recognized as foci of encephalomalacia within the same characteristic locations just described.

On MR imaging, contusions appear as poorly marginated areas of increased signal on proton density and T2-weighted sequences. They are recognized because of their characteristic distribution in the frontal and temporal lobes and often have a "gyral" morphology. Hemorrhage causes heterogeneous signal intensity that varies depending on the age of the lesion (Fig. 3.18). Hemosiderin staining from hemorrhage of any cause leads to markedly decreased signal intensity on T2WI, especially at higher field strengths. This signal loss can persist indefinitely as a marker of prior hemorrhage.

Intracerebral Hematoma. Occasionally, intraparenchymal hemorrhage is seen that is not necessarily associated with cortical contusion but rather represents shear-induced hemorrhage from the rupture of small intraparenchymal blood vessels. This lesion is known simply as an intracerebral hematoma. Intracerebral hematomas tend to have less surrounding edema than cortical contusions because they represent bleeding into areas of relatively normal brain. Most intracerebral hematomas are located in the frontotemporal white matter, although they have also been described in the basal ganglia. They are often associated with skull fractures and other primary neuronal lesions, including contusions and DAI. In the absence of other significant lesions, patients with intracerebral hematomas can remain lucid after their injury. When symptoms develop, they commonly result from the mass effect associated with an expanding hematoma. Intracerebral hematomas can also present late secondary to delayed hemorrhage,

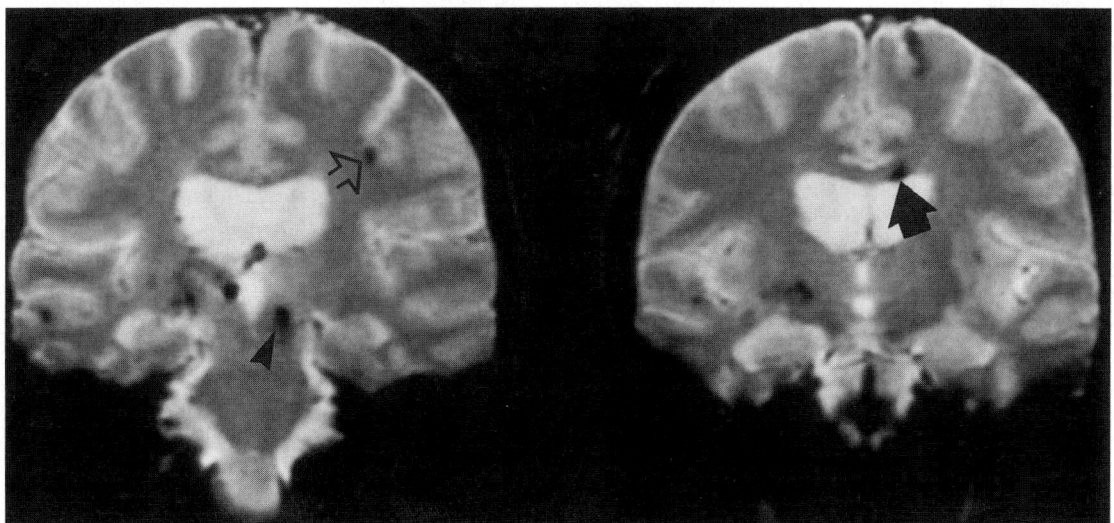

Figure 3.14. The MR Appearance of Chronic DAI. Coronal gradient-echo images in a patient with a history of prior severe head trauma demonstrate numerous hypointense foci in a distribution characteristic of DAI, including the gray–white junction (*open arrow*), corpus callosum (*closed arrow*), and cerebral peduncle (*arrowhead*). Evidence of remote hemorrhage is especially conspicuous on gradient-echo sequences. (Reprinted with permission from Gean AD. Imaging of Head Trauma. Philadelphia: Lippincott-Raven, 1994:235.)

which is another cause of clinical deterioration during the first several days after head trauma (Fig. 3.19).

Subcortical Gray Matter Injury is an uncommon manifestation of primary intra-axial injury and is seen as multiple, petechial hemorrhages primarily affecting the basal ganglia and thalamus. These represent microscopic perivascular collections of blood that may result from disruption of multiple small perforating vessels. These lesions are typically seen following severe head trauma.

Vascular Injuries as causes of intra- and extra-axial hematomas were discussed previously. Other types of traumatic vascular injury include arterial dissection or occlusion, pseudoaneurysm formation, and the acquired arteriovenous fistula. Arterial injury commonly accompanies fractures of the base of the skull. The internal carotid is the most often injured artery, especially at sites of fixation. These include its entrance to the carotid canal at the base of the petrous bone and at its exit from the cavernous sinus below the anterior clinoid process.

MR findings of vascular injury include the presence of an intramural hematoma or intimal flap with dissection, or the absence of normal vascular flow void with occlu-

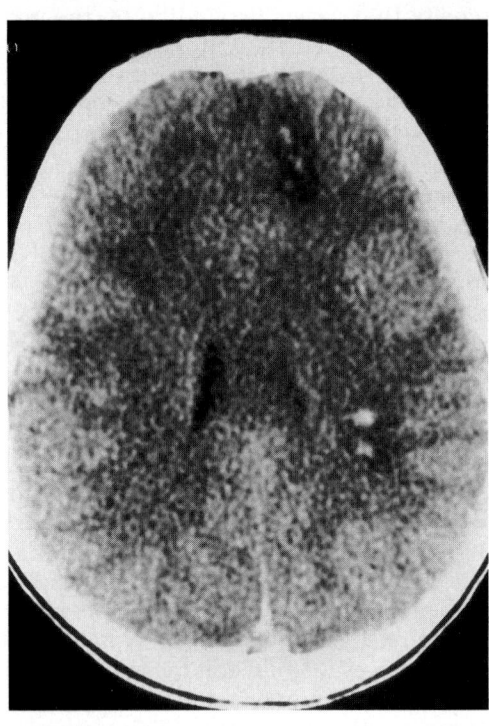

Figure 3.15. The CT Appearance of DAI. Noncontrast CT scan shows punctate high-attenuation foci with surrounding edema in the left frontal and parietal white matter consistent with hemorrhagic DAI. Additional lesions could be seen at other levels.

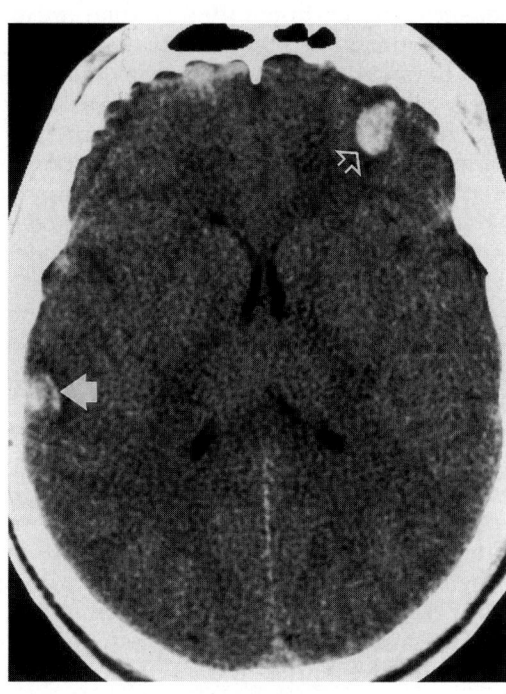

Figure 3.17. The CT Appearance of Cortical Contusion. Noncontrast CT scan reveals high-attenuation lesions involving the left frontal (*open arrow*) and right temporal (*closed arrow*) gray matter consistent with hemorrhagic cortical contusions.

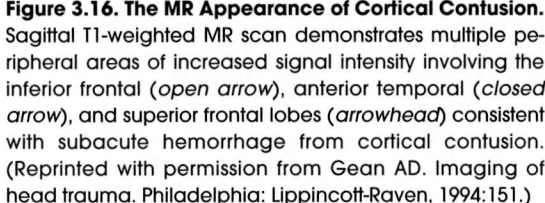

Figure 3.16. The MR Appearance of Cortical Contusion. Sagittal T1-weighted MR scan demonstrates multiple peripheral areas of increased signal intensity involving the inferior frontal (*open arrow*), anterior temporal (*closed arrow*), and superior frontal lobes (*arrowhead*) consistent with subacute hemorrhage from cortical contusion. (Reprinted with permission from Gean AD. Imaging of head trauma. Philadelphia: Lippincott-Raven, 1994:151.)

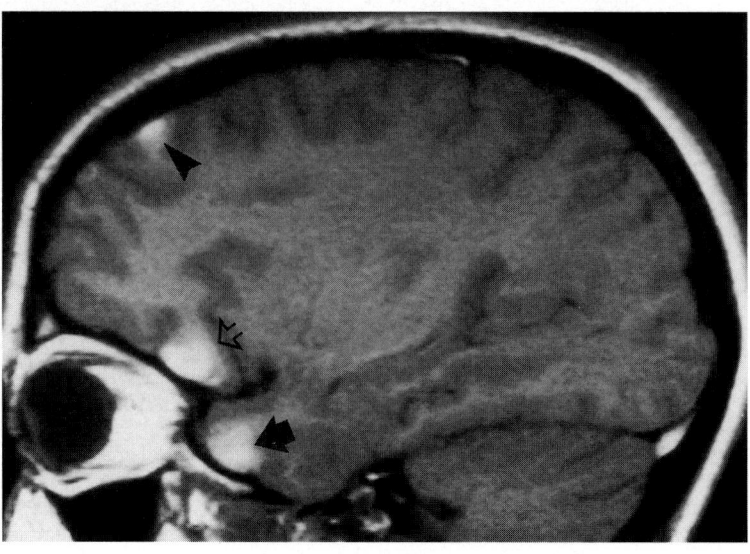

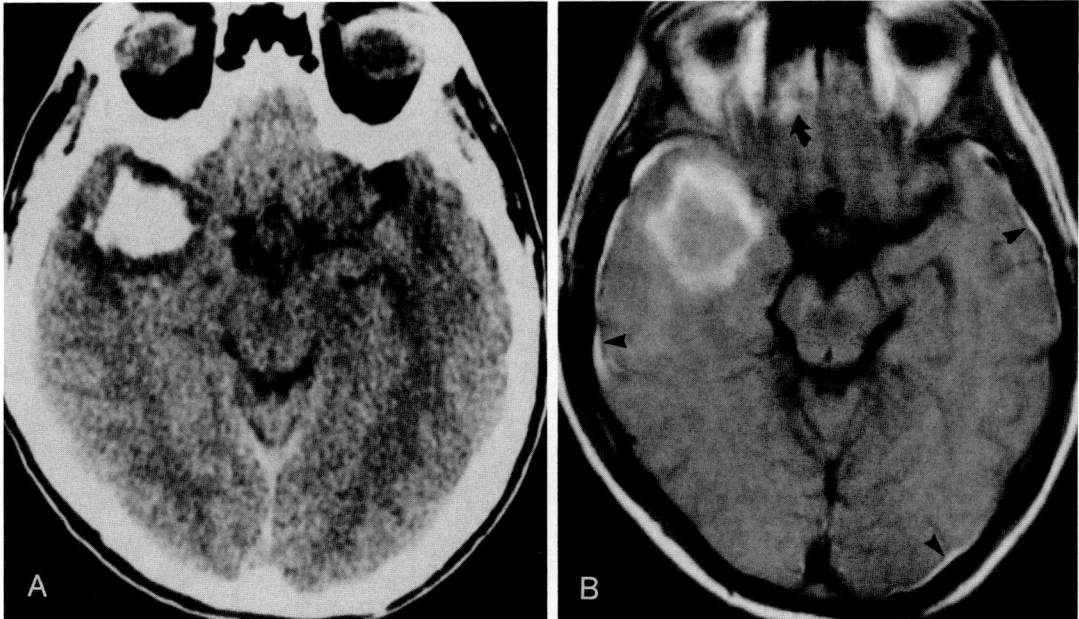

Figure 3.18. Intracerebral Hematoma. A. Axial CT scan demonstrates a high-attenuation mass within the right temporal lobe. **B.** The corresponding T1-weighted MR scan demonstrates a central region of isointensity consistent with acute hemorrhage (deoxyhemoglobin). The surrounding high signal intensity rim represents the conversion to methemoglobin, which begins to form at the periphery of a hematoma. High signal in the inferior right frontal lobe (*curved arrow*) represents an associated frontal contusion. A small amount of subdural blood is also present bilaterally and is hyperintense (*arrowheads*).

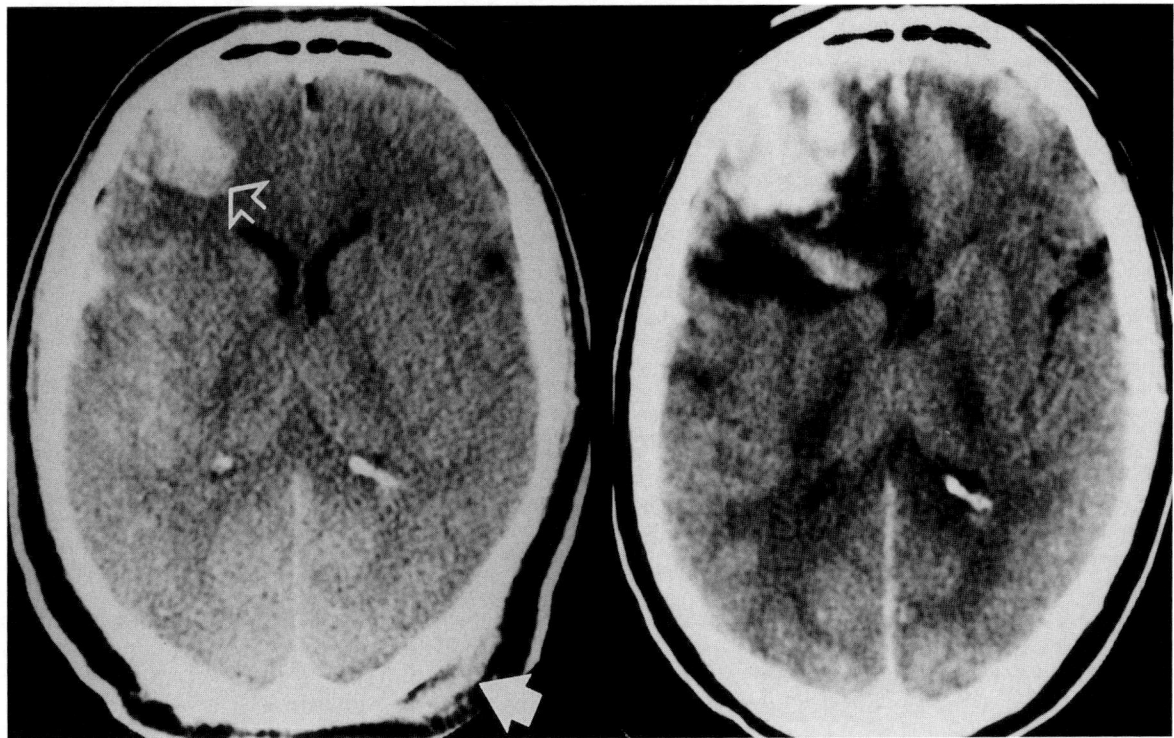

Figure 3.19. Delayed Hemorrhage. Admission CT scan **(left)** shows a small right frontal hematoma without significant mass effect (*open arrow*). Left parietal soft-tissue swelling indicates the site of impact (*closed arrow*). A follow-up CT scan **(right)** was performed when the patient's clinical condition deteriorated, and it demonstrates marked increase in the size of the hematoma with increased edema, mass effect, and compression of the ipsilateral frontal horn.

Figure 3.20. Carotid Cavernous Fistula.
A. A CT scan shows fullness in the right cavernous sinus (*open arrow*) and right proptosis, with swelling of the extraocular muscles (*closed arrows*) and preseptal soft tissues (*arrowheads*). **B.** Internal carotid angiogram in a different patient shows opacification of the cavernous sinus (*open arrow*) and jugular vein (*closed arrow*) during the arterial phase. (Reprinted with permission from Gean AD. Imaging of Head Trauma. Philadelphia: Lippincott-Raven, 1994:349.)

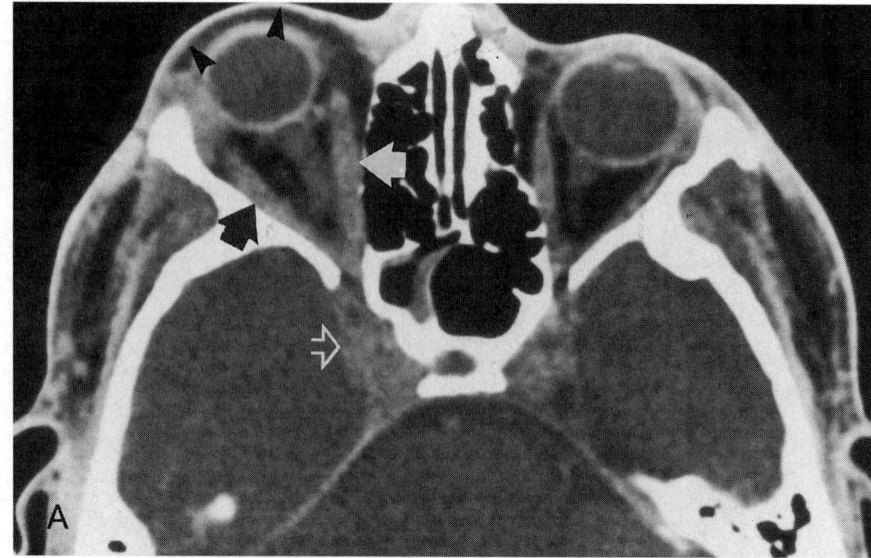

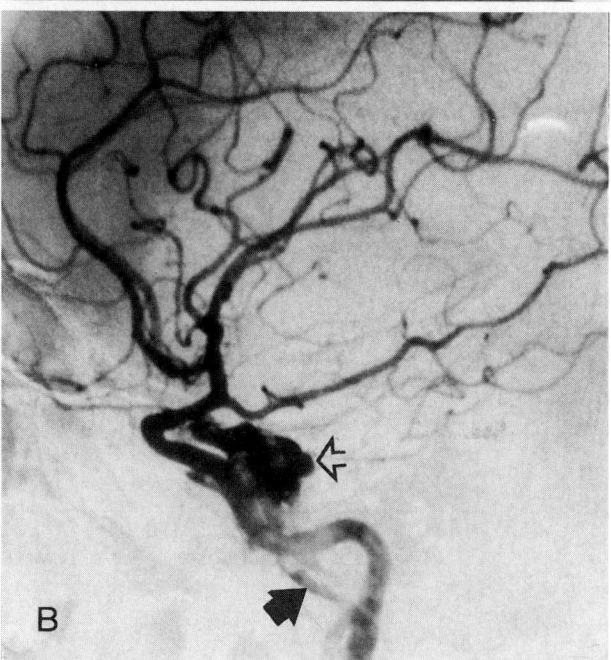

sion. An associated parenchymal infarction might also be seen. There is a potential role for MR angiography in evaluating patients with suspected traumatic vascular injury. Conventional angiograms are usually needed to confirm and delineate dissections and may also show spasm or pseudoaneurysm formation in injuries to the vessel wall.

The carotid cavernous fistula (CCF) is a communication between the cavernous portion of the internal carotid artery and the surrounding venous plexus. The lesion typically follows a full-thickness arterial injury, resulting in venous engorgement of the cavernous sinus and its draining tributaries (e.g., the ipsilateral superior ophthalmic vein and inferior petrosal sinus). Findings may be bilateral because venous channels connect the cavernous sinuses. The CCF most often results from severe head injury. Skull base fractures, especially those involving the sphenoid bone, indicate patients at in-

creased risk for associated cavernous carotid injury. The CCF may also result from ruptured cavernous carotid aneurysms. On MR, the CCF may manifest as enlarged superior ophthalmic vein, cavernous sinus, and petrosal sinus flow voids. There may be evidence of proptosis, swelling of the preseptal soft tissues, and enlargement of the extraocular musculature. Diagnosis usually requires selective carotid angiography with rapid filming to demonstrate the site of communication (Fig. 3.20). On occasion, patients present with findings weeks or months after the initial trauma.

Dural fistulas are also associated with trauma. For example, they may be caused by laceration of the middle meningeal artery with resultant meningeal artery to meningeal vein fistula formation. Drainage via meningeal veins prevents formation of an epidural hematoma. Patients may be asymptomatic or present with nonspecific complaints, including tinnitus.

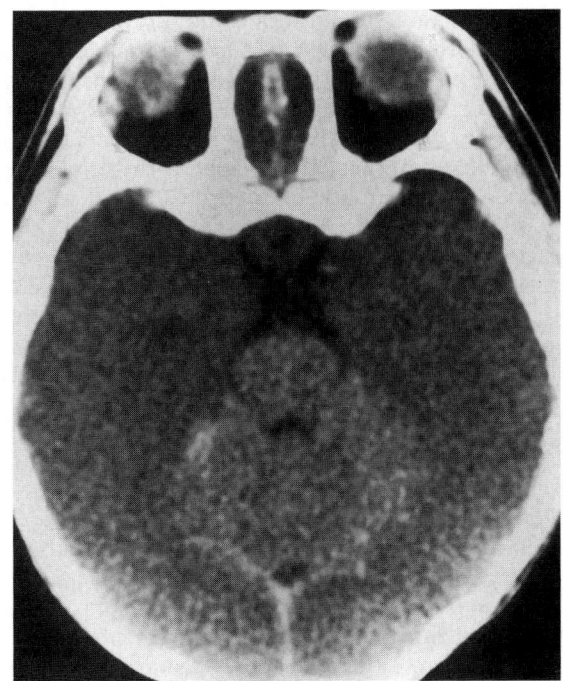

Figure 3.21. Diffuse Cerebral Edema. Noncontrast CT scan in an infant with diffuse cerebral edema following strangulation. There is a diffuse decrease in attenuation of the cerebral hemispheres with loss of gray–white differentiation. Sparing of the brainstem and cerebellum causes these structures to appear dense relative to the rest of the brain.

MECHANISMS OF PRIMARY HEAD INJURIES

Early research suggested that head injuries could be explained by areas of parenchymal compression and rarefaction caused by direct impact. Many authors still use the terms "coup" and contrecoup" to describe intracranial lesions that characteristically occur both on opposite the side of a blow to the head. More recently, however, Gentry and others have questioned the use of these terms, which they feel incorrectly imply that neuronal injury is caused by compression and rarefaction strains subsequent to direct impact.

Gennarelli et al. have shown in a primate model that all major types of intraaxial lesions, as well as subdural hematomas, can be produced purely by rotational acceleration of the head without direct impact. Only skull fractures and epidural hematomas require a physical blow to the head. Rotational acceleration causes damage by shear forces, rather than by compression-rarefaction strain. Compression-rarefaction strain is not felt to play a significant role in most head injuries.

The character of the accelerational force influences the type of injury produced. Cortical contusions and intracranial hematosis are more severe when the period of acceleration or deceleration is very short, whereas DAI and gliding contusions are associated with a longer acceleration or deceleration injury. Thus, DAI is more common in motor vehicle accidents while contusions and hematomas are more frequent in falls.

Secondary Head Injury

Diffuse Cerebral Swelling is a common manifestation of head trauma. It may occur either because of an increase in cerebral blood volume or an increase in tissue fluid content. Hyperemia refers to an increase in blood volume, whereas cerebral edema refers to an increase in tissue fluid. Both lead to generalized mass effect with effacement of sulci, suprasellar and quadrigeminal plate cisterns, and compression of the ventricular system. Effacement of the brainstem cisterns indicates severe mass effect and may herald impending transtentorial herniation.

Cerebral swelling from hyperemia is most commonly seen in children and adolescents. The pathogenesis is poorly understood but appears to be the result of loss of normal cerebral autoregulation. Hyperemia is recognized on CT as ill-defined mass effect, effacement of sulci, and normal attenuation of brain. Acute subdural hematomas are often associated with unilateral swelling of the ipsilateral hemisphere.

Diffuse cerebral edema occurs secondary to tissue hypoxia. Because of the increase in tissue fluid, edema causes decreased attenuation on CT images with loss of gray–white differentiation. The cerebellum and brainstem are usually spared and may appear hyperdense relative to the cerebral hemispheres (Fig. 3.21). Often, the falx and cerebral vessels appear dense, mimicking acute subarachnoid hemorrhage. Focal areas of edema are frequently seen in association with cortical contusions and may contribute significantly to mass effect.

Brain Herniation. Several forms of herniation are seen secondary to mass effect produced by primary intracranial injury. These are not specific for head trauma and can be seen secondary to mass effect produced by other causes as well, including intracranial hemorrhage, infarction, or neoplasm (Fig. 3.22).

Subfalcial herniation, in which the cingulate gyrus is displaced across the midline under the falx cerebri, is

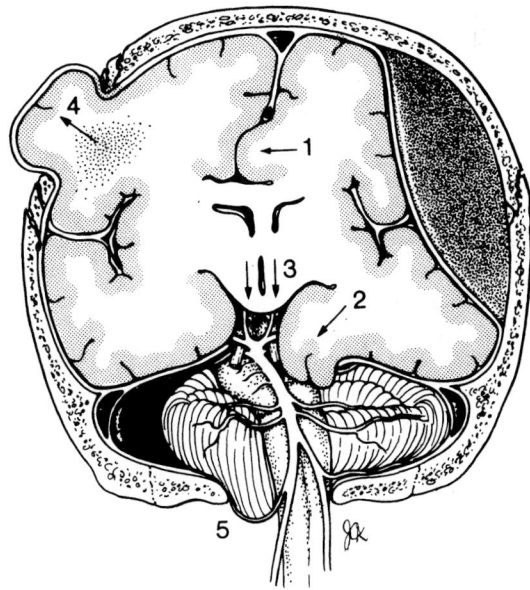

Figure 3.22. Types of Brain Herniation. Diagram of the major types of brain herniation. (*1*) Subfalcial herniation. (*2*) Uncal herniation. (*3*) Descending transtentorial herniation. (*4*) External herniation. (*5*) Tonsillar herniation. (Reprinted with permission from Gean AD. Imaging of Head Trauma. Philadelphia: Lippincott-Raven, 1994:264.)

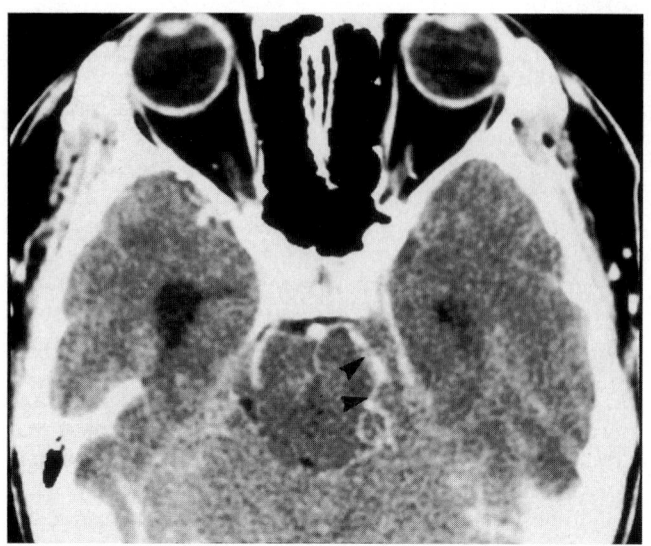

Figure 3.23. Uncal Herniation. Contrast-enhanced CT scan shows compression of the left aspect of the brainstem, displacement of the left posterior cerebral artery (PCA) (*arrowheads*), and effacement of the ambient and crural cisterns. The temporal horns of the lateral ventricles are dilated, indicating obstructive hydrocephalus. Compression of the PCA during uncal herniation can lead to a PCA infarct. (Reprinted with permission from Gean AD. Imaging of Head Trauma. Philadelphia: Lippincott-Raven, 1994:273.)

the most common form of brain herniation (see Fig. 3.7). Compression of the adjacent lateral ventricle may be seen on CT scans, as well as enlargement of the contralateral ventricle from obstruction at the level of the foramen of Monro. Both anterior cerebral arteries (ACAs) may be displaced to the contralateral side. These patients are at risk of ACA infarction in the distribution of the callosomarginal branch of the ACA, where it becomes trapped against the falx.

Uncal herniation, in which the medial aspect of the temporal lobe is displaced medially over the free margin of the tentorium, is also common (Fig. 3.23). Uncal herniation causes focal effacement of the ambient cistern and the lateral aspect of the suprasellar cistern. Rarely, displacement of the brainstem causes compression of the contralateral cerebral peduncle against the tentorial margin, resulting in peduncular hemorrhage or infarction. The focal impression on the cerebral peduncle is known as "Kernohan's notch." Mass effect on the third cranial nerve and compression of the contralateral cerebral peduncle cause a recognizable clinical syndrome characterized by a blown pupil with ipsilateral hemiparesis.

Transtentorial herniation. The brain can herniate either downward or upward across the tentorium. Descending transtentorial herniation is recognized by effacement of the suprasellar and perimesencephalic cisterns. Pineal calcification, usually seen at about the same level as calcified choroid plexus in the trigones of the lateral ventricles, is displaced inferiorly. Large posterior fossa hematomas can cause ascending transtentorial herniation, in which the vermis and portions of the cerebellar hemispheres can herniate through the tento-

rial incisura. This is much less common than descending transtentorial herniation. Posterior fossa hematomas can also cause herniation of the cerebellar tonsils downward through the foramen magnum. Finally, external herniation can occur in which swelling or mass effect causes the brain to herniate through a calvarial defect. This can be posttraumatic or occur at the time of craniotomy and prevent closure of the skull flap.

Hydrocephalus can occur after subarachnoid or intraventricular hemorrhage as a result of either impaired CSF reabsorption at the level of the arachnoid granulations or obstruction at the level of the aqueduct or fourth ventricular outflow foramina. Mass effect from cerebral swelling or an adjacent hematoma can also cause hydrocephalus by compression of the aqueduct or outflow foramina of the fourth ventricle. Asymmetrical lateral ventricular dilatation can be produced by compression of the foramen of Monro.

Ischemia or Infarction. Posttraumatic ischemia or infarction can result from raised intracranial pressure, embolization from a vascular dissection, or direct mass effect on cerebral vasculature from brain herniation or an overlying extra-axial collection. In addition, patients may suffer diffuse ischemic damage from acute reduction in cerebral blood flow or from hypoxemia secondary to respiratory arrest or status epilepticus. Patterns of infarction from focal mass effect include anterior cerebral artery infarction from subfalcial herniation, posterior cerebral artery infarction from uncal herniation, and posterior inferior communicating artery infarction from tonsillar herniation. Ischemia or infarction secondary to globally reduced cerebral perfusion tends to occur in characteristic "watershed zones" and is not specific for trauma (see chapter 4).

CSF Leak requires a dural tear and can occur after calvarial or skull base fractures. CSF rhinorrhea occurs subsequent to fractures in which communication develops between the subarachnoid space and the paranasal sinuses or middle ear cavity. CSF otorrhea occurs when communication between the subarachnoid space and middle ear occurs in association with disruption of the tympanic membrane. CSF leaks can be difficult to localize and can lead to recurrent meningeal infection. Radionuclide cisternography is highly sensitive for the presence of CSF extravasation; however, CT scanning with intrathecal contrast is required for detailed anatomic localization of the defect.

Leptomeningeal Cyst or "growing fracture" is caused by a traumatic tear in the dura, which allows an outpouching of arachnoid to occur at the site of a suture or skull fracture. This leads to progressive, slow widening of the skull defect or suture, presumably as a result of CSF pulsations. The leptomeningeal cyst appears as a lytic skull defect on CT or plain skull films, which can enlarge over time.

Encephalomalacia. Focal encephalomalacia consists of tissue loss with surrounding gliosis and is a frequent manifestation of remote head injury. It may be asymptomatic or serve as a potential seizure focus. CT demonstrates fairly well-defined areas of low attenuation with volume loss. There may be dilation of adjacent portions of the ventricular system (Figs. 3.24, 3.25). Encephalomalacia

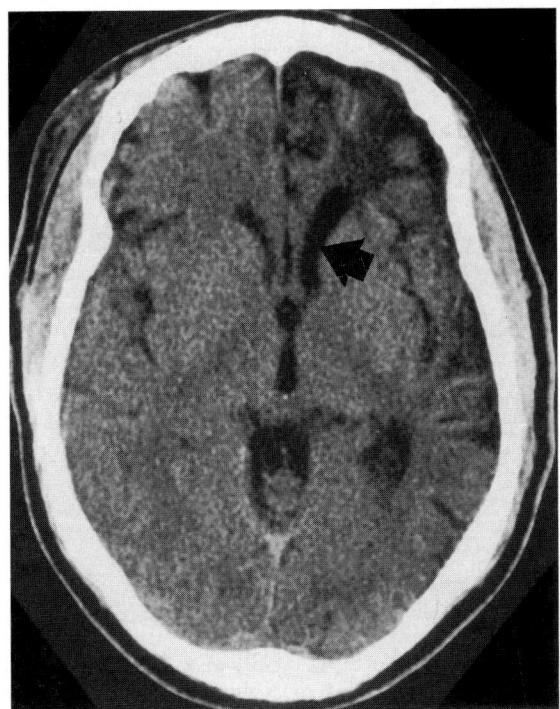

Figure 3.24. Posttraumatic Encephalomalacia. Axial CT shows a well-defined area of decreased attenuation involving gray and white matter of the left frontal lobe consistent with encephalomalacia. Dilation of the ipsilateral frontal horn (*arrow*) confirms the presence of tissue loss rather than a space-occupying lesion.

will follow CSF signal on MR sequences, except for gliosis, which appears as increased signal intensity on both proton-density and T2WI. The appearance of encephalomalacia is not specific for posttraumatic injury, but the locations are characteristic: anteroinferior frontal and temporal lobes. Focal volume loss along the white matter tracts associated with cell death is known as wallerian degeneration and may be seen on CT and especially MR studies.

Brainstem Injury

Primary. The most common form of primary brainstem injury is DAI, which affects the dorsolateral aspect of the midbrain and upper pons (Fig. 3.26). The superior cerebellar peduncles and the medial lemnisci are particularly vulnerable. Both the location and lack of sufficient amounts of hemorrhage make this lesion difficult to diagnose on CT scans. Brainstem DAI is nearly always seen in association with lesions of the frontal or temporal white matter and corpus callosum. This distinguishes brainstem DAI from a rare form of primary injury caused by direct impact of the free margin of the tentorium on the brainstem. Primary brainstem injury may also occur in the form of multiple petechial hemorrhages in the periaqueductal regions of the rostral brainstem (see previous discussion on subcortical gray matter injury). They are not associated with DAI, although they occur in a similar distribution. This form of injury represents disruption of penetrating brainstem blood vessels by shear strain and carries a grim prognosis.

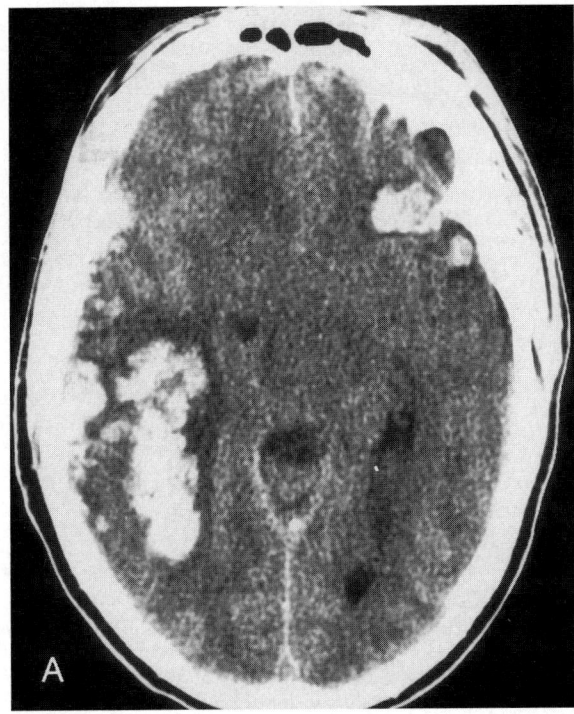
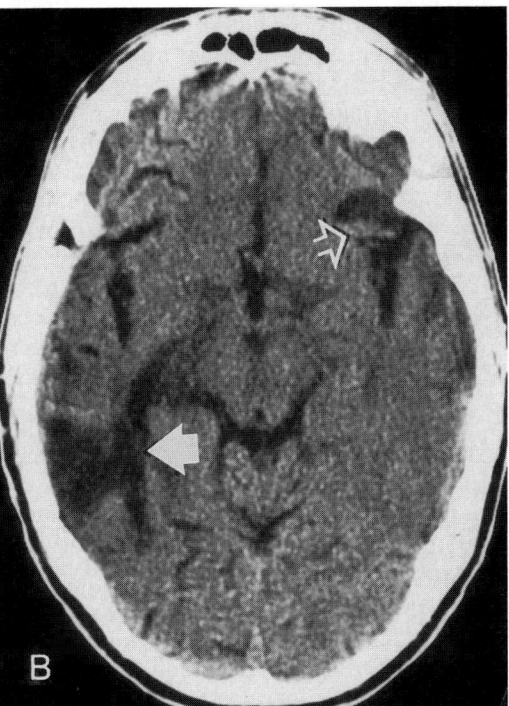

Figure 3.25. Posttraumatic Encephalomalacia. Admission **(A)** and follow-up **(B)** scans in a patient with severe head trauma show the interval development of left frontal (*open arrow*) and right posterior temporal (*closed arrow*) encephalomalacia in the same locations as the initial intracerebral hematomas. (Reprinted with permission from Gean AD. Imaging of Head Trauma. Philadelphia: Lippincott-Raven, 1994:507.)

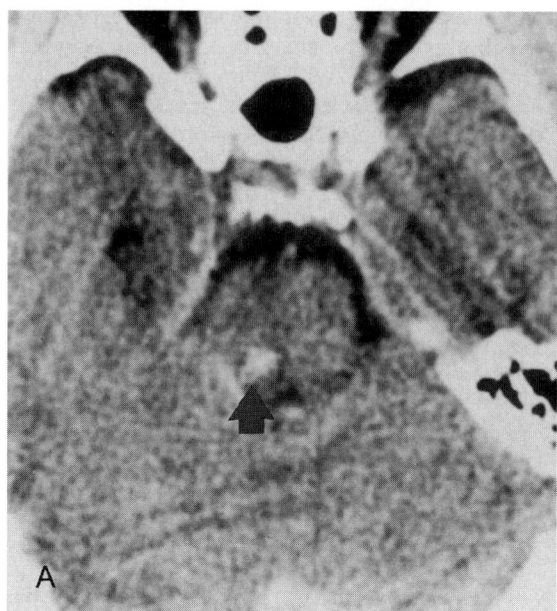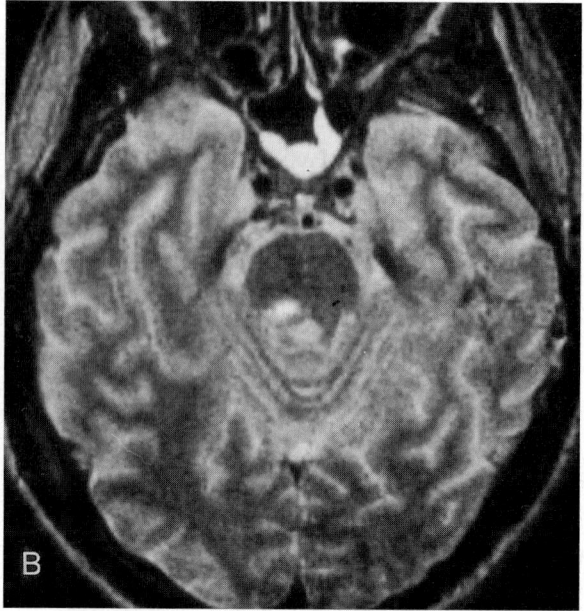

Figure 3.26. Brainstem DAI. A. Noncontrast CT scan shows a punctate focus of increased attenuation representing focal hemorrhage from DAI of the brainstem (*arrow*). Note the characteristic location in the dorsolateral aspect of the brainstem. **B.** T2-weighted MR scan in a different patient shows a hyperintense lesion in a similar location.

An extremely rare form of indirect primary brainstem injury is the pontomedullary separation or rent. As the name implies, this represents a tear in the ventral surface of the brainstem at the junction of the pons and medulla. There is a spectrum of severity ranging from a small tear to complete avulsion of the brainstem. Pontomedullary separation can occur without associated diffuse cerebral injury. This lesion is usually fatal.

Secondary brainstem injury includes infarction, hemorrhage, or compression of the brainstem as a result of adjacent or systemic pathology. Brainstem infarction from hypotension-induced cerebral hypoperfusion is usually seen in conjunction with supratentorial ischemic injury. The brainstem may be relatively spared in hypoxic injury. Mechanical compression of the brainstem usually occurs in the setting of uncal herniation. There may be visible displacement or a change in the overall shape of the brainstem as a result of the mass effect. Neurologic injury caused by brainstem compression may be reversible in the absence of intrinsic brainstem lesions.

Brainstem lesions that occur as a result of downward herniation, or hypoxia or ischemia, usually involve the ventral or ventrolateral aspect of the brainstem, in contrast to primary brainstem lesions, which are most common in the dorsolateral aspect of the brainstem. A characteristic secondary brainstem lesion is the Duret hemorrhage. This is a midline hematoma in the tegmentum of the rostral pons and midbrain seen in association with descending transtentorial herniation. It is believed to result from stretching or tearing of penetrating arteries as the brainstem is caudally displaced (Fig. 3.27). The brainstem infarct is another type of secondary brainstem injury that typically occurs in the central tegmentum of the pons and midbrain.

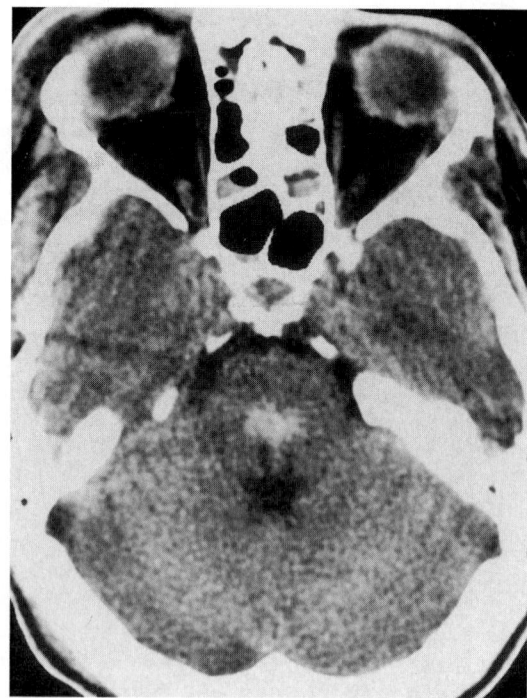

Figure 3.27. Duret Hemorrhage. Noncontrast CT scan performed 24 hours after severe head trauma shows a midline pontine hemorrhage. This type of secondary brainstem injury, known as the Duret hemorrhage, occurs in association with downward transtentorial herniation and can be distinguished from most primary brainstem injuries by its midline location (compare with Fig. 3.26). (Reprinted with permission from Gean AD. Imaging of Head Trauma. Philadelphia: Lippincott-Raven, 1994:282.)

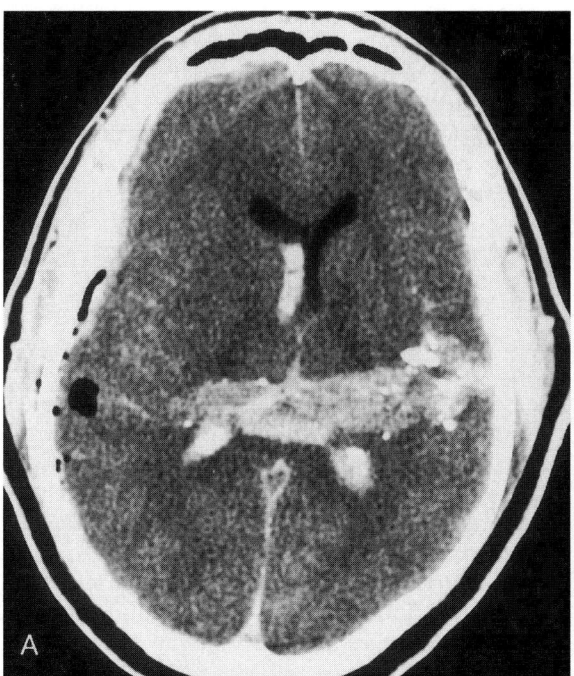

Figure 3.28. Gunshot Wound. A. Noncontrast CT scan shows hemorrhage delineating the bullet's path in this despondent southpaw. There is associated intraventricular and subarachnoid hemorrhage as well as pneumocephalus and a right subdural hematoma.

B. Bone window shows the typical beveled entry site (*arrow*) and scattered bullet fragments along the trajectory. (Reprinted with permission from Gean AD. Imaging of Head Trauma. Philadelphia: Lippincott-Raven, 1994:193.)

Penetrating Trauma

Unlike blunt head trauma in which diffuse injury often occurs secondary to acceleration-induced shear strain, in penetrating injury the damage is defined by the trajectory of the object. Penetrating sharp objects such as knives or glass cause tissue laceration along their course with resultant bleeding or infarction from vascular injury. Plain films or CT can be used to confirm and localize radiopaque intracranial foreign bodies. Leaded glass and metal are hyperdense on CT scans, whereas wood is hypodense.

Gunshot wounds are among the most common causes of penetrating head trauma. They can cause the type of injuries seen in nonpenetrating trauma as well, because significant blunt force occurs from the bullet's impact on the skull. Metallic foreign bodies such as bullet fragments often cause significant streak artifact, which can obscure underlying injury. Tilting the CT gantry to change the plane of section helps minimize this artifact. The entry and exit sites can often be distinguished by the direction of beveling of the calvarial defect or from the pattern of calvarial fracture. The bullet path can often be recognized on CT as a linear hemorrhagic strip (Fig. 3.28). Gunshot wounds in which the bullet crosses the midline or in which small fragments are seen displaced from the main bullet are associated with a poorer prognosis.

Additional complications of penetrating injury are caused by associated skull fractures and dural lacerations with resultant pneumocephalus, CSF leaks, and infection. Fragments of bone, skin, or hair that may be driven intracranially also increase the risk of subsequent abscess formation.

Predicting Outcome After Acute Head Trauma

The Glasgow coma scale (GCS), which stratifies patients with acute head trauma based on clinical findings including level of consciousness, brainstem reflexes, and response to pain, helps standardize assessment of the severity of injury (Table 3.1). Mild head injury refers to a GCS of 13–15, moderate head injury refers to a GCS of 9–12, and severe head injury is defined as a GCS of 8 or below. Although there is a direct correlation between the initial GCS score and subsequent morbidity and mortality, the Glasgow coma scale is limited in its ability to predict long-term outcome. Likewise, CT findings, although valuable in identifying injuries requiring acute intervention, do not correlate well with prognosis. There is growing evidence (13), however, that MR will be helpful in de-

Table 3.1. The Glasgow Coma Scale

Eye Opening	Best Motor	Best Verbal
4- spontaneous	6- obeys	5- oriented
3- to voice	5- localizes	4- confused
2- to pain	4- withdraws	3- inappropriate words
1- none	3- abnormal flexion	2- incomprehensible words
	2- extensure posturing	1- nothing
	1- flaccid	

The total score is the sum of the scores in each category.

termining a patient's prognosis after severe head injury. This reflects the advantage of MR over CT in detecting brainstem injury and DAI. MR studies have shown good correlation between initial GCS and the number and distribution of DAI lesions. Numerous DAI lesions and the presence of DAI in the corpus callosum or brainstem are associated with more severe clinical findings and low initial scores on the GCS. Perhaps more important is the finding (13) that the number of DAI lesions and the presence of brainstem injury or corpus callosum DAI are associated with poor long-term outcome. The number of cortical contusions is not related to outcome, except in cases with significant mass effect. There is also a poor correlation between the presence of an isolated epidural or subdural hematoma and long-term outcome, unless transtentorial herniation is also present.

Child Abuse

Nonaccidental trauma accounts for at least 80% of deaths from head trauma in children younger than 2 years of age (14). It is important to consider the possibility of child abuse and to recognize the characteristic features in these suspected cases.

Skull fractures represent the second most common skeletal injury in child abuse after long bone fracture. They are only found in approximately 50% of children with intracranial injuries from abuse (15,16). In patients with suspected intracranial injury, CT should be the initial imaging study. Skull films are rarely indicated, except perhaps for documentation of cranial injury in neurologically intact children with suspected child abuse.

Subdural hematomas are the most commonly recognized intracranial complication from child abuse. The association of subdural hematomas and retinal hemorrhages in children with metaphyseal long bone fractures was described as "whiplash shaken injury" by Caffey in 1946 (17). The mechanism was thought to be one of violent shaking, with generation of rotational and shear forces intracranially because of the weak neck musculature. The mechanism might include impact against a soft object such as a mattress, which has been shown experimentally (18) to increase the forces produced into the range that could cause coma, subdural hematomas, and primary brain injury, leading to the term "shaken impact injury."

Subdural hematomas in child abuse often are found in the posterior interhemispheric fissure. These are seen on CT as hyperdense collections with a flat medial border along the falx and an irregular convex lateral border. Subdural hematomas may also be found along the convexity, over the tentorial surface, at the skull base, or in the posterior fossa. Occasionally, low-density extra-axial fluid collections are seen in infants without any clear precipitating trauma or infection. These most often represent dilated CSF spaces, known as "benign enlargement of the subarachnoid space of infancy," but can mimic chronic subdural hematomas. They occur in neurologically intact infants 3–6 months old who present with enlarging head circumference. In this setting, they require no treatment and usually regress by age 2. An old term for this condition, "external hydrocephalus," has been abandoned by many because it fails to convey the benign nature of the condition. Epidural hematomas are not frequently seen in child abuse.

The most common intra-axial manifestation of head injury related to child abuse is diffuse brain swelling. The initial swelling is believed to be caused by vasodilation associated with loss of autoregulation. At this stage, the injury may be reversible despite dramatic findings on CT. CT scans show global effacement of the subarachnoid space and compressed ventricles. As the brain becomes edematous, the normal attenuation of gray and white matter may appear indistinguishable or even reversed. The cerebral hemispheres will demonstrate diffusely decreased attenuation. The brainstem, cerebellum, and possibly deep gray matter structures may be spared (see Fig. 3.21). Cerebral edema in the setting of shaking injury can also occur secondary to respiratory depression, apnea, and hypoxia. The other manifestations of intra-axial injury previously described in this chapter may also be seen in child abuse, including diffuse axonal injury and brainstem injury. Cortical contusions occur but are considered less common, possibly because the inner surface of the skull is relatively smooth in children. In infants, head trauma may lead to tears at the gray–white junction, especially in the frontal and temporal lobes.

Multiple injuries of various ages also strongly suggest child abuse. Chronic sequelae of head injury in children includes chronic subdural collections (which may occasionally calcify), global cerebral atrophy, and encephalomalacia. Although CT is the modality of choice for the evaluation of acute head injury in children, MR can help identify subdural collections of various ages or hemosiderin deposits from prior hemorrhages (Fig. 3.29). The ability of MR to identify these remote intracranial hemorrhages makes it an important tool in the evaluation of suspected child abuse. In some centers, it has been proposed as a necessary complement to the skeletal series. MR is also recommended when patients are clinically stable after head injury, to help determine the full extent of injury and prognosis.

FACIAL TRAUMA

Imaging Strategy

Plain Films. Many facial fractures can often be diagnosed by plain films alone and need no further imaging. Four views are usually adequate in the plain film evaluation of acute facial trauma. These are the Caldwell view, a shallow Waters' view, a cross-table lateral view, and a submental vertex view. When patients are acutely injured and unable to cooperate with upright imaging, the Caldwell and Waters' views can be obtained supine in the anteroposterior projection. Films obtained in the PA projection provide better bone detail and less magnification and may be helpful if the initial films are difficult to interpret. The lateral and submental vertex views are both obtained with a horizontal beam, thus enabling the detection of air-fluid levels.

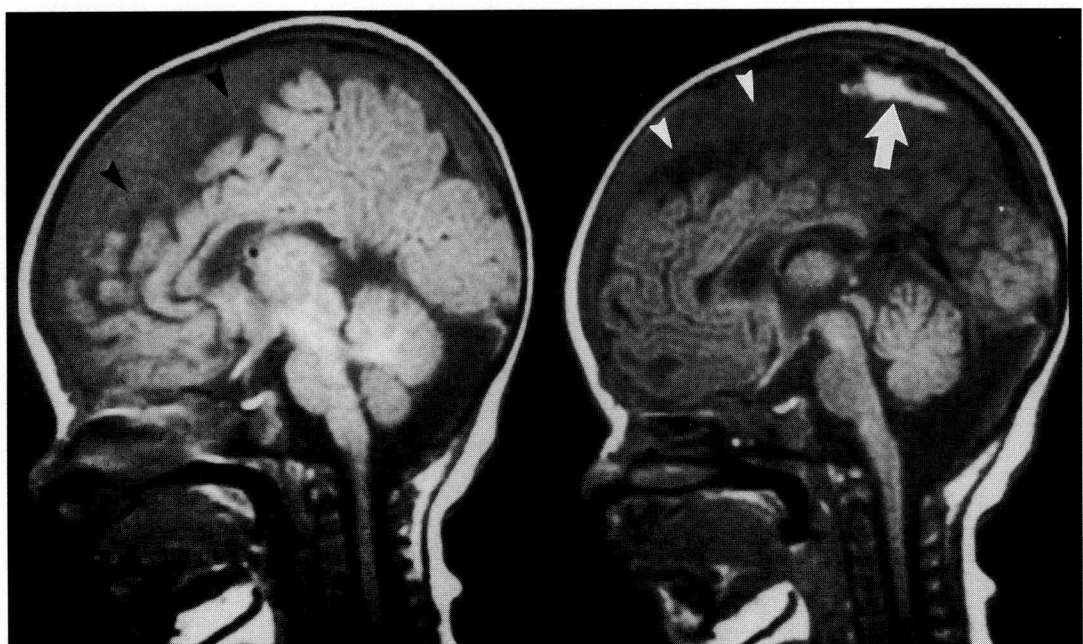

Figure 3.29. Subacute and Chronic Interhemispheric Subdural Hematomas. Midline sagittal and parasagittal T1-weighted MR scans in a child demonstrate a low signal intensity chronic subdural hematoma (*arrowheads*) and superimposed high signal intensity subacute hematoma (*arrow*). The presence of intracranial injury of different ages is strong presumptive evidence of child abuse. The appearance is not pathognomonic for child abuse, however, because subdural hematomas do have a propensity to rebleed.

CT is indicated when the clinical or plain film findings suggest complex facial fractures or complications such as extraocular muscle entrapment or optic nerve impingement. Patients with facial fractures frequently have concurrent intracranial injury, especially victims of motor vehicle accidents. Imaging of the potential intracranial injury takes precedence in the acute management of these patients. If CT of the facial bones is required in patients suspected of having concurrent intracranial injury, it is usually performed after CT imaging of the brain or delayed several days until the patient is clinically stable.

Three- to five-millimeter sections (1–1.5 mm for the orbits) are usually obtained through the facial bones in the axial plane using a bone algorithm. The field of view should extend from the orbital roof to the superior alveolar ridge. The frontal sinus or maxillary dentition can be included if fractures are suspected in these areas. The mandible should be included when maxillary alveolar or palatal fractures are seen because of the high incidence of associated mandibular fractures in this setting. A standard algorithm with soft-tissue windows can be used to evaluate potential nonosseous injury, especially in the orbits. If there is no concern for a cervical spine injury, patients also undergo scans in the direct coronal plane for better visualization of the orbital floors, palate, and floor of the anterior cranial fossa. Coronal reformations of axial or helical acquisitions may be used when patients are unable to tolerate direct coronal scanning. Contrast is unnecessary except in the rare circumstance in which vascular injury is being considered. Occasionally, three-dimensional reconstruction is used and may help plan operative repair of displaced or comminuted facial fractures.

MR. The facial bones are difficult to visualize on MR scanning because they and the adjacent aerated sinuses are relatively void of signal. CT is the preferred modality for cross-sectional evaluation of facial injuries primarily because it provides excellent bone detail. MR may be useful for injuries to orbital contents including the optic nerve, globe, and extraocular muscles. It is also useful for assessing potential vascular complications such as arterial dissections, pseudoaneurysms, and arteriovenous fistulas, and it is the best way to evaluate trauma to the temporomandibular joint.

Angiography may be indicated when clinical or radiographic evidence suggests a vascular injury. Vascular injuries are more frequent with penetrating trauma, such as that occurring from gunshot or stab wounds. Fractures that extend through the carotid canal also predispose to vascular injury and may require angiographic evaluation.

Soft-Tissue Findings

Indirect signs of facial injury on plain films can help provide objective evidence of trauma, localize the site of impact, and direct attention to areas of potential bony injury. Soft-tissue swelling is the most commonly seen plain film finding in facial trauma. It may help localize the site of impact but does not necessarily indicate associated facial fractures or other more severe injury.

Paranasal sinus opacification suggests the presence of an associated fracture, particularly when air-fluid levels are seen. Fluid levels are most commonly seen in the maxillary sinus but may also be seen in the frontal or sphenoid sinuses. The ethmoids may become opacified

Figure 3.30. Orbital Emphysema on Plain Film. Air in the left orbit can be seen outlining the optic nerve (*arrow*) in this shallow Waters' view. An orbital floor fracture is also evident (*arrowheads*).

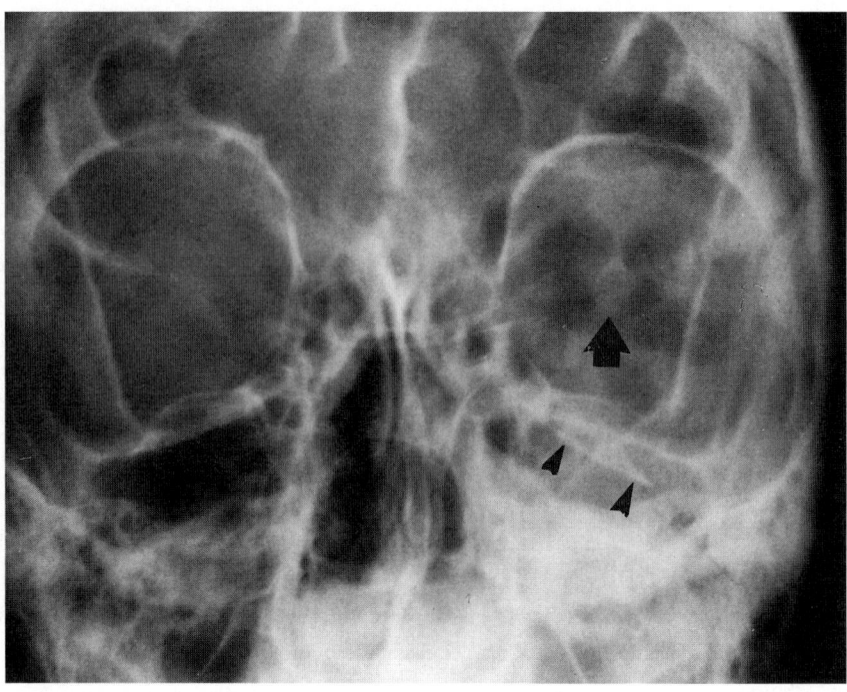

with acute hemorrhage but are less likely to demonstrate fluid levels on plain films, probably because they contain internal septations.

Air in the soft tissues is also suggestive of associated fractures, depending on location. Orbital emphysema is most commonly caused by fracture of the thin medial orbital wall. Orbital floor blow-out fractures can also cause orbital emphysema (Fig. 3.30).

Occasionally, facial films reveal important findings unrelated to fracture of the facial bones. For example, the films should be scrutinized for the presence of foreign bodies that may not be clinically apparent. The craniocervical junction and upper cervical spine should be examined when included on the film. Nasopharyngeal and prevertebral soft-tissue swelling can indicate hemorrhage from cervical or skull base fractures. Pneumocephalus or depressed skull fractures are also occasionally seen. Rarely, shift of pineal calcification can be detected, indicating the presence of intracranial mass effect. Though plain films are usually no longer indicated for evaluation of head trauma, it still pays to remain alert to indirect manifestations of head trauma when reviewing facial films.

Nasal Fractures

Nasal bone fractures are the most common fractures of the facial skeleton. They can occur as an isolated injury or in association with other facial fractures. Nasal trauma frequently results in a depressed fracture of one of the paired nasal bones, without associated ethmoidal injury. An anterior blow can fracture both nasal bones as well as the nasal septum. Associated fractures of the frontal process of the maxilla can be seen. Cartilaginous nasal injury cannot be diagnosed radiographically.

Nasal fractures are usually clinically evident and do not require radiologic diagnosis. Films of the nasal bone may document injury but are generally not useful for patient management and are often unnecessary. Fractures of the nasal bone may be transverse or longitudinal. Longitudinal fractures can be confused with the nasomaxillary suture and nasociliary grooves, which have the same orientation. Transverse fractures of the nasal bone are more common and are easily detected because they are oriented perpendicular to the normal suture line.

When films are obtained, remember to look for fractures of the anterior nasal spine of the maxilla, which may be associated with nasal fractures. One potentially serious injury that can be suggested on plain films or CT is a septal hematoma. Trauma to the septal cartilage may lead to hematoma formation between the perichondrium and cartilage, which can cause cartilage necrosis by disrupting the vascular supply. An organized hematoma can also cause breathing difficulty and may predispose to septal abscess formation.

Maxillary and Paranasal Sinus Fractures

Fracture of the maxillary alveolus is the most common isolated maxillary fracture. It frequently results from a blow to the chin that drives the teeth of the mandible into the maxillary dental arch. These fractures are usually demonstrated by dental films or panorex (panoramic radiographs), but can be seen on CT if the scan is extended inferior to the level of the palate. Associated fractures of the mandible are common with this form of injury, as predicted by the mechanism.

Fractures of the palatine process of the maxilla and horizontal plate of the palatine bone commonly occur in the sagittal plane near the midline (Fig. 3.31). Palatine fractures may also be seen in association with complex fractures of the midface.

The most common isolated sinus fracture involves the anterolateral wall of the maxillary antrum. The fracture

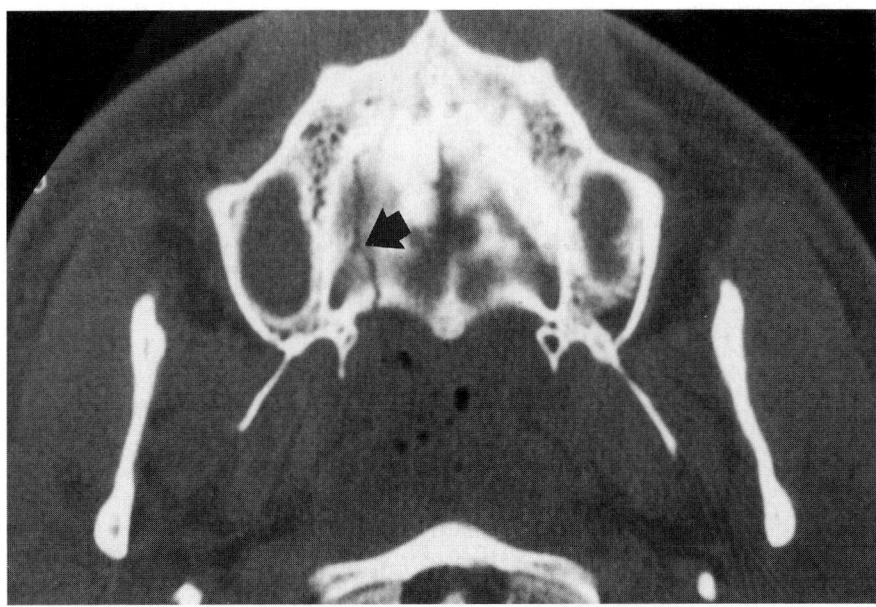

Figure 3.31. Palatine Fracture. Axial CT scan demonstrates a nondisplaced right palatine fracture in the characteristic parasagittal location (*arrow*). (Reprinted with permission from Gean AD. Imaging of Head Trauma. Philadelphia: Lippincott-Raven, 1994:439.)

may be seen directly or may be suspected by the finding of a maxillary sinus fluid level in the setting of acute trauma.

Isolated frontal sinus fractures can also occur and may be more serious if they extend intracranially. Frontal sinus fractures may be linear or comminuted and depressed. Open (compound) frontal sinus fractures involve the posterior sinus wall (Fig. 3.32). These can lead to CSF rhinorrhea and recurrent meningitis or intracerebral abscess formation. Pneumocephalus may be seen in association with these fractures. Fractures of the medial wall and superior rim of the orbit frequently involve the frontal sinus.

Fractures of the sphenoid sinus are often seen in association with fractures of the orbital roof, nasoethmoid complex, midface, or temporal bone. Nondisplaced sphenoid sinus fractures may be subtle on CT. Angiography should be considered if there is a suspicion of associated vascular injury involving the cavernous portion of the internal carotid artery.

Orbital Trauma

Fractures. The orbit is involved in a number of facial fractures including the tripod, Le Fort, and nasoethmoidal complex fractures. Isolated orbital wall fractures usually involve either the medial wall or orbital floor. Medial wall fractures are detected on plain films by the presence of orbital emphysema and opacification of the adjacent ethmoid air cells. Medial wall fractures can be directly visualized well with axial or coronal CT scans. Bone displacement is usually minimal, and muscle entrapment is unusual.

Orbital floor fractures are usually linear when seen in association with other facial fractures. These are rarely associated with entrapment. Comminuted orbital floor

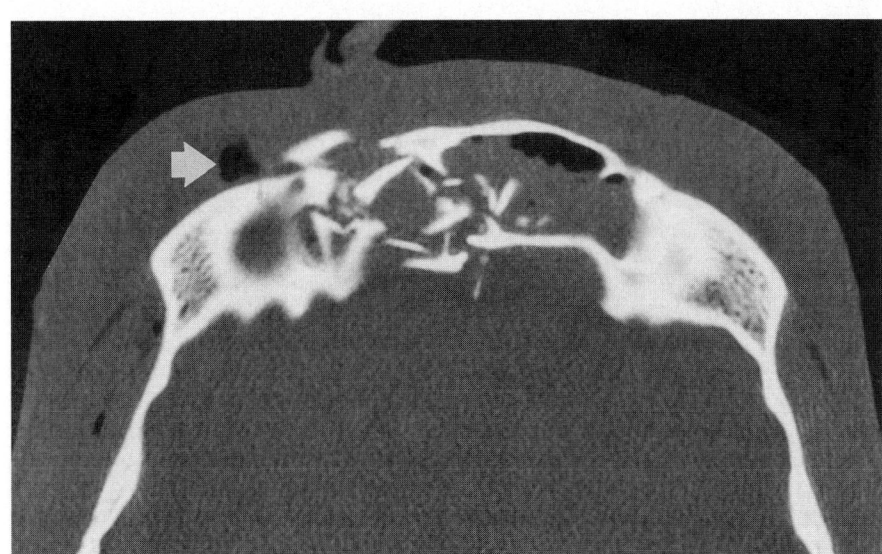

Figure 3.32. "Open" Frontal Sinus Fracture. Noncontrast CT scan demonstrates a severely comminuted fracture involving both walls of the frontal sinus (open fracture). The frontal sinus is opacified and subcutaneous air is present (*arrow*). Open fractures are prone to CSF leakage and meningitis or intracerebral abscess formation. (Reprinted with permission from Gean AD. Imaging of Head Trauma. Philadelphia: Lippincott-Raven, 1994:46.)

fractures, or blow-out fractures, may be seen as an isolated injury and result from a direct blow to the eye. Intraorbital pressure is acutely increased and relieved by fracture through the orbital floor (Fig. 3.33). The orbital rim remains intact in pure blow-out fractures. Blow-out fractures are often associated with herniation of orbital contents through the fracture. When the inferior rectus muscle is compromised, patients will experience persistent vertical diplopia. Mild or transient diplopia can occur simply as a result of periorbital edema or hemor-

rhage. Rarely, fragments from an orbital floor fracture buckle upward into the orbit, an injury referred to as a "blow-in" fracture.

Plain film findings suggestive of orbital floor blow-out fractures include orbital emphysema, a fluid level in the ipsilateral maxillary sinus, indistinct orbital floor on Waters' view, and soft tissue representing prolapsed orbital contents in the superior aspect of the maxillary sinus (Fig. 3.34). A bony spicule may be seen in the antrum, representing the inferiorly displaced fracture

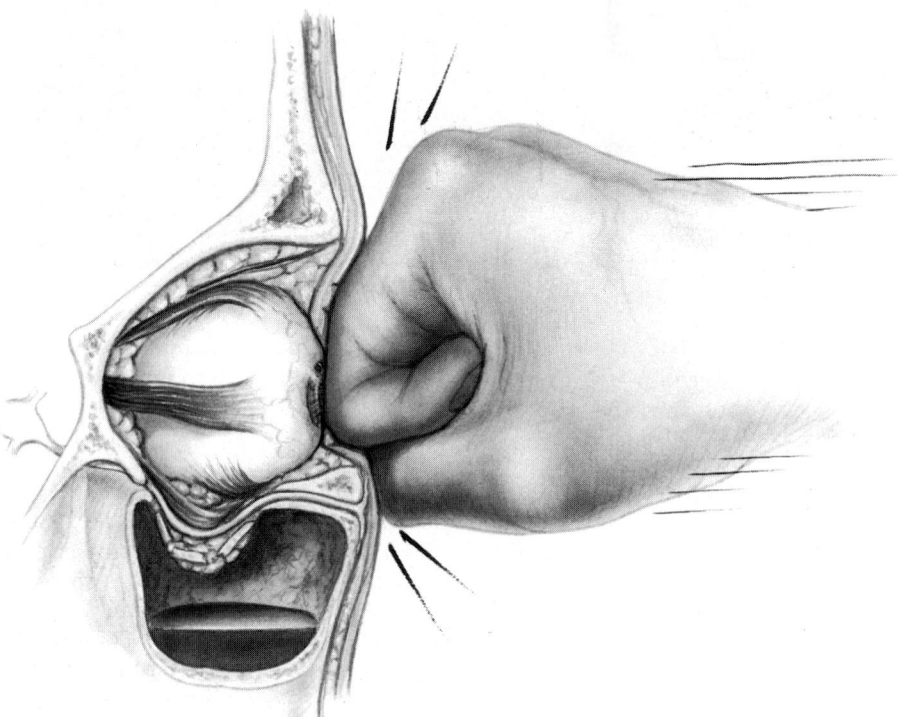

Figure 3.33. Diagram of Orbital Floor Blow-out Fracture. Sudden increase in intraocular pressure from a direct blow to the eye can lead to a comminuted fracture of the orbital floor, with herniation of orbital contents into the maxillary sinus. A fluid level in the sinus is often seen acutely secondary to bleeding. (Reprinted with permission from Gean AD. Imaging of Head Trauma. Philadelphia: Lippincott-Raven, 1994:478.)

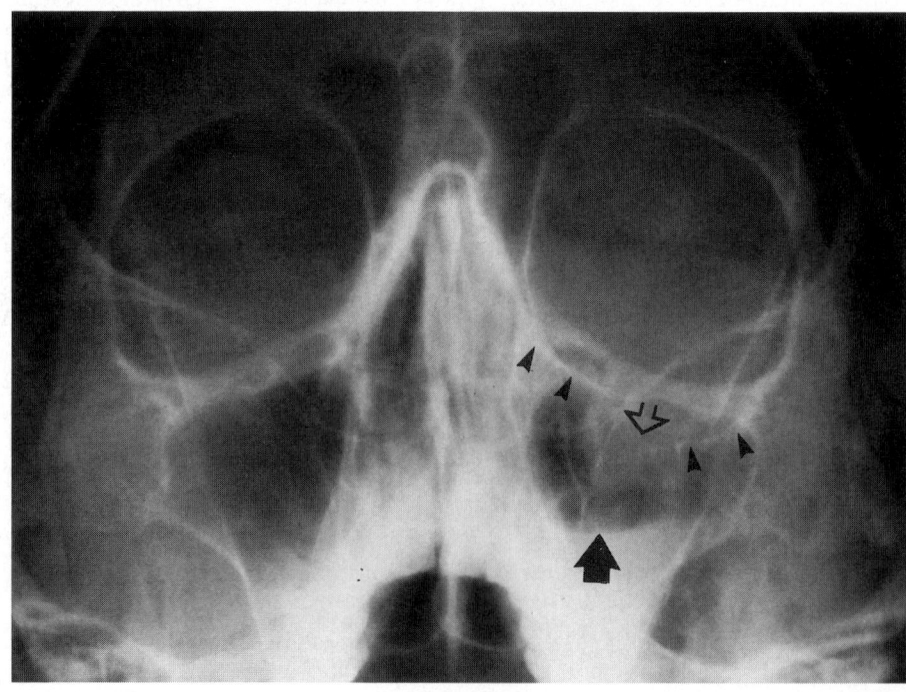

Figure 3.34. Orbital Floor Blow-out Fracture on Plain Film. Waters' view shows the major findings associated with an orbital floor blow-out injury: disruption of the orbital floor (*arrowheads*), soft-tissue mass in the superior aspect of the maxillary sinus (*open arrow*), and a maxillary sinus fluid level (*closed arrow*). (Reprinted with permission from Gean AD. Imaging of head trauma. Philadelphia: Lippincott-Raven, 1994:478.)

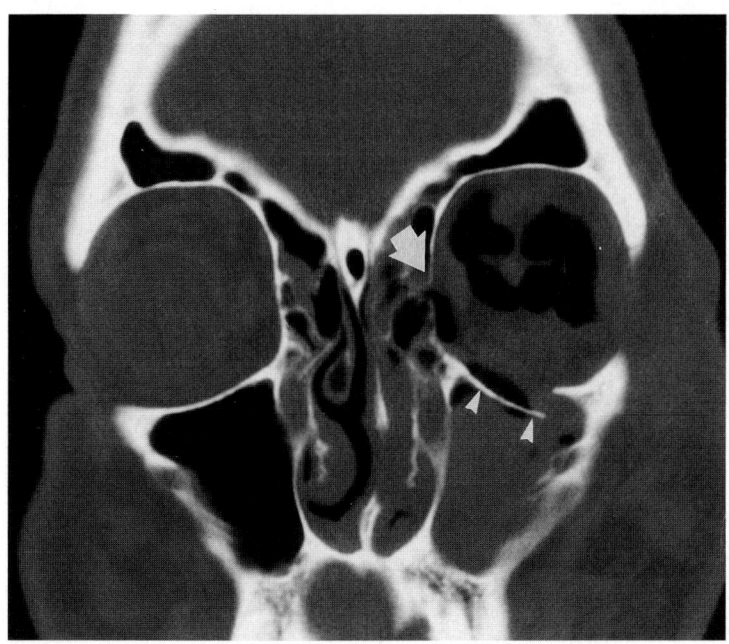

Figure 3.35. Orbital Floor Blow-out Fracture on CT Scan. Direct coronal CT scan shows a depressed left orbital floor fracture (*arrowheads*) with opacification of the ipsilateral maxillary sinus. Orbital air can be seen outlining the optic nerve (same patient as Fig. 3.30). A subtle medial wall fracture is also present (*arrow*), which likely accounts for the large amount of orbital emphysema in this case.

fragment. Blow-out fractures are best seen on direct coronal CT images (Fig. 3.35). These should be obtained with the patient lying prone. In the supine position, fluid and debris in the maxillary antrum will layer against the orbital floor and could obscure soft tissue herniating through the fracture.

Soft-Tissue Injury. Penetrating foreign bodies such as bullets, metal fragments, glass, or other sharp objects account for a significant amount of traumatic injury to the orbit. Thin-section CT is the method of choice for confirming the presence of foreign bodies and for this localization (Fig. 3.36). CT can usually clearly define the relationship of bone fragments or foreign bodies to critical structures such as the optic nerve, globe, or extraocular muscles (Fig. 3.37). MR carries a potential risk of further injury by causing motion of intraocular ferromagnetic metal.

Traumatic optic neuropathy is seen in a significant number of patients with severe head trauma and occasionally occurs in patients with relatively minor deceleration injury. Damage may be maximal initially, with unilateral blindness or decreased acuity, or may worsen in the first few days after the injury. When delayed worsening occurs, secondary optic nerve compression from edema or hemorrhage in the optic nerve sheath should be considered. Imaging studies, particularly CT scans, are indicated to detect fractures through the optic canal or orbital apex. Rarely, displaced fractures are responsible for direct injury to the optic nerve sheath. More commonly, these fractures are nondisplaced but serve as evidence of severe stress transmitted to the orbital apex. Primary optic nerve injury may occur as a result of deceleration strain causing damage to the delicate meningeal vessels or direct neural disruption. Secondary optic nerve injury may occur as a result of swelling of the optic nerve within the rigid bony canal, with subsequent mechanical compression and vascular compromise.

Fractures of the Zygoma

The zygoma, or "cheekbone," is one of the most common sites of injury in fractures that involve multiple facial bones. Zygomatic arch fractures may occur as an isolated finding, or as part of a zygomaticomaxillary complex ("tripod," "quadripod," or "trimalar") fracture. Comminution and depression are frequently seen with zygomatic arch fractures. On plain films, the zygomatic arch is best evaluated on the submental vertex view (Fig. 3.38). Deformity of the arch is a frequent finding in populations with a high incidence of facial trauma, and clinical examination may be required to differentiate acute from chronic injury.

Zygomaticomaxillary complex fractures usually result from a blow to the face. The zygoma articulates with the frontal, maxillary, sphenoid, and temporal bones. Fractures are somewhat variable, but typically involve the zygomatic arch, zygomaticofrontal suture, infraorbital rim, orbital floor, lateral wall of the maxillary sinus, and lateral wall of the orbit. Injury to the infraorbital nerve is common secondary to fracture of the infraorbital rim at the infraorbital foramen. Diastasis of the zygomaticofrontal suture may injure the lateral canthal ligament or suspensory ligaments of the globe. Many of the fractures associated with this injury can be seen on both plain films and CT scans (Fig. 3.39). Associated findings on plain films include opacification of the ipsilateral maxillary antrum and posterior displacement of the body of the zygoma on the submental vertex view with overlying soft-tissue swelling.

Fractures of the Midface (Le Fort Fractures)

Complex fractures of the facial bones are frequently classified according to the method of Le Fort, who developed his theory by inflicting facial trauma on cadavers and analyzing the results. He described three general

Figure 3.36. Intraocular Metallic Foreign Body. Axial **(A)** and coronal **(B)** CT scans confirm the presence of a metallic foreign body in the left globe.

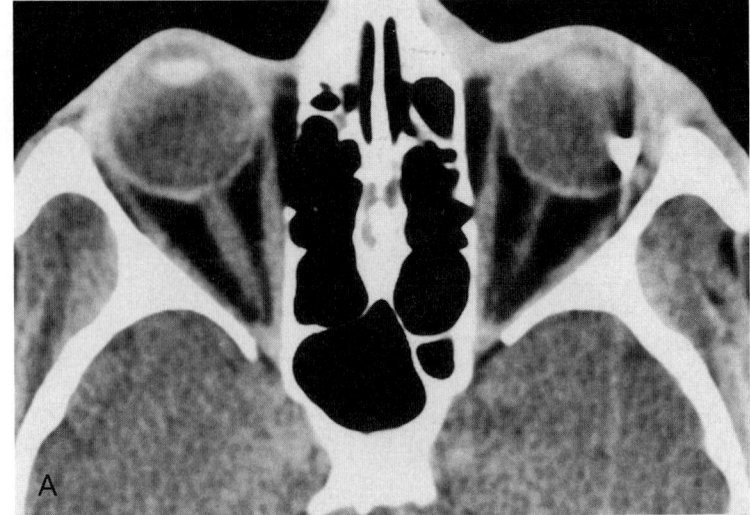

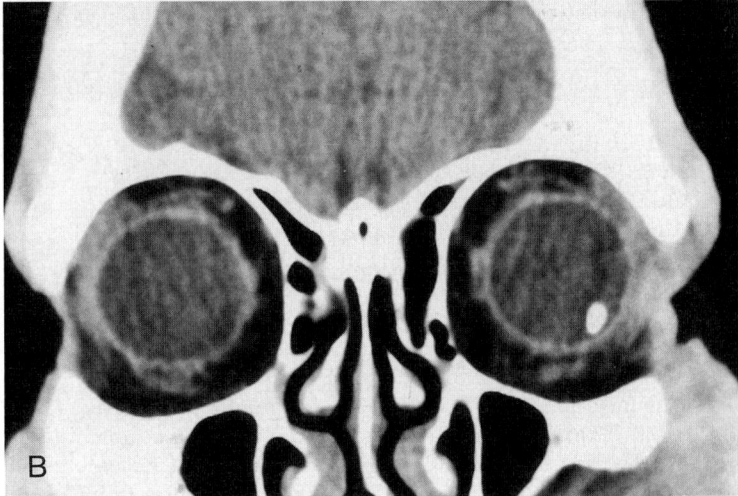

patterns of fractures that differ in location of the fracture plane across the face (Fig. 3.40) (19). The three Le Fort fractures initially described are bilateral processes. All involve the pterygoid plates, which help anchor the facial bones to the skull. Although there is great variability in complex facial fractures, and the classic Le Fort injuries are rarely seen in their pure form, they remain a convenient way to categorize and describe basic patterns of injury. Frequently, similar patterns of injury are seen on one side only and are known as "hemi-Le Forts." Combinations also occur, such as a Le Fort I pattern on one side and a Le Fort II pattern on the other.

Le Fort I, or "floating palate," fracture is a horizontal fracture through the maxillary sinuses. It extends through the nasal septum and walls of the maxillary sinuses into the inferior aspect of the pterygoid plates. The fracture plane is parallel to the plane of axial CT images but is recognized by the fracture of all walls of both maxillary sinuses (Fig. 3.41). It is well seen in the coronal plane. There may be an associated midpalatal or maxillary split fracture. The Le Fort I fracture is more often seen in the pure form than is either the Le Fort II or Le Fort III fractures. It occasionally may be accompanied by a unilateral zygomaticomaxillary complex fracture.

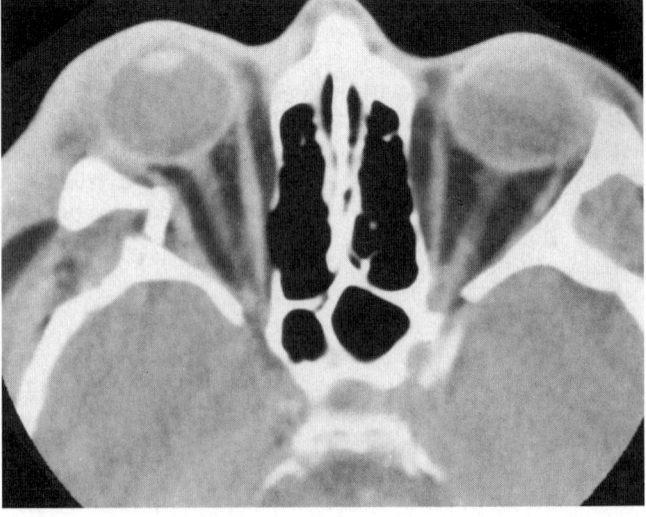

Figure 3.37. Lateral Orbital Wall Fracture With Impingement of Lateral Rectus Muscle. Noncontrast CT scan precisely localizes the site and degree of impingement on the right lateral rectus muscle in this patient with a comminuted fracture involving the zygomaticofrontal suture.

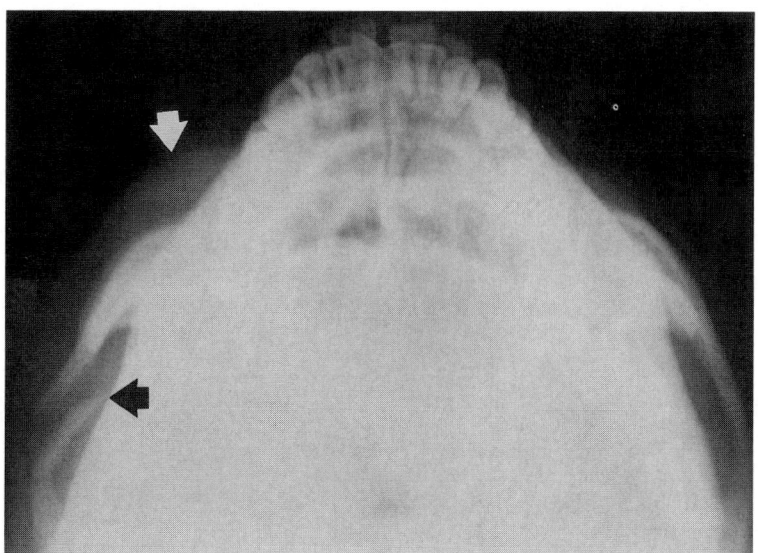

Figure 3.38. Right Zygomatic Arch Fracture. Submental vertex view shows a comminuted, depressed right zygomatic arch fracture (*black arrow*). Soft-tissue swelling anterior to the body of the zygoma is also seen (*white arrow*). (Reprinted with permission from Gean AD. Imaging of Head Trauma. Philadelphia: Lippincott-Raven, 1994:448.)

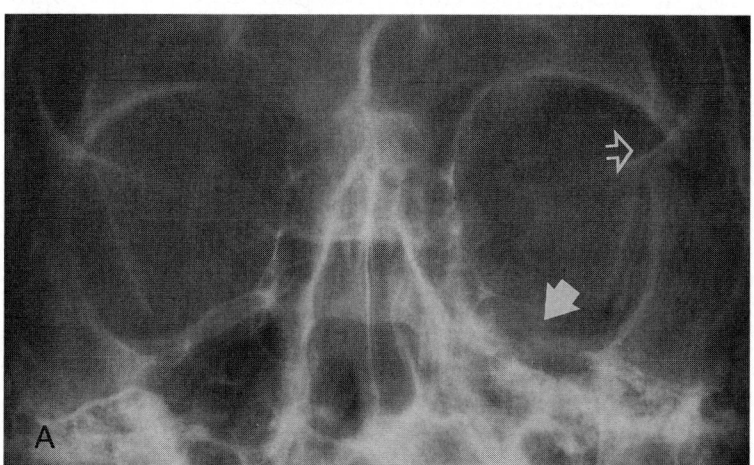

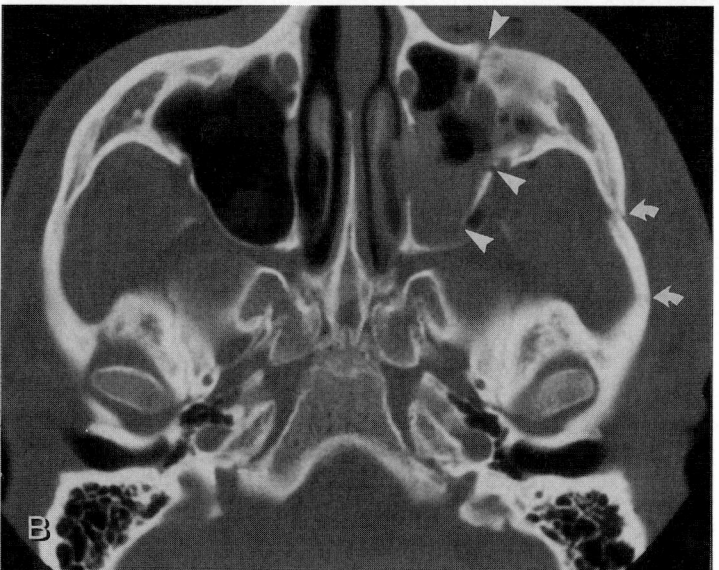

Figure 3.39. Zygomaticomaxillary Complex Fracture. **A.** Plain film shows diastasis of the left zygomaticofrontal suture (*open arrow*) and disruption of the orbital floor (*closed arrow*). An associated zygomatic arch fracture was seen on submental vertex view (not shown). **B.** A CT scan in a different patient shows comminuted left zygomatic arch fracture (*curved arrows*), with fractures of the anterior and posterolateral walls of the maxillary sinus (*arrowheads*). Associated signs of acute injury include soft-tissue swelling and partial opacification of the maxillary sinus. (Reprinted with permission from Gean AD. Imaging of Head Trauma. Philadelphia: Lippincott-Raven, 1994:452.)

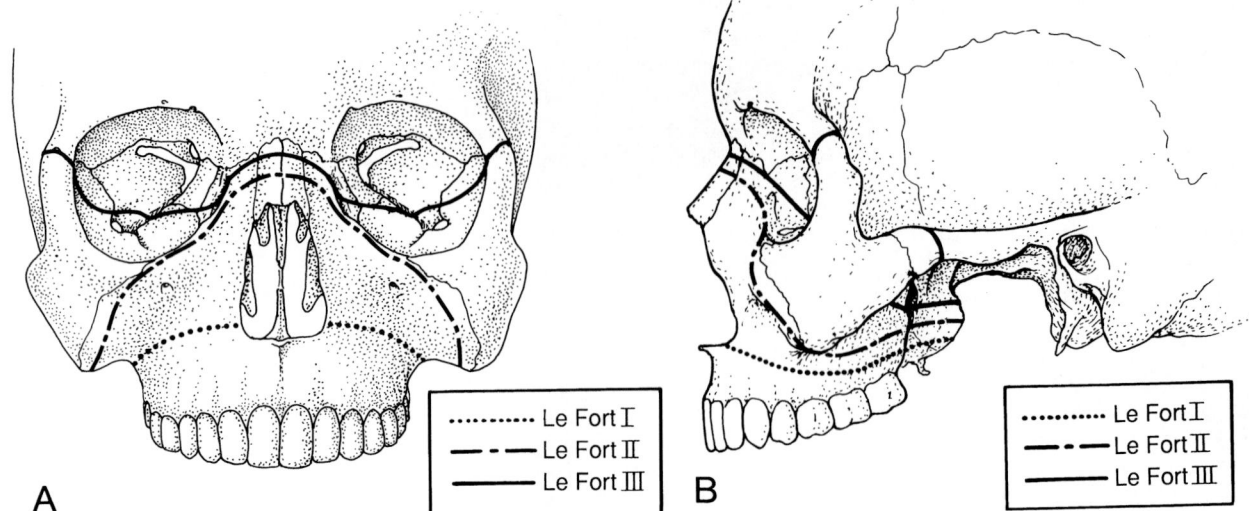

Figure 3.40. Diagram of Le Fort Fractures. Frontal **(A)** and lateral **(B)** projections demonstrate the patterns of facial fractures as originally described by Le Fort. (Reprinted with permission from Gean AD. Imaging of Head Trauma. Philadelphia: Lippincott-Raven, 1994:454.)

Figure 3.41. Le Fort I Fracture. Axial CT scan demonstrates comminuted fractures involving all walls of both maxillary sinuses, with associated fractures through the pterygoid plates (*black arrows*). Both nasolacrimal ducts are also disrupted (*white arrows*). Both maxillary antra are completely opacified. (Reprinted with permission from Gean AD. Imaging of Head Trauma. Philadelphia: Lippincott-Raven, 1994:456.)

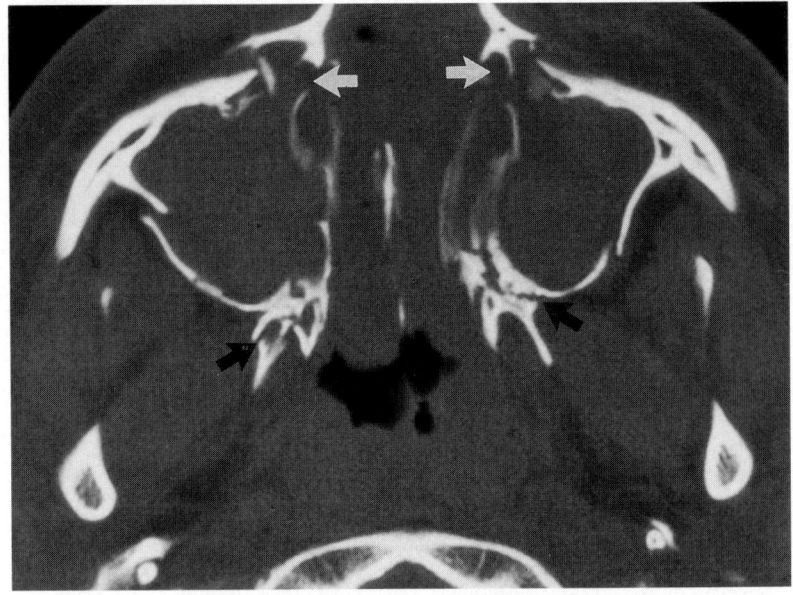

Le Fort II, or "pyramidal," fracture describes a fracture through the medial orbital and lateral maxillary walls. It begins at the bridge of the nose and extends in a pyramidal fashion through the nasal septum, frontal process of the maxilla, medial wall of the orbit, inferior orbital rim, superior, lateral and posterior walls of the maxillary antrum, and midportion of the pterygoid plates. The zygomatic arch and lateral orbital walls are left intact. The Le Fort II is usually associated with posterior displacement of the facial bones, resulting in a "dish-face" deformity and malocclusion. The infraorbital nerve is frequently injured. Le Fort II fractures are rarely seen in the pure form.

Le Fort III fracture, or "craniofacial dysjunction," is a horizontally oriented fracture through the orbits. It begins near the nasofrontal suture and extends posteriorly to involve the nasal septum, medial and lateral orbital walls, zygomatic arch, and base (superior aspect) of the pterygoid plates.

Patients with a Le Fort III fracture also have dish-face deformity and malocclusion. Injury to the infraorbital nerve is less commonly seen with Le Fort III than with Le Fort II fractures. A recognizable feature on plain films is the elongated appearance of the orbits on Waters' and Caldwell views.

When interpreting CT scans obtained for facial trauma, it is probably best to describe the specific bones that are fractured on either side of the face. When appropriate, the Le Fort injury that best describes the distribution of fractures may also be used to categorize complex fractures.

Nasoethmoidal Fractures

Nasoethmoidal complex injuries describe the constellation of findings seen as a result of a blow to the midface between the eyes. This term encompasses a wide variety of different fracture complexes that are best described by listing the specific fractures seen on CT scans. These injuries may include fractures of the lamina papyracea, inferior, medial, and supraorbital rims, frontal or ethmoid sinuses, orbital roofs, nasal bone and frontal process of the maxilla, and sphenoid bone (Fig. 3.42). These fractures have also been called orbitoethmoid or nasoethmoid–orbital fractures because of the importance of the often associated orbital injuries. There may be associated fractures of the skull base and clivus. Other findings include orbital and intracranial air, opacification of the ethmoid and frontal sinuses, and depression of the midface. Nasoethmoidal fractures can be suspected on plain films when the lateral view shows posterior displacement of the nasion. Thin-section CT helps evaluate the extent of the injury and helps localize bony fragments that might encroach on the optic nerve or canal.

Complications of nasoethmoidal complex fractures depend on the location and extent of injury. Patients with fractures involving the floor of the anterior cranial fossa are prone to develop CSF leaks because of the high frequency of associated dural lacerations. The olfactory nerves are frequently injured when fractures extend to the cribriform plate. As mentioned earlier, orbital injuries are often seen as a component of nasoethmoid fractures. The globes or optic nerves may be damaged by displaced medial orbital wall fracture fragments.

Mandibular Fractures

Mandibular fractures are extremely common in patients with maxillofacial injury. Plain films are used in the initial evaluation of patients with suspected mandibular injury. The mandibular series includes PA, lateral, Towne, and bilateral oblique projections. CT or panoramic radiographs (panorex films) can also be used to evaluate mandibular injury (Fig. 3.43).

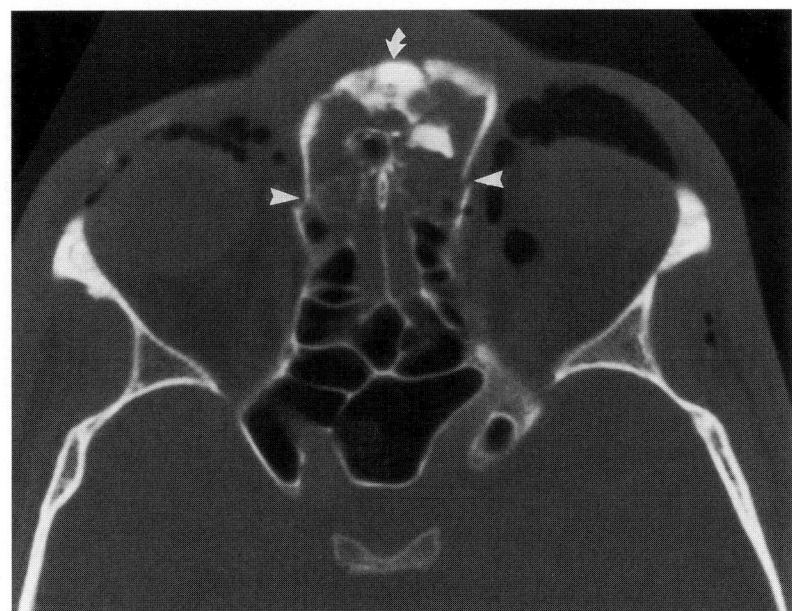

Figure 3.42. Nasoethmoidal Complex Fracture. Axial CT scan demonstrates a depressed fracture involving the root of the nose (*curved arrow*) and anterior ethmoids. Bilateral fractures of the medial orbital walls are also present (*arrowheads*) with bilateral orbital emphysema.

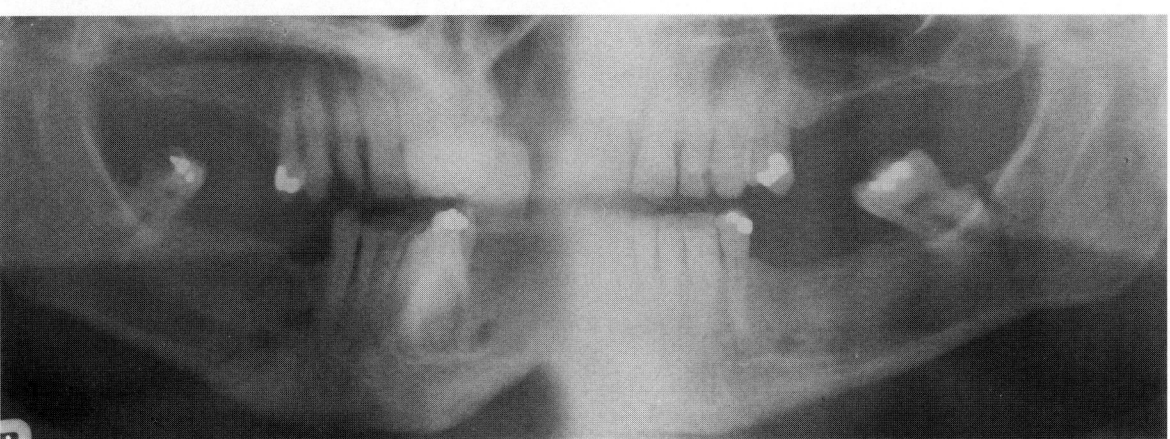

Figure 3.43. Panorex Film with Bilateral Mandibular Fractures. Fractures of the left mandibular angle (extending into the root of a molar tooth) and right horizontal ramus are both clearly seen on single panorex film. (Reprinted with permission from Gean AD. Imaging of Head Trauma. Philadelphia: Lippincott-Raven, 1994:431.)

Mandibular fractures can be considered either simple or compound. Simple fractures are most common in the ramus and condyle and do not communicate externally or with the mouth. Compound fractures are those that communicate internally through a tooth socket or externally through a laceration (Fig. 3.44). Fractures of the body of the mandible are almost always compound fractures. Pathologic mandibular fractures can occur at sites of infection or neoplasm. Mandibular fractures are frequently multiple or bilateral, and such fractures often involve the condyle (Fig. 3.45). Subcondylar fractures may be recognized on plain films by the "cortical ring" sign, a well-corticated density seen above the condylar neck on lateral views because of the horizontal axis of the fragment. A common pattern of injury is a unilateral condylar fracture with a contralateral fracture of the mandibular angle. The mandibular angle is also the most common site of isolated injury. Fractures of the ramus and coronoid processes are rare. Fractures through the symphysis or parasymphyseal region are common but difficult to diagnose on plain films because of the obliquity of the fracture plane. Fractures involving the dentoalveolar complex are also often missed on mandibular series

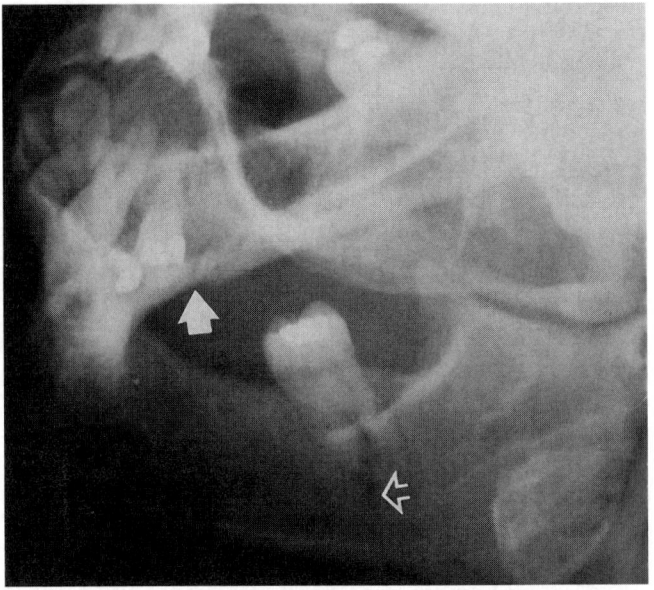

Figure 3.44. Compound Fracture of the Mandible. Oblique view of the mandible demonstrates a posterior ramus fracture extending through the adjacent tooth socket (*open arrow*). A contralateral fracture of the horizontal ramus is also present (*closed arrow*). (Reprinted with permission from Gean AD. Imaging of Head Trauma. Philadelphia: Lippincott-Raven, 1994:467.)

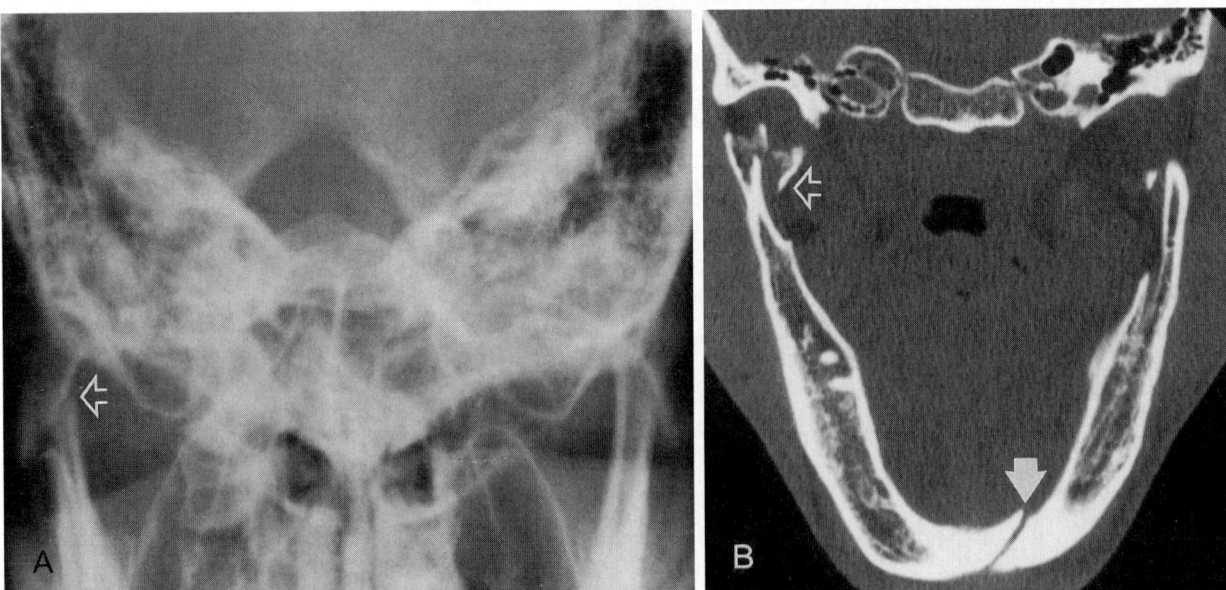

Figure 3.45. Mandibular Condylar Fracture. A. Plain film (Towne projection) shows a displaced right subcondylar fracture (*open arrow*). **B.** Axial CT in a different patient shows a right condylar fracture (*open arrow*) and an associated parasymphyseal fracture (*closed arrow*). The latter fracture is easily missed on plain films because of the oblique fracture plane. (Reprinted with permission from Gean AD. Imaging of Head Trauma. Philadelphia: Lippincott-Raven, 1994: 464.)

and require intraoral dental films or CT for evaluation. Bilateral fractures through the mandibular body or comminuted fractures can lead to airway obstruction from posterior displacement of the tongue and free mandibular fragment.

Suggested Readings

Intracranial Injury

Eelkema EA, Hecht ST, Horton JA. Head trauma. In: Latchaw RE, ed. MR and CT Imaging of the Head, Neck, and Spine. 2nd ed. St. Louis: CV Mosby, 1991:203–265.

Gean AD. Imaging of Head Trauma. New York: Raven Press, 1994.

Cranial and Skull Base Injury

Holland BA, Brant-Zawadzki M. High-resolution CT of temporal bone trauma. AJNR Am J Neuroradiol 1984;5:291–295.

Head Trauma in Child Abuse

Merten DF, Radkowski MA, Leonidas JC. The abused child: a radiological reappraisal. Radiology 1983;146:377–381.

Sato Y, Smith WL. Head injury in child abuse. Neuroimaging Clin North Am 1991;1:475–492.

Facial Trauma

DelBalso AM, Hall RE. Mandibular and dentoalveolar fractures. Neuroimaging Clin North Am 1991;1:285–303.

Kassel EE, Gruss JS. Imaging of midfacial fractures. Neuroimaging Clin North Am 1991;1:259–283.

Som PM. Sinonasal cavity. In: Som PM, Bergeron RT, eds. Head and Neck Imaging. 2nd ed. St. Louis: CV Mosby, 1991: 227–249.

References

1. Link TM, Schuierer G, Hufendiek A, et al. Substantial head trauma: value of routine CT examination of the cervicocranium. Radiology 1995;196:741–745.
2. Gentry LR, Godersky JC, Thompson B, et al. Prospective comparative study of intermediate-field MR and CT in the evaluation of closed head trauma. AJR Am J Roentgenol 1988;150:673–682.
3. Orrison WW, Gentry LR, Stimac GK, et al. Blinded comparison of cranial CT and MR in closed head injury evaluation. AJNR Am J Neuroradiol 1995;15:351–356.
4. Alsop DC, Murai H, Detre JA, McIntosh TK, Smith DH. Detection of acute pathologic changes following experimental traumatic brain injury suing diffusion-weighted magnetic resonance imaging. J Neurotrauma 1996;13:515–521.
5. Noguchi K, Ogawa T, Seto H, et al. Subacute and chronic subarachnoid hemorrhage: diagnosis with fluid-attenuated inversion-recovery MR imaging. Radiology 1997;203(1): 257–262.
6. Masters SJ. Evaluation of head trauma: efficacy of skull films. AJR Am J Roentgenol 1980;135:539–547.
7. Bell RS, Loop JW. The utility and futility of radiographic skull examination for trauma. N Engl J Med 1971;284: 236–239.
8. Hackney DB. Skull radiography in the evaluation of acute head trauma: a survey of current practice. Radiology 1991; 181:711–714.
9. Adams JH. Pathology of nonmissile head injury. Neuroimaging Clin North Am 1991;1:397–410.
10. Gentry LR. Temporal bone trauma. Neuroimaging Clin North Am 1991;1:319–340.
11. Gentry LR. Imaging of closed head injury. Radiology 1994; 191:1–17.
12. Gennarelli TA, Thibault LE, Adams JH, et al. Diffuse axonal injury and traumatic coma in the primate. In: Dacey RG Jr, Winn HR, Rimel RW, et al, eds. Trauma of the Central Nervous System. New York: Raven Press, 1985:169–193.
13. Gentry LR. Head trauma. In: Atlas SW, ed. Magnetic Resonance Imaging of the Brain and Spine. 2nd ed. Philadelphia: Lippincott-Raven, 1996:611–647.
14. Bruce DA, Zimmerman RA. Shaken impact syndrome. Pediatr Ann 1989;18:482–494.
15. Merten DF, Osborne DRS, Radkowski AM. Craniocerebral trauma in the child abuse syndrome: radiological observations. Pediatr Radiol 1984;14:272–277.
16. Zimmerman RA, Bilaniuk LT. Pediatric head trauma. Neuroimaging Clin North Am 1994;4:349–366.
17. Caffey J. Multiple fractures in the long bones of infants suffering from chronic subdural hematoma. AJR Am J Roentgenol 1946;56:163–173.
18. Duhaime AC, Gennarelli TA, Thibault LE, et al. The shaken baby syndrome. A clinical, pathological, and biomechanical study. J Neurosurg 1987;66:409–415.
19. Le Fort R. Etude experimental sur les fractures de la machoire superieure, parts I, II, III. Rev Chir (Paris) 1901:23: 208–227.

4
Cerebrovascular Disease

Howard A. Rowley

Stroke is a clinical term applied to any abrupt nontraumatic brain insult, literally "a blow from an unseen hand." Strokes are caused by either brain infarction (75%) or hemorrhage (25%) and must be distinguished from other conditions causing abrupt neurologic deficits. *Infarction* is a permanent injury that occurs when tissue perfusion is decreased long enough to cause necrosis, typically attributable to occlusion of the feeding artery. *Transient ischemic attacks* (TIA) are defined as transient neurologic symptoms or signs lasting less than 24 hours, which may serve as a warning sign of an infarction occurring in the next few weeks or months. TIAs are often the result of temporary occlusion of a feeding artery. *Hemorrhage* is seen when blood ruptures through the arterial wall, spilling into the surrounding parenchyma, subarachnoid space, or ventricles.

Stroke is the third leading cause of death in the United States and is a major source of long-term disability among survivors. Treatment of ischemic stroke has been largely preventive or supportive in the past, but the recent approval of intravenous thrombolysis for acute stroke and neuroprotective drug development have made rapid imaging and intervention a critical part of stroke management. The patient with hemorrhage may harbor an aneurysm, vascular malformation, or other condition, each having important differences in treatment options. The radiologist plays a critical role in the triage and evaluation of all patients suffering stroke. Selection of the proper imaging technique, recognition of early ischemic changes, differentiation of stroke from other brain disorders, and recognition of important stroke subtypes can have a significant impact on therapy and outcome.

This chapter reviews the pathophysiology of stroke, the time course of findings on computed tomography and magnetic resonance imaging, patterns of arterial and venous occlusions, and overall radiologic approach to evaluation of patients who have suffered stroke.

ISCHEMIC STROKE

Etiology. Despite our best clinical efforts, no clear source is ever identified in up to a quarter of patients with brain infarction. Among those with an established mechanism, approximately two thirds of infarcts are caused thrombi and one third by emboli. Thrombi are formed at sites of abnormal vascular endothelium, typically over an area of atherosclerotic plaque or ulcer. Large-artery thrombosis in the neck might or might not cause distal infarction, depending on the time course of occlusion and available collateral supply. Small vessel thrombi frequently occur in "end arteries" of the brain, accounting for approximately one fifth of infarcts ("lacunes"). Emboli may arise from the heart, aortic arch, carotid arteries, or vertebral arteries, causing infarction by distal migration and occlusion. There is obviously overlap between the thrombotic and embolic groups, as the majority of emboli begin as thrombi somewhere more proximal in the cardiovascular tree (hence the practical term, "thromboembolic disease"). Vasculitis, vasospasm, coagulopathies, global hypoperfusion, and venous thrombosis each account for 5% or less of acute strokes, but they are important to recognize because of differing treatment and prognosis. A given patient's age, medical history, and type of stroke seen will help establish the major etiologic considerations (Table 4.1).

Pathophysiologic Basis for Imaging Changes

Brain Metabolism and Selective Vulnerability. Neurons lead a precarious life. The brain consumes 20% of the total cardiac output to maintain its minute-to-minute delivery of glucose and oxygen. Because there are no significant long-term energy stores (e.g., glycogen, fat), disruption of blood flow for even a few minutes will lead to neuronal death. The extent of injury depends on both the duration and degree of vascular occlusion. Minor reduction in perfusion is initially compensated for by increased extraction of substrate, but injury becomes inevitable below a critical flow threshold (10–20 mL/100 g tissue/min versus normal 55 mL/100 g/min).

Certain cell types and neuroanatomic regions show selective vulnerability to ischemic injury. Gray matter normally receives three to four times more blood flow than

Table 4.1. Differential Diagnosis of Ischemic Stroke by Age

Pediatric	Young Adult	Elderly
Congenital heart disease	Cardiac emboli	Atherosclerosis
Blood dyscrasias	Atherosclerosis	Cardiac emboli
Meningitis	Drug abuse	Coagulopathy
Arterial dissection	Arterial dissection	Amyloid
Trauma	Coagulopathy	Vasculitis
ECMO	Vasculitis	Venous thrombosis
Venous thrombosis	Venous thrombosis	

ECMO, extracorporeal membrane oxygenation.

does white matter, and it is therefore more likely to suffer under conditions of oligemia. Some subsets of neurons (e.g., cerebellar Purkinje cells, hippocampal CA-1 neurons) are injured more readily than others, possibly because of greater concentrations of receptors for excitatory amino acids. The slower metabolizing capillary endothelial cells and white matter oligodendrocytes are more resistant to ischemia than is gray matter, but they will die when deprived of nutrients. Cells served by penetrating end arteries or those residing in the watershed zone between major territories have no alternate route for perfusion and are more prone to infarction. Damage will likely be more severe in a patient with an incomplete circle of Willis than in one with a complete arterial collateral pathway.

Imaging Findings in Acute Ischemia. Ischemia causes a cascade of cellular level events leading to the gross pathologic changes detected in clinical imaging. Failure of membrane pumps permits efflux of K^+ and simultaneous influx of Ca^{2+}, Na^+, and water. This leads to cellular ("cytotoxic") edema, observed clinically as increased water content in the affected region. *Increased brain water is the fundamental change that enables us to detect areas of infarction by CT and MR.* Even a small increase in water content causes characteristic decreased attenuation on CT, low signal on T1-weighted MR, and high signal on T2-weighted MR. This edema peaks 3 to 7 days postinfarction and is maximum in the gray matter. A smaller component of vasogenic edema also develops as the more resistant capillary endothelial cells lose integrity. In contrast, tumor-associated edema is primarily vasogenic and preferentially affects the white matter (see chapter 5).

Careful inspection of CT and MR images done within minutes to a few hours after vessel occlusion can give clues to ischemic injury, even before gross tissue edema or mass effect is seen. These "hyperacute" signs primarily relate to morphologic changes in the vessels rather than density or signal changes in the parenchyma. On CT, the actual thrombus may occasionally be seen in larger intracranial branches, resulting in the "hyperdense artery sign" (Fig. 4.1). On MR, the normal black signal of flowing blood within the lumen ("flow void") is immediately lost and may be replaced by abnormal signal representing clot (Fig. 4.2).

Loss of the flow void is best seen acutely in the large vessels (carotid siphon, vertebrobasilar vessels, middle cerebral branches). Dissolution of clot and improved collateral flow may occur within the first few days, leading to re-establishment of flow void on follow-up MR examinations.

Acute MCA Ischemia on CT: Insular Ribbon and Lentiform Nucleus Edema. CT scans done within 6 hours of middle cerebral artery occlusion will commonly exhibit the "insular ribbon sign," a subtle but important blurring of the gray–white layers of the insula attributable to early edema (Fig. 4.3). Early edema may also be most conspicuous in the putamen in proximal middle cerebral artery occlusions (lentiform nucleus edema sign). MR examinations in the first few hours may show a similar loss of gray–white borders and slight crowding of sulci in areas destined to undergo infarction. Swelling noted on T1-weighted images may precede T2 hyperintensity, which typically develops at 6 to 12 hours postictus. Beyond the first several hours, increased water in the infarcted tissue is most easily (and sometimes only) detected on T2-weighted sequences (Fig. 4.4).

CT Screening for Thrombolysis Careful but rapid interpretation of CT scans is particularly important in

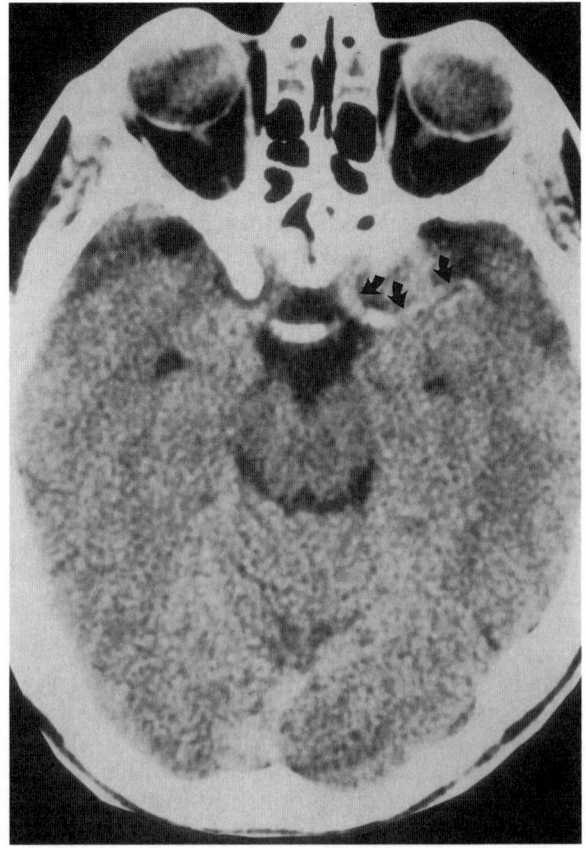

Figure 4.1. Hyperdense Artery Sign. Three hours postocclusion, high density is seen in the proximal left middle cerebral artery (*arrows*). Acute thrombus fills the lumen.

patients who are candidates for thrombolytic drug treatment (e.g., tissue plasminogen activator, t-PA). Administration of intravenous t-PA within 3 hours of stroke onset has been reported to improve neurologic outcome, provided that rigid inclusion and exclusion treatment criteria are met. The screening CT is examined to exclude patients with brain hemorrhage, masses, or other structural abnormalities that contraindicate thrombolysis. Early studies also suggest that patients with extensive edema on their initial CT scan may be at particularly high risk for reperfusion hemorrhage, so these patients must be excluded from thrombolytic treatment. Although universal guidelines are not agreed on, patients with edema affecting more than one third of the MCA territory should be excluded. More subtle baseline changes, such as an isolated insular ribbon sign or limited lentiform nucleus edema, are generally not considered contraindications for thrombolysis. Current work suggests that diffusion-weighted and perfusion-sensitive MR techniques may prove useful in the future for evaluation and triage in thrombolysis protocols. The treatment window of opportunity may also widen beyond 3 hours as neuroprotective drugs are introduced in clinical use.

Diffusion-Weighted MR in Acute Ischemia.
Diffusion-weighted imaging (DWI) uses a novel form of MR tissue contrast to detect noninvasively ischemic changes within minutes of stroke onset. Diffusion-weighted images are acquired by applying a strong gradient pair that sensitizes the images to microscopic (Brownian) water motion. Brain water diffusion rates fall rapidly during acute ischemia, recovering to normal over days or weeks in infarcted tissues. Because random water motion is slowed down in areas of acute ischemia, the early infarct stands out as bright signal on DWI, compared with dark signal (dephasing) in the normal areas. Patients suffering acute stroke may show clear DWI changes hours before any abnormality can be seen on spin-echo T2-weighted MR (Fig. 4.5). This can also be a useful way to distinguish new ischemic areas (high signal on DWI) from older lesions (normal or low signal on DWI). By using a series of different diffusion gradient strengths, the process may also be quantified in an apparent diffusion coefficient. Implementation is facilitated using echo-planar MR systems with their inherently faster, stronger gradients and rapid digitization equipment.

FLuid Attenuated Inversion Recovery (FLAIR) in Ischemia.
FLAIR allows heavy T2-weighting of the parenchyma and simultaneously suppresses free water signal from the cerebrospinal fluid. These techniques increase conspicuity of T2 changes in ischemia. FLAIR is

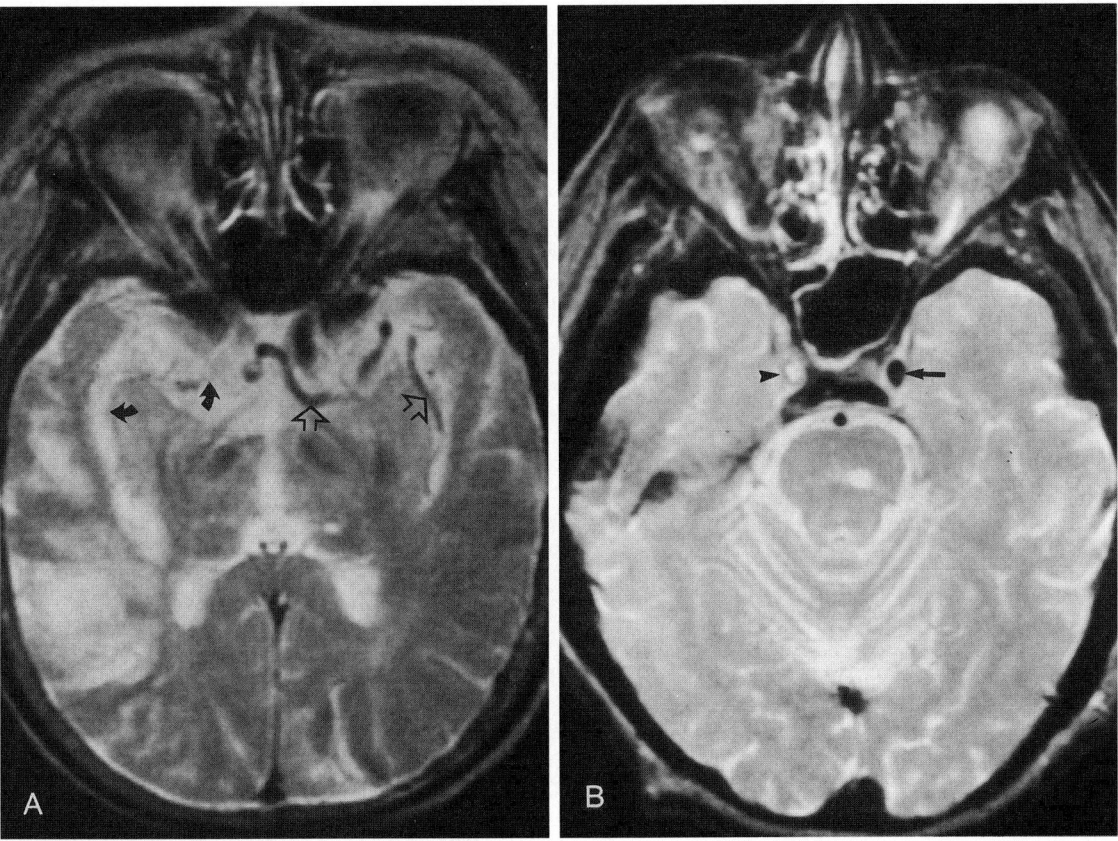

Figure 4.2. Loss of Flow Void. Six hours after right internal carotid occlusion **(A)**, there is a loss of vascular flow voids in the ICA and MCA branches (*arrows*) compared with the patent left side (*open arrows*). Hyperintensity is developing in the right posterior sylvian region, indicative of early edema on this T2WI. A section below **(B)** shows complete occlusion of the right ICA in its cavernous segment (*arrowhead*), with normal flow void preserved on the left (*arrow*). An older lacune in the pons is evident.

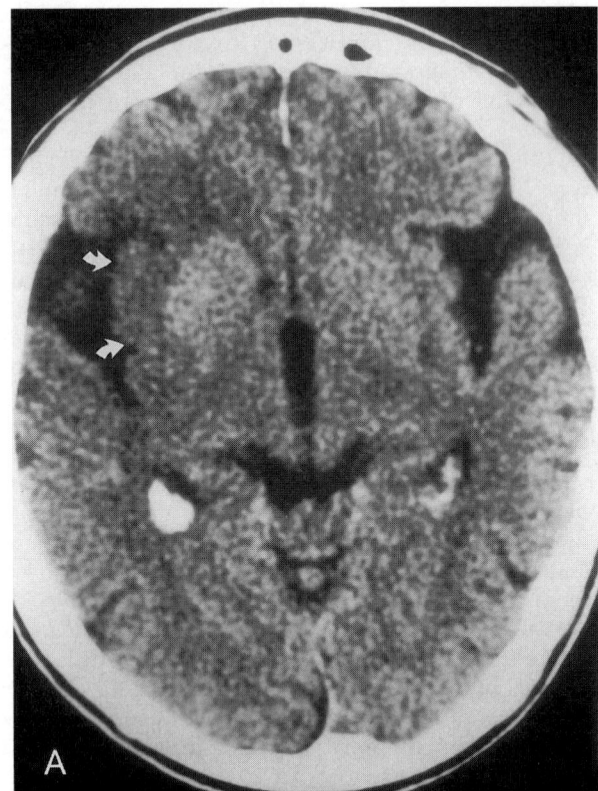

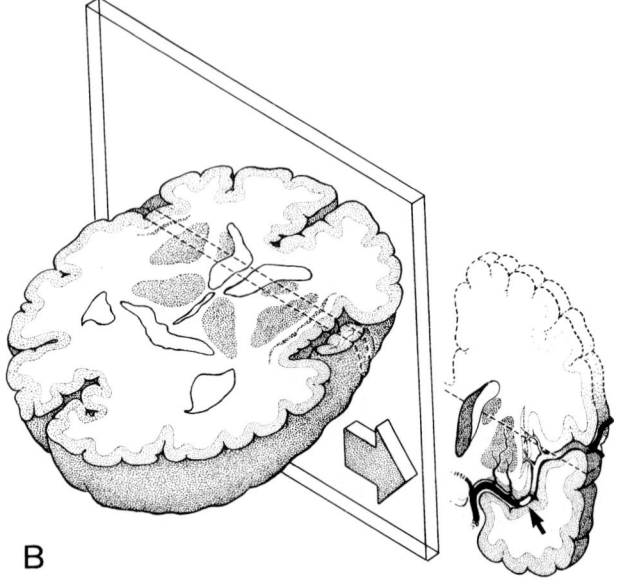

Figure 4.3. Insular Ribbon Sign. A. A noncontrast CT done 4 hours after right MCA occlusion shows decreased attenuation and loss of gray–white borders in the right insular region (*arrows*). **B.** Diagram of the insula in transverse and coronal planes. The insular cortex, claustrum, and extreme capsule are infarcted due to occlusion of the MCA (*arrow*) beyond the lateral lenticulostriate vessels. (Reprinted with permission from Truwit CL, Barkovich AJ, Gean-Marton A, et al. Loss of the insular ribbon: another early CT sign of acute middle cerebral artery infarction. Radiology 1990;176:805.)

Figure 4.4. Edema in Early Ischemia. Edema is detected as high signal intensity and mild mass effect in the entire right MCA territory on this T2-weighted transverse image obtained 2 days postocclusion. Partial effacement of the right lateral ventricle is evident.

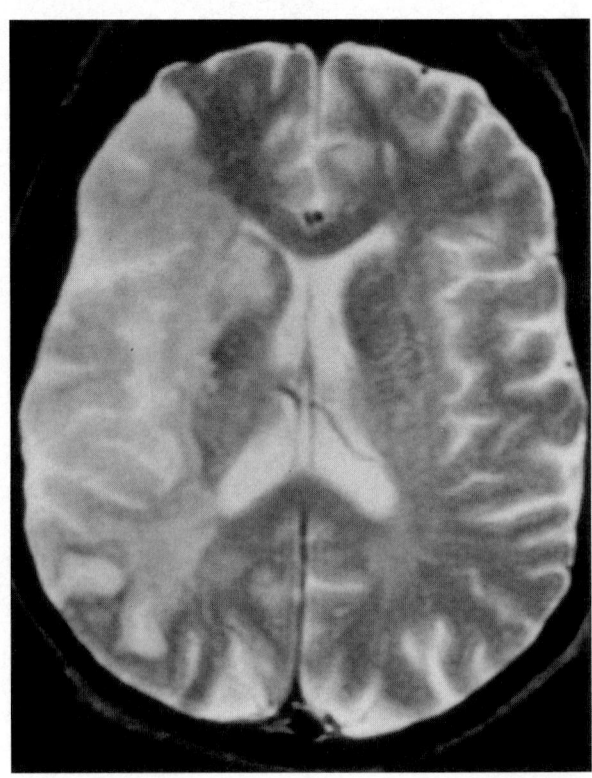

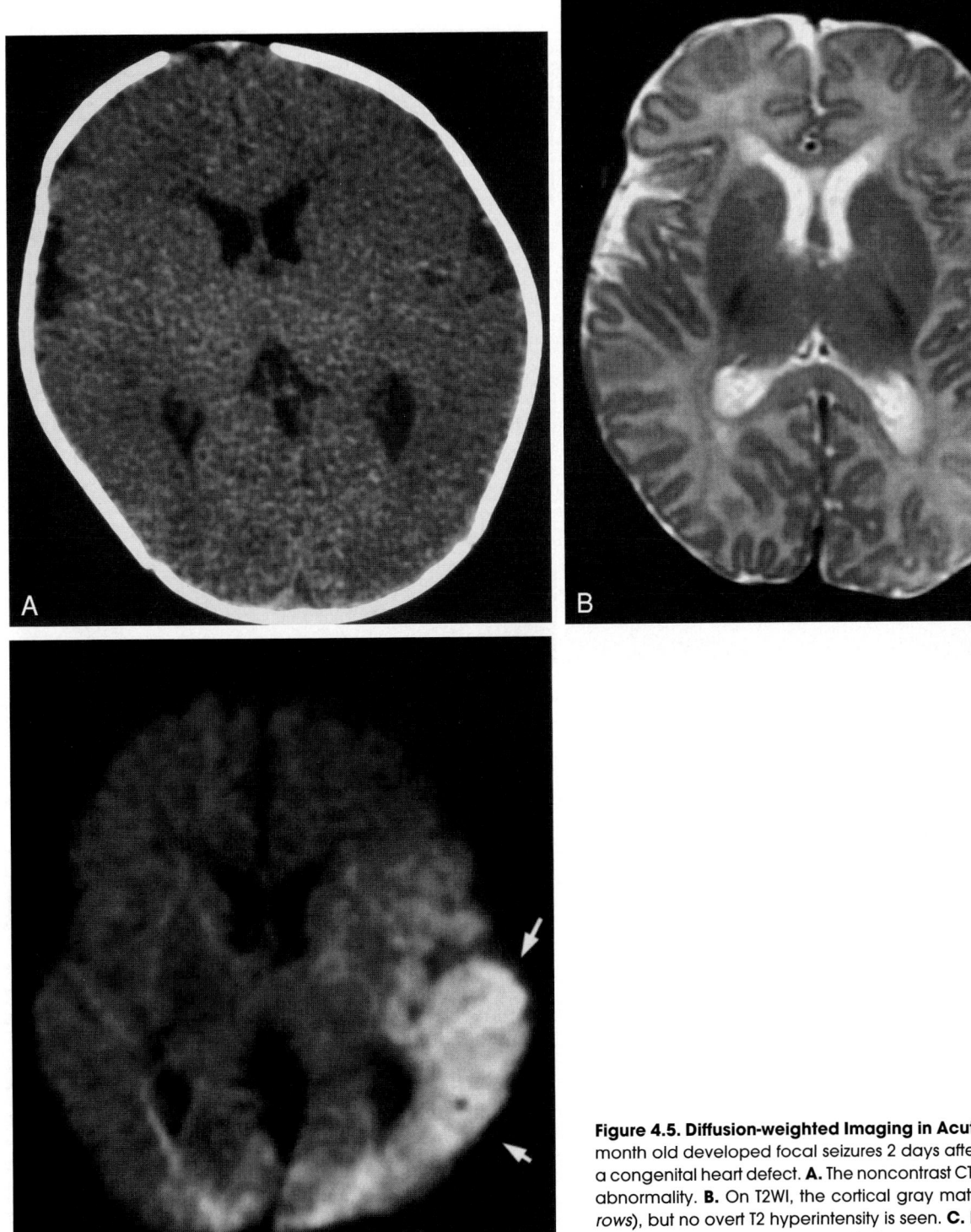

Figure 4.5. Diffusion-weighted Imaging in Acute Ischemia. This 1 month old developed focal seizures 2 days after surgery to repair a congenital heart defect. **A.** The noncontrast CT shows no obvious abnormality. **B.** On T2WI, the cortical gray matter is indistinct (*arrows*), but no overt T2 hyperintensity is seen. **C.** Diffusion-weighted image clearly show high signal in the posterior aspect of the left hemisphere, indicative of acute infarction (*arrows*).

not inherently better than T2 MR for early detection of ischemia but may be particularly helpful in detecting small lesions in the cortex or brainstem.

Subacute and Chronic Ischemia. In the subacute phase, edema leads to mass effect, ranging from slight sulcal effacement to marked midline shift with brain her-

niation, depending on the size and location of infarct. These changes peak at 3–7 days, with progressive brain softening (encephalomalacia) ensuing. One potential imaging pitfall, the "fogging effect," may be encountered on CTs done during the second week after infarction as edema and mass effect are subsiding. At this stage, de-

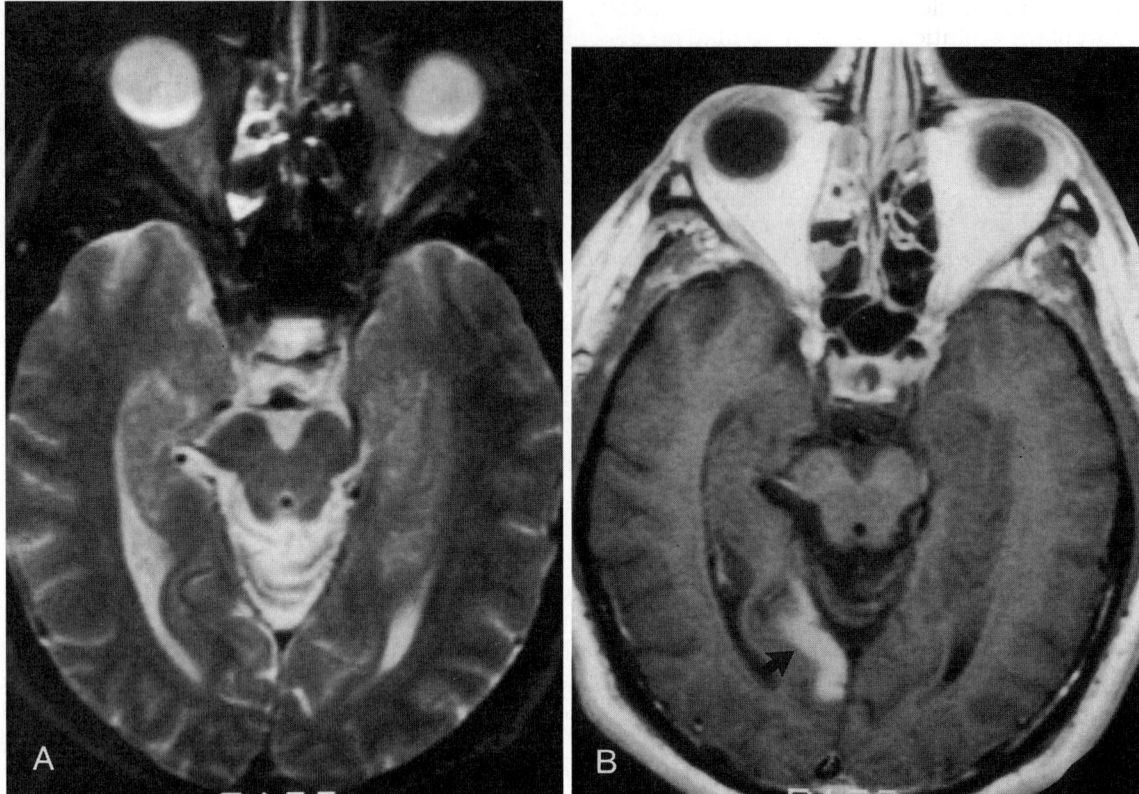

Figure 4.6. Fogging Effect in Subacute Infarction. As edema and mass effect subside, but before development of atrophy, infarcts may be inconspicuous on unenhanced CT or MR images. **A.** T2WI is essentially normal in the occipital regions 13 days after posterior cerebral artery infarction. **B.** T1WI after gadolinium show enhancement of the infarcted deep right occipital cortex (*arrow*).

crease in edema and accumulation of proteins from cell lysis balance each other such that brain morphology and density in the injured region can be nearly normal by CT. Fogging effects are much less of a problem on MR owing to its greater tissue sensitivity, particularly when contrast is used (Fig. 4.6). Edema or mass effect that persists beyond 1 month effectively rules out simple ischemia and should raise the possibility of recurrent infarction or an underlying tumor.

In the weeks and months after infarction, macrophages remove dead tissue, leaving a small amount of gliotic scar and encephalomalacia behind. Cerebrospinal fluid takes up the space previously occupied by the brain. The affected corticospinal tract atrophies (wallerian degeneration), leading to a shrunken appearance of the ipsilateral cerebral peduncle. If hemorrhage accompanied the infarct, hemosiderin may be seen grossly or detected as signal hypointensity by T2WI. Widening of adjacent sulci and "ex-vacuo" dilation of the ventricle occurs adjacent to the infarcted area (Fig. 4.7).

Hemorrhagic Transformation of Infarction

Reperfusion into infarcted capillary beds may secondarily lead to gross or microscopic hemorrhage, seen in many as half of infarcts. In most cases, this takes the form of microscopic leakage (diapedesis) of red blood cells, but on rare occasions, a frank hematoma will form.

Physical disruption of the capillary endothelial cells, loss of vascular autoregulation, and anticoagulation may all contribute to the development of these hemorrhages. Patients may develop headaches at the time of bleeding but commonly have no new symptoms, presumably because the hemorrhage occurs within brain areas that are already dead or dysfunctional. Hemorrhagic infarction is confined to the territory of the infarcted vessel, whereas primary hemorrhage does not necessarily respect vascular boundaries. Intraventricular extension is uncommonly seen with hemorrhagic transformation and should raise the possibility of another process (such as hypertensive bleeding or a ruptured arteriovenous malformation).

The peak time for hemorrhagic transformation is at approximately 1–2 weeks postinfarction. It is usually manifest as a serpiginous line of petechial blood following the gyral contours of the infarcted cortex. These dots of hemorrhage are often patchy and discontinuous. On CT, a faint line of high attenuation is observed, and on MR, bright signal is seen along the affected gyrus on the unenhanced T1WI because of methemoglobin (Fig. 4.8A). (Alternate explanations for this bright signal have been offered, including laminar necrosis or calcification related to infarction; the practical point is to recognize this appearance as a feature of ischemia.) The petechial gyral pattern is not seen in primary brain hemorrhage and can be helpful in confirming the underlying ischemic cause of a suspicious lesion. This is considered a normal part of the evolution of an infarct. Management in the presence of petechial hemorrhage is controversial, but most neurologists continue anticoagulation if there is a well-documented embolic source.

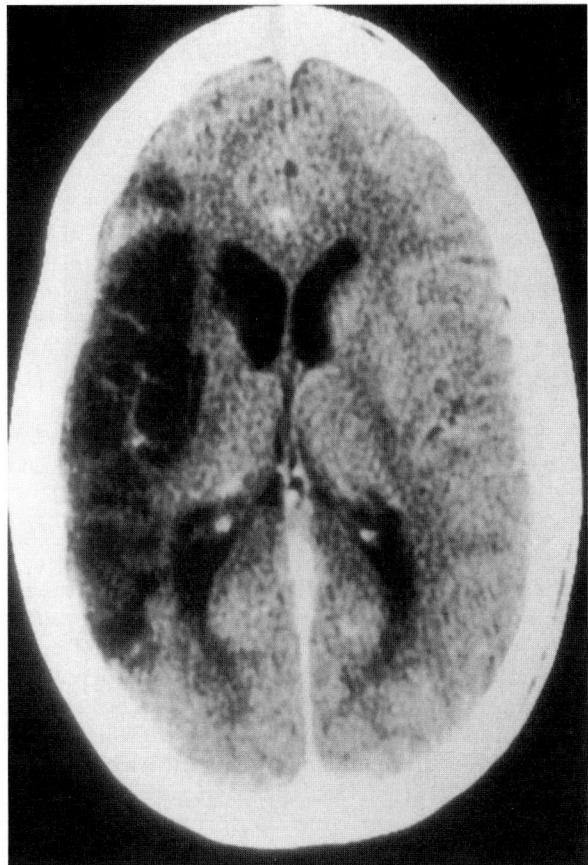

Figure 4.7. Chronic Infarction. Cystic encephalomalacia is present in the right MCA territory on CT 1 year after infarction. Note widening of the ipsilateral ventricle (ex-vacuo dilatation).

More extensive hemorrhagic transformation of the infarcted tissue may lead to the formation of a gross parenchymal hematoma. The blood does not conform to a gyrus and may form a clot indistinguishable from a primary hematoma. Large cortical infarcts are at somewhat higher risk for this type of change, compared with limited cortical or subcortical lesions. Catastrophic hemorrhagic transformation can also follow thrombolysis, particularly when treatment is delayed or the baseline CT shows extensive edema. In contrast to the petechial gyral transformation just described, gross parenchymal hematomas tend to occur earlier and are more commonly associated with clinical deterioration. Anecdotal evidence suggests that reperfusion of a large cortical infarct during the first 24 hours may pose an especially high risk of hematoma formation. Frank hematomas seen on infarct follow-up studies should be reported promptly because anticoagulation therapy is contraindicated, even when the finding is incidental.

Use of Contrast in Ischemic Stroke

CT Contrast. A noncontrast CT remains the radiologic examination of choice for assessment of suspected acute stroke. The unenhanced study is necessary to help triage the patient. It serves to rule out hemorrhage, may define patterns and extent of ischemic injury, shows areas of abnormal vascular calcification (e.g., giant aneurysms), and excludes mass lesions. This is important first-line information needed by the clinician faced with determining the need for lumbar puncture, vascular surgery, anticoagulation, thrombolysis, cardiac evaluation, or other therapies. All acute stroke CTs should, however, be reviewed on the monitor because the unenhanced study may rarely show the need for intravenous contrast. A nonstroke lesion such as a tumor, abscess, or an isodense subdural hematoma might be suspected on the noncontrast examination and then be shown to better advantage with contrast.

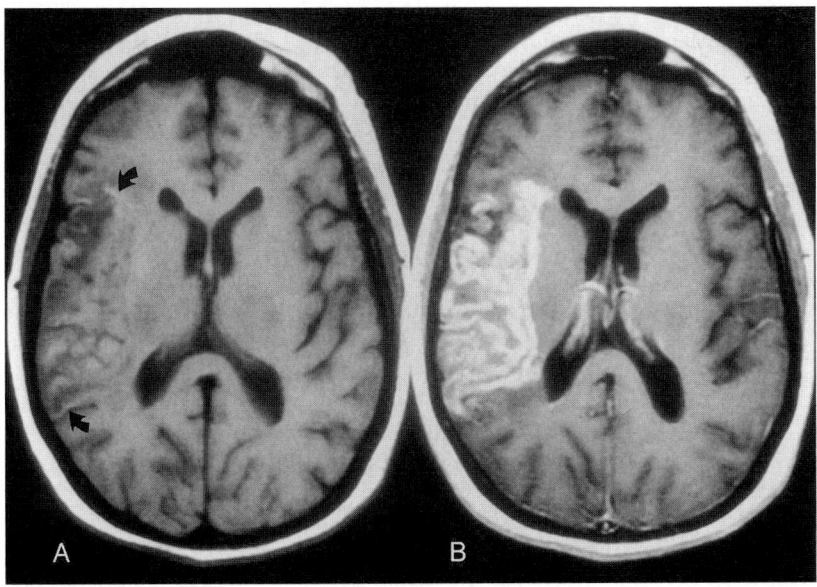

Figure 4.8. Petechial Hemorrhage and Gyral Enhancement in Subacute Infarction. A. Precontrast T1WI shows mild effacement of sulci in the right MCA territory. A few subtle areas of bright signal intensity scattered along the cortex indicate areas of petechial hemorrhage or laminar necrosis (*arrows*). **B.** Postcontrast T1WI demonstrates marked gyral enhancement, a hallmark of subacute infarction.

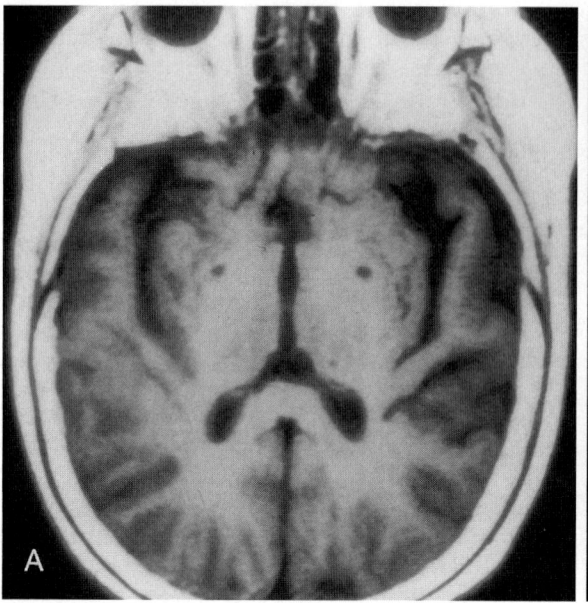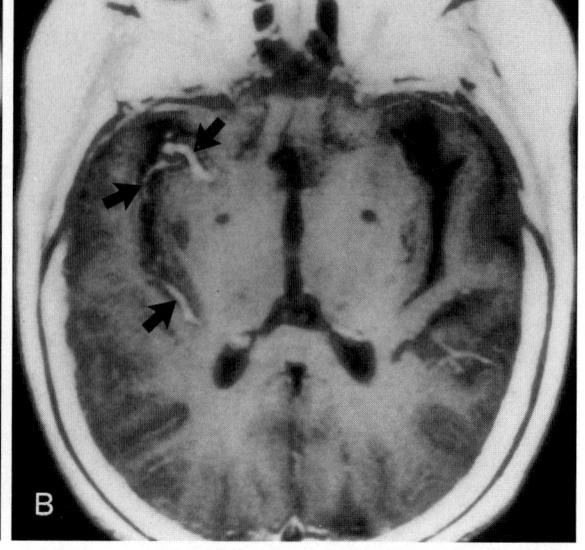

Figure 4.9. Intravascular Enhancement in Acute Infarction. Precontrast **(A)** and postcontrast **(B)** contrast T1-weighted transverse images in acute right MCA infarction. Mild sulcal effacement and prominent enhancement of sylvian branches of the MCA (*arrows*) is evident. Intravascular enhancement is seen only during the first 10 days after stroke.

The use of intravenous contrast for CT beyond the acute phase is slightly more controversial. Some radiologists believe contrast is contraindicated in brain infarction. They cite a slightly increased risk of seizures and other untoward central nervous system effects, presumably the result of a toxic effect of the contrast as it leaks through the abnormal blood–brain barrier. Most of these data, however, are based on studies using ionic contrast media. Others counter that this risk is exceedingly small and should not preclude its use. On the balance, use of nonionic contrast for CT seems reasonable when MR is not available and there is significant ambiguity about the diagnosis based on the noncontrast CT and clinical findings.

An intact blood–brain barrier normally excludes contrast from the brain. Leakage of macromolecular contrast agents through damaged vessels leads to local accumulation of iodine, seen as high attenuation (enhancement) of infarcted parenchyma. Blood–brain barrier breakdown underlies both hemorrhagic transformation and contrast enhancement of infarctions. Not surprisingly, then, these processes are seen at roughly the same time and often in combination. As with petechial gyral hemorrhage, a gyral pattern of enhancement (by CT or MR) is highly specific evidence of an underlying infarction. CT-detected enhancement of infarcted brain parenchyma typically begins at approximately 1 week, peaks at 7–14 days, often assumes a gyral pattern, and is less commonly observed in subcortical regions (Fig. 4.8B). Enhancement is seen in approximately half of patients during the first week and in approximately two-thirds between weeks 1 and 4. As gliosis ensues and the blood–brain barrier is repaired, enhancement fades and then resolves by 3 months.

MR Contrast. Most of the comments regarding the strategy, pathophysiology, and enhancement patterns for CT also generally hold true for contrast in MR. Intravenous gadolinium diethylenetriamine penta-acetic acid and similar recently released gadolinium agents are very well tolerated by patients who have suffered stroke and may give valuable information not readily available from the noncontrast MR. Stasis of gadolinium within vessels or leakage of contrast through an abnormal blood–brain barrier will shorten T1 relaxation of adjacent protons, leading to hyperintensity (enhancement) on T1WI. As with CT, a noncontrast MR sequence is mandatory before contrast is given, as both enhancement and subacute blood appear hyperintense on T1WI. (See *Hemorrhage.*)

Intravascular enhancement on MR is commonly seen in the infarcted territory during the first week. This may be attributable to slow flow or vasodilatation leading to stasis of gadolinium. The intravascular enhancement pattern may be detected within minutes of vessel occlusion, is seen in a majority of cortical infarcts at 1–3 days, and resolves by 10 days. The proximal trunks of more distally occluded arteries and leptomeningeal cortical channels are most prominently involved (Fig. 4.9). The area of vascular enhancement may extend beyond the T2 hyperintensity, possibly indicating recruitment of collateral supply at the ischemic border. Meningeal enhancement that attends meningitis, and dural enhancement seen postoperatively, can superficially resemble intravascular enhancement, but the distinction should be obvious on clinical grounds. MR intravascular enhancement helps identify early strokes, dates them to less than 11 days old, and has no obvious CT counterpart.

MR parenchymal enhancement occurs in a similar pattern to that seen on CT (and with the same time course seen by nuclear medicine infarct scans of the past). It may occur as early as day 1, but more typically begins after the first week, a time when intravascular enhancement is waning (Fig. 4.10). Virtually all cortical infarcts enhance by MR at 2 weeks. Elster has summarized this in his Rule of 3s: MR parenchymal enhancement peaks at 3 days to 3 weeks and resolves by 3 months.

The imaging time course for CT and MR examinations in brain infarction are summarized in Table 4.2.

Pattern Recognition in Ischemic Stroke

Familiarity with the major vascular territories can help distinguish between infarction and other pathologic processes. The clinical time course and localization should be consistent with the imaging findings, and all should correspond to a known vascular distribution. Stroke localization is not necessarily synonymous with "focal." An ischemic event may cause a pattern of damage that is diffuse (hypoxic-ischemic injury), multifocal (vasculitis, emboli), or focal (single embolism or thrombus). The vessels causing stroke may be large or small and may be on either the arterial or venous side. There is no such thing as a "funny" stroke; if it does not fit a vascular territory, then the differential diagnosis changes (Fig. 4.11).

The relation of vascular anatomy to functional neuroanatomy is at the heart of clinicoradiologic correlation in stroke. Classically, strokes and TIAs are divided into anterior (carotid territory) or posterior (vertebrobasilar territory) events. Patients with anterior circulation ischemia have been shown to benefit from carotid endarterectomy when the carotid is narrowed by at least 70% compared with its normal diameter. Surgery has not been proved beneficial for patients with lesser degrees of carotid stenosis or those with posterior territory TIAs, who therefore usually receive medical therapy (e.g., anticoagulation). Ischemia in the carotid territory may cause visual changes, aphasia, or sensorimotor deficits owing to retinal, cortical, or subcortical damage. Vertebrobasilar strokes are more likely to cause syncope, ataxia, cranial nerve findings, homonymous visual field deficits, and facial symptoms opposite those of the body. A given deficit can be predicted from the known functional topography of the cortex and its connections through the internal capsule (Fig. 4.12).

The patterns of injury observed after occlusion of large arteries in the anterior and posterior circulations, small arteries in any region, and of the dural venous channels are reviewed in turn.

Anterior (Carotid) Circulation

Internal Carotid Artery (ICA). Thromboembolic disease in the ICA may cause TIAs or infarction in its middle cerebral artery or anterior cerebral artery branches or in the watershed zone between them. Embolic occlusion of the ophthalmic branch of the ICA may cause transient monocular blindness (amaurosis fugax). Observation of any of these patterns should prompt a careful look at the carotid arteries. The extent and distribution of ischemia observed depend on the time course of occlusion, degree of oligemia, and available collateral supply. Complete carotid occlusions are occasionally found in asymptomatic patients with a well-developed collateral supply.

Atherosclerotic disease near the carotid bifurcation is responsible for the majority of ischemic events in the ICA territory. Arterial dissection, trauma, fibromuscular dysplasia, tumor encasement, prior neck radiotherapy, and connective tissue diseases may also cause significant carotid narrowing (Fig. 4.13). Hemodynamic effects begin to be seen when there is greater than 80% reduction in area or greater than 60% decrease in diameter. Lesions causing less severe narrowing may nonetheless become symptomatic when they serve as a nidus for thrombus formation or are unmasked by hypotension. Studies have shown a clear benefit of endarterectomy in symptomatic patients with greater than 70% stenosis, but not for those with less than a 30% narrowing. Ongoing studies should clarify the guidelines for the 30–70% group within the next few years.

Noninvasive screening of the carotid arteries may be achieved with either US or MR angiography (MRA). The choice of US versus MRA depends on the abilities of the available personnel and equipment. Sensitivity and specificity are as high as 85–90% for either technique. Both methods noninvasively identify patients with hemodynamically significant disease who might then be referred for conventional angiography. US is the most commonly used screening examination in most centers. It has the advantage of portability, generally lower costs, and can be performed in patients with contraindications to MR or MRA. US is more operator dependent than MRA and is unable to assess reliably portions of the distal ICA near the

Table 4.2. Imaging Time Course After Brain Infarction

Time	CT	MR
Minutes	No changes	Absent flow void Arterial enhancement (days 1–10) DWI: high signal
2–6 h	Hyperdense artery sign Insular ribbon sign	Brain swelling (T1) (No signal Δ yet)

6–12 h	Sulcal effacement
	  ± Decreased
	  attenuation
		T2 hyperintensity

12–24 h	Decreased attentuation	T1 hypointensity
3–7 d	Maximum swelling	Maximum swelling

3–21 d	Gyral enhancement
	  (peak: 7–14 d)
		Gyral enhancement
		  (peak: 3–21 d)
		Petechial methemoglobin

30–90 d	Encephalomalacia
	Loss of enhancement
	Resolution of
	  petechial blood
		Encephalomalacia
		Loss of enhancement
		Resolution of petechial
		  blood

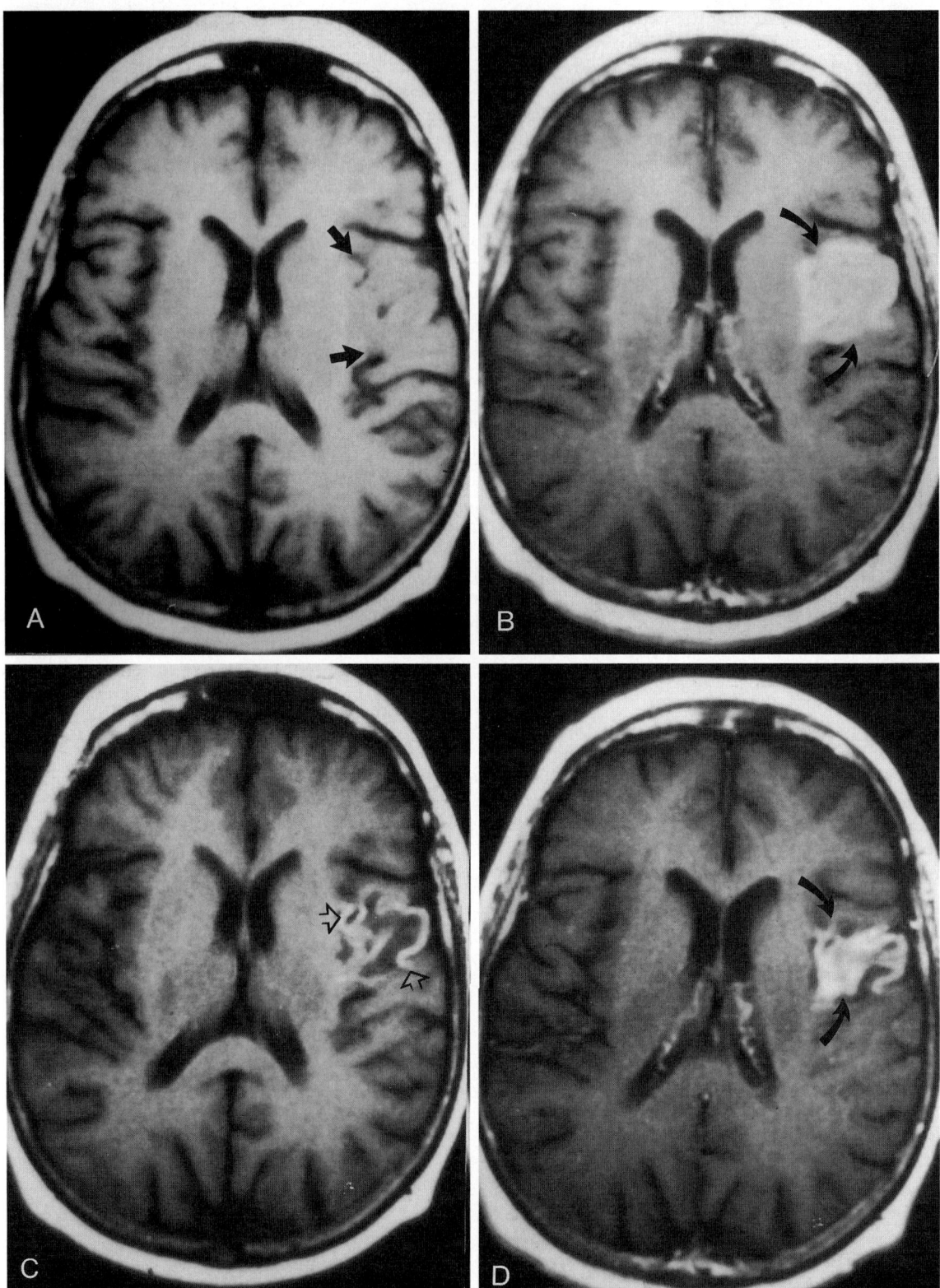

Figure 4.10. Evolution of petechial hemorrhage and parenchymal enhancement. Before and after contrast T1WI in left sylvian cortical infarction. The acute study **(A, B)** shows nonhemorrhagic swelling (*straight arrows*) with prominent cortical enhancement **(B,** *curved arrows*). At 2-month follow-up **(C, D)** petechial hemorrhage (*open arrows*) and decreasing parenchymal enhancement **(D,** *curved arrows*) are seen. Parenchymal enhancement resolves by 3 months.

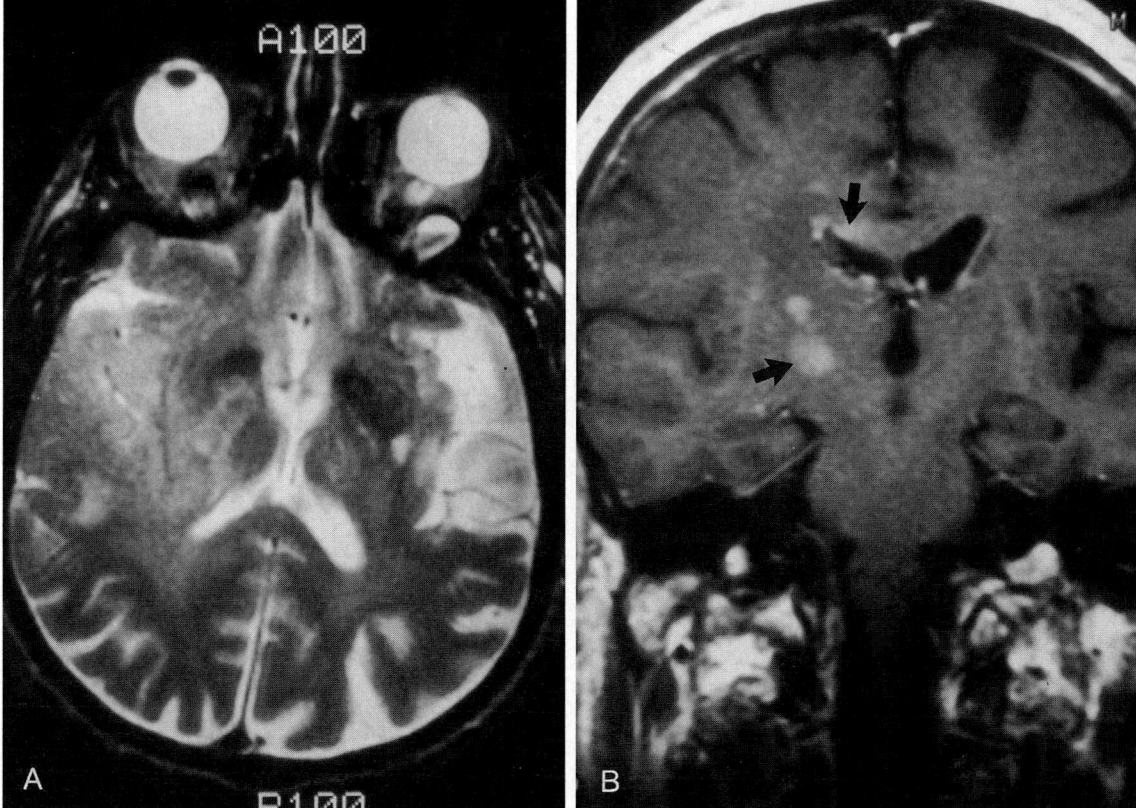

Figure 4.11. Glioblastoma Mimicking a Stroke. A. T2-weighted axial section shows edema primarily in the right MCA territory, but with additional involvement of the medial temporal lobe, thalamus, and periatrial regions. **B.** Postcontrast coronal T1WI shows patchy, nodular areas of enhancement in the basal ganglia and periventricular regions (*arrows*). Even with a strong clinical history for strokelike onset, the nonvascular distribution and atypical enhancement pattern effectively exclude underlying infarction. When in doubt, follow-up imaging studies will usually clarify the diagnosis.

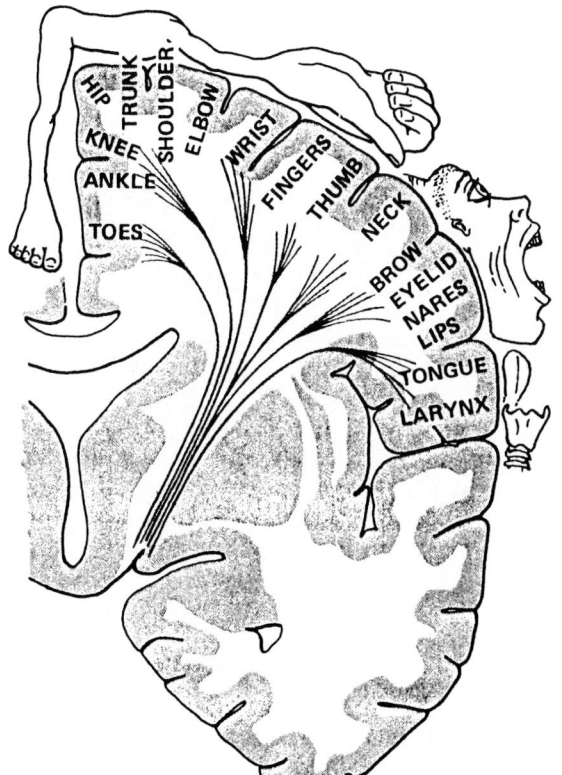

Figure 4.12. Homunculus. A coronal section through the precentral (motor) cortex depicts the topographic representation of the opposite side of the body. The face and hand areas are served by the MCA territory, the leg by the ACA. (Reprinted with permission from Gilman S, Winans SS. Essentials of clinical neuroanatomy & neurophysiology. Philadelphia: FA Davis Company, 1982:180.)

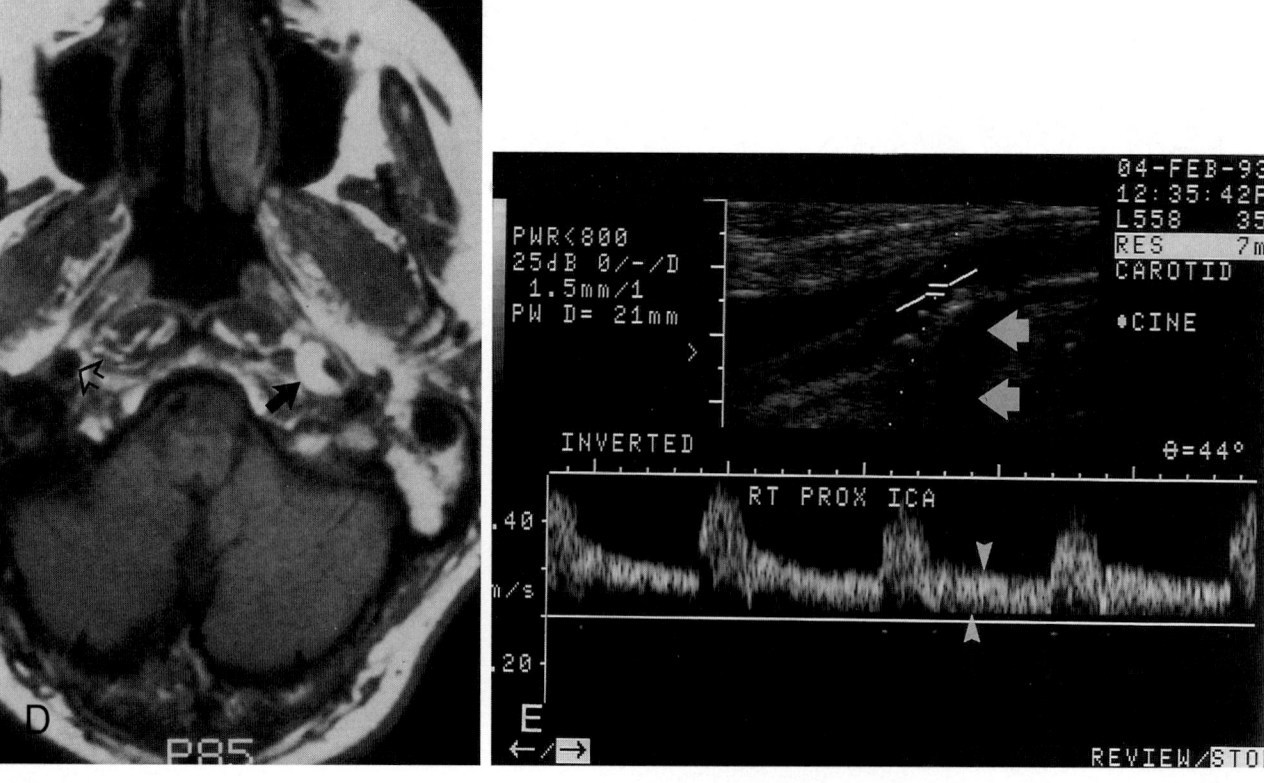

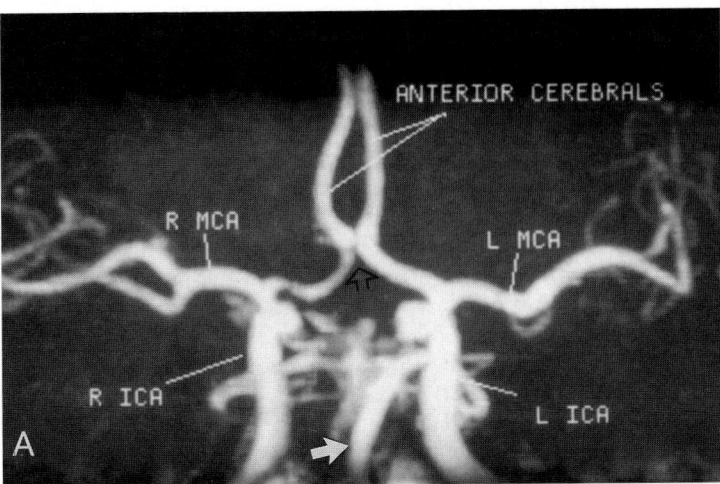

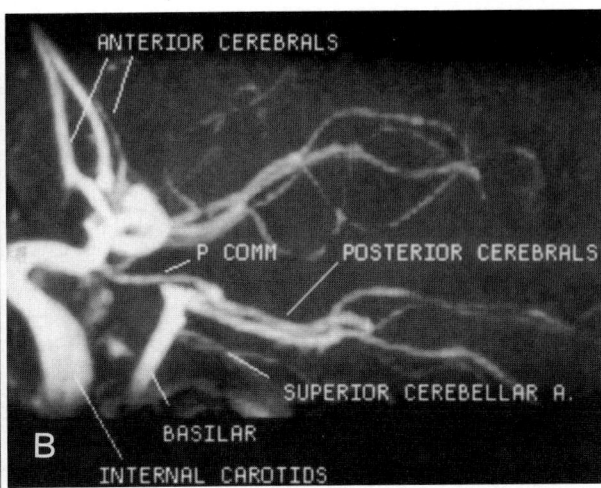

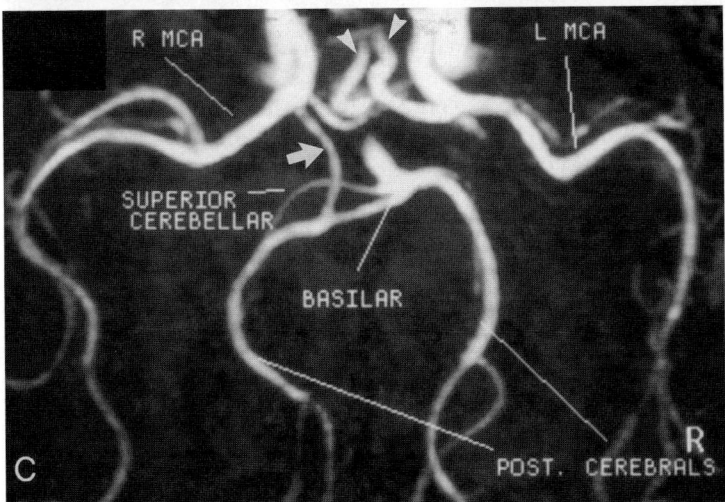

Figure 4.14. MR Angiography of the Normal Circle of Willis and Its Branches. A. The anterior (coronal) projection depicts the normal internal carotid arteries (ICA) with bifurcation into the ACA and MCA intracranial branches. The basilar artery and cerebellar branches project below (*arrow*). The anterior communicating artery is very short in this patient (*open arrow*). **B.** Lateral projection shows a single large posterior communicating artery (P COMM) connecting the anterior to posterior circulations. The superior cerebellar and posterior cerebral branches of the basilar artery are clearly shown. **C.** Submentovertex projection outlines the relationship of the major vessels to the circle of Willis. We are looking "down the barrel" of the ICAs and basilar artery. A single posterior communicating artery is again seen (*arrow*); the opposite side is likely hypoplastic. The anterior cerebrals project between the ICAs (*arrowheads*).

skull base. Transcranial Doppler sonography may extend the ability of US to examine the carotid siphon and intracranial branches. MRA can evaluate the entire course of the carotid and may be quickly performed in conjunction with the patient's brain MR study. It is a particularly good method for screening pediatric or elderly patients in whom conventional angiography may be technically more difficult.

Selective common carotid angiography remains the gold standard for carotid artery evaluation and is generally the method of choice for surgical planning. The study should cover the entire ICA, including cervical and cranial portions. Evaluation of the surgically inaccessible cranial segments (petrous, cavernous, and supraclinoid) is necessary to exclude high-grade intracranial

stenoses or "tandem" lesions which might contraindicate endarterectomy.

Anterior Cerebral Artery (ACA). The terminal bifurcation of the ICA is into the anterior and middle cerebral arteries (Fig. 4.14). The ACA is divided into three subgroups: *medial lenticulostriates* serve the rostral portions of the basal ganglia; *pericallosal* branches supply the corpus callosum; and *hemispheric* branches serve the medial aspects of the frontal and parietal lobes (Fig. 4.15). Approximately 5% of infarcts involve the ACA.

The medial lenticulostriates penetrate the anterior perforating substance to give variable supply to the anterior–inferior aspect of the internal capsule, putamen, globus pallidus, caudate head, and portions of the hy-

Figure 4.13. Carotid Disease. A. Atherosclerosis. Lateral view of the carotid bifurcation by conventional digital subtraction angiography. The diameter of the proximal ICA (*arrow*) is reduced approximately 60% compared with its normal caliber above. CCA, common carotid artery; ICA, internal carotid artery; ECA, external carotid artery and its branches. **B.** Atherosclerosis. Lateral maximum-intensity projection from a two-dimensional time-of-flight MR angiogram in the same patient shows a very similar pattern of flow-related enhancement. **C.** Carotid dissection with a tapering occlu-

sion in the ICA just above the bifurcation. **D.** Carotid dissection in another patient shows the "mural crescent sign" indicative of intramural thrombus in the petrous portion of the left ICA (*arrow*). Note the normal caliber flow void and scant amounts of fat surrounding the normal right ICA (*open arrow*) on T1WI. **E.** Carotid US shows calcified plaque with acoustic shadowing (*arrows*), vessel narrowing, and spectral broadening (*between arrowheads*) in a case of atherosclerosis.

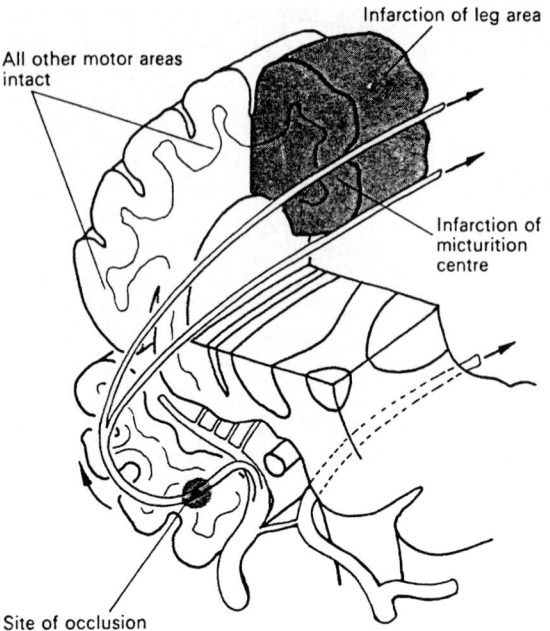

Figure 4.15. Anterior Cerebral Artery Occlusion. An ACA occlusion causes infarction of the paramedian frontal cortex responsible for motor and sensory function of the opposite leg (*stippled area*). If bilateral, incontinence and akinetic mutism may also be seen. (Reprinted with permission from Patten J. Neurological differential diagnosis. New York: Springer Verlag, 1996:137.)

pothalamus and optic chiasm. The largest of these vessels supplies the caudate head or anterior internal capsule region and is recognized as the recurrent artery of Heubner. Infarction in the medial lenticulostriate territory may cause problems with speech production (motor aphasia), facial weakness, and disturbances in mood and judgment.

Above the take-off of the lenticulostriates, the ACAs are interconnected by the anterior communicating artery. Each ACA ascends further, giving off branches to the frontal pole (orbitofrontal and frontopolar arteries). The ACAs terminate as a bifurcation into the (lower) pericallosal and (upper) callosomarginal branches. These arteries run parallel to the corpus callosum from front to back, giving supply to the medial cortex of the frontal and parietal lobes. As its name would imply, the pericallosal artery courses around and feeds the corpus callosum. ACA branching patterns are quite variable from one patient to the next, with approximately 10% having only one pericallosal branch, which supplies both hemispheres, an "azygous" ACA (Fig. 4.16).

Unilateral damage in the ACA hemispheric branches will cause preferential leg weakness on the opposite side of the body (Table 4.3). Bilateral ACA infarctions lead to incontinence and an awake but apathetic state known as akinetic mutism. Infarction of the corpus callosum can cause a variety of interhemispheric disconnection syndromes including ideomotor apraxia (inability to perform right hemisphere tasks when given cues from the dominant left hemisphere).

Middle Cerebral Artery. The MCA supplies more brain tissue than any other intracranial vessel and is host to almost two thirds of infarcts. Its offspring are the *lateral lenticulostriates*, which supply most of the basal ganglia region, and the *hemispheric branches*, which serve the lateral cerebral surface (Figs. 4.4, 4.17).

The lateral lenticulostriates arise from the proximal MCA as numerous small perforating end arteries distributed to the putamen, lateral globus pallidus, superior half of the internal capsule and adjacent corona radiata, and majority of the caudate. Isolated vascular lesions of the globus pallidus or putamen are commonly asymptomatic or may affect contralateral muscle tone and motor control. Lesions of the internal capsule or corona radiata may cause pure or mixed sensory and motor deficits on the opposite side of the body. Interruption of visual connections to the lateral geniculate nucleus results in a subtle type of contralateral homonymous hemianopsia. Rarely, the arcuate fasciculus pathway from Wernicke's to Broca's speech areas may be selectively infarcted, leading to a conduction aphasia (inability to repeat or read aloud, despite preserved comprehension and fluency).

The MCA loops laterally through the insula, where it bifurcates or trifurcates into its major cortical branches (Fig. 4.14A.). The insula itself is supplied by hemispheric branches, not by the lateral lenticulostriates. When the proximal MCA is occluded, this insular region is furthest from any potential collateral supply, probably explaining the early appearance of edema that gives rise to the "insular ribbon sign" (Fig. 4.3). The anterior hemispheric branches of the MCA supply the anterolateral tip of the temporal lobe (anterior temporal artery), the frontal lobe (operculofrontal arteries), and the motor and sensory

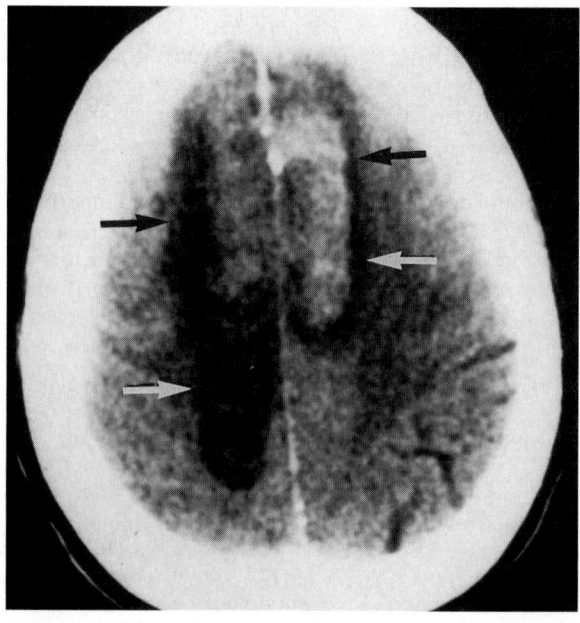

Figure 4.16. Hemorrhagic Infarction. Hemorrhagic infarction in a bilateral ACA distribution (*arrows*) shown by noncontrast CT. This was an embolic stroke, presumably occluding an azygous ACA.

Table 4.3. Functional Vascular Anatomy[a]

Vessel	Branch	Side	Deficit/Syndrome
ACA	Hemispheric	Either	Leg weakness
		Both	Incontinence, akinetic mutism
	Medial lenticulostriates	Either	Facial weakness
		Left	Dysarthria; ± motor aphasia
MCA	Hemispheric	Either	Face and arm > leg weakness
		Left	Motor aphasia (anterior lesion)
			Receptive aphasia (posterior lesion)
			Global aphasia (total MCA)
			Neglect syndromes
		Right	Visuospatial dysfunction
	Lateral lenticulostriates	Either	Variable lacunar syndromes
PCA	Hemispheric	Either	Hemianopsia
		Both	Cortical blindness
			Memory deficits
	Thalamoperforators	Either	Somnolence
			Sensory disturbances
Cerebellar	PICA, AICA, or SCA	Either	Ataxia, vertigo, vomiting; coma if mass effect ± brainstem deficits
Watershed	ACA/MCA/PCA	Either	"Man-in-a-barrel syndrome"
		Bilateral	Severe memory problems

[a] Assumes left hemisphere language dominance.
ACA, anterior cerebral artery; AICA, anterior inferior cerebellar artery; PICA, posterior inferior cerebellar artery; MCA, middle cerebral artery; PCA, posterior cerebral artery; and SCA, superior cerebellar artery.erior cerebellar artery; PICA, posterior inferior cerebellar artery; MCA, middle cerebral artery; PCA, posterior cerebral artery; and SCA, superior cerebellar artery.

strips (central sulcus arteries). Posterior hemispheric branches of the MCA supply the parietal lobe behind the sensory strip (posterior parietal artery), the posterolateral parietal and lateral occipital lobes (angular artery), and the majority of the temporal lobe (posterior temporal artery).

Occlusion of the rostral MCA branches of the dominant hemisphere will cause a motor (Broca) aphasia in which comprehension remains intact. Posterior branches in the dominant hemisphere supply Wernicke's area, causing a receptive aphasia when occluded. Posterior temporal branch occlusion may interrupt visual radiations, causing contralateral homonymous field defects. Involvement of either hemisphere's precentral gyrus (motor strip) will produce contralateral weakness that affects face and arm more than leg (Fig. 4.12). Contralateral cortical sensory loss occurs when the primary or association sensory cortex behind the central sulcus is affected. In the nondominant right hemisphere, posterior MCA infarcts commonly cause bizarre impairment in visualospatial abilities and sometimes neglect (or nonrecognition) of the left body. Complete occlusion of the MCA beyond the lenticulostriates causes a combination of these deficits: contralateral face and arm hemiparesis, field defect, and either neglect or global aphasia, depending on which hemisphere is affected. Leg weakness may also be seen when the MCA stem is occluded, because of internal capsule involvement. These relationships are summarized in Table 4.3.

Posterior (Vertebrobasilar) Circulation

Vertebral Arteries. The vertebral arteries usually originate from the subclavian arteries, ascend straight upward in the transverse foramina of C6–C3, turn sharply through the C2–C1-foramen magnum levels and unite anterior to the low medulla to form the basilar artery (Fig. 4.18). Atherosclerotic narrowing commonly affects the vertebral arteries at their origins and

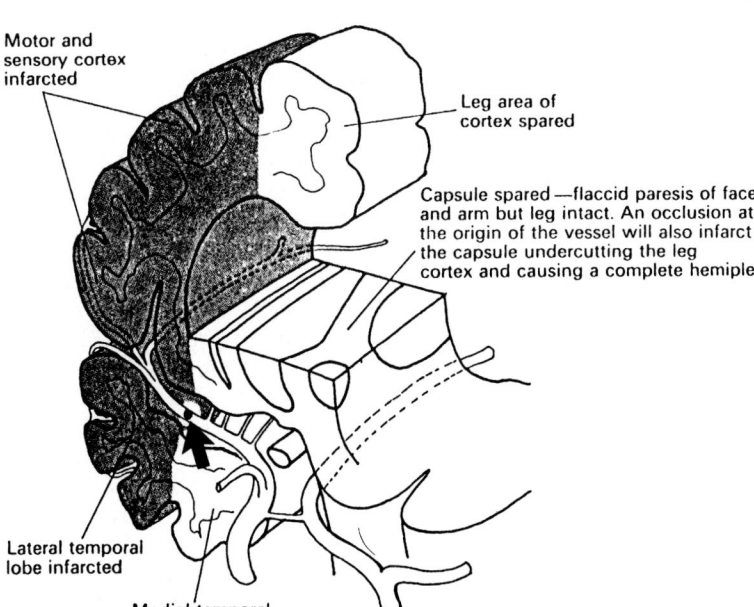

Motor and sensory cortex infarcted

Leg area of cortex spared

Capsule spared —flaccid paresis of face and arm but leg intact. An occlusion at the origin of the vessel will also infarct the capsule undercutting the leg cortex and causing a complete hemiplegia

Lateral temporal lobe infarcted

Medial temporal lobe spared

Figure 4.17. Middle Cerebral Artery Occlusion. An MCA occlusion distal to the lateral lenticulostriates (*large arrow*) causes infarction of the motor and sensory cortex of the arm and face (stippled area). More proximal occlusion will also affect the internal capsule, potentially adding leg deficits. (Reprinted with permission from Patten J. Neurological differential diagnosis. New York: Springer Verlag, 1996:138.)

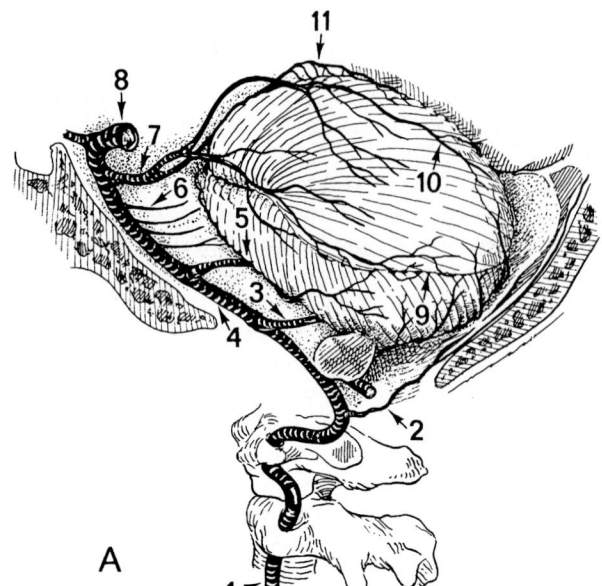
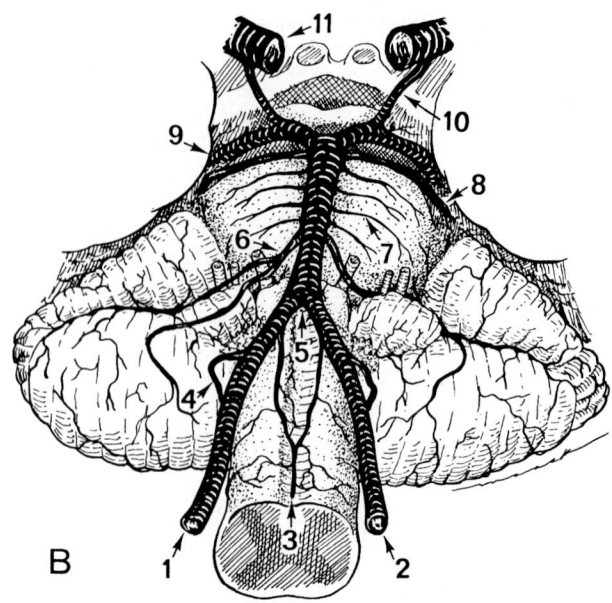

Figure 4.18. Vertebrobasilar Arteries. A. Lateral view. *1)* Left verte-bral, *2)* posterior meningeal, *3)* posterior inferior cerebellar (PICA), *4)* basilar, *5)* anterior inferior cerebellar (AICA), *6)* pontine perfora-tors, *7)* superior cerebellar (SCA), *8)* posterior cerebral (PCA), *9)* branches of the SCA and AICA in the horizontal fissure of the cere-bellum, *10)* SCA hemispheric branches, and *11)* superior vermian branches. **B.** Anterior view. *1)* Right vertebral, *2)* left vertebral, *3)* an-terior spinal, *4)* PICA, *5)* basilar, *6)* AICA, *7)* pontine, *8)* SCA, *9)* PCA, *10)* posterior communicating, and *11)* ICA. (Reprinted with permis-sion from Osborn AG. Introduction to cerebral angiography. Philadelphia: Harper & Row, 1980:380–381.)

may affect the basilar artery over variable lengths. Narrowing of the cervical portion of the vertebrals may be because compressive uncovertebral osteophytes. Rapid head turning (e.g., that experienced in motor ve-hicle accidents) may stretch the vertebrals at the C1–2 level, leading to arterial dissection. Any of these condi-tions may cause vertebrobasilar ischemia via throm-botic or embolic mechanisms. Endarterectomy or an-gioplasty are sometimes feasible for correction of atherosclerotic lesions but have not gained wide ac-ceptance. Anticoagulation and antiplatelet agents re-main the mainstay of treatment for vertebrobasilar ischemia.

Basilar Artery. The basilar is formed by the union of the two vertebral arteries. As it ascends between the clivus and brainstem, it sends large branches to the cere-bellum and smaller perforating vessels to the brainstem. The basilar ends at its bifurcation into the posterior cere-bral arteries just above the tentorium cerebelli. Occlusion of the basilar artery itself is usually rapidly fatal owing to infarction of respiratory and cardiac centers in the medulla. Occlusion of the perforating end arteries from the basilar artery causes focal brainstem infarction, usu-ally manifest as cranial nerve dysfunction, ataxia, som-nolence, and crossed motor or sensory deficits. These le-sions characteristically respect the midline of the brainstem and often extend to the ventral surface (Fig. 4.19). Metabolic disturbances (e.g., central pontine myeli-nolysis) and hypertensive hemorrhages (most commonly in the pons) tend to be more centrally or diffusely located. Large or multiple lesions in the pons can cause a night-

marish syndrome of quadriparesis with intact cognition, the "locked in" state.

Posterior Cerebral Artery. The basilar artery ends at its bifurcation into the PCAs at the midbrain level, just above the tentorial hiatus. The major branches of the PCA include midbrain and thalamic *perforating vessels*, *posterior choroidal arteries*, and *cortical branches* to the medial temporal and occipital lobes (Fig. 4.20). Ten to fifteen percent of infarcts occur in the PCA territory.

The proximal segments of the PCAs sweep postero-laterally around the midbrain, giving off small perfo-rating branches to the mesencephalon and thalamus along the way. Midbrain infarction causes loss of the pupillary light responses, impaired upgaze, and som-nolence resulting from damage of the quadrigeminal plate, third cranial nerve nuclei, and reticular activat-ing formation, respectively. Proximal PCA perforators also supply the majority of the thalamus and some-times portions of the posterior limb of the internal cap-sule. Thalamic infarction may cause a variety of dis-turbances, but contralateral sensory loss is the most common problem.

The posterior choroidal arteries arise from the proxi-mal PCA to supply the choroid plexus of the third and lateral ventricles, pineal gland, and regions contiguous with the third ventricle. Isolated posterior choroid in-farctions are rare due to rich collateral supply through the choroid plexus.

PCA cortical branches supply the inferomedial tem-poral lobe (inferior temporal arteries), superior occipital gyrus (parieto-occipital artery), and visual cortex of the occipital lobes (calcarine artery) (Fig. 4.21). Hemispheric PCA occlusions are usually from an embolic source. Inferomedial temporal infarction may cause memory deficits, which are severe when bilateral. Loss of the primary visual cortex causes complete loss of vision in the opposite visual field (homonymous hemianopsia).

In approximately 20% of patients, one or both of the proximal PCA segments may be hypoplastic or absent. In these cases, flow is derived from the ICA system via a prominent posterior communicating artery. This is commonly referred to as "fetal origin" of the PCA because embryologically, the PCA develops with the ICA. Given

that this is a fairly common variation, both vertebral and carotid disease should be considered when evaluating PCA infarctions.

Cerebellar Arteries. Headache, vertigo, nausea, vomiting, and ipsilateral ataxia are the hallmarks of cerebellar stroke; 85% are ischemic and 15% are primary hemorrhages. Clinically, it is difficult to distinguish which cerebellar subterritory is involved and whether it derives from infarction or hemorrhage. *Because of clinical urgency, acute evaluation of suspected cerebellar strokes should be performed by CT.* Cerebellar hemorrhages and any infarctions with significant mass effect are neurosurgical emergencies requiring posterior fossa decompression. Multiplanar MR

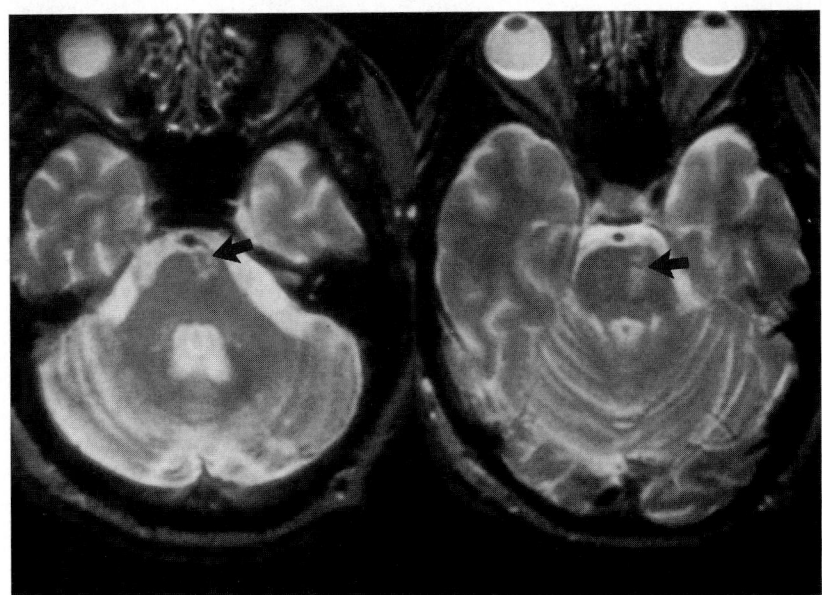

Figure 4.19. Brainstem Infarction. Adjacent transverse T2WI show a left paramedian pontine infarct (*arrows*) that respects the midline.

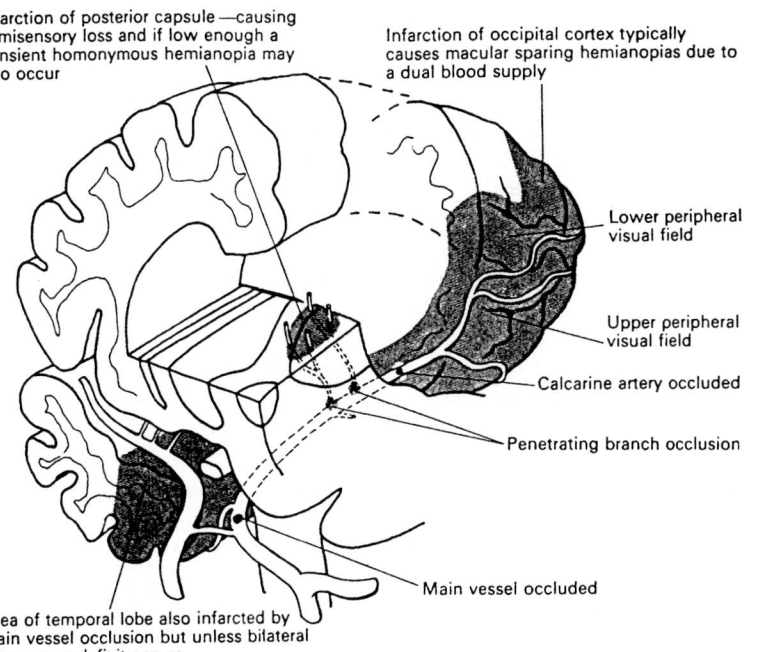

Infarction of posterior capsule —causing hemisensory loss and if low enough a transient homonymous hemianopia may also occur

Infarction of occipital cortex typically causes macular sparing hemianopias due to a dual blood supply

Lower peripheral visual field

Upper peripheral visual field

Calcarine artery occluded

Penetrating branch occlusion

Main vessel occluded

Area of temporal lobe also infarcted by main vessel occlusion but unless bilateral no memory deficit occurs

Figure 4.20. Posterior Cerebral Artery Occlusion. A PCA occlusion results in syndromes of memory impairment, opposite visual field loss, and sometimes hemisensory deficits. (Reprinted with permission From Patten J. Neurological differential diagnosis. New York: Springer Verlag, 1996:140.)

Figure 4.21. Posterior Cerebral Artery Infarction. Adjacent T2WI show involvement of the left occipital lobe and medial temporal lobe. The patient presented with a dense right homonymous visual field defect.

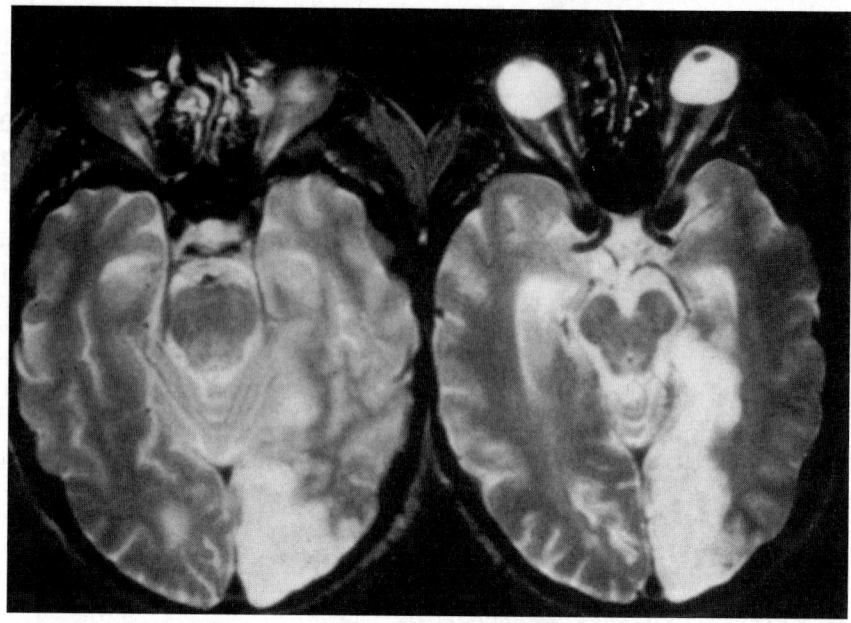

is preferred for evaluation beyond the acute phase, as beam-hardening artifacts degrade posterior fossa images on CT.

Even though deficits related to the cerebellar territories are hard to distinguish clinically, it is important to recognize characteristic distributions in order to elucidate stroke mechanisms. The correct order of cerebellar branches going from top to bottom is the *superior, anterior inferior,* and *posterior inferior* cerebellar arteries (Fig. 4.18).

Superior cerebellar arteries (SCA). The upper parts of the cerebellum are supplied by the SCA. These arise from the distal basilar as the last large branches beneath the tentorium cerebelli. The SCA territory includes the superior vermis, middle and superior cerebellar peduncles, and superolateral aspects of the cerebellar hemispheres (i.e., the "roof" of the cerebellum). Most SCA infarcts are embolic.

Anterior inferior cerebellar arteries (AICA). These arteries arise from the proximal basilar to supply the anteromedial cerebellum and sometimes part of the middle cerebellar peduncle. AICA is usually the smallest of the three major cerebellar hemisphere branches. Occlusion commonly causes ipsilateral limb ataxia, nausea, vomiting, dizziness, and headache.

Posterior inferior cerebellar arteries (PICA). The bottom of the cerebellum is supplied by the PICA. The PICA is the first major intracranial branch of the vertebrobasilar system, usually arising from the distal vertebral artery 1–2 cm below the basilar origin. Its territory is variable but often includes the dorsolateral medulla, inferior vermis, and posterolateral cerebellar hemisphere. PICA maintains a reciprocal relation with AICA above it. If the PICA is large, then the ipsilateral AICA is usually small, and vice versa. This arrangement is sometimes referred to as the AICA–PICA loop. PICA is usually the largest cerebellar hemispheric branch and the most commonly infarcted. Occlusions may occur from exten-

sion of a vertebral dissection that began at the C1–2 level (Fig. 4.22). If only the cerebellar hemisphere is affected, ipsilateral limb ataxia, nausea, vomiting, dizziness, and headache are seen, just as for AICA infarcts. Involvement of the medulla in PICA infarction adds elements of Wallenberg's syndrome, including ataxia, facial numbness, Horner's syndrome, dysphagia and dysarthria.

Watershed (Border Zone) Infarction

An episode of transient global hypoperfusion may result in bilateral infarctions in the watershed regions between arterial territories (also referred to as the border zones). Typical triggering events include cardiac arrest, massive bleeding, anaphylaxis, and surgery under general anesthesia. The border zones are regions perfused by terminal branches of two adjacent arterial territories (Fig. 4.23). When flow in one or both of the parent vessels falls below a critical level, the brain living in the watershed zone is the first to go. Unilateral watershed damage may be seen when carotid occlusion or stenosis is unmasked by global hypotension; in this case, the nonstenotic side recovers because of relative preservation of flow. Images show damage extending out from the "corners" of the lateral ventricles on higher sections (Fig. 4.24). Characteristic clinical findings include weakness isolated to the upper arms ("man in a barrel syndrome"), cortical blindness, and memory loss.

Small Vessel Ischemia

Lacunes are small subcortical infarcts that may occur in any territory. They account for 15–20% of all strokes. Lacunes are the 2–5 mm³ cavities (literally, "little lakes") left in the brain as the result of occlusion of a penetrating artery causing infarction and ensuing encephalomalacia. Patients usually have a history of long-standing hyperten-

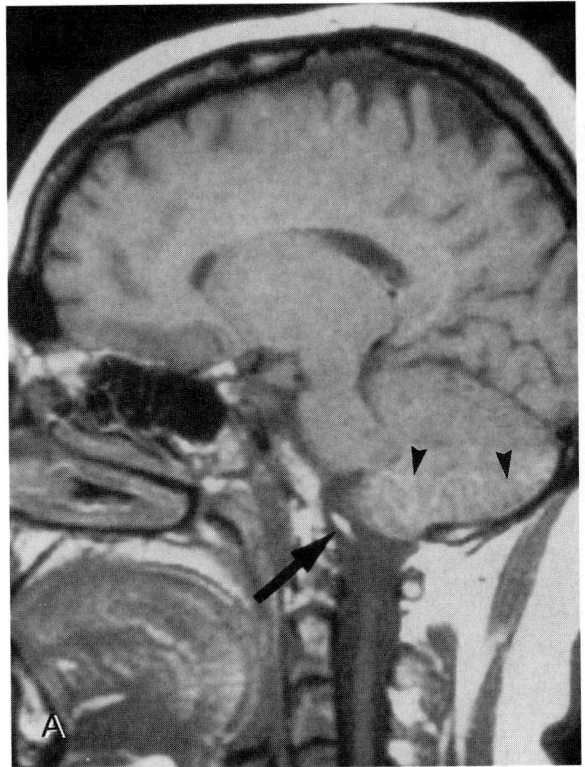

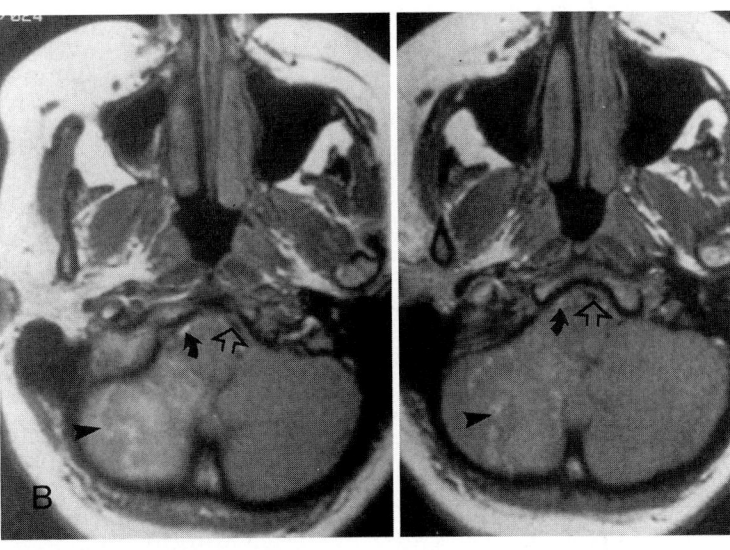

Figure 4.22. Vertebral Dissection with PICA Infarction. This patient developed neck pain and ataxia following a skiing accident. Sagittal **(A)** and transverse **(B)** T1WI without contrast show high signal in the occluded right vertebral artery (*closed arrows*) with preserved flow void in the left vertebral (*open arrows*). Hemorrhagic infarction is seen in the right PICA territory (*arrowheads*).

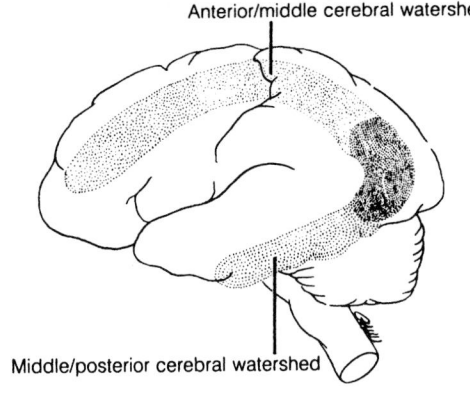

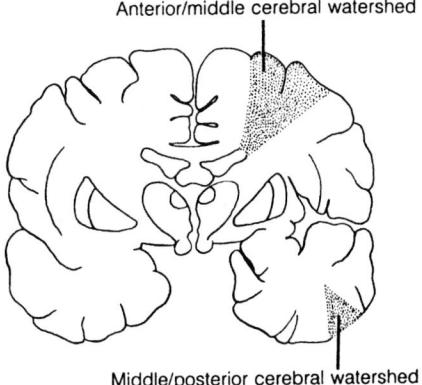

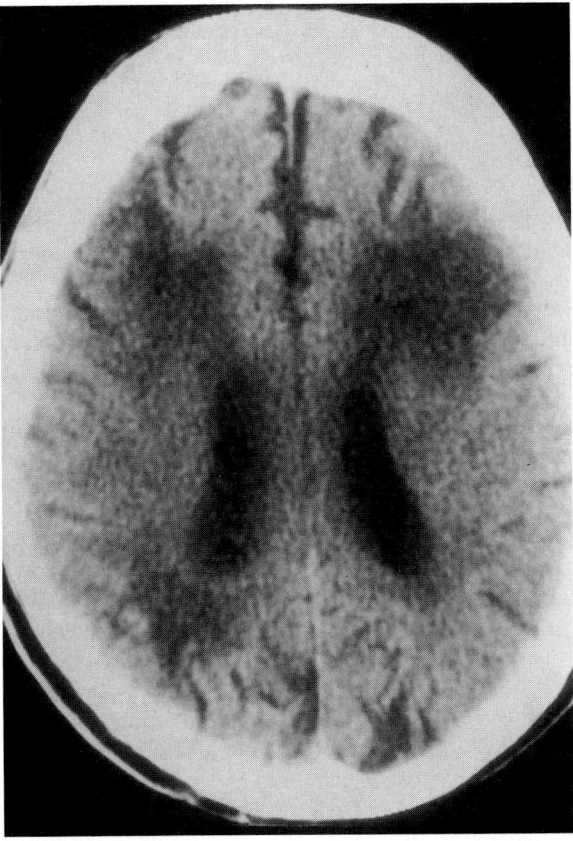

Figure 4.23. Watershed Ischemia. *Stippled* brain areas are served by terminal branches of adjacent parent arteries. The watershed zones are at highest risk of infarction when flow is reduced in one or both carotids. (Reproduced with permission from Simon RP, Aminoff MJ, Greenberg DA, eds. Clinical neurology. 3rd ed. Norwalk, CT: Appleton & Lange, 1996.)

Figure 4.24. Watershed Infarctions. This patient developed upper arm weakness and memory deficits after resuscitation from cardiac arrest. The ACA/MCA border zones show infarction bilaterally near the vertex.

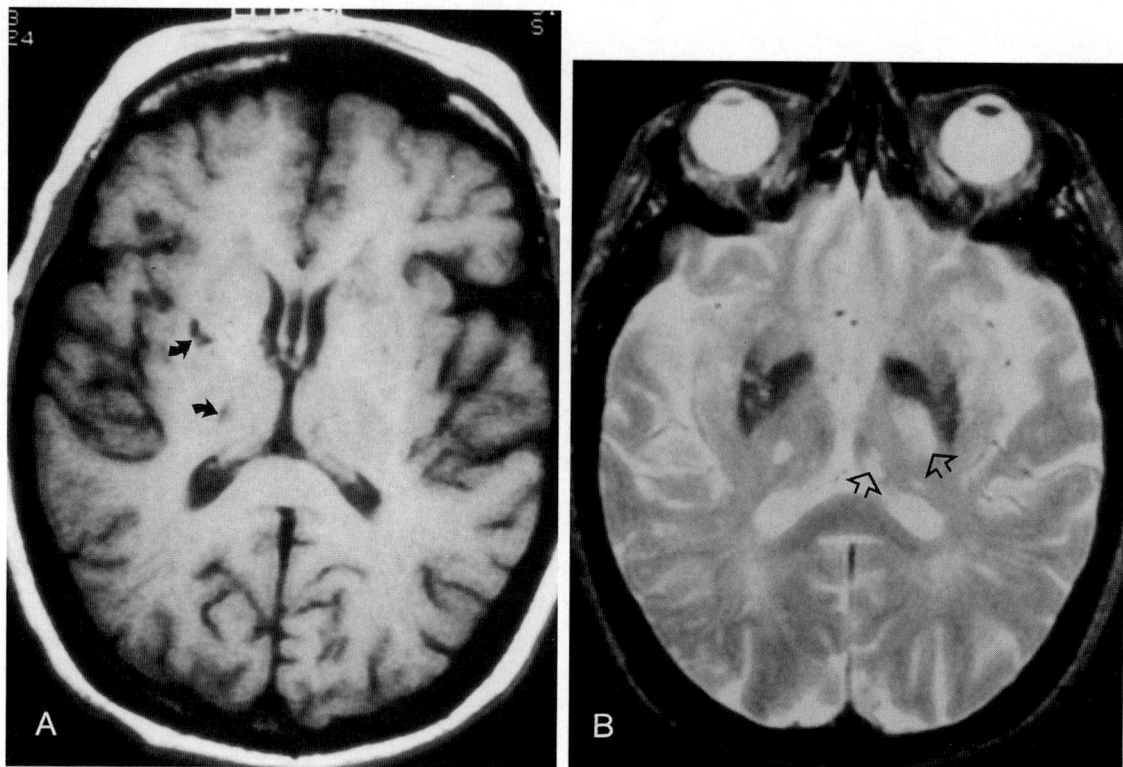

Figure 4.25. Lacunes. T1WI **(A)** and T2WI **(B)** show small holes of CSF intensity in the right thalamus and posterior putamen, likely representing old lacunes (*arrows*). New areas of edema and mass effect are seen in the left thalamus and inferior aspect of the internal capsule on the T2WI (*open arrows*). The latter correspond to an acute right hemiparesis and sensory deficit, indicating recent lacunar infarction. Bilateral hypointensity in the putamen and globus pallidus on the T2WI represents normal iron deposition associated with aging.

sion, leading to lipohyalinosis of the vessels and eventual thrombosis. TIAs precede the stroke in 60% of cases, and a stuttering course is common in the first 2 days. Pure motor or sensory syndromes may occur with these small lesions. Characteristic locations include the lenticular nucleus (37%), pons (16%), thalamus (14%), caudate (10%), and internal capsule (10%) (Fig. 4.25).

Internal capsule lacunes are an especially important subset of lacunes because they are quite common and cause characteristic syndromes. Axonal projections to and from the cortex must funnel through the internal capsule and brainstem, where even tiny lacunes may cause major deficits. The internal capsule receives supply from multiple small perforating arteries at the base of the brain, all of which are common sites for lacunar infarction and hypertensive hemorrhages. Its contributors include the ACA and MCA lenticulostriates, the ICAs anterior choroidal branch, and PCA thalamogeniculates. Isolated lesions of the anterior limb interrupt connections of the anterior frontal lobe but are usually clinically silent. Beginning at the genu and working back, the capsule carries corticobulbar, *head*, *arm*, and then *leg* fibers in a somatotopically organized fashion (Fig. 4.26). (Our little homunculus man, *HAL*, stands in the posterior limb with his head at the genu, reclining with his head directed medially as

he enters the cerebral peduncle.) Lesions in the posterior limb are clinically most important because they may cause severe sensory, motor, or mixed deficits. Lesions at the genu may disrupt speech production or swallowing, but they generally become apparent only when bilateral.

Lacunes Versus Perivascular Spaces. "Etat lacunaire" refers to a state of multiple lacunar infarctions. The term is still used in the literature and should be distinguished from the term "etat crible," which refers to enlarged perivascular spaces (Virchow-Robin spaces) that may develop around perforating vessels (Fig. 4.27). These normal spaces may simulate lacunes but have no associated neurologic deficit or other clinical relevance. By definition, Virchow-Robin spaces should follow CSF intensity on all MR sequences, have no associated mass effect, and occur along the path of a penetrating vessel. Common locations include the medial temporal lobes and inferior one third of the putamen and thalamus. Occasionally, they may be seen along the course of small medullary veins near the vertex (Fig. 4.28). Most perivascular spaces seen on MR are between 1 and 3 mm in diameter, but some may be 5 mm or larger. Enlarged perivascular spaces are observed as a normal variant in all age groups. Both increasing size and frequency are noted with increasing age.

Small-Vessel Ischemic Changes. Small foci of T2 hyperintensity are commonly seen scattered throughout the brains of older patients with or without clinical symptoms. These "UBOs" (unidentified bright objects) can cause considerable consternation. They are commonly associated with patchy or diffuse T2 hyperintensity in the centrum semiovale (Fig. 4.27). Pages could be filled with different authors' terms for related processes: small-vessel ischemic disease, senescent change, Binswanger's disease, multi-infarct dementia, and

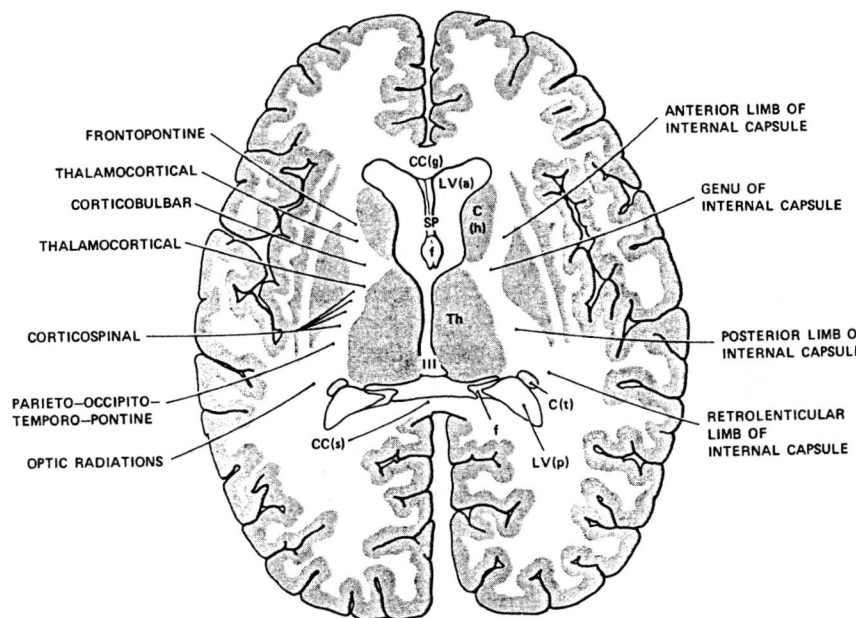

Figure 4.26. Somatotopy of the Internal Capsule. Transverse diagram showing the main parts of the internal capsule (*labeled on the **right***) and major fiber tracts passing through it (*labeled on the **left***). *CC(g)*, genu of the corpus callosum; *CC(s)*, splenium of the corpus callosum; *C(h)*, caudate head; *C(t)*, caudate tail; *f*, fornix; *LV(a)*, anterior horn of the lateral ventricle; *LV(p)*, posterior horn of the lateral ventricle; *SP*, septum pellucidum; *Th*, thalamus; *III*, third ventricle. (Reprinted with permission from Gilman S, Winans SS. Essentials of clinical neuroanatomy & neurophysiology. Philadelphia: FA Davis Company, 1982:188.)

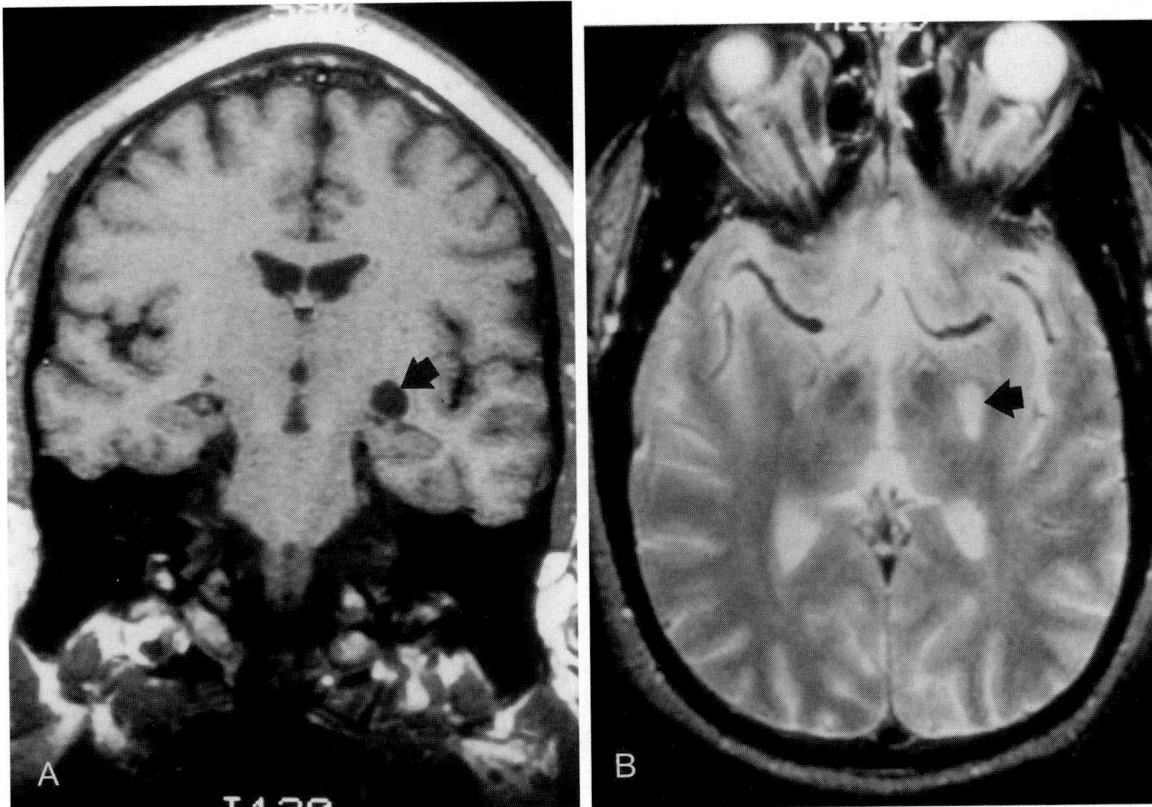

Figure 4.27. Virchow-Robin Spaces. Coronal T1WI **(A)** and transverse T2WI **(B)** show an enlarged but normal perivascular space (*arrows*) that exactly follows CSF intensity. There is no mass effect, and the patient had no symptoms referable to this region.

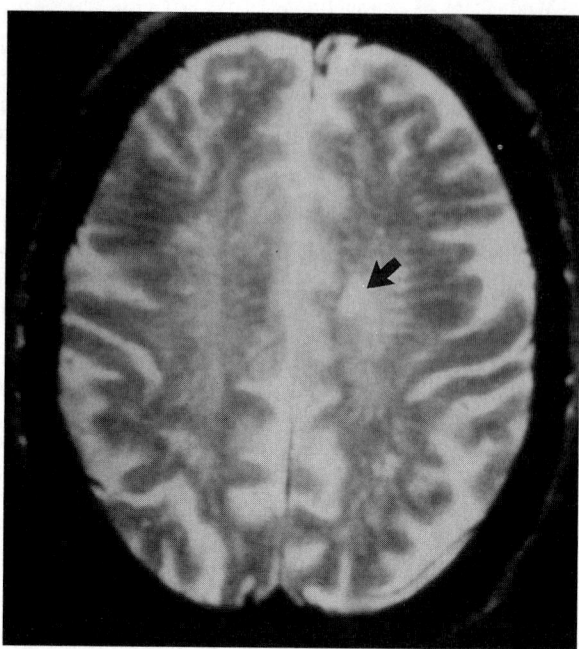

Figure 4.28. Small Vessel Ischemic Changes and Perivascular Spaces. Transverse T2WI at the level of the centrum semiovale shows numerous areas of hyperintensity. The radial, linear areas likely represent prominent CSF spaces around small medullary veins. A rounded lesion (*arrow*) indicates a site of probable small infarction.

leukoariosis, to name a few. There is no consensus on when these imaging changes should be considered abnormal and when they simply represent a normal part of the aging process. At one end of the spectrum are patients who have collected enough tiny infarcts over the years to impair brain function. Individually or in small numbers, these were presumably asymptomatic but in the aggregate lead to a multi-infarct dementia picture. At the other end of the spectrum are perfectly healthy patients who have presumably developed a speck of gliosis or occlusion of an inconsequential tiny vessel as a normal part of aging. The clinical findings must determine which of these patients with small-vessel ischemic changes needs further workup.

Vasculitis. Patchy inflammatory changes in arterial walls may lead to either large or small-vessel stroke. Vasculitis may be triggered by autoimmune disorders, drug exposure (heroin, amphetamines), polyarteritis nodosa, and idiopathic processes (e.g., giant cell arteritis). Vasculitic infarcts are often scattered across multiple vascular territories and may produce atypical patterns of damage. Varying stages of inflammation, necrosis, fibrosis, and aneurysms may be seen simultaneously.

Cases of suspected vasculitis are evaluated by conventional cut-film angiography, which provides the highest possible resolution. Views of the intracranial circulation and the external carotid artery are reviewed in search of irregular focal narrowing. Positive sites may then be selected for biopsy confirmation.

Sometimes the vessels affected are so small the angiogram is normal. In these cases, skin, nerve, muscle, or random temporal artery biopsy may be required to make the diagnosis. Diagnostic confirmation is important because many of the vasculitides respond to steroids or cytotoxic drugs.

Venous Infarction

Venous occlusion is an uncommon but important cause of stroke. Characteristically, venous infarcts occur in younger patients who present with headache, sudden focal deficits, and often seizures. Predisposing factors include hypercoagulable states, pregnancy, infection (spread from contiguous scalp, face, middle ear, or sinus), dehydration, meningitis, and direct invasion by tumor. Even though arterial supply is intact, blockage of outflow leads to stasis, deoxygenation of blood, and neuronal death. Continued perfusion into damaged, occluded vessels frequently leads to hemorrhage. Any dural sinus or cortical vein may be affected, but the commonest are transverse (lateral), superior sagittal, and cavernous sinus occlusions.

A pattern of hemorrhagic infarction in the deep cortical or subcortical regions is usually present. These lesions tend to be rounded and may spare some overlying cortex, as opposed to the classic wedge-shaped arterial occlusions, which grow larger toward the surface (Fig. 4.29). Venous infarctions may also be suspected when there is an apparent infarct not conforming to a known arterial territory.

The venous clot responsible may be seen indirectly as a filling defect in the superior sagittal sinus on contrast-enhanced CT, the "empty delta" sign (Fig. 4.30). The empty delta sign is usually present 1 to 4 weeks after sinus occlusion but may not be seen in the acute and chronic phases of the disease. Small venous occlusions are not reliably detected by CT. An appearance that mimics the empty delta sign has also been described in up to 10% of normal patients when CT scanning is delayed for more than 30 minutes after contrast infusion. This is probably the result of differential blood pool clearance and dural absorption of contrast, effectively highlighting the dural margins of a normal venous sinus.

A combination of spin-echo MR and MR venography probably provide the best imaging evaluation for dural sinus occlusion. On MR, venous sinus thrombosis is suspected when venous flow voids are lost and confirmed when actual clot is observed (Fig. 4.29). Normal but slowly flowing blood can sometimes cause high signal within veins, a potential MR pitfall in the diagnosis of venous occlusion. MR venography can be helpful in equivocal cases. A combination of spin-echo MR and MR venography probably provide the best imaging evaluation for dural sinus occlusion. Intravenous digital subtraction angiography in the venous phase remains a suitable alternative in areas where MR is unavailable; this is one of the few uses of this technique in which a large contrast bolus into the central venous system is followed digitally.

HEMORRHAGE

Hemorrhage occurs when an artery or vein ruptures, allowing blood to burst forth into the brain parenchyma or subarachnoid spaces. Although mixed patterns occur, hemorrhages are most conveniently divided into subarachnoid and parenchymal categories. Imaging studies are critical in determining the source of bleeding and in showing any associated complications. The location and pattern of hemorrhage help predict what the underlying lesion is and direct further workup.

Imaging of Hemorrhage

Hemorrhages are detected as a result of increased attenuation on CT and complex signal patterns related to iron oxidation on MR. In both cases, the formation of "clot," which has far less serum and therefore water than whole blood, also plays a role in the imaging findings. *A noncontrast CT should be performed when there is a question of acute hemorrhage, but MR is much more sensitive for evaluation of subacute or chronic hemorrhage* (Fig. 4.31).

The MR signal generated by blood depends on a complex interplay of hematocrit, oxygen content, type of hemoglobin and chemical state of its iron-containing moieties, tissue pH, protein content of any clot formed, and the integrity of red blood cell membranes. Dominant among these mechanisms is the oxidation state and location of iron species related to hemoglobin. Oxygenated hemoglobin is sequentially converted to deoxyhemoglobin, methemoglobin, and then hemosiderin over time. The magnetic properties of the resultant degradation products change the MR relaxation rates of adjacent

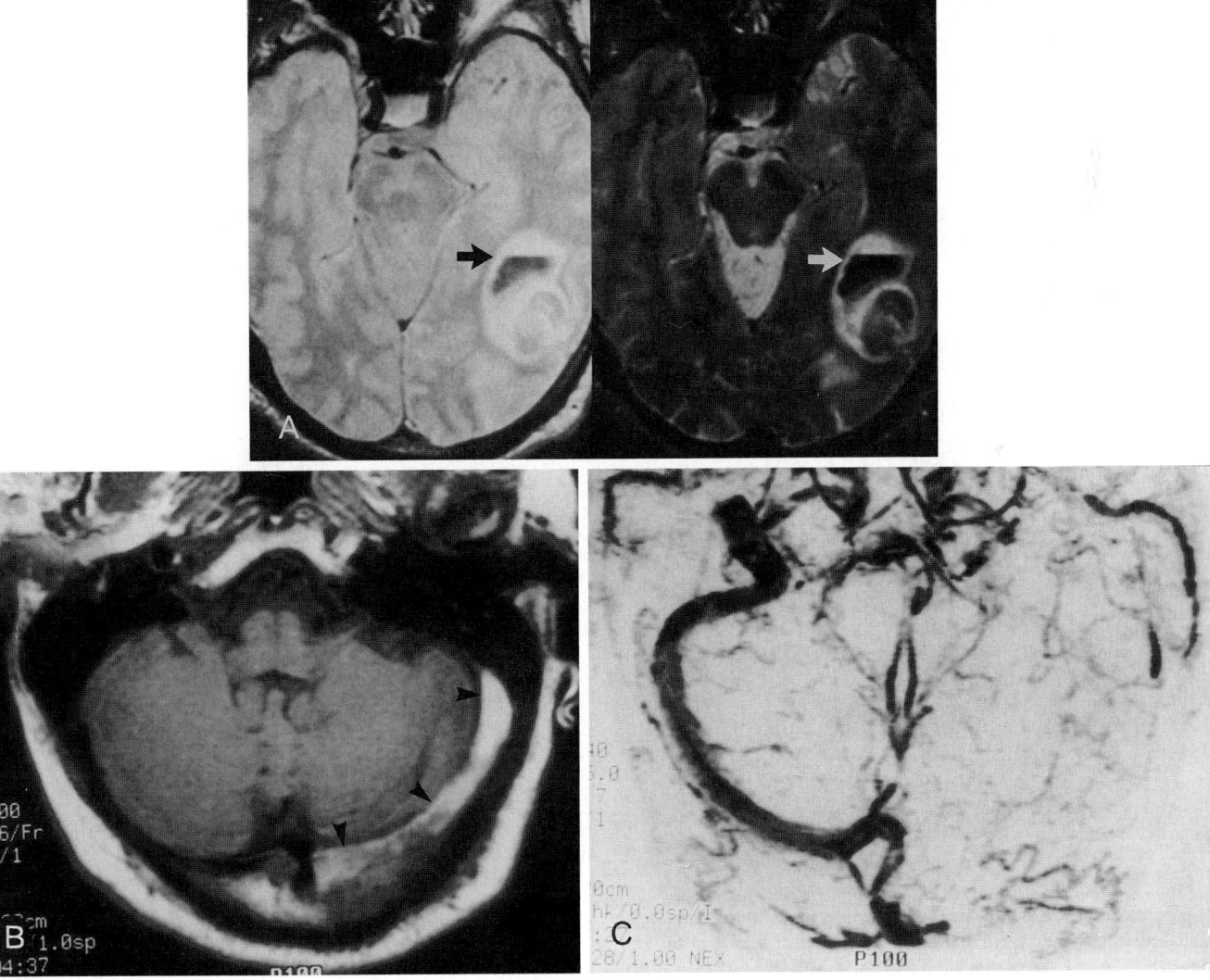

Figure 4.29. Transverse Sinus Occlusion with Venous Infarction. A. This patient presented with headache and new focal seizures. First and second echo T2WI show hemorrhage deep in the left posterior temporal region with layering of blood clot, the "hematocrit effect" (*arrow*). Signal intensities suggest a dependent layer of intracellular methemoglobin or deoxyhemoglobin with a supernatant of extracellular methemoglobin. A small amount of edema surrounds the hematoma. **B.** Transverse noncontrast T1WI through the posterior fossa shows hyperintensity in the left transverse sinus (*arrowheads*), consistent with thrombus containing methemoglobin. **C.** Submentovertex projection from a two-dimensional time-of-flight MR angiogram confirms normal flow on the right but lack of flow in the left transverse sinus.

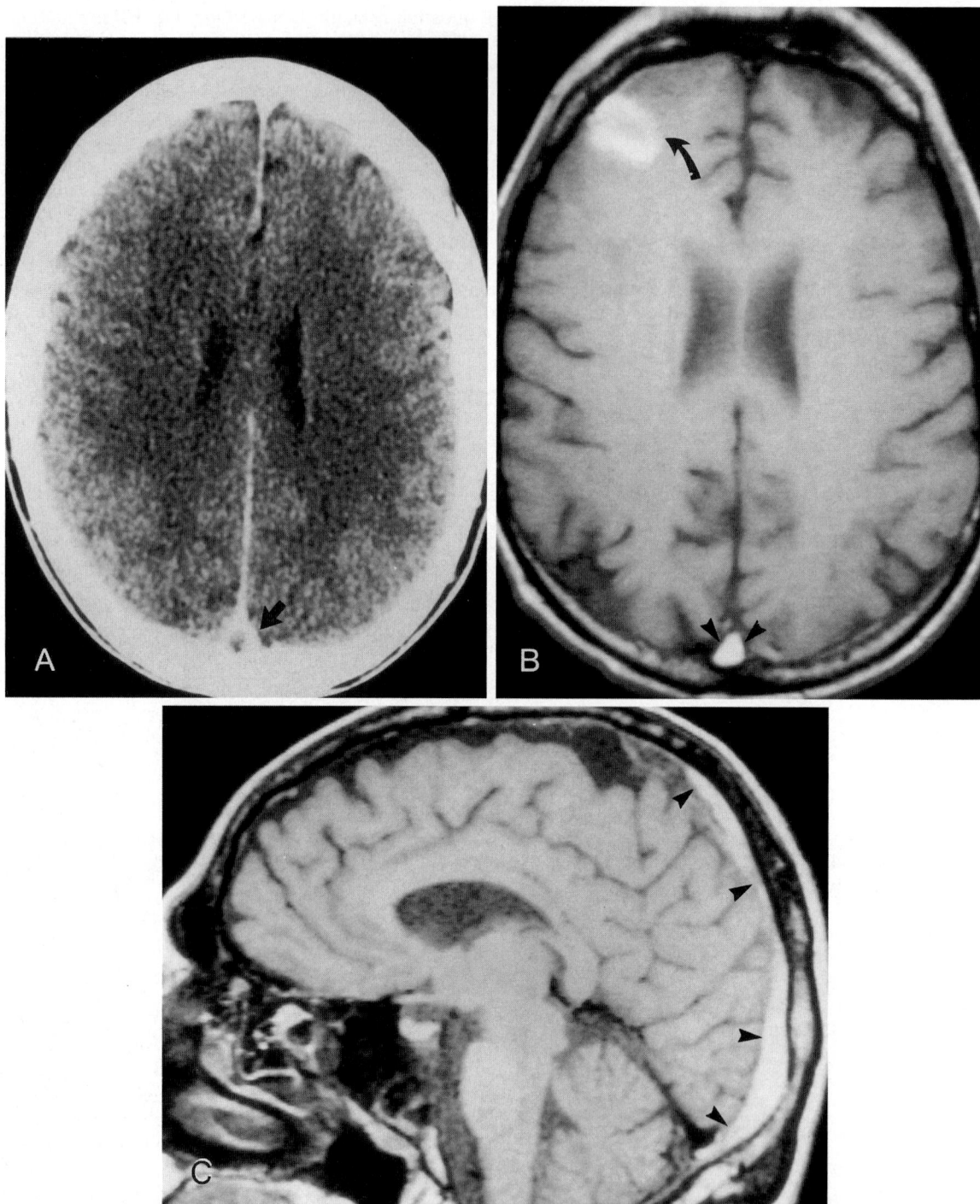

Figure 4.30. Superior Sagittal Sinus Thrombosis with Hemorrhagic Infarction. This patient was undergoing chemotherapy for lymphoma when he developed headache and was found to have papilledema. Venous occlusion was probably the result of dehydration. **A.** The initial contrast-enhanced CT shows a filling defect in the sagittal sinus—the "empty delta" sign (*arrow*). No hemorrhage was detected. He was treated with anticoagulants but presented 1 week later with worsening headaches. **B.** Follow-up axial noncontrast T1 MR shows high signal with mass effect in the right frontal lobe, indicative of hemorrhagic infarction (*curved arrow*). The normal flow void of the superior sagittal sinus has been replaced by high signal clot (*arrowheads*). Hyperintense blood on T1 indicates presence of methemoglobin. **C.** Sagittal T1 image confirms clot in the superior sagittal sinus (*arrowheads*).

protons, enabling the hemorrhage to be detected. A small halo of surrounding edema is common in the subacute phase of parenchymal bleeds, sometimes making interpretation of signal changes quite complex. High-field scanners and gradient-echo sequences tend to improve conspicuity of subacute and chronic blood products. The general pattern of MR signal changes seen over time on a 1.5-T magnet is summarized in Table 4.4 and in Figure 4.32. Individual cases may of course vary somewhat from these simplified guidelines owing to the multiple factors involved.

The complicated signal changes seen during the evolution of a hemorrhage can be understood within a context of physical chemistry. To change the signal characteristics of a tissue, hemorrhage must affect T1 or T2 relaxation. The sequential oxidation products of hemoglobin accomplish this due to changes in both magnetic properties and in molecular conformation. Iron within hemorrhage breakdown products changes the effective local magnetic field, a process known as magnetic susceptibility. This change in field is translated into an alteration in signal intensity because of acceleration or slowing of T1 and T2 relaxation rates. Changes in T1 relaxation occur only within a very short range (measured in angstroms), whereas T2 effects can be seen millimeters away.

Under normal conditions, circulating red blood cells contain a mixture of both oxyhemoglobin and deoxyhemoglobin forms. During transit through the capillary bed, tissues extract oxygen according to metabolic needs, converting oxyhemoglobin to deoxyhemoglobin in the process.

Neither of these forms have much detectable effect on T1 signal intensity in clinical images, but they may be distinguished due to their opposite effects on T2WI. *Oxyhemoglobin* is a diamagnetic compound containing ferrous (Fe^{2+}) ions, *detected as high signal intensity* on T2WI (particularly first echo). Deoxyhemoglobin also contains Fe^{2+} ions but is a paramagnetic substance. The magnetic susceptibility of deoxyhemoglobin causes accelerated dephasing of spins on T2 or T2*-weighted images (e.g., gradient-recalled echo sequences), which results in signal loss. *Deoxyhemoglobin* is therefore *hypointense* on heavily T2WI. These patterns are of altered T2 signal are occasionally encountered on clinical images of acute hemorrhage. Perhaps more importantly, dynamic magnetic susceptibility effects related to blood oxygenation form the basis for a number of emerging functional MR mapping methods (brain regions activated by a task recruit more blood flow and oxyhemoglobin, detected as a focal increase in T2* MR signal).

Table 4.4. Evolution of Hemorrhage by Magnetic Resonance Imaging

Time (d)	Red Blood Cells	Hemoglobin State	T1 Signal	T2 Signal
<1	Intact	Oxyhemoglobin	Iso/dark	Bright
0–2	Intact	Deoxyhemoglobin	Iso/dark	Dark
2–14	Intact	Methemoglobin (Intracellular)	Bright	Dark
10–21	Lysed	Methemoglobin (Extracellular)	Bright	Bright
≥21	Lysed	Hemosiderin/Ferritin	Iso/dark	Dark

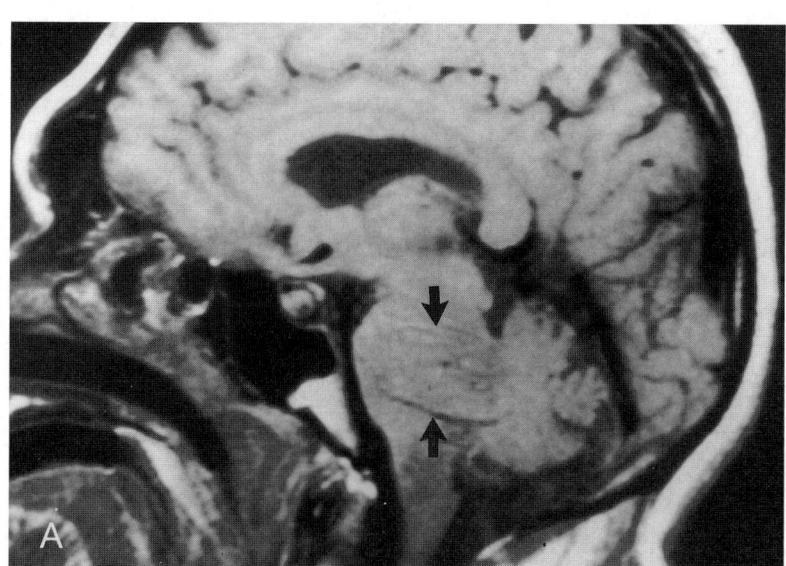
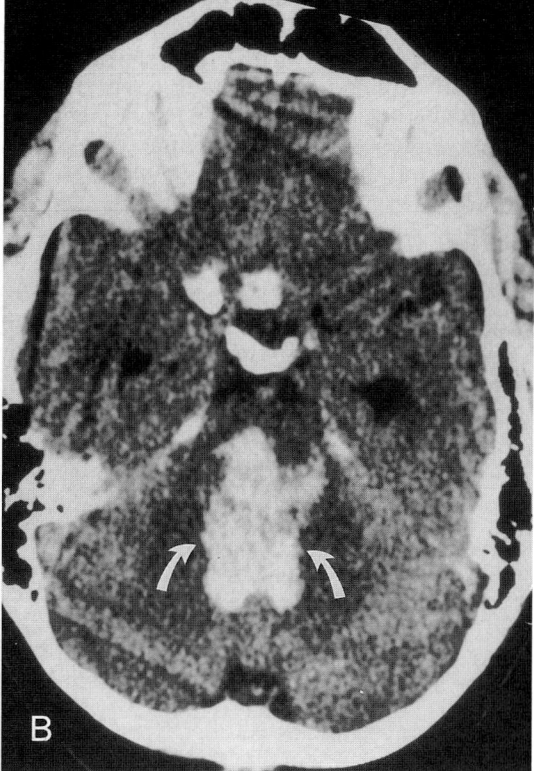

Figure 4.31. Insensitivity of MR to Hyperacute Blood. A patient who was undergoing anticoagulation treatment as a result of posterior fossa TIAs suddenly lost consciousness while hospitalized. **A.** Sagittal T1 MR done within an hour shows a suggestion of mass effect in the posterior pons and region of the fourth ventricle (*arrows*). Little if any signal change is seen, probably because the blood is still in the oxyhemoglobin and deoxyhemoglobin state. **B.** Noncontrast CT done immediately after MR confirms a very large hemorrhage (*curved arrows*).

Figure 4.32. Biochemical Evolution of Hemorrhage. Within minutes of hemorrhage, a hematoma consists of intact red blood cells containing oxyhemoglobin. Over several hours, the clot begins to retract and the hemoglobin is oxidized from oxyhemoglobin to deoxyhemoglobin to methemoglobin. Methemoglobin tends to form in a ring that converges from the periphery to the center over time. Red cells lyse, releasing methemoglobin into the surrounding fluid. Macrophages break down the iron products into hemosiderin and ferritin, leaving a stain at the periphery of older hematomas. (Reprinted with permission from Atlas SW. Magnetic resonance imaging of the brain and spine. New York: Raven Press, 1991:186.)

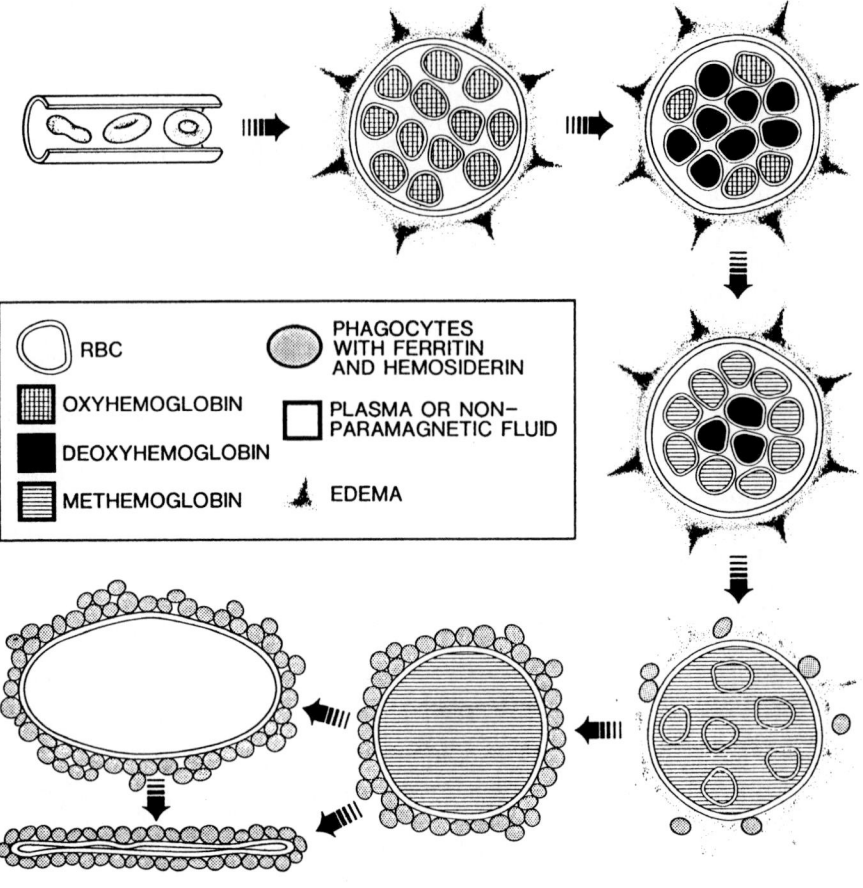

When hemorrhage occurs, oxyhemoglobin is converted to deoxyhemoglobin at a rate dependent on local pH and oxygen tension. This takes place for hours for parenchymal hematomas but can be considerably delayed when oxygen-containing CSF surrounds subarachnoid blood. This may explain why acute subarachnoid blood is relatively difficult to detect by MR. In parenchymal or extra-axial hematomas, further oxidation of deoxyhemoglobin leads to formation of methemoglobin, a ferric (Fe^{3+}) paramagnetic substance. This occurs over several days or longer, parallel in time course to lysis of red blood cells.

Methemoglobin causes a marked acceleration of T1 relaxation, leading to bright signal on T1WI (Fig. 4.8A). This T1 shortening occurs with both intracellular and extracellular methemoglobin. The influence of methemoglobin on T2 relaxation is more complicated and depends on whether it is intra-cellular or extracellular. Thus, methemoglobin contained within intact red cells is able to set up local field gradients between the cell and the protons outside; this magnetic susceptibility leads to signal loss on T2WI. After cell lysis methemoglobin is dispersed throughout the tissue water, the gradient is lost, and T2 relaxation similar to CSF is seen. T2WI of subacute hematomas therefore show a "hematocrit effect": a dependent layer of intact cells exhibiting dark signal and a plasma supernatant showing bright signal (Fig. 4.29A).

Further oxidation of hemoglobin and breakdown of the globin molecule leads to accumulation of hemosiderin in the lysosomes of macrophages. Hemosiderin causes the gross rust-colored stain at the edges of an old hematoma seen at surgery or autopsy, even years after the index event. It is a paramagnetic ferric (Fe^{3+}) containing substance that is insoluble in water. As a result, hemosiderin shows no appreciable T1 effects but very prominent T2 shortening (dark signal) due to magnetic susceptibility effects. An area of remote hemorrhage will commonly be seen as atrophy alone on CT or T1-weighted MR, but a dark rim along the cleft on T2WI implicates a prior bleed. Occasionally, large or recurrent subarachnoid hemorrhages will lead to diffuse hemosiderin deposition on the brain surface, a condition known as superficial hemosiderosis (or superficial siderosis).

Subarachnoid Hemorrhage

The subarachnoid space is the CSF-lined compartment that surrounds the blood vessels and communicates with the ventricular system. Subarachnoid hemorrhage (SAM) is most commonly the result of aneurysm rupture. Arteriovenous malformations of the brain or spinal cord and vascular malformations involving the dura may also cause SAH, but it is usually in combination with parenchymal or subdural bleeding, respectively. Previously normal vessels may rupture into the subarachnoid space when damaged by drugs, trauma, or dissection. SAH may also occasionally be seen in patients with marked thrombocytopenia or other severe coagulopathies.

Patients with aneurysms may develop symptoms attributable to either bleeding or local mass effect. Sudden, severe headache is the most common symptom of aneurysm rupture, sometimes described by patients as the worst headache of their life. Unruptured aneurysms or those with limited surrounding hemorrhage may also develop significant mass effect with or without headache. Classic presentations in this regard are the unilateral third nerve palsy resulting from a posterior communicating artery aneurysm, cavernous sinus syndrome from an internal carotid artery or parasellar aneurysm, and optic chiasmal syndrome (bitemporal field defect) from an anterior communicating artery aneurysm.

A patient who presents with SAH is very likely to harbor a ruptured congenital (berry) aneurysm (Fig. 4.33). One to two percent of us have aneurysms, thought to occur because of a congenital absence of the arterial media. Probably, many of these aneurysms remain asymptomatic, but those greater than 3–5 mm in diameter are at increased risk for rupture. Berry aneurysms often occur near branch points of the circle of Willis. Approximately 85% sprout from the anterior part of the circle of Willis, whereas 15% arise in the vertebrobasilar territory. Common locations include the anterior communicating (33%), the middle cerebral (30%), the posterior communicating (25%), and the basilar (10%) arteries.

Less commonly, the ophthalmic artery, cavernous ICA, or PICA is to blame. When distal branch aneurysms are seen, an episode of prior trauma or systemic infection should be considered (e.g., bacterial endocarditis with "mycotic" aneurysm). Other conditions associated with aneurysms include atherosclerosis, fibromuscular disease, and polycystic kidney disease. Management depends on the clinical situation and on location and size of the aneurysm. Treatment options include surgical clipping, interventional endovascular coil embolization, and combinations of the two (Fig. 4.34).

Even large acute SAHs easily seen by CT may be entirely missed on MR. CT is more than 90% sensitive for the detection of acute SAH, probably because of the increased density of clotted blood. Use of FLAIR sequences on MR can improve conspicuity of acute blood, but CT is still considered the imaging method of choice when clinical findings suggest the possibility of SAH. SAHs may be quite difficult to detect even by CT when the patient's hematocrit is low, the amount of hemorrhage small, or there is a delay in scanning. In these cases, detection of red blood cells or xanthochromia by lumbar puncture may be the only way to confirm a suspected SAH. The most sensitive places to look for SAH on CT are the dependent portions of the subarachnoid space where gravity causes the blood to settle—the interpeduncular fossa and the far posterior aspects of the occipital horns (Fig. 4.35). Prompt scanning is important, as dissolution of subarachnoid blood reduces CT sensitivity to 66% by day 3.

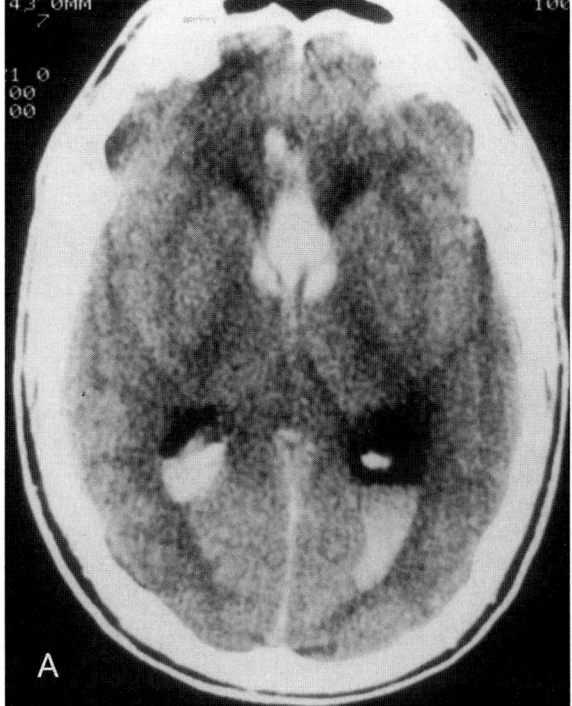

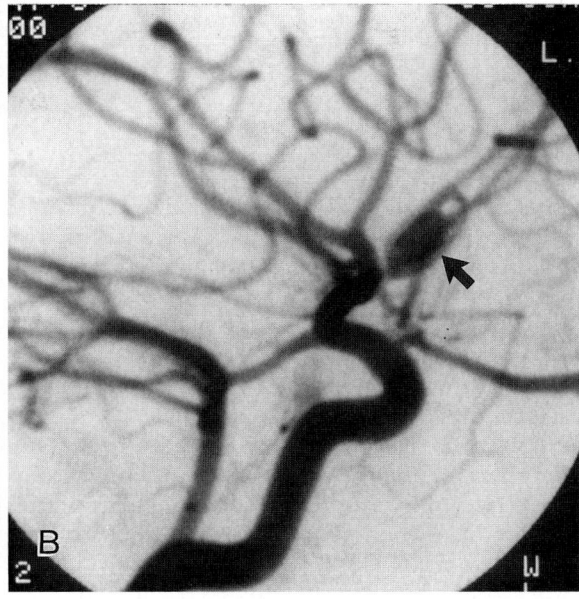

Figure 4.33. Ruptured Anterior Communicating Artery Aneurysm. This 21-year-old man collapsed immediately after snorting a line of cocaine. **A.** Noncontrast CT shows blood in the interhemispheric fissure and in the dependent portions of the lateral ventricles. Blood in the ventricles, cisterns, or layered in the sulci is subarachnoid by definition. **B.** Lateral view from a digital subtraction angiogram demonstrates a large anterior communicating artery aneurysm (*arrow*). Over half of all drug abusers with intracranial hemorrhage will be found to have an underlying aneurysm or AVM.

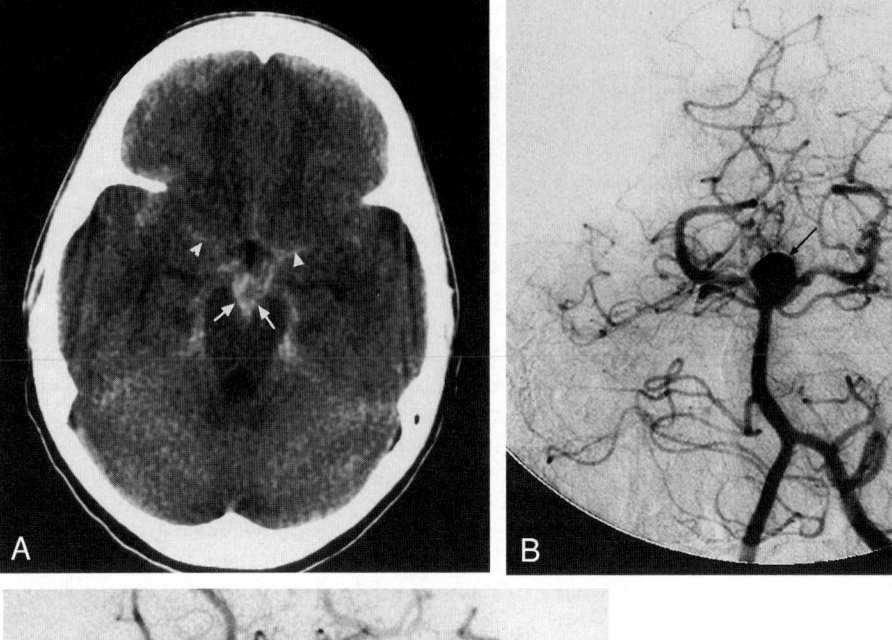

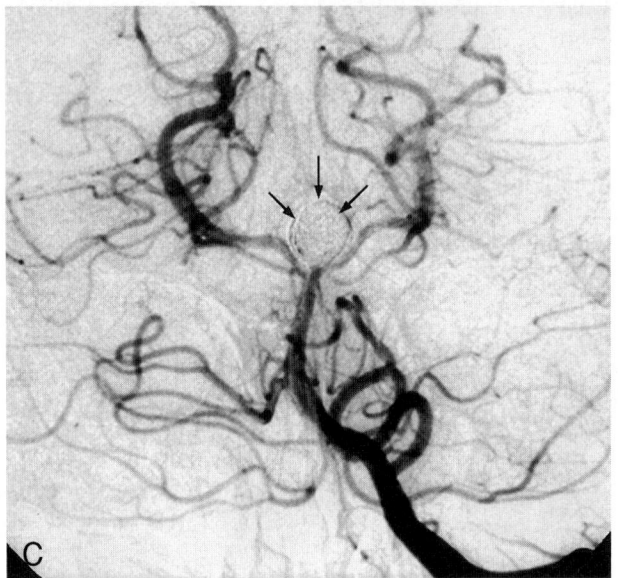

Figure 4.34. Endovascular Coil Treatment of a Basilar Tip Aneurysm. This 36-year-old patient presented with a severe headache. **A.** A noncontrast CT shows prominent subarachnoid hemorrhage in the interpeduncular fossa (*arrows*) and throughout the basilar cisterns (*arrowheads*). **B.** Angiogram, frontal view of a left vertebral injection shows a basilar tip aneurysm (*arrow*). **C.** Angiogram following endovascular placement of electrolytically detachable platinum coils shows obliteration of the aneurysm (*arrows*) with preservation of adjacent arterial branches.

Approximately 15–20% of patients with subarachnoid bleeding will have multiple aneurysms. Because of this multiplicity, a "four-vessel" angiogram is needed on the initial evaluation. Sometimes, special views or maneuvers are needed to make the offending aneurysm rear its ugly head (e.g., opposite common carotid compression to fill the anterior communicating artery). When multiple aneurysms are present, the one that is largest or more irregular, has focal mass effect, intra-aneurysmal clot, or shows a change on serial examinations is likely to be the culprit. Although MR angiography shows great promise for aneurysm evaluation in the future, it is not yet of proved reliability for the primary workup of a patient presenting with SAH. The combination of MR and MRA probably detects the vast majority of aneurysms greater than 3 mm in diameter, making it a reasonable screening tool for some at-risk patients (strong family histories, polycystic kidney disease, and so forth).

The location of blood in the subarachnoid spaces is imperfectly correlated with the location of a ruptured aneurysm, as subarachnoid blood can layer dependently. Sometimes, a parenchymal clot will surround the site of hemorrhage, or thrombus may be seen in the aneurysm itself. When the routine screening CT shows SAH, sometimes fine sections through suspicious areas will demonstrate the aneurysm. Within a few days, a focus of methemoglobin may pinpoint the bleeding site on MR. Unless there has been a massive SAH or rebleeding, subarachnoid blood is generally inconspicuous on CT at 1 week.

Intravenous contrast will also potentially improve aneurysm localization and characterization (e.g., Is there clot?). The condition of the patient and the philosophy of the surgeon determine which patients get contrast. Some surgeons operate within the first few days after hemorrhage, citing an early risk of rebleeding (20%) and the improved ability to manage hemodynamics aggressively once clipping is achieved. In this situation, contrast is not routinely administered because (a) the aneurysm needs to be characterized by angiography, not CT, for any surgical planning and (b) the contrast used for CT could limit the amount used in the subsequent angiogram or add to nephrotoxicity. Other centers routinely do the angiogram and operate after 10 days in order to avoid the period of maximal vasospasm (3–10 days). In this instance, contrast may be administered on a more routine basis. Use of spiral CT after intravenous contrast allows CT angiographic assessment for aneurysm screening, but like MRA, it is not generally considered definitive for management of the patient suffering acute stroke.

Follow-up studies are an integral part of SAH evaluation. The initial or subsequent CT may show communicating hydrocephalus requiring a ventriculostomy or shunt. Episodes of possible rebleeding are evaluated with noncontrast CT. Postsurgical angiography is used to assess adequacy of clip placement and to rule out vasospasm. Infarcts may also be seen in patients with elevated intracranial pressure or vasospasm and are the main pathologic finding in patients whose condition continues to deteriorate after the initial SAH.

Parenchymal Hemorrhage

Primary intraparenchymal hemorrhage occurs as a result of bleeding directly into the brain substance. Traumatic hemorrhages are not included in this section; they are discussed in chapter 3. Parenchymal bleeds generally have a higher initial mortality than infarcts, but on recovery, they show fewer deficits than would a similarly sized infarct. This is because hemorrhage tends to tear through and displace brain tissue but can be resorbed. A similarly sized infarct is made up of dead rather than just displaced neurons. The main differential considerations are hypertensive hemorrhage, vascular malformations, drug effects, congophilic angiopathy, and bloody tumors.

Hypertensive hemorrhages are seen in the putamen (35–50%), the subcortical white matter (30%), the cerebellum (15%), thalamus (10–15%), and pons (5–10%) (Fig. 4.36). As with lacunes, lipohyalinosis of vessels is thought to be the primary predisposing pathologic feature, although miliary aneurysms in the vessel wall may also play a role. Small hypertensive hemorrhages may resolve with few deficits. Bleeds in the posterior fossa, those with a large amount of mass effect, or hemorrhages extending into the ventricular system have a relatively poor prognosis.

Vascular malformations are far less frequently encountered than is hypertension, but they are a cause of hemorrhage that must be ruled out, especially in young patients. Vascular malformations develop because of a congenitally abnormal vascular connection that may enlarge over time. The relative frequency of vascular malformations as a cause of intracranial hemorrhage is approximately 5%. There are four main subtypes: arteriovenous malformations, cavernous malformations, telangiectasias, and venous malformations.

Arteriovenous malformations (AVMs) are the most

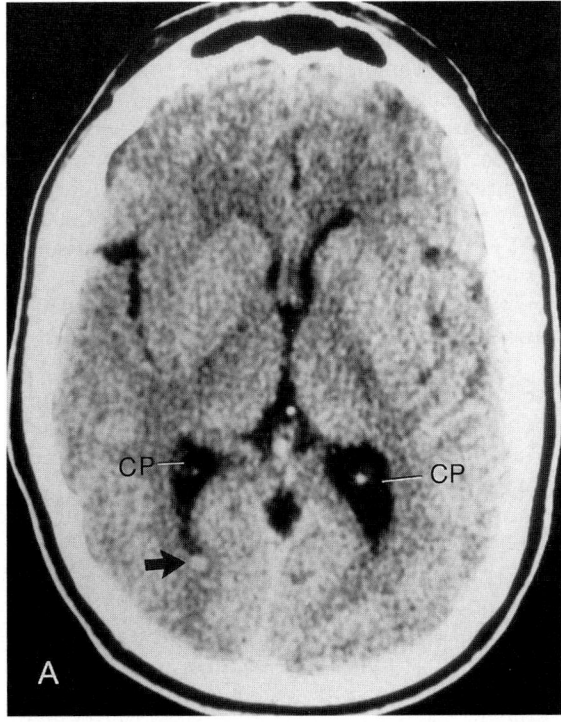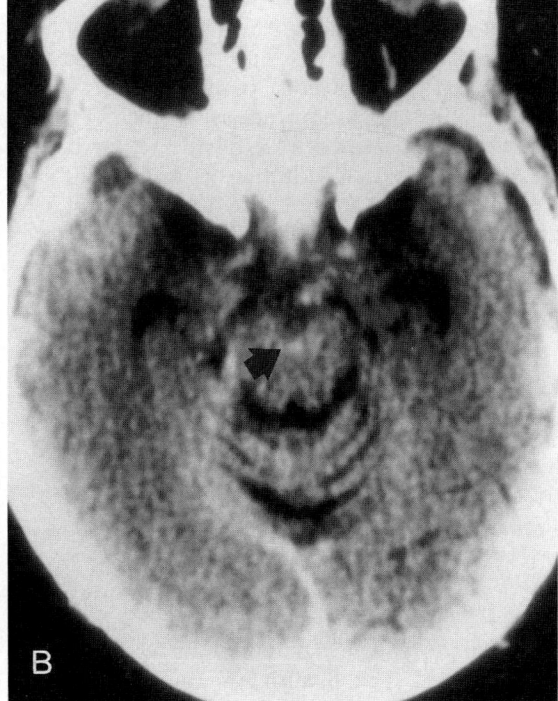

Figure 4.35. Subtle Subarachnoid Hemorrhage by CT. The most sensitive areas for detecting SAH are the dependent parts of the occipital horns **(A, arrow)** and the interpeduncular fossa **(B, arrow)**. The choroid plexus at the atrium of the lateral ventricle **(A, CP)** normally appears dense because of calcification or enhancement. The nondependent location of the choroid differentiates it from hemorrhage.

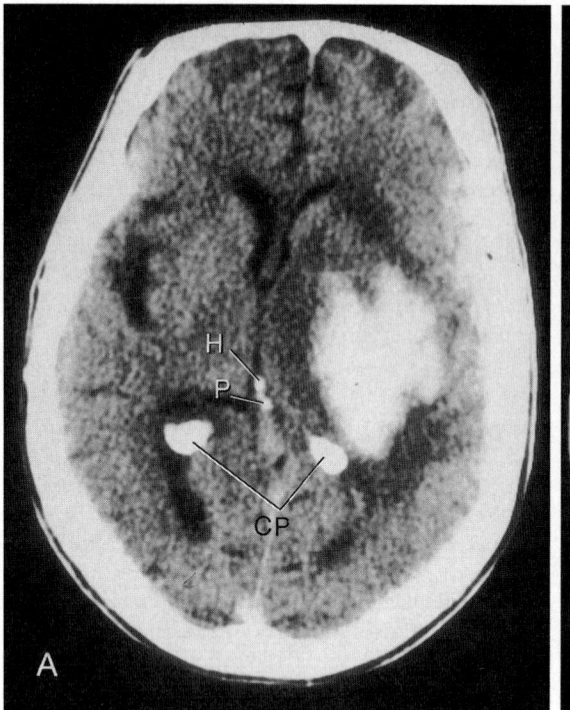
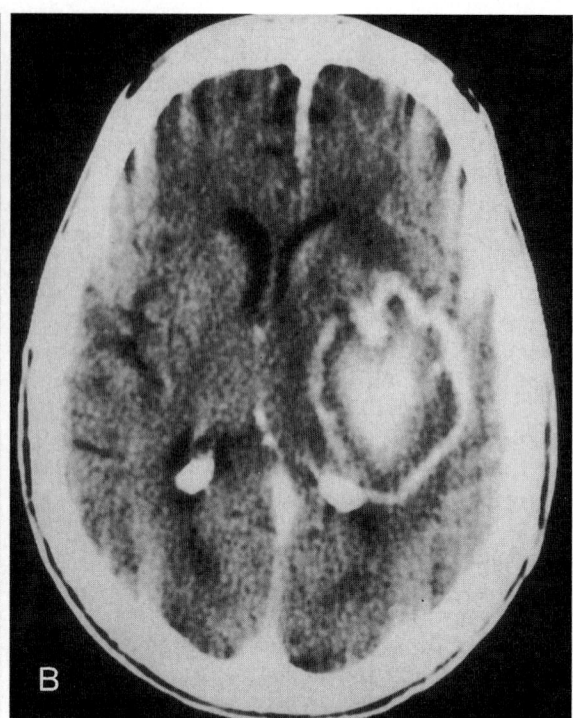

Figure 4.36. Hypertensive Putamenal Hemorrhage with Enhancement at 10 Days. The precontrast study **(A)** shows a large hematoma centered in the left putamen. Dense calcification of the choroid plexus (*CP*), pineal (*P*), and habenula (*H*) should not be mistaken for intraventricular extension. Moderate mass effect and a small amount of surrounding edema are evident. A ring of enhancement surrounds this benign hematoma **(B)**, likely the result of a vascular capsule. Resolving infarcts and hemorrhages normally show enhancement at the subacute phase.

common type of brain vascular malformation. AVMs are an abnormal tangle of arteries directly connected to veins without an intervening capillary network. Approximately 80–90% are supratentorial, but any area may be affected. Most patients present with hemorrhage or seizures. AVMs have a 2–3% annual risk of bleeding, but the risk may double or triple in the first year after an initial bleed. Treatment depends on the age of the patient, the patient's symptoms, and philosophy of the attending physicians. Embolization, surgery, and radiotherapy all may play a role.

Unruptured AVMs typically appear as a jumble of enlarged vessels without mass effect (Fig. 4.37). Noncontrast CT will show a mixed attenuation lesion, sometimes with evidence of calcification. MR demonstrates flow voids or complex flow patterns, sometimes leading to artifacts in the phase-encoding direction. T2- or T2*-weighted images may show dark signal intensity related to the AVM, a sign of prior hemorrhage with hemosiderin deposition. Intravenous contrast usually results in marked enhancement and, therefore, in increased conspicuity of the AVM on both CT and MR studies. Feeding arteries and draining veins may show impressive enlargement well beyond the center (nidus) of the AVM. Approximately 10% of AVMs will develop an associated aneurysm, generally on a feeding artery. Angiography remains the definitive method for evaluation of the AVMs anatomy.

Arteriovenous malformations can be difficult to detect soon after hemorrhage. Occasionally, the AVM will obliterate itself at the time of rupture, but more commonly, the resultant hematoma compresses and obscures many of the remaining vessels. Contrast studies may identify an enhancing portion of a vascular malformation adjacent to a hemorrhage. Normally acute hemorrhage will not take up contrast unless there is an associated vascular malformation. A subacute hematoma of any cause may enhance owing to a surrounding vascular capsule and should not be mistaken for an AVM (Fig. 4.36).

Cavernous malformations are thin-walled sinusoidal vessels (neither arteries nor veins) that may present with seizures or small parenchymal hemorrhages. These lesions may be asymptomatic and can occur on a familial basis. CT scans and angiography are usually normal. MR will show a reticulated, often enhancing lesion with dark rim (hemosiderin) on T2.

Venous malformations (or venous angiomas) are developmentally anomalous veins that drain the normal brain. They are seen in 1–2% of patients studied by contrast MR but may easily be missed on CT or noncontrast MR. The classic appearance is of an enlarged enhancing stellate venous complex extending to the ventricular or cortical surface. The MR appearance is usually diagnostic, but venous phase angiography may be needed in equivocal cases. Although these may bleed, treatment is somewhat controversial because they are commonly

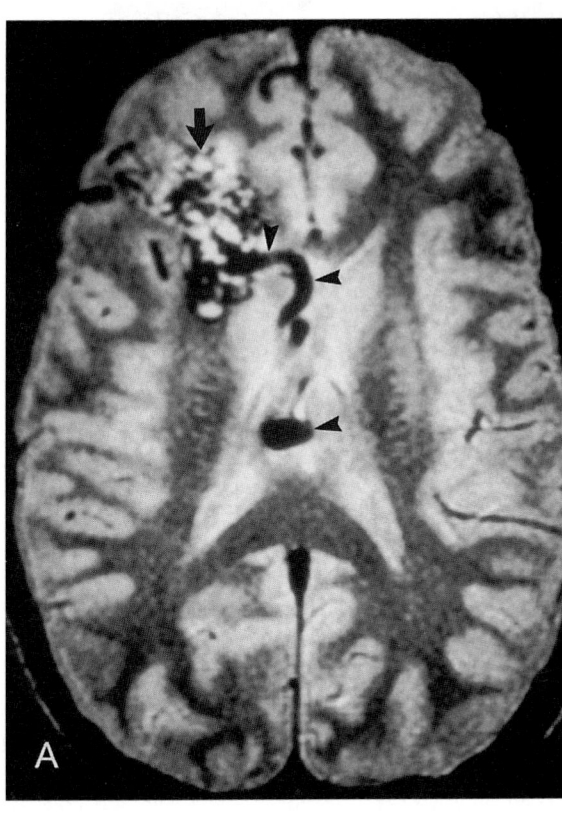

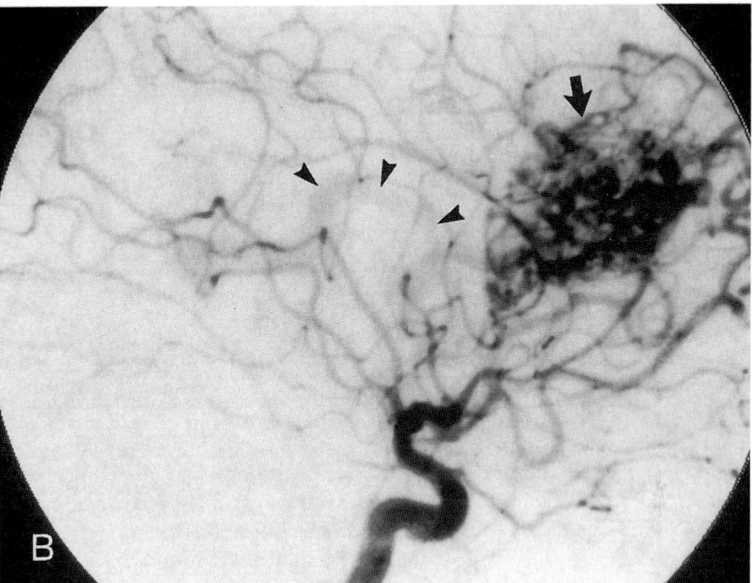

Figure 4.37. Right Frontal AVM. An MR was performed because of headaches. **A.** Transverse T2WI shows a large right frontal lesion (*arrow*) with a complex mixture of hyperintensity and hypointensity resulting from turbulent flow. A tortuous flow void headed toward the midline indicates a large draining vein (*arrowheads*). **B.** Digital subtraction angiography in the lateral projection (ICA injection) depicts the large frontal nidus (*arrow*) and tortuous draining vein (*arrowheads*).

seen in asymptomatic patients and are often the only venous drainage for a brain region.

Telangiectasias are dilated capillary-sized vessels usually diagnosed at autopsy. These are generally small, solitary lesions found incidentally by MR. No treatment is necessary.

Occult Cerebrovascular Malformations. CT and MR cannot always reliably distinguish among these subtypes of small, angiographically occult ("cryptic") vascular malformations. The generic term *occult cerebrovascular malformation* is used to describe telangiectasias, cavernous malformations, and small, thrombosed AVMs. Occult cerebrovascular malformations are usually inconspicuous on CT but may be detected as a small area of calcification. On MR, an occult cerebrovascular malformation should be suspected when focal heterogeneous signal (acute or subacute blood) is seen with a surrounding ring of hypointensity (hemosiderin) (Fig. 4.38). Venous malformations may provide drainage for occult cerebrovascular malformations, but no feeding vessels should be seen. Unless recently ruptured, an occult cerebrovascular malformation should show no mass effect or edema. If all these criteria are met, conventional angiography may be unnecessary.

Hemorrhage Resulting from Coagulopathies. Intracranial hemorrhage may also occur because of blood dyscrasias. Chronic oral anticoagulation increases by eightfold the risk of intracranial hemorrhage. The association is particularly true when the coagulation parameters are extended beyond the recommended therapeutic range.

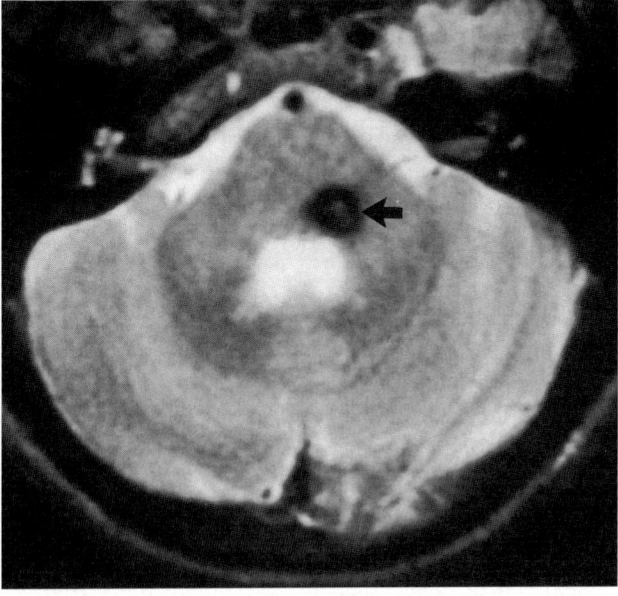

Figure 4.38. Pontine Occult Cerebrovascular Malformation. T2 transverse image shows a focal rim of marked hypointensity with slight central hyperintensity (*arrow*). The rim indicates ferritin or hemosiderin deposition, and the core represents subacute blood products or abnormal parenchyma related to the anomalous vessels.

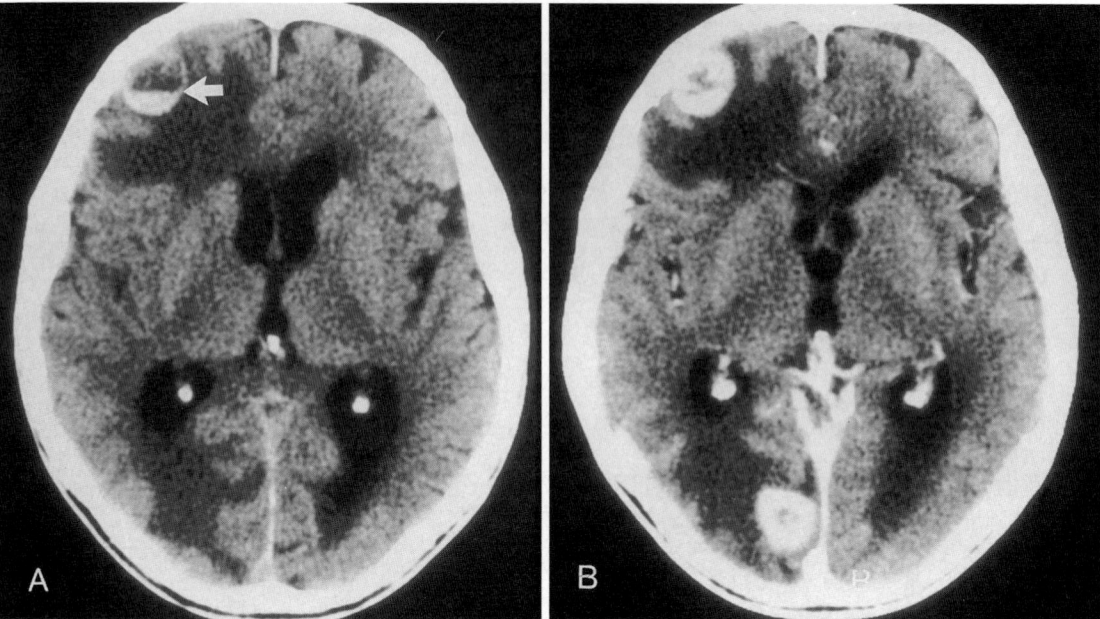

Figure 4.39. Hemorrhagic Metastases. This patient with oat cell carcinoma of the lung presented with new onset seizures. The precontrast CT **(A)** shows a rounded bloody mass in the right frontal lobe with a "hematocrit" layer (*arrow*). Marked white matter edema surrounds this lesion and is also seen in the right occipital lobe. Postcontrast scan **(B)** shows irregular ring enhancement of the bloody lesion, and a second discrete focus is identified in the occipital lobe. The degree of surrounding edema, focal and irregular enhancement, and nonvascular distribution implicate metastases and not stroke.

Drug-Associated Hemorrhage. Sympathomimetic drugs seem to provide an effective (if unintended) stress test for the presence of brain vascular anomalies (Fig. 4.33.). Drugs such as amphetamines and cocaine have been commonly associated with intracranial hemorrhage. Symptoms develop within minutes to hours following the use of the drug. The genesis may be related to transient hypertension or arteritislike vascular change similar to periarteritis nodosa. Up to 50% of drug abusers who suffer an intracranial hemorrhage have a demonstrable underlying structural cause such as an aneurysm or AVM.

Amyloid angiopathy or "congophilic" angiopathy is an increasingly recognized cause of intracranial hemorrhage, frequently lobar in nature. It is characterized by amyloid deposits in the media and adventitia of medium-sized and small cortical leptomeningeal arteries. It is not associated with systemic vascular amyloidosis. This angiopathy characteristically affects elderly individuals. Autopsy incidence rises steeply, ranging from 8% in the seventh decade of life to 22–35% in the eighth decade, 40% in the ninth decade, and 58% in persons older than 90 years. It is rarely seen in patients younger than 55 years. Cerebral amyloid angiopathy is associated with progressive senile dementia in approximately 30% of cases. Systemic hypertension is common in this age group but is not directly related to cerebral amyloid angiopathy. Amyloid is unique in that the associated cerebral infarcts and hemorrhages tend to occur in superficial locations rather than in the deep white matter and basal ganglionic areas. These affect the occipital and parietal lobes, where the angiopathy tends to predomi-

nate. More widespread, multifocal involvement can be seen in some cases, particularly when T2*-weighted MR sequences are used to make old hemorrhages more conspicuous. Amyloid angiopathy should come to mind when an elderly, frequently demented patient presents with new or recurrent superficial hemorrhages.

Primary Hemorrhage versus Hemorrhagic Neoplasm

Intracranial tumors are an uncommon but well-recognized cause of intracranial hemorrhage. They account for 1–2% of bleeds in autopsy series and as much as 6–10% in clinical radiologic series. Tumor necrosis, vascular invasion, and neovascularity may contribute to the pathogenesis of hemorrhagic neoplasms. Glioblastomas are the most common primary brain tumors to hemorrhage, whereas in the metastatic category, bronchogenic carcinoma, thyroid, melanoma, choriocarcinoma, and renal cell carcinoma often bleed (Fig 4.39).

It may be possible to distinguish between a hemorrhagic neoplasm and a primary (benign) intracranial hemorrhage on the basis of the MR findings. Intratumoral bleeds tend to be more complex and heterogeneous than benign hematomas. The expected evolution of blood products is commonly delayed with tumors, possibly because of profound intratumoral hypoxia. If a patient is scanned in the acute phase, lack of enhancement beyond the hematoma strongly supports a primary intracranial hemorrhage. If there is an enhancing component, then lesions such as tumor or AVM must be considered. In the subacute phase, a resolving hematoma may develop a thin area of ring enhancement of its own (Fig. 4.36). Both acute hemorrhage

Table 4.5. Features of Benign versus Malignant Intracranial Hemorrhage

Sign	Benign	Malignant
Evolution of blood products	Peripheral to central	Irregular, complex
Hemosiderin rim	Complete	Delayed, incomplete
Surrounding edema	Minimal/mild	Moderate/severe
Acute enhancement patterns	Minimal (unless AVM)	Moderate/severe

and hemorrhagic neoplasms may cause an edematous reaction, although in the tumors, edema is more predominant. In a benign intracranial hypertensive bleed, the edema should begin to substantially resolve within a week, whereas in the presence of a neoplasm, it should persist. With a resolving benign hematoma, a fully circumferential hemosiderin ring begins to develop at approximately 2 to 3 weeks' time on MR. In the hematoma associated with tumor, this hemosiderin ring may be absent or incomplete. These useful differential features are summarized in Table 4.5. Sometimes when the findings are ambiguous, a follow-up examination in 3 to 6 weeks will clarify the diagnosis, avoiding the need for a biopsy.

Primary Hemorrhage versus Hemorrhagic Transformation of Infarction

As discussed in the ischemia section, it may also be difficult to distinguish between primary intracranial hemorrhage and hemorrhagic infarction. In hemorrhagic infarction, arterial occlusion causes infarction of the parent vessel itself along with its brain territory. If clot dissolution occurs or if collateral flow ensues, blood may then be extruded from the damaged vessel wall. Hemorrhagic infarctions tend to be in classic vascular distributions and infrequently show much mass effect. They usually exhibit some degree of contrast enhancement, as blood–brain barrier breakdown is present by definition. They are not associated with intraventricular blood, which may accompany a primary bleed. Primary hemorrhage is characterized by disruption of the blood vessel wall, leading to extravasation of blood into the surrounding tissues, sometimes at a distance from the damaged vessel. Unlike hemorrhagic infarcts, primary hemorrhages may therefore cross vascular boundaries.

Suggested Readings

Atlas SW, ed. Magnetic Resonance Imaging of the Brain and Spine. 2nd ed. Philadelphia: Lippincott-Raven, 1996.

Atlas, SW. Intracranial vascular malformations and aneurysms. Radiol Clin North Am 1988;26:821–837.

Berman SA, Hayman LA, Hinck VC. Correlation of CT cerebral vascular territories with function: I. anterior cerebral artery. AJR Am J Roentgenol 1980;135:253–257.

Berman SA, Hayman LA, Hinck VC. Correlation of CT cerebral vascular territories with function: III. middle cerebral artery. AJNR Am J Neuroradiol 1984; 5:161–166.

Bousser M-G, Barnett HJM. Cerebral venous thrombosis. In: Barnett HJM, Mohr JP, Stein BM, Yatsu FM, eds. Stroke: Pathophysiology, Diagnosis and Management. New York: Churchill Livingstone, 1992:517–538.

Braffman BH, Zimmerman RA, Trojanowski JQ, et al. Brain MR: pathologic correlation with gross and histopathology. 1. Lacunar infarction and Virchow-Robin spaces. AJNR Am J Neuroradiol 1988; 9:621–628.

Brandt-Zawadski M, Atkinson D, Detrick M, et al. Attenuated inversion recovery (FLAIR) for assessment of cerebral infarction. Stroke 1996;27:1187–1191.

Brown JJ, Hesselink JR, Rothrock JF. MR and CT of lacunar infarcts. AJNR Am J Neuroradiol 1988;9:477–482.

Donnan GA, Davis SM, Chambers BR, et al. Streptokinase for acute ischemia stroke with relationship to time of administration. JAMA 1996;276:961–966.

Elster AD, Moody DM. Early Cerebral infarction: gadopentetate dimeglumine enhancement. Radiology 1990;177:627–632.

Fisher M, Prichard JW, Warach S. New magnetic resonance techniques for acute ischemic stroke. JAMA 1995;274:908–911.

Fisher M. Characterizing the target of acute stroke therapy. Stroke. 1997;28:866–872.

Gomori JM, Grossman RI. Mechanisms responsible for the MR appearance and evolution of intracranial hemorrhage. Radiographics 1988;8:427–440.

Hacke W, Kaste M, Fieschi C, et al. Intravenous thrombolysis with recombinant tissue plasminogen activator for acute hemispheric stroke: The European Cooperative Acute Stroke Study (ECASS). JAMA 1995;274:1017–1025.

Hayman LA, Berman SA, Hinck VC. Correlation of CT cerebral vascular territories with function: II. posterior cerebral artery. AJR Am J Roentgenol 1981;137:13–19.

Hayman LA, Taber KH, Ford JJ, Bryan RN. Mechanisms of MR signal alteration by acute intracerebral blood: old concepts and new theories. AJNR Am J Neuroradiol 1991;12:899–907.

Moulin T, Cattin F, Crepin-Leblond T, et al. Early CT signs in acute middle cerebral artery infarction: predictive value for subsequent infarct locations and outcome. Neurology 1996;47:366–375.

The National Institute of Neurological Disorders and Stroke rt-PA Stroke Study Group. Tissue plasminogen activator for acute ischemic stroke. N Engl J Med 1995;333:1581–1587.

Osborn AG. Introduction to Cerebral Angiography. Philadelphia: Harper & Row, 1980.

Savoiardo M, Bracchi M, Passerini A, Visciani A. The vascular territories in the cerebellum and brainstem: CT and MR Study. AJNR Am J Neuroradiol 1987;8:199–209.

Sorensen AG, Buonanno FS, Gonzalez RG, et al. Hyperacute stroke: evaluation with combined multisection diffusion-weighted and hemodynamically weighted echo-planar MR imaging. Radiology 1996;199:391–401.

Truwit CL, Barkovich AJ, Gean-Marton A, et al. Loss of the insular ribbon: another early sign of acute middle cerebral artery infarction. Radiology 1990;176:801–806.

Ulmer JL, Elster AD. Physiologic mechanisms underlying the delayed delta sign. AJNR Am J Neuroradiol 1991;12:647–650.

Vintners HV. Cerebral amyloid angiopathy, a critical review. Stroke 1987;18:311–324.

Warach S, Gaa J, Siewert B, et al. Acute human stroke studied by whole brain echo planar diffusion-weighted magnetic resonance imaging. Ann Neurol 1995;37:231–241.

Wolpert SM, Bruckmann H, Greenlee R, et al. Neuroradiologic evaluation of patients with acute stroke treated with recombinant tissue plasminogen activator. AJNR Am J Neuroradiol 1993;14:3–13.

Yuh WTC, Crain MR, Loes DJ, et al. MR imaging of cerebral ischemia: findings in the first 24 hours. AJNR Am J Neuroradiol 1991;12:621–629.

5

Central Nervous System Neoplasms

Kelly K. Koeller

Fortunately, neoplasms of the CNS are rare, with an incidence of approximately 20,000 new cases in the United States each year. For a disease entity that is comparatively uncommon, these lesions garner exceptional interest because of the dramatic and often catastrophic alteration these tumors produce in patients' lives. Approximately 15–20% of all intracranial neoplasms occur in patients younger than 15 years. Within this age range, 70% of these neoplasms are located within the posterior fossa, and metastatic lesions are rare. CNS tumors follow leukemia as the second most common type of all cancers in this group. In patients older than 15 years, approximately 70% of CNS neoplasms are supratentorial, and metastatic lesions are more common, comprising approximately 30% of all CNS neoplasms.

Although CNS neoplasms have been categorized classically (and with considerable controversy) according to their cell of origin by neuropathologists, it is most helpful for the radiologist to also consider the anatomic location of these lesions within the CNS. This chapter will consider CNS masses not only by their histologic composition but also by their differential diagnoses based on their specific locations.

CLASSIFICATION

Although modified several times, the basic classification scheme proposed by Bailey and Cushing in the 1920s remains the most widely used (1). Basically, this scheme recognizes seven cell types that give rise to CNS

neoplasms (Table 5.1). These include glial cells (composed of astrocytes, oligodendrocytes, and ependymal cells), nerve sheath cells (composed of Schwann cells and fibroblasts), mesenchymal tissue (composed of meninges, blood vessels, and bone), lymphocytes and leukocytes, germ cells, neuroepithelial cells, and finally endodermal, mesodermal, and ectodermal elements. Mature neurons do not divide and thus cannot produce neoplastic growth. Each of these cell types listed in Table 5.1 gives rise to a particular type of neoplasm. For instance, glial cells give rise to gliomas, of which astrocytomas are, by far, the most common. In addition, oligodendrogliomas and ependymomas are part of the glioma family. If the cell of tumor origin is not a glial cell, then the tumor is considered non-glial. These tumors include tumors of primitive bipotential precursors and nerve cells, nerve sheath tumors, mesenchymal tumors, lymphoreticular tumors and leukemia, tumors of maldevelopmental origin, and finally the phakomatoses. The histologic composition of these tumors is important to the radiologist because it directly impacts on the location of the tumor. Because glial tumors originate from glial cells, it is reasonable to deduce that these tumors must be of the brain parenchyma itself. Conversely, barring an invasive non-glial tumor, we will not see a non-glial tumor within the brain itself.

CLINICAL PRESENTATION

The clinical presentation of a CNS neoplasm is almost always related to either increased intracranial pressure, seizures, or a focal neurologic deficit secondary to the tumor mass (2).

Subfalcine Herniation. When the mass is located in certain key locations or when the mass is of sufficient size, portions of the brain itself may be pushed across the midline (subfalcine herniation) or through the tentorial incisura (uncal herniation and central descending transtentorial herniation). Subfalcine (or cingulate) herniation is the most common type of herniation. If the midline shift is 3 mm or greater, a significant subfalcine herniation has occurred. The falx is a very tough fibrous structure that is very resistant to any sort of displacement.

Uncal and Central Herniation. The uncus represents the hooked extremity of the parahippocampal formation of the medial temporal lobe. Uncal herniation often compromises the many tracts running through the brainstem as well as cranial nerves, particularly the oculomotor (III) nerves. Such compromise will result in ipsilateral pupillary dilation (or "blown pupil"). Effacement of the ambient cistern and contralateral hydrocephalus, which can be seen with imaging studies, are the hall-

Table 5.1. Intracranial Neoplasms and Their Cells of Origins

Type of Cell	Neoplasm
Glial Cells	
Astrocyte	Astrocytoma
Oligodendrocyte	Oligodendroglioma
Ependyma	Ependymoma
Non-glial Cells	
Nerve sheath cells	
Schwann cells	Schwannoma
Fibroblasts/Schwann cells	Neurofibroma
Mesenchymal cells	
Meninges	Meningioma
Blood vessels	Hemangioblastoma
Bone	Ostefocartilagenous tumors, Sarcoma
Lymphocytes, Leukocytes	**Primary**
	Non-Hodgkin's lymphoma
	Histiocytosis X
	Rare: Leukemia, Myeloma
	Secondary
	Lymphoma
	Myeloma
	Leukemia
Germ Cells	Germinoma
	Teratomatous types (embryonal carcinoma, yolk sac, teratoma, choriocarcinoma)
Neuroepithelial cells	Craniopharyngioma
	Rathke's cleft cyst
Endo-, Meso-, Ectoderm Elements	Epidermoid/Dermoid
	Lipoma
	Hamartoma

marks of uncal herniation (3). Central herniation (or central descending transtentorial herniation) is the downward displacement of the lower brainstem and cerebellum without horizontal displacement. Most commonly seen in bilateral or midline masses, central herniation results in complete obliteration of the cisternal spaces (4).

Hydrocephalus. The mass effect of an intracranial neoplasm may be sufficient by itself to produce increased intracranial pressure or hydrocephalus secondary to obstruction of the flow of CSF as it circulates through the ventricles and into the subarachnoid space. In either case, the increased pressure may produce a classic triad of headaches, nausea, and vomiting, and papilledema (caused by partial obstruction of the venous outflow from the optic nerve). This classic triad has a variable presentation, occurring early in the course, late in the course, or never (5). In addition, altered mental status, (particularly with bifrontal lobe tumors) or alterations in equilibrium (commonly seen in cerebellar or eighth cranial nerve tumors) may be present. Intracranial neoplasms usually present with an indolent course marked by progressive headache and focal neurologic deficit, but it may also present abruptly.

APPROACH TO A RADIOGRAPHIC ABNORMALITY

The detection of an intracranial abnormality on any imaging study should immediately cause the radiologist to ask three questions.

Mass? By far the most important question to ask is, "Is it a mass?" One must consider that abnormal signal intensity on either an MR or CT scan does not necessarily indicate a "mass." To call a lesion a "mass," it must have mass effect; that is, it must displace normal structures of the brain. Differentiation of a small neoplasm from a small infarct, however, may be very difficult. The clinical presentation may allow differentiation. When it does not, a follow-up imaging study (preferably an MR) in 3 weeks is often helpful. Virtually all (about 96%) of infarcts will be smaller in 3 weeks. If the lesion is the same size or larger at 3 weeks, a neoplasm should be favored. Also, as detailed in chapter 4, a subacute infarct will often show signs of subtle hemorrhage. In some circumstances, it may even be necessary to perform a second follow-up scan in 3 weeks after the first follow-up. Obviously, as the treatment of tumor and infarct are dramatically incongruous, the differentiation between a tumor and an infarct is critical to appropriate clinical management of the patient.

Intra-axial or Extra-axial? The second most important question to ask is, "Is the mass intra-axial or extra-axial?" An intra-axial mass is a mass that is of the brain itself (i.e., arises from brain parenchyma). An extra-axial mass refers to everything outside the brain (i.e., arachnoid, meninges, dural sinuses, skull, etc.). The ventricular system is also considered extra-axial. Determining the intra-axial or extra-axial origin of a mass allows the radiologist to formulate an appropriate differential diagnosis. Extra-axial lesions are characterized by "white matter buckling," or inward compression of the white matter (often with thinning of the fronds of the white matter) and maintenance of the gray-white matter interface (Fig. 5.1). An intra-axial mass, in contradistinction, expands the white matter, thickens its fronds, and blurs the gray-white matter interface. However, white matter buckling is not foolproof in differentiating extra-axial from intra-axial lesions. Where extensive white matter edema is present, buckling of the white matter may not occur. Thus, although the presence of white matter buckling is a helpful sign, its absence does not necessarily indicate that a lesion is intra-axial (6).

Tumor Margin? The third question often posed is, "Where's the tumor margin?" The answer is that it is not possible, unfortunately, by any imaging technique currently available to positively identify the margin of an intracranial neoplasm. By their very nature, virtually all glial malignancies will have—despite a grossly well-circumscribed appearance—some microscopic invasion into the surrounding brain parenchyma. The current wisdom is to treat the entire region of abnormal hyperintensity on T2WI, and not just the region described by enhancement on the T1-weighted postcontrast sequence (7).

Trying to make a histologic diagnosis from an MR or CT scan is fraught with hazard. However, rendering an intelligent analysis of the mass that includes an assess-

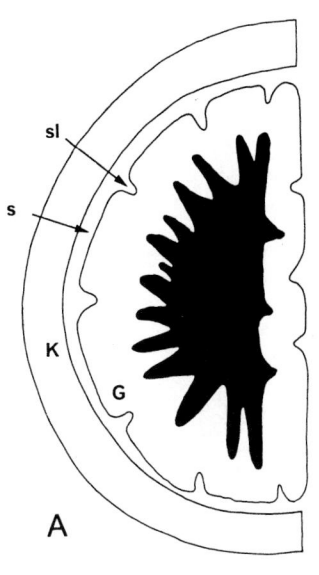
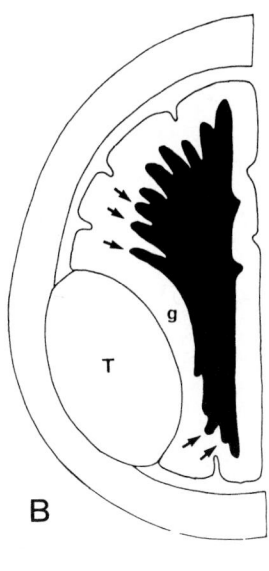
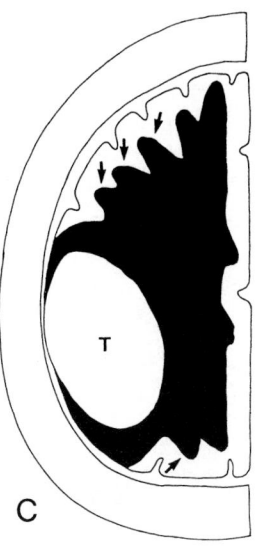

Figure 5.1. Extra- vs. Intra-axial Locations for Intracranial Lesions. The presence of "white matter buckling" may provide a valuable clue in determining whether an intracranial mass is intra-axial or extra-axial in location. **A.** Diagrammatic representation of normal axial image at level of centrum semiovale. Fronds of white matter (black area) insinuate themselves into cortical gray matter (*G*). *s*, subarachnoid space; *sl*, sulcus. **B.** Extra-axial tumor (*T*) crowds fronds of white matter producing white matter buckling. *g*, gray matter. **C.** Intra-axial tumor (*T*) expands white matter, thickening white matter fronds. Tumor is bathed by white matter edema. (From George AE, Russell EJ, Kricheff II. White matter buckling: CT sign of extra-axial intracranial mass. AJNR 1980(1): 425–430.)

ment of signal intensities and enhancement characteristics of the mass is possible. Therefore, presenting an accurate differential diagnosis is also possible.

IMAGING PROTOCOL

Imaging evaluation of intracranial neoplasms is best conducted by MR, which is far superior to CT because of its multiplanar capability, increased contrast resolution, and lack of ionizing radiation. CT is still superior to MR in the assessment of calcification although the use of gradient-recalled echo sequences increases the sensitivity of MR to calcification. CT is invaluable for the evaluation of bony abnormalities such as erosion of the skull base.

MR. A basic MR evaluation of a patient suspected of having an intracranial neoplasm includes a sagittal T1-weighted sequence followed by an axial T2-weighted sequence. An unenhanced T1-weighted sequence is performed to allow distinction between inherent T1 shortening, such as in hemorrhage, and contrast enhancement. Depending on the location of the tumor, either the axial or coronal plane is selected for this sequence. For temporal lobe and midline lesions, the coronal plane often provides the best delineation of the tumor. Whatever plane is chosen for the precontrast sequence, doing a postcontrast sequence in the same plane is imperative to accurately assess tumor enhancement. To assist neurosurgical planning, at least two imaging planes (usually axial and coronal) should be used for the postcontrast T1-weighted sequences. A sagittal postcontrast T1-weighted sequence will facilitate the placement of radiation ports. The performance of all of these sequences can be completed easily within one hour on current high-field (1.5T) units.

In the evaluation of posterior fossa lesions, imaging in all three orthogonal planes postcontrast is ideal. The postcontrast images should be performed with gradient-moment nulling (flow-compensating) technique, to decrease phase artifact generated by the dural sinuses (Fig. 5.2).

APPEARANCE OF TUMORS

The radiologic appearance of CNS tumors varies with cellular composition and the presence or absence of hemorrhage and calcification. On CT, intra-axial neoplasms usually appear as hypodense masses with a variable amount of surrounding white matter edema, the area of which roughly correlates with the aggressiveness of the tumor. On MR the mass is usually dark on T1 (T1 prolongation) and bright on T2 (T2 prolongation), with variable surrounding white matter edema. The presence of calcification within the tumor usually produces marked hypointensity on T1WI and T2WI. Because of the surface area of the crystals producing T1 shortening, however, calcification may occassionally appear bright on T1WI (8)

Nontumoral Hemorrhage. The appearance of intracranial parenchymal hemorrhage usually depends on the blood's age. In hyperacute (<6 hours) hemorrhage, the predominant oxyhemoglobin will produce T1 and T2 prolongation (dark on T1, bright on T2). When the hemorrhage has been present for 6–24 hours, the effect of deoxyhemoglobin predominates, and the lesion has mild T1 prolongation (dark on T1WI) and moderate T2 shortening (darker on T2WI). At approximately 3–4 days, methemoglobin begins to predominate, first being intracellular, producing T1 and T2 shortening (bright on T1WI, dark on T2WI) and then, as the red blood cells begin to lyse, becoming extracellular where the lesion has T1shortening and T2 prolongation (bright on T1WI and T2WI). In chronic hemorrhages (those older than 10–14 days), hemosiderin appears, producing a rim of extreme T2 shortening. This peripheral black rim occurs because of migrating macrophages that carry the hemosiderin to the periphery of the hemorrhage. On CT, acute hemorrhage (less than 1 week old) has increased attenuation (appearing bright) compared with brain tissue. By 1–3 weeks after the hemorrhage, the signal becomes isodense with brain parenchyma. After 3 weeks, the focus of hemorrhage will be hypodense to brain parenchyma, simulating the attenuation of CSF. This evolution of

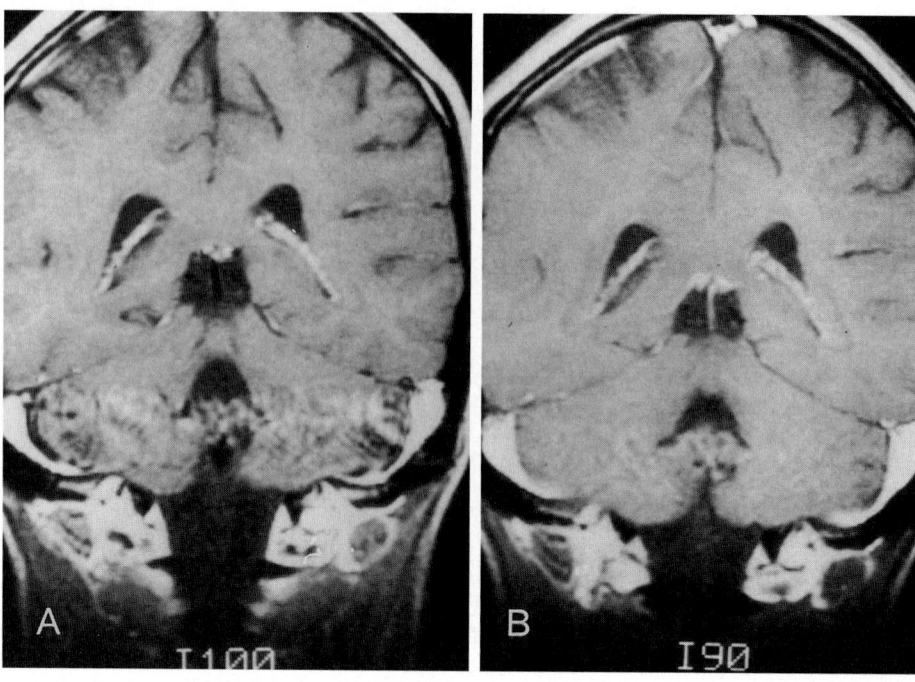

Figure 5.2. Flow Compensation in Posterior Fossa Imaging. Postcontrast images show the improvement in visualization of posterior fossa structures by employing flow compensation technique. **A.** Without flow compensation, significant phase artifact generated from the enhancing dural sinuses degrades the image. **B.** With flow compensation, the image is markedly improved.

blood breakdown products is illustrated in detail in chapter 4.

Tumoral Hemorrhage. The appearance of intratumoral hemorrhage reflects the heterogeneous nature of the tumor and is quite different than benign parenchymal hemorrhage. Intratumoral hemorrhage is often intermittent, producing a heterogeneous mixture of the various blood breakdown products just described. In addition, hemorrhage may occur in cystic or necrotic portions of the tumor, creating blood-blood or fluid-blood levels. Debris from the necrotic mass will also contribute to this heterogeneous mixture. Normal deoxyhemoglobin evolution is delayed, causing it to persist for longer than the usual 3–4 days after hemorrhage. The typical hemosiderin ring does not occur with intratumoral hemorrhage, probably owing to interference with the migration of the macrophages by viable tumor at the margins. In cases where confusion as to the nature of an intracranial hemorrhage exists, the presence of a nonhemorrhagic mass adjacent to the hemorrhage, the persistence of T2 prolongation (most likely representing edema or tumor itself), and mass effect all suggest intratumoral hemorrhage instead of a simple parenchymal hematoma (9). Gadolinium administration is often helpful in such cases because benign hematomas should not have as significant an enhancing rim as hematomas in tumors.

Hemorrhagic Neoplasms. Because of their high vascularity, certain neoplasms are noted for their propensity to hemorrhage. Choriocarcinoma among primary tumors and metastasis from melanoma, thyroid carcinoma, and renal carcinoma show this characteristic. In the setting of multiple hemorrhagic lesions within the brain, these tumors should be considered. Multiple cryptic arteriovenous malformations, either occurring *de novo* or secondary to radiation therapy, can have a similar appearance.

T1 Shortening. In addition to hemorrhage, two other entities may produce focal T1 shortening on MR scans. Lipomas or other neoplasms that contain fat (e.g., dermoid) will have marked T1 shortening and intermediate signal on T2WI following the signal intensity of subcutaneous fat. The presence of chemical shift artifact on T2WI associated with such a lesion helps confirm the presence of fat. Melanin, as seen in melanotic melanoma, also follows the same signal intensities as fat on T1WI and T2WI, distinguishing melanin from hemorrhage.

Hyperdense Neoplasms. Tumors of high cellular density—usually those with small cells such as lymphoma, pineoblastoma, neuroblastoma, or medulloblastoma—are usually hyperdense compared to brain tissue on CT. In addition, metastasis from melanoma, lung carcinoma, colon carcinoma, and breast carcinoma may be hyperdense. On MR, these same tumors typically are hypointense on T2WI with the appearance presumably being related to a high nucleus:cytoplasm ratio of the tumor cells, which produces less free water and thus less T2 prolongation. However, on occasion, isointensity or hyperintensity may be seen because of heterogeneity of the tumor matrix.

Enhancement. Contrast enhancement, whether from the iodinated contrast agents used in CT or the paramagnetic gadolinium agents used in MR, works on the same principle: breakdown of the blood-brain barrier. Unlike nonneural endothelium, the endothelium of the cerebral capillaries allows the passage of only small molecules through the tight junctions and narrow intercellular gaps. The macromolecules that comprise contrast agents are too large to pass this barrier under normal circumstances (10). The blood-brain barrier breaks down in many pathologic states, including intra-axial and extra-axial tumors (either primary or metastatic), inflammatory diseases, subacute infarcts, postoperative gliosis, and radiation necrosis. However, some tumors, particularly low-grade neoplasms, will not show enhancement, presumably because they form new capillaries that are quite similar to the native cerebral capillaries, thus leaving the blood-brain barrier intact. More aggressive neoplasms have fenestrated capillaries, allowing the passage of contrast media and facilitating image enhancement. However, that a lesion enhances only means that the blood-brain barrier breaks down. Therefore, the presence or absence of enhancement cannot always be used to categorically state that a lesion is malignant or benign (Fig. 5.3). In addition, some specialized areas of the brain, such as the choroid plexus, pituitary and pineal glands, tuber cinereum, and area postrema, have no blood-brain barrier and will normally enhance after administration of a contrast agent (10).

THE POSTOPERATIVE PATIENT

In the evaluation of the postoperative brain tumor patient, timing is essential. Ideally, these patients should have an MR scan performed within 72 hours after surgery to serve as a baseline scan for future follow-up. Scar tissue, which occurs in all patients who have had neurosurgical transgression of the blood-brain barrier, takes approximately 72 hours to fully develop and enhances after administration of contrast. Once formed, the scar tissue in the operative site and dura may persist for weeks to months. Because most malignant brain tumors have some enhancement, if the patient can be scanned within this 72 hour "window," enhancement can be interpreted as being secondary to residual tumor and not to granulation tissue. After 72 hours, distinguishing between enhancing tumor and enhancing scar tissue becomes difficult.

Safety. Postoperative neurosurgical patients are often not ideal candidates for scanning in an MR unit, and monitoring of vital signs is usually required to ensure their safety. If proper monitoring and life-support equipment (e.g., shielded pulse oximeter and oxygen) and personnel for MR are not available, a contrast-enhanced CT can be substituted.

THE FOLLOW-UP SCAN

Many malignant tumors can be treated by a combination of chemotherapy and radiation therapy following surgical debulking. Typical radiation doses are in the range of 5000–5400 rads, most often delivered in divided doses (approximately 180 rads each visit) over several weeks. As a consequence of these hefty doses, radiation injury may occur. This occurs in two forms: focal radiation necrosis and diffuse white matter injury. Radiation necrosis is seen on imaging studies as having mass effect and enhancement whereas diffuse radiation injury presents as T2 hyperintensity, without mass effect or enhancement, and is more commonly seen following whole-brain or large-volume radiation. Clinically, radiation necrosis occurs with focal neurologic deficits, but diffuse white matter injury is often asymptomatic (11). When radiation necrosis occurs in the vicinity of the operative site (and this is where it is most likely to occur), reliably distinguishing it from tumor recurrence by CT or MR is not possible (12). Positron emission tomography (PET) or SPECT-Thallium studies are effective in making this distinction (12). White matter hyperintensity on T2WI caused by diffuse radiation injury will conform to the selected radiation ports and should not be misinterpreted as vasogenic edema from the tumor.

SPECIFIC NEOPLASMS

It is hazardous, in many circumstances, to suggest a specific *histologic* diagnosis based on the imaging char-

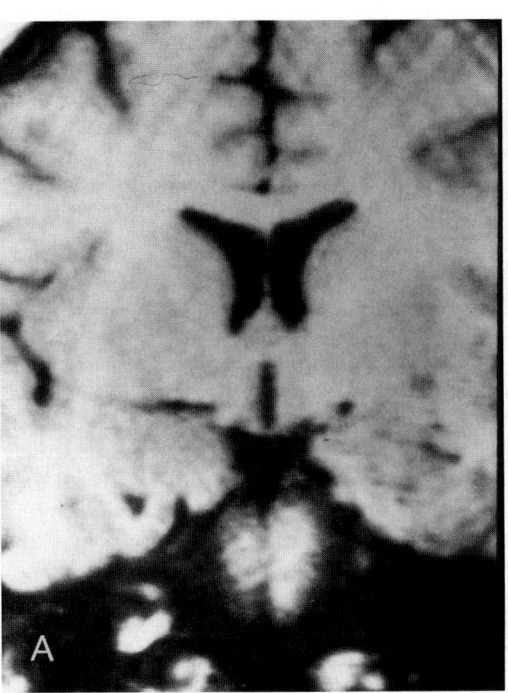 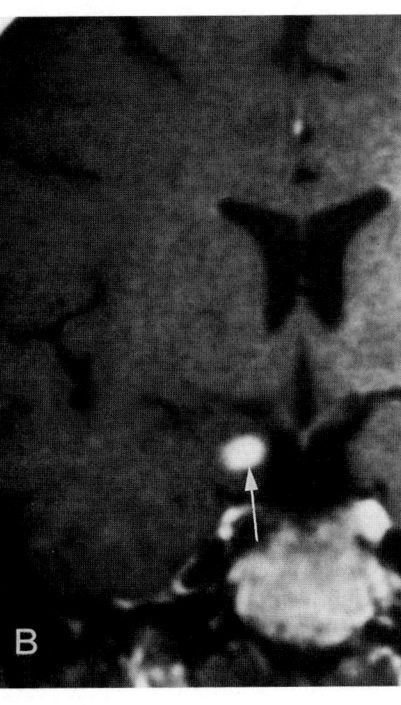

Figure 5.3. Enhancement: Benign or Malignant? Young adult female with long history of medically refractory seizures. Intense enhancement (*arrow*) of temporal lobe lesion pathologically proven to be a ganglioglioma, a low-grade neoplasm.

Table 5.2. Tumor Predominance by Gender

Females	Males
Meningioma (4:1)	Pineal germinoma (10:1)
Neurofibroma	Pineal parenchymal tumor (4–7:1)
Pineocytoma	Medulloblastoma (3:1)
Pituitary tumor	Glioblastoma multiforme (3:2)
	Choroid plexus papilloma (2:1)
	CNS lymphoma
	Hamartoma of the tuber cinereum

acteristics alone. However, taking into account other factors such as the location of these tumors (intra-axial, extra-axial, intraventricular, sellar, pineal region) and clinical information (age, sex, endocrinologic data, etc.), the differential diagnosis can be limited to just a few possibilities and sometimes a single most probable entity. Some intracranial tumors have a definite predilection for one sex; these are listed in Table 5.2.

Glial Tumors

Gliomas, which are derived from glial cells (astrocytes, oligodendrocytes, ependymal cells), account for 40–50% of all primary CNS neoplasms.

ASTROCYTOMAS

Astrocytomas comprise 70% of all gliomas. These neoplasms have been graded according to degree of histologic malignancy. Originally, astrocytomas were divided into four grades: grades 1 and 2 for low-grade tumors and grades 3 and 4 for high-grade tumors. Glioblastoma multiforme, the most malignant form of astrocytomas, was considered a grade 4 lesion. Today, there has been greater use of a three-tiered system with well-differentiated (fibrillary) astrocytoma at one end, anaplastic astrocytoma occupying an intermediate grade, and the highly malignant glioblastoma multiforme (GBM)/highly anaplastic astrocytoma (HAA) at the other. Glial tumors do not have a capsule and therefore are malignant. However, the low-grade fibrillary astrocytomas are usually so slow-growing and exhibit such nonaggressive behavior that patients with these tumors often do well with surgical resection alone. Prognosis for these tumors is measured in years.

Low-grade Tumors. The low-grade or "benign" astrocytoma and the high-grade or "malignant" astrocytoma have certain clinical and pathologic features that aid in distinguishing the two. Benign astrocytomas occur in younger patients, usually children and adults aged 20–40 years. These well-demarcated tumors have no necrosis or neovascularity, rarely hemorrhage, and are often cystic. They show calcification in 20% of cases and rarely have surrounding edema. On CT, they are hypodense with little or no enhancement. On MR, compared to gray matter, they are hypointense on T1WI, hyperintense on T2WI, and show minimal enhancement (Fig. 5.4).

High-grade Tumors. In contrast, the malignant astrocytoma usually occurs in patients older than 40

years. These tumors are poorly delineated microscopically although they may appear well-circumscribed grossly. Necrosis, hemorrhage, and neovascularity are common. Surrounding white matter edema is very common (Table 5.3). On CT, they are typically heterogeneous with intense enhancement, often in a ring-like pattern. On MR they are isointense to hypointense compared to gray matter on T1WI and hyperintense on T2WI. A ring-like pattern following contrast may be seen (Fig. 5.5).

Pathology. Astrocytomas demonstrate a paradox in their gross appearances. The well-differentiated low-grade astrocytomas insinuate themselves through the neurons and other supporting cells that make up the "scaffold" of the brain parenchyma, whereas the highly-malignant GBM is macroscopically better circumscribed. All astrocytomas are poorly circumscribed upon microscopic examination. All will show extension into normal brain tissue beyond the expected margin of the tumor noted on gross inspection. If necrosis is present, the pathologist considers the lesion to be a GBM/HAA; if necrosis is not present, the lesion is considered an anaplastic astrocytoma. As GBM and HAA have essentially the same biologic behavior, they can be considered synonymous.

Spread. Gliomas spread from their native site by one of four ways. They may spread by way of natural passages or along subpial or subependymal surfaces. They may spread via the white matter tracts, such as the corona radiata, corticospinal tracts, corpus collosum, and commissures. Finally, tumors may also spread across the meninges.

Glioblastoma Multiforme

Glioblastoma multiforme (GBM) is the most malignant type of and most common form of glioma. The peak age of incidence is 45–55 years, with males slightly more commonly affected. The deep white matter of the frontal lobe, the largest lobe in the brain, is the most common location followed by the temporal lobe and basal ganglia.

Imaging. The radiologic appearance reflects the pattern of necrosis, hemorrhage, and neovascularity seen pathologically. The classic appearance of a GBM on either CT or MR is an expansile mass with central necrosis, ring enhancement, and a large surrounding region of white matter edema (13). On non-contrast CT, GBMs are heterogeneous and lobulated with marked surrounding white matter edema. Calcification occurs occasionally, and necrosis and hemorrhage are common. The most common hemorrhagic neoplasms in the brain are GBM, metastasis, and oligodendroglioma (Table 5.4). On contrast-enhanced CT, more than 90% of GBMs will show at least some enhancement, usually in an irregular, occasionally nodular, ring-like pattern. On MR the tumor nidus commonly shows T1 and T2 prolongation (dark on

Table 5.3. Intra-axial Lesions with Marked Surrounding Edema

Metastasis	Radiation necrosis
Abscess	Hematoma (mild)
Glioma	

T1WI, bright on T2WI) compared with gray matter (Fig. 5.5). Because of cellular debris from the necrosis, the signal intensity of these "cystic areas" is usually slightly different than normal CSF.

Ring Enhancement. In addition to GBMs, many other lesions can present as ring-enhancing masses. A convenient method to remember these is by the mnemonic "magic doctor" (MAGIC DR) (Table 5.5). The first three

entities (metastasis, abscess, and glioma) are in order of frequency. The irregular ring of a neoplasm is often distinct from the smooth ring usually seen in cerebral abscesses (compare Fig. 5.5 with Fig. 6.3A). Furthermore, an abscess rim typically is hyperintense on T1WI and hy-

Table 5.4. Hemorrhagic Tumors

Glioblastoma multiforme—most common overall
Metastasis—second most common overall
Oligodendroglioma—second most common primary tumor

Table 5.5. Ring-enhancing Lesions ("Magic DR")

Metastasis
Abscess
Glioma
Infarct
Contusion
Demyelinating disease
Resolving hematoma

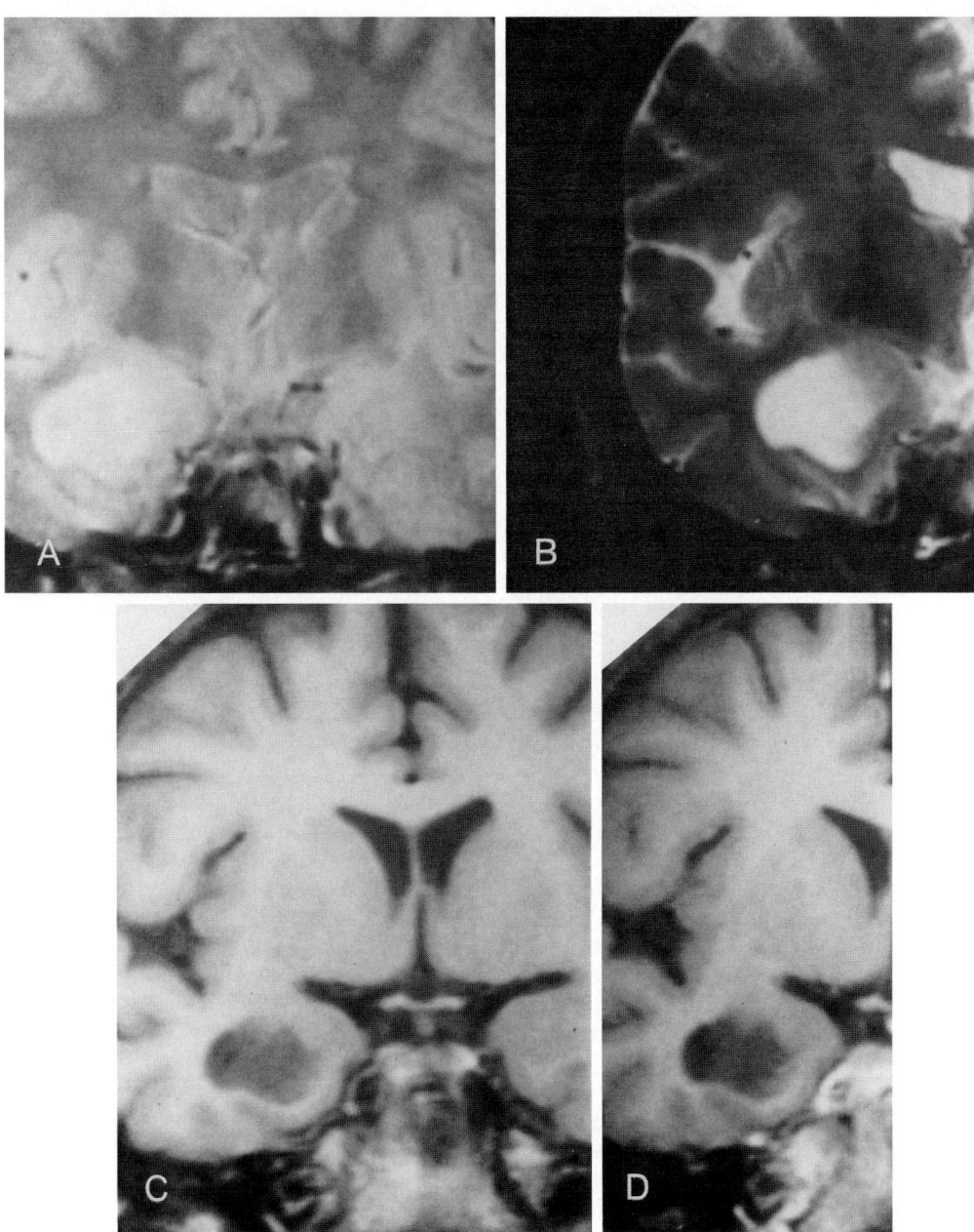

Figure 5.4. Typical Appearance of Low-grade Astrocytoma. A, B. Hyperintense well-defined temporal lobe mass on T2WI. Precontrast **(C)** and postcontrast **(D)** T1WI show hypointense mass without enhancement.

Figure 5.5. Glioblastoma Multiforme.
A,B. Axial T2WI show large areas of hy-perintensity predominantly in the left cerebral hemisphere. Note the dark rim lesions (*small arrows*) of anterior left temporal lobe and of left posterior peri-ventricular area. Also note abnormal hyperintensity (*large arrow*) extending across splenium of corpus collosum. **C,D.** Postcontrast T1WI through same levels as in **(A)** and **(B)** shows multiple enhancing lesions corresponding to ar-eas of T2 hyperintensity. Central area of hypointensity (*arrow*) within left tempo-ral lesion was proven pathologically to be necrosis, characteristic of GBMs.

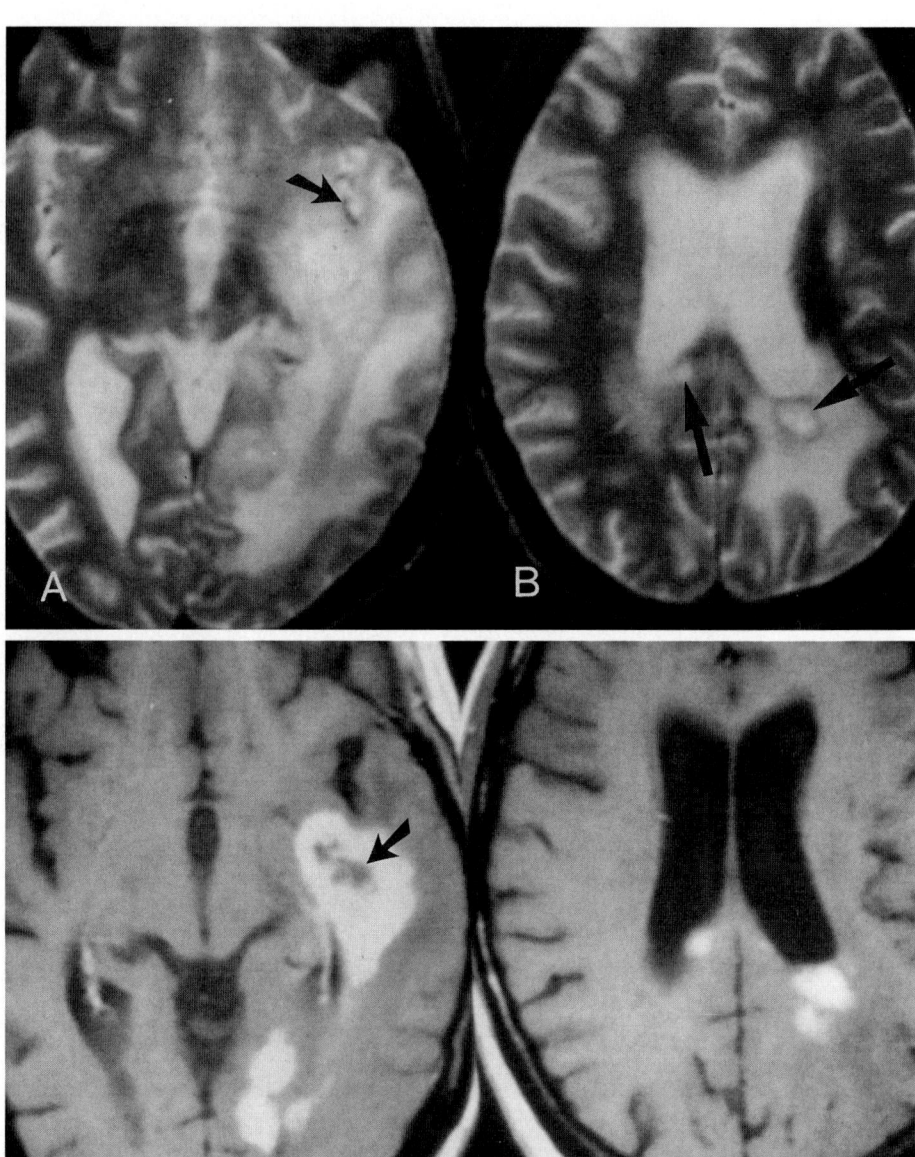

pointense on T2WI—features not commonly seen in tu-mors (14).

"Butterfly Glioma." Glioblastoma multiforme tends to be a highly vascular tumor, and multiple dark holes rep-resenting flow voids may be seen on T2WI. Glioblastoma multiforme is one of two entities (CNS lymphoma is the other) that may have bihemispheric spread through the corpus collosum. Because of the imaging appearance of these GBMs, they are known as "butterfly gliomas." White matter edema does not occur in the corpus collosum be-cause its commissural fibers do not conduct edema fluid. White matter or vasogenic edema also cannot travel through projection fibers of the internal capsule that run from the cerebral cortex to the lower centers. In the pres-ence of an intra-axial neoplasm, any T2 hyperintensity seen in the corpus collosum or internal capsule must be considered secondary to neoplastic spread.

Prognosis. For the highly malignant anaplastic astrocy-toma and GBM, chemotherapy and radiation therapy are standard treatment protocols at present. Following treat-ment, GBMs typically decrease in size in association with some symptomatic improvement. Treated lesions are often extensively necrotic and calcified. However, usually within 1 year after surgery, radioresistant cells left behind prolif-erate, causing the lesion to recur. Therefore, the prognosis for these patients is much worse than intermediate-grade moderately anaplastic astrocytomas (MOAA). Glioblastoma multiforme has an 8–12% 2-year survival rate, and MOAAs have 38–50% 2-year survival. New treatment modalities, such as gamma-knife surgery and more advanced chemotherapy protocols, may alter these dismal statistics.

Low-grade Astrocytoma

Low-grade astrocytoma is characterized by slow growth and a longer clinical course. Patients often have productive lives for many years after diagnosis. Intermediate grade anaplastic and low-grade astrocytomas account for 20–30% of all gliomas. Males are slightly more frequently affected and the peak incidence is between 30–40 years of age. In children, they usually occur in optic pathways, the hypothalamus, and the third ventricle. In adults, the lesions are supratentorial within the hemispheres themselves.

Pathology. Low-grade astrocytomas are pathologically divided into the low-grade fibrillary astrocytoma, the pilocytic (cerebellar cystic) astrocytoma, and the subependymal giant cell astrocytoma seen in tuberous sclerosis. Gemistocytic astrocytomas and pleomorphic xanthoastrocytomas are extremely rare. Approximately 10% of low-grade astrocytomas will degenerate into a more aggressive form (15).

Imaging. On CT and MR, these lesions have variable amounts of surrounding white matter edema and have variable mild and heterogeneous enhancement. Less than 50% will show enhancement. They may not have any abnormal T2 hyperintensity and may not even be apparent on either noncontrast or contrast-enhanced CT. Calcification (in 25% of cases) and hemorrhage may be present, but necrosis does not occur. Tumors are usually poorly marginated with mild mass effect (Fig. 5.4). The variable appearance occasionally makes distinction from an acute infarct difficult. In these cases, a follow-up scan can be crucial in separating the two.

Subependymal Giant Cell Astrocytoma. Subependymal giant cell astrocytoma has a strong association with tuberous sclerosis, occurring in as many as 10% of patients. It is very rare in patients who do not have this syndrome. Any mass discovered in the region of the foramen of Monro in a young patient should provoke investigation for other manifestations of tuberous sclerosis, such as subependymal and cortical hamartomas. Subependymal giant cell astrocytomas are benign and slow-growing with calcification a common feature. Because of their location within the foramen of Monro, these tumors almost always produce some degree of hydrocephalus. On MR, they are typically isointense to slightly hyperintense to gray matter on T1WI, and hyperintense to gray matter on T2WI, with some heterogeneity noted because of the calcification. With contrast, they usually enhance. Tuberous sclerosis is discussed in greater detail in the chapter on pediatric neuroimaging.

Juvenile pilocytic astrocytomas will be discussed in the section on posterior fossa tumors.

Gliomatosis Cerebri

Gliomatosis cerebri is a rare disease resulting from widespread infiltration of neoplastic astrocytes that may be in varying degrees of differentiation. Despite the diffuse involvement of the brain seen pathologically and on imaging studies, the clinical symptoms are often mild. Peak incidence is between 20–40 years of age. Frequently, the lesion appears to smolder for weeks to years before erupting into a full-blown GBM or highly anaplastic astrocytoma. Radiotherapy may temporarily improve the radiologic appearance and improve clinical symptoms. Because these are uncommon lesions, the long-term prognosis is not well defined but is probably poor.

Imaging. Invariably, the CT appearance of gliomatosis cerebri is normal because the lesions are isodense to normal brain parenchyma and do not enhance. However, on MR, the lesion is characterized by diffuse T1 and T2 prolongation throughout the white and gray matter, particularly the hypothalamus, basal ganglia, and thalami. Mass effect and enhancement are minimal (16). Distinction between the gray and white matter is often lost. This appearance can be quite similar to that seen in progressive multifocal leukoencephalopathy in immunocompromised patients.

Oligodendroglioma

Oligodendrogliomas account for approximately 5% of all gliomas (2–3% of all intracranial neoplasms). They are more common in adults with a peak age of 35–40 years. Slow growth with prolonged survival is characteristic. However, the postoperative survival rates are relatively poor, with 50% 5-year survival and 10–30% 10-year survival. The tumor is supratentorial in 85% of cases. Calcification is present pathologically in 100% of oligodendrogliomas and is seen in about 70% of CT studies (Table 5.6). However, it is important to remember that, because astrocytomas which calcify in about 25% of cases are far more common than oligodendrogliomas, a calcified tumor in the brain is more likely to be an astrocytoma rather than an oligodendroglioma. Hemorrhage and cysts occur approximately 20% of the time. Hematogenous or subarachnoid spread is uncommon. About half of the time, these tumors present as a heterogeneous mixed glioma (e.g., oligoastrocytoma).

Imaging. On MR, oligodendrogliomas are usually hypointense to gray matter on T1WI and hyperintense on T2WI. Surrounding edema is seen in only about one-third of cases. With contrast, about two-thirds show some enhancement although the degree of enhancement is variable. They are most commonly located in the frontal lobes and often extend to the cortex, where they may erode the calvarium. The appearance, in an adult, of a heterogeneous calcified mass within the periphery of a frontal lobe with calvarial erosion and relative absence of edema should suggest the diagnosis of an oligodendroglioma (17).

Posterior Fossa Neoplasms in Children

The posterior fossa is the most common site for intracranial neoplasms in the pediatric population. Medulloblastomas and cerebellar astrocytomas account for about two-thirds of all posterior fossa neoplasms in

Table 5.6. Calcified Glial Tumors: "Old Elephants Age Gracefully" (in order of frequency)

*O*ligodendroglioma
*E*pendymoma
*A*strocytoma
*G*lioblastoma multiforme

Table 5.7. Posterior Fossa Masses in Children

Tumor	Location (in relation to 4th ventricle)	Appearance
Medulloblastoma	Posterior (vermis)	Hyperdense on CT Hypointense on T1WI Variable on T2WI
Juvenile pilocytic astrocytoma	Lateral/Posterior	Cystic, with solid mural nodule which enhances intensely
Ependymoma	Within	Foraminal extension Heterogeneous—CT and MR Inhomogeneous enhancement
Brainstem glioma hypo-	Anterior	Expansile brainstem Isodense to hypodense on CT Hypointense on T1WI Hyperintense on T2WI

children with the ependymoma and brainstem glioma composing the remaining one-third (Table 5.7). Symptoms related to cerebellar dysfunction (ataxia, nausea, vomiting, etc.) dominate the clinical picture in all of these lesions.

MEDULLOBLASTOMA

The first problem with medulloblastomas is what to call them. Controversy among neuropathologists as to the exact nature of these neoplasms exists because of histologic similarities between several neoplasms seen in children. Medulloblastomas, called by some primitve neuroectodermal tumors, are the second most common pediatric brain tumor (second only to astrocytomas) and the most common pediatric posterior fossa tumor. Peak occurrences are from 4–8 years old and from 15–35 years. They may occur at any age, with 75% in patients less than 15 years of age. Males are more commonly affected. Clinical presentation is usually nausea, vomiting, and headaches. Medulloblastomas are found only in the posterior fossa, originating most commonly from the vermis, and extending into the fourth ventricle. Most adults with these tumors have them located within the cerebellar hemispheres. They are highly malignant, exhibiting rapid growth that almost always leads to hydrocephalus. Medulloblastomas are thought to arise from residual bipotential precursor cells of the germinal matrix.

Imaging. Medulloblastomas are usually solid hyperdense masses on CT. Cystic change or necrosis occurs in up to 50% of cases and calcification occurs in up to 20%. Hemorrhage is still rare. According to Barkovich (18), the most reliable way to differentiate these tumors from astrocytomas is on a noncontrast CT scan, where the astrocytoma will usually be hypodense and the medulloblastoma will almost never be hypodense. On MR, they are usually hypointense to gray matter on T1WI and have an extremely variable appearance on T2WI probably reflecting the varying nucleus to cytoplasm ratio. Cerebellopontine angle involvement is rare. Surrounding

edema is almost always seen. With contrast, there is intense and fairly homogeneous enhancement of the tumor (Fig. 5.6). Blurring of cerebellar folia on the midline sagittal MR image can be a helpful differentiating feature and reflects the infiltrative nature of these neoplasms (18).

Treatment. Therapeutically, these tumors are challenging because of their tendency to spread via the subarachnoid spaces, which occurs in as many as 50% of cases at the time of diagnosis. CSF metastases are found in the ventricular system, at the operative site, and in the thecal sac of the spinal canal. Postcontrast MR scans demonstrate lesions as brightly enhancing foci, "studding" the meninges. It is particularly important that MR evaluation of the spinal canal with gadolinium be performed preoperatively. Postoperative granulation tissue and hemorrhagic debris can create either the illusion of "drop" metastasis or mask true lesions during the first 6–8 weeks after surgery. Systemic metastasis may occur in approximately 5% with the skeleton being the most common site (19).

CEREBELLAR ASTROCYTOMA

Cerebellar astrocytomas occur with virtually identical incidence as medulloblastomas. Most are of a distinct subset, the juvenile pilocytic astrocytoma (JPA). Early morning headache and vomiting are typical early symp-

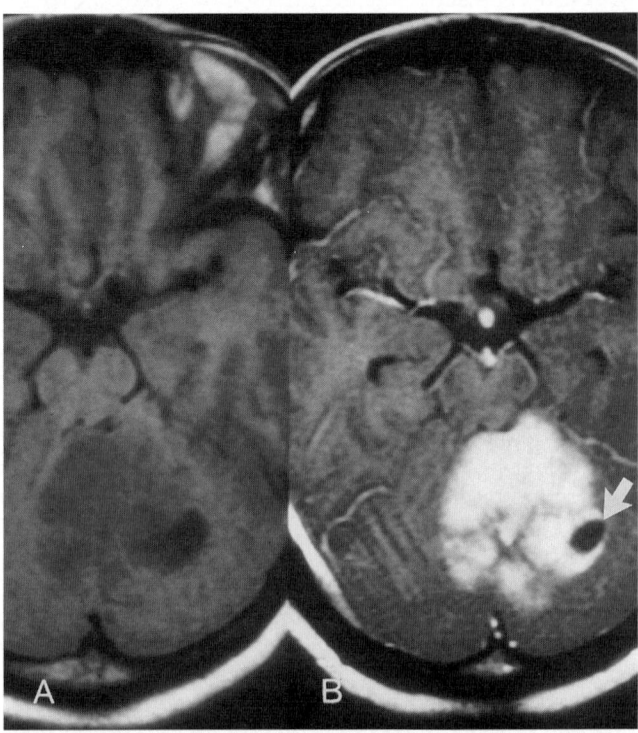

Figure 5.6. Medulloblastoma. Axial T1WI precontrast **(A)** and postcontrast **(B)** demonstrate fairly well circumscribed and intensely enhancing posterior fossa mass that lies in the region of the vermis and extends slightly into the left cerebellar hemisphere. Well-defined area of hypointensity (*arrow*) along left lateral margin of enhancing mass represents a cyst, a not uncommon feature of these tumors.

toms, and there is eventual development of ataxia if no intervention is sought. With neurofibromatosis, the frequency of these tumors increases (9). Although 60% are located within the posterior fossa, these tumors may also occur supratentorially where common locations include the optic pathways and cerebral hemispheres. Most (85%) of the posterior fossa tumors originate within the vermis but 30% extend into the cerebellar hemispheres.

Cystic and Solid. Two basic forms of these tumors exist. Half are cystic with a mural nodule; these have a benign character with a 94% 25-year survival. The other half present as solid masses with or without a necrotic center and are more aggressive with approximately 40% 5-year survival. Calcification occurs in 20% of cases, usually in the solid tumor types. Hemorrhage is very unusual.

Imaging. On CT, they present as a well-delineated vermian or hemispheric masses with the solid portions being isodense or hypodense to brain tissue. On MR, they are isointense or hypointense to gray matter on T1WI and hyperintense to gray matter on T2WI. The cystic portion usually contains proteinaceous fluid and therefore will not exactly follow the signal intensity of CSF. Surrounding edema is rare. The solid component of the tumor enhances to some degree, but is of variable intensity. The mural nodule of the cystic forms will enhance intensely (Fig. 5.7). On noncontrast MR, one should exercise caution in ascribing hypointensity on T1WI and hyperintensity on T2WI within a mass to be "cystic." Truly cystic lesions can only be confidently identified by the presence of fluid-fluid levels or wave pulsation.

Differential Diagnosis. The appearance of a cystic mass with an enhancing mural nodule should suggest two possible diagnoses, and the best discriminator between the two is the patient's age. Juvenile pilocytic astrocytoma much more commonly occur in children with a peak age from birth to 9 years. Hemangioblastomas occur at the peak age of 35 years and are the most common primary intra-axial neoplasm of the posterior fossa in adults. Other possible posterior fossa lesions include infection (especially toxoplasmosis), other cystic gliomas, and metastasis, which is the most common posterior fossa intra-axial tumor in adults.

EPENDYMOMA

Ependymomas comprise approximately 5–6% of all intracranial neoplasms and primarily occur in children and adolescents. A benign subtype of ependymoma known as subependymoma occurs in the middle-aged and elderly population; this subtype is characteristically intraventricular in location. Ependymomas are the most common spinal cord tumor. In children, 60–70% of ependymomas occur within the posterior fossa, with 70% of those centered within the fourth ventricle. The 30% that occur supratentorially are usually parenchymal in location. Symptoms, which are insidious in onset, are related to increased cerebellar pressure from obstruction of the fourth ventricle or cerebellar ataxia.

Pathology. Most tumors are benign. Most are solid but 20% of cases are composed of myxopapillary ele-

ments, making them soft and conforming to the shape of whatever structure they are within. Calcification occurs in 50%. Subarachnoid seeding is rare, and its presence should suggest the possibility of a malignant ependymoma. A characteristic feature of these tumors is extension through the foramen of Luschka into the cerebellopontine angle or through the foramen of Magendie into the cisterna magna and through the foramen magnum. This feature of extension helps differentiate ependymomas from the other pediatric posterior fossa masses. Difficult to cure, these tumors have a high recurrence rate with 25–50% 5-year survival.

Imaging. On CT, these tumors are isodense with a mixture of calcification, cystic change, and even hemorrhage that produces an overall heterogeneous appearance. This pattern is also seen on MR, where they are slightly hypointense to gray matter on T1WI and hyperintense to gray matter on T2WI. With contrast, inhomogeneous enhancement of the solid component occurs. A posterior fossa mass extending through the foramen magnum strongly favors the diagnosis (Fig. 5.8) (18).

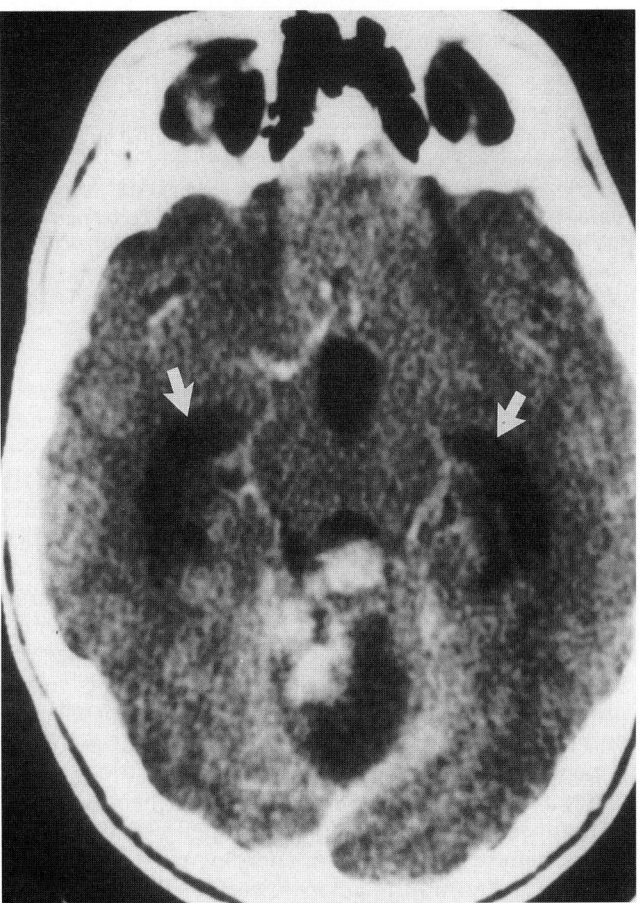

Figure 5.7. Juvenile Pilocytic Astrocytoma. Axial postcontrast CT scan shows heterogeneous posterior fossa mass with both cystic and solid enhancing components. Hydrocephalus, as evidenced by the dilated temporal horns (*arrows*), is also present. Hemangioblastomas may also appear as cystic posterior fossa masses with mural nodules. Age of the patient is a useful discriminator between JPAs (peak age 9 years) and hemangioblastomas (peak age 35 years).

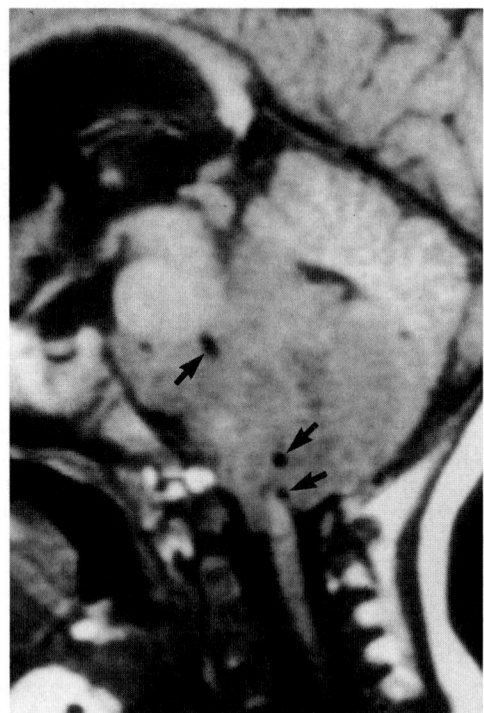

Figure 5.8. Ependymoma. Sagittal noncontrast T1WI in 4-year-old patient with ataxia. A lobulated mass extends inferiorly through the foramen magnum. The mass also extended through the foramen of Luschka (not shown). The tumor is centered within the fourth ventricle with only a small portion of the fourth ventricle still visible at the superior margin of mass. The dark holes (*arrows*) contained within the mass represent vessels surrounded by this soft tumor.

BRAINSTEM GLIOMA

These astrocytomas account for approximately 15% of all pediatric CNS neoplasms. No gender predilection exists, and the peak incidence is between 3–10 years of age. Like other astrocytomas, they infiltrate through the normal tracts and produce expansile enlargement of the brainstem, consequently creating cranial nerve palsies, pyramidal tract signs, and ataxia. Because of the nature of the tumor and of the delicate structures (e.g., cranial nerve nuclei) located within this region, chemotherapy and radiation therapy, rather than surgery, are the treatment options. However, brainstem gliomas nearly always recur within 2 years after completion of therapy, and the overall prognosis for patients with these tumors is poor (10–30% 5-year survival).

Key Features. Detection of brainstem gliomas may be difficult. Identification of three imaging features will prove helpful in suggesting the diagnosis. First, exophytic growth into the adjacent cisternal spaces occurs in approximately 60% of cases. Second, if the ventral portion of the pons extends anteriorly to the margin of the basilar artery (which normally lies within the midline indentation of the ventral pons), then abnormal enlargement of the pons is present and a cause should be identified. The differential diagnosis of pontine enlargement also includes encephalitis, tuberculoma, acute disseminated encephalomyelitis, infarction, resolving hema-

toma, and vascular malformation. The presence of blood breakdown products makes detection of one of the vascular causes straightforward on MR. However, encephalitis and tuberculoma cannot be distinguished from a brainstem glioma based on imaging characteristics alone. Third, alteration of the normal fourth ventricle contour provides a useful clue. The floor of the fourth ventricle may be flattened, the ventricle itself may be displaced posteriorly, and if there is involvement of the lateral recesses, the ventricle will be rotated. In cases in which the tumor grows exophytically into the cerebellar hemispheres, it may mimic a cerebellar astrocytoma. Occasionally, a brainstem glioma may involve not only the pons (the most common site) but also the medulla and even the cervical cord. When a brainstem glioma extends through the foramen magnum, it may resemble an ependymoma. However, ependymomas are separate from the brainstem, and they typically enhance more vigorously than brainstem gliomas.

Imaging. On CT, brainstem gliomas present as focal hypodense to isodense expansion with extremely variable enhancement that may change with time. The degree of enhancement does not correlate reliably with the grade of the tumor. The adjacent cisterns may be compressed. On MR, typical prolongation of T1 and T2 is seen (Fig. 5.9). The T2WI are of most value in assessing

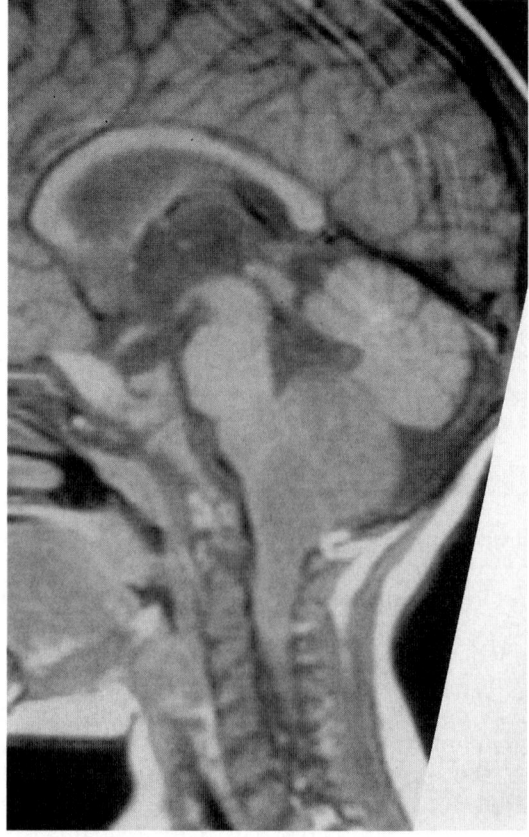

Figure 5.9. Brainstem Glioma. Midline sagittal T1WI in a young child with progressive ataxia. The large mass, slightly hypointense to normal surrounding brainstem, has large exophytic component and involves the upper cervical cord as well.

the true extent of the tumor because the signal hyperintensity of the tumor contrasts sharply with the relative low signal of normal white matter. Because of the slow growth of these tumors, hydrocephalus is not usually seen. Hemorrhage or cysts occur in approximately 25% of cases (18).

Non-glial Tumors

PRIMITIVE NEUROECTODERMAL TUMORS (PNET)

Classification of this tumor and differentiation from medulloblastoma is controversial. Because of the diverse heterogeneity of the cells that compose these neoplasms, neuropathologists have disagreed as to their exact nature. It is believed that they arise from bipotential precursor cells of the germinal matrix with the ability to differentiate along either glial or neuronal cell lines. Similar histology is also seen in other "-blastoma" lesions—ependymoblastoma, pineoblastoma, spongioblastoma, and neuroblastoma.

PNETs occur supratentorially in two-thirds of cases and are much more common in children than adults. However, the age distribution in some specific types of PNETs, such as neuroblastoma, may be more equally weighted between adult and pediatric populations (20). Along with teratomas, PNETs are one of the most common congenital intracranial neoplasms (Table 5.8). Primitive neuroectodermal tumors typically present with symptoms of increased intracranial pressure or seizures. Overall, they carry a very poor prognosis with a mean survival of only 5 months (21).

Pathology. The most common appearance is a large well-demarcated heterogeneous mass within the deep cerebral white matter. Heterogeneity is secondary to necrosis, hemorrhage, and calcification. Hydrocephalus is very common. A periventricular or intraventricular location is common with neuroblastoma (20). The solid portions of the tumor are usually hyperdense on CT and isointense to hypointense to gray matter on T2WI, probably reflecting decreased amounts of intracellular water. These tumors show at least some enhancement.

CNS LYMPHOMA

Primary CNS Lymphoma. The incidence and demographics of primary CNS lymphoma are changing rapidly as a consequence of AIDS. Once considered extremely rare as a primary neoplasm, this tumor (almost always a B-cell non-Hodgkin's lymphoma) now accounts for more than the previously reported 1% of all brain tumors. Also at increased risk are other immunocompromised patients, such as those who have undergone organ transplantation or those who have congenital immunodeficiencies. Confusion, lethargy, and memory loss are common. Most patients will have elevated protein and decreased glucose within the CSF, but positive cytology is rare. Despite being exquisitely sensitive to radiotherapy initially, primary CNS lymphoma virtually always reappears, leading some to call it the "vanishing" or "ghost" tumor. An impressive response to corticosteroids is quite also common, and withholding this medication until a biopsy can be completed is recommended to avoid false-negative results (22). Recent advances in combination radiotherapy and chemotherapy has led to some long-term survivals in this once uniformly fatal disease. However, the prognosis for AIDS patients with primary CNS lymphoma still lags behind those who do not have AIDS (23).

Imaging. The classic appearance of CNS lymphoma, particularly in those with AIDS, is multifocal well-demarcated enhancing lesions scattered within the cerebral white matter tracts, often in a periventricular distribution (Fig. 5.10). Most (85%) are supratentorial. Calcification and hemorrhage are rare. The lesions generate relatively little edema for their size. Subependymal spread is common and bihemispheric involvement via the corpus collosum (similar to "butterfly glioma") may be seen. Usually the enhancement is focal rather than ring-like, a pattern more commonly seen with toxoplasmosis (24).

Differentiating from Toxoplasmosis. Toxoplasmosis lesions do not exhibit subependymal spread and are more likely to be located within the corticomedullary junction or within the basal ganglia. Both lymphoma and toxoplasmosis lesions are hypointense to white matter on T1WI. However, hypointensity to white matter on T2WI or hyperdensity on CT (again refecting the high density of small cells) strongly suggests lymphoma. PET and SPECT-thallium scans reliably differentiate between primary CNS lymphoma and toxoplasmosis. When these modalities are not available, an empiric trial of anti-*Toxoplasma* therapy for three weeks is frequently employed, and the lesions are reassessed using CT or MR. If the lesions are not regressing in size, then a stereotactic biopsy may be performed to determine the diagnosis (25). Other considerations in the differential diagnosis include metastasis and focal cerebritis.

Secondary CNS Lymphoma. Secondary involvement of the brain by systemic lymphoma more commonly involves the leptomeninges instead of the brain parenchyma itself. Differential diagnosis in these cases would incude meningioma and leptomeningeal carcinomatosis.

METASTASIS

Metastasis to the CNS from extracranial sites accounts for approximately 32% of all intracranial neoplasms. Metastases may be intra-axial (most commonly from

Table 5.8. Congenital Brain Tumors in Infants Younger Than 60 Days of Age

Teratoma—most common, one-third to one-half of all tumors, two-thirds supratentorial
Primitive neuroectodermal tumors—curvilinear, sparse calcification
Astrocytoma
Choroid plexus papilloma
Ependymoma
Medulloepithelioma
Germinoma
Angioblastic meningioma
Ganglioglioma

Figure 5.10. CNS Lymphoma. A 69-year-old immunocompromised male with altered mental status of progressive nature. **A,B.** Post-contrast axial CT scans show multiple areas of enhancement in a predominantly periventricular distribution. Involvement of the genu of the corpus collosum and subependymal spread (within the frontal horns) are also seen.

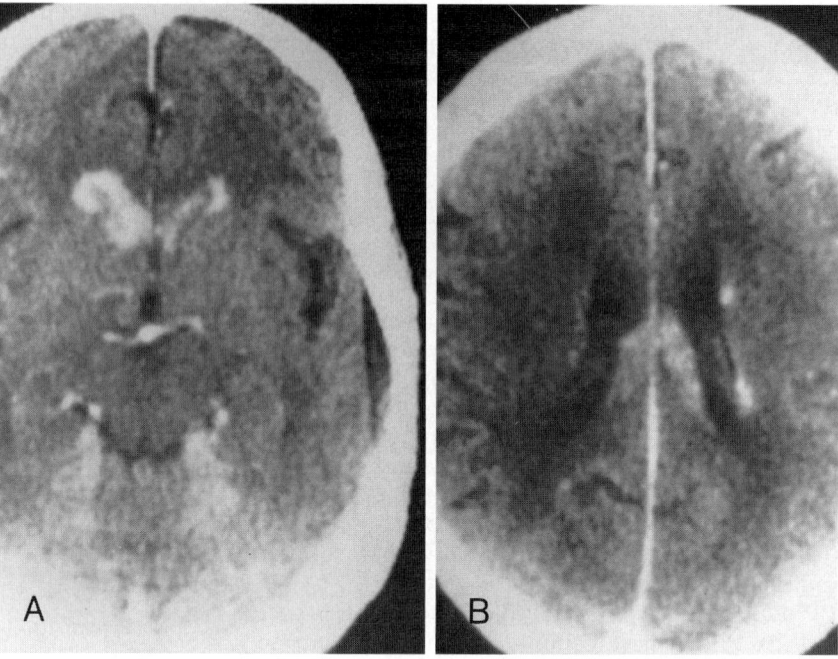

lung, breast, melanoma, and colon carcinomas), extra-axial, dural (most commonly breast carcinoma, lymphoma, prostate carcinoma, and neuroblastoma), or within the subarachnoid spaces or skull (Table 5.9). They may occur at any age but most frequently present in older age groups, often with seizures or focal deficits. Clinically silent metastases are most common in patients with oat cell carcinoma, lung carcinoma (especially adenocarcinoma), and melanoma (9).

Most (80–85%) metastatic lesions occur supratentorially, with the exception of renal cell carcinoma, which has a predilection for the posterior fossa. Although most metastases are mutiple, up to 30% are solitary (with melanoma, lung, and breast carcinoma the most likely primaries). Approximately 10% of metastases—especially those from melanoma, thyroid carcinoma, and renal cell carcinoma—are hemorrhagic (Fig. 5.11).

Imaging. The classic appearance of metastatic spread on CT or MR is one of mutiple foci, located at the corticomedullary junction, hypodense on CT, hypointense on T1WI, and variable signal intensity on T2WI with marked edema surrounding each lesion. As with vasogenic edema seen in other neoplastic processes, sparing of the cortical gray matter occurs. With contrast administration, there is intense enhancement, which is variable in its form (ring or nodular) (Fig. 5.12). Studies have documented the advantage of contrast, particularly gadolinium on MR, in the detection of more lesions compared to plain spin-echo images, contrast-enhanced CT (26), or even doube-dose delayed CT (27). The sensitivity of metastatic detection may be increased even further by high-dose gadolinium MR (28). These are important considerations because single metastases may be treated by surgical resection whereas mutiple lesions are more commonly treated by radiotherapy. Postcontrast MR is especially helpful in the detection of cortically based lesions that, presumably owing to a lack of interstitium,

Table 5.9. Most Common Metastasis to the CNS

Intra-axial	Extra-axial	Hemorrhagic
Lung CA	Breast CA	Melanoma
Breast CA	Lymphoma	Renal CA
Melanoma	Prostate CA	Thyroid CA
Colon CA	Neuroblastoma	Choriocarcinoma

do not demonstrate much edema in the surrounding parenchyma.

Dural Metastases. Dural (either epidural or subdural) metastases is the most common form of extra-axial spread, seen in 18% of autopsy series. When symptoms occur, they are most often secondary to compression of brain parenchyma or dural venous sinus thrombosis. Skull lesions, usually secondary to breast, lung, prostate, or renal carcinoma, give rise to epidural metastases. Subdural lesions are believed to result from hematogenous spread and, in the case of spine lesions, spread from pelvic tumors via Batson's plexus, the epidural collection of spinal veins (29). Epidural and subdural metastases both may have a biconvex shape, but they can be distinguished by the presence of adjacent skull involvement in the epidural metastases.

Leptomeningeal Spread. Leptomeningeal carcinomatosis deserves special mention because its radiographic appearance may exactly mimic meningitis. Characterized by cranial nerve palsies because of its involvement of the basilar cisterns, this lesion is the result of leptomeningeal spread by primary CNS malignancies, extracranial adenocarcinomas (especially those of lung or breast origin), leukemia, or lymphoma. Postcontrast MR is far more sensitive than contrast-enhanced CT in the detection of leptomeningeal enhancement. However, even with this technique, not all cases will be detected; thus, the presence of hydrocephalus in a patient with a

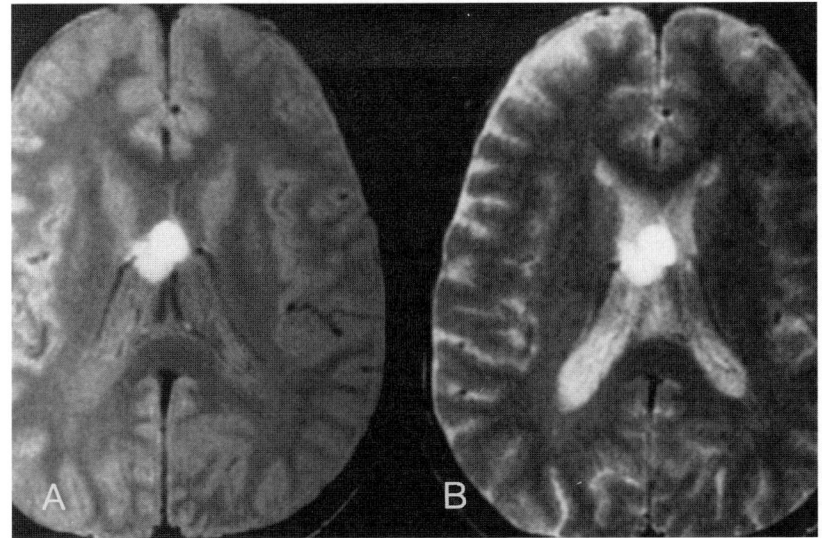

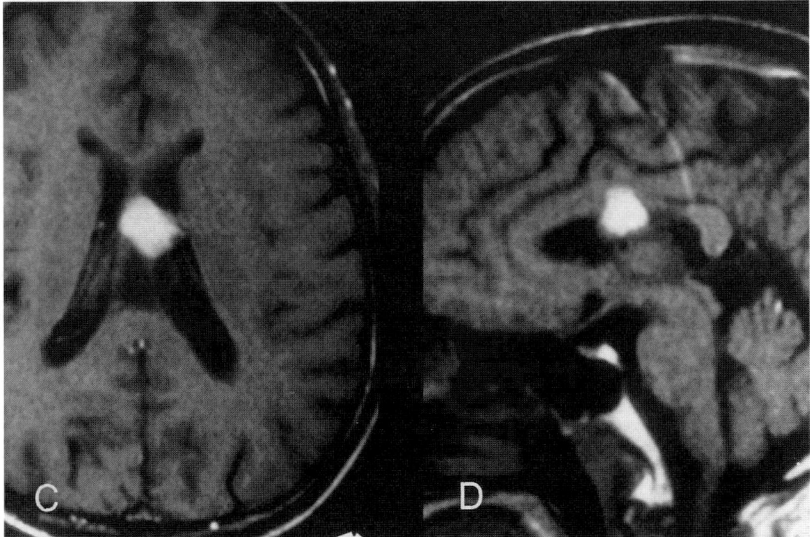

Figure 5.11. Thyroid Metastasis. An adult female with florid pulmonary metastases (not shown) from thyroid carcinoma and recent onset of headaches. Axial T2WI **(A)** first echo; **(B)**, second echo) show hyperintense mass of corpus collosum body. Hyperintensity persists on axial **(C)** and sagittal **(D)** T1WI (without contrast) confirming the hemorrhagic nature of the lesion. Melanoma and metastases from renal cell carcinoma and choriocarcinoma are the most common metastases to hemorrhage. Among primary tumors, GBM and oligodendroglioma are the most common to do so.

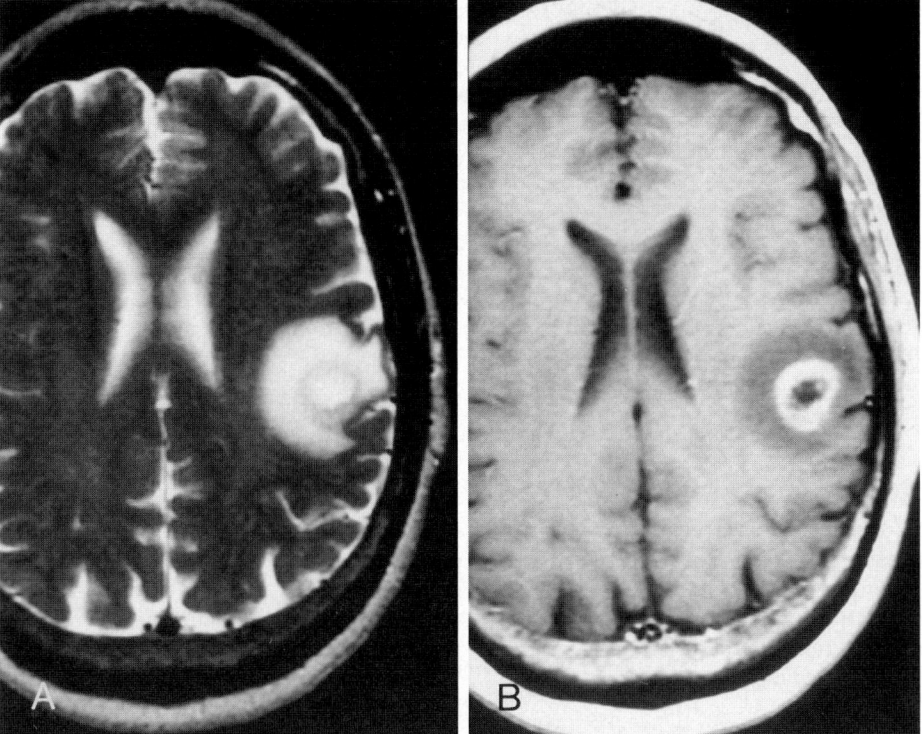

Figure 5.12. Cerebral Metastasis. Axial T2WI **(A)** shows prominent T2 prolongation consistent with vasogenic edema surrounding lesion within the left posterior frontal lobe. Note the mildly hypointense ring representing the margin of the mass. Postcontrast axial T1WI **(B)** shows intense ring-enhancement with central hypointense area. The irregular shape of the rim (compared with the usual smooth wall of an abscess) is a clue to the true nature of this lung metastasis.

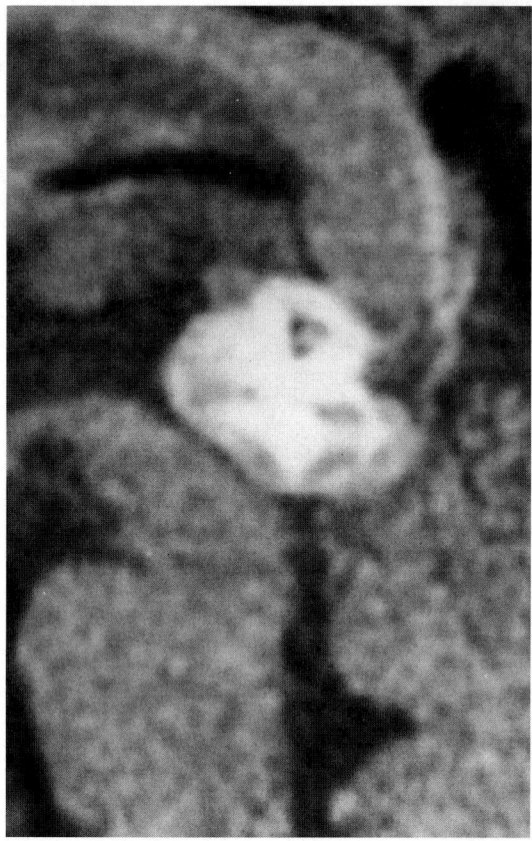

Figure 5.13. Pineal Germinoma. Postcontrast sagittal T1WI in a young adult male with onset of Parinaud's syndrome. The lobulated pineal mass shows heterogeneous enhancement. It is not possible to distinguish pineal germinomas from pineal parenchymal tumors on the basis of an imaging study alone.

known malignancy should suggest this diagnosis as a possibility (29).

Skull Lesions. Skull metastasis may present a special problem on MR imaging. As with metastases to the spinal vertebral bodies, the administration of contrast will often obscure lesions of the bone marrow that are easily visible on noncontrast T1-weighted sequences. For this reason, noncontrast T1WI should aways be obtained in cases of suspected skull metastasis. Although CT with bone windows is superior in detecting subtle bone erosion, MR, with its increased contrast resolution and mutiplanar capability, easily outperforms CT in the evaluation of epidural and intracranial extension of skull metastasis.

GANGLIOGLIOMA/GANGLIOCYTOMA

Gangliogliomas are composed of both glial cells and differentiated neurons. Gangliocytomas or ganglioneuromas are pure neuronal tumors without glial components. Both of these tumors are part of the spectrum of ganglion neoplasms that includes ganglioneuroblastoma, anaplastic ganglioglioma, and neuroblastoma, in increasing order of malignancy. Gangliogliomas and gangilocytomas, which account for approximately 1% of

all intracranial neoplasms, are relatively low-grade neoplasms with good prognoses, with a peak age of incidence between 10–20 years but occurring at any age. No gender predilection is noted. Clinical presentation, often with long-standing symptoms (belying their slow-growth), is in the form of focal seizures or hypothalamic dysfunction depending on their location (18). Although the temporal lobe is the most common location for these tumors, they may occur anywhere, even within the spinal cord. A gangliocytoma occurring in the cerebellum is termed "Lhermitte-Duclos disease" (28).

Imaging. On CT, these tumors are most often hypodense or isodense well-circumscribed lesions with little associated mass effect or surrounding edema. Calcification is a frequent (35%) feature. They are often peripheral in location. Enhancement is variable, ranging between absent to completely homogeneous. On MR, they are usuay hypointense to isointense relative to gray matter on T1WI and almost always hyperintense to gray matter on T2WI. There is nothing specific about this appearance.

Differential Diagnosis. When these tumors occur in the region of the hypothalamus, another consideration is hypothalamic glioma. When they occur peripherally, the differential diagnosis includes low-grade astrocytoma, oligodendroglioma, and dysembryoplastic neuroepithelial tumor (DNT), a benign tumor of neuroepithelial origin seen in patients with medically refractory partial seizures (30).

Pineal Region Masses

Germ cell tumors constitute the most common type of neoplasms of the pineal region, accounting for 60% of all pineal masses (Fig. 5.13). Pineal parenchymal tumors such as pineoblastoma (malignant) and pineocytoma (benign) compose 14% of pineal masses. The remaining 26% is divided among glioma (from adjacent brain parenchyma), meningioma (from the tentorium) (Fig. 5.14), and miscellaneous lesions such as arachnoid cyst, Vein of Galen aneurysm, lipoma, and pineal cyst (Table 5.10). No distinction can be made on imaging studies between germinomas and pineal parenchymal tumors (31). However, a calcified pineal mass in a female is more likely to be secondary to a pineocytoma whereas in a male this same appearance is more likely to be a germinoma. Anytime calcification in the pineal region exceeds 1 cm, a pathologic pineal process should be suspected.

Table 5.10. Pineal Region Masses

Germ Cell Tumors (60%)	Others
Germinoma	Pineal cyst
Teratoma	Glioma
Embryonal carcinoma	Meningioma (tentorial)
Endodermal sinus tumor	Vein of Galen aneurysm
Choriocarcinoma	Arachnoid cyst
	Lipoma
Pineal Parenchymal Tumors (14%)	
Pineocytoma	
Pineoblastoma	

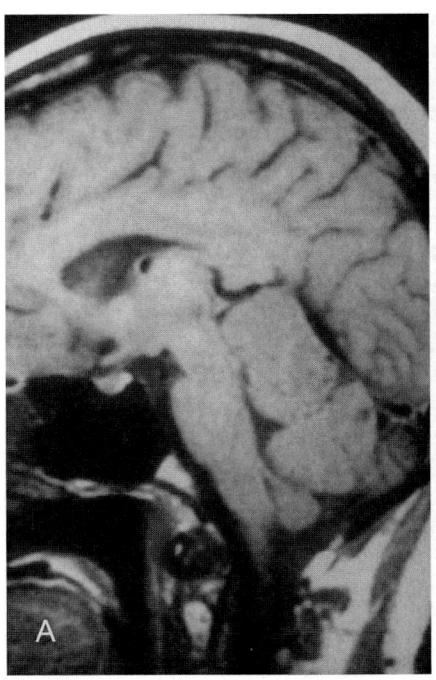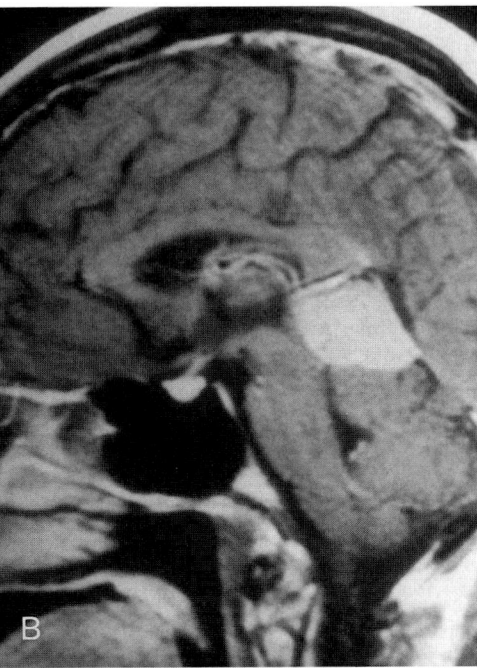

Figure 5.14. Tentorial Meningioma. Midline sagittal precontrast **(A)** and post-contrast **(B)** T1WI of dural-based intensely enhancing mass compressing the superior portion of the cerebellum and the tectum. The pineal gland itself is not evident, most likely being severely flattened by the expanding meningioma.

The size and location of the mass are important imaging characteristics to be conveyed to the neurosurgeon. If a lesion does not contain a large supratentorial component, the preferred infratentorial approach can be performed (32).

GERM CELL TUMORS

Germ cell tumors are well-defined, usually midline masses occurring most commonly (65%) in the region of the pineal where they account for approximately 60% of all pineal masses. **Germinomas** are by far the most common intracranial germ cell tumors. They also occur in the suprasellar region (35%) and are most commonly seen in chidren and young adults, with peak incidence during puberty. CSF dissemination is common. Histologically, germinomas are similar to testicular seminomas and ovarian dysgerminomas. For the pineal region, males are much more commonly affected than females (10:1). Typical clinical presentation is related to compression of the Sylvian aqueduct, producing hydrocephalus or compression of the superior colliculus, which produces Parinaud's syndrome. Curiously, in the case of suprasellar germinomas, there is no sex predilection. Tumors arise in the floor of the third ventricle and rarely extend into the basal ganglia. Because of compression of the optic chiasm and infundibulum, symptoms related to hypothalamic dysfunction (emotional disturbance, diabetes insipidus, precocious puberty, etc.) and visual changes are common.

In either the pineal or suprasellar regions, germinomas maintain the same appearance on CT: isodense to hyperdense well-circumscribed mass. "Engulfment" of the normal physiologic calcification is a feature of germinomas distinguishing them from pineal parenchymal tumors, which more commonly produce an "exploded" appearance of this calcification (33). On MR, hypointensity on T1WI and hyperintensity on T2WI is most common. Hypointensity on T2WI is occasionally present and favors the diagnosis of a germinoma over pineal tumor. As with pineal parenchymal tumors, intense enhancement on either CT or MR is the rule (Fig. 5.13). In the final analysis, no discriminating factors on imaging studies exist between pineal parenchymal tumors and germinomas that allow accurate differentiation.

Other Germ Cell Tumors. Teratomas, embryonal carcinoma, choriocarcinoma, and endodermal sinus tumor compose the remainder of the germ cell tumors and are all much less common compared to germinomas. Teratomas usually occur at an earlier age than germinomas and have a variable radiographic appearance and biologic behavior. Besides the pineal region (their most common location), teratomas also occur in the third ventricle and posterior fossa. Because they contain all three germ cell lines, they usually are extremely heterogeneous on CT and MR, containing a mixture of fat, calcification, and cysts. Hydrocephalus is frequent and enhancement is variable. A midline heterogeneous mass in a child should suggest this diagnosis.

Embryonal carcinoma, choriocarcinoma, and endodermal sinus tumor are highly malignant types of germ cell tumors. All are frequently hemorrhagic but have no specific radiographic features. Alpha fetoprotein (AFP) may be elevated in embryonal cell carcinoma, teratoma, or choriocarcinoma. Human chorionic gonadotropin (HCG) may be elevated in choriocarcinoma or teratoma. Germinomas are not associated with elevated HCG or AFP levels.

Microneurosurgical and stereotactic techniques allow relatively safe biopsy of suspicious pineal masses for much more accurate pathologic confirmation of the diagnosis (33).

PINEOCYTOMA/PINEOBLASTOMA

Pineoblastoma. Pineocytoma and pineoblastoma are true pineal tumors that account for 14% of all pineal masses. Pineoblastomas are histologically and radiographically similar to medulloblastomas and have been categorized as part of the PNET group by some neuropathologists. Highly malignant neoplasms, pineoblastomas occur primarily in young children although they may occur in patients up to 30 years of age. Rarely well-circumscribed, these tumors often demonstrate a lobular contour, local invasion, and frequent calcification. Intratumoral hemorrhage is rare. Similar to other PNETs, CSF spread is common. There is a rare variant in the form of "trilateral retinoblastoma" seen in patients who have bilateral retinoblastomas and a pineoblastoma.

Pineocytomas, on the other hand, most commonly occur in adults although they may occur at any age. In contrast with pineoblastomas, most are well-demarcated, noninvasive, and slow-growing; they are often calcified. Much less commonly than pineoblastomas, they may metastasize with CSF spread. On either CT or MR, they cannot be reliably differentiated from either pineal germinomas or from pineoblastomas.

Imaging. Both pineal parenchymal tumors are isodense to hyperdense on CT. On MR, they are usually isointense to hypointense on T1WI. Extensive variability in signal intensity of these tumors exists on T2WI, with most being isointense to hyperintense to gray matter. Both the native tumor and their metastases enhance intensely with contrast.

PINEAL CYSTS

Pineal cysts are common (approximately 40% in autopsy series) and have internal signal intensity similar to that of CSF (34). The lack of CSF pulsation may cause slightly higher signal on T1WI and on T2WI. No enhancement of the cyst itself is seen and no internal acrhitecture is noted. If the cyst is eccentric to the pineal gland itself, differentiating this lesion from a small pineal neoplasm may be difficult. These cysts may produce slight flattening of the superior colliculus but do not cause Parinaud's syndrome (paralysis of upward gaze) or hydrocephalus. Very rarely, they hemorrhage.

Sellar Masses

PITUITARY ADENOMAS

Pituitary adenomas account for approximately 10–15% of all intracranial tumors and constitute the most common sellar masses by far, being five times more common than craniopharyngiomas and Rathke's cleft cysts. Based on their size, they are considered either microadenomas ($\leq$10 mm) or macroadenomas (>10 mm). In general, approximately 75% of adenomas are hormonally active; most of these will be microadenomas. The other 25% are nonsecreting adenomas; most of these will be macroadenomas. A topographical relationship of the secretory cells within the pituitary gland exists and, depending on the clinical signs and symptoms,

this can be used to focus attention on particular sections of the gland. Prolactinomas and growth-hormone (GH)–secreting adenomas are more commonly located within the lateral aspects of the gland. Adenomas with secretion of ACTH, TSH, or FSH/LH are more common in the central region of the gland. Clinical symptoms are related to the type of hormone secreted. For instance, ACTH-producing tumors cause Cushing's disease and GH-producing tumors cause acromegaly in adults and gigantism in children. Prolactinomas are the most common (40–50%) of the secreting adenomas and are marked clinically by amenorrhea, galactorrhea, or impotence. A serum prolactin level of greater than 150 ng/ml almost always indicates a prolactinoma, and levels greater than 1000 ng/ml herald invasion into the cavernous sinus. Normal prolactin levels are less than 20 ng/ml.

Imaging. MR has supplanted CT as the best imaging modality to detect pituitary tumors. Microadenomas are usually detected best on coronal T1WI as focal areas of hypointensity (on noncontrast studies) compared to the rest of the pituitary gland (Fig. 5.15). Occasionally they may be isointense or even hyperintense on noncontrast studies. Other clues to the presence of a microadenoma should be sought; these include deviation of the infundibulum, asymmetric convexity of the pituitary gland, or mild down-sloping of the roof of the sphenoid sinus. In general, gadolinium contrast increases the conspicuousness of these often small neoplasms. Gadolinium contrast reveals these small tumors as hypointense foci within the gland on immediate postcontrast scans or as hyperintense foci on delayed (approximately 30 minutes) scans. In addition, the use of narrow windows is essential to optimize visualization of these small lesions.

Macroadenomas are never a problem to visualize on MR. When they are heterogeneous because of cyst formation or hemorrhage (Fig. 5.16), and differentiation from a craniopharyngioma or parasellar meningioma is difficult, the use of contrast may be helpful (Fig. 5.17). Macroadenomas most commonly present because of optic chiasm or nerve compression, hydrocephalus, cranial nerve palsies, or occasionally anterior pituitary dysfunction. These lesions are isointense to gray matter on T1WI and characteristically will produce "draping" of the optic chiasm over the top of the tumor. Invasion of the cavernous sinus can only be accurately stated when there is tumor tissue between the internal carotid artery flow void and the *lateral* wall of the cavernous sinus (29).

CRANIOPHARYNGIOMA / RATHKE'S CLEFT CYST

Both of these entities arise from squamous epithelial remnants of the anterior lobe of the pituitary gland, with the craniopharyngiomas derived from the pars tuberalis and Rathke's cleft cyst arising from the pars intermedia. However, whereas Rathke's cleft cysts are usually asymptomatic (seen in up to 33% of autopsies), craniopharyngiomas are frequently symptomatic because of their larger size. Symptoms related to increased intracranial pressure, optic nerve or chiasm compression, or hypothalamic symptoms are common. Two age peaks

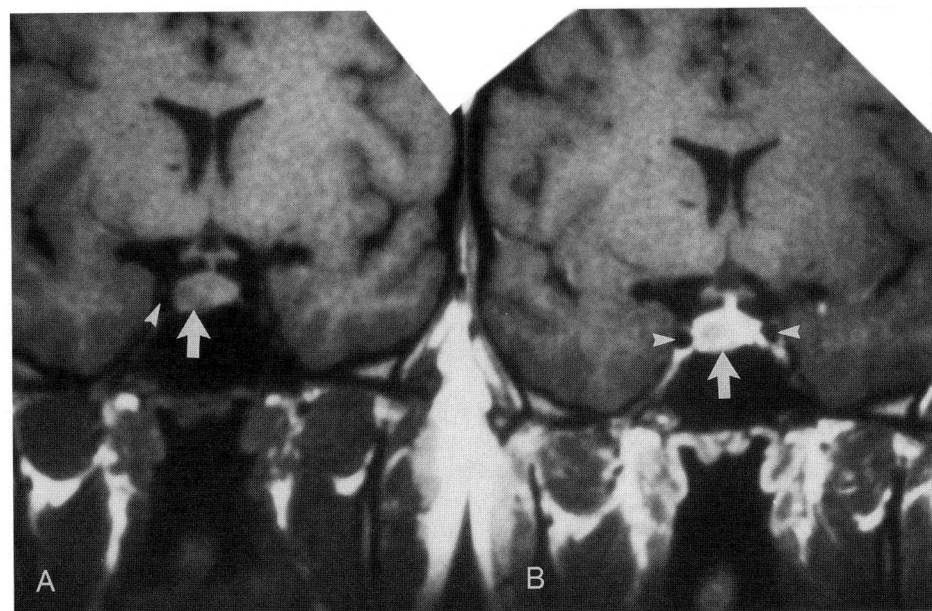

Figure 5.15. Pituitary Microadenoma.
A. Precontrast thin-section coronal T1WI through the sella in patient with elevated prolactin levels shows prominent right aspect of gland with slight hypointensity (*arrow*) compared to the normal pituitary gland to the left. Downsloping of the sphenoid roof is also seen. **B.** With contrast, the lesion is slightly more conspicuous, measuring 8 mm in transverse diameter. Note the normal flow voids (*arrowheads*) of the internal carotid arteries and normal enhancement of the cavernous sinuses.

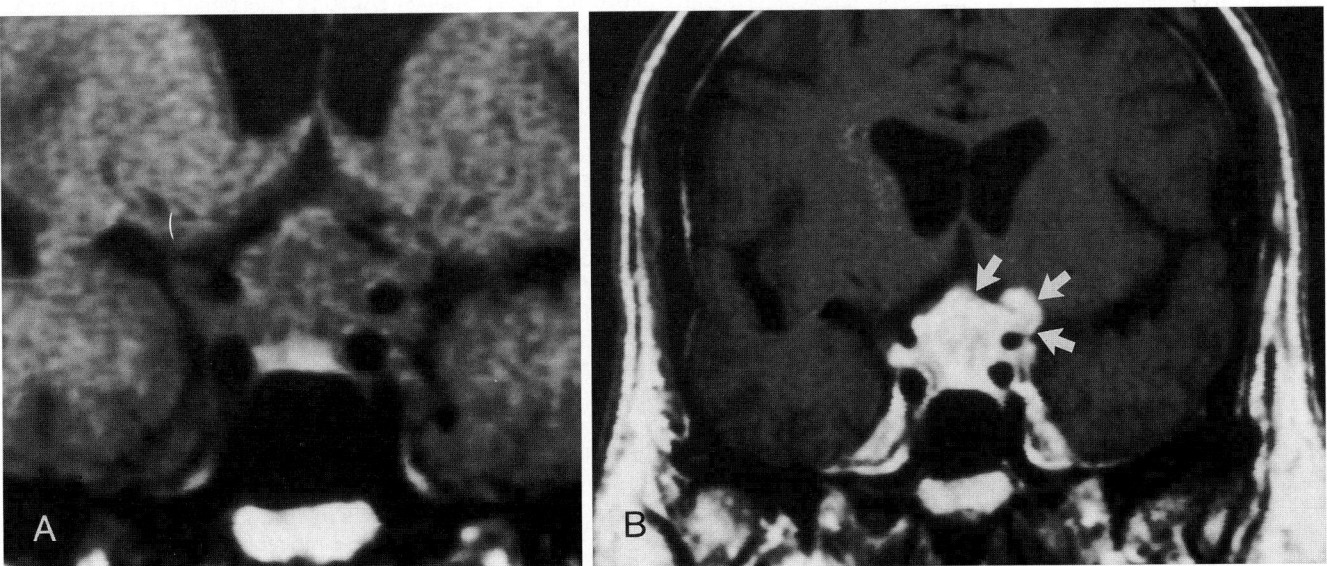

Figure 5.16. Pituitary Macroadenoma. Coronal T1WI without **(A)** and with **(B)** contrast show enhancing mass (*arrow*) extending beyond lateral margin of cavernous sinus and flow voids of left internal carotid artery.

for craniopharyngiomas are between 5–10 years old and 50–60 years old. They are the most common suprasellar masses in the pediatric population. Most craniopharyngiomas involve both intrasellar and suprasellar compartments (70%) whereas 20% are intrasellar only and 10% purely extrasellar. Solid and cystic components are typical with the fluid of the cyst often containing cholesterol crystals and grossly having the appearance of "crank-case oil."

Imaging. On CT, the classic appearance of a craniopharyngioma is a large cystic-appearing sellar/suprasellar mass with an enhancing rim and evidence of some calcification. In children, calcification is seen in up to 80% of cases (compared to 40% for adult cases). On MR,

because of the presence of the liquid cholesterol, the classic finding of hyperintensity on T1WI and T2WI, corresponding to the cystic portion, is most common (Fig. 5.18). However, some craniopharyngiomas will not contain fluid but instead will have a solid nodule that may be completely calcified. Enhancement of the rim and any soft tissue component is noted.

Rathke's cleft cyst. Either purely intrasellar (66%) or intrasellar and suprasellar (33%), these cysts have variable contents. Most commonly, a mucoid fluid fills the cyst. Less commonly, serous fluid or desquamated cellular debris occupies the cyst. Because of this variability, they may be hyperintense on T1WI and T2WI, appearing identical to craniopharyngiomas or they may be isointense to hypointense on either sequence because of cellular debris mimicking the appearance of a solid nodule. Rathke's cleft cysts show peripheral enhancement much less commonly than craniopharyngiomas.

A complete differential diagnosis (and time-tested mnemonic) for suprasellar masses is contained in Table 5.11.

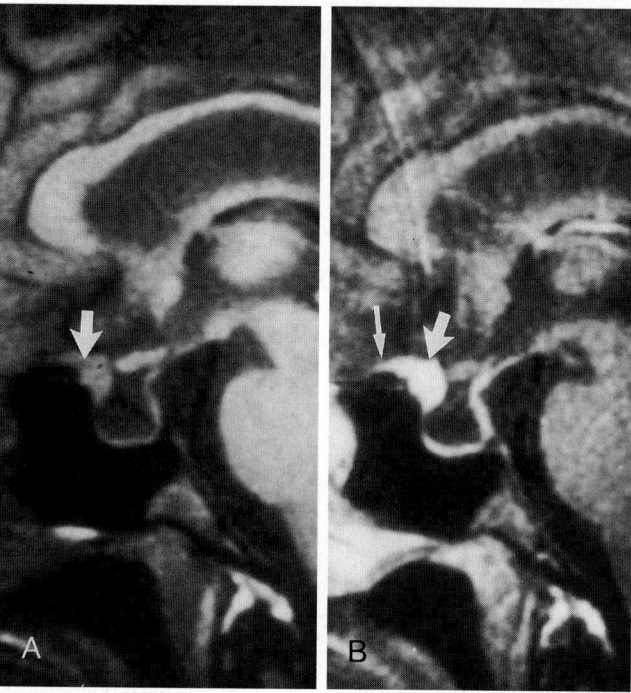

Figure 5.17. Tuberculum Sella Meningioma. Suprasellar enhancing mass (*arrows*) in region of tuberculum sella with extension along the planum sphenoidale (*small arrow*), a highly characteristic feature of parasellar meningiomas.

Nerve Sheath Tumors

There are three types of nerve sheath tumors: schwannomas (also known as neurilemomas or neurinomas), neurofibromas, and malignant nerve sheath tumors, which are very rare and will not be discussed further.

Schwannomas arise from Schwann cells, which form the myelin sheaths of axons. They are focal and encapsulated, and they affect the cranial nerves, most often the vestibulocochlear (VIII) nerve and trigeminal (V) nerve. They are often cystic, with hemorrhage and necrosis common. Comprising approximately 8% of all intracranial neoplasms, they are more common in adults. Virtually 100% of patients with bilateral acoustic schwannomas will have neurofibromatosis type II. Symptoms depend on the cranial nerve involved. For instance, sensorineural hearing loss is very common in acoustic schwannomas. Depending on the sizes and locations of schwannomas, hydrocephalus, brainstem compression, or neuropathy may be present.

On CT, these are isodense to hypodense masses that homogeneously enhance with contrast. On MR, it is advantageous to perform thin-section (3 mm) axial and coronal T1WI images through the basal cisterns to exclude these neoplasms, which demonstrate hypointensity to gray matter on T1WI and hyperintensity to gray

Table 5.11. Suprasellar Masses ("SATCHMO")

Sella tumor, **S**arcoid
Aneurysm, **A**rachnoid cyst
Teratoma
Craniopharyngioma
Hypothalamic glioma, **H**amartoma of tuber cinereum, **H**istiocytosis
Meningioma
Optic glioma

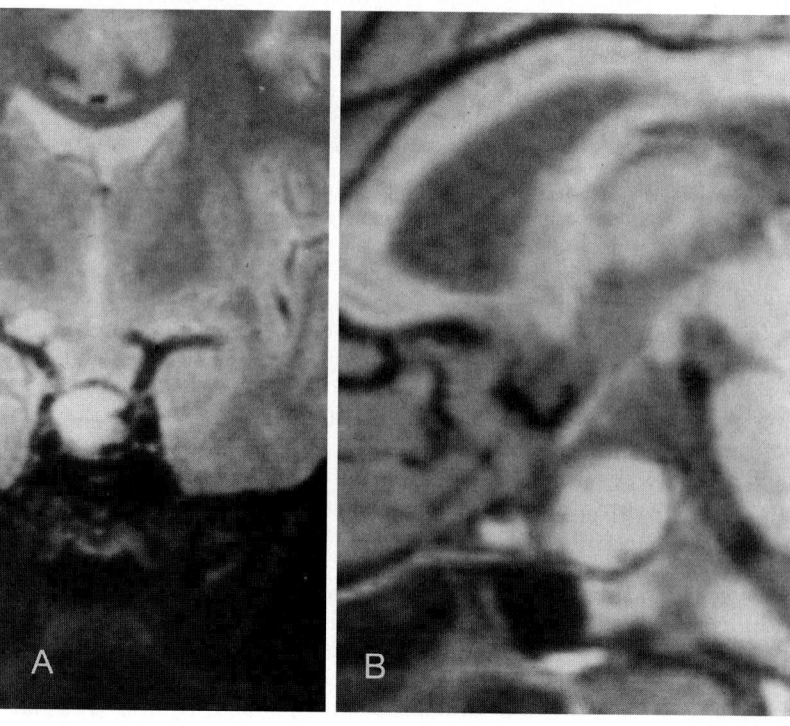

Figure 5.18. Craniopharyngioma. A. Coronal T2WI through the sella in patient with mild visual symptoms. A hyperintense intrasellar mass with suprasellar component is seen. **B.** Sagittal T1WI shows hyperintense signal is maintained consistent with the presence of liquid cholesterol characteristic of these tumors.

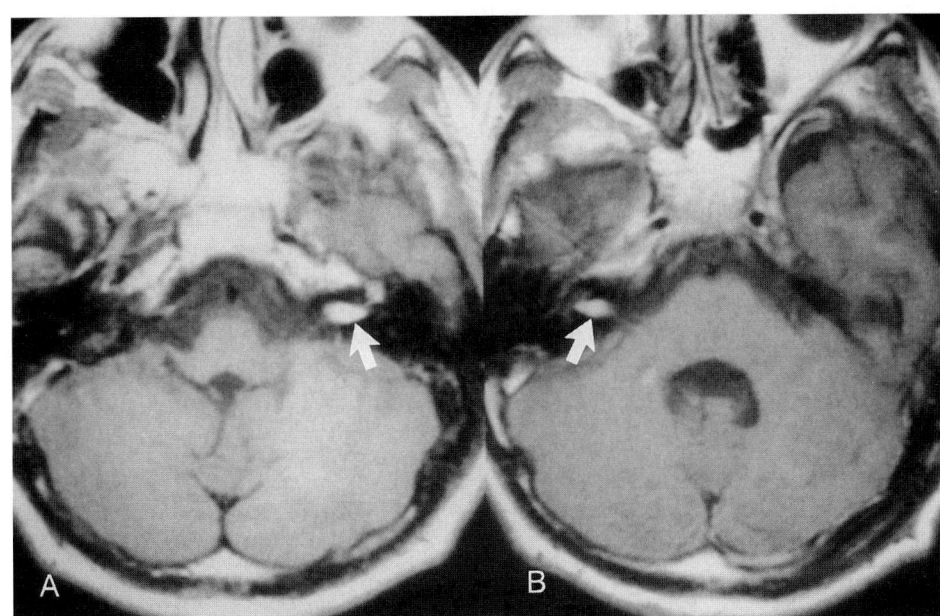

Figure 5.19. Acoustic Schwannoma. A,B. Postcontrast axial T1WI show bilateral intracanalicular acoustic schwannomas (*arrows*) in patient with neurofibromatosis type 2. Extension into the internal acoustic canal and lack of a broad dural base differentiate this entity from meningioma.

matter on T2WI. As with CT contrast, they enhance intensely with gadolinium. The larger a schwannoma is, the more likely it is to show heterogeneity because of cysts, hemorrhage, or necrosis.

Acoustic schwannomas are located within the internal auditory canal, either being completely intracanalicular or extending into the cerebellopontine angle. The internal auditory canal is frequently enlarged. Differentiation from a cerebellopontine meningioma may be difficult. The single most helpful imaging feature to distinguish an acoustic schwannoma from a meningioma is extension of the enhancement along the course of the seventh and eighth nerves, seen in approximately 80% of acoustic schwannoma cases (Fig. 5.19). Meningiomas very rarely demonstrate this feature and instead frequently will have a broad dural tail (Fig. 5.20). A precontrast or fat-suppressed sequence will detect the unlikely intracanalicular lipoma that appears identical to an acoustic schwannoma on postcontrast images. Other cerebellopontine angle lesions include epidermoid tumors (Fig. 5.21) and nonacoustic (cranial nerves V, IX–XI) schwannomas. A mnemonic for cerebellopontine angle lesions is given in Table 5.12.

Trigeminal schwannomas can be identified by their location within the pontine cistern at the midpons level between the trigeminal ganglion located in Meckel's cave (just posterolateral to the cavernous sinus) and the brainstem (Fig. 5.22). Extension through the ganglion and into the foramen ovale, foramen rotundum, or superior orbital fissure may be seen. Less commonly, schwannomas may also involve cranial nerves IX–XI.

Neurofibromas, on the other hand, arise from fibroblasts and Schwann cells, are fusiform, and involve the cutaneous exiting spinal nerves. They are rarely cystic, hemorrhagic, or necrotic. Neurofibromas, which are rarely solitary, are more commonly seen in the spine as part of neurofibromatosis types I and II. The most common clinical presentation is that of multiple radiculopathies or cord compression. These tumors are discussed in greater detail in chapter 8.

Tumors of Mesenchymal Origin

MENINGIOMA

Meningioma is the most common extra-axial neoplasm of adults and accounts for 15% of all intracranial neoplasms, second only to gliomas. The peak age of incidence is 50–60 years. For both intracranial (2:1) and intraspinal (4:1) meningiomas, females are more commonly affected. Because the tumors are hormonally sensitive, they may increase in size during pregnancy. Up to 9% are multiple and are associated with neurofibromatosis. Although rare in children unless associated with neurofibromatosis, pediatric meningiomas are more likely to be malignant. Most meningiomas are benign and slow-growing tumors that are most frequently found in parasagittal or convexity locations (50%). Other locations include sphenoid wing (20%), olfactory groove/ planum sphenoidale (10%), parasellar (10%), and a whole host of miscellaneous locations (10%) such as the ventricles (the most common site in children), tentorium, and optic nerve sheath. Approximately 2–3% occur within the spine, with the thoracic spine being the most common location.

Table 5.12. Cerebellopontine Masses ("AMEN")

Lesion	T1WI (compared to gray matter)	T2WI (compared to gray matter)	Gadolinium enhancement
Acoustic schwannoma (80%)	Hypo	Hyper	Yes
Meningioma (11%)	Iso to hypo	Iso to hyper	Yes
Ependymoma (4%)	Hypo	Hyper	Yes
Neuroepithelial cyst (arachnoid, epidermoid) (5%)	CSF	CSF	No

Iso = isointense relative to gray matter
Hypo = hypointense relative to gray matter
Hyper = hyperintense relative to gray matter
CSF = follows signal of cerebrospinal fluid

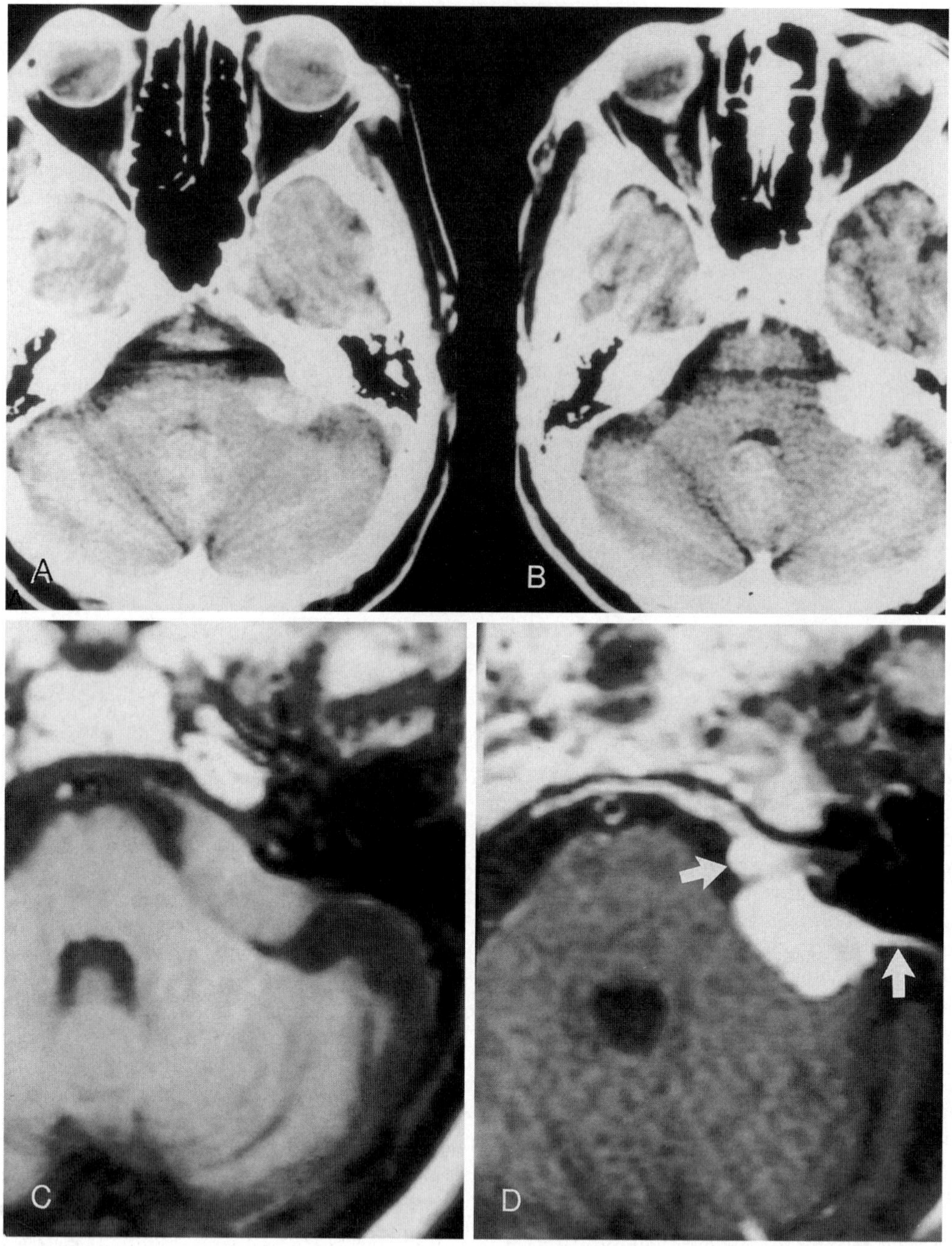

Figure 5.20. Cerebellopontine angle meningioma. Noncontrast **(A)** and postcontrast **(B)** CT scans show left cerebellopontine mass which intensely enhances. Noncontrast **(C)** and postcontrast **(D)** T1WI show extra-axial lesion with broad dural base and intense en-hancement. There is no extension along neurovascular bundle of internal acoustic canal. Note the dural tails (*arrows*) extending anteriorly and posteriorly within cerebellopontine angle.

Pathology. Meningiomas arise from meningothelial arachnoid cells (villi), probably with some contribution from dural fibroblasts and pial cells. Intraventricular meningiomas arise from arachnoidal cell rests within the choroid plexus. There are five basic types: meningothelial (syncytial), transitional, fibroblastic, hemangiopericytoma/angioblastic, and malignant meningioma. Two basic shapes (globular and en plaque) are seen.

Imaging—CT. Meningiomas present some of the most classic roentgenologic findings of any disease process.

Even on plain skull films, these tumors can be suspected by focal sclerosis, prominent dural grooves from enlarged middle meningeal arteries, and calcification. On CT, they are well-defined hyperdense (85%) masses with variable surrounding edema with intense and homogeneous enhancement (Fig. 5.23). Hyperostosis of the adjacent inner table is noted approximately 40% of the time. Calcification is seen in 10–20%. The key to diagnosis is the broad dural base of these extra-axial masses. Adjacent dural thickening (the "dural tail") (Figs.

5.17,5.20) is seen in approximately 60% of cases but is not specific for meningiomas and does not necessarily indicate involvement by meningioma tumor cells (35,36). Hemorrhage is rare but cysts are not uncommon.

Imaging—MR. On MR, meningiomas are characterized by isointensity to hypointensity to gray matter on T1WI and isointensity to hyperintensity to gray matter on T2WI. Hyperintensity on T2WI almost always correlates with a syncytial or angioblastic type of meningioma. Heterogeneity is the rule because of the presence of cysts, vessels, or calcification. Often, a hypointense rim is present around the tumor. Prominent pial blood vessel flow voids are frequently (80%) noted on MR and provide evidence of the extra-axial nature of the tumor. CSF clefts around the margin of the tumor also confirm the extra-axial location in 80% of cases. Invasion of the dural margin interface is highly specific for a dural process (29). Special attention should be given to possible involvement of the dural sinuses as this finding carries important significance in neurosurgical planning.

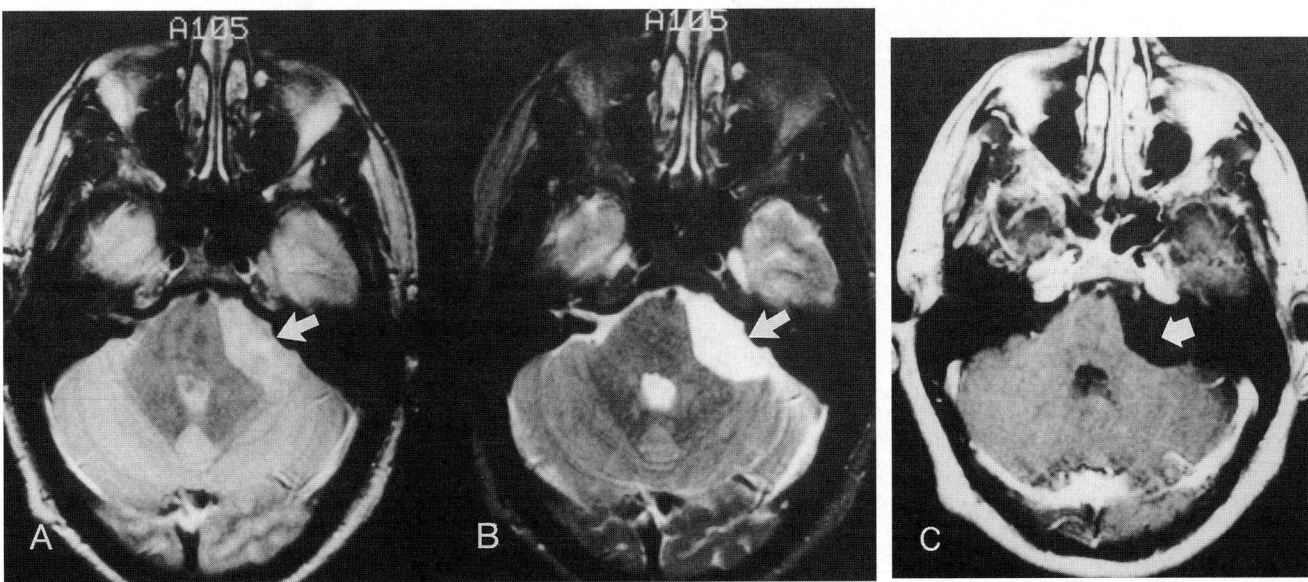

Figure. 5.21. Epidermoid. Axial T2WI **(A,** first echo; **B,** second echo) show left cerebellopontine angle mass *(arrows)* that closely follows signal intensity of CSF. Postcontrast T1WI **(C)** shows no enhancement of the extra-axial mass *(arrow)* which again has signal intensity similar to that of CSF.

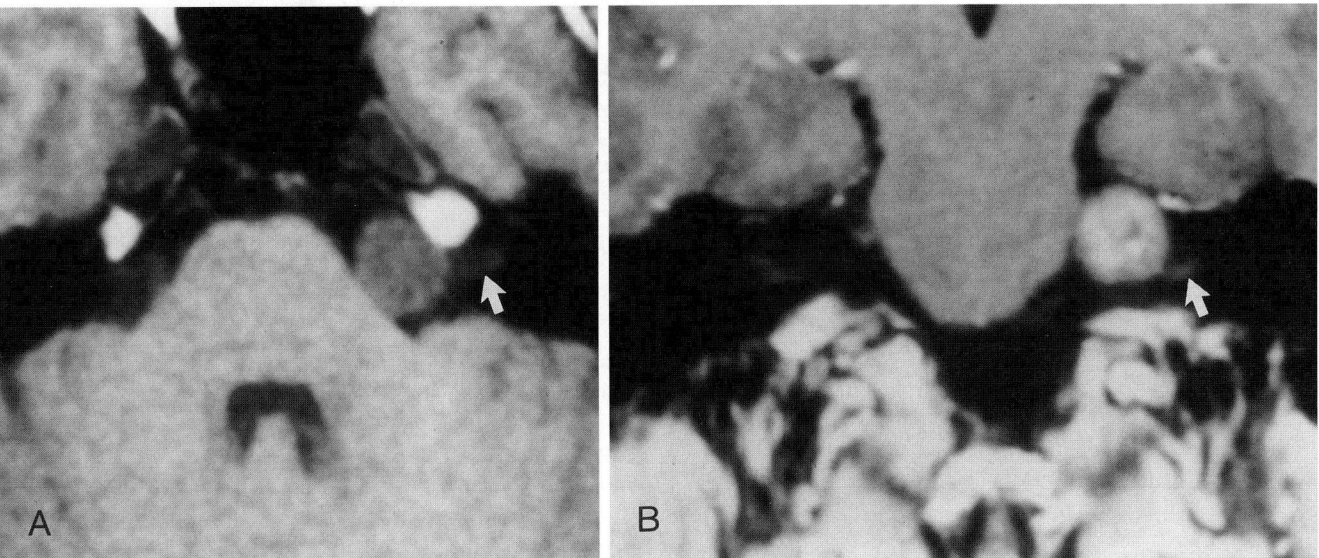

Figure 5.22. Trigeminal Schwannoma. A. Axial T1WI in patient with dizziness shows isointense mass in cisternal space near vicinity of internal auditory canal. Note the portion of seventh and eighth nerve complex *(arrow)* displaced by mass. **B.** Postcontrast coronal T1WI shows homogeneous enhancement. Again note the seventh and eighth nerve complex *(arrow)* displaced by this schwannoma from the trigeminal nerve.

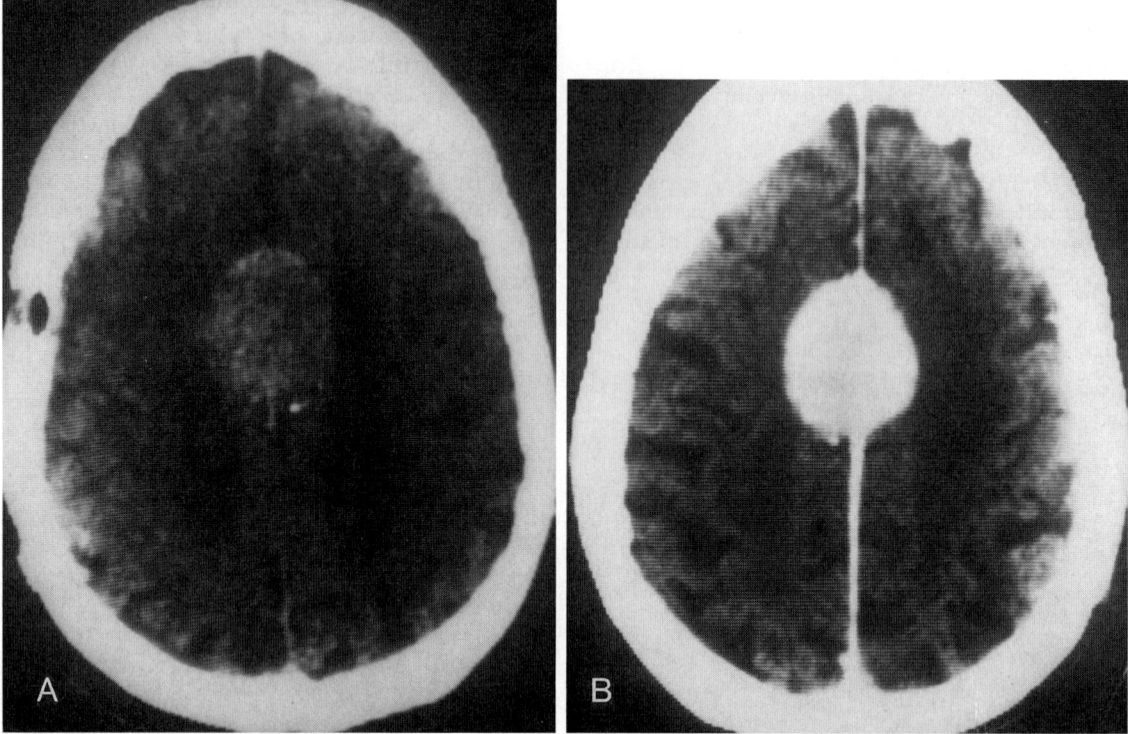

Figure 5.23. Meningioma. Precontrast **(A)** and postcontrast **(B)** CT images of falcine meningioma. On the precontrast study, the mass is hyperdense to normal brain parenchyma. With contrast, there is intense enhancement. One-half of all meningiomas occur parasagittally or along the convexity.

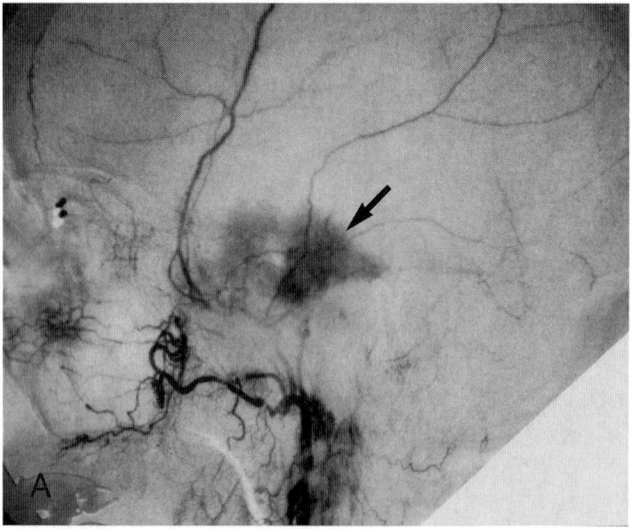
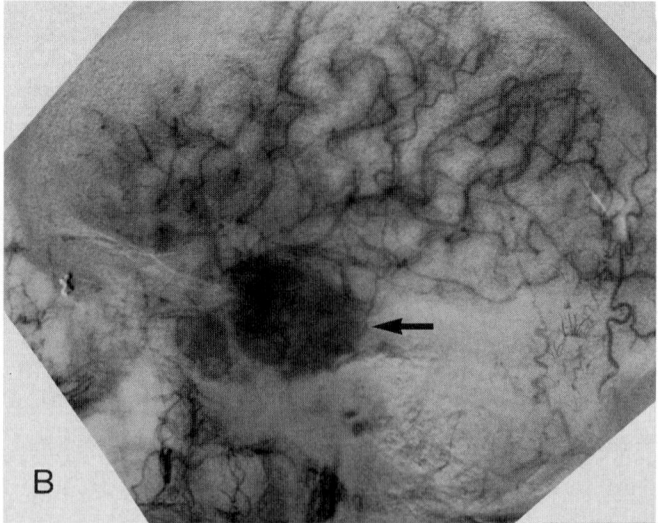

Figure 5.24. Meningioma on Angiogram. Selective external carotid injection, in which **(A)** demonstrates early blush (*arrow*) on arterial phase while **(B)** shows persistent staining on venous phase. This "coming early and staying late" has been called the "in-law sign."

Because of this feature, MR is superior to CT in overall evaluation of these tumors. Any diminution in the caliber of a dural sinus adjacent to a meningioma suggests involvement. Further evaluation with MR angiography or conventional angiography may confirm this finding and provide evidence for or against complete occlusion.

Angiography. Angiographically, meningiomas present a classic appearance. During the arterial phase, an early dense tumor blush with a radial arrangement of the vessels occurs. This blush persists well into the venous phase. Because the blush "comes early and stays late," some (not necessarily this author) have called this "the in-law sign" (Fig. 5.24). In addition, enlarged dural vessels and arteriovenous shunting may be noted. The most common blood supply to meningiomas is from branches of the external carotid artery, primarily the ter on T1WI and hyperintensity to gray matter on T2WI. Surrounding edema may be present, and serpiginous flow voids within the nodule may be seen. In the less common presentation of a solid mass, the margins are usually ill-defined and occasionally hemorrhage is present. Because of the highly vascular nature of the nodule, intense enhancement is the rule (Fig. 5.25). If CT or MR is negative in highly clinically suspicious cases, angiography may be helpful in revealing small (<1 cm) lesions.

Tumors of Maldevelopmental Origin

EPIDERMOID/DERMOID

Epidermoid and dermoid are uncommon congenital neoplasms that result from enclosure of ectodermal elements when the neural tube closes. Epidermoid tumors account for approximately 1% of all intracranial neoplasms whereas dermoid tumors, as intracranial masses, are much less common. Both are benign and characterized by slow growth. The peak age of incidence is between 40–50 years for epidermoids and 20–30 years for dermoids. Although epidermoids are made up of squamous epithelium alone, dermoids contain mesodermal elements as well. They both contain keratin but dermoid tumors are also composed of fat and calcification. Epidermoids are most often located off the midline at the skull base (i.e., cerebellopontine angle, parasellar, or the posterior fossa) whereas dermoids are characteristically midline masses, most common at the inferior vermis or at the vallecula. Epidermoids commonly are tightly adherent to and compress adjacent structures, most commonly the cranial nerves. Symptoms from dermoid tumors are secondary to obstruction of CSF pathways, chemical meningitis (secondary to rupture of the dermoid), or infection if associated with a sinus tract. A comparison of epidermoids and dermoids is given in Table 5.13.

Imaging. On imaging studies, the differing compositions produce different signal intensities. Epidermoid tumors are well-circumscribed lobulated masses that, because of the presence of solid cholesterol and/or CSF within the interstices of the tumor, most commonly have signal intensities on both CT and MR that follow that of CSF (hypodense on CT, hypointense on T1WI, and hy-

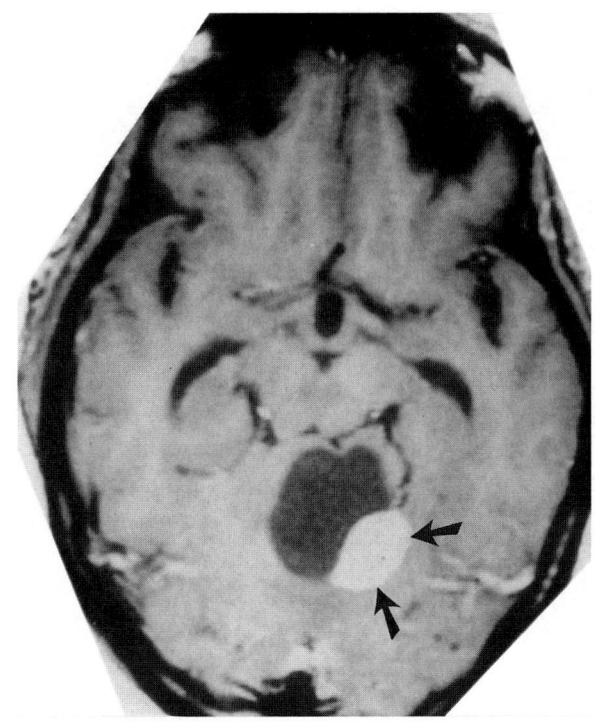

Figure 5.25. Hemangioblastoma. Classic appearance on postcontrast axial T1WI of cystic posterior fossa mass with intensely enhancing mural nodule (*arrow*), which represents the tumor itself.

middle meningeal artery. The anterior meningeal arteries (arising from the ophthalmic arteries) and the posterior meningeal arteries (arising from the vertebral arteries) also provide blood supply to these tumors. Pre-operative embolization of these vessels often facilitates neurosurgical resection.

Malignant variants of meningiomas are rare, occurring in approximately 1% of cases. It is not possible to reliably distinguish malignant from nonmalignant meningiomas based on imaging characteristics alone.

HEMANGIOBLASTOMA

Capillary hemangioblastomas are benign neoplasms of endothelial origin. Most common in young and middle-aged adults, they are the most common primary intra-axial neoplasm of the posterior fossa in adults. Approximately 4–20% occur as part of the von Hippel-Lindau syndrome (discussed in chapter 8), in which case they are often multiple. They most often occur in the cerebellar hemispheres, but other sites of involvement include the spinal cord (especially the cervical portion), medulla, and even the cerebral hemispheres (very rare). As they contain no capsule, recurrence is common if only partial resection is performed. Because the tumor nidus receives its blood supply from the pia mater, the nodule (which represents the tumor itself) is always superficial in location (37). Calcification is very rare.

Imaging. The classic appearance is a well-defined cystic mass with an intensely enhancing mural nodule (60% of cases). As many as 40% are entirely solid. On MR, they appear as cystic masses with hypointensity to gray mat-

Table 5.13. Epidermoid vs. Dermoid

Characteristics	Epidermoid	Dermoid
Frequency	Common	Uncommon
Peak Age	40–50	20–30
Germ Cells	Ectoderm	Ectoderm and mesoderm
Location	Off midline (cerebellopontine angle, parasellar, posterior fossa)	Midline (pericerebellar, suprasellar)
Imaging	Follows CSF most commonly, lobulated with interstices	Some portion will follow fat

Figure 5.26. Dermoid Tumor. Coronal T1WI **(A)** shows hyperintense suprasellar mass (*arrow*). With fat suppression technique **(B),** the signal of the dermoid becomes isointense following the signal of subcutaneous fat confirming the nature of the lesion.

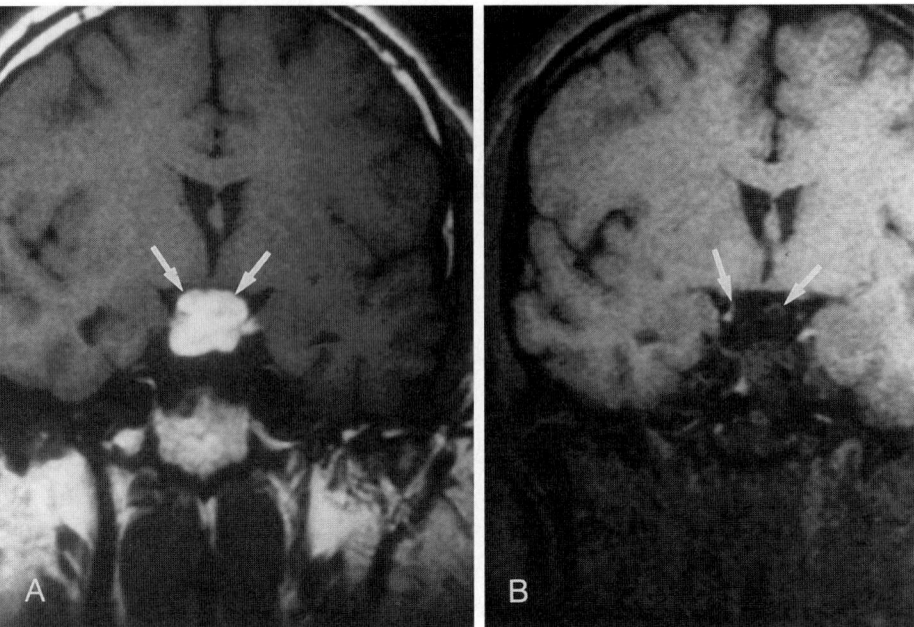

perintense on T2WI) (Fig. 5.21). Rim enhancement following contrast may be seen. On occasion, epidermoids contain enough liquid cholesterol (similar to craniopharyngioma) to produce T1 shortening (hyperintensity) of the mass (38). The primary differential diagnosis is an arachnoid cyst. If the diagnosis is in doubt, the definitive study is a cisternogram that demonstrates contrast filling the interstices of the epidermoid (producing a "cauliflower-like" appearance) whereas an arachnoid cyst will have a smooth margin. Sometimes this cauliflower appearance can be appreciated on thin-section T1WI.

Dermoid tumors, on the other hand, typically have signal characteristics that follow that of fat (low density on CT, hyperintense on T1WI, and intermediate to hypointense on T2WI, with signal suppression on fat-saturation images) (Fig. 5.26). They do not enhance unless infected. Heterogeneity of the mass may be seen because of calcification and other soft tissue components. The presence of a fat-fluid level is almost pathognomonic. If no heterogeneity is present, distinguishing dermoid tumors from lipomas is impossible. Occasionally, dermoids may rupture into the subarachnoid space, producing a chemical meningitis. In this situation, multiple foci of T1 shortening will be seen extra-axially, and the patient is almost always quite ill. In such situations, some fatalities have been reported. In the presence of an intracranial dermoid, the nasofrontal and occipital regions of the scalp should be evaluated to detect a sinus tract.

LIPOMA

Intracranial lipomas are usually asymptomatic and incidental findings on imaging studies. They occur in all ages and are most common in the midline, the corpus collosum, the quadrigeminal plate, and the suprasellar regions. Lipomas are thought to arise from incomplete resorption of the primitive meningeal tissue in the devel-

opment of the subarachnoid cisterns (9). Lipomas in the pericollosal region are commonly associated with agenesis of the corpus collosum (Fig. 5.27). As expected for a fatty mass, they exhibit low density on CT, occasionally containing calcification. On MR, they exhibit T1 and mild T2 shortening, following the signal intensity of subcutaneous fat. They do not enhance. The presence of either a chemical shift artifact or signal suppression on a fat saturation T1WI establishes the diagnosis.

ARACHNOID CYST

Arachnoid cysts account for approximately 1% of all intracranial masses and are congenital in nature. "Secondary" or "acquired arachnoid cysts" are in reality leptomeningeal cysts that result from a prior inflammatory process (meningitis, hemorrhage, etc.). True arachnoid cysts are created by secretion of CSF from the cells lining the cyst and are therefore intra-arachnoidal. They are most common (50%) in the middle cranial fossa where they may be quite large. Other sites include the frontal convexity, the suprasellar and quadrigeminal cisterns, and the posterior fossa. If they attain sufficient size to obstruct CSF flow or compress the brain, they become symptomatic.

Imaging. They follow the attenuation/signal intensity pattern for CSF on CT and MR. Remodeling of the adjacent bone may be seen. Hemorrhage may occur after trauma or spontaneously. Unless infection is present, no enhancement is noted.

Differential Diagnosis. The differential diagnosis for the posterior fossa arachnoid cyst includes enlarged cisterna magna, epidermoid, and Dandy-Walker malformation. Enlarged cisterna magna and epidermoid may be difficult to distinguish from an arachnoid cyst based on CT or MR. Intrathecal injection of iodinated contrast, which will fill the cisterna magna but not the arachnoid cyst, demonstrates the fronds of the epidermoid or the

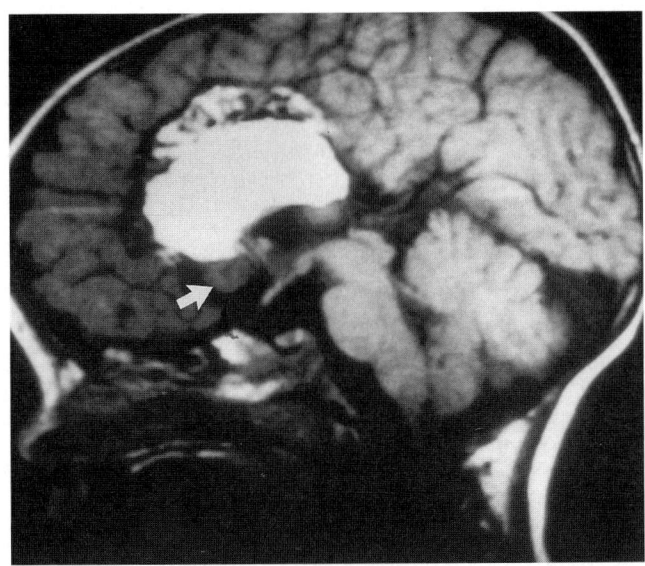

Figure 5.27. Lipoma with Agenesis of Corpus Callosum. Sagittal T1WI shows large hyperintense midline mass. The development of a lipoma in this location prevents normal development of the corpus collosum. Note that only a portion of the genu (*arrow*) is present while the remaining structures of the corpus collosum are absent.

arachnoid cyst's smooth margins. Dandy-Walker cysts are extensions of the fourth ventricle, and an arachnoid cyst will be separate from the fourth ventricle (18).

Neuroepithelial Tumors

COLLOID CYST

Colloid cysts characteristically occur in the anterior-superior third ventricle near the Foramen of Monro. Although they account for only 2% of all intracranial tumors, they are important because of their propensity to cause acute hydrocephalus as a consequence of their obstructing the foramina of Monro. The classic presentation is that of acute onset of a severe headache that can be reproduced by the patient tilting the head forward (Brun phenomenon). Occasional fatalities have been reported.

Pathology. Some colloid cysts are entirely cystic and others have a heterogeneous composition of old hemorrhage, cholesterol crystals, and various ions. They are believed to have an epithelial lining similar to respiratory mucosa (39).

Imaging. The imaging appearance is variable. On CT, most are hyperdense to brain tissue; on MR, hyperintensity on T1WI is most common (Fig. 5.28). Rim enhancement has been seen in as many as to 40%. Other lesions that occur in the anterior-superior third ventricle are listed in Table 5.14. Dense enhancement suggests a lesion other than colloid cyst (40).

CHOROID PLEXUS PAPILLOMA

Choroid plexus papilloma is a rare neuroepithelial tumor most common in the first decade but can also be seen in adults. They account for only approxi-

mately 0.5% of all intracranial neoplasms. The atrium of the lateral ventricle is the most common site in children, and the fourth ventricle is the most common site in adults. The clinical presentation of choroid plexus papilloma is often related to increased intracranial pressure and hydrocephalus, which occur because of the marked increase production of CSF by these tumors. CSF resorption is also reduced because of hemorrhage and increased protein content within the CSF. Malignant degeneration in the form of choroid plexus carcinoma occurs in approximately 10–20% of cases (41).

Imaging. On CT, these are well-defined masses that are isodense to hyperdense and typically have the shape of a cauliflower (Fig. 5.29). Engulfment of the glomus of the choroid plexus is said to be a distinguishing feature. Choroid plexus calcification in the first decade of life is atypical and suggests the possibility of a choroid plexus papilloma. On MR, they are isointense to gray matter on T1WI and hyperintense to gray matter on T2WI. These highly vascular tumors enhance markedly. Carcinomatous degeneration is suggested by heterogeneity or parenchymal invasion with white matter edema. Differential diagnoses for intraventricular masses based on age and location are provided in Tables 5.15 and 5.16.

Subarachnoid spread of either choroid plexus papilloma or choroid plexus carcinoma is possible. The

Table 5.14. Masses of the Antero-Superior Third Ventricle

Colloid cyst	Glioma
Meningioma	Vascular lesion
Choroid plexus papilloma	Granulomatous lesion
Hamartoma	

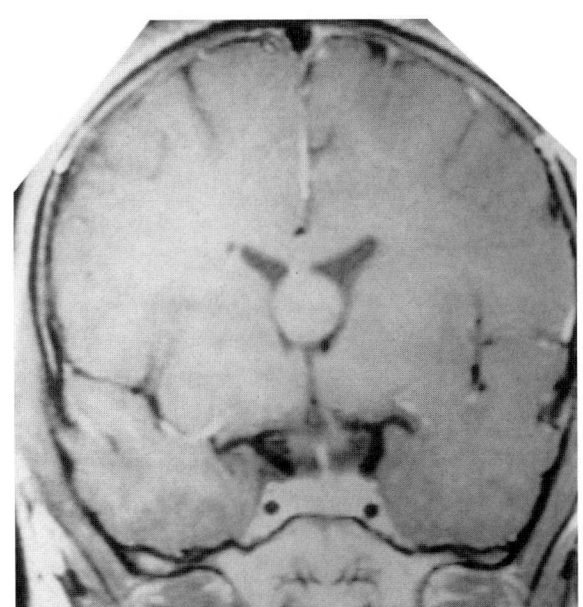

Figure 5.28. Colloid Cyst. Coronal T1WI shows the typical appearance and characteristic location in third ventricle.

Table 5.15. Most Common Lateral Ventricle Masses by Location and Age

Age (years)	Foramen of Monro	Body	Trigone
0–5		Primitive neuroectodermal tumor Teratoma Choroid plexus papilloma	Choroid plexus papilloma
6–30	Subependymal giant cell astrocytoma Juvenile pilocytic astrocytoma	Ependymoma Juvenile pilocytic astrocytoma	Ependymoma Oligodendroglioma
>30	Metastasis	Subependymoma Glioblastoma multiforme	Meningioma

Adapted from Jelinek J, Smirniotopoulos JG, Parisi JE et al. Lateral ventricular neoplasms of the brain: differential diagnosis based on clinical, CT, and MR findings. AJNR 1990;11:567–574.

Table 5.16 Intraventricular Masses

The Major Players

Astrocytoma—most common frontal horn lesion, least enhancement

Colloid cyst—foramen of Monro, most common III ventricle mass

Meningioma—most common atrial lesion

Ependymoma—most common body of lateral ventricle lesion

Medulloblastoma—IV ventricle (by direct extension), III and lateral by seeding

Craniopharyngioma—second most common III ventricle mass

Choroid plexus papilloma/carcinoma—lateral ventricle > III ventricle, enhance intensely

Others

Cysticercosis—IV > anterior III ventricle, change position with head tilting

Epidermoid—IV ventricle

Ependymal/Arachnoid cyst—III ventricle most common

Dermoid—IV ventricle and frontal horn

Subependymoma—IV ventricle, frontal horn

Arteriovenous malformations—lateral and IV ventricles

Teratoma

Adapted from Morrison G, Sobel DF, Kelly WM, et al. Intraventricular mass lesions. Radiology 1984;153:435–442.

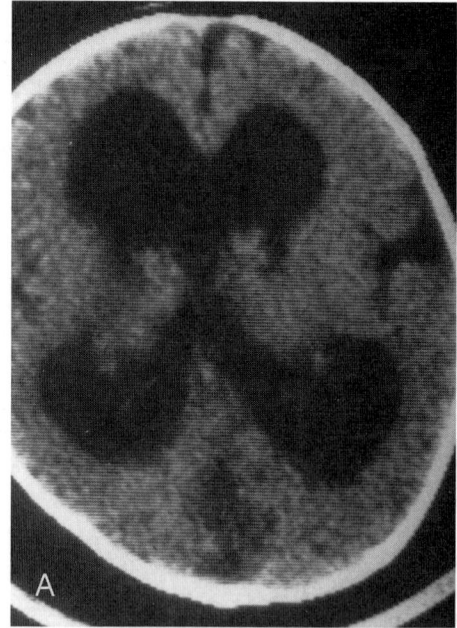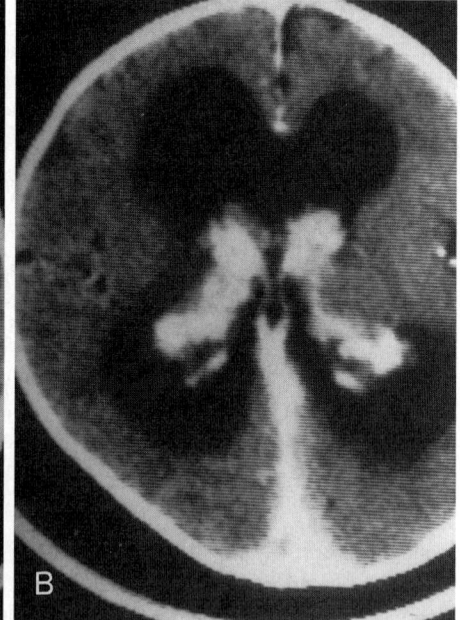

Figure 5.29. Choroid Plexus Papilloma. Precontrast **(A)** and postcontrast **(B)** CT scans. Note the enlarged ventricles and extremely prominent choroid plexus formation bilaterally. Hydrocephalus results from increased production of CSF and decreased resorption secondary to proteinaceous debris and hemorrhage.

prognosis of choroid plexus papilloma is quite favorable if resected early before irreversible damage secondary to hydrocephalus or repeated hemorrhage has occurred. The prognosis for choroid plexus carcinoma is more guarded.

HAMARTOMA OF THE TUBER CINEREUM

An "Aunt Minnie" in neuroradiology, these rare congenital malformations of normal neuronal tissue are more common in boys who usually have precocious puberty, seizures, developmental delay, and hyperactivity. They are well-circumscribed round or oval masses centered in the region of the tuber cinereum (at the base of the infundibulum). They do not calcify or hemorrhage. On CT and MR, they have the same signal intensity as brain tissue (possibly slightly hyperintense on T2WI) and do not enhance (Fig. 5.30) (18). Along with the characteristic location, a stalk connecting the mass with the tuber cinereum or mamillary bodies cinches the diagnosis.

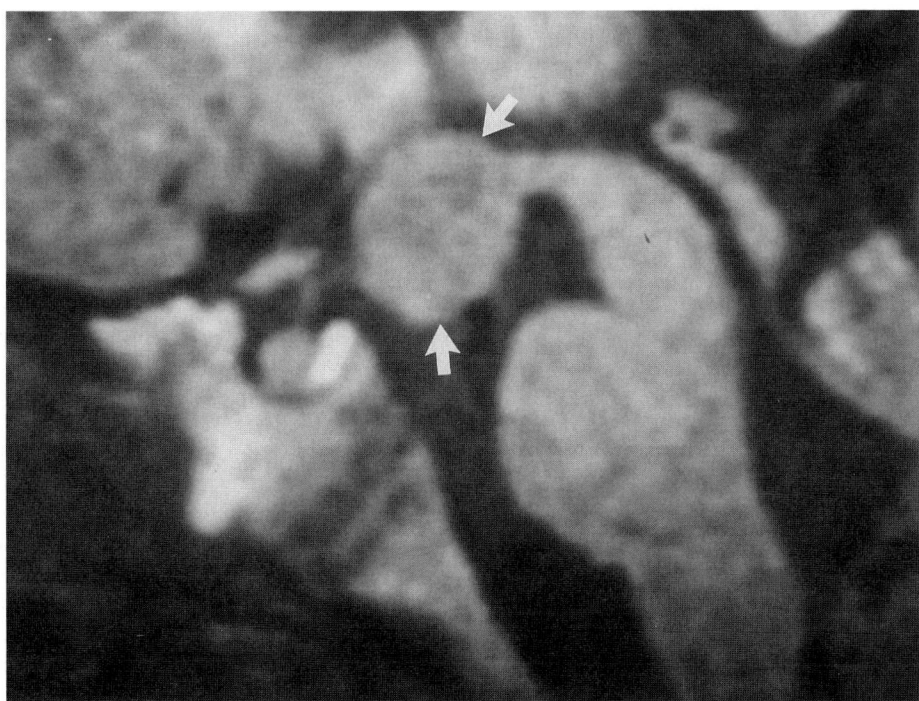

Figure 5.30. Hamartoma of Tuber Cinereum. This lesion was found in a young adult with diabetes insipidus. Hamartomas may vary in size from 1–2 mm to larger lesions such as this one (*arrow*).

References

1. Kleihues P, Burger PC, Scheithauer BW. Histological Typing of Tumors of the Central Nervous System. 2nd ed. Berlin: Springer-Verlag, 1993.
2. Netter FH. Nervous system. Vol. 1 of The CIBA Collection of Medical Illustrations. West Caldwell, NJ: CIBA Pharmaceutical, 1986:115.
3. Gean AD. Imaging of Head Trauma. 1st ed. New York: Raven Press, 1994:267–278.
4. Hahn F, Gurney J. CT signs of central descending transtentorial herniation. AJNR 1985;6:844–845.
5. Fetell MR, Stein BM. Tumors: general considerations. In: Rowland LP, ed. Merritt's Textbook of Neurology. Philadelphia: Lea & Febiger, 1989:275–367.
6. George AE, Russell EJ, Kricheff II. White matter buckling: CT sign of extra-axial intracranial mass. AJNR Am J Neuroradiol 1980;1:425–430.
7. Kelly PJ, Daumas-Duport C, Scheithauer BW, et al. Stereotactic histologic correlation of CT- and MR-defined abnormalities in patients with glial neoplasms. Mayo Clin Proc 1987;62:450–459.
8. Henkelman RM, Watts JF, Kucharczyk W. High signal intensity in MR images of calcified brain tissue. Radiology 1991;179:199–206.
9. Atlas SA. Intra-axial neoplasms. In: Atlas SA, ed. Magnetic Resonance Imaging of the Brain and Spine. New York: Raven Press, 1991:223–326.
10. Sage MR. Blood-brain barrier: Phenomenon of increasing importance to the imaging clinician. AJR Am J Roentgenol 1982;138:887–898.
11. Kahn D, Follett KA, Bushnell DL, et al. Diagnosis of recurrent brain tumor: value of 201Th SPECT vs. 18F-fluorodeoxy PET. AJR Am J Roentgenol 1994;163:1459–1465.
12. Valk PE, Dillon WP. Radiation injury of the brain. AJNR Am J Neuroradiol 1991;12:45–62.
13. Burger PC. Malignant astrocytic neoplasms: classification, pathologic anatomy, and response to therapy. Semin Oncol 1986;13:16–26.
14. Haimes AB, Zimmerman RD, Morgello S. MR imaging of brain abscess. AJNR Am J Neuroradiol 1989;10:279–291.
15. Russell DS, Rubenstein LJ. Pathology of tumors of the central nervous system. 5th ed. Baltimore: Williams & Wilkins, 1989.
16. Spagnoli MV, Grossman RI, Packer RJ, et al. Magnetic resonance imaging determination of gliomatosis cerebri. Neuroradiology 1987;29:15–18.
17. Lee Y-Y, Tassel PV. Intracranial oligodendrogliomas: imaging findings in 35 untreated cases. AJNR 1989;10:119–127.
18. Barkovich AJ. Pediatric Neuroimaging. 2nd ed. New York: Raven Press, 1995:321–437.
19. Olson EM, Tien RD, Chamberlain MC. Osseous metastasis in medulloblastoma: MRI findings in an unusual case. Clin Imaging 1991;15:286–289.
20. Davis PC, Wichman RD, Takei Y, et al. Primary cerebral neuroblastoma: CT and MR findings in 12 cases. AJNR Am J Neuroradiol 1990;11:115–120.
21. Buetow PC, Smirniotopoulos JG, Done S. Congenital brain tumors: a review of 45 cases. AJNR Am J Neuroradiol 1990; 11:793–799.
22. Hochberg FH, Miller DC. Primary central nervous system lymphoma. J Neurosurg 1988;68:835–853.
23. So YT, Beckstead JH, Davis RL. Primary central nervous system lymphoma in acquired immune deficiency syndrome: a clinical and pathological study. Ann Neurol 1986; 20:566–572.
24. Koeller KK, Smirnitopoulos JG, Jones RV. Primary central nervous system lymphoma: radiologic-pathologic correlation. Radiographics 1997;17:1497–1526.
25. Dina TS. Primary central nervous lymphoma versus toxoplasmosis in AIDS. Radiology 1991;179:823–828.
26. Sze G, Milano E, Johnson C, et al. Detection of brain metastasis: comparison of contrast-enhanced MR with unenhanced MR and enhanced CT. AJNR Am J Neuroradiol 1990;11:785–791.
27. Davis PC, Hudgins PA, Peterman SB, et al. Diagnosis of cerebral metastasis: double-dose delayed CT vs. contrast-enhanced MR imaging. AJNR Am J Neuroradiol 1991;12: 293–300.

28. Yuh WTC, Engelken JD, Muhonen MG, et al. Experience with high-dose MR imaging in the evaluation of brain metastasis. AJNR Am J Neuroradiol 1992;13:335–345.

29. Goldberg HI. Extra-axial brain tumors. In: Atlas SA, ed. Magnetic Resonance Imaging of the Brain and Spine. New York: Raven Press, 1991:327–378.

30. Koeller KK, Dillon WP. MR appearance of dysembryoplastic neuroepithelial tumors (DNT). AJNR 1992;1319–1325.

31. Castillo M, Davis PC, Takei Y, et al. Intracranial ganglioglioma: MR, CT, and clinical findings in 18 patients. AJNR 1990;11:109–114.

32. Edwards MSB, Hudgins RJ, Wilson CB, et al. Pineal region tumors in children. J Neurosurg 1988;68:689–697.

33. Ganti SR, Hilal SK, Stein BM, et al. CT of pineal region tumors. AJR 1986;146:451–458.

34. Lee DH, Norman D, Newton TH. MR imaging of pineal cysts. J Comput Assist Tomogr 1987;11:586–590.

35. Goldsher D, Litt AW, Pinto RS, et al. Dural "tail" associated with meningiomas on Gd-DTPA-enhanced MR images: characteristics, differential diagnostic value, and possible implications for treatment. Radiology 1990;176:447–450.

36. Tokumaru A, O'uchi T, Eguchi T, et al. Prominent meningeal enhancement adjacent to meningioma on Gd-DTPA-enhanced MR images: histopathologic correlation. Radiology 1990;175:431–433.

37. Lee SR, Sanches J, Mark AS, et al. Posterior fossa hemangioblastomas: MR imaging. Radiology 1989;171:463–468.

38. Gao P-Y, Osborn AG, Smirniotopoulos JG, et al. Epidermoid tumor of the cerebellopontine angle. AJNR 1992;13:863–872.

39. Kirsch C, Smirniotopoulos JG, Koeller KK. Colloid cysts: radiologic pathologic correlation with review of the Armed Forces Institute of Pathology (AFIP) experience and world literature. J International Neuroradiology (in press).

40. Waggenspack GA, Guinto FCJ. MR and CT of masses of the anterosuperior third ventricle. AJNR 1989;10:105–110.

41. Coates TL, Hinshaw DB, Peckman N, et al. Pediatric choroid plexus eoplasms: MR, CT, and pathologic correlation. Radiology 1989;173:81–88.

6
Central Nervous System Infections

Walter L. Olsen

PARENCHYMAL INFECTIONS
  Pyogenic Cerebritis and Abscess
  Mycobacterial Infections
  Fungal Infections
  Parasitic Infections
  Spirochete Infections
  Viral Infections
EXTRA-AXIAL INFECTIONS
  Meningitis
  Subdural and Epidural Infections
ACQUIRED IMMUNODEFICIENCY SYNDROME

CNS infections commonly require evaluation by radiologists. Because these infections often have dire neurologic consequences, early diagnosis and management is crucial. CT and MR have significantly aided this effort. For example, before CT, pyogenic abscesses of the brain carried a 30–70% mortality rate. The mortality rate has dropped to less than 5% in recent years, largely because of the ability of CT to diagnose the abscess accurately and to monitor the efficacy of treatment accurately. MR is playing an increasingly greater role in the evaluation of CNS infection because of improved sensitivity for detecting early infections. Because CT and MR are highly accurate, the choice of modality often depends on the clinical situation. Gravely ill patients are usually better evaluated by CT, which is faster, less susceptible to patient motion artifact, and permits closer patient monitoring. MR is generally preferable in the clinically stable patient.

PARENCHYMAL INFECTIONS

Pyogenic Cerebritis and Abscess

Pyogenic infections of the brain may develop by direct extension after trauma, surgery, sinusitis, dental infections, or otomastoiditis. Hematogenous infections occur even more frequently, especially in patients with lung infections, endocarditis, or congenital heart disease. Anaerobic bacteria are the most common organisms overall. Staphylococcus aureus is common after surgery or trauma. Gram-negative rod, pneumococcal, streptococcal, listerial, nocardial, and actinomycetic infections also occur with some frequency. With infections resulting from hematogenous spread, the frontal and parietal lobes (middle cerebral artery distribution) are most commonly involved, with the abscess centered at the gray–white junction. The frontal lobes are most com-

monly affected with spread of sinus infections. The temporal lobe or cerebellum are involved in patients with spread from otomastoiditis.

Clinical symptoms in patients with pyogenic brain infections may be mild or severe. Usually, there is headache. There may be varying degrees of lethargy, obtundation, nausea, vomiting, and fever. Fever is absent more than 50% of the time. Meningeal signs are present in only 30% of patients. Focal neurologic deficits, papilledema, nuchal rigidity, and seizures often develop rapidly, during the course of a few days. This is in distinction to tumors, in which these symptoms usually develop more slowly. There is often, but not invariably, an elevated white blood count. CSF findings are often nonspecific and are usually not obtained because of the risk of lumbar puncture in the setting of a brain mass.

Pathologically, there are four stages of evolution of a brain abscess, which correlate with the imaging findings.

Early Cerebritis. Within the first few days of infection, the infected portion of the brain is swollen and edematous. Areas of necrosis are filled with polymorphonuclear leukocytes, lymphocytes, and plasma cells. Organisms are present in both the center and periphery of the lesion, which has ill-defined margins. CT scans may be normal or show an area of low density (Fig. 6.1A). There may be mild mass effect and patchy areas of enhancement within the lesion. On MR, the lesion shows increased signal on proton density and T2WI, with low or isointensity on T1WI (Fig. 6.1B,C). Enhancement with gadolinium is inconstant at this stage. Use of high-dose (0.3 mmol/kg) gadolinium or magnetization transfer or both will increase the likelihood of detecting enhancement. A ring of enhancement is not present at this stage, distinguishing it from the later three stages. Unfortunately, these imaging features are nonspecific and can be seen with tumors or infarcts. The clinical features are most important in making the correct diagnosis. If the diagnosis can be made at this stage, nonsurgical treatment with antibiotics is often effective.

Late Cerebritis stage occurs within 1 or 2 weeks of infection. Central necrosis is increased, with fewer organisms detected pathologically. There is vascular proliferation at the periphery of the lesion, with more inflammatory cells, which represents the brain's effort to contain the infection. Not surprisingly, this results in thick, irregular contrast enhancement at the edges of the lesion on imaging studies (Fig. 6.2). Vasogenic edema is seen outside the enhancing rim at this stage as well. Delayed scans may show central filling in with contrast. No discrete low-signal capsule is evident on T2-weighted MR imaging, in distinction to some mature abscesses. This stage can also be treated effectively with antibiotic

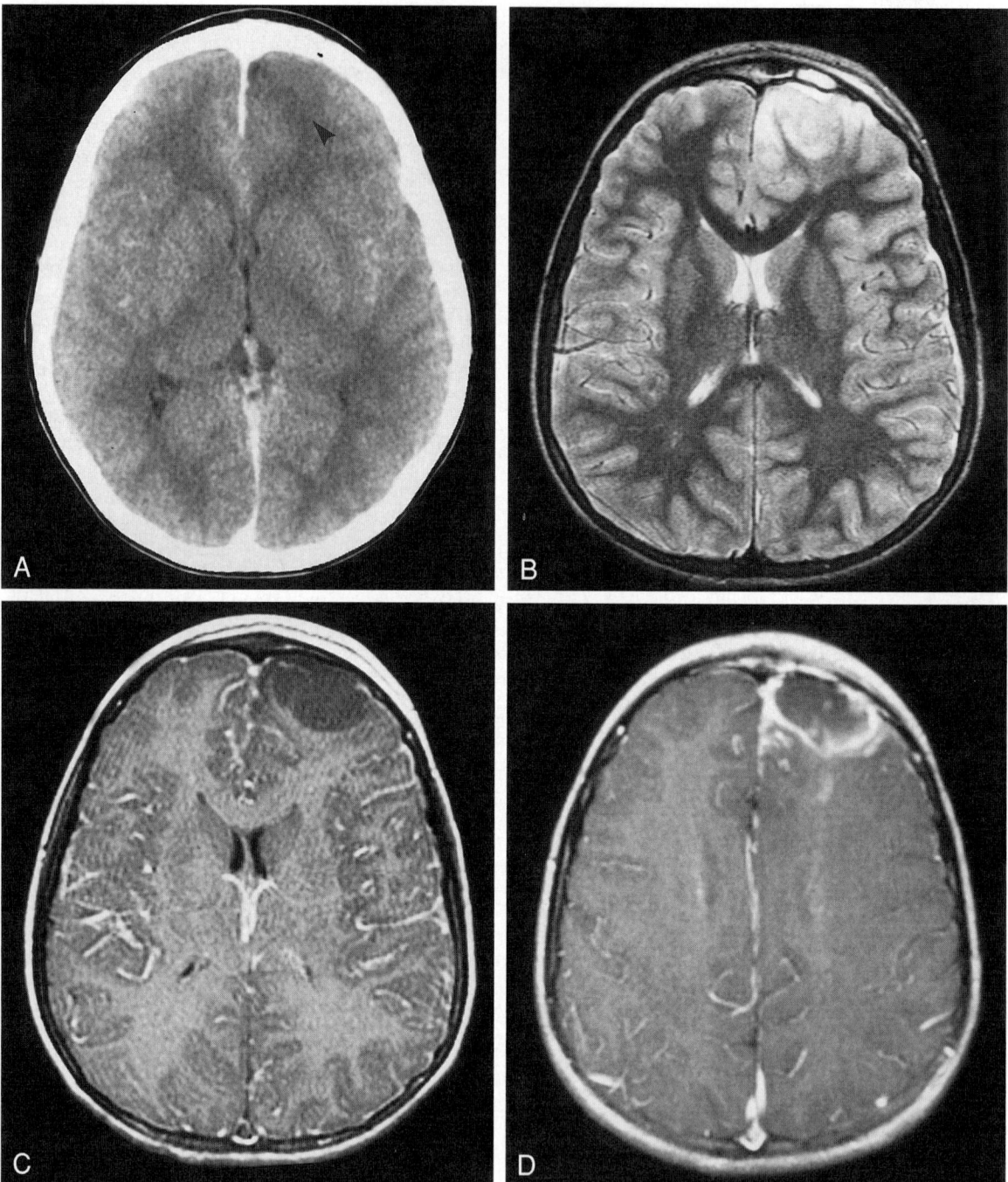

Figure 6.1. Early Cerebritis. A. A contrast CT scan shows a subtle area of decreased density in the left frontal lobe (*arrowhead*). **B.** The T2-weighted MR scan the next day shows high signal intensity in the left frontal lobe and left frontal sinusitis. **C.** The gadolinium-enhanced T1-weighted scan shows low signal intensity without enhancement, consistent with early cerebritis. **D.** Two weeks later a T1-weighted, gadolinium-enhanced scan shows a ring enhancing abscess.

therapy, but distinguishing late cerebritis from an early abscess or tumor can be difficult, and surgery is often performed.

Early Capsule. Within 2 weeks, the infection is walled off as a capsule of collagen and reticulin forms in the inflammatory, vascular margin of the infection. Macrophages, phagocytes, and neutrophils are also present in the capsule. The necrotic center contains very few organisms. This is the early capsule stage of brain

abscess formation. Contrast-enhanced CT and MR scans show a well-defined rim of enhancement (Fig. 6.3). The rim tends to be low in signal on T2-weighted MR. Centrally, there is necrosis (low density on CT; low signal on T1-weighted MR; high signal on intermediate and T2-weighted MR). There is prominent surrounding vasogenic edema.

Late Capsule. In the late capsule stage, the rim of enhancement becomes even more well defined and thin,

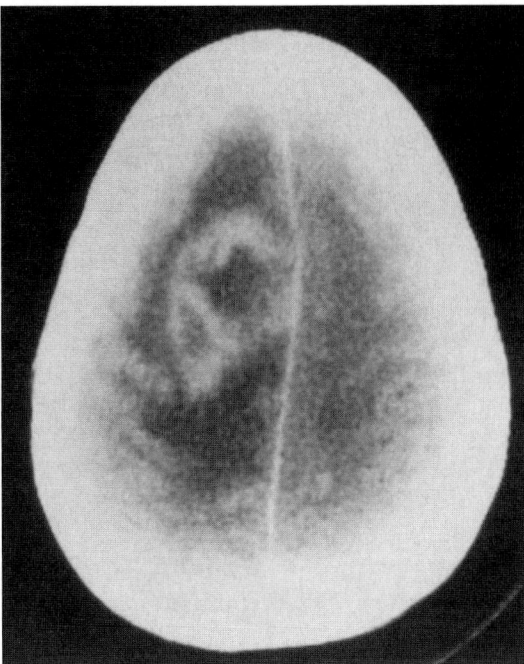

Figure 6.2. Late Cerebritis. This contrast-enhanced CT scan demonstrates irregular enhancement peripherally and low density centrally. There is surrounding low-density vasogenic edema. This is typical of the late cerebritis stage of pyogenic infection.

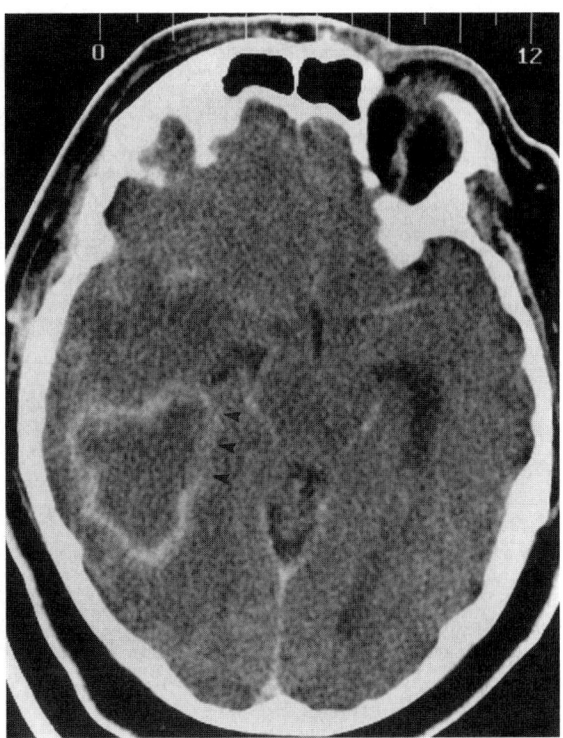

Figure 6.3. Pyogenic Cerebral Abscess. There is thin, smooth, well-defined contrast enhancement in the capsule of this right temporal lobe abscess imaged with CT. The enhancement is thinnest medially (*arrowheads*), which is typical of pyogenic abscesses. This patient had a dental infection and developed a headache that progressed to lethargy, weakness, and coma within a few days. Surgery revealed an actinomycete abscess.

reflecting more complete collagen in the abscess wall (Fig. 6.4). Multiloculation is common. The capsule often exhibits characteristic MR features that are helpful diagnostically at this stage. On T1WI, the capsule is usually isointense or hyperintense to white matter, and on T2WI, it is usually hypointense to white matter (Fig. 6.5). These signal characteristics suggest paramagnetic T1 and T2 shortening, similar to that seen in hematoma evolution (see chapter 4). Hemorrhage is not often found pathologically, and the paramagnetic effects may be secondary to the presence of free radicals produced by macrophages in the capsule. In any case, the MR appearance of the capsule is fairly specific for abscesses, as capsules are unusual in tumors. The medial aspect of the enhancing capsule is often (approximately 50% of the time) thinner than the lateral aspect (Figs. 6.3,6.4). This reflects decreased blood supply and fibroblast migration centrally, compared with cortically; the blood supply at the gray–white junction runs superficial to deep. This thin medial rim predisposes to intraventricular rupture with resulting ependymitis or ventriculitis (Figs. 6.4,6.5). CT or MR scans reveal enhancement of the ependymal lining of the ventricle and sometimes reveal abnormal density or signal intensity of the intraventricular CSF.

A solitary abscess is usually treated surgically. Often, a stereotactic needle aspiration followed by antibiotic therapy is performed, especially if the abscess is in an eloquent area of the brain. If there is significant mass effect, or if the lesion is in a relatively "safe" area, a formal drainage or resection is performed. If there are multiple abscesses, or if the patient is at high surgical risk, antibiotic therapy alone is used. Imaging studies should be performed frequently (about once a week) to monitor the

efficacy of treatment and to assess for complications such as ventriculitis, infarction, or hydrocephalus.

The differential diagnosis of pyogenic abscess includes tumor and resolving hematoma. The clinical features, combined with the appearance of a thin enhancing rim (thinnest medially), much edema, and paramagnetic effects in the capsule (with no blood products centrally) should strongly suggest a brain abscess. Multiple loculations and/or enhancement of the ependyma, if present, should clinch the diagnosis.

Septic Embolus. Infections that begin with a septic embolus may not have the typical appearance of an abscess. The embolus frequently causes an infarct that dominates the imaging findings. Depending on the size of the embolus, there may be a small rounded area of enhancement or a larger wedge-shaped cortical infarct. As with other embolic infarcts, hemorrhage may occur. Because of the nonviable, infarcted tissue with a poor blood supply, a typical capsule may not form. A thicker, more irregular ring of enhancement that persists within an area of infarction should suggest the diagnosis. Septic emboli may lead to mycotic aneurysm formation, which can result in intraparenchymal or subarachnoid hemorrhage.

Listeria monocytogenes is an anaerobic Gram-positive bacillus that primarily infects immunocompromised patients. The organism can cause meningitis, meningoencephalitis, and abscesses. Listerial rhombencephalitis in-

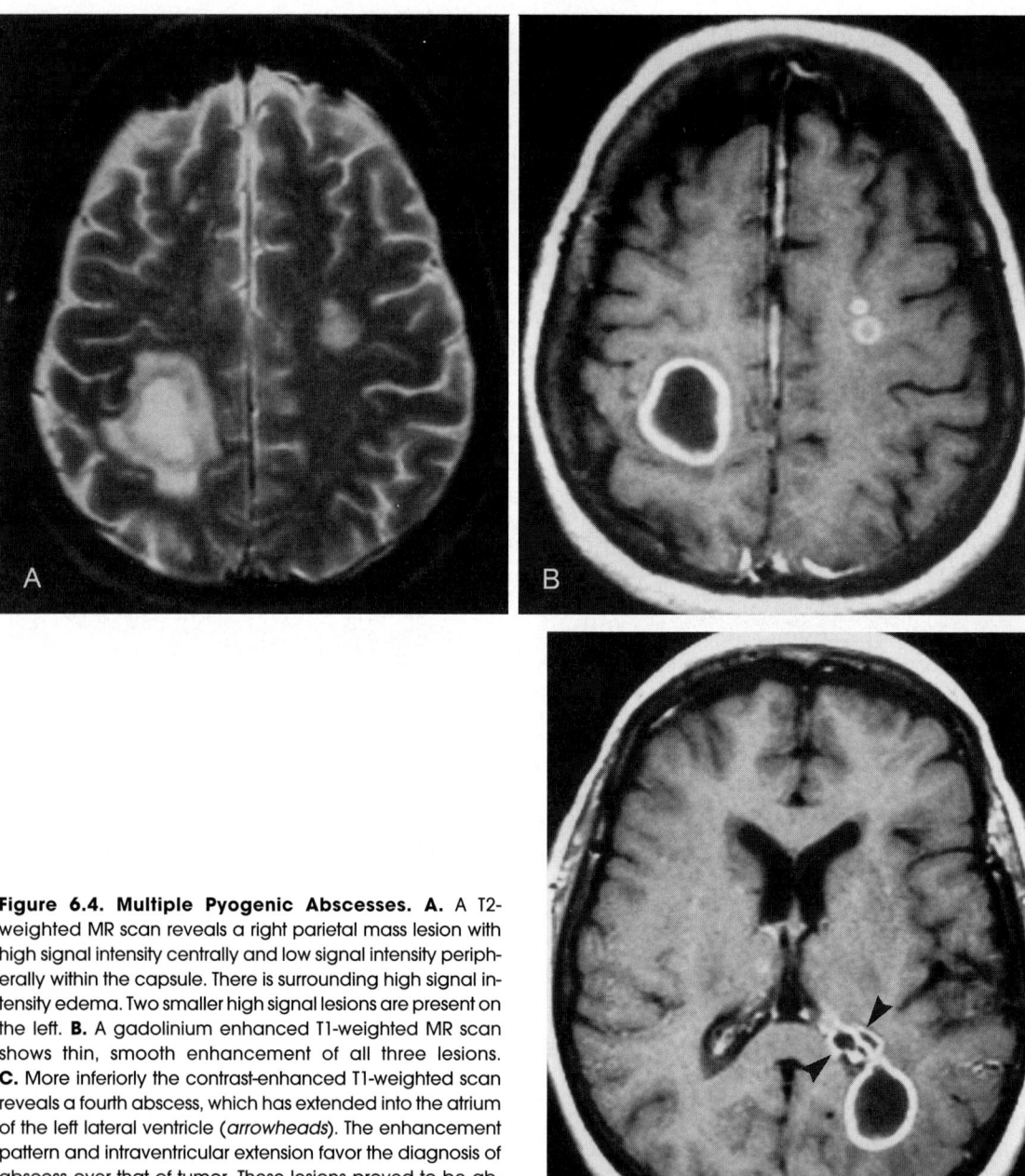

Figure 6.4. Multiple Pyogenic Abscesses. A. A T2-weighted MR scan reveals a right parietal mass lesion with high signal intensity centrally and low signal intensity peripherally within the capsule. There is surrounding high signal intensity edema. Two smaller high signal lesions are present on the left. **B.** A gadolinium enhanced T1-weighted MR scan shows thin, smooth enhancement of all three lesions. **C.** More inferiorly the contrast-enhanced T1-weighted scan reveals a fourth abscess, which has extended into the atrium of the left lateral ventricle (*arrowheads*). The enhancement pattern and intraventricular extension favor the diagnosis of abscess over that of tumor. These lesions proved to be abscesses that cultured anaerobic streptococcus. (Case courtesy of Dr. Vincent Burke, Atherton, California.)

volves the brainstem and cerebellum. MR scans reveal areas of abnormal signal and enhancement in the brainstem and cerebellar white matter tracts. The appearance is similar to acute disseminated encephalomyelitis (see discussion later in this chapter). Occasionally, otherwise healthy patients may develop this infection.

Mycobacterial Infections

The most common form of CNS mycobacterial infection is tuberculous meningitis, which is discussed later in this chapter. Focal mycobacterial infection of the brain occurs in two forms: tuberculoma and abscess. A tuberculoma is a granuloma with central caseous necrosis. A tuberculous abscess has similar characteristics as

a pyogenic abscess but develops in patients with impaired T-cell immunity.

Tuberculoma. In the early 1900s, one third of all brain mass lesions in England were tuberculomas. Because of improved prevention and treatment, these lesions are now unusual in industrialized countries. In developing areas of the world, tuberculomas account for as much as 15–30% of brain masses. Approximately 5–10% of patients with tuberculosis develop CNS disease. There is a predilection for the extremes of age, children and the elderly. The infection spreads to the brain hematogenously from the lungs. In developed countries, tuberculomas usually result from reactivation of quiescent disease, although only 50% of patients have a known history of previous tuberculosis. Most lesions in adults are supratentorial, involving the frontal or parietal lobes. Sixty percent of tuberculomas in children are in the posterior fossa, usually the cerebellum. Multiple lesions are common. Most tuberculomas are not associated with tuberculous meningitis. Clinical features include headache, seizures, papilledema, and focal neurologic signs. Fever is seen only rarely. The CSF is almost always abnormal, showing elevated protein and reduced glucose. An abnormal chest radiograph is present in up to 50% of patients. These lesions can be treated medically if there are characteristic clinical and imaging features. Surgery is often performed when the diagnosis is in doubt, for medical treatment failures, and for large lesions.

Noncontrast CT scans show one or more isodense or slightly hyperdense nodules or small mass lesions. Multiple lesions are present approximately 50% of the time. Thick rim enhancement is common postcontrast (Fig. 6.6A). The center of the tuberculoma is usually more dense than the fluidlike center of a pyogenic abscess, because of caseous necrosis. Smaller lesions may show a solid enhancement pattern. A "target" appearance with a central calcification surrounded by rim enhancement is an uncommon but helpful finding, strongly suggesting the diagnosis. Calcification is present in less than 5% of cases at the initial diagnosis, but it is commonly seen with treatment as the lesions resolve. Surrounding edema is variably present. On MR, tuberculomas usually have a low signal rim, reflecting

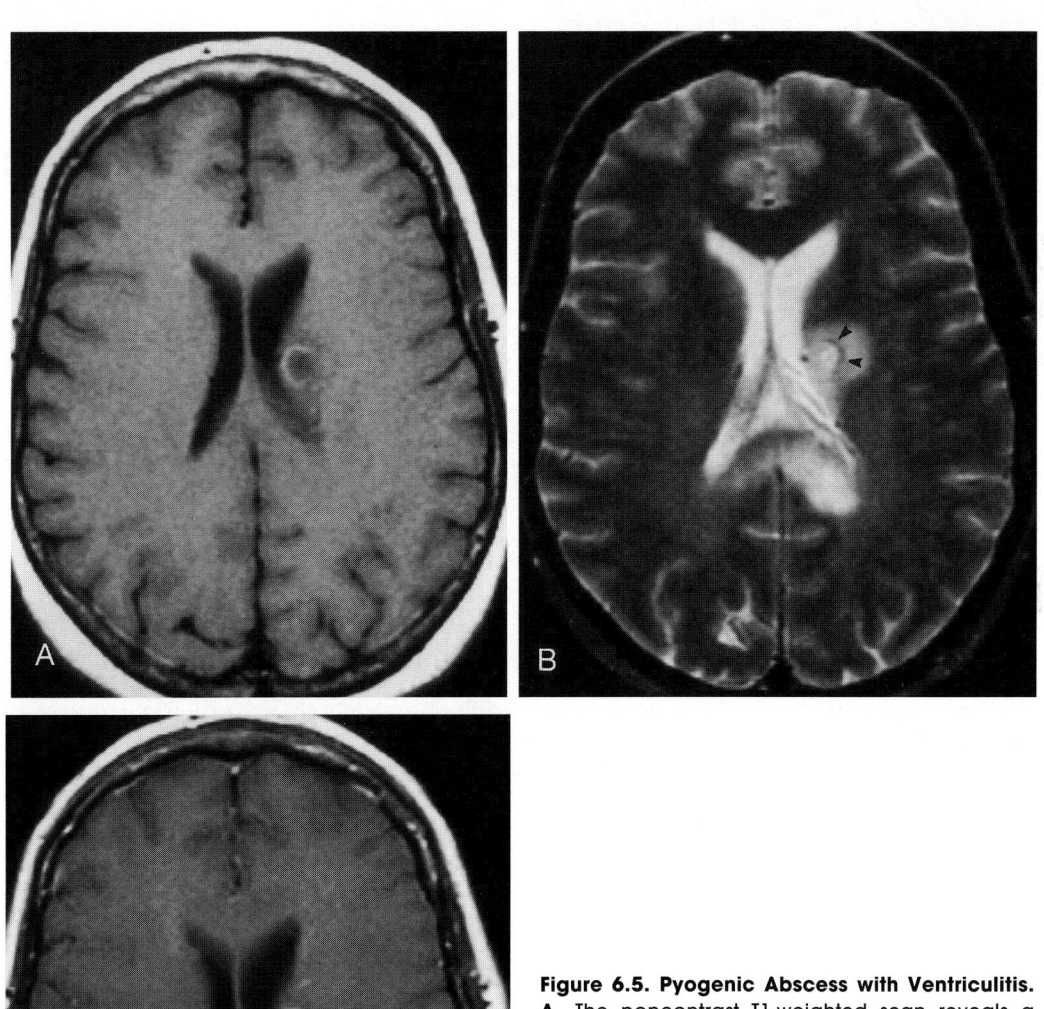

Figure 6.5. Pyogenic Abscess with Ventriculitis.
A. The noncontrast T1-weighted scan reveals a rounded lesion adjacent to the body of the left lateral ventricle. The medial rim of the lesion is high in signal, suggesting paramagnetic T1 shortening, often seen in the capsules of pyogenic abscesses. **B.** The T2-weighted scan shows the lateral aspect of the capsule to be of low signal (*arrowheads*). There is surrounding high signal edema, as well as edema posterior to the left lateral ventricle. **C.** After gadolinium contrast enhancement, the T1WI shows thin, smooth enhancement of the capsule, as well as enhancement of the ependyma of the left lateral ventricle (*arrowheads*), indicating intraventricular extension and ventriculitis.

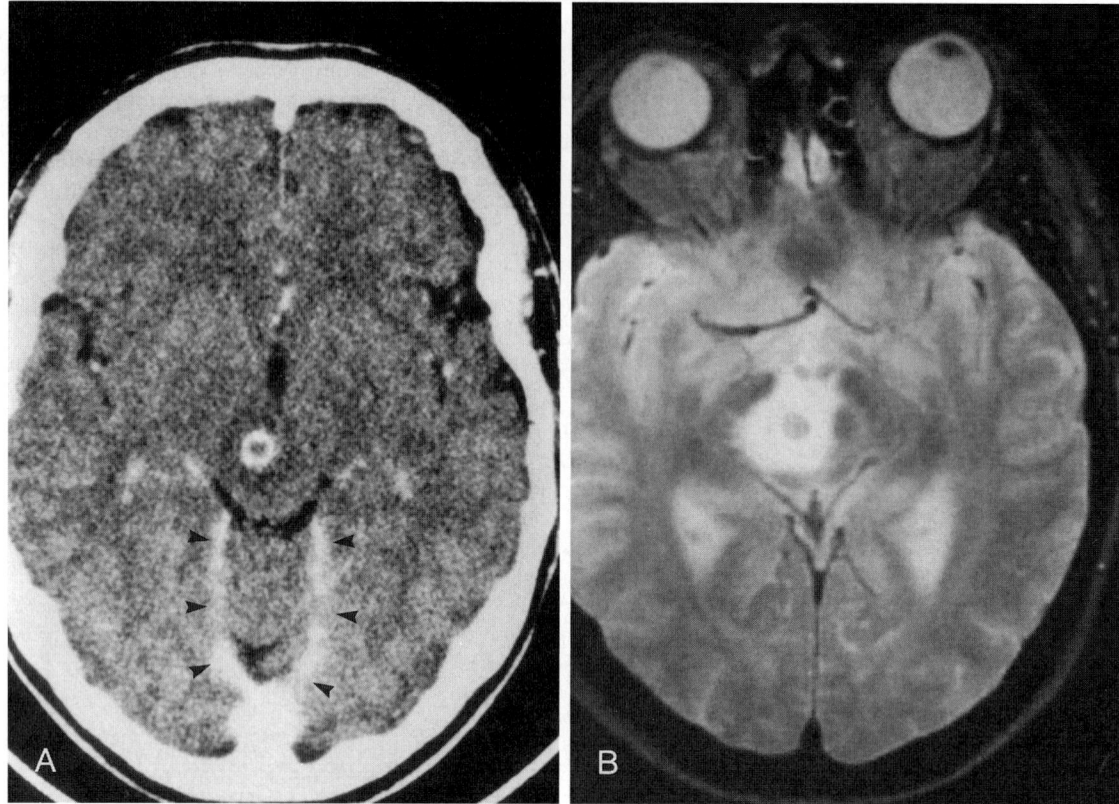

Figure 6.6. Midbrain Tuberculoma. A. The contrast enhanced CT scan shows a ring enhancing lesion in the right side of the midbrain with surrounding low-density edema. Most tuberculomas this size are solid or show thick rim enhancement. Thick enhancement of the tentorial edges is attributable to tuberculous meningitis (*arrowheads*), helping to distinguish this lesion from a pyogenic abscess. Meningitis is, however, often absent in patients with tuberculoma. **B.** The T2-weighted MR scan shows that the lesion is in the right red nucleus. The high signal edema is more apparent than on the CT scan, reflecting the increased sensitivity of MR in detecting alterations in brain water content.

the fibrous wall, which enhances markedly. Centrally, there may be high or low signal intensity with T2-weighted MR, depending on the water content of the caseation necrosis. Smaller lesions or those containing calcifications may be entirely low in signal, especially on T2WI (Fig. 6.6B). Surrounding edema is usually better seen with MR than with CT scans but is often mild. The differential diagnosis includes tumor, pyogenic abscess, fungal and parasitic infections, and sarcoidosis.

Tuberculous abscess is a rare complication, seen primarily in immunocompromised patients. Abnormal T-cell function prevents the normal host response of tuberculoma formation with caseous necrosis. Symptoms develop more rapidly than with tuberculomas. The imaging features are similar to those seen with pyogenic abscesses. The lesions are often large and multiloculated, in distinction to tuberculomas. Prominent edema and mass effect also distinguish tuberculous abscess from tuberculoma. Atypical mycobacterial infections are also more common in immunocompromised patients.

Fungal Infections

Fungal infections of the CNS can be grouped into endemic and cosmopolitan categories. Endemic fungal infections are geographically restricted. They can occur in immunocompetent and immunosuppressed patients. Cosmopolitan fungal infections occur worldwide, usually in immunosuppressed patients, infants, the elderly, or the chronically ill, with the exception of cryptococcosis, which also occurs in patients with normal immunity.

Endemic Fungal Infections. The most common endemic fungal infections in the United States are coccidiomycosis, North American blastomycosis, and histoplasmosis. These infections usually manifest as granulomatous meningitis, as is discussed later in this chapter. Focal parenchymal lesions are unusual. CNS involvement is a manifestation of disseminated infection, with hematogenous spread, usually from pulmonary disease.

Coccidiomycosis occurs in the southwestern United States. The spores are inhaled, with outbreaks occurring after groundbreaking for construction projects. Most infected patients are asymptomatic or have mild respiratory symptoms. Less than 1% of patients develop disseminated infection and meningitis. Focal parenchymal granulomas are rare.

Blastomycosis occurs in the Ohio and Mississippi River valleys. CNS involvement occurs in 6–33% of disseminated cases. Meningitis is the most frequent presentation, but parenchymal abscesses and granulomas occur more frequently than with coccidiomycosis. Epidural granulomas and abscesses also occur in the head

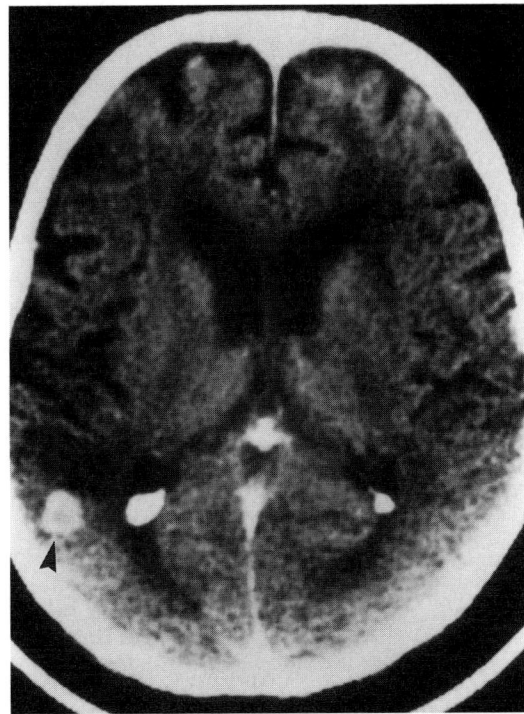

Figure 6.7. Histoplasmosis Granuloma. This patient had disseminated histoplasmosis with several lesions in the brain and spine. This contrast-enhanced CT scan shows a solidly enhancing lesion near the atrium of the right lateral ventricle (*arrowhead*). Most fungal granulomas are small and show either solid or thick rim enhancement. (Case courtesy of Dr. J. R. Jinkins, San Antonio, Texas.)

and spine, usually from direct extension from bone infection. Up to 40% of focal brain lesions are multiple.

Histoplamosis is usually a benign, asymptomatic infection, occurring in the Midwest and southern United States. Dissemination is unusual, and only a small percent of disseminated cases involve the CNS. Meningitis is most common, but multiple or solitary granulomas may occur. Abscesses are unusual.

As seen with CT or MR, most fungal granulomas are small and show solid or thick rim enhancement (Fig. 6.7). Fungal abscesses (as sometimes seen with blastomycosis) have a similar appearance to pyogenic abscesses, described earlier. Meningeal enhancement from meningitis is a common accompanying feature. Hydrocephalus is also common, especially with coccidiomycosis.

Cosmopolitan Fungal Infections. The most common cosmopolitan fungal infections are cryptococcosis, aspergillosis, mucormycosis, and candidiasis. These infections also usually present as meningitis, but focal parenchymal lesions are fairly common.

Aspergillosis involves the CNS in 60–70% of patients with disseminated disease. The infection may arise from hematogenous spread or by direct extension from an infected paranasal sinus, leading to meningitis or meningoencephalitis. Parenchymal disease usually takes the form of an abscess. Granulomas are unusual. The abscesses are often multiple and show irregular ring enhancement (Fig. 6.8). Subcortical or cortical infarcts and

hemorrhage from blood vessel invasion may occur. The mortality rate with invasive intracerebral aspergillosis is greater than 85%.

Mucormycosis. *Mucor* invades the brain usually by direct extension from the sinuses or nose or oral cavity, but hematogenous spread also occurs. Almost all patients are diabetic or otherwise immunocompromised. The mortality rate in treated diabetic patients is 65–75% and is worse in immunocompromised patients. Like aspergillosis, mucor tends to invade blood vessels. Imaging studies in patients with CNS mucormycosis will reveal single or multiple mass lesions with varying degrees of peripheral enhancement. The amount of enhancement depends on the compromised host's ability to fight the infection. Surrounding edema is variable in amount. Smaller lesions will show a solid enhancement pattern. The lesions are often in the base of the brain, adjacent to diseased sinuses. Infarcts, intra- or extra-axial hemorrhage, and meningeal enhancement can be seen with CT or MR. A lesion with peripheral enhancement, cortical sparing, and a nonvascular distribution is more likely to be a mucor abscess than an infarct, but often it is difficult to distinguish the two.

Candidiasis usually causes meningitis, but granulomas and small abscesses may occur. Spread to the CNS is usually hematogenous from the lung or GI tract. In cases of CNS candidiasis, meningeal enhancement or multiple small enhancing granulomas or microabscesses are usually seen. Infarcts, hydrocephalus, and large abscesses may also be identified.

Cryptococcosis is the most frequently reported CNS fungal infection. In approximately 50% of cases, it occurs in patients with normal immune function. This is also an extremely common infection in patients with AIDS, as is discussed later. Infection of the CNS occurs via hematogenous spread from the lungs. Serologies and CSF studies are valuable in making the diagnosis: approximately 90% of patients have antigen in the CSF or antibody in the serum, or both. The usual manifestation is meningitis. Granulomas can occur and are usually multiple. Abscesses are less common. CT scans in patients with cryptococcosis are usually normal, reflecting relatively mild meningeal involvement in most cases. Mass lesions are seen in approximately 10% of cases. Cryptococcomas are shown as small, usually multiple, solid enhancing, peripheral parenchymal nodules. Calcifications within a granuloma are occasionally seen. With the improved sensitivity of MR, meningeal and parenchymal lesions are seen more frequently than with CT. Leptomeningeal nodules are often only seen on T1-weighted contrast-enhanced MR as multiple tiny enhancing lesions near the basal cisterns and sulci. Diffuse meningeal enhancement is unusual. Granulomas may show either solid or ring enhancement.

Another characteristic cryptococcal lesion is the gelatinous pseudocyst. This is a cystic lesion, usually in the basal ganglia, representing enlarged Virchow-Robin spaces filled with the organism. These lesions are usually found only in immunocompromised patients (see Fig. 6.32). With CT, gelatinous pseudocysts are smooth, round, low-density masses in the basal ganglia that show no contrast enhancement.

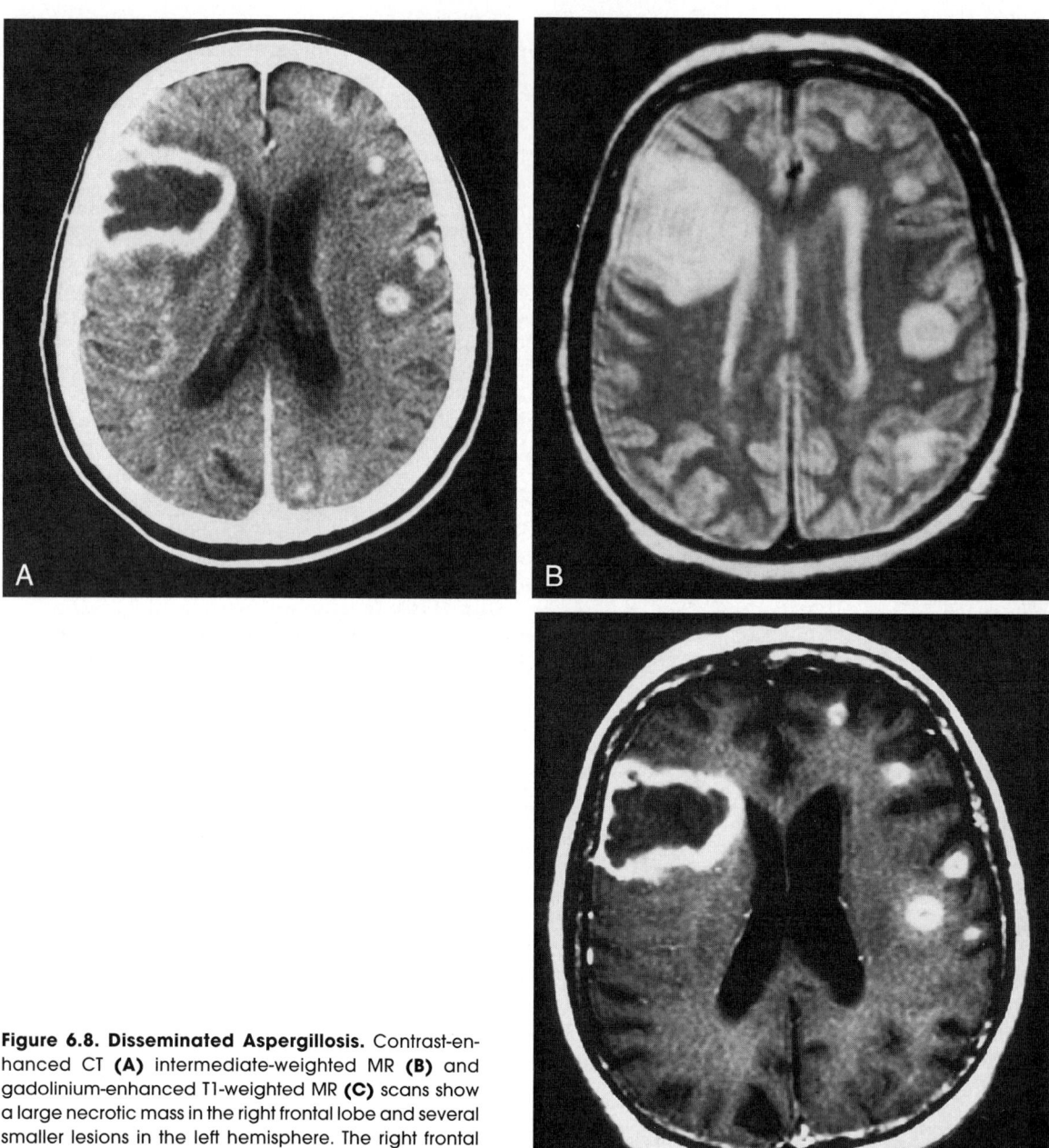

Figure 6.8. Disseminated Aspergillosis. Contrast-enhanced CT **(A)** intermediate-weighted MR **(B)** and gadolinium-enhanced T1-weighted MR **(C)** scans show a large necrotic mass in the right frontal lobe and several smaller lesions in the left hemisphere. The right frontal lobe lesion was surgically drained, and aspergillosis was found. The patient was a poorly controlled diabetic.

They are usually better seen with MR than with CT, as lesions nearly isointense with CSF on all sequences that do not enhance.

Parasitic Infections

Parasitic infections are common throughout much of the third world, but they are relatively uncommon in the industrialized nations. The most common infections likely to be encountered in the United States are cysticercosis, echinococcosis, toxoplasmosis, and rarely amebiasis. CNS involvement in malaria, trypanosomiasis, paragonimiasis, sparganosis, and schistosomiasis is rarely encountered here and is not discussed here.

Cysticercosis is caused by the larvae of the pork tapeworm, *Taenia solium.* Infestation occurs via the fecal–oral route. The eggs are shed by humans, the definitive host, and then ingested by the intermediate host, pigs or humans. The life cycle can be completed in the pig, but not in humans. The eggs form oncospheres (primary larvae) that hatch in the intestine and are hematogenously distributed throughout the body and form cysticerci (secondary larvae). The cysticerci cannot develop further in humans and eventually die. The cysticerci that reach the CNS may infest the parenchyma, meninges, ventricles, or spine. This disease is fairly frequently encountered in the southwestern United States in Latin American immigrants. Seizures occur in more than 90% of patients. Cysticercosis is the most common cause of seizures in Latin America. Encephalitic symptoms are also common. Treatment is with anticysticercus drugs such as praziquantel and albendazole.

Parenchymal cysticercosis is the most common type. Early in the infestation, during the tissue-invasion stage, CT or MR scans show edema or nodular enhancement or both. Later, the viable cysts appear as small (usually 1 cm or less in diameter), solitary or multiple rounded lesions that are low density on CT and isointense to CSF on MR (Fig. 6.9). The lesions are usually peripherally distributed near the gray–white junction or in the gray matter. A small marginal nodule representing the scolex is sometimes seen (Figs. 6.9B,6.10). There is usually no enhancement or edema at this vesicular stage. When the cyst dies, the fluid within it leaks into the surrounding brain, causing inflammation. This produces clinical symptoms of an acute encephalitis, which may be severe, depending on the number of lesions. Imaging studies now reveal ring enhancing lesions with surrounding edema (Fig. 6.10). The cyst fluid is of increased density on CT and increased signal compared with CSF on T1- and T2-weighted MR. As the dead cyst degenerates, it becomes smaller, showing nodular enhancement, and then calcifies. CT scans at this late stage show small, peripheral calcifications, with no edema or enhancement (Fig. 6.11). With MR, the calcifications are best seen on T2-weighted or T2*-weighted gradient-echo images, but they are better demonstrated by CT. Imaging with CT or MR is useful in staging and monitoring treatment. Once the cyst has degenerated, further drug therapy is not warranted.

Intraventricular cysticercosis is similar to the parenchymal variety in pathogenesis and appearance (Fig. 6.12). The cysts are usually isodense and isointense to CSF, making them difficult to visualize. MR is superior to CT for imaging, as subtle signal changes and lack of CSF pulsations within the cyst make them more visi-

ble. Enhancement might or might not be present, depending on the stage, similar to the parenchymal form. The cysts may obstruct the foramen of Monro, the third ventricle or aqueduct, resulting in hydrocephalus. If acute hydrocephalus occurs, death may rapidly ensue. Ventriculitis occurs if the cyst ruptures.

Meningeal infestation is known as meningobasal (because the basal cisterns are most frequently involved) or racemose (Latin for "clusters") cysticercosis. The cysts lack a scolex but may grow by proliferation of the cyst wall. The cysts may grow in grapelike clusters (Figs. 6.13,6.14) or conform to the shape of the cistern. No mural nodules or calcifications are seen. CT scans show CSF density cysts in the basal cisterns. MR reveals cysts that are isointense with CSF, often with mural enhancement or diffuse meningeal enhancement. Hydrocephalus is commonly observed.

Spinal cysticercosis is usually intradural, but can be either intramedullary or extramedullary. Intramedullary lesions are best seen with MR as solid or ring enhancing cord lesions similar to those seen in the brain parenchyma. Extramedullary cysts are analogous to the racemose form and, like most spine pathology, are also best evaluated with MR.

Echinococcosis, also known as hydatid disease, occurs in South America, Africa, Central Europe, the Middle East, and rarely in the southwestern United States. The etiologic agent is the dog tapeworm and the human is an intermediate host. Hydatid cysts are more frequently present in the lung and liver, but the brain is involved in 1–4% of cases. The cysts are usually solitary, unilocular, large, round, and smoothly marginated. They are most often supratentorial, in the middle cerebral artery territory. There may rarely be mural calcification. With CT, the fluid within the cyst is usually isodense with CSF. There is usually no surrounding edema or abnormal contrast enhancement, unless the cyst has

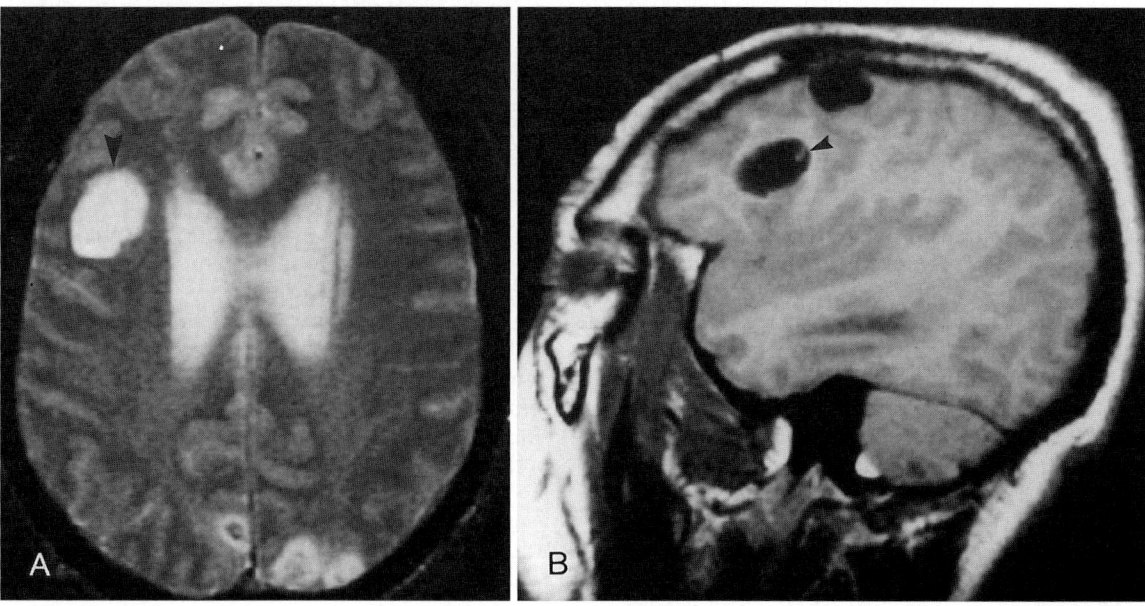

Figure 6.9. Cysticercosis. A. T2-weighted MR shows a right frontal lesion isointense with CSF (*arrowhead*). There is no surrounding edema, indicating that this is early in the course of the disease. Three smaller lesions are present posteriorly. **B.** The T1-weighted para-sagittal image in the same patient shows two cysticercal cysts that are isointense with CSF. A scolex is visible in one of the cysts (*arrowhead*).

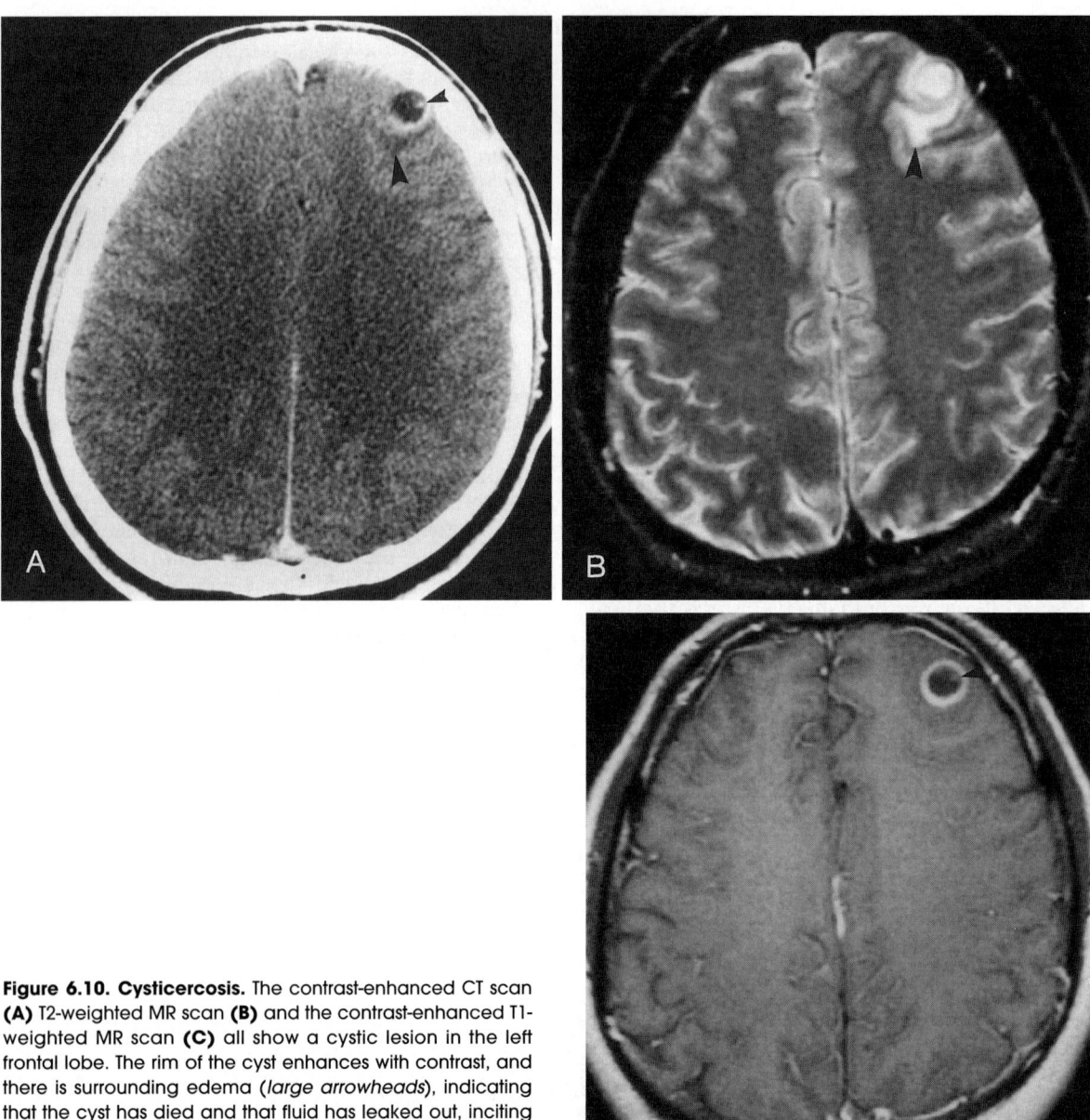

Figure 6.10. Cysticercosis. The contrast-enhanced CT scan **(A)** T2-weighted MR scan **(B)** and the contrast-enhanced T1-weighted MR scan **(C)** all show a cystic lesion in the left frontal lobe. The rim of the cyst enhances with contrast, and there is surrounding edema (*large arrowheads*), indicating that the cyst has died and that fluid has leaked out, inciting an inflammatory response. The scolex is visible (*small arrowheads*).

ruptured, leading to an inflammatory reaction. With MR, the lesions are usually nearly isointense with CSF.

Toxoplasmosis is caused by the protozoa *Toxoplasma gondii*, which occurs worldwide. The disease may be either congenital or acquired. The acquired form is seen primarily in immunocompromised patients and is very common in AIDS, as is discussed later in this chapter. The congenital form results when the mother eats poorly cooked meat or is infected from a cat during pregnancy. A diffuse encephalitis of the fetal brain ensues, usually causing severe destruction. The infant is usually born with microcephaly (Fig. 6.15), chorioretinitis, and mental retardation. Imaging studies reveal atrophy, dilated ventricles, and calcifications. The calcifications occur in the periventricular white matter, basal ganglia, and cerebral hemispheres. This is in distinction to congenital cytomegalovirus in which the calcifications are usually periventricular only.

Amebic meningoencephalitis is sometimes seen in the southern United States. The amebae enter the nasal cavity of patients swimming in infested freshwater ponds or pools. There is direct extension through the cribriform plate to the brain. A severe meningoencephalitis results, which is usually fatal. Imaging studies often underestimate the severity of the disease. Early in the infection, there may be meningeal or gray matter enhancement, or both. Later, there is diffuse cerebral edema. There are a few reports of single or multiple, ring or solid enhancing lesions with surrounding edema in patients with amebic brain abscesses. Amebic abscesses are more common in immunosuppressed patients.

Spirochete Infections

Neurosyphilis develops in approximately 5% of patients who are not treated for the primary infection.

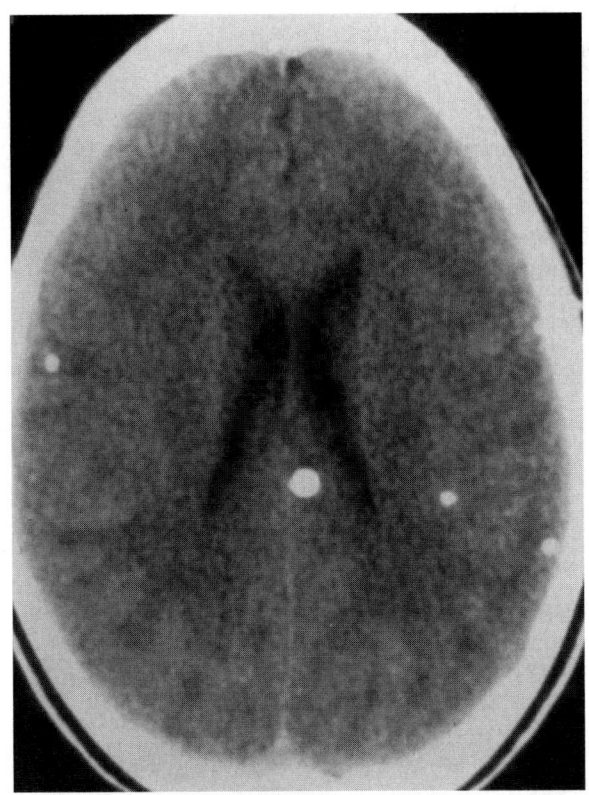

Figure 6.11. Late-stage Cysticercosis. This unenhanced CT scan shows multiple calcifications in the gray matter and gray–white junction, typical of old cysticercosis.

Involvement of the CNS usually occurs in the secondary or tertiary stages. Because of effective antibiotic therapy, the disease is rare. There has, however, been a significant increase in incidence since the AIDS epidemic. Neurosyphilis is more likely to develop in HIV-infected patients and the neurologic symptoms occur after a shorter latency period than in non-HIV–infected patients. Patients with neurosyphilis are usually asymptomatic. Symptomatic patients may have an aseptic meningitis, tabes dorsalis, general paresis, or meningovascular disease. Imaging studies are usually normal in patients with tabes dorsalis, but rarely gummas are found. These usually appear as small enhancing nodules at the surface of the brain with adjacent meningeal enhancement. Meningovascular syphilis presents as an acute stroke syndrome or a subacute illness with a variety of symptoms. Pathologically, there is thickening of the meninges and a medium-to-large vessel arteritis. Imaging studies reveal small infarcts of the basal ganglia, white matter, cerebral cortex or cerebellum (Fig. 6.16A). The infarcts may exhibit patchy or gyral enhancement, best seen with MR. Meningeal enhancement is unusual, but cranial nerve enhancement in patients with syphilitic cranial neuritis has been described. Angiography in patients with meningovascular neurosyphilis reveals multiple segmental constrictions and/or occlusions of large and medium-sized arteries, including the distal internal carotid, anterior cerebral, middle cerebral, posterior cerebral, and distal basilar arteries (Fig. 6.16B).

Lyme disease is a multisystem spirochetal infection caused by *Borrelia burgdorferi*. It is found worldwide in

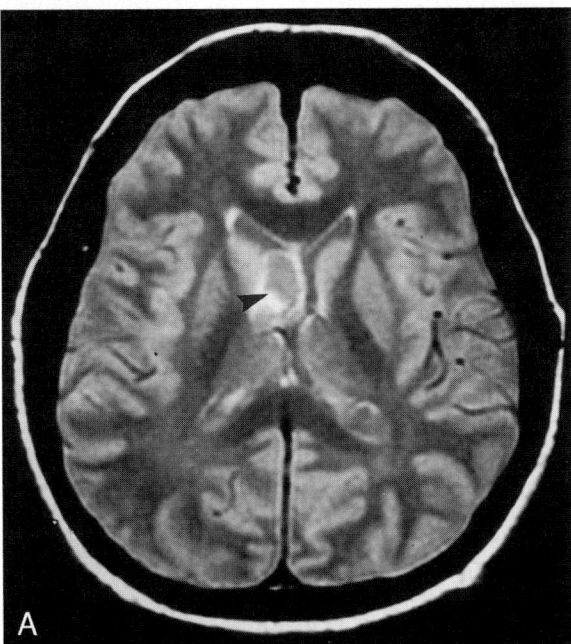
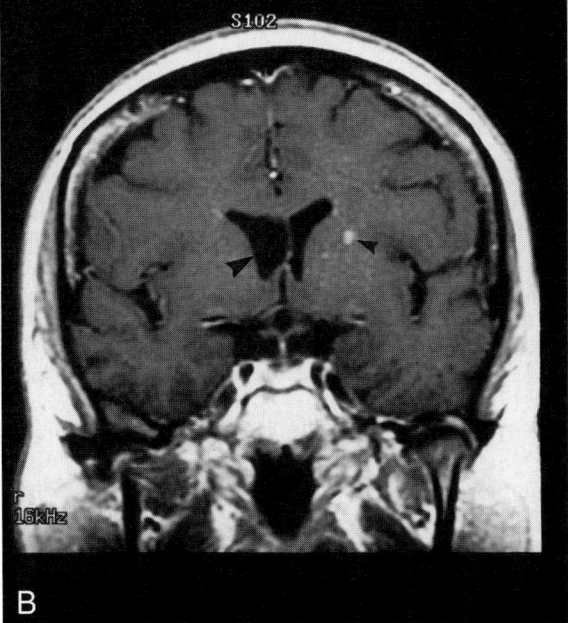

Figure 6.12. Intraventricular Cysticercosis. The intermediate-weighted axial **(A)** and gadolinium-enhanced T1-weighted coronal **(B)** scans show a cystic mass in the frontal horn of the right lateral ventricle (*large arrowheads*). The lesion is of slightly increased signal intensity compared with CSF in the ventricle. The scolex is of high signal intensity in the posterior aspect of the cyst in **(A)**. There is also a small parenchymal lesion in the left basal ganglia (*small arrowhead*).

Figure 6.13. Subarachnoid (Racemose) Cysticercosis. There are multiple cysts in a grapelike cluster in the basal cisterns on this parasagittal T1-weighted scan (*arrowheads*). These cysts lack a scolex, but they grow by proliferation of the cyst wall.

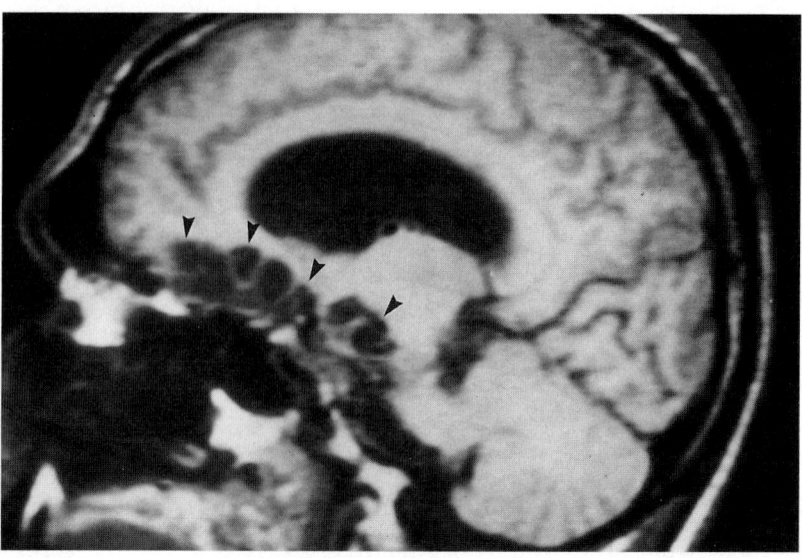

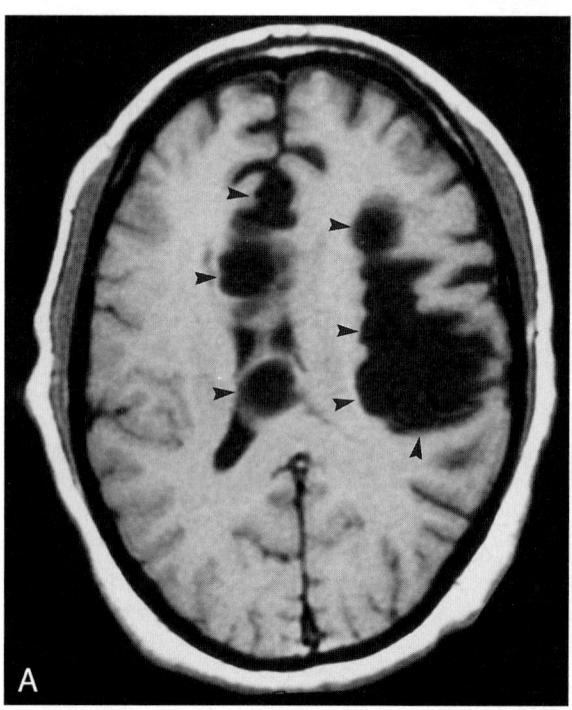

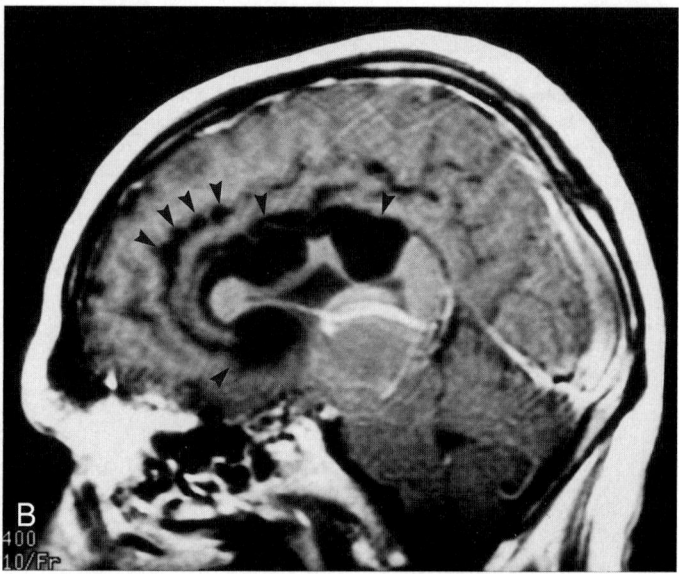

Figure 6.14. Subarachnoid (Racemose) Cysticercosis. The T1-weighted axial **(A)** and gadolinium-enhanced T1-weighted sagittal **(B)** scans show multiple nonenhancing cysts (*arrowheads*) in the left sylvian fissure, callosal sulcus, and cingulate sulcus. The corpus callosum is markedly distorted by the cysts.

deer, mice, raccoons, and birds. It is spread to humans via ticks, especially the deer tick. The disease occurs most frequently on the east coast, but Midwestern and west coast cases also occur. The disease begins as a flu-like illness, with a rash and an expanding skin lesion at the tick-bite site. In a small percentage of patients, cardiac, arthritic, or neurologic symptoms develop. Neurologic abnormalities are found in 10–15% of patients. A variety of symptoms, including peripheral and cranial neuropathies, radiculopathies, myelopathies, encephalitis, meningitis, pain syndromes, cognitive disorders, and movement disorders have been reported.

Treatment with antibiotics and corticosteroids may have variable results. MR is the modality of choice for imaging these patients. In patients with cranial neuritis, MR scans may show thick, enhancing cranial nerves. Cranial nerves III–VIII can be involved, with the facial nerve most commonly observed. In patients with parenchymal CNS Lyme disease, MR scans show multiple small white matter lesions similar to that seen with multiple sclerosis. The lesions can be found in the supratentorial and infratentorial white matter tracts. The lesions often enhance with contrast, in a nodular or ring pattern, depending on the size. There may be

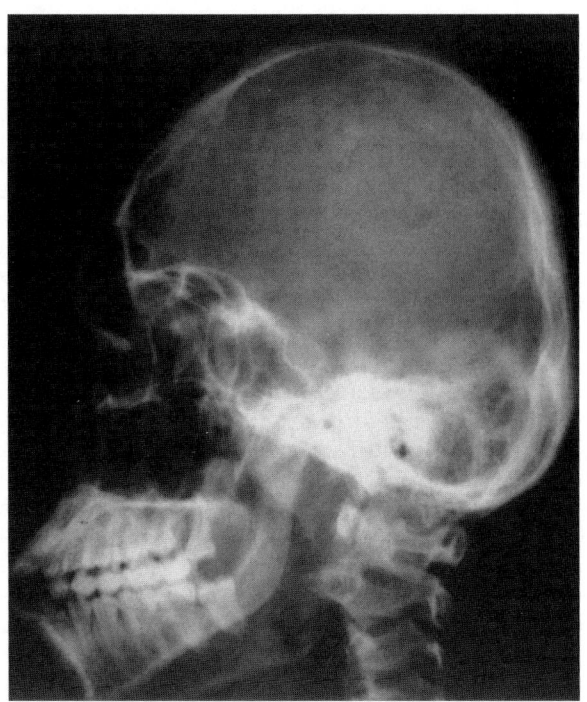

Figure 6.15. Microcephaly. A lateral skull film shows a small cranial vault, as can be seen in congenital toxoplasmosis or other TORCH (*T*oxoplasmosis; *O*ther, which includes syphilis; *R*ubella; *C*ytomegalovirus; and *H*erpes) infections.

meningeal enhancement. The differential diagnosis includes multiple sclerosis and other demyelinating processes.

Viral Infections

The most common viral infections of the CNS include cytomegalovirus, herpes simplex, varicella zoster, and the HIV. Rubella was once a devastating fetal viral infection, but it is now uncommon because of widespread immunization.

Cytomegalovirus is a DNA virus in the herpesvirus family. It causes symptomatic CNS disease primarily through congenital transmission. A maternal CMV infection results in transplacental transmission to the fetus in 30–50% of cases and symptomatic disease in 5%. Symptomatic neonates may have hepatosplenomegaly, jaundice, cerebral involvement (psychomotor retardation), chorioretinitis, and deafness. Mental retardation and deafness are present in 20% of cases. Intracranial manifestations of congenital CMV infection largely depend on when during gestation the infection occurs. Infection in the first trimester results in necrosis in the germinal matrix resulting in migrational anomalies. MR scans may show a spectrum of abnormalities, including agyria, polymicrogyria, and focal cortical dysplasia. Delayed myelination and cerebellar hypoplasia are also common findings. Patients infected later during gestation may have a normal gyral pattern, but delayed mye-

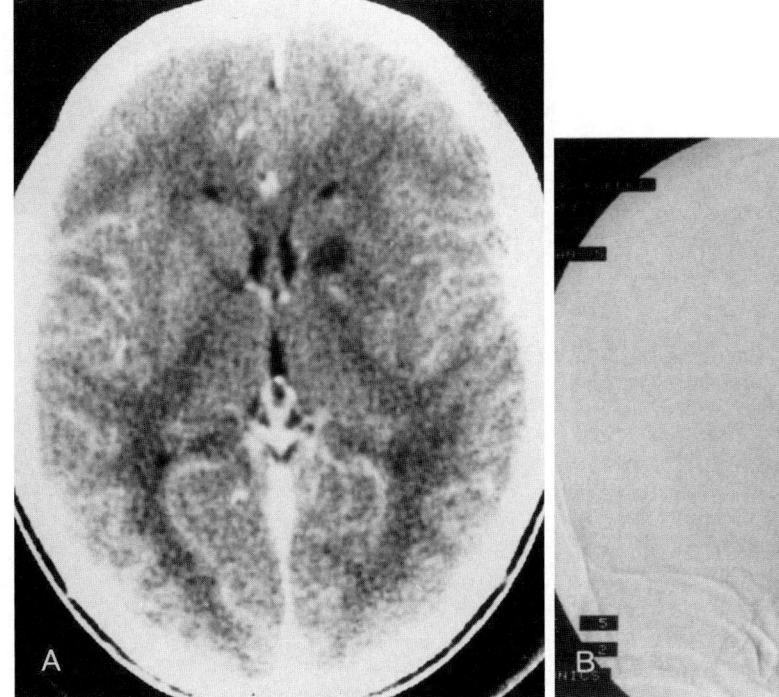

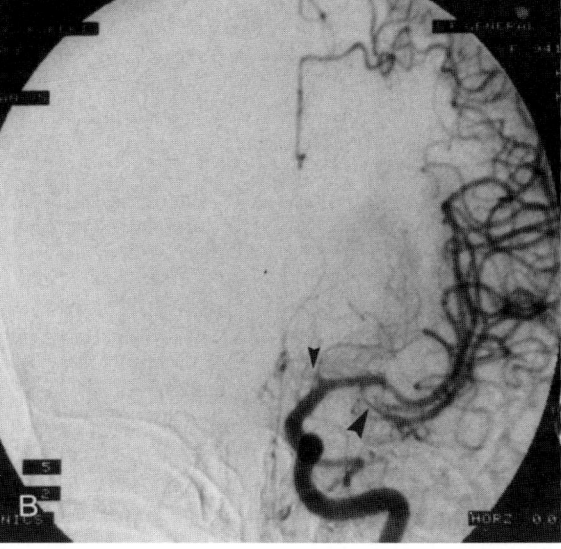

Figure 6.16. Meningovascular Syphilis. A. The contrast-enhanced CT scan reveals a small infarct in the left striate nucleus in this 21-year-old man with meningovascular syphilis. **B.** A left internal carotid arteriogram in the frontal projection on another patient with meningovascular syphilis shows occlusion of the left anterior cerebral artery (*small arrowhead*) and narrowing of branches of the left middle cerebral artery (*large arrowhead*). Both patients improved with penicillin therapy.

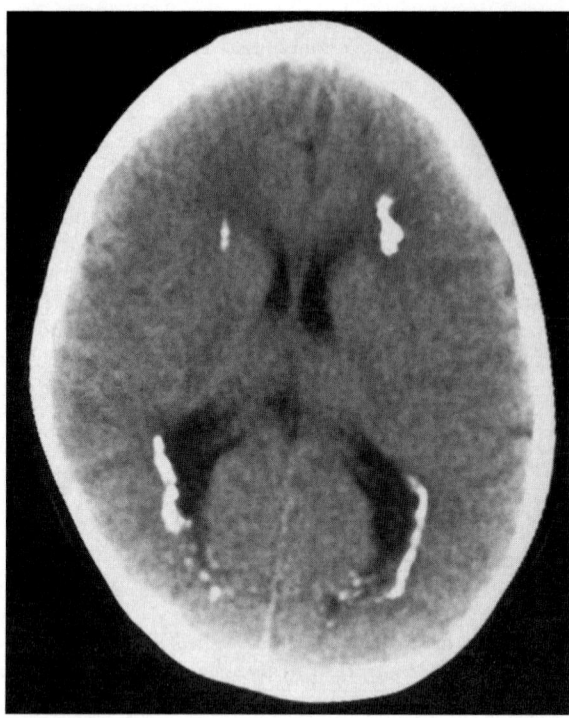

Figure 6.17. Congenital Cytomegalovirus Infection. A noncontrast CT scan shows multiple periventricular high-density calcifications. The calcifications in congenital CMV infection tend to be periventricular only, as in this case. With congenital toxoplasmosis, calcifications may be found throughout the brain.

lination and periventricular white matter lesions are often seen. The most common finding with CT scanning is periventricular calcifications (Fig. 6.17). These are detected better with CT than MR. There are usually no basal ganglia or cortical calcifications as are seen in congenital toxoplasmosis. Parenchymal atrophy and ventriculomegaly are common. The disease has been diagnosed in utero with obstetric sonography. Periventricular hyperechoic calcifications, preceded by hypoechoic periventricular ringlike zones, are characteristic findings. CMV infection in adults is unusual, except in immunosuppressed patients. (See *Acquired Immunodeficiency Syndrome*.).

Herpes simplex encephalitis occurs most frequently in neonates. The infant is usually infected during descent through the birth canal when the mother has genital (type II) herpes. Occasionally, there is transplacental transmission before delivery, but this usually results in spontaneous abortion. The infection causes a severe encephalitis that is either fatal or has grave neurologic consequences. The patient usually presents with seizures in the second to fourth week. If the patient survives, varying degrees of microcephaly, mental retardation, micropthalmia, enlarged ventricles, intracranial calcifications, and multicystic encephalomalacia may occur. Early in the course of the encephalitis, CT scans may reveal diffuse brain swelling or bilateral patchy areas of decreased density in the cerebral white matter and cortex, with relative sparing of the basal ganglia, thalami, and posterior fossa structures (Fig. 6.18A). Cranial sonography will

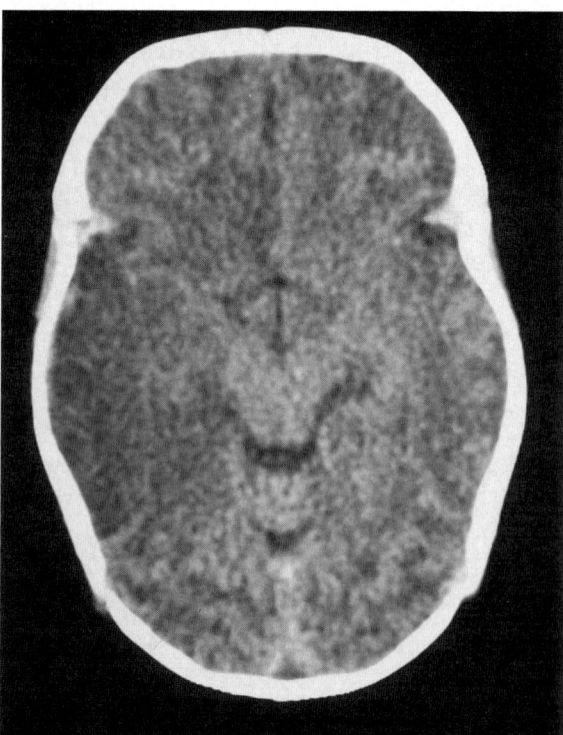

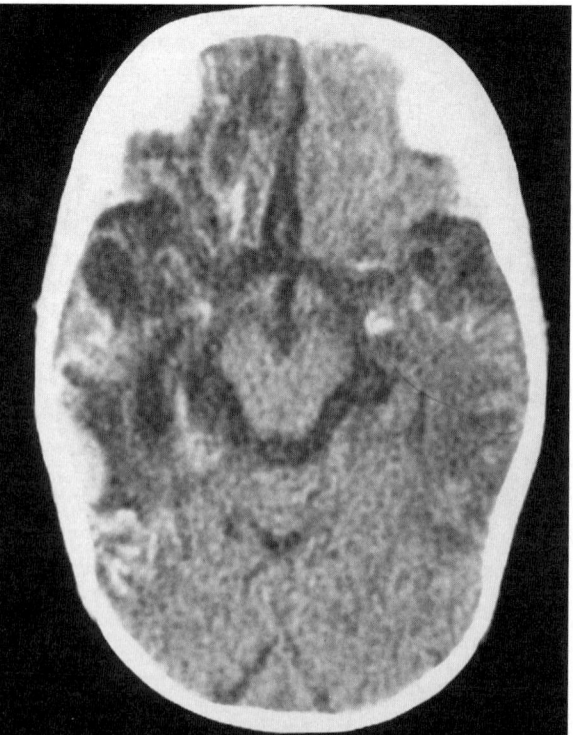

Figure 6.18. Neonatal Herpes. A. There is low density and swelling in the right temporal lobe and, to a lesser extent, in the frontal and left temporal lobes on the noncontrast CT scan of this 2-week-old child with herpes type II infection in the acute stage. **B.** Three weeks later, the noncontrast CT scan on this same infant reveals multiple areas of cystic encephalomalacia and widespread gray matter calcification, typical of late-stage neonatal herpes infection.

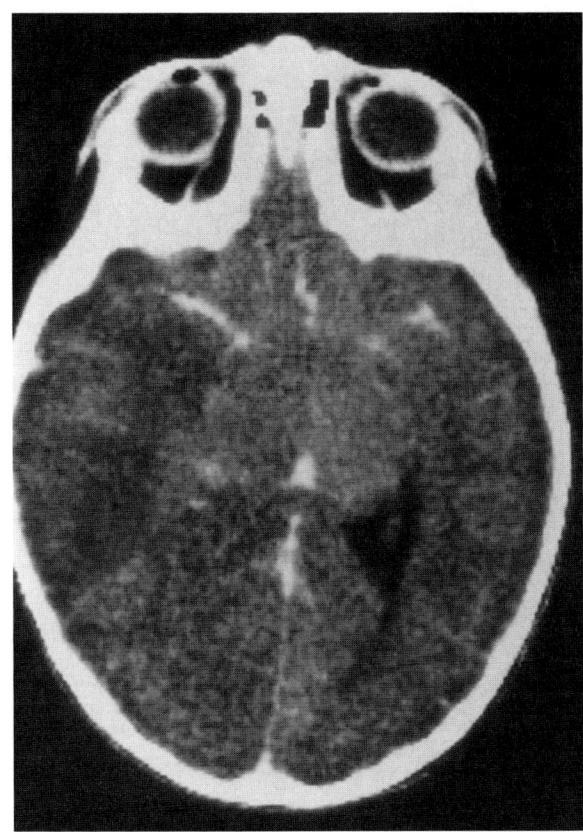

Figure 6.19. Adult Herpes Encephalitis. Both temporal lobes are of low density and appear swollen, especially on the right, on this contrast-enhanced CT scan. The appearance is similar to that of cerebral infarcts, but the clinical presentation is usually different.

show areas of increased echogenicity corresponding to these low-density zones. The low-density lesions progress to areas of necrosis, which are sometimes hemorrhagic and may eventually calcify. Multicystic encephalomalacia is the end result. Increased density in the cortical gray matter is characteristic in this late stage (Fig. 6.18B). With MR, there is decreased gray–white matter contrast early in the infection, reflecting gray-matter edema. Later, there is decreased signal on the T2WI within the thinned cortical gray matter.

In adults, herpes simplex infection may cause encephalitis or cranial neuritis. The infection usually is secondary to reactivation of latent herpes simplex type I. Patients with herpes encephalitis present with the gradual onset of personality changes, dysphasia, and focal neurologic deficits. Seizures and coma may occur. An inconstant but characteristic EEG finding is a localized spiked and slow wave pattern. Early diagnosis is crucial because there is a greater than 70% mortality rate in untreated patients. Unfortunately, CSF studies are often negative. Treatment is with acyclovir, which significantly reduces mortality, but many survivors have permanent deficits. CT scans show a poorly defined area of decreased density in one or both temporal lobes (Figs. 6.19,6.20A). The predilection for the temporal lobes is because the virus is usually latent within the Gasserian ganglion. The frontal lobes may also be involved. The in-

sular cortex is often involved, but the adjacent putamen is usually spared. There is usually swelling with mass effect. Streaky enhancement is variable. The CT findings are not usually seen before the fifth day of symptoms. With MR, the findings may be identified somewhat sooner. There is a nonspecific pattern of increased signal on the intermediate and T2WI in the temporal or frontal lobe(s), or both, with sparing of the putamen. This increased signal may be subtle and use of a T2-weighted *FL*uid *A*ttenuated *I*nversion *R*ecovery (FLAIR) sequence can help improve detection (Fig. 6.20B,C). Early on, meningeal enhancement may be seen. Later, there may be parenchymal enhancement or evidence of hemorrhage. The differential diagnosis includes middle cerebral artery infarct (which will often involve the putamen, unlike herpes), early bacterial cerebritis, and other types of viral encephalitis.

Varicella zoster rarely causes an encephalitis that is similar to that caused by herpes simplex. Another unusual manifestation is the syndrome of herpes zoster opthalmicus and delayed contralateral hemiparesis caused by cerebral angiitis. In this syndrome, there are cerebral infarcts resulting from a large and medium-sized vessel angiitis on the same side as opthalmic zoster skin manifestations. Imaging studies show typical infarcts, and angiography shows segmental areas of narrowing and/or beading of the arteries. Herpes zoster may also cause cranial neuritis, which may involve any of the cranial nerves. The most commonly involved is the facial nerve, resulting in the Ramsay Hunt syndrome. Clinically there is ear pain and a facial paralysis accompanied by a vesicular eruption about the ear. CT scans are usually normal, but MR may reveal increased contrast enhancement of the facial nerve.

Acute disseminated encephalomyelitis (ADEM) is an acute demyelinating disease that occurs after a viral infection, following a vaccination, or sometimes spontaneously. It probably has an autoimmune basis, as organisms are not isolated from brain tissue. Symptoms develop acutely with fever, headache, and meningeal signs. Seizures, focal neurologic deficits, stupor, and coma may develop. The mortality rate is 10–20%. When treated early with steroids, most patients make a full recovery. T2-weighted MR is much more sensitive than CT in identifying lesions of increased signal intensity in the white matter (Fig. 6.21). The brainstem, cerebellum, and basal ganglia are often involved. Optic neuritis is also common. The lesions are usually multiple, but few. There sometimes is solid or ring enhancement of the lesions. The appearance is similar to that seen in multiple sclerosis, but with a monophasic clinical course. The lesions regress with successful treatment, correlating with clinical improvement. Acute hemorrhagic leukoencephalitis is a severe variant of ADEM that is often fatal. Pathologically, there is perivascular hemorrhagic necrosis, primarily in the centrum semiovale. The major imaging feature is a rapid progression of white matter lesions during the course a few days.

Subacute sclerosing panencephalitis is caused by a variant of the measles virus. It typically occurs after a 6- to 10-year asymptomatic period in children and young adults who had measles before the age of 2 years.

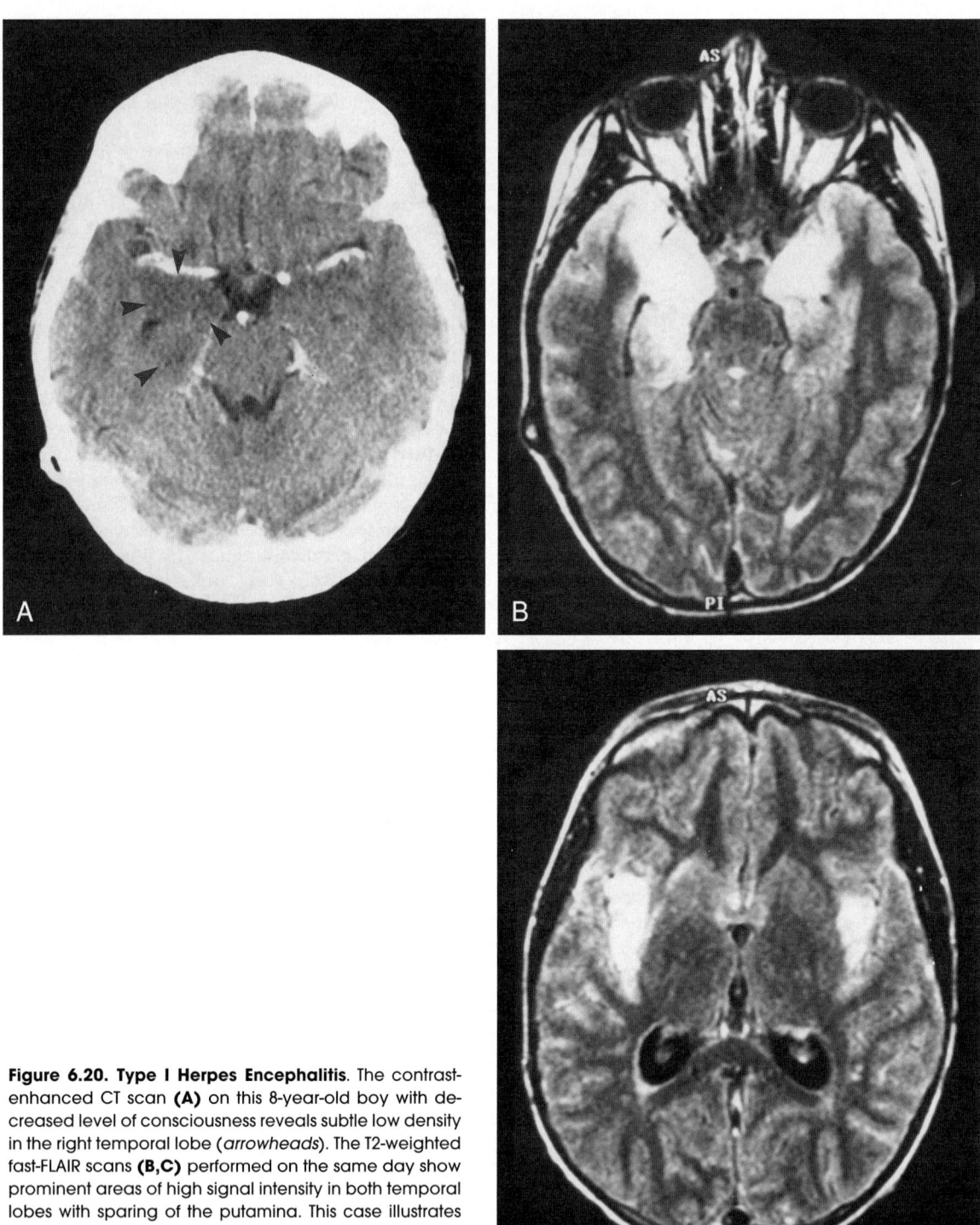

Figure 6.20. Type I Herpes Encephalitis. The contrast-enhanced CT scan **(A)** on this 8-year-old boy with decreased level of consciousness reveals subtle low density in the right temporal lobe (*arrowheads*). The T2-weighted fast-FLAIR scans **(B,C)** performed on the same day show prominent areas of high signal intensity in both temporal lobes with sparing of the putamina. This case illustrates why MR is the imaging modality of choice when herpes encephalitis is suspected.

The disease causes a progressive dementia, seizures, and paralysis, leading to death. There is no treatment. Imaging studies initially reveal focal lesions in the gray matter and subcortical white matter. Later, there are periventricular white matter lesions that may enhance. In the late stages, there is usually profound cortical atrophy.

Progressive multifocal leukoencephalopathy is a demyelinating disease caused by a papova virus (the

JC virus, not to be confused with the Creutzfeldt-Jakob agent, which is a prion). It occurs only in immunosuppressed patients and has an increased incidence in patients with AIDS as is later discussed.

Encephalitis can be caused by a variety of viruses not already discussed, including the togaviruses (arboviruses) that result in St. Louis, California, western equine, and eastern equine encephalitis, Epstein-Barr

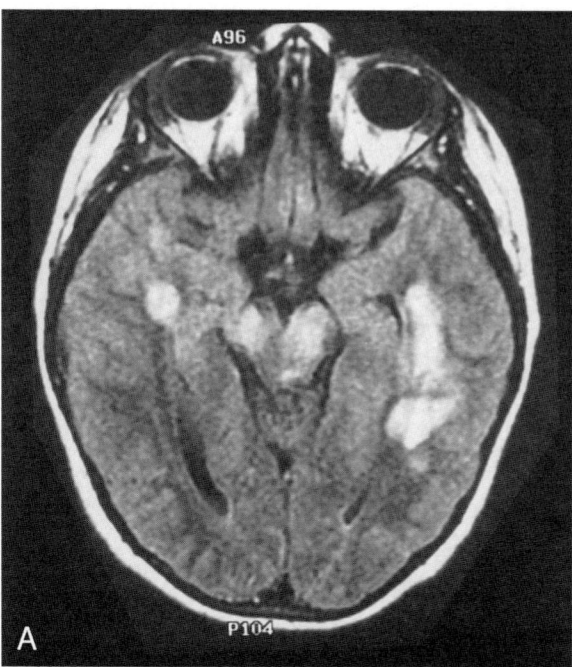
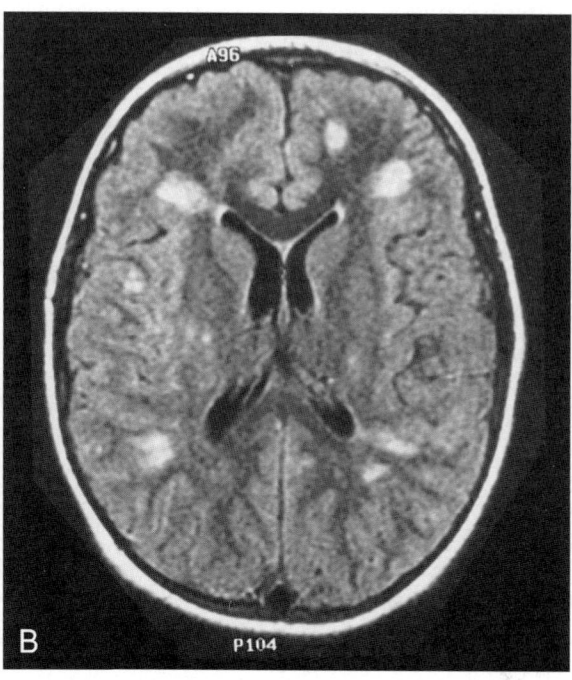
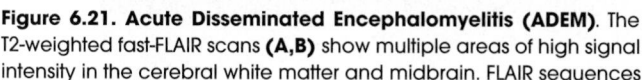

Figure 6.21. Acute Disseminated Encephalomyelitis (ADEM). The T2-weighted fast-FLAIR scans **(A,B)** show multiple areas of high signal intensity in the cerebral white matter and midbrain. FLAIR sequences are extremely sensitive for detecting white matter lesions. This 8-year-old child recovered fully after steroid therapy.

virus, mumps, measles, rubella, and enteroviruses. Rickettsia (Rocky Mountain spotted fever) and mycoplasma pneumoniae may also produce encephalitis. Japanese encephalitis is a viral encephalitis found in Asia. Bilateral hemorrhagic thalamic lesions are typical of this disease. Rasmussen's encephalitis is a devastating disease of childhood, most likely of viral etiology. There are intractable seizures and progressive neurologic deficits. The disease usually affects one cerebral hemisphere. Imaging studies show severe atrophy of the involved hemisphere. PET scans show the hemisphere to be hypometabolic.

Creutzfeldt-Jakob disease is caused by a transmissible protein called a prion or slow virus. Clinically, there is a rapidly progressive dementia, ataxia, and myoclonus, leading to death. The diagnosis is usually made on the basis of the clinical and EEG findings. Imaging studies are often normal, but serial studies may show rapid progress from normal to marked cortical atrophy during the course of months. With T2-weighted MR, bilaterally symmetrical, diffuse high signal abnormalities in the basal ganglia are often present. Increased signal and thinning of the periventricular white matter are also common findings.

EXTRA-AXIAL INFECTIONS

Meningitis

Meningitis can be caused by bacteria, mycobacteria, fungi, parasites, and viruses. Bacterial meningitis is caused by *Haemophilis influenzae* (in children), *Neisseria meningitidis* (in young adults), and *Streptococcus pneumoniae* (in older adults) in more than 80% of cases.

Escherichia coli, group B streptococcus, and *Listeria monocytogenes* occur commonly in neonates. The bacteria most commonly enter the meninges during a systemic bacteremia but can spread directly from infected sinuses or after surgery or trauma. Patients present with a relatively acute onset of fever, a stiff neck, and headache, followed by a decrease in mental status. CSF studies are usually diagnostic, and imaging studies are generally not required. CT scans may be performed in the emergency setting in acutely comatose patients or in patients with a nonspecific headache, but they are usually normal (Fig 6.22A). The inflammatory exudate caused by the meningitis may occasionally produce high density within the subarachnoid spaces, similar to that seen in subarachnoid hemorrhage.

The increased density is often more pronounced in the peripheral sulci than in the basal cisterns, unlike most cases of aneurysmal bleeding. Diffuse cerebral edema is sometimes seen (Fig. 6.22B). If contrast is given, there might or might not be meningeal enhancement. CT and MR are more often used later in the course of meningitis, when there are suspected complications such as hydrocephalus, cerebritis or abscess, ventriculitis, and venous or arterial infarctions. The hydrocephalus that may develop is usually of the communicating type, reflecting decreased function of the arachnoid villi in absorbing CSF. Subdural effusions may be seen in infants, especially with *H. influenzae* meningitis. With CT and MR, subdural effusions appear as thin collections, along the surface of the brain, isodense or isointense with CSF (Fig. 6.23). These sterile effusions can be identified with cranial sonography in infants. Echogenic sulci, ventriculomegaly, and abnormal parenchymal echogenicity have

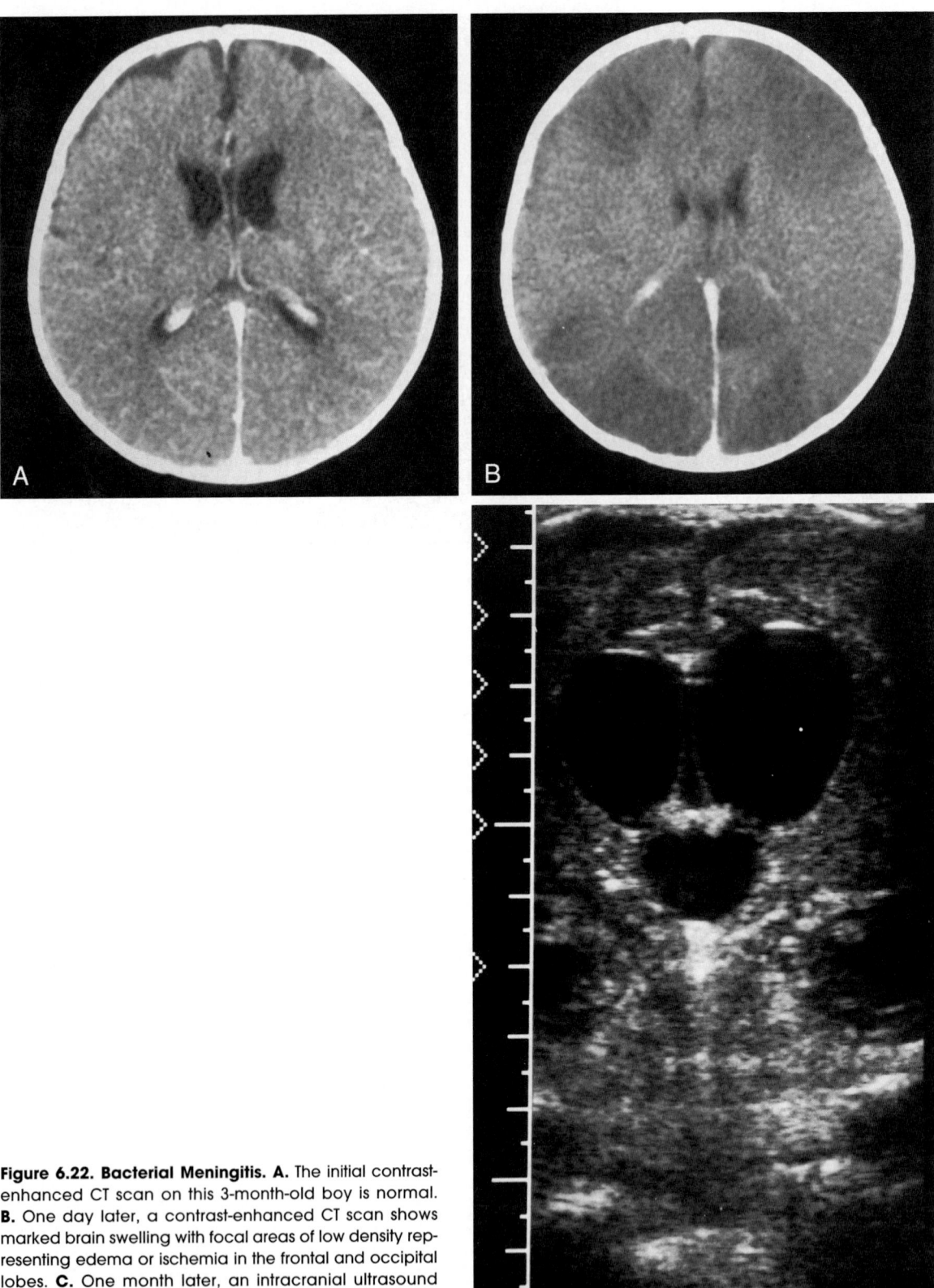

Figure 6.22. Bacterial Meningitis. A. The initial contrast-enhanced CT scan on this 3-month-old boy is normal. **B.** One day later, a contrast-enhanced CT scan shows marked brain swelling with focal areas of low density representing edema or ischemia in the frontal and occipital lobes. **C.** One month later, an intracranial ultrasound shows ventriculomegaly from marked cortical atrophy owing to widespread cortical destruction.

also been reported in infants with bacterial meningitis imaged with US (Fig. 6.22C).

Tuberculous meningitis is the most common form of CNS tuberculosis. Although it is usually caused by *Mycobacterium tuberculosis*, it may be caused by atypical mycobacteria, such as *M. avium–intracellulare*,

specifically in patients with AIDS. Tuberculous meningitis has a predilection for infants and children, but it is seen in all age groups. The disease spreads to the meninges hematogenously from the lungs, but the CXR is normal in 40–75% of patients. The tuberculin skin test is also frequently negative. Clinically, there is usually a

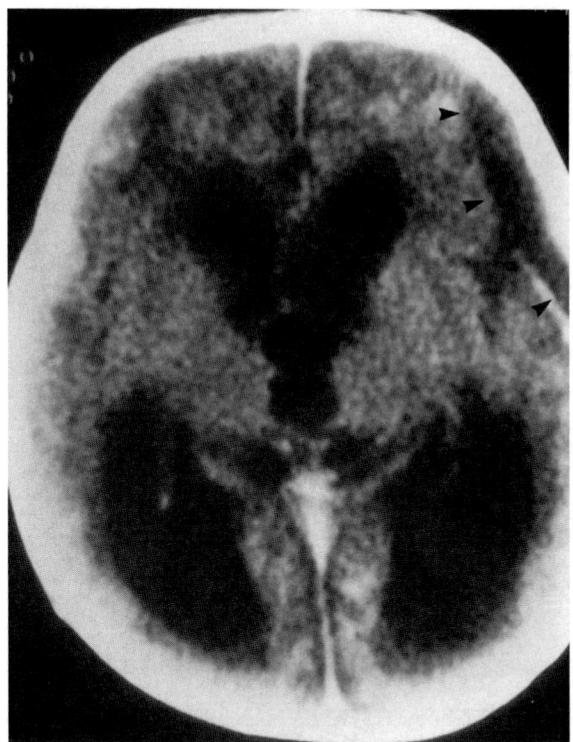

Figure 6.23. Subdural Effusion. A contrast-enhanced CT scan on this 6-year-old child with *Haemophilis influenzae* meningitis reveals a subdural collection nearly isodense with CSF (*arrowheads*). Subdural effusions are common with H. influenzae meningitis. There is also enlargement of the lateral and third ventricles because of communicating hydrocephalus, which is a common complication of meningitis.

subacute or insidious onset of headache, malaise, weakness, apathy, or focal neurologic findings. Imaging studies will show enhancing, thickened meninges, especially near the base of the brain (Fig. 6.24), unlike bacterial meningitis, in which the peripheral meninges are more often involved. The often marked thickening of the meninges also distinguishes tuberculous and other granulomatous meningitides from pyogenic meningitis. The thick exudate in the basal cisterns may extend into the Virchow-Robin spaces, causing a vasculitis. This frequently leads to infarcts, better detected with MR than with CT. Communicating hydrocephalus is another relatively common complication.

The differential diagnosis of tuberculous meningitis includes fungal meningitis, racemose cysticercosis, sarcoidosis, and carcinomatous meningitis.

Fungal meningitis usually causes thick meningeal enhancement in the basal cisterns, as with tuberculosis (Fig. 6.25). Enhancement is variable with cryptococcosis, depending on the immune status of the patient. Hydrocephalus is common, but infarcts and extension of fungal meningitis into the brain occur less frequently than with tuberculous or pyogenic meningitis (except in cases of aspergillosis and mucormycosis).

Racemose cysticercosis may show thick meningeal enhancement, but cystic lesions in the cisterns are also frequently found (see Figs. 6.13,6.14).

Sarcoidosis involves the CNS in up to 14% of patients at autopsy, but it only rarely causes neurologic

symptoms. It primarily affects the leptomeninges, so abnormal meningeal enhancement is seen with CT or MR. Focal parenchymal-enhancing mass lesions or nonenhancing small white matter lesions may also be seen.

Viral meningitis is caused most commonly by the enteroviruses but can be caused by mumps, togaviruses, herpes simplex, lymphocytic choriomeningitis virus, and HIV. Most patients do not require treatment, and neurologic deficits are uncommon. Imaging studies are typically normal.

Subdural and Epidural Infections

Extra-axial pyogenic infections may also involve the epidural or subdural spaces. An epidural abscess may be caused by penetrating injuries, surgery, sinusitis, mastoiditis, orbital infection, or, rarely, by hematogenous spread. CT scans show an inwardly convex, extra-axial collection with increased density compared with CSF (Fig. 6.26). The inner margin usually enhances with contrast. There may be adjacent sinusitis or skull abnormalities. MR is probably more sensitive in demonstrating these lesions and can do so in multiple planes. The strong dural attachments prevent rapid expansion of epidural abscesses. A subdural empyema, however, may spread rapidly throughout the subdural space, which is acutely life threatening. Cortical venous thrombosis resulting in venous infarcts is a common result of

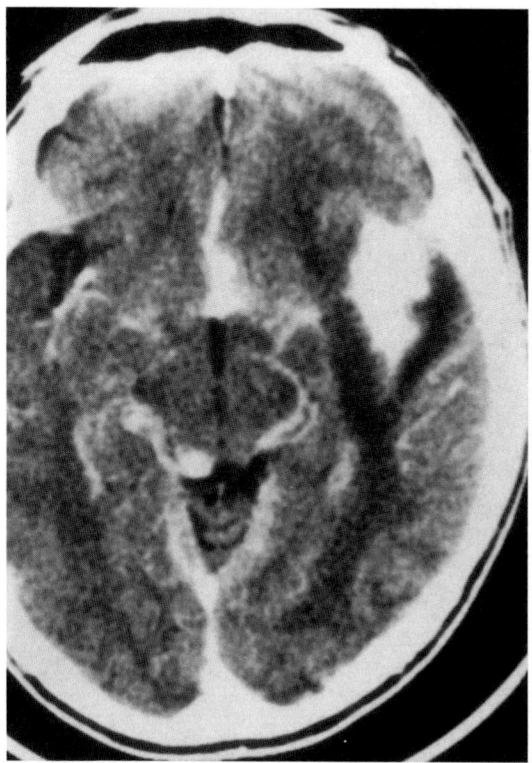

Figure 6.24. Tuberculous Meningitis. The contrast-enhanced CT scan shows marked abnormal contrast enhancement in the left sylvian fissure, interhemispheric fissure, ambient cistern, and along the tentorium. This thick, irregular enhancement in the basal cisterns is typical of a pachymeningitis such as TB or fungal meningitis. CT scans in patients with bacterial meningitis are usually normal or may reveal subtle increased density or enhancement in the peripheral sulci.

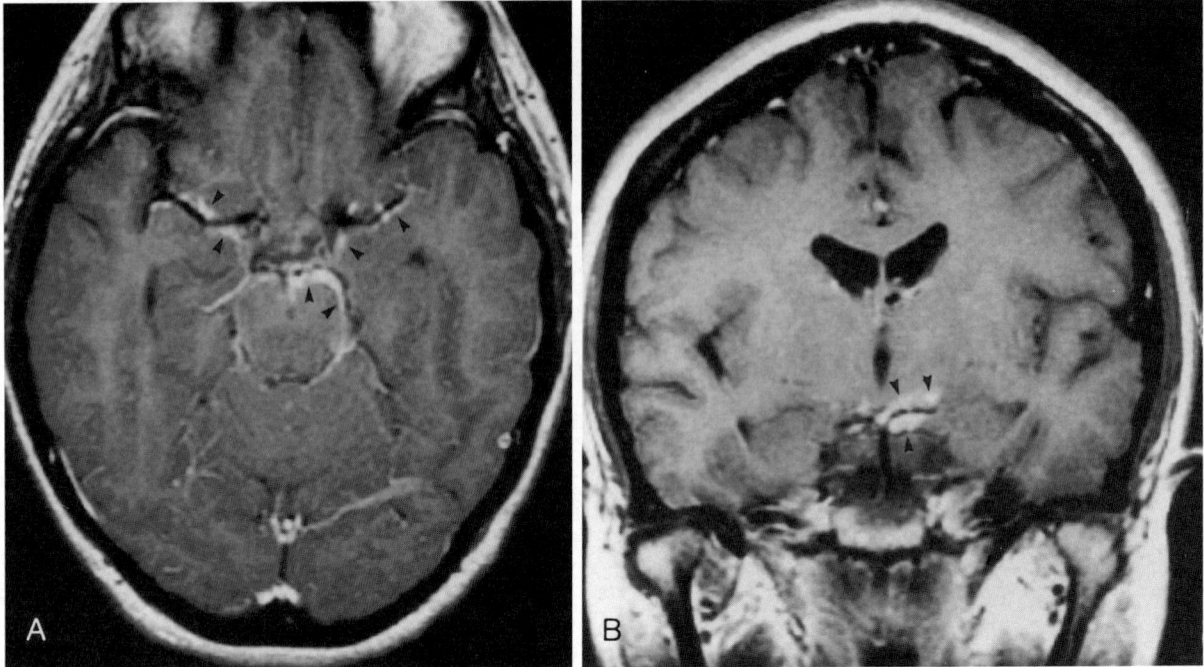

Figure 6.25. Coccidiomycosis Meningitis. Contrast-enhanced, T1-weighted axial **(A)** and coronal **(B)** scans reveal abnormal enhancement of the meninges in the basal cisterns (*arrowheads*).

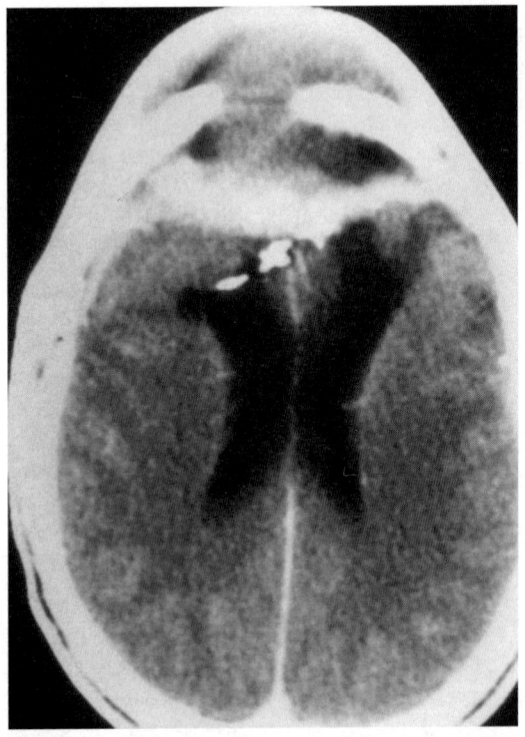

Figure 6.26. Epidural Abscess. This patient had a penetrating injury to the frontal bone several months before this contrast-enhanced CT scan. There is medium density pus extending through the calvarial defect into the epidural space. The inner margin enhances markedly. Surgical clips are present near the frontal horn of the right lateral ventricle.

these infections. Subdural empyemas are caused by the same conditions that produce epidural abscesses. Both CT and MR can demonstrate these subdural collections, which usually have enhancing inner margins. MR is more sensitive in showing smaller lesions because of the problem of partial volume averaging with the calvarium with CT. MR is also better at detecting venous thrombosis and venous infarcts.

Mild, smooth dural or meningeal enhancement may be seen after brain surgery and in patients with a ventriculostomy tube, especially with MR (Fig. 6.27). The enhancement can persist for years and should be considered benign in this clinical setting. It most likely reflects a chemical meningitis owing to perioperative hemorrhage.

ACQUIRED IMMUNODEFICIENCY SYNDROME

The CNS is a common site of involvement in patients with AIDS) Nearly 40% of patients with AIDS will develop neurologic symptoms, and 10% present with CNS disease as the earliest manifestation of the syndrome. In the advanced stages of the disease, 70–80% of patients with AIDS exhibit neurologic symptoms. A variety of infections and neoplasms may be diagnosed in these patients. The most common infections include HIV encephalitis, toxoplasmosis, cryptococcosis and other fungal infections, CMV and herpetic meningoencephalitis, mycobacterial infection, progressive multifocal leukoencephalopathy, and meningovascular syphilis. Primary CNS lymphoma is by far the most common tumor, but metastatic lymphoma, gliomas, and rarely Kaposi sarcoma may also occur.

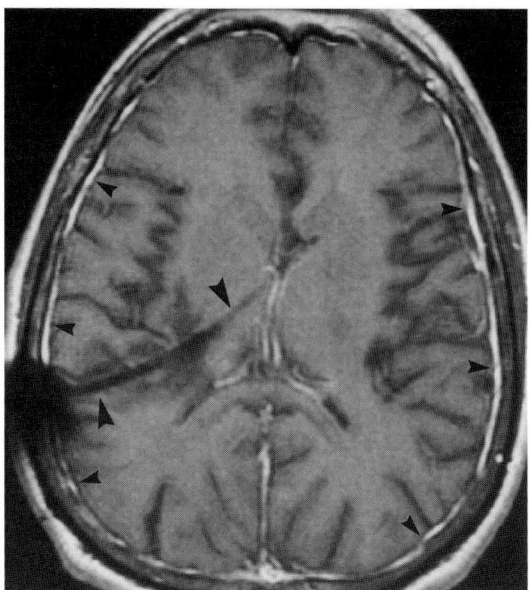

Figure 6.27. Benign Postoperative Meningeal Enhancement. Several years after brain surgery, this T1-weighted contrast enhanced MR scan reveals smooth, but definitely abnormal enhancement of the dura (*small arrowheads*). There were no signs of infection or tumor recurrence. A ventricular shunt tube is seen on the right (*large arrowheads*).

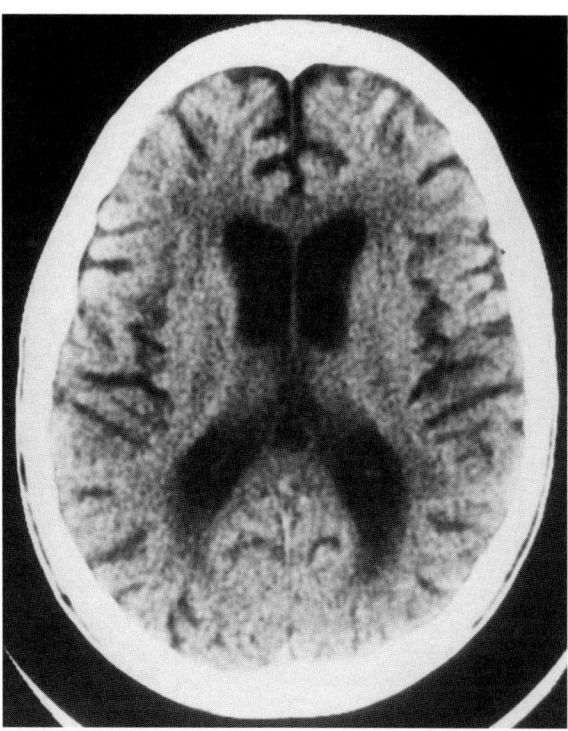

Figure 6.28. AIDS-related Atrophy. A noncontrast CT scan reveals enlarged ventricles and sulci in this 24-year-old patient with AIDS. This is the most common abnormality found on brain imaging of patients with AIDS. It often correlates with the AIDS dementia complex.

HIV Encephalitis. The etiologic agent in AIDS, HIV, is neurotropic, infecting the brain in up to 90% of patients at autopsy. Clinical symptoms of brain involvement by HIV occur in a minority of these patients. Pathologically, HIV infection results in vacuolation of the white matter, with areas of demyelination and multinucleated giant cells. The centrum semiovale is involved most severely, but all white matter tracts, including the brainstem and cerebellum, may be affected. The cortical gray matter is usually spared. Clinically, patients with HIV encephalitis may develop a subcortical dementia with cognitive, behavioral, and motor deterioration. This is known as the AIDS dementia complex, which occurs in approximately 7–15% of patients with AIDS. Infants and children with HIV encephalitis exhibit loss of developmental milestones, apathy, failure of brain growth, and spastic paraparesis. This is the most common form of CNS disease in pediatric patients with AIDS, as opportunistic infections and CNS are unusual.

Diffuse atrophy is the most common manifestation of HIV infection of the brain on neuroimaging studies (Fig. 6.28). This is largely central atrophy, reflecting the predominant white matter involvement. White matter lesions are also commonly seen in patients with the ADC. MR is significantly more sensitive than CT for detecting these abnormalities. A diffuse pattern of increased signal in the deep white matter or multiple small punctate white matter lesions on T2WI are the most common findings. The punctate lesions do not correlate well with symptoms and do not exhibit mass effect or abnormal contrast enhancement.

The most severe cases of HIV encephalitis show extensive bilateral areas of abnormal signal throughout the periventricular white matter, brainstem, and cerebellum (Fig. 6.29). In these severe cases, CT may also be abnor-

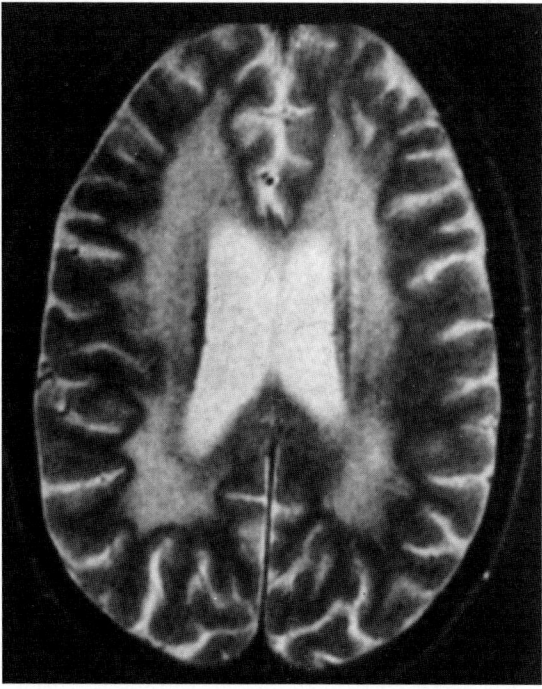

Figure 6.29. HIV Encephalitis. This young patient clinically had the AIDS dementia complex. The T2-weighted MR shows widespread abnormal high signal in the periventricular white matter.

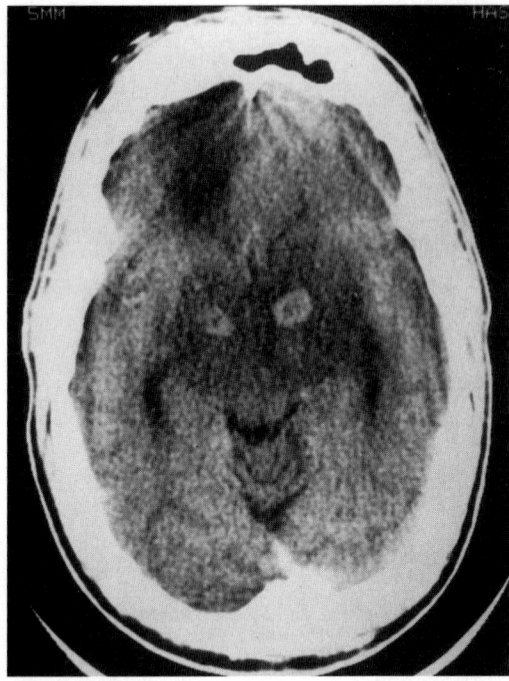

Figure 6.30. Toxoplasmosis. A contrast-enhanced CT scan reveals bilateral ring enhancing lesions in the basal ganglia of this patient with AIDS. There is marked surrounding low density edema. The basal ganglia are a common site for toxoplasmosis.

mal, showing low density without enhancement in the white matter. Such severe involvement usually correlates with symptoms of the AIDS demential complex. The clinical and imaging abnormalities may respond to treatment with anti-HIV drugs. Decrease metabolism has been demonstrated in the white matter of patients with ADC studied with localized phosphorus-31 nuclear magnetic resonance (NMR) spectroscopy. There is also a modest decrease in the magnetization transfer ratio (MTR) in HIV infected white matter. In infants and children with HIV infection, atrophy is the most common observation, followed by calcifications in the basal ganglia. White matter calcifications and low-density lesions are also sometimes seen.

Toxoplasmosis is the next most common CNS infection in AIDS occurring in approximately 13–33% of patients with CNS complications. *Toxoplasma gondii* is an obligate intracellular protozoan that is ubiquitous throughout the world, causing subclinical or mild infection in a large percentage of the population. In the United States, between 20–70% of the population are seropositive for toxoplasmosis. In patients with AIDS, CNS toxoplasmosis usually results from reactivation of the previously acquired infection. A necrotizing encephalitis usually results, with the formation of multiple thin-walled abscesses. Patients present clinically with headache, fever, lethargy, decreased level of consciousness, and focal signs that initially can be confused with the subacute encephalitis of HIV infection. Neuroimaging studies are crucial in patient management.

The typical appearance of CNS toxoplasmosis is that of multiple enhancing mass lesions with surrounding vasogenic edema (Figs. 6.30,6.31). The lesions are usually

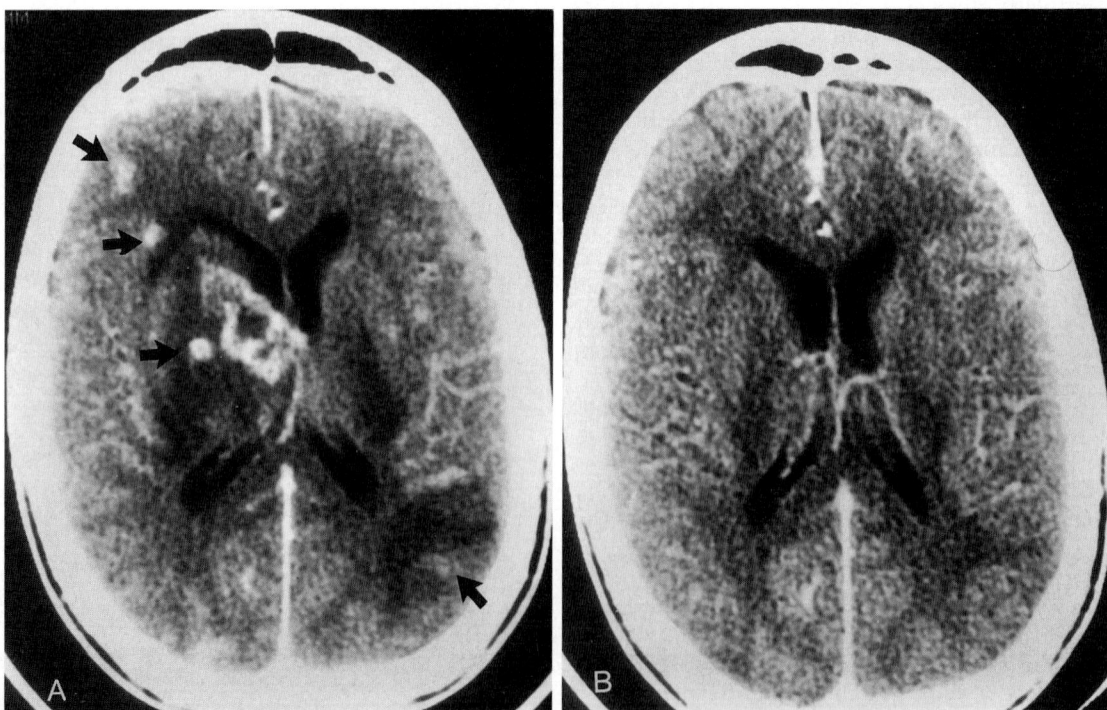

Figure 6.31. Toxoplasmosis. A. A contrast-enhanced CT scan shows a large right basal ganglia enhancing mass and several other small enhancing lesions (*arrows*). The small size and multiplic- ity of the lesions favors toxoplasmosis over lymphoma. **B.** After 2 weeks of antibiotic therapy, the contrast-enhanced CT scan reveals complete resolution of the lesions, typical for toxoplasmosis.

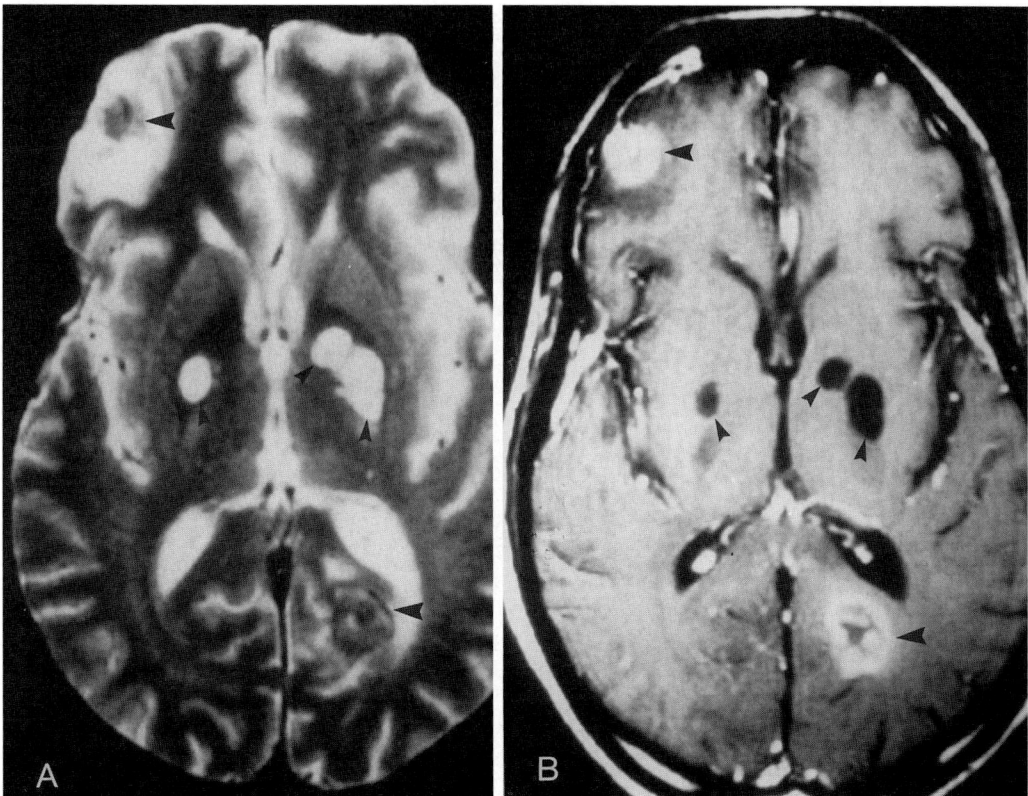

Figure 6.32. Cryptococcosis and Toxoplasmosis. A. The T2-weighted MR scan reveals multiple rounded lesions, isointense to CSF in the basal ganglia (*small arrowheads*). There is no surrounding edema. Darker lesions with surrounding edema are present in the right frontal and left occipital areas (*large arrowheads*). **B.** The contrast-enhanced T1-weighted MR scan again reveals the basal ganglia lesions to be isointense with CSF (*small arrowheads*). There is no contrast enhancement. The appearance of these lesions is typical of gelatinous pseudocysts of cryptococcosis. These lesions represent dilated Virchow-Robin spaces filled with cryptococcus organisms. The right frontal and left occipital lesions do enhance with contrast (*large arrowheads*), as is typical of toxoplasmosis.

relatively small, between 1 and 4 cm in diameter. The larger lesions usually exhibit ring enhancement, whereas the smaller lesions are usually solid. The lesions are usually of increased signal on precontrast T2WI, but there may be central areas of decreased signal from calcification or hemorrhage, especially after antibiotic treatment. The basal ganglia is a favored site, but white matter and cortical lesions are also common. The main differential consideration is primary CNS lymphoma, which is discussed later. A clinical and imaging response to antitoxoplasmosis antibiotics will usually distinguish between toxoplasmosis and lymphoma in most cases (Fig. 6.31). Biopsy is usually reserved for atypical cases or when there is no response to antibiotics. Other infections or tumors may occasionally mimic toxoplasmosis, but they are unusual. Fungal, mycobacterial, and amebic abscesses have been described. Bacterial abscesses are exceedingly rare in patients with AIDS.

Fungal Meningitis. Although fungal abscesses and granulomas are unusual, fungal meningitis is a common complication of AIDS, occurring in 5–15% of patients. Cryptococcosis is the most common fungal infection, although histoplasmosis, candidiasis, aspergillosis, and coccidiomycosis also occur. The meningitis caused by these agents is usually mild because of the diminished inflammatory response of the immunocompromised host. There is usually little or no enhancement of the meninges, and imaging studies are usually normal. The diagnosis is made when there are elevated cryptococcal antigen titers in the serum and CSF.

As already mentioned, cryptococcosis may sometimes present as dilated Virchow-Robin spaces filled with cryptococcus organisms, known as gelatinous pseudocysts. These cysts appear as rounded, smoothly marginated lesions in the basal ganglia that are nearly isodense and isointense to CSF (Fig. 6.32). There is no enhancement following contrast administration, which distinguishes these lesions from toxoplasmosis.

Progressive multifocal leukoencephalopathy (PML) is an infection of immunosuppressed patients caused by a papova virus (the JC virus). The incidence of PML in patients with AIDS is between 4–7%. It can also occur in other immunosuppressed patients, such as transplant recipients and leukemics, but it does not occur in patients with normal immunity. The infection causes demyelination and necrosis primarily involving white matter. Clinical symptoms include mental status changes, blindness, aphasia, hemiparesis, ataxia, and other focal findings. There is a progressive course to death within months. In non-AIDS immunosuppressed patients, PML has a predilection for the occipital lobes,

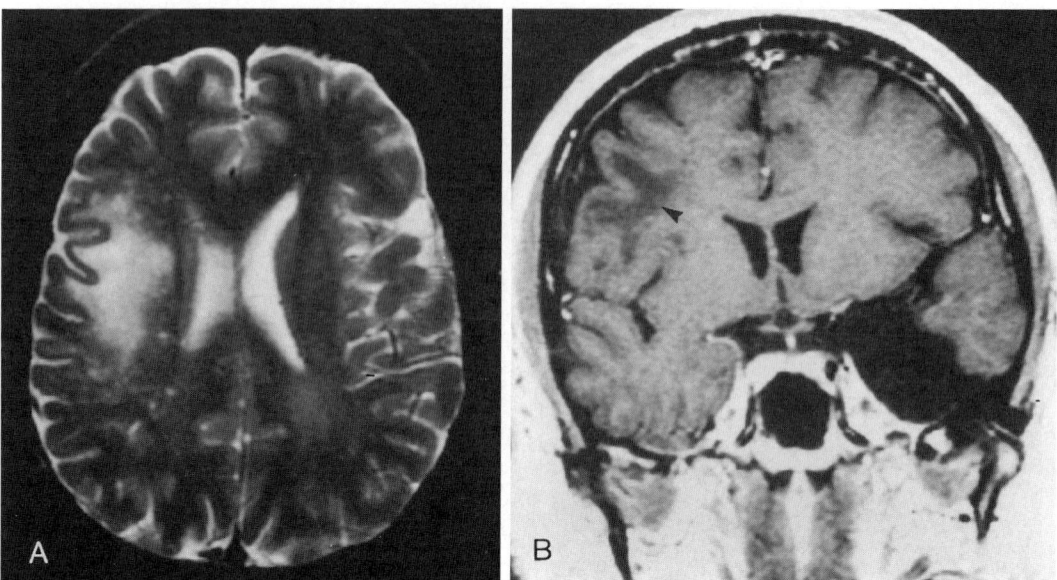

Figure 6.33. Progressive Multifocal Leukoencephalopathy. A. There is an area of abnormal high signal intensity in the right corona radiata on this T2WI. There is no significant mass effect. **B.** On the contrast-enhanced T1WI, the lesion is of low signal intensity (*arrow-* *head*) and does not enhance. These are typical features of PML, which was proved with biopsy in this patient with AIDS. Incidentally, a left temporal arachnoid cyst can be noted.

but in patients with AIDS, any part of the brain may be involved. Because it is primarily a white matter process, MR is superior to CT in showing the lesions of PML. MR reveals focal lesions of increased signal on T2WI and decreased signal on T1WI within the subcortical and deep white matter (Fig. 6.33). CT shows white matter lesions of decreased density. The lesions may be solitary or multifocal. Mass effect and contrast enhancement are almost always absent, which are important distinguishing features. Rarely, both gray and white matter or the basal ganglia are involved, simulating an infarct. The main differential diagnosis in the setting of AIDS is that of HIV encephalitis. Unlike PML, HIV encephalitis is usually more diffuse, less intense on T2WI, and does not extend to the gray–white junction.

Virus Infection. Pathologically, cytomegalovirus infection is a common CNS infection in patients with AIDS, but it does not usually result in frank tissue necrosis and is usually subclinical. There are may cases of pathologically proved CMV brain infection with normal CT and MR scans. CMV meningoencephalitis is occasionally imaged as areas of increased signal on T2-weighted MR in the periventricular white matter. Subependymal contrast enhancement, if present, is a valuable diagnostic sign. Rarely, CMV will present as a ring enhancing mass. Herpesvirus and varicella virus infection are also only occasionally imaged. In patients with AIDS, these viral infections often have a more benign clinical course and imaging appearance because of a diminished immune response.

Intracranial mycobacterial infections occur in a small percentage of patients with AIDS. Most of these patients are IV drug abusers with pulmonary tuberculosis. The chest radiographs are positive in approximately 65% of cases. There is a very high mortality rate (nearly 80%)

in these patients. Most patients present with meningitis. Imaging studies in these patients reveal communicating hydrocephalus or meningeal enhancement, or both. Tuberculomas occur in approximately 25% of patients with HIV-related CNS tuberculosis, but tuberculous abscesses are less common. Tuberculomas are usually smaller and have less edema than tuberculous abscesses.

Primary CNS lymphoma is by far the most common intracranial tumor in AIDS. Up to 6% of patients with AIDS will develop this tumor. It is the main differential diagnostic consideration, along with toxoplasmosis, when a mass lesion is found in patients with AIDS. Patients present with symptoms of a space-occupying lesion, as with toxoplasmosis. Solitary or multiple enhancing mass lesions are found with neuroimaging studies (Fig. 6.34). The lesions are usually centrally located within the deep white matter or basal ganglia, but cortical lesions also occur. There may be subependymal spread, or extension across the corpus callosum, which does not usually occur with toxoplasmosis. With MR imaging, there is variable signal intensity, with areas of low or high signal on T2WI, and isointense or low signal on T1WI. With CT, the lesions are often isodense with gray matter. The lesions almost always enhance with contrast, in either a ring or solid pattern. The imaging appearance is often indistinguishable from toxoplasmosis. The main distinguishing features are size and number. Toxoplasmosis is more frequently multiple, and the lesions are usually smaller than with lymphoma. Isointensity with white matter on T2-weighted MR and diffuse, homogeneous contrast enhancement favors lymphoma. High signal on T2-weighted MR (often with a low signal rim) and ring enhancement following contrast administration favors toxoplasmosis. Toxoplasmosis is also

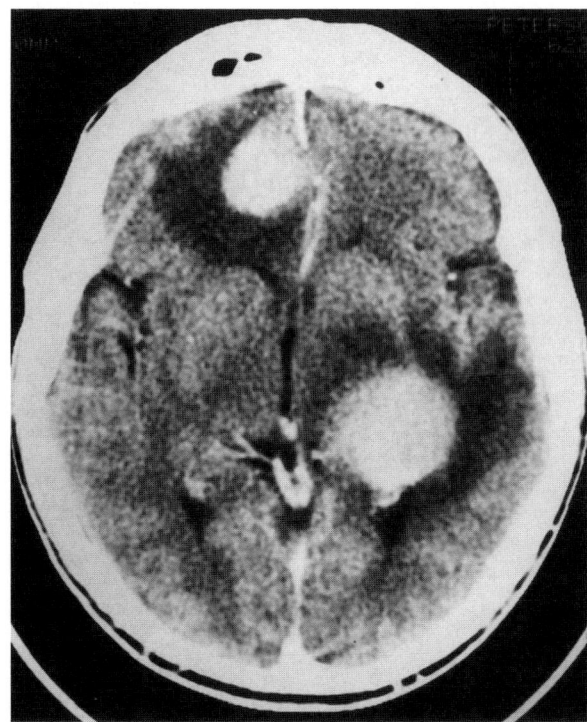

Figure 6.34. Primary CNS Lymphoma. There are two solidly enhancing mass lesions with surrounding edema on this CT scan of a patient with AIDS. The relatively large size and solid enhancement pattern are more suggestive of lymphoma than toxoplasmosis, as was proved in this case.

more common than lymphoma. There is a great deal of overlap in the imaging appearance of these two mass lesions, which can coexist in the same patient. For this reason, some authors advocate biopsy when enhancing mass lesions are found in a patient with AIDS. In most institutions, an empirical trial with antitoxoplasmosis antibiotics is usually attempted prior to biopsy. Clinical and radiologic improvement usually are seen within 2 weeks.

Suggested Readings

Ashdown BC, Tien RD, Felsberg GJ. Aspergillosis of the brain and paranasal sinuses in immunocompromised patients: CT and MR imaging findings. AJR Am J Roentgenol 1994; 162:155–159.

Barboriak DP, Provenzale JM, Boyko OB. MR diagnosis of Creutzfeldt-Jakob disease: significance of high signal intensity of the basal ganglia. AJR Am J Roentgenol 1994;162: 137–140.

Barkovich AJ, Lindan CE. Congenital cytomegalovirus infection of the brain: imaging analysis and embryologic considerations. AJNR Am J Neuroradiol 1994;15:703–715.

Brightbill TC, Ihmeidan IH, Donovan Post MJ, et al. Neurosyphilis in HIV-positive and HIV-negative patients: neuroimaging findings. NR Am J Neuroradiol 1995;16:703–711.

Brismar J, Gascon GG, Vult von Steyern K, et al. Subacute sclerosing panencephalitis: evaluation with CT and MR. NR Am J Neuroradiol 1996;17:761–772.

Caldemeyer KS, Smith RR, Harris TM, et al. MRI in acute disseminated encephalomyelitis. Neuroradiology 1994;36: 216–220.

Dousset V, Armand JP, Lacoste D, et al. Magnetization transfer study of HIV encephalitis and progressive multifocal leukoencephalopathy. NR Am J Neuroradiol 1997;18:895–901.

Dumas JL, Visy JM, Belin C, et al. Parenchymal neurocysticercosis: follow-up and staging by MRI. Neuroradiology 1997; 39:12–18.

Enzmann DR, ed. Imaging of Infections and Inflammations of the Central Nervous System: Computed Tomography, Ultrasound, and Nuclear Magnetic Resonance. New York: Raven Press, 1984.

Federle MP, Megibow A, eds. Radiology of AIDS. New York: Raven Press, 1988.

Fitz CR. Inflammatory diseases of the brain in childhood. NR Am J Neuroradiol 1992;13:551–567.

Haimes AB, Zimmerman RD, Morgello S, et al. MR imaging of brain abscesses. AJNR Am J Neuroradiol 1989;10:279–291.

Han BK, Babcock DS, McAdams L. Bacterial meningitis in infants: sonographic findings. Radiology 1985;154:645–650.

Mader I, Stock KW, Ettlin T, et al. Acute disseminated encephalomyelitis: MR and CT features. AJNR Am J Neuroradiol 1996;17:104–109.

Olsen WL. Neuroradiologic abnormalities in AIDS. Curr Probl Diagn Radiol 1988;17:89–100.

Rauch RA, Jinkins JR. Infections of the central nervous system. Curr Opin Radiol 1991;3:16–24.

Runge VM, Wells JW, Kirsch JE. Magnetization transfer and high-dose contrast in early brain infection on magnetic resonance. Invest Radiol 1995;30:135–143.

Sze G, Zimmerman RD. The magnetic resonance imaging of infections and inflammatory diseases. Radiol Clin North Am 1988;26:839–859.

Tien RD, Chu PK, Hesselink JR, et al. Intracranial cryptococcosis in immunocompromised patients: CT and MR findings in 29 cases. NR Am J Neuroradiol 1991;12:283–289.

Weingarten K, Zimmerman RD, Becker RD, et al. Subdural and epidural empyemas: MR imaging. AJNR Am J Neuroradiol 1989;10:81–87.

Whiteman M, Espinoza L, Donovan Post MJ, et al. Central nervous system tuberculosis in HIV-infected patients: Clinical and radiographic findings. AJNR Am J Neuroradiol 1995; 16:1319–1327.

7
White Matter and Neurodegenerative Diseases

Jerome A. Barakos

In contrast to gray matter, which contains neuronal cell bodies, white matter is composed of the long processes of these neurons. The axonal processes are wrapped by myelin sheaths, and it is the lipid composition of these sheaths for which white matter is named. In this chapter, a host of diseases, characterized by the involvement of white matter, is described. This is followed by a discussion of hydrocephalus and neurodegenerative disorders.

The marked sensitivity of T2-weighted magnetic resonance images allows white matter lesions to be readily detected. The difficulty that confronts the radiologist is that a wide gamut of diseases may involve the white matter and these lesions are often nonspecific in nature (1). An understanding of these white matter diseases, their clinical features, and parenchymal patterns of involvement are important in enabling the radiologist to generate a useful differential diagnostic list.

Cerebral white matter diseases are classified into two broad categories, demyelinating and dysmyelinating. **Demyelination** is an acquired disorder that affects normal myelin. The vast majority of white matter diseases, especially in the adult, falls into this category and is the principal focus of this chapter. In contrast, dysmyelination is an inherited disorder affecting the formation or maintenance of myelin. **Dysmyelination** is a rare condition usually identified in the pediatric age group and is discussed later in this chapter.

DEMYELINATING DISEASES

Demyelinating disease can be divided into four main categories based on etiology: *a)* primary, *b)* ischemic, *c)* infectious, and *d)* toxic and metabolic (Table 7.1).

Primary Demyelination

Multiple sclerosis (MS) is the classic example of a primary demyelinating disease. MS is characterized as a chronic, relapsing, often disabling disease affecting more than a quarter of a million people in the United States alone. The age of onset is between 20 to 40 years, with only 10% of cases presenting in individuals older than 50. There is a female predominance of almost 2 to 1. Several environmental factors have been associated with MS, such as higher geographic latitudes and upper socioeconomic status. The etiology of MS remains unclear.

Establishing a diagnosis of MS is challenging because no specific examination, laboratory test, or physical finding is diagnostic. Additionally, making a diagnosis of MS is portentous, as there are significant implications on many aspects of one's life. Making the diagnosis is now more important than ever because numerous therapies are available, including beta-interferon and copolymer-1, which can influence disease progression.

The classic clinical definition of MS is multiple central nervous system lesions separated in both time and space. Patients may present with virtually any neurologic deficit, but they most commonly present with limb weakness, paresthesia, vertigo, and visual or urinary disturbances. Important characteristics of MS symptoms are their multiplicity and tendency to vary over time. The clinical course of MS is characterized by unpredictable relapses and remissions of symptoms. The diagnosis can be supported with laboratory findings consisting of abnormal brainstem-evoked potentials and detection of oligoclonal antibody bands within the cerebrospinal fluid (2). Histopathologically, active MS lesions represent areas of selective destruction of myelin sheaths and perivenular inflammation, with sparing of the underlying axons. These lesions may occur throughout the white matter of the CNS, including the spinal cord. The inflammatory demyelination interrupts nerve conduction and nerve function, producing the symptoms of MS.

MR is the most sensitive indicator in the detection of MS plaques, but imaging findings alone should never be considered diagnostic. In clinically confirmed cases of MS, MR typically demonstrates lesions in more than 90% of cases. This compares with far less than 50% for computed tomography and 70% for laboratory tests such as brainstem-evoked potentials and CSF oligoclonal bands.

A variety of T2-weighted imaging techniques have been described in optimizing detection of white matter lesions. In addition to conventional spin-echo imaging, fast spin-echo, short tau inversion recovery, and fluid-attenuated inversion recovery (FLAIR) sequences have been described. As the name suggests, FLAIR imaging has the advantage of providing heavy T2-weighting while suppressing signal from CSF. As a result, FLAIR images provide improved lesion conspicuity of periventricular lesions, which may be obscured by the bright signal of CSF. Comparative studies have demonstrated that FLAIR imaging provides the best visualization of all supratentorial white matter lesions (3). The superiority of the FLAIR sequence does not hold up when imaging the posterior fossa and spine partly because of pulsation artifacts.

MS plaques are typically round or ovoid, with a periven-

Table 7.1. Classification of White Matter Diseases

Primary demyelination
  Multiple sclerosis
Ischemic demyelination
  Deep white matter infarcts
  Lacunar infarcts
  Vasculitis (including sarcoidosis and lupus)
  Dissection
  Thromboembolic infarcts
  Migrainous ischemia
  Moya-Moya disease
  Postanoxic
Infection-related demyelination
  Progressive multifocal leukoencephalopathy
  HIV encephalopathy
  Acute disseminated encephalomyelitis
  Subacute sclerosing panencephalitis
  Lyme disease
  Neurosyphilis
Toxic and metabolic demyelination
  Central pontine myelinolysis
  Marchiafava-Bignami syndrome
  Wernicke-Korsakoff syndrome
  Radiation injury
  Necrotizing leukoencephalopathy
Dysmyelination (inherited white matter disease)
  Metachromatic leukodystrophy
  Adrenal leukodystrophy
  Leigh's disease
  Alexander's disease

tricular or subcortical location (Fig. 7.1). Lesions are dark on T1WI and bright on T2WI. Only a fraction of MS plaques will demonstrate contrast enhancement. Lesions that enhance are thought to reflect new lesions, with active demyelination and disruption of the blood– brain barrier. In older lesions, in which no active inflammatory reaction exists, abnormal high signal on T2WI still persists and reflects residual scarring, that is, gliosis. Within the CNS, cells can mount only a limited response to neuronal injury. This typically manifests as a focal proliferation of astroglia at the site of injury, termed gliosis. In long-standing cases of MS, there is loss of deep cerebral white matter, with associated thinning of the corpus callosum.

MS lesions are nonspecific, and many of the diseases and conditions discussed in this chapter may have an identical appearance. Patients with migraines are especially challenging because both their symptoms and imaging findings may closely mimic those of MS. A pattern that is suggestive of MS is one of periventricular lesions that are ovoid and aligned perpendicular to the long axis of the ventricles. This pattern is the result of the alignment of the lesions along the perivenular spaces. Additional characteristic features include lesions that are confluent in nature and greater than 6 mm in diameter with a periventricular location.

In addition to the periventricular white matter, the cerebellar and cerebral peduncles as well as the corpus callosum and spinal cord are often affected in MS. Because ischemic changes uncommonly involve these locations, if periventricular lesions are accompanied by lesions in any of these areas, this dramatically increases the specificity for the diagnosis of MS. In other words, as ischemic changes rarely involve the cerebellar and cerebral peduncles, the presence of posterior fossa lesions is a useful differential diagnostic factor in suggesting MS. This is particularly important in patients older than 50 years because it is difficult to decide whether multifocal white matter lesions are the result of ischemia or a demyelinating process. Additional concepts for making this distinction are discussed in the next subsection (see Fig. 7.5).

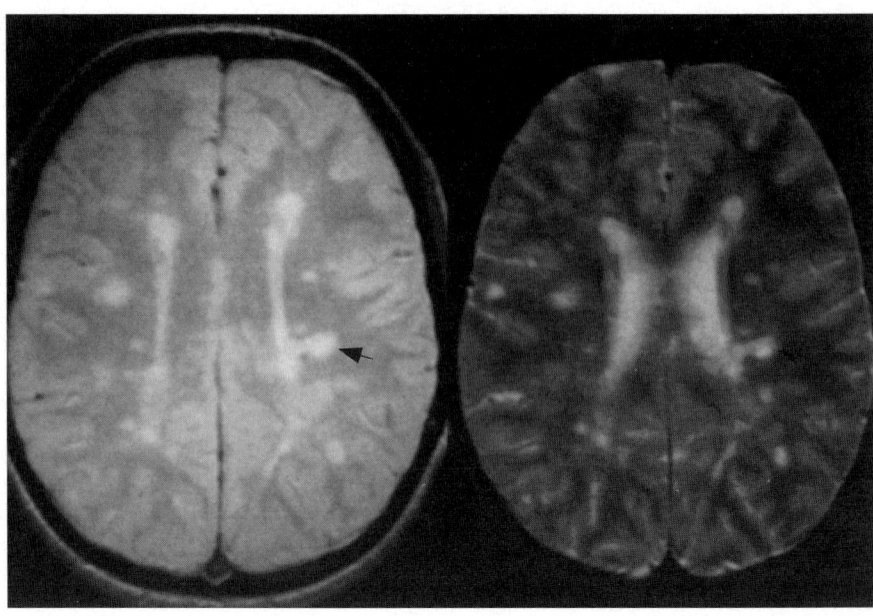

Figure 7.1. Multiple Sclerosis. First and second echo T2WI of a 23-year-old woman with MS demonstrate multiple periventricular and subcortical white-matter lesions. These lesions are ovoid, and many are perpendicular to the long axis of the ventricles (*arrow*). Although the findings are suggestive of MS, these lesions are nonspecific and indistinguishable from other demyelinating conditions such as Lyme disease and acute disseminated encephalomyelitis.

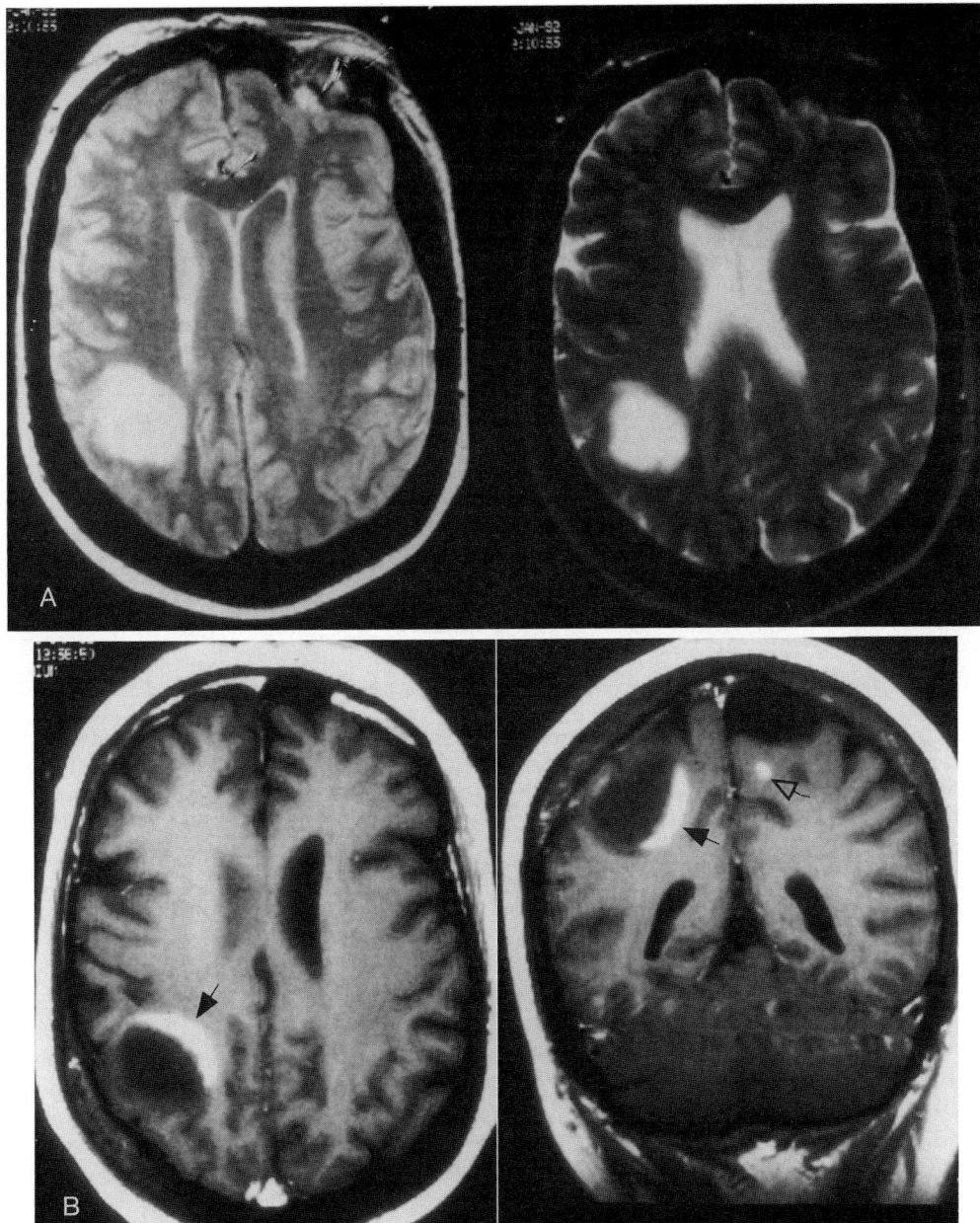

Figure 7.2. Multiple Sclerosis. MR images of a 34-year-old male with a history of right-sided weakness and sensory changes. **A.** First (*left*) and second (*right*) echo T2-weighted sequence reveals a large right parietal white matter lesion. The fact that the lesion is brighter than CSF on the first echo suggests that it is a solid parenchy-mal lesion rather than a simple cyst. **B.** Axial (*left*) and coronal (*right*) post-Gd T1WI reveal a crescentic rim of contrast enhance-ment (*arrow*) that reflects the advancing edge of demyelination. An additional active demyelinating lesion is seen in the opposite hemi-sphere open (*open arrow*).

MS lesions may also present as a large, conglomerate, deep white matter mass that can be mistaken for a neoplasm (Fig. 7.2) (4). A characteristic finding in these conglomerate MS plaques is that they often demonstrate a peripheral crescentic rim of contrast enhancement, which represents the advancing region of active demyelination. Detecting this pattern of enhancement, and searching carefully for other more characteristic periventricular lesions, are helpful in distinguishing a giant MS plaque from a neoplasm.

The spinal cord may also be involved with MS, and whenever a focal abnormality of the spinal cord is detected, a demyelinating MS plaque must be in the differential diagnosis (5). Demyelinating plaques may have mild mass effect as well as contrast enhancement, thus mimicking a neoplasm (see Figs. 10.5, 10.6). The majority of spinal cord MS lesions (70–80%) will have associated plaques in the brain. In the setting of a cord lesion, performing an MR scan of the head may confirm the diagnosis, thus avoiding a spinal cord biopsy.

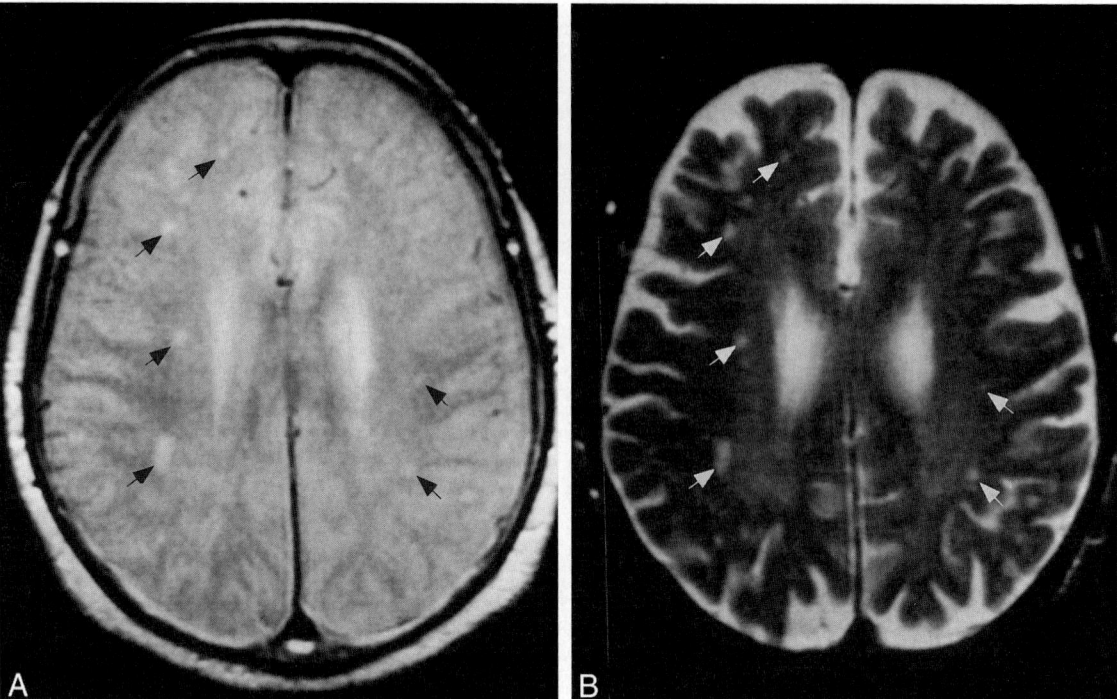

Figure 7.3. Ischemic Demyelination. Deep white matter ischemic lesions in a 67-year-old woman presenting with unrelated symptoms (headaches). Axial first **(A)** and second **(B)** echo T2WI demonstrate multiple punctate lesions involving the deep cerebral white matter (*arrows*). These lesions can be distinguished from Virchow-Robin spaces by their visibility on the first echo sequence. In contrast, perivascular spaces are of CSF signal intensity and would be isointense on the first echo and, thus, imperceptible.

Ischemic Demyelination

Although MR imaging is extremely sensitive in the detection of white matter lesions, a major difficulty in arriving at a diagnosis is that white matter lesions are often nonspecific. Thus, distinguishing MS lesions from other white matter lesions can be difficult. The most commonly encountered white matter lesions are ischemic in origin.

Age-related Demyelination. Small-vessel ischemic changes within the deep cerebral white matter are seen with such frequency in the older population (>60 years) that they can be considered a normal part of aging (Fig. 7.3) (6). This represents an arteriosclerotic vasculopathy of the penetrating cerebral arteries. The deep white matter is more susceptible to ischemic injury compared with the gray matter because it is supplied by long, small-caliber penetrating arteries. These vessels become narrowed by arteriosclerosis and lipohyaline deposits. The result is the formation of small ischemic lesions primarily involving the deep cerebral and periventricular white matter as well as the basal ganglia. The cortex, subcortical "U" fibers, central corpus callosum, medulla, midbrain, and cerebellar peduncles are usually spared because of their dual blood supply, which decreases their vulnerability to hypoperfusion. As previously described, if lesions are identified in these locations, a cause other than ischemia should be entertained.

Histologically, areas of infarction demonstrate axonal atrophy with diminished myelin. Early neuropathologists noted the areas of paleness associated with these changes and coined the term "myelin pallor." These white matter changes have received many names over the years. including leukoaraiosis, microangiopathic leukoencephalopathy, and subcortical arteriosclerotic encephalopathy. None of these terms are very satisfying, as they do not accurately reflect all the changes observed histologically and overstate the clinical significance of these lesions. A more appropriate term may simply be "age-related white matter ischemia." These small ischemic white matter lesions are often asymptomatic, and clinical correlation is always required before a diagnosis of subcortical arteriosclerotic encephalopathy or multi-infarct dementia (Binswanger's disease) is made (7). The white matter infarcts just described differ from lacunar infarcts. Lacunae refer to small infarcts (5–10 mm) occurring within the basal ganglia, typically the upper two thirds of the putamina. Both lacunar and deep white matter infarcts have similar etiologies and are the result of disease involving the deep penetrating arteries.

Small white matter lesions are more prominent in any patient with a vasculopathy, whether it is related to atherosclerosis (age, hypertension, diabetes, hyperlipidemia, coronary artery disease) or to a vasculitis (lupus, sarcoid, polyarteritis nodosa, Behçet's syndrome). In younger individuals, causes include vasculitis, embolic disease, hypoxia, dissection, and migrainous ischemia (Fig. 7.4). Differentiating these lesions related to ischemic changes from MS lesions can be difficult, especially in the older patient. This is important because 10% of patients who present with MS are older than 50 years of age. Clinical testing and history are helpful. Additionally, deep white matter infarcts tend to spare the subcortical arcuate fibers and the corpus callosum, both of which are often involved with MS. Involvement of the callosal–septal interface is relatively specific for MS (Fig. 7.5)(9).

Ependymitis Granularis is a normal anatomic finding that may mimic pathology (10). Ependymitis granularis consists of an area of high signal on the T2WI, along the tips of the frontal horns. These foci of signal range in width from several millimeters to a centimeter. Histologic studies of this subependymal area reveal a loose network of axons with low myelin count. This porous ependyma allows transependymal flow of CSF, resulting in a focal area of T2 prolongation. Unfortunately, this entity has been given a name that sounds more like a disease entity than a simple histologic observation.

Prominent Perivascular Spaces can also mimic deep white matter or lacunar infarcts. As blood vessels penetrate into the brain parenchyma, they are enveloped by CSF and a thin sheath of pia. These CSF-filled perivascular clefts are called Virchow-Robin spaces and present as punctate foci of high signal on T2WI (11). They are typically located in the centrum semiovale (high cerebral hemispheric white matter) and the lower basal ganglia at the level of the anterior commissure, where lenticulostriate arteries enter the anterior perforated substance. These perivascular spaces are typically 1–2 mm in diameter but can be considerably larger (Fig. 7.6). They can be seen as a normal variant at any age but become more prominent with increasing age as atrophy occurs.

An important means for differentiating a periventricular space from a parenchymal lesion is the use of the pro-

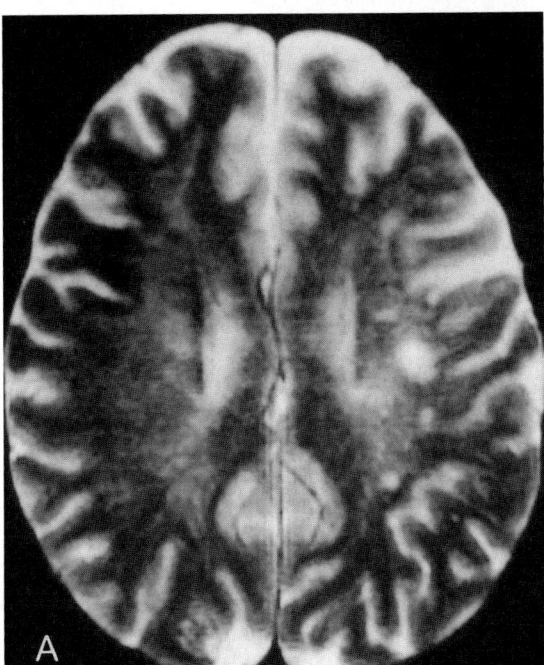

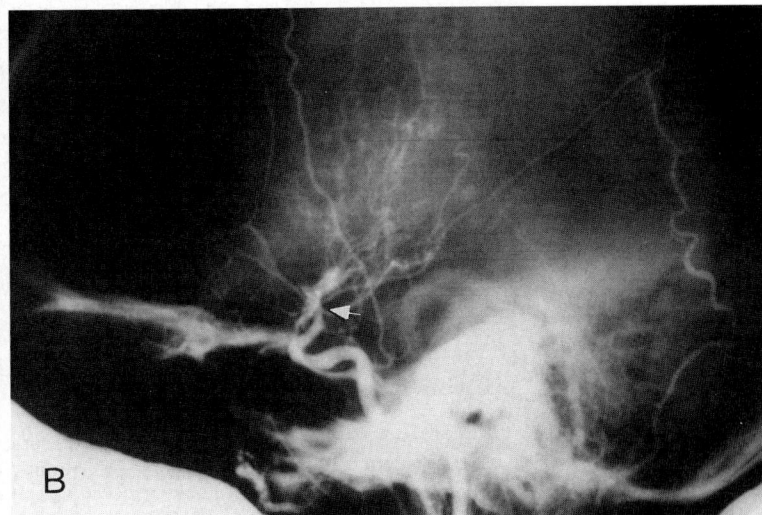

Figure 7.4. Vasculitis. T2WI **(A)** demonstrates left hemispheric white matter lesions in a 42-year-old woman. Although in a 60-year-old person, these lesions may simply represent age-related white matter ischemic changes, these findings are distinctly abnormal in a younger patient. Left internal carotid arteriogram **(B)** reveals severe supraclinoid stenosis (*arrow*), the result of vasculitis.

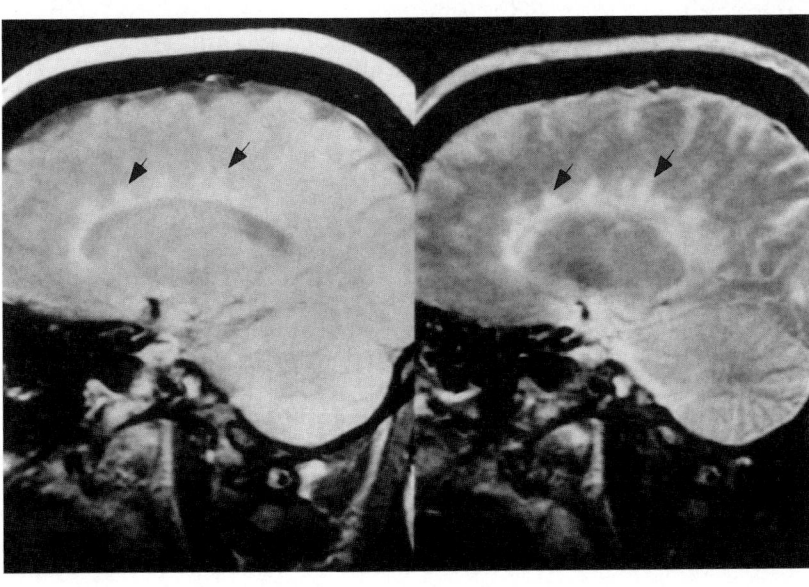

Figure 7.5. Multiple Sclerosis. Sagittal first and second echo T2WI of a 32-year-old woman with MS demonstrate a multitude of lesions involving the callosal–septal interface (*arrows*). This location is a characteristic site of MS involvement.

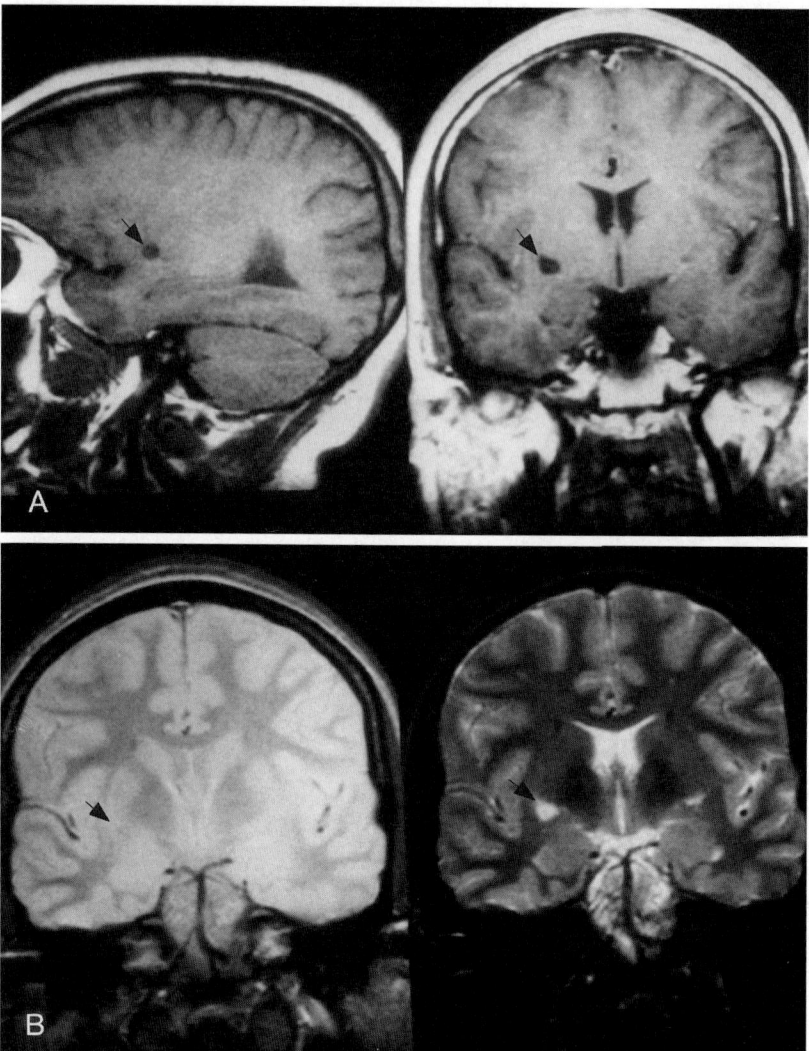

Figure 7.6. Virchow-Robin Spaces. A large perivascular space in a 32-year-old man (*arrow*) shown in sagittal and coronal T1WIs **(A)**, which demonstrate a well-rounded, right-sided lesion along the course of the lenticulostriate arteries as they enter the basal ganglia through the anterior perforated substance. Although perivascular spaces are typically 1–2 mm in diameter, they can be considerably larger. First and second echo coronal T2WIs **(B)** demonstrate that this lesion parallels the signal intensity of CSF on all imaging sequences and is almost imperceptible on the proton-density sequence (*arrow*). An old cavitated lacunar infarction may have a similar appearance but would be distinctly unusual in the inferior portion of the striatum. If differentiation is difficult, clinical history may be invaluable.

ton density–weighted (first echo T2WI) or FLAIR image (see Fig. 7.3). On the proton density–weighted sequence, CSF has similar signal intensity as white matter. A perivascular space is composed of CSF and will parallel CSF signal intensity on all sequences, that is, isointense on proton density sequence. In contrast, ischemic lesions, unless cavitated with cystic change, will be bright on the proton density sequence. Both a deep infarct and a perivascular space will be bright on the second echo T2WI, but only the infarct will remain bright on the first echo image. Similarly, on a FLAIR image, because fluid signal is attenuated, only true parenchymal lesions will yield abnormal signal. An additional differentiating feature is that lacunar infarcts, as already described, tend to occur in the upper two thirds of the corpus striatum and are usually larger than 5 mm. In contrast, periven-tricular spaces are typically smaller, bilateral, and often symmetric within the inferior third of the striatum.

Infection-related Demyelination

Various infectious agents may result in white matter disease, directly or indirectly, and most commonly are viral. Some of the more common agents are described here. For further discussion of viral-induced demyelination, see chapter 6.

Progressive Multifocal Leukoencephalopathy (PML) is seen with increased frequency because of an expansion in the population of those with AIDS. PML represents a reactivation of a latent JC papovavirus (12). This is usually seen in immunocompromised patients, particularly individuals with AIDS, lymphoma, organ

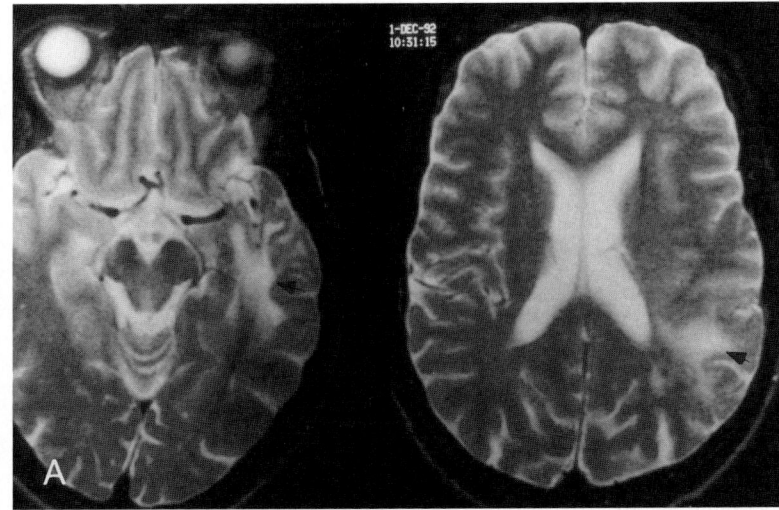
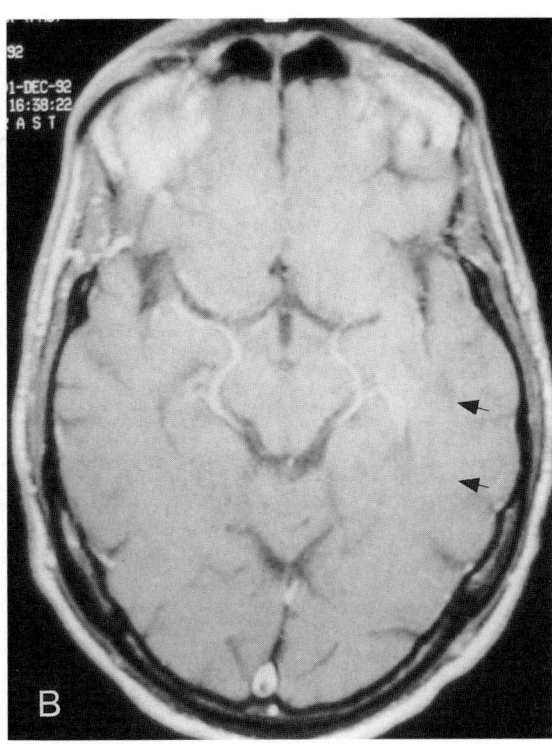

Figure 7.7. Progressive Multifocal Leukoencephalopathy. MR of 34-year-old man. T2WI **(A)** reveals abnormal signal in the subcortical white matter of the left temporal and parietal lobe (*arrows*). Characteristic features of PML include lack of mass effect without significant contrast enhancement or hemorrhage **(B)** (post-Gd T1WI). Rarely, mild contrast enhancement or petechial hemorrhage may be noted.

transplantation, and disseminated malignancies. The JC virus infects oligodendrocytes, resulting in widespread demyelination. PML typically involves the deep cerebral white matter, cerebellum, and brainstem. Lesions are characterized by a lack of mass effect, contrast enhancement, and hemorrhage (Fig. 7.7). Additionally, lesions appear as patchy asymmetric areas of demyelination with a predilection for the parietal region. These lesions rapidly progress and coalesce into larger confluent areas. Although most lesions involve supratentorial white matter, gray matter and infratentorial involvement are not uncommon. PML is relentlessly progressive, with death ensuing within several months from the time of onset.

HIV Encephalopathy. HIV involvement of the brain presents as a subacute encephalitis, referred to as AIDS dementia complex or diffuse HIV encephalopathy. This is characterized clinically by a progressive dementia without focal neurologic signs. The cause of HIV encephalopathy does not appear to be as the result of a direct infection of the neurons or macroglia (i.e., CNS support cells; astrocytes and oligodendrocytes). Instead, the active HIV infection develops in the microglia (brain macrophages). It is the resulting cytokines and excitatory compounds that are produced that have a toxic effect on adjacent neurons.

HIV encephalopathy most often results in mild cerebral atrophy without a focal abnormality. It is not uncommon for HIV encephalopathy to cause either focal or diffuse white matter hyperintensities on T2WI. Specifically, HIV white matter involvement tends to present as a subtle, diffuse T2 hyperintensity that often is bilateral and relatively symmetric. This supratentorial white matter signal abnormality is ill-defined and often involves a large area, in contrast to the dense lesions characteristic of PML (Fig. 7.8)(13). HIV encephalopathy

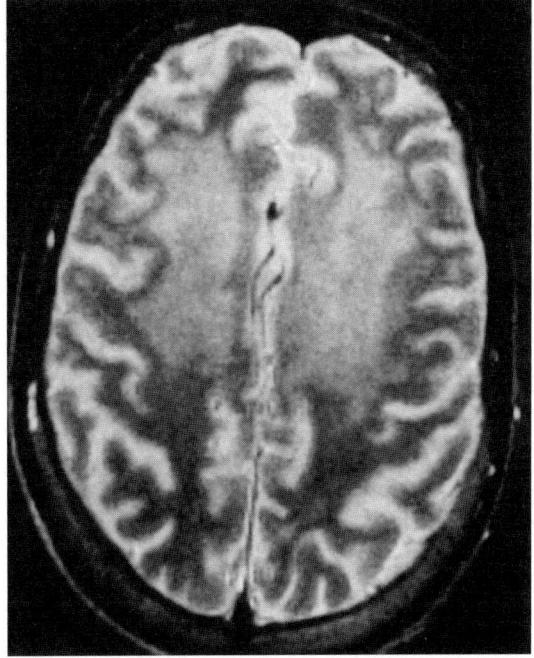

Figure 7.8. HIV Encephalopathy. T2WI of a 27-year-old man demonstrates diffuse hyperintensity of the deep cerebral white matter, as well as cortical atrophy. These findings represent the most common imaging abnormalities associated with HIV disease.

can also present with more focal punctate lesions. HIV lesions do not demonstrate contrast enhancement.

Demyelination may also occur as an indirect result of a viral infection. Specifically demyelination may follow a viral illness, the result of a viral-induced autoimmune response to white matter (14).

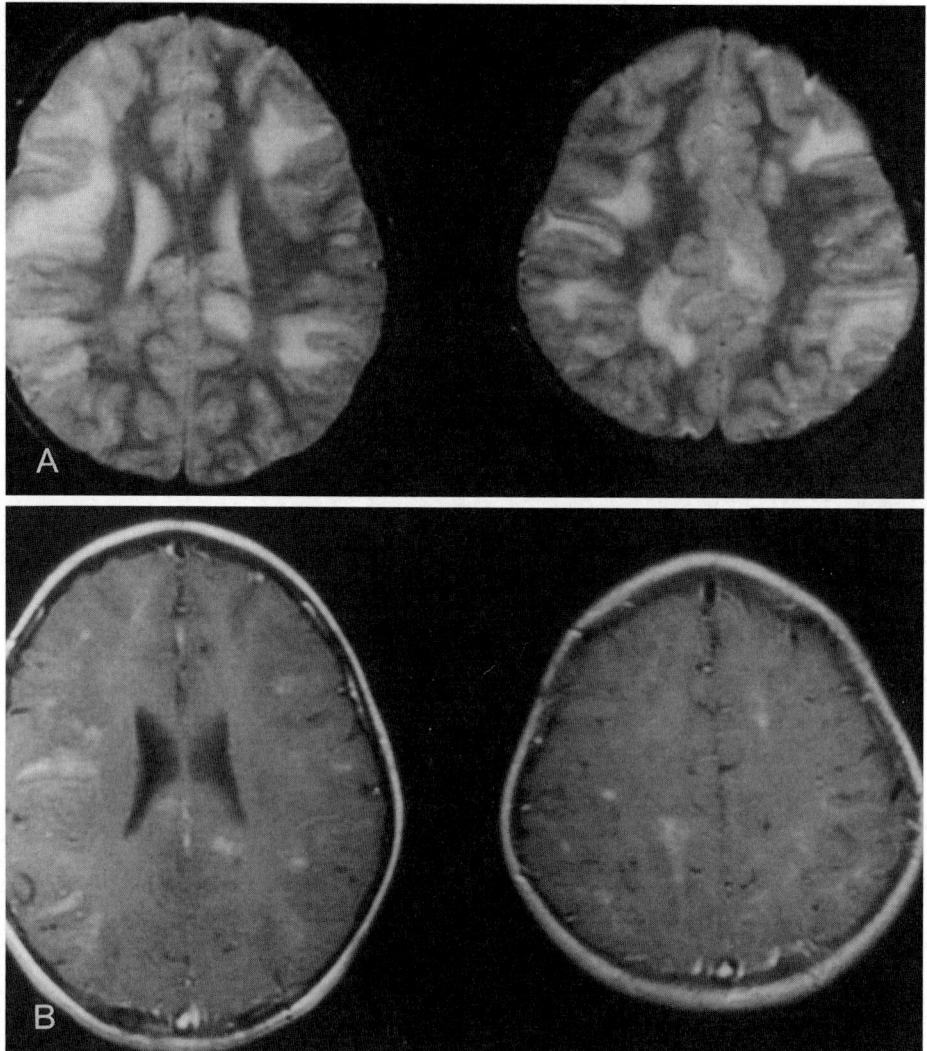

Figure 7.9. Acute Disseminated Encephalomyelitis. T2WI **(A)** and post-Gd T1WI **(B)** in a 7-year-old boy who presented with deteriorating mental status 1 week after viral gastroenteritis. Imaging reveals multiple enhancing subcortical white matter lesions. The finding that all lesions demonstrate enhancement is suggestive of a monophasic demyelinating process. The patient improved after treatment with steroids.

Acute Disseminated Encephalomyelitis (ADEM), postinfectious and postvaccinal encephalomyelitis, typically occurs after a viral illness or vaccination, with measles, rubella, and mumps being the most common agents (15). This condition is considered an immune-mediated inflammatory demyelinating disease. Demyelinating lesions associated with ADEM typically begin approximately 2 weeks after a viral infection, with the abrupt clinical onset of seizures and focal neurologic deficits. In the majority of cases, there is spontaneous resolution of symptoms, but permanent sequelae can be seen in up to 20% of patients, with some even progressing to death. Although occurring most commonly in children, any age can be affected. Lesions primarily involve white matter, but gray matter may also be affected. MR imaging demonstrates multifocal or confluent white matter lesions similar to those of MS (Fig 7.9). A differential feature is that ADEM is a monophasic illness, unlike MS, which has a remitting and relapsing course.

This is a feature often useful in differentiating ADEM from MS. Specifically, if the majority of the identified white matter lesions enhance, this suggests a monophasic process, that is, ADEM.

Subacute Sclerosing Panencephalitis (SSPE) represents a reactivated, slowly progressive infection caused by measles virus. Children between the ages of 5 and 12 years, who had measles usually before the age of 3, are typically affected. MR demonstrates patchy areas of periventricular demyelination as well as lesions of the basal ganglia. The disease course is variable and may be rapidly progressive or protracted.

Lyme Disease is caused by a spirochete infection (*Borrelia burgdorferi*) that results in white matter lesions that are indistinguishable from MS (Fig. 7.10)(16). The vector of transmission to humans is the ixodid tick (*Ixodes dammini*), which commonly infests deer and mice. The course of human infection, which has been divided into three stages, starts with a migrating erythe-

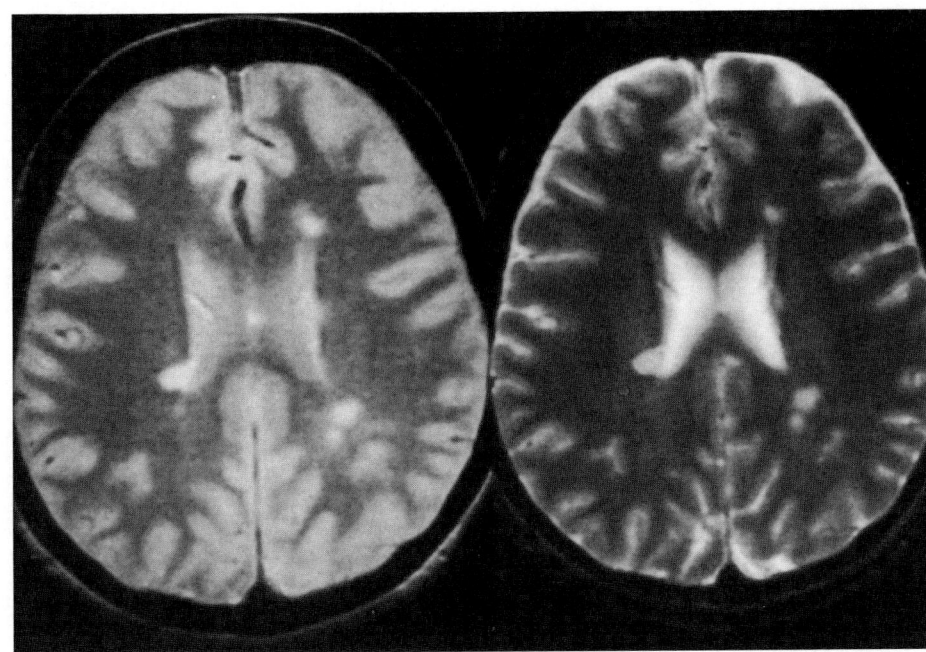

Figure 7.10. Lyme Disease. First and second echo T2WIs of a 30-year-old man demonstrate periventricular lesions mimicking MS. The patient presented several weeks after a migrating erythematous rash. Diagnosis was supported by serum spirochete-specific IgM immunofluorescence. Symptoms resolved after treatment with antibiotics.

matous rash. The most prominent neurologic symptoms occur during the second stage, several weeks after the onset of the rash, and include cranial nerve palsies, irritability, and memory and sleep disorders. Lyme disease is a clinical diagnosis, and laboratory tests should only be used to clarify diagnostic issues. The current standard for laboratory diagnosis includes a two-step approach using an initial immunoassay with a confirmatory Western blot. There are sensitivity and specificity problems with these laboratory tests, and meaningful results can usually be obtained if caution is used in their interpretation and if the clinical symptomatology, history, and examination are integrated with the laboratory results. Because treatment with antibiotics is both simple and curative, one must have a high index of suspicion for this entity in endemic areas when encountering white matter lesions similar to those of MS.

Toxic and Metabolic Demyelination

Central Pontine Myelinolysis is a disorder that results in characteristic demyelination of the central pons. This is most commonly seen in patients with electrolyte abnormalities, particularly involving hyponatremia, that are rapidly corrected giving rise to the term "osmotic demyelination syndrome" (17). This condition occurs most commonly in children and alcoholics with malnutrition. Occasionally, cases have been associated with diabetes, leukemia, and infections. Typical clinical presentation is that of a rapidly evolving corticospinal syndrome with quadriplegia and a "locked-in" state in which the patient is mute and unable to move, and occasionally comatose. Patients tend to be extremely ill and often have a very poor prognosis. MR characteristically demonstrates abnormal high signal on T2WI, corresponding to the regions of central pontine demyelination (Fig. 7.11). Additionally, extrapontine sites of involvement such as the basal ganglia and thalamus are not unusual.

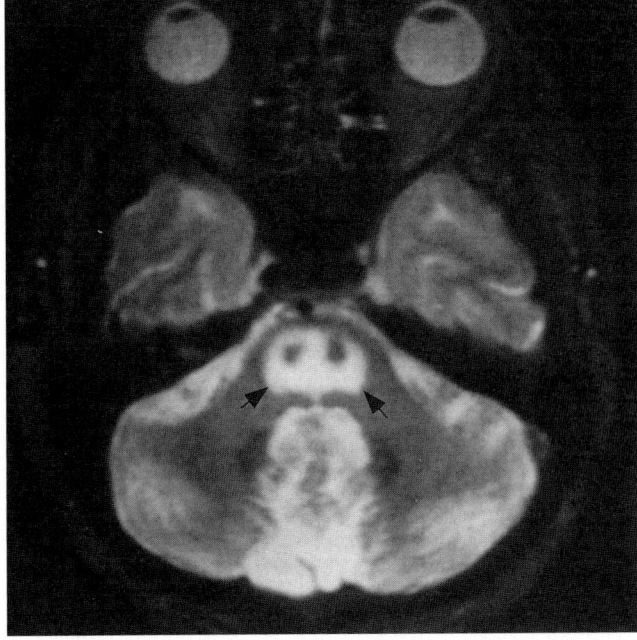

Figure 7.11. Central Pontine Myelinolysis. A 52-year-old alcoholic was admitted with a serum sodium of 110 mEq/mL. After rapid normalization of sodium, the patient became comatose. This T2WI demonstrates well-defined high signal within the central pons (*arrows*). Often, the central most corticospinal tracts remain preserved, giving rise to this characteristic pattern.

Marchiafava-Bignami Syndrome is a rare form of demyelination seen most frequently in alcoholics. This condition was first described in Italian red wine drinkers, but it has since been reported with other types of alcohol use as well as in nonalcoholics. The disease is characterized by demyelination involving the central fibers (medial zone) of the corpus callosum. Onset is

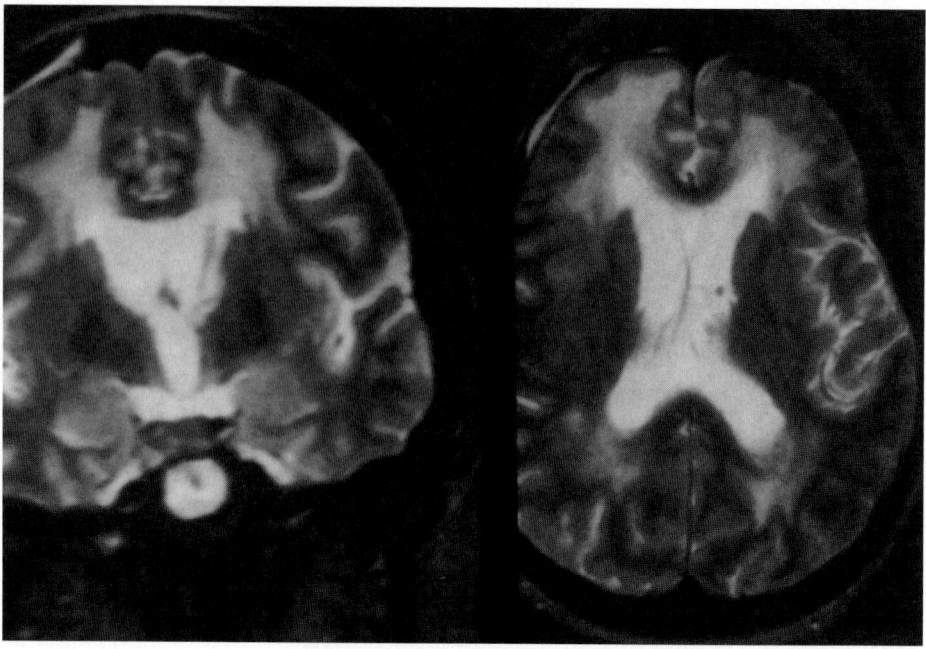

Figure 7.12. Radiation Leukoencephalitis. MR of a 57-year-old woman 1 year after whole brain radiation for metastatic breast carcinoma to the brain. T2-weighted coronal and axial images reveal confluent areas of high signal involving the periventricular white matter. The patient was entirely asymptomatic, returning for a routine follow-up examination.

usually insidious, with the most common symptom being nonspecific dementia. No adequate therapy exists, and the disease is usually slowly progressive, resulting in death.

Wernicke–Korsakoff Syndrome. Although pathologically indistinguishable, Wernicke and Korsakoff syndromes are clinically distinguishable, and both are the result of thiamine deficiency. In both cases, patients present with dementia. MR demonstrates lesions of the basal ganglia, thalamus, and brainstem with periaqueductal involvement. Additionally, atrophy of the mamillary bodies may be seen. In the acute phase, actual enhancement of the mamillary bodies may be identified. Except for the mamillary body involvement, these findings are very similar to Leigh's disease.

Radiation Leukoencephalitis. Radiation may result in damage to the white matter secondary to a radiation-induced vasculopathy. Radiation leukoencephalitis usually follows a cumulative dose in excess of 40 Gy delivered to the brain and occurs 6–9 months after treatment. Findings consist of areas of abnormal high signal on T2WI, typically involving confluent areas of white matter extending to involve the subcortical U fibers in the distribution of the irradiated brain (Fig. 7.12). Note that this represents an indirect effect of radiation on the brain and results from an arteritis (endothelial hypertrophy, medial hyalinization, and fibrosis) involving small arteries and arterioles.

Radiation Necrosis and Radiation Arteritis. In contrast to the rather benign nature of radiation leukoencephalitis, radiation necrosis and radiation arteritis are the major hazards related to CNS radiation. Both of these radiation effects are strongly dose related and are less commonly seen today because of greater fractionation of CNS radiation doses. Radiation necrosis may occur several weeks to years after irradiation and can be progressive and fatal. Radiation necrosis typically

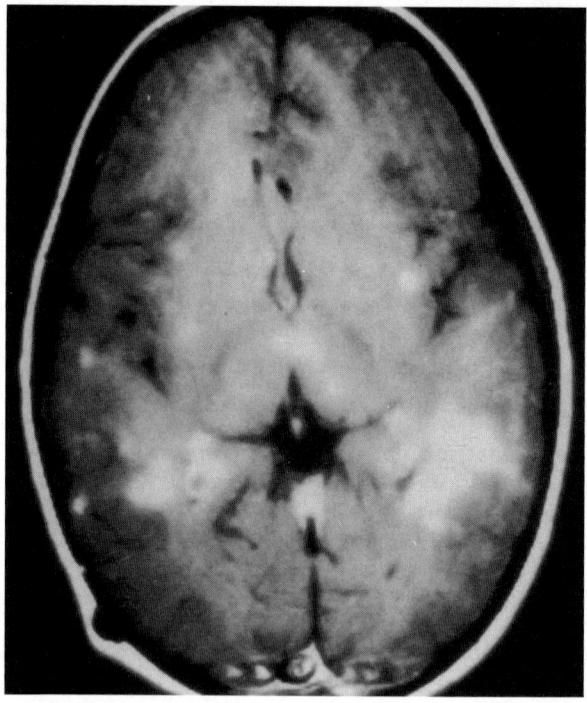

Figure 7.13. Radiation Necrosis. Radiation necrosis in a 7-year-old boy presenting 16 months after irradiation of a posterior fossa glioma. Post-Gd T1WI reveals multiple scattered foci of contrast enhancement. Review of radiation ports revealed that all lesions were confined to the port.

presents as an enhancing lesion, with mass effect and ring enhancement, or as multiple foci of enhancement, mimicking recurrent neoplasm (Fig. 7.13). Radiation may also induce telangiectasia within the radiation field, which may appear similar to cryptic vascular malformations (18).

Radiation necrosis is found most commonly in or near the irradiated tumor bed, but it sometimes is more remote from the tumor bed. It is theorized that the partially injured brain parenchyma within and adjacent to the tumor bed is more susceptible to radiation injury, thus accounting for the distribution of radiation necrosis. After resection of a brain neoplasm and subsequent radiation therapy, it can be very difficult to differentiate tumor recurrence from radiation-associated necrosis. In such cases, serial MR scans are required to evaluate for tumor recurrence and progression. The use of positron emission tomography (PET) has also been reported to be useful in distinguishing tumor recurrence from radiation necrosis, as the former will be active metabolically and the latter will not (Fig. 7.14).

Large vessels included within the radiation port may undergo radiation-induced endothelial hypertrophy, medial hyalinization, and fibrosis. The net result is a pro-

gressive vascular narrowing that may be obliterative in nature. This often involves the cavernous and supraclinoid portions of the carotid arteries in children who have undergone irradiation of the parasellar region for treatment of tumors, for example, craniopharyngiomas or optic and hypothalamic gliomas. The near complete obliteration of the supraclinoid carotid arteries results in cerebral and striatal ischemic changes. Occasionally, there may be a compensatory proliferation of lenticulostriate collaterals. When performing angiography, these collateral vessels present with a blush, which in Japan has been referred to as *Moya-Moya*, meaning, "puff of smoke." Moya-Moya disease classically refers to a supraclinoid obliterative arteriopathy, occurring primarily in children, which is idiopathic in nature.

When methotrexate chemotherapy (intrathecal or systemic) is administered in combination with CNS radiation, these agents may have a synergistic effect in caus-

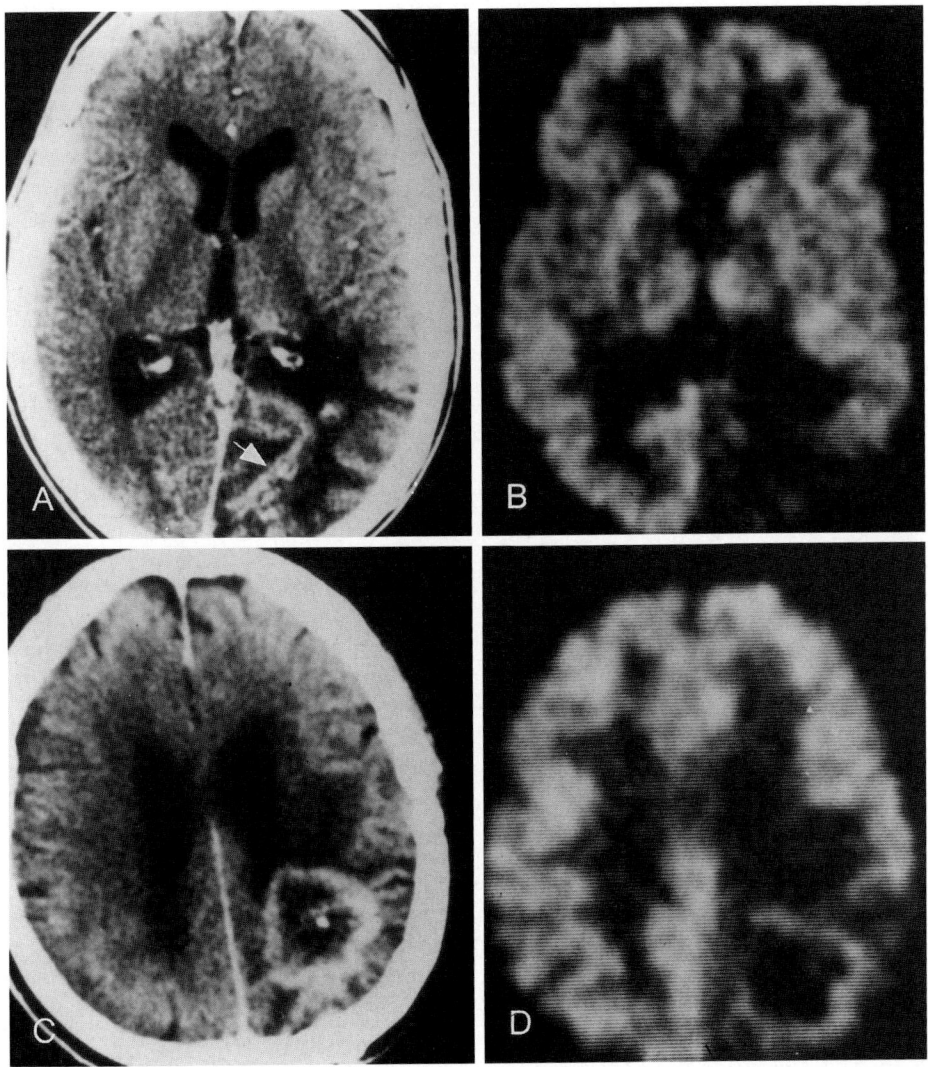

Figure 7.14. Tumor Recurrence. Contrast-enhanced CT and PET (¹⁸F-2-fluoro-2-d-deoxyglucose) scans. **A.** CT reveals a new linear area of enhancement (*arrow*) within the tumor bed 10 months following surgery and focal irradiation for a high-grade glioma. **B.** The PET demonstrates no significant activity in this area, suggesting that the enhancement represents radiation necrosis. **C.** A CT of a different patient 6 months after surgery and focal irradiation for a high-grade glioma reveals a focus of ring enhancement. **D.** The PET reveals increased metabolic activity in this region, suggesting recurrent tumor.

Table 7.2. Dysmyelinating Diseases

Disease	Head Size	Age of Onset (y)	White Matter Involvement	Gray Matter Involvement
Metachromatic leukodystrophy	Normal	Infantile form 1–2 years Juvenile form 5–7 years	Diffusely affected	None
Adrenoleukodystrophy	Normal	5–10	Symmetrical occipital and splenium of corpus callosum	None
Leigh's disease	Normal	<5	Focal areas of subcortical white matter	Basal ganglia and periaqueductal gray
Alexander's disease	Normal to large	≤1	Frontal	None
Canavan's disease	Normal to large	≤1	Diffusely affected	Vacuolization of cortical gray matter

ing marked white matter abnormalities. It is theorized that low-dose radiation alters the blood–brain barrier, allowing increased penetration of methotrexate to neurotoxic levels. This has been noted most frequently in children being treated for leukemia, and two specific conditions have been described. The first has been called **mineralizing microangiopathy**, which is seen in up to one third of these children. The result is diffuse destructive changes to the brain, characterized by symmetric corticomedullary junction and basal ganglia calcifications. There is also diffuse signal abnormality throughout the white matter. A more serious but less common complication of combined radiation and methotrexate therapy is called **necrotizing leukoencephalopathy.** This process results in widespread damage to the white matter, consisting of demyelination, necrosis, and gliosis. MR reveals large, diffuse, confluent areas of white matter signal abnormality with cortical sparing. Clinically, these children may have symptoms ranging from slight reduction in cognitive function to progressive dementia, seizures, hemiplegia, and coma.

DYSMYELINATING DISEASES

The disease processes that have been described up until this point are demyelinating, as they represent the destruction of normal myelin. In contrast, the dysmyelinating conditions, also referred to as leukodystrophies, are disorders where myelin is abnormally formed or cannot be maintained in its normal state because of an inherited enzymatic or metabolic disorder. Although most of these conditions are not treatable, establishing a diagnosis is valuable in providing a prognosis and enables parental genetic counseling. These conditions are characterized by the progressive destruction of myelin owing to the accumulation of various catabolites, depending on the specific enzyme deficiency. Children often present clinically with progressive mental and motor deterioration. Radiographically, these diseases present with diffuse white matter lesions that are very similar to one another; however, some distinguishing features do exist (Table 7.2). Factors that are helpful in differentiation include the age of onset, as well as the pattern of white matter involvement. Ultimately, biochemical and enzymatic analyses allow a specific diagnosis to be made. Dysmyelinating diseases are rather uncommon, and we focus on a few of the classic conditions.

Metachromatic leukodystrophy is the most common of the leukodystrophies. It is transmitted by an autosomal recessive pattern and is the result of a deficiency of the enzyme arylsulfatase A. The most common type is an infantile form, presenting at approximately 2 years of age with gait disorder and mental deterioration. There is steady disease progression, with death occurring within 5 years from the time of onset. MR demonstrates progressive symmetrical areas of nonspecific white matter involvement. Imaging findings are typically nonspecific.

Adrenal leukodystrophy is a sex-linked recessive condition and occurs only in boys. Typical age of onset is between 5 and 10 years. As the name implies, these patients often have symptoms related to the adrenal gland, such as adrenal insufficiency or abnormal skin pigmentation. Adrenal leukodystrophy has a striking predilection for the visual and auditory pathways, presenting with symmetrical involvement of the periatrial white matter with extension into the splenium of the corpus callosum (Fig. 7.15). The predilection for periatrial involvement results in early extension to the medial and lateral geniculate nuclei, which represent relays for the auditory and visual pathways, respectively. This accounts for the early presentation of visual and auditory symptomatology in these children.

Leigh's Disease, also called necrotizing encephalomyelopathy, commonly manifests in infancy or childhood (usually younger than 5 years). It has histopathologic findings similar to Wernicke's encephalopathy, hence the suspicion that it is related to an inborn defect in thiamine metabolism. Clinical findings are extremely variable and often nonspecific. Symmetrical focal necrotic lesions are found in the basal ganglia and thalamus as well as in the subcortical white matter (Fig. 7.16). Lesions may also extend into the midbrain, medulla, and posterior columns of the spinal cord. A characteristic finding is involvement of the periaqueductal gray matter. In contrast to Wernicke–Korsakoff syndrome, there is sparing of the mamillary bodies.

Alexander's and Canavan's Diseases are the rarest of the leukodystrophies and may appear as early as the first few weeks of life. Patients often have an enlarged brain and have macrocephaly on examination. Typically, these patients present with delayed developmental milestones. In Alexander's disease, white matter lesions often begin in the frontal white matter and progress posteriorly (Fig. 7.17).

CEREBROSPINAL FLUID DYNAMICS

In patients with acute hydrocephalus, transependymal flow of CSF may mimic periventricular white matter disease. CSF is produced predominately by the choroid plexus of the lateral, third, and fourth ventricles. CSF flows from the lateral ventricles into the third ventricle through the foramina of Monro and then by way of the cerebral aqueduct into the fourth ventricle. The CSF leaves the ventricular system via the lateral and medial fourth ventricular foramina, foramen of Luschka and Magendie, respectively. CSF then travels through the basilar cisterns and over the surfaces of the cerebral hemispheres. The principal site of absorption is into the venous circulation through the arachnoid villi, which project into the dural sinuses, primarily the superior sagittal sinus. Although the principal routes of CSF production and absorption are as just outlined, a significant amount of CSF may be both produced and reabsorbed via the ependymal lining of the ventricles. This transependymal flow of CSF can become an important means of CSF reabsorption during ventricular obstruction.

Hydrocephalus is caused by an obstruction of the CSF circulatory pathway and is classified into two principal types, noncommunicating and communicating. **Noncommunicating hydrocephalus** refers to an ob-

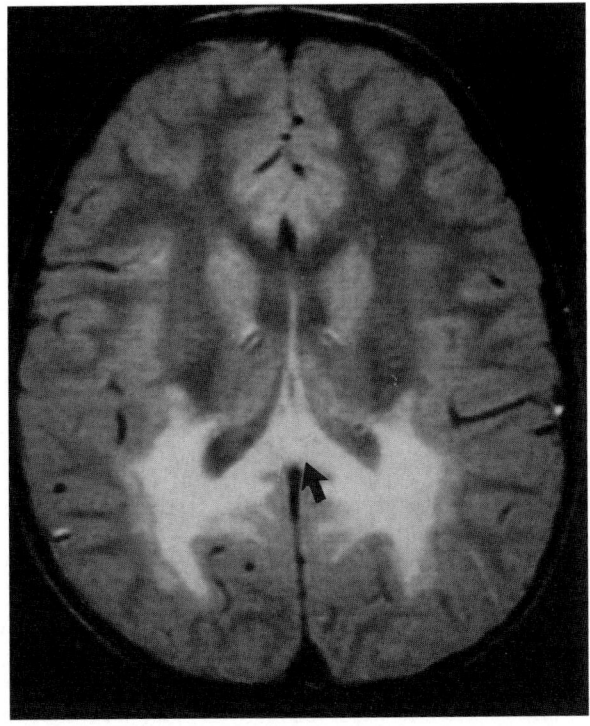

Figure 7.15. Adrenal Leukodystrophy. Adrenal leukodystrophy in a 6-year-old boy who presented with gradual gait disturbance and adrenal insufficiency. Axial T2WI reveals high signal within the periatrial and occipital white matter extending into the splenium of the corpus callosum (*arrow*).

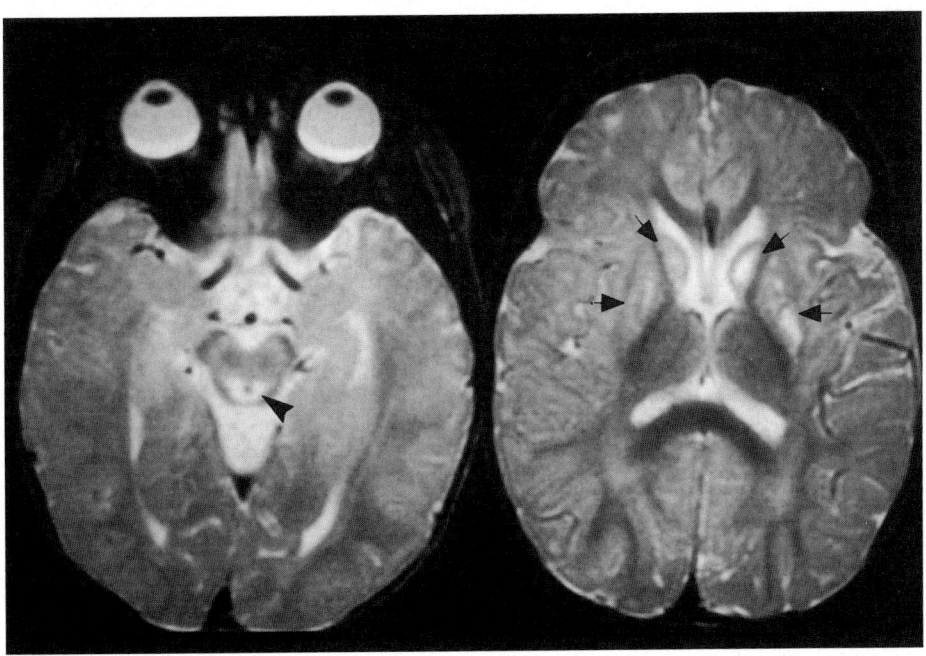

Figure 7.16. Leigh's Disease. Leigh's disease in a 2-year-old patient presenting with seizures. Axial T2WI demonstrates high signal in the caudate nuclei and in the putamina (*arrows*). The involvement of the periaqueductal gray matter (*arrowhead*) is suggestive of Leigh's disease.

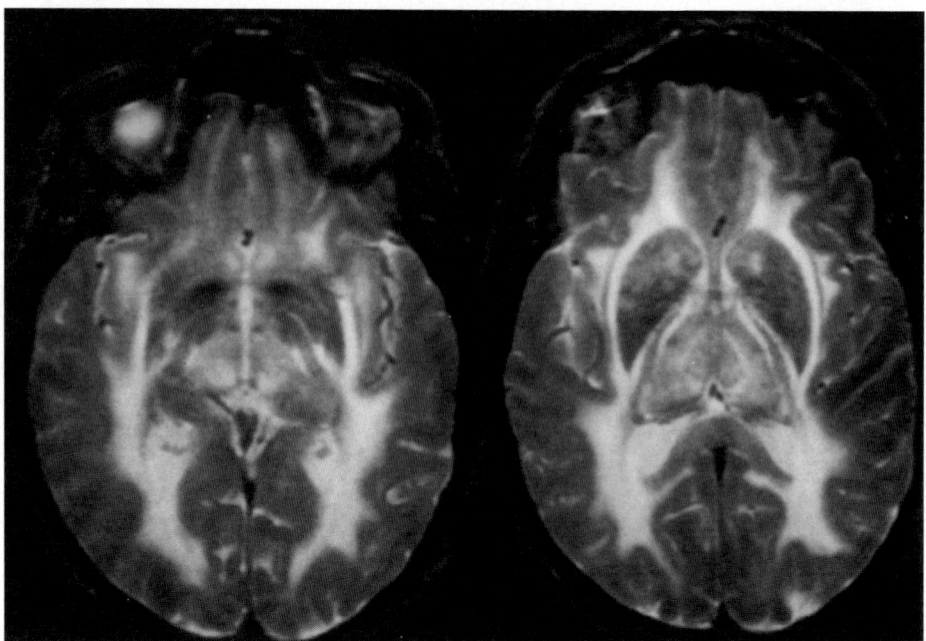

Figure 7.17. Alexander's Disease. A 16-month-old child presented with progressive spastic quadriparesis and macrocephaly. Axial T2WI reveal diffuse high signal extending throughout the deep cerebral white matter as well as both the internal and external capsules.

struction occurring within the ventricular system that prevents CSF from exiting the ventricles. In contrast, with **communicating hydrocephalus,** the level of obstruction is beyond the ventricular system, being located within the subarachnoid space. CSF is able to exit the ventricular system but fails to undergo normal resorption by the arachnoid villi. In theory, with communicating hydrocephalus most of the ventricular system is enlarged, whereas with noncommunicating hydrocephalus, dilation occurs up to the point of obstruction. The fourth ventricle often does not dilate because of the relatively confined nature of the posterior fossa. Communicating hydrocephalus will commonly demonstrate supratentorial ventriculomegaly with a normal appearing fourth ventricle. Although dilation of the fourth ventricle is suggestive of communicating hydrocephalus, it is not a reliable sign because obstruction at the outlet foramina of the fourth ventricle (Luschka and Magendie) may give a similar appearance.

In assessing for the presence of hydrocephalus, specific attention should be directed to the third ventricle and the temporal ventricular horns. Convex bowing of the lateral walls and inferior recesses of the third ventricle is characteristic for hydrocephalus (Fig. 7.18). As with fourth ventricular enlargement, however, this finding is seldom present. A far more sensitive indicator of hydrocephalus is enlargement of the temporal horns. Not uncommonly, the temporal horns will demonstrate enlargement, even before lateral ventricular involvement is evident. Bowing and stretching of the corpus callosum, easily detected on the sagittal images, are an additional finding that is suggestive of hydrocephalus.

Ex-Vacuo Ventriculomegaly. Distinction must be made between hydrocephalus and ex-vacuo ventriculomegaly. The latter represents an enlarged ventricular system that is simply the result of parenchymal atrophy. With atrophy, the loss of brain matter results in prominence of all CSF spaces, both cerebral sulci as well as ventricles. In contrast, with hydrocephalus the ventricles are enlarged out of proportion to the sulci. The third ventricle and temporal ventricular horns are particularly helpful in making this distinction. Both of these ventricular spaces are surrounded by tissue that is not typically subject to significant atrophy. The third ventricle is surrounded by the thalamus (gray matter), and there is a relative paucity of white matter within the temporal lobes. This is in contrast to the large amount of white matter surrounding the lateral ventricles, which may atrophy. Enlargement of the third ventricle with bowing of its lateral and inferior recesses, as well as temporal horn enlargement, suggests hydrocephalus.

Subarachnoid hemorrhage and meningitis are the most frequent causes of hydrocephalus and may result in either communicating or noncommunicating hydrocephalus, with obstruction at any level of the ventricular system, basilar cisterns, or at the arachnoid villi. The obstruction is because of adhesions and inflammation, and no obstructing mass is typically detected. Noncommunicating hydrocephalus can be the result of either an acquired or a congenital obstructive process. Benign congenital webs may form across the cerebral aqueduct, resulting in aqueductal stenosis. Additionally, the Chiari and Dandy-Walker malformations are believed to represent adhesions occurring during CNS development, at the outlet foramina of the fourth ventricle and posterior fossa. A variety of neoplasms may result in obstructive hydrocephalus, often in very characteristic locations. Colloid cysts typically block the anterior third ventricle; pineal tumors and tectal gliomas obstruct the aqueduct; and ependymomas and medulloblastomas interrupt CSF flow at the level of the fourth ventricle. Whenever hydrocephalus is detected, it is important to inspect the ventricles for an obstructing mass. A location that should be specifically evaluated is the cerebral aqueduct. On routine axial and sagittal images, a normal pulsatile flow void should be detected, otherwise the diagnosis of aqueductal stenosis should be considered.

The duration of hydrocephalus affects the imaging findings. In acute hydrocephalus, there is insufficient time for compensatory mechanisms, and a striking amount of transependymal CSF flow is noted. This results in a dramatic accumulation of high signal in the periventricular white matter on T2WI. In chronic forms of hydrocephalus, compensatory mechanisms of CNS production and resorption have occurred and the degree of transependymal flow is minimal (Fig. 7.19).

NEURODEGENERATIVE DISORDERS

Neurodegenerative disorders frequently have no known cause and result in progressive neurologic deterioration that is faster than expected given the patient's age.

Alzheimer's Disease is the most common neurodegenerative disease and the commonest cause of dementia (19). Neuroimaging studies demonstrate diffuse atrophy, which is the result of neuronal loss. Although overlap does exist with normal degrees of age-related atrophy, certain regions tend to be more severely affected with Alzheimer's disease (20). Specifically, the hippocampal formation and entire temporal lobes are consistently and heavily involved; therefore, marked enlargement of the temporal horns, suprasellar cisterns, and sylvian fissures may be useful in discriminating Alzheimer's disease from normal aging.

Parkinsonism is the most common basal ganglia disorder and one of the leading causes of neurologic disability in individuals older than age 60. This disease is characterized clinically by tremor, muscular rigidity, and loss of postural reflexes. Parkinsonism results from a deficiency of the neurotransmitter dopamine caused by dysfunction of the dopaminergic neuronal system, specifically the pars compacta of the substantia nigra. A variety of parkinsonian syndromes exist including Parkinson's disease, progressive supranuclear palsy, and striatonigral degeneration. Idiopathic Parkinson's disease is referred to as paralysis agitans and affects 2–3% of the population some time during their life. MR occasionally may reveal thinning of the pars compacta. The substantia nigra is made of the pars compacta (high-signal intensity band on T2WI) posteriorly, which is sandwiched between the pars reticularis anteriorly and the red nuclei posteriorly. With thinning of the pars compacta, the high-signal intensity band between the pars reticularis and the red nuclei is lost.

Normal Pressure Hydrocephalus (NPH) is a chronic, low-level form of hydrocephalus. The classic clinical triad is dementia, gait disturbance, and urinary incontinence. In this condition, the CSF pressure is within normal limits, but a slight gradient exists between the ventricular system and the subarachnoid space because of an incomplete subarachnoid CSF block. This most commonly results from a previous subarachnoid hemorrhage or meningeal infection. The result is diffuse ventriculomegaly, which is out of proportion to the degree of sulcal prominence. Differentiating mild hydrocephalus from atrophic ventriculomegaly can be very difficult. Studies (21) suggest that MR CSF velocity and stroke volume calculations can be used to predict which patients may have favorable response to ventriculoperi-

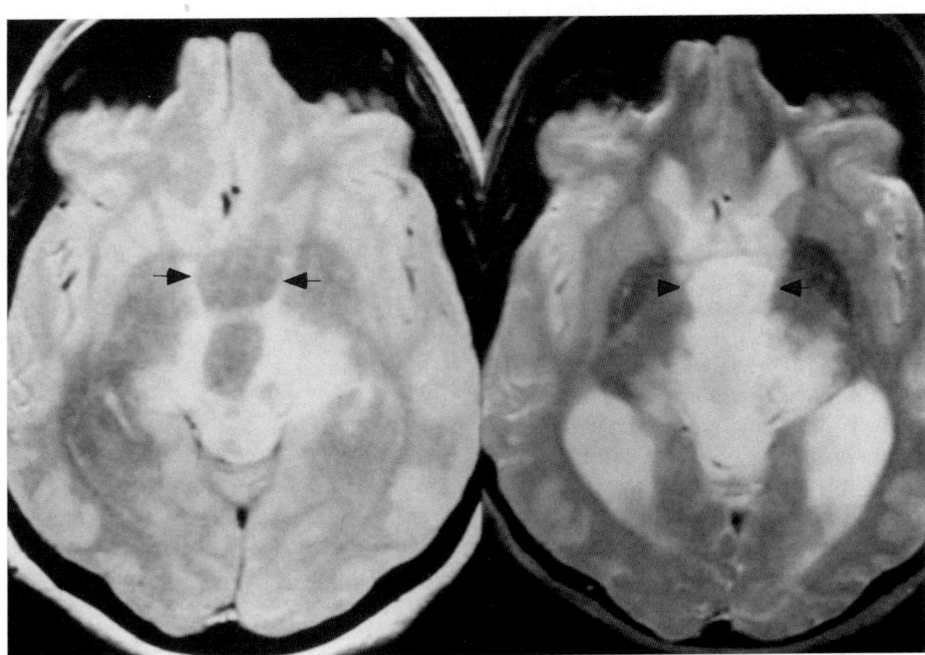

Figure 7.18. Hydrocephalus. Axial first and second echo T2WI in a 67-year-old patient with tuberculous meningitis. The ventricles clearly are dilated out of proportion to the cerebral sulci. This finding, in addition to the bowing of the inferior third ventricle recesses (*arrows*), is characteristic for hydrocephalus.

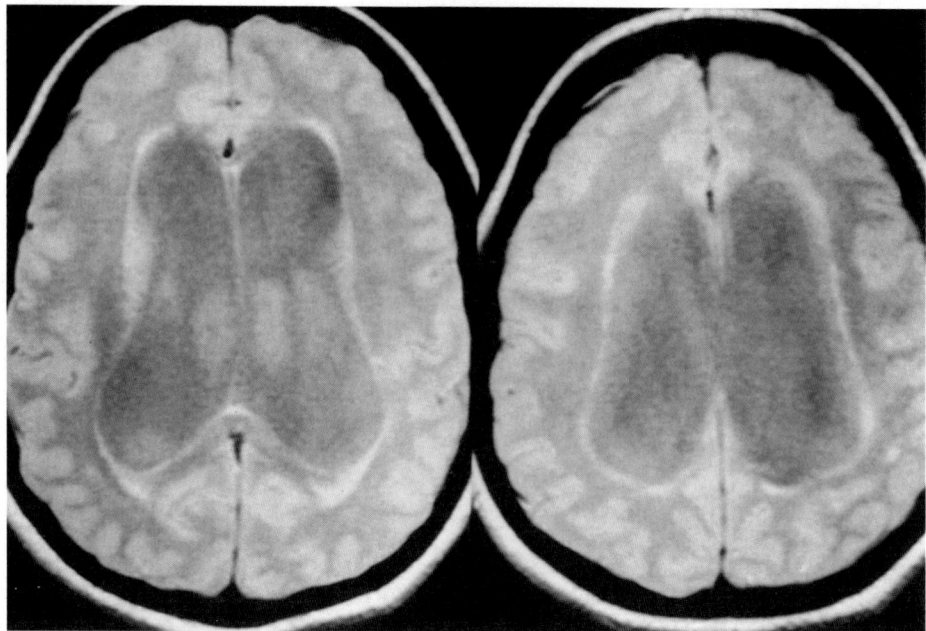

Figure 7.19. Chronic Hydrocephalus. Chronic hydrocephalus in a 40-year-old patient after traumatic subarachnoid hemorrhage. Only minimal periventricular transependymal CSF flow is identified on the axial proton-density images, reflecting the chronic nature of this pro-cess. As opposed to acute hydrocephalus, in which transependymal flow is common, sufficient time has elapsed for compensatory methods of CSF resorption to take place.

toneal shunting. In addition to cross-sectional studies, radioisotope studies may be of value. The classic findings on radioisotope cisternogram are early entry of the radiopharmaceutical into the lateral ventricles, with persistence at 24 and 48 hours, and considerable delay in the ascent to the parasagittal region. Differentiating normal pressure hydrocephalus from atrophic ventriculomegaly can be very difficult, and unfortunately, no imaging study is definitive in making this diagnosis. NPH is not a radiographic diagnosis, and close correlation of clinical and imaging findings is required in establishing the diagnosis. The definitive diagnosis of NPH is made on demonstrating clinical improvement following ventricular shunting.

The following are degenerative diseases of the extrapyramidal nuclei.

Huntington's Disease is a progressive hereditary disorder that appears in the fourth and fifth decades of life. This disease is characterized by a movement disorder (typically choreoathetosis), dementia, and emotional disturbance. Huntington's disease is inherited in an autosomal dominant pattern with complete penetrance. Although neuroimaging studies demonstrate diffuse cortical atrophy, the caudate nucleus and putamen are most severely affected. The caudate atrophy results in characteristic enlargement of the frontal horns, which take on a heart-shape configuration.

Wilson's Disease, also known as hepatolenticular degeneration, is an inborn error of copper metabolism that is associated with hepatic cirrhosis and degenerative changes of the basal ganglia. A deficiency of ceruloplasmin (serum transport protein of copper) results in deposition of toxic levels of copper in various organs. Patients present with varied neurologic and psychiatric findings including dystonia, tremor, and rigidity. The Kayser–Fleischer ring, an intracorneal deposit of copper, is virtually diagnostic of the disease when present (75% of cases). MR findings include diffuse atrophy with signal abnormalities involving the deep gray matter nuclei and deep white matter.

Besides these neurodegenerative diseases, abnormalities of the basal ganglia can have a wide range of causes. Toxins such as carbon monoxide or methanol poisoning may result in signal abnormalities of the basal ganglia, characteristically the globus pallidus. MR demonstrates low signal on T1WI and high signal on the T2WI. T1-shortening (high signal on T1WI) has been described within the basal ganglia and brainstem associated with hepatic dysfunction, such as hepatic encephalopathy as well as hyperalimentation. The cause of these findings has not been fully determined. Occasionally, calcification of the basal ganglia may also appear as high signal on the T1WI. This is the result of the hydration layer effect, where water molecules that are adjacent to the calcification have reduced relaxation times. This same effect causes T1 shortening with proteinaceous fluids. As a result, any condition that results in basal ganglia calcifications may demonstrate T1-shortening within the basal ganglia.

References

1. Scott TF. Diseases that mimic multiple sclerosis. Postgrad Med 1991;89:187–191.
2. Rolak LA. The diagnosis of multiple sclerosis. Neurol Clin 1996;14:27–43.
3. Bastianello S, Bozzao A, Paolillo A, et al. Fast spin-echo and fast fluid-attenuated inversion-recovery versus conventional

spin-echo sequences for MR quantification of multiple sclerosis lesions. AJNR Am J Neuroradiol 1997;18:699–704.

4. Dagher AP, Smirniotopoulos J. Tumefactive demyelinating lesions. Neuroradiology 1996;38:560–565.

5. Hittmair K, Mallek R, Prayer D, et al. Spinal cord lesions in patients with multiple sclerosis: comparison of MR pulse sequences. AJNR Am J Neuroradiol 1996;17:1555–1565.

6. Longstreth WT Jr, Manolio TA, Arnold A, et al. Clinical correlates of white matter findings on cranial magnetic resonance imaging of 3301 elderly people. The Cardiovascular Health Study. Stroke 1996;27:1274–1282.

7. Scheltens P, Barkhof F, Leys D, et al. Histopathologic correlates of white matter changes on MRI in Alzheimer's disease and normal aging. Neurology 1995;45:883–888.

8. Schmidt R, Hayn M, Fazekas F, et al. Magnetic resonance imaging white matter hyperintensities in clinically normal elderly individuals. Correlations with plasma concentrations of naturally occurring antioxidants. Stroke 1996;27:2043–2047.

9. Gean AD, Weinstein MA. New MR imaging findings in multiple sclerosis. Radiology 1991;179:591–594.

10. Sze G, De Armond SJ, Brant–Zawadzki M, et al. Foci of MRI signal (pseudo lesions) anterior to the frontal horns: histologic correlations of a normal finding. AJR Am J Roentgenol 1986;147:331–337.

11. Ogawa T, Okudera T, Fukasawa H, et al. Unusual widening of Virchow-Robin spaces: MR appearance. AJNR Am J Neuroradiol 1995;16:1238–1242.

12. Sarrazin JL, Soulie D, Derosier C, et al. MRI aspects of progressive multifocal leukoencephalopathy. J Neuroradiol 1995;22:172–179.

13. Walot I, Miller BL, Chang L, Mehringer CM. Neuroimaging findings in patients with AIDS. Clin Infect Dis 1996;22:906–919.

14. Lee WT, Wang PJ, Liu HM, et al. Acute disseminated encephalomyelitis in children: clinical, neuroimaging and neurophysiologic studies. Acta Paediatr Sin 1996;37:197–203.

15. Mader I, Stock KW, Ettlin T, Probst A. Acute disseminated encephalomyelitis: MR and CT features. AJNR Am J Neuroradiol 1996;17:104–109.

16. Oksi J, Kalimo H, Marttila RJ, et al. Inflammatory brain changes in Lyme borreliosis. A report on three patients and review of literature. Brain 1996;119:2143–2154.

17. Laubenberger J, Schneider B, Ansorge O, et al. Central pontine myelinolysis: clinical presentation and radiologic findings. Eur Radiol 1996;6:177–183.

18. Gaensler EH, Dillon WP, Edwards MS, et al. Radiation-induced telangiectasia in the brain simulates cryptic vascular malformations at MR imaging. Radiology 1994;193:629–636.

19. Xanthakos S, Krishnan KR, Kim DM, Charles HC. Magnetic resonance imaging of Alzheimer's disease. Prog Neuropsychopharmacol Biol Psychiatry 1996;20:597–626.

20. Hauser RA, Olanow CW. Magnetic resonance imaging of neurodegenerative diseases. J Neuroimaging 1994;4:146–158.

21. Bradley WG Jr, Scalzo D, Queralt J, et al. Normal-pressure hydrocephalus: evaluation with cerebrospinal fluid flow measurements at MR imaging. Radiology 1996;198:523–529.

8

Pediatric Neuroimaging

Todd E. Lempert

Specific areas of pediatric neuroimaging are sufficiently different from adult neuroimaging to warrant a separate discussion in this chapter. These areas are normal patterns of myelination, hypoxic ischemic brain injury, congenital lesions, migration anomalies, and phakomatoses (neurocutaneous syndromes).

MR has established itself as the procedure of choice for pediatric neuroimaging although specific situations in which US and CT remain advantageous will be described.

Sedation is usually required for children younger than 6 years old. Pediatric sedation protocols should be performed in conjunction with pulse oximetry monitoring at a minimum. A pediatric-equipped crash cart should be available along with personnel skilled in pediatric sedation techniques. Pediatric Advanced Life Support Training, a course offered by the American Heart Association, provides a useful review for radiologists.

NORMAL PATTERNS OF MYELINATION

Any discussion of pediatric neuroimaging must begin with normal myelination as a frame of reference. T1-weighted and T2-weighted sequences allow observation of the myelination process. T1WI provide a detailed view of actively myelinating structures in the first 8 months of life. Areas that become myelinated stand out as high signal on T1WI against a background of low signal intensity, unmyelinated white matter. This is because the myelin sheath (a lipid) is hydrophobic; therefore, myelinated white matter has a decreased amount of water, the source of mobile hydrogen protons, which form the basis of the MR signal. An oversimplified memory aid is to remember that myelinated white matter parallels the signal intensity of fat on T1-weighted and T2-weighted sequences. Heavily weighted T2-images (long TR/TE = 3000/120) are recommended for patients 0–12 months old. The water content of the infant brain is high, and heavily weighted T2 images are needed to discriminate between many brain structures that have similar long T2 relaxation times. The myelination landmarks given in Table 8.1 are based on sequences performed at 1.5 tesla. Other field strength magnets may show differing patterns of myelination with the patients age.

At birth, normal myelination by MR usually involves the dorsal lentiform nucleus, lateral geniculate nucleus, dorsal brainstem, cerebellar peduncles, ventrolateral thalamus, posterior limb of the internal capsule, and corticospinal tract extending into the perirolandic (precentral and postcentral) white matter (Fig. 8.1).

T1WI are useful for assessing myelination in patients 8 months or younger; thereafter, the T2WI become more important. Myelination usually proceeds from dorsal to ventral, from caudad to cephalad, and from central to peripheral.

Evaluation of every pediatric brain image obtained by MR should begin with an assessment of myelin development. This important step helps determine the presence or absence of myelination delay and provides a framework for interpretation of suspected neuropathology.

The anterior limb of the internal capsule demonstrates high signal intensity on T1WI by 3 months (Fig. 8.2). The corpus callosum provides the next set of landmarks with the splenium becoming high signal on T1WI by 4 months and the genu by 6 months. At 6 months the splenium becomes low signal intensity on T2WI, but the unmyelinated peripheral white matter remains high signal (Fig. 8.3). With growth, the deep white matter gradually assumes the adult low signal intensity on T2WI, with some high signal intensity persisting in the terminal myelination zones on T2WI (Figs. 8.4, 8.5).

Delayed Myelination. The differential diagnosis of delayed myelination includes a wide variety of disorders, including in utero insult (hypoxic ischemia or infection), metabolic/nutritional disorders, and leukodystrophy (Pelizaeus-Merzbacher disease). Delayed myelination also exhibits excellent correlation with clinical measures of developmental delay.

In utero insults cause delayed myelination in both premature and term neonates. Look for other findings of hypoxic ischemic injury (HII) in conjunction with myelination delay. Nutritional deficiencies owing to diet or malabsorption syndromes cause myelination delay because of an inadequate supply of myelin precursors. Similarly, inborn errors of metabolism (amino and organic acidopathies) cause delayed myelination.

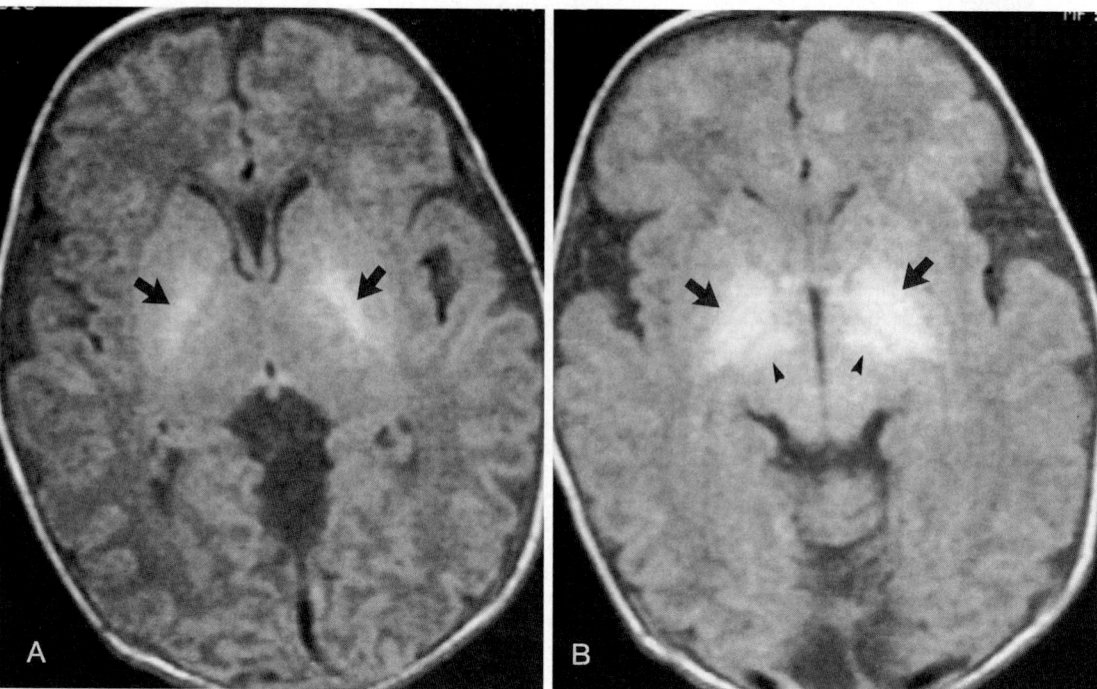

Figure 8.1. Normal Myelination—Newborn. T1WI of a newborn infant. **A.** The level of the internal capsule shows normal high signal intensity of the posterior limb of the internal capsule (*arrows*). Note the absence of high signal intensity in the anterior limb. **B.** At a slightly lower level, the ventral lateral thalamus (*arrowheads*) and lentiform-nuclei (*arrows*) are high signal intensity, consistent with myelination in these areas present at birth.

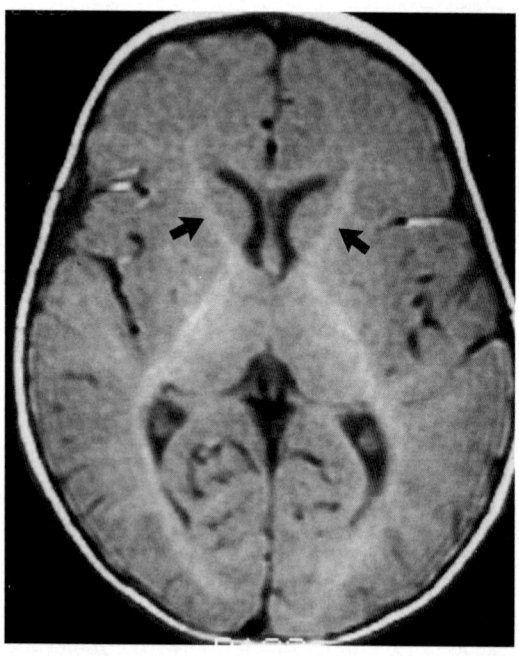

Figure 8.2. Normal Myelination—3 Months. Axial T1WI of a 3-month-old infant. The level of the internal capsule shows extension of high signal into the anterior limb of the internal capsule, reflecting a progressive myelination of this region (*arrows*).

Table 8.1. Myelination Landmarks by Age

Age (months)	Location/Appearance
Newborn	Dorsal brainstem, ventrolateral thalamus, lentiform nucleus, central corticospinal tracts: high signal, T1WI
	Posterior limb internal capsule posterior portion: low signal, T2WI
3	Anterior limb internal capsule: high signal, T1WI
	Cerebellar white matter: high signal, T1WI
4	Splenium of corpus callosum: high signal, T1WI
	Centrum semiovale: high signal, T1WI
6	Genu of corpus callosum: high signal, T1WI
	Splenium of corpus callosum: low signal, T2WI
8	Subcortical white matter: high signal, T1WI
	Genu: low signal, T2WI
11	Anterior limb internal capsule: low signal, T2WI
14	Occipital white matter: low signal, T2WI
16	Frontal white matter, low signal, T2WI
18	Adult appearance except for terminal myelination zones periatrial, adjacent to frontal horns

Pelizaeus-Merzbacher Disease is a rare X-linked leukodystrophy that demonstrates an arrest of myelin development usually in the neonatal period. It can mimic other causes of delayed myelination because it shows lack of myelin formation only, not myelin formation followed by destruction (typical of many other leukodystrophies). A follow-up scan can be helpful in detecting a pattern of arrested myelination such as Pelizaeus-Merzbacher disease.

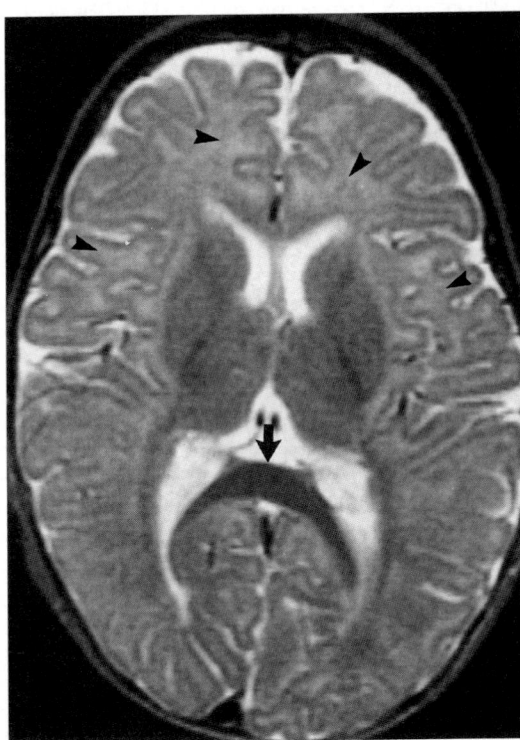

Figure 8.3. Normal Myelination—6 Months. Axial T2WI of a 6-month-old infant at the level of the corpus callosum. The splenium of the corpus callosum is low signal intensity on T2WI (*arrow*), but the unmyelinated deep and superficial cerebral white matter is high signal intensity (*arrowheads*).

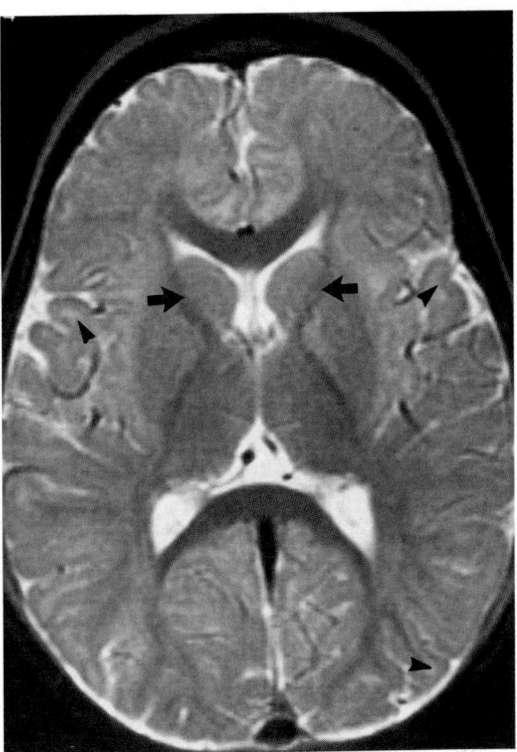

Figure 8.4. Normal Myelination—11 Months. Axial T2WI of an 11-month-old infant at the level of the atria of the lateral ventricles. Note that the anterior limb of the internal capsule is now low signal on T2WI (*arrows*). There has been progressive myelination of central white matter (low signal) but the subcortical white matter (*arrowheads*) is still unmyelinated and high signal intensity.

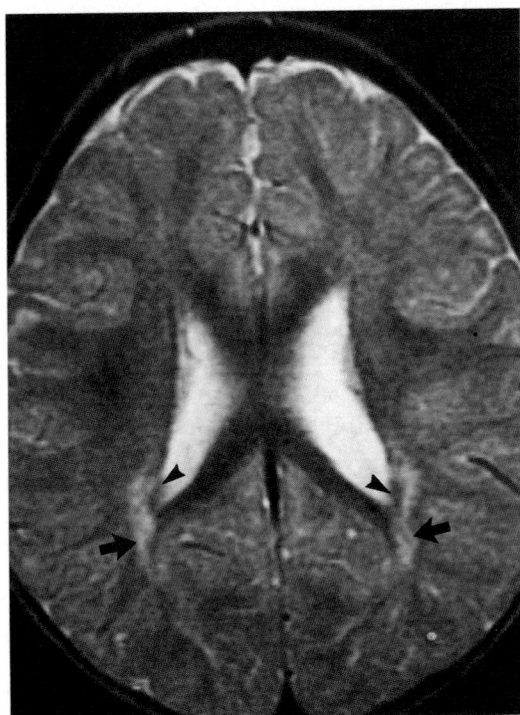

Figure 8.5. Normal Myelination—18 Months. Axial T2WI of a normal 18-month-old infant. The process of normal myelination is essentially complete except for terminal myelination zones, which show persistent high signal (*arrows*) in the periatrial region. A thin hypointense band of white matter separates the terminal myelination zone from the atrial margin (*arrowheads*).

"Developmental delay" is a nonspecific term, used because of the large percentage of cases of myelination delay with no known cause that are related to a clinical diagnosis of developmental retardation (developmental function < 80% of chronologic age).

In summary, if a particular MR scan shows myelination delay (corrected for any prematurity), a careful search for additional clues may yield a diagnosis.

HYPOXIC ISCHEMIC BRAIN INJURY

Unfortunately, hypoxic ischemic brain injury (HII) is very common in the pediatric population, and as neonatology continues to advance, more cases will be seen because ischemic brain injury is related to prematurity and its complications. Knowledge of brain development and the reproducible patterns of brain damage can help answer questions about the severity of the insult and the timing of the injury. Patterns of brain injury can be divided into first and second trimester, late third trimester and perinatal, and postnatal. These patterns are summarized in Table 8.2.

The first and second trimesters of embryonic growth are characterized by rapid development of key brain structures. Hypoxic ischemic insults to the developing brain at this time are often severe and may arrest or alter further brain development. HII can be divided into focal HII and diffuse HII. Focal HII causes an arrest/alter-

Table 8.2. Imaging of Hypoxic Ischemic Brain Injury

Time	Deep Gray	Cortex	Other
1st Trimester	Spared	Cortical dysplasias Hydranencephaly	
<26 Weeks	Spared	Spared	Periatrial Injury No gliosis Ex vacuo enlargement
>28 Weeks	Spared	Spared	Periatrial gliosis: high signal, T2W1
Term	Spared	Watershed infarcts Ulegyria	Variable deep, superficial white matter gliosis and atrophy Myelination delay Injury to hippocampus, pons

ation in brain development manifested as focal cell migration disorders. Diffuse HII leads to generalized damage as seen in hydranecephaly and cortical dysplasias.

Hydraencephaly represents ischemic infarction of both cerebral hemispheres and is believed to be caused by early occlusion of both carotid arteries, or possibly a severe inutero infection. The pattern of destruction is characterized by little or no supratentorial brain tissue (Fig. 8.6). Another pattern that mimics this appearance is early severe hydrocephalus although in cases of hydrocephalus, a thin rind of cortical gray matter is usually evident. In hydraencephaly, on the other hand, there is usually nearly complete infarction of all supratentorial cerebral tissues in the vascular distribution of the carotid arteries with preservation of the thalami and cerebellum.

HII is a common type of insult (along with in utero infection) that causes disorders of the neuronal migration and cortical dysplasias. This is because any severe insult to the developing brain can lead to an arrest of normal neuronal migration. Disorders of neuronal migration are described in "Migration Anomalies."

Injuries in the second and third trimester correlate with the location of arterial border zones, which are areas uniquely sensitive to watershed infarction. These border zones usually move centrifugally as the brain develops. The zones start in the immediate periventricular region and move outward into more peripheral white matter and cortical gray matter. Hence, injuries to second-trimester and third-trimester fetuses are characterized by ischemic infarction in the periarterial and, less commonly, periventricular border zones. These areas of peritrigonal white matter undergo neuronal loss, which leads to atrophy. The resulting atrial margin is often crenulated where necrotic periventricular white matter cysts have been incorporated. The loss of white matter leads to ex vacuo enlargement of the atria. Fetuses younger than 26 weeks do not exhibit a significant response to gliosis. Therefore, HII to fetuses younger than 26 weeks causes periventricular (periatrial) white matter thinning and atrial enlargement (Fig. 8.7).

Periventricular Leukomalacia. After 26 weeks, the brain responds to HII by gliosis in the periatrial region. Damage to the periventricular region is termed "periventricular leukomalacia." This is best seen on proton-density–weighted images. Periventricular leukomalacia can be differentiated from the normal peritrigonal terminal myelination zones by noting an extension of high signal on T2WI to the ventricular margin. This is owing to a loss of the normal thin myelinated white matter roof (tapetum) of the atrium of the lateral ventricle. Periatrial white matter thinning and atrial enlargement are also evident (Fig. 8.8).

In the late third trimester and perinatal period, continuing centrifugal extension of the arterial border zones sensitive to watershed infarction occurs. Infants born at term who sustain insults during this period will demonstrate infarcts in the peripheral white matter and cortex (Fig. 8.9). Watershed infarction occurs at border zone regions between arterial distributions of major cerebral vessels.

The important border zones are a) in the parasagittal cerebrum, between anterior and middle cerebral arteries, which leads to an appearance of bilateral infarcts in the paramedian cortex and subsequent gliosis of subcortical white matter, and b) the posterior convexity, between the anterior, middle, and posterior cerebral arteries. HII shows bilateral parieto-occipital watershed infarcts. The medial surface between the anterior and posterior cerebral arteries is another important zone. Other brain areas affected by HII include the mesial temporal lobes (hippocampus). The temporal lobe infarcts may evolve to cause ex vacuo enlargement of the temporal horn of the lateral ventricle and/or mesial temporal sclerosis. Mesial temporal sclerosis is a condition characterized by neuronal loss and gliosis confined to the hippocampus, leading to partial complex seizures. A remodeling of subcortical infarcts occurring in the depths of sulci that spare the overlying gyri form a characteristic pattern of mushroom-shaped gyri called ulegyria.

The brainstem may be affected with selective neuronal loss of cranial nerve nuclei or neurons of the pons (pontosubicular necrosis). The Purkinje cells of the cerebellum also are sensitive to HII.

Term infants with HII can also demonstrate gliosis of affected periventricular white matter, ex vacuo ventricular enlargement, and resulting apposition of sulci to the ventricular surface because of white matter loss, a pattern seen in infants with periventricular leukomalacia. Associated sequelae of HII include delayed myelination and thinning of large white matter tracts such as the corpus callosum.

Remember, term infants will primarily show peripheral damage corresponding to peripheral border zones. Periatrial damage, white matter loss, and delayed myelination are associated findings. Thus, the patterns of in utero HII can be correlated with gestational age (Table 8.2).

Hypoxic Ischemic Injury and the Premature Infant

Premature infants present special challenges because often their brains are developmentally immature when

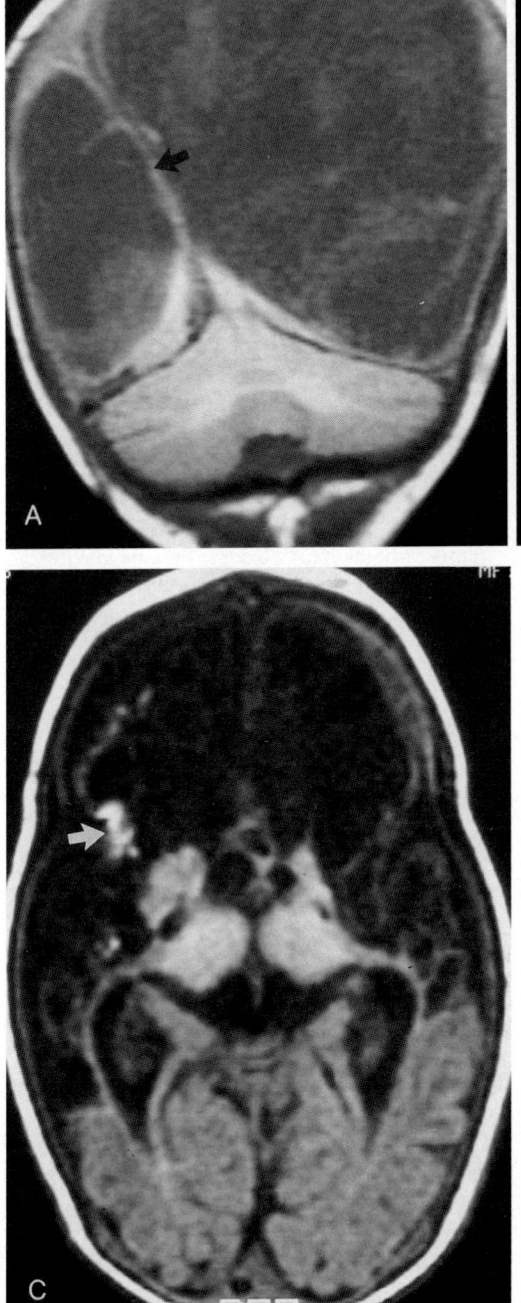

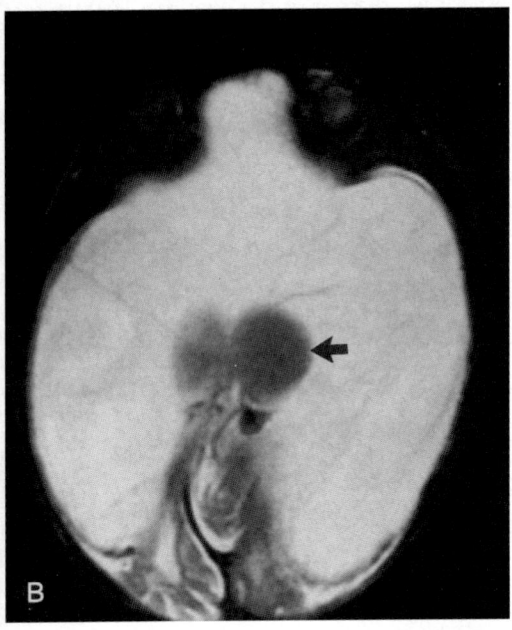

Figure 8.6. Hydranencephaly. A. Coronal T1WI. Hydranencephaly reflects varying degrees of infarction of both cerebral hemispheres. Note that the anterior circulation is completely infarcted with only a thin rim of leptomeningeal connective tissue (no cortex). Some cerebral tissue supplied by the posterior circulation has been spared. The presence of the falx (*arrow*) excludes holoprosencephaly as the diagnosis. **B.** Axial T2WI of the same case. Note that the brainstem is preserved (*arrow*). **C.** Axial T1WI of a different case with similar findings to the hydranencephaly case seen in **(A)** and **(B)**. Note that there is some sparing of the posterior temporal lobes. The presence of punctate foci of high signal (*arrow*) reflecting dystrophic calcification indicate that the initial insult was an in utero infection, probably of the TORCH (toxoplasma; other, which includes syphilis; rubella, cytomegalovirus; and herpes) group. This case illustrates the common final pathway of early severe in utero brain destruction, whether the inciting event was ischemic or infectious.

imaged. The first step is to understand the degree of prematurity and subtract the intervening time interval. For example, if we image an infant who is 2 months old but was delivered 2 months premature, the expected appearance would be of a newborn term infant. Premature infants are also special because extrauterine life places many severe stresses on the developmentally immature brain. Premature infants still have periventricular border zones of sensitivity to HII. Damage to the periventricular regions, leading to varying degrees of periven-

tricular leukomalacia, is common in premature infants. In severe cases, white matter undergoes cystic necrosis and subsequently becomes incorporated into the margins of the ventricle.

Germinal Matrix Hemorrhage. The germinal matrix, a zone of proliferating, richly vascularized neuroectodermal cells, is also exquisitely sensitive to injury. The response of this region to disturbances in cardiorespiratory function—whether caused by apnea, hypoxia, acidosis, bradycardia, unstable blood pressure, or im-

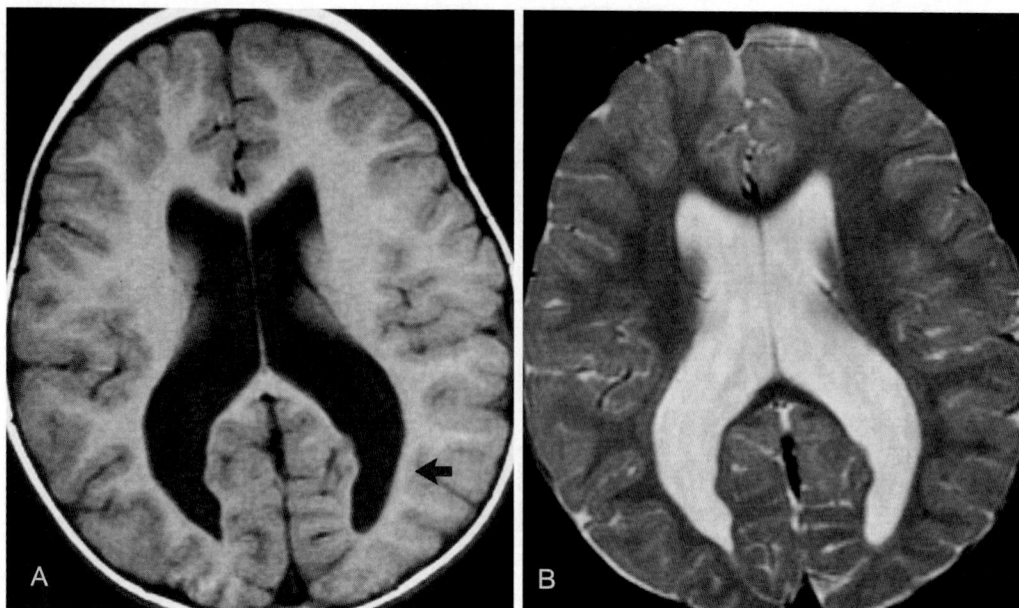

Figure 8.7. Hypoxic Ischemic Injury at Less Than 26 Weeks Gestation. A. Axial T1WI of a child who sustained an HII at less than 26 weeks of gestation, resulting in injury to the periatrial white matter. This is reflected in ex vacuo enlargement of the atria of the lateral ventricles. The severe periatrial white matter thinning has resulted in close apposition of a sulcus to the ventricular margin (*arrow*). **B.** The lack of periventricular gliosis is consistent with an insult occurring at 26 weeks of gestation age or less.

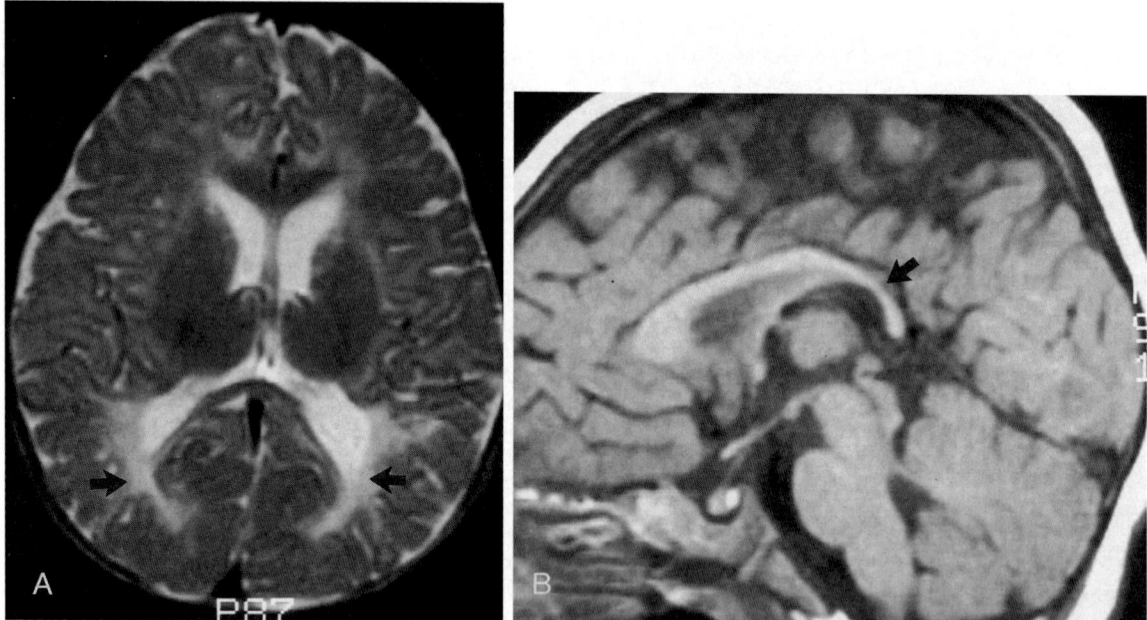

Figure 8.8. Periventricular Leukomalacia. A. Axial T2WI of a child who sustained an in utero HII later than 26 weeks of gestation age, resulting in periventricular leukomalacia. Note the high signal intensity due to gliosis in the periatrial region (*arrows*) that extends to the ventricular margin. **B.** Hypoxic ischemic injury causes white matter injury and subsequent white matter loss, as evidenced by thinning of the posterior corpus callosum (*arrow*), on this sagittal T1WI.

paired cerebral blood flow autoregulation—leads to rupture and hemorrhage of fragile blood vessels within the germinal matrix. Premature infants at risk for germinal matrix hemorrhage are best evaluated by serial neonatal neurosonography, which is reviewed in chapter 39. Isolated germinal matrix hemorrhage, termed "grade I subependymal hemorrhage," has the typical sonographic acute appearance of an echogenic focus directly anterior to the caudothalamic notch (see Fig. 39.17). The original hemorrhage eventually matures, either by disappearing entirely or evolving into a subependymal cyst. Bleeding may occur in the germinal matrix alone extend to the parenchyma, or rupture into the ventricle (see Fig. 39.18).

Term infants rarely have subependymal hemorrhage because, developmentally, their germinal matrix has involuted and their arterial border zones have moved peripherally. This situation elicits a number of useful rules.

1. Isolated periventricular leukomalacia in the term infant is only rarely caused by birth-related hypoxic ischemic events.
2. Gliosis in the periatrial region (seen best on proton-density scans) is caused by injury to the developing brain at 28 weeks' gestational age or older.
3. Ex vacuo atrial enlargement without gliosis reflects injury prior to 26 weeks.

Profound versus Partial Hypoxic Ischemic Brain Injury

Differing injury patterns can be detected by MR, which distinguishes between term infants subjected to severe hypoxic ischemic insults, and those with milder or partial episodes of hypoxia/anoxia. Examples of profound hypoxic ischemic events include full cardiorespiratory arrest and complete placental abruption. The MR appearance will vary depending on the age of the patient and whether the injury is evaluated acutely, subacutely, or in the chronic phase.

Profound Perinatal HII tends to damage central brain areas but spares the cerebral cortex. Evaluated acutely (immediate to 3 days) by CT, these infants may show injury to deep gray matter structures (basal ganglia and thalamus) with relative cortical sparing. In newborn infants, this may lead to the peculiar appearance of deep gray matter structures becoming isodense to surrounding white matter, a very subtle abnormality (Fig. 8.10).

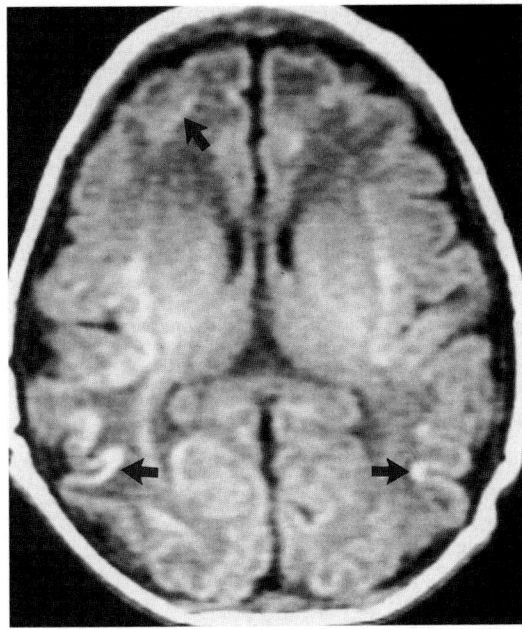

Figure 8.9. Perinatal Hypoxic Ischemic Injury. T1WI of a term infant who sustained partial HII injury in the perinatal period. Peripheral (cortical) hemorrhagic petechial infarcts (*arrows*) are seen in anterior and posterior watershed distributions.

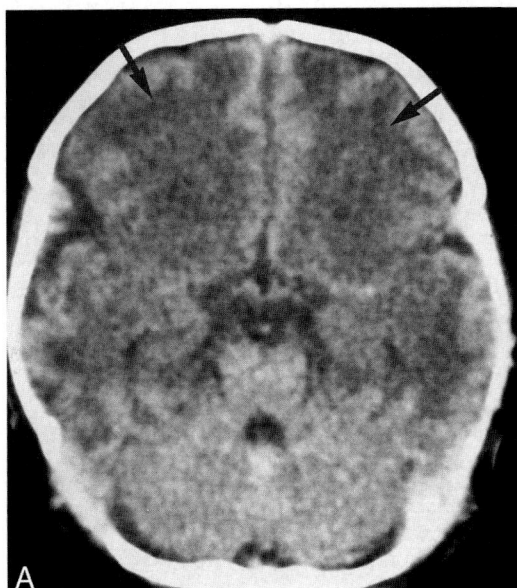
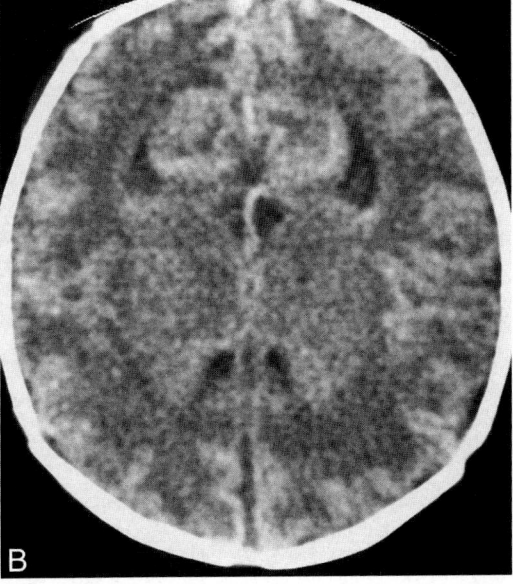

Figure 8.10. Prolonged Hypoxic Ischemic Injury on CT. This two-day-old infant sustained a prolonged hypoxic ischemic injury. **A.** CT scan obtained soon after the event demonstrates diffuse low attenuation of the supratentorial brain, especially the subcortical white matter (*arrows*), caused by edema. The clue to the severe nature of the injury is the relative "white" appearance of the cerebellum. The cerebellum is more resistant to ischemia than the supratentorial brain. **B.** Axial images at the level of the basal ganglia show gener-alized diminished attenuation of the basal ganglia due to edema. Note the indistinctness of the posterior limbs of the internal capsule relative to the thalamus and lentiform nucleus. This is subtle evidence for injury to the ventrolateral thalamus. Follow-up scans taken at one month demonstrated severe postischemic injury and encephalomalacia to the supratentorial cortex, lentiform nucleus, and thalamus.

Profound HII in the perinatal period evaluated acutely (up to 3 weeks) by MR will show mottled, globular high signal on T1WI in the basal ganglia (posterolateral lentiform), and ventral/lateral thalamus (Fig. 8.11). These same areas show mottled low signal intensity on

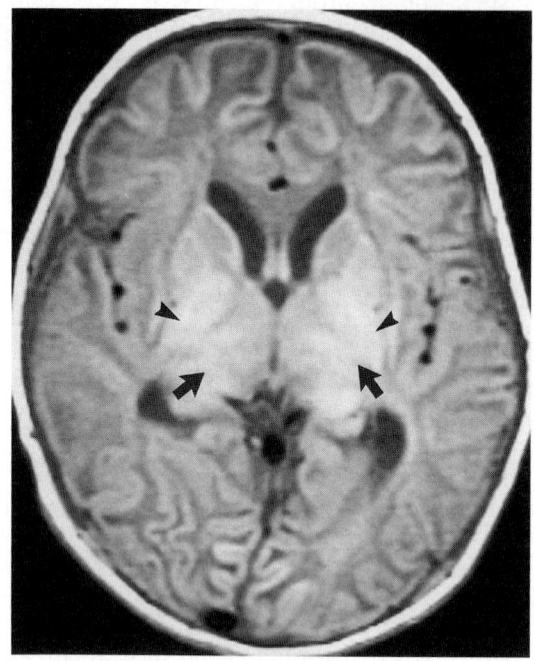

Figure 8.11. Profound Perinatal HII—Acute. Axial T1WI of a term infant evaluated acutely by MR. Mottled high signal intensity is seen in the posterolateral lentiform nuclei (*arrowheads*) and ventrolateral thalami (*arrows*). These high signal intensity areas most likely represent blood breakdown products.

T2WI. The signal intensity abnormalities may reflect hemorrhagic byproducts. Additionally, similar signal intensity abnormalities may be present in the tegmentum of the midbrain, lateral geniculate nuclei, and hippocampi (Fig. 8.12). The cortical damage is not often readily apparent in the acute phase. Spin-echo T2WI taken in the first few days will show an apparently normal cortex and subadjacent white matter. Careful inspection of proton-density–weighted images is helpful in identifying cortical edema, resulting in loss of the gray matter-white matter interface, which is indicative of injury.

In the subacute period (3 weeks–3 months), the signal intensity of the basal ganglia damage may be variable on T2WI. Damage to the cortex and white matter becomes more evident.

Profound HII in the perinatal period evaluated chronically (>3 months) predominantly shows evolving injury to central gray matter: the posterolateral lentiform nuclei and ventral/lateral thalami. The small area of cortex involved is the perirolandic cortex (precentral and postcentral gyri). The affected areas evaluated chronically have evolved in their appearance because of atrophy and gliosis (high signal on T2WI) (Fig. 8.13). Table 8.3 summarizes the imaging findings in profound perinatal HII.

The basal ganglia regions are also extremely sensitive to toxic and metabolic processes and will exhibit a relatively nonspecific response to these nonhypoxic insults as well (Fig. 8.14).

Profound postnatal HII tends to injure a much larger proportion of cerebral cortex, with relative sparing of the perirolandic cortex. Postnatal HII damages the corpus striatum (globus pallidas, putamen, and caudate) and tends to spare the thalamus (Table 8.4).

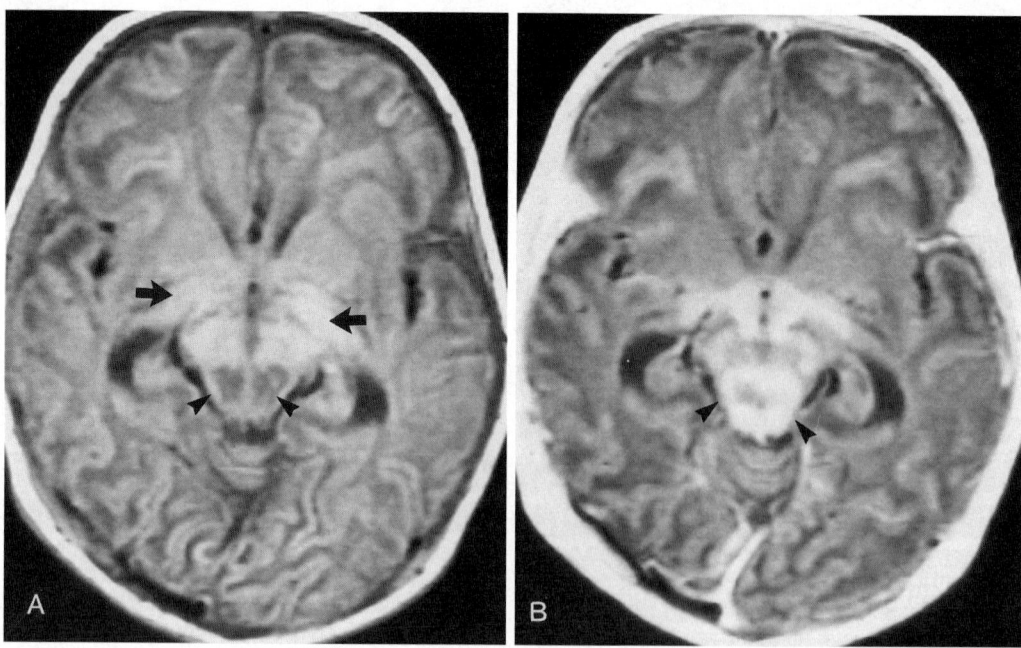

Figure 8.12. Profound Perinatal HII—Acute. A. T1WI of the level of the midbrain (same case as in Figure 8.11). Mottled high signal intensity is seen in the lateral geniculate nuclei (*arrows*) and abnormal low signal is seen in the midbrain tegmentum (*arrowheads*). The actively myelinating regions such as the midbrain tegmentum are particularly susceptible to injury. **B.** Axial T1WI following gadolinium administration shows blood-brain barrier breakdown caused by ischemia in the midbrain tegmentum (*arrowheads*).

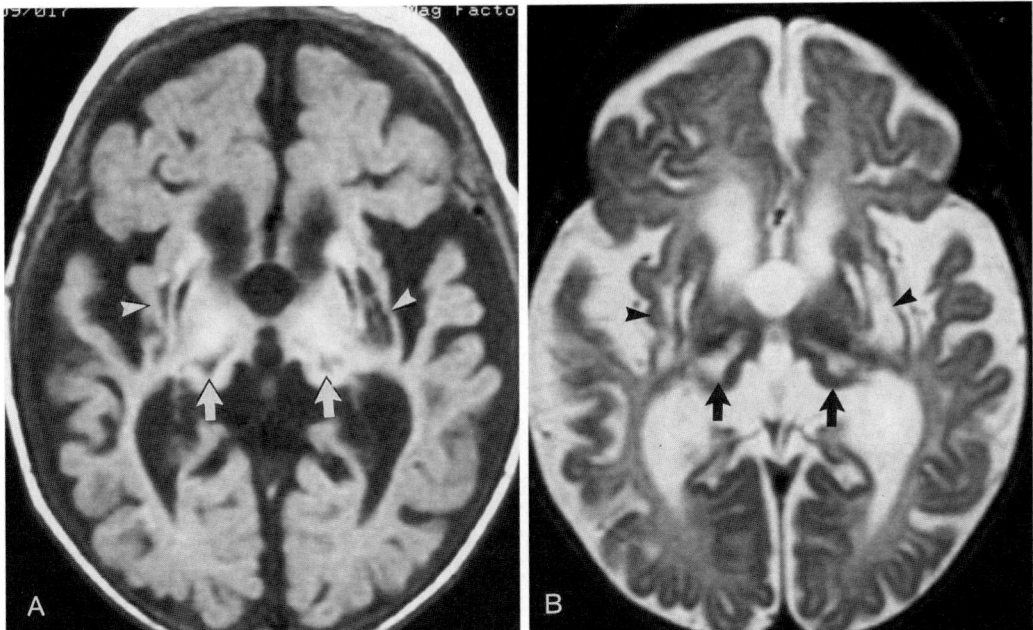

Figure 8.13. Profound Perinatal HII—Chronic. Profound perinatal HII in a term infant evaluated chronically shows the evolving changes on MR. **A.** T1WI shows neuronal loss in the posterolateral lentiform (*arrowheads*) and ventrolateral thalami (*arrows*). Marked periatrial white matter atrophy is also seen. **B.** T2WI shows high signal intensity in the posterolateral lentiform (*arrowheads*) and ventrolateral thalami (*arrows*) caused by neuronal loss and gliosis.

Table 8.3. Imaging of Profound Perinatal Hypoxic Ischemic Injury

Time	Deep Gray (PLL, VLT)	Cortex	Other
Acute	Isodense to white matter on CT Mottled high signal, T1WI Mottled low signal, T2WI	Normal—may see blurred gray/white junction on protein density images	
Subacute	Variable signal, T1WI, T2WI	Perirolandic cortex: high signal T1WI, low signal T2WI	Atrophy: hippocampi, lateral geniculate, midbrain tegmentum Deep, superficial perirolandic white matter gliosis and atrophy, high signal on T2WI, variable myelination delay
Chronic	High signal, T2WI	Perirolandic cortex: high signal T2WI Thinned gyri, atrophy	Atrophy: hippocampi, lateral geniculate, midbrain tegmentum Deep, superficial perirolandic white matter gliosis and atrophy, high signal on T2WI, variable myelination delay

PLL, posterolateral lentiform; *VLT,* ventrolateral thalamus.
Adapted from Barkovich AJ. MR and CT evaluation of profound neonatal and infantile asphyxia. AJNR Am J Neuroradiol 1992;13:959–972.

Partial Perinatal HII. Partial or milder hypoxic ischemic events in the perinatal period usually spare central brain areas and damage more peripheral gray matter. These peripheral infarcts are often located in watershed zones as previously described. The peripheral infarcts will often progress over time to petechial gyral hemorrhage and eventually to areas of cortical thinning. Marked diminution and high signal on T2WI of the subcortical and deep white matter is also seen.

Acute hypoxic ischemic damage can be difficult to discern in newborn infants. Some helpful hints follow:

1. Unmyelinated white matter is bright on T2WI, making infarcts less apparent.

2. T1WI can be a source of confusion. Do not confuse normal active myelination (basal ganglia, thalami, cerebral peduncles, and perirolandic white matter) with the petechial hemorrhage owing to profound HII. Petechial hemorrhage occurs in the putamina and thalami as punctate clumps on T1WI and as blurred normal margins between the posterior limb of the internal capsule and the thalamus on T2WI. Subtle punctate hyperintensity of a gyrus may indicate petechial hemorrhage on T1WI.

3. Cerebral edema is often not well seen on MR. A CT may be more appropriate.

4. An extremely useful sign of infarction is the loss of normal grya matter hypointensity amidst a sea of hyperintense (unmyelinated) white matter on T2WI.

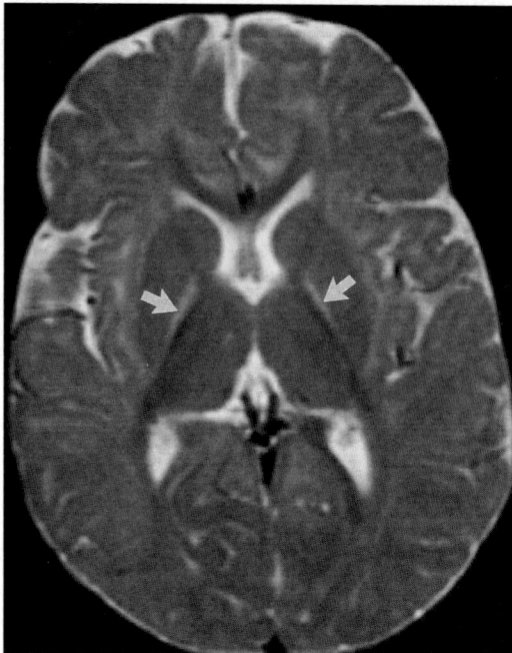

Figure 8.14. Non-HII Basal Ganglia Injury. A child's axial T2WI at the level of the basal ganglia. A wide variety of metabolic and inflammatory insults can affect the basal ganglia. In this case, neonatal kernicterus has damaged the basal ganglia (globus pallidus) (*arrows*) and the subthalamic nuclei (not shown), a somewhat different pattern than HII. This case illustrates the relatively nonspecific response of the basal ganglia to *non*hypoxic ischemic injury. (Courtesy of Dr. Majeed Al-Mateen.)

Prolonged partial HII in the perinatal period evaluated acutely may show a global pattern of injury and severe low density of the cerebral hemispheres on CT, owing to diffuse edema. The cerebellum is relatively resistant to injury, leading to the "white cerebellum" sign (Fig. 8.10). The CT sign shows a normal cerebellum appearing relatively white against a background of edematous supratentorial brain. MR appears relatively insensitive to signs of edema in infants, and CT is still the preferred modality for assessing supratentorial brain edema. A correlate to the CT is still the preferred modality for assessing supratentorial brain edema. However, a correlate to the CT white cerebellum sign has been described. This is the "dark-cerebellum sign" on MR. The normal cerebellum appears uniformly dark compared with the relatively hyperintense ischemic supratentorial brain.

Summary. The developing brain shows continually shifting areas of brain vulnerability to HII and changing brain response. A general knowledge of these regions and the evolving response of the damaged brain is necessary to sort out differing patterns of brain injury. US is the best modality for demonstrating germinal matrix hemorrhage, and CT is useful in demonstrating early signs of brain edema and hemorrhage. MR is able to demonstrate many of the characteristic conditions associated with HII, including selective neuronal loss, watershed infarction, selective thalamic and basal ganglia necrosis, pontosubicular necrosis, hippocampal necrosis, periventricular leukomalacia, white matter thinning, and delayed myelination.

CONGENITAL LESIONS

Congenital lesions cannot be lumped into convenient categories by appearance. Most are "Aunt Minnies," i.e., unique in their appearance. Some of the entities that share common features are clustered together.

Septo-optic Dysplasia is defined as hypoplasia of the optic nerves and absence of the septum pellucidum. Complete or partial absence of the septum pellucidum can be seen. There is also variable hypoplasia of the optic nerves. A fundoscopic examination of the optic nerves is often a helpful correlate (Fig. 8.15). Endocrine abnormalities are common, as are associated migration anomalies and periventricular cysts.

Holoprosencephaly is a spectrum of disorders related to unsuccessful cleavage of the developing brain. Holoprosencephaly also presents with orbital hypotelorism and varying degrees of facial dysmorphism.

Alobar Holoprosencephaly. The alobar form is a severe malformation with a dismal prognosis. This type of holoprosencephaly is distinctive, consisting an anterior rind of brain tissue and a posterior monoventricle that communicates with a dorsal cyst. The thalami are fused, and the septum pellucidum, corpus callosum, and falx are absent (Fig. 8.16).

This form of holoprosencephaly only needs to be discriminated from two other entities—hydranencephaly (Fig. 8.6), which represents bilateral in utero cerebral hemisphere infarction, and severe hydrocephalus, with secondary pressure atrophy of the septum pellucidum. A reliable discriminating sign of alobar holoprosencephaly id the tips of the upside-down U-shaped mantle of brain tissue. These ends of the "U," known as the hippocampal ridges, are best seen in the axial plane.

Semilobar Holoprosencephaly is less severe and shows partial fusion of the hemispheres. The corpus callosum and the septum pellucidum are absent or dysgenic. There is a high association with migration anomalies (abnormalities of cortical development) (Fig. 8.17). The posterior portion of the interhemispheric fissure and falx are usually formed in cases of semilobar holoprosencephaly.

Lobar Holoprosencephaly is characterized by a normal-appearing brain. Typically, a frontal interhemispheric fissure is partially absent. The absent septum pellucidum and the relatively normal brain gives this entity an overlap with septo-optic dysplasia. The body and

Table 8.4. Imaging of Profound Postnatal Hypoxic Ischemic Injury

Deep Gray Matter	Cortex	Other
Damage to corpus striatum: high signal on T2WI	Majority of cortex injured: high signal on T2WI	Atrophy: hippocampi, lateral geniculate
Relative sparing of thalami	Relative sparing of perirolandic cortex	
	Thinned gyri	

Adapted from Barkovich AJ. MR and CT evaluation of profound neonatal and infantile asphyxia. AJNR Am J Neuroradiol 1992;13:959–972.

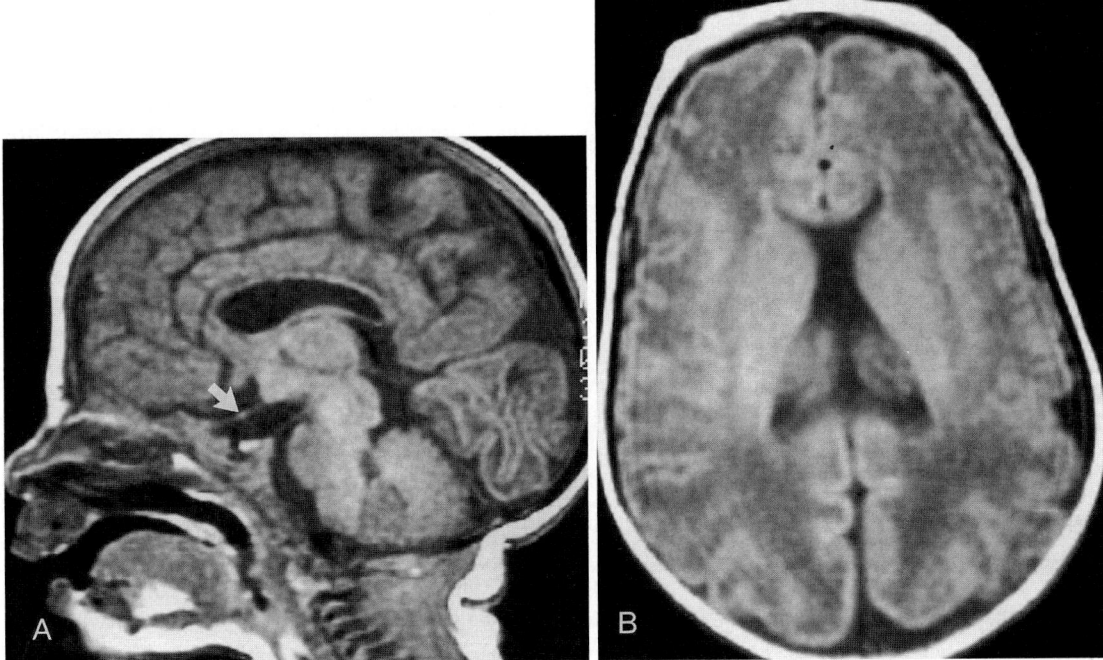

Figure 8.15. Septo-optic Dysplasia. A. Sagittal T1WI shows a hypoplastic optic nerve (*arrow*), an inconstant finding on MR imaging of septo-optic dysplasia. **B.** Axial T1WI shows absence of the septum pellucidum, characteristic of septo-optic dysplasia.

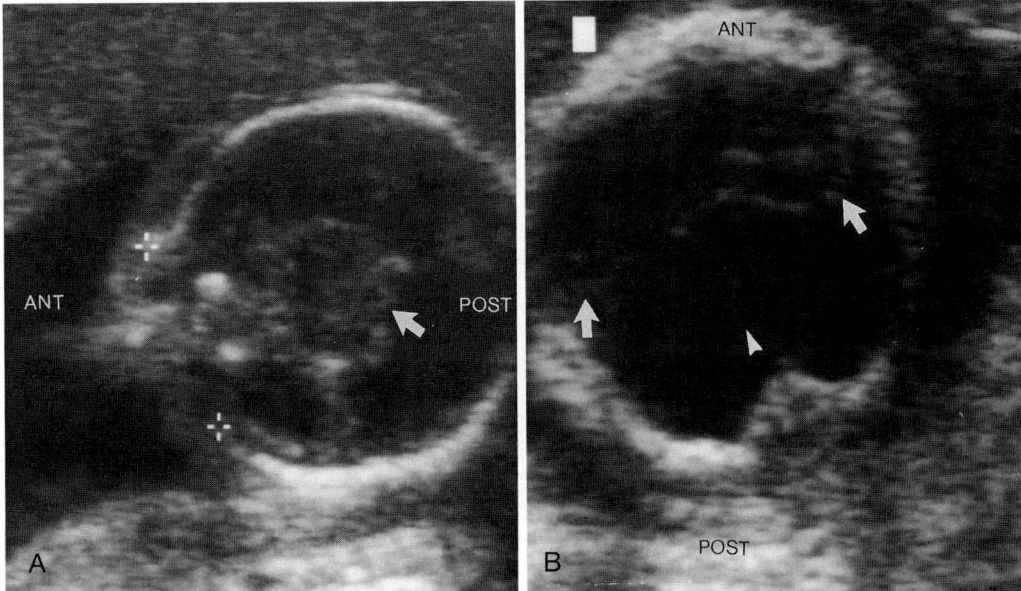

Figure 8.16. Alobar Holoprosencephaly. A. An axial obstetrical US through the fetal brain demonstrates the in utero appearance of alobar holoprosencephaly. This severe disorder consists of a monoventricle with absence of the septum pellucidum, corpus callosum, and falx. The thalami are fused (*arrow*). The white markers are placed at the orbits to measure the degree of hypotelorism. **B.** An axial image at a slightly higher level shows the posterior tips of the mantle of cerebral tissue, termed "hippocampal ridges" (*arrows*), characteristic of holoprosencephaly. This mantle is displaced forward within the calvarium by the posterior monoventricle. The monoventricle communicates with the cerebrospinal fluid space called the dorsal sac (*arrowhead*).

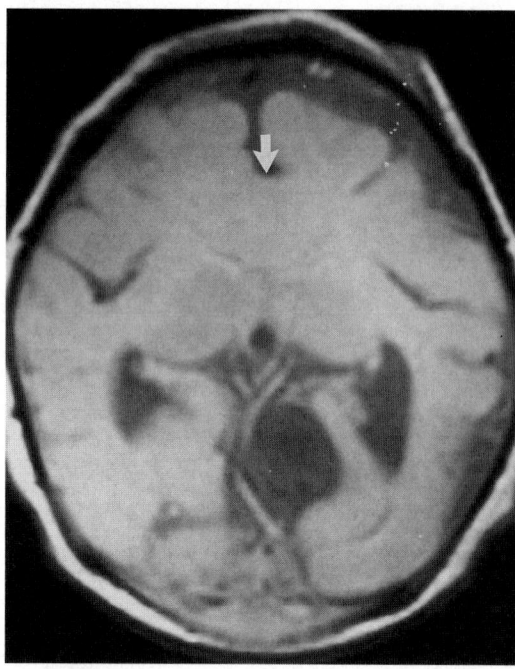

Figure 8.17. Semilobar Holoprosencephaly. An MR image of semilobal holoprosencephaly shows partial fusion of the anterior cerebral hemispheres (*arrow*).

splenium of the corpus callosum are usually present with the genu and rostrum absent (dysgenic corpus callosum).

The absence of the septum pellucidum is a constant helpful feature of the holoprosencephalies. Any portion of a visible septum pellucidum excludes holoprosencephaly and should prompt consideration of severe hydrocephalus or agenesis of the corpus callosum. Remember, absence of the septum pellucidum is strongly associated with other malformations, including anomalies of the face and cerebral cortex (schizencephaly, polymicrogyria, and pachygyria). Coronal T1 images are helpful in demonstrating a narrow portion of hemisphere fusion, confirming the diagnosis of holoprosencephaly.

Agenesis of the Corpus Callosum. The corpus callosum forms from front to back and myelinates from back to front. These facts help discriminate a number of callosal anomalies and myelination questions. Following these principles, partial agenesis of the corpus callosum will result in formation of the genu but absence of the dorsal body and splenium.

Two conditions deviate from the typical callosal agenesis appearance. Both secondary destruction of the corpus callosum and holoprosencephaly can result in nonsequential segments of absent callosum. The resultant dysgenic callosal pattern thus yields valuable clues regarding brain development and a correct diagnosis. For example, a callosum *only* missing a genu segment may indicate an insult to the brain after development of the corpus callosum, or it may indicate lobar holoprosencephaly (if the septum is absent), which exhibits disorganized callosal development.

The imaging appearance is variable, ranging from complete to partial absence of callosal tissue. Concomitant with the absence of the corpus callosum is failure to form the cingulate sulcus. Without the supporting white matter fibers, alteration of the ventricles occurs with "steer-horn frontal ventricles" in the coronal plane or a "racing car" ventricular appearance in the axial plane (Fig. 8.18). This is due to redirection of longitudinal callosal fibers (Probst bundles) along the medial ventricular walls. An interhemispheric cysts may be seen, frequently in communication with the third ventricle.

A description of a potential pitfall in interpretation is important. Occasionally, callosal hypogenesis will be accompanied by relative prominence of the hippocampal commissure. The hippocampal commissure should not be mistaken for the splenium, erroneously signaling "atypical callosal hypogenesis" or callosal dysgenesis.

Lipomas of the Corpus Callosum have imaging criteria similar to other intracranial lipomas in other locations. Lipomas are high signal intensity on T1WI, and they cause chemical shift artifact along the frequency encoding direction of the scan. T2WI show a diminution in signal intensity although some fast-spin echo sequences will have high signal intensity from fat. Lipomas do not cause mass effect, and vessels course through these lesions unperturbed. Lipomas of the corpus callosum are associated with callosal anomalies (Fig. 8.19). Other common locations of intracranial lipomas include the pericallosal, quadrigeminal, and suprasellar cisterns. Less common locations include cerebellopontine angle, sylvian fissure, cerebellar vermis (Fig. 8.20), and the lamina terminalis.

Cephaloceles represent the inability of the skull and dura to close over the brain, leading to a herniation of intracranial contents through the defect. Meningoceles reflect herniation of the leptomeninges alone, and encephaloceles are associated with herniation of brain and leptomeninges. Occipital encephaloceles are the most common. Other locations include frontoethmoidal, parietal, and sphenoidal regions. The brain remaining inside the calvarium is typically stretched and distorted toward the defect. Frontoethmoidal encephaloceles are associated with craniofacial anomalies (including hypertelorism), and a higher incidence of callosal abnormalities (Figs. 8.21, 8.22).

Sphenoid encephaloceles are often occult and present as nasopharyngeal masses that contain variable amounts of herniated third ventricle, hypothalamus, and optic chiasm.

MIGRATION ANOMALIES

This group of disorders reflects varying patterns of arrested migration of neurons toward the brain surface. Many of the discrete layers of the cortex are formed by directed migration of specific neurons from the subependymal regions outward. Cells destined to become cortical gray matter end up in the wrong place following arrested migration. These abnormal areas can become foci of seizure activity.

"Lissencephaly" and "Agyria" are synonymous terms for the most severe disorder in this spectrum:

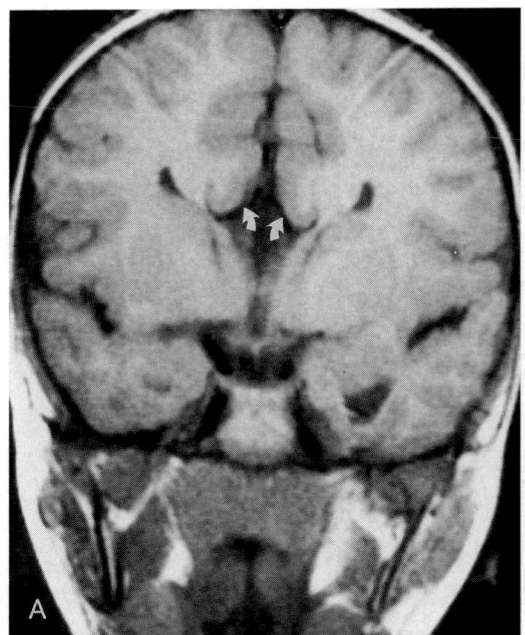 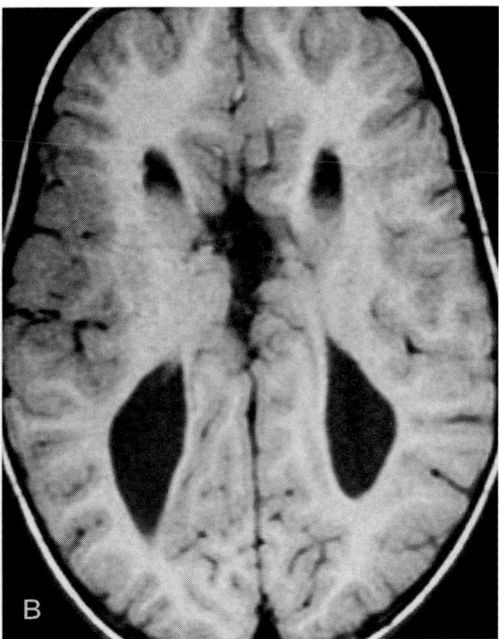

Figure 8.18. Agenesis of the Corpus Callosum. A. Coronal T1WI shows steer-horn shape of the frontal horns of the lateral ventricle. There is absence of the midline corpus callosal tissue and cingulate sulcus (*arrows*). **B.** Axial T1WI of the same case showing the "racing car" configuration of the ventricles. The frontal horns look like the front wheels, and the atria of the lateral ventricles look like the larger rear tires on a racing car.

absence of gyri. The lack of sulcation gives a smooth figure-of-eight appearance to the brain. The cortex is abnormally thick (Fig. 8.23) and multilayered. The premature infant's brain can mimic the appearance of lissencephaly. However, the history of prematurity and the normal-thickness cortex distinguish the premature infant.

Polymicrogyria and Pachygyria are both milder disorders of neuronal migration than agyria; however, they are similar in appearance and prognosis. These entities are called cortical dysplasias. For simplicity's sake, lesions with these characteristics can be described as representing either polymicrogyria or pachygyria, but pachygyria is seen as broad, thick gyri, with shallow sulci. Polymicrogyria is characterized by a thick mantle of gray matter with multiple small gyri. Underlying white matter gliosis in polymicrogyria can sometimes help differentiate it from pachygyria. In both polygyria and pachygyria, the normal interdigitating fingers of subcortical white matter are absent. These anomalies produce an abnormally thickened cortex with little or no sulcation, but in distinction to lissencephaly, they are more focal (Figs. 8.24,8.25). Cortical dysplasias also show anomalous cortical venous drainage, which should not be confused with the abnormal vessels seen in arteriovenous malformations. Because polymicrogyria and pachygyria reflect an in utero insult resulting in arrested cell migration, other associated anomalies are common. These include heterotopic gray matter, schizencephaly, and callosal hypogenesis. Sometimes a whole hemisphere contains polymicrogyric and pachymicrogyric changes. This condition is termed "hemimegalencephaly."

Heterotopic Gray Matter. Disrupted migration of neurons can result in trapped nests of gray matter deep

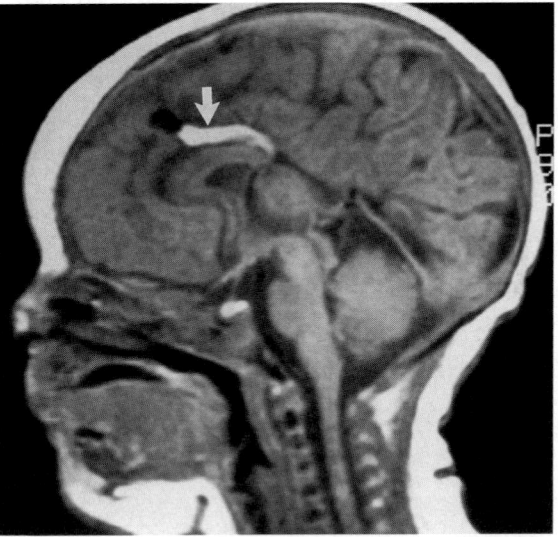

Figure 8.19. Lipoma of the Corpus Callosum. A Sagittal T1WI shows a high signal intensity lipoma of the corpus callosum (*arrow*) with accompanying hypogenesis of the posterior body and splenium of the corpus callosum. (Courtesy of Dr. Robin Shanahan.)

within the brain. These islands of gray matter can be seen anywhere between the ependymal surface and the subcortical white matter. These foci are termed "heterotopic gray matter." Heterotopic gray matter appears isointense to normal gray matter on all imaging sequences. These lesions do not enhance with gadolinium and do not calcify (Fig. 8.26). The only really important mimic of heterotopic gray matter are the lesions seen in

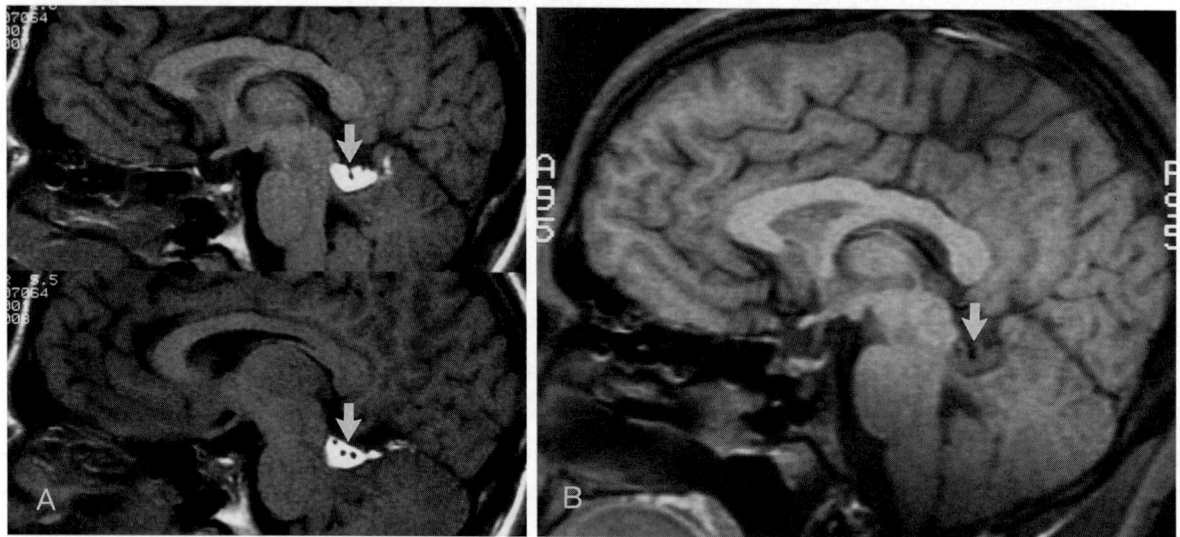

Figure 8.20. Lipoma of the Cerebellar Vermis. A. Sagittal T1WI shows a lipoma of the superior vermis (*arrows*). Note that a vessel courses through the lipoma unperturbed. **B.** A fat-saturation T1WI shows the suppression of fat signal from the image, confirming the diagnosis of lipoma (*arrow*).

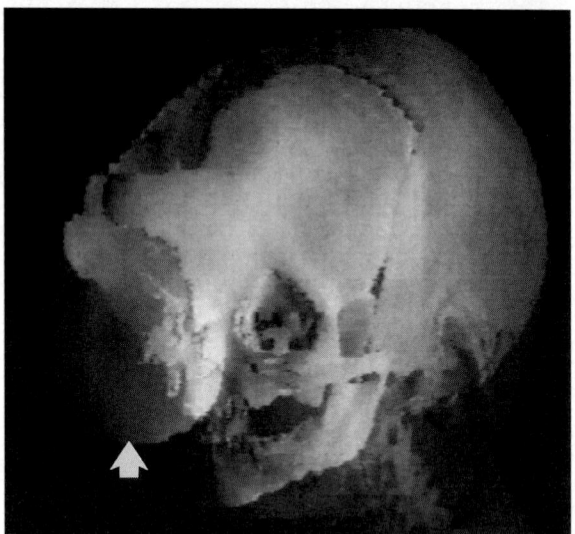

Figure 8.21. Frontal Encephalocele. A three-dimensional reformation CT image of a dramatic frontal encephalocele shows the calvarial defect and a soft-tissue sac (*arrow*) herniating out through the defect.

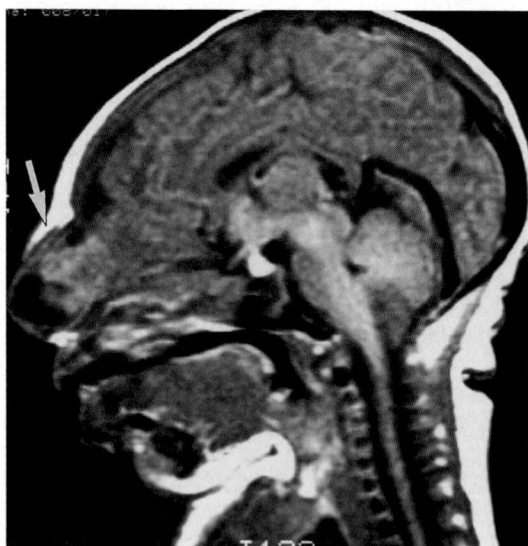

Figure 8.22. Frontal Encephalocele. T1-weighted MR image of a frontal encephalocele shows herniation of brain and meninges through the defect (*arrow*). (Courtesy of Dr. Michael Taekman.)

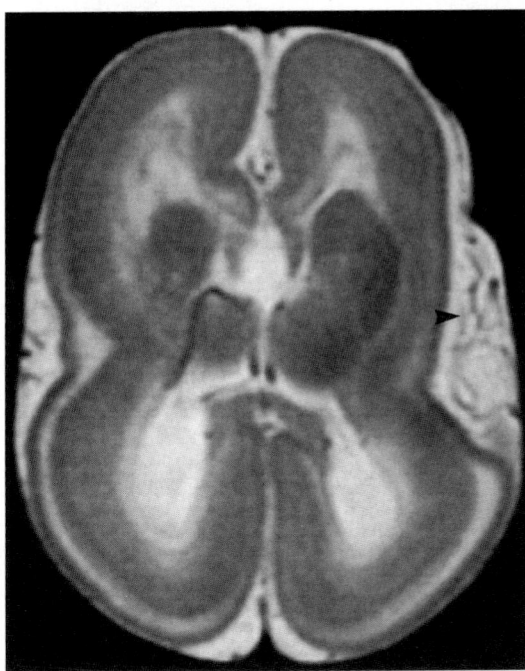

Figure 8.23. Lissencephaly. Axial T2WI of lissencephaly. The brain has a smooth agyric appearance with an abnormally thickened multilayered cortex. The anomalous cortical venous drainage pattern is also seen (*arrowhead*).

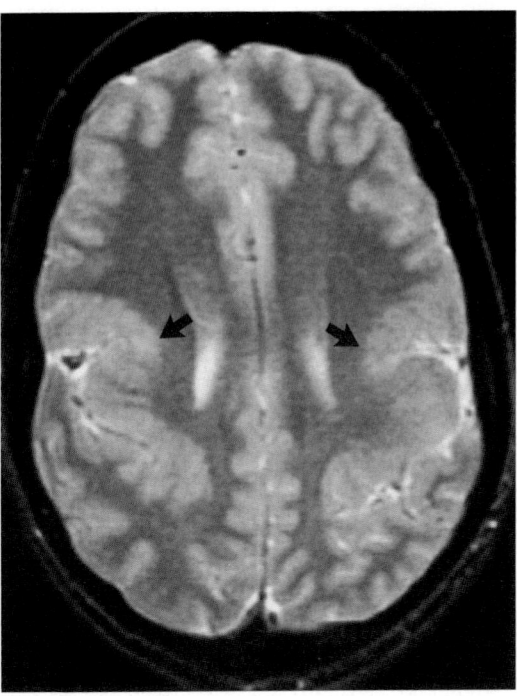

Figure 8.24. Polymicrogyria. Bilateral areas of focal cortical thickening with deep clefting are seen in both hemispheres in this case of polymicrogyria (*arrows*).

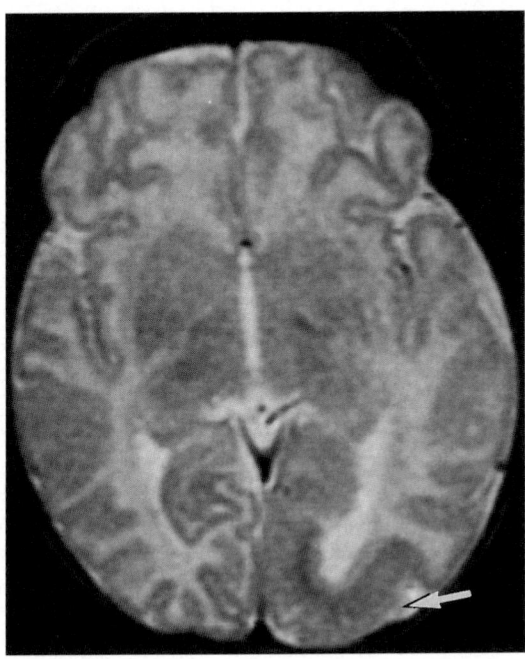

Figure 8.25. Pachygyria. A more focal area of smooth cortical thickening is seen in this more subtle case of focal pachygyria (*arrow*).

tuberous sclerosis, which do calcify. Most heterotopic gray matter is nodular, although band heterotopias can be seen.

Schizencephaly represents abnormal gray matter—lined clefts that deeply invaginate the brain. A pial/

ependymal seam communicates with the ventricle. All other clefts that do not extend to the ventricle are polymicrogyric clefts. Multiple imaging planes are often necessary to optimally visualize the clefts. The clefts can be either open lip or closed lip in appearance (Fig 8.27).

All of the migration anomalies can present with seizures as the clinical manifestation. When imaging a child for seizures, careful examination for mass lesions should be followed by scrutiny for anomalies of neuronal migration. If a gyrus looks suspiciously thickened, image it again in another plane. Schizencephaly is differentiated from porencephalic cysts by the presence of a gray matter-lined cleft. Porencephalic cysts are lined by a thin layer of white matter.

Chiari II Malformations involve the brain and spine. Chiari II malformations are the serious neural tube disorders that are screened for in maternal prenatal US and alphafetoprotein programs. Starting from the head down of the fetus, the key abnormalities are described.

Supratentorial Brain. Nearly all patients will present with hydrocephalus. Most cases show partial or complete agenesis of the corpus callosum. The falx cerebri is often fenestrated, resulting in herniation of individual gyri across the midline. The massa intermedia (midline rounded mass of gray matter connecting the thalami on sagittal images) is enlarged. The posterior cingulate gyrus is often dysplastic.

Posterior Fossa. Most of the hindbrain findings in Chiari II malformation derive from a diminutive posterior fossa with brain structures squeezed superiorly, inferiorly, and anteriorly. The cerebellum is squeezed up against the tentorium, down through the foramen magnum (tonsillar

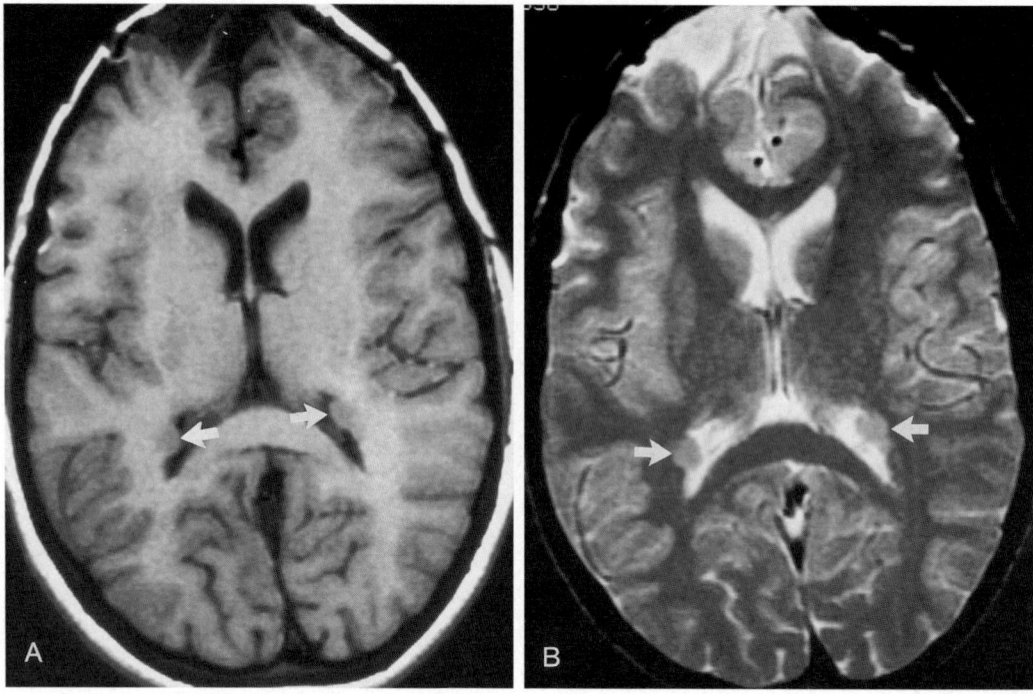

Figure 8.26. Heterotopic Gray Matter. A. T1WI demonstrates heterotopic gray matter (*arrows*) along the ependymal surface of the ventricle. Damage to the frontal lobes was secondary to trauma.

B. A T2WI at the same level again shows the heterotopic nodules that parallel gray matter signal in all sequences (*arrows*).

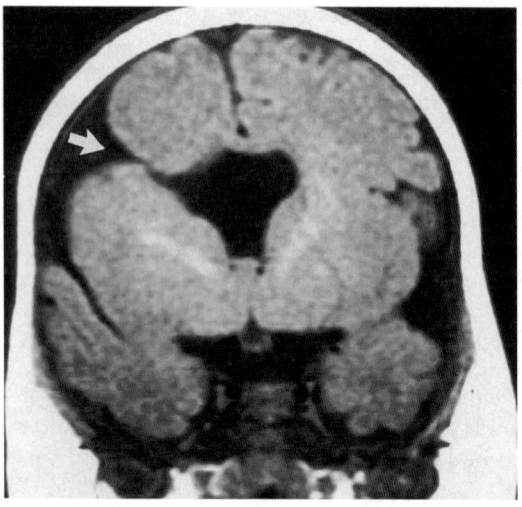

Figure 8.27. Schizencephaly. An open-lip schizencephaly is seen on the coronal T1WI. The cleft is lined by thickened polymicrogyric gray matter (*arrow*).

herniation), and forward around the brainstem. The fourth ventricle is squeezed into a small vertical slit. The pons and medullar are also squeezed inferiorly, and with fixed attachments of the upper cervical spinal cord, a cervicomedullary kink often develops as the medulla buckles down past the tethered cord (Fig. 8.28).

Spine. Most Chiari II malformations present with myelomeningocele. A myelomeningocele represents a failure to close the caudal end of the neural tube during development. This splayed open neural tube also fails to induce a dural or bony covering (Fig. 8.29).

Chiari I Malformations consist of cerebellar tonsillar ectopia (tonsils extend >5 mm below the foramen magnum). Although patients may be asymptomatic, alterations of cerebrospinal fluid dynamics at the level of the forament magnum are believed to promote cervical spinal cord syrinx in some patients (Fig. 8.30). Similarly, Chiari II malformations are associated with cord syrinx (Fig. 8.31).

Cystic Lesions of the Posterior Fossa. A simple working classification of cystic posterior fossa malformations is to consider them within the spectrum of Dandy-Walker malformations. In distinction to Chiari malformations, Dandy-Walker malformations are characterized by a large posterior fossa (a high tentorial insertion). The posterior fossa is filled by a cystically dilated fourth ventricle that exerts mass effect (Fig. 8.32). Hypoplasia or absence of the cerebellar vermis and cerebellar hemispheres are associated findings.

Hydrocephalus is also common in this disorder, as is callosal hypogenesis. From this definition follow the other entities within the spectrum: Dandy-Walker variant and megacisterna magna.

A Dandy-Walker variant shows a normal-sized posterior fossa, hypoplasia or absence of the vermis and cerebellar hemispheres, but no significant mass effect. Megacisterna magna shows a normal-sized posterior fossa and relatively normal cerebellar hemispheres and vermis. Characterized by a prominent cisterna magna cerebrospinal fluid space without mass effect, megacisterna magna is thus distinct from retrocerebellar arachnoid cysts and epidermoid neoplasms. Mass lesions cause an inward convex bowing of brain tissues at their interface, and long-standing masses will cause smooth erosion of the inner table of the skull.

THE PHAKOMATOSES

The phakomatoses are syndromes that are grouped together because they all share neurologic and cutaneous manifestations.

Neurofibromatosis is divided into type I (von Recklinghausen's disease), with distinct neurocutaneous manifestations, and neurofibromatosis II (NF-II) (Table 8.5). *Neurofibromatosis I* (NF-I) is characterized by skin lesions ("café au lait" spots), neurofibromas, and ocular findings. The findings in the brain consist of tumors and nonneoplastic lesions in the white matter and globus pallidus. Neurofibromatosis I is associated with a high incidence of gliomas. The most common gliomas involve the optic pathways. A typical tumor causes fusiform enlargement of the optic nerve (Fig. 8.33). However, the chiasm, optic tracts, and optic radiations can also become involved. Typically, the tumors show poor or no contrast enhancement, consistent with a low histologic grade. Parenchymal involvement along optic pathways is seen

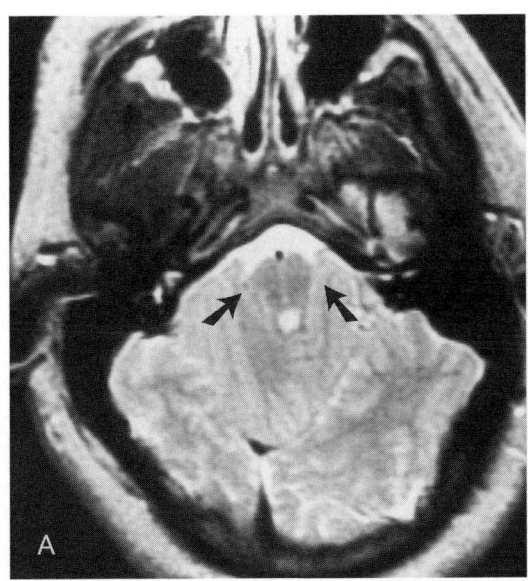
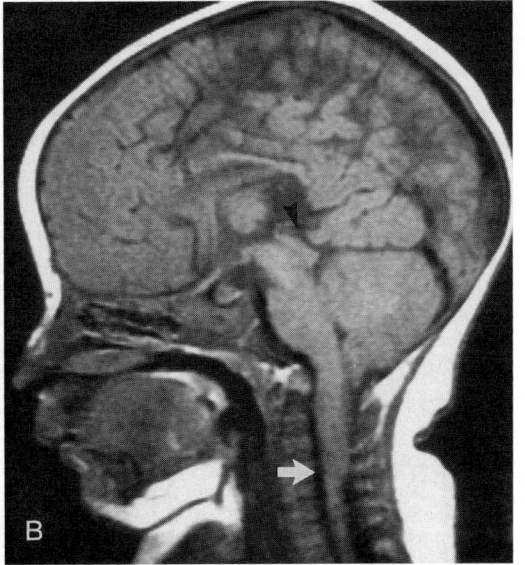

Figure 8.28. Chiari II Malformation. A. Axial T1WI of a Chiari II malformation demonstrates how the small posterior fossa squeezes the cerebellum around the brainstem (*arrows*). **B.** Sagittal T1WI shows breaking of the tectum (*arrowhead*) and downward displacement of the cerebellar tonsils. A cervicomedullary kink is identified (*arrow*). (Courtesy of Dr. John Zovickian.)

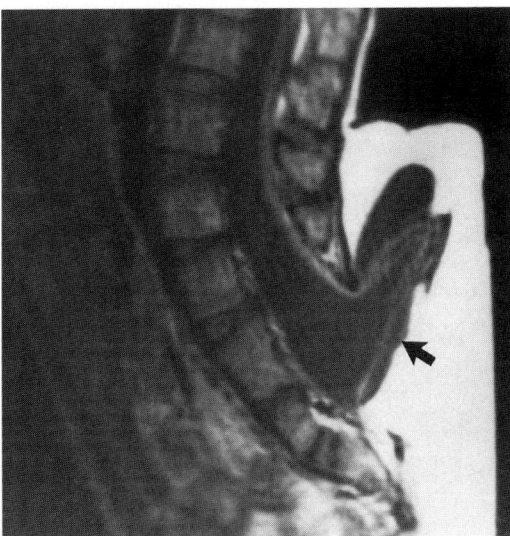

Figure 8.29. Myelomeningocele. Sagittal T1WI of a myelomeningocele in a case of Chiari II malformation. The myelomeningocele sac (*arrow*) contains neural tissue and meninges and protrudes through the dysraphic posterior elements of the lumbar spine.

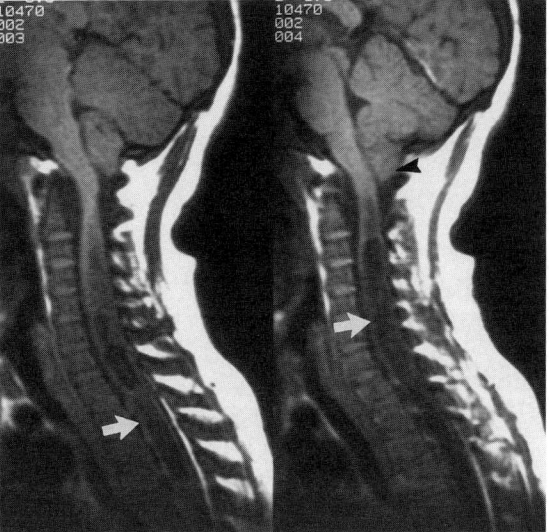

Figure 8.30. Chiari I Malformation—Syrinx. Altered cerebrospinal fluid flow dynamics around the foramen magnum from tonsillar ectopia (*arrowhead*) in this Chiari I malformation has resulted in cervical cord syrinx (*arrows*).

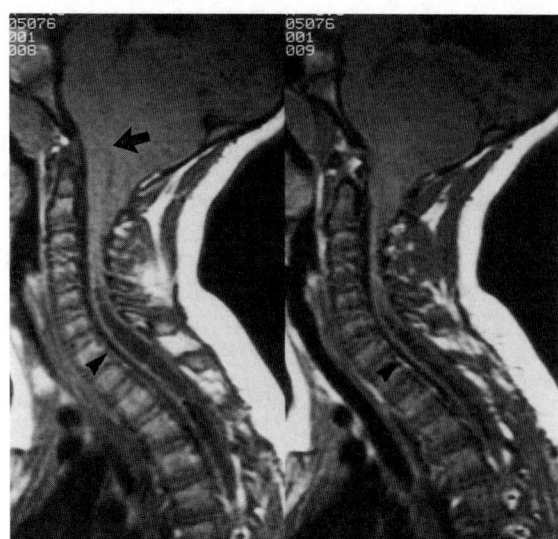

Figure 8.31. Chiari II Malformation—Syrinx. Sagittal T1WI show features of Chiari II malformation with syrinx formation in the cervical cord (*arrowheads*). Note the more crowded appearance of the posterior fossa as compared with the Chiari I malformation shown in Figure 8.30. The cisterna magna is obliterated and the fourth ventricle (*arrow*) is effaced.

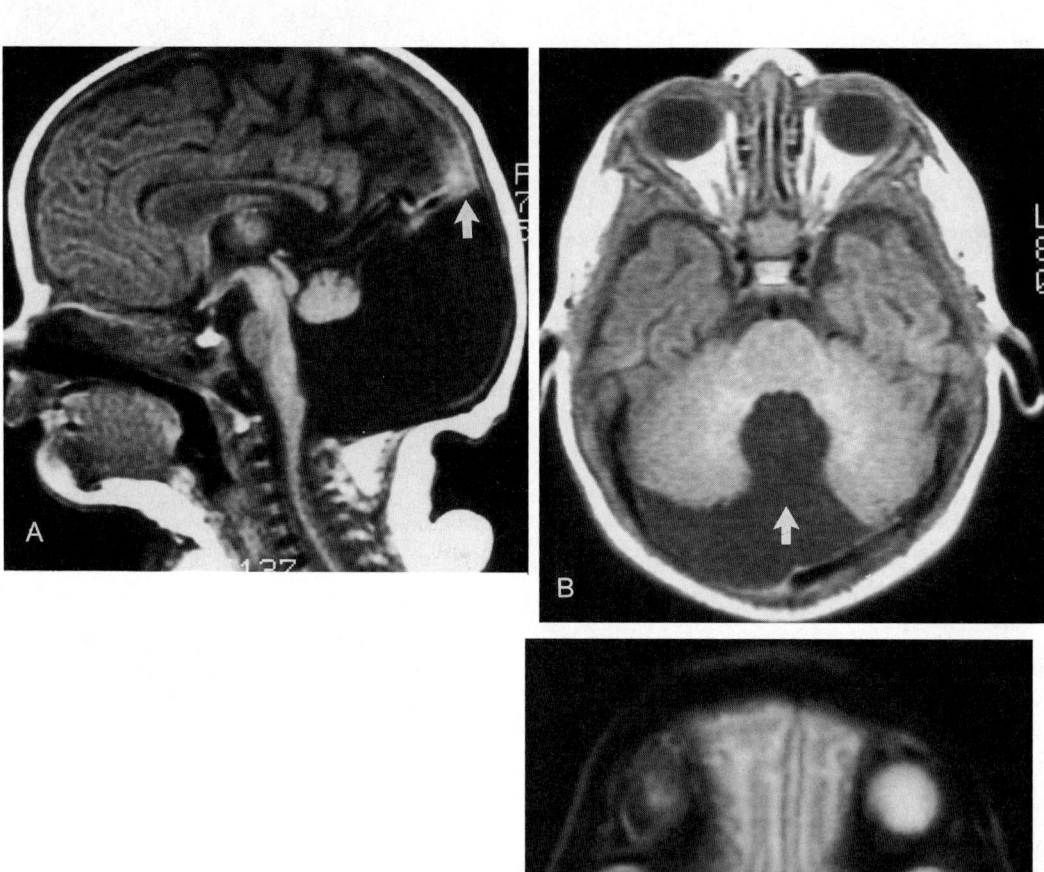

Figure 8.32. Dandy-Walker Malformation. A. Dandy-Walker malformation characteristically demonstrates a cystic dilated fourth ventricle and vermian agenesis, as demonstrated on this sagittal T1WI. The posterior fossa is enlarged, as seen by a high torcular insertion (*arrow*). **B.** Axial T1WI shows the cystically dilated fourth ventricle (*arrow*). **C.** This case demonstrates some of the features of Dandy-Walker malformation, but there is asymmetric hypoplasia of the right cerebellar hemisphere.

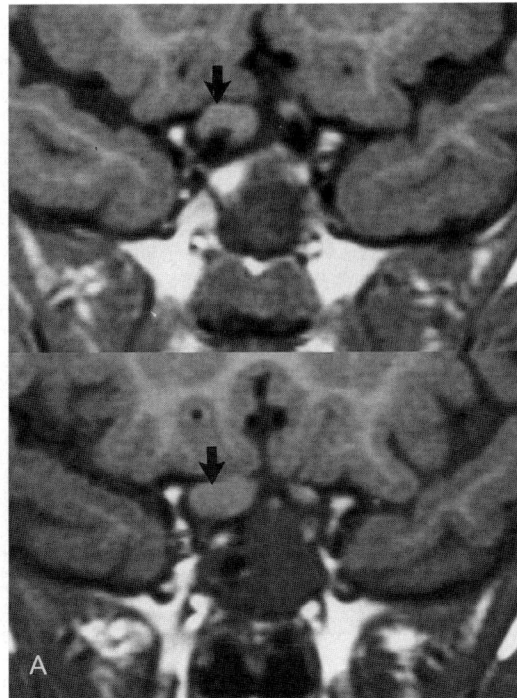

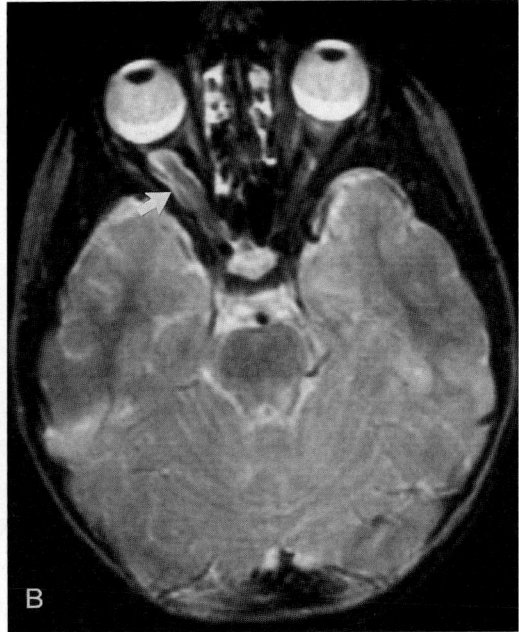

Figure 8.33. Neurofibromatosis—Optic Glioma. A. Optic nerve gliomas in NFI are fusiform enlargements of the nerve on thin-section coronal T1WI (*arrows*). **B.** An axial T2WI at the midorbit level shows the fusiform enlargement of the right optic nerve (*arrow*). (Courtesy of Dr. Gamal Boutros.)

Table 8.5. Neurofibromatosis: Type I versus Type II

	Neurofibromatosis I von Recklinghausen's	Neurofibromatosis II*
Epidemiology		
Incidence	1/4000	1/50,000
Age at presentation	Childhood	young adult
Affected chromosome	17	22*
CNS Findings		
Acoustic schannomas	No	Yes*
Meningiomas	No	Yes
Spinal glial tumors	No	Yes
White matter changes	Yes	No
Dural ectasia	Yes	No
Optic & other gliomas	Yes	Yes
Skeletal Findings		
Sphenoid dysplasia	Yes	No
Thinning long bone cortex (ribbon ribs)	Yes	No
Other Findings		
Plexiform neurofibromas	Yes	No
Café au lait spots	Typically 6 or more	Rare
Iris hamartoma (Lisch nodules)	Yes	No
Vascular stenoses	Yes	No

* For NF II, use the number 2 as your mnemonic: NF 2 patients typically have 2 (bilateral) acoustic schwannomas and an abnormal chromosome 22.

as hyperintense signal on T2WI. Other parenchymal gliomas are also seen (Fig. 8.34).

Hyperintense foci in deep cerebral and cerebellar white matter are commonly seen on T2WI. These lesions wax and wane when analyzed over serial scans, do not cause mass effect, and do not enhance (Figs. 8.35, 8.36). In general, the lesions regress with increasing age. Lesion progression in a child older than 10 years warrants close follow-up to rule out neoplastic transformation. Significant enlargement, new mass effect, and gadolinium enhancement may herald degeneration into gliomas. The exact histology of these lesions is not known. The globus pallidi also exhibit abnormal hyperintense signal on both T1WI and T2WI.

Neurofibromatosis I has other manifestations, which include plexiform neurofibromas (rope-like masses of neural tissue in subcutaneous soft tissues), vascular lesions, aneurysms, ectasias stenoses, moya-moya syndrome, spinal lesions (neurofibromas, meningoceles, scoliosis), and osseous lesions (sphenoid/lambdoid dysplasia, pseudoarthrosis, rib abnormalities).

Neurofibromatosis II (NF-II), also called neurofibromatosis, differs considerably from NF I. The key features of NF II are bilateral acoustic schwannomas and meningiomas (Fig. 8.37). Neurofibromatosis II also has spinal manifestations, which include neurofibromas, meningiomas, ependymomas, and schwannomas of other cranial nerves.

Tuberous Sclerosis is another distinctive neurocutaneous disorder. The skin lesions are adenoma sebaceum and ash-leaf spots. Brain lesions consist of subependy-

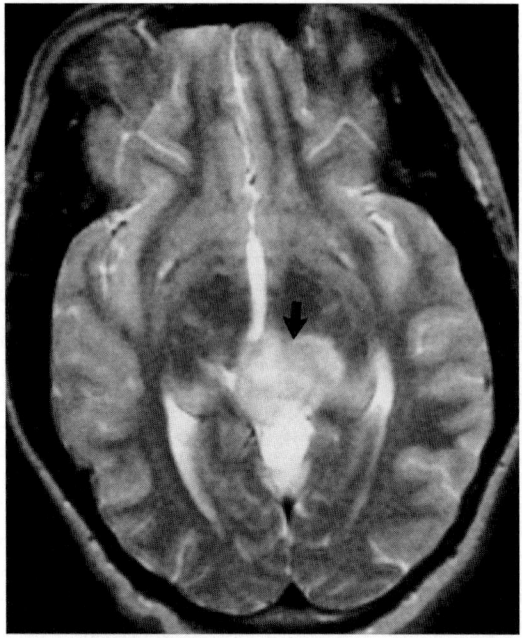

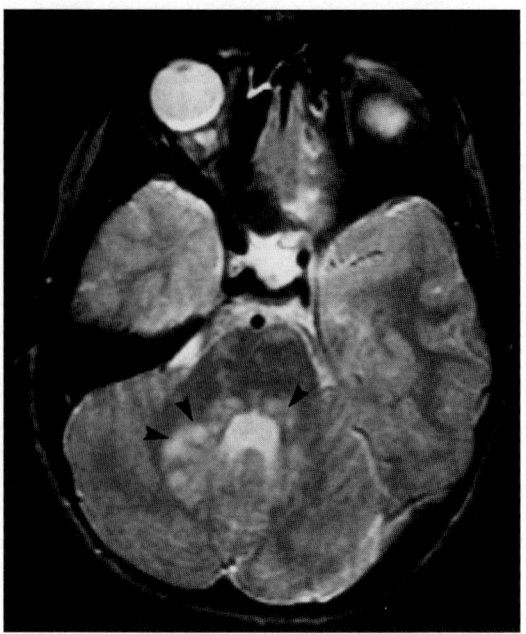

Figure 8.34. Neurofibromatosis—Glioma. Axial T2WI shows an exophitic tectal glioma (*arrow*) in this patient with NFI.

Figure 8.35. Neurofibromatosis—Nonneoplastic Lesions. T2WI of patient with NFI shows multifocal area of hyperintense signal in both middle cerebellar peduncles (*arrowheads*).

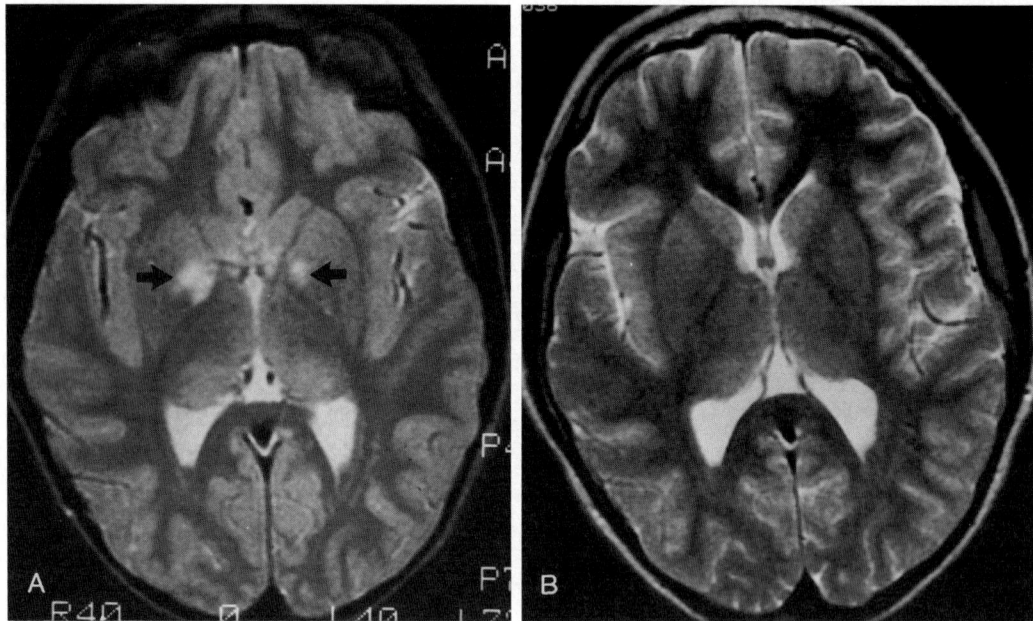

Figure 8.36. Neurofibromatosis—Nonneoplastic Lesions. A. Hyperintense foci on T2WI are seen in the basal ganglia in this patient with NFI (*arrows*). **B.** The lesions are seen to regress on a 4-year follow-up scan.

mal hamartomas and cortical tubers (Fig. 8.38). Some of the subependymal nodules near the foramen of Monro can enlarge, cause mass effect, and invade brain tissue. Locally aggressive nodules are called subependymal "giant cell" astrocytomas (Fig. 8.39).

Both cortical and subepndymal lesions can undergo age-dependent calcification. Subependymal nodules represent hamartomas, and before calcification, they tend to parallel white matter signal on MR images. Sub-

ependymal nodules are distinct from heterotopic gray matter in their signal characteristics and tendency to calcify. Calcified nodules may be isointense or hyperintense on T1WI. Enhancement of nodules at the foramen of Monro does not determine malignant transformation to a giant cell astrocytomas, rather look for brain invasion to make this distinction. Cortical tubers are usually hypointense on T1WI and hyperintense on T2WI, and they may calcify.

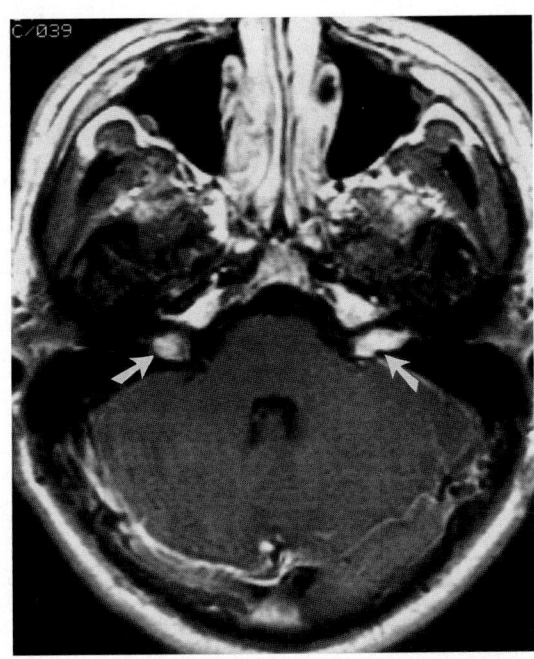

Figure 8.37. Neurofibromatosis II. Axial T1-weighted postgadolinium image in a patient with neurofibromatosis type II shows bilateral enhancing acoustic schwannomas of the eighth cranial nerves (*arrows*). (Courtesy of Dr. Ronald Shallat.)

Sturge-Weber Syndrome, or encephalotrigeminal angiomatosis, features angiomatous lesions of the skin and meninges. The facial lesion (a skin angioma called a port-wine nevus) appears in the ophthalmic division of the fifth cranial nerve. The pathologic entity seen in the brain is pial angiomatosis. These pial angiomas undergo age-dependent calcification and appear on CT scans as gyral cortical calcifications. The pial angiomatous results in chronic ischemia of the gray matter, leading to gyral atrophy and underlying gliosis.

Another sequela of pial angiomatosis is alteration of normal superficial cortical venous drainage with concomitant enlargement of deep and subependymal veins (Fig. 8.40). These dilated subependymal veins can mimic arteriovenous malformations. Gadolinium enhancement can reveal the full extent of pial angiomatosis and is helpful in cases where calcification atrophy has not yet occurred (Fig. 8.41). Young children may show subtle hypointensity of the underlying white matter on T2WI without calcification of the cortex. Ipsilateral choroid plexus hypertrophy is another feature of this entity (Fig. 8.42). Use gradient-recalled echo technique on MR images to accentuate the presence of calcium (Fig. 8.43).

von Hippel-Lindau Syndrome is an inherited disorder consisting of retinal angiomas, and cerebellar and spinal hemangioblastomas. Hemangioblastomas are considered benign neoplasms, and the presence of multifocal spinal cord nodules near the pia-arachnoid surface represents multicentric tumors, not drop metastasis.

Characteristic features of cerebellar hemangioblastomas include a well-circumscribed cystic lesion with an

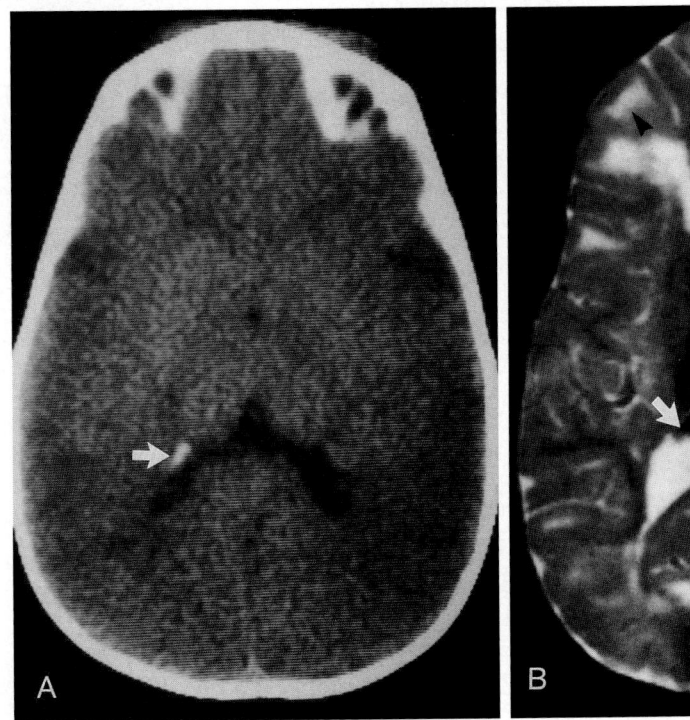
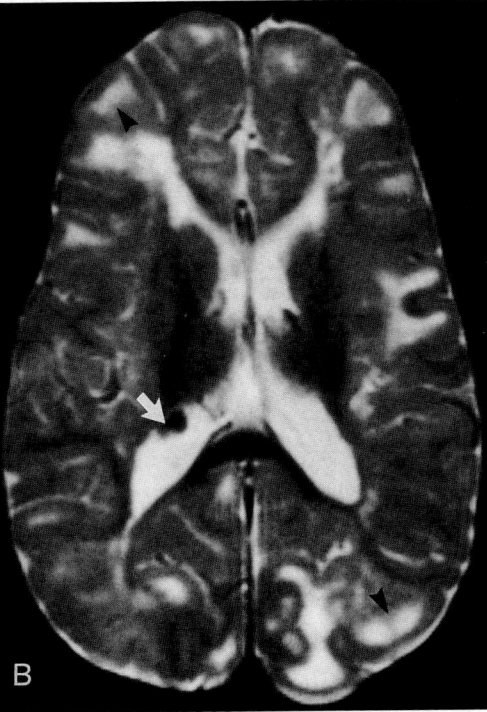

Figure 8.38. Tuberous Sclerosis. A. An axial slice from a CT in a patient with tuberous sclerosis shows a single calcified ependymal tuber (*arrow*). **B.** T2 weighted MR shows the same ependymal tuber seen on the CT scan. The tuber is seen as low signal intensity nodule (*arrow*). The subcortical tubers are also well demonstrated (*arrowheads*).

Figure 8.39. Tuberous Sclerosis. A. In another case of tuberous sclerosis, the sagittal T1WI demonstrates a giant cell astrocytoma arising in the region of the foramen of Monro (*arrow*). **B.** Axial T2WI of a giant cell astrocytoma with concomitant hydrocephalus. The lesion (*arrows*) is heterogeneous signal intensity.

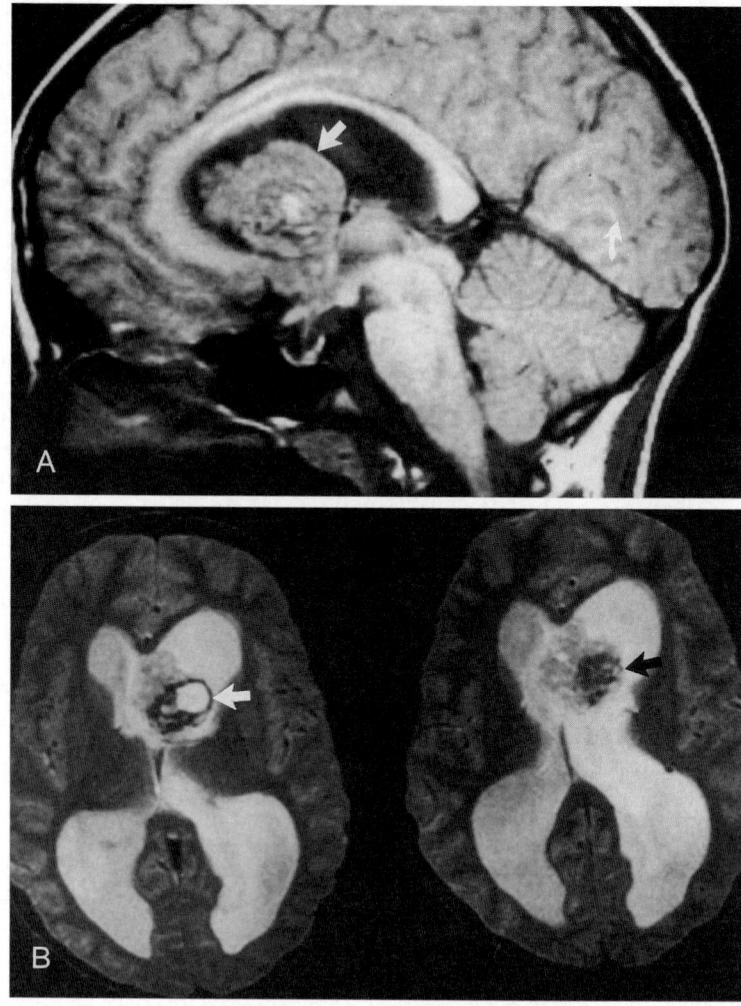

Figure 8.40. Sturge-Weber Syndrome. Axial T2WI illustrates the dilated ependymal veins seen in Sturge-Weber syndrome. The veins (*arrow*) are serpentine flow voids bordering the ependymal surface of the ventricle .

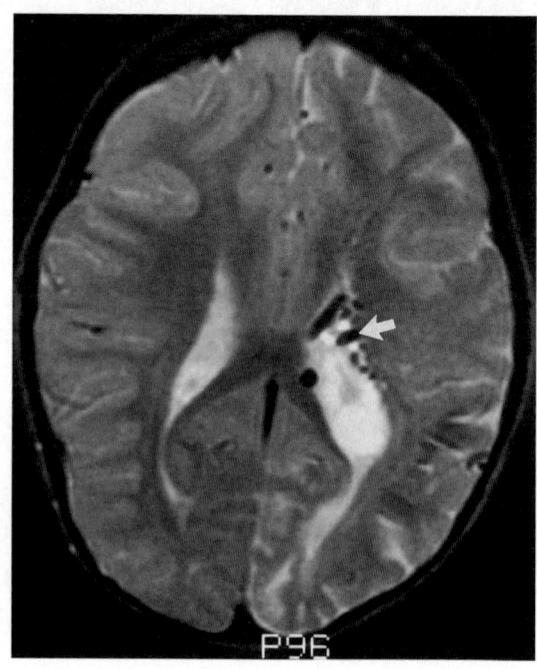

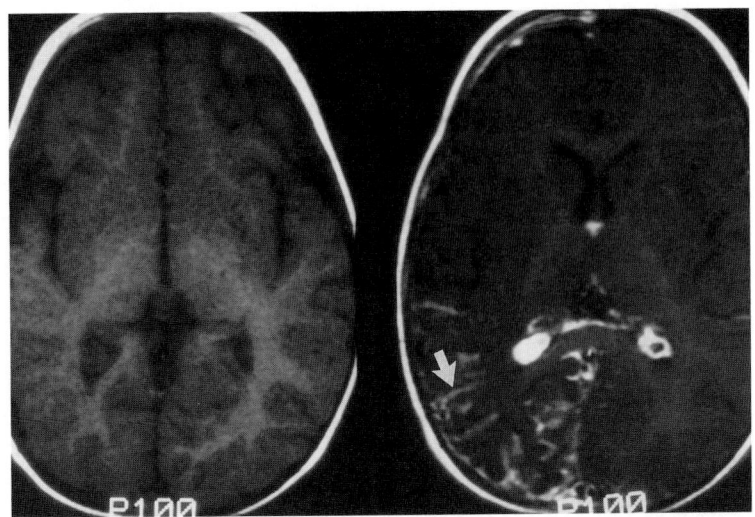

Figure 8.41. Sturge-Weber Syndrome. A young patient with Sturge-Weber syndrome with before (left) and after (right) gadolinium T1WI demonstrating the full extent of pial angiomatosis (*arrow*). Gadolinium may be particularly useful in younger patients who do not yet demonstrate cortical calcifications. (Courtesy of Dr. Jean Hayward.)

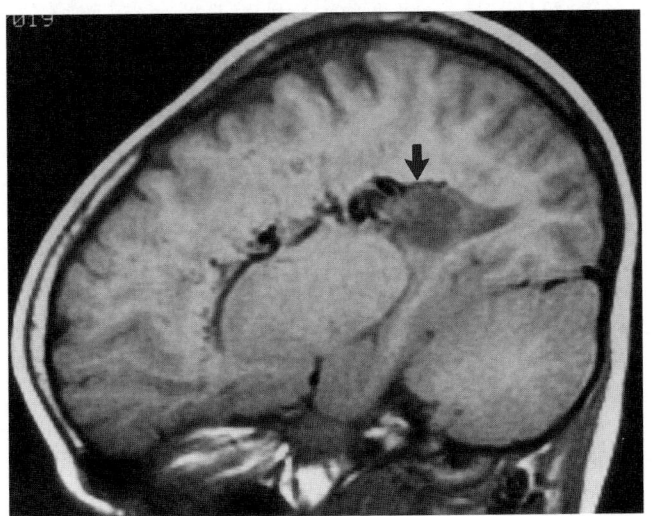

Figure 8.42. Sturge-Weber Syndrome. Sagittal T1WI of a patient with Sturge-Weber syndrome shows ipsilateral choroid plexus hypertrophy (*arrow*).

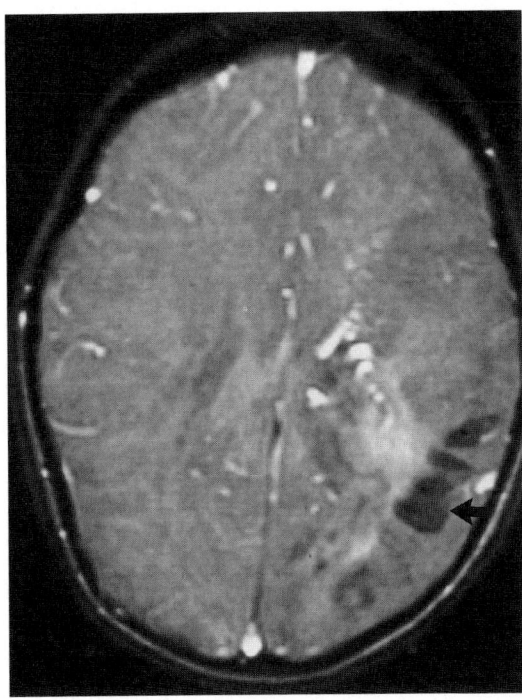

Figure 8.43. Sturge-Weber Syndrome. Gradient-recalled echo images accentuate the magnetic susceptibility artifact associated with the cortical calcifications (*arrow*) of Sturge-Weber syndrome.

enhancing mural nodule. Other appearances include solid tumors, solid masses with central cysts, and a singular cyst (Figs. 8.44, 8.45). Another helpful finding is a large blood vessel leading to the nodule. The small multifocal hemangioblastoma nodules are seen near the pial surface of the cerebellum or spinal cord (Fig. 8.46).

Although they are considered benign neoplasms, hemangioblastomas recur at rates of up to 25%. Additionally, these vascular lesions are prone to sudden spontaneous hemorrhage. Gadolinium-enhanced MR imaging is the examination of choice for preoperative evaluation. Other associations with von Hippel-Lindau syndrome include renal cell carcinoma, and angiomas of the liver and kidney.

Figure 8.44. von Hippel-Lindau Syndrome. Axial T1WI in a patient with von Hippel-Lindau syndrome. The left image is pregadolinium and the right image is postgadolinium injection. Some of the lesions are cystic, and one of the enhancing foci (*arrow*) was seen to represent a mural nodule on a lower image.

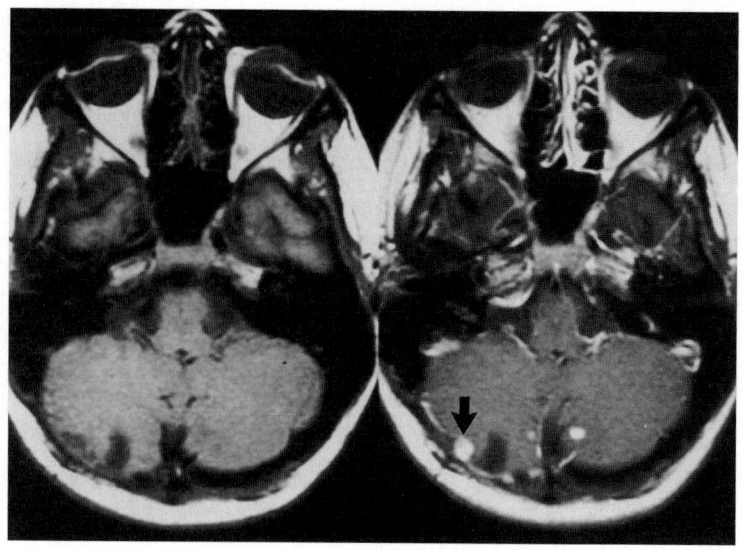

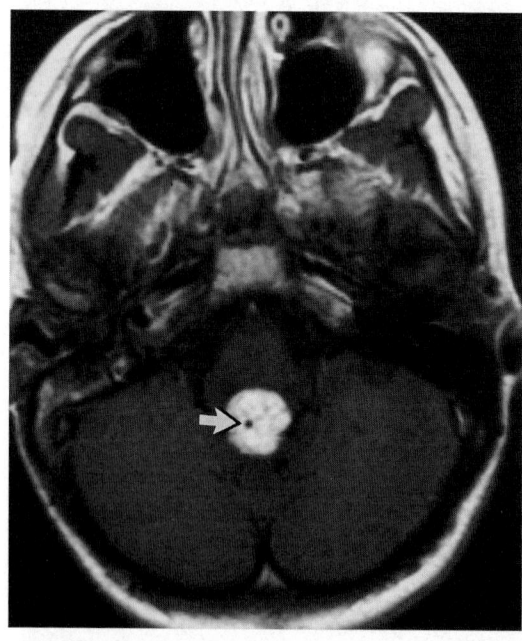

Figure 8.45. von Hippel-Lindau Syndrome. Von Hippel-Lindau syndrome has a variable appearance, as demonstrated in this case of a solid-enhancing mass in the fourth ventricle. A central speck of hypointensity represents a blood vessel (*arrow*). (Courtesy of Dr. Nora Wu.)

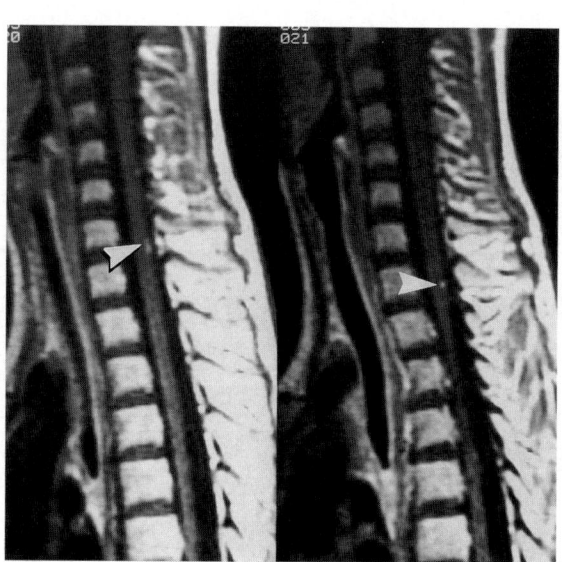

Figure 8.46. von Hippel-Lindau Syndrome—Spinal Cord Hemangioblastoma. Multicentric pial-based hemangioblastomas (*arrowheads*) are seen on T1-weighted, gadolinium-enhanced thoracic spine images as punctate-enhancing foci.

Suggested Readings

Barkovich AJ. Pediatric Neuroimaging. 2nd ed. New York: Raven Press, 1995.

Barkovich AJ. MR and CT evaluation of profound neonatal and infantile asphyxia. AJNR 1992;13:959–972.

Barkovich AJ, Truwit CL. Brain damage from perinatal asphyxia. AJNR 1990;11:1087–1096.

Barkovich AJ, Beatrice LH, et al. Prediction of neuromotor outcome in perinatal asphyxia: evaluation of MR scoring systems. AJNR 1998;19:143–149.

Brodsky MC, Glasier CM. Optic nerve hypoplasia: clinical significance of associated central nervous system abnormalities on magnetic resonance imaging. Arch Ophtalmol 1993; 111:66–74.

Rorke LB, Zimmerman RA. Prematurity, and destructive lesions in utero. AJNR 1992;13:517–536.

Smirniotopoulos JG, Murphy FM. The phakomatoses. AJNR 1992;13:725–746.

Truwit CL, Lempert TE. Pediatric Neuroimaging: A Casebook Approach. DPS Press, distributed by Williams & Wilkins, Baltimore, 1992.

9
Head and Neck Imaging

Jerome A. Barakos

"Head and neck" is a collective term used to describe the extracranial structures, including the sinonasal cavity, skull base, pharynx, oral cavity, larynx, neck, orbit, and temporal bone. The head and neck region encompasses a tremendous spectrum of tissues in a compact space with almost every organ system represented, including the digestive, respiratory, nervous, osseous, and vascular systems. Because of this anatomic complexity, the head and neck region is an area approached with considerable trepidation. However, accurate assessment of this area can be accomplished by understanding both the normal anatomy and the scope of pathologic entities that may occur. We will begin our discussion by considering lesions of the paranasal sinuses and nasal cavity. This will be followed by a review of the skull base, the deep spaces of the neck, lymph nodes, orbit, and finally congenital head and neck lesions.

IMAGING METHODS

Both HRCT and MR can be used to display exquisitely the normal and pathologic anatomy of the head and neck (1,2). Although each modality has advantages and disadvantages, the selection of CT versus MR is often based on which technique the patient is more likely to tolerate. If a patient has difficulty handling their oral secretions because of prior head and neck surgery, particularly following tracheotomy or partial glossectomy, they may have significant hardship lying still for the time required for MR scanning. In such cases, the rapid imaging time of spiral CT is more likely to yield a study unmarred by motion artifact.

Because calcification is better depicted with CT, this is the modality of choice when looking for obstructing salivary ductal calculi, or for the detection of fractures. In contrast, MR provides outstanding sensitivity for the discrimination of soft tissues, and often better demonstrates the full extent of pathology. At the same time, the superior tissue contrast discrimination of MR allows for enhanced diagnostic specificity. The direct multiplanar capability of MR may also provide for improved evaluation of pathologic entities. For example, because of the axial orientation of the palate, floor of mouth, and skull base, sagittal and coronal imaging are invaluable in optimally assessing these areas.

PARANASAL SINUSES AND NASAL CAVITY

Sinusitis

Inflammatory disease is the most common pathology involving the paranasal sinuses and nasal cavity. Mild mucosal thickening, primarily within the maxillary and ethmoid sinuses, is not uncommon and may be seen in asymptomatic individuals. In contrast, acute sinusitis is characterized by the presence of air-fluid levels and is typically caused by a viral upper respiratory tract infection. In chronic sinusitis, changes include mucoperiostal thickening as well as osseous thickening of the sinus walls. Soft-tissue findings suggestive of sinusitis are most readily detected on the T2WI, as they are often high in signal. An exception is chronic sinus secretions that have become so desiccated that they yield no signal, and may mimic an aerated sinus. These sinus concretions and the bony wall thickening associated with chronic sinusitis will be most easily appreciated on CT.

Endoscopic sinonasal surgery, used for the evaluation and treatment of inflammatory sinonasal disease, is being performed with increasing frequency (3). Direct coronal sinus CT provides exquisite definition of sinonasal anatomy and provides pre-endoscopic sinus assessment (Fig. 9.1). Knowledge of the anatomy of the lateral wall of the nasal cavity and routes of mucociliary drainage of the paranasal sinuses is critical to understanding patterns of inflammatory sinonasal disease. A major area of mucociliary drainage is the middle meatus, known as the osteomeatal unit. It is important to note that disease limited to the infundibulum of the maxillary ostium will result in isolated obstruction of the maxillary sinus. In contrast, a lesion located in the hiatus semilunaris (middle meatus) results in obstruction of the ipsilateral

Figure 9.1. Osteomeatal Unit (OMU). Line drawing in coronal plane demonstrates the anatomy of the OMU. Lines with arrows show the normal route of mucociliary clearance. Infundibular (*dashed line*) and OMU (*solid line*) patterns of obstruction are shown. Coronal CT far surpasses plain sinus films in evaluating problems of the OMU for potential relief through endoscopic surgery. (From RW Babbel, HR Harnsberger, J Sonkens, S Hunt. Recurring patterns of inflammatory sinonasal disease demonstrated on screening sinus CT. AJNR 1992;13:903–912.)

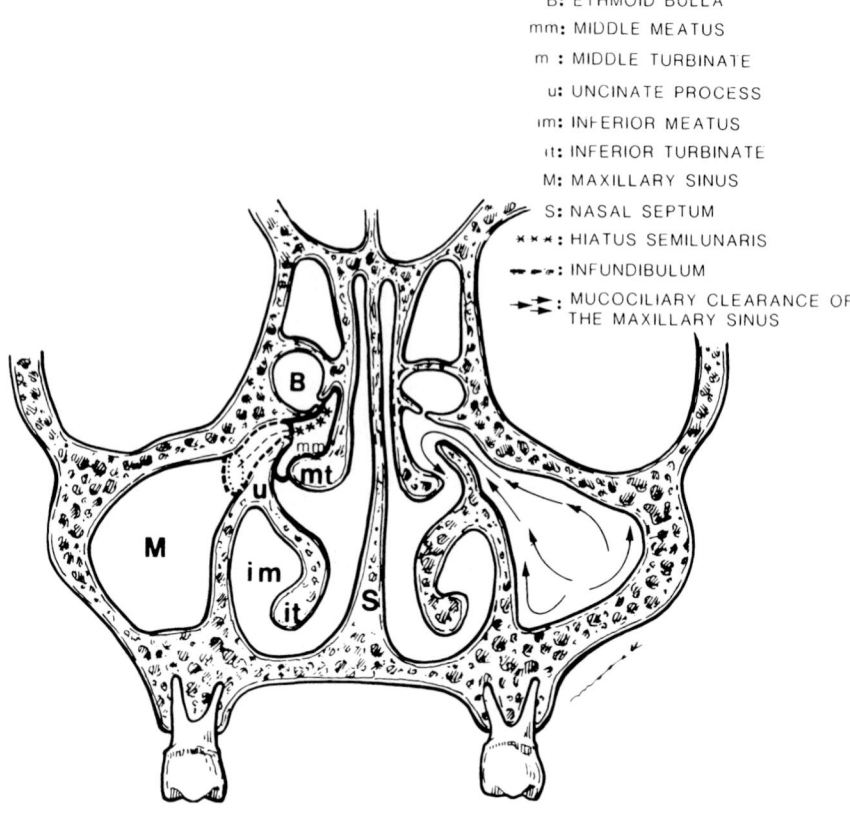

B: ETHMOID BULLA
mm: MIDDLE MEATUS
m : MIDDLE TURBINATE
u: UNCINATE PROCESS
im: INFERIOR MEATUS
it: INFERIOR TURBINATE
M: MAXILLARY SINUS
S: NASAL SEPTUM
×××: HIATUS SEMILUNARIS
▪▪▪: INFUNDIBULUM
→: MUCOCILIARY CLEARANCE OF THE MAXILLARY SINUS

maxillary sinus, anterior and middle ethmoid air cells, and the frontal sinus. This last pattern of sinonasal disease has been described as the osteomeatal pattern of obstruction. This pattern is significant because it indicates that one's attention should be directed to identifying the offending lesion within the hiatus semilunaris, rather than simply describing diffuse sinus disease.

Several common complications are associated with sinusitis, including inflammatory polyps, mucous retention cysts, and mucoceles.

Inflammatory Polyps. Chronic inflammation leads to mucosal hyperplasia, which results in mucosal redundancy and polyp formation. Most often these polyps blend imperceptibly with the mucoperiosteal thickening and cannot be clearly differentiated. When an antral polyp expands to the point where it prolapses through the sinus ostium, it is referred to as an antrochoanal polyp. Although these polyps may not be associated with chronic sinusitis, they are similar to inflammatory polyps in that they represent areas of reactive mucosal thickening. Their characteristic appearance is that of a soft-tissue mass extending from the maxillary sinus to fill the ipsilateral nasal cavity and nasopharynx. Often the ostium of the maxillary sinus will be enlarged in relation to the mass effect of the polyp. The importance in recognizing such a lesion is that if it is surgically snared like a nasal polyp, without regard for its antral stalk, it will recur.

Mucous Retention Cysts simply represent obstructed mucous glands within the mucosal lining. These lesions have a characteristic rounded appearance, measuring one to several cm in diameter, with the maxillary sinus being most commonly involved. These lesions are commonly recognized in asymptomatic individuals.

Mucocele is similar to a retention cyst, but instead of a single mucous gland becoming obstructed, the entire sinus is obstructed. This typically occurs because of a mass obstructing the draining sinus ostium. The characteristic feature of a mucocele is frank expansion of the sinus with associated bony thinning and remodeling. The frontal sinus is the sinus most commonly affected, but any sinus may be involved. If the mucocele becomes infected, it demonstrates peripheral enhancement and is called a mucopyocele.

Tumors

Inverting Papilloma. A variety of papillomas occur within the nasal cavity, but most attention has focused on the inverting papilloma. These papillomas are named based on their histologic appearance. In this condition, the neoplastic nasal epithelium inverts and grows into the underlying mucosa. These papillomas are not believed to be associated with allergy or chronic infection because they are almost invariably unilateral in location. Inverting papillomas occur exclusively on the lateral nasal wall centered on the hiatus semilunaris. Because an increased association with squamous cell carcinoma exists, it is recommended that these lesions be surgically resected with wide mucosal margins.

Juvenile Nasopharyngeal Angiofibroma are typically seen in adolescent males presenting with epistaxis. The tumor arises from fibrovascular stroma of the nasal wall adjacent to the sphenopalatine foramen. This is a benign tumor that can be very locally aggressive. In an adolescent male presenting with a nasal mass and epistaxis, it is important to have a high clinical suspicion for this lesion, as life-threatening hemorrhage may result if a biopsy or limited resection is attempted. The tumor characteristically fills the nasopharynx and bows the posterior wall of the maxillary sinus forward. The tumor enhances markedly with contrast administration on CT, differentiating the lesion from the rarer lymphangioma. Preoperatively, interventional radiology may play a role in embolization of these lesions, making them less vascular and facilitating surgical resection.

Malignancies. The tissues within the paranasal sinuses and nasal cavity that give rise to malignancies include squamous epithelium, lymphoid tissue, and minor salivary glands. The corresponding malignancies are therefore squamous cell carcinoma, lymphoma, and minor salivary tumors. Because the entire upper aerodigestive tract is lined with squamous epithelium, it follows that *squamous cell carcinoma* is the most common malignancy (80–90%) of not only the paranasal sinuses and nasal cavity, but of the entire head and neck. Squamous cell carcinoma of the sinuses is often clinically silent until it is quite advanced. Early symptoms are usually related to obstructive sinusitis. Imaging findings consist of an opacified sinus with associated bony wall destruction. These findings are nonspecific, and do not allow differentiation from non-Hodgkin's lymphoma or a minor salivary gland malignancy. The presence of constitutional symptoms with prominent head and neck or systemic adenopathy may suggest the diagnosis of lymphoma.

Minor salivary glands are dispersed throughout the upper aerodigestive tract, but are most highly concentrated in the palate. Any of these minor salivary glands found throughout the head and neck may give rise to salivary neoplasms. In contrast to parotid gland salivary neoplasms, the majority of which are benign, most minor salivary neoplasms are malignant. The most common salivary malignancies include adenoid cystic carcinoma, adenocarcinoma, and mucoepidermoid carcinoma.

An *esthesioneuroblastoma* is an additional malignancy that should be mentioned when describing lesions of the nasal cavity. The esthesioneuroblastoma is a tumor that arises from the neurosensory receptor cells of the olfactory nerve and mucosa. Thus, this lesion may originate anywhere from the cribiform plate to the turbinates. This tumor is often quite destructive by the time of diagnosis and is found high within the nasal vault (Fig. 9.2). Involvement of the cribiform plate with extension into the anterior cranial fossa is not uncommon.

In assessing the size and extent of sinonasal cavity pathology, it is often difficult to differentiate the offending lesion from associated obstructed sinus secretions. In such instances, heavily T2-weighted sequences are of value because, in general, sinus secretions will be brighter than the malignancy, which is often isointense with respect to muscle.

SKULL BASE

The skull base extends from the nose anteriorly to the occipital protuberance posteriorly and is composed of

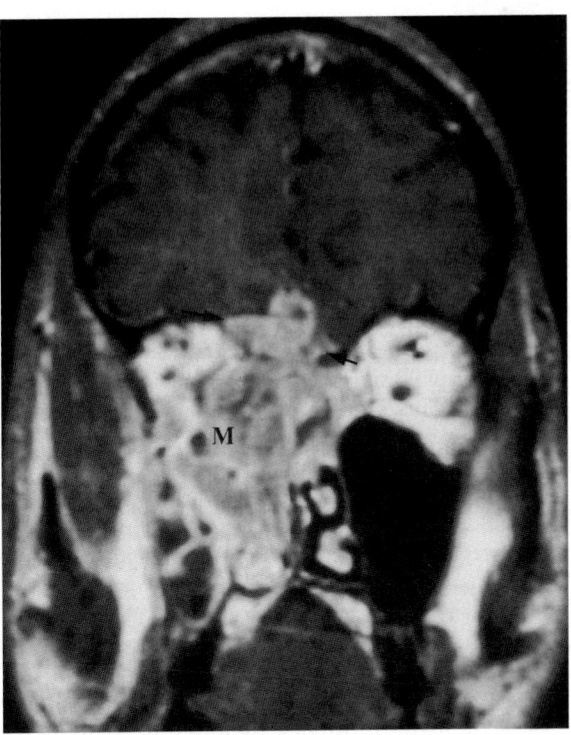

Figure 9.2. Esthesioneuroblastoma. Coronal fat-suppressed post-gadolinium T1WI. A large destructive mass (*M*) in the nasal cavity extends through the cribriform plate into the anterior cranial fossa (*arrows*). This degree of frank bony destruction is unusual for squamous cell carcinoma and lymphoma.

five bones: the ethmoid, sphenoid, occipital, temporal, and frontal bones (4). The skull base contains many foramina through which both vascular and neural structures pass. Because the skull base has an undulating surface with a horizontal orientation, coronal or sagittal images are valuable in its evaluation.

Tumors of the Skull Base

Tumors may arise that are intrinsic to the skull base. Additionally, an extrinsic lesion may extend to involve the skull base either from above or below. Any lesion from the paranasal sinuses and nasal cavity already described may extend to involve the skull base. Other lesions that may extend to involve the skull base include paragangliomas, neural sheath tumors (schwannoma and neurofibroma), and meningiomas. Although various primary malignant neoplasms of the skull base are described in the following, most malignant lesions of the skull base are metastatic in origin.

Primary Malignant Neoplasms are relatively uncommon, comprising only about 2–3% of skull base tumors. The three most common primary malignant tumors are chondrosarcoma, osteogenic sarcoma, and chordoma. *Chondrosarcomas* are malignant tumors that develop from cartilage. Because the skull base is preformed in cartilage, there is a predilection for chondrosarcoma to involve the skull base. A preferred site of origin is parasellar in location at the petroclival junction. *Osteogenic sarcoma* is typically the result of prior radiation therapy or malignant transformation of Paget's disease. *Chordoma* is a bone neoplasm that arises from remnants of the primitive notochord. These tumors may be found anywhere along the craniospinal axis; typically 35% of lesions involve the clivus, 50% the sacrum, and 15% the vertebral bodies. Radiographically, this lesion is characterized as a midline destructive bony lesion with predilection for the spheno-occipital synchondrosis. On a sagittal image, the spheno-occipital synchondrosis is occasionally seen as a horizontal line in the midclivus, midway between the sella and the basion (tip of clivus). The skull base, like any bone, may also be affected by metastases, myeloma, plasmacytoma, fibrous dysplasia, and Paget's disease.

Lesions of the jugular foramen are most commonly paragangliomas and are discussed below in the carotid space section. These patients commonly present with pulsatile tinnitus and a conductive hearing loss. These tumors are best initially evaluated with CT. If extension into the jugular fossa is identified, MR is valuable in defining the full extent of the lesion. CT often demonstrates moth-eaten destruction of the bone surrounding the jugular fossa, with MR revealing the typical heterogeneous "salt and pepper" signal related to numerous flow voids. Malignant tumors are often indistinguishable from paragangliomas on CT, but most fail to demonstrate flow voids on MR. Other lesions of the jugular fossa include schwannomas (arising from cranial nerves IX–XI), and meningiomas. These lesions cause a smooth expansion of the jugular foramen with marked enhancement. Additionally, schwannomas may demonstrate cystic components.

Temporal Bone

Although a thorough discussion of the temporal bone is beyond the scope of this chapter, we will focus on some highlights. The most common diseases involving the temporal bone are inflammatory in nature, and include cholesteatomas (5). Eustachian tube dysfunction with resultant decreased intratympanic pressure is believed to be the principal defect responsible for inflammatory disease of the middle ear and mastoid.

Cholesteatoma is an epidermoid cyst composed of desquamating stratified squamous epithelium. These cysts enlarge because of the progressive accumulation of epithelial debris within their lumen. They may be either congenital (2%) or acquired (98%). Congenital cholesteatomas originate from epithelial rests within or adjacent to the temporal bone. Acquired cholesteatomas originate from the stratified squamous epithelium of the tympanic membrane. These begin as localized tympanic membrane retraction pockets. The diagnosis of a cholesteatoma is based on the detection of a soft-tissue mass within the middle ear cavity, typically with associated bony erosion. The superior portion of the tympanic membrane (pars flaccida) retracts easily and is the most common sight for formation of an acquired cholesteatoma. Cholesteatomas arising in this area originate within Prussak's space (superior recess of the tympanic membrane), which is located medial to the pars flaccida between the scutum and the neck of the malleus. Thus

a finding of soft tissue in this region with subtle erosion of the scutum and medial displacement of the ossicles is characteristic of a cholesteatoma. Note that when fluid or inflammatory pathology is present, such as with an otitis media, these changes cannot be differentiated from cholesteatoma, as they have similar densities.

Although most cholesteatomas can be easily diagnosed otoscopically, the clinician cannot judge the size and full extent of the lesion. As a result, CT plays an important role in determining the size of the lesion, as well as the status of the ossicles, the labyrinth, the tegmen, and the facial nerve. MR has a limited role in the evaluation of erosive lesions of the temporal bone because the lack of landmarks does not allow localization of the process, and gives no information concerning the status of the ossicles and other bony structures.

Cholesterol Granuloma, also known as giant cholesterol cyst, is a type of granulation tissue that may involve the petrous apex. These lesions represent petrous apex air cells that have become partially obstructed, and are filled with cholesterol debris and hemorrhagic fluid. Because of their hemorrhagic components, these lesions are characterized by high signal on both T1-weighted and T2-weighted sequences.

SUPRAHYOID HEAD AND NECK

The suprahyoid head and neck is traditionally divided into compartments that include the nasopharynx, oropharynx, and oral cavity (6). Understanding the division between these spaces is essential to accurately determine and describe the full extent of mucosal lesions.

The term *nasopharynx* is frequently misused as a nonspecific term to describe any area in the upper aerodigestive tract. In fact, the nasopharynx refers to a very specific portion of the pharynx. The nasopharynx lies above the oropharynx, and is divided from the oropharynx by a horizontal line drawn along the hard and soft palates. Posteriorly the nasopharynx is bounded by the pharyngeal constrictor muscles and anteriorly by the nasal cavity at the nasal choana (paired funnel-shaped openings between the nasal cavity and the nasopharynx). Below the hard palate lie the *oral cavity* and *oropharynx*. These two areas are divided by a ring of structures that includes the circumvallate papillae (located along the posterior aspect of the tongue), tonsillar pillars, and the soft palate.

These traditional compartments (nasopharynx, oropharynx, and oral cavity) are important for describing the spread of superficial, mucosal-based lesions. In contrast to this division, multiple facial planes divide the deep head and neck into spaces that form true compartments. It is important to realize that these deep spaces are unrelated to the traditional division of the head and neck, and traverse the neck without regard to the traditional divisions. Therefore, when describing deep head and neck lesions, the traditional pharyngeal subdivisions are of limited value. Most radiologists have adapted a spatial approach to the head and neck as described next, popularized by H. Ric Harnsberger.

The deep anatomy of the head and neck is subdivided by layers of the deep cervical fascia into the following spaces:

a) superficial mucosal, b) parapharyngeal, c) carotid, d) parotid, e) masticator, f) retropharyngeal, and g) prevertebral. When evaluating a patient with pathology in the deep head and neck, it is important to determine within which space the pathology lies. Because only a limited number of structures are located within each compartment, these are the structures from which pathology will arise. Therefore, only specific pathology will be found within these separate fascial spaces, markedly limiting the differential diagnosis. For example, the principal structures within the parotid space are the parotid gland and parotid lymph nodes. Consequently, if a parotid space mass is identified, the diagnosis is primarily limited to either a parotid tumor or nodal disease. Each of these seven spaces will be reviewed in detail (Table 9.1). Note that although this spatial division is popular with radiologists, the surgeons and otolaryngologists occasionally use different terms, e.g., retrostyloid space instead of carotid space.

Superficial Mucosal Space

The superficial mucosal space includes all structures on the airway side of the pharyngobasilar fascia. The principle constituent of this space is the mucosa of the upper aerodigestive tract, which consists of squamous epithelium, submucosal lymphatics, and hundreds of minor salivary glands. The pharyngobasilar fascia represents the superior aponeurosis of the superior pharyngeal constrictor muscle, which inserts into the skull base. This tough fascia separates the mucosal space from the surrounding parapharyngeal space. Lesions originating within the superficial mucosal space may invade deep to the mucosal surface, resulting first in lateral displacement and then obliteration of the parapharyngeal space. However, many early lesions that begin within the mucosal space present as only mild mucosal irregularities or asymmetries (Fig. 9.3). This space is easily evaluated by the clinician and thus the radiologist should have a low threshold for suggesting the presence of abnormalities within this space. In children there is frequently prominent adenoidal tissue that fills the nasopharynx. Even in adults, following an upper respiratory infection, prominent mucosal tissue may be noted, and is of little concern as long as there is no invasion of deep facial places and no associated adenopathy (Fig. 9.4).

Table 9.1. Deep Compartments of the Head and Neck

Compartment (Space)	Contents	Pathology
Mucosal	Squamous mucosa Lymphoid tissue (adenoid, lingual tonsils) Minor salivary glands	Nasopharyngeal carcinoma Squamous cell carcinoma Lymphoma Minor salivary gland tumors Juvenile angiofibroma Rhabdomyosarcoma
Parapharyngeal	Fat Trigeminal nerve (V3) Internal maxillary artery Ascending pharyngeal artery	Minor salivary gland tumor Lipoma Cellulitis/abscess Schwannoma
Parotid	Parotid gland Intraparotid lymph nodes Facial nerve (VII) External carotid artery Retromandibular vein	Salivary gland tumors Metastatic adenopathy Lymphoma Parotid cysts
Carotid	Cranial nerves IX–XII Sympathetic nerves Jugular chain nodes Carotid artery Jugular vein	Schwannoma Neurofibroma Paraganglionoma Metastatic adenopathy Lymphoma Cellulitis/abscess Meningioma
Masticator	Muscles of mastication Ramus and body of mandible Inferior alveolar nerve	Odontogenic abscess Osteomyelitis Direct spread of squamous cell carcinoma Lymphoma Minor salivary tumor Sarcoma of muscle or bone
Retropharyngeal	Lymph nodes (lateral and medial retropharyngeal) Fat	Metastatic adenopathy Lymphoma Abscess/cellulitis
Prevertebral	Cervical vertebrae Prevertebral muscles Paraspinal muscles Phrenic nerve	Osseous metastases Chordoma Osteomyelitis Cellulitis Abscess

Benign Lesions. The most common benign lesions arising in the mucosal space are Thornwald cysts and lesions related to minor salivary gland tissue. *Thornwald cysts* are found in the midline and have high intensity on T2WI (Fig. 9.5). They are believed to be remnants of notochordal tissue aberrantly located in the nasopharynx, and have an incidence of approximately 1–2% in normal patients. Lesions arising from minor salivary glands in-

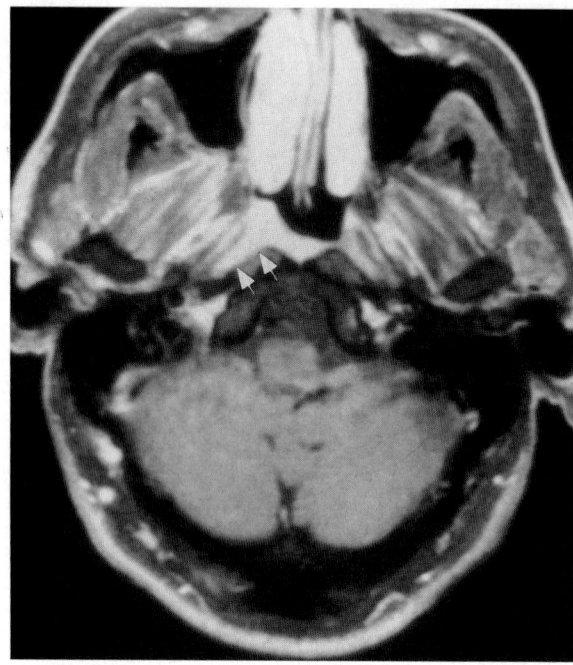

Figure 9.3. Squamous Cell Carcinoma. Axial postgadolinium fat-suppressed T1WI through the level of the nasopharynx. Contrast-enhancing soft tissue fills the right fossa of Rosenmüller (*arrows*). Although this lesion does not obviously invade the underlying parapharyngeal tissues, submandibular nodal metastases were present. This example underscores the point that even mild asymmetries of the mucosal space may represent a malignancy.

clude retention cysts and benign neoplasms. *Retention cysts* represent obstructed glands similar to those found within the paranasal sinuses. The most common benign neoplasm is the benign mixed cell tumor (pleomorphic adenoma). Both of these lesions present as well-circumscribed, rounded lesions that have high signal intensity on T2WI.

Malignant Lesions. The most common malignant neoplasms of the mucosa are squamous cell carcinoma, non-Hodgkin's lymphoma, and minor salivary gland malignancies; of these, squamous cell carcinoma is by far the most common. Unfortunately, these malignancies all appear similar on CT and MR. Initially there is mass effect, often associated with lateral compression or obliteration of the parapharyngeal space, followed by invasion of the skull base. An early triad of radiographic findings consists of *a)* superficial nasopharyngeal mucosal asymmetry, *b)* ipsilateral retropharyngeal adenopathy, and *c)* mastoid opacification. Mastoid opacification is an important early warning sign (Fig. 9.6). This finding is easily detected on T2WI and suggests potential dysfunction of the eustachian tube, frequently the result of tumor infiltration of the tensor and veli palatini muscles. This finding directs the radiologist to carefully evaluate the mucosa of the nasopharynx. Note that both the nasopharynx and the mastoid air cells are included on every head MR scan, and these areas should not be overlooked on routine head studies.

Fat-suppressed, fast spin-echo T2 and contrast-enhanced imaging are useful in detecting and defining the extent of pathology. Additionally, these sequences allow the detection of subtle perineural spread of neoplasms, particularly along cranial nerves extending into the skull base. This is particularly important with adenoid cystic carcinoma, which has a marked propensity for perineural spread and is the most common minor salivary gland malignancy (Fig. 9.7).

Squamous Cell Carcinoma is the most common malignancy of the upper aerodigestive tract. However, a par-

Figure 9.4. Adenoidal Hypertrophy. Axial first and second echo T2 images in a 5-year-old child. Prominent adenoidal tissue (*open arrows*) fills the nasopharynx, expanding the fossa of Rosenmüller bilaterally. Additionally, lateral pharyngeal nodes (*arrowheads*) are clearly visualized. These findings are typical for a child. The age of the patient and the lack of infiltration into the underlying soft tissues indicate that these are normal findings.

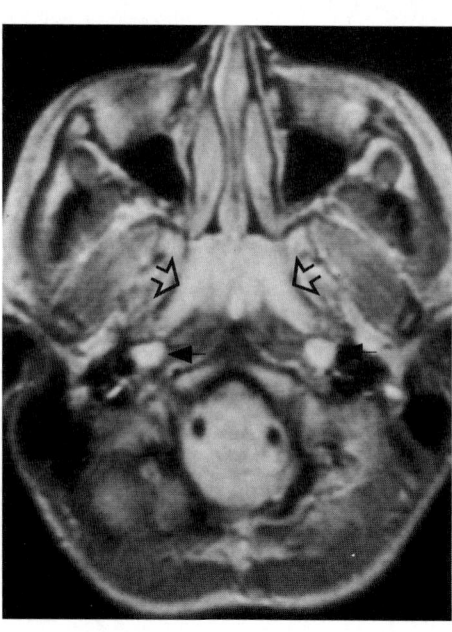
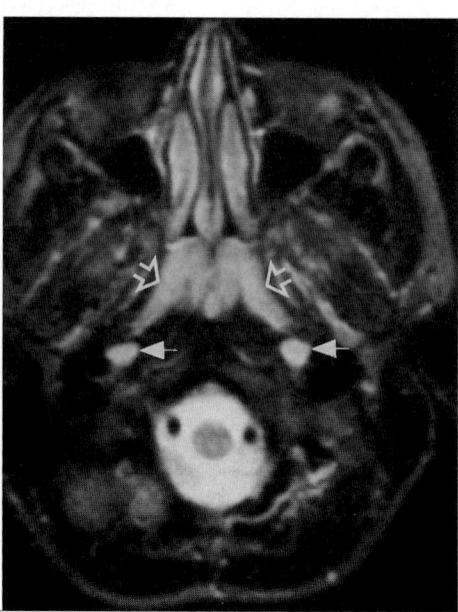

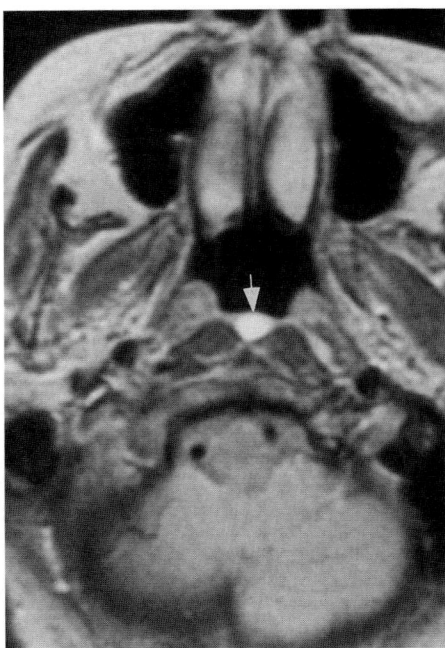
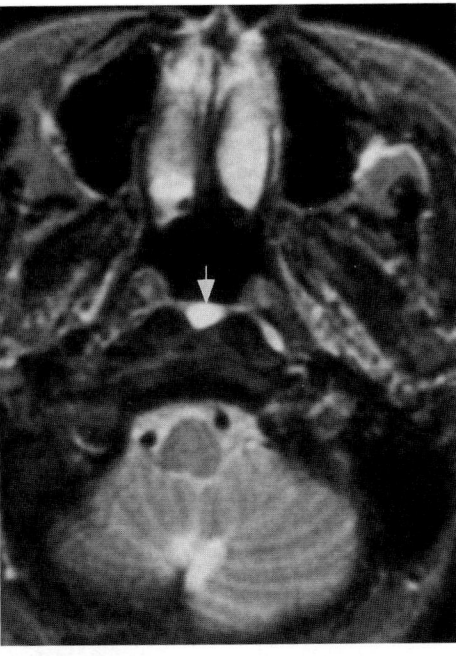

Figure 9.5. Thornwald's Cyst. Axial first and second echo T2WI. A high signal intensity lesion appears in the superficial mucosa (*arrows*). This midline location is characteristic of a Thornwald's cyst, and is found in 1–2% of the normal population.

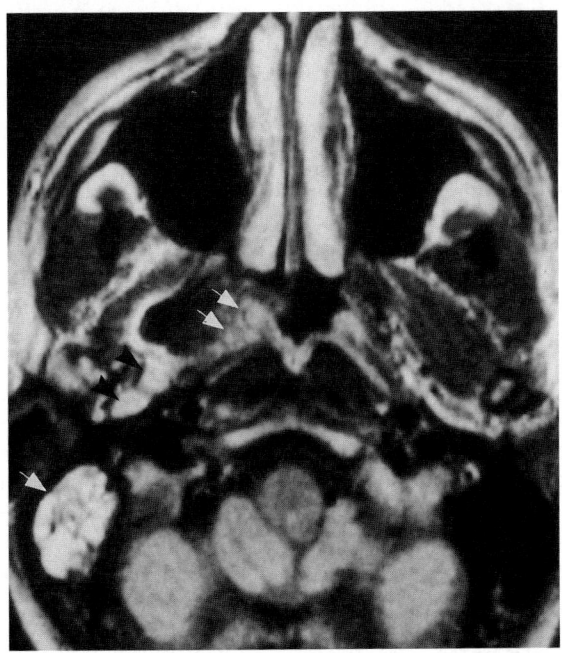

Figure 9.6. Nasopharyngeal Malignancy. Axial postgadolinium T1WI. The triad of nasopharyngeal malignancy consists of a) mucosal mass (*double white arrows*) of the lateral nasopharynx (fossa of Rosenmüller), b) lateral retropharyngeal nodes (*arrowheads*), and c) mastoid opacification (*white arrow*). Mastoid opacification is the result of dysfunction of the eustachian tube due to the nasopharyngeal mass.

ticular variant of squamous cell carcinoma occurs within the nasopharynx, and is termed nasopharyngeal carcinoma. *Nasopharyngeal carcinoma* has several unique features that distinguish it from squamous cell carcinoma. Although squamous cell carcinoma is common in the Caucasian population, nasopharyngeal carcinoma is not, with an incidence of about 1 in 100,000 people per year. This is in contrast to rates 20 times higher in Asia,

particularly in southern regions of China. Although smoking and alcohol abuse are often associated with squamous cell carcinoma, they have no causal association with nasopharyngeal carcinoma. However both environmental and genetic factors do appear to play a role in the genesis of nasopharyngeal carcinoma. Specifically, immunoglobulin-A antibodies to the Epstein-Barr virus have been associated with nasopharyngeal carcinoma.

Lymphoma involving the mucosa cannot be differentiated by imaging from squamous cell or minor salivary gland carcinoma. However, non-Hodgkin's lymphoma frequently has systemic manifestations, with extranodal and extralymphatic sites of involvement that are atypical for these other malignancies. Thus, the presence of a mucosal mass in association with bulky supraclavicular and mediastinal adenopathy as well as splenomegaly would be suggestive of lymphoma.

Parapharyngeal Space

The parapharyngeal space is a triangular, fat-filled compartment that extends from the skull base to the submandibular gland region. It is located at the center of the surrounding spaces, and is compressed or infiltrated in a characteristic fashion by masses originating from the various spaces. The primary importance of the parapharyngeal space is that it serves as an important landmark of mass effect in the deep face. When a lesion occurs in any of the four surrounding spaces, there will be characteristic impressions on the parapharyngeal fat space, which will suggest the space of tumor origin.

The parapharyngeal space is surrounded by the carotid space posteriorly, parotid space laterally, masticator space anteriorly, and the superficial mucosal space medially. Therefore, the parapharyngeal space will be compressed on its medial surface by masses originating from the mucosal surface, anteriorly displaced by carotid sheath masses, medially displaced by parotid masses, and posteriorly and medially displaced by masses within the masti-

Figure 9.7. Recurrent Adenoid Cystic Carcinoma. Coronal postgadolinium fat-suppression T1WI of a 50-year-old patient, status-post resection of nasal septum and turbinates for adenoid cystic carcinoma. A recurrent mass (*M*) extends into the right pterygopalatine fossa (*arrows*). Adenoid cystic carcinoma has a marked propensity for perineural spread, which allows the tumor to extend rapidly into noncontiguous spaces. Once the tumor enters the pterygopalatine fossa, it may extend into the orbit via the inferior orbital foramen, into the cavernous sinus via the foramen rotundum, and into the infratemporal fossa via the pterygomaxillary fissure. Once in the cavernous sinus, tumor can travel back along the cisternal portion of the trigeminal nerve into the brain stem.

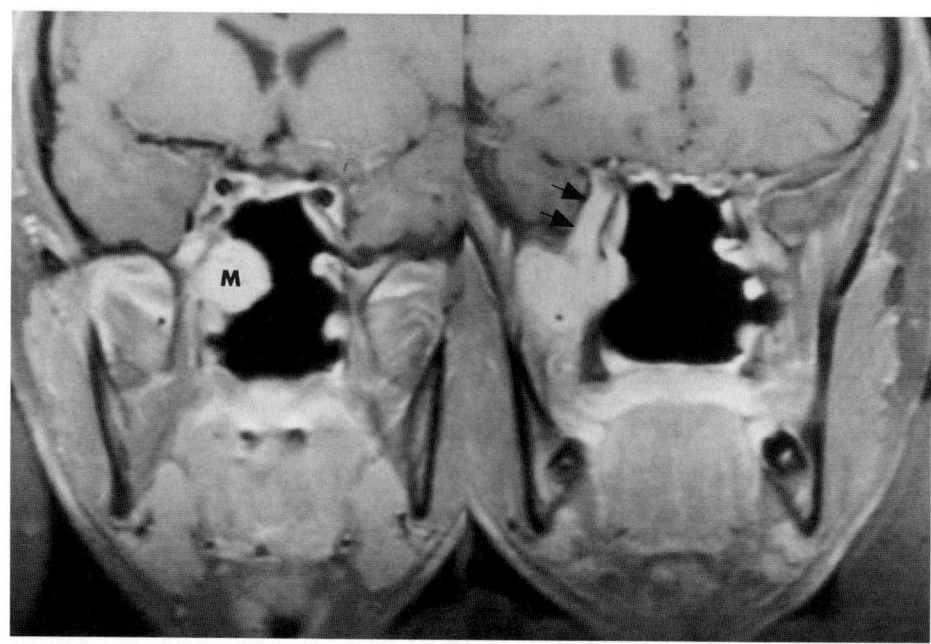

cator space. Thus, by assessing the location and displacement pattern of the parapharyngeal space, one can assign a space of origin to a deep facial mass (Fig. 9.8).

Carotid Space

Masses of the carotid space deviate the parapharyngeal space anteriorly, and separate or anteriorly displace

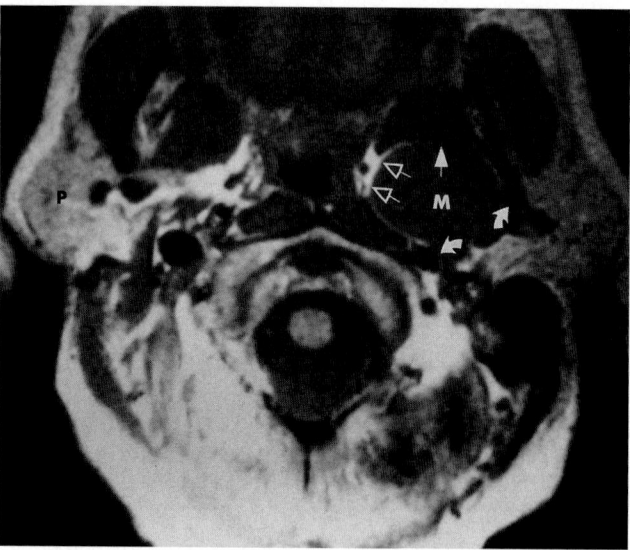

Figure 9.8. Parotid Benign Mixed Cell Adenoma (Pleomorphic Adenoma). Axial T1WI through the level of the oropharynx. A mass (*M*) displaces the parapharyngeal space medially (*open white arrows*) and the masticator space anteriorly (*white arrow*). The stylomandibular notch, from the carotid space to the mandible (*curved arrows*), is widened characteristic of a deep lobe parotid lesion. Conversely, a lesion originating from the carotid space would result in narrowing of the stylomandibular notch. The lesion is sharply demarcated from the normal parotid tissue (*P*).

the carotid and jugular vein. They sometimes displace the styloid process anteriorly, which narrows the stylomandibular notch (the space between the styloid process and the mandible). This is a characteristic feature that distinguishes these lesions from deep parotid space lesions, which widen the stylomandibular notch.

Pseudomasses. When evaluating carotid space tumors, there are several pseudomasses of the carotid space that must be taken into account. These pseudomasses are vascular variants that may be mistaken for masses both clinically and radiographically. Asymmetry of the internal jugular veins is the most common variation in the vascular anatomy of the neck. Marked asymmetry between the size of the left and right jugular veins is common, with the right vein typically being the larger of the two. Additionally, the jugular veins may demonstrate considerable variability in the degree of signal within their lumen, ranging from bright to signal void. The intraluminal bright regions should not be mistaken for thrombosis. It is important to follow the signal on serial images to visualize the tubular nature, thus confirming that the signal represents vasculature; otherwise it may easily be mistaken for adenopathy. Tortuosity of the carotid artery may present as a submucosal pulsatile mass in the pharynx. This variation, which is frequently seen in the elderly, is easily detected on CT or MR and obviates the need for further diagnostic work-up unless a post-traumatic aneurysm is suspected.

Tumors. Most carotid space masses are benign neoplasms which arise from nerves located within the carotid sheath. The most common lesions are paragangliomas and nerve sheath tumors such as schwannomas and neurofibromas. *Paragangliomas* are vascular tumors that arise from neural crest cell derivatives. These lesions are named according to the nerves from which they arise and their location of origin. When arising from the carotid body at the carotid bifurcation, they are called carotid body tumors (Fig. 9.9). Paragangliomas

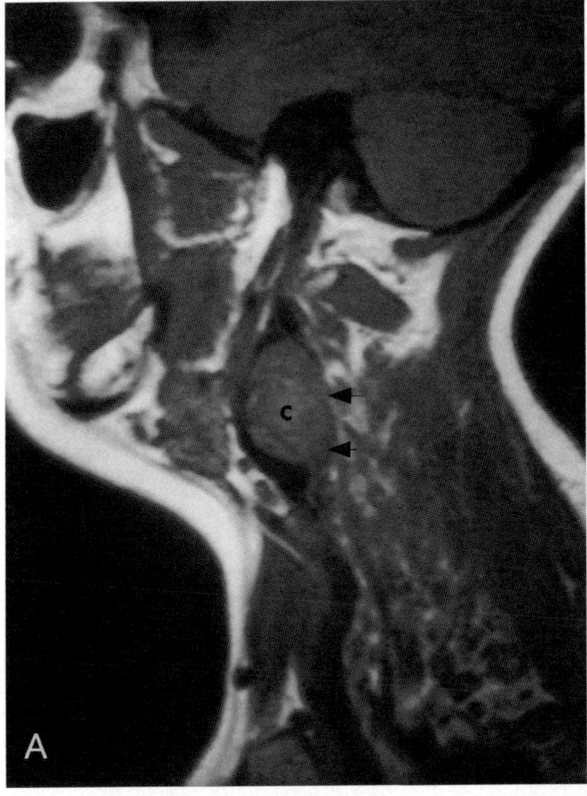

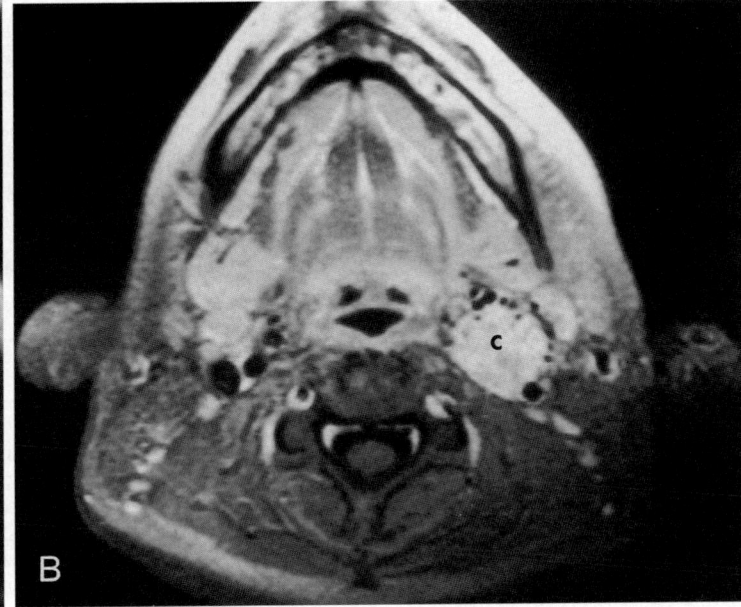

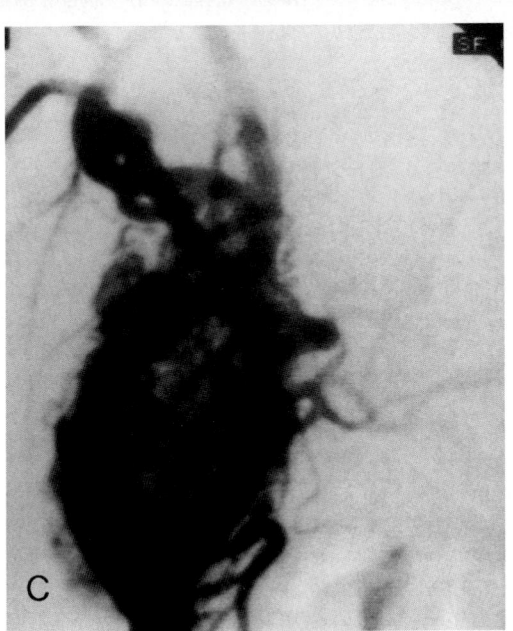

Figure 9.9. Carotid Body Tumor. Sagittal T1WI **(A)**, axial postgadolinium fat-suppression T1WI **(B)**, and angiogram **(C)**. A vascular mass located between the carotid bifurcation, with splaying of the internal and external carotid arteries, is characteristic of a carotid body tumor. The multiple flow voids in the axial image supports the diagnosis of a paraganglioma. The angiogram confirms the marked vascularity of this lesion. Angiography is helpful in providing preoperative embolization, which makes the lesion less vascular and easier to remove surgically.

may also arise from the ganglion of the vagus nerve (glomus vagale), along the jugular ganglion of the vagus nerve (glomus jugulare), and around Arnold's and Jacobson's nerves in the middle ear (glomus tympanicum).

Clinically, patients with paragangliomas present with a painless, slowly progressive neck mass that may be pulsatile with an associated bruit. Because these lesions are located within the carotid sheath, there are often associated slowly progressive cranial neuropathies (cranial nerves IX–XII) (Fig. 9.10). Paragangliomas are often multiple (5–10%) and, in familial cases, are multiple 25–33% of the time. Therefore, if a lesion is detected, it is essential to look for a second one.

Angiographically, paragangliomas are very vascular, with a strong blush in the capillary phase. Treatment often consists of surgical resection. Interventional radiology plays an important role, permitting preoperative embolization. On CT scanning, paragangliomas and neuromas are both densely enhancing, and are typically indistinguishable. In contrast, on MR, paragangliomas are characterized by multiple flow voids and prominent

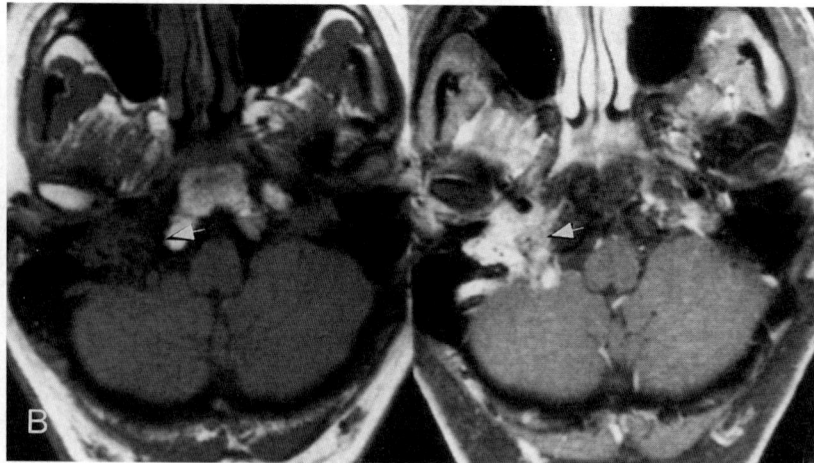

Figure 9.10. Glomus Jugulare Tumor. A. Axial contrast-enhanced CT. Fatty atrophy of the right tongue (hypoglossal nerve palsy)(*black arrows*) and patulousness of the right oropharynx (vagus nerve palsy)(*white arrow*) are evident. Dysfunction of multiple lower cranial nerves suggests involvement of the skull base where cranial nerves IX through XII arise in close proximity. **B.** Axial T1WI with fat suppression, pre-(left)gadolinium and post-(right)gadolinium. A contrast-enhancing mass (*arrows*) extending through the right jugular foramen into the posterior fossa is indicative of glomus jugulare tumor.

enhancement, but neuromas usually do not demonstrate flow voids and can be cystic (Figs. 9.11,9.12). These features reflect the typically more vascular nature of paragangliomas. Note that these findings are not pathognomonic for paragangliomas, because very vascular schwannomas may also have associated flow voids on occasion.

Lymph nodes are the next most common source of pathology. In fact, the principal malignancy of the carotid space is squamous cell nodal metastasis. A major nodal chain, the deep cervical jugular, is located within the carotid space. Any pathology that involves lymph nodes (metastases, lymphoma, infection, benign hyperplasia) may therefore be found within the carotid space.

Parotid Space

Masses arising from the deep lobe of the parotid gland will deviate the parapharyngeal space medially. Unlike carotid space masses, deep parotid masses push the styloid process and carotid vessels posteriorly. This results in characteristic widening of the stylomastoid foramen (Fig. 9.8). The structures within the parotid space that may give rise to pathology include the parotid gland and lymph nodes. The parotid gland is the only salivary gland to have lymph nodes contained within its capsule. This reflects the embryogenisis of the parotid gland, the late encapsulation of which results in the presence of 10–20 nodes within the gland parenchyma. Consequently, pathology of the parotid space includes salivary gland tumors and nodal disease.

Parotid Tumors. Most parotid tumors are benign (80%), and most of these are benign mixed cell tumors (pleomorphic adenomas) or Warthin's tumors (benign salivary gland tumors). Malignant tumors, which account for 20% of all parotid lesions, include adenocystic carcinoma, adenocarcinoma, squamous cell carcinoma, and mucoepidermoid carcinoma. MR and CT imaging cannot with certainty differentiate benign from malignant disease. Both may present as well-circumscribed lesions. Tumor homogeneity, indistinct margins, and signal intensity are poor predictors of histology. Nevertheless, both CT and MR are useful in portraying the relationship of the tumor to surrounding normal anatomy, and for verification of the location of a nonpalpable parotid mass before biopsy. A feature clearly suggestive of malignancy is infiltration into deep neck structures such as the masticator or parapharyngeal space. Clinical involvement of the facial nerve is another ominous finding suggestive of malignancy.

The presence of multiple lesions within the parotid space may be seen with several conditions including either inflammatory or malignant adenopathy. Another possibility is the Warthin's tumor (benign salivary gland tumor), which is multiple 10% of the time. Parotid cysts have been seen in collagen vascular disease, and more recently described in patients with acquired immunodeficiency syndrome (AIDS)(Fig. 9.13). These parotid cysts, also known as lymphoepithelial cysts, are believed to be the result of partial obstruction of the terminal ducts by surrounding lymphocytic infiltration.

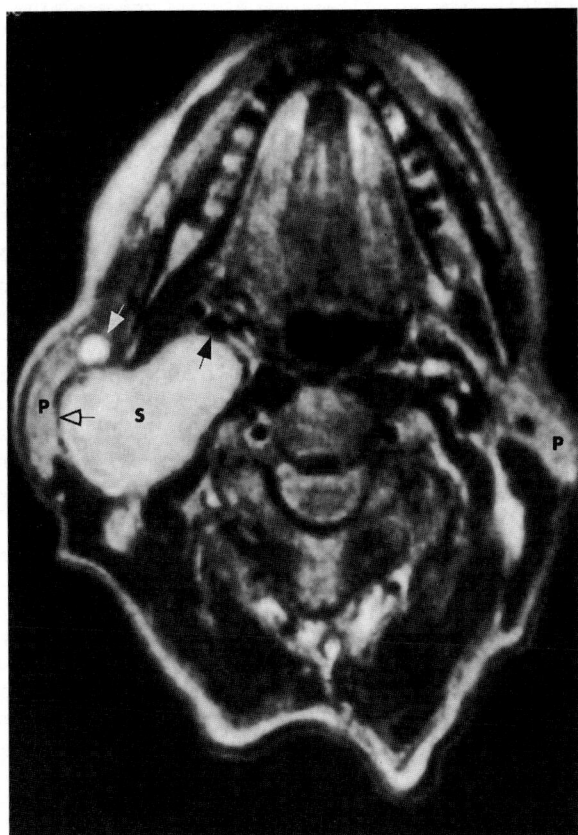

Figure 9.11. Schwannoma. Axial T2WI through the floor of the mouth. A homogeneous mass (*S*) displaces the carotid space anteriorly (*black arrow*) and the parotid space (*P*) laterally (*open arrow*). Anterior displacement of the carotid artery is characteristic of a carotid space mass. The lack of associated flow voids suggests that this lesion is a schwannoma, as opposed to a paraganglioma. High signal within the right retromandibular vein (*white arrow*) is due to partial compression. Normal flow void is seen in the opposite retromandibular vein.

Masticator Space

The masticator space is formed by a superficial layer of the deep cervical fascia that surrounds the muscles of mastication and the mandible. It extends from the angle of the mandible superiorly to the skull base, and over the temporalis muscle. The muscles of mastication include the temporalis, medial and lateral pterygoid, and the masseter. In addition, branches of the trigeminal nerve and the internal maxillary artery are located within this space. Masses of the masticator space displace the parapharyngeal space medially and posteriorly.

Most masses of the masticator space are infectious in origin. They usually result from either dental caries or are secondary to dental extraction. A mass will often surround the mandible, and may extend along the temporalis muscle. Additionally, pseudotumors of the masticator space are common and include accessory parotid glands as well as marked muscle hypertrophy due to bruxism. Occasionally, an accessory parotid gland may occur along the anterior surface of the masseter muscle and can be mistaken for a mass. Asymmetry of the mus-

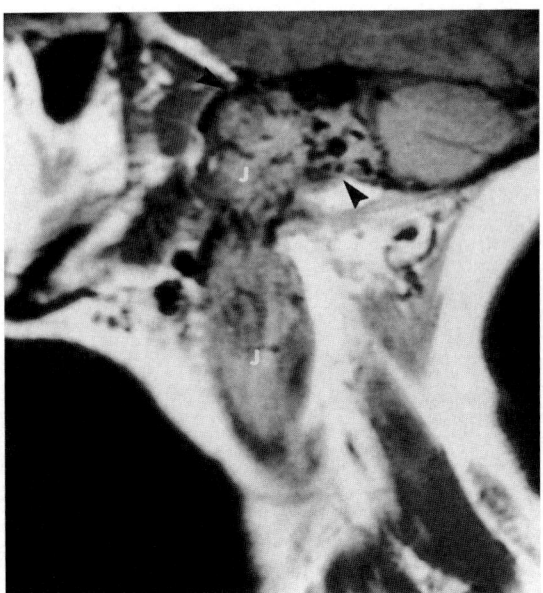

Figure 9.12. Glomus Jugulare. Sagittal T1WI through the carotid space. A large mass (*J*) extends from the carotid space through the jugulare foramen (*arrowhead*) into the posterior fossa. The presence of numerous flow voids is suggestive of a vascular lesion such as a paraganglioma.

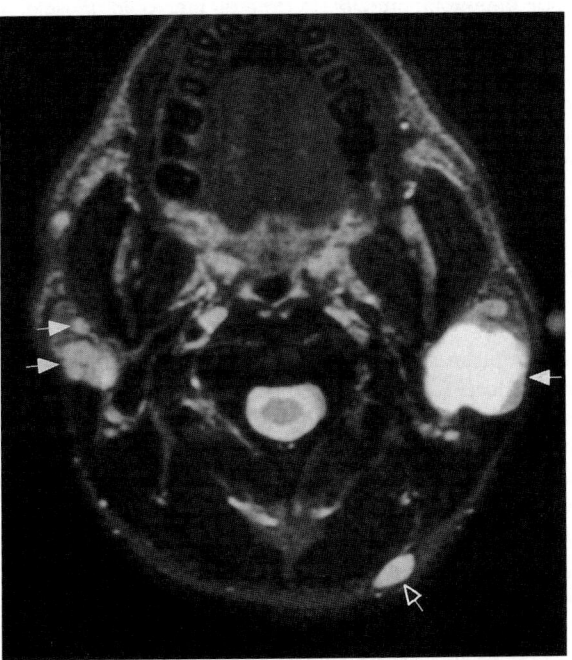

Figure 9.13. AIDS-related Parotid Cysts. Axial T2WI through the level of the oropharynx. Multiple cysts are seen within the parotid glands bilaterally (*arrows*). These result from lymphatic obstruction due to HIV. Incidentally, a sebaceous cyst is noted in the left posterior neck (*open arrow*).

cles of mastication may result from unilateral atrophy resulting from compromise of the mandibular division of the fifth cranial nerve (V3). This is most commonly seen in patients with head and neck neoplasms with perineural extension along the trigeminal nerve.

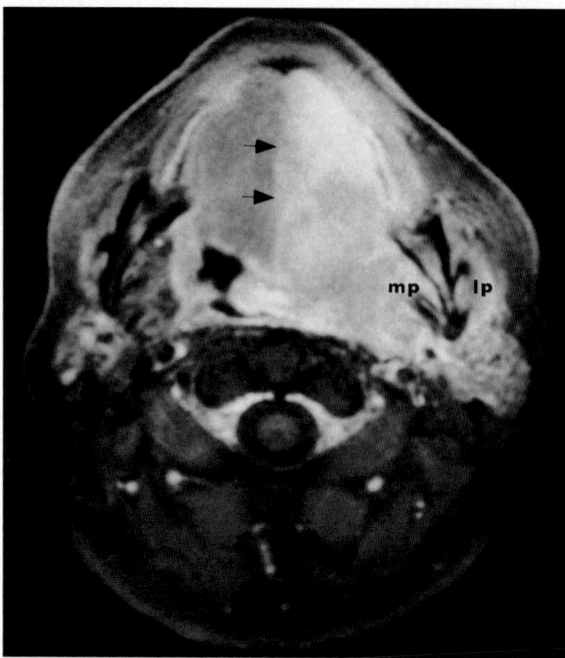

Figure 9.14. Squamous Cell Carcinoma of the Tongue. Axial post-gadolinium fat-suppression T1WI through the level of the oropharynx. A left tongue base squamous cell carcinoma extends posteriorly along the oropharyngeal wall into the masticator space. *mp*, medial pterygoid muscle; *lp*, lateral pterygoid muscle. Malignancies of the masticator space are most frequently the result of the direct posterior extension of oropharyngeal squamous cell carcinoma. In this example, the left half of the tongue (*arrows*) is diffusely enhancing, indicating denervation myositis, due to involvement of the hypoglossal nerve. Later, the muscles will atrophy and become replaced by fat.

Primary Malignancies of the masticator space are very uncommon. Malignancies of this space most often result from the extension of oropharyngeal or tongue base squamous cell carcinoma to involve the muscles of mastication (Fig. 9.14). In addition, tumor or infection from oropharyngeal or nasopharyngeal lesions may spread along the third division of the fifth cranial nerve, allowing the tumor to spread through the foramen ovale into the cavernous sinus (Fig. 9.15). From this location, tumor may extend posteriorly along the cisternal portion of the trigeminal nerve to the brainstem. Primary malignancies of the masticator space include sarcomas arising from muscle, chondroid, or nerve elements. In addition, sarcomas of the bone such as osteosarcoma and Ewing's sarcoma may be seen. Non-Hodgkin's lymphoma will occasionally involve the mandible or extraosseous soft tissues of the masticator space.

Retropharyngeal Space

The retropharyngeal space is a potential space that lies posterior to the superficial mucosal space and pharyngeal constrictor muscles, and anterior to the prevertebral space. A mass within this space results in characteristic posterior displacement of the prevertebral muscles. The fascial planes in this area are complex, but

can be considered as forming a single compartment for simplicity. This space is significant because it serves as a potential conduit for the spread of tumor or infection from the pharynx to the mediastinum (Fig. 9.16). In contrast to the carotid and parotid spaces, in which inflammatory disease and metastases account for a minority of lesions, most retropharyngeal space lesions are due to infection or nodal malignancy. This space is most often involved with nodal malignancy because of lymphoma or metastatic head and neck squamous cell carcinoma. These tumors frequently affect the retropharyngeal nodes, which are divided into a medial and lateral group. The lateral retropharyngeal nodes, also known as nodes of Rouviére, are normal when seen in younger patients but must be viewed with suspicion in older individuals (>30 years). In addition, head and neck infections may sometimes extend into the retropharyngeal space via lymphatics. Neck infections are most often the result of tonsillitis, dental disease, trauma, endocarditis, and systemic infections such as tuberculosis. With the advent of antibiotics, infections occur much less commonly, but are often seen in immunosuppressed patients. On routine T1-weighted and T2-weighted sequences it can be difficult to differentiate an abscess from cellulitis, as both can be isointense to muscle on T1 and hyperintense on T2. Gadolinium is of value in making this differentiation, as an abscess will demonstrate a rim of contrast enhancement surrounding a liquefied center.

Prevertebral Space

The prevertebral space is formed by the prevertebral fascia, which surrounds the prevertebral muscles. Masses of the prevertebral space displace the prevertebral muscles anteriorly. This allows prevertebral lesions to be easily differentiated from retropharyngeal processes, which will displace these muscles posteriorly. The structures that give rise to the preponderance of pathology in this space are the cervical vertebral bodies. Any process that involves the vertebral bodies, such as tumor (metastasis, chordoma, etc.) or osteomyelitis may extend anteriorly to involve this space (Fig. 9.11).

Transpacial Diseases

Occasionally, masses may not be localized to one of the spaces described above. Such masses are often secondary to lesions involving anatomic structures that normally traverse spaces of the head and neck, e.g., lymphatics, nerves and vessels. Examples include the following three categories: *a*) lymphatic masses (lymphangioma); *b*) neural masses (neurofibroma, schwannoma) and *c*) vascular masses (hemangioma). Differentiation between these subtypes can occasionally be made by virtue of signal intensity characteristics. For instance, neurofibromas may have a characteristic low intensity center on T1, and often involve more than one peripheral nerve. This is distinctly different from both lymphatic and vascular masses. Lymphangiomas and hemangiomas are congenital abnormalities that look quite similar on MR. Both entities have increased signal intensity on T2WI and are infiltrative. Hemangiomas may

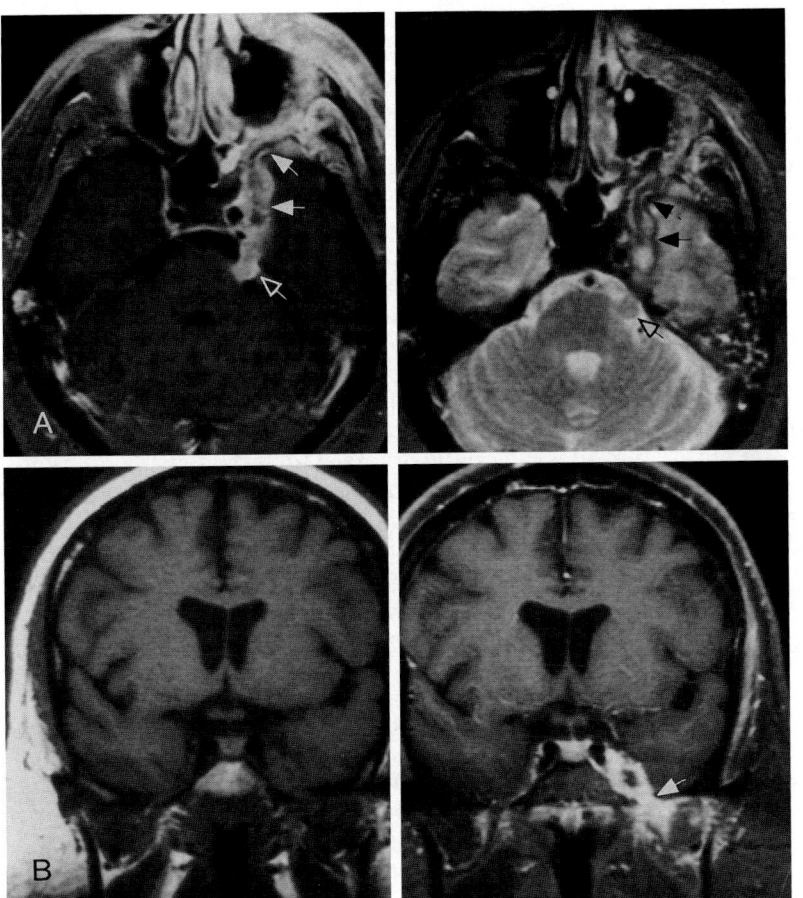

Figure 9.15. Masticator Space Infection. A. Axial postgadolinium fat-suppression T1WI (left) and T2WI (right) through the level of the nasopharynx. Soft-tissue infiltration involves the left malleolar soft tissues, and extends along the maxillary division of the trigeminal nerve (V2)(*arrows*) into the cavernous sinus. From the cavernous sinus, contrast-enhancing tissue extends along the cisternal portion of the trigeminal nerve (*open arrows*) to the brain stem. **B.** Coronal T1WI, pregadolinium (left) and post-gadonlinium (right) fat-suppression. Contrast enhancement is seen filling the cavernous sinus and extending through the foramen ovale (*arrow*) into the masticator space along the mandibular division of the trigeminal nerve (V3). Findings are due to mucormycosis infection in an immunocompromised host (ketoacidotic diabetic).

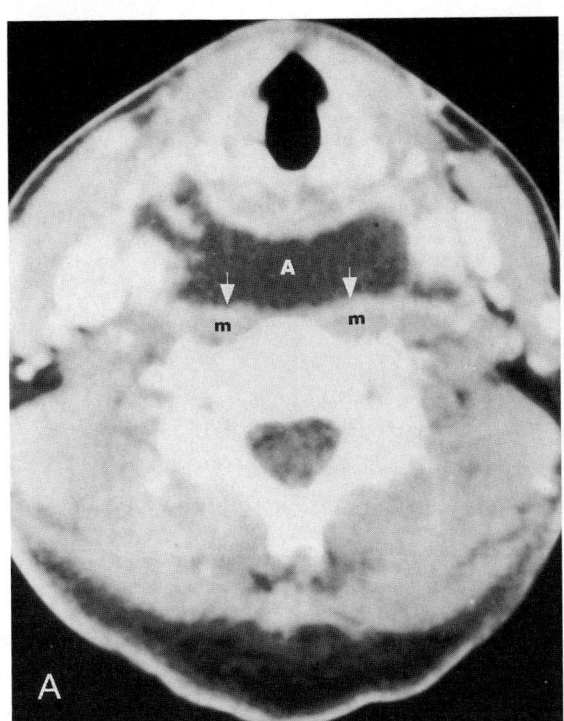

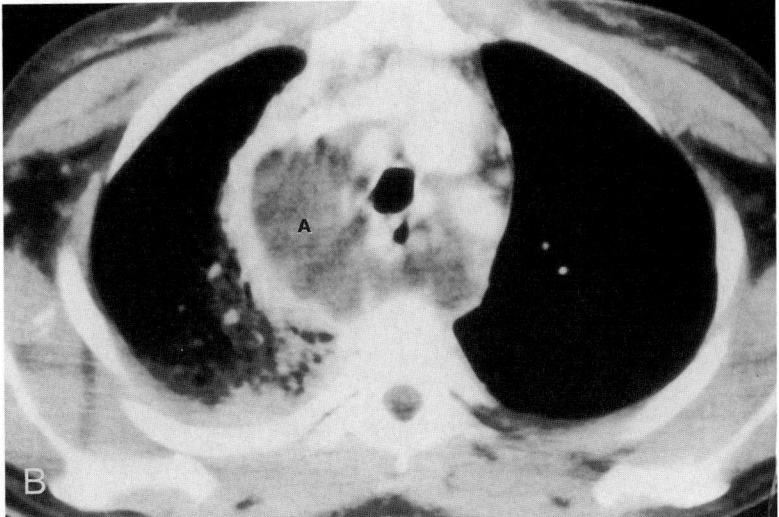

Figure 9.16. Retropharyngeal Abscess. Axial postcontrast CT through the level of the larynx **(A)** and the upper mediastinum **(B).** A large fluid collection (*A*) extends from the retropharyngeal space into the upper mediastinum. The posterior displacement of the prevertebral muscles (*m*)(*arrows*) identifies this collection as being retropharyngeal as opposed to prevertebral.

have phleboliths, which may only be detected on CT. Lymphangiomas tend to have heterogeneous signal intensity with evidence of blood degradation products. Both entities should be considered in a patient with a history of chronic facial swelling, and who has CT or MR evidence of an infiltrative process that traverses several spaces.

LYMPH NODES

Once a primary neoplasm of the head and neck is detected, the assessment of lymph nodes is a vital part of tumor staging. The presence of a single ipsilateral malignant node reduces the patient's expected survival by 50%, with extracapsular nodal extension reducing survival an additional 50%. Thus, the detection and evaluation of nodal disease is paramount for prognostic reasons as well as for therapeutic planning. CT and MR play a vital role in the staging of head and neck neoplasms, especially because clinical staging has many shortcomings. The full size and extent of the primary neoplasm can rarely be accurately determined clinically. Additionally, at least 15% of malignant nodes are clinically occult because of their deep location, and thus are not palpable by the clinician. The overall error rate in assessing the presence of adenopathy by palpation is between 25 and 33%. Thus, CT or MR is vital in obtaining the most accurate pretreatment planning information.

There are at least 10 major lymph node groups in the head and neck. Knowledge of the location of these cervical lymph node chains and the usual modes of spread of head and neck disease is essential for successful analysis of CT and MR scans (7). However, a complete discussion of all the head and neck nodal chains is beyond the scope of this text. We will focus on the principal lymph node group of the neck, the internal jugular chain. The internal jugular nodal chain serves as the final common afferent pathway for lymphatic drainage of the entire head and neck. This nodal chain follows the oblique course of the jugular vein beneath and adjacent to the anterior border of the sternocleidomastoid muscle. The jugulodigastric node is the highest node of the internal jugular chain. It is located where the posterior belly of the digastric muscle crosses this chain, near the level of the hyoid bone. The jugulodigastric lymph node is immediately posterior to the submandibular gland, and provides lymphatic drainage from the tonsil, oral cavity, pharynx, and submandibular nodes.

The jugulodigastric node and submandibular nodes may normally measure up to 1.5 cm in diameter; in contrast, all other nodes of the head and neck are considered abnormal if greater than 1.0 cm in diameter. When an enlarged node is encountered, differentiation between a benign reactive node and a malignant one can be difficult. Several features that suggest malignancy are *a*) peripheral nodal enhancement with central necrosis, *b*) extracapsular spread with infiltration of adjacent tissues, and *c*) a matted conglomerate mass of nodes. Nodal size itself is a less reliable indicator of malignancy, but is used because the other more reliable differentiating features are frequently not present.

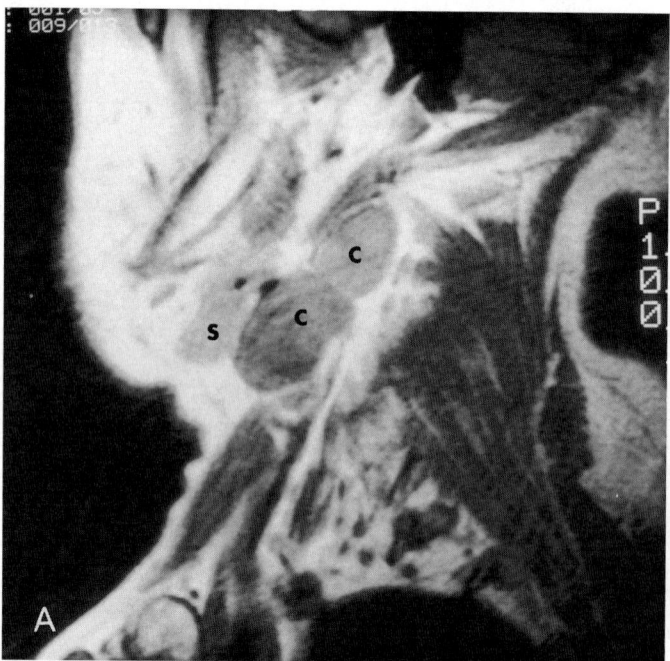 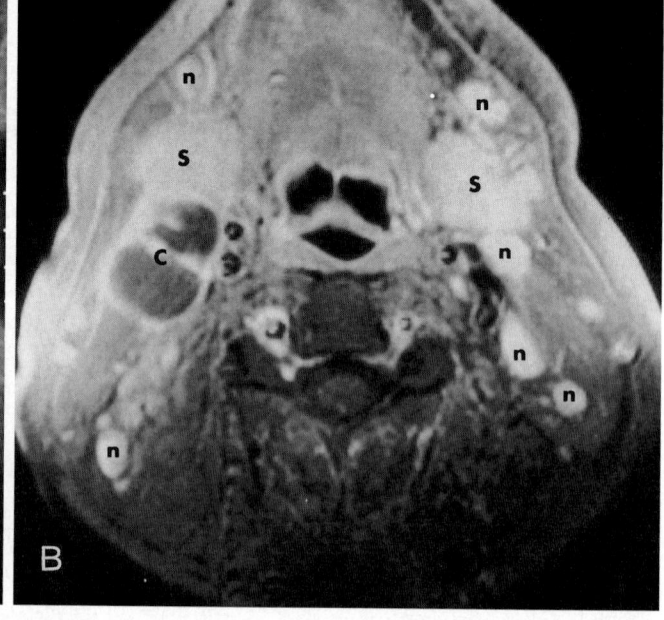

Figure 9.17. Squamous Cell Carcinoma—Cystic Node Metastasis. Sagittal T1WI **(A)** and axial postgadolinium fat-suppression T1WI **(B)**. A 43-year-old patient presented with a 6-month history of a right-sided neck mass that would swell during upper respiratory tract infections. Images reveal a multiseptated cystic lesion (*c*) in the right jugular nodal chain. On biopsy, this proved to be a squamous cell, cystic nodal metastasis. Although this lesion may appear similar to a branchial cleft cyst, the presence of multiple additional nodes (*n*) is unusual. A branchial cleft cyst may exhibit a thickened wall with septations, depending on current or previous infections. *S*, submandibular glands. Note that the jugulodigastric node is easily identified by its characteristic location; situated immediately posterior to the submandibular gland.

If size criteria alone are used, approximately 70% of enlarged nodes are secondary to metastatic disease and 30% are caused by benign reactive hyperplasia. Note that the features described as characteristic for malignancy are the same as for infection, and the two cannot be differentiated by imaging (Fig. 9.17). Fortunately, this distinction is often easily made clinically.

Lymph nodes can be accurately detected with either spiral CT or MR. Contrast enhanced spiral CT provides for rapid thin section imaging of the neck with minimal motion artifact. With MR imaging, lymph nodes are well visualized on fat-suppressed fast spin echo T2WI. Lymph nodes can also be identified on T1WI as well as postcontrast fat-suppressed T1WI. Lymph nodes typically demonstrate homogeneous signal intensity, whether on T1WI or T2WI. Any heterogeneity in signal, especially the presence of cystic change or necrosis, is consistent with metastatic disease. Note that a fatty central hilus is a normal finding. Shape is also a differentiating feature, as a rounded shape suggests neoplastic nodal infiltration with associated expansion. In contrast, if a node is enlarged but maintains its normal reniform configuration, it is less likely to represent metastatic disease.

ORBIT

Both CT and MR are valuable for imaging of the orbit, each with distinct merits (8,9). When evaluating for calcification, such as in retinoblastoma in a child with leukocoria, or for bony fracture following trauma, CT is the modality of choice. MR on the other hand, with its multiplanar capability and superior soft-tissue discrimination, has proven to be of tremendous value in orbital imaging. For most orbital abnormalities, including evaluation of the visual pathways, MR is the procedure of choice.

Understanding the spatial anatomy of the orbit is valuable because knowledge of the contents of the spaces provides insight into the naturally occurring lesions that develop within each space. The retrobulbar space contains both the extraconal and the intraconal spaces, which are separated by the muscle cone. This muscle cone is formed by the extraoccular muscles (superior, inferior, medial and lateral rectus; superior oblique; and levator palpebrae superior) and a fibrous septum. Together these structures form a cone with its base at the posterior of the globe and apex at the superior orbital fissure. When identifying an intraconal lesion, an essential issue is whether the lesion arises from the optic nerve sheath complex or is extrinsic to it. The optic nerve sheath complex is composed of the optic nerve and the surrounding perioptic nerve sheath. The optic nerve is an extension of the brain enveloped by cerebrospinal fluid (CSF) and leptomeninges, which form the optic nerve sheath. Therefore, the CSF space which envelops the optic nerve is continuous with the intracranial subarachnoid space. If a lesion arises from the optic nerve sheath complex, the most common lesion is either an optic nerve glioma or optic sheath meningioma.

Optic Nerve Glioma is the most common tumor of the optic nerve, and typically occurs during the first decade of life (Fig. 9.18) (10). There is a high association with neurofibromatosis type-1, particularly when there is bilateral optic nerve involvement. Histologically, these lesions are low-grade pilocytic astrocytomas. The characteristic imaging finding is that of enlargement of the optic nerve sheath complex. The enlarged sheath complex may be tubular, fusiform, or eccentric with kinking. Some optic nerve gliomas have extensive associated thickening of the perioptic meningies. Histologically, this reflects peritumoral reactive meningeal change that has been termed "arachnoidal hyperplasia" or "gliomatosis." This finding is often seen in patients with neurofibromatosis.

Optic Sheath Meningiomas arise from meningoendothelial cells of the arachnoid layer of the optic nerve sheath. These lesions assume a circular configuration and grow in a linear fashion along the optic nerve. Optic sheath meningiomas demonstrate a characteristic "tram track" pattern of linear contrast enhancement because

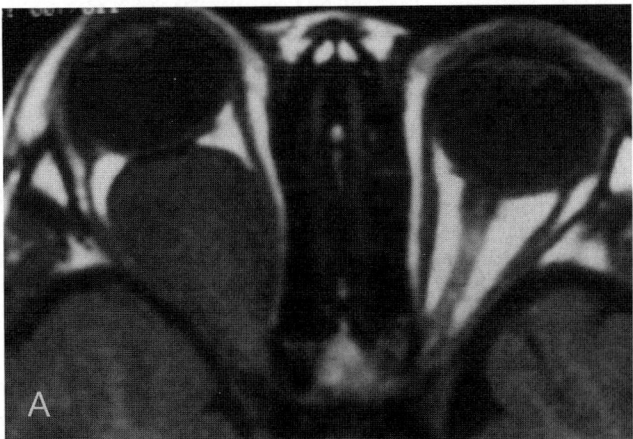

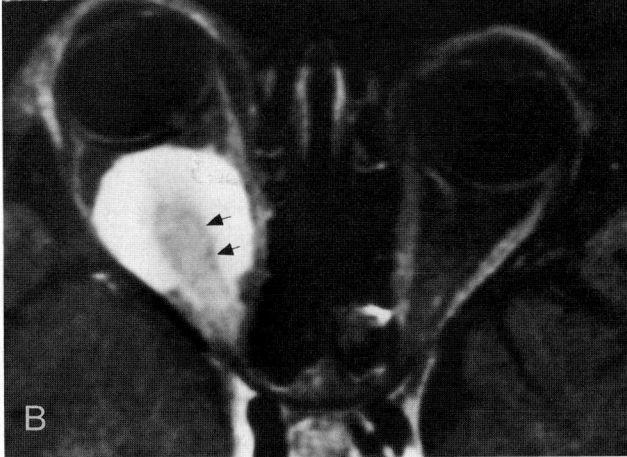

Figure 9.18. Optic Nerve Glioma. Axial pregadolinium **(A)** and postgadolinium **(B)** fat-suppressed T1WI through the orbits. A large mass involves the right optic nerve. Following the administration of contrast, the enlarged optic nerve (*arrows*) is visible coursing through markedly thickened optic sheath soft tissue. This soft tissue represents arachnoidal hyperplasia, which is a finding associated with optic gliomas in patients with neurofibromatosis.

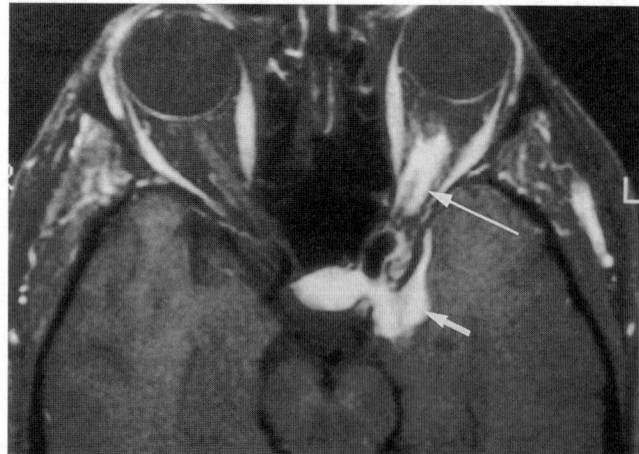

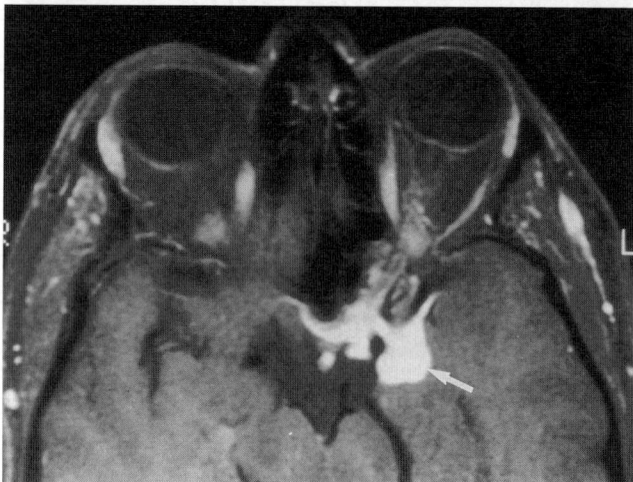

Figure 9.19. Optic Sheath Meningioma. Axial postgadolinium fat-suppression T1WI through the orbits. "Tram track" enhancement involves the left optic nerve sheath (*long arrow*), and a tumor (*short arrows*) extends into the middle cranial fossa. The "tram track" enhancement and the dural tail within the middle cranial fossa are characteristic of a meningioma.

the nerve sheath enhances and not the nerve itself. MR easily displays any tumor extension along the optic nerve sheath through the orbital apex (Fig. 9.19). In contrast to optic nerve gliomas, meningiomas may invade and grow through the dura, resulting in an irregular and asymmetrical appearance. Additionally, optic sheath meningiomas may be extensively calcified, whereas optic nerve gliomas rarely have any calcification. In patients with sarcoid, leukemia or lymphoma, cellular infiltrates may deposit within the perioptic nerve sheath CSF space. In such cases, contrast enhancement of the perioptic nerve sheath space may mimic the "tram track" appearance of a nerve sheath meningioma.

Vascular Lesions. A variety of vascular lesions may develop in the orbit. The four lesions we will consider include capillary hemangioma, lymphangioma, cavernous hemangioma, and varix. These lesions are readily distinguished by a combination of imaging and clinical findings, including the patient's age. Capillary hemangiomas develop in infants (younger than 1 year), and are diagnosed within the first weeks of life. Although these lesions may grow rapidly in size, they typically plateau during the first year or two, then regress spontaneously. On imaging studies, a capillary hemangioma appears as an infiltrative soft-tissue complex, often with multiple vascular flow voids. In contrast, lymphangiomas are one of the most common orbital tumors of childhood, and occur in an older group of children (3–15 years). Lymphangiomas are characterized by their propensity to bleed, and often contain blood degradation products. An acute hemorrhage may result in marked expansion of the lesion with sudden proptosis (Fig. 9.20). MR reveals a multiloculated, lobular mass with characteristic signal heterogeneity caused by blood degradation products (Fig. 9.21). The older age of presentation, combined with the characteristic heterogeneous signal related to blood products, allows differentiation from the capillary hemangiomas. Cavernous hemangiomas are one of the most common orbital masses in adults. In contrast to the other vascular lesions of the orbit, hemangiomas are characterized as a sharply circumscribed, rounded mass

Figure 9.20. Lymphangioma. Axial T2WI reveals a cystic retrobulbar lesion (*arrows*) with a hematocrit effect (serum layered above red blood cells). Hemorrhage into a lesion is a characteristic feature of lymphangiomas, and may be responsible for the rapid development of proptosis.

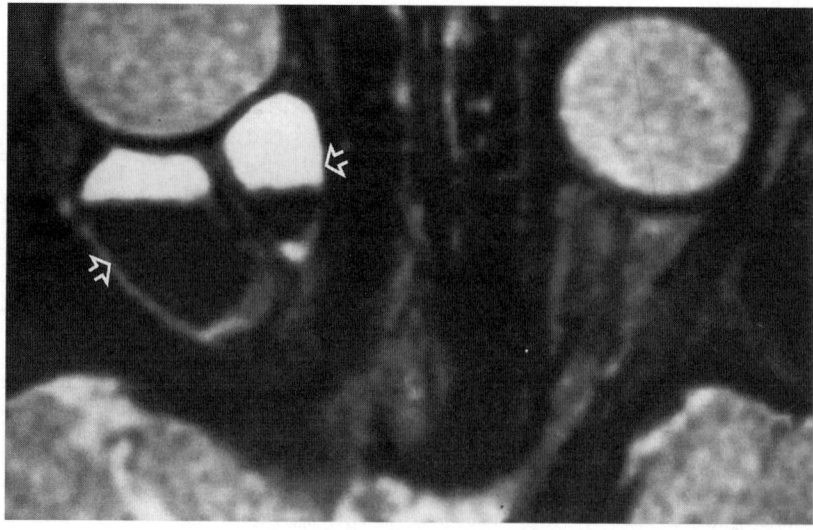

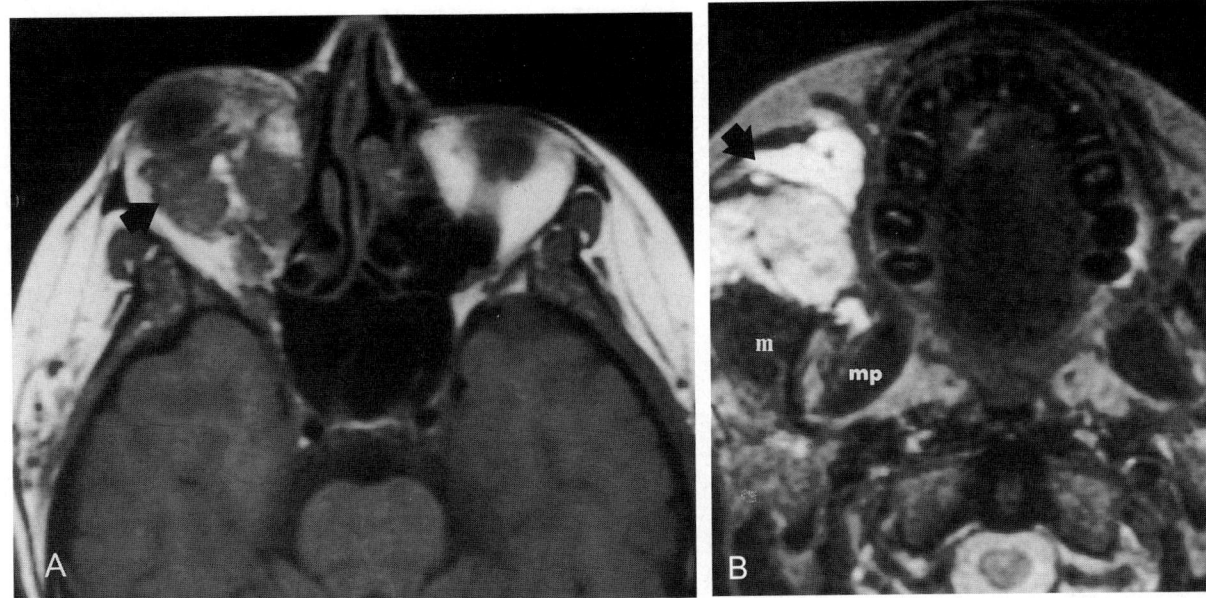

Figure 9.21. Lymphangioma. Axial T1WI **(A)** through the orbit and T2WI **(B)** through the midface. A heterogeneous lesion (*arrows*) extends from the right orbit through the inferior orbital fissure into the masticator space. The heterogeneous signal of this lesion as well as its tendency to extend across fascial spaces is characteristic for lymphangioma. *m*, masseter muscle; *mp*, medial pterygoid muscle.

(Fig. 9.22). These lesions demonstrate diffuse enhancement, sometimes with a mottled pattern. The venous varix is an enormously dilated vein that is characterized by its marked change in size with the Valsalva maneuver.

Superior Ophthalmic Vein is well visualized on MR studies. Pathology includes thrombosis and enlargement. Thrombosis often occurs in conjunction with cavernous sinus thrombosis and presents as loss of the normal flow void with signal intensity related to the age of the thrombus. Enlargement of the superior ophthalmic vein may also be seen with cavernous carotid fistulas (Figs. 9.23, 9.24). Cavernous carotid fistulas represent direct or indirect communication between the internal carotid artery and the venous cavernous sinus. These are either spontaneous or posttraumatic, and may present with pulsating exophthalmos and bruit.

Pseudotumor and Lymphoma are two important orbital lesions that may present with similar imaging findings (11). Idiopathic inflammatory pseudotumor is a poorly characterized condition, which results from an inflammatory lymphocytic infiltrate. This is the most common cause of an intraorbital mass lesion in the adult population. Pseudotumor is often rapidly developing, and presents with painful proptosis, chemosis and ophthalmoplegia. In contrast, lymphoma tends to present with painless proptosis. Lymphoma is the third most common adult orbital mass lesion, following pseudotumor and cavernous hemangioma. On imaging studies, both lymphoma and pseudotumor appear as diffusely infiltrating lesions capable of involving and extending into any retrobulbar structures (Fig. 9.25). Several reports have suggested that T2 shortening of the tumor (dark on T2) is suggestive of pseudotumor (Fig. 9.26). Nevertheless, the distinction between these two entities frequently remains very difficult clinically, radiographically, and even histopathologically.

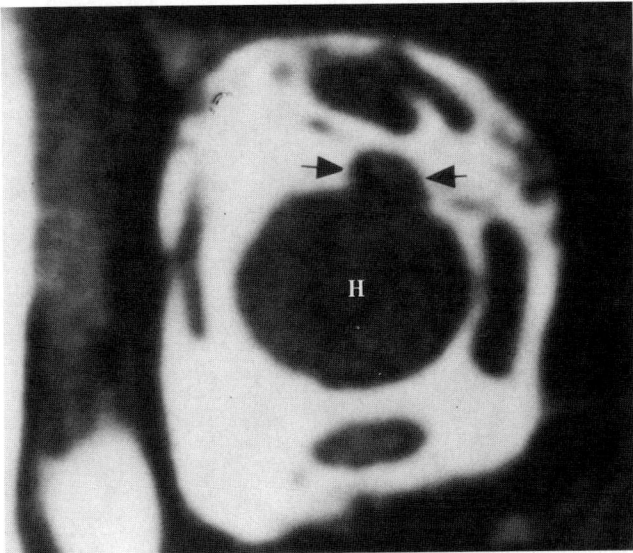

Figure 9.22. Cavernous Hemangioma. Coronal T1WI through the mid-orbit. A well-circumscribed retrobulbar mass (*H*) is identified. The optic nerve is clearly separate from the mass (*arrows*). The well-circumscribed nature of this mass is characteristic of a cavernous hemangioma, the most common orbital mass in adults.

It is reported that a trial dose of steroids may be valuable in differentiating these two entities. Steroids are reported to have a lasting effect on eliminating the pseudotumor lesion. However, the cytolytic effect of steroids on lymphoma may also have a similar but short-lived response that may initially be confounding. Additionally, when a diffusely infiltrative orbital mass is encountered in a young child, rhabdomyosarcoma should be a consideration.

Figure 9.23. Carotid Cavernous Fistula. Axial T1WI through the superior orbit. Following a remote head injury, this patient presented with right chemosis. A large flow void is identified within the right cavernous sinus (*white arrows*). The right superior ophthalmic vein is abnormally dilated (*open arrows*), but the left vein is normal (*black arrows*). Dilatation of the superior ophthalmic vein is an important clue to the presence of a carotid cavernous fistula.

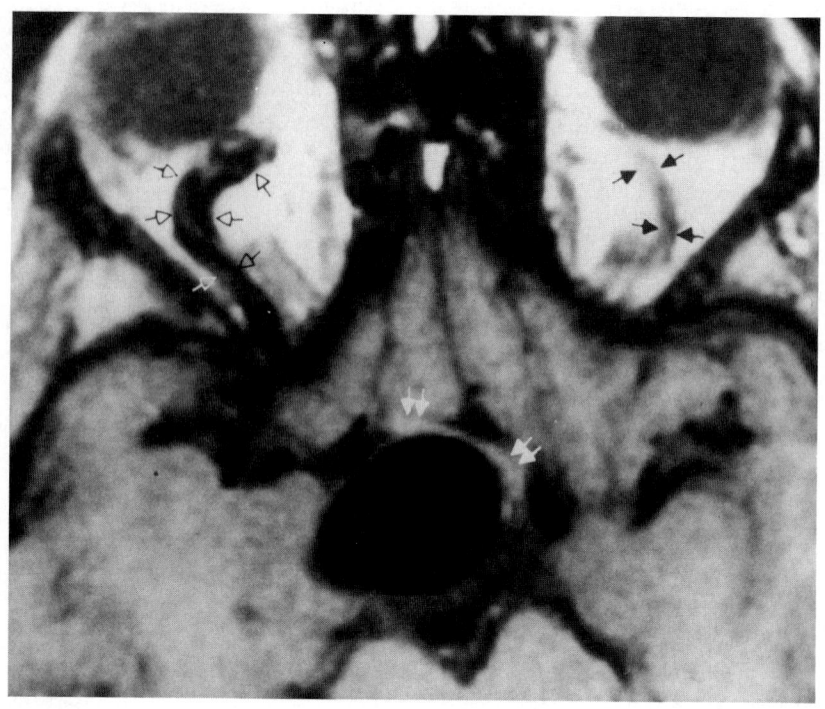

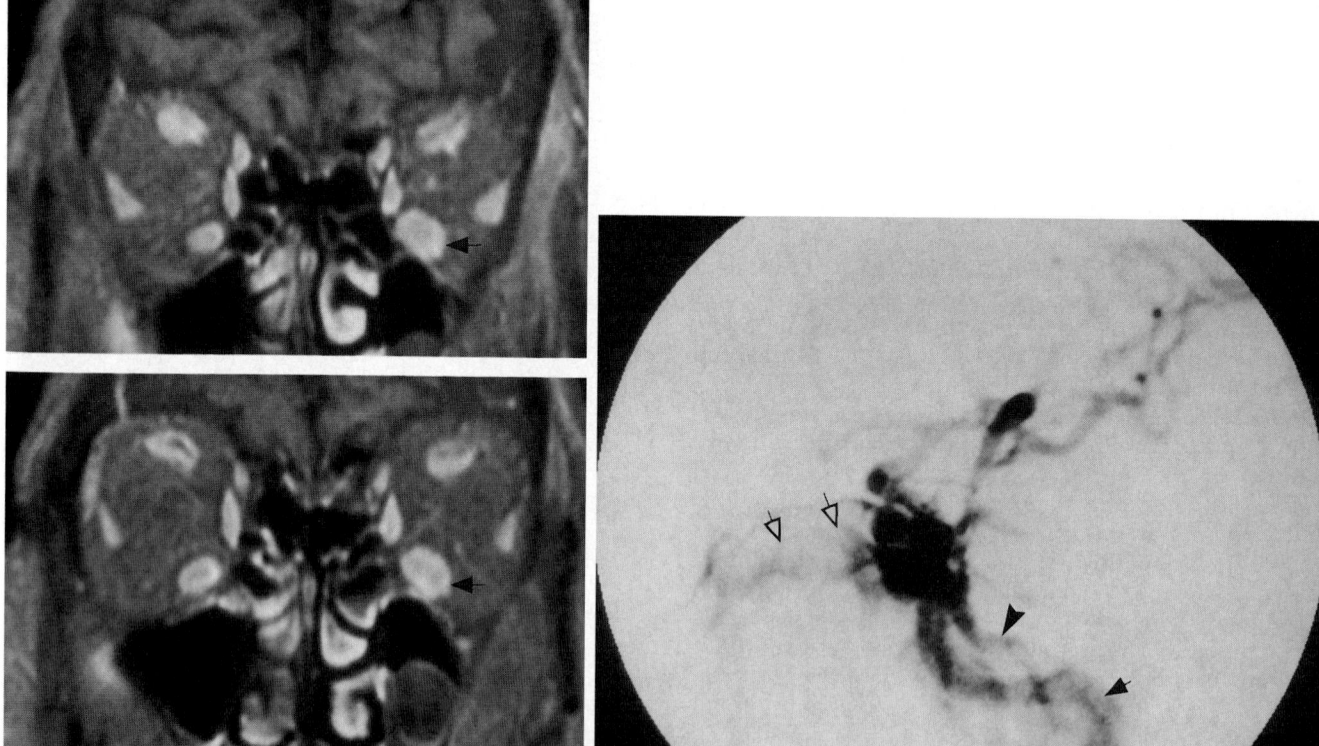

Figure 9.24. Cavernous Carotid Fistula. A. Coronal postgadolinium fat-suppression T1WI. A 35-year-old patient presented with left proptosis and deteriorating vision. Coronal images revealed mild enlargement of the left inferior rectus muscle (*arrows*). Clinical symptoms were consistent with thyroid ophthalmopathy. At surgery for optic sheath decompression, massive blood loss ensued. **B.** Coronal projection, left internal carotid artery injection (*arrow*). Contrast is identified rapidly filling the cavernous sinus (*open arrows*) and inferior petrosal sinus (*arrowhead*). The cavernous sinuses and superior ophthalmic veins were entirely normal on retrospective MR evaluation. This is a case of spontaneous cavernous carotid fistula without significant drainage into the superior ophthalmic veins. Extraocular muscle enlargement has many possible causes, one of which is venous congestion due to a cavernous carotid fistula.

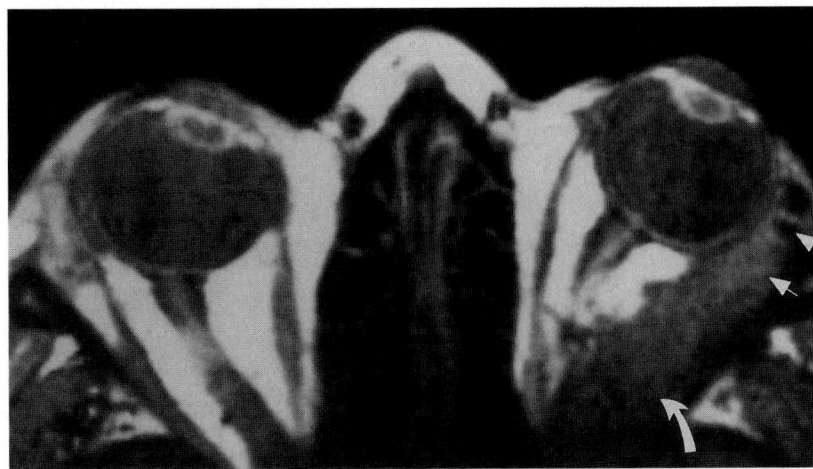

Figure 9.25. Pseudotumor. Axial T1WI through the orbits. A diffusely infiltrating lesion (*curved arrow*) extends along the lateral rectus muscle to its tendinous insertion on the globe (*short arrows*). This feature distinguishes pseudotumor from thyroid ophthalmopathy, in which the muscle insertion is spared.

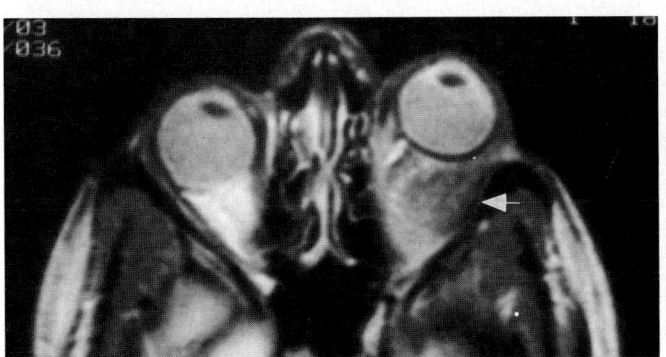

Figure 9.26. Pseudotumor. Axial first **(A)** and second echo **(B)** T2WIs of a patient with painful proptosis and chemosis. A soft-tissue mass (*arrow*) is seen in the left orbit with associated proptosis. This lesion demonstrates T2 shortening (dark on T2) on the heavily T2- weighted sequence **(B)**. This finding is useful in differentiating lymphoma from pseudotumor, which may present with a similar clinical picture.

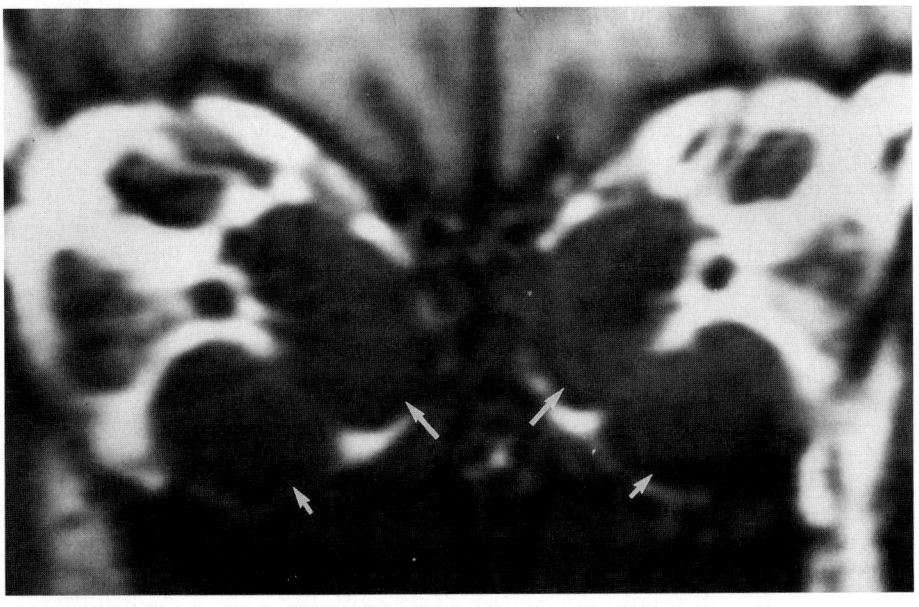

Figure 9.27. Thyroid Ophthalmopathy. Coronal T1WI through the midorbits. Marked extraocular muscle enlargement is identified, involving primarily the medial (*long arrows*) and inferior (*short arrows*) rectus muscles. Thyroid ophthalmopathy is the most common cause of proptosis in the adult. Severe muscle hypertrophy may result in orbital apex compression and loss of vision.

Thyroid Ophthalmopathy (Graves' disease) is a common lesion, and is the most frequent cause of unilateral or bilateral proptosis in the adult. This condition is the result of an inflammatory infiltration of the orbital muscles and orbital connective tissues. Most patients will have clinical or laboratory evidence of hyperthyroidism, but 10% will not; these are referred to as "euthyroid ophthalmopathy." Imaging findings consist of enlargement of the extraocular muscles with sparing of the tendinous attachments to the globe (Fig. 9.27). This is in contrast to pseudotumor, which typically involves the muscle attachments to the globe. The muscles involved in decreasing order of frequency are the inferior, medial, superior, and lateral rectus. Eighty percent of patients have bilateral muscle involvement. In some cases of thyroid ophthalmopathy, the extraocular muscles may be normal, and exophthalmos is the result of increased retrobulbar fat.

Lacrimal Gland. The extraconal space primarily contains fat and the lacrimal gland. However, many lesions involving the extraconal space are the result of tumor or inflammation extending from surrounding structures. These may include most of the lesions described above, as well as sinus-related inflammation. In contrast, lesions arising from within the extraconal space are primarily lacrimal in origin. Lesions of the lacrimal gland are very nonspecific, but can be divided into inflammatory (e.g., sarcoid, Sjögren's syndrome) and neoplastic types. Neoplasms of the lacrimal gland include epithelial and lymphoid tumors. Epithelial tumors are any of the lesions that arise from the salivary glands, such as benign mixed cell tumor or adenoid cystic carcinoma. Lymphoid tumors include lymphoma and pseudotumor. Although none of these lesions have specific imaging findings, dermoid is one lesion that does have a characteristic finding, consisting of a fat-fluid level (Fig. 9.28).

CONGENITAL LESIONS

In children, neck masses tend to be benign, including both congenital (thyroglossal duct cysts, branchial cleft cysts, and lymphangiomas/cystic hygromas) and inflammatory lesions (12). When malignancy is entertained, the most common lesion in the pediatric age group is lymphoma, followed by rhabdomyosarcoma.

Thyroglossal Duct Cysts account for about 90% of congenital neck lesions and usually are found in children, but may be seen in adults. The thyroglossal duct represents an epithelial-lined tract along which the primordial thyroid gland migrates. This tubular structure originates from the foramen cecum (at the tongue base), extends anterior to the thyrohyoid membrane and strap muscles, ends at the level of the thyroid isthmus. The duct normally involutes by 8–10 weeks of gestation.

Because the duct is lined with secretory epithelium, any portion of the thyroglossal duct that fails to involute may give rise to a cyst or sinus tract. Additionally, thyroid glandular tissue can arrest anywhere along the course of the thyroglossal duct, giving rise to ectopic thyroid tissue. Seventy-five percent of thyroglossal duct cysts are midline, and most are located at or below the level of the hyoid bone in the region of the thyrohyoid membrane. In fact, thyroglossal duct cysts are the most common midline neck mass.

Surgery is the treatment of choice for these lesions because they may become infected. These lesions tend to recur if incompletely resected. Therefore, sagittal MR is ideal for determining the full extent of the lesion prior to surgery. On CT and MR, these lesions appear as cystic masses with a uniformly thin peripheral rim of capsular enhancement, with occasional septations (Fig. 9.29). Differential diagnostic considerations include necrotic anterior cervical nodes, thrombosed anterior jugular vein, abscess, or obstructed laryngocoele.

Branchial Cleft Cysts. Structures of the face and neck are derived from the branchial cleft apparatus, which consists of six branchial arches. A branchial cleft cyst, sinus, or fistula may develop if there is failure of the cervical sinus or pouch remnants to regress. Although branchial abnormalities can arise from any of the pouches, the majority (95%) arise from the second branchial cleft. The course of the second branchial cleft begins at the base of the tonsillar fossa, and extends between the internal and external carotid arteries. Thus, second branchial cleft cysts are typically found along this pathway, anterior to the middle portion of the sternocleidomastoid muscle and lateral to the internal jugular vein at the level of the carotid bifurcation. The usual clinical presentation is that of a painless neck mass along the anterior border of the sternocleidomastoid muscle, presenting during the first to third decade. These lesions tend to vary in size over time, often enlarging with upper respiratory tract infections.

Branchial cleft cysts are readily identified on CT and MR as well-circumscribed cystic lesions. Wall thickness, irregularity, and enhancement are related to active or prior infections. With MR, the T1-weighted signal characteristics of the cyst may be either hypointense or hy-

Figure 9.28. Dermoid. Axial T1WI. A well-circumscribed mass in the lateral orbit demonstrates a fat-fluid level (*arrow*) characteristic for a dermoid.

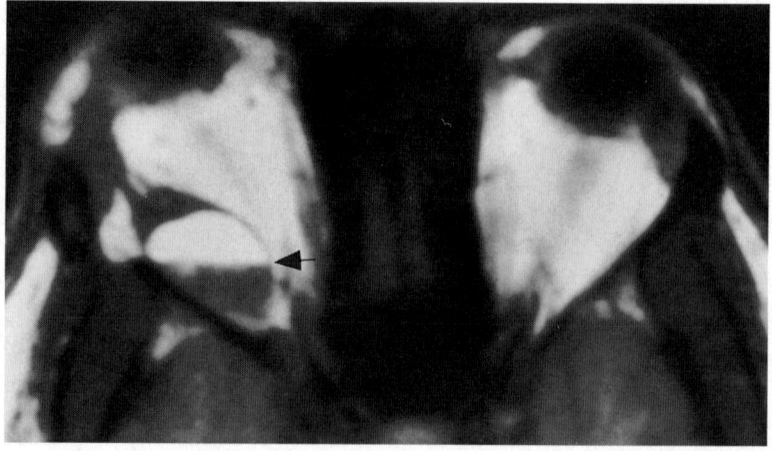

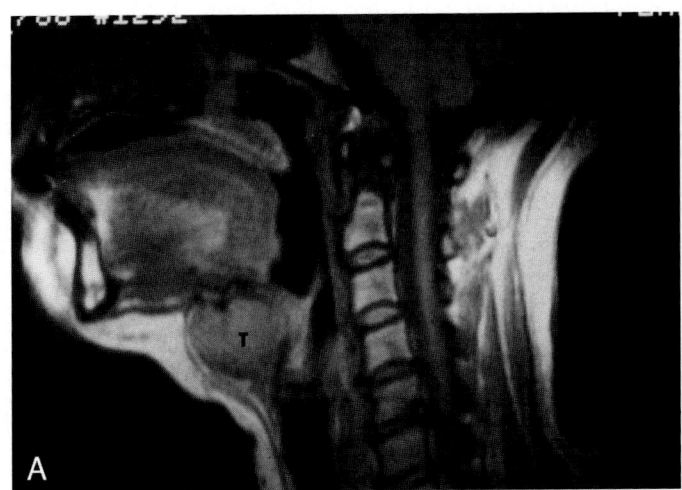
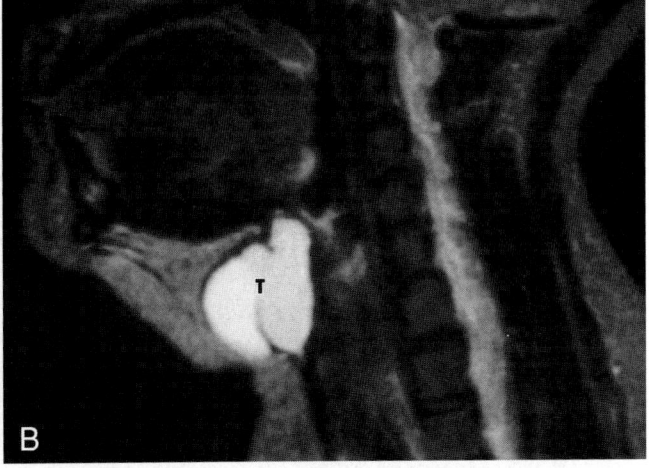

Figure 9.29. Thyroglossal Duct Cyst. Sagittal T1WI **(A)** and T2WI **(B).** A well-defined, multilobulated cystic mass (*T*) is seen below the tongue base. A cystic lesion in this location is highly suggestive of a remnant of the thyroglossal duct. Imaging in the sagittal plane is important in defining the full craniocaudal extent of the lesion.

perintense (Fig. 9.30). This signal variability is related to proteinacious cyst contents. Differential diagnostic considerations include necrotic nodes, abscesses, cystic neural lesions, and thrombosed vessels.

Lymphangiomas are congenital malformations of the lymphatic channels. These lesions are benign and nonencapsulated. Histologically they are classified as capillary, cavernous, or cystic. Any of these histologic types can be found in a given lesion, but the preponderance of a certain type dictates how the lesion is classified. The capillary lymphangiomas are composed of capillary-sized, thin-walled lymphatic channels. In contrast, cavernous lymphangiomas are composed of moderately dilated lymphatics with a fibrous adventitia. Cystic hygromas represent enormously dilated lymphatic channels.

The lymphatic system develops from primitive embryonic lymph sacs that are in turn derived from the venous system. If these sacs fail to communicate with the venous system, they dilate due to accumulation of lymphatic fluid. Thus, lymphangiomas represent sequestrations of the primitive embryonic lymph sacs. If this defect is localized, the result is an isolated cystic hygroma. However, extensive defects in this lymphovenous communication are incompatible with life, and result in fetal hydrops. Various congenital malformation syndromes occur in association with fetal cystic hygromas, including Turner's syndrome, fetal alcohol syndrome, Noonan's syndrome, and several chromosomal aneuploidies. Most lymphangiomas present by 2 years of age (90%), with 50% presenting at the time of birth. This early presentation reflects that the time of greatest lymphatic development occurs in the first 2 years of life.

Lymphangiomas and cystic hygromas appear as painless compressible neck masses that, if large enough, will transilluminate. The lesions commonly occur in the posterior triangle of the neck. On imaging studies, these lesions are multiloculated cystic masses with septations (Fig. 9.31); they also have a propensity to hemorrhage into themselves. This may result in a dramatic, acute increase in the size of the lesion. On imaging studies, one

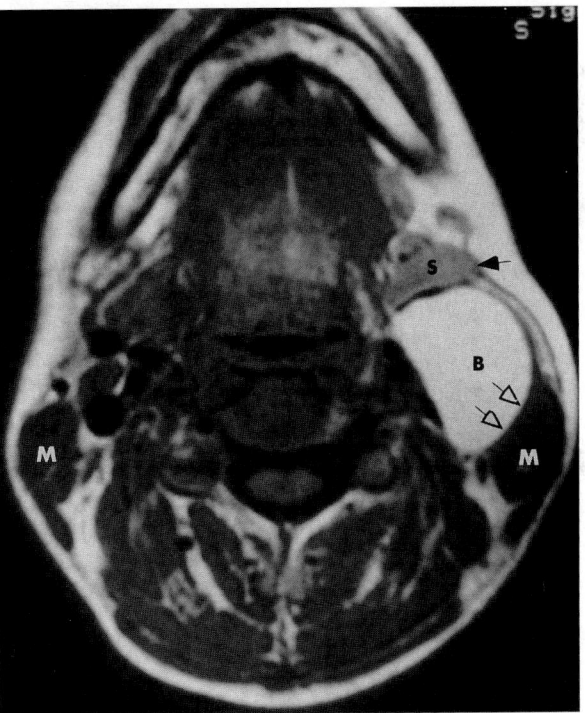

Figure 9.30. Branchial Cleft Cyst. Axial T1WI through the floor of the mouth. A well-rounded, noninfiltrating lesion (*B*) is seen anterior to the left sternocleidomastoid muscle (*M*), which is displaced posteriorly (*open arrows*). The submandibular gland (*S*) is displaced anteriorly (*arrow*). This lesion is at the level of the carotid bifurcation. This combination of features is characteristic of a branchial cleft cyst. Branchial cleft cysts may display high signal on the T1WI, the result of T1 shortening effect due to proteinacious fluid.

can expect a hemorrhage-fluid level or heterogeneous signal characteristics associated with blood degradation products. Because these lesions are easily compressible, they tend not to displace adjacent soft-tissue structures, and this may prove a helpful differentiating feature from other cystic lesions, such as necrotic lymph nodes.

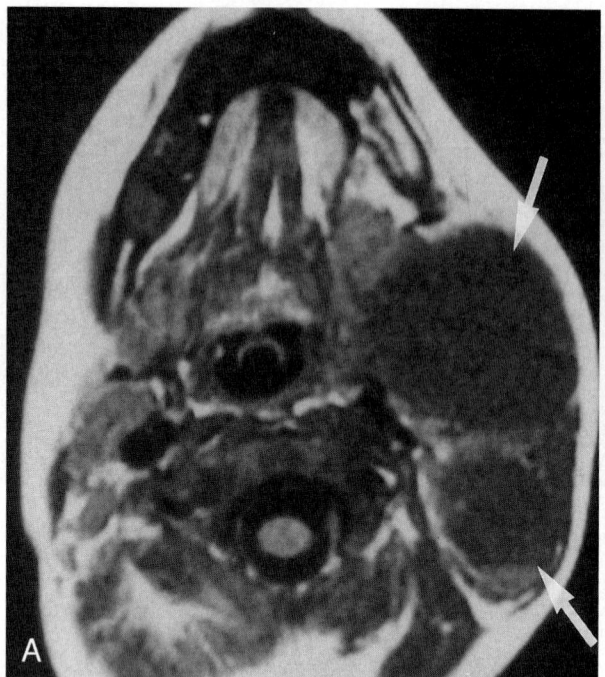
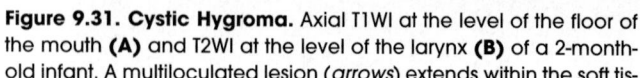
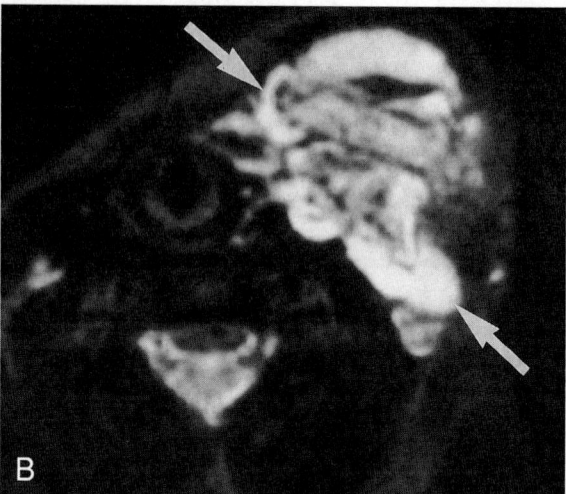

Figure 9.31. Cystic Hygroma. Axial T1WI at the level of the floor of the mouth **(A)** and T2WI at the level of the larynx **(B)** of a 2-month-old infant. A multiloculated lesion (*arrows*) extends within the soft tissues of the anterior neck. The transpacial nature of this lesion and its heterogeneous T2 signal is characteristic of a cystic hygroma or lymphangioma.

References

1. Castelijns JA, van den Brekel MW. Magnetic resonance imaging evaluation of extracranial head and necktumors. Magn Res Quarterly 1993;9:113–128.
2. Hudgins PA. Contrast enhancement in head and neck imaging. Neuroimag Clin North Am 1994;4:101–115.
3. Mafee MF. Modern imaging of paranasal sinuses and the role of limited sinus computerized tomography; considerations of time, cost and radiation. Ear Nose Throat J 1994; 73:532–542.
4. Lustrin ES, Robertson RL, Tilak, S. Normal anatomy of the skull base. Neuroimag Clin North Amer 1994;4:465–478.
5. Casselman JW. Temporal bone imaging. Neuroimag Clin North Am 1996;6:265–289.
6. Hasso AN, Nickmeyer, CA. Magnetic resonance imaging of soft tissues of the neck. Topics Magn Res Imag 1994;6:254–274.
7. van den Brekel MW, Castelijns JA, Snow GB. Imaging of cervical lymphadenopathy. Neuroimag Clin North Amer 1996;6:417–434.
8. Mafee MF, Ainbinder D, Afshani E, et al. The eye. Neuroimag Clin North Am 1996;6:29–59.
9. Warner MA, Weber AL, Jakobiec FA. Benign and malignant tumors of the orbital cavity including the lacrimal gland. Neuroimag Clin North Am 1996;6:123–142.
10. Barnes PD, Robson CD, Robertson RL, Poussaint TY. Pediatric orbital and visual pathway lesions. Neuroimag Clin North Am 1996;6:179–198.
11. Weber AL, Jakobiec FA, Sabates NR. Lymphoproliferative disease of the orbit. Neuroimag Clin North Am 1996; 6:93–111.
12. Vazquez E, Enriquez G, Castellote A, et al. US, CT, and MR imaging of neck lesions in children. Radiographics 1995; 15:105–122.

10
Nondegenerative Diseases of the Spine

Erik H.L. Gaensler

This chapter focuses on nondegenerative diseases of the spinal cord, meninges, and paraspinous soft tissues, and is divided into sections covering inflammation, infection, neoplasms, vascular diseases, congenital malformations, and trauma (1–5). The spine is composed of vertebrae, which house the spinal cord and proximal spinal nerves, and thereby represents a "border zone" between the central nervous system (CNS) and musculoskeletal system (this is true politically as well as anatomically—with both neurosurgeons and orthopaedic surgeons claiming the spine as their province). Disc degeneration and spinal stenosis are covered in chapter 11. Primary osseous tumors involving the vertebrae are covered in section IX.

Common Clinical Syndromes

The clinical syndromes produced by degenerative disease and nondegenerative disease can be indistinguishable. Patients with spine disorders present with focal or diffuse back pain, radiculopathy, or myelopathy. Focal back pain without neurologic compromise or fever is not usually an emergency and is virtually an epidemic in our society, with tremendous implications in terms of lost productivity. Focal back pain can be caused by a wide variety of both degenerative and nondegenerative processes. In the low back, the causes most commonly are orthopaedic, such as muscle and ligament strain, facet joint disease, or discogenic disease that does not compromise the nerve roots. However, vertebral metastases or infectious discitis may also cause focal back pain. Because degenerative disease of the spine is far more common than nondegenerative disease, nondegenerative processes may initially be overlooked, with disastrous consequences. Therefore, a good clinical history that

specifically addresses any previous cancers, or ongoing fevers and chills, is crucial in raising the suspicion for a nondegenerative process. When history and physical findings are nonspecific—as often is the case—imaging procedures become central to the diagnosis.

In patients with spinal neurologic findings, one should attempt to distinguish between the clinical syndromes of myelopathy and radiculopathy because they differ in significant respects, including degree of urgency. Important distinctions between radiculopathy and myelopathy are summarized in Table 10.1.

Myelopathy results from compromise of the spinal cord itself, caused by mechanical compression, intrinsic lesions, or inflammatory processes loosely grouped under the term "myelitis." Classic symptoms include bladder and bowel incontinence, spasticity, weakness, and ataxia. With cord compression, a motor or sensory level may develop, and knowing this level may prove helpful in focusing the imaging examination. However, the lesion may be several vertebral bodies higher than the apparent dermatomal sensory level, particularly in the thoracic region. Myelopathy often presents without a clear sensory level, and complete screening of the cord from the cervicomedullary junction to the conus may be required. This is easily accomplished with modern phased array coils.

The spinal cord, like the brain, has limited healing powers. In fact, the spinal cord in many respects is less tolerant of injury than the brain. A small benign mass, such as a 2-cm epidural hematoma or meningioma, may permanently damage the cord because of the small diameter of the spinal canal. A similar-sized mass may be asymptomatic within the voluminous calvarium. The "plasticity" of the brain, whereby remaining cortex can assume the function of injured areas through a complex network of redundant axons, is well documented, particularly in younger patients. The spinal cord, which consists of long linear neuronal tracts, has far less plasticity. After 24 hours of acute cord compression, little hope remains for significant recovery of function. Therefore, an acute myelopathy is an emergency, and the radiologist should do everything to facilitate prompt imaging, preferably with MR, for reasons that will be discussed.

Radiculopathy results from impingement of the spinal nerves, either within the canal, lateral recesses, or neural foramina. This compromise, typically because of mass effect, results in specific dermatomal sensory deficits and muscle group weakness. These are outlined in any neurology or physical diagnosis text, and are worth knowing. The most common causes of pain and neurologic defect are disc herniations, spinal stenosis,

Table 10.1. Myelopathy vs. Radiculopathy

Cause	Myelopathy	Radiculopathy
Typical disease processes	Spinal cord compromise Extramedullary disease: cord compression due to epidural mass effect Intramedullary disease: tumor, inflammation, AVMs, SDAVFs*	Spinal nerve compromise Osteophytic spurring (especially cervical-spine) Disc herniations Extramedullary and paraspinous tumors and inflammatory processes compromising nerve roots
Neurologic findings	Ataxia Bowel and bladder incontinence Babinski's sign	Weakness and diminished reflexes in specific muscle groups, dermatomal sensory deficits
Accuracy of clinical localization	Often poor; lesion may be several levels higher than anticipated	Usually quite good
Urgency for imaging (of acute presentations)	High—little recovery expected with deficits untreated >24 hour	Low—short delay for conservative treatment usually entails little risk
Preferred imaging modality	MR has no substitute as the initial screening exam	CT, especially with intrathecal contrast is still excellent, particularly in cervical spine

* Spinal dural arteriovenous fistula.

and in the cervical spine, uncovertebral joint spurring. Of course, malignant and infectious processes compromise spinal nerves but overall are less common. The peripheral nervous system, unlike the CNS, has significant ability to withstand injury and to regenerate. Therefore, pure radicular symptoms, although at times excruciatingly painful, rarely represent a surgical emergency. Extensive epidural neoplasms and infections may present with mixed myelopathic and radicular signs. These patients must be imaged with the urgency of a pure cord syndrome.

Imaging Methods

Plain Radiographs of the spine were once the initial test in every spine evaluation, but with newer techniques this is no longer logical or cost-effective. Radiographs continue to be the mainstay for ruling out trauma to the vertebral column, and other acute screening settings. Plain films are indispensable for correct localization in the operating room. Radiographs have a great deal of useful information to offer when evaluating degenerative processes, particularly with extensive osteophyte formation in the cervical spine. Flexion and extension plain films were once the only dynamic imaging technique for assessment of spine stability. MR now also can be done in flexion and extension, which can be useful in evaluating cord compression that is positional (see Fig. 10.8).

In nondegenerative disease, careful attention should be paid to the integrity of the vertebral bodies and pedicles, frequent sites of metastases. However, early infiltrative changes in the marrow space, easily seen on MR, cannot be detected by plain films. The classic radiographic findings of widened interpedicular distance with tumors, and midline bony spurs with diastematomyelia, are rarely seen except on board examinations.

Myelography. The definitive indications for plain film myelography are limited; these include complex postoperative cases and patients in whom MR is contraindicated because of MR-incompatibile implanted devices.

Screening for dilated vessels from spinal dural arteriovenous fistulas remains a rare but useful application for myelograpy (see Fig 10.53B) Water-soluble nonionic contrast media have low toxicity and have replaced metrizamide, an older agent although the term "metrizamide myelogram" has stuck. Pantopaque (iophendylate), an even older oil-based iodinated medium, is almost never used. *Ionic contrast agents are absolutely contraindicated for myelography* because they can result in severe inflammation, seizures, arachnoiditis, and death.

The recommended dosage of nonionic contrast in adults depends on the region to be studied, the size of the patient, and the size of thecal sac. A convenient and conservative rule of thumb in adults is not to exceed 3 g of intrathecal iodine, which works out to 17 ml of 180 mg/ml, 12.5 ml of 240 mg/ml, or 10 ml of 300 mg/ml, three of the standard concentrations. In general, lumbar myelography should be performed using contrast media with a concentration between 180–240 mg/ml, and cervical and/or thoracic myelography should be performed with 200–300 mg/ml. The smaller the area of the subarachnoid space, the denser the contrast must be for good plain films. With the high contrast sensitivity of CT, 180 mg/ml is more than adequate, and small doses (5 ml) or dilution of the full dose with time (3–4 hours delay if a full dose is given) is required for proper iodine concentration to avoid CT artifacts although with modern CT scanners, these are minimal. Full-dose plain film myelography was already in decline before MR because of CT myelography, which can be done with lower doses of intrathecal contrast.

Myelography begins with a lumbar puncture, with the patient in prone position under fluoroscopy. The preferred puncture site depends on the clinical findings, and usually is the midlumbar region, inferior to the posterior elements of L-2 or L-3. This injection level will avoid most disc herniations and spinal stenosis, which are worse at lower levels, as well as the conus, which in adults lies between T-12/L-1 and L-1/L-2 disc spaces. Care should be taken to place the needle near the midline in order to reduce the chances of an extra-arachnoid injection or spearing of an exiting nerve root. Contrast should be injected only after spontaneous CSF backflow is established. The complications of poor needle placement include subdural and epidural injection. Examples of these complications are well illustrated in older neuroradiology textbooks, and have medicolegal implications. Therefore, if in doubt where the contrast is going, stop, take frontal and lateral plain films, and examine them carefully. Avoid any air bubbles in the tubing system because they can cause filling defects easily confused with drop metastases. If tumor or infection is suspected, collect adequate CSF for chemistry, cultures, and cytology if this has not already been done. For routine degenerative cases, CSF examination has not proved worthwhile.

C1-2 punctures are rarely required and are inherently more dangerous than lumbar injection because direct injury to the cord or a low-lying posterior inferior cerebellar artery loop can occur. The puncture is best done under lateral fluoroscopy, placing the needle in the posterior third of the spinal canal between C-1 and C-2. Classic indications include known blocks caudally or the need for dense opacification of the cervical and upper thoracic spinal canal for plain films. Today, one of the rare good reasons for a C1-2 puncture would be complete spine block in the midthoracic region identified by lumbar myelography, with the need to define the upper extent of the block—in a patient with a pacemaker precluding MR. If the pacemaker were not an issue, MR would be the study of choice. MR is far quicker, more comfortable, and, most importantly, safer for the patient. Even if there is no technical complication with a myelogram, patients with spine block can deteriorate from the subtle fluid and pressure shifts that inevitably accompany needle placement in the subarachnoid space, a syndrome known as "spinal coning." The multiple steps in the evaluation of spine block by plain film myelography followed by CT are shown in Figure 10.1. Contrast this with the simplicity and elegance of MR as shown in Figure 10.2. In oncologic cases, MR has the additional benefit of excellent evaluation of the marrow space—not available with CT.

Space-occupying lesions of the spinal canal are classified according to their location as intramedullary, intradural-extramedullary, and extradural. This distinction, which can be made on myelography as well as on CT and MR, is critical in formulating a differential diagnosis. Intramedullary lesions are usually confined to the spinal cord itself, but may be exophytic.

Extramedullary lesions are by definition outside the cord, but they may be either intradural or extradural. A summary of the radiologic appearance and differential diagnosis for each lesion location is outlined in Table 10.2. Remember that the lesion must be seen in at least two (and preferably three) 90° orthogonal planes because large intradural lesions may simulate an extradural mass on any single view. Similarly, bilateral extradural disease can flatten the cord, increasing its apparent anteroposterior dimension in sagittal view, giving the false impression of an intramedullary mass (Fig. 10.3). Correlation with axial imaging is invaluable in this re-

gard. Also remember that lateral lesions such as lateral disc herniations may be completely missed by myelography. In most cases today, a CT is performed after myelography.

CT. The decline of plain film myelography for degenerative disease was initially because of CT, especially CT with intrathecal contrast, which is superior to myelography in diagnostic accuracy. However, CT is now steadily being replaced by MR for most screening examinations of the spine. Low-dose CT myelography remains the gold standard in cases where the limits of the thecal sac or nerve root sleeves must be precisely defined, such as in complex postoperative states. Small leptomeningeal (drop) metastases can be identified; however, MR with gadolinium has largely replaced CT myelography as the initial screening examination for drop metastases. In the cervical spine, CT remains the most reliable way to assess foraminal stenosis.

CT has been less effective in depicting intramedullary diseases of the spinal cord such as primary tumors, myelitis, and syringohydromyelia. These conditions are better evaluated with MR. For example, a nonexpansile multiple sclerosis (MS) plaque will escape detection on any imaging examination except MR.

MR has done for the spinal canal what CT did for the calvarium, allowing for the first-time a noninvasive "look inside." Therefore, it has become the examination of choice for any disorder of the spine resulting in myelopathy. The key to MR's success has been its superior soft-tissue contrast (including the ability to evaluate the marrow compartment), multiplanar capabilities, noninvasiveness, and high sensitivity to gadolinium enhancement, recently heightened further by fat-saturation techniques.

MR scanning techniques for the spine continue to improve, and with the wide variety of imaging systems available, recommending specific protocols in a general text makes little sense. A few general guidelines follow. Surface coils are an absolute must to obtain adequate signal to noise in most systems. Motion suppression techniques, such as anterior radiofrequency saturation bands, gradient moment nulling, and cardiac/respiratory gating, are critical to reduce motion artifact. This is particularly important on T2 spin-echo images of the cervical and thoracic spine, which remain the standard for evaluating intrinsic cord disease. "Fast spin-echo" (FSE) sequences have replaced conventional spin echo for spine work, with great time savings and little cost when only degenerative disease is present. FSE technique, hovever, is poor for marrow evaluation, but this can be overcome by using fat saturation with the T2WI, a technique widely used in musculoskeletal MR to search for marrow edema.

Gradient-echo images are also poor for marrow space evaluation, because of susceptibility effects from the bony trabeculae, and are of little use in evaluating nondegenerative spinal disease except when searching for blood-breakdown products (see Fig. 10.65). Short TR inversion recovery (STIR) probably offers the highest sensitivity for marrow space edema, but conventional STIR is time-consuming, with poor signal to noise. "Fast inversion recovery" techniques, however, have recently been perfected, and these compete with T2 FSE with fat

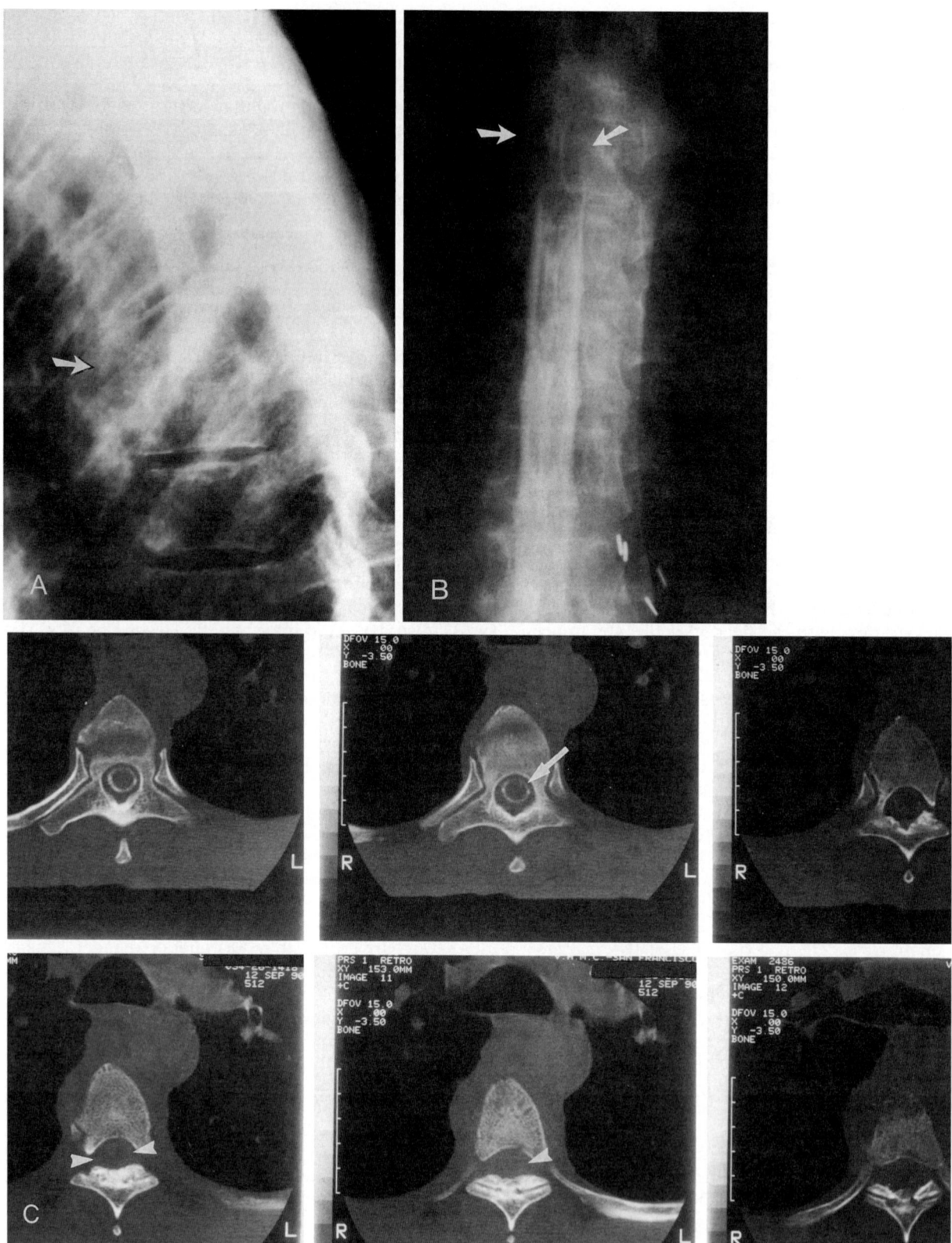

Figure 10.1. Acute Cord Compression. Middle-aged patient with acute myelopathy and midthoracic back pain, worked up the "old-fashioned" way. **A.** Plain film done in the emergency department shows compression fracture of a midthoracic vertebrae (*arrow*). **B.** Lumbar myelogram shows complete block to contrast in the midthoracic vertebrae (*arrows*). A portable C-arm fluoroscope then had to be obtained to do a C1-2 puncture, followed by a cervical and upper thoracic myelogram (not shown). **C.** Upper thoracic CT- myelogram images show gradual effacement of the subarachnoid space (*arrow*), which disappears at site of the block (*arrowheads*). **D.** Sagittal reconstruction enables assessment of the entire process in a single image, showing cord compression centered around an abnormal disc space (*arrow*), consistent with infection, which was proven at laminectomy. Note the gradual effacement of the sub-arachnoid space (*arrowheads*). Total elapsed time for procedures **A–D** was 3 hours—not bad for this technique!

saturation as the optimum marrow screening exam (see Figs. 10.37, 10.43). Ultrathin section imaging (<1 mm) without interslice gaps is now performed with three-dimensional Fourier transformation and now rivals CT for thin-slice profiles, critical in the cervical spine for examination of the foramina.

Some pitfalls with spinal MR, however, do exist. These include motion sensitivity, imprecise detection of calcium, and occasional false-negatives with contrast examinations. Despite motion compensation techniques, both physiologic and patient motion remain problematic.

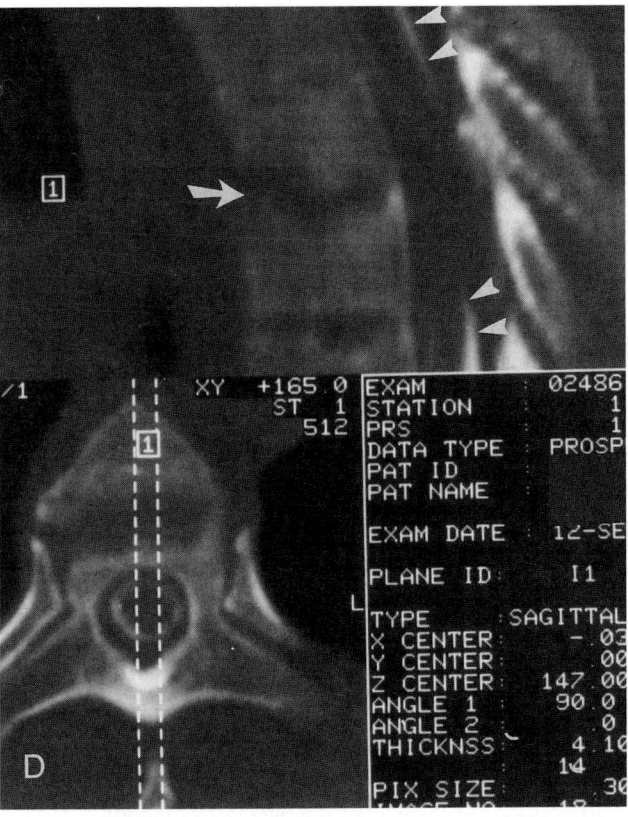

Figure 10.1.D.

Patient movement exaggerates osseous encroachment of the spinal canal and neural foramina because far more movement occurs during the 8 minutes it may take to do a three-dimensional Fourier transformation cervical spine axial image than a 2-second CT slice. Spin-echo MR techniques are usually inferior to CT in the detection of subtle calcification. This may be important in defining small osteophytic spurring, ossification of the posterior longitudinal ligament, identifying retropulsed bone fragments following trauma, or characterizing calcification in tumors. Because of susceptibility effects, gradient recalled techniques may overestimate the size of calcific structures. Gadolinium is essential in the evaluation of infection and intrathecal metastases, but it may obscure vertebral metastases by making them isointense with surrounding marrow fat (Fig. 10.4). Also, evaluating hemorrhage on postcontrast images is difficult. Always obtain a precontrast T1 "scout" image to avoid these two pitfalls.

Spinal Angiography is technically demanding, dangerous in untrained hands, and difficult to interpret. There is no reliable spinal "circle of Willis" allowing collateral flow from multiple sources although some variable interconnected vascular arcades exist. Therefore, an inadvertent catheter-induced complication can have tragic consequences. Excellent texts exist on spinal angiography, but this area has increasingly become the province of interventional neuroradiologists, who can both diagnose and treat spinal arteriovenous malformations—the main indication for spinal angiography.

Nuclear Medicine Bone Scans give a comprehensive view of the skeleton when searching for metastases. If a new focus of vertebral isotope uptake is noted and plain films do not show an abnormality, MR is used because of its excellent delineation of the marrow space and any associated spinal cord compression. Bone scans are highly sensitive but quite nonspecific because both degenerative and nondegenerative processes will show increased uptake. When such patients are referred for MR, it is critical to be aware of the bone scan findings in order to protocol the examination appropriately.

US has limited applications for evaluating the spine because in adults the posterior elements obscure the po-

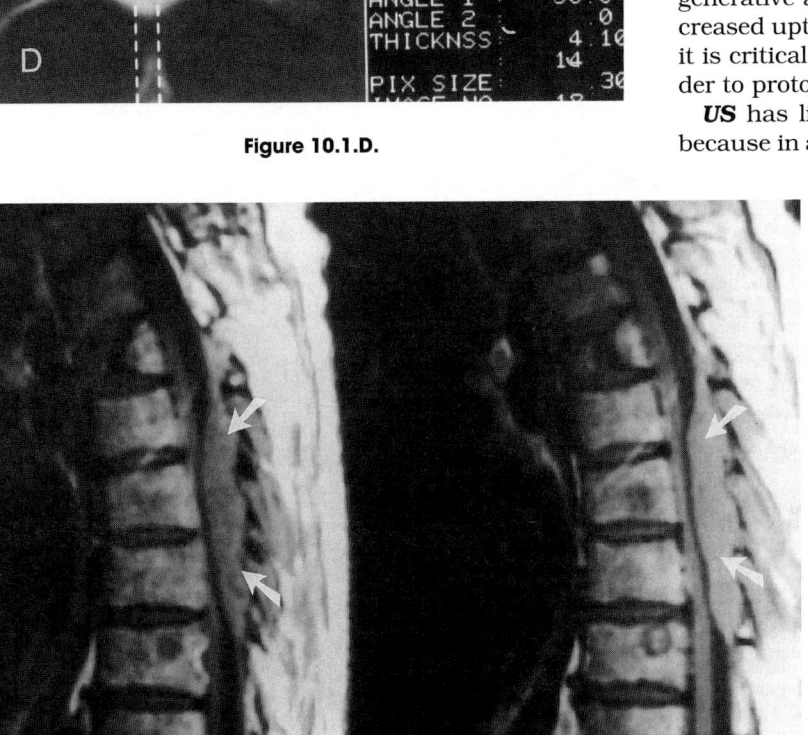

Figure 10.2. Acute Cord Compression—MR. Evaluation of a thoracic cord compression, the easy way—compare with Figure 10.1. A middle-aged patient presented to a physician's office with acute myelopathy. This emergency MR using T1 sagittal and axial sequences took 20 minutes, was completely noninvasive, and gives excellent detail of the marrow space, unavailable on CT. The epidural soft tissue mass (*arrows*) proved to be lymphoma.

Table 10.2. Differential Diagnosis of Spinal Lesions by Location

LOCATION AND IMAGING APPEARANCE

DIFFTENTIAL DIAGNOSIS

A. INTRADURAL   INTRAMEDULLARY

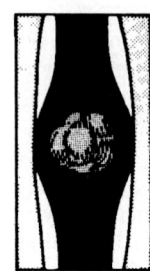 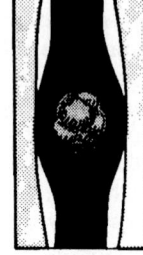 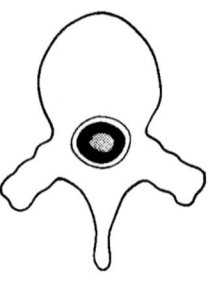

AP   Lateral   Axial

Ependymoma
Astrocytoma
Hemanigioblastoma
Lipoma/(Epi)Dermoid
Syringohydromyelia
Intramedullary AVM
Rare site: met/abscess

Cord appears widened in all views. The CSF space appears thinned on all sides in all views.

B. INTRADURAL   EXTRAMEDULLARY

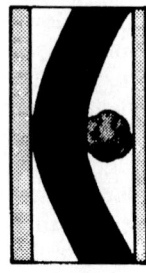 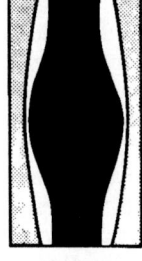 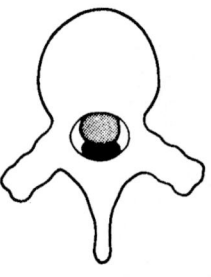

AP   Lateral   Axial

DIFFERENTIAL DIAGNOSIS

Meningioma
Schwannoma/neurinoma
Neurofibroma
Hemangiopericytoma
Lipoma/(Epi) Dermoid
Arachnoid cyst/adhesion
Drop/leptomeningeal met
Veins (extramed AVM)

The contrast/CSF forms acute angles with the mass (which may have a dural attachment—"marble on the carpet"). This results in a "meniscus" around the mass, and a widened contrast column between the cord and the mass on one side, with effacement of the CSF on the other.

C. EXTRADURAL

DIFFERENTIAL DIAGNOSIS

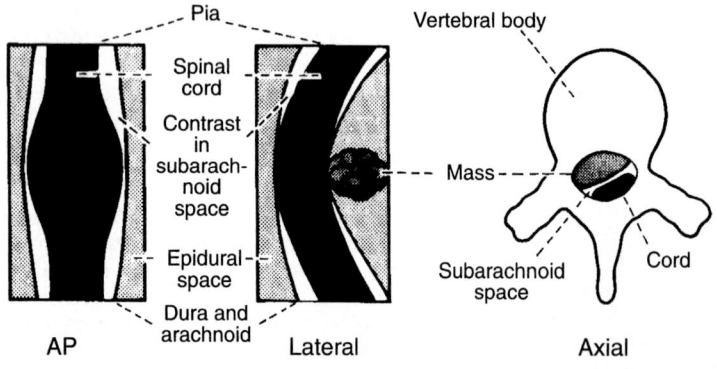

AP   Lateral   Axial

Degenerative
  Herniated disc
  Synovial cyst
  Osteophyte
  Rheumatoid pannus
Nondegenerative
  Metastasis
  Abscess
  Hematoma
  1° tumor expansion
    or invasion
  Epidural lipomatosis

The dura and the sac will be displaced together, away from the mass. The CSF angles around the mass will be obtuse with a "marble under the carpet" appearance. The cord may be widened in one plane by pressure from the mass, with contrast material thinned on both sides of the cord.

Adapted from Latchaw, 1991, with permission.

Adapted from Latchaw RE, ed. MR and CT of the Head, Neck, and Spine. 2nd ed. St. Louis: Mosby, 1991.

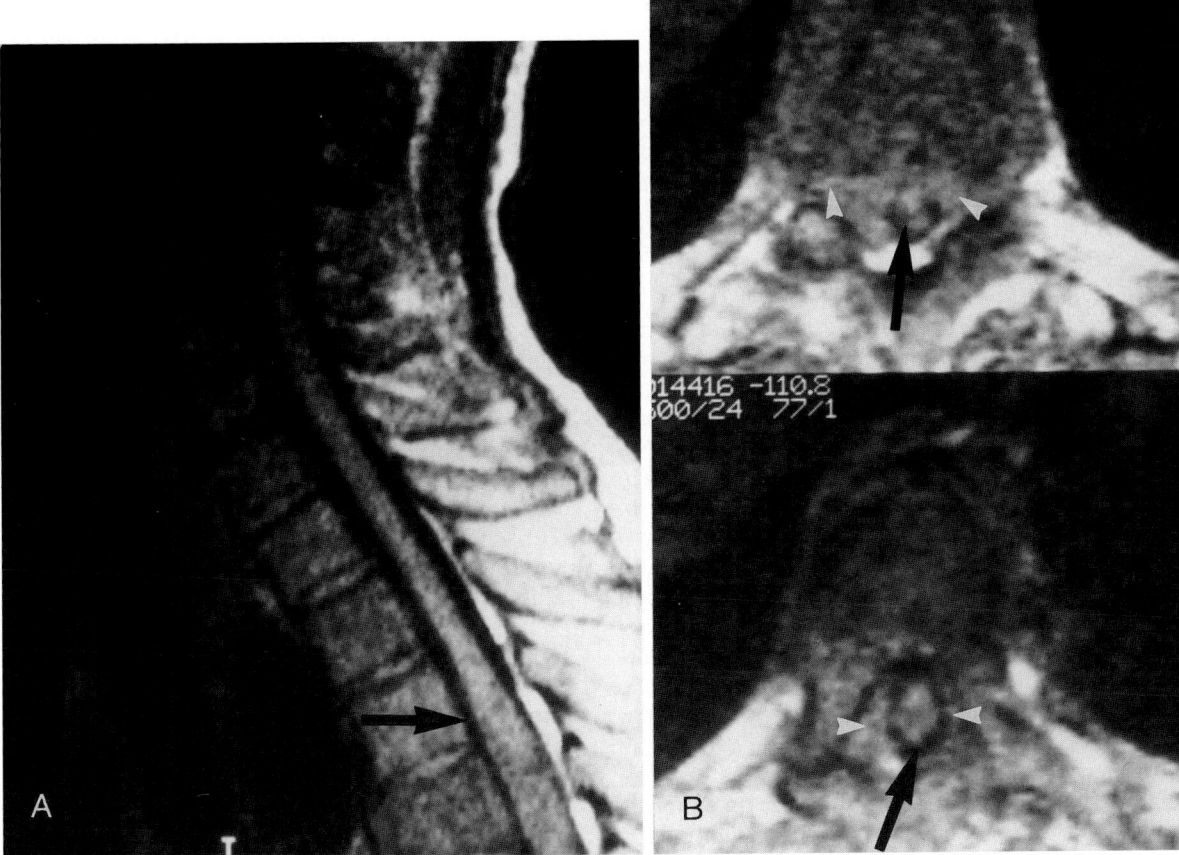

Figure 10.3. Extramedullary Tumor. This patient presented with myelopathy with an upper thoracic sensory level. **A.** On this midline sagittal image, the spinal cord appears widened (*arrow*), suggestive of an intramedullary lesion. The patient was unable to stay still for additional images. **B.** Subsequent reimaging in the axial plain shows that the extramedullary tumor (*arrowheads*) has flattened the cord (*arrow*) from its sides, increasing its anteroposterior dimensions, giving the spurious impression of an intramedullary expansile process on the midline sagittal images. The moral is the same as on plain films: always look at pathology in two (preferable 90° opposed) orthogonal planes.

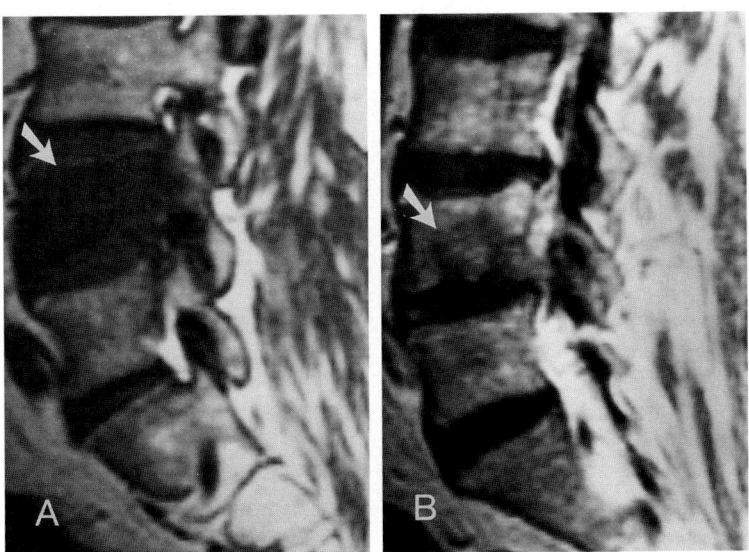

Figure 10.4. Gadolinium-enhanced Imaging Potential Pitfalls. A. Infiltration of the entire L-4 vertebral body (*arrow*) on this unenhanced lumbar MR is readily apparent. **B.** After contrast administration, the area involved with metastatic tumor (*arrow*) has enhanced to isointensity with the remaining normal vertebrae, and is far less conspicuous. The lesion still could be visualized with fat saturation or STIR techniques, despite the gadolinium, but why do things the hard way? Moral: always obtain a precontrast image when using gadolinium in the spine.

tential acoustic window. However, in neonates the unossified posterior elements provide a window through which spinal anomalies can be evaluated, and excellent work has been done in this highly specialized area. Once the laminae have been removed surgically, intraoperative US has proven to be an excellent tool for the evaluation of the spinal cord for tumor, syrinx, and other intramedullary processes, thus minimizing the need for cord exploration.

INFLAMMATION

This section focuses on inflammatory diseases that cause myelopathy, principally through direct involvement of the spinal cord (6–12). The mechanisms of many of these disorders is not fully understood, and they are sometimes lumped under the term "myelitis." Myelitis may be focal or diffuse. When both clinical and pathologic findings are confined to distinct level(s), the term "transverse myelitis" may be used. This is not really a specific disease, but rather a category of diseases, and few agree on exactly what processes should be grouped under "transverse myelitis." On the whole, carefully describing the imaging findings and giving specific differential diagnoses is better than invoking such nonspecific terms in MR reports. Strictly speaking, a distinction should be made between processes affecting the gray matter, termed "poliomyelitis," and those affecting the white matter, or leukomyelitis. In practice, these terms are rarely heard, and poliomyelitis become synonymous with the colloquial "polio," a specific syndrome caused by a specific picornavirus, against which we all hopefully have been vaccinated.

Multiple Sclerosis is the most common spinal cord "inflammatory" disorder. The epidemiology and pathophysiology of MS are reviewed in detail in chapter 7. Multiple sclerosis of the brain and spinal cord are similar regarding the patient profile, with the hallmark of the disease being multiple neurologic deficits separated both anatomically and temporally. When spinal MS predominates, it follows a progressive clinical course, in contrast to the relapsing/remitting pattern more characteristic with brain involvement. The majority of MS patients have mixed presentations, with both brain and spinal cord involvement. Although imaging can be helpful, the diagnosis ultimately rests on clinical grounds.

MS plaques appear as areas of increased signal in the white matter of the spinal cord, typically within the white matter of the anterior and posterior columns and lateral spinothalamic tracts. The best screening study is a gated sagittal T2-weighted series, where MS plaques appear as areas of increased signal intensity, usually without significant change in cord diameter, which is why cord MS plaques are often occult myelographically. Occasionally, subtle cord expansion in the acute phase may exist because of edema, (Fig. 10.5) and "burnt out" MS plaques can present as myelomalacia (literally cord softening or atrophy).

As in the brain, plaque enhancement may be present, which correlates with acute lesion activity (Fig. 10.6). Because the white matter is on the "outside" of the cord, MS plaques tend to be peripheral (Fig 10.6B). However, edema and enhancement can extend into the central gray matter as well, probably because of perivenular inflammatory changes. Differentiation from a glial tumor may be difficult although MS plaques typically are under two vertebral segments in length, and involve less than half the cross-sectional area of the cord. When a small bright intramedullary lesion is seen on T2WI (Fig 10.5 B), MR of the brain to search for concomitant MS plaques is a more useful next step than contrast administration. The brain and spinal cord are composed of the same tissue types, are physically connected, and share the CSF. Therefore, a good general rule is when presented with a diffuse spinal process, either in-

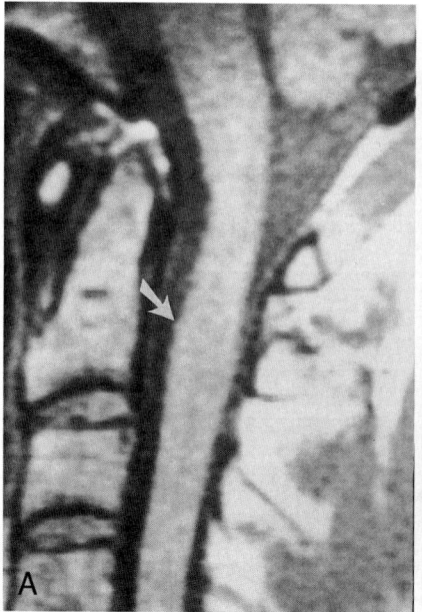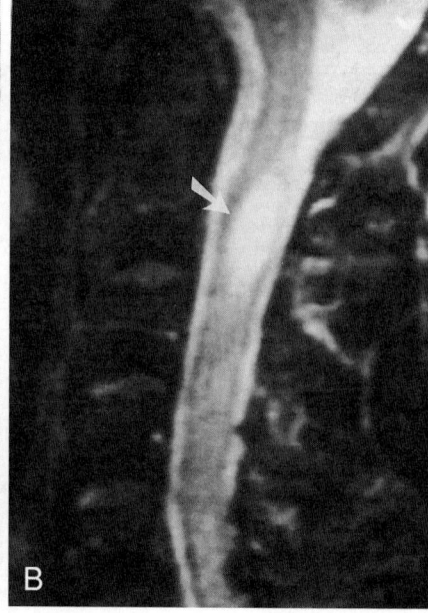

Figure 10.5. Multiple Sclerosis. A solitary lesion (*arrow*) shows subtle cord expansion on T1WI **(A)**, and **(B)** becomes bright on T2WI, because of edema. Differential considerations included an intramedullary tumor, and the diagnosis of MS was supported by the confirmation of concomitant periventricular lesions classic for MS on brain MR.

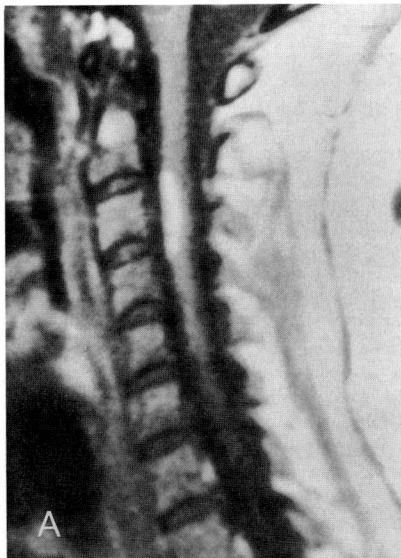

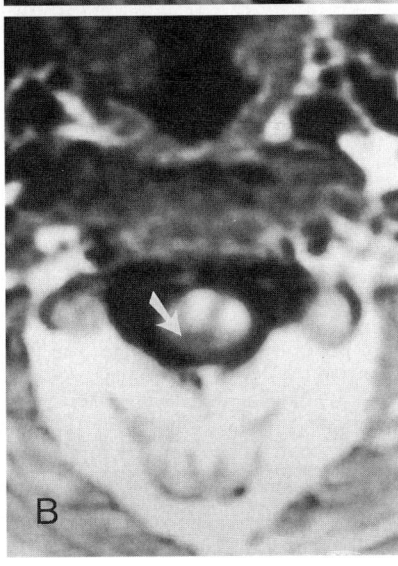

Figure 10.6. Multiple Sclerosis. Considerable swelling and enhancement of the spinal cord is noted on these postcontrast sagittal (**A**) and axial (**B**) images. Note how the central gray matter (*arrow*) is displaced posteriorly by the inflammatory changes in the anterior white matter.

tramedullary or leptomeningeal, remember to look "upstairs" because the same process may be occurring in the brain.

Lupus Erythematosis. Other CNS inflammatory processes are seen in both the brain and spinal cord. A classic example is systemic lupus erythematosus (SLE), where a necrotizing arteritis causes cord ischemia and injury. Antibodies may also damage neuronal elements directly. The spinal cord will show diffuse areas of increased signal intensity with cord swelling on T2WI. Enhancement is less frequently seen (Fig. 10.7). SLE "lesions" have less well defined margins than the discrete plaques of MS and may show dramatic improvement with corticosteriods. MS plaques, in contrast, represent areas of focal myelin destruction, and although the

symptoms improve with corticosteroids, the MR findings improve less dramatically.

Rheumatoid Arthritis (RA) is another "collagen-vascular" disease that can compromise the spinal cord; however, the mechanism is different. Focal inflammatory changes termed "pannus" destroy the transverse ligament of C-1, allowing the odontoid to slide posteriorly relative to C-1 and compressing the cord, particularly in flexion (Fig. 10.8). Therefore, the injury in RA is due to an extramedullary, extradural "mass" rather an intramedullary lesion. A soft-tissue mass at the C1-2 articulation with instablility does not necessarily imply RA; a fibrous pseudotumor has been described in the same location in association with os odontoideum, and this can develop in response to any chronically unstable spinal anatomy, including an ununited Type 1 dens fracture.

The remaining list of inflammatory conditions of the spinal cord is long and parallels the differential considerations in the brain. Chemotherapy, radiation, electrical burns, and lightning are physical factors that can injure the cord.

Radiation Myelitis is similar to radiation injury to the brain: peak incidence occurs roughly 6–12 months after initial treatment, with affected areas demonstrating increased signal intensity on T2WI, with variable enhancement (Fig. 10.9). Radiation myelitis can lead to paralysis, and fear of this complication is usually the limiting factor in radiotherapy for vertebral body metastases. Radiation has a very characteristic effect on the vertebral bodies. The normal erythropoietic marrow is destroyed and replaced by fat, making the vertebrae very homogeneously bright on T1WI (Fig. 10.10). In growing children, cellular repopulation of the vertebral marrow may occur, with stunted growth of the affected vertebrae because of radiation injury to the epiphyses being the main finding (Fig. 10.11).

Acute Viral Illnesses are associated with myelitis in a number of ways, some of which are well described and others which are still poorly understood. The "polio" virus causes direct injury to the anterior horn cells. Herpes zoster is invisible to imaging when latent, but cord swelling and enhancement have been reported with acute "shingles" outbreaks, appearing at spinal levels corresponding to the dermatologic outbreak. Measles provokes an autoimmune reaction that can damage the cord, which has been studied experimentally as a model for MS, and is termed "subacute sclerosing panencephalitis." Acute disseminated encephalomyelitis, described in chapter 7, is a monophasic postviral syndrome, which also affects spinal cord as its name, "encephalo*myelitis*," suggests.

These patients typically have sudden high fevers (presumably viral in origin), followed within four weeks by rapid onset of motor, sensory, and usually autonomic dysfunction, referable to a specific spinal cord level. Many neurologists reserve the catch-all term "transverse myelitis" for this clinical presentation, which may be due to an autoimmune process. The imaging findings typically are a focal area of cord swelling with high signal on T2WI, with variable enhancement. It is difficult not to draw comparisons with Guillain-Barré syndrome, a pro-

Figure 10.7. Systemic Lupus Erythematosus. An MR in a 40-year-old patient with new myelopathy. The spinal cord shows ill-defined areas of edema on **(A)** T2WI and **(B)** gradient echo image (*arrows*). Postcontrast images **(C)** show mild enhancement (*arrow*). The brain was free of abnormalities.

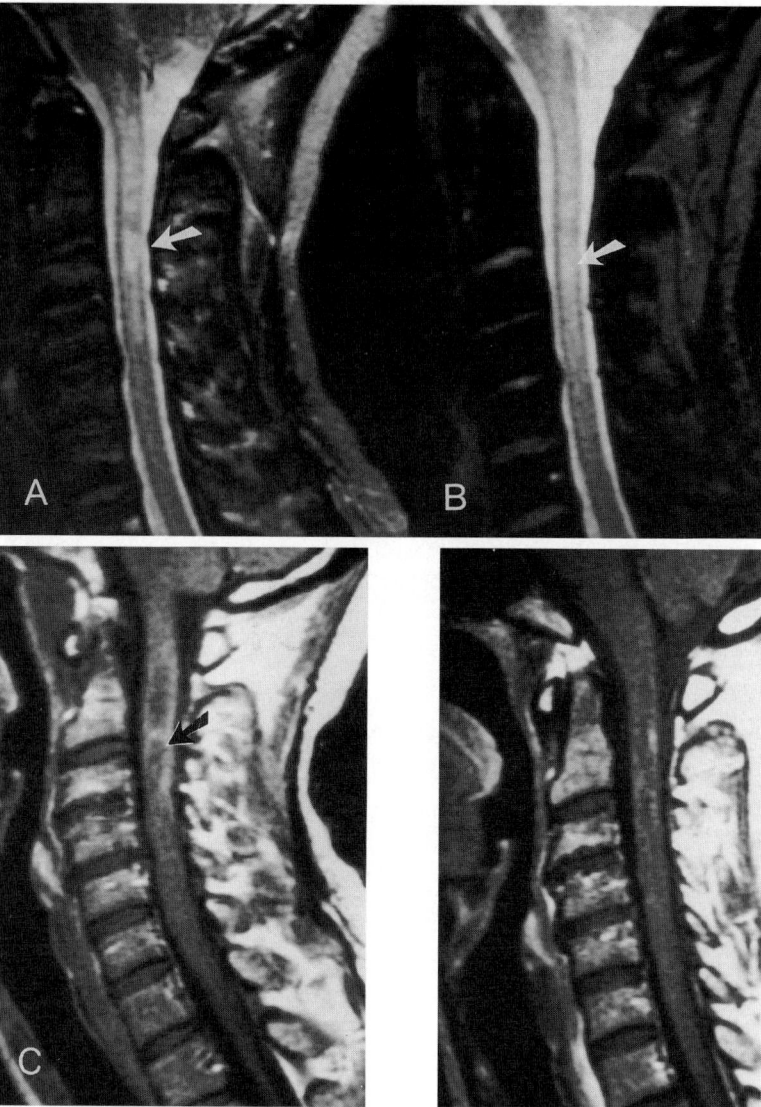

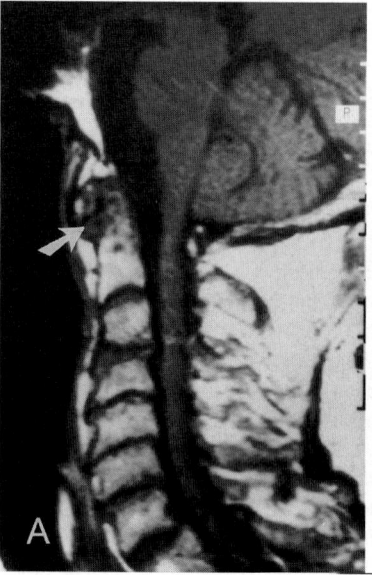
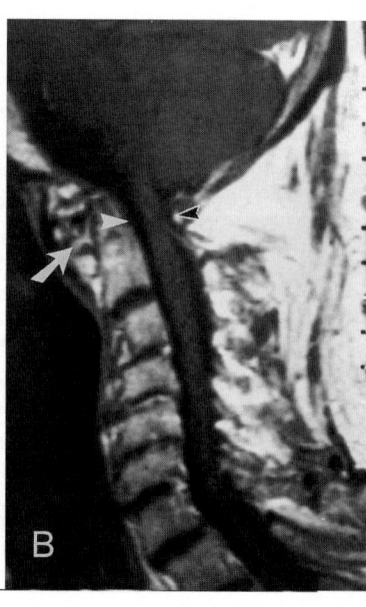

Figure 10.8. Rheumatoid Arthritis. A. This elderly patient had myelopathy caused by atlantoaxial instability secondary to pannus (*arrow*), which has destroyed the transverse ligament of C-1. In extension, no cord impingement is seen. **B.** In flexion, the dens has borderline mass effect on the cord (*arrowheads*). The pannus enhances vigorously with contrast (*arrow*).

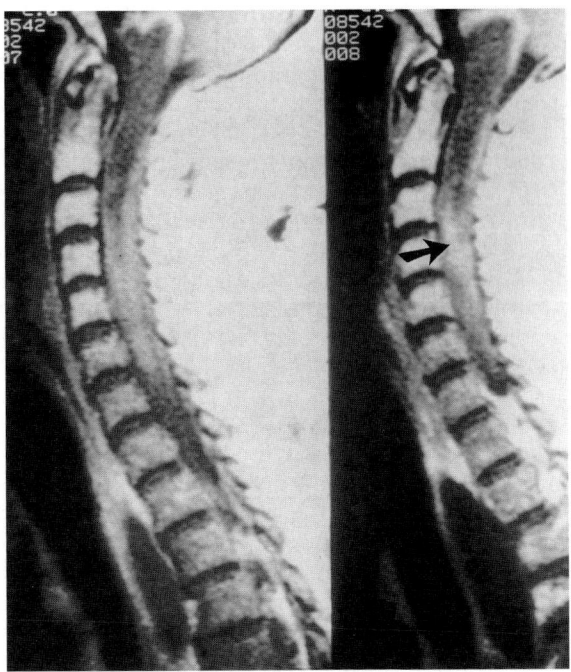

Figure 10.9. Radiation Myelitis. Intramedullary enhancement (*arrow*) is noted in this patient who received radiation therapy to the neck.

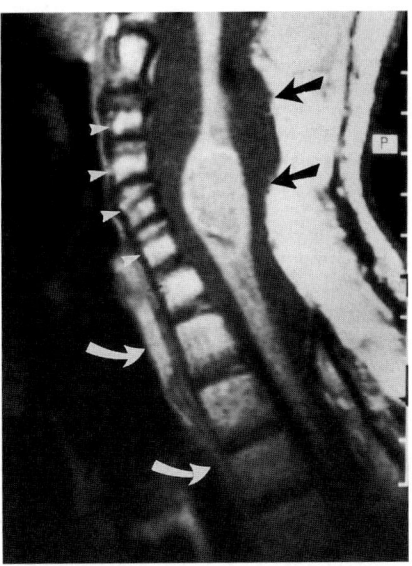

Figure 10.11. Radiation Effect. This child is status postlaminectomy (*arrows*) and radiation for an intramedullary astrocytoma. Note the growth retardation of the vertebrae within the x-ray therapy field (*arrowheads*), as compared with vertebrae left outside the field (*curved arrows*). The epiphyseal plates of vertebrae, like any other rapidly dividing tissue, are highly sensitive to radiation injury.

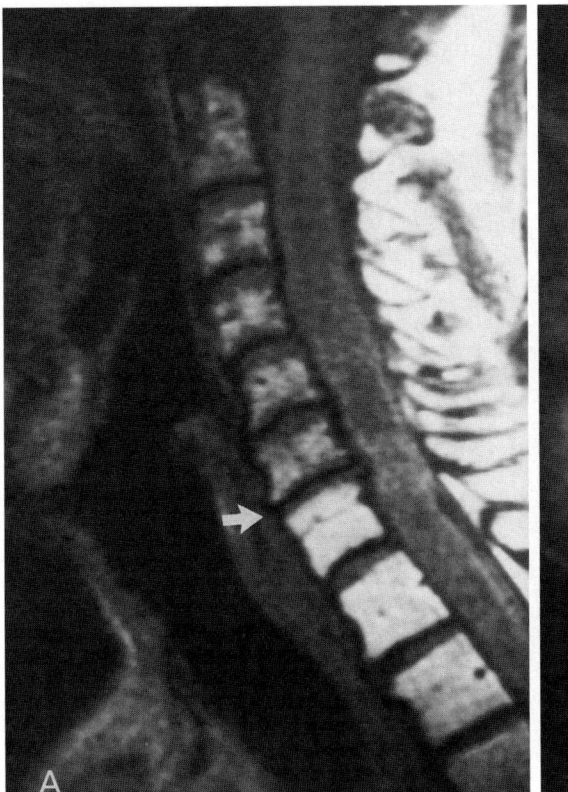

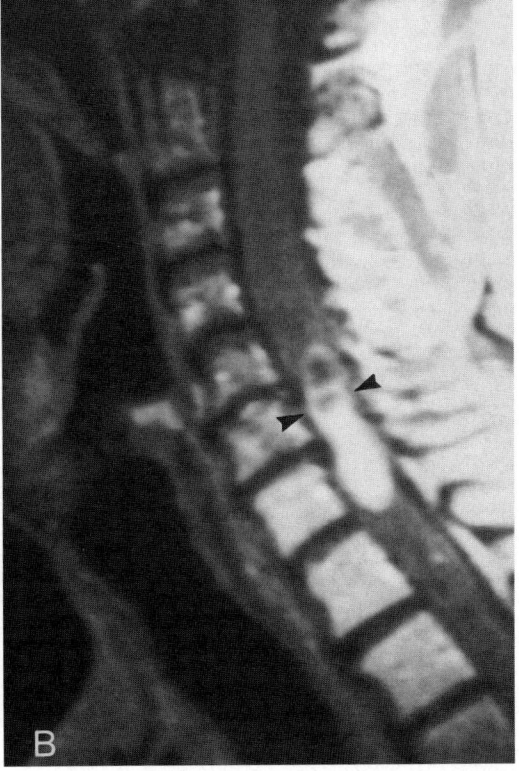

Figure 10.10. Acute Myelopathy—Intramedullary Metastasis. This patient, who had received radiation to the chest for an apical lung tumor, developed an acute myelopathy. **A.** The upper cervical vertebrae outside the field show normal marrow. The margin of the radiation port can be seen in the lower cervical spine (*arrow*). Below this margin, the cervical and upper thoracic vertebrae show a typi-cal bright fat-replaced "postradiation appearance" on T1WI. **B.** Postcontrast images show an enhancing lesion at the port margin (*arrowheads*) that proved to be an intramedullary lung metastasis. Note that the enhancement is much denser and more focal than seen with radiation myelitis in Figure 10.11.

gressive ascending motor weakness that affects more than one limb but involves peripheral nerves rather than the spinal cord. Guillain-Barré has occurred after vaccinations, and it evolves over a maximum of four weeks. Sometimes, enhancement of the spinal nerves is seen although this finding of "radiculitis" is nonspecific and can even be seen in disc disease.

Another puzzle is a myelopathy seen in patients with AIDS, with vacuolar changes in the spinal cord. Whether this is due to the HIV itself or concomitant infections such as cytomegalovirus is unclear. The role of MR in these enigmatic syndromes is more to exclude other treatable conditions, such as unsuspected cord compression, than to make a highly specific diagnosis. However, one must not dismiss a case of noncompressive myelopathy with cord edema as idiopathic transverse myelitis until a thorough search for treatable causes, including spinal vascular malformations (see Fig. 10.53), has been performed.

Neurosarcoidosis. Inflammatory conditions involving pia and arachnoid have a similar differential diagnosis whether they involve cerebral or spinal leptomeninges. A classic example is neurosarcoidosis, which can present as diffuse leptomeningeal granulomatous nodules, which typically enhance (Fig. 10.12). This appearance is similar to that of carcinomatous and infectious meningitis, which will be discussed, and the distinction must be made on clinical grounds. Sarcoid can also present with intramedullary or vertebral body granulomatous changes.

Pantopaque Arachnoiditis. One "physical agent" that causes leptomeningeal irritation is Pantopaque, which was used in myelography. Patients can develop delayed arachnoiditis, which manifests itself as adhesions within the cauda equina. The normally free-layering roots become adherent to each other or to the peripheral wall of the thecal sac, giving the sac a "bald" appearance on myelography or T2WI. Although this agent is rarely used today, keep this complication in mind in patients whose plain spine films show the telltale pearly white beads of residual Pantopaque. On MR, these droplets appear bright on T1WI because of their lipid content.

INFECTION

Infections involving the spine can be classified according to their cause or anatomic location. Both approaches are useful. Certain infections, such as pediatric pyogenic meningitis, are so dramatic in their presentation that there is little need for imaging because emergent lumbar puncture and CSF analysis are the cornerstones of diagnosis. Other processes, such as fungal osteomyelitis in the immunocompromised cancer patient, can be quite subtle, and imaging plays a crucial (if not always successful) role in differentiating spinal infection from tumor (13–16). Evaluation of the pathologic vertebral body is a constant challenge, and the many "rules of thumb" sprinkled throughout this chapter are summarized in Table 10.3.

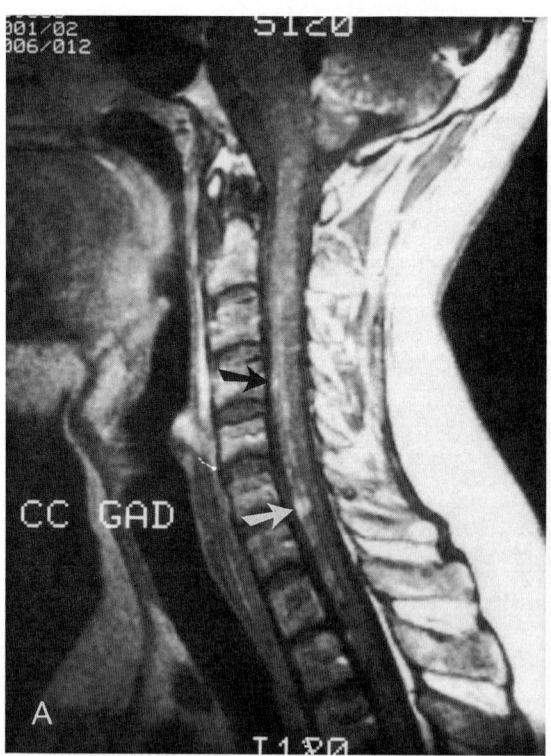

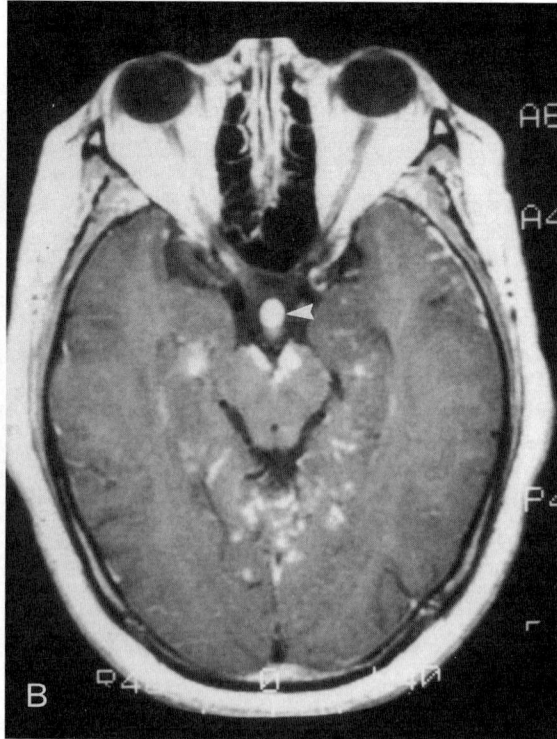

Figure 10.12. Neurosarcoidosis. A. Multiple nodular enhancing areas are seen involving both the leptomeninges and the cord (*arrows*). **B.** A concomitant scan of the brain reveals similar findings involving leptomeninges as well as the pituitary stalk (*arrowhead*). Accumulation of granulation tissue in this region is the source of the "suprasellar mass" associated with sarcoid.

Table 10.3. Imaging Evaluation of the Pathologically Collapsed Vertebral Body

Criteria	Infection	Neoplasm	Osteoporosis
Number of vertebrae affected, and pattern	Single vertebral involvement rare Usually at least two vertebrae around an affected disc (pyogenic) or intact disc with subligamentous spread (tuberculosis or fungus)	Isolated or noncontiguous involvement common	Typically >1 vertebrae
Portions of vertebra affected	Destruction greatest at endplates Posterior elements relatively spared	Irregular vertebral body involvement Entire vertebra often infiltrated Pedicles typically affected	Anterior "wedge" deformity of the vertebral body Posterior elements spared
Marrow signal	Decreased on T1 Increased on T2 Abnormal marrow signal centered around disc in osteomyelitis/discitis complex	Decreased on T1 Increased on T2 Entire vertebral body usually infiltrated with pathologic compression fracture	Normal (unless acute) Portions of vertebral body retain normal marrow even with acute compression fracture
Disc integrity	Pyogenic: disc involved and enhances Nonpyogenic: disc spared	Discs typically spared (prostate cancer an exception)	Discs spared
Epidural component (if present)	Granulation tissue (best seen post-gadolinium) extends several levels above and below the affected vertebrae	Focal mass usually only at level of affected vertebra(e) Lymphoma an exception, with more extensive epidural mass	None, unless acute fracture with hematoma
Caveats	Discogenic vertebral sclerosis can mimic the osteomyelitis complex on T1-weighted images (but not on enhanced scans)	Gadolinium enhancement may obscure metastases, by reducing their conspicuity relative to fat	Acute compression fractures show marrow edema, and can be difficult to distinguish from pathologic fracture (although posterior elements are usually spared) A follow-up scan in 2–6 months helps make the distinction.

In most spine infections, the organism is seeded via the arterial route, rather than transvenously, as was once believed. As with most bacteremia, the source of the organism is usually the skin, gastrointestinal tract, or lungs. Exceptions are in children with spinal dysraphism, or immediate postoperative patients, where a direct portal for infection exists.

Osteomyelitis/Discitis. In adults, the most common initial site of hematogenous infectious "seeding" is the vertebral body, particularly the portions near the endplates, which have the richest blood supply. Vertebral osteomyelitis then develops (Fig. 10.13), which can be self-limiting. However, if pyogenic infection breaks through the endplates into the disc, discitis ensues, with inevitable infection of the adjacent vertebral body, creating an "osteomyelitis/discitis complex" (Fig. 10.14). This pattern is highly suggestive of infection, and it is unusual with neoplasms (Table 10.3). The epidural space can also be seeded hematogenously, but more often is involved by direct extension. Once the disc and epidural space are involved, extension into the paraspinous soft tissues, such as the psoas muscle, often occurs. The disc itself has a relatively poor blood supply in adults, but in children, blood vessels supply the growing disc and penetrate the endplate providing a route for hematogenous primary infection.

Epidural Abscess. The dura presents a relative barrier to infection, which tends to spread in a craniocaudad fashion within the epidural space, extending as many as three to four interspaces away from the vertebral abnormality, which is unusual with neoplasms (Table 10.3). Epidural abscesses have little room to expand axially, given the confines of the spinal canal, and thus can lead to cord compression (Fig. 10.15).

Subdural Empyemas are rare and are usually associated with surgery or other violation of the dura. This is fortunate because subdural infections could rapidly spread through the arachnoid layer, resulting in meningitis. Infection of the subarachnoid space is termed "meningitis," whether it is in the brain or spinal canal. Indeed, the theory of a lumbar puncture is that there is continuous mixing of the CSF, with the fluid in the lumbar recesses being representative of the fluid bathing the brain. The clinical presentation of meningitis is discussed in detail in chapter 6. Meningitis typically is caused by direct hematogenous seeding of the CSF rather than contiguous spread of adjacent vertebral infection unless there is a disruption of the leptomeninges on a congenital or acquired basis. Postcontrast MR is the most sensitive imaging examination for meningitis in both the brain and the spine, but the finding of leptomeningeal enhancement often appears relatively late in the infection's course, and sometimes not at all. Therefore, *a negative enhanced MR does not exclude*

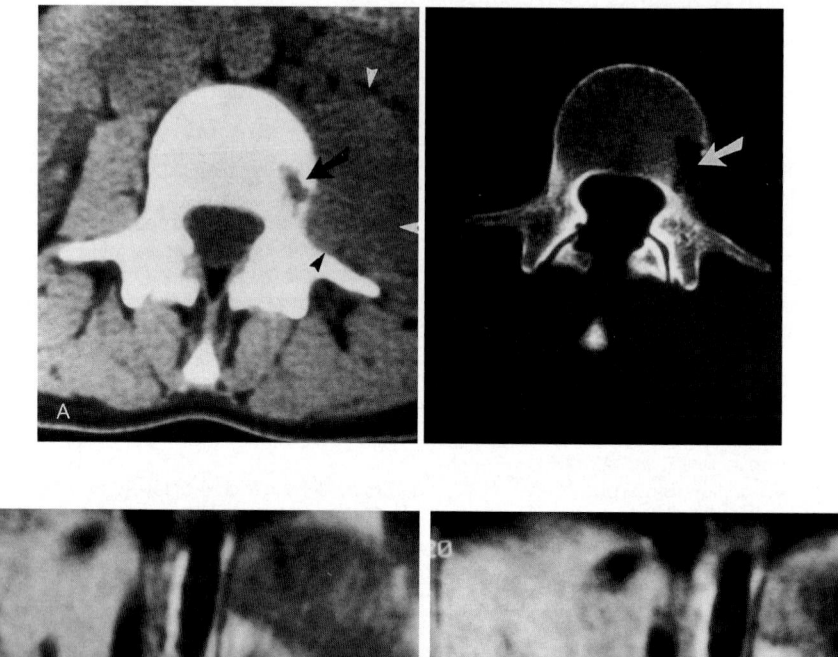

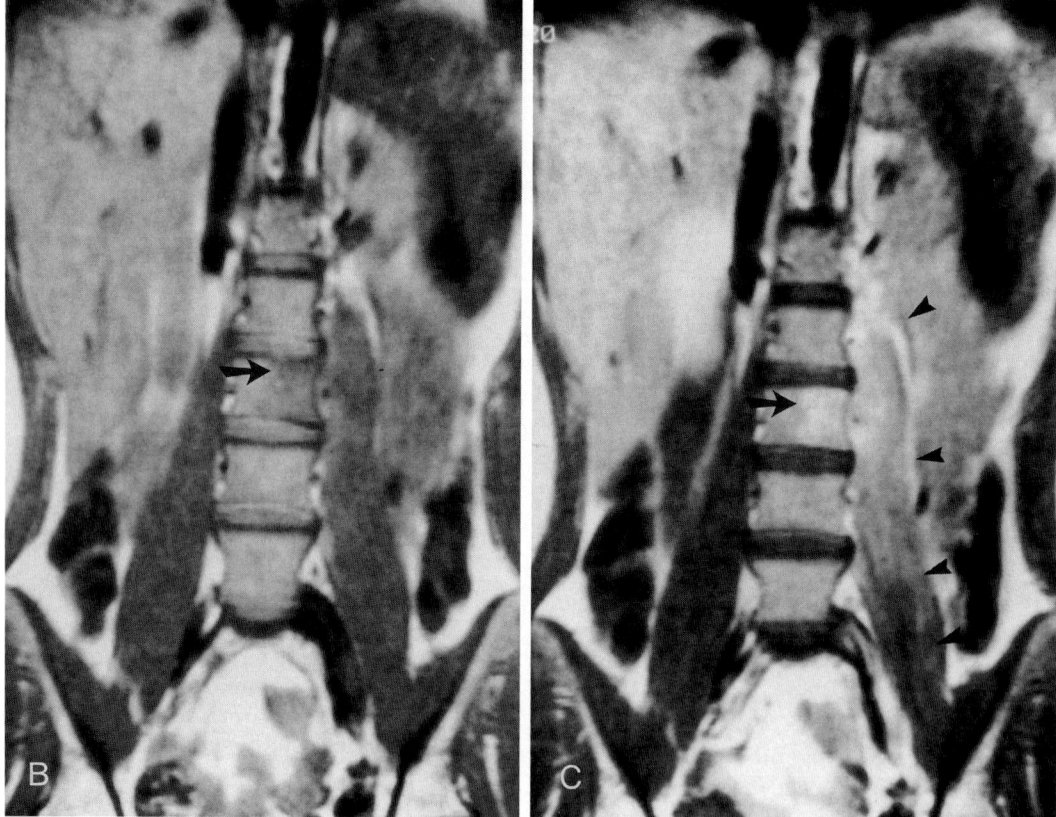

Figure 10.13. Early Osteomyelitis. This young athlete who developed back pain had a slightly elevated sedimentation rate, with negative blood cultures and negative plain films, and a bone scan showing increased uptake at L-3. **A.** A CT, filmed with different windows, shows a destructive process within the vertebral body (*arrow*), which extends into the left psoas muscle (*arrowheads*), which is enlarged. **B.** The unenhanced T1WI in coronal plane shows decreased signal intensity within the left-sided marrow space of L-3, consistent with edema (*arrow*). **C.** Postcontrast T1WI shows marked enhancement within the affected portion of L-3 (*arrow*) and the left psoas (*arrowheads*), which is enlarged and enhances all the way into the pelvis. This pattern would be unusual for a tumor. Biopsy yielded *S. aureus*. The discs appear spared, which is atypical for *S. aureus*. Note how well the coronal plane shows both the spine and paraspinous tissues over a large area. This plane is underused but is very effective in imaging of nondegenerative diseases.

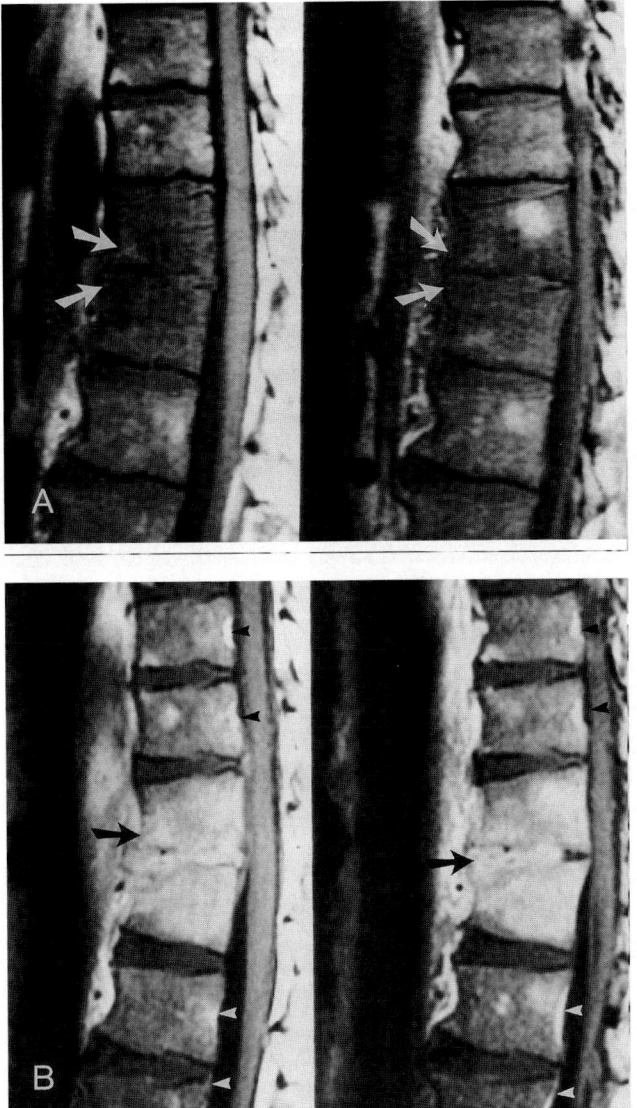

Figure 10.14. Osteomyelitis with Discitis. A. T1-weighted sagittal images show decreased signal in a pair of vertebral body endplates (*arrows*) centered around an abnormal disc. **B.** The disc (*arrow*) enhances intensely, confirming discitis. This "osteomyelitis/discitis complex" is classic for pyogenic infection and virtually rules out neoplasm. Note basivertebral venous plexus (*arrowheads*), which normally becomes bright after gadolinium, due to normal venous enhancement. This basivertebral plexus enhancement confirms that gadolinium was given, much as nasal mucosal enhancement does in the head. Enhanced basivertebral veins should not be mistaken for epidural infection or tumor.

meningitis—and should never delay or be a substitute for a lumbar puncture.

Spinal Cord Abscesses are rare and usually the result of direct seeding of the cord from overwhelming sepsis. Given the difficulty of myelography in an acutely ill patient and the relative insensitivity of the technique for small intramedullary lesions, the imaging literature on this topic historically has been sketchy, with most data from autopsy reports. MR now allows a direct look inside the cord in these patients. Spinal cord pyogenic abscesses, not surprisingly, appear similar to those in the brain: bright on T2WI, with rim enhancement (Fig. 10.16).

Plain films cannot identify a spinal infection unless some disc or bone destruction has occurred, which may take 4–8 weeks, with the earliest sign being erosion of the vertebral endplates. Because older patients often have significant loss of vertebral body and disc height because of degenerative processes, evaluation of plain films is difficult—even after months of symptoms. Late in the infectious course, the endplates may become sclerotic bone as healing occurs, sometimes leading to fusion across the obliterated disc space. Radionuclide bone scans can turn positive in infection far sooner than plain films, but these suffer from the same ambiguity: degenerative and nondegenera-

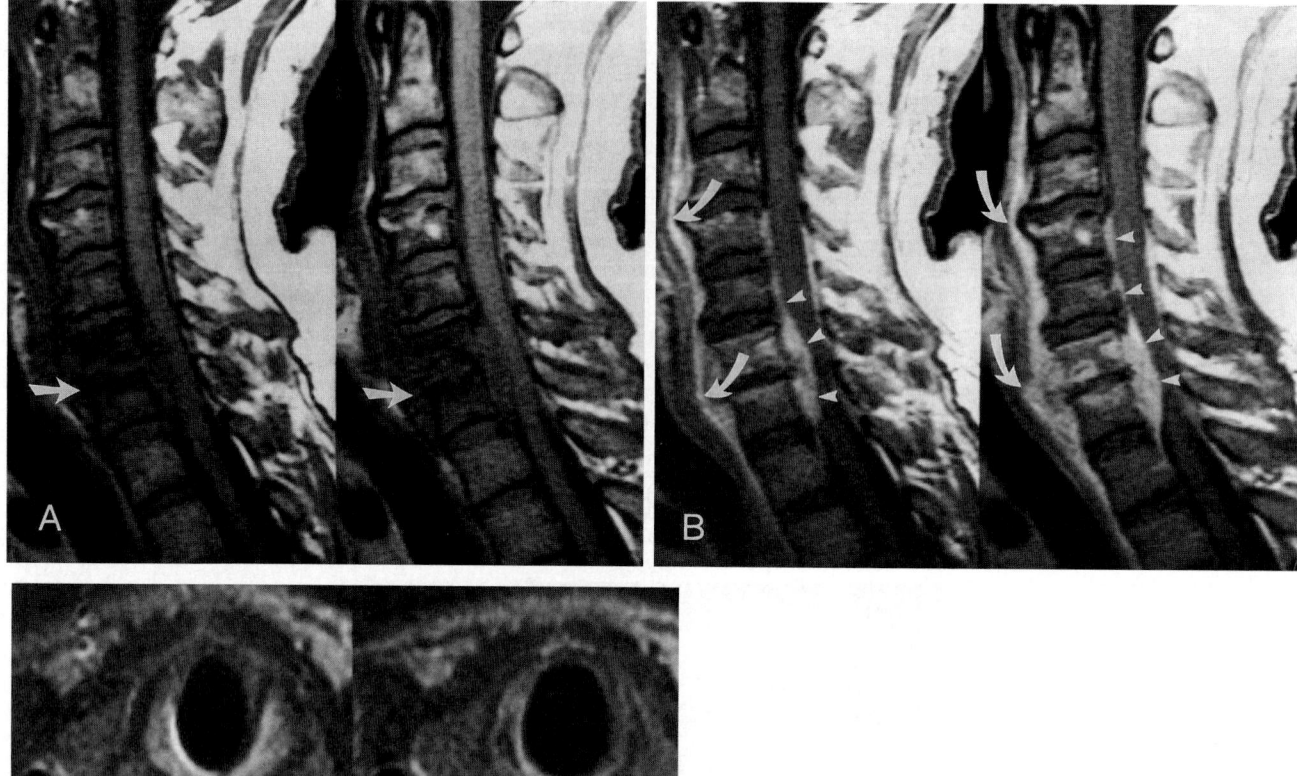

Figure 10.15. Osteomyelitis with Discitis and Epidural Abscess. T1-weighted sagittal images before **(A)** and after **(B)** contrast, show an osteomyelitis-discitis complex, centered around an abnormal enhancing disc (*arrow*). Considerable enhancing tissue is seen within the epidural space (*arrowheads*) as well as anterior to the spine, involving the anterior longitudinal ligament (*curved arrows*). Ligamentous involvement extends several vertebral bodies away from the area of infiltrated marrow favors infection, which is unusual for metastatic tumor. **C.** Axial images confirm compression of the cord (*arrows*).

tive processes can look the same. Indium-labeled white cell studies and gallium scans are more specific for infection but relatively insensitive for small foci of vertebral osteomyelitis.

CT is useful for paraspinous disease, such as psoas infection, which may be associated with vertebral osteomyelitis and epidural abscess (Fig. 10.13). However, CT does not show the contents of the spinal canal adequately unless intrathecal contrast is used. MR can demonstrate the initial replacement of the fatty marrow by osteomyelitis; therefore, MR has become the preferred technique of examination. Gadolinium-enhanced images are extremely helpful in confirming discitis. In the evaluation of the extent of epidural involvement, fat suppression is a useful adjunct as the epidural fat is inherently bright (Fig. 10.17).

Pyogenic Infections

Staphylococcus aureus is by far the most common cause of spine infection in adults, followed by Gram-negative bacteria, particularly *Escherichia coli, Pseudomonas,* and *Klebsiella. Salmonella* is seen in association with sickle cell disease. As already mentioned, the vertebrae are seeded hematogenously in most cases, resulting in osteomyelitis that then spreads to the disc space and adjacent vertebral body. This process typically results in severe back pain that, unlike degenerative conditions, is unrelieved by any positional maneuvers. Fevers, chills, leukocytosis, and an elevated sedimentation rate may be present. However, the early and haphazard use of antibiotics for any "malaise" may mask these findings. Blood cultures are often negative, mandating disc biopsy, which also has a surprisingly low yield. *Staphylococcus aureus* produces enzymes that rapidly "digest" discs. This has led to the plain film "pearl" that destruction of the disc space implies pyogenic infection. Tuberculous spondylitis, in contrast, typically spares the disc.

On MR, however, the converse of this pearl does not always hold up: *Staphylococcus* infections can be detected as early as the isolated osteomyelitis phase, as marrow edema with enhancement, before any discitis has developed (Fig. 10.13). Once the infection has broken through to the disc, intense contrast enhancement confirms the discitis (Fig. 10.14) and usually shows subligamentous spread to the vertebra on the other side of the disc. Infection can course along the anterior and posterior longitudinal ligaments, extending several vertebral body levels away from the affected disc. As the infection progresses, epidural involvement—with or without pathologic fracturing of the vertebra—can lead to cord com-

pression (Fig. 10.15). Epidural infection can have a variable appearance, ranging from rounded rim-enhancing areas, which yield frank pus at surgery, to more oblong stretches of thickened granulation tissue.

Nonpyogenic Infections

The most important nonpyogenic infections of the spine are tuberculosis and fungal diseases. These disorders present a diagnostic challenge for several reasons. First, they typically have an indolent course and do not present with the acute pain and leukocytosis that are the hallmark of pyogenic infections. Second, the population most at risk for nonpyogenic infections, aside from in certain endemic areas, is the immunosuppressed. Patients who are immunocompromised because of chemotherapy are at risk for metastases from their pri-

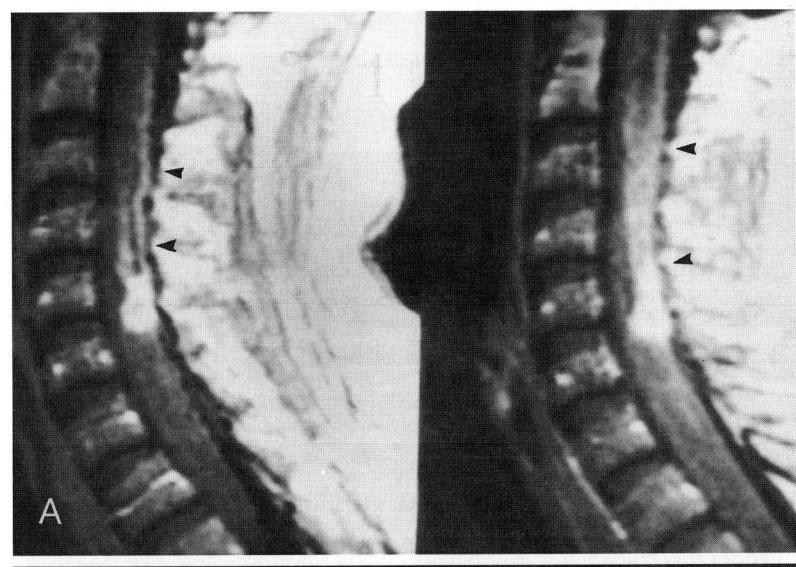
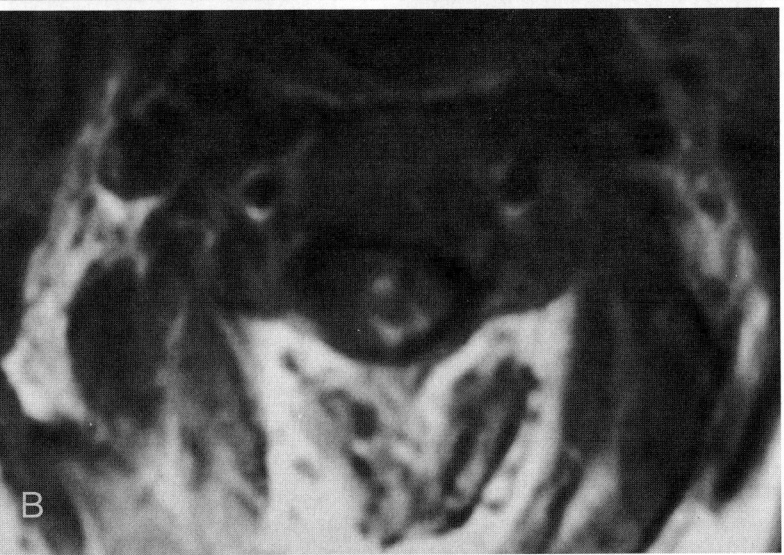

Figure 10.16. Spinal Cord Abscess. Sagittal **(A)** and axial **(B)** enhanced images through the cervical spine show intramedullary enhancement in this patient with overwhelming sepsis, who developed myelopathy. Results of a laminectomy (*arrowheads*) and biopsy revealed abscess.

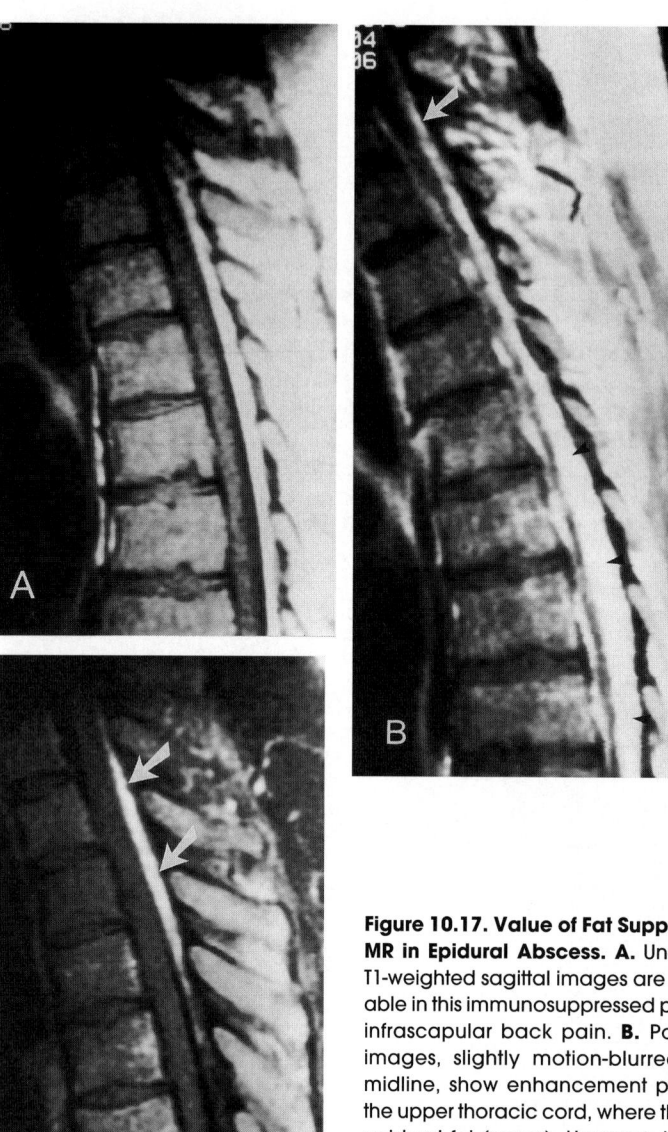

Figure 10.17. Value of Fat Suppression on MR in Epidural Abscess. A. Unenhanced T1-weighted sagittal images are unremarkable in this immunosuppressed patient with infrascapular back pain. **B.** Postcontrast images, slightly motion-blurred and off midline, show enhancement posterior to the upper thoracic cord, where there is little epidural fat (*arrow*). However, in the middle and lower thoracic spine, it is difficult to distinguish enhancement from normal epidural fat (*arrowheads*). **C.** Fat-suppression images reveal the true extent of the epidural abscess (*arrows*).

mary tumor, and AIDS patients are at risk for lymphoma involving the spine. In both settings, therefore, a pathologic fracture with mild epidural mass effect easily can represent either infection or neoplasm. The dichotomy of the potential treatments, antibiotics versus radiation, mandates a definitive diagnosis that often requires biopsy. Sometimes, however, the radiologist can steer the workup in such a way that invasiveness of this biopsy is minimized, or can detect findings so characteristic of a given disease that biopsy is not necessary (Table 10.3). Figure 10.18 illustrates such a case as it evolved, from plain films to CT, and finally MR.

Tuberculosis of the Spine, or Pott's disease, causes slow collapse of one or usually more vertebral bodies, spreading underneath the longitudinal ligaments (Fig. 10.19). The result is an acute kyphotic or "gibbus" de-

formity. This angulation, coupled with epidural granulation tissue and bony fragments, can lead to cord compression. Unlike pyogenic infections, the discs tend to be preserved. Psoas abscess without severe pain or frank pus is common, leading to the expression "cold abscess." As with other extrapulmonary tuberculosis, the chest film may be unrevealing, with the source being a primary lung lesion that is clinically silent. Unfortunately, the incidence of tuberculous spondylitis, as with other forms of tuberculosis, is on the rise, with new strains with multiple drug resistances developing. In many parts of the world, tuberculosis is the most common cause of vertebral body infection, with the majority of cases seen in patients younger than age 20. Tuberculosis can also affect the meninges of the spine, causing an intense pachymeningitis that enhances dramatically (Fig. 10.20).

Fungal Infections can be particularly difficult to differentiate from malignant processes, with the classic problem being *Candida* and *Aspergillus* in the oncology patient. Coccidioidomycosis and blastomycosis have specific endemic areas, but with widespread travel, geographic borders have less meaning. Coccidioidomycosis

(Fig. 10.18) is common in the southwestern United States, and blastomycosis in the southeast. Both are common in Africa and South America, with some variation in strains. Another distinction is that coccidioidomycosis, like tuberculosis, spares the discs whereas blastomycosis, like actinomycosis, can destroy

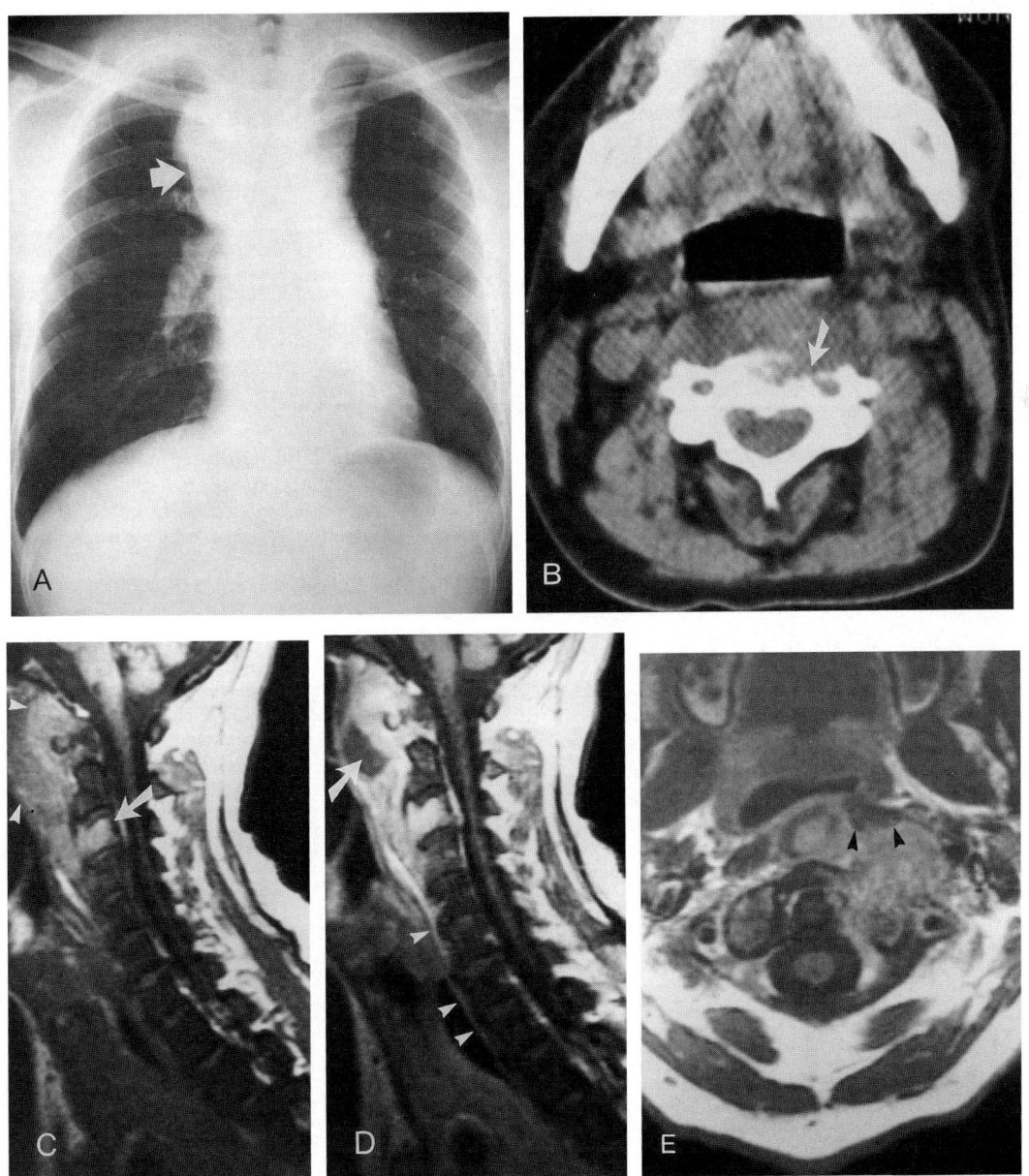

Figure 10.18. Coccidioidomycosis Osteomyelitis with Prevertebral Abscess. This 26-year-old patient presented with history of 3 months of fevers, weight loss, and chills. **A.** Chest film shows an anterior mediastinal mass (*arrow*) suspicious for lymphoma. **B.** A CT confirmed mediastinal adenopathy and showed destructive changes in C-3 (*arrow*), which are atypical for lymphoma. **C.** A T1-weighted image shows abnormal low signal in all of the cervical vertebrae, owing to anemia of chronic disease, likely accompanied by increased marrow iron. The C-3 vertebral body (*arrow*) is infiltrated with fluid. In a normal patient it would be the darkest verte-

bral body; here it is the brightest. An anterior mass (*arrowheads*) is noted in the prevertebral space. **D.** After contrast, the prevertebral mass (*arrow*) shows central low signal, consistent with necrosis or abscess. Note the dense enhancement of the anterior longitudinal ligament (*arrowheads*) well into the lower cervical spine, suggestive of infection. This proved to be coccidioidomycosis. **E.** An axial image proves that the mass is in the prevertebral space rather than the retropharyngeal space by showing the longus colli muscle (*arrowheads*) displaced forward.

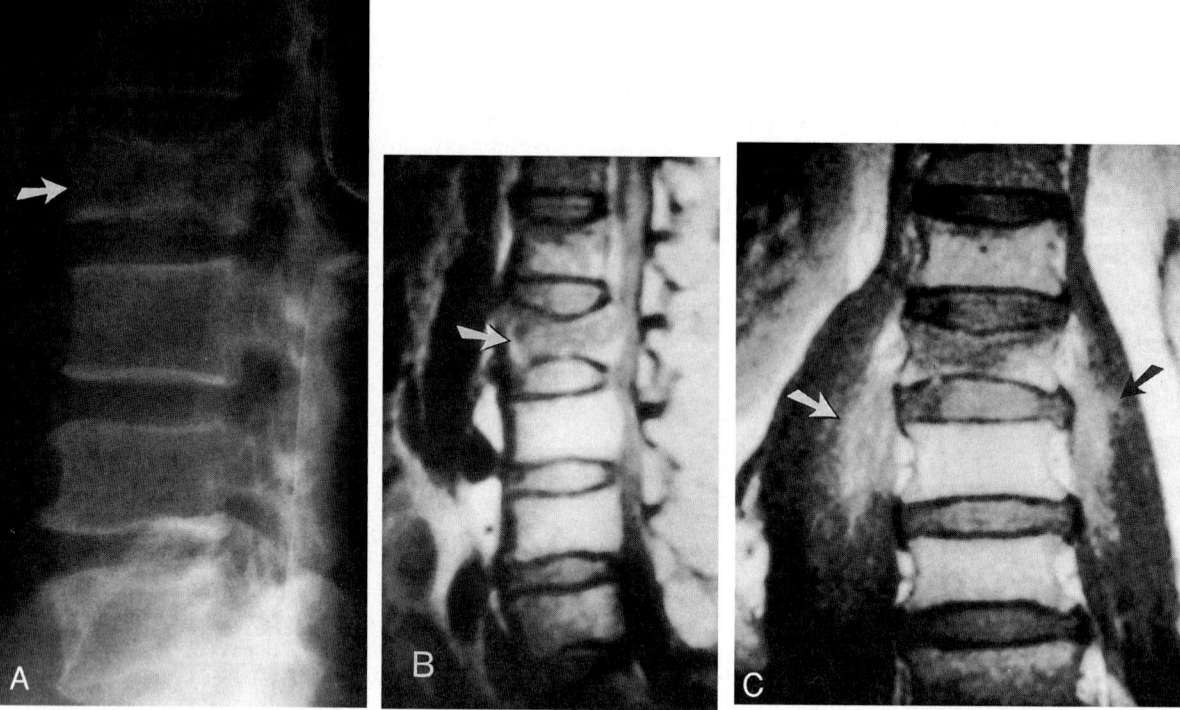

Figure 10.19. Tuberculous Osteomyelitis. A. Plain film shows loss of height of L-2 (*arrow*), with subtle sclerotic changes. **B.** Enhanced T1WI show abnormal marrow throughout L-2 (*arrow*), consistent with a pathologic fracture, making neoplasm or infection prime suspects. Acute compression fractures usually show anterior "wedg-ing," and chronic compression fractures have normal marrow. **C.** Coronal enhanced images reveal bilateral psoas infiltration (*arrows*), but normal discs, consistent with a nonpyogenic infection such as tuberculosis. Metastatic tumor rarely infiltrates the psoas in such a diffuse fashion.

Figure 10.20. Tuberculous Meningitis. A. Sagittal T1 un-enhanced image through the cervical spine shows rela-tively homogenous signal intensity tissue filling the spinal canal, making it difficult to decide if the process is in-tramedullary or extramedullary. **B.** Postcontrast image demonstrates enhancing granulation tissue filling the sub-arachnoid space (*arrows*). This patient had similar pachy-meningitis surrounding the brain, yet was surprisingly in-tact clinically, typical for tuberculous meningitis, which is less angioinvasive and consequently less destructive than pyogenic meningitis.

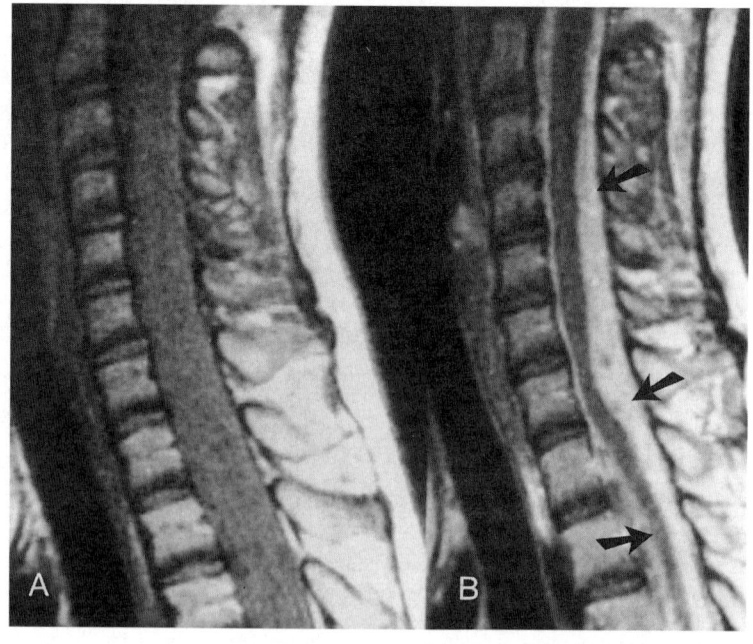

the discs and the ribs. *Cryptococcus*, usually associated with meningitis, also affects the vertebrae, causing well-defined osteolytic changes.

Other infectious agents can occasionally affect the spine. Cysticercosis can involve the CSF pathways at any point, and has been noted in the lumbar recesses. Recently, intramedullary toxoplasmosis has been described in AIDS patients. *Echinococcus* will occasionally affect the vertebral bodies. Viral and postviral syndromes are discussed in the section "Inflammation."

NEOPLASMS

MR, unique in its ability to detect nonexpansile tumors of the spinal cord, is the only reliable noninvasive method for detection of spinal canal tumors that do not affect bone. When formulating the differential diagnosis for a spinal tumor, establishing the location of the lesion as intramedullary, intradural extramedullary, or extradural is important, as described previously in the section "Myelography" and in Table 10.2. Having determined the "compartment," consider the patient's age when ranking the lesions occurring in that compartment in order of likelihood (16–21). In children, 38% of symptomatic spinal canal lesions are developmental. Meningiomas constitute 25% of all intraspinal lesions in adults but are rare in children. These figures exclude bony and epidural metastases, which are the most common neoplastic conditions involving the adult spine. MR is also an excellent tool for evaluating these osseous metastases (Fig. 10.21). Signal alterations from tumor infiltration within the normal bright marrow fat on T1WI usually precede any bony changes detectable on plain film or CT, and MR is probably the earliest reliable method (aside from bone marrow biopsy) for detecting the presence of metastatic disease of the spine. Technetium bone scanning, however, remains the most cost-effective tool for whole-body screening.

Intramedullary Masses

The classic plain film finding of an intramedullary mass, widening of the interpedicular distance due to slow expansile forces, is seen in less than 10% of cases. Because bony changes are relatively rare, plain CT is not useful for intramedullary tumors. Even with intrathecal contrast, the crucial internal details of the cord are not visualized. Astrocytomas and ependymomas are the two most common primary intramedullary tumors, but the distinction between them is difficult to make, even with high-quality MR. Both are expansile, low in signal intensity on T1WI, and bright on T2WI, with variable enhancement. Both have an increased incidence in neurofibromatosis. Although some guidelines, based on in-

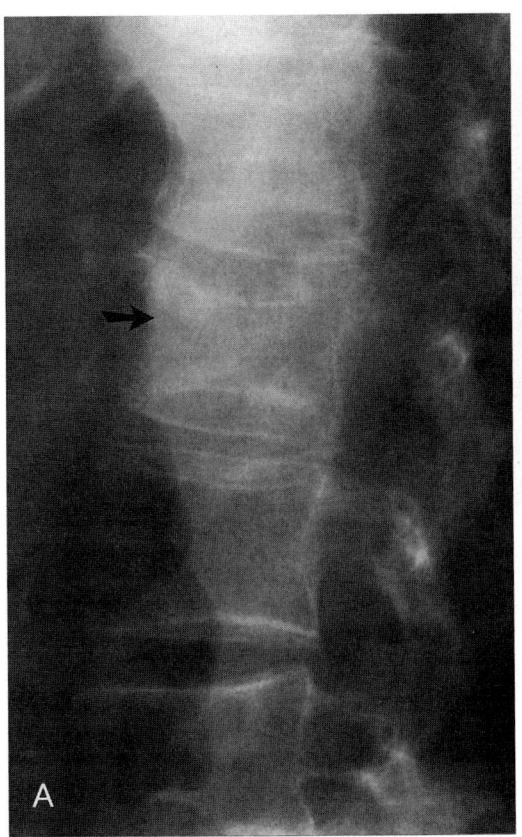

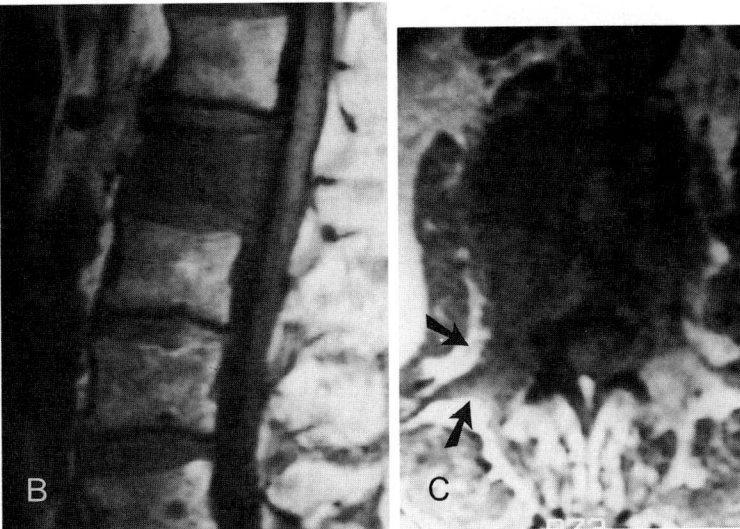

Figure 10.21. Prostate Metastasis. A. Plain film in this elderly male with acute lower back pain reveals a compression deformity at L-1 (*arrow*), which could represent either a benign or pathologic compression fracture. Sagittal **(B)** and axial **(C)** T1WI reveal infiltration of the entire vertebral body marrow space, including the right pedicle (*arrows*), a pattern that is highly indicative of metastasis. Biopsy results revealed prostate carcinoma.

volvement of the entire cord diameter and longer cord segments (favors astrocytoma) and presence of cysts and hemorrhage (favors ependymoma), have been proposed to distinguish between the two types of tumors, in any single case they are rarely a substitute for biopsy. Gadolinium contrast is useful to identify tumor nidus and to document spread of tumor along CSF pathways, or drop metastases.

Hemangioblastomas, on the other hand, are very distinctive, with a focal vascular blush at their nidus and angiographic signs being virtually pathognomonic. Syringomyelia, although not a neoplasm, presents as an intramedullary mass on plain film myelogram and is therefore traditionally included in this gamut. Abscesses (Fig. 10.16), metastases (Fig. 10.10), lipomas (Fig. 10.58), and teratomas will present on rare occasions as intramedullary masses.

Ependymomas are the most common spinal cord tumor. Peak incidence is in the third through sixth decades, with a predominance in males. These slow-growing neoplasms arise from ependymal cells lining the central canal of the cord or cell rests along the filum. Histologically, these tumors are usually benign, but a complete curative excision may be impossible with the intramedullary types. Sixty percent are seen within the conus and filum terminale. Associated hemorrhage can be seen, especially on MR, and cystic areas are common (Fig. 10.22). The filum terminale ependymomas typically have a myxopapillary histology, and because of their location a reasonably specific diagno-

sis can be made. These often can be excised completely, particularly if they are well encapsulated (Fig. 10.23).

Astrocytoma. Most (75%) astrocytomas occur in the cervical and upper to midthoracic cord, and presentation in the conus and filum is rarer than with ependymomas. Fusiform cord widening, hyperintensity on T2WI, and contrast enhancement often extend over several vertebral body segments (Fig. 10.24). They usually have a lower histologic grade than astrocytomas in the brain. As in the brain, there is considerable histologic variability, and the unusual variants, such as protoplasmic astrocytoma, can also involve the spinal cord. Peak incidence is in the third or fourth decade. They may be exophytic and at times may even appear largely extramedullary. Brainstem gliomas will sometimes extend through the medulla into the rostral cervical spine.

Hemangioblastomas occur in the spine as well as the posterior fossa. Both types have a high association with von Hippel-Lindau syndrome. These rare tumors, with their characteristic densely enhancing nidus, represent 2% of intraspinal neoplasms. Forty percent are extramedullary and 20% are multiple. The nidus shows vascular hypertrophy, and may be mistaken for an arteriovenous malformation (AVM). However, intramedullary AVMs do not typically show a related cyst or cord expansion (Fig. 10.25).

Syringohydromelia. Hydromyelia refers to dilation of the central canal of the spinal cord, which is lined by ependyma. Syringomyelia, on the other hand, is a cavity

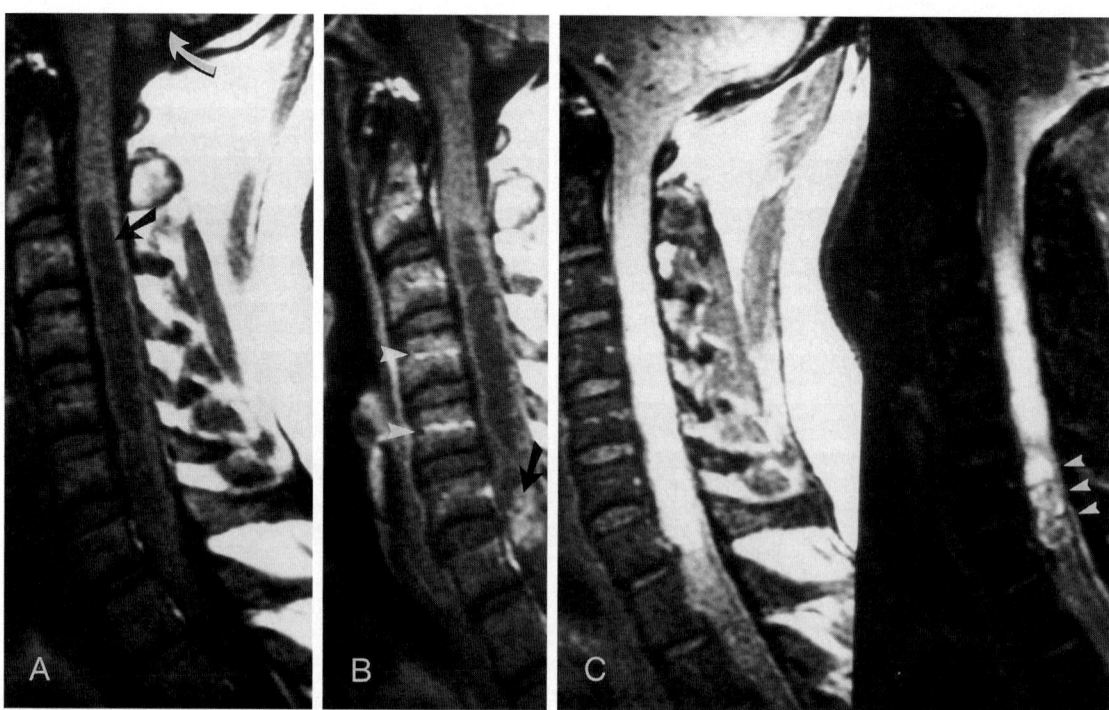

Figure 10.22. Ependymoma. A. T1WI shows a cavity (*arrow*) within the cervical cord, but the cerebellar tonsils (*curved arrow*) are normal in position, so this cannot be a Chiari I (contrast with Fig. 10.26). **B.** Postcontrast image shows an enhancing nodule (*arrow*) at the lower pole of the intramedullary cavity. Note the normal enhancement of the basivertebral plexus (*arrowheads*). **C.** T2WI show blood-breakdown products at the lower end of the cavity (*arrowheads*), suggestive of hemorrhage within the tumor.

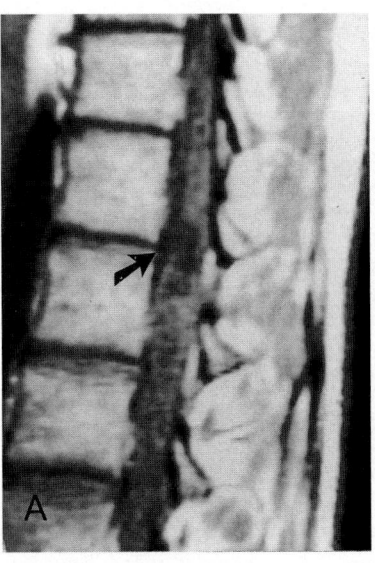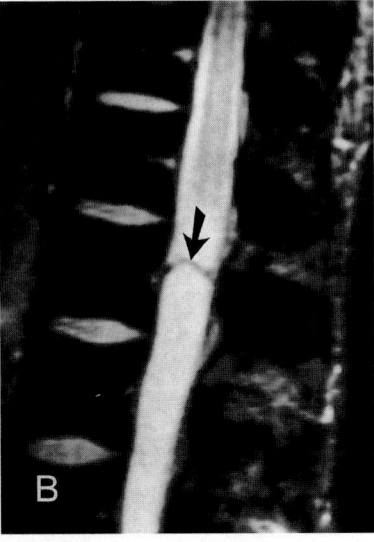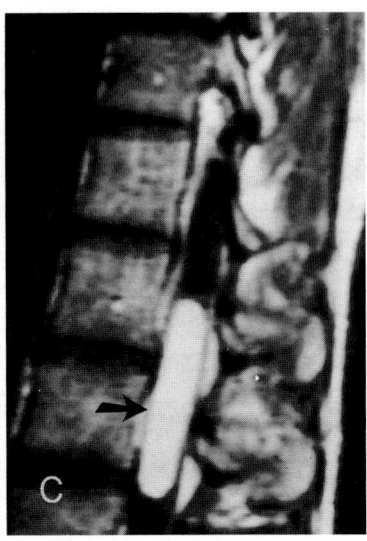

Figure 10.23. Myxopapillary Ependymoma of the Filum Terminale. A. This 29-year-old patient presented with lower extremity radicular complaints. T1-weighted sagittal images show an irregular appearance to the conus (*arrow*) and surrounding CSF, but no distinct mass. **B.** Sagittal gradient refocused echo images demon-

strates a low signal "rim" (*arrow*), suggesting an intraspinal mass. **C.** Postcontrast images confirm an enhancing encapsulated intraspinal mass (*arrows*) abutting the conus. A complete resection was performed and the patient has done well.

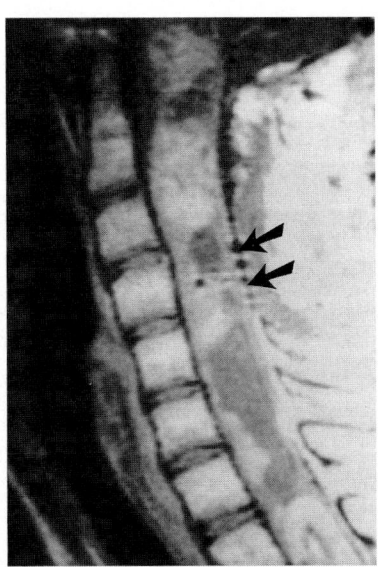

Figure 10.24. Astrocytoma. Astrocytoma of the cervical spine in a child with NF-1. Patient has undergone a laminectomy (*arrows*) in an attempt at decompression.

The preferred imaging method is T1WI in the sagittal and axial planes, along with sagittal T2WI. Be aware that high signal truncation (Gibbs) artifacts can superimpose themselves over the cord, mimicking a syrinx, particularly when a low-resolution matrix, such as 128×128, is used. A syrinx cavity should have very well defined margins, and its contents should follow CSF signal intensity. Always suspect tumor as a cause of unexplained syrinx. Unless a definite benign cause is apparent, such as prior history of cord contusion or the low cerebellar tonsils of a Chiari I (Fig. 10.26), give gadolinium to search for a tumor nidus. If the syrinx borders are indistinct and the signal is brighter than CSF on T1WI and darker than CSF on T2WI, you may be dealing with severe central cord edema. It is critical to establish the full extent of the cavity for potential shunting; thus, if on a cervical spine examination, a cord cavity extends into the thoracic spine, follow it down, or the patient will inevitably need to return to complete the examination. With CT myelography, contrast often enters into a syrinx cavity with delayed images. Occasionally, this technique is useful in establishing the degree to which a cord cavity communicates with the CSF.

Intradural/Extramedullary Masses

Meningioma is the most common intradural tumor in the thoracic region, and represents roughly 25% of all adult intraspinal tumors. Most (80%) occur in women, with an average age of 45. Multiple meningiomas, as in the brain, raise the question of neurofibromatosis. The usual location is extramedullary-intradural although an extradural component may exist. Dense calcification can

outside the central canal lined by glial cells. Distinction between these two conditions is difficult on imaging studies, given that the lining of the cavity cannot be examined histologically. The preferred generic term covering either, "syringohydromyelia," is a bit of a tongue-twister, and the abbreviated "syrinx" is often used for both conditions. The cause of a syrinx can be developmental, such as in the Arnold-Chiari malformations. However, trauma and tumors, as well as inflammatory and ischemic conditions, can also cause a syrinx.

Figure 10.25. Hemangioblastoma. A. Sagittal T1WI show expansion of the upper cervical cord due to a low signal central mass (*arrow*), which has a darker inferior component suggestive of a cyst (*arrowheads*). This cavity must be investigated further because it lacks sharp margins and does not follow CSF signal (compare to Fig. 10.26). **B.** Postcontrast image shows an intensely enhancing nodule (*arrow*) at the level of the foramen magnum, classic for a hemangioblastoma. (Courtesy of Dr. William P. Dillon, University of California, San Francisco.)

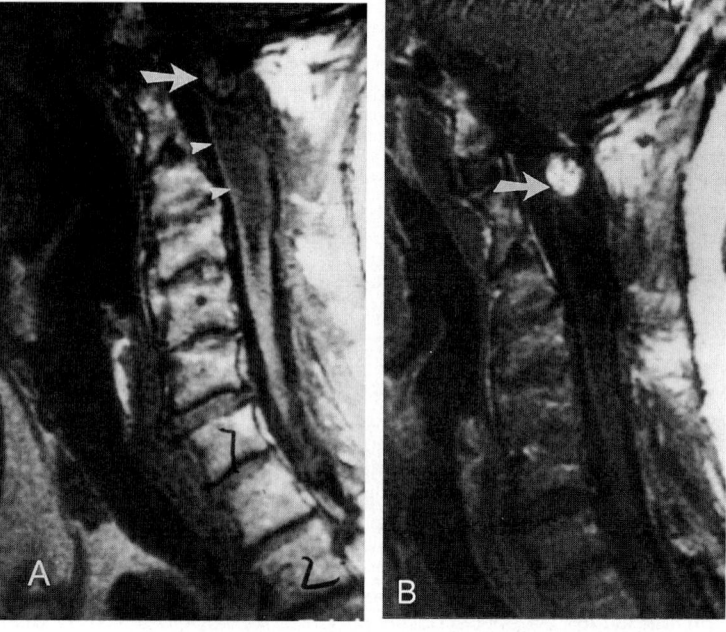

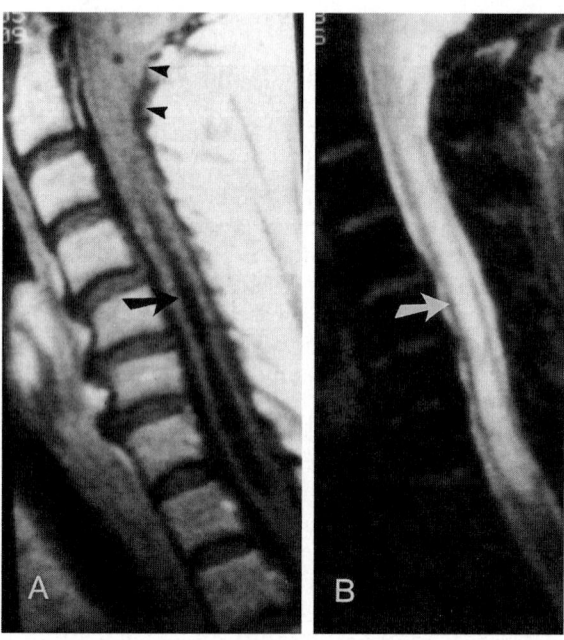

Figure 10.26. Syrinx. A. T1WI. **B.** T2WI. This intramedullary lesion (*arrow*) shows the classic features of a benign syrinx: The margins of the intramedullary cavity are sharp and the intramedullary contents follow CSF signals on all sequences. The cause of the syrinx, the low cerebellar tonsils of the Chiari malformation (*arrowheads*), is also seen.

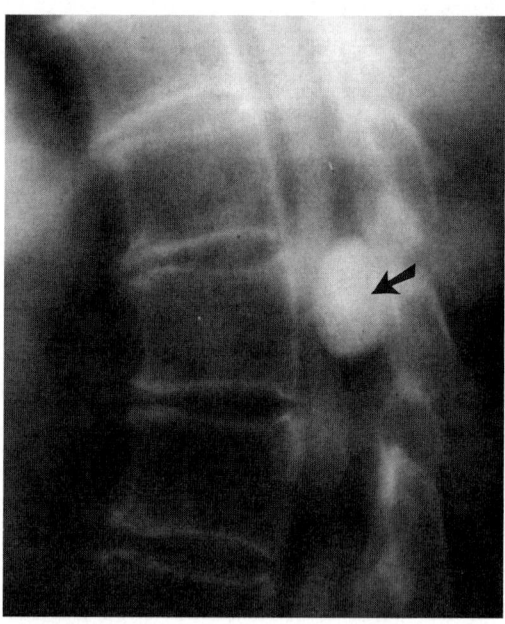

Figure 10.27. Meningioma. This myelogram was performed using air as contrast, a "pneumomyelogram." A densely calcified dorsal intradural extramedullary mass (*arrow*) seen indenting the cord proved to be a meningioma. (Courtesy of Dr. Van Halbach, University of California, San Francisco.)

occur, as in a meningioma in the brain (Fig. 10.27). CT and MR characteristics are similar to that of intracranial meningiomas, with homogenous enhancement (Fig. 10.28). The main differential consideration is usually schwannoma, which often will extend through a neural foramen and lacks a broad dural base. Given that

meningiomas and schwannomas are both relatively common, comprising together over half of intraspinal tumors, occasional mistakes are made in image interpretation. Luckily, these errors are of little consequence because both types of lesions must be resected if causing symptomatic mass effect.

Nerve Sheath Tumors include schwannoma (also known as neurinomas, neurolemmoma, neuroma) and neurofibromas. Schwannoma is the preferred term because pathologically these tumors are composed of Schwann cells. They are the most common intraspinal mass, comprising 29% of the total. Schwannomas usually originate from the dorsal sensory nerve roots, but remain extrinsic to the nerve, causing symptoms by mass effect. Most are solitary, with a peak presentation in the fifth decade although with MR more are being discovered as in-

cidental findings in younger patients (Fig. 10.29). Extension into the neural foramen is a frequent finding, especially in the cervical and thoracic regions. Part of the tumor will be intraspinal, and part will be extraspinal, with the waist at the neural foramen, giving the classic "dumbbell" appearance (Fig. 10.30). In the lumbar region, schwannomas usually remain within the dural sac (Fig. 10.29).

Spinal neurofibromas are almost always associated with neurofibromatosis (NF) Type 1. They are less often multiple than the schwannomas of NF-2. Spinal neurofi-

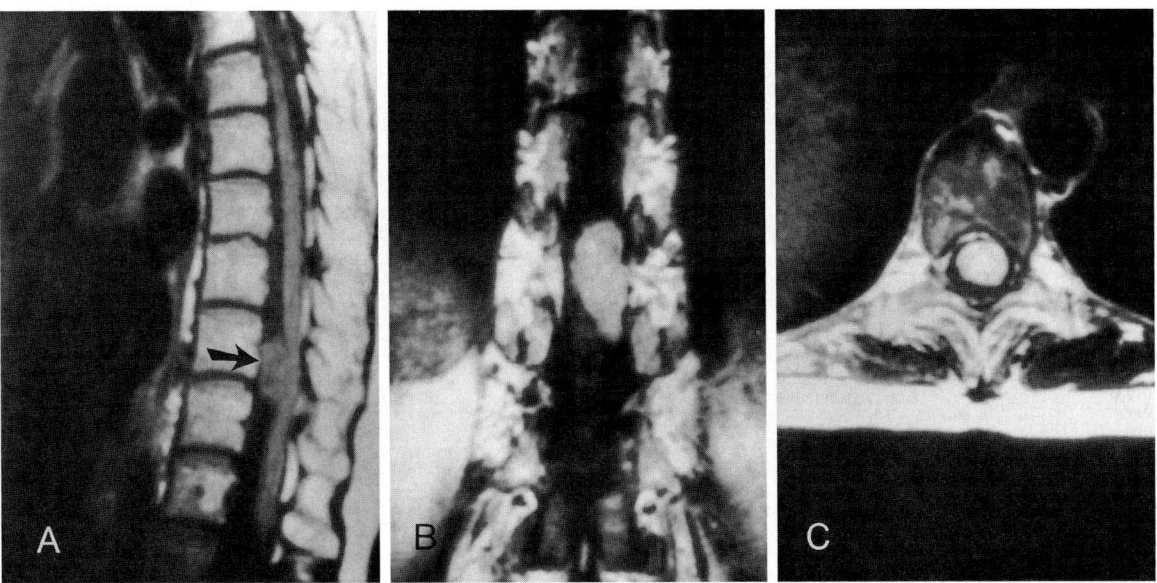

Figure 10.28. Meningioma. A. Sagittal T1WI shows a well-defined anterior extradural intraspinal mass, with a broad dural base (*arrow*). Coronal **(B)** and axial **(C)** images show severe cord compression and the dense enhancement characteristic of meningioma.

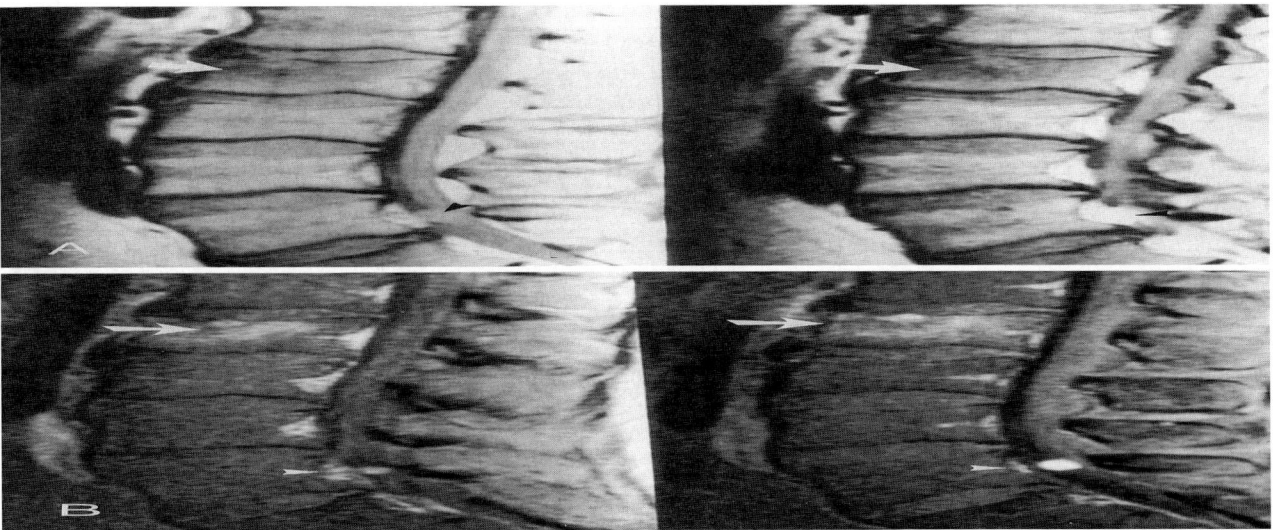

Figure 10.29. Schwannoma. A. This patient had acute focal back pain after an accident, resulting in an acute compression fracture of the superior aspect of L-2, which shows marrow edema (*arrow*). A small intraspinal mass was also noted at L-5 (*arrowhead*). **B.** This lesion enhanced with contrast (*arrowhead*). Unchanged on follow-up examination, this lesion likely represents a small schwannoma. Note enhancement of the L-2 compression fracture (*arrow*), which is highlighted on this fat-saturation image.

bromas can have a plexiform configuration, extending out through multiple adjacent neural foramina (Fig. 10.31). Pathologically, neurofibromas (unlike neurinomas) contain fibrous and myxoid tissue, infiltrate the nerve without encapsulated margins, and have a malignant potential. Radiographically, however, these two types of nerve sheath tumors are often indistinguishable. Both can be intradural or extradural in location. In patients with NF-1, look for the additional findings of kyphoscoliosis, rib dysplasia (ribbon ribs), and scalloping of the posterior vertebral body because of dural ectasia (Fig. 10.32). As in the brain, both schwannomas and neurofibromas enhance.

Heterogeneous enhancement with areas of low signal is more characteristic of a neurofibroma.

Intrathecal (Drop) Metastases. The classic cause of spinal intradural extramedullary metastases is subarachnoid seeding of primary CNS tumors, such as posterior fossa medulloblastomas, ependymomas, and pineal region neoplasms. Tumor cells in the posterior fossa exfoliate into the CSF and "drop" down into the spinal canal, seed the arachnoid, and grow into small nodules, giving rise to the term "drop metastases" (Fig. 10.33). However, any tumor spreading via the CSF pathways of the brain can involve the spinal leptomeninges.

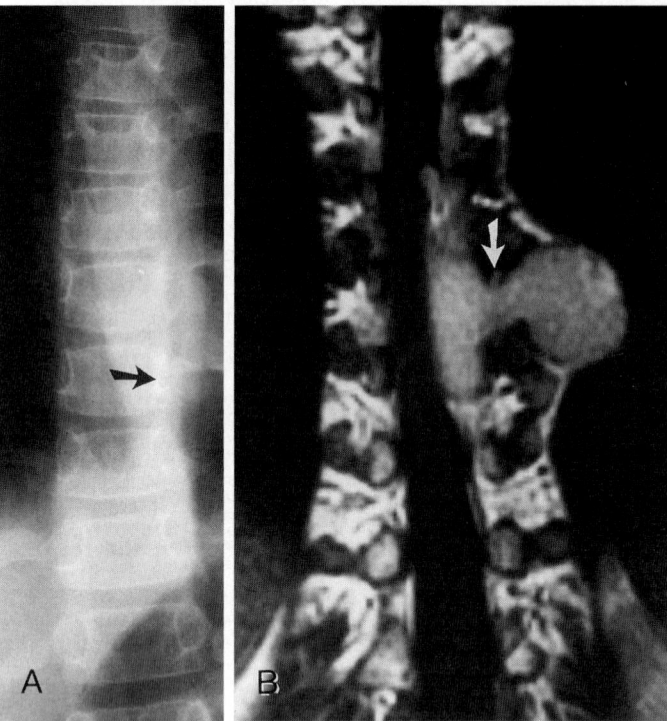

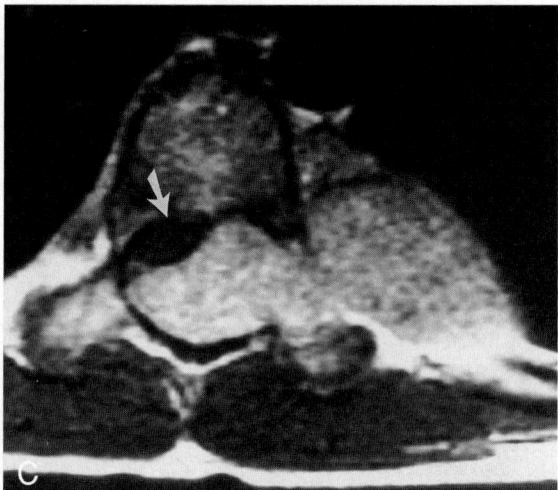

Figure 10.30. Dumbell Neurofibroma. A. Plain thoracic anteroposterior film shows erosion of a left-sided pedicle (*arrow*). **B.** Coronal T1WI demonstrates a huge neurofibroma with both intraspinal and extraspinal components in the classic dumbbell configuration with the waist at the neural foramen (*arrow*). **C.** Axial image is helpful in identifying the position of the spinal cord (*arrow*) and in assessing the degree of cord compression.

Figure 10.31. Cervical Neurofibromatosis. A. The cervical canal is widened with scalloping of the posterior aspects of the vertebrae caused by dural ectasia and multiple neurofibromas (*arrows*). **B.** Post-contrast coronal images reveal multiple enhancing intraspinal masses, consistent with neurofibromas, which extend out the neural foramina (*arrows*), consistent with a plexiform neurofibroma.

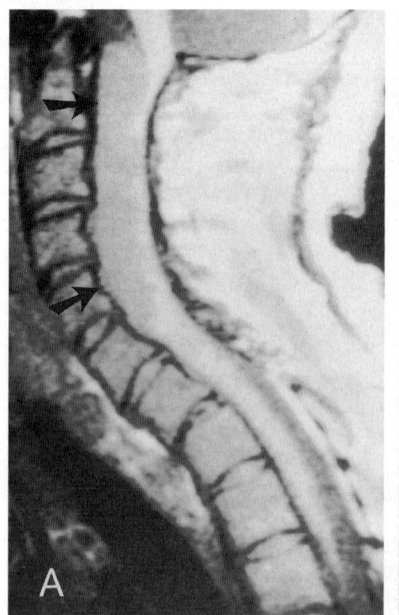

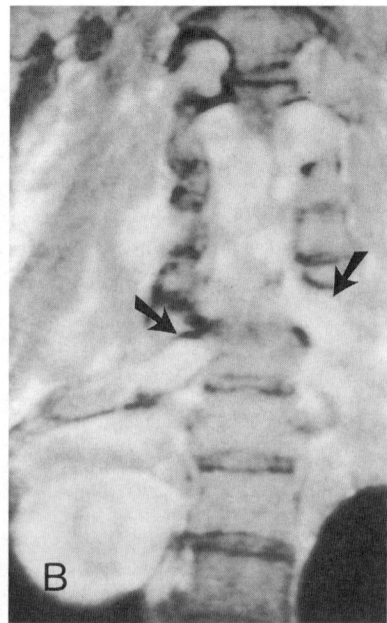

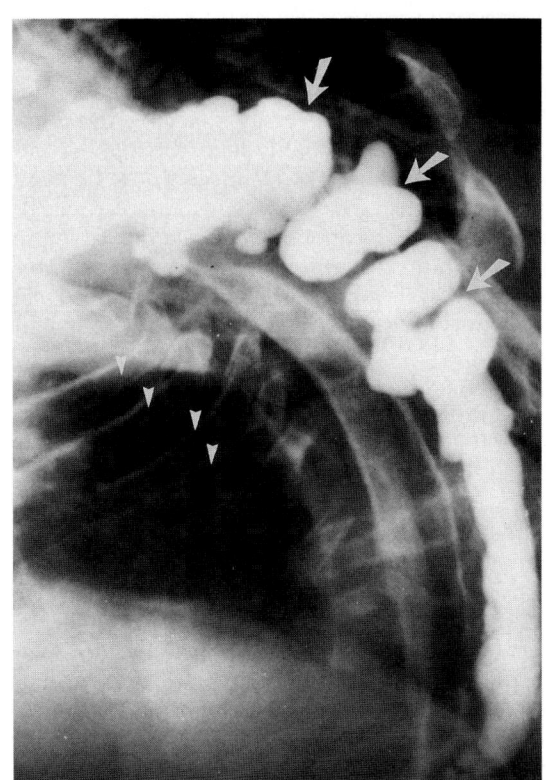

Figure 10.32. Neurofibromatosis. Myelogram shows severe dural ectasia due to neurofibromatosis (*arrows*). Note also the "ribbon ribs" (*arrowheads*).

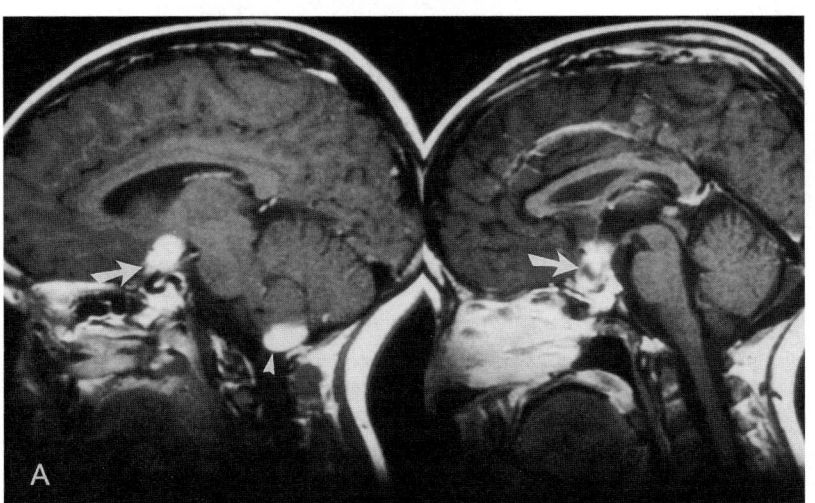

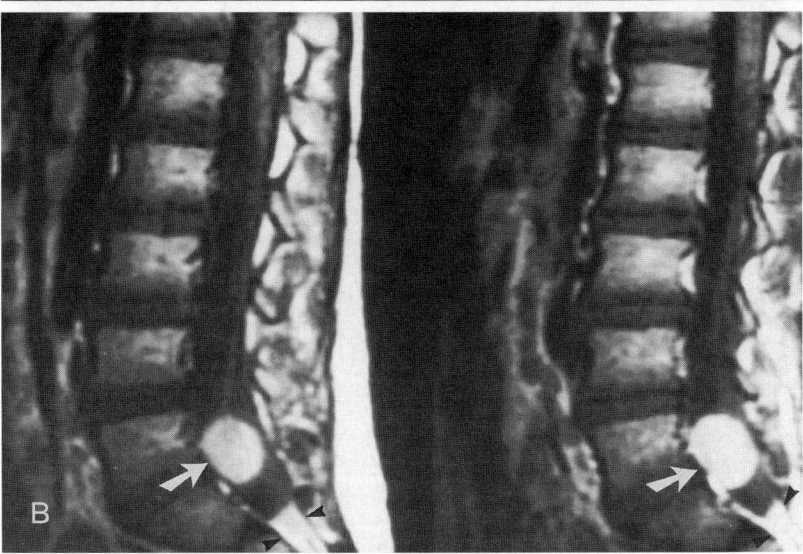

Figure 10.33. Central Nervous System Drop Metastases. A. A sagittal enhanced midline T1WI through the brain shows a suprasellar juvenile pilocytic astrocytoma (*arrow*), with a metastasis that has reached the cerebellar tonsils via the CSF (*arrowhead*). **B.** A sagittal enhanced lumbar T1WI shows a large intraarachnoid metastatic nodule posterior to L-5 (*arrow*). High signal tissue is also seen posterior to S-2 (*arrowheads*). If it were clinically necessary to confirm that this sacral area represents tumor rather than epidural fat, fat-saturation images would be useful.

Solid tumors, such as breast and lung carcinoma, can metastasize to the subarachnoid space. Leukemias, which will be discussed, probably have the highest rate of infiltration of the meninges of any non-CNS tumor. These leptomeningeal metastases can cause considerable inflammation, and patients can present with signs of meningeal irritation, leading to the term "carcinomatous meningitis." Systemic lymphoma (particularly T-cell lymphomas) and carcinomas can also spread to the CSF pathways.

Leptomeningeal metastases classically appear as multiple intradural nodules causing filling defects on myelography (Fig. 10.34) or CT myelograms. Because it is noninvasive, MR with gadolinium enhancement is now the preferred method for screening. Indeed, enhanced MR is probably better than myelography because thin, smooth sheets of intrathecal tumor cells, described by pathologists as "cake-frosting" on the cord and roots, may be difficult to detect on a myelogram because there is no discrete mass (Fig. 10.35). As these tumor layers thicken, widening of the cord contour may occur, mimicking an intramedullary mass from a myelographic standpoint. The differential diagnosis includes infectious meningitis, and in the immunocom-

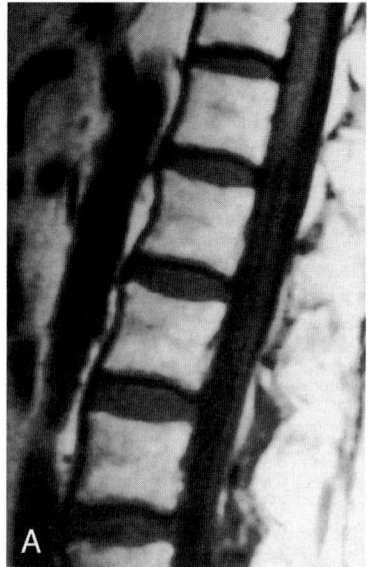

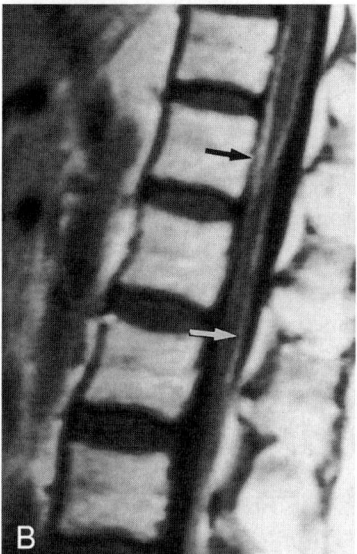

Figure 10.35. Carcinomatous Meningitis. A. Sagittal unenhanced T1WIs in this breast cancer patient are unremarkable. **B.** Enhanced images through the conus show fine sheets of enhancing tumor coating the distal cord and cauda equina (*arrows*). This thin diffuse "cake frosting" type of leptomeningeal tumor involvement may be hard to detect myelographically.

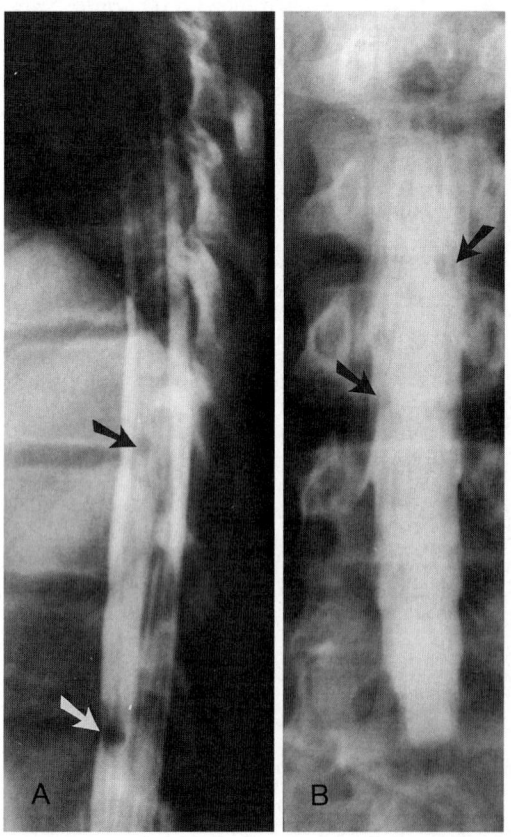

Figure 10.34. Intrathecal Metastases. Lateral **A.** and anteroposterior **B.** myelographic images show multiple nodular filling defects within the subarachnoid space (*arrows*), consistent with nodular leptomeninigeal metastases, in this case of lung carcinoma. (Courtesy of Dr. Anton Pogany, Berkeley, CA.)

promised patient, diffuse leptomeningeal enhancement requires CSF analysis to distinguish between tumor and infection.

Blood in the subarachnoid space may be bright on T1WI, and in the immediate postoperative period, obtaining pregadolinium images is essential to ensure that trace methemoglobin is not mistaken for enhancing drop metastases. Subarachnoid and subdural blood in the spinal canal can cause leptomeningeal irritation and enhancement, further confusing the postoperative "rule out drop metastasis" scan. These problems are easily avoided by obtaining a *preoperative* enhanced MR

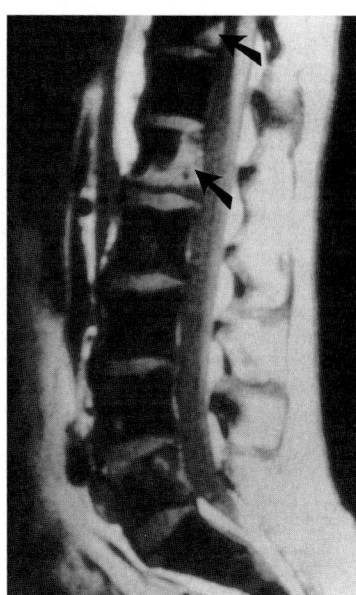

Figure 10.36. Prostate Cancer. The spine appears quite dark on these standard sagittal T1WI, with only occasional islands of normal marrow fat (*arrows*). The vertebrae remained dark on T2WI (not shown). Plain films (not shown) showed dense bony sclerosis, consistent with the "ivory vertebrae" of prostate metastases.

Metastases therefore appear as low signal areas on T1WI or high signal areas on T2WI because of their higher water content as compared with fat. Prostate cancer and other densely sclerotic metastases can be somewhat confusing on MR unless one appreciates that areas of intensely sclerotic bone may be dark on all sequences (Fig. 10.36). Historically, unenhanced T1WI were the mainstay of vertebral body evaluation, but today newer sequences that provide different T2 effects are more sensitive for marrow space pathology.

With gradient-refocused images, the metastases should also be bright, but susceptibility effects from the bony trabeculae reduce their conspicuity, making these sequences less useful. Fast versions of STIR, and T2 FSE with fat saturation are ideal for increasing the conspicuity of abnormal marrow (Figs. 10.37, 10.43). As with other metastases, neovascularity develops to supply the expanding mass of intravertebral tumor cells, which is why vertebral metastases can enhance intensely; however, this may reduce their conspicuity against background fat (Fig. 10.4) unless fat saturation is used.

scan of the spine in any patient at risk for spinal drop metastases, such as a child with medulloblastoma. Once such a child has been sedated and contrast given for the brain, a complete spinal scan will only take another 15 minutes or so, and will save a lot of consternation postoperatively when the case requires staging for adjunctive chemotherapy and radiation.

Extradural Masses

Metastases. After disc herniations and other degenerative processes, neoplasm is the second most common cause of extradural mass; however, in immunosuppressed patients, and certain parts of the world, infections may outnumber neoplasms as a source of extradural mass effect. Primary vertebral tumors such as chordomas, giant cell tumors, hemangiomas, and sarcomas behave like any other extradural mass in terms of myelographic findings and must be kept in the differential diagnosis. The most common extradural neoplasm, however, is metastatic spread of solid tumors such as breast, lung, and prostate carcinoma. Most metastases, like infection, reach the vertebrae via arterial seeding although prostate carcinoma may preferentially ascend to the lumbar region via Batson's venous plexus. The vertebral marrow space, like the liver and the lungs, "filters" a great deal of blood and is a fertile ground for metastatic deposits.

As these deposits grow, they replace normal marrow, which contains considerable fat and is bright on T1WI.

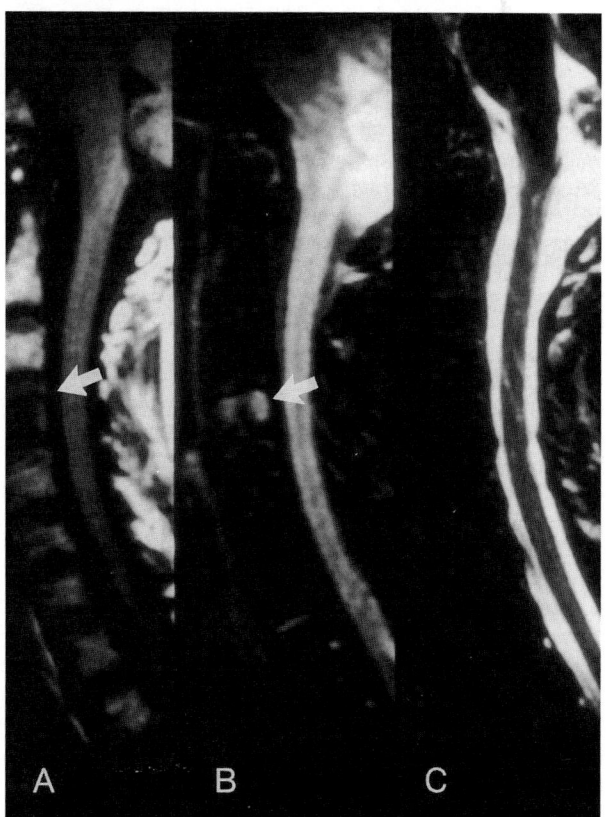

Figure 10.37. Value of Inversion Recovery in the Evaluation of Metastases. This patient has breast carcinoma. **A.** Vertebrae C-2 and C-3 are bright consistent with radiation; C-4 (*arrow*) is quite dark, raising the question of metastasis; C-5 and below are intermediate in signal, and may or may not be normal. **B.** This STIR image shows high signal, consistent with metastasis limited to C-4 (*arrow*). **C.** Fast spin echo sequence with T2-weighting shows little useful information on the marrow, one of the shortcomings of this technique. (Courtesy of Dr. Rahul Mehta, Stanford, CA.)

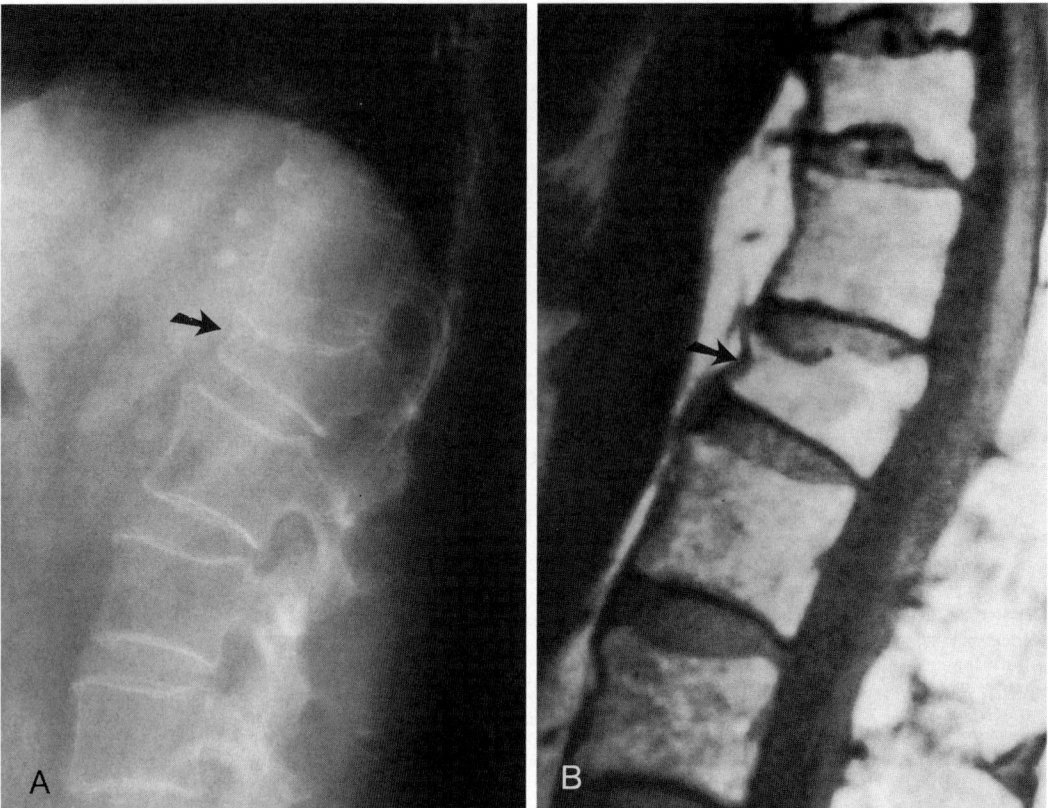

Figure 10.38. Benign Compression Fracture. A. Plain films show a compression fracture of L-1 (*arrow*). The vertebral body shows a classic wedge deformity, with greater loss of height anteriorly than posteriorly, with intact pedicles on the anteroposterior view (not shown). This configuration is suggestive of a benign compression fracture. **B.** T1 sagittal MR shows normal marrow signal in the affected vertebrae (*arrow*), confirming a benign cause of the compression fracture, such as osteoporosis.

Once a tumor has infiltrated the cortex, spread to the epidural space can occur, which along with compression fractures, may lead to cord compromise. Certain signs (summarized in Table 10.3) help determine whether a compression fracture is caused by infection or tumor or is merely secondary to osteoporosis (Fig. 10.38). In general, metastases differ from pyogenic infection in that they involve the vertebrae diffusely but noncontiguously, sparing the discs, with epidural mass and enhancement limited to the levels of the pathologic vertebrae (Fig. 10.39). Marked involvement of the pedicles is another sign of metastases (Fig. 10.40). Exceptions include disc-sparing nonpyogenic infections, notorious for mimicking tumor, and lymphoma, which may have extensive epidural infiltration.

Direct Extension of Paraspinous Tumor. Retroperitoneal and mediastinal tumors can invade the vertebral column and spinal canal by direct extension. Neuroblastoma and its relatives ganglioneuroma and ganglioneuroblastoma arise from primitive paraspinous neural remnants, which are similar to fetal neuroblasts.

These tumors frequently involve the spinal canal, infiltrating through the neural foramina (Figs. 10.41, 10.42). Any paraspinous tumor can do likewise, including lymphomas, apical lung (Pancoast) tumors, and a variety of retroperitoneal and mediastinal carcinomas and sarcomas.

Hematologic malignancies affecting the spine include leukemia, myeloma, and lymphoma.

Leukemias change the appearance of the vertebrae in the characteristic fashion of diffuse, even replacement of the marrow with tumor (Fig. 10.43, also see 10.67). Solid leukemic infiltrates, or chloromas, can involve the epidural space and cause cord compression. Studies that have tracked the MR appearance of the marrow in these patients through induction chemotherapy, radiation, bone marrow transplantation, and repopulation with normal marrow cells are referenced and worth reviewing when evaluating such cases (Fig. 10.44)(20).

Multiple Myeloma can present as a diffuse and homogeneous low signal in the spine on T1WI, but more typi-

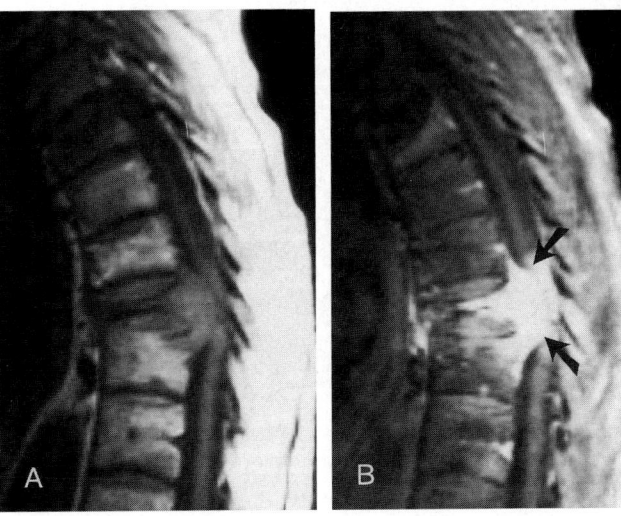

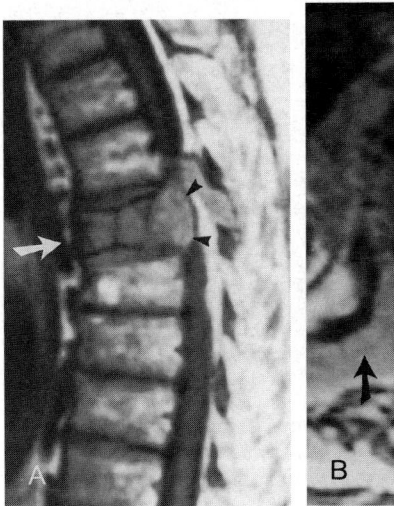
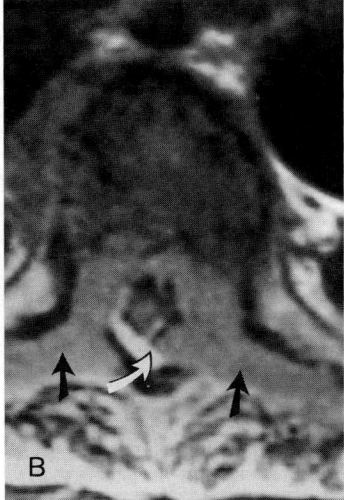

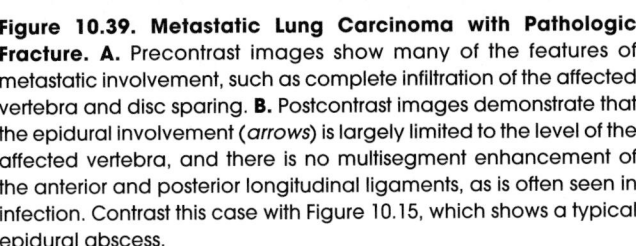

Figure 10.39. Metastatic Lung Carcinoma with Pathologic Fracture. A. Precontrast images show many of the features of metastatic involvement, such as complete infiltration of the affected vertebra and disc sparing. **B.** Postcontrast images demonstrate that the epidural involvement (*arrows*) is largely limited to the level of the affected vertebra, and there is no multisegment enhancement of the anterior and posterior longitudinal ligaments, as is often seen in infection. Contrast this case with Figure 10.15, which shows a typical epidural abscess.

Figure 10.40. Multiple Myeloma. Sagittal **(A)** and axial **(B)** MR images show several features associated with neoplastic infiltration in a midthoracic vertebra (*large arrows*). The affected vertebra is completely involved, the discs are spared, and the epidural mass (*arrowheads*) is limited to the level of affected vertebra. The pedicles and lamina are infiltrated and expanded, (*small arrows*) and the epidural fat (*curved arrow*) is displaced rather than infiltrated. None of these signs alone confirms a neoplastic process, but taken together they are highly suggestive of metastatic tumor.

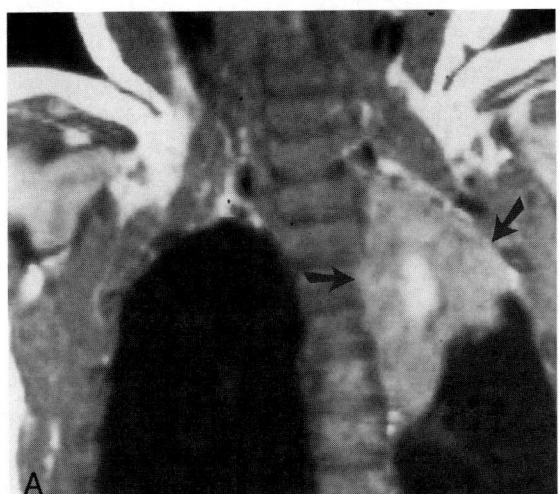
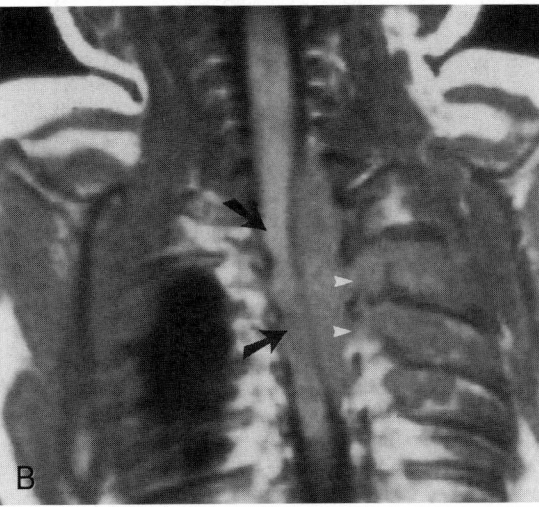

Figure 10.41. Neuroblastoma. A. This patient presented with flaccidity of the lower extremities and an apical paraspinous chest mass (*arrows*). **B.** The myelopathy is easily explained by cord compression (*arrows*) caused by neuroblastoma infiltrating into the spinal canal via multiple neural foramina (*arrowheads*).

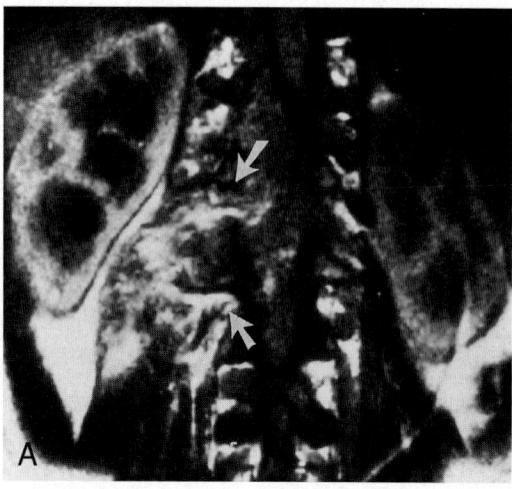
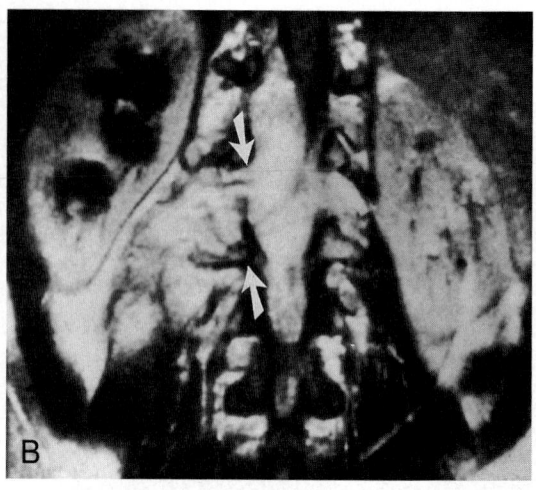

Figure 10.42. Ganglioneuroblastoma. A. This tumor is believed to represent a more "mature" or differentiated form of tumor of the sympathetic nervous system than neuroblastoma. It shares a similar paraspinous distribution and a tendency to dumbbell into the spinal canal (*arrows*) via the neural foramina. **B.** Note the diffuse enhancement with gadolinium.

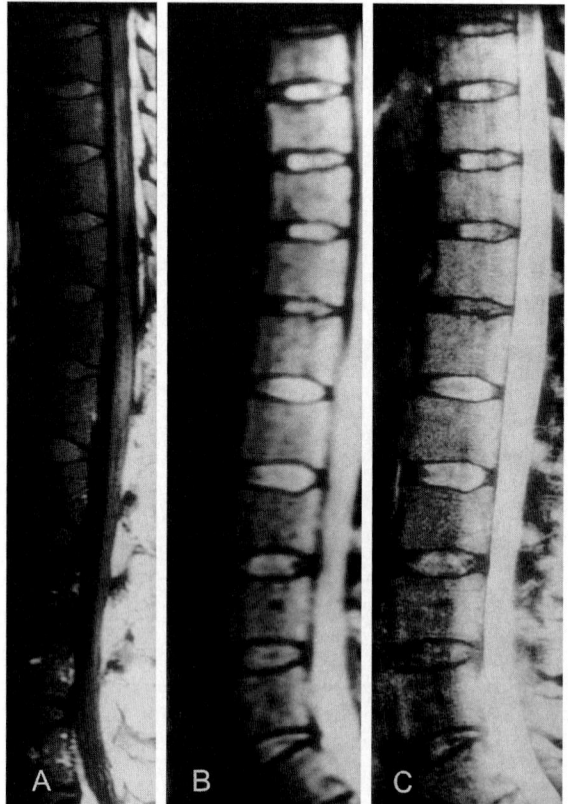

Figure 10.43. Three MR Techniques for Evaluating the Marrow in Leukemia. A. T1WI shows diffuse homogenous infiltration of the marrow, which is dark, as leukemic cells, high in water content, have replaced the normal marrow fat. Normal marrow should be brighter than the discs on T1-weighted spin echo images. **B.** Short TR inversion recovery images (STIR), make this "watery" marrow bright. **C.** "Fast inversion recovery" produces the same effect as conventional STIR in a fraction of the time. (Courtesy of Dr. Rahul Mehta, Stanford, CA.)

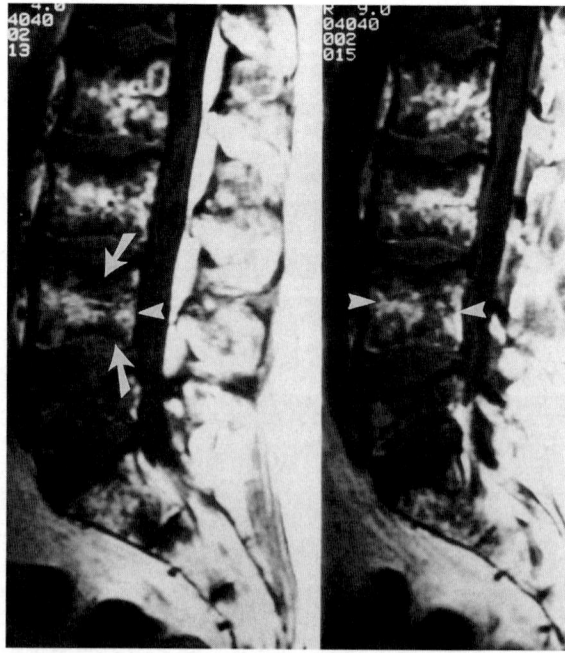

Figure 10.44. Bone Marrow Transplantation. Marrow repopulation is occurring in this patient after bone marrow transplantation. The new hematopoietic marrow, dark on T1WI, has settled in the areas of the vertebrae adjacent to the endplates (*arrow*), probably due to the rich arterial supply to these regions. The center of the vertebrae (*arrowheads*) shows less new active marrow ingrowth and more fat, and consequently, is bright on T1WI.

cally shows multiple focal defects. Occasionally, a plasmacytoma is noted. Myelofibrosis will present as very dark marrow space on T1WI and remains dark on T2WI because there is "dry" fibrous tissue rather than "wet" tumor replacing the marrow (Fig. 10.45). Patients with hemoglobinopathies such as sickle cell disease may have

areas of extramedullary hematopoiesis that are often paraspinous and can infiltrate into the spinal canal causing cord compression.

Lymphoma is a another "hematologic" tumor, with protean imaging manifestations that can serve as the topic for an entire monograph—and have! The classification schemes for lymphoma are complex and not terribly helpful in understanding the presentations in the spine. Lymphomas may present as primary spinous or paraspinous lesions, with pathologic vertebral involvement and compression (Fig. 10.46). The related epidural and paraspinous mass is usually far more extensive than most metastatic disease from solid tumors, and can mimic the appearance of epidural infection. Lymphomas involving mediastinum and retroperitoneum can insidiously invade the spinal canal via the neural foramina. Given that CT remains the dominant technique for following lymphoma in the chest and abdomen, subtle intraspinous disease can easily be missed, and any lymphoma patient with back pain should be evaluated by MR (Fig. 10.47).

VASCULAR DISEASES

Spinal Cord Infarction. Vascular diseases of the spine and spinal cord can be divided into cord infarctions and vascular malformations (22–24).

Spinal "strokes" are quite rare compared with cerebrovascular accidents. The classic scenario is a patient who becomes paralyzed after major thoracic surgery, such as repair of a thoracic aortic aneurysm. The affected segments of the cord will appear bright on T2WI, with enhancement, similar to a brain infarct, followed by the development of myelomalacia. The spinal gray mat-

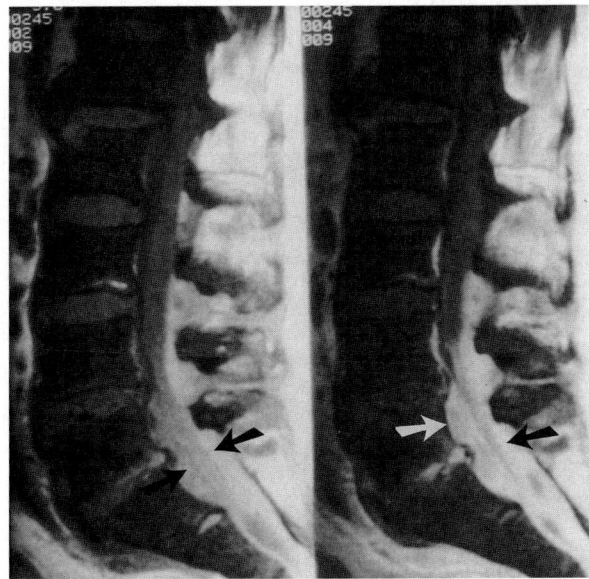

Figure 10.45. Myelofibrosis. This patient has very dark marrow compartment on these enhanced T1WI caused by myelofibrosis, which has replaced the normal erythropoetic marrow. Because there is no increased water in this marrow condition, the marrow remained dark on T2WI. Note the enhancing epidural abscess (*arrows*).

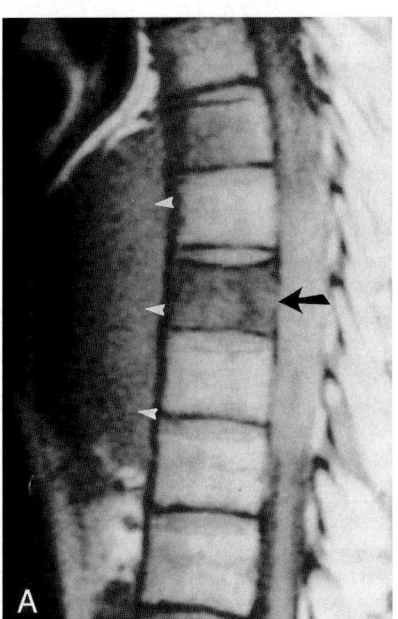
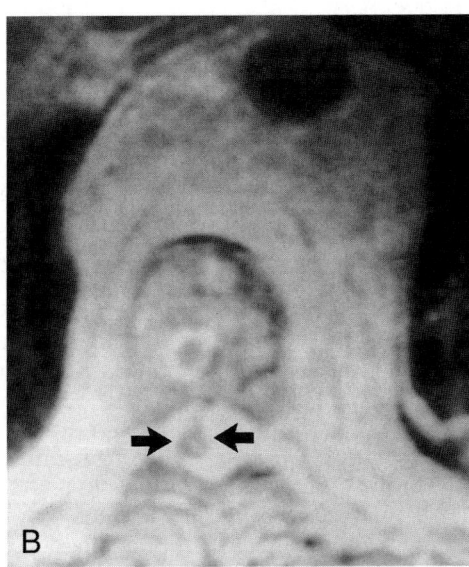
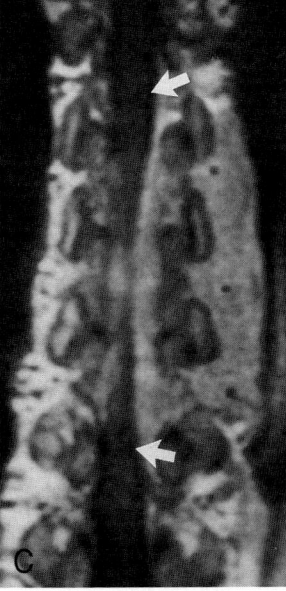

Figure 10.46. Lymphoma. A. Sagittal T1WI shows a large posterior mediastinal mass (*arrowheads*), with infiltration of a midthoracic vertebral body (*arrow*). **B.** Axial images show the cord (*arrow*) and the degree of compression. **C.** A coronal image nicely shows the craniocaudal extent of spinal canal compromise (*arrows*). Lymphoma adjacent to the spine is always a threat for cord compression.

Figure 10.47. Lymphoma Infiltrating the Spinal Canal—Difficulty of CT Visualization. A. This patient with lymphoma was imaged for new back pain. Left renal involvement is obvious (*white arrow*), and left psoas infiltration is also noted (*arrowhead*). Spinal canal involvement (*curved arrow*), even in retrospect, is equivocal. **B.** The MR clearly demonstrates involvement of the spinal canal (*arrows*). Anytime a patient with paraspinous tumor presents with back pain, MR is the study of choice.

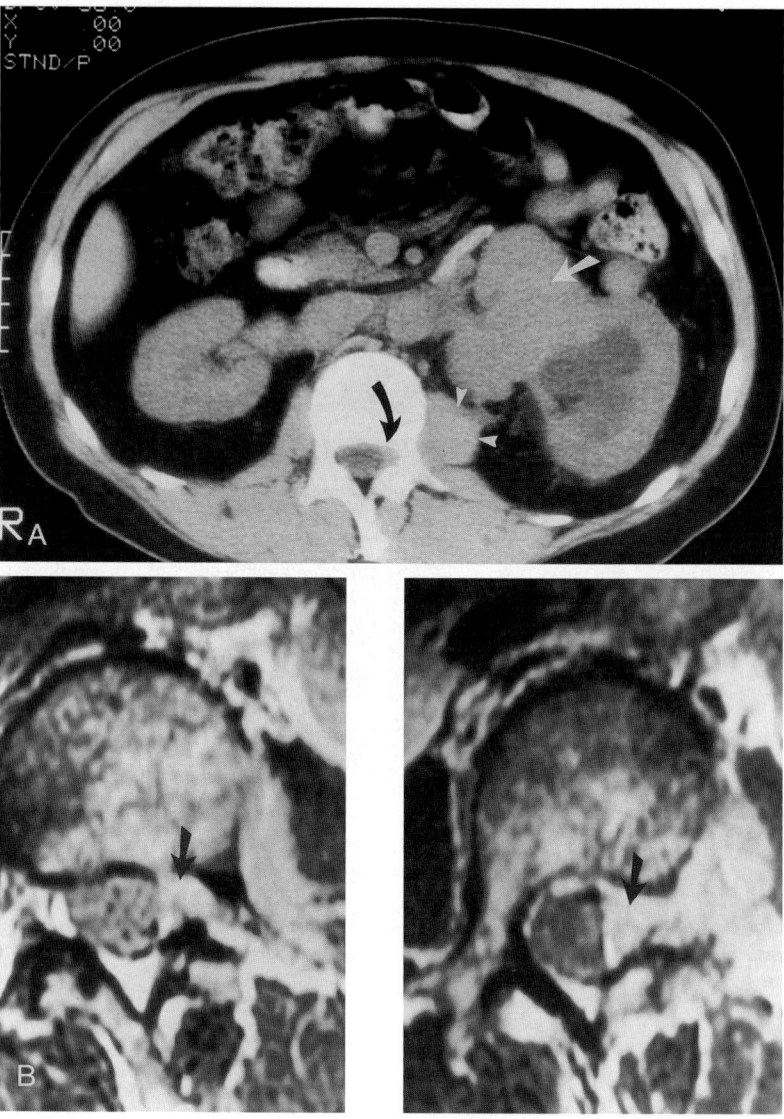

ter in an infarct will enhance to a greater degree than the white matter as occurs in the brain (Fig. 10.48). These findings were difficult to assess prior to MR, when the diagnosis was made solely on clinical grounds. Obviously, when a patient in the recovery room after aortic surgery is paraplegic, it does not require great insight to consider a cord infarct. More subtle, however, are cases where atherosclerotic disease or severe degenerative disease leads to thromboembolic cord infarctions, and infarcts must be considered in the differential of unexplained myelopathy.

Spinal AVM. Spinal stroke can also be related to spinal AVMs. These lesions are of growing interest for two reasons. First, the development of superselective, interventional neuroangiographic and microsurgical techniques has improved understanding and treatment of the lesions. Second, MR has allowed widespread screening of patients with unexplained myelopathy, leading to the discovery of more patients with spinal AVMs.

"Arteriovenous malformation" is used here as a generic term to encompass any abnormal vascular complex, which necessarily violates a number of rather complicated spinal AVM classification systems, where true AVMs represent a specific subtype. For a more in-depth discussion, the excellent article by Rosenblum is recommended (23). For a first pass at this topic, it is worth going back to the initial question one should ask about any spinal lesion: Is the location intramedullary, intradural extramedullary, or extradural? Although an oversimplification, this approach provides a good initial analysis of spinal AVMs.

Intramedullary AVMs have a congenital "nidus" of abnormal vessels within the cord substance, which cause symptoms by hemorrhage or ischemia because of steal phenomenon. These typically present in young patients with hemorrhage, leading to acute paraparesis. Some are high flow, with visible signal voids within the cord substance (Fig. 10.49). Others escape detection even with angiography, and MR is the primary means for their

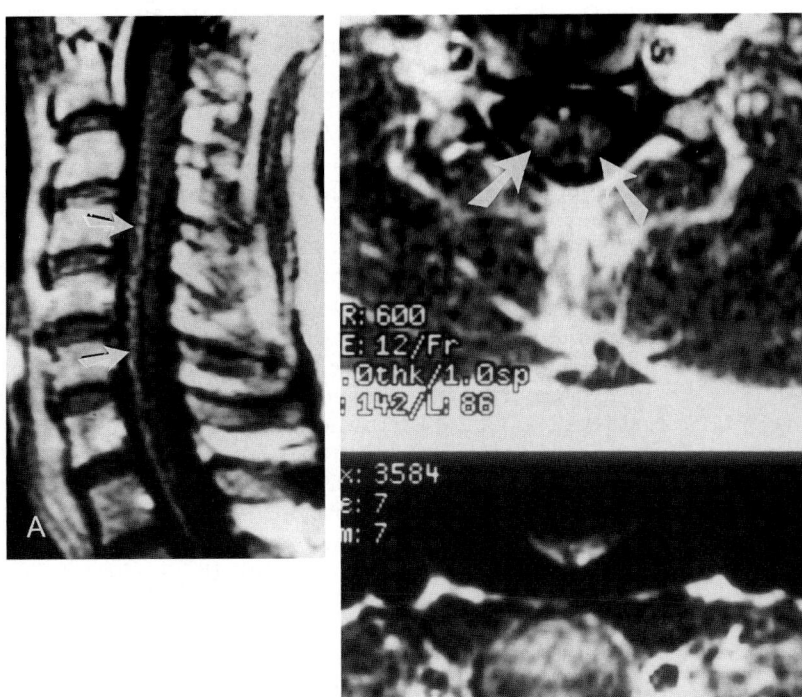

Figure 10.48. Spinal Stroke. This patient who presented with acute myelopathy, has increased signal in the cervical cord seen on T2WI. Postcontrast sagittal **(A)** and axial **(B)** images show enhancement of the central gray matter (*arrows*), a finding highly suggestive of infarct.

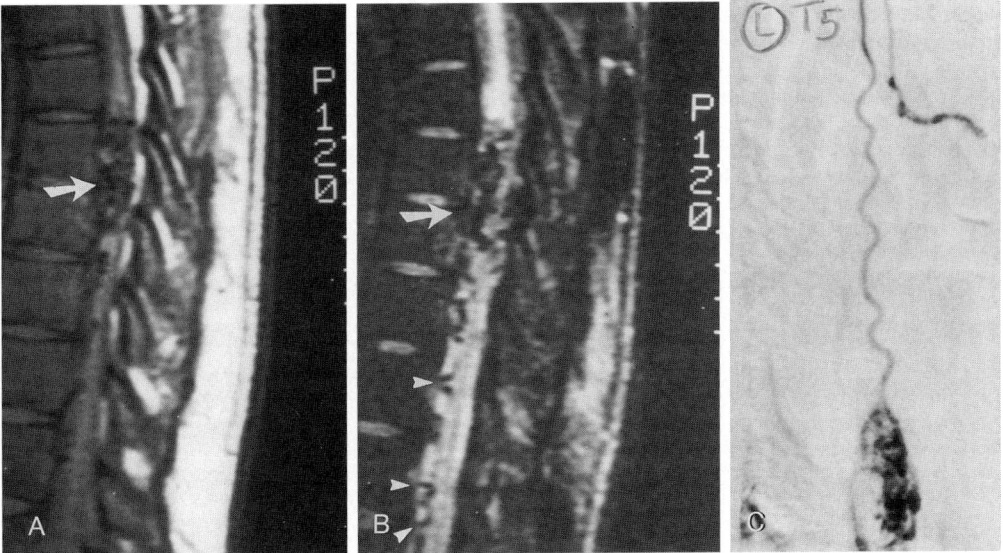

Figure 10.49. Intramedullary AVM. Sagittal proton density **(A)** and T2WI **(B)** show multiple serpentine signal voids within the midthoracic spinal cord (*arrow*), consistent with an intramedullary AVM. A long draining vessel is also noted in the subarachnoid space (*ar-*rowheads*). **C.** Spinal angiogram injecting the left T-5 intercostal artery confirms the MR findings. (Courtesy of Dr. Grant Hieshima, University of California, San Francisco.)

identification, similar to occult vascular malformations in the brain (Fig. 10.50).

Extramedullary AVMs are located in the pia or the dura. When in the dura, they can be as far from the cord as the nerve root sleeves. The lesion is typically an arteriovenous fistula, a direct connection between an artery and vein without an intervening nidus of congenitally

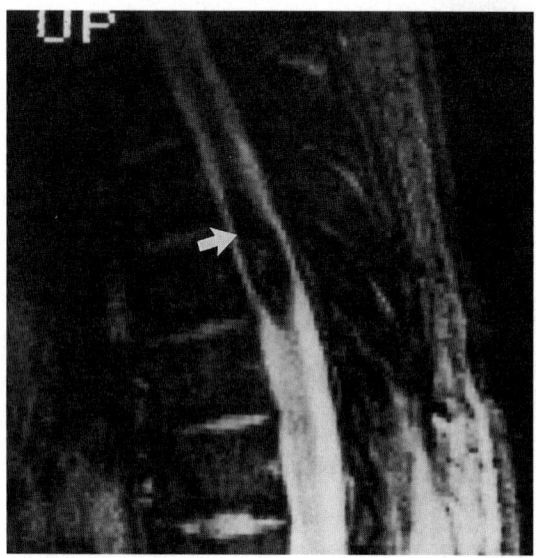

Figure 10.50. Occult Vascular Malformation. An intramedullary area of decreased signal was present on all sequences, but was most prominent on this gradient series (*arrow*). No abnormal vessels were seen on MR or angiography, consistent with an occult vascular malformation, which was confirmed surgically.

abnormal vasculature. The direct arterial inflow into the local venous system through the fistula, undamped by the resistance of a capillary bed, raises pressure within the coronal venous plexus draining the spinal cord, which is valveless (Fig. 10.51). Spinal dural arteriovenous fistulas, or SDAVFs as they are known, cause symptoms through venous hypertension and congestion of the cord with edema. This edema can be detected on MR as increased signal on T2WI, typically within an enlarged conus (see Fig. 10.53A), which often enhances. The reason for cord enhancement in SDAVFs is not fully understood but probably results from breakdown of the blood-brain barrier because of either chronic infarction or capillary leak phenomenon secondary to venous hypertension (25,26). Regardless of the explanation, enhancement of the cord with SDAVFs is yet another reason why a postcontrast scan should be obtained in any patient with unexplained myelopathy.

The dilated vessels of the coronal venous plexus sometimes can be visualized by MR, but this is quite technique-dependent. With older imaging systems, normal CSF flow created tubular flow voids that mimicked vessels, leading to false-positive examinations (Fig. 10.52). Now, various motion-suppression techniques have reduced this problem, but the sensitivity of MR for these small veins remains moderate at best. In the face of an equivocal MR, the best screening examination, short of spinal angiography, is supine thoracic high-dose plain film myelography. The dilated veins of the coronal venous plexus appear as serpentine filling defects in the dorsal subarachnoid space on myelography (Fig. 10.53B). An additional advantage of myelography is the potential to identify the primary arterialized vein fed by the fistula, a landmark that can greatly facilitate the angiographer's search for the arterial supply to fistula (Fig.

Figure 10.51. Anatomy of a Spinal Dural Arteriovenous Fistula. The fistula is an abnormal direct connection between an artery and a vein in the dura of the nerve root sleeve. The fistula results in reversal of flow in the draining vein (*arrow*), which in turn feeds the coronal venous plexus with arterial blood under high pressure. The coronal venous plexus dilates, becoming visible to imaging studies, and the cord has difficulty draining its blood because of this fistula-induced venous hypertension, and it becomes edematous and bright on T2WI (see Fig. 10.53). (From Rosenblum B, Oldfield EH, Doppman JL, et al. Spinal arteriovenous malformations: a comparison of dural arteriovenous fistulas and intradural AVMs in 81 patients. J Neurosurg 1987;67:796.)

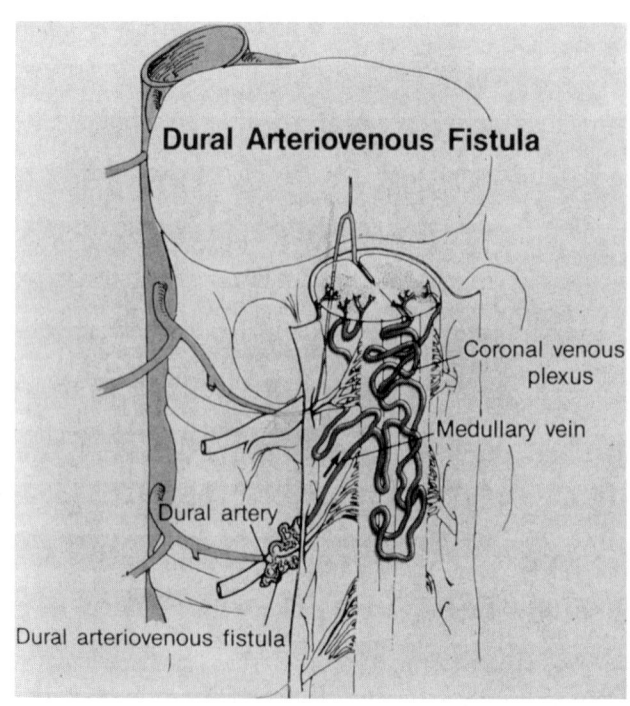

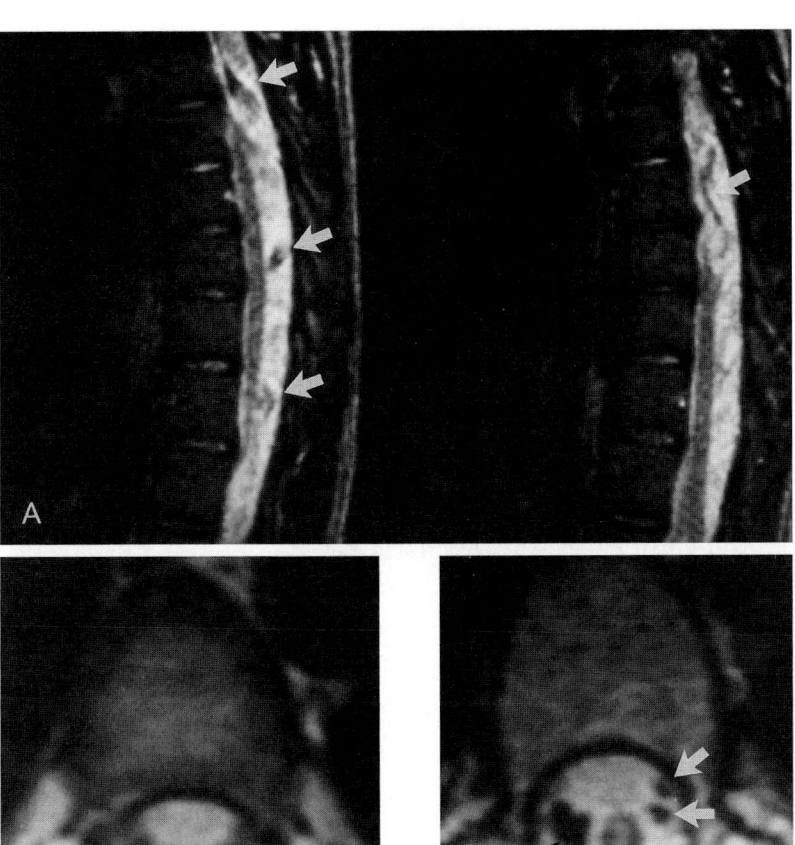

Figure 10.52. False-positive Dilated Spinal Veins.
A. Sagittal T2WI show multiple large tubular signal voids in the subarachnoid space (*arrows*), without cord edema. **B.** Axial images show flow voids that are most prominent in the lateral aspects of the spinal canal (*arrows*), areas of maximal velocity of CSF pulsation. All of the signal voids seen here are caused by CSF pulsation rather than abnormal vessels in the subarachnoid space. The scan was repeated with cardiac gating and these "abnormalities" disappeared.

10.53C). Focused MR angiography (MRA) has succeeded in depicting known dilated spinal veins, but given the small field of view need for good MRA, it remains problematic as a spinal vascular screening exam.

CONGENITAL MALFORMATIONS

MR has become the primary method for investigation of children born with neural axis defects involving either the brain or the spine. Pediatric brain malformations, and the combined brain and spine malformation of the Chiari II syndrome, are discussed in detail in chapter 8 (see Figs. 8.28, 8.29, 8.31). The Chiari I syndrome was mentioned in the discussion of syringohydromyelia (see Fig 8.30). This section briefly addresses the remaining range of congenital spine problems, emphasizing those that are not immediately apparent at birth which may present in adulthood. The references listed are recommended for a more complete discussion of these disorders, which easily are as complex as the remaining topics of this chapter combined (27–28).

In the spine, neural tube defects that are open or have associated dermal defects are usually detected by US done prenatally or at birth. Anomalies of neural tube closure where the covering skin is intact are more subtle and range from asymptomatic nonfusion of the laminae and spinous processes to severe cord tethering with spinal lipomas (Fig. 10.54). A picture is worth a thousand words in understanding the range of presentations of spinal dysraphism, and Figure 10.55, adapted from Barkovich's text, serves as an introduction to this complex topic (25). It is worth remembering that developmental lesions are the most common cause of pediatric intraspinal masses, and T1WI are preferred for evaluating fine anatomic detail as well as the fat components seen in many of these disorders. The standard pediatric spine examination for congenital anomalies, therefore, includes T1-weighted sagittal and axial images; T2WI are less critical. If there is a "sacral dimple" or other skin defect, tape a marker (such as a vitamin E capsule) over it, to ensure that the defect is identifiable on the scan.

Tethered Cord. When the cord is truly tethered, the conus will be low in position although determining the

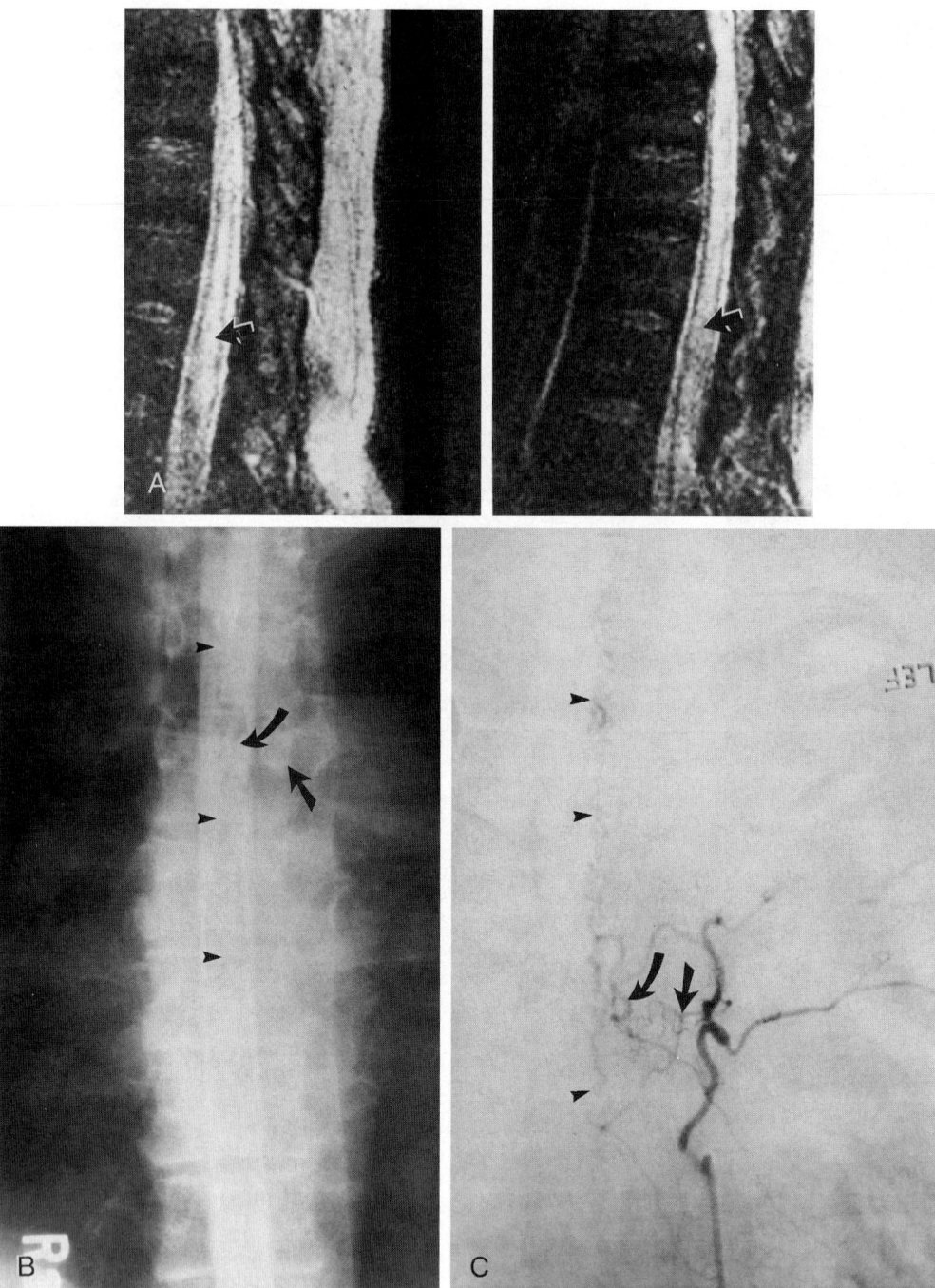

Figure 10.53. Spinal Dural Arteriovenous Fistula. A. This 45-year-old patient had progressive myelopathy, and this T2-weighted series showed increased signal in the conus (*arrow*), consistent with edema. MR was equivocal for abnormal vessels in the subarachnoid space. **B.** A supine thoracic myelogram demonstrates abnormal vessels causing filling defects in the contrast column posterior to the cord (*arrowhead*). The largest vessel (*curved arrow*) appears to exit the spinal canal just below the left T-5 pedicle (*arrow*), and rep-resents the arterialized vein fed by the fistula. The myelogram, therefore, suggests a promising site to begin spinal angiography. **C.** A spinal angiogram demonstrates the dural fistula (*arrow*) and the arterialized vein with reversal of flow (*curved arrow*) that has led to dilation of the entire coronal venous plexus (*arrowheads*). Note how the subarachnoid vessels seen on the angiogram and myelogram are superimposable. Compare to the diagram shown in Figure 10.51.

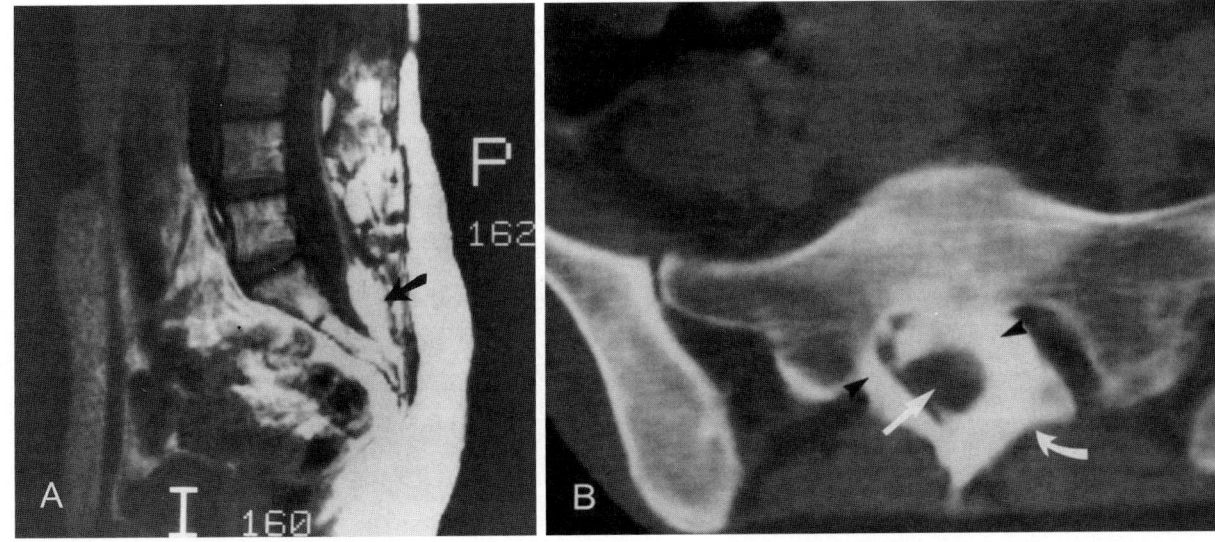

Figure 10.54. Spinal Lipoma. A. Sagittal T1WI shows a dorsal intraspinal lipoma (*arrow*) at S-1. **B.** An axial CT myelogram demonstrates that the distal lipoma (*arrow*) is intrathecal, surrounded by enhanced CSF (*arrowheads*), with an incomplete posterior sacrum (*curved arrow*), consistent with spinal dysraphism. This defect is illustrated schematically in Figure 10.55A.

exact position of the conus is often difficult because the roots of the cauda equina, when tethered, form a taut mass in the posterior lumbar canal, obscuring the conus/cauda junction (Fig. 10.56). Not every lumbar intradural fatty deposit implies pathologic tethering, and small fibrolipomas of the filum terminale may be noted on MR examinations in patients with normal conus position and no symptoms of cord tethering (Fig. 10.57). These patients must be followed throughout their lives before such fibrolipomas can be dismissed as incidental because symptoms of cord tethering occasionally can present well into adulthood. Before describing the conus as low in position, recall that the conus in a newborn is normally at L-2 and typically ascends one to two vertebral segments as the child grows.

Intramedullary Lipomas can be seen in patients with normal or bifid spinal canals and, as with brain lipomas, may be discovered incidentally. Usually thoracic, these lipomas are more common in males, and when symptomatic, present with myelopathy in young adulthood (Fig. 10.58). If any cysts, hemorrhage, or debris are seen in association with the fat, suspect a teratoma. Dermoid and epidermoid tumors occur intraspinally, with imaging characteristics similar to their presentations in the brain. Both may be associated with dorsal dermal sinus tracts. Intraspinal teratomas are a distinct entity from sacrococcygeal teratoma, a pediatric lesion with a high malignant potential, often associated with other anomalies.

Caudal Regression Syndrome. A number of other sacral anomalies have been grouped under the "caudal regression syndrome," where the distal spine and sacrum may be hypoplastic or absent and the conus has a blunted appearance (Fig. 10.59). Caudal regression is believed to be caused by an insult to the mesoderm during the fourth gestational week, and associated cardiac and renal anomalies are common. A high association with maternal diabetes exists. However, subtle forms, such as partial sacral agenesis, may not be discovered until adulthood. The distal spine is also the site of a number of CSF-filled, arachnoid-lined cystic lesions with associated bony deformity, ranging from small perineural (Tarlov's) cysts (Fig. 10.60) to huge anterior sacral meningoceles. The latter is distinct from posterior meningocele, which, like a myelomeningocele, results from failure of neural tube closure rather than leptomeningeal diverticulation. Arachnoid cysts in the spine present as masses that are relatively isointense to CSF. As in the brain, the primary differential diagnostic consideration is an epidermoid. Either can occur in the lumbar spine as a rare complication of lumbar puncture (Fig. 10.61).

Many unsuspected spinal abnormalities present as curvature of the spine, or scoliosis. Most adolescents with curvature of the spine have idiopathic scoliosis, but when the onset is earlier or more severe or plain scoliosis films show a vertebral anomaly (Fig. 10.62), MR is indicated to rule out an intraspinal abnormality. These cases are collectively known as "congenital scoliosis," and the primary cause, such as cord tethering, must be addressed before the spine undergoes mechanical straightening (Fig. 10.63).

Text cont. on p. 276

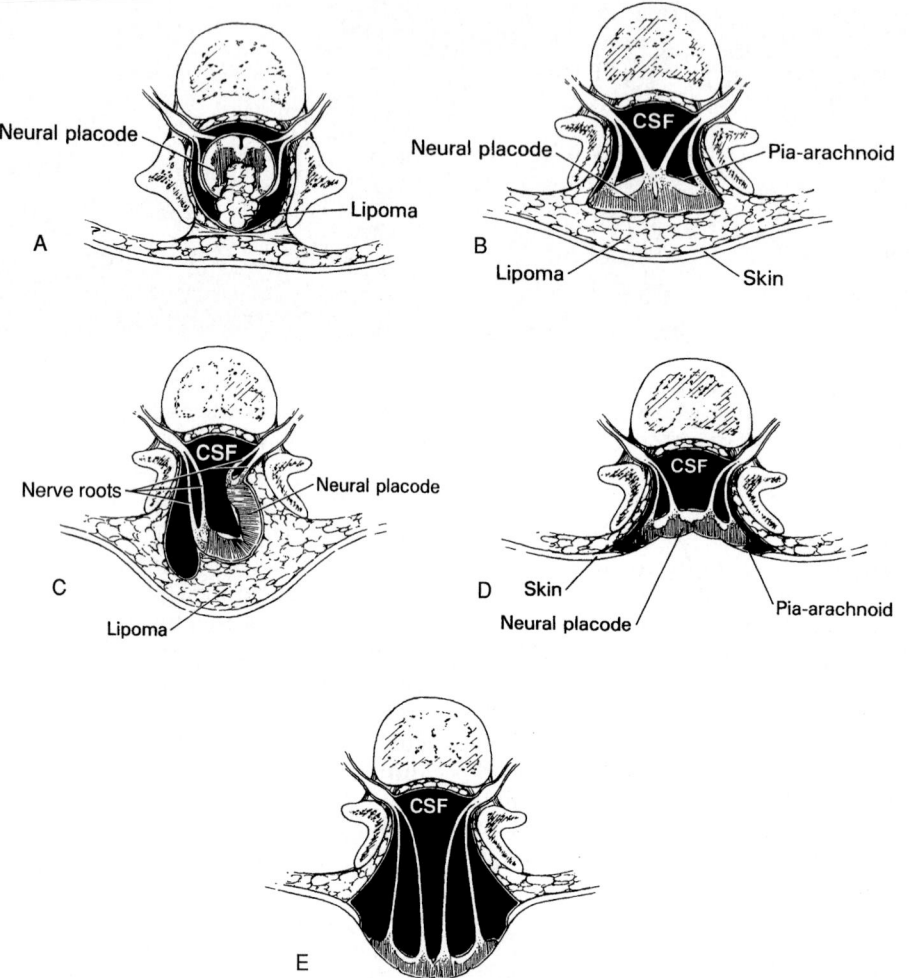

Figure 10.55. Spinal Dysraphism. This series of drawings from Barkovich's text nicely illustrates the range of appearances of spinal dysraphism. In all of these conditions, there has been failure of the lips of the neural folds to close in the midline dorsally, forming a tube. The incompletely fused plaque of neural tissue is referred to as the neural "placode." When the placode is covered by intact skin and subcutaneous fat, without dorsal herniation of neural tissue, the defect **(A,B)** may be overlooked in the newborn examination, giving rise to the term "occult spinal dysraphism." **A. Spinal lipoma.** The dorsal spinal cord has failed to close, with an intradural lipoma situated between the lips of the unfused placode. The MR and CT appearance of this defect is shown in Figure 10.54. **B. Lipomyelocele.** The dorsal dura is incomplete. The subarachnoid space lies ventral to the placode, which is covered by pia and arachnoid on its internal surface. The subcutaneous fat is contiguous with a lipoma, which is adherent to the dorsal surface of the placode.

C. Lipomyelomeningocele. This is similar to the lipomyelocele **B**, except there the subarachnoid space is dilated, causing the placode to bulge posteriorly. In this image, the lipoma is asymmetric and extends into the canal on the left, rotating the placode and causing discrepancy in the length of the nerve roots, which complicates surgical repair. Lipomyelomeningoceles are seen in conjunction with rostral craniospinal abnormalities in the Chiari II syndrome, illustrated in Figure 8.31 and 8.33. **D. Myelocele.** The neural placode is contiguous with the skin, and will be obvious on newborn examination. The ventral aspect of the placode has the same anatomy as the lipomyelocele. **E. Meningomyelocele.** The ventral subarachnoid space is dilated, displacing the placode posteriorly (as in lipomyelomeningocele). Otherwise, the defect is identical to a myelocele. (From Barkovich AJ. Pediatric Neuroimaging. New York: Raven Press, 1990:240,248.)

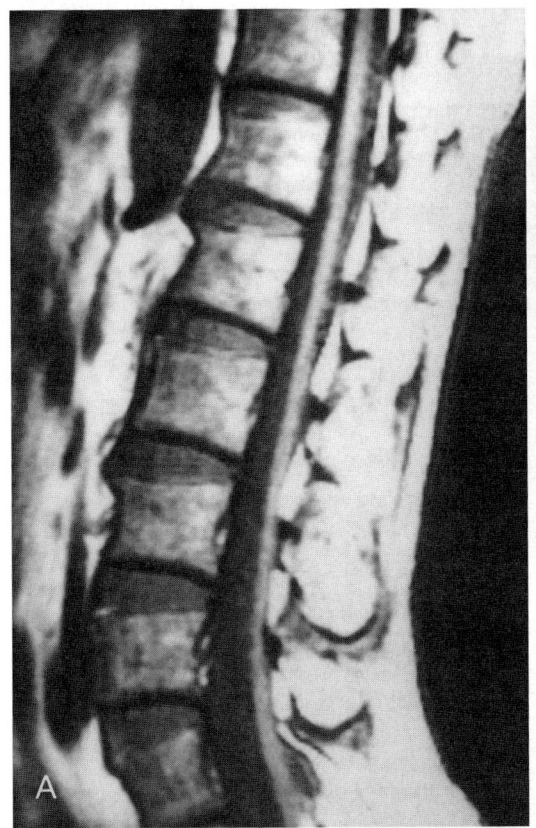

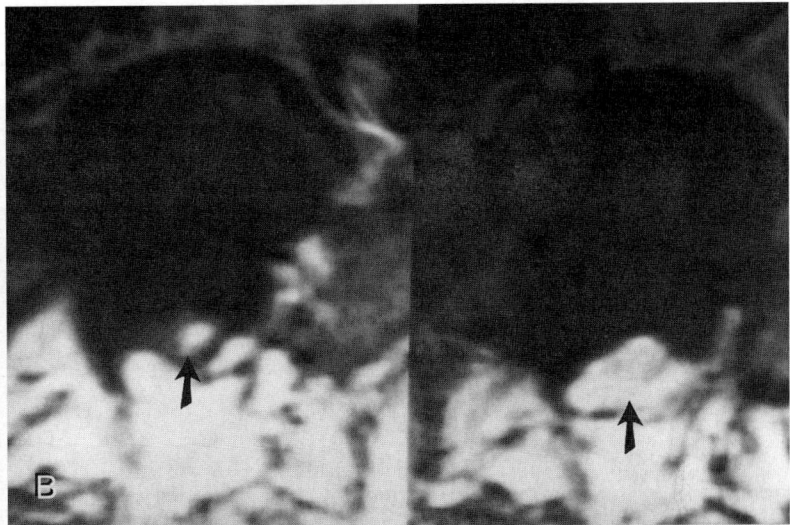

Figure 10.56. Adult Cord Tethering. This young adult presented with a gait disorder. **A.** The position of the conus on sagittal plane is difficult to determine with certainty because of the clumping of the roots posteriorly, but it is definitely very low. **B.** Axial T1WI demonstrate spinal dysraphism with a lipoma (*arrows*), consistent with cord tethering.

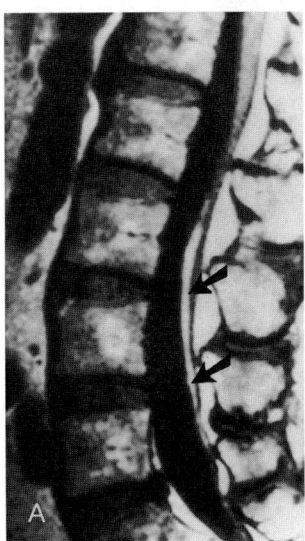

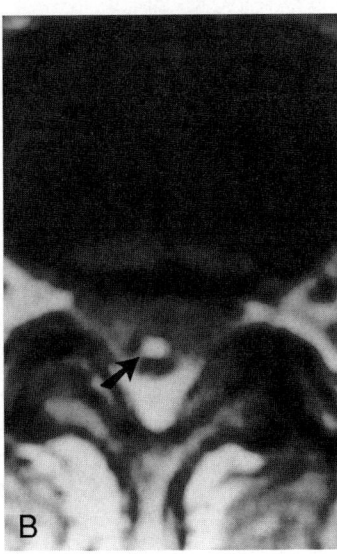

Figure 10.57. Fibrolipoma of the Filum Terminale. A. A sagittal T1WI shows that the conus is normal in position, but the filum terminale shows high signal consistent with fat (*arrows*). **B.** Axial T1WI confirms the intrathecal position of the thickened fatty filum (*arrow*).

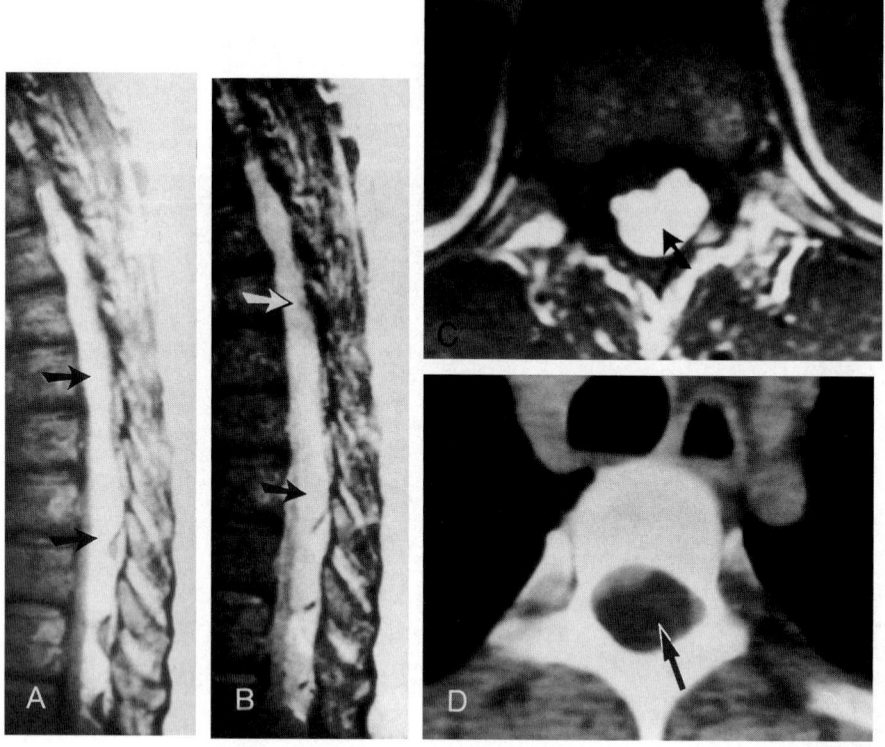

Figure 10.58. Intrathecal Lipoma Noted Incidentally After Trauma. A. Sagittal T1WI shows a high signal intraspinal mass (*arrows*), which appears to be intramedullary. Possible diagnoses include lipoma and hemorrhage in the methemoglobin state. A fat-saturated T1WI would be ideal for making this distinction. **B.** T2WI shows relative signal drop-off within the mass (*arrows*), more consistent with fat than methemoglobin. **C.** Axial T1WI shows the lipoma (*arrow*) is central within the canal, and is probably intramedullary. **D.** The CT demonstrates a low attenuation mass, confirming a lipoma (*arrow*).

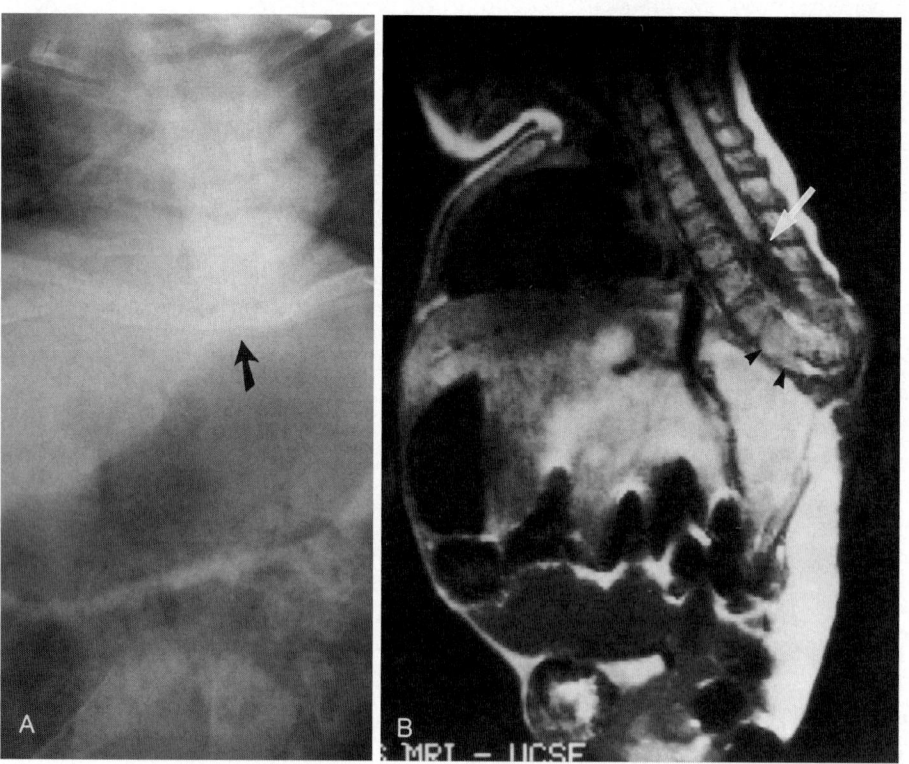

Figure 10.59. Severe Caudal Regression Syndrome. A. Plain film of the abdomen shows absence of the spinal column below T-8 (*arrow*). **B.** Sagittal T1WI shows a characteristic blunted appearance of the distal cord (*arrow*), and fusion of the caudal vertebrae (*arrowheads*), the lowest of which is dysplastic. (From Barkovich AJ. Pediatric Neuroimaging. New York: Raven Press, 1990:242.)

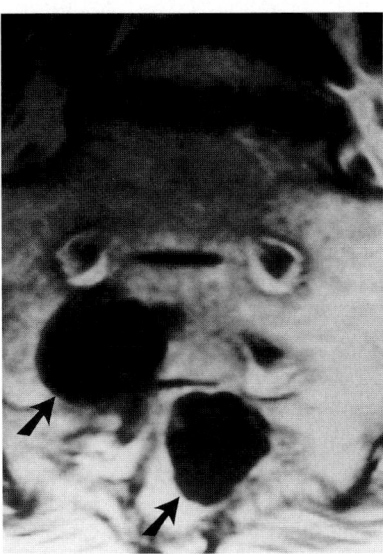

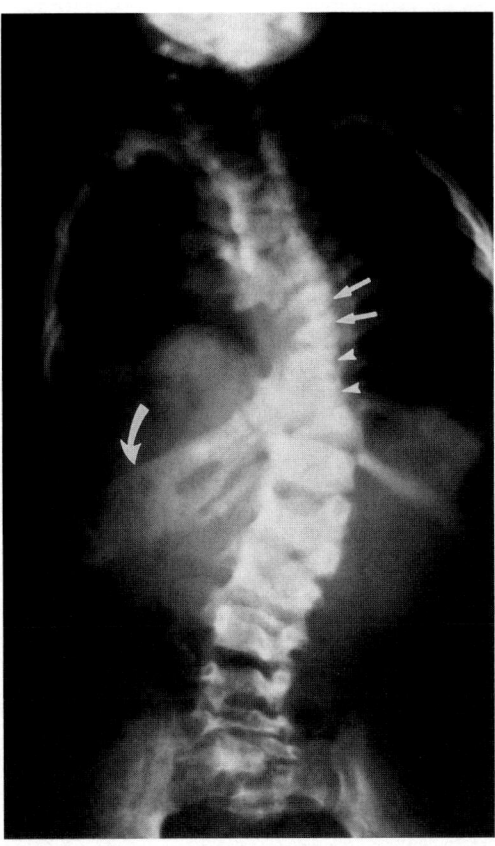

Figure 10.60. Sacral Cysts. Leptomeningeal-lined sacral cysts have been classified many different ways. The spectrum includes intrasacral meningoceles, anterior sacral meningoceles, and perineural (Tarlov's) cysts (*arrows*), shown here in this T1WI through the sacrum. These are often asymptomatic but can result in radicular compression.

Figure 10.62. Congenital Scoliosis. This plain film shows hemivertebrae (*arrows*), block vertebrae (*arrowheads*), and fused ribs (*curved arrow*), leaving no doubt that this is congenital rather than idiopathic scoliosis. An MR would be valuable to evaluate the spinal cord for position and possible mass effect.

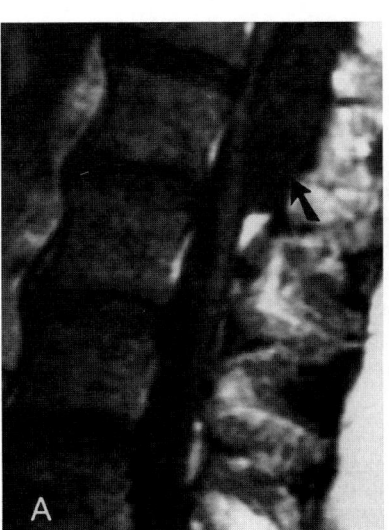
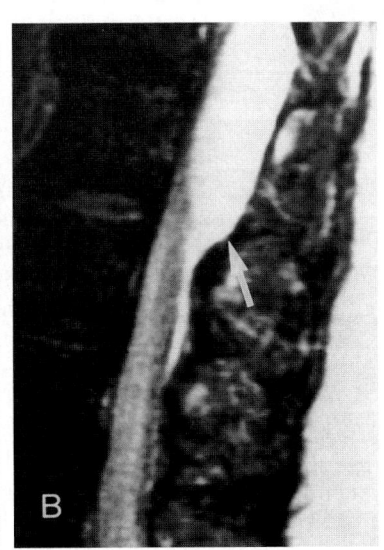

Figure 10.61. Arachnoid Cyst. A. Sagittal T1WI shows a mass isointense to CSF (*arrow*) posterior to the proximal cauda equina, displacing it forward. **B.** This mass becomes brighter than the remainder of the CSF on the T2WI (*arrow*). This proved to be an arachnoid cyst. These can be congenital or related to prior inflammation or injury. Epidermoid is the main differential consideration.

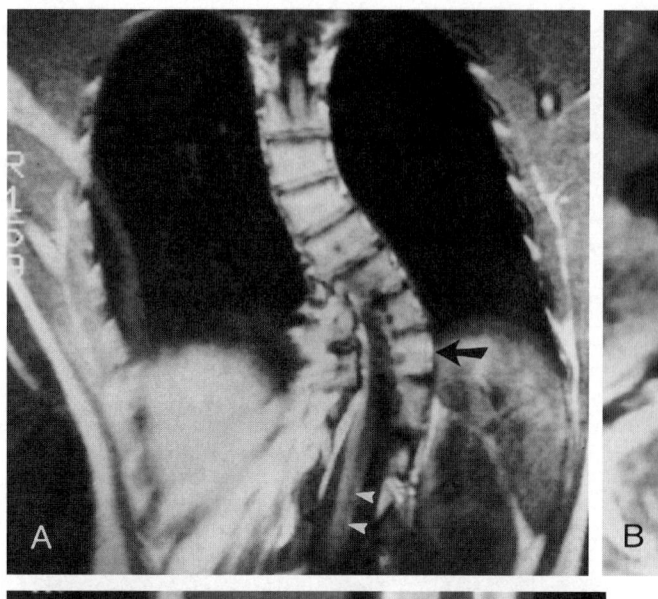

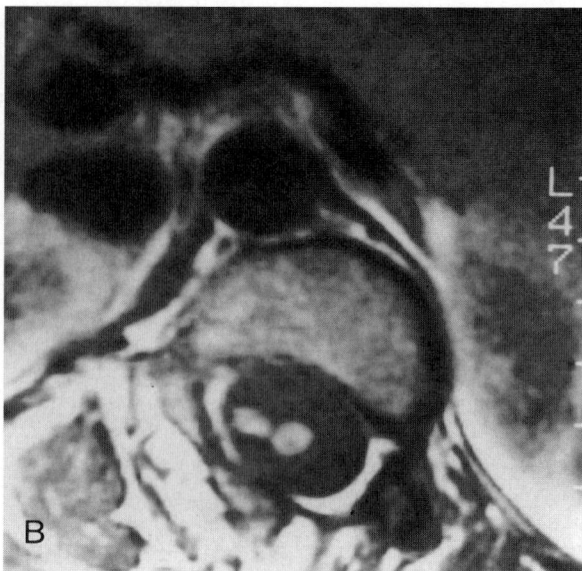

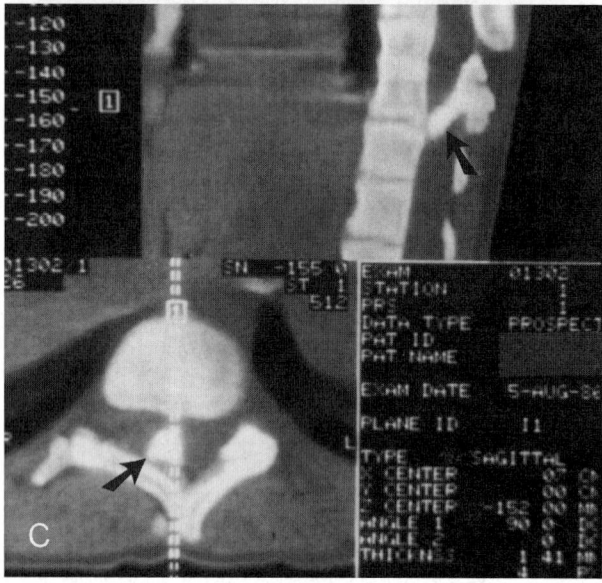

Figure 10.63. Diastematomyelia. This 15-year-old patient with progressive scoliosis, despite bracing, was a candidate for surgery. Plain films had been unrevealing. **A.** Coronal MR shows the levoscoliosis with its apex (*arrow*) near the thoracolumbar junction. Distal to this apex, the cord appears separated into two distinct parallel portions (*arrowheads*). **B.** Axial images confirm a split cord, or diastematomyelia. MR is not good at assessing bony content of the midline fibrocartilagenous spur. (**A** and **B** from Brant-Zawadzki M, Norman D. Magnetic resonance imaging of the central nervous system. New York: Raven Press, 1987.) **C.** A CT scan with sagittal reconstruction on a similar patient confirms a dense, bony midline spur (*arrows*). This spur was also visible on plain film.

TRAUMA

In the acute trauma patient, spine alignment must be evaluated immediately to rule out fractures. Unstable fractures can compromise the diameter of the spinal canal, leading to cord compression and paralysis. Plain films, therefore, are the study of choice in the emergency department because they can be obtained quickly and inexpensively, without significant interruption of other resuscitation efforts. When complex spine fractures are seen on plain films, CT studies often help define the relationship of the bone fragments. CT of the cervical spine is particularly useful in detecting injury to the foramen transversarium, which houses the vertebral artery, a vessel that can be compromised by cervical trauma. Spine fractures and their evaluation are critical topics for radiology residents and others responsible for emergency radiology to master (see chapter 43).

Some discussion, however, is needed concerning the immediate and delayed consequences of vertebral trauma to the spinal cord and spinal nerves, that cannot properly be evaluated on plain films or with noncontrast CT. These include cord contusion, epidural hematoma (and their sequela, such as myelomalacia and syringohydromyelia), and nerve root avulsion (29–31).

Cord Contusion. The spinal cord, like the brain, lies suspended in a bath of CSF, contained by arachnoid membranes, dura, and bone. The cord, again like the brain, is subject to significant impact against its surrounding bony suit of armor during abrupt acceleration and deceleration injuries. In the brain, contusions appear at the site of a blow and 180° opposite, in the classic coup-contrecoup pattern. Certain bony sites, such as the planum sphenoidale, traumatize adjacent brain because of their irregular coutour. In the spine, contusions

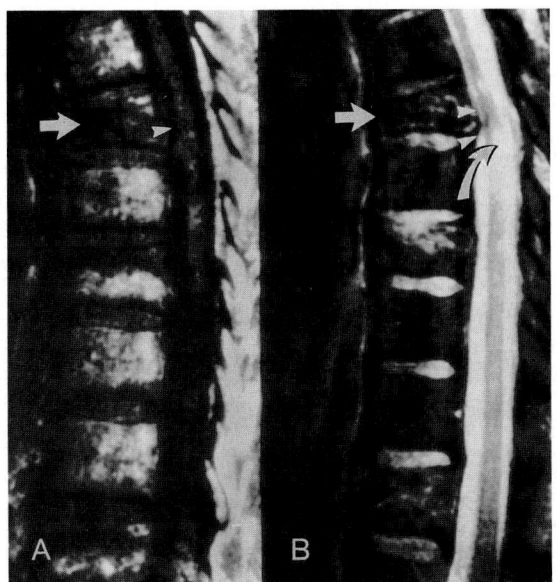

Figure 10.64. Spinal Contusion. A. Compression fracture (*arrow*) with narrowing of the spinal canal (*arrowheads*) caused by retropulsed bony fragments. **B.** Intramedullary edema (*curved arrow*), seen on this T2WI, is a poor prognostic factor in this setting. The presence of a hematoma is associated with an even poorer outcome. Fortunately, none is evident.

usually occur at sites of fractures, secondary to bony impingement and cord compression (Fig. 10.64). However, spinal cord contusions may occur in the absence of spinal fractures because of hyperflexion or hyperextension, resulting in myelopathy (Fig. 10.65). The presence of cord edema, and particularly of cord hemorrhage, has been established as poor a prognostic factor in spinal cord injury patients evaluated by MR. Therefore, T2-weighted or gradient-echo images are a critical portion of any MR protocol for spine trauma. Certain types of injury, such as sudden distraction forces along the long axis of the spine, can lead to cord avulsion (Fig. 10.66).

If the spinal cord is injured, myelomalacia results and further changes can occur because of CSF flow patterns. An area of myelomalacia can enlarge with CSF entry, particularly if adhesions disturb CSF flow and evolve into a posttraumatic syrinx. The expanding syrinx can cause further neurologic deficit and thus require shunting.

Epidural Hematoma. As in the head, extra-axial or, more appropriately, "extramedullary" hematomas can follow trauma, with certain important distinctions. Subdural hematomas are rare in the spine (and usually related to coagulopathies [Fig. 10.67]), although epidural hematomas are far more common. The reverse is true in the calvarium, as discussed in chapter 3.

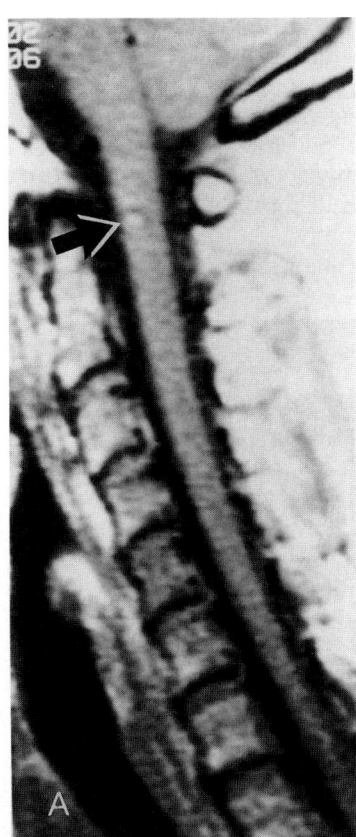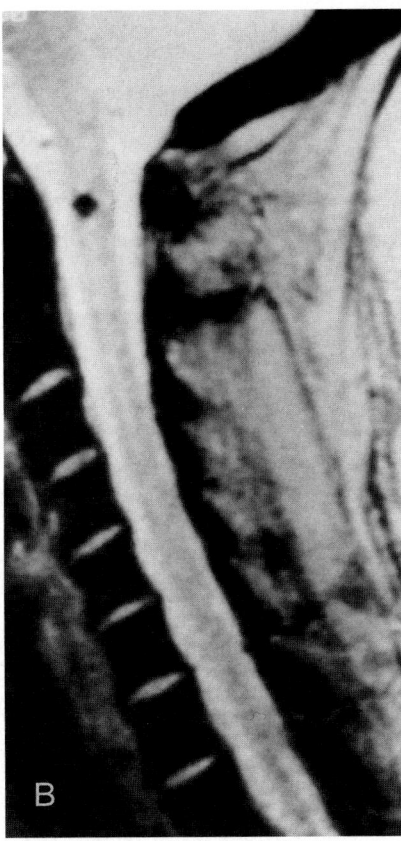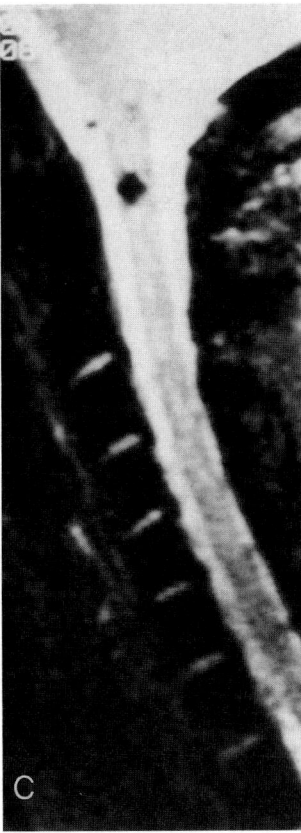

Figure 10.65. Cord Hematoma. A. Sagittal T1WI show a tiny focus of methemoglobin with a dark rim (*arrow*) in the cord posterior to the dens. The dark rim "blooms" on the first **(B)** and second **(C)** echoes of the gradient refocused sequence, consistent with hemosiderin.

This distinction can be explained by differences in venous anatomy between the skull and the spine because the majority of posttraumatic bleeding is venous. In the bony calvarium, the dura is functionally the periosteum, with no potential space between the dura and bone for low-pressure venous blood to accumulate. Bleeding under arterial pressure will create an epidural hematoma by stripping the dura away from the inner table. In the spine, the dura is separated from the bone by epidural fat. In the ventral spinal canal, the epidural space also contains a rich plexus of veins, which drains the vertebral bodies. Trauma, with or without vertebral fracture, can tear these veins, resulting in an epidural hematoma. These hematomas grow with time, leading to cord compression in the setting of normal plain films. CT may detect these epidural hematomas in the lumbar spine, where there is some fat to provide contrast, but generally will not demonstrate an epidural hematoma in the cervical or thoracic spine unless intrathecal contrast is given. MR is the study of choice, given its ability to image the contents of the spinal canal noninvasively and depict blood-breakdown products (Fig. 10.68).

Nerve Root Avulsion. Most of these traumatic complications have been discussed in terms of their effects on the spinal cord. It should be remembered that epidural hematomas and contusions can also affect nerve roots and cause radicular problems. An additional form of direct trauma to the spinal nerve roots is avulsion from their connection to the cord. In the spinal canal, the most common site for root avulsion is the cervical spine, probably because of its wide range of motion during accidents. The roots serving the brachial plexus and upper extremities are typically affected, with obvious neurologic deficits. Birth trauma, typically traction on the shoulder, is one of the classic causes of nerve root avulsion at the cervicothoracic junction. This can result in an Erb's palsy on the affected side—the shoulder will be adducted and internally rotated, the elbow extended and pronated, and the wrist flexed, all due to injury to the C5, C6, and C7 roots. The clinical diagnosis can be confirmed by MR or CT myelography. Typically, CSF will leak out into the epidural space through the rent in the arachnoid and dura from the missing nerve, as can be seen in Figure 10.69. The thoracic spinal nerves (other

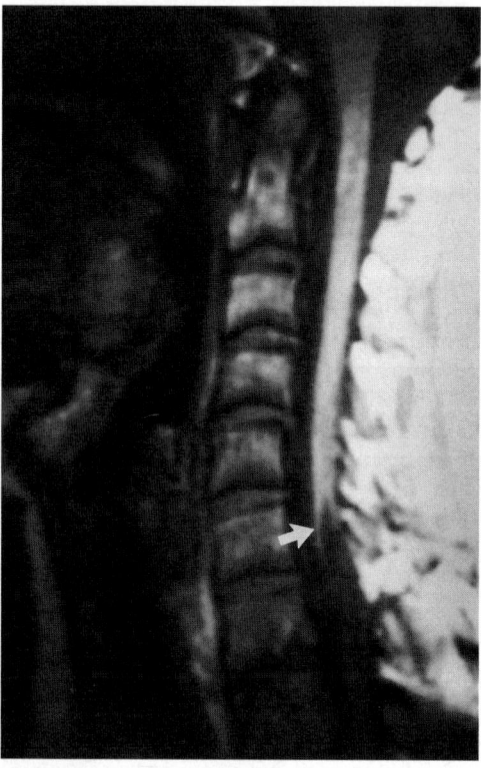

Figure 10.66. Cord Avulsion. The junction of the cervical and thoracic cord is a weak point where tearing can occur in injuries that stretch the cord (*arrow*).

Figure 10.67. Spinal Hematoma. A spinal subdural hematoma (*arrows*) occurred spontaneously in this thrombocytopenic leukemia patient. Note the low marrow signal consistent with leukemia, and the constriction of the thecal sac (*curved arrow*) by the hematoma. The hematoma is difficult to distinguish from epidural fat (*arrowheads*) on the T1WI **(A)**, but becomes more obvious as the epidural fat darkens on the T2WI **(B)**.

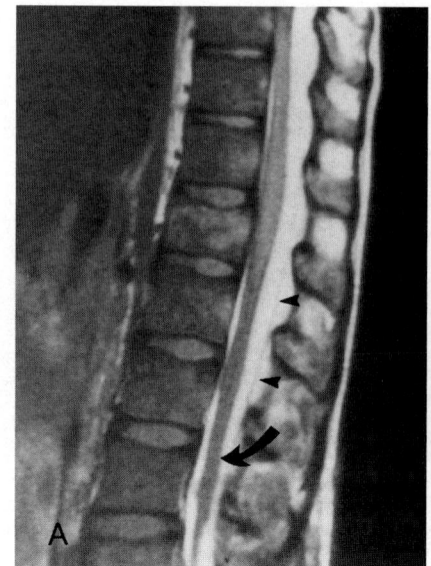
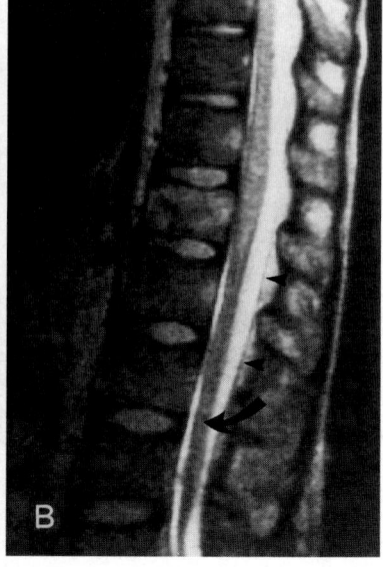

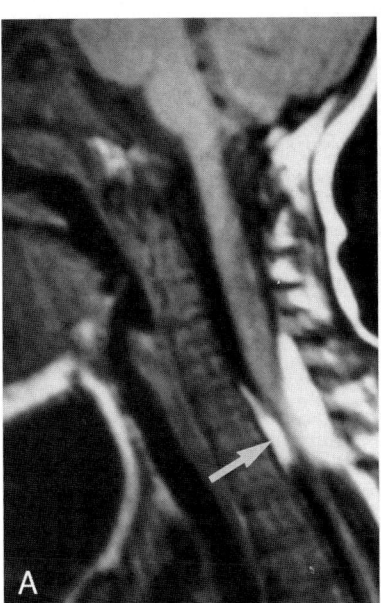
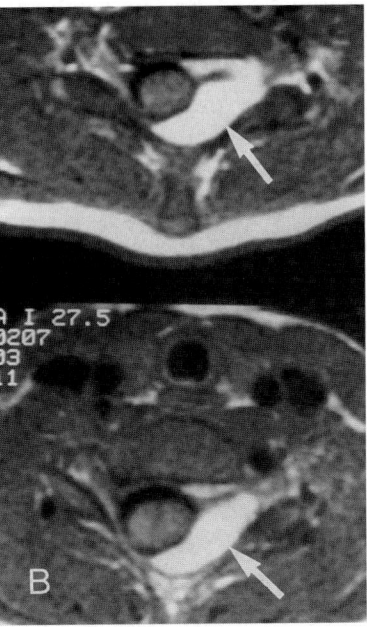

Figure 10.68. Epidural Hematoma. T1 sagittal **(A)** and axial **(B)** images show a bright epidural mass (*arrows*) consistent with a hematoma in the methemoglobin stage. An epidural hematoma can occur in the face of normal plain films and must be suspected if neurologic compromise exists.

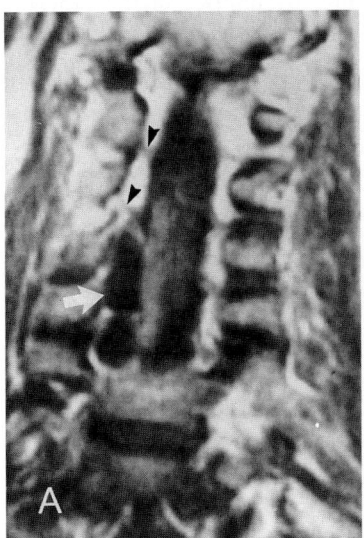
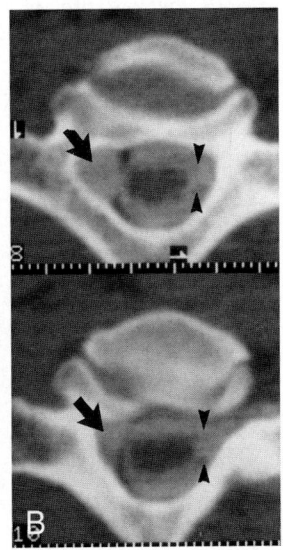

Figure 10.69. Nerve Root Avulsion. A. Coronal T1 image shows a low signal collection in the right epidural space in the midcervical spine (*arrow*), consistent with CSF that has leaked through avulsed nerve root sleeves. Intact spinal nerves (*arrowheads*) are seen in the upper cervical canal bilaterally traversing through the normal epidural fat. **B.** A CT myelogram confirms the absence of the right-sided nerve roots and the CSF leak (*arrow*). Note the normal roots on the left outlined by myelographic contrast (*arrowheads*).

the neurologic complications of trauma. MR has increased our understanding of spinal cord injury, and it facilitates prediction of long-term outcome.

References

1. Atlas S, ed. Magnetic Resonance Imaging of the Brain and Spine. New York: Raven Press, 1996:chapters 24–28.
2. Enzmann DR, DeLaPaz RL, Rubin JB, eds. Magnetic Resonance of the Spine. St Louis: Mosby, 1990.
3. Kricun R, Kricun ME. MRI and CT of the Spine: A Case Study Approach. New York: Raven, 1994.
4. Modic MT, Masaryk TM, Ross JS. Magnetic Resonance Imaging of the Spine. St. Louis: Mosby, 1994.
5. Rao KCVG, Williams JP, Lee PCP, et al. MRI and CT of the Spine. Baltimore: Williams & Wilkins, 1994.
6. Tartaglino LM, Friedman DP, Flanders AE. Multiple sclerosis in the spinal cord: MR appearance and correlation with clinical parameters. Radiology 1995;195:725–732.
7. Reijnierse M, Bloem JL, Dijkmans BAC, et al. Cervical spine in rheumatoid arthritis: relationship between neurologic signs and morphology on MR images and radiographs. Skeletal Radiol 1996; 25:113–118.
8. Provenzale JM, Barboriak DP, Gaensler EHL, et al. Lupus-related myelitis: serial MR findings. AJNR Am J Neuroradiol 1994;15:1911–1917.
9. Tartaglino LM, Croul SE, Flanders AE, et al. Idiopathic acute transverse myelitis: MR imaging findings. Radiology 1996;201:661–669.
10. Friedman DP. Herpes zoster myelitis: MR appearance. AJNR Am J Neuroradiol 1992;13:1404–1406.
11. Quencer RM, Post MJD. Spinal cord lesions in patients with AIDS. Neuroimag Clin North Am 1997;7:359–373.
12. Wang PY, Shen WC, Jan JS. Serial MRI changes in radiation myelopathy. Neuroradiology 1995;37:374.
13. Thrush A, Enzmann DR. MR Imaging of infectious spondylitis. AJNR Am J Neuroradiol 1990;11:1171–1180
14. Post MJD, Sze G, Quencer RM, et al. Gadolinium-enhanced MR in spinal infection. J Comput Assist Tomogr 1990;14:721–729.

than T1) and nerves of the lumbar cauda equina rarely undergo avulsion. Given the small field of view needed, thin, highly T2 weighted (1–2mm) axial images give excellent detail, and can be reconstructed into "MR-myelograms," much like MR angiograms.

Although MR is often not practical in the acute setting, it has become a superb noninvasive tool for evaluating

15. Smith AS, Weinstein MA, Mizushima A, et al. MR imaging characteristics of tuberculous spondylitis vs. vertebral osteomyelitis. AJNR 1989;10:619–625.

16. Sloof JL, Kernohan JW, MacCarty CS. Primary Intramedullary Tumors of the Spinal Cord and Filum Terminale. Philadelphia: WB Saunders, 1964.

17. Dillon WP, Norman DN, Newton TH, et al. Intradural spinal cord lesions: Gd-DTPA-enhanced MR imaging. Radiology 1989;170:229–237.

18. Fine MJ, Kritcheff IL, Freed D, et al. Spinal cord ependymomas: MR imaging features. Radiology 1995;197:655–658.

19. Egelhoff JC, Bates DJ, Ross JS, et al. Spinal MR findings in neurofibromatosis types 1 and 2. AJNR Am J Neuroradiol 1992;13:1071–1077.

20. Stevens SK, Moore SG, Amylon MD. Repopulation of marrow after transplantation: MR imaging with pathologic correlation. Radiology 1990;175:213–218.

21. Yuh WTC, Zachar CK, Barloon TJ, et al. Vertebral compression fractures: distinction between benign and malignant causes with MR imaging. Radiology 1989;172:215–218.

22. Cuenod CA, Laredo JD, Chevret S, et al. Acute vertebral collapse owing to osteoporosis or malignancy: appearance on unenhanced and gadolinium-enhanced MR images. Radiology 1996;199:541–549.

23. Rosenblum B, Oldfield EH, Doppman JL, et al. Spinal arteriovenous malformations: a comparison of dural arteriovenous fistulas and intradural AVMs in 81 patients. J Neurosurg 1987;67:795–802.

24. Ernst RJ, Gaskill-Shipley M, Tomsik TA, et al. Cervical myelopathy associated with intracranial dural arteriovenous fistula: MR findings before and after treatment. AJNR 1997;18;1330–1334

25. Friedman DP, Flanders AE. Enhancement of gray matter in anterior spinal infarction. AJNR Am J Neuroradiol 1992;13:983–985.

26. Mawad ME, Rivera V, Crawford S, et al. Spinal cord ischemia after the resection of thoracoabdominal aneurysms: MR findings in 24 patients. AJNR Am J Neuroradiol 1990;11:987–991.

27. Barkovich AJ. Congenital anomalies of the spine. In: Barkovich AJ, ed. Pediatric Neuroimaging. New York: Raven Press, 1995, pp. 477–540.

28. Raghavan N, Barkovich AJ, Edwards MSB, et al. MR imaging in the tethered spinal cord syndrome. AJNR Am J Neuroradiol 1989;10:27–36.

29. Silberstien M, Tress BM, Hennessy O. Delayed neurologic deterioration in the patient with spine trauma: role of MR imaging. AJNR Am J Neuroradiol 1992;13:1373–1381.

30. Flanders AE, Spetell CM, Tartaglino LM. Forecasting motor recovery after cervical cord injury: value of MR imaging. Radiology 1996;201:649–655.

31. Gasparotti R, Ferraresi S, Pinelli L, et al. Three-dimensional MR myelography of traumatic injuries of the brachial plexus. AJNR Am J Neuroradiol 1997;18:1733–1742.

11

Lumbar Spine: Disc Disease and Stenosis

Clyde A. Helms

Imaging Methods
Disc Disease
SPINAL STENOSIS
POSTOPERATIVE CHANGES
BONY ABNORMALITIES

Imaging Methods

Imaging the lumbar spine for disc disease and stenosis has evolved in the past 10 years from predominantly myelography-oriented examinations to plain CT and MR examinations. Multiple studies have shown that myelography is not as accurate as CT or MR (1–3), yet myelography continues to be performed. Little justification exists for using a lumbar myelogram to determine disc disease or stenosis in this era.

Although few differences between CT and MR have been noted concerning diagnostic accuracy in the lumbar spine, MR will give more information and a more complete anatomic depiction than will CT. Whether the additional information afforded by an MR examination will prove to be clinically useful remains to be seen. For example, MR can determine if a disc is degenerated by showing loss of signal on T2WIs (Fig. 11.1). CT cannot provide this information, but it hardly matters because no treatment is currently given solely for a degenerated disc. In fact, degenerative discs have been reported in asymptomatic children who deny a history of back pain (4).

At present, MR is clearly superior to CT in imaging the lumbar spine in only one aspect: evaluating the back postoperatively. The use of gadolinium has greatly aided the differentiation of postoperative fibrosis from recurrent disc protrusion. The single area in which CT has been shown to be superior to MR in the lumbar spine is in diagnosing spondylolysis. Pars defects can be very difficult to appreciate with MR, yet they are easily seen with CT. CT and MR are seemingly diagnostically equivalent for disc disease and spinal stenosis.

To achieve a high degree of accuracy, the proper imaging protocols must be observed. With CT scans, thin-section (3–5 mm) axial images should be obtained from the midbody of L-3 to the midbody of S-1 in a contiguous manner, i.e., no skip areas or gaps should be present (Fig. 11.2). One of the leading causes of failed back surgery is missed free fragments. Skip areas will often allow a free fragment to remain undiagnosed. Angling the gantry parallel to the endplates is not necessary, and image reformations are not helpful in the routine evaluation of disc disease and stenosis.

The MR imaging protocol is similar to that of CT in that thin-section axial images should be obtained from the midbody of L-3 to the midbody of S-1 (Fig. 11.3). Angling of the plane of imaging to be parallel to the endplates is not necessary, and contiguous images without skip areas are considered mandatory. Even though sagittal images will be obtained, free fragments and areas of stenosis are often seen on the axial images to better advantage than on the sagittal images. Other entities that can be overlooked if gaps are present in the axial imaging protocol include conjoined nerve roots, pars defects (spondylolysis), and lateral recess stenosis. These entities occur dorsal to the vertebral body, away from the disc level; thus, axial images limited to the disc level will not show them.

Both T1 (or proton density)-weighted and T2 (or T2*)-weighted images should be obtained in the sagittal and the axial planes. Attempting to shorten the study by foregoing one of the T2 sequences is not recommended. The addition of T2 axial images will increase diagnostic accuracy and the confidence with which diagnoses are made.

Disc Disease

DISC PROTRUSIONS

Terminology plays a large role in how radiologists describe disc bulges or protrusions. Since the advent of CT in the 1970s, disc bulges have been described by their morphology. A broad-based disc bulge has been said to be a bulging annulus fibrosus, and a focal disc bulge is a herniated nucleus pulposus. These interpretations are no more than 90% accurate. More significantly, most surgeons are not concerned with what name is applied to a disc bulge; they do not treat a bulging annulus differently than a herniated nucleus pulposus. They treat the patient's symptoms and have to decide if the disc bulge is responsible for those symptoms. Up to 50% of the asymptomatic population have disc protrusions (5); hence, just seeing a disc bulge on CT or MR does not mean it is clinically significant.

Both CT and MR have a high degree of accuracy in delineating disc protrusions and showing if neural tissue is impressed (Fig. 11.4). MR can also show if annular fibers of the disc are disrupted, a so-called extrusion. Although CT cannot be used to diagnose extrusions, clinicians treat extrusions the same way they treat protrusions (annular fibers intact).

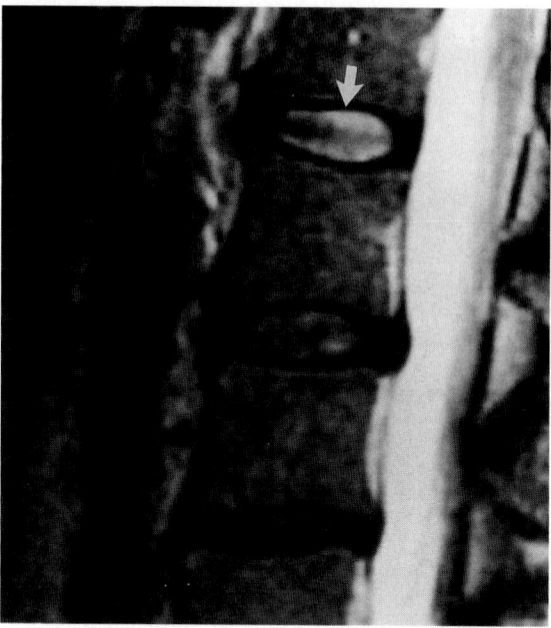

Figure 11.1. Desiccated Disc. A sagittal T2WI (TR, 4000; TE, 102) shows the L2-3 and L3-4 discs to be abnormally low in signal, indicating disc dessication and degeneration. Compare with the normal L1-2 disc (*arrow*), which has high signal.

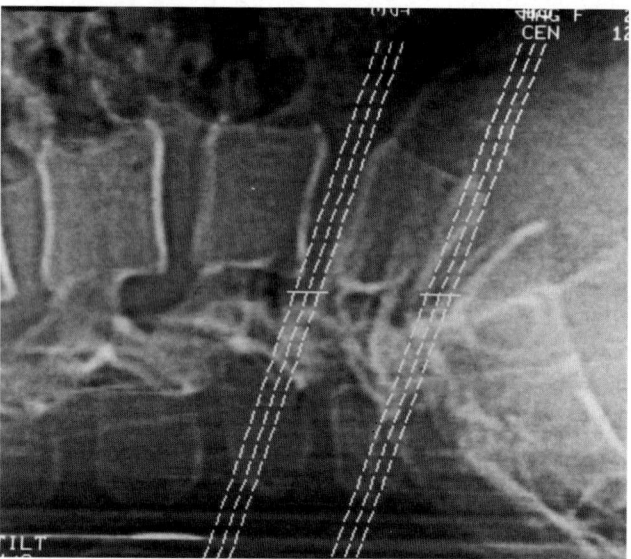

Figure 11.2. Inadequate Technique—Skip Areas. This CT scout film has cursors placed through the L4-5 and L5-S1 disc spaces. This allows large gaps or skip areas that can result in missed free fragments of discs. Also, the L3-4 disc space should be imaged.

FREE FRAGMENTS

A type of disc extrusion critical to diagnose is the free fragment or sequestration. Missing free fragments is one of the most common causes of failed back surgery (6). The preoperative diagnosis of a free fragment contraindicates chymopapain, percutaneous discectomy, and, for many surgeons, microdiscectomy. At the very least, the presence of a free fragment means the surgeon must explore more cephalad or caudally during the surgery in

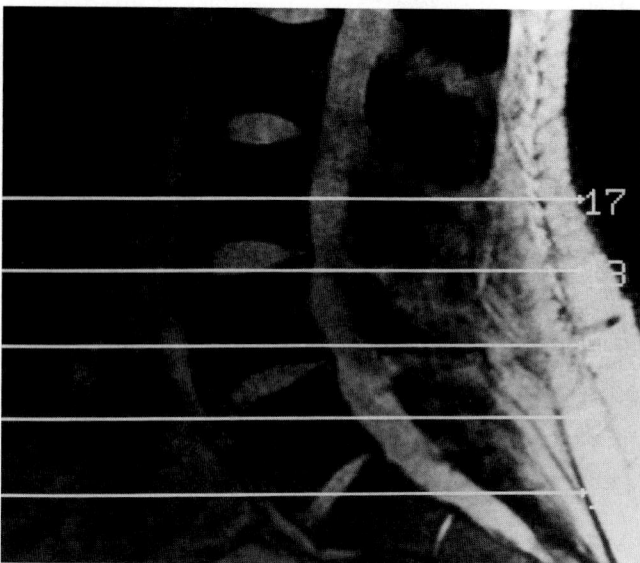

Figure 11.3. Proper MR Technique. This MR scout with cursors placed contiguously from the body of L-3 to S-1 allows complete coverage of the lower lumbar spine in the axial plane.

order to remove the free fragment. As free fragments can be very difficult to diagnose clinically, imaging is critical in the evaluation of the spine for any patient contemplating surgery. At times it can be difficult to ascertain if a disc that has extruded is still attached to the parent disc or is really "free." If disc material is above or below the level of the disc space, whether it is attached really does not matter. Chymopapain and percutaneous discectomy would still be contraindicated and many surgeons would not perform or, at the very least, would modify their microdiscectomy. The key element is recognizing that disc material is present away from the level of the disc space.

Free fragments are diagnosed on CT by the presence of a soft tissue density with a higher attenuation value than the thecal sac (Fig. 11.5). A conjoined root (a normal variant of two roots exiting the thecal sac together; seen in 1–3% of the population [7]) (Fig. 11.6) or a Tarlov cyst (a normal variant referring to a dilated nerve root sleeve) can have a similar appearance to a free fragment, but these will have attenuation values similar to the thecal sac.

Free fragments are diagnosed on MR by noting disc material that has moved away from the disc space (Fig. 11.7). Up to 80% of free fragments will have high signal on T2WI even though the parent disc may be low signal (8). Free fragments migrate either cephalad or caudally, with no documented preference.

It is imperative to obtain contiguous axial images without large skip areas or gaps when imaging with both CT and MR in order to not miss free fragments.

LATERAL DISCS

Discs will occasionally protrude in a lateral direction, causing the nerve root that has already exited the central canal to be stretched (Fig. 11.8). Although not com-

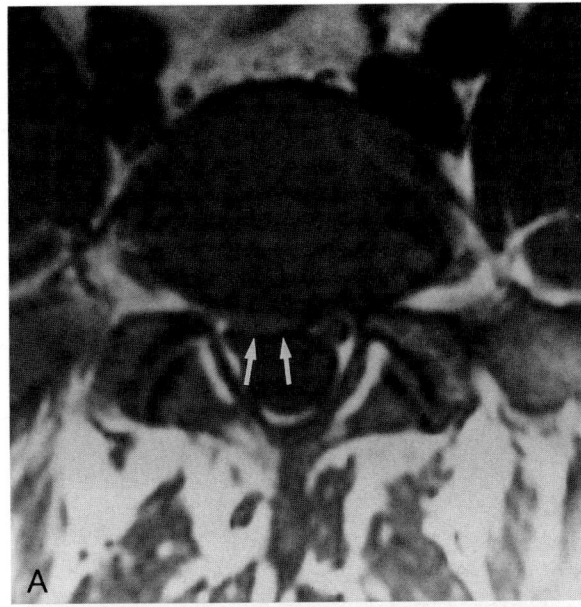

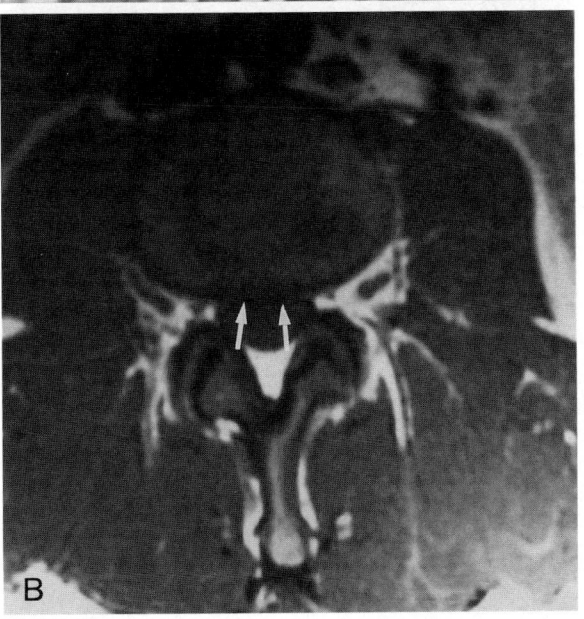

Figure 11.4. Disc Protrusions. Axial T1WI (TR, 800; TE, 20) show focal **(A)** (*arrows*) and broad-based **(B)** disc protrusions (*arrows*). Either of these could be a herniated disc or a bulging annulus fibrosis. Because these are both showing impression of the thecal sac, they could each cause symptoms.

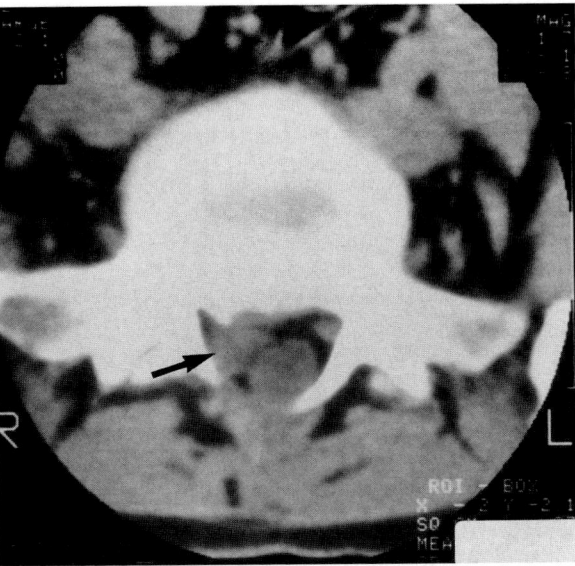

Figure 11.5. Free Fragment (CT). A soft tissue mass is seen in the right lateral recess (*arrow*), which has a CT attenuation value of 24.1 Hounsfield units; however, sampling of the thecal sac gave a measurement of only 4.6 CT units. Thus, the soft tissue mass is of higher density than the thecal sac and represents a free fragment of disc material, which is also called a sequestration.

mon (<5% of cases), these discs are frequently overlooked and are known to be a source of failed back surgery (9). Because they affect the already exited root, they can clinically mimic symptoms of a disc protrusion from one level more cephalad (Fig. 11.9). For example, in a patient who has multilevel disc disease and symptoms referable to the L3-4 disc, the disc protrusion is usually a posterior bulge that impresses the L-4 nerve root. However, a lateral disc at L4-5 could impress the L-4 nerve root and cause the same symptoms. If not noticed, surgery could be performed at the L3-4 disc, which is the wrong level. Notifying the surgeon that the disc is lateral

to the neuroforamen is also important because a standard surgical approach through the lamina might not allow removal of a lateral disc.

Lateral discs are best identified on axial images. Sagittal images will often show a lateral disc occluding a neuroforamen, but many times a lateral disc will not extend into the foramen and the sagittal images will appear normal.

SPINAL STENOSIS

By definition *spinal stenosis* is encroachment of the bony or soft tissue structures in the spine on one or more of the neural elements, with resulting symptoms. It is classically divided into congenital and acquired types; however, even the most severe forms of congenital stenosis do not cause symptoms unless a component of acquired stenosis (usually degenerative disease of the facets and the discs) is present. A more useful classification of stenosis is on an anatomic basis: central canal, neuroforaminal, and lateral recess. One must realize that stenosis and disc disease are often present concomitantly, and clinically differentiating the two can be challenging. As with disc disease, any imaging findings must be matched with clinical findings. It is not unusual to have a patient with stenosis that appears severe on images, but who has no symptoms.

CENTRAL CANAL STENOSIS

Although measurements were once considered very useful in the determination of central canal stenosis, they are no longer considered a valid indicator of dis-

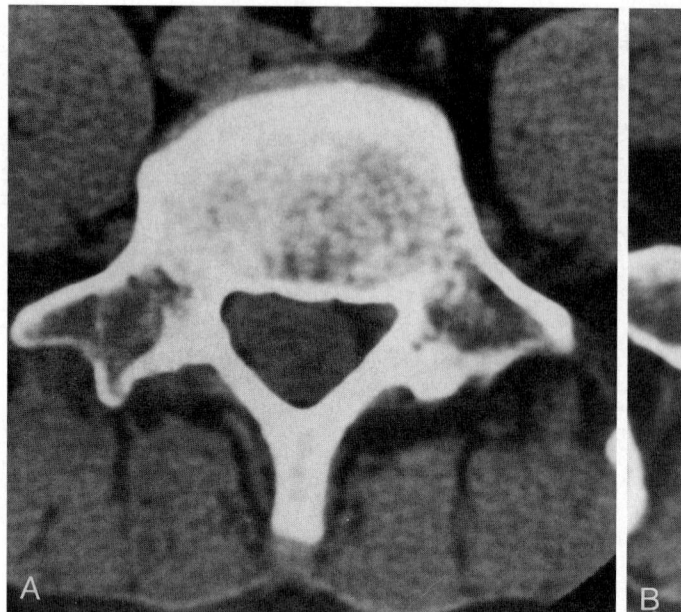
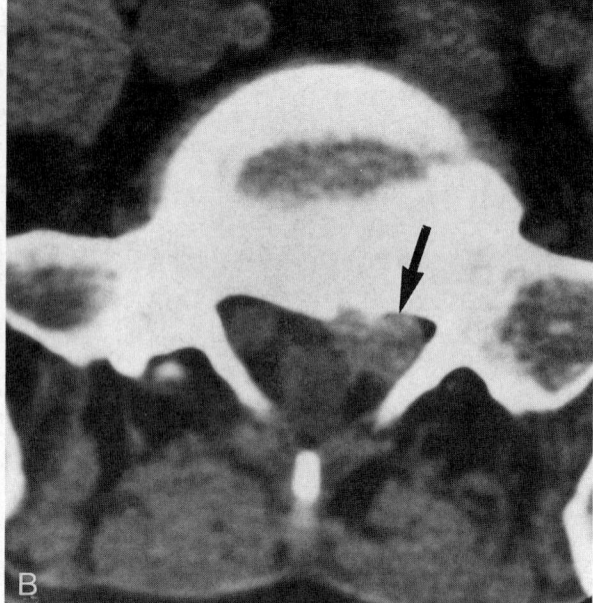

Figure 11.6. Conjoined Root and Free Fragment. A. A soft tissue mass is seen in the right L-5 lateral recess, which has CT attenuation values identical to the thecal sac. This is a conjoined nerve root.

B. In the same patient, a soft tissue mass is present in the left S-1 lateral recess (*arrow*), which has a density greater than the adjacent thecal sac. This is a free fragment.

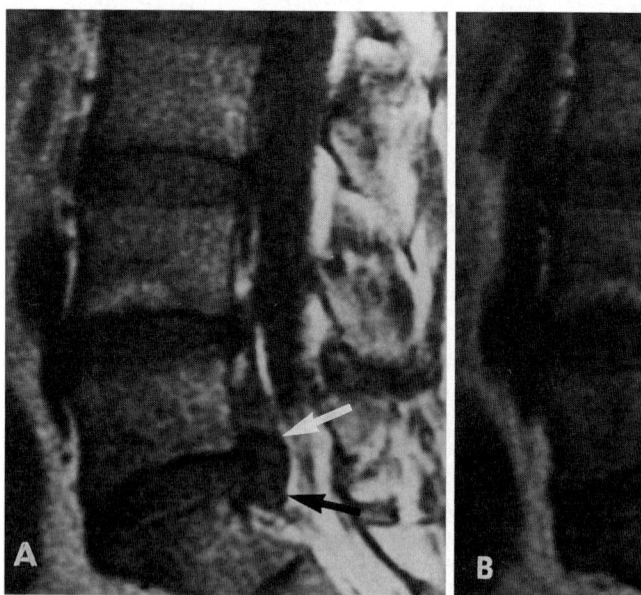
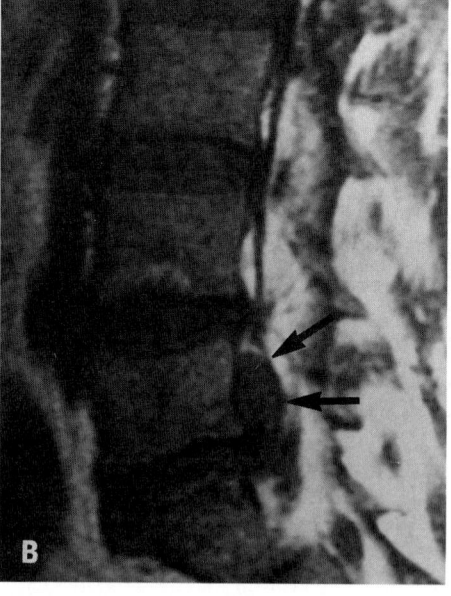

Figure 11.7. Free Fragment. A. A sagittal T1-weighted (TR, 500; TE, 20) MR image shows a large amount of disc material bulging posteriorly at the disc space (*arrows*). **B.** The adjacent slice shows disc material that has migrated cephalad (*arrows*) and now lies posterior to the L-5 vertebral body. This is a large free fragment.

ease. Instead, simply noting whether the thecal sac is compressed or round will reliably determine central canal stenosis (Fig. 11.10). A subjective assessment as to whether the compression (usually in an anteroposterior direction) is mild, moderate, or severe is all that is necessary for evaluating the central canal.

The most common cause of central canal stenosis is degenerative disease of the facets with bony hypertrophy that encroaches on the central canal (Fig. 11.11). This is also the most common cause of lateral recess stenosis. When the facets undergo degenerative joint disease (DJD), they often have some slippage, which results in buckling of the ligamentum flavum. This has been termed "ligamentum flavum hypertrophy" and is a common cause of central canal stenosis (Fig. 11.12). Frequently, mild disc bulging is associated with minimal facet hypertrophy and ligamentum flavum hypertrophy. This combination can result in severe focal central canal stenosis. Both CT and MR will show these bony and soft tissue changes.

Less common causes of central canal stenosis include bony overgrowth from Paget's disease, achondroplasia, posttraumatic changes, and severe spondylolisthesis.

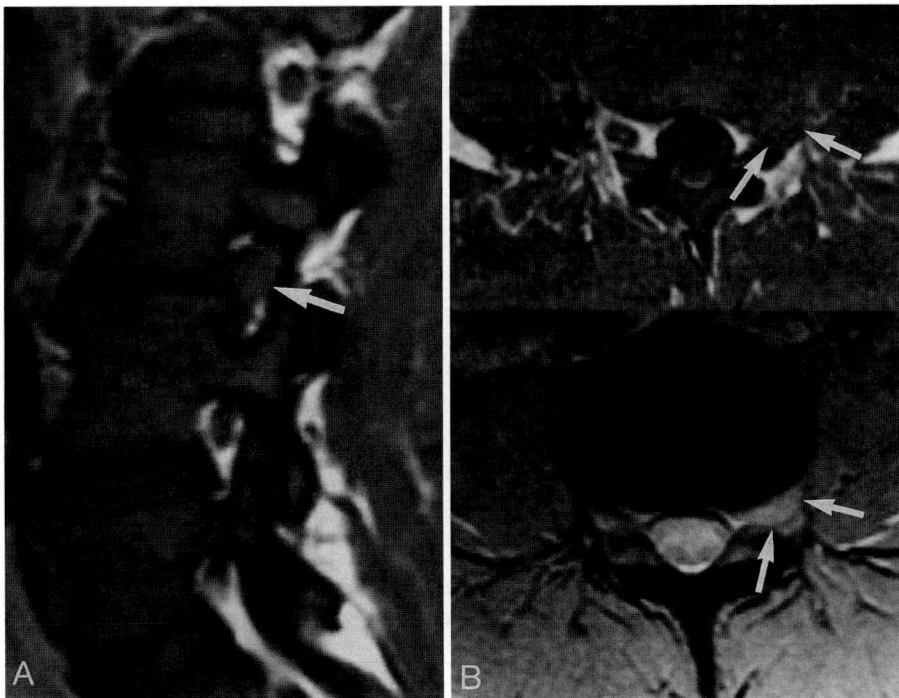

Figure 11.8. Lateral Disc (MR). A. A sagittal T1-weighted (TR, 600; TE, 30) MR image through the left neuroforamen shows a low signal structure in the L-4 neuroforamen (*arrow*), which is a lateral disc protrusion. **B.** Axial T1-weighted (upper) (TR, 600; TE, 30) and T2* image (lower) (TR, 600; TE, 30; 30°) show the lateral disc (*arrows*) in the left neuroforamen.

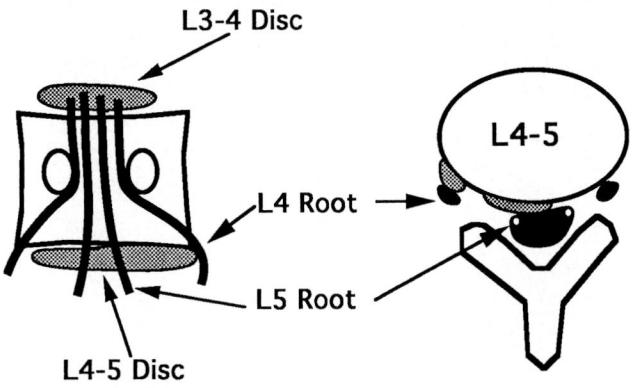

Figure 11.9. Schematic of Lateral Disc. This schematic illustrates how a posterior L4-5 disc protrusion affects the L-5 nerve root, yet a lateral L4-5 disc affects the L-4 root.

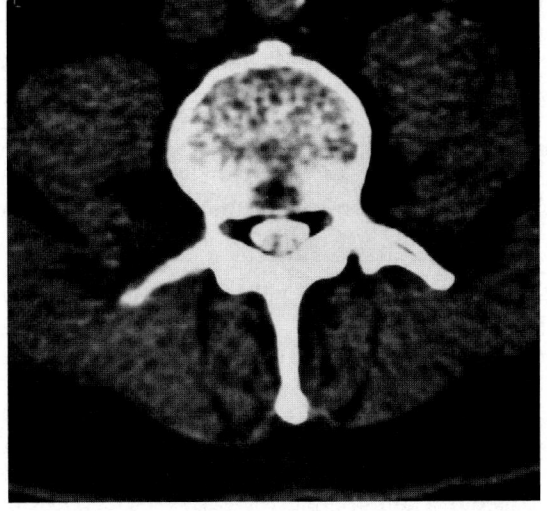

Figure 11.10. Central Canal Stenosis. A CT-myelogram demonstrates absence of the normally round thecal sac caused by central canal stenosis. It is not necessary to perform a myelogram to see flattening of the thecal sac; a plain CT or MR will show this equally well.

NEUROFORAMINAL STENOSIS

Degenerative joint disease of the facet with bony hypertrophy is the most common cause of neuroforaminal stenosis; however, encroachment on the nerve root in the neuroforamen can be seen with free disc fragments, postoperative scar, and from a lateral disc protrusion.

The neuroforamen are best evaluated on axial images, just cephalad to the disc space. The disc space lies at the inferior portion of the neuroforamen, and the exiting nerve root lies in the superior or cephalad portion of the neuroforamen. Although the neuroforamen can be clearly seen on sagittal MR images, care must be taken to evaluate the entire neuroforamen and not just the 4 or 5 mm of one sagittal image.

LATERAL RECESS STENOSIS

The lateral recesses are the bony canals in which the nerve roots lie after they leave the thecal sac and before they enter the neuroforamen. Hypertrophy of the superior articular facet from DJD is the most common cause of encroachment on the lateral recesses; however, as with the neuroforamen, disc fragments and postoperative scar can cause nerve root impingement.

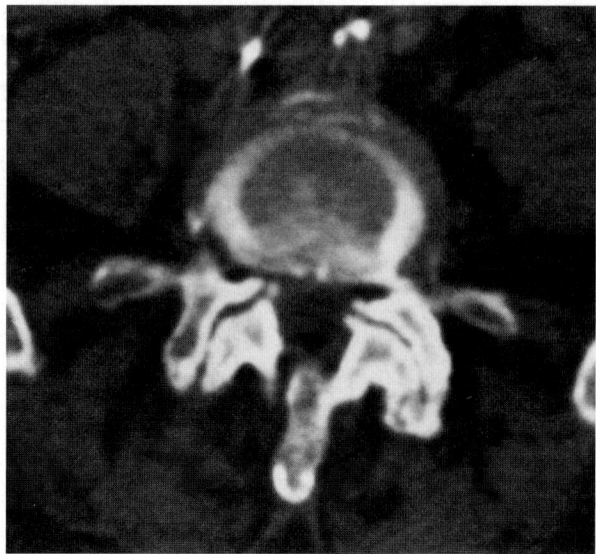

Figure 11.11. Facet Hypertrophy Causing Stenosis. This CT shows marked facet degenerative disease with hypertrophy of the facets causing lateral recess and central canal stenosis.

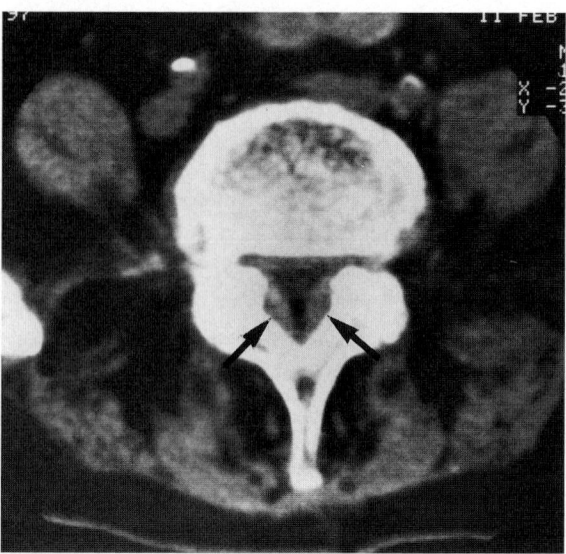

Figure 11.12. Ligamentum Flavum Hypertrophy. Inward bulging of the ligamentum flavum (*arrows*) is shown on this CT scan. Central canal stenosis from ligamentum flavum hypertrophy is common.

SPONDYLOLYSIS AND SPONDYLOLISTHESIS

Defects in the bony pars interarticularis (spondylolysis) are commonly found in asymptomatic individuals, yet they can be a source of low back pain and instability. Prior to disc surgery or other back surgery, the identification of any spondylolysis is imperative. Because spondylolysis can mimic back pain from other pathology, it must be preoperatively assessed. If necessary, it can then be surgically addressed at the same time. Failure to note and evaluate spondylolysis is a known source of failed back surgery.

CT is superior to MR imaging at identifying spondylolysis (10). Although MR will show spondylolysis defects, these defects can sometimes be very difficult to see. As previously mentioned, this is the only area in which CT is clearly superior to MR in evaluating the lumbar spine. Spondylolysis is identified on the axial images through the midvertebral body as a break in the normally intact bony ring of the lamina (Fig. 11.13).

Spondylolisthesis (forward slippage of one vertebral body on a lower one) occurs from either slippage of two vertebral bodies following bilateral spondylolysis or from DJD of the facets with slippage of the facets. Bilateral spondylolysis can result in a large amount of slippage, but facet DJD will usually result in only minimal slippage. If spondylolisthesis is severe, the result can be central canal stenosis, neuroforaminal stenosis, or both.

A grading scale that is widely used to describe the degree of spondylolisthesis is the Meyerding grading scale. The more caudal vertebral body is divided into fourths, and the posterior corner of the more cephalad vertebral body is marked at the position where it has slipped forward. If it has slipped forward only into the first quarter of the more caudal vertebral body, it is a grade 1 spondylolisthesis; slippage into the second quarter is a grade 2, and so on (Fig. 11.14).

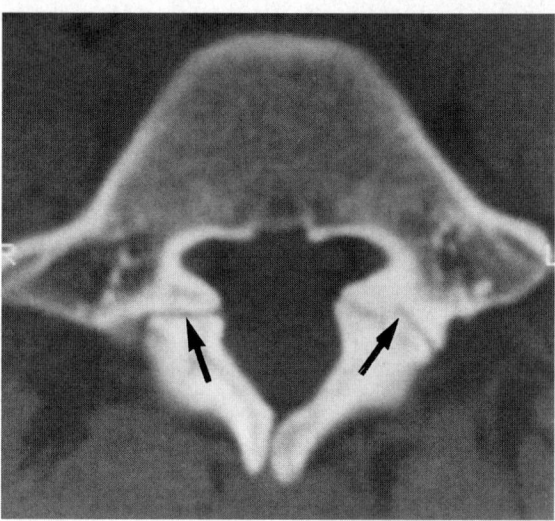

Figure 11.13. Spondylolysis (CT). A CT scan through the midvertebral body reveals a break bilaterally (*arrows*) in the bony lamina, which indicates bilateral spondylolysis.

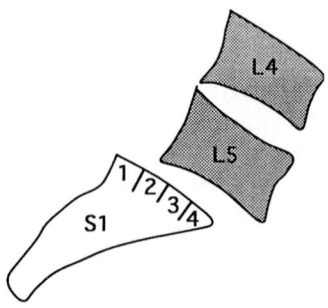

Figure 11.14. Schematic of the Spondylolisthesis Grading Scale. This schematic shows the grading scale used to gauge the degree of spondylolisthesis. This example would be a grade 2 spondylolisthesis because the posterior edge of the slipped L-5 vertebral body lies above the second quadrant of the S-1 vertebral body.

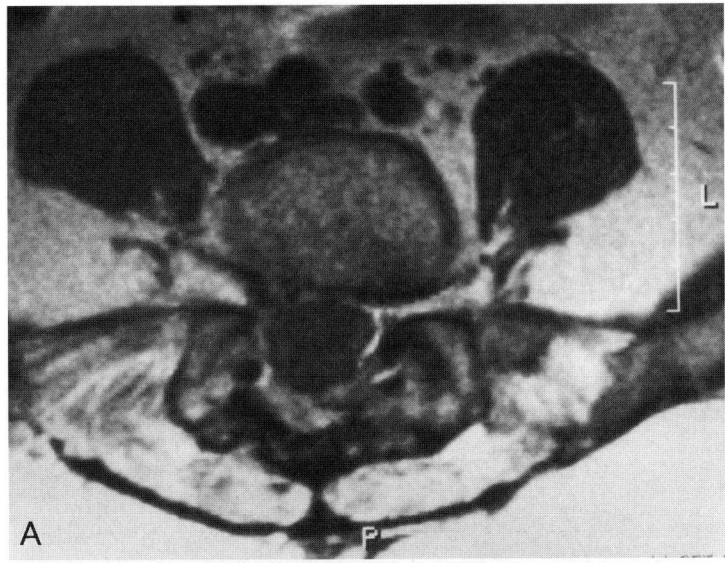

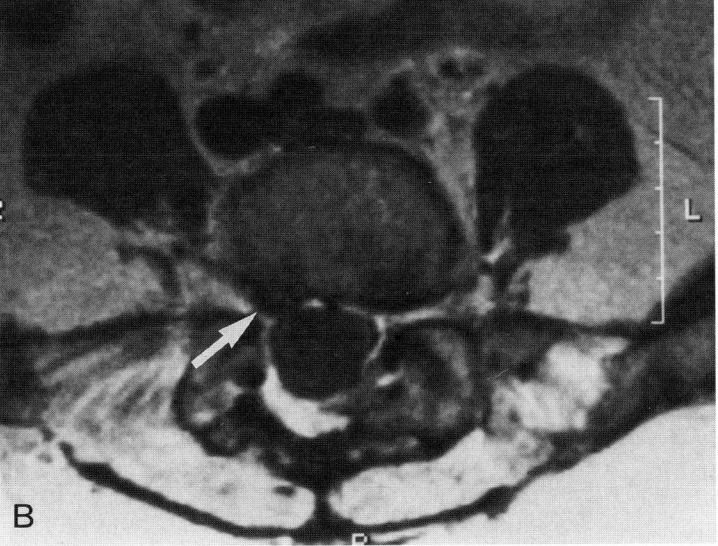

Figure 11.15. Postoperative Scar Enhancement with Gadolinium. A. A T1-weighted axial image (TR, 600; TE, 30) shows soft tissue around the thecal sac in this postoperative patient. This could represent scar, but it makes evaluation for recurrent disc protrusion difficult. **B.** A T1-weighted axial image (TR, 600; TE, 30) through the same level following administration of gadolinium-pentetic acid (Gd-DTPA) intravenously shows enhancement of the scar tissue surrounding the thecal sac. In addition, a focal right-sided disc protrusion can be identified (*arrow*).

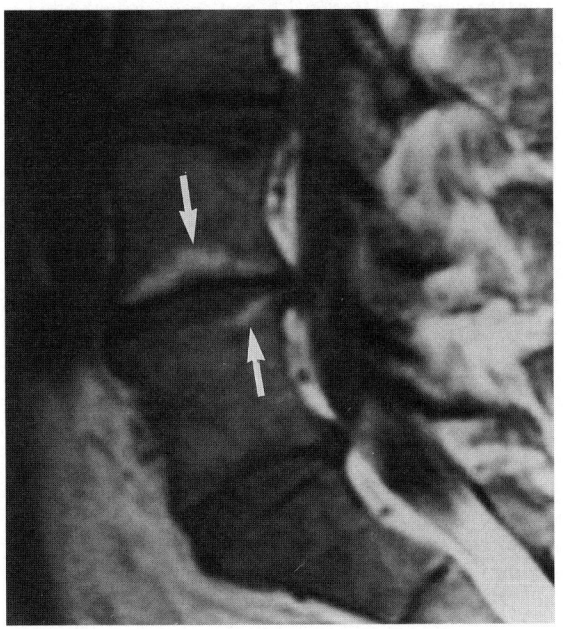

Figure 11.16. Type 2 Marrow Changes. A sagittal T1WI (TR, 600; TE, 11) in a patient with degenerative disc disease shows bands of fatty marrow parallel to the L4-5 endplates (*arrows*) which are type 2 marrow changes, seen often with degenerative disc disease.

POSTOPERATIVE CHANGES

Failed back surgery is unfortunately common. It has many causes including inadequate surgery (including missed free disc fragments), postoperative scarring, failure of bone grafting for fusion, and recurrent disc protrusion. CT is useful in evaluating bone grafts, but it is not reliable for differentiating postoperative scar from disc material. However, MR has been particularly useful in distinguishing scar from disc material (11).

The use of intravenous gadolinium will allow virtual certainty in distinguishing scar tissue from a disc. Scar tissue will enhance following the administration of gadolinium, whereas disc material will have only some minimal peripheral enhancement, presumably owing to inflammation (Fig. 11.15).

BONY ABNORMALITIES

Parallel bands of high or low signal adjacent to the vertebral body endplates are often seen with MR imaging in association with degenerative disc disease. The most common appearance is of high-signal bands on T1WI that remain high on T2WI (Fig. 11.16). This represents fatty marrow conversion. It was seen in 16% of cases in the first report in the literature (1) and was termed type 2. Type 1 changes are seen as low-signal bands parallel to the endplates on T1WI that get brighter on T2WI. This represents an inflammatory or granulomatous response to degenerative disc disease. The type 2 changes were reported in 4% of cases, and these must be distinguished from disc space infection. In disc space infection, the disc should be bright on the T2WI (Fig. 11.17); for a degenerative disc to have high signal on T2 WI is unusual. Type 3 changes are parallel bands of low signal adjacent to the endplates on both T1WI and T2WI. Type 3 changes represent bony sclerosis seen on plain films.

MR imaging and CT have changed diagnostic imaging of the lumbar spine from a painful, invasive study to a highly accurate, noninvasive study that provides a more complete anatomic depiction than plain films or myelography. Although MR has no ionizing radiation and is widely available, it can be much more expensive than CT and does not currently increase the accuracy of diagnosis for disc disease or spinal stenosis.

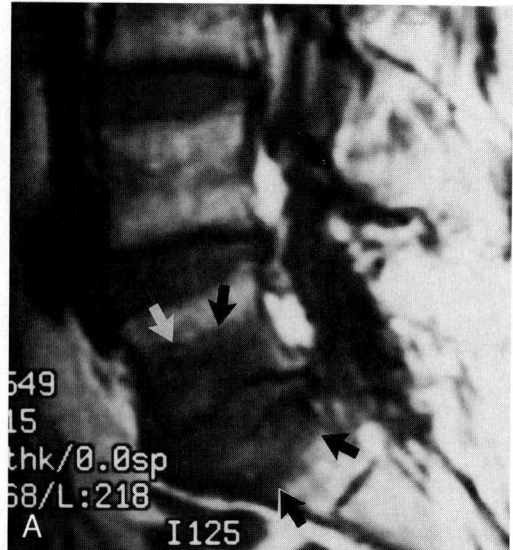

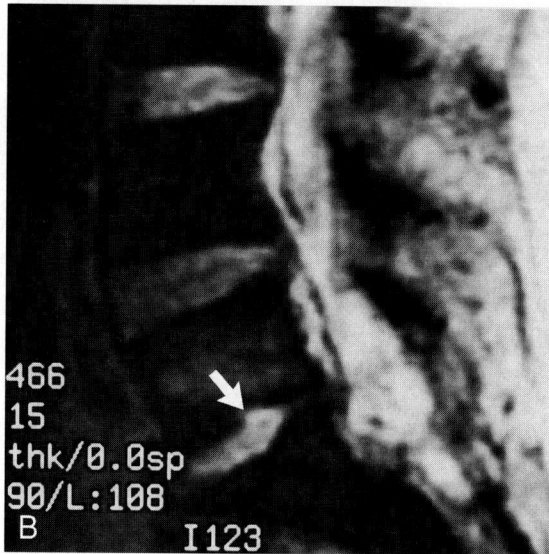

Figure 11.17. Disc Infection. A. A sagittal T1WI (TR 549; TE 15) shows bands of low signal adjacent to the L5-S1 disc (*arrows*). This is the typical appearance for Type 1 changes seen with degenerative disc disease. **B.** A T2* image (TR 466; TE 15θ 15°) show high signal in the disc (*arrow*) rather than low signal (dessication). This was a disc infection.

References

1. Modic M, Masaryk T, Ross J, et al. Imaging of degenerative disk disease. Radiology 1988;168:177–186.
2. Hesselink J. Spine imaging: history, achievements, remaining frontiers. AJR Am J Roentgenol 1988;150:1223–1230.
3. Sartoris DJ, Resnick D. Computed tomography of the spine: an update and review. CRC Crit Rev Diagn Imaging 1987; 27:271–296.
4. Tertti M, Salminen J, Paajanen H, et al. Low-back pain and disk degeneration in children: a case-control MR imaging study. Radiology 1991;180:503–507.
5. Jensen MC, Brant-Zawadzki MN, Obuchowski N, et al. Magnetic resonance imaging of the lumbar spine in people without back pain. N Engl J Med 1994;331(2):69–73.
6. Onik G, Mooney V, Maroon J, et al. Automated percutaneous discectomy: a prospective multi-institutional study. Neurosurgery 1990;26:228–233.
7. Helms CA, Dorwart RH, Gray M. The CT appearance of conjoined nerve roots and differentiation from a herniated nucleus pulposus. Radiology 1982;144:803–807.
8. Masaryk T, Ross J, Modic M, et al. High-resolution MR imaging of sequestered lumbar intervertebral disks. AJR Am J Roentgenol 1988;150:1155–1162.
9. Winter DDB, Munk PL, Helms CA, et al. CT and MR of lateral disc herniation: typical appearance and pitfalls of interpretation. J Canad Assoc Radiol 1989;40:256–259.
10. Grenier N, Kressel HY, Schiebler ML, et al. Isthmic spondylolysis of the lumbar spine: MR imaging at 1.5 T. Radiology 1989;170:489–494.
11. Ross J, Masaryk T, Schrader M, et al. MR imaging of the postoperative spine: assessment with gadopentetate dimeglumine. AJR Am J Roentgenol1990;155:867–872.

Section III   CHEST

Section Editor:
Jeffrey S. Klein

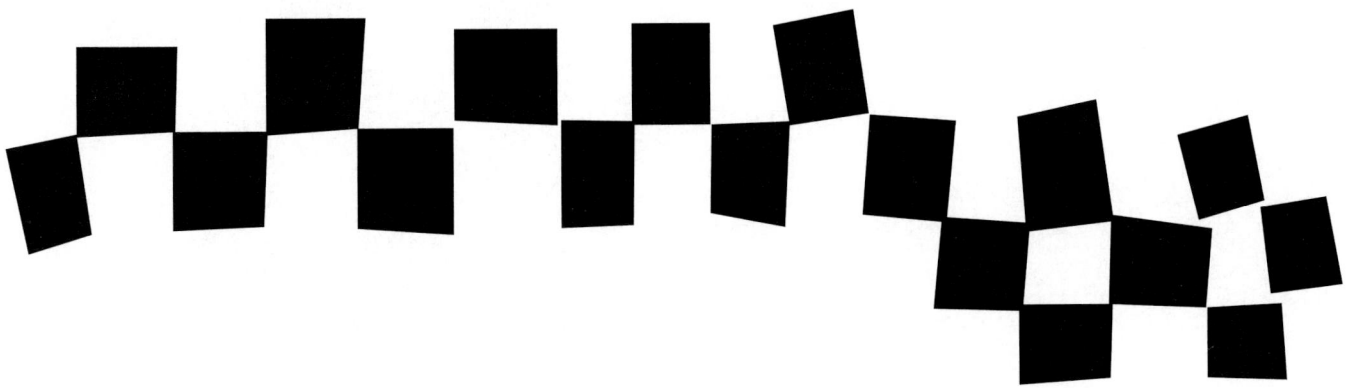

12
Methods of Examination and Normal Anatomy

Peter Dietrich
Jeffrey S. Klein

Many imaging techniques are available to the radiologist for the evaluation of thoracic disease (1). The decision of which imaging procedures to perform depends on many factors, the most important of which are the availability of various modalities and the type of information sought. Although the indications for the use of certain modalities such as CT and ventilation/perfusion lung scanning are well elucidated, the indications for other imaging techniques such as MR continue to evolve. Although the imaging algorithm for specific problems may seem relatively straightforward, a dogmatic approach to the individual patient should be discouraged. For example, a thin section CT showing a suspicious solitary pulmonary nodule might be followed directly by a thoracotomy, or rather, in selected patients, by transthoracic needle biopsy. This type of flexible approach will often streamline the diagnostic workup and ultimately lead to better patient care.

IMAGING MODALITIES

Conventional Chest Radiography. PA and lateral chest radiographs are the mainstay of thoracic imaging. Conventional radiographs should be performed as the initial imaging study in all patients with thoracic disease. These films are obtained in most radiology departments on a dedicated chest unit capable of obtaining radiographs with a focus to film distance of 6 feet, a high kVp (140 kVp) technique, a grid to reduce scatter, and a phototimer to control the length of exposure (2).

The recognition of proper radiographic technique on frontal radiographs involves assessment of four basic features: penetration, rotation, inspiration, and motion. Proper penetration is present when faint visualization of the intervertebral disc spaces of the thoracic spine exists and discrete branching vessels can be identified through the cardiac shadow and the diaphragms. Rotation is as-

sessed by noting the relationship between a vertical line drawn midway between the medial cortical margins of the clavicular heads and one drawn vertically through the spinous processes of the thoracic vertebrae. Superimposition of these lines (the former in the midline anteriorly and the latter in the midline posteriorly) indicates a properly positioned, nonrotated patient. An appropriate deep inspiration in a normal individual is present when the apex of the right hemidiaphragm is visible below the tenth posterior rib. Finally, the cardiac margin, diaphragm, and pulmonary vessels should be sharply marginated in a completely still patient who has suspended respiration during the radiographic exposure (Fig. 12.1).

Portable Radiography. Portable anteroposterior (AP) radiographs are obtained when patient transport to the radiology department, usually in the critical care setting, is not feasible (3). Portable radiographs help monitor a patient's cardiopulmonary status; assess the position of various monitoring and life support tubes, lines, and catheters; and detect complications related to the use of these devices.

There are technical and patient-related limitations of portable bedside radiography. The limited maximal kVp of portable units requires longer exposures to penetrate cardiomediastinal structures, resulting in greater motion artifact, especially in patients who are on ventilators and are unable to hold their breath. Because critically ill patients are difficult to position for portable radiographs, the patients are often rotated. Inaccuracies in directing the x-ray beam perpendicular to the patient lead to excessively kyphotic or lordotic radiographs. The short focus-to-film distance (typically 40 inches) and AP technique result in magnification of intrathoracic structures. This increases the apparent cardiac diameter by 15–20%; the upper limit of normal for the cardiothoracic ratio on AP radiographs is 57%. The supine position of critically ill patients results in a high position of the diaphragm resulting in smaller lung volumes and compression of the lower lobes. The normal gravitational effect of evening out of blood flow between upper and lower zones with the patient supine makes assessment of pulmonary venous hypertension difficult. The increase in systemic venous return to the heart produces a widening of the upper mediastinum or "vascular pedicle." The detection of small or moderate pleural effusions is difficult because of their posterior location in a supine patient. Similarly, detecting a pneumothorax may be difficult because free intrapleural air rises to a nondependent position producing a subtle anteromedial or inferior radiolucency. A device called the inclinometer accurately records the position of the bedridden patient

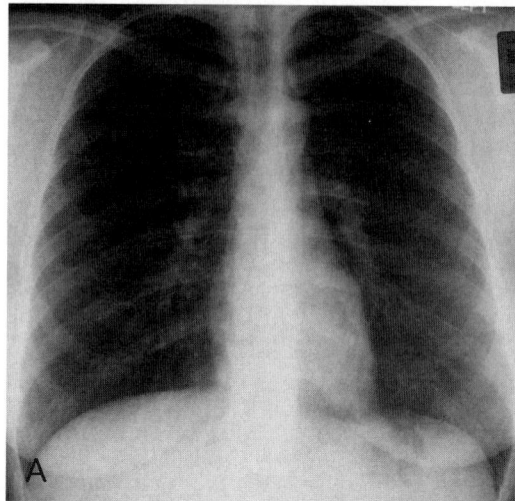
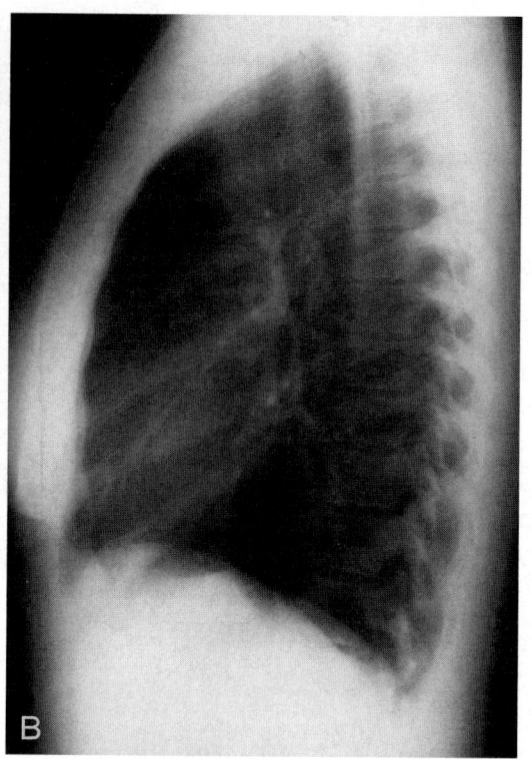

Figure 12.1. Normal PA (A) and Lateral (B) Radiographs of the Chest.

from supine to completely upright. This device, which clips on to the portable film cassette, allows the radiologist to precisely calculate the patient's position at the time of the radiograph, which helps assess the distribution of pulmonary blood flow, pleural effusions and pneumothorax.

Lateral Decubitus Radiography. Radiographs of the chest obtained with a horizontal x-ray beam while the patient lies in the decubitus position can demonstrate small, free-flowing pleural effusions. As little as 50 ml of fluid can be demonstrated by this technique (Fig. 12.2). Decubitus films can be used to visualize the nondependent lung when a pleural effusion obscures the lower lobe. Similarly, a small pneumothorax can be seen on decubitus films in the nondependent lung when an upright film cannot be obtained. Normally the downside diaphragm assumes a higher position than the upside one. Air trapping can be demonstrated in the dependent lung in patients with check valve bronchial obstructions who are unable to cooperate for inspiratory/expiratory radiographs or chest fluoroscopy.

Expiratory Radiography. Films obtained after maximal expiration to residual volume may be performed to detect focal or diffuse air trapping or to aid in the detection of a small pneumothorax. The increased sensitivity of expiratory films for pneumothorax is because of the increased opacity and decreased volume of the lung after exhalation. This creates a greater difference in radiographic density between air in the pleural space and the lung. The lung will also be displaced away from the chest wall, thereby aiding in recognition of the visceral pleural line.

Apical Lordotic Radiography is usually performed to improve visualization of the lung apices, which are ob-scured on routine PA radiographs by the clavicles and first costochondral junctions. The lordotic film projects these anterior bony structures superiorly, providing an unimpeded view of the apices. This projection is also used occasionally to enhance the visualization of middle lobe atelectasis by placing the inferiorly displaced minor fissure in tangent with the x-ray beam and by increasing the AP thickness of the atelectatic middle lobe.

Chest Fluoroscopy. Real-time visualization of the chest is useful in several situations. In the evaluation of a nodular opacity seen on only one view, the fluoroscopic observation of the opacity can demonstrate whether it represents a pseudotumor caused by the vertebral lamina, osteophytes, vertebral transverse processes, healed rib fractures, skin lesions, nipples, or other external objects. This determination may obviate the need for CT or oblique chest films. In a patient with an elevated diaphragm on frontal radiograph, diaphragmatic movement can be assessed fluoroscopically to detect paralysis.

Digital Chest Radiography. The main advantages of digital chest radiography are superior contrast resolution and the ability to transmit and view radiographs on a monitor ("soft copy" format) where contrast levels and windows can be manipulated to enhance visualization of various regions in the chest. This latter feature and the inherent wider lattitude of digital chest radiography help compensate for the technical limitations of portable chest radiographs; thus, digital radiography has had a great impact in this respect. Disadvantages include limited spatial resolution and the high cost of most digital units.

CT and High-Resolution CT. CT and in particular helical (spiral) CT has revolutionized the field of thoracic imaging. Single breath-hold helical scanning allows optimal contrast enhancement without respiratory misregistration inherent in incremental scanning. Techniques matching narrow collimation with increased pitch provide optimal spatial resolution with maximal scan coverage on a single breath-hold. Routine helical chest CT protocols include single breath-hold acquisitions obtained at near total lung capacity following three maximal respirations. Iodinated contrast agents are routinely administered intravenously to optimize the evaluation of mediastinal vascular disease or hilar lymphadenopathy, to distinguish a central hilar mass from peripheral at-

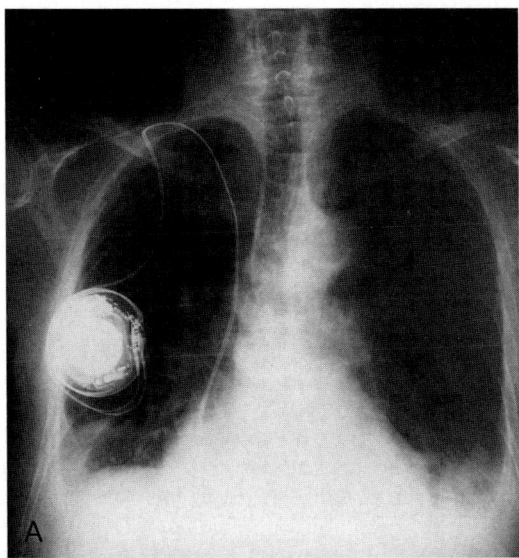
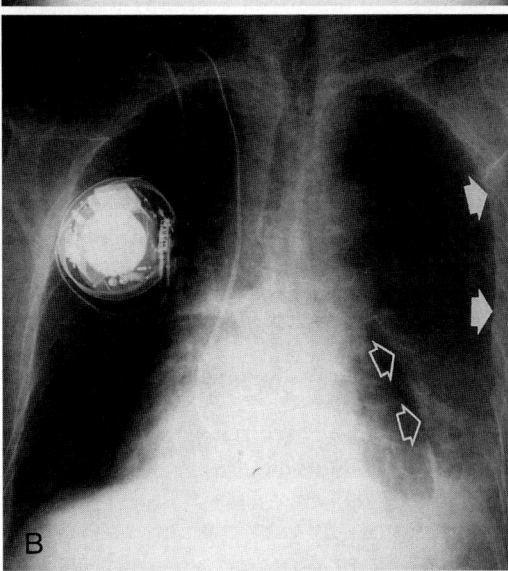

Figure 12.2. Lateral Decubitus Film for the Detection of Pleural Effusion. An upright radiograph **(A)** in a patient recovering from pulmonary edema shows blunting of both lateral costophrenic sulci. A left lateral decubitus film **(B)** demonstrates free-flowing effusion laterally on the downside (*solid arrows*) and within the lateral aspect of an incomplete oblique fissure (*open arrows*). Note the clearing of fluid from the right lateral costophrenic sulcus with the patient in the opposite decubitus position, with fluid layering medially along the mediastinal pleural surface.

electatic lung, or to assess complex peripheral parenchymal and pleural disease.

The field of view for image reconstruction is determined by measuring the widest transverse diameter of the as seen on the CT scout view. An edge enhancing computer reconstruction algorithm ("bone" or "sharp" algorithm) improves the spatial resolution of parenchymal structures and is used for all types of thoracic CT. Each pixel comprising the CT image is assigned a value expressed in CT or H units, which is based on the density of the voxel relative to water (arbitrarily assigned a value of 0 H). The resultant image is composed of a 512×512 matrix of pixels and can be photographed to film in a 12 on 1 format for interpretation and storage or can be displayed on a computer terminal. In this way the radiologist can manipulate the upper and lower range of H units displayed (window width or WW) and the value of the median shade of gray (window level or WL). Routine settings for CT photography and display of mediastinal structures is WW = 400, WL = 40 and for the lungs is WW = 1500, WL= −600.

Volumetric scans are routinely reconstructed at intervals equal to the collimation width (i.e., 5-mm intervals for a 5-mm collimated helical scan) but an infinite number of images can be reconstructed from the raw data set. Single breath-hold acquisitions using 1-mm or 3-mm collimation allow for accurate characterization of the density and margins of a solitary pulmonary nodule. Images reconstructed at intervals of one-half the collimation width and viewed on a workstation in a cine or paging format help distinguish small lung nodules from vertically oriented pulmonary vessels. Narrow collimated acquisitions (3–5 mm) obtained in a single breath-hold with overlapping reconstructions are used for tracheobronchial disease and allow for two-dimensional and three-dimensional renderings of central airway lesions. Rapid single breath-hold scanning during maximal pulmonary vascular and aortic contrast enhancement helps detect subtle hilar adenopathy and is being used with greater frequency for the detection of pulmonary emboli and assessing aortic dissection, aneurysm, and laceration.

HRCT technique involves incremental thinly collimated scans (1–2 mm) obtained at evenly spaced intervals through the thorax in the evaluation of diffuse parenchymal lung disease and bronchiectasis. As with all chest CT, a high spatial frequency or edge-enhancing reconstruction algorithm is used. Scan time is limited to minimize the effects of respiratory and cardiac motion. Expiratory HRCT scans are useful for the detection of air trapping in patients with small airways disease. Normal and abnormal HRCT findings are reviewed in chapter 18.

The major advantages of CT are superior contrast resolution and the cross-sectional display format. Superior contrast resolution allows for the detection of calcification within solitary pulmonary nodules and the depiction of mediastinal masses or lymph nodes within mediastinal fat. IV contrast enhancement is an additional method of improving contrast resolution and identifying and evaluating vascular structures (e.g., pulmonary emboli, aortic dissection). The cross-sectional display eliminates the superimposition of structures and allows visualization of parenchymal nodules as small as 3 mm. In addition, suspect hilar or parenchymal opacities seen on only a single view by conventional radiography are easily localized.

The clinical indications for thoracic CT will vary among institutions. The indications for thoracic CT and HRCT are shown in Tables 12.1 and 12.2.

MR. Routine thoracic MR involves spin-echo, T1-weighted and T2-weighted imaging sequences in the axial plane; coronal and sagittal planes are used in selected cases. Numerous techniques including EKG gating are used to control cardiac and cardiovascular motion and improve image quality. Respiratory motion is minimized by performing rapid single breath-hold acquisitions or by using respiratory compensation techniques. Contrast-enhanced MR with IV injection of paramagnetic agents is not routinely performed but is used investigationally for the evaluation of pulmonary embolism.

The major advantages of MR are the superior contrast resolution between tumor and fat, the ability to characterize tissues based on T1 and T2 relaxation times, the ability to scan in direct sagittal and coronal planes, and the lack of need for IV iodinated contrast (4). The signal void produced by flowing blood in vascular structures helps identify the mediastinal and hilar vessels, detect

Table 12.2. Indications for Thoracic HRCT

Indication	Example
Solitary pulmonary nodule	Breath-hold volumetric exam with thin collimation for accurate density determination without respiratory misregistration
Detect lung disease in a patient with pulmonary symptoms or abnormal pulmonary function studies and a normal or equivocal chest film	Emphysema Extrinsic allergic alveolitis Small airways disease Immunocompromised patient
Evaluate the diffusely abnormal chest film	
A baseline for evaluating patients with chronic diffuse infiltrative lung disease for follow-up changes with therapy	Cystic fibrosis Sarcoidosis Interstitial lung disease Histiocytosis X Adult respiratory distress syndrome
To determine approach (type and location) of biopsy	Bronchoscopy vs. VATS or needle biopsy
Hemoptysis	Routine HRCT incremental scans plus single breath-hold volumetric examination of the central airways

Table 12.1. Indications for Thoracic CT

Indication	Example
Evaluation of an abnormality identified on conventional radiographs	Densitometry of a solitary pulmonary nodule Localization and characterization of a hilar or mediastinal mass
Staging of lung cancer	Assess the extent of the primary tumor, and the relationship of the tumor to the pleura, chest wall, airways, and mediastinum Detect hilar and mediastinal lymph node enlargement
Detection of occult pulmonary metastases	Extrathoracic malignancies with a propensity to metastasize to the lung (osteogenic sarcoma, breast and renal cell carcinoma) or mediastinal nodes (lymphoma); CT is the most sensitive imaging technique to detect subradiographic nodules or lymph node enlargement, respectively
Distinction of empyema from lung abscess	Contrast enhanced CT can usually distinguish a peripheral lung abscess from loculated empyema
Detection of central pulmonary embolism	Breath-holding and using high contrast injection rates and thin collimation assuring maximal pulmonary arterial enhancement
Detection and evaluation of aortic dissection	Detection and localization of extent including aortic branch involvement

vascular invasion by tumor, detect intraluminal tumor or thrombus, and distinguish vascular structures from nodes or masses without the need for IV contrast. In addition, the ability to obtain images along the long axis of the aorta and the advent of cine MR techniques have made MR the primary modality for the imaging of most congenital and acquired thoracic vascular disorders. Direct coronal scans are of benefit in imaging regions that lie within the axial plane and are therefore difficult to depict by CT. For this reason, superior sulcus tumors, subcarinal and aortopulmonary window lesions, and certain hilar masses are better depicted by MR than CT. MR is superior to CT in the diagnosis of chest wall or mediastinal invasion because of the high contrast between tumor and chest wall fat and musculature, and tumor and mediastinal fat respectively. The characterization of tissues by their T1 and T2 relaxation times allows for the diagnosis of fluid-filled cysts, hemorrhage, and hematoma formation. The ability to distinguish tumor from fibrosis, based on T1 and T2 relaxation times, has proven particularly useful in the follow-up of patients irradiated for Hodgkin's disease. MR is currently unable to distinguish benign from malignant masses or lymph nodes.

The major disadvantages of thoracic MR scanning are the limited spatial resolution, the inability to detect calcium, and the difficulties in imaging the pulmonary parenchyma. MR is also more time-consuming and expensive than CT. These factors, along with the ability of CT to provide superior or equivalent information in most situations, have limited the use of thoracic MR for most noncardiovascular thoracic disorders. The primary indications for thoracic MR are listed in Table 12.3.

Table 12.3. Indications for MR of the Thorax

Evaluation of thoracic aortic aneurysm
Evaluation of aortic dissection in stable patients
Assessment of superior sulcus tumors
Determining vascular invasion by lung cancer
Evaluation of mediastinal and chest wall invasion of lung cancer
Staging of lung cancer patients unable to receive IV iodinated contrast
Evaluation of posterior mediastinal masses

US. Transthoracic US is now commonly used for the detection, characterization, and sampling of pleural, peripheral parenchymal, and mediastinal lesions (see chapter 39). The aspiration of small pleural effusions visualized on real-time US is preferable to blind thoracentesis. Similarly, sampling of visible pleural masses in patients with malignant effusions can diminish the number of negative pleural biopsies. The aspiration of pleural-based masses and abscesses can be safely performed by US-guided needle placement into the lesion through the point of contact between the mass and pleura. Large anterior medistinal masses that have a broad area of contact with the parasternal chest wall may have biopsies done to them without trangressing the lung.

Real-time US may be preferable to fluoroscopy in confirming phrenic nerve paralysis because of its lack of ionizing radiation, portability, and the ability to detect subpulmonic and subphrenic fluid collections which may cause diaphragmatic elevation.

Ventilation/Perfusion Lung Scanning. The nuclear medicine examinations utilized in the evaluation of noncardiac thoracic disease are ventilation/perfusion (V/Q) lung scintigraphy and gallium scintigraphy. V/Q scanning is used almost exclusively for the diagnosis of pulmonary embolism although quantitative V/Q imaging may be useful in the planning of bullectomy, lung volume reduction surgery for emphysema, and lung transplantation. Gallium-67 scanning of the chest is used in detecting pulmonary infection (e.g., *Pneumocystis carinii* pneumonia in a patient with a normal radiograph) or inflammation (e.g., disease activity in idiopathic pulmonary fibrosis) and in evaluating suspected sarcoidosis.

Pulmonary Arteriography involves catheterization of the right heart via upper or lower extremity veins and fluoroscopically guided selective placement of a pigtail-tip catheter into the pulmonary arteries, followed by contrast injection and rapid filming. The main indication for pulmonary arteriography is the evaluation of suspected pulmonary embolism, particularly when noninvasive imaging is unable to provide a confident diagnosis. Additional indications include the evaluation of congenital pulmonary vascular disease, particularly pulmonary arteriovenous malformations, and rarely, the detection of a pulmonary artery pseudoaneurysm in the patient with massive hemoptysis. The decrease in the amount of contrast necessary to opacify pulmonary vessels and superior contrast resolution are advantages of digital subtraction pulmonary angiography (DSPA) over conventional angiography although inferior spatial resolution and misregistration artifact caused respiratory and cardiac motion limit its use for pulmonary embolism diagnosis.

Thoracic Aortography involves the placement of a multiple side hole catheter into the aorta via the femoral, axillary, or brachial artery followed by power injection of contrast and rapid filming. Many conditions previously evaluated with thoracic aortography, particularly congenital aortic anomalies and aortic dissection, are presently better evaluated with CT, MR, or US. However, there are several indications for this procedure, with the most common being the detection of thoracic aortic or arch vessel laceration following blunt chest trauma. Additional indications include the evaluation of selected patients with aortic dissection or aneurysm and for the diagnosis of aortitis.

Bronchial Arteriography via a transfemoral arterial route with transcatheter arterial embolization is performed for the evaluation and treatment of massive or recurrent hemoptysis, most commonly from bronchiectasis, neoplasm, or mycetoma.

Transthoracic Needle Biopsy guided by CT, fluoroscopy, or US is a diagnostic technique utilized in selected patients with pulmonary, pleural, or mediastinal lesions (5).

Percutaneous Catheter Drainage of intrathoracic air or fluid collections, performed by imaging-guided placement of small bore multihole catheters, is used for the treatment of empyema, pneumothorax, malignant pleural effusion, and other intrathoracic fluid collections (3).

NORMAL LUNG ANATOMY

Tracheobronchial Tree (Fig. 12.3). The trachea is a hollow cylinder composed of a series of C-shaped cartilaginous rings. The rings are completed posteriorly by a flat band of muscle and connective tissue called the posterior tracheal membrane. The tracheal mucosa consists of a pseudostratified, ciliated columnar epithelium which contains scattered neuroendocrine (APUD) cells. The submucosa contains cartilage, smooth muscle, and seromucous glands. The left lateral wall of the distal trachea is indented by the transverse portion of the aortic arch.

The trachea is approximately 12 cm long in adults, with an upper limit of normal coronal tracheal diameter of 25 mm in men and 21 mm in women. In cross-section, the trachea is oval or horseshoe-shaped with a coronal-to-sagittal diameter ratio of 0.6–1.0. A narrowing of the coronal diameter producing a coronal:sagittal ratio of <0.6 is termed a "saber sheath trachea" and is seen in patients with chronic obstructive pulmonary disease.

On chest radiographs, the trachea is seen as a vertically oriented cylindical lucency extending from the cricoid cartilage superiorly to the main bronchi inferiorly. A slight tracheal deviation to the right after entering the thorax can be a normal radiographic finding. The interface of the right upper lobe with the right lateral tracheal wall is called the right paratracheal stripe (Fig. 12.4A). This stripe should be uniformly smooth and should not exceed 4 mm in width; thickening or nodularity reflects disease in any of the component tissues, including medial tracking pleural effusion. The left lat-

Figure 12.3. Prevailing Pattern of Segmental Bronchi. *B1* apical (upper lobe), *B2* posterior (upper lobe), *B3* anterior (upper lobe), *B4* lateral (middle lobe) and superior lingula), *B5* medial (middle lobe) and inferior (lingula), *B6* superior (lower lobe), *B7* medial basilar (lower lobe), *B8* anterio (lower lobe), *B9* lateral basilar (lower lobe), *B10* posterior (lower lobe). (From Yamashita H. Roentgenologic Anatomy of the Lung. Tokyo: Igaku-Shoin, 1978. Used with permission.)

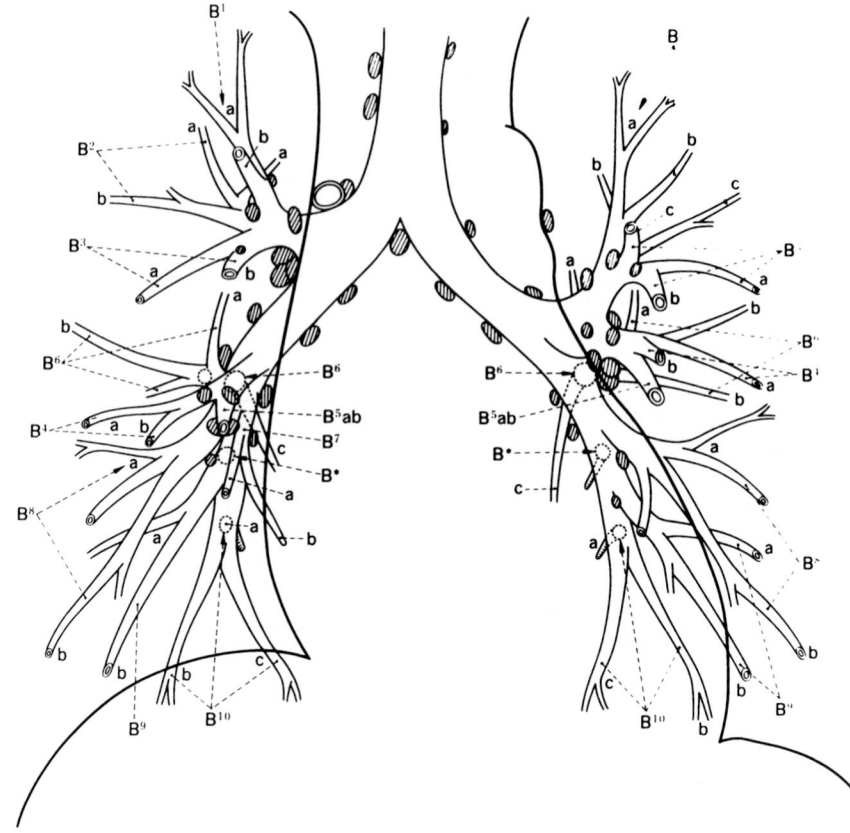

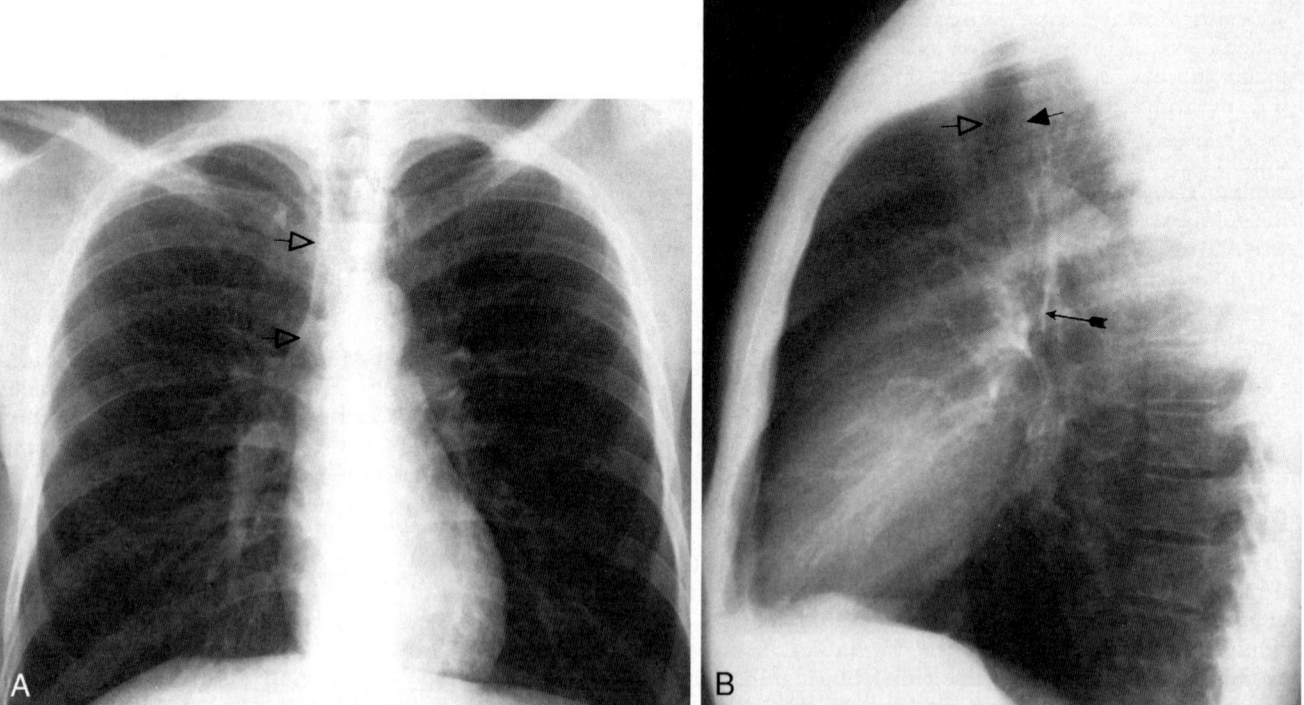

Figure 12.4. Trachea. A. The right paratracheal stripe (*open arrows*) is composed of the right lateral tracheal wall, a small amount of mediastinal fat, paratracheal lymph nodes, and the visceral and parietal pleural layers of the right upper lobe. **B.** Left lateral chest film shows the anterior (*open arrow*) and posterior (*short solid arrow*) walls of the trachea. The posterior wall of the bronchus intermedius (*long solid arrow*) is readily visible on lateral radiographs as it crosses the end-on view of the left upper lobe bronchus.

eral wall is surrounded by mediastinal vessels and fat and is not normally visible radiographically. The posterior trachea can be visualized on the lateral chest (Fig. 12.4B). The presence of air in the esophagus produces the tracheoesophageal stripe, which represents the combined thickness of the tracheal and esophageal walls and intervening fat. This stripe should measure less than 5 mm; thickening is most commonly seen with esophageal carcinoma.

The bronchial system exhibits a branching pattern of asymmetric dichotomy, with the daughter bronchi of a parent bronchus varying in diameter, length, and the number of divisions. The main bronchi arise from the trachea at the carina, with the right bronchus forming a more obtuse angle with the long axis of the trachea. The bronchi are composed of tissues that are similar to the trachea. The right main bronchus is considerably shorter than the left (2.2 cm vs. 5.0 cm mean length). The lobar bronchi, which lie partly within the mediastinum and partly in the lung, are visible on frontal chest radiographs as hollow cylinders silhouetted by the solid cylinders of central pulmonary vessels, or as ring shadows when seen end on. The segmental bronchi that course horizontally (anterior segmental upper lobe, superior segmental lower lobe) may be seen as small ring shadows within the pulmonary parenchyma when viewed end on. The tracheal and main, lobar, and segmental bronchial anatomy as seen on CT is shown in (Fig. 12.5).

Lobar and Segmental Anatomy (Figs. 12.3, 12.6). The right lung is divided by invaginations of the visceral pleura (interlobar fissures) into three lobes. The right upper lobe branches into three segments: anterior, apical, and posterior. The middle lobe is a triangularly shaped structure marginated by the minor fissure superiorly and the lower half of the major fissure posteroinferiorly. The middle lobe bronchus arises from the intermediate bronchus and divides into medial and lateral segmental branches, with blood supply to the middle lobe supplied by a branch of the right interlobar pulmonary artery. The right lower lobe is marginated by lower half of the major fissure anterosuperiorly and is supplied by the right lower lobe bronchus and pulmonary artery. It is subdivided into a superior and four basal segments: anterior, lateral. posterior, and medial.

The left lung is divided into upper and lower lobes by the left major fissure. The left upper lobe is analogous to the combined right upper and middle lobes. The left upper lobe is subdivided into four segments: anterior, apicoposterior and the superior and inferior lingular segments. Arterial supply to the anterior and apicoposterior segments parallels the bronchi and is via branches of the upper division of the left main pulmonary artery. The superior and inferior lingular arteries are proximal branches of the left interlobar pulmonary artery, analogous to the middle lobe blood supply. The left lower lobe is marginated by the major fissure anterosuperiorly and has a superior and three basal segments: anteromedial, lateral, and posterior.

Respiratory Portion of Lung. Distal to the terminal bronchioles, the bronchi lose their cartilage and become respiratory bronchioles. The respiratory bronchioles contain a few alveoli along their walls and give rise to the gas-exchanging units of the lung: the alveolar ducts and alveolar sacs. The pulmonary alveolus is lined by two types of epithelial cells (pneumocytes). Type I pneumocytes are flattened squamous cells that cover 95% of the alveolar surface area and are invisible by light microscopy. These cells are incapable of mitosis or repair. The more rare type II pneumocytes are cuboidal cells that are visible under light microscopy and are capable of mitosis. Type II pneumocytes are the source of new type I pneumocytes, and provide a mechanism for repair following alveolar damage. These cells are also thought to be the source of alveolar surfactant, a phospholipid that lowers the surface tension of alveolar walls and prevents alveolar collapse at low lung volumes.

Pulmonary Subsegmental Anatomy. The secondary pulmonary lobule and the acinus, which comprise the functional gas-exchanging portion of the lung, are the basic units of lung structure. The secondary pulmonary lobule is defined as that subsegment of lung supplied by three to five terminal bronchioles and separated from adjacent secondary lobules by intervening connective tissue (interlobular) septa. The lung subtended from a terminal bronchiole is termed a "pulmonary acinus" and is composed of a series of respiratory bronchioles, alveolar ducts, and alveolar sacs. Therefore, the secondary lobule is comprised of three to five pulmonary acini, which are marginated by interlobular septa.

The normal subsegmental anatomy of the lung is visible only by HRCT of the lung and is detailed in chapter 18.

Fissures. The interlobar pulmonary fissures represent invaginations of visceral pleura deep into the substance of the lung (Fig. 12.6)(6). These fissures may completely or incompletely separate the lobes from one another. An incomplete fissure has important consequences regarding interlobar spread of parenchymal consolidation, collateral air drift in patients with lobar bronchial obstruction, and the appearance of pleural effusion in supine patients. The fissures are well delineated on HRCT (Fig. 12.7).

Most individuals have two interlobar fissures on the right and one on the left. The fissures are complete laterally and incomplete medially, fusing with the adjacent lobe. The minor fissure is complete in about one-fourth of individuals but fuses with the RUL in about one-half. The inferior fissure of the RML is well developed, and very little fusion occurs between the RML and RLL. This oblique fissure is complete in less than one-third of individuals, with fusion between the lobes most common along the posteromedial portion of the fissure. The left major fissure is similar to the right, with fusion along the posterior aspect in approximately one-third of individuals.

The major and minor fissures are best visualized on lateral radiographs. Variable portions of the major fissures are seen as obliquely oriented thin white lines coursing anteroinferiorly from posterior to anterior. The left major fissure usually begins more superiorly and has a slightly more vertical course than the right major fis-

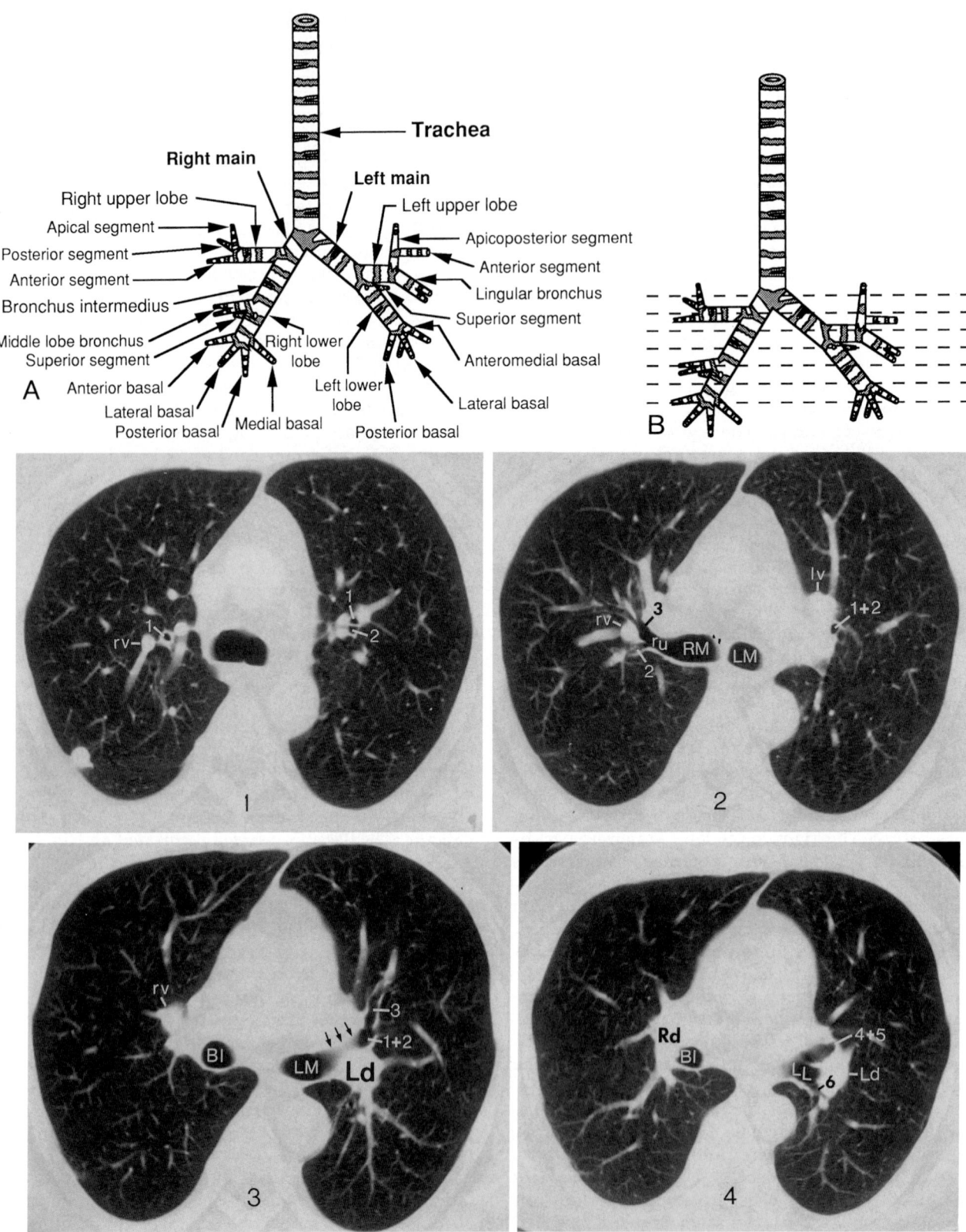

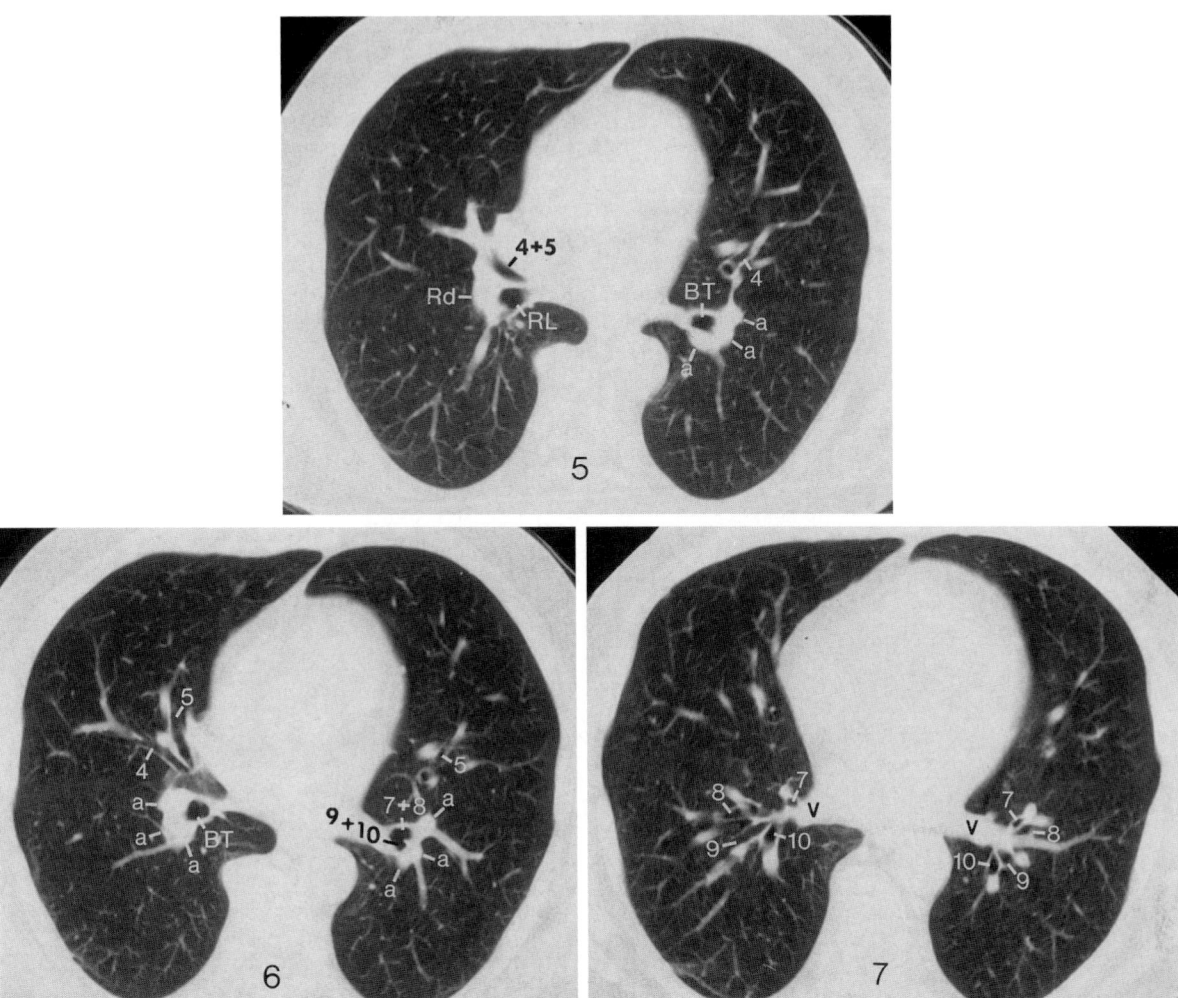

Figure 12.5 Tracheobronchial and Hilar Anatomy. A. Diagram of trachea and bronchi. **B.** Diagram showing bronchial and hilar anatomy as depicted by CT. **1. Level of tracheal carina.** Right apical bronchus (*1*); right superior posterior pulmonary vein (*rv*); left apicoposterior bronchus (*1* and *2* on the left). **2. Level of right upper lobe bronchus.** Right main bronchus (*RM*); right upper lobe bronchus (*ru*); right upper lobe anterior (*3*) and posterior (*2*) segmental bronchi; right superior pulmonary vein (*rv*); left main bronchus (*LM*); left apicoposterior segmental bronchus (*1+2*); left superior pulmonary vein (*lv*). **3. Level of left upper lobe bronchus, superior division.** Bronchus intermedius (*BI*); right superior pulmonary vein (*rv*); left main bronchus (*LM*); superior division of left upper lobe bronchus (*small arrows*); left upper lobe anterior (*3*) and apicoposterior (*1+2*) segmental bronchi; left descending pulmonary artery (*Ld*). **4. Level of left upper lobe bronchus, inferior (lingular) division.** Bronchus intermedius (*BI*); right descending pulmonary artery (*Rd*); lingular bronchus (*4+5*); left lower lobe

bronchus (LL); left lower lobe superior segmental bronchus (*6*); left descending pulmonary artery (*Ld*). **5. Level of middle lobe bronchus.** Middle lobe bronchus (*4+5*); right lower lobe bronchus (*RL*); right descending pulmonary artery (*Rd*); lingular superior segmental bronchus (*4*); left lower lobe basal trunk (*BT*); left lower lobe segmental arteries (*a*). **6. Level of lower lobe basal trunks.** Lateral (*4*) and medial (*5*) segmental bronchi of the middle lobe; right lower lobe basal trunk (*BT*); right lower lobe basal segmental arteries (*a*, on right); lingular segmental bronchus (*5*); left lower lobe antero-medial segmental bronchus (*7+8*); left lower lobe lateral and posterior basal segmental bronchi (*9+10*); left lower lobe basal segmental arteries (*a*, on left). **7. Level of basal segmental bronchi.** Right lower lobe medial (*7*, on right), anterior (*8*, on right), lateral (*9*, on right), and posterior (*10*, on right) basal segmental bronchi; right inferior pulmonary vein (*v*, on right); left lower lobe medial (*7*, on left), anterior (*8*, on left), lateral (*9*, on left), and posterior (*10*, on left) basal segmental bronchi; left inferior pulmonary vein (*v*, on left).

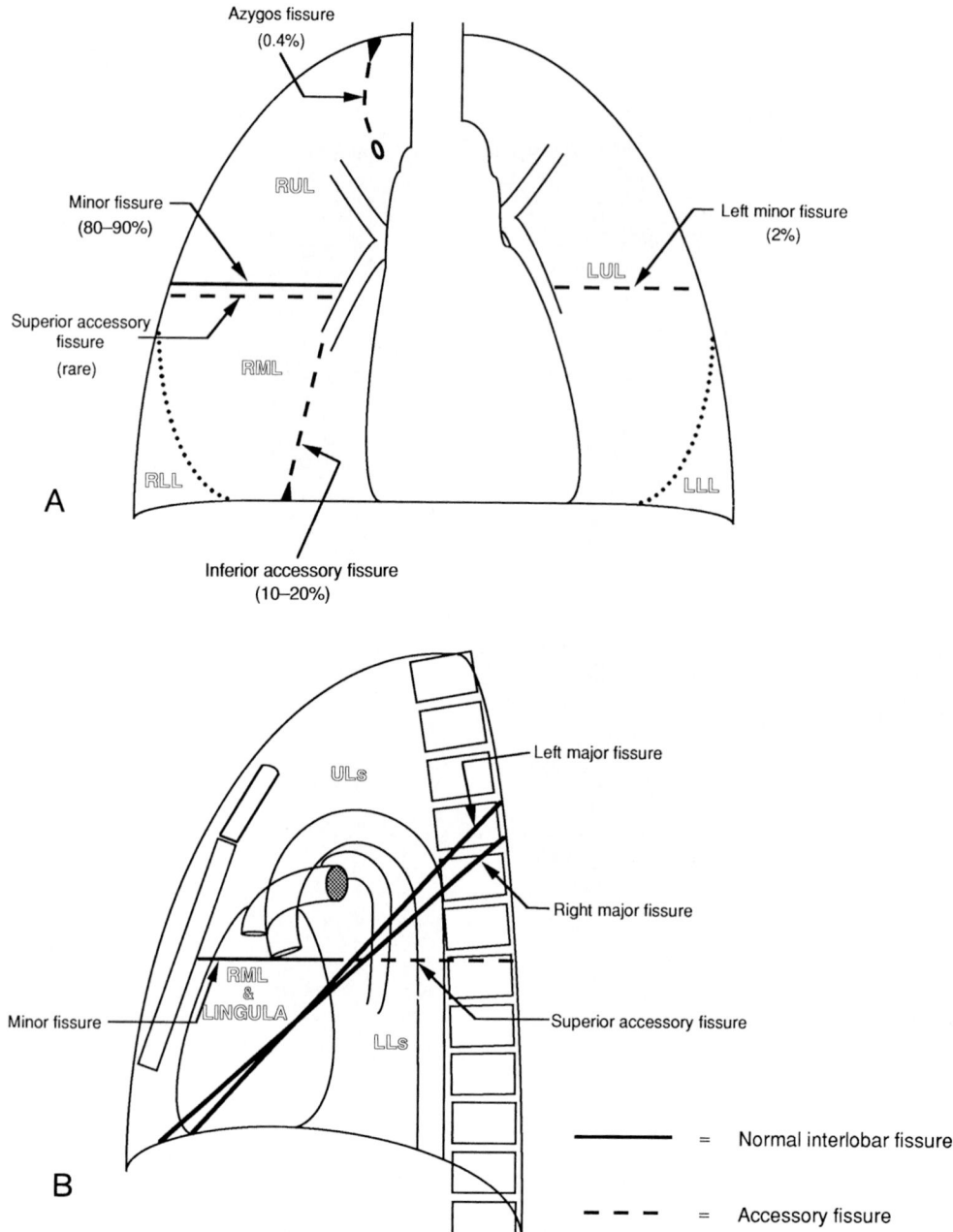

Figure 12.6. Normal Lobar and Fissural Anatomy. A. Frontal view. **B.** Lateral view. *RUL,* right upper lobe; *LUL,* left upper lobe; *RML,* right middle lobe; *RLL,* right lower lobe; *LLL,* left upper lobe; *ULs,* upper lobes; *LLs,* lower lobes.

sure. Occasionally, the fissure is recognized as a sharp edge as it marginates a homogeneous air-space filling process. At the points of intersection with the diaphragm, the inferior aspects of the major fissures often have a triangular configuration, with the apex of the triangle pointing toward the fissure. This appearance is caused by the presence of a small amount of fat within the inferior aspect of the fissure. On frontal radiographs, the major fissures are not usually visualized because of their oblique course relative to the x-ray beam. Occasionally, the superolateral aspects of the major fissures are seen as curvilinear edges in the upper thorax with a ground-glass opacity superolaterally and a lu-

cency inferomedially. This appearance is caused by the intrusion of extrapleural fat into the superolateral portion of the fissure. Rarely, the superolateral portion of the major fissure may be seen as a thin line projecting superomedial to the hilar shadows. This latter appearance occurs when the upper portion of the major fissure is brought in tangent to the x-ray beam because of lordotic positioning or from lower lobe atelectasis. The minor fissure projects at the level of the right fourth rib and is seen as a thin undulating line on frontal radiographs in approximately 50% of individuals. On lateral radiograph, the minor fissure is often seen as a thin curvilinear line with a convex superior margin extending anteri-

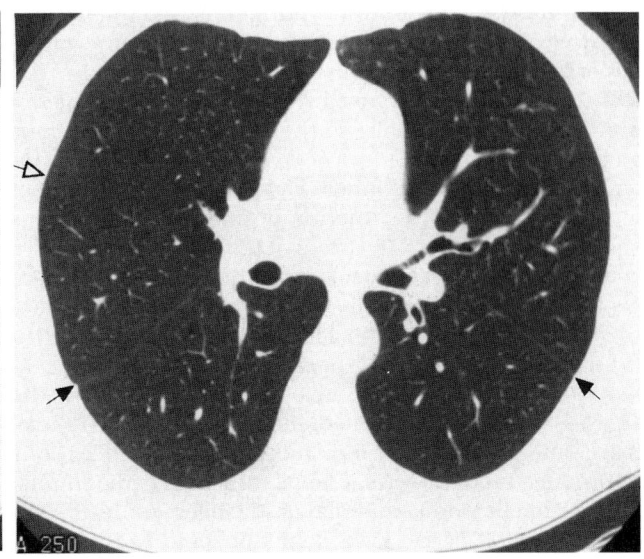

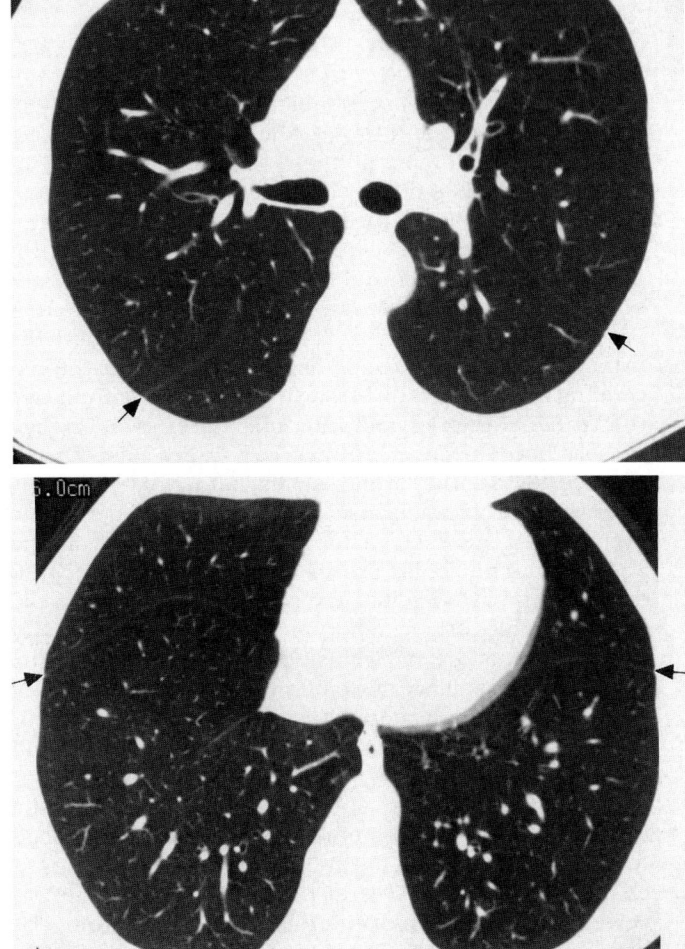

Figure 12.7. Fissural Anatomy on HRCT. The oblique fissures appear as thin curvilinear lines (*solid arrows*) concave anteriorly in the upper thorax **(A)**, flat lines in the midthorax **(B)**, and convex anterior lines in the lower chest **(C)**. The apex of the domed minor fissure is seen as an avascular zone in the midthorax (*open arrow* in **B**).

orly from the right major fissure. Not uncommonly, the posterior aspect of the minor fissure extends posterior to the margin of the right major fissure, an illusion explained by the concomitant visualization of the posterolateral aspect of the minor fissure and the anteromedial aspect of the undulating major fissure.

The inferior accessory fissure is the most common accessory fissure, found in approximately 10–20% of individuals. This fissure, which separates the medial basal from the remaining basal segments of the lower lobe, is often incomplete (Fig. 12.6). It may be seen on frontal radiographs as a thin curvilinear line extending superiorly from the medial third of the hemidiaphragm toward the lower hilum. The inferior accessory fissure has been misidentified as the inferior pulmonary ligament (invisible on normal chest radiographs) and is responsible for the juxtaphrenic peak described in upper lobe volume loss. A small triangle of extrapleural fat, seen at its point of insertion on the diaphragm, helps identify the inferior accessory fissure. An inferior accessory fissure can be seen on CT through the lower thorax, where it is identified as a curvilinear line extending anterolaterally from

just in front of the inferior pulmonary ligament toward the major fissure. The azygos fissure is seen in 0.5% of individuals (Fig. 12.6). It is comprised of four layers of pleura (two visceral, two parietal) and represents an invagination of the right apical pleura by the azygos vein, which has incompletely migrated to its normal position at the right tracheobronchial angle. The azygos fissure appears as a vertical curvilinear line, convex laterally, which extends inferiorly from the lung apex, ending in a teardrop, which is the azygos vein. The significance of this fissure is its ability to limit the spread of apical segmental consolidation to the azygos lobe (that portion of the apical segment delineated by the azygos fissure) and to exclude pneumothorax from the apical portion of the pleural space. The superior accessory fissure separates the superior segment from the basal segments of the lower lobe. On the right side it may be distinguished from the minor fissure on lateral radiographs as it extends posteriorly from the major fissure to the chest wall. The left minor fissure is a rarely seen normal variant that separates the lingula from the remaining portions of the upper lobe.

Ligaments. The inferior pulmonary ligament is a sheet of connective tissue that extends from the hilum superiorly to a level at or just above the hemidiaphragm. It is thus comprised of fused visceral and parietal pleura and binds the lower lobe to the mediastinum and runs alongside the esophagus. The ligament contains the inferior pulmonary vein superiorly and a variable number of lymph nodes. The inferior pulmonary ligament is sometimes seen on CT through the lower thorax as a small laterally directed beak of mediastinal pleura adjacent to the esophagus (Fig. 12.8). The tethering effect of this ligament on the lower lobe accounts for the medial location and triangular appearance of lower lobe collapse. The ligament may also act as a barrier to the spread of pleural and mediastinal fluid, and it may marginate medial pleural or mediastinal air collections to produce a characteristic appearance on radiographs. As pleural effusion accumulates, the ligament keeps the medial portion of the lower lobe anchored to the mediastinum acting as a hinge around which the lateral portion of the lower lobe can rotate.

The sublobar septum (Fig. 12.8) is sometimes mistaken for the inferior pulmonary ligament. It is a linear structure seen on CT near the inferior pulmonary ligament extending into the lung from the mediastinal pleura.

The pericardiophrenic ligament is a triangular density extending toward the lung that is seen along the posterior aspect of the right heart border on lung windows on chest CT (Fig. 12.8). Representing a reflection of pleura over the inferior portion of the phrenic nerve and peri-

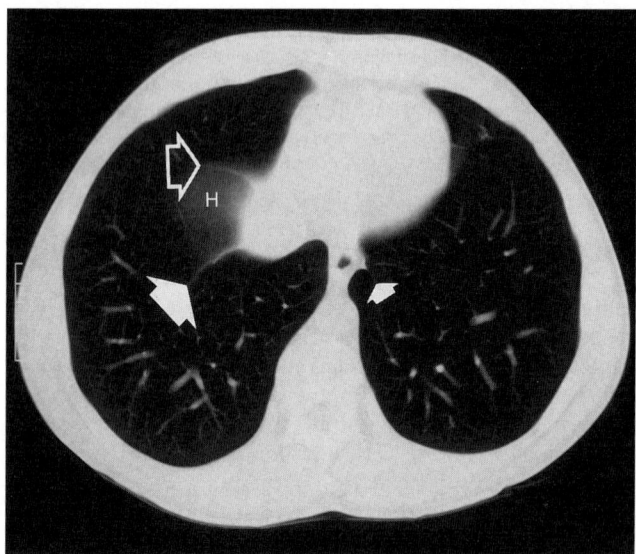

Figure 12.8. Inferior Pulmonary and Pericardiophrenic Ligaments. A CT just above the diaphragm demonstrates a thin line (*small solid arrow*) extending posterolaterally at the level of the esophagus that represents the sublobar septum extending to the inferior pulmonary ligament. On the right, a curvilinear line (*large solid arrow*) extending from just lateral to the inferior vena cava represents the right pericardiophrenic ligament containing branches of the phrenic nerve and pericardiophrenic vessels. More anteriorly, a thin line (*open arrow*) is seen just above the apex of the right hemidiaphragm (*H*) which represents fat within the inferior aspect of the major fissure.

cardiophrenic vessels, this ligament is distinguished from the sublobar septum by its more anterior location and by its characteristic ramifications as branches of the nerve and vessel reflect over the hemidiaphragm.

Pulmonary Arteries. The pulmonary artery (Fig. 12.9A) is an elastic artery that arises from the right ventricle anterior to the ascending aorta and courses superiorly, posteriorly, and toward the left before bifurcating into right and left main pulmonary arteries. The left pulmonary artery is a direct continuation of the main pulmonary artery. Within the left hilum, it envelopes the upper margin of the left main bronchus, at which point it divides into the upper and lower lobe arteries. The right pulmonary artery courses laterally toward the right from the main pulmonary artery. It then travels anterior to the tracheal carina and immediately posterior to the ascending aorta, and it divides within the pericardium into the truncus anterior and interlobar arteries. Many accessory branches of the pulmonary artery exist. As the arteries divide, they diminish in caliber. At the same level that the bronchi lose their cartilage and become bronchioles, the elastic arteries lose their elastic lamina and become muscular arteries. At a diameter of 70–80 microns, the arteries lose their muscular layer and become arterioles. The capillary network of the pulmonary arterial circulation, which envelopes the alveoli, is the most prolific capillary system in the body. Thickening of the alveolocapillary membrane from edema fluid or fibrosis impedes gas exchange and results in dyspnea and hypoxemia.

Bronchial Arteries. The bronchial arteries are the primary nutrient vessels of the lung. They supply blood to the bronchial walls to the level of the terminal bronchioles. In addition, several mediastinal structures receive a variable amount of blood supply from the bronchial circulation. These include the tracheal wall, middle third of the esophagus, visceral pleura, mediastinal lymph nodes, vagus nerve, pericardium, and thymus.

The origin of the bronchial arteries is quite variable. The bronchial arteries arise from the proximal descending thoracic aorta between the level of the third and eighth thoracic vertebral bodies. Most commonly, one right-sided and two left-sided arteries arise. The right bronchial artery usually arises from the posterolateral wall of the aorta in common with an intercostal artery as an intercostobronchial trunk. This artery typically arises at the T5-6 level, which corresponds radiographically to the level of the tracheal carina. The left bronchial arteries arise individually from the anterolateral aorta at or about the same level; the left bronchial arteries occasionally arise from an intercostal artery. Approximately two-thirds of the blood from the bronchial arterial system returns to the pulmonary venous system via the bronchial veins. The remainder, which include veins draining the large bronchi, tracheal bifurcation, and mediastinum, drain into the azygos or hemiazygos systems.

Pulmonary Veins. Pulmonary veins (Fig. 12.9B) arise within the interlobular septa from the alveolar and visceral pleural capillaries. The veins travel in connective tissue envelopes separate from the bronchoarterial trunks. The pulmonary veins, which may number from three to eight, drain into the left atrium.

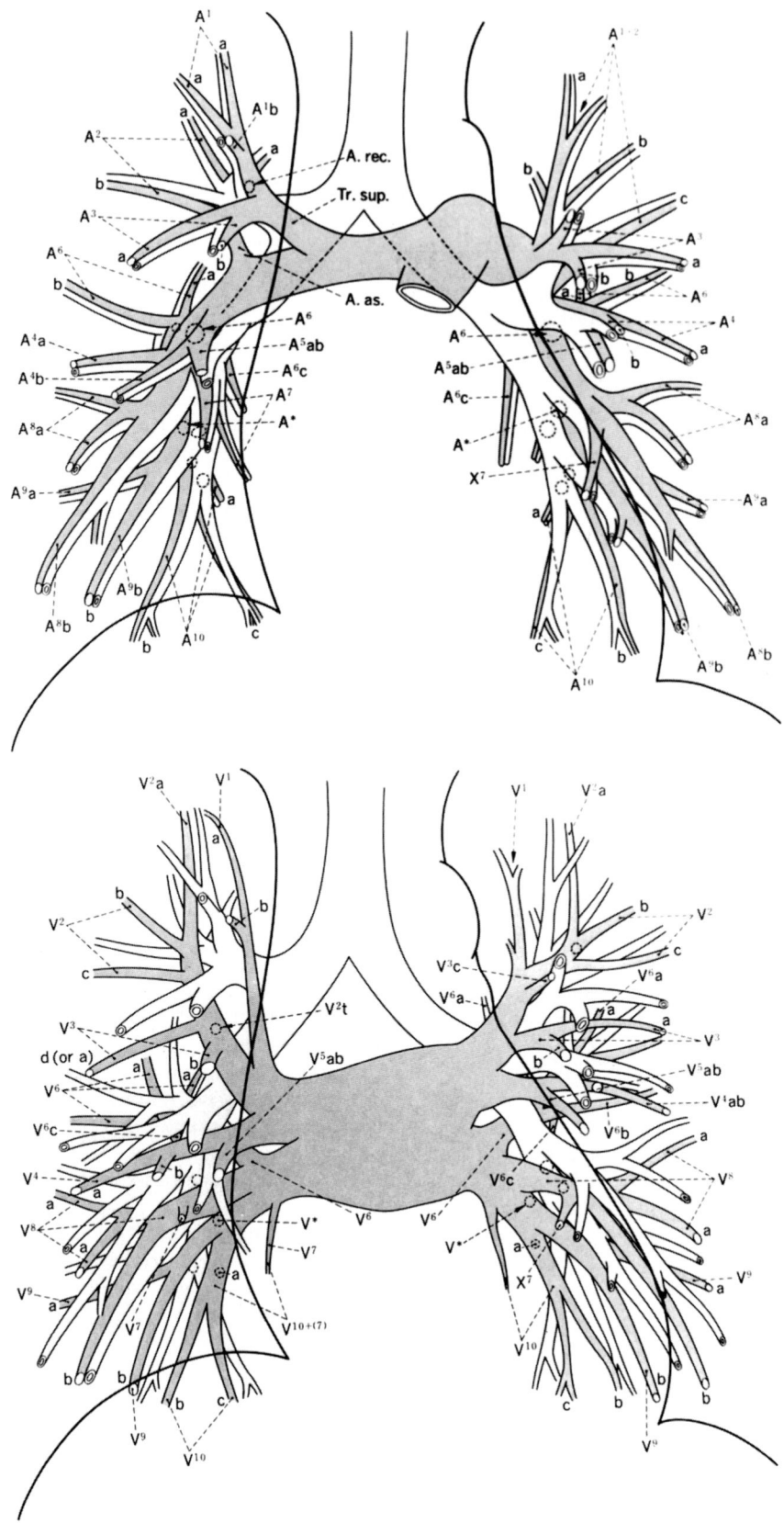

Figure 12.9. Prevailing Pattern of Segmental Arteries and Veins. A. The branches of the right and left pulmonary arteries accompany and divide in parallel with the corresponding lobar, segmental, and subsegmental bronchi. *A1* apical (upper lobe), *A2* posterior (upper lobe), *A3* anterior (upper lobe), *A4* lateral (middle lobe) and superior (lingula), *A5* medial (middle lobe) and inferior (lingula), *A6* superior (lower lobe), *A7* medial basal (lower lobe), *A8* anterior basal (lower lobe), *A9* lateral basal (lower lobe), *A10* posterior basal (lower lobe). Note that the right upper lobe receives an accessory branch from the proximal right interlobar pulmonary artery (*A.as*). **B.** Prevailing pattern of pulmonary veins. Note that the veins do not follow the segmental bronchi and arteries. *V1* apical (upper lobe), *V2* posterior (upper lobe), *V3* anterior (upper lobe), *V1+2* apical posterior (left upper lobe), *V4* lateral (middle lobe) and superior (lingula), *V5* medial (middle lobe) and inferior (lingula), *V6* superior (lower lobe), *V7* medial basal (right lower lobe), *V8* anterior basal (right lower lobe), *V9* lateral basal (lower lobe), *V8+9* medial anterior basal (left lower lobe), *V10* posterior basal (lower lobe). (From Yamashita H. Roentgenologic Anatomy of the Lung. Tokyo: Igaku-Shoin, 1978. Used with permission.)

Pulmonary Lymphatics help clear fluid and particulate matter from the pulmonary interstitium. Two major lymphatic pathways can be found in the lung and pleura. The visceral pleural lymphatics, which reside in the vascular (innermost) layer of the visceral pleura, form a network over the surface of the lung that roughly parallels the margins of the secondary pulmonary lobules. These peripheral lymphatics penetrate the lung to course centrally within interlobular septa along with the pulmonary veins toward the hilum. The parenchymal lymphatics originate in proximity to the alveolar septa ("juxta-alveolar lymphatics") and course centrally with the bronchoarterial bundle. The perivenous and bronchoarterial lymphatics communicate via obliquely oriented lymphatics located within the central regions of the lung. These communicating lymphatics and their surrounding connective tissue, when distended by fluid, account for the radiographic appearance of Kerley's A lines.

Pulmonary Interstitium is the scaffolding of the lung, providing support for the airways and pulmonary vessels (Fig. 12.10)(6). It begins within the hilum and extends peripherally to the visceral pleura. The interstitial compartment that extends from the mediastinum and envelopes the bronchovascular bundles is termed the "axial interstitium." The axial fiber system continues distally as the centrilobular interstitium along with the arterioles, capillaries, and bronchioles to provide support for the air-exchanging portions of the lung. The subpleural interstitium and interlobular septa are parts of the peripheral interstitium that divides secondary pulmonary lobules. The pulmonary veins and lymphatics lie within the peripheral interstitium. The intralobular interstitium is a thin network of fibers that bridge the gap between the centrilobular and peripheral compartments.

Edema involving the axial interstitium is recognized radiographically as peribronchial cuffing. Pathologic involvement of the intralobular interstitium is difficult to discern radiographically, but it may account for some cases of so-called "ground-glass" opacity on chest radiographs and HRCT scans. Thickening of portions of this intersitium is occasionally seen as intralobular lines on HRCT. Radiographically, edema of the peripheral and subpleural interstitium accounts for Kerley's B lines (or interlobular lines on HRCT) and "thickened" fissures on chest radiographs.

POSTEROANTERIOR CHEST RADIOGRAPH

A firm knowledge of the normal anatomy displayed on the frontal (usually posteroanterior) chest radiograph is key to detecting and localizing pathologic conditions and to avoid mistaking normal structures for pathologic findings.

Soft Tissues of the chest wall consist of the skin, subcutaneous fat, and muscles. The lateral edges of the sternocleidomastoid muscles are readily visible in most patients. The visualization of normal fat in the supraclavicular fossae and the companion shadows of skin and subcutaneous fat paralleling the clavicles helps exclude mass, adenopathy, or edema in this region. The inferolateral edge of the pectoralis major muscle is normally seen curving toward the axilla. Congenital absence of the pectoral muscle creates relative radiolucency on the affected side and should not be mistaken for a contralateral increase in opacity. Both breast shadows should be evaluated routinely to detect evidence of prior mastectomy or distorting mass. The soft tissues lateral to the bony thorax should be smooth, symmetric homogeneous densities.

Bones. The thoracic spine, ribs and costal cartilages, clavicles, and scapulae are routinely visible on frontal chest radiographs. The bodies of the thoracic vertebrae should be vertically aligned, with endplates, pedicles, and spinous processes visualized. Twelve pairs of symmetric ribs should be seen; the upper ribs have smooth superior and inferior cortical margins, and the middle and lower ribs have flanged inferior cortices where the intercostal neurovascular bundles run. Cervical ribs, identified in approximately 2% of individuals, may be associated with symptoms of thoracic outlet syndrome. Companion shadows paralleling the inferior margins of the first and second ribs represent extrapleural fat, which may be abundant in obese individuals. Costal cartilage calcification is seen in a majority of adults and increases in prevalence with advancing age. Men typically show calcification at the upper and lower margins whereas the majority of women develop central cartilaginous calcification.

Lung-Lung Interfaces. A familiarity with the normal mediastinal interfaces is key to the interpretation of frontal chest radiographs (2). The lung-mediastinal interfaces are seen as sharp edges where the lung and adjacent pleura reflect off of various mediastinal structures. The lung-lung interfaces as seen on frontal radiographs relate directly to the space available in three regions viewed on the lateral film: the retrosternal space, the retrotracheal triangle, and the retrocardiac space (Fig. 12.11).

The retrosternal air space reflects contact of the anterosuperior aspect of the upper lobes (Fig. 12.11). On frontal radiographs the anterior junction line is seen as a thin vertical line that overlies the thoracic spine (Fig.

THE LUNG INTERSTITIUM

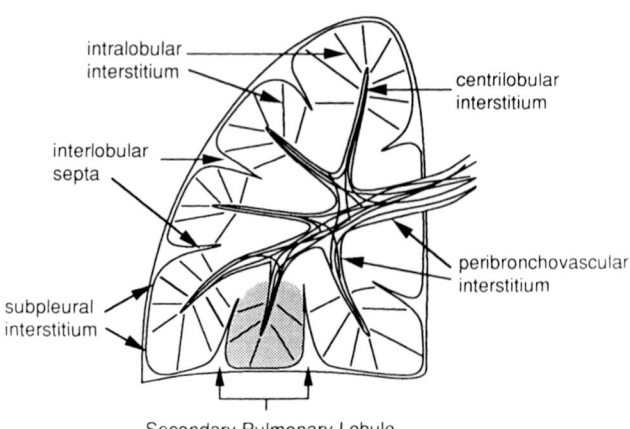

Figure 12.10. Diagram of the Pulmonary Interstitium.

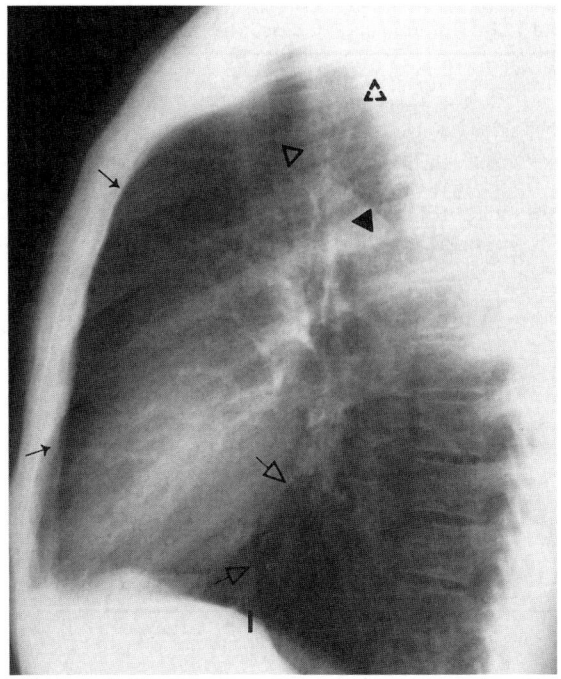

Figure 12.11. Radiolucent Spaces on Lateral Chest Radiograph. The retrosternal space is demarcated anteriorly by the posterior margin of the sternum (*small arrows*) and the heart and ascending aorta posteriorly and accounts for the anterior junction line seen on frontal radiographs. The retrotracheal triangle is marginated by the posterior wall of the trachea anteriorly (*open triangle*), spine posteriorly (*broken triangle*) and aortic arch inferiorly (*solid triangle*). The retrocardiac space is demarcated anteriorly by the posterior cardiac margin (*upper open arrow*) and the inferior vena cava (*I, lower open arrow*).

12.12). The anterior junction anatomy is an inferior extension of the upper lobe reflections off the innominate veins, with the latter producing an inverted V-shaped retromanubrial opacity. No anterior junction line occurs when abundant anterior mediastinal fat precludes retrosternal contact of the upper lobes.

A second potential lung-lung interface is seen on the lateral chest radiograph as the retrotracheal triangle, a radiolucent region representing contact of the posterosuperior portions of the upper lobes (Fig. 12.11) If the retrotracheal space available is small, only a right paraesophageal interface is visualized on the PA view (Fig. 12.13). If the space is large, a posterior junction line is seen (Figs. 12.12, 12.13)(Table 12.4).

The third potential lung-lung interface occurs in the retrocardiac space (Fig. 12.11). If this space is large, the azygoesophageal recess of the right lower lobe can abut the preaortic recess of the left lower lobe to produce an *inferior* posterior junction line (Fig. 12.13).

Lung-Mediastinal Interfaces (Table 12.5). The right lateral margin of the superior vena cava is commonly seen as a straight or slightly concave interface with the right upper lobe, extending from the level of the clavicle to the superior margin of the right atrium. Prominence or convexity of the caval interface may represent caval dilatation or lateral displacement by a dilated or tortuous aortic arch or other mediastinal mass.

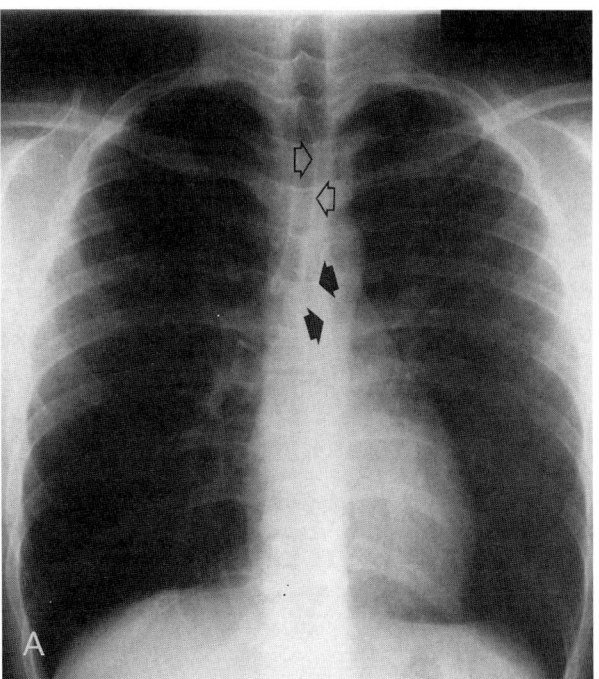

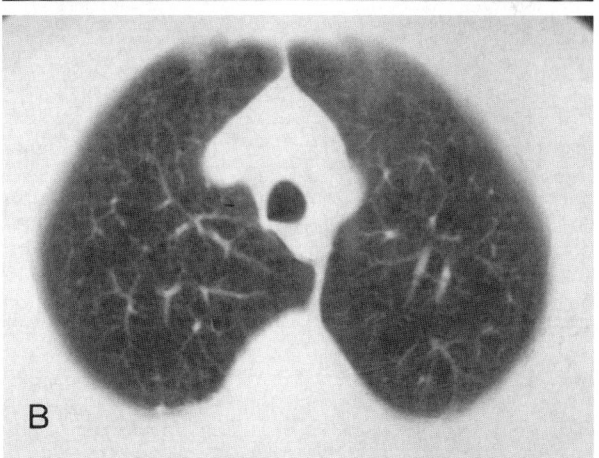

Figure 12.12. Anterior and Posterior Junction Lines. A. PA chest film shows both anterior (*solid arrows*) and posterior (*open arrows*) junction lines. **B.** CT through the upper thorax in another patient shows the anterior junction line in the retrosternal space, and the posterior junction line lies in the retrotracheal space.

Along the right upper mediastinum, the right upper lobe contacts the right lateral tracheal wall in a majority of individuals. This produces the right paratracheal stripe (Fig. 12.4A). The thickness of this line, measured above the level of the azygos vein, should not exceed 4 mm. Thickening or nodularity of the paratracheal stripe is seen in abnormalities of the tissues comprising the strip, including tracheal tumors, paratracheal lymph node enlargement, and right pleural effusion (Fig. 12.2).

The arch of the azygos vein separates the right paraesophageal from the upper azygoesophageal space (Fig. 12.13). Measurements for the azygos vein must take into account the position of the patient (i.e., supine or upright) and the intrathoracic pressure at the time the film was exposed. The measurement should be made

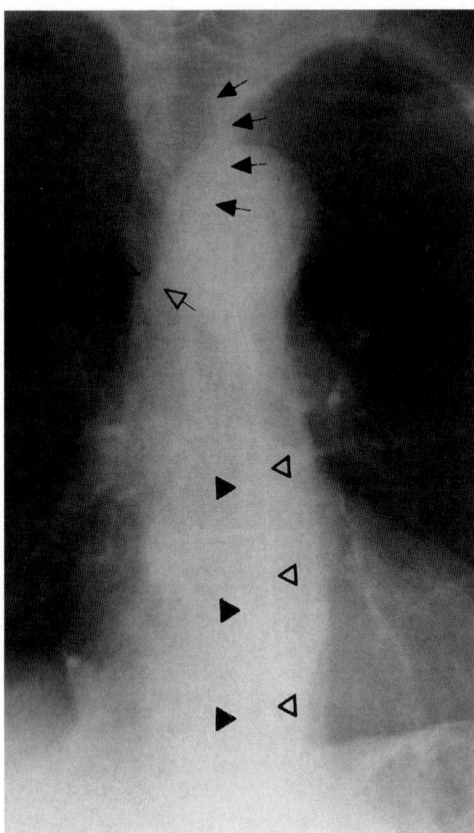

Figure 12.13. Lung-Lung Interfaces on Frontal Radiograph. Coned-down view of a PA film shows the right paraesophageal interface (*solid arrows*). The azygous arch (*open arrows*) separates the supra-azygous lung from the infra-azygous lung, which creates the azygoesophageal recess interface (*solid triangles*). The retrocardiac left lung creates the preaortic recess interface (*open triangles*).

Table 12.4. Anterior and Posterior Junction Lines

Line	Features
Anterior junction line	Obliquely oriented from right superior to left inferior
	Extends from upper sternum to base of heart
Posterior junction line	Vertically oriented in the midline
	Extends from upper thoracic spine to level of azygous and aortic arches

Table 12.5. Normal Lung-Mediastinal Interfaces

Right-sided	Right paraesophageal interface
	Superior vena cava/Right paratracheal stripe
	Anterior arch of the azygous vein
	Right paraspinal interface
	Azygoesophageal recess
	Lateral margin of right atrium
	Confluence of right pulmonary veins (right border of left atrium)
	Lateral margin of inferior vena cava
Left-sided	Lateral margin of left subclavian artery
	Transverse aortic arch
	Left superior intercostal vein (''aortic nipple'')
	Aortopulmonary window interface
	Aortopulmonary interface
	Lateral margin of main pulmonary artery
	Preaortic recess
	Left paraspinal interface
	Left atrial appendage
	Left ventricle
	Epipericardial fat pad

through the midpoint of the azygos arch perpendicular to the right main bronchus. The supine position or performance of the Mueller maneuver (forced inspiration against a closed glottis) will increase azygos venous diameter. In general, a diameter of greater than 10 mm on a PA radiograph should raise the possibility of mass, adenopathy or dilatation of the azygos vein; the latter may be seen in patients with right heart failure, obstruction of venous return to the heart, or a congenital venous anomaly such as azygos continuation of the inferior vena cava. An increase in diameter of the azygos vein from prior comparable radiographs is more important than the actual measurement.

The azygoesophageal recess interface is a vertically oriented interface overlying the thoracic spine. (Fig. 12.13). Although normally straight or concave in contour, the middle third of the interface may have a slight rightward convexity at the level of the right inferior pulmonary veins. Convexity of the superior third of the interface should suggest subcarinal lymph node enlargement or a bronchogenic cyst. Convexity of the middle third of this recess is usually due to the confluence of right pulmonary veins or the right border of the left atrium. Left atrial dilatation will enlarge and laterally displace this interface, producing a double-density composed of the right lateral borders of both right and left atria. Convexity of the inferior third most commonly is caused by a sliding hiatal hernia. Occasionally, a tortuous descending aorta or enlarged paraesophageal lymph nodes can cause this recess to be convex to the right in its lower third. When air is present in the distal portion of the esophagus and the azygoesophageal recess interfaces with the right lateral wall of the esophagus, a line (the right inferior esophagopleural stripe) rather than an edge is seen.

The paraspinal interface is a straight, vertical interface extending the length of the right hemithorax and represents contact of the right lung with a small amount of tissue lateral to the thoracic spine. It is inconsistantly visualized on the right side. A focal convexity of this interface suggests spinal or paraspinal disease.

The right heart projects just to the right of the lateral margin of the thoracic spine on a normal PA radiograph (Fig. 12.1). This portion of the heart is the lateral margin of right atrium, which creates a smooth convex interface with the medial segment of the middle lobe. Individuals with pectus excavatum have leftward cardiac displacement and may not demonstrate this interface. In patients with right atrial dilatation, this interface becomes more prominent, extending well into the right lung.

The right lateral border of the inferior vena cava may be seen at the level of the right hemidiaphragm as a concave lateral interface. The inferior vena caval interface is best visualized on lateral radiographs (Fig. 12.1). This interface may be absent in patients with azygos continuation of the inferior vena cava.

In the uppermost portion of the left mediastinum, one or more interfaces may be recognized cephalad to the aortic arch. The interface most often visualized is the subclavian artery (Fig. 12.14). It is unusual for the left upper lobe to interface with the left lateral wall of the trachea to form the left paratracheal stripe because the subclavian artery and adjacent fat usually intervene.

The transverse portion of the aortic arch (aortic knob) creates a small convex indentation on the left lung in normal individuals (Fig. 12.14). As the aorta elongates and dilates with age, this interface projects more laterally and lung may be seen to encircle a greater circumference of the knob.

In approximately 5% of individuals, the left superior intercostal vein may be seen on frontal radiographs as a rounded or triangular opacity that focally indents the lung immediately superolateral to the aortic arch. This density, termed the "aortic nipple," represents the superior intercostal vein as it arches anteriorly from its paraspinal position around the aortic arch to drain into the posterior aspect of the left innominate vein. This

structure, which normally measures less than 5 mm, may enlarge with elevation of right atrial pressure or with congenital or acquired obstruction of venous return to the right heart.

Immediately inferior to the aortic arch, the left upper lobe contacts the mediastinum to produce the aortopulmonary window interface (Fig. 12.14). This interface is usually straight or concave toward the lung; the latter appearance is seen with a tortuous aorta, emphysema, or congenital absence of the left pericardium. A convex lateral interface should suggest mass or lymph node enlargement in the aortopulmonary window.

A mediastinal-pleural interface termed the "aortopulmonary interface" is occasionally seen in the left upper mediastinum superimposed on the aortic knob and extending inferiorly toward the main pulmonary artery. This interface represents the left upper lobe contacting mediastinal fat in a plane just anterolateral to the aortic arch and extending inferiorly toward the left hilum. Convexity or lobulation of this interface may be caused by mediastinal lipomatosis, lymph node enlargement, or mass in this region of the mediastinum.

Immediately inferior to the aortopulmonary window is the left lateral border of the main pulmonary artery (Fig. 12.14). The interface of this structure may be convex, straight, or concave toward the lung. Enlargement of the main pulmonary artery is seen as an idiopathic condition in young women, caused by poststenotic dilatation in valvular pulmonic stenosis, or in conditions that cause increased flow or pressure in the pulmonary arterial system such as left-to-right intracardiac shunts.

The preaortic recess interface is seen in a small percentage of normal individuals as a reflection of the left lower lobe with the esophagus anterior to the descending aorta, extending vertically from the undersurface of the aortic knob a variable distance toward the diaphragm. This interface is the left-sided analog of the azygoesophageal recess interface.

The left paraspinal interface represents the reflection of the left lung off of paraspinal soft tissues, which largely consist of fat but also contain the sympathetic chain, proximal intercostal vessels, intercostal lymph nodes, and hemiazygos and accessory hemiazygos veins. The left paraspinal interface, in contrast to the right paraspinal interface, is seen in a majority of individuals. The reason for this is that the left-sided descending thoracic aorta produces an interface between the left lower lobe and paraspinal soft tissues that is oriented in the sagittal plane. This interface lies farther lateral to the lateral margin of the spine than the right paraspinal reflection owing to an increased amount of left paraspinal fat below the level of the aortic arch. Neurogenic tumors, hematoma, paraspinal abscess, lipomatosis, and medial pleural effusion can cause lateral displacement of this interface.

The left atrial appendage forms a concave interface immediately below the main pulmonary artery (Fig. 12.14). Straightening or convexity of this interface is most commonly seen in rheumatic mitral valve disease but may be seen in patients with left atrial enlargement of any cause.

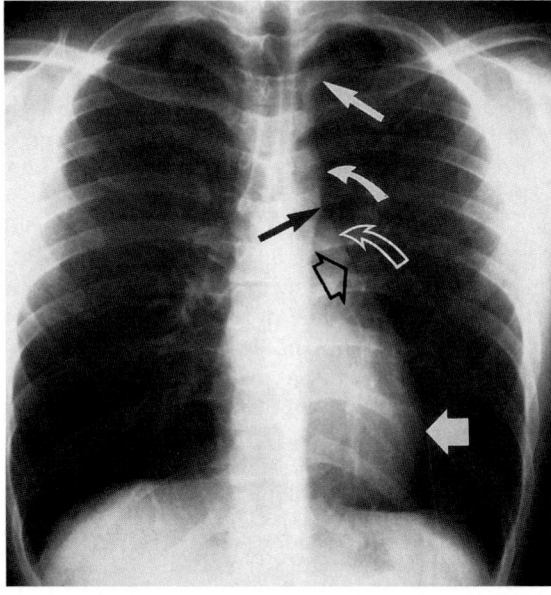

Figure 12.14. Lung-Mediastinal Interfaces—Left Side. PA chest radiograph shows the normal contours along the left mediastinum (from superior to inferior): left subclavian artery (*long straight white arrow*), aortic knob (*curved white arrow*), aortopulmonary window (*straight black arrow*), main pulmonary artery (*curved open white arrow*), left atrial appendage (*open black arrow*), and left ventricle (*solid white arrow*).

The left ventricle comprises most of the left heart border. A gentle convex margin with the lingula is normal (Fig. 12.14). Abnormalities of the left ventricular contour will be discussed in detail in the section on cardiovascular disease.

Fat adjacent to the cardiac apex may create a focal bulge in the left cardiac contour that obscures the heart border at the left cardiophrenic angle. This epipericardial fat pad, which is usually unilateral or more prominent on the left, is most often seen in obese patients and those on corticosteroids. A typical appearance on the lateral radiograph is usually diagnostic; CT is helpful in equivocal cases.

The Lungs (Fig. 12.14). The opacity of the lungs as visualized radiographically is attributable solely to the presence of the pulmonary vasculature and enveloping interstitial structures. The intraparenchymal pulmonary arteries course vertically from the hilar pulmonary arteries, sometimes allowing distinction from the pulmonary veins, which are more horizontally oriented. The arteries are solid cylinders with slightly indistinct margins that branch with the hollow cylinders of the airways. They gradually diminish in caliber as they travel distally in tandem with the bronchi, which are not visible radiographically. The pulmonary veins can often be traced horizontally to the left atrium but are otherwise indistinguishable from pulmonary arteries. In the upright individual, the lower lobe arteries and veins are larger in caliber than the upper lobe vessels due to the effects of gravity on pumonary blood flow. The normal dark gray opacity of the upper lungs increases inferiorly in females due to summation of overlying breast tissue. The opacity of the lung may be increased by processes that render the interstitium or air spaces opaque or decreased by any process associated with diminished blood flow to the lung or destruction of parenchymal structures.

Diaphragm. The diaphragm is the major inspiratory muscle comprised of muscular origins along the costal margins and insertions into the membranous dome. The right hemidiaphragm overlies the liver and the left hemidiaphragm overlies the stomach and spleen. On frontal radiographs exposed in deep inspiration, the apex of the right hemidiaphragm typically lies at the level of the sixth anterior rib, approximately one-half interspace above the apex of the left hemidiaphragm (Fig. 12.14). A scalloped appearance to the hemidiaphragm is not uncommon. Focal bulges in the diaphragmatic contour are usually caused by acquired diaphragmatic eventration (thinning).

Upper Abdomen. Portions of the liver, spleen, and gastric findus are routinely visualized on most frontal chest radiographs. Abnormalities of abdominal situs may be identified by noting the location and appearance of the liver, stomach, and spleen. Enlargement of the liver may cause right diaphragmatic elevation and right lateral compression of the stomach. Intrahepatic air may be seen within the biliary tree, portal vein, or a hepatic abscess. Calcified hepatic lesions such as echinococcal cysts or calcified gallstones overlying the lower portion of the liver may be visible. A mass arising within the gastric fundus can occasionally be seen as a soft tissue opacity protruding into a gas-filled gastric lumen. Splenomegaly may be identified by noting a soft tissue mass in the left upper quadrant that displaces the stomach medially and the splenic flexure of the colon inferiorly.

LATERAL CHEST RADIOGRAPH

The normal lateral chest film is a challenge because of summation of the right hemithorax over the left. (Fig. 12.1). However, knowledge of normal lateral radiographic anatomy can greatly aid in detection and localization of parenchymal and cardiomediastinal processes (7,8).

Soft Tissues. Air outlining the anterior axillary folds may render the anterior edge of these skin folds visible overlying the superior aspect of the thorax. The edges are seen as bilateral opacities that are concave anteriorly and can be followed through the level of the thoracic inlet to merge with the soft tissues of the arms.

Bones. The anterior margins of the scapulae may be seen overlying the superior and posterior aspect of the thorax. They are identified by their location, duplicity, and typical straight edge, which is oriented obliquely from superoposterior to anteroinferior. They should be identified so as to be subtracted from the analysis of the retrotracheal triangle. The thoracic spine is readily visualized on the lateral chest radiograph. The vertebral bodies should be aligned along their anterior and posterior cortical margins, forming a gradual kyphosis.

Lung Interfaces. The retrotracheal triangle is a posterosuperior radiolucent region (Fig. 12.11). Opacities in the upper lobes, retrotracheal masses (e.g., aberrant subclavian artery or posterior thyroid goiter), or esophageal masses may produce an abnormal opacity in this region. The posterior edge of the retrotracheal triangle may interface with a thin soft tissue stripe immediately anterior to the thoracic spine in this region. A thickness exceeding 3 mm should prompt an evaluation for spinal disease.

The posterior half of the aortic arch may be visible on lateral radiograph as the base of the retrotracheal triangle (Fig. 12.11). If the descending aorta is tortuous, its posterior and occasionally anterior margin may be followed for varying distances depending upon where the aorta returns to a prespinal position to traverse the aortic hiatus and enter the abdomen. Rarely, the superior margin of the arch of the azygos vein is visible overlying the lower aspect of the aortic arch. In certain individuals, the posterior edges of the arteries arising from the aortic arch may be visible in relation to the tracheal air column. The innominate artery appears as a convex posterior curvilinear opacity projecting through the upper tracheal air column, and the left subclavian artery projects just behind the tracheal air column and has a straight posterior edge. The left common carotid artery is not normally visible because it is embedded in mediastinal fat and does not contact the left lung.

The appearance of the retrosternal space depends on the shape of the sternum and the amount of anterior mediastinal fat. On well-penetrated lateral radiographs, the body of the sternum is readily visible (Fig.12.11). Immediately behind the body of the sternum, the lung interfaces with a small amount of retrosternal fat to produce the thin retrosternal stripe. Sternal fracture, infection, or tumor can distort or thicken this stripe. Enlargement of internal mammary lymph nodes (e.g., lymphoma or metastatic breast carcinoma) or arteries (e.g., coarctation of the aorta) produces masses seen projecting through the concavities seen between the costal cartilages. Occasionally, the parasternal interfaces are relatively straight and summate on the retrosternal line simulating thickening of the retrosternal stripe. Inferiorly, the left lung may be excluded from contacting the anteromedial chest wall by a round or triangular opacity that represents the cardiac apex and adjacent extapleural fat. This impression on the anterior surface of the lingula has been termed the "cardiac incisura" and should not be mistaken for a mass. CT will prove helpful in equivocal cases. A mass arising within the anterior mediastinum may encroach on this retrosternal clear space. These masses may not be visible on the frontal radiograph.

In 20% of normal individuals, a thin curvilinear white line may be seen paralleling the anteroinferior cardiac margin. This line is visible when epicardial fat and fat in the anterior mediastinum outline the inner and outer edges of the visceral and parietal pericardium respectively. Normally less than 2 mm in thickness, this pericardial stripe suggests pericardial effusion when the thickness increases.

The posterior aspect of the inferior vena cava is visible in a majority of individuals as a concave posterior or straight edge visible at the posteroinferior cardiac margin just above the diaphragm (Fig. 12.11). In a small percentage of patients, the cava has a convex interface with the lung, which should not be mistaken for a mass or lymph node enlargement.

The hemidiaphragms appear as parallel domed structures on lateral radiographs (Fig. 12.1). At maximal inspiration, the posterior portion lies at a more inferior level than the anterior portion, creating a deep posterior costophrenic sulcus and a more shallow anterior sulcus. Several methods of distinguishing the right from left hemidiaphragm on the lateral view exist. The right hemidiaphragm is more commonly seen in its entire anteroposterior extent than the left because the heart excludes the left lung from contacting the anterior aspect of the left hemidiaphragm. On a well-positioned left lateral chest radiograph, with the right side of the thorax farther from the x-ray cassette than the left, the right anterior and posterior costophrenic sulcus should project beyond the corresponding left-sided sulci due to x-ray beam divergence. Identifying the right and left costophrenic sulci should allow identification of the corresponding hemidiaphragms. The presence of air in the stomach or splenic flexure projecting above one hemidiaphragm and below another identifies the more cephalad structure as the left hemidiaphragm. Occasionally, when the right and left major fissures are distinguishable (the left is more vertically oriented than the right), tracing a major fissure to

its point of contact with the diaphragm will allow identification of that hemidiaphragm.

ANATOMY OF THE THORACIC INLET

The thoracic inlet is the junction between the neck and mediastinum proper. It parallels the plane of the first rib and therefore slopes upward from anterior to posterior. The anatomy of the thoracic inlet is best depicted by CT and MR (Fig. 12.15)(Table 12.6). The most anterior aspect of the thoracic inlet is occupied by the thymus gland. The thymus extends inferiorly into the anterior

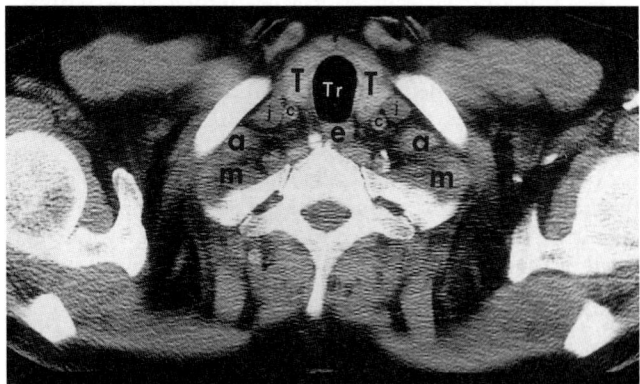

Figure 12.15. Normal Anatomy of the Thoracic Inlet. *Tr,* trachea; *t,* thyroid; *e,* esophagus; *j,* internal jugular vein; *c,* common carotid artery; *a,* anterior scalene muscle; *m,* middle scalene muscle.

Table 12.6. Contents of the Thoracic Inlet and Mediastinum

Compartment	Contents
Thoracic inlet	Thymus
	Confluence of right and left internal jugular and subclavian veins
	Right and left carotid arteries
	Right and left subclavian arteries
	Trachea
	Esophagus
	Prevertebral fascia
	Phrenic, vagus, recurrent laryngeal nerves
Anterior mediastinum	Internal mammary vessels
	Internal mammary and prevascular lymph nodes
	Thymus
Middle mediastinum	Heart and pericardium
	Ascending and transverse aorta
	Main and proximal right and left pulmonary arteries
	Confluence of pulmonary veins
	Superior and inferior vena cava
	Trachea and main bronchi
	Lymph nodes and fat within mediastinal spaces
Posterior mediastinum	Descending aorta
	Esophagus
	Azygous and hemiazygous veins
	Thoracic duct
	Sympathetic ganglia and intercostal nerves
	Lymph nodes

mediastinum, where it appears in adults as a triangular or bilobed fatty structure, with varied amounts of residual glandular tissue in younger adults. The right and left subclavian veins enter the thorax from the axillae anterior to the anterior scalene muscle to join the right and left internal jugular veins at the anterolateral aspect of the thoracic inlet to form the right and left brachiocephalic veins, respectively. The subclavian arteries occupy the lateral aspect of the thoracic inlet, behind the corresponding subclavian veins. They curve laterally to exit the thorax at a slightly higher level than the veins enter, coursing behind the anterior scalene muscles toward the axillae. The carotid arteries course vertically within the anterior portion of the thoracic inlet, anterolateral to the trachea, posteromedial to the subclavian and brachiocephalic veins, and immediately behind the thymus. The trachea occupies a midline position within the thoracic inlet, immediately surrounded anteriorly by the carotid, laterally by the subclavian arteries, and posteriorly by the upper esophagus. The esophagus lies in a prevertebral location immediately behind the posterior tracheal membrane. The thoracic duct lies to the left and posterolateral to the esophagus, arching forward above the left subclavian artery to enter the posterior aspect of the left internal jugular and subclavian veins at their confluence to form the left brachiocephalic vein. The right and left superior intercostal veins run vertically immediately anterolateral to the upper thoracic spine. The prevertebral fascia is a thin connective tissue membrane that is inseparable from the anterior longitudinal ligament of the upper thoracic spine. The phrenic and vagus nerves are not visible on CT scans, but run together in the space between the subclavian arteries and brachiocephalic veins. The recurrent laryngeal nerves lie on each side within the tracheoesophageal groove.

NORMAL MEDIASTINAL ANATOMY

The mediastinum is a narrow, vertically oriented structure that resides between the medial parietal pleural layers of the lungs, and contains central cardiovascular, tracheobronchial structures, and the esophagus enveloped in fat with intermixed lymph nodes (Table 12.6)(9). Several schemes have been described to divide the mediastinum into separate compartments. The most commonly used classification is the anatomic method, in which a line drawn through the sternal angle anteriorly and fourth thoracic intervertebral space posteriorly divides the mediastinum into superior and inferior compartments. The inferior mediastinum is further subdivided into anterior, middle, and posterior compartments. This division of the mediastinum is purely arbitrary as no true anatomic boundaries between the three compartments exist. However, by using the most easily recognizable mediastinal structure—the heart—as the focal point, the relationship of mediastinal masses to the heart allows for simple and consistent compartmentalization. Furthermore, this division of the mediastinum corresponds to easily recognizable regions as seen on the lateral chest radiograph. A minor variation of the anatomic method, in which there is no superior and in-

ferior division and the anterior, middle, and posterior compartments extend vertically from the thoracic inlet superiorly to the diaphragm inferiorly, is most practical for radiologists and is used here (Fig. 12.16). Within each compartment are readily identifiable structures and a number of spaces, in free communication with one another, that contain fat and lymph nodes. The structures and spaces native to each compartment and their normal appearance are reviewed here.

Anterior Mediastinum. The anterior (prevascular) mediastinal compartment includes all structures behind the sternum and anterior to the heart and great vessels, and it also includes the internal mammary vessels and lymph nodes, thymus, and the brachiocephalic veins (Table 12.6). The internal mammary vessels reside within the parasternal fat and lie on either side of the sternum. Normal lymphs nodes accompany the vessels but are not routinely visualized on CT. The interface of the retrosternal space with the anterior portion of right and left lungs may be visualized on lateral chest radiographs. The thymus is a triangular or bilobed structure that is maximal in size at puberty and then undergoes gradual fatty involution. In most individuals older than 35 years of age, the thymus is predominantly fatty with

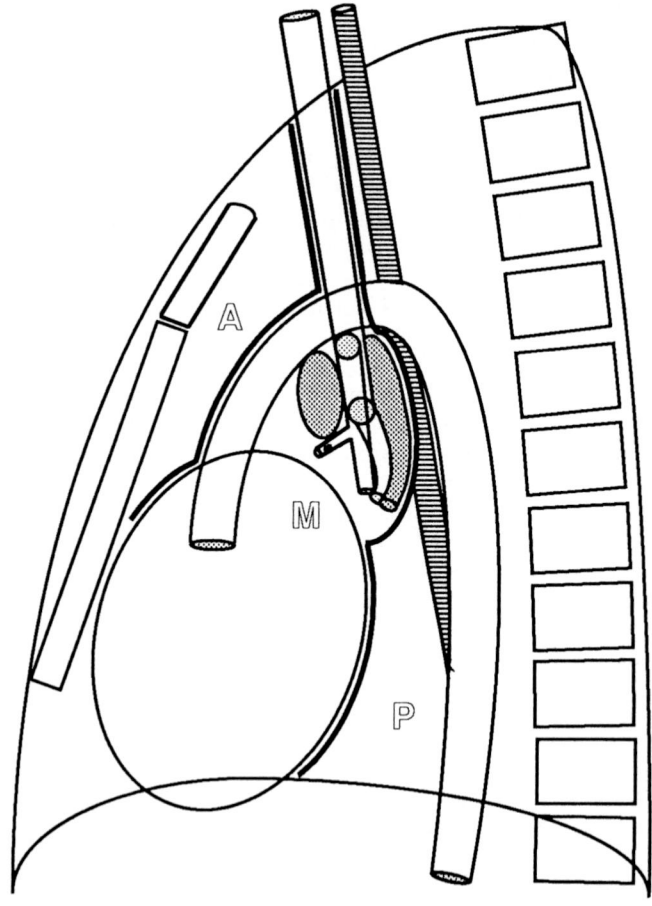

Figure 12.16. Mediastinal Compartments as Defined on Lateral View. *A*, anterior mediastinum; *M*, middle mediastinum; *P*, posterior mediastinum.

little or no intermixed glandular (soft tissue) component (Fig. 12.17A). The margins of the gland in an adult should be flat or concave toward the lung. The left lobe is commonly larger than the right. Anatomically, the thymus lies in the prevascular space, which is continuous with the retrosternal space anteriorly. It lies immediately anterior to the superior vena cava, aortic arch and great vessels, the main pulmonary artery, and more inferiorly, the heart. The prevascular space generally retains the triangular configuration of the involuted thymus. Normal lymph nodes may be visible on CT within the fat of the prevascular space. Beginning at the level of the aortic arch in most individuals, the anterior portion of the prevascular space tapers to form a thin, vertically oriented linear density that represents the anterior junction line. The right and left brachiocephalic veins occupy the posterior aspect of the prevascular space at the level of the root of the great vessels. The right brachiocephalic vein is seen on CT as a round density due to its vertical orientation whereas the crossing left brachiocephalic vein appears oval or tubular in configuration.

Middle Mediastinum. The middle (vascular) mediastinal compartment is comprised of the pericardium and its contents, the aortic arch and proximal great arteries, central pulmonary arteries and veins, trachea and main bronchi, and lymph nodes (Table 12.6). The hila may be considered as extensions of the middle mediastinal compartment. Superiorly, at the level of the crossing left brachiocephalic vein, the brachiocephalic, left common carotid, and left subclavian arteries surround the trachea with the large brachiocephalic artery directly anterior, the small left common carotid artery anterolateral, and the intermediate-sized subclavian artery directly lateral to the tracheal air column (Fig. 12.17A). More inferiorly, the superior vena cava and the oval-shaped, obliquely oriented aortic arch surround the trachea anteriorly (Fig. 12.17B). Immediately below the aortic arch, through the level of the ascending and descending aorta, are four middle mediastinal spaces that surround the trachea and carina (Fig. 12.17C). The right paratracheal space, a narrow space that contains lymph nodes and a small amount of fat, appears as the right paratracheal stripe on frontal chest radiographs. This space extends from the thoracic inlet superiorly to the azygos vein inferiorly. At this level, the pretracheal space is seen between the trachea posteriorly and the posterior margin of the ascending aorta anteriorly. In addition to fat and small lymph nodes, this space, which is contiguous with the precarinal space inferiorly, contains the retroaortic portion of the superior pericardial recess. The pretracheal space is traversed during routine transcervical mediastinoscopy. The retrotracheal space's thickness is highly variable in the anteroposterior dimension, depending on the degree of invagination of the right upper lobe behind the upper trachea. To the left of the trachea lies the aortopulmonary window. The borders of the aortopulmonary window are as follows: the aortic arch superiorly; the left pulmonary artery inferiorly; the distal trachea, left main bronchus, and esophagus medially; the mediastinal pleural surface of the left upper lobe laterally; the posterior surface of the ascending aorta anteriorly; and the anterior surface of the proximal descending aorta posteriorly. This space contains fat, lymph nodes, the ligamentum arteriosum, and the left recurrent laryngeal nerve.

Continuing inferiorly, the main and left pulmonary arteries occupy the left anterolateral portion of the middle mediastinum (Fig. 12.17D). The tracheal carina forms the posterior margin of the middle mediastinum. The right upper lobe bronchus is seen just below the tracheal carina. More inferiorly, the right pulmonary artery is seen coursing toward the right and slightly posteriorly just behind the ascending aorta and anterior to the bronchus intermedius (Fig. 12.17E). The subcarinal space is outlined posteriorly by air in the azygoesophageal recess and anteriorly by the posterior aspect of the transverse right pulmonary artery. The left superior pulmonary vein lies immediately anterior to the left main and upper lobe bronchi.

The main pulmonary artery can be followed inferiorly to the level of the outflow tract of the right ventricle. At this level, the right and left atrial appendages and the top of the left atrium proper may be seen (Fig. 12.17F). Also at this level, the right superior pulmonary vein lies anterior to the middle lobe bronchus, which in turn lies immediately anterior to the right lower lobe bronchus. Inferiorly, the right atrium proper, right ventricle, and left ventricle are identified (Fig. 12.17G).

ATS Nodal Stations. To provide greater uniformity in the nodal staging of bronchogenic carcinoma and thereby help guide diagnostic and therapeutic efforts in this disease, the American Thoracic Society (ATS) has devised a standard classification scheme for mediastinal lymph nodes (see Fig. 13.8).

Posterior Mediastinum. The posterior (postvascular) mediastinal compartment lies behind the pericardium and includes the esophagus, descending aorta, azygous and hemiazygous veins, thoracic duct, and intercostal and autonomic nerves (Table 12.5). The esophagus lies posterior or posterolateral to the trachea from the level of the thoracic inlet superiorly to the tracheal carina inferiorly. From the thoracic inlet to the level of the aortic arch, the right and left upper lobe of lung meet behind the esophagus and anterior to the spine to form the narrow posterior junction line seen on CT through the upper thorax and appearing as a vertical line through the tracheal air column on frontal radiographs. The esophagus then maintains a constant relationship with the descending thoracic aorta, usually lying anteromedial to the aorta (Figs. 12.17, 12.18) down to the level of the aortic hiatus, where the aorta is in a direct prevertebral position and the esophagus crosses the aorta anteriorly to exit the thorax via the esophageal hiatus. There are lymph nodes around the descending aorta that are not normally visible. The descending aorta lies anterolateral to the thoracic spine at the level of the aortopulmonary window. In young adults the aorta maintains this position to the level of the aortic hiatus of the diaphragm, where it lies directly in the midline. In older patients and those with a tortuous or dilated aorta, the vessel lies more laterally and protrudes into the left lower lobe as it descends, carrying the esophagus with it before return-

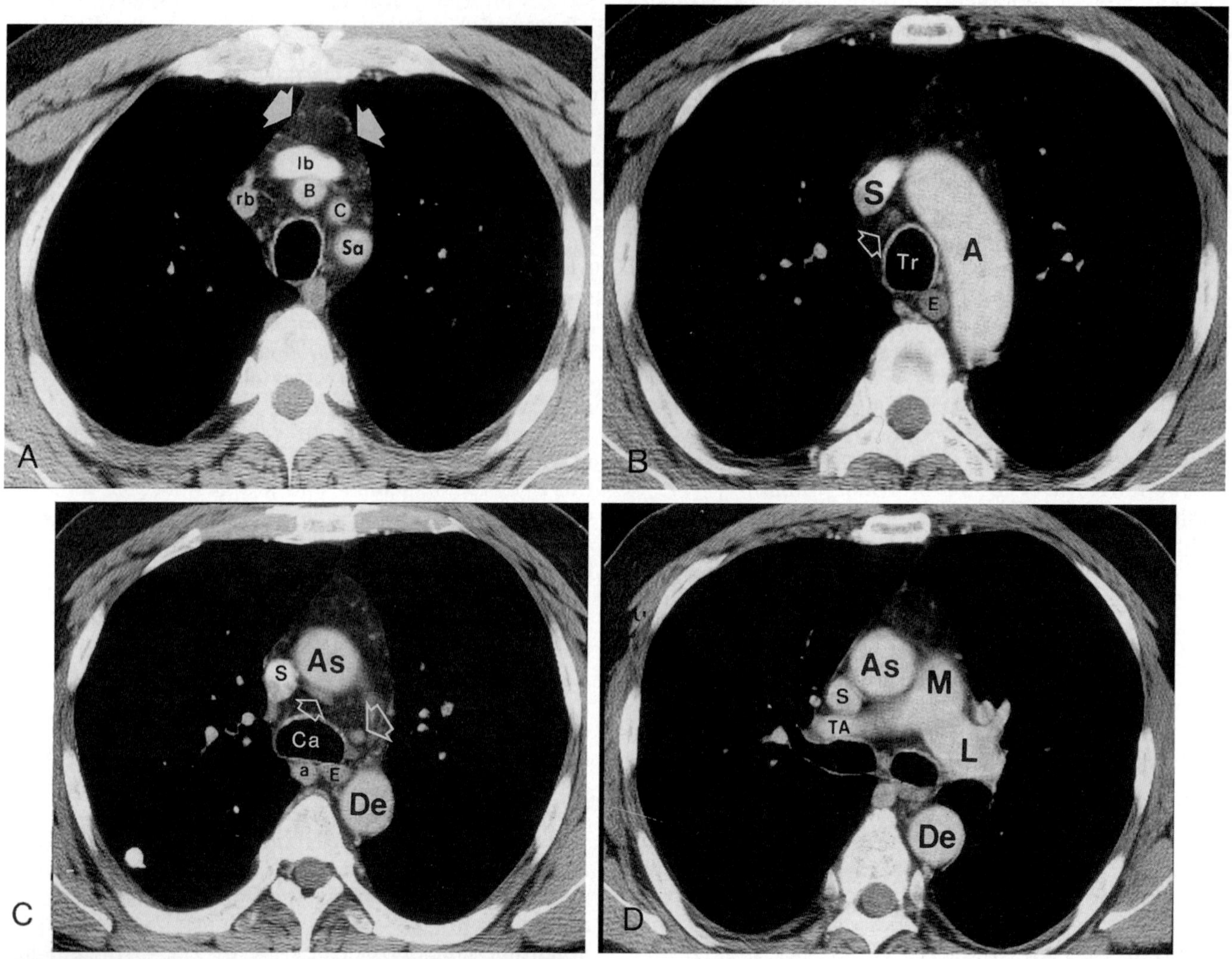

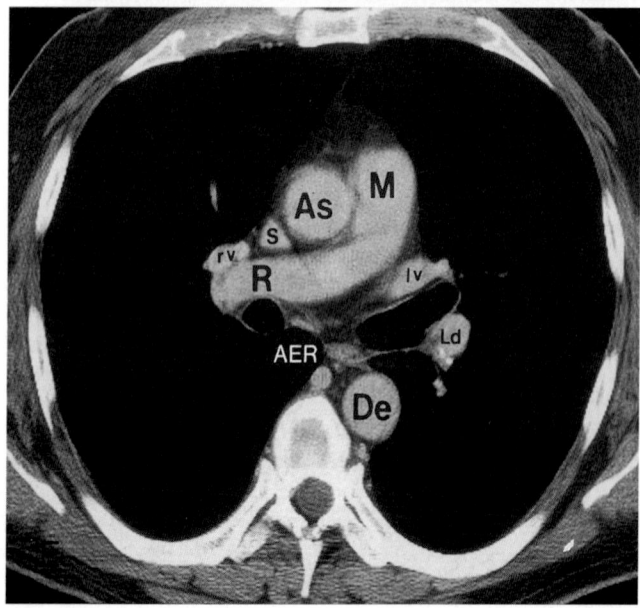

**Figure 12.17. Normal Mediastinal and Hilar Anatomy on CT.
A. Supra-aortic level.** CT scan demonstrates the triangular appearance of the fatty thymus (*arrows*) occupying the anterior mediastinum. *lb*, left brachiocephalic vein; *rb*, right brachiocephalic vein; *B*, brachiocephalic artery; *C*, common carotid artery; *Sa*, left subclavian artery. **B. Aortic arch level.** Four main structures are identified at this level. *A*, aortic arch; *S*, superior vena cava; *Tr*, trachea; *E*, esophagus. Normal-sized lymph nodes are seen in the retrocaval, pretracheal space (*open arrow*). **C. Aortopulmonary window level.** The aortopulmonary window contains fat and small lymph nodes (*large open arrow*). The retroaortic portion of the superior pericardial recess is seen as a crescent-shaped fluid-filled structure (*small open arrow*). *As*, ascending aorta; *De*, descending aorta; *S*, superior vena cava; *Ca*, tracheal carina; *a*, azygos vein; *E*, esophagus. **D. Main and left pulmonary artery level.** *As*, ascending aorta; *S*, superior vena cava; *De*, descending aorta, *M*, main pulmonary artery; *L*, left pulmonary artery; *TA*, truncus anterior branch of right pulmonary artery. **E. Right pulmonary artery and azygoesophageal recess level.** *M*, main pulmonary artery; *R*, right pulmonary artery; *As*, ascending aorta; *De*, descending aorta; *S*, superior vena cava; *rv*, right superior pulmonary veins; *lv*, left superior pulmonary veins; *Ld*, left descending pulmonary artery; *AER*, azygoesophageal recess.

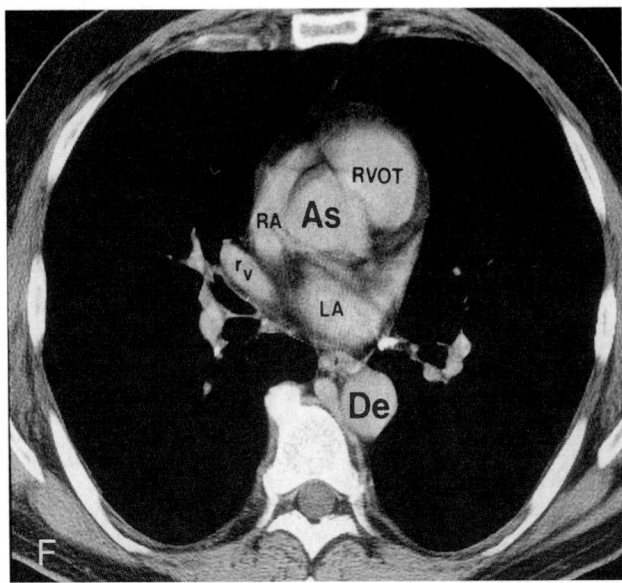

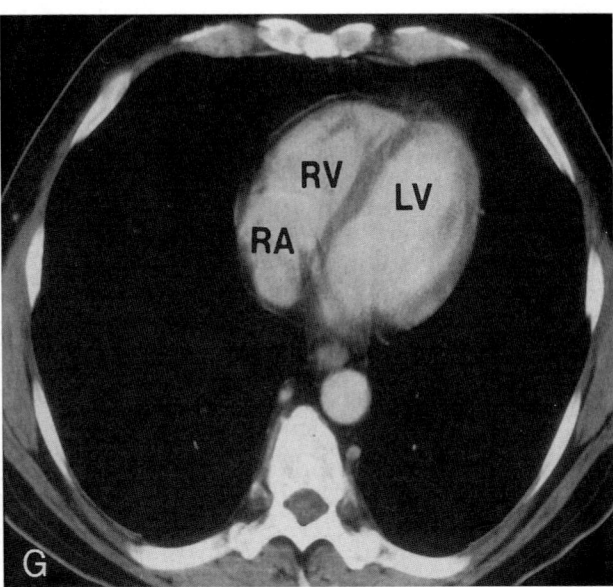

Figure 12.17. (*Continued*) F. Right ventricular outflow tract/atrial appendages. *RVOT*, right ventricular outflow tract; *RA*, right atrium; *LA*, left atrium; *rv*, right superior pulmonary vein; *As*, ascending aorta; *De*, descending aorta. **G. Ventricles and intraventricular septum.** *RA*, right atrium; *RV*, right ventricle; *LV*, left ventricle.

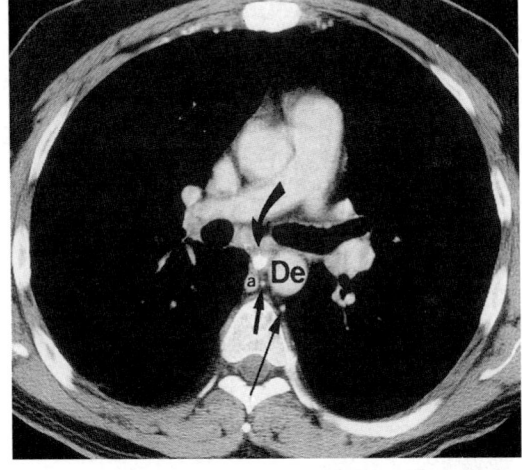

Figure 12.18. Posterior Mediastinal Anatomy. A CT scan shows a contrast-filled esophagus (*curved arrow*) anteromedial to the proximal descending aorta (*De*). Also visible within the posterior mediastinum are the azygos vein (*a*), hemiazygos vein (*long arrow*), and thoracic duct (*short arrow*).

ing to a midline position at the level of the aortic hiatus. The azygos and hemiazygos veins lie on the right and left sides respectively, posterolateral to the descending aorta within a fat-containing space that contains the thoracic duct and the sympathetic chains, structures not normally visible, and small lymph nodes (Fig. 12.18). Inferiorly, this space is continuous with the retrocrural space, and laterally with the paraspinal space, which contains the intercostal arteries, veins, and lymph nodes.

NORMAL HILAR ANATOMY

Frontal View. The hilum represents the junction of the lung with the mediastinum and is composed of up-

per lobe pulmonary veins and branches of the pulmonary artery and corresponding bronchi (Fig. 12.19). These are all enveloped by small amounts of fat with intermixed lymph nodes.

The shape of the right hilum on frontal radiograph has been likened to a sideways V, with the opening pointing to the right (Fig. 12.19A,B). The upper portion of the V is composed primarily of the truncus anterior and the posterior division of the right superior pulmonary vein. The superior pulmonary vein forms the lateral margin of the upper portion of the right hilum. The anterior and posterior segmental divisions of the right upper lobe bronchus and artery are often seen at the superolateral margin of the upper right hilum. The right descending artery forms the lower half of the V as it descends lateral to the bronchus intermedius. The right inferior pulmonary vein crosses the lower right hilar shadow but does not contribute to its opacity (Figs. 12.5B,12.19A).

On CT the upper portion of the right hilum is composed of the right superior pulmonary vein, truncus anterior division of the right pulmonary artery, and the right upper lobe bronchus. The right upper lobe pulmonary vein courses vertically, anterolateral to the truncus anterior (Fig. 12.17D–F). The right upper lobe bronchus is an eparterial bronchus because it lies above the right pulmonary artery. The lower portion of the right hilum is composed of the right descending pulmonary artery laterally and the bronchus intermedius and proximal right lower lobe bronchus medially (Fig. 12.17E,F). The right inferior pulmonary vein courses horizontally to empty into the right lateral border of the left atrium below the lower margin of the hilum medial to the right basal trunk bronchus.

The upper left hilar shadow is composed centrally of the distal left main pulmonary artery and more peripherally of one or more branches of its left upper lobe divi-

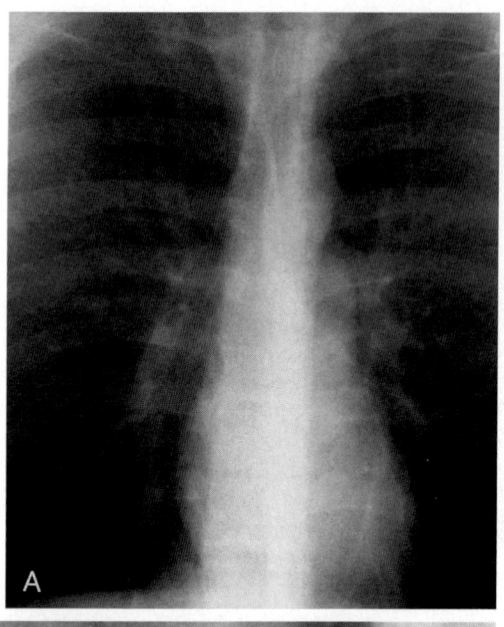

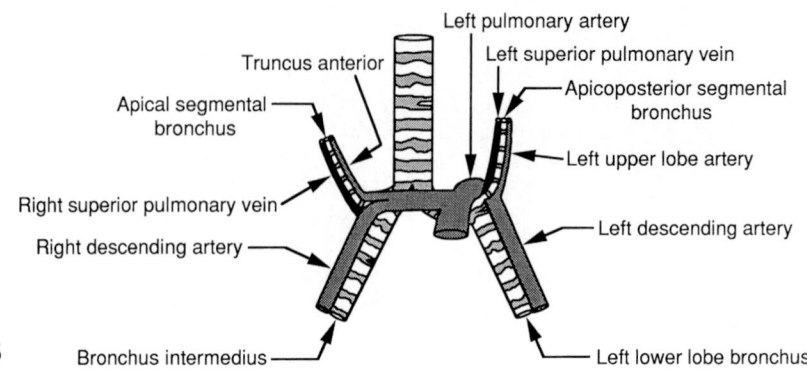

Figure 12.19. Normal Frontal and Lateral Hilar Anatomy. A. Coned-down frontal view. **B.** Diagram of frontal hilar anatomy. **C.** Coned-down left lateral view. **D.** Diagram of left lateral hilar anatomy.

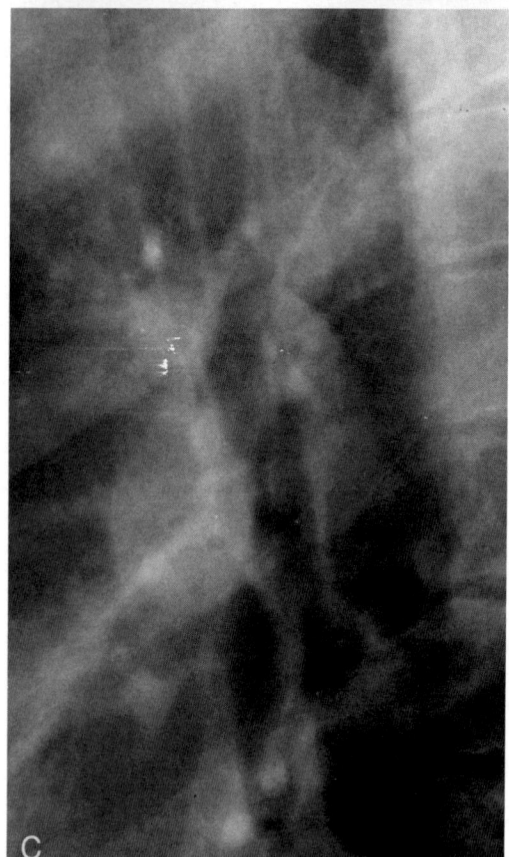

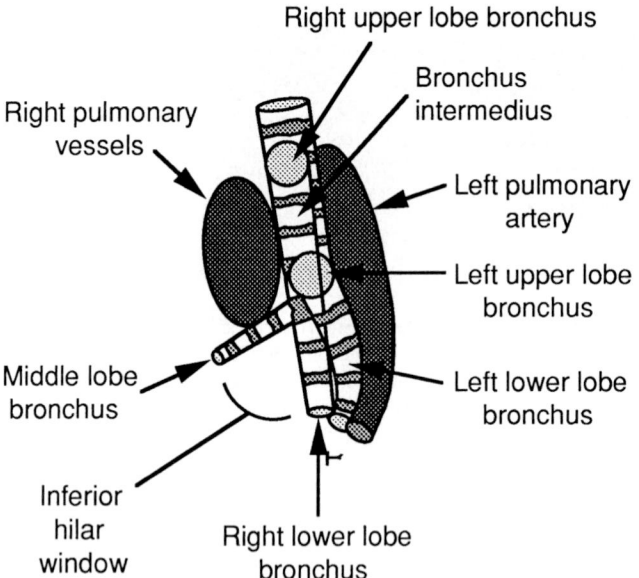

sion and the posterior division of the left superior pulmonary vein (Fig. 12.19C,D). Either the superior pulmonary vein or apicoposterior branch of the artery may form the lateral margin of the upper hilar shadow. The left upper lobe bronchus is readily identified within the central aspect of the hilar shadow because the left pulmonary artery encircles it. The anterior segmental bronchus and its accompanying artery may be seen end-on at the lateral margin of the upper left hilar shadow.

The descending artery forms the lower portion of the left hilar shadow as it descends behind the left heart. The adjacent left lower lobe bronchus is inconstantly visualized because it lies somewhat anterior and medial to the artery.

On CT of the upper left hilum, the left superior pulmonary vein courses anterior to the left pulmonary artery and, more inferiorly, anterior to the left upper lobe bronchus to empty into the superolateral aspect of the left atrium (Fig. 12.17D–F). The left pulmonary artery arches posteriorly, superiorly, and to the left, over the left main and upper lobe bronchi, to bifurcate into upper and lower lobe arteries (Fig. 12.17D). The number and size of the branches of the upper division of the left pulmonary artery are variable. The left main and upper lobe bronchi are encircled anteriorly, superiorly, and posteriorly by the left main and proximal interlobar pulmonary artery and are therefore hyparterial bronchi (Fig. 12.17D,E). The lower portion of the left hilum is composed of the left descending artery, which is posterolateral to the left lower lobe bronchus (Fig. 12.17E). The left inferior pulmonary vein courses horizontally at a level slightly behind that of the right inferior vein to empty into the left atrium just medial to the left basal trunk bronchus.

As seen on frontal radiographs, the right and left pulmonary arteries comprise the predominant portion of the hilar opacity, with the superior pulmonary veins, lobar bronchi, bronchopulmonary lymph nodes, and a small amount of fat contributing little to the overall hilar density (Fig. 12.19A). In more than 90% of normal individuals, the left hilar shadow is higher than the right. This is because the left pulmonary artery, which comprises the predominant portion of the left hilar shadow, ascends over the left main and upper lobe bronchus, but the right pulmonary artery lies inferior to the right upper lobe bronchus. In the remainder of individuals, the right and left hila lie at the same level; a right hilum that lies above the left suggests volume loss in the right upper or left lower lobe.

Left Lateral View. On a true lateral radiograph, the right and left hilar shadows are not completely superimposed and comprise a combination of the right and left pulmonary arteries and the superior pulmonary veins (Fig. 12.19C,D). The anterior aspect of the hilar shadow is composed of the transverse portion of the right pulmonary artery, which produces a vertically oriented oval opacity projecting immediately anterior to the bronchus intermedius. The confluence of right superior pulmonary veins overlaps the lower portion of the right pulmonary artery and contributes to its opacity. Superiorly and posteriorly, the comma-shaped left pulmonary artery passes above and behind the round or oval lucency representing the horizontally oriented left upper lobe bronchus summating on a portion of the left mainstem bronchus; the artery then descends behind the left lower lobe bronchus. The confluence of left superior pulmonary veins, which lie behind the level of the right superior pulmonary vein, creates an opacity that occupies the posteroinferior aspect of the composite hilar shadow. The avascular aspect of the composite hilar shadow, inferior to the shadow of the right pulmonary artery and veins and anterior to the descending left pulmonary artery and left superior vein, is called the inferior hilar window. This region is roughly triangular in shape with its apex at the junction of the left upper and lower lobe bronchi and its base directed anteriorly and inferiorly. The right middle lobe and lingular veins cross the inferior hilar window but, because of their small size, do not contribute significant opacity to this area.

The vascular structures of the composite hilar shadow

are suspended around the central bronchi (Fig. 12.19). Beginning superiorly, the right upper lobe bronchus is seen in approximately 50% of individuals as an end on round lucency at the upper margin of the composite hilar shadow. Recognition of this bronchus, when not visible on prior radiographs, should suggest a mass or lymph node enlargement around the bronchus. The posterior wall of the bronchus intermedius is a thin vertical line, 2 mm or less in thickness, extending inferiorly from the posterior aspect of the right upper lobe bronchus. The line is seen in 95% of patients and extends inferiorly to bisect the end-on lucency of the left upper lobe bronchus on a properly positioned lateral film. This structure is rendered visible because air within the intermediate bronchus anteriorly and lung within the azygoesophageal recess posteriorly outlines its posterior wall. Thickening or nodularity of this line is seen in bronchogenic carcinoma, pulmonary edema, or enlargement of azygoesophageal recess lymph nodes. The left upper lobe bronchus, which is seen in 75% of individuals, lies no more than 4 cm directly inferior to the right upper lobe bronchus. This bronchus is visualized with greater frequency than the right upper lobe bronchus because it is silhouetted by the left pulmonary artery superiorly and posteriorly, the left superior pulmonary vein posteroinferiorly, and the superior aspect of the left atrium inferiorly, and the right upper lobe bronchus is contacted only by the right main pulmonary artery anteroinferiorly and the azygous arch superiorly. The left upper lobe bronchus is identified by noting the concave anterior curvilinear density of the anterior wall of the left lower lobe bronchus extending inferiorly from its anteroinferior wall. The intersection of the posterior wall of the bronchus intermedius with the left upper lobe bronchus also helps identify the latter structure. Below the oval lucency of the left upper lobe bronchus, the basal trunk of the left lower lobe bronchus can sometimes be identified with its anterior wall visible as a white line, outlined by air in the bronchial lumen and air in the lung. The left lower lobe bronchus is seen immediately below and continuous with the horizontal left upper lobe bronchus. The basal trunk bronchus of the right lower lobe lies slightly anterior to the left lower lobe bronchus and has a straight anterior wall. It may be seen extending inferiorly from the lucency of the right upper lobe bronchus, but it is less commonly visualized than the left.

The appearance of the hila changes with slight degree of rotation. If the patient is rotated slightly right side back and left side forward, the more posteriorly positioned left pulmonary artery will be summated on the more anterior right main pulmonary artery and hila are termed "closed." On the other hand, if the rotation is slightly left side back and right side forward, the left pulmonary artery is further separated from the right and the hila are termed "open." If the patient is in a true lateral position, the beam divergence will magnify the right-sided structures and simulate minimal "closing" of the hila. The relationship of the right-sided bronchus intermedius to the round hole of the end on left upper lobe bronchus can be helpful in evaluatiing differences in rotation between serial lateral views on the same patient.

Analyzing this normal hilar relationship is helpful in determining the side of the posterior costophrenic sulcus if the ribs are not completely superimposed.

PLEURAL ANATOMY

The pleura is a serosal membrane that envelopes the lung and lines the costal surface, diaphragm, and mediastinum (10). It is composed of two layers, the visceral and the parietal pleura, which join at the hilum. Blood supply to the parietal pleura is via the systemic circulation, but the visceral pleura is supplied by the pulmonary circulation. The parietal pleura is contiguous with the chest wall and diaphragm and therefore extends deep posteriorly into the costophrenic sulci, and the visceral pleura is adherent to the surface of the lung. The pleural space is a potential space between the two pleural layers, and normally contains a small amount of fluid (<5 cc) that reduces friction during breathing.

The normal costal, diaphragmatic, and mediastinal pleura is not visible on plain radiographs or CT. On HRCT, a 1–2-mm stripe may be seen lining the intercostal spaces

between adjacent ribs (Fig. 12.20). This "intercostal stripe" represents the combination of the two pleural layers, the endothoracic fascia, and the innermost intercostal muscle (Fig. 12.21). Internal to the ribs, the normal pleura is not seen and the inner cortex of rib appears to contact the lung. The presence of soft tissue density between the inner rib and the lung, best appreciated on HRCT studies, indicates pleural thickening. The innermost intercostal muscle is anatomically absent in the paravertebral area; if a thin line is visible between the lung and paravertebral fat or rib, it represents a combination of the two pleural surfaces and the endothoracic fascia.

The normal radiographic and CT appearance of the fissures and the inferior pulmonary ligament are discussed earlier in this chapter.

CHEST WALL ANATOMY

The radiographic anatomy of the soft tissues and bony structures of the chest wall were discussed in the section on the normal frontal radiograph. CT provides detailed anatomic information about the normal chest wall and axillae. Although the bilateral symmetry of the chest wall on CT usually allows for the detection of pathologic conditions, a detailed knowledge of normal cross-sectional chest wall and axillary anatomy is key to accurate localization and characterization of disease processes. The CT anatomy from six representative levels is shown in Figure 12.22.

ANATOMY OF THE DIAPHRAGM

The diaphragm is composed of striated muscle and a large central tendon separating the thoracic and abdominal cavities. The diaphragmatic muscle arises anteriorly from the posterior aspect of the xiphoid process, anterolaterally, laterally, and posterolaterally from the sixth to twelfth costal cartilages and ribs. The diaphragmatic crura originate from the upper lumbar vertebrae and course to the posterior aspect of the central tendon. They have no direct action on the rib cage (Fig. 12.23). The diaphragm has three normal openings and two potential gaps. The aortic hiatus lies in the midline immediately behind the diaphragmatic crura and anterior to the twelth thoracic vertebral body. The aorta, thoracic duct, and azygos and hemiazygous veins traverse this opening. The esophageal hiatus usually lies slighty to the left of midline, cephalad to the aortic hiatus, and transmits

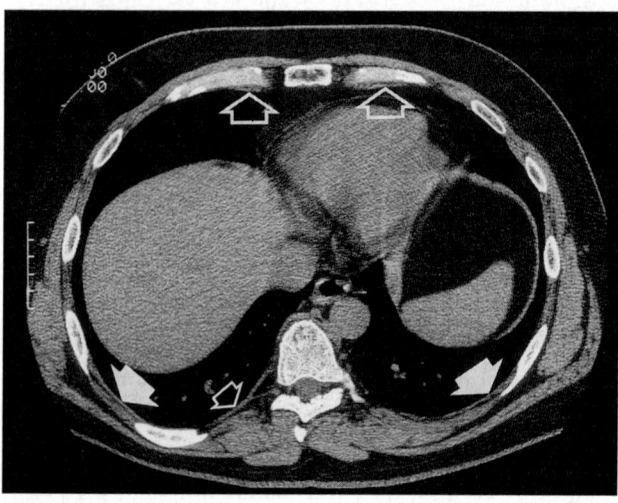

Figure 12.20. HRCT of the Pleura. HRCT through the lung bases demonstrates normal intercostal stripes *(solid arrows)* that are separated from the intercostal muscles by a layer of fat. An intercostal vein *(small open arrow)* is seen in the paravertebral region. Anteriorly, the transversus thoracic muscles *(large open arrows)* line in the parasternal pleural surface.

Figure 12.21. Normal Pleural and Chest Wall Anatomy. The visceral pleura is 0.1–0.2 mm thick and is composed of a single layer of mesothelial cells and its associated fibroelastic fascia called the subpleural interstitium that is part of the peripheral interstitial network. The parietal pleura is 0.1 mm thick and is composed of a single layer of mesothelial cells lining a loose connective tissue layer containing systemic capillaries, lymphatics, and sensory nerves. Outside the parietal pleura is the fibroelastic endothoracic fascia separated from the pleura by a thin layer of extrapleural fat. The endothoracic fascia lines the ribs and intercostal muscles.

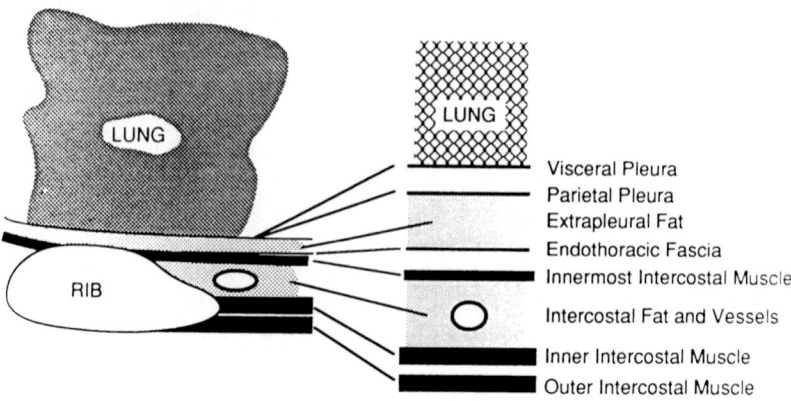

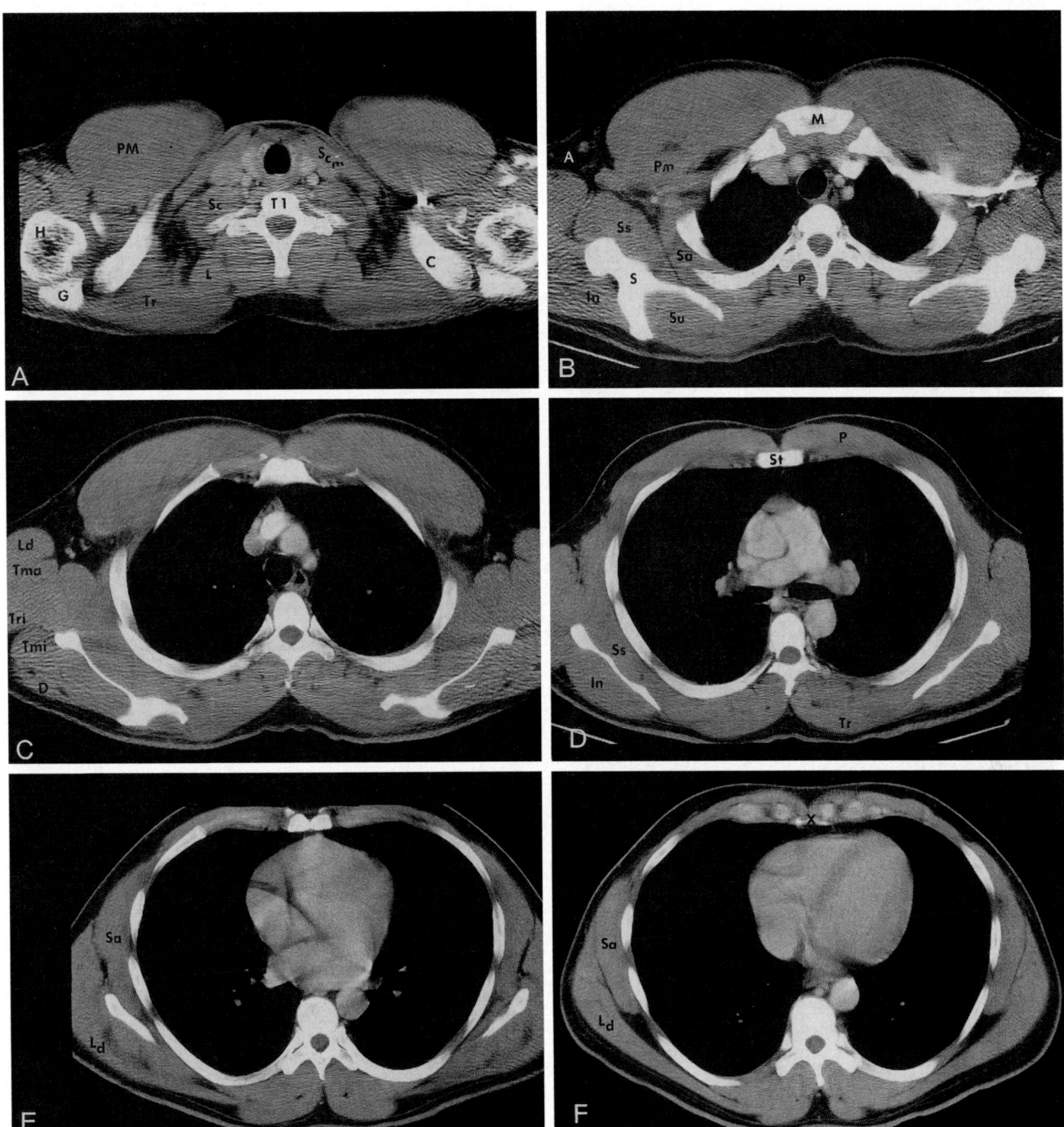

Figure 12.22. Normal Chest Wall Anatomy on CT. A. Level of the thoracic inlet. *PM*, pectoralis major muscle; *Tr*, trapezius muscle; *L*, levator scapulae muscle; *Sc*, scalene muscle; *Scm*, sternocleidomastoid muscle; *H*, humeral head; *G*, glenoid; *C*, distal clavicle; *T1*, first thoracic vertebral body. **B. Level of the axillary vessels.** *Pm*, pectoral minor muscle; *Sa*, serratus anterior muscle; *Su*, supraspinatus muscle; *In*, intraspinatus muscle; *Ss*, subscapularis muscle; *P*, paraspinal muscles; *M*, manubrium of the sternum. *S*, body of the scapula; *A*, axilla with normal lymph nodes. **C. Level of the ster-** nomanubrial joint. *Ld*, latissiumus dorsi muscle; *Tma*, teres major muscle; *Tri*, long head of the triceps muscle; *Tmi*, teres minor muscle; *D*, deltoid muscle. **D. Level of the body of the sternum.** *P*, pectoralis muscles; *Ss*, subscapularis muscle; *In*, intraspinatus muscle; *Tr*, trapezius muscle; *St*, body of the sternum. **E. Level of tip of scapula.** *Ld*, latissimus dorsi muscle; *Sa*, serratus anterior muscle. **F. Level of the xiphoid process.** *Ld*, latissimus dorsi muslce; *Sa*, serratus anterior muscle; *X*, xiphoid process of the sternum.

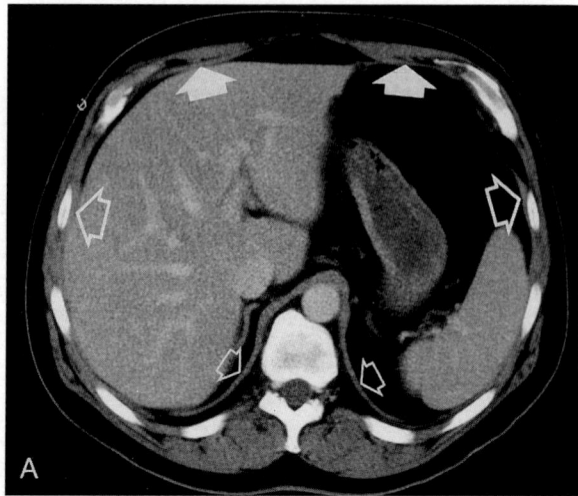

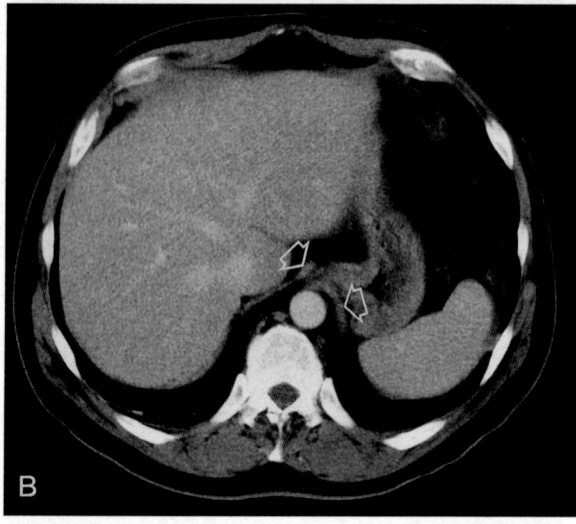

Figure 12.23. Normal Anatomy of the Diaphragm on CT. A. A scan through the upper abdomen demonstrates the crura of the diaphragm posteriorly (*small open arrows*), the costal origins of the diaphragm laterally (*large open arrows*), and the costal cartilaginous origins anterolaterally (*solid arrows*). **B.** More inferiorly, the esophageal hiatus is seen between the crura (*open arrows*).

the esophagus and vagus nerves. The inferior vena cava pierces the central tendon of the diaphragm at the level of the eighth thoracic intervertebral disc space. The foramina of Morgagni are triangular gaps in the muscles of the anteromedial diaphragm. This cleft is normally occupied by fat and the internal mammary vessels; it is a site of potential intrathoracic herniation of abdominal contents. The foramina of Bochdalek are defects in the closure of the posterolateral diaphragm at the junction of the pleuroperitoneal membrane with the septum transversum. Hernias through the foramina of Morgagni and Bochdalek are discussed in chapter 20.

The radiographic appearance of the diaphragms on frontal and lateral chest radiographs is discussed in preceding sections. The domes of the diaphragms appear as rounded opacities on either side of the chest on CT at the level of the base of the heart. In some patients scanned on deep inspiration, the diaphragm has an undulating or nodular appearance from contraction of slips of diaphragmatic muscle. This appearance is seen with increasing frequency in older patients and is more common on the left than the right. Posteriorly, the superior aspects of the diaphragmatic crura are seen. The crura are curvilinear opacities that arise from the upper two to three lumbar vertebrae, and their associated esophageal and aortic openings within the bundles of the crura are well visualized on CT (Fig. 12.23). Continuing inferiorly into the upper abdomen, the inferior aspects of the diaphragmatic crura may have a rounded appearance in cross-section and should not be mistaken for enlarged retrocrural lymph nodes. Review of contiguous CT images will allow proper identification of these structures.

References

1. Wilkinson GA, Fraser RG. Roentgenography of the chest. Appl Radiol 1975;4:41–53.
2. Ravin CE, Chotas HG. Chest radiography. Radiology 1997; 204:593–600.
3. Wandtke JC. Bedside chest radiography. Radiology 1994; 192:282–284.
4. Webb WR, Sostman HD. MR imaging of thoracic disease: clinical uses. Radiology 1992;182:621–630.
5. Westcott JL. Percutaneous transthoracic biopsy. Radiology 1988;169:593–601.
6. Raasch BN, Carsky EW, Lane EJ, et al. Radiographic anatomy of the interlobar fissures: a study of 100 specimens. AJR Am J Roentgenol 1982;138:1043.
7. Proto AV, Speckman JM. The left lateral radiograph of the chest 1. Med Radiogr Photogr 1979;55:30–74.
8. Proto AV, Speckman JM. The left lateral radiograph of the chest 2. Med Radiogr Photogr 1980;56:38–64.
9. Heitzman ER. The Mediastinum: Radiologic Correlations with Anatomy and Pathology. Berlin: Spinger-Verlag, 1988: 311–349.
10. Im JG, Webb WR, Rosen A, et al. Costal pleura: appearances at high-resolution CT. Radiology 1989;171:125–131.

13

Mediastinum and Hila

Jeffrey S. Klein

This chapter will review the radiologic approach to mediastinal masses, diffuse mediastinal disease, and hilar abnormalities.

MEDIASTINAL MASSES

Localized mediastinal abnormalities are common diagnostic challenges for the radiologist. Patients with mediastinal masses tend to present in one of two fashions: with symptoms related to local mass effect or invasion of adjacent mediastinal structures (stridor in a patient with thyroid goiter), or incidentally, with an abnormality on routine chest radiograph. Occasionally, a mediastinal mass is discovered in the course of an evaluation for known malignancy (a patient with non-Hodgkin's lymphoma) or for a condition such as myasthenia gravis, in which there is an association with thymoma. CT and MR are the primary cross-sectional modalities used to evaluate mediastinal masses (Table 13.1).

For the purposes of the following discussion, the mediastinum is divided into superior (thoracic inlet) and inferior components, with the inferior mediastinum subdivided into anterior, middle, and posterior compartments as described in chapter 12.

Thoracic Inlet Masses

The thoracic inlet is the region of the upper thorax marginated by the first rib, and it represents the junction between the neck and thorax. Masses in this region commonly present as neck masses or with symptoms of upper airway obstruction owing to tracheal compression. Thyroid masses, lymphomatous nodes, and lymphangiomas are the most common thoracic inlet masses (Table 13.2).

Thyroid Masses. In a small percentage of patients with cervical thyroid goiters, thyroid carcinomas, or enlarged glands from thyroiditis, extension of the thyroid through the thoracic inlet into the superior mediastinum may occur. These lesions are usually discovered as incidental findings on chest radiographs; a minority of patients will present with symptoms of dyspnea or dysphagia caused by tracheal or esophageal compression. Thyroid goiters arising from the lower pole of the thyroid or the thyroid isthmus can enter the superior mediastinum anterior to the trachea (80%) or to the right and posterolateral to the trachea (20%).

On chest radiographs, an anterosuperior mediastinal mass typically deviates the trachea laterally and either posteriorly (anterior masses) or anteriorly (posterior masses). Coarse, clumped calcifications are common in thyroid goiters. Radioiodine studies should be performed as the initial imaging procedure although false-negatives do occur. CT usually shows characteristic findings: *a)* well-defined margins, *b)* continuity of the mass with the cervical thyroid, *c)* coarse calcifications, *d)* cystic or necrotic areas, *e)* baseline high CT attenuation (owing to intrinsic iodine content), and *f)* intense enhancement (>25 H) owing to the hypervascularity of most thyroid masses and prolonged enhancement (caused by active uptake of iodine from contrast media) following intravenous contrast administration (Fig. 13.1)(1). MR is useful in depicting the longitudinal extension of thyroid goiters without the use of intravenous contrast (Fig. 13.2).

Parathyroid Masses. In approximately 2% of patients, the parathyroid glands do not separate from the thymus in the neck and thus descend with the gland into the anterosuperior mediastinum. These glands can be found near the thoracic inlet in or about the thymus. This is important in the small percentage of patients with persistent clinical and biochemical evidence of hyperparathyroidism following routine neck exploration and parathyroidectomy. Most of these ectopic parathyroid lesions are small (<3 cm) adenomas; rarely, they represent hyperplastic glands or parathyroid carcinoma. When US and nuclear medicine studies have failed to localize a lesion in the neck, CT, MR, or Tc-99m sestamibi scanning may be useful in detecting mediastinal lesions (Fig. 13.3).

Lymphangiomas. These uncommon masses are tumors comprised of dilated lymphatic channels. The cystic or cavernous form (cystic hygroma) is most commonly discovered in infancy and is often associated with chromosomal abnormalities including Turner's syndrome and trisomies 13, 18, and 21. In infants, these lesions extend from the neck into the anterior mediastinum; less commonly, they may arise primarily within the anterior mediastinum in older patients. Histologically, these tumors contain cystic spaces lined by epithelium filled with clear straw-colored fluid. Although these lesions are benign histologically, they usually insinuate themselves

Table 13.1. Utility of CT and MR in the Evaluation of Mediastinal Masses

Indication for Study	Modalities
Confirming the presence of a mass vs. tortuous vascular structures	CT = MR
Localization of mass to anterior, middle, or posterior compartment	CT = MR
Suspected aneurysm or vascular anomaly	MR > CT
Tissue characterization of mass	
Dectection of fluid	CT = MR = US (for anterior masses)
Detection of calcium	CT
Distinction of tumor from fibrosis	MR
Relationship to adjacent structures	
Vascular invasion	CT = MR
Tracheal involvement	CT > MR
Involvement of spinal canal	MR > CT
Thoracic inlet lesions	MR > CT
Contraindication to iodinated contrast	MR > CT
Percutaneous biopsy of mediastinal mass	CT
	US for anterior mediastinal masses

between vascular structures and the trachea. This makes complete surgical resection of lymphangiomas difficult, and they frequently recur. CT demonstrates a well-defined cystic mass within the thoracic inlet or superior mediastinum. MR typically shows a mass of high signal intensity on T2WI owing to its fluid content.

Anterior Mediastinal Masses

A number of neoplasms and nonneoplastic conditions arise in the anterior mediastinum and produce anterior mediastinal masses. These include thymic neoplasms, lymphoma, germ cell neoplasms, and primary mesenchymal tumors (Table 13.3).

Thymoma is the second most common primary mediastinal neoplasm in adults after lymphoma. A neoplasm that arises from thymic epithelium, a thymoma contains varying numbers of intermixed lymphocytes. The admixture of epithelial cells and lymphocytes, which varies with each tumor, gives rise to the histologic subtyping of thymoma as predominantly lymphocytic, mixed lymphoepithelial, and predominantly epithelial types. In the predominantly lymphocytic form, in which there are few interspersed epithelial tumor cells, the histologic differentiation from lymphoma may be difficult. No correlation exists between the histologic features of thymoma and malignant behavior; surgical and pathologic evidence of capsular and local invasion is the best predictor.

The average age at diagnosis of thymoma is 45–50; these lesions are rare in patients younger than 20. Although most often associated with myasthenia gravis, thymoma has been associated with other autoimmune diseases such as pure red cell aplasia and hypogammaglobulinemia. Of patients with myasthenia gravis, 10–28% have a thymoma, and a larger percentage of patients with thymoma (30–54%) have or will develop myasthenia.

On chest radiographs, thymomas are seen as round or oval, smooth or lobulated soft tissue masses arising near the origin of the great vessels at the base of the heart (Fig. 13.4)(2). CT is best for characterizing thymomas and detecting local invasion preoperatively. As a result of its firm consistency, thymomas characteristically maintain their shape where they contact the sternum anteriorly and heart and great vessels posteriorly. Cystic areas are not uncommon, and calcification is detected in 25% of cases (Fig. 13.4). Invasion of tumor through the thymic capsule ("invasive" or "malignant" thymoma) is present in 33–50% of patients. In the majority of these patients, this determination cannot be made by CT or MR and may even be difficult to determine on examination of the resected specimen. Local invasion of pleura, lung, pericardium, chest wall, diaphragm, and great ves-

Table 13.2. Thoracic Inlet Masses

Thyroid mass	Goiter
	Malignancy
	Thyromegaly due to thyroiditis
Parathyroid mass	Hyperplasia
	Adenoma
	Carcinoma
Lymph node mass	Lymphoma
	Hodgkin's
	Non-Hodgkin's
	Metastases
	Inflammatory
	Tuberculosis
Lymphangioma	

Table 13.3. Anterior Mediastinal Masses

Thymic masses	Thymoma
	Thymic cyst
	Thymolipoma
	Thymic hyperplasia
	Thymic neuroendocrine tumors
	Thymic carcinoma
	Thymic lymphoma
Lymphoma	Hodgkin's
	Non-Hodgkin's
Germ cell neoplasms	Teratoma
	Seminoma
	Embryonal cell carcinoma
	Endodermal sinus tumor
	Choriocarcinoma
Thyroid mass	Goiter
	Tumor
	Thyroiditis
Ectopic parathyroid mass	Hyperplasia
	Adenoma
	Carcinoma
Mesenchymal tumor	Lipoma
	Hemangioma
	Leiomyoma
	Liposarcoma
	Angiosarcoma

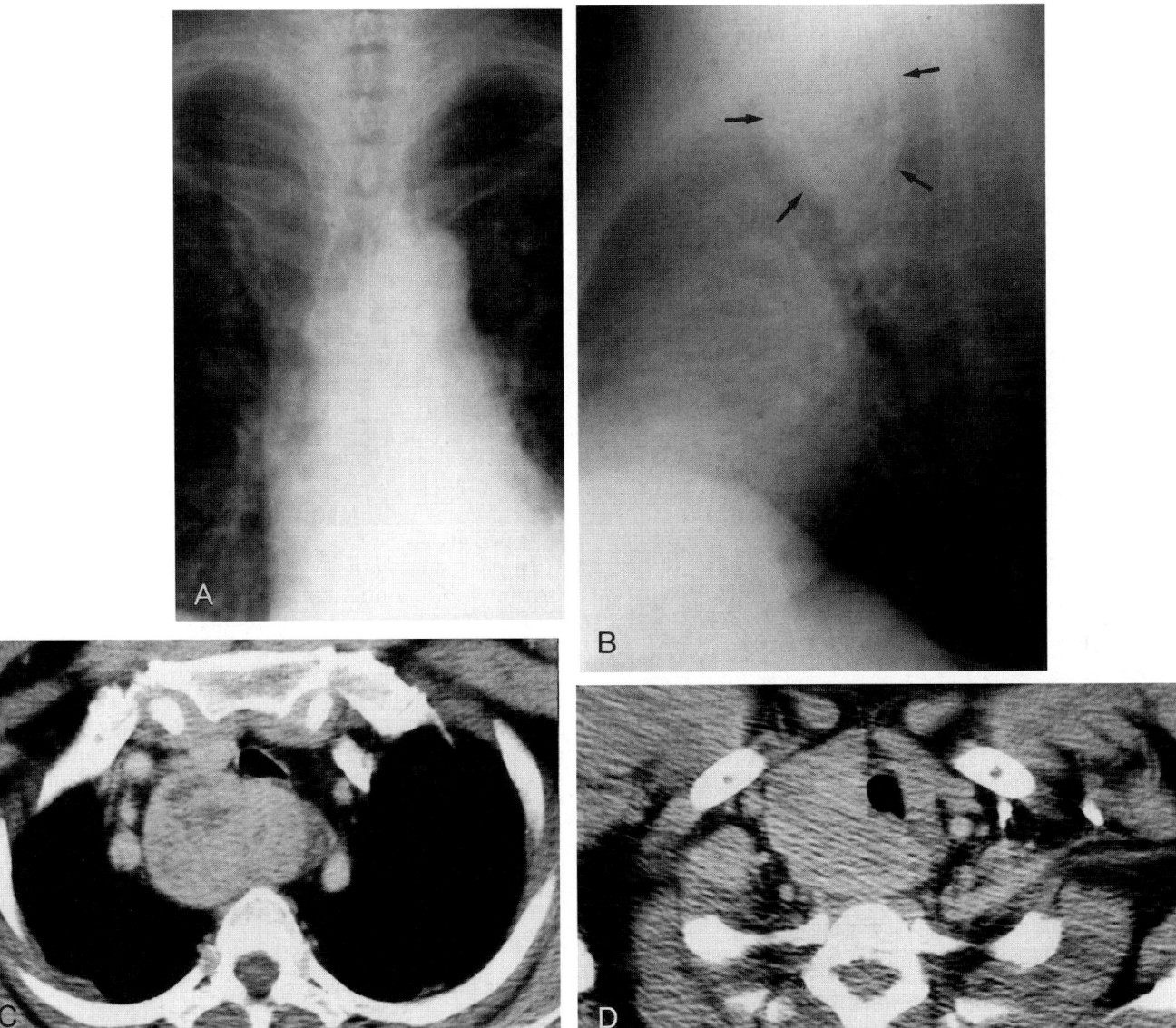

Figure 13.1. Thyroid Goiter. PA **(A)** and lateral **(B)** radiographs show a right superior mediastinal mass (*arrows*) compressing the trachea from posteriorly. **C.** Contrast-enhanced CT at the level of the sternoclavicular joints shows inhomogeneous increased attenua-tion and enlargement of the thyroid gland which extends retrotra-cheally. **D.** More superiorly, the mass is contiguous with the right lobe of an enlarged gland.

sels occurs in decreasing order of frequency in 10–15% of patients. Contiguity of a thymoma with the adjacent chest wall or mediastinal structures cannot be used as reliable evidence of invasion of these structures. Drop metastases to dependent portions of the pleural space are a recognized route of spread of thymoma that has invaded the pleura. Extrathoracic metastases are rare although transdiaphragmatic spread of pleural tumor into the retroperitoneum has been described. For these reasons, imaging the entire thorax and upper abdomen is important in any patient with suspected invasive disease.

In patients with myasthenia gravis being evaluated for thymoma, CT can demonstrate tumors that are invisible on conventional radiographs. However, very small thymic tumors may not be distinguishable from a normal or hy-perplastic gland with CT, particularly in younger patients who have a large amount of residual thymic tissue.

Thymic cysts may be congenital or acquired lesions. Congenital thymic cysts are rare lesions that contain thin or gelatinous fluid and are characterized histologi-cally by an epithelial lining with thymic tissue in the cyst wall. The latter feature distinguishes thymic cysts histo-logically from other congenital cystic lesions within the anterior mediastinum. Acquired thymic cysts have been associated with previous thoracotomy and concurrent or previously treated Hodgkin's disease. Large cysts will be evident as soft tissue masses on conventional radio-graphs, and CT or MR will demonstrate the cystic nature of the lesion. A history of Hodgkin's disease or confirma-tory needle aspiration of the cyst will allow conservative management in most patients. If the distinction between a true thymic cyst and cystic degeneration of a thymoma, lymphoma, or germ cell neoplasm is impossible on clinical and radiographic grounds, a biopsy should be done or the lesion should be resected.

Thymolipoma is a rare, benign thymic neoplasm that consists primarily of fat with intermixed rests of normal thymic tissue. These masses are asymptomatic and therefore are typically large when first detected. Chest radiographs show a large anterior mediastinal mass that, because of its pliable nature, tends to envelope the heart and diaphragm. CT demonstrates a fatty mass with interspersed soft tissue densities. Resection is curative.

Thymic Carcinoid. Neuroendocrine tumors of the thymus are rare malignant neoplasms believed to arise from thymic cells of neural crest origin (APUD or Kulchitsky cells). The most common histologic type is carcinoid tumor that, as with similar lesions arising within the bronchi, ranges in differentiation and behavior from typical carcinoid to atypical carcinoid to small cell carcinoma. Approximately 40% of patients have Cushing's syndrome as a result of ACTH secretion by the tumor; these patients have smaller lesions at time of diagnosis because they present early with signs of corticosteroid excess. The carcinoid syndrome is uncommon. This lesion is indistinguishable from thymoma on plain radiographs and CT.

Thymic hyperplasia is defined as enlargement of a thymus that is normal on gross and histological examination. This rare entity occurs primarily in children as a rebound effect in response to an antecedent stress, discontinuation of chemotherapy, or treatment of hypercortisolism. An association with Grave's disease has also been noted. The term "thymic hyperplasia" has been used incorrectly to describe the histologic findings of lymphoid follicular hyperplasia of the thymus found in 60% of patients with myasthenia gravis. In contrast to most cases of true thymic hyperplasia, lymphoid hyperplasia does not produce thymic enlargement. Most patients with thymic hyperplasia have normal or diffusely enlarged glands on CT; occasionally, thymic hyperplasia will present as a mass that is radiographically indistin-

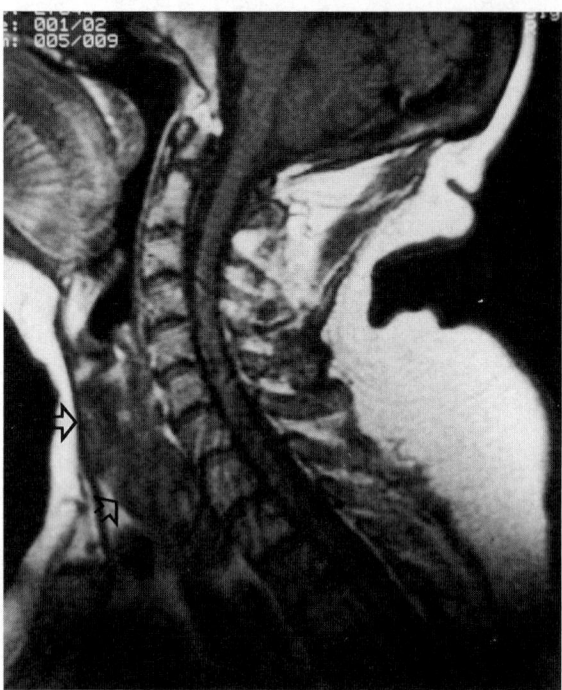

Figure 13.2. MR of Thyroid Goiter. Midline sagittal T1-weighted MR in a patient with thyroid goiter shows the enlarged gland (*arrows*) extending inferiorly into the superior mediastinum. Note the absence of the trachea on this midline image caused by lateral deviation by the goiter.

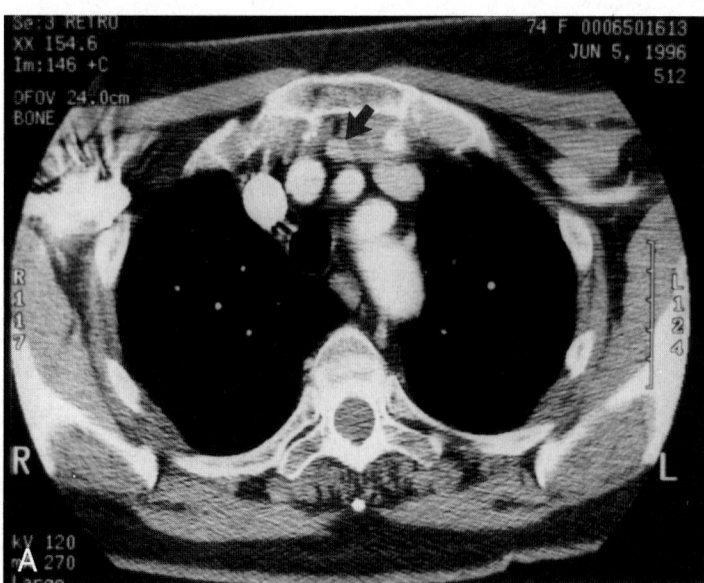

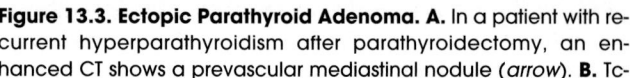

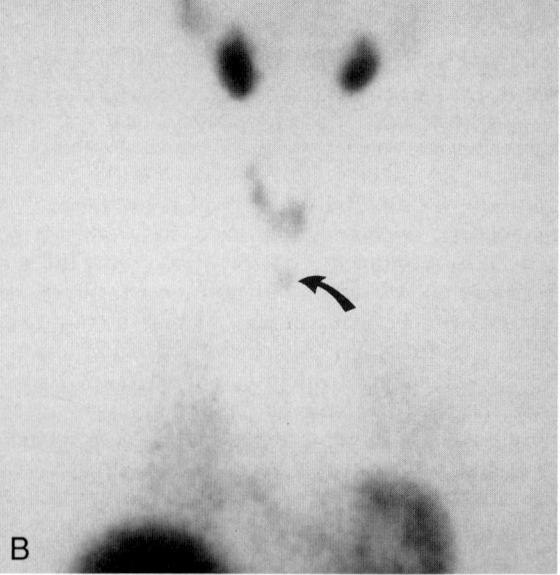

Figure 13.3. Ectopic Parathyroid Adenoma. A. In a patient with recurrent hyperparathyroidism after parathyroidectomy, an enhanced CT shows a prevascular mediastinal nodule (*arrow*). **B.** Tc- 99m sestamibi scan shows a focal area of increased activity in the superior mediastinum (*arrow*) corresponding to the nodule on CT.

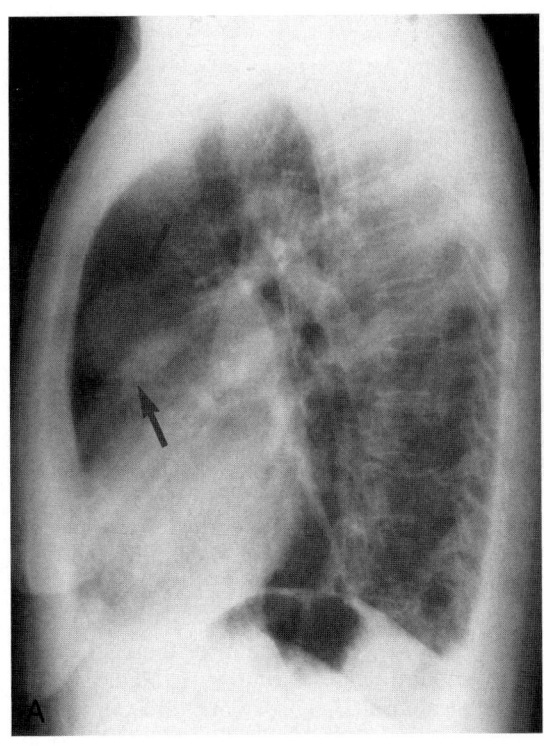
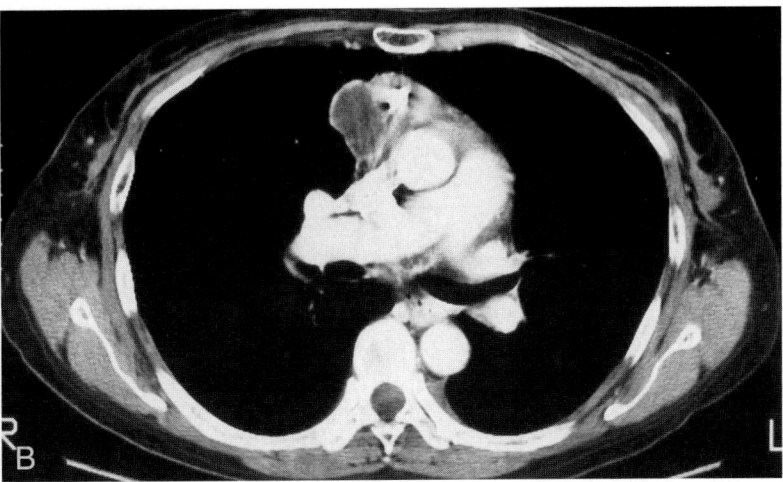

Figure 13.4. Thymoma. A. Lateral chest radiograph reveals a round anterior mediastinal mass (*arrow*). **B.** CT confirms a cystic anterior mediastinal mass with eccentric calcification. Sternotomy revealed an invasive thymoma.

guishable from thymoma. Most cases can be resolved by noting a decrease in size on follow-up studies, thereby obviating the need for biopsy.

Thymic carcinoma is a rare malignant neoplasm of the thymus diagnosed when the epithelial elements of a thymic mass show characteristic findings of cellular atypia and numerous mitoses. This lesion is distinguished from invasive thymoma, which, although malignant in behavior, lacks the histological and cytological features of carcinoma. The most common histologic subtype is squamous cell carcinoma. Most thymic carcinomas are solid lesions that on CT or MR have invaded the mediastinum or lung at the time of diagnosis.

Thymic Lymphoma. The thymus is involved in 40–50% of patients with the nodular sclerosing subtype of Hodgkin's disease. The radiographic appearance is indistinguishable from other solid neoplasms arising within the thymus. The presence of lymph node enlargement in other portions of the mediastinum or anterior chest wall involvement, best seen on T2-weighted MR images, should suggest the diagnosis.

Lymphoma is the most common primary mediastinal neoplasm in adults, and it is either Hodgkin's disease or non-Hodgkin's lymphoma, Hodgkin's disease involves the thorax in 85% of patients at time of presentation. The majority (90%) of patients with intrathoracic involvement have mediastinal lymph node enlargement; this most commonly involves the anterior mediastinal and hilar nodal groups. The anterior mediastinum is the most frequent site of a localized nodal mass in patients with Hodgkin's disease, particularly those with the nodular sclerosing type (Fig. 13.5)(3). Isolated enlargement of mediastinal or hilar nodes outside the anterior mediastinum should suggest an alternative diagnosis.

Only 25% of patients with Hodgkin's lymphoma have disease limited to the mediastinum at the time of diagnosis. Non-Hodgkin's lymphoma (NHL) involves the thorax in 40% of patients at presentation. In contrast to Hodgkin's disease, only 50% of patients with NHL and intrathoracic disease have mediastinal nodal involvement and only 10% of all patients have disease limited to the mediastinum (4). Lymphoma involving a single mediastinal or hilar nodal group is much more common in NHL than in Hodgkin's disease. Non-Hodgkin's lymphoma most commonly involves middle mediastinal and hilar lymph nodes; juxtaphrenic and posterior mediastinal nodal involvement is uncommon but is seen almost exclusively in NHL. Patterns of pulmonary parenchymal involvement in lymphoma are discussed in the section on neoplasms.

Although Hodgkin's disease spreads in a fairly predictable pattern from one nodal group to an adjacent group, NHL is felt to be a multifocal disorder for which patterns of involvement are unpredictable. Localized intrathoracic Hodgkin's disease is usually treated with radiation therapy, with 90% response rates. More widespread Hodgkin's disease and NHL are treated with chemotherapy, with better response rates for Hodgkin's disease than for NHL.

On plain radiographs, lymphoma involving the anterior mediastinum is indistiguishable from thymoma or germ cell neoplasm and presents as a lobulated mass projecting to one or both sides (Fig. 13.5A). Calcification in untreated lymphoma is extremely uncommon, and its presence within an anterior mediastinal mass should suggest another diagnosis. Involvement of other lymph nodes in the mediastinum or hila makes lymphoma more likely. An enlarged spleen displacing the gastric air

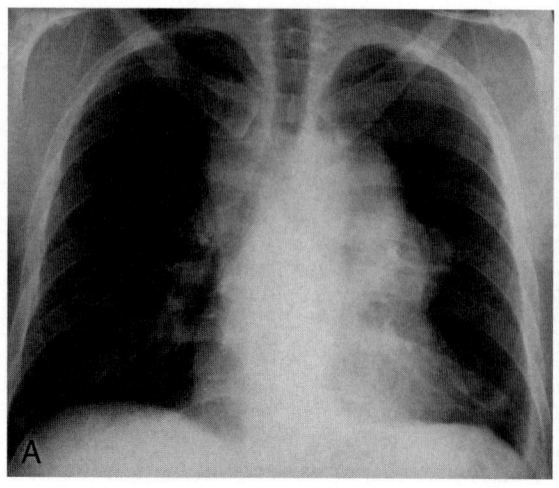 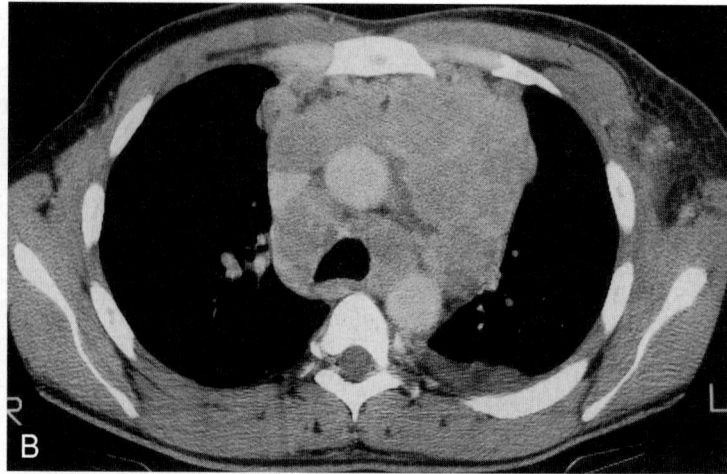

Figure 13.5. Hodgkin's Lymphoma. A. PA chest radiograph in a 35-year-old male shows a large, lobulated mediastinal mass. **B.** Contrast-enhanced CT at the level of the aortic arch shows bulky anterior and middle mediastinal lymphadenopathy.

bubble medially, seen in the upper abdominal portion of the frontal chest film, provides an additional clue to the diagnosis.

CT is performed in virtually all patients with lymphoma. The advantages of chest CT include the ability to better characterize and localize masses seen on chest radiographs; detection of subradiographic sites of involvement that can alter disease staging, prognosis, and therapy; guidance for transthoracic or open biopsy; monitoring response to therapy; and detecting relapse. The appearance of nodal involvement in lymphoma varies; most commonly, discrete enlarged solid lymph nodes or conglomerate masses of nodes are seen (Fig. 13.5B). Central necrosis, seen in 20% of patients, has no prognostic significance. Nodal calcification is rare in the absence of previous mediastinal radiation or systemic chemotherapy. Parenchymal involvement is usually the result of direct extranodal extension of tumor from hilar nodes along the bronchovascular lymphatics; this is better appreciated on axial CT images than on chest radiographs. Likewise, a tumor extending from the mediastinum to the pericardium, subpleural space, and chest wall is best appreciated on CT or MR. On MR, untreated lymphoma appears as a mass of uniform low signal intensity on T1WI, and uniform high signal intensity or intermixed areas of low and high signal intensity on T2WI. The areas of low signal intensity on T2-weighted scans of untreated patients may be caused by foci of fibrotic tissue in nodular sclerosing Hodgkin's disease.

Both CT and MR have been used to monitor response of lymphoma to therapy. Although CT can accurately assess tumor regression and detect relapse within nodal groups outside the treated region, the ability to distinguish residual tumor from sterilized fibrotic masses is limited. Residual soft tissue masses have been reported in as many as 50% of patients, most commonly with nodular sclerosing Hodgkin's disease, and are more common when the pretreatment mass is large. Some patients with residual masses on CT or MR will have tumor recurrence within 6–12 months following the completion of therapy. In general, the appearance of high sig-

nal intensity regions on T2-weighting more than 6 months after treatment should suggest recurrence. Radionuclide scintigraphy with gallium-67, particularly SPECT, is now considered the routine method of assessing disease activity within nodal masses of patients with lymphoma (Fig. 13.6).

Germ Cell Neoplasms, which include teratoma, seminoma, choriocarcinoma, endodermal sinus tumor, and embryonal cell carcinoma, arise from collections of primitive germ cells that arrest in the anterior mediastinum on their journey to the gonads during embryologic development. Because they are histologically indistinguishable from germ cell tumors arising in the testes and ovaries, the diagnosis of a primary malignant mediastinal germ cell neoplasm requires exclusion of a primary gonadal tumor as a source of mediastinal metastases. A key in distinguishing primary from metastatic mediastinal germ cell neoplasm is the presence of retroperitoneal lymph node involvement in metastatic gonadal tumors.

The most common benign mediastinal germ cell neoplasm is teratoma (5). Teratomas may be cystic or solid. The cystic, or mature, teratoma is the most common type of teratoma seen in the mediastinum. In contrast to a dermoid cyst, which is an ovarian neoplasm containing only elements derived from the ectodermal germinal layer, a cystic teratoma of the mediastinum commonly contains tissues of ectodermal, mesodermal, and endodermal origins. For this reason, it is inaccurate to use the term "dermoid cyst" to describe cystic mediastinal germ cell neoplasms. Solid teratomas are usually malignant. Most germ cell neoplasms are detected in patients in their third or fourth decade of life. Although benign tumors have a slight female preponderance (female/male=60%/40%), malignant tumors are seen almost exclusively in men.

Radiographically, these tumors have a distribution similar to that of thymomas. Although the majority are located in the anterior mediastinum, up to 10% are found in the posterior mediastinum. Benign lesions are often round or oval and smooth in contour; an irregular, lobulated, or ill-defined margin suggests malignancy. Calcification is present in 33–50% but is nonspecific unless in the form of a tooth. At CT, benign teratomas are usually cystic and may contain soft tissue, bone, teeth, fat or, rarely, fat/fluid levels. Seminoma, choriocarcinoma, and endodermal sinus (yolk sac) tumors are malignant lesions seen primarily in young men. Seminoma is the most common malignant germ cell neoplasm, accounting for 30% of these tumors. The radiographic findings are nonspecific. CT typically shows a large lobulated soft tissue mass that may contain areas of hemorrhage, calcification, or necrosis (Fig. 13.7). Elevated serum alpha-feto protein (AFP) or human chorionic gonadotropin (hCG) are helpful in differential diagnosis, and clinical and CT evidence of gynecomastia is an additional clue.

Thyroid Masses. Although masses arising from the thyroid can present as anterior and superior mediastinal masses, these lesions are best considered as thoracic inlet masses as discussed previously.

Mesenchymal Tumors. Benign and malignant tumors arising from the fibrous, fatty, muscular, or vascular tissues of the mediastinum may present as mediastinal masses, most commonly in the anterior mediastinum. Lipomas can occur in any location in the mediastinum but are most often anterior. The diagnosis is made by recognition of a well-defined mass of uniform fatty attenuation (< –50 H). The presence of soft tissue elements should raise the possibility of a thymolipoma or liposarcoma; the latter may show evidence

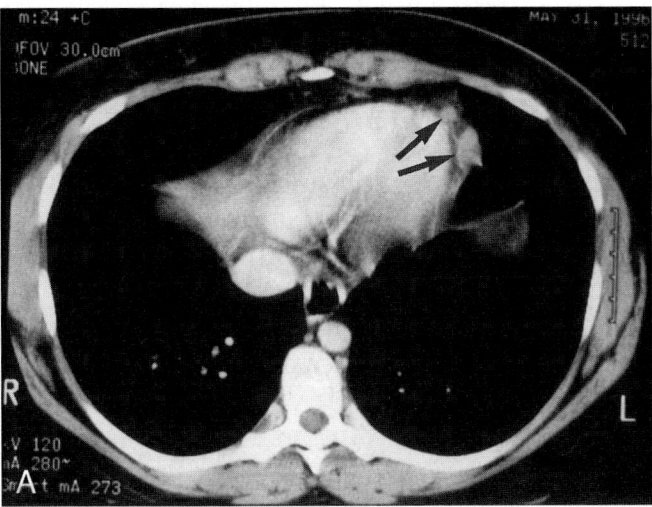
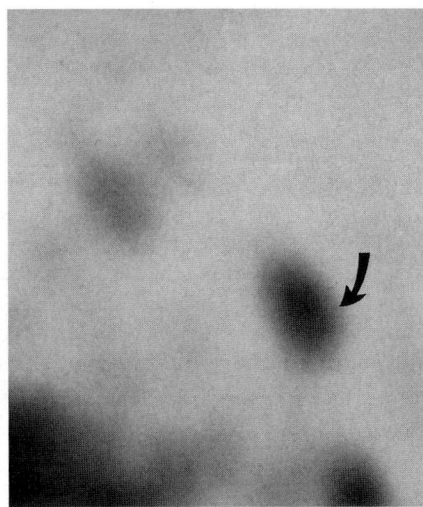

Figure 13.6. Gallium Scanning for Recurrent Hodgkin's Lymphoma. A. In a patient with treated mediastinal Hodgkin's lymphoma, a CT scan at the level of the heart shows enlarged left pericardial lymph nodes (*arrows*). **B.** Coronal SPECT gallium scan demonstrates focal increased uptake (*arrow*) corresponding with the CT findings. Thoracoscopic biopsy confirmed recurrent Hodgkin's lymphoma.

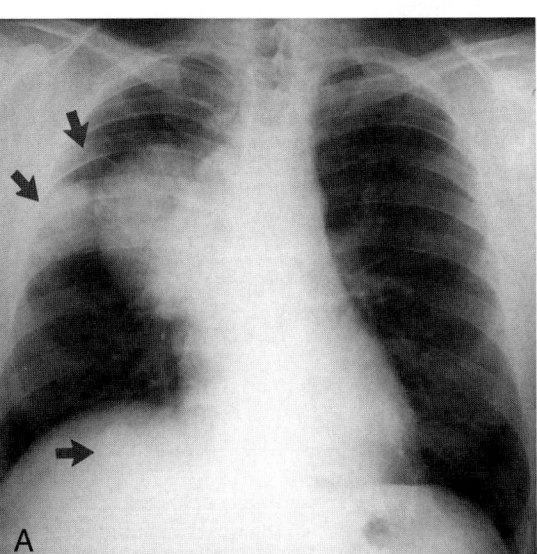
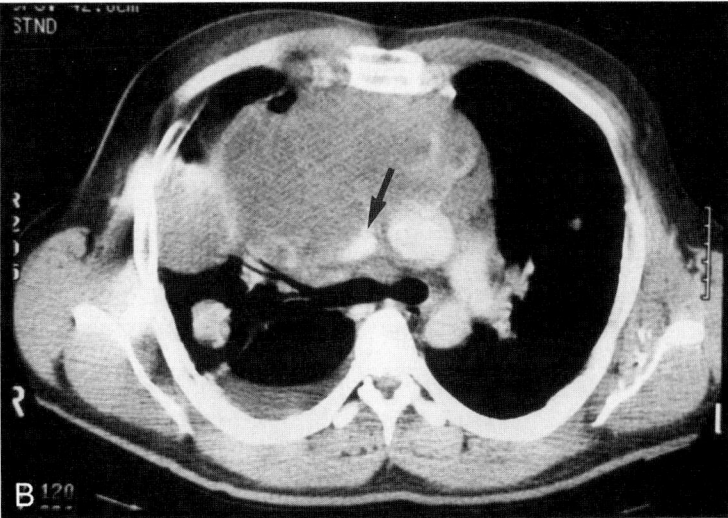

Figure 13.7. Malignant Germ Cell Tumor. A. PA chest radiograph in a 38-year-old male reveals a right mediastinal mass with a discrete right lung nodules (*arrows*). **B.** Contrast-enhanced CT demonstrates a large anterior mediastinal mass invading the superior vena cava (*arrow*) with right lung nodules and a small pleural effusion. CT-guided biopsy showed choriocarcinoma.

of invasion of adjacent structures at the time of diagnosis. Fat within a mature teratoma or transdiaphragmatic herniation of omental fat is easily distinguished from a lipoma.

Hemangiomas are benign tumors composed of vascular channels that may be associated with the syndrome of hereditary hemorrhagic telangiectasia. A pathognomonic sign on chest radiographs is the recognition of phleboliths within a smooth or lobulated soft tissue mass. Angiosarcomas are rare malignant vascular neoplasms that are indistinguishable from other invasive neoplasms arising within the anterior mediastinum.

Leiomyomas are rare benign neoplasms that arise from smooth muscle within the mediastinum. Similarly, fibromas and mesenchymomas (tumors that contain more than one mesenchymal element) can appear as anterior mediastinal masses.

Middle Mediastinal Masses

Lymph Node Enlargement and Masses. Most middle mediastinal lymph node masses (Table 13.4) are malignant, representing metastases from bronchogenic carcinoma, extrathoracic malignancy, or lymphoma. Benign causes of middle mediastinal lymph node enlargement include sarcoidosis, mycobacterial and fungal infection, angiofollicular lymph node hyperplasia (Castleman's disease), and angioimmunoblastic lymphadenopathy.

On plain radiographs, several findings suggest that a middle mediastinal mass represents lymph node enlargement. The presence of multiple bilateral mediasinal masses that distort the lung/mediastinal interface is relatively specific for lymph node enlargement. Solitary masses resulting from lymph node enlargement tend to be elongated and lobulated rather than spherical because usually more than a single node in a vertical chain of nodes is involved. Occasionally, calcification can be detected within enlarged lymph nodes on plain radiographs; CT is more sensitive in detecting nodal calcification and its distribution within lymph nodes, as will be described in the following.

One of the prime indications for performing thoracic CT is to detect the presence of enlarged mediastinal lymph nodes. CT is most often obtained to confirm an abnormal chest radiographic finding or to evaluate a patient with suspected mediastinal disease despite normal radiographs (a patient with a suspicious solitary pulmonary nodule or with cervical Hodgkin's disease). The ability of CT to image in the axial plane and its inherent high contrast resolution allows for the recognition of abnormally enlarged lymph nodes not evident on chest radiographs. Abnormal lymph nodes are seen as round or oval soft tissue masses that measure >1.0 cm in their short axis diameter. Although CT is unable to distinguish between benign inflammatory nodes and those involved by malignancy based upon size criteria alone, CT can provide useful information about the internal density of the nodes (Table 13.5).

A standardized classification system for hilar and mediastinal lymph nodes has recently been advanced by the American Thoracic Society (Fig. 13.8)(6). This

Figure 13.8. American Thoracic Society Nodal Stations.

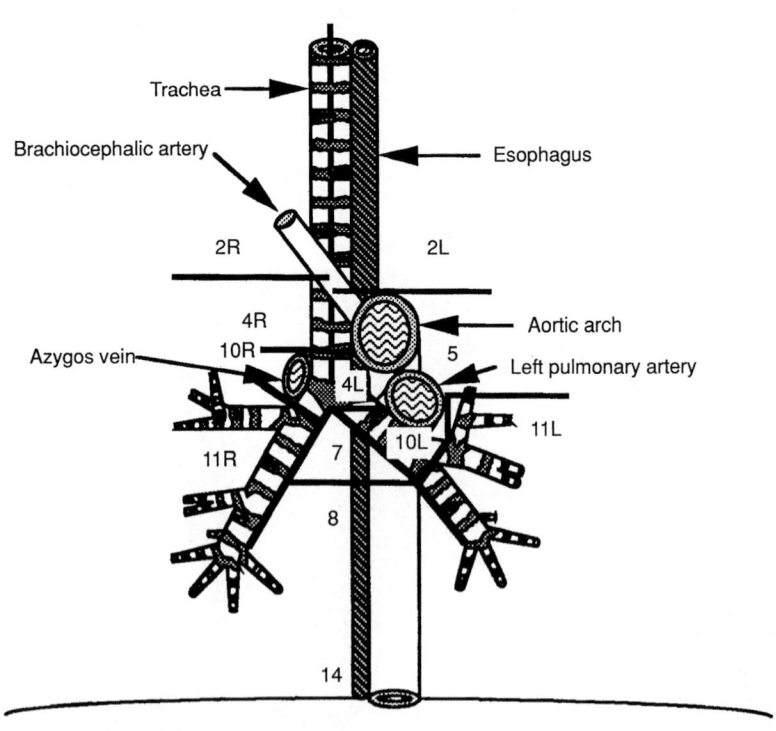

2R	=	Right upper paratracheal nodes	8 =	Paraesophageal nodes
2L	=	Left upper paratracheal nodes	10R =	Right tracheobronchial nodes
4R	=	Right lower paratracheal nodes	10L =	Left peribronchial nodes
4L	=	Left lower paratracheal nodes	11R =	Right lobar or segmental nodes
5	=	Aortopulmonary nodes	11L =	Left lobar or segmental nodes
7	=	Subcarinal nodes	14 =	Peridiaphragmatic nodes

Table 13.4. Middle Mediastinal Masses

Lymph node masses	Malignancy
	Bronchogenic carcinoma
	Lymphoma
	Leukemia
	Kaposi's sarcoma
	Extrathoracic malignancy
	Head and neck tumors (squamous
	cell carcinoma of skin, larynx,
	thyroid carcinoma)
	Genitourinary tumors (renal cell
	carcinoma, seminoma)
	Breast carcinoma
	Melanoma
	Infection
	Bacteria
	Anaerobic lung abscess
	Anthrax
	Plague
	Tularemia
	Tuberculosis
	Fungi
	Histoplasmosis
	Coccidioidomycosis
	Cryptococcosis
	Viral infection
	Measles
	Mononucleosis
	Idiopathic
	Sarcoidosis
	Castleman's disease
	Angioimmunoblastic lymphadenopathy
Foregut and mesothelial cysts	Bronchogenic cyst Pericardial cyst

Tracheal and central bronchial neoplasms	Malignant
	  Carcinoid tumor (bronchi)
	  Adenoid cystic carcinoma (trachea)
	  Squamous cell carcinoma

Diaphragmatic hernias	Foramen of Morgagni hernia Traumatic hernia

Vascular lesions	Arterial
	  Double arch/right arch
	  Tortuous innominate/subclavian artery
	  Aneurysm of the aortic arch
	Venous
	  Dilated azygous vein
	  Dilated hemiazygous vein
	  Dilated SVC
	  Left sided SVC
	  Dilated left superior intercostal vein
	  Dilatation of the main pulmonary artery

scheme correlates with easily identifiable CT and anatomic landmarks and is most important when reporting lymph node enlargement in patients with bronchogenic carcinoma.

MR is as sensitive as CT in detecting enlarged mediastinal lymph nodes. Advantages of MR include the absence of iodinated contrast, easy distinction between vascular and soft tissue structures, exquisite contrast resolution between mediastinal nodes and fat on T1-weighted sequences, and the ability to image in the direct coronal or sagittal plane. The latter feature is an ad-

vantage in those mediastinal regions that parallel the axial plane (subcarinal space, aortopulmonary window) and therefore tend to suffer from partial volume averaging effects on CT. The major disadvantages of MR at present are the inability to detect nodal calcification, high cost, and limited spatial resolution; the latter can result in an inability to distinguish between a group of normal-sized nodes and a single enlarged node, thereby leading to false-positive results.

In addition to the detection and characterization of enlarged mediastinal nodes, CT can help guide diagnostic nodal tissue sampling. This is usually most helpful in the setting of suspected bronchogenic carcinoma, where accurate staging of mediastinal nodal disease is important for prognostic purposes and treatment planning. The recognition of enlarged subcarinal or pretracheal nodes on CT may suggest biopsy via transcarinal Wang needle or mediastinoscopy, respectively.

As previously mentioned, mediastinal lymph node enlargement is common in Hodgkin's disease and non-Hodgkin's lymphoma. Lymphoma accounts for 20% of all mediastinal neoplasms in adults, and most patients with intrathoracic lymphoma have concomitant extrathoracic disease. In most patients, the nodal enlargement is bilateral but asymmetric. Nodular sclerosing Hodgkin's disease commonly results in lymph node enlargement predominantly within the anterior mediastinum and thymus. Isolated posterior nodal enlargement is usually seen only in patients with non-Hodgkin's lymphoma.

Leukemia, particularly the T-lymphocytic varieties, can cause intrathoracic lymph node enlargement. The lymph node enlargement is usually confined to the middle mediastinal and hilar nodes.

The most common source of metastases to middle mediastinal nodes is bronchogenic carcinoma. In the majority of patients, symptoms or plain radiographic findings suggest the presence of a primary tumor in the lung. In a small percentage of patients, particularly those with small cell carcinoma, the primary carcinoma may be inconspicuous or invisible on plain radiographs, with nodal metastases being the only visible abnormality. Lymph node enlargement is often unilateral on the side

Table 13.5. Density of Mediastinal/Hilar Nodes on CT

Calcification	
Central	Mycobacteria
	Fungus
Peripheral (eggshell)	Silicosis
	Sarcoidosis
Hypervascular	Carcinoid tumor/small cell carcinoma
	Kaposi's sarcoma
	Metastases
	Renal cell carcinoma
	Thyroid carcinoma
	Castleman's disease
Necrosis	Mycobacteria
	Fungus
	Metastases
	Squamous cell carcinoma
	Seminoma
	Lymphoma

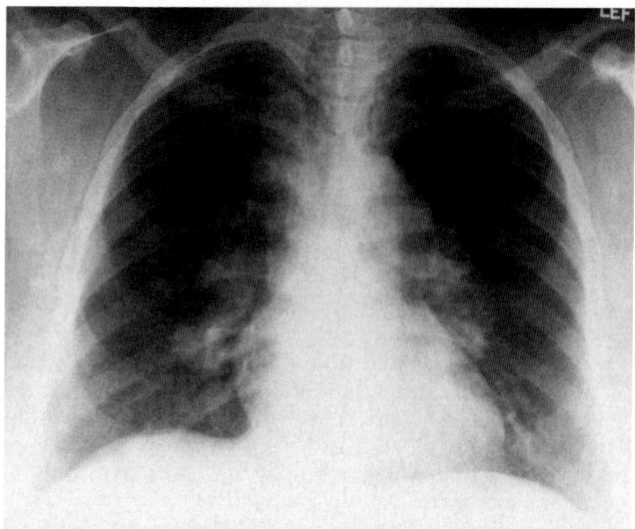

Figure 13.9. Lymphadenopathy in Sarcoidosis. PA radiograph in a 56-year-old female with sarcoidosis reveals discrete hilar, paratracheal, and aortopulmonary window lymphadenopathy.

of the visible pulmonary or hilar abnormality. Paratracheal and aorticopulmonary nodes are most commonly involved. Because the accuracy of CT in predicting the presence or absence of mediastinal lymph node metastases is approximately 60–70%, biopsy of enlarged mediastinal lymph nodes should be performed before foregoing a possibly curative resection. A more thorough discussion of mediastinal nodal involvement in bronchogenic carcinoma may be found in chapter 16.

Lymph node metastases from extrathoracic malignancies can result in mediastinal node enlargement, either with or without concomitant pulmonary metastases. These mediastinal nodal metastases may result from inferior extension of neck masses (thyroid carcinoma, head and neck tumors), extension along lymphatic channels from below the diaphragm (testicular or renal cell carcinoma, gastrointestinal malignancies), or hematogenous (breast carcinoma, melanoma, Kaposi's sarcoma)(7).

Mediastinal lymph node enlargement is very common in patients with sarcoidosis, occurring in 60–90% of patients at some stage of their disease. Nodal enlargement is typically bilateral, symmetric, and involves the hila as well as the mediastinum; this usually allows for differentiation of sarcoidosis from lymphoma and metastatic disease. In sarcoidosis, the enlarged nodes produce a lobulated appearance on chest radiographs and CT because the enlarged nodes do not coalesce (Fig. 13.9). This is in contrast to lymphoma and nodal metastases in which the intranodal tumor extends through the nodal capsule to form conglomerate enlarged nodal masses. Right and left paratracheal lymph nodes are typically involved; anterior or posterior mediastinal nodal enlargement has been described with greater frequency recently, likely because of the improved sensitivity of CT for detecting nodal involvement in these regions.

A variety of infections—most commonly histoplasmosis, coccidioidomycosis, cryptococcosis, and tuberculo-

sis (Fig. 13.10)—can cause mediastinal nodal enlargement. Typically these patients have parenchymal opacities on chest radiographs, but isolated lymph node enlargement may be seen, particularly in children and young adults. Bacterial infections such as anthrax, bubonic plague, and tularemia are uncommon causes of lymph node enlargement. Typically, symptoms and signs of acute infection are present, and chest radiographs will show evidence of pneumonia. Bacterial lung abscesses also may be associated with reactive lymph node enlargement. Hilar and mediastinal lymph nodes may be enlarged in patients with measles pneumonia and infectious mononucleosis.

Angiofollicular lymph node hyperplasia (Castleman's disease) is characterized by enlargement of hilar and mediastinal lymph nodes, predominantly in the middle and posterior mediastinal compartments. In the more common hyaline vascular type, the disease is localized to one lymph node region and presents as an asymptomatic mediastinal soft tissue mass. Histologically, there is replacement of normal nodal architecture with multiple germinal centers and multiple small vessels with hyalinized walls that course perpendicularly towards the germinal centers to give a characteristic "lollipop" appearance on light microscopy. The vascular nature of these masses accounts for the intense enhancement seen on contrast-enhanced CT or angiography. Calcification within these masses has been described. These lesions are cured by resection.

Angioimmunoblastic lymphadenopathy, a rare disorder seen in older adults, is characterized by constitutional symptoms, lymphadenopathy, hepatosplenomegaly, and skin rash. Hemolytic anemia and hypergammaglobulinemia may be seen. Histologically, the enlarged nodes contain a chronic inflammatory infiltrate and are hypervascular. Chest radiographs and CT show hilar and mediastinal lymph node enlargement indistinguishable

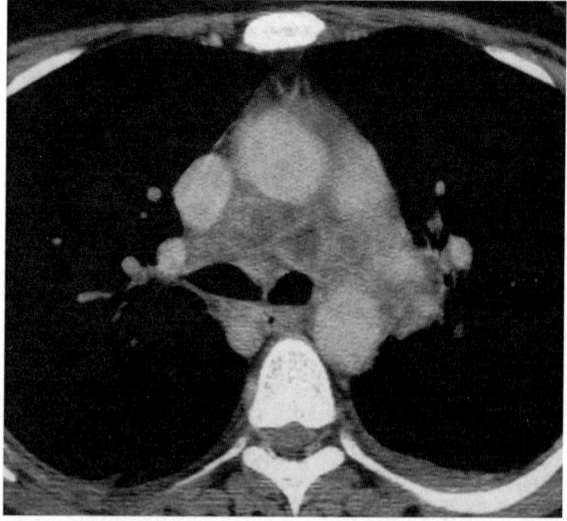

Figure 13.10. Tuberculous Lymphadenopathy. Contrast-enhanced CT at the level of the tracheal carina demonstrates enlarged precarinal and left peribronchial lymph nodes with central necrosis and peripheral enhancement. Material obtained by mediastinoscopy revealed *Mycobacterium tuberculosis*.

from other etiologies. As with Castleman's disease, the vascular nature of the involved lymph nodes accounts for the contrast enhancement seen on CT. These patients manifest signs of immunodeficiency similar to those associated with the acquired immunodeficiency syndrome with one-third developing high-grade lymphoma and many succumbing to opportunistic infections such as *Pneumocystis carinii* pneumonia and cytomegalovirus inclusion disease.

Foregut and Mesothelial Cysts are common mediastinal lesions that typically present as asymptomatic masses on routine chest radiographs in young adults. CT and MR show findings characteristic of the cystic nature of these lesions.

Congenital bronchogenic cysts result from anomalous budding of the tracheobronchial tree during development. To be characterized as bronchogenic in origin, the wall of the cyst must be lined by a respiratory epithelium with pseudostratified columnar cells and contain seromucous glands; some may contain cartilage and smooth muscle within their walls. Distinguishing between bronchogenic and enteric cysts based on their location and pathologic appearance is often difficult; the term "foregut cyst" has been used to describe those lesions that cannot be specifically characterized. The majority of bronchogenic cysts (80–90%) arise within the mediastinum in the vicinity of the tracheal carina. Most mediastinal lesions are asymptomatic; occasionally, compression of the tracheobronchial tree or esophagus may produce dyspnea, wheezing, or dysphagia. Rarely, mediastinal cysts become secondarily infected after communication with the airway or esophagus, or cause symptomatic compression after rapid enlargement following hemorrhage. Bronchogenic cysts are seen as soft tissue masses in the subcarinal or right paratracheal space on frontal chest radiographs; less common sites of involvement include the hilum, posterior mediastinum, and periesophageal region. They appear as a single, smooth, round or elliptical mass; a minority are lobulated in contour. CT is the method of choice for the diagnosis of a mediastinal cyst. If a well-defined, thin-walled mass of fluid density (0–10 H) is seen that fails to enhance following intravenous contrast administration, it can be assumed to represent a benign cyst (8). High CT numbers (>40 H) suggesting a solid mass can be seen when the cyst is filled with mucoid material, milk of calcium, or blood. Calcification of the cyst wall has been described but is uncommon. MR shows characteristic low signal intensity on T1WI and high signal intensity on T2WI (Fig. 13.11). The presence of proteinaceous material within the cyst will shorten T1

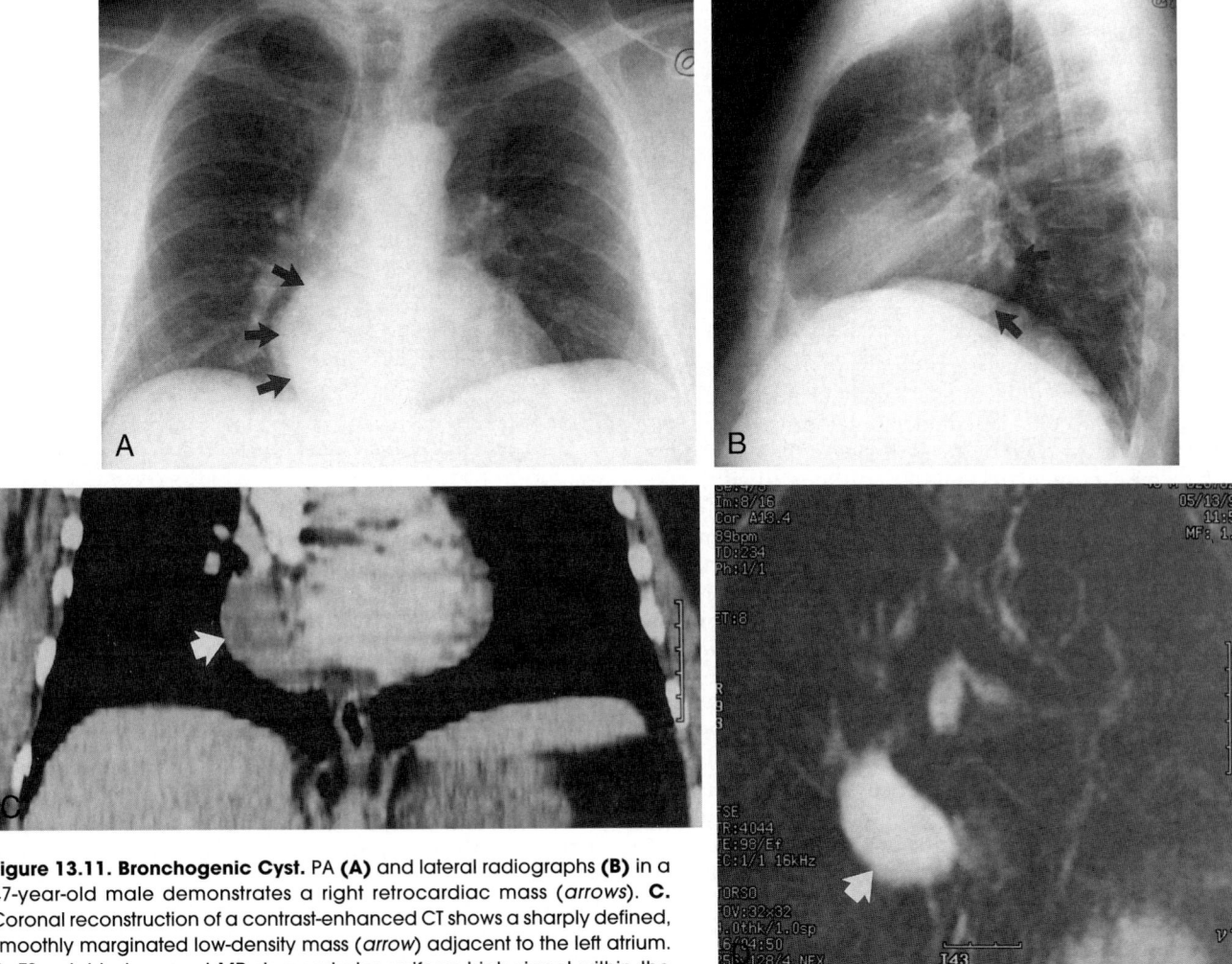

Figure 13.11. Bronchogenic Cyst. PA **(A)** and lateral radiographs **(B)** in a 47-year-old male demonstrates a right retrocardiac mass (*arrows*). **C.** Coronal reconstruction of a contrast-enhanced CT shows a sharply defined, smoothly marginated low-density mass (*arrow*) adjacent to the left atrium. **D.** T2-weighted coronal MR demonstrates uniform high signal within the mass (*arrow*).

relaxation times, yielding high signal intensity on T1WI. In many patients, resection is required for definitive diagnosis. Both transbronchoscopic and precutaneous needle aspiration and drainage are used successfully for the diagnosis and treatment of these lesions.

Pericardial cysts arise from the parietal pericardium and contain clear serous fluid surrounded by a layer of mesothelial cells. They most commonly arise in the anterior cardiophrenic angles, with right-sided lesions being twice as common as left; approximately 20% arise more superiorly within the mediastinum. These lesions usually present as incidental, asymptomatic, round or oval masses in the cardiophrenic angle. Their pliable nature can be demonstrated with a change in patient position. CT typically shows a unilocular cystic mass adjacent to the heart; MR or US via a subxiphoid approach show findings characteristic of a simple cyst. As with bronchogenic cysts, there have been reports of cysts with high-attenuation on CT that on resection are filled with proteinaceous or mucoid material.

Tracheal and Central Bronchial Masses commonly produce upper airway symptoms with obstructive pneumonitis and atelectasis and rarely present as asymptomatic mediastinal masses. Occasionally, central airway masses present as radiographic abnormalities when they distort the tracheal air column or mediastinal contour. These masses are discussed in chapter 19.

Diaphragmatic Hernias, which may present as pericardiac masses, are discussed in chapter 20.

Vascular Lesions. Congenital or acquired anomalies of the heart and great vessels are common middle mediastinal masses, and are discussed in chapter 25.

Posterior Mediastinal Masses

Neurogenic Tumors (Table 13.6). Posterior mediastinal masses arising from neural elements are classified by their tissue of origin. Three groups have been recognized: tumors arising from intercostal nerves (neurofibroma, schwannoma), sympathetic ganglia (ganglioneuroma, ganglioneuroblastoma, and neuroblastoma), or paraganglionic cells (chemodectoma, pheochromocytoma). Tumors in each of these three groups may be benign or malignant neoplasms (9). Although neurogenic tumors can occur at any age, they are most common in young patients. Neuroblastoma and ganglioneuroma are most common in children, and neurofibroma and schwannoma more frequently affect adults.

Histologically, both neurofibroma and schwannoma are comprised of spindle cells that arise from the Schwann cell. Although neurofibroma is an encapsulated tumor that contains interspersed neurons, schwannoma is not encapsulated and contains no neuronal elements. Both tumors are more common in patients with neurofibromatosis. Multiple lesions in the mediastinum, particularly bilateral apicoposterior masses, are virtually diagnostic of neurofibromatosis. A small percentage of schwannomas (10%) are locally invasive (malignant schwannoma).

Radiographically, intercostal nerve tumors appear as round or oval paravertebral soft tissue masses. CT

Table 13.6. Posterior Mediastinal Masses

Neurogenic tumors	Peripheral (intercostal) nerves
	Neurofibroma
	Schwannoma
	Sympathetic ganglia
	Ganglioneuroma
	Ganglioneuromablastoma
	Neuroblastoma
	Paraganglion cells
	Chemodectoma
	Pheochromocytoma
Esophageal lesions	Duplication (enteric) cyst
	Diverticulum
	Neoplasm
	Leiomyoma
	Squamous cell carcinoma
	Esophageal dilatation
	Achalasia
	Scleroderma
	Peptic stricture
	Carcinoma
	Paraesophageal varices
	Hiatal hernia
	Sliding
	Paraesophageal
Foregut cysts	Enteric
	Neurenteric
Vertebral lesion	Trauma
	Paraspinal hematoma
	Infection
	Paraspinal abscess
	Tuberculosis
	Staphylococcus
	Tumor
	Metastases (bronchogenic, breast, renal cell carcinoma)
	Multiple myeloma
	Lymphoma
	Degenerative disease (osteophytosis)
	Extramedullary hematopoiesis
Lateral thoracic meningocele	
Pancreatic pseudocyst	

shows a smooth or lobulated paraspinal soft tissue mass that may erode the adjacent vertebral body or rib (Fig. 13.12). CT demonstration of tumor extension from the paravertebral space into the spinal canal via an enlarged intervertebral foramen is characteristic of a "dumbbell" neurofibroma. MR is the modality of choice for imaging a suspected neurofibroma. In addition to the occasional demonstration of both intra-spinal and extra-spinal canal components, MR of neurofibromas shows typical high signal intensity on T2WI.

Tumors that arise from the sympathetic ganglia represent a continuum from the histologically benign ganglioneuroma found in adolescents and young adults to the highly malignant neuroblastoma seen almost exclusively in children younger than the age of five. These tumors generally present as elongated, vertically oriented paravertebral soft tissue masses with a broad area of contact with the posterior mediastinum (Fig. 13.13). These findings may help distinguish these lesions from neurofibromas, which usually maintain an acute angle with the vertebral column and posterior mediastinum and therefore tend to show sharp superior and inferior margins on the lateral chest radiograph. Large masses may erode vertebral bodies or ribs. Calcification, seen in up to 25% of cases, is a helpful diagnostic feature of these tumors but does not help distinguish benign from malig-

nant neoplasms. Because these tumors often produce catecholamines, urinary levels of vanilylmandelic acid or metanephrines, which are byproducts of catecholamine metabolism, may be elevated. Prognosis depends on the histological features of the tumor and the patient's age and extent of disease at the time of diagnosis.

Paraganglionomas are tumors that arise in the aorticopulmonary paraganglia of the middle mediastinum or the aorticosympathetic ganglia of the posterior mediastinum. They are divided into nonfunctioning neo-

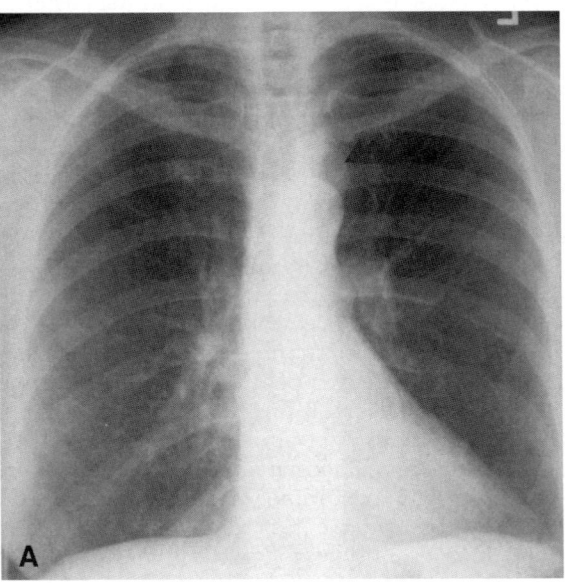
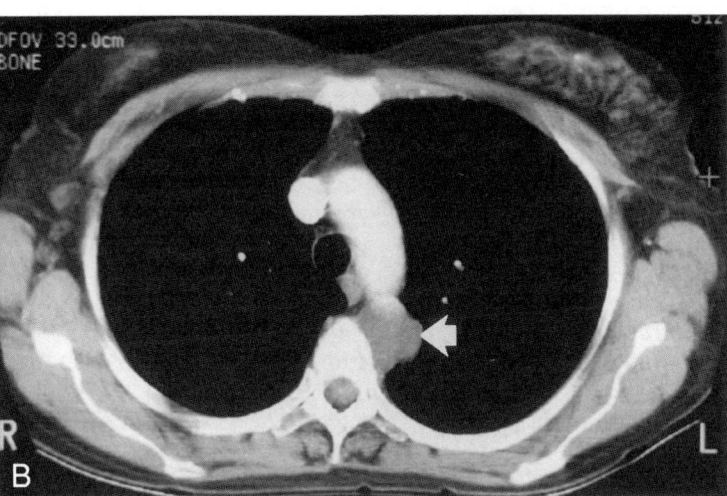

Figure 13.12. Neurofibroma. A. Frontal chest radiograph shows a left upper mediastinal mass. **B.** Contrast-enhanced CT confirms the presence of a left paravertebral soft tissue mass (*arrow*). Surgical resection confirmed a neurofibroma.

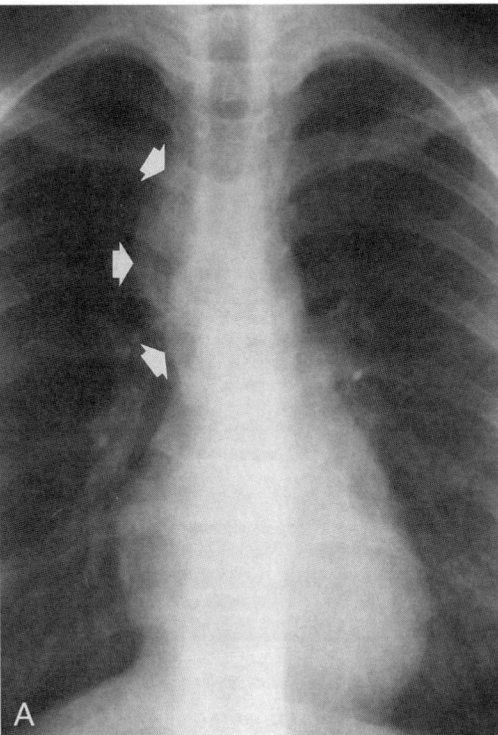
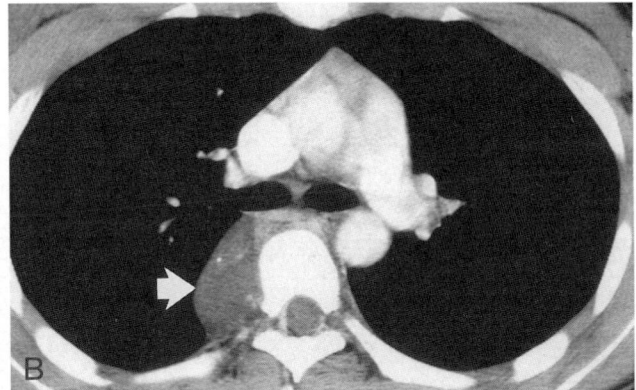

Figure 13.13. Ganglioneuroma. A. PA radiograph in a 15-year-old female reveals an oval, vertically oriented, right-sided mediastinal mass (*arrows*). **B.** Contrast-enhanced CT shows a low attenuation posterior mediastinal mass with calcification. This is a surgically proven ganglioneuroma.

plasms (chemodectomas), which occur almost exclusively in or about the aortopulmonary window, and functioning neoplasms (pheochromocytomas), which are found in the posterior sympathetic chain or in or about the heart or pericardium. Approximately 2% of all pheochromocytomas arise in the mediastinum. The posterior mediastinum is the site of fewer than 25% of mediastinal paraganglionomas, with the majority arising in the anterior or middle mediastinum. Radiographically, these tumors are indistinguishable from other neurogenic tumors. However, most patients have hypertension and biochemical evidence of excess catecholamine production. CT and angiography demonstrate hypervascular masses; radionuclide MIBG scanning is diagnostic in functioning tumors.

Esophageal Lesions. As most of the intrathoracic esophagus is intimately associated with the thoracic spine and descending thoracic aorta, lesions in the mid or distal one-third of the esophagus may present as posterior mediastinal masses. Common presenting symptoms include dysphagia and aspiration pneumonia, although many patients will be asymptomatic.

The majority of esophageal neoplasms, excluding lesions arising at the esophagogastric junction, are squamous cell carcinomas. Unlike benign neoplasms of the posterior mediastinum, these lesions, when seen on chest radiographs, are rarely asymptomatic. Typically these patients have a history of dysphagia and significant weight loss. Difficulty in detecting asymptomatic lesions and the absence of a serosa account for the advanced stage of most esophageal carcinoma at presentation and a five year survival rate of less than 20%. Most patients with esophageal carcinoma have abnormal plain radiographic findings including an abnormal azygoesophageal interface (Fig. 13.14), widening of the mediastinum (due to the tumor itself or a dilated esophagus proximal to the obstructing lesion), abnormal thickening of the tracheoesophageal stripe, and tracheal

deviation and compression. The diagnosis is usually made on barium esophagram and confirmed by endoscopic biopsy. CT scanning has proved accurate for staging esophageal carcinoma: findings include an intraluminal mass, thickening of the esophageal wall, loss of fat planes between the esophagus and adjacent mediastinal structures (usually the trachea with upper esophageal lesions and the descending aorta with lower esophageal lesions), and evidence of nodal and distant metastases.

Several benign esophageal neoplasms, including leiomyoma, fibroma, and lipoma, can present as smooth, solitary mediastinal masses projecting laterally from the posterior mediastinum on frontal chest radiographs. They usually involve the lower third of the esophagus from the level of the subcarinal space to the esophageal hiatus. Initial evaluation is with barium studies, which show a smooth, broad-based mass forming obtuse margins with the esophageal wall. CT demonstrates a smooth, well-defined soft tissue mass adjacent to the esophagus without obstruction. The absence of esophageal dilatation above the mass helps distinguish benign tumors from carcinoma.

Pulsion diverticula arising at the cervicothoracic esophageal junction or distal esophagus are false diverticula representing mucosal outpouchings through defects in the muscular layer of the esophagus. A large proximal pulsion diverticulum (Zenker's) may extend through the thoracic inlet and appear as a retroesophageal superior mediastinal mass containing an air-fluid level on upright chest radiographs. A distal pulsion diverticulum appears as a juxtadiaphragmatic mass with an air-fluid level projecting to the right of midline. Barium swallow is diagnostic.

A dilated esophagus caused by functional (achalasia, scleroderma) or anatomic (stricture, carcinoma) obstruction may produce a mass that courses vertically over the length of the mediastinum, projecting toward the right side on frontal chest radiograph. An air-fluid level on upright films is usually present. A completely air-filled di-

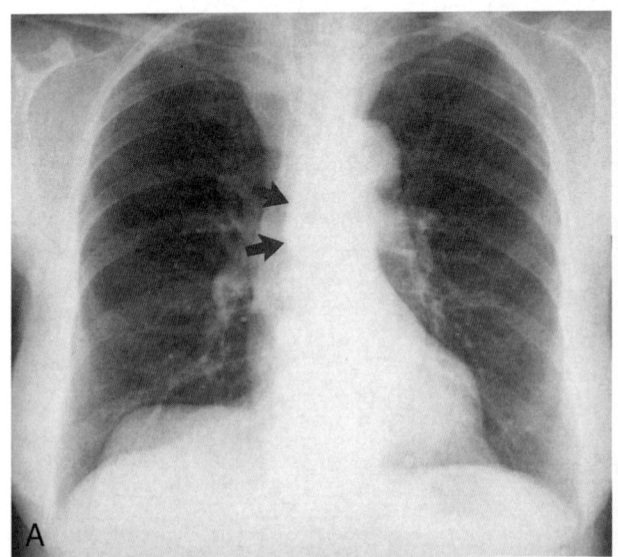
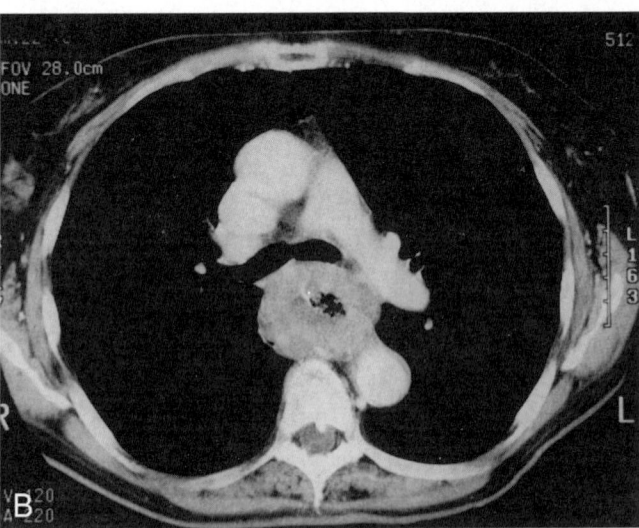

Figure 13.14. Esophageal Carcinoma. A. PA radiograph in an 81-year-old female with dysphagia show an abnormal convexity in the upper azygoesophageal recess (*arrows*). **B.** CT through the tracheal carina shows marked circumferential thickening of the esophagus. Endoscopic biopsy confirmed esophageal carcinoma.

lated esophagus appears as a thin curvilinear line along the medial right thorax because the right lateral wall of the esophagus is outlined by intraluminal air medially and the right lung laterally. Barium study or CT will confirm the diagnosis of a dilated esophagus; determination of the cause of obstruction often requires endoscopy or esophageal manometry.

Esophageal varices may produce a round or lobulated retrocardiac mass in patients with portal hypertension. The diagnosis is usually made by endoscopic recognition of submucosal varices involving the distal esophagus. The varices are readily recognized on contrast CT, MR, or portal venography.

A common cause of a mass in the posteroinferior mediastinum is a hiatal hernia. This results from a separation of the superior margins of the diaphragmatic crura and stretching of the phrenicoesophageal ligament. The stomach is by far the most common structure in the hernia sac; the gastric cardia (sliding hernia) or fundus (paraesophageal hernia) may be involved. Rarely, omental fat, ascitic fluid, or a pancreatic pseudocyst herniates through the esophageal hiatus into the mediastinum. The characteristic location at the esophageal hiatus and the presence of a rounded density containing an air or air-fluid level on upright films is diagnostic. Barium swallow or CT will confirm the diagnosis.

Enteric/Neurenteric Cysts. Enteric cysts are fluid-filled masses lined by enteric epithelium. Esophageal cysts usually arise intramurally or immediately adjacent to the esophagus. When an enteric cyst has a persistent communication with the spinal canal (canal of Kovalevski) and is associated with congenital defects of the thoracic spine (anterior spina bifida, hemivertebrae, or butterfly vertebrae), it is termed a "neurenteric cyst." CT or MR can confirm the cystic nature of these masses. If the cyst communicates with the gastrointestinal tract, it may contain air or an air-fluid level or opacify with contrast during an upper GI series.

Vertebral Abnormalities. A variety of conditions that affect the thoracic spine may manifest as posterior mediastinal masses. These lesions typically produce lateral deviation of the paraspinal reflection on frontal radiographs. Often, the bony origin of these lesions is not obvious on the initial examination, making distinction from neurogenic tumors and other posterior mediastinal masses difficult.

Neoplastic, infectious, metabolic, traumatic, or degenerative processes of the thoracic spine may produce a paraspinal mass by one of four mechanisms: expansion of vertebral body or posterior elements (multiple myeloma, aneurysmal bone cyst); extraosseous extension of infection, tumor, or marrow elements (infectious spondylitis, metastatic carcinoma, extramedullary hematopoiesis, respectively); pathologic fracture and paraspinal hematoma formation (any destructive neoplastic or inflammatory process, trauma); or protrusion of degenerative osteophytes. Neoplastic processes are usually easily identified by expansion and destruction of vertebral bodies with sparing of intervertebral discs. Bronchogenic, breast, or renal cell carcinoma are the most common primary sites of thoracic spinal metastases. Infectious spondylitis is distinguished from neo-

plastic processes by the presence of a paravertebral mass centered at the point of maximal bone destruction. In patients with a paravertebral abscess secondary to tuberculosis or bacterial infection, narrowing of the adjacent disk space and destruction of vertebral endplates are important clues to the diagnosis. Extramedullary hematopoiesis is seen almost exclusively in conditions associated with ineffective production or excessive destruction of erythrocytes such as thalassemia major, congenital spherocytosis, and sickle cell anemia. It is recognized by noting expansion of the medullary space and cyst formation within long bones, ribs, and vertebral bodies with associated lobulated paraspinal soft tissue masses. These masses, which represent hyperplastic bone marrow that has extruded from the vertebral bodies and posterior ribs, are typically seen in the lower thoracic and upper lumbar region. Traumatic injuries to the thoracic spine are usually obvious from the patient's history and recognition of spine fracture on conventional and spiral CT studies (of the spine). Degenerative disc disease may produce a localized paraspinal mass on frontal radiographs. Well-penetrated films will show the characteristic inferolaterally projecting osteophytes at the level of the mass, which are most commonly right-sided due to the inhibitory effect of the pulsating descending aorta on left-sided osteophyte formation.

Lateral thoracic meningoceles represent an anomalous herniation of the spinal meninges through an intervertebral foramen, resulting in a paravertebral soft tissue mass. Most meningoceles are discovered in middle-aged patients as asymptomatic masses. They are slightly more common on the right and are multiple in 10% of cases. A high association between lateral thoracic meningoceles and neurofibromatosis exists. A meningocele is the most common posterior mediastinal mass in patients with neurofibromatosis; conversely, approximately two-thirds of patients with meningoceles have neurofibromatosis. Chest radiographs typically reveal a round, well-defined paraspinal mass that is indistinguishable from a neurofibroma. Additional clues to the diagnosis include rib erosion, enlargement of the adjacent neural foramen, vertebral anomalies, or kyphoscoliosis. When a lateral meningocele is associated with kyphoscoliosis, it is usually found at the apex of the scoliotic curve on the convex side. MR demonstration of a herniated subarachnoid space is the diagnostic technique of choice; conventional or CT myelography, which demonstrates filling of the meningocele with contrast, is reserved for equivocal cases.

Miscellaneous Conditions. As described in the section on hiatus hernias, a pancreatic pseudocyst rarely produces a posterior mediastinal mass by extending cephalad from the retroperitoneum through the esophageal or aortic hiatus of the diaphragm. The diagnosis relies on CT demonstration of continuity of a predominantly cystic mass with its retroperitoneal portion. The presence of a left pleural effusion is a further clue to the diagnosis. Hernias through the foramen of Bochdalek that produce a posterior mediastinal mass are discussed in chapter 20.

Malignant lymph node enlargement may rarely produce a recognizable paraspinal mass. This is most often

Table 13.7. Diffuse Mediastinal Widening

Smooth	Mediastinal lipomatosis
	Malignant infiltration
	Lymphoma
	Small cell carcinoma
	Adenocarcinoma
	Mediastinal hemorrhage
	Arterial bleeding
	Traumatic aortic arch/great vessel
	laceration
	Aneurysmal rupture
	Venous bleeding
	SVC/right atrial laceration
	Mediastinitis
	Acute (suppurative)
	Chronic (sclerosing) mediastinitis
	Histoplasmosis
	Tuberculosis
	Idiopathic
Lobulated	Lymph node enlargement (see Table 14.4)
	Thymic mass (see Table 13.3)
	Germ cell neoplasm (see Table 13.3)
	Vascular lesions
	Tortuosity of great vessels
	SVC occlusion (dilated venous collaterals)
	Malignancy
	Sclerosing mediastinitis
	Catheter-induced thrombosis
	Neurofibromatosis

seen in non-Hodgkin's lymphoma and metastatic lung cancer; other mediastinal or extrathoracic sites of involvement are invariably present.

Despite the advances in detection and characterization of mediastinal masses with cross-sectional imaging, most patients will require tissue sampling for definitive diagnosis. However, the radiologist can use the information provided by CT or MR to help limit the differential diagnosis and thereby guide the appropriate evaluation and treatment. In a large percentage of cases where tissue sampling is required, this can be accomplished by CT-guided or US-guided transthoracic biopsy.

DIFFUSE MEDIASTINAL DISEASE

The differential diagnosis of diffuse widening of the mediastinum is reviewed in Table 13.7.

Mediastinal infection is an uncommon condition that may be divided into acute and chronic forms based upon cause, clinical features, and radiologic findings. The distinction between acute and chronic infection is important because the treatment and prognosis are considerably different.

Acute mediastinitis is caused by bacterial infection that most often develops following esophageal perforation or is a complication of cardiothoracic surgery. Esophageal perforation may complicate esophageal instrumentation (e.g., endoscopy, biopsy, dilatation, or stent placement), penetrating chest trauma, esophageal carcinoma, foreign body or corrosive ingestion, or vomiting. Spontaneous esophageal perforation following prolonged vomiting is termed "Boerhaave's syndrome". In this condition, a vertical tear occurs along the left pos-

terolateral wall of the distal esophagus, just above the esophagogastric junction, leading to signs and symptoms of acute mediastinitis. Less commonly, acute mediastinitis may develop from intramediastinal extension of infection in the neck, retropharyngeal space, lungs, pleural space, pericardium, or spine.

The clinical presentation of acute mediastinitis is usually dramatic and is characterized by severe retrosternal chest pain, fever, chills, and dysphagia, often accompanied by evidence of septic shock. Physical examination may reveal findings associated with pneumomediastinum, with subcutaneous emphysema in the neck and an apical, systolic crunching sound on chest auscultation ("Hamman's sign").

The most common chest radiographic findings are widening of the superior mediastinum in 66% and pleural effusion in 50% of patients. Specific findings such as mediastinal air or air-fluid levels are less common. When mediastinitis occurs in association with Boerhaave's syndrome, pneumoperitoneum and left hydropneumothorax may be seen.

When esophageal perforation is suspected, an esophagram should be performed to detect leakage of contrast into the mediastinum and to localize the exact site of perforation. In a patient not at risk for aspiration, a water-soluble contrast agent is administered initially. Once gross contrast extravasation has been excluded, barium is then given for superior radiographic detail. The sensitivity of the esophagram for detecting contrast leakage is highest when the study is obtained within 24 hours of the perforation.

Chest CT is the radiologic study of choice for the diagnosis of acute mediastinitis (10). CT findings include extraluminal gas, bulging of the mediastinal contours, and focal or diffuse soft tissue infiltration of mediastinal fat. Localized fluid collections suggest focal abscess formation (Fig. 13.15). Associated findings include mediastinal venous thrombosis, pneumothorax, pleural effusion or empyema, subphrenic abscess, and vertebral osteomyelitis.

Although the clinical and radiographic diagnosis of mediastinitis is often straightforward, it may be difficult in postoperative patients who have undergone recent me-

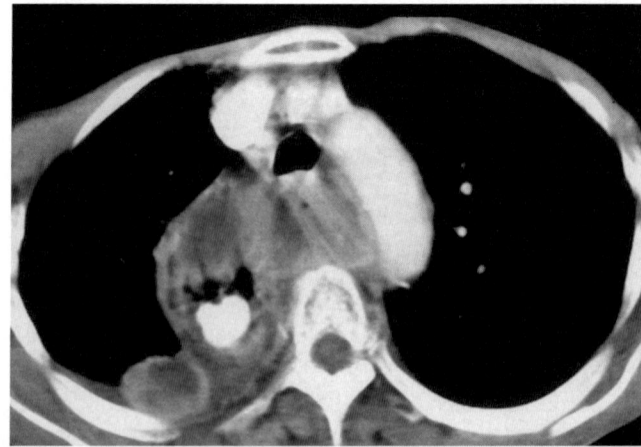

Figure 13.15. Mediastinitis with Abscess Formation. A CT scan in a patient with esophageal carcinoma demonstrates extraluminal contrast from a recent barium esophagram with enhancing mediastinal fluid collections representing abscess formation.

dian sternotomy. In these patients, infiltration of mediastinal fat and focal air or fluid collections may be normal findings on postoperative CT scans performed days to weeks following the removal of intraoperatively placed mediastinal drains. In such patients, the progression of findings on follow-up CT scans will correctly identify the majority of those with postoperative mediastinal infection.

The prognosis for patients with acute mediastinitis varies with the underlying cause and the extent of mediastinal involvement at the time of diagnosis. Esophageal perforation is associated with the poorest outcome, with the mortality approaching 50%. A delay in diagnosis and treatment of the mediastinal infection of greater than 24 hours is associated with a significant increase in overall morbidity and mortality.

In addition to its sensitivity in the diagnosis of mediastinitis, CT can be used to guide treatment and predict outcome. Those patients with evidence of extensive mediastinal infection, seen on CT as diffuse infiltration of the mediastinal fat without evidence of abscess formation, have a mortality approaching 50%. In contrast, patients with discrete mediastinal abscesses amenable to surgical or percutaneous drainage, or with small localized abscesses amenable to antibiotic therapy alone, have a more favorable prognosis. In addition, patients with mediastinal abscesses and contiguous empyema or subphrenic abscess may respond favorably to drainage of these extramediastinal collections.

Chronic Sclerosing (Fibrosing) Mediastinitis. The hallmarks of chronic sclerosing mediastinitis are chronic inflammatory changes and mediastinal fibrosis. The most common cause of this rare condition is granulomatous infection, usually secondary to Histoplasma capsulatum. Tuberculous infection, radiation therapy, and drugs (methysergide) are less common causes. Idiopathic mediastinal fibrosis, which is probably an autoimmune process, is related to fibrosis in other regions including the retroperitoneum, intraorbital fat, and thyroid gland.

Several theories have been advanced to explain the pathogenesis of sclerosing mediastinitis due to histoplasmosis. The most widely accepted theory suggests that affected patients develop an idiosyncratic hypersensitivity response to a fungal antigen that "leaks" from infected mediastinal lymph nodes.

Clinically, this condition occurs in adults and presents with a variety of symptoms dependent upon the extent of fibrosis and the mediastinal structures compromised by the fibrotic process. The superior vena cava is the most commonly affected structure, with involvement in more than 75% of symptomatic patients. The superior vena cava syndrome manifests with headache; epistaxis; cyanosis; jugular venous distention; and edema of the face, neck, and upper extremities. The most serious and potentially fatal manifestation of sclerosing mediastinitis is obstruction of the central pulmonary veins producing pulmonary edema, which may mimic severe mitral stenosis. Patients with involvement of the tracheobronchial tree may have cough, dyspnea, wheezing, hemoptysis, and obstructive pneumonitis. Dysphagia or hematemesis can be seen with esophageal involvement. Less commonly, pulmonary arterial hypertension and cor pulmonale can develop from narrowing of the pulmonary arteries.

The most common finding noted on chest radiographs is asymmetric lobulated widening of the upper mediastinum, most often on the right (Fig. 13.16). When the process is secondary to granulomatous infection, enlarged calcified lymph nodes may be seen. Narrowing of the tracheobronchial tree

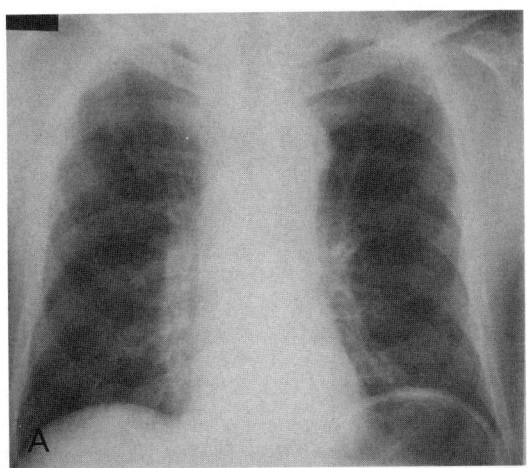

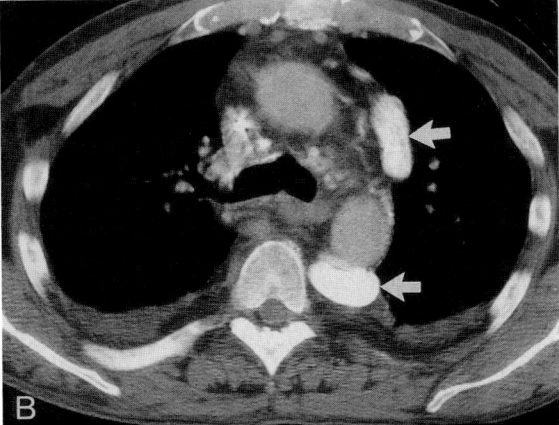

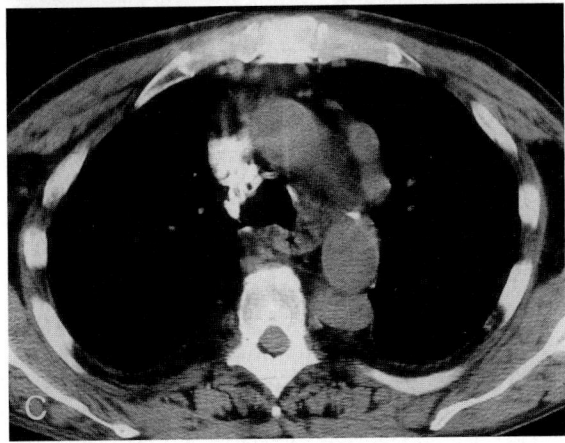

Figure 13.16. Sclerosing Mediastinitis from Histoplasmosis. A. PA chest film in an asymptomatic 68-year-old man shows lobulated widening of the upper mediastinum. **B.** Contrast-enhanced CT reveals marked dilatation of the left superior intercostal vein (*arrows*), high attenuation material in and around the superior vena cava, and numerous collaterals within the mediastinal fat. **C.** A noncontrast scan at approximately the same level reveals mediastinal cacification obliterating the superior vena cava.

may be evident. The sequelae of vascular involvement may be seen, including oligemia from pulmonary arterial compression or venous hypertension and pulmonary edema from involvement of the central pulmonary veins. Postobstructive atelectasis or consolidation may also be seen.

CT is the modality of choice for the diagnosis and assessment of chronic sclerosing mediastinitis. Enlarged lymph nodes with calcification are the most common finding (Fig. 13.16C). The fibrotic infiltration of the mediastinal fat characteristic of this condition is seen as abnormal soft tissue density replacing the normal mediastinal fat with obliteration of the normal mediastinal interfaces. CT delineates the degree of involvement of the mediastinal vessels, trachea, and central bronchi. In patients with significant SVC involvement, collateral venous channels within the mediastinum and chest wall are well demonstrated (Fig. 13.16B).

MR is superior to CT in the assessment of vascular involvement. The ability to examine the mediastinal vessels in both axial and coronal planes without the need for intravenous contrast helps detect vascular compromise. A significant disadvantage of MR is the inability to detect nodal calcification, a finding that is key to the diagnosis. For this reason, MR is most often used as an adjunct to CT when findings of vascular involvement are equivocal.

A definitve diagnosis of chronic sclerosing mediastinitis and the establishment of the underlying cause are difficult. Skin tests for histoplasmosis and tuberculosis may add additional information but are usually not helpful. The precise diagnosis—and more importantly the distinction from infiltrating malignancy—usually requires biopsy.

Mediastinal Hemorrhage. Injury to mediastinal vessels resulting from blunt or penetrating thoracic trauma is the most common cause of mediastinal hemorrhage. Blunt chest trauma most often occurs in the setting of a motor vehicle accident when rapid deceleration and thoracic cage compression produce shearing effects at the aortic isthmus. Iatrogenic trauma, usually from attempts at central line placement, can also cause mediastinal hemorrhage. Spontaneous hemorrhage may develop in patients with a coagulopathy or with aortic rupture from aneurysm or dissection (Fig. 13.17). Chronic hemodialysis, radiation vasculitis, and bleeding into a mediastinal mass are rare causes of mediastinal hemorrhage.

In the nontraumatic setting, the symptoms and signs of mediastinal hemorrhage are often mild or absent. The patient may complain of retrosternal chest pain radiating toward the back. Rarely, superior vena cava compression may result in the SVC syndrome. Extension of blood from the mediastinum superiorly into the retropharyngeal space may result in neck stiffness, odynophagia, or stridor.

The main radiographic finding in mediastinal hemorrhage of any cause is a focal or diffuse widening of the mediastinum that obscures the normal mediastinal contours (11). In mediastinal hemorrhage, the mediastinum develops a flat or slightly convex outward contour, unlike the round, lobulated, or irregular contour seen with enlarged lymph nodes or a localized mediastinal mass. Blood extending from the mediastinum into the pleural or extrapleural space produces a free-flowing effusion or a loculated extrapleural collection, respectively. Rarely, extension of blood into the lungs via the bronchovascular interstitium produces interstitial opacities that mimic pulmonary edema. Serial radiographs may show rapid

changes in mediastinal or pleural fluid collections in patients with persistent hemorrhage. CT demonstrates abnormal soft tissue within the mediastinum that obliterates the normal interfaces between the mediastinal fat, vessels, and airways. Freshly clotted blood is high in attenuation and is usually easily appreciated on helical CT (Fig. 17B). CT is also superior to plain radiography in demonstrating the extramediastinal extent of hemorrhage and is useful in demonstrating associated thoracic injuries in patients studies following blunt chest trauma.

Mediastinal lipomatosis is a benign, asymptomatic condition characterized by excessive deposition of fat in the mediastinum. Predisposing conditions include obesity, Cushing's disease, and corticosteroid therapy. However, this entity is unassociated with identifiable conditions in approximately 50% of patients.

On plain radiographs, the most common finding is smooth, symmetric widening of the superior mediastinum. If the amount of fat deposition is marked, the mediastinum

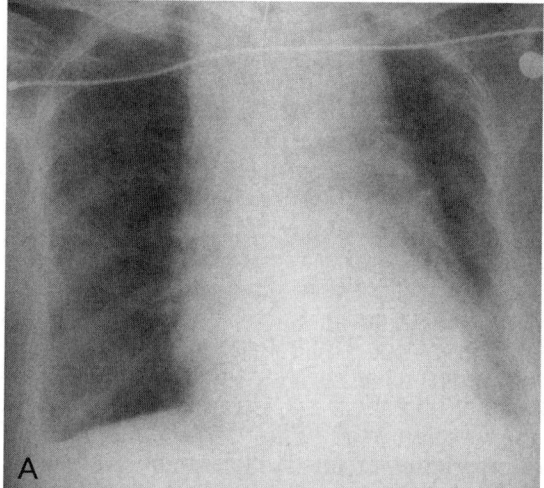
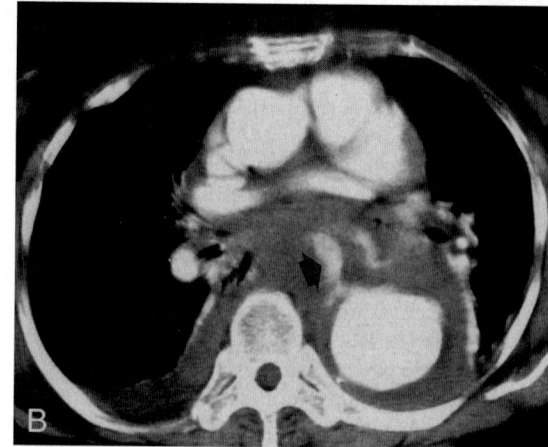

Figure 13.17. Mediastinal Hematoma from Ruptured Thoracic Aortic Aneurysm. A. Portable chest radiograph in an 83-year-old woman with chest pain shows marked mediastinal widening. **B.** Contrast-enhanced CT demonstrates aneurysmal dilatation of the descending aorta with active extravasation (*arrow*) into a large mediastinal hematoma. The patient was not a surgical candidate and expired shortly after the study.

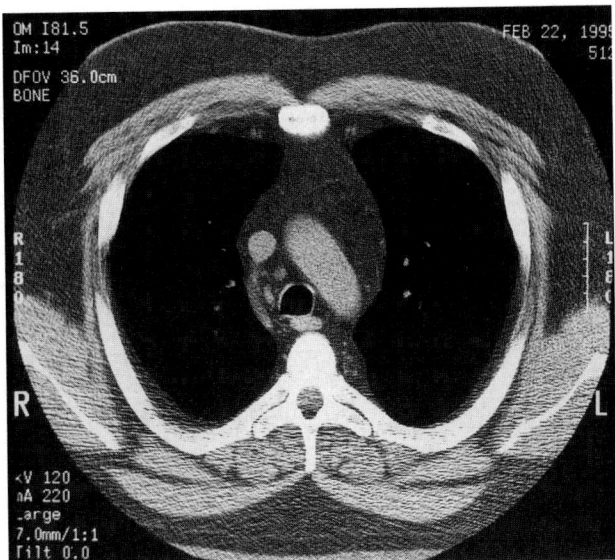

Figure 13.18. Mediastinal Lipomatosis. Unenhanced CT at the level of the aortic arch shows abundant mediastinal fat producing uniform widening of the mediastinum.

may show lobulated margins. Unlike mediastinal tumor infiltration or hemorrhage, which usually cause tracheal deviation or narrowing, the trachea remains midline in position in mediastinal lipomatosis. Fat may also accumulate in the paraspinal regions, chest wall, and cardiophrenic angles; the latter produces enlargement of the epipericardial fat pads, which is a clue to the proper diagnosis.

CT provides a definitive diagnosis by demonstrating abundant, homogeneous, unencapsulated fat that bulges the mediastinal contours (Fig. 13.18). Displacement or compression of mediastinal structures, particularly the trachea, is notable by its absence. Heterogeneity within the fat suggests other primary or superimposed conditions such as neoplastic infiltration, infection, hemorrhage, or fibrosis.

Multiple symmetric lipomatosis is a rare entity that resembles simple mediastinal lipomatosis radiographically. The distinction between these two conditions is made by the distribution of abnormal fat and mass effect on mediastinal structures. In multiple symmetric lipomatosis, the cardiophrenic angles, paraspinal areas, and the anterior mediastinum are spared; periscapular lipomas may also be seen. The trachea is often compressed or displaced by fat in patients with this condition whereas this is not seen in simple lipomatosis.

Malignancy. Malignant involvement of the mediastinum is typically seen as discrete masses or lymph node enlargement. Rarely, diffuse soft-tissue infiltration of the mediastinal fat may occur, either alone or in association with focal lesions. Plain radiographs are nonspecific, usually demonstrating mediastinal widening. CT shows soft-tissue infiltration of the normal mediastinal fat and obliteration of the normal tissue planes. This pattern is most common with extracapsular spread of lymphoma or small cell carcinoma of the lung. The latter disease has a high propensity to invade mediastinal structures and therefore may present with symptoms of airway obstruction or superior vena cava syndrome.

Pneumomediastinum is the presence of extraluminal gas within the mediastinum. Possible sources of such gas include the lungs, trachea, central bronchi, esophagus, and extension of gas from the neck or abdomen (Table 13.8)(12).

Air from the lungs is the most common source of pneumomediastinum. The mechanism of pneumomediastinum formation involves a sudden rise in intrathoracic and intra-alveolar pressure that leads to alveolar rupture. The extra-alveolar air first collects within the bronchovascular interstitium and then dissects centrally to the hilum and mediastinum (the Macklin effect)(Fig. 13.19). Less commonly, the air may dissect

Table 13.8. Pneumomediastinum

Intrathoracic source	Alveoli
	Valsalva maneuver
	Positive pressure ventilation
	Esophagus
	Boerhaave's syndrome
	Endoscopic interventions (biopsy, dilatation, sclerotherapy)
	Carcinoma
	Tracheobronchial tree
	Bronchial stump dehiscence
	Tracheobronchial laceration
	Fistula formation
	Tracheal/esophageal malignancy
	Infection (tuberculosis, histoplasmosis)
Extrathoracic source	Recent sternotomy/thoracotomy
	Pneumoperitoneum/pneumoretroperitoneum
	Subcutaneous emphysema in neck
	Stab wound
	Laryngeal fracture

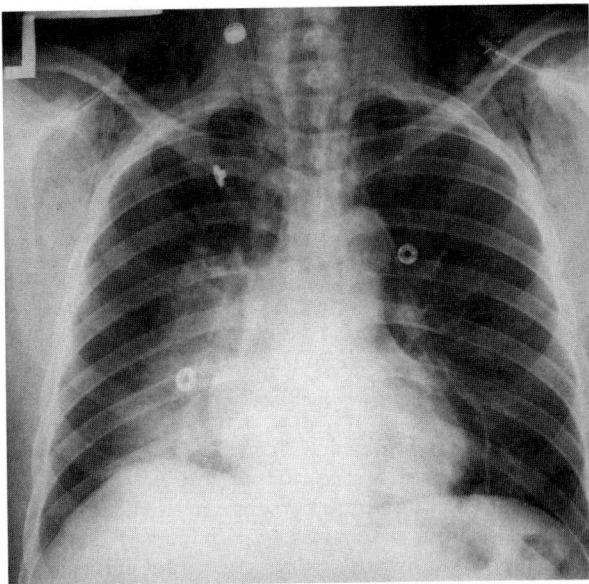

Figure 13.19. Pneumomediastinum. In a patient with an intractable cough due to right lower lobe pneumonia, a frontal radiograph shows mediastinal gas outlining the left heart and extending into the upper mediastinum and neck.

peripherally toward the subpleural interstitium and rupture through the visceral pleura to produce a pneumothorax.

Pneumomediastinum most commonly complicates mechanical ventilation in patients with ARDS because the combination of positive pressure ventilation and abnormally stiff lungs predisposes to alveolar rupture. Spontaneous pneumomediastinum can occur with deep inspiratory or Valsalva maneuvers during strenuous exercise; childbirth; inhalation of drugs such as marijuana, nitrous oxide, and crack cocaine; and weightlifting. Patients with asthma are prone to pneumomediastinum related to the airways obstruction that characterizes this disease. Prolonged vomiting from any cause may lead to sufficiently high intrathoracic pressures to produce pneumomediastinum. In patients with diabetic ketoacidosis, the increased respiratory effort that accompanies attempts at correcting the underlying metabolic acidosis can lead to pneumomediastinum. Blunt chest trauma can result in pneumomediastinum caused by an abrupt increase in intra-alveolar pressure and shearing forces affecting the alveolar walls.

Pneumomediastinum arising from the tracheobronchial tree or esophagus usually results from traumatic disruption of these structures. The marked shearing forces that develop with blunt trauma may lead to fracture of the trachea or mainstem bronchi. Penetrating trauma to the tracheobronchial tree is usually iatrogenic and may follow endotracheal intubation, bronchoscopy, or tracheostomy. Rarely, neoplasms or inflammatory lesions (e.g., tuberculosis) may erode through the tracheal wall and into the peritracheal fat. Esophageal rupture is most often spontaneous, usually in the setting of severe, prolonged vomiting (Boerhaave's syndrome). In addition to pneumomediastinum, a left hydropneumothorax and pneumoperitoneum may be present in this condition. Spontaneous esophageal rupture may occur during childbirth, during a severe asthmatic episode, or with blunt chest trauma. Endoscopic procedures, stent placement, esophageal dilatation, corrosive ingestion, and carcinoma may lead to esophageal perforation. Mediastinal gas may be produced by bacterial organisms in acute mediastinitis.

Air within the soft tissues of the neck from penetrating trauma or laryngeal fracture may lead to pneumomediastinum by extending inferiorly through the retropharyngeal and prevertebral spaces, or along the sheaths of the great vessels. Deep-space infections in the neck can spread along the same fascial planes and lead to mediastinitis. "Ludwig's angina" describes the substernal chest pain caused by the intramediastinal extension of such infections. Rarely, pneumomediastinum develops as air dissects superiorly from the retroperitoneum through the aortic hiatus or from the peritoneal cavity along the internal mammary vascular sheaths.

The symptoms associated with pneumomediastinum vary with the underlying cause, the extent of mediastinal air, and the presence of mediastinitis. Mediastinal air without infection is usually asymptomatic and does not require treatment. In some patients with spontaneous pneumomediastinum, there may be substernal, pleuritic-type chest pain of sudden onset that can be related to a specific inciting incident such as vomiting or Valsalva maneuver. Dyspnea may be present. In adults, mediastinal air under pressure usually escapes into the neck producing crepitus over the neck, supraclavicular regions, and chest wall. Rarely, mediastinal air under pressure may produce a tension pneumomediastinum in which the clinical findings are those of cardiac tamponade. Patients with mediastinitis and pneumomediastinum are usually seriously ill with chest pain, high fevers, dyspnea, and signs of sepsis. The radiographic findings of pneumomediastinum are reviewed in chapter 14.

THE HILA

Hilar abnormalities are first appreciated on conventional posteroanterior and lateral chest radiographs. CT and MR are used to confirm and characterize hilar masses or to detect subradiographic involvement of the hila, the latter most often in patients with bronchogenic carcinoma.

Unilateral Hilar Enlargement

Malignancy (Table 13.9). A hilar mass usually represents bronchogenic carcinoma or confluent lymph node metastases. Unilateral hilar enlargement may be the presenting radiographic feature of squamous cell carcinoma, where the hilar mass represents the central extension of an endobronchial tumor from its origin within a segmental bronchus (see Fig. 16.8). Concommitant hilar lymph node involvement may contribute to the hilar enlargement in some of these patients. Approximately 20% of patients with squamous cell carcinoma have a hilar mass on chest radiograph. In contrast, patients with adenocarcinoma and large cell carcinoma more commonly present with a peripheral pulmonary nodule or mass. In many patients, the hilar mass may be obscured by adjacent lung collapse or obstructive pneumonitis.

Unilateral hilar enlargement caused by metastatic lymph node involvement is most often seen in small cell carcinoma (Fig. 13.20). The propensity of this tumor for early invasion of the bronchial submucosa and peribronchial lymphatics accounts for the high incidence of widespread hematogenous and hilar and mediastinal lymph node metastases at the time of diagnosis. Plain film evidence of enlarged hilar lymph nodes caused by metastases from adenocarcinoma of lung or large cell carcinoma are seen in only 10–15% of patients. Contrast-enhanced CT or MR is more sensitive for detecting enlarged hilar nodes and should be performed in all patients to guide further staging procedures and for proper preoperative or treatment planning.

Metastases to hilar and mediastinal lymph nodes from extrathoracic malignancies are uncommon, occurring in approximately 2% of patients. The malignancies that are most often associated with intrathoracic nodal metastases are genitourinary (renal and testicular), head and neck (skin, larynx, and thyroid), breast, and melanoma (7). In renal cell carcinoma and seminoma, lymphatic spread of tumor to retroperitoneal nodes and up the thoracic duct to the posterior mediastinum is the mode of

Table 13.9. Unilateral Hilar Enlargement

Lymph node enlargement	
Malignancy	Bronchogenic carcinoma
	Lymph node metastases
	Bronchogenic carcinoma
	Head and neck malignancy
	Squamous cell carcinoma of skin, larynx
	Thyroid carcinoma
	Breast carcinoma
	Melanoma
	Genitourinary malignancy
	Renal cell carcinoma
	Testicular neoplasm
	Lymphoma
Infection	Tuberculosis
	Histoplasmosis
	Coccidioidomycosis
	Pneumonic plaque
	Tularemia
	Anaerobic lung abscess
	Measles
	Mononucleosis
Pulmonary artery enlargement	Valvular pulmonic stenosis
	Pulmonary artery aneurysm
	Infection
	Tuberculosis (Rasmussen's aneurysm)
	Left-to-right shunts
	Patent ductus arteriosis
	Atrial and ventricular septal defects
	Arteritis (see below)
	Tetrology of Fallot
	Central pulmonary embolus
	Chronic thromboembolic disease
	Pulmonary arteritis
	Behcet's disease
	Hughes-Stovin syndrome
	Takayasu's arteritis
Cyst	Bronchogenic cyst

as intrathoracic lymph node enlargement, with 35% showing hilar or middle mediastinal lymph node enlargement, some as an isolated finding.

Infection. Unilateral hilar or mediastinal lymph node enlargement is a characteristic feature in primary pulmonary tuberculosis in distinction to postprimary tuberculosis; an exception is the severely immunocompromised patient with AIDS. Isolated lymph node enlargement as a manifestation of primary tuberculosis is more common in children than in adults. There is almost always concommitant parenchymal disease in immunocompetent patients with lymph node enlargement.

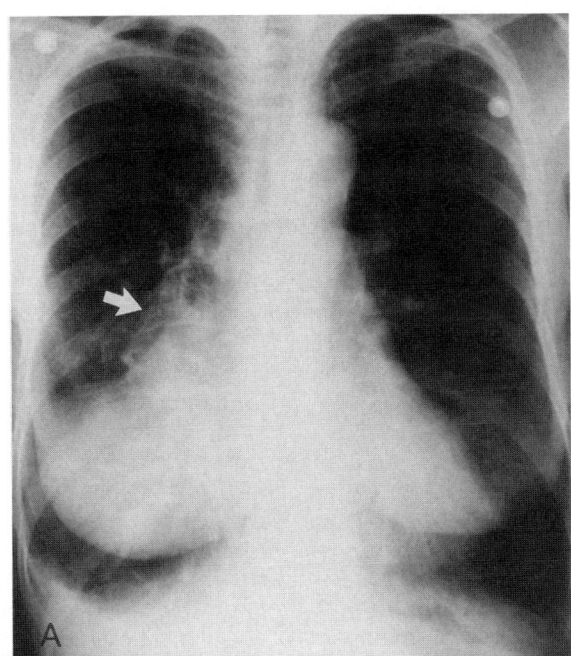
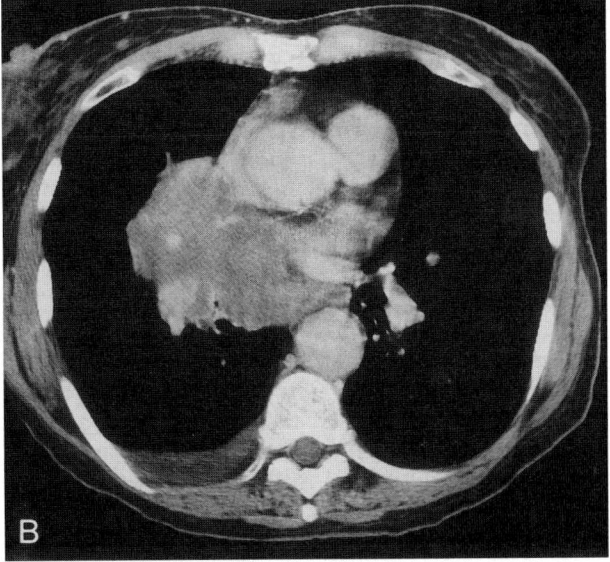

Figure 13.20. Hilar Nodal Metastases from Small Cell Carcinoma of Lung. A. A frontal radiograph in a patient with small cell carcinoma of lung shows emphysema and a right hilar mass (*arrow*) with middle lobe atelectasis and a right pleural effusion. **B.** CT shows a large right hilar and mediastinal mass occluding the middle and lower lobe bronchi.

spread to thoracic nodes. Although no direct communication occurs between the thoracic duct and anterior mediastinal lymph nodes, reflux of tumor emboli through incompetent valves may allow tumor spread to hilar, paratracheal, and intraparenchymal lymphatics. Head and neck tumors reach the mediastinum via lymphatic spread from cervical lymph nodes. Intrathoracic nodal metastases from breast carcinoma are often seen late in the course of disease, often years after the initial diagnosis. Malignant melanoma is the extrathoracic neoplasm with the highest incidence of intrathoracic nodal metastases; patients with nodal disease will almost invariably have radiographic evidence of parenchymal metastases.

Although 75% of patients presenting with Hodgkin's lymphoma have evidence of intrathoracic lymph node enlargement, isolated unilateral hilar lymph node enlargement is uncommon. The thoracic manifestations in non-Hodgkin's lymphoma differ in primary pulmonary lymphoma as compared to lymphoma that primarily involves extrathoracic sites with secondary pulmonary involvement. Thoracic involvement in primary pulmonary lymphoma is largely limited to parenchymal and pleural disease, but secondary pulmonary lymphoma manifests

Fungal infections such as histoplasmosis and coccidioidomycosis may present with hilar lymph node enlargement, typically associated with patchy or lobar airspace consolidation in the ipsilateral lung (see Fig. 17.10). A variety of bacterial infections have been associated with unilateral hilar lymph node enlargement and include plague, tularemia, and anaerobic lung abscess. Tularemia (*Francisella tularensis*) causes parenchymal consolidation in association with hilar lymph node enlargement and pleural effusion.

The viral infections most commonly associated with hilar lymph node enlargement are infectious mononucleosis and measles pneumonia. The thorax is infrequently involved in mononucleosis, but hilar lymph node enlargement is the most common manifestation of intrathoracic disease. Lymph node enlargement may accompany the reticular interstitial opacities of typical measles pneumonia, or may be associated with nodular, segmental, or lobar opacities and pleural effusion in atypical measles pneumonia.

Pulmonary Artery Enlargement. Although unilateral hilar enlargement is most often caused by a mass or enlarged lymph nodes, abnormal enlargement of the right or left pulmonary artery may also cause hilar prominence. Vascular disorders producing unilateral pulmonary artery enlargement include post-stenotic dilatation from valvular or postvalvular pulmonic stenosis, pulmonary artery aneurysms, and distension of the pulmonary artery by thrombus or tumor. Patients with congenital valvular pulmonic stenosis may develop post-stenotic dilatation or aneurysms of the main and left pulmonary arteries from the jet effect of blood upon these vessels. Rarely, stenoses resulting from pulmonary artery vasculitis, congenital rubella, or William's syndrome may lead to post-stenotic dilatation of a pulmonary artery. Aneurysms of the central pulmonary arteries are usually associated with congenital heart disease such as pulmonic stenosis and left-to-right shunts from ventricular septal defect and patent ductus arteriosis. Rare vasculitides such as Behcet's disease and the Hughes-Stovins syndrome may present with pulmonary artery aneurysms. A large pulmonary embolus lodging in the proximal portion of a pulmonary artery may cause proximal dilatation. Obviously, these patients are symptomatic and will show characteristic findings on perfusion lung scan, helical CT, and pulmonary arteriography.

Bronchogenic cyst is an uncommon cause of a hilar mass. CT and MR will show a round, smooth, thin-walled cyst, usually found in an asymptomatic young adult. Because the hilum is an unusual location for a bronchogenic cyst and distinction from a necrotic tumor or lymph node mass cannot be made radiographically, these lesions should be removed or a biopsy should be done.

Bilateral Hilar Enlargement

Bilateral hilar enlargement is caused by either enlargement of hilar lymph nodes or the central pulmonary arteries (Table 13.10).

Malignancy. The malignancies producing bilateral hilar lymph node enlargement are similar to those producing unilateral enlargement. In distinction to unilateral nodal enlargement, metastases are uncommon causes of bilateral hilar nodal enlargement. The most frequent solid tumors producing bilateral hilar disease are small cell carcinoma of lung and malignant melanoma.

Bilateral hilar lymph node involvement by lymphoma is more common in Hodgkin's disease than non-Hodgkin's's lymphoma. Hilar involvement is virtually never seen without concomitant anterior mediastinal nodal enlargement in Hodgkin's disease whereas non-Hodgkin's's lymphoma may produce isolated hilar disease.

The most common chest radiographic manifestation of leukemic involvement of the thorax is hilar and mediastinal lymph node enlargement, which is seen in as many as 25% of patients. Lymph node enlargement is much more common in the lymphocytic than the myelogenous form, particularly in chronic lymphocytic leukemia.

Infection. Mediastinal and hilar lymph node enlargement from infection is most often seen in tuberculous and fungal infection with histoplasmosis and coccidioidomycosis. In these diseases, the lymph node enlargement may be unilateral or bilateral. With bilateral disease, the enlargement is asymmetric in distinction to sarcoidosis, which is typically symmetric. Bacterial infection from *Bacillus anthracis* (anthrax) and *Yersinia pestis* (plague) may produce bilateral hilar enlargement. In anthrax infection, the lymph node enlargement is often associated with lower lobe, patchy air-space opacities. The bubonic form of plague may produce marked hilar and mediastinal adenopathy without pneumonia. Recurrent bacterial infection complicating cystic fibrosis is often associated with bilateral hilar lymph node enlargement, and distinction from pulmonary artery enlargement due to the pulmonary hypertension may be difficult.

Sarcoidosis is associated with bilateral hilar lymph node enlargement in 80% of patients. Most of these patients have concomitant paratracheal lymph node enlargement, and nearly half have concomitant radiographic parenchymal disease. The pattern of lymph node involvement in sarcoidosis has been termed the 1-2-3 sign, with 1 = right paratracheal, 2 = right hilar, and

Table 13.10. Bilateral Hilar Enlargement

Lymph node enlargement	Malignancy (see Table 13.2)
	Infection (see Table 13.2)
	Inflammatory disease
	Sarcoidosis
	Berylliosis
	Angioimmunoblastic lymphadenopathy
	Inhalational disease
	Silicosis
Pulmonary artery enlargement	Pulmonary arterial hypertension
	Left-to-right intracardiac shunt
	High output state
	Anemia
	Thyrotoxicosis
	Cystic fibrosis

Table 13.11. Small Hilum (Hila)

Unilateral	Absence or hypoplasia of the pulmonary artery
	Hypoplastic or hypogenetic lung
	Swyer-James syndrome
	Lobar atelectasis
	Lobar resection
	Compression/invasion of the pulmonary artery
	Cyst
	Neoplasm
	Fibrosing mediastinitis
Bilateral	Emphysema
	Obstruction to pulmonary flow
	Fibrosing mediastinitis
	Tetrology of Fallot
	Valvular pulmonic stenosis
	Ebstein's anomaly

3 = left hilar lymph node enlargement. The enlarged nodes produce symmetric, lobulated hilar masses on plain film because the enlarged nodes remain separate (Fig. 13.9). In 20% of patients, the involved lymph nodes will calcify; usually the calcifications are punctate in appearance, but occasionally peripheral "egg-shell" calcification is seen. In some patients, the involved nodes can be seen to enhance after contrast administration on CT. In the majority of patients, the enlarged nodes resolve within 2 years of discovery; in a small percentage, the nodes remain enlarged for many years.

Berylliosis and Silicosis. The hilar and mediastinal lymph node enlargement of chronic berylliosis is radiographically indistinguishable from sarcoidosis. Similarly, silicosis can produce hilar and mediastinal lymph node enlargement; eggshell calcification of hilar nodes is highly suggestive of this entity although peripheral nodal calcification may also be seen with sarcoidosis, histoplasmosis, or amyloidosis.

Bilateral pulmonary artery enlargement is seen with increased flow or increased resistance in the pulmonary circulation. The conditions associated with bilateral pulmonary arterial enlargement are reviewed in chapter 15.

Small Hilum (Hila)

Bilaterally small hila (Table 13.11) can be seen in some adults with severe pulmonary overinflation from emphysema or in those with diminished pulmonary blood flow caused by congenital pulmonary outflow obstruction (Tetralogy of Fallot, Ebstein's anomaly).

The most common cause of a small hilum is atelectasis or resection of a portion of lung, leaving a small residual hilar artery supplying the remaining lobe or lobes. Hypoplasia of the pulmonary artery, often with associated abnormalities of the ipsilateral lung (hypogenetic lung syndrome, Swyer-James syndrome), is another cause of a small hilum. Less commonly, invasion of the proximal pulmonary artery by mediastinal tumor or obstruction of the pulmonary artery caused by fibrosing mediastinitis can produce a diminutive hilar shadow. In any patient in whom a small hilum is a new radiographic finding, a CT should be performed to assess the mediastinum for central obstructing lesions. The left hilum can appear small in patients in whom the hilar shadow is obscured by the upper left heart margin or by fat in the region of the aortopulmonic interface. In these cases, the lateral radiograph will usually show a normal-sized left pulmonary artery.

References

1. Glazer GM, Axel L, Moss AA. CT diagnosis of mediastinal thyroid. AJR. Am J Roentgenol. 1992;138:495–498.
2. Chen J, Weisbrod GL, Herman SJ. Computed tomography and pathologic correlations of thymic lesions. J Thorac Imag 1988;3:61–65.
3. Filly R, Blank N, Castellino RA. Radiographic distribution of intrathoracic disease in previously untreated patients with Hodgkin's disease and non-Hodgkin's lymphoma. Radiology 1976;120:277–281.
4. Castellino RA. The non-Hodgkin's lymphomas: practical concepts for the diagnostic radiologist. Radiology 1991;178:315–321.
5. Rosado-de-Christenson ML, Templeton PA, Moran CA. Mediastinal germ-cell tumors: radiologic-pathologic correlation. Radiographics 1992;12:1013–1020.
6. Friedman PJ. Lung cancer: update on staging classifications. AJR Am J Roentgenol 1988;150:261–264.
7. McLoud TC, Kalisher L, Stark P, et al. Intrathoracic lymph node metastases from extrathoracic neoplasm. AJR Am J Roentgenol 1978;131:403–407.
8. Nakata H, Nakayama C, Komoto T, et al. Computed tomography of mediastinal bronchogenic cysts. J Comput Assist Tomogr 1982;6:733–738.
9. Reed JC, Haller KK, Feigin DS. Neural tumors of the thorax: subject review from the AFIP. Radiology 1978;126:9–17.
10. Carrol CL, Jeffrey RB, Federle MP, et al. CT evaluation of mediastinal infections. J Comput Assist Tomogr 1989;11:449–454.
11. Woodring JH, Loh FK, Kryscio RJ. Mediastinal hemorrhage: an evaluation of radiographic manifestations. Radiology 1984;151:15–21.
12. Gray JM, Hanson GC. Mediastinal emphysema: etiology, diagnosis, and treatment. Thorax 1966;21:325–332.

14
Radiographic Findings in Chest Disease

Jeffrey S. Klein

RADIOGRAPHIC FINDINGS IN LUNG DISEASE

Parenchymal lung disease can be divided into those processes that produce an abnormal increase in density of all or a portion of the lung on chest radiographs (pulmonary opacity) and those that produce an abnormal decrease in lung density (pulmonary lucency). The normal density of lung is due to the relative proportion of air to soft tissue (blood or parenchyma) in the ratio of 11 to 1. Therefore, processes that increase the relative amount of soft tissue will create a significant decrease in this ratio and be more easily discernable than diffuse processes that destroy blood vessels and parenchyma and cause little change in this ratio, thereby producing only small decreases in the overall lung density. CT, by virtue of superior contrast resolution, is more sensitive to subtle decreases in overall radiographic density than plain radiography.

Abnormal pulmonary opacities consist of air space filling opacities, opacities resulting from atelectasis, interstitial opacities, nodular or mass-like opacities, and branching opacities (Table 14.1). These patterns accurately represent pulmonary pathologic processes in correlative radiographic-pathologic studies, and are a practical means of generating a differential diagnosis based on the known patterns of parenchymal involvement in a wide variety of pulmonary diseases.

Pulmonary Opacity

AIR SPACE DISEASE

Radiographic Findings. The radiographic characteristics of air space disease are listed in Table 14.2. Air space patterns of opacity develop when the air normally present within the terminal air spaces of the lung is replaced by material of soft tissue density such as blood, transudate, exudate, or neoplastic cells. A segmental distribution of disease may be seen in a process such as pneumococcal pneumonia, which begins in the terminal air spaces and spreads from involved to uninvolved air spaces via interalveolar channels (pores of Kohn) and channels bridging preterminal bronchioles with alveoli (canals of Lambert). Initially, the opacity is poorly marginated as the air space filling process extends in an irregular fashion to involve adjacent air spaces, creating an irregular interface with the x-ray beam. Not uncommonly, air-space nodules, which are poorly marginated rounded opacities 6–8 mm in diameter, may be seen at the leading edge of an air space filling process. These nodules represent filling of acini or other sublobular structures, and are most often seen in diffuse alveolar pulmonary edema and transbronchial spread of cavitary tuberculosis.

A characteristic of air space filling processes is the tendency of air space shadows to coalesce as they extend through the lung (1). When the air spaces are rendered opaque by the presence of intra-alveolar cellular material and fluid, the normally aerated bronchi become visible as tubular lucencies called air bronchograms (Fig. 14.1). Occasionally, small intra-acinar bronchi or groups of uninvolved alveoli may be visible within an air space nodule as air bronchiolograms or air alveolograms respectively. Rarely, severe interstitial disease encroaching on the air spaces may produce an air bronchogram; this is most typically seen in "alveolar" sarcoid. When the air space filling process extends to the interlobar fissure, it appears as a sharply marginated lobar opacity.

A pattern of parenchymal opacity that reliably represents an air space filling process is the "bat's wing" or "butterfly" pattern of disease. In this pattern, dense opacities occupy the central regions of lung and extend laterally to abruptly marginate before reaching the peripheral portions of the lung, hence the term "bat's wing" (see Fig. 15.2). To date, no explanation exists for this distribution of disease, which appears almost exclusively in patients with pulmonary edema or hemorrhage. Another feature of air space filling processes is the tendency to rapidly change in appearance over short intervals of time. The development or resolution of parenchymal opacities within hours usually indicates an air space filling process; prominent exceptions include atelectasis and interstitial pulmonary edema. The differential diagnosis of diffuse confluent air space opacifiies is reviewed in Table 14.3.

CT/HRCT Findings. The CT and HRCT findings of air space disease are similar to those described on plain

Table 14.1. Patterns of Parenchymal Opacity

Type	Example
Air space (alveolar) filling	Pneumococcal pneumonia
Interstitial opacities	
Reticular	Idiopathic pulmonary fibrosis
Reticulonodular	Sarcoidosis
Nodular	Miliary tuberculosis
Linear	Interstitial pulmonary edema
Nodule/mass	Granuloma
	Bronchogenic carcinoma
Linear/tubular opacities	
Linear/curvilinear	Subsegmental atelectasis
	Parenchymal scar
Branching	Allergic bronchopulmonary aspergillosis
Atelectasis	Endobronchial neoplasm

Table 14.2. Radiographic Characteristics of Air Space Disease

Lobar or segmental distribution
Poorly marginated
Air space nodules
Tendency to coalesce
Air bronchograms
Bat's wing (butterfly) distribution
Rapidly changing over time

Table 14.3. Diffuse Confluent Air-Space Opacities—Differential Diagnosis

Type	Example
Pulmonary edema	Cardiogenic
	Fluid overload/renal failure
	Noncardiogenic (ARDS)(See Table 15.2)
Pneumonia	Pneumocystis carinii
	Gram negative bacteria
	Influenza
	Fungi
	Histoplasmosis
	Aspergillosis
Hemorrhage	See Table 15.3
Neoplasm	Bronchoalveolar cell carcinoma
	Lymphoma
Alveolar proteinosis	Acute silica inhalation
	Lymphoma
	Leukemia
	AIDS

chest radiograph. These are as follows: *a)* lobar, segmental, and/or lobular distribution of disease; *b)* poorly marginated opacities that tend to coalesce; *c)* air space nodules; and *d)* air bronchograms. A lobar or segmental distribution of disease is easily appreciated on cross-sectional imaging. CT and HRCT are further capable of showing individually opacified lobules, termed a "patchwork quilt" appearance, seen in many air space processes, most classically bronchopneumonia (see Fig. 17.3). Coalescence of opacities, commonly seen in pulmonary edema and pneumonia, is best assessed on serial CT studies. With isolated air space disease, the interlobular septa are normal or obscured. As with plain films, the presence of air space nodules provides further evidence of an air space process. On HRCT studies, these nodules are usually seen within the peribronchiolar (centrilobular) region of the pulmonary lobule. Air bronchograms or bronchiolograms are usually better appreciated on CT and HRCT than on plain radiographs because of superior contrast resolution and the cross-sectional nature of CT. This is particularly true in those regions of the lung where bronchi course in the transverse plane (anterior segments of upper lobes, middle lobe and lingula, and superior segments of the lower lobes).

ATELECTASIS

General Principles and Mechanisms. Atelectasis literally means incomplete expansion. It is used to describe any condition in which lung volume loss occurs and is usually but not invariably associated with an in-

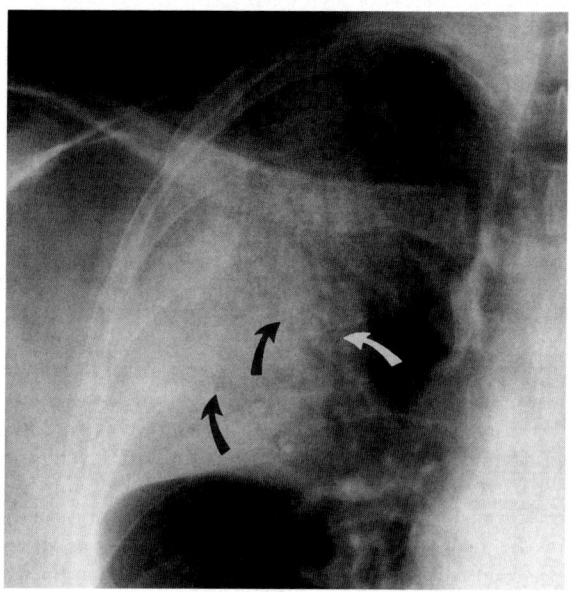

Figure 14.1. Air Bronchograms in Air Space Disease. Coned-down view of the right upper lobe in a patient with *Pneumococcal* pneumonia shows homogeneous lobar air space disease delineated inferiorly by the minor fissure. Note the presence of air bronchograms (*arrows*) within the opacified lobe.

crease in radiographic density. There are four basic mechanisms of atelectasis (Table 14.4).

The most common form of atelectasis is *obstructive or resorptive atelectasis,* which is secondary to complete endobronchial obstruction of a lobar bronchus with distal resorption of gas. Incomplete bronchial obstruction more often produces air trapping from a check-valve effect rather than atelectasis because air enters but cannot exit the lung. Complete obstruction of a central bronchus may not produce atelectasis if collateral air flow to the obstructed lung (via pores of Kohn, canals of

Lambert, or incomplete interlobar fissures) allows the lung to remain inflated. An obstructed lobe or lung containing 100% oxygen, as may be seen in some mechanically ventilated patients, will collapse more rapidly (sometimes within minutes) than a lung containing ambient air. This occurs because oxygen is rapidly absorbed from the alveolar spaces into alveolar capillaries. Bronchogenic carcinoma, foreign bodies, mucus plugs, and malpositioned endotracheal tubes are the most common causes of endobronchial obstruction and secondary resorptive atelectasis.

Passive or relaxation atelectasis results from the mass effect of an air or fluid collection within the pleural space on the subjacent lung. Because the natural tendency of the lung is to collapse when dissociated from the chest wall, pleural collections will produce atelectasis. The degree of atelectasis depends on the size of the pleural collection, presence or absence of pleural adhesions, and the underlying lung's condition. A large pleural collection in a normal pleural space will produce virtual complete collapse of a normal lung, which will be seen as a small, dense, rounded opacity retracted to a perihilar location. Alternatively, if the underlying lung is abnormal (consolidated or has interstitial disease), it may show only minimal volume loss. A large pleural or chest wall mass or an elevated diaphragm can also produce passive atelectasis. *Compressive atelectasis* is a form of passive atelectasis in which an intrapulmonary mass compresses adjacent lung parenchyma; common causes include bullae, abscesses, and tumors.

Processes resulting in parenchymal fibrosis reduce alveolar volume and produce *cicatricial atelectasis.* Localized cicatricial atelectasis is most often seen in association with chronic upper lobe fibronodular tubercu-losis. The radiographic appearance is that of severe lobar volume loss with scarring, bronchiectasis, and compensatory hyperinflation of adjacent lung. Diffuse cicatricial atelectasis is seen in interstitial fibrosis of any cause. An overall increase in lung density with reticular opacities and diminished lung volumes is characteristic of this condition.

Adhesive atelectasis occurs in association with surfactant deficiency. Type II pneumocytes, the cells responsible for surfactant production, may be injured as a result of as a result of general anesthesia, ischemia, or radiation damage. Surfactant deficiency causes increased alveolar surface tension that results in diffuse alveolar collapse and volume loss. Radiographs show a diminution in lung volume that may be associated with an increase in density.

Radiographic Signs of Atelectasis. Lobar atelectasis is described in Table 14.5 (2). The only direct radiographic finding of lobar atelectasis is the displacement of an interlobar fissure. Several indirect findings of atelectasis exist, most of which reflect attempted compensation for the volume loss (Fig. 14.2). Diminished aeration results in increased density in the affected portion of lung. Shift of mediastinal and hilar structures toward the affected lung is a common finding in lobar atelectasis. Tracheal displacement and hilar elevation are common in upper lobe atelectasis, and hilar depression, cardiac shift, and elevation of the hemidiaphragm may be seen with lower lobe atelectasis. Shift of the entire mediastinum is typical of collapse of an entire lung. Compensatory hyperinflation represents an attempt by the normal portion of the lung to occupy a greater than

Table 14.4. Types of Pulmonary Atelectasis

Type	Example
Obstructive (resorptive)	Bronchogenic carcinoma (endobronchial)
Passive (relaxation)	Pleural effusion Pneumothorax
Compressive	Bulla
Cicatricial	Postprimary tuberculosis Radiation fibrosis
Adhesive	Respiratory distress syndrome of the newborn

Table 14.5. Radiographic Signs in Lobar Atelectasis

Direct Signs	Indirect Signs
Displacement of interlobar fissure	Increased density of atelectatic lung Ipsilateral mediastinal shift Hilar elevation (upper lobe atelectasis) or depression (lower lobe atelectasis) Compensatory hyperinflation of adjacent lobe(s) Shifting granuloma Small hemithorax

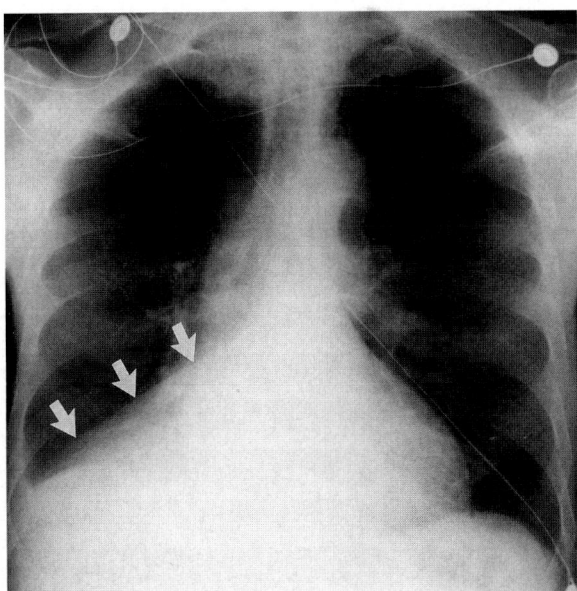

Figure 14.2. Lobar Atelectasis. Upright frontal chest radiograph in a postoperative patient with right lower lobe atelectasis shows a homogeneous triangular opacity in the right lower lung partially obscuring the right hemidiaphragm. The upper margin of the collapsed lobe is marginated by the inferiorly displaced major fissure (*arrows*). Bronchoscopy retrieved a mucous plug from the right lower lobe bronchus and the lobe subsequently re-expanded.

normal portion of one or both hemithoraces in response to atelectasis. Usually developing with chronic volume loss and not seen in acute collapse, this mechanism is seen as increased lucency with attenuation of pulmonary vascular markings. In complete lung or upper lobe atelectasis, the contralateral upper lobe may herniate across the midline, bowing the anterior junction line toward the affected side. A characteristic but seldom seen plain radiographic finding of compensatory hyperinflation is the "shifting granuloma" in which a preexisting granuloma in an adjacent aerated lung changes position as it moves toward the collapsed lobe. In chronic atelectasis of a lung, a hemithorax size decrease with approximation of the ribs may be seen. The absence of an air bronchogram distinguishes resorptive lobar atelectasis from lobar pneumonia, particularly if the atelectatic lobe is only slightly diminished in volume. Compensatory hyperinflation in patients with long-standing atelectasis is best appreciated on CT because of its superior contrast resolution and cross-sectional nature.

Segmental Atelectasis. Atelectasis of one or several segments of a lobe is difficult to determine on plain radiographs. The appearance ranges from a thin linear opacity to a wedge shaped opacity which does not abut an interlobar fissure. Segmental atelectasis is better appreciated on CT.

Subsegmental (plate-like) Atelectasis. Band-like linear opacities representing linear atelectasis are commonly associated with disorders in which diaphragmatic movement is diminished. This is seen in patients with pleuritic chest pain, postoperative patients, or patients with massive hepatosplenomegaly or ascites. Subsegmental atelectasis tends to occur at the lung bases. The linear shadows are 2–10 cm in length and are typically oriented perpendicular to the costal pleura (Fig. 14.3). Pathologically these areas of linear collapse are deep to invaginations of visceral pleura formed by incomplete fissures or scars.

Rounded Atelectasis. This is an uncommon form of atelectasis in which the collapsed lung forms a round

mass in the lower lobe. This condition is most closely associated with asbestos related pleural disease, but may be seen in any condition associated with an exudative (proteinaceous) pleural effusion. The process develops when pleural adhesions form in the resolving phase of a pleural effusion and cause the adjacent lung to roll up into a ball as it reexpands. The round opacity is often found along the inferior and posterior costal pleural surface adjacent to an area of pleural fibrosis or plaque formation. Plain radiographs reveal a well-defined pleural-based mass between 2–7 centimeters in size adjacent to an area of pleural thickening in the lower lung. The identification of a curvilinear bronchovascular bundle, or "comet tail," entering the anterior inferior margin of the mass as seen on lateral radiographs or tomograms is characteristic. The CT appearance of round atelectasis is characteristic (Fig. 14.4). The round or wedge-shaped mass forms an acute angle with the pleura and is seen adjacent to an area of pleural thickening, usually in the inferior and posterior thorax. The "comet tail" of vessels and bronchi is seen curving between the hilum and the apex of the mass. The atelectatic lung enhances following IV contrast administration. When the characteristic CT findings are seen in a patient with a known history of asbestos exposure, the appearance is diagnostic and no further evaluation is necessary. However, any doubt regarding the diagnosis remains, a biopsy should be done on the lesion to exclude malignancy.

The characteristics of lobar atelectasis have been described. A triangular configuration with the apex at the pulmonary hilum is common to all types of lobar atelectasis. The displaced fissures typically assume a bowed configuration convex toward the collapse. The changes of lobar atelectasis are best appreciated on CT.

Right Upper Lobe Atelectasis. In right upper lobe atelectasis, the lung collapses superiorly and medially with superomedial displacement of the minor fissure and anteromedial displacement of the upper half of the major fissure, producing a right upper paramediastinal density on frontal radiographs. An obstructing central mass may

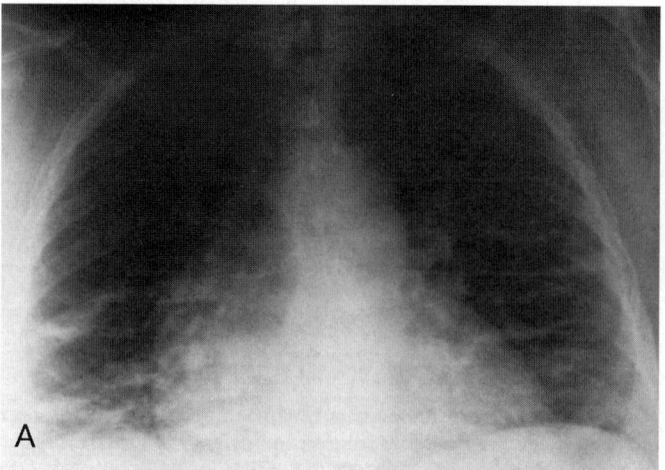
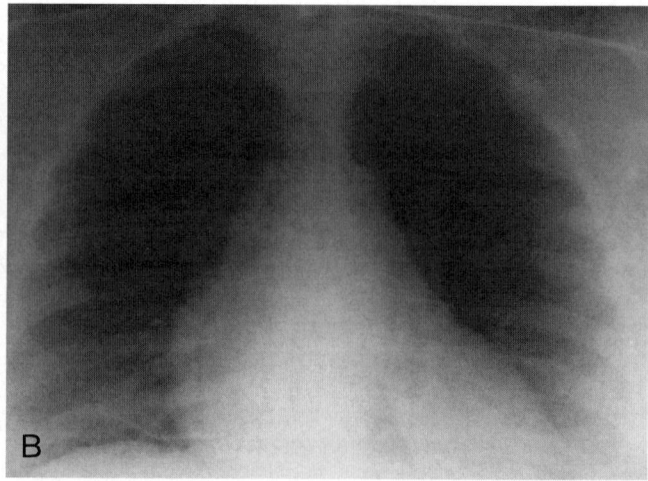

Figure 14.3. Subsegmental (plate-like) Atelectasis. Frontal chest radiograph in a woman 1 day following a cholecystectomy shows diminished lung volumes and numerous bilateral middle and lower zone linear opacities coursing perpendicular to the costal pleura representing areas of subsegmental atelectasis. The opacities resolved within several days.

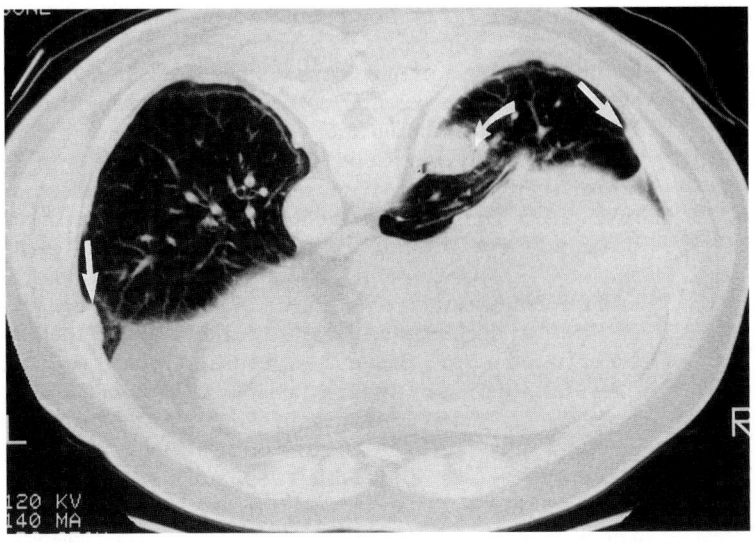

Figure 14.4. Round Atelectasis. Prone CT scan through the lung bases in a patient with asbestos-related pleural disease and rounded atelectasis shows a triangular opacity in the posteromedial right lower lobe associated with pleural thickening. Note the bronchus at the apex of the triangle (*curved arrow*). Bilateral pleural plaques are also evident (*straight arrows*).

produce a central convexity along the interface of the collapsed lobe with the overinflated middle lobe. The continuity of a central convexity with the peripheral concave interface between the collapsed upper lobe and aerated lung produces the "S-sign of Golden." The trachea is deviated toward the right, and the right hilum and hemidiaphragm are elevated. "Tenting," or "peaking," of the diaphragm is occasionally seen and represents fat within the inferior aspect of a stretched inferior accessory fissure. The left upper lobe may herniate across the midline anteriorly toward the right. The lateral radiograph may reveal a triangular opacity with its apex at the hilum and base against the apicoposterior costal pleural surface. Compensatory hyperinflation of the middle and lower lobes may be seen in chronic atelectasis. An atypical appearance of atelectasis, in which the collapsed right upper lobe maintains contact with the lateral costal pleural surface and collapses laterally rather than medially, has been described and is termed "peripheral right upper lobe atelectasis." In this form of atelectasis, the superior segment of the right lower lobe is interposed medial to the collapsed upper lobe, producing a well-marginated density laterally that mimics pleural disease on frontal radiographs. Scarring from tuberculosis, endobronchial tumor, and mucus plugging are common causes of right upper lobe atelectasis.

Middle Lobe Atelectasis produces inferior displacement of the minor fissure and superior displacement of the major fissure. Because of the minimal thickness of the collapsed middle lobe and the oblique orientation of the inferiorly displaced minor fissure, the detection of middle lobe atelectasis on frontal radiographs is difficult. The only finding on frontal radiographs may be a vague density over the right lower lung with obscuration of the right heart margin. The lateral radiograph shows a typical triangular density with its apex at the hilum (Fig. 14.5). A lordotic frontal radiograph, which projects the minor fissure tangent to the frontal x-ray beam, will depict the atelectatic middle lobe as a triangular opacity, which is sharply marginated superiorly by the minor fissure, with its apex directed laterally. Middle lobe atelec-

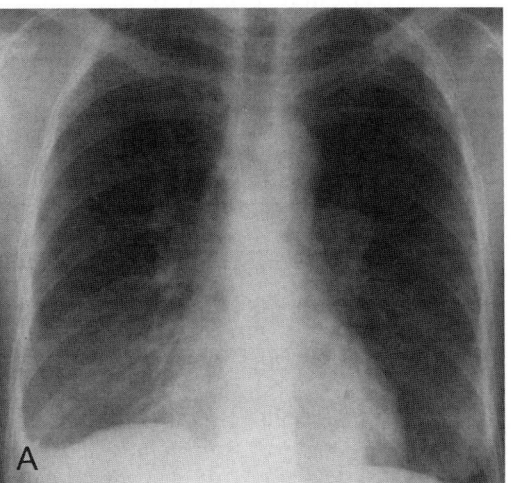

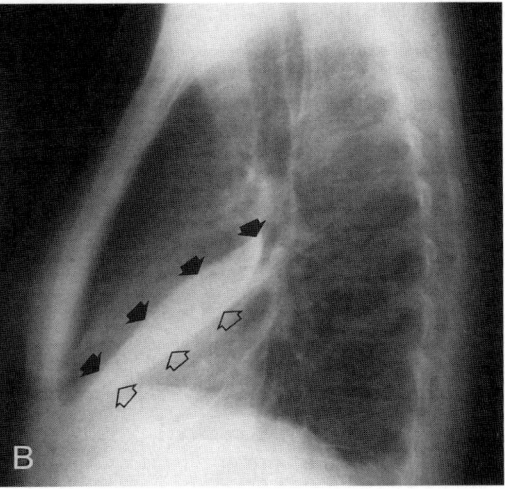

Figure 14.5. Middle Lobe Atelectasis. A. A frontal radiograph demonstrates a vague opacity in the right lower lung obscuring the right heart border and a small right pleural effusion. **B.** The lateral film shows the typical triangular opacity of middle lobe atelectasis overlying the cardiac shadow. The upper (*solid arrows*) and lower (*open arrows*) margins of the opacity represent the displaced minor and inferior portion of the right major fissure respectively.

tasis is most often cicatricial and follows middle lobe infection with secondary fibrosis and bronchiectasis.

Right Lower Lobe Atelectasis. The right lower lobe collapses toward the lower mediastinum because of the tethering effect of the inferior pulmonary ligament. This results in inferior displacement of the upper half of the major fissure and posterior displacement of the lower half, producing a triangular opacity in the right lower paravertebral space that obscures the medial right hemidiaphragm on frontal radiographs (Fig. 14.2). The lateral margin of this triangular opacity is formed by the displaced major fissure. The right hemidiaphragm may be elevated. The right interlobar pulmonary artery is obscured within the opaque collapsed lower lobe, a finding that helps distinguish the triangular opacity of right lower lobe atelectasis from a medial pleural effusion, which laterally displaces and does not obscure the interlobar artery. On lateral radiographs, a vague triangular opacity with its apex at the hilum and base over the posterior portion of the right hemidiaphragm and posterior costophrenic sulcus may be seen. Mucous plugs, foreign bodies, and endobronchial tumors are the most common causes.

Left Upper Lobe Atelectasis has a different appearance from right upper lobe atelectasis as a result of the absence of a minor fissure. The left upper lobe collapses anteriorly, maintaining a broad area of contact with the anterior costal pleural surface. The major fissure shifts anteriorly and is seen marginating a long, narrow band of increased opacity paralleling the anterior chest wall on lateral radiographs. The diagnosis on frontal radiographs may be difficult. A veil of increased opacity can be seen over the left upper thorax and obscuration of the left heart margin. The apex of the left hemithorax remains lucent because of hyperinflation of the superior segment of the left lower lobe. Leftward tracheal displacement, hilar and diaphragmatic elevation, and leftward bulging of the anterior junction line from an overinflated right upper lobe are additional clues to the diagnosis. An uncommon finding on the frontal radiograph in left upper lobe atelectasis is a crescent of air ("Luftsichel") along the left upper mediastinum, which represents a portion of the overinflated superior segment of the left lower lobe interposed between the aortic arch medially and the collapsed upper lobe laterally (see Fig. 16.8). Postinflammatory cicatrization and endobronchial tumor are the common causes of left upper lobe atelectasis.

Left Lower Lobe Atelectasis is similar in appearance to atelectasis of the right lower lobe. A triangular opacity in the left lower paramediastinal region with loss of the medial retrocardiac diaphragmatic outline is seen on frontal radiographs. In addition, the left hilum is displaced inferiorly and the interlobar artery is obscured. The diaphragm may be elevated and the heart shifted toward the left. Compensatory hyperinflation of the left upper lobe may be seen. The left lower lobe commonly is atelectatic in patients with large hearts and in postoperative patients, particularly those who have had coronary bypass surgery.

Combined Middle and Right Lower Lobe Atelectasis may be seen with obstruction of the bronchus intermedius by a mucous plug or tumor. The radiographic appearance on the frontal radiograph is characteristic, with a homogeneous triangular opacity sharply marginated superiorly by the depressed minor fissure and obscuration both of the right heart border and the right hemidiaphragm. Cardiac and mediastinal shift toward the right is common.

Lung Atelectasis. Collapse of an entire lung is most often seen with obstructing masses in the main bronchus. The lung is opacified with an absence of air bronchograms. The trachea and heart are shifted toward the side of collapse, with herniation of the contralateral anteromedial lung across the midline to widen the retrosternal space on lateral radiograph and bulge the anterior junction line on frontal radiograph. The chest wall may show approximation of the ribs in chronic collapse. Compensatory diaphragmatic elevation in left lung atelectasis may be recognized by noting superior displacement of the gastric air bubble or splenic flexure of colon.

INTERSTITIAL DISEASE

Interstitial opacities are produced by processes that thicken the interstitial compartments of the lung. Water, blood, tumor, cells, fibrous tissue, or any combination of these may render the interstitial space visible on radiographs. Interstitial opacities are usually divided into reticular, reticulonodular, nodular, and linear patterns on plain radiographs (Fig. 14.6)(Table 14.6)(3). The predominant pattern of opacity produced by an interstitial process depends on the nature of the underlying disease and the portion of the interstitium affected.

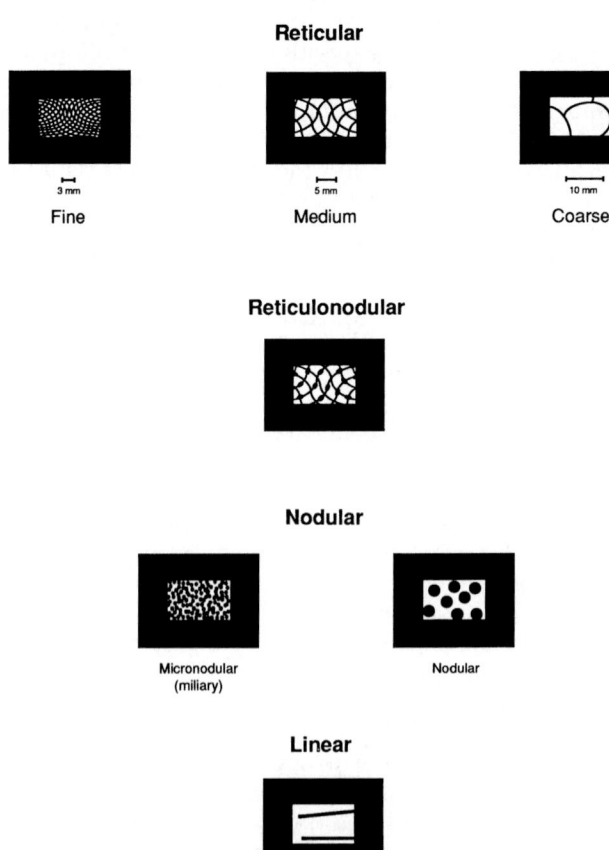

Figure 14.6. Patterns of Interstitial Opacity on Chest Radiographs.

Table 14.6. Causes of Chronic Interstitial Lung Disease

Predominantly Linear

Chronic interstitial edema
Lymphangitic carcinomatosis
Interstitial fibrosis of any etiology

Predominantly Reticular or Reticulonodular

Postinfectious scarring	Tuberculosis (postprimary)
	Histoplasmosis (chronic)
	Coccidioidomycosis (chronic)
	Pneumocystis carinii
Chronic interstitial edema	Mitral valve disease
Collagen vascular disease	Rheumatoid lung
	Scleroderma
	Dermatomyositis/polymyositis
	Ankylosing spondylitis
	Mixed connective tissue disease
	Idiopathic pulmonary hemorrhage
Granulomatous disease	Sarcoidosis
	Eosinophilic granuloma
Neoplasm	Lymphangitic carcinomatosis
	Lymphoma
	Lymphocytic interstitial pneumonitis (LIP)
Inhalational	Asbestosis
	Silicosis
	Coal worker's pneumoconiosis
	Berylliosis
	Hypersensitivity pneumonitis (chronic phase)
	Chronic aspiration
Drug reaction	Nitrofurantoin
	Chemotherapeutic agents
	Amiodarone
	Radiation pneumonitis (chronic)
Idiopathic	Idiopathic pulmonary fibrosis
	Lymphangioleiomyomatosis
	Tuberous sclerosis
	Neurofibromatosis
	Amyloidosis (alveolar septal form)

Predominantly Nodular

Miliary infection	Tuberculosis
	Fungi
	Histoplasmosis
	Coccidioidomycosis
	Cryptococcosis
	Virus
	Varicella (healed)
Pneumoconiosis	Silicosis
	Coal worker's pneumoconiosis
	Heavy metal dust
Granulomatous disease	Sarcoidosis
	Eosinophilic granuloma
	Talc granulomatosis
Neoplasm	
Primary	Synchronous bronchogenic carcinoma
	Lymphoma
	Hodgkin's
	Non-Hodgkin's
	Lymphomatoid granulomatosis
Metastatic	Bronchogenic carcinoma
	Thyroid carcinoma
	Renal cell carcinoma
	Breast carcinoma
	Melanoma
	Choriocarcinoma
	Osteogenic carcinoma
Idiopathic	Alveolar microlithiasis
	Amyloidosis (nodular form)

Radiographic Findings. A *reticular pattern* refers to a network of curvilinear opacities that usually involves the lungs diffusely. The subdivision of reticular opacities into fine, medium, and coarse opacities refers to the size of the lucent spaces created by these intersecting curvilinear opacities (Fig. 14.6). A fine reticular pattern, also known as a ground glass pattern, is seen in processes that thicken or line the parenchymal interstitium of the lung to produce a fine network of lines with intervening lucent spaces 1–2 mm in diameter. Diseases most commonly producing this appearance include interstitial pulmonary edema and usual interstitial pneumonitis (UIP) (see Fig. 18.14). Medium reticulation, also termed "honeycombing," refers to reticular interstitial opacities where the intervening spaces are 3–10 mm in diameter. This pattern is most commonly seen in pulmonary fibrosis involving the parenchymal and peripheral interstitial spaces. Coarse reticular opacities with spaces 1 cm in diameter are seen most commonly in diseases producing cystic spaces as a result of parenchymal destruction. The most common interstitial diseases associated with coarse reticulation are idiopathic pulmonary fibrosis, sarcoidosis, and histiocytosis X of the lung.

Reticulonodular opacities may be produced by the overlap of numerous reticular shadows or by the presence of both nodular and reticular opacities. In the latter situation, the nodules are usually caused by granulomata or small tumor deposits in the interstitium. Sarcoidosis and lymphangitic carcinomatosis are diseases that may give rise to true reticulonodular opacities.

Nodular opacities represent small, rounded lesions within the pulmonary interstitium. In contrast to air space nodules, interstitial nodules are homogeneous (they lack air bronchiolograms or air alveolograms) and are well defined because their margins are sharp and they are surrounded by normally aerated lung. In addition, unlike air space nodules, which tend to be uniform in diameter (~8 mm), interstitial nodules may be micronodular (<1 mm), small (1–5 mm), medium (5–10 mm) or large (>10 mm). A micronodular or miliary pattern is seen predominantly in granulomatous processes (e.g. miliary tuberculosis or histoplasmosis)(see Fig.17.8), hematogenous pulmonary metastases (most commonly thyroid and renal cell carcinoma), and pneumoconioses (silicosis)(see Fig. 18.10). Medium and large nodules are most often seen in metastatic disease to the lung, commonly from breast carcinoma or colorectal malignancy.

A linear pattern of interstitial opacities is seen in processes that thicken the axial (bronchovascular) or peripheral interstitium of the lung. Because the axial interstitium surrounds the bronchovascular structures, thickening of this compartment produces parallel linear opacities radiating from the hila when visualized in length or peribronchial "cuffs" when viewed end on. A central distribution of linear interstitial disease is most often seen with interstitial pulmonary edema or "increased markings" emphysema. This pattern of interstitial disease may be impossible to distinguish from airways diseases, such as bronchiectasis and asthma, which primarily thicken the walls of airways. Thickening of the peripheral interstitium of the lung produces linear opacities that are either obliquely oriented 2–6 cm long,

Table 14.7. Causes of Pulmonary Lucency

Localized	Cavity
	Cyst
	Bulla
	Bleb
	Pneumatocele
Diffuse	
Unilateral	Technical factors
	Grid cutoff
	Patient rotation
	Extrapulmonary disorder
	Soft tissue abnormalities
	Absent pectoralis muscle
	Mastectomy
	Contralateral pleural effusion/thickening
	Pneumothorax
	Pulmonary disease
	Diminished pulmonary blood flow
	Hypoplastic lung/pulmonary artery
	Obstruction of pulmonary artery
	Pulmonary embolism
	Mediastinal/hilar tumor
	Fibrosing mediastinitis
	Diminished pulmonary blood flow and
	hyperinflation
	Lobar atelectasis/resection
	Swyer-James syndrome
	Endobronchial tumor/foreign body
	producing a check valve effect
Bilateral	Technical factors
	Overpenetrated radiograph
	Diminished pulmonary blood flow
	Congenital pulmonary outflow
	obstruction
	Mediastinal tumor
	Pulmonary arterial hypertension
	Chronic thromboembolic disease
	Fibrosing mediastinitis
	Diminished pulmonary blood flow and
	hyperinflation
	Emphysema
	Asthma

less than 1 mm thick lines that course through the substance of the lung toward the hila (Kerley's A lines) or shorter (1–2 cm) thin lines that are peripheral and course perpendicular to and contact the pleural surface (Kerley's B lines). Kerley's A lines correspond to thickening of connective tissue sheets within the lung that contain lymphatic communications between the perivenous and bronchoarterial lymphatics, whereas Kerley's B lines represent thickened peripheral subpleural interlobular septa (see Fig. 15.1)(4). A linear pattern of disease is seen in pulmonary edema, lymphangitic carcinomatosis, and acute viral or atypical bacterial pneumonia. The HRCT findings of interstitial lung disease are reviewed in chapter 18.

PULMONARY NODULE

A pulmonary nodule refers to a discrete rounded opacity within the lung measuring less than 3 cm in diameter. A round opacity >3 cm in diameter is termed a "pul-

monary mass." A solitary pulmonary nodule presents a common diagnostic dilemma that will be discussed in chapter 16.

BRANCHING OPACITIES

Mucoid Impaction. Branching tubular opacities that are distinguished from normal vascular shadows invariably represent mucous-filled, dilated bronchi and are termed "bronchoceles," or mucoid impaction. Their appearance has been likened to that of a gloved finger or the shape of the letters V or Y, depending upon the length of airway and number of branches involved. When in a central perihilar location, these bronchoceles are a result of nonobstructive bronchiectasis, as occurs in patients with cystic fibrosis or allergic bronchopulmonary aspergillosis, or by postobstructive bronchiectasis distal to an endobronchial tumor or a congenitally atretic bronchus. In the latter condition, a typical location immediately distal to the expected location of the apical segmental bronchus and a hyperlucent segment or lobe distal to the bronchocele owing to collateral air drift should suggest the diagnosis. Peripheral bronchoceles are most often seen in cystic fibrosis and posttuberculous bronchiectasis.

Pulmonary Lucency

Abnormal lucency of the lung may be localized or diffuse (Table 14.7). Focal radiolucent lesions of the lung include cavities, cysts, bullae, blebs, and pneumatoceles (Fig. 14.7). These lesions are usually recognized by the identification of the wall that marginates the lucent lesion.

Focal pulmonary lucent lesions

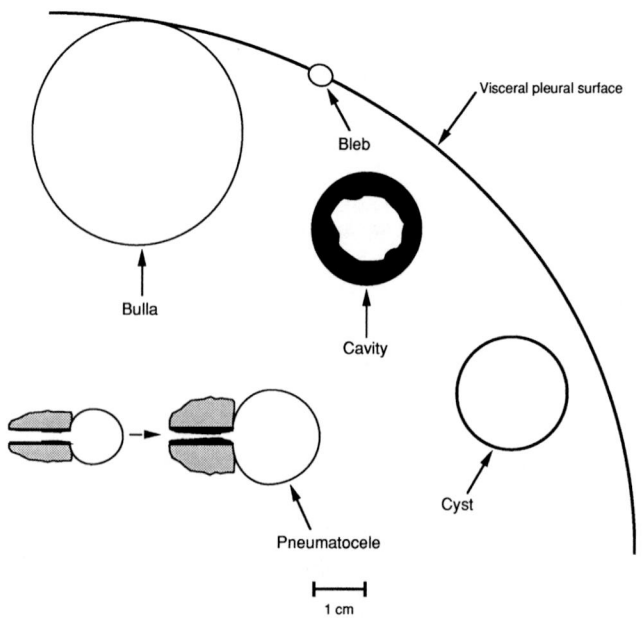

Figure 14.7. Focal Lucent Pulmonary Lesions.

FOCAL RADIOLUCENT LESIONS

A *cavity* forms when a pulmonary mass undergoes necrosis and communicates with an airway, leading to gas within its center. The wall of a cavity is usually irregular or lobulated and, by definition, is greater than 1 mm thick. Lung abscess and necrotic neoplasm are the most common cavitary pulmonary lesions. A *bulla* is a gas collection within the pulmonary parenchyma that is greater than 1 cm in diameter and has a thin wall less than 1 mm thick. It represents a focal area of parenchymal destruction (emphysema) and may contain fibrous strands, residual blood vessels, or alveolar septa. An *air cyst* is a term used to describe any well-circumscribed intrapulmonary gas collection with a smooth thin wall greater than 1 mm thick. Although some of these lesions will have a true epithelial lining (bronchogenic cyst that communicates with a bronchus), most do not and likely represent postinflammatory or posttraumatic lesions (5). A *bleb* is a collection of gas less than 1 cm in size within the layers of the visceral pleura. It is usually found in the apical portion of the lung. These small gas collections are not seen on plain radiographs, but may be visualized on chest CT where they are indistinguishable from paraseptal emphysema. Rupture of an apical bleb can cause spontaneous pneumothorax. *Pneumatoceles* are thin-walled gas-containing structures that represent distended air spaces distal to a check-valve obstruction of a bronchus or bronchiole. Often these are secondary to staphylococcal pneumonia. A *traumatic air cyst* results from pulmonary laceration following blunt trauma. These lesions resolve within 4–6 months. *Bronchiectatic cysts* are usually multiple-rounded thin-walled lucencies found in clusters in the lower lobes, and they represent saccular dilatations of airways in varicose or cystic bronchiectasis.

DIFFUSE PULMONARY HYPERLUCENCY

Unilateral pulmonary hyperlucency must be distinguished from differences in lung density caused by technical factors or overlying soft tissue abnormalities. Grid cutoff from a combination of lateral and near or far focus-grid decentering may lead to a graduated increase in density across the width of the chest film, simulating unilateral hyperlucency. Rotation of the patient will produce an increase in density over the lung rotated away from the film cassette. A left anterior oblique radiograph obtained with a posteroanterior beam will show increased density over the right hemithorax, simulating pleural disease on the right or hyperlucency on the left. Congenital absence of the pectoralis muscle (Poland's syndrome) or mastectomy can produce apparent hyperlucency.

True unilateral hyperlucent lung results from decreased blood flow to the lung. Diminished blood flow may result from a primary vascular abnormality, shunting of blood away from a lung that traps air, or a combination of the two. Hypoplasia of the right or left pulmonary artery produces a lung that is hyperlucent and diminished in size. A similar appearance may be produced by lobar resection or atelectasis, where the remaining lobe or lung hyperinflates to accommodate the

hemithorax, thereby attenuating pulmonary vessels and producing hyperlucency. Pulmonary arterial obstruction may be secondary to extrinsic compression or invasion by a hilar mass or to pulmonary embolism. A check-valve effect from an endobronchial tumor or foreign body can produce air trapping, resulting in shunting of blood and unilateral hyperlucency. The Swyer-James syndrome or unilateral hyperlucent lung is a condition that follows adenoviral infection during infancy (see Fig. 19.14). An asymmetric obliterative bronchiolitis with severe air trapping on expiration and secondary unilateral pulmonary artery hypoplasia produces the hyperlucency in this condition. Finally, asymmetric involvement of lung by emphysema can produce a hyperlucent lung; this is most common with severe bullous disease.

Bilateral hyperlucent lungs may be simulated by an overpenetrated film or in an image taken of a thin patient. As with unilateral hyperlucency, true bilateral hyperlucent lungs are the result of diminished pulmonary blood flow. This may be the result of congenital pulmonic stenosis, most commonly associated with the tetralogy of Fallot, or secondary to an acquired obstruction of the pulmonary circulation as in pulmonary arterial hypertension or chronic thromboembolic disease. Pulmonary emphysema results in hyperinflation with air trapping on expiration, destruction of the pulmonary microvasculature, and attenuation of lobar and segmental vessels, thereby producing bilateral hyperlucency (6). Asthma produces transient air trapping and diffuse bilateral vascular attenuation resulting in both hyperinflation and hyperlucency.

RADIOGRAPHIC FINDINGS OF MEDIASTINAL DISEASE

Mediastinal Masses

Posteroanterior and lateral chest radiographs are often the radiologic studies that lead to the discovery of a mediastinal mass. Mediastinal masses are recognized on frontal radiographs by the presence of a soft tissue density that causes unilateral or bilateral displacement of the normal lung-mediastinal interface or displaces adjacent mediastinal structures. The lung-mass interface typically is well defined laterally where it is convex with the adjacent lung, and it creates obtuse angles with the lung at its superior and inferior margins. This latter characteristic is diagnostic of an extrapulmonary, intramediastinal lesion although the occasional medial pleural mass may be indistinguishable from a mediastinal lesion. Lateral displacement of trachea or heart may be seen with large mediastinal masses, sometimes first recognized by displacement of an indwelling endotracheal tube, nasogastric tube, or intravascular catheter. The presence of calcification, fat, or, rarely, a fat/fluid level (as in a cystic teratoma) can limit the differential diagnosis of a mediastinal mass.

A thoracic CT or MR will be performed on virtually every patient with a mediastinal mass. Transthoracic US is occasionally useful, particularly in the evaluation of cardiac and vascular masses but its value is mostly limited to providing real-time imaging guidance during transthoracic needle biopsy.

CT, MR, and transthoracic US provide important information in the evaluation of mediastinal masses. The vascular origin of a mediastinal mass is readily apparent on contrast-enhanced CT, MR, and, occasionally, transthoracic or transesophageal US. The recognition of fat within a mediastinal mass on CT or MR limits the differential diagnosis to a small number of entities including diaphragmatic hernia, lipoma, teratoma, epicardial fat pad, and thymolipoma. A fat-fluid level is virtually diagnostic of a mature teratoma. Although calcification is occasionally detected radiographically within mediastinal masses, CT is considerably more sensitive and provides more specific characterization of the calcification. The presence of coarse calcification within an anterior mediastinal mass should suggest the diagnosis of a teratoma (especially if a tooth is seen) or thymoma (coarse calcification). Curvilinear rim-like calcification should suggest a cyst or aneurysm. Conversely, the presence of calcification within an untreated mediastinal mass virtually excludes the diagnosis of lymphoma.

Although frontal and lateral chest radiographs usually localize a mediastinal mass to one of three mediastinal compartments (anterior, middle, or posterior—see chapter 12), CT and MR provide more precise information regarding the location of the mass. This not only helps narrow the differential diagnosis but is key in guiding further diagnostic procedures (Fig. 14.8). For example, a posterior mediastinal mass intimately related to the esophagus is evaluated by esophagoscopy and transesophageal biopsy, but a subcarinal mass is best approached by bronchoscopy and transcarinal needle aspiration biopsy.

Mediastinal Widening

Described as a smooth, uniform increase in the transverse diameter of the mediastinum, mediastinal widening is often difficult to distinguish between technical factors, including anteroposterior technique, supine positioning, and rotation or true mediastinal disease as a cause of diffuse mediastinal widening on frontal chest radiographs. Clues to to the presence of disease include change in mediastinal width from prior frontal radiographs, mass effect upon adjacent mediastinal structures (tracheal deviation or displacement of an indwelling nasogastric tube or central venous catheter), increased density of the mediastinum, and obscuration of the normal mediastinal contours, most specifically the aortic knob and paratracheal stripe. Although normal measurements have been developed for mediastinal width, such great individual variability exists that absolute measurements are somewhat useless.

Pneumomediastinum and Pneumopericardium

The diagnosis of pneumomediastinum is usually made by findings on conventional radiographs. Small amounts of extraluminal air appear as linear or curvilinear lucencies within the confines of the mediastinum (see Fig. 13.19). Larger collections may be seen outlining the cardiac silhouette, mediastinal vessels, tracheobronchial tree or esophagus. The most common finding is air outlining the left heart border, where a curvilinear lucency representing pneumomediastinum is paralleled by a thin curvilinear opacity representing the combined thickness of the visceral and parietal pleura of the lingula. Another

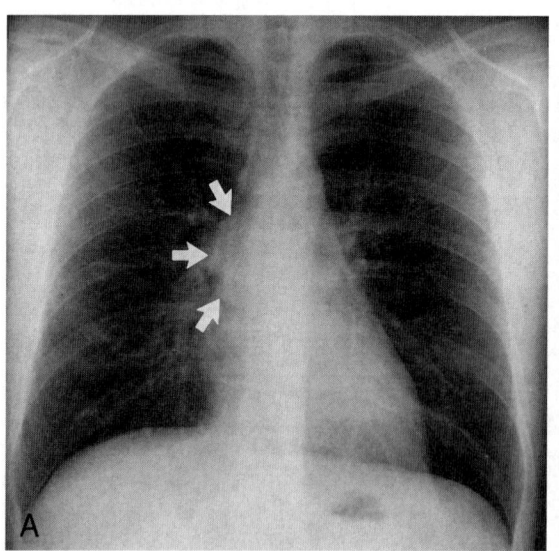

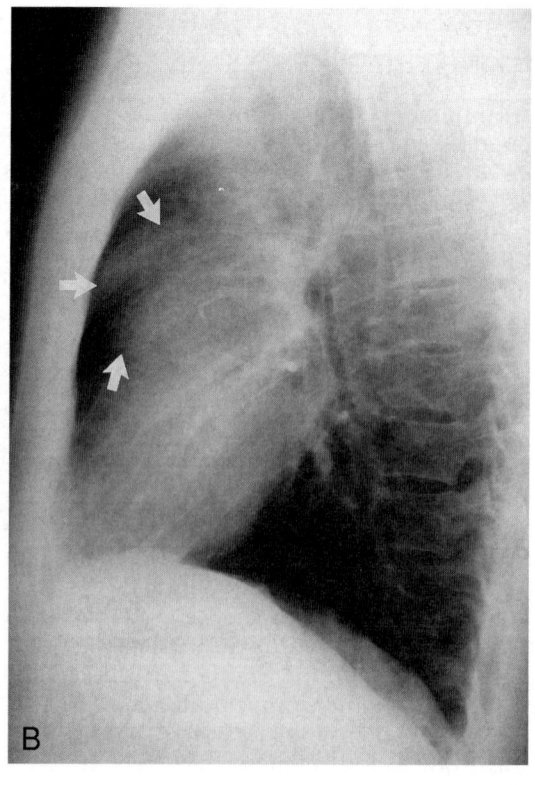

Figure 14.8. Anterior Mediastinal Mass Due to Seminoma. Frontal **(A)** and lateral **(B)** chest radiographs in a 35-year-old man with a history of cough and fatigue demonstrate a lobulated mass (*arrows*) in the right anterior mediastinum. A CT-guided biopsy showed seminoma.

sign of pneumomediastinum is the "continuous diaphragm" sign, in which air dissects between the pericardium above and central diaphragm below to allow visualization of the central portion of the diaphragm in contiguity with the right and left hemidiaphragms, each of which is outlined by air in the lower lobes respectively. Although this sign is fairly specific for pneumomediastinum, pneumopericardium may produce a similar finding. Small amounts of mediastinal air are often more easily appreciated on the lateral film, with air outlining the aortic root or main or central pulmonary arteries.

Pneumomediastinum should be distinguished from three entities that may mimic some of the radiographic findings and have significantly different causes and therapeutic implications: pneumopericardium, medial pneumothorax, and Mach bands. Air in the pericardial sac is limited by the normal pericardial reflections and extends superiorly to the proximal ascending aorta and main pulmonary artery. Additionally, pneumopericardium is often secondary to an infectious process with associated pericardial fluid and thickening, which will produce an air fluid level on horizontal beam radiographs. Air within the pericardial sac will rise to a nondependent position on decubitus positioning, unlike mediastinal air, which is nonmobile. The differentiation of pneumomediastinum from a medial pneumothorax is also aided by decubitus views because pleural air will rise nondependently along the lateral pleural space. In contrast to pneumothorax, pneumomediastinum may outline intramediastinal structures (pulmonary artery, trachea) and is often bilateral. However, the distinction between pneumomediastinum and pneumothorax may be impossible, and the two conditions often coexist, particularly during the neonatal period. Paramediastinal lucent bands created by Mach effect are easily distinguished from pneumomediastinum. The lateral margin of lucent Mach bands consist of lung parenchyma as opposed to the thin pleural line seen with mediastinal air. These bands represent an optical illusion that disappears when the interface between mediastinal soft tissues and lung is covered.

RADIOLOGIC FINDINGS OF HILAR DISEASE

Posteroanterior Radiograph. Signs of hilar abnormality on frontal films caused by enlarged bronchopulmonary lymph nodes or hilar mass include the following: hilar enlargement, increased hilar density, lobulation of the hilar contour, and distortion of central bronchi (7). An abnormal hilum is most easily appreciated by comparison with the contralateral hilum and by review of prior chest radiographs. An enlarged right or left hilum appears as widening of the hilar shadow with convexity or lobulation of its margins (Fig. 14.9). A left hilar mass may be difficult to detect on frontal radiographs because the lower portion of the left hilum is often obscured by the upper portion of the left cardiac shadow. CT will often show a left hilar mass not evident on plain radiographs. The normally sharp right hilar angle, formed by the intersection of the lower lateral aspect of the right superior pulmonary vein with the upper lateral aspect of

the right interlobar pulmonary artery, is blunted or obscured by a right hilar mass. An increase in density of the hilar shadow is seen with a hilar mass lying primarily anterior or posterior to the normal hilar vascular shadows. In such patients the enlarged hilar nodes will produce an increase in density on frontal view and a lobulated appearance when viewed in profile on the lateral radiograph.

Two pitfalls are common in the detection of a hilar mass. An abnormally dense hilum due to an overlying intrapulmonary mass superimposed on the normal hilar shadow (the "hilum overlay" sign) may be difficult to distinguish from an intrinsic hilar abnormality. The lateral radiograph or CT will clarify the abnormality. In addition, a well-penetrated radiograph will show a normal in-

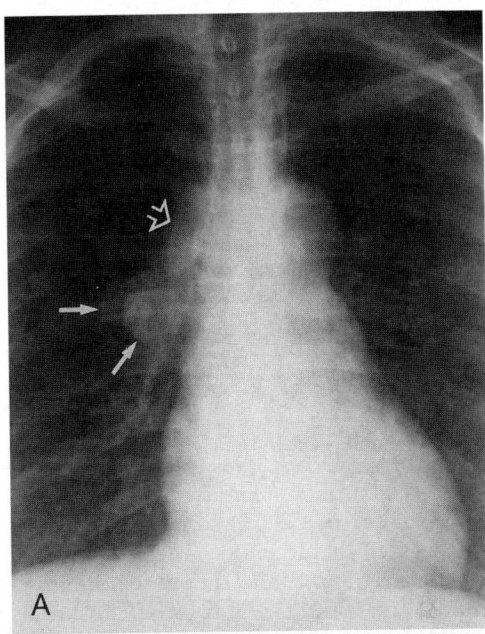

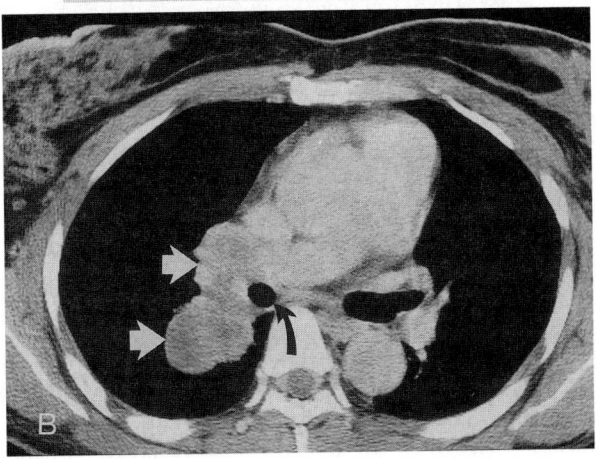

Figure 14.9. Hilar Lymph Node Enlargement on Frontal Radiograph. A. A PA radiograph in a 49-year-old woman with metastatic renal cell carcinoma demonstrates a lobulated enlargement and increased density of the right hilum (*solid arows*) with concomitant paratracheal lymph node enlargement (*open arrow*). **B.** A CT scan through the hila shows the lobulated soft-tissue mass (*short arrows*) within the right hilum surrounding the bronchus intermedius (*curved arrow*).

terlobar pulmonary artery in those with a mass superimposed on the hilar shadow whereas an intrahilar mass obscures the shadow of the normal interlobar pulmonary artery. A mass in the lower right hilum on frontal radiographs may be simulated by the end-on projection of a horizontally oriented right interlobar artery. This is common in patients with low lung volumes or exaggerated thoracic kyphosis. Comparison with prior radiographs will usually resolve the matter, with CT reserved for equivocal cases.

Bronchogenic carcinoma involving the lobar bronchi or bronchus intermedius may produce lumenal narrowing of the bronchi with enlargement of the hilar shadow. Occasionally, an endobronchial mass produces an abrupt cutoff of the bronchial air column, which is invariably associated with lobar atelectasis or obstructive pneumonitis. The walls of the right and left main and lobar bronchi are seen on frontal radiographs as they are completely encircled by branches of the right and left pulmonary arteries and upper lobe pulmonary veins. In a small percentage of normal individuals, the right or left anterior segment upper lobe bronchi are visualized as end-on ring shadows at the superolateral margin of the hila. The presence of a soft tissue density greater than 5 mm in thickness lateral to an anterior segmental bronchus is suspicious for mass or adenopathy in this region because the posterior division of the superior vein that lies immediately lateral to the anterior segmental bronchus should not exceed this thickness. Abnormal thickening of the walls of the main or lobar bronchi is a prominent feature of hilar abnormality on lateral chest films.

Enlargement of the right or left hilar shadow from pulmonary artery dilatation is produced by increased flow or increased pressure in the pulmonary arterial circulation. Pulmonary artery dilatation is usually assessed by measurement of the right interlobar pulmonary artery on PA radiographs. The margins of this vessel are readily visible, with the lateral margin outlined by air in the lower lobe and the medial margin outlined by air in the bronchus intermedius. The upper limit of normal for the transverse diameter of the proximal right interlobar artery, measured on a PA radiograph at a level immediately lateral to the proximal portion of the bronchus intermedius, is 16 mm in males and 15 mm in females (which equals the diameter of a dime). A dilated right pulmonary artery is most easily distinguished from a hilar mass by noting smooth enlargement of the right hilar shadow with concomitant left and main pulmonary artery enlargement (see Fig. 15.11). The enlarged right and left pulmonary arteries produce a minimal increase in hilar density without distortion of the adjacent bronchus intermedius or left lower lobe bronchus respectively. An additional feature of arterial enlargement is the ability to trace dilated intrapulmonary branches of the interlobar artery proximally to the lateral margins of the dilated interlobar vessel (the "hilum convergence" sign).

Lateral Radiograph. The lateral radiograph can confirm the impression of hilar abnormality seen on frontal radiographs and may demonstrate a mass when the frontal radiograph is normal. A knowledge of the normal lateral hilar anatomy enhances the ability to detect hilar masses on the lateral radiograph, increasing the sensitivity of plain radiographs for detecting hilar abnormalities. Hilar masses that lie predominantly anterior or posterior to the hilar vessels are best visualized on the lateral view. Because the lateral radiograph is a composite of both hilar shadows, the cumulative density of bilateral hilar masses may produce a significant increase in the normal density of the composite shadow, which is more easily appreciated on the lateral than the frontal view.

The radiographic findings of a hilar mass on lateral radiograph are similar to those seen on the frontal view. These are an abnormal size of, or a lobulated contour to, the normal vascular shadows, the presence of soft tissue in a region normally radiolucent, an increase in density of the composite hilar shadow, and abnormalities of the central bronchi. An increase in the size and density of the composite hilar shadow is best appreciated by comparison with prior radiographs and is usually seen with bilateral hilar lymph node enlargement from sarcoidosis. Hilar lymph node enlargement produces lobulation of the normally smooth outlines of the right and left main pulmonary arteries. Additional findings unique to the lateral radiograph suggest the presence of a hilar mass and may allow lateralization of the hilar abnormality. Because the right upper lobe bronchus is visualized on the lateral radiograph in only a minority of individuals, visualization of the right upper lobe bronchial lumen, particularly if it was invisible on a prior lateral radiograph, is strong evidence of mass or adenopathy in the upper right hilum. The intermediate stem line, which represents the posterior wall of the bronchus intermedius, is seen in a majority of normal individuals as a thin vertically oriented line on the lateral radiograph. A thickness greater than 3 mm or lobulation of the wall indicates an abnormality of the bronchus (bronchitis, bronchogenic carcinoma), edema of the axial interstitium (pulmonary edema, lymphangitic carcinomatosis), or enlargement of lymph nodes in the posterior aspect of the lower right hilum.

The normal anatomy of the inferior hilar window has been reviewed in chapter 12. The identification of a soft tissue mass greater than 1 cm in diameter within this radiolucent region is an accurate indicator of unilateral or bilateral hilar mass. Occasionally, the silhouetting of the anterior wall of the left lower lobe bronchus, recognized as a concave anterior curvilinear structure contiguous with the anterior aspect of the left upper lobe bronchus, allows lateralization of a mass to the left lower hilum (Fig. 14.10). The added opacity of a mass within the normally radiolucent inferior hilar window produces an oval opacity to the composite hilar shadow on lateral radiographs.

Dilatation of the right and left main pulmonary arteries is recognized on lateral radiographs as an enlargement of the normal hilar vascular shadows. This is most easily appreciated on lateral radiographs obtained with the right chest rotated 10° anterior to the left chest.

CT and MR. Helical CT is the most sensitive method of detecting and localizing enlarged hilar (bronchopulmonary) lymph nodes and masses. Contrast enhancement of the hilar vessels allows for ready identification of enlarged vascular structures or nonenhancing enlarged nodes (defined as nodes that exceed 10 mm in short axis diameter) or masses. Hilar masses are seen on axial or coronal spin-echo MR as round masses of low or intermediate signal intensity, in distinction to the signal void of flowing blood within hilar vessels or of air in bronchi. Coronal MR may be superior to CT in the detection of enlarged hilar lymph nodes because it displays the hilar vessels, which are oriented in the cephalocaudad direction, in length rather than in cross-section. Displacement or distortion of the hilar vessels provides indirect evidence of hilar disease. Tumor invasion of a branch of the pulmonary artery or vein within the hilum produces a filling defect within the vessel on contrast-enhanced CT or intraluminal signal on MR. The density characteristics of hilar masses on CT can help provide important information for differential diagnosis; for example, a round, cystic hilar mass with imperceptible walls in an asymptomatic young person is typical of a bronchogenic cyst.

Enlarged hilar lymph nodes can be detected by CT without the use of IV contrast. A detailed knowledge of the normal hilar vascular and bronchial anatomy as seen on CT is necessary for the identification of subtle hilar contour abnormalities. In those portions of the hilum where lung directly contacts a wall of a bronchus, thickening or lobulation of the normal thin linear shadow of the bronchial wall indicates hilar abnormality. This is particularly well seen where the right and left lower lobes contact the posterior walls of the bronchus intermedius and the left upper lobe bronchus respectively (Fig. 14.11). Lymph node enlargement in these regions is obscured on frontal radiographs by the overlying cardiac and hilar vascular shadows. CT is more sensitive

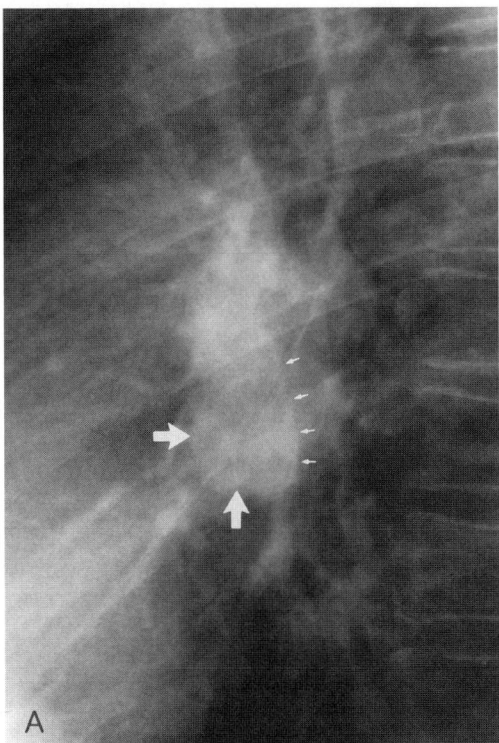

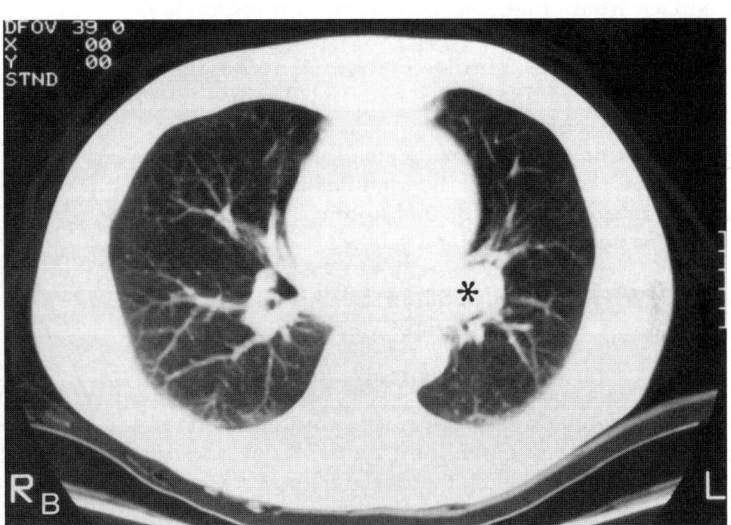

Figure 14.10. Hilar Mass within the Inferior Hilar Window. A. A coned-down view of a lateral radiograph in a patient subsequently found to have a plasmacytoma of the left hilum shows a mass (*large arrows*) within the inferior hilar window obliterating the anterior wall of the left lower lobe bronchus (*small arrows*). **B.** A CT scan through the lower hila confirms the presence of a left hilar mass (*).

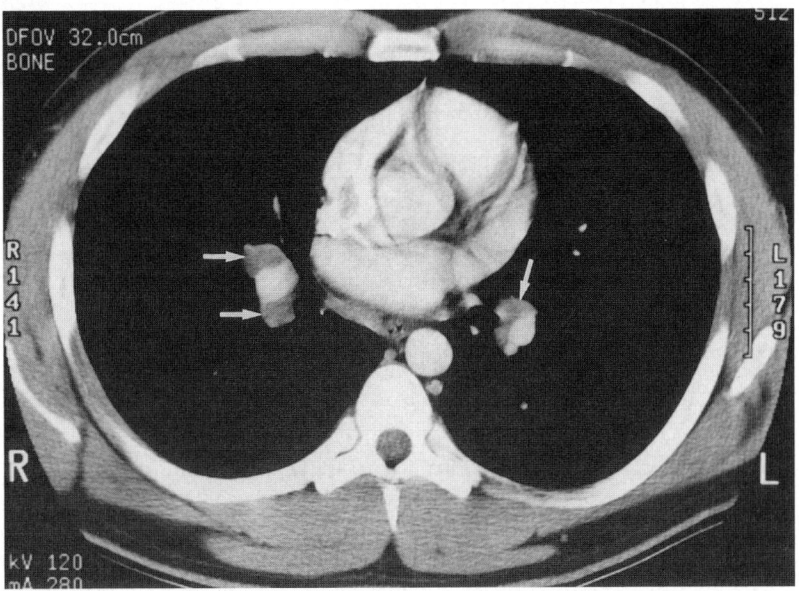

Figure 14.11. Enlarged Hilar Nodes on CT. Enhanced CT in a patient with biopsy-proven sarcoidosis demonstrates bilateral hilar lymph node enlargement (*arrows*).

than plain radiographs or MR in the detection of soft tissue masses within lobar or proximal segmental bronchi. In most patients with an endobronchial mass, a large extraluminal component produces a radiographically visible hilar soft tissue mass and obstructive atelectasis.

Enlarged hilar lymph nodes may have different appearances on CT. Enlargement of discrete lymph nodes, most commonly seen in sarcoidosis, appears as multiple distinct round masses (Fig. 14.11). When tumor or an inflammatory process extends through the nodal capsule to involve contiguous nodes, a single large mass of confluent lymph nodes is produced; it may be difficult to distinguish from a primary hilar bronchogenic carcinoma. This latter appearance is most often seen in hilar nodal metastases from small cell carcinoma of lung or lymphoma (see Fig. 16.9).

As in enlargement of mediastinal lymph nodes, the CT density of enlarged hilar nodes can provide clues to the diagnosis (see Table 13.5).

Small Hilum. An abnormally small hilum indicates a diminution in the size of the right or left pulmonary artery. The implications of this finding in one or both hila are discussed in chapter 13.

RADIOGRAPHIC FINDINGS IN PLEURAL/CHEST WALL DISEASE

Pleural Effusion

The radiographic appearance of pleural effusions depends on the amount of fluid, the patient's position during the radiographic examination, and the presence or absence of adhesions between the visceral and parietal pleura. Small amounts of pleural fluid initially collect between the lower lobe and diaphragm in a subpulmonic location. As more fluid accumulates, it spills into the posterior and lateral costophrenic sulci. A moderate amount of pleural fluid (>175 ml) in the erect patient will have a characteristic appearance on the frontal radiograph, with a homogeneous lower zone opacity seen in the lateral costophrenic sulcus with a concave interface toward the lung. This concave margin, known as a pleural meniscus, appears higher laterally than medially on frontal radiographs because the lateral aspect of the effusion, which surrounds the costal surface of the lung, is tangent to the frontal x-ray beam. Similarly, the meniscus of pleural fluid as seen on lateral radiographs peaks anteriorly and posteriorly (Fig. 14.12)(8).

In patients with suspected pleural effusion, a lateral decubitus film with the affected side down is the most sensitive technique to detect small amounts of fluid. With this technique, pleural fluid collections as small as 5 ml may be seen layering between the lung and lateral chest wall. Although a moderate-sized free flowing collection should be obvious on upright radiographs, a large pleural effusion can cause passive atelectasis of the entire lung, producing an opaque hemithorax. Distinguishing the latter condition from collapse of an entire lung may be difficult. Although a massive effusion should produce contralateral mediastinal shift, a collapsed lung without pleural effusion will show shift toward the opaque side. In some patients, CT or US may be necessary to distinguish pleural fluid from collapsed lung.

CT is quite sensitive in the detection of free pleural

fluid. On axial scans, pleural fluid layers posteriorly with a characteristic meniscoid appearance and has a CT attenuation value of 0–20 H. Small effusions may be difficult to differentiate from pleural thickening, fibrosis, or dependent atelectasis, and decubitus scans are useful in this distinction. The pleural and peritoneal spaces are oriented in the axial plane at the level of the diaphragm. This may cause some difficulty in localizing the fluid to one or both spaces. Fluid in either the pleural or peritoneal space can displace the liver and spleen medially, away from the chest wall. A key to distinguishing ascites from pleural fluid on axial CT scans is to observe the relationship of the fluid to the diaphragmatic crus. Pleural fluid in the posterior costophrenic sulcus will lie posteromedial to the diaphragm and displace the crus laterally. In contrast, peritoneal fluid lies within the confines of the diaphragm and therefore will displace the crus me-

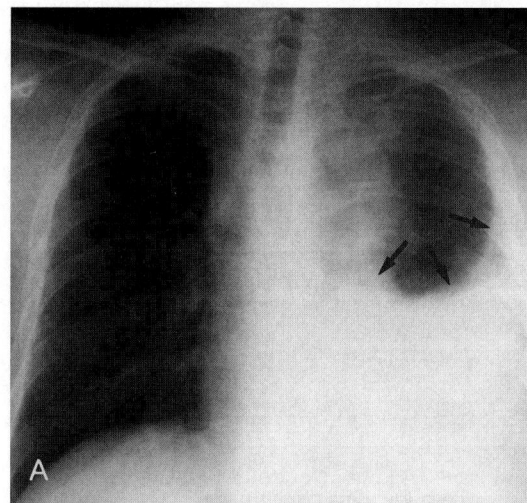

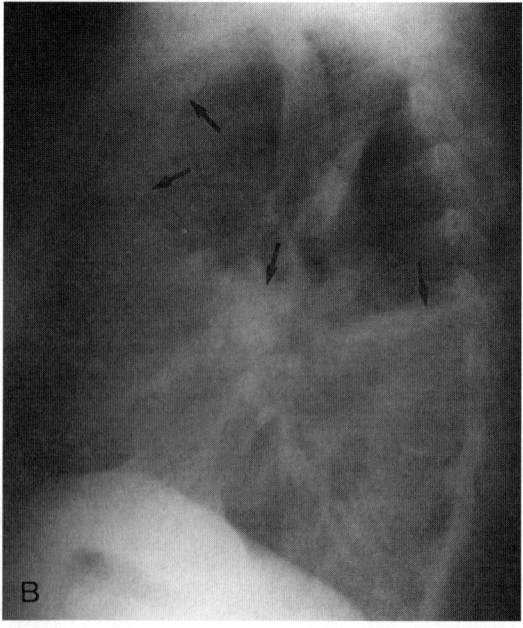

Figure 14.12. Pleural Effusion on Chest Radiographs. Posteroanterior **(A)** and lateral **(B)** chest radiographs demonstrate the typical meniscoid appearance (*arrows*) in a patient with a left pleural effusion due to mediastinal Hodgkin's lymphoma.

dially. Another useful distinguishing feature is the quality of the interface of the fluid with the liver or spleen. Intraperitoneal fluid will show a distinct, sharp interface with the liver and spleen as it directly contacts these organs whereas pleural effusions will have a hazy, indistinct interface with these viscera due to the interposed hemidiaphragms. Because the peritoneal space does not extend posterior to the bare area of the liver, right-sided fluid extending posteromedially must be pleural. A large effusion will allow the inferior edge of adjacent atelectatic lower lobe to float in the fluid, creating a curvilinear opacity that can be misinterpreted as the diaphragm separating pleural fluid from ascites. This "pseudodiaphragm" is recognized as a broad band that does not extend far laterally or anteriorly and is contiguous superiorly with atelectatic lung containing air bronchograms (Fig. 14.13). US is paticularly useful in detecting free-flowing pleural effusions, which are usually seen as anechoic collections at the base of the pleural space surrounding atelectatic lung (see chapter 39).

Pleural fluid may become loculated between the pleural layers to produce an appearance indistinguishable from a pleural mass. Fluid loculated within the costal pleural layers appears as a vertically oriented elliptical opacity with a broad area of contact with the chest wall, producing a sharp convex interface with the lung when viewed in tangent. CT is commonly used to detect and localize loculated pleural fluid collections. The characteristic finding is a sharply marginated lenticular mass of fluid attenuation, conforming to the concavity of the chest wall, which forms obtuse angles at its edges and compresses and displaces the subjacent lung. Multiple fluid locules can mimic pleural metastases or malignant

mesothelioma radiographically; CT or US can confirm the fluid characteristics of these pleural "masses."

Pleural fluid may extend into the interlobar fissures, producing characteristic findings. Free fluid within the minor fissure is usually seen as smooth, symmetric thickening on frontal radiograph. Fluid within the major fissure is normally not visible on frontal radiographs as the fissures are viewed en face. An exception is fluid extending into the lateral aspect of an incomplete major fissure, which produces a curvilinear density extending from the inferolateral to the superomedial aspect of the lung. Fluid loculated between the leaves of visceral pleura within an interlobar fissure results in an elliptical opacity oriented along the length of the fissure. These loculated collections of pleural fluid are termed "pseudotumors" and are most often seen within the minor fissure on frontal radiographs in patients with congestive heart failure. The tendency for these opacities to disappear rapidly with diuresis has led to the term "vanishing lung tumor." Although a characteristic appearance on plain radiographs is usually sufficient for diagnosis, the CT demonstration of a localized fluid collection in the expected location of the major or minor fissure is confirmatory.

An uncommon appearance of pleural effusion is seen when fluid accumulates between the lower lobe and diaphragm; this is termed a "subpulmonic effusion." Although small amounts of pleural fluid normally accumulate in this location, it is uncommon for larger effusions to remain subpulmonic without spilling into the posterior and lateral costophrenic sulci. A subpulmonic effusion may be difficult to appreciate on upright chest radiographs because the fluid collection mimics an ele-

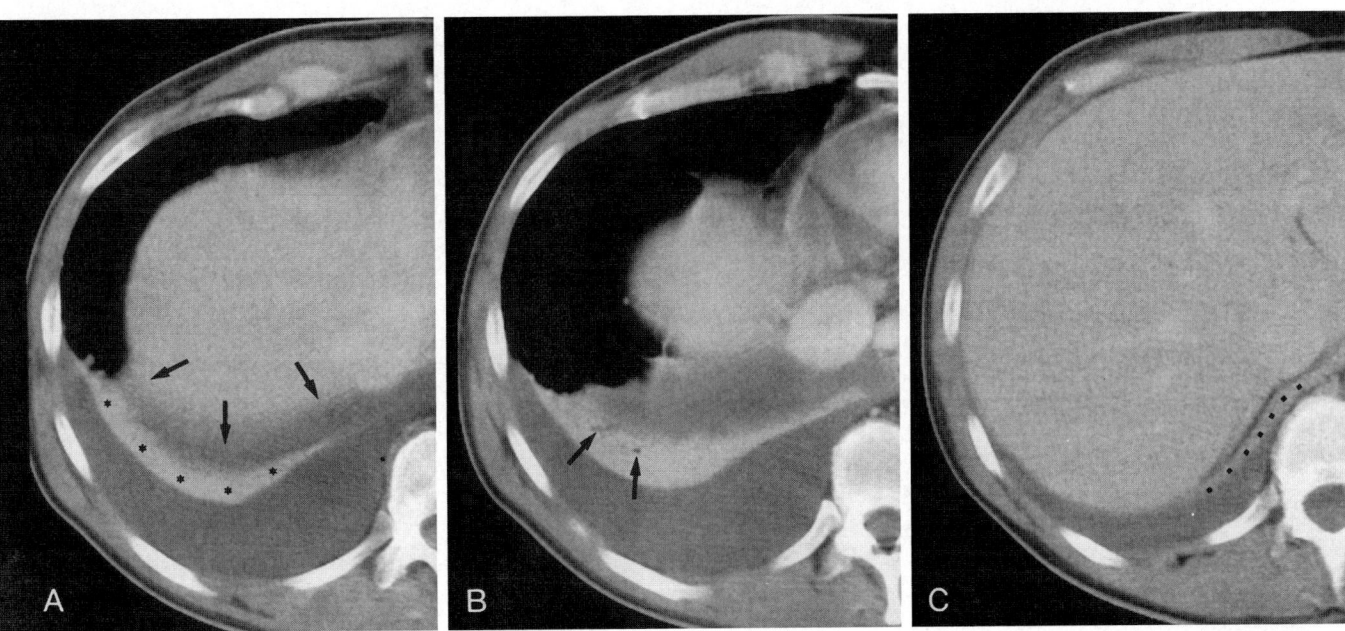

Figure 14.13. Subpulmonic Pleural Effusion on CT. A. A CT scan through the lower chest shows fluid surounding an enhancing broad curvilinear structure (*asterisks*). The fluid creates an ill-defined interface with the liver (*arrows*). **B.** A scan 1 cm more cephalad shows that the curvilinear density represents the tip of an atelectatic right lower lobe containing air bronchograms (*arrows*). **C.** More inferiorly, the crus of the diaphragm (*dotted structure*) is displaced laterally by posteromedial pleural fluid.

vated hemidiaphragm. Clues to its presence on frontal radiographs include the following: apparent elevation of the diaphragm, which is new; lateral peaking of the hemidiaphragm, which is accentuated on expiration; a minor fissure that is close to the diaphragm (right-sided effusions); and an increased separation of the gastric air bubble from the base of the lung (left-sided effusions). Despite the atypical subpulmonic accumulation of fluid with the patient upright, the effusion will layer dependently on lateral decubitus radiographs (Fig. 14.14).

The radiographic detection of pleural effusion in the supine patient can be difficult because fluid accumulates in a dependent location posteriorly. The most common finding is a hazy opacification of the affected hemithorax with obscuration of the hemidiaphragm and blunting of the lateral costophrenic angle. Fluid extending over the apex of the lung may produce a soft tissue cap with a concave interface inferiorly, and medial fluid may cause an apparent mediastinal widening.

Pneumothorax

The classic radiographic finding of pneumothorax on upright chest films is visualization of the visceral pleura as a curvilinear line that parallels the chest wall, separating the partially collapsed lung centrally from pleural air peripherally (Fig. 14.15). An expiratory radiograph aids the detection of a small pneumothorax by increasing the volume of intrapleural air relative to lung, thereby displacing the visceral pleural reflection away from the chest wall and exaggerating the differences in density of pneumothorax (black) to lung (gray) at end expiration. In a small percentage of patients, a pneumothorax will be visible only on a lateral or decubitus film or a frontal radiograph obtained during full inspiration. This suggests that when a strong clinical suspicion of pneumothorax exists and the frontal expiratory radiograph is normal, a lateral or inspiratory film may be beneficial for proper diagnosis.

The detection of a pneumothorax is difficult when chest films are obtained in the supine position. Approximately 30% of pneumothoraces present on supine radiographs remain undetected. Because many portable radiographs are obtained with the patient supine, the recognition of a pneumothorax on a supine film is particularly important in the critically ill patient who is at high risk from iatrogenic trauma or barotrauma. In a supine patient, the most nondependent portion of the pleural space is anterior or anteromedial. Small pneumothoraces will initially collect in these regions and will fail to produce a visible pleural line. The affected hemithorax may appear hyperlucent. Anteromedial air may sharpen the borders of me-

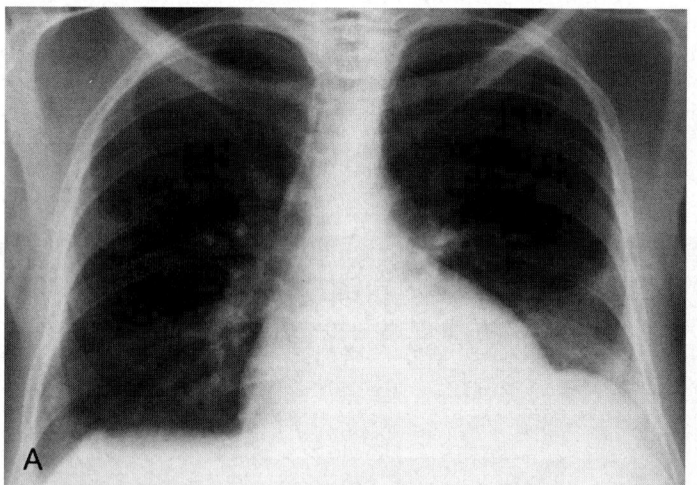
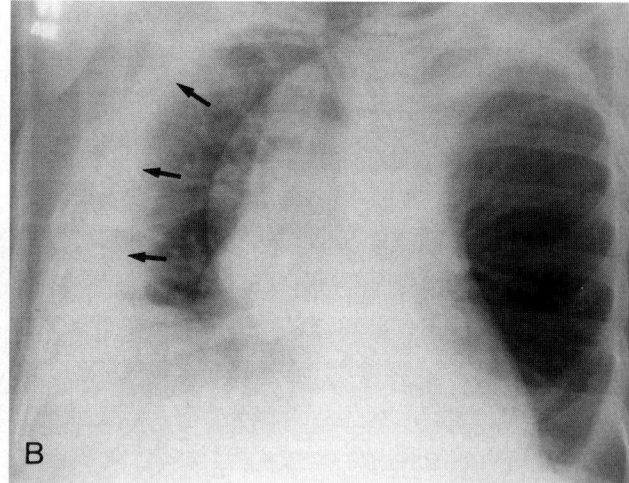
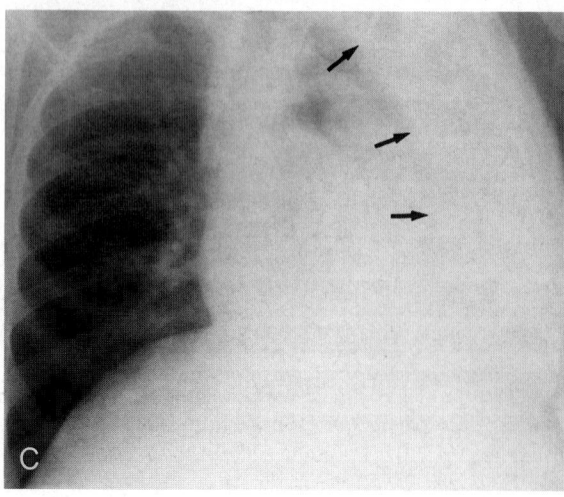

Figure 14.14. Bilateral Subpulmonic Pleural Effusions. A. An upright posteroanterior radiograph in a 41-year-old woman with ascites demonstrates apparent elevation of both hemidiaphragms. Right **(B)** and left **(C)** decubitus films demonstrate dependent layering of the subpulmonic pleural fluid (*arrows*).

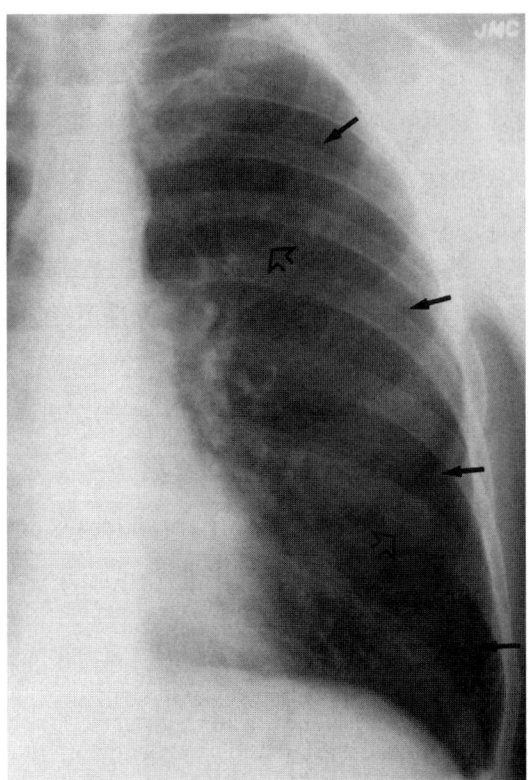

Figure 14.15. The Visceral Pleural Line in Pneumothorax. A coned-down view of an upright PA radiograph in a patient with a spontaneous pneumothorax demonstrates the curvilinear visceral pleural line (*solid arrows*) separating the lung medially from the chest wall laterally. Note the presence of thin-walled cysts (*open arrows*) from *Coccidioides* infection, which are most likely responsible for the pneumothorax.

diastinal soft tissue structures, resulting in improved visualization of the cardiac margin and aortic knob. The lateral costophrenic sulcus may appear abnormally deep and hyperlucent, a finding known as the "deep sulcus" sign. Visualization of the anterior costophrenic sulcus due to anterior and inferior air produces the "double diaphragm" sign because the dome and anterior portions of the diaphragm are outlined by lung and pleural air respectively. When an anterior pneumothorax is suspected on a supine radiograph, an upright film, lateral decubitus film with the affected side up, or CT scan should be obtained (Fig. 14.16).

Subpulmonic pneumothoraces are rare. Radiographically, a localized area of hyperlucency is seen inferiorly with the visceral pleural line paralleling the hemidiaphragm. Loculated pneumothoraces develop as the result of adhesions between visceral and parietal pleura, and may be found anywhere in the pleural space. CT is often necessary for diagnosis.

Several entities produce a curvilinear line or interface or hyperlucency on chest radiographs that must be distinguished from a pneumothorax. Skin folds resulting from the compression of redundant skin by the radiographic cassette can produce a curvilinear interface that simulates the visceral pleural line. A skin fold produces an edge or interface with atmospheric air, in distinction to the visceral pleural line seen in a pneumothorax. The interface produced by a skin fold rarely continues over the lung apex and is often seen to extend beyond the chest wall. Pulmonary vascular opacities may be followed peripheral to the skin-fold interface. Bullae may simulate pneumothorax by producing localized or unilateral hyperlucency. They are marginated by thin curvilinear walls that are concave rather than convex to the chest wall. The distinction of pneumothorax from bullous disease may be difficult but is usually evident by the

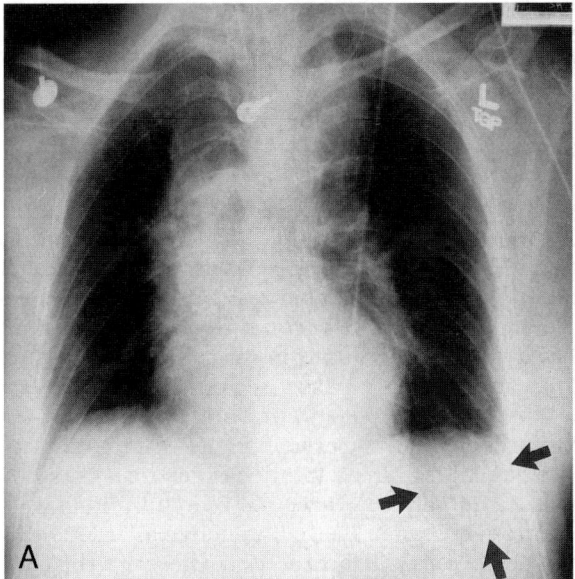

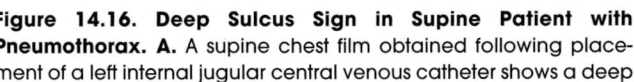

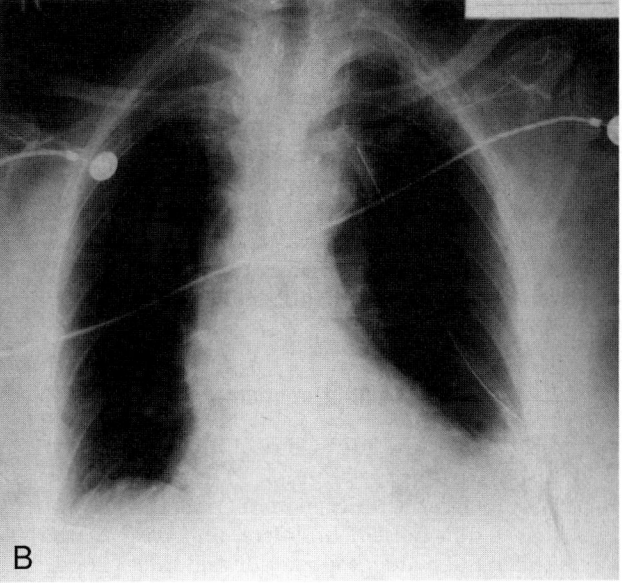

Figure 14.16. Deep Sulcus Sign in Supine Patient with Pneumothorax. A. A supine chest film obtained following placement of a left internal jugular central venous catheter shows a deep sulcus sign at the left base (*arrows*) representative of a pneumothorax. **B.** A film obtained after left thoracostomy tube placement shows that the deep sulcus sign has resolved.

clinical presentation. However, because this distinction has important therapeutic implications, certain patients may require CT.

CT is more sensitive than conventional radiographs in the detection of pneumothorax because of its cross-sectional nature and superior contrast resolution. The CT demonstration of linear parenchymal bands of tissue traversing large avascular areas helps distinguish bullae from loculated pneumothoraces. CT may be used to detect and drain loculated pneumothoraces in critically ill patients.

Localized Pleural Thickening

Radiographically, localized pleural thickening is seen as a flat, smooth, slightly raised soft tissue opacity extending over one or two intercostal spaces and displacing the lung from the innermost cortical margin of the ribs when viewed in tangent. Localized pleural thickening viewed en face is usually undetectable radiographically because the lesion does not significantly attenuate the x-ray beam and does not present a raised edge to be recognized as a distinct opacity. An exception is the presence of pleural calcification, which can usually be recognized as discrete, thin, linear or curvilinear calcific opacities paralleling the inner surface of the ribs when viewed end-on or as geographic areas of increased density with round or lobulated borders when viewed en face. Focal areas of pleural fibrosis are best appreciated on conventional and high-resolution CT scans, on which they are easily distinguished from deposits of subpleural fat by their density.

Two additional radiographic findings mimic the appearance of focal pleural thickening. The apical cap is a curvilinear subpleural opacity less than 5 mm thick with a sharp or slightly irregular inferior margin that represents nonspecific fibrosis of the apical lung and adjacent visceral pleura. Although it is usually bilateral and symmetric, slight asymmetry in thickness is not uncommon. Any growth of the opacity, significant asymmetry, inferior convexity of the opacity, rib destruction, or symptoms should prompt a CT or MR examination followed by biopsy to exclude an apical neoplasm (Pancoast's or superior sulcus tumor). The companion shadows of the inferior aspects of the first and second ribs are smooth apical linear opacities that parallel the lower cortical margins of the first two ribs and represent the pleural layers and subpleural fat viewed in tangent. These are most prominent in obese individuals and should not be mistaken for pleural fibrosis.

Diffuse Pleural Thickening

Fibrothorax appears as a thin, smooth band of soft tissue with a sharp internal margin seen immediately beneath and parallel to the inner margin of the ribs and intercostal spaces. It is usually unilateral and extends over large areas of the dependent (posterior and inferior) portions of the pleural space. Anterior or posterior costal pleural thickening creates a veil-like opacity without sharp margins when viewed en face on frontal radiographs. Blunting of the lateral costophrenic sulcus may

be seen on frontal radiographs, and sparing of the posterior costophrenic sulcus and an absence of layering fluid on decubitus positioning help distinguish pleural fibrosis from a small effusion. Fibrothorax spares the interlobar fissures and mediastinal pleura. CT and HRCT are more sensitive than conventional radiographs in the detection of pleural thickening. The diminished volume of the affected hemithorax seen with extensive fibrothorax is more easily appreciated on axial CT images than on frontal radiographs (see Fig. 20.8). CT and HRCT provide unimpeded views of the underlying lung in patients with diffuse pleural thickening, allowing detection of associated interstitial pulmonary fibrosis. This is important in evaluating patients with suspected asbestosis and in assessing the extent of pulmonary disease in patients being considered for pleurectomy.

Pleural and Extrapleural Lesions

The shape and margins of a peripheral opacity as seen on conventional radiographs help define the opacity as parenchymal, pleural, or extrapleural. Pleural masses form obtuse angles with the adjacent normal pleura, in distinction to peripheral lung lesions, which usually contact the normal pleura at acute angles. Pleural and extrapleural masses are usually vertically orientated elliptical opacities. Pleural lesions have smooth, well-defined margins because they compress normal lung. These smooth margins are best appreciated on radiographic projections with the x-ray beam tangent to the interface between the mass and the lung. Another feature of pleural lesions is the clarity of the margin of the lesion on frontal and lateral radiographs; a mass sharply outlined by lung on one view but poorly marginated on the orthogonal view should suggest a pleural or extrapleural process. In distinction, intraparenchymal lesions are surrounded by air and will have similar margins on both views. Pleural lesions, unlike parenchymal lesions, do not change position with respiratory motion. Lung disease is often confined to a lobe whereas pleural disease may extend across fissures. Pedunculated pleural lesions such as fibromas are rare but can present with radiographic features of both pleural and parenchymal lesions.

Despite these features, the distinction of pleural from peripheral parenchymal lesions may be difficult. This distinction has important diagnostic implications; although parenchymal processes are best evaluated by examination of expectorated sputum or by bronchoscopy, pleural lesions will require thoracentesis or pleural biopsy. CT is often used to distinguish between pleural and parenchymal disease (see chapter 20). A peripheral lesion that is completely surrounded by lung on CT is intraparenchymal, the exception being the rare pleural lesion arising within an interlobar fissure. Peripheral lung masses usually have irregular margins and may contain air bronchograms. Those parenchymal lesions that contact the pleura will form acute angles with the chest wall as on plain films. The CT appearance of pleural and extrapleural or chest wall lesions are similar. Both pleural and extrapleural lesions are sharply defined and form obtuse angles with the chest wall (see Fig. 20.9); rib destruction or subcutaneous mass are the only findings that localize an extrapulmonary lesion to the chest wall. When a peripheral parenchymal lesion invades the pleura, determining the origin of the mass may be impossible. CT can further characterize peripheral lesions by their density; a smooth fatty mass is almost certainly a pleural lipoma whereas a homogeneous pleural or extrapleural soft tissue mass is most likely a fibroma or neurogenic tumor (see Fig. 20.10). The signal intensity on T1-weighted and T2-weighted spin-echo MR images may be useful in the characterization of focal pleural masses. On T1WI and T2WI, loculated fluid collections will show homogeneous low and high signal, respectively. Lipomas will show homogeneous high signal intensity on T1WI and intermediate signal intensity on T2WI whereas fibromas are typically of intermediate and high signal intensity, respectively, as a result of the high cellularity of these tumors.

Chest Wall Lesions

Chest wall lesions become evident radiographically when a) they extend into the thorax and become outlined by displaced lung, b) there is bone displacement or destruction by the mass, or c) they protrude externally from the skin surface to be outlined by air in the atmosphere. CT, MR, and US are all useful in assessing the characteristics of chest wall lesions. Although CT and MR are most useful in determining the extent of intrathoracic involvement by chest wall lesions, US is the least expensive and easiest method of characterizing the nature of pal-

pable chest wall lesions, particularly if the lesions are thought to be vascular or cystic in nature. The radiographic findings of chest wall lesions related to specific bony or soft tissue components of the chest wall are detailed in the section on chest wall disease in chapter 20.

Diaphragm

Radiographic findings of diaphragmatic disorders include elevation and depression of the diaphragm and abnormalities of diaphragmatic contour. The diagnostic considerations of diaphragmatic disease are reviewed in chapter 20.

References

1. Felson B. The roentgen diagnosis of disseminated pulmonary alveolar diseases. Semin Radiol 1967;2:3–21.
2. Proto AV, Tocino I. Radiographic manifestations of lobar collapse. Semin Roentgenol 1980;15:117–173.
3. Felson B. Disseminated interstitial diseases of the lung. Ann Radiol 1966;9:325.
4. Kerley P. Radiology in heart disease. BMJ 1933;2:594–597.
5. Godwin JD, Webb WR, Savoca CJ, et al. Multiple thin-walled cystic lesions of the lung. AJR 1980;135:593–604.
6. Simon G. Radiology and emphysema. Clin Radiol 1964;15:293–306.
7. Muller NL, Webb WR. Imaging of the pulmonary hila. Invest Radiol 1985;20:661–671.
8. Raasch BN, Carsky EW, Lane EJ, et al. Pleural effusion: explanation of some typical appearances. AJR 1982;139:899–904.

15
Pulmonary Vascular Disease

Jeffrey S. Klein

PULMONARY EDEMA
PULMONARY HEMORRHAGE
PULMONARY EMBOLISM
PUMONARY ARTERIAL HYPERTENSION

PULMONARY EDEMA

Basic Principles. Under normal conditions, the interstitial space of the lung is kept dry by pulmonary lymphatics located within the axial and peripheral interstitium of the lung. The lymphatics drain the small amounts of transudated fluid that enters the interstitial spaces as an ultrafiltrate of plasma. Because no lymphatic structures are located immediately within the alveolar walls (parenchymal interstitium), filtered interstitial fluid is drawn to the lymphatics by a pressure gradient from the alveolar interstitium to the axial and peripheral interstitium. When the rate of fluid accumulation in the interstitium exceeds the lymphatic drainage capabilities of the lung, fluid accumulates first within the interstitial space. As the amount of extravascular fluid increases, fluid accumulates in the corners of the alveolar spaces. Progressive fluid accumulation eventually produces flooding of the alveolar spaces, resulting in air-space pulmonary edema. Although interstitial edema may leave the gas-exchanging properties of the lung unaffected, flooding of the alveolar spaces leads to impaired oxygen and carbon dioxide exchange.

Excess fluid accumulation in the lung is caused by one of three basic mechanisms. The most common mechanism involves a change in the normal Starling's forces that govern fluid movement in the lung. Because normal fluid movement is determined by the differences in hydrostatic and oncotic pressure between the pulmonary capillaries and surrounding alveolar interstitium, an inbalance in these forces may lead to pulmonary edema. Pulmonary edema is most commonly caused by increased capillary hydrostatic pressure from left heart failure; however, diminished plasma oncotic pressure or diminished interstitial hydrostatic pressure may be contributing factors. Another mechanism involves an absence or obstruction of the normal pulmonary lymphatics, leading to the excess accumulation of interstitial fluid. Lastly, numerous disorders can injure the capillary endothelium and alveolar epithelium, producing an increase in capillary permeability that allows protein-rich fluid to escape from the capillaries and into the pulmonary interstitium.

Radiographic Findings in pulmonary edema can be divided into interstitial and air-space components. The radiographic appearance of interstitial pulmonary edema is caused by thickening of the various components of the interstitial spaces by fluid (1). Thickening of the axial interstitium results in lost definition of the intrapulmonary vascular shadows, peribronchial cuffing, and tram tracking. Edema within alveolar septa is not discernable as discrete opacities but produces a ground-glass opacification in the perihilar and lower lung zones, regions where fluid accumulates in the early phases of edema. Involvement of peripheral and subpleural interstitial structures produces Kerley's lines and subpleural edema. Kerley's A and B lines represent thickening of central connective tissue septa and peripheral interlobular septa, respectively, and Kerley's C lines represent a network of thickened interlobular septa (Fig. 15.1). Subpleural edema is the accumulation of fluid within the innermost (interstitial) layer of the visceral pleura and is best seen on lateral radiograph as smooth thickening of the interlobar fissures. The radiographic changes of interstitial pulmonary edema may progress to those of air-space edema or, if successfully treated, may resolve within 12–24 hours.

Air-space pulmonary edema develops when progressive fluid accumulates in the interstitial spaces and spills into the alveoli. The chest radiograph typically shows symmetric bilateral air-space opacities that are confluent and predominate in the mid and lower lung zones. Air-space nodules and the findings of interstitial edema (Kerley's B lines and subpleural edema) may be seen peripherally. An uncommon form of air-space pulmonary edema, seen most commonly in left heart failure or renal failure, is the "bat's-wing" or "butterfly" distribution of disease. In this situation, the air-space opacification is sharply confined to the central, parahilar regions of lung with sparing of the peripheral or subpleural regions (Fig. 15.2). The reason for this distribution of edema is unknown. As with interstitial edema, the air-space opacities of alveolar edema change rapidly, often within hours. The differential diagnosis of diffuse air-space opacities has been reviewed (see Table 14.2).

Although not commonly used to image the patient with pulmonary edema, CT and HRCT demonstrate fairly characteristic findings in this disorder. Thickening of subpleural, septal, and bronchovascular structures are well depicted on HRCT. Mild parenchymal edema produces a ground-glass pattern around the hila. Early alveolar edema is seen as centrilobular air-space nodules surrounding the arteries within the lobular core, and severe alveolar edema produces dense perihilar air-space opacification. Cardiomegaly, pulmonary venous distention, and pleural effusions are associated findings in cardiogenic or fluid overload edema.

Atypical Radiographic Appearances. Several conditions may cause atypical radiographic appearances of pul-

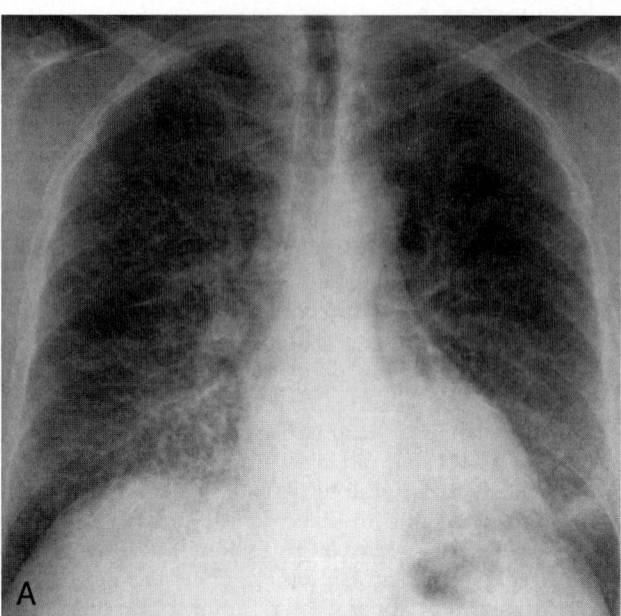

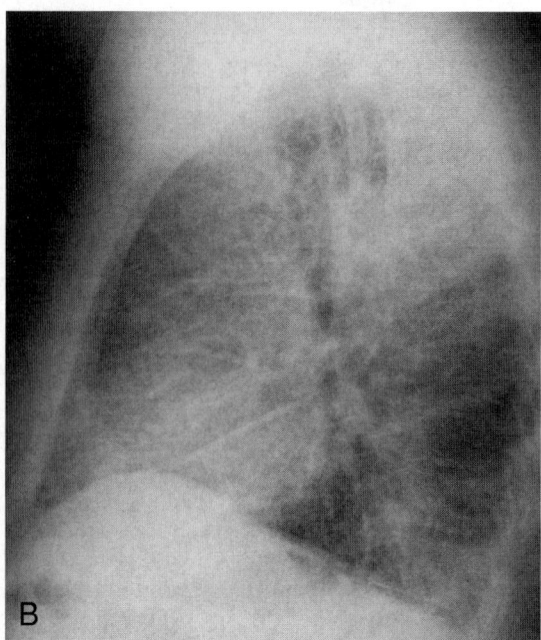

Figure 15.1. Interstitial Pulmonary Edema caused by Cardiac Disease. PA **(A)** and lateral **(B)** chest films in a 65-year-old man with an anterior wall myocardial infarction shows bilateral linear opaci- ties (Kerley's A, B, and C lines) representing interstitial pulmonary edema. Note the prominence of upper lobe vessels indicating concommitant pulmonary venous hypertension.

monary edema. Because the distribution of edema is affected by gravity, edema fluid accumulates posteriorly or unilaterally in patients maintaining a prolonged supine or decubitus position, respectively. The diagnosis of unilateral edema is suggested by typical radiographic and clinical findings of pulmonary edema in one lung that resolve rapidly or redistribute with changes in patient positioning. Another cause of asymmetric or unilateral pulmonary edema is an interruption in the blood supply to one lung. This may be seen in pulmonary artery hypoplasia or in an acquired obstruction to pulmonary arterial blood flow such as central pulmonary embolus or extrinsic compression of the pulmonary artery from tumor or fibrosis. In these conditions, the lung with diminished pulmonary blood flow is "protected" from the transudation of fluid and the development of pulmonary edema. Bronchogenic carcinoma, lymphoma, or other causes of unilateral lymph node enlargement can impede normal lymphatic drainage and predispose a patient to unilateral pulmonary edema. Similarly, unilateral pulmonary venous obstruction from tumor or fibrosing mediastinitis will predispose a patient to edema on the affected side. Unilateral pulmonary edema may develop in the lung reexpanded by the rapid evacuation of a large pleural fluid collection or pneumothorax. This is known as reexpansion pulmonary edema and is discussed in a subsequent section.

Alveolar pulmonary edema localized to the right upper lung may be seen in patients with severe mitral regurgitation. The mechanism of edema formation is likely caused by preferential regurgitant flow of blood into the right upper lobe pulmonary vein across the superiorly and posteriorly oriented mitral valve. These patients will usually have typical radiographic findings of interstitial edema elsewhere in the lungs (Fig. 15.3).

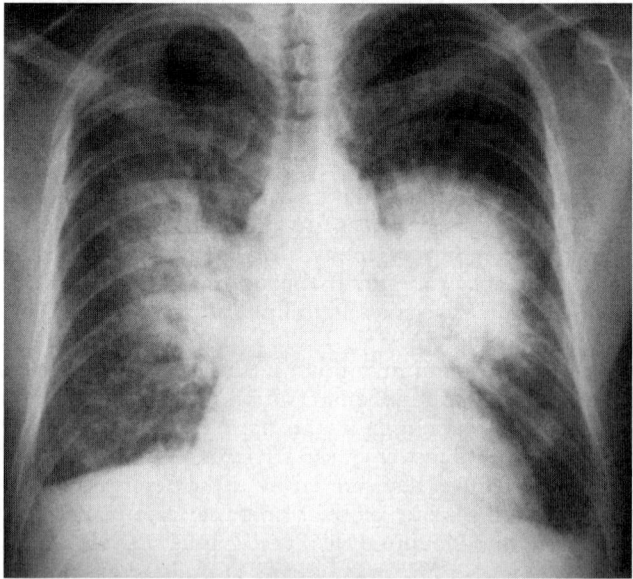

Figure 15.2. Perihilar "Bat's Wing" Pulmonary Edema. Frontal chest radiograph in a 32-year-old man with a dilated cardiomyopathy reveals dense bilateral perihilar air-space opacification caused by pulmonary edema.

Patients with pulmonary emphysema may have unusual appearances of alveolar edema. Areas of bulla, most commonly in the apical portions of the lungs, are spared from the development of alveolar edema because the pulmonary blood flow to these regions has already been obliterated by the emphysematous process. These emphysematous regions within adjacent areas of air-

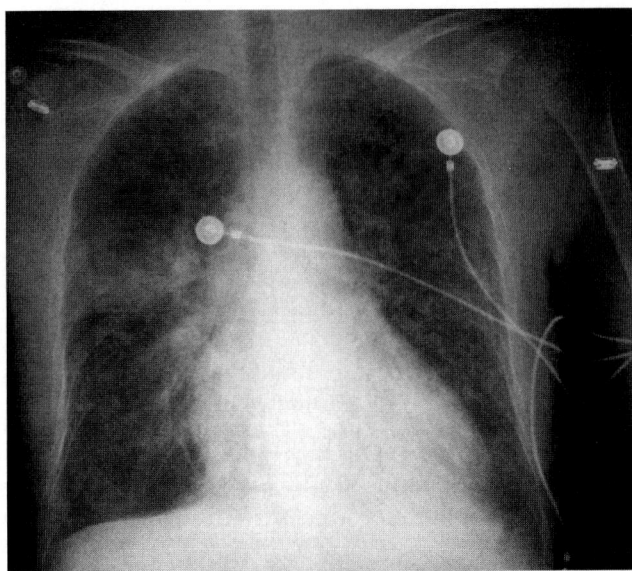

Figure 15.3. Interstitial and Right Upper Lung Pulmonary Edema. In a 64-year-old woman with unstable angina and mitral regurgitation on echocardiography, PA chest radiograph shows diffuse interstitial pulmonary edema with localized right upper lobe air-space opacification, the latter secondary to ischemic mitral valvular dysfunction.

space opacification can simulate cavity formation and may be difficult to distinguish radiographically from necrotizing pneumonia or pneumatocele formation. Comparison with previous radiographs and correlation with the clinical course will aid in making the proper diagnosis.

Hydrostatic Pulmonary Edema (normal capillary permeability) is the most common form of pulmonary edema. Patients with acute or chronic renal failure may develop pulmonary edema because of increased pulmonary capillary hydrostatic pressure. The elevated hydrostatic pressure is caused by a combination of hypervolemia and left ventricular dysfunction with resultant pulmonary venous and capillary hypertension. Volume overload without renal failure may also produce pulmonary edema by a hydrostatic mechanism. Decreased capillary oncotic pressure, present in patients with hypoalbuminemia secondary to the nephrotic syndrome or liver failure, is not considered to be an independent risk factor for the development of pulmonary edema, but is a cofactor in several conditions.

Hydrostatic pulmonary edema is usually caused by pulmonary venous hypertension secondary to congestive heart failure. Thus, identification of the radiographic findings of pulmonary venous hypertension and pulmonary edema will provide the diagnosis. The majority of these patients will have left ventricular failure or mitral valve disease. A list of the causes of mechanical or functional obstruction to pulmonary venous return is found in Table 15.1.

The radiographic findings of pulmonary venous hypertension are enlargement of pulmonary veins and redistribution of pulmonary blood flow to the upper lung zones (2). Pulmonary venous enlargement is seen as progressive dilatation of horizontally oriented pulmonary veins on serial chest radiographs. The redistribution of pulmonary blood flow results from lower zone pulmonary venous constriction and increased resistance to lower zone blood flow with resultant preferential flow through upper lobe vessels. Therefore, in pulmonary venous hypertension in the upright patient, the upper zone vessels are equal to or greater in diameter than the lower zone vessels. This is the opposite of the normal appearance in which the lower zone vessels are larger than the upper zone vessels owing to the normal gravitational effects on pulmonary blood flow. It should be noted that conditions other than pulmonary venous hypertension can cause distention of upper zone pulmonary vessels, including left-to-right shunts and basilar lung disease. The association of upper zone vascular prominence with findings of left ventricular failure (cardiomegaly, pulmonary edema, and pleural effusion) usually allows for the correct diagnosis (Fig. 15.1).

The sequence of events following the development of pulmonary venous hypertension has been studied in patients with acute cardiac decompensation following myocardial infarction. Several studies have correlated the radiographic findings of pulmonary venous hypertension in the erect patient with measurements of pulmonary capillary wedge pressure (PCWP) using flow-directed balloon occlusion (i.e., Swan-Ganz) catheters. When PCWP is normal (8–12 mm Hg), the chest radiograph is normal. Mild elevation of PCWP (12–18 mm Hg) produces constriction of lower lobe vessels and enlargement of upper lobe vessels. Progressive elevation of PCWP (19–25 mm Hg) leads to the findings of interstitial pulmonary edema: loss of vascular definition, peribronchial cuffing, and Kerley's lines. PCWP above 25 mm Hg produces alveolar filling with radiographic findings of bilateral air-space opacities in the perihilar and lower lung zones.

The causes of pulmonary venous hypertension may be divided radiographically into those associated with a normal heart size and those with cardiomegaly. Severe, long-standing obstruction to left ventricular outflow (e.g., aortic stenosis) is usually associated with a normal heart size unless the left ventricle has failed. Chronic left ventricular failure is invariably associated with cardiomegaly although acute left ventricular decompensation, as in acute myocardial infarction or acute aortic re-

Table 15.1. Causes of Pulmonary Venous Hypertension and Pulmonary Edema

Obstruction to LV outflow	Aortic coarctation
	Aortic stenosis
	Hypoplastic left heart syndrome
Left ventricular failure	
Mitral valve disease	Mitral stenosis
	Mitral insufficiency
Left atrial myxoma	
Cor triatriatum	
Obstruction of pulmonary veins	
Central pulmonary veins	Fibrosing mediastinitis
	Pulmonary vein stenosis
	Pulmonary venous thrombosis
Intrapulmonary veins	Pulmonary venoocclusive disease

Table 15.2. Etiologies of Adult Respiratory Distress Syndrome

Septicemia	Gram-negative bacteria
Shock	
Major surgery	
Burns	
Acute pancreatitis	
Disseminated intravascular coagulation	
Drugs	Narcotics
	Heroin
	Crack cocaine
	Aspirin
Inhalation of noxious fumes	Nitrogen dioxide (silo-filler's dx)
	Hydrocarbons
	Smoke
	Chlorine
	Phosgene
Aspiration of fluid	Fresh or salt water near drowning
	Gastric fluid aspiration (Mendelson's syndrome)
Fat embolism	
Amniotic fluid embolism	

gurgitation, may show a normal heart size. Obstruction or incompetence at the level of the mitral valve (e.g., mitral stenosis or regurgitation, left atrial myxoma) may only show left atrial enlargement without ventricular dilatation. Obstruction of the central pulmonary veins (i.e., fibrosing mediastinitis, pulmonary vein thrombosis) is usually associated with the radiographic findings of pulmonary venous hypertension and pulmonary edema with a normal heart size. Intrapulmonary venous obstruction (i.e., pulmonary venoocclusive disease) may show only pulmonary edema, but often the diagnosis is delayed until pulmonary arterial hypertension has developed (Table 15.1).

Injury Edema. Rapidly progressive respiratory failure caused by leakage of protein-rich edema fluid into the lung resulting from damage to the pulmonary microcirculation may develop as a complication of a variety of systemic conditions. This condition is termed the **adult respiratory distress syndrome** (ARDS)(3). The edema associated with this syndrome is called lung injury or increased capillary permeability edema as compared to the normal alveolocapillary permeability of hydrostatic edema. A long list of pulmonary and nonpulmonary disorders have been associated with ARDS (Table 15.2); the most common are shock, severe trauma, burns, sepsis, narcotic overdose, and pancreatitis. Although the precise pathogenesis of capillary permeability edema has yet to be completely elucidated, current evidence suggests that recruitment and activation of neutrophils in the lung with release of enzymes and oxygen radicals are key factors in the development of capillary endothelial damage.

The pathologic changes associated with ARDS are those of diffuse alveolar damage and are common to all patients regardless of the underlying cause. Within 12–24 hours following the initial insult (stage 1 ARDS), damage to capillary endothelium produces engorged capillaries and proteinaceous interstitial edema. Within

the first week (stage 2), the injury to type I pneumocytes leads to the flooding of alveoli with edema fluid and proteinaceous and cellular debris, which form hyaline membranes lining the distal airways and alveoli. In stage 3 ARDS, type II pneumocytes proliferate in an attempt to reline the denuded alveolar surfaces, and fibroblastic tissue proliferates within the air spaces. This fibroblastic tissue may resolve and leave minimal scarring or, particularly in those with severe disease and long-standing oxygen requirements, result in extensive interstitial fibrosis.

Radiographically, ARDS follows a predictable pattern. Chest radiographs become abnormal 12–24 hours following the onset of dyspnea and demonstrate patchy, peripheral air-space opacities. These opacities coalesce during the next several days to produce confluent bilateral air-space opacities with air bronchograms (Fig. 15.4). Radiographic improvement in the opacities may be seen within the first week, but this is often owing to the effects of increasing positive pressure ventilation rather than true histologic improvement. After 1 week, the air-space opacities gradually give way to a coarse reticulonodular pattern that may resolve over the course of several months or remain unchanged, in which case the pattern represents irreversible pulmonary fibrosis (i.e., honeycombing). Pneumonia complicating ARDS is difficult to diagnose radiographically, but it should be suspected when a focal area of air-space opacification or a significant pleural effusion develops during the course of the disease. Likewise, the superimposition of left ventricular failure may be impossible to recognize but is suggested by rapid clinical and radiographic deterioration associated with changes in measured PCWP and the protein content of edema fluid. Pneumomediastinum and pneumothorax may result as a complication of positive pressure ventilation to stiff lungs and should be sought on portable chest radiographs.

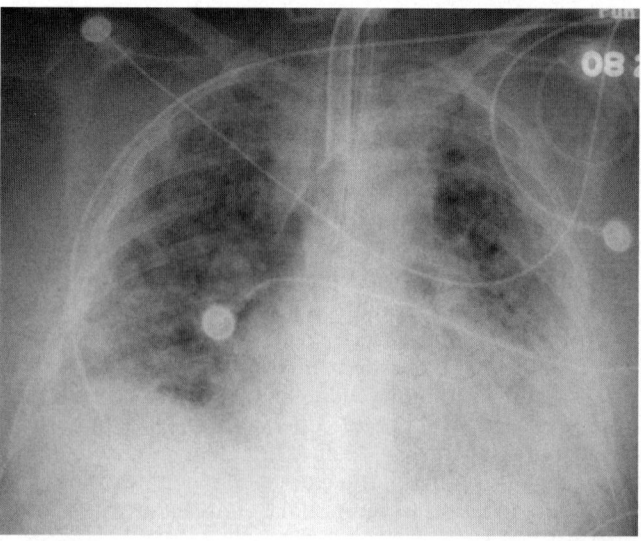

Figure 15.4. Increased Permeability (Lung Injury) Edema in ARDS. Portable chest radiograph in a 46-year-old woman with severe pancreatitis and respiratory failure reveals bilateral air-space opacification with a somewhat peripheral distribution representing diffuse alveolar damage and permeability edema.

Radiographic Distinction of Hydrostatic from Permeability Edema. Beyond identifying the presence of pulmonary edema, the ability to distinguish between types of pulmonary edema has significant diagnostic and therapeutic import. Measurements of PCWP and transbronchial sampling of pulmonary edema fluid are techniques that accurately distinguish hydrostatic from increased capillary permeability edema. In hydrostatic edema, PCWP measurements are elevated and a protein-poor transudative edema fluid is present, but in increased capillary permeability edema, PCWP is normal and proteinaceous edema fluid is seen. Milne and colleagues have described the findings on the chest radiograph used to distinguish cardiac and overhydration edema from increased capillary permeability edema (4). In pulmonary edema associated with chronic cardiac failure, the heart is usually enlarged with an inverted (redistributed) pulmonary blood flow pattern. The distribution of edema is even from central to peripheral over the lower lung zones. The vascular pedicle, which represents the mediastinal width at the level of the superior cava and left subclavian artery, is widened (>53 mm on PA radiograph), reflecting increased circulating blood volume. Lung volumes are diminished because of decreased pulmonary compliance from edema. Peribronchial cuffing, Kerley's lines, and pleural effusions represent interstitial and intrapleural transudation of fluid, respectively.

Overhydration or renal failure edema has some features in common with chronic cardiac failure and may be indistinguishable radiographically. Capillary permeability edema can sometimes be distinguished from hydrostatic edema. A more peripheral distribution of edema with a normal heart size and normal vascular pedicle width, the latter indicating normal circulating blood volume, are findings typical of capillary permeability edema.

It should be noted that certain factors may render radiographic distinction of types of pulmonary edema difficult. Radiographs of supine patients will make evaluation of pulmonary blood flow distribution and vascular pedicle width difficult. The presence of severe alveolar edema will obscure the underlying vascular markings. Many patients with capillary permeability edema will be overhydrated in attempts to maintain circulating blood volume, producing complex radiographic findings.

Neurogenic Pulmonary Edema following head trauma, seizure, or increased intracranial pressure is a complex phenomenon that appears to involve both hydrostatic and increased permeability mechanisms. Massive sympathetic discharge from the brain in these conditions produces systemic vasoconstriction and increased venous return with resultant increase in left ventricular diastolic pressure and hydrostatic pulmonary edema. However, the finding of protein-rich edema fluid and normal PCWP in some patients suggests that increased permeability may be a contributing factor.

High-Altitude Pulmonary Edema develops in certain individuals after rapid ascent to altitudes above 3500 meters. Edema typically develops within 48–72 hours of ascent and appears to reflect a varied individual response to hypoxemia in which scattered areas of pulmonary arterial spasm result in transient pulmonary arterial hypertension. This produces an overflow of blood at high pressure to uninvolved areas, resulting in damage to the capillary endothelium and increased permeability edema, which is patchy in distribution. Rapid resolution usually occurs within 24–48 hours after the administration of supplemental oxygen or a return to sea level.

Reexpansion Pulmonary Edema. Rapid reexpansion of a lung after collapse lasting more than 48 hours may result in the development of unilateral pulmonary edema. Marked increases in negative pleural pressure following pleural tube placement, impaired pulmonary lymphatic drainage following prolonged lung collapse, and ischemia-induced surfactant deficiency resulting in the need for high negative pleural pressure to reexpand the collapsed lung are proposed mechanisms. Recent evidence points toward prolonged collapse, producing ischemia and hypoxemia within the lung, which promotes anaerobic metabolism and free-radical formation. Reperfusion of the lung upon reexpansion then leads to lung injury and permeability edema. Gradual reexpansion of the lung by slow removal of pleural air or fluid over a 24–48 hour period and supplemental oxygen administration help limit the incidence and severity of this complication.

Acute Upper Airway Obstruction. Pulmonary edema may be seen during or immediately following treatment of acute upper airway obstruction. The proposed mechanism involves the creation of markedly negative intrathoracic pressure by attempts to inspire against an extrathoracic airway obstruction, producing transudation of fluid into the lung. No distinguishing radiographic features exist.

Amniotic Fluid Embolism. A severe and often fatal form of pulmonary edema may develop in a pregnant woman when amniotic fluid gains access to the systemic circulation during labor. There is an association of this entity and fetal distress and demise as the mucin within fetal meconium plays a key role in the pathogenesis of this disorder. Embolic obstruction of the pulmonary vasculature by mucin and fetal squames within the amniotic fluid leads to sudden pulmonary arterial hypertension and cor pulmonale with decreased cardiac output and pulmonary edema. An anaphylactoid reaction and DIC from factors within the amniotic fluid contribute to the shock state. Radiographically, bilateral confluent air-space opacities are indistinguishable from pulmonary edema of other causes. In severe cases, secondary enlargement of the central pulmonary arteries and right heart occurs as a manifestation of cor pulmonale. The diagnosis can be confirmed premortem by identification of fetal squames and mucin in blood samples obtained from indwelling pulmonary artery catheters.

Fat Embolism. The embolization of marrow fat to the lung is a common complication occurring 24–72 hours after the fracture of a long bone (e.g., femur). Within the lung, the fat is hydrolyzed to its component fatty acids, which cause increased pulmonary capillary permeability and hemorrhagic pulmonary edema. Radiographically, confluent air-space opacities tend to be peripheral and

Table 15.3. Causes of Pulmonary Hemorrhage

Spontaneous	Thrombocytopenia
	Hemophilia
	Anticoagulant therapy
Trauma	Pulmonary contusion
Embolic disease	Pulmonary embolism
	Fat embolism
Vasculitis	Autoimmune
	Goodpasture's
	Idiopathic pulmonary hemorrhage
	Wegener's granulomatosis
	Infectious
	Gram negative bacteria
	Influenza
	Aspergillus
	Mucormycosis
Drugs	Penicillamine

have a lower zone predominance. The diagnosis is made by recognizing findings of systemic fat embolism (petechial rash, CNS depression) and pulmonary changes in the appropriate time period following trauma. Most patients have a mild course with minimal respiratory compromise, but a minority will develop progressive respiratory failure leading to death.

PULMONARY HEMORRHAGE

Hemorrhage or hemorrhagic edema of the lung can result from trauma, bleeding diathesis, infections (invasive aspergillosis, mucormycosis, Pseudomonas, influenza), drugs (penicillamine), pulmonary embolism, fat embolism, ARDS, and autoimmune diseases (Table 15.3)(5). The autoimmune diseases that can cause pulmonary hemorrhage include Goodpasture's syndrome, idiopathic pulmonary hemorrhage, Wegener's granulomatosis, systemic lupus erythematosis, rheumatoid arthritis, and polyarteritis nodosa.

AUTOIMMUNE DISEASES

Goodpasture's Syndrome is an autoimmune disease characterized by damage to the alveolar and renal glomerular basement membranes by a cytotoxic antibody. The antibody is directed primarily against renal glomerular basement membrane and cross-reacts with alveolar basement membrane to produce the renal injury and pulmonary hemorrhage characteristic of this disorder. Young adult males are most commonly affected and present with cough, hemoptysis, dyspnea, and fatigue. The pulmonary complaints usually precede clinical evidence of renal failure. Chest films show bilateral coalescent air-space opacities that are radiographically indistinguishable from pulmonary edema (Fig. 15.5). Within several days, the air-space opacities resolve, giving rise to reticular opacities in the same distribution. Complete radiographic resolution is seen within 2 weeks except in patients with recurrent episodes of hemorrhage in whom the reticular opacities persist and represent pulmonary fibrosis. The diagnosis is made by immunofluorescent studies of renal

or lung tissue, which show a smooth, wavy line of fluorescent staining along the basement membrane. The overall prognosis is poor; however, the use of immunosuppressive drugs and plasmaphoresis has improved survival.

Idiopathic Pulmonary Hemorrhage. The pulmonary manifestations of idiopathic pulmonary hemorrhage are clinically and radiographically indistinguishable from those of Goodpasture's syndrome. In distinction to Goodpasture's syndrome, this disorder is most common in children, with an equal sex distribution. The diagnosis is one of exclusion and is suggested when pulmonary hemorrhage and anemia are found in a patient with normal renal function and urinalysis, and absence of antiglomerular basement membrane antibodies.

Other Autoimmune Diseases. Wegener's granulomatosis, systemic lupus erythematosis, rheumatoid arthritis, and polyarteritis nodosa are autoimmune disorders associated with a systemic immune complex vasculitis (6). The development of pulmonary hemorrhage in these diseases is secondary to small vessel pulmonary arteritis and capillaritis that results in spontaneous hemorrhage. The pulmonary manifestations of these diseases are discussed in subsequent sections.

Differentiation of Pulmonary Hemorrhage from pulmonary edema or pneumonia may be difficult, particularly because many causes of pulmonary edema and pneumonia may have a significant hemorrhagic component. The rapid development of air-space opacities associated with a dropping hematocrit and hemoptysis should suggest the diagnosis. Hemoptysis, however, is not always present. Associated renal disease, hematuria, or findings of a collagen vascular disorder or systemic vasculitis may provide additional clues. The distinction of pulmonary hemorrhage from pneumonia is made by the absence of fever or purulent sputum and the finding of a normal or elevated carbon monoxide diffusing capacity. This latter determination is directly related to the volume

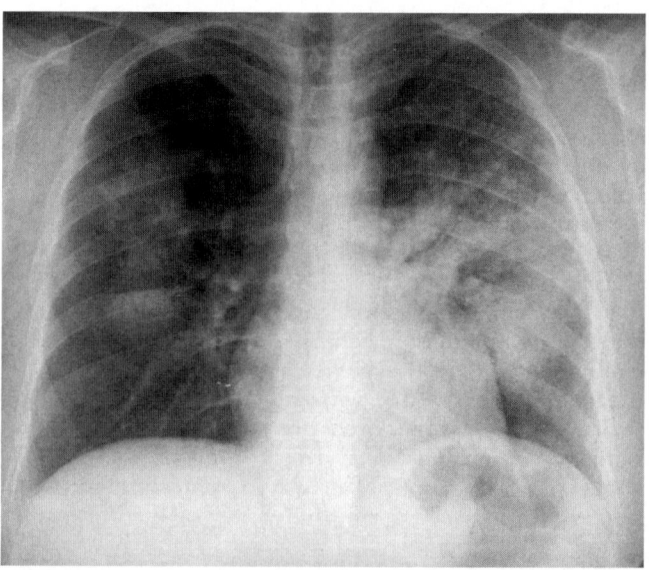

Figure 15.5. Pulmonary Hemorrhage in Goodpasture's Syndrome. PA chest film in a patient with Goodpasture's syndrome shows asymmetric bilateral air-space disease presenting intra-alveolar blood.

of gas-exchanging intravascular and extravascular intrapulmonary red blood cells and is therefore elevated in pulmonary hemorrhage or hemorrhagic edema but decreased in pneumonia. The presence of hemosiderin-laden macrophages in sputum, bronchoalveolar lavage fluid, or tissue specimens is evidence of chronic or recurrent intrapulmonary hemorrhage. A rapid radiographic improvement of the air-space opacities in pulmonary hemorrhage is common and may aid in diagnosis.

PULMONARY EMBOLISM

In the United States more than 600,000 cases of pulmonary embolism (PE) occur each year, with one-third of episodes causing or contributing to death. In patients surviving for 1 hour after the initial episode, 71% do not have PE diagnosed; this is associated with a 30% mortality rate. Alternatively, in the 29% of patients correctly diagnosed and treated for PE, there is an 8% mortality rate. These data suggest that empiric treatment for all patients with suspected PE is warranted. However, the high (up to 30%) incidence of hemorrhagic complications associated with anticoagulant therapy requires that an accurate diagnosis of pulmonary embolism be made.

The radiologist plays a central role in the diagnostic evaluation of the patient with suspected PE. This section will briefly review the nonimaging aspects of patient evaluation and then detail the various imaging modalities available to the radiologist. A practical algorithm that serves as a useful guide to the workup of each patient with suspected PE will be provided.

Clinical and Laboratory Findings. The majority of patients with PE have a variety of symptoms including dyspnea (84%), pleuritic chest pain (74%), anxiety (59%), and cough (53%). However, in certain groups of patients at high risk for PE, asymptomatic embolization occurs. For example, in patients undergoing elective total hip or knee re-

placement, 4% will develop postoperative PE as documented on pulmonary angiography. Physical examination may reveal tachypnea (respiratory rate >16/min), rales, and a prominent pulmonary component of the second heart sound. Unfortunately, these findings are entirely nonspecific. Only 20% of patients presenting to an emergency department with pleuritic chest pain will be found to have PE.

Laboratory tests commonly used in suspected PE include the measurements of PaO_2 and electrocardiography. Although less than 10% of patients with PE have a PaO_2 greater than 90 mm Hg, hypoxemia is common in a variety of disorders and is therefore nonspecific. Similarly, the absence of an alveolar-arterial oxygen gradient (A-aO_2) does not exclude the diagnosis. The electrocardiographic finding of an $S_1Q_3T_3$; right bundle branch block, right axis deviation, and right ventricular hypertrophy—all signs of cor pulmonale—are likewise inaccurate for the diagnosis of PE.

RADIOLOGIC DIAGNOSIS

A number of imaging techniques are routinely employed in the evaluation of the patient with suspected pulmonary embolism. These include the chest radiograph, ventilation/perfusion lung scintigraphy, helical CT, and pulmonary angiography. Noninvasive methods of imaging deep venous thrombosis (DVT) include compression and Doppler ultrasound of the legs and magnetic resonance venography of the extremities and pelvis. The relatively noninvasive nature and high accuracy of these techniques to diagnose DVT and an increasing familiarity with their performance and interpretation among radiologists has led to their widespread use in the workup of PE. A practical algorithm for the radiologic evaluation of PE is shown in Fig. 15.6.

Chest Radiograph is the first examination obtained in all patients with suspected PE. Although the majority

Figure 15.6. Algorithm for the Radiologic Evaluation of Pulmonary Thromboembolism.

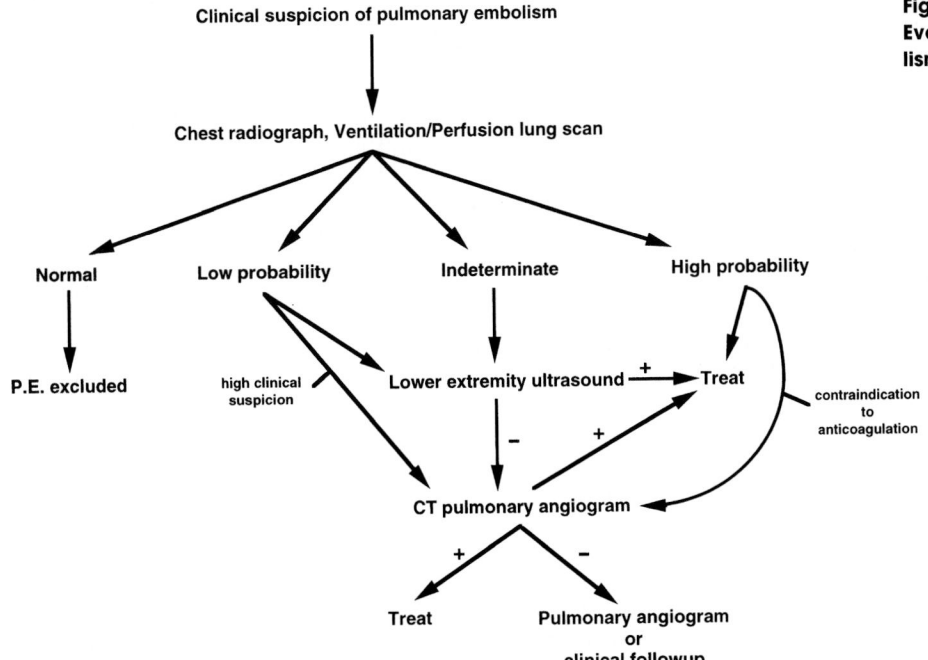

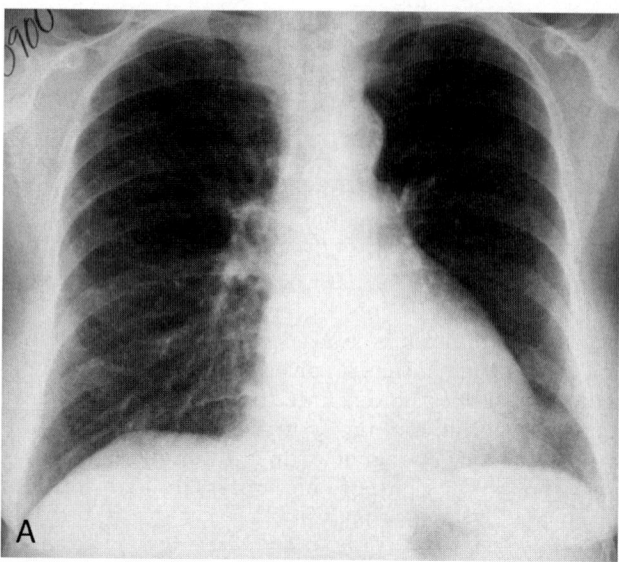

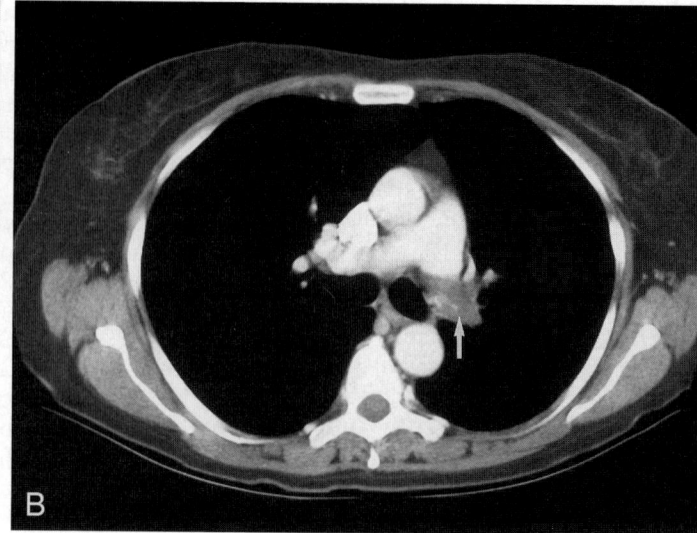

Figure 15.7. Westermark's Sign in Pulmonary Embolism. A. PA chest radiograph in a 64-year-old woman with sudden onset of dyspnea shows hyperlucency of the left lung. **B.** Helical CT pulmonary angiogram demonstrates thrombus (*arrow*) within the left main pulmonary artery.

of patients with PE will have abnormal radiographs, a significant percentage of patients will have normal chest radiographs. The radiographic findings include cardiac, pulmonary arterial, parenchymal, pleural, and diaphragmatic changes (7).

Cardiac, or more precisely right heart, enlargement is an uncommon finding seen with massive or extensive PE producing cor pulmonale. Enlargement of the central pulmonary arteries from pulmonary arterial hypertension may also be seen but is more commonly a late sequela of chronic thromboembolic disease. The most common radiographic findings in embolism without infarction are localized peripheral oligemia with or without distended proximal vessels (Westermark's sign) and peripheral air-space opacification or linear atelectasis (Fig. 15.7). The air-space opacification represents localized pulmonary hemorrhage produced by bronchial and pulmonary venous collateral flow to the obstructed region and is seen with peripheral but not central emboli. Volume loss in the lower lung from adhesive atelectasis owing to ischemic injury to type II pneumocytes and secondary surfactant deficiency may produce diaphragmatic elevation and the development of linear atelectasis.

Less than 10% of all PE result in lung infarction. Collateral bronchial arterial and retrograde pulmonary venous flow prevent infarction in most patients. The distinction between embolism without and with infarction is usually impossible radiographically and is of limited importance as treatment is identical. Infarction from embolism occurs with greater frequency in patients with underlying heart failure because of limited collateral bronchial arterial flow to the ischemic region. In PE with infarction, the cardiac, pulmonary arterial, and peripheral vascular changes are indistinguishable from those seen in embolism without infarction. Radiographic features that suggest infarction include the presence of a small pleural effusion and the development of a pleural-

based, wedge-shaped opacity (Hampton's hump). This opacity, typically found in the posterior or lateral costophrenic sulcus of the lung, is wedge-shaped, homogeneous, and lacking air bronchograms. The blunted apex of the wedge points toward the occluded feeding vessel, and the base is against the pleural surface (Fig. 15.8). This wedge-shaped opacity is often obscured by surrounding areas of hemorrhage in the early phases following infarction and becomes more obvious with time as the peripheral areas of hemorrhage resolve. A distinction between embolus with and without infarction is usually made by noting changes in the radiographic opacities with time. In embolism without infarction, the air-space opacities should resolve completely within 7–10 days, and infarcts resolve over the course of several weeks or months and usually leave a residual linear parenchymal scar and/or localized pleural thickening.

None of the aforementioned radiographic findings, either alone or in combination, are useful in making a definitive diagnosis of PE. Conversely, a completely normal radiograph may be seen in up to 40% of patients with emboli. The prime uses of the chest radiograph in the evaluation of PE are detecting conditions that mimic PE clinically, such as pneumonia or pneumothorax, and aiding the interpretation of the ventilation/perfusion lung scan.

Ventilation/Perfusion (V/Q) Lung Scintigraphy. The IV administration of macroaggregates of albumin radiolabeled with technetium has given the radiologist a noninvasive method of assessing the patency of the pulmonary circulation. The sensitivity of this technique allows for the confident exclusion of pulmonary embolism when a technically adequate perfusion scan is normal. The addition of ventilation scanning increases the specificity of an abnormal perfusion scan and is always performed in conjunction with the perfusion scan when possible.

Perfusion lung scanning is performed by intravenous injection of 5 millicuries of Tc-99m macroaggregated albumin with the patient supine. Images are then obtained in eight projections: AP, PA, right and left lateral, and right and left anterior and posterior oblique views. If perfusion abnormalities are present, a ventilation scan using Krypton-81m, Xenon-133, or aerosolized Tc-99m DTPA is then performed. The use of Krypton-81m and Tc-99m DTPA allow for comparable oblique projections identical to the perfusion scan. Perfusion defects can then be characterized as ventilation/perfusion matches (absent ventilation/absent perfusion) or mismatches (normal ventilation/ absent perfusion). Ventilation/perfusion mismatch is the hallmark of pulmonary embolism.

Although V/Q scanning is commonly used in the evaluation of the patient with suspected PE, its use for the diagnosis of PE is limited. First, only a minority of patients (27% in the PIOPED [Prospective Investigation of Pulmonary Embolism Diagnosis] study) undergoing V/Q studies will have either a normal or high probability study, results that clinicians can confidently rely on to guide treatment decisions (8). Second, significant interobserver variability occurs in the interpretation of V/Q studies. Finally, few well-constructed prospective studies have evaluated the accuracy of various patterns of V/Q abnormality in predicting the likelihood of PE.

Several diagnostic schemes have been proposed to assign PE probability (as determined by pulmonary angiography) given specific combinations of ventilation, perfusion, and concurrent chest radiographic findings. The V/Q scan interpretation categories published with the results of the PIOPED study have become the standard for radiologists interpreting V/Q studies. A normal V/Q scan effectively excludes PE because of the high sensitivity of the test. Patients with high-probability scans, particularly for those with a strong clinical suspicion for embolic disease, can be confidently treated for PE. Patients with intermediate or indeterminate (due to extensive obstructive lung disease) probability scans have a 30–40% incidence of pulmonary embolism. Likewise, those with a low probability V/Q scan and a high clinical suspicion for PE should have further noninvasive imaging of the deep venous system or pulmonary arteries. See chapter 56 for an expanded discussion of pulmonary scintigraphy.

Despite its limitations, V/Q scanning can provide useful information and remains the primary noninvasive screening modality for detecting pulmonary embolism. As compared with the evolving modalities of CT or MR pulmonary angiography, large experience with the technique exists. Although uncommon, a normal perfusion study excludes embolism whereas a high-probability V/Q study, in the appropriate clinical setting, allows for a confident enough diagnosis of PE to initiate anticoagulant therapy. Additionally, the localization of regions of absent perfusion helps guide selective pulmonary angiography.

Helical CT Pulmonary Angiography. Dedicated CT angiography of the central pulmonary arteries using a helical acquisition technique, thin collimation (2–5 mm), and rapid infusion of intravenous contrast (3–5 cc/second for a total of 100–120 cc) has proven sensitive in the detection of segmental, lobar, and main pulmonary arterial emboli (9). Emboli are recognized as intraluminal filling defects or as nonopacifiying vessels (Figs. 15.8B,15.9). At present the technique is limited by an inability to reliably detect emboli limited to subsegmental vessels. The exact role of this technique in the evaluation of pulmonary embolism continues to evolve; it is unclear if it will replace ventilation/perfusion lung scanning as a screening technique for pulmonary embolism or whether it will be used in lieu of conventional angiography.

Pulmonary Angiography is the gold standard in the diagnosis of pulmonary embolism (10). Selective film-screen pulmonary angiography can reliably detect pulmonary emboli at the segmental level. More sensitive techniques, such as balloon occlusion cineangiography

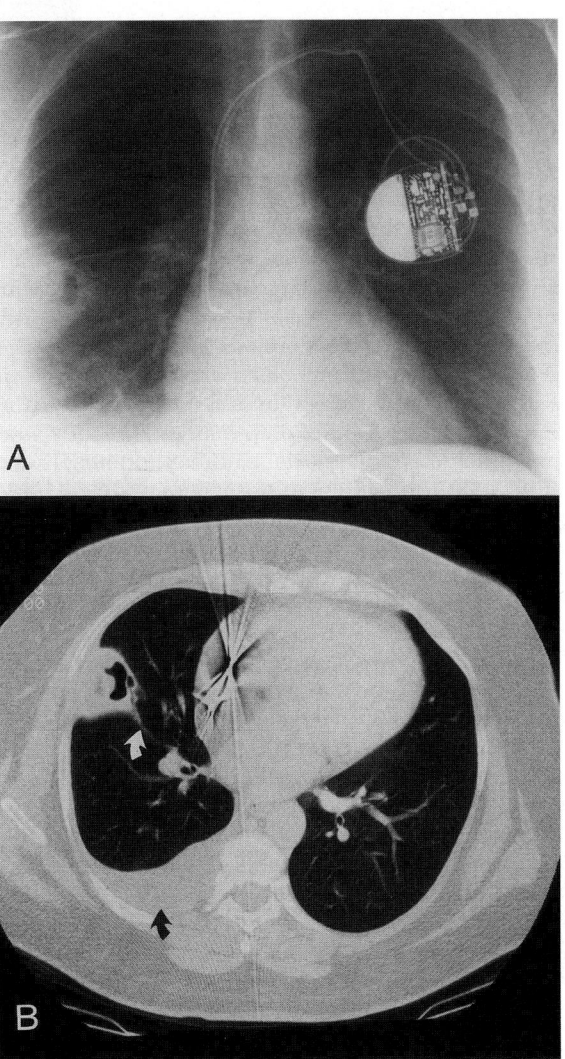

Figure 15.8. Pulmonary Infarct (Hampton's Hump). A. Frontal radiograph in a 56-year-old woman with cardiomyopathy, deep venous thrombosis, and pulmonary embolism shows a peripheral wedge-shaped opacity with cavitation in the right, lower lung. **B.** CT shows a smooth, cavitating, pleural-based mass representing an infarct, fed by a branch of the middle lobe pulmonary artery (*white arrow*). An associated right pleural effusion (*black arrow*) is a common finding in pulmonary infarct.

Figure 15.9. Pulmonary Embolism on CT. CT pulmonary angiogram in a 74-year-old woman demonstrates filling defects within the right main (*black arrow*) and left interlobar (*white arrow*) pulmonary arteries representing bilateral pulmonary emboli.

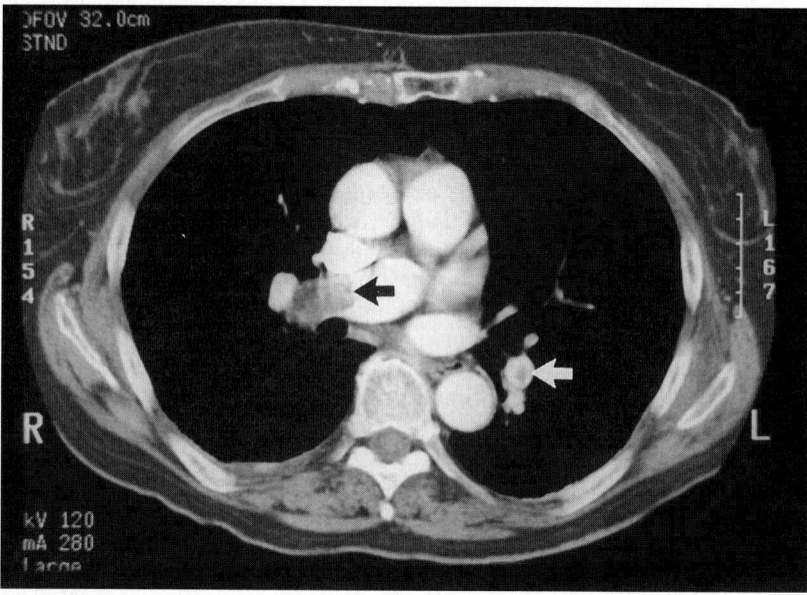

and magnification angiography, can detect emboli as small as 2 mm in diameter. The accuracy of pulmonary arteriography in the diagnosis of PE is high. Based upon clinical follow-up of patients with negative studies, the sensitivity of pulmonary angiography is 98–99%, with almost 100% specificity for positive angiographic studies.

The indications for pulmonary angiography in the diagnosis of pulmonary embolism are listed in Table 15.4. The most common indication is a patient with an indeterminate or intermediate probability V/Q study who requires a definitive diagnosis. Although no absolute contraindications to pulmonary angiography exist, several conditions do place the patient at an increased risk from the procedure. These include a previously documented idiosyncratic reaction to contrast, right ventricular failure, renal insufficiency, and left bundle branch block (LBBB). When any of these conditions exist in a patient referred for pulmonary angiography, an attempt at correcting these factors (e.g., premedication for contrast reaction or pacemaker placement for LBBB) should be undertaken. Alternatively, these patients may undergo noninvasive imaging for proximal deep venous thrombosis using US, impedance plethysmography, or MR venography. See chapter 24 for a detailed discussion of pulmonary angiography

PE is diagnosed on pulmonary angiography when an intraluminal filling defect or the trailing end of an occluding thrombus is outliined by contrast (Fig. 15.10). Secondary signs including a prolonged arterial phase, diminished peripheral perfusion, and delay in the venous phase are nonspecific and are not used to diagnose PE. Once thrombus is unequivocally identified, the study is terminated. The only exception would be a patient who is considered a candidate for surgical thrombectomy or thrombolytic therapy, for which precise knowledge of the laterality, location, and extent of thrombus is required.

The overall complication rate of pulmonary angiography is 2–5% and can be divided into those related to contrast administration and those secondary to car-

Table 15.4. Indications for Pulmonary Angiography in Suspected Pulmonary Embolism

Indeterminate V/Q scan
High clinical suspicion for PE and a low probability V/Q scan
High probability V/Q scan and a relative or absolute contraindication to anticoagulation
Patient with diagnosis of PE who is considered for fibrinolytic therapy or embolectomy
CT pulmonary angiogram negative or inconclusive and suspicion for PE remains high

diac catheterization and intrapulmonary arterial contrast injection. Many of these complications, such as myocardial and endocardial injury and cardiac perforation, were associated almost exclusively with the use of angled, sharp-tipped catheters. These traumatic complications are rare now that the vast majority of angiographers use pigtail-tipped catheters. Mortality from pulmonary angiography is less than 0.5% and is usually related to sudden right ventricular failure from transient elevation of pulmonary artery pressure secondary to contrast injection. Death from pulmonary angiography is seen almost exclusively in critically ill patients and those with preexisting severe pulmonary arterial hypertension (pulmonary artery systolic pressure >70 mm Hg) or right ventricular dysfunction (right ventricular end diastolic pressure >20 mmHg). However, there is no significant increase in the incidence of major, nonfatal reactions in patients with pulmonary arterial hypertension. In addition, the majority of patients with severe right ventricular dysfunction have uneventful studies. When one considers the added safety of selective contrast injections using nonionic contrast agents and the high mortality of untreated pulmonary embolism in this population, pulmonary angiography should be performed in these patients when indicated.

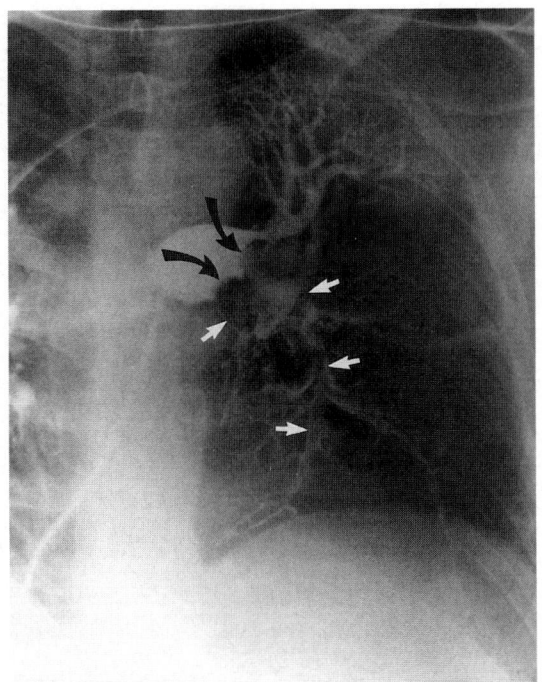

Figure 15.10. Pulmonary Embolism on Pulmonary Arteriogram. A frontal radiograph from a left pulmonary arteriogram reveals a large intraluminal filling defect within the main and left interlobar pulmonary artery diagnostic of pulmonary embolism. Note the typical meniscus of contrast outlining the trailing edge of the thrombus (*curved black arrows*) and a rim of contrast around the body of the thrombus (*small white arrows*).

Noninvasive Imaging for Deep Venous Thrombosis. The use of US and MR for the diagnosis of DVT has altered the conventional approach to the evaluation of pulmonary thromboembolic disease. Because 90% of PE arise from the lower extremities and because the treatment for proximal (i.e., above the knee) DVT is identical to that for proven PE, a confident diagnosis of proximal DVT can provide an endpoint in patient evaluation for thromboembolic disease. Although contrast venography requires venipuncture and contrast administration and is associated with discomfort and possible thrombophlebitis, US and MR have no known associated risks. US is used in the majority of patients with nondiagnostic ventilation/perfusion studies that are referred for a diagnosis of pulmonary thromboembolism. The US diagnosis of DVT is reviewed in chapter 40.

When performed by skilled personnel, compression US has a sensitivity of 90–95% and a specificity of 95–98% for the diagnosis of acute DVT when compared to contrast venography. False-negative studies occur when DVT is limited to the calf; this is not a serious limitation of the technique as these thrombi do not lead to significant pulmonary emboli. False positive studies are seen most often in patients with prior DVT. Studies show that as many as 50% of patients with occlusive DVT have findings on follow-up compression US studies performed within 15 months of the acute episode that can mimic the findings of acute DVT. Pelvic masses compressing the iliac veins can make compression of the femoral vein

difficult, thereby mimicking acute DVT on US examination. In addition to providing an accurate diagnosis of the presence of DVT, US offers the advantage of imaging the nonvenous structures in the leg, allowing the radiologist to diagnose conditions that may simulate DVT clinically such as Baker's cysts, enlarged lymph nodes, pseudoaneurysms, and pelvic masses compressing the iliac vein.

Although accurate for the diagnosis of proximal deep venous thrombosis, a negative compression US study does not exclude pulmonary embolus. Thus, patients with a negative US study should undergo pulmonary angiography.

MR venography provides an alternative for the noninvasive diagnosis of DVT. Studies using 2-D time-of-flight MR venography have shown high sensitivity and specificity for the diagnosis of DVT as compared to contrast venography. MR may provide the added benefit of determining the age of a thrombus based on its T1 and T2 relaxation times, thereby allowing distinction between acute and chronic DVT. Evaluation of the iliac veins and superior vena cava is possible as is the identification of pelvic masses that may compress the iliac vein and mimic DVT.

The usefulness of radionuclide scanning for the diagnosis of DVT remains equivocal. Intrapedal Tc-99m MAA and intravenous I-125 fibrinogen have met with variable success. Indium 111-labeled platelets have been used to successfully diagnose patients with venographically proven DVT although the 24-hour delay necessary to increase the sensitivity of the test is unacceptable to most clinicians. Another difficulty is that patients receiving heparin may have false-negative examinations. More recently, labeled monoclonal antithrombus antibodies, either to platelets or thrombus itself, have been used for the diagnosis of DVT; however, their use in this setting remains investigational.

PULMONARY ARTERIAL HYPERTENSION

Pulmonary arterial hypertension (PAH) is defined as a systolic pressure in the pulmonary artery exceeding 30 mm of mercury, measured either directly by catheterization of the pulmonary artery or estimated by echocardiography. The diagnosis of PAH is usually evident from the clinical history, physical findings, and appearance on chest radiographs. The typical radiographic findings of PAH are an enlarged main artery and hilar pulmonary arteries that taper rapidly toward the lung periphery (Fig. 15.11)(11). Associated enlargement of the right ventricle, seen on lateral radiographs as prominence of the anterosuperior cardiac margin with obliteration of the retrosternal air space, is an additional clue to the diagnosis. Occasionally, hypertension-induced atherosclerotic lesions in the large elastic arteries can produce mural calcifications on radiographs, a rare finding that is specific for PAH. A useful measurement for enlargement of the central pulmonary arteries, usually indicating PAH in the absence of a left-to-right shunt, is a transverse diameter of the proximal interlobar pulmonary artery on posteroanterior chest radiograph exceeding 16 mm. Another specific indicator of PAH is a transverse

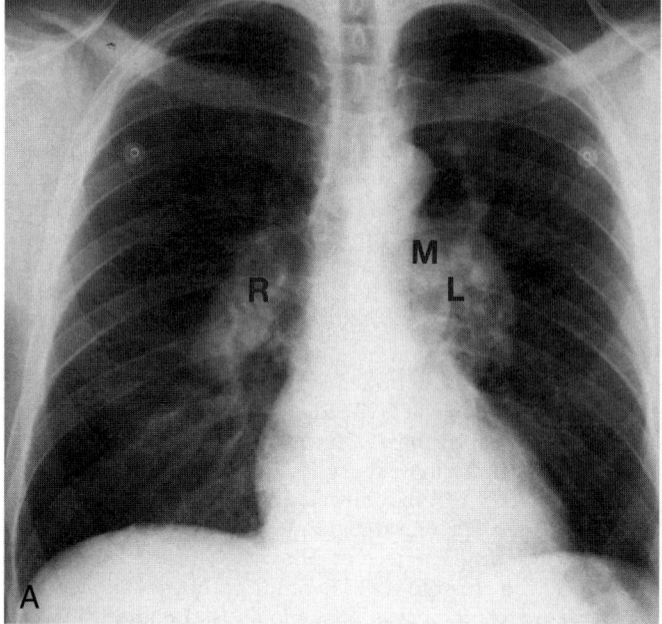
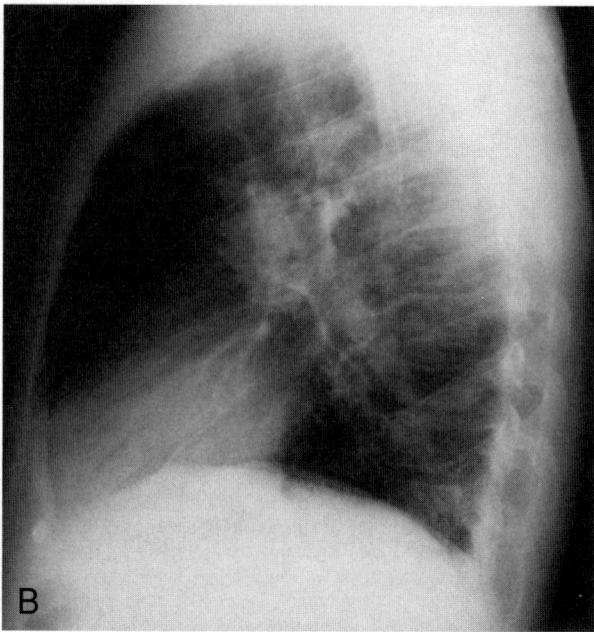

Figure 15.11. Pulmonary Arterial Hypertension. PA **(A)** and lateral **(B)** chest radiographs in a 32-year-old woman with pulmonary hypertension from chronic pulmonary thromboembolic disease shows enlarged main (*M*), right (*R*), and left (*L*) pulmonary arteries with diminutive peripheral vessels.

measurement of the main pulmonary artery on CT or MR that exceeds 28.6 mm. However, a normal measurement of the main or right interlobar pulmonary artery does not exclude PAH because patients with mild or even moderate elevation of pulmonary artery pressure may have normal-sized arteries. Those patients with long-standing PAH will develop right ventricular hypertrophy, with eventual right ventricular dilatation and failure (cor pulmonale). In addition, MR may also demonstrate intraluminal signal during the early diastolic phase of the cardiac cycle, a finding indicative of turbulent flow caused by increased vascular resistance sometimes seen with marked elevation of pulmonary artery pressure.

In addition to PAH, enlargement of the central pulmonary arteries may be seen in conditions associated with increased flow through the pulmonary circulation. This occurs in patients with a high cardiac output, such as those with anemia, thyrotoxicosis, or left-to-right shunts. The latter includes atrial and ventricular septal defect, patent ductus arteriosus, and partial anomalous pulmonary venous return. Early in the course of left-to-right shunts, the pulmonary artery pressure is normal or slightly elevated as pulmonary vascular resistance decreases to compensate for the increased flow. In these patients, both central and peripheral pulmonary arteries become enlarged, producing "shunt vascularity" on chest radiographs. Later, usually in young adulthood, the muscular pulmonary arterioles develop medial hyperplasia and intimal fibrosis, with resultant increased pulmonary vascular resistance. When this occurs, the chest radiograph demonstrates findings typical of PAH indistinguishable from PAH due to other causes.

An increase in resistance to pulmonary blood flow is the most common cause of PAH. The disorders produc-

ing increased pulmonary vascular resistance are pulmonary venous hypertension, parenchymal lung disease, chest wall deformity, diffuse pleural fibrosis, pulmonary arterial disease, and idiopathic pulmonary vascular disease. The most common cause of chronic elevation of pulmonary venous pressure is mitral stenosis although any impedence to pulmonary venous return to the left heart can produce venous hypertension. Less common entities in this group include chronic left ventricular failure, atrial myxoma, cor triatriatum, and pulmonary vein stenosis or occlusion. In addition to the characteristic pulmonary arterial changes of PAH, patients may show left ventricular dilatation in left ventricular failure or left atrial enlargement in mitral stenosis or cor triatriatum. The radiographic signs of pulmonary venous hypertension and pulmonary edema may be seen early in the course of these disorders but are often absent by the time PAH has developed.

Parenchymal lung disease, particularly centrilobular emphysema and diffuse interstitial fibrosis, are common causes of PAH. The mechanisms by which these disorders produce increased vascular resistance include chronic hypoxemia and reflex vasoconstriction and the development of irreversible changes in pulmonary arteriolar caliber with widespread obliteration of the pulmonary vascular bed. The radiographic findings of emphysema and interstitial fibrosis are usually evident on plain radiographs by the time PAH has developed.

Chronic hypoxemia from alveolar hypoventilation is the likely mechanism for PAH that complicates pleural fibrosis, kyphoscoliosis, and the obesity-hypoventilation syndrome. Pleural thickening and kyphoscoliosis are readily evident radiographically. The obesity-hypoventilation (Pickwickian) syndrome is associated with marked truncal obesity and lungs that are diminished in volume (mostly because of diaphragmatic elevation) but are normal in appearance.

Disorders of the pulmonary arteries producing PAH include pulmonary emboli, vasculitis, and the pulmonary arteriopathy resulting from long-standing increased pulmonary blood flow from the left-to-right shunt. Occlusion of lobar and segmental vessels producing pulmonary arterial hypertension can result from failure of pulmonary thromboemboli to lyse or completely recanalize. The diagnosis of large vessel thromboembolic pulmonary hypertension is usually made by demonstrating large mismatches on ventilation/perfusion lung scanning, with pulmonary arteriography showing occlusion or stenosis of multiple lobar or segmental pulmonary arteries. Radiographically, regions of peripheral oligemia may be seen, but more often the lungs are normal in appearance. Rarely, pulmonary vasculitis resulting from diseases such as rheumatoid lung disease or Takayasu's arteritis can produce obliteration of the pulmonary vasculature and lead to PAH.

Idiopathic or primary pulmonary hypertension encompasses diseases or the pulmonary arterioles and venules that are not attributable to other causes and have characteristic histologic findings. Plexogenic pulmonary arteriopathy, recurrent microscopic pulmonary embolism, and pulmonary veno-occlusive disease are the three diseases that comprise this category. Plexogenic pulmonary arteriopathy is a disease of young women in whom medial hypertrophy and intimal fibrosis obliterate the muscular arteries. Dilated vascular channels within the periphery of the obliterated vessel produce the plexogenic lesions seen on biopsy in virtually all patients with this disease. Progressive dyspnea and fatigue develop with characteristic physical findings of PAH and cor pulmonale. In plexogenic pulmonary arteriopathy, pulmonary perfusion scans typically show normal perfusion or small, nonsegmental, peripheral perfusion defects, allowing distinction from large vessel thromboembolic disease. Microembolic disease is clinically and radiographically indistinguishable from plexogenic arteriopathy. In this entity, plexogenic lesions within arterioles are absent. Perfusion scans are more likely to show small perfusion defects in this disorder. The presence of small microemboli histologically is not a distinguishing feature because in situ thrombosis within diseased arterioles can have a similar appearance. In pulmonary veno-occlusive disease, the obliteration of small intrapulmonary venules results in interstitial pulmonary edema. The transmission of increased pressure to the arterial side leads to medial hypertrophy and obliteration of vessel lumina with resultant arterial hypertension. Chest radiographs often show interstitial or air-space pulmonary edema with a normal heart size. The radiographic signs of pulmonary venous hypertension are absent, and the pulmonary capillary wedge pressure (PCWP) is usually normal. Perfusion lung scanning is usually normal or shows small, peripheral, nonsegmental defects. The combination of pulmonary edema with a normal heart size, absent findings for pulmonary venous hypertension, normal PCWP, and the insidious onset of dyspnea should suggest this diagnosis rather than left heart failure, mitral valve disease, or large pulmonary venous occlusion. A definitive diagnosis can only be made by characteristic findings on open lung biopsy. The prognosis is universally poor, with most patients succumbing to their disease within 2 years of diagnosis.

References

1. Pistolesi M, Miniati M, Milne ENC, et al. The chest roentgenogram in pulmonary edema. Clin Chest Med 1985; 6:315-344.
2. Turner AF, Lau FYK, Jacobson G, et al. A method for the estimation of pulmonary venous and arterial pressures from the routine chest roentgenograms. AJR Am J Roentgenol 1972;116:97–106.
3. Iannuzzi M, Petty TL. The diagnosis, pathogenesis, and treatment of adult respiratory distress syndrome. J Thorac Imag 1986;1:1–10.
4. Milne ENC, Pistolesi M, Miniati M, et al. The radiologic distinction of cardiogenic and noncardiogenix edema. AJR Am J Roentgenol 1985;144:879–894.
5. Albelda SM, Gefter WB, Epstein DM, et al. Diffuse pulmonary hemorrhage: a review and classification. Radiology 1985;154:289–297.
6. Leatherman JW. Immune alveolar hemorrhage. Chest 1987;91:891–897.
7. Buckner CB, Walker CW, Purnell GL. Pulmonary embolism: chest radiographic abnormalities. J Thorac Imag 1989; 4:23–27.
8. The PIOPED investigators. Value of the ventilation/perfusion scan in acute pulmonary embolism: results of the prospective investigation of pulmonary embolism diagnosis (PIOPED). JAMA 1990;263:2753–2759.
9. Remy-Jardin M, Remy J, Wattinne L, Giraud F. Central pulmonary thromboembolism. Diagnosis with spiral volumetric CT with the single breath-hold technique-comparison with pulmonary angiography. Radiology 1992;185: 381–387.
10. Stein PD, Athanasoulis C, Alavi A, et al. Complications and validity of pulmonary angiography in acute pulmonary embolism. Circulation 1992;85:462–468.
11. Ravin CE. Pulmonary vascularity: radiographic considerations. J Thorac Imag 1988;3:1–8.

16
Pulmonary Neoplasms

Jeffrey S. Klein
Austin Wand

   Lesions Presenting as SPNs
BRONCHOGENIC CARCINOMA
   Cytologic and Pathologic Features
   Radilologic Staging of Lung Cancer
TRACHEAL AND BRONCHIAL MASSES
METASTATIC DISEASE TO THE THORAX
NONEPITHELIAL PARENCHYMAL MALIGNANCIES AND
   NEOPLASTIC-LIKE CONDITIONS

THE SOLITARY PULMONARY NODULE

General Considerations. The radiologic evaluation of a solitary pulmonary nodule (SPN) is one of the most common and most difficult diagnostic dilemmas in thoracic radiology (1). Before embarking on a detailed diagnostic evaluation of a SPN, one must determine if the nodular opacity seen on the chest radiograph is real or artifactual. This may require repeat radiographs, occasionally with nipple markers, to identify a nipple shadow appearing as a nodule. If the opacity is judged to represent a real lesion, the radiologist must then determine whether it is a solitary pulmonary nodule. First, is the lesion truly solitary? Not uncommonly, a dominant pulmonary nodule on chest radiographs is associated with smaller nodules or nodules that are obscured by the heart or the hemidiaphragms. A careful search on PA and lateral chest radiographs will identify most of these patients although helical CT may be necessary to identify additional nodules not seen on chest radiographs. Multiple pulmonary nodules of similar size and appearance are almost always metastases or granulomas, and these require a different evaluation from that of a solitary lesion.

Second, is the lesion intrapulmonary? Intrapulmonary lesions are discrete opacities that are completely circumscribed by aerated lung on both frontal and lateral radiographs. A pleural or mediastinal lesion may be outlined by lung when it projects inward. However, the base of the lesion, which forms obtuse angles with the lung, is not outlined by lung where it arises from the pleura or mediastinum. Skin or chest wall lesions can also mimic intrapulmonary nodules as they project outward to be outlined by air, but these are not completely circumscribed where they arise from the chest wall (the breast is a good example). Some skin lesions are completely circumscribed by air, but a careful physical examination of the patient, usually following the chest radiograph, will

reveal the surface lesion responsible for the "nodule" seen on chest film (Fig. 16.1). One of the most troublesome skin "lesions" to distinguish from a true pulmonary nodule is the nipple shadow. This is usually readily identified by obtaining films in the PA, lateral, and 5° oblique (from the PA) projections with nipple markers, or by performing chest fluoroscopy. A sclerotic bone lesion or healing rib fracture can simulate a new pulmonary nodule; oblique radiographs or fluoroscopy will often help localize these lesions to a rib. Occasionally, CT will be necessary for confident localization of a nodular density seen on plain radiographs.

Finally, is the lesion a nodule? A nodule is a discrete round or oval opacity; linear or angular opacities are not nodules and represent scars or areas of linear atelectasis. When a focal opacity is seen in the lung apices, an apical lordotic film or CT may be necessary to distinguish a linear from a nodular opacity. A round opacity greater than 3 cm in diameter is termed a mass. Because the majority of lung masses in patients over the age of 35 represent bronchogenic carcinoma, these lesions are not considered SPNs.

Once a solitary pulmonary nodule has been identified, the radiologist should initiate a series of investigations to determine whether the nodule is definitely benign or suspicious for malignancy (i.e., indeterminate). This stepwise approach is summarized in Fig. 16.2.

Clinical Factors. Before considering the radiologic characteristics used to distinguish benign from indeterminate nodules, important clinical factors may be helpful in making this distinction. In a patient younger than the age of 35 years, particularly a nonsmoker, without a history of malignancy, a SPN is invariably a granuloma, hamartoma, or inflammatory lesion. These nodules can be followed with plain radiographs to confirm their benign nature. Patients older than 35 years have a significant incidence of malignant SPNs, with approximately 50% of noncalcified SPNs in patients older than 50 years of age malignant at thoracotomy. Therefore, as a rule, a SPN in a patient older than 35 years should never be followed radiographically without tissue confirmation unless a benign pattern of calcification or the presence of intralesional fat is identified on radiographs or HRCT, or there has been radiographically documented lack of growth over a minimum of 2 years. Exceptions to this rule include the following: a history of cigarette smoking or asbestos exposure or both raises the level of concern for malignancy in a patient with a SPN. Alternatively, if the patient is from an area where histoplasmosis or tuberculosis is endemic, the likelihood of a granuloma is greater and in such patients, a conservative approach may be warranted. Finally, the finding of a SPN in a pa-

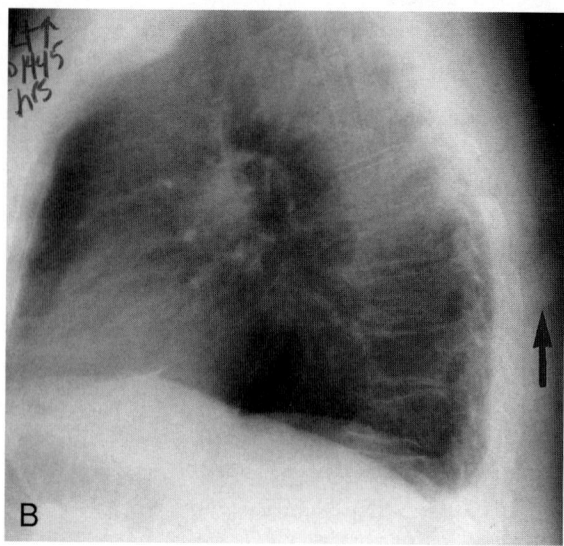

Figure 16.1. Skin Lesion Simulating SPN. A. PA chest radiograph shows a nodular opacity (*arrows*) projecting over the right mid-lung. **B.** Lateral film shows a skin lesion projecting from the posterior chest wall (*arrow*). Physical examination confirmed the presence of a skin hemangioma.

tient with an extrathoracic malignancy raises the possibility of a solitary pulmonary metastasis. If the lung is the sole site of metastatic disease, distinguishing between a primary bronchogenic carcinoma and a pulmonary metastasis is usually not important because many surgeons will resect a solitary pulmonary metastasis. An SPN that arises more than 2 years after the diagnosis of an extrathoracic malignancy is almost always a primary lung tumor rather than a metastasis; breast carcinoma and melanoma are notable exceptions to this rule.

Growth Pattern. Pulmonary malignancies grow at a relatively predictable rate. The growth rate of an SPN is usually expressed as the doubling time, or the time it takes for a nodule to double its volume. For a sphere, this corresponds to a 25% increase in diameter. Although some benign lesions (mostly hamartomas and histoplasmomas) may exhibit a growth rate similar to that of malignant lesions, the absence of growth or an extraordinarily slow or rapid rate of growth is reliable evidence that a SPN is benign. Studies show that bronchogenic carcinoma has a doubling time of between 1 month and 2 years. Therefore, a doubling time of less than one month or greater than 2 years reliably characterizes a lesion as benign. Infectious lesions and rapidly growing metastases from choriocarcinoma, seminoma, or osteogenic sarcoma comprise the majority of rapidly growing solitary nodules whereas lack of growth or a doubling time exceeding 2 years is seen in hamartomas and histoplasmomas. However, there are also exceptions to this rule. A giant cell carcinoma, a subtype of large cell carcinoma, pulmonary carcinosarcomas and pulmonary blastomas may have a doubling time of less than 1 month. Even more common pulmonary malignancies such as the occasional adenocarcinoma or carcinoid tumors may have a doubling time of greater than 2 years. Any malignancy that hemorrhages into its substance will

appear to enlarge rapidly. Two important caveats to using the growth rate of a SPN to determine benignity exist. The first is that the growth rate of a SPN which is not visible on prior radiographs cannot be estimated because noncalcified nodules less than 1 cm in diameter are not usually visible on conventional radiographs. Most importantly, with few exceptions, a patient older than 35 with a noncalcified SPN should not be evaluated prospectively to determine benignity by following the growth rate on serial chest radiographs. The assessment of growth rate to determine benignity should only be used retrospectively in comparing the size of an SPN with prior radiographs from at least 2 years ago.

If a decision is made to simply follow an SPN radiologically, either because of an overwhelming likelihood of benignity or because the patient cannot tolerate an invasive diagnostic procedure, the lesion should be followed by chest radiographs or limited thin-section CT at intervals of 3–6 months for a minimum of 2 years.

Size. Although size does not reliably discriminate benign from malignant SPNs, the larger the lesion the greater the likelihood of malignancy. Masses exceeding 4 cm in diameter are usually malignant. However, the converse does not hold true; many pulmonary malignancies are less than 2 cm in diameter at the time of diagnosis.

Margin (Border) Characteristics. The appearance of the edge of an SPN is a helpful sign in determining the nature of the lesion. The edge characteristics are best evaluated on thin-section CT because this technique is considerably more accurate than plain radiographs. A round, smoothly marginated nodule is most likely a granuloma or hamartoma although a rare primary pulmonary malignancy such as a carcinoid tumor, adenocarcinoma, or a solitary metastasis may have a perfectly smooth margin. A notched or lobulated margin is strongly suggestive but not diagnostic of malignancy. Pathologic examination has shown that the lobulated edge of a malignant nodule represents mounds of tumor extending into the adjacent lung. A spiculated margin is highly suspicious for malignancy (Fig. 16.3). The term "corona radiata" has been used to describe this appearance, in which linear densities radiate from the edge of a nodule into the adjacent lung. Pathologically, these linear radiations represent reoriented connective tissue (interlobular) septa drawn into the tumor by the cicatrizing (scarring) nature of many malignant lung tumors. Tumor extension from the nodule, or fibrosis and edema of these connective tissue septa may thicken these linear densities. However, spiculation is not specific for malignancy because benign processes that produce cicatrization can have an identical appearance. Benign lesions that may show a spiculated margin include lipoid pneumonia, organizing pneumonia, tuberculomas, and the mass lesions of progressive massive fibrosis in complicated silicosis. A peripherally situated pulmonary nod-

ule may contact the costal pleura or interlobar fissure via a linear opacity known as a "pleural tail." As with the corona radiata, the recognition of this line, although suggestive of malignancy (particularly bronchioloalveolar cell carcinoma), is not specific and may be seen in peripheral granulomas.

Three additional characteristics of the border of an SPN help identify the nature of the lesion. The presence of small "satellite" nodules around the periphery of a dominant nodule is strongly suggestive of benign disease, particularly granulomatous infection. The identification of feeding and draining vessels emanating from the hilar aspect of an SPN is pathognomonic of a pulmonary arteriovenous malformation (AVM). Contrast-enhanced helical CT scanning through the nodule or MR is diagnostic. A posttraumatic pulmonary artery pseudoaneurysm will show marked contrast enhancement and contiguity with the feeding artery on CT. Finally, the

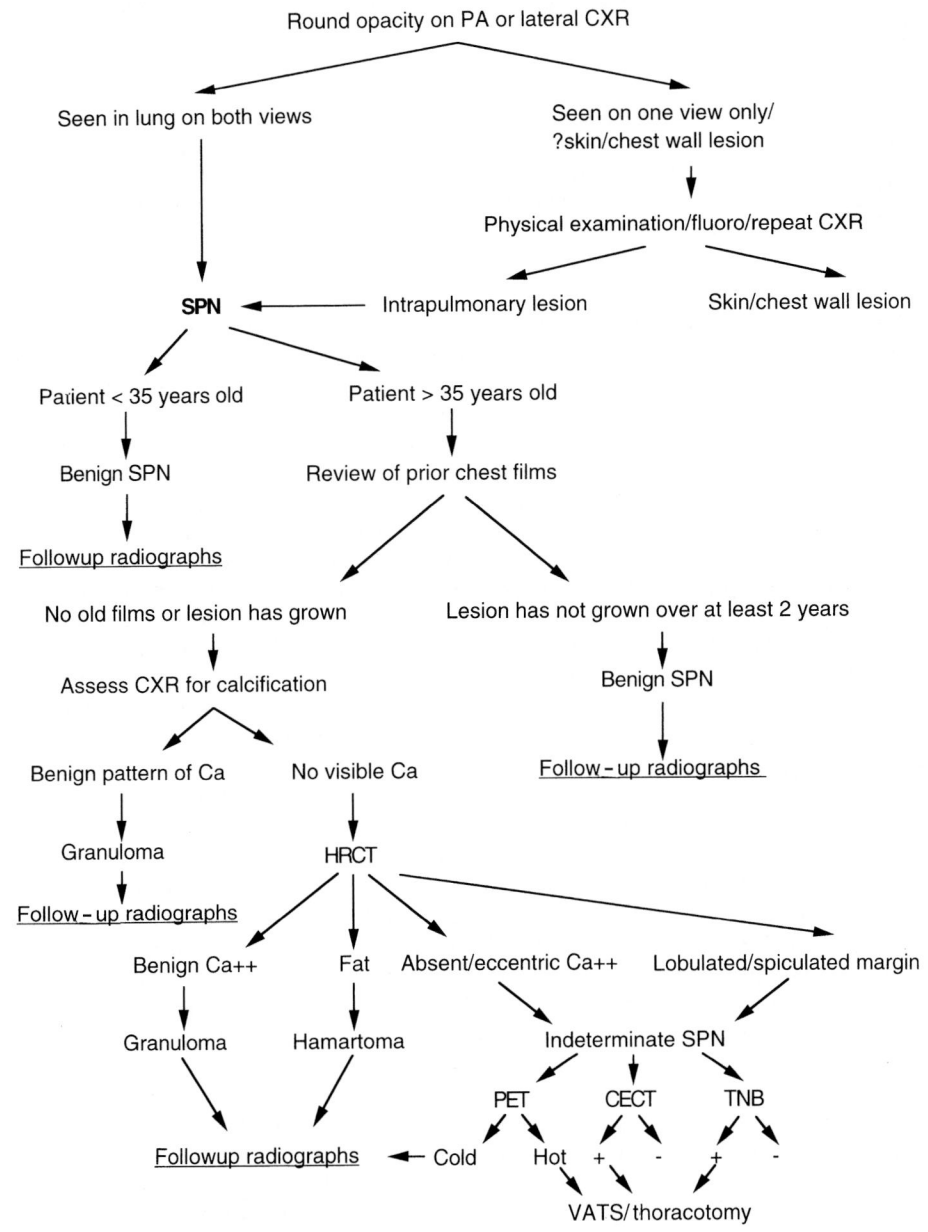

Figure 16.2. Algorithm for Approach to the SPN. *Ca*, calcification; *TNB*, transthoracic needle biopsy; *CXR*, chest x-ray; *PET*, positron emission tomography; *CECT*, contrast-enhanced CT.

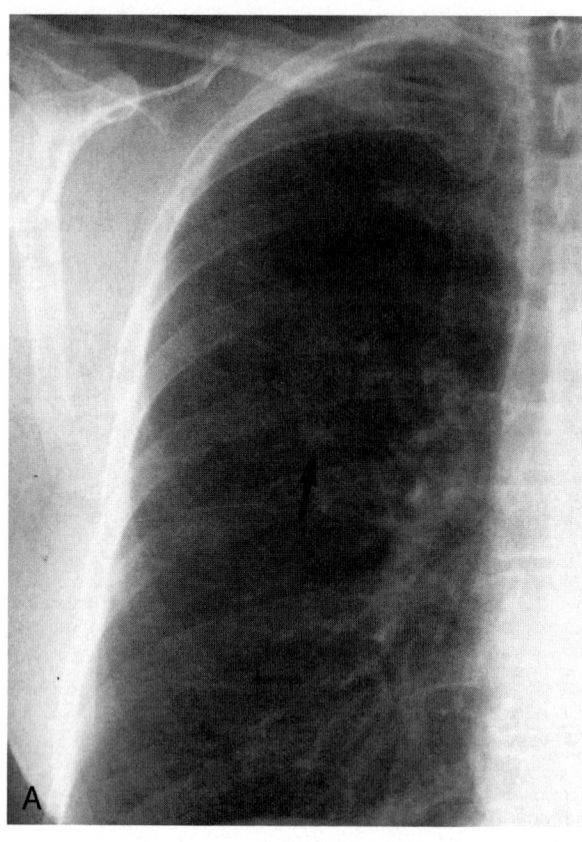

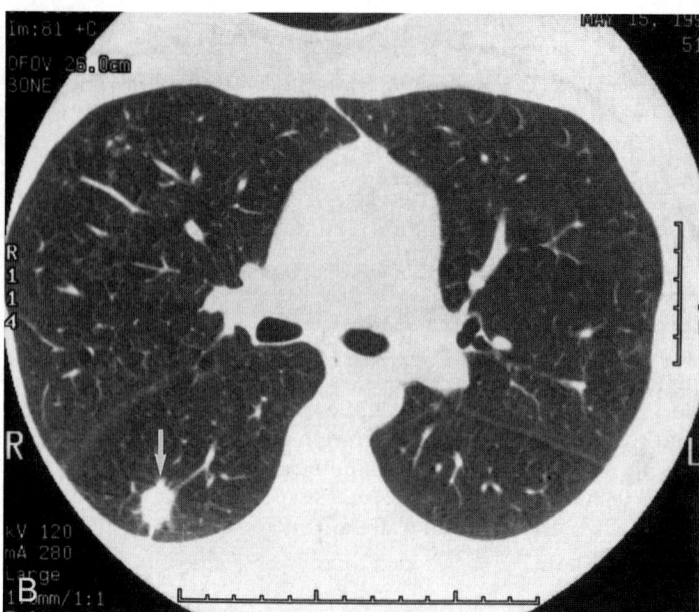

Figure 16.3. Adenocarcinoma Presenting as SPN. A. Coned-down view of PA radiograph shows right mid-lung nodule (*arrow*). **B.** Thin-section CT shows 12-mm nodule with spiculated margins (*arrow*) in the superior segment of the right lower lobe. Transthoracic needle biopsy revealed adenocarcinoma.

presence of a halo of ground-glass opacity circling an SPN in an immunocompromised, neutropenic patient should suggest the diagnosis of invasive pulmonary aspergillosis.

Density. The internal density of an SPN is probably the single most important factor in characterizing the lesion as benign or indeterminate. Lesions that are calcified usually are benign. Four patterns of calcification reliably indicate the benignity of an SPN (Fig. 16.4). These patterns can be identified on plain chest radiographs, but thin-section CT is often necessary to detect and characterize the calcification. *Complete or central calcification* within an SPN is specific for a healed granuloma from tuberculosis or histoplasmosis. *Concentric or laminated calcification* indicates a granuloma and allows confident exclusion of neoplasm (Fig. 16.5). *Popcorn calcification* within a nodule is diagnostic of a pulmonary hamartoma in which the cartilaginous component has calcified (Fig. 16.6).

One must remember that calcification within an SPN is synonymous with a benign lesion only if the calcification follows one of the four patterns of benign calcification shown in Figure 16.4. Approximately 10% of malignant nodules contain calcification on CT. A bronchogenic carcinoma that arises in an area of previous granulomatous infection may engulf a preexisting calcified granuloma as it enlarges. In this situation, the calcification will be eccentric in the nodule, allowing distinction from a centrally calcified granuloma. Malignant pulmonary neoplasms may demonstrate small or microscopic foci of calcification, particularly adenocarcinomas that produce

mucin or psammoma bodies. The rare solitary pulmonary metastasis from osteosarcoma or chondrosarcoma may contain calcium, but the diagnosis in these patients will usually be obvious clinically.

Although benign patterns of calcification may be detected on plain radiographs or HRCT, some benign nodules contain microscopic calcifications that are not readily evident on visual inspection of the images. This has led to the use of quantitative CT nodule densitometry to detect the presence and distribution of microscopic calcification within SPNs. Two quantitative techniques have been utilized: 1) comparing the CT density of the SPN with that of a reference nodule containing a quantity of calcium sufficient to characterize as benign, placed in a chest phantom, and 2) determining the absolute CT numbers of an SPN by obtaining a computer generated pixel display through the center of the nodule (2). The latter method obviates the need for an anthropomorphic chest phantom and is most often utilized. A mean CT value exceeding 200 H in at least 10% of the pixels within a nodule is reliable evidence of the presence of benign calcification. As with visible calcification, the calcification detected by densitometry must be either central or evenly distributed throughout the nodule to be considered benign. The use of nodule densitometry has significantly reduced the percentage of patients considered to have indeterminate SPNs by visual inspection alone, thereby decreasing the number of thoracotomies performed for benign lesions.

The identification of fat within an SPN is diagnostic of a pulmonary hamartoma. A discussion of the radiographic and CT features of a pulmonary hamartoma can be found in the section on Neoplastic and Nonneoplastic Lesions Presenting as SPNs.

It is important to remember that not all SPNs require CT densitometry. A nodule with a diameter greater than 3 cm, showing lobulated or spiculated margins, or is cavitary has such a high likelihood of malignancy regardless of its internal density that the results of HRCT densitometry could only be misleading. Likewise, the demon-

stration of an air bronchogram or bubbly lucencies within an SPN is highly suspicious for adenocarcinoma, particularly bronchioloalveolar cell carcinoma. Such SPNs, along with those small, well-defined solid lesions lacking benign calcification or fat on HRCT, are suspicious enough for malignancy to be considered indeterminate.

Contrast-enhanced CT and PET. Recent studies have demonstrated the utility of dynamic, contrast-

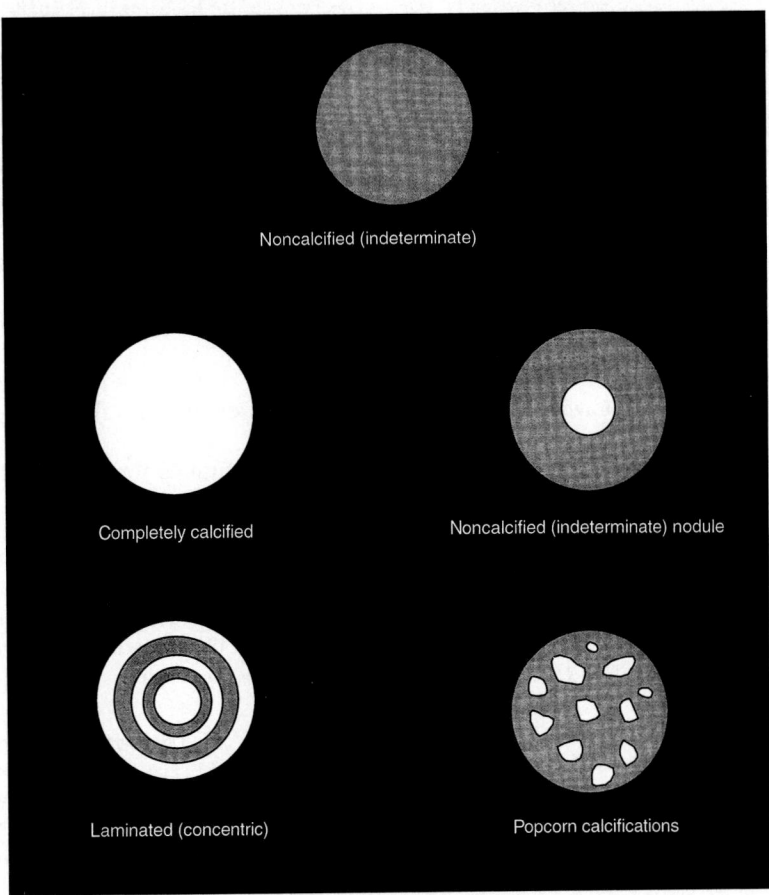

Figure 16.4. Benign Patterns of Calcification within an SPN.

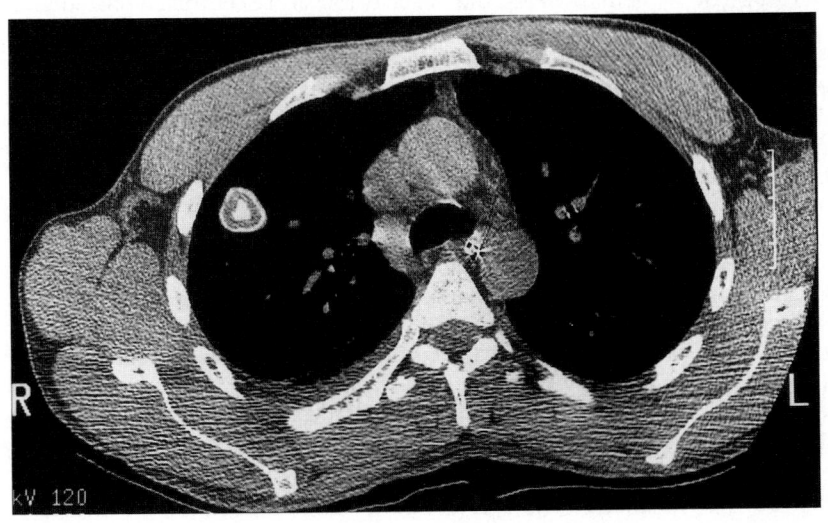

Figure 16.5. Laminated Calcification in an SPN. Thin-section CT in a 37-year-old man shows a pattern of laminated calcification, likely representing a granuloma from histoplasmosis.

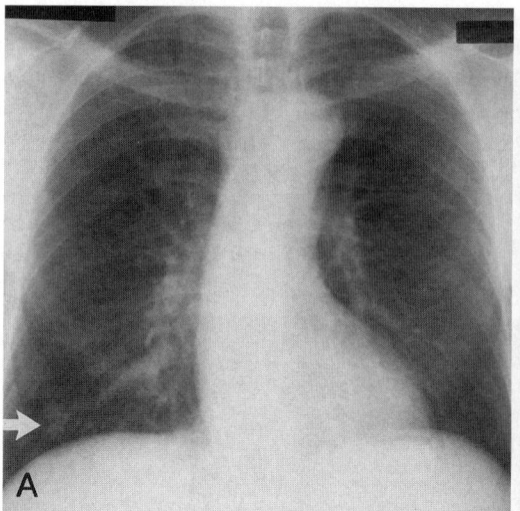
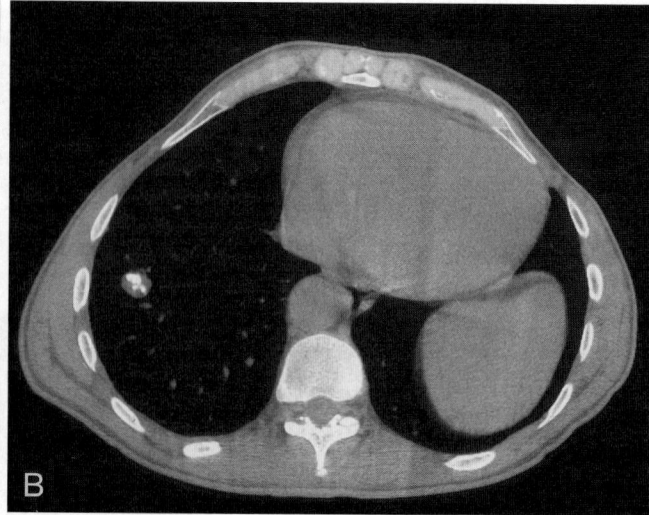

Figure 16.6. Hamartoma. A. Routine chest radiograph in a 48-year-old man demonstrates a well-defined nodule in the right lower lobe (*arrow*) with calcification. **B.** Thin-section CT shows a smoothly marginated nodule containing coarse "popcorn" calcifications typical of a pulmonary hamartoma.

enhanced CT in the evaluation of SPNs, with virtually all malignant lesions demonstrating an increase in attenuation of at least 20 H after contrast administration (3). Despite the encouraging preliminary results, few institutions perform contrast-enhanced CT in this manner. Similarly, positron emission tomography (PET) using Fluorine-18-labeled fluordeoxyglucose (FDG) has shown a high accuracy in the distinction of benign and malignant SPNs (4). The limited availability of PET scanners and high cost of examination has limited the application of this technique.

Management Decisions. Patients with indeterminate SPNs should undergo either transthoracic biopsy or resection. When the lesion is very likely to be malignant, it is reasonable to forego biopsy and proceed directly to thoracotomy and resection. However, there are several reasons to perform a preoperative biopsy on an indeterminate SPN. The primary reason to biopsy an indeterminate SPN is to make the diagnosis of a benign lesion, thereby avoiding an unnecessary thoracoscopy or thoracotomy. This would most benefit the patient with a reasonable likelihood of having a benign lesion. Factors suggesting benignity include: age under 35, non-smoker, patient from an area endemic for tuberculosis or histoplasmosis, nodule <2 cm with smooth margins, and a doubling time of less than 30 days or greater than two years. The other major indication for the biopsy of an indeterminate SPN is a patient with limited pulmonary reserve who is a poor surgical candidate for pulmonary resection. In these patients, a biopsy can provide a diagnosis and guide nonoperative therapy. As most SPNs are peripherally situated in the lung, transthoracic needle biopsy (TNB) is the procedure of choice for tissue sampling. Peripheral lesions requiring biopsy that are too small for successful transthoracic needle biopsy (i.e. lesions <5 mm diameter) can be sampled with video-assisted thoracoscopic surgery (VATS). Patients with SPNs that are centrally situated with a large bronchus entering the lesion should undergo transbronchoscopic biopsy.

An SPN that is judged to be benign based on patient age, growth rate, presence of benign calcification, or those with a specific benign diagnosis provided by TNB should be followed carefully with radiographs for a minimum of two and preferably three years to confirm their benign nature. The radiographic followup consists of PA and lateral chest radiographs or limited thin-section CT at 6-month intervals.

Lesions Presenting as SPNs

The differential diagnosis of an SPN is shown in Table 16.1. In addition to bronchogenic carcinoma (particularly adenocarcinoma) and granulomas (e.g. tuberculosis and histoplasmosis), there are a number of entities that may produce a solitary pulmonary nodule. Many of these entities are discussed elsewhere in the text.

Carcinoid Tumors. While carcinoid tumors may present as SPNs, the majority (80%) are central endobronchial lesions that present with atelectasis or obstructive pneumonitis. A detailed discussion of carcinoid tumors can be found in the section on malignant pulmonary neoplasms.

Pulmonary Hamartoma is a benign neoplasm composed of an abnormal arrangement of the mesenchymal and epithelial elements found in normal lung. Histologically these lesions contain cartilage surrounded by fibrous connective tissue with variable amounts of fat, smooth muscle, and seromucous glands; calcification and ossification is seen in 30%. These tumors are seen most commonly in the fourth to fifth decade of life. Approximately 90% of hamartomas arise within the pulmonary parenchyma, accounting for approximately 5% of all solitary pulmonary nodules.

These lesions usually present as incidental findings on chest radiographs. While the diagnosis is often suggested on plain radiographs, CT is obtained in most pa-

Table 16.1. Solitary Pulmonary Nodule or Mass

Neoplasm	Bronchogenic carcinoma
	Hamartoma
	Bronchial adenoma
	Granular cell myoblastoma
	Mesenchymal neoplasms
	Leiomyoma/leiomyosarcoma
	Fibroma
	Lipoma
	Neurofibroma
	Lymphoma
	Solitary metastasis
	Colon carcinoma
Infection	Septic embolus
	Staphylococcus
	Round pneumonia
	Pneumococcus
	Legionella
	Nocardia
	Fungi
	Lung abscess
	Infectious granuloma
	Tuberculosis
	Histoplasmosis
	Coccidioidomycosis
	Cryptococcosis
	Parasitic
	Echinococcal cyst
	Amebic abscess
Collagen vascular disease	Necrobiotic nodule (rheumatoid lung)
	Wegener's granulomatosis
Vascular	Infarct
	AVM
	Pulmonary artery aneurysm
	Hematoma
Airways	Congenital foregut malformations
	Bronchogenic cyst
	Sequestration
	Mucocele
	Infected bulla
Miscellaneous	Amyloidoma
	Round atelectasis

tients. A confident diagnosis of hamartoma can be made when HRCT shows a nodule <2.5 cm in diameter, demonstrates a smooth or lobulated border and contains focal fat. Calcification, when present, is in the form of multiple clumps of calcium dispersed throughout the lesion ("popcorn" calcification)(Fig. 16.6). As a rule, hamartomas that contain calcium also contain fat. While hamartomas tend to grow slowly, the presence of characteristic HRCT findings allows for observation alone. Rapid growth, pulmonary symptoms, or a size greater than 2.5 cm warrants transthoracic biopsy or resection.

Non-Hodgkin's Lymphoma. Primary pulmonary lymphoma arising from the bronchus-associated lymphoid tissue (BALT) are low-grade B-cell lymphomas that present in adults in their fifties. The most common radiographic finding is an SPN or focal air-space opacity (Fig. 16.7). The diagnosis is made by immunohistochemistry and flow cytometry of resected specimens or of aspirated cells obtained by transthoracic needle biopsy.

Granular Cell Myoblastoma is a benign neoplasm arising from neural elements in the central airways or parenchyma. The skin is the most common site for these tumors. These tumors may present as SPNs or as endobronchial masses.

Leiomyoma/Leiomyosarcoma, Fibroma, Neurofibroma. Arising from the smooth muscle of the airways or pulmonary vessels, leiomyomas and leiomyosarcomas are rare neoplasms that present as endobronchial or intrapulmonary lesions with equal frequency. Radiographically, the parenchymal lesions are sharply marginated smooth or lobulated nodules or masses. The histologic distinction of benign from malignant lesions is difficult. Similarly, fibromas and neurofibromas appearing as SPNs lack distinguishing radiographic features.

Lipomas are rare intrapulmonary lesions, arising more commonly within the tracheobronchial tree to produce atelectasis. The demonstration of fat attenuation on CT is diagnostic.

Hemangiopericytoma is a connective tissue tumor arising within the lung from the pericyte, a cell associated with the arteriolar and capillary endothelium. On chest radiographs, these lesions are seen as SPNs and are indistinguishable from bronchogenic carcinoma.

Plasma Cell Granuloma (Inflammatory Pseudotumor) of Lung refers to a localized chronic inflammatory response to an unknown agent in the lung. It is characterized histologically by an abundance of plasma cells. There are no distinguishing radiographic features.

Lipoid Pneumonia. The inadvertent aspiration of mineral oils ingested by elderly patients to treat constipation may produce a localized pulmonary lesion. Patients with gastroesophageal reflux or disordered swallowing mechanisms are at particular risk. Radiographically, a focal area of air-space opacification or a solid mass may be seen in the lower lobes. A spiculated appearance to the edge of the mass is not uncommon, as the oil may produce a chronic inflammatory reaction in the surrounding lung that leads to fibrosis. While CT can demonstrate fat within the lesion, most patients with the mass-like form of this entity require resection for definitive diagnosis.

Bronchogenic Cyst. Fluid filled cystic lesions of the lung may produce an SPN. Intrapulmonary bronchogenic cysts are uncommon causes of SPNs; 90% of these lesions are found in the middle mediastinum. The characteristic finding is a sharply marginated cyst on CT or MR in a young patient, although distinction from an infected bullae, solitary echinococcal cyst, mucocele, or thin-walled lung abscess may be impossible. Superinfection of a lung bulla may produce an SPN or mass. In such patients, the radiographic or CT appearance of an intra-parenchymal air/fluid level within a thin walled localized air collection (usually in an upper lobe), with typical bullous changes in other portions of lung, usually allows for the proper diagnosis.

BRONCHOGENIC CARCINOMA

Bronchogenic carcinoma is one of several neoplasms that may arise within the lung (Table 16.2). It is now the leading cause of death from malignancy in the United States and most industrialized countries for both men

Figure 16.7. Non-Hodgkin's Lymphoma Presenting as an SPN. CT scan in a 73-year-old patient with carcinoma of the breast shows a smoothly marginated 2-cm nodule (*arrow*) in the middle lobe. A diagnosis of low-grade non-Hodgkin's lymphoma (BALToma) was made by transthoracic needle biopsy.

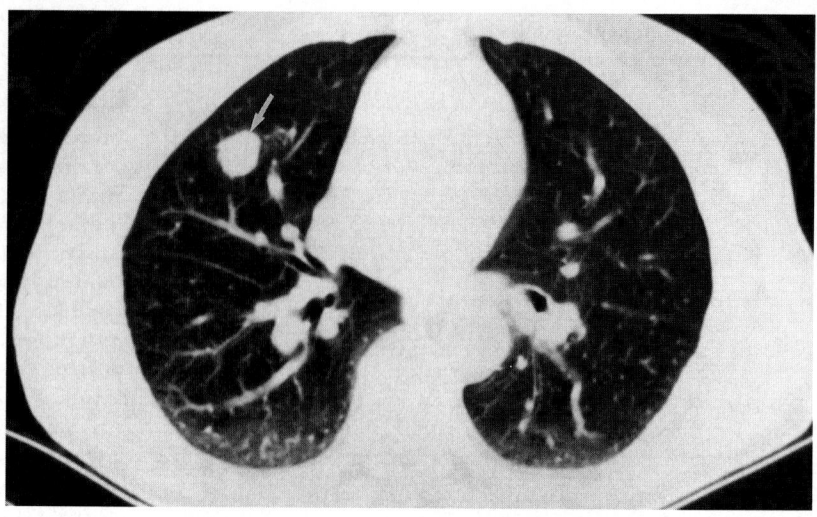

Table 16.2. Pulmonary Neoplasms

Benign
   Epithelial
      Squamous cell papilloma
      Pleomorphic adenoma (benign mixed tumor)
   Mesenchymal
      Hamartoma
      Lipoma
      Neurofibroma
      Leiomyoma
      Granular cell myoblastoma
      Hemangiopericytoma
Malignant
   Epithelial
      Bronchogenic carcinoma
      Carcinoid tumor
      Bronchial gland carcinoma
         Mucoepidermoid carcinoma
         Adenoid cystic carcinoma (cylindroma)
   Epithelial/mesenchymal
      Pulmonary blastoma
      Carcinosarcoma
   Lymphoid
      Non-Hodgkin's lymphoma
      Hodgkin's lymphoma

and women, having surpassed breast cancer in women in recent years (5). Although survival rates for lung cancer are poor, radiology plays a central role in diagnosis and management and may ultimately contribute to improved survival rates. This section will review the key pathological, epidemiological, and radiological features of bronchogenic carcinoma with an emphasis on the radiological staging of this disease.

Cytologic and Pathologic Features

Bronchogenic carcinoma is a malignant neoplasm that arises from bronchial or alveolar epithelium. Ninety-nine percent of malignant epithelial neoplasms of the lung arise from the bronchi or lung, while less than 0.5% arise from the trachea. Bronchogenic carcinoma is divided into four main histologic subtypes based on their gross and microscopic features: adenocarcinoma, squamous cell carcinoma, small cell carcinoma, and large cell carcinoma (Table 16.3)(6).

Adenocarcinoma is now the most common type of lung cancer, accounting for approximately one-third of all bronchogenic carcinomas. Whereas these tumors were once found to occur overwhelmingly in the lung periphery, they are now found in the central portions of the

Table 16.3. Subtypes of Bronchogenic Carcinoma

Type	Incidence	Radiologic Features	Treatment	5-Year Survival
Adenocarcinoma	35%	Peripheral nodule Peripheral mass	I-IIIa = surgery IV = XRT/chemo	17%
Squamous cell	25%	Hilar mass Atelectasis	I-IIIa = surgery IV = XRT/chemo	15%
Small cell	25%	Hilar mass Mediastiastinal mass	Chemotherapy	5%
Large cell	15%	Large peripheral mass	I-IIIa = surgery IV = XRT/chemo	11%

XRT, radiation therapy

lungs in about one-fourth of cases. These tumors arise from bronchiolar or alveolar epithelium and have an irregular or spiculated appearance where they invade adjacent lung. Fibrosis in and about the tumor is common. These gross features usually produce an ill-defined pulmonary nodule or central mass on chest radiographs (Fig. 16.3). Histologically, adenocarcinoma demonstrates gland formation and mucin production. A subtype of adenocarcinoma, bronchioloalveolar cell carcinoma (BAC), has unique pathologic features. This tumor is characterized by growth along preexisting bronchiolar and alveolar walls ("lepidic growth") without invasion or distortion of these structures. When localized, BAC appears as a solitary pulmonary nodule or as a focal area of ground-glass opacity on CT. Diffuse disease, which represents either multifocal origin of disease or transbronchial spread of tumor, may present as air-space opacification simulating pneumonia or as diffuse bilateral nodular air-space opacities.

Squamous Cell Carcinoma is the second most common subtype of bronchogenic carcinoma, accounting for approximately one-fourth of all cases. This tumor arises centrally within a lobar or segmental bronchus. Grossly, these tumors are polypoid masses that grow into the bronchial lumen while simultaneously invading the bronchial wall. The central location and endobronchial component of the tumor accounts for the presenting symptoms of cough and hemoptysis and for the common radiographic findings of a hilar mass with or without obstructive pneumonitis or atelectasis (Fig. 16.8). Central necrosis is common in large tumors; cavitation may be seen if communication has occurred between the central portion of the mass and the bronchial lumen. Histologically, squamous cell carcinoma is characterized by invasion of the bronchial wall by nests of malignant cells with abundant cytoplasm. The formation of keratin pearls and intercellular bridges, seen in well-differentiated tumors, is specific for this tumor.

Small Cell Carcinoma accounts for 25% of bronchogenic carcinomas and arises centrally within main or lobar bronchi. These tumors are the most malignant neoplasms arising from bronchial neuroendocrine (Kulchitsky) cells and are alternatively referred to as Kulchitsky cell cancers or KCC-III. Typical carcinoid tumors (KCC-I) represent the least malignant type and atypical carcinoid tumors (KCC-II) are intermediate in aggressiveness. Small cell carcinomas exhibit a small endobronchial component, invading the bronchial wall and peribronchial tissues early in the course of disease. This produces a hilar or mediastinal mass with extrinsic bronchial compression and obstruction. Invasion of submucosal and peribronchial lymphatics leads to local lymph node enlargement (Fig. 16.9) and hematogenous dissemination that are almost invariable at the time of presentation. Microscopically, these malignant cells are tightly clustered with nuclei molded together because of the scant amount of cytoplasm. This lesion is distinguished from carcinoid tumor histologically by the presence of mitoses. Electron microscopy demonstrates the presence of intracytoplasmic neurosecretory granules.

Large Cell Carcinoma accounts for 15% of bronchogenic carcinomas and is occasionally diagnosed when a non–small cell bronchogenic carcinoma lacks the histologic characteristics of squamous cell carcinoma or adenocarcinoma. Histologic features include large cells with abundant cytoplasm and prominent nucleoli. This tumor arises peripherally as a solitary mass and is often large at the time of presentation (Fig. 16.10).

Epidemiology. The majority of patients with bronchogenic carcinoma are cigarette smokers who are older than 40 years of age. Men are most commonly affected; however, the percentage of female lung cancer patients has risen steadily in parallel with the increased prevalence of heavy cigarette smoking among women. The overall five-year survival rate for all patients with lung cancer is 10–15%.

In additon to cigarette smoke, well-recognized risk fac-

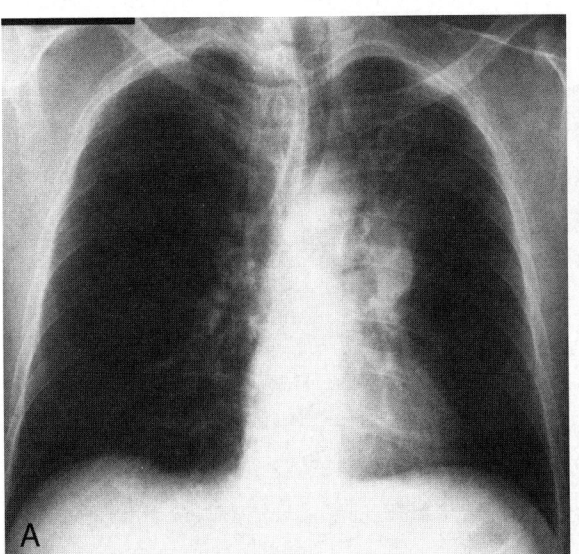
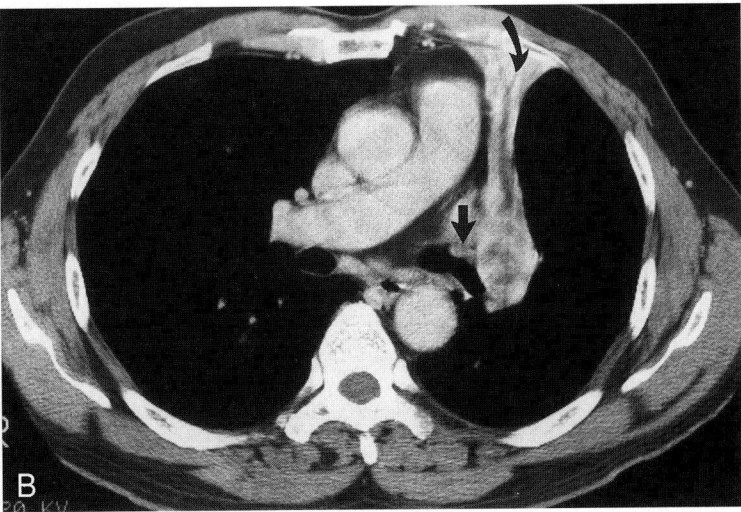

Figure 16.8. Squamous Cell Carcinoma. A. PA chest film in a 58-year-old male smoker with hemoptysis shows a left hilar mass with left upper lobe atelectasis. **B.** Enhanced CT shows the left hilar mass occluding the left upper lobe bronchus with an endobronchial component (*straight arrow*). Note the presence of mucus bronchograms within the atelectatic lung (*curved arrow*).

tors for the development of bronchogenic carcinoma include asbestos exposure, previous Hodgkin's lymphoma, radon exposure, viral infection, and diffuse interstitial or localized lung fibrosis. Cigarette smoke is by far the leading cause of lung cancer with approximately 87% of cases attributed to smoking. The relationship between cigarette smoke and bronchogenic carcinoma is irrefutable, with the intensity of smoking (number of pack years) showing the greatest positive correlation with development rates of malignancy. Lung cancer is uncommon in nonsmokers, and cigarette smoking is associated with a 10-fold to 30-fold increase in the incidence of bronchogenic carcinoma as compared to nonsmokers. Cessation of smoking decreases the risk of developing lung cancer with the greatest decline found in those with the longest smoking cessation interval. Carcinogens in cigarette smoke pro-

duce cellular atypia and squamous metaplasia of the bronchiolar epithelium that may precede malignant transformation. Small cell carcinoma and squamous cell carcinoma are the two histologic subtypes with the strongest association with cigarette smoking in men, and cigarette smoking in women is associated with an increased incidence of all histologic subtypes.

A subset of cigarette smokers are at particular risk of developing lung cancer. Young adult smokers with bullous lung disease usually develop their lung cancers at an earlier age than the general population of smokers. Proposed theories include greater susceptibility of the lining of the bulla to metaplastic transformation and impaired ventilation within the bulla, leading to prolonged exposure to the carcinogens in cigarette smoke.

Asbestos exposure is associated with an increased incidence of bronchogenic carcinoma, malignant pleural mesothelioma, laryngeal carcinoma, and esophagogastric carcinoma. Bronchogenic carcinoma may follow prolonged exposure, usually 20 years or greater in duration, from the mining or processing of asbestos fibers. A long latency period from the initial asbestos exposure, usually 35 years or longer, is necessary for the development of bronchogenic carcinoma. Although asbestos exposure alone is associated with a four fold increase in the incidence of bronchogenic carcinoma, concomitant cigarette smoking, perhaps by acting as a co-carcinogen, is associated with a 40-fold to 50-fold increase in the incidence as compared to the nonexposed, nonsmoking individual.

Patients previously treated for mediastinal Hodgkin's disease with radiation, chemotherapy, or a combination of the two, have an eightfold increase in lung cancer beginning 10 years after treatment. Exposure to inhaled radioactive material, particularly radon, is associated with the development of small cell carcinoma of lung 20 years or more after the exposure.

The link between viral infection and bronchogenic carcinoma comes chiefly from the study of Jaagsietke, a disease of sheep that closely resembles bronchioloalveolar

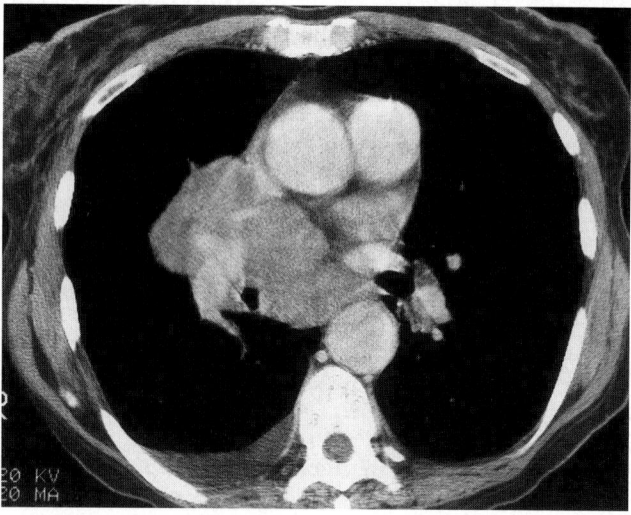

Figure 16.9. Small Cell Carcinoma. CT at the level of the bronchus intermedius demonstrates a large mass in the right hilum invading the middle mediastinum and subcarinal region. Cytologic examination of the associated right pleural effusion revealed small cell carcinoma.

Figure 16.10. Large Cell Carcinoma. CT in a 53-year-old man reveals a right lung mass extending to the right hilum and invading the left atrium (*arrow*). CT-guided transthoracic biopsy showed large cell carcinoma.

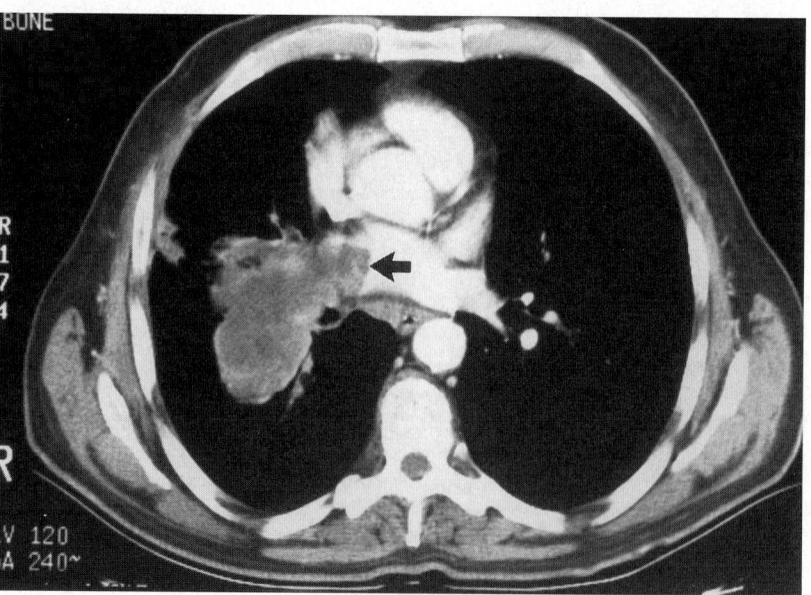

cell carcinoma of the lung in humans. This disease is caused by a retroviral infection, leading to speculation that a similar pathogenesis exists in humans with this subtype of adenocarcinoma.

It has been suggested that local lung scarring as a result of inflammation or infarction can induce the development of a "scar carcinoma," most commonly adenocarcinoma. Because adenocarcinoma can produce fibrous tissue, whether the "scar" is the result or cause of the carcinoma is unclear. Nevertheless, there are patients in whom a focal scar can be identified on prior radiographs in the region of a carcinoma. Diffuse interstitial fibrosis in patients with scleroderma has been associated with an increased incidence of bronchogenic carcinoma, particularly bronchioloalveolar cell carcinoma. Similarly, adenocarcinoma occurs with greater than expected frequency in patients with interstitial fibrosis associated with rheumatoid lung disease.

Radiographic Findings in Bronchogenic Carcinoma depend on the subtype of cancer (7) and the stage of disease at the time of diagnosis. The two most common findings are a solitary pulmonary nodule (size between 2 mm and 3 cm) or mass (3 cm or larger in size) and a hilar mass with or without bronchial obstruction. All cell types can present with a pulmonary nodule. Because squamous and small cell carcinoma arise from central bronchi, the majority of these types of bronchogenic carcinoma produce a hilar mass (Figs. 16.8, 16.9). The hilar mass represents either the extraluminal portion of the bronchial tumor or hilar lymph node enlargement from metastatic disease. Extension of the hilar lesion into the mediastinum or the presence of mediastinal nodal metastases can produce a smooth or lobulated mediastinal mass. Marked mediastinal nodal enlargement producing a lobulated mediastinal contour is characteristic of small cell carcinoma. Extensive replacement of the mediastinal fat by either primary tumor or extracapsular nodal extension may produce diffuse mediastinal widening, with loss of the mediastinal fat planes and compression or invasion of the trachea or central bronchi, esophagus, and mediastinal vascular structures as seen on contrast-enhanced CT or MR.

Obstruction of the bronchial lumen by the endobronchial component of a tumor can result in several different radiographic findings. The most common finding is resorptive atelectasis or obstructive pneumonitis of lung distal to the obstructing lesion. Resorptive atelectasis is recognized by the classic findings of lobar or whole lung collapse whereas obstructive pneumonitis results in minimal or no atelectasis or occasionally an increase in the volume of the affected portion of lung. An abnormal increase in lobar or whole lung volume is recognized radiographically by a bulging interlobar fissure marginating the obstructed lobe or by mediastinal shift respectively, and is termed "drowned lung." Occasionally, the mass producing lobar atelectasis creates a central convexity in the normally concave contour of the collapsed lobe, producing the "S-sign of Golden" (Fig. 16.8). Most commonly, the opacity of the obstructed lung obscures the underlying central lesion. The lung with obstructive pneumonitis is not infected, but rather shows a chronic inflammatory infiltrate and alveolar filling with lipid-laden macrophages; the latter finding accounts for the descriptive terms golden or endogenous lipoid pneumonia. Additional radiographic features of atelectasis that should suggest obstruction by tumor include obliteration of the main or proximal lobar bronchial air column, hilar mass, combined middle and lower lobe atelectasis, and atelectasis or opacification that persists beyond 3–4 weeks. CT confirms the presence of lobar atelectasis and typically demonstrates mucus bronchograms within the lung distal to the obstructing lesion (Fig. 16.8). The central mass is readily distinguished from vascular structures, with narrowing or occlusion of the bronchial lumen best seen on images viewed at lung windows. The central tumor is usually distinguished from atelectatic lung by the contrast between the perfused but nonventilated enhancing lung and the low-attenuation, nonenhancing central mass. An uncommon manifestation of bronchial obstruction by bronchogenic carcinoma is the development of mucoid impaction (mucocele). This represents mucus within dilated segmental bronchi distal to the obstructing neoplasm. The appearance has been likened to a gloved hand, with the dilated bronchi representing the fingers of the glove (see Fig. 19.9). Radiographic visualization of the mucocele requires collateral ventilation to the obstructed lobe or segment.

Tumors that arise from bronchiolar or alveolar epithelium, namely adenocarcinoma and large cell carcinoma, commonly produce a solitary pulmonary nodule or mass on chest radiography. The radiographic evaluation of the solitary pulmonary nodule, in particular the size, growth rate, shape, margins, and internal density, has been reviewed in detail earlier in this chapter. A notched, lobulated, or spiculated margin to the nodule is common in bronchogenic carcinoma (Fig. 16.3). The radially spiculated appearance of a peripheral nodule has been termed "corona radiata." Although it was initially thought to be pathognomonic for malignancy, the finding of a corona radiata is nonspecific and can be seen in granulomas. The edge characteristics of a solitary pulmonary nodule are best appreciated on thin-section HRCT images through the lesion.

Cavitation of solitary malignant nodules is uncommon. The walls of cavitating neoplasms are thicker and more nodular than inflammatory lesions. The presence of air bronchograms or bubbly lucencies within a nodule or mass is highly suggestive of an adenocarcinoma, particularly bronchioloalveolar cell carcinoma. Eccentric calcification within nodules may represent dystrophic calcification of necrotic regions, granulomas engulfed by an enlarging tumor, or calcification of mucin or psammoma bodies secreted by tumor cells in adenocarcinomas.

The size and growth pattern of an SPN are important characteristics. Masses greater than 3 cm in diameter seen in adults older than 35 years of age are overwhelmingly malignant. The volume doubling time (equivalent to a 25% increase in diameter) for a malignant nodule usually ranges from 1 month (some squamous cell and large cell carcinomas) to 24 months (certain bronchioloalveolar cell carcinomas). However, this rule has exceptions and should only be used for retrospective evaluation of interval growth and not used to follow a newly discovered and potentially resectable lesion.

Pancoast's (superior sulcus) tumor is a peripheral neoplasm arising in that portion of the lung apex indented superiorly by the subclavian artery. Although they can be of any cell type, these lesions are usually squamous cell carcinomas or adenocarcinomas. The presenting symptoms are related to invasion of adjacent structures, with arm pain and muscular atrophy attributable to brachial plexus involvement, Horner's syndrome from involvement of the sympathetic chain, and shoulder pain from chest wall invasion (Fig. 16.11). The chest radiographic finding of an apical density may be mistaken for a pleuroparenchymal fibrous cap, which is a common finding in older individuals. Apical thickness exceeding 5 mm, asymmetry of the apical opacities of greater than 5 mm, enlargement on serial radiographs, or evidence of rib destruction should prompt further evaluation with helical CT or MR. The presence of a mass with an inferior convex margin toward the lung and the presence of rib or vertebral body destruction are uncommon plain film findings. CT demonstrates the apical region to better advantage and is best for determining the extent of chest wall and vertebral invasion. Coronal and sagittal MR is useful for determining the relationship of the mass to the subclavian artery, brachial plexus, and spinal canal (Fig. 16.11).

Air-space opacification caused by bronchogenic carcinoma is an uncommon radiographic finding in the absence of an obstructing endobronchial lesion. BAC may produce air-space opacification as malignant cells grow along the preexisting parenchymal lattice while producing large amounts of mucus. The majority (60–90%) of BACs are localized and appear as solitary pulmonary nodules. CT often shows air-filled bronchi within the lesion and a pleural tail extending from the tumor toward the pleural surface. The diffuse form may present as lobar or multilobar air-space opacification, or as diffuse bilateral air-space nodules. These latter appearances may be indistinguishable from pneumonia or edema although the clinical findings, chronicity of the process, and cytologic examination of sputum and bronchoalveolar lavage specimens should provide the correct diagnosis. The production of copious amounts of mucus by these tumors may be an occasional clinical feature. An additional finding on contrast-enhanced CT in patients with the diffuse form of BAC is the so called "CT angiogram" sign within consolidated areas (Fig. 16.12). In these patients, filling of the air spaces with mucoid material produced by the malignant cells creates low-density air-space opacification surrounding the enhanced pulmonary arteries that traverse the consolidated regions. However, the CT angiogram sign is not specific for BAC and may be seen in other air-space filling diseases including lymphoma and lipoid pneumonia.

The SVC syndrome results from obstruction of the superior vena cava from compression or invasion by mediastinal tumor, particularly small cell carcinoma or lymphoma. Lung cancer is the most common cause of SVC syndrome. A discussion of this entity is found in chapter 13.

A malignant pleural effusion is an exudative fluid collection in a patient with proven malignancy that shows malignant cytology on thoracentesis or tumor on pleural biopsy. Although the presence of a pleural effusion in patients with bronchogenic carcinoma is associated with a poor prognosis, it is not synonymous with malignant pleural involvement because central lymphatic obstruction and postobstructive infection can produce benign effusions in patients with malignancy. Smooth or lobulated pleural thickening or a discrete pleural mass suggests malignant pleural involvement. Contrast-enhanced CT may demonstrate pleural thickening or

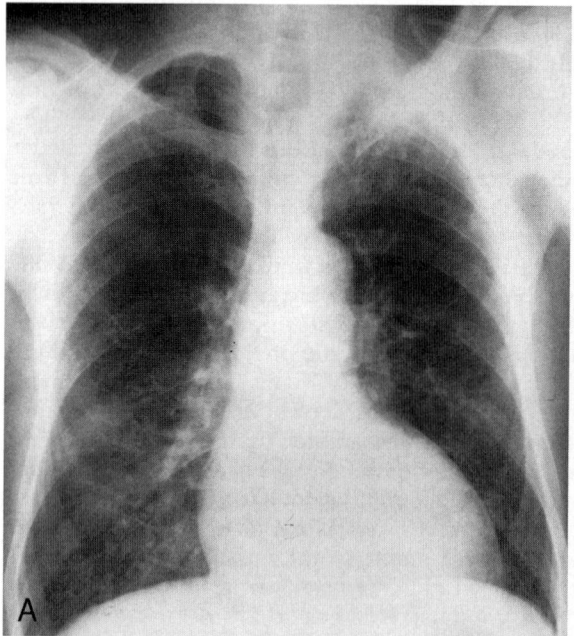
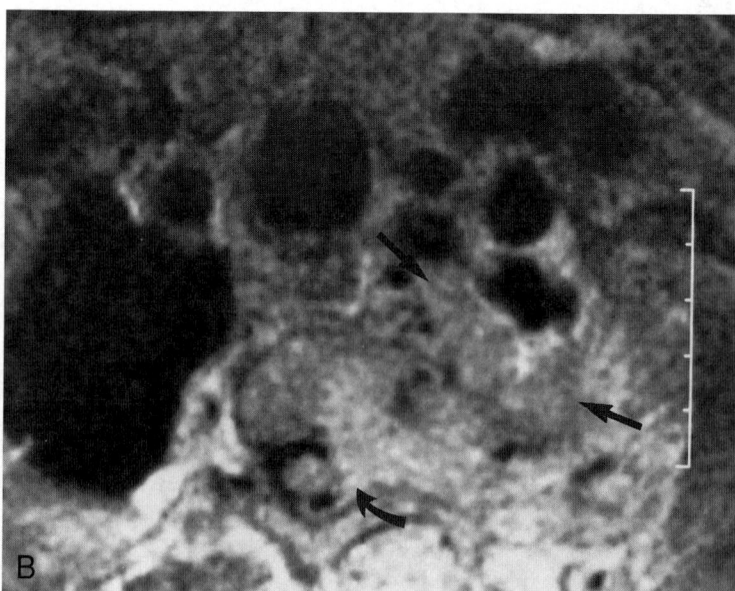

Figure 16.11. Superior Sulcus (Pancoast's) Tumor. A. PA chest film in a 56-year-old man with left shoulder and back pain reveals a left apical opacity. **B.** T1-weighted MR through the lung apices shows a left apical mass (*straight arrows*) with invasion of the spinal canal (*curved arrow*). Biopsy showed squamous cell carcinoma.

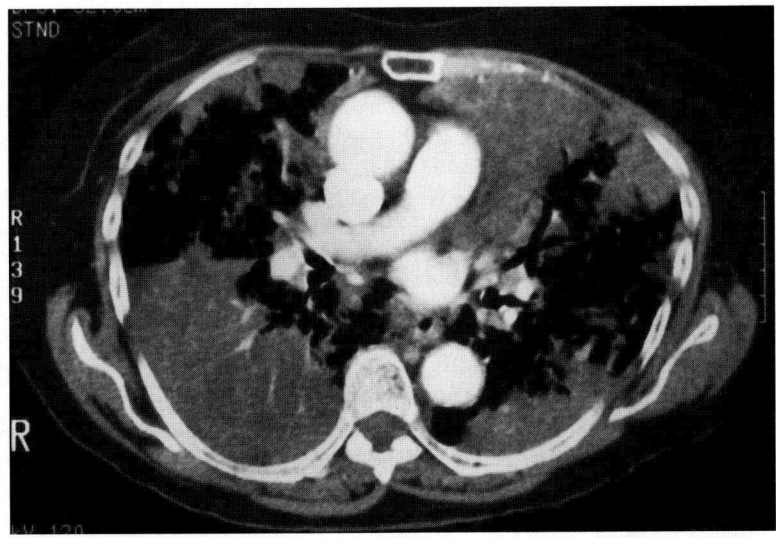

Figure 16.12. Bronchioloalveolar Cell Carcinoma. Enhanced CT in an 82-year-old woman with progressive dyspnea shows bilateral low-attenuation airspace opacification with visible pulmonary vessels ("CT angiogram sign"). Examination of sputum cytology showed bronchioloalveolar cell carcinoma.

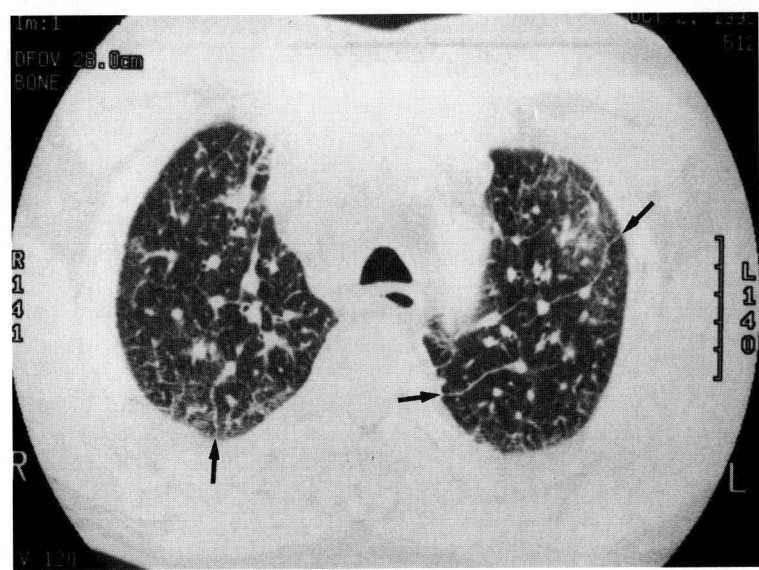

Figure 16.13. Lymphangitic Carcinomatosis. HRCT through the upper lobes in a patient with colon carcinoma shows smooth and nodular thickening of the interlobular septa (*arrows*) representing lymphangitic carcinomatosis. The diagnosis was confirmed by transbronchial biopsy.

mass obscured by pleural fluid on plain radiographs. The use of CT in the diagnosis of pleural and chest wall invasion is discussed in the section on lung cancer staging. Chest wall invasion is detected radiographically by the presence of an extrathoracic soft tissue mass or rib destruction. CT is more sensitive in detecting subtle bone destruction, but MR is best for detecting invasion of chest wall fat or muscle, particularly in superior sulcus tumors. Diaphragmatic elevation and paralysis may be seen with malignant invasion of the phrenic nerve. Progressive enlargement of the cardiac silhouette may be seen in patients with a malignant pericardial effusion; echocardiography and pericardiocentesis are diagnostic.

Lymphangitic carcinomatosis represents invasion of the lymphatic channels of the lung by tumor. Invasion of lymphatics or neoplastic involvement of hilar and mediastinal nodes leads to retrograde (centrifugal) lymphatic flow with dilatation of lymphatic channels, interstitial deposits of tumor, and fibrosis. Radiographically, the typical findings are linear and reticulonodular opacities

with peribronchial cuffing and subpleural edema or pleural effusion. In bronchogenic carcinoma, invasion and obstruction of lymphatics at the site of tumor may produce a segmental or lobar distribution of opacities. Lymphangitic spread to hilar and mediastinal lymph nodes produces unilateral lymph node enlargement with interstitial opacities, and hematogenous dissemination of tumor to the pulmonary capillaries with secondary lymphatic invasion leads to bilateral interstitial abnormalities. Unilateral or asymmetric involvement of the lungs by lymphangitic tumor suggests lung cancer rather than an extrapulmonary site. (Fig. 16.13). HRCT best demonstrates the characteristic smooth or beaded thickening of the interlobular septa and bronchovascular interstitium.

Diagnostic Evaluation in Bronchogenic Carcinoma.
Although prevention of lung cancer is the best and most cost-effective solution to the problem of lung cancer mortality, this is not achievable as long as the addictive habit of cigarette smoking is not entirely eliminated. Early de-

tection and treatment has the potential to improve survival rates from this deadly disease. Screening with periodic chest radiographs in high-risk patients has not been shown to be effective because chest radiographs only detect lesions exceeding 1 cm in diameter. Improvements in CT technology have led to the development of spiral (helical) CT scanners. As a result of its cross-sectional format and volumetric data acquisition, spiral CT is capable of routinely detecting lesions as small as 3 mm in diameter. In studies comparing conventional with spiral CT, the latter has detected a greater number of pulmonary nodules. Several preliminary clinical studies have demonstrated promising results for cancer detection using low-dose spiral CT acquisition techniques. The potential drawback of increased radiation exposure with CT as compared to chest radiography for lung cancer screening has been minimized by reducing exposure factors (mA of 30–50 vs. 120). The higher cost of CT versus conventional radiography remains an obstacle to widespread screening. However, cost savings from early diagnosis and treatment is an additional benefit of screening high-risk patients.

Functional imaging may ultimately be the best opportunity for early lung cancer detection. Radioisotope-labeled monoclonal antibodies have the potential for demonstrating early lung cancer but are not yet clinically feasible. Fluorine-18-labeled fluordeoxyglucose (FDG) PET scans have been shown to have a very high sensitivity and moderately high specificity in detecting malignant tumors. FDG is a glucose precursor that is incorporated into metabolically active cells but not further metabolized. Because malignant tumors have a higher rate of glucose metabolism than most benign processes, increased FDG uptake is suggestive of malignancy. The current threshold for lung cancer detection appears to be a lesion size of 1 cm. This technique is not limited to primary tumor detection. PET scans using FDG reliably discriminates between malignant and benign lymph nodes exceeding 1 cm in diameter. Sensitivities and specificities of approximately 90% and 99% respectively have been reported for lymph node staging using this technique (8). This is in contrast to CT and MR, for which the accuracy for lymph node metastases is 60–70%. The limited availibility of PET scanners and cyclotron-produced FDG precludes its widespread use for lung cancer staging.

Efforts to diagnose lung cancer should also attempt to stage the patient whenever possible so that management decisions, particularly regarding resectability, can be made expeditiously. Cytologic examination of sputum or bronchoalveolar lavage fluid is simple and inexpensive and is most useful in central tumors. Bronchoscopy with endobronchial biopsy is useful for the visualization and biopsy of main or lobar bronchial lesions, with bronchoscopically guided transcarinal Wang needle biopsy used to sample subcarinal masses. CT-guided or fluoroscopically guided transthoracic biopsy of peripheral masses can establish a diagnosis in more than 90% of patients with lung cancer. Radiologically guided sampling of hilar or mediastinal masses in patients with negative bronchoscopic examinations can provide material for cancer diagnosis and staging. Where available, FDG PET scans may complement CT and MR scans and decrease the need for more invasive staging procedures.

CT is obtained in all patients with possible bronchogenic carcinoma to guide efforts at tissue sampling. The detection of distal lesions in the adrenal gland, liver, or bones with biopsy of accessible lesions can provide both diagnostic and staging information. The relationship of the tumor to the central airways determines the utility of transbronchoscopic endobronchial or endotracheal biopsy, and the detection of large subcarinal nodes can direct transcarinal biopsy with a Wang needle. The pleura may be evaluated for thickening, masses, or effusions, suggesting that thoracentesis or closed pleural biopsy is the appropriate initial diagnostic procedure. Thoracotomy with resection of a peripheral lesion is appropriate in suspicious solitary lesions lacking clinical or CT evidence of unresectable nodal, mediastinal, pleural, or extrathoracic metastases. In some cases, patient's with peripheral lesions may benefit from more limited surgery using video-assisted thoracscopic surgery (VATS). Radiology may occasionally play a role in VATS by guiding placement of localizing needles and wires preoperatively using CT or intraoperative sonographic guidance.

Radiologic Staging of Lung Cancer

The primary role of the radiologist in imaging the patient with bronchogenic carcinoma is to determine the anatomic extent or stage of the tumor (9). This has prognostic importance and determines the resectability of the lesion. In patients with small cell carcinoma, which is almost invariably not a surgically curable disease, patients are divided into two groups: those with disease limited to one hemithorax (limited disease) and those with contralateral lung or extrathoracic spread (extensive disease). The staging of non–small cell bronchogenic carcinoma is based on the extent of the primary tumor (T), the presence of nodal involvement (N), and evidence of distant metastases (M). Using this TNM classification, lung cancer is divided into four stages. This TNM scheme has recently been modified (Table 16.4)(10). The major distinction in lung cancer staging is the division of patients with stage I-IIIa (resectable) from stage IIIb and IV (unresectable) disease (Table 16.5). Stage IIIa disease represents T3 disease (i.e., localized tumor invasion of the pleura, chest wall, diaphragm, or pericardium or tumor extending into the proximal main bronchus with sparing of the tracheal carina), associated with ipsilateral hilar nodal involvement (N1), or a T1 or T2 lesion associated with mediastinal or subcarinal nodal involvement (N2). The surgical techniques used for stage IIIa disease include en-bloc resection of locally invaded chest wall, pleura, or pericardium; resection of proximal main bronchial tumors by resecting distal trachea and reimplanting the contralateral main bronchus into the proximal trachea; and mediastinal and subcarinal lymph node dissection with resection of the lung. Stage IIIb disease represents invasion of tracheal carina, mediastinum, major cardiovascular structures, esophagus, or vertebral body (T4), separate tumor nodules in the same lobe (T4), malignant pleural effusion (T4), or contralateral hilar or mediastinal, scalene or supraclavicular nodal involvement (N3). The presence of distant metastases or separate tumor nodules in different lobes is classified as M1 or stage IV disease.

Table 16.4. TNM Classification of Lung Cancer

Primary Tumor (T)

Tx	Malignant Cells in Sputum Without Identifiable Tumor
T0	No evidence of primary tumor
T1	Tumor <3 cm in diameter, surrounded by lung or visceral pleura, arising distal to a main bronchus
T2	Tumor >3 cm in diameter; any tumor invading the visceral pleura; any tumor with atelectasis or obstructive pneumonitis of less than an entire lung; the tumor must be >2 cm from the tracheal carina
T3	Any tumor with localized chest wall, diaphragmatic, mediastinal pleural or pericardial invasion; the tumor may be <2 cm from the carina but cannot involve the carina
T4	Any tumor that invades the mediastinum or vital mediastinal structures including the heart, great vessels, trachea, carina, or vertebral body; separate tumor nodules in the same lobe; presence of a malignant pleural effusion

Nodal Metastases

N0	No evidence of nodal metastases
N1	Metastasis to ipsilateral peribronchial or hilar nodes, including involvement by contiguous spread of tumor
N2	Metastasis to ipsilateral mediastinal or subcarinal nodes
N3	Metastasis to contralateral mediastinal or hilar nodes, or scalene or supraclavicular nodes

Distant metastases (M)

M0	No evidence of distant metastases
M1	Distant metastases; separate tumor nodules in different lobes

Table 16.5. Clinical Staging of Lung Cancer Based on TNM Classification

Stage	TNM
Ia	T1 **N0** M0
Ib	T2 **N0** M0
IIa	T1 **N1** M0
IIb	T2 **N1** M0
	T3 N0 M0
IIIa	T1 or T2 **N2** M0
	T3 N1 or **N2** M0
IIIb	AnyT **N3** M0
	T4 AnyN M0
IV	AnyT AnyN **M1**

Primary Tumor (T). *Chest Wall Invasion.* Tumors invading the chest wall (including the superior pulmonary sulcus), diaphragm, mediastinal pleura, pericardium, or proximal main bronchus are considered resectable by many surgeons and are classified as T3 lesions (Fig. 16.14). In patients with superior sulcus tumors, verte-

bral body or mediastinal invasion or involvement of the brachial plexus or subclavian artery above the lung apex precludes surgical resection. Lower-grade superior sulcus tumors can be treated by local irradiation followed by en-bloc resection of the tumor and chest wall, which has reasonable survival rates.

Rib destruction and an extrathoracic soft tissue mass are the only plain film findings specific for chest wall invasion; pleural thickening adjacent to a lung mass is nonspecific and need not indicate chest wall invasion. The CT diagnosis of chest wall invasion can be difficult; however, CT should be obtained if this is suspected. CT findings suggestive of chest wall invasion are obtuse angles at the point of contact of the tumor and pleura, greater than 3 cm of contact between tumor and pleura, pleural thickening adjacent to the mass, and infiltration of extrapleural fat. Extrathoracic extension of the mass or rib destruction are specific but insensitive CT findings for chest wall invasion (Fig. 16.14). Additional techniques that have been described to assess parietal pleural invasion by tumor include assessment of respiratory movement on dynamic expiratory CT and the use of diagnostic pneumothorax.

MR is equal to CT in its ability to diagnose chest wall invasion (11). T2WI show excellent contrast between tumor and chest wall muscle and fat, and these are used in selected cases to detect chest wall invasion. MR also detects early obliteration of the high-signal extrapleural fat that may be an early finding in chest wall invasion. Coronal MR images are useful in superior sulcus tumors to determine chest wall, brachial plexus, or subclavian artery involvement.

Mediastinal Invasion. Tumor invasion of the mediastinum with involvement of the heart, great vessels, trachea, or esophagus (T4 tumor) precludes resection. Localized invasion of the mediastinal pleura or pericardium (T3 tumor) does not prevent resection, but ex-

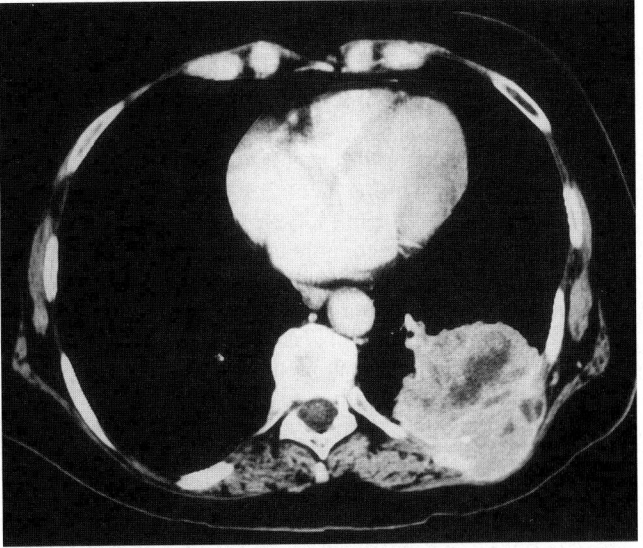

Figure 16.14. T3 Tumor with Localized Chest Wall Invasion. CT through a large left lower lobe adenocarcinoma shows invasion of the posterior chest wall. A portion of the chest wall was removed en-bloc with the tumor.

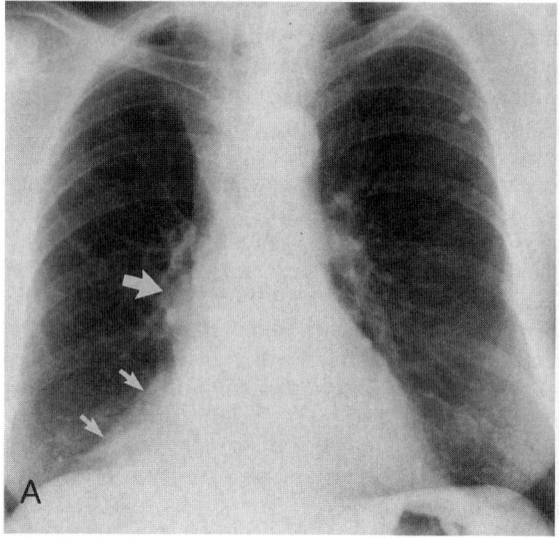
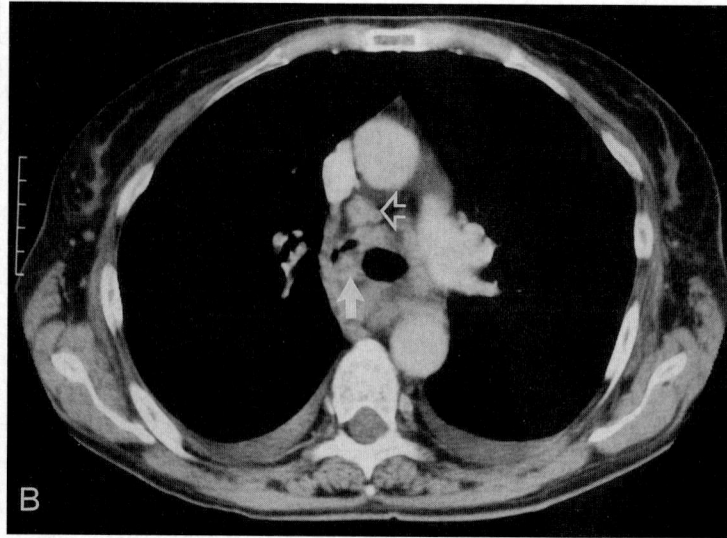

Figure 16.15. Tracheal Carinal Involvement in Squamous Cell Carcinoma. A. A frontal chest radiograph in a middle-aged woman with hemoptysis shows a mass in the lower right hilum (*large arrow*) with right lower lobe atelectasis (*small arrows*). **B.** CT demonstrates a mass surrounding the main bronchi, with irregular narrowing of the right main bronchial lumen and infiltration of the tracheal carina (*arrow*). An enlarged precarinal lymph node (*open arrow*) and small bilateral pleural effusions are also seen. Bronchoscopy revealed invasion of the tracheal carina by squamous cell carcinoma.

tensive invasion with replacement of mediastinal fat does.

On plain radiographs, a mediastinal mass, mediastinal widening, or diaphragmatic elevation (from phrenic nerve involvement) suggests invasion. As with the diagnosis of chest wall invasion, CT demonstration of tumor mass in contiguity with the mediastinal pleura or thickening of the mediastinal pleura does not necessarily indicate mediastinal extension or unresectability. However, a significant mediastinal mass contiguous with a lung tumor, which compresses mediastinal vessels or esophagus or replaces mediastinal fat, strongly suggests this diagnosis. Other findings that may suggest mediastinal invasion include: *a)* obliteration of the fat plane adjacent to the descending aorta or other mediastinal vessels, *b)* tumor contacting more than one-fourth of the circumference of the aortic wall, or *c)* tumor contacting more than 3 cm of the mediastinum. If none of these findings are present, the tumor is potentially resectable even though 29% of resectable lesions lacking any of these findings are found to invade the mediastinum locally (12).

As with CT, MR is incapable of accurately demonstrating mediastinal pleural invasion or minimal invasion of mediastinal fat. Mediastinal invasion can be diagnosed with a reasonable degree of accuracy when fat planes are significantly obliterated or mediastinal vessels are compressed or displaced. In a recent study, MR was significantly more accurate than CT in diagnosing mediastinal invasion, but this result was based on a small number of patients who had invasion (11). Other studies show no significant advantage of MR over CT for this purpose. MR is occasionally performed when vascular invasion is suspected and is likely more accurate than CT in this regard.

Central Airway Involvement. Tumors extending into a main bronchus within 2 cm of the tracheal carina (T3

tumor) are resectable. Although tracheal carinal involvement (T4 tumor)(Fig. 16.15) can be treated by carinal resection with end-to-side anastamosis of the remaining bronchus to the tracheal stump ("sleeve pneumonectomy"), most surgeons would consider this unresectable tumor. Although plain films can occasionally demonstrate a mass within the main bronchus or trachea, CT is more accurate in assessing the relationship of the mass to the tracheal carina (Fig. 16.15B). However, CT is known to underestimate the mucosal or submucosal extent of tumor as seen bronchoscopically. Therefore, any patient with a central lesion should undergo bronchoscopy to determine the proximal extent of tumor unless CT shows obvious carinal or tracheal invasion.

Pleural Effusion. Malignant pleural effusion (T4 tumor) precludes curative resection of tumor. In a patient with bronchogenic carcinoma, pleural effusion can occur for numerous reasons including pleural invasion, obstructive pneumonia, and lymphatic or pulmonary venous obstruction by tumor. Although the presence of effusion associated with lung cancer indicates a poor prognosis, only those patients with tumor cells in the pleural fluid or on pleural biopsy are considered unresectable. Other patients with effusion are considered to have "resectable" lesions, despite the poor prognosis. Plain radiographs, including decubitus films, are sufficient to diagnose a pleural effusion. Thoracentesis with cytologic examination and/or pleural biopsy is necessary for definitive diagnosis of malignant pleural involvement. Pleural thickening greater than 1 cm thickness, lobulated pleural thickening, or circumferential pleural thickening (i.e., involvement of the mediastinal pleura) on CT or MR strongly suggests pleural invasion.

Lymph Node Metastases (N). Selected patients with ipsilateral mediastinal or subcarinal node metastases are classified as N2 and are considered potentially resectable. However, patients with N2 nodal disease (i.e., stage IIIa lung cancer) have a significantly worse prognosis than patients with stage IIIa disease due to a T3 lesion. Those patients with N2 disease from nonbulky, intracapsular nodal metastases limited to one mediastinal nodal station have the best 5-year survival rates following extensive mediastinal nodal dissection. Contralateral hilar or mediastinal, supraclavicular, or infraclavicular nodal metastases represent N3 disease and are unresectable (Fig. 16.16).

The detection of a large mediastinal mass on chest radiograph in a patient with lung cancer requires mediastinoscopic or transthoracic biopsy confirmation of tumor invasion before the patient can be deemed unresectable. A normal chest radiograph or the suggestion of hilar or mediastinal adenopathy should prompt a chest CT to assess the status of the lymph nodes. No single measurement allows completely accurate distinction of normal from malignant nodes because malignant involvement does not always enlarge the lymph node (producing false negative findings and reducing sensitivity),

and enlarged nodes in patients with lung cancer may represent reactive hyperplasia rather than tumor replacement (producing false-positive findings and reducing specificity). If a small nodal diameter (5 mm) is used as the dividing point between benign and malignant, sensitivity will be excellent but specificity will be low. However, choosing a large nodal diameter (2 cm) increases specificity but decreases sensitivity. Most radiologists use a short axis nodal diameter of 1 cm because this value achieves the best compromise of sensitivity and specificity.

Recent studies show that CT is relatively inaccurate in determining the nodal status of the patient with lung cancer. Both sensitivity and specificity for nodal metastases, using a short axis diameter of 1 cm or greater as abnormal, are approximately 60–65% on a patient by patient basis, and may be even lower when looking at individual nodal stations (13). Although CT cannot be considered accurate enough to determine with certainty whether or not mediastinal lymph nodes are involved by tumor, it can provide information of value in guiding invasive staging procedures such as mediastinoscopy,

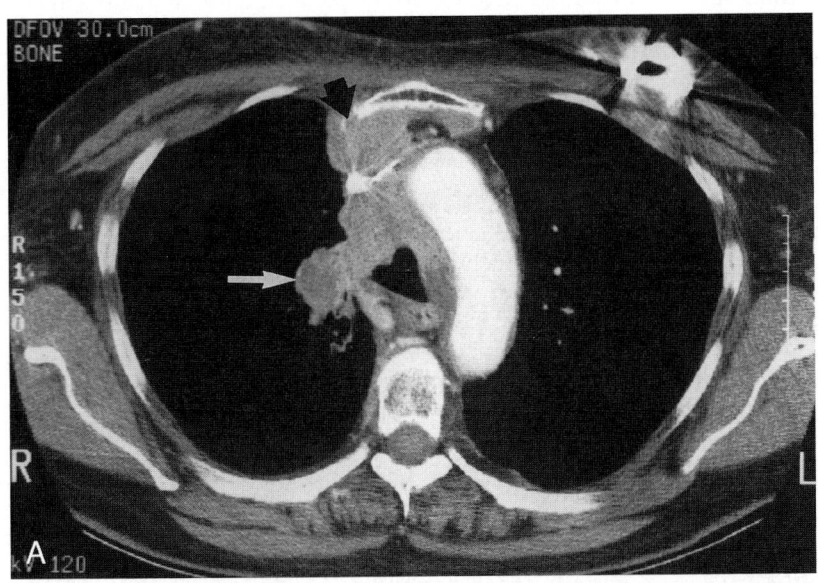

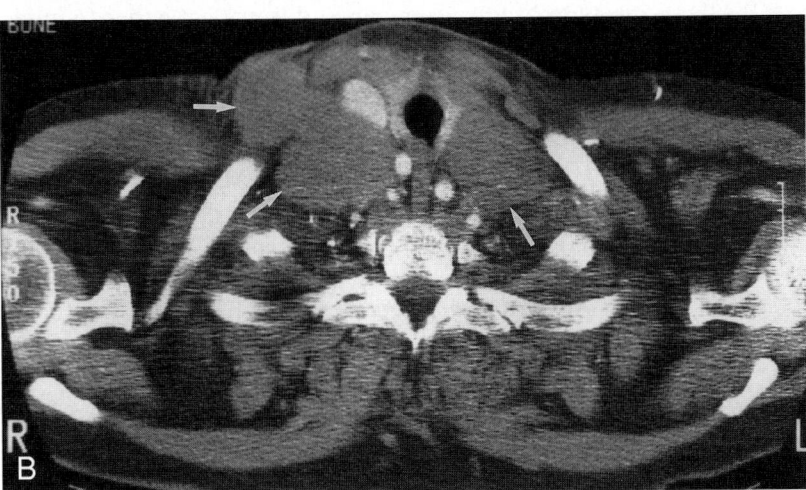

Figure 16.16. N3 Nodal Metastases in Bronchogenic Carcinoma. A. CT through the aortic arch in a 57-year-old man shows a right hilar mass (*white arrow*) invading the distal trachea and mediastinal fat (T4 tumor). There are enlarged prevascular lymph nodes (N2)(*black arrow*). **B.** CT at the supraclavicular level shows marked bilateral supraclavicular lymphadenopathy (*arrows*) representing N3 disease.

transcarinal Wang biopsy, and transthoracic or open biopsy. As discussed earlier, CT and FDG-PET scans can provide complementary information in cases in which the latter is available.

In most institutions, mediastinoscopy plays a complementary role to CT in the nodal staging of lung cancer. Most patients with enlarged mediastinal nodes on CT that are accessible to trancervical mediastinoscopy (pretracheal, anterior subcarinal, and right tracheobronchial nodes) should have mediastinoscopy and biopsy. Whether patients with negative CT studies for nodal enlargement should undergo mediastinoscopy depends on the local surgical practice. In patients with small, peripheral lung nodules, mediastinal metastases are uncommon, and thoracotomy may be warranted without prior CT or mediastinoscopy, but this remains controversial. Patients with borderline pulmonary function benefit most from mediastinoscopy because a positive mediastinoscopic biopsy almost certainly precludes any attempt at resection.

The accuracy of MR is equal to that of CT in the diagnosis of mediastinal lymph node metastases. Specific advantages and disadvantages of MR in characterizing mediastinal lymph nodes exist. Clusters of normal size nodes may be mistaken for a single enlarged nodal mass because of the limited spatial resolution of MR. MR is incapable of demonstrating calcification within nodes, which is diagnostic of benign lymph node disease. However, aortopulmonary window and subcarinal nodes are best demonstrated on coronal MR images because CT demonstration of nodes in these regions is limited by partial volume averaging with adjacent cardiovascular structures. Although the true promise of MR may be in the distinction of benign from malignant lymph nodes based on T1 and T2 relaxation values, this is not yet possible.

Metastatic Disease (M). Each patient with proven lung cancer should be carefully evaluated for the presence of distant metastases (M1). Unequivocal evidence of metastases can obviate an unnecessary thoracotomy. Common sites of extrathoracic spread in patients with lung cancer include lymph nodes, liver, adrenal gland, bone, and brain. Metastases to the opposite lung, although intrathoracic, are also considered in this category. Involvement of these sites probably represents hematogenous spread of tumor from the lung.

Chest and upper abdominal CT is part of the initial evaluation in virtually all patients evaluated for bronchogenic carcinoma. This is adequate for assessing the liver, spleen, adrenal glands, and upper abdominal lymph nodes for evidence of metastases. US or MR may be used to distinguish soft tissue hepatic masses from incidental cysts. Technetium-99m-methylene diphosphonate radionuclide bone scanning is used in patients with an elevated serum alkaline phosphatase. Plain films are obtained to assess specific foci of abnormally increased bone tracer uptake or to evaluate localized bone pain.

Imaging of the brain is routinely performed in patients with symptoms or signs suggesting intracranial metastases. This usually involves MR or contrast-enhanced head CT. Head scanning in patients without clinical evidence of CNS involvement is somewhat more controversial. Because virtually all patients with isolated or asymptomatic brain metastases are found to have adenocarcinoma or large cell carcinoma, patients with these subtypes of bronchogenic carcinoma should have head CTs regardless of the clinical findings in order to identify silent metastases. Patients with positive findings can be spared an unnecessary thoracotomy.

Approximately 60–65% of patients with small cell carcinoma have metastatic disease at the time of diagnosis. Because patients with small cell carcinoma are likely to have gross or microscopic metastatic foci at presentation, these patients are not candidates for curative surgical resection. However, accurate staging of these patients for extrathoracic involvement determines prognosis and allows for proper assessment of response to chemotherapy. An additional reason for extrathoracic staging of small cell carcinoma is the ability to manage localized bone or soft tissue involvement with radiation or resection.

Adrenal masses are seen in approximately 10% of patients undergoing staging CT examinations for bronchogenic carcinoma. However, approximately 5% of normal individuals are known to have benign adrenal cortical adenomas. In fact, isolated adrenal masses in patients with non–small cell bronchogenic carcinoma are twice as likely to be adenomas than metastases. In many patients the adrenal mass is the the only extrathoracic site of abnormality, making accurate diagnosis of the adrenal mass crucial in determining management.

Recent investigators have focused on the ability of chemical shift MR imaging to distinguish between adenomas and malignant (primary or metastatic) adrenal lesions. This technique is based on the presence of lipid protons within the cytoplasm of adrenal adenomas and their absence in metastases. By selecting an appropriate TE that places lipid and water protons out of phase (i.e., a TE = 2.3 msec or an odd whole multiple thereof), the signal of adenomas will decrease as compared to in-phase images (i.e., a TE of 4.6 msec or an odd whole multiple thereof) while metastases will remain constant or increase in signal (14). The ability of unenhanced CT to detect fat within adenomas has been used with a high specificity if the attenuation of the lesion is less than 18 H.

Despite these noninvasive techniques in the characterization of isolated adrenal masses, a definitive diagnosis in lung cancer patients is critical either to guide potentially curative thoracic resection or to withhold this option. This may require tissue sampling of the adrenal mass with CT-guided percutaneous needle biopsy.

TRACHEAL AND BRONCHIAL MASSES

Tracheal Neoplasms. Intratracheal masses may be divided into neoplastic (15) and non-neoplastic masses. Primary tracheal tumors are rare. However, 90% of all primary tracheal tumors in adults are malignant. The majority of primary tracheal malignancies arise from tracheal epithelium or mucous glands (90%) or from the mesenchymal elements of the tracheal wall (10%). Squamous cell carcinoma is the most common primary tracheal malignancy, accounting for at least 50% of all malignant tracheal neoplasms (Fig. 16.17). These tu-

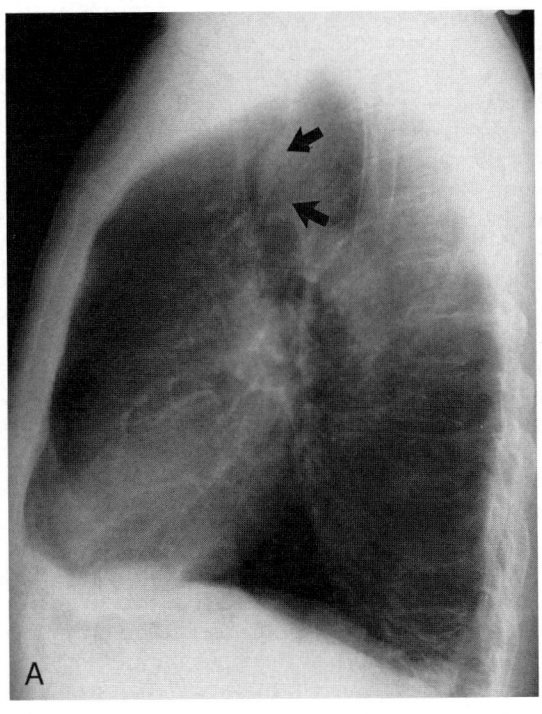

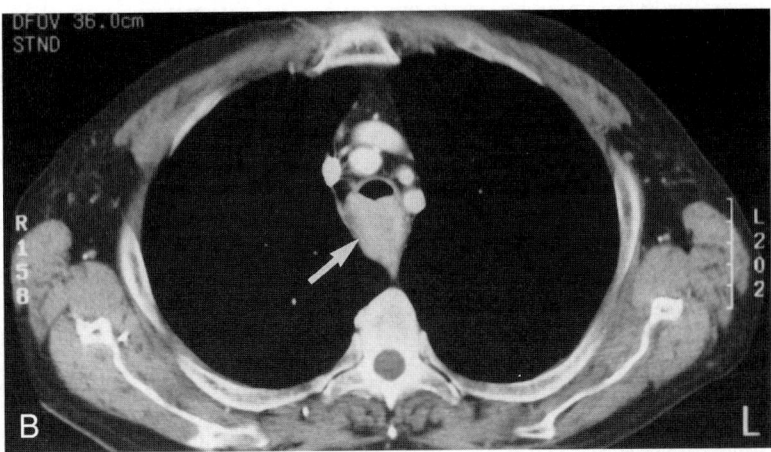

Figure 16.17. Squamous Cell Carcinoma of the Trachea. A. Lateral chest radiograph in a 68-year-old man shows a mass in the mid-trachea (*arrows*). **B.** CT demonstrates an enhancing mass (*arrow*) in the posterior trachea with narrowing of the tracheal lumen. Bronchoscopic biopsy showed squamous cell carcinoma.

mors affect middle-aged male smokers and are associated with laryngeal, bronchogenic, or esophageal malignancies in up to 25% of cases. The majority arise in the distal trachea within 3–4 cm of the tracheal carina, with the cervical trachea the next most common site. Cough, hemoptysis, dyspnea, and wheezing are common presenting symptoms. Patients may be mistakenly treated for asthma before the correct diagnosis is made. Adenoid cystic carcinoma (formerly called cylindroma) is a malignant neoplasm that arises from tracheal salivary glands and accounts for 40% of primary tracheal malignancies. This neoplasm involves the posterolateral wall of the distal two-thirds of the trachea or main or lobar bronchi.

The diagnosis of a primary tracheal malignancy is rarely made prospectively on chest radiographs although well-penetrated radiographs can demonstrate distortion of the tracheal air column by a mass. CT typically shows a lobulated or irregular soft tissue mass that eccentrically narrows the tracheal lumen and has a variable extraluminal component (Fig. 16.17B). Masses greater than 2 cm in diameter are likely to be malignant, and those less than 2 cm are more likely benign. Calcification is uncommon. Resectability of these lesions depends on the length of tracheal involvement and the extent of mediastinal invasion at the time of diagnosis. CT is particularly well suited for determining mediastinal involvement and has become the modality of choice for imaging tracheal neoplasms. The prognosis in patients with squamous cell carcinoma is poor because up to 50% of patients have mediastinal extension of tumor at the time of diagnosis. Although adenoid cystic carcinoma has a better prognosis, these slow-growing lesions are locally invasive with a tendency toward late recurrence and metastases.

A variety of other lesions comprise the remainder of primary tracheal malignancies and include mucoepidermoid carcinoma, carcinoid tumor, adenocarcinoma, lymphoma, small cell carcinoma, leiomyosarcoma, fibrosarcoma, and chondrosarcoma. Chondrosarcoma arises from tracheal cartilage and is identified by the presence of calcified chondroid matrix within the tumor.

The trachea may be secondarily involved by malignancy either by direct invasion or hematogenous spread. Laryngeal carcinoma may extend below the vocal cords to involve the cervical trachea. Tumors tend to recur at the tracheostomy site in patients who have undergone total laryngectomies for carcinoma. Papillary and follicular carcinoma are the most common types of thyroid malignancy to invade the trachea. Squamous cell carcinoma of the upper third of the esophagus can invade the posterior tracheal wall and may produce a tracheoesophageal fistula. Bronchogenic carcinoma may involve the trachea by direct proximal extension from central bronchi, by extranodal spread of tumor from metastatic pretracheal or paratracheal lymph nodes or by direct invasion of large right upper lobe tumors. CT is best at demonstrating tumor invasion of the tracheal wall and the extent of intraluminal mass. Extrathoracic primary tumors most often associated with hematogenous endotracheal metastases are carcinomas of the breast, kidney, and colon, and melanoma. These lesions may appear on CT as irregular thickening of the tracheal wall or as well-defined, localized masses indistinguishable from benign tracheal tumors.

Chondroma, fibroma, squamous cell papilloma (Fig. 16.18), hemangioma, and granular cell myoblastoma are the most common benign tracheal tumors in adults. A chondroma arises from the tracheal cartilage and produces a well-circumscribed endoluminal mass. CT may demonstrate stippled cartilaginous calcification within the mass. Fibromas are sessile or pedunculated fibrous

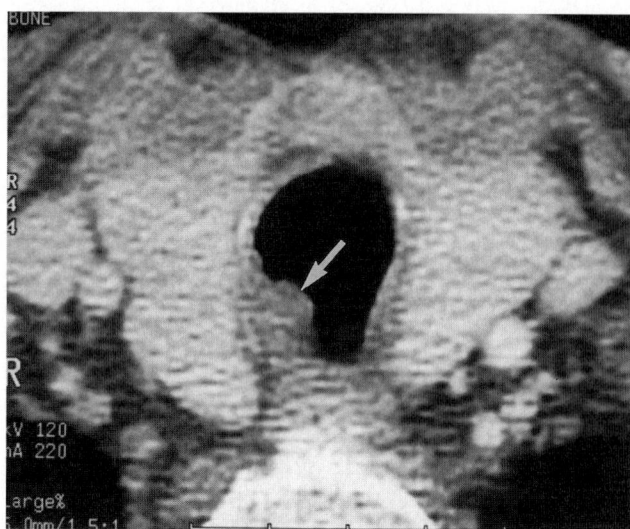

Figure 16.18. Squamous Cell Papilloma. Magnified view of CT at the level of the thyroid in a 48-year-old man with laryngotracheal papillomatosis shows a mural nodule (*arrow*) along the right posterolateral wall of the trachea representing a squamous cell papilloma.

masses arising in the cervical trachea. Squamous cell papilloma is a mucosal lesion caused by infection with human papilloma virus. This disease typically produces multiple laryngeal masses in children born to women with venereal warts (condylomata acuminata). The trachea, bronchi, and lungs may become involved over time. These lesions usually regress by adolescence and therefore are uncommon causes of a solitary tracheal lesion in adults. Hemangiomas are seen in the cervical trachea almost exclusively in infants and young children, appearing as focal masses on CT. Granular cell myoblastoma is a neoplasm that arises from neural elements in the tracheal or bronchial wall. These lesions usually involve the cervical trachea or main bronchi. CT shows a broad-based or pedunculated soft tissue mass that may invade the tracheal wall and has a tendency toward local recurrence.

Non-neoplastic Intratracheal Masses from ectopic intratracheal thyroid or thymic tissue have been reported and are radiographically indistinguishable from intratracheal neoplasms. Intratracheal thyroid is seen in females with extratracheal goiters. The intratracheal tissue is likewise goitrous and most commonly found in the posterolateral wall of the cervical trachea, although any portion of the trachea may be involved. Mucus plugs may appear as intratracheal masses in patients with excess sputum production or diminished clearance mechanisms. They are typically low-attenuation masses on CT that change position or disappear after an effective cough.

Primary Malignant Neoplasms of the Central Bronchi include carcinoma, carcinoid tumor, and bronchial gland tumors (adenoid cystic carcinoma and mucoepidermoid carcinoma). Carcinoid and bronchial gland tumors account for approximately 1% of all tracheobronchial neoplasms; 90% of these lesions arise in the bronchi or lung, and the remainder arise within the

trachea. Carcinoid tumor accounts for nearly 90%, adenoid cystic carcinoma 8%, and mucoepidermoid 2% of these lesions. However, adenoid cystic carcinoma accounts for 90% and carcinoid 10% of all malignant tracheal neoplasms excluding bronchogenic carcinoma. The use of the term "bronchial adenoma" to describe these lesions is misleading as these are malignant tumors that tend to locally invade and metastasize to regional lymph nodes.

Carcinoid tumors arise from neuroendocrine (APUD or Kulchitzky) cells within the airways. There is a spectrum of histologic differentiation and malignant behavior in tumors of Kulchitzky cell origin, ranging from the low-grade malignant typical carcinoid (KCC-I) to atypical carcinoid (KCC-II) to the highly malignant small cell carcinoma (KCC-III). Eighty percent of bronchial carcinoid tumors arise within central bronchi and present with cough, dyspnea, wheezing, recurrent episodes of atelectasis or pneumonia, or hemoptysis (Fig. 16.19). The hemoptysis may be massive and is attributable to the highly vascular nature of these lesions. The average age at diagnosis is 50. Histologically, these tumors show sheets or trabeculae of uniform cells separated by a fibrovascular stroma. The cells may contain intracytoplasmic inclusions; immunohistochemistry will reveal a variety of neuroendocrine products including serotonin, vasoactive intestinal polypeptide, ACTH and ADH. Carcinoid syndrome is seen in fewer than 3% of cases.

Radiologically, central bronchial carcinoids present with atelectasis or pneumonia secondary to large airway obstruction. A hyperlucent lobe or lung of diminished volume may result from incomplete obstruction or collateral airflow with reflex hypoxic vasoconstriction; this finding is also rarely seen in bronchogenic carcinoma. Carcinoids arising within the lung have a propensity to involve the right upper and middle lobes and appear as well-defined smooth or lobulated nodules or masses.

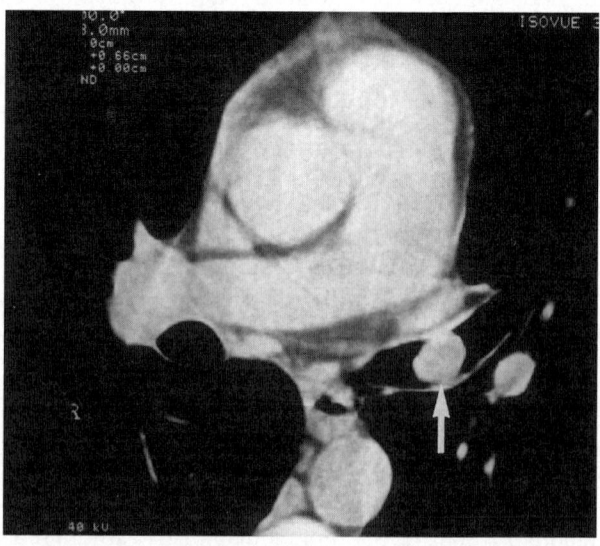

Figure 16.19. Bronchial Carcinoid. CT through the left upper lobe bronchus in a 35-year-old man shows a smooth endoluminal mass (*arrow*) at the junction of the left main and upper lobe bronchi. Bronchoscopic biopsy showed carcinoid tumor, which required a left pneumonectomy for curative resection.

Calcification or ossification is seen in 10% of pathologic specimens but is rarely visualized on plain radiographs. CT is ideally suited to demonstrate the relationship of the mass to the central airways. The typical appearance on CT is a smooth or lobulated soft tissue mass within a main or lobar bronchus (Fig. 16.19)(16). The presence of a small intraluminal and large extraluminal soft tissue component has given rise to the descriptive term "iceberg tumor." Atypical carcinoids tend to have more irregular margins and inhomogeneous contrast enhancement and are much more likely to be associated with hilar and mediastinal lymph node metastases. In some cases, the presence of small punctate peripheral calcifications or marked contrast enhancement on CT may allow distinction from bronchogenic carcinoma.

Prognosis in patients with typical bronchial carcinoid is excellent, with a 5-year survival rate of 90%. Regional lymph node metastases, seen in approximately 5% of operative specimens, lower the 5-year survival rate to 70%. Atypical carcinoids are associated with metastases in up to 70% of cases although these may appear many years after discovery of the primary tumor. The 5-year survival rate in these patients is less than 50%.

Pulmonary Hamartoma is a benign neoplasm comprised of disorganized epithelial and mesenchymal elements normally found in the bronchus or lung. Histologically, these lesions contain cartilage surrounded by fibrous connective tissue with variable amounts of fat, smooth muscle, and seromucous glands; calcification and ossification is seen in 30%. Of these lesions, 90% arise within the pulmonary parenchyma; less than 10% are endobronchial. Endobronchial hamartomas are usually pedunculated lesions with fatty centers covered by fibrous tissue that contain little cartilage. Patients are usually diagnosed in their forties. Central bronchial hamartomas present with cough or upper airway obstruction. CT shows a soft tissue mass that is usually indistinguishable from a bronchial carcinoid.

METASTATIC DISEASE TO THE THORAX

The spread of extrapulmonary neoplasm to the lung may occur by direct invasion of the pulmonary parenchyma or as a result of hematogenous dissemination, with the latter mechanism much more common (17). Rarely, a tumor can disseminate throughout the lungs via the tracheobronchial tree, as in laryngotracheal papillomatosis and some cases of bronchioloalveolar cell carcinoma. Transpleural spread of tumor can be seen in cases of invasive thymoma.

Direct Invasion of the lung may occur with mediastinal, pleural, or chest wall malignancies. The most common mediastinal malignancies to invade the lung are esophageal carcinoma, lymphoma, and malignant germ cell tumors, or any malignancy metastasizing to mediastinal or hilar lymph nodes. Malignant mesothelioma and metastases to the pleura or chest wall can extend through the pleura to invade the adjacent lung.

Hematogenous Metastases to the lung may be seen with any tumor that gains access to the superior or inferior vena cava or the thoracic duct because the pulmonary artery is the final common pathway for these channels. Although only a minority of tumor emboli survive within the pulmonary interstitium; those that do produce one of two morphologic and radiographic appearances: pulmonary nodules or lymphangitic carcinomatosis.

Pulmonary Nodules are the most common manifestation of hematogenous metastases to the lung. They are most commonly seen in carcinomas of the lung, breast, kidney, thyroid, colon, uterus, and head and neck. Although most patients have multiple nodules, metastasis can present as a solitary pulmonary nodule. SPNs due to metastasis are typically smooth in contour whereas primary bronchogenic tumors are lobulated or spiculated. The likelihood that an SPN represents a solitary metastasis in a patient with a synchronous extrathoracic malignancy is slightly less than 50%; SPNs in patients with prior malignancies are almost always primary bronchogenic tumors or granulomas. However, the site of the primary tumor may affect the likelihood that an SPN is a metastasis. Carcinoma of the rectosigmoid colon, osteogenic sarcoma, renal cell carcinoma, and melanoma are more likely to give solitary pulmonary metastases. It should be cautioned that what may appear as a solitary metastasis on plain radiographs may be only one of multiple pulmonary nodules as shown by chest CT.

Nodular pulmonary metastases are usually smooth or lobulated lesions that are found in greater numbers in the peripheral portions of the lower lobes because of greater pulmonary blood flow to these regions. Because helical CT is considerably more sensitive than plain radiographs, conventional whole lung tomography, and incremental CT in detecting lung nodules, it is the modality of choice for the evaluation of pulmonary metastases There are no characteristic features of nodular metastases that allow distinction among different primary neoplasms. Similarly, the distinction between metastases and granulomas is usually impossible although there are three findings on CT that may help in this regard. First, the demonstration of a feeding vessel entering the central aspect of a well-defined peripheral pulmonary nodule stongly suggests hematogenous metastases; however, this may be seen in other blood-borne pulmonary processes such as pulmonary infarcts and septic emboli. Second, the demonstration of calcification within multiple pulmonary nodules, in the absence of a history of a primary bone forming neoplasm such as osteogenic sarcoma or chondrosarcoma, is diagnostic of granulomas. Although primary mucinous adenocarcinomas of the colon and ovary may rarely produce calcification within pulmonary metastases, these microscopic calcifications are usually too small to be detected even on CT. Finally, in patients with miliary nodular opacities, the presence of one or more larger nodules interspersed with uniformly sized miliary nodules is highly suggestive of metastases from melanoma or carcinoma of the lung, thyroid, or kidney.

The diagnosis of nodular pulmonary metastases is usually presumptive. It is based on the demonstration of multiple pulmonary nodules in a patient with a known malignancy that has a propensity for lung metastases who lacks evidence of a granulomatous process. In some patients, particularly those with solitary pulmonary nodules and no evidence of additional sites of metastases or those with a history of a prior localized malignancy, a biopsy of the nodule should be performed. In selected patients, resection of a solitary pulmonary metastasis or several peripheral metastases may be undertaken. CT is the best imaging modality to conduct follow-up studies on the response of metastases to chemotherapy, with resolution of nodules indicating a positive response. An important caveat is that persistent nodular opacities representing sterilized tumor deposits may be seen following successful treatment of metastatic choriocarcinoma or seminoma. In these patients, follow-up CT scans will demonstrate a lack of growth of these "sterile" nodules.

Lymphangitic Carcinomatosis (LC). Although direct parenchymal lymphatic invasion and obstruction of hilar and mediastinal lymph nodes by bronchogenic carcinoma is the most common cause of unilateral lymphangitic carcinomatosis, extrapulmonary malignancies may invade pulmonary lymphatics after hematogenous dissemination to both lungs to produce interstitial deposits of tumor. In LC, the tumor cells invade the lymphatics within the peribronchovascular and peripheral interstitium, resulting in lymphatic dilatation, interstitial edema, and fibrosis. The most common extrathoracic malignancies to produce LC are carcinomas of the breast, stomach, pancreas, and prostate. Occasionally, LC will present in a patient without a known primary malignancy. Most patients with LC have slowly progressive dyspnea and a nonproductive cough.

The chest radiographic findings in LC complicating extrathoracic malignancy correlate with the involvement of the peribronchovascular and peripheral interstitium seen pathologically. Peribronchial cuffing and linear opacities, particularly Kerley's B lines, are characteristically seen. Coarse reticulonodular opacities may also be present. Concomitant hilar and mediastinal lymph node enlargement need not be present.

The predominant HRCT findings in lymphangitic carcinomatosis are thickening of interlobular septa and the subpleural interstitium (see Fig. 16.13)(18). Although nodular thickening of the septa, reflecting tumor nodules, is characteristic of LC, it is seen in only a minority of patients. The thickened septal lines do not distort the pulmonary lobule, a feature that helps distinguish LC from interstitial fibrosis, which characteristically distorts the normal lobular shape. Visibility of the intralobular bronchioles or prominence of the centrilobular vessel is frequently seen, as is thickening of the peribronchovascular interstitium within the central (parahilar) portions of the lung. The findings may be unilateral or even limited to one lobe, particularly when LC occurs secondary to bronchogenic carcinoma. Because most patients with LC have pathologic involvement of the peribronchovascular interstitium, the diagnosis is best made by transbronchial biopsy. In a patient with the appropriate history, the HRCT appearance of lymphangitic spread may be specific enough to obviate the need for transbronchial biopsy. Occasionally, the HRCT study will demonstrate the typical findings of LC when the plain radiograph is normal or equivocal.

NONEPITHELIAL PARENCHYMAL MALIGNANCIES AND NEOPLASTIC-LIKE CONDITIONS

Lymphoma. Parenchymal involvement in Hodgkin's disease is two to three times more common than in non-Hodgkin's lymphoma. Parenchymal abnormalities in Hodgkin's lymphoma usually produce linear and coarse reticulonodular opacities that directly extend into the lung from enlarged hilar lymph nodes. Extensive areas of parenchymal involvement can produce mass-like opacities and areas of air-space opacification. Atelectasis in Hodgkin's disease is rarely caused by extrinsic nodal compression of the bronchi but rather develops from an obstructing endobronchial tumor. Extension into the subpleural lymphatics may produce subpleural plaques or masses visible only by CT. Although parenchymal involvement in Hodgkin's disease does not occur in the absence of hilar and mediastinal nodal disease (excluding patients who have undergone mediastinal irradiation), non-Hodgkin's lymphoma may involve the parenchyma without concomitant nodal disease in up to 50%. The parenchymal involvement most often appears as masses or air-space opacities (Fig. 16.7); the latter may simulate lobar pneumonia. Coarse reticulonodular opacities may be seen and, rarely, a solitary pulmonary nodule is the sole manifestation of intrathoracic disease. Most cases of primary pulmonary non-Hodgkin's lymphoma arise from the bronchus-associated lymphoid tissue (BALT) and represent low-grade B-cell lymphomas.

Pseudolymphoma. This term describes a localized nonneoplastic reactive proliferation of lymphocytes in the lung. Histologically, the distinction from well-differentiated lymphoma may be difficult; the demonstration of a polyclonal population of lymphocytes with multiple germinal centers and the absence of lymph node enlargement are necessary for the diagnosis. A more appropriate term for this disorder is "nodular lymphoid hyperplasia" because it produces a sharply marginated pulmonary nodule or mass radiographically. The mass may contain air bronchograms as alveoli are compressed by large numbers of interstitial lymphocytes. Pseudolymphoma is usually associated with a good prognosis although it may develop into lymphoma in patients with Sjogren's syndrome.

Lymphocytic Interstitial Pneumonitis (LIP) or diffuse lymphoid hyperplasia is an infiltration of the pulmonary interstitium by mature lymphocytes that is histologically indistinguishable from nodular lymphoid hyperplasia. Patients with Sjogren's syndrome, hypogammaglobulinemia, and AIDS are at particular risk for this condition. Radiographically, a predominantly lower lobe reticulonodular and linear pattern of disease is seen, often with intermixed areas of air-space opacification. Some patients with this disorder develop frank pulmonary lymphoma or interstitial fibrosis; others resolve with the administration of corticosteroid treatment. In children with AIDS, the course of LIP is often indolent.

Lymphomatoid Granulomatosis was originally thought to represent a distinct histological entity but has recently been reclassified as a form of pulmonary lymphoma. Histologically, multiple round nodules containing lymphocytes infiltrate small vessels to produce an obliterative vasculitis. These findings are similar to

Wegener's granulomatosis although well-formed granulomas are rare in lymphomatoid granulomatosis. CNS and skin involvement are common but renal failure is not present. Radiographically, there are multiple nodular opacities with a lower lobe predilection. Cavitation is common and results from ischemic necrosis. This condition is a lymphatic malignancy and is treated with chemotherapy. The prognosis is poor, with 50% of patients developing frank lymphoma. Overall 5-year survival is approximately 20%.

Leukemia. Although leukemic involvement of the lung is found in approximately one-third of patients at autopsy, clinical or radiographic evidence of parenchymal infiltration is uncommon during life. The majority of pulmonary disease in leukemic patients is caused by pneumonia complicating immunosuppression, edema from cardiac disease, or hemorrhage due to thrombocytopenia. Parenchymal involvement in leukemia usually takes the form of interstitial infiltration by leukemic cells, with resultant peribronchial cuffing and reticulonodular opacities on chest radiograph. Focal accumulation of leukemic cells can produce a chloroma and the radiographic appearance of an SPN. An unusual pulmonary manifestation of leukemia is pulmonary leukostasis, which is seen in acute leukemia or those in blast crisis in whom the peripheral white blood cell count exceeds 100,000–200,000/cm^3. In this condition, the white cell blasts clump within the pulmonary microvasculature to produce dyspnea. Approximately 50% of affected patients have normal radiographs, and the remainder demonstrate a diffuse reticulonodular pattern of disease.

Kaposi's Sarcoma (KS) of the lung is a common complication of AIDS. Pulmonary involvement almost invariably follows skin, oropharyngeal, and/or visceral involvement. The histological features are characteristic: clusters of spindle cells with numerous mitotic figures are separated by thin-walled vascular channels containing red blood cells. The tumor involves the tracheobronchial mucosa and the peribronchovascular, alveolar, and subpleural interstitium of the lung. Radiographically,

Kaposi's sarcoma produces small-sized to medium-sized, poorly marginated nodular and coarse linear opacities that extend from the hilum into the mid-lung and lower lung. CT shows the typical peribronchovascular location of the opacities and may demonstrate air bronchograms traversing mass-like areas of confluent disease (Fig. 16.20). A bloody pleural effusion is present in up to 50% of patients; this is attributed to lesions within the subpleural interstitium of the lung. Hilar and mediastinal lymph node enlargement is found in 20% of patients. Important diagnostic features of pulmonary Kaposi's sarcoma are the slow rate of progression of disease (usually over many months) and the absence of fever or pulmonary symptoms despite extensive parenchymal disease. Bleeding from endobronchial or parenchymal lesions may produce focal or diffuse air-space opacities that are difficult to distinguish from complicating bacterial pneumonia or *Pneumocystis carinii* infection.

The diagnosis of pulmonary Kaposi's sarcoma is usually made indirectly by the visualization of typical endobronchial lesions in a patient with characteristic chest radiographic findings. Combined thallium and gallium lung scanning has been used successfully to distinguish KS from pneumonia and non-Hodgkin's lymphoma. Although pneumonia is both gallium and thallium avid, lymphoma is gallium avid only and KS is thallium avid only.

Pulmonary Blastoma is a rare malignant tumor affecting children and young adults. The tumors are comprised of both mesenchymal and glandular elements of lung, with an appearance that simulates fetal lung at 10–16 weeks' gestation. Those tumors composed predominantly of glandular elements are also called fetal adenocarcinomas, and tumors with malignant mesenchyme alone are referred to as cystic and pleuropulmonary blastomas of childhood. Tumors with mixed malignant epithelial and mesenchymal components are called biphasic blastomas. Pulmonary blastomas are difficult to distinguish histologically from carcinosarcomas. Radiographically, these tumors are extremely large at presentation. Diagnosis is made by resection of the le-

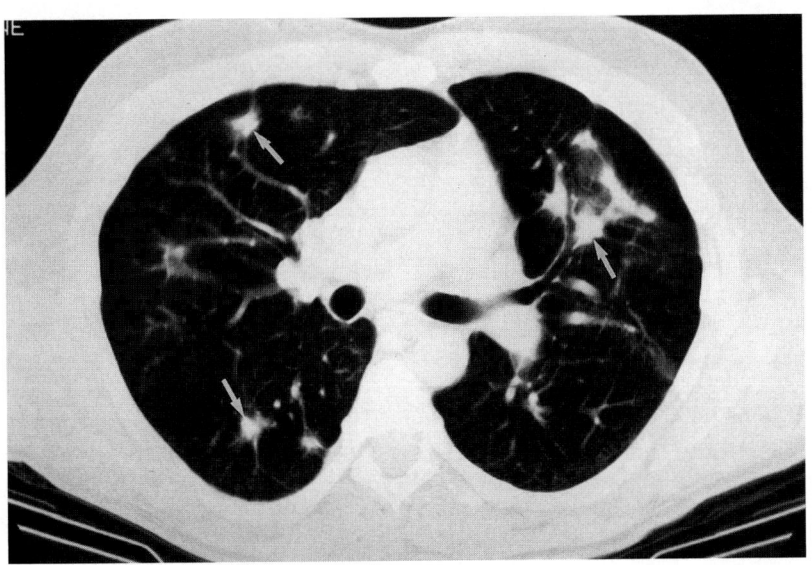

Figure 16.20. Kaposi Sarcoma. CT in a 41-year-old man with AIDS and cutaneous lesions reveals bilateral irregularly marginated nodules (*arrows*) with a peribronchovascular distribution. The presence of pulmonary involvement with Kaposi sarcoma was confirmed by bronchoscopy.

sion. The prognosis is poor because many lesions have metastasized at the time of diagnosis.

A variety of other rare neoplasms and non-neoplastic tumors may affect the lung. Because many of these present as a nodule or mass on chest radiographs, they are reviewed in the section on the SPN.

References

1. Webb WR. Radiologic evaluation of the solitary pulmonary nodule. AJR Am J Roentgenol 1990;154:701–708.
2. Siegelman SS, Khouri NF, Leo FP, et al. Solitary pulmonary nodule: CT assessment. Radiology 1986;160:307–312.
3. Swensen SJ, Brown LR, Colby TV, et al. Lung nodule enhancement at CT: prospective findings. Radiology 1996; 201:447–455.
4. Knight SB, Delbeke D, Stewart JR, Sandler MP. Evaluation of pulmonary lesions with FDG-PET. Chest 1996;109:982–988.
5. Travis WD, Lubin J, Ries L, et al. United States lung carcinoma incidence trends. Cancer 1996; 77:2464–2470.
6. Quinn D, Gianlupi A, Broste S. The changing radiographic presentation of bronchogenic carcinoma with refence to cell types. Chest 1996;110:1474–1479.
7. Byrd RB, Carr DT, Miller WE, et al. Radiographic abnormalities in carcinoma of the lung as related to histological cell type. Thorax 1969;24:573–575.
8. Steinert HC, Hauser M, Allemann F, et al. Non–small cell lung cancer: nodal staging with FDG PET versus CT with correlative lymph node mapping and sampling. Radiology 1997;202:441–446.
9. Klein JS, Webb WR. Radiologic staging of lung cancer. J Thorac Imag 1991; 7:29–47.
10. AJCC Cancer Staging Manual. 5th ed. Philadelphia: Lippincott-Raven, 1997, pp. 127–137.
11. Webb WR, Gatsonis C, Zerhouni EA, et al. CT and MR imaging in staging non–small cell bronchogenic carcinoma: report of the Radiologic Diagnostic Oncology Group. Radiology 1991;178:705–713.
12. Glazer HS, Kaiser LR, Anderson DJ, et al. Indeterminate mediastinal invasion in bronchogenic carcinoma: CT evaluation. Radiology 1989;173:37–42.
13. McLoud TC, Bourgouin PM, Greenberg RW, et al. Bronchogenic carcinoma: analysis of staging in the mediastinum with CT by correlative lymph node mapping and sampling. Radiology 1992;182:319–323.
14. Schwartz LH, Panicek DM, Koutcher JA, et al. Adrenal masses in patients with malignancy: prospective comparison of echo-planar, fast spin-echo, and chemical shift MR imaging. Radiology 1995;197:421–425.
15. Weber AL, Grillo HC. Tracheal tumors: a radiological, clinical, and pathological evaluation of 84 cases. Radiol Clin North Am 1978;16:227–246.
16. Magid D, Siegelman SS, Eggleston JC, et al. Pulmonary carcinoid tumors: CT assessment. J Comput Assist Tomogr 1989;13:244–247.
17. Coppage L, Shaw C, Curtis AM. Metastatic disease to the chest in patients with extrathoracic malignancy. J Thorac Imag 1987;2:24–37.
18. Stein MG, Mayo J, Müller NL, et al. Pulmonary lymphangitic spread of carcinoma. Radiology 1987;162: 371–375.

17
Pulmonary Infection

Todd Peebles
Jeffrey S. Klein

INFECTION IN THE NORMAL HOST

The bronchopulmonary system is open to the atmosphere and therefore is relatively accessible to airborne microorganisms. Multiple host defense mechanisms exist at the level of the pharynx, trachea, and central bronchi. When these mechanisms do not work properly, pathogenic organisms can penetrate to the small distal bronchi and the pulmonary parenchyma. Once the invading organisms penetrate the parenchyma, both the cellular and humoral immune systems become active. This response may manifest clinically and radiographically as pneumonia, and in a normal host will often lead to eradication or at least suppression of the infecting organisms. If the immune response is impaired, a lower respiratory tract infection may cause a very severe illness and often death, despite appropriate antibiotic therapy.

Mechanisms of Disease and Radiographic Patterns. Microorganisms responsible for producing pneumonia enter the lung and cause infection by three potential routes: via the tracheobronchial tree; via the pulmonary vasculature; or via direct spread from infection in the mediastinum, chest wall, or upper abdomen Infection via the tracheobronchial tree is usually secondary to inhalation or aspiration of infectious microorganisms, and can be divided into three subtypes based on gross pathologic appearance and radiographic patterns: lobar pneumonia, lobular or bronchopneumonia, and interstitial pneumonia. As will be discussed later in this chapter, certain organisms will typically produce one of these three patterns although considerable overlap may occur.

Lobar pneumonia is typical of pneumococcal pulmonary infection. In this pattern of disease, the inflammatory exudate begins within the distal air spaces. The inflammatory process spreads via the pores of Kohn and canals of Lambert to produce nonsegmental consolidation. If untreated, the inflammation may eventually involve an entire lobe (Fig. 17.1). Because the airways are usually spared, air bronchograms are common and significant volume loss is unusual (see Table 14.1).

Bronchopneumonia is the most common pattern of disease and is most typical of staphylococcal pneumonia. In the early stages of bronchopneumonia, the inflammation is centered primarily in and near lobular bronchi. As the inflammation progresses, exudative fluid extends peripherally along the bronchus to involve the entire pulmonary lobule. Radiographically, multifocal opacities that are roughly lobular in configuration produce a "patchwork quilt" appearance owing to the interspersion of normal and diseased lobules (Fig. 17.2). Although bronchopneumonia is the most common cause of multifocal, patchy air-space opacities, a broad list of differential diagnostic considerations exists (see Table 14.2). Exudate within the bronchi accounts for the absence of air bronchograms in bronchopneumonia. With coalescence of affected areas, the pattern may resemble lobar pneumonia.

In interstitial pneumonia, seen in viral and mycoplasma infection, inflammatory thickening of bronchial and bronchiolar walls and the pulmonary interstitium occurs. This results in a radiographic pattern of airways thickening and reticulonodular opacities (see Table 14.3). Air bronchograms are absent because the alveolar spaces remain aerated. Segmental and subsegmental atelectasis from small airways obstruction is common.

The spread of infection to the lung via the pulmonary vasculature usually occurs in the setting of systemic sepsis. The pattern of parenchymal involvement is patchy and bilateral. The lung bases are most severely involved because blood flow is greatest in the dependent portions of the lungs. Pulmonary infection from direct spread results in a localized parenchymal process adjacent to an extrapulmonary source of infection. If an organism causes extensive parenchymal necrosis, abscess formation may result.

Bacterial Pneumonia

GRAM-POSITIVE BACTERIA

Streptococcus pneumoniae (Pneumococcus). S. pneumoniae is a gram-positive organism that may cause infection in healthy individuals but is much more commonly seen in the elderly, alcoholics, and other compromised hosts. Patients with sickle cell disease or who have undergone splenectomy are at particular risk for severe pneumococcal pneumonia.

Pneumococcal pneumonia begins in the lower lobes or the posterior segments of the upper lobes. Initially the terminal airways are affected, but rather than remaining localized to this site, there is rapid development of an air-space inflammatory exudate. The spread of infection to contiguous air spaces via interalveolar connections ac-

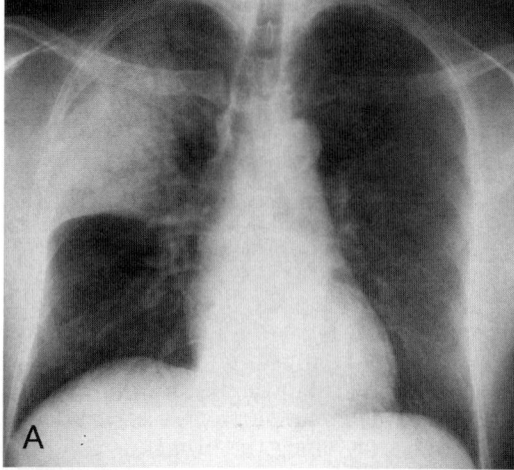

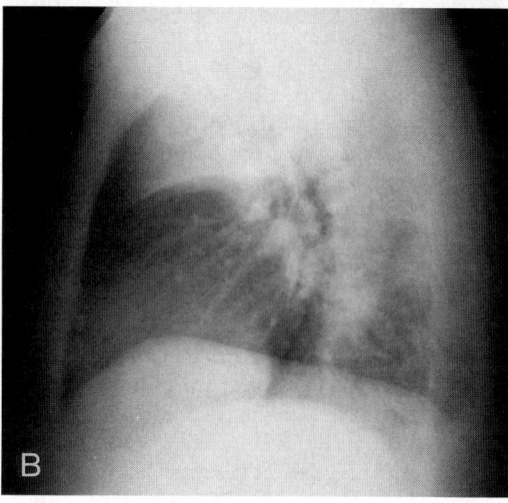

Figure 17.1. Lobar Pneumonia from Pneumococcus. Postero-anterior **(A)** and lateral **(B)** radiographs in a 57-year-old man with fever, chills, and productive cough demonstrate air-space opacification in the right upper lobe with air bronchograms. Sputum culture was positive for *Streptococcus pneumoniae*.

counts for the nonsegmental distribution and homogeneity of the resultant consolidation.

The typical radiographic appearance of acute pneumococcal pneumonia is lobar consolidation (Fig. 17.1). Air bronchograms are usually evident. Cavitation in pneumococcal pneumonia is rare, with the exception of infections due to serotype III. Uncomplicated parapneumonic effusion or empyema may be seen in up to 50% of patients. With appropriate therapy, complete clearing may be seen in 10–14 days. In older patients or those with underlying disease, complete resolution may take 8–10 weeks.

Patients with pneumococcal pneumonia occasionally present with atypical radiographic patterns of disease (1). Patchy lobular opacities similar to those seen with bronchopneumonia or, rarely, a reticulonodular pattern may be seen. In some patients, the atypical appearance may relate to the presence of preexisting lung disease (e.g., emphysema), partial treatment, or an impaired immune response (e.g., AIDS). In children, pneumococcal

pneumonia may present as a spherical opacity ("round pneumonia") simulating a parenchymal mass.

Staphylococcus aureus. Staphylococcal pneumonia is most common in hospitalized and debilitated patients. It may also develop following hematogenous spread to the lung in patients with endocarditis, patients with indwelling catheters, and intravenous drug users. Community-acquired infection may complicate influenza or other viral pneumonias.

S. aureus typically produces a bronchopneumonia and appears radiographically as patchy opacities (Fig. 17.3). In severe cases, the opacities may become confluent to produce lobar opacification. Because the inflammatory exudate fills the airways, air bronchograms are rarely seen. In adults, the process is often bilateral and may be complicated by abscess formation in 25–75% of patients. In patients who develop pulmonary infection from hematogenous seeding, one sees multiple, bilateral, poorly defined nodular opacities that eventually become more sharply defined and cavitate. Parapneumonic effusion and empyema is common. Pneumatocele formation is common in children and may lead to pneumothorax. Pneumatoceles may be distinguished from abscesses by their thin walls, rapid change in size, and tendency to develop during the late phase of infection.

Streptococcus pyogenes. Acute streptococcal pneumonia is rarely seen today although it can occasionally complicate viral infection or streptococcal pharyngitis. The radiographic appearance is similar to staphylococcal pneumonia, with lobular or segmental lower lobe opacities. The process may be complicated by abscess formation and cavitation; empyema is relatively common.

GRAM-NEGATIVE BACTERIA

Gram-negative bacteria are increasingly important causes of pneumonia in hospitalized patients, accounting for more than 50% of nosocomial pulmonary infections. Although gram-negative organisms may be isolated from only a small percentage of healthy individuals, the isolation rate in hospitalized and severely ill patients ranges from 40–75%. The organisms most often responsible for pneumonia include members of the Enterobacteriaceae family (*Klebsiella, E. coli, Proteus*), *Pseudomonas aeruginosa, Hemophilus influenzae,* and *Legionella pneumophila* (2).

The radiographic appearance of gram-negative bacterial pneumonia varies from small, ill-defined nodules to patchy areas of opacification that may become confluent and resemble lobar pneumonia. Involvement is usually bilateral and multifocal, and the lower lobes are most frequently affected. Abscess formation and cavitation are relatively common. Parapneumonic effusion is common and is often complicated by empyema formation.

Klebsiella pneumoniae. Klebsiella pneumonia occurs predominantly in older alcoholic males and debilitated hospitalized patients. Radiographically, it appears as a homogeneous lobar opacification containing air bronchograms. Three features help distinguish it radiographically from pneumococcal pneumonia: 1) the volume of the involved lobe may be increased by the exuberant inflammatory exudate, producing a bulging

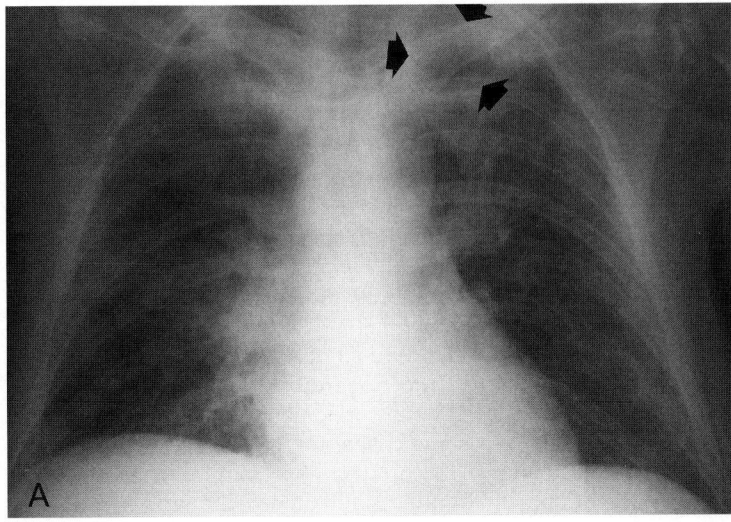

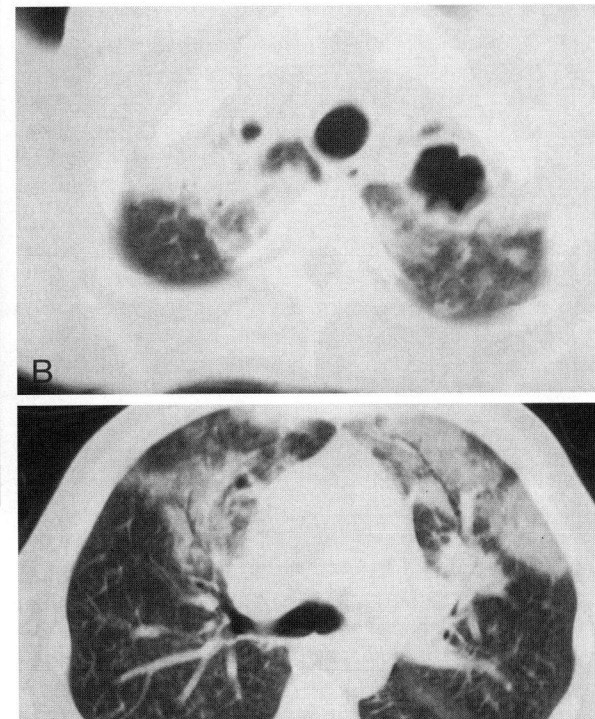

Figure 17.2. *Pseudomonas aeriguinosa* **Pneumonia. A.** Frontal radiograph in an HIV-positive male with fever and progressive respiratory symptoms shows multifocal air-space opacities with dense apical opacification with cavitation (*arrows*). **B.** A CT through the apices shows air-space opacification with left apical cavitation. **C.** A CT at the level of the tracheal carina shows air-space disease in the anterior segments of right and left upper lobes with sparing of the dependent portions of lung. Bronchoscopy revealed *Pseudomonas.*

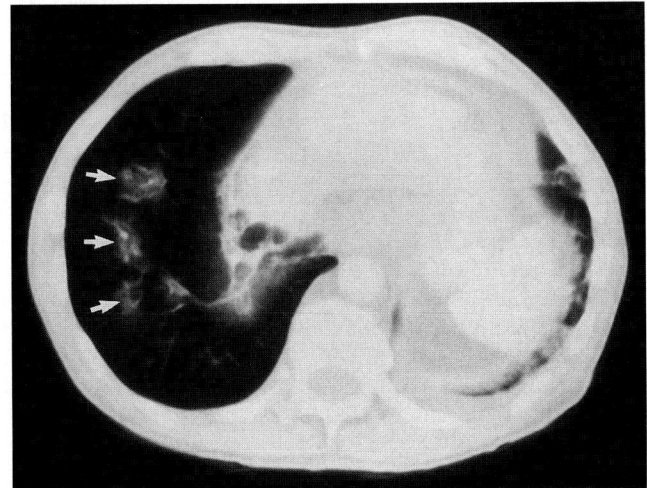

Figure 17.3. *Staphylococcus aureus* **Bronchopneumonia.** A CT through the right lung base shows multiple air-space opacities in a lobular distribution. Sputum cultures showed *Staphylococcus aureus* pneumonia.

interlobar fissure, 2) an abscess with cavity formation develops, which is uncommon in pneumococcal pneumonia, and 3) a higher incidence of pleural effusion and empyema exists. Pulmonary gangrene may be seen but is uncommon.

Hemophilus influenzae. In adults, *H. influenzae* in-

fection is most common in patients with COPD, alcoholism, diabetes mellitus, and an anatomic or functional splenectomy. It most often causes bronchitis although it may extend to produce bilateral lower lobe bronchopneumonia.

Pseudomonas aeruginosa. Pseudomonas pneumonia most often affects debilitated patients, particularly those requiring mechanical ventilation. There is a high mortality rate associated with the disease. The radiographic pattern of parenchymal involvement depends on the method by which the organisms reach the lung. Patchy opacities with abscess formation which mimic staphylococcal pneumonia are common when the infection reaches the lung via the tracheobronchial tree (Fig. 17.2). Diffuse, bilateral, ill-defined nodular opacities usually reflect hematogenous dissemination. Pleural effusions are common and are usually small.

Legionella pneumophila. Legionnaire's disease is due to *L. pneumophila,* a gram-negative bacillus commonly found in air-conditioning and humidifier systems. This infection affects older men. Community-acquired infection is seen in patients with COPD or malignancy, but nosocomial infection primarily affects immunocompromised patients or those with renal failure or malignancy.

The characteristic radiographic pattern is air-space opacification that is initially peripheral and sublobar. In some patients, the air-space opacities appear as a round pneumonia. The infection progresses to lobar or multilobar involvement despite the initiation of an-

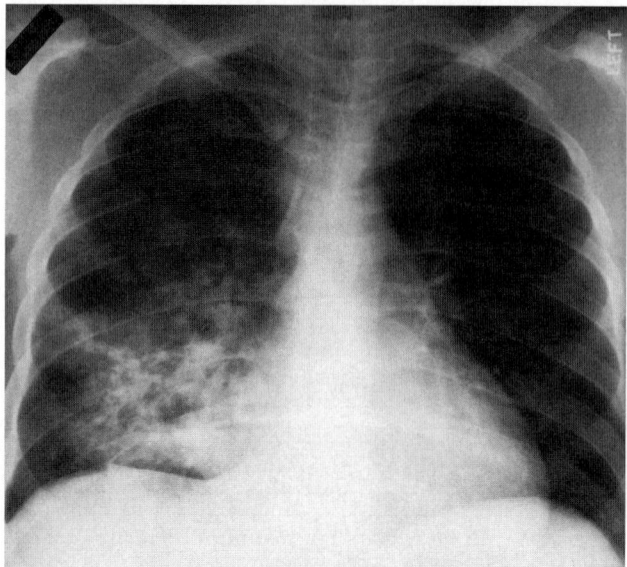

Figure 17.4. Legionella Pneumonia in an Immunocompromised Patient. Frontal chest radiograph in a 35-year-old man with AIDS demonstrates a middle lobe air-space opacification with areas of cavitation. Bronchoscopy showed *Legionella pneumophila* pneumonia.

tibiotic therapy. At the peak of the disease, the parenchymal involvement is usually bilateral. Pleural effusions are seen in approximately 30% of patients. Cavitation is not seen except in the immunocompromised patient (Fig. 17.4). The radiographic resolution of pneumonia is often prolonged and may lag behind symptomatic improvement.

ANAEROBIC BACTERIAL INFECTION

The majority of anaerobic lung infections arise from aspiration of infected oropharyngeal contents (3). Approximately 25% of patients give a history of impaired consciousness, and many are alcoholic. The most common organisms responsible are the gram-negative bacilli *Bacteroides* and *Fusobacterium*; however, the majority of pulmonary infections are polymicrobial. All anaerobic pulmonary infections produce a similar radiographic appearance. The distribution of parenchymal opacities reflects the gravitational flow of aspirated material. When aspiration occurs in the supine position, the posterior segments of the upper lobes and superior segments of the lower lobes are predominantly involved, but aspiration in the erect position leads to involvement of basal segments of the lower lobes. The typical radiographic appearance is peripheral lobular and segmental air-space opacities. Cavitation within areas of consolidation is relatively common, and discrete lung abscesses may be seen in 50% of patients. Hilar and/or mediastinal lymph node enlargement may be seen in those with lung abscesses. Empyema, with or without bronchopleural fistula formation, is a common complication seen in up to 50% of patients.

ATYPICAL BACTERIAL INFECTIONS

Actinomycosis. *Actinomyces israelii* is an anaerobic gram-positive filamentous bacterium that is a normal inhabitant of the human oropharynx. It causes disease when it gains access to devitalized or infected tissues, which facilitate its growth. Actinomycosis most commonly follows dental extractions, manifesting as mandibular osteomyelitis or a soft tissue abscess. The lungs may be infected by aspiration of infectious oral debris or, less commonly, by direct extension from the primary site of disease.

The radiographic pattern of actinomycosis is often indistinguishable from nocardiosis. Findings consist of nonsegmental air-space opacities in the periphery of the lower lobes. In some cases, the infection manifests as a localized mass-like opacity that mimics bronchogenic carcinoma. If therapy is not instituted, a lung abscess may develop. Thoracic actinomycosis is characterized by its ability to spread to contiguous tissues without regard for normal anatomic barriers. Extension into the pleura will cause empyema, and chest wall involvement is characterized by osteomyelitis of the ribs and chest wall abscess. Involvement of the ribs is seen as wavy periosteal reaction or lytic rib destruction (4). If the pleuropulmonary disease becomes chronic, extensive fibrosis may be seen. Rarely, the disease is disseminated and a miliary pattern is seen.

Mycoplasma pneumonia is an organism with both bacterial and viral characteristics and is considered as a separate group. It is probably the most common nonbacterial cause of pneumonia and accounts for 10–30% of all community-acquired pneumonia. Affected patients usually have a subacute illness of 2–3 weeks duration. Symptoms include fever, nonproductive cough, headache, and malaise. Unusual physical findings include bullous myringitis and rash.

In the early stages of infection, interstitial inflammation causes a fine reticular pattern on the chest radiograph. This may progress to patchy segmental air-space opacities that may coalesce to produce lobar consolidation (Fig. 17.5). The process is often unilateral and tends to involve the lower lobes. Pleural effusion may be seen in the consolidative form of disease, and occurs most commonly in children. Lymph node enlargement is uncommon but may be seen in children. Radiographic resolution may require 4–6 weeks.

MYCOBACTERIAL INFECTIONS

Mycobacterium tuberculosis is an aerobic, acid-fast bacillus. Two principal forms of tuberculous pulmonary disease are recognized clinically and radiographically: primary tuberculosis (TB) and reactivation or postprimary disease. The inflammatory response to *M. tuberculosis* differs from the normal response to bacterial organisms in that it involves cell-mediated immunity (delayed hypersensitivity). Initially, droplet nuclei laden with bacilli are inhaled and implant in a subpleural location. In most patients, the bacilli are phagocytized and killed by alveolar macrophages. If the bacilli overcome host immune response, an inflammatory focus is estab-

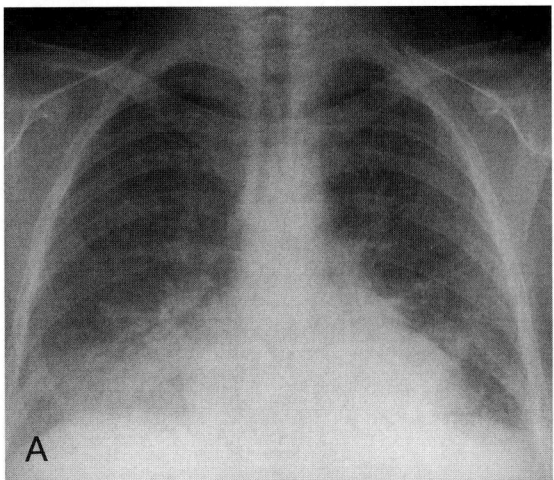

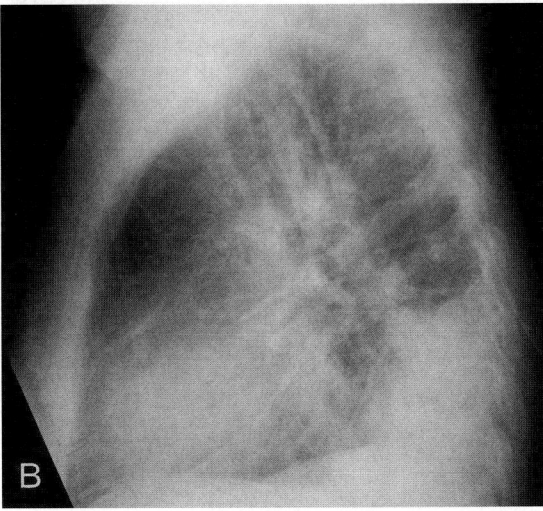

Figure 17.5. Mycoplasma Pneumonia. Posteroanterior **(A)** and lateral **(B)** radiographs in a 21-year-old woman demonstrate mixed diffuse interstitial and bibasilar air-space opacities. Immunofluorescent staining of induced sputum samples revealed *M. pneumoniae.*

lished. The macrophages are then transformed into epithelioid cells, which aggregate to form granulomas. The granulomas are usually well formed by 1–3 weeks, coinciding with the development of delayed hypersensitivity. The granulomas typically demonstrate central caseous necrosis, thereby distinguishing them from the granulomas seen in sarcoidosis. Inflammation and enlargement of draining hilar and mediastinal lymph nodes is common in primary disease, particularly in children and immunocompromised patients.

In primary infection, the parenchymal disease and adenopathy may completely resolve or a residual focus of scarring or calcification may occur. In some situations, usually in infants younger than 1 year of age, local parenchymal disease progresses, and is termed "progressive primary tuberculosis." More commonly, the disease will be contained by the granulomatous response and recur years later ("reactivation," or postprimary tuberculosis) in the setting of weakened host defenses from aging, alcoholism, diabetes, cancer, or HIV infection.

Postprimary TB develops under the influence of hypersensitivity, with caseous necrosis seen histologically.

Primary tuberculosis has classically been a disease of childhood although the incidence of primary disease has increased because of the HIV epidemic. Most patients with primary TB are asymptomatic and have no radiographic sequelae of infection. In some patients a Ranke complex, consisting of a calcified parenchymal focus (the Ghon lesion) and nodal calcification, is seen. If the patient is symptomatic, a nonspecific focal pneumonitis occurs and is seen as small, ill-defined areas of segmental or lobar opacification (Fig. 17.6). The parenchymal consolidation may mimic a bacterial pneumonia, but the clinical and radiographic course is much more indolent. Cavitation is relatively uncommon in the immunocompetent patient (5). The pulmonary focus may resolve completely or persist as a Ghon lesion or a Ranke complex. Tuberculomas are discrete nodular opacities that may develop in primary TB but are much more common in postprimary disease. Unilateral pleural effusions are seen in 25% of cases and are usually associated with parenchymal disease. If a tuberculous empyema develops, it may break through the parietal pleura to form an extrapleural collection (empyema necessitans). Unilateral hilar or mediastinal lymph node enlargement is common, particularly in children, and may be the sole radiographic manifestation of infection. Bilateral hilar or mediastinal lymph node enlargement may be seen but is uncommon and almost invariably assymetric in distinction to lymph node enlargement in sarcoidosis. During the primary tuberculous infection, there is hematogenous dissemination of the organism to regions with a high partial pressure of oxygen; these include the lung apices, renal medullae, and bone marrow. These microscopic foci are clinically silent and serve as a source of reactivation disease.

Postprimary Tuberculosis. Patients with postprimary TB often present with cough and constitutional symp-

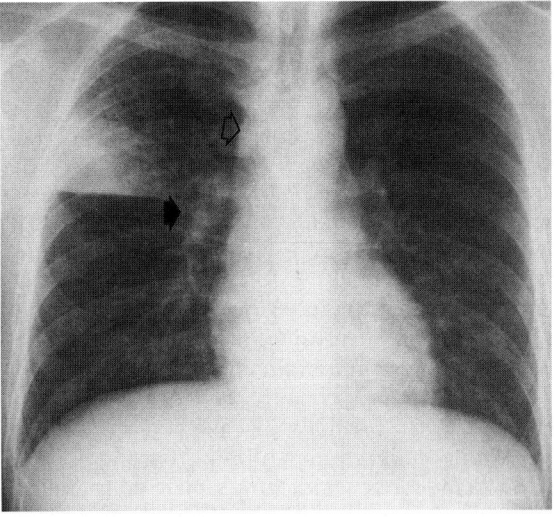

Figure 17.6. Primary Tuberculosis. A PA chest radiograph in a 32-year-old homeless man shows air-space disease within the anterior segment of the right upper lobe with right hilar *(solid arrow)* and paratracheal *(open arrow)* lymph node enlargement. Sputum stains and cultures revealed *M. tuberculosis.*

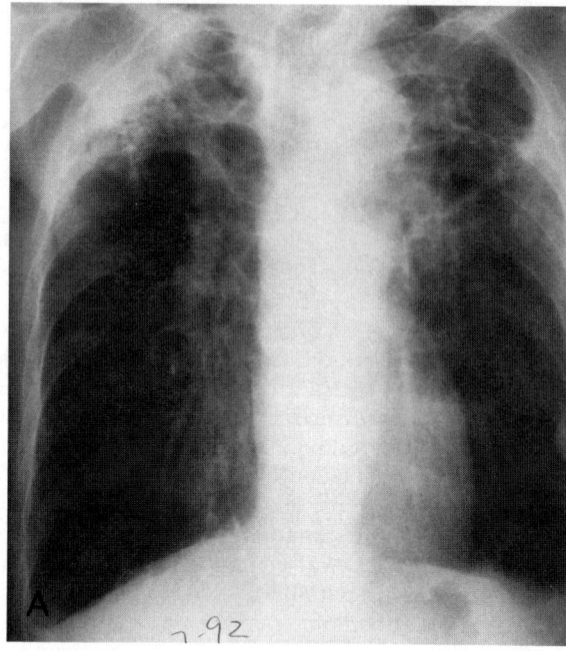

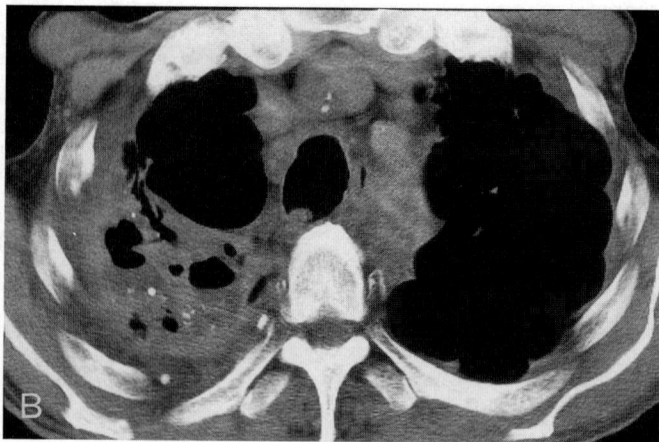

Figure 17.7. Postprimary (Reactivation) Tuberculosis. A. Frontal chest film in a 69-year-old Asian immigrant with a cough and severe wasting reveals hyperinflation with marked fibrotic and cavitary disease in the upper lobes with severe volume loss. **B.** A CT through the lung apices demonstrates consolidative and cavitary changes with air-fluid levels and pleural and parenchymal calcifications. Sputum cultures were positive for *M. tuberculosis.*

toms including chills, night sweats, and weight loss. Reactivation occurs in the apical and posterior segments of the upper lobes and the superior segments of the lower lobes. Ill-defined patchy and nodular opacities are commonly seen. Cavitation is an important radiographic feature of postprimary infection and indicates active and transmissable disease (Fig. 17.7). The cavitary focus may cause transbronchial spread of organisms and result in a multifocal bronchopneumonia. Erosion of a cavitary focus into a branch of the pulmonary artery can produce an aneurysm (Rasmussen's aneurysm) and cause hemoptysis. With appropriate antimicrobial treatment, the disease is controlled by a granulomatous response. Parenchymal healing is associated with fibrosis, bronchiectasis, and volume loss (cicatrizing atelectasis) in the upper lobes.

There are several late complications of pulmonary TB. Interstitial fibrosis can cause pulmonary insufficiency and secondary pulmonary arterial hypertension. Hemoptysis may be secondary to bronchiectasis, mycetoma formation in an old tuberculous cavity, or erosion of a calcified peribronchial lymph node (broncholith) into a bronchus. Bronchostenosis is a result of healed endobronchial TB.

Miliary Tuberculosis. Miliary TB may complicate either primary or reactivation disease. It results from hematogenous dissemination of tubercle bacilli and produces diffuse bilateral two to three millimeter pulmonary nodules (Fig. 17.8). Miliary disease is associated with a high mortality and requires prompt therapy.

Atypical Mycobacterial Infection. Several nontuberculous mycobacteria may cause pulmonary disease (6), with the most common organisms responsible for pulmonary disease being *M. avium-intracellulare* (MAI) or *M. kansasii.* Disease in nonimmunocompromised patients typically affects those with underlying COPD. The radiographic features are often indistinguishable from reacti-

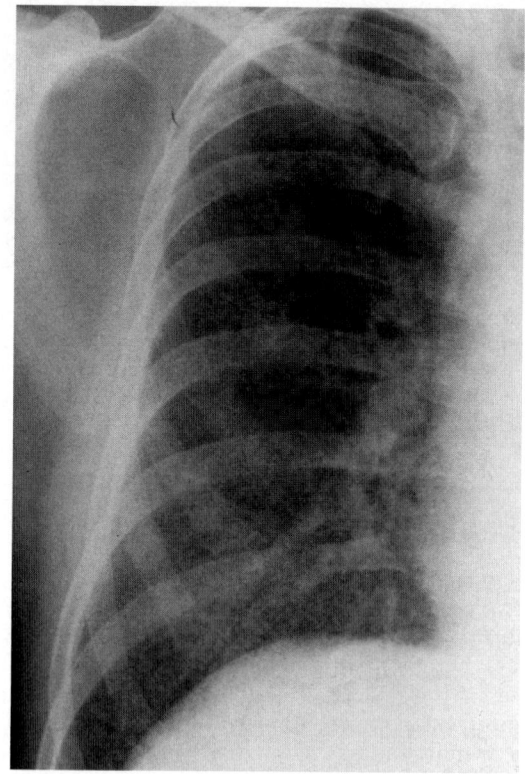

Figure 17.8. Miliary Tuberculosis. A coned-down view of a frontal radiograph demonstrates innumerable micronodular opacities characteristic of micronodular (miliary) interstitial disease. Transbronchial biopsy demonstrated caseating granulomas containing acid-fast bacilli.

vation TB, with chronic fibrocavitary opacities involving the upper lobes. Although cavitation is common, pleural effusion, lymph node enlargement, and miliary spread are distinctly unusual. A second pattern of disease with MAI has recently been described in middle-aged and elderly females, with small peribronchial nodules and bronchiectasis seen in a middle lobe and lingular distribution. Although the disease caused by nontuberculous mycobacteria tends to be more indolent than that seen with *M. tuberculosis*, effectively treating it is often difficult.

Viral Pneumonia

Viruses are a major cause of upper respiratory tract and airways infection, but pneumonia is relatively uncommon. The diagnosis of viral pneumonia is often one of exclusion. Chest radiographic features are nonspecific, usually demonstrating a pattern of bronchopneumonia or interstitial opacities (7). Resolution is usually complete, but permanent sequelae may be seen, including bronchiectasis, bronchiolitis obliterans (which may produce the unilateral hyperlucent lung or Swyer-James syndrome), and interstitial fibrosis.

Influenza. In adults, the most common cause of viral pneumonia is influenza. Outbreaks of influenza can occur in pandemics, epidemics, or sporadically. In most patients, the disease is confined to the upper respiratory tract, but in elderly persons or those with underlying cardiopulmonary disease, a severe hemorrhagic pneumonia may develop. In adults with influenzal pneumonia, bilateral lower lobe patchy air-space opacification often occurs. In children, a diffuse interstitial reticulonodular pattern is more commonly seen. Bacterial superinfection with *Streptococcus* or *Staphylococcus* contributes to a fulminating course that may result in death. The development of lobar consolidation, pleural effusion, or cavitation suggests bacterial superinfection.

Varicella-zoster. The varicella-zoster virus, which causes chickenpox and shingles, may produce a severe pneumonia in adults. Patients on immunosuppressive therapy or with lymphoma are at greatest risk. Chest radiographs characteristically show diffuse bilateral ill-defined nodular opacities 5–10 mm in diameter. These opacities usually resolve completely although in some patients they involute and calcify to produce innumerable small (2–3 mm) calcified nodules (Fig. 17.9).

Fungal Infection

Fungal infections are now seen with increased frequency, owing to an increase in the incidence of disease caused by pathogenic fungi in healthy hosts and the emergence of opportunistic species in immunnocompromised hosts. Fungi can cause pulmonary disease by several mechanisms. Some fungi, including *Histoplasma capsulatum*, *Coccidioides immitis*, and *Blastomyces dermatitidis*, are primary pathogens and most commonly infect normal hosts. Other fungi, most notably *Aspergillus*, *Candida*, and *Cryptococcus*, are opportunistic pathogens in immunocompromised individuals. In all cases, the fungi elicit a necrotizing granulomatous reaction. The high mortality of untreated invasive infection and the

availability of effective antifungal therapy with intravenous amphotericin B and the oral azoles (e.g., fluconazole, intraconazole) has made the early and accurate diagnosis of fungal infection imperative. A number of serologic assays (complement fixation, immunodiffusion) and histologic methods are available for the accurate diagnosis of fungal infection.

Histoplasmosis. *Histoplasma capsulatum* is endemic to certain areas of North America—most notably the Ohio, Mississippi, and the St. Lawrence River Valleys—and Mexico. The overwhelming majority (95–99%) of infections caused by *H. capsulatum* are asymptomatic. A routine chest film demonstrating multiple well-defined, calcified nodules <1 cm in size, with or without calcified hilar or mediastinal lymph nodes, may be the only indication of prior infection.

Acute histoplasma infection most often presents with the abrupt onset of flu-like symptoms. The chest radiograph in such patients may be normal or may show nonspecific changes, including subsegmental air-space opacities with or without associated hilar lymph enlargement. If the patient inhales a large inoculum of organisms, widespread, fairly discrete nodular opacities 3–4 mm in diameter are seen with hilar adenopathy. Alternatively, acute histoplasmosis may result in a solitary, sharply defined nodular opacity less than 3 cm in diameter, which is termed a "histoplasmoma." Histoplasmomas are most common in the lower lobes and frequently calcify.

H. capsulatum can also cause chronic pulmonary disease, usually in patients with underlying emphysema. Unilateral or bilateral upper lobe cicatrizing atelectasis with marked hilar retraction may mimic the radiographic findings seen in postprimary tuberculosis. Similarly, chronic upper lobe fibrocavitary disease may be seen. Involvement of the mediastinum by chronic

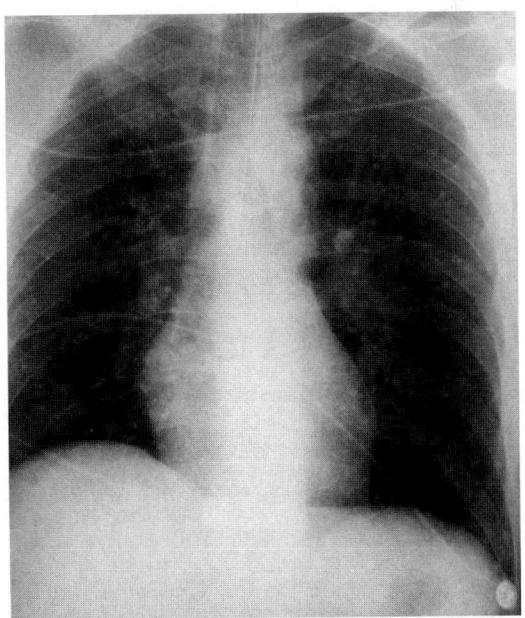

Figure 17.9. Healed Varicella Pneumonia. Frontal chest radiograph in a 38-year-old man shows multiple small calcified nodules representing healed varicella pneumonia.

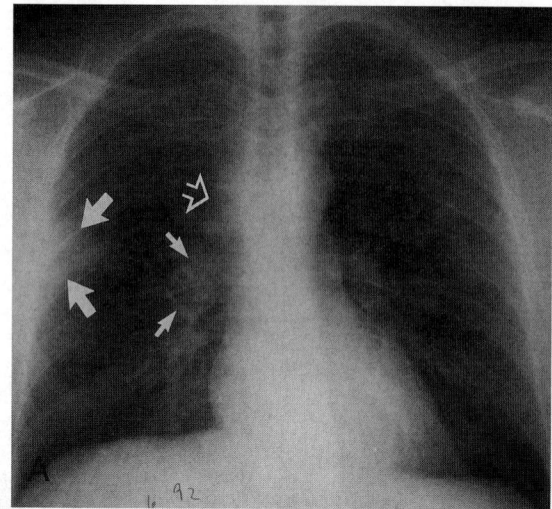

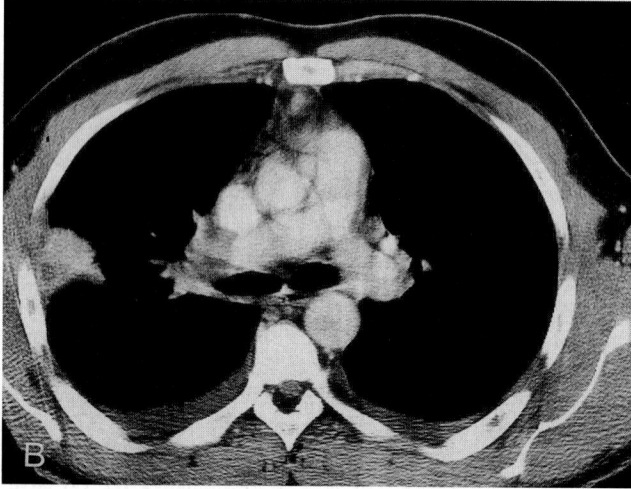

Figure 17.10. Primary Coccidioides Infection. A. Frontal radiograph in a 42-year-old man reveals a pleural-based, wedge-shaped opacity in the peripheral portion of the right upper lobe (*large arrows*) with enlarged right hilar (*small arrows*) and paratracheal (*open arrow*) nodes. **B.** A CT confirms the presence of right hilar nodal enlargement and shows a small focus of necrosis within the parenchymal lesion. Fluoroscopically guided transthoracic biopsy of the peripheral lung lesion revealed coccidioidomycosis.

granulomatous inflammation may lead to fibrosing mediastinitis whereas endobronchial disease can produce bronchostenosis.

Asymptomatic blood-borne dissemination of *H. capsulatum* is common as judged by the frequency of calcified splenic granulomas in residents of endemic areas. Clinically apparent disseminated histoplasmosis, however, is extremely rare and is usually seen in infants or immunocompromised adults. The chest film most commonly shows widespread 2–3 mm nodules indistinguishable from those of miliary tuberculosis; however, reticular opacities and patchy areas of consolidations may also be seen.

Coccidioidomycosis. *Coccidioides immitis* is endemic to the southwestern United States and San Joaquin Valley of California. The four types of clinical and radiographic *Coccidioides* pulmonary infection are acute, per-

sistent, chronic progressive, and disseminated coccidioidomycosis. Acute coccidiodomycosis develops in 40% of infected adults. These patients develop a self-limiting viral-type illness, which is referred to as valley fever when associated with erythema nodosum and arthralgias. The chest radiograph may be normal or show focal or multifocal segmental air-space opacities that resolve over several months. Hilar and mediastinal adenopathy and pleural effusions may be seen in association with parenchymal disease (Fig. 17.10).

Patients whose symptoms or radiographic abnormalities persist longer than 6–8 weeks are considered to have persistent coccidioidomycosis. The radiographic features of persistent pulmonary disease include coccidioidal nodules or masses (coccidioidomas), persistent areas of consolidation, and miliary nodules. Coccidioidal nodules are areas of round pneumonia, usually located in the subpleural regions of the upper lobes. These nodules tend to cavitate rapidly and produce characteristic thin-walled cavities. In chronic progressive disease, upper lobe fibrocavitary disease similar to postprimary tuberculosis and histoplasmosis is seen. Disseminated (miliary) coccidioidomycosis is relatively rare and usually affects immunocompromised patients and non-Caucasians (Fig. 17.11).

Blastomycosis. North American blastomycosis, caused by *B. dermatitidis*, is a chronic systemic disease primarily affecting the lungs and skin. Its geographic distribution overlaps that of histoplasmosis, extending farther to the east and north. The pulmonary infection is often asymptomatic. Symptomatic infection resembles that of an acute bacterial pneumonia. The radiographic findings in pulmonary blastomycosis are nonspecific. The most common manifestation of disease is homogeneous nonsegmental air-space opacification with a propensity for the upper lobes. A less common presentation is single or multiple masses that cavitate in 15% of cases. Pulmonary masses occur in patients with prolonged symptoms (>1 month) and may mimic bronchogenic carcinoma. A third pattern of disease is diffuse reticulonodular opacities. Pleural effusion and lymph node enlargement are uncommon. A disseminated miliary form may be seen in immunocompromised hosts.

Aspergillus. *Aspergillus* species is responsible for a spectrum of pulmonary disease in humans. *Aspergillus* pulmonary disease includes aspergilloma or mycetoma formation within preexisting cavities, semi-invasive (chronic necrotizing) aspergillosis in patients with mildly impaired immunity, invasive pulmonary aspergillosis in the neutropenic lymphoma or leukemia patient, and allergic bronchopulmonary aspergillosis in the hyperimmune patient.

An aspergilloma (mycetoma, fungus ball) is a ball of hyphae, mucus, and cellular debris that colonizes a preexisting bullae or a parenchymal cavity created by some other pathogen or destructive process. Invasion into adjacent lung parenchyma does not occur unless host defense mechanisms are compromised. The mycetoma is usually asymptomatic, but may cause hemoptysis that may be massive (>350 cc/24 hours). An aspergilloma is seen as a solid, round mass within an upper lobe cavity, with an "air crescent" separating the mycetoma from the cavity wall (Fig. 17.12) The mycetoma is usually free within the cavity and can be seen to roll dependently on decubitus radiographs or CT. Progressive apical pleural thickening adjacent to a cavity is a common radiographic finding and should prompt a search for a complicating mycetoma.

Semi-invasive and invasive aspergillosis are discussed in the section on infections in immunocompromised patients, and allergic bronchopulmonary aspergillosis is reviewed in chapter 19.

Parasitic Infection

Parasitic infections of the lung are relatively uncommon in the United States. However, increasing travel to countries where parasites are endemic, the immigration of people from these regions to the United States, and an increasing number of immunocompromised patients requires a familiarity with these infections. In general, parasitic diseases of the thorax are manifested by either a direct invasion of lungs and pleura or, less commonly, a hypersensitivity reaction.

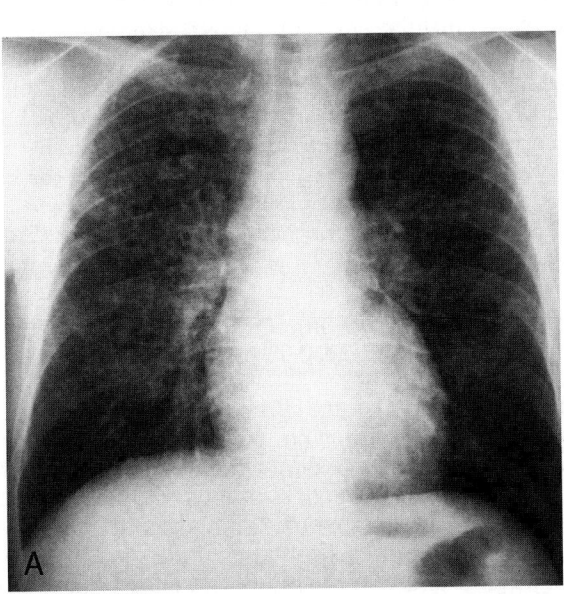
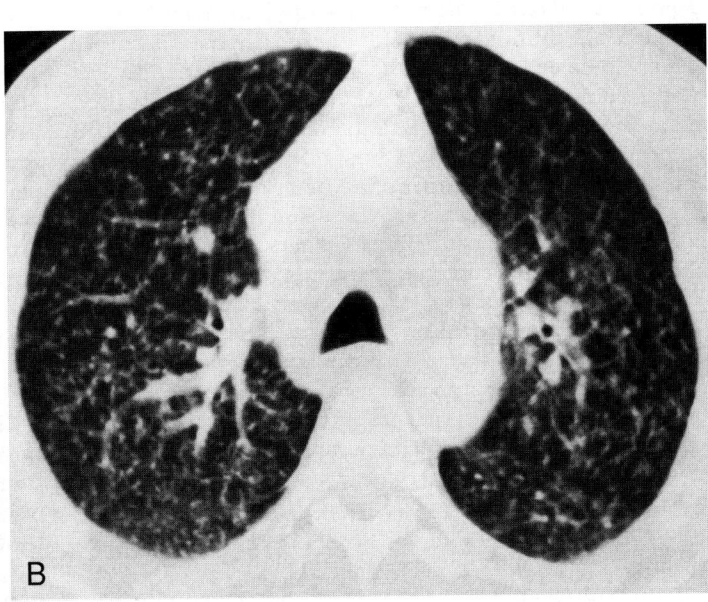

Figure 17.11. Disseminated (Miliary Coccidioidomycosis). A. Frontal radiograph in a 42-year-old patient with AIDS shows miliary nodulation with enlarged hilar and mediastinal nodes. **B.** CT confirms the presence of diffuse nodular and reticular opacities. Transbronchial biopsy showed *Coccidioides* infection.

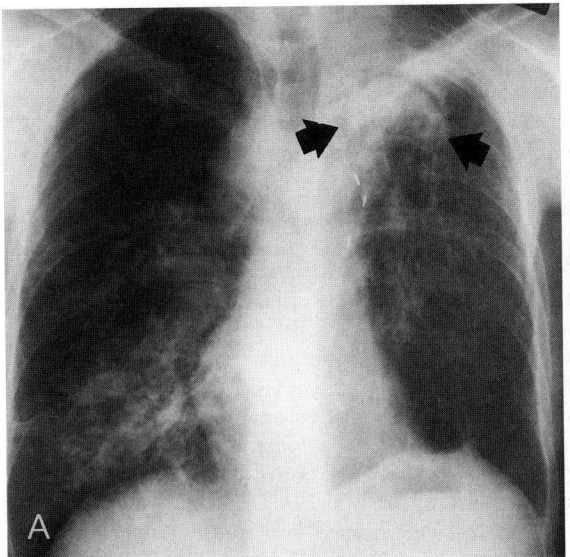
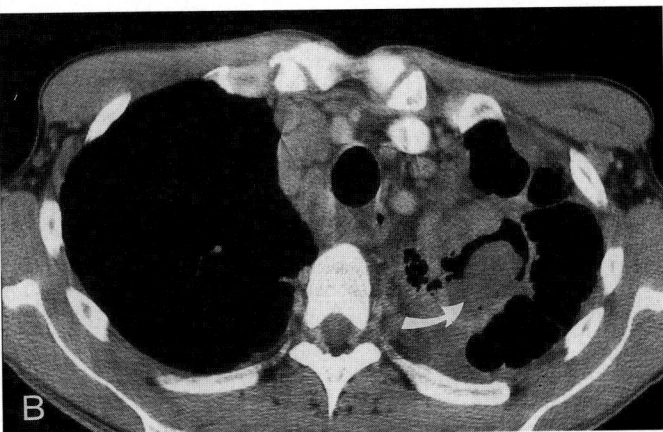

Figure 17.12. Aspergilloma. A. PA chest radiograph in a 32-year-old man with long-standing bullous disease from sarcoidosis and prior left upper lobectomy for aspergilloma. A mass (*arrows*) is seen in the left upper lung capped by a crescent of air with adjacent apical pleural thickening. **B.** A CT shows a low-density mass representing a mycetoma (*curved white arrow*) within a pre-existing cavity. Sputum showed heavy *Aspergillus*.

Amebiasis. Symptomatic infection with *Entamoeba histolytica* is usually confined to the GI tract and liver. If the infection remains confined to the subphrenic space, a right pleural effusion and basilar atelectasis may result from local diaphragmatic inflammation. The most common method of pleuropulmonary involvement by amebiasis is by the direct intrathoracic extension of infection from a hepatic abscess. This transdiaphragmatic spread of organisms may extend into the right pleural space to produce an empyema or may involve the right lower lobe to produce an amebic pneumonia or lung abscess.

Hydatid Disease (Echinococcosis) of the Lung. *Echinococcus granulosus* is the cause of most cases of human hydatid disease. The disease is endemic in sheep-raising areas and is relatively uncommon in the United States. Dogs are the usual definitive hosts, with sheep acting as intermediate hosts. When a human becomes an accidental intermediate host, disease may result. The larval organisms travel to the liver and lungs and, if they survive host defenses, encyst and gradually enlarge. Pulmonary echinococcal cysts are composed of three layers: an exocyst (chitinous layer), which is a protective membrane; an inner endocyst, which produces the daughter cysts; and a surrounding capsule of compressed, fibrotic lung known as the pericyst.

Pulmonary echinococcal cysts characteristically present as well-circumscribed, spherical soft-tissue masses. In distinction to hepatic cysts, lung cysts do not have calcified walls. The cysts range in size from 1–20 cm, with a predilection for the lower lobes and the right side. Although most cysts remain asymptomatic, patients may present when the cyst develops a communication with the bronchial tree. If the pericyst ruptures, a thin crescent of air will be seen around the periphery of the cyst, producing the "meniscus" or "crescent" sign. If the cyst itself ruptures, the contents of the cyst are expelled into the airways producing an air-fluid level. On occasion, the cyst wall may be seen crumpled and floating within a noncollapsed pericyst, producing the pathognomonic "sign of the camalote" or "water lily" sign. Rarely, a cyst will rupture into the pleural space producing a large pleural effusion.

Paragonimiasis results from infection with the lung fluke *Paragonimus westermani.* The organism is found predominantly in the Far East and is usually acquired by eating raw crabs or snails. Infestation of the lung may be asymptomatic or may present with cough, hemoptysis, dyspnea, and fever. In 20% of affected patients, the chest radiograph is normal. The most common radiographic finding is multiple cysts with variable wall thickness. These cystic opacities may become confluent, and are often associated with focal atelectasis and subsegmental consolidation. Dense linear opacities representing the burrows of the organisms may be identified. Because the flukes penetrate the pleura, effusions are common and may be massive.

Schistosomiasis. Human schistosomiasis is caused by three blood flukes: *Schistosoma mansoni, S. japonicum,* and *S. haematobium.* It is one of the most important parasitic infestations of humans worldwide although it is rarely acquired in the United States. The life cycle of the fluke is complex, with human infestation acquired through contact with infested water. The larvae penetrate the skin or oropharyngeal mucosa and travel via the venous circulation to the pulmonary capillaries. As the larvae pass through the lungs, an allergic response may develop, which presents radiographically as transient air-space opacities (eosinophilic pneumonia) that resolve spontaneously. The larvae then pass through the pulmonary capillaries into the systemic circulation. *S. japonicum* and *S. mansoni* eventually migrate to the mesenteric venules while *S. haematobium* migrates to bladder venules. The mature flukes produce ova, which may embolize to the lungs where they implant in and around small pulmonary arterioles. The organism induces granulomatous inflammation and fibrosis, which leads to an obliterative arteriolitis resulting in pulmonary hypertension and cor pulmonale. Radiographically, a diffuse fine reticular pattern is most commonly seen in association with dilatation of the central pulmonary arteries. Small nodular opacities resembling miliary TB may be seen as granulomata form around ova.

INFECTION IN THE IMMUNOCOMPROMISED HOST AND AIDS

Immunocompromise is defined as a decrease in the normal host defense mechanisms that fight infection. Immunocompromised patients include those with HIV infection or underlying hematologic malignancy and those receiving chemotherapeutic and immunosuppressive therapy. The types of pulmonary infection seen in the immunocompromised patient depend on the specific defect(s) in host defense mechanisms. Although the majority of pulmonary complications in immunocompromised patients are infectious in nature, noninfectious complications of disease can account for up to 25% of lung disease in this population. The accurate identification of the predominant radiographic pattern of abnormality in the immunocompromised patient helps limit the differential diagnostic considerations (Tables 17.1, 17.2)(8).

Bacterial Pneumonia. Bacteria are the most common cause of pneumonia in immunocompromised hosts. In HIV-infected patients, bacterial pneumonia occurs early in the course of infection with an incidence four times that seen in the normal population. The most common organisms causing pneumonia in HIV patients are *S. pneumoniae* and *H. influenzae.* Uncommon causes of bacterial pneumonia in the AIDS population include *Moraxella cattharalis, Rhodococcus equi,* and *Rochalimaea hensalae* (bacillary angiomatosis). In the non–HIV immunocompromised patient, *Staphylococcus aureus* and gram-negative aerobes including Klebsiella, Proteus, *E. coli,* Pseudomonas, Enterobacter, and Serratia are the most common bacterial pathogens. Bacterial pneumonia is characterized by focal segmental or lobar air-space opacities. Cavitation is more frequent in the immunocompromised population compared with normal individuals and may occur as multiple microabscesses. Multilobar involvement and diffuse pneumonia may occur and is distinctly unusual in normal individuals. Pleural effusions and empyema are uncommon.

Table 17.1. Radiographic Patterns of Abnormality in Non–HIV Immunocompromised Patients

Pattern	Potential etiology
Lobar/segmental consolidation	Gram-negative bacteria
	Gram-positive bacteria
	Legionella
Nodules +/– cavitation	Fungi
	Aspergillus species
	Coccidioides imitis
	Cryptococcus neoformans
	Mucor species
	Nocardia asteroides
	Legionella micdadei
	Neoplasm
	Other
Diffuse lung disease	*Pneumocystis carinii*
	Viral pneumonia
	Fungi
	Toxoplasma gondii
	Strongyloides stercoralis
	Drug reaction
	Hemorrhage
	Radiation pneumonitis
	NSIP
	Lymphangitic carcinoma

Modified from McLoud TC, Naidich DP. Radiol Clin North Am 1992;30(3):525–554.

Renal transplant recipients and patients on highdose corticosteroids are at increased risk of pneumonia caused by *Legionella pneumophila* and *Legionella micdadei* (Pittsburgh agent). *L. pneumophila* causes multilobar focal areas of consolidation, sometimes with cavitation and pleural effusion. The Pittsburgh agent causes a characteristic appearance of multiple, well-circumscribed, centrally cavitating nodules.

Nocardia is a gram-positive, branching filamentous bacillus that is weakly acid-fast. *N. asteroides* is the most important cause of pulmonary disease. It is usually an opportunistic infection in patients on immunosuppressive therapy, those with lymphoma or leukemia, and patients with alveolar proteinosis.

The most frequent radiographic presentation is a homogeneous, nonsegmental air-space opacity or a mass. Cavitation is frequent, and infection may extend into the pleural space and chest wall to produce empyema and osteomyelitis, respectively. Hilar lymph nodes may be enlarged. Treatment is with sulfur antibiotics.

Tuberculosis. The incidence of tuberculosis has increased considerably since the onset of the AIDS epidemic. Most cases are caused by reactivation of previously acquired disease. The diagnosis of TB in immunocompromised hosts is complicated because skin reactivity and sputum analysis are less sensitive in immunocompromised hosts and the yield of bronchoalveolar lavage is decreased in this patient population. The chest radiographic findings depend on the stage of HIV infection and the degree of immune dysfunction that can be estimated by the CD4 count. In the early stages of AIDS (CD4 >200 cells/mm^3), a postprimary pattern of upper lobe fibrocavitary disease indistinguishable from

that seen in the immunocompetent patient is most common. Later in the course of AIDS (CD4 50–200 cells/mm^3), the radiographic features most often associated with primary disease are seen and include lobar consolidation, mediastinal and hilar lymphadenopathy, and pleural effusion (9). Rim-enhancing nodes with central necrosis on CT are a characteristic finding and should strongly suggest tuberculosis in a patient with AIDS. In advanced AIDS (CD4 <50 cells/mm^3), the radiographic findings are atypical and are characterized by diffuse reticular or nodular (miliary) opacities.

Mycobacterium avium-intracellulare (MAI) infection is the most common nontuberculous mycobacterial infection in AIDS patients. The disease primarily affects the GI tract, but disseminated disease can involve the chest. Lymphadenopathy is the major radiographic manifestation but nonspecific focal air-space opacity or diffuse nodular opacities may be seen. Infection by *M. kansasii* may produce an identical pattern to post primary tuberculosis.

Viral Pneumonia is uncommon in AIDS and other immunocompromised patients with defects in cell-mediated immunity.

Cytomegalovirus (CMV) is a common cause of viral pneumonia in patients with impaired cell-mediated immunity, specifically renal transplant recipients and lymphoma. It is an uncommon cause of pneumonia in the AIDS population. Chest radiographs exhibit diffuse, bilateral lower lobe reticular or nodular opacities.

Table 17.2. Radiographic Patterns of Abnormality in AIDS Patients

Pattern	Potential Etiology
Normal	*P. carinii* pneumonia (PCP)
	TB or fungal infection
	NSIP
Focal lung disease	Bacterial pneumonia
	P. carinii pneumonia
	Mycobacterial/fungal infection
	Non-Hodkin's lymphoma
Diffuse lung disease	*P. carinii* pneumonia
	PCP + other infection (CMV, MAI, MTB, fungus)
	M. tuberculosis
	Fungal infection
	NSIP
	LIP
	Kaposi's sarcoma
Nodules	Non-Hodgkin's lymphoma
	Kaposi's sarcoma
	Septic emboli
	Mycobacterial/fungal infection
Adenopathy	Mycobacterial or fungal infection
	Kaposi's sarcoma
	Non-Hodgkin's lympoma
	P. carinii (uncommon)
Pleural effusion	Kaposi's sarcoma
	Mycobacterial/fungal infection
	Non-Hodgkin's lympoma
	Pyogenic empyema
	P. carinii (uncommon)

Modified from McLoud TC, Naidich DP. Radiol Clin North Am 1992; 30(3):525–554.

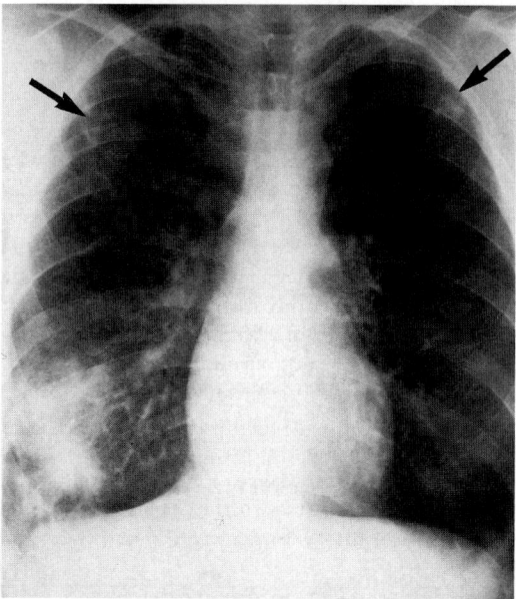

Figure 17.13. Invasive Aspergillosis. PA radiograph in an immuno-compromised patient with aspergillus infection reveals right lower lobe opacification and bilateral upper lobe nodules with cavitation (*arrows*).

Aspergillosis. Invasive *Aspergillus* infection usually occurs in severely immunocompromised patients with neutropenia, most commonly those with leukemia or those receiving chemotherapy or corticosteroids. It occurs less frequently in those with AIDS, usually in the terminal stages of disease. The radiographic manifestations range from large nodular opacities to diffuse parenchymal consolidation (Fig. 17.13). The organism usually invades blood vessels, thus causing infarction. Much of the observed opacity represents hemorrhage and edema. If pleural effusion develops, it usually indicates empyema. Cavitation, in the form of an air crescent, is not usually evident on chest films early in the course of disease, but it characteristically develops when the patient's complement of circulating neutrophils returns to a normal level. CT, particularly HRCT, is useful for the early diagnosis of invasive aspergillosis. The demonstration of a zone of relative decreased attenuation surrounding a dense mass-like opacity has been termed the "CT halo sign" and is relatively specific for invasive aspergillosis in a neutropenic patient (Fig. 17.14). The halo represents a region of edema and hemorrhage where an air crescent will develop, separating the region of infected, necrotic lung from normal parenchyma.

Semi-invasive aspergillosis is an unusual form of *Aspergillus* pulmonary infection seen in patients with mild degrees of immunosuppression. The organism invades previously diseased lung tissue, thus producing slowly progressive air-space opacification or chronic cavitary disease.

Coccidioidomycosis in AIDS and other immunocompromised hosts is usually manifested by disseminated infection rather than the localized granulomatous disease seen in normal hosts. Pulmonary involvement is usually diffuse and produces miliary nodules, diffuse nodules, or reticu-

lonodular opacities (Fig. 17.11). Hilar and mediastinal lymphadenopathy and pleural effusions are uncommon.

Cryptococcosis. *Cryptococcus neoformans* is a budding yeast commonly found in soil and bird droppings. Cryptococcus is the most common cause of fungal infection in the AIDS population but can affect any immunocompromised patient. In some patients, particularly those with AIDS, the organism disseminates from its portal of entry in the lung to involve the central nervous system, bones, and mucocutaneous tissues. Meningitis is the most serious consequence of infection. There are several chest radiographic patterns of disease: single or multiple nodules or masses (which mimic bronchogenic carcinoma) (Fig. 17.15), single or multiple patchy air-space opacities, and multiple small nodules (which mimic miliary TB). Cavitation, lymphadenopathy, and pleural effusion are more commonly seen in AIDS patients than in those without AIDS.

Candidiasis. *Candida albicans* is an unusual cause of pneumonia in the immunocompromised patient. Patients with severe neutropenia due to lymphoma or leukemia in the late stages of disease are most susceptible. The diagnosis is often difficult because *Candida* is a common colonizer in immunocompromised patient and its presence is often associated with other opportunistic infections. Chest radiographs in patients with *Candida* pneumonia show diffuse bilateral, nonsegmental air-space or interstitial opacities. Miliary nodules may be seen but cavitation, adenopathy, and pleural effusion are uncommon features.

Mucormycosis is a rare cause of pneumonia in immunocompromised patients with lymphoma, leukemia, or diabetes. Pulmonary infection is commonly accompanied by paranasal sinus infection, which may extend to involve the brain or meninges. Chest radiographic appearances include a solitary nodule or mass or focal air-space opacity that may cavitate. Pleural effusion is uncommon.

Pneumocystis carinii Pneumonia. *P. carinii* is a fungus commonly found in human lungs although clinically sig-

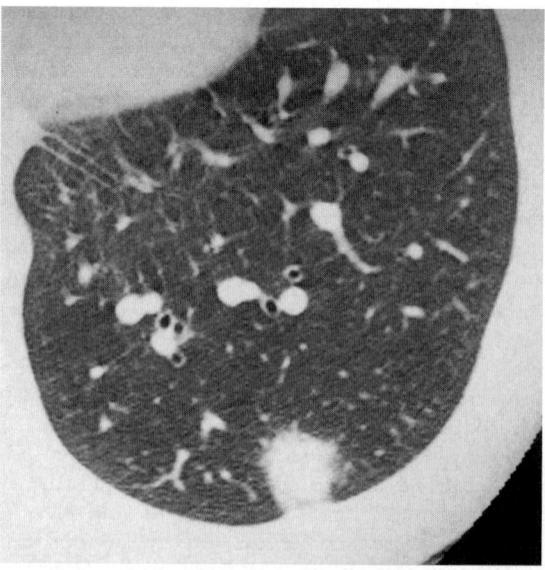

Figure 17.14. HRCT of Invasive Aspergillosis (the "CT Halo" Sign). Coned-down view of an HRCT through the left lower lobe in a patient receiving high-dose corticosteroid therapy shows a nodule with a halo of ground-glass opacity characteristic of invasive aspergillosis.

nificant pneumonia is seen only in immunocompromised individuals. *P. carinii* pneumonia (PCP) is most common in AIDS patients, affecting more than 75% of individuals usually in the late stages of HIV infection (CD4 <200). Organ transplant recipients on immunosuppressive drugs (particularly corticosteroids) and patients with lymphoreticular malignancies are also at increased risk for infection.

The chest radiograph may be normal in the early phase of disease. In such patients, gallium scanning or high-resolution CT of the lung may provide evidence of subradiographic disease. As the disease progresses, a fine reticular or ground-glass pattern develops, particularly in the parahilar regions (Fig. 17.16)(10). Progressive disease leads to confluent symmetric air-space opacification. Pleural effusion or lymph node enlargement is distinctly uncommon (<5%), and should suggest an alternative or additional diagnosis. The diagnosis of PCP in AIDS is made by methenamine silver staining of induced sputum samples or bronchoalveolar lavage fluid specimens.

Several atypical radiographic features of PCP have been described. PCP may manifest as single or multiple pulmonary nodules, simulating fungal infection or malignancy such as Kaposi's sarcoma. Thin-walled cysts or pneumatoceles may develop during the course of disease and are responsible for an increased incidence of spontaneous pneumothorax complicating PCP (Fig. 17.17).

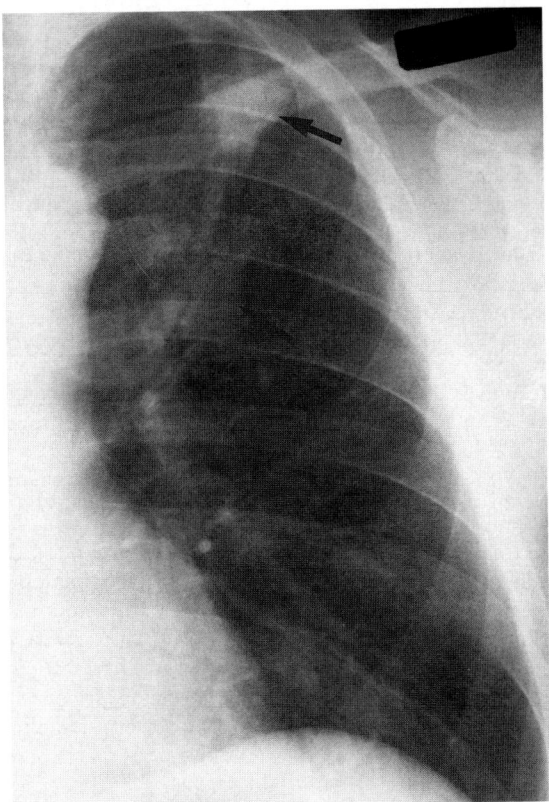

Figure 17.15. Cryptococcus in AIDS. Coned-down view of the left upper lobe in a 45-year-old AIDS patient shows two left upper lobe nodules (*arrows*). Stains of a transthoracic needle biopsy aspirate showed cryptococcal pneumonia.

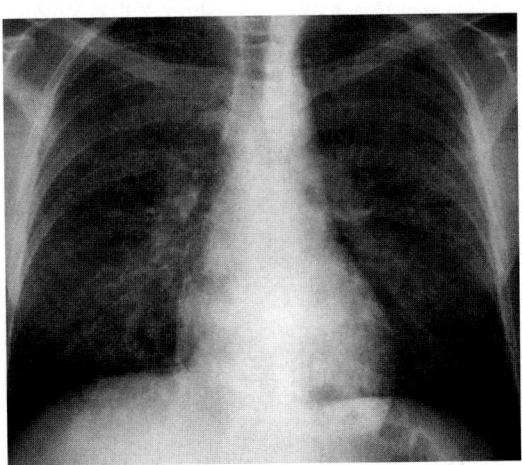

Figure 17.16. *Pneumocystis carinii* **Pneumonia.** Frontal radiograph in a 36-year-old man with HIV infection shows bilateral symmetric fine reticular or ground-glass opacities. Stains of induced sputum revealed *P. carinii*.

Figure 17.17. Lung cysts in *Pneumocystis carinii* **Pneumonia.** CT in a patient with documented *Pneumocystis carinii* pneumonia shows scattered areas of ground-glass opacity with variably sized thin-walled cysts. Note the subpleural location of the large left upper lobe cyst.

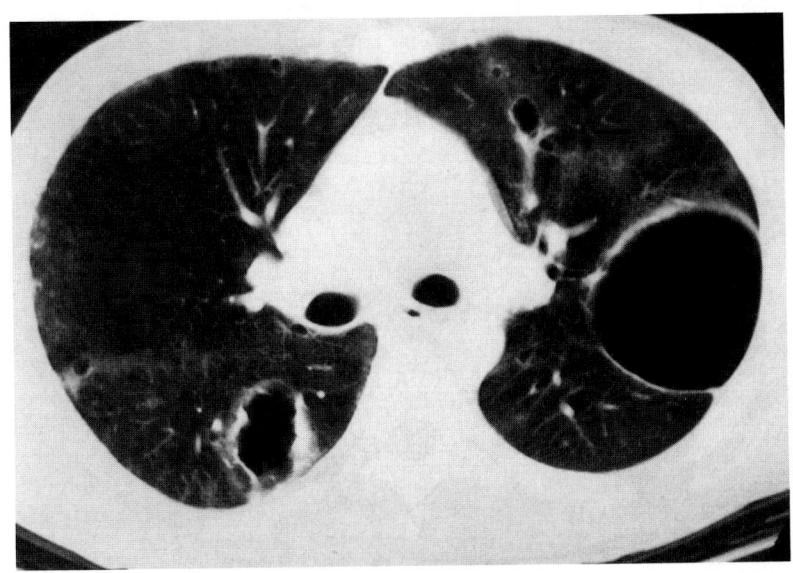

Patients receiving prophylaxis with inhaled aerosolized pentamidine are prone to develop predominantly upper lobe PCP, which simulates postprimary tuberculosis. Rare cases of miliary PCP simulating TB or disseminated fungal infection have been reported. Patients receiving systemic prophylaxis with Bactrim are also at risk for extrapulmonary pneumocystis infection. Systemic pneumocystis infection usually involves the liver, spleen, kidney, and lymph nodes, and appears on CT or US as microabscesses or punctate calcifications.

Toxoplasmosis. *Toxoplasma gondii* is an obligate intracellular protozoan whose definitive host is the cat. Humans acquire the organism by ingestion of material contaminated by oocyst-containing stool. Toxoplasmosis has been estimated to exist in a chronic asymptomatic form in 50% of the population of the United States. Disease can be recognized in four clinicopathologic forms: congenital, ocular, lymphatic, and generalized. Pulmonary involvement is usually seen in the generalized form of the disease that affects immunocompromised hosts including those with AIDS, organ transplant recipients, and patients with leukemia or lymphoma.

The radiographic findings in pulmonary toxoplasmosis include diffuse reticular opacities that resemble acute viral pneumonia. Less commonly, air-space opacities with air bronchograms may be seen. Hilar and mediastinal lymph node enlargement is common, but pleural effusion is rare. With generalized disease, most often seen in patients with AIDS, diffuse bilateral small nodular opacities may be seen.

References

1. Kantor HG. Many radiologic faces of pneumococcal pneumionia. AJR Am J Roentgenol 1981;137:1213–1220.
2. Pierce AK, Sandford JP. Aerobic gram-negative bacillary pneumonias: state of the art. Am Rev Respir Dis 1974;110: 647–658.
3. Bartlett JG, Finegold SM. Anaerobic infections of the lung and pleural space. Am Rev Respir Dis 1974;110:56–77.
4. Kwong JS, Müller NL, Godwin JD, et al. Thoracic actinomycosis: CT findings in eight patients. Radiology 1992;183: 189–192.
5. Choyke PL, Sostman HD, Curtis AM, et al. Adult-onset pulmonary tuberculosis. Radiology 1983;148:357–362.
6. Contreras MA, Cheung OT, Sanders DE, et al. Pulmonary infection with nontuberculous mycobacteria. Am Rev Respir Dis 1988;137:149–152.
7. Conte P, Heitzman ER, Markarian B. Viral pneumonia: roentgen pathologic correlations. Radiology 1970;95: 267–272.
8. McLoud TC, Naidich DP. Thoracic disease in the immunocompromised patient. Radiol Clin North Am 1992;30: 525–554.
9. Shah RM, Kaji AV, Ostrum BJ, Friedman AC. Interpretation of chest radiographs in AIDS patients: usefulness of CD4 lymphocyte counts. Radiographics 1997;17:47–58.
10. McGuiness G. Changing trends in the pulmonary manifestations of AIDS. Radiol Clin North Am 1997;35:1029–1082.

18
Interstitial Lung Disease

Anne S. Hayton
Jeffrey S. Klein

Interstitial lung disease represents a broad spectrum of disorders that primarily affect the pulmonary interstitium (Table 18.1). These diseases present in a variety of manners, most typically with symptoms of progressive dyspnea. However, some patients present with minimal or no symptoms, and the disease is discovered either incidentally or during radiologic screening for interstitial disease associated with collagen vascular disease. Restrictive lung disease and hypoxemia on pulmonary function tests are characteristically present. The radiographic findings produced by interstitial disease are reviewed in chapter 14. High-resolution CT (HRCT) has revolutionized the diagnosis of interstitial lung disease and HRCT's role in the evaluation of interstitial disease is detailed in this chapter.

HRCT OF THE PULMONARY INTERSTITIUM

Normal Anatomy. HRCT provides the most direct radiographic method for assessment of the pulmonary interstitium. The general use of HRCT is in the evaluation of chronic interstitial lung disease, and this is outlined in Table 18.2(1). The pulmonary interstitium is the scaffolding of the lung, providing support for the airways, gas-exchanging units, and vascular structures. A continuous network of connective tissue fibers, the pulmonary interstitium begins at the lung hilum and extends peripherally to the visceral pleura (see Fig. 12.10). The central interstitial compartment extending from the mediastinum peripherally and enveloping the bronchovascular bundles is termed the "axial," or "bronchovascular," interstitium. The axial interstitium is contiguous with the interstitium surrounding the small centrilobular arteriole and bronchiole within the secondary pulmonary lobule where it is called the "centrilobular" interstitium. The most peripheral component of the interstitium is the subpleural or peripheral interstitium, which lies between the visceral pleura and the lung surface. Invaginations of the subpleural interstitium into the lung parenchyma form the borders of the secondary pulmonary lobules and represent the interlobular septa. Extending between the centrilobular interstitium within the lobular core and the interlobular septal/subpleural interstitium in the lobular periphery is a fine network of connective tissue fibers that support the alveolar spaces called the intralobular, parenchymal, or alveolar interstitium.

The secondary pulmonary lobule is defined as that subsegment of lung supplied by three to five terminal bronchioles and separated from adjacent secondary lobules by intervening connective tissue (interlobular septa) (Fig. 18.1). Each terminal bronchiole further subdivides into respiratory bronchioles, alveolar ducts, alveolar sacs, and alveoli. The unit of lung subtended from a single terminal bronchiole is called a pulmonary acinus. The centrilobular artery and preterminal bronchiole are located in the center of the secondary lobule. Pulmonary veins and lymphatics run at the margins of lobules within the interlobular septa, with lymphatics and connective tissue found within the contiguous subpleural interstitium. The secondary pulmonary lobule is typically polyhedral in shape, with each side ranging from 1.0–2.5 cm in length. The interlobular septa are most prominent over the periphery of the lung where they are readily seen on HRCT. At the surface of the lung, these septa are short structures that course perpendicular to the pleural surface and completely separate adjacent lobules. Within the parahilar portions of the lung, the interlobular septa are longer and more obliquely oriented, and they incompletely marginate the secondary lobules.

Normal HRCT Findings. HRCT can demonstrate much of the normal anatomy of the secondary pulmonary lobule. Interlobular septa are normally 0.1-mm thick and can be seen in the lung periphery, particularly along the anterior and mediastinal pleural surfaces (Fig. 18.2). Centrilobular arteries (1 mm in diameter) are V-shaped or Y-shaped structures on HRCT seen within 5–10 mm of the pleural surface. Normal intralobular (0.7 mm) and acinar (0.3–0.5mm) arteries are commonly seen. Normal airways are visible only to within 3 cm of the pleura. With a diameter of 1 mm and a wall thickness of 0.15 mm, the centrilobular bronchiole is not normally visible on HRCT. Pulmonary veins (0.5 cm) are occasionally seen as linear or dot-like structures within 1–2 cm

Table 18.1. The Alphabet Soup of Interstitial Lung Disease

Abbreviation	Disease
AIP	Acute interstitial pneumonia
BOOP	Bronchiolitis obliterans organizing pneumonia
COP	Cryptogenic organizing pneumonia
CWP	Coal worker's pneumoconiosis
DIP	Desquamative interstitial pneumonia
EG	Eosinophilic granuloma
IPF	Idiopathic pulmonary fibrosis
LIP	Lymphocytic interstitial pneumonitis
LAM	Lymphangioleiomyomatosis
NF	Neurofibromatosis
NIP	Nonspecific interstitial pneumonia
PMF	Progressive massive fibrosis
RB-ILD	Respiratory bronchiolitis-associated interstitial lung disease
SLE	Systemic lupus erythematosis
TS	Tuberous sclerosis
UIP	Usual interstitial pneumonia

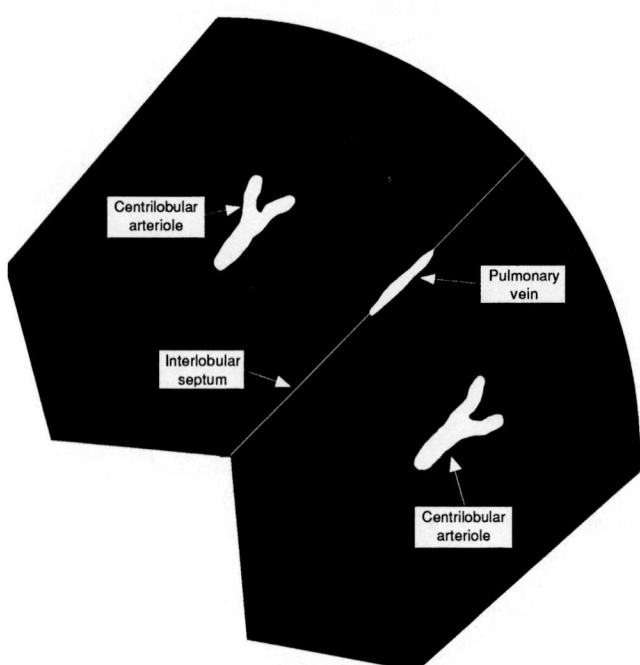

Figure 18.1. Diagram of the Normal Secondary Pulmonary Lobule.

Table 18.2. Utility of High Resolution CT in the Evaluation of Chronic Interstitial Lung Disease

1. Detection of clinically suspected parenchymal abnormality when the chest radiograph is normal or shows questionable abnormality
2. Characterization of parenchymal abnormalities
3. Biopsy planning:
   Determination of route for biopsy, ie. transbronchial, open lung or bronchoalveolar lavage
   Targeting biopsy to area(s) of active disease, avoiding areas of end-stage fibrosis
4. Monitoring of response to therapy or progression of disease

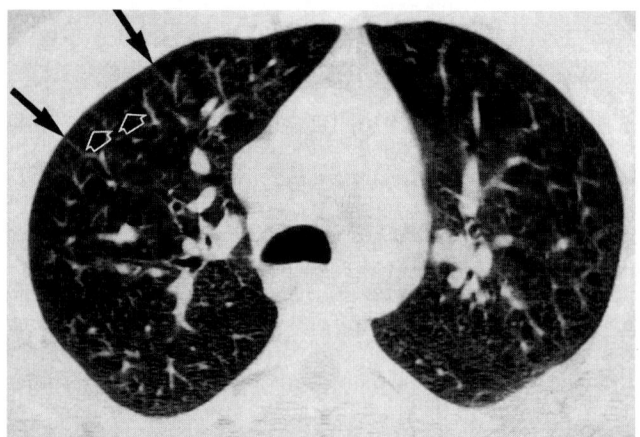

Figure 18.2. HRCT of Normal Lobular Anatomy. Normal interlobular septa (*solid black arrows*) and centrilobular arteries (*open white arrows*) are clearly visible.

of the pleura; when visible, they indicate the location of interlobular septa. The peribronchovascular, centrilobular, and intralobular interstitial compartments are not normally visible on HRCT.

HRCT Signs of Disease

The signs of interstitial lung disease on HRCT are illustrated in Figure 18.3, and their differential diagnosis is listed in Table 18.3 (2).

Interlobular (Septal) Lines. Septal thickening is most often seen as thin, short 1–2-cm lines oriented perpendicular to and intersecting the costal pleura. These lines are best visualized in the subpleural and juxtadiaphragmatic regions of the lung where they outline the anterior and posterior margins of secondary lobules. In the central regions of the lung, the thickened septa can completely envelope lobules to produce polygonal structures. Although septa can be seen in normal individuals, these lines are thicker (>1 mm) and more numerous in patients with diseases primarily affecting the interlobular interstitium such as interstitial pulmonary edema, idiopathic pulmonary fibrosis (IPF), and lymphangitic carcinomatosis (Fig. 18.4). Interlobular lines on HRCT are the equivalent of Kerley's B lines seen in the infero-

lateral portions of the lungs on frontal radiographs. Within the central regions of the lung, long (2–6 cm) linear opacities representing obliquely oriented connective tissue septa can be seen; these are the equivalent of radiographic Kerley's A lines.

Intralobular Lines. In some patients, a lattice of fine lines is seen within the central portion of the pulmonary lobule radiating out toward the thickened lobular borders to produce a "spokewheel" or "spider web" appearance. These lines are not normally visible on HRCT and represent thickening of the intralobular or parenchymal interstitium. Intralobular lines usually represent fibrosis and are most commonly seen in IPF and other forms of usual interstitial pneumonia. However, intralobular

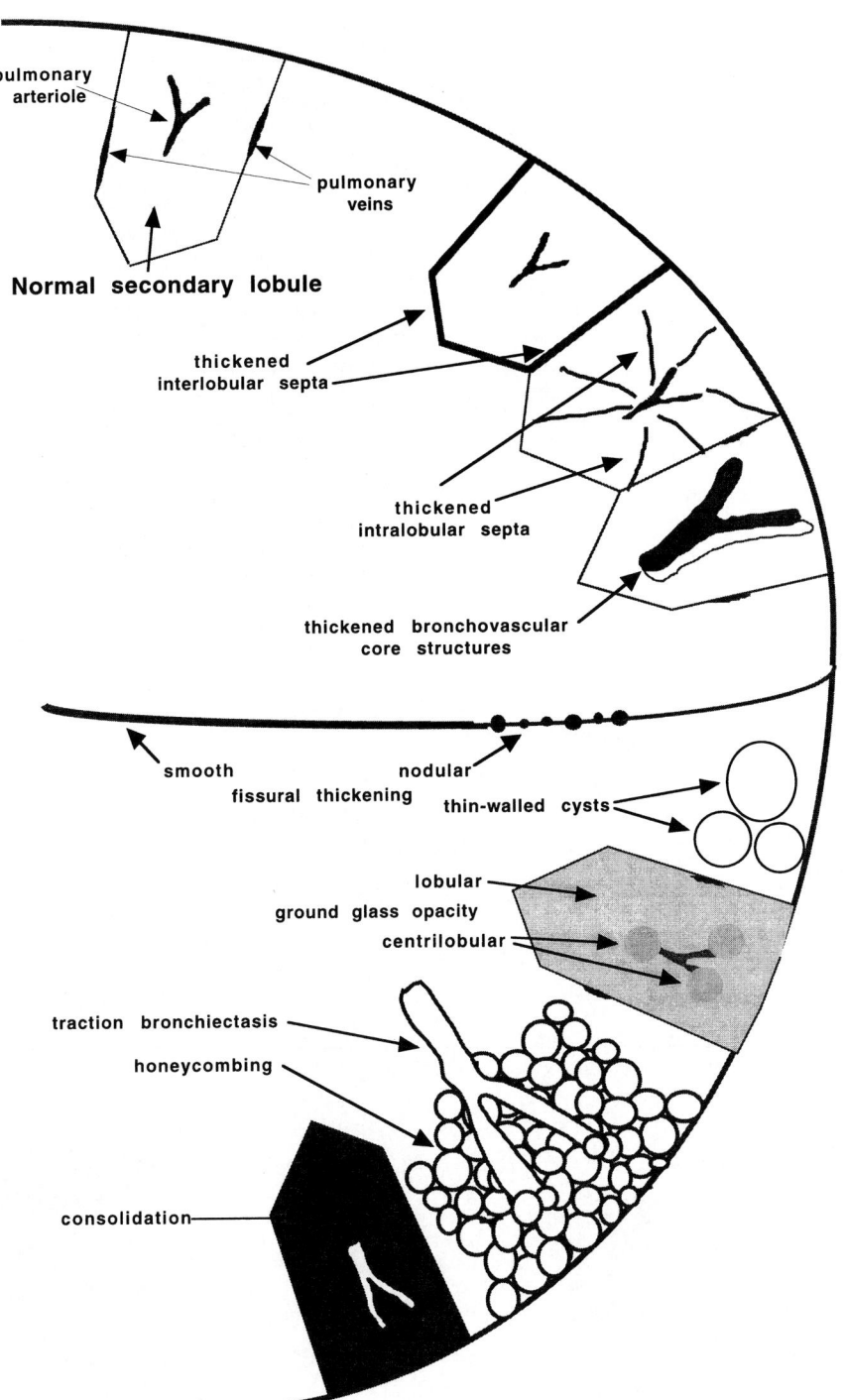

Figure 18.3. HRCT Findings in Interstitial Lung Disease. (Reprinted with permission from The Radiologist, Baltimore: Williams & Wilkins, 1998 in press.)

lines can also be seen in other infiltrative diseases such as pulmonary alveolar proteinosis (Fig. 18.5).

"Thickened" Fissures. The apparent thickening of interlobar fissures in patients with interstitial lung disease is usually a direct extension of the thickening of interlobular septa to involve the subpleural interstitium of the lung. Although such a process normally involves all pleural surfaces equally, the "thickening" is usually best appreciated on the fissures, where two layers of visceral pleura—and therefore two layers of subpleural interstitium—are seen outlined on either side by aerated lung. The fissural thickening can be smooth or nodular.

Smooth fissural thickening is virtually indistinguishable from a small amount of pleural fluid within the fissure, and it is most commonly seen with pulmonary edema. Nodular fissural thickening is commonly seen in sarcoidosis and lymphangitic carcinomatosis (Fig. 18.4), where the nodules lie within the subpleural lymphatics.

Thickened Bronchovascular Structures of the lung results from thickening of the peribronchovascular interstitium. This produces apparent enlargement of perihilar vascular structures and thickening of bronchial walls, which is the HRCT equivalent of peribronchial cuffing and tram tracking seen radiographi-

Table 18.3. Differential Diagnostic HRCT Features in Interstitial Lung Disease

HRCT Finding	Differential Diagnosis	HRCT Finding	Differential Diagnosis
Interlobular (septal) lines	Interstitial edema Lymphangitic carcinomatosis Sarcoidosis Idiopathic pulmonary fibrosis (and other forms of UIP)	Irregular lung interfaces Micronodules–random distribution	Pulmonary edema IPF (UIP) Sarcoidosis Miliary tuberculosis or histoplasmosis Hematogenous metastases
Intralobular lines	IPF (UIP) Asbestosis Alveolar proteinosis Hypersensitivity pneumonitis (chronic)	 Micronodules–	Silicosis/Coal worker's pneumoconiosis (CWP) Eosinophilic granuloma (EG) Sarcoidosis
''Thickened'' fissures	Pulmonary edema Sarcoidosis Lymphangitic carcinomatosis	perilymphatic distribution Ground glass opacities	Lymphangitic carcinomatosis Silicosis/CWP Usual interstitial pneumonia (UIP)
Peribronchovascular interstitial thickening	Pulmonary edema (smooth) Sarcoidosis (nodular) Lymphangitic carcinomatosis (smooth or nodular)		Desquamative interstitial pneumonia (DIP) Acute interstitial pneumonia (AIP) Hypersensitivity pneumonitis
Centrilobular nodules	Hypersensitivity pneumonitis BOOP/COP Respiratory bronchiolitis-associated interstitial lung disease (RB-ILD)		Bronchiolitis obliterans organizing pneumonia (BOOP/COP) RB-ILD Hemorrhage
Subpleural lines	Asbestosis IPF (UIP)		Pneumocystis carinii pneumonia Cytomegalovirus pneumonia Alveolar proteinosis
Parenchymal bands	Asbestosis IPF (UIP) Sarcoidosis	Architectural distortion Traction bronchiectasis	UIP/IPF Sarcoidosis Silicosis/CWP
Honeycombing	IPF (UIP) Asbestosis Hypersensitivity pneumonitis (chronic) Sarcoidosis	Conglomerate mass	Sarcoidosis Silicosis Coal worker's pneumoconiosis (CWP) Radiation fibrosis
Thin-walled cysts	Eosinophilic granuloma (EG) Lymphangioleiomyomatosis (LAM) Tuberous sclerosis Neurofibromatosis (pneumatocele) (emphysema)	Consolidation	Bronchiolitis obliterans organizing pneumonia (BOOP/COP) Sarcoidosis Acute interstitial pneumonia (AIP) Usual interstitial pneumonia (UIP)

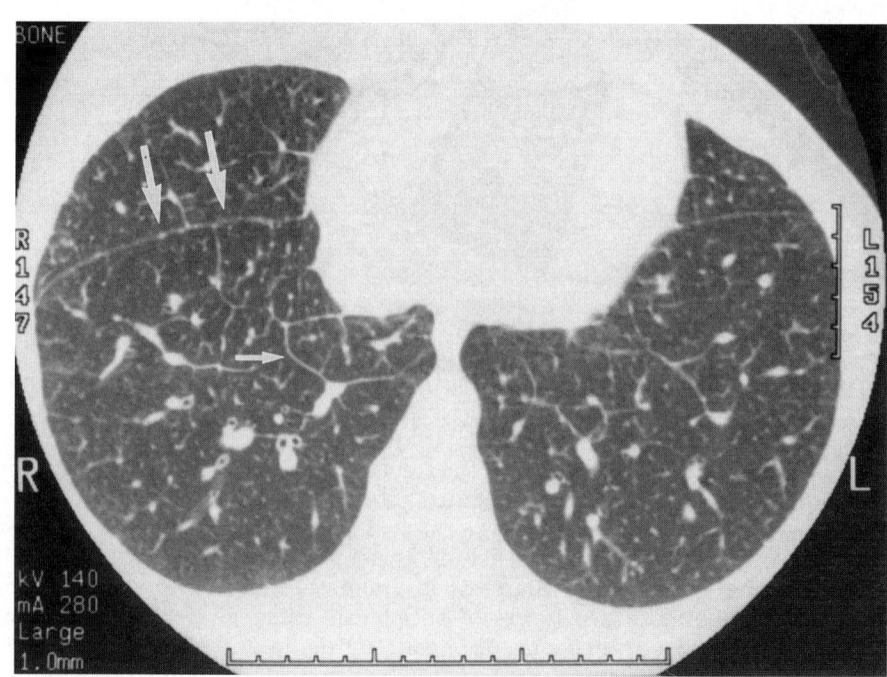

Figure 18.4. Interlobular Septal Lines in Lymphangitic Carcinomatosis. HRCT scan through the lower lobes in a patient with lymphangitic carcinomatosis shows thickened interlobular septa (*small arrow*). Note the presence of nodular fissural thickening (*large arrows*), another common finding in this disorder.

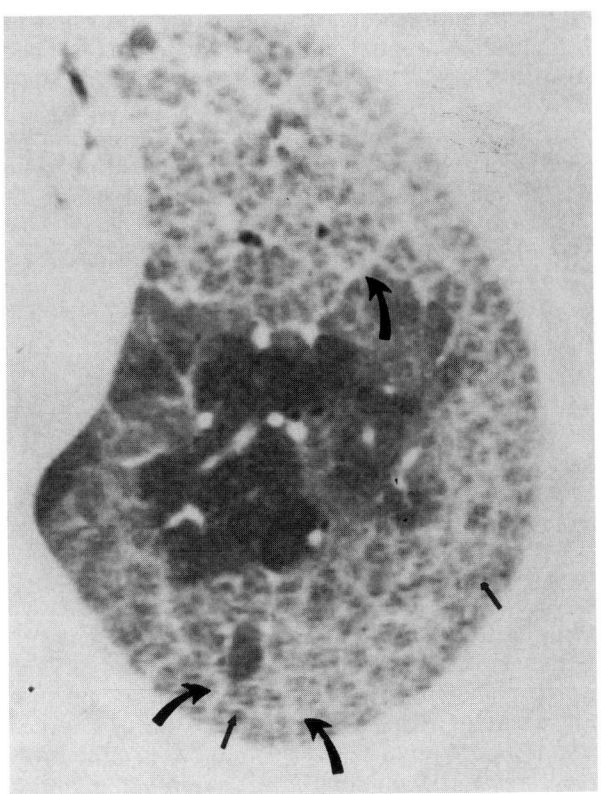

Figure 18.5. Intralobular Lines in Pulmonary Alveolar Proteinosis. An HRCT in a patient with pulmonary alveolar proteinosis shows thickening of intralobular (*small arrows*) and interlobular (*curved arrows*) lines associated with widespread ground-glass opacity.

cally. Although pulmonary edema causes smooth thickening of the peribronchovascular interstitium, nodular or irregular thickening can be seen in sarcoidosis (Fig. 18.6) or usual interstitial pneumonitis (UIP). Lymphangitic carcinomatosis can result in either smooth or irregular peribronchovascular thickening; however, the former is more common.

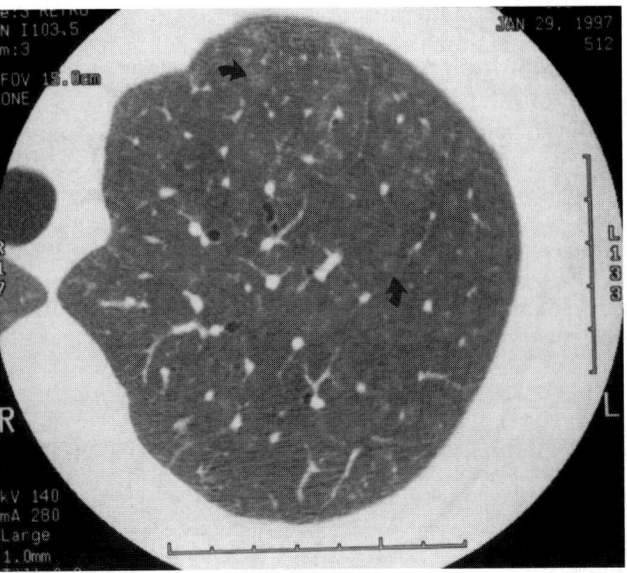

Figure 18.7. Centrilobular Ground-glass Nodules in Subacute Hypersensitivity Pneumonitis. HRCT shows the typical poorly defined centrilobular nodules (*arrows*) of subacute hypersensitivity pneumonitis (bird fancier's lung).

Centrilobular (Lobular Core) Abnormalities. Thickening of the axial interstitium within the lobular core produces an abnormal prominence of the dot-like or branching centrilobular arteriole. Diseases that commonly produce this appearance include pulmonary edema, lymphangitic carcinomatosis, and UIP. The centrilobular bronchiole is not normally seen on HRCT but may be rendered visible as a result of lumenal dilatation or centrilobular interstitium thickening. Small airways disease can produce centrilobular bronchiolar abnormalities seen on HRCT as fluid-filled, dilated, branching, Y-shaped structures producing a "tree-in-bud" appearance. Ill-defined centrilobular nodules represent disease of the bronchiole and adjacent parenchyma and can be seen in subacute hypersensitivity pneumonitis (Fig. 18.7),

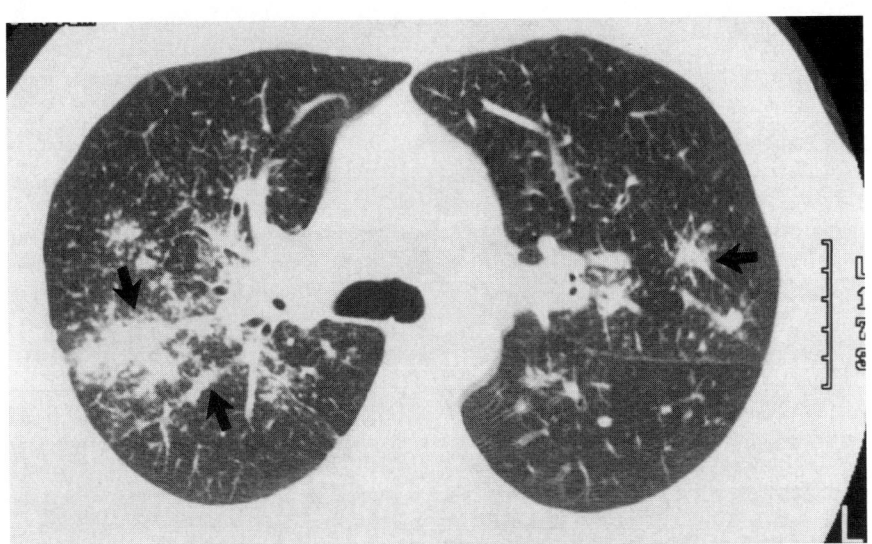

Figure 18.6. Thickened Bronchovascular Structures in Sarcoidosis. In a patient with sarcoidosis, an HRCT shows nodular thickening of the bronchovascular structures (*arrows*) that represents granulomatous inflammation of the axial interstitium.

bronchiolitis obliterans organizing pneumonia (BOOP), and other disorders.

Subpleural Lines. These 5–10-cm long curvilinear opacities are found within 1 cm of the pleura and parallel the chest wall. They are most frequent in the posterior portions of the lower lobes and remain unchanged on prone scans This finding, which probably represents an early phase of lung fibrosis, should be distinguished from a similar line that results from atelectasis in the dependent portion of the lungs in normal individuals. Subpleural lines are most often seen in patients with asbestosis and, less commonly, IPF.

Parenchymal Bands are nontapering linear opacities 2–5 cm in length that extend from the lung to contact the pleural surface. These fibrotic bands can be distinguished from vessels and thickened septa by their length, thickness, course, absence of branching, and their association with regional parenchymal distortion. Parenchymal bands are usually seen in asbestosis, IPF, and sarcoidosis.

Honeycombing, seen as small (6–10 mm) cystic spaces with thick (1–3 mm) walls most often in the posterior subpleural regions of the lower lobes, represents end-stage pulmonary fibrosis of various causes. Pathologically, the cysts are lined by bronchiolar epithelium and are the result of bronchiolectasis. Most patients show additional signs of interstitial disease including thickened interlobular and intralobular lines, parenchymal bands, irregularity of lung interfaces, and areas of ground-glass opacification. Honeycombing is frequently seen in IPF (and other forms of UIP), chronic hypersensitivity pneumonitis (Fig. 18.8), and occasionally sarcoidosis.

Thin-walled Cysts are a common manifestation of late stages of eosinophilic granuloma of lung (EG) and lymphangioleiomyomatosis (LAM). These cysts are slightly larger in diameter (10 mm) than honeycomb cysts, are more uniform in size, and have thinner walls. Honeycomb cysts usually have shared walls, and the cysts of EG and LAM do not. The cysts of EG and LAM are evenly distributed from central to peripheral portions of the upper lobes (Fig. 18.9), with or without lower lobe involvement whereas honeycombing occurs in the subpleural regions of the lower lobes. Although normal lung may be found in the intervening spaces between the cysts of EG and LAM, honeycombing uniformly destroys lung and produces distortion of lung interfaces and traction bronchiectasis, features not found in EG and LAM.

Irregularity of Lung Interfaces. A common HRCT sign of interstitial disease, irregularity of the normally smooth interface between the bronchovascular bundles

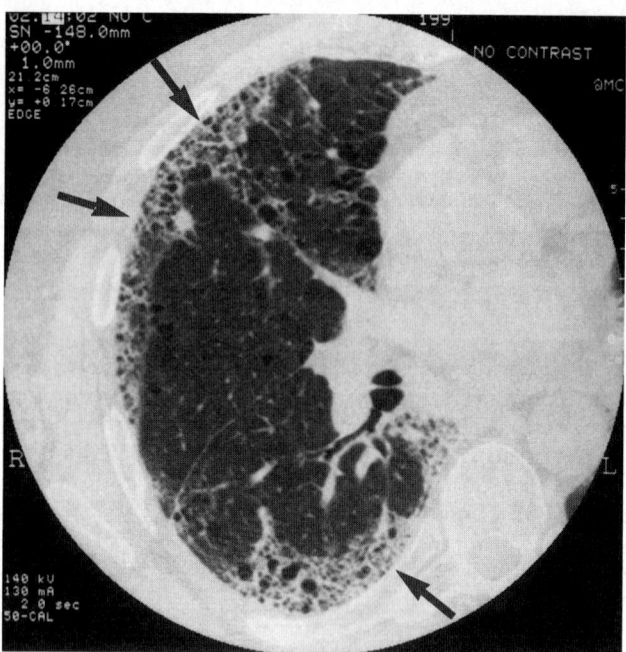

Figure 18.8. Honeycomb Lung in Chronic Hypersensitivity Pneumonitis. HRCT in a patient with farmer's lung shows peripheral honeycombing (*arrows*) indicative of end-stage pulmonary fibrosis.

Figure 18.9. Thin-walled Cysts in Lymphangioleiomyomatosis. An HRCT of a patient with LAM shows multiple variably sized round thin-walled cysts.

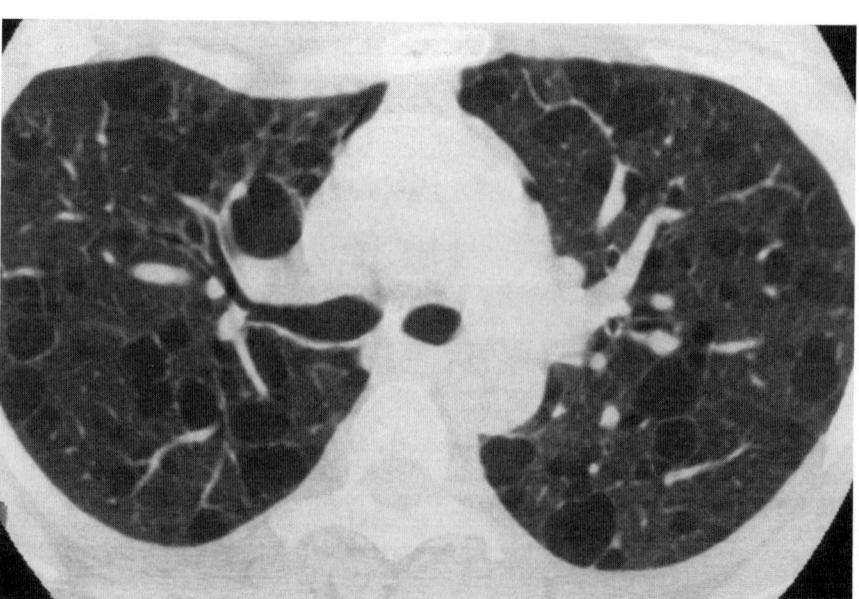

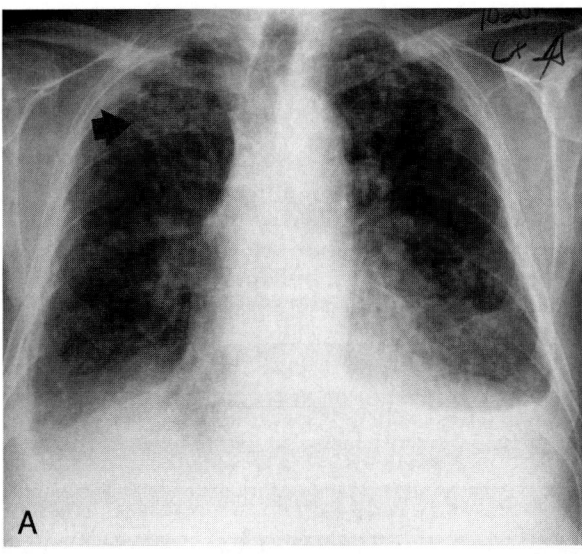 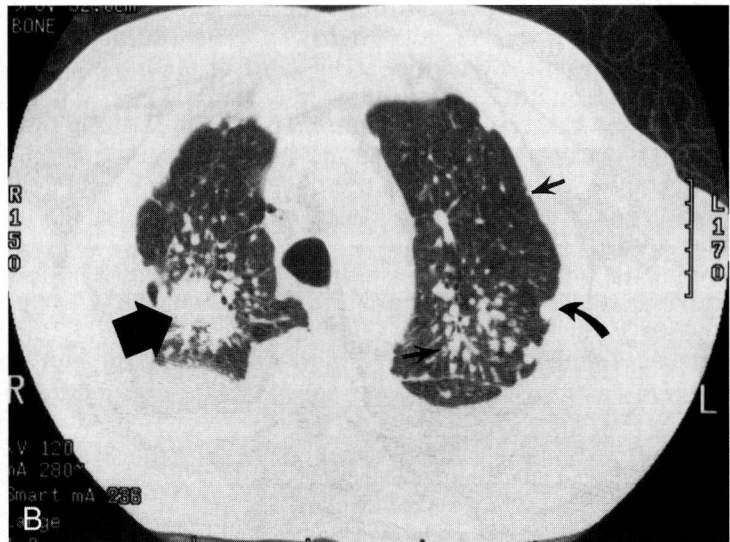

Figure 18.10. Nodules and a Conglomerate Mass in Silicosis. A. A PA radiograph of a 79-year-old patient with silicosis shows diffuse nodules as well as a conglomerate mass in the right upper lobe (*arrow*). **B.** An HRCT through the upper lobes shows peribronchovascu-

lar and subpleural micronodules (*small arrows*), larger nodules (*curved arrow*), and a conglomerate mass representing progressive massive fibrosis (PMF) in the right upper lobe (*large arrow*). The pleural effusions are due to concommitant congestive heart failure.

and the surrounding lung reflects edema or fibrosis of the axial interstitium, or infiltration by granulomas (Fig. 18.6) or tumor. Similarly, irregularity of the interface between fissures or pleural surfaces and adjacent lung indicates peripheral interstitial disease. Pulmonary edema, IPF, and sarcoidosis are the most common causes of irregular lung interfaces.

Micronodules. These 1–3 mm, sharply marginated, round opacities seen on HRCT represent conglomerates of granulomas or tumor cells within the interstitium. These are most often seen in sarcoidosis, EG, silicosis (Fig. 18.10), miliary tuberculosis or histoplasmosis, metastatic adenocarcinoma, and lymphangitic carcinomatosis. They may be seen along the central bronchovascular structures (sarcoidosis, EG), within interlobular septa or subpleural interstitium (sarcoidosis, lymphangitic carcinomatosis, silicosis), or within the substance of the pulmonary lobules (metastatic adenocarcinoma, miliary granulomatous infection). Nodules predominating in the peribronchovascular, interlobular, and subpleural regions, those portions of the interstitium where the lymphatics lie, are said to have a "perilymphatic" distribution. Because it may be difficult to distinguish vertically oriented small upper and lower lobes vessels from interstitial nodules on HRCT, contiguous thick (10 mm) scans are often helpful.

Ground-glass or Hazy Increased Density. Multifocal areas of increased density can sometimes be identified in patients with diffuse interstitial lung disease. These regions, which often respect lobular borders, are distinguished from typical air-space opacification by their granular appearance with maintained visibility of pulmonary vessels and the absence of air bronchograms. These opacities are most often produced by thickening of the alveolar septa with or without lining of the alveolar spaces by inflammatory exudate or fluid. Diseases commonly associated with this appearance include the early,

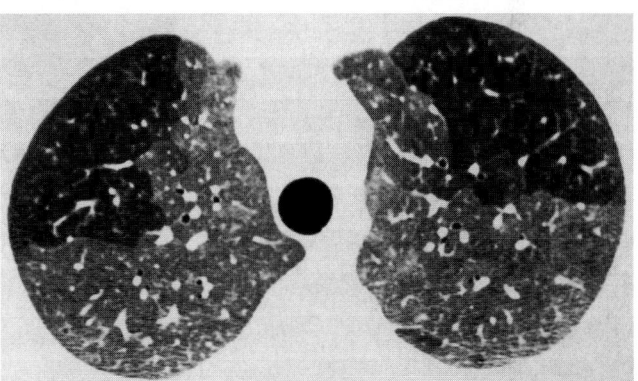

Figure 18.11. Ground-glass Opacity in Acute Hypersensitivity Pneumonitis. An HRCT through the upper lobes shows confluent ground-glass opacity in a patient with hypersensitivity pneumonitis. Note that the pulmonary vessels are still visible within the areas of abnormality.

active phase of UIP, desquamative interstitial pneumonia (DIP), *Pneumocystis carinii* pneumonia, acute hypersensitivity pneumonitis (Fig. 18.11), and interstitial pulmonary edema. The ground-glass densities are occasionally confined to the immediate centrilobular regions of the pulmonary lobules, where they appear as fuzzy nodular densities that outline the normally invisible centrilobular bronchiole (Fig. 18.7). This reflects involvement of the peribronchovascular interstitium and surrounding alveoli by an inflammatory process and is seen in hypersensitivity pneumonitis, BOOP, and panbronchiolitis. The presence of ground-glass opacities is important because it often implies an active inflammatory process or edema that is reversible and warrants aggressive treatment. However, ground-glass abnormality associated with a predominant pattern of honeycombing can represent microscopic pulmonary fibrosis.

Architectural Distortion and Traction Bronchiectasis. Processes that result in extensive parenchymal fibrosis can distort the normal architecture of the lung, creating irregularities of the lung-mediastinal, lung-pleural, and lung-vascular interfaces. Parenchymal distortion is often better appreciated on HRCT than on plain radiographs. Sarcoidosis and UIP (Fig. 18.12) are the diseases most commonly associated with architectural distortion.

A finding commonly associated with architectural distortion is traction bronchiectasis, where fibrosis causes traction on the walls of bronchi, resulting in irregular dilatation. Although this usually involves segmental and subsegmental bronchi, it also can be seen at the intralobular level where traction bronchiolectasis contributes to honeycombing. Traction bronchiectasis is most commonly seen in IPF (Fig. 18.12) and other forms of UIP, but it is also common in long-standing sarcoidosis.

Conglomerate Masses. In some patients with extensive pulmonary fibrosis, masses of fibrotic tissue develop in the parahilar regions of the upper lobes, often associated with peripheral bullous. On CT and HRCT, these masses are seen to contain crowded vessels and dilated bronchi. These conglomerate masses are most often seen in patients with end-stage sarcoidosis but

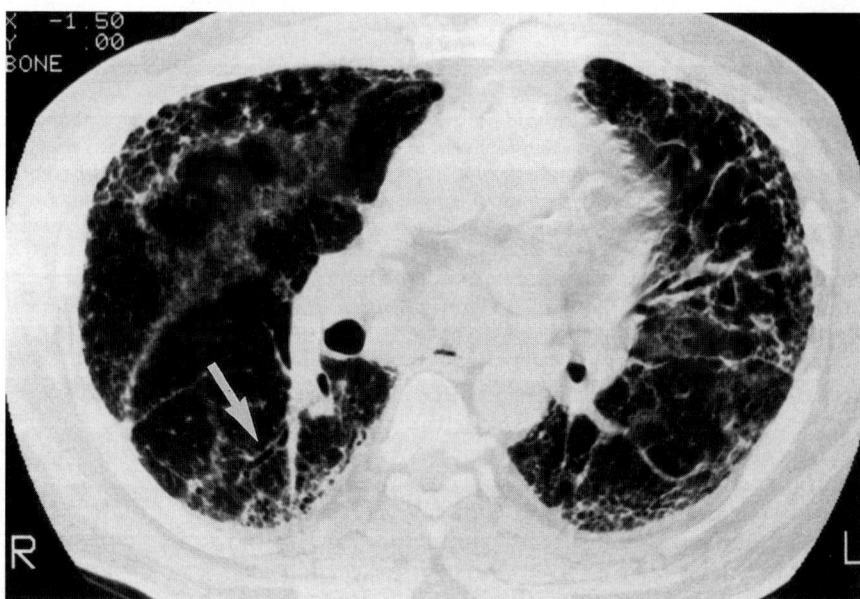

Figure 18.12. Architectural Distortion and Traction Bronchiectasis in Idiopathic Pulmonary Fibrosis (IPF). An HRCT through the lower lobes shows peripheral honeycombing, traction bronchiectasis (*arrow*) and resultant architectural distortion.

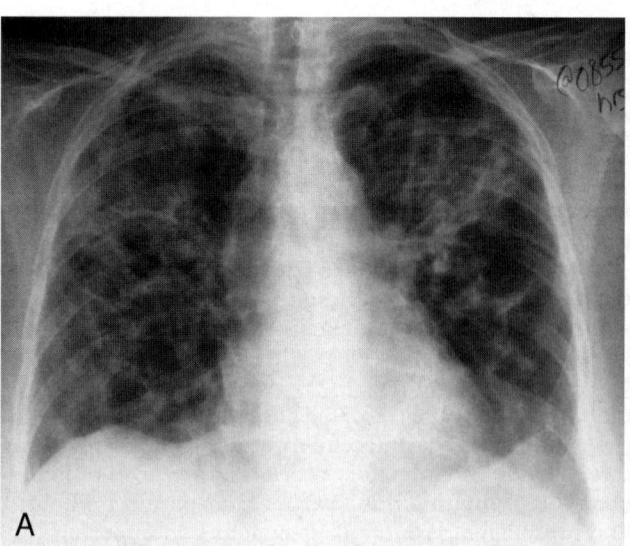
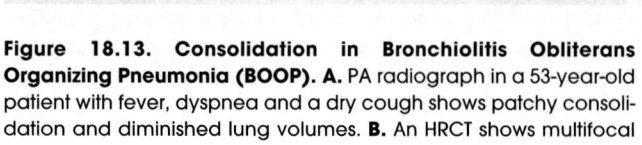
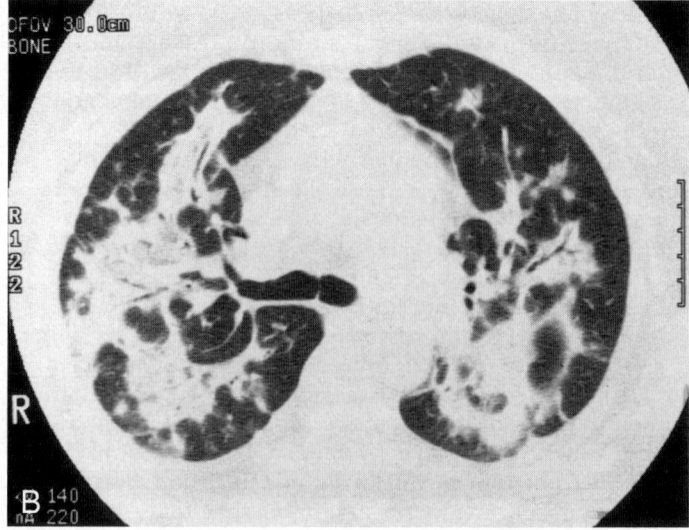

Figure 18.13. Consolidation in Bronchiolitis Obliterans Organizing Pneumonia (BOOP). A. PA radiograph in a 53-year-old patient with fever, dyspnea and a dry cough shows patchy consolidation and diminished lung volumes. **B.** An HRCT shows multifocal areas of consolidation in a peribronchial distribution. Note air bronchograms with mild bronchial dilatation within the consolidated areas. An open lung biopsy showed BOOP.

can occur in complicated silicosis with progressive massive fibrosis (Fig. 18.10) or radiation fibrosis following treatment of Hodgkin's lymphoma or lung cancer. A similar finding can sometimes be seen in IV drug users when a granulomatous fibrosis results as a response to intravenous talc or starch mixed with narcotics.

Consolidation refers to increased lung density that obscures underlying blood vessels with air bronchograms commonly present. This finding can be seen with any air-space filling process (Fig. 18.13) but occasionally occurs in interstitial diseases such as UIP and sarcoidosis.

CHRONIC INTERSTITIAL LUNG DISEASE

Chronic interstitial lung disease usually results from diffuse inflammatory processes that primarily affect the axial and parenchymal interstitium of the lung. A wide variety of disease processes can result in diffuse damage to the pulmonary interstitium (see Table 14.6) (3). Careful evaluation of all available radiologic studies and correlation with clinical findings and laboratory data are essential to the accurate diagnosis of chronic interstitial lung disease (Table 18.4). However, the majority of patients with interstitial lung disease will require histologic examination of lung tissue for definitive diagnosis.

Table 18.4. Differential Diagnostic Features in Chronic Interstitial Lung Disease

Finding	Differential Diagnosis	Finding	Differential Diagnosis
Upper zone distribution	Tuberculosis (postprimary) Chronic fungal infection 　Histoplasmosis 　Coccidioidomycosis Sarcoidosis Eosinophilic granuloma Silicosis Ankylosing spondylitis Hypersensitivity pneumonitis (chronic) Radiation fibrosis from treatment of 　head and neck malignancy	Hilar/mediastinal lymph node enlargement	Sarcoidosis Lymphangitic carcinomatosis Lymphoma Hematogenous metastases Tuberculosis Fungal infection Silicosis
Lower zone distribution	Idiopathic pulmonary fibrosis Asbestosis Rheumatoid lung Scleroderma Neurofibromatosis Dermatomyositis/polymyositis Chronic aspiration	Pleural disease	Asbestosis (plaques) Lymphangitic carcinomatosis (effusion) Rheumatoid lung disease 　(effusion/thickening) Lymphangioleiomyomatosis (chylous 　effusion)
Normal or increased lung volumes	Sarcoidosis Eosinophilic granuloma Lymphangioleiomyomatosis Tuberous sclerosis Interstitial disease superimposed on 　emphysema	Abnormalities of soft tissues and bony thorax	Skin nodules 　Neurofibromatosis Subcutaneous calcifications 　Dermatomyositis 　Scleroderma Erosion of distal clavicles 　Rheumatoid lung 　Scleroderma Rib lesions 　Ribbon ribs/erosion of inferior rib 　　margins 　Neurofibromatosis Erosion of superior margins 　Rheumatoid lung 　Scleroderma Kyphoscoliosis 　Neurofibromatosis Lytic bone lesions 　Metastases 　Eosinophilic granuloma
Honeycombing	Idiopathic pulmonary fibrosis Sarcoidosis Eosinophilic granuloma Rheumatoid lung Scleroderma Pneumoconiosis Hypersensitivity pneumonitis Chronic aspiration Radiation fibrosis		
Miliary nodules	Tuberculosis Fungi 　Histoplasmosis 　Coccidioiodomycosis 　Cryptococcosis Silicosis Metastases 　Thyroid carcinoma 　Renal cell carcinoma 　Bronchogenic carcinoma 　Melanoma 　Choriocarcinoma Sarcoidosis Eosinophilic granuloma		

Chronic Interstitial Pulmonary Edema

Chronic elevation of pulmonary venous pressure may result in increased interstitial markings on plain radiographs. The interstitial thickening is caused by distention of pulmonary lymphatics and chronic interstitial edema, which may lead to fibrosis. Most commonly, this is seen in patients with long-standing mitral stenosis or left ventricular failure. Radiographically, peribronchial cuffing, tram tracking, poor definition of vascular markings, and linear or reticular opacities may be seen. Redistribution of blood flow to the upper lobes, a manifestation of pulmonary venous hypertension, and prominence of the fissures caused by subpleural edema and fibrosis are concomitant findings. Honeycombing is not a feature of chronic pulmonary venous hypertension; its presence in a patient with cardiac disease should suggest another cause of pulmonary fibrosis (e.g., amiodarone lung toxicity).

Connective Tissue Disease

These disorders cause immunologically mediated inflammation and damage to connective tissues throughout the body. The most common thoracic manifestations of this group of heterogeneous disorders are vasculitis and interstitial fibrosis although the pleura, chest wall, diaphragm, and heart may also be affected (4).

Rheumatoid Lung Disease (Table 18.5). Rheumatoid arthritis produces a chronic arthritis of peripheral joints. Extra-articular manifestations are seen in up to 75% of patients. In contrast to the disease as a whole, pulmonary involvement is more common in men. The pleuropulmonary manifestations of rheumatoid disease typically follow the onset of joint disease, and are seen in patients with high serum rheumatoid factor titers and eosinophilia. However, in up to 15% of patients, pleuropulmonary involvement precedes the joint disease.

The most common radiographic manifestation of parenchymal lung involvement is an interstitial pneumonitis and fibrosis that histologically is a form of UIP. This begins as an alveolitis (inflammation of the alveolar interstitium) seen radiographically as fine reticular or ground-glass opacities with a lower-zone predominance. Gradual progression to end-stage pulmonary fibrosis with the development of a bibasilar medium or coarse

reticular or reticulonodular pattern (honeycombing) occurs (Fig. 18.14). HRCT is more sensitive in detecting the earliest parenchymal changes than conventional radiographs and is also more sensitive in depicting the development of interstitial fibrosis (Fig. 18.15). Predominant upper lobe fibrosis and cavity or bulla formation are rare. This less common pattern of lung involvement is indistinguishable from that seen with ankylosing spondylitis; thus, it must be distinguished from postprimary fibrocavitary tuberculosis by acid fast staining of sputum.

Less common parenchymal manifestations of rheumatoid disease are lung nodules and changes attributable to BOOP. Necrobiotic (rheumatoid) nodules in the lung can produce peripheral, well-defined nodular opacities on chest radiographs that are indistinguishable from the subcutaneous rheumatoid nodules seen on the extensor surfaces of the elbows and knees in these patients. The lung nodules commonly evolve into thick-walled cavities that wax and wane in parallel with the flares of arthritis. Similar nodules may develop in the lungs of coal miners and silica or asbestos workers with rheumatoid arthritis as a hypersensitivity response to inhaled dust particles (Caplan's syndrome). Caplan's syndrome is indistinguishable radiographically from the necrobiotic nodules of simple rheumatoid disease although the presence of the associated characteristic small, nodular or irregular parenchymal opacities of simple pneumoconiosis helps make this distinction. BOOP and bronchiolitis obliterans

Table 18.5. Manifestations of Rheumatoid Lung Disease

Manifestation	Radiographic Findings
Serositis	
Pleuritis	Pleural effusion, thickening
Pericarditis	Pericardial effusion
Interstitial pneumonitis	Pulmonary fibrosis (basilar predominance)
Necrobiotic nodules	Multiple peripheral cavitating nodules
Caplan's syndrome	Multiple peripheral cavitating nodules
Bronchiolitis obliterans	Hyperinflation
Pulmonary arteritis	Pulmonary arterial hypertension and right heart enlargement
	Pulmonary hemorrhage

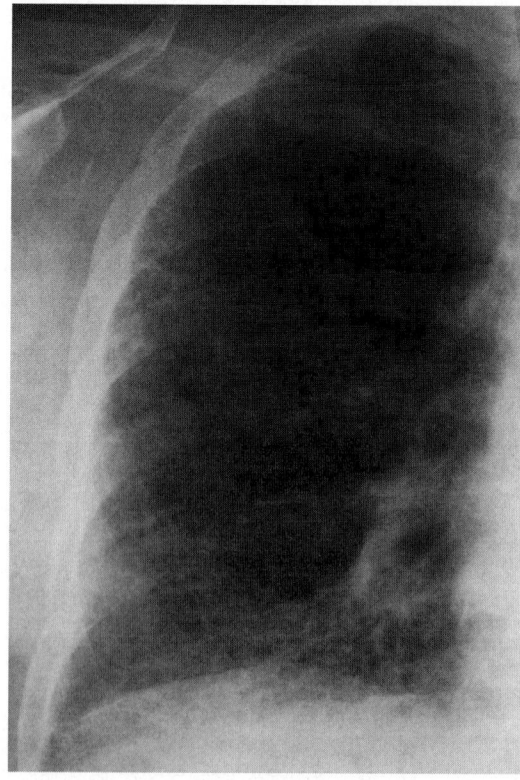

Figure 18.14. Honeycombing in Rheumatoid Lung. A coned-down view of the right lung in a patient with end-stage rheumatoid lung disease demonstrates a medium reticular process with thin-walled cysts representing honeycomb lung. Note the predominant subpleural distribution of disease.

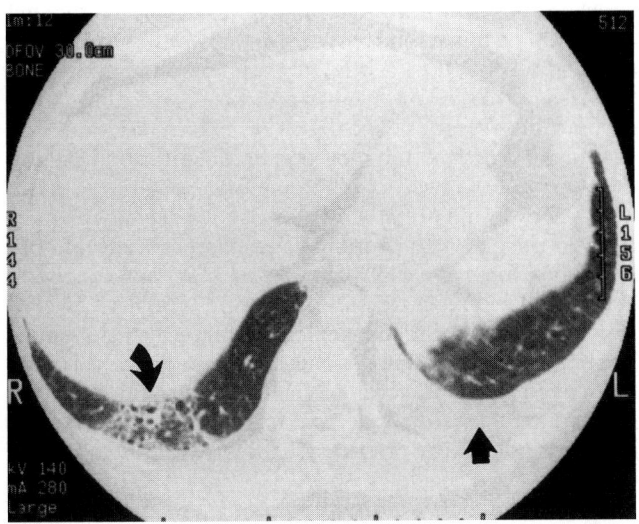

Figure 18.15. Rheumatoid Lung Disease. An HRCT through the lung bases in a patient with rheumatoid arthritis shows a focal area of honeycombing at the periphery of the right lung base (*curved arrow*). Note also the left pleural effusion (*straight arrow*), a frequent finding in rheumatoid disease.

(constrictive bronchiolitis) are associated with rheumatoid disease. The clinical, functional, and radiographic findings are similar to BOOP or bronchiolitis obliterans associated with SLE, drugs, or viral infection.

Pleuritis is the most common thoracic manifestation of rheumatoid disease and is found in 20% of patients. As with pulmonary involvement, there is a male predilection for pleural disease. Unilateral or bilateral pleural effusions that are exudative and have a characteristically low glucose concentration may be seen.

Enlargement of the central pulmonary arteries and right ventricular dilatation may be seen on chest radiographs in patients with pulmonary arterial hypertension. This is an uncommon manifestation of rheumatoid disease that usually develops secondary to diffuse interstitial fibrosis. Rarely, the pulmonary arteries are involved as a part of the systemic vasculitis seen in extraarticular rheumatoid disease. No parenchymal abnormalities are associated with rheumatoid pulmonary arteritis.

Abnormalities that may be seen in the chest walls of individuals with rheumatoid arthritis include tapered erosion of the distal clavicles, rotator cuff atrophy with a high-riding humeral head, bilateral symmetric narrowing of the glenohumeral joint space with or without superimposed degenerative joint disease, and superior rib notching or erosion.

Systemic Lupus Erythematosis. This disease of young and middle-aged females typically involves inflammation of multiple organs mediated by autoantibodies and circulating immune complexes. The thorax is commonly affected and may be the initial site of involvement. The thoracic disease is often limited to the pleura and pericardium; however, the lung, heart, diaphragm, and intercostal muscles are affected in as many as one-third of patients. In the pleura and pericardium, a fibrinous serositis produces painful pleural and pericardial effusions that are exudative in nature. Radiographically, the pleural effusions are small-sized or moderately sized and can be unilateral or bilateral. The effusions usually resolve with corticosteroid therapy. Pleural fibrosis, seen in a majority of patients with long-standing disease, results in diffuse pleural thickening.

Pulmonary involvement may take the form of acute lupus pneumonitis or chronic interstitial disease. Acute lupus pneumonitis is characterized by rapid onset of fever, dyspnea, and hypoxemia, which occasionally requires mechanical ventilation. These patients have pathological changes indistinguishable from those seen in ARDS, with diffuse alveolar damage producing an exudative intraalveolar edema with hyaline membrane formation. Radiographically, rapidly coalescent bilateral air-space opacities are seen, but the typical HRCT finding is one of ground-glass opacity. These findings are difficult to distinguish from those seen in diffuse alveolar hemorrhage associated with pulmonary vasculitis, severe pneumonia related to immunosuppressive therapy, or pulmonary edema secondary to renal failure. The diagnosis of acute lupus pneumonitis is made by excluding pneumonia and pulmonary edema and by noting an improvement following the initiation of immunosuppressive therapy.

Radiographic evidence of IPF is distinctly uncommon in SLE but fibrosis is said to be present pathologically in one-third of patients. When seen radiographically, the pattern is one of bibasilar reticular opacities indistinguishable from those seen in rheumatoid lung disease or scleroderma. Therefore, the presence of severe interstitial fibrosis in a patient with clinical features of SLE should prompt consideration of the diagnosis of an overlap syndrome (mixed connective tissue disease). As with rheumatoid lung disease and scleroderma, HRCT is the most sensitive technique for demonstrating early interstitial disease.

Additional chest radiographic findings in SLE include elevation of the hemidiaphragms with decreased lung volumes and resultant bibasilar areas of linear atelectasis. Diaphragmatic elevation is present in as many as 20% of patients and is the result of diaphragmatic weakness from a primary myopathy unrelated to corticosteroid therapy. Rarely, the central pulmonary arteries are enlarged from pulmonary arterial hypertension secondary to pulmonary vasculitis. Pulmonary embolism with or without infarction may produce peripheral parenchymal opacities and results from deep venous thrombosis, which develops in the presence of a circulating lupus anticoagulant. BOOP has been described in patients with SLE but is indistinguishable clinically and radiographically from lupus pneumonitis because both conditions produce parenchymal opacities that are steroid-responsive. Although superior rib erosions may be seen, they are indistinguishable from similar findings in rheumatoid arthritis or scleroderma.

Scleroderma produces inflammation and fibrosis of the skin, esophagus, musculoskeletal system, heart, lungs, and kidneys in young and middle-aged females. The cause and pathogenesis are unknown. The lungs are involved pathologically in nearly 90% of patients, but only 25% have respiratory symptoms or radiographic evidence of pulmonary involvement. Pulmonary function testing is more sensitive than conventional radiography in the diagnosis of lung disease and shows the typical diminished lung volumes, preserved flow rates, and low diffusing capacity of interstitial pulmonary fibrosis. Pathologically, the sequence of parenchymal and radiographic changes is indistinguishable from rheumatoid lung disease, IPF, and other forms of UIP. Severe pulmonary involvement is reflected radiographically as a coarse reticular or reticulonodular pattern involving the subpleural regions of the lower lobes. The most common HRCT findings are interlobular septal thickening, ground-glass opacities, and honeycombing (Fig. 18.16). HRCT is more sensitive than chest radiographs in detecting early interstitial disease. Progressive loss of lung volume is seen with advancing pulmonary fibrosis. The development of large (1–5 cm) subpleural lower lobe cysts may cause spontaneous pneumothorax.

Pulmonary arterial hypertension with enlarged central pulmonary arteries and right ventricular dilatation, seen in up to 50% of patients with scleroderma, may be seen in the absence of interstitial fibrosis. In these patients, thickening and obliteration of small muscular pulmonary arteries and arterioles are responsible for the development of pulmonary arterial hypertension. Pleural effusions are significantly less common in scleroderma than in rheumatoid disease or SLE and may be a helpful distinguishing feature radiographically. Pleural thickening is more often attributable to extension of pulmonary interstitial fibrosis into the interstitial layer of the pleura than to pleuritis.

Several additional chest radiographic findings may be seen in patients with scleroderma. Eggshell calcification of mediastinal lymph nodes has been reported although it is more common in silicosis and sarcoidosis. A dilated, air-filled esophagus may be identified on the upright chest radiograph and is a manifestation of esophageal dysmotility from smooth muscle atrophy and fibrosis. An air-fluid level within a dilated esophagus suggests secondary distal esophageal stricture formation from chronic reflux esophagitis. The functional or anatomic esophageal obstruction may result in aspiration with the development of lower lobe pneumonia. Because patients with scleroderma are at a greater risk for developing lung cancer, particularly bronchioloalveolar cell carcinoma, the appearance of a mass or persistent air-space opacity should raise this possibility. Patients with the CREST syndrome (subcutaneous **c**alcification, **R**aynaud's phenomenon, **e**sophageal dysmotility, **s**clerodactyly, and **t**elangiectasia), a variant of scleroderma, may have radiographically visible calcifications within the subcutaneous tissues of the chest wall. Superior rib notching or erosion may be seen.

Dermatomyositis/Polymyositis. These disorders involve an autoimmune inflammation and destruction of skeletal muscle that produces proximal muscle pain and weakness (polymyositis), occasionally associated with a skin rash (dermatomyositis). The thoracic manifestations of these diseases include respiratory and pharyngeal muscle weakness and an associated interstitial pneumonitis. Interstitial pneumonitis, indistinguishable from that associated with rheumatoid lung disease, SLE, scleroderma, or IPF, is seen in 5–10% of patients. A fine reticular interstitial pattern in acute disease leads to a chronic, coarse reticular or reticulonodular process that is predominantly basilar in distribution. Most patients with polymyositis and interstitial lung disease have clinical manifestations of rheumatoid arthritis or scleroderma, and these patients often respond favorably to corticosteroids. As with scleroderma, the early parenchymal changes may be subradiographic but can be demonstrated on HRCT studies through the lower lobes (Fig. 18.17). Additional chest radiographic findings in polymyositis reflect the involvement of skeletal muscle. Small lung volumes with diaphragmatic elevation and basilar linear atelectasis are sec-

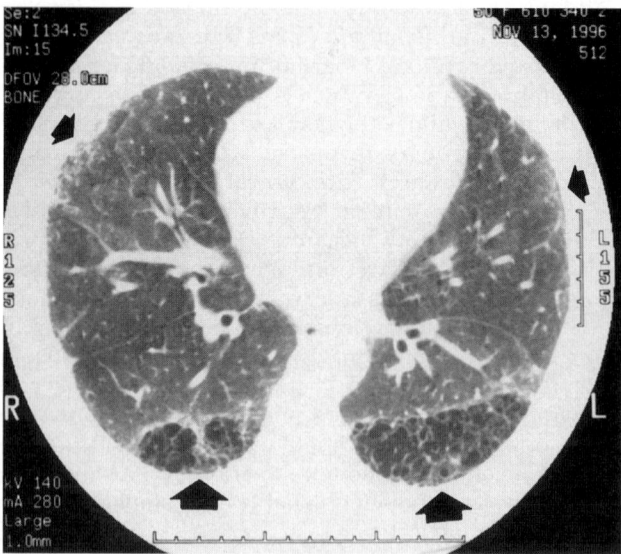

Figure 18.16. Scleroderma. An HRCT of a patient with scleroderma demonstrates minimal interstitial disease in the periphery of the middle lobe and lingula (*small arrows*) with honeycombing in the posterior subpleural portions of the lower lobes (*large arrows*).

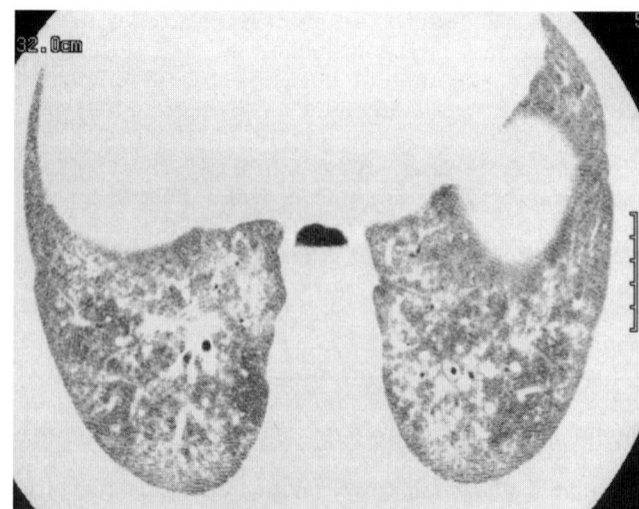

Figure 18.17. Polymyositis. An HRCT through the lung bases shows reticulation and nodules, reflecting interstitial pneumonitis in a patient with polymyositis.

ondary to diaphragmatic and intercostal muscle involvement. Pharyngeal and upper esophageal muscle weakness predispose patients to aspiration pneumonia. The chest radiograph should be examined carefully for lung masses because bronchogenic carcinoma accounts for a significant percentage of the malignancies that are seen with a higher than normal frequency in patients with dermatomyositis or polymyositis.

Sjogren's Syndrome. This autoimmune disorder of middle-aged women is characterized by the sicca syndrome of dry eyes (keratoconjunctivitis sicca), dry mouth (xerostomia), and dry nose (xerorhinia), which result from lymphocytic infiltration of the lacrimal, salivary, and mucous glands, respectively. Most patients with the sicca syndrome have associated manifestations of other collagen vascular diseases such as rheumatoid arthritis, scleroderma, or SLE.

The chest is involved in approximately one-third of patients with Sjogren's syndrome with or without associated collagen vascular disease. The most common manifestation is interstitial fibrosis indistinguishable from that seen with other collagen vascular disorders. Involvement of tracheobronchial mucous glands leads to thickened sputum with mucus plugging and recurrent bronchitis, bronchiectasis, atelectasis, and pneumonia. HRCT demonstrates both interstitial opacities and the presence of small airways involvement with bronchiolectasis and a tree-in-bud appearance. Pleuritis and pleural effusion are less common.

Patients with Sjogren's syndrome are at increased risk for developing lymphocytic interstitial pneumonitis (LIP) and non-Hodgkin's pulmonary lymphoma. The radiographic appearance of LIP is coarse reticular or reticulonodular opacities in the lower lobe that are indistinguishable from interstitial fibrosis. The development of lymphoma in these patients should be suspected when nodular or alveolar opacities develop in the lung in association with mediastinal lymph node enlargement.

Ankylosing Spondylitis. Approximately 1–2% of individuals with ankylosing spondylitis develop pulmonary disease in the form of upper lobe pulmonary fibrosis. The fibrotic changes are commonly associated with the development of bullae and cavities, which are prone to mycetoma formation with aspergillus. The diagnosis should be suspected in a young to middle-aged male with characteristic spine changes (kyphosis, spinal ankylosis) seen in association with abnormally increased lung volumes and upper lobe fibrobullous disease, the latter of which simulates postprimary fibrocavitary tuberculosis.

Overlap Syndromes and Mixed Connective Tissue Disease. Some patients with collagen vascular disease have features of more than one of the recognized syndromes previously discussed in this chapter. These patients are classified as having an overlap syndrome, with thoracic manifestations characteristic of the other disorders. Patients with a distinct form of overlap syndrome, called mixed connective tissue disease, have clinical features of SLE, scleroderma, and polymyositis and have serum antibodies to extractable nuclear antigen. The thoracic manifestations of mixed connective tissue disease include IPF, pulmonary arterial hypertension due to plexogenic pulmonary arteriopathy, and pleural effusion and thickening from a fibrinous pleuritis typical of SLE.

Idiopathic Chronic Interstitial Pneumonias

The idiopathic interstitial pneumonias are a group of disorders characterized by an inflammatory process in the lung which can result in pulmonary fibrosis. These histologic terms provide the most precise method of classifying these disorders and include usual interstitial pneumonia (UIP), acute interstitial pneumonia (AIP), desquamative interstitial pneumonia (DIP), bronchiolitis obliterans organizing pneumonia (BOOP), respiratory bronchiolitis-associated interstitial lung disease (RB-ILD), and nonspecific interstitial pneumonia (NIP). Unfortunately, confusion arises when clinical terms are used interchangeably with the aforementioned histologic terms in describing these disorders. When possible (when the histology is known), using the histologic term to describe a particular disorder is most accurate while reserving clinical terms such as IPF or rheumatoid lung for interstitial disease associated with specific clinical diseases for which histology is unavailable.

Usual Interstitial Pneumonia. UIP is the most common of the idiopathic interstitial pneumonias. It is likely the result of a repetitive injury to the lung. The initial response in the lung is inflammation followed by repair and eventually fibrosis. The pathologic abnormalities seen in UIP represent a spectrum of findings, characterized in the early stage of disease by marked proliferation of macrophages in the alveolar air spaces associated with a mild and uniform thickening of the interstitium by mononuclear cells. Late in the course of disease, the pathologic findings are characterized by thickening of the alveolar interstitium by mononuclear inflammatory cells and fibrous tissue. A distinguishing histologic feature of UIP is that the different stages of disease are seen simultaneously within different portions of the lung.

Patients with UIP typically present in the fifth to seventh decades with a slight preponderance in males. Presenting symptoms include progressive dyspnea or a nonproductive cough. Pulmonary function tests show restrictive disease and a decreased diffusing capacity for carbon monoxide (DLCO). Most cases of UIP are sporadic, but as many as 30% of patients with UIP have an associated collagen vascular or immunologic disorder. Most often rheumatoid arthritis, this disorder can also be SLE, scleroderma, or dermatomyositis/polymyositis.

The radiographic manifestations of UIP parallel the pathologic changes. In the early phase of disease, the chest radiograph may appear normal despite the presence of clinical symptoms and abnormalities on pulmonary function testing. The earliest radiographic changes are bibasilar fine to medium reticular opacities or ground-glass density (Fig. 18.18). As the disease progresses, a coarse reticular or reticulonodular pattern is seen and almost invariably leads to the formation of honeycomb cysts (3–10mm diameter) and progressive loss of lung volume. Extensive pulmonary fibrosis may be associated with findings of pulmonary arterial hypertension. Upper lobe bullae may be seen and predispose to the development of spontaneous pneumothorax. Hilar lymph

Figure 18.18. Usual Interstitial Pneumonia (UIP). A. A PA radiograph in a patient with UIP demonstrates bilateral coarse reticular opacities and diminished lung volumes. **B.** An HRCT through the mid lungs shows honeycombing in a peripheral, subpleural distribution. Traction bronchiectasis is evident (*arrow*).

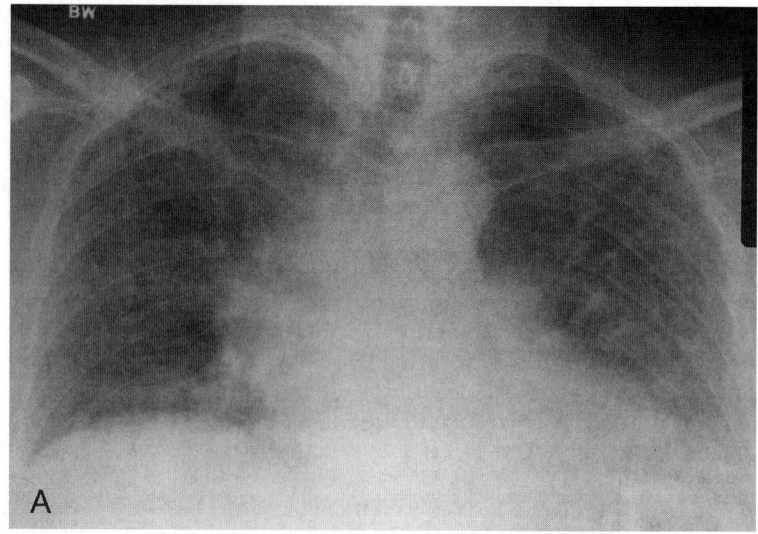

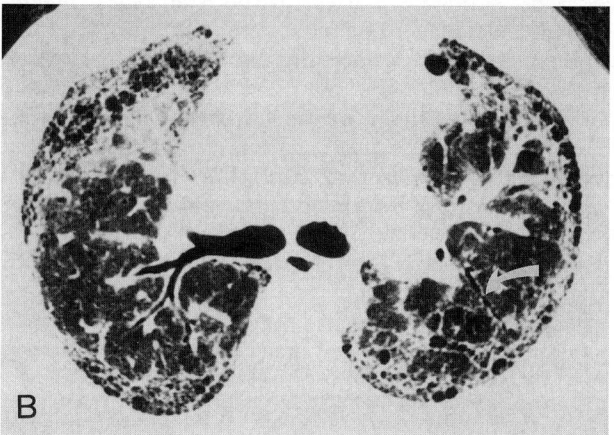

node enlargement and pleural effusions have been described but are rare and should suggest an alternative diagnosis.

The HRCT findings in UIP differ with the stage of the disease and vary from one lung region to another. Patients with active, inflammatory areas of disease, as demonstrated histologically by interstitial and intra-alveolar inflammatory changes, show areas of ground-glass density on HRCT. As fibrosis develops, findings include irregular septal or subpleural thickening (in contrast to the smooth septal thickening seen with edema or lymphangitic spread of carcinoma), intralobular lines, irregular interfaces, honeycombing, and traction bronchiectasis (Fig. 18.12). The changes are typically most severe in the peripheral and basal portions of the lungs, which can be helpful in differential diagnosis (Fig. 18.18). Mildly enlarged mediastinal lymph nodes are often seen.

In most patients, the disease progresses inexorably with an overall mean survival of less than 5 years. Patients with early, active disease (positive gallium scan, ground-glass or air-space opacities radiographically) may benefit from immunosuppressive therapy with corticosteroids or cyclophosphamide, but those with end-stage fibrosis (honeycombing) will not. Most patients succumb to respiratory failure, often precipitated by infection or cardiac disease. There is an increased incidence of bronchogenic carcinoma, with adenocarcinoma the most common histologic subtype.

Desquamative Interstitial Pneumonia. DIP describes a histologic pattern characterized by the accumulation of macrophages within alveolar spaces. Of patients with DIP, 90% are cigarette smokers. Although focal areas of macrophage accumulation can be seen as a component of UIP, the finding in DIP is diffuse and temporally homogeneous. Although histologically distinct entities, DIP and UIP are thought by many to represent different ends of the spectrum of the same disease process, with DIP representing the early phase of UIP. However, distinguishing clinical features support the concept of two distinct entities. DIP affects younger individuals, with a mean age at diagnosis of 42 years. Most important, DIP is more steroid-responsive than UIP and therefore carries a more favorable prognosis; the median survival for patients with DIP is 12 years compared with 4 years for UIP.

DIP cannot be reliably distinguished from UIP radiographically. The typical radiographic findings in DIP are bibasilar reticular opacities with normal or minimally diminished lung volumes. Ground-glass opacities are seen in only 33% of cases although honeycombing is seen in 12–33%. Up to 22% of patients have a normal chest radiograph. HRCT shows ground-glass opacities, most often seen within the peripheral aspects of the bases (Fig. 18.19). Irregular linear opacities, honeycombing, and traction bronchiectasis can be seen, but these are much less common than in UIP. Ground-glass abnormalities often improve or completely resolve with corticosteroid therapy.

Acute Interstitial Pneumonia. Also known as the Hamman-Rich syndrome, AIP is an acute, aggressive form of idiopathic interstitial pneumonitis and fibrosis. Patients with AIP typically present with a brief history of cough, fever, and dyspnea that progresses rapidly to severe hypoxemia and respiratory failure requiring mechanical ventilation. The pathologic manifestations of AIP are those of ARDS and the disease has also been termed idiopathic ARDS. The histologic findings are those of diffuse alveolar damage with minimal mature collagen deposition. A characteristic of the process is that it is diffuse and temporally homogeneous.

Chest radiographs and HRCT scans show findings of ARDS with diffuse ground-glass opacity and consolidation with air bronchograms (5). On CT, a gradient of increasing density from anterior to posterior lung can be seen. Linear opacities, honeycombing, and traction bronchiectasis are uncommon. As in other forms of ARDS, mortality rates range from 60–90%. Fibrosis can develop but usually stabilizes and does not progress beyond the recovery phase.

Bronchiolitis Obliterans Organizing Pneumonia. BOOP is a disorder characterized by the widespread deposition of granulation tissue (fibroblasts, collagen, and capillaries) within small airways and peribronchiolar air spaces. Most cases are idiopathic, but a number of conditions have been associated with this disorder. These include viral infection (influenza, adenovirus, measles), toxic fume inhalation (sulfur dioxide, chlorine), collagen vascular disease (rheumatoid arthritis and SLE), organ transplantation (bone marrow, lung, and heart-lung), drugs, and chronic aspiration. The idiopathic form of this entitiy is also termed "cryptogenic organizing pneumonia" (COP).

Patients with BOOP often have a subacute illness with a several-month history of nonproductive cough and dyspnea. The physical examination may reveal rales or wheezes. Pulmonary function tests usually show a restrictive pattern of disease with diminished lung volumes and normal to increased flow rates. The DLCO is significantly decreased. Pathologically, a mononuclear cell exudate in the bronchioles and surrounding alveoli organizes to form intrabronchiolar and intralveolar granulation tissue. Characteristics of this disease include the uniformity of the histologic changes and the absence of parenchymal distortion and fibrosis; these features help distinguish BOOP from UIP, which can have similar clinical, functional, and radiographic features.

Radiographs in patients with BOOP reveal patchy bilateral air-space or ground-glass opacities (Fig. 18.13A) with some patients showing scattered nodular opacities. The most common HRCT finding is patchy consolidation or ground-glass opacity, with either a subpleural or peribronchial pattern of distribution (Fig. 18.13B). Small, ill-defined peribronchial nodules are less commonly seen. Bronchiectasis and bronchial wall thickening are commonly seen in the involved areas of lung.

The diagnosis of BOOP can only be made by recognizing the characteristic histologic changes on open lung biopsy. The distinction of BOOP from IPF may be difficult but is important as BOOP has a more favorable prognosis and usually responds rapidly to corticosteroid therapy. BOOP complicating heart-lung transplantation has a worse prognosis but may respond favorably to immunosuppressive therapy.

Respiratory Bronchiolitis-associated Interstitial Lung Disease. Respiratory bronchiolitis is a disorder seen only in cigarette smokers and is characterized by inflammation within and around the respiratory bronchioles. The histology of RB-ILD overlaps with that of DIP, and some authors have suggested that it is an early form of DIP. Patients with RB-ILD are typically young and heavy smokers who have mild cough and dyspnea. Pulmonary function tests show restrictive or mixed restrictive-obstructive patterns. Symptoms respond to smoking cessation or steroid therapy, and no progression to end-stage fibrosis occurs.

The chest radiograph is normal in up to 21% of cases of RB-ILD. Diffuse linear and nodular opacities are often seen as is bibasilar atelectasis. The most common HRCT findings

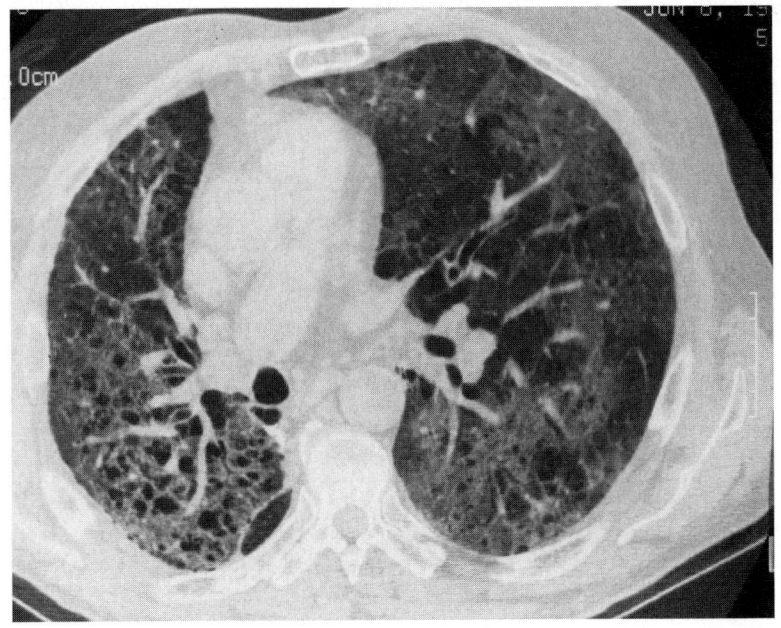

Figure 18.19. Desquamative Interstitial Pneumonia (DIP). An HRCT shows ground-glass opacities superimposed on findings of emphysema in a smoker with DIP. Right-sided volume loss is due to prior resection for bronchogenic carcinoma.

are scattered ground-glass opacities and small centrilobular nodules, often with an upper lobe predominant distribution (Fig. 18.20). Linear opacities are rare and honeycombing is not seen. Emphysema is often a concomitant finding.

Nonspecific Interstitial Pneumonia. NIP is a recently introduced term, used to describe interstitial pneumonias that cannot be otherwise classified as UIP, DIP, AIP, BOOP, or RB-ILD. Many cases of NIP are seen in association with collagen vascular disease. Most cases will show areas of ground-glass opacity or consolidation on HRCT (Fig. 18.21). Bronchial dilatation and linear opacities may also be seen, but honeycombing is rare. NIP is usually steroid-responsive.

Other Chronic Interstitial Lung Diseases

Neurofibromatosis (NF) is an autosomal dominant neurocutaneous syndrome that has two types: type I or von Recklinghausen's disease, and type II. The classic manifestations of NF I are cutaneous "café au lait" spots and neurofibromas of cutaneous and subcutaneous peripheral nerves and nerve roots. In addition, the skeletal, vascular, and pulmonary systems are often involved. The condition is also associated with a variety of neo-

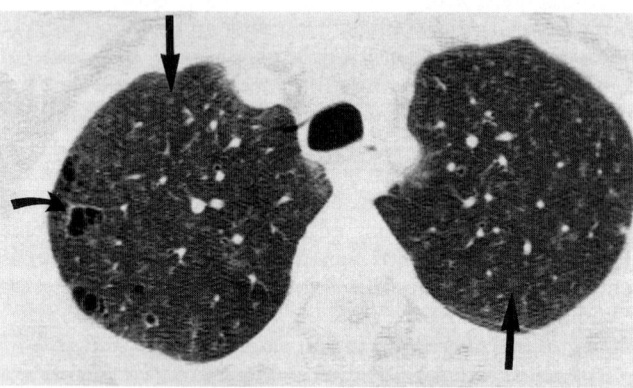

Figure 18.20. Respiratory Bronchiolitis-associated Interstitial Lung Disease (RB-ILD). An HRCT through the upper lobes in a smoker with RB-ILD shows small centrilobular ground-glass nodules (*straight arrows*) and concomitant emphysema (*curved arrow*).

Figure 18.21. Nonspecific Interstitial Pneumonia (NIP). A 10-mm axial CT of a 57-year-old man with cough and dyspnea shows multifocal consolidation and ground-glass opacities. Open lung biopsy demonstrated NIP.

plasms, including meningiomas, optic gliomas, neurofibrosarcomas, and pheochromocytomas.

Radiographically, several thoracic manifestations of NF I can be noted. Cutaneous and subcutaneous neurofibromas may be seen along the chest wall or projecting over the lungs. The spine may show a kyphoscoliosis with scalloping of the posterior aspect of the vertebral bodies due to dural ectasia. "Ribbon rib" deformities and rib notching may be seen. Mediastinal masses in patients with NF I include neurofibromas, lateral thoracic meningoceles, and extra-adrenal pheochromocytomas.

Parenchymal lung disease is seen in approximately 20% of patients with NF I. The findings include diffuse interstitial fibrosis and bulla formation. The interstitial fibrosis is predominantly lower zonal and bilaterally symmetric. Bullae usually develop in the upper zones with asymmetric involvement of the lungs. Pulmonary symptoms are usually minimal or absent, with pulmonary function tests showing a mixed obstructive/restrictive pattern. A small number of patients will develop respiratory failure due to pulmonary fibrosis with secondary development of pulmonary arterial hypertension and cor pulmonale.

Tuberous Sclerosis. TS is an autosomal dominant neurocutaneous syndrome with variable expression. The classical clinical triad of TS is seizures, mental retardation, and adenoma sebaceum. Additional manifestations include intracranial calcifications, cerebral cortical and periventricular hamartomas, renal angiomyolipomas, cardiac rhabdomyomas, retinal phakomas, and sclerotic bone lesions.

Pulmonary involvement in TS is rare and is seen in approximately 1% of cases. Patients with pulmonary TS are usually older and have a lower incidence of seizures and mental retardation. The pulmonary involvement is indistinguishable clinically, pathologically, and radiographically from that seen in LAM. Pathologically, smooth muscle proliferation occurs in the peribronchovascular and parenchymal interstitium of the lung. Small adenomatoid nodules measuring several millimeters in diameter may be seen scattered throughout the lungs.

Radiographically, symmetric bilateral reticular or reticulonodular opacities can be seen. In the later stages of disease, a pattern of coarse reticular or small cystic opacities

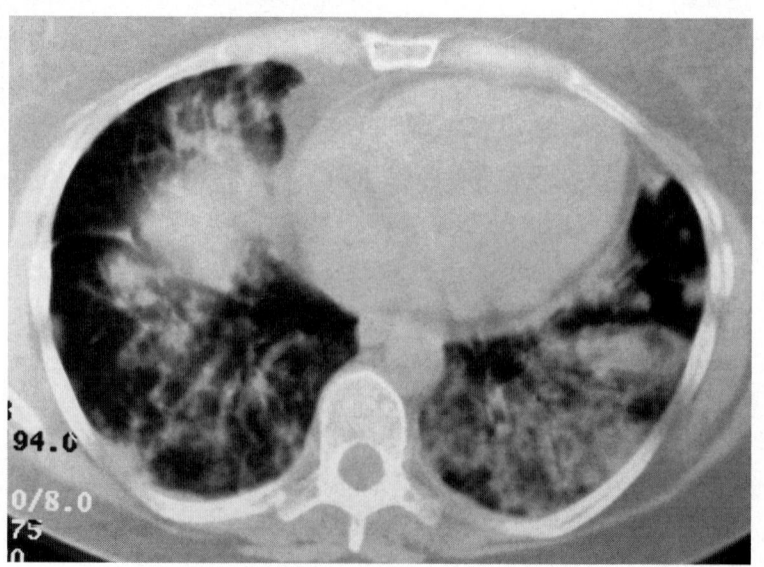

may be seen. The cysts are uniform in size and less than 1 cm in diameter. HRCT is best at depicting the presence of thin-walled pulmonary cysts and can help detect associated extrapulmonary abnormalities including renal angiomyolipomas and periventricular tubers. A helpful feature in distinguishing TS from other chronic interstitial lung diseases is the normal to increased lung volumes in patients with TS due to small airways obstruction and expiratory air trapping. In distinction to eosinophilic granuloma of the lung and sarcoidosis, which have a predominant upper zone distribution of disease, pulmonary TS affects the entire lung uniformly. Pneumothorax is common and results from the rupture of a subpleural cyst. Pleural effusions are uncommon. The pulmonary involvement often leads to pulmonary arterial hypertension and cor pulmonale, which are associated with a high mortality.

Lymphangioleiomyomatosis. LAM is an uncommon condition that is seen exclusively in women. The average age at diagnosis is 43 years. Although LAM shares many features with pulmonary tuberous sclerosis, it is not an inherited condition and lacks the extrapulmonary features of TS.

On gross pathologic examination, replacement of the normal lung architecture by cysts can be seen in patients with advanced LAM. These cysts, which range from 0.2–2.0 cm in diameter, are separated by thickened interstitium containing numerous interlacing bundles of smooth muscle. Smooth muscle proliferation is also seen within the walls of pulmonary veins, bronchioles, and lymphatics. The smooth muscle proliferation within lymphatic channels causes lymphatic obstruction and dilatation that may lead to the development of chylothorax, chyloperitoneum, or chylopericardium. Similarly, smooth muscle proliferation within mediastinal and retroperitoneal lymph nodes may result in nodal enlargement. The perilymphatic smooth muscle proliferation and nodal enlargement help distinguish LAM pathologically from the pulmonary involvement of tuberous sclerosis.

The patient with LAM is typically a woman of childbearing age who presents with progressive dyspnea or a spontaneous pneumothorax. Hemoptysis may be seen in some patients, presumably related to pulmonary venous obstruction by the smooth muscle proliferation.

The chest radiograph may be normal early in the disease. Eventually, symmetric bilateral fine reticular or reticulonodular opacities are seen. The late radiographic pattern is one of cysts and honeycombing; the cysts usually have thinner walls than those seen with IPF or NF (Fig. 18.22A). As in TS, the lung volumes are typically normal or increased. Large, recurrent chylous pleural effusions may be unilateral or bilateral. Spontaneous pneumothorax is also a common finding and may be bilateral.

HRCT demonstrates thin-walled cysts distributed throughout the lungs (Fig. 18.22B). In less severely involved areas, the intervening lung is normal. Interlobular septal thickening is mild or absent. Although thin-walled cysts are seen in a variety of other diseases, most notably emphysema and eosinophilic granuloma, the HRCT findings, when seen in a patient with a characteristic history (a female with dyspnea, spontaneous pneumothorax, and chylous pleural effusions) are diagnostic.

The prognosis of patients with symptomatic LAM is poor, with approximately 70% of patients dying within 5 years. In some patients, the administration of antipro-gesterone agents such as tamoxifen may slow the progression of disease.

Alveolar Septal Amyloidosis. Amyloidosis encompasses a group of diseases characterized by the extracellular deposition of insoluble fibrillary proteins termed "amyloid." Amyloid represents a number of proteins that are distinctive biochemically but similar physically in that their polypeptide chains form beta-pleated sheets. Amyloidosis has traditionally been divided into four forms: *1)* primary, in which there is no associated chronic disease or in which there is an underlying plasma cell disorder; *2)* secondary, in which an underlying chronic abnormality such as tuberculosis is present; *3)* familial, which is very uncommon and usually localized to nervous tissue; and *4)* senile, which affects many organs in patients over 70 years of age. A more recently developed classification scheme is based on the specific protein comprising amyloid. In this scheme, the most important forms are amyloid L (AL), usually seen with plasma cell dyscrasias and associated with the deposi-

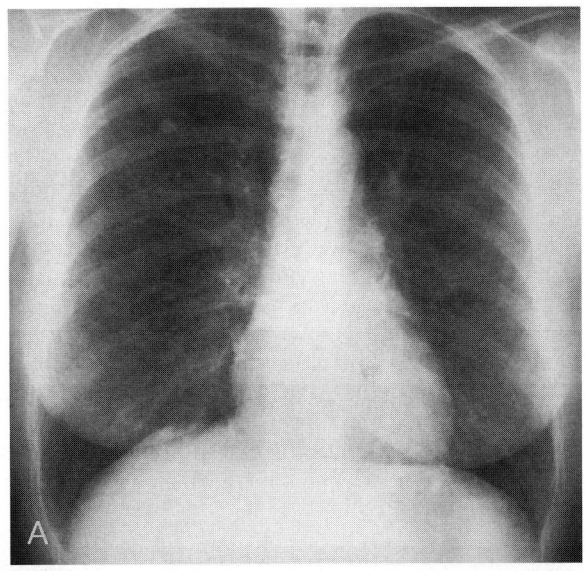

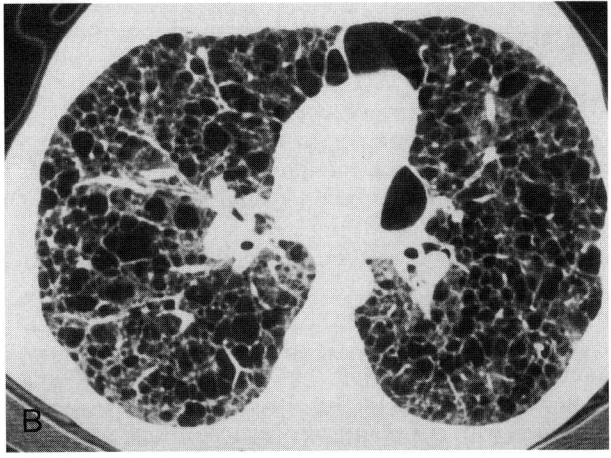

Figure 18.22. Lymphangioleiomyomatosis (LAM). A. A PA radiograph in a 36-year-old patient with LAM shows diffuse coarse reticular opacities with normal lung volumes. **B.** An HRCT in another patient with LAM shows almost complete replacement of the parenchyma by fairly uniform thin-walled cysts.

tion of immunoglobulin light chains, and amyloid A (AA), occurring in patients with chronic inflammatory diseases such as familial Mediterranean fever and certain neoplasms including Hodgkin's disease.

The three major patterns of amyloid deposition within the lungs and airways are tracheobronchial, nodular parenchymal, and diffuse parenchymal (alveolar septal). In most cases these patterns occur independently but they may overlap.

In alveolar septal amyloidosis, the amyloid is deposited in the parenchymal interstitium and within the media of small blood vessels. Within the alveolar septa, amyloid deposits are located between the endothelial cells lining the septal capillaries and the alveolar epithelium; inflammatory cells are typically absent.

This process is usually seen in older patients who have symptoms of chronic progressive dyspnea. Recurrent hemoptysis may also be caused by medial dissection of the involved pulmonary arteries. Radiographically, patients with parenchymal alveolar septal disease show evidence of interstitial disease, with fine reticular or reticulonodular opacities that may become more coarse and confluent over time. The radiographic appearance simulates that seen in silicosis or sarcoidosis.

The diagnosis is made on lung biopsy by the identification amorphous eosinophilic material thickening the alveolar septa that appears apple green in color when stained with Congo red and viewed under polarized light. No effective treatment exists.

Chronic Aspiration Pneumonia. Patients who repeatedly aspirate may develop chronic interstitial abnormalities on chest radiographs. With repeated episodes of aspiration over months to years, a residuum of irregular reticular interstitial opacities may persist, probably representing peribronchial scarring. A reticulonodular pattern may be seen caused by granulomas forming around food particles. These chronic interstitial abnormalities can be observed in between episodes of acute aspiration pneumonitis.

INHALATIONAL DISEASE

Pneumoconiosis

The term "pneumoconiosis" is used to describe the non-neoplastic reaction of the lungs to inhaled inorganic dust particles (6). The inorganic dust pneumoconioses result from the inhalation and retention of asbestos, silica, or coal particles within the lung. With time, the accumulation of these particles leads to two types of pathologic reaction that may be seen alone or in combination: fibrosis, which may be focal and nodular or diffuse and reticular, and the aggregation of particle-laden macrophages. The organic dust inhalational syndromes, which are discussed at the end of this section, are not associated with the retention and accumulation of particles within the lungs. Instead, the organic dusts induce a hypersensitivity reaction known as hypersensitivity pneumonitis or extrinsic allergic alveolitis.

Asbestosis. "Asbestos" is the generic term for a group of fibrous silicates that are resistant to heat and various chemical insults. Asbestos is divided into two major sub-

groups: the serpentines and the amphiboles. The serpentines are curly, flexible, and smooth; the only commercially important serpentine is chrysotile. The amphiboles have straight, needle-like fibers; this subgroup includes crocidolite and amosite. The different types of asbestos fibers vary in their potential to cause disease, with the amphiboles having a greater fibrogenic and carcinogenic potential than the serpentines. At present, more than 90% of the asbestos used in the United States is chrysotile.

Asbestos inhalation may cause disease of the pleura, parenchyma, airways, and lymph nodes. Pleural disease is the most common of these, and it usually manifests as parietal pleural plaques. Other pleural manifestations include pleural effusion, localized visceral pleural fibrosis, diffuse pleural fibrosis and mesothelioma. The pleural manifestations of asbestos exposure are discussed in more detail in chapter 20. The pulmonary parenchymal manifestations of asbestos inhalation include interstitial fibrosis (asbestosis), rounded atelectasis, and bronchogenic carcinoma.

Asbestosis is defined as a diffuse parenchymal interstitial fibrosis caused by the inhalation of asbestos fibers. The development of asbestosis depends on both the length and severity of exposure, and clinical manifestations are usually not apparent for 20–40 years following initial exposure. Pathologically, a large number of "asbestos bodies" will be seen in lung tissue. This characteristic structure consists of a core transparent asbestos fiber surrounded by a variably thick coat of iron and protein. Asbestos bodies are usually found within interstitial fibrous tissue or air spaces, and only rarely in pleural plaques. The number of asbestos bodies and fibers per gram of digested lung tissue is roughly proportional to the degree of occupational exposure and the severity of interstitial fibrosis. On gross examination of affected lungs, fibrosis is most prominent in the subpleural regions of the lower lobes. Microscopically, the appearance varies from a slight increase in interstitial collagen to complete obliteration of normal architecture and formation of thick fibrous (parenchymal) bands and cystic spaces (honeycombing).

The majority of patients with asbestos-related pleuropulmonary disease are asymptomatic. Patients beyond the early stages of interstitial fibrosis will often experience shortness of breath and a restrictive pattern on pulmonary function tests. These patients are also at risk to develop asbestos-associated neoplasia, particularly bronchogenic carcinoma and pleural mesothelioma, and require close clinical follow-up.

The radiographic findings in asbestosis occur in two forms: small and large opacities. Small opacities may be reticular, nodular, or a combination of the two. The changes produced on chest radiographs are divided into three stages. The earliest finding is a fine reticulation predominantly in the lower lung zones that is a manifestation of early interstitial pneumonitis and fibrosis. With time, the small, irregular opacities become more prominent, creating a coarse reticular pattern of disease. In later stages, the reticular opacities may extend into the mid and upper lung zones, with progressive obscuration of the cardiac and diaphragmatic margins and progressive diminution of lung volumes. Large opacities, measuring greater than 1 cm in diameter, are invariably associated with widespread interstitial fibrosis and pleural plaques. These large opacities show a lower zone predominance and may be well-defined or ill-defined and multiple.

HRCT is a sensitive indicator of both the pleural and parenchymal changes associated with clinical asbestosis (7). Interlobular septal thickening is the most common HRCT finding in asbestos-exposed individuals. Intralobular septal thickening and small centrilobular dot-like opacities, the latter due to peribronchiolar fibrosis, are also common. Many cases will progress to honeycombing. Many of these HRCT findings overlap with those of UIP (Figs. 18.12–18.18), but patients with asbestosis may also have pleural disease, which may help distinguish between these two entities. Additionally, ground-glass opacity is relatively uncommon in asbestosis compared with IPF and other forms of UIP.

Identification of intrafissural plaques, especially if they contain calcification, is also possible with HRCT. Characteristic CT features of focal lung masses in asbestos-exposed individuals may allow for conservative management of these lesions. For example, a wedge-shaped or round mass adjacent to focal pleural thickening, with evidence of lobar volume loss and a "comet tail" bronchovascular bundle coursing into it, can be confidently diagnosed as rounded atelectasis by HRCT.

Silicosis. Silica is an abundant mineral composed of regularly arranged molecules of silicon dioxide. It is ubiquitous in the earth's crust, and exposure to a high concentration may lead to pathologic and radiologic changes. Occupations associated with such levels of exposure include mining, quarrying, foundry work, ceramic work, and sandblasting.

Two distinct histopathologic reactions to inhaled silica are silicotic nodules and silicoproteinosis. Silicotic nodules measure from 1–10 mm in diameter, and are comprised of dense concentric lamellae of collagen. They are typically most numerous in the upper lobes and parahilar regions of lung; calcification or ossification of the nodules is common. Coalescence of these nodules produces areas of progressive massive fibrosis (PMF). Progressive massive fibrosis may occupy an entire lobe, with areas of emphysema often seen adjacent to these masses. Focal necrosis is common within the central portions of these large conglomerate lesions, often the result of ischemia or superinfection by tuberculosis or anaerobic bacteria. Silicoproteinosis is a different manifestation of the disease, usually occurring in individuals exposed to very high concentrations of silica, and is characterized by filling of alveolar spaces with lipoproteinaceous material similar to that seen in idiopathic alveolar proteinosis. There is little collagen deposition associated with this reaction, and the well-defined collagenous nodule is not typically seen. Patients with both fibrotic silicosis and acute silicoproteinosis have an increased susceptibility to tuberculosis.

Exposure of 10–20 years is required for the radiographic changes of silicosis to develop. The classic radiographic appearance consists of multiple, well-defined nodules ranging from 1–10 mm in diameter. These nodules, which calcify in approximately 20% of cases, are diffuse and demonstrate an upper zone predominance. A reticular pattern of disease may be seen preceding or associated with the nodular pattern; this pattern is sometimes the earliest radiographic finding. This pattern of reticulonodular opacities is often referred to as "simple" silicosis, in contrast to the large conglomerate opacities which characterize "complicated" silicosis (Fig. 18.10) (8). Representing areas of progressive massive fibrosis, these conglomerate opacities most commonly develop in the peripheral portions of the upper and middle lung zones. The opacities migrate toward the hila, leaving areas of emphysema between the pleural surface and the areas of progressive fibrosis. These conglomerate areas may cavitate, often in association with superimposed tuberculous infection. Hilar lymph node enlargement may be seen at any stage, and these hilar nodes often demonstrate peripheral "eggshell" calcification. A variant of the classic radiographic form of the disease is seen in patients with acute heavy exposure to silica, usually sandblasters, who develop acute silicoproteinosis. This presents radiographically with diffuse air-space disease and is indistinguishable in appearance from idiopathic alveolar proteinosis. These patients are also predisposed to superinfection with *Nocardia*, which may produce mass-like consolidation and chest wall involvement.

Clinically, the diagnosis of silicosis is based on identification of a diffuse reticular, nodular, or reticulonodular pattern on the chest radiograph in a patient with an appropriate exposure history. Patients may be asymptomatic for many years but may worsen functionally in conjunction with progression of the radiographic changes. The pulmonary fibrosis and associated restrictive functional impairment of silicosis may progress even after removing the individual from the offending environment.

Coal Worker's Pneumoconiosis. The inhalation of large amounts of carbon-containing inorganic material may cause significant pulmonary disease. The exposure levels required to cause this disease occur almost exclusively in the workplace. Because the most common occupation producing this entity is coal mining, the resultant disease is termed "coal worker's pneumoconiosis" (CWP).

CWP has two characteristic pathologic findings: the coal dust macule and PMF. The coal dust macule results from the deposit of carbonaceous material within the lung. Coal dust macules are round or stellate nodules ranging in size from 1–5 mm. Composed of pigment-laden macrophages with minimal or absent collagen formation, they are found within the interstitium adjacent to respiratory bronchioles and are scattered throughout the lungs with a predilection for the apices. The coal dust macule or nodule is the hallmark of simple CWP, but is usually not associated with functional impairment. In fact, radiographic abnormalities may be absent in simple CWP. Complicated CWP is characterized by the presence of PMF. PMF is defined as nodular or mass-like lesions exceeding 2–3 cm in diameter that are composed of irregular fibrosis and pigment. PMF is most common in the posterior segments of the upper lobes and superior segments of the lower lobes. The conglomerate masses may cross interlobar fissures. Central cavitation is common and is most often caused by infarction from obliteration of pulmonary vessels by the fibrotic masses. Occasionally, superinfection of the masses by tuberculosis or fungus accounts for central necrosis and cavitation. The mass lesions of complicated CWP are similar to those seen in complicated silicosis. It should be noted that despite their name, the lesions of PMF may not progress with time and are not necessarily massive in size.

Patients with CWP usually present with respiratory difficulties only when PMF has developed because those with simple pneumoconiosis are typically asymptomatic. In complicated CWP, progressive dyspnea with cor pulmonale and right heart failure occur. Because many coal workers also smoke cigarettes, the development of centrilobular emphysema and chronic bronchitis may complicate the clinical picture.

Radiographically, simple CWP presents typically as upper zone reticulonodular or small nodular opacities. A purely reticular pattern may also be seen, especially in the early stages of the process. The nodules range from 1–5 mm in diameter and correspond to conglomerates of coal dust macules seen pathologically. The lesions are indistinguishable radiographically from the nodules of simple silicosis. In as many as 10% of coal miners, some of these nodules will calcify centrally. This is in distinction to the diffuse calcification of silicotic nodules. The nodular opacities of simple CWP do not progress once coal dust exposure has ceased. The lesions of complicated pneumoconiosis (PMF) range in size from 2 cm to an entire lobe and are seen in the upper portion of the lungs. PMF usually begins peripherally as a mass with a smooth, well-defined lateral border and an ill-defined medial border. PMF gradually "migrates" toward the hilum, creating a zone of emphysema between the opacities and the chest wall. These lesions may mimic primary carcinoma, particularly if a background of nodular opacities is not appreciated. The PMF seen with CWP may develop years after exposure to coal dust has ceased and may progress in the absence of further exposure.

Certain complicating factors may alter the radiographic appearance of CWP. Tuberculosis is relatively common in patients with CWP and may produce central cavitation in some patients with PMF. Caplan's syndrome or "rheumatoid pneumoconiosis," seen in coal workers with rheumatoid arthritis, is characterized radiographically by nodular opacities 0.5–5 cm in diameter that develop rapidly and appear in crops. The nodules are more sharply defined and seen more peripherally than the masses of PMF. These lesions are not specific for CWP and may be seen in patients with silicosis or asbestosis.

Miscellaneous Pneumoconioses. A variety of inorganic dusts other than asbestos, silica, and coal dust can cause pleuropulmonary disease but are far less common. Chronic berylliosis results in a reaction that mimics sarcoidosis, and is discussed in the section on granulomatous diseases. Aluminum workers may develop disabling pulmonary fibrosis after years of exposure to aluminum dust, usually from bauxite mining. Radiographic changes include fine to coarse reticular or reticulonodular opacities distributed throughout the lungs with greatly diminished lung volumes and marked pleural thickening. Apical bullae, which produce spontaneous pneumothorax, may be seen. Hard metal pneumoconiosis, formerly called giant cell interstitial pneumonitis, may result from exposure to cobalt and tungsten alloys and lead to interstitial pneumonitis with varying degrees of fibrosis. The chest radiograph demonstrates a reticulonodular pattern that may be very coarse and, if advanced, may be associated with small cystic shadows. Lymph node enlargement may be seen.

Hypersensitivity Pneumonitis

Hypersensitivity pneumonitis or extrinsic allergic alveolitis is an immunologic pulmonary disorder associated with the inhalation of one of the antigenic organic dusts. These dusts must be of small particle size in order to penetrate into the alveolar spaces and incite a host inflammatory response. A wide variety of etiologic agents have been implicated, including many thermophilic bacteria, true fungi, and various animal proteins. Some of the more common disease entities include farmer's lung, which follows exposure to moldy hay; humidifier lung, which follows exposure to water reservoirs contaminated by thermophilic bacteria; and bird fancier's lung, which results from exposure to avian proteins in feathers and excreta.

The development of hypersensitivity pneumonitis depends on the size, number, and immunogenicity of the inhaled organic particles and the immune response of the host. Two forms of the disease are distinguished by their clinical presentation and immunopathogenesis. Acute disease develops 4–6 hours following exposure to the inciting antigen, and is mediated by a type III (immune complex) reaction. Typical symptoms include cough, dyspnea, and fever. Chronic disease is often insidious and commonly results in interstitial pulmonary fibrosis. Patients with chronic disease often have malaise, chronic cough, and progressive dyspnea. This form of disease appears to be mediated by a type IV (cell-mediated) immune reaction.

The histopathologic features of the different types of hypersensitivity pneumonitis are usually indistinguishable, except in rare situations in which antigenic material can be identified in the pathologic preparations. The pathologic features are dependent on the intensity of exposure to the allergen and on the disease stage at time of tissue biopsy is obtained. Early findings include capillary congestion and inflammation within alveolar septae. In later stages of acute disease, bronchiolitis and alveolitis with granuloma formation is present. With repeated antigenic exposure, a progressive increase in interstitial fibrosis occurs, which is initially patchy in distribution but may progress to diffuse interstitial fibrosis.

The radiographic changes of hypersensitivity pneumonitis parallel the pathologic findings. The chest radiograph may be normal early in the acute stage of disease. Within hours, fine nodular or ground-glass opacities develop, most often in the lower lobes; progressive air-space opacification may simulate pulmonary edema. Within hours to days, the opacities resolve and the chest radiograph becomes normal. With continued or repeated exposures, the chest radiograph will remain abnormal between acute episodes. The chronic changes appear as diffuse coarse reticular or reticulonodular opacities in the middle and upper lung zones; a honeycomb pattern with loss of lung volume may be seen. The diagnosis of hypersensitivity pneumonitis should be considered when repeated episodes of rapidly changing ground-glass or air-space opacification are seen in a patient with underlying coarse interstitial lung disease. Hilar or mediastinal lymph node enlargement and pleural effusion are uncommon findings in patients with hypersensitivity pneumonitis.

HRCT may be very helpful in the diagnosis of hypersensitivity pneumonitis, particularly in the subacute phase, when chest radiographs may be normal or quite nonspecific. The most common findings in the acute phase of the disease are air-space opacities, and the subacute phase is characterized by patchy areas of ground-glass opacity and poorly defined ("fuzzy") centrilobular nodules (Figs. 18.7,18.11)(9). These findings may be superimposed, and both show a predominance in the middle and lower lung zones. In the chronic phase of the disease, findings are those of fibrosis: interlobular and intralobular interstitial thickening, honeycombing, and traction bronchiectasis (Fig. 18.8). Distribution of disease is varied, but sometimes there is relative sparing of the costophrenic angles, which may help distinguish hypersensitivity pneumonitis from IPF and other forms of UIP.

The diagnosis of hypersensitivity pneumonitis is made by eliciting a history that suggests a temporal relationship between the patient's symptoms and certain exposures. The intermittent exposure of susceptible persons to high concentrations of antigen leads to recurrent episodes that typically begin 4–6 hours following exposure. The symptoms usually persist for 12 hours and then resolve spontaneously if the exposure has been terminated. Repeated exposure to the inciting antigen will result in acute exacerbations with typical symptoms and radiographic findings. Chronic disease is more difficult to diagnose and develops when there is a continuous low level of exposure to the antigen. The prognosis for patients whose disease is recognized at an early stage is good if the offending agent can be removed from the patient's environment. In the more insidious chronic form of disease, the diagnosis is often delayed and considerable interstitial fibrosis may be present at the time of diagnosis. These patients usually suffer from chronic respiratory insufficiency.

GRANULOMATOUS DISEASES

Sarcoidosis

Sarcoidosis is a multisystem granulomatous disease of unknown cause characterized histologically by noncaseating granulomas that may progress to fibrosis. The disease is seen more commonly in blacks than whites and is rare in Asians. African-American women are at particular risk for this disease. Most patients are 20–40 years of age at the time of diagnosis. However, because patients with this disease are often asymptomatic, many cases are never identified.

The cause of sarcoidosis is unknown although an inhaled infectious agent such as *Mycobacterium, Yersinia,* or a virus has been suggested. Whatever the causative agent, the underlying pathogenesis involves activation of pulmonary macrophages that in turn recruit mononuclear cells to the pulmonary interstitium leading to the formation of granulomas. The activated macrophages also stimulate proliferation of T-helper lymphocytes in the lung, which induces an overactivity of B lymphocytes resulting in the hypergammaglobulinemia characteristically seen in this disease. The excess number of T-helper lymphocytes in the lung may be detected in bronchoalveolar lavage fluid of patients with sarcoidosis, and is helpful in the differential diagnosis of this condition.

The pathologic changes of sarcoidosis follow a fairly predictable pattern. The earliest changes involve the pulmonary interstitium, with the development of a nonspecific lymphocytic and histiocytic infiltrate. This progresses to the formation of microscopic granulomas. The granulomas contain palisading epithelioid histiocytes with intermixed multinucleated giant cells, and in contrast to tuberculous granulomas are typically noncaseating. The giant cells in the granulomas may contain dark-staining lamellated structures within their cytoplasm called Schaumann's bodies, which are characteristic of sarcoidosis. The granulomas are found most commonly within the axial (peribronchovascular) and peripheral or subpleural interstitium of the lung, but may involve the parenchymal (alveolar) interstitium and airway mucosa; the airway lesions may be visualized bronchoscopically. Involvement of the axial interstitium of the lung accounts for the high (approximately 90%) diagnostic yield of blind transbronchial biopsy in sarcoidosis because this technique usually provides samples of the bronchial wall, the surrounding axial interstitium, and adjacent air spaces. The small granulomas usually resolve after months or years. In some patients, the microscopic granulomas coalesce to form larger nodules. Rarely, these nodules grow to form large well-defined masses or poorly marginated opacities containing air bronchograms and simulating an air-space filling process. In this "alveolar" form of sarcoidosis, the air spaces are not filled with material but rather are compressed and obliterated by the exuberant granuloma formation within the surrounding interstitium.

In 20% of patients, fibrous tissue is deposited at the periphery of the granulomas and eventually grows inward to replace the granulomas resulting in interstitial fibrosis. The fibrosis progresses over time, with the development of broad bands of fibrous tissue extending from the hilar regions toward the lung apices, producing hilar elevation and distortion of the hilar vessels and upper mediastinum. Masses of fibrous tissue may develop in the perihilar regions of the upper lobes with peripheral areas of emphysema or cyst formation. These cysts predispose patients to spontaneous pneumothoraces and provide a site for mycetoma formation.

Lymph node involvement in sarcoidosis is characterized by replacement of the normal nodal architecture with granulomas indistinguishable from those found in the pulmonary parenchyma. As with parenchymal involvement, these may regress, coalesce, or undergo fibrosis.

The clinical presentation may be dominated by pulmonary or extrapulmonary manifestations of the disease, but a considerable percentage of patients are asymptomatic and are identified by incidental findings on chest radiographs. Pulmonary symptoms are present in 25% of patients and include dyspnea and a nonproductive cough. Common extrapulmonary findings include fever, malaise, uveitis, and erythema nodosum. In a minority of patients, involvement of liver, heart, kidneys, or CNS may dominate the clinical picture.

Common laboratory findings in sarcoidosis include hypercalcemia, hypergammaglobulinemia, and elevated serum angiotensin converting enzyme (ACE) levels. Cutaneous anergy to PPD reflects an abnormality of delayed hypersensitivity found in these patients. Pulmonary function tests vary from normal in those with minimal or no parenchymal disease to a severe restrictive pattern with low diffusing capacity in patients with end-stage pulmonary fibrosis.

RADIOGRAPHIC FINDINGS

Lymph Node Enlargement. Enlargement of mediastinal and hilar lymph nodes is found in 80% of patients with sarcoidosis, and is associated with radiographically normal lungs in slightly more than half of these patients (10). The typical appearance on chest radiographs is right paratracheal and bilateral symmetric hilar lymph node enlargement (Fig. 18.23). The symmetric enlargement is a key feature that allows distinction from malignancy and tuberculosis, conditions that usually produce unilateral or asymmetric lymph node enlargement. Left

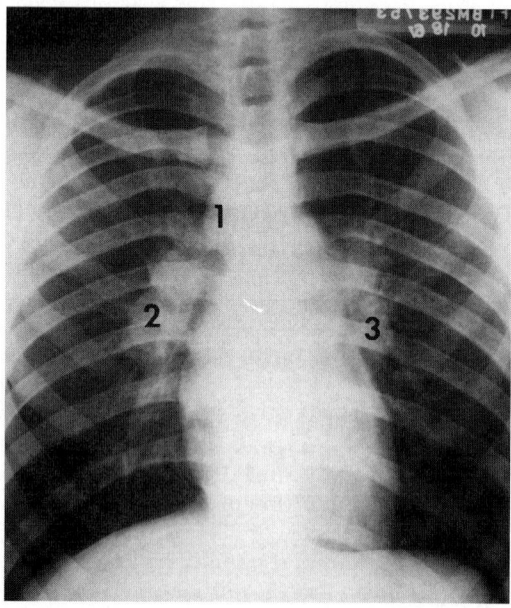

Figure 18.23. Sarcoidosis. A PA radiograph in an asymptomatic 26-year-old shows marked enlargement of right paratracheal (*1*), right hilar (*2*), and left hilar (*3*) lymph nodes characteristic of sarcoidosis.

paratracheal lymph node enlargement is common as determined by CT although enlargement of these nodes is usually not appreciated on radiographs because this region is obscured by the aorta and great vessels on frontal radiographs. The enlarged nodes tend to have a lobulated contour as the individual nodes remain discrete. Mediastinal (paratracheal) lymph node enlargement without concomitant hilar enlargement is uncommon and should suggest lymphoma or metastatic disease. Similarly, unilateral hilar nodal enlargement is unusual, seen in only 5% of individuals. Involvement of anterior mediastinal, posterior mediastinal, subcarinal, and aortopulmonary lymph nodes occurs with greater frequency than previously thought, owing to the ability of CT to detect nodes in regions that are invisible on plain radiographs. Involved nodes may show contrast enhancement.

The enlarged lymph nodes regress within 2 years in 75% of affected patients. A small percentage of patients will have persistent lymph node enlargement for years. The development of parenchymal opacities concomitant with the resolution of lymph node enlargement is a helpful feature in differentiating sarcoidosis from lymphoma, in which enlarged lymph nodes do not regress when parenchymal abnormalities develop. Calcification of involved lymph nodes is common, seen in up to 20% of patients, and may involve only the periphery of the node ("eggshell" calcification).

Lung Disease. The lung is involved radiographically in only 40–50% of patients with sarcoidosis, despite the nearly 90% yield from transbronchial biopsy of the lung. The earliest finding is a diffuse micronodular pattern identical in appearance to miliary tuberculosis, which represents the superimposition of microscopic granulomas. This pattern, which is rarely identified radiographically, may precede the development of hilar lymph node enlargement. The most common parenchymal abnormality is bilateral symmetric reticulonodular opacities, which have a predilection for the middle and upper lung zones (Fig. 18.24). The reticulonodular opacities represent the combination of granulomas and fibrosis. CT shows most nodules to lie predominantly in a peribronchovascular and subpleural location. The appearance of reticulonodular opacities never precedes the enlargement of hilar and mediastinal lymph nodes.

In approximately 10% of patients, the coalescence of granulomas can produce one of two unusual radiographic manifestations of parenchymal sarcoidosis. Exuberant interstitial granulomas can obliterate adjacent air spaces producing poorly defined air-space opacities that may contain air bronchograms. In some cases, intra-alveolar inflammation and granulomas contribute to the alveolar pattern of disease. These air-space opacities are primarily seen in the peripheral portions of the middle lung zone, thereby simulating eosinophilic pneumonia radiographically. The presence of reticulonodular opacities elsewhere in the lung or concomitant symmetric hilar and mediastinal lymph node enlargement, best seen on CT and HRCT, provide important clues to the diagnosis.

Nodular or mass-like sarcoidosis develops in a manner similar to alveolar disease. These masses can be quite

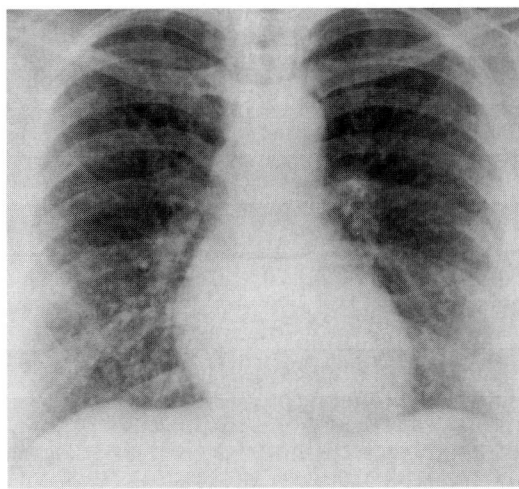

Figure 18.24. Sarcoidosis. A PA chest film in a 39-year-old black female with mild dyspnea shows extensive bilateral reticulonodular opacities. Transbronchial biopsy showed noncaseating granulomas typical of sarcoidosis.

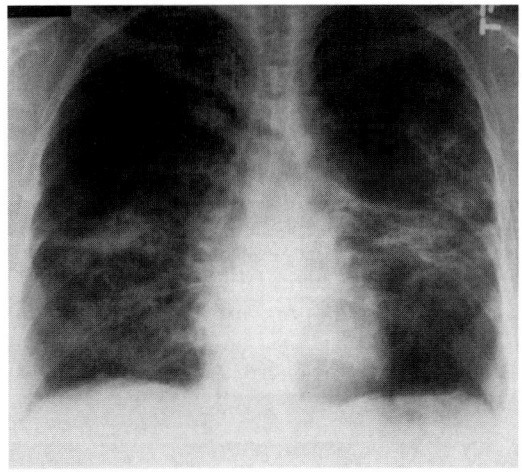

Figure 18.25. Bullous Changes in Sarcoidosis. In a 49-year-old woman with long-standing sarcoidosis, a PA chest film shows extensive middle and lower zone coarse interstitial opacities and biapical bullous disease.

large and typically have a sharp margin. Air bronchograms are often demonstrated on CT and HRCT; cavitation is extremely rare.

Pulmonary fibrosis develops in 20% of patients with long-standing parenchymal involvement. The chest radiograph shows coarse linear opacities extending obliquely from the hila toward the upper and middle lung zones. There is considerable distortion and elevation of the hila with scalloping of the lung-mediastinal interface. Occasionally, conglomerate masses of fibrosis form in the upper perihilar regions, which simulate the progressive massive fibrosis of complicated silicosis. On CT, these masses contain air bronchograms with traction bronchiectasis. Distortion and obstruction of the airways from fibrosis can lead to secondary air trapping with resultant alveolar septal disruption and bullae formation. An increase in radiographic lung volumes may accompany these cystic changes, a finding that is characteristic of bullous sarcoidosis (Fig. 18.25). Mycetomas can develop within the cysts and cause massive hemoptysis from erosion into bronchial arteries. Cysts may also rupture into the pleural space and produce spontaneous pneumothoraces.

Pleural Changes. Pleural thickening or effusion occurs in approximately 7% of patients with sarcoidosis and is caused by a granulomatous inflammation of the visceral and parietal pleura.

Miscellaneous Findings. Endobronchial granulomas can result in fibrosis of the bronchial wall and bronchostenosis. Pulmonary arterial hypertension is an uncommon finding and is usually secondary to long-standing pulmonary fibrosis.

HRCT Findings. HRCT is clearly more sensitive than chest radiographs in detecting the parenchymal abnormalities in sarcoidosis. A variety of HRCT findings have been described in this disease, which represent both the granulomatous and fibrotic response seen histologically. The most frequent finding is the presence of interstitial nodules, 3–10 mm in diameter, seen as nodular thick-

ening of the peribronchoarterial (axial) interstitium and interlobular septa or as subpleural nodules. The nodules correlate closely with the coalescing noncaseating granulomas seen microscopically on tissue specimens. Septal thickening, thickening of bronchovascular bundles, architectural distortion, lung cysts, honeycombing, and central conglomerate masses with crowded and ectatic bronchi are findings indicative of fibrosis from long-standing disease (Fig. 18.6). Segmental or mass-like air-space opacities, termed "alveolar" sarcoid, usually indicate active disease and resolve with corticosteroid therapy. Likewise, the finding of patchy areas of ground-glass density correlates with increased uptake on gallium scans and may indicate an active alveolitis. Several recent papers have showed good correlation between conventional and HRCT findings and pulmonary function tests.

Radiographic Staging of Sarcoidosis. The chest radiographic manifestations of sarcoidosis have been divided into five stages (Table 18.6).

These stages usually parallel the course of disease and are useful for prognostic purposes. Stage 1 disease is associated with a 75% rate of resolution whereas only 30% of patients with stage 2 and 10% of patients with stage 3 disease resolve.

The diagnosis of sarcoidosis is usually based on the histologic demonstration of noncaseating granulomas involving multiple organs. Tissue is most often obtained

Table 18.6. Radiographic Staging of Sarcoidosis

Stage	Radiographic Findings
0	Normal chest radiograph
1	Bilateral hilar lymph node enlargement
2	Bilateral hilar lymph node enlargement and parenchymal disease
3	Parenchymal disease only
4	Pulmonary fibrosis

by bronchoscopically guided transbronchial biopsy, which provides a diagnosis in up to 90% of patients. Biopsy of organs likely to be involved in this disease, such as the liver and scalene lymph nodes, will provide a diagnosis in a majority of patients. Percutaneous needle biopsy can provide diagnostic tissue specimens in those with mass-like pulmonary lesions. In certain situations, the diagnosis of sarcoidosis is made on a constellation of chest radiographic findings and characteristic eye or skin changes. In such patients, gallium scintigraphy showing a pattern of increased uptake in the hilar lymph nodes, lung, and salivary glands may be used as a confirmatory test. Gallium scanning has also been used to assess the degree of disease activity.

Berylliosis

Although berylliosis is actually an inhalational lung disease, it is discussed here because of the clinical, pathologic, and radiographic similarities to sarcoidosis. This uncommon disease produces noncaseating granulomas in multiple organs, with primary lung involvement. The radiographic features of berylliosis are indistinguishable from sarcoidosis. Hilar and mediastinal lymph node enlargement and bilateral reticulonodular opacities are the most common findings. As with sarcoidosis, progression to end-stage interstitial fibrosis with honeycombing or upper lobe bullous disease may occur, with the latter predisposing the patient to aspergilloma formation and spontaneous pneumothorax.

Langerhans' Cell Histiocytosis of Lung

This entity includes three disorders with similar pathologic features that differ in the age at the time of diagnosis, mode of presentation, specific organs involved, and prognosis. These diseases are felt to be related to an acquired immunological defect. Eosinophilic granuloma (EG) is the form of this disease affecting adults, with predominant involvement of lung and bones. The disease most commonly affects young adults without a sex predilection. There is a very high association between pulmonary involvement and cigarette smoking.

Pathologically, EG of lung demonstrates multiple small nodules that are found predominantly in the axial interstitial tissues of the upper and mid lung zones around small bronchioles. The nodules represent granulomas composed predominantly of cells with eosinophilic cytoplasm previously called histiocytosis X cells and now known as Langerhans' cells. These cells are normally found in the skin and appear to proliferate in the lung and other organs in response to an unidentified antigenic stimulus. In some patients, the nodular phase of disease may be preceded by an exudative phase with filling of the alveolar spaces with a cellular exudate containing the Langerhans' cells. The small peribronchiolar nodules may coalesce to form larger nodules which may cavitate, or they may extend to infiltrate the alveolar septa and induce an interstitial inflammatory reaction. The nodules may resolve completely, but in most patients, the central portions of the nodules undergo fibro-

sis, producing a stellate nodular lesion characteristic of pulmonary EG histologically. In the late stages, characteristic findings include fibrosis and the development of small uniform, thin-walled cysts. Larger peripheral cysts or bullae may develop in the apical regions, presumably as a result of bronchiolar obstruction by fibrosis with distal air trapping.

Pulmonary symptoms are present in two-thirds of patients with EG of lung at presentation. Cough and the gradual onset of dyspnea are the most common complaints. Pleuritic chest pain may indicate the development of a spontaneous pneumothorax from rupture of a subpleural cyst. The physical examination is typically unremarkable. Pulmonary function tests reflect the fibrosis and cystic changes seen in this disorder, with characteristic restrictive and obstructive patterns of disease and a diminished diffusing capacity.

The radiographic findings in EG of lung usually follow a predictable pattern. Although the earliest changes in EG of lung are associated with filling of alveoli, the radiographic demonstration of air-space opacities is uncommon. The earliest findings are small-sized to medium-sized nodular opacities that have an upper and middle lung zone distribution (Fig. 18.26). In some cases the nodules coalesce to form larger nodules or masses that rarely cavitate. The nodular pattern may resolve completely or be replaced by a predominantly reticulonodular or reticular pattern that represents the fibrotic phase of the disease. Late stages of the disease are characterized by a coarse reticular pattern with intermixed thin-walled cysts. These cysts account for the relative preservation or increase in lung volumes typical of EG, which is a distinguishing feature of this disease. Hilar or mediastinal lymph node enlargement is distinctly uncommon, a feature that helps distinguish EG from sarcoidosis. Pneumothorax from rupture of a cyst or bulla

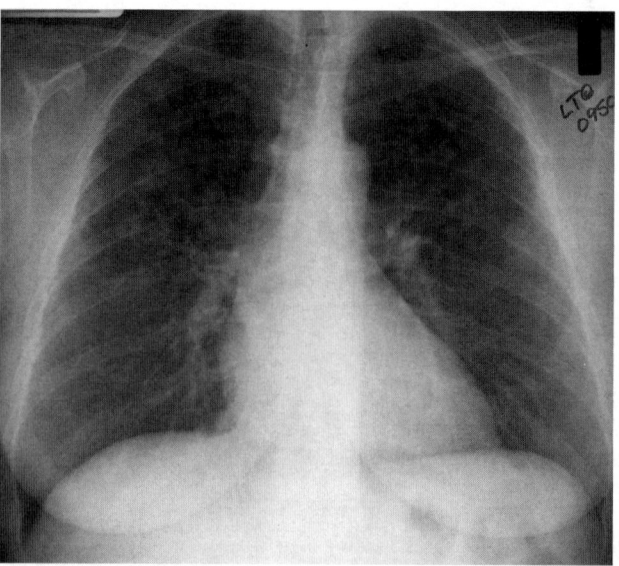

Figure 18.26. Eosinophilic Granuloma (Langerhans' Cell Histiocytosis) of Lung. PA radiograph in a 52-year-old woman with eosinophilic granuloma shows a nodular pattern with a middle and upper zone predominance.

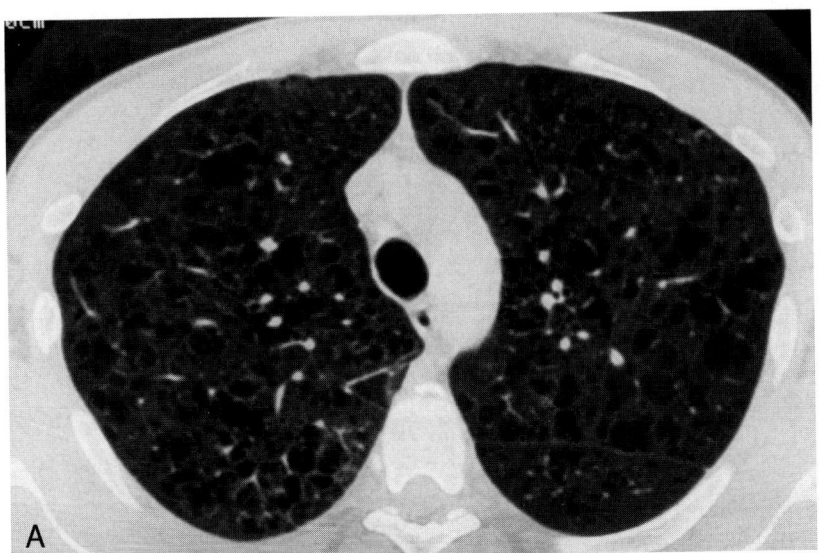

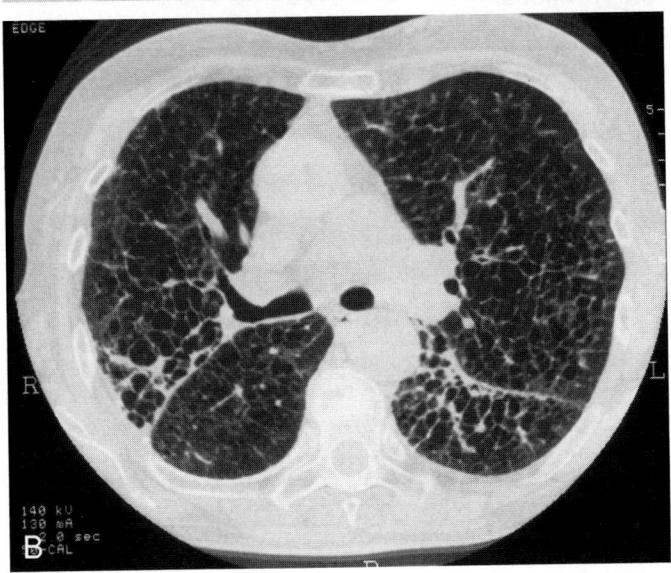

Figure 18.27. Eosinophilic Granuloma on HRCT. A. HRCT in a 39-year-old smoker with EG shows multiple cysts with thin but well-defined walls. **B.** In another patient with EG, the cysts are more extensive with little normal intervening parenchyma. Note the irregular shape of many of these cysts.

is the presenting finding or develops during the course of disease in up to 25% of patients. Pleural effusion in the absence of a pneumothorax is rare. Extrapulmonary manifestations include well-defined lytic rib or vertebral lesions.

The parenchymal changes of EG are best demonstrated on HRCT. HRCT in patients with a relatively short duration of symptoms (<6 months) shows well-defined interstitial nodules of varying size, sometimes with cavitation, and cyst formation in the upper lungs. More long-standing disease is characterized by larger cysts (Fig. 18.27) and honeycombing. It was recently demonstrated that nodules and thick-walled cysts can transform into thin-walled cysts, suggesting that the sequence of evolution of EG lesions is as follows: nodule → cavitated nodule → thick-walled cyst → thin-walled cyst (11). The distinguishing features between EG and emphysema are the presence of nodules (with or without cavitation) and thin-walled cysts in EG that lack a constant relationship to the centrilobular core structures. The

HRCT distinction of EG from LAM in a female is more difficult; an upper zone distribution and the presence of nodules favors EG.

The diagnosis of EG of lung is made by noting the characteristic stellate nodular lesions with Langerhans' cells on open lung biopsy specimens. The treatment for symptomatic patients is corticosteroid therapy although more than half of the patients with lung disease stabilize or improve spontaneously.

Wegener's Granulomatosis

This is a systemic autoimmune disorder characterized pathologically by a necrotizing granulomatous vasculitis involving the upper and lower respiratory tracts and kidneys. The characteristic lesions in the lungs are discrete nodules or masses of granulomatous inflammation with central necrosis and cavitation. The lesions involve pulmonary vessels, accounting for the high incidence of central necrosis and for the occasional presentation with pulmonary hemorrhage. Mucosal and submucosal le-

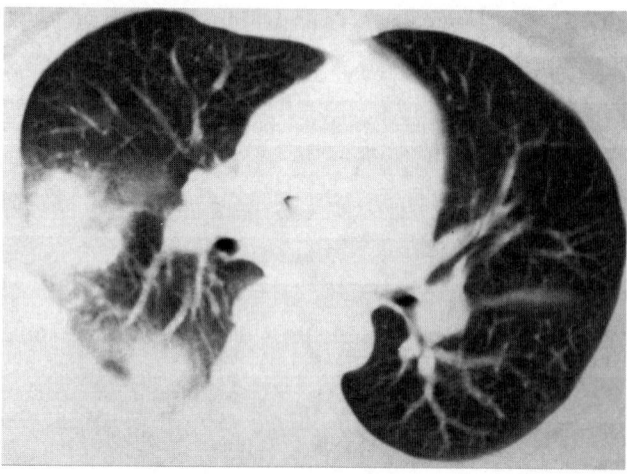

Figure 18.28. Wegener's Granulomatosis. A CT examination in a patient with Wegener's granulomatosis shows several large masses with indistinct margins in the right lower lobe.

sions may be present in the tracheobronchial tree and are seen almost exclusively in females.

Most patients with Wegener's granulomatosis are middle-aged, with a slight male predominance. The respiratory tract is affected in 100% of patients, with symptoms usually dominated by the sinus and nasal mucosal involvement. Pulmonary involvement may be asymptomatic or manifested by cough, dyspnea, or chest pain. Presentation with pulmonary hemorrhage and hemoptysis may mimic other pulmonary-renal syndromes such as Goodpasture's and idiopathic pulmonary hemorrhage. Renal involvement usually follows involvement of the respiratory tract and is seen in almost 90% of patients.

The characteristic chest radiographic features of lung involvement in Wegener's granulomatosis are multiple sharply marginated nodules or masses (Fig. 18.28); solitary lesions are seen in up to one-third of patients. Irregular, thick-walled cavitary lesions are seen in 50% of patients during the course of disease. Localized or diffuse areas of air-space opacification may be seen, representing either hemorrhage or pneumonia, the latter often due to complicating *Staphylococcus aureus* infection. Tracheal or bronchial lesions may be present and are usually best appreciated on CT where they appear as calcified mucosal or submucosal deposits producing irregular narrowing of the airway lumen. The airway lesions are not associated with parenchymal disease, but endobronchial lesions may produce distal atelectasis. Pleural effusion from pleural involvement is not uncommon. Pneumothorax may result from rupture of a cavi-

tary lesion into the pleural space. Lymph node enlargement is not seen in this disease.

The diagnosis of Wegener's granulomatosis should be made on biopsy of involved tissues, usually nasal mucosa or lung, which show the granulomatous inflammation and vasculitis characteristic of this disease. The pathologic changes in the kidneys are often nonspecific; therefore, renal biopsy is often nondiagnostic. This disease usually responds dramatically to cyclophosphamide (cytoxan) therapy. Some patients with disease limited to the chest respond to oral Bactrim. Untreated patients invariably die of renal failure or, less commonly, progressive respiratory disease. High serologic titers for the presence of antineutrophil cytoplasmic antibody are specific for the diagnosis of Wegener's granulomatosis although a negative test does not exclude the diagnosis, particularly in patients with limited or inactive disease.

References

1. Padley S, Gleeson F, Flower CDR. Review article: current indications for high resolution computed tomography scanning of the lungs. BJR 1995;68:105–109.
2. Webb WR, Muller NL, Naidich DP. HRCT findings of lung disease. In: High Resolution CT of the Lung. 2nd ed. Philadelphia: Lippincott-Raven, 1996:41–108.
3. McAdams HP, Rosado-de-Christenson ML, Wehunt WD, et al. The alphabet soup revisited: the chronic interstitial pneumonias in the 1990's. Radiographics 1996;16:1009–1033.
4. Fraser RS, Pare JAP, Fraser RG, et al. Diseases of altered immunologic activity. In: Diagnosis of Diseases of the Chest. Vol 2. 3rd ed. Philadelphia: WB Saunders, 1989:1189–1240.
5. Armstrong P, Wilson AG, Dee P. Pulmonary diseases of unknown origin and miscellaneous lung disorders. In: Imaging of Diseases of the Chest. 2nd ed. St Louis: Mosby, 1995:568–608.
6. Armstrong P, Wilson AG, Dee P. Inhalational lung diseases. In: Imaging of Diseases of the Chest. 2nd ed. St Louis: Mosby, 1995:426–460.
7. Aberle DR, Gamsu G, Ray CS. High-resolution CT of benign asbestos-related diseases: clinical and radiographic correlation. AJR Am J Roentgenol 1988;151:883–891.
8. Begin R, Ostiguy G, Groleau S, et al. Computed tomography scanning of the thorax in patients at risk of or with silicosis. Semin Ultrasound CT MR 1990;11:380–392.
9. Lynch DA, Rose CS, Way D, et al. Hypersensitivity pneumonitis: sensitivity of high-resolution CT in a population-based study. AJR Am J Roentgenol 1992;159:469–472.
10. Kirks DR, McCormick VD, Greenspan RH. Pulmonary sarcoidosis: roentgenologic analysis of 150 patients. AJR Am J Roentgenol 1973;117:777–786.
11. Brauner MW, Grenier P, Tijani K, et al. Pulmonary Langerhans' cell histiocytosis: evaluation of lesions on CT scans. Radiology 1997;204:497–502.

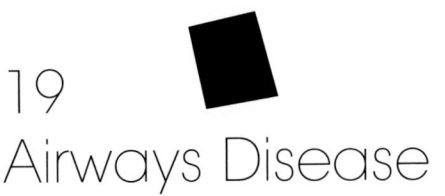

19
Airways Disease

Jeffrey S. Klein

TRACHEA AND CENTRAL BRONCHI

Congenital Tracheal Anomalies

Tracheal agenesis, cartilaginous abnormalities of the trachea, tracheal webs and stenosis, tracheoesophageal fistulas, and vascular rings and slings present as breathing and feeding difficulties in the neonatal and infancy period. These uncommon congenital lesions are discussed in chapter 51.

Tracheoceles are true diverticula that represent herniation of the tracheal air column through a weakened posterior tracheal membrane. These lesions occur almost exclusively in the cervical trachea because the pressure gradient from the extrathoracic trachea to the atmosphere with the Valsalva maneuver favors their formation in this region. Tracheoceles are usually asymptomatic and easily recognized on fluoroscopy, CT, or contrast tracheogram.

Tracheal Bronchus, or bronchus suis, so-called because it is the normal pattern of tracheal branching in pigs, consists of an accessory bronchus to all or a portion of the right upper lobe, which arises from the right lateral tracheal wall within 2 cm of the tracheal carina (Fig. 19.1). However, it most often supplies the apical segment of the right upper lobe. While it is usually an incidental finding on chest CT in 0.5–1.0% of the population, tracheal bronchus has an association with congenital tracheal stenosis and an aberrant left pulmonary artery. Most patients are asymptomatic.

Focal Tracheal Disease

Focal disorders of the trachea may produce narrowing or dilatation of the tracheal lumen (Table 19.1)(1). Focal narrowing may be produced by extrinsic or intrinsic mass lesions, retraction, or inflammatory disorders of the tracheal wall.

Extrinsic Compression/Narrowing. The most common causes of extrinsic mass effect on the trachea are an intrathoracic goiter and a large paratracheal lymph node mass. In older individuals, a tortuous or aneurysmal transverse portion of the aortic arch may cause right lateral deviation of the distal intrathoracic trachea. Extrinsic mass effect can also be seen with congenital vascular anomalies such as an aberrant left pulmonary artery and aortic ring, or a large mediastinal bronchogenic cyst. Because the tracheal cartilage provides resiliency, extrinsic masses displace the trachea without narrowing its lumen. Traction deformity of the trachea is usually seen in cicatrizing processes that asymmetrically affect the lung apices, most commonly chronic tuberculosis and histoplasmosis. Occasionally, the distal trachea is narrowed in patients with sclerosing mediastinitis; however, this disorder normally affects the central bronchi.

Focal Tracheal Stenosis. Focal tracheal or central (main and proximal lobar) bronchial narrowing may result from inflammatory disorders that affect the tracheal or central bronchial walls. Cartilaginous damage or the development of granulation tissue and fibrosis from a tracheostomy or at the site of a previously inflated endotracheal tube balloon cuff can cause focal tracheal narrowing. The tracheal stenosis has a typical hourglass deformity on frontal radiographs. Those patients with tracheomalacia from cartilage damage may only manifest narrowing during phases of the respiratory cycle when extratracheal pressure exceeds intratracheal pressure. Therefore, patients with extrathoracic tracheomalacia—most often at the site of a prior tracheostomy, demonstrate tracheal narrowing on inspiration—but patients with intrathoracic tracheomalacia, usually from prior endotracheal intubation, have tracheal narrowing on expiration. Postintubation stenosis is rare with the low-pressure, high-volume endotracheal tube cuffs in current use. Wegener's granulomatosis can produce a necrotizing granulomatous inflammation of the trachea and central bronchi, leading to focal cervical tracheal narrowing or, in advanced disease, narrowing of the entire length of the trachea. The diagnosis of tracheal involvement by Wegener's granulomatosis is made by the radiographic demonstration of tracheal narrowing in association with upper airway and renal involvement, and characteristic findings on biopsy. Cyclophosphamide therapy administered early in the course of the disease may reduce inflammation and improve tracheal narrowing. Sarcoidosis involving the central airways may rarely cause focal tracheal or bronchial stenosis.

Figure 19.1. Tracheal Bronchus. Endoluminal rendering of a helical CT data set reveals an anomalous bronchus (*arrow*) arising from the right lateral tracheal wall above the tracheal carina (*C*). *R*, right main bronchus; *L*, left main bronchus.

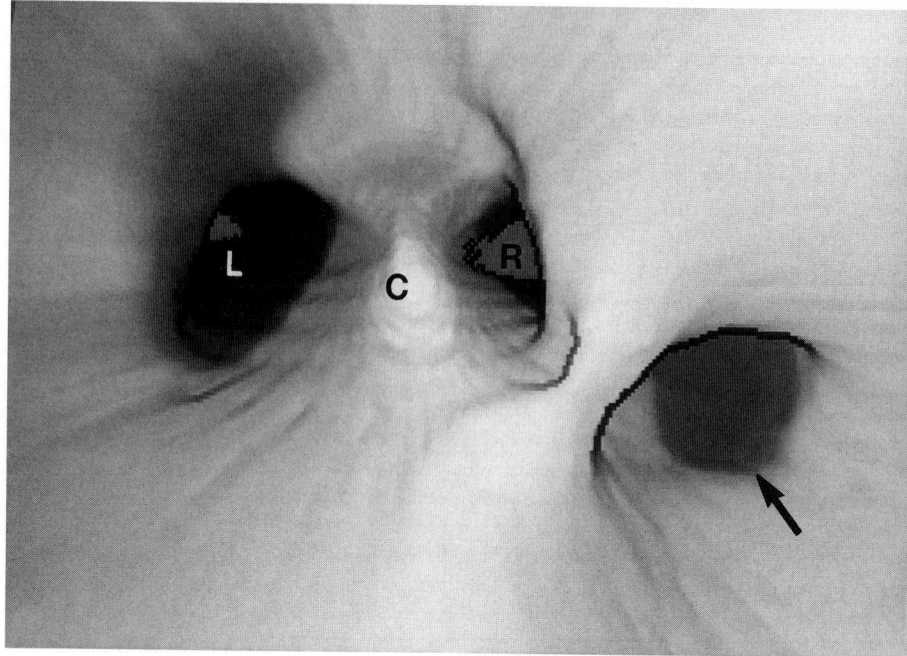

A number of infectious processes may result in tracheal or bronchial inflammation and stenosis. Endotracheal and endobronchial tuberculosis is usually associated with cavitary tuberculosis, in which the production of large volumes of infected sputum predisposes patients to tracheal and central bronchial infection. Upper tracheal inflammation and stenosis may result from histoplasmosis and coccidioidomycosis. Invasive tracheobronchitis from *Aspergillus*, *Candida*, and mucormycosis has been described in immunodeficient patients. Scleroma is a chronic granulomatous disorder caused by infection with *Klebsiella rhinoscleromatis*. This disease is uncommon in the United States and is seen most commonly in people of lower socioeconomic status in Central and South America and Eastern Europe. The infection begins as an inflammation of the nasal mucosa and paranasal sinuses, extending inferiorly to involve the larynx, pharynx, and trachea in a minority of patients. In its chronic phase, intense granulation tissue and fibrosis leads to nasal cavity, pharyngeal, laryngeal, and upper tracheal stenosis; the latter is seen in less than 10% of patients. Radiographically, the upper trachea shows irregular nodular narrowing that may extend to involve the length of the trachea. The diagnosis is made on biopsy, which reveals granulation tissue containing large foamy histiocytes filled with the causative organism (Mikulicz cells). Antibiotic treatment is effective if administered in the early phases of infection before extensive fibrosis has developed.

Tracheal and Bronchial Masses are mostly neoplasms and are discussed in chapter 16.

Focal Tracheal Dilatation is caused by congenital or acquired abnormalities of the elastic membrane or cartilaginous rings of the trachea. Localized tracheal dilatation may be seen with tracheoceles, acquired tracheomalacia related to prolonged endotracheal intubation, or as a result of tracheal traction from severe unilateral upper lobe parenchymal scarring.

Diffuse Tracheal Disease

Diffuse disorders of the trachea manifest as either narrowing or dilatation of the tracheal lumen. Diffuse tracheal narrowing may be seen with saber-sheath trachea, amyloidosis, tracheobronchopathia osteochondroplastica, relapsing polychondritis, Wegener's granulomatosis, or tracheal scleroma (Table 19.2)(2). The latter two conditions may cause diffuse tracheal narrowing, but more commonly the involvement is limited to the cervical trachea. These conditions are discussed in the section on focal tracheal narrowing.

DIFFUSE TRACHEAL NARROWING

Saber-Sheath Trachea is a fixed deformity of the intrathoracic trachea in which the coronal diameter is diminished to less than two-thirds of the sagittal diameter (3). The tracheal wall is uniformly thickened, and calcification of the cartilaginous rings is present in most cases. This entity exclusively affects older males with functional evidence of chronic obstructive pulmonary disease. The tracheal narrowing likely reflects the chronic transmission of increased intrapleural pressure seen in obstructive lung disease and tracheal injury from chronic cough. The characteristic findings are seen on frontal radiographs and CT (Fig. 19.2).

Amyloidosis is characterized by the deposition of a fibrillar protein-polysaccharide complex in various organs and may involve the airways as part of localized or systemic disease. Submucosal deposits in the tracheobronchial tree are more commonly a manifestation of localized disease, and may be associated with nodular or

Table 19.1. Causes of Focal Tracheal Disease

Narrowing	**Extrinsic**
	Thyroid goiter
	Paratracheal lymph node mass
	Asymmetric or unilateral upper lobe fibrosis
	Tuberculosis
	Histoplasmosis
	Intrinsic
	Tracheomalacia
	Endotracheal tube cuff
	Tracheostomy site
	Wegener's granulomatosis
	Sarcoidosis
	Infection
	Tuberculosis
	Fungus
	Histoplasmosis
	Coccidiomycosis
	Aspergillosis
	Scleroma
Masses	**Neoplasm**
	Malignant
	Primary
	Squamous cell carcinoma
	Adenoid cystic carcinoma (cylindroma)
	Metastatic
	Direct invasion
	Laryngeal carcinoma
	Thyroid carcinoma
	Esophageal carcinoma
	Bronchogenic carcinoma
	Hematogenous (endobronchial)
	Breast carcinoma
	Renal cell carcinoma
	Colon carcinoma
	Melanoma
	Benign
	Chondroma
	Fibroma
	Squamous cell papilloma
	Hemangioma
	Granular cell myoblastoma
	Non-neoplastic
	Ectopic thyroid or thymus
	Mucus
Dilatation	Tracheoceles
	Tracheomalacia
	Upper lobe fibrosis

Table 19.2. Causes of Diffuse Tracheal Disease

Tracheal Narrowing	Saber sheath trachea
	Amyloidosis
	Tracheobronchopathia osteochondroplastica
	Relapsing polychondritis
	Wegener's granulomatosis
	Tracheal scleroma
Tracheal Dilatation	Tracheobronchomegaly (Mournier-Kuhn syndrome)
	Tracheomalacia
	Interstitial pulmonary fibrosis

alveolar septal deposits in the lungs. Mass-like circumferential deposits that irregularly narrow the tracheal lumen are best demonstrated on CT and can result in recurrent atelectasis and pneumonia. Calcification of these deposits occurs in only 10% of cases. The diagnosis is made by the presence of typical protein-polysaccharide deposits demonstrated on Congo red stains of tracheal or bronchial wall biopsy specimens.

Tracheobronchopathia Osteochondroplastica is a rare disorder characterized by the presence of multiple submucosal osseous and cartilaginous deposits within the trachea and central bronchi of elderly men. The lesions arise as enchondromas from the tracheal and bronchial cartilage and project internally to produce nodular submucosal deposits that irregularly narrow the tracheal lumen and have a characteristic appearance and feel on bronchoscopy. The diagnosis is usually made on bronchoscopy and CT, where calcified plaques can be seen involving the anterior and lateral walls of the trachea. Sparing of the membranous posterior wall of the trachea, which lacks cartilage, is a helpful feature that distinguishes this entity from tracheobronchial amyloid. Although usually asymptomatic, patients may have recurrent infection related to bronchial obstruction by the masses.

Relapsing Polychondritis is a systemic autoimmune disorder that commonly affects the cartilage of the earlobes, nose, larynx, tracheobronchial tree, joints, and large elastic arteries. Early in the disease, tracheal wall inflammation associated with cartilage destruction leads to an abnormally compliant and dilated trachea. Later in the disease, fibrosis leads to diffuse, fixed narrowing of the tracheal lumen. Respiratory complications secondary to involvement of the upper airway cartilage account for nearly 50% of all deaths from this condition. The diagnosis is made by noting recurrent inflammation at two or more cartilaginous sites, most commonly the pinnae of the ear (producing cauliflower ears) and the bridge of the nose (producing a saddlenose deformity). Radiographs and CT show diffuse, smooth thickening of the wall of the trachea and central bronchi with narrowing of the lumen.

DIFFUSE TRACHEAL DILATATION

Tracheobronchomegaly (Mournier-Kuhn syndrome) is a congenital disorder of the elastic and smooth muscle components of the tracheal wall (4). An association with the Ehlers-Danlos syndrome, a congenital defect in collagen synthesis, and cutis laxa, a congenital defect in elastic tissue, has been reported. The disease is found almost exclusively in men younger than 50 years of age. Abnormal compliance of the trachea and central bronchi leads to central bronchial collapse during coughing. The airways obstruction impairs mucociliary clearance, predisposing the patient to recurrent episodes of pneumonia and bronchiectasis. Symptoms are indistinguishable from those associated with chronic bronchitis and bronchiectasis. On frontal radiographs, the trachea and central bronchi measure greater than 3.0 cm and 2.5 cm, respectively, in coronal diameter. The trachea has a corrugated appearance owing to herniation of tracheal mucosa and submucosa between the tracheal cartilages.

Figure 19.2. Saber Sheath Trachea in COPD. HRCT scans just above **(A)** and at the tracheal carina **(B)** in a 65-year-old man with COPD reveals coronal narrowing of the trachea representing a saber sheath tracheal deformity. Note additional findings associated with cigarette smoking: centrilobular emphysema and bronchial wall thickening representing chronic bronchitis.

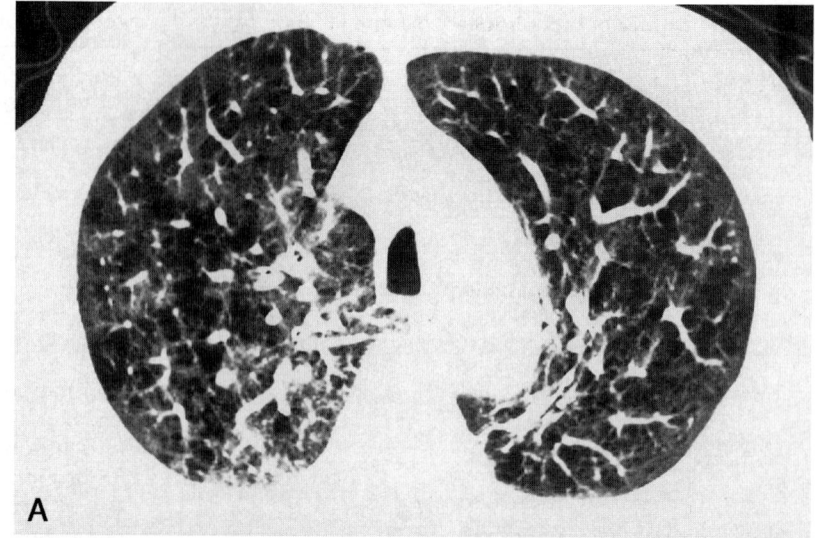

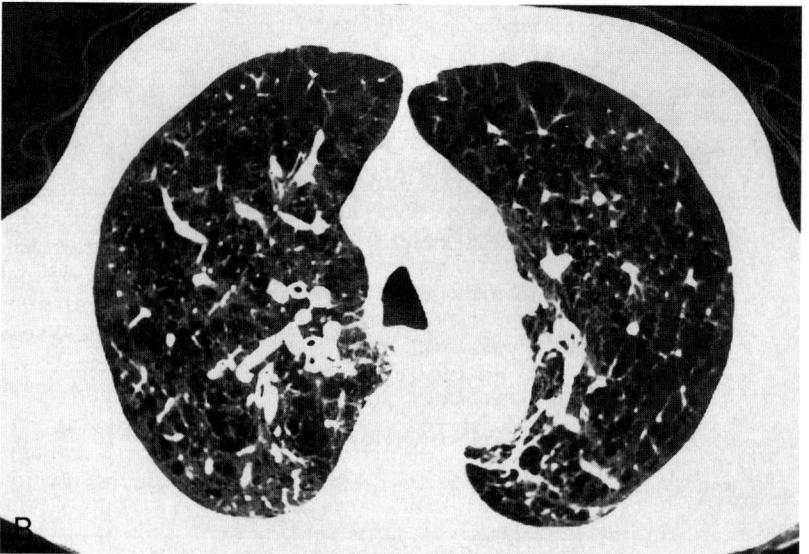

The lungs are typically hyperinflated and may demonstrate bulla.

Tracheobronchomalacia with diffuse tracheal and central bronchial dilitation may result from a congenital or acquired defect of tracheal cartilage. The most common causes of acquired tracheomalacia are chronic obstructive pulmonary disease, chronic bronchitis, cystic fibrosis, and relapsing polychondritis. Symptoms and radiographic findings are similar to those of tracheobronchomegaly.

In some patients with long-standing interstitial pulmonary fibrosis, diffuse tracheal dilatation may be seen. The cause of the tracheal dilatation may relate to longstanding elevation in transpulmonary pressures caused diminished lung compliance or to chronic coughing.

Tracheal and Bronchial Injury

Injury to the trachea or main bronchi is most often seen with blunt chest trauma from a deceleration-type injury. Concomitant aortic laceration, great vessel injury, and rib (particularly an upper anterior rib), sternum, scapula, or vertebral fracture typically dominate the clinical picture. The mechanism of injury is forceful compression of the central tracheobronchial tree against the thoracic spine during impact. The fractures usually involve the proximal main bronchi (80%) or distal trachea (15%) within 2 cm of the tracheal carina; the peripheral bronchi are involved in 5% of cases. Horizontal laceration or transection parallel to the tracheobronchial cartilage is the most common form of injury.

The diagnosis of tracheobronchial injury is often first suggested on early posttrauma chest radiographs by the presence of pneumothorax and pneumomediastinum, particularly in a patient not receiving mechanical ventilation (Fig. 19.3)(5). Typically, the pneumothorax does not respond to chest tube drainage because there is a large air leak at the site of airway interruption. The subtended lung remains collapsed against the lateral chest wall ("fallen lung" sign)(Fig. 19.3). An aberrant endotracheal tube or overdistended balloon cuff are further clues to the presence of an unsuspected tracheobronchial disruption. As many as one-third of tracheobronchial injuries have a delayed diagnosis; these patients may present with a collapsed lung or pneumonia

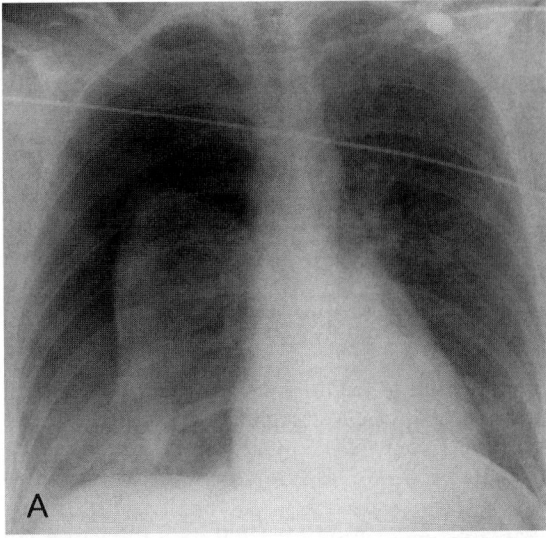

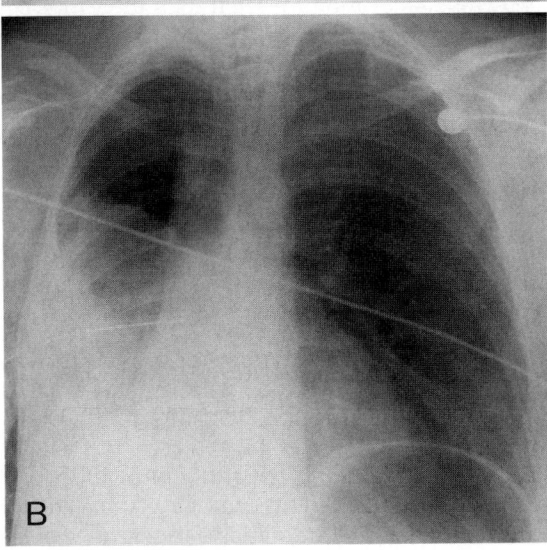

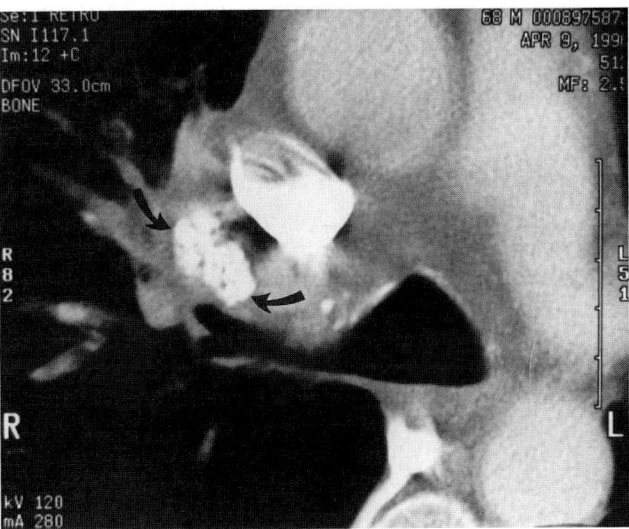

Figure 19.4. Broncholithiasis. Coned-down view of a CT in a 68-year-old man with hemoptysis shows calcified lymph nodes (*arrows*) adjacent to the anterior segment right upper lobe bronchus. Bronchoscopy shows calcified nodes eroding in the bronchus, accounting for the hemoptysis.

Figure 19.3. Transection of the Right Main Bronchus. A. An upright chest film shows a broken right clavicle with a large right pneumothorax and pneumomediastinum in a 24-year-old woman struck by a car. **B.** A film obtained following chest tube placement shows a persistent pneumothorax. A large air leak was noted from the tube. Bronchoscopy revealed complete disruption of the right main bronchus, which was confirmed at thoracotomy.

secondary to bronchial stenosis. Definitive diagnosis is by bronchoscopy. Helical CT with three-dimensional reconstruction with shaded surface display or contrast bronchography may be useful in patients who develop bronchial occlusion or stenosis as a result of a delayed diagnosis.

Penetrating tracheal injuries usually involve the cervical trachea and result from gunshot or stab wounds to the neck. Injury to the intrathoracic trachea is usually associated with a fatal penetrating cardiovascular injury.

Broncholithiasis

Broncholithiasis, the presence of calcified material within the tracheobronchial tree, develops from erosion of a calcified peribronchial lymph node into the

bronchial lumen (Fig. 19.4). Most calcified lymph nodes result from granulomatous lymph node inflammation due to histoplasmosis or tuberculosis. Broncholiths may occlude the airway and lead to bronchiectasis, obstructive atelectasis, or pneumonia. Patients are often asymptomatic but may have cough productive of stones or calcified material (lithoptysis). Hemoptysis may develop from erosion of the broncholith into a bronchial vessel.

CHRONIC OBSTRUCTIVE PULMONARY DISEASE

Disorders of the trachea and main bronchi are discussed in chapter 13. The diseases known collectively as chronic obstructive pulmonary disease (COPD) include asthma, chronic bronchitis, bronchiectasis, and emphysema. The common pathophysiology in this group of diseases is obstruction to expiratory airflow.

Asthma and Chronic Bronchitis

Asthma is an airways disorder characterized by the rapid onset of bronchial narrowing with spontaneous resolution or improvement as a result of therapy. Numerous inciting factors and agents have been identified. Many patients have allergy histories and develop episodic bronchial constriction from excessive IgE production when exposed to antigenic stimuli. This results in bronchial smooth muscle contraction, bronchial wall inflammation, and excessive mucus production. These responses narrow the bronchial lumen and produce symptoms of coughing, wheezing, and dyspnea.

The radiographic findings in uncomplicated asthma primarily result from diffuse airways narrowing. Hyperinflation producing increased lung volume, flattening or inversion of the diaphragm, attenuation of the peripheral vascular markings, and prominence of the retrosternal air space is the result of expiratory air trapping (6). Bronchial wall inflammation and thickening appears radiographically as peribronchial cuffing and tram tracking. In some patients, the hila are prominent from transient pulmonary arterial hypertension due to hypoxic vasoconstriction (Fig. 19.5).

There are several reasons to obtain a chest radiograph in patients with asthma. Tracheal and central bronchial narrowing from extrinsic or intrinsic lesions may produce dyspnea and wheezing and be mistaken for asthma. Bacterial pneumonia may induce airway hyperreactivity and present as an acute asthmatic attack. Complications of asthma may be detected on chest radiographs obtained during and following the asthmatic episode. Mucus plugs can cause bronchial obstruction and resorptive atelectasis; pneumonia can develop in these collapsed regions. Expiratory airflow obstruction with resultant alveolar rupture and dissection of air medially may produce pneumomediastinum. If the extra-alveolar air dissects peripherally to the subpleural space to form subpleural blebs, pneumothorax may result. Both pneumomediastinum and pneumothorax may be exacerbated in ventilated patients receiving high positive pressure ventilation.

Chronic Bronchitis is a clinical and not a radiographic diagnosis. It is defined as the excess production and expectoration of sputum that occurs on most days for at least 3 consecutive months in at least 2 consecutive years. The majority of individuals with chronic bronchitis are cigarette smokers. Morphologically, the lower lobe bronchi are most often affected, with thickening of their walls from mucus gland hyperplasia. The ratio of mucus gland thickness to bronchial wall thickness is known as the Reid index; an abnormally high index (>50%) correlates strongly with symptoms of excess mucus production. Of patients with a history of chronic bronchitis, 50% have normal chest films. Some patients show peribronchial cuffing or tram tracks when the

thick-walled and mildly dilated bronchi are viewed end on or in length respectively. Other patients have "dirty chests," in which the peripheral lung markings are accentuated. This radiographic appearance has no definite pathologic correlate but may represent small airways disease or prominent pulmonary arteries from pulmonary arterial hypertension complicating associated centrilobular emphysema. CT in patients with chronic bronchitis may show bronchial wall thickening (Fig. 19.2B).

Bronchiectasis

Bronchiectasis is defined as an abnormal permanent dilatation of bronchi. Morphologically, bronchiectasis is divided into three groups: cylindrical, varicose, and saccular (cystic). Cylindrical bronchiectasis is characterized by mild diffuse dilatation of the bronchi. Varicose bronchiectasis is cystic bronchial dilatation interrupted by focal areas of narrowing, its appearance has been likened to a string of pearls. Cystic bronchiectasis is seen as clusters of bronchi with marked, localized saccular dilatation. Bronchiectasis may be localized or generalized. Localized bronchiectasis is most commonly a result of prior tuberculosis; generalized bronchiectasis is seen in patients with cystic fibrosis. Patients usually have a history of chronic sputum production and recurrent lower respiratory infections. Hemoptysis associated with enlargement of bronchial arteries is common and may be massive and life-threatening.

The chest radiographic findings of bronchiectasis are typically nonspecific. Scarring, volume loss, and loss of the sharp definition of the normal bronchovascular markings are present in the affected regions. Parallel linear shadows representing the walls of cylindrically dilated bronchi seen in length may be visualized. Cystic bronchiectasis has a characteristic appearance of multiple peripheral thin-walled cysts, with or without air-fluid levels, that cluster together in the distribution of a bronchovascular bundle. The findings are peripheral in most cases of localized bronchiectasis; central bronchiectasis is seen only in allergic bronchopulmonary aspergillosis, cystic fibrosis, bronchial atresia, or acquired central bronchial obstruction.

CT has all but eliminated the need for contrast bronchography in the evaluation of bronchiectasis. In the diagnosis of bronchiectasis, using thin-section CT scans at regular intervals has shown an accuracy exceeding 95% compared to bronchography (7). The CT appearance of bronchiectasis depends on the site of involvement and the type of bronchiectasis. In the upper and lower lobes, all bronchi are imaged in cross-section, and their luminal diameter can be directly compared to the accompanying pulmonary arteries. Cylindrical bronchiectasis in these regions appears as multiple, dilated, thick-walled circular lucencies, with the adjoining smaller artery giving each dilated bronchus the appearance of a "signet ring." In the midlung, where the bronchi course horizontally, the appearance is that of parallel linear opacities or "tram tracks." Mucoid impaction within dilated upper or lower lobe bronchi may be mistaken for lung nodules unless one observes the vertical nature of the opacity on se-

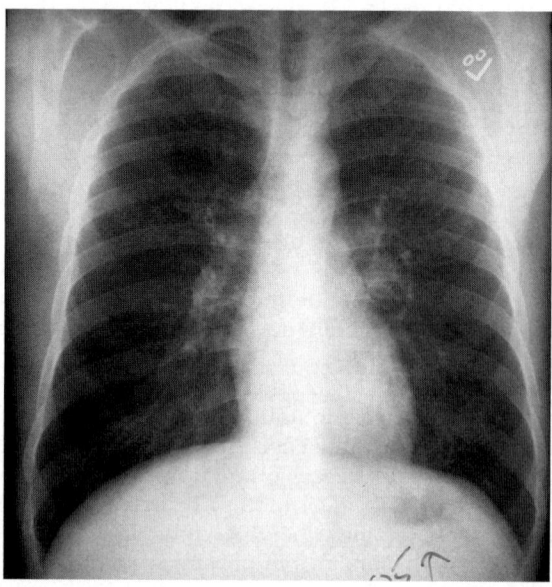

Figure 19.5. Asthma. PA chest radiograph in a 27-year-old man suffering an acute asthma exacerbation reveals hyperinflation, bronchial wall thickening, and hilar prominence.

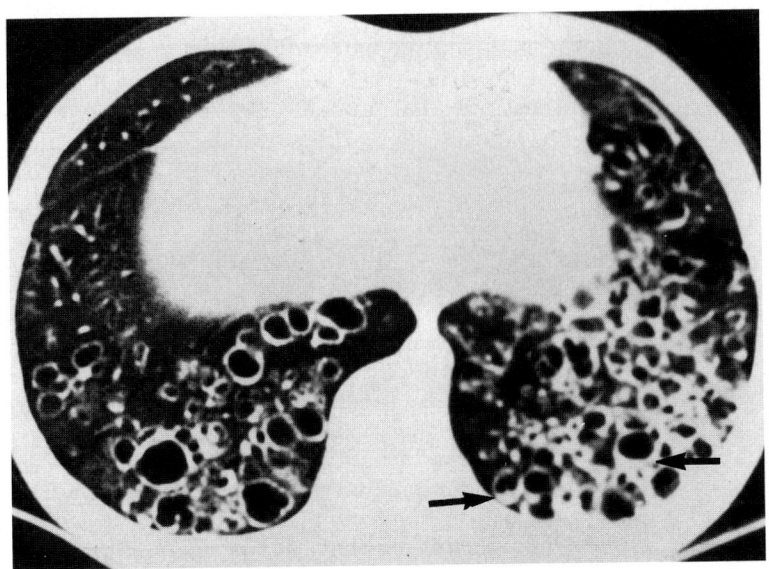

Figure 19.6. Cystic Bronchiectasis. CT through the lower lobes in a 12-year-old boy with severe postinfectious bronchiectasis shows clustered, thin-walled cysts representing dilated bronchi in cross-section. Note the presence of dependent fluid within several left lower lobe bronchi (*arrows*).

quential axial images. In the midlung regions, impacted bronchi sectioned in length are recognized as branching finger-like opacities. Cystic bronchiectasis in any region is easily recognized as clusters of rounded lucencies often containing air-fluid levels; this appearance has been likened to a "cluster of grapes" (Fig. 19.6). Varicose bronchiectasis cannot be differentiated from cylindrical bronchiectasis unless sectioned longitudinally in the midlung regions, where the pattern of dilatation simulates the contour of a caterpillar.

Bronchography remains the gold standard for diagnosing and evaluating the extent of bronchiectasis. However, its invasive nature and associated complications, particularly in patients with limited pulmonary reserve, preclude its routine use for evaluating bronchiectasis. Because it is noninvasive and highly accurate, CT has replaced bronchography for the diagnosis of bronchiectasis. Scans obtained at 10-mm intervals with 1.5-mm collimation and a high spatial resolution reconstruction algorithm are used to detect the presence and extent of disease. Currently, bronchography is limited to those patients considered for curative resection who appear to have localized disease by CT examination.

Bronchiectasis is caused by a variety of disorders, all of which predispose the bronchi to chronic inflammation with resultant cartilage damage and dilatation (Table 19.3).

Cystic Fibrosis is a hereditary disease of young Caucasians characterized in the lung by the production of abnormally thick, tenacious mucus. The thick mucus plugs the small airways and leads to bronchial obstruction and infection. A vicious cycle of recurrent infection, most often with *Pseudomonas aeruginosa* or *Staphylococcus aureus*, eventually causes severe bronchiectasis. The bronchiectasis is associated with functional airways obstruction and dyspnea. Hemoptysis, sometimes massive, may complicate the bronchiectasis and may require treatment by transcatheter bronchial artery embolization. Chest radiographs in affected adults show hyperinflation with predominantly upper lobe bronchiectasis and mucus plugging. Distal at-

Table 19.3. Specific Causes of Bronchiectasis

Localized	Tuberculous scarring, upper lobes (postprimary disease)
	Bronchial disease
	Extrinsic compression
	Enlarged hilar nodes
	Bronchial stenosis/occlusion
	Bronchial atresia
	Tuberculosis
	Sarcoidosis
	Prior bronchial injury
	Endobronchial mass
	Carcinoid tumor
	Bronchogenic carcinoma
	Foreign body
Diffuse	Cystic fibrosis
	Dysmotile cilia syndrome
	Congenital immunodeficiency
	Postinfectious
	Adenovirus (Swyer-James)
	Measles
	Pertussis
	Chronic aspiration
	Allergic bronchopulmonary aspergillosis
	Interstitial pulmonary fibrosis (traction bronchiectasis)

electasis and obstructive pneumonitis are common findings. The pulmonary hila may be prominent from enlarged lymph nodes because of chronic infection or from vascular dilatation associated with pulmonary arterial hypertension. The diagnosis rests on a positive family history and a sweat test showing an abnormally high concentration of chloride. Improvements in antibiotic therapy and pulmonary physiotherapy have increased long term survival, but the overall prognosis remains poor, with most patients succumbing to respiratory insufficiency in young adulthood. Recently, the use of inhaled recombinant DNAase to reduce the viscosity of tracheobronchial secretions has brought symptomatic and functional improvement to a number of patients. Lung or heart-lung transplantation is an option in selected individuals.

Dysmotile Cilia Syndrome is a disorder in which the epithelial cilial motion is abnormal and ineffective. A variety of structural cilial abnormalities may be found, the most common of which is an absence of the outer dynein arms of the peripheral microtubules of the cilia. The abnormality may result in rhinitis, sinusitis, bronchiectasis, dysmotile spermatozoa and sterility, situs inversus, and dextrocardia. The triad of sinusitis, situs inversus, and bronchiectasis is known as Kartagener's syndrome. Chest radiographs show diffuse bronchiectasis and hyperinflation; situs inversus is seen in approximately 50% of patients (Fig. 19.7). The diagnosis is made on the basis of the clinical and radiographic findings, along with studies of cilial anatomy and motion on samples obtained from nasal biopsy.

Postinfectious. A severe childhood pneumonia, usually the sequela of infection with adenovirus, measles, or pertussis (the latter two are commonly seen in nonimmunized Asian immigrants), may cause severe bronchial damage and recurrent infection with resultant bronchiectasis (Fig. 19.6). In some patients, childhood bronchitis and bronchiolitis are associated with obstructive airways disease and an underdeveloped lung; the latter is known as the Swyer-James syndrome.

Allergic Bronchopulmonary Aspergillosis (ABPA) represents a hypersensitivity reaction to *Aspergillus* and is characterized clinically by asthma, blood eosinophilia, bronchiectasis with mucus plugging, and circulating antibodies to *Aspergillus* antigen. An immediate (type I) hypersensitivity reaction to *Aspergillus* antigen accounts for acute episodes of wheezing and dyspnea whereas an immune complex mediated (type III) hypersensitivity within the lobar bronchi leads to bronchial wall inflammation and proximal bronchiectasis. Affected patients invariably have an allergic history and a high association with cystic fibrosis exists. Patients with this disorder have recurrent episodes of coughing, wheezing, and expectorating mucus plugs. The chest radiograph is diagnostic and shows proximal, predominantly upper lobe bronchiectasis. The dilated bronchi may be seen as dilated, air-filled tubules or as broad, branching opacities characteristic of mucoid impaction within the dilated bronchi. CT and HRCT are helpful in characterizing the opacities as dilated bronchi (Fig. 19.8). Corticosteroids are the treatment of choice.

Bronchial Obstruction. Bronchiectasis can develop distal to an endobronchial obstruction caused by neoplasm, atresia, or stenosis. Slow-growing central bronchogenic neoplasms that have a large endoluminal component (e.g., carcinoid tumor) may obstruct the distal bronchi and produce bronchiectasis with mucus plugging (mucoceles) (Fig. 19.9). Similarly, bronchial atresia or bronchostenosis from trauma or chronic bronchial infection (i.e., endobronchial tuberculosis) can lead to distal bronchial dilatation. The plain radiographic recognition of mucocele formation in patients with endobronchial obstruction relies on adequate collateral ventilation to the lung supplied by the obstructed airway. Unfortunately, in most patients, collapse of lung around the dilated, mucus-filled bronchi precludes diagnosis on plain radiographs. CT will show the central airway obstruction and dilated mucus bronchograms, and can help guide bronchoscopic examination and biopsy.

Peribronchial Fibrosis. "Traction bronchiectasis" is a term used to describe the effect of severe pulmonary fibrosis on the peripheral airways. Airways traversing regions of parenchymal fibrosis and honeycombing often become irregularly dilated as their walls are retracted by the fibrotic process. This occurs most commonly in the upper lobes in patients with long-standing tuberculosis and in the subpleural regions of the lower lobes in patients with end-stage idiopathic pulmonary fibrosis. Because the accompanying fibrosis precludes visualization of the dilated bronchi radiographically, traction bronchiectasis is best appreciated on HRCT studies of the lung.

Emphysema

Definition and Subtypes. Emphysema is a pathologic diagnosis defined as an abnormal, permanent enlargement of the air spaces distal to the terminal bronchiole, accompanied by destruction of alveolar walls, and without obvious fibrosis. The pathologic classification of emphysema is based on the portion of the secondary pulmonary lobule affected (8). Centrilobular emphysema is the most common and is characterized by air-space distention in the central portion of the lobule, with sparing of the more distal portions of the lobule. This form of emphysema affects the upper lobes to a greater extent than the lower lobes (Fig. 19.10). Panlobular emphysema results in uniform distention of the air spaces throughout

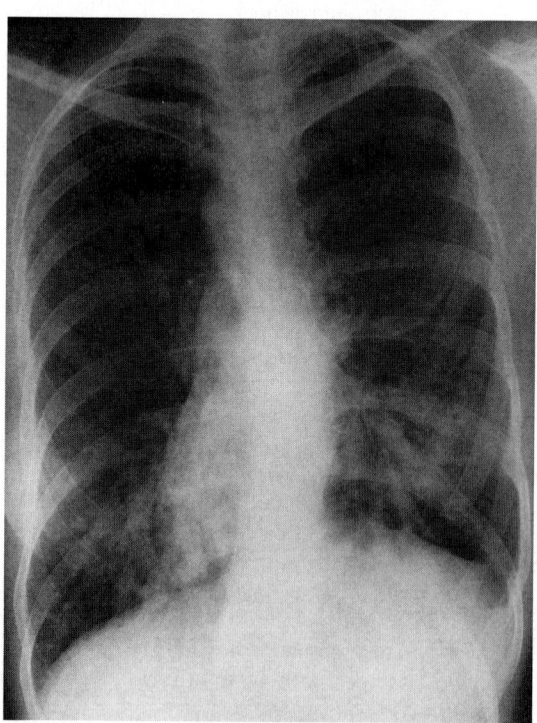

Figure 19.7. Bronchiectasis in Kartagener's Syndrome. PA chest film in a 32-year-old man with long-standing sinusitis, dextrocardia, and situs inversus reveals bilateral lower lobe bronchiectasis.

the substance of the lobule from the central respiratory bronchioles to the peripheral alveolar sacs and alveoli. In contrast to centrilobular emphysema, this form has a predilection for the lower lobes (Fig. 19.11). Paraseptal emphysema is seen as selective distention of peripheral air spaces adjacent to interlobular septa, with sparing of the centrilobular region. This form of emphysema is most often seen in the immediate subpleural regions of the upper lobes (Fig. 19.10). Paraseptal emphysema may coalesce to form apical bullae; rupture of these bullae into the pleural space may cause spontaneous pneumothorax. Paracicatricial or irregular emphysema refers to destruction of lung tissue associated with fibrosis that bears no consistent relationship to a given portion of the lobule. It is most often seen in association with old granulomatous inflammation (Fig. 19.12).

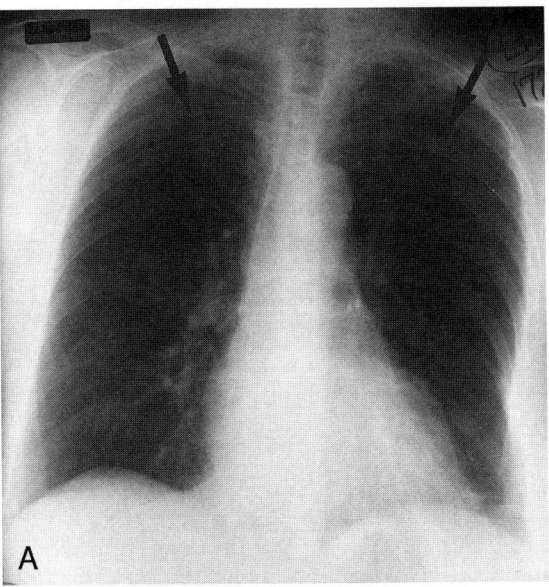
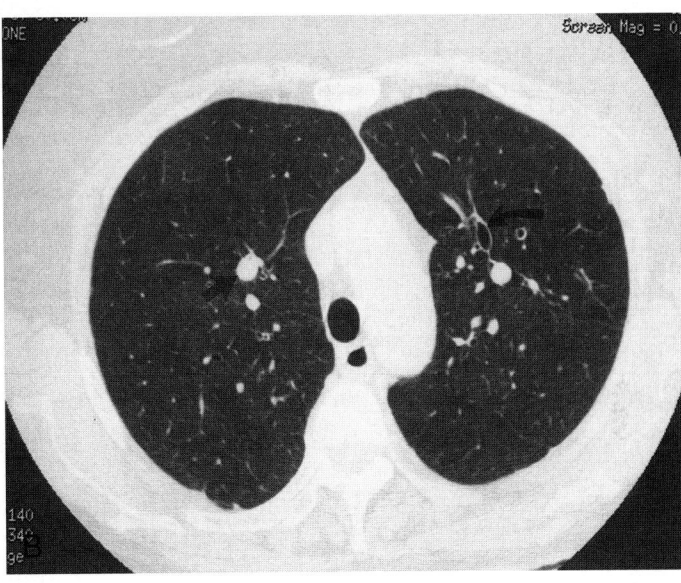

Figure 19.8. Allergic Bronchopulmonary Aspergillosis (ABPA). A. PA chest radiograph in a 68-year-old woman with asthma and eosinophilia shows tubular upper lobe opacities (*arrows*). **B.** HRCT reveals dilated mucus-filled (*straight arrows*) and air-filled (*curved arrow*) proximal bronchi characteristic of ABPA.

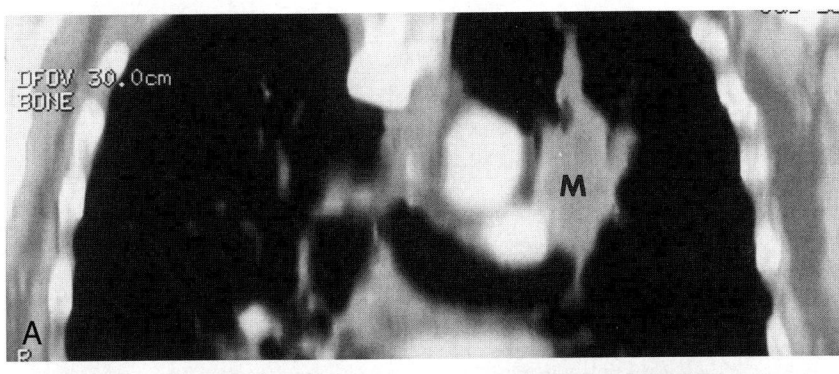

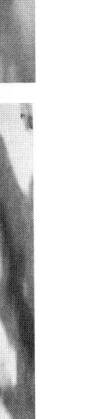

Figure 19.9. Mucocele from Bronchial Carcinoid. A. Coronal reformatted CT shows a mass (*M*) obstructing the left upper lobe bronchus. **B.** Coronal maximum intensity projection (MIP) shows branching, dilated, mucus-filled bronchi paralleling arterial branches in the apicoposterior segment of the left upper lobe. Bronchoscopy revealed carcinoid tumor.

Figure 19.10. Centrilobular and Paraseptal Emphysema. HRCT through the upper lobes shows scattered low attenuation regions (*straight arrows*) representing centrilobular emphysema. Paraseptal emphysema (*curved arrows*) is seen in the subpleural regions.

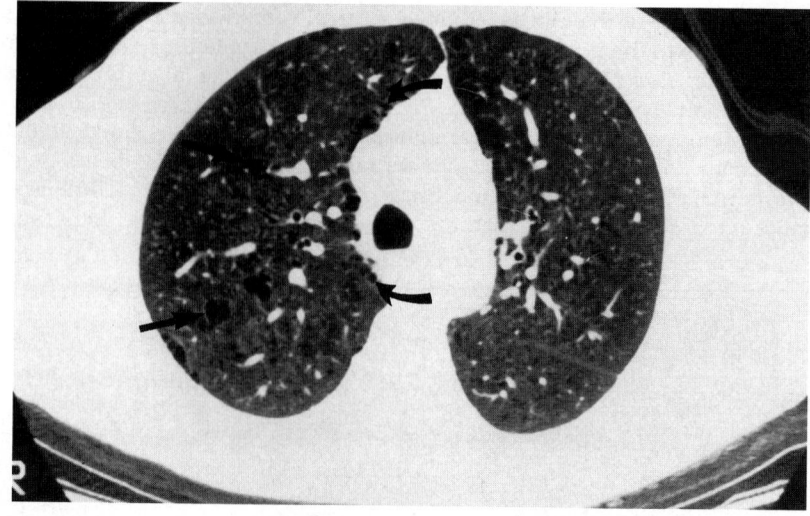

Figure 19.11. Panlobular Emphysema. HRCT through the lower lobes shows uniform destruction of secondary pulmonary lobules.

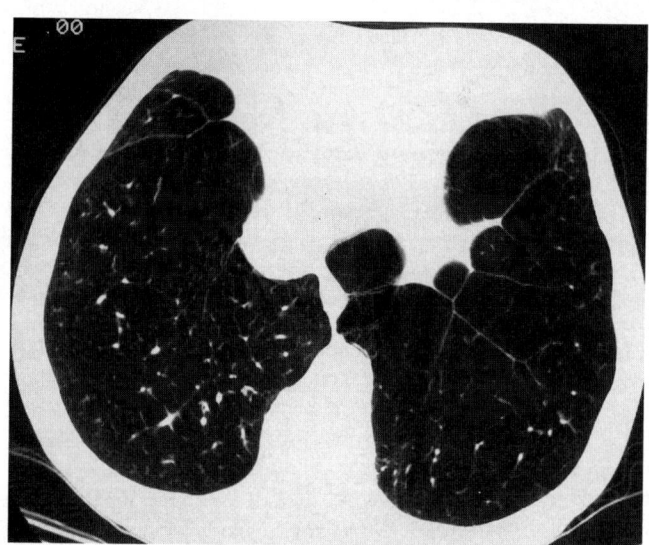

Figure 19.12. Paracicatricial Emphysema. HRCT in a patient with focal right lower lobe postinflammatory scarring and bronchiectasis shows focal hyperlucency (*arrows*), which represents paracicatricial emphysema.

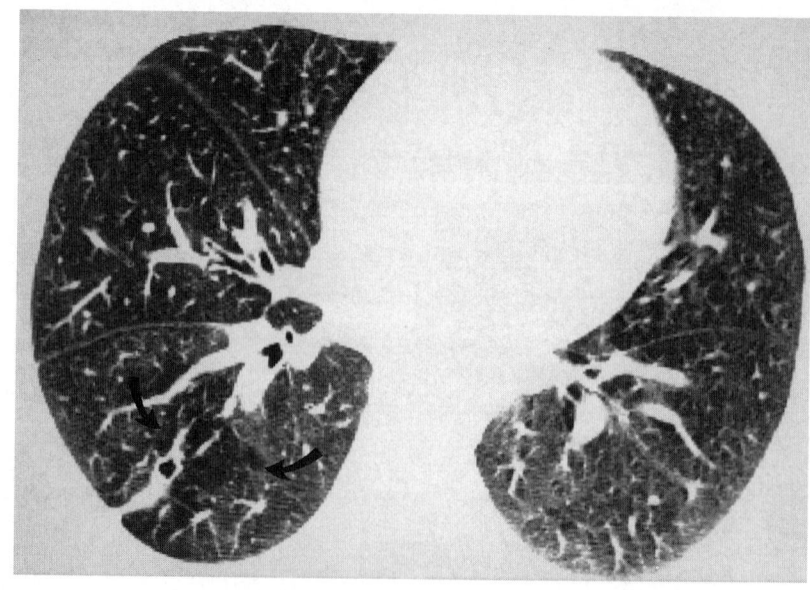

Etiology and Pathogenesis. The most common causative factor for the development of emphysema is cigarette smoking. This is associated predominantly with centrilobular emphysema but may be a contributing factor in the development of panlobular emphysema. The pathogenesis of centrilobular emphysema is complex and has not been completely elucidated. Cigarette smoke leads to excess neutrophil deposition in the lung. This results in the release of proteases (e.g., elastase) and antiprotease inhibitors, which in turn leads to destruction of alveolar septa. Inflammation and obstruction of small airways likely contributes to distal air-space distention and alveolar septal disruption. The association between deficiency of the serum protein alpha-1-antitrypsin (alpha-1-protease inhibitor) and the development of panlobular emphysema is well established. This disease is inherited as an autosomal recessive trait. Individuals homozygous for both recessive genes (ZZ phenotype) develop panlobular emphysema by middle age. Heterozygotes (MZ phenotype) have only a slightly increased incidence of emphysema. Cigarette smoking, by producing excess antiprotease inhibitors, can accelerate the development of emphysema in patients with the ZZ and MZ phenotypes.

Clinical Findings and Functional Abnormalities. As a definitive diagnosis of emphysema requires tissue, the diagnosis during life is based on a combination of clinical, functional, and radiographic findings. The vast majority of patients with emphysema are long term cigarette smokers. Symptoms associated with emphysema include dyspnea and a productive cough, the latter is attributed to chronic bronchitis which often accompanies centrilobular emphysema. The functional hallmarks of emphysema are decreased airflow and diffusing capacity. Expiratory airflow obstruction is expressed as a decrease in the volume of air expired in the first second of a forced expiratory maneuver from total lung capacity (FEV_1) and a decrease in the ratio of FEV_1 to the total volume of air expired during a forced expiratory maneuver (FEV_1/FVC). Airflow obstruction is secondary to increased airways resistance and decreased driving pressure (i.e., elastic recoil). In patients with moderate to severe emphysema, the predominant factor limiting expiratory airflow is the decreased elastic recoil that results from parenchymal destruction. Airflow obstruction, however, is not invariably present in patients with mild emphysema. Diffusing capacity, measured by the diffusion of carbon monoxide from the alveoli into the bloodstream during a single breath hold ($DL_{CO}SB$), assesses the integrity and surface area of the alveolocapillary membrane. The diffusing capacity in persons with emphysema is decreased because the volume of pulmonary parenchyma available for gas exchange is diminished. The severity of the emphysema correlates well with the $DL_{CO}SB$. Although an abnormal diffusing capacity is more sensitive than abnormal spirometry in diagnosing emphysema, it is nonspecific. Because $DL_{CO}SB$ depends on both the surface area available for gas diffusion and the number and hemoglobin content of red blood cells within the pulmonary capillaries, any process affecting these factors can alter the measurement of $DL_{CO}SB$. For example, a decreased $DL_{CO}SB$ can be seen in any disease that diminishes the volume of pulmonary capillaries

available for gas diffusion (e.g., pulmonary embolism), interferes with gas exchange across the alveolocapillary membrane (e.g., interstitial pulmonary fibrosis), or produces airway obstruction thereby diminishing the gas-exchanging air spaces (i.e., cystic fibrosis). Furthermore, some patients with mild to moderate morphologic emphysema can have a normal $DL_{CO}SB$.

Radiologic Evaluation. Frontal and lateral chest radiographs are the initial radiographic examinations obtained in patients with suspected emphysema. The plain radiographic findings of emphysema are listed in Table 19.4 (9). Hyperinflation is the most important plain radiographic finding and reflects the loss of lung elastic recoil. It is the radiographic equivalent of an abnormally increased total lung capacity (TLC). The abnormal increase in lung volumes is best detected by noting inferior displacement and flattening of the normally convex superior hemidiaphragms, right or obtuse angles to the normally acute-angled costophrenic sulci, and an increase in the anteroposterior chest diameter, which is best appreciated by noting an increase in the depth of the retrosternal clear space. Absent or attenuated peripheral vascular markings result from parenchymal destruction and obliteration of peripheral pulmonary arteries traversing emphysematous areas (Fig. 19.11). When the characteristic thin walls of bullae are seen marginating the peripheral avascular regions, emphysema can be diagnosed with certainty. Increased radiolucency of the lungs caused by pulmonary hyperinflation and attenuation of peripheral vascular markings is difficult to detect because it is subject to various patient and technical factors and is thus an inaccurate indicator of the presence of emphysema. The effects of emphysema and chronic hypoxemia on the right side of the heart may be appreciated as enlargement of the central pulmonary arteries and right ventricles in those with complicating pulmonary arterial hypertension and cor pulmonale. The use of the term "chronic obstructive pulmonary disease" (COPD) to describe patients with the plain radiographic findings of emphysema is inaccurate

Table 19.4. Radiographic Findings in Pulmonary Emphysema

Finding	Explanation
Diffuse hyperlucency (panlobular)	Destruction of pulmonary capillary bed and alveolar septa
Flattening and depression of the hemidiaphragms; increased retrosternal air space (panlobular > centrilobular)	Hyperinflation due to loss of elastic recoil of lung
Bulla	Thin-walled region of confluent (panlobular > centrilobular) emphysematous destruction
Enlarged central pulmonary arteries; right heart enlargement (centrilobular)	Loss of pulmonary capillary bed; associated chronic hypoxemia causes increased pulmonary vascular resistance
Increased peripheral vascular markings (centrilobular)	? small airways disease ? increased pulmonary vascularity

and should be discouraged. COPD is a functional diagnosis, and the chest radiograph depicts anatomy only. In fact, patients with radiographic findings of hyperinflation and vascular attenuation, although invariably having emphysema morphologically, can rarely lack functional evidence of airflow obstruction and therefore do not have COPD.

Many patients with severe centrilobular emphysema have minimal or absent hyperinflation on chest radiographs, and images usually show increased lung markings rather than peripheral vascular attenuation. These observations have led to the description of two major groups of patients with emphysema, each with distinctive radiographic patterns. Patients with predominant panlobular emphysema show hyperinflated lungs with peripheral vascular attenuation and a normally sized heart and central pulmonary vessels. Bullae are common in this form of emphysema. This pattern of emphysema has been termed "arterial deficiency" emphysema. Clinically, these patients are described as "pink puffers" because of their tachypnea and normal partial pressure of oxygen. Those with centrilobular emphysema show mild hyperinflation and increased linear parenchymal markings that represent the small airways thickening of chronic bronchitis seen concomitantly in these patients. Bullae are uncommon in this form of emphysema. This radiographic pattern of emphysema has been termed "increased markings" emphysema. As a result of chronic hypoxemia, these individuals develop secondary polycythemia and are described as "blue bloaters." Although most patients do not fit neatly into one or the other category either clinically or radiographically, familiarity with these two patterns will facilitate correctly diagnosing the majority of patients with moderately severe or severe centrilobular or panlobular emphysema.

Widespread, extensive emphysema may be accurately diagnosed on chest radiographs, but mild disease is often not evident radiographically. Chest CT has allowed for the diagnosis of emphysema in the absence of chest radiographic findings of hyperinflation or parenchymal abnormalities. Because of its cross-sectional nature and high contrast resolution, CT is ideally suited to the diagnosis of emphysema. Early reports on using CT to diagnose emphysema depended on recognizing either large avascular areas or regions with abnormally low H attenuation numbers. Recently, improvements in detectors, shorter scan times, and the ability to perform HRCT have allowed better characterization of centrilobular emphysema. Centrilobular emphysema is now seen as discrete, well-defined areas of abnormal low attenuation that lack definable walls and is situated centrally within the secondary pulmonary lobule adjacent to the bronchovascular bundle. HRCT, with its thin collimation technique and high spatial resolution, can detect mild centrilobular emphysema that may be missed on conventional 10-mm collimated CT due to partial volume averaging of small emphysematous areas within the thickness of the scan section.

Treatment of Emphysema. Advances in operative techniques now provide two surgical options for the treatment of emphysema. Recently, a surgical technique first developed in the 1950s, volume reduction surgery, has been reintroduced as a method of relieving patient dyspnea by resecting severely emphysematous regions of lung and improving respiratory mechanics. This experimental technique is currently undergoing a multicenter prospective trial to determine its value in patients with debilitating emphysema. An alternative surgical technique available to treat patients with emphysema, particularly younger patients with alpha-1 antitrypsin deficiency, is single-lung or double-lung transplantation.

BULLOUS LUNG DISEASE

Bullae are thin-walled cystic spaces that exceed 1 cm in diameter and are found within the lung parenchyma (Fig. 19.13). Three morphologic types have been described: type 1 bullae, which are apical, subpleural rounded gas collections without septations containing a narrow neck; type 2 bullae, which are also subpleural but have wide necks and contain strands of residual tissue; and type 3 bullae, which are morphologically similar to type 2 bullae but are located deep within the lung substance. Bullae most often represent confluent areas of emphysematous lung and may be seen as part of generalized emphysema. However, in a minority of patients, bullae are unassociated with emphysema. For example, the increased lung weight and chronically elevated transpleural pressure in patients with lower lobe interstitial pulmonary fibrosis predisposes bullae formation.

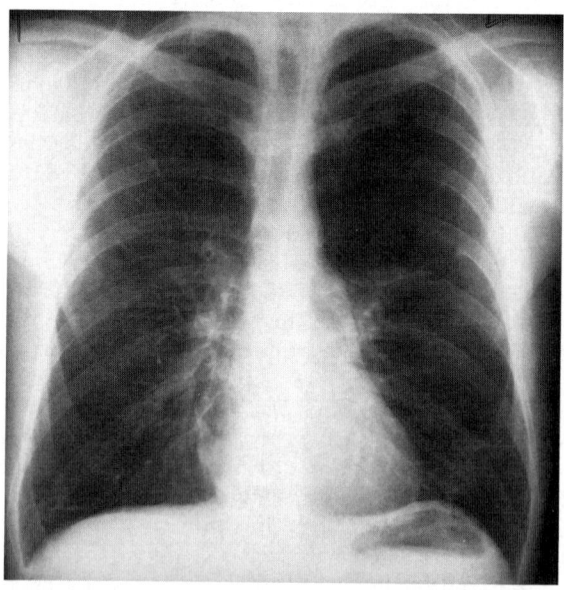

Figure 19.13. Bullous Lung Disease. PA chest film in a 27-year-old man shows left lung and right upper lobe bullae, representing vanishing lung disease.

Table 19.5. Causes of Primary Bullous Lung Disease

Familial	Ehler's-Danlos syndrome
Vanishing lung disease	Intravenous drug use
Marfan's syndrome	HIV infection

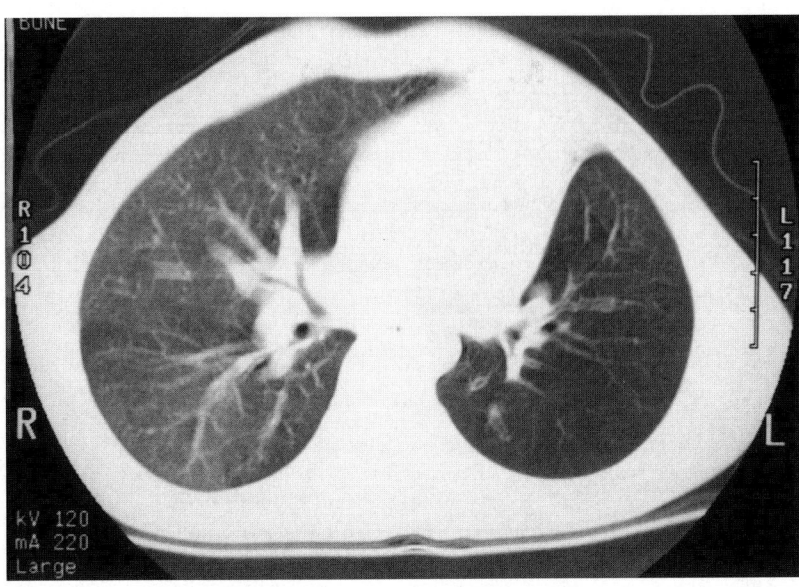

Figure 19.14. Unilateral Hyperlucent Lung (Swyer-James) Syndrome. CT in a 7-year-old boy with a history of neonatal pneumonia shows a small hyperlucent left lung with attenuated vascularity and central bronchiectasis.

Bullae may also be seen in diseases such as sarcoidosis, pulmonary histiocytosis X, and ankylosing spondylitis, which cause chronic upper lobe fibrosis. In these diseases, chronic bronchiolar obstruction leads to distal air-space distention, alveolar septal disruption, and bullae development.

Primary bullous disease (Table 19.5) is a group of disorders in which bullae are isolated lesions without intervening areas of emphysema or interstitial lung disease. Primary bullous lung disease may be familial and has been found in association with Marfan's or Ehler's-Danlos syndromes, IV drug users, HIV infection, and the vanishing lung syndrome, which is an accelerated form of paraseptal emphysema seen in young adult males (Fig. 19.14). Most patients are asymptomatic unless large bullae compress normal parenchyma and cause compressive atelectasis and dyspnea. Radiographically, isolated bullae have an upper lobe distribution and appear as rounded, thin-walled lucencies of varying size. These lesions can become huge as a result of air trapping and cause depression of the ipsilateral lung and hemidiaphragm. They may even produce contralateral mediastinal shift. CT is useful in evaluating the extent of bullous disease and the amount of compressed pulmonary tissue.

Spontaneous pneumothorax is a complication that occurs when a subpleural bulla ruptures into the pleural space. These patients may be difficult to manage; persistent air leaks lead to prolonged and often unsuccessful closed tube drainage of the pleural space and reexpansion of the lung. When a bulla becomes secondarily infected, chest radiographs or CT will demonstrate an air-fluid level within the bulla that resolves over several weeks with the administration of antibiotics. A cancer may rarely develop within the wall of a bulla. Symptomatic patients and those with enlarging bullae should be considered for bullectomy. Radioisotope lung perfusion studies may be performed preoperatively to assess the amount of perfused and potentially functional lung parenchyma compressed by the bullae.

SMALL AIRWAYS DISEASE

Bronchiolitis refers to an inflammation of the small noncartilaginous airways. Infectious bronchiolitis, a disease of young children caused by respiratory syncytial virus or adenovirus, produces respiratory distress and radiographic hyperinflation indistinguishable from asthma. Bronchiolitis in adults can be infectious, such as in Asian panbronchiolitis. However, bronchiolar and peribronchial inflammation is more commonly a result of heavy cigarette smoking. This latter disease is termed "respiratory bronchiolitis-associated interstitial lung disease" (RB-ILD) and presents with signs and symptoms of interstitial lung disease. RB-ILD is reviewed in chapter 18.

Bronchiolitis Obliterans, also known as constrictive bronchiolitis, is a subacute disease characterized pathologically by a mononuclear cell inflammatory process within the walls of respiratory bronchioles that leads to the formation of granulation tissue, which plug small airways. This results in dyspnea and functional airways obstruction. This disorder may be idiopathic or secondary to viral infection, toxic fume inhalation, drug reaction, collagen vascular disorders, organ transplantation, or chronic aspiration. Lung, heart-lung, and bone marrow transplant patients are particularly prone to bronchiolitis obliterans. Bronchiolitis obliterans in the adult may be the result of an early childhood lower respiratory infection with adenovirus, in which case it is called unilateral hyperlucent lung or the Swyer-James syndrome. In the Swyer-James syndrome, the bronchiolitis causes diffuse small airways obliteration, air trapping, alveolar walls destruction, and emphysema due to overdistention of peripheral air spaces. Because postinfectious bronchiolitis obliterans affects the lungs asymmetrically and usually occurs during a period of lung growth and development, the affected lung is typically small and hyperlucent, and the ipsilateral pulmonary artery is hypoplastic. Most patients with the Swyer-James syndrome are asymptomatic, but some patients

Figure 19.15. Bronchiolitis Obliterans (Constrictive Bronchiolitis). Inspiratory **(A)** and expiratory **(B)** HRCT scans in a 59-year-old woman with rheumatoid arthritis and airflow obstruction shows mosaic attenuation on the inspiratory scans with regional air trapping on expiration, representing small airways disease (bronchiolitis obliterans).

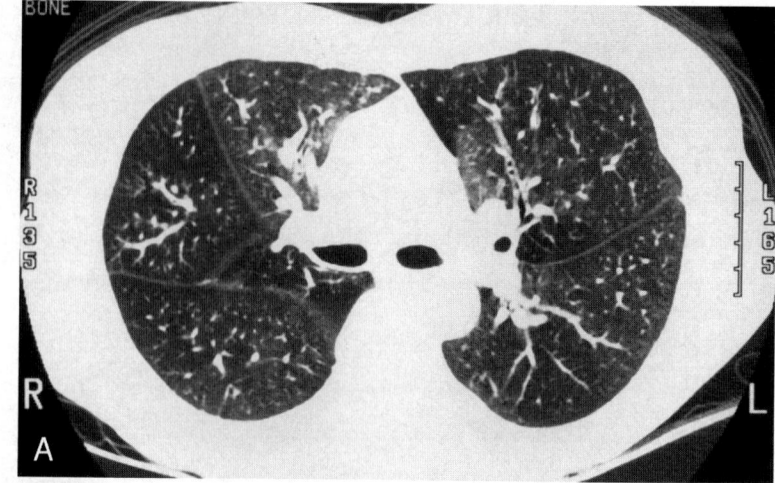

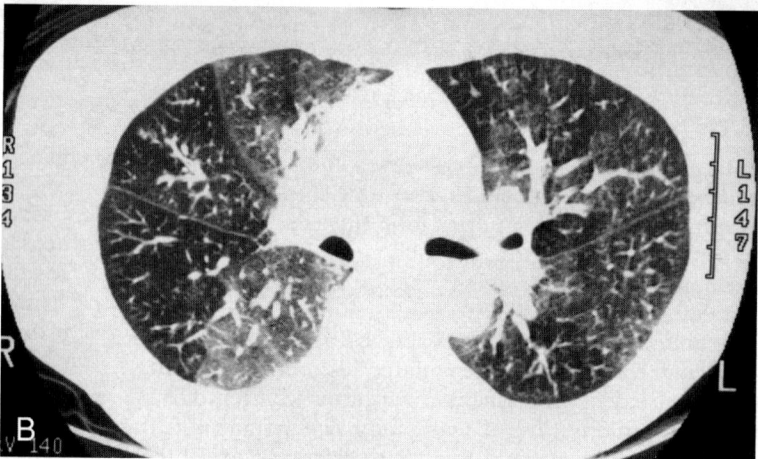

complain of dyspnea or recurrent lower respiratory tract infections.

The chest radiograph in patients with pure bronchiolitis obliterans may be normal despite the presence of severe dyspnea and functional evidence of airflow obstruction. The most common radiographic abnormality in this disorder is diffuse reticulonodular opacities with associated hyperinflation. Central bronchiectasis has been described, particularly in those with bronchiolitis obliterans developing as a complication of heart-lung transplantation. In patients with the Swyer-James syndrome, the affected lung is normal or small in volume, and marked unilateral air trapping is seen on fluoroscopy or expiratory films. The air trapping is caused by bronchiolar obstruction with collateral air drift to the distal air spaces on inspiration; this air drift cannot escape on expiration. The ipsilateral hilum is small and the pulmonary vasculature reduced, accounting for the hyperlucency seen radiographically and on CT (Fig. 19.14). Perfusion lung scanning shows decreased perfusion of the affected lung whereas the ventilation study shows decreased ventilation with markedly delayed radioisotope washout. This latter finding helps distinguish the Swyer-James syndrome from primary central pulmonary artery occlusion or hypoplastic lung, conditions in which ventilation is maintained.

HRCT in Small Airways Disease. HRCT is a sensitive indicator of the presence of small airways disease (10).

Both direct and indirect findings that allow detection of this process may be evident on HRCT. The direct sign of small airways disease is centrilobular opacities, which represent diseased preterminal bronchioles. This is seen on HRCT as sharply defined or ground-glass nodules or Y-shaped or V-shaped tubular branching opacities centrally situated within the secondary pulmonary lobule within 1 cm of the pleural surface. Pathologically, the opacities reflect dilatation and mucus plugging of small bronchioles or peribronchiolar inflammation and fibrosis.

The indirect signs of small airways disease result from expiratory air trapping and are most easily seen on HRCT. Those portions of lung most severely affected by small airways disease are poorly ventilated and perfused and appear relatively hyperlucent adjacent to areas of normal lung. This results in an appearance on HRCT termed "mosaic attenuation," which is virtually indistinguishable from the changes seen in primary pulmonary arterial occlusive disease. Furthermore, infiltrative processes such as *Pneumocystis carinii* pneumonia and desquamative interstitial pneumonitis, which produce patchy ground-glass opacification, also result in a mosaic attenuation appearance on HRCT. Using both inspiratory and expiratory HRCT scans helps distinguish between these various disorders. In a patient with mosaic attenuation, attenuated vessels within the lucent regions of lung indicates that the lucent regions are abnormal because of decreased perfusion. This finding allows distinction from ground-glass opacification, in which the caliber of vessels in normal and abnormal lung are comparable. The presence of small airways disease is confirmed on expiratory HRCT by noting air trapping within the hyperlucent regions (Fig. 19.15).

References

1. Takasugi JE, Godwin JD. The airway. Semin Roentgenol 1991;26:175–190.
2. Berkman YM. The trachea: the blind spot in the chest. Radiol Clin North Am 1984;22:539–562.
3. Greene R, Lechner GL. "Saber-sheath" trachea: a clinical and functional study of marked coronal narrowing of the intrathoracic trachea. Radiology 1975;115:265–268.
4. Woodring JH, Howard RS, Rehm SR. Congenital tracheobronchomegaly (Mournier-Kuhn syndrome): a report of 10 cases and review of the literature. J Thorac Imag 1991; 6:1–10.
5. Unger JM, Schuchmann GG, Grossman JE, et al. Tears of the trachea and main bronchi caused by blunt trauma: radiologic findings. AJR Am J Roentgenol 1989;153: 1175–1180.
6. White CS, Cole RP, Lebetsky HW, et al. Acute asthma: admission chest radiography in hospitalized adult patients. Chest 1991;100:14–16.
7. Grenier P, Maurice F, Musset D, et al. Bronchiectasis: assessment by thin-section CT. Radiology 1986;161:95–99.
8. Bergin C, Muller N, Miller RR. CT in the qualitative assessment of emphysema. J Thorac Imag 1986;1:94–103.
9. Pratt PC. Radiographic appearance of the chest in emphysema. Invest Radiol 1987;22:927–929.
10. Lynch DA. Imaging of small airways disease. Clin Chest Med 1993;14:623–634.

4

Pleura, Chest Wall, Diaphragm, and Miscellaneous Chest Disorders

Jeffrey S. Klein

PLEURA

Pleural Effusion

Pleural Fluid Physiology and Pathophysiology. The normal volume of fluid in the pleural space is approximately two milliliters. The formation of pleural fluid follows Starling's law and depends on hydrostatic and oncotic forces in both the systemic capillaries of the parietal pleura and the pleural space (1). Under normal conditions, pleural fluid is formed by filtration from systemic capillaries in the parietal pleura and resorbed via the parietal pleural lymphatics.

Pleural effusions may be classified by their gross appearance (bloody, chylous, purulent, serous), the causative disease (Table 20.1), or by the pathophysiology of abnormal pleural fluid formation (transudative versus exudative). This latter differentiation is made by measuring the protein, LDH, and glucose concentration of the pleural fluid obtained by thoracentesis. Conditions associated with elevated plasma hydrostatic pressure or a decrease in plasma oncotic pressure will produce a trans-

udative pleural effusion characterized by: *a)* pleural/serum protein ratio of less than 0.5, *b)* pleural/serum LDH ratio of less than 0.6, and *c)* pleural LDH of less than 200 IU/L. Left heart failure is the most common cause of pleural effusion resulting from an increase in hydrostatic pressure, which in turn results from pulmonary venous and capillary hypertension. Fluid overload from renal failure, pregnancy, and constrictive pericarditis are additional causes of hydrostatic pleural effusion. The hypoproteinemia associated with liver disease is the most common cause of a transudative effusion; additional causes are the nephrotic syndrome, severe malnutrition, and protein losing enteropathy. An exudative pleural effusion, characterized by: *a)* pleural/serum protein ratio of 0.5, *b)* pleural/serum LDH ratio of greater than 0.6, and *c)* pleural LDH of 200 IU/L, is the result of increased pleural capillary permeability. Peripheral pulmonary or pleural processes that inflame the pleura (pneumonia, serositis) or directly invade the pleura (malignancy) are the most common causes of pleural exudates.

SPECIFIC CAUSES OF PLEURAL EFFUSION

Congestive Heart Failure is the condition most commonly associated with a transudative pleural effusion. The effusions are usually bilateral and larger on the right side (2). An isolated right effusion is twice as common as an isolated left effusion.

Parapneumonic Effusion and Empyema. A parapneumonic effusion is defined as an effusion associated with pneumonia. Peripheral parenchymal infection produces an exudative pleural effusion by causing visceral pleural inflammation that increases pleural capillary permeability. Inflammatory thickening of the pleural membranes with lymphatic obstruction may also be a contributing factor. Empyema results when the parenchymal infection extends into the pleural space. Parenchymal infections that typically result in empyema formation are bacterial pneumonia, septic emboli, and lung abscess, whereas fungal, viral, and parasitic infections are uncommon causes. Less commonly, infection may extend into the pleural space from the spine, mediastinum, and chest wall.

Forty percent of bacterial pneumonias have an associated pleural effusion. Staphylococcus aureus and gram negative pneumonias are the most common cause of parapneumonic effusion and empyema. The natural history of parapneumonic effusions may be divided into three stages (3). Stage 1 is an exudative stage; visceral pleural inflammation causes increased capillary permeability and pleural fluid accumulation. Most of these sterile exudative effusions resolve with appropriate antibiotic therapy. A stage 2 parapneumonic effusion is a fibrinopurulent pleural fluid collection containing bacteria and neutrophils. Fibrin deposition on the visceral and parietal pleura impairs fluid resorption and produces loculations. If the infection is not treated, the loculations will impair attempts at closed pleural fluid drainage. A stage 3 parapneumonic effusion develops 2–3 weeks after initial pleural fluid formation and is characterized by the ingrowth of fibroblasts over the pleura that produces pleural fibrosis and entraps the lung. Dystrophic calcification of the pleura may develop following resolution of the pleural infection.

Tuberculous pleural effusion or empyema resulting from the rupture of subpleural caseating granulomas may complicate pulmonary infection or occur as the primary manifestation of disease. Effusions in TB are more common in young adults with pulmonary disease and in HIV-positive individuals with severe immunodeficiency. The pleural fluid is characteristically straw colored with greater than 70% lymphocytes and a low glucose concentration.

Radiographically, empyema most often appears as a loculated pleural fluid collection. On CT, it is elliptical in shape and is seen most often within the posterior and inferior pleural space. The collection conforms to and maintains a broad area of contact with the chest wall. The distinction of empyema from peripheral lung abscess has important therapeutic implications; empyemas require external drainage while lung abscesses usually respond to postural drainage and antibiotic therapy. Contrast-enhanced chest CT is most useful in making this distinction (Fig. 20.1)(Table 20.2)(4). Detecting an empyema may be difficult when there is extensive parenchymal consolidation. In these cases, CT and US are useful in detecting parapneumonic fluid collections and guiding diagnostic thoracentesis and pleural drainage.

Neoplasms. Pleural effusion may be seen with benign or malignant intrathoracic tumors. The tumors most commonly associated with pleural effusion are, in order of frequency, lung carcinoma, breast carcinoma, pelvic tumors, gastric carcinoma, and lymphoma. Pleural fluid

Table 20.1. Etiology of Pleural Effusions

Infectious	Bacterial/mycobacterial
	Viral
	Fungal
	Parasitic
Cardiovascular	Heart failure
	Pericarditis
	Superior vena cava obstruction
	Postcardiac surgery
	Myocardial infarction
	Pulmonary embolism
Neoplastic	Bronchogenic carcinoma
	Metastases
	Lymphoma
	Pleural or chest wall neoplasms (mesothelioma)
Immunologic	Systemic lupus erythematosus
	Rheumatoid arthritis
	Sarcoidosis (rare)
	Wegener's granulomatosis
Inhalational	Asbestos
Trauma	Blunt or penetrating chest trauma
Abdominal disease	Cirrhosis
	Pancreatitis
	Subphrenic abscess
	Acute pyelonephritis
	Ascites (from any cause)
	Splenic vein thrombosis
Miscellaneous	Drugs
	Myxedema
	Ovarian tumor

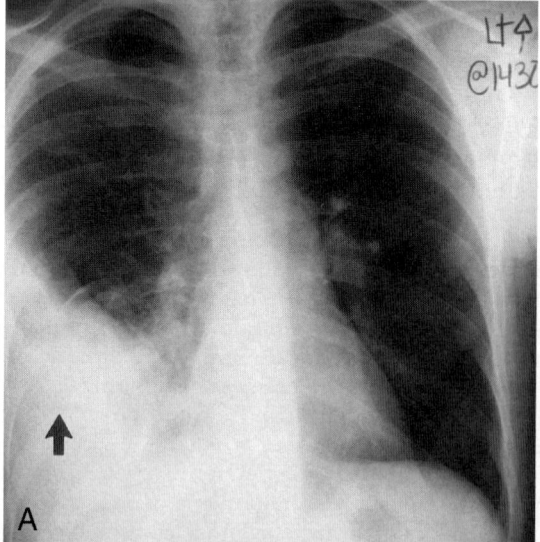
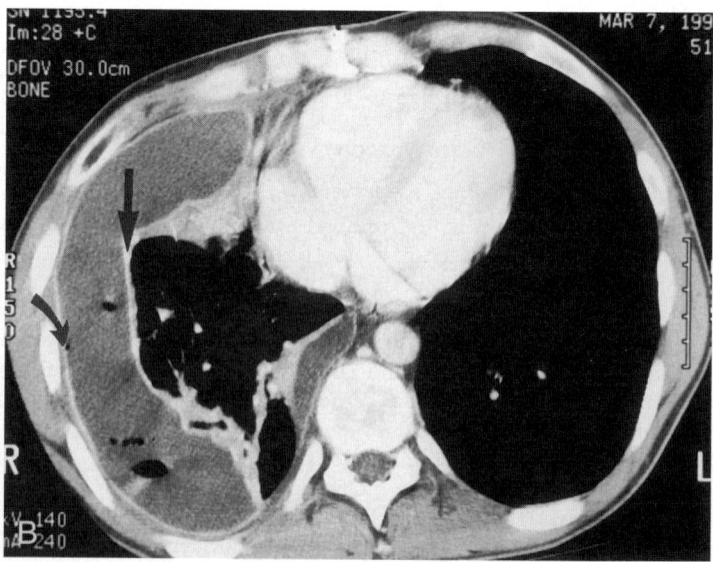

Figure 20.1. Empyema on CXR and CT. A. A PA chest film in a patient with a recent right lower pneumonia demonstrates an oval opacity in the right lateral costophrenic sulcus containing gas (*arrow*). **B.** An enhanced CT shows a circumferential pleural fluid collection with enhancing visceral (*straight arrow*) and parietal (*curved arrow*) pleural layers representing an empyema. Note the contained gas pockets indicating loculations within the collection itself.

may result from pleural involvement by tumor or from lymphatic obstruction anywhere from the parietal pleura to the mediastinal nodes. The effusions are exudative and may be bloody. Demonstrating malignant cells on cytologic examination of pleural fluid obtained at thoracentesis is necessary for the diagnosis of a malignant effusion. Closed or thoracoscopic biopsy is reserved for patients with negative cytologic examination. Clues to the presence of a malignant pleural effusion include smooth or lobulated pleural thickening, mediastinal or hilar lymph node enlargement or mass and solitary or multiple parenchymal nodules. CT is useful in demonstrating pleural masses or underlying parenchymal lesions in those with large effusions (Fig. 20.2).

Trauma. Blunt or penetrating trauma to the chest including iatrogenic trauma from thoracotomy, thoracostomy, or placement of central venous catheters may result in a hemothorax. Hemothorax results from laceration of vessels within the lung, mediastinum, chest wall, or diaphragm. Intrapleural blood coagulates rapidly, and septations form early. In some individuals, pleural motion causes defibrination that lyses the clotted blood. In the acute setting, pleural fluid of high CT

attenuation (>80 H) may be seen; associated rib fractures or subcutaneous emphysema should suggest the diagnosis. An acute hemothorax is treated with thoracostomy tube drainage, while thoracotomy is generally reserved for persistent bleeding or hypotension.

Esophageal perforation from prolonged vomiting (Boerhaave's syndrome) or as a complication of esophageal dilatation may produce a pleural effusion, most commonly on the left side. Extravascular placement of a central line can result in a hydrothorax when intravenous solution is inadvertently infused into the pleural or extrapleural space.

Collagen Vascular and Autoimmune Disease. Systemic lupus erythematosus has a reported incidence of pleural effusions ranging from 33–74%. These exudative effusions are a result of pleural inflammation and patients present with pleuritic chest pain. In some cases, the nephrotic syndrome associated with systemic lupus erythematosus may produce transudative effusions. Cardiomegaly is a common chest radiographic finding, and may be caused by pericardial effusion, hypertension, renal failure, or lupus-associated endocarditis or myocarditis.

Pleural effusion is the most common intrathoracic manifestation of rheumatoid arthritis and is most frequently seen in male patients following the onset of joint disease (Fig. 20.3). The effusions occur independent of pulmonary parenchymal involvement but may develop following intrapleural rupture of peripheral rheumatoid nodules. The effusions of rheumatoid arthritis are exudative, with a lymphocytosis, low glucose concentration, and low pH (<7.2). Rheumatoid effusions may persist unchanged for years.

Autoimmune syndromes producing pleural and pericardial effusions have been described following myocardial infarction (Dressler's syndrome) or cardiac surgery (postpericardiotomy syndrome). Both are characterized by fever, pleuritis, pneumonitis, and pericarditis devel-

Table 20.2. Empyema vs. Lung Abscess on CT

Feature	Empyema	Abscess
Shape	Oval Oriented longitudinally	Round
Margin	Thin, smooth (''split pleura'' sign)	Thick, irregular
Angle with chest wall	Obtuse	Acute
Effect on lung	Compression	Consumption
Treatment	External drainage	Antibiotics Postural drainage

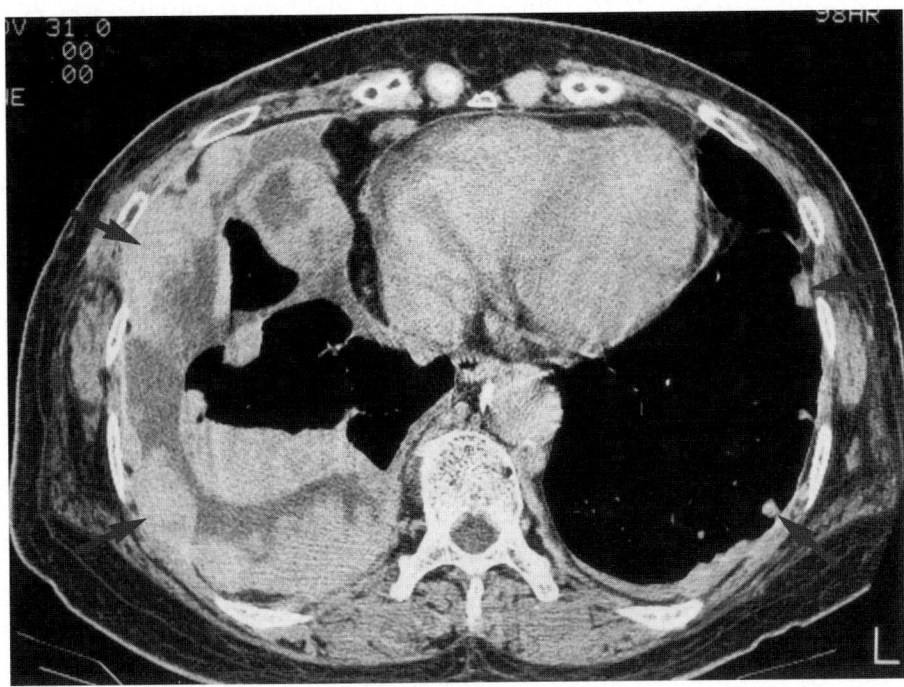

Figure 20.2. Malignant Pleural Effusion: CT Diagnosis. HRCT in a patient with breast carcinoma and a right pleural effusion on chest radiographs demonstrates multiple bilateral pleural nodules and masses *(arrows)* representing pleural metastases. The diagnosis was confirmed by US-guided right pleural biopsy.

oping within days to weeks of the precipitating event. The radiographic findings include enlargement of the cardiac silhouette, pleural effusions, and parenchymal air-space opacities. A serosanguinous exudative pleural effusion is seen in over 80% of patients. Treatment with nonsteroidal anti-inflammatory drugs usually results in symptomatic and radiographic improvement.

Abdominal Disease. Radioisotope studies have demonstrated that peritoneal fluid may enter the pleural space via transdiaphragmatic lymphatic channels or through defects in the diaphragm. The lymphatic channels are larger on the right side, accounting for the higher incidence of right sided effusions associated with ascites or liver failure.

Acute or chronic pancreatitis can cause pleural effusions which are most often left-sided because of the

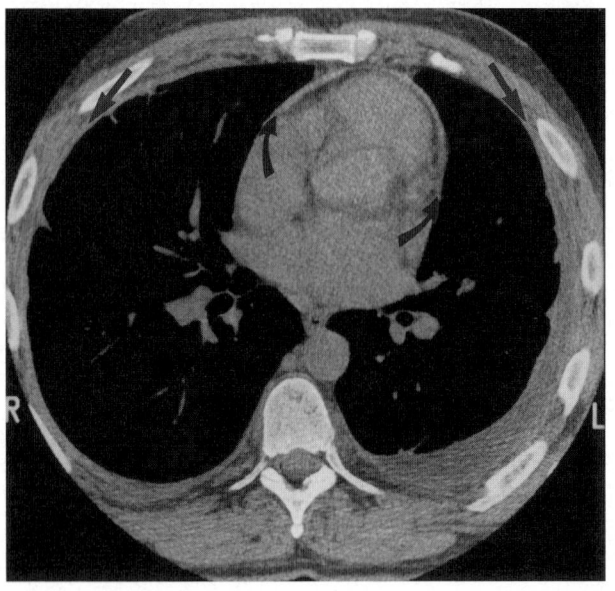

Figure 20.3. Serositis in Rheumatoid Arthritis. HRCT in a 43-year-old man with rheumatoid arthritis reveals bilateral pleural thickening (*straight arrows*) and small dependent effusions with pericardial thickening (*curved arrows*).

Figure 20.4. Chylous Pleural Effusion due to Hodgkin's Lymphoma. Enhanced CT scan in a 42-year-old man with nodular sclerosing Hodgkin's lymphoma shows a large anterior mediastinal mass associated with a moderate left and small right pleural effusions. Chylous fluid was obtained at left-sided thoracentesis.

proximity of the pancreatic tail to the left hemidiaphragm. The effusion associated with acute pancreatitis is typically exudative and may be bloody. Pleural effusion from chronic pancreatitis may cause pleuritic chest pain and shortness of breath. Rupture of the pancreatic duct can lead to a pancreaticopleural fistula. A high amylase concentration in the pleural fluid should suggest the pancreas as the etiology of the effusion, although an elevated amylase may be seen in pleural effusions due to malignancy or esophageal perforation.

Subphrenic abscesses complicating abdominal surgery or perforation of a hollow viscus can cause diaphragmatic paresis, basilar atelectasis, and pleural effusion. Patients with a pleural effusion associated with upper abdominal pain, fever, and leukocytosis should have CT or US examination and, when feasible, percutaneous catheter drainage of the abscess.

An association between benign pleural effusions and pelvic tumors has long been recognized. First described with ovarian fibroma (Meigs' syndrome), a number of pelvic and abdominal tumors including pancreatic and ovarian malignancy, lymphoma, and uterine leiomyomas have been found to cause pleural effusion. The effusions in Meigs' syndrome are usually transudative and resolve after removal of the pelvic tumor.

Chylothorax is a pleural collection containing triglycerides in the form of chylomicrons and results from perforation of the thoracic duct, which communicates with the pleural space. The thoracic duct originates from the cisterna chyli at the level of the first lumbar vertebra and ascends along the right paravertebral space, entering the thorax via the aortic hiatus. The duct crosses from right to left at the level of the sixth thoracic vertebra to lie alongside the upper esophagus. At the level of the left subclavian artery, the duct arches anteriorly to empty into the confluence of the left internal jugular and subclavian veins. Disruption of the upper duct caused by direct trauma or obstruction with rupture produces a left chylothorax, while injury to the lower intrathoracic duct produces a right chylothorax. The most common causes of chylothorax are malignancy, iatrogenic trauma, and tuberculosis (Fig. 20.4). The radiographic appearance is

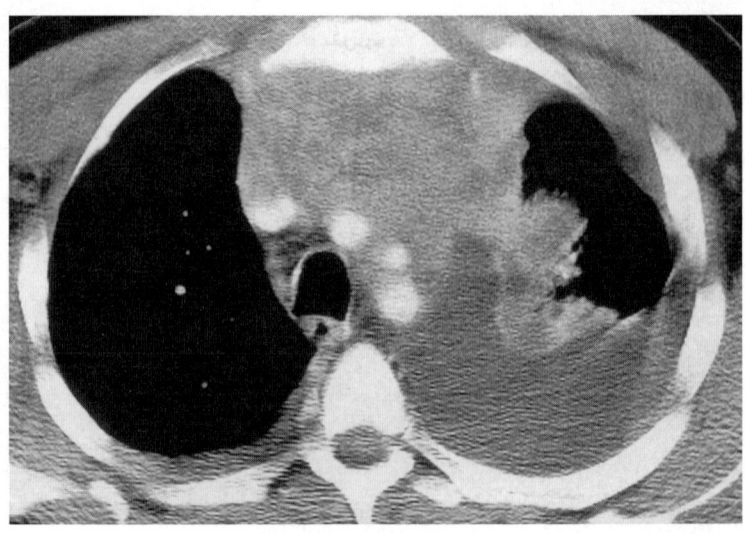

indistinguishable on plain radiographs and CT from other causes of free flowing effusions. The diagnosis is confirmed by triglyceride levels exceeding 110 mg/dl in the pleural fluid.

Pulmonary Embolism. Infarction complicating pulmonary embolism is a well-recognized cause of pleural effusion. The effusion may be associated with elevation of the ipsilateral diaphragm and peripheral wedge-shaped opacities (Hampton's hump). The pleural effusion is typically a small, unilateral, serosanguinous exudate.

Drugs may cause pleural effusions as a result of pleural inflammation (methysergide) or by producing a lupus-like syndrome (phenytoin, isoniazid, hydralazine, procainamide). Nitrofurantoin has been associated with an immunological reaction that causes pleuropulmonary disease with eosinophilia.

Management of Pleural Effusion. Transudative pleural effusions are managed by treatment of the underlying disorder because the pleura is intrinsically normal in these diseases. Patients with stage 1 parapneumonic effusions do not require specific treatment of the effusion, and are managed by antibiotic therapy directed at the causative organism. Stages 2 and 3 parapneumonic effusions and frank empyema require drainage with either catheters or tubes. Although intrapleural fibrinolytic therapy with streptokinase or urokinase will help a certain subset of patients with complex parapneumonic effusions, some will require open pleural drainage by video-assisted thoracoscopic surgery (VATS) or formal thoracotomy with decortication.

Malignant pleural effusions most often require closed drainage and pleural sclerosis, with talc (the agent of choice), doxycycline, or bleomycin. Some patients may benefit from VATS drainage and sclerosis with intrapleural talc. Patients with chylothorax require therapy directed at the underlying etiology (lymphoma, tuberculosis); those patients with traumatic disruption of the thoracic duct often require surgical ligation of the duct.

Patients with pleural effusions from trauma, pulmonary embolism, autoimmune disorders, and drug reactions often require no specific therapy. An exception is the postpericardiotomy (Dressler's syndrome), which is treated with nonsteroidal antiinflammatory agents.

Bronchopleural Fistula

A bronchopleural fistula is a communication between the lung and the pleural space, which often originates from a peripheral airway. A bronchopleural fistula from a bronchus results in an empyema, while an air leak from peripheral air spaces may cause an intractable pneumothorax. Bronchopleural fistulas often develops from dehiscence of a bronchial stump following lobectomy or pneumonectomy, or as the result of a necrotizing pulmonary infection. Presenting symptoms include fever, cough, and dyspnea; large air leaks may be noted in patients with pleural drains. Radiographically, a bronchopleural fistula presents as a loculated intrapleural air and fluid collection (Fig. 20.5). The development of an air-fluid level in the postpneumonectomy space or a drop

in the air-fluid level during the early postoperative period, associated with shift of the mediastinum back towards the midline, should suggest the diagnosis. CT is useful in evaluating patients with suspected bronchopleural fistula and empyema. It can distinguish a hydropneumothorax from a peripheral lung abscess and occasionally demonstrates the actual fistulous communication.

Postpneumonectomy Space

Following pneumonectomy, the residual space gradually fills with fluid and appears radiographically as an opaque hemithorax with ipsilateral mediastinal shift. The radiographic findings suggesting bronchopleural fistula formation complicating pneumonectomy are decribed above. CT and MR are useful in evaluating the postpneumonectomy space for evidence of tumor recurrence, and may help in the diagnosis of postoperative bronchopleural fistula and empyema.

Pneumothorax

Pneumothorax results from air entering the pleural space, and may be traumatic or spontaneous. Spontaneous pneumothorax is further subdivided into a primary form, which has no identifiable etiology, and a secondary form that is associated with underlying parenchymal lung disease (Table 20.3)(5). Patients with a pneumothorax typically present with the sudden onset of dyspnea and pleuritic chest pain.

Traumatic Pneumothorax. Trauma is the most common cause of pneumothorax. Penetrating injuries can produce pneumothorax by introducing air from the atmosphere into the pleural space or by laceration of the visceral pleura resulting in an air leak from the lung. Gun shot and knife wounds to the chest and upper abdomen, central line placement, thoracentesis, transbronchial biopsy, and percutaneous needle biopsy are common penetrating injuries that cause traumatic pneumothorax. Blunt chest trauma may cause pneumothorax by two different mechanisms: *a)* an acute increase in intrathoracic pressure results in extraalveolar interstitial air due to alveolar disruption that tracks peripherally and ruptures into the pleural space, and *b)* laceration of the tracheobronchial tree can produce a pneumothorax with a large bronchopleural fistula. In patients with rib fractures, the free edge of the fractured ribs can project inward to lacerate the lung and cause pneumothorax.

Primary Spontaneous Pneumothorax most often occurs in young or middle aged men. A familial incidence and a propensity for taller individuals has been noted. Affected patients often have blebs or bullae within the lung apices, which are responsible for the development of recurrent pneumothoraces. Treatment of the initial episode is with closed tube drainage, with thoracoscopic bullectomy reserved for recurrent episodes or persistent air leak.

Secondary Spontaneous Pneumothorax. Multiple entities have been associated with secondary spontaneous pneumothorax. Most of these disorders have as-

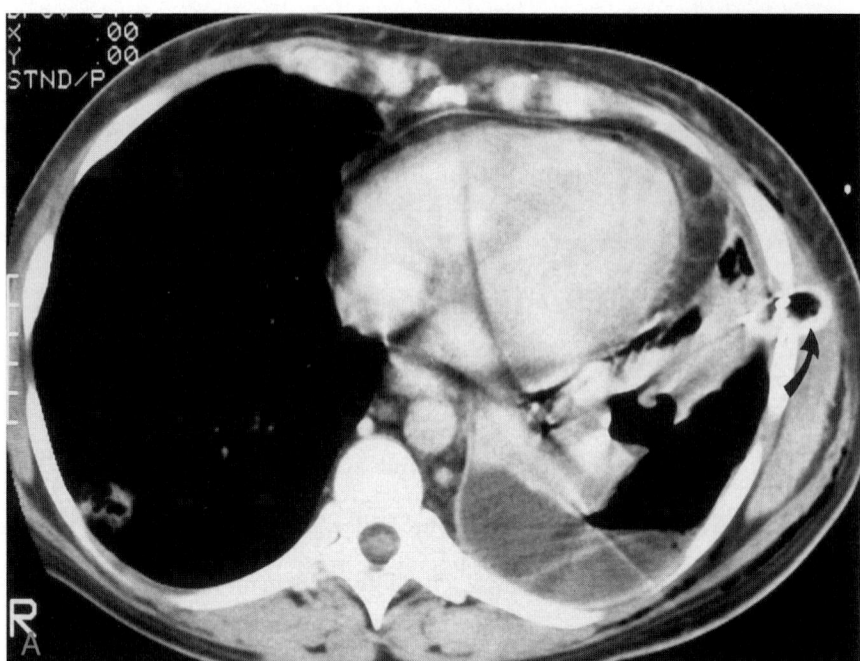

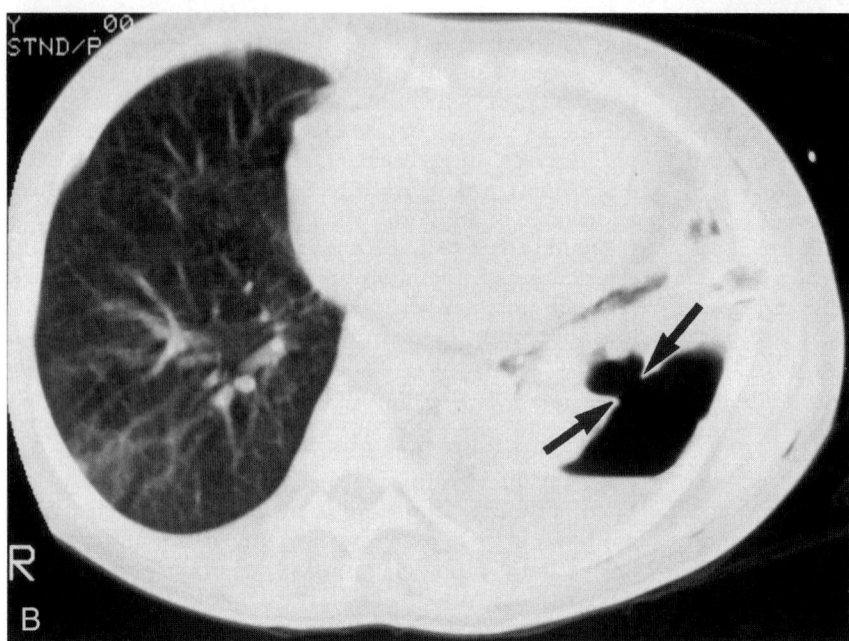

Figure 20.5. Bronchopleural Fistula and Empyema Complicating Septic Emboli. A. An enhanced CT scan in a 43-year-old woman with septic emboli complicating intravenous drug use reveals a posterior pleural air-fluid collection associated with left lower lobe consolidation. Note chest tube entering thorax laterally (*curved arrow*). **B.** The same scan at lung windows shows the left lower lobe cavity communicating with the pleural space via a breach in the visceral pleura (*straight arrows*). A properly positioned chest tube drained infected fluid and demonstrated a continuous air leak.

sociated blebs, bullae, cysts, or cavities, although in some patients the lungs are intrinsically normal. In the majority of the latter, there is usually a history of sudden increases in intrathoracic pressure. Chronic obstructive pulmonary disease is the most common predisposing disease. Acute obstruction to expiration from bronchoconstriction (asthma) or the performance of the Valsalva maneuver (crack cocaine or marijiuana smoking, transvaginal childbirth) may cause spontaneous pneumothorax. Pneumothorax may complicate cystic lung changes in sarcoidosis, Langerhan's histiocytosis of lung, and lymphangioleiomyomatosis. Necrotizing pneumonia or lung abscess caused by gram-negative or anaerobic bacteria, tuberculosis, or *Pneumocystis carinii* pneumonia can lead to pneumothorax, particularly in the mechanically ventilated patient. Metastases to the lung are an infrequent cause of pneumothorax, and rarely are a presenting feature of disease. In these cases, pneumothorax develops when necrotic subpleural metastases rupture into the pleural space. Sarcomas, particularly osteogenic sarcoma, lymphoma, and germ cell malignancies are the most common primary malignancies to produce spontaneous pneumothorax. Marfan's syndrome is the most common connective tissue disease producing pneumothorax, which usually results from the rupture of apical bullae. Other connective tissue diseases that can produce pneumothorax are Ehlers-Danlos and cutis laxa.

Mechanically ventilated patients are particularly at risk for pneumothorax due to the administration of pos-

Table 20.3. Etiology of Pneumothorax

Trauma	Iatrogenic
	Thoracic/abdominal surgery
	Percutaneous interventional procedures
	Lung/pleural biopsy
	Thoracentesis
	Central line placement
	Aberrant feeding tube placement
	Mechanical ventilation
	Esophagoscopic biopsy/dilatation
	Bronchoscopic biopsy
	Noniatrogenic
	Penetrating injury
	Stab wound
	Gunshot wound
	Blunt injury
	Tracheobronchial disruption
	Esophageal rupture
	Rib fractures
Spontaneous	Primary (Idiopathic)
	Secondary
	Obstructive airways disease
	Asthma
	Emphysema
	Infection
	Cavitating pneumonia
	Lung abscess
	Septic emboli
	Pneumatoceles
	Pulmonary infarction (rare)
	Neoplasm
	Bronchogenic carcinoma
	Pleural or chest wall neoplasm
	Metastases
	Cystic lung disease
	Sarcoidosis
	Eosinophilic granuloma
	Cystic fibrosis
	Tuberous sclerosis
	Lymphangioleiomyomatosis
	Catamenial pneumothorax
	Connective tissue disorders
	Marfan's syndrome
	Ehlers-Danlos syndrome
	Cutis laxa

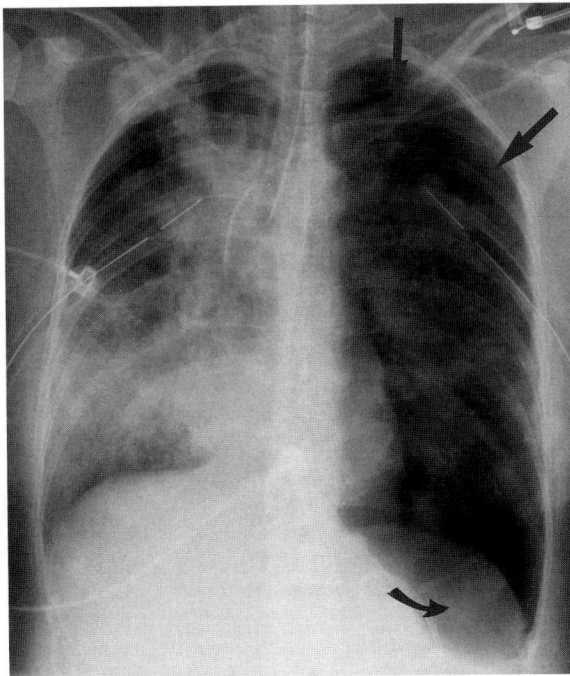

Figure 20.6. Pneumothorax Complicating ARDS. PA chest film in a 41-year-old woman with ARDS and recurrent pneumothoraces reveals a left apical (*straight arrows*) and subpulmonic (*curved arrow*) pneumothorax despite the presence of a chest tube.

itive pressure, emphysema, underlying or complicating necrotizing pneumonia, and frequent line placements and other invasive procedures (Fig. 20.6). Not uncommonly, patients with ARDS develop small peripheral cystic air spaces that can rupture into the pleural space. When these are seen to develop on serial chest radiographs, impending pneumothorax can be suggested.

A particularly rare type of recurrent pneumothorax that occurs with menstruation is catamenial pneumothorax. This condition affects women in their fourth decade, and is most likely caused by the cyclical necrosis of pleural endometrial implants that create an air leak between the lung and pleura. Rarely, air entering the peritoneal cavity during menstruation gains access to the pleural cavity via diaphragmatic defects. The predilection for right-sided pneumothoraces in this disorder indicates a key role for right sided diaphragmatic defects. The pneumothoraces tend to be small and re-

solve spontaneously. Catamenial pneumothorax is managed by preventing menstruation with the administration of oral contraceptives.

Tension Pneumothorax is a critical condition that most often results from iatrogenic trauma in mechanically ventilated patients. Tension pneumothorax results from a check-valve pleural defect that allows air to enter but not exit the pleural space. This leads to a pleural air collection that has a pressure exceeding atmospheric pressure, causing complete collapse of the underlying lung and impairing venous return to the heart. Clinically, patients present with tachypnea, tachycardia, cyanosis, and hypotension. Radiographically, the involved hemithorax is expanded and hyperlucent, with a medially retracted lung, ipsilateral diaphragmatic depression or inversion, and contralateral mediastinal shift (Fig. 20.7). Remembering that contralateral mediastinal shift from pneumothorax does not invariably indicate tension is important because a relative inequality in the degree of negative intrapleural pressure can produce shift in the absence of tension. Therefore, tension pneumothorax remains a clinical diagnosis. Immediate evacuation of the pleural space should be performed with a needle, catheter, or large bore thoracostomy tube.

Focal Pleural Disease

Focal pleural disease may be divided into localized pleural thickening, pleural calcification, or pleural mass (Table 20.4)(6).

Localized Pleural Thickening from fibrosis is usually the end result of peripheral parenchymal and pleu-

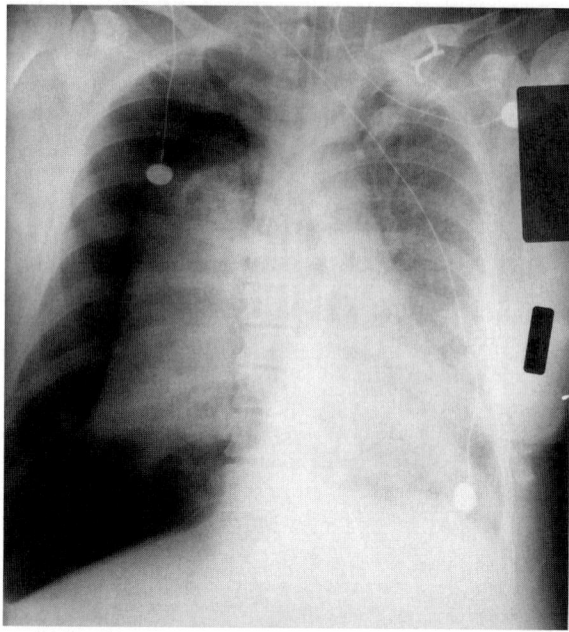

Figure 20.7. Tension Pneumothorax. Portable chest film in a 43-year-old woman with ARDS shows a large right pneumothorax with mediastinal shift and ipsilateral diaphragmatic depression suggesting tension. Air was evacuated under pressure during emergent placement of a right chest tube.

Table 20.4. Focal Pleural Disease

Opacities that mimic focal pleural thickening	Apical cap
	Companion shadows of first and second ribs
	Subpleural deposits of fat
Thickening	Pneumonia
	Pulmonary infarct
	Trauma
	Asbestos exposure (bilateral)
Calcification	Visceral pleura
	Hemothorax
	Empyema (tuberculosis)
	Parietal pleura
	Asbestos exposure (bilateral)
Pleural/Extrapleural Mass	Neoplasm
	Benign
	Fibroma
	Lipoma
	Neurofibroma
	Malignant
	Metastases (usually multiple)
	Mesothelioma (usually diffuse pleural thickening)
	Loculated pleural effusion/empyema
	Hematoma

ral inflammatory disease, with pneumonia the most common cause. Additional causes include pulmonary embolism with infarction, asbestos exposure, trauma, prior chemical pleurodesis, and drug-related pleural disease.

Pleural Calcification is most often unilateral and involves the visceral pleura. It is usually the result of prior

hemothorax or empyema (e.g. tuberculous), although pleural thickening of any cause may calcify. Asbestos exposure can cause bilateral calcified parietal pleural plaques. Visceral pleural calcification from pleural hemorrhage or infection are indistinguishable radiographically. Initially, the calcification is punctate, but it often progresses to become sheet-like. CT is particularly useful in detecting pleural calcification (Fig. 20.8). The presence of fluid within calcified pleural layers seen on CT suggests an active empyema, and is most often seen in patients with prior tuberculosis. The use of CT and HRCT in the evaluation of asbestos related focal pleural disease and calcification is discussed in a subsequent section.

Pleural Mass. Focal pleural masses are usually benign neoplasms such as fibromas and lipomas; loculated pleural fluid can mimic a pleural mass radiographically.

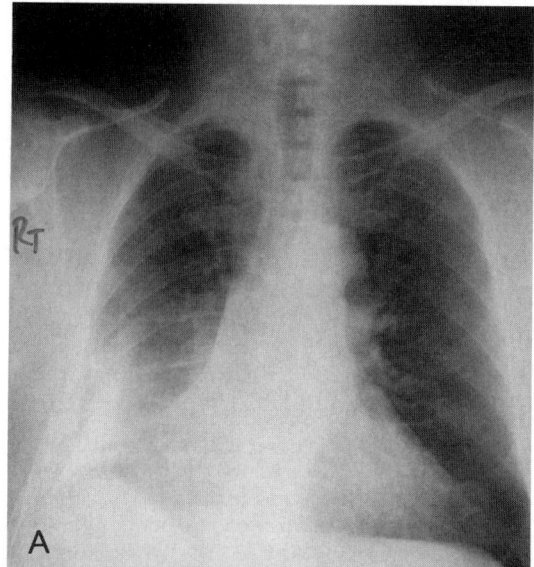

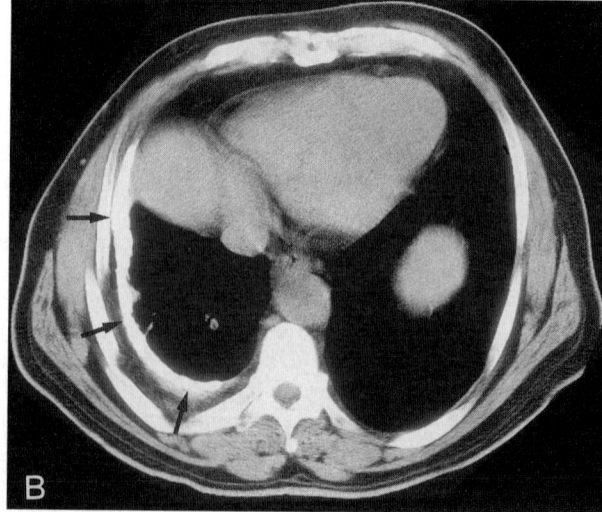

Figure 20.8. Pleural Calcification Due to Tuberculosis. A. PA chest radiograph in a 61-year-old man with prior tuberculosis demonstrates a small right hemithorax and a dense opacity inferolaterally. **B.** A CT scan through the lung bases shows a thick rind of pleural calcification (*arrows*) surrounding a contracted lung.

Thoracic lipomas may arise in the chest wall or subpleural fat. Subpleural lipomas produce a pleural mass and can change shape during respiration or with changes in patient positioning because of their pliable nature. Homogeneous fat attenuation on CT scan (-30 to -100 H) is diagnostic (Fig. 20.9). Pleural fibromas, now referred to as localized fibrous tumors of pleura, are uncommon benign pleural tumors (Fig. 20.10)(6). They appear as well defined, spherical or oblong masses that arise from the visceral pleura in 80% of cases. These tumors are occasionally attached to the pleura by a narrow pedicle, a finding that is virtually pathognomonic and accounts for changes in intrapleural location seen with changes in patient positioning in some individuals. An association between pleural fibroma and hypertrophic pulmonary osteoarthropathy and hypoglycemia is recognized. Unlike malignant mesothelioma, there is no association between benign mesothelioma and asbestos exposure.

Diffuse Pleural Disease

Diffuse pleural disease represents either diffuse pleural fibrosis (fibrothorax), pleural malignancy, or multi-loculated pleural effusion (Table 20.5)(7); the latter has been discussed in a preceding section.

Fibrothorax (diffuse pleural fibrosis) is defined as pleural thickening extending over greater than one-fourth of the costal pleural surface. Fibrothorax most commonly results from the resolution of an exudative pleural effusion, (including asbestos-related effusions), empyema, or hemothorax. It may also be seen as a sub-pleural extension of diffuse interstitial fibrosis. The fibrothorax can encompass the entire lung and produce entrapment. When this causes a restrictive ventilatory defect, pleurectomy (decortication) may be necessary to restore function to the underlying lung.

Pleural Malignancy. Metastatic disease to the pleura commonly causes irregular or lobulated pleural thickening, usually in association with a pleural effusion. The ma-

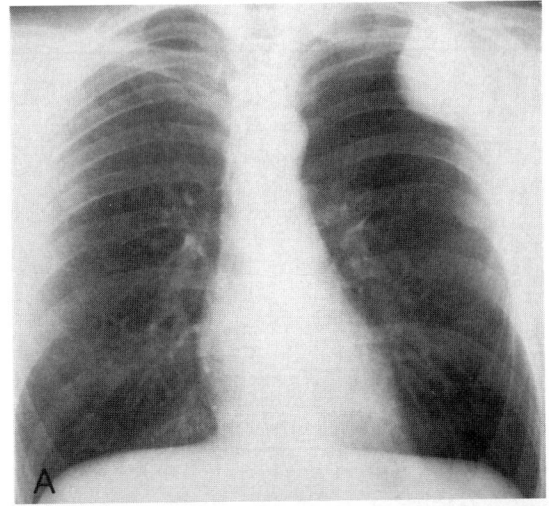

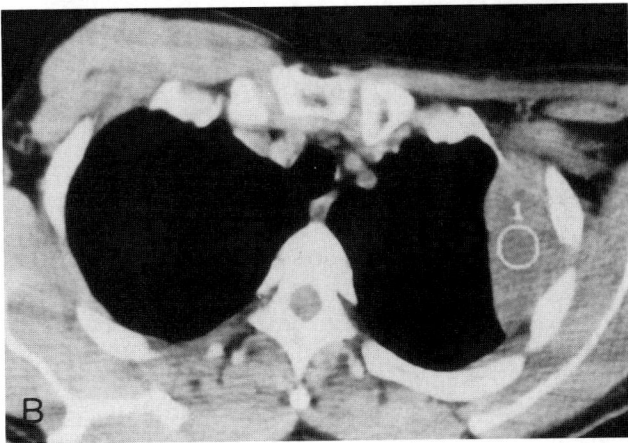

Figure 20.10. Localized Fibrous Tumor of Pleura. A. Posteroanterior radiograph in a 37-year-old man reveals a superolateral pleural mass. **B.** A CT scan shows a sharply-defined soft tissue mass forming obtuse margins with the lung. Note the incidental finding of absence of the left pectoralis major muscle. Thoracotomy revealed a benign fibrous tumor.

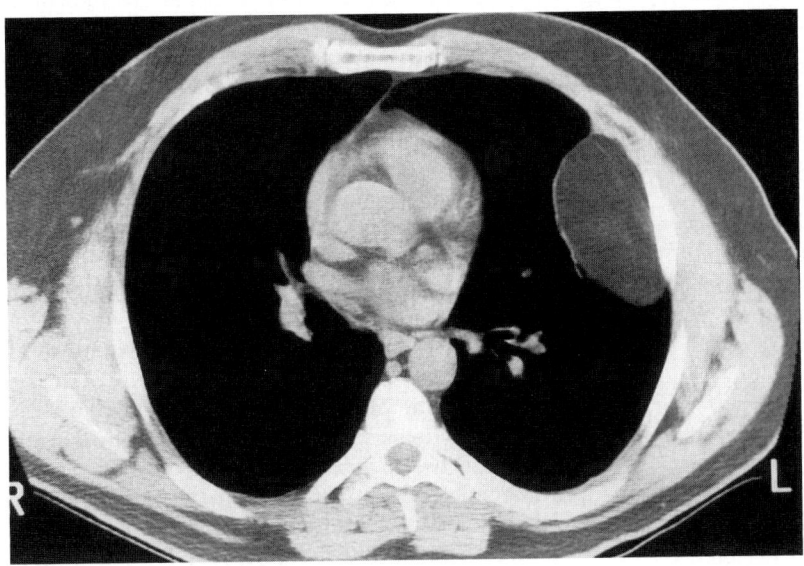

Figure 20.9. Pleural Lipoma. CT scan in a patient with an asymptomatic mass discovered as an incidental chest radiographic finding shows a left anterolateral pleural-based mass with homogeneous fatty attenuation representing a lipoma.

Table 20.5. Diffuse Pleural Disease

Smooth thickening	Pleural fibrosis
	Hemothorax
	Prior empyema or exudative effusion (including asbestos exposure)
	Interstitial pulmonary fibrosis
	Pleural effusion (particularly on supine radiographs)
Lobulated	Primary
	Mesothelioma
	Metastatic
	Adenocarcinoma of lung, breast, ovary, kidney, GI tract
	Invasive thymoma
	Lymphoma (subpleural deposits)
	Multiloculated pleural effusion/empyema

lignant tumors with a propensity to metastasize to the pleura include adenocarcinomas of the lung, breast, ovary, kidney, and gastrointestinal tract. Malignant mesothelioma is seen almost exclusively in asbestos exposed individuals.

Malignant pleural disease (either metastatic adenocarcinoma or mesothelioma) usually presents radiographically as multiple discrete pleural masses or lobulated pleural thickening (Fig. 20.2). The pleural lesions are obscured by an associated malignant pleural effusion in many patients. Contrast-enhanced CT can distinguish solid pleural masses from loculated pleural fluid, and can show discrete pleural masses or thickening in those with large effusions. In contrast to benign pleural thickening, malignant pleural disease is more likely when the pleural thickening on CT is circumferential and nodular, greater than one centimeter in thickness, and/or involves the mediastinal pleura (8). Mesothelioma is radiographically indistinguishable from metastatic pleural disease and will be discussed in the section on asbestos-related pleural disease. Chest wall invasion by pleural tumor, seen as rib destruction or soft tissue infiltration of the subcutaneous fat and musculature, is better appreciated on CT or MR than on plain films. The diagnosis of malignant pleural disease is made by cytologic examination of fluid obtained at thoracentesis, closed or thoracoscopically guided pleural biopsy, or by thoracotomy.

Asbestos-related Pleural Disease

Prolonged exposure to the inorganic fibers generically known as asbestos can result in a variety of pleural and pulmonary disorders. Benign pleural disease is the most common thoracic manifestation of asbestos inhalation and includes pleural plaques, pleural effusions, and diffuse pleural fibrosis. Rounded atelectasis is reviewed in chapter 14. Malignant asbestos-related pleural disease is manifested as malignant mesothelioma.

BENIGN ASBESTOS-RELATED PLEURAL DISEASE

Pleural Plaques are the most common benign manifestation of asbestos inhalation. These plaques develop 20–30 years after the initial asbestos exposure, and are

more frequent with increasing length and severity of exposure. Asbestos plaques are found on the parietal pleura, most commonly over the diaphragm and lower posterolateral chest wall. The mediastinal pleural surface and costophrenic sulci are characteristically spared. The plaques are discrete, bilateral, slightly raised (2–10 mm in thickness) foci of pleural thickening that are pearly white and shiny in gross appearance. Histologically, the plaques are comprised of dense bands of collagen. Punctate or linear calcification within the plaques is common, and is more frequent as the plaques enlarge. Asbestos bodies (short, straight asbestos fibers coated with iron and protein that microscopically look like small dumbbells) are not seen within the plaques. Visceral pleural plaques, seen as discrete flat regions of pleural thickening within the major fissures on HRCT, are most commonly associated with interstitial fibrosis. Most patients with isolated asbestos-related pleural plaques are asymptomatic.

Detecting pleural plaques on conventional radiographs is best performed with 45° oblique views that profile the anterolateral and posterolateral plaques. When viewed en face, the calcified plaques appear as geographic areas of opacity that have been likened to a Holly leaf (Fig. 20.11). CT and HRCT studies are extremely sensitive in detecting calcified and noncalcified pleural plaques in asbestos exposed individuals and can distinguish pleural plaques and diffuse pleural fibrosis from subpleural fat deposits that may mimic pleural disease on conventional radiographs (Fig. 20.12). Although plaques are invariably bilateral on gross examination of the pleural space in affected individuals, it is not unusual to see unilateral plaques (most often left sided) on conventional radiographs or HRCT.

Pleural Effusion occurs 10–20 years after the initial exposure and is the earliest manifestation of asbestos-related pleural disease. The development of asbestos-related effusions appears to be dose-related. The effusions are usually small, unilateral or bilateral, exudative, and may be bloody. The diagnosis of a benign asbestos pleural effusion is one of exclusion and, in addition to a history of exposure, requires the exclusion of tuberculosis or pleural malignancy (i.e., mesothelioma or metastatic adenocarcinoma). A long latency period between the initial exposure and the development of pleural effusion (>20 years) should prompt a diagnostic evaluation for malignant mesothelioma. While most asbestos-related pleural effusions resolve spontaneously, up to one-third recur and some develop diffuse pleural fibrosis.

Diffuse Pleural Thickening or fibrosis may follow asbestos-related pleural effusion or result from the confluence of pleural plaques. Diffuse asbestos pleural thickening is defined as smooth, flat pleural thickening extending over one-fourth of the costal pleural surface. In distinction to pleural plaques that affect the parietal pleura alone, diffuse pleural fibrosis involves both the parietal and visceral pleura. Radiographically, diffuse pleural thickening is seen as a smooth thickening of the pleura involving the lower thorax with blunting of the costophrenic sulci. CT and HRCT are useful to determine the extent of pleural thickening, involvement of the interlobar fissures, and to detect underlying fibrotic or em-

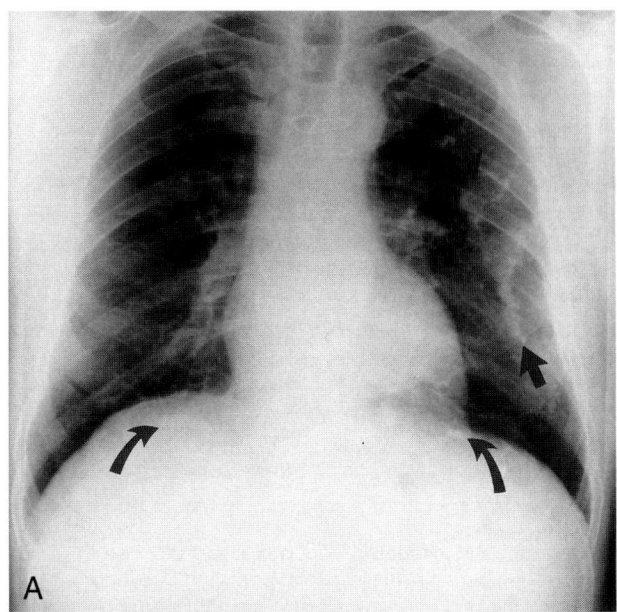

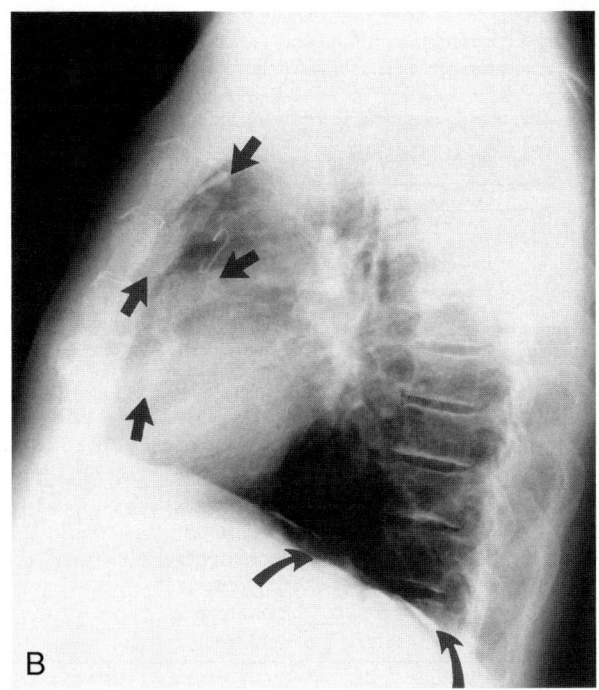

Figure 20.11. Calcified Pleural Plaques. PA **(A)** and lateral **(B)** chest films in a 64-year-old man shows bilateral diaphragmatic (*curved arrows*) and anterolateral (*straight arrows*) pleural plaques reflecting prior asbestos exposure.

physematous lung disease (Fig. 20.12). Diffuse pleural fibrosis can result in symptomatic restrictive lung disease.

MALIGNANT ASBESTOS-RELATED PLEURAL DISEASE

Malignant Mesothelioma is a rare malignant pleural neoplasm associated with asbestos exposure. Unlike other pleural and parenchymal manifestations of asbestos, it does not appear to be dose-related. Mesothelioma most often occurs 30–40 years after the

initial exposure. Although the incidence increases with heavy exposure, malignant mesothelioma may also develop after minimal exposure and contrasts with the linear relationship between the development of benign asbestos pleural disease and the dose of asbestos exposure. Crocidolite is the fiber type most often implicated in the development of malignant mesothelioma. This tumor grows by contiguous spread from the pleural space into the lung, chest wall, mediastinum, and diaphragm; distant metastases are not uncommon.

Malignant mesothelioma most often appears radiographically as thick (>1 cm) and lobulated diffuse pleural thickening (7). Calcification is seen in only 20% of tumors, although calcified pleural plaques may be seen in uninvolved areas of the pleura. A pleural effusion is often present, and if large, it may obscure the pleural tumor. Malignant involvement of the mediastinal pleural surface may prevent contralateral mediastinal shift despite extensive pleural tumor volume and effusion, a finding that may help distinguish mesothelioma from metastatic disease. CT is the imaging modality of choice in the evaluation of malignant mesothelioma, and depicts the extent of pleural involvement and invasion of the chest wall and mediastinum (Fig. 20.13). Diaphragmatic invasion by tumor, best assessed by coronal MR scans, is important only in those patients who are considered for resection (Fig. 20.14). Adenopathy is seen in the ipsilateral hilum and mediastinum in approximately 50% of patients. While the radiologic findings may be highly suggestive of mesothelioma, metastatic pleural malignancy can have a similar appearance and histologic confirmation is necessary.

The diagnosis of malignant mesothelioma is made histologically using specimens, and often requires the use of special stains. The malignant cells may be of the spindle or epithelial type or a combination of both. The epithelial type of malignant mesothelioma may be indistin-

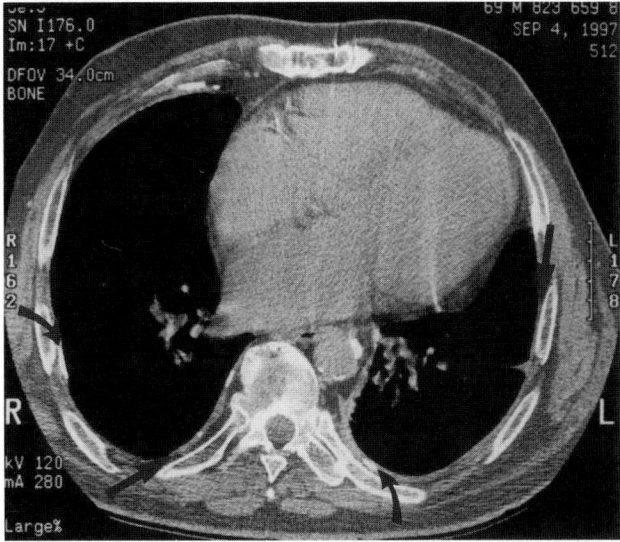

Figure 20.12. Pleural Plaques and Diffuse Pleural Thickening from Asbestos Exposure. HRCT in a 69-year-old man with benign asbestos-related pleural disease demonstrates bilateral thickening (*straight arrows*) and calcified pleural plaques (*curved arrows*).

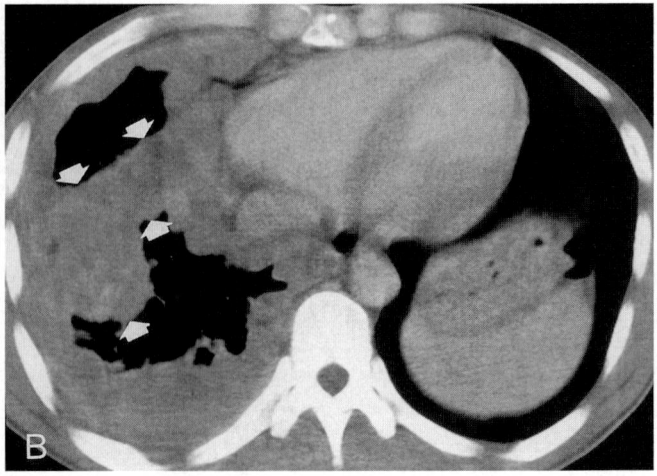

Figure 20.13. Malignant Mesothelioma. A. A posteroanterior chest radiograph in a 34-year-old man evaluated for a positive PPD reveals lobulated right pleural thickening encompassing the right lung. **B.** A CT scan through the lung bases demonstrates a circumferential pleural soft tissue process traversing the major fissure (*arrows*). US-guided pleural biopsy revealed malignant mesothelioma.

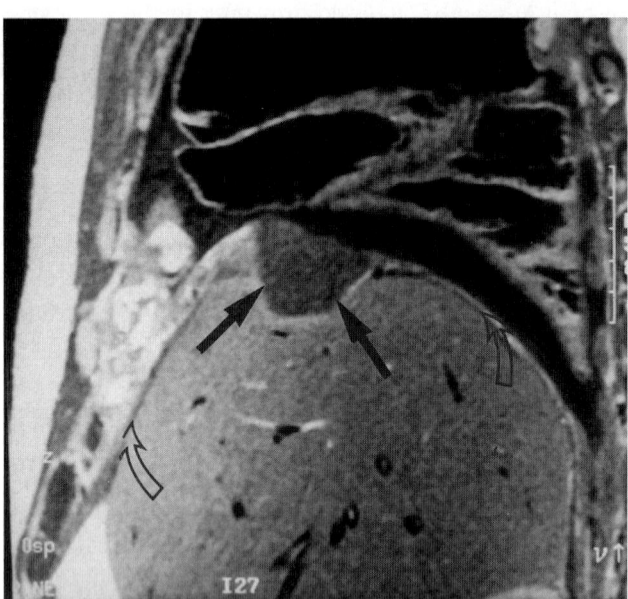

Figure 20.14. Diaphragmatic Invasion of Malignant Mesothelioma on MR. Sagittal T1-weighted MR scan through the dome of the right hemidiaphragm in a 53-year-old man with known pleural mesothelioma shows a basilar pleural mass (*straight arrows*) invading through the right diaphragm (*curved arrows*) into the liver. Laparoscopy confirmed the MR findings that rendered the patient unresectable.

Table 20.6. Chest Wall Lesions

Tumors	Benign
	Mole
	Nevus
	Wart
	Neurofibroma
	Lipoma
	Hemangioma
	Desmoid
	Malignant
	Fibrosarcoma
	Liposarcoma
	Metastases
	Melanoma
	Bronchogenic carcinoma
Infection (abscess)	Staphylococcus
	Tuberculosis
Trauma	Hematoma

guishable from adenocarcinoma on light microscopy. PAS staining of the cellular cytoplasm following diastase digestion of the tissue specimen detects the presence of intracellular neutral mucins that is found in 80% of patients with metastatic adenocarcinoma to the pleura. Alcian blue staining of the cytoplasm following tissue pretreatment with hyaluronidase detects the presence of intracellular acid mucins and is diagnostic in 50% of patients with the epithelial type of malignant mesothelioma. Positive keratin staining helps diagnose the spindle cell type of mesothelioma and distinguishes this form of mesothelioma from fibrosarcoma.

While surgical resection by pleurectomy or extrapleural pneumonectomy may benefit selected patients with limited disease and good pulmonary reserve, the median survival from the time of diagnosis is only 6 to 12 months.

CHEST WALL

Disorders of the soft tissues or bony structures of the chest wall may come to attention because of local symptoms or physical findings, during evaluation of pulmonary or pleural disease, or as an incidental finding on radiographic studies (Table 20.6).

Soft Tissues

Congenital absence of the pectoralis muscle (Fig. 20.10B) results in hyperlucency of the affected hemithorax on frontal radiographs. Poland's syndrome is an autosomal recessive disorder characterized by unilateral absence of the sternocostal head of the pectoralis major, ipsilateral syndactyly, and rib anomalies. There may be associated aplasia of the ipsilateral breast. Patients who have had a mastectomy will also show unilateral hyperlucency. In those who have undergone a modified radical mastectomy, the horizontally-oriented inferior edge of the hypertrophied pectoralis minor muscle may be identified on frontal radiographs.

A variety of skin lesions such as moles, nevi, warts, neurofibromas, and accessory nipples may produce a nodular opacity on frontal radiographs which mimicks a solitary pulmonary nodule. Examination of the skin surface should be performed in any patient with a new nodular opacity seen on chest radiographs, and repeat radiographs obtained with a radioopaque marker over the skin lesion will confirm the nature of the opacity and avoid unnecessary followup radiographs and chest CT.

Chest wall abscesses may present as localized, painful, fluctuant subcutaneous masses. Staphylococcus and tuberculosis are the most common organisms responsible. The diagnosis is usually obvious clinically. Chest radiographs demonstrate a poorly defined opacity on the frontal radiograph when the abscess involves the anterior or posterior chest wall. CT shows a localized fluid collection with an enhancing wall, and is used to determine the location and extent of the collection prior to open drainage.

Soft tissue neoplasms of the chest wall are rare (9). They are most often detected clinically as a mass protruding from the chest wall, and appear as nonspecific extrathoracic soft tissue masses on chest radiographs. The most common benign neoplasm of the chest wall is a lipoma. Lipomas may be intrathoracic, extrathoracic, or project partially within and outside the thorax (dumbbell lipoma). CT shows a sharply circumscribed mass of fatty density (Fig. 20.15), while MR shows characteristic high and intermediate signal intensity on T1WI and T2WI respectively. A desmoid tumor is a rare fibroblastic tumor arising within striated muscle that is histologically benign but has a tendency for local invasion. Desmoids are most common in the abdominal wall musculature of multiparous women, but may arise in the chest wall musculature following local trauma. Hemangiomas are uncommon chest wall tumors. While often indistinguishable from other soft tissue tumors radiographically, the recognition of phleboliths, hypertrophy of involved bones, or the identification of vascular channels on contrast enhanced CT or MR studies should suggest the diagnosis.

Fibrosarcomas and liposarcomas are the most common malignant soft tissue neoplasms of the chest wall in adults. Malignant tumors often present with symptoms of localized chest wall pain and a visible, palpable mass. Patients who have received chest wall radiation are at particular risk for developing sarcomas. Radiographically, these soft tissue masses are often associated with bony destruction. CT best depicts the bone destruction and intrathoracic component of tumor, while MR shows the extent of tumor and delineates tumor from surrounding muscle and subcutaneous fat (8).

The Bony Thorax

RIBS

Congenital Anomalies (Table 20.7). The most common congenital anomalies of the ribs are bony fusion and bifid ribs, neither of which have clinical significance. Intrathoracic ribs are extremely rare congenital anomalies where an accessory rib arises from a vertebral body or the posterior surface of a rib and extends inferolaterally into the thorax, usually on the right side. Osteogenesis imperfecta and neurofibromatosis may be associated with thin wavy "ribbon" ribs. A relatively common congenital anomaly is the cervical rib, which arises from the seventh cervical vertebral body. Cervical ribs are usually asymptomatic, although in a minority of individuals with the thoracic outlet syndrome, the rib or associated fibrous bands can compress the subclavian artery and produce secondary ischemic symptoms or compress the subclavian vein and brachial plexus producing pain, weakness, and swelling of the upper extremity. Surgical resection of the cervical rib can relieve the symptoms in selected patients.

Rib Notching is seen in a variety of pathologic conditions. Inferior rib notching is much more common than superior rib notching, and is caused by enlargement of one or more of the structures that lie in the subcostal grooves (intercostal nerve, artery, or vein). The notching predominantly affects the posterior aspects of the ribs bilaterally and may be narrow, wide, deep, or shallow.

The most common cause of bilateral inferior rib notching is coarctation of the aorta distal to the origin of the left subclavian artery. In this condition, blood circumvents the aortic obstruction and reaches the descending aorta via the subclavian, internal mammary, and inter-

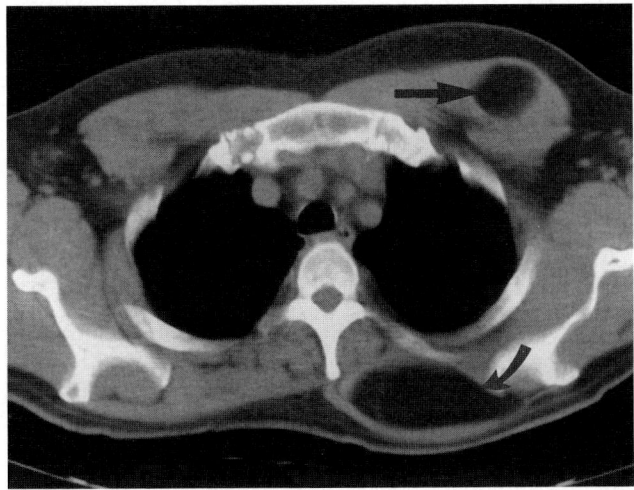

Figure 20.15. Chest Wall Lipomas. Unenhanced CT scan shows sharply circumscribed homogeneous fatty masses in the left pectoral (*straight arrows*) and rhomboid major (*curved arrows*) muscles.

Table 20.7. Rib Lesions

Congenital	Fusion anomalies
	Cervical rib
	Ribbon ribs
	Rib notching
	Inferior
	Coarctation of the aorta
	Tetralogy of Fallot
	Superior vena caval obstruction
	Blalock-Taussig shunt (unilateral right)
	Neurofibromatosis
	Superior
	Paralysis
	Collagen vascular disease
	Rheumatoid arthritis
	Systemic lupus erythematosis
Trauma	Healing rib fracture
Non-neoplastic tumors	Fibrous dysplasia
	Eosinophilic granuloma
	Brown tumor
Neoplasms	Benign
	Osteochondroma
	Enchondroma
	Osteoblastoma
	Malignant
	Primary
	Chondrosarcoma
	Osteogenic sarcoma
	Fibrosarcoma
	Metastatic
	Multiple myeloma
	Metastases
	Breast carcinoma
	Bronchogenic carcinoma
	Renal cell carcinoma
	Prostate carcinoma
Osteomyelitis	Staphylococcus aureus
	Tuberculosis
	Actinomycosis
	Nocardiosis

costal arteries. The increased blood flow in the intercostal arteries produces tortuosity and dilatation of these vessels, which erodes the inferior margins of the adjacent ribs. Other causes of aortic obstruction that can lead to inferior rib notching include aortic thrombosis and Takayasu's aortitis. Congenital heart diseases associated with decreased pulmonary blood flow may be associated with rib notching as the intercostal arteries enlarge in an attempt to supply collateral blood flow to the oligemic lungs. Superior vena cava obstruction can cause increased flow through intercostal veins and produce rib notching.

Patients with aortic coarctation develop rib notching gradually; it is most common in adolescents and is rare in children under the age of seven. The first two ribs are uninvolved because the first and second intercostal arteries arise from the superior intercostal branch of the costocervical trunk of the subclavian artery, and therefore do not communicate with the descending thoracic aorta. Coarctation may produce unilateral left rib notching when the aortic narrowing occurs proximal to an aberrant right subclavian artery. Unilateral right sided

notching occurs when the coarctation is proximal to the left subclavian artery. Additional causes of unilateral inferior rib notching include subclavian artery obstruction and surgical anastamosis of the proximal subclavian artery to the ipsilateral pulmonary artery (Blalock-Taussig procedure)

Multiple intercostal neurofibromas in neurofibromatosis type I is the most common nonvascular cause of inferior rib notching. The neurofibromas appear as multiple extrapleural soft tissue masses, most often seen in the upper paravertebral regions. Other thoracic bony manifestations of neurofibromatosis include ribbon ribs, thoracic kyphoscoliosis, and scalloping of the posterior aspect of the vertebral bodies caused by dural ectasia.

Superior rib notching is much less common than inferior rib notching. The pathogenesis of superior rib notching is unknown, although a disturbance of osteoblastic and osteoclastic activity and the stress effect of the intercostal muscles are proposed mechanisms. Paralysis is the most common condition associated with superior rib notching. Other etiologies include rheumatoid arthritis, systemic lupus erythematosis, and rarely, marked tortuosity of the intercostal arteries from severe, long standing aortic obstruction.

Trauma. Rib fractures may result from blunt or penetrating trauma to a normal rib cage or from minimal trauma to abnormal ribs such as those affected by metastases. An acute rib fracture is seen as a thin vertical lucency; malalignment of the superior and inferior cortices of the rib may occasionally be the only radiographic finding. The tendency to affect the posterolateral aspects of the ribs explains the utility of obtaining ipsilateral posterior oblique radiographs for suspected fracture, as this projection best displays the fracture line. In any patient with an acute rib fracture, a careful search should be made for associated pneumothorax, hemothorax, and pulmonary contusion or laceration. Because the first three ribs are well protected by the clavicles, scapulae, and shoulder girdles, fracture of these ribs indicates severe trauma and should prompt a careful evaluation for associated great vessel and visceral injuries. Fracture of the tenth, eleventh, or twelth ribs may be associated with injury to the liver or spleen. Severe blunt trauma to the rib cage in which multiple contiguous ribs are fractured in more than one place is termed a "flail chest." This results in a free segment of the chest wall that moves paradoxically inward on inspiration and outward on expiration. Healing rib fractures will demonstrate callus formation, which may be exuberant in patients receiving corticosteroids. Multiple contiguous healed rib fractures, particularly if bilateral, should suggest chronic alcoholism or a prior motor vehicle accident.

Non-neoplastic Lesions. The ribs are the most common site of involvement by monostotic fibrous dysplasia. The typical appearance is an expansile lesion in the posterior aspect of the rib with a lucent or ground glass density; rarely, the lesion is sclerotic. Multiple rib involvement from polyostotic fibrous dysplasia can result in severe restrictive pulmonary disease. Eosinophilic granuloma can cause lytic lesions in patients less than 30 years of age. These are usually solitary lytic lesions that can be expansile but do not have sclerotic margins; this latter feature helps distinguish these lesions from fibrous dysplasia. Brown tumors from hyperparathyroidism can also produce lytic rib lesions.

Neoplasms. Primary osteochondral neoplasms or metastatic disease can involve the ribs. Osteochondromas are the most common benign neoplasm of ribs, followed in relative frequency by enchondromas and osteoblastomas (Fig. 20.16). Primary malignant neoplasms of the ribs in adults are uncommon. Chondrosarcoma is the most common primary rib malignancy, with osteogenic sarcoma and fibrosarcoma less common (Fig. 20.17). Rib involvement from multiple myeloma or metastatic carcinoma can produce solitary or multiple lytic lesions and is much more common than primary tumors. Myeloma can also cause permeative bone destruction indistinguishable from severe osteoporosis. The diagnosis of myeloma is made by identification of a monoclonal spike on serum protein electrophoresis and typical findings of abnormal aggregates of plasma cells on bone marrow biopsy. The most common metastatic lesions to ribs are from bronchogenic and breast carcinoma, which produce multiple lytic lesions when dissemination is hematogenous or localized rib destruction when invasion is by direct contiguous spread. Expansile lytic rib metastases are seen most commonly from renal cell and thyroid carcinoma. Sclerotic rib metastases are most commonly seen in breast and prostate carcinoma.

Infection. Chest wall infection and osteomyelitis of the ribs usually develops from contiguous spread from the lung, pleural space, and vertebral column. Less commonly, infection complicates penetrating chest trauma or spreads to the ribs hematogenously. Pleuropulmonary infections that may traverse the pleural space and produce a chest wall infection include tuberculosis, actinomycosis, and nocardiosis. Radiographs may demonstrate bone destruction, periostitis, and subcutaneous emphysema; bone scans can detect subradiographic bone involvement. CT can demonstrate bone destruction, soft tissue swelling, and abscesses within the chest wall. Additionally, CT may show involvement of the adjacent pleural space, lung, sternum, or vertebral column.

Costal Cartilages. Ossification of the costal cartilages is a normal finding on frontal chest radiographs in adults. Female costal cartilage ossification involves the

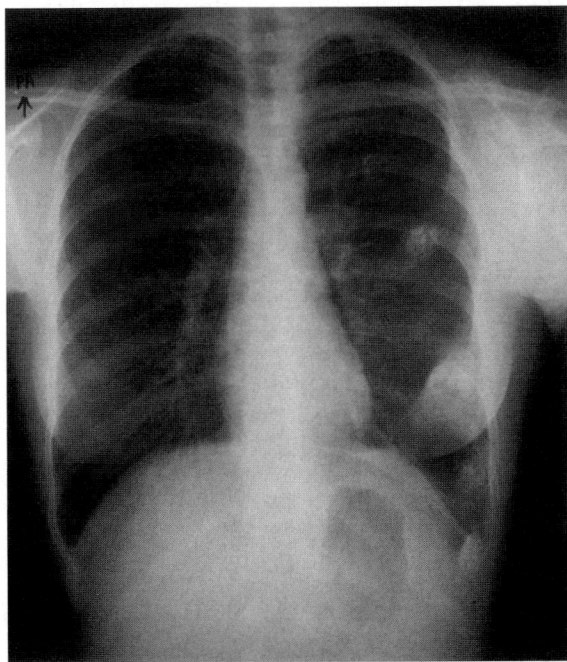

Figure 20.16. Multiple Enchondromas of Ribs. PA chest film in a 23-year-old woman with multiple enchondromatosis and Maffucci's syndrome shows enchondromas within multiple left ribs.

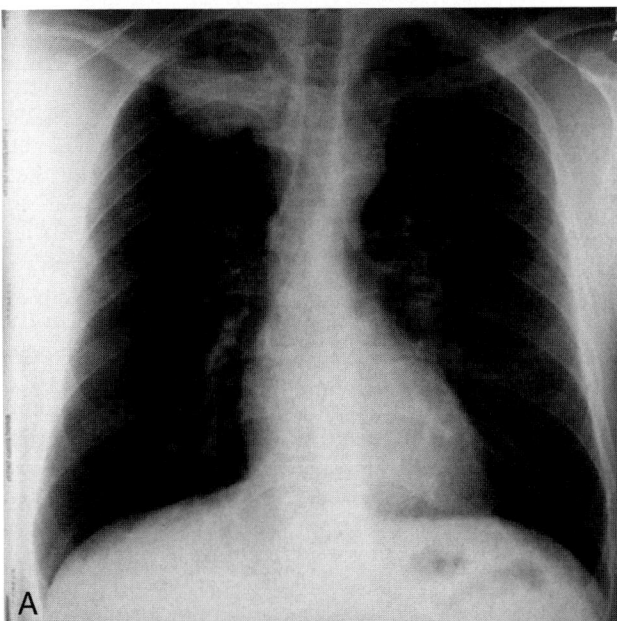

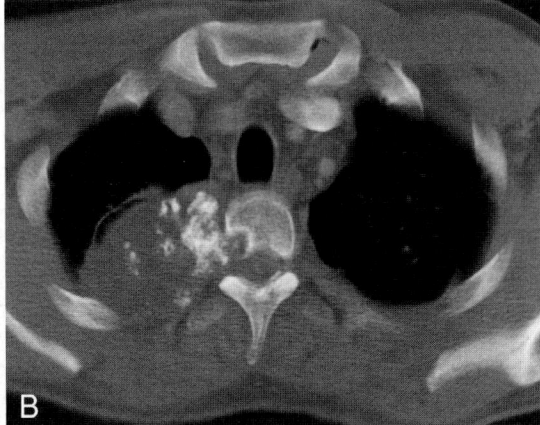

Figure 20.17. Chrondrosarcoma of Rib. A. PA chest radiograph in a 37-year-old man with a 3 month history of right shoulder pain demonstrates a right apical extrapulmonary mass. **B.** A CT scan reveals a bone-forming mass arising from the right third costotransverse junction with erosion of the adjacent vertebral body. This chondrosarcoma was successfully resected by a combined thoracic and neurosurgical approach.

central portion of the cartilage, extending from the rib towards the sternum in the shape of a solitary finger, while male costal cartilage ossification involves the peripheral portion of the cartilage and has the appearance of two fingers ("peace" sign). These typical patterns of male and female costal cartilage ossification are seen in 70% of patients, and do not apply to the first rib.

Scapula. Scapular abnormalties visible on frontal radiographs include congenital, posttraumatic, and neoplastic lesions. Sprengel's deformity is a congenital anomaly in which the scapula is hypoplastic and elevated. The association of Sprengel's deformity with an omovertebral bone, fused cervical vertebrae, hemivertebrae, kyphoscoliosis, and rib anomalies is termed the Klippel-Feil syndrome. Scapular fractures may result from direct trauma to the upper back and shoulder or from impaction of the humeral head into the glenoid. A winged scapula is identified when the scapula is superiorly displaced from its normal position and the inferior portion is posteriorly displaced from the chest wall, thereby foreshortening its appearance on the frontal radiograph. This deformity results from disruption in the innervation of the serratus anterior muscle, which maintains the scapula against the chest wall. Metastatic disease to the scapula is recognized by the presence of lytic destructive lesions; bronchogenic and breast carcinomas are the most common primary malignancies.

Clavicle. A variety of diseases can affect the clavicle. The clavicle is involved in cleidocranial dystostosis, in which there is partial or complete aplasia of the clavicle. The distal third of the clavicle is commonly fractured in blunt trauma. Rheumatoid arthritis and hyperparathyroidism are associated with erosion of the distal clavicles. The distal clavicle is sharply defined in rheumatoid arthritis and tapers to a point, whereas in hyperparathyroidism it is often widened and irregular. Additional findings in rheumatoid arthritis include narrowing of the glenohumeral joint and a high-riding humeral head due to rotator cuff atrophy. Primary malignant neoplasms of the clavicle include Ewing's or osteogenic sarcoma. Metastases to the clavicle are usually associated with lesions in other portions of the bony thorax. Osteomyelitis of the clavicle is uncommon and is most often seen in intravenous drug users. Paget's disease can involve the clavicle but there is often concommitant pelvic bone and calvarial involvement

Thoracic Spine. Disorders of the thoracic spine are discussed in the section on musculoskeletal disease. Numerous thoracic spine abnormalities are visible on chest radiographs. Congenital anomalies including hemivertebrae, butterfly vertebra, spina bifida, and scoliosis can be seen on well penetrated frontal radiographs. Vertebral compression fractures due to trauma, osteoporosis, or metastases are best seen on lateral radiographs and may produce an exaggerated kyphosis. Large bridging osteophytes may mimic a paraspinal mass on frontal radiographs or a pulmonary nodule on lateral films. Vertebral osteomyelitis is seen as destruction of vertebral bodies and intervertebral discs, often associated with a paraspinal abscess. Chronic anemia in patients with thalassemia major or sickle cell disease may have pre- or paravertebral masses of extramedullary hematopoiesis, which represent herniated hyperplastic bone marrow. Sickle cell anemia produces a characteristic appearance of H-shaped or Lincoln-log vertebrae on lateral chest radiographs which is pathognomonic of this disease. Similarly, a rugger-jersey appearance to the thoracic spine on lateral chest films suggests renal osteosclerosis.

Sternum. Developmental sternal deformities include pectus excavatum (funnel chest), pectus carinatum (pigeon breast), and abnormal segmentation (9). In pectus excavatum, the sternum is inwardly depressed and the ribs protrude anterior to the sternum. It often has an autosomal dominant pattern of inheritance but may occur sporadically. Pectus excavatum is commonly associated with congenital connective tissue disorders such as Marfan's syndrome, Poland's syndrome, osteogenesis imperfecta, and congenital scoliosis. Most patients are asymptomatic. A clinically insignificant systolic murmur can result from compression of the right ventricular outflow tract, although some patients with pectus deformities and systolic murmurs have mitral valve prolapse. Pectus excavatum has a characteristic appearance on frontal chest radiograph. The heart is displaced to the left and the combination of the depressed soft tissues of the anterior chest wall and the vertically oriented anterior ribs results in loss of the right heart border. The findings on frontal radiographs may be mistakenly attributed to middle lobe opacification from pneumonia or atelectasis. The typical inward depression of the mid and lower sternum is seen on lateral chest radiographs. CT helps define the deformity and its effect on the heart and mediastinal structures.

Pectus carinatum is an outward bowing of the sternum which may be congenital or acquired. The congenital form is seen more commonly in boys and in families with a history of chest wall deformities or scoliosis. Congenital atrial or ventricular septal defects and severe childhood asthma account for the majority of the acquired cases of pectus carinatum. Affected patients are asymptomatic. The characteristic outward bowing of the sternum with deepening of the retrosternal air space is seen on lateral radiographs.

Severe blunt trauma to the chest, most often associated with deceleration injury from a motor vehicle accident, can result in fracture or dislocation of the sternum. Sternal body fracture and sternomanubrial dislocation are associated with a 25–45% mortality from concomitant injuries to the aorta, diaphragm, heart, tracheobronchial tree, and lung. Sternal films or lateral radiographs will show the fracture and often demonstrate a retrosternal hematoma; CT may be useful in those patients with normal plain films and a high suspicion of sternal injury.

A prior median sternotomy is the most common sternal abnormality seen on conventional radiographs and chest CT. Circular wires encompassing the sternum are seen spaced along its length within the interspaces between costal cartilages. The vertical lucency representing the sternotomy may heal but in many patients bony union does not occur. In the early postoperative period, a retrosternal hematoma may be seen that normally resolves within the first several weeks. The radiologist plays a key role in the evaluation of possible sternal wound infection. Plain film evidence of bony destruction or air in the sternal incision appearing days to weeks after sternotomy are specific but insensitive findings for osteomyelitis. Bone scans are not particularly useful as there will be increased radionuclide uptake for months following sternotomy. CT is the modality of choice in the evaluation of sternal wound infection. The CT findings of sternal osteomyelitis include bone destruction, peristernal soft tissue mass, enhancing fluid collection, and gas. The extent of infection, specifically associated mediastinitis, can also be determined.

Diaphragm

Unilateral Diaphragmatic Elevation. The differential diagnosis of unilateral diaphragmatic elevation is listed in Table 20.8. Eventration of the diaphragm is a congenital absence or underdevelopment of diaphragmatic musculature. This produces a localized elevation of the anteromedial portion of the right hemidiaphragm on frontal radiographs in older individuals, indistinguishable from the rare foramen of Morgagni hernia. Complete diaphragmatic eventration is usually left sided and is indistinguishable radiographically from diaphragmatic paralysis (Fig. 20.18).

Unilateral diaphragmatic paralysis is usually caused by surgical injury or neoplastic involvement of the phrenic nerve, which affects the right and left hemidiaphragms with equal frequency. Idiopathic phrenic nerve dysfunction resulting from a viral neuritis is a common cause of diaphragmatic paralysis in males and is usually right sided. A positive fluoroscopic or ultrasonographic sniff test (paradoxical superior movement of the diaphragm with sniffing that results from the effects of negative intrathoracic pressure on a flaccid diaphragm during inspiration) is diagnostic.

Table 20.8. Unilateral Diaphragmatic Elevation

Eventration	
Diminished lung volume	Congenital
	Hypoplastic lung
	Acquired
	Lobar/lung atelectasis
	Pulmonary resection
Paralysis	Idiopathic
	Iatrogenic phrenic nerve injury
	Phrenic crush (tuberculosis)
	Intraoperative
	Malignant invasion of phrenic nerve
	Bronchogenic carcinoma
	Inflammation of diaphragmatic
	muscle
	Pleuritis
	Lower lobe pneumonia
	Subphrenic abscess
Upper abdominal mass	Hepatomegaly or liver mass
	Splenomegaly
	Gastric/colonic distention
	Ascites (usually bilateral)
	Diaphragmatic hernia*
	Subpulmonic pleural effusion*

* Apparent diaphragmatic elevation

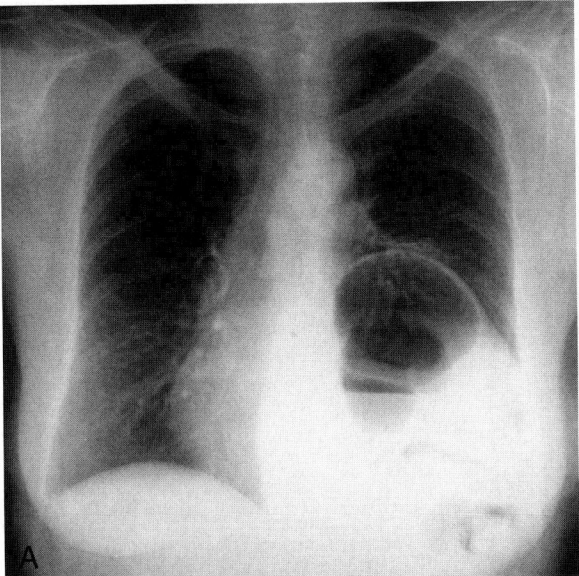
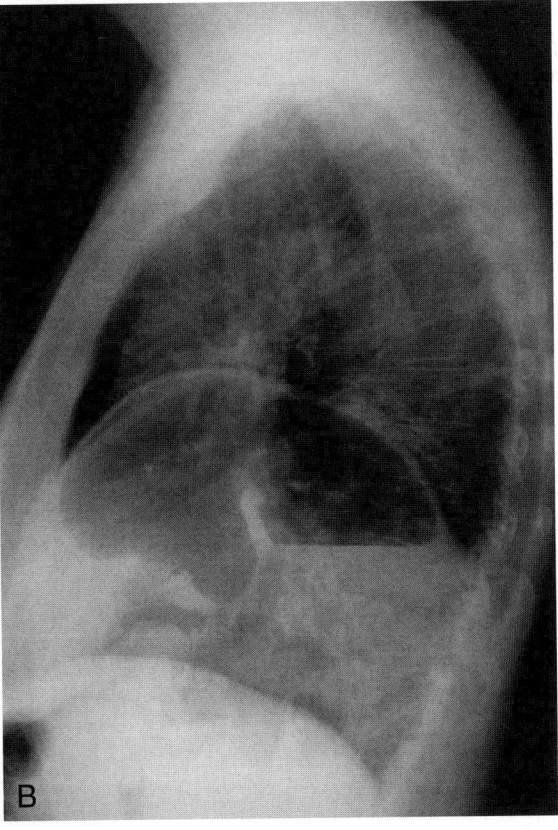

Figure 20.18. Eventration of the Diaphragm. PA **(A)** and lateral **(B)** chest radiographs in an asymptomatic 61-year-old woman reveals marked elevation of the left hemidiaphragm representing diaphragmatic eventration.

Chronic loss of lung volume, particularly from collapse or resection of the lower lobe, results in diaphragmatic elevation. This is also a common sequela of chronic cicatrizing atelectasis of the upper lobe from tuberculosis.

An enlarged liver or hepatic mass can produce right hemidiaphragmatic elevation by direct pressure on the undersurface of the hemidiaphragm. Similarly, an enlarged spleen, gas-distended stomach or enlarged splenic flexure can produce an elevated left hemidiaphragm. Irritation of the superior surface of the hemidiaphragm by a pleural or pleural-based parenchymal process (e.g., infarct, pneumonia), or of the undersurface of the diaphragm by a subphrenic abscess, hepatitis, or cholecystitis may cause the diaphragm to become flaccid, leading to elevation. A subpulmonic effusion may simulate an elevated hemidiaphragm.

Bilateral Diaphragmatic Elevation that is not effort related may be caused by a neuromuscular disturbance or intrathoracic or intra-abdominal disease. Radiographically, the diaphragms are elevated on both frontal and lateral views. Bibasilar linear atelectasis or passive lobar or segmental lower lobe atelectasis may be seen.

Bilateral phrenic nerve disruption or intrinsic diaphragmatic muscular disease will produce bilateral diaphragmatic paralysis and elevation. Common disorders include cervical cord injury, multiple sclerosis, and the myopathy associated with systemic lupus erythematosis. In these patients, fluoroscopic or real time US imaging of the diaphragms demonstrates a positive sniff test.

Lung restriction due to interstitial fibrosis, bilateral pleural fibrosis, or chest wall disease (most commonly from obesity) can produce bilateral diaphragmatic elevation. An increase in intraabdominal volume, most often from ascites, hepatosplenomegaly, or pregnancy can restrict diaphragmatic motion. These conditions may be distinguished from bilateral paralysis by observing normal but diminished inferior excursion of the diaphragms on fluoroscopy, US, or inspiratory/expiratory radiographs.

Diaphragmatic Depression. Depression and flattening of one hemidiaphragm is seen with unilateral overinflation of a lung, usually as a compensatory mechanism

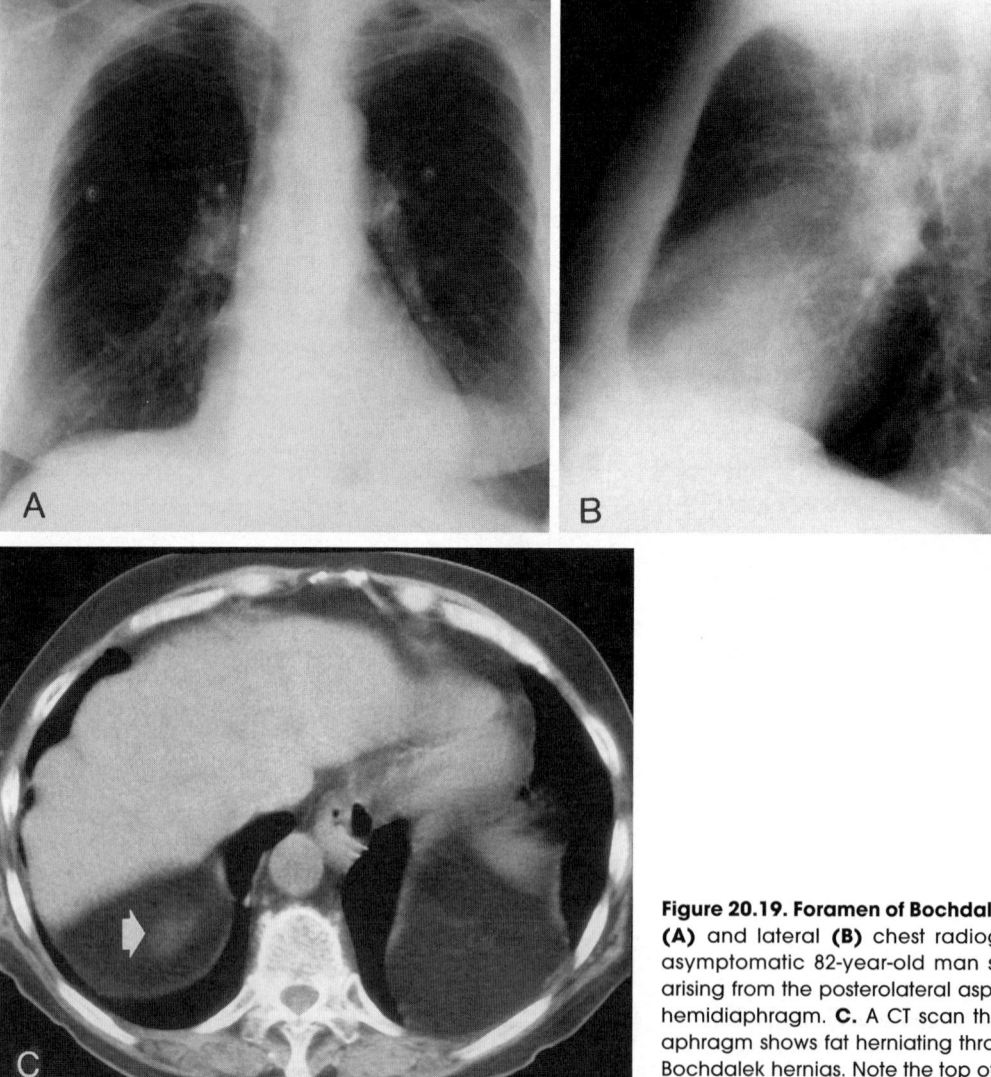

Figure 20.19. Foramen of Bochdalek hernia. PA **(A)** and lateral **(B)** chest radiographs in an asymptomatic 82-year-old man show a mass arising from the posterolateral aspect of the left hemidiaphragm. **C.** A CT scan through the diaphragm shows fat herniating through bilateral Bochdalek hernias. Note the top of the right kidney within the herniated fat (*arrow*).

when the contralateral lung is small, or as a result of a large ipsilateral pneumothorax. Distinction between these two entities is usually possible by the clinical history and by characteristic findings in those with pneumothorax. A tension pneumothorax may cause inversion of the hemidiaphragm. Bilateral diaphragmatic depression is either a permanent finding as a result of abnormally increased lung compliance in patients with emphysema, or is a transient finding in those with asthma and expiratory air trapping.

Diaphragmatic Hernias. There are three types of congenital diaphragmatic hernia. The most common is the esophageal hiatal hernia, which represents herniation of a portion of the stomach through the esophageal hiatus. These are usually seen as incidental asymptomatic masses on chest radiographs, although some patients may have symptoms of gastroesophageal reflux or, rarely, severe pain from strangulation of the herniated stomach. Hiatal hernias are seen projecting behind the heart on frontal chest radiographs in the immediate supradiaphragmatic region of the posterior mediastinum. An air-fluid level may be seen in the hernia. An esophagram is confirmatory. CT shows widening of the esophageal hiatus and depicts the contents of the hernia sac, which often includes stomach, omental fat, and, rarely, ascitic fluid.

The foramen of Bochdalek is a defect in the hemidiaphragm at the site of the embryonic pleuroperitoneal canal. Large hernias through Bochdalek's foramen present in the neonatal period with hypoplasia of the ipsilateral lung and respiratory distress. In adults, small hernias through this foramen are common and are predominantly seen on the left side, presumably because of the protective effect of the liver that prevents herniation of right infradiaphragmatic fat through the right foramen of Bochdalek. The hernia typically appears as a posterolateral mass above the left hemidiaphragm, although it can occur anywhere along the posterior diaphragmatic surface. CT shows the diaphragmatic defect with herniation of retroperitoneal fat, omentum, spleen, or kidney (Fig. 20.19)(10).

A defect in the parasternal portion of the diaphragm, the foramen of Morgagni, is the least common type of diaphragmatic hernia. A Morgagni's hernia is invariably right sided and appears as an asymptomatic cardiophrenic angle mass. The diagnosis is made by noting herniation of omental fat, liver, or transverse colon through the paracardiac portion of the right hemidiaphragm on CT scans through the lung bases. The presence of omental vessels within a fatty paracardiac mass is diagnostic (Fig. 20.20). Coronal MR or US can demonstrate the diaphragmatic defect, distinguishing this entity from partial eventration of the hemidiaphragm.

Traumatic herniation of abdominal contents through a tear or rupture of the central or posterior aspect of the hemidiaphragm may follow blunt thoracoabdominal trauma or penetrating injury (10). The left side is affected in over 90% of cases because the liver dissipates the traumatic forces and protects the right hemidiaphragm from injury. Radiographically, the diagnosis should be suspected when the left hemidiaphragmatic contour is indistinct or elevated, or when gas-filled loops of bowel or stomach are seen in the left lower thorax following severe trauma. Early diagnosis is often difficult, as associated thoracic and abdominal injuries may obscure the clinical and radiographic findings. The diagnosis is often made long after the traumatic episode, with symptoms caused by intestinal obstruction with strangulation (pain, vomiting, fever) or compression of the left lung (cough, dyspnea, chest pain). In addition to the stomach, small intestine, colon, omentum, spleen, kidney, and the left lobe of liver can also herniate through the defect. The diagnosis is usually made by upper or lower GI contrast studies demonstrating bowel herniating into the thorax through a constricting diaphragmatic defect. The resultant narrowing or "waist" of the herniated intestine as it traverses the diaphragmatic defect differentiates a hernia from simple diaphragmatic elevation. Large diaphragmatic defects may be demonstrated on volumetric helical CT with coronal and sagittal reconstructions, which also characterizes the herniated tissues and detects associated visceral injuries (Fig. 20.21). US or MR are difficult to obtain in the acute trauma setting but allow direct coronal and sagittal imaging of the diaphragm and therefore are occasionally useful (Fig. 20.21B)(11).

Diaphragmatic Tumors. Primary diaphragmatic tumors are rare, with an equal incidence of benign and malignant lesions. Benign lesions include lipomas, fibromas, Schwannomas, neurofibromas, and leiomyomas. Echinococcal cysts and extralobar sequestrations may be found within the diaphragm. Fibrosarcomas are the most common primary malignant diaphragmatic lesion. Radiographically, they appear as focal extrapulmonary masses obscuring all or part of the hemidiaphragm, and are indistinguishable from masses arising within the diaphragmatic pleura. CT may show the origin of the mass, although the relationship of the mass to the diaphragm is best appreciated on coronal MR images or transabdominal US. Direct invasion of the diaphragm by lower lobe bronchogenic carcinoma, mesothelioma, or a subphrenic neoplasm is much more common than primary diaphragmatic malignancy.

CONGENITAL LUNG DISEASE

Bronchogenic cysts represent anomalous outpouchings of the primitive foregut that no longer communicate with the tracheobronchial tree. They are commonly present as asymptomatic mediastinal masses and are discussed in detail in chapter 13.

Cystic adenomatoid malformation (CAM) is a lesion usually seen in newborn infants, although it occasionally presents in childhood or early adulthood. Three pathologic subtypes of CAM have been described. The most common subtype is comprised of one or several large cysts that are lined by respiratory epithelium with scattered mucus glands, smooth muscle and elastic tissue in their walls. Multiple smaller cystic structures are present in the intervening lung between the larger cysts. Radiographically, these lesions often appear as round air-filled masses that exert mass effect on the adjacent lung and mediastinum (Fig. 20.22). A CAM in the left lower lobe may be difficult to distinguish from a congenital diaphragmatic hernia. Delayed clearance of fetal fluid in the newborn may give the radiographic appearance of an intrapulmonary soft tissue mass. These lesions may be identified on prenatal US examination.

Bronchial Atresia. In this condition, a developmental stenosis or atresia of a lobar or segmental bronchus produces bronchial obstruction with resultant distal bronchiectasis. Most patients are asymptomatic and are first recognized by typical findings on frontal chest radiographs, namely a rounded, oval, or branching central lung opacity representing the obstructed mucus filled dilated bronchus (mucocele) with hyperlucency in that portion of lung supplied by the atretic bronchus. The

overinflated lobe or segment results from air trapping in the obstructed lung as air enters by collateral air drift on inspiration but cannot empty through the proximal tracheobronchial tree on expiration. The most common site of involvement is the apicoposterior segment of the left upper lobe, followed by the segmental bronchi of the right upper and middle lobes. The combination of a central mucocele with peripheral hyperlucency in a young, asymptomatic patient is virtually diagnostic of this disorder.

Congenital lobar emphysema may develop from a variety of disorders that produce a check valve bronchial obstruction. These include extrinsic compression by me-

Figure 20.20. Foramen of Morgagni Hernia. Frontal **(A)** and lateral **(B)** chest radiographs in a 60-year-old woman reveals a large mass in the right cardiophrenic angle. **C.** CT scan at the level of the diaphragm shows a fatty pericardiac mass containing omental vessels. **D.** A more inferior scan demonstrates an abnormally high transverse colon (*arrow*), which is characteristic of this entity.

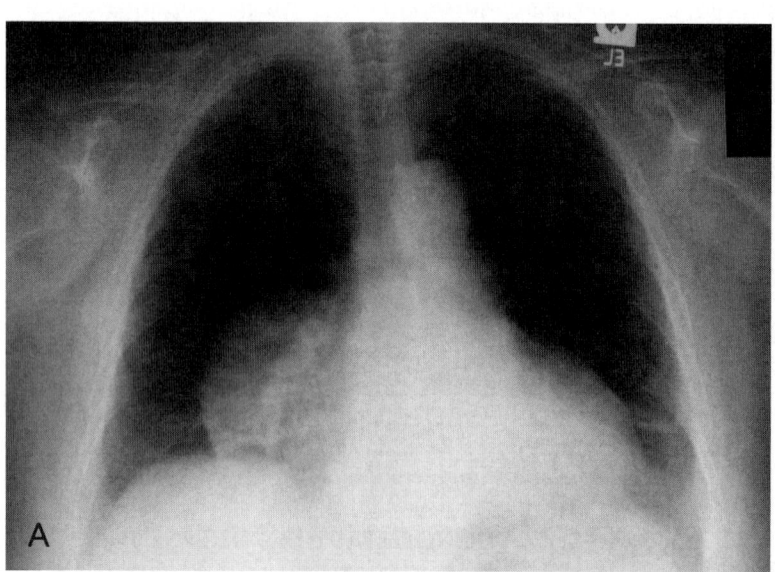

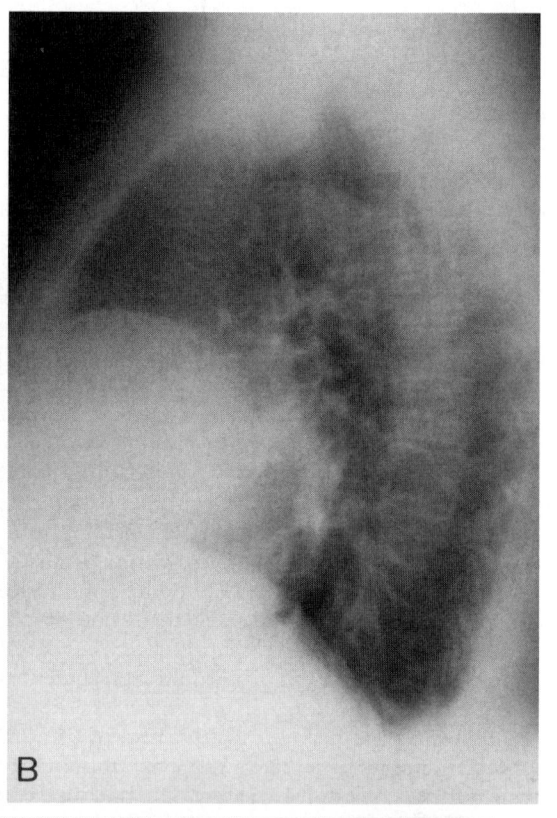

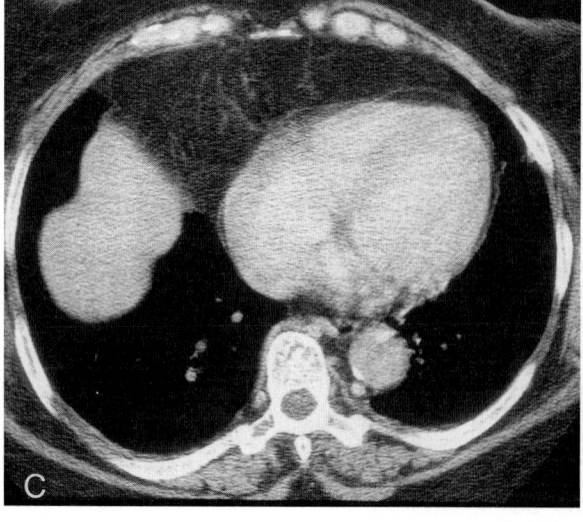

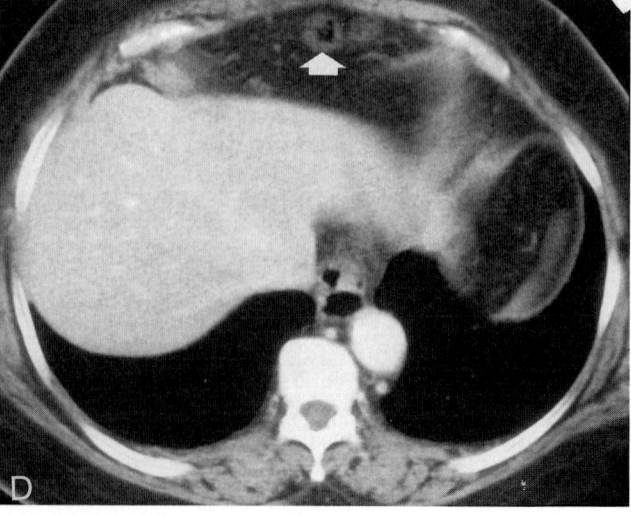

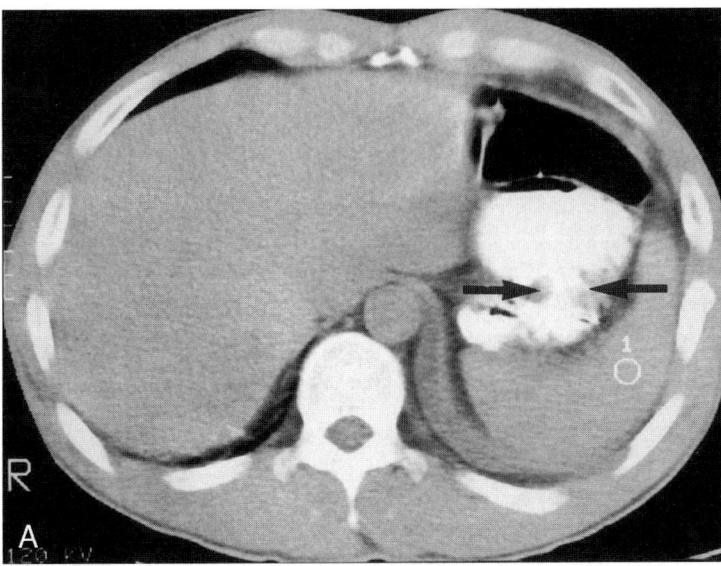
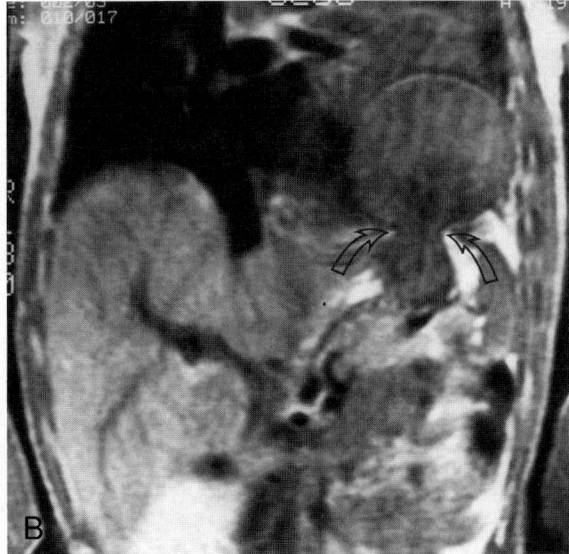

Figure 20.21. Traumatic Diaphragmatic Hernia. A. CT scan through the upper abdomen in a 34-year-old man who sustained blunt abdominal trauma 4 days earlier shows an area of concentric narrowing in the gastric fundus (*straight arrows*). **B.** Coronal MR obtained one week later shows intrathoracic gastric herniation through a central diaphragmatic defect (*curved arrows*).

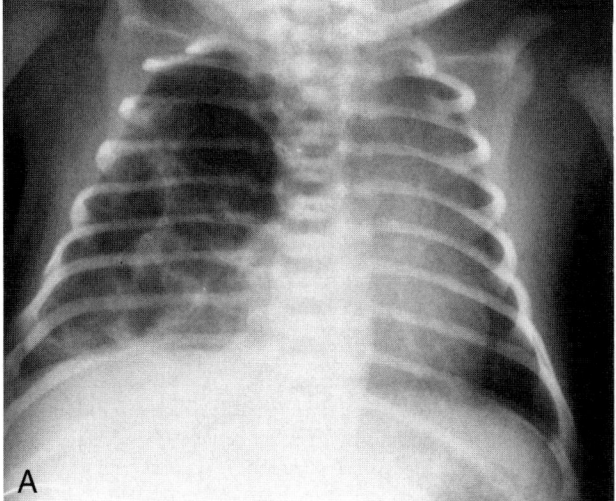
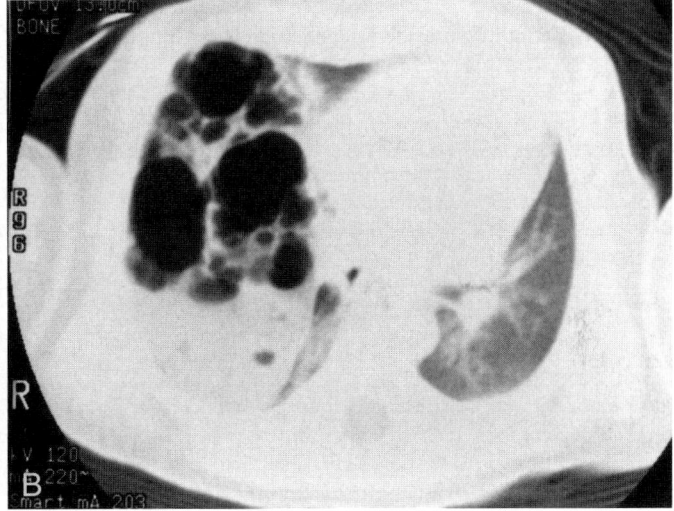

Figure 20.22. Congenital Cystic Adenomatoid Malformation (CCAM). **A.** Frontal chest radiograph in a newborn shows a multicystic mass in the right mid and lower lung. **B.** CT scan demonstrates a complex mass occupying the middle and right lower lobes with air-filled cysts and a solid component posteriorly. Surgery revealed a CCAM of the middle lobe.

diastinal bronchogenic cysts, anomalous left pulmonary artery, congenital deficiency of bronchial cartilage, and congenital or acquired bronchial stenosis. The bronchial obstruction leads to air trapping on expiration with resultant overinflation of distal lung. In order of decreasing frequency, the left upper lobe, right middle lobe, and right upper lobe are the most common sites of involvement. Respiratory difficulties are usually evident within the first month of life, with a minority presenting later. Radiographically, hyperlucency of the affected lobe is seen with compression of adjacent lung, diaphragmatic depression and contralateral mediastinal shift (Fig. 20.23). These findings are accentuated on expiratory films or on decubitus films obtained with the affected side down. CT, particularly when performed in expiration or with the affected side down, shows a hyperlucent overexpanded lobe with attenuated blood vessels (Fig. 20.23B)(12). Because many of these cases are not truly congenital but rather arise in the neonatal period from acquired abnormalities and overinflation of normal alveoli without destruction of alveolar walls is seen pathologically, the term "neonatal lobar hyperinflation" has been used to more appropriately describe this syndrome. Treatment is surgical for symptomatic patients, while relatively asymptomatic patients are observed for spontaneous resolution.

The findings in bronchial atresia and congenital lobar emphysema are reviewed in Table 20.9.

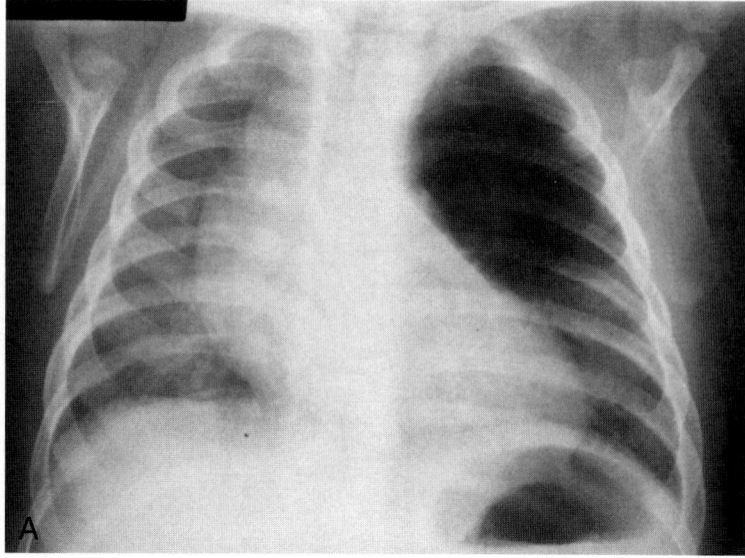
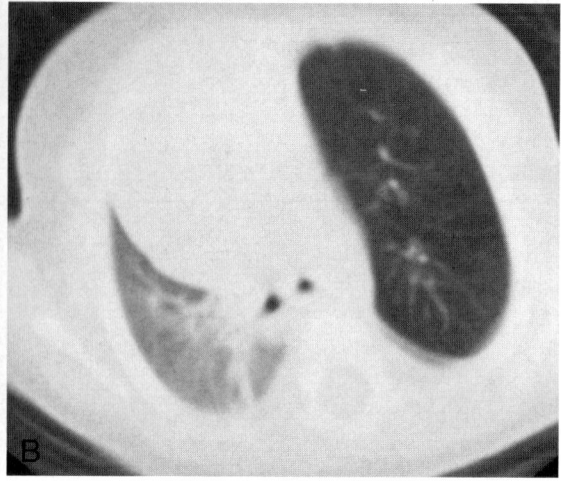

Figure 20.23. Congenital Lobar Emphysema. A. Frontal chest radiograph in a 1-year-old male shows a hyperlucent left upper lobe producing contralateral mediastinal shift. **B.** CT scan confirms the presence of an overexpanded and hyperlucent left upper lobe representing congenital lobar emphysema.

Table 20.9. Bronchial Atresia vs. Congenital Lobar Emphysema

	Bronchial Atresia	Congenital Lobar Emphysema
Age at presentation	Teens-young adults	Neonatal period
Symptoms	Asymptomatic	Respiratory distress
Location	LUL>RUL>RML	LUL>RML>RUL
Radiographic/ CT findings	Hyperlucent segment with mucocele	Hyperlucent lobe Diaphragmatic depression Mediastinal displacement
Treatment	None	Resection

LUL, left upper lobe; RUL, right upper lobe; RML, right middle lobe.

Table 20.10. Pulmonary Sequestration

	Intralobar Sequestration	Extralobar Sequestration
Frequency (of all sequestrations)	Common (75%)	Uncommon (25%)
Age at presentation	Young adult	Neonate/infant
Mode of presentation	Recurrent pneumonia	Asymptomatic
Location	Left lower lobe (60%) Right lower lobe (40%)	Left lower lobe (90%) Right lower lobe (10%)
Pleural covering	Within visceral pleura	Separate pleural layer
Associated congenital anomalies	Rare	Common (diaphragmatic eventration/hernia)
Radiographic appearance	Cystic lung mass w/ or w/o air/fluid levels	Solid peridiaphragmatic mass
Arterial supply	Single vessel from peridiaphragmatic aorta	Multiple small systemic/ pulmonary arteries
Venous drainage	Pulmonary (left-to-right shunt)	Systemic (left-to-right shunt)

Bronchopulmonary Sequestration. This congenital abnormality results from the independent development of a portion of the tracheobronchial tree that is isolated from the normal lung and maintains its fetal systemic arterial supply. Grossly, the sequestered lung is cystic and bronchiectatic. These patients most often present with recurrent pneumonia from recurrent infection in the sequestered lung, although some (mostly extralobar sequestrations) are discovered as asymptomatic posterior mediastinal masses on routine radiographs.

Pulmonary sequestration is divided into intralobar and extralobar forms (Table 20.10). Intralobar sequestration is contained within the visceral pleura of the normal lung. Extralobar sequestration is enclosed by its own visceral pleural envelope and may be found adjacent to the normal lung or within or below the diaphragm. Most patients with intralobar sequestration present with pneumonia, while extralobar sequestration is usually asymptomatic and is seen as an incidental finding in a neonate with other severe congenital anomalies. Intralobar sequestration is more common than the extralobar type by a ratio of 3:1.

While both forms are found in the lower lobes, extralobar sequestration is predominantly left sided (90%), while one-third of intralobar sequestrations are right sided. A major differentiating feature between the two types is the arterial supply to and venous drainage from the sequestered lung. An intralobar sequestration is supplied by a single large artery arising from the infradiaphragmatic aorta and enters the sequestered lung via the pulmonary ligament. The venous drainage is via the pulmonary veins. In contrast, extralobar sequestration receives several small branches from systemic and occasionally pulmonary arteries, with venous drainage into the systemic venous system (inferior vena cava, azygos or hemiazygos veins).

Radiographically, sequestration appears as a solid posterior mediastinal mass or as a solitary or multicystic air collection (13). Air-fluid levels are seen when infection has produced communication of the sequestered lung with the normal tracheobronchial tree. The definitive diagnosis is made by the demonstration of abnormal systemic arterial supply to the abnormal lung, which is usually accomplished by thoracic aortography, contrast-enhanced helical CT, US, or coronal MR and MR angiography (Fig. 20.24). Arteriography is usually reserved for preoperative patients in whom precise demonstration of the origin and number of the systemic feeders is necessary.

Hypoplastic Lung is a developmental anomaly resulting in a small lung. It occurs secondary to congenital pulmonary arterial deficiency or from compression of the developing lung in utero from a variety of causes. Grossly the lung is small with a decrease in the number and size of airways, alveoli, and pulmonary arteries. Radiographically, the small lung and hemithorax is associated with ipsilateral diaphragmatic elevation and mediastinal shift with herniation of the hyperinflated contralateral lung anteriorly towards the affected side. Hypoplastic lung can simulate total lung collapse radiographically, but can usually be distinguished on clinical grounds and review of prior radiographic studies that show a small lung without evidence of pleural or parenchymal scarring.

Hypogenetic Lung-Scimitar Syndrome, a variant of the hypoplastic lung, is characterized by an underdeveloped right lung with abnormal venous drainage of the lung to the inferior vena cava just above or below the right hemidiaphragm. The systemic venous drainage of the lung produces an extracardiac left-to-right shunt. The anomalous vein, which drains all or most of the right lung, may be seen as a vertically oriented curvilinear density shaped like a scimitar in the medial right lower lung, thereby giving this syndrome its common name of scimitar syndrome (Fig. 20.25). The anomalies of venous drainage and lobar bronchial anatomy (usually bilateral left-sided [hyparterial] bronchial branching) has given rise to the term congenital pulmonary venolobar syndrome. The right pulmonary artery is invariably hypoplastic, with supply to all or part of the lung (usually the lower lobe) from the systemic circulation. Associated anomalies include eventration of the right hemidiaphragm, horseshoe lung (congenital fusion of the right and left lungs posteroinferiorly), and cardiac anomalies such as atrial septal defect (most common), coarctation of the aorta, patent ductus arteriosus, and tetralogy of Fallot. The frontal chest radiographic findings are diagnostic and include a small right hemithorax with diaphragmatic elevation or eventration, dextroposition of the heart, and herniation of left lung anteriorly into the right hemithorax. The classic appearance of a solitary scimitar vein is seen in only one-third of cases, with the remainder having multiple small draining veins. Although plain film findings are usually diagnostic, CT or MR shows the abnormal draining vein and associated abnormalities. Most patients are asymptomatic, but some may present with recurrent infection, symptoms related to a left-to-right shunt, or from the associated cardiac anomalies.

Arteriovenous Malformation. Pulmonary arteriovenous malformations (AVMs) are abnormal vascular masses in which a focal collection of congenitally weakened capillaries dilate to become a tortuous complex of vessels fed by a single pulmonary artery and drained by a single pulmonary vein. Most pulmonary AVMs do not come to attention until early adulthood. They are detected either incidentally, as part of a screening evaluation in patients with hereditary hemorrhagic telangiectasia (a condition that is present in approximately 80% of all patients with pulmonary AVMs), or because of a variety of symptoms. The most common pulmonary symptoms are hemoptysis and dyspnea, the latter

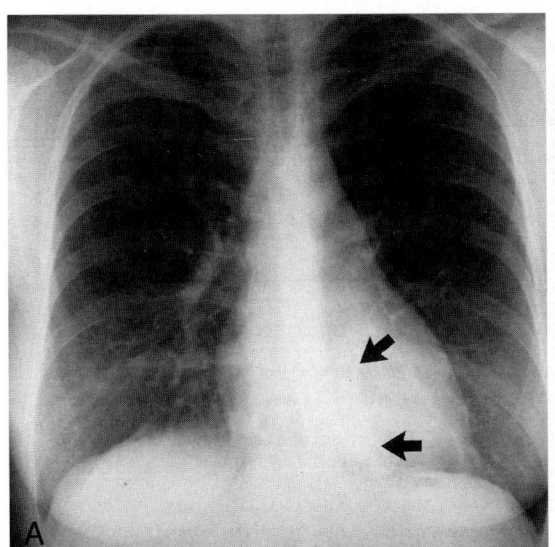
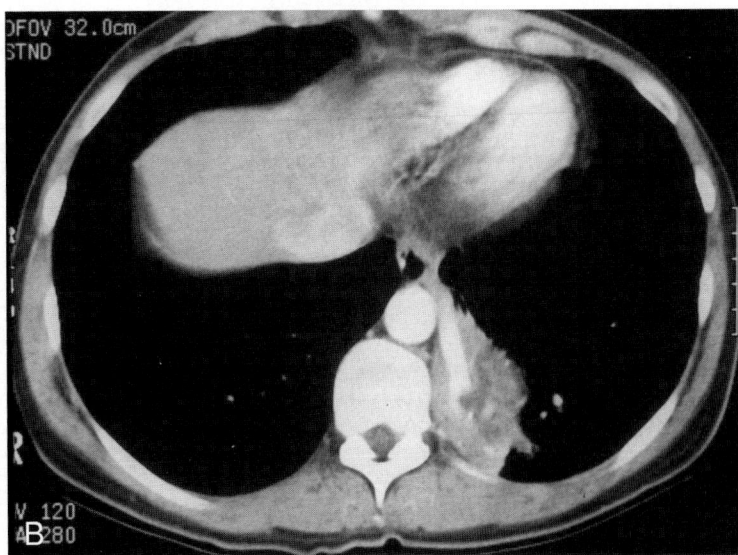

Figure 20.24. Intralobar Pulmonary Sequestration. A. Frontal chest film in a 27-year-old woman with recurrent left lower lobe pneumonia shows a retrocardiac left lower lobe opacity (*arrows*). **B.** Contrast-enhanced helical CT shows paraspinal consolidation with a large feeding artery, which was seen to arise from the celiac axis on more inferior scans. An intralobar sequestration was resected by a left thoracotomy.

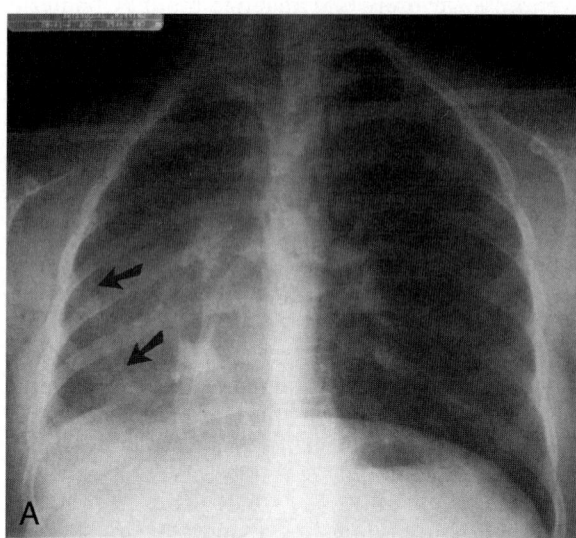

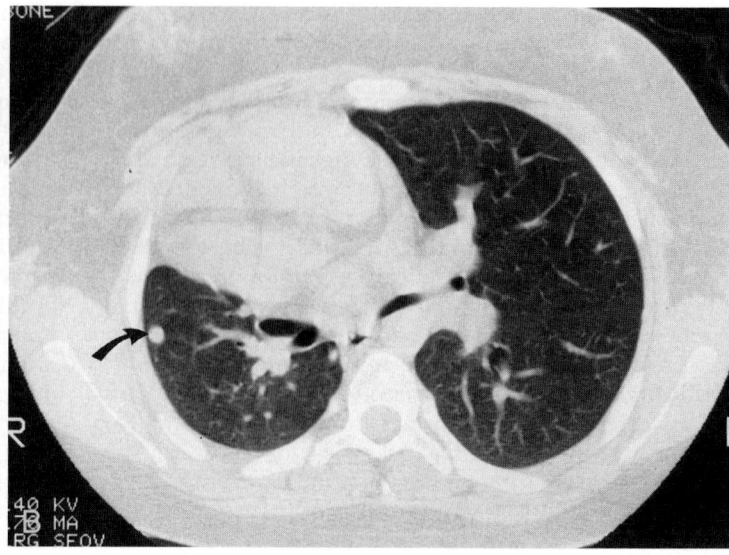

Figure 20.25. Congenital Pulmonary Venolobar (Scimitar) Syndrome. A. PA chest radiograph in an asymptomatic 16-year-old female shows a small right lung with rightward cardiomediastinal shift. A curvilinear opacity is visible in the lower lung laterally (*ar-* *rows*). **B.** CT scan shows an anomalous vessel (*curved arrow*) within a small right lung that represents the scimitar vein, seen on more inferior scans draining into the inferior vena cava.

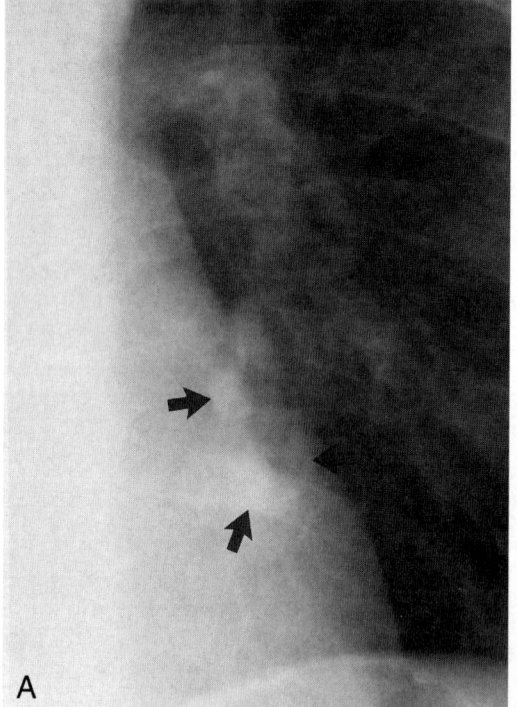

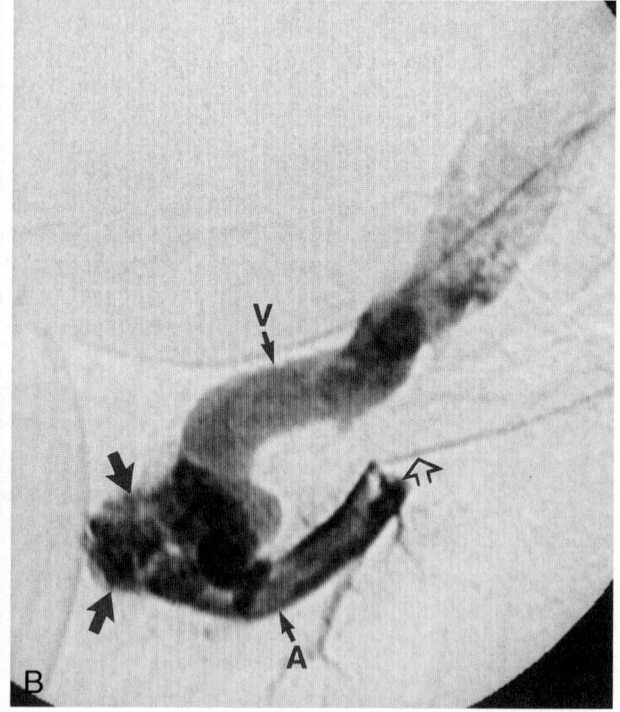

Figure 20.26. Arteriovenous Malformation. A. Coned-down view of the left lower lobe from a PA radiograph shows a curvilinear opacity (*arrows*) in the retrocardiac region. **B.** Selective pulmonary arte- riogram with catheter (*open arrow*) in feeding artery (*A*) shows the malformation (*solid arrows*) and draining vein (*V*).

attributable to hypoxia due to the intrapulmonary right-to-left shunt. Non-pulmonary symptoms most often relate to central nervous system disease. Stroke may occur from paradoxical right-to-left cerebral emboli or from thrombosis resulting from secondary polycythemia caused by chronic hypoxemia. Brain abscess may develop from paradoxical septic emboli.

The chest radiograph of a pulmonary AVM usually shows a solitary pulmonary nodule, most often located in the subpleural portions of the lower lobes. Approximately one-third of patients have multiple lesions. The lesion is often lobulated and has feeding and drainings vessels emanating from the mass and extending toward the hilum (Fig. 20.26). The morphology of the lesions is best demonstrated on helical CT with retrospective overlapping reconstructions viewed in a cine format. The feeding and draining vessels can be demonstrated by contrast-enhanced CT or MR. Angiography is reserved for preoperative evaluation and for patients undergoing therapeutic transcatheter embolization with spring coils or detachable occlusion balloons, which is the treatment of choice for patients with multiple AVMs.

TRAUMATIC LUNG DISEASE

Pulmonary Contusion usually follows blunt chest trauma and typically develops adjacent to the site of impact. Blood and edema fluid fill the alveoli of the lung within the first 12 hours after trauma, producing scat-

tered areas of air-space opacification that may rapidly become confluent and may be difficult to distinguish from aspiration pneumonia (Fig. 20.27). Patients may have shortness of breath and hemoptysis; blood can usually be suctioned from the endotracheal tube. The typical radiographic course is stabilization of opacities by 24 hours and improvement within two to seven days. Progressive opacities seen more than 48 hours after trauma should raise the suspicion of aspiration pneumonia or developing ARDS.

Pulmonary Laceration, Traumatic Lung Cyst, and Pulmonary Hematoma. Pulmonary laceration is a common sequela of penetrating or blunt chest trauma. In the latter situation, it represents a shearing injury to the substance of the lung. The elastic properties of the lung

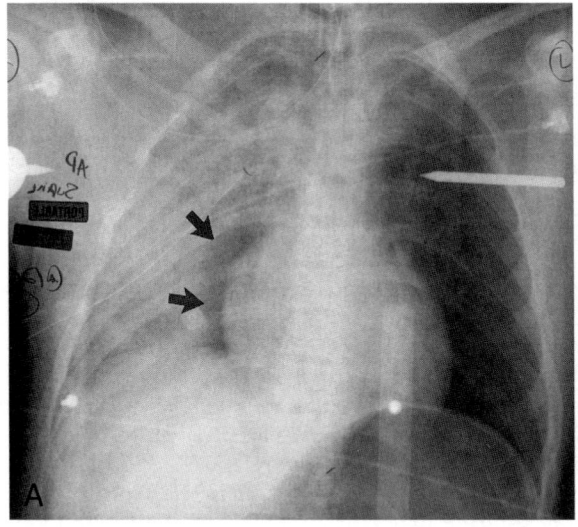
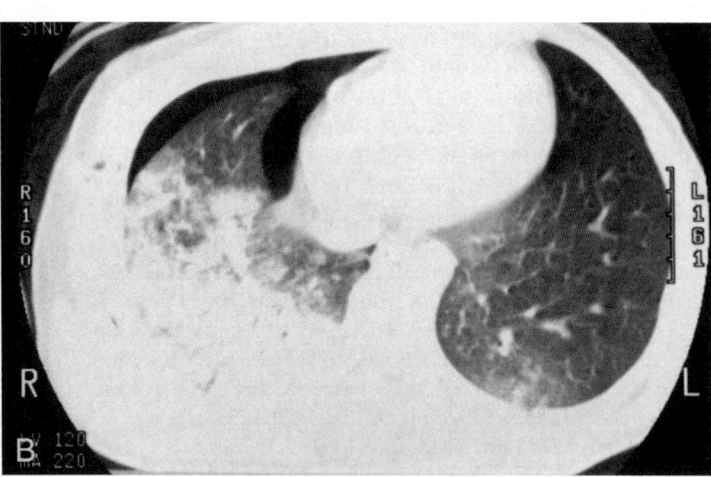

Figure 20.27. Pulmonary Contusion. A. Upright portable chest film in a 37-year-old man involved in a motor vehicle accident shows extensive right lung air-space opacification with an inferomedial lucency (*arrows*). **B.** CT scan shows middle and right lower lobe con-

solidation representing lung contusion and an anterior pneumothorax, the latter accounting for the lucency seen on the portable chest radiograph.

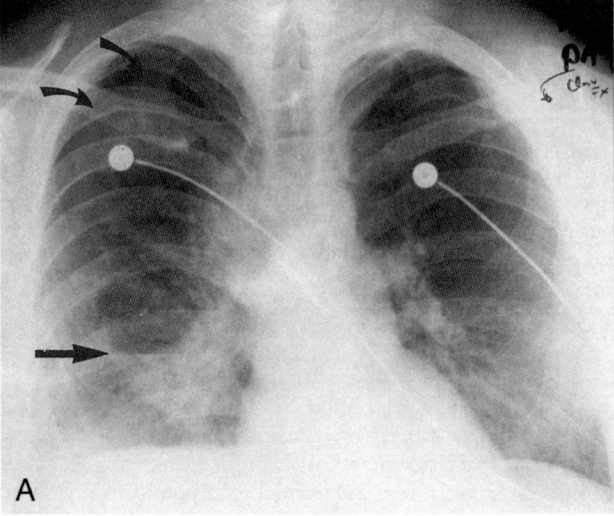
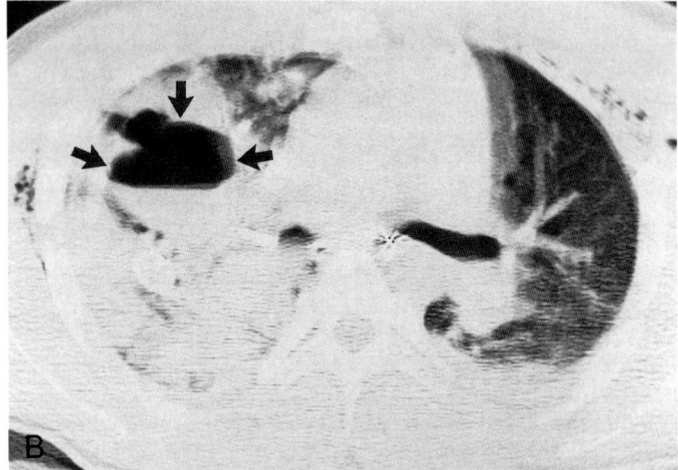

Figure 20.28. Traumatic Lung Cyst. A. Upright portable chest film in a 37-year-old man who was trampled by a bull shows a localized air-fluid level (*straight arrow*) in the lower right lung and an associ-

ated pneumothorax (*curved arrows*). **B.** A CT scan shows extensive right lung contusion with a middle lobe traumatic lung cyst (*arrows*).

quickly transform the linear laceration into a rounded air cyst. These cysts may be filled with varied amounts of blood as a result of laceration of pulmonary capillaries and those that are completely filled with blood are more appropriately termed pulmonary hematomas. On radiographs and CT, these cysts appear as rounded lucencies that may contain air or an air-fluid level (Fig. 20.28)(14). Initially, these cysts are often obscured by the adjacent contused lung, only to be recognized after resorption of the blood. The cysts tend to shrink gradually over a period of weeks to months. The term traumatic air cysts rather than pneumatoceles should be used for these lesions, the latter term is reserved for air cysts that result from a check-valve overdistention of distal lung as seen in staphylococcal pneumonia.

ASPIRATION

Aspiration Pneumonia and pneumonitis are terms used to describe the different pulmonary inflammatory responses to aspirated material. As was discussed in the chapter on infection, aspiration pneumonia decribes a mixed anaerobic infection resulting from the aspiration of infected oropharyngeal contents. The aspiration of oropharyngeal or gastric secretions may also occur in a "pure" form uncomplicated by anaerobic infection, producing an aspiration pneumonitis.

Aspiration of oropharyngeal or gastric secretions, with or without food particles, is not an uncommon event. It is seen in debilitated patients with chronic diseases, in patients with tracheal or gastric tubes, in unconscious patients, and in those who have suffered strokes, seizures or trauma. More chronic and less easily recognizable forms of aspiration may occur in patients with anatomic abnormalities of the upper gastrointestinal tract (Zenker's diverticulum, esophageal stricture) or functional disorders (gastroesophageal reflux, neuromuscular dysfunction).

Gastric fluid is highly irritating to the lungs and often stimulates explosive coughing and associated deep inspirations, which leads to widespread distribution of the fluid throughout both lungs and into the peripheral air spaces. The hydrochloric acid contained in gastric fluid causes direct damage to both the bronchiolar lining and the alveolar wall. The severity of the resultant pneumonitis depends on several factors. The severity of aspiration pneumonitis is increased with a pH of the aspirated fluid greater than 2.5, large volume of aspirated fluid, large particulate matter in the aspirated fluid, and young age all associated with an increased. The massive aspiration of gastric contents is known as Mendelson's syndrome. When the aspirate includes particulate material, the particles are distributed by gravity and may incite a granulomatous foreign body-type reaction.

Three basic radiographic patterns of aspiration pneumonitis have been observed; extensive bilateral air-space opacification (Fig. 20.29), diffuse but discrete air-space nodular opacities, and irregular parenchymal opacities that are not obviously air-space filling in nature (15). Parenchymal involvement is most often bilateral with a predilection for the basal and perihilar regions. When a significant amount of admixed food is present, the opac-

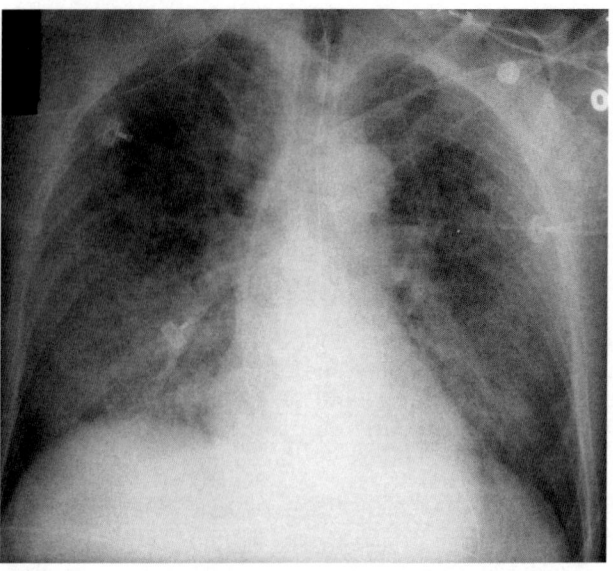

Figure 20.29. Aspiration Pneumonitis. Portable chest radiograph in a 43-year-old man who had a witnessed aspiration and developed ARDS demonstrates diffuse bilateral air-space opacification.

ities are usually posterior and segmental. Atelectasis is often present, presumably resulting from airways obstruction by food particles. The radiographic appearance may worsen over the first few days, but then demonstrates rapid improvement. A worsening of the radiographic appearance at this stage suggests development of a complicating infection, ARDS, or pulmonary embolism.

Chronic Aspiration Pneumonitis. Patients who repeatedly aspirate may develop chronic interstitial abnormalities on chest radiographs. With repeated episodes of aspiration over months to years, irregular reticular interstitial opacities may persist, probably representing peribronchial scarring. A reticulonodular pattern may be seen caused by granulomas forming around food particles. These chronic interstitial abnormalities can be observed in between episodes of acute aspiration pneumonitis.

DRUG-INDUCED LUNG DISEASE

Drugs can induce a variety of adverse effects in the lung (16,17). The majority of cases of drug-induced lung disease are iatrogenic, though accidental or intentional drug overdoses may result in severe pulmonary disease. The changes are often difficult to distinguish from infection, pulmonary edema, or a pulmonary manifestation of the disease being treated.

Mechanisms of Drug Reaction

Acute Reactions. There are a limited number of ways for drugs to produce acute pulmonary disease. An acute pulmonary reaction may involve a hypersensitivity response to a metabolite of the drug combined with an endogenous protein. Antibody production directed against this haptene-protein complex leads to antibody-mediated immediate or immune complex hypersensitivity reactions. In the lung, this produces bronchospasm or eosinophilic pneumonia, usually associated with fever, skin rash, and blood eosinophilia. Radiographically, fleeting peripheral patchy air-space opacities are seen, which develop hours to days after the initiation of drug therapy. The opacities often respond to corticosteroid therapy. The penicillin and sulfanomide antibiotics are the drugs most often associated with hypersensitivity reactions.

The other common acute lung reaction to administered drugs is a diffuse alveolar damage that is histologically identical to the early changes of ARDS. Opiates including heroin and crack cocaine and chemotherapeutic agents, particularly busulfan and chlorambucil, are most commonly associated with this reaction. Radiographically, the lungs show acute interstitial or air-space opacities which are indistinguishable from those of pulmonary edema although the heart size is usually normal (Fig. 20.30). Characteristically, the edema clears as rapidly as it appeared.

Acute pulmonary hemorrhage and infarction may occur secondary to drug-induced pulmonary vasculitis, while diffuse hemorrhage may complicate anticoagulation therapy with coumadin or thrombocytopenia following intensive chemotherapy administered prior to bone marrow transplantation. Penicillamine therapy has been associated with pulmonary hemorrhage in patients with rheumatoid arthritis via an unknown mechanism. Affected individuals typically have hemoptysis and a falling hematocrit that is associated with the rapid development of diffuse bilateral air-space opacities. The diagnosis is usually confirmed by noting bloody fluid return on bronchoalveolar lavage. The lavage also shows an increased percentage of alveolar macrophages containing hemosiderin deposits. The opacities of diffuse pulmonary hemorrhage resolve completely without residual scarring, while the focal opacities of pulmonary infarcts may leave pleuroparenchymal scars.

Chronic Reactions. Chronic pulmonary or pleural disease generally develops weeks to months after initial exposure to the offending drug, but can be delayed for years. The most common form of chronic lung toxicity from drugs is that of a chronic interstitial pneumonitis, with subsequent development of pulmonary fibrosis in the healing phase of this disorder. The drugs most commonly implicated in this form of lung disease are amiodarone, and nitrofurantoin and the chemotherapeutic agents cytoxan, bleomycin, and methotrexate. Radiographically, there are bilateral predominantly lower lobe coarse reticular and linear opacities with diminished lung volumes. In patients undergoing chemotherapy for malignancy, the findings are difficult to distinguish from lymphangitic carcinomatosis, pulmonary hemorrhage, or opportunistic pneumonia, while pulmonary edema is the major differential diagnosis in patients on amiodarone therapy. The diagnosis is usually made by excluding one of these other processes. Pulmonary nodules are an uncommon manifestation of chronic lung injury from bleomycin or cytoxan, and in this situation, is radiographically indistinguishable from pulmonary metastases.

A number of drugs have been associated with a lupus-like syndrome that is often indistinguishable from systemic lupus erythematosis. Procainamide, hydralazine, and isoniazid are the drugs most commonly producing a lupus like reaction. Pleural and pericardial effusions are common. Basilar interstitial disease has been described but is uncommon.

Bronchiolitis obliterans is a small airways inflammatory process that results in granulation tissue within bronchioles. This reaction can result from a variety of insults including aspiration, organ transplantation, viral infection, collagen vascular disease, and drugs. Penicillamine administered in patients with rheumatoid arthritis is the drug most often associated with this reaction. This entity is described in more detail in chapter 19.

A chronic granulomatous vasculitis may develop as a response to particulate substances such as talc or starch mixed with illicit intravenous drugs. This can lead to obliteration of the pulmonary vasculature producing pulmonary hypertension and right ventricular failure. Radiographically, the lungs may show an interstitial pattern of disease, with enlargement of the central pulmonary arteries and right heart. The radiographs may rarely show central conglomerate masses indistinguishable from progressive massive fibrosis of silicosis or end stage sarcoidosis.

Hilar and mediastinal lymph node enlargement on chest radiographs is an uncommon manifestation of drug toxicity. Dilantin and methotrexate are the main drugs associated with this rare complication. The lymphadenopathy is usually part of a systemic hypersensitivity reaction, and regresses with removal of the offending agent.

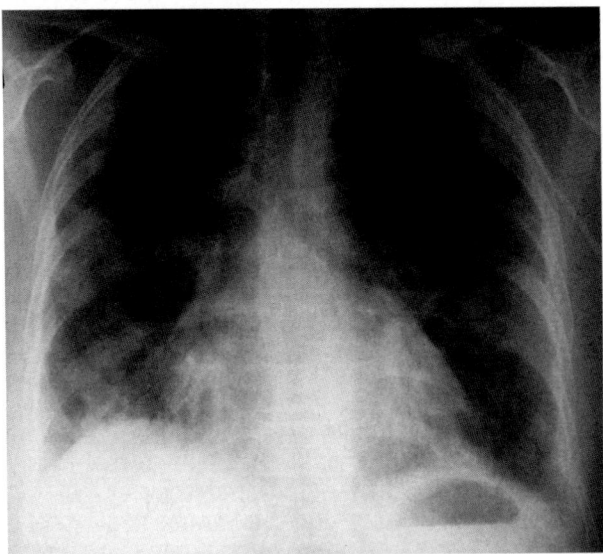

Figure 20.30. Bleomycin Lung Toxicity. Frontal radiograph in a patient receiving bleomycin chemotherapy for non-Hodgkin's lymphoma shows patchy bilateral air-space opacities associated with mild cardiomegaly and small pleural effusions. After empiric therapy for congestive heart failure failed to provide clinical or radiographic improvement, both bronchoscopic and open lung biopsies were necessary and revealed a diagnosis of diffuse alveolar damage caused by bleomycin.

Specific Drug Toxicities

Nitrofurantoin is an oral antibiotic used widely in the treatment of urinary tract infections. There are two distinct patterns of nitrofurantoin-associated pulmonary reaction: acute and chronic. The acute form, seen in approximately 90% of cases, most likely represents a hypersensitivity reaction. The chest film demonstrates interstitial or mixed alveolar/interstitial infiltrates with a basal predominance, often accompanied by small pleural effusions. The chronic form occurs after weeks to years of continuous therapy and is probably caused by direct toxic damage. Interstitial pneumonitis and fibrosis indistinguishable from idiopathic pulmonary fibrosis is seen pathologically. The chest radiograph demonstrates reduced lung volumes and diffuse reticular pattern with relative basal predominance.

Bleomycin is a cytotoxic antibiotic used in the treatment of lymphoma, squamous cell carcinoma, and testicular cancer. Bleomycin-induced lung disease is related to the cumulative dosage of the drug. Free oxygen radicals within the lung are felt to play a major role in the lung injury and account for the deleterious effects of supplemental oxygen administration in patients with bleomycin toxicity. The typical radiographic pattern is that of bilateral lower lobe reticular opacities. A minority of patients will demonstrate acute patchy or confluent air-space opacities as a result of a hypersensitivity reaction to the drug or diffuse alveolar damage (Fig. 20.29). The reticular or air-space opacities tend to have a basal predominance. Solitary or multiple pulmonary nodules is an unusual radiographic appearance of bleomycin lung toxicity that is indistinguishable radiographically from pulmonary metastases; the lesions generally disappear following cessation of the drug.

Alkylating Agents. Drugs such as busulfan, which is used in the treatment of myeloproliferative disorders, and cyclophosphamide (Cytoxan), used widely in the treatment of malignancies and autoimmune disease, can cause clinically recognizable pulmonary toxicity in 1–4% of patients. Pathologic findings include organizing intraalveolar exudate, fibrosis, and the presence of large atypical type II pneumocytes. Radiographically, a diffuse reticular pattern with basal predominance is seen; airspace opacities may be present and are more common with busulfan than from cyclophosphamide.

Methotrexate is an antimetabolite used for the treatment of malignancies and autoimmune diseases such as rheumatoid arthritis and psoriasis. In contrast to bleomycin and the alkylating agents, methotrexate usually causes reversible pulmonary disease resulting from a hypersensitivity reaction rather than direct toxic damage to the lung. However, diffuse alveolar damage leading to restrictive lung disease is seen in approximately 10% of cases and appears radiographically as a diffuse reticular pattern.

Amiodarone. This antiarrhythmic agent is an important cause of drug-induced pulmonary damage, affecting approximately 5% of individuals on chronic therapy. Amiodarone is concentrated in the lung and has a long tissue half-life. The exact mechanism of lung damage is unknown, but relates to the accumulation of phospholipids that disturb metabolic functions in the lung. Pathologically, there is inflammation and fibrosis of the alveolar septae, with an accumulation of lipid-laden alveolar macrophages and hyperplasia of type II pneumocytes.

Pulmonary toxicity begins months to years after the initiation of therapy. Patients typically present with dyspnea or a non-productive cough that may be difficult to distinguish from congestive heart failure or pneumonia. The chest film typically shows a diffuse reticular pattern caused by interstitial fibrosis. In addition, multiple peripheral airspace opacities may be seen, often with an upper lobe predominance. Gallium lung scanning is often used to detect subradiographic pulmonary involvement from amiodarone toxicity and distinguish this from pulmonary edema. Amiodarone should be withdrawn or the dose diminished at the earliest sign of toxicity, as the drug has an extraordinarily long half life (approximately 90 days). The cessation of amiodarone at an early stage of toxicity, with occasional use of corticosteroids usually provides relief.

RADIATION-INDUCED LUNG DISEASE

The pulmonary effects of external irradiation, most commonly administered for palliation of unresectable bronchogenic carcinoma or the treatment of mediastinal Hodgkin lymphoma, depend on several variables. The volume of lung treated will affect the incidence of radiation injury; the greater the volume irradiated, the more likely radiation injury will ensue. Most radiation treatment is limited to less than one third to one half of the lung, as an equivalent dose administered to an entire lung or both lungs would cause serious lung injury. The total dose and the method of fractionation will affect the incidence of radiation injury. Doses of less than 2000 rads rarely produce lung injury, while doses exceeding 3000 rads have a significant incidence of radiation pneumonitis. Administration of a single large dose is more deleterious than fractionation of a similar total dose over the course of several weeks. There is variation in the susceptibility to radiation among individuals; a given dose may cause pneumonitis in one patient while another remains unaffected. The concomitant use of chemotherapeutic agents, particularly bleomycin, or the withdrawal of corticosteroid therapy may accentuate the deleterious effects of radiation.

The mechanism of radiation-induced lung injury is not completely understood, but the acute effects involve injury to capillary endothelial and pulmonary epithelial cells that line the alveoli. This diffuse alveolar damage produces a cellular, proteinaceous intraalveolar exudate and hyaline membranes that is indistinguishable histologically from ARDS. These changes develop four to twelve weeks following the completion of therapy. While most patients with acute radiation pneumonitis are asymptomatic, dyspnea and a nonproductive cough may be present. Radiographically, a sharply marginated, localized area of air-space opacification is seen which does not conform to lobar or segmental anatomic boundaries and directly corresponds to the radiation port (18). Adhesive atelectasis of the involved portion of lung is common, as the radiation produces a loss of surfactant by damaging type II pneumocytes. The pneumonitis may resolve completely with or without the administration of corticosteroids, or may progress to pulmonary fibrosis. Pulmonary fibrosis corresponds histologically to a reparative phase with regeneration of type II pneumocytes, reorganization of the parenchyma, ingrowth of granulation tissue, and eventually interstitial fibrosis. Fibrosis appears as coarse linear opacities or occasionally as a homogeneous parenchymal opacity with severe cicatrizing atelectasis of the involved portion of the lung. The sharp margination of the parenchymal fibrotic changes may be difficult to appreciate on plain radiographs but is usually obvious on cross-sectional CT or MR studies. Fibrotic tissue is characteristically low signal on T2-weighted MR sequences, a finding that is helpful in distinguishing fibrosis from recurrent tumor, which is typically high signal on T2WI. The parenchymal changes are usually stable by one year following radiation therapy. Pleural thickening caused by fibrosis is a common finding. Small pleural and pericardial effusions may be seen but are uncommon.

The diagnosis of radiation pneumonitis is usually made by excluding infection or malignancy as a cause of the patient's symptoms and by the presence of typical radiographic findings following a course of radiation therapy to the chest. This distinction may require bronchoalveolar lavage (BAL) and transbronchial biopsy. An increased number of lymphocytes in the BAL fluid and the absence of malignant cells confirms the diagnosis. The demonstration of air-space opacification on CT that conforms to a known portal of radiation is usually sufficient for the diagnosis. Gallium scanning may be used to detect subradiographic radiation-induced lung inflammation.

EOSINOPHILIC LUNG DISEASE

This term refers to a heterogeneous group of allergic diseases characterized by excess eosinophils in the lung and occasionally blood. Fraser and Pare have classified these diseases into three groups: idiopathic, those of known etiology, and autoimmune or collagen vascular disorders (Table 20.11).

Idiopathic Eosinophilic Lung Disease

The idiopathic disorders associated with eosinophilic lung disease include simple pulmonary eosinophilia, chronic eosinophilic pneumonia, and the hypereosinophilic syndrome.

Simple Pulmonary Eosinophilia, also known as Loeffler's syndrome, is a transient pulmonary process characterized pathologically by pulmonary infiltration with an eosinophilic exudate. Most patients have a history of allergy, most commonly asthma. The characteristic radiographic findings are peripheral, homogeneous ill-defined areas of air-space opacification that may parallel the chest wall (Fig. 20.31); this latter feature is best appreciated on CT. The opacities in Loeffler's syndrome have been described as fleeting because a tendency for rapid clearing in one area with new involvement in other areas exists. A dry cough, dyspnea, and peripheral blood eosinophilia are common but are not invariably present. The diagnosis is based on the combination of pulmonary symptoms, blood eosinophilia, and characteristic radio-

Table 20.11. Eosinophilic Lung Disease

Idiopathic	Simple pulmonary eosinophilia (Loeffler's syndrome)
	Chronic eosinophilic pneumonia
	Hypereosinophilic syndrome
Known etiology	Drugs
	Antibiotics
	Penicillins
	Nitrofurantoin
	Nonsteroidal antiinflammatory agents
	Aspirin
	Chemotherapeutic agents
	Bleomycin
	Methotrexate
	Parasites
	Filaria
	Strongyloides
	Ascaris
	Hookworm
Autoimmune disease	Wegener's granulomatosis
	Sarcoidosis
	Rheumatoid lung disease
	Polyarteritis nodosa
	Allergic angiitis and granulomatosis (Churg-Strauss syndrome)

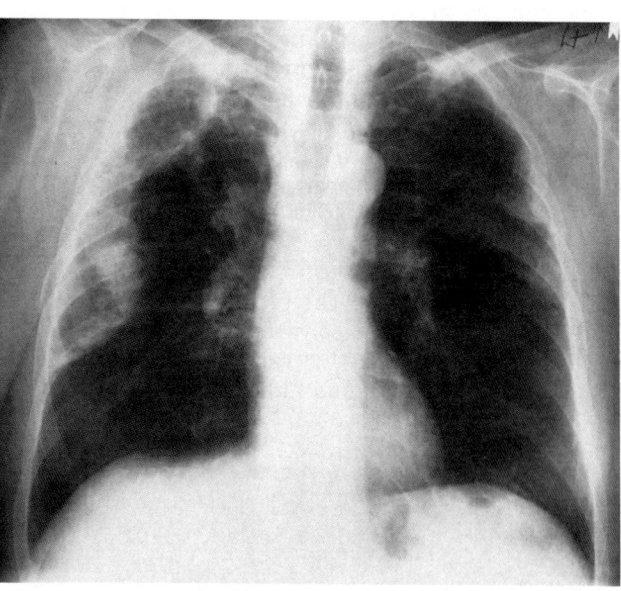

Figure 20.31. Eosinophilic Pneumonia. In a 38-year-old man with asthma, shortness of breath, and peripheral eosinophilia, a frontal chest film demonstrates bilateral peripheral air-space opacities. The patient's symptoms and the radiographic findings improved rapidly following initiation of corticosteroid therapy.

graphic findings. Most patients having a self-limiting illness that resolves spontaneously within four weeks.

Chronic Eosinophilic Pneumonia. Patients with symptoms and radiographic abnormalities that last greater than one month are considered to have chronic eosinophilic pneumonia. The clinical and radiographic features are similar to Loeffler's syndrome, although there is a distinct predilection for women. Patients are usually symptomatic with fever, malaise, and dyspnea. The pulmonary symptoms and radiographic opacities respond dramatically to corticosteroid therapy and improve within four to seven days, although relapse on discontinuation of treatment is common.

Hypereosinophilic Syndrome is a systemic disorder with a male predominance that is characterized by multi-organ damage from eosinophilic infiltration of tissues. Blood eosinophilia is prolonged and marked in this condition. The major chest radiographic findings are associated with cardiac involvement and secondary congestive heart failure and include cardiomegaly, pulmonary edema, and pleural effusions. Pulmonary parenchymal infiltration with eosinophils may produce interstitial or air-space opacities.

Eosinophilic Lung Disease of Identifiable Etiology

Pulmonary eosinophilia of known etiology includes drug and parasite induced eosinophilic lung disease. Drugs associated with pulmonary eosinphilia include nitrofurantoin and the penicillins. The parasitic infections most commonly responsible are filaria and the roundworms *Ascaris lumbricoides* and *Strongyloides stercoralis*. These parasites may produce pulmonary eosinophilia as they migrate through the alveolar capillaries and into the alveoli during their tour of the body. These disorders are usually indistinguishable clinically and radiographically from Loeffler's syndrome.

Autoimmune Disease. A number of autoimmune disorders are associated with eosinophilic pulmonary infiltrates. These include Wegener's granulomatosis, sarcoidosis, rheumatoid lung disease, polyarteritis nodosa, and allergic angiitis and granulomatosis. The first three disorders have a variety of thoracic manifestations and are discussed elsewhere. The predominant chest radiographic findings seen in polyarteritis nodosa represent hemorrhage caused by a vasculitis involving the bronchial arterial circulation; this condition is discussed

in chapter 15. Allergic angiitis and granulomatosis (Churg-Strauss syndrome) is a multi-system disorder in which asthma, blood eosinophilia, necrotizing vasculitis, and extravascular granulomas are invariable features. Pulmonary involvement, as seen radiographically or pathologically, is indistinguishable from chronic eosinophilic pneumonia.

PULMONARY ALVEOLAR PROTEINOSIS

Pulmonary alveolar proteinosis (PAP) is a rare disease in which the lipoproteinaceous material surfactant deposits in abnormal amounts within the air spaces of the lung. PAP has a predilection for males in their twenties to forties, although the disease has been reported in children. In adults, PAP has been associated with acute exposure to large amounts of silica dust (acute silicoproteinosis), most commonly in sandblasters, and immunocompromised patients with lymphoma, leukemia, or AIDS. These conditions are associated with an acquired defect of alveolar macrophages which fail to phagocytize surfactant, resulting in the accumulation of surfactant within the alveolar spaces. Pathologically, the alveoli are filled with a lipoproteinaceous material that stains deep pink with periodic acid Schiff. The interstitium is usually not involved, but some patients may have chronic interstitial inflammation and fibrosis.

Patients with PAP are often asymptomatic, although some complain of progressive dyspnea and a nonproductive cough. The absence of orthopnea is an important clinical feature distinguishing PAP from pulmonary edema secondary to congestive heart failure.

The typical radiographic finding in alveolar proteinosis is bilateral symmetric perihilar air-space opacification indistinguishable in appearance from pulmonary edema. Air-space nodules are commonly seen at the periphery of the confluent opacities. Cardiomegaly, pleural effusions, and evidence of pulmonary venous hypertension are notably absent. CT and HRCT scans typically shows geo-

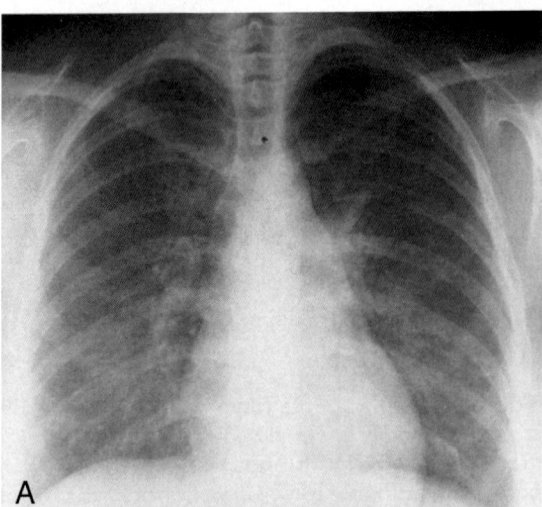
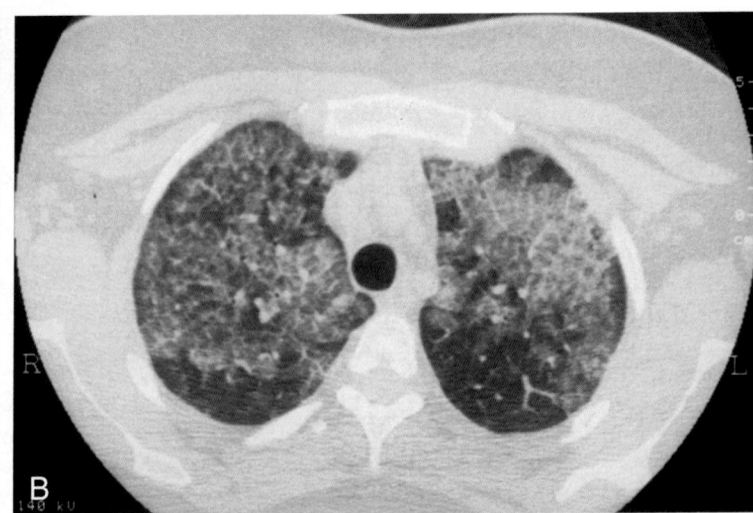

Figure 20.32. Pulmonary Alveolar Proteinosis (PAP). A. Frontal chest radiograph in a 34-year-old man with PAP demonstrates subtle bilateral ground glass opacities. **B.** A CT scan viewed at lung windows shows a mixed pattern of ground glass attenuation superimposed on thickened inter- and intralobular lines which has been termed "crazy paving" and is characteristic of this disorder.

graphic ground glass opacities superimposed on thickened interlobular and intralobular septa, a pattern that has been described as "crazy paving" and is relatively specific for this entity (Fig. 20.32)(19).

Patients with PAP are particularly prone to superinfection of the lung with nocardia, aspergillus, cryptococcus, and atypical mycobacteria. The factors responsible for this propensity may include macrophage dysfunction and the favorable culture medium of intraalveolar lipoproteinaceous material. Infection by one of these organisms should be suspected in any patient with PAP who develop symptoms of pneumonia or radiographic findings of focal parenchymal opacification or cavitation and pleural effusion. CT helps in the early detection of opportunistic infection because pneumonia or abscess formation may be obscured by the underlying process on plain radiographs.

Prior to the advent of bronchoalveolar lavage, one-third of patients died from respiratory failure or opportunistic infections, while the remaining two-thirds either stabilized or resolved spontaneously. Repeated bronchoalveolar lavage with saline has significantly reduced the mortality from this disease. The duration of treatment with BAL varies; some patients require repetitive long term therapy, while others resolve after a single treatment.

ALVEOLAR MICROLITHIASIS

Alveolar microlithiasis is a rare disorder characterized by the deposition of minute calculi within the alveolar spaces. Although alveolar microlithiasis can affect individuals of any age without sex predilection, there is a very high incidence of this disease in siblings. The underlying abnormality responsible for the formation of these calculi, known as calcispherytes, is unknown. These are small calculi measuring less than one millimeter in diameter and are composed of calcium phosphate. Pathologically these calculi are found within normal alveoli; interstitial fibrosis may develop in long-standing disease. The radiographic findings are specific: confluent bilateral dense micronodular opacities are seen which, because of their high intrinsic density, produce the so-called "black pleura sign" at their interface with the chest wall. Apical bullous disease is common and may lead to spontaneous pneumothorax. The diagnosis is made by a history of alveolar microlithiasis in a sibling of an affected individual and typical radiographic findings. Biopsy is usually unnecessary. The majority of patients are asymptomatic at presentation despite the marked radiographic abnormalities, a feature that is characteristic of this disorder. Most patients develop progressive respiratory insufficiency, although some remain stable for years. There is no effective treatment.

ALVEOLAR SEPTAL AMYLOIDOSIS

Amyloidosis encompasses a group of diseases characterized by the extracellular deposition of insoluble fibrillary proteins termed amyloid. Amyloid represents a number of proteins that are distinctive biochemically but similar physically in that their polypeptide chains form beta-pleated sheets. Amyloidosis has traditionally been divided into four forms: a) primary, in which there is no associated chronic disease or in which there is an underlying plasma cell disorder; b) secondary, in which an underlying chronic abnormality such as tuberculosis is present; c) familial, which is very uncommon and usually localized to nervous tissue; and d) senile, which affects multiple organs in patients over 70. More recently, a classification scheme has been developed that is based on the specific protein comprising amyloid. In this scheme, the most important forms are amyloid L (AL), usually seen with plasma cell dyscrasias and associated with the deposition of immunoglobulin light chains, and amyloid A (AA), occurring in patients with chronic inflammatory diseases such as familial Mediterranean fever and certain neoplasms including Hodgkin disease.

There are three major patterns of amyloid deposition within the lungs and airways: tracheobronchial, nodular parenchymal, and diffuse parenchymal (alveolar septal). These patterns usually occur independently, but there can be overlap between them. The diffuse parenchymal form of pulmonary amyloidosis is discussed here; the tracheobronchial form is discussed in the section on the trachea in chapter 19.

In alveolar septal amyloidosis, amyloid is deposited in the parenchymal interstitium and within the media of small blood vessels. Within the alveolar septa, amyloid deposits are located between the endothelial cells lining the septal capillaries and the alveolar epithelium; inflammatory cells are typically absent. This process is usually seen in older patients who have symptoms of chronic progressive dyspnea. Recurrent hemoptysis may be present and may be caused by medial dissection of the involved pulmonary arteries.

Radiographically, patients with parenchymal alveolar septal disease show evidence of interstitial disease, with fine reticular or reticulonodular opacities that may become more coarse and confluent over time. The radiographic appearance simulates silicosis or sarcoidosis. HRCT demonstrates thickening of interlobular septa and bronchovascular structures, findings that simulate lymphangitic carcinomatosis.

The diagnosis is made on lung biopsy by the identification amorphous eosinophilic material thickening the alveolar septa that appears apple green in color when stained with Congo red and viewed under polarized light. There is no effective treatment.

References

1. Light RW. Pleural diseases. 2nd ed. Phiadelphia: Lea and Febiger, 1990:9–19.
2. Peterman TA, Brothers SK. Pleural effusions in congestive heart failure and in pericardial disease. N Engl J Med 1983; 309–313.
3. Light RW. Parapneumonic effusions and empyema. Clin Chest Med 1985;6:55–62.
4. Stark DD, Federle MP, Goodman PC, et al. Differentiating lung abscess and empyema: radiography and computed tomography. AJR Am J Roentgenol 1983;141:163–167.
5. Light RW. Management of spontaneous pneumothorax. Am Rev Respir Dis 1993;148:245–248.

6. Pugatch RD, Spirn PW. Radiology of the pleura. Clin Chest Med 1985;6:17–32.

7. Muller NL. Imaging of the pleura. Radiology 1993;186:297–309.

8. Leung AN, Muller NL, Miller RR. CT in the differential diagnosis of diffuse pleural disease. AJR Am J Roentgenol 1990;154:487–492.

9. Jafri SZH, Roberts JL, Bree RL, et al. Computed tomography of chest wall masses. Radiographics 1989;9:51–68.

10. Gale ME. Bochdalek hernias: prevalence and CT characteristics. Radiology 1985;156:449–452.

11. Demos TC, Solomon C, Popsniak HV, et al. Computed tomography in traumatic defects of the diaphragm. Clin Imag 1989;13:62–67.

12. Markowitz RI, Mercurio MR, Vahjen GA, et al. Congenital lobar emphysema: the roles of CT and V/Q scans. Clin Pediatr 1989;28:19–23.

13. Fitch SJ, Tonkin ILD. Imaging of pulmonary sequestration. AJR Am J Roentgenol 1990;154:241–249.

14. Wagner RB, Crawford WO Jr, Schimpf PP. Classification of parenchymal injuries of the lung. Radiology 1988;167:77–82.

15. Landay MJ, Christensen EE, Bynum LJ. Pulmonary manifestations of acute aspiration of gastric contents. AJR Am J Roentgenol 1978;131:587–592.

16. Cooper JAD, White DA, Matthay RA. Drug induced pulmonary disease. Part 1. Cytotoxic drugs. Am Rev Respir Dis 1986;133:321–340.

17. Cooper JAD, White DA, Matthay RA. Drug induced pulmonary disease. Part 2. Non-cytotoxic drugs. Am Rev Respir Dis 1986;133:488–505.

18. Bell J, McGivern D, Bullimore J, et al. Diagnostic imaging of post-irradiation changes in the chest. Clin Radiol 1988;39:109–119.

19. Godwin JD, Muller NL, Takasugi JE. Pulmonary alveolar proteinosis: CT findings. Radiology 1988;169:609–613.

Section IV   BREAST RADIOLOGY

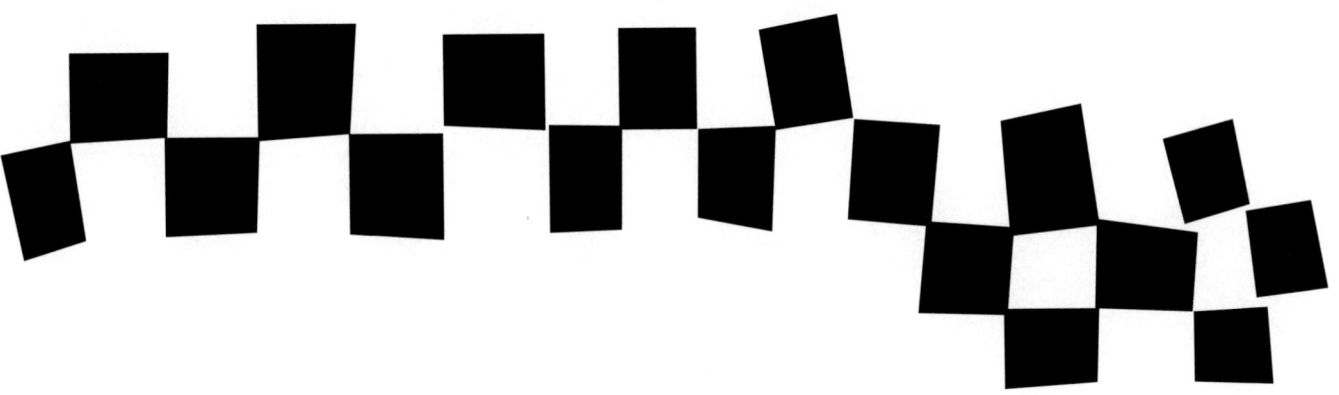

21   Breast Imaging
Karen K. Lindfors

21
Breast Imaging

Karen K. Lindfors

Breast imaging is used for two purposes. The first purpose is to screen asymptomatic women for early breast cancer. The second purpose is to evaluate breast abnormalities in symptomatic patients or patients with indeterminate screening mammograms. Screening is accomplished with standard two-view mammography, but diagnostic evaluation often requires the additional use of special mammographic views, breast US, and interventional procedures.

SCREENING FOR BREAST CANCER

Breast cancer survival is influenced by the size of the tumor and the lymph node status at the time of diagnosis. Small tumors with negative axillary lymph nodes have survival rates greater than 90%. Such cancers are detected far more often with screening mammography than with physical examination. It follows that screening mammography should lower mortality from breast cancer. Several randomized controlled trials have proved the efficacy of this technique.

In 1963, the Health Insurance Plan of New York (HIP) invited 31,000 women aged 40–64 years to participate in four annual screenings for breast cancer by mammography and physical examination. This study group was compared with a control group of women who received routine medical care. Nine years after beginning the study, there was a 29% reduction in breast cancer mortality in the group receiving annual screening (1).

Other trials of mammographic screening were begun in the late 1970s and early 1980s. Five of these were carried out in Sweden and were similar in design. They were population based, meaning that all women living within a specific geographic area who were within the age range being studied were included in the trial. Breast cancer mortality was compared between women invited to screening and those not invited (controls). When the data from all centers were combined, the reduction in breast cancer mortality among women aged 40–74 years was 24% in the group invited to mammographic screening (2).

Controversy arose when the results of screening trials were stratified by age. A clear benefit with mammographic screening was seen for women aged 50–69 years, but early results showed no significant reduction in breast cancer mortality for screened women in their forties. Unfortunately, none of the trials was properly designed or performed for the evaluation of women aged 40–49 years as a separate group. The individual trials lacked sufficient numbers of women in their forties to provide the statistical power required to demonstrate a reduction in mortality early in the follow-up period of the trials. Even when all the world's trials are combined, the total number of women participating amount to fewer than 180,000, yet to prove a 25% reduction in mortality at 5 years, nearly 500,000 participants would be required (3).

Meta analyses can be used to combine the results of different studies, thereby increasing the number of deaths and women-years (number of women × number of years of follow-up) in study and control groups. The most recent meta analysis of five population-based Swedish mammographic screening trials performed after longer follow-up (11–15 years) shows a statistically significant reduction in breast cancer mortality of 29% among screened women in their forties (4). Additionally, two individual Swedish trials have now shown statistically significant reductions in breast cancer mortality among women in their forties who undergo mammographic screening. After 12 years of follow-up, the Gothenburg trial (5) has shown a 44% reduction in mortality and the Malmo trial (6) has shown a 36% reduction.

It is clear that relative breast cancer mortality reductions among women in their forties who undergo mammographic screening appear later than they do in older women. This is probably the result of *a*) a lower incidence of breast carcinoma among younger women, *b*) the small numbers of women aged 40–49 years in the screening trials, *c*) a greater proportion of noninvasive cancers in screened women in their forties requiring a longer period of follow-up to determine mortality owing to the early stage at diagnosis, and *d*) the lower effectiveness in detecting aggressive tumors at favorable stages when there are intervals of more than 1 year between screens (used in most trials).

The actual benefit of screening mammography for women of all ages is likely to exceed that demonstrated by the randomized clinical trials. Breast cancer mortality data for all women invited for screening, regardless of whether they actually underwent mammography, were used in calculating the reduction of mortality attributable to screening. Compliance rates for obtaining mammography among trial invitees ranged from 61–89%. The technology used for mammography has improved greatly since the time that the trials began; earlier detection of breast cancer has resulted (4).

Detection of breast cancer at an early stage also provides the option of treatment that may be less disfiguring and toxic; women with small tumors may be candidates for breast-conserving surgery. Chemotherapy, radiation therapy, and axillary dissection may not be necessary in some mammographically detected cancers.

Screening Guidelines

Updated data from the randomized, controlled trials of mammographic screening, as well as information from large community-based screening programs, encouraged the American Cancer Society (ACS)(7) and the National Cancer Institute (NCI)(8) to revise their guidelines for breast cancer screening in 1997. ACS guidelines for breast cancer screening are shown in Table 21.1. Both clinical examination and mammography are essential components of a screening program because all cancers are not seen mammographically. False-negative mammograms occur in 9–16% of breast cancers; these cancers are generally detected by physical examination. The ACS also recommends the practice of monthly breast self-examination by all women.

The NCI advises that women at average risk for breast cancer who are 40 years old or older a bit should undergo screening mammography every 1–2 years. The optimum interval between screens is currently the focus of considerable debate, particularly for women in their 40s. Studies (9–11) of cancers that occur between screens have shown that a greater proportion of breast cancers grow faster in younger women than in older women. It is for this reason that the ACS has recommended *annual*

mammographic screening for women aged 40 and older, yet the chance of being diagnosed with breast cancer between the ages of 40 and 49 years is 1 in 66 women or 1.5%, and the chance of dying from breast cancer is 0.3%. Although it is clear that annual mammographic screening is more effective in reducing breast cancer deaths for women in their 40s, economic considerations may favor biennial screening.

For women aged 50 and older, there is some additional benefit gained by annual compared with biennial screening, but it is not as great as that gained by annual mammography for women aged 40–49 years (9,11). Because the incidence of breast cancer increases with age, the efficiency of mammographic screening increases as women get older. There is no recommended age at which mammographic screening should cease. For elderly women, general health status and quality of life should be considered when deciding whether to undergo mammography.

The NCI also advises women at high risk for development of breast cancer to seek expert advice regarding the advisability of beginning regular mammographic screening before age 40 and the periodicity of mammography once they reach age 40. Factors known to increase a woman's risk include *a*) a personal history of breast cancer; *b*) laboratory evidence that the woman is a carrier of the BRCA1 or BRCA2 genetic mutation. These mutations confer an estimated risk of 85% for development of breast cancer by age 70; *c*) having a mother, sister, or daughter with breast cancer; *d*) atypical or precancerous lesions diagnosed on a previous breast biopsy; and *e*) nulliparity or having a first child at age 30 or older.

When adopting a screening policy, the physician must remember that all women are at risk for developing breast cancer. The ACS estimates that one woman in every eight will develop the disease during her lifetime. The majority of women who contract breast cancer will not have histories that place them at higher risk.

Screening Outcomes

What are the expected outcomes in a group of 1000 asymptomatic women undergoing bilateral screening mammography for the first time? Approximately 80 of these women will be recalled for additional studies. These may include magnification or other special mammographic views and US. Biopsy will be recommended in approximately 16 of these women, and cancer will be found in approximately 6 of them. With subsequent screenings of the same women, the numbers of cancers found will decrease and the positive predictive value, or percentage of women undergoing biopsy who actually have cancer, should increase.

The goal of screening asymptomatic women is to find breast cancer in its earliest stages, when survival is greatest. In a well-established screening program, more than 50% of cancers will be minimal; minimal cancers are defined as those that are noninvasive or those that are invasive but less than 1 cm in size with negative nodes. Greater than 80% of breast cancer discovered by screening mammography should be node-negative (12,13).

Table 21.1. American Cancer Society Guidelines for Breast Cancer Screening

Age	Clinical Examination	Mammography
20–39	Every 3 years	Not recommended
40 and over	Annually	Annually

Optimal effectiveness of a breast cancer screening program requires the use of physical examination in addition to mammographic screening. Nine to 16 percent of cancers are not visualized mammographically; such cancers are discovered on physical examination. The minimum size of breast cancers that can be felt on physical examination averages between 1.5 and 2 cm.

False-negative mammograms can occur for a variety of reasons. The palpable abnormality may not be included on a film. Dense breast parenchyma may obscure visualization of a mass. The filming technique may be suboptimal for visualization of an abnormality. The particular tumor type may not be visible mammographically or there may be observer error in the interpretation of the mammogram. A negative mammogram should not deter further diagnostic evaluation of a clinically palpable mass.

Some breast cancers arise in the interval between screening examinations. The number of such cancers depends on the frequency of screening. Interval cancers tend to be more advanced at diagnosis when compared with those diagnosed at screening (10); they may be biologically more aggressive. Additionally, a previous negative mammogram or the knowledge that screening will be performed regularly may be a disincentive for patients to perform breast self-examination or to seek immediate medical care for a breast mass found in the interval between screens. Physicians must stress that any breast mass requires immediate attention, regardless of whether the patient has had a recent negative mammogram.

Radiation Risk

An increased susceptibility to breast cancer has been documented among women exposed to high doses of radiation (1–20 Gy). The survivors of the atomic bomb explosions in Japan, patients undergoing radiation therapy, and sanitoria patients undergoing multiple chest fluoroscopies for monitoring of tuberculosis therapy are all groups with an increased incidence of breast cancer. Such data raises questions about the risk incurred from the low doses of radiation received during screening mammography ($\approx$2 mGy).

A controlled study of the effects of low doses of radiation, such as those received during mammography, would require large numbers of women in both the study and control groups. Nearly 100 million patients in each group would be required in order to provide statistically significant data. Clearly, this would not be practical or possible. As such, estimates or risk have been hypothesized by extrapolation from data obtained at higher doses using a linear dose–response model.

The latest follow-up data from the Japanese atomic bomb survivors have shown progressively decreasing radiation risk with increased age at exposure. Women exposed in their youth and teens suffered the highest increase in risk. No increased risk was demonstrable for women aged 40 or older at exposure. Studies of the other populations sustaining significant breast radiation exposure have also supported a diminished risk with advancing age at exposure. Estimated lifetime risk of breast cancer death from a single mammogram in women aged 40–49 years is approximately 2 in 1 million. In women aged 50–59, this risk is reduced to fewer than 1 in 1 million; progressive reductions in risk are seen at older ages (14).

These theoretical risks should be weighed against the risk of dying from spontaneous breast cancer, which would be approximately 700 per million in women aged 40–49 years and 1000 per million in women aged 50–59. This risk increases steadily with advancing age.

The Use of Other Imaging Modalities for Breast Cancer Screening

Mammography is the only imaging modality with proved capability to screen asymptomatic women for breast cancer. Other modalities have been investigated for their potential in screening, but none can approach the sensitivity and specificity of mammography.

In the mid-1970s, when there were questions regarding the radiation risk from mammography, US was investigated as a screening technique. US units that would scan the entire breast were developed; however, studies revealed that up to 42% of all breast cancers were not visualized by US. The results were even worse for cancers smaller than 1 cm in diameter; in one study, 92% of these were not seen sonographically (15). In follow-up studies of patients who had suspicious abnormalities by US, but negative mammograms and normal physical examinations, no cancers were found (16). These data have led to the conclusion that there is no role for US in screening for breast cancer. US is useful only in diagnosis or further characterization of a specific lesion detected by mammography or physical examination; its primary utility is in distinguishing simple cysts from solid masses in the breast. This distinction is of great importance, as simple cysts are invariably benign.

Recent technical advances have led to increasing interest in magnetic resonance imaging as a possible detection technique for breast cancer in certain populations. Recent data suggest that MR can reveal lesions that are missed by conventional mammography in radiographically dense breasts. The cost of MR, as well as the time it takes to perform, will probably prohibit its use as a general screening tool, but the technique may prove useful in specific cases.

Other imaging technologies, such as positron-emission tomography and radionuclide scintigraphy, are also being explored for use in breast cancer detection and diagnosis. Currently, mammography remains the single best test for early detection of breast cancer; it is the "gold standard" by which all other potential screening modalities must be measured.

EVALUATION OF THE SYMPTOMATIC PATIENT

Bilateral mammography should be the first imaging study performed in patients older than 30 years of age who present with breast masses that are suspicious for carcinoma. The mass should be indicated by placing a radiopaque marker over the site. This will assist the radiologist in a targeted mammographic evaluation of this area and will also ensure that the palpable abnormality corresponds to the mammographic abnormality, if one is visualized. Such correlation is important in ensuring that the surgical biopsy of a palpable abnormality will encompass the mammographically suspicious area.

The primary reason for performing mammography in a patient with a suspicious palpable mass is to assess the affected breast for multifocal disease and the contralateral breast for suspicious abnormalities that should be biopsied concurrently. Mammography may also be helpful in definitively diagnosing the palpable abnormality as benign, thus avoiding biopsy.

Mammography should be performed before any intervention. A hematoma, resulting from percutaneous fine-needle aspiration biopsy, can look similar to a small carcinoma. When such procedures have been performed prior to mammography, it is best to perform a follow-up mammogram 4 to 6 weeks later.

If mammography is negative in a patient with a clinically evident mass and dense breasts, US is often suggested as a subsequent imaging study. US can determine whether the mass represents a simple cyst. Simple cysts are virtually never malignant and do not require aspiration unless the patient has pain related to the cyst. US cannot provide a specific diagnosis for a solid or complex mass.

Alternatively, definitive diagnosis of a palpable mass can usually be made by performing a fine-needle aspiration of the mass with a 22-gauge needle. When a simple cyst is present, the aspiration is both diagnostic and therapeutic, as all of the fluid can be withdrawn. In solid or complex masses, a cytologic examination of the cells removed at aspiration will yield the diagnosis.

In younger patients who present with breast masses, mammography must be used more judiciously. This more cautious approach is based on data from the atomic bomb survivors in Japan showing an excess risk of breast cancer in younger women exposed to high doses of radiation. These data, combined with the low incidence of breast cancer in young women (less than 1% of breast cancer occurs in women less than 30 years old), suggest that a restricted use of mammography is prudent. Some experts also believe that dense breast tissue, which is more common in younger women, limits the sensitivity of mammography, but studies have shown that mammography can demonstrate up to 90% of cancers in women younger than 35 years (17).

Women less than 30 years of age who have a focal suspicious palpable abnormality are frequently first evaluated with US. If the US is negative and the patient is older than age 20, a single oblique view of the affected breast is performed to assess for suspicious microcalcifications, which would not be visualized by US. Women less than age 20 should not undergo mammography.

If fine-needle aspiration is available, it may be used in lieu of imaging studies when young patients have suspicious palpable masses. In the extremely rare circumstance of a diagnosis of carcinoma, mammography can be performed subsequently. The radiologist should be aware that a previous needle aspiration may confound the mammographic assessment of the affected area, but it will not compromise assessment of surrounding or contralateral tissues.

Increased awareness of breast cancer has led many clinicians to request more imaging studies in young women. Breast imaging cannot replace careful clinical evaluation of the breasts. If there is no suspicious focal abnormality, imaging studies will not be helpful; they may subject the patient to unnecessary risk.

TECHNICAL CONSIDERATIONS IN BREAST IMAGING

Because both high-contrast and high-spatial resolution are needed for optimal mammography, standard radiographic equipment cannot be used for this examination. Mammography must be performed on a unit dedicated to this purpose. Mammographic equipment and technique differ from standard radiography in several ways. The anode material used to generate the x-rays in most dedicated mammography units is molybdenum. This allows the production of lower energy x-rays, which in turn produces greater contrast between soft tissue structures. The structures of the breast do not differ greatly in their inherent contrast, so these low kilovolt or "softer" photons are extremely important in producing a high-contrast image. Some newer units also have rhodium anodes that can be used to increase the contrast in denser breasts, while keeping radiation dose and time of exposure low.

The radiologist must be able to discern tiny microcalcifications on mammograms; some of these calcifications may be 0.1 mm or less in size. The small focal spot size used in mammography units, a longer distance from the x-ray source to the image, and special high resolution, single intensifying screens used with single emulsion film, contribute to the creation of images with high resolution.

All mammographic units are equipped with compression paddles that squeeze the breast against the film holder. Good compression of the breast is essential to high-quality mammography for several reasons. Compression spreads overlapping breast structures so that true masses can be differentiated from summation shadows that occur because of overlapping soft tissues. The breast is immobilized during compression, so motion unsharpness or blurring owing to patient movement is minimized. Geometric unsharpness, caused by the finite focal spot dimension, is minimized by bringing the breast structures closer to the film. Compression renders the breast nearly uniform in thickness, so the film density of tissues near the nipple will be similar to those near the chest wall. Radiation dose can be reduced by good compression; a thinner breast requires fewer photons for penetration. Beam attenuation is also reduced.

Some women find breast compression uncomfortable, but most can tolerate it once the benefits are explained. During routine mammography the breast is compressed for a few seconds while each film is taken. Many units are equipped with automated compression devices so the technologist can release the tension immediately after the film is exposed.

Other factors are also important to consider in the production of high-quality mammograms. These include other equipment features such as type of x-ray generator, beam filtration, grid use, as well as film-intensifying

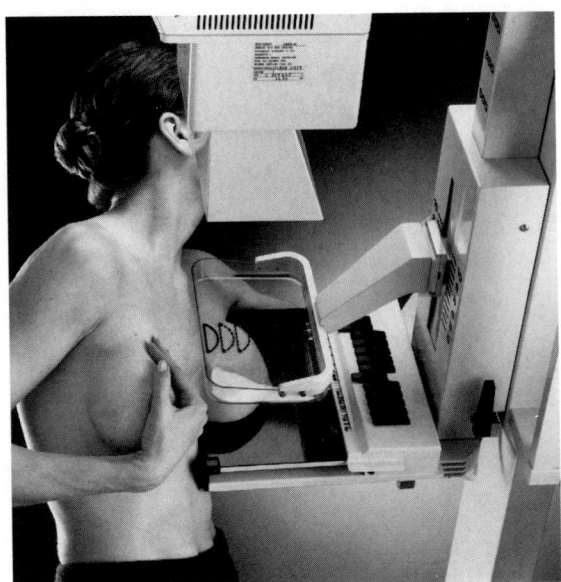

Figure 21.1. Patient Positioning for a MLO View. (Reproduced with permission from General Electric Medical Systems, Milwaukee, Wisconsin.)

screen combinations and the film processing system. All of these factors are interrelated and must be optimized to produce technically acceptable films of the breast.

Quality Assurance

It is the responsibility of radiologists to ensure that the highest quality of breast imaging is performed at their facilities. All standards mandated by the Mammography Quality Standards Act (MQSA) must be met. MQSA was passed into law by Congress in 1992 to ensure that all women receive optimal mammography services. The law requires that every practice become accredited by the Food and Drug Administration (FDA). Specified standards for personnel (radiologists, technologists, and physicists), equipment used, radiation dose, and quality assurance practices are stipulated. Once FDA accreditation is granted, an annual survey by a physicist must be performed to ensure that the practice continues to meet quality control and equipment standards. All facilities performing mammography are inspected annually by an FDA inspector. Each radiologist who interprets mammograms must be fully informed of the MQSA regulations. Failure to comply with the law can result in sanctions or even closure of the mammography facility.

Mammographic Positioning for Screening

Mammography can be performed with the patient seated or standing. Most screening practices prefer the standing position because it allows faster throughput and is less cumbersome. Patients are able to lean into the unit to a greater degree when standing, thus enabling more of the posterior breast tissues to be imaged. Recumbent imaging is possible but quite difficult; its use should be restricted to problem-solving situations.

Two views of each breast are generally used for screening mammography in the United States. Several European countries use a single mediolateral oblique (MLO) view for screening examinations, but authorities in this country have shown that one-view examinations would lead to an excessive number of patients being called back for additional views. Asking large numbers of patients to return for such views would result in unacceptable levels of patient anxiety and cost. The standard views for screening mammography are the MLO view and the craniocaudal (CC) view.

MLO View. The MLO view, when properly positioned, depicts the greatest amount of breast tissue. It is the most useful view in mammography. In those countries using single-view screening, the MLO view is preferred. To perform an MLO view, the x-ray tube and film holder, which are fixed with respect to one another, are moved to an angle that parallels the orientation of the patient's pectoralis major muscle. The technologist is given flexibility in choosing the angle so that the greatest amount of breast tissue possible can be imaged. The angle is generally between 40° and 60° from the horizontal.

The patient is asked to relax her arm and chest muscles and to lean into the machine. The breast is placed on the film holder and compression is applied from the superomedial direction, the same direction from which the x-ray photons will pass through the breast. The breast must be pulled anteriorly and spread in a superior–inferior direction as much as possible to minimize overlapping structures and to maximize the amount of tissue imaged. The nipple should be in profile. Compression must be applied vigorously (Fig. 21.1). By convention in the MLO view, a marker indicating the side (left or right) and type of view is placed near the axillary tissues of the breast.

A properly positioned MLO mammogram should show the pectoralis major muscle down to the level of a line drawn perpendicular to the muscle through the nipple (posterior nipple line). The nipple should be in profile so that the subareolar area can be adequately evaluated. The inframammary fold should be visible to ensure that the inferior portion of the breast has been imaged (Fig. 21.2).

CC View. For the CC view, the unit is placed in the vertical position so that the x-ray tube is perpendicular to the floor. Photons will travel from the anode, located superior to the breast, to the film underneath the breast. The breast is placed on the film holder, pulled anteriorly, and spread horizontally before the compression plate is applied to the superior skin surface (Fig. 21.3). The nipple should again be in profile. The chest wall should rest against the film holder. The markers indicating the side imaged and type of view should be placed near the skin close to the lateral aspect of the breast.

When evaluating a CC mammogram, optimal positioning can be ensured when pectoralis muscle is seen centrally on the film and the nipple is in profile (Fig. 21.4). The pectoralis muscle can be visualized in about 30% of patients on the CC view. An alternative method of ensuring appropriate visualization of posterior tissues is to measure the distance from the nipple to the edge of the film through the central axis of the breast; this distance

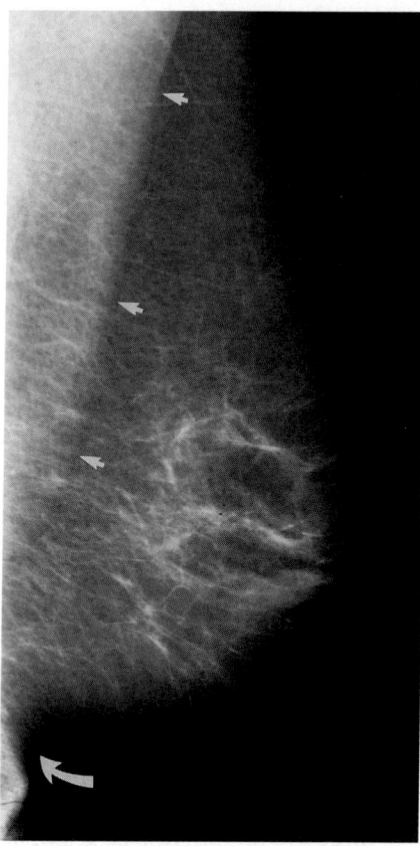

Figure 21.2. Normal MLO View of Left Breast. The pectoralis muscle (*white arrows*) is seen from the axilla to below the level of the posterior nipple line. The inframammary fold (*curved arrow*) is well seen, and the nipple is in profile.

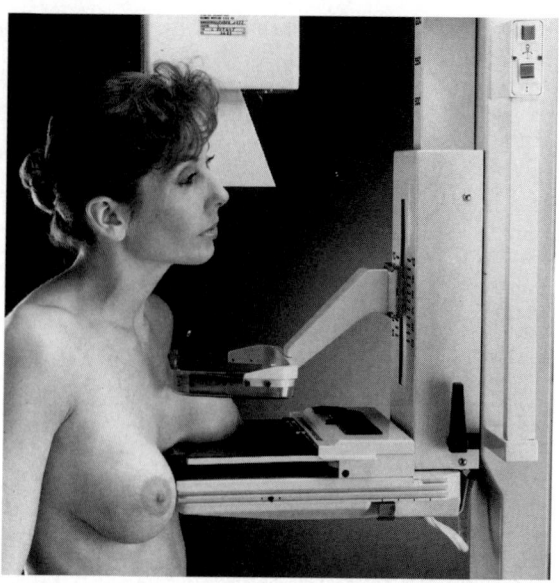

Figure 21.3. Patient Positioning for the CC View. (Reproduced with permission from General Electric Medical Systems, Milwaukee, Wisconsin.)

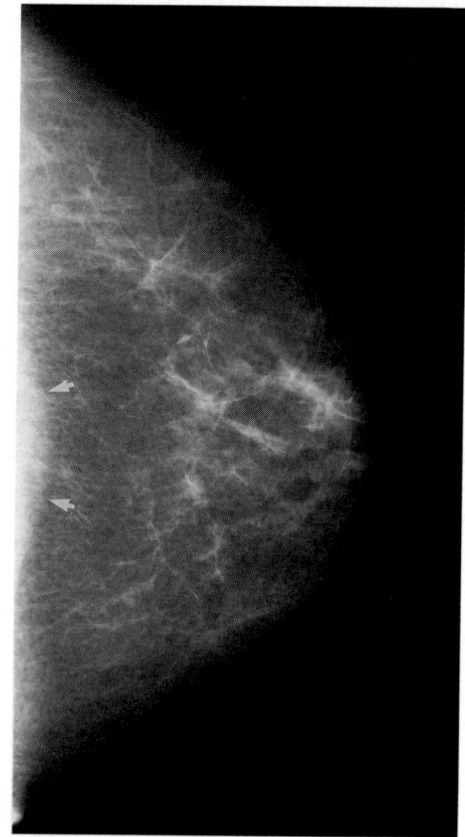

Figure 21.4. Normal CC View of the Left Breast. Note that the nipple is in profile and the pectoralis muscle (*arrows*) is seen posteriorly, indicating optimal visualization of breast tissue.

should be within 1 cm of the length of the posterior nipple line as seen on the MLO view.

Interpreting the Mammogram

For interpretation, CC and MLO mammograms should each be hung together in a mirror-image configuration. This will enable the radiologist to scan the breasts for symmetry. Viewing conditions are extremely important to optimal mammographic film reading. The room must be darkened. All adjacent-view box light should be blocked out. Dedicated mammography film alternators and view boxes can do this automatically. If standard view boxes or alternators are used, exposed blackened film can be cut to mask out unwanted light.

A magnifying lens should be used to examine each film thoroughly. All visible parenchyma should be scanned systematically with magnification. This will enable visualization of tiny microcalcifications and will ensure that the radiologist has examined all parts of the breast in detail.

If previous mammograms are available, they should be compared to the current study so that the radiologist can evaluate the examination for any changes in the mammographic appearance of the breasts. In turn, current questionable areas can be evaluated for their stability.

In most practices, patients are asked to complete a brief history form that includes questions relevant to breast health and cancer risk. Knowledge of the patient's history will be helpful in assessing the malignant potential and likely diagnosis of a particular mammographic finding. The risk of malignancy is much greater in a 60-year-old woman than in a 30-year-old woman. A woman with a personal or close family history of breast cancer is at greater risk for development of malignancy, and the interpretation of mammographic findings should be tailored accordingly. Other information such as previous surgical biopsies or hormone replacement intake must also be taken into account during interpretation of the mammogram.

Correlation with the physical examination is also extremely important so that false-negative reports can be minimized. All palpable lesions should be marked and assessed mammographically. Special views can image palpable lesions that occur in locations not included on standard mammography. The mammographer can also be certain that the mass felt corresponds to the mammographic abnormality. Areas of asymmetrical tissue seen mammographically can be assessed for palpable abnormalities, which may render them more suspicious for malignancy.

Classic mammographic signs of malignancy are spiculated masses or pleomorphic clusters of microcalcifications; however, only about 40% of all occult breast carcinoma presents in these ways (18). In the remainder of cases, more subtle or indirect signs of malignancy are present. The radiologist must look at each mammogram with great care, using all available diagnostic techniques so that false-negative diagnoses are minimized. This charge must be balanced against the need to minimize false-positive diagnoses. Each time a woman is subjected to a surgical biopsy, financial and emotional costs as well as risks are incurred.

Diagnostic Evaluation of the Indeterminate Mammogram

In the majority of cases, a two-view screening mammogram will provide a conclusive interpretation, but when the results of mammography are indeterminate, further evaluation is necessary; additional mammographic views (Table 21.2) (19) or US may be required for clarification. The workup must be tailored to the specific situation.

Projections other than the standard CC and MLO views may help to visualize a lesion that is seen only in one standard view or that is obscured by surrounding parenchyma. Tangential views of the skin can be used to establish a dermal location for calcifications or superficial masses. Dermal abnormalities do not represent breast cancer.

Further characterization of an abnormality can be accomplished with spot compression and magnification views. The compression plate used is much smaller than that used in standard views, therefore greater force can be applied, which results both in further spreading of any overlying tissue and in bringing the abnormality closer to the film for increased detail. Magnification also produces finer detail, which enables more accurate assessment of the morphology of microcalcifications and the borders of masses.

Well-defined or partially obscured masses can be evaluated with US. A high-frequency (7–10 MHz), hand-held linear array transducer is most commonly used. A targeted evaluation of the mammographically visible abnormality is performed. Simple cysts are easily distinguishable from complex or solid masses. This differentiation is extremely important, as simple cysts are always benign and require no further workup, whereas noncystic masses may represent cancers.

ANALYZING THE MAMMOGRAM

Masses

Complete assessment of a mammographically visible, potentially malignant mass requires several steps. First, the radiologist must decide whether the mass is real. The left and right breasts must be compared in each view.

Most women have reasonably symmetric parenchyma;

Table 21.2. Diagnostic Mammographic Views

View	Abbreviations	Purpose
90° lateral	ML (mediolateral) or	Localizing lesion seen in one view
	LM (lateral medial)	Demonstrate milk of calcium due to its gravity dependency.
Spot compression	—	Determine whether lesion is real or is a summation shadow.
Spot compression with magnification	M	Better definition of margins or masses and morphology of calcifications.
Exaggerated craniocaudal	XCCL	Show lesions in outer aspect of breast and axillary tail not seen on CC view.
Cleavage view	CV	Show lesions deep in posteromedial breast not seen in CC view.
Tangential	TAN	Verify skin lesions.
		Show palpable lesions obscured by dense tissue.
Roll view	RM (rolled medial) or	Verify true lesions.
	RL (rolled lateral)	Determine location of lesion seen in one view by seeing how location changes.
Lateromedial oblique	LMO	Improved visualization of superomedial tissue.
		Improved tissue visualization and comfort for women with pectus excavatum, recent sternotomy, prominent pacemaker.
Implant displacement	ID	Improved visualization of native breast tissue in women with implants.

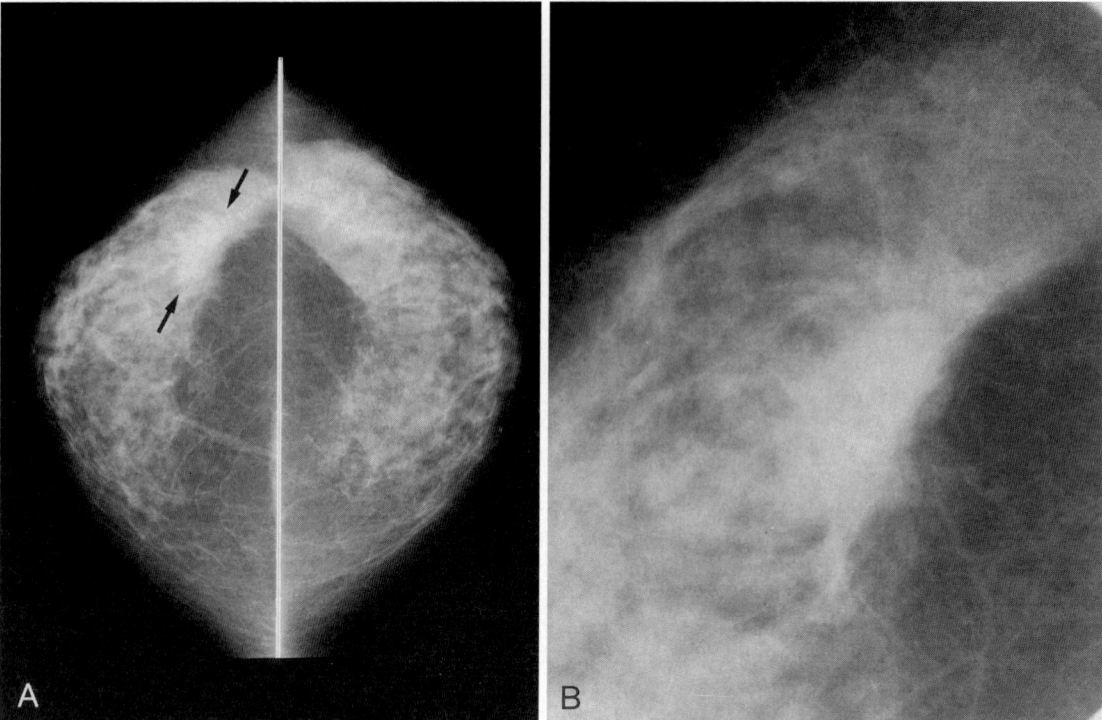

Figure 21.5. Infiltrating Duct Carcinoma. A. Craniocaudal views of both breasts, showing an asymmetrical area of increased density in the outer aspect of the right breast (*arrows*). **B.** Magnification compression view shows this to be a true mass with defined, convex borders and increasing density toward its center.

however, at least 3% of women have areas of asymmetrical, but histologically normal, breast tissue. When attempting to distinguish asymmetrical normal breast tissue from a true abnormality, the radiologist must look for the mammographic features of a mass. Masses have convex borders and become denser toward the center. They distort the normal breast architecture. True masses are seen in multiple projections and can still be visualized when focal compression is used (Fig. 21.5).

Asymmetrical breast parenchyma has an amorphous quality. On spot compression, the tissue spreads apart and fat can be seen interspersed with the denser breast structures in a pattern of normal architecture (Fig. 21.6). The appearance of asymmetrical tissue varies significantly from one mammographic projection to another.

When evaluating the breast for a possible mass, it is important to correlate the mammographic findings with the physical examination. When a suspicious palpable abnormality corresponds to the area of asymmetry seen on mammography, a biopsy should be undertaken. In a study (20) of 221 patients with mammographically visible asymmetries, only 3 patients had malignancies and all 3 had suspicious, palpable abnormalities corresponding to the visualized asymmetries.

Summation shadows that resemble masses on mammography can be produced by overlapping breast tissue. They are visible in only one view and usually disappear when focal compression spreads the tissues apart.

Once the radiologist has concluded that a mass is present, its margins, density, location, and size should be assessed. The number of mammographically visible

masses and their similarities or differences should be analyzed. Previous films should be compared with the current study to look for new masses or an increase in the size of a mass. It is impossible to evaluate one characteristic independent of the others.

MARGINS

The margins of a mass are probably the most important characteristics to be assessed. Overlying breast parenchyma often obscures margin analysis, but liberal use of magnification compression views, in multiple projections, will aid the radiologist.

Spiculated Margins

Breast carcinoma classically appears as a spiculated mass on mammography (Fig. 21.7); however, less than 20% of nonpalpable cancers present as such (18). Most spiculated-appearing breast cancers will be infiltrating ductal carcinoma; however, tubular and lobular carcinomas can present as such. Tubular carcinomas are more well-differentiated histologically and carry a better prognosis. Lobular carcinomas comprise about 10% of all invasive carcinomas. They are not mammographically distinguishable from invasive ductal carcinomas, although they are frequently more subtle. Single rows of lobular cancer cells can infiltrate surrounding tissues, so they generally cause less tissue distortion.

A very limited differential exists for a spiculated mass. **Fat necrosis** from a previous surgical biopsy can appear spiculated (Fig. 21.8).

Scars from previous breast surgery should be carefully marked with radiopaque wires. Comparison should be made with previous films, both to determine the location of the abnormality that underwent biopsy and to assess for any increase in size of the presumed scar. Many scars will regress with time, but others will be stable in appearance and size. Any increase in size should be viewed with suspicion, and biopsy should be undertaken.

Radial scar or complex sclerosing lesion can also present as a spiculated lesion. These are spontaneous lesions that are benign and consist histologically of central sclerosis and varying degrees of epithelial proliferation, represented by strands of fibrous connective tissue.

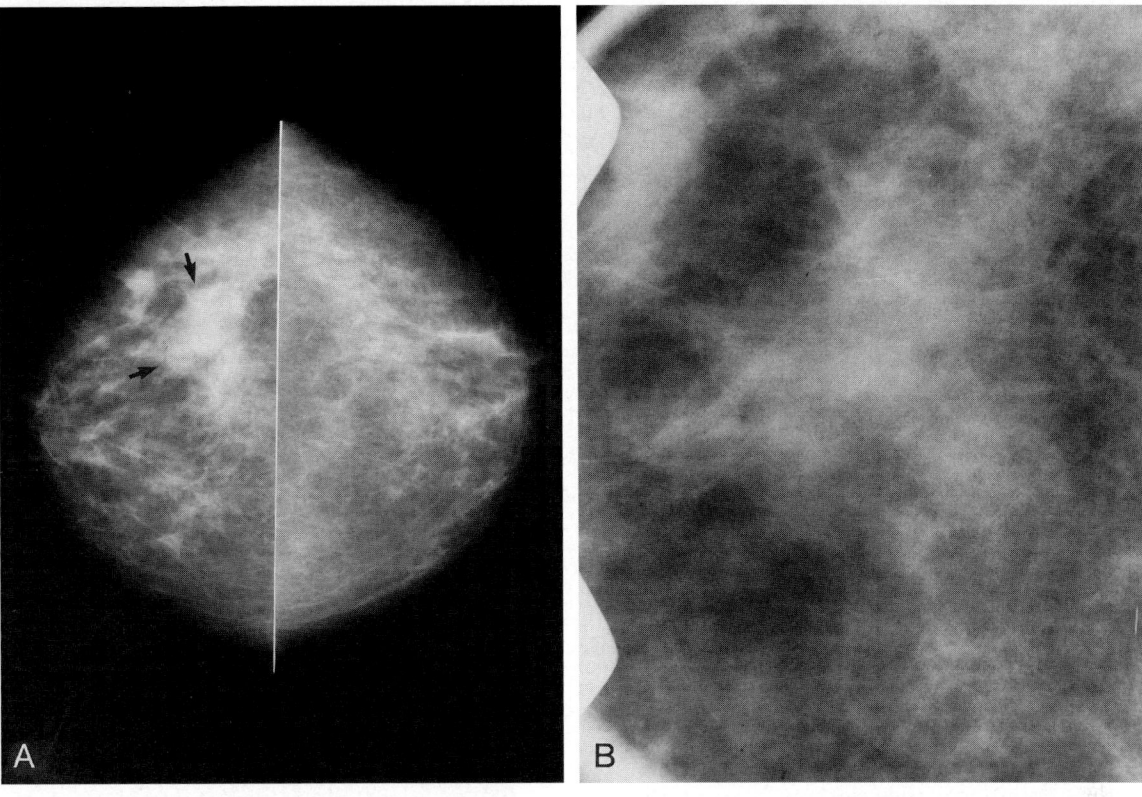

Figure 21.6. Asymmetrical Breast Parenchyma. A. CC views of both breasts in an asymptomatic woman. An area of asymmetrical density is seen in the outer aspect of the right breast (*arrows*). **B.** Compression magnification view demonstrates normal breast architecture in the area of increased density. These findings are consistent with histologically normal, but asymmetrical, mammary parenchyma.

Figure 21.7. Classic Breast Carcinoma. This spiculated breast mass is an infiltrating duct carcinoma.

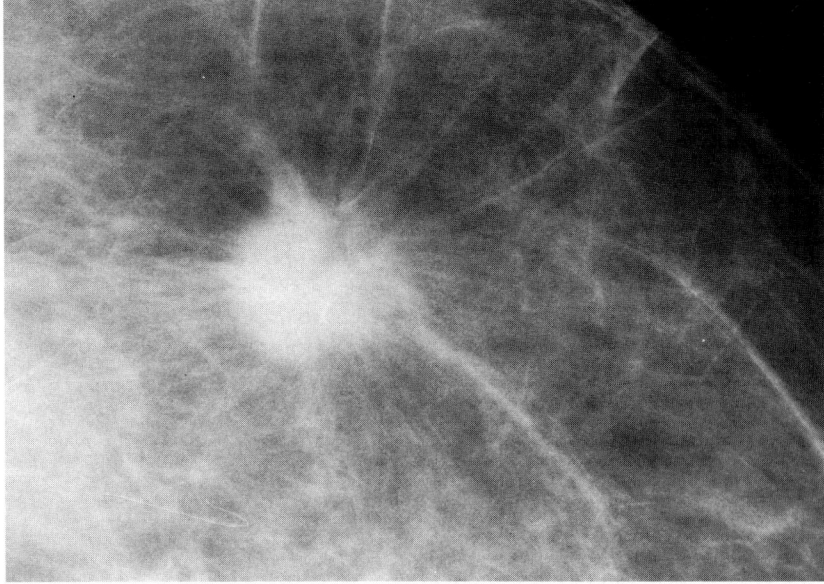

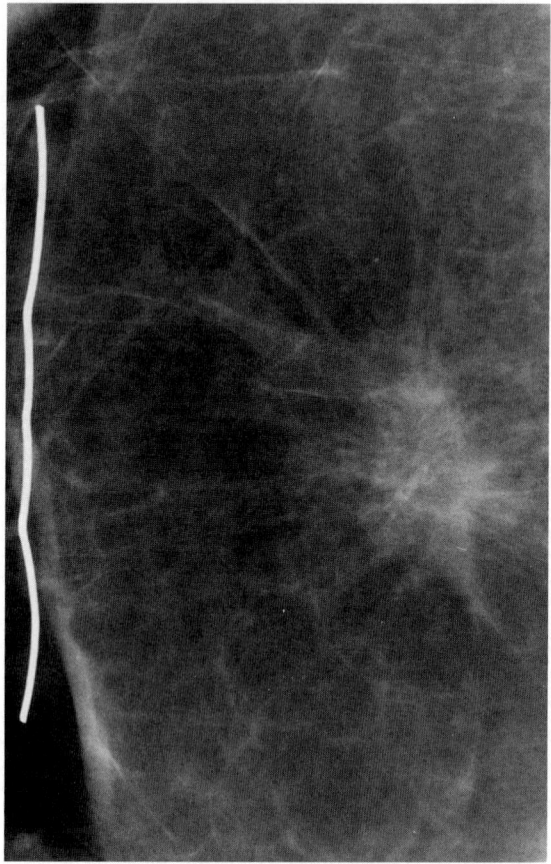

Figure 21.8. Postsurgical Fat Necrosis. This spiculated mass had been stable for 7 years. The radiopaque wire indicates the scar on the patient's skin from the previous lumpectomy.

Histologic differentiation of these lesions from carcinoma is mandatory.

Indistinct (Ill-defined) Margins

Breast carcinoma can also present as a round mass with indistinct or ill-defined borders (Fig. 21.9). Benign lesions that can present as such include abscess, hematoma, and focal fibrosis.

Breast abscesses are most commonly seen in a sub-areolar location in lactating women (Fig. 21.10). Clinically, there is associated pain, swelling, and erythema.

Spontaneous hematomas are seen in women on anticoagulant therapy or in those with blood dyscrasias. They can also be secondary to trauma, needle aspiration, or surgery. Correlation with the patient's history and physical examination will be helpful in discerning whether a lesion represents a hematoma. If doubt persists as to the nature of a possible hematoma, short-interval follow-up mammograms (4–6 wk later) to demonstrate resolution will be helpful (Fig. 21.11).

Circumscribed (Well-Defined) Margins

Circumscribed masses are almost always benign; however, up to 5% of masses that appear well circumscribed

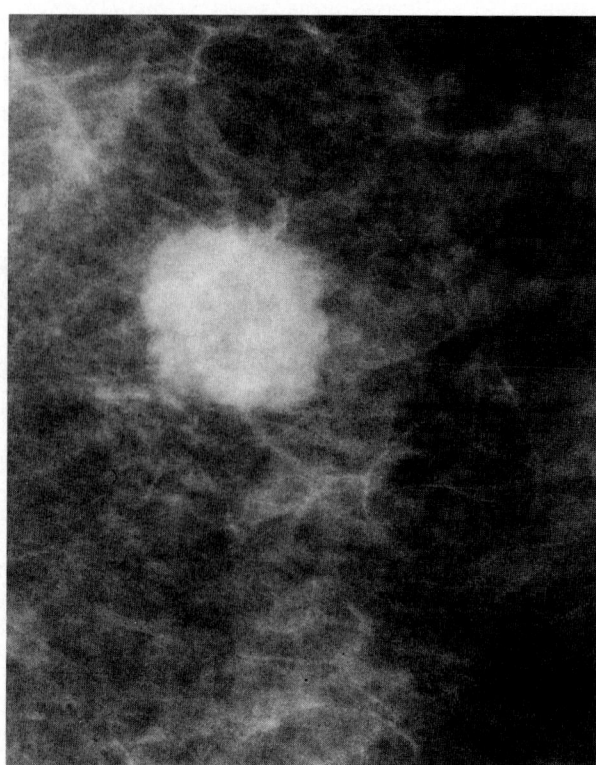

Figure 21.9. Infiltrating Duct Carcinoma. Infiltrating duct carcinoma presenting as a round mass with indistinct, microlobulated borders.

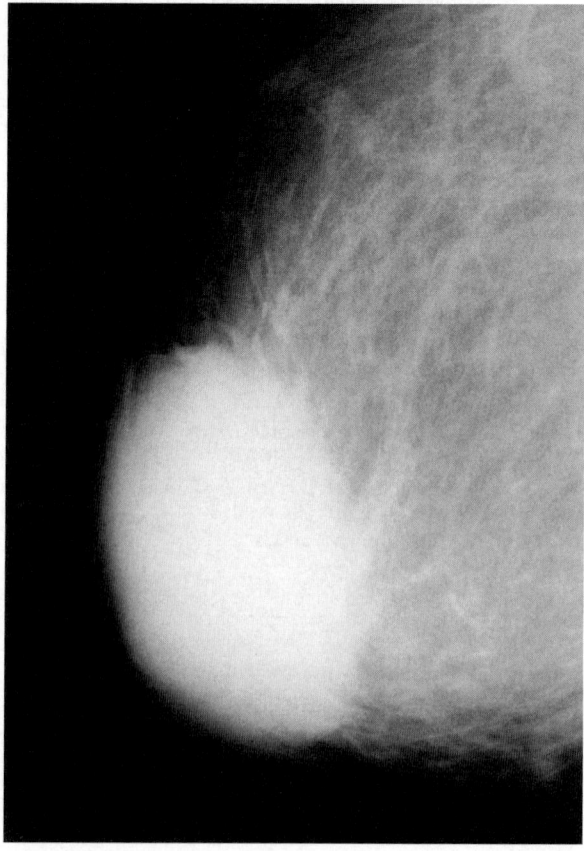

Figure 21.10. Large Subareolar Abscess. The indistinct borders of the mass are the result of surrounding inflammation.

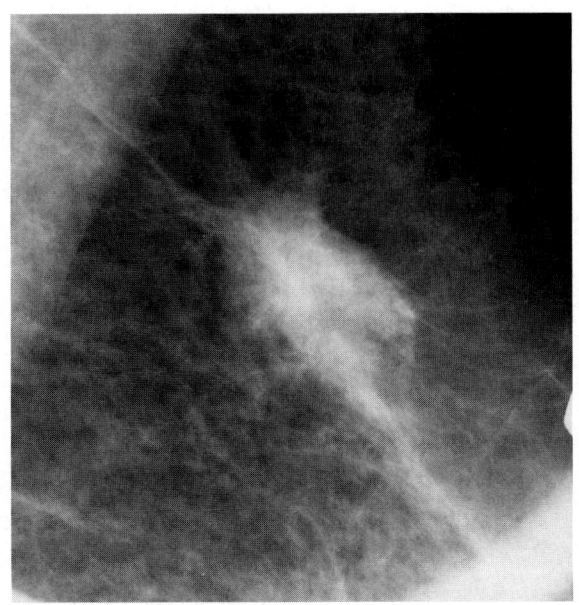

Figure 21.11. Infiltrating Duct Carcinoma. Magnification view of a palpable abnormality in the upper outer quadrant. The patient had undergone a negative FNAB the previous day; the mammographic differential diagnosis included hematoma and carcinoma. Follow-up mammogram 6 weeks later demonstrated no resolution. Surgical biopsy showed infiltrating duct carcinoma.

on conventional mammograms may represent carcinomas (21). The "halo sign," which is a partial or complete radiolucent ring surrounding a mass, is not helpful in determining benignity. Sonography should be used to assess circumscribed masses prior to any additional mammographic views; if a simple cyst is diagnosed by US, no further imaging workup is required. Magnification compression views will greatly assist in clarifying the nature of borders of an apparently well-circumscribed, solid mass. Masses that appear well circumscribed on conventional views may have indistinct or microlobulated margins on compression magnification views (22); such masses should undergo biopsy. If a solid mass appears circumscribed on magnification views and there are no previous mammograms available for comparison, the mass can generally be characterized as one that has a high probability of being benign. Such masses are frequently subjected to a course of follow-up mammography. The first of these surveillance mammograms should be performed 6 months after the original study.

Cysts are the most common well-circumscribed masses seen in women between the ages of 35 and 50 years (Fig. 21.12). They are rare after menopause unless hormone replacement therapy has been instituted. Cysts can be accurately diagnosed by US and are virtually never malignant. A high-frequency (generally, 5–10

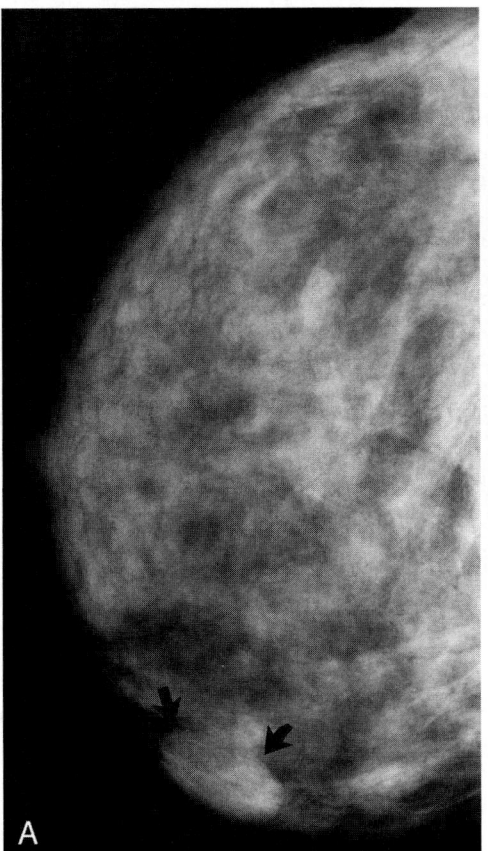

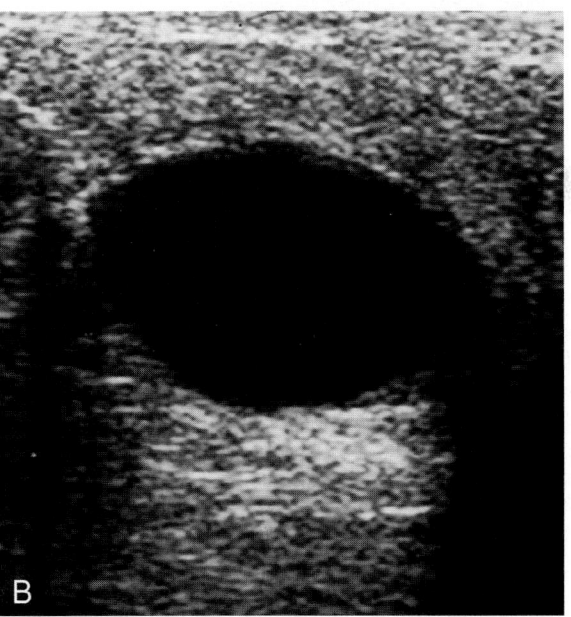

Figure 21.12. Simple Breast Cyst. A. Craniocaudal mammogram demonstrates a 1.5-cm mass in a 50-year old-woman (*arrows*). The mass is at least partially well circumscribed. **B.** US of the mass demonstrates a round, anechoic structure with well-defined margins and enhanced through transmission of sound. These features are diagnostic of a simple cyst.

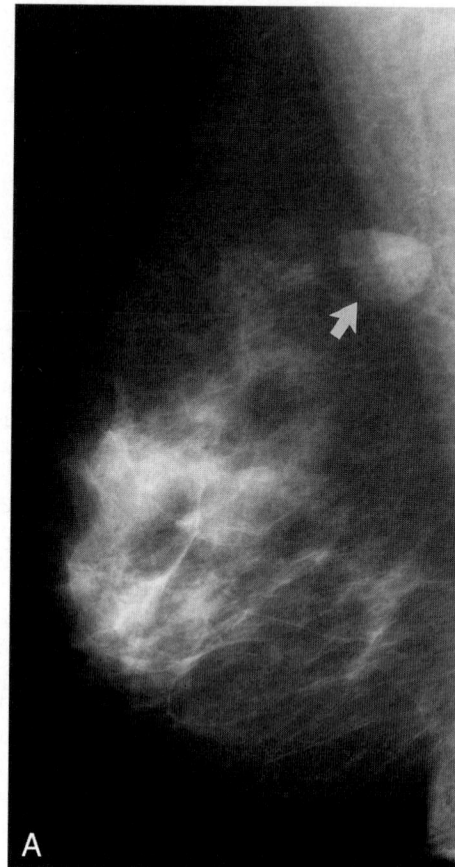

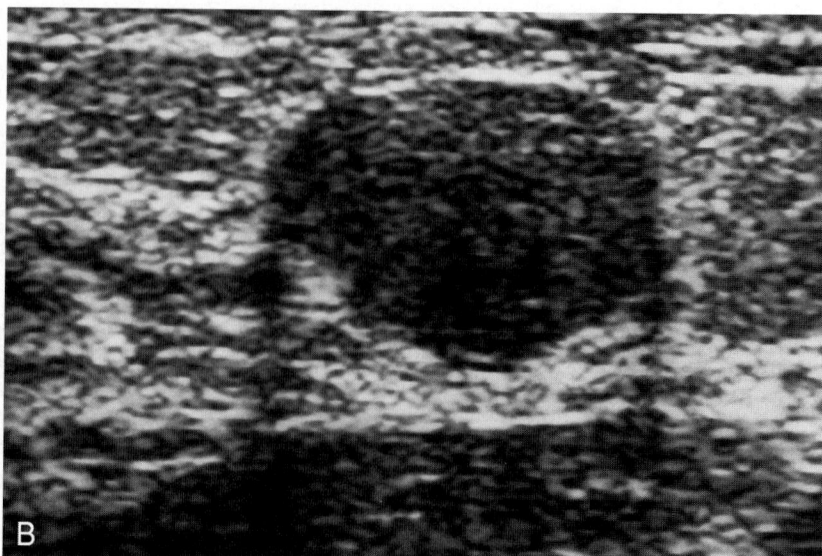

Figure 21.13. Fibroadenoma. A. MLO view of a 1.8-cm partially well defined mass (*arrow*). **B.** US demonstrates a solid hypoechoic mass with a macrolobulated well-defined margin.

MHz) US transducer is used in a targeted examination of the mass in question. On sonography, cysts are round or oval, smooth-walled, anechoic, and produce enhanced through transmission of sound. They can frequently be deformed with gentle pressure from the transducer. It is essential that the focal zone and gain of the US unit be optimally adjusted for the lesion so that cysts can be accurately diagnosed sonographically. The cyst must be thoroughly examined in two projections to rule out any irregularities or masses emanating from the walls.

Fibrosis is another manifestation of fibrocystic change that can be seen mammographically. It can be quite focal, giving it the appearance of a well-defined mass on the films. Such areas of focal fibrosis may also present with ill-defined borders, making them difficult to differentiate from carcinomas.

Fibroadenomas are the most common well-defined solid masses seen on mammography (Fig. 21.13). They are homogenous but frequently show large, coarse calcifications. They may have a lobulated contour, but there are usually only a few large lobulations. If a fibroadenoma is not calcified, it cannot be distinguished from a cyst by mammography. Sonography will allow characterization of fibroadenomas as solid hypoechoic masses. The peak age of patients with clinically detected fibroadenomas is 20 to 30 years; however, fibroadenomas are seen into the eighth decade. They rarely appear or grow after menopause.

Primary breast malignancies to be considered when a well-defined density is visualized on mammography are *infiltrating duct carcinoma, papillary carcinoma, mucinous carcinoma,* and *medullary carcinoma.*

Lymphoma, either primary or metastatic, may also present as a well-circumscribed mass.

Metastatic disease to the breast from other sources may present as a well-circumscribed nodule. The most common primary cancer to produce breast metastases is melanoma, but a large variety of other primary sites have also been reported to metastasize to the breast. When these malignancies are encountered, magnification compression views of the abnormality often demonstrate some irregularity to the contour of the mass (Fig. 21.14).

DENSITY

Density is relevant to analysis of mammographically detected masses when these masses contain lucent areas indicative of fat. Breast masses that clearly contain fat are benign. The assessment of density in homogeneous nonfatty masses is not useful in the prediction of benignity or malignancy.

Fat Density. Benign breast lesions that are purely fat density include oil cysts from fat necrosis, lipomas, and sometimes galactoceles. **Oil cysts** are generally the result of trauma (Fig. 21.15). They are round lucent lesions surrounded by a thin capsule; often they are multiple and can demonstrate rim calcifications. **Lipomas** are similar to oil cysts in appearance; they are also lucent with a surrounding capsule. The surrounding breast architecture may be distorted because of the mass effect of

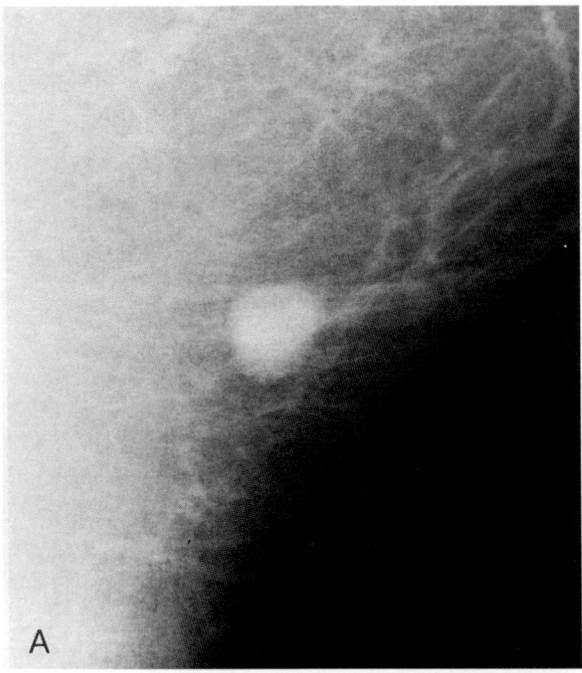

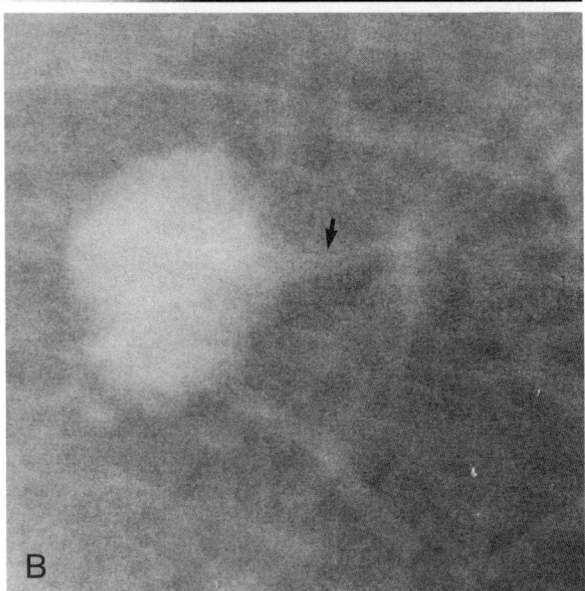

Figure 21.14. Infiltrating Duct Carcinoma. A. A well-circumscribed, 8-mm mass that had increased in size compared with a study done 1 year previously. **B.** Magnification view shows a spiculation anteriorly (*arrow*). Infiltrating duct carcinoma was proved at biopsy.

the lipoma. **Galactoceles** usually occur in lactating or recently lactating women and are probably the result of an obstructed duct. If the inspissated milk is of sufficient fat quantity, these lesions will appear lucent; they can also be of mixed fat or water density.

Mixed Fat and Water Density. Other benign masses that are mixed fat and water density are **hamartomas**, which are rare benign tumors, and intramammary lymph nodes. **Intramammary lymph nodes** are frequently seen on mammograms. They are generally located in the upper outer quadrant in the posterior three fourths of the breast parenchyma. They

normally contain a fatty center or a lucent notch, representing fat in the hilus of the node (Fig. 21.16). Fat-fluid levels can occasionally be seen on MLO mammograms in galactoceles and postsurgical hematomas.

LOCATION

Breast cancers can occur in any location within the breast. The location of a lesion is helpful in mammographic diagnosis in only two situations. The first occurs when the mammographer is considering an intramammary lymph node in the differential. The second occurs when a lesion can be localized to the skin..

Intramammary nodes visualized on mammograms are almost always located in the upper outer quadrant of the breast. They have been noted in other locations in autopsy series, and there are rare case reports of visualization of such nodes by mammography in other locations in the breast.

Skin Lesions. If a lesion is located only on the skin, it does not represent a breast carcinoma. Frequently, however, skin lesions project over the parenchyma and can appear to be within the breast. Such lesions are usually recognizable by air trapping around the edges or in the interstices. This air trapping can produce a dark halo around one edge (Fig. 21.17). Air trapping will not be evident with flat, pigmented skin lesions or sebaceous cysts.

It is helpful to examine the patient and place a ra-

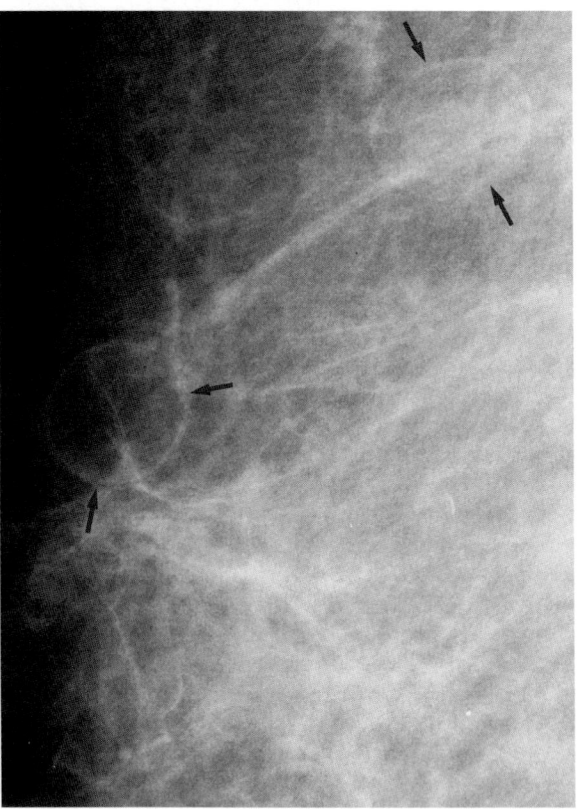

Figure 21.15. Oil Cysts. Multiple lucent masses with thin capsules (*arrows*) are characteristic of oil cysts. The patient had suffered trauma to the breast.

Figure 21.16. Intramammary Lymph Node. Intramammary lymph node with a characteristic lucent center (*arrow*) and well-circumscribed margins. The node was located in the upper outer quadrant.

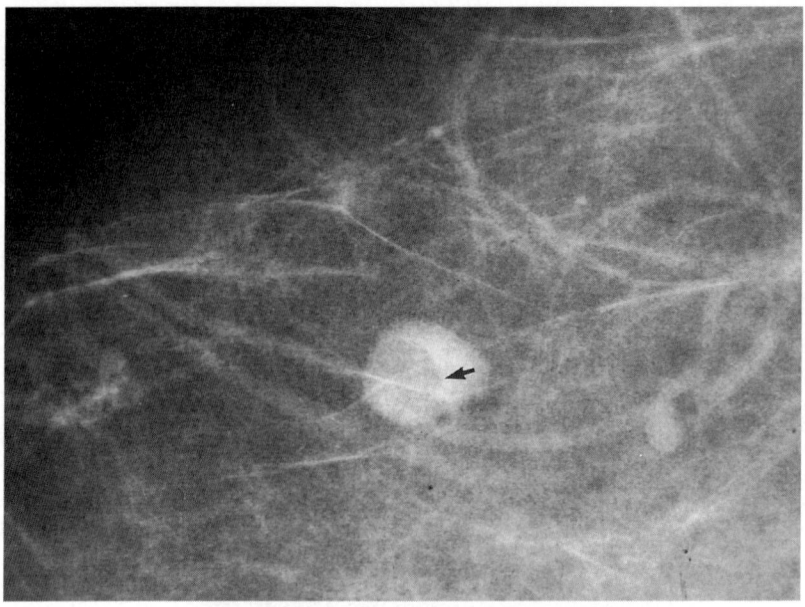

diopaque marker on any skin lesions or possible sebaceous cysts. The technologist can then perform a repeat film in the projection that the lesion was visualized. If necessary, this view can be followed by a tangential view to demonstrate that the lesion is located in the skin.

SIZE

By itself, the size of a mammographically discovered mass is not particularly helpful in determining its etiology. A spiculated or ill-defined mass should undergo biopsy no matter what its size. When the mammographer is dealing with a circumscribed mass that has a much lower chance of being malignant, size may play a role in determining the next step in the workup. US is not usually helpful when lesions are less than about 3–5 mm in size, particularly in fatty breasts. Frequently, patients with such lesions will be asked to return in 6 months for a follow-up study to assess for interval growth. If the lesion increases in size, further investigation with US and possible biopsy can be performed. After the first 6-month follow-up, stable lesions should be followed at yearly intervals for a minimum of 3 years.

Larger, clinically occult masses require both US to prove they are solid and magnification views to prove they are circumscribed before surveillance mammography is suggested. Some experts advocate a size upper limit of 1–1.5 cm for masses that are to undergo follow-up, but recent research (23) has shown that nonpalpable, circumscribed breast masses can be managed by periodic mammographic surveillance regardless of size. Generally, a 6 month follow-up of the affected breast is advocated; this is followed by a bilateral mammogram 6 months later and then annual mammography for at least 3 years to document stability.

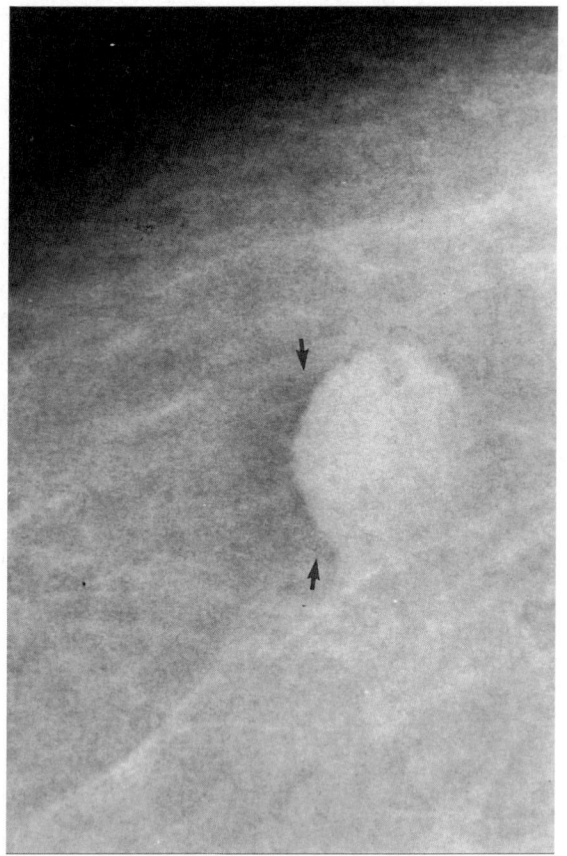

Figure 21.17. Skin Nevus. The dark halo produced around one edge is the result of air trapping (*arrows*).

NUMBER OF MASSES

Multiple Masses. In many cases, multiple well-defined round masses will be seen on mammography. When evident, such masses are also frequently bilateral. Multiple, bilateral round masses are usually benign.

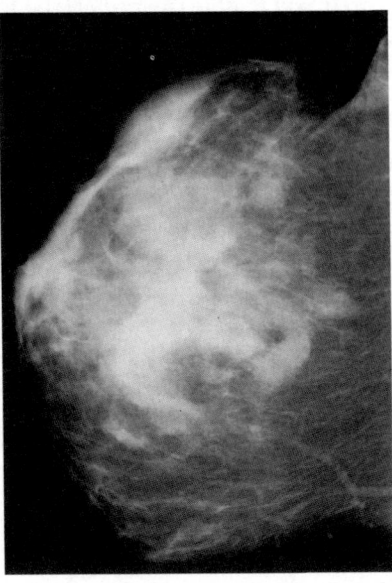 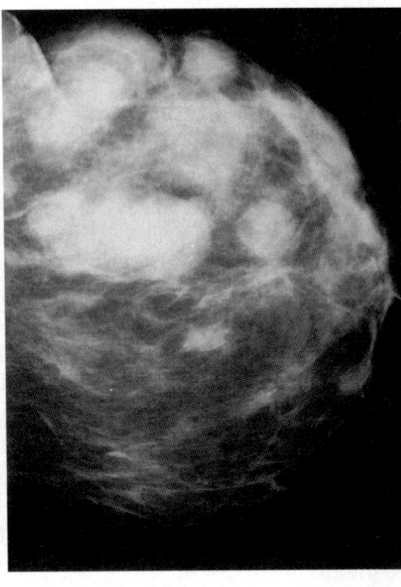

Figure 21.18. Multiple Benign Masses. Bilateral CC views show multiple large round masses in both breasts. The patient was asymptomatic. Differential diagnosis was cysts or fibroadenomas.

They most often represent **cysts** or **fibroadenomas**, although **multiple papillomas** can also present in this way (Fig. 21.18). In patients with a history of previous malignancy, **metastasis** may also be considered, although metastatic disease is much more commonly unifocal.

All lesions should be evaluated carefully. Benign and malignant lesions can coexist in the same breast. A lesion with a different, suspicious morphology should prompt a biopsy.

When evaluating the patient with similar-appearing multiple, bilateral, rounded breast masses, it is not generally advisable to use US. US is confusing and frequently demonstrates hypoechoic areas that, although disconcerting to the radiologist, do not prove to be malignant. **Multifocal primary breast cancers** generally present as obvious, ill-defined or stellate lesions that are suspicious in appearance (Fig. 21.19).

Calcifications

Clustered, pleomorphic microcalcifications, with or without an associated soft tissue mass, are a primary mammographic sign of breast cancer. Such calcifications are seen in more than half of all mammographically discovered cancers; about one third of all nonpalpable cancers are manifest by calcifications alone, without an associated mass (18).

The calcifications associated with malignancy are dystrophic; they are the result of abnormalities in the tissues. Some malignant calcifications occur in necrotic tumor debris; others are the result of calcification of stagnant secretions that are trapped in the cancer (24).

Calcifications are a frequent finding on mammographic examinations. In the majority of cases, such calcifications will turn out to be benign and their origin will be easily identifiable. There is, however, a significant overlap in the appearance of benign and malignant cal-

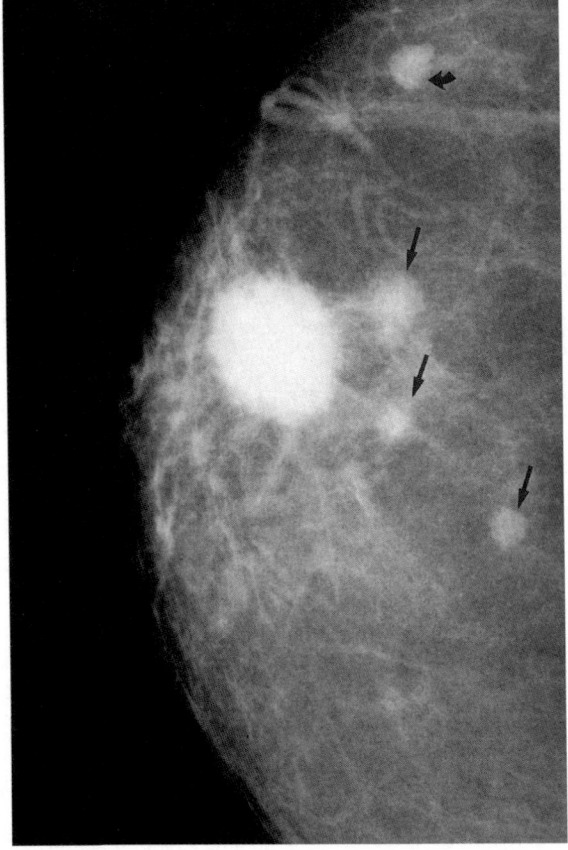

Figure 21.19. Multifocal Carcinoma. Craniocaudal View. The largest mass was palpable. The others were discovered by mammography (*straight arrows*). The more well-defined nodule (*curved arrow*) probably represented an intramammary lymph node.

cifications. Only 25–35% of all calcifications that undergo biopsy will prove to be malignant.

The importance of technically optimal mammography cannot be overstated when calcifications are being studied. The film exposure must be appropriate; an underexposed film can hide calcifications in a background of white breast tissue. Slight overpenetration of films is optimal for detection of calcifications. Magnification views will be extremely helpful for assessing the malignant potential of a group of calcifications.

Careful analysis of the form, size, distribution, and number of calcifications, as well as any association with

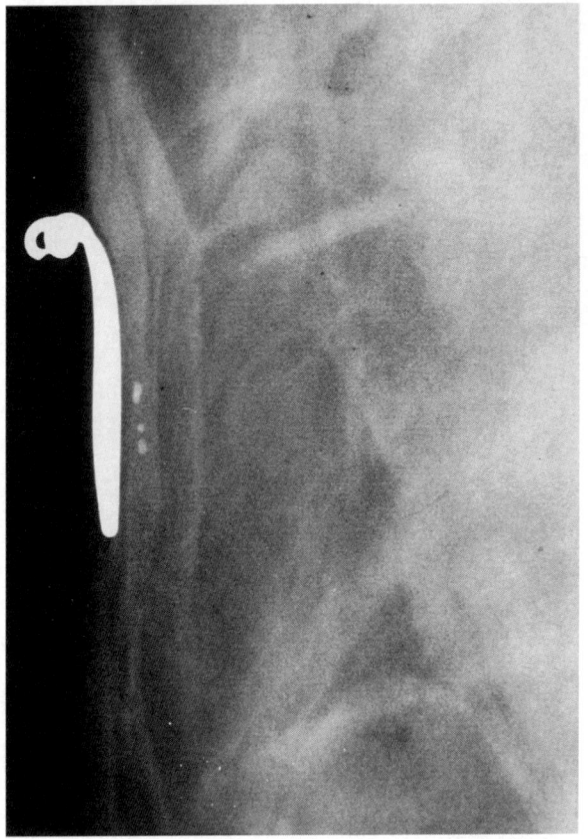

Figure 21.20. Skin Calcifications. Tangential view showing calcifications to be in the skin. A radiopaque marker had been placed on the skin at the site of the calcifications. This was done to facilitate positioning for the tangential view.

Figure 21.21. Eggshell Calcifications in Oil Cysts. These are large calcifications with lucent centers that are benign.

other soft tissue structures, will enable the radiologist to determine which calcifications are unequivocally benign and which require biopsy or follow-up studies.

FORM

Benign Calcifications. Some shapes of calcifications can be easily identified as benign. Any calcification with a lucent center should not cause concern. Calcifications with lucent centers are often located in the skin. A skin marker can be placed over the calcifications, and a subsequent tangential view can be taken to confirm their location in the skin (Fig. 21.20). Calcifications with lucent centers are also seen as a result of fat necrosis. Such calcifications can be smooth and round or they can be eggshell-type calcifications in the walls of an oil cyst (Fig. 21.21).

Calcifications that layer into a curvilinear or linear shape on 90° lateral films, yet appear as smudged clusters on CC views, are also representative of a benign process (Fig. 21.22). Such calcifications represent sedimented calcium ("milk of calcium") within the fluid of tiny breast cysts. Similar benign calcifications can also be seen within larger cysts and oil cysts. Sedimented calcium is a common finding in approximately 5% of women who present for mammography.

Other benign calcifications that are easily recognizable by their form include arterial calcifications, the calcifications in a degenerating fibroadenoma, and calcifications associated with secretory disease. Arterial calcifications generally present as tubular parallel lines of calcium (Fig. 21.23). Occasionally, early arterial calcification can present a diagnostic problem, but this can usually be resolved by looking for soft tissue of the vessel in association with the calcification. Magnification in multiple projections can be helpful (Fig. 21.24).

Fibroadenomas can calcify in various patterns. Sometimes, the calcifications are indeterminate, but the

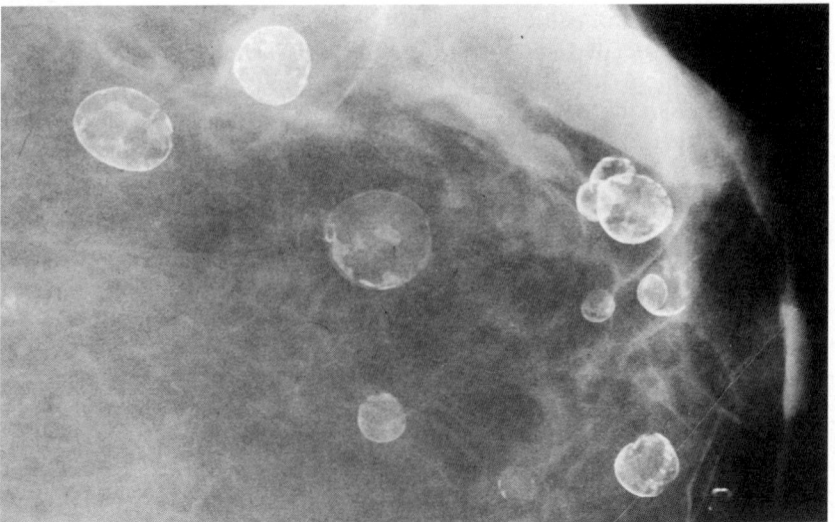

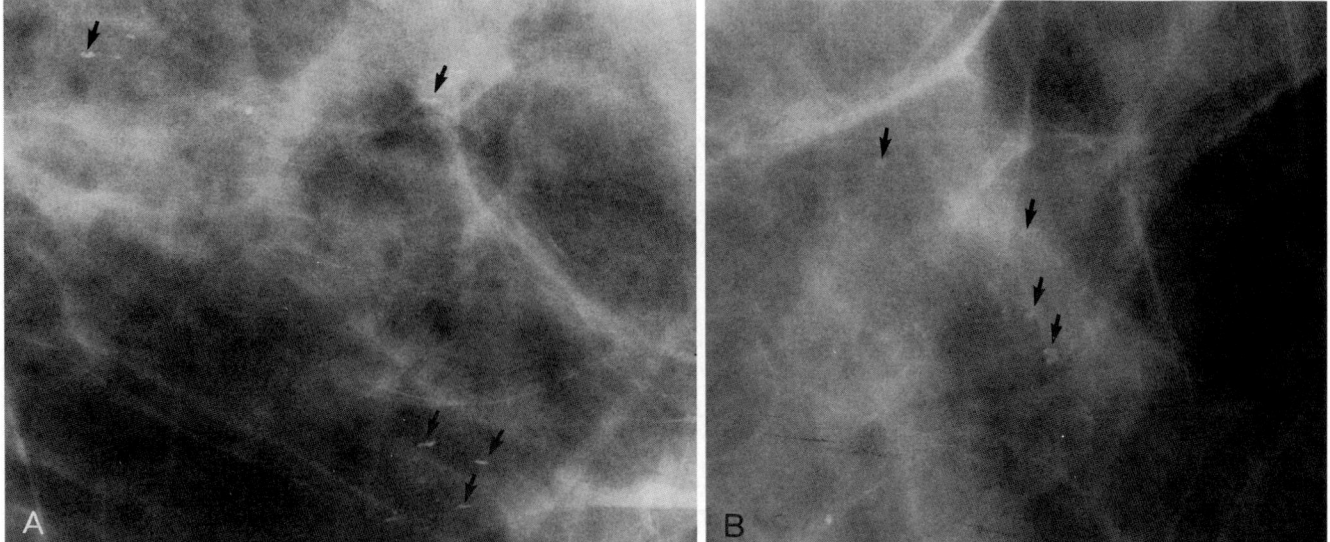

Figure 21.22. Milk of Calcium in Breast Cysts. A. Magnification of a 90° lateral mammogram showing diffuse linear calcifications (*arrows*). **B.** CC magnification view of the same area showing smudged, rounded calcifications (*arrows*). This change in configuration between views is typical of sedimented calcium. The calcium is layering in the bottom of microcysts, so it appears as a line or meniscus when viewed from the side in the lateral projection. When viewed from the top, these calcifications simply appear smudged and rounded.

Figure 21.23. Arterial Calcifications. Arterial calcifications in the breast are identified by their location in the wall of a tortuous vessel.

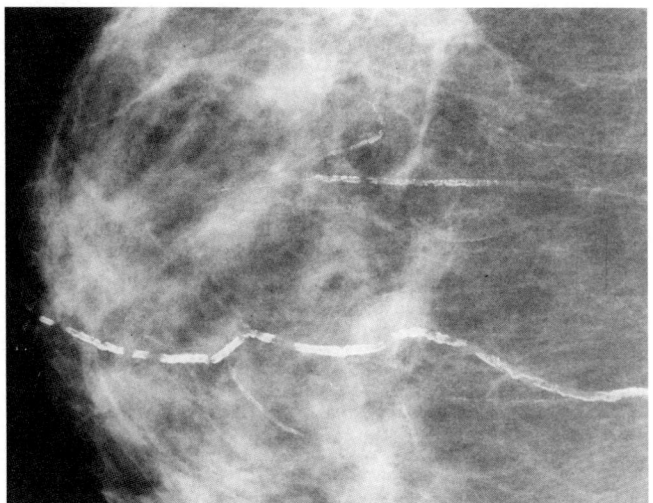

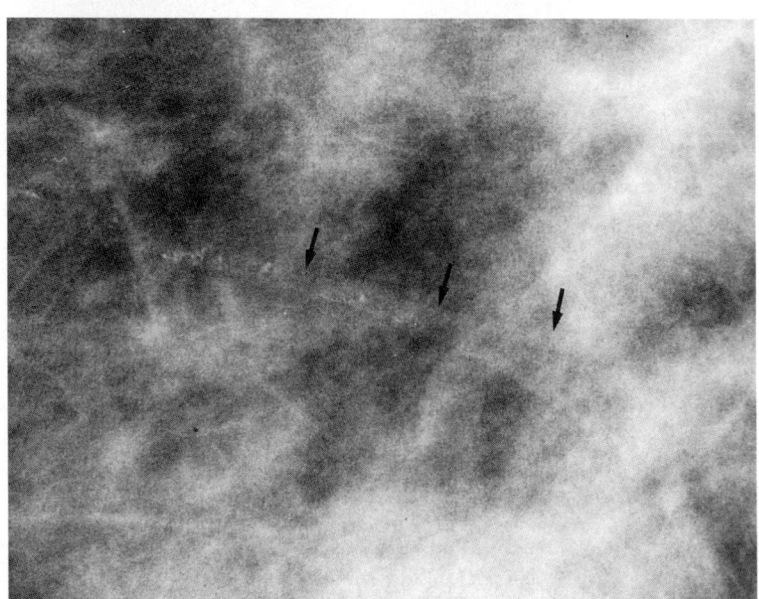

Figure 21.24. Early Arterial Calcification. Magnification view. The calcification can be seen clearly in the walls of an artery (*arrows*). The soft tissue of the artery was difficult to appreciate on the conventional views.

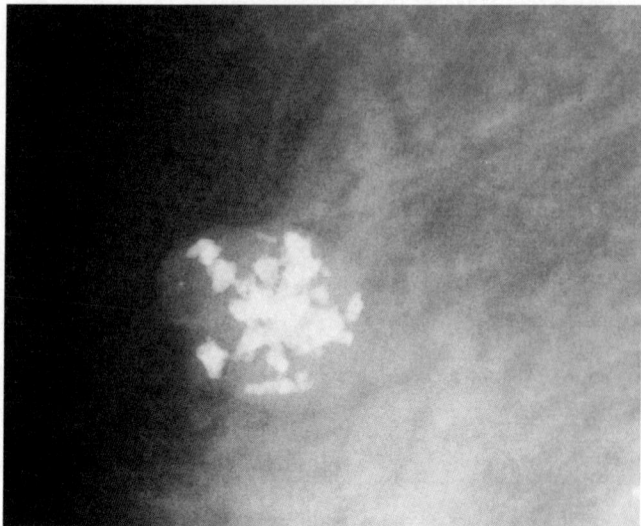

Figure 21.25. Fibroadenoma. Typical large, coarse, irregular calcifications are seen in a fibroadenoma.

classic calcifications associated with an atrophic fibroadenoma are large, coarse, and irregular in shape (Fig. 21.25).

Secretory Disease. The calcifications associated with secretory disease are smooth, long, thick linear calcifications that radiate toward the nipple in a generally orderly pattern (Fig. 21.26). These calcifications are located in ectatic ducts. When periductal inflammation has occurred, these calcifications may appear more lucent centrally because calcium is deposited in the tissues adjacent to the ducts.

Malignant calcifications vary in shape and size (Fig. 21.27). The margins of the calcifications are jagged and irregular. Malignant calcifications are often branching. Ductal carcinoma in situ (DCIS), or noninvasive breast cancer, is most often detected mammographically as a result of such calcifications. Groups of pleomorphic calcifications that appear more linear of "dot–dash" in appearance are more commonly associated with the comedocarcinoma type of intraductal carcinomas (Fig. 21.28). The cribriform and micropapillary types are often manifest by more punctate- or granular-appearing calcifications. The morphology of the calcification cannot be used to predict the subtype of DCIS because there is considerable overlap in the forms of the calcification associated with each subtype; frequently, multiple DCIS subtypes exist together in the same lesion. In the comedocarcinomas, the calcifications can be an approximate indication of the size of the tumor, although the extent of disease is often greater than mammographically predicted. In the noncomedo varieties, correlation is even poorer. The biologic behavior of these subtypes also differs; comedocarcinomas are the most likely to recur (25).

Pleomorphic microcalcifications in association with a malignant soft tissue mass can also indicate areas of extensive intraductal component within or adjacent to the invasive tumor. It is especially important to recognize malignant calcifications occurring in tissues surrounding invasive cancers so that they can be excised with the invasive tumor. Such extensive intraductal component-positive cancers also have a greater tendency to recur.

Indeterminate Calcifications. Morphologically indeterminate calcifications account for the majority of mammographically generated biopsies of calcifications (Fig. 21.29). Such calcifications are most often associated with fibrocystic change. Diagnoses included under the general category of fibrocystic disease are fibrosis adenosis, sclerosing adenosis, epithelial hyperplasia, cysts, apocrine metaplasia, and atypical hyperplasia. Occasionally, biopsy of indeterminate calcification will yield a diagnosis of lobular carcinoma in situ (LCIS), also called lobular neoplasia. Although not an invasive cancer, LCIS places a woman at higher risk for development of invasive breast cancer. Mammographically, LCIS has no distinct features. If it is clinically occult, it is most often found serendipitously adjacent to a focus of mammographically indeterminate, but histologically benign, calcifications.

DISTRIBUTION

Calcifications that are widely scattered and seen bilaterally are usually indicative of a benign process, such as sclerosing adenosis or adenosis. Multiple, bilateral clusters of calcifications that appear morphologically similar are also usually benign. Careful analysis with a magnifying lens is essential in these cases so that a morphologically dissimilar cluster is not overlooked. Such calcifications should be thoroughly examined with magnification views.

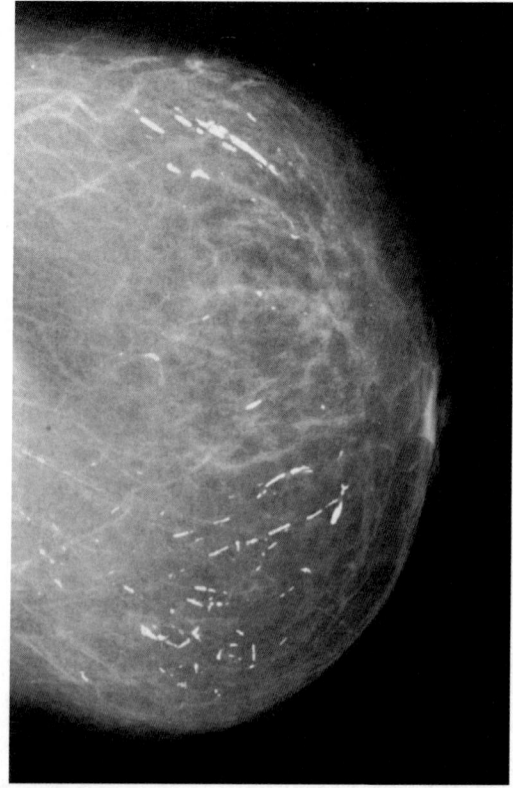

Figure 21.26. Secretory Calcifications. Craniocaudal view demonstrates long and thick calcifications in ectatic ducts that radiate toward the nipple.

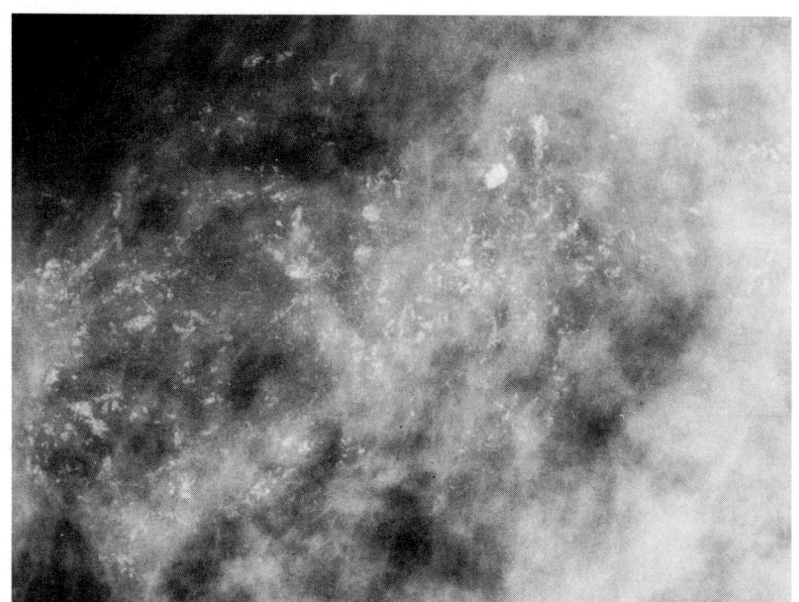

Figure 21.27. Malignant Calcifications. Magnification view of infiltrating ductal carcinoma. Note the irregular forms as well as the variety of sizes and shapes.

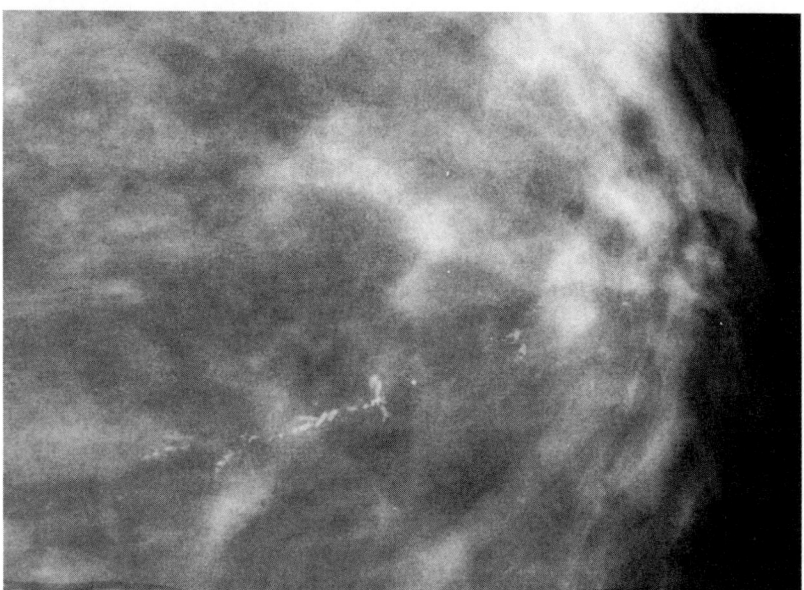

Figure 21.28. Malignant Calcifications. Dot–dash or "casting" calcifications of the comedo subtype of DCIS. Note the pleomorphism in the size and shape of the calcifications. (Reproduced with permission from Kline TS, Kline IK. Guides to aspiration biopsy of the breast. New York: Igaku-Shoin, Medical Publishers, 1989:201.)

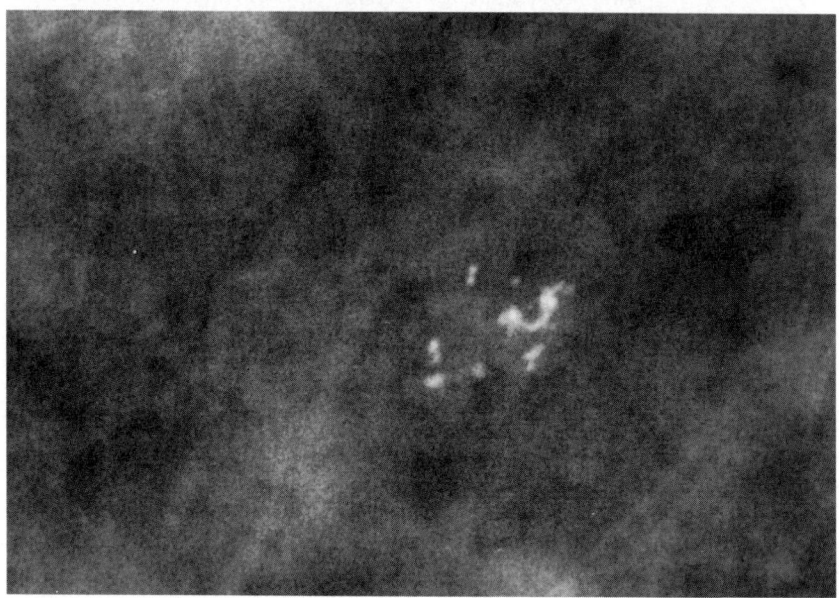

Figure 21.29. Indeterminate Calcifications. Magnification view of cluster of calcifications. There is some irregularity in shape and variation in size, but these calcifications were benign. They were associated with fibrocystic change.

Figure 21.30. Architectural Distortion Representing Breast Carcinoma. Note how the cancer pulls the surrounding parenchyma toward it (*arrows*).

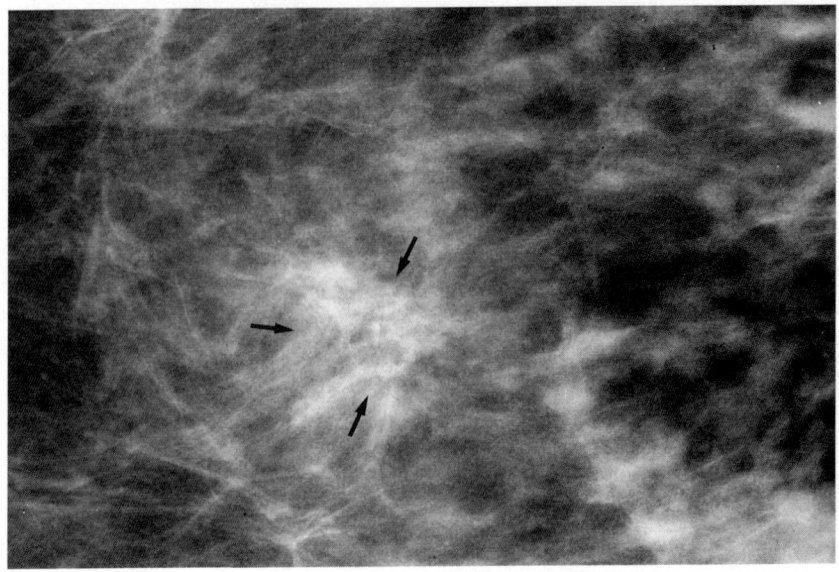

Malignant calcifications usually occur in tight clusters within a small volume of tissue, but DCIS can produce calcifications that encompass large areas of the breast. Calcifications that are morphologically suspicious or indeterminate and occupy a segment of the breast should undergo biopsy.

SIZE

Malignant calcifications are generally less than 0.5 mm in size. Because the calcifications associated with carcinoma are so small, they are frequently referred to as microcalcifications. Within a cluster, there will be a variety of sizes.

Benign calcifications are often larger. When benign disease produces clusters of calcifications, the size of these calcifications is usually similar.

NUMBER

Calcifications associated with malignancy are generally quite numerous. The greater the number of calcifications, the more likely they are associated with malignant disease. Establishing the lower limit of the number of calcifications in a cluster that would require biopsy is extremely difficult. Assessment of the morphology of these calcifications by magnification views will influence this decision more than the actual number of calcifications.

Architectural Distortion

Breast cancer is occasionally heralded by distortion in the normal architecture of the breast (Fig. 21.30). Differential diagnosis includes fat necrosis related to scarring from previous surgery and a complex sclerosing lesion, also known as radial scar. On close inspection, fat may be seen interspersed with fibrous elements in the center of fat necrosis or complex sclerosing lesions, but this appearance is not specific for benignity. Similar findings can be seen in malignant lesions. Biopsy is necessary for differentiation.

Increased Density of Breast Tissue

Hormone Therapy. Increasing parenchymal density of breast tissue can be bilateral or unilateral. Bilateral increased density is usually the result of estrogen replacement therapy in postmenopausal women. Such hormone therapy can give the breasts a more glandular, premenopausal appearance. Intrinsic hormonal fluctuations in premenopausal, pregnant, or lactating women may cause similar changes in the density of the breasts. Hormonally related changes in breast density are not associated with skin thickening.

Inflammatory Carcinoma. A unilateral increase in breast density with associated skin thickening may result from several processes. The most ominous of these is inflammatory carcinoma of the breast (Fig. 21.31). Clinically, this disease is manifest by a warm, erythematous, firm, tender breast. Histologically, the dermal lymphatics are diffusely involved. Mammographically, a focal mass may be seen within the dense tissue, but often the breast appears homogeneously dense. Inflammatory carcinoma of the breast is a locally advanced disease that carries a poor prognosis.

Radiation Therapy. A unilateral increase in parenchymal density with skin thickening can also be seen in patients who have undergone radiation therapy to the breast. Radiation changes are most pronounced during the first 6 months following therapy. They usually resolve gradually during a period of years.

Diffuse mastitis can produce a generalized skin thickening and increase in breast density. Clinical differentiation from inflammatory carcinoma is usually possible.

Obstruction to the lymphatic or venous drainage from metastatic disease, surgical removal, or thrombosis can produce a unilateral increase in breast density with skin thickening resulting from edema. The anasarca associated with congestive heart failure, renal failure, cirrhosis, or hypoalbuminemia most often presents as bilateral increased breast density with skin thickening; however, asymmetrical involvement of the breasts can occur.

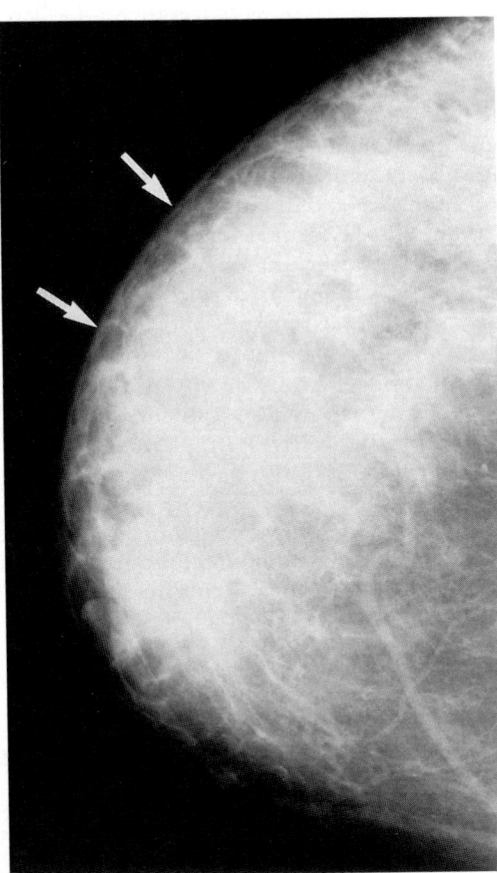

Figure 21.31. Inflammatory Carcinoma. Craniocaudal view demonstrates a diffuse increase in parenchymal density, along with skin thickening laterally (*arrows*).

Correlation of physical examination findings and history will usually allow differentiation of the various causes of an increase in breast density.

Axillary Adenopathy

Axillary lymph nodes are frequently visualized on the MLO mammogram. Normally, they are less than 2 cm in size and have lucent centers or notches resulting from fat in the hilum. Fatty infiltration of the nodes themselves can cause lucent enlargement and replacement.

Pathologic axillary nodes are homogeneously dense and enlarged. A variety of processes can result in replacement of normal nodal architecture. Malignant involvement of axillary nodes can be the result of primary breast cancer, metastatic disease, or lymphoma (Fig. 21.32). Axillary nodes can also become pathologically enlarged because of inflammation. Patients with rheumatoid arthritis, systemic lupus erythematosus, scleroderma, and psoriasis may also have axillary adenopathy.

Coarse calcifications in axillary nodes may reflect granulomatous disease. Microcalcifications are occasionally seen in nodes involved with metastatic breast cancer. Gold deposits, seen in patients being treated for rheumatoid arthritis, are occasionally seen in axillary nodes and may be confused with calcifications.

The Augmented Breast

More than 1.5 million women in the United States have undergone augmentation mammoplasty. Imaging of the augmented breast poses unique challenges. Special techniques must be used both to screen for breast cancer and to evaluate the patient for possible complications related to the implant.

Various types of implants have been used in augmentation procedures. They include silicone envelopes filled with saline or with viscous silicone gel, as well as double-lumen implants containing an inner core of silicone gel surrounded by an outer envelope filled with saline. Silicone is more radiopaque than saline, although neither allows adequate visualization of immediately surrounding tissue.

Implants can be placed either anterior (prepectoral) or posterior (subpectoral) to the pectoralis muscle. A fibrous capsule develops around the implant. Patients having prepectoral implants are subject to a greater risk of fibrous and calcific contractures around the implant. Such contractures are not only painful and deforming, but they also make mammography more difficult.

Screening mammography in the woman with implants requires the use of at least two extra views of each breast. Standard MLO and CC views are performed with

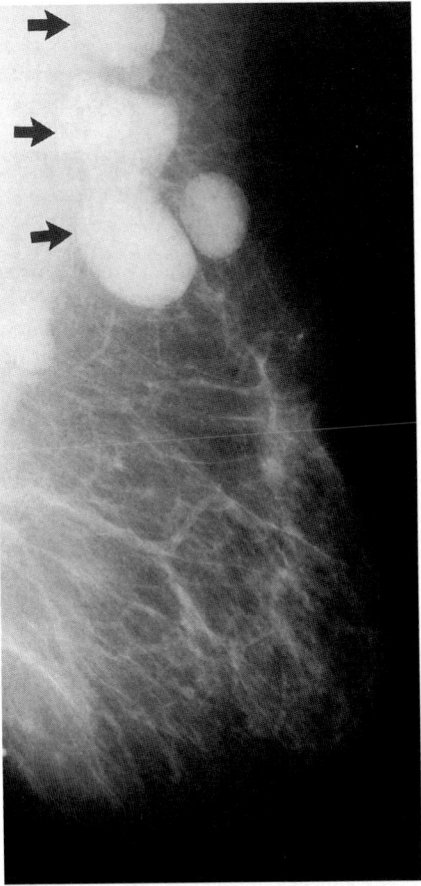

Figure 21.32. Lymphoma. Hodgkin's disease involves the axillary lymph nodes. The nodes are homogeneous, dense, and enlarged (*arrows*).

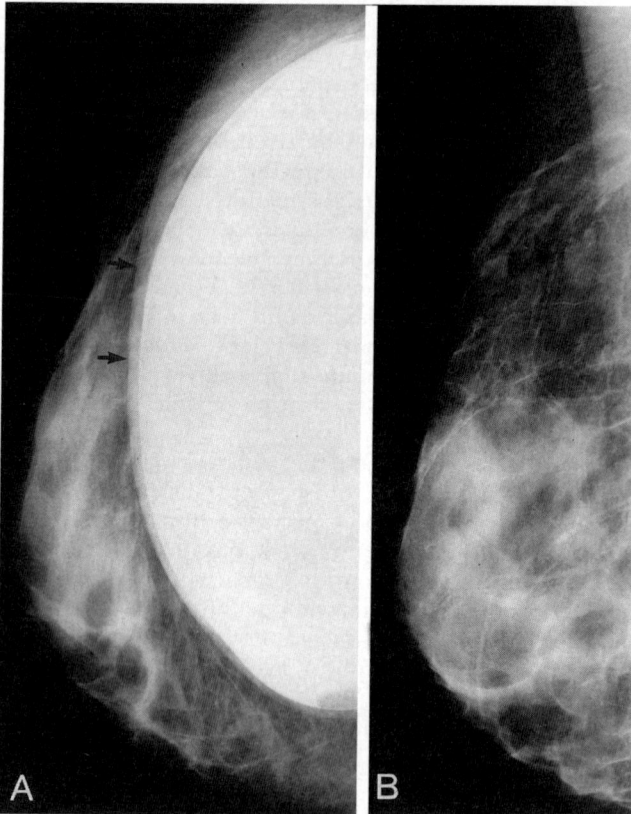

Figure 21.33. Breast Implants. A. Standard MLO view of a patient with a subpectoral silicone implant. Note the pectoralis muscle (*arrows*) anterior to the implant. **B.** Mediolateral oblique implant displacement view on the same patient. The implant has been displaced posteriorly, out of view, while the compression has been applied anteriorly.

moderate compression. Then the implants are displaced posteriorly against the chest wall while the breast tissue is pulled anteriorly and more vigorously compressed (Fig. 21.33). The compression paddle keeps the implant from migrating into the field of view. Greater compression of anterior tissues allows more optimal imaging (Fig. 21.34). Both MLO and CC views are repeated using this technique. These modified views are called implant displacement views (26).

Implant displacement views are more difficult to accomplish in patients with prepectoral implants with associated capsular contractures around the implant. The implants are not easily displaced, and so less of the anterior breast tissue is depicted on the modified views. In such cases, a 90° lateral view may also be helpful in screening.

Although some breast tissue may be obscured in patients with implants, these women, when in the appropriate age groups, deserve the same careful screening examinations at the same intervals as patients without implants. The indeterminate mammogram in a patient with implants should be evaluated in a manner similar to that in a patient without implants.

Women who have undergone augmentation mammoplasty may also present with abnormalities related to

their implants. These include capsular contractures, herniations of the implant through rents in the capsules, implant rupture with free (extracapsular rupture) or contained (intracapsular rupture) silicone, and deflation of saline implants. Many patients will present for breast imaging subsequent to noticing a change in implant contour or size (Fig. 21.35). Mammography is generally the first examination performed if the woman is older than the age of 30; however, mammography is not useful in the detection of intracapsular silicone implant ruptures because the silicone is contained within the fibrous capsule that has developed around the implant. Extracapsular silicone implant ruptures can sometimes be detected by mammography, but often the free silicone is obscured by the overlying implant or is in an area of the breast of chest wall not imaged on the mammogram (27).

Other imaging modalities can be used for the assessment of implant complications. MR is the most accurate in identifying silicone implant rupture and in localizing free silicone (Figs. 21.36, 21.37) (28). US is also used to detect implant rupture but has a lower sensitivity (70%) than does MR (94%) (29). Specificity with both US and

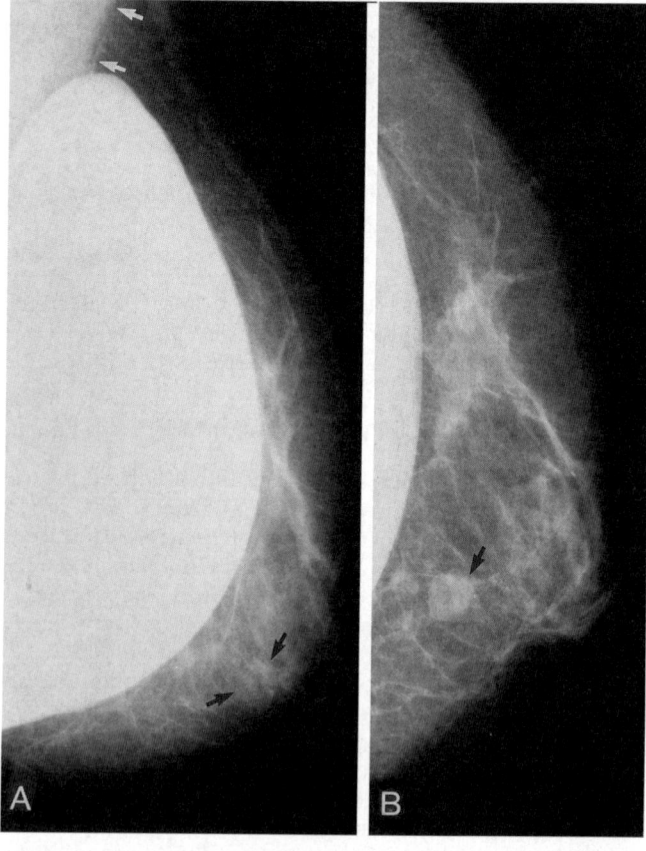

Figure 21.34. Infiltrating Duct Carcinoma. A. Standard MLO view in a patient with prepectoral silicone implants. Note the pectoralis muscle (*white arrows*) extending posterior to the implant. A poorly defined 1-cm mass (*black arrows*) was noted in the subareolar tissues. **B.** MLO implant displacement view in the same patient. The subareolar mass (*black arrow*) is more clearly defined because of greater compression of the tissues anterior to the implant. Histologic examination of the mass showed infiltrating duct carcinoma.

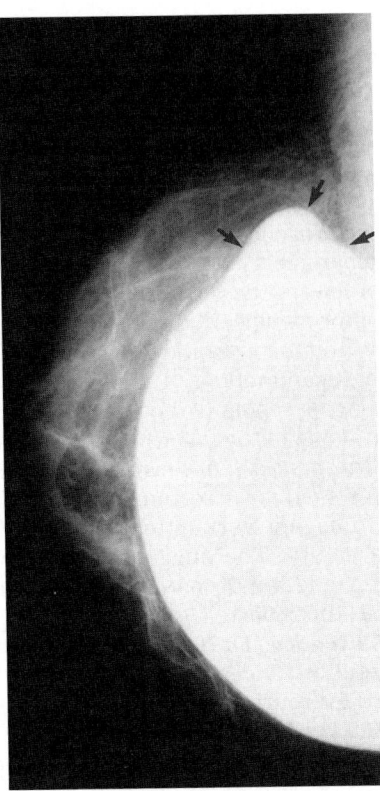

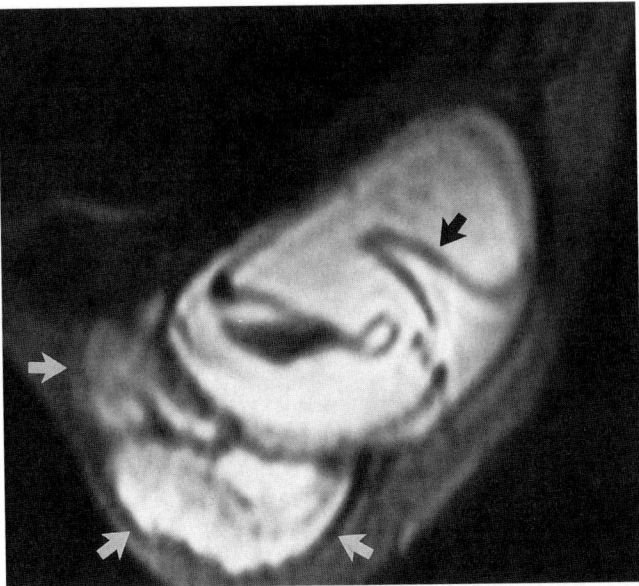

Figure 21.37. MR of an Extracapsular Silicone Implant Rupture. Axial T2-weighted, fat suppressed, image shows free silicone (*white arrows*) in the anteromedial breast tissue. The collapsed implant shell (*black arrow*) is seen within the silicone that remains within the fibrous capsule surrounding the implant.

Figure 21.35. Ruptured Implant. Standard MLO view of a patient with prepectoral silicone implants. The patient had noted a new mass superolaterally in her breast. The mammogram shows an extracapsular rupture with silicone outside the implant capsule (*arrows*) that corresponded to the palpable abnormality.

MR are similar (92–97%). The success of US in the assessment of implant integrity greatly depends on the operator; an experienced radiologist must scan the breasts in a methodical manner.

The Male Breast

The most common indication for breast imaging in men is a palpable asymmetrical thickening or mass. Gynecomastia is usually the cause. Breast cancer is rare, but it can occur.

Normal male breast appears on mammography as a mound of subcutaneous fat without glandular tissue (Fig. 21.38). The nipple is small.

Gynecomastia generally appears as a triangular or flame-shaped area of subareolar glandular tissue that points toward the nipple. Fat is interspersed with parenchymal elements. A gradual merging of the more glandular elements with the fat occurs at the deep margin (Fig. 21.39). Gynecomastia can be unilateral or bilateral. When bilateral, it is most frequently asymmetrical. Many causes have been reported, including ingestion of a variety of drugs, such as reserpine, cardiac glycosides, cimetidine, and thiazides, as well as marijuana. Testicular, adrenal, and pituitary tumors are associated with gynecomastia. Chronic hepatic disease, by virtue of reduced ability to clear endogenous estrogens, can also cause male breast enlargement.

Male breast cancer is mammographically similar to that found in women. It can have a variety of appearances, including an ill-defined, spiculated, or circumscribed mass (Fig. 21.40). Microcalcifications can occur.

Comparison with Previous Films

The importance of comparing current mammograms with previous films cannot be overstated. In one series, de-

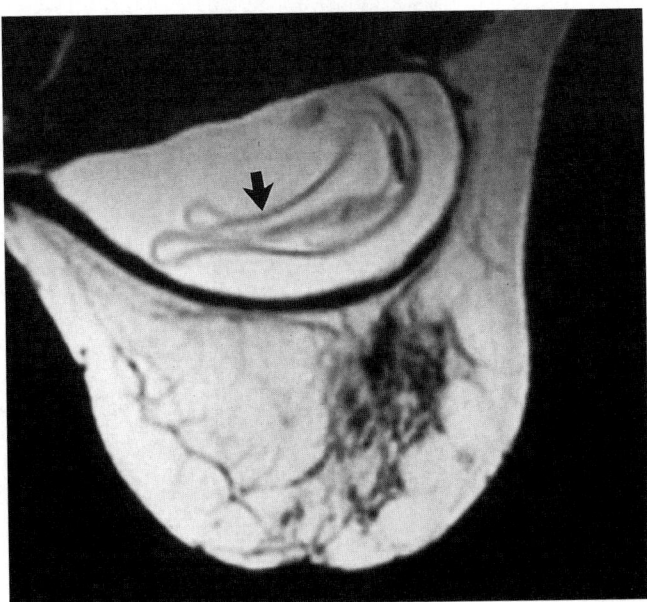

Figure 21.36. MR of Intracapsular Silicone Implant Rupture. Axial T2-weighted fast spin echo image shows multiple low intensity curvilinear lines within the implant (*arrow*), which represent the collapsed implant shell (linguine sign). There is no extracapsular silicone, and the mammogram showed a normal appearing implant.

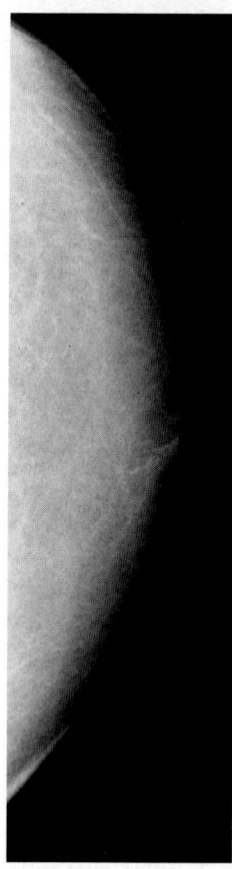

Figure 21.38. Male Breast. Relatively normal male breast, which is a mound of subcutaneous fat. Note the lack of glandular tissue.

veloping densities accounted for 6% of nonpalpable breast carcinomas (17). Comparison with previous films will allow detection of subtle changes, in turn suggesting the need for further evaluation of such areas at an earlier time than might be possible if no comparison had been made (Fig. 21.41). It must be remembered that benign masses may appear or enlarge over time. In fact, in the majority of cases, interval change will be benign, but such changes should be fully evaluated by correlation with the history and physical examination, as well as the use of ancillary testing methods such as US, aspiration, and biopsy.

Malignant masses that were stable in size for up to 4.5 years have been reported. Although such a long period of stability is unusual, these reports emphasize the need for suspicious-appearing lesions to undergo biopsy regardless of their apparent lack of change in size on serial films. Such lesions may have been overlooked or misinterpreted on a previous study.

Any new microcalcifications or increase in number of such calcifications deserve special consideration. Appropriate workup with magnification views will allow analysis of the morphology of such calcifications. Any calcifications that are not clearly benign deserve biopsy.

THE RADIOLOGIC REPORT

The radiologic report should be clear and concise. The American College of Radiology has developed a standard-

ized format and terminology called the Breast Imaging Reporting and Data System (BI-RADS) (30). All mammography reports should begin with description of the overall breast composition so that the referring clinician can gauge the sensitivity of the mammographic examination. The breast should be characterized as *a)* composed almost entirely of fat, *b)* containing scattered fibroglandular densities, *c)* heterogeneously dense, which may lower the sensitivity of mammography, or *d)* extremely dense breast tissue, which lowers the sensitivity of mammography. A description of the significant findings on the mammogram should follow, and there should be comparison to any previous available examinations. The most important part of the breast imaging report is the final assessment, which should fall into one of the following six categories:

BI-RADS Category (0): **Assessment incomplete.** This category is reserved for screening examinations that require further imaging workup to fully characterize a potential abnormality. The suggested additional studies such as US or additional mammographic views should be specified in the report.

BI-RADS Category (1): **Negative.** No significant findings are present on a negative mammogram. The patient should return for routine screening.

BI-RADS Category (2): **Benign finding.** There is a benign finding such as a lipoma, oil cyst, galactocele, in-

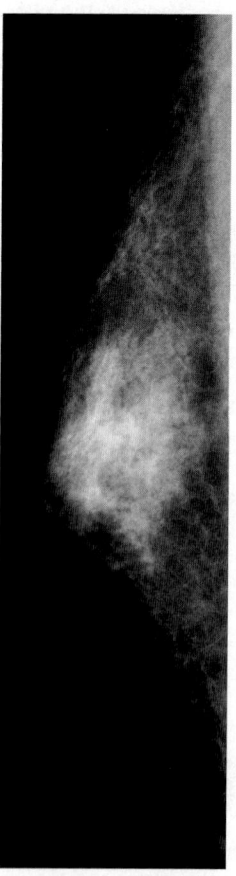

Figure 21.39. Gynecomastia. MLO view of a man with breast enlargement. Glandular tissue is seen in the subareolar area. This tissue gradually intersperses with the fat and does not appear as a mass.

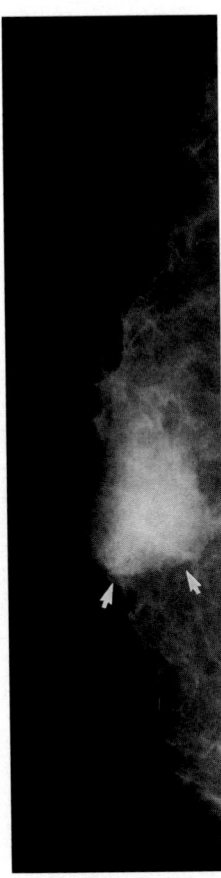

Figure 21.40. Male Breast Cancer. MLO view of the breast in a male. The mass has a defined interface with the surrounding fat (*arrows*). (Courtesy of Patricia Bell, MD, Auburn, California.)

tramammary lymph node, hamartoma, fibroadenoma, cyst, scattered round calcifications of adenosis, arterial calcifications, sedimented calcium within microcysts, secretory calcifications, duct ectasia, skin calcifications, or multiple bilateral well-circumscribed masses representing cysts or fibroadenomas. These patients should return for routine screening.

***BI-RADS Category (3):* Probably benign.** The findings that should be included in this category are circumscribed masses, asymmetrical parenchymal densities that are not associated with palpable masses and, occasionally, clusters of smooth, round similar-appearing microcalcifications. The probability that such abnormalities represent cancer is less than 2% (31); therefore, most mammographers recommend a plan of careful follow-up. The first follow-up mammogram of the affected breast should be performed 6 months after discovery of the abnormality. If the abnormality is stable, a bilateral study should be performed 6 months later and then a follow-up should occur at yearly intervals for a period of at least 3 years. Progression of a cancerous lesion depends on tumor biology and doubling time; hence, the necessity of a lengthy follow-up. Some cancers may grow slowly, and others may change rapidly.

***BI-RADS Category (4):* Suspicious abnormality.** Included in this category are lesions that are not classically malignant but are suspicious enough to warrant biopsy. The probability that such a lesion will represent malignancy is approximately 25–35% in most practices in the United States.

***BI-RADS Category (5):* Highly suggestive of malignancy.** These are lesions that have a high probability of being malignant and should undergo biopsy. Spiculated masses and pleomorphic clusters of calcifications are included in this category.

Clinicians must be cautioned that mammography has a false-negative rate of 9–16%; therefore, a negative mammogram should not preclude biopsy of a clinically suspicious mass.

INTERVENTIONAL PROCEDURES FOR NONPALPABLE LESIONS

Mammographically suspicious abnormalities require histologic or cytologic examination for definitive diagnosis. If the abnormality is clinically occult, an image-guided localization can be performed by the radiologist; this procedure is followed by an excisional biopsy. Although open surgical biopsy is the traditional method used for definitive diagnosis, percutaneous, image-directed aspiration or core biopsies performed in the radiology department are now an accepted alternative.

Localization of Occult Breast Lesions

If an excisional biopsy of a mammographically suspicious, but nonpalpable, abnormality is to be performed, a localization will be required so that the surgeon is accurately directed to the lesion. Many methods for localization have been described. In choosing a technique, the radiologist should decide which method will allow sufficient accuracy so that the lesion can be removed without sacrificing large volumes of breast tissue. Malignancy will be found in only 25–35% of all biopsies performed for mammographically suspicious abnormalities. Because the majority of biopsies will be benign, it is extremely important to preserve as much breast tissue as possible.

Localizations can be performed using needle-wire systems or dye injection. There are several commercially available needle-wire systems. All allow placement of a wire through an introducing needle that has been positioned in the breast at the site of the abnormality. The wires differ mainly in the configuration of the anchoring end.

Injection of blue dye is a less frequently used method of localization. A needle is placed at the site of the abnormality, and dye is injected. If there is a delay between the time of injection and surgery, diffusion of the dye through the tumors can occur, resulting in a biopsy specimen that may be larger than necessary. Methylene blue, formerly in common usage for localizations, also interferes with estrogen receptor analysis.

Most mammographic units are equipped with a compression paddle that contains either one large hole marked on the edge with a grid, or a series of smaller holes marked with letters or numbers. The seated patient is placed in the mammographic unit so that the le-

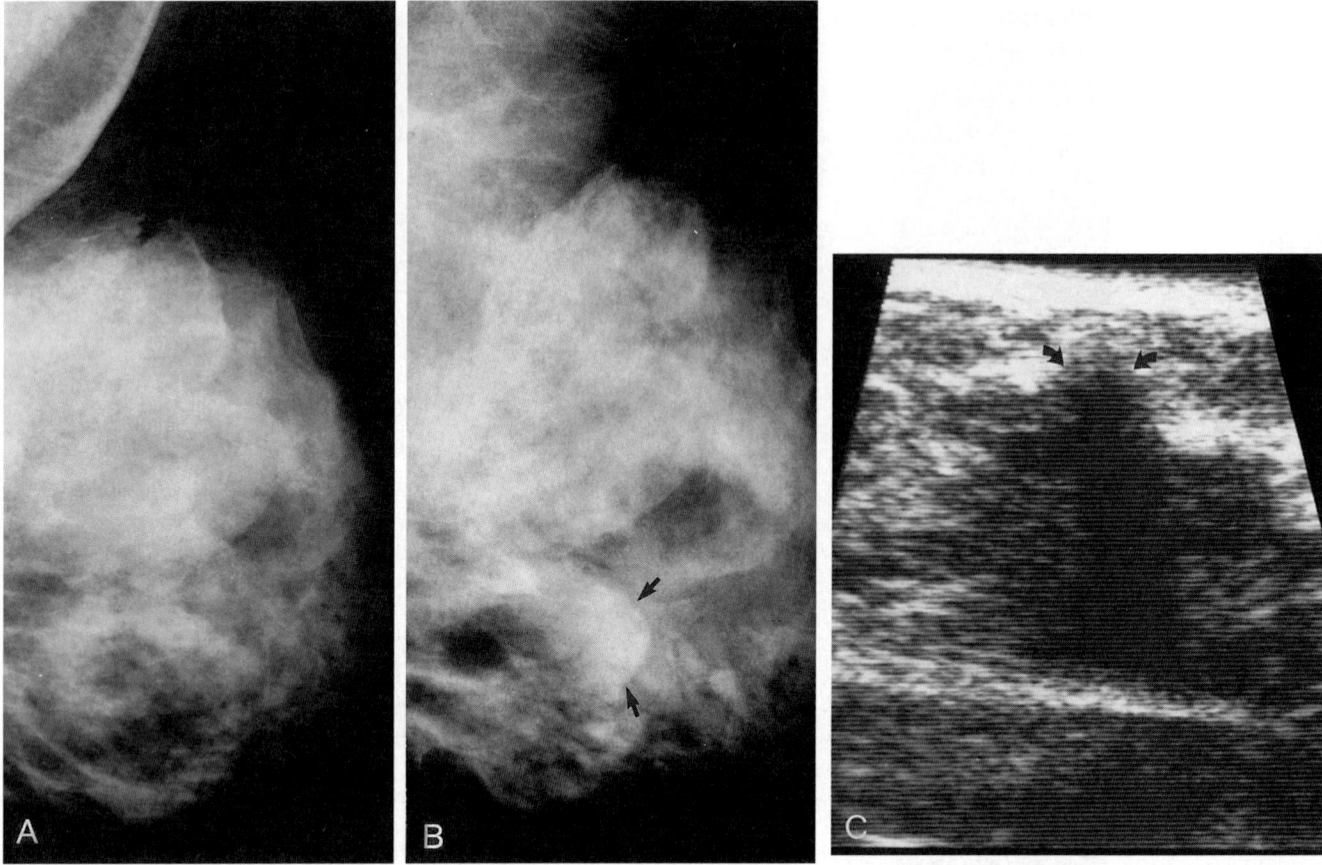

Figure 21.41. Infiltrating Duct Carcinoma. A. MLO mammogram shows dense mammary parenchyma but no evidence of malignancy. **B.** Mammogram 1 year later shows development of a subtle new mass (*arrows*). **C.** US of the mass shows a shadowing, solid lesion (*arrows*). Biopsy demonstrated infiltrating duct carcinoma. (Courtesy of Patricia Bell, MD, Auburn, California.)

sion to be localized is located under a hole in the compression plate. The breast is then filmed to determine the exact location of the abnormality. A needle is inserted parallel to the x-ray beam and through the abnormal area. The position of the needle with respect to the lesion is then checked by taking another film. If the needle position is satisfactory, the patient, with needle in place, is carefully removed from the mammography unit so that the tube can be rotated 90°. The patient is then positioned in the unit and compressed along an axis parallel to the needle. A film is taken to assess the depth of the needle tip with respect to the lesion. The needle must be in the lesion or deep to it in order to proceed. This ensures a fixed relationship between the localizer and the lesion. Once the depth of the needle tip is satisfactory, the wire can be inserted through the needle and the needle withdrawn, leaving the wire in place (Fig. 21.42). Alternatively, dye can be injected through the needle and then the needle can be withdrawn. The patient is then sent to the operating room for surgical biopsy (32).

Once the biopsy has been performed, the excised tissue should be sent for x-ray. This ensures that the mammographic abnormality has been removed. In a small number of cases (1–5%), localization will fail and the lesion will not be removed. In most of these cases, the localization will have to be repeated.

Most localizations are performed under mammo-

graphic guidance, but US can also be used to guide such procedures. The technique used is similar to that for US-guided percutaneous biopsy. A high-frequency transducer is placed over the lesion, and the needle is introduced obliquely or vertically under real-time monitoring. When the tip is seen in the lesion, the wire can be inserted or the dye injected. Wire position should be confirmed by mammography.

US is most useful in guiding a localization when the abnormality is seen well in one projection but is obscured by dense tissue in the second. It may also be useful when lesions are located in areas of the breast that are difficult to position within the hole in the localized compression paddle. US can only be used when the lesion can be visualized. Microcalcifications cannot be imaged, and not all soft tissue masses are well delineated by US.

Percutaneous Biopsy

Increasing use of mammographic screening has led to the discovery of greater numbers of potentially malignant but clinically occult breast lesions. In the past, excisional biopsy was the only method for definitive diagnosis, but the development of imaging guided percutaneous core biopsy of the breast now provides a more cost-effective alternative (33). Nearly all mammographically detected nonpalpable suspicious lesions are amenable to core biopsy either with stereotactic or US guidance.

Core biopsy has emerged as the preferred technique for diagnostic evaluation of nonpalpable mammographically detected lesions; it is superior to fine needle aspiration biopsy for the following reasons:

1. Histologic evaluation of core biopsy specimens can be performed by all pathologists, whereas cytologic diagnosis of fine needle aspirates requires that the pathologist have special expertise and training.
2. The amount of tissue obtained from core biopsies is usually sufficient for diagnosis; insufficient material for diagnosis is a frequent problem with fine needle aspiration.
3. Differentiation of invasive from noninvasive carcinomas is usually possible with core biopsy, whereas, it is not possible with fine needle aspiration cytology.

Indications for core biopsy are similar to those for surgical biopsy. A full breast imaging workup must be completed before core biopsy is recommended. Core biopsy should not be substituted for short interval follow-up of probably benign lesions, as this approach is not cost-effective and may induce increased anxiety in some

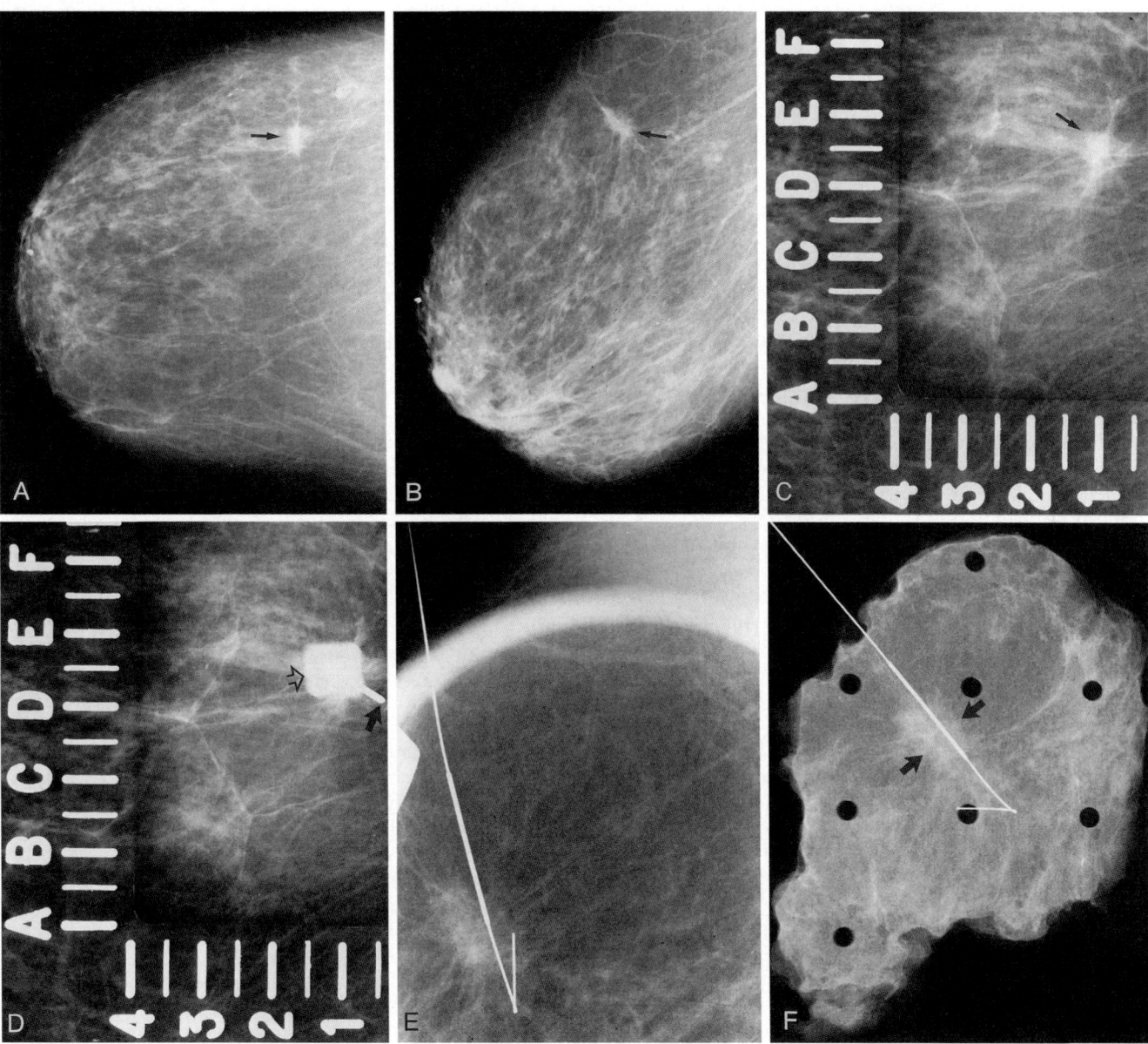

Figure 21.42. Needle Localization. Craniocaudal **(A)** and mediolateral **(B)** mammograms show a highly suspicious spiculated mass in the upper outer quadrant (*arrows*). **C.** Localization was performed by placing the fenestrated compression plate over the lesion (*arrow*) and then placing a needle parallel to the x-ray beam through the lesion. **D.** The hub of the needle (*open arrow*) is superimposed on the lesion; the tip (*solid arrow*) is at the posterior edge. A film is then taken in the 90° orthogonal projection, and once the depth is adjusted, the hook wire is passed through the needle. **E.** A film in the same projection demonstrates the final depth of the wire. **F.** The excised tissue is sent for specimen x-ray to confirm that the abnormality (*arrows*) has been removed. Histologic examination in this case revealed invasive lobular carcinoma.

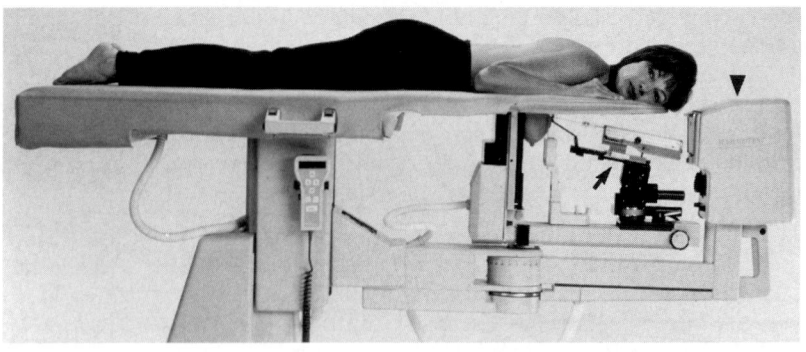

Figure 21.43. Dedicated Stereotactic Biopsy Unit. The x-ray tube (*arrowhead*) moves independent of the compressed breast, so stereo images can be obtained. The needle guide (*arrow*) is adjusted so that the needle will be centered in the lesion. (Reproduced with permission from Fischer Imaging Corporation, Denver, Colorado.)

women. Core biopsy is not recommended for lesions that are suspicious for radial scars because of the high prevalence of adjacent proliferative changes such as atypical ductal hyperplasia, ductal carcinoma in situ, and rarely tubular carcinoma; such adjacent lesions might not be sampled at core biopsy. Technical difficulties such as inadequate visualization of the lesion may occasionally preclude the use of a core biopsy.

Core biopsies can be guided by stereotactic images or by US (34). Currently, there are two types of stereotactic units available. One can be added onto a standard mammography machine but has limited working space and requires a seated patient. The other is a prone dedicated unit that is more costly but offers the advantages of having the patient in a prone position so as to minimize movement and vasovagal reactions (Fig. 21.43). A stereotactic unit allows the x-ray tube to move independently of the compressed breast. The lesion is centered in the aperture within the compression plate and images at negative and positive 15° are obtained. Calculation of the amount of deviation of the lesion in these two views allows the exact determination of the depth of the lesion. The needle guide is adjusted for exact positioning of the needle in three dimensions to the center of the lesion. After the injection of local anesthetic, a small skin incision is made to permit needle entry into the breast. Positioning of the needle is verified with stereotactic views, and biopsies are taken (Fig. 21.44).

When US is used, the needle can be observed in real time as the biopsy is performed (Fig. 21.45). Adequate sonographic visualization of the lesion is essential if core biopsy is to be performed with US guidance. Most microcalcifications and some masses, particularly those in fatty replaced breasts, cannot be visualized and, hence, cannot be biopsied using US. Aspiration of fluid cannot be performed through a core biopsy needle. Many lesions chosen for US guided biopsy will be atypical cysts; in such cases, it is prudent to attempt aspiration with a 22-gauge needle. If fluid is not obtained, a core biopsy can be performed.

Either a 14-gauge automated push-button biopsy gun or a 14-gauge or 11-gauge vacuum-assisted needle can be used for a core biopsy. The standard 14-gauge needle works by a spring action mechanism that fires the needle through the lesion. The inner cannula containing the tissue notch is projected through the lesion first, and then the cutting cannula is fired over it so that a small core of tissue is retained within the specimen notch.

With the vacuum-assisted devices, suction is used to bring the tissue into the specimen notch of the needle, which is then cut by an inner rotating cannula. Vacuum-assisted devices generally require only a single needle pass to obtain multiple specimens, whereas standard core biopsy requires multiple passes, one for each specimen. The vacuum-assisted needle offers improved ability to sample microcalcifications adequately when compared with the standard biopsy gun (35).

The accuracy of core biopsy in diagnosing breast carcinoma approaches that of surgical biopsy with reported sensitivities of 85–100% and specificities of 96–100% (36). To achieve such high sensitivities and specificities, it is essential that the mammographic appearance of the lesion be correlated with the pathologic diagnosis. If there is discordance, repeat core biopsy or excisional biopsy should be performed. In cases in which atypical hyperplasia is diagnosed by core biopsy, excisional biopsy should be performed as 18–48% of these lesions will ultimately prove to be carcinoma (37). Excisional biopsy is also necessary when a noninvasive carcinoma is diagnosed by core biopsy in cases in which breast conserving therapy is desired; 20% of such lesions will ultimately prove to have areas of invasion, and definitive therapy, thus, may be altered (38).

Other Interventional Procedures

Aspiration of sonographically atypical cysts can be performed for confirmation of the diagnosis using either US or mammographic guidance. The majority of such lesions will be smooth-walled masses that are atypical either because they lack through transmission or because the fluid within them is not anechoic. In such cases, a 22-gauge needle can be inserted using a technique similar to that used for core biopsy. If fluid is withdrawn, the lesion should be totally aspirated. After aspiration, air can be insufflated into the cyst cavity. This may prevent recurrence. If fluid cannot be withdrawn, the lesion is presumably solid, and core biopsy can be performed.

In cases in which there is irregularity or nodularity of the cyst wall by sonography, some mammographers advocate pneumocystography for confirmation. Core biopsy of the nodule or wall should be undertaken in these cases even though intracystic carcinomas are rare. Cytologic evaluation of aspirated fluid is unreliable for diagnosis.

Galactography can be used to investigate the cause of a spontaneous nipple discharge. The procedure in-

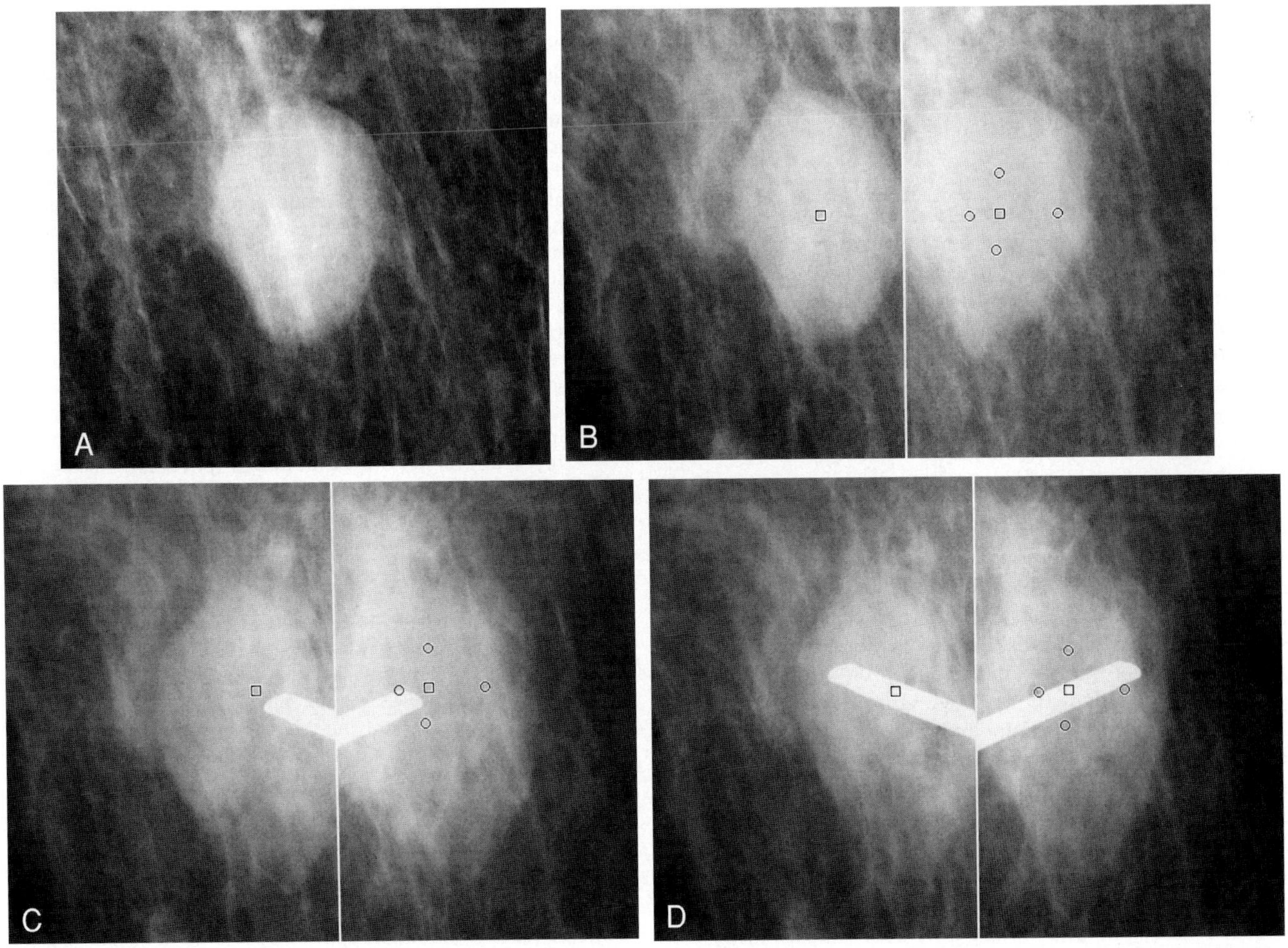

Figure 21.44. Stereotactic Core Biopsy. A. On the scout view, the lesion is centered in the aperture of the compression paddle. **B.** Stereo views at −15° and +15° are obtained, and the center of the lesion is marked in both views with the *square target mark.* Additional targets are then plotted (*circular marks*). **C.** After injection of local anesthetic, a 14-gauge core biopsy needle is inserted and prefire stereo images are obtained to verify appropriate posi-

tioning of the needle; the needle should be inserted to a depth that is 5 mm short of the targeted center of the lesion. **D.** After the core needle is fired, stereo images are obtained to verify that the needle has pierced the lesion. The specimen is then removed, and subsequent biopsies are taken. In this case, the histologic diagnosis was fibroadenoma.

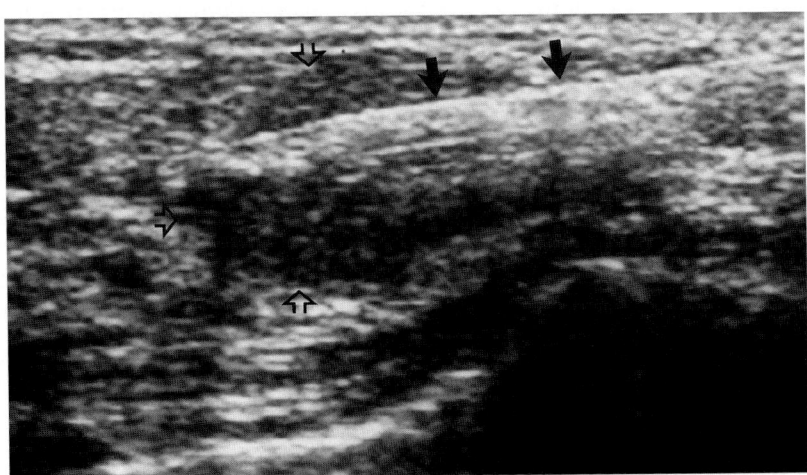

Figure 21.45. US-Guided Core Biopsy. Longitudinal US of a solid hypoechoic mass (*open arrows*) pierced by a 14-gauge core biopsy needle (*solid arrows*).

volves the injection of contrast material into a duct, after which films are taken to look for intraductal tumors. These are most frequently papillomas and less commonly carcinomas. The utility of this study is controversial. If the patient has a bloody discharge, some surgeons prefer to inject the discharging duct with methylene blue in the operating room before dissecting along it. Others use preoperative galactography to evaluate bloody discharge and believe that if the galactogram is negative, the patient can be observed. The use of galactography in the evaluation of a unilateral, spontaneous serous discharge is similarly controversial, as both bloody and serous fluid can be associated with small cancers that may not be visible mammographically (39).

CONCLUSION

Breast cancer represents a significant public health problem. More than 180,000 new cases are diagnosed and nearly 45,000 women die of the disease each year in the United States. Early detection with screening mammography is the only proved way to lower mortality from breast cancer. Diagnostic accuracy can be increased with the use of special mammographic views, US, and percutaneous biopsy techniques. Other modalities, such as MR and positron-emission tomography, are under study to determine their potential utility in detection and diagnosis of breast diseases. Use of breast imaging has increased during the last decade, and mortality from breast cancer has begun to decline. Our challenge, as radiologists, is to maintain the highest standards of quality in performance and interpretation of breast imaging studies; it is also to encourage all women to take regular advantage of these life-saving techniques.

References

1. Shapiro S. Evidence on screening for breast cancer from a randomized trial. Cancer 1977;39:2772–2782.
2. Nyström L, Rutqvist LE, Wall S, et al. Breast cancer screening with mammography: overview of Swedish randomized trials. Lancet 1993;341:973–978.
3. Kopans DB. Screening mammography and the controversy concerning women aged 40–49 years. RSNA syllabus: a categorical course in breast imaging. Oak Brook, IL: Radiological Society of North America 1995:39–49.
4. Hendrick RE, Smith RA, Rutledge JH, et al. Benefit of screening mammography in women age 40–49: a new meta-analysis of new randomized controlled trial results. J Natl Cancer Inst Monogr 1997;22:87–92.
5. Bjurstam N, Bjornel L, Duffy SW. The Gothenburg Breast Cancer Screening Trial: preliminary results on breast cancer mortality for women aged 39–49. J Natl Cancer Inst Monogr 1997;22:53–55
6. Andersson I, Janzon L. Reduced breast cancer mortality in women under age 50: updated from the Malmö mammographic screening program. J Natl Cancer Inst Monogr 1997;22:63–68.
7. Leitch AM, Dodd GD, Costanza M, et al. American Cancer Society guidelines for the early detection of breast cancer: update 1997. Cancer 1997;47:150–153.
8. National Cancer Institute (Bethesda, MD). National Cancer Advisory Board recommendations on mammography. Available at: http://WWW.NCI.NIH.GOV/; gopher://gopher.nih.gov:70/0R0 -20327-/clin/cancernet/facts/detection/Questions%20and%20Answers%20About%20Mammography%20Screening). Issued March 27, 1997.
9. Tabar L, Larsson LG, Andersson I, et al. Breast-cancer screening with mammography in women aged 40–49 years. Int J Cancer 1996;68:693–699.
10. Tabar L, Fagerberg G, Day NE, et al. What is the optimum interval between mammographic screening examinations? An analysis based on the latest results of the Swedish two-county breast cancer screening trial. Br J Cancer 1987;55:547–551.
11. Kerlikowske K, Grady D, Barclay J, et al. Effect of age, breast density, and family history on the sensitivity of first screening mammography. JAMA 1996;276:33–38.
12. Curpen BN, Sickles EA, Sollitto RA, et al. The comparative value of mammographic screening for women 40–49 years old versus women 50–64 years old. AJR Am J Roentgenol 1995;164:1099–1103.
13. Linver MN, Paster SB. Mammography outcomes in a practice setting by age: prognostic factors, sensitivity, and positive biopsy rate. J Natl Cancer Inst Monogr 1997;22:113–117.
14. Feig SA, Ehrlich SM. Estimation of radiation risk from screening mammography: recent trends and comparison with expected benefits. Radiology 1990;174:638–647.
15. Sickles EA, Filly RA, Callen PW. Breast cancer detection with sonography and mammography: comparison using state-of-the-art equipment. AJR Am J Roentgenol 1983;140:843–845.
16. Kopans DB, Meyer JE, Lindfors KK. Whole-breast US imaging: four-year follow-up. Radiology 1985;157:505–507.
17. de Paredes ES, Marsteller LP, Eden BV. Breast cancers in women 35 years of age and younger: mammographic findings. Radiology 1990;177:117–119.
18. Sickles EA. Mammographic features of 300 consecutive nonpalpable breast cancers. AJR Am J Roentgenol 1986;146:661–663.
19. US Department of Health and Human Services. Clinical practice guideline, quality determinants of mammography, screening and diagnostic views. AHCPR publ. no. 95-0632. Washington, DC: U.S. Government Printing Office, October 1994:25–31.
20. Kopans DB, Swann CA, White G, et al. Asymmetric breast tissue. Radiology 1989;171:639–643.
21. Marsteller LP, de Paredes ES. Well-defined masses in the breast. Radiographics 1989;9:13–37.
22. Sickles EA. Breast masses: mammographic evaluation. Radiology 1989;173:297–303.
23. Sickles EA. Nonpalpable, circumscribed, noncalcified solid breast masses: likelihood of malignancy based on lesion size and age of patient. Radiology 1994;192:439–442.
24. Bassett LW. Mammographic analysis of calcifications. Radiol Clin North Am 1992;30:93–105.
25. Harris JR, Lippman ME, Veronesi U, et al. Breast cancer [second of three parts]. N Engl J Med 1992;327:390–398.
26. Eklund GW, Busby RC, Miller SH, et al. Improved imaging of the augmented breast. AJR Am J Roentgenol 1988;151:469–473.
27. Destouet JM, Monsees BS, Oser RF, et al. Screening mammography in 350 women with breast implants: prevalence and findings of implant complications. AJR Am J Roentgenol 1992;159:973–978.
28. Gorczyca DP, Schneider E, DeBruhl ND, et al. Silicone breast implant rupture: comparison between three-point Dixon and fast spin-echo MR imaging. AJR Am J Roentgenol 1994;162:305–310.

29. DeBruhl ND, Gorczyca DP, Ahn CY, et al. Silicone breast implants: US evaluation. Radiology 1993;189:95–98.

30. American College of Radiology. Breast imaging reporting and data system (BI-RADS™). 2nd ed. Reston, VA: American College of Radiology, 1995.

31. Sickles EA. Periodic mammographic follow-up of probably benign lesions: results in 3,184 consecutive cases. Radiology 1991;179:463–468.

32. Kopans DB, Lindfors K, McCarthy KA, et al. Spring hookwire breast lesion localizer: use with rigid-compression mammographic systems. Radiology 1985;157 537–538.

33. Lindfors KK, Rosenquist CJ. Needle core biopsy guided with mammography: a study of cost-effectiveness. Radiology 1994;190:217–222.

34. Parker SH, Burbank F. A practical approach to minimally invasive breast biopsy. Radiology 1996;200:11–20.

35. Meyer JE, Smith DN, DiPiro PJ, et al. Stereotactic breast biopsy of clustered microcalcifications with a directional, vacuum-assisted device. Radiology 1997;204:575–576.

36. Bassett L, Winchester DP, Caplan RB, et al. Stereotactic core-needle biopsy of the breast: a report of the joint task force of the American College of Radiology, American College of Surgeons, and College of American Pathologists. Cancer 1997;47:171–190.

37. Jackman RJ, Burbank F, Parker SH, et al. Atypical ductal hyperplasia diagnosed at stereotactic breast biopsy: improved reliability with 14-gauge, directional vacuum-assisted biopsy. Radiology 1997;204:485–488.

38. Liberman L, Dershaw DD, Rosen PP, et al. Stereotaxic core biopsy of breast carcinoma: accuracy at predicting invasion. Radiology 1995;194:379–381.

39. Fajardo LI, Jackson VP, Hunter TB. Interventional procedures in diseases of the breast: needle biopsy, pneumocystography and galactography. AJR Am J Roentgenol 1992;158:1231–1238.

Section V CARDIOVASCULAR RADIOLOGY

Section Editor:
David K. Shelton Jr.

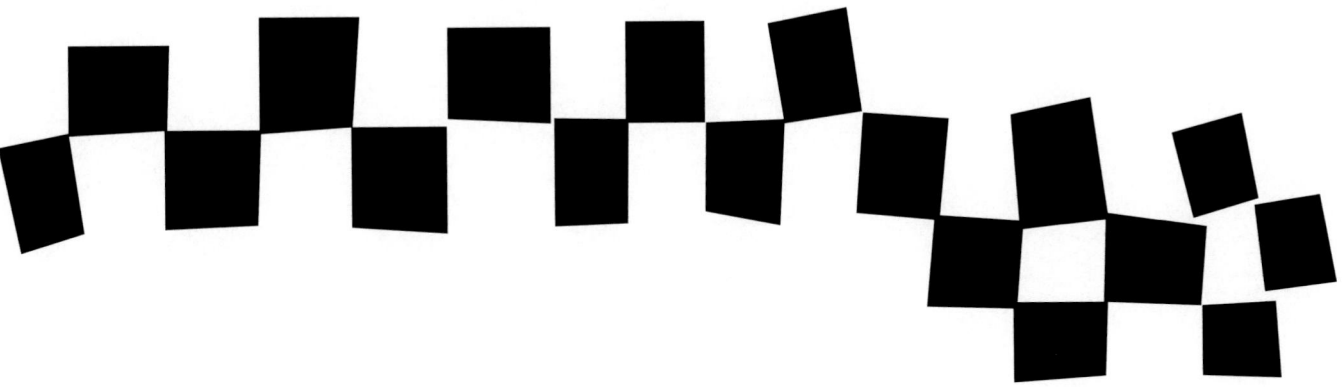

22
Cardiac Anatomy, Physiology, and Imaging Modalities

David K. Shelton Jr.
Michael Galloway

IMAGING METHODS

Thorough knowledge of cardiac anatomy and physiology is important as a basis for cardiac imaging. Comprehensive knowledge of cardiac imaging also requires consideration of virtually all the available imaging modalities. Chest radiography provides the initial evaluation of most cardiac patients. A barium esophagram provides additional information because of the close relationship of the esophagus to cardiac structures. Fluoroscopy increases the detectability of coronary and valvular calcification as well as provides dynamic and positional information. Transthoracic echocardiography, including pulse wave and color flow Doppler, and transesophageal echocardiography provide additional detailed imaging of internal cardiac anatomy and function. Nuclear cardiology, positron emission tomography, and pharmacologic testing provide key functional, perfusion, and physiologic information. Cardiac and coronary angiography, although invasive, provide detailed anatomic information that can lead directly to interventional or surgical therapy. CT and ultrafast CT with the use of IV iodinated contrast material are capable of providing critical information, particularly for pericardial or intracardiac disease. Recent technological advances in the latter

also allow detection of premature coronary calcification, which may have prognostic implications. MR adds three-dimensional tomographic and motion studies of the myocardium, valves, and chambers without using ionizing radiation or intravascular contrast. Cardiac imaging requires familiarity with all imaging techniques and their associated physics, three-dimensional cardiac anatomy, cardiac physiology, and cardiac disease processes.

ANATOMY

The four-chambered heart lies primarily in the anterior left hemithorax with the left ventricle (LV) lying on the left hemidiaphragm (Figs. 22.1, 22.2). The right atrium (RA) extends to the right of midline as it receives systemic blood from the superior vena cava (SVC), inferior vena cava (IVC), and coronary sinus. The RA and right ventricle (RV) lie primarily anterior to the planes of the left atrium (LA) and left ventricle. The RV is the most anterior chamber and abuts the sternum (Fig. 22.3). The LA is subcarinal and midline in the thorax, being supplied by the right and left surperior and inferior pulmonary veins.

Frontal Projection. The right border of the cardiac silhouette is formed primarily by the RA, with the SVC entering superiorly and the IVC often seen at its lower margin (Figs. 22.1, 22.3). The left border of the heart is created primarily by the LV and LA appendage. The pulmonary artery (PA), aortopulmonary window, and aortic knob extend superiorly.

Lateral Projection. The RV is border forming anteriorly adjacent to the sternum, with its outflow tract extending superiorly and posteriorly (Fig. 22.2). The LA is border forming in the high posterior, subcarinal region. The LV is border forming inferiorly and posteriorly.

Right Atrium. The RA is divided into two portions. The smooth posterior wall develops from the sinus venosus, with the attached SVC and IVC in continuity posteriorly (Fig. 22.4). The trabeculated anterior wall is derived from the embryonic RA. The RA appendage extends superiorly and medially from the SVC opening. The crista terminalis is a muscular ridge that runs from the mouth of the SVC and fades inferiorly to the mouth of the IVC. It divides the two portions of the atrium and corresponds to an external sulcus terminalis. The medial wall of the RA is the interatrial septum, which contains a smooth, central dimpled area called the fossa ovalis. Inflow from the SVC, IVC, and coronary sinus enters the smooth posterior portion of the right atrium. The SVC has a free opening, whereas the IVC is partially guarded by a thin eustachian valve, which is occasionally absent

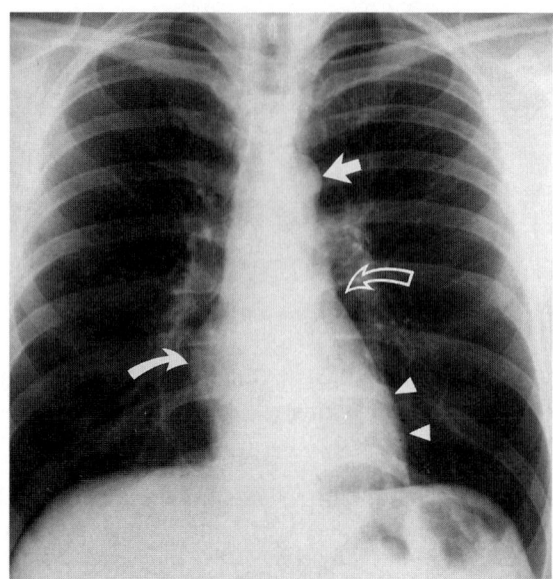

Figure 22.1. Normal PA Chest Radiograph. Frontal view of the chest demonstrates normal heart size, contours and chamber size. The hila and pulmonary vascularity are normal. The LV (*arrowheads*) is border forming on the left. The RA (*curved arrow*) is border forming on the right. The aortic knob (*arrow*) is of normal contour, and the PA (*open arrow*) is concave.

or perforated (network of Chiari). The large draining coronary vein or coronary sinus enters the RA anterior and medial to the IVC. Its opening is guarded by the thebesian valve between the orifice of the IVC and the tricuspid valve.

Right Ventricle. The RV (Figs. 22.4, 22.5) lies anterior to the left ventricular outflow tract and wraps around it and to the left. The right ventricular outflow is directed superiorly, posteriorly, and to the left. The RV is divided into a posterior or inferior portion (inflow or sinus portion), which is heavily trabeculated and a less trabeculated anterior or superior portion (outflow tract or pulmonary conus). The two portions of the RV are divided by the crista supraventricularis, which is a muscular ridge with a septal band called the moderator band. This band is present in more than 40% of patients, connects the interventricular septum to the anterior papillary muscle, and contains the right bundle branch. The infundibulum (conus arteriosus) is the smooth cephalic portion of the RV that leads to the pulmonary trunk.

Pulmonary Arteries. The muscular pulmonary conus extends to the semilunar, tricuspid pulmonary valve, with the pulmonary trunk extending superiorly and to the left. The left PA extends posteriorly as a continuation of the main PA, coursing over the top of the left main stem bronchus, then descending posteriorly. The right PA extends horizontally to the right, bifurcates within the pericardial sac, and exits the right hilum as the truncus anterior and interlobar arteries. The right upper lobe bronchus is eparterial, meaning that it lies above the right PA. The left main stem bronchus is hyparterial, meaning that it lies below the PA.

The ligamentum arteriosum arises from the superior, proximal left PA and crosses through the aorticopul-

monary window to the floor of the aorta. The ligamentum arteriosum is the remnant of the ductus arteriosus, which closes functionally in the first 24 hours and closes anatomically by 10 days. Desaturated blood from the right heart circulates through the lungs and returns as oxygenated blood through the right and left superior and inferior pulmonary veins into the LA.

LEFT ATRIUM. The LA is the highest and most posterior chamber (Fig. 22.6). Its smooth walls are nestled between the right and left bronchi, and its posterior wall abuts the anterior wall of the esophagus. The left atrial appendage is a small pouch that projects superiorly and to the left and is smoother and longer than the right atrial appendage. The left atrial appendage extends anterior to the left superior pulmonary veins and is commonly seen on MR and CT scans. The foramen ovale within the interatrial septum remains nominally patent in up to 25% of adults. Its inferior margin is a remnant of the septum primum and may be somewhat scalloped. The mitral valve is located anterior and inferior to the body of the LA, with the mitral valve leaflets extending into the LV.

LEFT VENTRICLE. The mitral valve is the conduit for blood flow from the LA to the LV and is in the high posterior "valve plane" of the LV (Figs. 22.5, 22.6). The anterior or septal leaflet of the mitral valve lies near the interventricular septum and extends to the posterior (noncoronary) cusp of the aortic valve. The smaller posterior mitral leaflet lies posteriorly and to the left. The

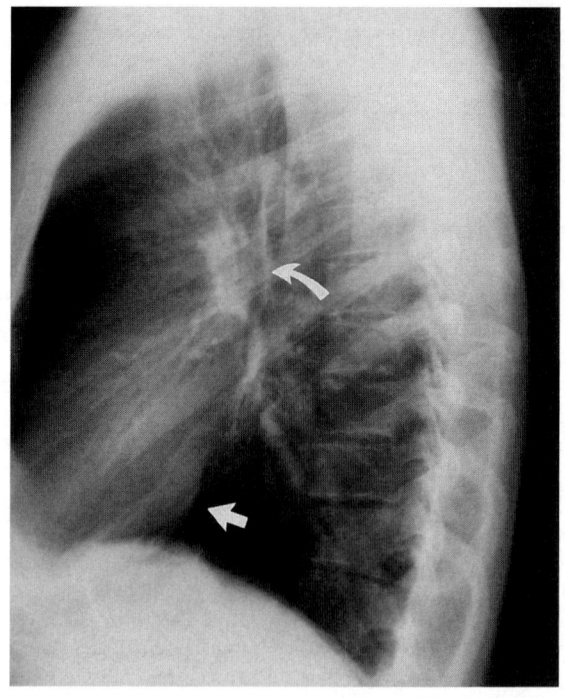

Figure 22.2. Normal Lateral Chest Radiograph. This well-positioned left lateral chest radiograph demonstrates the right ribs projected posterior to the left ribs because of divergence of the x-ray beam. The right and left bronchi are overlapped, and the sternum is seen in the lateral view. The true lateral projection allows evaluation of the IVC intersection (*arrow*) with the LV. There is no evidence of posterior displacement of the left bronchus (*curved arrow*) to indicate left atrial enlargement. There is no evidence of right ventricular encroachment into the retrosternal clear space.

chordae tendineae are strong fibrous cords that extend from the mitral leaflets to the papillary muscles of the LV. The inflow portion of the LV is posterior to the anterior leaflet of the mitral valve. The outflow portion of the LV is anterior and superior to the anterior mitral leaflet. The interventricular septum has a high membranous portion that is contiguous with the aortic root. The more muscular inferior portion of the septum extends to the left ventricular apex. The esophagus passes immediately posterior and is in contact with the muscular wall of the LV.

Aorta. The outflow tract of the LV leads into the aortic root through the aortic valve which is composed of right, left, and posterior (noncoronary) cusps. The sinuses of Valsalva are the reservoirs created by the closure of the aortic valve and from which the right and left coronary arteries arise. The posterior wall of the aorta is continuous with the anterior leaflet of the mitral valve and more superiorly abuts the anterior wall of the LA. The anterior wall of the aorta is continuous with the interventricular septum. After coursing superiorly and then to the left, the aorta gives off the right innominate artery, left common carotid artery, and left subclavian artery. The aortic arch is the transverse portion of the aorta that abuts the left wall of the trachea, causing a characteristic indentation.

Conduction System. The sinoatrial node consists of specialized neuromuscular tissue that measures approximately 5–20 mm and is located on the anterior endocardial surface of the RA just above the SVC and right atrial appendage junction, near the crista terminalis. Electrical propagation spreads to both atria via Purkinje-like fibers and is recorded as the P wave on an electrocardiogram. The atrioventricular node is a 2×5 mm region of neuromuscular tissue on the endocardial surface, along the right side of the interatrial septum, just inferior to the ostium of the coronary sinus. The impulse is collected and delayed approximately 0.7 seconds in the atrioventricular node before passing into the bundle of His. The bundle of His is a 20-mm–long tract extending down the right side of the membranous interventricular septum. The bundle of His bifurcates into a right and left bundle before arborizing through the two ventricles via the Purkinje system. The interventricular septum activates from superior to inferior with the anterior or septal RV being the first to activate and the posterior or basal LV being the last to activate. This information is particularly

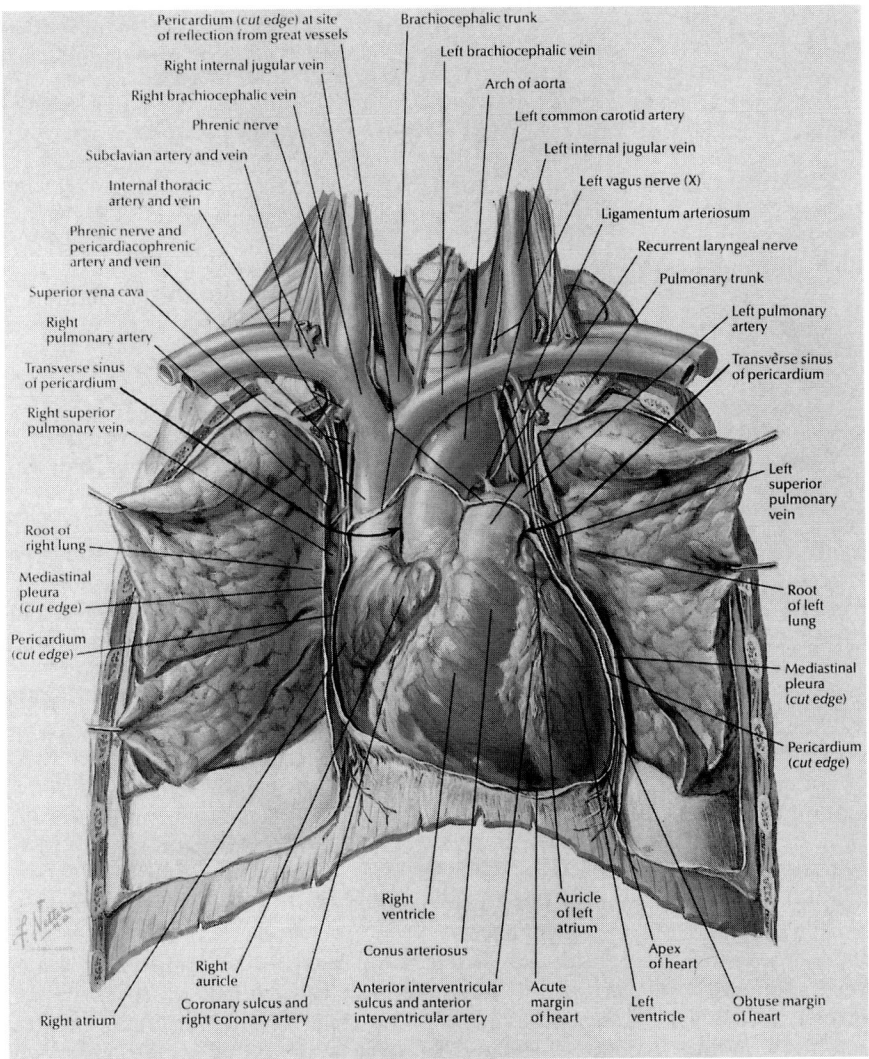

Figure 22.3. Cardiothoracic Anatomy: Frontal View of the Heart After Cutaway of the Chest Wall, Pleural Surfaces, and Pericardial Surface. Note the relationship of the RA, RV, left atrial appendage, and LV to the great vessels. (Reproduced with permission. Drawing by Frank H. Netter, MD, from *Atlas of human anatomy.* The CIBA collection of medical illustrations, clinical symposia. West Caldwell, NJ: CIBA-Geigy Corp, 1989.)

Figure 22.4. Cutaway Views of the Right Atrium and Right Ventricle. (Reproduced with permission. Drawing by Frank H. Netter, MD, from *Atlas of human anatomy*. The CIBA collection of medical illustrations, clinical symposia, 1989.)

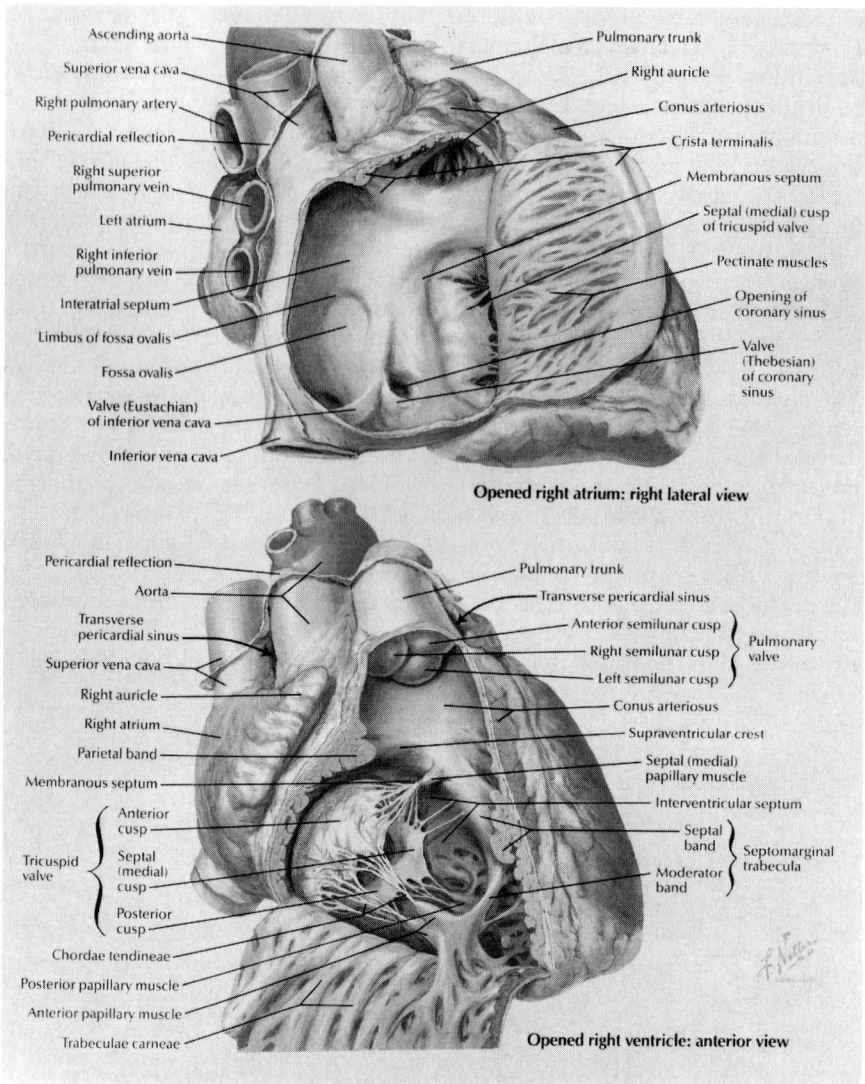

Opened right atrium: right lateral view

Opened right ventricle: anterior view

useful when evaluating phase analysis or phase propagation in gated cardiac scintigraphy.

CARDIAC CATHETERIZATION

Left-sided catheterization is normally accomplished via arterial puncture in the femoral or brachial artery (Fig. 22.7). It is typically used for aortography, coronary and coronary bypass graft angiography, ventriculography, and evaluation for patent ductus arteriosus. Right-sided catheterization is typically accomplished by venous puncture in the femoral or brachiocephalic vein (Fig. 22.8). It is used for pulmonary angiography, catheterization of the RA and RV, or evaluation of shunt lesions such as an atrial septal defect.

Important considerations include determination of the catheter course to help diagnose atrial septal defects, ventricular septal defects, patent ductus arteriosus, or persistent left SVC. During catheterization, oxygen saturation percentages are commonly determined, along with pressure measurements and pressure gradients (Table 22.1). Contrast is injected to demonstrate additional de-

tails of anatomy, as well as to evaluate for valvular lesions, chamber size, ventricular function, and wall motion.

Right atrial pressures are normally 2–5 mm Hg and oxygen saturation is 65–75%. Elevated right atrial pressures are seen with right heart failure, decreased compliance, and tricuspid valve disease. A 7% or greater increase in saturation from the IVC to the RA is considered evidence of a left-to-right shunt (ASD).

Right ventricular pressures are typically 25 systolic and 0–5 diastolic mm Hg. Elevated systolic pressures are seen with pulmonary hypertension, pulmonic valve stenosis, and congenital heart lesions such as transposition and truncus arteriosus. Diastolic pressures increase with right heart failure. Saturations should be nearly the same as right atrial saturations. A 5% increase in saturation from RA to RV suggests a ventricular septal defect.

Pulmonary arterial pressures are normally 25 systolic and 10 diastolic mm Hg, with a mean pulmonary artery pressure of 15 mm Hg. A significant pressure gradient (>10 mm Hg) across the valve implies pulmonic valve stenosis. Increased pressures are seen with shunt lesions, pulmonary vascular disease, and pulmonary venous obstruction. Pulmonary arterial saturation should be approximately the same as right ventricular saturation, with a 3% difference considered significant for a shunt lesion.

Pulmonary capillary wedge pressure is typically 2–8 mm Hg and approximates the left atrial pressure unless there is evidence of pulmonary venous obstruction. Elevations in the left atrial or wedge pressure are usually seen with mitral stenosis and left-sided congestive heart failure. Normal left atrial saturation is approximately

94%, and a decrease greater than 5% implies a right-to-left shunt.

Left ventricular pressures are 120 systolic and 0–5 diastolic mm Hg. Decreased systolic pressures are seen with shock and congestive heart failure. Elevated systolic pressures imply systemic hypertension or outlet obstruction. Increased diastolic pressure is seen with congestive heart failure. Decreased saturation at the left ventricular level would imply a right-to-left shunt. Aortic pressure is normally 120 systolic and 80 diastolic, with a mean pressure of 70–100 mm Hg.

With each systolic contraction, the average stroke volume of each ventricle is 70 mL of blood (Table 22.2). End diastolic volume is normally 125–150 mL for the LV and 165 mL for the RV. A normal cardiac output is 4–5 L/min, with a normal cardiac index of 2.8–4.0 L/min/m^2 of body surface area. The normal ejection fraction is 50–75% for the LV and 45–55% for the RV. Typical end diastolic volumes are 57 mL for the RA and 50 mL for the LA. Coronary blood flow averages approximately 224 mL/min and increases up to sixfold during exercise.

Aortic Valve. The normal aortic valve orifice is 3 cm^2. Symptoms result from aortic stenosis usually when either the orifice is less than 0.7 cm^2 or when it is less than

Table 22.1. Normal Values for Cardiac Catheterization

Site	Pressures (mm Hg)	Saturation (%)
Vena cava	5	60–65
Right atrium	2–5	65–75
Right ventricle	25/0	70
Pulmonary artery	25/10	73
Left Atrium	2–8	94–98
Left Ventricle	120/0–5	94–98
Aorta	120/80	94–98

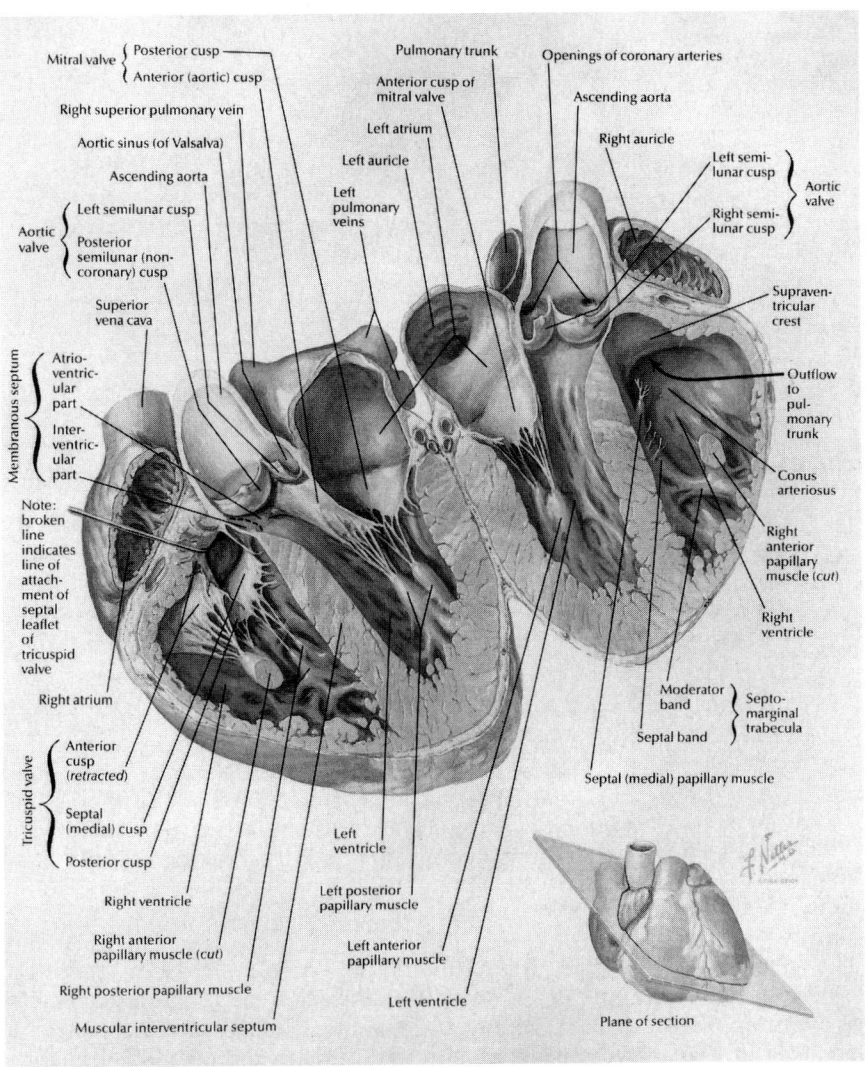

Figure 22.5. Bisection Through the Heart Simulating a Four-Chamber View. (Reproduced with permission. Drawing by Frank H. Netter, MD, from *Atlas of human anatomy*. The CIBA collection of medical illustrations, clinical symposia, 1989.)

Figure 22.6. Cutaway views of the LV and LA. (Reproduced with permission. Drawing by Frank H. Netter, MD, from *Atlas of human anatomy*. The CIBA collection of medical illustrations, clinical symposia, 1989.)

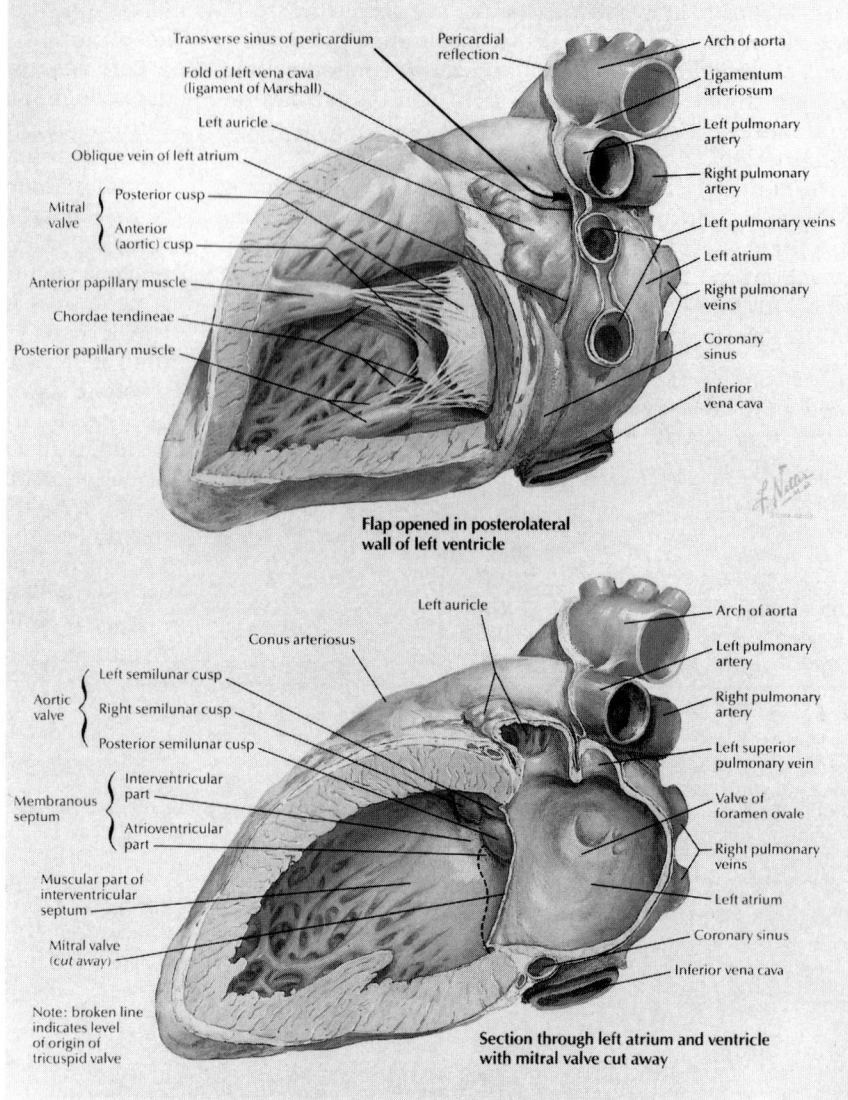

Transverse sinus of pericardium
Fold of left vena cava (ligament of Marshall)
Left auricle
Oblique vein of left atrium
Mitral valve — Posterior cusp — Anterior (aortic) cusp
Anterior papillary muscle
Chordae tendineae
Posterior papillary muscle
Pericardial reflection
Arch of aorta
Ligamentum arteriosum
Left pulmonary artery
Right pulmonary artery
Left pulmonary veins
Left atrium
Right pulmonary veins
Coronary sinus
Inferior vena cava

Flap opened in posterolateral wall of left ventricle

Conus arteriosus
Left auricle
Aortic valve — Left semilunar cusp — Right semilunar cusp — Posterior semilunar cusp
Membranous septum — Interventricular part — Atrioventricular part
Muscular part of interventricular septum
Mitral valve (cut away)
Note: broken line indicates level of origin of tricuspid valve
Arch of aorta
Left pulmonary artery
Right pulmonary artery
Left superior pulmonary vein
Valve of foramen ovale
Right pulmonary veins
Left atrium
Coronary sinus
Inferior vena cava

Section through left atrium and ventricle with mitral valve cut away

Table 22.2. Average Physiologic Data for Cardiac Chambers

Parameter	Left Chambers	Right Chambers
Atrial end diastolic volume	50 mL	57 mL
Ventricular end diastolic volume	125–150 mL	165 mL
Ejection fraction	50–75%	45–55%
Stroke volume	70 mL	70 mL
Cardiac output	4–5 L/min	4–5 L/min
Cardiac index	2.8–4 L/min/m²	2.8–4 L/min/m²

1.5 cm^2 if there is aortic stenosis and insufficiency. Mild stenosis is indicated by a pressure gradient across the aortic valve greater than 25 mm Hg, moderate stenosis by a gradient greater than 40–50 mm Hg, and severe stenosis by a gradient exceeding 80 mm Hg.

Mitral Valve. The mitral valve orifice usually measures 4–6 cm^2. Mild mitral stenosis occurs with an orifice less than 1.5 cm^2, moderate mitral stenosis at less than 1.0 cm^2, and severe mitral stenosis at less than 0.5 cm^2.

Pulmonic stenosis is considered significant if the right ventricular systolic pressure exceeds 70 mm Hg.

Pulmonary artery hypertension is defined as a mean pulmonary artery pressure of more than 25 mm Hg.

CHEST RADIOGRAPHY

The chest radiograph remains the mainstay for imaging of the heart and lungs. There are many approaches to reading the radiograph. Although most radiologists initiate the process with "global perception," it is important to develop a checklist scan technique. This discussion concerns adult PA and lateral radiographs.

Cardiac Silhouette

Size. The cardiothoracic ratio should not exceed 0.5 on a 72-in. erect PA radiograph or 0.6 on a portable or anteroposterior (AP) examination. Other factors should be considered, such as fat pads and pectus deformity.

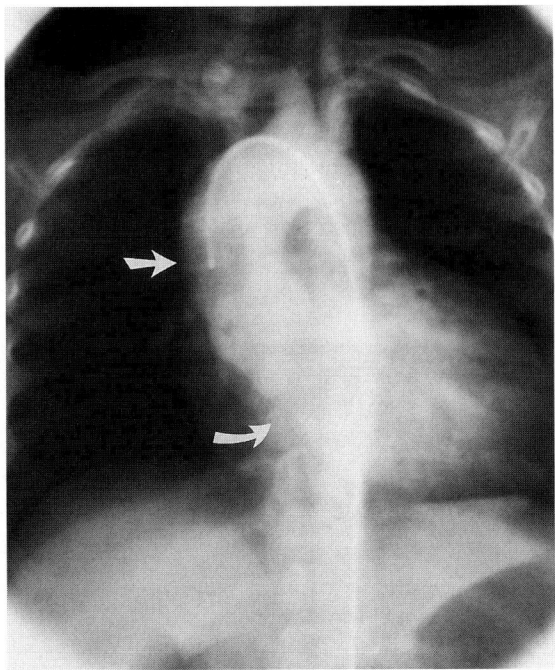

Figure 22.7. Aortogram via Transfemoral Approach. The catheter is placed in the mildly dilated ascending aorta (*straight arrow*). Notice the reflux of contrast from the aortic valve into the LV (*curved arrow*) in this patient with aortic insufficiency.

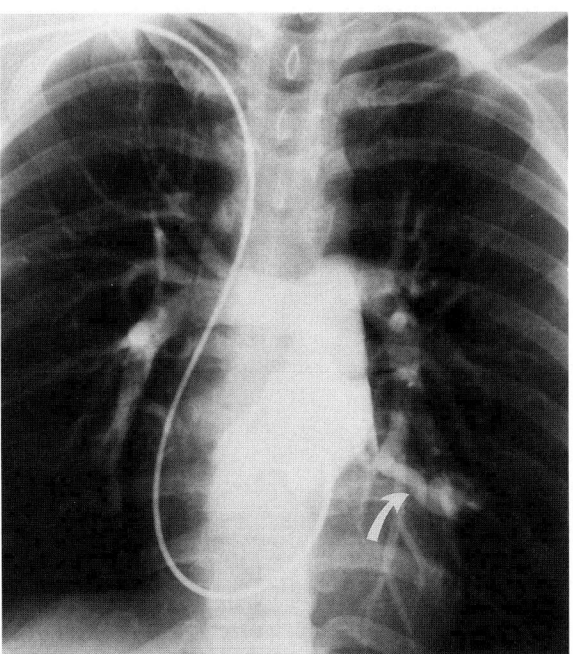

Figure 22.8. Right Heart Catheterization via the Right Subclavian Vein. The catheter is positioned in the pulmonary conus. Contrast fills the main, right, and left pulmonary arteries. Note the arteriovenous malformation with a large feeding artery (*arrow*).

Shape. Various contour effects can be clues to underlying disease. "Water bottle" configuration occurs with pericardial effusion or generalized cardiomyopathy. Left ventricular or "Shmoo" configuration (after Al Capp's Shmoo) describes lengthening and rounding of the left heart border with a downward extension of the apex resulting from left ventricular enlargement. "Hypertrophy" configuration describes increased convexity of the left heart border and apex. Right ventricular hypertrophy and enlargement tends to lift the apex and create a more horizontal vector to the cardiac axis. Hypertrophy of either ventricle usually causes little enlargement of the silhouette unless dilatation is also present. Hypertrophy typically results from increased afterload, whereas dilation occurs with failure or diastolic overload. "Straightening" of the left heart border is seen with rheumatic heart disease and mitral stenosis.

"Moguls of the Heart." Skiing the moguls of the heart refers to the left mediastinal outline beginning at the aortic knob. A prominent knob is a clue to ectasia, aneurysm, or hypertension. Notching or "figure 3" sign of the aorta suggests coarctation (Fig. 22.9). The second mogul is the main PA segment. Excessive convexity is seen with poststenotic dilatation, chronic obstructive pulmonary disease, PA hypertension, left-to-right shunts, and pericardial defects. Severe concavity suggests right-to-left shunts. The third mogul is a prominent left atrial appendage that in 90% of cases indicates prior rheumatic carditis (Fig. 22.10). It rarely is seen with other causes of left atrial enlargement. The fourth mogul is a bulge just above the cardiophrenic angle, seen with infarction or ventricular aneurysm. A fifth

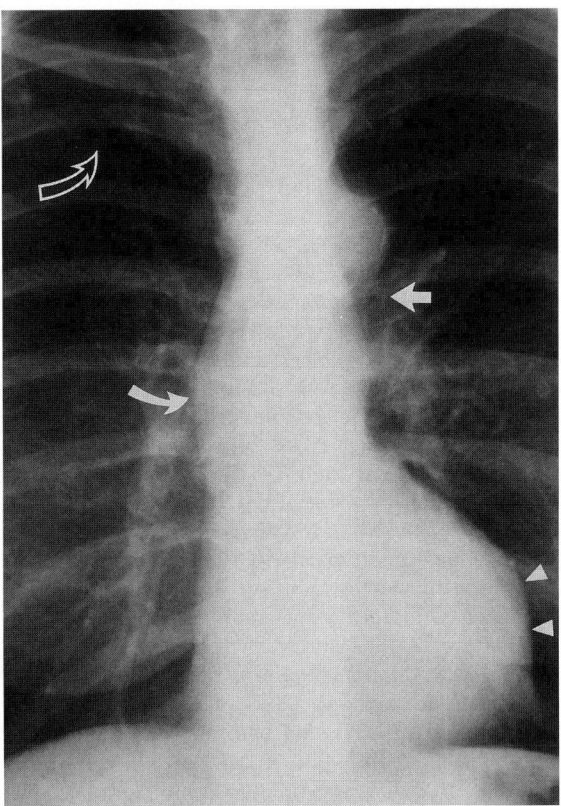

Figure 22.9. Aortic Coarctation. Notice the "figure 3 sign" or notching of the aorta near the aortic knob (*straight arrow*). The ascending aorta (*curved arrow*) is prominent, and the LV is excessively rounded (*arrowheads*). Rib notching is noted along the right fifth rib margin inferiorly (*curved open arrow*).

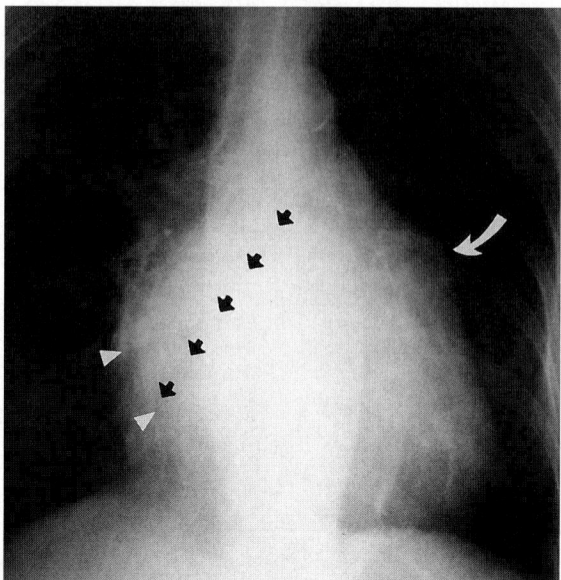

Figure 22.10. Rheumatic Heart Disease. The left atrial appendage is strikingly prominent (*curved arrow*). Splaying of the carina and a double density along the right heart border indicates left atrial enlargement (*arrowheads*). When the distance from the lateral margin of the LA to the midpoint on the under surface of the left bronchus exceeds 7 cm, left atrial enlargement is likely (*black arrows*).

bulge at the cardiophrenic angle is caused by pericardial cysts, prominent fat pads, or adenopathy.

Chamber Enlargement

Left atrial enlargement is best confirmed by measuring the distance from the midinferior border of the left main stem bronchus to the right lateral border of the left atrial density (see Fig. 22.10). This distance is less than 7 cm in 90% of normal patients and is greater than 7 cm in 90% of patients with left atrial enlargement, as proved by echocardiography. This measurement can be approximated by placing one's right fifth finger under the left bronchus and while keeping the fingers closed, determining whether the LA is seen beyond one's four fingertips; if so, the LA is enlarged. Less sensitive signs of left atrial enlargement include splaying of the carinal angle, uplifting of the left main stem bronchus, and prominence of the left atrial appendage. On occasion, the enlarged LA will displace the descending aorta to the left. Massive left atrial enlargement can result in the LA becoming border forming on the right side, so-called atrial escape. On lateral views, an enlarged LA will displace the left bronchus posteriorly, with the bronchi creating right and left legs for the "walking man sign." An enlarged LA also impresses against the esophagus.

Right atrial enlargement is more difficult to define on chest radiographs than left atrial enlargement, but fortunately, it is less common. Clues include a prominent atrial bulge too far to the right of the spine (more than 5.5 cm from the midline on a well-positioned PA radiograph). Another sign is elongation of the right atrial convexity to exceed 50% of the mediastinal or cardiovascular shadow. Right atrial enlargement usually accompanies right ventricular enlargement.

Left Ventricular Enlargement. On the PA view, an enlarged LV creates an elongated left heart border with the apex pointing downward. Prominent rounding of the inferior left heart border is also seen (Fig. 22.11). The lateral view shows an enlarged LV extending behind the esophagus. The Hoffman-Rigler sign for left ventricular enlargement exists when the LV extends more than 1.8 cm posterior to the posterior border of the IVC at a level 2 cm cephalad to the intersection of the LV and IVC (Fig. 22.12). This sign requires a true lateral radiograph and

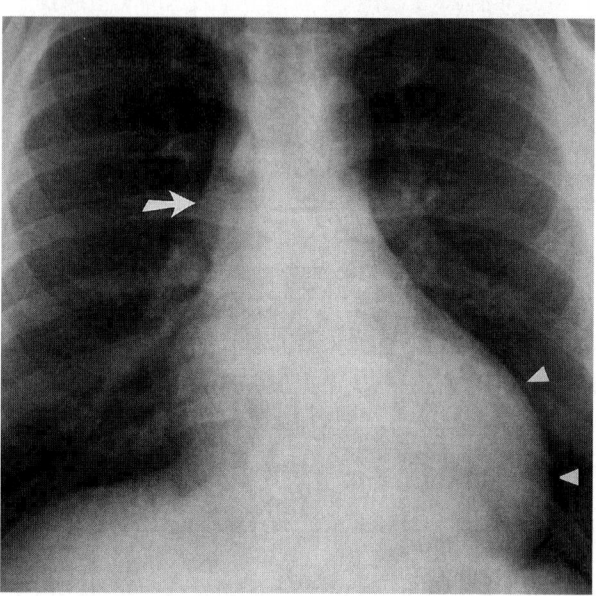

Figure 22.11. Left Ventricular Enlargement. Prominence of the LV with rounding along the inferior heart border and an apex that is pointing downward (*arrowheads*) is indicative of "left ventricular configuration." The ascending aorta (*arrow*) is dilated because of aortic stenosis and insufficiency.

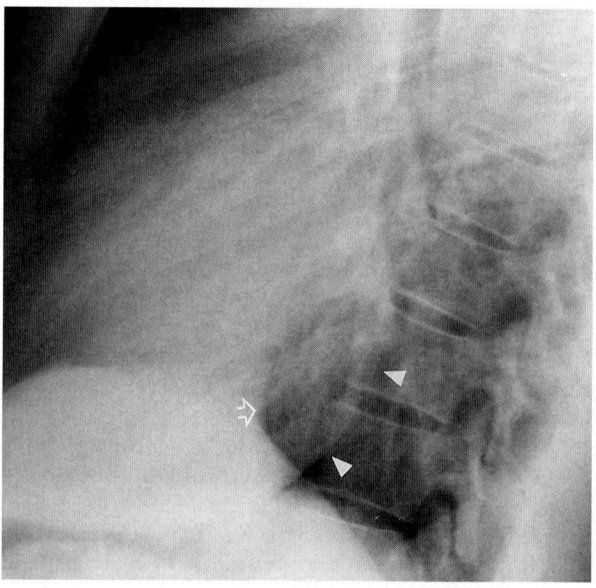

Figure 22.12. Left Ventricular Enlargement. The posterior margin of the LV (*arrowheads*) projects prominently behind the IVC (*open arrow*) and overlaps the thoracic spine. The Hoffman-Rigler sign is positive.

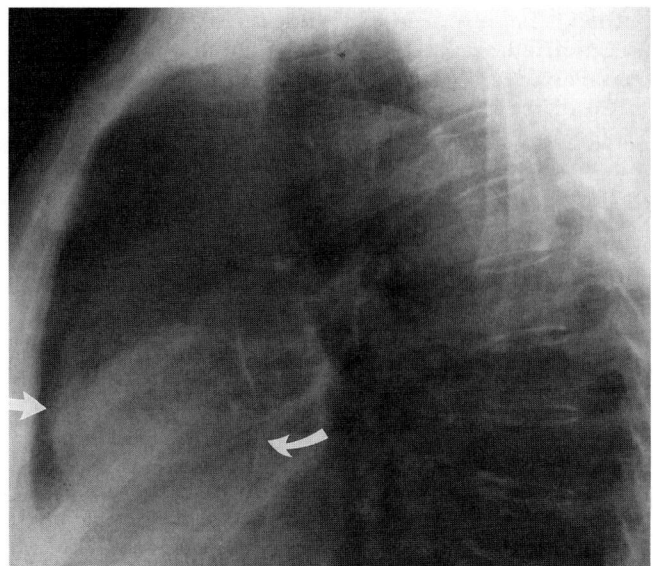

Figure 22.13. Calcified Aortic Aneurysm. The ascending aorta is enlarged in this patient with a syphilitic calcified aortic aneurysm. The anterior margin is identified by soft-tissue prominence (*straight arrow*) overlapping the retrosternal clear space. The posterior margin is identified by calcification in the wall (*curved arrow*).

can be false-positive if the lateral view is obliqued or there is volume loss in either lower lobe. This sign can be quickly applied by using one of the "2-cm fingertips" for a quick check without a ruler.

Right ventricular enlargement is not as easily detected as left-sided enlargement. If the heart is enlarged and Rigler's sign does not show left ventricular enlargement, then consider right-sided enlargement. If the RV fills too much of the retrosternal clear space or "climbs" more than one third of the sternal length, then right ventricular enlargement is likely. Indirect signs such as enlargement of the pulmonary outflow tract or hilar arteries add confidence.

Abnormal Mediastinal Contours

Aorta. Dilatation of the ascending aorta as a result of poststenotic dilatation is seen in approximately 80% of patients with aortic stenosis (Fig. 22.11). It can also be seen in patients older than 50 when there is tortuosity of the entire aorta or systemic hypertension. Ascending aortic aneurysm (calcific with syphilis, not calcified with Marfan's syndrome) is another possibility (Fig. 22.13). A ductus bump adjacent to the aortic knob is an indication of patent ductus arteriosus.

Azygos vein dilatation (>6 mm on upright PA or >1 cm on supine radiograph) is seen with intravascular volume expansion, elevated central venous pressure, and right heart failure (see Fig. 23.17). Additional causes include the Valsalva maneuver, pregnancy, renal failure, vena cava obstruction, or azygos continuation of the IVC. Dilatation of the SVC often accompanies volume expansion or elevated central venous pressure but is more difficult to detect with certainty.

Cardiac Calcifications

Coronary Calcification. Radiographs commonly demonstrate coronary artery calcification in a 3-cm triangle along the upper left heart border, called the "CAC" (coronary artery calcification) triangle (Figs. 22.14, 23.1). If chest pain and coronary calcification are present, there is a 94% chance the patient will have occlusive coronary artery disease at angiography. Fluoroscopic detection of coronary calcification actually has higher sensitivity and specificity in screening asymptomatic individuals than does exercise tolerance testing. In symptomatic patients, the detection of coronary calcification approaches exercise tolerance testing in sensitivity and exceeds exercise tolerance testing in specificity. More than 82% of the patients with fluoroscopically demonstrated coronary artery calcification and positive exercise tolerance testing have significant coronary artery disease at angiography. Calcifications have more significance when seen in patients less than 60 years of age. Heavier and more extensive calcification correlates with more severe coronary disease. Detection of coronary calcification helps to differentiate patients with ischemic, from those with nonischemic, cardiomyopathy.

Valvular calcification is seen in 85% of patients with acquired valvular disease but is rarely detected in patients less than 20 years of age. Aortic valve calcification

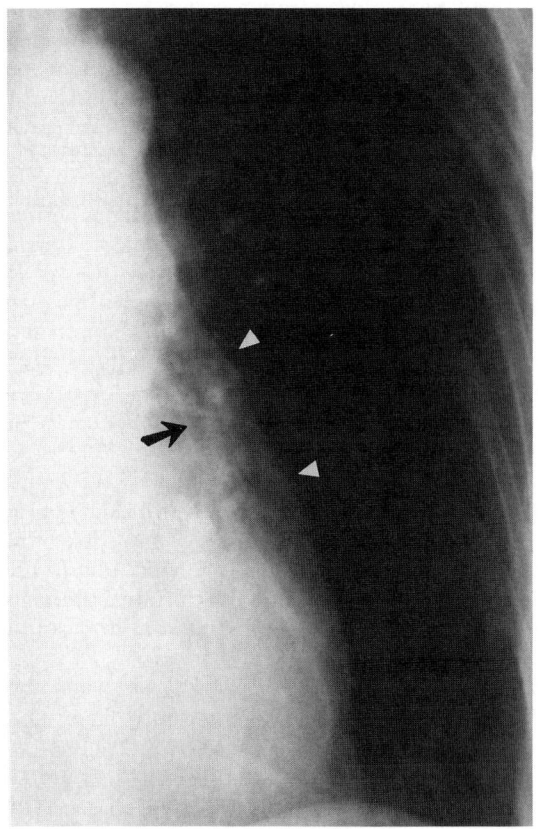

Figure 22.14. Coronary Artery Calcification. The calcification (*arrow*) is most commonly detected in the coronary artery calcification triangle along the upper left heart margin (*arrowheads*). The presence of coronary artery calcification may be indicative of coronary stenosis and ischemic heart disease.

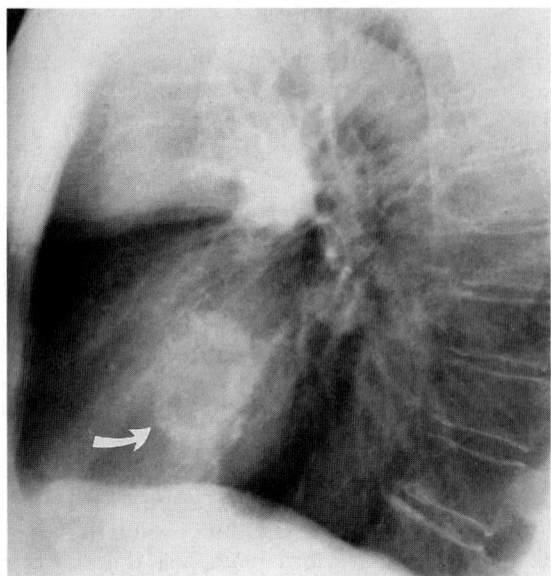

Figure 22.15. Mitral Annulus Calcification. Ovoid calcification of the mitral annulus (*arrow*) is secondary to atherosclerosis and is commonly associated with mitral insufficiency. Mitral calcification is best seen on a lateral radiograph.

is highly specific for valve disease. Calcific aortic stenosis is most often degenerative in origin and is usually seen in elderly males. Extensive aortic annulus calcification is atherosclerotic in nature and has been associated with conduction blocks.

Mitral valve calcification is highly suggestive of rheumatic valvular disease and is seen on chest radiograph in approximately 40% of patients with mitral stenosis. It is even more common in patients with stenosis and regurgitation. Atherosclerotic calcification of the mitral annulus occurs in approximately 10% of the elderly population (Fig. 22.15). It appears as circular, ovoid, or C- or J-shaped calcification in the mitral annulus and can lead to mitral valve incompetence.

Sinus of valsalva aneurysm calcification is seen as a curvilinear density anterior and lateral to the ascending aorta.

Calcified ligamentum arteriosum is seen as a linear calcification in the aortopulmonary window connecting the top of the left PA to the floor of the aortic arch.

Calcified LA. Thin curvilinear calcification in the wall of the LA is usually associated with mitral stenosis, left atrial enlargement, atrial fibrillation, and left atrial thrombus.

Calcified pericardium is typically anterior and inferior in location. It can be single or double layered and is associated with a high incidence of constrictive pericardial hemodynamics. Causes include viral, hemorrhagic, and tuberculous pericarditis as well as postsurgical scarring.

Calcified Infarct. Dystrophic calcification may occur in the myocardial wall from prior myocardial infarction.

Calcified ventricular aneurysm. Thin curvilinear calcification anterolaterally near the apex is most often seen with true aneurysms. Posterior curvilinear calcifi-

cation is usually seen in pseudoaneurysms (Fig. 22.16).

Calcified thrombus is seen as clumpy calcification in the LA or, less commonly, in the LV.

Calcified Pulmonary Arteries. Thin eggshell-like calcification in the walls of the pulmonary arteries is virtually diagnostic of long-standing pulmonary arterial hypertension (see Figs. 23.15,23.16).

Tumors. Rounded or stippled calcifications are seen occasionally in atrial myxomas and rarely in other cardiac neoplasms (see Fig. 23.29).

Pulmonary Vascularity

The lungs have dual blood supply with pulmonary arteries and systemic bronchial arteries.

Pulmonary Arteries. Increased circulation from left-to-right shunts results in enlargement of the main and hilar pulmonary arteries with increased blood flow to the upper and lower lobes. Asymmetrical blood flow can be seen with pulmonary hypoplasia, Swyer-James syndrome, and congenital lesions such as pulmonary stenosis (increased to the left lung) or tetralogy of Fallot (increased to the right lung).

Bronchial arteries arise from the aorta and penetrate into the lungs, traveling with the bronchi. Tetralogy of Fallot and pseudotruncus arteriosus result in a shift to bronchial circulation. Bronchial arteries are also important in Rasmussen's aneurysms from tuberculosis and systemic hypervascularity of any chronic infection.

Pulmonary arterial hypertension (Fig. 22.17) results in *a*) dilated main PA, *b*) right-sided cardiac enlargement, *c*) central enlargement of left and right pulmonary arteries, *d*) rapid pruning of the peripheral pulmonary arteries, *e*) decreased peripheral pulmonary circulation, *f*) calcification of the central pulmonary arteries, and *g*) secondary enlargement of the azygos vein.

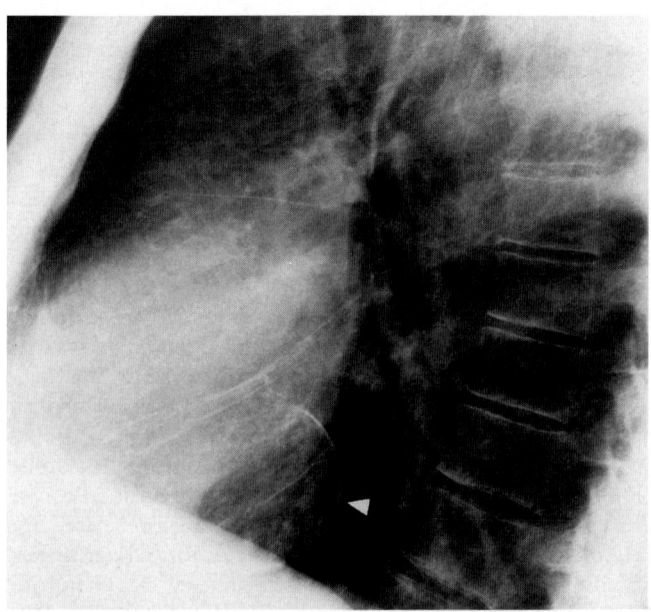

Figure 22.16. Calcified Ventricular Pseudoaneurysm. Thin, curvilinear calcification along the LV (*arrowhead*) is indicative of a ventricular pseudoaneurysm.

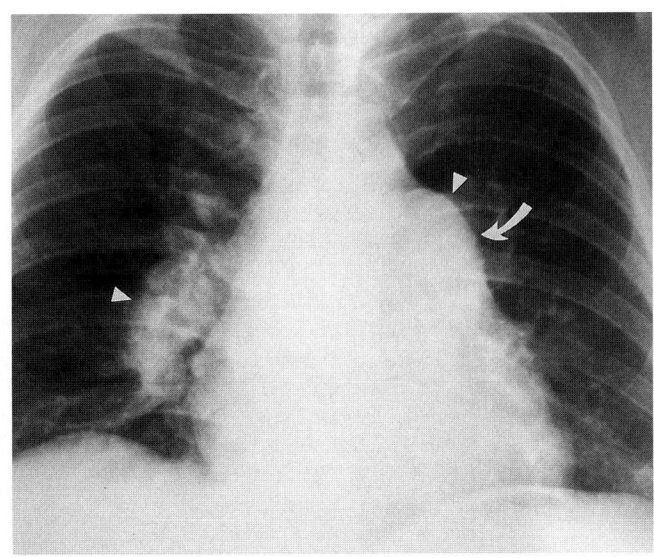

Figure 22.17. Idiopathic Pulmonary Hypertension. The main (*curved arrow*), right, and left (*arrowheads*) pulmonary arteries are dilated. The pulmonary arteries taper rapidly and peripheral pulmonary vascularity is decreased.

Pulmonary aneurysms and peripheral pulmonic stenosis can also cause unusual enlargements of the pulmonary arteries and may be seen in Williams syndrome, Marfan's syndrome, and collagen disorders.

Pulmonary venous hypertension (Fig. 22.18) results from mitral stenosis, mitral regurgitation, or elevated left ventricular pressure (aortic stenosis or congestive heart failure). The normal vessel caliber in the lower lobes is greater than that in the upper lobes by a 3:2 ratio because of hydrostatic pressure and the high compliance of the venous system. Elevated venous pressure causes progressive, edematous perivascular cuffing, which occurs first in the lower vessels, which have higher hydrostatic pressures. Perivascular edema in the lower lobes results in decreased compliance and progressive cephalization of blood flow. The chest radiograph shows decreased caliber of lower lobe vessels and increased caliber of upper lobe vessels. Cephalization of blood flow is the earliest radiographic sign of congestive heart failure and pulmonary venous hypertension. Cephalization begins at 10–13 mm Hg wedge pressure. Equalization of upper to lower pulmonary blood flow occurs at 14–16 mm Hg. Reversal of the normal distribution with the upper lobe vessels distended and the lower lobe vessels constricted occurs at 17–20 mm Hg. Hilar fullness, "Viking helmet sign" in the hila, and filling out of the right hilar angle commonly accompany reversed flow distribution.

Pulmonary Edema. Interstitial edema with Kerley A, B, and C lines and thickened pulmonary fissures occurs at 20–25 mm Hg wedge pressure (Fig. 22.19). Kerley lines represent thickened interlobular septa: A lines are long straight lines radiating toward the hila; B lines are horizontal lines connecting to the pleural surface near the costophrenic angle; and C lines are random reticular lines seen throughout the lungs. Alveolar edema begins

at 25–30 mm Hg wedge pressure (Fig. 22.20). Chronic failure "toughens" the interstitium (often resulting in hemosiderosis and pulmonary ossification) and can add an additional 5 mm Hg protective zone prior to developing interstitial or alveolar edema. These progressive signs of failure have been classified as stages 1–4 (Table 22.3).

Congestive Heart Failure. Radiographic findings include *a)* cardiomegaly, *b)* left ventricular and left atrial enlargement, *c)* cephalization of blood flow, *d)* azygos vein and SVC distension, *e)* perivascular cuffing with haziness and unsharpness of the pulmonary vessels, *f)* peribronchial cuffing with thickening of the bronchial walls seen as small "Cheerios" when viewed end on, *g)* Kerley lines, *h)* thickening of the pulmonary fissures, *i)* subpleural edema, *j)* pleural effusions, usually larger in

Table 22.3. Signs of Progressive Cardiac Failure

Stage	Sign	Wedge Pressure (mm Hg)
1	Progressive cephalization	10–20
2	Interstitial edema and septal lines	20–25
3	Alveolar edema, often in bat wing perihilar distribution	>25–30
4	Chronic or severe pulmonary venous hypertension resulting in hemosiderosis, pulmonary ossification, and chronic interstitial disease such as from long-standing mitral stenosis	>30–35

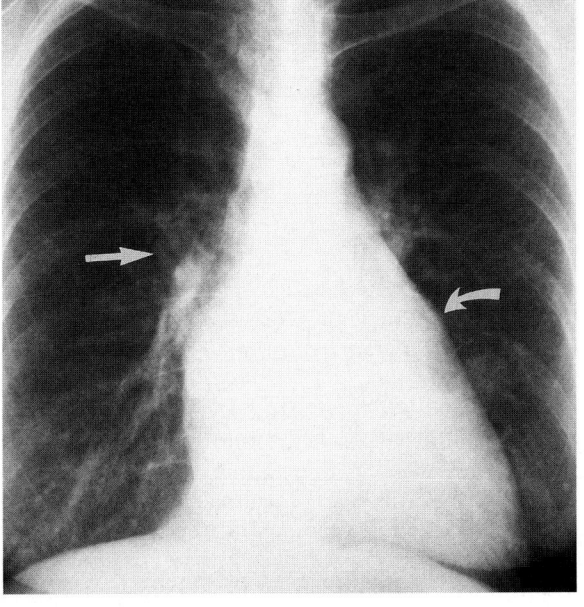

Figure 22.18. Pulmonary Venous Hypertension. Cephalization of blood flow is evident in this patient with mitral stenosis and enlarged left atrial appendage (*curved arrow*). The lower lobe vessels are constricted, and the upper lobe vessels are distended. Fullness in the hilar angle (*straight arrow*) is because of enlargement of the superior pulmonary veins crossing between the interlobar artery and the upper lobe artery.

Figure 22.19. Interstitial Edema. The edema is indicated by prominent Kerley lines. Thickening of the fissures (*arrow*) is also present, along with prominence of the LV and LA and cephalization of blood flow.

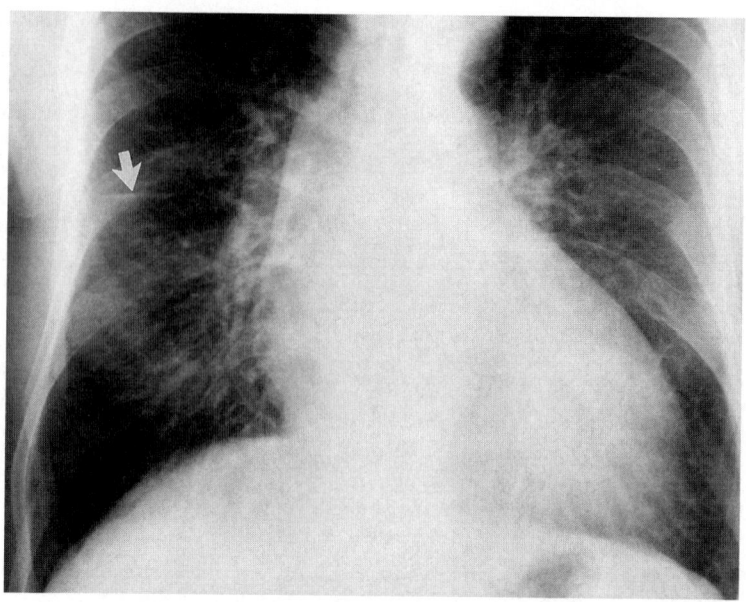

Figure 22.20. Alveolar Pulmonary Edema. Classic bat wing or butterfly perihilar alveolar infiltrates are present in a symmetrical cloudlike pattern.

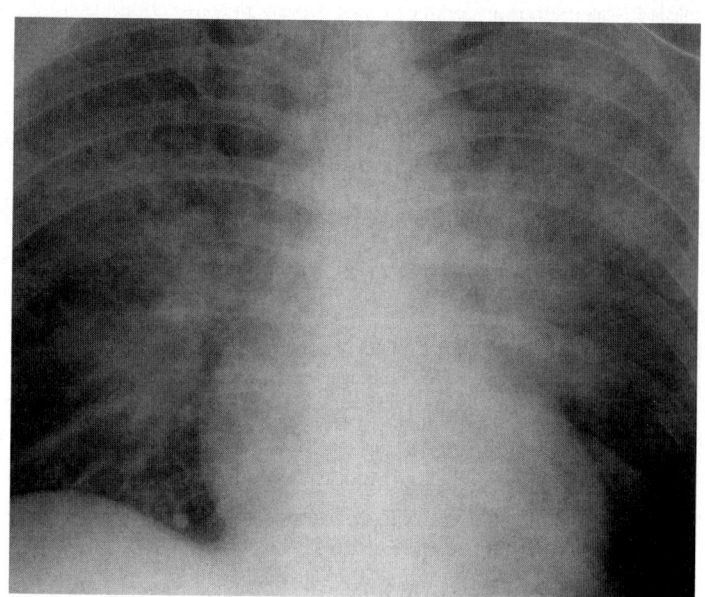

the right hemithorax, and *k*) alveolar edema in a "bat wing" or "butterfly" distribution, also often more pronounced on the right.

Right Heart Failure. The most common cause of right heart failure is left heart failure. Elevated left-sided pressures manifest in the pulmonary circuit and then the right side of the heart. Long-standing venous hypertension leads to pulmonary arterial hypertension. Elevated right-sided pressures cause right ventricular hypertrophy and dilatation, as well as systemic venous dilatation involving azygos vein, SVC, and jugular veins. Dilatation of the right heart can also cause tricuspid valve incompetence. Right heart failure protects the pulmonary circuit by accumulating edema and fluid outside the lungs, similar to the old therapeutic maneuver of rotating tourniquets.

Right heart failure may also occur with the dilated car-

diomyopathies, including viral and alcoholic cardiomyopathy. When right heart failure is the result of pulmonary disease such as chronic obstructive pulmonary disease, destructive lung disease, or primary pulmonary hypertension, the term *cor pulmonale* is used.

The Pericardium

The pericardium is composed of one continuous fibrous membrane that is folded back on itself, creating two layers. The inner layer of visceral pericardium or epicardium is closely attached to the myocardium and subepicardial fat. The outer layer or parietal pericardium is thicker and is often referred to simply as the pericardium.

Pericardial Effusion. Between the visceral and parietal layers is the pericardial space, which usually contains 20

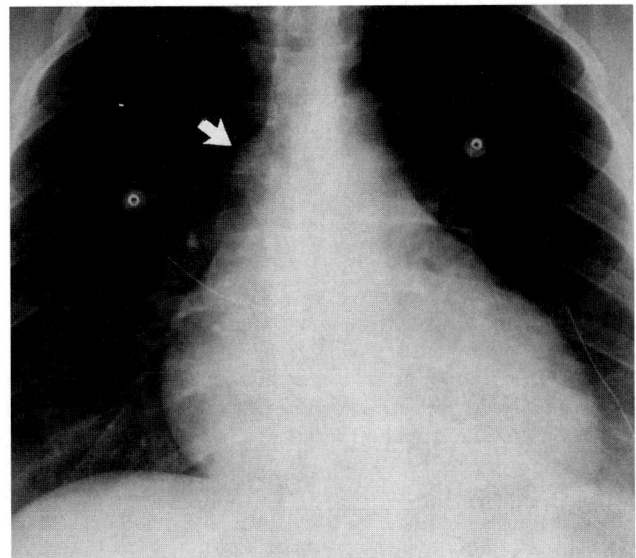

Figure 22.21. Pericardial Effusion. Water-bottle configuration of the cardiac silhouette is indicative of pericardial effusion or dilated cardiomyopathy. This patient with systemic lupus erythematosus has an enlarged azygos vein (*arrow*), decreased pulmonary vasculature, and clear lung parenchyma.

mL of serous fluid. More than 50 mL of fluid is clearly abnormal, but 200 mL is required for detection by plain film radiography. Mediastinal and epicardial fat enable the pericardium to be visualized as a thin arcuate line paralleling the anterior heart border in the retrosternal region. A pericardial stripe exceeding 2–3 mm is indicative of pericardial thickening or effusion. Unfortunately, the thickened pericardial stripe can be seen on the lateral radiograph in only about 15% of patients with pericardial effusion. The "differential density sign" refers to a lucent margin along the left heart border on the PA radiograph or along the posterior cardiac border on the lateral radiograph. It is seen in up to 63% of patients with pericardial effusion but is less specific than the thickened pericardial stripe. Large pericardial effusions cause the heart to appear on frontal radiographs in the shape of a sac of water sitting on a tabletop (Fig. 22.21).

Pneumopericardium appears on plain films as radiolucency surrounding the heart and separated from the lung by a thin white line of pericardium (Fig. 22.22). Air may also be seen outlining the pulmonary arteries or the undersurface of the heart. Pneumopericardium can be caused by trauma, infection, or pneumomediastinum. Firm attachment of the pericardium to the ascending aorta just above the main PA acts to contain the pneumopericardium.

Other Signs of Cardiac Disease

Situs Anomalies. Careful attention should be directed at the location of the aortic arch, gastric fundus, heart, pulmonary fissures, and the branching pattern of the bronchi. Normal anatomic positioning is termed *situs solitus. Situs inversus* means that the patient's entire anatomic arrangement is reversed in a right-to-left direction as a "mirror image." Situs inversus is associated

with a 5–10% incidence of congenital heart disease, compared with less than 1% incidence for situs solitus. *Dextrocardia* indicates that the heart is in the right hemithorax. The apex of the heart lies to the right, with the long axis of the heart directed from left to right. *Kartagener's syndrome* is a combination of situs inversus with dextrocardia, bronchiectasis, and sinusitis (Fig. 22.23). The latter findings are because of the abnormal mucosal cilia.

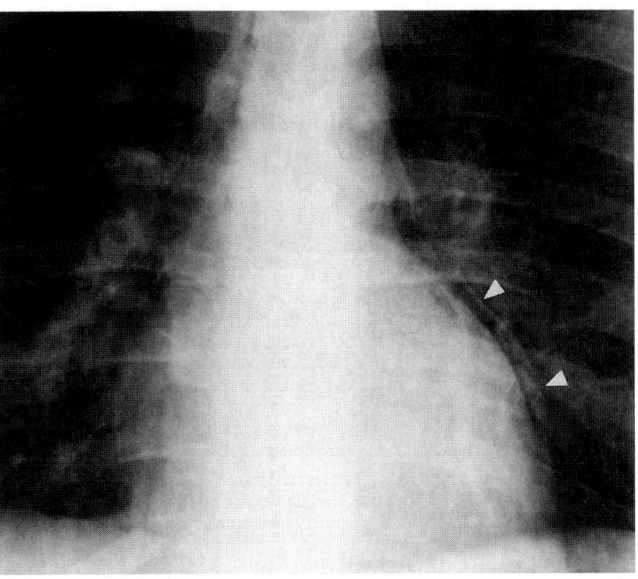

Figure 22.22. Pneumopericardium. Air within the pericardial sac enables visualization of the pericardium (*arrowheads*), seen as a thin white line paralleling the left heart border.

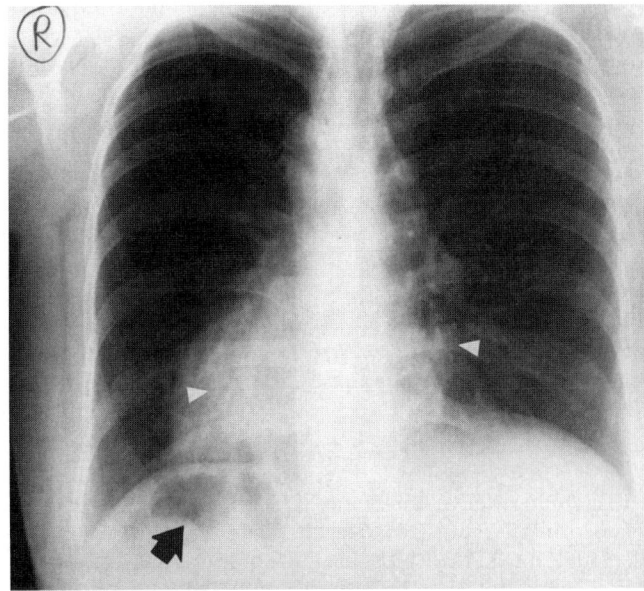

Figure 22.23. Kartagener's Syndrome. Situs inversus is evident with dextrocardia and the gastric air bubble (*black arrow*) on the patient's right. Evidence of bronchiectasis is present behind the heart and in the left lower lobe (*arrowheads*).

Dextroposition means the heart is shifted toward the right hemithorax. It is associated with hypoplastic right lung and an increased incidence of congenital heart disease, particularly left-to-right shunts. *Dextroversion* means the cardiac apex is to the right, but the stomach and aortic knob remain on the left. The LV remains on the left but lies anterior to the RV.

Dextrocardia with situs ambiguous and polysplenia is also called "bilateral left-sidedness." Each lung contains only two lobes and hyparterial bronchi. Bilateral SVCs are also common. The incidence of congenital heart disease is increased, most commonly that of atrial septal defect or anomalous pulmonary venous return. Dextrocardia with asplenia is referred to as "bilateral right-sidedness" because of bilateral minor fissures and three lobes in each lung. The cardiac anomalies are usually more complex and severe than in polysplenia.

Bony Abnormalities. Postoperative changes of sternotomy suggest prior cardiac surgery and the presence of cardiac disease. Sternal fractures from motor vehicle accidents are associated with a 50% incidence of cardiac contusion. Hypersegmentation of the sternum (more than four to five segments) is present in 90% of patients with Down syndrome and offers a clue to the presence of endocardial cushion defect or complete atrioventricular canal. Wavy retrosternal linear opacities suggest dilated internal mammary arteries associated with coarctation of the aorta. Pectus excavatum is associated with an increased incidence of mitral valve prolapse and Marfan's syndrome. A barrel-shaped chest with pectus carinatum is associated with ventricular septal defects and complete atrioventricular canal. Scoliosis with a "shield chest" is seen with Marfan's syndrome, aortic valve disease, coarctation, and aortic dissection.

The presence of 11 or fewer ribs is highly associated with Down syndrome and atrioventricular canal. "Ribbon ribs" or bifurcated ribs and an overcirculation pattern suggest truncus arteriosus, whereas their association with an undercirculation pattern suggests tetralogy of Fallot. Rib notching and inferior rib sclerosis indicate collateral circulation through intercostal arteries and occurs with coarctation of the aorta and Blalock-Taussig operations. The third through the eighth ribs are most commonly involved. Fractures of the first and second ribs indicate high-velocity blunt trauma has occurred, and there is an increased risk of aortic injury.

The spine offers clues to the presence of aortic valve disease when changes of ankylosing spondylitis, neurofibromatosis, or rheumatoid arthritis are present. Scoliosis is associated with an increased incidence of congenital heart disease.

NUCLEAR CARDIOLOGY

Cardiac nuclear medicine is a central modality in cardiac imaging and is covered in detail in chapter 57. Perfusion scans with thallium or new technetium agents are useful for diagnosing coronary ischemia and myocardial infarcts. Normal perfusion scans appear in the shape of a horseshoe in the vertical and long axes and in the shape of a doughnut in the short axis (see Fig. 57.1). The scans are accomplished during rest, with controlled exercise or with pharmacologic stress with IV dipyridamole. The stress and redistribution or rest images appear identical in normal patients. Hypoperfused segments on stress images, which fill in on rest, are indicative of ischemia. Hypoperfused segments on both rest and stress images are usually infarcts or scars. Myocardial infarction scanning can be accomplished using rest perfusion agents for "cold spot" imaging or technetium pyrophosphate for "hot spot" imaging (see Figs. 23.8, 23.9). The new antimyosin antibodies have also shown great promise for diagnosing and sizing myocardial infarction.

Electrocardiogram-gated myocardial blood pool studies examine wall motion and allow left ventricular ejection fraction calculations. Ventricular function, aneurysms, and valvular disease may be studied with volume curves and functional images. Right ventricular ejection fraction calculations require first-pass examinations because of anatomic overlap of the RV with the atria in the left anterior oblique projection. First-pass cardiac studies can also diagnose SVC obstruction and left-to-right cardiac shunts. Right-to-left cardiac shunts can be evaluated and quantified with technetium macroaggregated albumin or microspheres.

SPECT imaging greatly improves the diagnostic capabilities of perfusion imaging and infarct scans. Positron emission tomography is a new technology with increased resolution compared with SPECT. Positron emission tomography can assess cardiac metabolism as well as perfusion, enhancing its ability to evaluate cardiomyopathies, ischemia, infarction, and "hibernating" or viable myocardium.

ECHOCARDIOGRAPHY

Echocardiography includes M-mode, real-time two-dimensional US, range-gated and color flow Doppler, and transesophageal US. Transesophageal echocardiography uses a nasogastric probe with a steerable ultrasonic beam that views the heart and aorta from the close posterior position provided by the esophagus (Fig. 22.24). M-mode echocardiograms are produced by a narrow ultrasonic beam that is directed at cardiac structures and observed over time or is swept across an area of anatomy (see Figs. 22.25–22.27). The returning echoes produce a time–motion study of cardiac structures. With a transthoracic technique, anterior structures are usually displayed at the top of the image. The thickness and motion of the myocardium can be evaluated throughout the cardiac cycle. Pericardial effusions are shown as an echo-free space adjacent to the myocardium (Fig. 22.25). Large pleural effusions create an echolucent space posterior to the LV and pericardium. The RA and atrial septum are not well seen by M-mode echocardiography.

The interventricular septum appears as a band of echoes near the midplane. It normally thickens and moves toward the posterior wall of the LV during systole (Fig. 22.25). Paradoxic septal motion may be seen in pericardial effusion, with cardiac tamponade, chronic obstructive pulmonary disease, asthma, atrial septal defects pulmonary hypertension, LBBB, and septal ischemia. The interventricular septum measures less than

10–11 mm at end diastole and is compared with the thickness of the posterior wall of the LV for asymmetric or concentric hypertrophy.

The aortic root lies immediately posterior to the RV and measures 8–12 mm in neonates and 20–40 mm in adults (Fig. 22.26). The thin parallel aortic walls move anteriorly during systole. The aortic root is dilated with aortic stenosis, aortic insufficiency, tetralogy of Fallot, and aortic aneurysm. The thin aortic cusps seen within the aortic root should open widely during systole and should not reverberate.

The LA is seen posterior to the aortic root (Fig. 22.26).

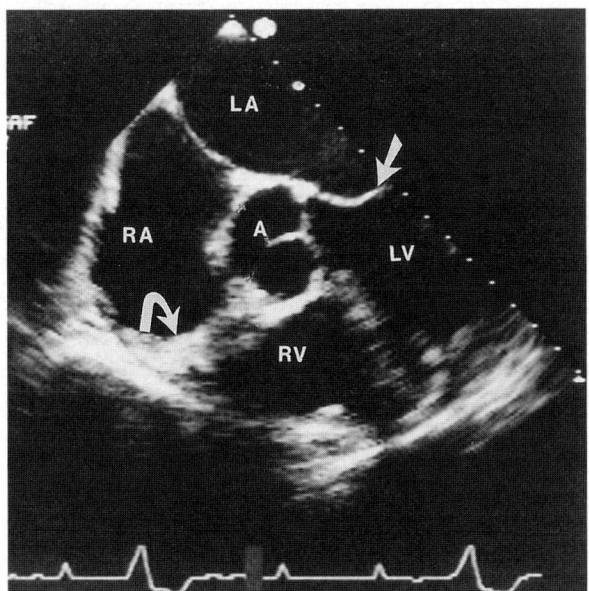

Figure 22.24. Transesophageal Echocardiogram. A five-chamber view of the heart is provided by an US probe within the esophagus. The probe is behind the *LA* and is depicted at the top of the image. All four chambers and the aortic valve are seen in one plane, the "five-chamber view." The *LA* and *RA* are separated by the interatrial septum. The aortic valve (*A*) is readily identified in the midplane. The *RV* and *LV* are separated by the interventricular septum. The tricuspid valve (*curved arrow*) is seen between the *RA* and *RV*, and the mitral valve (*straight arrow*) is seen between the *LA* and *LV*.

The normal size is no larger than 40 mm during diastole in adults. The LA is free of internal echoes and has a thin posterior wall that merges with the thicker left ventricular wall.

The LV lies inferior and lateral to the LA and is an echo-free space except for the thin chordae tendineae and the echogenic projections of the papillary muscles. The left ventricular posterior wall thickens during systole and contracts anteriorly. The transverse diameter of the LV does not normally exceed 5.7 cm during diastole. The wall measures approximately the same as the ventricular septum (10–11 mm).

The mitral valve produces a saw-toothed or M-shaped pattern posterior to the interventricular septum (Fig. 22.27). The anterior leaflet is the dominant echo and is continuous with the posterior wall of the aortic root. Immediately posterior to the anterior leaflet is the W-shaped pattern of the posterior leaflet. The two leaflets close during systole. The echo pattern of the anterior leaflet should be carefully scrutinized for evidence of thickening, delay in closure (seen with mitral stenosis), vegetations, prolapse, myxoma, or high-frequency vibration secondary to aortic regurgitation (Austin Flint phenomena). The specific points of the mitral waveform are (Fig. 22.27) the following:

A point: **A**trial contraction with peak anterior opening motion

B point: notch **B**etween the A and C points representing elevated LVEDP

C point: **C**losure of the mitral valve occurs with contraction of the LV during systole

D point: early **D**iastole when mitral valve begins to open

E point: maximal **E**xcursion of the valve opening. This is the peak of early diastolic opening and the most anterior position of the valve during diastole.

F point: most posterior point of early diastolic **F**illing prior to atrial contraction

The E–F slope is a function of left atrial emptying rate and should be steep. With mitral stenosis, the slope will be flattened and look more squared off than M-shaped. With valve thickening and calcification, the squared-off part appears thickened.

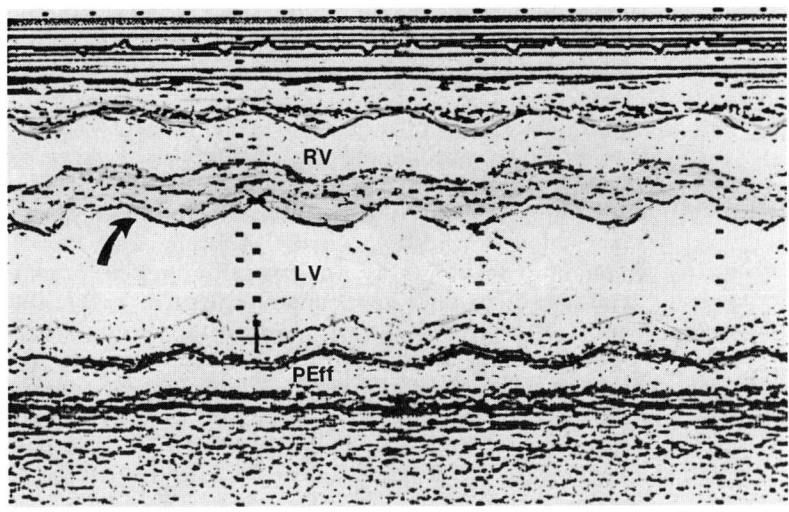

Figure 22.25. Pericardial Effusion. An M-mode echocardiogram with the ultrasonic probe at the top of the image demonstrates the *RV*, interventricular septum (*curved arrow*), and *LV*. Note the normal myocardial contractility with the interventricular septum contracting toward the posterior left ventricular wall during systole. A pericardial effusion (*PEff*) is seen as an echolucent space posterior to the left ventricular wall.

Figure 22.26. Aortic Root. An M-mode echocardiogram demonstrates anterior movement of the anterior (*curved arrow*) and posterior (*straight arrow*) walls of the aortic root during systole. The *RV* is seen anterior to the aortic root and the *LA* is seen posterior to the aortic root. Aortic valve motion can be seen within the aortic root.

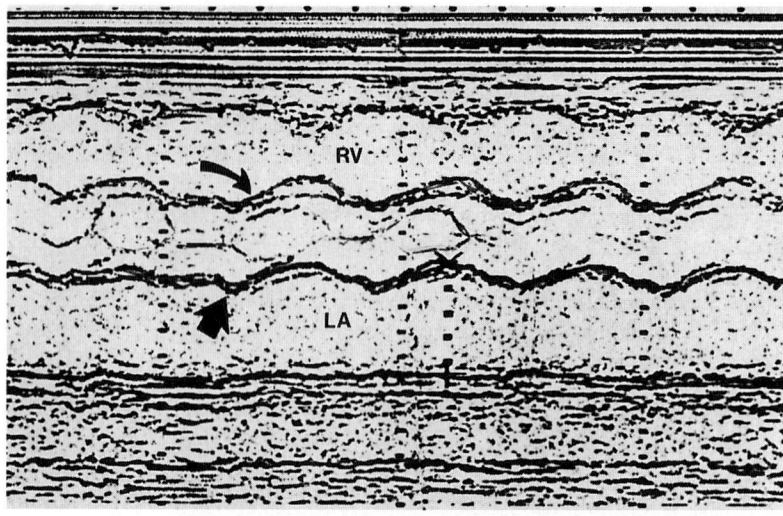

Figure 22.27. Normal Mitral Valve. An M-mode echocardiogram demonstrates the right ventricular cavity and left ventricular cavity separated by a band of echoes representing the interventricular septum (*arrow*). The moving mitral valve can be seen within the left ventricular cavity. Because of plane of section, the full systolic motion of the myocardium is not well visualized. The points of the mitral waveform are *labeled with letters.*

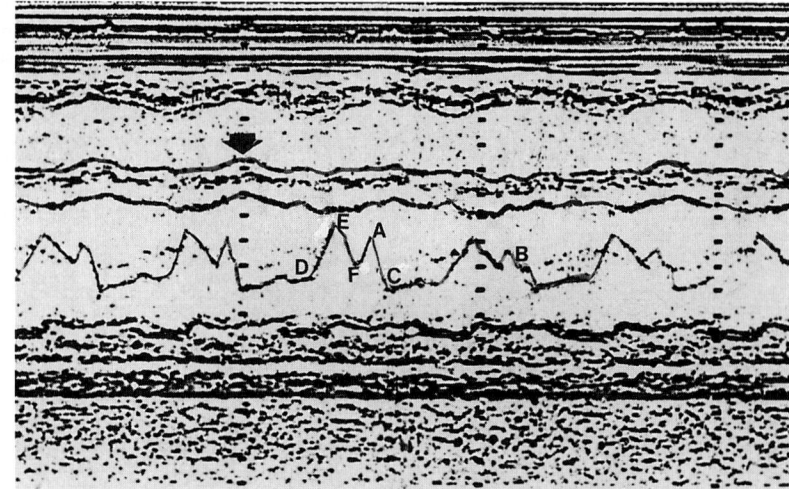

The tricuspid valve is identified by locating the mitral valve and rotating the transducer medially. It has an M-shaped echo pattern similar to that of the mitral valve. The E–F slope is decreased with tricuspid stenosis and is increased with Ebstein's anomaly, tricuspid regurgitation, and atrial septal defect.

The pulmonic valve is rather difficult to evaluate by M-mode echocardiography. The diameter of the pulmonary trunk is similar to that of the aortic root. Pulmonary valve motion is similar to aortic valve motion, except that only the posterior leaflet is well seen and there may be a small "A wave" because of atrial contraction.

CORONARY ANGIOGRAPHY

Selective catheterization of the coronary arteries was first accomplished in 1959 by Sones with the use of a flexible, tapered tip catheter using a cut-down procedure on the brachial artery. In 1966, Amplatz used J-shaped, preformed catheters with better torque control from a transfemoral approach. In 1968, Judkins used separate preformed catheters for the right and left coronary arteries. After selective catheterization of the coronary artery, hand injections of contrast verify the size and flow of the artery. The left coronary artery generally requires 7–9 mL of contrast at 4–6 mL/s, whereas 6–8 mL at 3–5 mL/s is sufficient for the smaller right coronary artery. Pressure limits for power injectors should be set at less than 150 psi. The catheter tip should not be left wedged in the coronary ostium, as this might occlude blood flow.

Complications of coronary angiography include hematoma, pseudoaneurysm, and fistula formation at the puncture site, arrhythmias including premature ventricular contractions, heart block and asystole, myocardial infarction, stroke, emboli, and death. Indications for coronary arteriography include *a*) confirmation of an anatomic cause for angina, *b*) identification of high-risk lesions, *c*) evaluation of asymptomatic patients with abnormal exercise tolerance test or occupational risk, *d*) preoperative evaluation for cardiac surgery, *e*) evaluation of patients with coronary artery bypass grafts for stenosis or occlusion, and *f*) after myocardial infarction, for evaluation of interventional therapy.

Coronary Anatomy

The right coronary artery (RCA) arises from the right coronary cusp, and the left coronary artery (LCA) arises from the left coronary cusp. Approximately 85% of patients are right dominant, meaning that the RCA supplies the posterior descending artery and the posterior and inferior surface of the myocardium. In 10–12% of patients, the LCA is dominant and supplies the inferior and posterior surface. Approximately 4–5% of patients are codominant. The LCA measures 0.5–1.5 cm in length before it divides beneath the left atrial appendage (Figs. 22.28, 22.29). The left anterior descending artery (LAD) extends anteriorly in the interventricular groove. The cir-

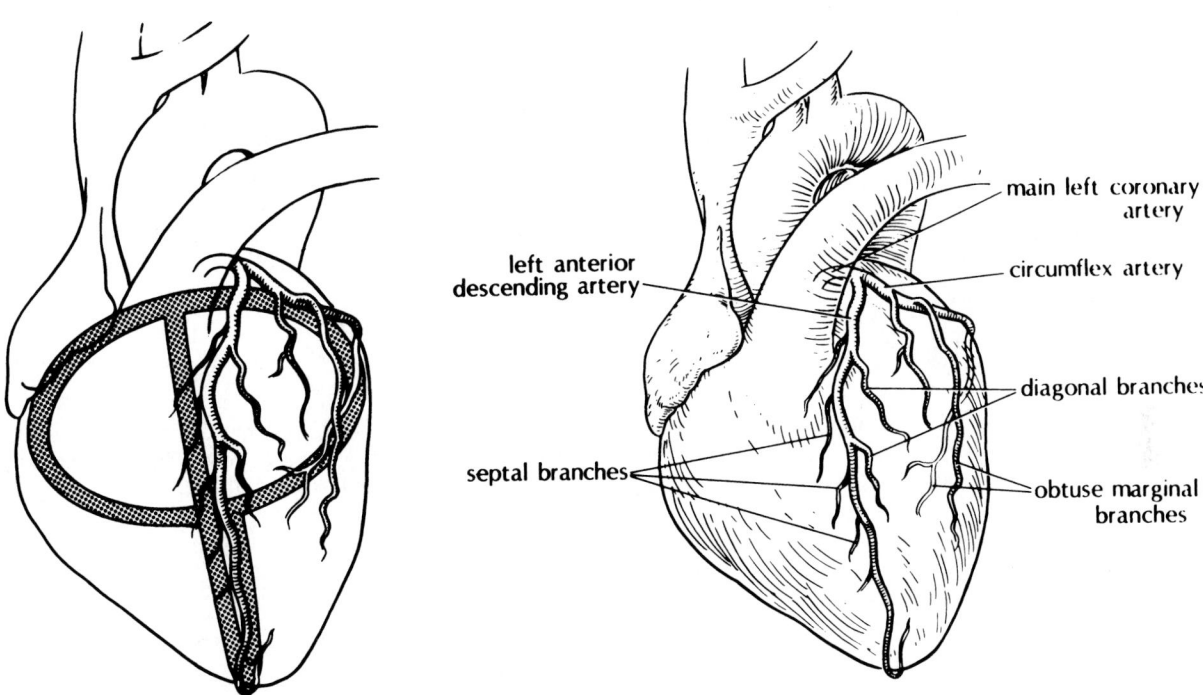

Figure 22.28. Left Coronary Artery in the Left Anterior Oblique Projection. The LCA divides into the circumflex artery that makes up the *left side of the circle*, and the left anterior descending artery that makes up the *anterior portion of the loop*. Obtuse marginal branches extend from the circumflex artery; diagonal and septal branches extend from the left anterior descending artery. (Reproduced with permission from Kubicka RA, Smith C. How to interpret coronary arteriograms. Radiographics 1986;6:661–701.)

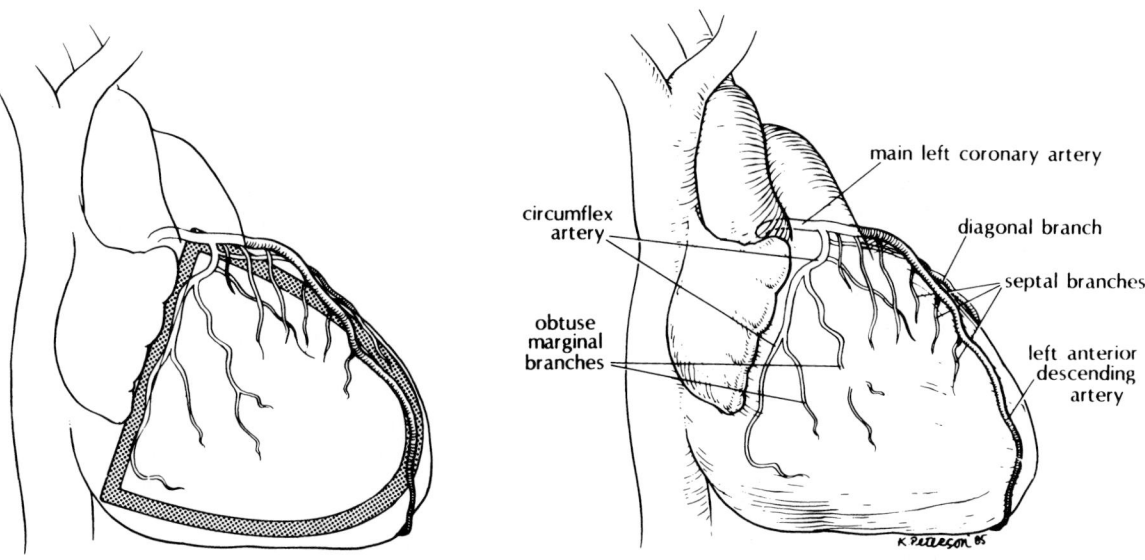

Figure 22.29. Left Coronary Artery in the Right Anterior Oblique. The *loop* is more open in this projection, whereas the *circle* is superimposed. The left anterior descending artery makes up the *anterior portion of the loop*. The circumflex artery and its obtuse marginal branches make up the *left side of the circle*. (Reproduced with permission from Kubicka RA, Smith C. How to interpret coronary arteriograms. Radiographics 1986;6:661–701.)

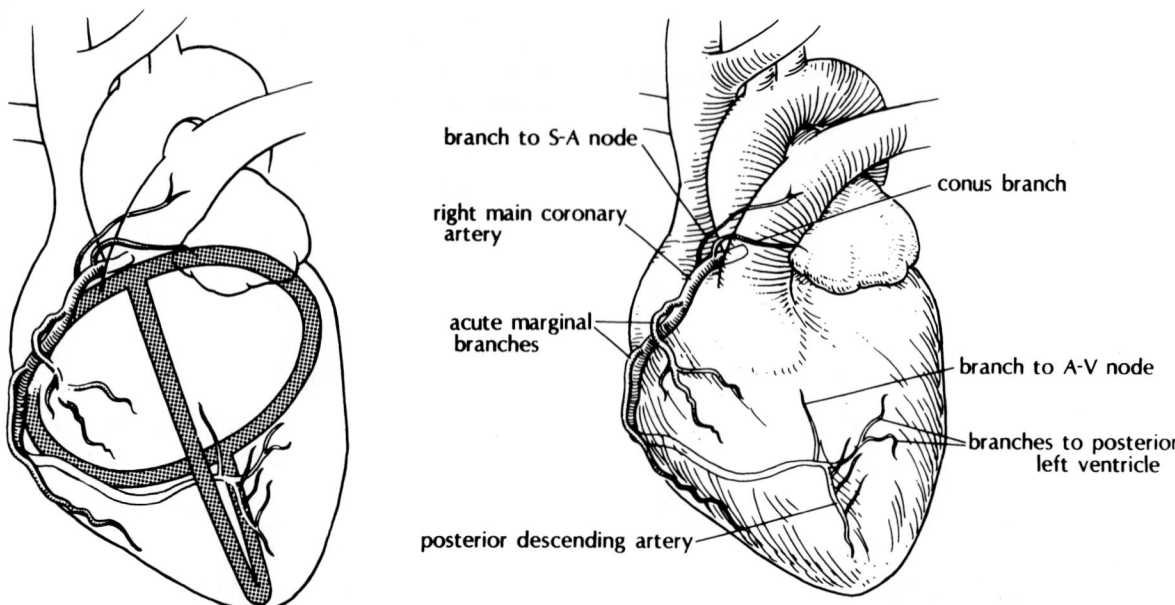

Figure 22.30. Right Coronary Artery in the Left Anterior Oblique Projection. The *right portion of the circle* represents the RCA and the *posterior portion of the loop* represents the posterior descending artery. *S-A,* sinoatrial; *A-V,* atrioventricular. (Reproduced with permission from Kubicka RA, Smith C. How to interpret coronary arteriograms. Radiographics 1986;6:661–701.)

cumflex artery extends laterally and posteriorly under the left atrial appendage to the atrioventricular groove. An occasional third branch is the ramus intermedius, which extends as a first diagonal branch (d1) or a first marginal branch (m1).

The LAD gives off several septal branches that penetrate into the septum. One or more diagonal branches extend toward the anterolateral wall. Occasionally, a conus branch comes off after the first septal branch and extends to the right ventricular infundibulum. The circumflex artery gives off one or more obtuse marginal branches that supply the lateral wall of the LV.

The RCA passes anterior and to the right between the PA and the RA (Figs. 22.30, 22.31). Its first branch is a conus branch to the pulmonary outflow tract. The second branch is the sinus node branch with a smaller branch to the RA. Muscular branches extend into the right ventricular myocardium. At the posterior turn, a large acute marginal branch is often given off anteriorly toward the diaphragmatic surface of the RV. The RCA then extends posteriorly in the atrioventricular sulcus and makes a 90° turn toward the apex in right dominant systems. As the posterior descending artery, it supplies branches to the diaphragmatic myocardium and the posterior one third of the interventricular septum. The digital RCA may also give off a variable number of posterolateral ventricular branches.

The coronary arteries can be visualized as a circle and loop, with the atrioventricular groove being the circle and the interventricular septum being the attached loop (Figs. 22.28–22.31). In the right anterior oblique projection, the circle is superimposed on itself and the loop is in profile. In the left anterior projection, the circle is more open and the loop is foreshortened. In the left anterior craniad view, there is a better, elongated view of the left main coronary artery, LAD, and ramus intermedius. For additional details on the circle and loop concept, please refer to the excellent primer on this subject by Kubicka and Smith (1).

Coronary Pathology

Fixed Coronary Stenosis. A 75% reduction in cross-sectional area is required to cause a significant reduction in blood flow (see Fig. 23.4). A 50% reduction in diameter corresponds to a 75% reduction in cross-sectional area. Other significant findings include coronary calcification, ulcerative plaques, and aneurysm formation. Collateral flow typically develops when there is greater than 85% stenosis.

Catheter spasm is most often seen in the RCA as a smooth transient narrowing, 1–2 mm distal to the catheter tip. The patient usually remains asymptomatic.

Prinzmetal variant angina is angina secondary to prolonged coronary spasm. IV ergonovine may be used in a provocative test to incite coronary spasm, typical symptoms, and electrocardiographic changes. Prinzmetal angina is usually treated medically.

Kawasaki syndrome is an inflammatory condition of the coronary arteries, probably attributable to a prior viral syndrome, that results in coronary stenosis and coronary aneurysms, occasionally persisting into adulthood.

Myocardial bridging describes a normal variant in which the coronary arteries penetrate and then emerge from the myocardium rather than running along the surface of the epicardium. This causes arterial constriction during systole, which reverts to normal flow during diastole.

Anomalies of the coronary arteries include multiple coronary ostia with more than one coronary artery arising directly from one coronary cusp, a single coronary

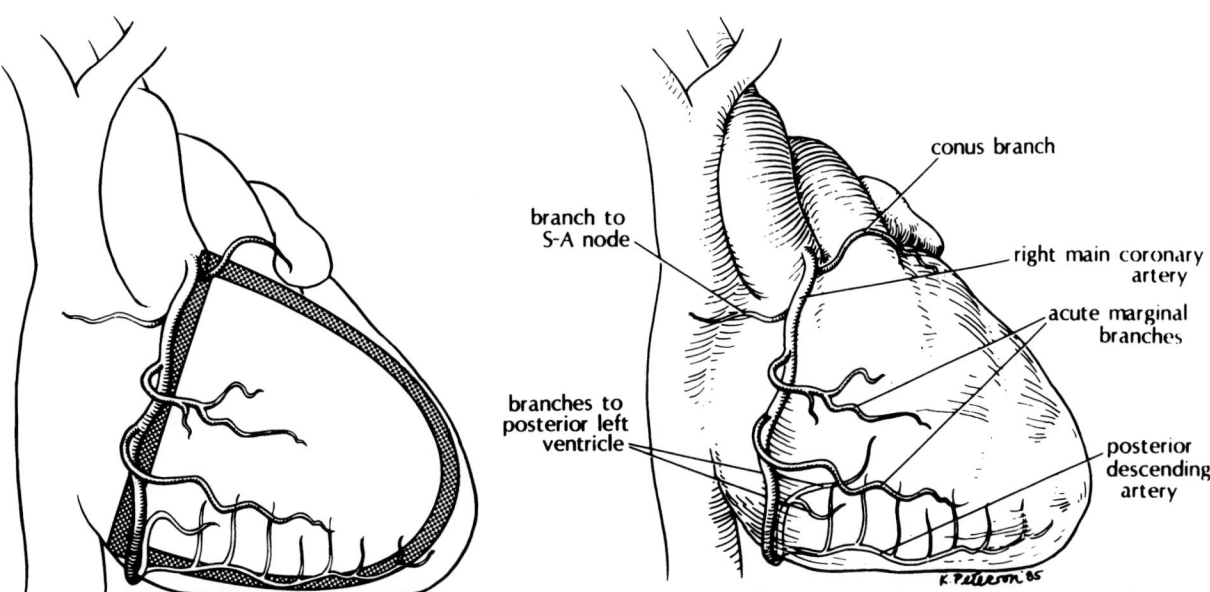

Figure 22.31. Right Coronary Artery in the Right Anterior Oblique Projection. The RCA forms the atrioventricular *circle*. The *loop* is more opened in this projection with the posterior descending artery making up its inferior margin. *S-A*, sinoatrial. (Reproduced with permission from Kubicka RA, Smith C. How to interpret coronary arteriograms. *Radiographics* 1986;6:661–701.)

artery, and origination of the LCA from the PA (Fig. 22.32).

Therapeutic Considerations

The primary modes of therapy for coronary artery disease include many efficacious medical regimens, percutaneous coronary angioplasty and stenting, and coronary artery bypass graft surgery. Coronary artery bypass grafting usually uses native internal mammary arteries or saphenous vein grafts. Surgical bypass has been shown to prolong life in left main coronary artery disease and three-vessel disease. Percutaneous coronary angioplasty (see Fig. 23.5) is considered useful for both single vessel and multivessel disease and has an 85–90% initial success rate. Restenosis remains a significant problem in up to 50% of cases, typically occurring within the first 6 months. Angioplasty is typically accomplished by balloon dilation of the stenotic lesion over a guidewire. Angioplasty is considered successful when the stenosis is reduced to less than 50% of diameter narrowing, although long-term prognosis is better when there is less than a 30% residual stenosis. Directional and rotational atherectomy and atherectomy with the transluminal extraction catheter and laser angioplasty are additional percutaneous techniques that are currently used in certain specific situations.

CARDIAC ANGIOGRAPHY

Angiography of the heart in adults most often involves left-sided catheterization via arterial puncture with retrograde examination of the aorta, LV, and LA. Selective catheterization of the coronary arteries is also accomplished from the arterial side. Right heart angiography

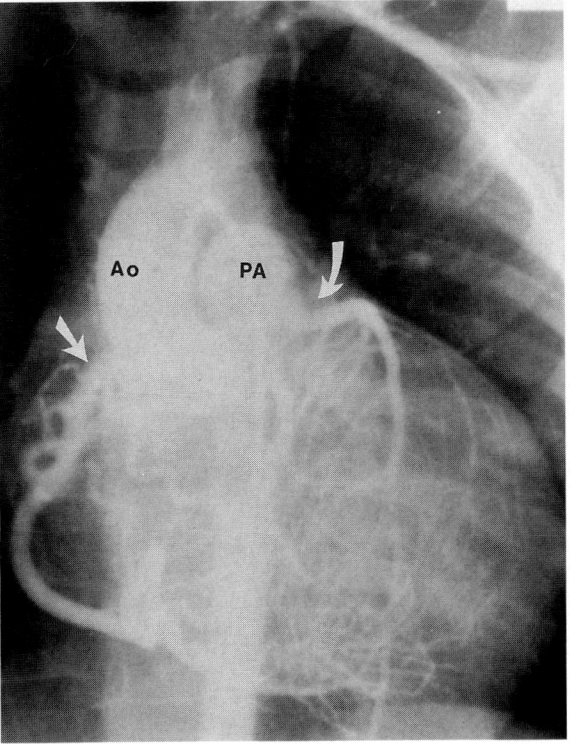

Figure 22.32. Aberrant LCA. The catheter in the ascending aorta (*Ao*) opacifies a dilated RCA (*straight arrow*). The LCA (*curved arrow*) arises from the pulmonary artery (*PA*) and is filled in a retrograde fashion via collateral flow from the RCA.

uses puncture of a neck or femoral vein with catheter placement in the RA, RV, pulmonary outflow tract, or PA. Additionally, the LA or LV may be seen on delayed or "levo-phase" views from a right-sided injection. It is also possible to access the left side during right heart catheterization by puncturing the atrial septum. End-hole catheters are used for pressure measurements, and pigtail or multiple side-hole catheters are used for intracardiac injections to avoid contrast injection into the myocardium itself. Blood flow is estimated with standard oximetry, thermodilution and indicator dilution techniques.

Wall motion is evaluated globally and regionally. *Hypokinesia* describes diminished contractility or less systolic motion than normal. *Akinesia* means no systolic wall motion. *Dyskinesia* means there is paradoxic wall motion during systolic contraction. *Asynchrony* refers to cardiac motion that is out of phase with the remainder of the myocardium.

Ventricular aneurysms appear as a bulge in the wall that moves paradoxically compared with other areas of the LV (Fig. 22.33). True aneurysms are lined by thinned, scarred myocardium and are typically located near the apex or anterolateral wall. Pseudoaneurysms are focal, contained ruptures that are often larger but have narrower ostia, and are most commonly located at the inferior and posterior aspect of the LV. Intramural thrombi may be seen in up to 50% of ventricular aneurysms.

CT AND ULTRAFAST CT

CT is useful in evaluating aortic aneurysms, aortic dissections, central pulmonary thrombosis (Fig. 22.34), intracardiac masses and thrombi (Fig. 22.35),

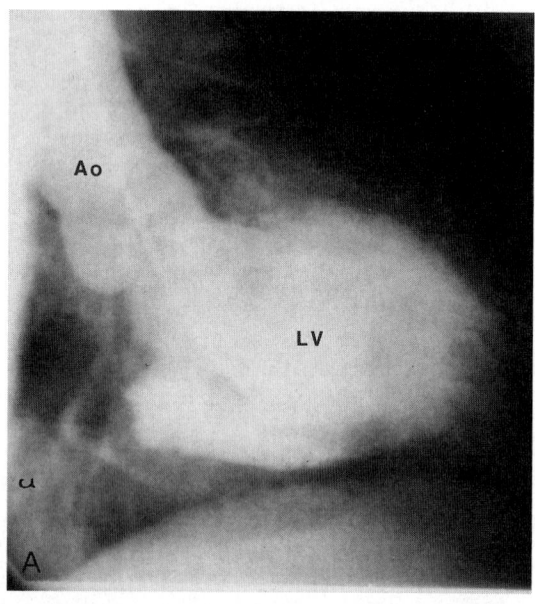
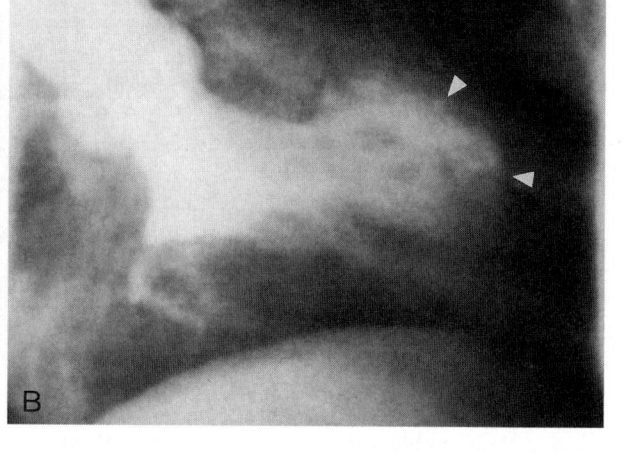

Figure 22.33. Left Ventricular Aneurysm. Diastole **(A)** and end systole **(B)**. The left ventriculogram (*LV*) is accomplished with the pigtail catheter entering the LV from the aortic root (*Ao*). A paradoxic bulge near the apex (*arrowheads*) indicates a left ventricular aneurysm.

Figure 22.34. Pulmonary Artery Embolus. Contrast-enhanced CT examination shows a filling defect within the right PA (*arrowheads*). Disappearance with time confirms an embolus. Primary neoplasms or metastatic emboli may cause a similar filling defect.

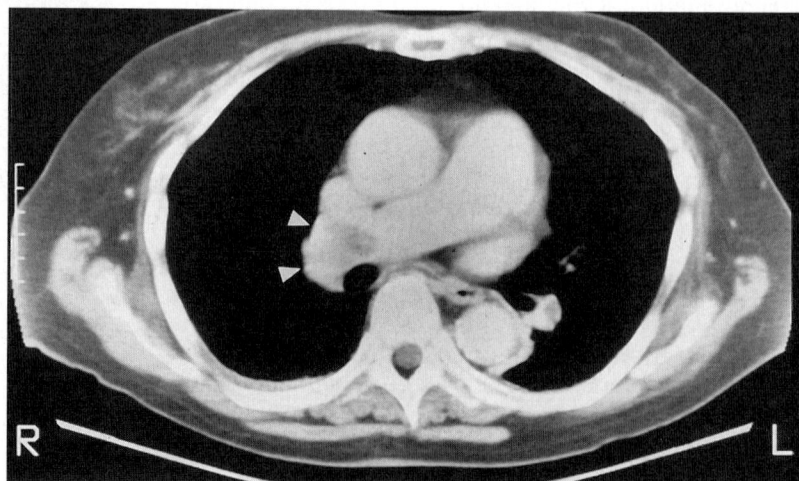

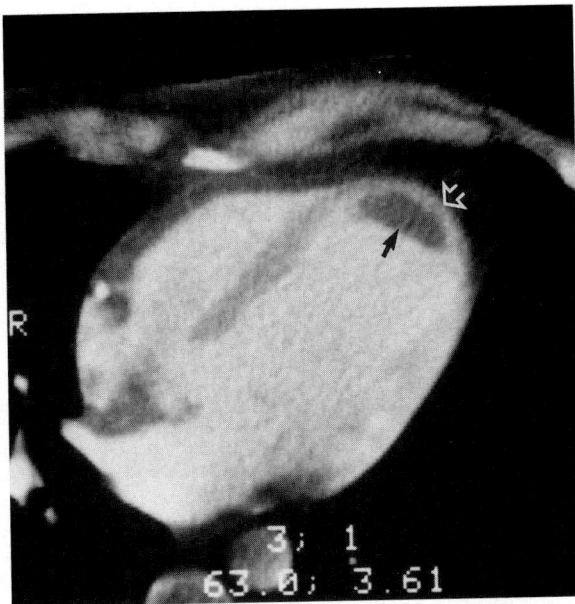

Figure 22-35. Ultrafast CT. Contrast enhanced, electron beam CT shows intraventricular clot (*black arrow*), thinned myocardium (*white arrow*), and akinesis, secondary to anteroapical infarct. (Courtesy of William Stanford, MD, Professor of Radiology, University of Iowa.)

pericardial thickening, fluid collections, and pericardial calcifications. Optimal contrast enhancement is required for most studies. Ultrafast CT offers the advantage of high-speed scanning to stop action and eliminate motion artifact. Angled couch views supplement standard axial imaging. With cardiac gating, cine-CT can provide wall motion studies and valve evaluation. Ultrafast CT has also been used to screen for coronary artery calcification and to document patency of coronary bypass grafts.

CARDIAC MR

Cardiac MR combines many of the capabilities of the other imaging modalities into one examination. These include excellent static anatomic images and dynamic motion studies for function. Cardiac MR applications include congenital heart disease, aortic and PA disease, pericardial disease, ventricular function, valvular function, cardiomyopathies, and cardiac masses. Cardiac pacemakers are considered contraindications, but most prosthetic valves can be safely studied.

The best anatomic depiction is accomplished on spin-echo T1WI in which the moving blood produces a signal void or "black blood" appearance (Fig 22.36). Gradient-echo or fast-field echo images impart bright signal to coherently flowing blood, creating a "white blood" appearance similar to contrast studies (Fig. 22.37). Electrocardiographic gating can be used similar to gated cardiac blood pool scintigraphy. Slice-specific information is acquired with reference to specific phases within the cardiac cycle. With gradient

recalled echo technique applied, motion studies can show flowing blood as well as myocardial contractility.

MR images are acquired as tomographic slices through any selected plane. The planes may be angled to match cardiac or vascular anatomy. Tissue characterization of the myocardium is accomplished using T1WI and T2WI, contrast enhancement, and spectroscopy. This may be useful for neoplastic, infiltrative, or inflammatory conditions of the myocardium.

Cardiac MR motion studies provide functional information including wall motion analysis, systolic wall thickening, chamber volumes, stroke volumes, right and left ventricular ejection fractions, and valve evaluation (Fig. 22.38). Flowing blood becomes turbulent and loses its coherence when it passes through stenotic or regurgitant valves. The high-velocity stenotic jet or regurgitant flow is displayed as a wedge-shaped puff of dark turbulent flow readily identified on the white blood background with the gradient-echo technique (see Figs. 23.22, 23.23). Visual and region-of-interest grading can be accomplished for stenotic or regurgitant flow based on distance, area, or regurgitant volume (see chapter 23). The regurgitant fraction is calculated by comparing the right and left stroke volumes. Velocity-encoded cine-MR techniques, using phase analysis, can calculate flow velocities and flow volumes in addition to the regurgitant volumes. These techniques can be used in lieu of angiography for many cases. Understanding MR signal characteristics and details of three-dimensional cardiac anatomy displayed in different tomographic planes is critical to the accurate utilization of cardiac MR.

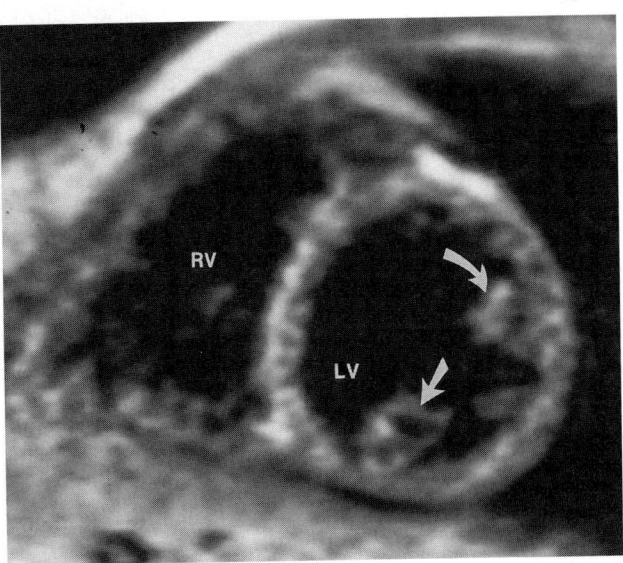

Figure 22.36. Spin-echo MR. A tomographic slice in the short axis projection demonstrates the *RV*, interventricular septum, and *LV*. The anterior (*straight arrow*) and posterior (*curved arrow*) papillary muscles are seen within the left ventricular cavity. The spin-echo technique creates a black blood appearance because of the signal void of moving blood.

Figure 22.37. Fast-Field Echo MR. The fast-field echo technique creates a white blood depiction that shows flowing blood and turbulence during motion studies. The end diastole image (*straight arrow*) has the largest ventricular size. The end systole image (*curved arrow*) has the smallest ventricular cavity and the thickest wall.

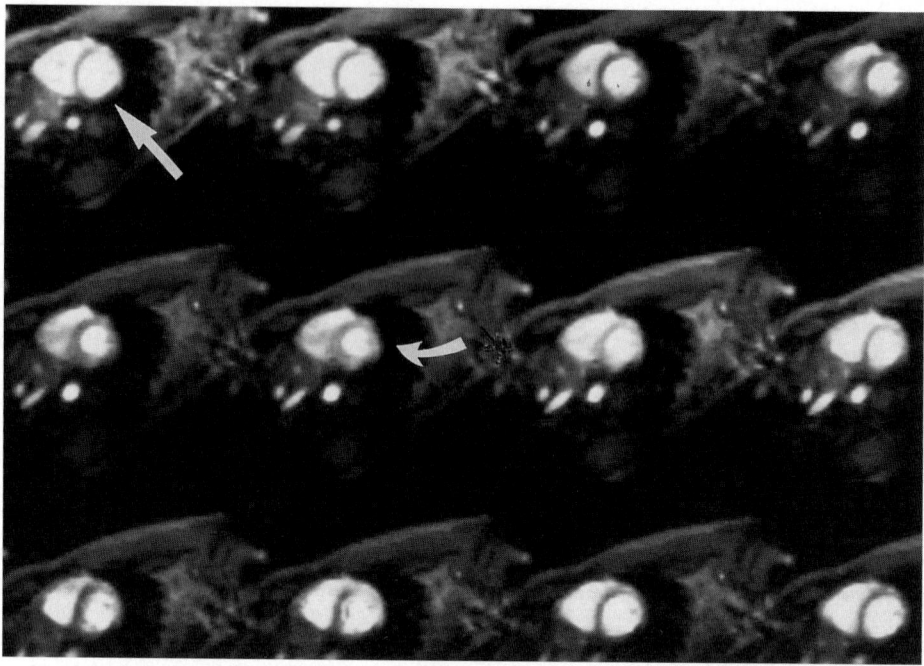

Figure 22.38. MR Ejection Fraction Technique. Regions of interest are drawn on the diastolic image (*straight arrow*) and the end systolic image (*curved arrow*) of each slice. An area ejection fraction (EF) is then calculated for each slice. Volume ejection fraction calculations are calculated using sequential slices that include the entire ventricular volume. *EDV*, end diastolic volume; *ESV*, end systolic volume; *SV*, stroke volume; *CO*, cardiac output; *ED*, end diastole; *ES*, end systole.

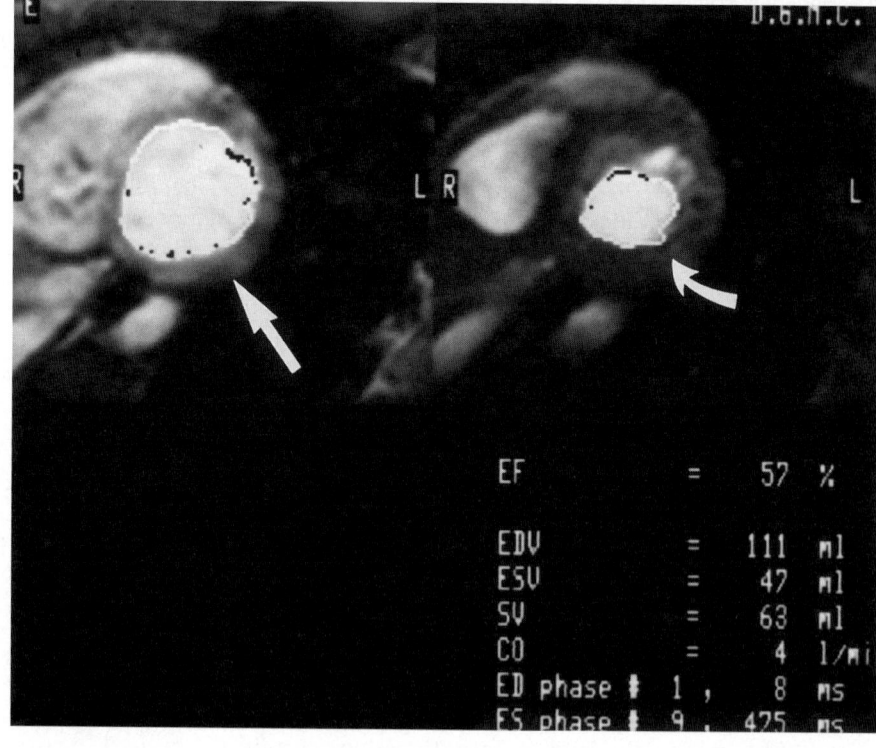

Reference

1. Kubicka RA, Smith C. How to interpret coronary arteriograms. Radiographics 1986;6:661–701.

Suggested Readings

Brundage BH. Comparative Cardiac Imaging. Rockville, MD: Aspen Publications, 1990.

Budhoff MJ, et al. Ultrafast computed tomography as a diag-

nostic modality in the detection of coronary artery disease. Circulation 1996; 93: 898–904.

Chapman S, Nakielny R. Aids to Radiological Diagnosis. 2nd ed. London: WB Saunders, 1990.

Dahnert W. Radiology Review Manual. 3rd ed. Baltimore: Williams & Wilkins, 1996.

Feigenbaum H. Echocardiography. 5th ed. Philadelphia: Lea & Febiger, 1994.

Gedgaudas E, Moffer JH, Castaneda-Zuniga WR, Amplatz K. Cardiovascular Radiology. Philadelphia: WB Saunders, 1985.

Gutierrez. Cardiovascular Magnetic Resonance Imaging. St. Louis: Mosby 1991.

Higgins CB. Essentials of Cardiac Radiology and Imaging. Philadelphia: JB Lippincott, 1992.

Kelley MJ. Chest Radiography for the Cardiologist. Cardiology clinics. Philadelphia: WB Saunders, 1983.

Kotler MN, Steiner RM. Cardiac imaging: non technologies and clinical applications. Cardiovascular Clinics, vol 17, no. 1. Philadelphia: Davis Co, 1986.

Kubicka RA, Smith C. How to interpret coronary arteriograms. Radiographics 1986;6:661–701.

Marcus ML, Schelbert HR, Skorton DJ, Wolf GL. Cardiac Imaging—A Companion to Braunwald's Heart Disease. Philadelphia: WB Saunders, 1991.

Miller DD, Burns RG, Gill JB, Ruddy TD. Clinical Cardiac Imaging. New York: McGraw-Hill, 1988.

Miller SW, ed. Symposium on advances in cardiac imaging. Radiol Clin North Am 1985;23:587–793.

Miller SW, ed. Cardiopulmonary imaging. Radiol Clin North Am 1989;27:1059–1266.

Netter FH. Atlas of Human Anatomy. The CIBA Collection of Medical Illustrations. West Caldwell, NJ: CIBA-Geigy Corp, 1989.

Pohost GM. Cardiovascular Applications of Magnetic Resonance (American Heart Association Ser.) Armonk, NY: Futura Publishing, 1993.

Putnam CE. Cardiopulmonary Imaging. Radiol Clin North Am. Philadelphia: WB Saunders, 1983.

Ravin CE, Cooper C. Review of Radiology. 2nd ed. Philadelphia: WB Saunders, 1993.

Taveras JM, Ferrucci JT. Radiology. Philadelphia: WB Saunders, 1993.

Wolfe CL. Cardiac Imaging. Cardiology Clinics. Philadelphia: WB Saunders, 1989.

23
Cardiac Imaging in Acquired Diseases

David K. Shelton Jr.
Michael Galloway

Cardiac disease remains among the most common problems affecting patient morbidity and mortality today, despite many important dietary, pharmaceutical, interventional, and surgical advances. Most acquired cardiac diseases can be classified under six general categories: ischemic heart disease, cardiomyopathies, pulmonary vascular disease, acquired valvular disease, cardiac masses, and pericardial disease. Use of plain film, fluoroscopy, US, CT, MR, nuclear imaging, and angiocardiography must be integrated with knowledge of specific disease processes.

ISCHEMIC HEART DISEASE

Coronary Artery Disease

Coronary artery disease is the most common cause of mortality in the United States, with approximately one American dying every minute. Six million to seven million Americans have active symptoms related to ischemic heart disease. Approximately 300,000 coronary artery bypass graft (CABG) surgeries are performed per year in the United States, with a similar number of percutaneous transluminal coronary angioplasties (PTCA).

Clinical Presentations include *a*) stable angina, *b*) unstable angina (often preinfarction), *c*) acute myocardial infarction, *d*) congestive heart failure secondary to chronic ischemia or prior infarction sequelae, *e*) arrhythmias, and *f*) sudden death. Clinical symptoms are caused by luminal abnormalities of the coronary arteries including *a*) atheromatous disease, *b*) coronary thrombosis, *c*) intraluminal ulceration and hemorrhage, *d*) vasoconstriction, and *e*) coronary ectasia and aneurysm.

Risk Factors for development of atherosclerotic coronary artery disease include elevated serum cholesterol, tobacco smoking, diabetes, hypertension, sedentary life style, age, male gender, and heredity. Aggravating conditions include aortic stenosis, ventricular hypertrophy, cardiomyopathy, coronary embolism, congenital anomalies, Kawasaki syndrome, and anemia. Noninvasive imaging is often used as a screening test. Selective coronary angiography with ventriculography is usually required to determine coronary anatomy and to direct the specific therapy.

A typical imaging workup includes chest radiography, nuclear medicine perfusion scans, and consideration for coronary angiography. Indications for coronary angiography include angina refractory to medical therapy, unstable angina, high-risk occupation such as pilot, and abnormal electrocardiograms or stress perfusion tests. Coronary angiography is considered following myocardial infarction when PTCA or intracoronary thrombolysis are being deliberated. Additional indications include development of mechanical dysfunction, progressive congestive failure, refractory ventricular arrhythmias, and follow-up of IV thrombolytic agents.

Coronary Artery Calcification occurs in the intima and is directly related to advanced atheromatous disease and coronary narrowing (Fig. 23.1, see Fig. 22.14). Coronary calcification is detected at angiography in 75% of patients with 50% diameter stenosis. Only 11% of men without significant coronary artery disease have coronary calcification. In the asymptomatic population, the detection of coronary calcification has a predictive accuracy of 86%. In symptomatic patients, coronary calcification is seen in 50% of patients with single-vessel disease, 77% of those with two-vessel disease, and 86% of those with three-vessel disease. Fluoroscopically detected coronary calcification in the presence of anginalike chest pain is associated with coronary stenosis 94% of the time. Overall, fluoroscopic detection of coronary artery calcification has a 73% sensitivity and 84% specificity for symptomatic patients. Exercise tolerance testing has a sensitivity of 76–88% and a specificity of 43–77%. Exercise testing with planar thallium imaging has a sensitivity and a specificity of approximately 85%. Use of ultrafast CT has improved the sensitivity for detecting coronary artery calcification to approximately 77–95% (Fig. 23.2).

Myocardial Perfusion Scanning, using thallium, Tc-99m-sestamibi, Tc-99m-tetrofosmin, or Tc-99m-teboroxime, is one of the primary imaging modalities for detecting myocardial ischemia. Stress images are obtained with exercise or pharmacologic agents such as adenosine dipyridamole. SPECT has increased the sensitivity to 90–94% and the specificity to 90–95%. The hallmark for segmental ischemia is a perfusion defect on

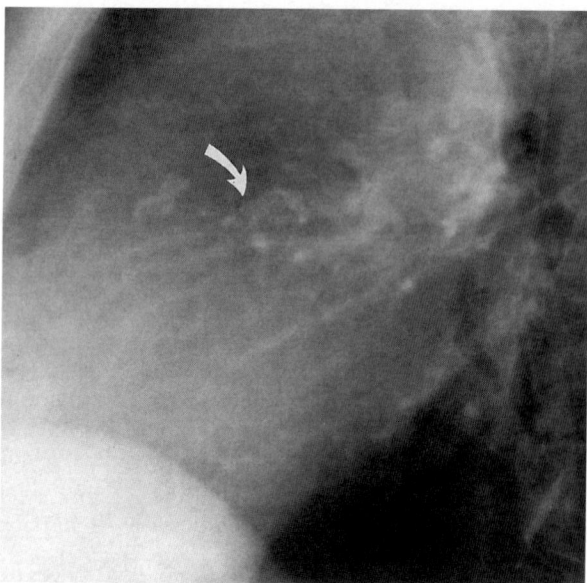

Figure 23.1. Coronary Artery Calcification. Lateral chest radiograph demonstrates coronary artery calcification (*arrow*).

stress testing that fills in during rest examination (Fig. 23.3). A defect that appears stable during both stress and rest examinations is usually an infarction. "Hibernating" regions of viable myocardium associated with tight coronary stenosis may appear as fixed defects on sestamibi or tetrofosmin images or on redistribution thallium images obtained 4 hours after stress.

Stress Echocardiography using either exercise or pharmacologic stress modalities has also become a widely accepted method to detect significant (>50–70%) coronary artery stenosis. With the advent of digital image acquisition and cine-loop playback, prestress echocardiographic views can be simultaneously compared with views taken either immediately postexercise or at peak pharmacologic doses. Development of new segmental wall motion abnormalities or worsening of resting abnormalities suggests stress-induced ischemia. One advantage of these techniques is that they also allow prior assessment of resting wall motion abnormalities that are consistent with either profoundly ischemic, stunned, hibernating, or infarcted myocardium.

The overall sensitivity of exercise echocardiography is 76–97% using pharmacologic stress agents; the sensitivity is 72–96% with dobutamine, approximately 85% with adenosine, and 52–56% with standard dose dipyridamole. The sensitivities for these tests are lowest for single-vessel disease and improve incrementally for two- and three-vessel disease. Stress echocardiography has a specificity of 66–100%.

Gated Blood Pool Scintigraphy will demonstrate exercise-induced wall motion abnormalities in 63% of patients with significant coronary artery disease. With exercise, the ejection fractions normally increase by at least 5%. Failure of ejection fraction to increase with exercise is an indication of myocardial dysfunction. Using these two findings, exercise gated blood pool scintigraphy has a sensitivity of 87–95% and a specificity of 92% for coronary artery disease.

Coronary Angiograms should be evaluated for the percent of stenosis, the number of vessels involved, focal versus diffuse disease, coronary anatomy, ectasia or aneurysm, coronary calcification, and collateral flow (Fig. 23.4). Collaterals may include epicardial, intramyocardial, atrioventricular, intercoronary, or intracoronary vessels (i.e., "bridging collateral"). The angiographer must count the number of major epicardial vessels with greater than 50% diameter narrowing. Patients are divided into one-vessel, two-vessel, or three-vessel disease on the basis of involvement of the right or left main coronary artery, left anterior descending artery and left circumflex artery. A 50% diameter narrowing roughly predicts a 75% cross-sectional area reduction, which is the physiologic point at which flow is restricted enough to result in ischemia. Reliability for estimating the percent diameter narrowing depends on the observer, projection, resolution, and presence of coronary calcification or ectasia. The degree of coronary disease may be assessed using percent stenosis of each individual coronary artery or of 5-mm segments of the coronary arteries. The right coronary artery is 10-cm long, the left main coronary artery is 1-cm long, the left anterior descending (LAD) is 10-cm long, and the left circumflex is 6-cm long, for a total of 27 cm. These may be divided into fifty-four 5-mm segments. This scoring system allows the interpreter to quantify the number of 5-mm segments with stenoses in

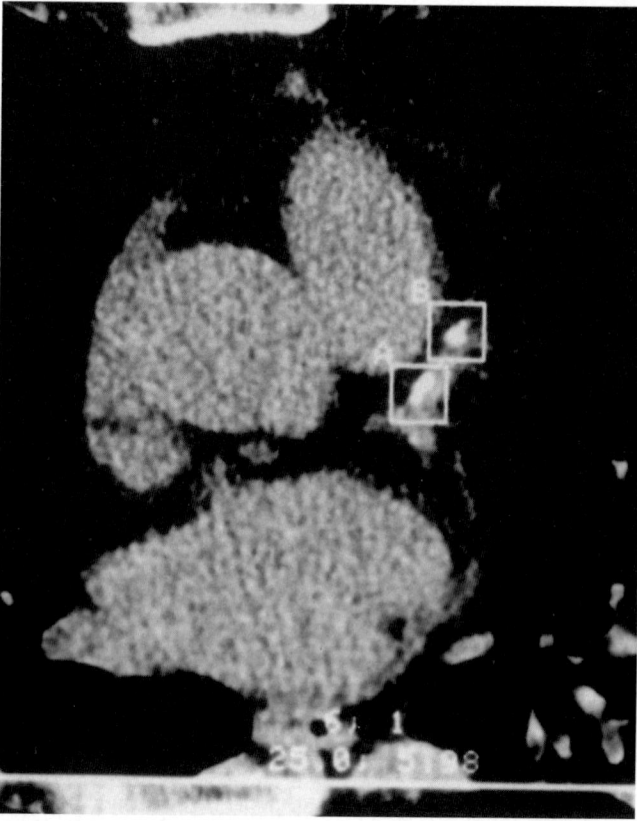

Figure 23.2. Coronary Calcification. Calcification is seen in LAD with regions of interest (*white boxes*) placed for quantification. Electron beam CT, 100 ms, 3-mm slice, without contrast. (Courtesy of William Stanford, MD, Professor of Radiology, University of Iowa.)

Figure 23.3. Myocardial Perfusion Scan. SPECT images of the LV in short axis projection demonstrate a defect (*arrows*) in the inferior wall of the LV during stress, which is well perfused on the rest images. This is strong evidence of ischemic heart disease utilizing Tc-99m-sestamibi as the radionuclide and pharmacologic stress testing with dipyridamole.

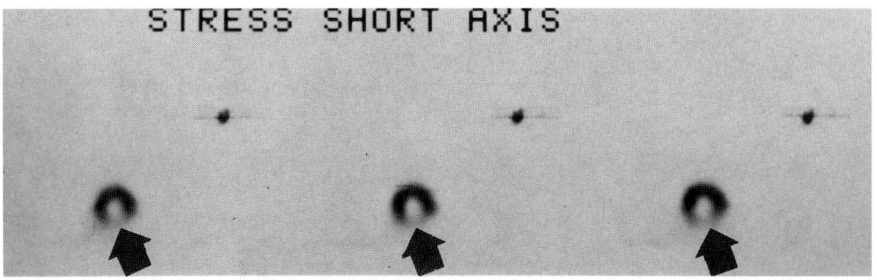

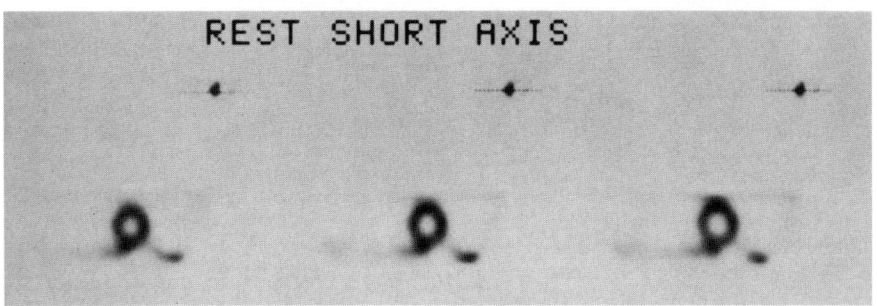

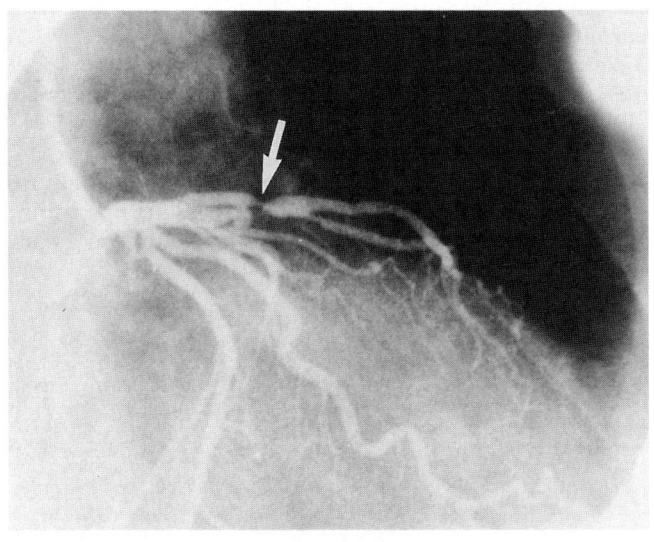

Figure 23.4. Coronary Stenosis. An 80% stenotic lesion (*arrow*) is identified in the left anterior descending artery. This patient was experiencing classic angina.

the 0–25%, 25–50%, 50–75%, and 75–100% ranges. The significance of 30–70% lesions is often clarified by correlation with stress-induced perfusion scintigraphy.

Percutaneous transluminal angioplasty has traditionally been reserved for localized lesions in one- or two-vessel disease (Fig. 23.5), but recent published series comparing PTCA with CABG in multivessel disease reveal no difference in the endpoints of death and myocardial infarction. The PTCA group, however, requires a significantly higher number of repeat procedures during follow-up. Coronary artery bypass grafting, with the use of saphenous vein grafts or internal mammary arteries, is usually reserved for more complex or longer-segment disease. CABG markers are usually placed at the anas-

tomotic site to help the angiographer during future selective angiography. Use of the internal mammary artery has better long-term results than saphenous vein grafts and has been correlated with increased survival. Recurrence of symptoms after CABG may be because of occlusion, graft stenosis, or progression of native vessel disease. Graft stenoses and acute occlusions may be amenable to percutaneous interventional techniques.

Echocardiography is useful in detecting some of the long-term complications of ischemic disease, including ventricular aneurysm, thinning of myocardium, akinesia, or dyskinesia. Aneurysms are best seen at the apex and septum. Mural thrombi may also be diagnosed but are difficult to visualize at the apex. Stress echocardiography with either exercise or pharmacologic stress techniques is increasingly used to evaluate for ischemia.

CT is capable of establishing the patency of coronary artery bypass grafts. Ultrafast CT has a 93% sensitivity, 89% specificity, and 92% accuracy for establishing patency of the CABG grafts. This has also shown to be extremely sensitive for detecting coronary calcification. Ultrafast CT with contrast can evaluate wall motion, thrombi, old infarcts, aneurysm, and pericardial abnormalities.

MR can be used *a*) to define the location and size of previous myocardial infarctions, *b*) to demonstrate complications of previous infarctions, *c*) to establish the presence of viable myocardium for possible revascularization, *d*) to differentiate acute versus chronic myocardial infarction, *e*) to evaluate regional myocardial wall motion and systolic wall thickening (Fig. 23.6), *f*) to demonstrate global myocardial function with right ventricular and left ventricular ejection fractions, *g*) to demonstrate regional myocardial perfusion, and *h*) to evaluate papillary muscle and valvular abnormalities. Gadolinium-enhanced T1WI demonstrate areas of ischemia and reperfusion after myocardial infarction. MR with spectroscopy targeting myocardial phosphate

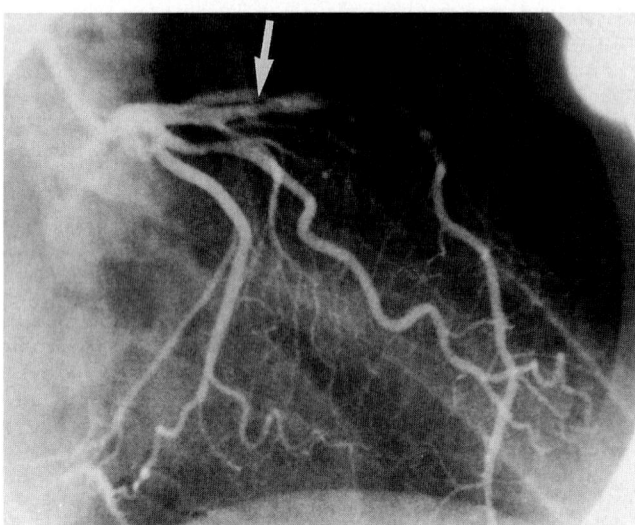

Figure 23.5. Percutaneous Transluminal Angioplasty. Marked improvement in the LAD lesion (*arrow*) seen in Figure 23.3 is evident following PTCA. The angina symptoms resolved.

metabolism can distinguish acute from chronic ischemia and reperfused, infarcted myocardium from reperfused, viable myocardium. With spin-echo imaging, MR has a 78% accuracy for establishing patency of CABGs. Cine MR with gradient echo has a sensitivity of 88–93%, specificity of 86–100%, and overall accuracy of 89–91% for patency of coronary artery bypass grafts.

Myocardial Infarction

After acute infarction, the chest radiograph will initially show a normal heart size in 90% of cases. Cardiomegaly and congestive failure will eventually develop in 60–70%, more frequently with anterior wall infarction, multivessel disease, or left ventricular aneurysm. Increasing stages of pulmonary venous hypertension, particularly alveolar edema, are associated with worsened prognosis.

Complications of myocardial infarction include the following.

Cardiogenic Shock implies that systolic pressure is less than 90 mm Hg and is typically associated with acute pulmonary edema and worsened prognosis.

Atrioventricular Block is common especially after inferior wall infarcts resulting from either ischemia or injury to the atrioventricular nodal branch of the right coronary artery or increased vogal tone. Complete heart block occurs with larger infarcts and has a worse prognosis.

Right Ventricular Infarction occurs in approximately 33% of inferior wall infarctions. Symptoms are caused by the reduction in right ventricular ejection infarction, which returns to normal within 10 days in approximately 50% of cases. The diagnosis may be established using technetium pyrophosphate (PYP) radionuclide scans. Complications include cardiogenic shock, elevated right atrial pressure, and decreased pulmonary artery pressure. Right precordial EKG leads can also assist in making the diagnosis.

Myocardial Rupture (3.3% of infarcts) may occur 3–14 days after infarction. The mortality rate approaches 100% and accounts for 13% of myocardial infarction deaths. The chest radiograph shows acute cardiac enlargement secondary to leakage of blood into the pericardium. Rupture of the interventricular septum (1%) typically occurs between days 4 and 21, usually as a complication of anterior myocardial infarction and LAD disease. Mortality is 24% within 24 hours and 90% within 1 year. Swan-Ganz catheter measurements show an acute increase in saturation in the RV, although the wedge pressures may be normal. Chest radiographs show acute pulmonary vascular engorgement and right-sided cardiac enlargement because of left-to-right shunt. Pulmonary edema is not a typical feature. Echocardiography readily demonstrates the septal defect.

Papillary Muscle Rupture (1%) is suggested by abrupt onset of mitral regurgitation, with acute pulmonary edema on the radiograph. Typically, the LV is only minimally enlarged, whereas the LA enlarges quickly. Inferior infarcts are associated with posteromedial papillary rupture. Anterior infarcts less commonly affect the anterolateral papillary muscle. Mortality is 70% within 24 hours and 90% within 1 year. Echocardiography confirms the diagnosis.

Ventricular Aneurysm develops in approximately 12% of survivors from myocardial infarction. Ventricular aneurysms may also be caused by Chagas' disease or trauma and are rarely congenital—usually seen in young black males. Aneurysms present with congestive failure, arrhythmias, and systemic emboli. *True aneurysms* are broad-mouthed, localized outpouchings that do not contract during systole (see Fig. 22.33). They are typically

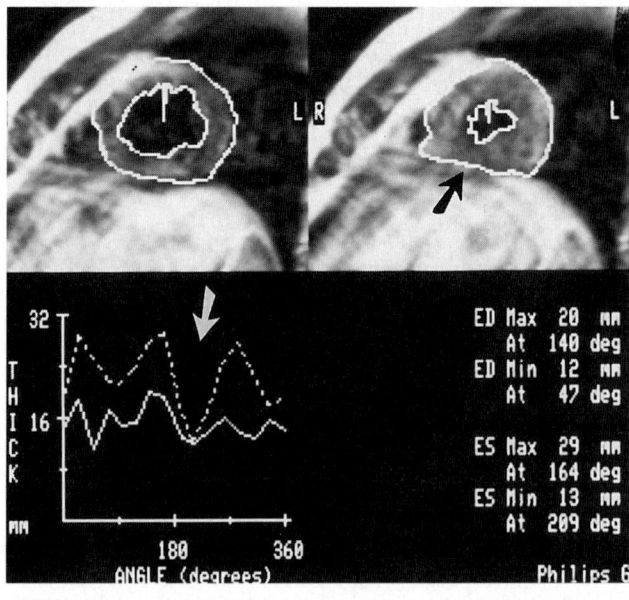

Figure 23.6. Wall Motion MR Evaluation. Short axis tomographic views of the LV are used for evaluation of systolic wall thickening. Regions of interest are drawn around the myocardium in diastole (**left**) and systole (**right**). The inferior wall (*black arrow*) demonstrates hypokinesia and poor systolic wall thickening. The functional graph (**below**) confirms the findings (*white arrow*). The patient had a previous inferior wall myocardial infarction.

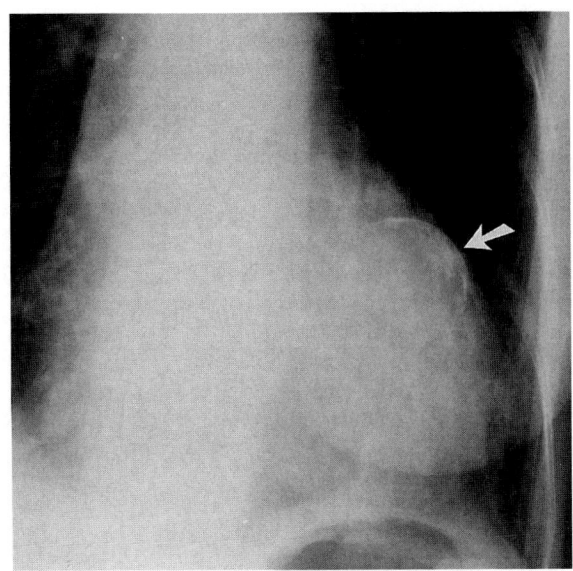

Figure 23.7. Left Ventricular Aneurysm. A localized calcified bulge (*arrow*) is seen along the left heart border, secondary to prior myocardial infarction complicated by left ventricular aneurysm.

anterior or apical and result from LAD disease. The chest radiograph shows a localized bulge along the left cardiac border and may show rimlike calcification in the wall (Fig. 23.7). Fluoroscopy detects up to 50%, whereas 96% are detected by radionuclide ventriculography or myocardial perfusion scan. Echocardiography, contrast-enhanced CT, and MR are also accurate at detecting true aneurysms.

Pseudoaneurysms are contained myocardial ruptures consisting of a localized hematoma surrounded by adherent pericardium. Causes include infarction and trauma. Patients are at high risk for delayed rupture. Pseudoaneurysms are typically posterolateral or retrocardiac in location and have smaller mouths than true aneurysms. MR is the most accurate at detecting pseudoaneurysms, but they can also be seen with echocardiography.

Dressler's Syndrome (4%) is also known as the postmyocardial infarction syndrome and is similar to the postpericardiotomy syndrome complicating cardiac surgery. Onset is typically 1 week to 3 months postinjury (peak at 2–3 weeks), but relapses occur up to 2 years later. Presentation includes fever, chest pain, pericarditis, pericardial effusion, and pleuritis with pleural effusion usually more prominent on the left. Dressler's syndrome responds well to anti-inflammatory medications.

Infarct Imaging

The indications for myocardial infarct imaging include late admission, equivocal enzymes, equivocal electrocardiogram, recent cardiac surgery or trauma, and suspicion of right ventricular infarction.

Radionuclide Imaging. "Cold spot" imaging is accomplished with thallium or technetium perfusion agents (Fig. 23.8). Sensitivity is 96% within 6–12 hours, but only 59% for remote infarction. Acute infarction can

not be distinguished from remote infarction. "Hot spot" infarct imaging uses Tc-PYP, Tc-tetracycline, Tc-gluco-heptonate, indium-111 antimyosin antibodies, or F-18 sodium fluorine (Fig. 23.9). Pyrophosphate uptake occurs in myocardial necrosis as a result of PYP complexing with calcium deposits. The PYP scans turn positive at 12 hours, have peak sensitivity at 48–72 hours, and revert to normal by 14 days. Persistent abnormal uptake implies a poor prognosis or developing aneurysm. Cardiomyopathies and diffuse myocarditis show diffuse increased uptake. Contusions and radiation myocarditis show increased regional uptake.

Ultrafast CT with contrast demonstrates poor perfusion of the infarcted segment immediately after administration of contrast. After a delay of 10–15 minutes, the normal myocardium washes out, leaving a contrast enhanced periphery of the infarcted zone.

MR demonstrates prolongation of T1 and T2 times secondary to edema of the acutely infarcted segment. Edema occurs within 1 hour after infarct and may be associated with myocardial hemorrhage. MR has a 93% sensitivity, 80% specificity, and 87% accuracy for acute myocardial infarction. The infarcted region is best delineated by high signal on T2WI; however, surrounding edema tends to overestimate the size of the infarct. T1WI with gadolinium demonstrate the acutely ischemic region and will help to differentiate reperfusion from occlusive myocardial infarction. Regional wall thinning and lack of systolic thickening are the best evidence of the size of the infarcted segment (Figs. 23.6,23.10). Scar tissue will not contract, whereas viable myocardium will contract and thicken by at least 2 mm. Very high grade

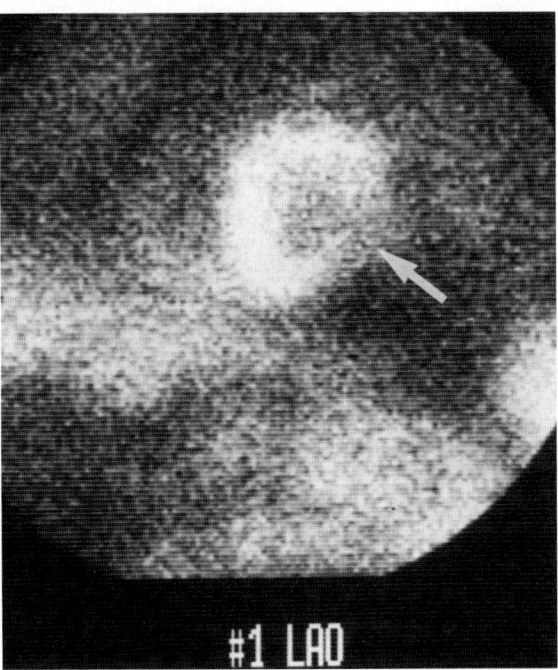

Figure 23.8. Myocardial Infarction. Resting, planar thallium image in the left anterior oblique projection demonstrates a defect in the inferoposterior wall (*arrow*), consistent with a myocardial infarction. Cold spot imaging can be accomplished within 6 hours of the acute event.

Figure 23.9. Myocardial Infarct Scan. Hot spot imaging was accomplished using PYP. Notice the uptake in the anterolateral wall of the myocardium (*arrows*), which is almost as "hot" as the sternum (*curved arrow*). Images are obtained in right anterior oblique (*RAO*), left lateral (*LT LAT*), anterior (*ANT LT*), and left anterior oblique (*LAO*) projections.

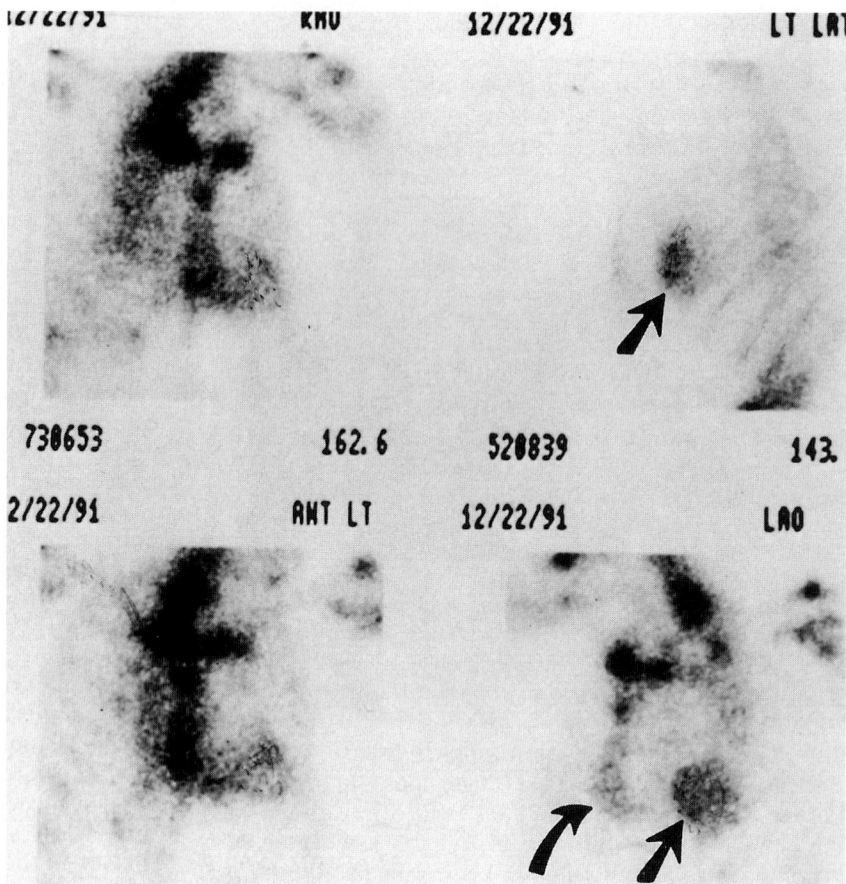

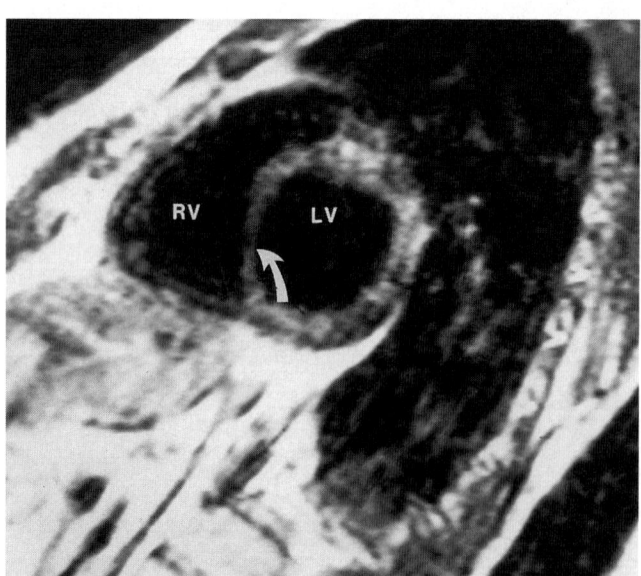

Figure 23.10. Old Septal Infarction. Spin-echo MR demonstrates fixed thinning of the myocardial wall (*arrow*) attributable to prior myocardial infarction. *RV*, right ventricle; *LV*, left ventricle.

stenotic lesions may result in chronically ischemic myocardium with altered metabolism. This "hibernating myocardium" may act like postinfarction scar, but it remains viable and may improve in function with revascularization. Unfortunately, it also remains at risk for acute infarction. "Stunned myocardium" describes postischemic, dysfunctional myocardium without complete necrosis, which is potentially salvageable.

Echocardiography demonstrates hypokinesis, akinesis, or dyskinesis in previously infarcted myocardial segments; however, this cannot be distinguished from stunned or hibernating myocardium. Global hypokinesis can also be seen with cardiomyopathic processes. Thinned, hyperechoic walls with resting wall motion abnormalities suggest transmural scar. Use of echocardiographic microbubble contrast can enhance the infarcted region by highlighting perfused areas, resulting in a negative contrast effect at the site of the infarct.

CARDIOMYOPATHIES

The prevalence of cardiomyopathies is approximately 8 cases per 100,000 population in developed countries. One percent of cardiac deaths in the United States is attributable to cardiomyopathy. The mortality rate in males is twice that in females, and in blacks, is twice that of whites. In developing countries and in the tropics, the prevalence and mortality rates are much higher, probably because of nutritional deficiency, genetic factors, physical stress, untreated hypertension, and infection, especially Chagas' disease.

The cardiomyopathies are a group of anomalies with three basic features: *a*) failure of the heart to maintain its architecture, *b*) failure of the heart to maintain normal electrical activity, and *c*) failure of the heart to maintain cardiac output. General features of cardiomyopathies include cardiomegaly; congestive heart failure, often with relatively clear lungs; dilated left and right ventricles with elevated end-diastolic pressures and decreased contractility; and decreased ejection fractions. These findings are only seen in the later stages of hypertrophic and restrictive cardiomyopathies. Causes of congestive heart failure are listed in Table 23.1.

The cardiomyopathies may also be divided into dilated, hypertrophic, restrictive, and right ventricular forms (Table 23.2).

Dilated Cardiomyopathy

In the western world, dilated cardiomyopathy accounts for 90% of all cardiomyopathies (Fig. 23.11). The term "congestive cardiomyopathy" should be reserved for a subgroup of the dilated cardiomyopathies, for which the etiology is unknown. Specific causes for dilated car-

diomyopathies should be pursued as the specific therapy may vary: *a)* ischemic cardiomyopathy (the most common cause) because of chronic ischemia, prior infarction or anomalous coronary arteries, *b)* long-term sequelae of myocarditis (Coxsackie virus most commonly), *c)* toxins (ethanol and adriamycin), *d)* metabolic (mucolipidosis, mucopolysaccharidosis, glycogen storage disease), *e)* nutritional deficiencies (thiamin and selenium), *f)* infants of diabetic mothers, and *g)* muscular dystrophies.

Clinical presentation is related to congestive heart failure, although the initial presentation may include cardiac arrhythmias, conduction disturbances, thromboembolic phenomena, or sudden death. Presentation may also differ, depending on left-sided dominance, right-sided dominance, or biventricular involvement.

Chest radiograph commonly demonstrates global cardiomegaly. Larger heart sizes are associated with worse prognosis. Coronary artery calcification may be a clue to ischemic cardiomyopathy. Gated myocardial scintigraphy shows decreased left ventricular ejection fraction, prolonged pre-ejection period, shortened left ventricular

Table 23.1. Causes of Congestive Heart Failure

Myocardial
  Cardiomyopathy (dilated, restrictive, hypertrophic)
  Myocarditis
  Postpartum cardiomyopathy
Coronary
  Transient ischemia
  Chronic ischemic cardiomyopathy
  Prior infarct or aneurysm
Endocardial
  Fibrosis
  Löffler syndrome
Valvular
  Stenosis
  Regurgitation
Pericardial
  Effusion
  Constrictive
Vascular
  Hypertension
  Pulmonary emboli
  Arteriovenous fistula
  Vasculitis
Extracardiac
  Endocrinopathy (thyroid, adrenal)
  Toxic
  Anemic
  Metabolic

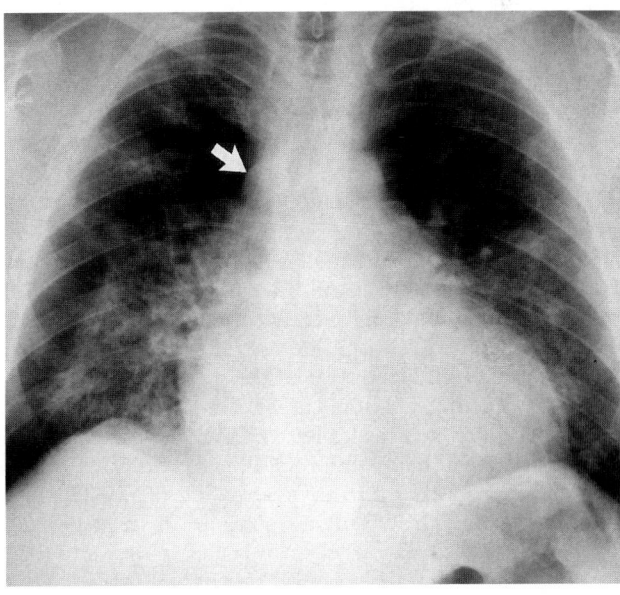

Figure 23.11. Dilated Cardiomyopathy. The typical appearance of a dilated cardiomyopathy is demonstrated with a water-bottle configuration and dilatation of the azygos vein (*arrow*). Pulmonary infiltrates are the result of pulmonary edema and capillary leak in this patient with viral myocarditis.

Table 23.2. Types of Cardiomyopathies

Type	Ventricular Wall	Ventricular Cavity	Contractility	Compliance
Dilated	LV thin	LV dilated	Decreased	Normal to decreased
Hypertrophic	LV thick	LV normal to decreased	Increased	Decreased
Restrictive	Normal	Normal	Normal to decreased	Severely decreased
Uhl's anomaly	RV thin	RV dilated	Decreased	Normal to decreased

LV, left ventricle
RV, right ventricle

ejection time, and a decreased rate of ejection. Echocardiography shows a dilated LV with global hypokinesia, thinning of the left ventricular wall and interventricular septum, decreased myocardial thickening, left atrial enlargement, and often right ventricular hypokinesia. MR shows dilatation of the specific chambers, decreased thickness of the myocardium with nonuniformity seen in prior infarctions, pericardial effusions, right and left ventricular ejection fractions, stroke volumes, wall-stress physiology, and quality of systolic wall thickening.

Hypertrophic Cardiomyopathy

Hypertrophic Cardiomyopathy may be familial (60%), autosomal dominant with variable penetrance, associated with neurofibromatosis and Noonan's syndrome, or secondary to pressure overload. The hypertrophic cardiomyopathies are divided into two basic types: a) *concentric hypertrophy,* which may be diffuse, midventricular, or apical in distribution, and b) *asymmetrical septal hypertrophy,* also known as *idiopathic hypertrophic subaortic stenosis* (Fig. 23.12). Either form may cause some degree of muscular outflow obstruction with a systolic pressure gradient. Systemic hypertension may cause left ventricular hypertrophy followed by dilation, pulmonary venous hypertension, and increased risk of coronary artery disease.

The clinical presentation includes angina, syncope, arrhythmias, and congestive heart failure. Sudden death occurs in up to 50% of patients. The overall mortality rate is 2–3% per year.

On chest radiography, 50% of patients with hypertrophic cardiomyopathy will have a normal chest radiograph and 30% have left atrial enlargement, commonly because of mitral regurgitation. Echocardiographic features include a) hypertrophy of the interventricular septum (>12–13 mm), b) abnormal ratio of thickness of the interventricular septum to left ventricular posterior wall (>1.3:1), c) systolic anterior motion of the mitral valve with mitral regurgitation, d) narrowing of the left ventricular outflow tract during systole, e) high velocity across the left ventricular outflow tract with delayed systolic peaks on Doppler examination, f) midsystolic closure of the aortic valve, and g) normal or hyperkinetic left ventricular function.

Restrictive Cardiomyopathy

Restrictive Cardiomyepathy is the least frequent form of cardiomyopathy. Etiologies include infiltrative disorders such as amyloid, glycogen storage disease, mucopolysaccharidosis, hemochromatosis, sarcoidosis, and myocardial tumor infiltration. In the tropics, endomyocardial fibrosis is highly prevalent. A rare form of endomyocardial fibrosis associated with eosinophilia is called Löffler's endocardial fibrosis. Restrictive cardiomyopathy should be considered when patients present with symptoms of congestive failure without radiographic evidence of cardiomegaly or ventricular hypertrophy (Fig. 23.13). The primary differential diagnosis is constrictive pericardial disease that can be differentiated by CT or MR.

Signs and symptoms are related to congestive failure, arrhythmias, and heart block. In late stages, the electrocardiogram shows low voltage. Pathophysiology includes impaired diastolic function with decreased ventricular compliance, poor diastolic filling, and elevation of right and left ventricular filling pressures. Early in the progression of the disease, ventricular systolic function is normal or near normal. There may be a significant decline in later stages.

The chest radiograph often shows a normal-sized heart with pulmonary congestion. Left atrial enlargement and pulmonary venous hypertension may be present. The PYP nuclear scans demonstrate hot spots in abnormal areas of myocardium in 50–90% of patients. Echocardiography may show decreased systolic and diastolic function with normal to decreased ejection fractions. Mild left ventricular wall hypertrophy is often present with a granular or "snowstorm" appearance to the myocardium, especially noted in the case of cardiac amyloidosis. MR shows high signal in the myocardium on T2WI in patients with amyloidosis and sarcoidosis.

Figure 23.12. Hypertrophic Cardiomyopathy. Gradient-echo MR demonstrates marked left ventricular hypertrophy on these short axis views of the LV. Note the asymmetric thickening of the septum (*arrow*) compared with the remainder of the left ventricular myocardium. Diastole is on the **left** and systole is on the **right.**

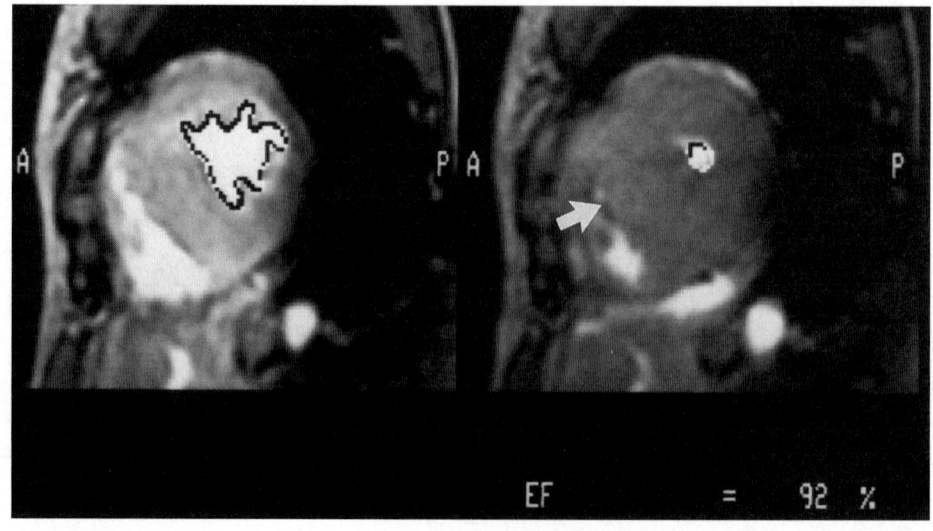

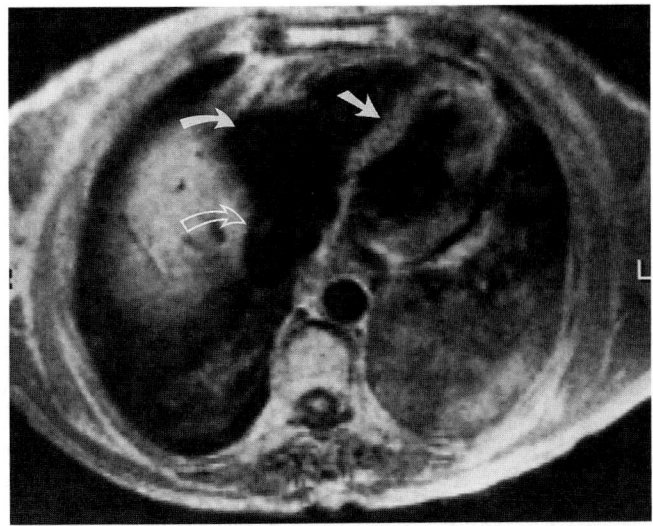

Figure 23.13. Restrictive Cardiomyopathy. Spin-echo MR demonstrates a variable high-density signal within the myocardium, a dilated RA (*closed curved arrow*), and an enlarged inferior vena cava (*open curved arrow*). The interventricular septum has an abnormal contour (*straight arrow*) because of high right ventricular pressures in this biopsy-proved case of amyloid cardiomyopathy.

The atria are enlarged because of elevated diastolic pressures, but ventricular volumes are often normal. Mitral regurgitation and tricuspid regurgitation are readily depicted with gradient-echo cine MR and Doppler echocardiography. The inferior vena cava and superior vena cava may be greatly dilated.

Right Ventricular Cardiomyopathies

Cor Pulmonale is defined as right ventricular failure secondary to pulmonary parenchymal or pulmonary arterial disease. It may be considered a secondary form of right ventricular cardiomyopathy. Etiologies include *a)* destructive pulmonary disease such as pulmonary fibrosis and chronic obstructive pulmonary disease; *b)* hypoxic pulmonary vasoconstriction resulting from chronic bronchitis, asthma, central nervous system hypoxia, and upper airway obstruction; *c)* acute and chronic pulmonary embolism; *d)* idiopathic pulmonary hypertension; and *e)* extrapulmonary diseases affecting pulmonary mechanics such as chest deformities, morbid obesity (*pickwickian syndrome*), and neuromuscular diseases.

The end result is alveolar hypoxia leading to hypoxemia, pulmonary hypertension, elevated right ventricular pressures, right ventricular hypertrophy, right ventricular dilation, and right ventricular failure. Symptoms include marked dyspnea and decreased exercise endurance out of proportion to pulmonary function tests. Blood gases demonstrate hypoxemia and hypercapnia.

The chest radiograph shows a normal-sized heart or mild cardiomegaly (Fig. 23.14). Right ventricular and right atrial enlargement may be present. The main and central pulmonary arteries are prominent, and the periphery is oligemic. The interlobar artery typically mea-

sures more than 16 mm. The lungs show signs of chronic obstructive pulmonary disease, emphysema, or pulmonary fibrosis. Nuclear scintigraphy shows right ventricular enlargement with decrease in the right ventricular ejection fraction on first pass examination. Echocardiography and MR show right ventricular and right atrial enlargement with thickening of the anterior right ventricular wall. M-mode echocardiography of the tricuspid valve shows a diminished A wave and flat E–F slope. Therapy is aimed at the underlying pulmonary disorder.

Uhl's Anomaly was initially described as a congenital disorder with "parchment-like thinning" of the RV. More recently it has been described as an acquired disorder in infants or adults and is called "arrhythmogenic right ventricular dysplasia." This rare form of cardiomyopathy is limited to dilation of the RV with marked thinning of the anterior right ventricular wall. Clinical presentation includes syncope, recurrent ventricular tachycardia, and premature death from early congestive failure or arrhythmias. Familial occurrence has been reported, and males outnumber females by 3:1. Ventricular ejection fractions are commonly reduced to less than half of normal, with mild reductions in the left ventricular ejection fraction.

PULMONARY VASCULAR DISEASE

Enlargement of the Pulmonary Outflow Tract is seen in congenital heart disease with left-to-right shunts. Outflow tract prominence without evidence of a shunt lesion is usually the result of poststenotic dilatation secondary to pulmonary stenosis, pulmonary arterial hypertension, Marfan's syndrome, Takayasu's arteritis, or idiopathic dilatation of the pulmonary artery.

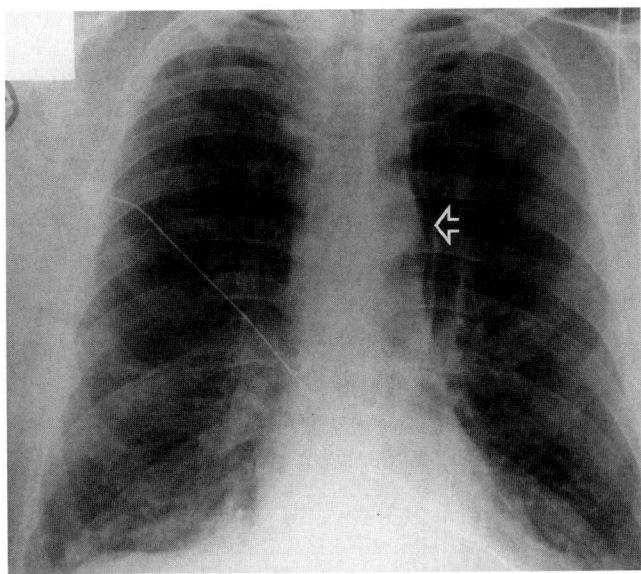

Figure 23.14. Cor Pulmonale. A posteroanterior chest radiograph demonstrates marked hyperinflation caused by chronic obstructive pulmonary disease. The anterior junction line (*arrow*) is herniated to the left of the aortic knob because of marked emphysema in the anterior segment of the right upper lobe.

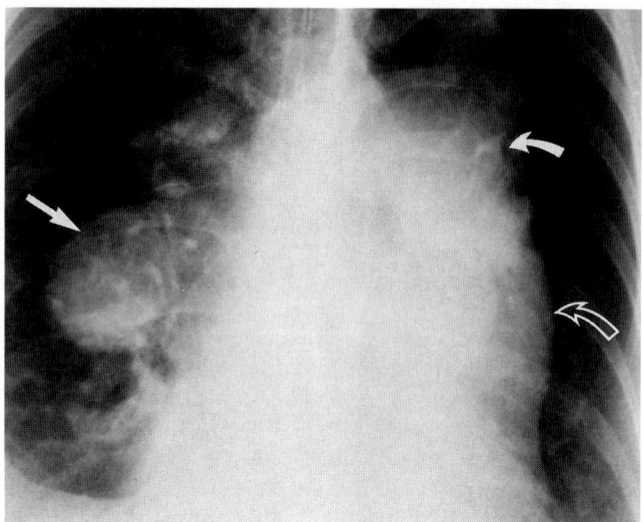

Figure 23.15. Pulmonary Arterial Hypertension. The main pulmonary artery (*curved arrow*), left pulmonary artery (*open arrow*), and right pulmonary artery (*straight arrow*) are extremely enlarged. Faint calcification is seen in the right pulmonary artery. The patient had schistosomiasis with resultant vasculitis and pulmonary arterial hypertension.

Idiopathic dilatation of the pulmonary artery demonstrates a dilated main pulmonary artery, normal peripheral pulmonary arteries, and normal, balanced circulation. This entity is much more common in females and is often associated with a mild systolic ejection murmur, but without evidence of pulmonary stenosis.

Pulmonary Arterial Hypertension should be considered whenever the main pulmonary artery and left and right pulmonary arteries are enlarged (Fig. 23.15). Signs of right atrial and ventricular enlargement or hypertrophy are often present. Systolic right ventricular and pulmonary artery pressures exceed 30 mm Hg. Other findings include rapid tapering and tortuosity of the pulmonary arteries. The peripheral lung zones appear clear. Calcification within the pulmonary arterial walls is virtually diagnostic of pulmonary arterial hypertension (Fig. 23.16).

The differential diagnosis for pulmonary arterial hypertension includes long-standing pulmonary venous hypertension (mitral stenosis), Eisenmenger's physiology (from long-standing left-to-right shunts), pulmonary emboli, vasculitides (such as rheumatoid arthritis or polyarteritis nodosa), and primary pulmonary hypertension. Polyarteritis nodosa is a necrotizing vasculitis involving the medium-sized pulmonary arteries. Radiographic findings include small pulmonary arterial aneurysms, focal stenoses, small infarctions and signs of pulmonary hypertension. Primary pulmonary hypertension is most common in women in their third and fourth decades. Histologic examination reveals plexiform and angiomatoid lesions with no evidence of emboli or venous abnormalities. Symptoms include dyspnea, fatigue, hyperventilation, chest pain, and hemoptysis.

Increased Pulmonary Blood Flow is caused by high output states and left-to-right shunts. High output

states include volume loading, pregnancy, peripheral shunt lesions (arteriovenous malformations), hyperthyroidism, anemia, and leukemia (Fig. 23.17). The main and central pulmonary arteries are enlarged with increased circulation to the lower lobes, upper lobes, and peripheral lung zones. Bronchovascular pairs show enlargement of the vascular component. The most common shunts in the adult are the acyanotic lesions including atrial septal defect, ventricular septal defect, patent ductus arteriosus, and partial anomalous pulmonary venous return. Cyanotic lesions with increased blood flow to the lungs include transposition of the great vessels, truncus arteriosus, total anomalous pulmonary venous return, and endocardial cushion defects. Ventricular

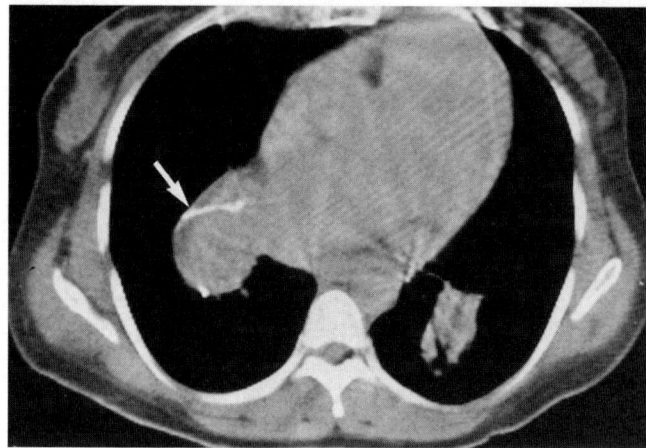

Figure 23.16. Pulmonary Arterial Hypertension. Noncontrast CT demonstrates calcification in the wall of the right pulmonary artery (*arrow*).

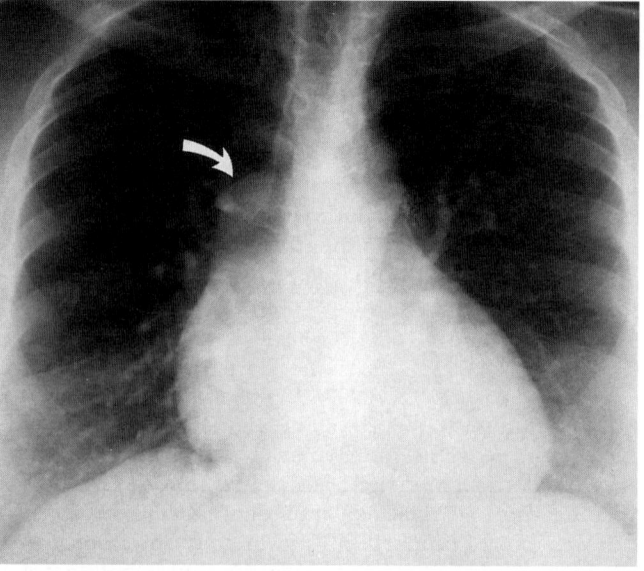

Figure 23.17. High Output Failure. Chest radiograph demonstrates cardiomegaly, vascular engorgement, and distension of the azygos vein in this pregnant patient with severe anemia. The azygos vein (*arrow*) is a good marker of intravascular volume expansion or elevated central venous pressures.

septal defects with left-to-right shunting may occur acutely following myocardial infarction.

Decreased Pulmonary Blood Flow with a small heart is caused by chronic obstructive pulmonary disease, hypovolemia, malnourishment, and Addison's disease. When the cardiac silhouette is enlarged, the differential diagnosis includes cardiomyopathy, pericardial tamponade, Ebstein's anomaly, and right-to-left shunts from congenital heart disease.

Asymmetrical Pulmonary Blood Flow may be evident on chest radiography, angiography or nuclear medicine pulmonary perfusion scans (Fig. 23.18 and see Fig. 23.25). This may result from either decreased or increased blood flow to one lung, Pulmonary valvular stenosis often results in increased blood flow to the left lung. With resultant left pulmonary artery dilatation, tetralogy of Fallot may cause increased blood flow to the right lung. Surgical shunts, such as the Blalock-Taussig procedure, increase blood flow to one lung. Decreased blood flow to one lung occurs in peripheral pulmonic stenosis (see Fig. 23.25), interruption of the pulmonary artery, scimitar syndrome, pulmonary hypoplasia, Swyer-James syndrome, pulmonary emphysema, pulmonary embolism, fibrosing mediastinitis, or carcinoma affecting one artery. When examining a chest radiography, one must be careful to exclude technical artifacts such as lateral decentering and soft-tissue asymmetry such as mastectomy. The balance of circulation and size of the central pulmonary arteries should be compared as well as the size of the bronchovascular pairs.

Pulmonary Venous Hypertension may be identified on radiographs, pulmonary angiograms, or nuclear medicine perfusion scans (Fig. 23.19 and see Fig. 22.18). Pulmonary venous hypertension is considered mild with wedge pressures of 10–13 mm Hg, moderate with equalization of upper and lower lobe blood flow and wedge pressures of 14–16 mm Hg, or severe with the upper lobe vessels being distended more than the lower lobe vessels and wedge pressure 17–20 mm Hg. Progressive cephalization is accompanied by progressive secondary enlargement of the pulmonary arteries and filling out of the hilar angles. The most common cause of pulmonary venous hypertension is elevation of left atrial pressures secondary to left ventricular failure (Table 23.3).

ACQUIRED VALVULAR HEART DISEASE

Mitral Stenosis in the adult is usually caused by rheumatic heart disease, with 50% of patients giving a history of rheumatic fever. Rarely, an atrial myxoma may mimic mitral stenosis. The incidence of mitral stenosis is higher in females by a ratio of 8:1. *Lutembacher's syndrome* is a combination of mitral stenosis with a pre-existing atrial septal defect, resulting in marked right-sided enlargement.

The normal mitral valve area is 4–6 cm^2. With mild mitral stenosis (mitral valve area <1.5 cm^2), the chest radiograph may be normal and left atrial pressures will be elevated only during exercise. Moderate mitral stenosis (valve area <1.0 cm^2) produces signs of left atrial enlargement and pulmonary venous hypertension (see Fig. 23.18). Dyspnea on exertion is common. Severe mitral stenosis (valve area <0.5 cm^2) has marked left atrial enlargement, right ventricular enlargement, Kerley's lines, pulmonary edema, and, occasionally, calcification in the left atrial wall. Patients are often dyspneic at rest, with resting left atrial pressure exceeding 35 mm Hg. Palpitations and atrial fibrillation with risk of atrial thrombi and systemic emboli are also common. Long-standing pulmonary venous hypertension leads to pulmonary arterial hypertension. Stages of progression of mitral stenosis are *a)* stage 1: pulmonary venous hypertension with hilar angle loss; *b)* stage 2: interstitial edema

Table 23.3. Causes of Pulmonary Venous Hypertension

Left ventricular failure
Mitral stenosis
Mitral regurgitation
Aortic stenosis
Aortic regurgitation
Pulmonary veno-occlusive disease
Congenital heart disease

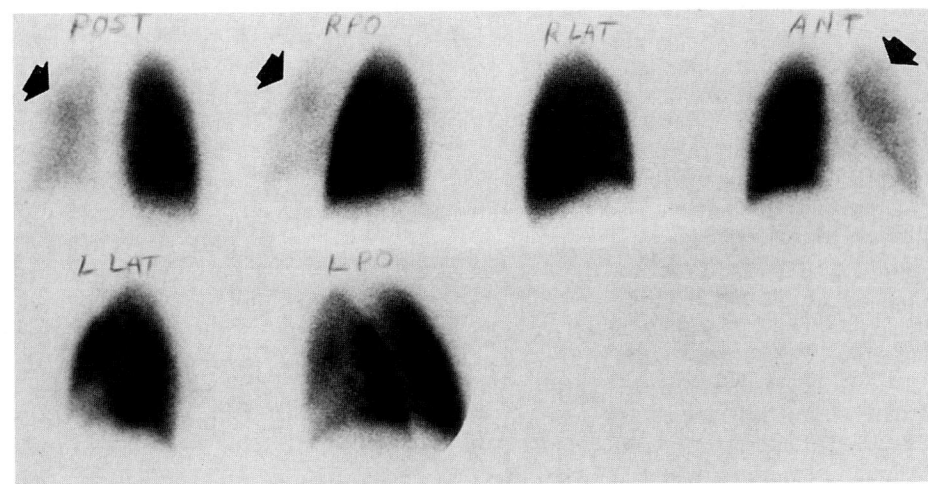

Figure 23.18. Asymmetrical Pulmonary Blood Flow. ^{99m}Tc macroaggregated albumin pulmonary perfusion lung scan demonstrates marked reduction in the pulmonary blood flow to the left lung (*arrow*) in comparison with the right lung. A subtle left hilar mass was causing compression of the left pulmonary artery. *POST,* posterior; *RPO,* right posterior oblique; *RLAT,* right lateral; *ANT,* anterior; *LLAT,* left lateral; *LPO,* left posterior oblique.

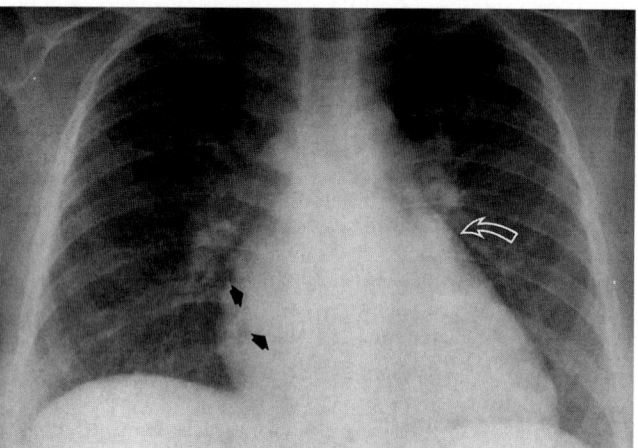

Figure 23.19. Moderate Mitral Stenosis. A chest radiograph demonstrates mild cardiomegaly with straightening of the left heart border, prominence of the left atrial appendage (*open arrow*), and evidence of left atrial enlargement (*arrows*). Cephalization of blood flow and enlargement of the pulmonary arteries indicate pulmonary venous and pulmonary arterial hypertension.

with Kerley's lines; *c*) stage 3: alveolar edema; and *d*) stage 4: chronic, recurrent congestive failure, hemosiderin deposits, and ossification or calcifications in the lung.

The chest radiograph is often characteristic with a long, straight, left heart border, left atrial enlargement, prominence of the left atrial appendage, cephalization of blood flow indicating pulmonary venous hypertension, pulmonary arterial hypertension, left atrial calcification, mitral valve calcification, prominent main pulmonary artery, right ventricular enlargement with filling of the retrosternal clear space, and dilatation of the inferior vena cava. Echocardiography shows a decreased E–F slope on M-mode, slow left ventricular filling, left atrial enlargement, thickened mitral valve, decreased excursion of the mitral valve with a narrow mitral orifice, parallel movement of the anterior and posterior leaflets, and atrial fibrillation. Gated nuclear angiograms are useful for following the left ventricular ejection fraction. MR grades the valvular disease and determines chamber volumes and ejection fractions. Velocity-encoded cine MR quantifies peak velocity and instantaneous blood flow. The peak gradient across the stenotic valve can be calculated when the echo times (TE) are less than 7 milliseconds, allowing measurements of velocities up to 6 m/s. Mitral commissurotomy or balloon valvuloplasty may be performed if the leaflets are pliable and not heavily calcified. Mitral valve replacement should be considered before left ventricular failure occurs.

Mitral Regurgitation associated with rheumatic heart disease used to be the most common hemodynamically significant form of mitral regurgitation in adults. Today, mitral regurgitation is more commonly the result of initial valve prolapse followed by infarct ischemia–related papillary muscle dysfunction and rupture (Table 23.4).

The radiograph shows left atrial enlargement that is greater than that seen with pure mitral stenosis (Fig. 23.20). Left ventricular enlargement is also present. Pulmonary venous hypertension is less prominent than

Table 23.4. Causes of Mitral Regurgitation

Rheumatic heart disease
Congenital heart disease
Mitral valve prolapse
Ruptured chordae tendineae
Infectious endocarditis
Papillary muscle rupture
Mitral annulus calcification

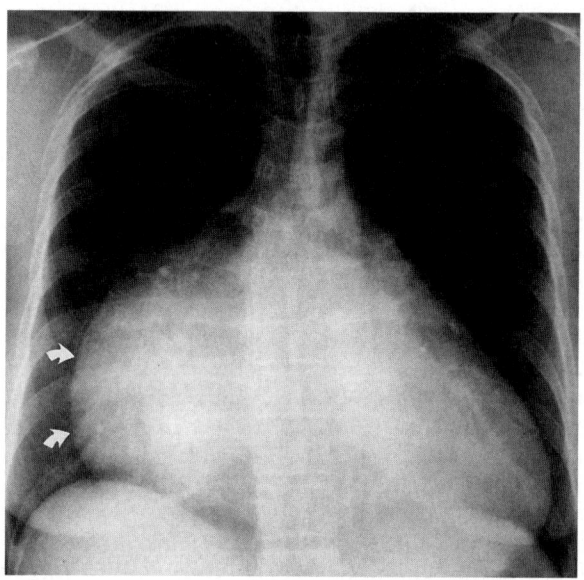

Figure 23.20. Mitral Regurgitation. A chest radiograph demonstrates marked left atrial enlargement with "atrial escape" where the LA (*arrows*) becomes border forming along the right cardiac silhouette. Note the marked carinal splaying because of this massive left atrial enlargement.

in mitral stenosis. The radiograph is near normal with mild mitral regurgitation, shows atrial enlargement and pulmonary venous hypertension with moderate disease, and shows progressive left atrial enlargement, left ventricular enlargement, pulmonary venous hypertension, and pulmonary edema with severe mitral regurgitation.

Echocardiography shows left atrial enlargement, left ventricular enlargement and bulging of the atrial septum to the right. Nuclear angiogram shows a dilated LV with an elevated left ventricular ejection fraction because of the hyperdynamic status. MR using gradient echo and gated cine mode shows the regurgitant jet projecting from the LV into the LA during systole. The regurgitant jet may be graded visually as mild, moderate, or severe based on the distance it extends toward the back wall. Grade 1 regurgitation is defined as turbulent flow extending less than one-third the distance to the back wall, grade 2 is less than two-thirds the distance to the back wall, and grade 3 is more than two-thirds of the distance to the back wall. The regurgitant fraction can be calculated by comparing the right and left ventricular stroke volumes, which are normally equal. The regurgitant fraction is equal to the right ventricular stroke volume minus the left ventricular stroke volume, divided by right ventricular stroke volume. Gated blood pool scintigraphy is used to follow the ejection fraction to optimize the timing of valve replacement. Echocardiography can be used to follow both the ejection fraction and left ventricular volumes.

Mitral Valve Prolapse is an interesting entity that has also been called "floppy mitral valve" or Barlow syndrome. It is seen in 2–6% of the general population and is more common in young women. It has an autosomal dominant transmission and is more common in patients with straight backs, pectus excavatum, and narrow anteroposterior diameters of the chest. Patients may be asymptomatic or have symptoms as a result of arrhythmias. A "honking" type of murmur or a murmur with midsystolic click is characteristic. The chest radiograph is usually normal, although occasionally patients will develop mitral regurgitation, left atrial enlargement, and pulmonary venous hypertension. Echocardiography demonstrates a characteristic bulging of the anterior or posterior leaflets usually beginning during midsystole when the valve should remain closed. This may also take the appearance of a pansystolic "hammock" type of leaflet bowing. Some patients develop myxomatous thickening of the mitral valve leaflets.

Aortic Stenosis is caused by partial fusion of the commissures between the aortic valve cusps. Bicuspid aortic valve is found in 1–2% of the population and is present in 95% of congenital aortic stenosis. *Bicuspid aortic valve* is most common in males and is present in 25–50% of patients with aortic coarctation. Sixty percent of patients older than 24 years of age have calcification within the bicuspid valve. *Calcific or degenerative aortic stenosis*, on the other hand, is usually seen in older patients with systemic hypertension. Aortic valve calcification is best seen on the lateral or right anterior oblique chest radiographs and implies an aortic gradient greater than 50 mm Hg. Noncalcific stenosis is usually because of rheumatic heart disease and coexists with mitral valve disease. The radiograph typically shows left ventricular hypertrophy with poststenotic dilatation of the aorta (Fig. 23.21). The ascending aorta is not normally seen on

frontal chest radiographs in patients less than 40 years of age. The echocardiogram shows dense aortic valve echoes, a dilated aortic root, hyperdynamic function, and left ventricular hypertrophy. A bicuspid valve may be directly visualized. The aortic valve area is normally 2.5–3.5 cm^2. Symptoms typically occur when the valve area is less than 0.7 cm^2 or is less than 1.5 cm^2 if there is combined aortic stenosis and aortic insufficiency. Mild aortic stenosis is associated with a 13–14 mm orifice and greater than 25 mm Hg gradient. Moderate aortic stenosis has an 8–12 mm orifice and greater than 40–50 mm Hg gradient. Severe stenosis occurs at a less than 8-mm orifice with a gradient greater than 100 mm Hg. Cardiac MR and echocardiography show increased ventricular muscle mass with hypertrophy (Fig. 23.22). MR and blood pool scintigraphy show decreased left ventricular ejection fraction, increased left ventricular emptying time, decreased rate of ejection, and a normal left ventricular filling rate.

Symptoms progress from angina to syncopal episodes to congestive failure with the possibility of sudden death with severe stenosis. Therapy is usually valve replacement, although some cases are amenable to valvuloplasty.

Aortic Insufficiency is primary when it is attributable to aortic valve disease or is secondary when it is the result of aortic root disease (Table 23.5). Physical examination reveals a water-hammer pulse, a decrescendo diastolic murmur, and, occasionally, when severe or directed toward the anterior mitral leaflet, an Austin-Flint murmur owing to vibrations of the mitral valve by regurgitant flow.

Chest radiograph shows a dilated, calcified aortic root with a normal heart size in mild disease. With moderate disease, the LV and cardiac silhouette enlarge. With severe disease, left atrial enlargement and congestive heart failure develop. Symptoms include dyspnea on exertion, fatigue, and symptoms of congestive failure.

Echocardiography and MR show the dilated aortic root, regurgitant aortic flow, diastolic flutter of the interventricular septum or anterior mitral leaflet (Austin-

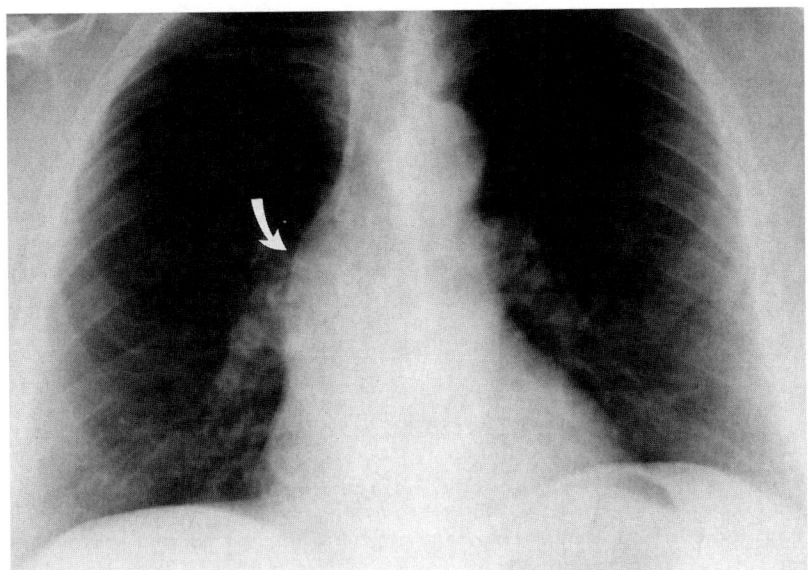

Figure 23.21. Aortic Stenosis. Note the enlarged ascending aorta (*arrow*), highly suggestive of poststenotic dilatation in this patient with normal heart size.

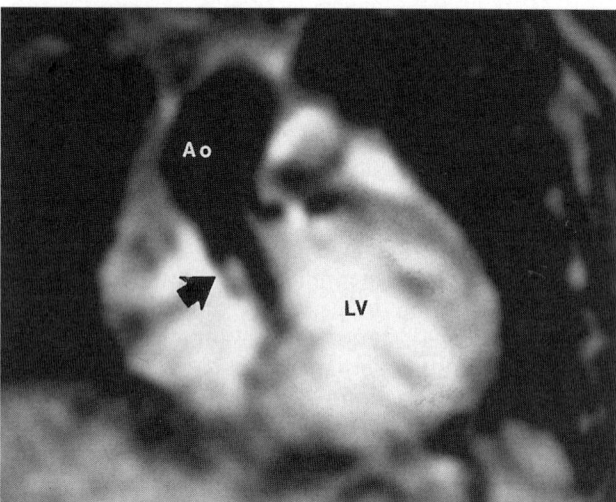

Figure 23.22. Aortic Stenosis. Gradient-echo MR coronal plane image of the ascending aorta (*AO*), aortic valve (*arrow*) and left ventricle (*LV*). Note the signal void in the entire ascending aorta as a result of marked turbulence caused by severe aortic stenosis.

Table 23.5. Causes of Aortic Insufficiency

Valvular
   Congenital
   Rheumatic
   Infectious endocarditis
   Trauma
Aortic Root
   Syphilis
   Dissecting aneurysm
   Marfan's syndrome
   Rheumatoid arthritis
   Reiter's syndrome
   Relapsing polychondritis
   Giant cell arteritis
Subvalvular
   Aneurysm of sinus of Valsalva
   Subaortic stenosis
   High ventricular septal defect

Flint phenomena), left ventricular dilation, increased wall motion, increased ejection fraction, and early mitral valve closure (Fig. 23.23). The ratio of the regurgitant flow width to the aortic root is helpful for grading the severity. Ventricular function may be followed by echocardiography, nuclear scintigraphy, or MR.

Supravalvular Aortic Stenosis is the result of a localized hourglass-type narrowing above the valve, a discrete fibrous-type membrane, or a diffuse hypoplastic tubular configuration of the ascending aorta. Supravalvular aortic stenosis is often associated with peripheral pulmonary stenosis and valvular or subvalvular aortic stenosis. This combination of findings is found with Marfan's syndrome or Williams syndrome. The coronary arteries are dilated because of the elevated systolic pressure and narrowing of the aortic root (<20 mm). The aortic cusps themselves are normal.

Subvalvular/Subaortic Stenosis may be a fixed anatomic defect or a dynamic functional obstruction. Fixed subaortic stenosis is associated with congenital heart disease, especially ventricular septal defect, in 50% of cases. Type 1 subaortic stenosis is a thin membrane located less than 2 cm below the valve. Type 2 is a thick, collar-type constriction. Type 3 subaortic stenosis is an irregular, fibromuscular type of narrowing. Type 4 is a funnellike constriction of the left ventricular outflow tract. The mitral valve is normal.

The functional type of subaortic stenosis has also been called asymmetrical septal hypertrophy, idiopathic hypertrophic subaortic stenosis, or hypertrophic obstructive cardiomyopathy. The appearances vary slightly. Findings may be evident with nuclear scintigraphy, but they are more obvious on echocardiography and MR. The interventricular septum is significantly thicker than the left ventricular free wall in 95% of patients. The left and right ventricular cavities are normal or small in 95% of patients. Systolic anterior motion of the mitral valve is best seen on echocardiography but may also be identified with MR. Asymmetrical septal hypertrophy may partially obstruct outflow in systole. The aortic cusp may flutter or partially close during systole. Mitral regurgitation is a common secondary finding attributable to abnormal mitral valve position or papillary muscle attachment.

Pulmonic Stenosis is seen in 8% of congenital heart disease and is uncommon as an acquired disease in adults. Symptoms may be secondary to cyanosis or heart failure. A systolic ejection murmur is heard over the sternal border. The chest radiograph often shows dilatation of the main left pulmonary arteries with increased flow into the left lung (Fig. 23.24). Right ventricular hypertrophy or enlargement is seen on chest radiographs, MR, and echocardiography. Systolic doming of the pulmonic valve is secondary to incomplete opening and is best seen on echocardiography. Rarely, calcification may be identified in the pulmonic valve.

Valvular pulmonic stenosis is caused by partial commissural fusion in 95% of cases. Symptoms typically

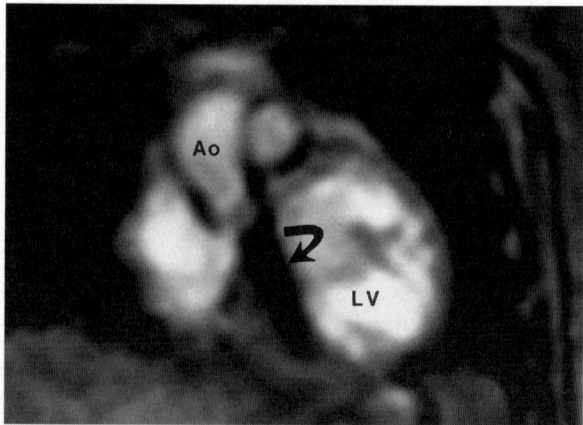

Figure 23.23. Aortic Regurgitation. Gradient-echo MR coronal plane image through the ascending aorta (*AO*) and left ventricle (*LV*) demonstrates regurgitant flow from the aortic valve into the LV (*arrow*).

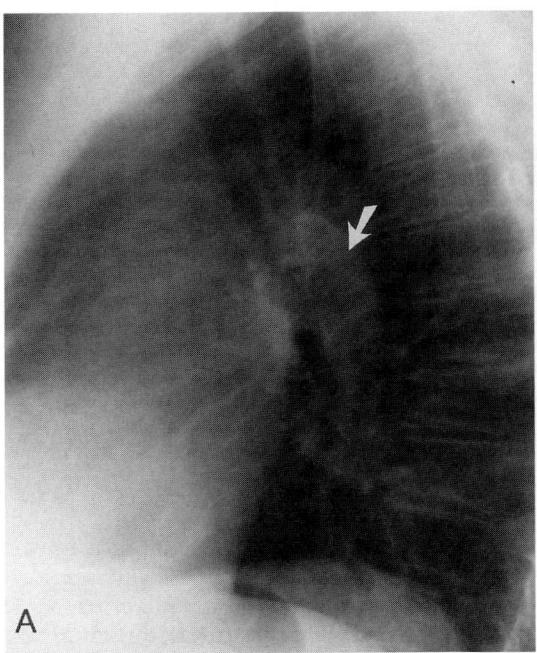

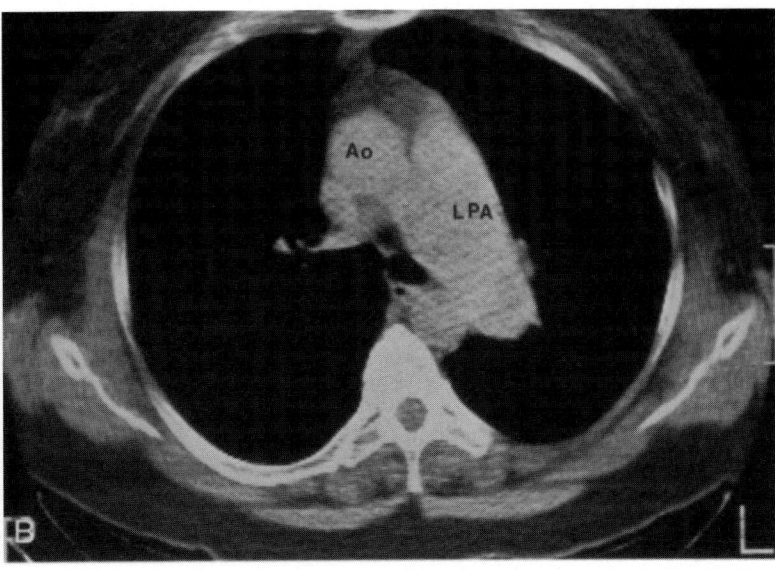

Figure 23.24. Pulmonary Stenosis. A. Lateral chest radiograph demonstrates marked poststenotic dilatation of the left pulmonary artery (*arrow*). **B.** CT through the ascending aorta (*Ao*) demonstrates marked dilatation of the left pulmonary artery (*LPA*).

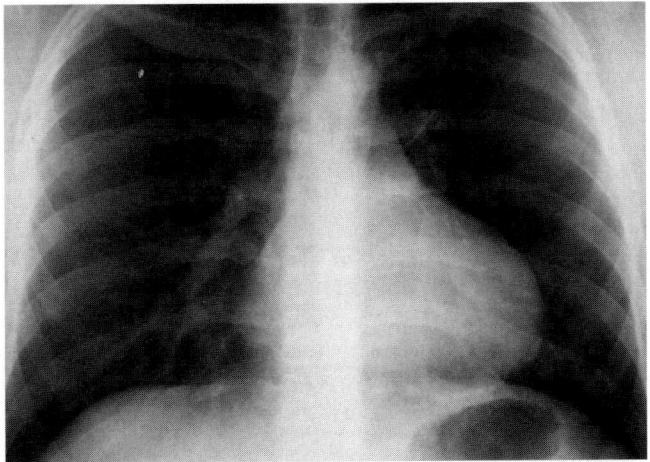

Figure 23.25. Peripheral Pulmonary Stenosis. A chest radiograph demonstrates classic right ventricular configuration indicative of RV hypertrophy. Asymmetric blood flow is noted with decreased markings in the left lung because of peripheral stenosis.

start in childhood and progress into adulthood. A pulmonic click is common, and the electrocardiogram often shows right ventricular hypertrophy. On angiography, a jet of contrast may be seen extending well into the left pulmonary artery. In dysplastic pulmonic stenosis (5% of cases) the cusps are immobile, thick, and redundant. There is no click and typically no poststenotic dilatation.

Infundibular or subvalvular stenosis is common with tetralogy of Fallot and often occurs with ventricular septal defects. Because of the location of the stenosis, preferential flow goes to the right lung.

Peripheral pulmonic stenosis or supravalvular stenosis commonly (up to 60%) accompanies pulmonary

valvular stenosis. Sites of narrowing include the main pulmonary artery, bifurcation, lobar, and segmental arteries (Fig. 23.25). Associated syndromes include Williams syndrome, tetralogy of Fallot, Ehlers-Danlos syndrome, and postrubella syndrome. Postrubella syndrome is associated with intrauterine growth retardation, deafness, cataracts, mental retardation, and patent ductus arteriosus. Williams syndrome is associated with hypercalcemia, elfin facies, mental retardation, and supravalvular aortic stenosis. Ehlers-Danlos syndrome is a defect in collagen formation associated with joint laxity, skin stretchability, aneurysms, and mitral regurgitation.

Pulmonic Insufficiency is very uncommon in adults and is usually the result of subacute bacterial endocarditis. Pulmonic insufficiency demonstrates regurgitant flow into the RV.

Bacterial Endocarditis. Patients predisposed to subacute bacterial endocarditis (SBE) include those with rheumatic heart disease, mitral valve prolapse, aortic stenosis, aortic regurgitation, bicuspid aortic valves (50% of aortic SBE), mitral stenosis, mitral regurgitation, congenital heart disease (especially ventricular septal defect and tetralogy of Fallot), or prosthetic valves (4% of SBE), and drug addicts. IV drug abusers are particularly at risk for tricuspid valve involvement. Tricuspid valve disease is suspected when multiple septic pulmonary emboli are seen on chest radiography. *Streptococcus viridans* was previously reported as the most common bacterial etiology; however, *Staphylococcus aureus* has now become the most common bacterial agent. *Serratia* and *Pseudomonas* organisms are also common offenders, particularly in certain geographic locations. *Candida* is the most common fungal agent, followed by *Aspergillus*.

Valve vegetations can be detected in 50–90% of pa-

Figure 23.26. Subacute Bacterial Endocarditis. Indium-labeled white cell scan shows migration of indium-labeled white cells to the area of severe aortic endocarditis. Note the marked increased activity (*arrows*) to the left and posterior to the sternum (*curved arrow*) on these anterior (*ANT*) and left anterior oblique (*LAO*) views of the chest. *L*, liver. *S*, spleen.

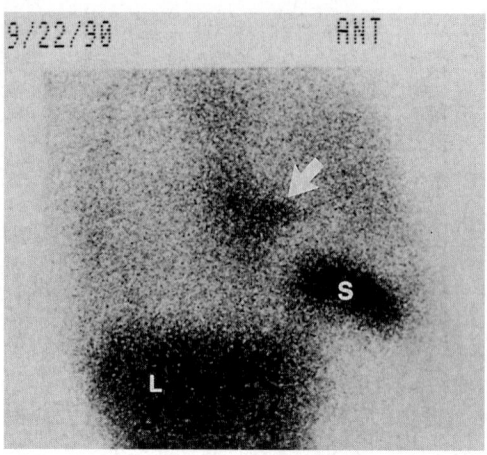 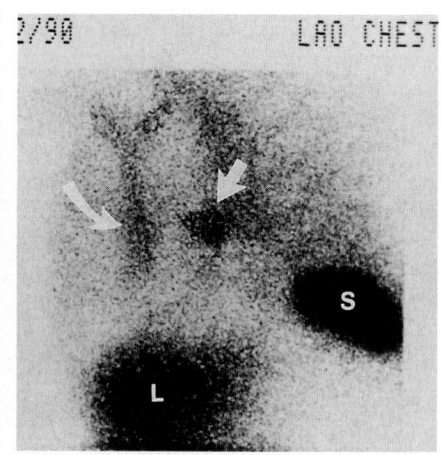

tients with known bacterial endocarditis. The vegetations cause excessive vibration of the valves during systole, and the leaflets may appear slightly thickened or fuzzy. The actual vegetations may be seen to prolapse when the valve is closed. The vegetations may cause valvular incompetence or acute valvular destruction. The vegetations, or chronic areas of thickening, may remain even after successful antibiotic therapy. It is difficult to discern acute infective vegetations from chronic changes. Infections of prosthetic valves result in exaggerated valve motion, partial valvular obstruction, loosening of the sutures, and perivalvular leak or frank dehiscence. MR and transesophageal echocardiography are quite good at detecting perivalvular or perisutural leaks. Noninfectious vegetations and focal valve thickenings may be seen with carcinoid syndrome (right heart valves), *Libman-Sack's vegetations* of systemic lupus erythematosus, *Lambl's excrescences* (focal benign thickening), and myxomatous degeneration.

Other forms of endocarditis include *Chagas' disease*, which is common in South America and Africa. Chagas' disease is a late sequelae of acute myocarditis involving the parasite *Trypanosoma cruzi*. This may result in cardiomyopathy or ventricular aneurysm. Patients with AIDS may also develop an endocarditis and cardiomyopathy, possibly because of viral infections. Indium-labeled white cell scans or gallium scans may prove useful in patients for whom echocardiography is inconclusive or in whom secondary endocardial or aortic abscess is suspected (Fig. 23.26).

CARDIAC MASSES

Cardiac masses include thrombi, primary benign tumors, primary malignant tumors, and metastatic tumors. Lipomatous hypertrophy, moderator bands, and papillary muscles may simulate cardiac masses. Because most cardiac masses do not deform the outer contours of the heart, chest radiography is typically not useful, except for the occasional calcific mass. Nuclear scintigraphy, CT, and cardiac angiography identify intracardiac masses. Echocardiography is usually the initial mode of evaluation, and MR may be helpful when there is uncertainty.

Thrombi are the most frequent cause of an intracardiac mass and are most common in the LA and LV, where they present a risk of systemic emboli. Intra-atrial thrombi are usually associated with atrial fibrillation, often secondary to rheumatic heart disease. Thrombosis commonly occurs along the posterior wall of the LA. Clots within the left atrial appendage are difficult to detect on transthoracic echocardiography but are readily identified with transesophageal echo (Fig. 23.27) and MR. Left ventricular thrombi are usually secondary to recent infarction or ventricular aneurysm (Fig. 23.28). The differentiation of tumor versus clot is best done with MR using gradient-echo techniques. Clots typically have low signal, whereas tumors have intermediate signal. Neoplasms appear as nonenhancing masses on CT or MR. Cine-mode gradient-echo MR is useful for determining the morphology of the lesion. Intracardiac lipomas or lipomatous hypertrophy have characteristic bright signal on T1WI and remain relatively bright on T2WI. Fat

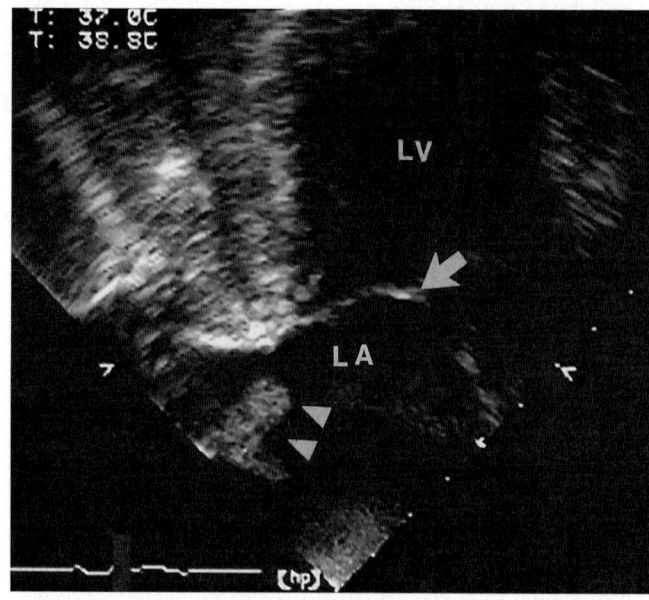

Figure 23.27. Left Atrial Thrombus. Transesophageal echo shows echogenic thrombus (*arrowheads*) in the left atrium (*LA*). The mitral valve (*arrow*) and the left ventricle (*LV*) are well seen.

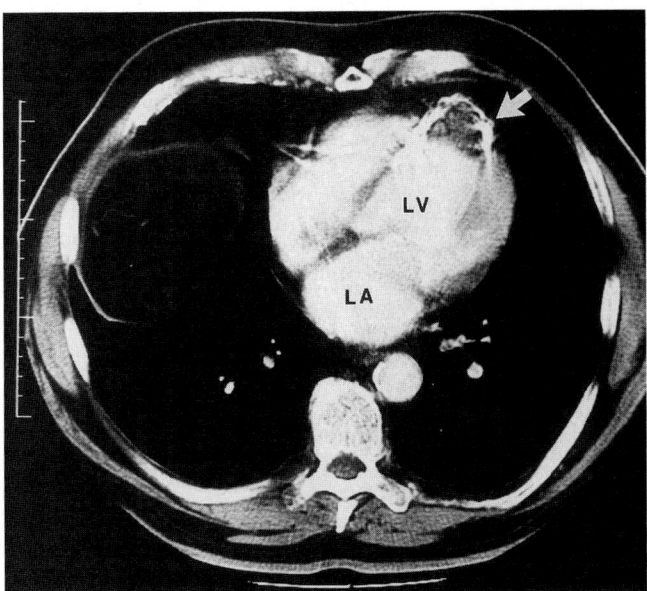

Figure 23.28. Left Ventricular Thrombus. Contrast enhanced CT through the left ventricle (*LV*) demonstrates calcification in an apical, left ventricular aneurysm (*arrow*). Note the nonenhancing low-density thrombus within the aneurysm. *LA*, left atrium.

saturation sequences help to make the specific diagnosis of lipoma, which is the second most common benign tumor.

Benign Tumors. Atrial myxoma makes up 50% of primary cardiac tumors and is the most common primary benign tumor. It occurs most frequently in patients in the 30- to 60-year age range and is often accompanied by fever, anemia, weight loss, embolic symptoms (27%), or syncope. Most (75–80%) myxomas are in the LA and may mimic rheumatic valvular disease (Fig. 23.29). Cardiomegaly, left atrial enlargement, pulmonary venous hypertension, and ossific pulmonary nodules may be seen. Enlargement of the left atrial appendage is uncommon. Echocardiogram and MR show the atrial filling defect that may prolapse into the LV during diastole. Left atrial myxomas may be pedunculated and are usually lobulated. On M-mode echo, the E–F slope is typically decreased with numerous echoes seen behind the mitral valve.

Other benign tumors include lipoma, rhabdomyoma (Fig. 23.30) (found in 50–85% of tuberous sclerosis patients), fibromas (12% of which may calcify), and the rare teratoma. Hydatid cysts typically show a bulge along the left heart border, with associated curvilinear calcification, and are at risk for rupture into the pericardium or myocardium.

Malignant Tumors. Metastatic cardiac tumors are 10 to 20 times more common than primary cardiac tumors. Breast, lung, melanoma, and lymphoma are the most common neoplasms to metastasize to the heart. MR is excellent for detecting direct extension, intracardiac metastases and pericardial involvement. Angiosarcoma is the most common primary malignant cardiac tumor, followed by rhabdosarcoma, liposarcoma, and other sarcomas.

PERICARDIAL DISEASE

Pericardial Effusion is the most common abnormality of the pericardium. The normal pericardial stripe is 2–3 mm on chest radiograph and CT and less than 4 mm on MR. Plain films show thickening of the pericardial stripe or differential density sign in up to 63% of patients with pericardial effusions. The water-bottle configuration is seen in chronic effusions. Fluoroscopy shows decreased cardiac pulsations. The normal pericardium contains approximately 20 mL of fluid, whereas it takes approximately 200 mL to be detectable by plain film. Echocardiography detects very small quantities (<50 mL) of pericardial fluid, usually as a posterior sonolucent collection (Fig. 23.31). Small effusions (<100 mL) will appear as anterior and posterior sonolucent regions. Moderate-sized effusions (100–500 mL) demonstrate a sonolucent zone around the entire ventricle. Very large effusions (>500 mL) extend beyond the field of view and may be associated with the "swinging heart" inside the pericardium. CT is useful in detecting loculated pericardial effusions. MR may characterize the fluid. Simple serous fluid appears dark on T1WI (probably because of fluid motion) and bright on gradient-echo images. Complicated or hemorrhagic effusions appear bright on T1WI and dark on gradient-echo imaging (probably because of susceptibility artifact). The differential diagnosis for pericardial effusions is listed in Table 23.6.

Cardiac Tamponade refers to cardiac chamber compression by pericardial effusion under tension, compromising diastolic filling. *Pulsus paradoxus* describes an exaggeration of the usual drop in systolic pressure greater than 10 mm Hg during inspiration. This occurs as a result of septal shift and paradoxic septal motion during right ventricular filling. Clinical examination shows marked jugular venous distension, distant heart sounds, and a pericardial rub. The chest

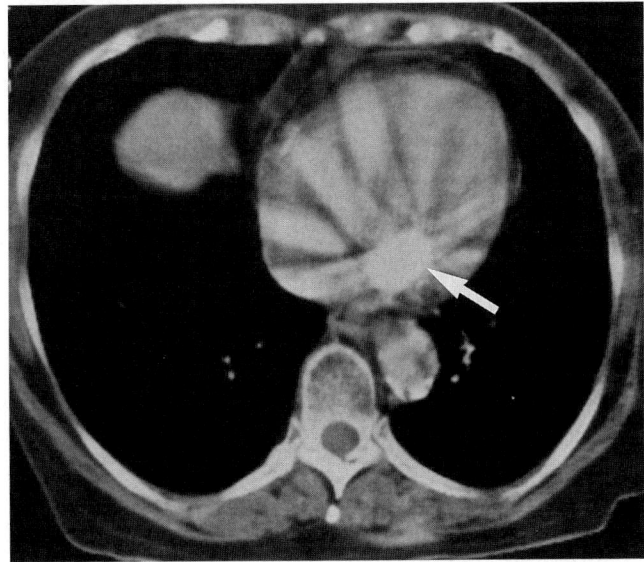

Figure 23.29. Left Atrial Myxoma. CT demonstrates a densely calcified mass (*arrow*) within the LA, indicative of left atrial myxoma.

Figure 23.30. Left Ventricular Rhabdo-myoma. Coronal spin-echo MR through the aorta (*Ao*) and LV demonstrates a large polypoid mass near the outflow tract of the LV (*arrow*). This patient had tuberous sclerosis, and a presumptive diagnosis of ventricular rhabdomyoma was made. Note the good delineation of the right atrium (*RA*) and right ventricle (*RV*).

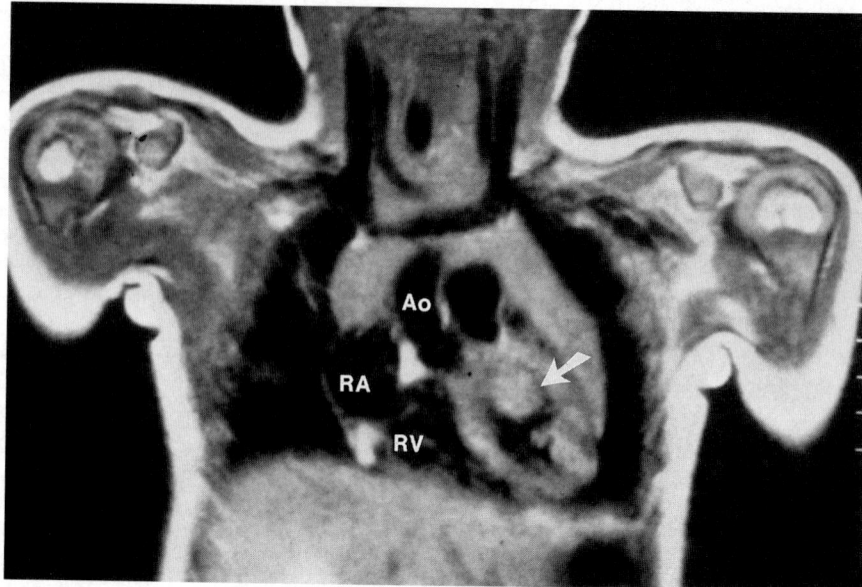

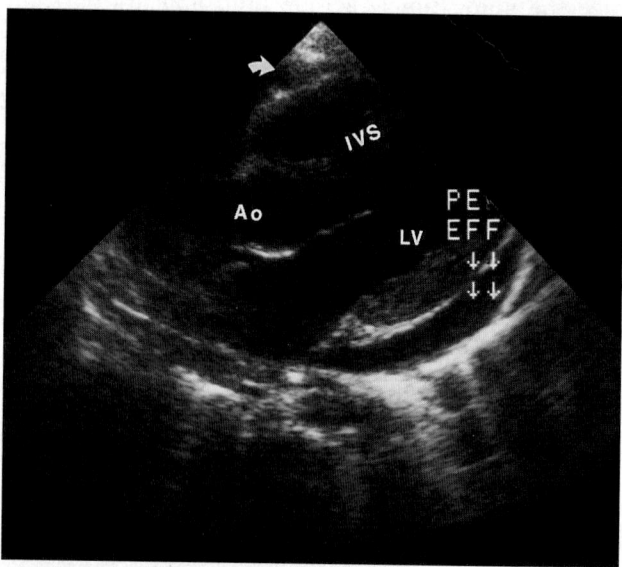

Figure 23.31. Pericardial Effusion. Longitudinal echocardiogram through the interventricular septum (*IVS*), aortic root (*Ao*), and left ventricle (*LV*) demonstrates a pericardial effusion (*PE EFF*). A smaller anterior effusion is also noted (*arrow*).

Table 23.6. Causes of Pericardial Effusion

Idiopathic
Infectious
　Viral (Coxsackie, echovirus, adenovirus)
　Bacterial (*Staphyloccocus, Streptococcus, Haemophilus influenzae*)
　Fungal (*Candida, Aspergillus, Nocardia*)
　Mycobacterial
Autoimmune
　Systemic lupus erythematosus
　Rheumatoid arthritis
　Scleroderma
　Dressler's and postpericardiotomy syndromes
　Radiation induced
Neoplastic
　Lymphoma, lung, breast metastases
Drug Induced
　Procainamide, hydralazine, phenytoin
Metabolic
　Uremia
　Myxedema
　Cholesterol
Miscellaneous
　Congestive heart failure
　Aortic dissection
　Sarcoidosis
　Pancreatitis
　Trauma

radiograph shows rapid enlargement of the cardiac silhouette with relatively normal-appearing vascularity. Echocardiography typically shows the septal shift, paradoxic septal motion, diastolic collapse of the RV, and cyclical collapse of the atria.

Constrictive Pericardial Disease is the result of fibrous or calcific thickening of the pericardium, which chronically compromises ventricular filling through restriction of cardiac motion. Age of onset is usually 30–50 years, and the incidence in men exceeds that in females by 3:1. The most common cause is postpericardiotomy. Other etiologies include virus (Coxsackie B), tuberculosis, chronic renal failure,

rheumatoid arthritis, neoplastic involvement, and radiation pericarditis. Calcification is seen on radiographs in up to 50% of patients. Pleural effusions and ascites are common, and there may be an associated protein-losing enteropathy. Clinical findings include ankle edema, neck vein distension, pulsus paradoxus, pericardial diastolic knock, and ascites. Chest radiographs show normal to mildly enlarged cardiac silhouette with small atria, dilated superior and inferior vena cava and azygos vein, and a flat or straightened right heart border. Echocardiography shows thickened pericardium, abnormal septal motion, and increased left ventricular ejection fraction with small end-diastolic volume. Small effusions may be seen with "effusive constrictive pericarditis," which has both thickening and effusion.

CT is particularly good at demonstrating pericardial thickening (>3 mm) in difficult cases (Fig. 23.32). Reflux of contrast into the coronary sinus, a bowed interventricular septum, flattening of the RV, ascites, pleural effusions, and pericardial calcifications may also be seen. MR shows pericardial thickening (>4 mm); dilatation of the RA, inferior vena cava, and hepatic veins; sigmoid septal shift; and narrowing of

the RV. Abnormal flow mechanics may also be seen in the vena cava and atria. The finding of an abnormally thick pericardium is important in differentiating constrictive pericardial disease from restrictive cardiomyopathy.

Pericardial Cysts are most common in the cardiophrenic angles, right more common than left (Fig. 23.33). They are usually asymptomatic and are more frequent in males. The cysts are attached to the parietal pericardium, are lined with epithelial or mesothelial cells, contain clear fluid, and range in size from 3–8 cm. They occasionally communicate with the pericardial space. Computed tomography attenuation numbers are 20–40 H (Fig. 23.33). MR demonstrates characteristic low signal on T1WI and bright signal on T2WI. The differential diagnosis for a cardiophrenic angle mass includes pericardial cyst, fat pad, lipoma, enlarged lymph nodes, diaphragmatic hernia, and ventricular aneurysm.

Congenital Absence of the Pericardium (Fig. 23.34) is more common in males than females by 3:1. The age at diagnosis is infancy through age 81. Complete left-sided absence (55%) is more common than foraminal defects (35%) or total absence (10%). Associated conditions include bronchogenic cysts, ventricular septal defects, diaphragmatic hernias, and sequestrations. With complete absence, the heart is shifted toward the left with a prominent bulge of the right ventricular outflow tract, main pulmonary artery, and left atrial appendage. Insinuation of the lung into the anteroposterior window and beneath the heart is characteristic. Decubitus views show a widely swinging cardiac silhouette. Partial absence of the pericardium risks strangulation of cardiac structures, with the possibility of sudden death. Surgical closure of partial defects is usually recommended.

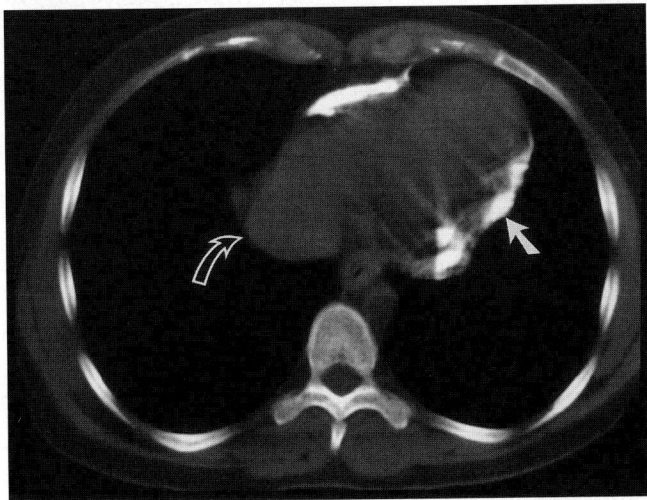

Figure 23.32. Constrictive Pericarditis. Nonenhanced CT demonstrates pericardial calcification (*closed arrow*) and a dilated inferior vena cava (*open arrow*). Note the distortion of the ventricles.

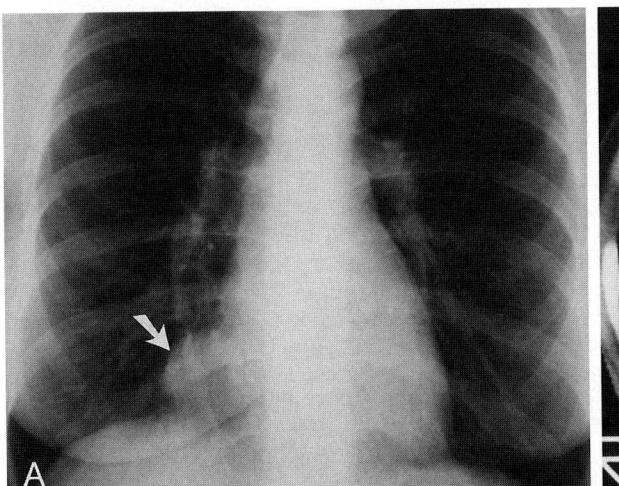
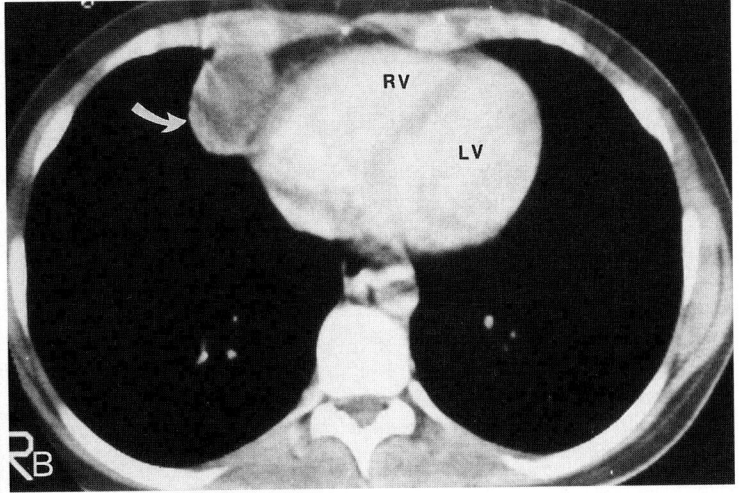

Figure 23.33. Pericardial Cyst. A. Chest radiograph demonstrates a soft-tissue mass in the right cardiophrenic angle (*arrow*). **B.** Contrast-enhanced CT demonstrates water density within the nonenhancing mass in the cardiophrenic angle, consistent with pericardial cyst. *RV*, right ventricle; *LV*, left ventricle.

Figure 23.34. Partial Absence of the Pericardium. A. Chest radiograph demonstrates a prominence of the main pulmonary artery (*closed arrow*) and an unusual bulge along the left heart border (*open arrow*). **B.** Coronal spin-echo MR confirms enlargement of the main pulmonary artery (*closed arrow*) and shows herniation of the left atrial appendage (*open arrow*). *Ao*, ascending aorta; *LA*, left atrium; *RA*, right atrium.

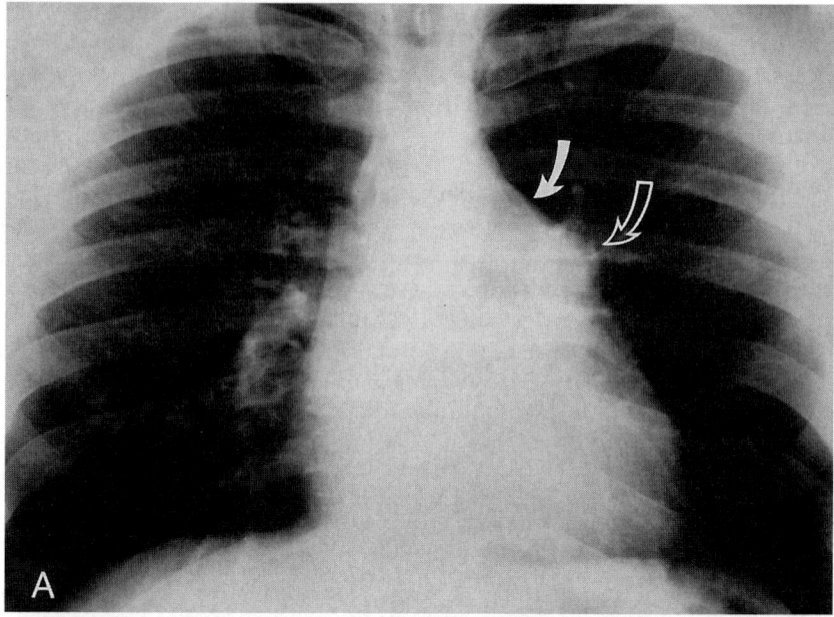

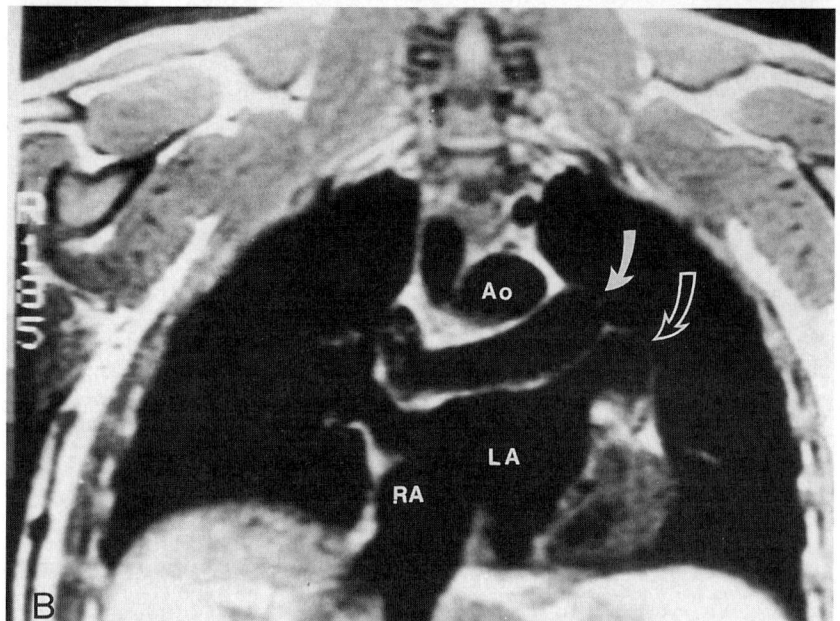

Suggested Readings

Brundage BH. Comparative Cardiac Imaging. Rockville, MD: Aspen Publications, 1990.

Chapman S, Nakielny R. Aids to Radiological Diagnosis. 2nd ed. London: WB Saunders, 1990.

Dahnert W. Radiology Review Manual. 3rd ed. Baltimore: Williams & Wilkins, 1996.

Duerinckx AJ, Higgins CB, Pettigrew RI. MRI of the Cardiovascular System. New York: Raven Press, 1994.

Eisenberg RL. Chest and Cardiac Imaging. New York: Raven Press, 1993.

Feigenbaum H. Echocardiography. 5th ed. Philadelphia: Lea & Febiger, 1994.

Gedgaudas E, Moffer JH, Castaneda-Zuniga WR, Amplatz K. Cardiovascular Radiology. Philadelphia: WB Saunders, 1985.

Higgins CB. Essentials of Cardiac Radiology and Imaging. Philadelphia: JB Lippincott, 1992.

Higgins CB, Hricak H, Helms CA. Magnetic Resonance Imaging of the Body. Lippincott: Raven Philadelphia, 1997.

Kelley MJ. Chest Radiography for the Cardiologist. Cardiology clinics. Philadelphia: WB Saunders, 1983.

Kubicka RA, Smith C. How to interpret coronary arteriograms. Radiographics 1986;6:661–701.

Marcovite PA, Armstrong WF. Accuracy of dobutamine stress echocardiography in detecting coronary artery disease. Am J Cardiol 1992;1269–1273.

Marcus ML, Schelbert HR, Skorton DJ, Wolf GL. Cardiac Imaging—A Companion to Braunwald's Heart Disease. Philadelphia: WB Saunders, 1991.

Miller SW, ed. Advances in Cardiac Imaging. Radiology Clinics of North America. Philadelphia: WB Saunders, 1985.

Miller SW, ed. Cardiopulmonary Imaging. Radiology Clinics of North America. Philadelphia: WB Saunders, 1989.

Miller SW. Cardiac Radiology—The Requisites. St. Louis: Mosby, 1996.

Putnam CE. Cardiopulmonary Imaging. Radiol clinics of North America. Philadelphia: WB Saunders, 1983.

Ravin CE, Cooper C. Review of Radiology. 2nd ed. Philadelphia: WB Saunders, 1993.

Taveras JM, Ferrucci JT. Radiology. Philadelphia: WB Saunders, 1993.

Wolfe CL. Cardiac Imaging. Cardiology clinics. Philadelphia: WB Saunders, 1989.

Zaret BL, Beller GA. Nuclear Cardiology. St. Louis: Mosby, 1993.

24
Vascular Radiology

John E. Williams
Mylon W. Marshall

IMAGING METHODS

Conventional and Digital Angiography. Imaging of the vascular system is unique in that for many years it was largely limited to the relatively invasive modality of conventional angiography (CA). With the advent of intravenous and intra-arterial digital subtraction angiography (DSA), significant improvements were made in decreasing overall patient risk; however these new modalities are relatively invasive. During the last two decades, CT, US, and MR have demonstrated remarkable capability in vascular imaging and satisfy the need for noninvasive, screening techniques.

CA uses film-screen imaging in combination with rapid film changers and has the advantage of superb spatial resolution (six line-pairs per millimeter versus two line-pairs per millimeter for DSA). DSA uses digital images acquired both immediately before and after the injection of iodinated contrast with subsequent electronic subtraction of the noncontrast (mask) images from those containing contrast. Its advantage lies in better contrast resolution, decreased examination time, and lower contrast dose. It is severely degraded by motion artifact if the patient moves between the precontrast and postcontrast images. For lower extremity imaging, most angiographers use "step-tables" with CA and DSA acquisition technique. This involves synchronous contrast injection in the distal aorta with regular, sequential movements of the table relative to the image intensifier. Rapid filming or digital image acquisition is carried out at each table stop, thus gaining maximal contrast use while imaging both lower extremities simultaneously. In addition, most modern angiographic suites use "C-arm" mounted image intensifier units coupled to both the digital imaging train and rapid film changer. This facilitates oblique imaging to visualize the anatomy optimally and obviates the need to move the patient, which may be difficult in certain situations. DSA and CA provide images of the vessel lumen. They provide little information about extraluminal pathology and are best used in addressing specific questions for pretreatment planning, during percutaneous intravascular intervention, and when noninvasive imaging is equivocal or fails to provide adequate information.

Carbon dioxide (CO_2) DSA imaging, which uses CO_2 as an intravascular contrast agent has become increasingly popular with the advent of more refined DSA equipment. Because CO_2 dissolves rapidly in blood (solubility $20\times$ room air or oxygen) and is completely eliminated on a single pass through the pulmonary circulation, it demonstrates minimal systemic or organ specific toxicity, making it an attractive vascular contrast agent. CO_2 imaging takes advantage of the difference in density between the gas within the vessel and the adjacent soft tissues. Water-soluble contrast mixes with blood to provide vascular contrast, whereas CO_2 provides contrast by displacing blood. This may lead to "fragmentation" of the gas column, with only segments of the vessel lumen visualized on sequential DSA images. This disadvantage can be overcome by using a software "stacking" or "image summation" program that effectively summates a series of masked images at the same anatomic location to produce a final composite image of the entire vessel lumen (1).

Because CO_2 exhibits the property of buoyancy, the more non-dependent structures are better opacified. This is best illustrated with lateral imaging of the abdominal aorta with the patient in the usual supine position. The anteriorly located celiac, superior mesenteric and inferior mesenteric arteries are usually well seen, while the posterior lumbar arteries are typically not visualized. The patient positioned with the vascular territory of interest placed non-dependently to take advantage of this feature. For instance, the patient's feet can be elevated slightly (15–20°) to enhance filling of the lower extremity vessels, or the patient rolled into a slight decubitus position for imaging of the renal arteries. Buoyancy must also be considered when timing repeated injections or imaging in low flow states to avoid completely replacing the blood volume in a given vascular territory resulting in tissue ischemia due to "vapor lock" phenomenon. This is prevented by appropriate delay between injections, use of the smallest volume necessary, and change in patient positioning. Another potential problem related to buoyancy is incomplete filling of the vessel lumen and underestimation of luminal size. Injection rates and volumes must be optimized to completely fill the vessel lumen.

The most common applications for CO_2 imaging are in patients with renal insufficiency or history of severe iodinated contrast reaction. CO_2 can be substituted for other intravascular contrast agents in any situation, except arterial imaging in the chest, head, and neck because of potential for neurotoxicity. Caution should be exercised with use in patients with severe obstructive airway disease (1).

CT and MR provide excellent visualization of vessels and their relationship to surrounding structures. CT depicts the vessel lumen optimally only when contrast enhancement is used. CT angiography uses a bolus contrast injection with helical CT acquisition and subsequent three-dimensional reconstruction to display either a two- or three-dimensional representation of the vessels being imaged in virtually any projection.

MR, with its inherent multiplanar imaging capability, is well suited for evaluation of the thoracic and abdominal aorta and may be used with or without contrast enhancement. The MR characteristics of flowing blood depend on velocity, turbulence, and direction of flow. In general, MR demonstrates the vessel lumen as "black blood" or flow void on routine cardiac-gated spin-echo imaging and as "bright blood" with gradient refocused techniques. MR angiography takes advantage of the inherent contrast produced by unsaturated protons within flowing blood relative to the stationary saturated protons within the soft tissues in *time of flight* imaging, and a second property of flowing blood as it interacts with specialized gradients imposed on the main magnetic field in *phase contrast* imaging. These two methods produce images similar to those obtained with contrast angiography once specialized processing algorithms have been applied to the raw data. Data for either technique may be obtained using two-dimensional (images obtained in "sequential slice" mode) or three-dimensional (images obtained in "slab" or "volume" mode). These data are then postprocessed typically using the *maximum intensity pixel* algorithm, which can then be displayed in multiple planes. MRA is limited by motion artifact, scan time, flow artifacts at severe stenoses, and methemoglobin in thrombosed vessels that produces bright signal that may simulate flowing blood (2).

US use in vascular imaging is reviewed in chapter 40. Intravascular ultrasound (IVUS) is an emerging technology that involves mounting of a high-frequency transducer (12.5–40 MHz) on a catheter shaft and imaging the vessel from an intraluminal position. This modality is currently best used for therapeutic interventional procedures such as balloon angioplasty and intravascular stent placement. IVUS is highly accurate in assessing vessel diameter, percent stenosis, plaque and vessel wall composition, location of branch vessels, evaluation of stents and stent grafts, and visualization of intimal flaps (3).

THORACIC AORTA

Anatomy

Arteries are composed of three layers: a thin lining known as the *intima*, a relatively thick muscular layer called the *media*, and an outer layer termed the *adventitia*. These are not typically differentiated by imaging modalities.

The thoracic aorta extends from the aortic valve to the diaphragmatic hiatus and is divided into three main sections: ascending aorta, arch, and descending aorta. The ascending portion extends to the origin of the innominate artery, is subdivided into the sinus and tubular regions, and lies predominately within the pericardial sac. The three aortic valve leaflets have corresponding dilatation within the sinus region of the aorta known as the sinuses of Valsalva. Two of the sinuses give rise to the right and left coronary arteries and are termed right and left coronary sinuses. The remaining sinus is termed the noncoronary sinus and is located posteriorly. At the junction of the sinus and tubular portions, the aorta has a diameter of approximately 3–4 cm in the adult. At no point is the descending larger than the ascending aorta (4).

The aortic arch extends from the innominate artery origin to the insertion of the ligamentum arteriosum. It courses from right anterolaterally to left posterolaterally in front of the trachea at the level of T-4. In the "classic origin" pattern seen in 70% of the population, it gives rise to the innominate, left common carotid, and left subclavian arteries (Fig. 24.1A). The most common variant pattern (22%) is a common trunk for the innominate and left common carotid arteries (5). Another variant (5%) is an arch origin of the left vertebral artery that arises between the left common carotid and left subclavian arteries (Fig. 24.1B). The arch between the left subclavian origin and the ligamentum attachment is termed

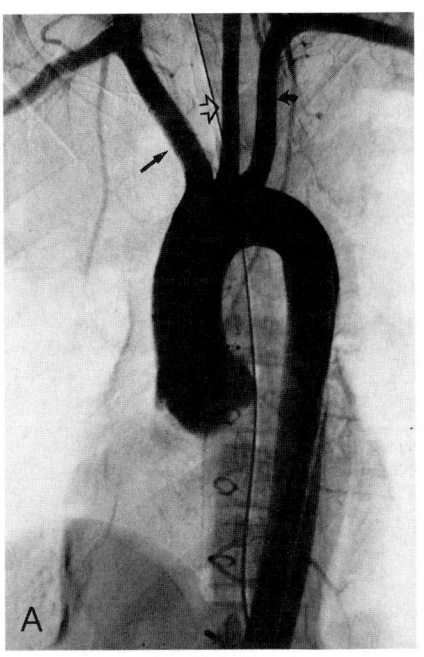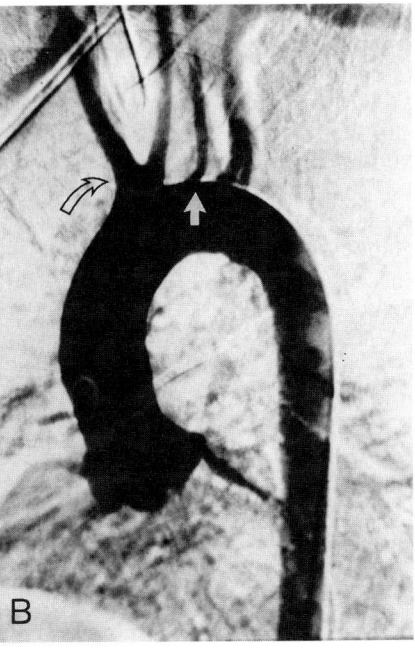

Figure 24.1. Normal Aortic Arch and Variants.
A. Aortogram with "classic" origin pattern of the great vessels; right brachiocephalic artery (*straight black arrow*), left common carotid artery (*open black arrow*), and left subclavian artery (*curved black arrow*). **B.** Normal variant aortic arch anatomy with common origin of the right brachiocephalic artery and left common carotid artery (*curved open black arrow*) and the origin of the left vertebral artery from the aortic arch (*white arrow*).

the *isthmus*. The diameter of the aorta may narrow slightly at the isthmus.

The descending portion comprises the remainder of the thoracic aorta. A *ductus diverticulum* is a normal variant fusiform dilatation along the ventromedial aspect of the proximal descending aorta adjacent to the ligamentum (Fig. 24.2) (5). Usually nine pairs of intercostal arteries arise from the posterior descending aorta at intercostal spaces 3–11. The superior two intercostal arteries arise from the superior intercostal artery, which is a branch of the costocervical trunk. The bronchial arteries have an extremely variable anatomy and arise from the posterolateral descending aorta usually from the level of T-4 through T-7. The most common patterns are three arteries (usually one right and two left) seen in 40%, single arteries bilaterally in 30%, and four arteries seen in 25% of cases.

Angiographic Technique

The most common and safest route of access to study the thoracic aorta is the common femoral artery (CFA). If the femoral approach is not feasible, the right axillary artery is the most useful for studying the ascending and arch regions, and the left axillary artery allows easier access to the descending thoracic and abdominal aorta. An alternative access route to the abdominal aorta is a translumbar direct puncture of the abdominal aorta with the patient in the prone position.

The CFA is palpated below the inguinal ligament, with the skin puncture site located near the inferior margin of the femoral head. The artery lies along the junction of the medial and middle thirds of the femoral head. After sterile preparation and drape and administration of local anesthetic, a small skin incision is made. While palpating the artery, the opposite hand is used to puncture the artery by passing the needle at approximately 45° to the skin surface. With the double-wall technique, the needle

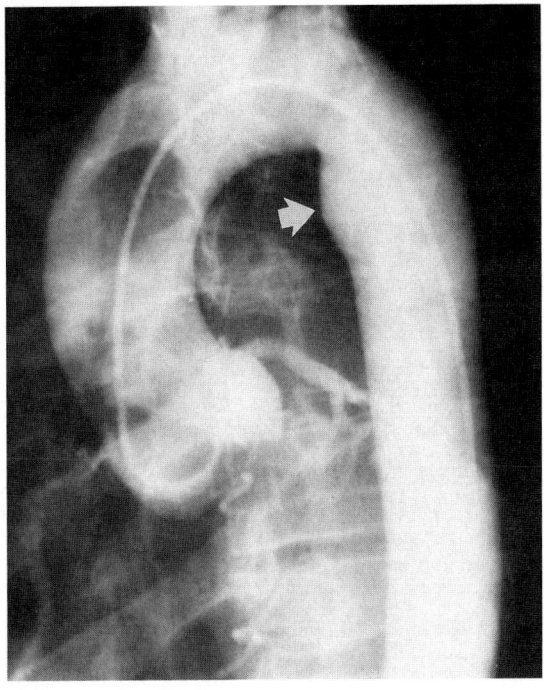

Figure 24.2. Ductus Diverticulum. Thoracic aortogram demonstrates normal variant fusiform dilatation (*arrow*) of the proximal descending aorta in the region of the ligamentum arteriosum.

is passed through both walls of the artery. The stylet is removed and the cannula withdrawn until pulsatile return is obtained. The single-wall technique involves puncturing the artery with a hollow needle through the anterior wall only. After brisk, pulsatile flow is seen, a guide wire is carefully passed through the needle and used to guide dilators and eventually the catheter into the artery. This is termed the Seldinger technique for percutaneous arterial access. Fluoroscopic visualization is used to advance guidewires and catheters so as to prevent subintimal passage. A test hand injection of contrast through a newly positioned catheter is always performed to ensure intraluminal placement within the desired vessel. The catheter is carefully flushed with heparinized saline throughout the procedure to prevent thrombus formation within the catheter. After the procedure, the catheter is removed and hemostasis is obtained at the puncture site using manual compression.

For imaging of the thoracic aorta, a pigtail catheter is placed approximately 1–2 cm above the aortic valve or within the descending aorta if this is the area of interest.

The 45° left anterior oblique projection best displays the arch and great vessel origins. Orthogonal views are usually required. Biplane imaging can be used initially with supplemental projections to best demonstrate the anatomy of interest. When using DSA, either the contrast volume or the concentration can be reduced (Table 24.1).

General Risks and Contraindications. The complication rates for the three most commonly used sites for arterial access are femoral (1.7%), translumbar (2.9%),

Table 24.1. Angiographic Techniques

Procedure	Catheter	Injection Rate (ml/second/ total volume contrast)	Filming Rate (films/ second/total seconds)
Thoracic aorta	Pigtail	30/60 (CA) 20/40 (DSA)[a]	3/3; 1/6[b] 3 frames per second
Abdominal aorta	Pigtail	25/50 (CA) 15/30 (DSA)[a]	2/4; 1/6[b] 2 frames per second
Bilateral lower extremity runoff	Pigtail	10/70 (CA) 8/42 (DSA)[a]	2/3; 1/3 2 frames per second
Common carotid	Simmons Headhunter	6/10 (CA) 5/9 (DSA)[a]	2/4; 1/6[b] 3 frames per second
Internal carotid	Simmons Headhunter	5/10 (CA) 4/8 (DSA)[a]	2/4; 1/6[b] 3 frames per second
Subclavian	Simmons Headhunter	6/18 (CA) 4/16 (DSA)[a]	2/4; 1/8 2 frames per second
Renal	Cobra Simmons	6/12 (CA) 4/8 (DSA)[a]	2/4; 1/6 2 frames per second
Celiac	Cobra/Simmons	10/50 (CA)	2/3; 1/4; 0.5/10[c]
SMA	Cobra/Simmons	8/48 (CA) 6/42 (DSA)[a,d]	2/3; 1/4; 0.5/10[c] 2 frames per second
SMA portogram	Cobra/Simmons	8/60 (CA) 6/42 (DSA)[a,d]	1/10; 0.5/10[c] 2 frames per second
IMA	Cobra/Simmons	3/18 (CA)	2/3; 1/4; 0.5/10[c]
Superior venacavagram	Pigtail	15/30 (CA) 10/20 (DSA)[a]	2/3; 1/3[b] 2 frames per second
	Multiside-hole straight catheters	Manual injection[e] 50 cc total volume (CA) 40 cc total vol. (DSA)[a]	2/3; 1/8 2 frames per second
Inferior venacavagram	Pigtail	20/40 (CA) 15/30 (DSA)[a]	2/3; 1/3[b] 2 frames per second
Pulmonary	Pigtail Grollman Balloon catheter	20/40 (CA) 15/30 (DSA)[a]	3/3; 1/6[b] 3 frames per second

[a] May use either reduced rates or amounts of "full-strength" (76%) contrast as presented here, or same rates/amounts as CA using "half-strength" dilute (30%) contrast.
[b] These techniques are for single plane imaging; for biplane these values may need to be doubled depending on the type of equipment being used (e.g., 6/3; 2/6).
[c] The designation "0.5/10" denotes exposing 1 film every other second for a total of 10 seconds.
[d] May require glucagon 1 mg IV to reduce bowel motion for DSA imaging.
[e] Simultaneous injection of bilateral antecubital approach with catheters in axillary veins. This techniques used for suspected SVC obstruction.

and axillary (3.3%). Complications can be categorized into those related to direct vascular trauma and those secondary to contrast media. The most common problem is puncture-site bleeding, which is of special concern in hypertensive patients. Other vascular injuries include subintimal dissection because of guidewire or catheter trauma and thrombus formation within or around the catheter. Both can lead to local vessel or distal embolization. These complications necessitate further percutaneous intervention or surgery and may, in the extreme, lead to limb loss (6).

Complications related to iodinated contrast administration include renal toxicity and idiosyncratic reactions. Factors predisposing to contrast-related acute renal dysfunction include dehydration, diabetes mellitus, pre-existing renal insufficiency, multiple myeloma, and hyperuricemia. Most cases of renal toxicity are self-limiting and resolve completely. The best preventive measure is adequate patient hydration. Idiosyncratic, anaphylactoid reactions are classified as mild, moderate, and severe and are less prevalent with use of low-osmolality contrast agents and with intra-arterial than with intravenous use. Most reactions are mild to moderate (5% of contrast administrations), with manifestations ranging from nausea and vomiting to hives, urticaria, and mild bronchospasm. These require little or no treatment. More severe reactions (0.1% of contrast administrations) are marked bronchospasm and cardiovascular collapse, which require immediate life-saving intervention. Death attributable to iodinated contrast occurs in approximately 0.001% of cases. Risk factors that predispose to reactions include prior contrast reaction, atopic history, patient anxiety, and age less than 1 year or greater than 60 years. Prophylaxis with corticosteroids and diphen-

hydramine decrease the risk of idiosyncratic reaction by 50% in high-risk patients (7).

Congenital Anomalies

Left arch/aberrant right subclavian artery is the most common arch anomaly, being found in 1% of individuals. It is rarely symptomatic. The right subclavian artery arises as a fourth branch of the arch and must cross the mediastinum to reach the right arm. It crosses behind the esophagus in 80% of cases, between the trachea and esophagus in 15%, and anterior to the trachea in 5% (Fig. 24.3A) (5). A dilatation at the origin of the anomalous vessel is termed an *aortic diverticulum*, or *diverticulum of Kommerell* (Fig. 24.3B) (8). This dilatation represents the residua of the right arch of the embryonic double arch system. If large, it may cause significant posterior impression on the esophagus and result in dysphagia (9). In 10% of patients, congenital heart disease is present, with coarctation and tetralogy of Fallot being the most common anomalies. Plain films demonstrate widening of the superior mediastinum and anterior deviation of the trachea. MR and CT demonstrate a higher than normal arch with a more anteroposterior orientation in addition to the aberrant vessel coursing through the mediastinum (9). Arteriography is rarely needed.

Right arch/aberrant left subclavian artery (Fig. 24.3B) is much less common (0.1% of individuals). Either the arch or the aberrant vessel may cause a posterior impression on the esophagus. Congenital heart disease is present in 12% of cases, with tetralogy of Fallot, atrial septal defect, and coarctation being the most common abnormalities (5).

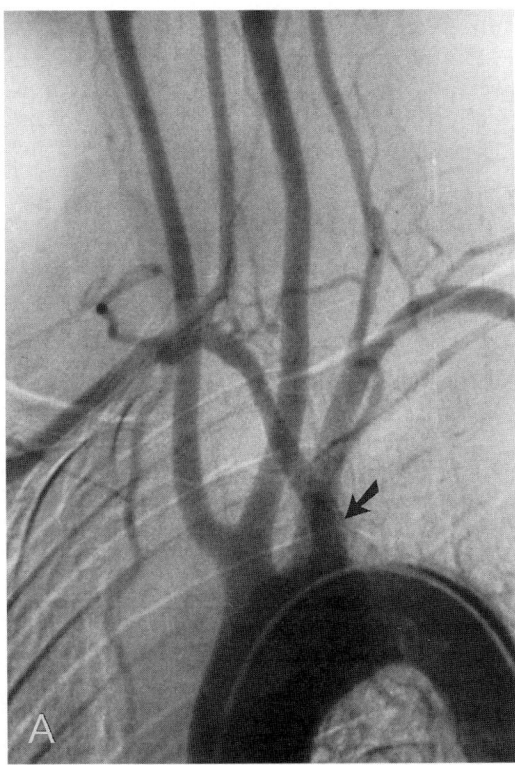

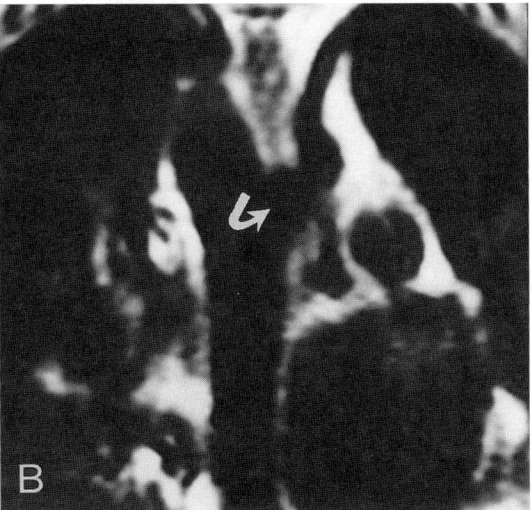

Figure 24.3. Congenital Anomalies of the Aortic Arch. A. Left arch/aberrant right subclavian artery: Aortogram shows origin of the right subclavian artery distal to the left subclavian artery (*arrow*). Note normal variant common origin of the right brachiocephalic artery and left common carotid artery. **B.** Right arch/aberrant left subclavian artery: Coronal MR demonstrates a diverticulum of Kommeral at the origin of the aberrant left subclavian artery (*arrow*).

Right arch with mirror image branching is a mirror image of the normal left arch branching system and thus has no retroesophageal component. There is a 98% association with congenital heart disease, with 90% of those being tetralogy of Fallot (9).

Coarctation is a primary abnormality of the media with eccentric narrowing of the aortic lumen resulting from infolding of the aortic wall. It occurs more commonly in males (4 : 1) and is extremely rare in blacks. The more common *localized* type is characterized by short-segment narrowing near the ligamentum arteriosum just distal to the left subclavian artery. The aortic isthmus may be narrowed proximal to the coarctation. Approximately 70% are associated with congenital cardiac anomalies, the most common being bicuspid aortic valve. Other associated congenital defects include patent ductus arteriosus, ventricular septal defect, and Berry aneurysms involving the circle of Willis. Coarctation is also often seen in patients with Turner's syndrome (8).

Plain films show the characteristic "3 sign" formed by an indentation in the contour of the descending aorta just below the knob in the frontal projection, which represents the area of the coarctation and poststenotic dilatation. Rib notching along the inferior aspect of ribs 3–9 is the result of dilatation and tortuosity of the intercostal arteries, which act as collateral pathways to the poststenotic descending aorta (Fig. 24.4A)(8). The first two to three intercostal arteries are not involved because of their origin proximal to the coarctation. Rib notching implies long-standing obstruction and may not be seen in young children. Coarctation occurring proximal to the left subclavian artery produces unilateral *right* rib notching. If an aberrant right subclavian artery arises distal to a coarctation, collateral flow would be provided via the left internal mammary or intercostal system, resulting in unilateral *left* rib notching (8, 9). Other findings are dilatation of the prestenotic aorta and brachiocephalic vessels, left ventricular hypertrophy, and linear retrosternal soft tissue densities resulting from dilated internal mammary arteries providing collateral flow.

The *diffuse* type is a long-segment hypoplastic narrowing distal to the origin of the innominate artery (Fig. 24.3B). This is typically identified in infancy or early childhood depending on severity of the stenosis and has a higher association with cardiac anomalies (bicuspid aortic valve in 85%)(8). The prognosis tends to be worse than the local type.

The abdominal aorta is involved in coarctation in 2% of cases. The *congenital* form is a developmental fusion anomaly of the paired primitive dorsal aorta, whereas the *acquired* form is the result of idiopathic inflammatory conditions, postradiation vasculitis, rubella syndrome, and neurofibromatosis. Imaging will demonstrate smooth diffuse or segmental narrowing, or diffuse hypoplasia of the abdominal aorta.

MR is currently the initial imaging modality of choice for aortic coarctation. Parasagittal imaging in the 30–40° left anterior oblique plane with cardiac gating will demonstrate both the ascending and descending aorta. This accurately defines the site and extent of the stenosis and collateral vessels. Cine MR enhances routine imaging and provides hemodynamic information. MR precludes the need for angiography in selected cases and provides an excellent method for postsurgical evaluation.

Two-dimensional echocardiography is also useful for diagnosis and follow-up of thoracic coarctations, especially in infants. In addition, it accurately evaluates the congenital cardiac defects associated with coarctation. Transabdominal US with color Doppler is useful in evaluating abdominal coarctation.

Angiography provides excellent visualization of the extent of aortic involvement and remains the most accurate in defining collateral vessel anatomy, which can be extremely valuable at the time of surgery. In addition, accurate pressure gradient measurements can be acquired.

Pseudocoarctation (aortic kink) of the thoracic aorta is a misnomer, as it is a mild form of coarctation. The infolding occurs near the ligamentum arteriosum, similar

Figure 24.4. Coarctation of the Aorta. A. Frontal chest radiograph shows inferior rib notching (*straight arrows*) and "3" sign (*curved arrow*). **B.** Aortic arch injection with "diffuse" type of coarctation (*curved arrow*), distal to the left subclavian artery.

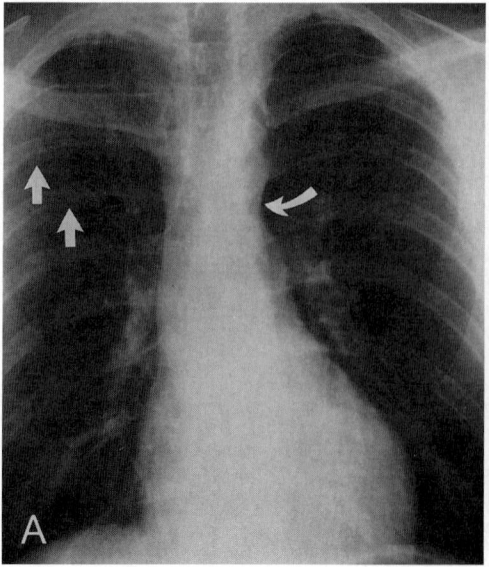
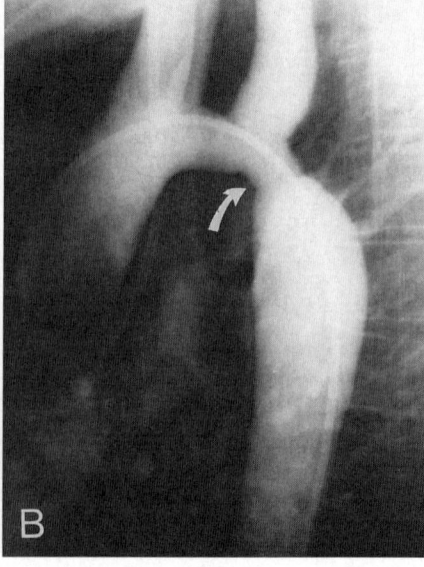

to the localized form of coarctation. Patients are asymptomatic because of the lack of a hemodynamically significant stenosis with <10 mm Hg pressure gradient across kink. The ascending aorta is elongated with a high, transverse arch and redundant descending portion distal to the kink. Plain film findings are similar to "true" coarctation, with the exception that rib notching and other evidence of collateral vessel formation is absent. In adults, as the aorta becomes more elongated and tortuous, the segment distal to the kink may resemble an enlarging left upper mediastinal mass. There is a similar incidence of associated bicuspid aortic valve.

Aortic Trauma

Aortic transection results from sudden deceleration injury in high-speed motor vehicle accidents or falls. The laceration may involve all three layers of the aortic wall (40% of cases) or only the intima; most often in the transverse orientation (5). The mechanism of injury is a combination of shearing and torsional forces at points of relative fixation along the course of the aorta. The most common site for injury is the aortic isthmus near the attachment of the ligamentum arteriosum (85% of cases), followed by the ascending aorta and aortic root with fixation at the valve plane (9%), and at the diaphragmatic hiatus (2%). This is a highly lethal injury, with a 90% mortality before reaching the hospital (10). Of those who survive but are not diagnosed and treated, 80% die within 1 hour, 85% die within the first 24 hours, and 98% die within 3 months. *Chronic pseudoaneurysms* are formed when a periaortic hematoma is contained by the adventitia or the mediastinal connective tissues. Clinical findings are nonspecific and include asymmetrical peripheral pulses, chest pain, and dyspnea. Relative hypertension in the upper extremities after aortic laceration is known as acute traumatic coarctation but is rarely seen.

Catheterization of the thoracic aorta should be performed extremely cautiously as the region of the isthmus is crossed. Any resistance to passing the J-wire or catheter is suspect for aortic laceration. Contrast should be injected gently by hand. The cusps of the aortic valve must be opacified to ensure a complete examination, and biplane conventional filming at a rapid rate should be used whenever possible. It is imperative that at least two views be obtained. DSA is not recommended. Conventional filming offers superior spatial resolution, large field of view, and decreased susceptibility to the motion artifact. Comprehensive examination encompasses the entire aorta including the proximal arch vessels and celiac axis.

Chest Radiograph. The supine films that are usually obtained in an acute trauma situation commonly show mediastinal widening suggestive of hemorrhage. An upright view with optimal inspiration should be obtained whenever possible. Several findings suggest aortic injury (Table 24.2) (10, 11). Any one of these alone has limited value in predicting vascular injury, although they do

Table 24.2. Chest Radiograph Findings with Blunt Chest Trauma and Aortic Injury

Indistinct aortic knob[a]
Abnormal aortic contour[a]
Nasogastric tube displaced to the right[a]
Trachea displaced to the right[a]
Left mainstem bronchus displaced inferiorly[a]
Left apical pleural cap
Fractures of first or second ribs
Mediastinum-to-chest width ratio > 0.25[b]
Mediastinum widened > 8 cm[b]
Pneumothorax
Pulmonary contusion

[a] Combination of these factors may have greatest sensitivity.
[b] Artifactual widening may resolve with upright positioning and optimal inspiration, although this may not be feasible in the setting of acute trauma.

suggest significant thoracic trauma (Fig. 24.5A). The most reliable signs of aortic injury are abnormal aortic contour, ill-defined aortic knob, tracheal and nasogastric tube deviation, and depression of the left mainstem bronchus. A near-normal chest film may be seen in the presence of serious aortic injury although the absence of the four criteria essentially excludes aortic injury (10, 11). The consequences of a missed diagnosis are so ominous that high clinical suspicion based on mechanism of injury alone or any plain film abnormality dictates the need for further imaging. Other causes of mediastinal widening in the patient suffering trauma include venous mediastinal bleeding and complications of central venous catheter placement.

CT Screening evaluation to exclude aortic injury now includes contrast-enhanced helical CT. Signs of aortic injury include mediastinal hemorrhage (surrounding or adjacent to the aorta), abrupt change in aortic or branch vessel contour, aortic pseudoaneurysm, intimal flap, pseudocoarctation (diminished caliber of the descending aorta), and contrast extravasation. If the mediastinum is normal or hemorrhage is limited to the anterior mediastinum or localized at the site of a spine fracture, aortic injury is unlikely (12). Currently, MR is not applicable in the acute setting of aortic trauma.

Aortography findings include subtle intimal tears (seen in 10%)(Fig. 24.5B,C), complete transection, traumatic aneurysms (common)(Fig. 24.5D), posttraumatic dissection (10%), and posttraumatic coarctation. Multiple injuries are present in up to 20% of patients. A *ductus diverticulum* (Fig. 24.2) is a normal variant bulging of the anteromedial aortic isthmus in the region of the ligamentum arteriosum seen in 10% of the population. It is differentiated from aortic injury by its smooth transition with the aorta, lack of intimal irregularity, and absence of delayed washout of contrast material.

Aneurysms

Aneurysms are localized dilatation of the vessel wall and are classified as *true aneurysms* (all three layers intact) or *false/pseudoaneurysms* (disruption of all three layers with containment provided by surrounding con-

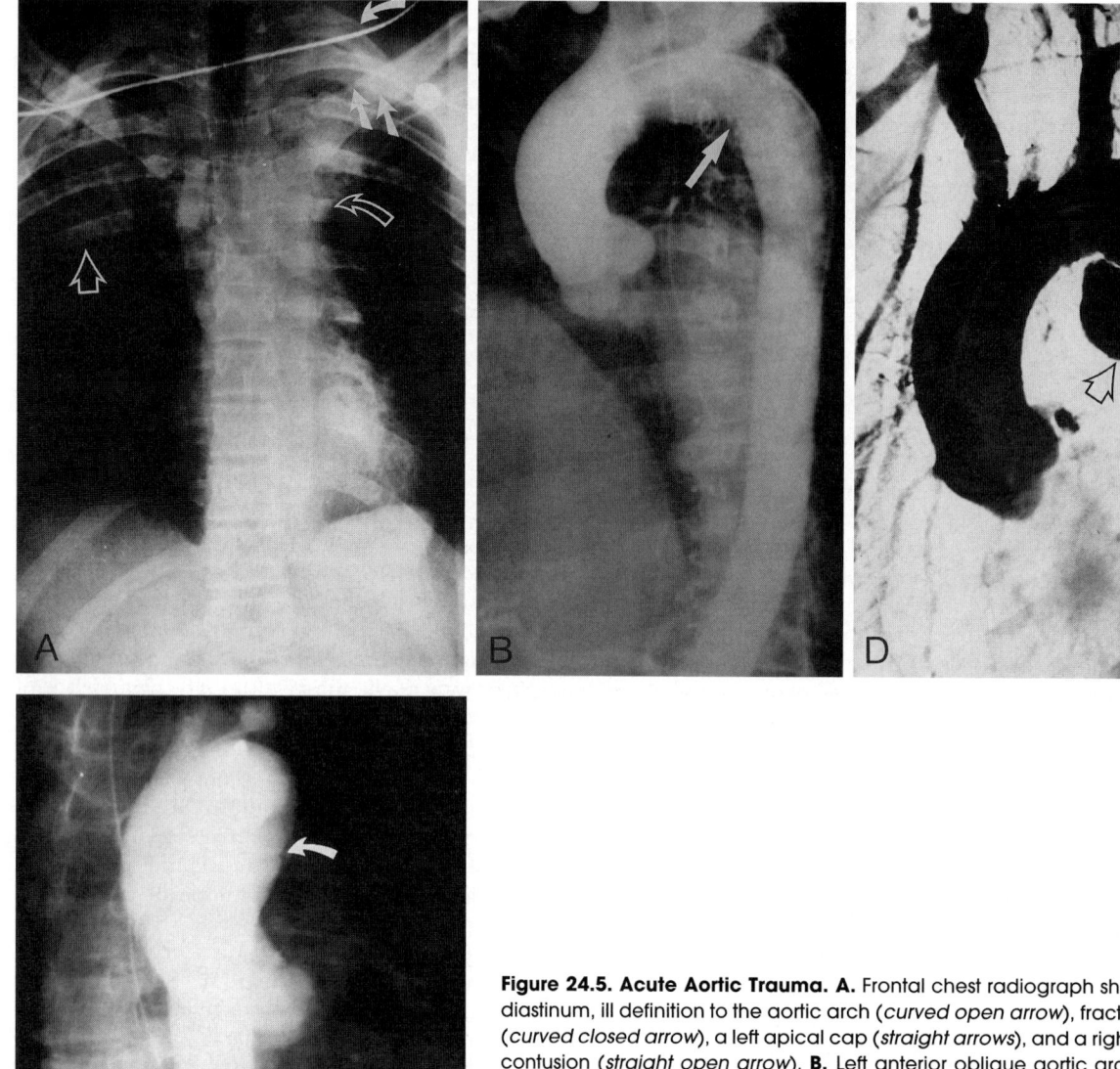

Figure 24.5. Acute Aortic Trauma. A. Frontal chest radiograph shows a widened mediastinum, ill definition to the aortic arch (*curved open arrow*), fracture of the left first rib (*curved closed arrow*), a left apical cap (*straight arrows*), and a right apical pulmonary contusion (*straight open arrow*). **B.** Left anterior oblique aortic arch injection demonstrates subtle irregularity of the intimal contour in the region of the ligamentum arteriosum attachment (*straight arrow*). **C.** Right anterior oblique projection of the aortogram in (**B**) confirms intimal injury manifested by a linear lucency (*curved arrow*). **D.** A contained rupture or pseudoaneurysm is seen at the level of aortic laceration (*open arrow*).

nective tissue). Most thoracic aneurysms are asymptomatic (4). Symptoms are usually the result of aneurysm size and mass effect: stridor and dysphagia because of tracheobronchial and esophageal compression, superior vena cava (SVC) syndrome because of venous compression, and hoarseness because of recurrent laryngeal nerve compression. Substernal chest pain occurs in approximately 25% of patients with aneurysms.

Chest radiographs demonstrate contour abnormality and tortuosity of the aorta and calcifications within the vessel wall (Fig. 24.6A). Differentiation from other mediastinal masses may require CT or MR.

Both CT and MR demonstrate vessel diameter, mural thrombus, calcifications, degree of luminal patency, and mass effect on adjacent mediastinal structures (4). CT is superior to MR in demonstrating calcifications within the wall. Both modalities are used to detect leaking or

ruptured aneurysms. CT shows increased soft-tissue density resulting from mediastinal hematoma and associated left pleural effusion. Direct extravasation is rarely seen. MR demonstrates signal intensities typical for acute or subacute blood products within the mediastinal soft tissues. MR has the advantage of better defining the relationship of the aneurysm with the arch vessels as a result of its ability to directly image in the sagittal plane.

Angiography is reserved for preoperative planning when it is vital to know the relationship of the aneurysm to the great vessels, coronary arteries, and the vascular supply to the spinal cord. Imaging of the abdominal aorta may also be needed and requires a greater volume of contrast (70–80 ml). Angiography is unreliable in accurately assessing aneurysm size in the presence of mural thrombus because only the patent portion of the lumen is visualized.

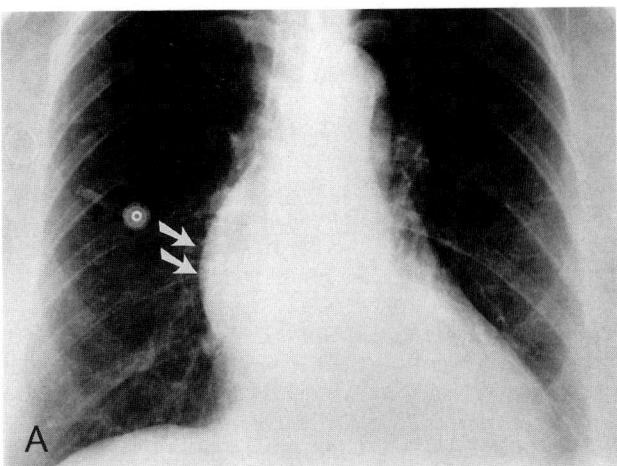

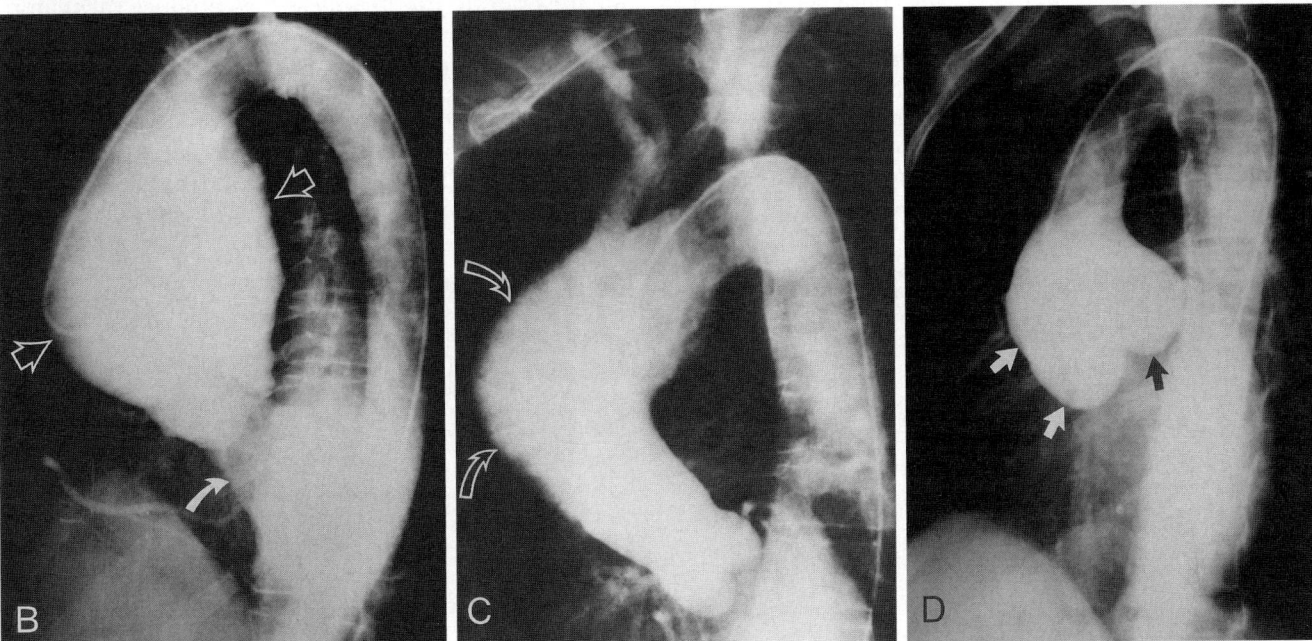

Figure 24.6. Ascending Aortic Aneurysms. A. Chest radiograph shows abnormal convexity to the right cardiac contour defined by a thin curvilinear calcification (*straight arrows*) representing aneurysmal dilation of the ascending aorta. **B.** Marked dilatation of the ascending aorta (*open arrows*) with associated aortic valvular regurgitation (*curved arrow*) is the result of syphilis. **C.** Atherosclerotic aneurysm (*arrows*) of the ascending aorta. **D.** "Tulip bulb" aortic root (*arrows*) is characteristic of Marfan's syndrome.

TYPES OF ANEURYSMS

Atherosclerotic aneurysms (Fig. 24.6C) are caused by impairment of the vasa vasorum blood supply to the aortic wall, with subsequent degeneration and loss of muscle fibers within the media. Most are fusiform with irregular walls resulting from mural thrombus and are most common in the distal arch and descending aorta (4). Calcifications of atherosclerotic disease are typically discontinuous, curvilinear, and plaquelike. The risk of aneurysm rupture is related to size. Those measuring <5cm in diameter rupture very rarely; those >10 cm rupture at a rate in excess of 40%. The 1-year survival for patients with aneurysms greater than 10 cm is 60%, with a 5-year survival rate of 19%. A rapidly expanding aneurysm of any size carries a poorer prognosis (4).

Syphilitic aneurysms are a late sequelae of the disease seen in 10–15% of untreated patients (4). They are attributable to an obliterative endarteritis of the vasa vasorum following obstruction of these vessels by the treponeme. This results in necrosis of the media, with weakening of the vessel wall and subsequent aneurysm formation. Scarring and contracture of the aortic wall produces wrinkling of the intima known as "tree-barking" (4). Involvement of the ascending aorta occurs in 36% of cases, transverse arch in 34%, descending arch in 25%, and descending aorta in 5% (4). Isolated abdominal aortic involvement is rare. Those involving the aortic root tend to be asymmetrical and saccular. Characteristic thin, "pencillike" calcifications within the media are present in 15% of cases. Syphilis also causes aortic valve insufficiency (Fig. 24.6B) because of either aneurysm or valvulitis. Death results from aneurysm rupture in 40% of cases.

Mycotic aneurysms are similar to those seen with syphilis but are the result of a bacterial infection in the vessel wall. The bacteria can gain access to the vessel wall by seeding via the vasa vasorum during generalized septicemia, secondary infection of a pre-existing atheromatous plaque, or direct invasion from an extravascular source. Predisposing factors include bacterial endocarditis, intravenous drug abuse, aortic surgery, and any immunocompromised state (4). Mycotic aneurysms occur most commonly in the ascending aorta and sinuses of Valsalva, are almost always saccular, and rarely contain calcifications. They account for 3% of all abdominal aortic aneurysms.

Marfan's syndrome is an autosomal dominant connective tissue disorder that has ocular, skeletal, and cardiovascular manifestations resulting from abnormal collagen production. Cystic medial necrosis in the aorta results in vascular elastic fiber fragmentation and weakening of vessel wall. Cardiovascular involvement (aorta, pulmonary artery, mitral valve, splanchnic vessels) is present in 60% of cases and responsible for 93% of the deaths. Aortic involvement alone is responsible for 55% of the deaths. Aortic manifestations include aneurysms (predominately ascending), dissection, dilatation of the aortic sinuses, and coarctation. The characteristic symmetrical dilatation of the sinuses of Valsalva is termed sinotubular dilatation or "tulip bulb aorta" (Fig. 24.6D). This finding differentiates Marfan's from atherosclerotic aneurysm; however, other processes such as aortitis can have a similar appearance. Aortic dilatation leads to aortic valvular insufficiency when the aortic root exceeds 6 cm.

Ehlers-Danlos syndrome is a group of heritable connective tissue disorders characterized by skin and joint hyperextensibility, soft-tissue calcifications, and vascular fragility. The ecchymotic or arterial type (type IV) is rare and typified by fragile thin skin, which, in contrast to the other forms, is not hyperextensible. Arterial manifestations include aortic aneurysms, aortic dissections, and pulmonary arterial ectasia. Because of the extreme vascular fragility that may be present, arteriography is *contraindicated* and other imaging modalities (CT, MR, possibly IVDSA) are used.

Congenital aneurysms are the result of discontinuity in the media pathologically similar to intracranial aneurysms. These comprise 2% of thoracic aortic aneurysms and predominately involve the sinuses of Valsalva (4). Congenital aneurysms usually are asymptomatic prior to rupture unless they produce valvular insufficiency or encroach on adjacent structures (left coronary artery or right ventricular outflow tract). The right sinus aneurysms typically rupture into the right ventricular outflow tract, and the noncoronary sinus aneurysms rupture into the right atrium. Both of these lesions result in left-to-right shunts. Other less common sites of rupture are the left atrium, left ventricle, or peri-

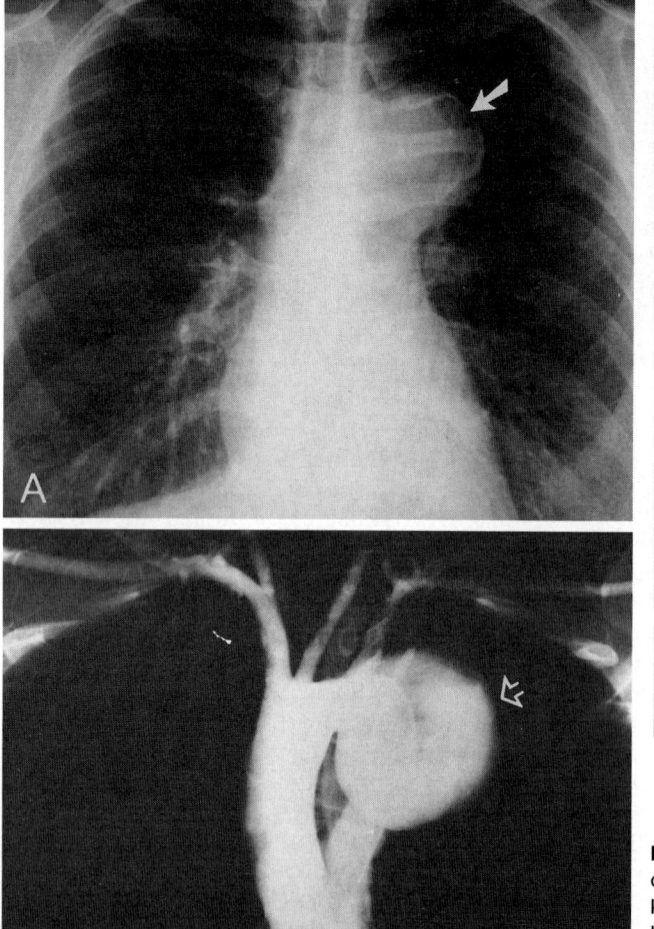

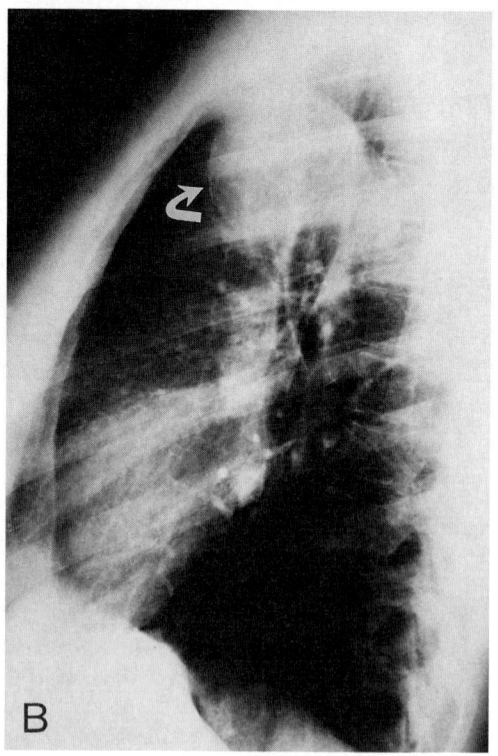

Figure 24.7. Chronic Pseudoaneurysm. A. A chest radiograph shows a double density aortic knob with abnormally convex contour (*arrow*). **B.** Lateral projection reveal thin curvilinear calcification of the enlarged aortic arch (*curved arrow*). Calcification is a sign of chronic pseudoaneurysm. **C.** Aortic arch angiogram defines the large pseudoaneurysm (*open arrow*).

cardial space. The chest radiograph findings are usually normal but may show enlargement of the aortic root or a contour abnormality along the right heart border. Calcification is rare and differentiates congenital sinus of Valsalva aneurysm from one attributable to bacterial endocarditis.

Posttraumatic/Postsurgical Pseudoaneurysms. With the increase in aortocoronary bypass, postoperative aneurysms are increasing in frequency. In addition, blunt chest trauma, particularly deceleration injuries, may result in aneurysms. These are properly termed pseudoaneurysms, as the aneurysm wall does not contain all three layers. Posttraumatic pseudoaneurysms occur most commonly in the region of the ligamentum arteriosum and appear on plain film as left upper mediastinal mass (Fig. 24.7). They frequently demonstrate wall calcification but uncommonly contain mural thrombus. Because of the tendency for rupture, these lesions are usually treated surgically. Postoperative thoracic aneurysms and dissections usually involve the ascending aorta, whereas postoperative abdominal aneurysms are usually located at the proximal or distal graft sites. CT and MR can be used to confirm the diagnosis. Angiography is usually required for preoperative evaluation.

Aortic Dissection

A dissection is defined as a separation of the layers of the vessel wall initiated either by a tear in the weakened intima or by rupture of a vasa vasorum with subintimal hemorrhage into a diseased aortic media. This may also be termed a *dissecting hematoma*. A natural cleavage plane exists between the middle and outer thirds of the media. The defect in the media can be congenital (Marfan's) or acquired. Predisposing factors include hypertension, bicuspid aortic valve, coarctation, pregnancy (accounting for 50% of dissections in women less than 40 years of age), scoliosis, pectus excavatum, trauma (rare), and prior aortic surgery. Dissections originating in the abdominal aorta are rare.

Death from aortic dissection is usually because of retrograde dissection into the pericardium causing cardiac tamponade, massive aortic regurgitation, or rupture into the pleural space. If signs of rupture are present, the mortality approaches 70%, and surgery is indicated regardless of type. Dissections involving the ascending aorta usually require surgery (13). Those involving only the descending aorta exhibit a mortality rate of 10% and may be managed medically.

Aortic dissection is more common between the ages of 30 and 85 years and is more common in men in a ratio of 3:1 (5). A history of hypertension is obtained in 60% of cases. Dissection is often (75%) signaled by sudden, severe, tearing substernal chest pain with radiation to the back. Neurologic symptoms resulting from involvement of the cranial or spinal vessels are present in 25% of cases and aortic valvular murmurs are present in 65%. Asymmetrical pulses in the upper extremities are often found if the arch is involved, and the femoral pulses are absent in 25% of cases.

Two classification systems in broad use describe the regions of the aorta involved and have bearing on prognosis and management (Fig. 24.8) (13).

DeBakey:

Type I (30%) involves the ascending aorta, arch, and variable portion of the descending aorta. Treatment is surgical.

Type II (20%) is limited to the ascending aorta and carries the worst prognosis. Treatment is surgical.

Type III (50%) originates near the isthmus distal to the left subclavian artery origin. This lesion carries the best prognosis. Treatment is medical or surgical.

Stanford:

Type A (60%) involves the ascending aorta, with variable involvement of the arch and descending aorta. Treatment is surgical.

Type B (40%) is limited to the arch and descending aorta, similar to DeBakey type III. Treatment is medical or surgical.

Technical Considerations. The femoral approach is used if the femoral pulse is normal or near normal. If not, the axillary approach is used. Lead with a floppy tip straight or J-guidewire to avoid extending the dissection. *Do not force* the catheter or guidewire at any time. When in doubt, stop and perform a gentle hand injection. The false channel is recognized by inability to advance the guidewire within the aorta. When advancing the guidewire, it may pass imperceptibly between true and false lumen. The false channel may be entered initially if the dissection extends to the groin. Position within the false lumen is confirmed with test contrast injection. If attempts to manipulate wire into the true lumen are unsuccessful, then judicious contrast injection may be performed to identify the re-entry point. The pigtail catheter is positioned above the aortic valve, and biplane imaging performed. Imaging of the abdominal aorta may be necessary to determine the distal extent of the dissection.

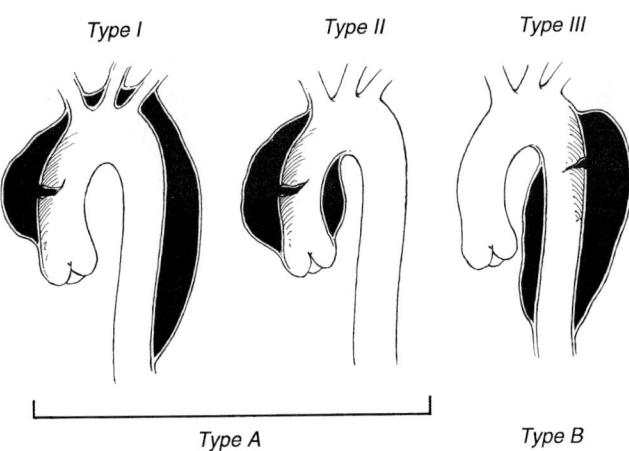

Figure 24.8. Classification Schemes of Aortic Dissection. DeBakey types I, II, and III and Stanford types A and B.

Delayed imaging is necessary to allow opacification of the false channel.

Chest Radiograph. Mediastinal widening is the most common finding (80%), followed by a double aortic contour or "double aortic knob sign" (40%) (5,13). Other findings include diffuse enlargement of the aorta with ill definition or irregularity of the contour, inward displacement of intimal calcification >10 mm, tracheal displacement to the right, pleural effusion (more common on the left and suggestive of leakage), pericardial effusion, and cardiac enlargement. All findings are nonspecific but

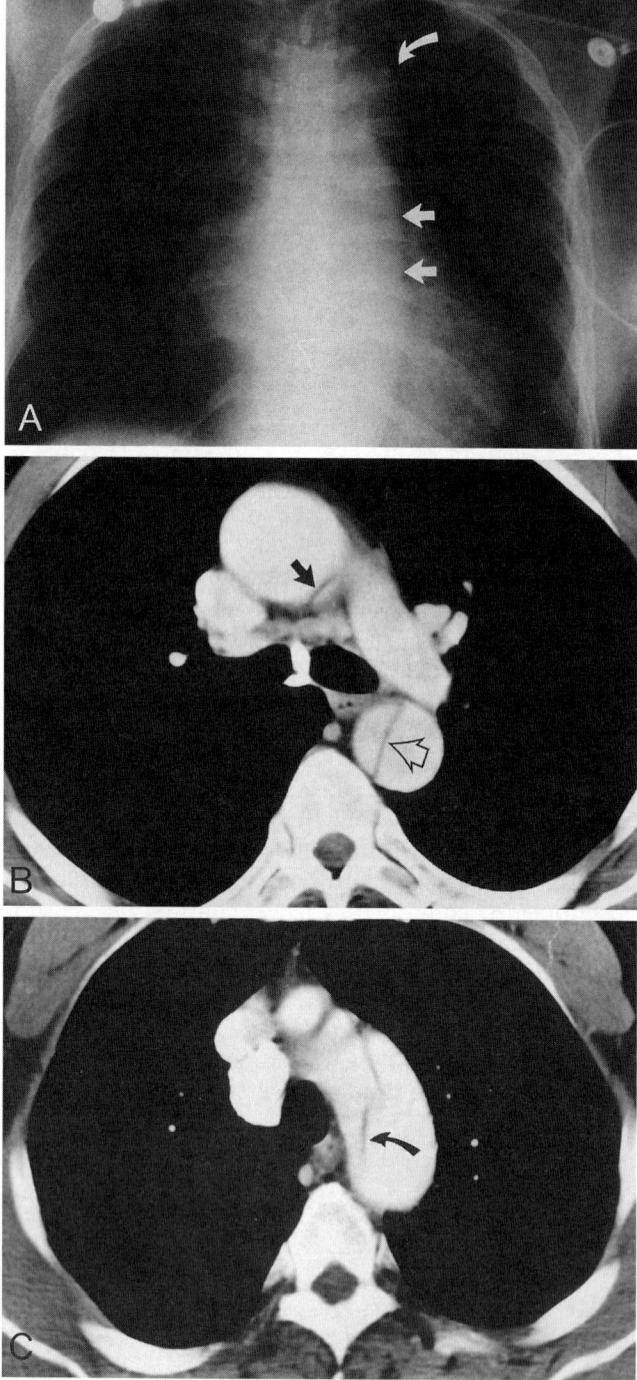

Figure 24.9. Type I (Stanford A) Aortic Dissection. A. Chest film shows widened superior mediastinal contour with "double aortic knob sign" (*curved white arrow*). Irregularity of the descending aortic contour is also seen (*straight arrows*). **B.** Contrast enhanced CT at the level of the left pulmonary artery shows the intimal flap within the ascending (*closed arrow*) and descending aorta (*open arrow*). The larger false lumen compresses the true lumen. **C.** An image cephalad to **B** defines the two channels within the aortic arch, separated by the intimal flap (*curved arrow*).

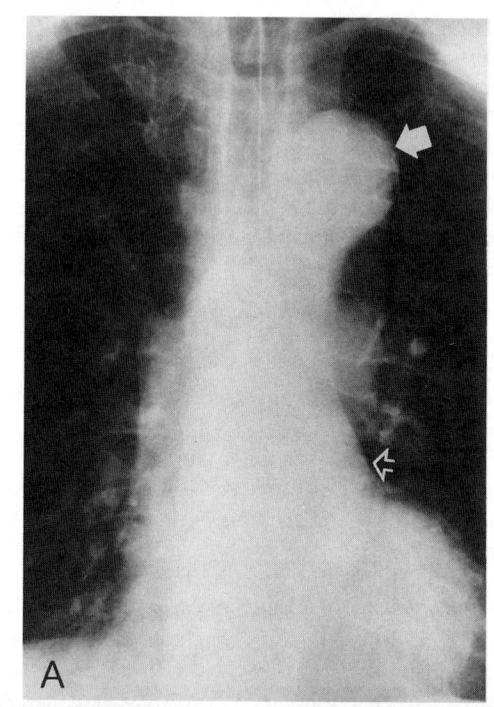

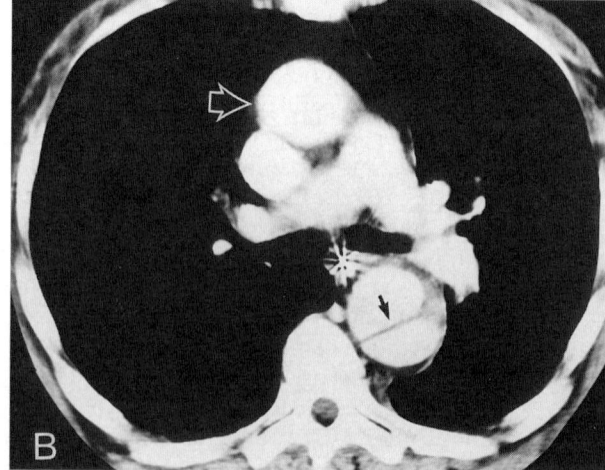

Figure 24.10. Type III (Stanford B) Aortic Dissection. A. Chest radiograph shows a prominent aortic knob (*open arrow*) that, with appropriate clinical history, is suspicious for aortic dissection. **B.** A CT at the level of the main pulmonary artery shows a well-defined intimal flap in the descending aorta (*arrow*) with a normal ascending aorta (*open arrow*).

serve to prompt further workup in the appropriate clinical setting (Figs. 24.9A, 24.10A).

CT evaluates dissection with accuracy exceeding 90%. Bolus contrast-enhanced helical scanning is used. Delayed scanning aids in the identification of the false channel. Noncontrast scanning is not recommended.

The intimal flap is seen as a linear filling defect within the aortic lumen, and a "double barrel" appearance to aorta is produced by opacification of both the true and false lumen (Figs. 24.9B,C and 24.10B). The false lumen may exhibit delayed opacification; may compress the true lumen, so the false lumen appears larger; and may contain thrombus (25%). Other findings include an increase in aortic diameter (>5 cm), hemopericardium, and hemothorax.

MR is extremely accurate with sensitivities and specificities exceeding 90% (13). The high accuracy of MR and CT may obviate the need for angiography in some cases. Both are primary imaging modalities in the postoperative patient and in the evaluation of chronic dissection (10%

of cases). Routine spin-echo imaging will demonstrate findings similar to those obtained on CT. The intimal flap will be outlined by "dark blood" (Fig. 24.11A), whereas GRE MR will delineate the flap surrounded by "bright blood" (13). The appearance will vary with the presence of thrombus or exceptionally slow flow within the false channel (Fig. 24.11B).

Aortography is the procedure of choice in the evaluation of acute dissection. Its importance in preoperative planning is to demonstrate the extent of the dissection, site of intimal tears, aortic valve regurgitation, coronary artery involvement, and filling of branch vessels (Fig. 24.11C,D) (13). The classic finding (87%) is a "double barrel" aorta with an interposed intimal flap. The intimal flap usually begins in the right anterolateral ascending aorta and spirals to the left posterolateral aspect of the descending aorta into the abdomen. The left renal artery is frequently supplied by the false lumen, and the left iliac artery is more commonly involved when the dissection extends distally. Flow within the false lumen is slow,

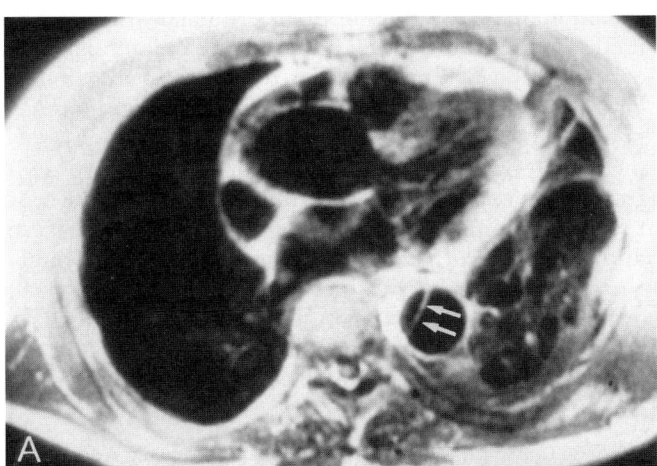

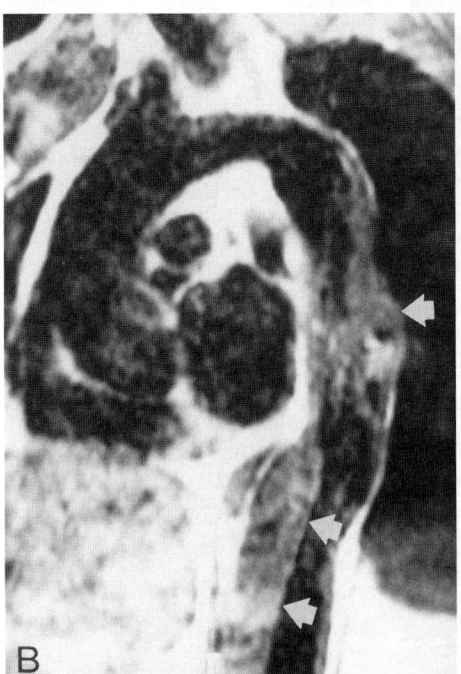

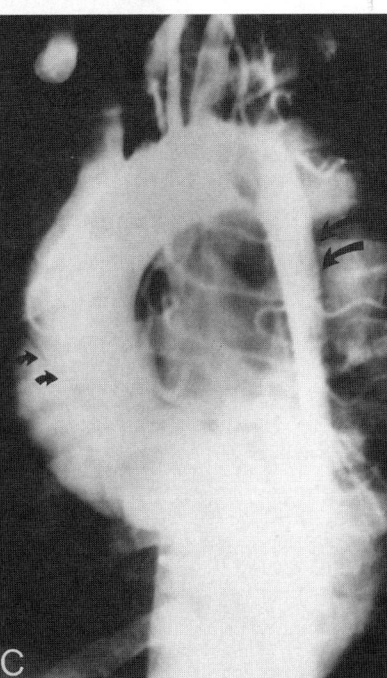

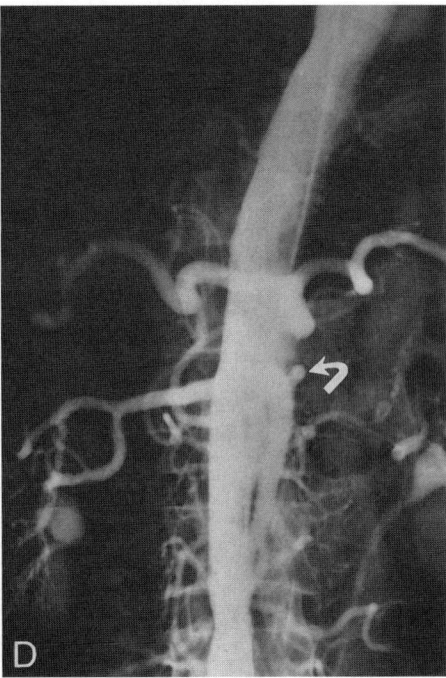

Figure 24.11. Aortic Dissection. A. Axial MR shows an intimal flap (*small arrows*) within the descending (type III/Stanford B dissection). The flap is outlined by dark flow void. **B.** An oblique sagittal MR in the same patient depicts a spiraling false lumen defined by intermediate signal owing to slow flowing blood. **C.** Aortic arch injection in another patient with a type I/Stanford A dissection shows the intimal flap beginning within the ascending aorta (*small curved arrows*) and extending into the descending aorta. The true lumen is flattened (*large curved arrows*). **D.** The left renal artery (*curved white arrow*) shows no filling on this phase of the angiogram. Blood is now supplied by the false lumen.

leading to late filling of branch vessels having their origin from this lumen. Thrombus in the false channel (25% of patients) appears as thickening of the aortic wall up to 1 cm. The true lumen is compressed and narrowed by the false channel in 85% of cases deviating the course of the catheter.

Aortitis

Aortitis is inflammation of the aortic wall that results from inflammatory arthropathies (rheumatoid, ankylosing spondylitis, scleroderma, SLE, Reiter's disease, and Behçet's disease), infection (suppurative, syphilis, and TB), radiation, rheumatic fever, and unknown causes (idiopathic aortitis).

Takayasu's disease ("pulseless disease") is an idiopathic, systemic, granulomatous vasculitis that principally affects the aorta and its major branches and less commonly affects the pulmonary arteries (50% of cases). Takayasu's is most common in young women (F:M = 9:1). The acute stage is manifested by fever, myalgia, arthralgia, and malaise and is commonly misdiagnosed. The fibrotic stage is recognized by pulse deficits, claudication, bruits, renovascular hypertension, and other symptoms of vascular insufficiency (14).

Chest radiographs show calcification in the aortic wall, a hallmark finding in young women. Arteriography shows long- or short-segment, smooth narrowing of the proximal branches of the aorta, with similar narrowing of the thoracic and abdominal aorta (Fig. 24.12). Classification is based on distribution of disease (15). *Type 1* demonstrates stenoses involving the aortic arch and arch branch vessels. *Type 2* involves the descending thoracic aorta, abdominal aorta and middle-sized abdominal aortic branch arteries. *Type 3* combines involvement of the aortic arch and abdominal aorta. *Type 4* combines involvement of the pulmonary artery and aorta. Associated aneurysms are seen in 10–15% of cases.

SYSTEMIC ARTERIES AND ABDOMINAL AORTA

Anatomy

Neck. The *right common carotid* artery arises from the bifurcation of the innominate artery. The *left common carotid* usually arises directly from the aortic arch, although it has a common origin with the innominate in approximately 20% of individuals. The common carotid arteries bifurcate into the *internal* and *external* carotid arteries (Fig. 24.13). The ICA courses posterolateral to the ECA initially, then crosses to ascend slightly medial to the ECA. The *vertebral* arteries are the first branches of the subclavian arteries, with the left the same size or larger than the right in 75% of cases. They ascend within the transverse foramen of C2–C6.

Upper Extremity. The right subclavian arises from the innominate artery, and the left subclavian arises directly from the aortic arch. Both extend to lateral aspect of the first rib and give rise to the following major branches in order: *vertebral; internal mammary* (arises opposite the vertebral artery and descends to anastomose with the intercostal arteries and the superior epigastric artery); *thyrocervical trunk* (gives rise to inferior thyroid, superficial cervical, and suprascapular artery); and *costocervical trunk* (branches into superior intercostal supplying intercostal arteries 1–3, deep cervical, and possibly a small branch to the spinal). The axillary artery continues from the lateral aspect of the first rib giving rise to the *anterior* and *posterior humeral circum-*

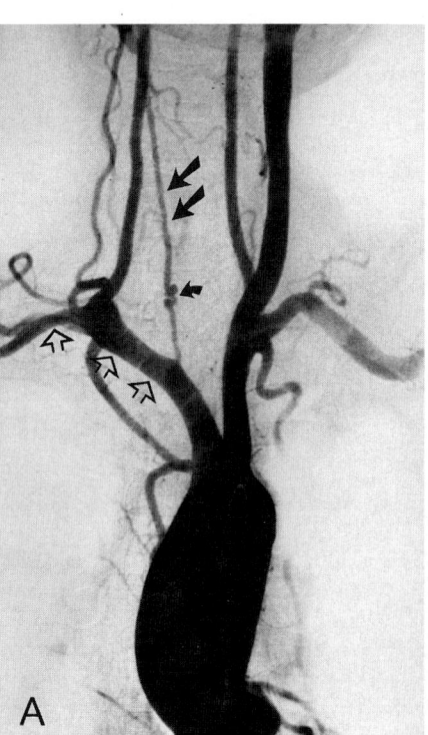

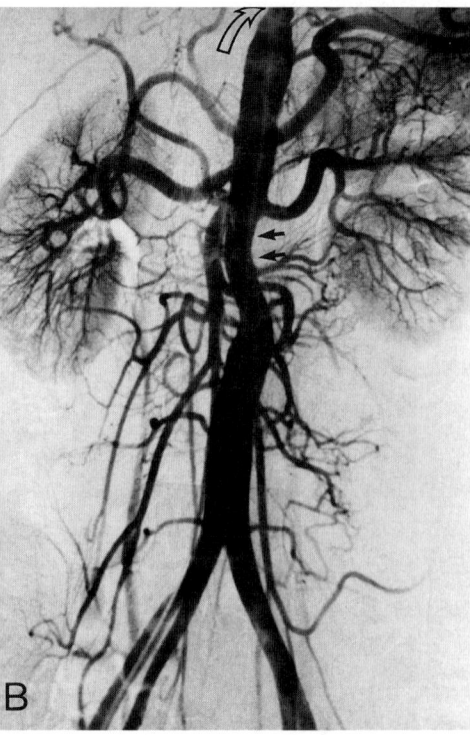

A

B

Figure 24.12. Takayasu's Arteritis. A. Aortic arch injection shows diffuse narrowing of the brachiocephalic and right subclavian arteries (*open arrows*) and right common carotid artery (*closed straight arrows*). An aneurysm (*curved arrow*) of the right common carotid artery is also evident. **B.** Abdominal aortogram shows areas of focal smooth narrowing in the proximal abdominal aorta (*curved arrow*) and just distal to the superior mesenteric artery origin (*straight arrows*).

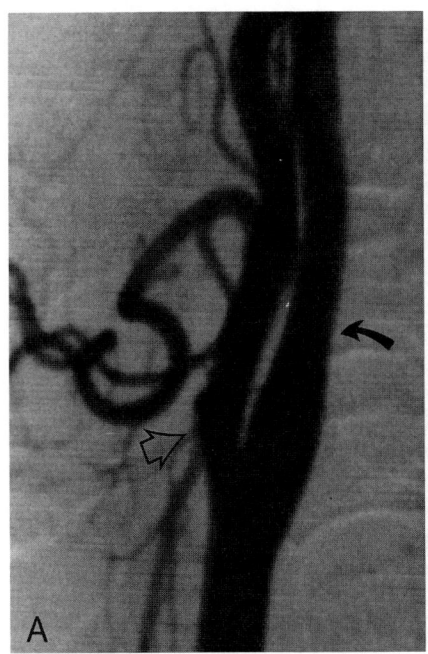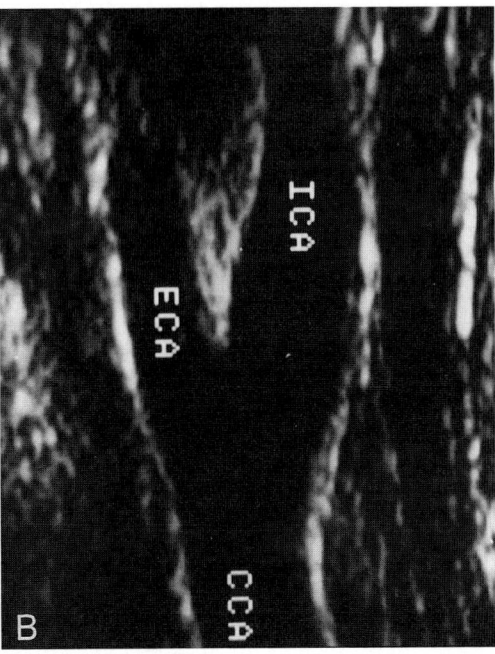

A   B

Figure 24.13. Normal Carotid Artery.
A. Common carotid artery injection with normal internal carotid (*curved arrow*) and external carotid (*straight open arrow*) arteries. **B.** Longitudinal US view from the posterolateral neck shows similar anatomy to that of the arteriogram. *ICA*, internal carotid artery; *ECA*, external carotid artery; *CCA*, common carotid artery.

flex arteries. The brachial artery courses along the medial aspect of the arm with the median and ulnar nerves and branches into the *radial* and *ulnar arteries* near the elbow joint. Just distal to its origin, the ulnar artery gives rise to the *common interosseus* artery, which terminates in the distal forearm. If it continues into the hand, it is termed a *persistent median* artery, which is seen in approximately 4%. The radial and ulnar artery form the *deep* and *superficial palmar arches* in the hand. The deep arch (complete in 95%) is formed predominantly by the radial, and the chief contributor to the superficial arch (complete in 80%) is the ulnar artery (16).

Abdominal Aorta. The abdominal aorta begins at the diaphragmatic hiatus and extends to its bifurcation into the right and left common iliac arteries at L4 (Fig. 24.14). It measures less than 2.5 cm in diameter and tapers gradually to 1.5–2 cm at the bifurcation. Main branches are the celiac axis (at the level of T12), superior mesenteric artery (T12–L1), inferior mesenteric artery (L3), all of which arise from the ventral aorta, and the paired renal arteries (L2), which arise laterally. A single artery to each kidney is present in two thirds of the population, and multiple renal arteries occur in the remainder. Other branch vessels are the paired phrenic, adrenal, and gonadal arteries and four pairs of lumbar arteries. All arise from the lateral or posterolateral aorta.

Lower Extremity. The *common iliac* artery originates at the aortic bifurcation and extends to the pelvic brim, where it bifurcates into the *external* and *internal iliac* arteries (Fig. 24.15). The internal iliac (hypogastric) artery divides into an anterior trunk (*superior and inferior vesicle, middle hemorrhoidal, internal pudendal, obturator, inferior gluteal, and uterine/prostatic* arteries) and a posterior trunk (*iliolumbar, lateral sacral, and superior gluteal* arteries). The external iliac courses to the inguinal ligament, giving off the *deep circumflex iliac* and

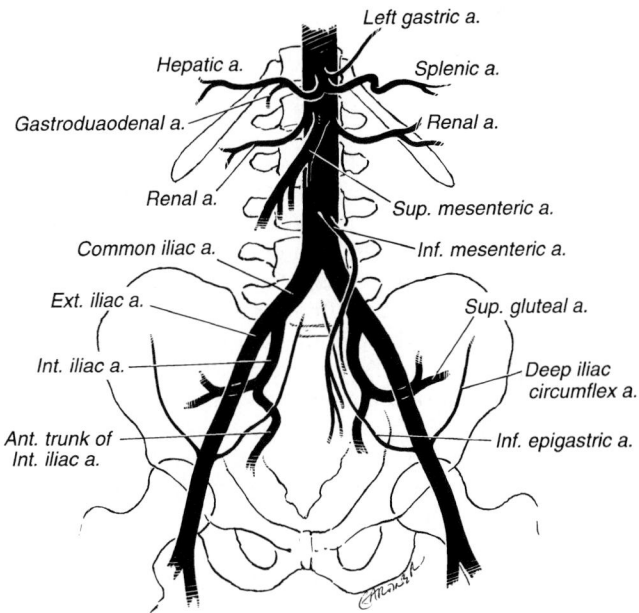

Figure 24.14. Normal Abdominal Aorta and Major Arterial Branch Anatomy.

the *inferior epigastric* arteries at that level. These branches are the angiographic markers for the division between the external iliac and *common femoral* artery. The common femoral artery bifurcates into the *profunda femoris* and *superficial femoral* (SFA) arteries near the inferior margin of the femoral head (Fig. 24.15). The SFA courses in the anteromedial thigh to the adductor canal becoming the *popliteal* artery, giving off several small muscular branches along the way. The popliteal artery travels in the popliteal fossa between the medial and lateral heads of the gastrocnemius muscle and terminates below the knee as the "trifurcation" vessels. In most cases, this is not a true trifurcation but an initial bifur-

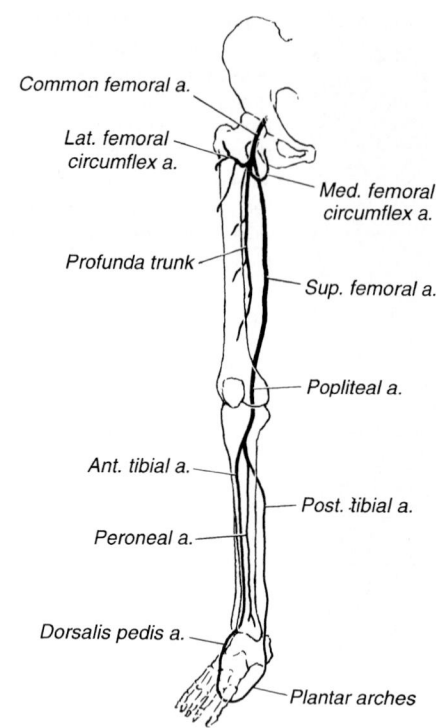

Common femoral a.

Lat. femoral
circumflex a.

Med. femoral
circumflex a.

Profunda trunk

Sup. femoral a.

Popliteal a.

Ant. tibial a.

Post. tibial a.

Peroneal a.

Dorsalis pedis a.

Plantar arches

Figure 24.15. Normal Lower Extremity Arterial Anatomy.

cation into *anterior tibial* artery and a short *tibioperoneal trunk* that divides into the *peroneal* and *posterior tibial* (AT) artery. The AT passes over the interosseous membrane below the knee to descend in the anterior compartment of the lower leg and continue into the foot as the *dorsalis pedis* (PT) artery. The peroneal terminates above the ankle, and the PT continues behind the medial malleolus and into the plantar aspect of the foot, giving off the *medial* and *lateral plantar* arteries. The *persistent sciatic* artery is a rare congenital variant seen as an enlarged inferior branch of the internal iliac artery that exits the pelvis posteriorly and joins the distal SFA near the adductor canal. The proximal SFA may be absent or hypoplastic.

Angiographic Technique

The upper extremities and neck vessels are usually examined from the femoral approach using selective catheters placed into each individual vessel. Selective catheterization of the right common carotid or vertebral arteries is occasionally not feasible because of tortuosity or origin disease. The catheter may then be placed in the proximal subclavian or innominate artery, and a blood pressure cuff placed on the ipsilateral arm. The cuff is inflated to systemic arterial pressure just before the injection in order to divert the majority of the flow into the vessel of interest.

Imaging of the abdominal aorta is performed using a pigtail catheter placed at the T11–T12 interspace and using either DSA or biplane CA (see Table 24.1). The lateral view is best for demonstrating the origins of the celiac axis and superior and inferior mesenteric vessels. The renal artery origins are optimally visualized with

oblique imaging, usually right posterior oblique projection, with the pigtail catheter placed at the L1–L2 interspace. Selective injection of the renal artery is required for evaluation of intrarenal branch disease.

The lower extremities are typically examined simultaneously with a pigtail catheter placed just proximal to the aortic bifurcation, and step-table or full-length film changer is used. Accurate timing of step-table movements and exposure speed can be gauged using a small contrast injection (5–10 ml) with either fluoroscopic visualization or 1 frame per second digital imaging over the knee. The time interval from onset of injection to arrival of the bolus at the knee is used to compute the optimum imaging rate. Selective evaluation of either lower extremity can be performed by passing a catheter over the bifurcation to the contralateral leg or by selectively catheterizing the ipsilateral common femoral artery.

Flow Enhancement. Several pharmacologic agents and manual maneuvers are used to enhance sluggish flow in the distal extremities to evaluate vessel patency optimally. Tolazoline (*Priscoline*) is a powerful vasodilator with direct, local effect lasting approximately 15 minutes when injected intra-arterially. The dose is 25–50 mg diluted in 5–10 ml normal saline and injected slowly through the catheter for 90 seconds. Adverse effects include hypertension, tachycardia, myocardial infarction, and arrhythmias. Several runs in different projections may be performed per administration. *Nitroglycerin* is a vascular smooth muscle relaxant with direct, local effects when injected via the catheter. The dose is 100–200 μg administered as a bolus. Caution must be exercised to prevent inducing hypotension. *Papaverine* is another direct acting, smooth muscle relaxant administered intra-arterially. It is useful in cases of spasm. The dose is 30 mg diluted in 10 ml normal saline and administered slowly for 60–90 seconds. Papaverine should not be mixed with alkalinized (lactated Ringer's) or heparin-containing solutions because of drug precipitation. *Reactive hyperemia* is induced by application of a blood pressure cuff to the proximal extremity and inflated to above systolic arterial pressure for 5–7 minutes. After release of the cuff, reactive vasodilatation enhances flow to the distal extremity. Similar results can be obtained through the application of warm, moist towels to the foot or hand. Both methods are effective but are inconvenient, time consuming, and uncomfortable for the patient.

Trauma

Abdominal Aortic Injury

Blunt abdominal aortic injury is most commonly associated with acute deceleration injuries in motor vehicle accidents. Clinical symptoms are often obscured by other intra-abdominal or musculoskeletal injuries. The loss of groin pulses, or more peripheral embolic symptoms, are suspicious for injury to the abdominal aorta. Aortic branch vessels are injured more commonly than the aorta itself.

Angiographic findings include intimal irregularity or flap, laceration with false aneurysm or retroperitoneal hematoma, posttraumatic dissection, and thrombosis. Penetrating trauma has the potential complication of arteriovenous fistula if adjacent arterial and venous structures are injured.

Peripheral Vascular Injury

Penetrating trauma from gunshot and stab wounds is the cause of 90% of peripheral vascular injury. Blunt

Table 24.3. Manifestations of Peripheral Vascular Trauma

Intimal tear
Spasm
Extrinsic compression
Contrast extravasation
Occlusion
Pseudoaneurysm
Arteriovenous fistula

trauma with long-bone fractures and dislocations are additional causes. Dislocations cause stretch injuries that result in spasm, intimal flap, or complete vessel disruption. Physical examination may be normal or reveal a cold, pulseless, ischemic extremity or pulsatile bleeding. Only 40% of patients with arterial injury show any pulse abnormality on physical examination.

The angiographic findings of peripheral vascular trauma are listed in Table 24.3 (Fig. 24.16). Diffuse or focal vessel narrowing may be caused by hypotensive vasospasm and should not be mistaken for vascular injury. If arterial narrowing is seen in the absence of contrast extravasation, the injection may be repeated following the intra-arterial administration of one of the vasodilating agents described. This will serve to (a) eliminate nontraumatic vasospasm unrelated to vessel injury, (b) reveal an underlying intimal tear or mural hematoma, or (c) exclude the possibility of extrinsic compression from hematoma if the spasm clears. In addition, this will improve opacification of more distal vessels and facilitate detection of distal injury. Vessel occlusion may be at-

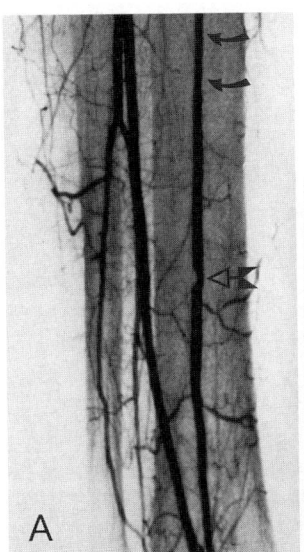

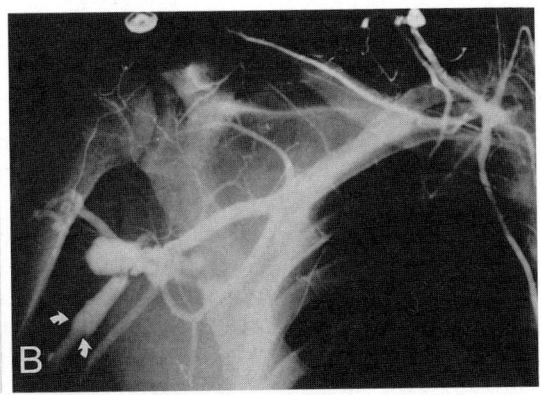

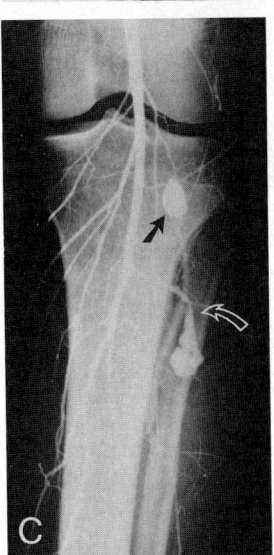

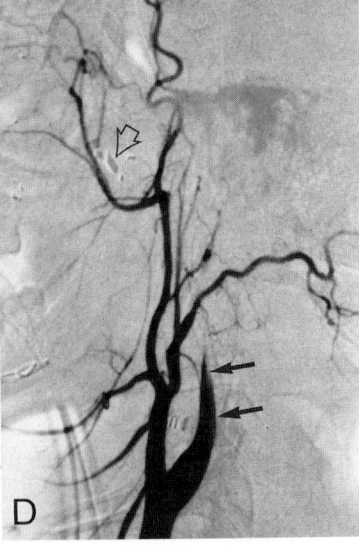

Figure 24.16. Manifestations of Peripheral Arterial Trauma. A. Stab wound to the lower leg caused an eccentric defect (*open arrow*) indicative of intimal injury in posterior tibial artery. Note proximal area of spasm (*curved arrows*). **B.** A gun shot wound to the right shoulder caused a pseudoaneurysm of the axillary artery (*straight black arrow*) and an arteriovenous fistula with opacification of the vein (*curved arrows*) in early arterial phase. **C.** A gun shot wound fractured the proximal fibula and caused a pseudoaneurysm (*curved arrow*). The *black arrow* points out the bullet. **D.** The smoothly bordered tapering of the internal carotid artery (*straight arrows*) is typical of traumatic dissection caused by a gun shot wound. Retained bullet fragments are evident (*open arrow*).

tributable to intimal flap, "recoil" spasm following complete transection of the vessel, extrinsic compression by bone or hematoma, or thromboembolization from a more proximal vascular injury. In cases of arterial extravasation in areas difficult to access surgically such as the pelvis and segmental renal arteries, transcatheter embolization may be used (17).

DSA is the imaging modality of choice in extremity trauma because of superior contrast resolution, decreased contrast load, and real-time image projection. General anesthesia or intravenous sedation may be necessary when a trauma patient is unable to cooperate fully during image acquisition to avoid motion artifacts that may obscure vessel injury. If a question of intimal injury exists on DSA examination, CA with its superior spatial resolution may be used. Tachycardia and rapid blood flow in trauma victims necessitate larger contrast volume and faster injection and filming rates.

Aneurysms

Abdominal Aortic Aneurysms (AAA) are defined as dilatation of the abdominal aorta greater than 3 cm. They occur in 2–6% of the population, most commonly in white men (M:F = 8 : 1) older than age 60. Most AAA are asymptomatic and are detected incidentally on physical examination or imaging studies of the abdomen (18). Potential symptoms are abdominal pain, abdominal mass, and distal embolization. Most AAA are atherosclerotic in origin.

TYPES OF ANEURYSMS

Atherosclerosis. Most (90%) AAA involve the infrarenal aorta (19). Vasa vasorum in the infrarenal aorta are insufficient to provide adequate metabolic support. This creates a dependency on diffusion to sustain the vessel wall. Lipids and collagen deposited in the media

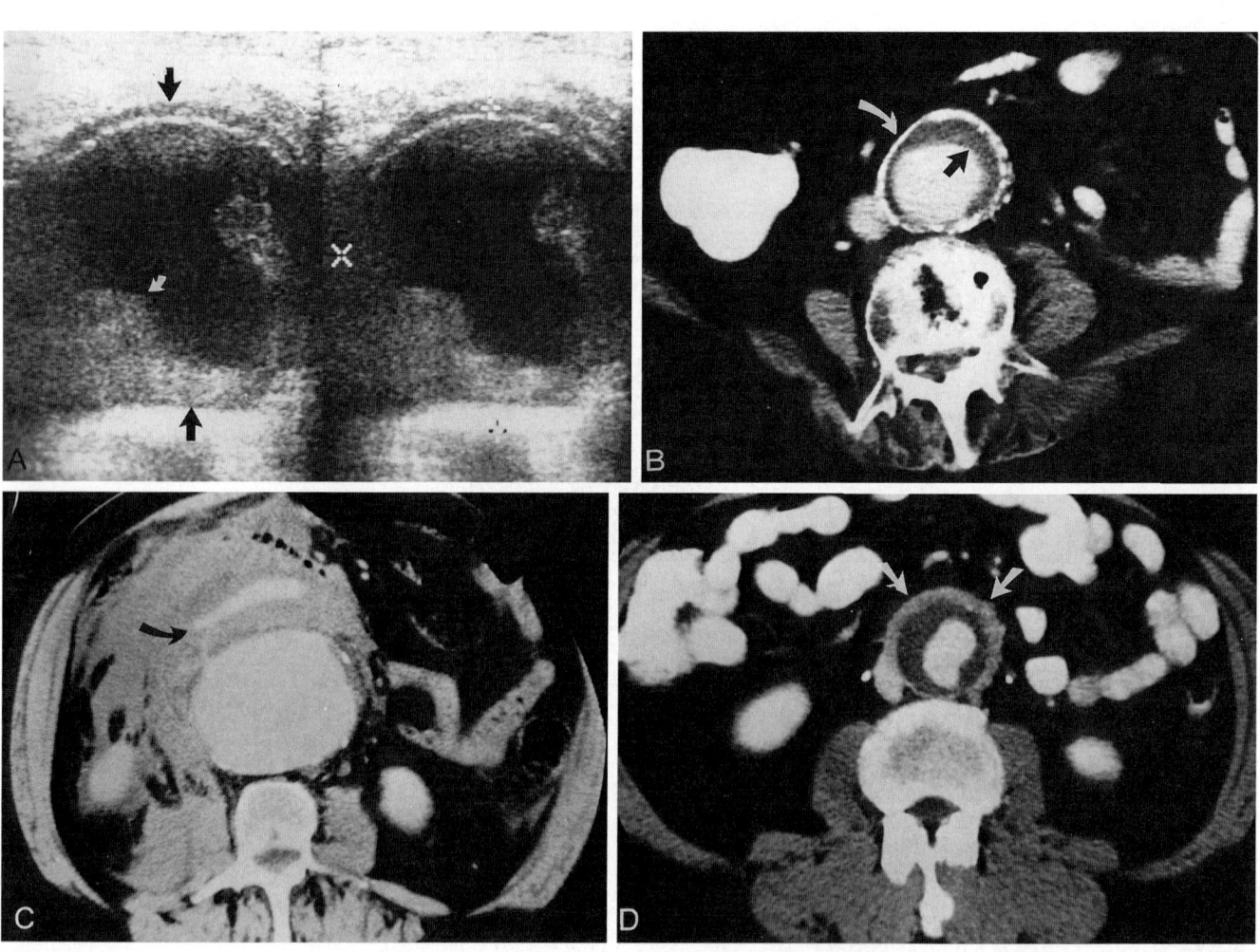

Figure 24.17. Abdominal Aortic Aneurysm. A. Transverse US images show an aneurysm with irregular intraluminal thrombus (*curved arrow*). Measurement of the anteroposterior diameter is illustrated (*black arrows*). **B.** Contrast-enhanced CT shows extensive mural calcification (*curved arrow*) and intraluminal thrombus (*straight arrow*). **C.** A ruptured aneurysm manifests as a crescentic collection of contrast (*curved arrow*) in the midst of extensive blood in the retroperitoneum and mesentery. **D.** Enhanced CT image shows an aortic aneurysm with surrounding enhancing irregular soft tissue (*arrows*) indicative of an inflammatory aneurysm.

interfere with the diffusion process and cause vessel wall ischemia, weakening, and progressive dilatation. As the vessel diameter increases, flow within the aneurysm becomes slower and more turbulent, leading to deposition of mural thrombus (Fig. 24.17A,B), which may occlude branch vessels, notably the inferior mesenteric artery and lumbar arteries (19).

Most AAA are *fusiform* (concentric dilatation) (Fig. 24.18) as opposed to *saccular* (asymmetric dilatation). Aneurysms enlarge at a rate of 2–4 mm/year. Extension into the common iliac arteries occurs in 69% of cases (19). Isolated iliac artery aneurysms are rare. Complications of AAA include rupture (Fig. 24.17C), peripheral embolization (blue toe syndrome), thrombosis, and infection. The incidence of aneurysm rupture increases with size as follows: <4 cm = 10%, 4–7 cm = 25%, 7–10 cm = 45%, and >10 cm = 60% (20). Rupture usually occurs into the left retroperitoneal space with rare instances of rupture into the adjacent gastrointestinal tract (*aortoenteric fistula*) and inferior vena cava (*aortovenous fistula*). Most aortoenteric fistulas are related to prosthetic aortic grafts and most (80%) involve the duodenum (18).

Chronic contained rupture is a break in the aneurysm wall with leak restrained by the retroperitoneal soft tissues. CT demonstrates a hematoma adjacent to the aneurysm. Continued flow into the contained hematoma is diagnostic of pseudoaneurysm.

Inflammatory aneurysms are a small subset of AAA (10%) characterized by perianeurysmal fibrosis of unclear etiology. Fibrosis is seen on CT as a thick, contrast-enhancing rind surrounding the aneurysm. It may obstruct the ureters (25%), left renal vein, inferior vena cava, duodenum, small bowel, or sigmoid colon (Fig. 24.17D). US demonstrates a hypoechoic ring surrounding the aneurysm. Evidence suggests this represents an autoimmune phenomenon that may respond to corticosteroids (18).

Infected (mycotic) aneurysms are rare and result from primary infection of the aortic wall, secondary infection of a pre-existing AAA, or contiguous spread from an adjacent abscess. The clinical presentation consists of sudden appearance of a pulsatile abdominal mass with fever. CT demonstrates a noncalcified, saccular aneurysm with periaortic fluid, gas, or vertebral osteomyelitis. *Staphylococcus* is the most common organism, followed by Gram-negative bacteria and *Salmonella*. Indium-labeled white cell radionuclide imaging is useful in differentiating this from other types of AAA (18).

IMAGING OF AAA

US is the imaging modality of choice in the initial evaluation, screening, and follow-up of AAA, with accuracy rates exceeding 98% (19). Asymptomatic AAA measuring less than 4–5 cm in diameter are followed with serial US until size or symptoms dictate the need for surgery. US detects intraluminal thrombus (Fig. 24.17A), accurately sizes the aneurysm, and detects extension into the iliac arteries. US is limited by obesity and overlying bowel gas, and detection of renal artery involvement is difficult.

Plain films demonstrate mural calcification with aneurysmal dilatation in 50-86% of AAA (Fig. 24.18).

CT surpasses US in defining the relationship of the aneurysm to the renal arteries and to surrounding structures (Fig. 24.17B). CTA with three-dimensional reconstruction is a useful adjunct for treatment planning. CT is the imaging modality of choice for the evaluation of suspected rupture (Fig. 24.17C), leaking aneurysm, and perianeurysmal fibrosis (Fig. 24.17D) (18). MR matches CT in accuracy and is particularly useful when there is a contraindication to iodinated contrast (19).

Angiography is used in the preoperative evaluation of AAA for defining the number of renal arteries and their

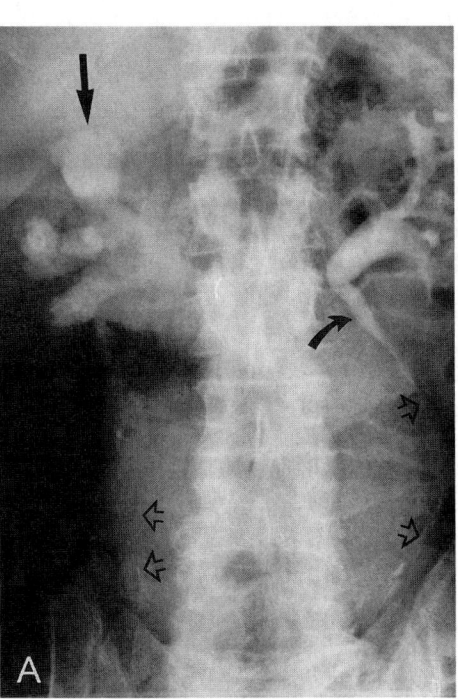
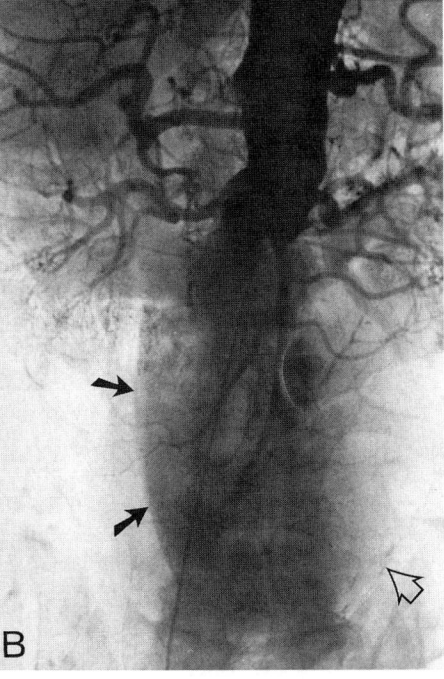

Figure 24.18. Abdominal Aortic Aneurysm. A. An intravenous pyelogram enhances the plain film findings of an aneurysm. The ureters are laterally displaced (*curved arrow*) and the right kidney is partially obstructed (*long arrow*). Mural calcification (*open arrows*) is well seen. **B.** Aortogram shows faint enhancement of this large aneurysm. The smooth borders (*straight arrows*) are common with thrombus lining the vessel lumen. Mural calcification is displaced from the contrast-enhanced lumen (*open arrow*). Note the lack of filling of lumbar arteries.

relationship to the aneurysm, and the patency of renal, mesenteric, external iliac, and common femoral arteries. The findings modify the surgical approach. Angiography demonstrates a smooth, featureless aortic lumen, which may not be widened depending on the amount of mural thrombus present (19).

Extremity Aneurysms. Lower extremity aneurysms are most commonly atherosclerotic. Upper extremity aneurysms are more commonly the result of trauma.

Popliteal aneurysms constitute two thirds of all extremity aneurysms, are commonly bilateral (60%), and are associated with aneurysms at other sites in 75% of cases (Fig. 24.19). *Femoral* aneurysms are bilateral in 60%, associated with AAA in 85% of cases and with popliteal aneurysms in 45%. Presenting symptoms include limb ischemia owing to aneurysm thrombosis, distal embolization, and gangrene.

US is used for initial evaluation except for the subclavian aneurysms, for which CT or MR are better suited. Angiography is usually required for the preoperative evaluation to determine the status of the peripheral vessels for bypass grafting.

Arteriomegaly (diffuse vascular ectasia, arteria magna, ectatic atherosclerosis) is an unusual manifestation of aneurysmal disease, with diffuse, generalized dilatation of the aortoiliac and femoral vessels (Fig. 24.19). It is associated with multiple aneurysms and characteristically

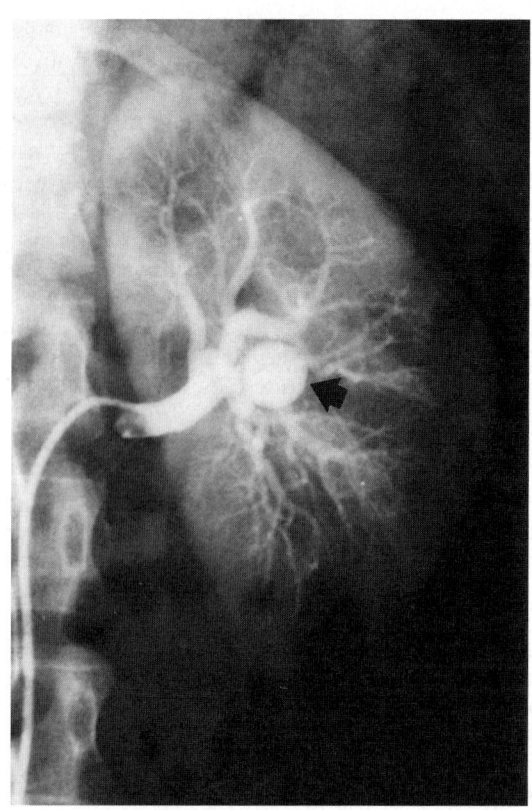

Figure 24.20. Renal Artery Aneurysm. This large aneurysm (*arrow*) of a segmental renal artery can be complicated by hypertension, hemorrhage, thrombosis, or arteriovenous fistula formation.

produces severe tortuosity in the iliac arteries. Because of the capacious vascular system, increased amounts of contrast and prolonged imaging times are required.

Renal artery aneurysms are uncommon and usually detected incidentally. Two-thirds are located at the main renal artery bifurcation with the remainder in the segmental branches (Fig. 24.20). They are bilateral in 20%. Etiologies include atherosclerosis, congenital, fibromuscular dysplasia, polyarteritis nodosa, mycotic, and posttraumatic pseudoaneurysms. Calcification in the wall of the aneurysm may be seen on plain film but is best demonstrated on unenhanced CT and is associated with a low incidence of rupture. Noncalcified aneurysms have a 25% incidence of rupture.

Splenic artery aneurysms account for 60% of visceral artery aneurysms. Most are solitary (70%) and located in the distal third of the artery (80%). Patients are usually asymptomatic. They are most common in women (4 : 1) and have an increased rupture rate in pregnancy. Aneurysm rupture has a mortality of 25% but occurs in only 2% of cases not associated with pregnancy. Aneurysms that are symptomatic, enlarging, associated with pregnancy or in women of child-bearing age, or are >2.0 cm in diameter usually require treatment. The two-thirds of aneurysms that contain calcification have a lower risk of rupture (20).

Other visceral artery aneurysms involve the hepatic artery (20%), SMA (5%), celiac artery (4%), gastric, pancreaticoduodenal and other branch arteries (10%), IMA

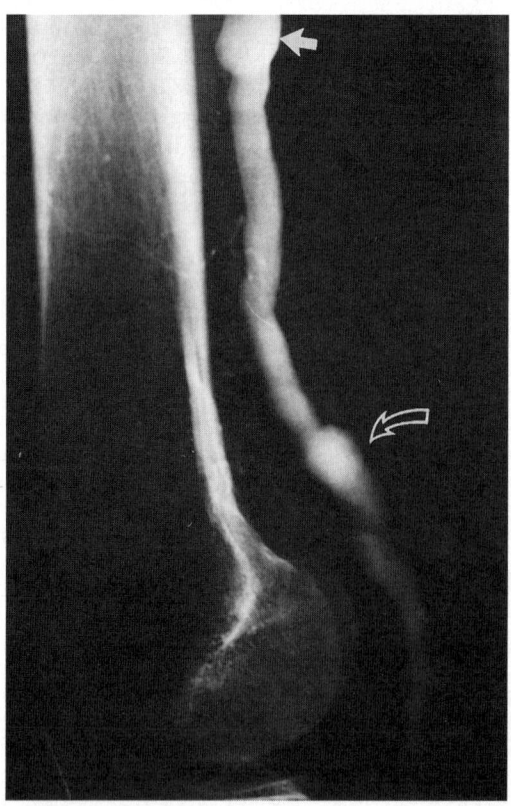

Figure 24.19. Popliteal Artery Aneurysm. Lateral view of a lower extremity arteriogram shows a distal SFA aneurysm (*straight arrow*), a proximal popliteal artery aneurysm (*curved arrow*), and arteriomegaly.

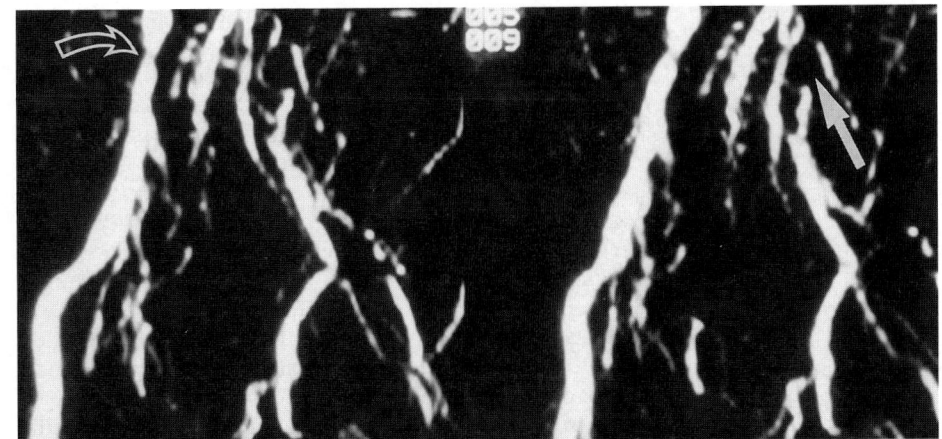

Figure 24.21. Iliac Arterial Occlusive Disease. Peripheral arterial two-dimensional MRA shows stenosis of the right common iliac artery (*curved arrow*) and complete occlusion of the left common iliac artery (*straight arrow*).

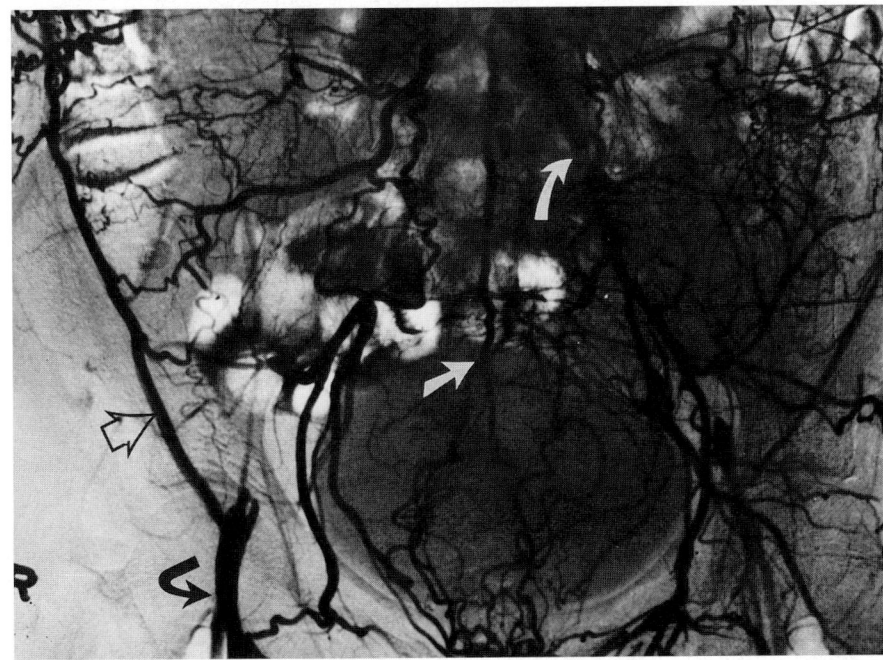

Figure 24.22. Collateral Pathways. Aortic injection demonstrates multiple collateral vessels in the presence of severe iliac occlusive disease. The left common iliac artery is occluded (*curved white arrow*). The right common iliac artery is not defined. The right femoral artery (*curved black arrow*) is reconstituted by collateral flow from the deep iliac circumflex artery (*open arrow*). Enlarged collateral vessels are seen throughout the pelvis. The median sacral artery (*straight arrow*) is visualized.

(rare). Most require treatment because of the high propensity to rupture (21).

Arterial Occlusive Disease

Imaging in arterial occlusive disease relies predominantly on contrast angiography. US is used for screening and follow-up, with the examination directed to specific areas of interest. MR angiography (MRA) is steadily improving as a screening modality (Fig. 24.21). It has shown greatest promise in the cervical carotid system (Fig. 24.15C) (22).

Collateral Pathways. With severe arterial stenosis or occlusion, collateral channels develop to bypass the obstruction and provide flow to the ischemic area. Small, pre-existing arterial communications enlarge in response to increased load requirements (Fig. 24.22). The more chronic the occlusion and the more severe the stenosis, the larger and more numerous are these ac-

cessory vessels. Knowledge of the anatomy of collateral pathways is important in planning catheter placement for optimal opacification of the vessels below the obstruction. For example, unilateral occlusion of the common and internal iliac artery may result in the ipsilateral intercostal or internal mammary arteries supplying the majority of flow to the leg. Placing the catheter at the aortic bifurcation would not opacify that extremity. The catheter should be placed at a level that would fill the collateral vessels.

The major collateral pathways for occlusive disease of the lower extremity are outlined in Tables 24.4 and 24.5. Other important collateral pathways in the lower extremity are *a*) the profunda femorus artery providing collateral flow around SFA or popliteal obstruction and *b*) the peroneal artery supplying collateral flow for disease in the anterior or posterior tibial artery.

Collateral supply for the renal artery may come from periureteral and peripelvic collaterals supplied by lumbar, subcostal, adrenal, and internal iliac arteries that

Table 24.4. Collateral Pathways for Aortic or Bilateral Common Iliac Occlusion

Internal mammary →Superior epigastric →Inferior epigastric →External iliac

SMA to IMA →Superior to middle hemorrhoidal →Internal iliac →External iliac

Intercostals and lumbars →Superior gluteal & ileolumbar →Internal iliac →External iliac

Intercostals & lumbars →Deep circumflex iliac →External iliac

Arrows indicate direction of flow.
Adapted from Kadir S: Diagnostic angiography. Philadelphia: WB Saunders, 1986.

Table 24.5. Collateral Pathways for Unilateral Common Iliac Occlusion

Intercostals & lumbars →Iliolumbar →Internal iliac →External iliac

Contralateral internal iliac →Lateral sacrals →Ipsilateral internal iliac →External iliac

Abdominal aorta →Testicular →Internal iliac →External iliac

Contralateral femoral →External pudendal →Ipsilateral external pudendal →Femoral

Intercostals and lumbars →Superficial circumflex iliac →Lateral femoral circumflex →Femoral

Reconstituted internal iliac →Superior/inferior gluteal/obturator →Medial femoral circumflex →Femoral

Arrows indicate direction of flow.
Adapted from Kadir S: Diagnostic angiography. Philadelphia: Saunders, 1986.

anastomose with the distal renal artery and branches. These collaterals produce multiple extraluminal impressions on the contrast-filled ureter.

Subclavian Steal Syndrome. If the obstruction of the subclavian artery is proximal to the origin of the vertebral artery, reversal of flow in the ipsilateral vertebral artery may occur to provide blood to the affected arm. Flow is diverted from the intracranial circulation to the subclavian artery, causing vertigo, syncope, paresthesias, and dysarthria in addition to upper extremity claudication. Subclavian steal syndrome most commonly affects men (M:F = 3:1) and the left side. Causes are atherosclerosis, vasculitis, tumor compression, and congenital vascular anomaly. Angiography demonstrates delayed, retrograde flow in the ipsilateral vertebral artery with late opacification of the subclavian artery. Reversal of flow in the vertebral artery on duplex US carotid examination suggests the diagnosis.

Atherosclerosis is the most frequent cause of chronic occlusive disease of the systemic arterial system. Intimal plaques, resulting from smooth muscle proliferation and extracellular lipid and collagen deposition, project into the vessel lumen, creating stenoses. Complex plaques result from calcification, ulceration, and intraplaque hemorrhage and thrombosis. Stenoses tend to occur at vessel bifurcations, at acute bends, and where vessels are deformed by overlying ligaments and joints. The lesions appear angiographically as irregular areas of concentric or eccentric luminal narrowing. Poststenotic dilatation may occur distal to severe stenosis. Stenosis may progress to complete vessel occlusion, with throm-

bosis forming above the lesion and propagating proximally to the next patent branch.

Clinical manifestations include claudication (intermittent pain or cramping owing to exercise-induced muscle ischemia), rest pain, coolness, and numbness, nonhealing ulcers, and gangrene. The severity of the symptoms is closely related to the measurement of the ankle to arm systolic blood pressure ratio (ankle-brachial index). The level of claudication correlates with the level of occlusive disease. Thigh and butt claudication indicates aortoiliac disease, and isolated calf claudication indicates SFA or popliteal involvement. Examination of the pulses indicates the level of disease and assists in choosing the best approach for angiography.

The disease is more common in men older than 50 years of age, postmenopausal women, and diabetics. Diabetics typically have more severe distal calf vessel disease with an earlier age of onset. *Leriche's syndrome* is aortic or bilateral common iliac occlusion manifest by bilateral lower extremity claudication and impotence.

Atherosclerotic disease can occur anywhere in the arterial system, but it is most common in the lower extremities and cervical carotid arteries. In the lower extremities, the superficial femoral artery, aortoiliac vessels, trifurcation vessels, and popliteal arteries are most commonly involved. Most carotid lesions involve the carotid bifurcation and proximal internal carotid

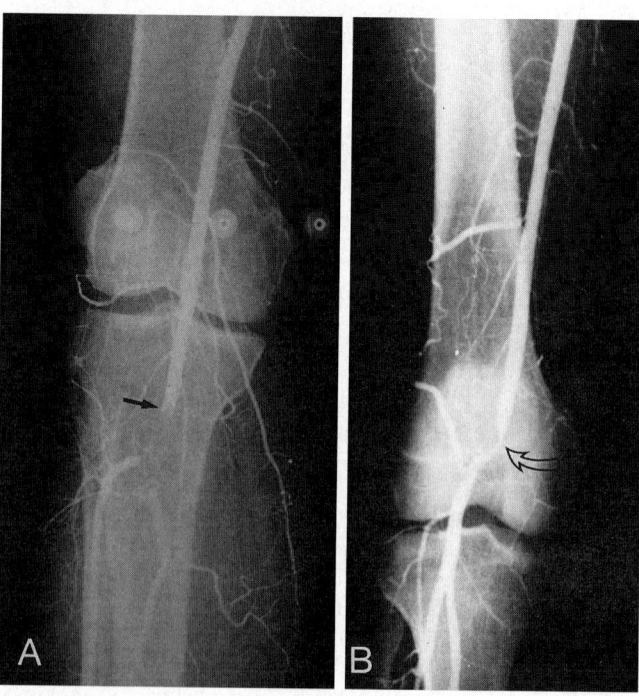

Figure 24.23. Popliteal Artery Occlusive Disease. A. Flow within the popliteal artery abruptly terminates of flow is noted. A filling defect with subtle convex superior margin (*straight arrow*) is typical for embolic occlusion. **B.** Smooth bordered narrowing (*arrow*) is typical of popliteal artery entrapment syndrome.

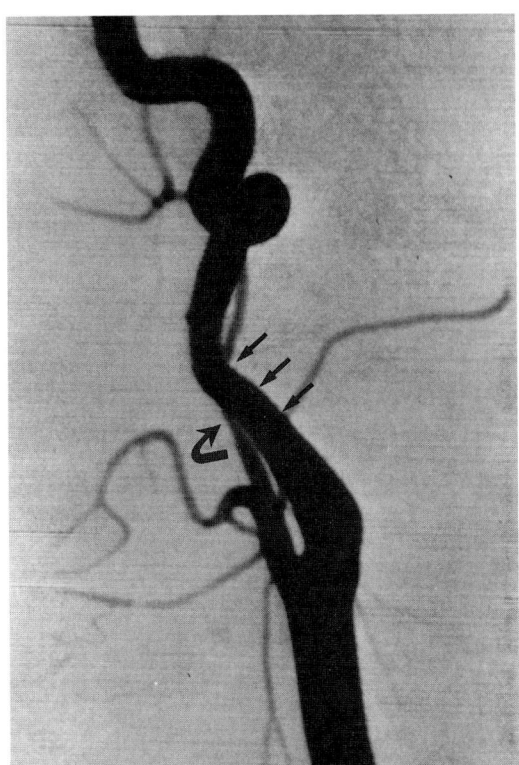

Figure 24.24. Radiation Vasculitis. Carotid arteriogram in a 30-year-old patient who underwent radiation for rhabdomyosarcoma at age 5 shows the chronic sequelae of radiation with smooth tapering of the internal carotid artery (*straight arrows*) and external carotid artery (*curved arrow*). A normal bifurcation helps differentiate this from atherosclerotic disease.

artery. Upper extremity involvement is less common and is usually confined to the subclavian artery.

Thromboembolism is a common cause of extremity arterial occlusion. Emboli originate from the heart or from aneurysms and impact at branch points and at preexisting stenoses. The characteristic angiographic appearance is abrupt vessel occlusion with a superior convex meniscus (Fig. 24.23A).

Radiation-induced injury produces three patterns of pathologic change: a) intimal damage with resultant mural thrombosis usually occurring within 5 years postradiation, b) fibrotic occlusion occurring within 10 years postradiation, and c) accelerated atherosclerotic changes with periarterial fibrosis with latent onset of 20 years or more (23). Angiography shows smooth, long-segment stenoses occurring in areas atypical for atherosclerotic disease and confined within a radiation port (Fig. 24.24). Duplex US may demonstrate the periarterial fibrosis associated with stenosis.

Fibromuscular dysplasia most commonly involves the renal artery (Fig. 24.25A) and uncommonly the middle or distal internal carotid artery (3%) or the iliac artery (<1%)(Fig. 24.25 B,C)(23, 24). Carotid lesions are associated with intracranial aneurysms (25%) and with FMD involving the renal artery.

Adventitial cystic disease refers to mucin-containing cysts that develop within the subadventitial layer of the vessel wall. Progressive accumulation of mucin within the cyst compresses the lumen, causing smooth eccentric or concentric stenoses. The artery is usually normal both proximal and distal to the lesion. This condition is more frequent in men and should be considered as a cause of claudication in young patients. Most cases involve the popliteal artery. CT and MR document the cystic component of the lesion. Treatment consists of surgical excision and bypass grafting (25).

VASCULITIC SYNDROMES

Buerger's disease (thromboangiitis obliterans) is an inflammatory vasculitis typically affecting men less than 40 years of age who almost invariably have a history of smoking. It is an obliterative process of intimal hyperplasia and thrombosis usually limited to the small and medium-sized arteries and veins, most commonly in the lower extremity. Rest pain involving the feet and hands may progress to ulceration and gangrene. The angiographic findings are bilateral distal extremity occlusions, luminal irregularities, skip lesions, and abrupt segmental narrowings. Characteristic "corkscrew" collaterals with normal-appearing major artery and occluded distal arteries are virtually diagnostic (Fig. 24.26) (14).

Temporal arteritis (giant cell arteritis) is an uncommon granulomatous vasculitis typically affecting white women older than 50 years old. The clinical presentation is a prodromal flulike illness with eventual jaw claudication, visual symptoms, myalgias, and tenderness of the superficial temporal artery. The sedimentation rate is markedly elevated. The diagnosis is confirmed on biopsy of the temporal artery. The most commonly affected arteries are the distal subclavian or axillary arteries, femoral arteries, distal forearm, and distal external carotid branches. Common carotid, proximal subclavian, and innominate artery involvement has not been seen (14). Involvement is usually bilateral and symmetrical. The lesions are typically long, smooth segments of stenosis with tapering at both end and abundant collaterals.

Takayasu's arteritis is also a giant cell arteritis, with lesions similar to those of temporal arteritis, but their distribution is distinguishing. Takayasu's typically involves the proximal brachiocephalic and carotid arteries and rarely extends beyond the carotid bifurcation (see Fig. 24.12). Aortic involvement seen in Takayasu's is not seen in temporal arteritis (14).

Collagen Vascular Diseases

Rheumatoid arthritis, systemic lupus erythematosus, and scleroderma affect the small and medium-sized arteries of the distal upper extremities. Involvement is typically bilateral and symmetrical, with progressive, concentric vessel narrowing leading to occlusion with poorly developed collaterals. The vasospastic disorder, *Raynaud's phenomenon*, is frequently associated.

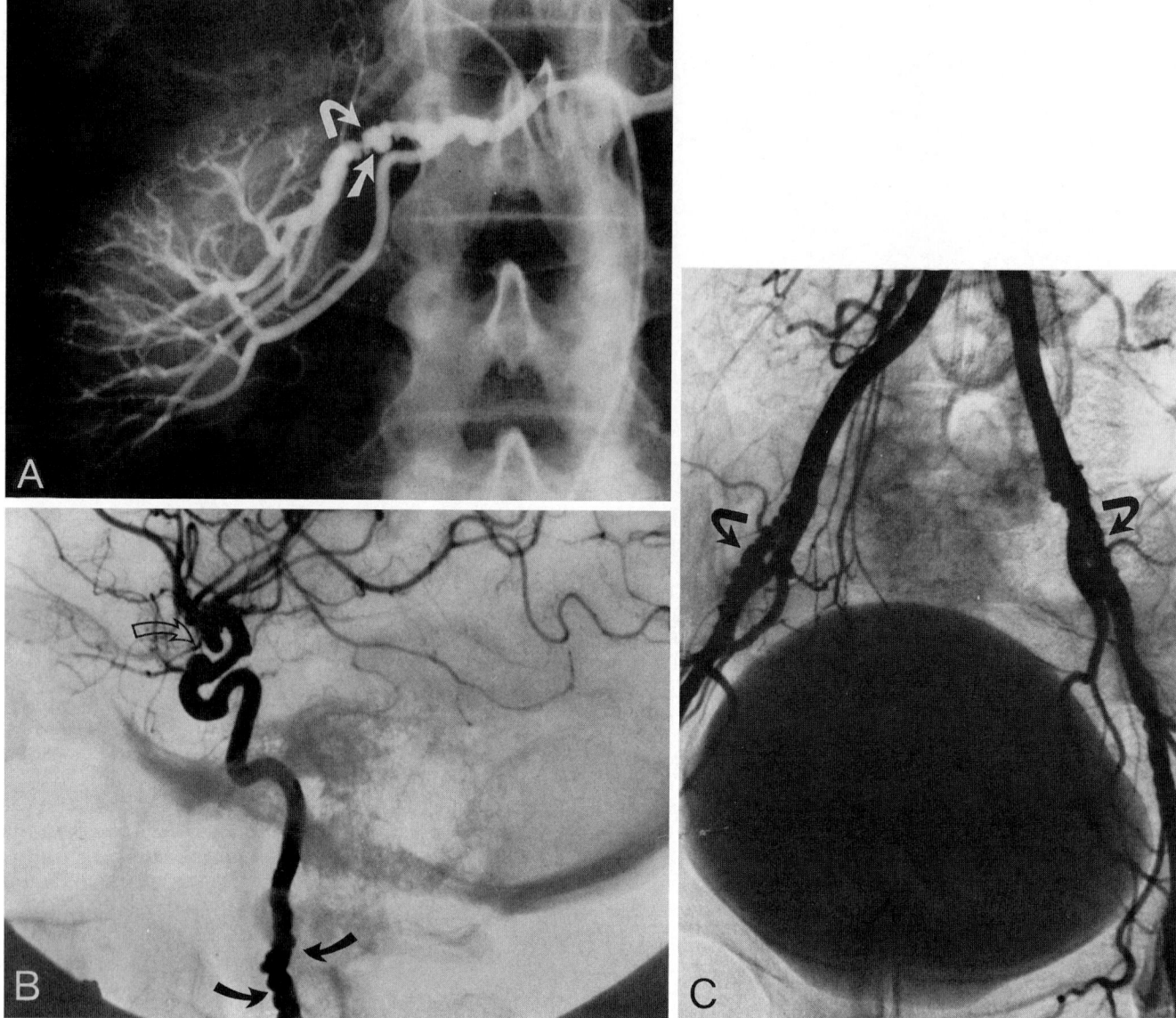

Figure 24.25. Fibromuscular Dysplasia. A. Right renal artery injection shows the beaded appearance of medial fibromuscular dysplasia (*curved arrow*) with aneurysm formation (*straight arrow*). **B.** The cervical carotid artery (*curved black arrows*) shown with an associated intracranial aneurysm (*curved open arrow*). **C.** Iliac arteries (*curved arrows*) are less commonly involved with FMD.

ENTRAPMENT SYNDROMES

Thoracic outlet syndrome comprises a group of anatomic abnormalities in which the artery, vein, or nerve are compressed as they pass through three areas of possible constriction: *(a)* the *interscalene triangle* formed by the anterior and middle scalene muscles and the first rib, *(b)* the *costoclavicular space* formed by the clavicle above and the first rib below, and *(c)* the *pectoralis minor tunnel* formed by the pectoralis minor tendon and the coracoid process. Compression results from congenital (cervical rib, abnormal first rib or muscle insertion) or acquired (muscular hypertrophy, aberrant

healing of rib or clavicle fracture, tumor) etiologies. The most common is the scalenus anticus syndrome resulting from an abnormal insertion of the anterior scalene on the first rib.

Symptoms include numbness, paresthesias, pain, sensory and motor deficits, and coolness, which are exacerbated in certain positions. If the artery is involved, the radial pulse on the affected side may diminish or cease when the symptomatic position (arm abduction or neck extended and head turned) is assumed. Venous involvement results in intermittent cyanosis, edema, and thrombosis.

Angiography is performed both in the neutral position

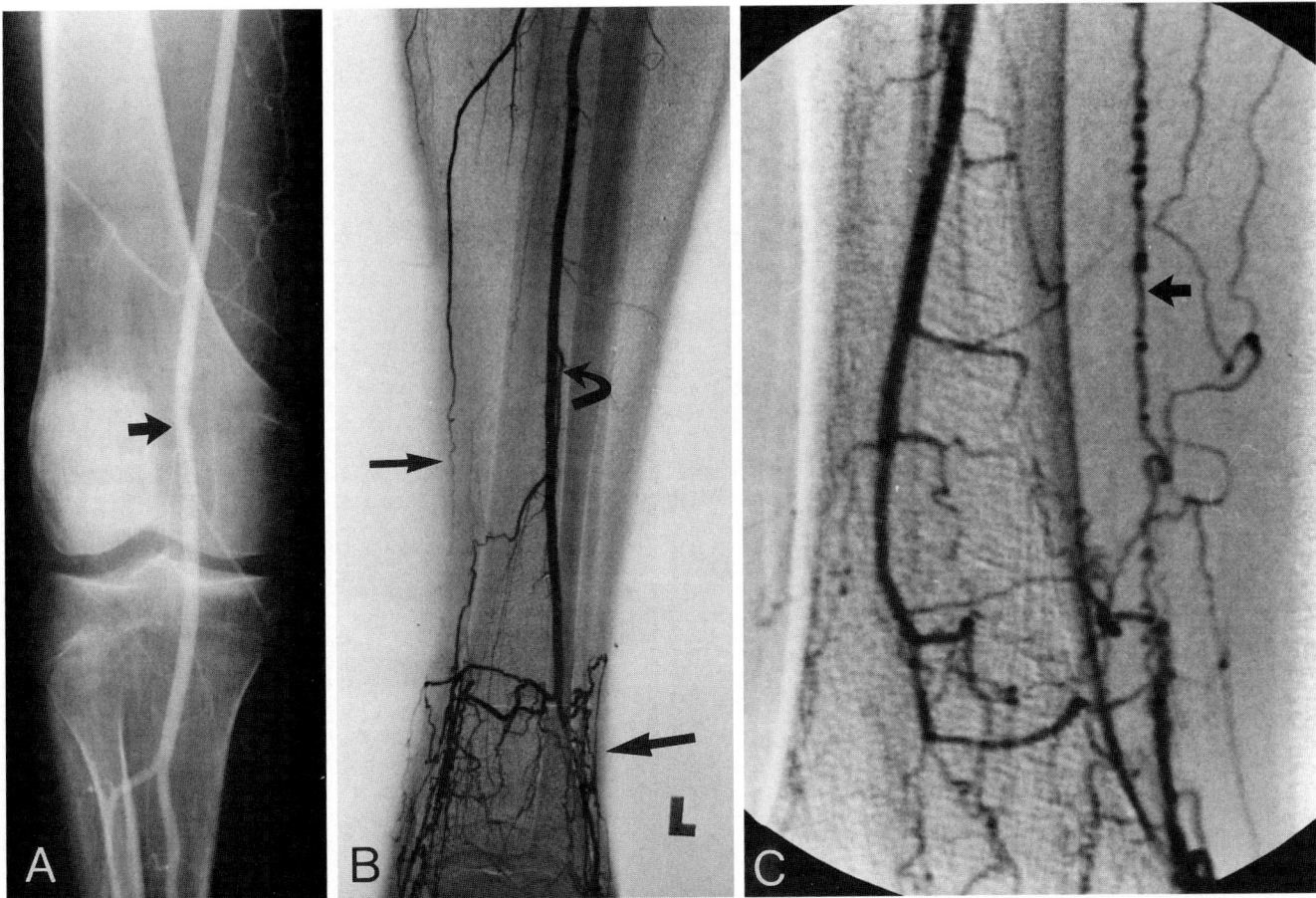

Figure 24.26. Burger's Disease A. A 37-year smoker with foot pain has normal superficial femoral and popliteal arteries (*arrow*). **B.** Distal arterial disease with "corkscrew" vessels (*straight arrows*) are diagnostic findings specific for this entity. Only the peroneal artery (*curved arrow*) is visualized. The anterior and posterior tibial arteries are occluded. **C.** An arteriogram of the opposite leg shows corkscrew vessels (*arrow*) just above the ankle.

with arms at the sides and in the position that reproduces the patient's symptoms (Fig. 24.27). Both arteriography and venography may need to be performed if symptoms dictate. Most patients with arterial involvement will have fusiform dilatation of the artery distal to the level of compression. Other findings include focal stenosis, aneurysm, and distal embolization.

Popliteal entrapment syndrome occurs with compression of the popliteal artery because of the abnormal medial course of the popliteal artery in relation to the medial head of the gastrocnemius muscle, an abnormal insertion of the muscle itself, or compression by the popliteus muscle. Bilateral disease is seen in 20% of cases, with males more commonly affected (M:F = 8:1). Symptoms of unilateral calf claudication in a young male may be sudden in onset. Classic angiographic findings include medial deviation of the popliteal artery and stenosis (see Fig. 24.23B). Stress views (active plantar flexion against resistance) may be necessary to evoke the findings. Other findings include popliteal artery thrombosis and aneurysm formation.

Vascular Grafts

Vascular grafts are used for the treatment of lower extremity occlusive disease and abdominal aortic aneurysms. The grafts frequently encountered are the *aortobifemoral* (Fig. 24.28) and *aortobi-iliac* grafts, which extend from the infrarenal aorta to the femoral or proximal external iliac arteries. Extra-anatomic grafts extend from the axillary artery to the ipsilateral common femoral, with an accompanying graft extending to the contralateral femoral artery, and are known as *"ax-fem/fem-fem"* grafts. Puncturing synthetic grafts can be difficult and is usually performed using a single-wall technique. Because of the resistance of the graft material and the fibrosis present in the groin, overdilatation may be required and a sheath placed. If no sheath is used, all catheters should be straightened over a guidewire before being removed.

Femoropopliteal ("fem-pop") grafts are used to bypass infrainguinal disease and extend from the common femoral to the popliteal artery either above or below the

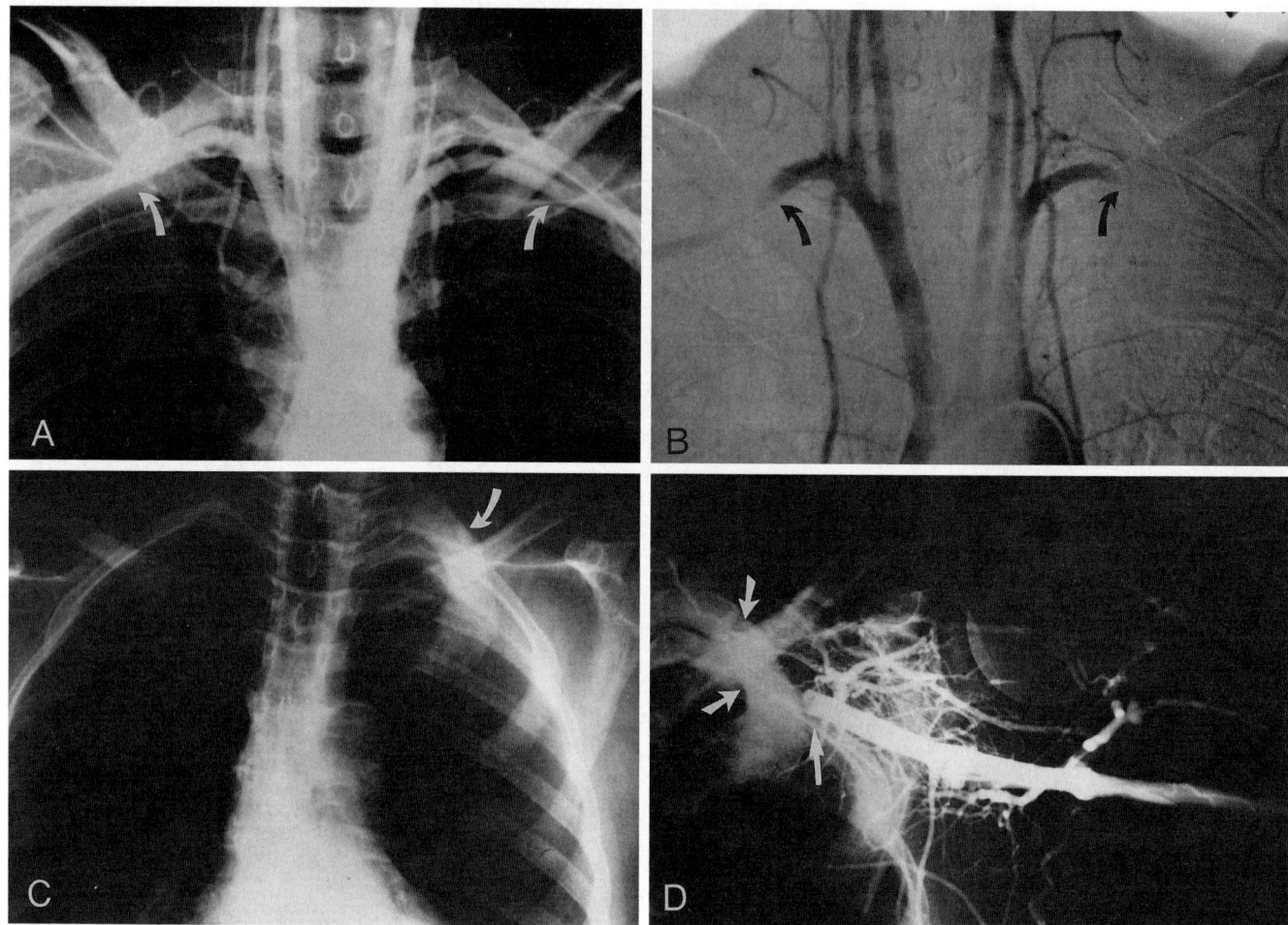

Figure 24.27. Thoracic Outlet Syndrome. A. Aortic arch injection in the neutral position shows normal opacification of the subclavian arteries (*curved white arrows*). **B.** With abduction of both arms, flow is partially occluded in both subclavian arteries (*curved black arrows*). **C.** Frontal chest radiograph shows bony expansion and scle-rosis of the left first rib due to Paget's disease (*curved arrow*). **D.** Upper extremity venogram demonstrates abrupt occlusion at the lateral margin of the enlarged first rib (*short arrows*). The meniscoid filling defect indicates thrombus (*long arrow*).

knee. A variant is the *"fem-distal"* graft, which bypasses to one of the trifurcation vessels at a variable distance into the calf. They are composed of either synthetic material or autologous vein. If the vein is removed and reversed end for end, negating the function of the valves, it is termed *reverse saphenous vein*. If the vein is left in place and the proximal and distal ends anastomosed to the respective arteries (after valve excision using a valvulotome), it is termed *in situ vein graft* .

Graft complications include thrombosis, pseudoaneurysm (Fig. 24.28B), infection, postoperative hemorrhage, and graft-enteric fistula (26). Duplex US is used to evaluate grafts below the inguinal ligament, with angiography reserved for when a complication is suspected and intervention is planned. Grafts within the abdomen and pelvis are best evaluated by CT. Graft infections typically demonstrate perigraft fluid and gas. Pseudoaneurysms occur at the graft anastomoses.

RENAL OCCLUSIVE DISEASES

Atherosclerosis is the most common cause (65%) of renal artery stenosis (Fig. 24.29). It is bilateral in 40% and occurs most frequently in patients more than 50 years old. The stenoses usually occur at the ostium and within the proximal third of the artery. Renal artery disease is nearly always associated with aortic disease and osteal involvement is attributable to atherosclerotic plaque within the aorta extending across the renal artery orifice. Isolated branch vessel disease is uncommon and is typically associated with main renal artery involvement.

Renal vein renin sampling can be used to assess the hemodynamic significance of renal artery stenosis and predict those patients who will respond favorably to angioplasty or surgery. Selective catheterization is performed to obtain venous samples for serum renin assay

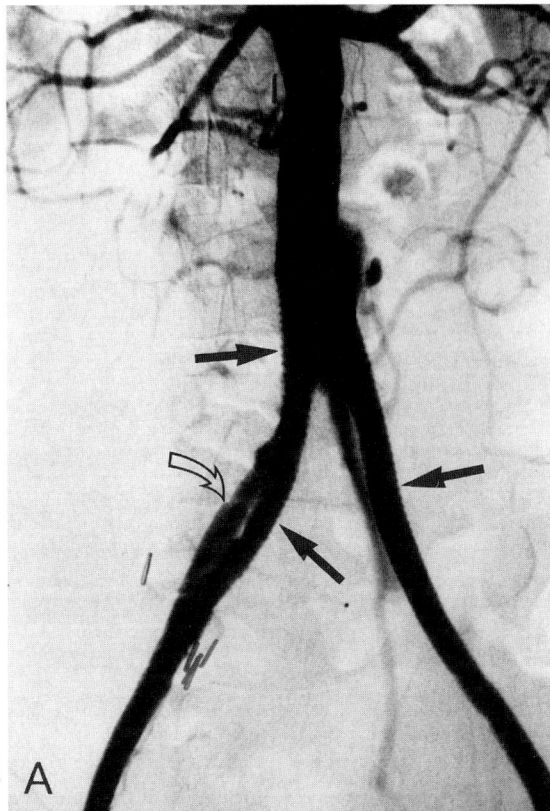

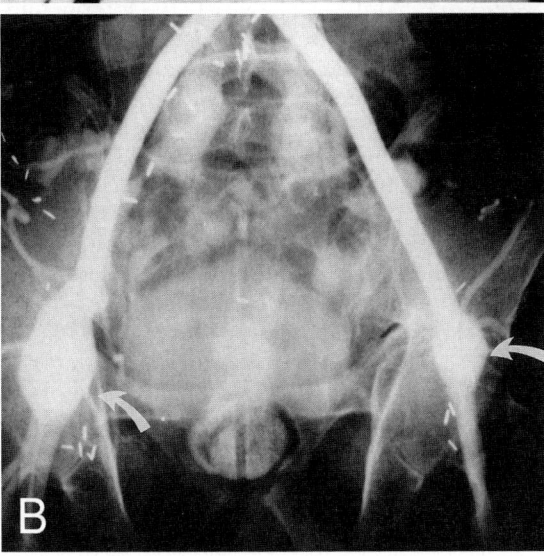

Figure 24.28. Vascular Grafts. A. Aortobifemoral graft. The regularly irregular surface of the graft (*straight arrow*) is typical. The diseased native right common iliac artery is also opacified (*curved arrow*). **B.** Bilateral pseudoaneurysms are seen at the distal anastomosis.

from each renal vein and from the IVC. The ischemic kidney produces increased levels of renin while suppressing renin production from the other kidney. The study is performed with the patient remaining supine prior to the procedure (upright posture increases renin production), adhering to a salt-restricted diet, and receiving no anti-

hypertensive medications. (A renin level ratio (renal vein to arterial [or IVC] renin) from the ischemic kidney of >0.5 is abnormal. The renin level ratio from a normal kidney is near zero. A ratio of renin levels from the ischemic side compared with the unaffected side of >1.5:1 is also considered a positive test (27). Angioplasty success rates are 80% for nonostial lesions and <40% for ostial lesions.

Fibromuscular dysplasia is responsible for 30% of renal artery stenoses. Most lesions occur in young females and more affect the right renal artery. Involvement is bilateral in 65% of cases. FMD includes a heterogeneous group of lesions of unknown pathogenesis that affects the intima, media, or adventitia of the artery. Classification is based on the primary site of involvement in the arterial wall: intimal hyperplasia, medial fibroplasia, fibromuscular hyperplasia, and subadventitial fibroplasia (28). Medial fibroplasia accounts for 75% of cases. It has a classic "string of beads" appearance on angiography, which represents alternating weblike stenoses and aneurysms (see Fig. 24.25A). The middle and distal main renal artery is most frequently involved. The proximal renal artery is rarely involved alone. FMD is the most common cause of hypertension in children. Angioplasty success rates approach 98%.

Neurofibromatosis causes renal artery stenosis by extrinsic compression of the renal artery by neurofibromata or from disorganized intimal and medial proliferation at the renal artery orifice or in the proximal renal artery. Angiography demonstrates smooth or nodular stenoses with or without associated aneurysms. Hypertension secondary to neurofibromatosis is seen mainly in children.

Polyarteritis nodosa is a rare necrotizing vasculitis that affects the small and medium-sized arteries of multiple organs, most commonly the renal (85%) and hepatic (65%) arteries. Characteristic subcutaneous nodules are seen in 15% of cases. The major angiographic findings are multiple, small, saccular "microaneurysms"; occlu-

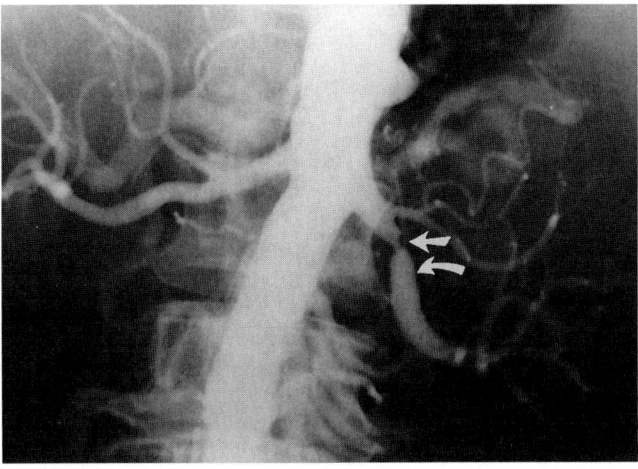

Figure 24.29. Atherosclerotic Renal Artery Stenosis. Stenosis of the proximal left renal artery (*straight arrow*) with mild poststenotic dilatation (*curved arrow*) is typical of atherosclerotic stenosis.

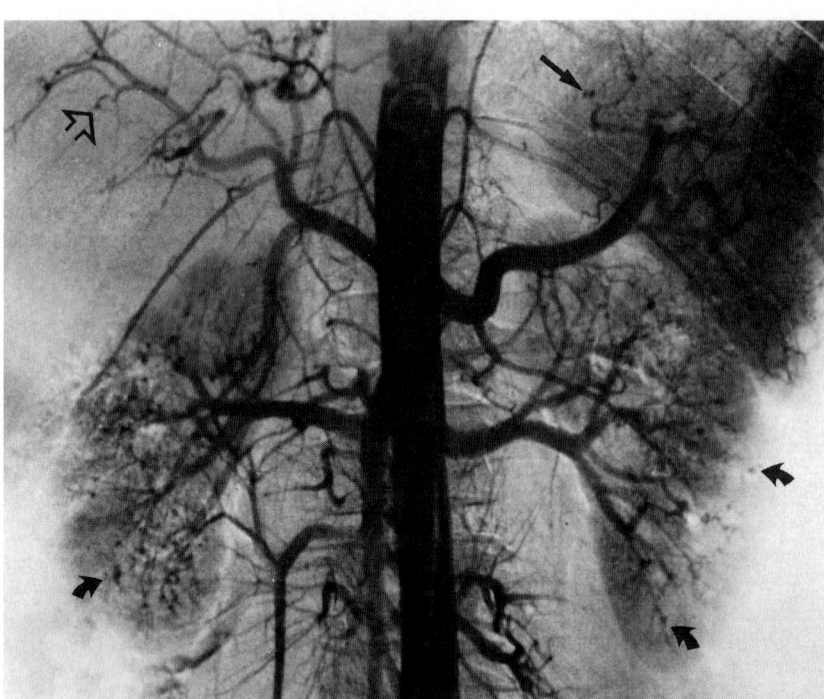

Figure 24.30. Polyarteritis Nodosa. Abdominal aortogram shows multiple microaneurysms in both kidneys (*curved arrows*). The hepatic (*open arrow*) and splenic (*straight arrow*) arteries are also involved.

sions; and irregular stenoses throughout the abdominal viscera (Fig. 24.30) (14). Microaneurysms are seen in 50% of patients, range in size from 1 to 12 mm, and are typically located at branch points. The differential diagnosis of the microaneurysms includes Wegener's granulomatosis, systemic lupus erythematosus, rheumatoid vasculitis, and drug abuse (14).

MESENTERIC VESSELS

Anatomy

Arterial. The *celiac axis, superior mesenteric* (SMA), and *inferior mesenteric* (IMA) arteries are the main arterial supply to the gastrointestinal tract (Fig. 24.31). The celiac axis originates at the T12 level, giving rise to the *splenic, common hepatic,* and *left gastric* arteries (Fig. 24.31A). The *common hepatic* becomes the *proper hepatic* artery after giving off the *gastroduodenal* artery, which then branches into the *superior pancreaticoduodenal* (anterior and posterior) and *right gastroepiploic* arteries. The *left gastroepiploic* artery and *short gastric* arteries are distal branches of the splenic artery. The *right gastric* artery is a small artery with variable origin, usually from the proper or left hepatic artery. The left gastric artery supplies the distal esophagus and the majority of the stomach running along the lesser curvature. The gastroepiploic arteries form an anastomosing arc along the greater curvature of the stomach, supplying the bulk of the remainder of gastric flow. A common normal variant is the *replaced right hepatic* artery that originates from the SMA in 10% of individuals.

The SMA originates at the T12–L1 level and supplies the entire small intestine and the proximal two thirds of the colon (Fig. 24.31B). The first branch is the *inferior pancreaticoduodenal* artery, which freely anastomoses with the superior pancreaticoduodenal artery to supply the duodenum. The remaining branches in order of origin are the *jejunal, ileal, middle colic, right colic,* and terminal *ileocolic* arteries. The middle colic divides into the left and right branches, which freely anastomose with the respective right and left colic arteries. The ileocolic supplies the terminal ileum and cecum; the right colic supplies the ascending colon and hepatic flexure; and the middle colic supplies the transverse colon.

The IMA originates at the L3 level and gives rise to the *left colic, sigmoid,* and *superior hemorrhoidal (rectal)* arteries (Fig. 24.31C). The superior hemorrhoidal branches freely anastomose with the hemorrhoidal branches of the internal iliac system.

Collateral communications of the mesenteric vessels are *(a) marginal artery of Drummond,* which provides anastomosis between the right colic, right and left branches of the middle colic, and the left colic arteries. It is found along the mesenteric border of the colon and is an important collateral supply in IMA occlusions (Fig. 24.32); *(b) Riolan's arc* is a variable communication between the SMA and IMA located more centrally in the mesentery than the marginal artery; *(c)* arc *of Beuhler* is a short, ventral artery between the main celiac and SMA. representing a persistent fetal communication.

Portal Venous Anatomy. The venous drainage of the gastrointestinal tract generally follows the arterial anatomy. The *superior mesenteric* vein joins the *splenic* vein to form the main *portal* vein (Fig. 24.33). The *inferior mesenteric* vein joins the splenic vein just to the left of this junction. The *left* and *right gastric (coronary)* veins drain directly into the portal vein. Normal antegrade flow in the portal venous system is termed *hepatopetal* flow.

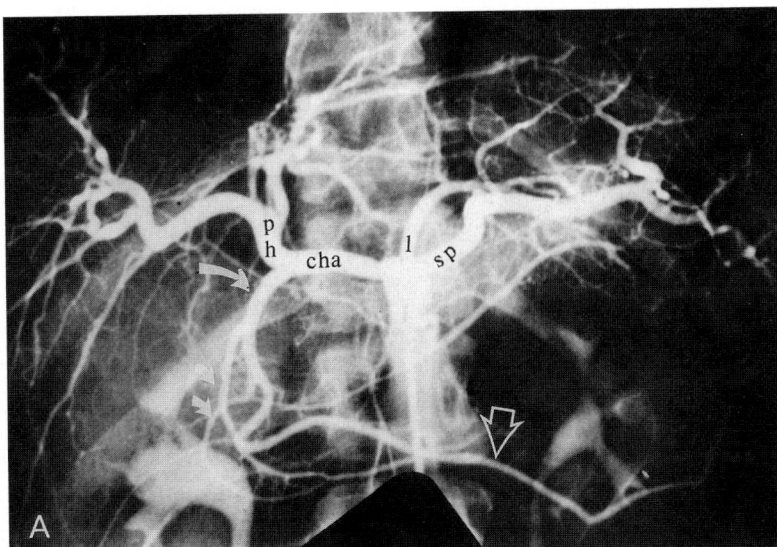

Figure 24.31. Normal Mesenteric Arteries. A. Celiac axis injection shows its major branches: common hepatic artery (*cha*), splenic artery (*sp*), and left gastric artery (*l*). The common hepatic artery continues as the proper hepatic artery (*ph*) after formation of the gastroduodenal artery (*large curved white arrow*). The gastroduodenal artery gives off the pancreaticoduodenal arcade (*small curved white arrows*) and continues as the right gastroepiploic artery (*open arrow*). **B.** Superior mesenteric artery injection shows the middle colic artery (*short straight arrow*), right colic artery (*large straight arrow*), and the ileocolic artery (*curved arrow*). **C.** Inferior mesenteric artery injection shows left colic branches (*straight arrow*), sigmoid branches (*curved open arrow*), and superior hemorrhoidal artery (*curved arrow*).

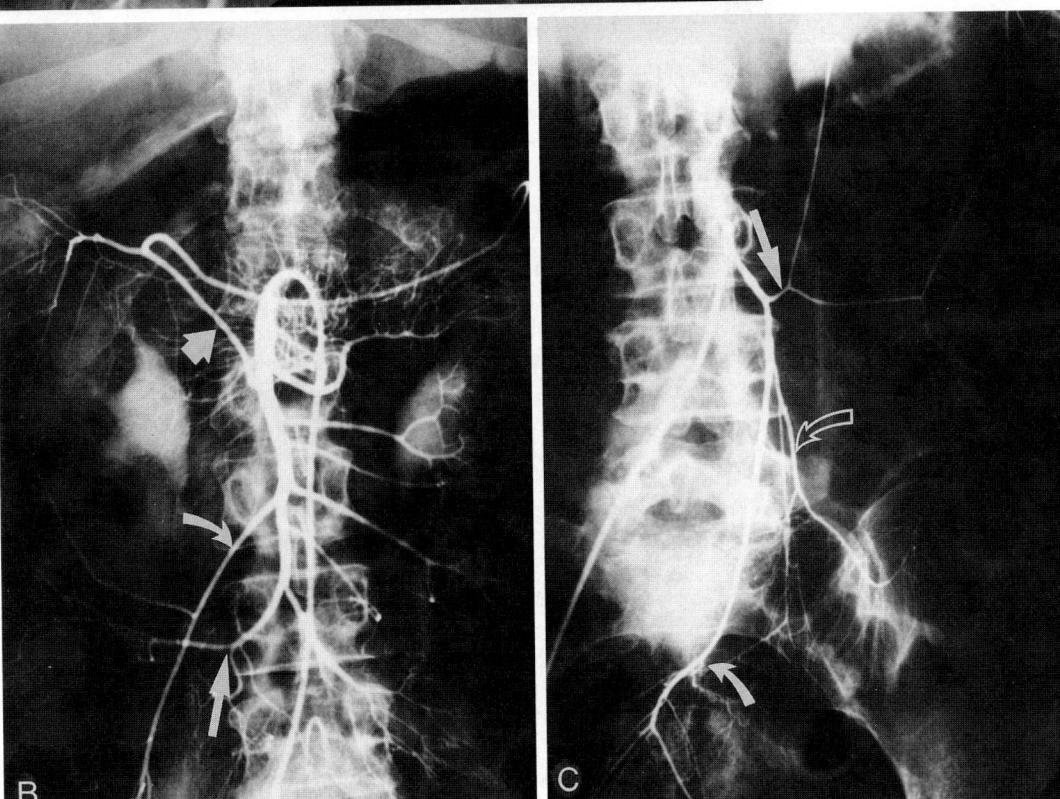

Reversal of flow is termed *hepatofugal* flow and represents flow through portosystemic communications (e.g., coronary vein to azygous system, resulting in esophageal varices).

Angiographic Technique

Selective injections of the individual vessels are required for accurate evaluation of the mesenteric arterial system (see Table 24.1). A lateral abdominal aortogram is performed to evaluate the patency of the proximal mesenteric vessels and to assess for anatomic variants. Imaging of the portal venous system may be accomplished in two ways. The first involves selective celiac or SMA injections, with late imaging to visualize the venous phase. Opacification may be enhanced with the direct arterial administration of tolazoline (Priscoline) 25–50 mg into the SMA to dilate end arterioles and facilitate flow into the venous system. Left anterior oblique (15°) positioning projects vessels off the spine and better profiles the main portal branches. The second method for portal venous imaging requires direct transhepatic puncture of the portal vein and is uncommonly used for purely diagnostic purposes.

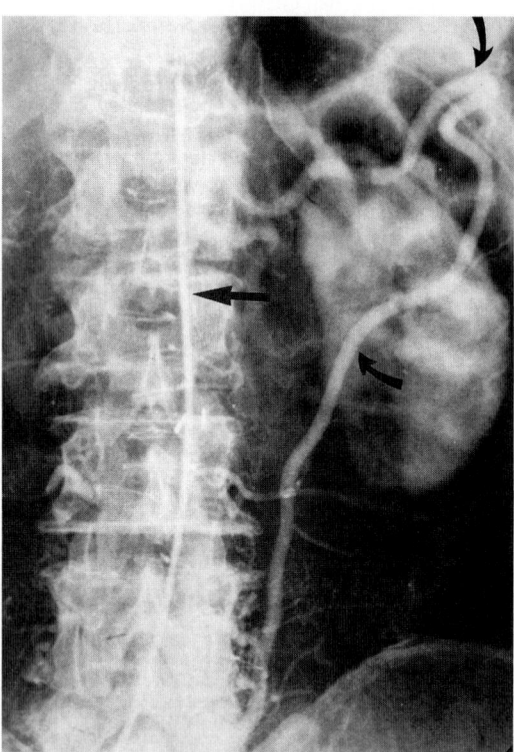

Figure 24.32. Marginal Artery of Drummond. The marginal artery of Drummond (*curved arrows*) provides collateral blood supply for an occluded inferior mesenteric artery. A catheter is seen within the aorta (*straight arrow*).

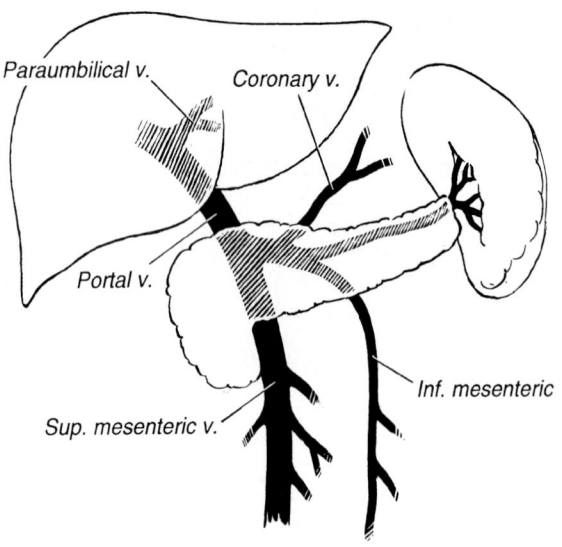

Figure 24.33. Portal Venous Anatomy.

Gastrointestinal Hemorrhage

The evaluation of gastrointestinal bleeding includes nasogastric (NG) tube aspirate, esophagogastric duodenoscopy, colonoscopy, radionuclide imaging (tagged-RBC and sulfur colloid), and angiography. The applica-

tion of these modalities depends on the likely source of bleeding and the clinical status of the patient. Hemodynamically unstable patients may require emergency angiography or surgery or both, whereas the stable patient is able to undergo a more controlled, systematic evaluation and treatment. For suspected upper GI bleeding (source proximal to the ligament of Treitz), the evaluation begins with NG aspirate and endoscopy. For lower GI bleeding (LGI), evaluation by colonoscopy or radionuclide imaging (Fig. 24.34; see Fig. 25.16) localizes the site of bleeding and guides the angiographic examination to the most likely vascular territory. Interventional procedures for the treatment of GI bleeding are discussed in chapter 25.

The most reliable angiographic sign of GI bleeding is contrast extravasation, which is seen as an amorphous contrast collection that persists through the venous phase. If the bleeding rate is rapid enough, the extravasated contrast may outline mucosal folds. The *"pseudovein"* sign is a linear collection of contrast between mucosal folds that simulates an enlarged vein (see Fig. 25.16). Bleeding must occur at a rate of at least 0.5ml per minute to be identified by angiography (29).

Upper Gastrointestinal Bleeding

Mallory-Weiss tear is a longitudinal split in the mucosa located on the posterolateral aspect of the esophagogastric junction, usually on the gastric side. These account for approximately 14% of UGI bleeds and are usually associated with severe vomiting and excessive alcohol consumption (29). Patients present with excruciating epigastric and left chest pain and may develop pneumothorax and pneumomediastinum if the injury is transmural. Arterial supply is left gastric, inferior phrenic, or short gastric arteries. Treatment is vasopressin with 88% success or embolization (29,30).

Acute hemorrhagic gastritis accounts for 27% of UGI bleeds and is usually seen in critically ill patients after surgery, burns, or trauma or in alcoholics. The angiographic appearance is a diffusely hyperemic mucosa with multiple punctate foci of contrast extravasation. Arterial supply is left gastric, gastroepiploic. Treatment is vasopressin with 84% success or embolization (29).

Gastric ulcers cause 10% of acute UGI bleeding (see Fig. 25.15). Angiography shows a single focus of contrast puddling or the "pseudovein" sign as contrast flows from the bleeding site between gastric rugae. Arterial supply is left gastric or gastroepiploic. Treatment is surgery, embolization, and vasopressin (29).

Duodenal peptic ulcer is the cause of UGI bleeding in 25% of cases. The NG aspirate may be negative, and a small percentage of patients present with LGI bleeding. Other causes of duodenal bleeding include vascular malformations, visceral aneurysms, and neoplasm. Arterial supply is gastroduodenal and inferior pancreaticoduodenal. Both the celiac and SMA may have to be studied. Treatment is surgery or embolization (29). Vasopressin is not effective because of rich collateral supply from both SMA and celiac.

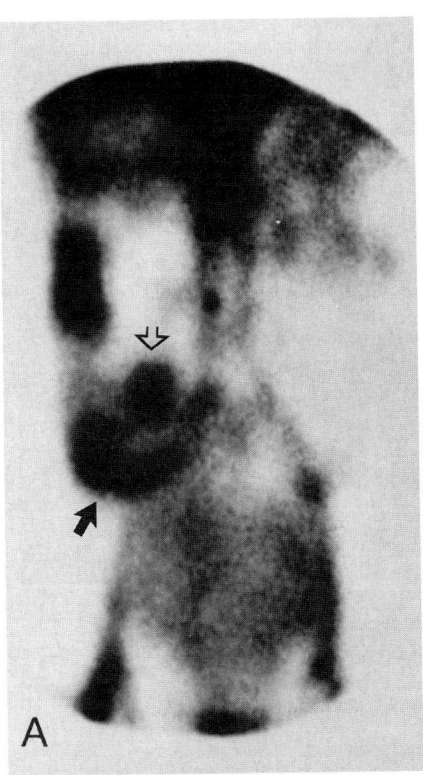
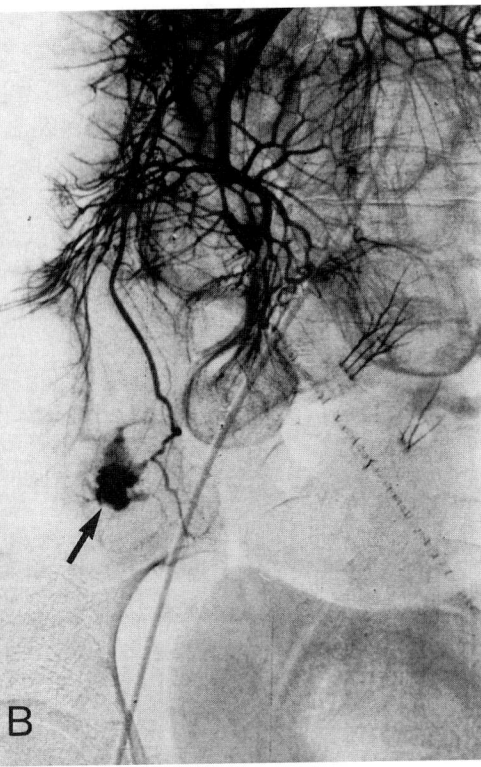

Figure 24.34. Bleeding Meckel's Diverticulum. A. A radionuclide tagged red blood cell study shows focal activity in the right lower quadrant of the abdomen (*open arrow*). Tracer activity is also seen in the terminal ileum (*closed arrow*) and ascending colon. **B.** An SMA arteriogram shows focal extraluminal pooling of contrast (*arrow*) in what was found at surgery to be a Meckel's diverticulum containing ectopic gastric mucosa.

Postsurgical anastomoses after gastric bypass procedures (e.g., gastrojejunostomy) may be complicated by erosive ulcers on the jejunal side. Because of the distorted anatomy after surgery, several vessels may need to be studied. Arterial supply is usually SMA. Treatment is vasopressin or cautious embolization. Vascular supply may be altered by surgery.

Lower Gastrointestinal Bleeding

SMALL BOWEL

Tumor is the most common cause for bleeding from the small bowel, responsible for 20–50% of the cases. Angiography depicts tumor neovascularity (enlarged, bizarre, irregular vessels with A–V shunting) with or without contrast extravasation. Treatment is surgery or embolization.

Aortoenteric fistula accounts for 10% of small bowel bleeding and is usually a complication of AAA surgery as soon as 3 weeks postoperatively. The duodenum is involved in 80% of cases where it crosses over the aorta. Gas in the retroperitoneal soft tissues in the region of the anastomosis is suggestive of fistula (26). Angiography shows an anterior nipplelike projection from the aortic graft anastomosis or, rarely, contrast extravasation at the fistula site. Angiography is performed using an aortic injection, not selective injections of the SMA. Treatment is urgent surgery (29).

Diverticula of the small bowel are an uncommon (6%) cause of small bowel bleeding. They are located along the mesenteric border of the bowel. The jejunum is a more common bleeding source than the ileum. Bleeding is typically slow and difficult to diagnose angiographically. Treatment is vasopressin, surgery, or embolization (30).

Meckel's diverticulum, the omphalomesenteric duct remnant, is found along the antimesenteric border in the distal ileum. Patients present with painless bleeding attributable to an ileal ulcer adjacent to the heterotopic gastric mucosa contained in the diverticulum (see Fig. 24.34). A radionuclide Meckel's scan is more sensitive than angiography, as this demonstrates the gastric mucosa. Treatment is vasopressin and then surgery.

Inflammatory bowel disease is identified angiographically as diffuse hyperemia, arteriovenous shunting, and oozing. Treatment is vasopressin and surgery.

Vascular malformations are responsible for 20% of small bowel bleeding. They may be solitary or multiple, as seen in Rendu-Osler-Weber syndrome, and usually present as a chronic, recurrent bleed.

COLORECTAL

Colonic diverticula are the most common cause of LGI bleeding. Although diverticula are much more common in the left colon, a bleeding diverticulum is three times more likely to found in the right colon. Treatment is vasopressin (90% success at controlling bleeding, with a 20% rebleed rate), surgery, or embolization (29).

Angiodysplasia is a vascular malformation located most commonly located in the right colon along the antimesenteric border. It is seen in patients older than 55 years of age and is responsible for 50% of colonic bleeding in the older age group. Angiodysplasia may be found in up to 15% of patients without a history of GI bleeding. Unless bleeding is detected, it is a diagnosis of exclusion after other causes (diverticula, ulcers, neoplasm, or colitis) have been excluded. Classic angiographic features

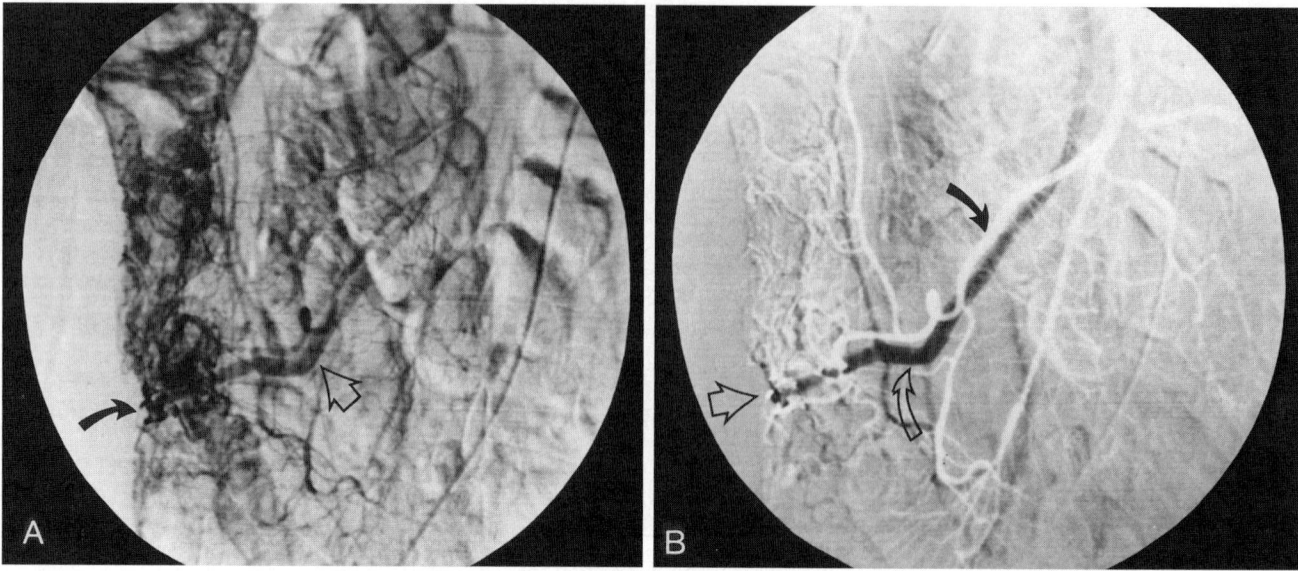

Figure 24.35. Colonic Angiodysplasia. A. A tangle of vessels within the ascending colon (*curved arrow*) with an associated enlarged draining vein (*open arrow*) are angiographic findings typical of angiodysplasia. **B.** Subtraction technique demonstrates to better advantage the feeding artery (*curved closed arrow*) and draining vein (*curved open arrow*) with the tangle of vessels on the antimesenteric border of the colon (*open straight arrow*).

are early opacification of an enlarged draining vein, persistent dense opacification of the vein, and vascular tufts along the antimesenteric border of the cecum or ascending colon (Fig. 24.35). Treatment is surgery (29).

Portal Hypertension

Bleeding from gastric and esophageal varices accounts for 17% of acute, massive upper GI hemorrhage (29). Varices are venous channels that become massively dilated and tortuous in an attempt to circumvent flow around the diseased liver (Fig. 24.36). Common collaterals are the coronary veins, which anastomose with the azygous system in the submucosa of the distal esophagus and gastric cardia. These abnormal vascular structures thin the overlying mucosa, project into the esophageal lumen, and are prone to erode and bleed. These are termed "uphill" varices as opposed to "downhill" varices seen with superior vena cava obstruction.

In up to 60% of patients with documented varices, the source of bleeding may be attributable to other causes, usually ulcer disease or gastritis (29). Endoscopy is necessary to confirm the diagnosis and perform endoscopic therapy if possible. When endoscopic sclerotherapy of variceal bleeding is not feasible or is unsuccessful, a transjugular intrahepatic portosystemic shunt can be placed and the varices embolized if necessary (see chapter 25) (30).

Mesenteric Ischemia

This entity comprises a group of disorders that have a common endpoint: bowel necrosis (Table 24.6). The mortality rate approaches 70%. Arterial embolism and

thrombosis account for 50% of cases, with nonocclusive ischemia accounting for 25% (31). Emboli usually have a cardiac source, with angiography demonstrating the classic reverse meniscus sign in the lumen of the SMA 4–6 cm from its origin. Arterial thrombosis occurs on a background of pre-existing severe atherosclerotic occlusive disease of the celiac and SMA. Symptoms of postprandial abdominal pain, weight loss, and altered bowel habits are typical. Treatment is usually surgical, although direct intrarterial infusion with vasodilators such as papaverine (30–50 mg/h) can be used in cases of nonocclusive ischemia or preoperatively to optimize bowel perfusion and maximize recovery (32).

Mesenteric venous occlusion generally affects the medium-sized veins of the middle small bowel and accounts for approximately 10% of cases. Nonocclusive ischemia is the result of conditions that produce low flow states such as hypotension, dehydration, and low cardiac output. The bowel responds with disproportionate vasoconstriction leading to ischemia. Angiography confirms diffuse vasoconstriction without underlying structural abnormality. Both mesenteric venous thrombosis

Table 24.6. Classification of Mesenteric Ischemia

Acute Ischemia
  Arterial embolism
  Arterial thrombosis
  Venous thrombosis
  Nonocclusive ischemia
  Colonic ischemia
Chronic ischemia

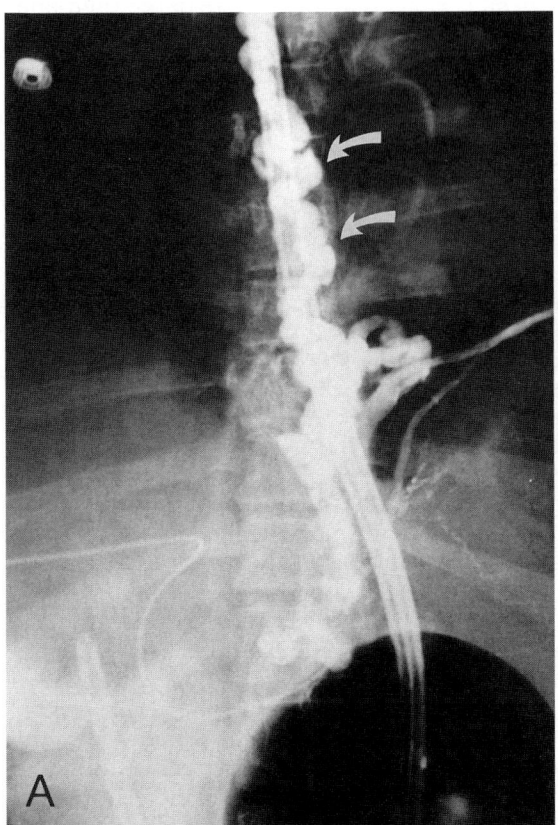

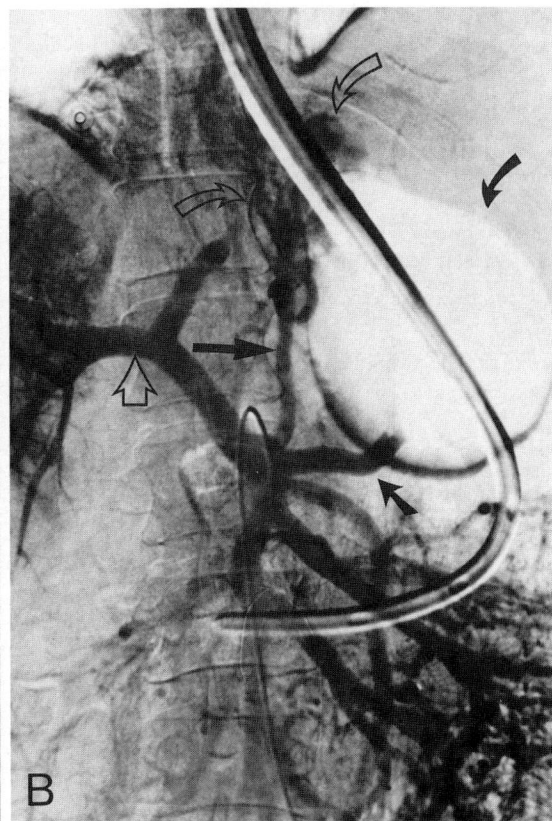

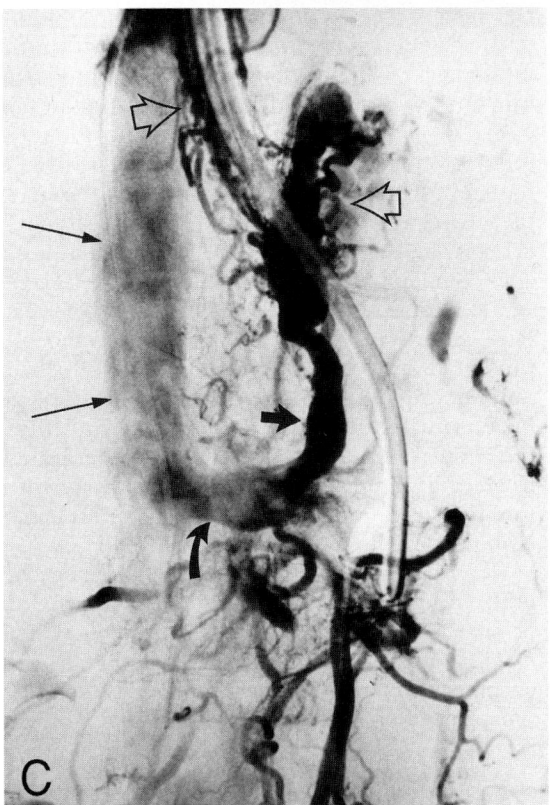

Figure 24.36. Portal Hypertension with Varices.
A. Transhepatic injection of the coronary vein shows typical configuration for "uphill" varices (*arrows*) in this patient with portal hypertension and variceal hemorrhage.
B. Portal venous filling (*open straight arrow*) following
SMA injection demonstrates esophageal and gastric fundal varices (*curved open arrows*) supplied by the coronary vein (*large straight arrow*). An occlusion balloon
(*curved closed arrow*) is expanded within the stomach
to temporarily stop variceal hemorrhage. The balloon
occludes the splenic vein (*small straight arrow*).
C. Multiple esophageal and gastric fundal varices
(*open straight arrows*) fill the left renal vein (*curved
arrow*) and IVC (*long thin arrows*), creating a splenorenal shunt.

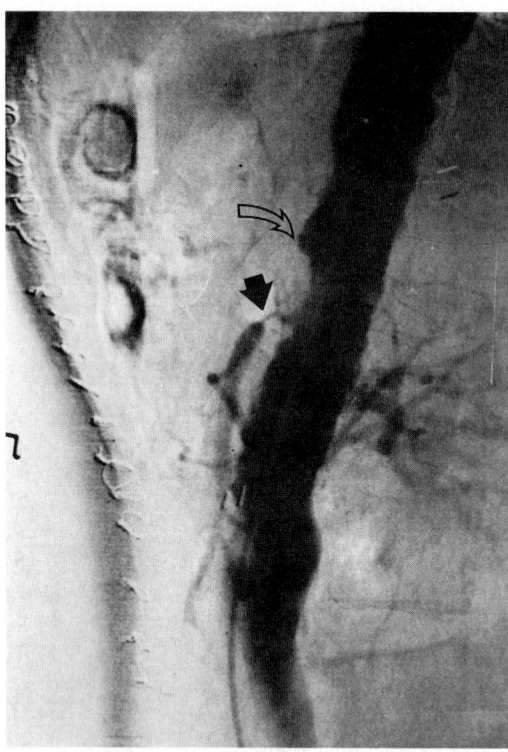

Figure 24.37. Mesenteric Ischemia. A lateral projection of an aortogram shows severe atherosclerotic disease with occlusion of the celiac trunk (*curved arrow*) and severe stenosis of the origin of the SMA (*straight arrow*). The IMA was also occluded.

and nonocclusive ischemia can present with GI bleeding. Chronic etiologies include atherosclerosis (Fig. 24.37), fibromuscular dysplasia, and various vasculitides (31).

CENTRAL VEINS

Anatomy

The superior vena cava (SVC) is formed by the junction of the short, vertically oriented right and longer obliquely oriented left bracheocephalic veins at the level of T1. The SVC contains no valves, measures 7 cm in length, and is usually less than 2 cm in diameter. It descends along the right side of the mediastinum and ends in the right atrium at the level of T3. The trachea, right mainstem bronchus, right main pulmonary artery, and the innominate artery lie posterior and to the left of the SVC. Anteriorly and to right, the SVC is bordered by lung and mediastinal fat. The major tributary of the SVC is the azygous vein, which enters the dorsal aspect at its midpoint.

The inferior vena cava (IVC) is formed by the junction of the right and left common iliac veins at L5. It ascends to the right of the abdominal aorta and anterior to the spine to enter the right atrium at about T8. A rudimentary valve (*eustachian valve*) is present just before its entrance into the right atrium. The main tributaries of the IVC are the hepatic (T10), renal (L2), right adrenal and gonadal, and lumbar veins.

The azygous venous system is an asymmetrically paired paravertebral venous complex that provides an important collateral communication between the SVC and IVC. This system is divided into the *azygous* and *hemiazygous* veins, which lie to the right and the left of the spine, respectively. Both are continuations of the ascending lumbar and subcostal veins and begin at the L1 level. The azygous follows the aorta through the diaphragm to the T6 level, where it arches anteriorly over the right main stem bronchus to join the SVC. The hemiazygous ascends into the chest and traverses the midline to join the azygous vein at approximately T8.

CT and MR are the best noninvasive methods for evaluating both congenital and pathologic entities involving the vena cava and azygous systems. Venography may be reserved for cases in which more anatomic detail and functional characteristics are required or as a precursor to intervention.

Venographic Technique

For imaging of the IVC, the most common access site is the common femoral vein. The common femoral vein is located just medial to the artery and is entered by localizing the arterial pulse and passing the needle just medial to it. Having the patient perform the Valsalva maneuver distends the vein and improves the probability of access. A syringe partially filled with saline is used to provide gentle aspiration as the needle is both advanced to ensure the artery is not penetrated and withdrawn until free return is encountered, confirming placement in the vein. Guidewires and catheters are then used in a manner similar to the technique described for the arterial system (see Table 24.1).

The SVC is imaged through access within the antecubital fossa of one or both upper extremities with simultaneous injection or via the internal jugular (IJ) vein (see Table 24.1). Slight Trendelenburg's position distends the jugular vein. Direct US guidance may be used to confirm patency of the IJ while permitting anterior single-wall puncture and avoiding injury of the adjacent carotid artery. The IJ may be entered either lateral to the sternocleidomastoid muscle within the midneck or at the apex of the sternal and clavicular heads of this same muscle more inferiorly. US guidance for the more inferior approach helps avoid puncture of the subclavian artery and pneumothorax. Care must be taken not to allow the needle and catheters to remain open to air with access in the central venous system above the diaphragm because the negative intrathoracic pressure may introduce air into the vascular system, causing a pulmonary artery air embolism.

The SVC may be imaged through access from the groin, and the IVC may be imaged from IJ, subclavian, or antecubital access. A pigtail catheter is usually used if injection is performed directly in the cava or selective catheters are used if injections are performed from a more peripheral site (see Table 24.1)

Congenital Anomalies

Left superior vena cava occurs in 0.3% of the population and is a persistence of the left anterior cardinal vein. The left SVC descends through the left mediastinum anterior to the aorta and left main pulmonary artery to join the coronary sinus, which drains into the right atrium. The coronary sinus is enlarged to accommodate the increased flow. A double SVC (left SVC with a normal right SVC) is the most common variation (85%). One third of these will have a transverse anastomosis between the paired cavas. A single left SVC is rare and is associated with congenital heart disease (33).

Azygous continuation of the IVC is attributable to absence of the intrahepatic portion of the IVC because of failure of the right subcardinal vein to anastomose with

the hepatic veins. The hepatic veins drain into the right atrium via the posthepatic segment of the IVC. The renal and iliac veins drain via the azygous and hemiazygous veins into the SVC. Findings include dilatation of the azygos vein, azygos arch, and the SVC (Fig. 24.38). Hemiazygous continuation is much less common and may drain via the normal communication with the azygos vein, through a persistent left SVC, or by the accessory hemiazygous system (34).

Duplicated IVC is present in 3% of the population and is a persistence of both right and left supracardinal

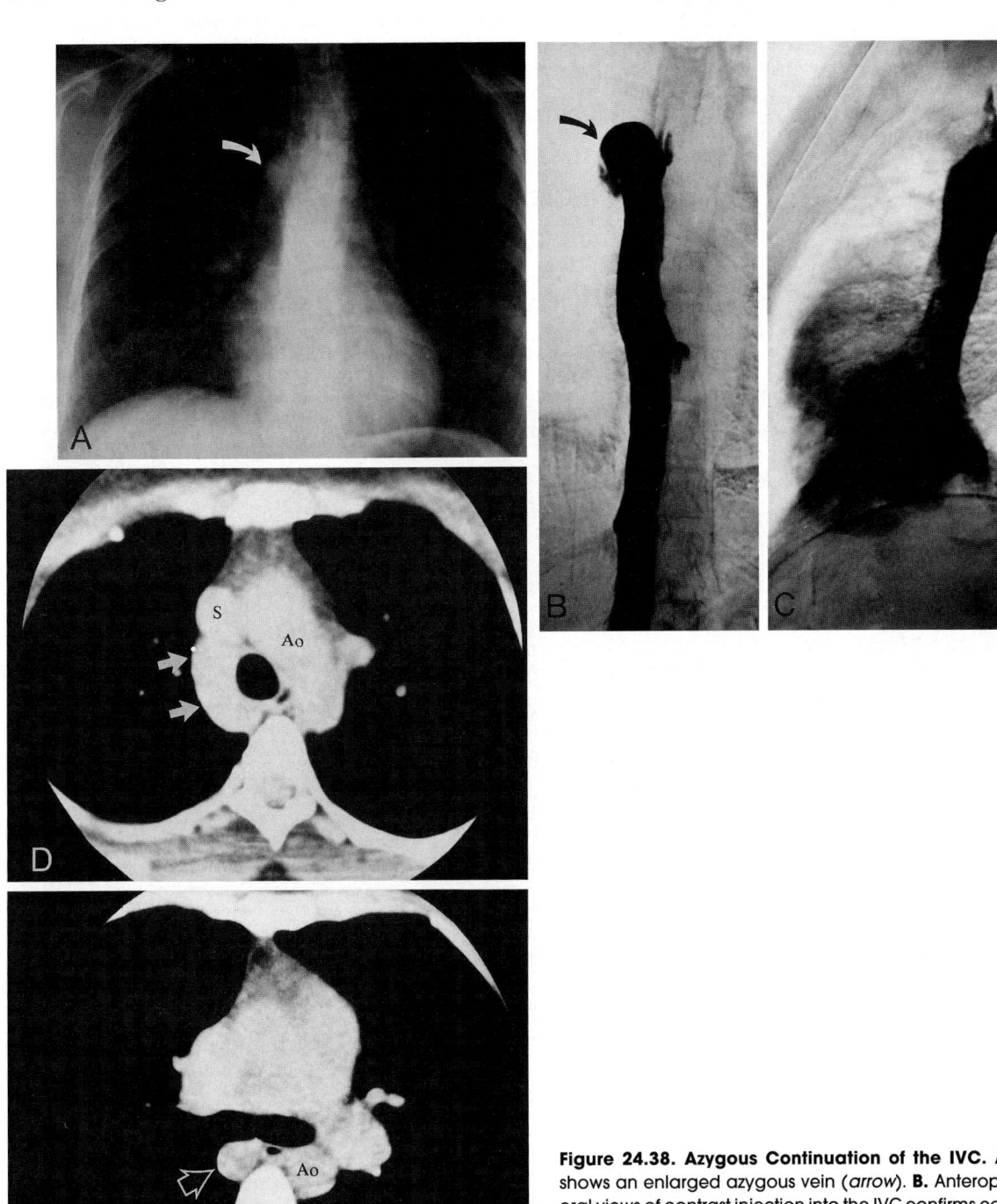

Figure 24.38. Azygous Continuation of the IVC. A. Frontal chest film shows an enlarged azygous vein (*arrow*). **B.** Anteroposterior and **(C)** lateral views of contrast injection into the IVC confirms continuation of the IVC into an enlarged azygous vein (*arrow*). **D.** Contrast-enhanced chest CT shows an enlarged azygous vein (*arrows*) joining the SVC (*s*). *Ao*, aorta. **E.** A CT slice inferior to **(D)** demonstrates the enlarged but normally positioned azygous vein (*open arrow*).

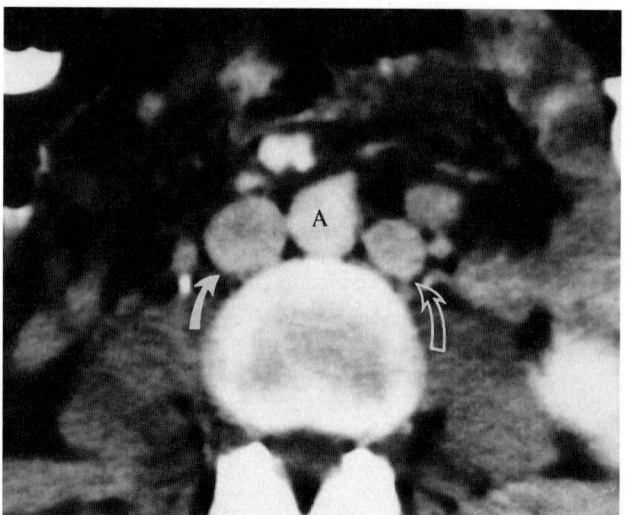

Figure 24.39. Duplicated Inferior Vena Cava. Contrast-enhanced CT of the abdomen shows vessels (*curved arrows*) on either side of the aorta (*A*) consistent with duplication of the inferior vena cava. More inferior images showed each vessel was contiguous with its respective common iliac vein.

veins. The left IVC is a continuation of the left iliac vein and ascends to the left of the aorta before crossing over to join the right IVC, usually via the left renal vein (Fig. 24.39).

Left IVC without a right IVC occurs in 0.2% of the population and, similar to the duplicated IVC, crosses the midline at the level of the renal veins and ascends normally into the intrahepatic segment.

Retroaortic/Circumaortic Left Renal Vein. The retroaortic left renal vein (2%) crosses behind the aorta instead of its usual path anterior to the aorta. The presence of both retroaortic and preaortic renal vein forms the circumaortic left renal vein (8%) encircling the aorta to join the IVC.

Occlusive Disorders

SVC obstruction results from extrinsic compression or intraluminal thrombosis. The marked venous hypertension in the head and upper extremities is known as *superior vena cava syndrome*. Clinical findings are dilatation of the veins of the head and upper extremities;

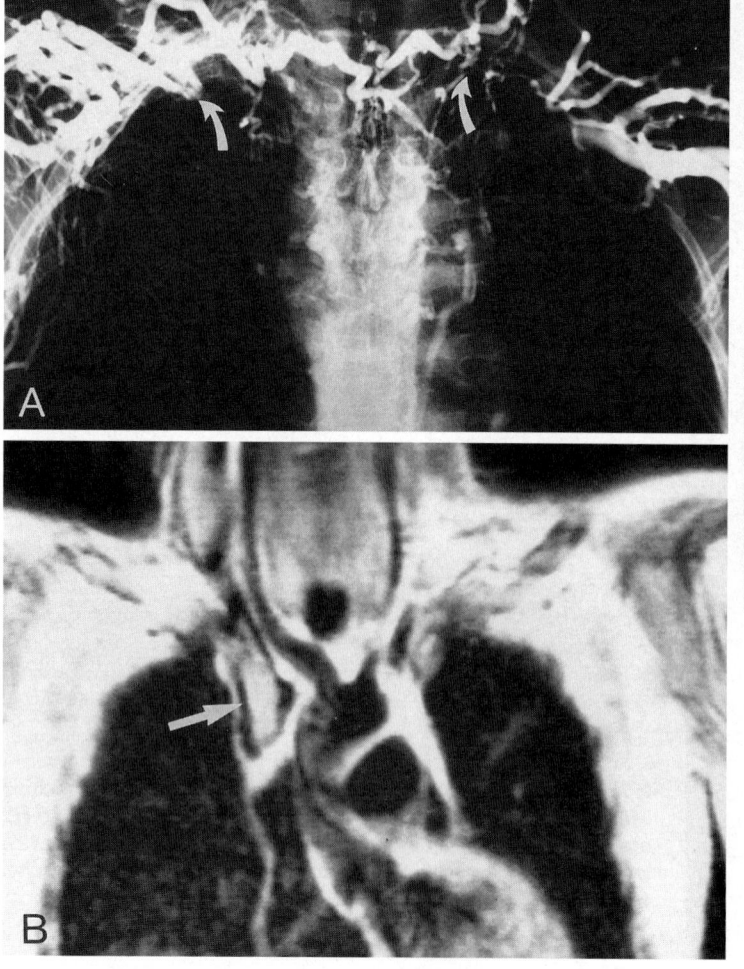

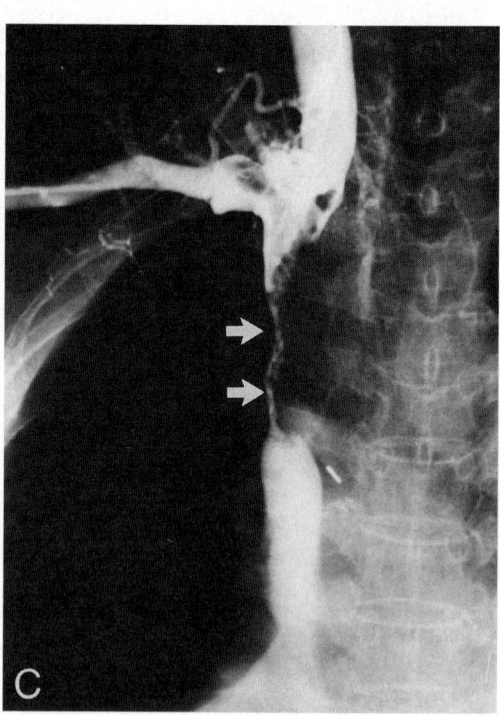

Figure 24.40. Superior Vena Cava Obstruction.
A. Dilated and tortuous collateral veins (*arrows*) carry venous return from the upper extremities. **B.** Coronal MR shows bright signal from thrombus (*arrow*) within the SVC. **C.** Contrast injection into the right subclavian vein reveals near complete obstruction of the SVC caused by tumor invasion (*arrows*).

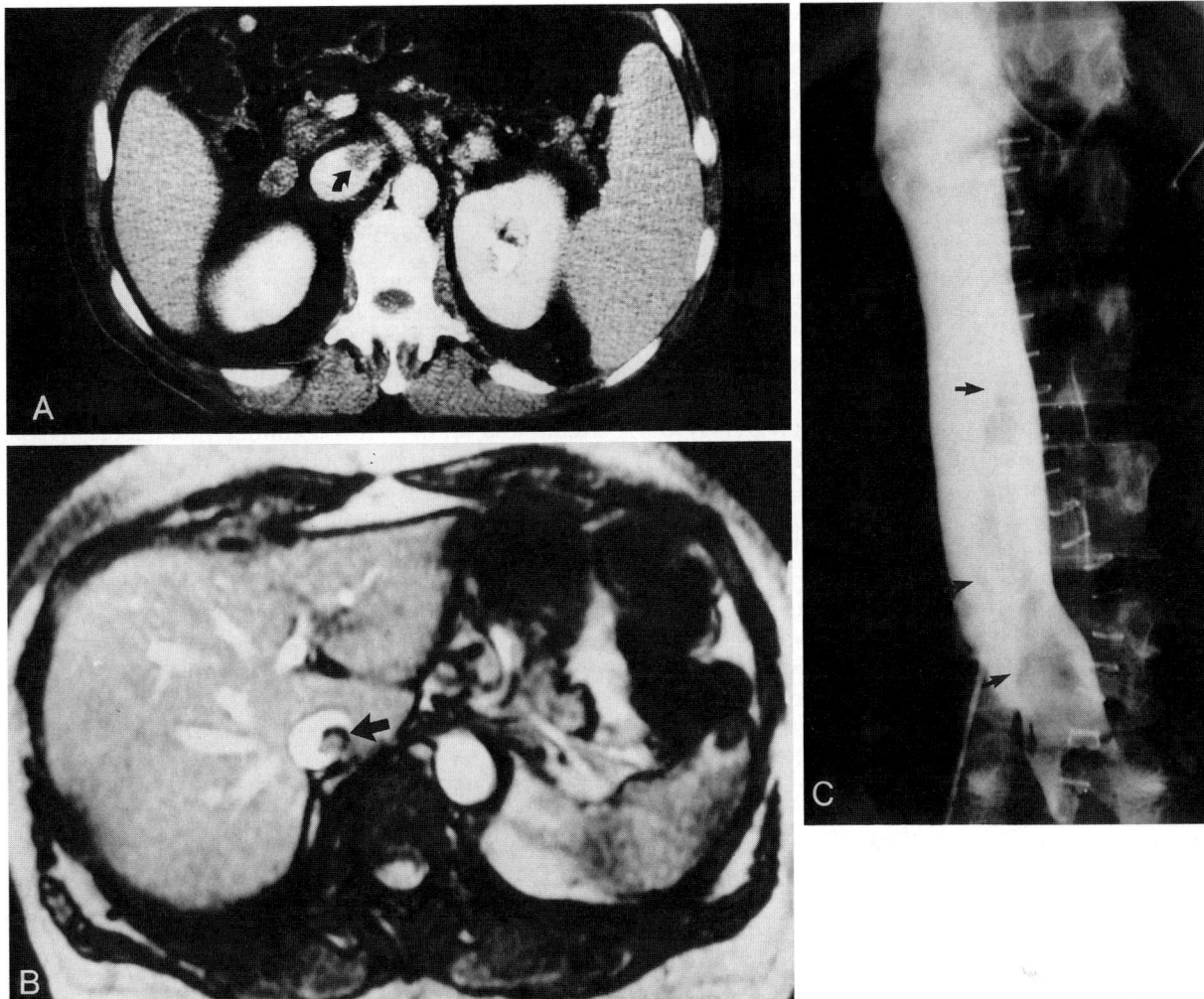

Figure 24.41. Inferior Vena Cava Thrombus. A. Contrast-enhanced CT shows an intraluminal clot within the IVC (*arrow*). **B.** Gradient recalled echo MR shows thrombus within the IVC as an ovoid focus of intermediate signal surrounded by a crescent of dark signal (*arrow*). **C.** Inferior vena cavagram reveals extensive thrombus propagating from the left iliac vein (*arrows*).

edema and plethora of the face, neck, and upper torso; cyanosis and conjunctival edema; dizziness, syncope, and headaches; and respiratory distress owing to airway edema. If obstruction occurs slowly, a compensatory collateral network via any one or combination of the azygos, internal mammary, vertebral, or lateral thoracic veins will develop and the clinical complex may not be readily apparent (Fig. 24.40).

Causes of SVC obstruction include malignancy, thrombosis from long-term central venous catheters, mediastinal granulomatous disease, aortic aneurysm, and fibrosing mediastinitis. Malignancy is by far the most common cause (65–97% of cases) and may extrinsically compress or directly invade the lumen or occlude the lumen by tumor thrombus. The most common causes are bronchogenic carcinoma, lymphoma, and metastatic disease, especially that resulting from breast carcinoma (35).

IVC obstruction is also most commonly the result of tumor. Renal cell carcinoma extends in the IVC via the renal veins. Adrenal and hepatic tumors may invade the lumen and lymphadenopathy extrinsically compresses the IVC. Nonneoplastic causes include thrombus extension from the lower extremities (Fig. 24.41), thrombosis of caval filters, coagulopathy, congestive heart failure, infection, and Budd-Chiari syndrome. Extrinsic nonneoplastic causes include hepatomegaly, massive ascites, retroperitoneal fibrosis, and inflammatory AAA. Functional obstruction can result from compression by the gravid uterus or a large abdominal mass.

PERIPHERAL VEINS

Anatomy

Upper Extremity. The upper extremity is drained predominantly by the superficial venous system. The *basilic* vein courses along the ulnar aspect of the forearm and medial upper arm to continue as the axillary vein. The *cephalic* vein lies along the radial aspect of the forearm and ascends on the anterolateral upper arm to join the axillary vein below the clavicle. The deep system consists of small, paired veins that follow the arteries and empty into the basilic vein. The axillary vein becomes the subclavian vein at the lateral border of the first rib.

Lower Extremity. The lower extremity is drained primarily by the deep venous system that consists of paired veins in the calf that follow the arteries both in course and name (Fig. 24.42). The paired *anterior tibial, posterior tibial,* and *peroneal* veins in the calf join to form a single *popliteal* vein below the joint line of the knee. The popliteal vein continues into the thigh as the *superficial femoral* vein, which is then joined by the *profunda femorus* vein to form the *common femoral* vein at the inferior margin of the femoral head. The popliteal and superficial femoral vein are occasionally duplicated.

The superficial system is composed of the *greater* and *lesser saphenous* veins. The lesser begins at the lateral ankle and courses over the posterior calf to join the popliteal or greater saphenous veins. The greater saphenous vein originates near the medial malleolus and ascends the anteromedial leg to empty into the common femoral vein (CFV) at the inguinal ligament. Multiple small communicating veins between the superficial and deep system in the calf and lower thigh are called *perforating* veins. These contain valves and are responsible for directing flow from the superficial to the deep system. The CFV enters the pelvis medial to the common femoral artery and continues as the *external iliac* vein.

Imaging of the venous system is usually performed to detect deep venous thrombosis and relies predominately on duplex US (see chapter 40), supplemented by contrast venography. Radionuclide venography may be performed in conjunction with ventilation perfusion lung scanning.

Contrast Venogram Technique

Lower extremity venography uses a non–weight-bearing technique. The patient stands on a box on the unaffected leg with the table tilted 30–45°. A dorsal vein on the medial aspect of the foot is cannulated (ideally directed toward the toes to facilitate filling of the deep system), and an intravenous infusion of heparinized saline is begun. A tourniquet is applied at the ankle to assist in forcing the contrast into the deep system. Intravenous injection of 90–120 ml of 60% contrast is performed, with imaging of the leg and pelvis on film or fluoroscopy. Filling of the iliac system and IVC is facilitated by having the patient perform the Valsalva maneuver while the calf is gently massaged.

Upper extremity venography is performed for the evaluation of axillary or subclavian vein obstruction. An antecubital vein is cannulated, and contrast is injected under fluoroscopic control with spot film or DSA imaging.

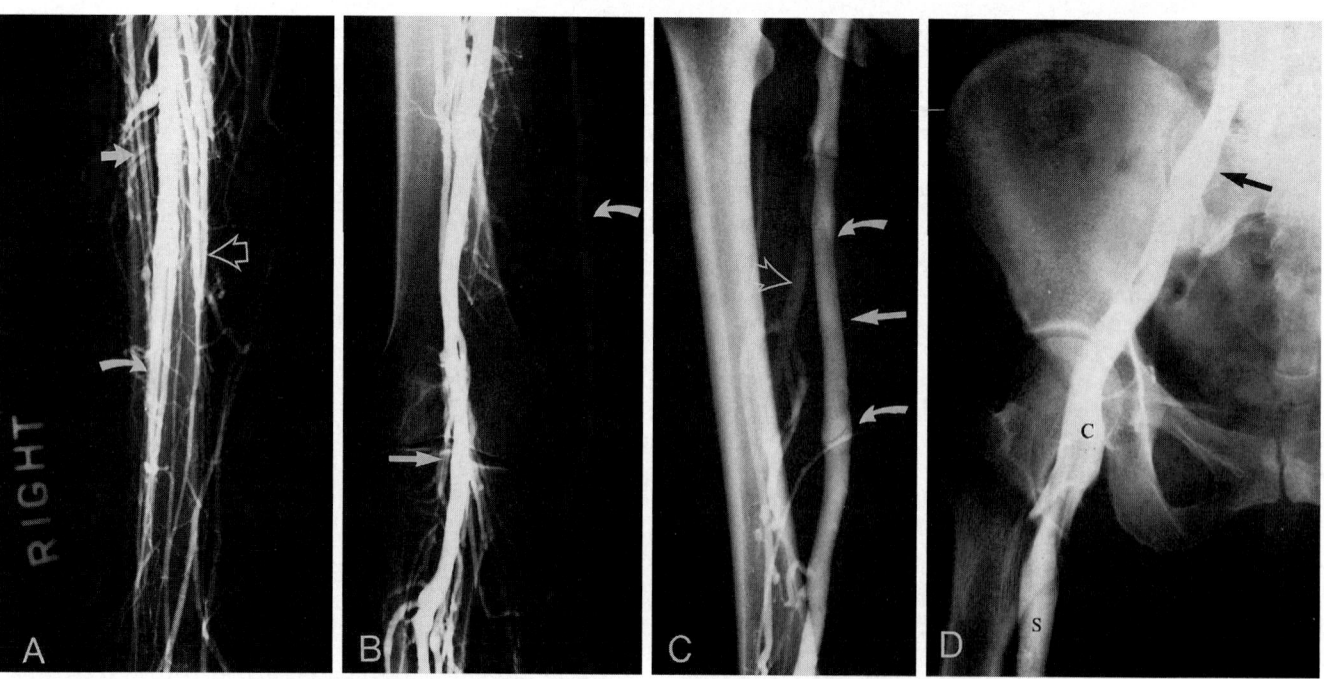

Figure 24.42. Normal Lower Extremity Venogram. A. Three pairs of calf veins are homogeneously opacified after contrast injection into a dorsal foot vein. Anterior tibial veins (*straight arrow*). Posterior tibial veins (*open arrow*). Peroneal veins (*curved arrow*). **B.** The trifurcation vessels form the popliteal vein (*straight arrow*). Faint opacification of the greater saphenous vein (*curved arrow*) is also seen.

C. The superficial femoral vein (*straight arrow*) is well opacified with multiple valves evident (*curved arrows*). The profunda femoral vein (*open arrow*) is faintly visualized. **D.** A "dump" shot shows normal filling of the iliac veins (*arrow*). *S,* superficial femoral vein. *CFV,* common femoral vein.

Deep Venous Thrombosis

Lower Extremity. The true prevalence of DVT is unknown, as it is a disease that remains asymptomatic in many patients. One third of patients with PE who exhibit no signs of DVT will have lower extremity thrombus. In addition, the clinical diagnosis of DVT is errant in 50% of cases (36). Risk factors for DVT include prolonged immobilization, advanced age, pregnancy, oral contraceptive use, obesity, surgery (especially abdominal and orthopedic), severe trauma, myocardial infarction, congestive heart failure, malignancy, polycythemia, and previous DVT. In most patients, the thrombus originates in the calf; in patients who undergo hip surgery, DVT is more likely to develop in the iliofemoral system (37). *May-Thurner syndrome* is compression of the left common iliac vein by the anteriorly crossing right common iliac artery. The constant, pulsatile compression is thought to induce intimal scarring and weblike adhesions within the vein, resulting in chronic left leg swelling and risk of venous thrombosis (see Figs. 25.5 and 25.9) (38).

Upper extremity DVT is much less common than lower extremity, but its incidence is increasing as a result of frequent use of indwelling central venous catheters. Other causes include trauma, thoracic outlet syndrome, central obstruction (see Fig. 24.27), tumor, or radiation. Effort thrombosis (*Paget-Schroetter syndrome*) is spontaneous axillosubclavian vein thrombosis following vigorous exercise, with compression of the vein during forced abduction. DVT within the upper extremity may be a source for pulmonary emboli (36).

Imaging. The only conclusive finding of acute DVT on contrast venography is a persistent intraluminal filling defect within the vein lumen (Fig. 24.43). Findings that are highly suggestive of DVT include abrupt termination of the contrast column in the vein, inability to opacify a vein, and collateral formation. The more chronic the obstruction, the more collaterals may be detected. Signs of clot organization and *chronic DVT* include eccentric mural filling defect; recanalization with establishment of an irregular, eccentric channel; loss of valves; persistent occlusion; and incompetent perforating veins and varicosities.

Postphlebitic syndrome is a manifestation of chronic DVT with valve destruction and an inefficient recanalized venous system. Chronic venous stasis disease causes distinctive skin changes (hyperpigmentation and induration), pain, swelling, varicosities, and venous stasis ulcers, typically at the ankles.

Phlegmasia cerulea dolens is a grave condition resulting from extensive DVT of the iliofemoral system. Marked elevation of venous pressure in the extremity leads to progressive swelling with compromise of the arterial circulation, resulting in gangrene.

PULMONARY ARTERIES

Anatomy. The main pulmonary artery is confined within the pericardium. It measures 3 cm in diameter and 5cm in length and extends from the pulmonic valve to its bifurcation into the right and left pulmonary arteries, which each measure 2 cm in diameter. The RPA courses posterior to the ascending aorta and SVC to divide into an ascending (truncus anterior) branch that supplies the upper lobe and a descending (interlobar artery) branch that supplies the middle and lower lobe. The LPA is the continuation of the MPA as it arcs over the left mainstem bronchus. It follows the curve of the aortic arch to which it is connected by the ligamentum arteriosum. The LPA divides into an ascending branch supplying the upper lobe and a descending branch supplying the lingula and lower lobe. Normal PA pressures average 25/8 mm Hg.

Imaging. The choice of imaging method for the pulmonary arteries depends on the condition being evaluated. For embolic disease, plain film and radionuclide ventilation-perfusion (V/Q) scanning is followed by angiography if required. For vascular abnormalities, plain film supplemented by CT and MR may be all that is required. Angiography is for uncertain diagnosis, if more detailed anatomic information is needed, or if surgical or percutaneous intervention is planned.

Angiographic Technique

The usual access site is the common femoral vein, although the right internal jugular vein or antecubital veins may be used. Catheters for pulmonary angiography have a pigtail configuration and a special curve that allows easy maneuverability through the heart. Balloon

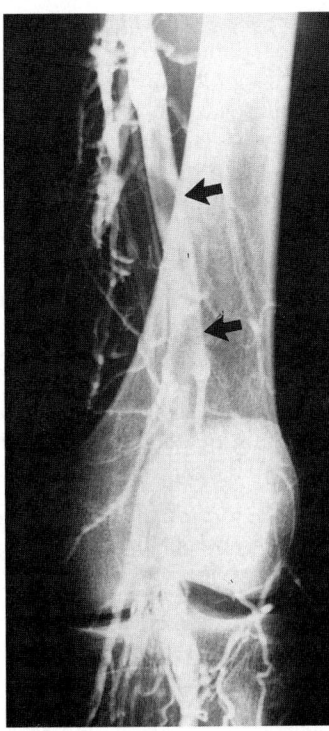

Figure 24.43. Lower Extremity Deep Venous Thrombosis. Left leg venogram shows a serpentine intraluminal filling defect (*arrows*) indicative of thrombus within the popliteal vein.

Table 24.7. Relative Contraindications for Pulmonary Angiography

Pulmonary artery pressure > 70 mm Hg
Right ventricular end-diastolic pressure > 20 mm Hg
Left bundle branch block
Bleeding abnormalities
History of contrast reaction
Renal insufficiency

occlusion catheters are used in selected cases when detailed visualization is required or standard LPA or RPA injections are contraindicated. Tip-deflecting wires may be necessary for negotiating large right heart chambers or congenital septal abnormalities. The catheter is passed through the tricuspid valve, right ventricle, and pulmonic valve into the MPA. As it is passed through the RV, careful cardiac monitoring is needed to detect catheter-induced, life-threatening dysrhythmias. The catheter is directed into the LPA or RPA, and imaging is performed in full inspiration using CA or DSA (see Table 24.1). Biplane CA is preferred, supplemented by posterior oblique positioning.

Precautions/Contraindications. *Pulmonary artery hypertension* with systolic pressures >70 mm Hg is a relative contraindication to angiography (Table 24.7). Subselective hand injections may be necessary to prevent the complication of acute right heart failure or cor pulmonale. In the presence of *left bundle branch block,* catheter manipulation in the right ventricle may induce right bundle branch block, leading to life-threatening complete heart block. Patients with left bundle branch block require placement of a temporary pacemaker prior to pulmonary angiography.

Congenital Anomalies

Unilateral agenesis of the pulmonary artery is an uncommon anomaly associated with systemic arterial supply, small hemithorax, elevated hemidiaphragm, and shift of the mediastinum to the affected side. Ipsilateral rib notching may be evident owing to hypertrophy of the intercostal arteries to supply the lung. V/Q scanning demonstrates absence of perfusion with normal ventilation. CT and MR document the absent pulmonary artery.

Aberrant left pulmonary artery or *pulmonary sling* is attributable to an abnormal origin of the LPA from either the distal MPA or the RPA. The aberrant artery courses over the right mainstem bronchus back across the mediastinum between the trachea and esophagus to the left hilum. Imaging findings include a small left hilum, right-sided mediastinal mass, anterior indentation of the barium-filled esophagus, and obstructive emphysema of the right lung if the right mainstem bronchus is compressed.

Pulmonary Embolism

Accurate diagnosis of PE is essential because the mortality rate for untreated patients is 30%, versus 8% for treated PE. The clinical diagnosis is rarely straightforward because most patients present with nonspecific signs and symptoms (38). The most common source for emboli is DVT of the lower extremities. The risk of PE when a diagnosis of DVT is confirmed depends on the site of involvement. Untreated calf DVT has less than a 10% incidence of PE, whereas clot within or above the popliteal vein places the patient at 50% risk of PE (36). However, 30% of cases with confirmed PE have no evidence of lower extremity DVT. Death from PE is usually associated with obstruction of greater than 50% of the pulmonary arterial bed. This creates a sudden rise in pulmonary vascular resistance and pulmonary arterial pressure leading to acute right ventricular failure (38).

Chest Radiograph. Most patients have nonspecific abnormalities on the chest radiograph. The utility of the chest radiograph is to exclude other conditions that mimic PE clinically (e.g., pneumothorax, pneumonia, rib fracture) and to aid in the interpretation of the V/Q scan (38).

V/Q scans are interpreted in degrees of probability of having PE (see chapter 56). The V/Q scan can be used to direct the pulmonary angiogram to the most likely effected area.

Angiography is performed when less-invasive methods fail to provide a definitive diagnosis (Table 24.8). It should *not* be performed when the V/Q scan is normal. Angiography is most sensitive in the first 24 hours of clinical symptoms because clot fragmentation diminishes detection of PE. Most emboli are found in the lower lobes, especially in the posterior segment (38).

The definitive findings are an intraluminal filling defect or a vessel cutoff, with thrombus extending into the contrast column (Fig. 24.44). Magnification technique may be necessary to demonstrate small, distal emboli. Nonspecific signs include areas of decreased perfusion, prolonged arterial phase, delayed venous phase, and tortuous peripheral vessels. The diagnosis of PE should not be based on these findings alone. as these may be seen in chronic obstructive pulmonary disease, bronchial asthma, mitral stenosis, and left ventricular failure. *Chronic PE* (1% of cases) represents the residua of unresolved emboli. It is manifested angiographically by stenoses, webs, and irregular tapering of the artery. These changes result in increased vascular resistance and pulmonary hypertension (38).

MR and CT have successfully demonstrated large central emboli as filling defects in the pulmonary arteries

Table 24.8. Indications for Pulmonary Angiography

Inadequate information from less invasive studies
    Intermediate probability V/Q scan
    Low probability V/Q scan with high clinical suspicion
    Underlying disease process that may cause false-positive V/Q scan
    Need for more detailed vascular anatomy
Possible adjustment of planned therapy
    Planned thrombolytic therapy
    Contraindication to anticoagulation with high probability V/Q scan
    Contemplate cava filter placement for recurrent PE

Figure 24.44. Pulmonary Embolism. A. RPA injection shows multiple intraluminal filling defects owing to pulmonary emboli (*arrows*). **B.** Contrast-enhanced CT reveals tumor thrombus from renal carcinoma at in the left pulmonary artery (*lpa*). **C.** Other causes of pulmonary arterial obstruction include encasement by tumor. The LPA is narrowed (*arrow*) by surrounding bronchogenic carcinoma.

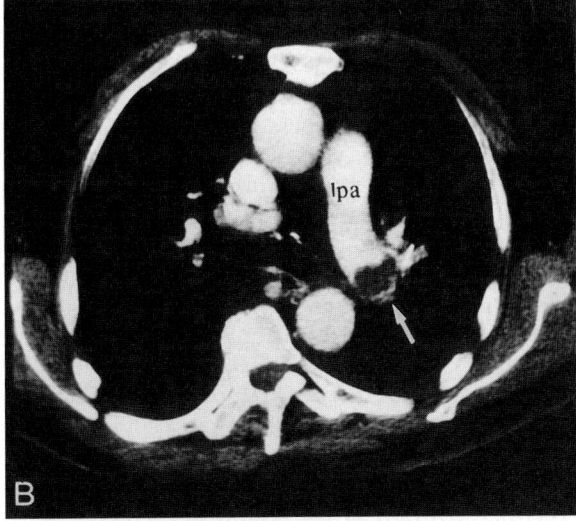

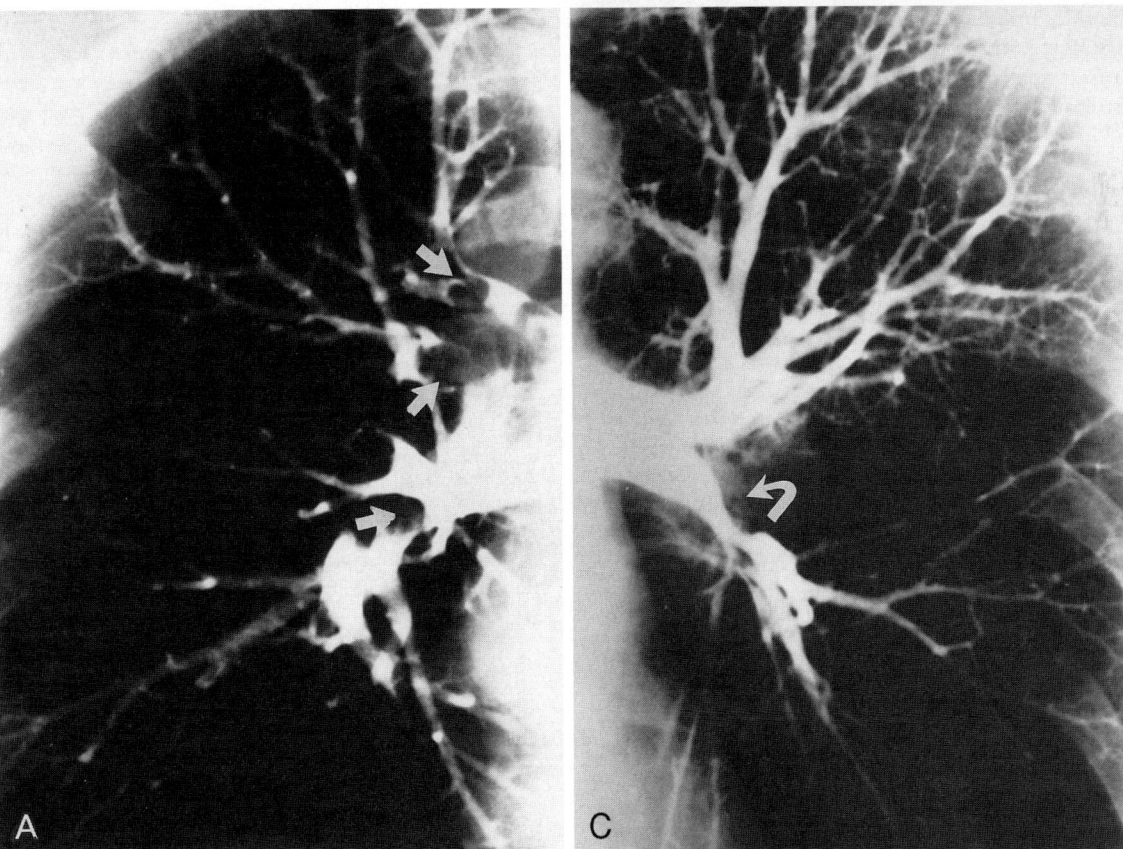

(Fig. 24.44B). Both are limited by spatial resolution and will miss small peripheral emboli (38).

Nonembolic Pathology

Pulmonary arteriovenous malformation (AVM) or pulmonary arteriovenous fistulas are abnormal communication between the pulmonary artery and vein, creating a right-to-left shunt. Although these fistulous communications may be acquired (trauma or infection), the majority are congenital. Most commonly, a single artery and vein in the lower lobe are involved; however, more complex lesions involve multiple vessels. One-third are multiple. Nearly 60% of patients with multiple pulmonary AVMs have associated extrathoracic hemangiomas or telangiectasias in a condition known as *hereditary hemorrhagic telangiectasia* or *Rendu-Osler-Weber syndrome.* Of patients with the syndrome, 15% have pulmonary AVMs. Complications include cyanosis, hemoptysis, thrombocytopenia, paradoxical embolus, and brain abscess.

Findings include lobulated masses of variable size usually located within the inner third of the lung adjacent to the hila. The feeding artery and draining vein may be detected. CT and MR are useful for documenting multiple lesions and further defining the anatomy. Angiography is reserved for equivocal cases and for planning of embolization or surgery.

Aneurysms. Mycotic aneurysms result from chronic TB (Rasmussen's aneurysm), septic emboli, and necrotizing pneumonias. They may rupture into a bronchus and cause hemoptysis. Dilated central pulmonary arteries may be seen with long-standing pulmonary hypertension, left-to-right cardiac shunts, and connective tissue disorders.

Occlusive Disorders. Narrowing and occlusion of the pulmonary arteries may be because of arteritis (e.g., Takayasu's), primary or metastatic pulmonary neoplasms (see Fig. 24.44C), extrinsic compression from granulomatous or neoplastic hilar nodes, or fibrosing mediastinitis. *Coarctation* of the pulmonary artery may be located either centrally or peripherally. The congenital type usually presents centrally and is associated with pulmonary valve stenosis and other cardiac abnormalities. Acquired coarctations seen in the postrubella syndrome can be either central or peripheral.

References

1. Kerns SR, Hawkins IF. Carbon dioxide digital subtraction angiography: expanding applications and technical evolution. AJR Am J Roentgenol 1995;164:735–741.

2. Sheppard S. Basic concepts in magnetic resonance angiography. Radiol Clin North Am 1995;33:91–113.

3. Benenati JF. Intravascular ultrasound: the role in diagnostic and therapeutic procedures. Radiol Clin North Am 1995;33:31–50.

4. Posniak HV, Demos TC, Marsan RE. Computed tomography of the normal aorta and thoracic aneurysms. Semin Roentgenol 1989;24:7–21.

5. Kadir S. Diagnostic Angiography. Philadelphia: WB Saunders, 1986:124–171.

6. Hessel SJ, Adams DF. Complications of angiography. Radiology 1981;138:273–281.

7. Cohan RH, Dunnick NR. Intravascular contrast media: adverse reactions. AJR Am J Roentgenol 1987;149:665–670.

8. Jaffe RB. Radiographic manifestations of congenital anomalies of the aortic arch. Radiol Clin North Am 1991;29:319–334.

9. Predy TA, McDonald V, Demos TC, Moncada R. CT of congenital anomalies of the aortic arch. Semin Roentgenol 1989;24:96–111.

10. Dee PM. The radiology of chest trauma. Radiol Clin North Am 1992; 30:291–306.

11. Marnocha KE, Maglinte DDT. Plain-film criteria for excluding aortic rupture in blunt chest trauma. AJR Am J Roentgenol 1985;144:19–21.

12. Mirvis SE, Kethirkamuganathan S, Miller BH, et al. Traumatic aortic injury: diagnosis with contrast-enhanced thoracic CT—five-year experience at a major trauma center. Radiology 1996;200:413–422.

13. Petsanick JP. Radiologic evaluation of aortic dissection. Radiology 1991;180:297–305.

14. Stanson AW. Roentgenographic findings in major vasculitic syndromes. Rheum Dis Clin North Am 1990;6:293–308.

15. Ishikawa K. Diagnostic approach and proposed criteria for the clinical diagnosis of Takayasu's arteriopathy. J Am Coll Cardiol 1988;12:964–972.

16. Rose SC, Kadir S. Arterial anatomy of the upper extremities. In: Kadir S, ed. Atlas of normal and variant angiographic anatomy. Philadelphia: WB Saunders, 1991.

17. Rose SC, Moore EE. Angiography in patients with arterial trauma: correlation between angiographic abnormalities, operative findings, and clinical outcome. AJR Am J Roentgenol 1987;149:613–619.

18. Bower TC, Cherry KJ, Pairolero PC. Unusual manifestations of abdominal aortic aneurysms. Surg Clin North Am 1989;69:745–754.

19. Bandyk DF. Preoperative imaging of aortic aneurysms. Surg Clin North Am 1989;69:721–735.

20. Darling RC, Messina CR, Brewster DC, et al. Autopsy study of unoperated abdominal aortic aneurysms. Circulation 1977;56:161–164.

21. Graham LM, Rubin JR. Visceral arterial aneurysms. In: Strandness DE, van Breda A, ed. Vascular diseases: surgical and interventional therapy. New York: Churchill Livingstone, 1994.

22. Mulligan SA, Matsuda T, Lanzer P, et al. Peripheral arterial occlusive disease: prospective comparison of MR angiography and color duplex US with conventional angiography. Radiology 1991;178:695–700.

23. Smullens SN. Surgically treatable lesions of the extracranial circulation, including the vertebral artery. Radiol Clin North Am 1986;24:453–460.

24. Wesen CA, Elliott BM. Fibromuscular dysplasia of the carotid arteries. Am J Surg 1986;151:448–451.

25. McAnespey D, Rosen RC, Cohen JM, et al. Adventitial cystic disease. J Foot Surg 1991;30:160–165.

26. Vogelzang RL, Limpert JD, Yao JST. Detection of prosthetic vascular complications: comparison of CT and angiography. AJR Am J Roentgenol 1987;148:819–823.

27. Pickering TG, Sos TA, Vaughan ED, et al. Predictive value and changes of renin secretion in hypertensive patients with unilateral renovascular disease undergoing successful renal angioplasty. Am J Med 1984; 76:398–403

28. Tegtmeyer CJ, Selby JB, Hartwell GD, et al. Results and complications of angioplasty in fibromuscular disease. Circulation 1991;83:I155–I161.

29. Kadir S, Ernest CB. Current concepts in angiographic management of gastrointestinal bleeding. Curr Prob Surg 1983;20:281–343.

30. Rosen RJ, Sanchez G. Angiographic diagnosis and management of gastrointestinal hemorrhage: current concepts. Radiol Clin North Am 1994;32:951–962.

31. Hunter GC, Guernsey JM. Mesenteric ischemia. Med Clin North Am 1988;72:1091–1115.

32. Morse SS, Clark RA. Management of nonocclusive and occlusive mesenteric ischemia. In: Kadir S, ed. Current practice of interventional radiology. Philadelphia: BC Decker, 1991.

33. Cormier MG, Yedlicka JW, Gray RJ, Moncada R Congenital anomalies of the superior vena cava: a CT study. Semin Roentgen 1989;24:77–83.

34. Dudiak CM, Olson MC, Posniak HV. Abnormalities of the azygos system: CT evaluation. Semin Roentgen 1989;24:47–55.

35. Yedlicka JW, Schultz K, Moncada R, Flisak M. CT findings in superior vena cava obstruction. Semin Roentgen 1989;24:84–90.

36. Ferris EJ. Deep venous thrombosis and pulmonary embolism: correlative evaluation and therapeutic implications. AJR Am J Roentgenol 1992;159:1149–1155.
37. Ferris EJ, Lim WN, Smith PL, Casali R. May-Thurner syndrome. Radiology 1983;147:29–31.
38. Dunnick NR, Newman GE, Perlmutt LM, Braun SD. Pulmonary embolism. Curr Prob Diagn Radiol 1988;17: 203–227.

Suggested Readings

Kadir S. Atlas of Normal and Variant Angiographic Anatomy. Philadelphia: WB Saunders, 1991.
Kadir S. Diagnostic Angiography. Philadelphia: WB Saunders, 1986.
Strandness DE, van Breda A. Vascular Diseases: Surgical and Interventional Therapy. New York: Churchill Livingstone, 1994.
Taveras JM, Ferrucci JT. Radiology. Philadelphia: WB Saunders, 1997.

25
Interventional Radiology

Mylon W. Marshall
John E. Williams

GENERAL PRINCIPLES

Interventional radiology is a field that has expanded the diagnostic applications of imaging to include methods of treating disease. Now a distinct specialty, the services of interventional radiologists have become indispensable in the modern delivery of health care. Among the most common diseases treated by interventionalists are vascular occlusive disease, life-threatening hemorrhage, renal and biliary obstruction, a variety of tumors, and complications of cancer. In addition, interventionalists are not uncommonly called on to find solutions to difficult clinical problems in patients with few, if any, therapeutic alternatives. If the site of disease is accessible using imaging guidance, it is potentially treatable by interventional methods.

Classification of interventions into *vascular* and *nonvascular* procedures is convenient. Vascular procedures generally involve methods of restoring or improving blood flow by various means of vascular recanalization, controlling hemorrhage or abnormal vascularity by transcatheter embolization, and placing vascular access catheters and other implantable devices. Needle biopsy and abscess drainage are nonvascular interventional procedures common in everyday radiologic practice. Other nonvascular interventions entail catheter-based therapy in organ systems such as bile ducts, genitourinary structures, GI tract, and pleural space.

Patient Care

Radiologists performing interventional procedures take an active role in the clinical management of patients (1). Before the procedure, this involves evaluation of the patient, assessment of indications and contraindications, and consultation with the referring physician. After establishing an indication, a targeted history and physical examination of the patient should be performed. Knowledge of pertinent laboratory results such as coagulation parameters, blood counts, renal and liver function, and electrolytes is necessary depending on the procedure. Availability of blood products may be indicated in anemic patients or patients at high risk for developing a bleeding complication. Emergent transfusion of packed red blood cells could become necessary. Transfusion of platelets or fresh frozen plasma before, during, or after the procedure may be required if coagulation parameters are abnormal. Severe uncorrectable coagulopathies are contraindications to virtually all percutaneous procedures. Prior imaging studies should be reviewed because they are often critical in planning the approach and execution of the intervention. When an indication is established, informed consent for the procedure is obtained prior to administration of conscious sedation. Risks and benefits of the procedure as well as of conservative and surgical options are thoroughly explained to the patient.

Proper care of the patient during the procedure is mandatory. IV access must be established in virtually all patients because emergency administration of fluids and medications may become necessary. Prophylactic antibiotics are indicated in some cases, such as abscess drainage, biliary procedures, genitourinary procedures, and other instances in which the risk of bacteremia is high. The skin access site is prepared by shaving and surgical scrub with povidone-iodine solution. Local anesthesia with 1–2% lidocaine or 0.25% bupivacaine hydrochloride is administered prior to needle puncture. *Conscious sedation* is the use of IV medications for patient comfort, sedation, and pain control. Commonly used agents include benzodiazepines such as midazolam (Versed) for sedation and analgesics such as fentanyl citrate (Sublimaze), meperidine hydrochloride (Demerol), or morphine sulfate for pain control. Use of these potent drugs during interventional procedures requires familiarity with managing their adverse reactions. The patient must be continuously monitored with electrocardiograpy, blood pressure, and pulse oximetry. A trained assistant, such as an interventional nurse, must be available to assume primary responsibility for monitoring the patient. Because the majority of patients receive conscious sedation as well as iodinated contrast, the radiologist must be familiar with their use and anticipate adverse reactions. In addition, it is crucial to recognize quickly and be prepared to treat a variety of procedural complications.

After the procedure, immediate and long-term follow-up of the patient is necessary to evaluate clinical success as well as to detect complications. Attention to detail in

Table 25.1. Lesion Appropriateness for Arterial Percutaneous Transluminal Angioplasty

Category	Description
1	Ideal lesions for PTA, which is considered the treatment of choice.
2	Still very amenable to PTA. These lesions may be slightly longer or more calcified than the most ideal lesions.
3	Less appropriate for PTA. PTA can be performed if the patient is not a surgical candidate or if there is insufficient vein available for bypass.
4	Poor candidates for PTA. In some cases, PTA may have a limited role if there is no surgical alternative.

the clinical care of patients is essential to the success of interventional procedures.

VASCULAR INTERVENTION

Percutaneous Transluminal Angioplasty

Percutaneous transluminal angioplasty (PTA) is a versatile procedure in which a stenosed blood vessel is dilated by inflating a catheter-mounted balloon. Under fluoroscopic observation, the balloon catheter is placed over a guidewire into position using an angiogram as a "road map." The PTA concept predates modern angioplasty balloons by a decade. In 1964, Dotter and Judkins (2) first described percutaneous dilation of a stenotic artery using successive dilations with incrementally larger diameter catheters. This has come to be known as the "Dotter technique." Charles Dotter has come to be regarded as the father of interventional radiology for this and other innovative ideas involving percutaneous catheter-based procedures.

The angioplasty balloon catheter has undergone technical improvements and modifications since its introduction by Gruntzig in 1974. Materials have improved, with the end result of causing less trauma to vascular endothelium. Guidewire technology has similarly advanced. There are a variety of balloon characteristics and guidewire combinations that can be exploited. For example, low-profile balloon catheters and small-caliber guidewires are useful in treating small vessel stenoses for which standard sizes would be too large. A high-pressure balloon may be the only method of successfully treating an otherwise resistant, fibrous venous stenosis. Hydrophilic coatings permit easier negotiation of difficult or highly diseased areas by reducing friction. Such coatings have been applied to balloons, catheters, and guidewires. Despite the variety of products available, the concept remains unchanged since its inception: percutaneous treatment of stenotic blood vessels with the use of a catheter-based system using radiologic guidance.

Clinical indications for PTA vary according to site of disease. Depending on disease distribution and severity, PTA can provide definitive therapy or serve as an adjunct to surgery for improving patency of vascular bypass. In the lower extremities, symptoms of chronic ischemia that justify intervention include lifestyle-limiting claudication, rest pain, or tissue devitalization such as nonhealing ulcers or gangrenous changes. In the upper extremities, symptomatic vertebral steal or upper-extremity claudication are indica-

tions for PTA. Dilatation of significant renal artery stenosis for renovascular hypertension or renal insufficiency is efficacious. Renal PTA is the treatment of choice for fibromuscular dysplasia, transplant renal artery stenosis, and most atherosclerotic stenoses. PTA is potentially useful in virtually any vascular system in which hemodynamically significant stenoses result in clinically significant symptoms.

Guidelines for appropriate application of PTA have been developed by the Society of Cardiovascular and Interventional Radiology. Appropriateness is determined by considering the risk-to-benefit ratio of PTA compared with surgery for symptomatic ischemia and is based on lesion characteristics and location. This classification addresses the likelihood of achieving a successful outcome while minimizing complications (Table 25.1) (3).

Classifying a lesion varies according to the vessel under consideration, but several general principles can be appreciated. Factors that predict a successful angioplasty result include *a) length of the stenosis*—shorter lesions (<3 cm) have better outcomes than do longer ones (>7 cm); *b) lesion morphology*—concentric stenosis are better than eccentric; and *c) calcification or ulceration*—heavily calcified lesions do not respond as well (3). In general, PTA of large arteries yields better results than does treatment of smaller caliber arteries.

Mechanism. The mechanism of PTA is multifactorial. Controlled vessel injury occurs by stretching the vessel wall, irreversibly disrupting medial elastic fibers. This prevents elastic recoil, a major cause of PTA failure. Fracture of the plaque and underlying intima also occurs (Fig. 25.1). A cleft in the lesion forms, which extends through the intima and into the media. This can often be seen angiographically as

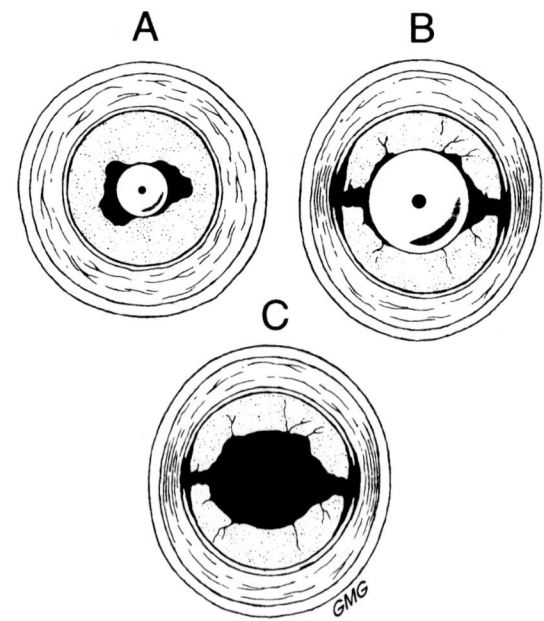

Figure 25.1. Angioplasty Mechanism. A. Cross section of an artery narrowed by atherosclerotic plaque. A balloon is positioned within the vessel lumen. **B.** When the balloon is inflated, it fractures the plaque and a portion of the intima. There is also stretching of the media, which is necessary to prevent elastic recoil. **C.** The diameter of the arterial lumen is larger following PTA. (Adapted from Cope C, Burke DR, Meranze S. Atlas of interventional radiology. Philadelphia: JB Lippincott Company, 1990.)

linear contrast collections outside main vessel lumen (Fig. 25.2C). Healing and remodeling occur during a period of months, resulting in a larger diameter vessel lumen (4).

Various pharmacologic agents play an adjunctive role in both PTA and vascular stent placement. Aspirin prevents platelet aggregation at the PTA site. It is administered at least one day prior to the procedure, and the patient is continued on oral daily aspirin (325 mg) indefinitely. Before

balloon dilatation, systemic heparin administration is often given to prevent acute thrombotic complications. A standard adult dose is 50–100 U/kg. Adequacy of anticoagulation can be monitored by periodic assessment of activated clotting times (ACT) during the procedure, which can guide the need for more heparin as well as the timing of catheter removal. An ACT of greater than 200 is considered adequate anticoagulation in most instances. Vascular anti-

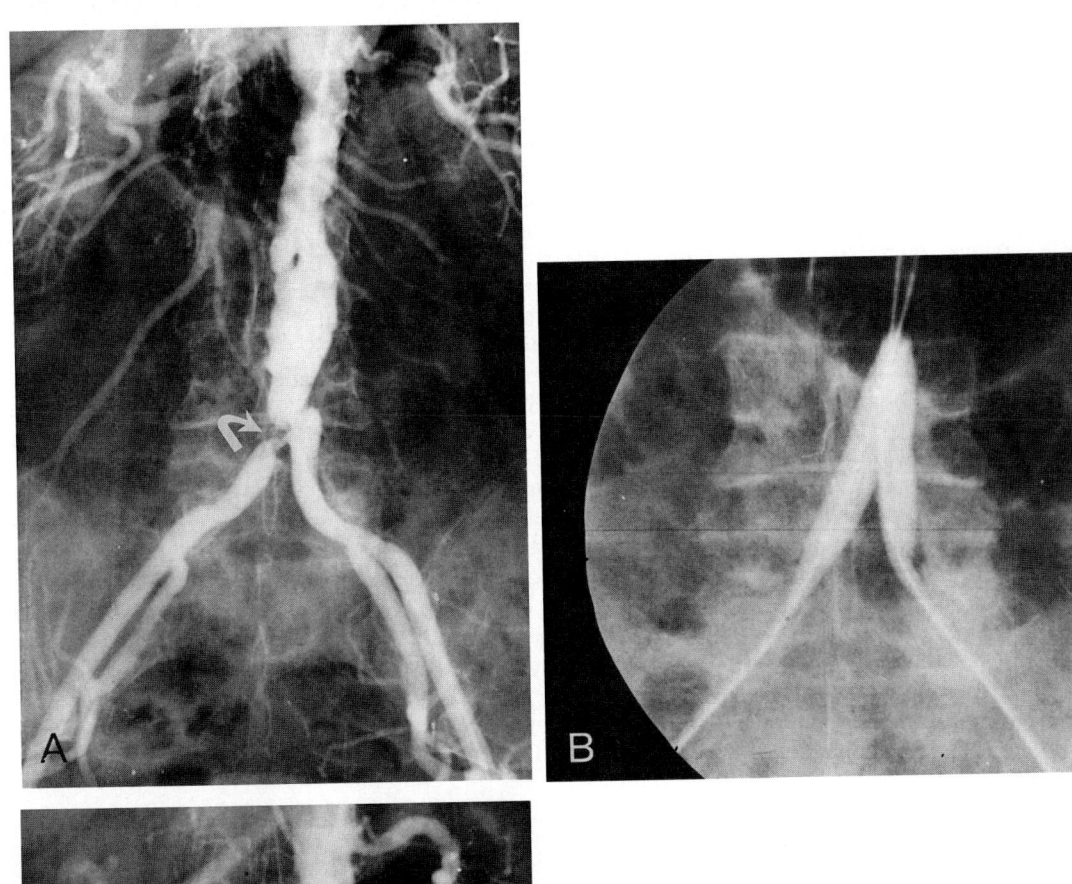

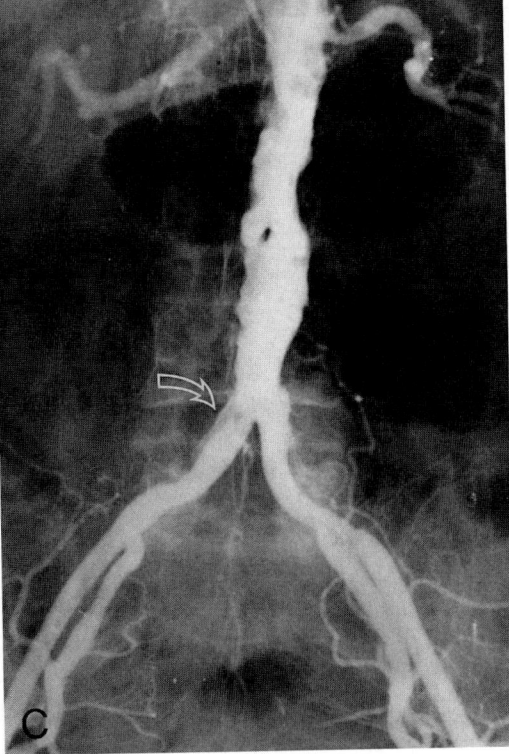

Figure 25.2. Common Iliac Artery Occlusive Disease and Angioplasty. **A**. Aortic injection shows a tight stenosis at the origin of the right common iliac artery (*arrow*). **B**. To provide support for the angioplasty balloon and protection of the contralateral common iliac artery, a "kissing" balloon technique is utilized for angioplasty. **C**. Postangioplasty result shows improved patency of the right iliac artery (*arrow*). Note the intimal cleft representing a normal intimal "crack" seen with angioplasty.

spasmodics are also useful. Nifedipine is a calcium channel blocker that prevents vasospasm. It is given sublingually in 10-mg doses 15–20 minutes prior to PTA of vessels particularly prone to vasospasm such as renal, tibial, vertebral, or upper-extremity arteries. Intra-arterial nitroglycerine (100 μg), papaverine (30 mg), or tolazoline (25 mg) may be used to treat vasospasm. Blood pressure response and heart rate must be closely monitored when using these drugs (5).

Procedure. The lesion is carefully crossed with a guidewire, followed by advancement of a diagnostic catheter. Once across the lesion, contrast can be injected through the catheter to confirm an intraluminal position. The catheter is exchanged over a guidewire for the angioplasty balloon catheter. Care is taken to determine the optimal C-arm fluoroscopy obliquity before PTA or stent placement. The lesion is precisely localized using digital road-mapping techniques, external radio-opaque markers, or bony landmarks. The balloon is centered across the lesion and slowly inflated with a dilute contrast–saline mixture under fluoroscopic control (Fig. 25.2B). The lesion initially deforms the balloon, forming a "waist" on the balloon, until a pressure is achieved great enough to dilate the lesion fully. The patient usually feels a mild to moderate amount of pain during inflation. Lack of pain may indicate underdilation, and severe pain, which does not subside on balloon deflation, may herald vascular rupture. Duration and pressure of inflation are not standardized. It is important to achieve a pressure high enough to overcome elastic recoil.

After balloon deflation and removal, contrast is injected to assess the result. The guidewire is left in place across the PTA site *at all times* in case further intervention, such as redilation or stent placement, is required. If the result is satisfactory, pressure measurements may be taken to assess the hemodynamic result in most vessels.

Balloon Sizing. PTA balloons are sized by length (in centimeters) and diameter (in millimeters). The nominal balloon diameter is chosen by measuring the diameter of a normal segment of artery near the lesion or a comparable normal segment in the contralateral artery. The balloon length should be long enough to span the lesion but short enough to minimize exposure of normal endothelium to the traumatic effects of balloon inflation. A measurement uncorrected for magnification on a cut-film angiographic image is chosen because this will result in overdilatation of the lesion by a factor of 10–20%, a desired effect in most cases. PTA of the aorta is an instance in which overdilatation should not be performed. The aorta and other vessels with large diameters are more prone to rupture owing to their increased wall tension (Law of La Place). Vessel sizing on newer angiographic equipment can be made using digital images by automated calibration to a known quantity such as French size of the catheter or distance of the radiographic source to the target.

Complications of PTA include intimal dissection, thrombosis, distal embolization, and vessel rupture; fortunately, the latter is rare. Patients on chronic steroid therapy and those with certain collagen diseases such as Ehlers-Danlos type IV are at greater risk of rupture. Risks of diagnostic angiography such as contrast reactions, renal failure, and puncture site hematoma also apply.

Results. Aortoiliac PTA has been extensively studied and achieves excellent technical and long-term outcomes (Fig. 25.2). Technical success and 1-year patency rates are approximately 90%, and 5-year patency is approximately 70% (5). Technical success in femoropopliteal PTA (Fig. 25.3) is also good at 80–90%. One-year patency is 60%, and 5-year patency is approximately 40% (6). Tibial PTA is useful in the setting of severe is-

Figure 25.3. Superficial Femoral Artery Atherosclerotic Stenosis. A. Atherosclerotic changes of the superficial femoral artery are seen with a focal dominant tight stenosis (*arrow*). **B.** After angioplasty, there is resolution of the stenosis (*arrows*).

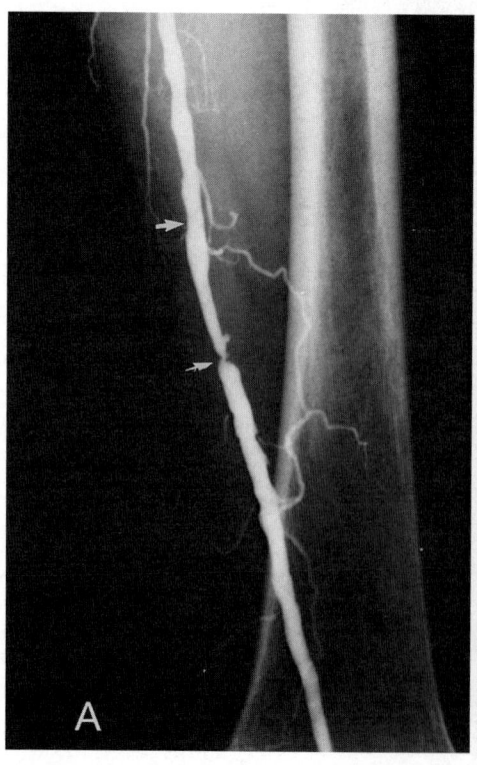
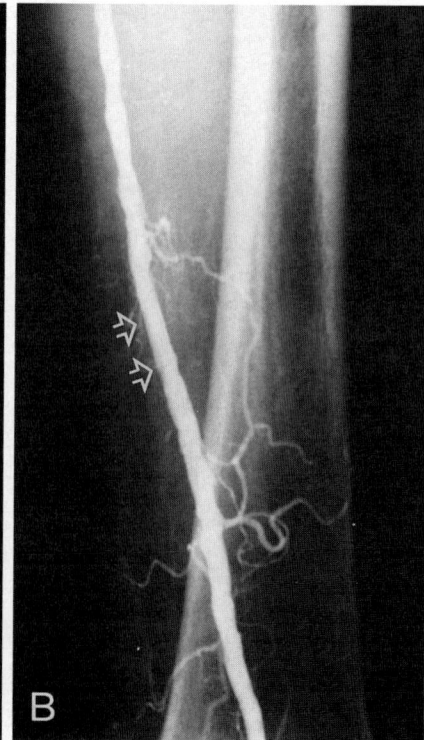

chemia causing rest pain, tissue ulceration, or gangrene. The majority of patients undergoing PTA for limb salvage are diabetic. Reported 2-year limb salvage rates range from approximately 40–80% (7,8). In patients with renovascular hypertension, renal PTA is technically successful in approximately 90% of cases. There is an approximately 90% benefit in fibromuscular dysplasia and a 70% benefit in atherosclerotic disease. Roughly half of patients with chronic renal insufficiency show improvement in serum creatinine levels (5).

Vascular Stents

Stents are medical devices that are used to provide support to living tissue during repair and healing of injury. Stents vary in their design, means of deployment, and physical characteristics. Intravascular stents have in common a cylindrical shape and a meshwork of metal struts. When they are deployed in a vessel, the struts must be adequately embedded into the vessel wall. This promotes rapid re-endothelialization and improves long-term patency (9). The most widely used intravascular stents are the two that are FDA-approved for iliac artery stenting at the time of this writing, the Palmaz stent (Johnson & Johnson Interventional Systems, Warren, NJ) and the Wallstent (Schneider, Minneapolis, MN). The *Palmaz stent* (Fig. 25.4), constructed of stainless steel, is rigid and strong. It is mounted on an angioplasty balloon, which expands with balloon inflation. It can be very accurately positioned at the target location under fluoroscopic observation. The *Wallstent* (Fig. 25.5), first approved for use in the biliary system, is made of a stainless steel alloy. It is a self-expanding stent premounted on a catheter, deployed by retracting a rolling membrane that constrains it. The Wallstent is flexible and can be placed in curved or tortuous vessel segments. Because it will re-expand when compressed, it is often used in vessels exposed to potential external forces such as the arms, legs, and neck. Both the Palmaz stent and the Wallstent are available in a wide variety of lengths and diameters. Other stent designs are in widespread use outside of the United States and will likely be approved for intravascular use in this country in the near future.

Indications. The development of vascular stents during the past several years is a major advance, improving angioplasty results. Use of an intravascular stent is often able to convert a suboptimal PTA result, due to intimal dissection or elastic recoil, into a success. Residual stenosis, a resting pressure gradient greater than 5 mm Hg, and significant intimal dissection following PTA are accepted indications for stent placement after PTA. Restenosis of a lesion previously treated with either PTA or atherectomy is another common indication for intravascular stenting. Indications for primary stenting (use of a stent without a trial of PTA) are less well defined. Primary stenting of chronic iliac occlusions is well accepted (10), and there is wide agreement that primary stenting of iliac artery stenoses is justified (Fig. 25.6). Use of stents is contraindicated in the setting of PTA-induced vascular rupture or if there is ongoing infection with bacteremia. *Stent-grafts* are stents covered by vascular graft material that renders them nonporous. These devices will play a future role in nonsurgical repair of vascular rupture. Such devices are also useful in the treatment of aneurysms and currently are being evaluated in the treatment of abdominal aortic aneurysms (11).

Results. Stent placement improves immediate PTA outcomes by treating flow limiting dissections and reducing residual postintervention pressure gradients to near zero. In addition, primary iliac stenting appears to improve long-term patency (12). Primary patency of Palmaz stents in iliac arteries is approximately 90% at 1 year, 85% at 2 years, and 70% at 4 years (13). Growing evidence for Wallstent placement in iliac arteries indicates comparable results (14). In the superficial femoral arteries, primary stenting offers no advantage over PTA alone (15). Primary renal artery stenting of ostial atherosclerotic renal artery stenoses is probably justified, although restenosis rates are high (16).

Thrombolysis

Peripheral vascular thromboembolism causing occlusion can result in major morbidity or mortality if not accurately diagnosed and appropriately treated. In acute lower extremity ischemia, prompt restoration of blood flow is of paramount importance. The time available to achieve reperfusion varies with the severity of ischemia. Surgical intervention is indicated in severely ischemic limbs with motor and sensory loss because a delay in revascularization will lead to certain amputation. Because more time is necessary to achieve reperfusion using transcatheter techniques, thrombolysis is used in cases in which the extremity is less profoundly ischemic (Fig. 25.7).

Thrombolysis is the process of clot dissolution. Thrombolytic agents are delivered directly into a thrombus or an embolus with an intravascular catheter. Catheter-directed thrombolysis is used to treat native arterial or bypass graft thrombosis, embolic occlusions, thrombosed hemodialysis access shunts, and deep venous thrombosis. It is an effective and well-established method of restoring blood flow in acute and subacute thrombotic occlusion. Classic signs and symptoms include rest pain, absent pulses, a pale, cool extremity, sensory impairment, and paralysis if ischemia is profound. Once blood flow is re-established, an underlying "culprit" lesion such as a stenosis is often found. This lesion, responsible for precipitating thrombosis, must be treated. This can often be achieved with percutaneous techniques such as angioplasty or stent placement. Surgical revascularization may also be indicated depending on the nature of the underlying problem. Occasionally, no culprit lesion is uncovered. Thrombosis in these cases may be related to hypercoagulability, hypotension, or external compression of the graft.

Contraindications to thrombolytic therapy include active bleeding, recent GI hemorrhage, intracranial tumor, recent stroke or neurosurgery, and irreversible extremity ischemia. A number of relative contraindications exist such as recent major surgery or biopsy, recent trauma or CPR, severe uncontrolled hypertension, coagulopathy, and pregnancy.

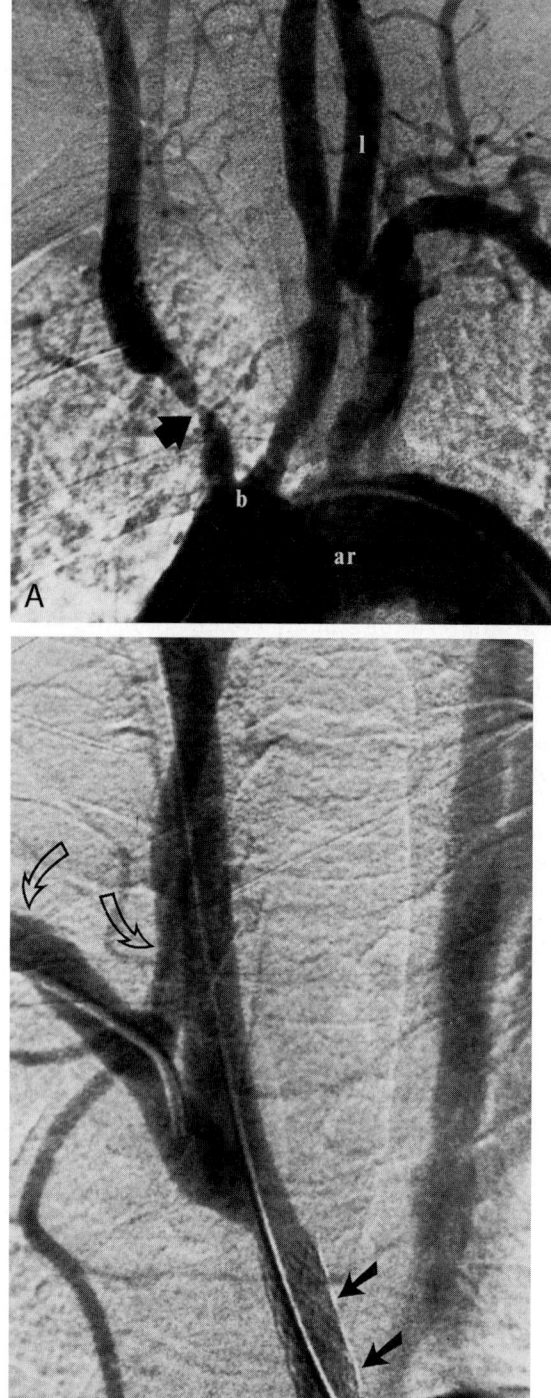

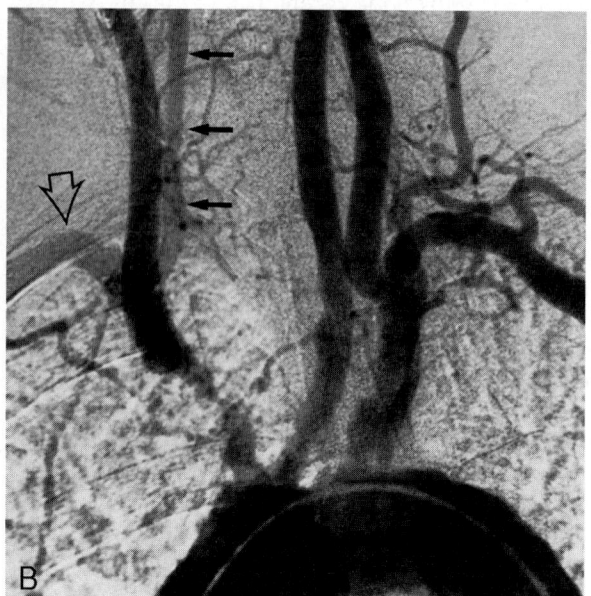

Figure 25.4. Brachiocephalic Artery Stent. A. This patient with severe right brachiocephalic artery stenosis also had severe left internal carotid artery stenosis (not shown). *ar,* aortic arch; *b,* bovine left common carotid origin; *l,* left vertebral artery with compensatory enlargement. **B.** Subclavian steal is evident on a delayed image. There is retrograde filling of the right vertebral artery (*arrows*) and reconstitution of the right subclavian artery (*open arrow*). **C.** After Palmaz stent placement (*arrows*), the stenosis has resolved. Antegrade flow has been re-established in the right vertebral and subclavian arteries (*open arrows*). (Courtesy of Pat Vogel, Sacramento, California.)

A basic understanding of the clotting cascade is helpful in the discussion of thrombolytic agents. Thrombin, formed by intrinsic or extrinsic coagulation pathways, converts fibrinogen to fibrin. Interaction of fibrin with platelets, vascular endothelium, and other substances results in fibrin cross-linking with clot formation. Plasmin, derived from plasminogen, disrupts fibrin cross-

links to achieve clot dissolution. Several pharmacologic agents are in use that exploit the action of plasmin. *Urokinase* is the most often used for peripheral thrombolysis. A human protein with a half-life of approximately 17 minutes, it directly activates plasminogen to form plasmin, causing clot lysis. Recombinant tissue plasminogen activator (rt-PA), another direct plasminogen activator, is widely used in the emergency treatment of myocardial infarction. Streptokinase is an indirect plasminogen activator. Although effective, it is currently used less frequently than urokinase primarily because of allergic complications and a relatively unpredictable dose response.

Procedure. A diagnostic angiogram is performed to determine the location and extent of thromboembolus and underlying atherosclerotic disease. The occluded vessel is catheterized and a guidewire traversal test is performed (17). This maneuver, in which the guidewire is used to test the firmness of the occluded segment, provides important prognostic information. Success with thrombolytic therapy is highest with soft thrombus, through which the guidewire passes easily, enabling catheter placement directly into the thrombus. The like-

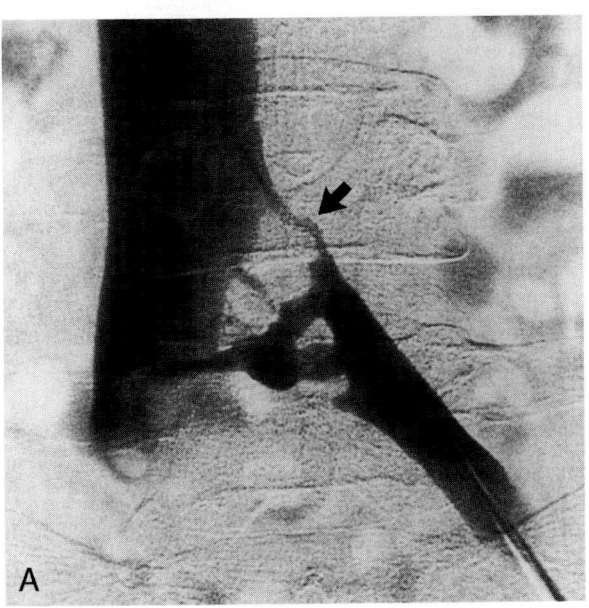
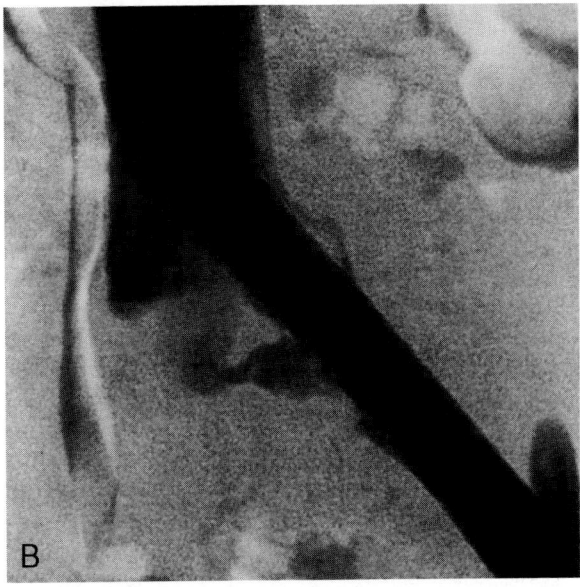

Figure 25.5. Venous Stent. A. Left iliac vein origin is irregularly stenosed with a weblike appearance. Known as May-Thurner syndrome, this condition is caused by extrinsic compression of the crossing right common iliac artery. **B.** A venous stent has been placed to treat the stenosis.

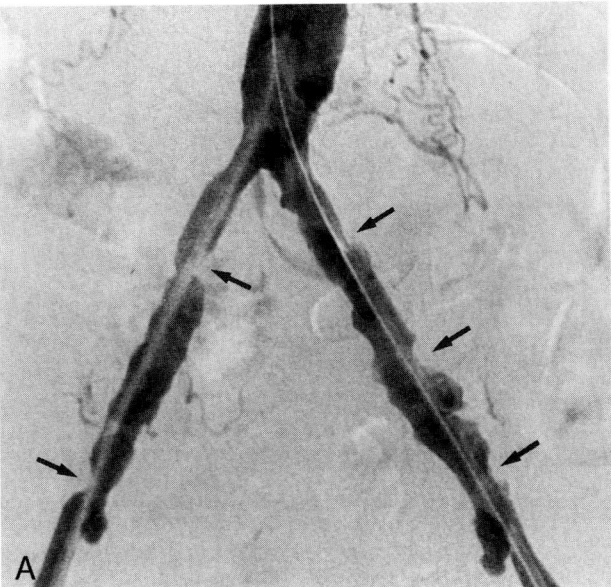
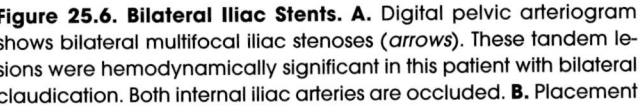
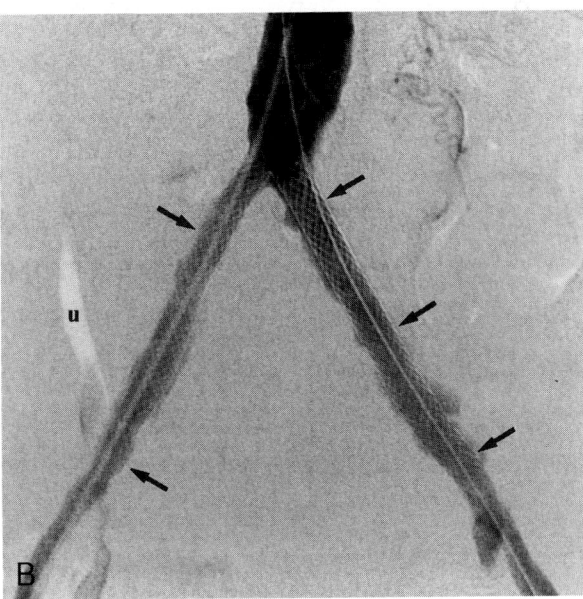

Figure 25.6. Bilateral Iliac Stents. A. Digital pelvic arteriogram shows bilateral multifocal iliac stenoses (*arrows*). These tandem lesions were hemodynamically significant in this patient with bilateral claudication. Both internal iliac arteries are occluded. **B.** Placement of bilateral iliac self-expanding Wallstents (*arrows*) results in angiographic and hemodynamic improvement. Single stents were used in each artery. *u,* ureter. (Courtesy of Pat Vogel, Sacramento, California.)

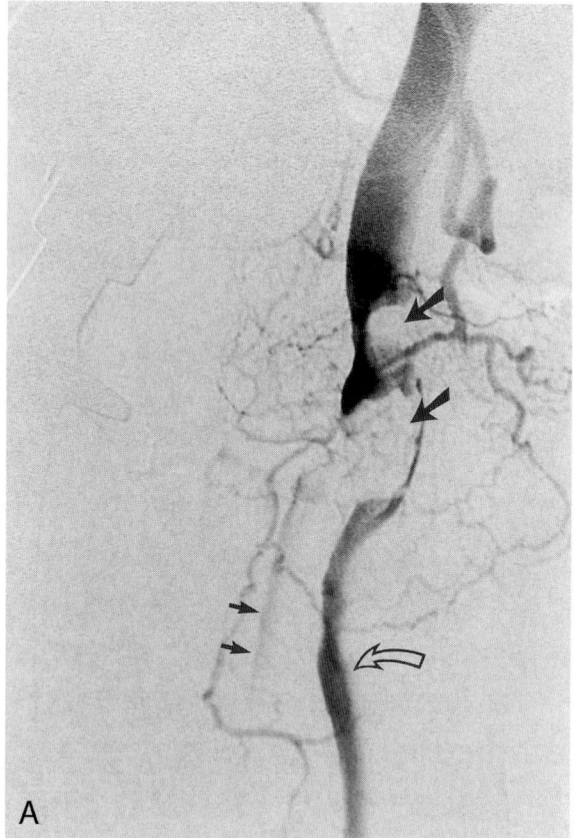

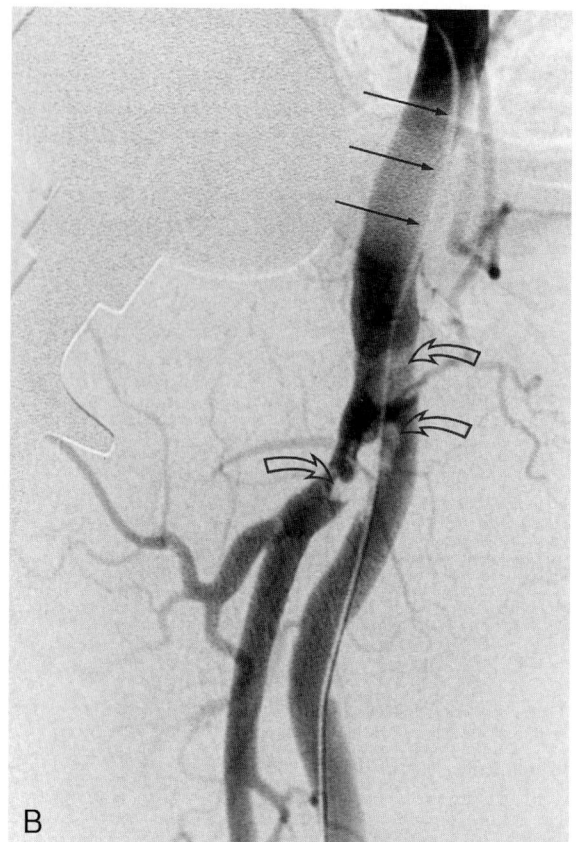

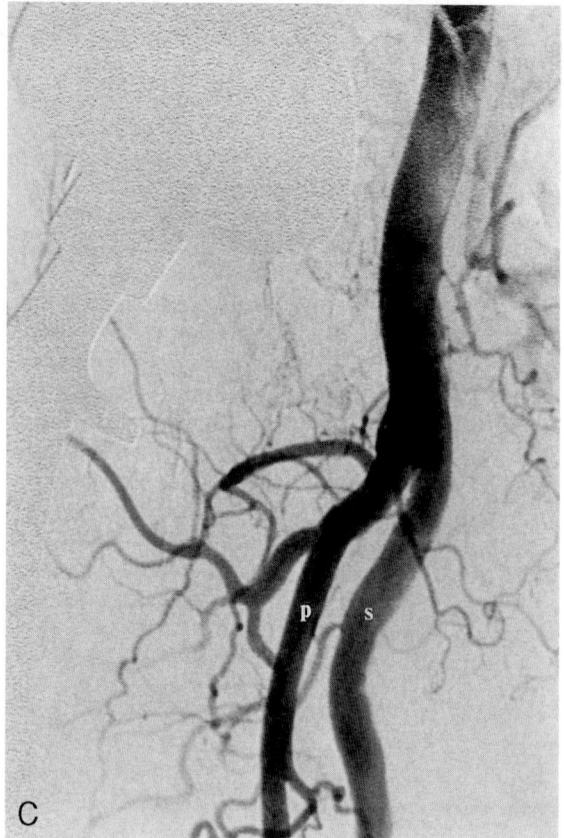

Figure 25.7. Common Femoral Artery Embolus. A. A large embolus (*large black arrows*) has lodged at the common femoral bifurcation in this patient with an acutely ischemic lower limb. Minimal flow is present in the profunda femoris artery (*small black arrows*) and superficial femoral artery (*curved open arrow*) distal to the embolus. **B.** After 12 hours of thrombolytic infusion, the embolus is significantly smaller (*curved open arrows*) and flow has improved distal to the embolus. *Black arrows* depict location of the guidewire. **C.** The embolus has completely resolved after 36 hours of infusion. No further intervention was necessary. *p*, profunda femoris artery; *s*, superficial femoral artery.

lihood of technical success is reduced when guidewire passage is not possible. A short trial of thrombolysis may be helpful because this may soften the clot enough to allow guidewire placement.

Several urokinase dosing protocols are used. Doses vary depending on the institution, physician preference, and clinical circumstances. Generally, doses range from 800–1000 U/min (50,000–60,000 U/h) to 4000 U/min (240,000 U/h). Doses closer to the lower rate are often considered *low dose*, whereas those in the higher range are *high dose* (17–19). Infusion rates are often individualized, with adjustments made as thrombolysis progresses or clinical conditions change. Anticoagulation with systemic heparin is also necessary to prevent pericatheter thrombus formation and rethrombosis. Close clinical monitoring for bleeding complications, heparin effect with PTT levels, and status of the affected limb is important during the course of the infusion. This requires an intensive care setting in most centers.

The infusion of urokinase through a catheter embedded in the thrombus helps prevent a *systemic lytic state*, which occurs when serum fibrinogen levels begin to drop to precipitously low levels. This condition significantly increases the risk of a bleeding complication. As a general guideline, when serum fibrinogen levels drop to less than 150 μg/mL without clinical evidence of bleeding, the dose should be reduced by half. If the level falls to 100 μg/mL or less, thrombolytic infusion is terminated for a period until fibrinogen levels rise again. Saline may be infused to maintain catheter patency. If a serious bleeding complication occurs, thrombolytic therapy is discontinued. Reversal of the lytic state with administration of fresh frozen plasma should be considered.

As with all areas of interventional radiology, materials and techniques have evolved over time. Thrombolytic infusions were first performed as a therapeutic extension of diagnostic angiography, using the diagnostic end-hole catheter embedded in the thrombosed vessel to administer thrombolytic agents. Later, coaxial infusions were popularized with the advent of infusable wires. This allowed longer segments of clot to be infused. Today, a variety of multisidehole catheters, as well as infusable wires or microcatheters, are available for use. Multisidehole catheters can be used alone or in a coaxial manner with an infusable wire.

Complications. The most common *complication* of thrombolysis is bleeding such as a puncture-site hematoma. Transfusion or operative repair are required in less than 10% of cases. Major abdominal, retroperitoneal, or thoracic hemorrhage occur in less than 5% of cases. The incidence of intracranial hemorrhage is less than 1% (20). Pericatheter thrombus formation, distal embolization, and compartment syndrome are other potential complications. Anticipation, early recognition, and appropriate treatment of complications reduce their clinical impact and increase the likelihood of achieving a good outcome.

The clinical success rate for arterial thrombolysis for acute ischemia is 85–90% (21). Acute upper extremity ischemia also responds well to thrombolysis (22) (Fig. 25.8).

Venous Thrombolysis for the treatment of acute deep venous thrombosis (DVT) is growing in acceptance. Complications of lower extremity DVT include leg swelling and pain, debilitating lower extremity edema because of chronic venous insufficiency, and pulmonary embolus. Left iliofemoral DVT is more common than right due to *May-Thurner syndrome* (Fig. 25.9). Indwelling central venous catheters or malignant central venous stenoses can be complicated by upper-extremity venous thrombosis. Primary axillosubclavian thrombosis, also known as *Paget-Schroetter syndrome*, also results in upper-extremity venous thrombosis. It is precipitated by extrinsic subclavian vein narrowing resulting from normal variations in anatomy such as a cervical rib, slips of fascia, or hypertrophied musculature.

Transcatheter techniques, widely used in the arterial system, have been applied in the deep venous system to address these complications (Fig. 25.10). Treatment of DVT in this manner is based on rationale that traditional anticoagulation therapy prevents further thrombosis but does nothing to actually treat the existing clot burden. Directly recanalizing acute venous occlusions leads to more rapid resolution of symptoms than is achieved with traditional therapy. It also greatly increases the likelihood that valve function will be preserved, preventing long-term morbidity associated with lower extremity venous insufficiency. Chronic venous insufficiency results from valvular damage that occurs when deep venous thrombosis heals slowly over time with fibrosis and retraction of clot adherent to valve cusps. A greater than 90% rate of recanalization in lower extremity DVT, with complete resolution of acute symptoms in approximately 80% of patients, has recently been reported with transcatheter thrombolysis (23).

Embolization

Transcatheter embolization is indicated as definitive or adjunctive therapy in a wide variety of clinical situations. Its most dramatic use is in the setting of uncontrolled bleeding when medical and surgical therapy are unsuccessful or inappropriate. Not only can embolization control bleeding and often avoid or minimize surgery, but it is sometimes the only way a life can be saved.

Traumatic injuries, tumor rupture, GI bleeding, massive hemoptysis, postpartum hemorrhage, and epistaxis are among the most important indications for embolization to control active hemorrhage. Primary treatment of arteriovenous malformations (AVMs), testicular varicoceles, hypersplenism, and selected hepatic tumors are other applications of transcatheter embolization. Preoperative embolization is useful to minimize blood loss during surgery in some cases (Fig. 25.11).

In addition to general contraindications for angiography, a unique contraindication to bear in mind is the inability to achieve safe access to the target vessel. An unstable catheter position imposes a high likelihood for nontarget embolization (24).

Procedure. After identifying hemorrhage on an arteriogram, embolization is performed by positioning a catheter tip selectively into the bleeding vessel. Assessment

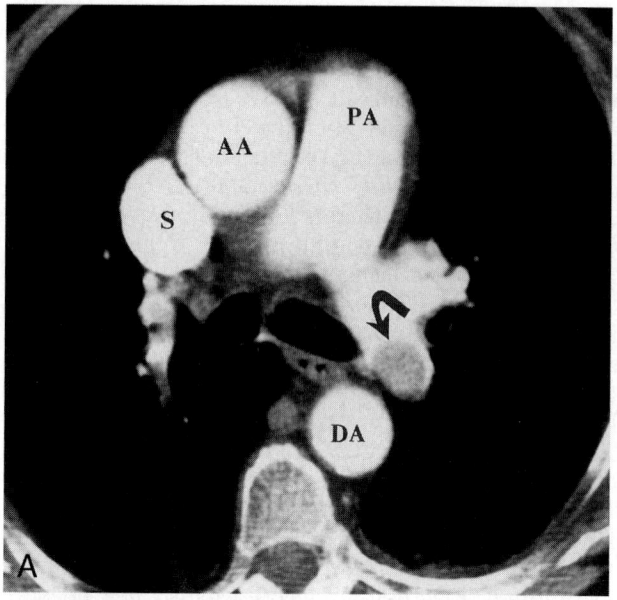

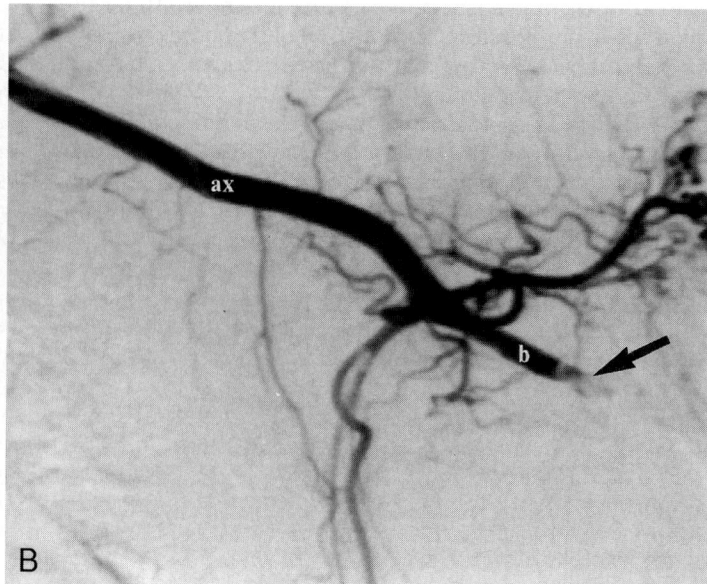

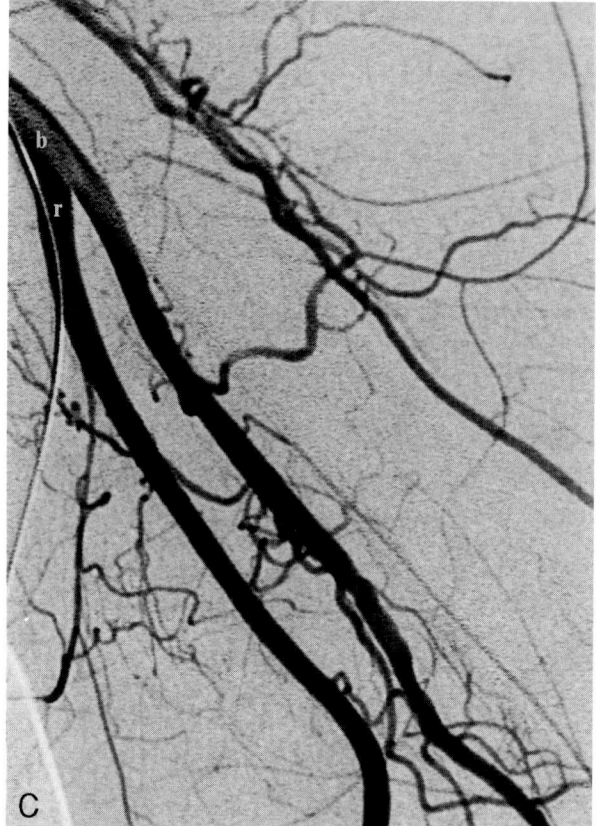

Figure 25.8. Embolism Through Patent Foramen Ovale. A. Helical CT of pulmonary arteries demonstrates pulmonary embolus (*curved arrow*). The patient presented with hypoxia and arm ischemia. **B.** The proximal brachial artery (*b*) is occluded by an acute embolus (*arrow*). Pulmonary embolus resulted in acute elevation of pulmonary pressures, allowing systemic embolization through a patent foramen ovale. **C.** Complete thrombolysis has been achieved. Note high origin of the radial artery (*r*) from the proximal brachial artery (*b*). *AA*, ascending aorta; *ax*, axillary artery; *DA*, descending aorta; *S*, superior vena cava. (Courtesy of Pat Vogel, Sacramento, California.)

of the bleeding site with regard to collateral blood flow to the affected organ is critical because the vessel is sacrificed. Embolization of end arteries with no potential for collateral flow will result in tissue necrosis. A vascular sheath is used during embolization to preserve access should the catheter become occluded. Once a stable catheter position is achieved, an embolic agent is carefully delivered through the catheter under fluoroscopic control. Keep in mind that flow dynamics change as em-

bolization progresses. It is best to avoid "overembolization" of the vessel. Nontarget embolization can be avoided by achieving a secure catheter position within the target vessel and by adhering to meticulous technique during embolization (25).

Selection of the appropriate embolic material is based on knowledge of the materials available and the clinical scenarios in which they are used. In certain situations, a combination of agents is useful. Materials in widespread use are particulate agents, sclerosants, and metallic coils. Agents are classified by the size of vessel that is occluded and by whether the occlusion is temporary or permanent (26).

Gelfoam (Upjohn, Kalamazoo, MI) is a widely used temporary agent that is absorbed by the body during the course of several days to several weeks. It is available in spongy sheets or as a powder. The powder form is no longer recommended for use because of high rates of tissue infarction. Gelfoam sheets are cut into variably sized pieces ranging from 1–2-mm squares to larger "torpedoes." It can also be used in a slurry form, which is quick and easy to prepare. Gelfoam causes a panarteritis and promotes thrombosis. It is useful in controlling hemorrhage in situations in which the organ involved is expected to undergo normal healing, given adequate collateral blood flow (Fig. 25.12). Examples include traumatic pelvic and extremity hemorrhage and benign causes of upper GI bleeding in otherwise healthy patients.

Permanent agents include coils, polyvinyl alcohol foam, and absolute ethanol. Detachable balloons and glue are also permanent agents but are not routinely available. *Polyvinyl alcohol foam* is available in multiple particle sizes, ranging from 100 to 1000 μm. The particles occlude at the arteriolar level. The smaller the particle size, the more peripheral it will lodge in the arteriole. Smaller particle sizes are very effective embolic agents but increase the risk for tissue necrosis. A robust inflammatory response occurs with vessel thrombosis, fibroblast invasion, and formation of dense fibrous connective tissue. Although classified as permanent, recanalization can occur over time. It is useful in treating various tumors and some forms of hemorrhage.

Tissue sclerosants are liquid agents that cause vessel thrombosis, endothelial denudation, and tissue necrosis. The chief examples are alcohol (dehydrated ethanol) and sodium tetradecyl sulfate (Sotradecol). These agents are useful in treating venous malformations, certain tumors,

or other entities for which capillary level occlusion is desired. Flow must be slowed sufficiently to allow prolonged contact with the vessel wall. An occlusion balloon can be used to slow down blood flow. Dehydrated ethanol is not radiopaque and can be very painful. These agents are not used in the emergency treatment of active bleeding.

Coils achieve a physiologic result analogous to surgical vessel ligation. Some are designed for placement through a 5F diagnostic catheter, whereas others must be delivered with a 3F microcatheter (Fig. 25.13). They are fashioned from stainless steel or platinum wire segments of various calibers and are manufactured to assume a variety of predetermined shapes and diameters when fully deployed. Coils must be carefully chosen on the basis of the diameter of the vessel to be embolized to avoid complications. Nominal coil sizes describe the diameter of the coil loops when fully deployed, as well as length of the coil wire when completely straightened. The size of the catheter lumen determines the caliber of the coil that can be used. Polyester fibers are often attached to the coil surface to promote thrombosis. Coils are considered permanent occlusive devices and are useful in trauma and selected other bleeding emergencies (25). Coils should not be used when recurrent hemorrhage is likely, such as in the treatment of massive hemoptysis, as their use prevents future access to the vessel should rebleeding occur. Coils are also used in the treatment of testicular varicoceles (Fig. 25.14) and pulmonary AVMs.

Complications of embolization include pain, target organ ischemia, nontarget embolization, and abscess formation. Examples of nontarget embolization include spinal or bowel infarction during renal embolization, stomach or duodenal infarction during liver chemoembolization, and escape of embolic material into arterial circulation during embolization of pulmonary AVMs. Target ischemia results in symptoms because of devascularization in the vicinity of the target organ such as bowel ischemia during subselective mesenteric emboli-

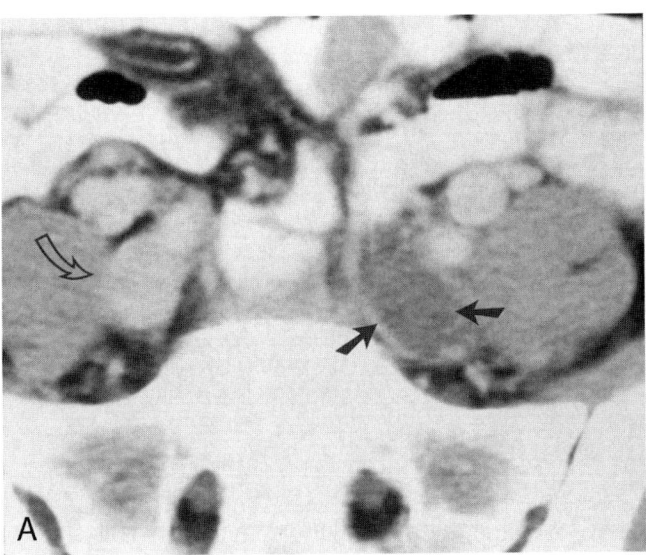

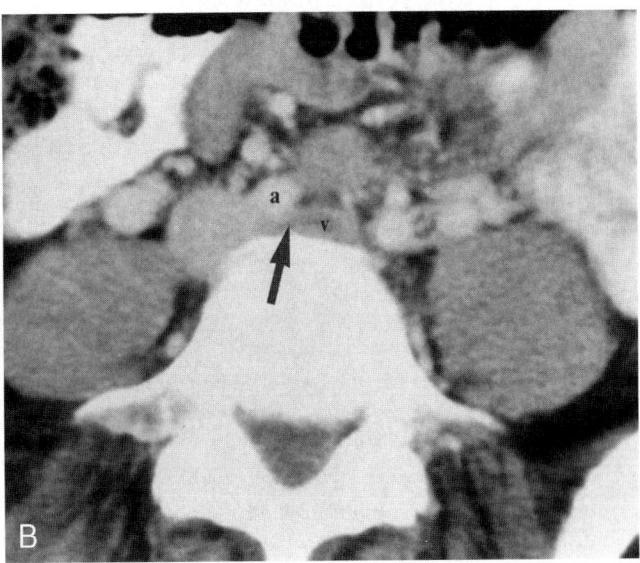

Figure 25.9. May-Thurner Syndrome. A. CT at the level of the sacroiliac joints shows the left iliac vein filled with low-density thrombus (*arrows*). The right iliac vein is patent (*curved open arrow*). **B.** A CT section 3-cm cephalad reveals extrinsic compression of the left iliac vein origin (*arrow*) by the right common iliac artery (*a*). *v*, proximal left common iliac vein.

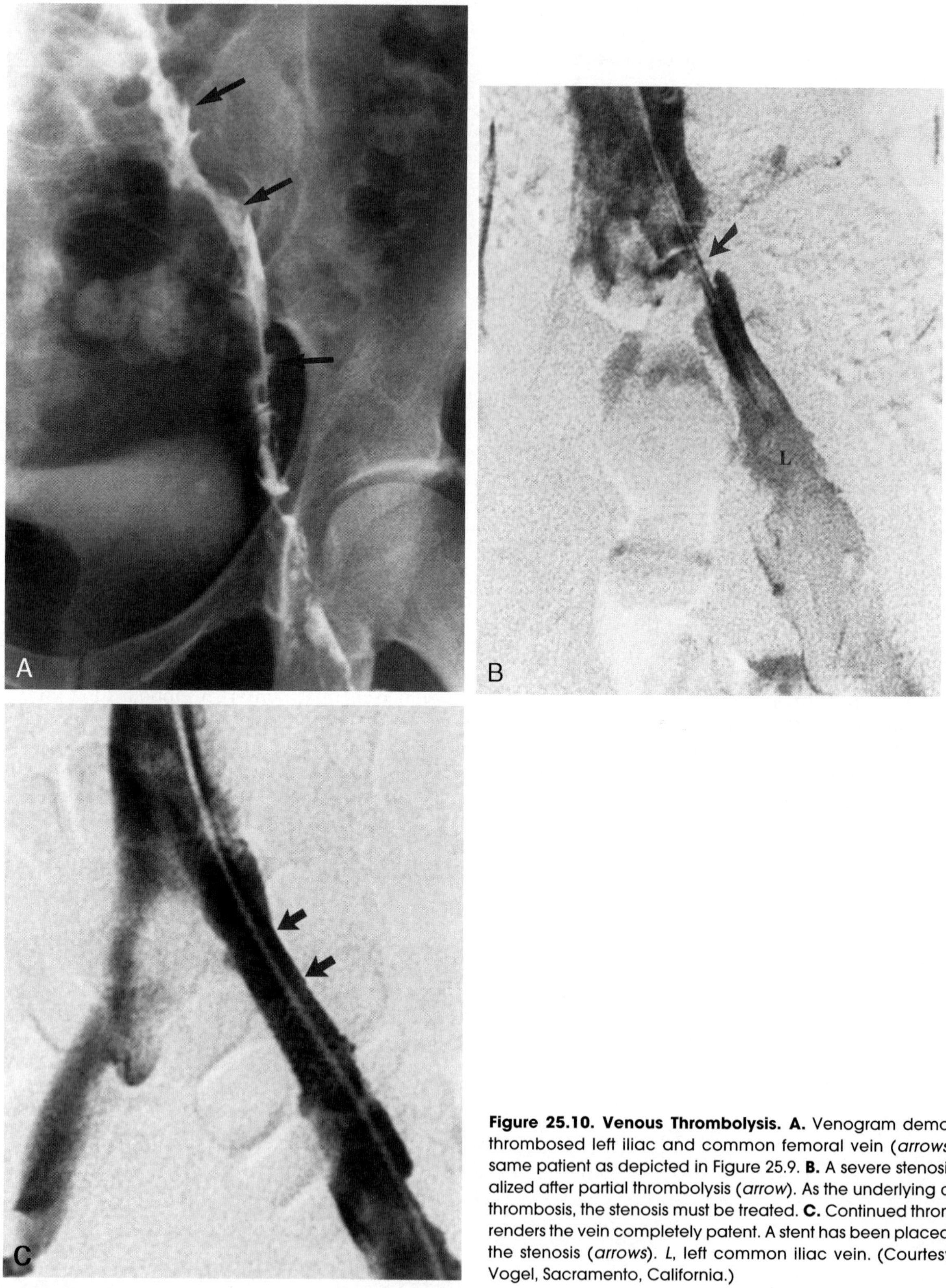

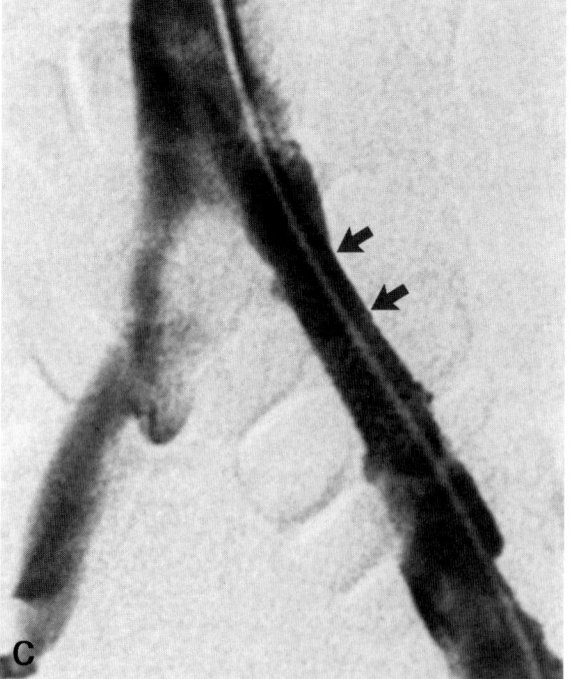

Figure 25.10. Venous Thrombolysis. A. Venogram demonstrates thrombosed left iliac and common femoral vein (*arrows*) in the same patient as depicted in Figure 25.9. **B.** A severe stenosis is visualized after partial thrombolysis (*arrow*). As the underlying cause of thrombosis, the stenosis must be treated. **C.** Continued thrombolysis renders the vein completely patent. A stent has been placed to treat the stenosis (*arrows*). *L*, left common iliac vein. (Courtesy of Pat Vogel, Sacramento, California.)

zation. Abscesses are uncommon, primarily encountered with embolization of solid organs such as the spleen (24). *Postembolization syndrome* commonly occurs with embolization of large tumors. Characterized by pain, fever, nausea, and leukocytosis, this condition is usually self-limiting with resolution of symptoms within several days. Treatment is supportive and includes adequate analgesia and hydration with IV fluids.

Generalizations regarding the efficacy of transcatheter embolization are difficult to make because of the wide variety of diseases treated. In the setting of trauma, bleeding is controlled 80–100% of the time (25,27).

Acute GI bleeding is a life-threatening emergency. Upper endoscopy and colonoscopy are often the initial and only diagnostic tests necessary. If a bleeding site is identified endoscopically, it can sometimes be controlled by local injection of vasospastic drugs, or surgery can be performed if appropriate. Tagged red blood cell nuclear scans are useful for diagnosis if endoscopic diagnosis is not definitive. Arteriography is usually reserved for problem solving, such as in cases in which the bleeding site cannot be localized either endoscopically or with a nuclear medicine scan. Active extravasation from the stomach or duodenum can be safely embolized in otherwise healthy patients (Fig. 25.15). Caution must be exercised in patients with severe atherosclerosis or prior GI surgery because of a higher risk of ischemic complications. Primary embolization of the bowel distal to the ligament of Treitz carries a greater risk than does more proximal embolization. It is often reserved for patients who have failed a trial of vasopressin infusion or for patients who are not good surgical candidates.

Vasopressin infusion is often used for the control of acute lower GI bleeding. It causes splanchnic vasoconstriction and GI smooth muscle contraction. Fewer complications occur if it is used selectively by intra-arterial injection. Complications include hypertension, myocardial infarction, arrhythmias, bowel infarction, peripheral ischemia, catheter-related thrombosis, and antidiuretic hormone side effects. The therapeutic infusion dose is 0.2–0.4 U/min. When initiating therapy, patients are placed on an infusion of 0.2 U/min for 20–30 minutes via a selective catheter in the superior or inferior mesenteric artery, depending on the bleeding site. A repeat angiogram is then performed to assess the following: *a)* control of bleeding, *b)* degree of vasospasm, and *c)* venous return from the area being infused (Fig. 25.16). The latter two features are very important, as overconstriction of arterial branches and inadequate venous return

will cause bowel ischemia. The dose is incrementally increased until bleeding stops or the maximum dose is reached. That dose is continued for 6–12 hours. If bleeding remains controlled, the dose is reduced by half in another 6–12 hours. Finally, saline infusion is substituted for vasopressin for an additional 6–12 hours. If there is no further bleeding, the catheter is removed (28).

Inferior Vena Cava Filters

Inferior vena cava (IVC) filters are percutaneously placed devices used in patients with deep venous thrombosis (DVT) to prevent fatal pulmonary emboli (PE). Filters are positioned within the IVC to trap clot fragments that embolize from the lower extremities or pelvis (Fig. 25.17). The indications for filter placement are DVT or PE in patients who have contraindications to anticoagulation, recurrent PE despite adequate anticoagulation, and complications that prevent continued anticoagulation. Other circumstances in which IVC filters may be indicated are large free-floating clots, progression of DVT in adequately anticoagulated patients, or failure of an existing IVC filter. Prophylactic filter placement may be warranted in certain patients who are temporarily at high risk for PE, such as patients with severe pelvic trauma. Retrievable or temporary IVC filters will be better suited for this application when they become available. Filter placement in young patients or in patients with long life expectancies is discouraged because of the long-term risk of caval thrombosis and other delayed complications (Fig. 25.18) (29).

Procedure. An IVC-gram is performed before filter placement to assess *a)* presence of IVC thrombus, *b)* IVC size (if it is too large, the filter will not anchor properly, resulting in immediate or delayed filter migration), *c)* number and location of renal veins or large venous collaterals, and *d)* presence of caval and renal vein anomalies (30). Selective injections may be necessary to evaluate fully the venous anatomy. Filters are best placed in the IVC immediately below the most inferior renal vein origin to provide continuous flow across the dome of the filter. The continuous streaming of blood from the renal veins aids in preventing clot propagation above the filter (Fig. 25.17B). Filters may be inserted from either a femoral or internal jugular vein approach, preferably from the right, although the left femoral and jugular veins may be used if other sites are occluded or otherwise unsuitable. Flexible filters should be used for left-sided approaches because these veins, particularly the left internal jugular vein, present a more tortuous path. Placement of the filter above the renal veins is occasionally necessary, such as when clot extends cephalad to the renal veins. After filter deployment, a cavagram or plain film of the abdomen is obtained to document filter position.

Four filter types are approved and in widespread use: Greenfield (Medi-tech/Boston Scientific, Watertown, MA), LGM-Vena Tech (B. Braun Vena-Tech, Evanston, IL), Simon nitinol (Nitinol Medical Technologies, Woburn, MA), and Bird's Nest (Cook, Bloomington, IN). The *Greenfield filter* was the first IVC filter used percutaneously. Modifications of the original design have been

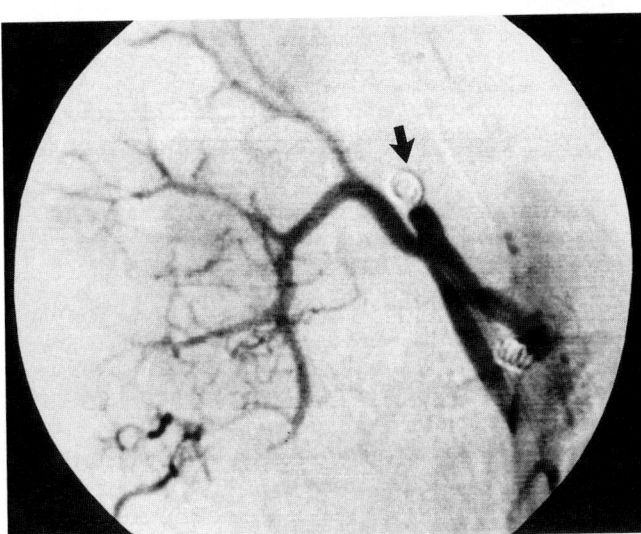

Figure 25.11. Preoperative Embolization. Placement of an embolization coil (*arrow*) within the renal artery prior to surgery for a renal cell carcinoma is a method of embolization used to reduce potential surgical bleeding complications.

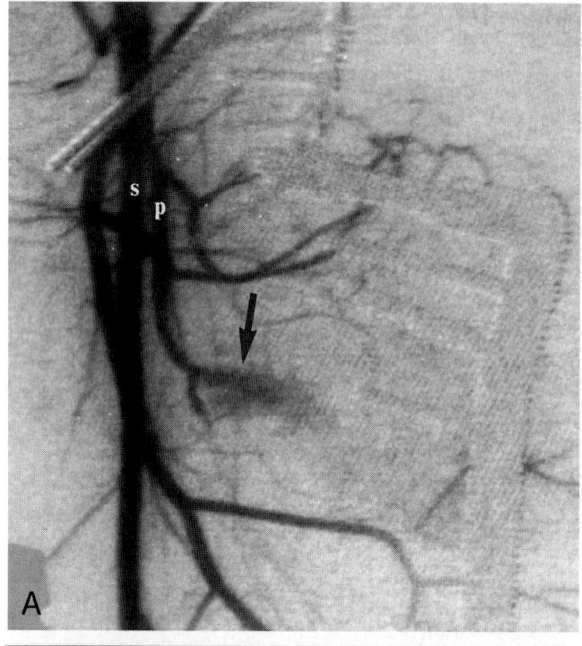

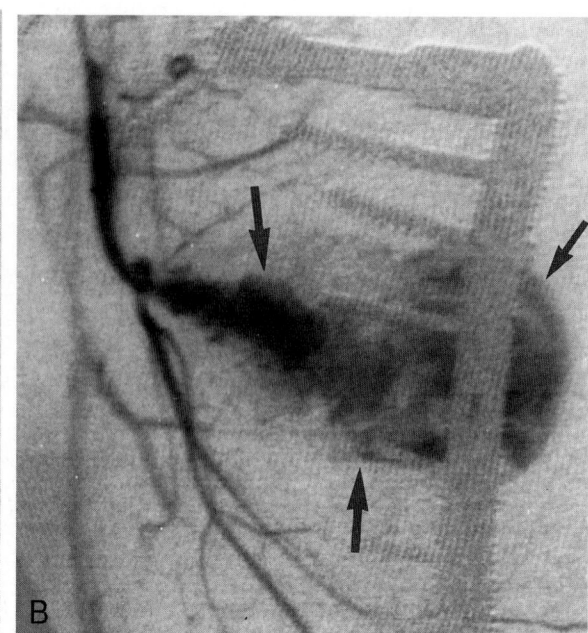

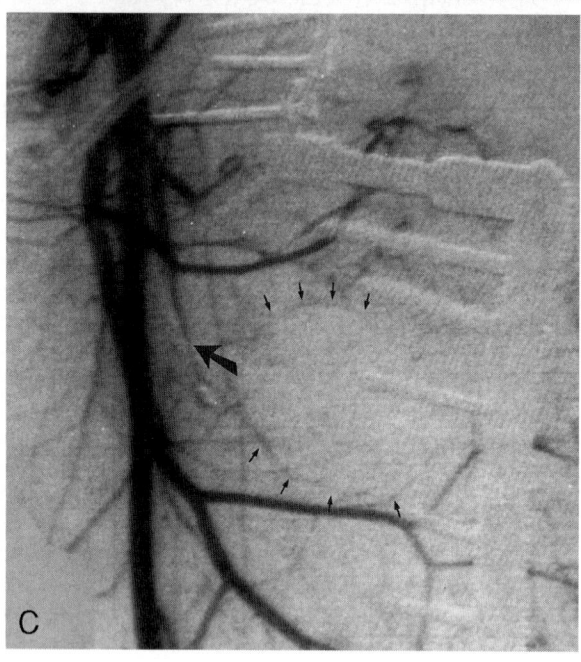

Figure 25.12. Massive Hemorrhage. A. Active extravasation from profunda femoris artery branch after hip surgery (*arrows*). **B.** *Arrows* demonstrate massive arterial bleeding on a selective injection of the profunda femoris artery. **C.** Bleeding has stopped after embolization (*arrow*). Note mass effect on arterial branches (*small arrows*) caused by the hematoma. *p*, profunda femoris artery; *s*, superficial femoral artery. (Courtesy of Sue Hanks, Los Angeles, California.)

made, the most important being miniaturization of the original 24 French delivery system to the current 12 French sheath size. A recent improvement is an over-the-wire Greenfield, the first such filter on the market. *Vena Tech* filters are similar in profile and physical characteristics to the Greenfield. One of its advantages is excellent self-centering. The *Simon nitinol filter* is very flexible and has the smallest sized introducer system (9 French). It is the only filter that allows placement from an arm vein. All filters, with the notable exception of the *Bird's Nest*, must be placed within a segment of the IVC that measures 28 mm or less in diameter. A Bird's Nest filter can be placed into a larger inferior vena cava, provided it does not exceed 40 mm in diameter. The Bird's Nest filter is also relatively flexible. An alternative to con-

sider if the IVC is larger than 28 mm is placement of bilateral iliac vein filters. MR is safely performed with minimal artifact with titanium and nitinol filters. Stainless steel filters, however, will cause considerable artifact. Patients with these filters should avoid MR for several weeks until the filter has been completely incorporated into the caval wall (31).

The rate of recurrent PE for IVC filters is 2–5%. A symptomatic caval thrombosis rate of approximately 3–8% has been reported, depending on filter type (31). Complications include filter migration, tilting or malpositioning, caval perforation, IVC thrombosis, and puncture-site thrombosis. The frequency of the latter complication has been significantly reduced since the development of smaller delivery systems.

Dialysis Grafts

More than 100,000 patients in the United States require hemodialysis, and this population of patients continues to grow. Problems relating to adequate access for hemodialysis contribute significantly to the medical care

required by these patients (32). The role of the interventionalist in treating occluded or failing dialysis grafts has increased in the past decade. A high success rate, a low complication rate, and the ability to treat underlying lesions have made interventional techniques an attractive alternative to surgical thrombectomy. Grafts have a fi-

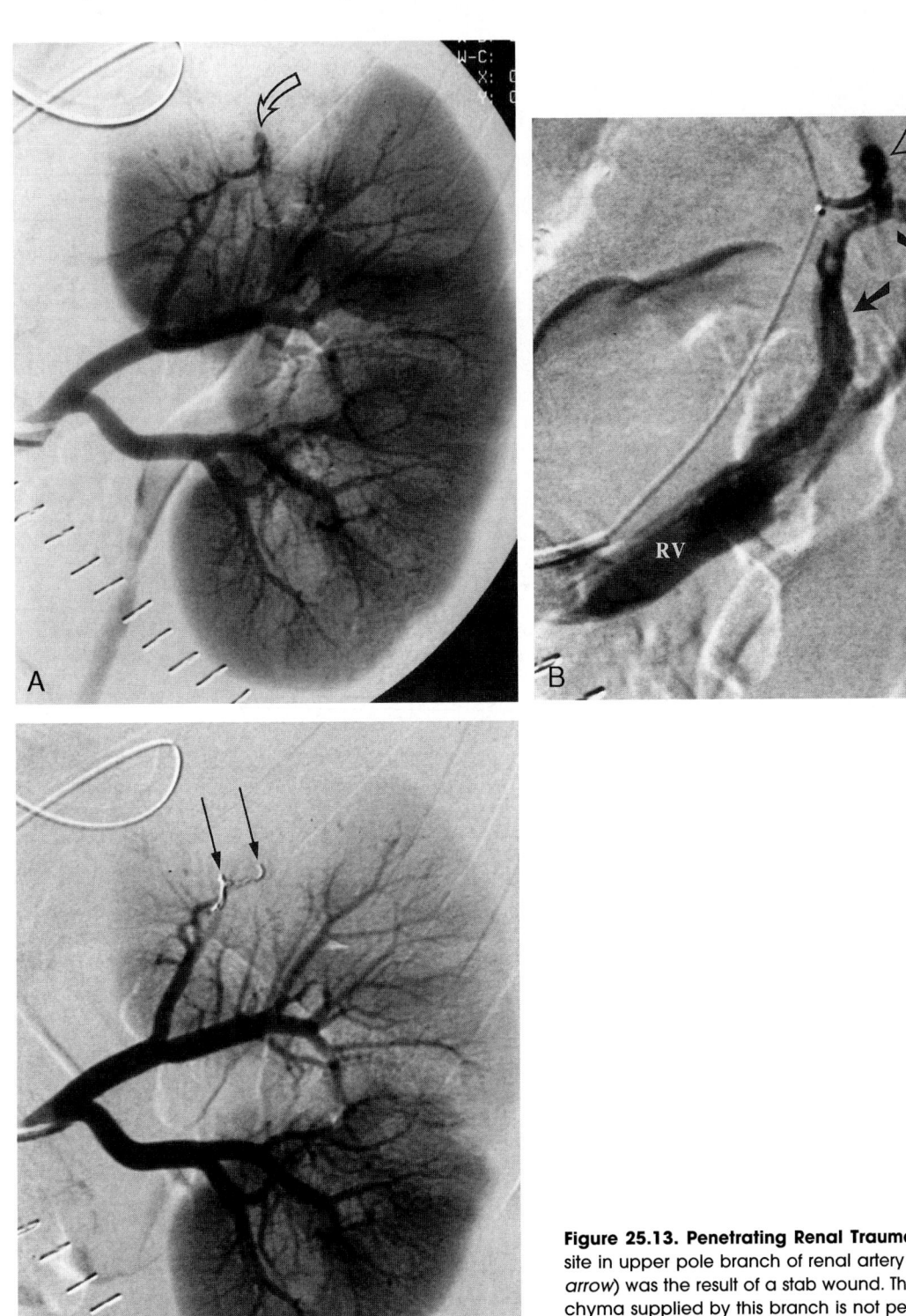

Figure 25.13. Penetrating Renal Trauma. A. Bleeding site in upper pole branch of renal artery (*curved open arrow*) was the result of a stab wound. The renal parenchyma supplied by this branch is not perfused. **B.** Subselective injection through a microcatheter reveals a small pseudoaneurysm (*open arrow*) with an arteriovenous fistula (*arrows*). **C.** Hemostasis is achieved after microcoil embolization (*arrows*). *RV*, renal vein. (Courtesy of Micheal Katz, Los Angeles, California.)

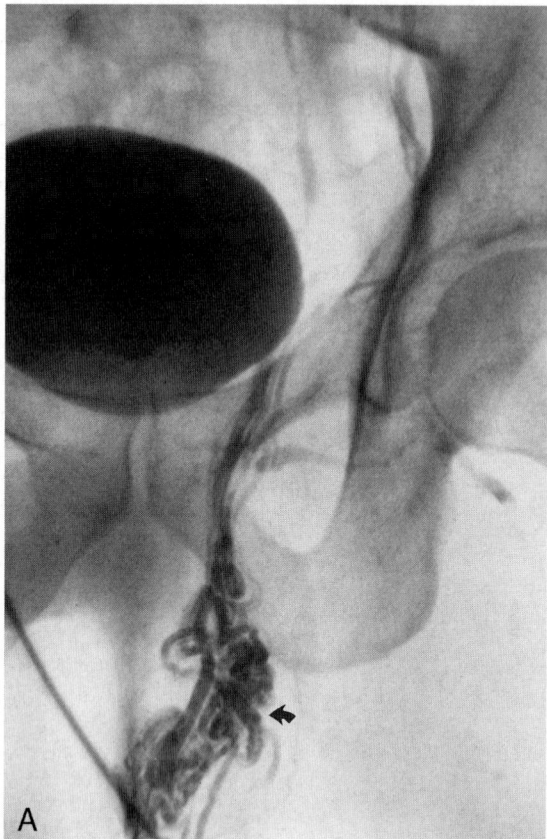
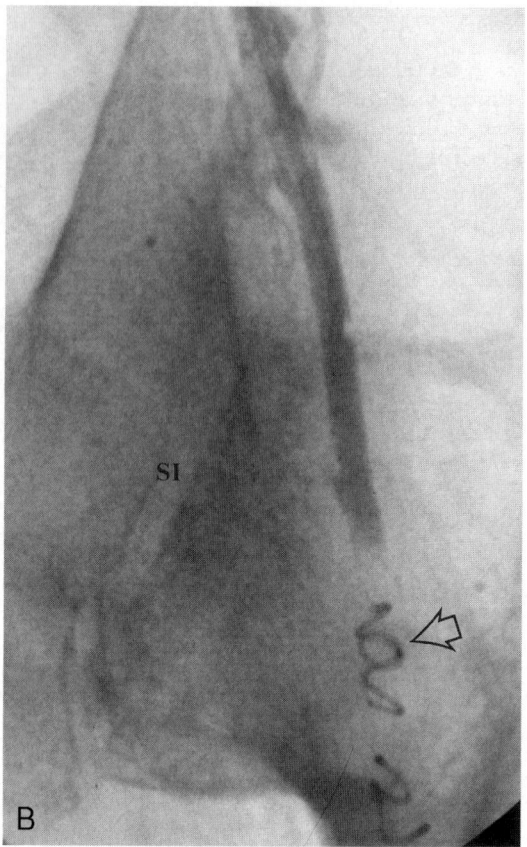

Figure 25.14. Varicocele Embolization. A. Testicular varicocele. A network of dilated venous structures is seen in the left hemiscrotum (*arrow*). **B.** Coil embolization of left internal spermatic vein (*arrow*) results in therapeutic occlusion. Coils are placed above the inguinal ligament. *SI*, sacroiliac joint.

nite life span, with an average patency of 20 months (32). Because the number of potential access sites, as well as the patency of each site, is limited, the life of each graft must be preserved for as long as possible. Interventional techniques are ideally suited for the periodic maintenance required to extend the patency of dialysis grafts.

Two surgical methods are used to create long-term hemodialysis access. The most common type of access today is the *arteriovenous bridge graft*, which is created with synthetic PTFE in the subcutaneous tissues of the forearm. Upper-arm sites are used only when forearm sites have been exhausted. Lower-extremity sites are used when upper-extremity sites are exhausted but are less desirable because of their proximity to the groin. Grafts may be constructed in a straight or looped configuration (Fig. 25.19). The graft material creates a bridge between artery and vein, permitting adequate flow rates for hemodialysis. The *Brescia-Cimino fistula* is a native arteriovenous fistula formed by an anastomosis between the radial artery and the cephalic vein at the wrist. The "arterialized" section of vein proximal to the anastomosis in the forearm is then used for dialysis access. Although Brescia-Cimino fistulas have better patency rates than PTFE grafts, they are not as common because many patients have unfavorable anatomy for their creation (33).

Dialysis access failure presents clinically with thrombosis, inadequate flow rates at dialysis, or elevated venous pressures and abnormal urea recirculation discovered at dialysis. Intervention is contraindicated in fistulas that have thrombosed within 1–2 weeks of surgical construction, or when there is suspected graft infection, severe allergy to iodinated contrast, or contraindications to urokinase. Recent surgical thrombectomy is not an absolute contraindication to thrombolysis.

Pharmacomechanical Thrombolysis is probably the most popular thrombolytic technique. It achieves more rapid thrombolysis than infusion alone, as well as having a higher success rate. Pharmacomechanical thrombolysis entails administration of urokinase with pulse-spray technique combined with mechanical means of thrombus fragmentation and maceration such as angioplasty, catheter disruption, or balloon displacement (33). Recently, dedicated devices for mechanical thrombolysis have been developed. The main advantage of mechanical thrombolysis is that complications of fibrinolytic drugs, primarily bleeding, can be avoided. Shorter procedure times and the potential for decreased cost are also claimed. Examples of recently approved mechanical devices in use include the Amplatz thrombectomy device (Microvena, White Bear Lake, MN), the Angiojet rheolytic catheter (Possis Medical, Minneapolis, MN), the Cragg thrombolytic brush (MicroTherapeutics, San Clemente, CA), and the Arrow-Trerotola device (Arrow International, Reading, PA) (34).

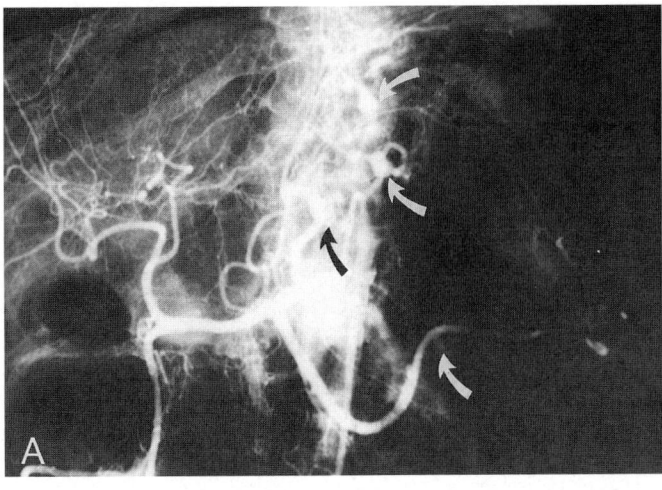
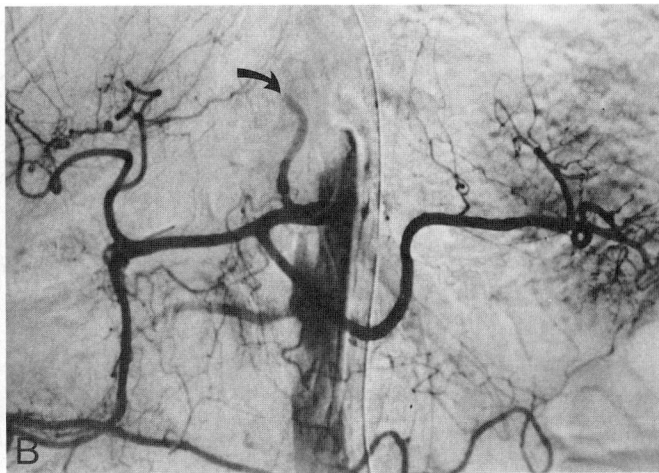

Figure 25.15. Bleeding Gastric Ulcers. A. Celiac artery injection shows multiple areas of extraluminal contrast within the stomach (*arrows*). These represent multiple foci of bleeding gastric ulceration.

B. The same patient, after embolization of the left gastric artery (*arrow*). The gastric bleeding has been successfully controlled.

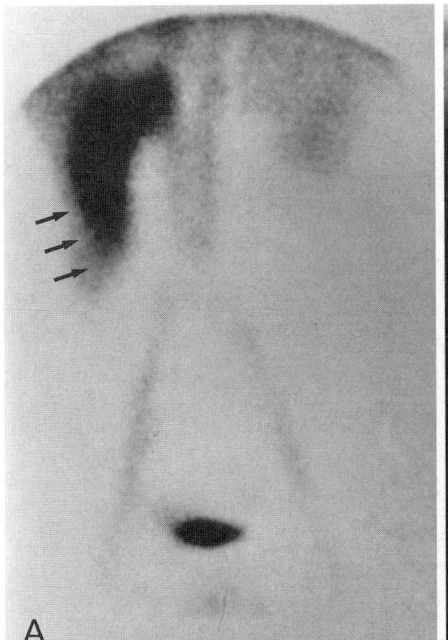
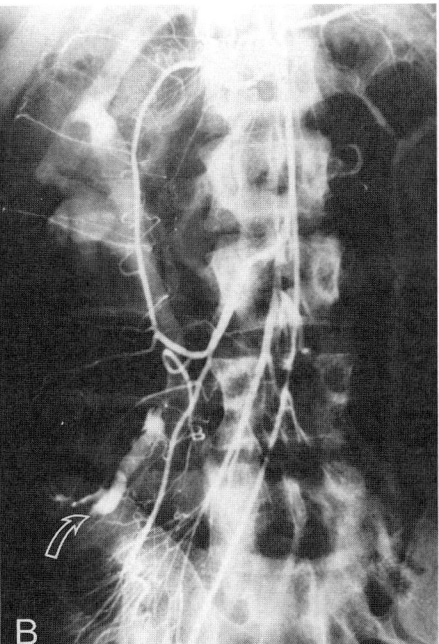
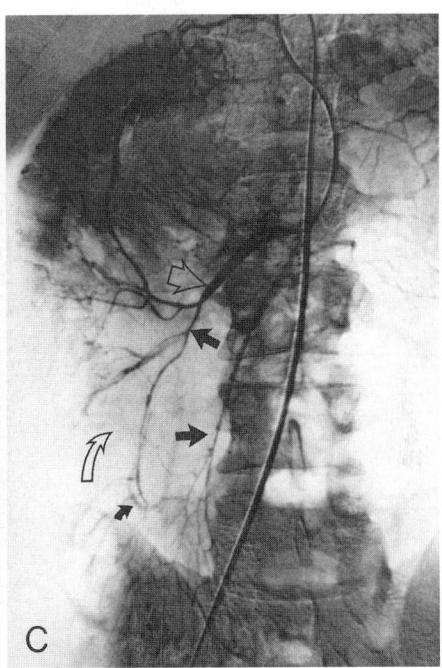

Figure 25.16. Lower GI Bleeding. A. A tagged red blood cell scan shows accumulation of radiotracer in the region of the hepatic flexure (*arrows*). The primary site of bleeding is not delineated. **B.** An SMA arteriogram demonstrates extravasation of contrast in the right lower quadrant within a bleeding diverticulum with a "pseudovein

sign" (*arrow*). **C.** After administration of intra-arterial vasopressin, repeat SMA injection reveals no further bleeding (*curved open arrow*). Note attenuation of vessels in response to the vasopressin infusion (*straight arrows*), with a sudden decrease in caliber (*open arrow*). *Small curved arrow* shows preservation of venous return.

Infusion catheters are placed in both the arterial and venous limbs of the graft so that the catheters overlap within the graft. Thrombolysis of the entire graft is possible with this crossed catheter configuration (33). The underlying cause of thrombosis requires treatment following clot lysis. A stenosis at the venous anastomosis is the most common underlying lesion, which is treated with angioplasty (Fig. 25.20). Not uncommonly, high-pressure balloons are needed to dilate resistant venous

stenoses. The entire graft, both anastomoses, and venous outflow from the arm to the SVC must then be evaluated. Graft failure may result from stenosis or occlusion anywhere along this course. The next most frequent sites of stenosis are the outflow arm veins, followed by the central veins. Intragraft lesions and arterial anastomotic stenoses are less common. A lysis-resistant thrombus, known as an *arterial plug*, is commonly present at or near the arterial anastomosis. This resistant

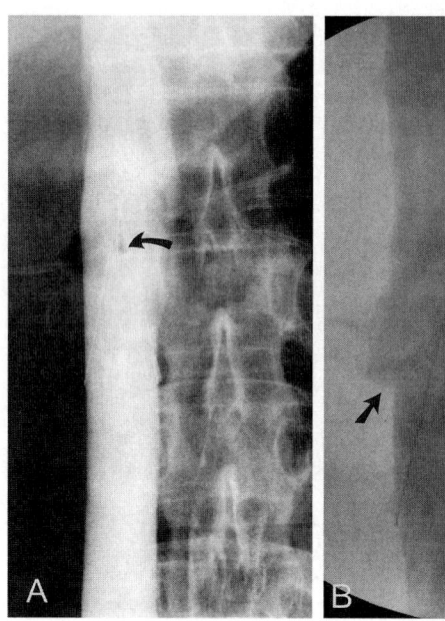

Figure 25.17. Inferior Vena Cava Filter. A. Inferior vena cavagram shows a small thrombus within the filter (*arrow*). **B.** Subtraction image from a contrast injection into the IVC shows ideal placement of a Greenfield filter. Placement just inferior to the renal veins (*arrows*) limits potential dead space for thrombus formation due to continuous renal vein inflow.

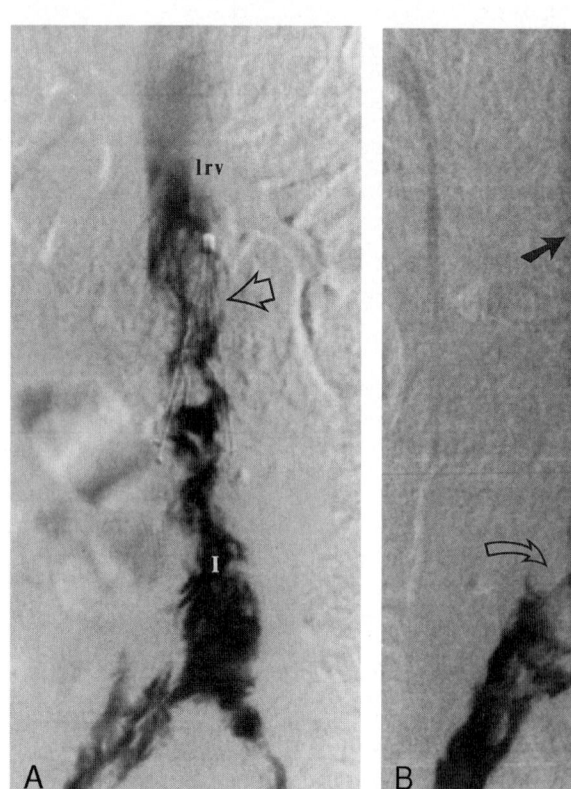

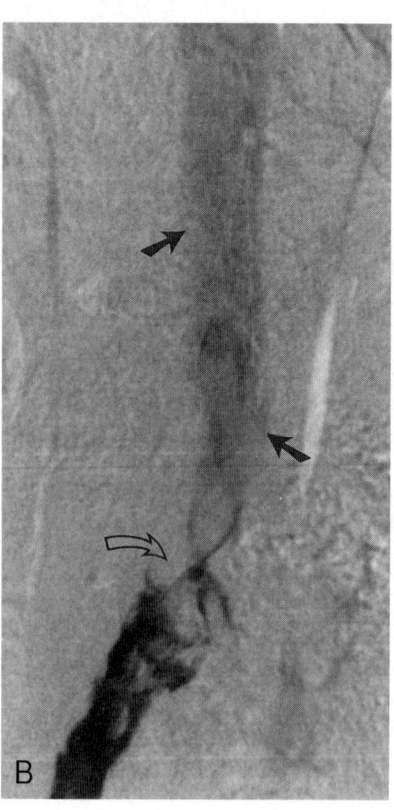

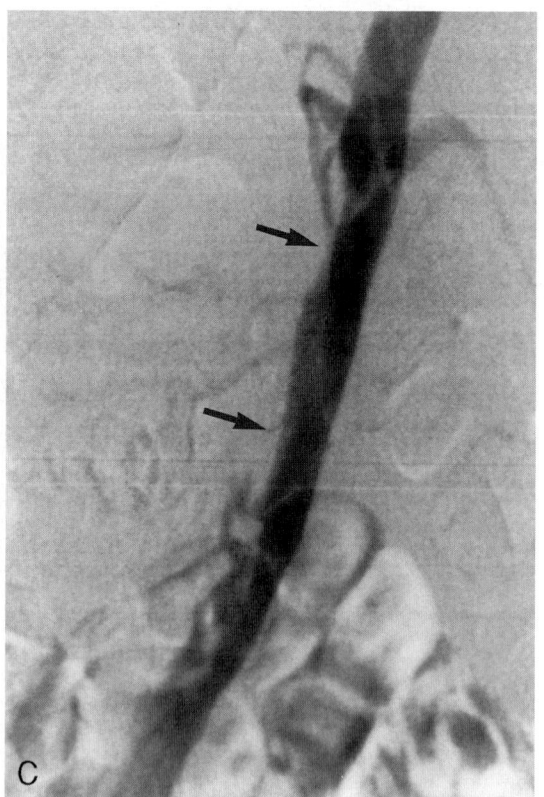

Figure 25.18. IVC Filter Thrombosis. A. Thrombosis of the inferior vena cava (I) complicating Greenfield IVC filter placement (*open arrow*). The patient presented with severe lower extremity and scrotal edema. The filter fulfilled its purpose of preventing a fatal PE. Note inflow of unopacified blood from the left renal vein (*lrv*). **B.** Re-canalization of the IVC (*arrows*) with residual iliac thrombosis (*open curved arrow*) after 18 hours of thrombolysis. **C.** Right iliac thrombus has resolved after balloon angioplasty and an additional 12-hour infusion (*arrows*). (Courtesy of Vance McCollom, Oklahoma City, Oklahoma.)

plug is removed using mechanical methods. A balloon of appropriate size is gently inflated in the artery past the arterial anastomosis. The plug is then mechanically displaced by pulling the inflated balloon into the graft. Fogarty balloons are well suited for this maneuver. The plug, now within the graft, can be removed or macerated with an angioplasty balloon. The procedure may be complete at this point, although more urokinase is sometimes needed if the residual clot volume is substantial. Release of very small fragments of thrombus into the central circulation occurs frequently and appears to be relatively safe in the absence of a right-to-left shunt or significant underlying pulmonary insufficiency.

Results. The various percutaneous methods for dialysis graft recanalization result in a success rate of 75–100%. The long-term outcomes are similar to thrombosed grafts that are managed surgically (34).

Hemodynamically significant central venous stenoses or occlusions are not uncommon in patients who have had indwelling central venous catheters, particularly in the subclavian or left internal jugular veins. These are difficult problems in management. Angioplasty is the first-line treatment option, but lesions often recur or do not respond at all. In patients in whom angioplasty has failed, placement of central venous stents is considered

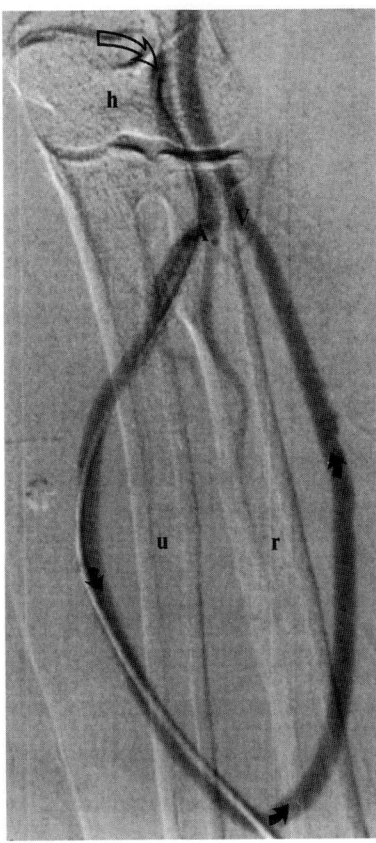

Figure 25.19. PTFE Dialysis Graft. Typical angiographic appearance of a PTFE forearm loop graft. Direction of blood flow is depicted by *black arrows*. Guidewire tip (*curved open arrow*) is in the proximal radial artery. Note close proximity of arterial and venous anastomoses. *A*, arterial anastomosis; *h*, humerus; *r*, radius; *u*, ulna; *V*, venous anastomosis.

(35). Particular care must be taken in placing these stents owing to the risk of central migration to the heart.

Venous Access

As the number of treatments for cancer, AIDS, and other chronic diseases has increased, so has the need for long-term IV access. Using imaging guidance for venous puncture and catheter positioning gives the radiologist several advantages over traditional blind access and placement. Initial access may be obtained with US or fluoroscopy. Rigorous sterile technique must be used to minimize infection. A brief overview of venous access devices follows (36).

Tunneled Central Catheters. The external portion of these central venous catheters is placed in a subcutaneous tunnel between the venous entry and skin exit sites on the chest wall. A polyester-fiber cuff attached to the catheter is placed within the tunnel. With tissue ingrowth, the cuff provides an anchor for the catheter, as well as a barrier to infection. These catheters are useful when long-term IV therapy is required. Groshong, Broviac, and Hickman catheters are examples.

Dialysis catheters are dual-lumen catheters with proximal "arterial" and distal "venous" lumens. The end holes are positioned at different levels to prevent recirculation during hemodialysis. The catheters might or might not be tunneled, depending on the length of time the patient needs it (Fig. 25.21). Blood is withdrawn from the arterial port at hemodialysis, and the dialysate is readministered into the venous port. High flow rates, in the range of 250–300 cc/min or greater, are necessary for successful hemodialysis. Flow through the catheter is related to its length as well as its lumen size.

Peripherally Inserted Central Catheters (PICC lines) are placed through an arm vein, with the tip positioned centrally in the distal superior vena cava. Trained nurses place most of these catheters in patients with easily accessible veins. If placement is difficult or unsuccessful, the interventional radiologist may place these catheters using fluoroscopic or US guidance. Flow rates are limited. Most PICC lines cannot be used for bolus CT injections.

Implantable Ports are placed in a soft-tissue pocket in either the arm or chest for access with a noncoring needle. Like tunneled catheters, they are used in patients requiring long-term IV access. Advantages over tunneled catheters include no external catheter to manage, reduced risk of infection, and convenience. Activities such as swimming are possible with these devices once the skin incision has completely healed. Disadvantages include repeated needle punctures each time the port is accessed.

Complications. Radiologists who place central venous catheters must be prepared to manage complications. Immediate complications include air embolism, pneumothorax, arterial injury, brachial nerve injury, and cardiac arrhythmias (37). Most of these can be avoided by using imaging guidance for venous access and catheter placement and using 21-gauge needles for venipuncture. Suspended respiration, Trendelenburg positioning, or other methods of increasing intrathoracic

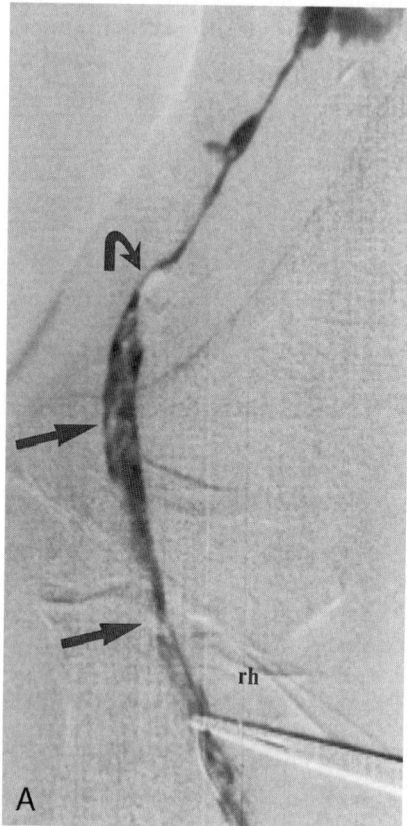

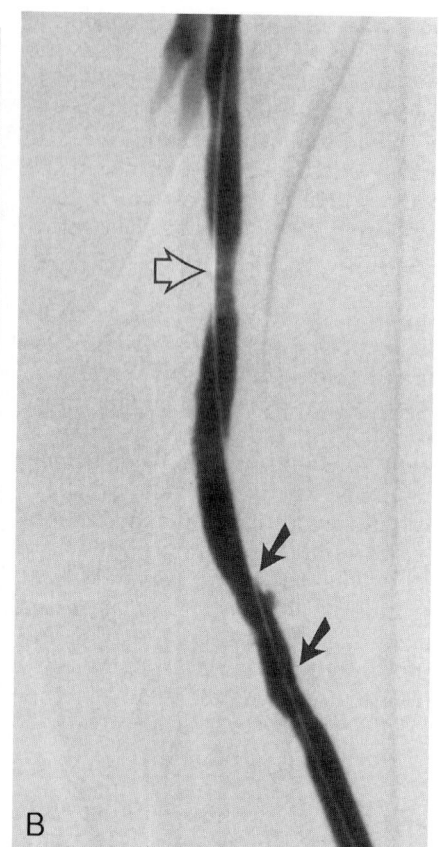

Figure 25.20. Venous Anastamotic Stenosis. A. Digital venogram of clotted dialysis graft (*arrows*) with typical severe stenosis at the venous anastomosis (*curved arrow*). **B.** After pharmacomechanical thrombolysis, there is resolution of graft thrombosis (*arrows*). Rapid flow is re-established after balloon angioplasty of the venous anastomosis (*open arrow*). *rh*, radial head.

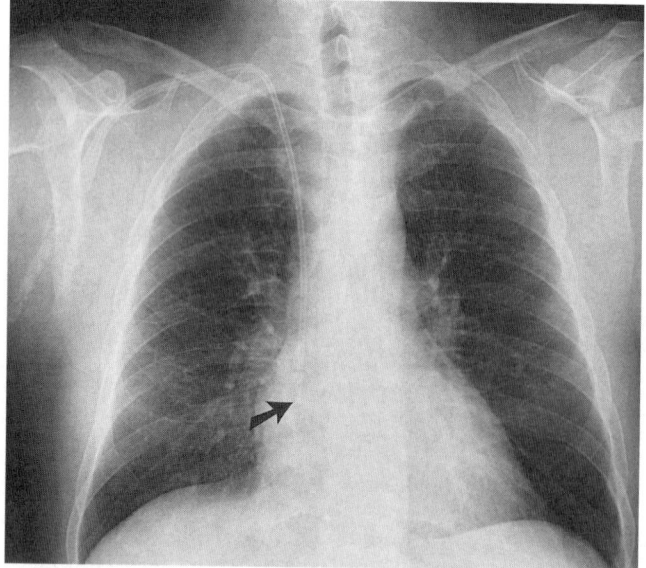

Figure 25.21. Tunneled Central Venous Catheter. A dual lumen dialysis catheter has been placed using the right internal jugular vein for access. The tip is in an appropriate position in the upper right atrium (*arrow*). The relatively smooth curve achieved by accessing the inferior right internal jugular vein improves flow rates at dialysis.

pressure during catheter insertion can aid in avoiding air embolism, which can be fatal.

Infection, thrombosis, and fracture or migration of catheter fragments are the most frequent long-term complications. Infection can be systemic, resulting from colonization of the intravascular portion of the catheter. Local infection of the subcutaneous tunnel or pocket can also occur. The catheter can often be salvaged with a trial of antibiotic therapy if the infection is not severe. Prompt catheter removal is necessary in more serious infections, such as purulent local infection or sepsis. Thrombosis resulting in a malfunctioning catheter can often be successfully managed with minidose urokinase administration or a short infusion of urokinase. A fibrin sheath universally forms around the catheter and is often the cause of catheter obstruction when it surrounds the tip. Stripping this off the catheter with a gooseneck snare is an effective means of restoring catheter function (38). If arm or facial swelling occurs as a result of venous thrombosis, catheter-directed thrombolysis can be performed. Malpositioned catheters or catheter fragments owing to fracture and migration can be percutaneously managed with gooseneck snares (39). Other retrieval devices such as baskets or forceps are occasionally needed to retrieve embolized catheter fragments. Long-term sequelae of indwelling catheters include central venous stenosis or occlusion. Use of the right internal jugular vein appears to reduce the frequency of this complication (40).

Some patients with chronic diseases depend on continuous, permanent central venous access. If traditional access sites such as the subclavian or internal jugular vein are no longer available because of occlusion, alternate locations may be considered. Access into collateral venous structures, hepatic veins, or directly into the inferior vena cava will allow placement of central venous catheters in most of these patients (36).

Transjugular Intrahepatic Portosystemic Shunt (TIPS)

Cirrhosis and portal hypertension are serious conditions with high mortality rates. Variceal hemorrhage and liver failure are the major causes of death in these patients. Definitive treatment with liver transplantation is not available to many patients because of limited donor supply. Several treatment options are available for control of variceal hemorrhage. Among these is the *transjugular intrahepatic portosystemic shunt* procedure. The concept of TIPS can be credited to Rosch et al. (41), who, in 1969, reported on shunt creation in dogs. Two decades later, it has expanded options available in the management of portal hypertension and plays a major role in the treatment of variceal bleeding.

Indications for TIPS are portal hypertension complicated by acute variceal bleeding uncontrolled with sclerotherapy, and recurrent variceal bleeding untreatable with medical management and sclerotherapy. TIPS also shows promise in patients with refractory ascites (42).

Contraindications include severe right-sided heart failure with elevated central venous pressure, polycystic liver disease, and severe liver failure. Relative contraindications include portal vein thrombosis, vascular liver masses, systemic infection, and poorly controlled hepatic encephalopathy (43).

Procedure. The preferred access is the right internal jugular vein (Fig. 25.22). A catheter is advanced over a guidewire and used to select the right hepatic vein. A venogram is performed to assess the adequacy of the hepatic vein for TIPS creation. A 9 French sheath is then placed, through which the TIPS needle is passed. The needle is carefully brought into the selected hepatic vein over the guidewire. The portal vein is punctured and a guidewire is placed, creating a connection between the hepatic vein and portal vein through the liver parenchyma. A catheter is placed into the splenic vein so that the size and flow dynamics of the varices can be determined with portography. A balloon catheter is inflated in the parenchymal tract (Fig. 25.23A), followed by placement of a bridging metallic stent. Wallstents are the most common stent used because of their flexibility and because they are FDA approved for this application. The resulting portosystemic pressure gradient is measured, with a target gradient of 12 mm Hg or less. Occasionally,

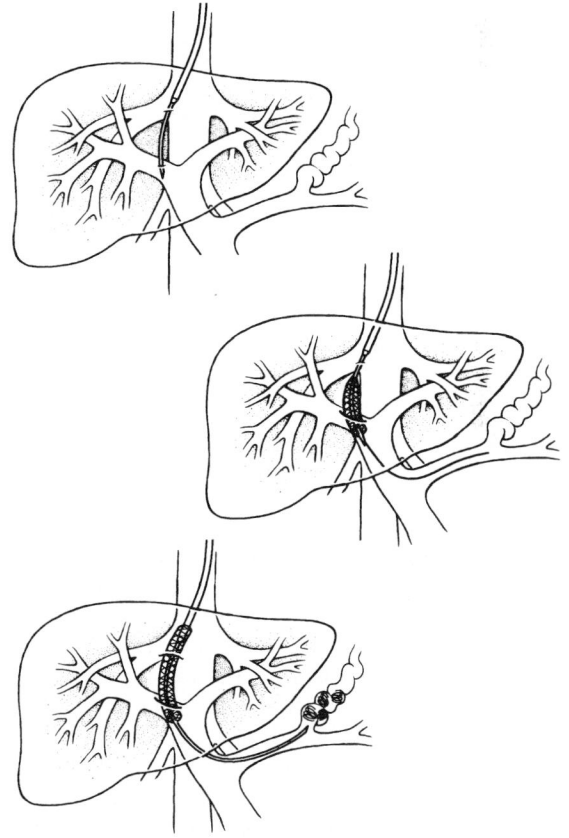

Figure 25.22. TIPS: Step by Step. A. Needle is shown passing from the proximal right hepatic vein into right portal vein 2–3 cm from the portal vein bifurcation. Note corkscrew appearance to the dilated coronary vein. **B.** After balloon angioplasty of the tract, a flexible Wallstent is being deployed to bridge the parenchymal tract. **C.** The stent is completely deployed, creating the shunt. The coronary vein is embolized with coils in patients with ongoing or recent active bleeding. (Adapted from Zemel G, Becker GJ, Bancroft JW, et al. Technical advances in transjugular intrahepatic portosystemic shunts. Radiographics 1992;12:615–622.)

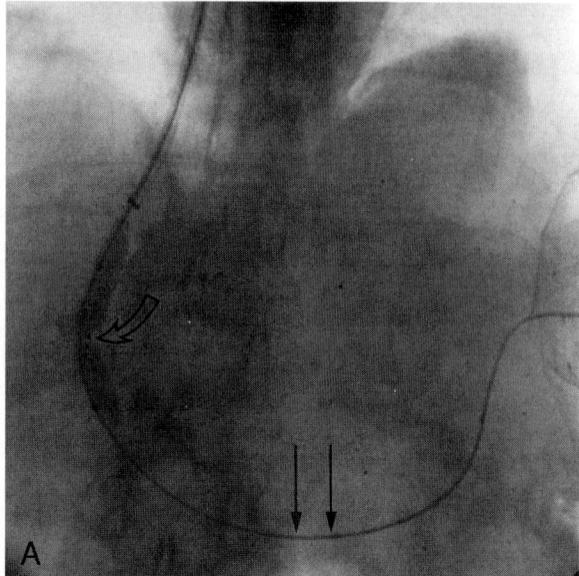

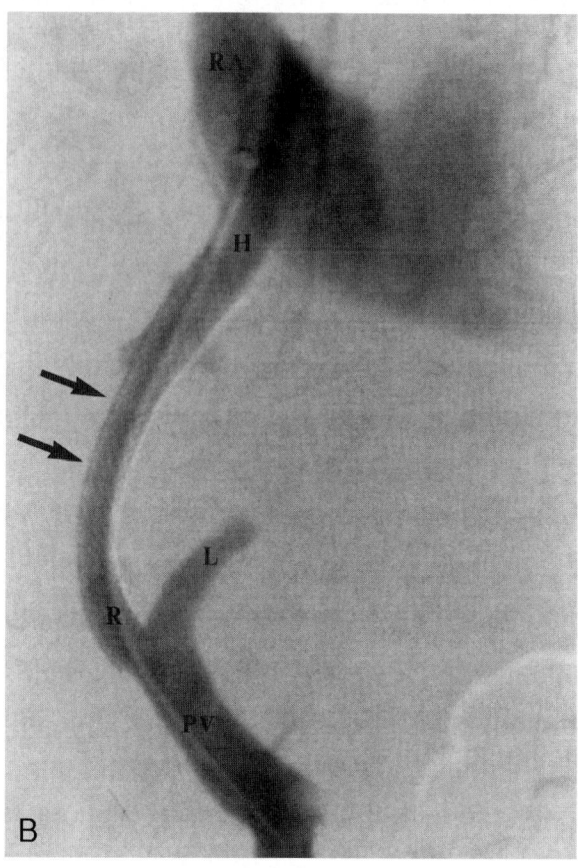

Figure 25.23. TIPS. A. After obtaining access to the portal circulation, a guidewire is placed in the splenic vein (*arrows*). An angioplasty balloon is used to dilate the parenchymal tract. Note the typical "waist" on the balloon (*curved open arrow*) due to the fibrous portal vein wall. This is a convenient landmark to guide subsequent stent placement. **B.** Portogram after shunt creation with a Wallstent shows rapid flow through the shunt (*arrows*). Note lack of intrahepatic portal venous opacification, indicating TIPS-induced hepatofugal flow in the intrahepatic portal venous branches. *H*, right hepatic vein; *L*, left portal vein; *PV*, main portal vein; *R*, right portal vein; *RA*, right atrium.

the portosystemic gradient remains high, with a technically successful TIPS. Further intervention may be necessary in these cases, especially if varices continue to opacify with contrast on portography. A final portal venogram is obtained when the target portosystemic gradient is achieved (Fig. 25.23B). If the patient has experienced recent or ongoing hemorrhage from esophageal varices, coronary vein embolization is justified (44).

Access to the portal vein with the transhepatic needle is often difficult, and many methods for targeting the portal vein have been described. These include real-time sonography, placement of transhepatic portal vein guidewires, portal vein catheterization via a recanalized paraumbilical vein, placement of a microcoil adjacent to the portal vein using US guidance, conventional or MR portography, and performance of a wedged hepatic venogram with iodinated contrast or CO_2. Wedged portography using CO_2 is relatively safe, requires no additional percutaneous needle punctures, and consistently results in visualization of the portal vein target (45) (Fig. 25.24). Care must be taken not to inject forcefully, as perforation of the liver capsule has been reported (46).

Results. Immediate technical success is high, ranging from 95% to 100%. Thirty-day mortality is reported in up to 15% of cases. Most deaths are in patients seriously ill prior to TIPS creation. Fatal peritoneal hemorrhage has been reported, but it appears to be a rare event. Injuries

may occur to the hepatic artery or portal vein. New or worsening encephalopathy is a relatively common complication, occurring up to 25% of the time (43). Encephalopathy can be treated medically in the majority of these patients. In a large multicenter prospective trial, recurrent bleeding occurred in 16% of patients. All rebleeding episodes in these patients related to portal hypertension were successfully treated with reintervention (47).

Long-term durability of TIPS is suboptimal without periodic follow-up and reintervention when necessary. Primary shunt patency has been reported in a prospective series to be 75% at 6 months, 50% at 1 year, and 32% at 2 years. Periodic Doppler US surveillance of these patients is required (see chapter 40). If shunt or portal vein velocities decrease from baseline, a venogram is performed. Failure is attributable primarily to intimal hyperplasia in the shunt or in hepatic veins, which results in flow-limiting stenoses. These lesions can be successfully treated with angioplasty or stent placement. Such reintervention results in a 1-year assisted primary patency of 85% (48).

NONVASCULAR INTERVENTION

Percutaneous Biopsy

Percutaneous image-guided biopsies may be performed using any imaging modality that adequately visualizes the lesion and allows safe and accurate guidance. The most common imaging modalities used are CT, US, and fluoroscopy. The advantages of percutaneous needle biopsy are its safety, cost-effectiveness, and relatively short procedural and recovery times. A percutaneous biopsy is indicated when the diagnosis will alter the patient's treatment, the lesion is visualized on an imaging study, and a safe access route can be achieved.

Needles. Many types of biopsy needles are available. Factors influencing needle selection include organ of involvement, amount and character of tissue required for diagnosis, availability, and operator preference. The main characteristics to consider are needle gauge, tip configuration, and whether the tissue obtained is primarily intended for cytologic or histologic evaluation. Fine needle aspiration (FNA) uses 20-to-23-gauge needles to obtain specimens for cytologic analysis or fluid sampling. These needles are useful in patients at high risk for bleeding, for sampling vascular lesions, or for passing through bowel interposed between the needle and target. Larger 14- to-19-gauge cutting needles obtain core biopsies for histologic analysis. They are often used when the type of malignancy is unknown, particularly if lymphoma is suspected (Fig. 25.25). Core biopsies may be needed to confirm benignancy.

Needle tips may be beveled, as in conventional and spinal needles, or modified in various ways to improve tissue-cutting capability. Examples include Franseen, Westcott, Turner, and Crown needles. These often obtain a core of tissue even when thin-gauge needles are used. Biopsy guns are spring-driven devices used to obtain core samples. A slotted stylet is mechanically advanced a preset depth into a target lesion when the device is fired. A coaxial outer cannula with cutting capability follows nearly instantaneously around the slotted stylet. The core of tissue recovered in the slot is well suited for histologic analysis.

Procedure. The safest route should be determined by study of the imaging examinations. In general, the best needle path is the shortest one (Fig. 25.26). Exceptions include vascular lesions in the liver, which should be biopsied through normal hepatic parenchyma even though this results in a longer needle path. Normal liver parenchyma will tamponade bleeding and reduce the risk of significant hemorrhage. Longer needle paths may also be necessary in some lung lesions to avoid crossing a fissure. Bony structures can impede the needle path and require repositioning of the patient or complex angulation of the needle.

Percutaneous biopsy may be performed using single- or double-needle techniques. Single-needle technique involves repeated separate needle passes into the lesion until sufficient diagnostic material is obtained. In the coaxial technique, a larger-caliber outer needle is placed into or at the edge of the lesion, and then a smaller-caliber inner needle is passed through the larger needle to acquire the sample. The outer needle serves as a guide and allows multiple passes into the lesion. The tandem technique involves placing a small-gauge needle as a guide needle. Once the appropriate angle and position of the guide needle are achieved, a biopsy needle is passed parallel to the guide needle to sample the lesion (49).

Image-guided percutaneous biopsy can be performed in the neck, chest, abdomen, retroperitoneum, pelvis,

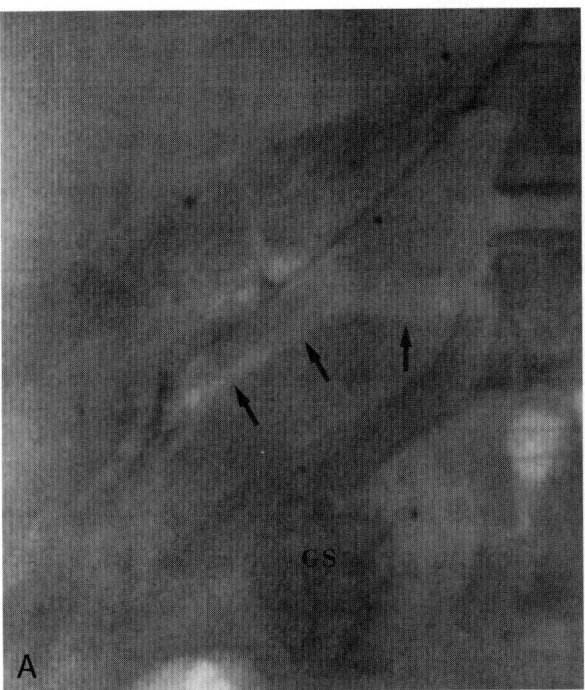
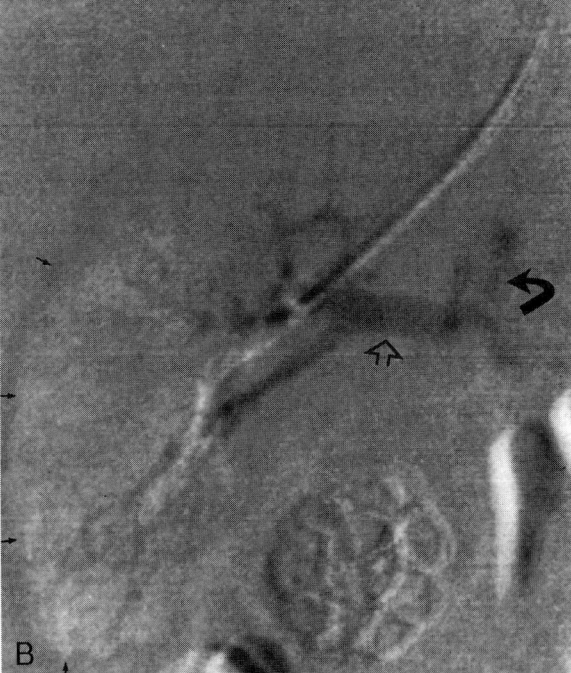

Figure 25.24. Wedged CO_2 Portogram. A. Unsubtracted wedged transhepatic portogram using CO_2 as contrast agent (*arrows*). Contrast injection was performed with an occlusion balloon catheter in the right hepatic vein. **B.** Subtracted image from the same CO_2 portogram. There is excellent delineation of portal vein anatomy. The bifurcation into right (*open arrow*) and left (*curved arrow*) portal vein is clearly shown. *Small arrows* outline liver margin. *GS*, gallstones.

Figure 25.25. Anterior Mediastinal Mass. A biopsy needle has been placed into a retrosternal anterior mediastinal mass. The needle path is medial to the internal mammary vessels (*white arrowheads*). *Black arrow* shows needle tip, which is positively identified by the black streak artifact distal to it. *A*, ascending aorta; *D*, descending aorta; *L*, left pulmonary artery; *S*, superior vena cava.

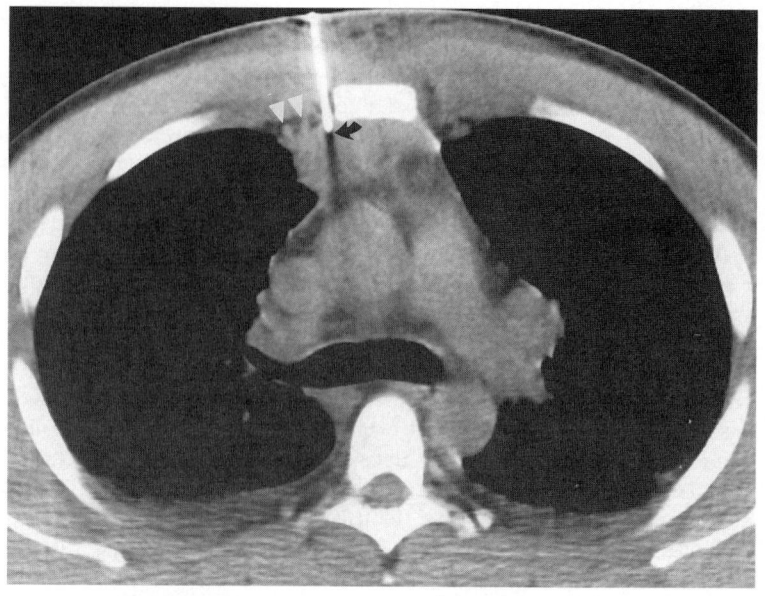

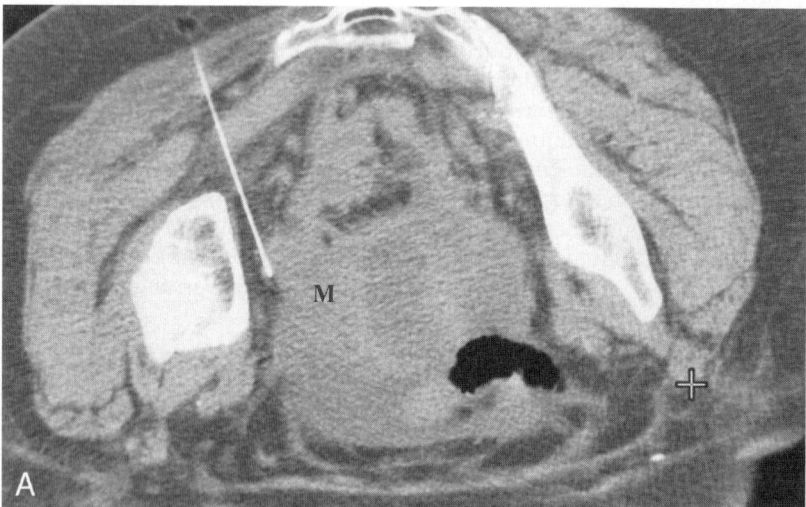

Figure 25.26. Pelvic Tumor. A. With the patient prone, a needle traverses the sacrosciatic notch for biopsy of a pelvic mass (*M*). **B.** Enlarged left periaortic lymph node (*arrow*) in the same patient. Needle tip is 1–2 mm beyond the anterior margin of the node and was retracted slightly before tissue sampling. *a*, abdominal aorta; *I*, inferior vena cava.

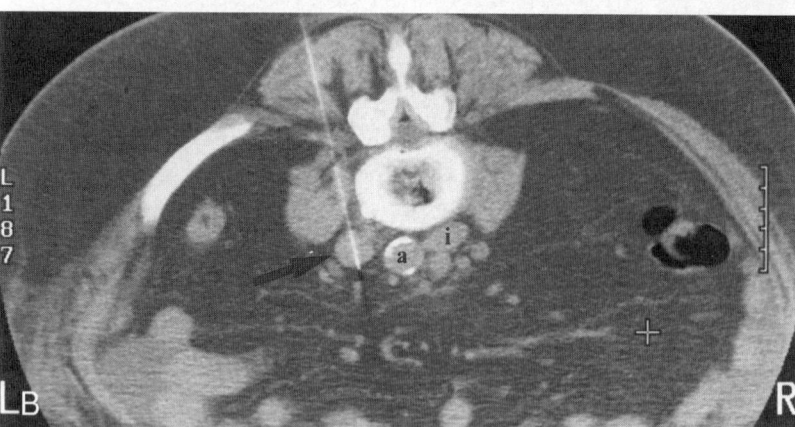

and extremities. Principles are similar, although organ-specific considerations exist.

Liver. Small, deep liver masses or lesions located at the dome of the liver may be difficult to biopsy with CT guidance. US guidance allows the steep needle path-

ways necessary to reach these lesions and to avoid crossing the lung parenchyma. US allows continuous real-time visualization of the needle, whereas CT guidance requires time-consuming rescanning with each repositioning of the needle. Transjugular liver biopsy is a useful technique in patients with bleeding diatheses or extensive ascites. A sheath is placed into a hepatic vein using internal jugular vein access. To perform the biopsy, a long needle is passed through the wall of the hepatic vein into the hepatic parenchyma. If bleeding occurs, it is into the patient's own hepatic vein, preventing blood loss from the patient's circulation. Significant bleeding can occur if the liver capsule is traversed by the needle. Liver biopsy with embolization of the percutaneous tract is an alternative to transjugular biopsy in patients with increased bleeding risk.

Adrenal masses are biopsied under CT guidance unless they are large enough to be seen by US. The patient is positioned to avoid crossing the pleural space en route to the lesion. The prone position requires angling the needle superiorly to avoid transgression of the lung in the posterior sulcus. A supine transhepatic approach may be used for right adrenal masses. A lateral decubitus position, with the side of the lesion down, is helpful because the dependent diaphragm and pleura will be displaced cephalad.

Lung biopsy is useful for tissue characterization of lung nodules and masses. FNA is often preferred to core biopsy because of lower risk of pneumothorax. A needle path should be chosen to avoid the increased risk of pneumothorax associated with crossing a fissure. CT and fluoroscopy are the most common imaging modalities used for lung biopsy. US can be used for peripheral lesions in contact with the pleura. Lesions completely surrounded by air are not seen with US.

Pneumothorax is the most frequent complication of percutaneous lung biopsy. Chest radiographs are obtained immediately and 2–3 hours after the procedure. A pneumothorax that is symptomatic or exceeds 50% is treated with a small-caliber catheter. The catheter is placed in the second or third anterior intercostal space in the midclavicular line and is positioned near the apex of the pleural cavity. As with any intercostal procedure, the neurovascular bundle must be avoided by placing the catheter over the top of the rib. Asymptomatic patients with no pneumothorax or with small, stable pneumothoraces may be discharged home with instructions to return to the hospital if symptoms develop (50). Air embolus is an extremely rare complication resulting from air entering a pulmonary vein and embolizing into the systemic circulation. Air embolism is prevented by suspending respiration and avoiding coughing during needle passage.

Results. Accuracy rates for abdominal and pelvic biopsy range from 66–100%, with a complication rate of up to 3% (49). Percutaneous lung biopsy achieves an accuracy of 80–95% in malignant lesions and 70–80% in benign lesions (50). Pneumothorax rates vary from 15–40% and require chest tube placement in 5–20% of cases (51). Patients with COPD are at higher risk using either imaging modality.

Abscess and Fluid Drainage

Needle aspiration of fluid collections is used to determine the nature of the fluid or the presence of infection. Catheter drainage is effective in the treatment of ab-

scesses and in palliation of symptoms resulting from other fluid collections such as pancreatic pseudocysts, hematomas, lymphoceles, and recurrent pleural effusions (52).

A safe access route must be determined prior to catheter placement. US or CT guidance can be used for the entire procedure but are best suited for initial access. Tract dilation and catheter placement is best performed under fluoroscopy to observe directly dilators and catheters as they are passed over the guidewire. Transgression of vascular structures, the pleural space, and bowel must be avoided. Deep pelvic abscesses are sometimes difficult to access safely with a percutaneous route because of surrounding vital structures. Use of transrectal or transvaginal catheter placement has been advocated as potential alternatives (Fig. 25.27).

The patient is positioned for optimal access, usually supine, with patient comfort kept in mind. Because catheters are left in place for several days or weeks, the skin exit site should be positioned to allow the patient to lie comfortably in bed. In lung abscess drainage, the lung containing the abscess should be placed in the dependent position. Otherwise, there is risk of infecting the noninvolved lung by tracheobronchial spillage, a potential catastrophe (53).

When performing diagnostic fluid aspiration, use a small-gauge needle initially and insert it during suspended respiration. Withdraw a small amount of fluid for Gram stain, culture, and other required tests. If no fluid is obtained, a larger needle should be tried, as the fluid may be too viscous for a thin needle. One should not remove too much fluid initially if a catheter is to be placed because access may be lost as the cavity collapses away from the needle tip.

Drainage catheters are available in many diameters, ranging from 6 French to 20 French or larger. Cysts and seromas can be drained with smaller catheter sizes, whereas more viscous fluid will require larger catheters. If the fluid contains solid-appearing debris, large-bore catheters will be necessary. Multiple catheters may be needed if the collection is multiloculated.

Procedure. Catheters may be placed using the trocar technique, sheath-needle technique, or Seldinger technique. The trocar technique is usually used when fluid collections are large and the route of entry does not pose significant risk of injury to vital structures. Sheath-needle and Seldinger techniques are over-the-wire methods of tract dilation followed by catheter placement (Fig. 25.28). They are used when the access window is narrower or when risk for injury to adjacent structures is higher. The collection is evacuated at the time of initial catheter placement. Irrigation with saline until the return is cleared of particulate debris may aid in the prevention of subsequent catheter occlusion. If irrigation is performed, care must be taken to avoid overdistension of the cavity, as this may precipitate hematogenous seeding and sepsis. The catheter is attached to a gravity drainage bag or low suction.

Daily monitoring of catheter function and the patient's clinical response is performed to assess the need for follow-up imaging and catheter removal. The catheter should be gently irrigated at least once a day with sterile

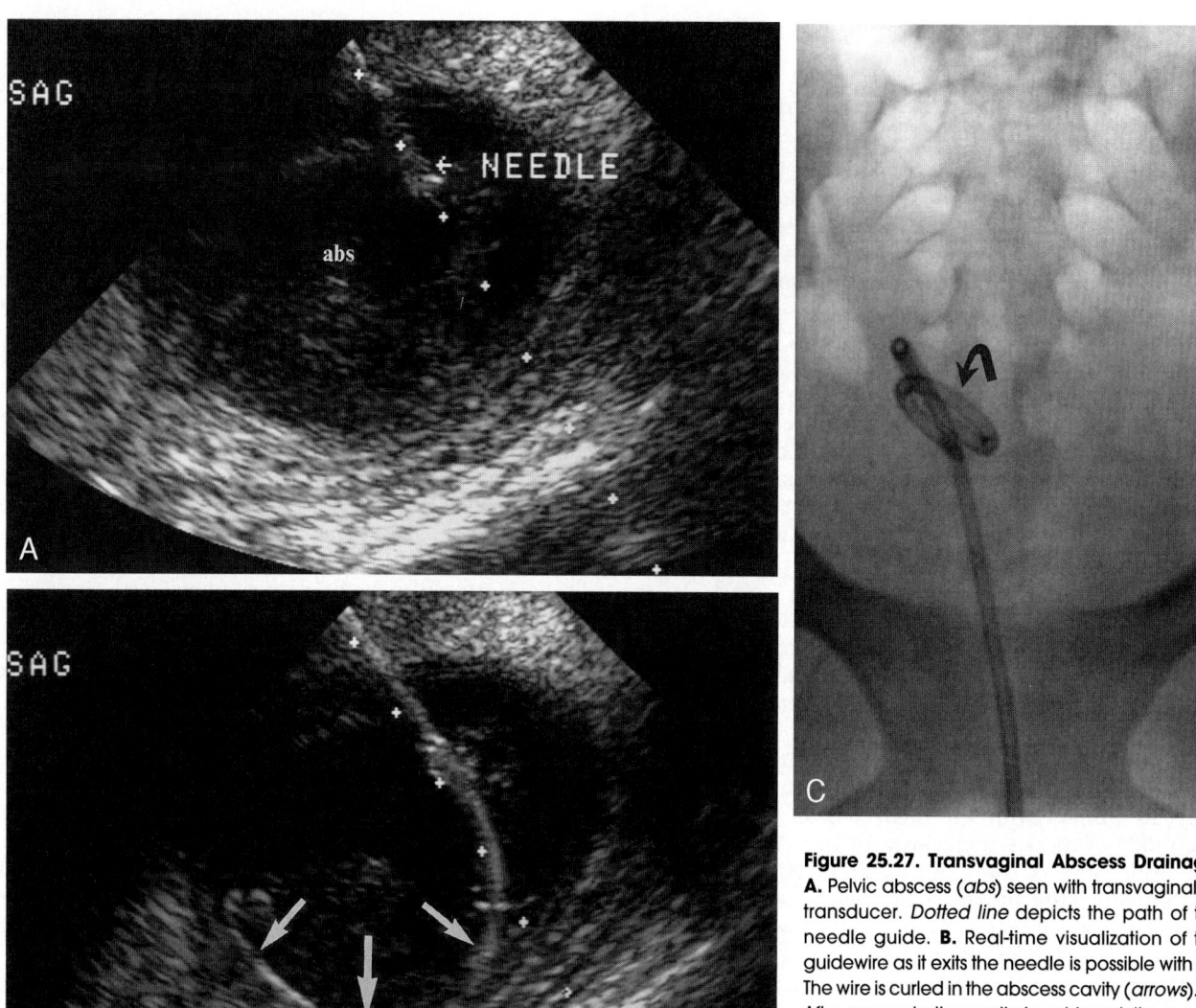

Figure 25.27. Transvaginal Abscess Drainage.
A. Pelvic abscess (*abs*) seen with transvaginal US transducer. *Dotted line* depicts the path of the needle guide. **B.** Real-time visualization of the guidewire as it exits the needle is possible with US. The wire is curled in the abscess cavity (*arrows*). **C.** After access to the cavity is achieved, the procedure is completed under fluoroscopic guidance. Because suturing is not feasible with transvaginal or transrectal catheters, a catheter with a locking pigtail (*curved arrow*) is necessary. (Courtesy of Fred Joseph, Travis Air Force Base, California.)

saline. More frequent irrigation is often required in viscous or debris-filled fluid collections. Temperature curves, vital signs, and drainage volumes are monitored.

Defervescence should occur within a couple of days with adequate drainage. Leukocytosis may be slower to resolve than fever. If fever persists, a repeat CT scan to check for undrained fluid collections is performed. Additional catheters may be needed, or the catheter may be manipulated under fluoroscopic guidance to achieve better positioning. Administration of intracavitary urokinase may be considered for multiloculated collections or collections with thick fibrous strands (54). Drainage volumes should decrease progressively in several days to a week. Sudden decreases in catheter output usually indicate a mechanical catheter problem such as kinking or obstruction, and a sudden increase is suspicious for a fistulous communication. Diversion of bile or urine flow may be necessary if fistulous communication with these structures is present. Abscesses associated with fistulas require longer periods for drainage.

Catheter Removal is determined by resolution of infectious signs and symptoms in conjunction with a catheter output of less than 10–20 cc in a 24-hour period. A CT scan or a contrast sinogram is performed if clinical indicators are equivocal. If a fistula has been discovered during the course of drainage, a sinogram of the fistula or sinus tract is performed to document healing.

Cure rates with percutaneous abscess drainage are 90–95% for simple, unilocular abscesses. In multilocular, viscous, or debris-filled abscesses, cure rates drop to 70–85% (52). There is often still a benefit to percutaneous drainage even if a cure cannot be achieved. Operative intervention can be delayed until the patient is more stable, permitting an elective procedure in a "cleaner" surgical field (52). Recurrence of the abscess is usually the result of a persistent abnormal communication or leak, premature catheter removal, or drainage of an infected tumor. The overall complication rate is approximately 10% (55).

Genitourinary Intervention

Percutaneous Nephrostomy is the most common intervention performed in the genitourinary system. Nephrostomy catheters are used to relieve mechanically obstructed renal collecting systems in both native and transplant kidneys (Fig. 25.29). Nephrostomy tube placement is the preferred method of urinary diversion for treatment of urinary leaks and fistulas. Access into the renal collecting system is also needed for tract creation in percutaneous stone removal, dilation of ureteral strictures, antegrade ureteral stent placement, and performance of a Whitaker test. Optimal guidance for nephrostomy placement is with use of real-time US. If US is not readily available, fluoroscopy may also be used if the renal outline is visible or if the patient's renal function allows safe administration of IV contrast for collecting system opacification.

The patient is placed in a prone or prone-oblique position. A thin needle is directed along an oblique posterolateral pathway through the posterior flank. Needle entry into a posterior calyx in the middle or lower pole of the kidney is required (Fig. 25.30). The skin entry site should be below the 12th rib. The needle path should avoid renal hilar vessels, pleural space, liver, spleen, and colon. Uncommonly, a portion of the liver, spleen, or colon is posteromedial and lies in the needle path. For this reason, review of prior cross-sectional imaging studies is valuable. Real-time US guidance is also useful in this regard. Careful planning of the skin entry site and needle path will allow successful, uncomplicated nephrostomy placement in the majority of cases (56,57).

Respiration is suspended during advancement of a thin noncutting needle toward the selected calyx. A decrease in resistance is noted when the collecting system is entered. The stylet is removed to observe reflux of urine, and a 0.018-in. guidewire is carefully advanced into the collecting system under fluoroscopic control.

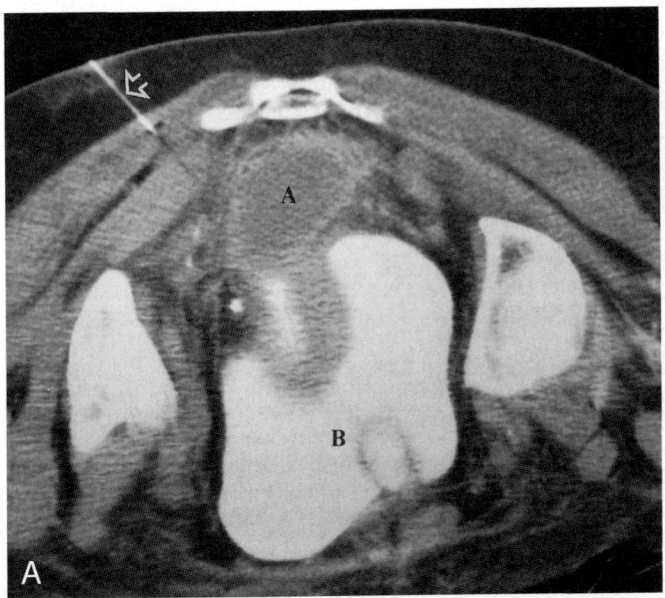

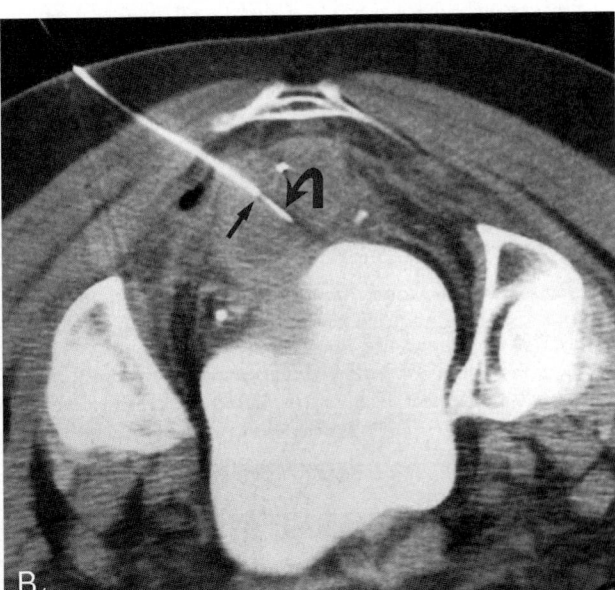

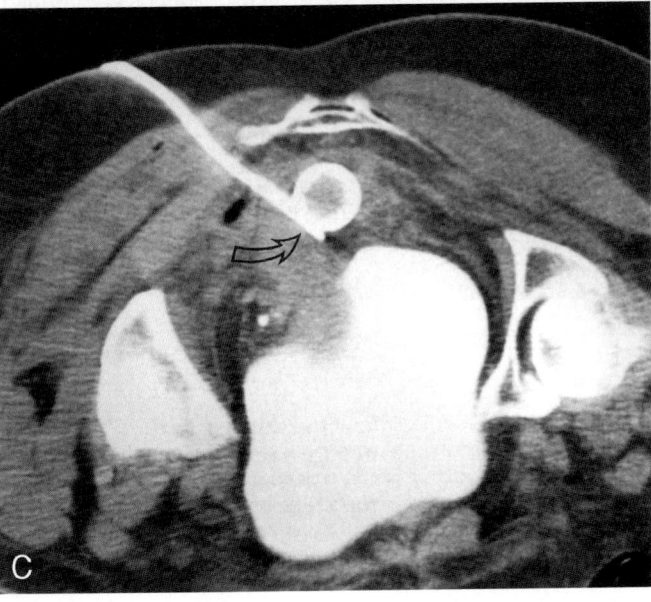

Figure 25.28. Presacral Abscess. A. Using a transgluteal path with the patient prone, a localizing needle (*open arrow*) has been placed. This patient with sepsis had undergone recent abdominoperineal resection. The needle course is too steep, as it does not target the center of the abscess. **B.** A second needle has been placed at a slightly shallower angle, using the course of the first needle as a guide. A guidewire (*curved arrow*) exits the needle tip (*arrowhead*) and is looped within the abscess. **C. A pigtail catheter** with self-retaining loop is placed in the abscess (*curved open arrow*) after tract dilatation. *A*, abscess; *B*, urinary bladder.

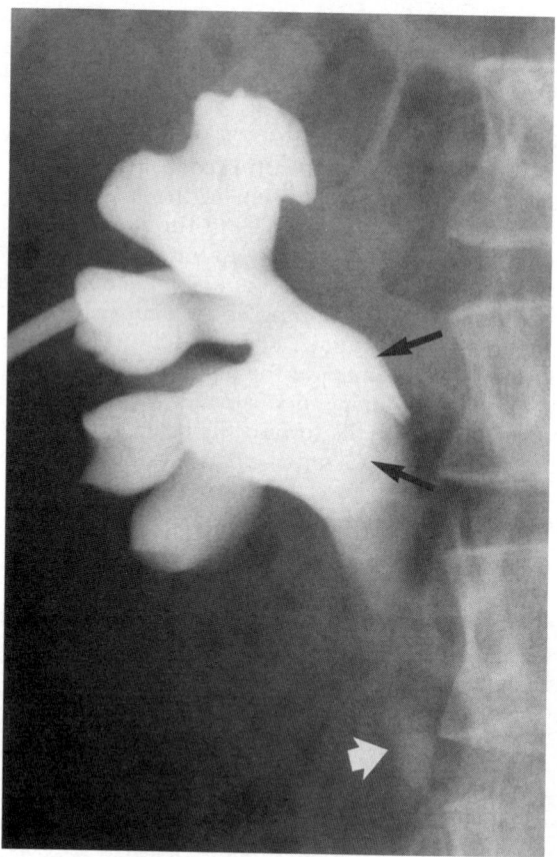

Figure 25.29. Percutaneous Nephrostomy Tube. In this patient with urosepsis, a percutaneous nephrostomy catheter with a self-retaining loop (*black arrows*) has been placed in the right renal pelvis. Note hydronephrosis secondary to an obstructing proximal ureteral stone (*white arrow*). Access is via the middle rather than lower pole calyx in anticipation of antegrade ureteral stent placement.

Little resistance should be encountered. If the calyx entered is appropriate for catheter placement, exchange for a 0.035-in. wire is made by means of a dilator system. The tract is dilated to the appropriate French size, and the nephrostomy tube is placed. Catheter position is confirmed with a small volume contrast injection, and the tube is left to external drainage. Antegrade pyelography may be performed at the time of initial tube placement or may be delayed for several days to allow decompression and resolution of infection if present.

Antibiotics are continued if infection is present. The patient is monitored for complications and tube function. The tube is flushed with 5–10 cc sterile saline every 4 hours if blood clots obstruct drainage. Blood-tinged urine is normally seen for up to 48 hours after nephrostomy placement. Grossly bloody urine indicates possible vascular injury. If vital signs or hemoglobin levels suggest ongoing blood loss, the patient should be evaluated for perinephric or retroperitoneal hematoma or renal arterial injury. If active arterial bleeding is confirmed, transcatheter embolization can be performed, with a high success rate.

Whitaker test is a diagnostic study that evaluates the physiologic significance of a dilated renal collecting sys-

tem in a patient who is still able to produce urine. When it is not clear whether the patient has an obstruction, the pressure gradient from the dilated renal pelvis to the bladder is measured using manometry. A dilute saline–contrast mixture is perfused into the renal pelvis at a rate of 10 cc/min while measuring the pressure gradient. A gradient of 15 cm of water or less is normal, whereas higher gradients are indicative of obstruction (58).

Ureteral Stents are catheters with multiple sideholes and a pigtail configuration at both ends. One end is positioned in the renal pelvis and the other in the bladder (Fig. 25.31). They are commonly known as "double J" stents. Ureteral stents can be placed in either an antegrade or retrograde fashion (59). Cystoscopic retrograde stent placement by a urologist is preferred. If unsuccessful, percutaneous antegrade placement is performed by an interventional radiologist. Indications for ureteral stent placement include ureteral obstructions resulting from malignancies of the bladder, prostate, cervix, and other pelvic structures; benign obstruction from strictures or stone disease; and traumatic laceration or transection of the ureter (Fig. 25.32). Associated urinomas respond well to percutaneous aspiration or drainage.

Percutaneous Nephrolithotomy (PCNL) is the percutaneous treatment of renal calculi. A team approach between interventional radiologist and urologist is common and benefits patient care. Using a nephrostomy tract for access, a large sheath (up to 30 French) is placed into the collecting system. Stones can then be removed or fragmented using a variety of urologic instruments. The application of extracorporeal shock-wave lithotripsy (ESWL) and ureteroscopic techniques for the primary treatment of nephrolithiasis has grown, resulting in a decrease in the frequency of PCNL. A definite role for PCNL remains in the management of difficult cases in which the stone burden is too extensive for ESWL or when ESWL and ureteroscopy have failed. Access to the renal collecting system must be planned to permit complete stone removal. Multiple access sites and sessions are sometimes necessary in patients with large stone burdens, such as staghorn calculi. Success depends on stone distribution in the collecting system, overall stone burden, and type of urologic instruments available (60).

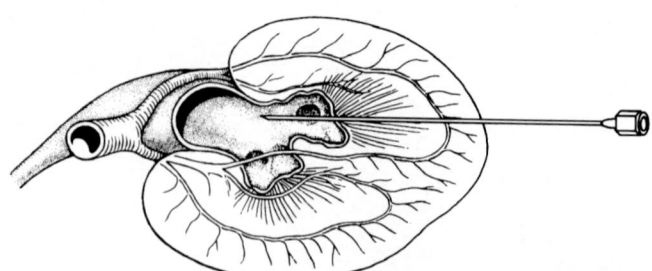

Figure 25.30. Needle Entry Into Posterior Calyx. Cross section of kidney demonstrating needle path for percutaneous nephrostomy placement. Needle entry into a posterior calyx poses the least risk of hemorrhage because it courses in the avascular plane of Brodel. (Redrawn from Kandarpa K, Aruny JE. Handbook of Interventional Radiologic Procedures 2nd ed. Boston: Little, Brown, and Company, 1996.)

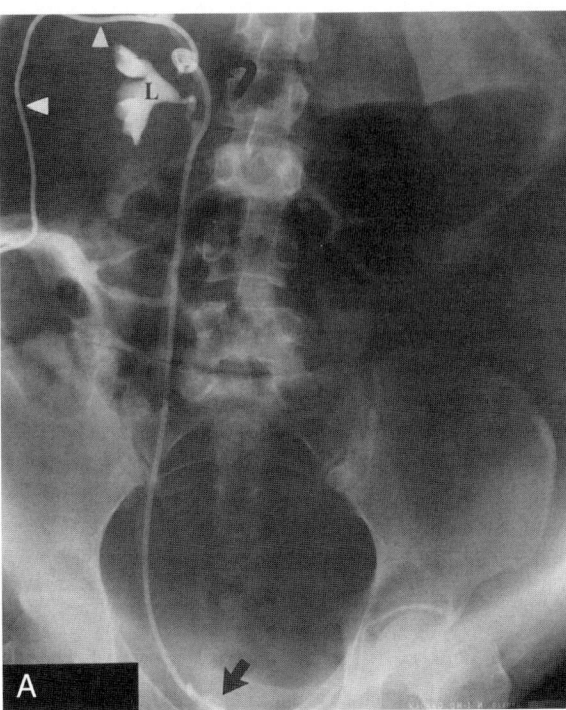

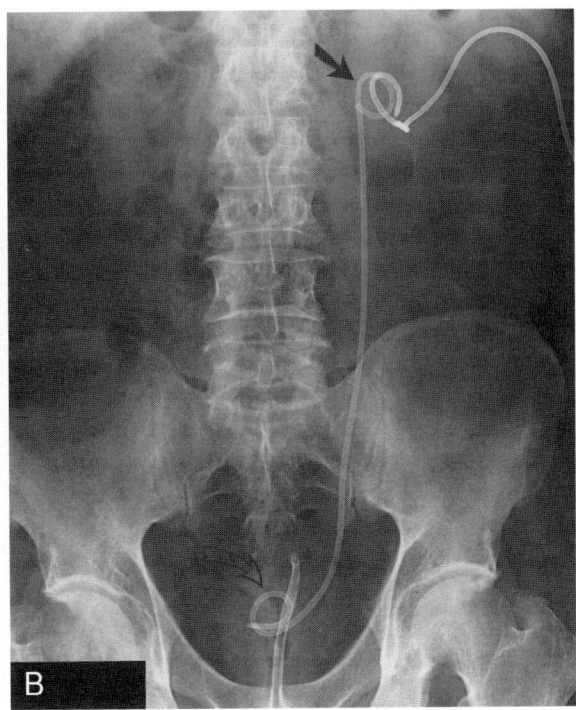

Figure 25.31. Ureteral Stents. A. Ureteral injury was sustained during pelvic surgery. Antegrade placement of ureteral stent requires successful negotiation of the disrupted ureter with a guidewire. Proximal stent is within the upper pole moiety of a duplicated renal collecting system (*curved black arrow*); distal end is in the bladder (*straight black arrow*). A nephrostomy tube (*white arrowheads*) has been left for external drainage of urine. **B.** Abdominal radiograph in a different patient with antegrade ureteral stent placed because of obstructing bladder carcinoma. There is more room for pigtail formation in both the renal pelvis (*black arrow*) and bladder (*open arrow*) than was the case in **(A)**. Note Cudet catheter in the bladder. L, lower pole moiety of renal collecting system.

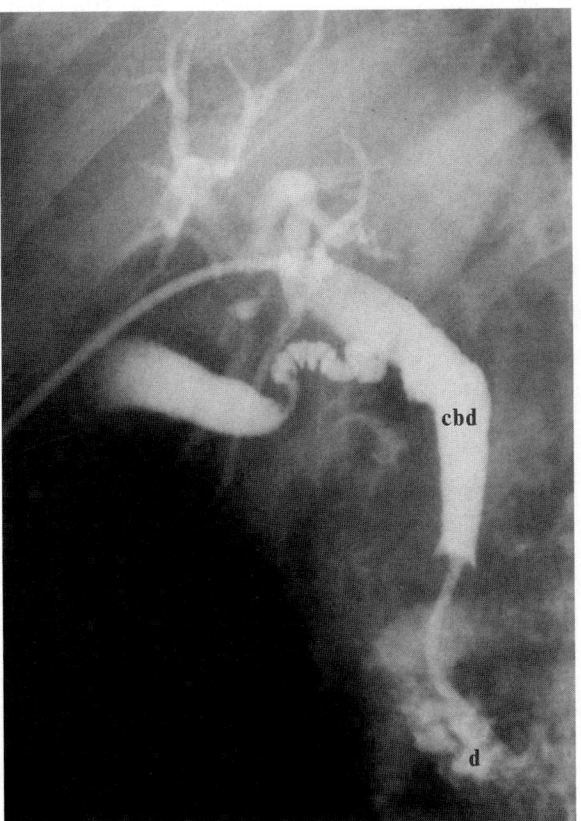

Figure 25.32. Transhepatic Biliary Drain. An internal-external biliary drainage catheter is in place. The catheter enters a right intrahepatic biliary duct and traverses the obstructing lesion in the common bile duct (*cbd*). The pigtail is within the second portion of the duodenum (*d*). Note abrupt margin of the obstructing ampullary tumor.

Fallopian Tube Recanalization is performed in women with infertility and proximal fallopian tube occlusion. With the patient in a lithotomy position, a speculum is inserted using sterile technique. A 5 French transcervical catheter is used to perform selective contrast injection of the fallopian tubes to document tubal occlusion. A 0.035-in. guidewire or 3 French microcatheter is guided into the occluded tube under fluoroscopic control. This maneuver renders the fallopian tube patent in 75–95% of cases. Intrauterine pregnancy rates range from 20% to more than 50% (61).

Biliary Intervention

Biliary intervention includes transhepatic cholangiography, brush biopsy, drainage procedures, stenting, and percutaneous stone removal. Indications center on the need to evaluate and treat causes of biliary obstruction with or without superimposed cholangitis.

Transhepatic Cholangiography (THC) entails the injection of contrast into the biliary ductal system with a thin noncutting needle introduced transhepatically. The procedure is less frequently performed today because of widespread use of ERCP as well as US. It is indicated in patients requiring contrast evaluation of the biliary tree if endoscopic methods fail. In patients with previous biliary-enteric bypass procedures such as hepaticojejunostomy or choledochojejunostomy, endoscopic access to the bile ducts difficult, if not impossible.

Right duct puncture is the traditional access method. The thin needle is passed into the liver, with skin entry in the midaxillary line inferior to the 10th rib. The needle is steadily advanced during suspended respiration under fluoroscopic visualization toward the pedicle of T12. Small volumes of dilute contrast are injected while slowly withdrawing the needle until a bile duct is opacified. Cholangiography is then performed.

Percutaneous biliary procedures pose a particularly high risk for inducing bacteremia and sepsis. Extreme care must be applied to avoid overdistension of the bile ducts. If drainage is to be performed, it is sometimes appropriate to defer definitive cholangiography until decompression of the ducts has been achieved. Other complications include hemobilia, vascular injury (Fig. 25.33), and peritonitis (62).

Percutaneous Biliary Drainage is performed to relieve symptomatic biliary obstruction when endoscopic drainage is not possible (63,64). Common benign causes include cholangitis, pancreatitis, and iatrogenic strictures. The primary malignant causes are pancreatic carcinoma, ampullary carcinoma, and cholangiocarcinoma. Access to the biliary system is obtained as described for THC. Left ductal access is an alternative in patients with a left lobe that is accessible for percutaneous puncture. US guidance is particularly useful for this approach. Methods of drainage can be classified as external, internal, and internal–external. *External drainage* is performed by placing a drainage catheter into obstructed bile ducts and attaching the catheter to an external gravity drainage bag. Close monitoring of fluids and electrolytes is necessary. Bile output can be substantial, resulting in serious electrolyte disturbances and dehydration if fluids and electrolytes are not adequately replenished. *Internal–external drainage* catheters have multiple sideholes that are able to bridge the obstructing lesion. The proximal sideholes are positioned above the obstruction, and the distal sideholes are placed into the duodenum. This allows internal drainage of bile as well as the potential for external drainage (Fig. 25.34). *Internal drainage* is achieved with internalized stents placed across the obstructing lesion. Advantages of internal drainage include the ability to remove external catheters completely. These are often bothersome to the patient. A disadvantage is loss of percutaneous access to the biliary system.

Numerous stents for internal biliary drainage are available. These fall into two groups: metal and plastic. Plastic stents are unable to expand in size and have lower patency rates because of their smaller internal diameter. They can be removed endoscopically when they

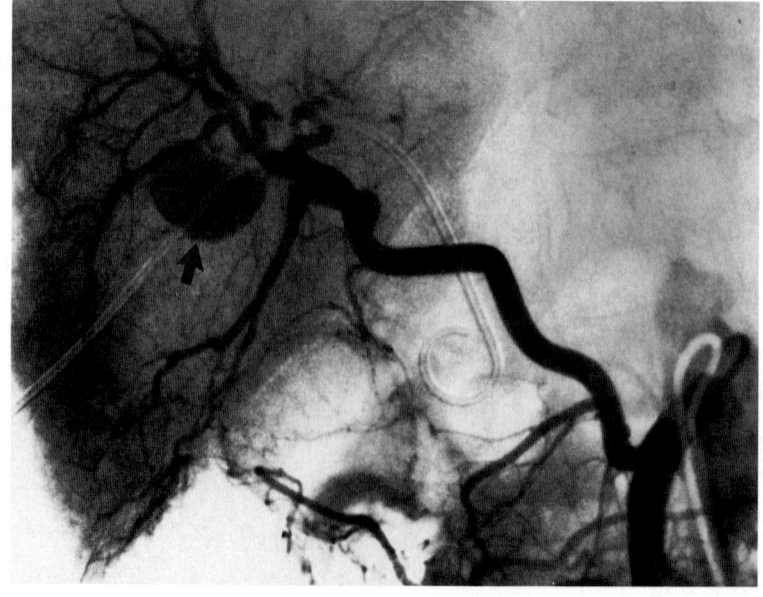

Figure 25.33. Hepatic Artery Pseudoaneurysm. A pseudoaneurysm (*arrow*) arising from a right hepatic artery branch. This was a complication of biliary drainage catheter placement. The catheter can be faintly seen on this subtracted image. Often the drainage catheter must be removed over a guidewire before arteriography in order to demonstrate hemorrhage because the catheter provides a tamponade effect.

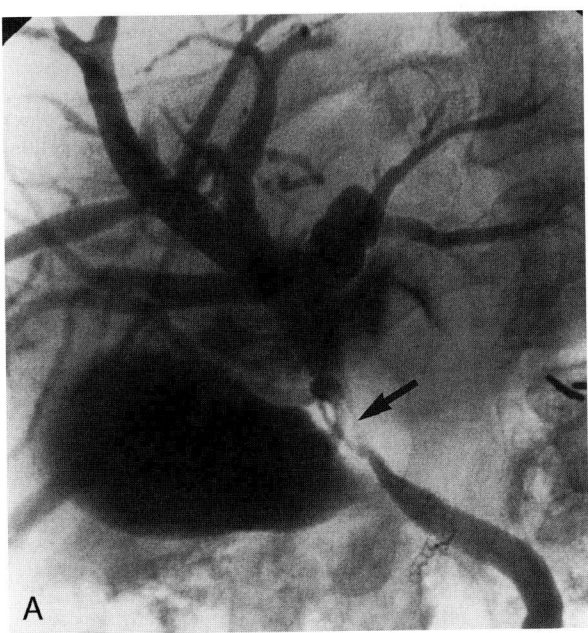

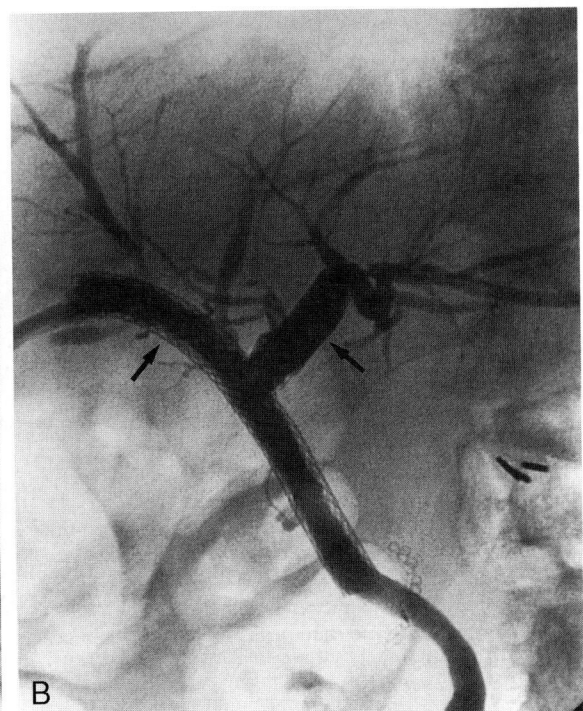

Figure 25.34. Internal Biliary Stents. A. Cholangiogram demonstrates intrahepatic biliary dilatation caused by neoplastic obstruction at the hilar level (*arrow*). The right and left intrahepatic ductal systems are isolated from one another. **B.** Metallic biliary stents (*arrows*) have been placed at the bifurcation into right and left ducts in a T-configuration. There is complete decompression of the biliary system. (Courtesy of Greg Smith, Atlanta, Georgia.)

become occluded. Metal stents cannot be removed, but their patency rates are higher as a result of their greater expansion ratio, which enables them to achieve significantly larger diameters (65,66). Metal stents are essentially permanent devices that inevitably become obstructed. They are primarily used for palliation in patients with short life expectancies (Fig. 25.34).

A relatively new area of biliary intervention has emerged since the introduction of laparoscopic cholecystectomy in 1989. Iatrogenic biliary injuries are more common with laparoscopic cholecystectomy than with open cholecystectomy. Minor biliary complications of laparoscopic cholecystectomy include bilomas and biliary ascites. Abscesses occur if these bile collections become infected. These minor complications respond well to percutaneous drainage. Major injuries include ligation, laceration, or transection of the ducts. Delayed strictures may also occur. Treatment of these complications involves external biliary diversion in addition to drainage of bilomas or abscesses. Ultimately, operative repair with choledochojejunostomy or hepaticojejunostomy is necessary if feasible. Feasibility is related to the level of ductal injury in relation to the common hepatic duct bifurcation, as well as the presence of variant ductal anatomy (67).

Cholecystostomy is indicated in patients with acute cholecystitis who are not operative candidates. Acalculous cholecystitis in critically ill patients is the most common scenario. US is the guidance method of choice for gallbladder puncture. A small catheter is placed in the gallbladder lumen for bile drainage. The ideal access is a transhepatic tract through the bare area of the liver in the gallbladder fossa, which minimizes the risk of bile leakage into the peritoneal cavity. Cultures are obtained but are of questionable value. Successful treatment is evaluated by following the patient's clinical response to drainage. The catheter must be left in place 2–3 weeks before removal regardless of the clinical response. Earlier removal may lead to leakage of bile into the peritoneal cavity and precipitate bile peritonitis (68).

Interventional radiology continues to grow in variety and complexity. These procedures benefit patients by reducing recovery time, minimizing surgical scarring, and decreasing overall morbidity. Along with laparoscopic surgery and endoscopic interventions, interventional procedures are examples of *minimally invasive therapy* that have emerged as alternatives to more invasive open surgical procedures. Technological advancement in materials, in design of endoprostheses, and in sophistication of imaging equipment is an ongoing process. Interventional radiology occupies a leading role in the expansion of minimally invasive techniques with the goal of providing continuous improvement to the quality of patient care.

References

1. Barth KH, Matsumoto AH. Patient care in interventional radiology: a perspective. Radiology 1991;178:11–17.
2. Dotter CT, Judkins MP. Transluminal treatment of arteriosclerotic obstructions: description of a new technic and a preliminary report of its application. Circulation 1964;30:654–670.

3. Standards of practice committee of the society of cardiovascular and interventional radiology: guidelines for percutaneous transluminal angioplasty. Radiology 1990;177:619–626.

4. Castaneda-Zuniga WR, Formanek A, Tadavarthy M, et al. The mechanism of balloon angioplasty. Radiology 1980;135:565–571.

5. Becker GJ, Katzen BT, Dake MD. Noncoronary angioplasty. Radiology 1989; 170:921–940.

6. Johnston KW. Femoral and popliteal arteries: reanalysis of results of balloon angioplasty. Radiology 1992; 183:767–771.

7. Brown KT, Moore ID, Getrajdman GI, Saddekni S. Infrapopliteal angioplasty: long-term follow-up. J Vasc Interv Radiol 1993;4:139–144.

8. Schwarten DE, Cutliff WB. Arterial occlusive disease below the knee: treatment with percutaneous transluminal angioplasty performed with low-profile catheters and steerable guide wires. Radiology 1988;169:71–74.

9. Palmaz JC, Rivera FJ, Encarnacion C. Intravascular stents. In: Najarian JS, Delaney JP, eds. Advances in Vascular Surgery. Chicago: Year Book, 1993:107–134.

10. Vorwerk D, Guenther RW, Schurmann K, et al. Primary stent placement for chronic iliac artery occlusions: follow-up results in 103 patients. Radiology 1995;194:745–749.

11. Katzen BT. Endovascular stent grafts: the beginning of the future, or the beginning of the end? J Vasc Interv Radiol 1996;7:469–476.

12. Richter GM, Roeren TK, Noeldge G, et al. Balloon-expandable stent placement versus PTA in iliac artery stenoses and occlusions: long-term results of a randomized trial. J Vasc Interv Radiol 1992;3:9.

13. Palmaz JC, Laborde JC, Rivera FJ, et al. Stenting of the iliac arteries with the Palmaz stent: experience from a multicenter trial. Cardiovasc Intervent Radiol 1992;15:291–297.

14. Martin EC, Katzen BT, Benenati JF, et al. Multicenter trial of the Wallstent in the iliac and femoral arteries. J Vasc Interv Radiol 1995;6:843–849.

15. Saproval MR, Long AL, Raynaud AC, et al. Femoropopliteal stent placement: long-term results. Radiology 1992;184:833–839.

16. Rees CR, Palmaz JC, Becker GJ, et al. Palmaz stent in atherosclerotic stenoses involving the ostia of the renal arteries: preliminary report of a multicenter trial. Radiology 1991;181:507–514.

17. McNamara TO, Fischer JR. Thrombolysis of peripheral arterial and graft occlusions: improved results using high-dose urokinase. AJR Am J Roentgenol 1985;144:769–775.

18. LeBlang SD, Becker GJ, Benenati JF, et al. Low-dose urokinase regimen for the treatment of lower extremity arterial and graft occlusions: experience in 132 cases. J Vasc Interv Radiol 1992;3:475–483.

19. Cragg AH, Smith TP, Corson JD, et al. Two urokinase dose regimens in native and graft occlusions: initial results of a prospective, randomized clinical trial. Radiology 1991;178:681–686.

20. Gardiner GA, Sullivan KL. Complications of regional thrombolytic therapy. In: Kadir S, ed. Current Practice of Interventional Radiology. Philadelphia: BC Decker, 1991:87–91.

21. McNamara TO, Bomberger RA, Merchant RF. Intra-arterial urokinase as the initial therapy for acutely ischemic lower limbs. Circulation 1991:83(suppl I):I-106–I-119.

22. Widlus DM, Venbrux AC, Benenati JF, et al. Fibrinolytic therapy for upper-extremity arterial occlusions. Radiology 1990;175:393–399.

23. Semba CP, Dake MD. Iliofemoral deep venous thrombosis: aggressive therapy with catheter-directed thrombolysis. Radiology 1994;191:487–494.

24. Drooz AT et al. for the SCVIR Standards of Practice Committee. Quality improvement guidelines for percutaneous transcatheter embolization. J Vasc Interv Radiol 1997;8:889–895.

25. Katz MD, Hanks SE. Arteriography and transcatheter treatment of extremity trauma. In: Baum S, Pentecost MJ, eds. Abrams Angiography. Boston: Little Brown and Co, 1997:857–868.

26. Coldwell DM, Stokes KR, Yakes WF. Embolotherapy: agents, clinical applications, and techniques. Radiographics 1994;14:623–643.

27. Panetta T, Sclafani SJA, Goldstein AS, Phillips TF. Percutaneous transcatheter embolization for arterial trauma. J Vasc Surg 1985;2:54–64.

28. Zuckerman DA, Bocchini TP, Birnbaum EH. Massive hemorrhage in the lower gastrointestinal tract in adults: diagnostic imaging and intervention. AJR Am J Roentgenol 1993;161:703–711.

29. Ferris EJ, McCowan TC, Carver DK, McFarland DR. Percutaneous inferior vena caval filters: follow-up of 7 designs in 320 patients. Radiology 1993;188:851–856.

30. Dorfman,GS. Percutaneous inferior vena caval filters. Radiology 1990;174:987–992.

31. Grassi CJ. Inferior vena cava filters: analysis of five currently available devices. AJR Am J Roentgenol 1991;156:813–821.

32. Gray RJ. Percutaneous intervention for permanent hemodialysis access: a review. J Vasc Interv Radiol 1997;8:313–327.

33. Valji K. Transcatheter treatment of thrombosed hemodialysis access grafts. AJR Am J Roentgenol 1995;164:823–829.

34. Trerotola SO. Mechanical thrombolysis of hemodialysis grafts. 1997 SCVIR Scientific Syllabus 126–130.

35. Trerotola SO. Interventional radiology in central venous stenosis and occlusion. Semin Intervent Radiol 1994;11:291–304.

36. Denny DF. Placement and management of long-term central venous access catheters and ports. AJR Am J Roentgenol 1993;161:385–393.

37. Lund GB. Complications from long-term tunneled venous access catheters. Semin Intervent Radiol 1994;11:340–348.

38. Crain MR, Mewissen MW, Ostrowski GJ, et al. Fibrin sleeve stripping for salvage of failing hemodialysis catheters: technique and initial results. Radiology 1996;198:41–44.

39. Nazarian GK, Myers TV, Bjarnason H, et al. Applications of the amplatz snare device during interventional radiologic procedures. AJR Am J Roentgenol 1995;165:673–678.

40. Cimochowski GE, Worley E, Rutherford WE, et al. Superiority of the internal jugular over the subclavian access for temporary dialysis. Nephron 1990; 54:154–161.

41. Rosch J, Hanafee W, Snow H. Transjugular portal venography and radiologic portacaval shunt: an experimental study. Radiology 1969; 92:1112–1114.

42. Ochs A, Rossle M, Haag K, et al. The transjugular intrahepatic portosystemic stent-shunt procedure for refractory ascites. New Engl J Med 1995;332:1192–1197.

43. Kerlan RK, LaBerge JM, Gordon RL, Ring EJ. Transjugular intrahepatic portosystemic shunts: current status. AJR Am J Roentgenol 1995; 164:1059–1066.

44. Zemel G, etc: Technical advances in transjugular intrahepatic portosystemic shunts. Radiographics 1992;12:615–622.

45. Saxon RR, Keller FS. Technical aspects of accessing the portal vein during the TIPS procedure. J Vasc Interv Radiol 1997;8:733–744.

46. Semba CP, Saperstein L, Nyman U, Dake MD. Hepatic laceration from wedged venography performed before transjugular intrahepatic portosystemic shunt placement. J Vasc Interv Radiol 1996;7:143–146.

47. Coldwell DM, Ring EJ, Rees CR, et al. Multicenter investigation of the role of transjugular intrahepatic portosystemic shunt in the management of portal hypertension. Radiology 1995;196:335–340.

48. Haskal ZJ, Pentecost MJ, Soulen MC, et al. Transjugular intrahepatic portosystemic shunt stenosis and revision: early and midterm results. AJR Am J Roentgenol 1994;163:439–444.

49. Charboneau JW, Reading CC, Welch TJ. CT and sonographically guided needle biopsy: current techniques and new innovations. AJR Am J Roentgenol 1990;154:1–10.

50. Westcott JL. Percutaneous transthoracic needle biopsy. Radiology 1988;169:593–601.

51. Mueller PR, vanSonnenberg E. Interventional radiology in the chest and abdomen. N Engl J Med 1990; 322:1364–1374.

52. vanSonnenberg E, Agostino HB, Casola G, et al. Percutaneous abscess drainage: current concepts. Radiology 1991;181:617–626.

53. vanSonnenberg E, Agostino HB, Casola G, et al. Lung abscess: CT-guided drainage. Radiology 1991;178:347–351.

54. Vogelzang RL, Tobin RS, Burnstein S, et al. Transcatheter intracavitary fibrinolysis of infected extravascular hematomas. AJR Am J Roentgenol 1987;148:378–380.

55. Society of cardiovascular and interventional radiology standards of practice committee: quality improvement guidelines for adult percutaneous abscess and fluid drainage. J Vasc Interv Radiol 1995;6:68–70.

56. Barbaric ZL. Percutaneous nephrostomy for urinary tract obstruction. AJR Am J Roentgenol 1984;143:803–809.

57. Farrell TA, Hicks ME. A review of radiologically guided percutaneous nephrostomies in 303 patients. J Vasc Interv Radiol 1997;8:769–774.

58. Whitaker RH, Chir M. The Whitaker test. Urol Clin North Am 1979;6:529–539.

59. Mitty HA, Train JS, Dan SJ. Placement of ureteral stents by antegrade and retrograde techniques. Radiol Clin North Am 1986;24:587–600.

60. LeRoy AJ. Diagnosis and treatment of nephrolithiasis: current perspectives. AJR Am J Roentgenol 1994;163:1309–1313.

61. Thurmond AS. Selective salpingography and fallopian tube recanalization. AJR Am J Roentgenol 1991;156:33–38.

62. Hamlin JA, Friedman M, Stein MG, Bray JF. Percutaneous biliary drainage: complications of 118 consecutive catheterizations. Radiology 1986;158:199–202.

63. Ferrucci JT Jr, Mueller PR, Harbin WP. Percutaneous transhepatic biliary drainage. Radiology 1980;135:1–13.

64. McLean GK, Burke DR. Role of endoprostheses in the management of malignant biliary obstruction. Radiology 1989;170:961–967.

65. Venbrux AC, Osterman FA Jr. Percutaneous management of benign biliary strictures. Semin Intervent Radiol 1996;13:207–214.

66. Winkelbauer F, Kontrus M, Thurner S. Plastic versus metallic biliary endoprostheses. Semin Intervent Radiol 1996;13:253–261.

67. Slanetz PJ, Boland GW, Mueller PR. Imaging and interventional radiology in laparoscopic injuries to the gallbladder and biliary system. Radiology 1996;201:595–603.

68. Vogelzang RL. Percutaneous cholecystostomy: current concepts and practice. Semin Intervent Radiol 1996;13:215–227.

Section VI GASTROINTESTINAL TRACT

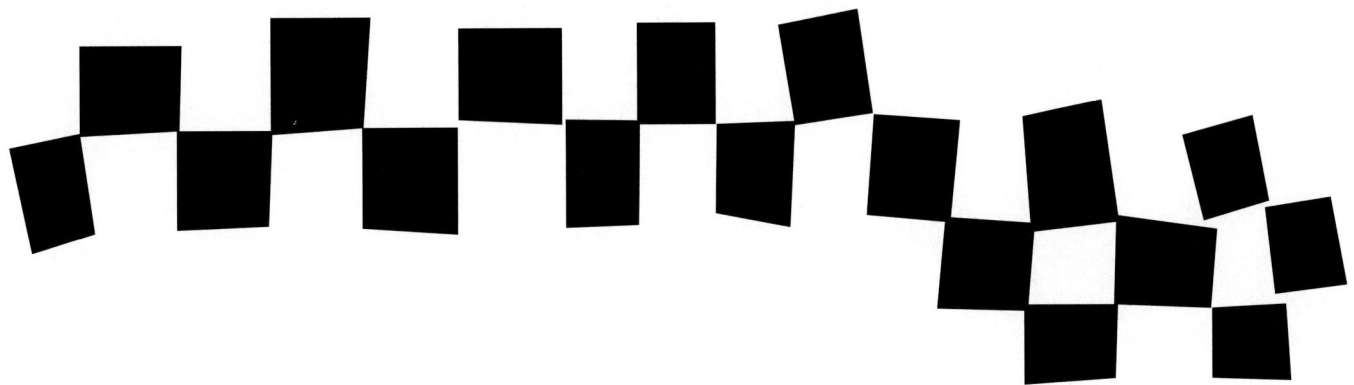

26
Abdomen and Pelvis

William E. Brant

IMAGING METHODS

Plain film radiographs of the abdomen are important for the assessment of the acute abdomen and to serve as "scout" films prior to contrast studies. US, CT, and MR provide comprehensive evaluation of the abdomen including the peritoneal cavity, retroperitoneal compartments, abdominal and pelvic organs, blood vessels, and lymph nodes.

COMPARTMENTAL ANATOMY OF THE ABDOMEN AND PELVIS

Knowledge of the complex compartmental anatomy of the abdomen and pelvis is fundamental to understanding the effects of pathologic processes and to correct interpretation of imaging studies (1). Understanding the shape and extent of anatomic compartments and their normal variations may clarify imaging findings that would otherwise be incomprehensible or lead to misdiagnosis. Fundamental considerations include constant anatomic landmarks, ligaments and fascia that define compartments, and normal variations in size and appearance of the various compartments and recesses. Identifying the precise compartment that an abnormality is in determines to a great extent the origin of the abnormality.

The peritoneal cavity is divided into the greater peritoneal cavity and the lesser peritoneal cavity (the lesser sac) (Fig. 26.1). Within both portions of the peritoneal cavity are numerous recesses in which pathological processes tend to loculate (2). The **right subphrenic space** communicates around the liver with the anterior subhepatic and posterior subhepatic space (Morison's pouch). Morison's pouch (the right hepatorenal fossa) is the most dependent portion of the abdominal cavity in a supine patient and it collects ascites, hemoperitoneum, metastases, and abscesses. The right subphrenic and subhepatic spaces communicate freely with the pelvic peritoneal cavity via the right paracolic gutter.

The **left subphrenic space** communicates freely with the left subhepatic space, but is separated from the right subphrenic space by the falciform ligament and from the left paracolic gutter by the phrenicocolic ligament. The left subphrenic (perisplenic) space distends with fluid from ascites and with blood from splenic trauma. It is a common location for abscesses and for disease processes of the tail of the pancreas. The left subhepatic space (gastrohepatic recess) is affected by diseases of the duodenal bulb, lesser curve of the stomach, gallbladder, and left lobe of the liver.

Free fluid, blood, infection, and peritoneal metastases commonly settle in the pelvis because the pelvis is the most dependent portion of the peritoneal cavity (in the upright patient) and communicates with both sides of the abdomen.

The **falciform ligament** consists of two closely applied layers of peritoneum extending from the umbilicus to the diaphragm in a parasagittal plane (3). The caudal free end of the falciform ligament contains the ligamentum teres, which is the remnant of the obliterated umbilical vein. Paraumbilical veins (portosystemic collateral vessels) that form in the falciform ligament are a specific sign of portal hypertension. The reflections of the falciform ligament separate over the posterior dome of the liver to form the coronary ligaments which define the **"bare area"** of the liver not covered by peritoneum (Fig. 26.2A). The coronary ligaments reflect between the liver and diaphragm and prevent access of ascites and other intraperitoneal processes from covering the bare area of the liver.

The **lesser omentum**, composed of the gastrohepatic and hepatoduodenal ligaments, suspends the stomach and duodenal bulb from the inferior surface of the liver. The lesser omentum separates the gastrohepatic recess of the left subphrenic space from the lesser sac (Figs. 26.1, 26.2). The lesser omentum transmits the coronary veins (which dilate as varices) and contains lymph nodes (which enlarge with involvement by gastric carcinoma and lymphoma). The **lesser sac** is the isolated peritoneal compartment between the stomach and the pancreas (4). It communicates with the rest of the peritoneal cavity (the greater sac) only through the small foramen of Winslow. Pathologic processes in the lesser sac usually occur because of disease in adjacent organs (pancreas, stomach) rather than spread from elsewhere in the abdominal cavity. The lesser sac is normally collapsed but can become huge when filled with fluid.

Figure 26.1. Anatomy of the Peritoneal Cavity.
A. Diagram of an axial cross-section of the abdomen illustrates the recesses of the greater peritoneal cavity and the lesser sac. **B.** CT scan of a patient with a large amount of ascites nicely demonstrates the greater peritoneal cavity and the lesser sac. The lesser sac (*LS*) is bounded by the stomach (*St*) anteriorly, the pancreas (*P*) posteriorly, and the gastrosplenic ligament (*open arrow*) laterally. The falciform ligament (*curved arrow*) separates the right (*rsp*) and left (*lsp*) subphrenic spaces. Fluid from the greater peritoneal cavity extends into Morison's pouch (*long arrow*) between the liver and the right kidney. Fluid in the gastrohepatic recess (*) separates the stomach from the liver (*L*). *S*, spleen; *gb*, gallbladder; *RK*, right kidney; *IVC*, inferior vena cava; *Ao*, aorta; *LK*, left kidney.

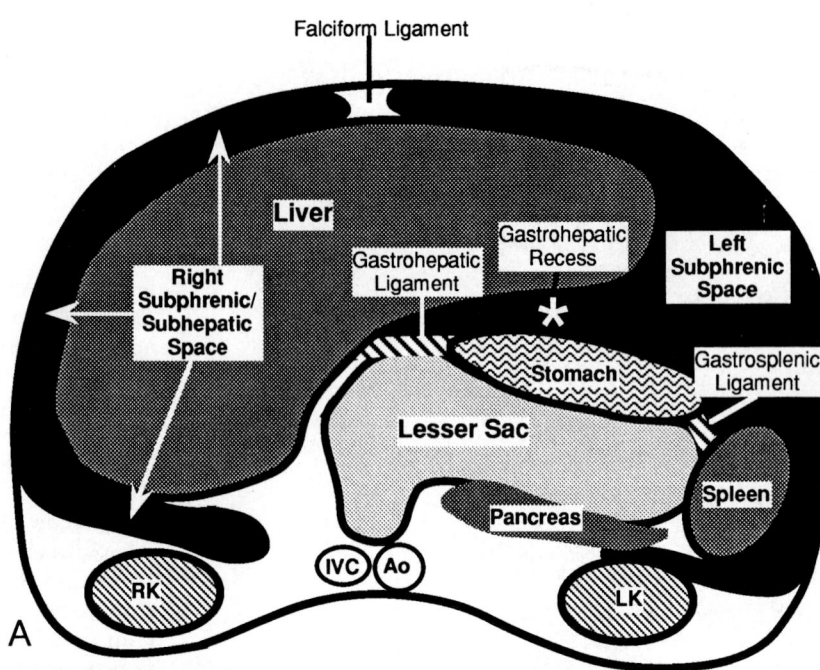

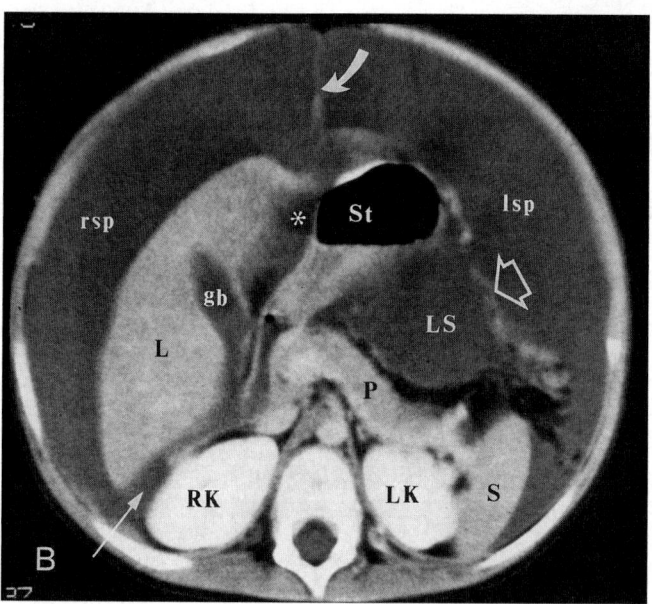

The **greater omentum** is a double layer of peritoneum that hangs from the greater curvature of the stomach and descends in front of the abdominal viscera separating bowel from the anterior abdominal wall (Fig. 26.2) (5). The greater omentum encloses fat and a few blood vessels. It serves as fertile ground for implantation of peritoneal metastases, and assists in loculation of inflammatory processes of the peritoneal cavity (abscesses, tuberculosis).

The retroperitoneal space between the diaphragm and the pelvic brim is divided into anterior pararenal, perirenal, and posterior pararenal compartments by the anterior and posterior renal fascia (Fig. 26.3) (1,6–8). The **anterior pararenal space** extends between the posterior parietal peritoneum and the anterior renal fascia. It is bounded laterally by the lateroconal fascia. The pancreas, duodenal loop, and ascending and descending

portions of the colon are within the anterior pararenal space. Disease in the anterior pararenal space usually originates from these organs (pancreatitis, perforating/penetrating ulcer, diverticulitis).

The anterior and posterior renal fascia encompass the kidney, adrenal gland, and perirenal fat within the **perirenal space**. The anterior renal fascia is thin and consists of one layer of connective tissue (9). The posterior renal fascia is thicker, consisting of two layers of connective tissue (Fig. 26.3). The anterior layer of the posterior renal fascia is continuous with the anterior renal fascia. The posterior layer of the renal fascia is continuous with the lateroconal fascia, forming the lateral boundary of the anterior pararenal space. The anterior and posterior layers of the posterior renal fascia may be separated by inflammatory processes, such as pancreatitis, extending from the anterior pararenal space. The renal fascia is bound to

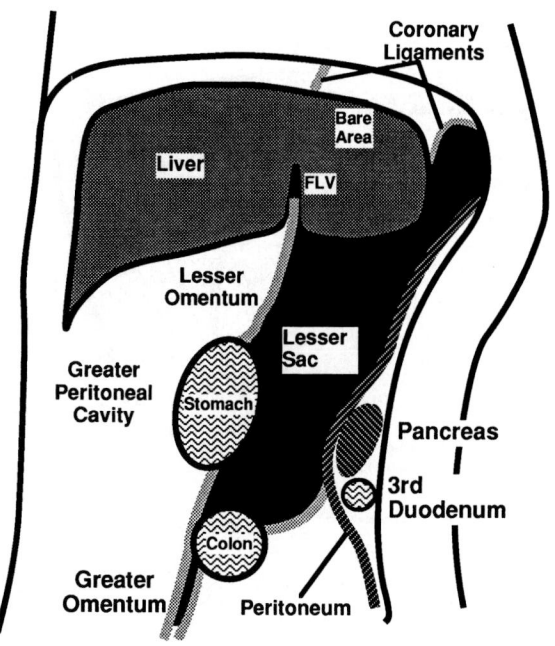

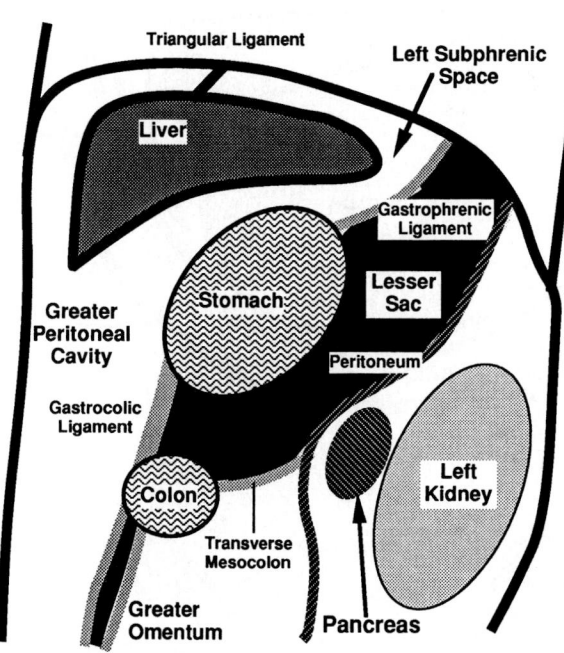

Figure 26.2. The Lesser Sac. Sagittal plane diagrams of the medial **(A)** and lateral **(B)** aspects of the lesser sac illustrate its position posterior to the stomach and anterior to the posterior parietal peritoneum covering the pancreas. Note that projections of the lesser sac extend to the diaphragm, resulting in the potential for disease processes in the lesser sac to cause pleural effusions. The coronary ligaments reflect between the liver and the diaphragm producing a bare area of liver not covered by peritoneum.

the fascia surrounding the aorta and vena cava usually preventing spread of disease to the contralateral perirenal space. However, disease processes arising from the perivascular space may extend into the perirenal space (hemorrhage from aortic aneurysm rupture, lymphoma). Fluid collections in the perirenal space are usually renal in origin (infection, urinoma, hemorrhage). Bridging septa

extend between the renal fascia and the renal capsule tend to cause loculations of fluid processes in the perirenal space. The right perirenal space is open superiorly to the bare area of the liver allowing spread of disease processes (infection, tumor) between the kidney and liver (7).

The **posterior pararenal space** is a potential space, usually filled only with fat, extending from the posterior renal fascia to the transversalis fascia. The posterior pararenal fat continues into the flank as the properitoneal fat "stripe" seen on plain films of the abdomen. The compartment is limited medially by the lateral edges of the psoas and quadratus lumborum muscles. Isolated fluid collections are rare and most commonly caused by spontaneous hemorrhage into the psoas muscle as a result of anticoagulation therapy.

The **pelvis** is divided into three major anatomic compartments (Fig. 26.4). The peritoneal cavity extends to the level of the vagina, forming the pouch of Douglas (**cul-de-sac**) in females (Fig. 26.5), or to the level of the seminal vesicles, forming the rectovesical pouch in males. The broad ligaments reflect over the uterus, fallopian tubes, and parametrial uterine vessels and serve as the anterior boundary of the rectouterine pouch of Douglas. The cul-de-sac is the most dependent portion of the peritoneal cavity and collects fluid, blood, abscesses, and intraperitoneal drop metastases. The **extraperitoneal space of the pelvis** is continous with the retroperitoneal space of the abdomen, extends to the pelvic diaphragm, and includes the retropubic space (of Retzius). Pathologic processes from the pelvis spread preferentially into the retroperitoneal compartments of the abdomen. The **perineum** lies below the pelvic diaphragm and includes the ischiorectal fossa (Fig. 26.6).

FLUID IN THE PERITONEAL CAVITY

Fluid in the peritoneal cavity originates from many different sources and varies greatly in composition. Ascites is serous fluid in the peritoneal cavity most commonly caused by cirrhosis, hypoproteinemia, or congestive heart failure. Exudative ascites results from inflammatory processes such as abscess, pancreatitis, peritonitis, or bowel perforation. Hemoperitoneum results from trauma, surgery or spontaneous hemorrhage. Neoplastic ascites is associated with intraperitoneal tumors. Urine, bile, and chyle may also spread freely within the peritoneal cavity.

Plain films diagnosis of ascites requires that at least 500 cc of fluid be present. Findings are: *a)* diffuse increase in density of the abdomen (gray abdomen), *b)* indistinct margins of the liver, spleen, and psoas muscles, *c)* medial displacement of gas-filled colon, liver, and spleen away from the properitoneal flank stripe, *d)* bulging of the flanks, *e)* increased separation of gas-filled small bowel loops, and *f)* "dog's ears" appearance of symmetric densities in the pelvis due to fluid spilling out of the cul-de-sac on either side of the bladder.

CT demonstrates fluid density in the recesses of the peritoneal cavity (Figs. 26.1B, 26.5). The CT density of the fluid gives a clue as to its composition. Serous ascites has attenuation values near water (−10 to +10 H). Exudative ascites is usually above +15 H, but acute bleeding into the peritoneal cavity averages +45 H.

Figure 26.3. Retroperitoneal Compartmental Anatomy. Diagrams illustrate two normal variations of the reflections of the posterior parietal peritoneum around the descending colon. In **(A)** the colon is entirely retroperitoneal and in **(B)** the peritoneum forms a deep pocket lateral to the colon, allowing intraperitoneal fluid to extend far posteriorly. Fluid or disease processes in the anterior pararenal space from the pancreas or colon may also extend posteriorly to the kidney by separating the two layers of the posterior renal fascia.

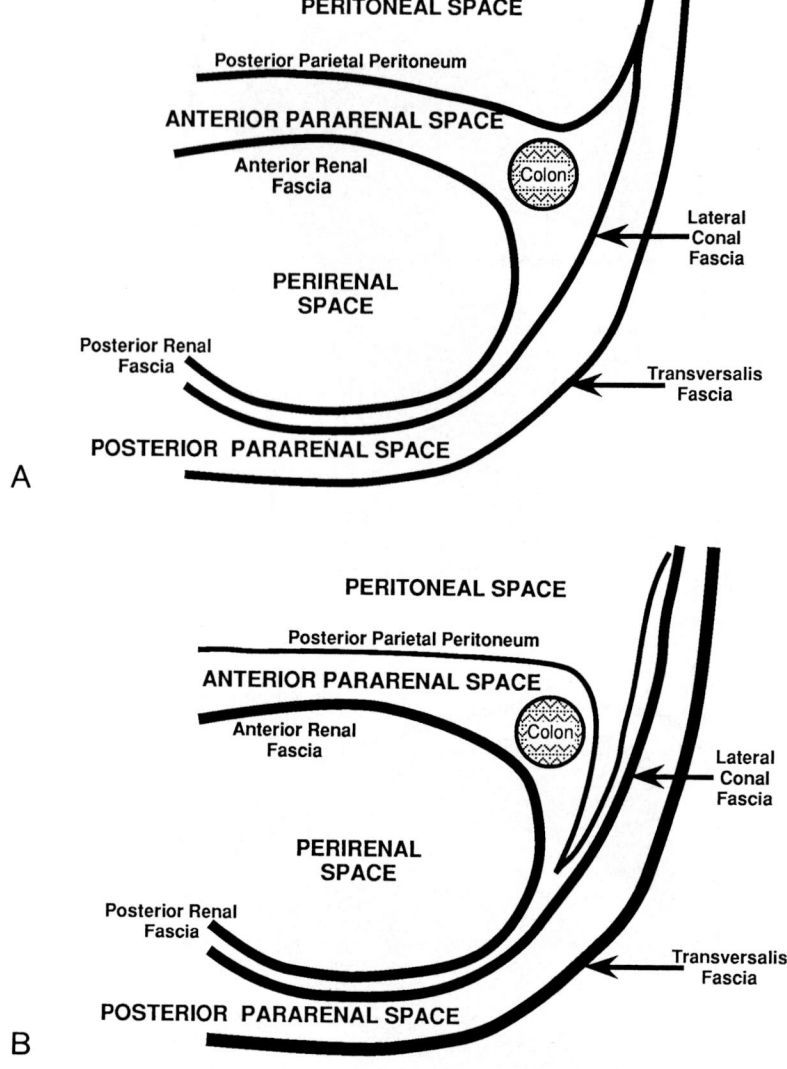

Figure 26.4. Compartmental Anatomy of the Pelvis. Diagram in the coronal plane illustrates the major anatomic compartments of the pelvis.

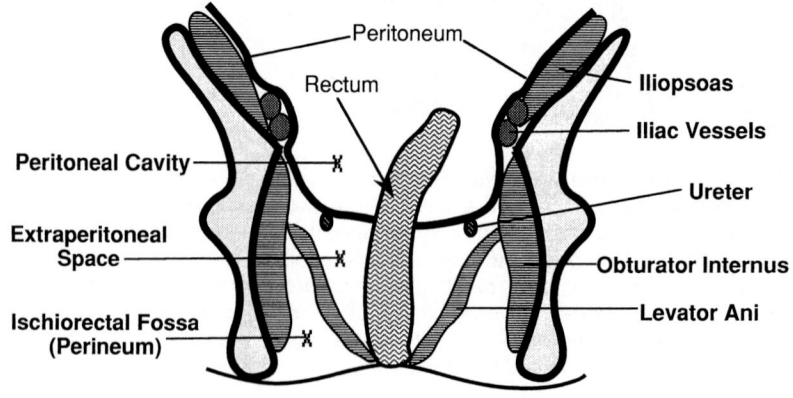

US is sensitive to small amounts of fluid in the peritoneal recesses (see Fig. 36.1). Care must be taken to examine the most gravity-dependent portions of the peritoneal cavity (Morison's pouch and the pelvis). Simple ascites is anechoic, and exudative, hemorrhagic, or neoplastic ascites often contains floating debris. Septations in ascites are associated with an inflammatory or malignant process.

MR shows limited specificity for defining the type of fluid present. Serous fluid is low intensity on T1WI and markedly increased in intensity on T2WI. Hemorrhagic fluid shows high signal intensity on both T1WI and

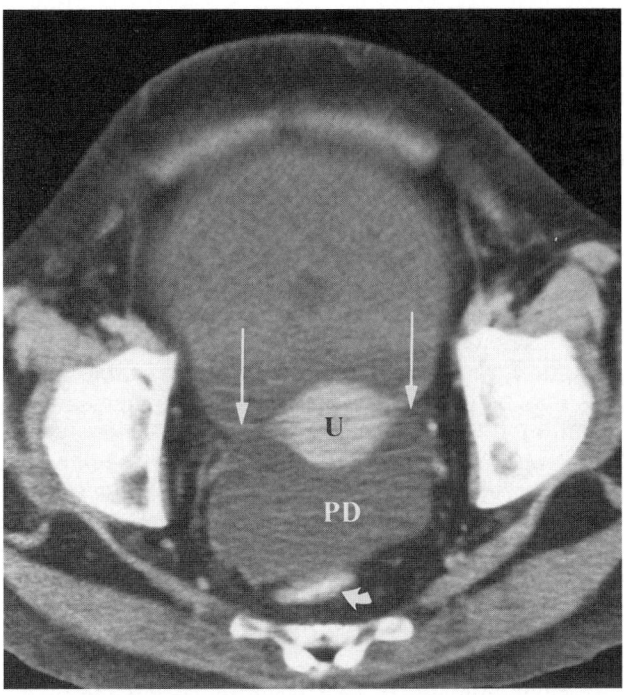

Figure 26.5. Pouch of Douglas. A CT of the pelvis in a woman with abundant ascites demonstrates fluid distension of the pouch of Douglas (*PD*) (cul-de-sac) posterior to the uterus (*U*) and anterior to the rectum (*curved arrow*). The broad ligament (*long arrows*) is outlined by fluid anteriorly and posteriorly.

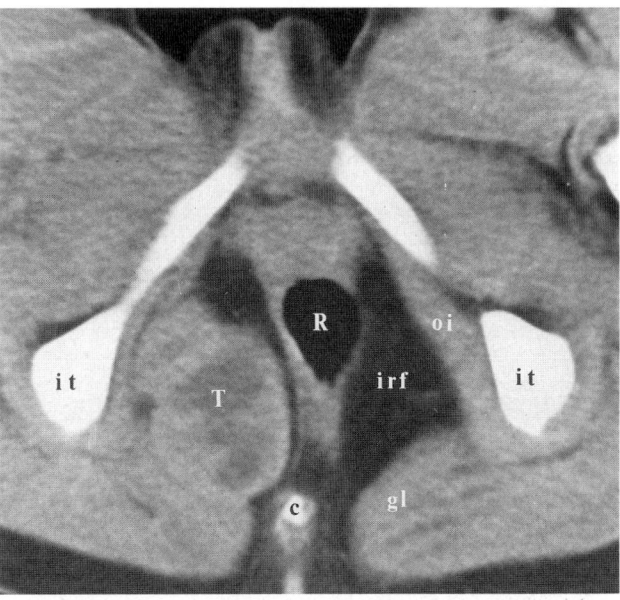

Figure 26.6. Perineal Tumor. A CT scan of a 12-year-old girl with a history of a rhabdomyosarcoma of the right leg demonstrates a tumor metastasis (*T*) in the right ischiorectal fossa. The left ischiorectal fossa (*irf*) shows its normal appearance as a triangle of fat bordered by the rectum (*R*), obturator internus muscle (*oi*) and the gluteus muscles (*gl*). The ischiorectal fossa is entirely below the levator ani and is part of the perineum. *c*, tip of the coccyx. *it*, ischial tuberosities.

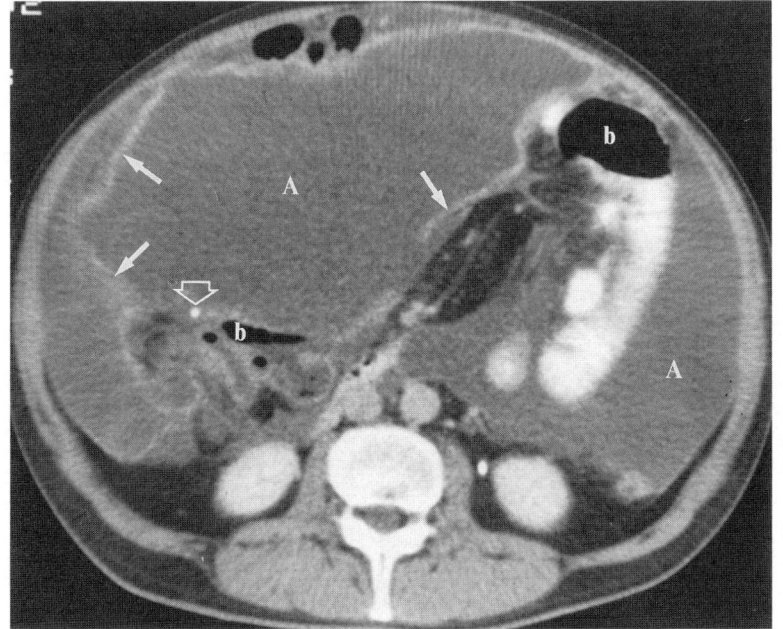

Figure 26.7. Pseudomyxoma Peritonei. A CT scan of a 65-year-old male with a ruptured appendiceal mucocele demonstrates copious ascites (*a*) with prominent septations (*closed arrows*) and mass effect displacing bowel loops (*b*). Punctate calcifications (*open arrow*) are also present on peritoneal surfaces.

T2WI. Serous ascites is commonly bright on gradient-echo images due to fluid motion.

Pseudomyxoma Peritonei refers to gelatinous ascites that occurs as a result of intraperitoneal spread of mucin-producing cells caused by rupture of appendiceal mucocele or intraperitoneal spread of mucinous adenocarcinoma of the ovary, colon, or rectum (10). Plain films may demonstrate punctate or ring-like calcifications scattered through the peritoneal cavity. CT demonstrates mottled densities, septations, and calcifications within the fluid (Fig. 26.7). The mucinous fluid is typically loculated and causes mass effect on the liver and bowel. US demonstrates intraperitoneal nodules that range from hypoechoic to strongly echogenic.

PNEUMOPERITONEUM

Free air within the peritoneal cavity is a valuable sign of bowel perforation, most commonly caused by duodenal or gastric ulcer perforation. However, additional causes of pneumoperitoneum include trauma, recent surgery or laparoscopy, and infection of the peritoneal cavity with gas-producing organisms. Postoperative pneumoperitoneum usually resolves in 3–4 days. Serial films demonstrate a progressive decrease in the amount of air present. Failure of progressive resolution or an in-crease in the amount of air present suggests a leak of bowel anastomosis or sepsis. Pneumoperitoneum in the absence of a ruptured viscus may occur with air introduced through the female genital tract by orogenital insufflation or associated with pulmonary emphysema, alveolar rupture, and dissection of air into the peritoneal cavity.

Plain film evidence of pneumoperitoneum is best seen on radiographs obtained with the patient in the standing or sitting position. Upright lateral chest radiographs are the most sensitive for free air. Small amounts of air are clearly demonstrated beneath the domes of the diaphragm. Left lateral decubitus and cross-table lateral views may be used with very ill patients to demonstrate air outlining the liver. Signs of pneumoperitoneum on supine radiographs include (Fig. 26.8) the following: a) gas on both sides of the bowel wall (Rigler's sign), b) gas outlining the falciform ligament, c) gas outlining the peritoneal cavity (the "football sign"), and d) triangular or linear localized extraluminal gas in the right upper quadrant (11).

On CT, small amounts of extraluminal gas may be confused with gas within the bowel (Fig. 26.9) and be surprisingly difficult to recognize. Images should be examined at lung windows (window level −600 H, window width 1000 H) to detect free intraperitoneal air.

ACUTE ABDOMEN

The differential diagnosis of patients presenting with acute abdominal pain is extremely broad (Table 26.1). Accurate and efficient diagnosis requires cooperation between the referring physician and the radiologist to select the imaging method most likely to provide the correct diagnosis. Routine assessment of the acute abdomen commonly includes the "acute abdomen series," which consists of an erect posterior-anterior chest radiograph, and supine and erect radiographs of the abdomen. The chest

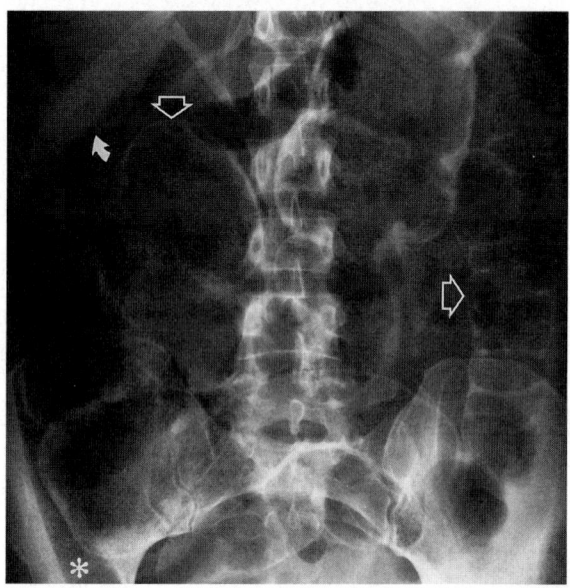

Figure 26.8. Pneumoperitoneum: Plain Film. Supine radiograph in a patient with a perforated gastric ulcer demonstrates visualization of both sides of the bowel wall (*open arrows*), free air outlining the edge of the liver (*curved arrow*), and free air outlining the pericolic gutter (*).

Figure 26.9. Pneumoperitoneum: CT. Without careful inspection, free air (*straight arrow*) in the peritoneal cavity is easily overlooked. Note that air within bowel loops (*curved arrows*) is surrounded by a distinct bowel wall and that free air is not.

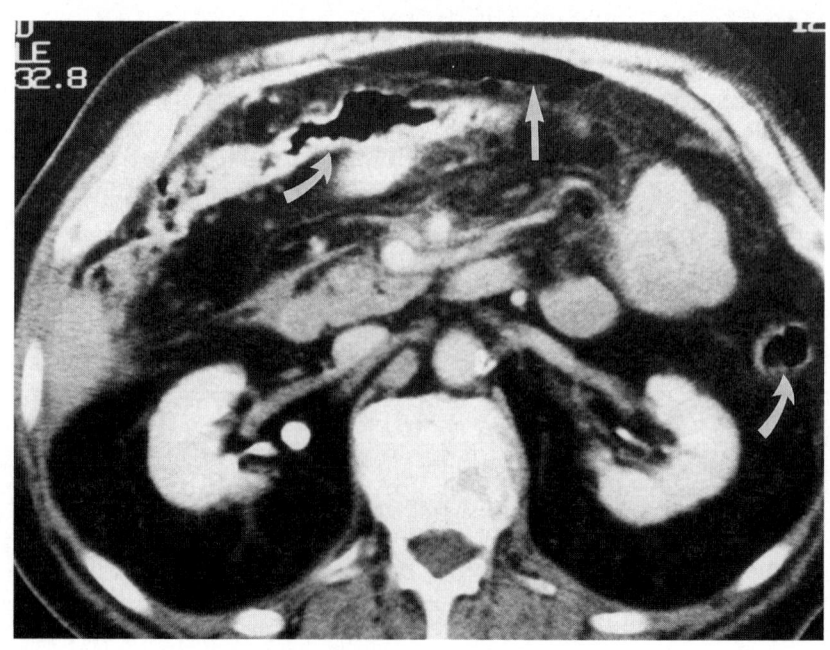

Table 26.1. Common Causes of Acute Abdomen

Appendicitis	Peritonitis
Acute cholecystitis	Intraperitoneal abscess
Acute pancreatitis	Retroperitoneal abscess
Acute diverticulitis	Bowel obstruction
Acute ulcerative colitis	Urinary tract infection
Pseudomembranous colitis	Urinary tract obstruction
Amebiasis	Pelvic inflammatory diseases
Acute intestinal ischemia	

radiograph provides optimal detection of pneumoperitoneum and intrathoracic diseases that may present with abdominal complaints. The supine abdominal film permits diagnosis of many acute abdominal conditions, and the erect abdominal film adds confidence to the diagnosis. US and CT provide valuable diagnostic information, but their precise role is debated due to cost considerations (12,13).

Mechanical bowel obstruction means stasis of bowel contents above a focal lesion. The obstruction may be due to obturation (occlusion by a mass in the lumen), stenosis due to intrinsic bowel disease, or compression of the lumen by extrinsic disease. Ileus means stasis of bowel contents. The goal of imaging is to confirm the presence of obstruction, identify its level, and demonstrate its cause. Radiographs can confirm the presence of bowel obstruction 6–12 hours before the diagnosis can usually be made clinically.

Normal Abdominal Gas Pattern. Interpretation of plain abdominal radiographs routinely includes assessment of gas, fluid, soft tissue, fat, and calcium densities. Normal gas in the abdomen (see Fig. 1.2B) is predominantly swallowed air. Air-fluid levels are seen in normal patients commonly in the stomach, often in the small bowel, and never in the colon distal to the hepatic flexure. Normal air-fluid levels in the small bowel should not exceed 2.5 cm in length. Small bowel air usually appears as multiple small, random gas collections scattered throughout the abdomen. Small bowel gas is increased in patients who chronically swallow air or drink carbonated beverages. A normal intestinal gas pattern varies from no intestinal gas to gas within 3–4 variably shaped small intestinal loops measuring less than 2.5–3 cm in diameter. The normal colon contains some gas and fecal material and varies in diameter from 3–8 cm, with the cecum having the largest diameter. The term "nonspecific abdominal gas pattern" has no precise meaning and should be abandoned (14).

Dilated Bowel. Small bowel is dilated when it exceeds 2.5–3.0 cm in diameter. The colon is dilated when it exceeds 5 cm in diameter, and the cecum is dilated when it exceeds 8 cm diameter. In adults, dilated small bowel can usually be differentiated from dilated large bowel by assessment of location and anatomic features. Small bowel is more central in the abdomen and is characterized by valvulae conniventes, which cross the entire diameter of the lumen (Fig. 26.10). Dilated small bowel rarely exceeds 5 cm in diameter although large bowel is not considered dilated until it exceeds 5 cm diameter. Large bowel is more peripheral in the abdomen and is characterized by haustra that extend only part way across the lumen.

Large bowel contains fecal material that has a characteristic mottled appearance. Large bowel usually exceeds 5 cm when dilated. The cecum, which has the largest normal diameter of the large bowel, always dilates to the greatest extent irrespective of the site of obstruction.

Adynamic Ileus. The word "ileus" means stasis and does not differentiate mechanical obstruction from nonmechanical stasis. The terms "adynamic ileus," "paralytic ileus," and "nonobstructive ileus" are used interchangeably and refer to stasis of bowel contents because of decreased or absent peristalsis. Common causes of adynamic ileus are listed in Table 26.2. Adynamic ileus typically demonstrates diffuse symmetric, predominantly gaseous, distension of bowel. The small bowel, stomach, and colon are proportionally dilated without an abrupt termination. More loops are dilated than with obstruction. Occasionally adynamic ileus may result in a gasless abdomen with dilated loops of bowel that are filled only with fluid. US is useful in confirming de-

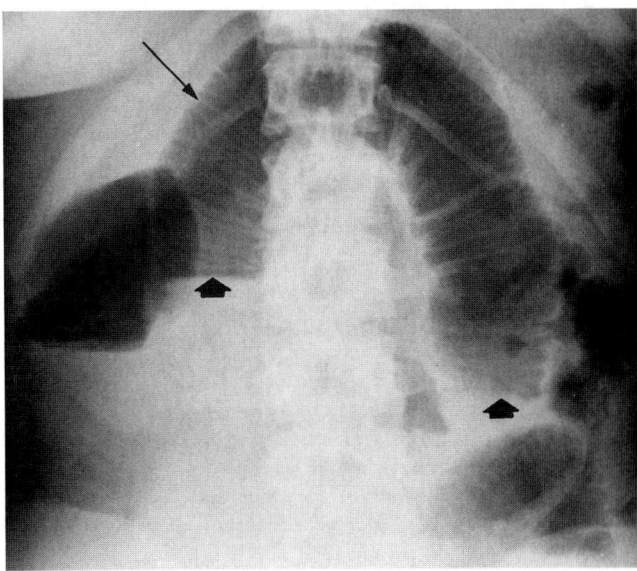

Figure 26.10. Small Bowel Obstruction. Erect radiograph of the abdomen reveals dilated air-filled loops of small bowel containing air-fluid levels at different heights within the same loop (*arrowheads*). Note the valvulae conniventes (*long arrow*) that extend across the entire diameter of the bowel lumen. The small bowel obstruction was due to adhesions.

Table 26.2. Common Causes of Adynamic Ileus

Drugs
  Atropine, glucagon, morphine, barbiturates, phenothiazines
Metabolic causes
  Diabetes mellitus, hypothyroidism, hypokalemia, hypercalcemia
Inflammation
  Intraluminal: gastroenteritis
  Extraluminal: peritonitis, pancreatitis, appendicitis, cholecystitis, abscess
Postoperative: resolves in 4–7 days
Posttrauma
Postspinal injury

creased or absent peristalsis, although examination may be difficult if large amounts of gas are present.

Sentinel Loop refers to a segment of intestine that becomes paralyzed and dilated as it lies next to an inflamed intraabdominal organ. In essence, it is a short segment of adynamic ileus that appears as an isolated loop of distended intestine that remains in the same general position on serial films. A sentinel loop alerts one to the presence of an adjacent inflammatory process. A sentinel loop in the right upper quadrant suggests acute cholecystitis, hepatitis, or pyelonephritis. In the left upper quadrant, pancreatitis, pyelonephritis, or splenic injury may be suspected. In the lower quadrants, diverticulitis, appendicitis, salpingitis, cystitis, or Crohn's disease are causes of a sentinel loop.

Toxic Megacolon is a manifestation of fulminant colitis characterized by extreme dilation of all or a portion of the colon. In this state, peristalsis is absent and the large bowel loses all tone and contractility. The patient has progressive abdominal distension and is toxic, febrile, and obtunded. Bowel sounds and bowel movements are absent. The bowel wall becomes like "wet blotting paper," and the risk of perforation is extreme. Mortality approaches 20% in toxic megacolon. Acute ulcerative colitis is the most common cause of toxic megacolon (Table 26.3).

Plain films demonstrate distension of the colon with absent haustra. Dilation of the transverse colon up to 15 cm diameter is often the most striking observation. The diagnosis is suggested when the diameter of the colon exceeds 6.5 cm and the mucosa appears abnormal. Pseudopolyps due to islands of edematous mucosa surrounded by extensive ulceration appear as soft tissue nodules within the air-distended colon. CT demonstrates a distended colon filled with air and fluid. The wall of the colon is thin but has an irregular nodular contour; air may be seen within the colon wall. Barium enema is absolutely contraindicated because of risk of perforation.

Bowel Obstruction. When bowel obstruction occurs, the lumen of the bowel proximal to the obstruction progressively dilates because of continued secretions, swallowed fluid, air, and food, and eventual cessation of absorption. Stasis results in the overgrowth of bacteria and production of toxins that may injure the mucosa. Compromise of blood supply may occur because of distension of the bowel wall and increased intraluminal pressure. A variety of terms used clinically must be understood (14). **Complete obstruction** means the lumen is totally occluded, but **partial obstruction** means some bowel contents pass through. **Simple obstruction** refers to blockage of the luminal contents without interference of blood supply. **Strangulation obstruction** means that the blood supply to the bowel wall is impaired. Most strangulation obstructions are **closed-loop obstructions** which means blockage of a bowel loop segment at both ends. This occurs with incarcerated hernias and volvulus.

SMALL BOWEL OBSTRUCTION

Small bowel obstruction accounts for 20% of surgical admissions for acute abdominal pain and 80% of all intestinal tract obstruction. The causes of small bowel obstruction are listed in Table 26.4. In the Western world, postsurgical adhesions account for 75% of small bowel obstruction, whereas in developing nations, 80% of small bowel obstruction are caused by incarcerated hernia, but only 10% are caused by adhesions. Patients present clinically with crampy abdominal pain, abdominal distention, and vomiting.

Plain films are diagnostic in only 50–60% of cases (14). Findings of small bowel obstruction (Fig. 26.10) are as follows: *a*) dilated loops of small bowel (>3 cm) disproportionate to more distal small bowel or colon, and *b*) small bowel air-fluid levels that exceed 2.5 cm in length. The level of obstruction is determined by dilated loops above the obstruction and normal or empty loops below the obstruction. Stepladder or hairpin loops of small bowel are most characteristic. Air-fluid levels at differing heights within the same loop are strong evidence of obstruction. Small bubbles of gas trapped between folds in dilated, fluid-filled loops produce the "string of pearls" sign. Inguinal hernias, easily overlooked clinically in the obese, may be evident on radiographs.

CT has become the imaging method of choice when the diagnosis is equivocal (14,15). CT offers the advantage of revealing the cause of obstruction in 70–90% of cases. CT diagnosis is based upon demonstration of a transition site between small bowel loops dilated with fluid or air and collapsed bowel loops distal to the obstruction (Fig. 26.11). A potential pitfall is the common finding of a collapsed descending colon even in patients with adynamic ileus. Bowel obstruction should not be diagnosed in this setting unless an obstructing lesion is visualized at the splenic flexure. Abrupt beak-like narrowing, without other lesion evident, is indicative of adhesions as the cause of obstruction. Other causes, including tumor, abscess, inflammation, hernia, intussusception, etc., have characteristic findings.

Enteroclysis is recommended in patients with nonacute symptoms or suspected partial obstruction.

Strangulation Obstruction is associated with changes in the bowel wall and mesentery due to impairment of blood supply (15,16). CT findings are: *a*) circumferential wall thickening (>3 mm), *b*) edema of the bowel wall (target or halo appearance of lucency in the bowel wall), *c*) lack of enhancement of the bowel wall (most specific sign), *d*) haziness or obliteration of the mesenteric vessels, *e*) infiltration of the mesentery with fluid or hemorrhage. Because most cases are due to closed loop obstruction,

Table 26.3. Causes of Toxic Megacolon

Ulcerative colitis: 75% of cases	Amebic colitis
Pseudomembranous colitis	Ischemic colitis
Crohn's colitis	Bacterial colitis: cholera, typhoid

Table 26.4. Causes of Small Bowel Obstruction

Adhesions	**Volvulus**
Postsurgical	**Gallstone ileus**
Postinflammatory	**Parasites**
Incarcerated hernia	Bolus of ascaris
Malignancy: usually metastatic	**Foreign body**
Intussusception	

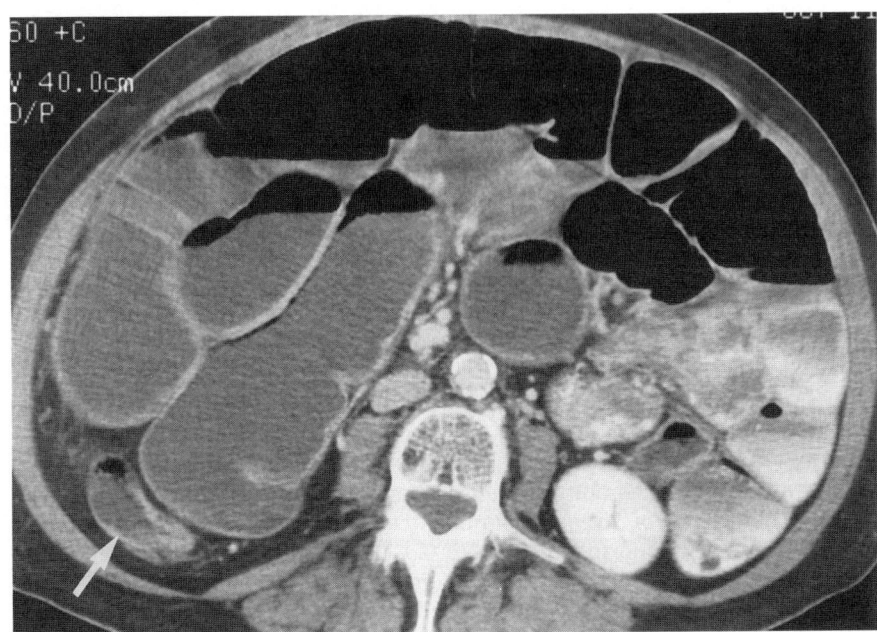

Figure 26.11. Small Bowel Obstruction. CT demonstrates dilated fluid and air filled loops of small intestine. A transition to nondilated bowel is evident in the distal ileum. No obstructing mass is seen. Adhesions obstructing the distal ileum were found at surgery.

findings of that condition are commonly present as well.

Closed Loop Obstruction is indicated by the following CT signs: *a)* radial distribution of dilated small bowel with mesenteric vessels converging toward a focus of torsion, *b)* U-shaped or C-shaped dilated small bowel loop, *c)* "beak" sign at the site of torsion seen as fusiform tapering of a dilated bowel loop, *d)* "whirl" sign of tightly twisted mesentery seen with volvulus (15,16).

Intussusception is a major cause of small bowel obstruction in children, but is less common in adults. In adults, intussusception is often chronic, intermittent, or subacute, and is usually caused by a polypoid tumor, such as lipoma. Additional causes are malignant tumor, Meckel's diverticulum, lymphoma, mesenteric nodes, and foreign bodies. Enteroenteric intussusception occurs with small bowel tumors and sprue. Ileocolic intussusception is usually idiopathic in children, but is caused by a mass in adults. Colocolic intussusception is common in adults but rare in children. Plain films in intussusception demonstrate small bowel obstruction and a soft tissue mass. Barium studies demonstrate barium trapped between the intussusceptum and the receiving bowel forming a coiled spring appearance. CT is usually diagnostic, demonstrating a characteristic target-like intestinal mass. On transverse section, the inner central density is the invaginating loop surrounded by fat density mesentery that is enveloped by the receiving loop (Fig. 26.12). US exhibits a similar "donut" configuration

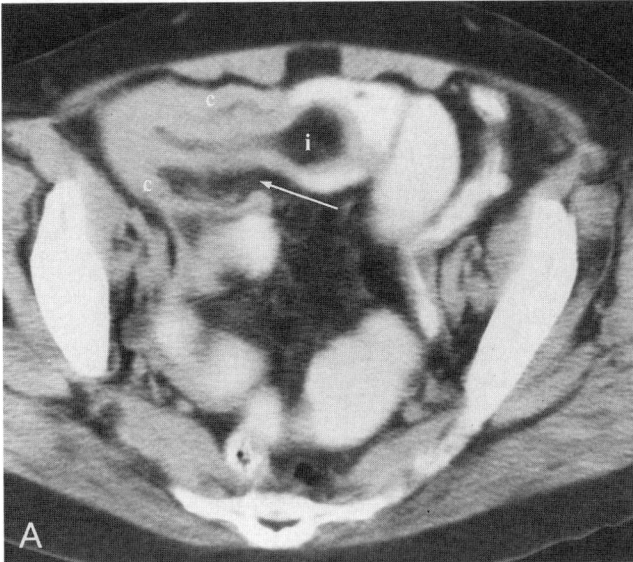

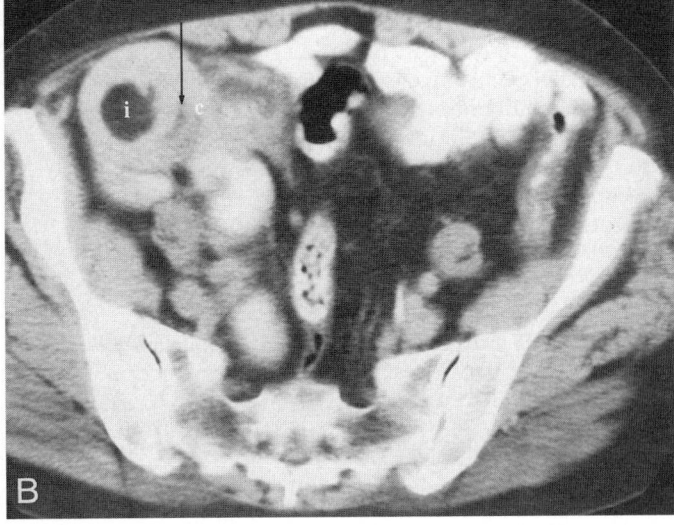

Figure 26.12. Intussusception. A. A CT scan demonstrates loop of ileum (*i*) invaginating into the cecum (*c*). Note the fat density (*arrow*) of the mesentery of the small bowel invaginating into the cecum adjacent to the ileal loop. **B.** A CT image at a higher level demonstrates a cross-section of the invaginating ileum (*i*) and the receiving cecum (*c*). Fat density (*arrow*) within the lumen of the cecum represents the invaginating ileal mesentery. (Case courtesy of Dr. Jim C. Chen, Roseville, CA.)

of alternating hyperechoic and hypoechoic rings representing alternating mucosa, muscular wall, and mesenteric fat tissues in cross-section.

Gallstone Ileus should be suspected in any elderly female with small bowel obstruction. It is the cause of 24% of small bowel obstruction in patients over age 70. Because it is a disease of the elderly, insidious in onset, and difficult to diagnose, mortality is increased five fold over mortality for small bowel obstruction due to adhesions. Bowel obstruction is caused by a large gallstone that erodes through the gallbladder wall and passes into the intestine, usually creating a cholecystoduodenal fistula. The gallstone most commonly lodges in the distal ileum. Specific radiographic signs are present in only about half the patients. Rigler's triad consists of the following: *a*) dilated small bowel loops (80% of cases), *b*) air in the biliary tree or gallbladder (67%), and *c*) calcified gallstone in an ectopic location (50%). Barium studies should include instillation of contrast into the duodenum to demonstrate passage of barium into the biliary tree. Nonopaque obstructing gallstones are demonstrated as an intraluminal mass.

LARGE BOWEL OBSTRUCTION

Large bowel obstruction is predominantly a condition of older adults, accounting for about 20% of all bowel obstruction. The cecum dilates to the greatest extent, irrespective of the site of large bowel obstruction. When the cecum exceeds 10 cm in diameter, it is at high risk for perforation with attendant risks of peritonitis and septic shock. The common causes of large bowel obstruction are listed in Table 26.5. Most colonic obstruction occur in the sigmoid colon where the bowel lumen is narrower and stool is more formed.

Plain films are commonly diagnostic in large bowel obstruction, demonstrating dilation of the colon from the cecum to the point of obstruction. The colon distal to the obstruction is devoid of gas. When the ileocecal valve is competent, the small bowel usually contains little gas; the colon is unable to decompress into the small bowel and gaseous distension of the cecum is progressive. When the ileocecal valve is incompetent, gaseous distension of the small bowel is often present; the colon can decompress into the ileum and jejunum, and risk of perforation of the cecum is reduced. Air-fluid levels distal to the hepatic flexure are strong evidence of obstruction unless the patient has had an enema.

Table 26.5. Causes of Large Bowel Obstruction

Colon carcinoma (50–60%)
Metastatic disease, especially pelvic malignancies
Diverticulitis
Volvulus
Fecal impaction
Amebiasis
Ischemia
Adhesions

Barium enema confirms the presence of obstruction and demonstrates the site, and frequently the cause, of obstruction.

Sigmoid Volvulus is most common in the elderly and in individuals on high-residue diets. The sigmoid colon twists around its mesentery, resulting in a closed-loop obstruction. The proximal colon dilates while the rectum empties. On plain films, the sigmoid colon appears as a large gas-filled loop without haustral markings, arising from the pelvis and extending high into the abdomen and often to the diaphragm (Fig. 26.13). The three white lines formed by the lateral walls of the loop and the summation of the two opposed medial walls of the loop converge inferiorly into the left iliac fossa. Barium enema demonstrates obstruction that tapers to a beak at the point of the twist. Mucosal folds spiral into the beak at the point of obstruction. Sigmoid volvulus causes 3–8% of large bowel obstruction in adults and has a reported mortality of 20–25%.

Cecal Volvulus. Twisting of the cecum usually occurs in the ascending colon above the ileocecal valve. Plain films demonstrate a massively dilated bowel loop projecting into the left middle or upper abdomen, usually with a single air-fluid level. The small bowel is distended while the distal colon is decompressed. The distal ileum encircles the cecum as it rotates. A contrast enema

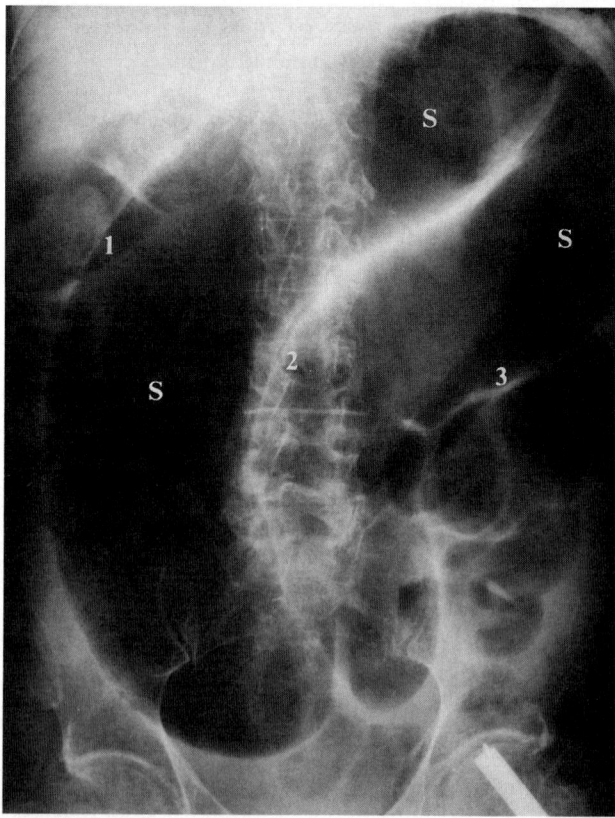

Figure 26.13. Sigmoid Volvulus. Plain radiograph demonstrates the characteristic massive dilation of the sigmoid colon (*S*) arising from the pelvis and extending to the left diaphragm. The three lines representing the walls of the twisted loop converging to the left lower quadrant are evident (*1, 2, 3*).

demonstrates a beak-like termination at the point of obstruction in the ascending colon. Cecal volvulus causes 1–3% of large bowel obstruction in adults and occurs most frequently in the elderly. Mortality rates of 20–40% are reported because of delays in diagnosis.

Fecal Impaction is the most common cause of large bowel obstruction in elderly and bedridden patients. Plain films demonstrate a large mass of stool having a characteristic mottled appearance in the distal colon. Following disimpaction, a barium enema should be performed to search for an obstructing carcinoma that may have caused the fecal impaction.

ABDOMINAL CALCIFICATIONS

Intraabdominal calcifications may be an important sign of intraabdominal disease and should be searched for on every plain film examination of the abdomen.

Vascular Calcifications are common in the aorta (Fig. 26.14) and iliac vessels (see Fig. 26.16) of older individuals. Plaque-like vascular calcifications overlie the lumbar spine and sacrum and commonly require detailed inspection to detect. Aneurysms of the aorta are manifest by luminal diameter exceeding 3 cm as measured between calcifications in the aortic wall (Fig. 26.14). Ring-like calcified aneurysms most commonly involve the splenic or renal arteries. *Phleboliths* are calcified thrombi in veins most commonly visualized in the lateral aspects of the pelvis. They are round or oval calcifications up to 5 mm size that commonly contain a central lucency.

Calcified Lymph Nodes result most commonly from granulomatous diseases such as tuberculosis or histoplasmosis. The calcification is usually mottled and 10–15 mm in size. Mesenteric nodes are the most commonly calcified.

Gallstones and Gallbladder. Only about 15% of gallstones contain sufficient calcium to be identified on plain film. Most calcified gallstones contain calcium bilirubinate and have a laminated appearance with a dense outer rim and more radiolucent center. When multiple gallstones are present, they are commonly faceted. Calcifications in the gallbladder wall (porcelain gallbladder) are plaque-like and oval in configuration conforming to the size and shape of the gallbladder (see Fig. 27.23). Milk of calcium bile is a suspension of radiopaque crystals within gallbladder bile. Layering of the suspension can be demonstrated on erect films.

Urinary Calculi. About 85% of urinary calculi are visible on plain film. They range in size from punctate up to several centimeters. Most characteristic are the staghorn calculi, which assume the shape of the renal collecting system (Fig. 26.15). Renal calculi are differentiated from gallstones by oblique projections that confirm their posterior position, as opposed to the more anterior positions of gallstones. Ureteral calculi may be seen anywhere along the course of the ureter, but are most common at the areas of narrowing: the ureteropelvic junction, the pelvic brim, and the vesicoureteral junction. Bladder calculi are single or multiple, commonly laminated, may be any size, and usually lie near the midline of the pelvis (Fig. 26.16). Calculi within bladder diverticula may be eccentric to the bladder.

Liver and Spleen Granulomas are usually multiple, small, and dense. They are healed foci of tuberculosis, histoplasmosis, or other granulomatous disease.

Appendicoliths and Enteroliths are concretions within the lumen of the bowel. Most are round or oval and have concentric laminations. Appendicoliths are

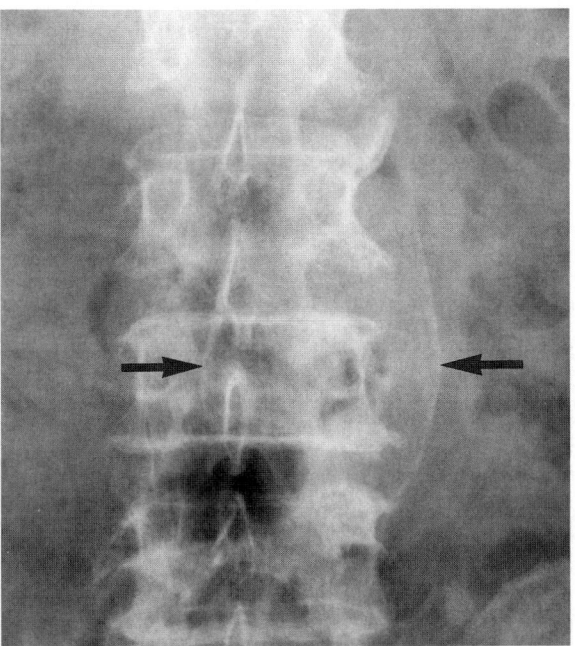

Figure 26.14. Abdominal Aortic Aneurysm. Plain radiograph demonstrates an aneurysm of the abdominal aorta evidenced by wide separation of calcifications in the aortic wall (*arrows*). Calcification in the wall overlying the spine may be difficult to visualize. A film taken with the patient in left posterior oblique position will project the aorta away from the spine and make visualization of wall calcifications easier.

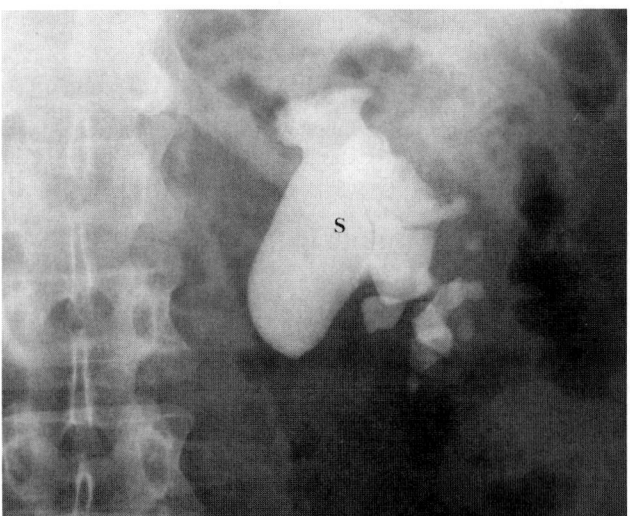

Figure 26.15. Staghorn Calculus. A plain radiograph reveals a large calculus occupying the collecting system of the left kidney and assuming its shape. Staghorn calculi (*S*) are usually composed of struvite and form in the presence of chronic urinary infection.

strongly indicative of acute appendicitis in patients with acute abdominal pain (see Fig. 32.19). Enteroliths are most common in the colon and often due to calcium deposition on an undigestible material such as a fruit pit.

Calcified Adrenal Glands are associated with adrenal hemorrhage in the newborn, tuberculosis, and Addison's disease. The calcification is mottled and in the location of the adrenal glands on either side of the first lumbar vertebra (see Fig. 33.10).

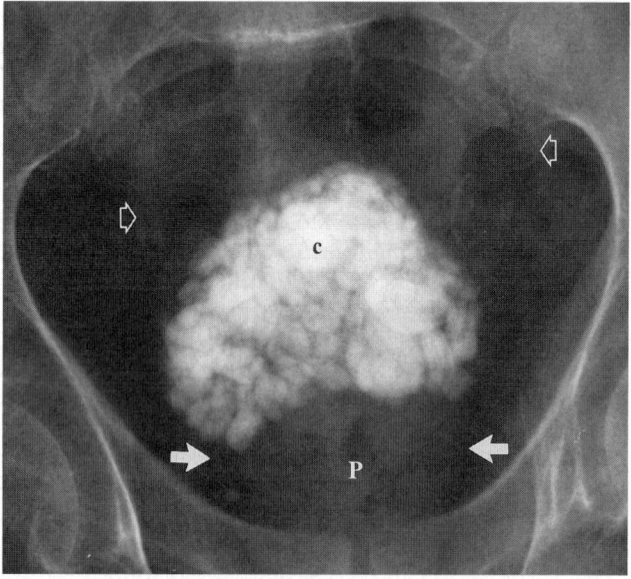

Figure 26.16. Bladder Calculi. Numerous calculi (*c*) in the bladder are evident on this plain radiograph of the pelvis. The large prostate (*P*, between *closed arrows*), responsible for urinary stasis leading to stone formation, makes a mass impression on the layering stones. Also evident are atherosclerotic calcifications in the iliac arteries (*open arrows*).

Figure 26.17. Peritoneal Metastases. A CT scan demonstrates intraperitoneal spread of a rhabdomyosarcoma. The tumor is implanted on the omentum (*o*), causing the appearance of "omental cake" as the thickened omentum floats in ascites (*A*) between bowel loops and the abdominal wall. A calcified metastasis (*arrow*) is implanted on the peritoneal surface.

Pancreatic Calcification is associated with chronic alcohol-induced pancreatitis and hereditary pancreatitis. The calcifications are due to pancreatic calculi and are usually coarse and of varying size (see Fig. 28.8).

Calcified Cysts may be found in the kidneys, spleen, liver, appendix, and the peritoneal cavity. Calcification in the wall of a cyst is curvilinear or ring-shaped. *Echinococcus* cysts commonly calcify and may be found in any intraabdominal organ as well as within the peritoneal cavity.

Tumor Calcification. A wide variety of different tumors of abdominal organs may contain calcifications. The coarse "popcorn" calcification of uterine leiomyomas is most characteristic (see Fig. 35.11). Benign cystic teratomas may form teeth or bone (see Fig. 35.15). Calcified peritoneal metastases of ovarian or colon mucinous cystadenocarcinoma may outline the peritoneal cavity (see Fig. 35.6A). Renal cell carcinoma calcifies in up to 25% of cases.

Soft-tissue Calcifications may be seen with hypercalcemic states, idiopathic calcinosis, and old hematomas. Calcified injection granuloma from quinine, bismuth, and calcium salts of penicillin are commonly evident in the buttocks. Cysticercosis causes characteristic "rice-grain" calcifications in muscles.

TUMORS OF THE PERITONEAL SURFACE

Peritoneal Mesothelioma is an uncommon primary tumor of the peritoneal membrane (17). Approximately 20–30% of mesotheliomas arise from the peritoneum, but most of the remainder arise from the pleura. All are closely associated with asbestos exposure. CT demonstrates nodular, irregular peritoneal and omental thickening and masses which merge to large plaques and cake-like thickening of the omentum, "omental cake." Adjacent bowel may be invaded and become fixed. US demonstrates the sheet-like superficial masses. Rare

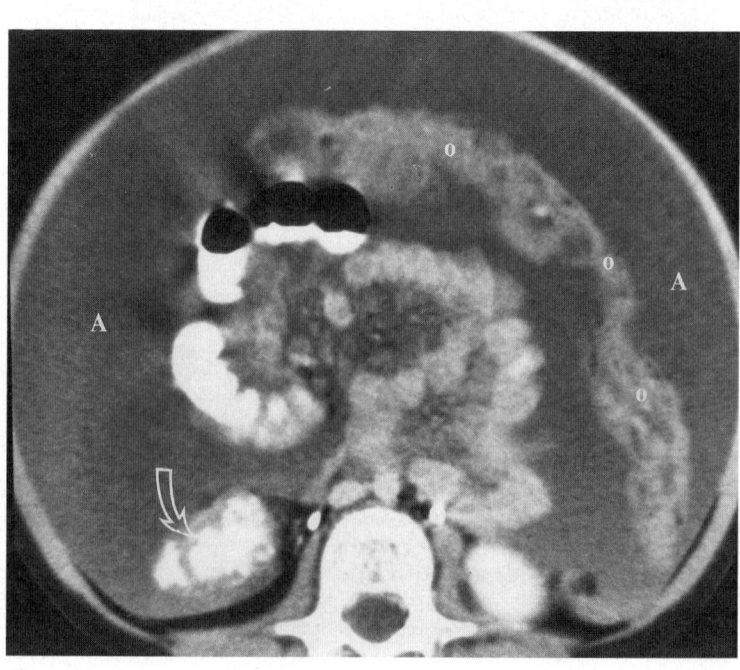

multilocular cystic forms of the tumor also occur. Prognosis is poor with most patients dying within one year of diagnosis.

Peritoneal Metastases are most commonly associated with ovarian, colon, stomach, or pancreas carcinoma (17,18). The preferential sites for tumor implantation are the pelvic cul-de-sac, right paracolic gutter, and the greater omentum (see Fig. 35.6). CT (Fig. 26.17) demonstrates tumor nodules on peritoneal surfaces, "omental cake," which displaces bowel away from the anterior abdominal wall, tumor nodules in the mesentery, thickening and nodularity of the bowel wall due to serosal implants, and ascites that is commonly loculated. US may directly visualize the peritoneal tumors, and demonstrates secondary signs of malignant ascites including echogenic debris in the fluid, septation, and matted bowel loops (see Fig. 37.19).

ABDOMINAL ABSCESS

Abscesses occur within the peritoneal cavity because of spillage of contaminated material from perforated bowel or as a complication of surgery, trauma, pancreatitis, or AIDS. Development of an abscess is commonly insidious, and the clinical presentation is often nonspecific and confusing. The pelvis is the most common site for abscess formation (Table 26.6).

Plain film findings include soft tissue mass, collection of extraluminal gas, viscus displacement, localized or generalized ileus, elevation of the diaphragm, pleural effusion, and pulmonary basilar changes. A focal collection of extraluminal gas is the most specific sign of abscess but is unfortunately uncommon.

CT shows a loculated fluid collection (see Fig. 36.2A) often with internal debris and fluid-fluid levels. The walls of the fluid collection are often thick and irregular. Gas within the fluid collection is strong evidence of abscess. Fascia adjacent to the abscess is thickened, and fat surrounding the abscess may be increased in density and contain soft tissue strands due to inflammation.

US demonstrates a focal fluid collection often containing echogenic fluid, floating debris, and septations (see Fig. 36.2B). However, completely anechoic fluid collections may also be infected. A thickened wall is usually evident. Gas within the fluid collection is evidenced by echogenic foci producing comet-tail or reverberation artifacts. CT-directed or US-directed aspiration confirms the diagnosis, provides material for culture, and offers the opportunity for percutaneous catheter drainage.

Table 26.6. Location of Abdominal Abscesses

Site	%
Pelvis	66
Subphrenic	18
Subhepatic	8
Infracolic	5
Lesser sac	3

LYMPHADENOPATHY

A wide variety of neoplastic and inflammatory diseases result in abdominal lymphadenopathy. CT, US, and MR can evaluate the entire abdominopelvic lymphatic system and have replaced lymphangiography in most clinical settings. The abdomen and pelvis contain more than 230 lymph nodes, and lymphangiography fails to evaluate many lymph node groups including mesenteric, retrocrural, portal, and celiac nodes. Unfortunately, none of the cross-section imaging methods can demonstrate tumor involvement of a lymph node by alteration of internal architecture. Criteria for pathologic involvement is based primarily on alterations in node size (Table 26.7).

Short axis measurements of lymph node size are preferred to determine abnormal enlargement. Morphologic patterns of pathologic lymphadenopathy include single enlarged nodes, multiple separate lobulated enlarged nodes, or bulky conglomerate masses of lymph nodes. Calcification in enlarged nodes may be seen with inflammatory adenopathy, mucinous carcinomas, sarcomas, and treated lymphoma. Patients who have had previous lymphangiograms may also show high density nodes on CT.

CT to detect adenopathy requires optimal contrast opacification of blood vessels and the gastrointestinal tract (19). Normal nodes are oblong in shape, homogeneous in configuration, and have short axis diameters below the limits listed in Table 26.7. Most pathologically enlarged nodes have CT densities slightly less than skeletal muscle. Low density nodal metastases are commonly seen with nonseminomatous testicular carcinoma, tuberculosis, and occasionally lymphoma.

Table 26.7. Abdominal and Pelvis Lymphadenopathy: Upper Limits of Normal Node Size by Location

Node Location	Maximum Dimension (mm)	Comments
Retrocrural	6	May enlarge from disease above or below the diaphragm
Retroperitoneal	10	Multiple nodes 8–10 mm in size are usually abnormal
Gastrohepatic ligament	8	Must differentiate lymphadenopathy from coronary varices
Porta hepatis	6	May cause biliary obstruction
Celiac and Superior mesenteric artery	10	Also called preaortic nodes
Pancreaticoduodenal	10	Commonly involved by lymphoma and GI carcinoma
Perisplenic	10	Involved by lymphoma and GI carcinoma
Mesenteric	10	In the small bowel mesentery
Pelvic	15	Most commonly involved by pelvic tumors

US is almost equal to CT in accuracy for detection of lymphadenopathy, however, a skillful dedicated examination is required (20). Lymphoma typically produces hypoechoic or even anechoic lymphadenopathy (see Fig. 36.3). Masses of retroperitoneal nodes may silhouette segments of the normally echogenic wall of the aorta (the "sonographic silhouette sign"). The "sandwich sign" refers to entrapment of mesenteric vessels by masses of enlarged lymph nodes in the mesentery.

MR usually provides excellent differentiation of lymph nodes from blood vessels because of flow void within vessels. However, because of the current lack of an effective gastrointestinal contrast agent, loops of bowel are commonly confused with masses of nodes. On T1WI, lymph nodes show low signal intensity compared to surrounding fat. On T2WI, lymph nodes show high signal intensity compared to muscle. Fat saturation technique highlights pathologic adenopathy (Fig. 26.18).

Hodgkin's Lymphoma is responsible for 20–40% of all lymphoma and is characterized histologically by the presence of the Reed-Sternberg cell (21). Hodgkin's lymphoma has a bimodal age distribution most commonly affecting patients aged 25–30 and over 70 years. At presentation, abdominal adenopathy is present in about 25% of cases. The spleen is involved in about 40% of cases and the liver in about 8%. Involvement of the gastrointestinal tract and urinary tract is much less common with Hodgkin's than with non-Hodgkin's lymphoma. Lymphoma staging is by the Ann Arbor classification (Table 26.8).

Non-Hodgkin's Lymphoma is responsible for 60–80% of lymphoma. Non-Hodgkin's lymphoma is a heterogeneous group of disorders with a confusing array of changing names and classifications (22). Non-Hodgkin's lymphomas are particularly common in patients with AIDS and other immunocompromised states. The non-Hodgkin's lymphomas commonly involve extranodal sites including the gastrointestinal and urinary tract. At presentation, abdominal adenopathy is present in about 50% of cases. The spleen is involved in about 40% of cases (Fig. 24.20) and the liver in about 14%. Non-Hodgkin's lymphoma is also staged by the Ann Arbor staging classification (Table 26.8).

RETROPERITONEAL FIBROSIS

Retroperitoneal fibrosis is a rare condition manifest by formation of a fibrous plaque in the lower retroperi-

Table 26.8. Staging of Lymphoma: Ann Arbor Staging Classification

Stage	Description
I	Involves single lymph node region
Ie	Involves single extralymphatic organ or site
II	Involves two or more lymph node regions on the same side of the diaphragm
IIe	Involves a localized extralymphatic organ or site and one or more lymph node regions on the same side of the diaphragm
III	Involves lymph node regions on both sides of the diaphragm
IIIs	Also involves the spleen
IIIe	Also involves extralymphatic organ or site
IIIse	Also involves extralymphatic organ or site and the spleen
IV	Diffuse or disseminated involvement of one or more extralymphatic organs or tissues
Suffix **A**	Absence of fever, night sweats, unexplained weight loss of 10% or more of body weight in previous 6 months
Suffix **B**	Presence of above

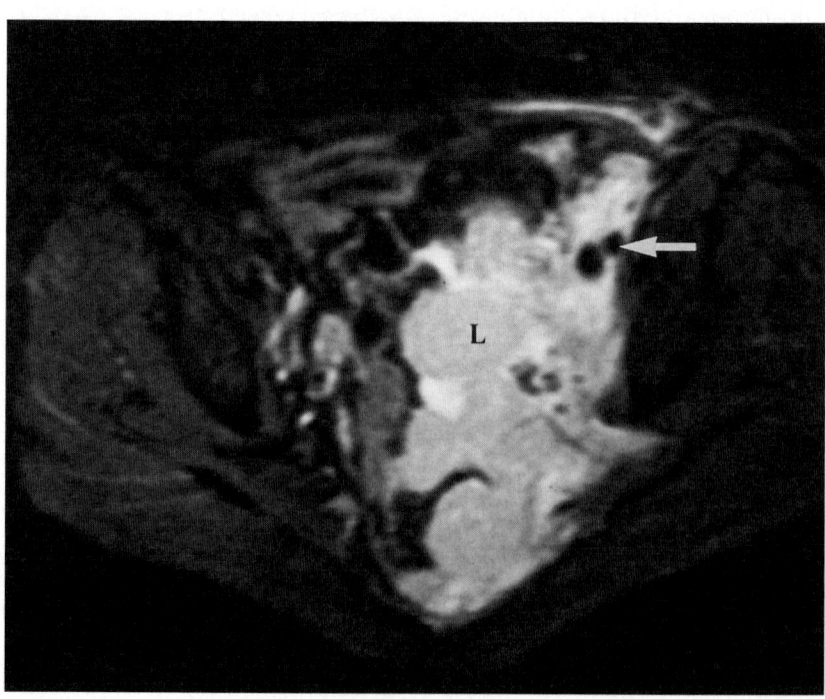

Figure 26.18. Lymphoma. Inversion recovery MR demonstrates a confluent mass of lymphoma nodes (*L*) with high signal intensity surrounded by low signal intensity fat and muscle. The iliac vessels (*arrow*) are encased by adenopathy.

toneum that encases and compresses the aorta, inferior vena cava, and ureters (23). Two-thirds of cases are idiopathic. Methysergide, an ergot prescribed for migraine headache, is a cause of 12% of cases. Small foci of metastatic malignancy that elicit a fibrotic reaction in the retroperitoneum account for another 8–10%. Inflammatory aneurysms, which induce a rind of perianeurysmal fibrosis, are responsible for 5–10% of cases. Other possible causes include tuberculosis, syphilis, actinomycosis, and fungi. About 15% of patients have additional fibrosing processes including mediastinal fibrosis, Riedel fibrosing thyroiditis, sclerosing cholangitis, and fibrotic orbital pseudotumors. The fibrotic plaque is usually located over the anterior surfaces of the L4 and L5 vertebrae. In the early stages the plaque is highly cellular and edematous; when mature, it consists of dense hyalinized collagen with few cells. Cases induced by malignancy have a few malignant cells scattered within the collagen.

The hallmark of retroperitoneal fibrosis on excretory urography is smooth extrinsic narrowing of one or both ureters in the region of L4-5. Proximal hydronephrosis commonly results from impairment of ureteral peristalsis. The process may extend into the pelvis and cause a teardrop configuration to the bladder and narrowing of the sigmoid colon. Venography and aortography demonstrate smooth extrinsic narrowing of the vena cava and aorta.

CT demonstrates a fibrous plaque that envelops the cava, aorta, and often the ureters. The plaque may be midline or asymmetric, well-defined or poorly defined, localized or expansive.

On MR the plaque is typically of low signal intensity on both T1WI and T2WI. Plaque that shows high signal intensity on T2WI should be considered supicious for malignancy as a cause, although early edematous plaques may have the same appearance.

On US, retroperitoneal fibrosis is easily confused with lymphoma in the retroperitoneum. Both show confluent hypoechoic masses encasing the cava and aorta. Typically, lymphoma extends behind the vessels and displaces them anteriorly, but retroperitoneal fibrosis does not.

AIDS IN THE ABDOMEN

AIDS in the abdomen is characterized by multiple coexisting diseases with multicentric involvement. Up to 90% of patients with AIDS develop complaints related to the gastrointestinal or hepatobiliary systems. Genitourinary tract disease affects 38–68% of AIDS patients. Manifestations of infectious and neoplastic processes in AIDS patients are effectively demonstrated by abdominal imaging techniques (Table 26.9).

AIDS is a disease of impaired cellular immunity caused by the retrovirus designated human immunodeficiency virus (HIV). The disease is characterized by multiple opportunistic infections and aggressive malignancies, most commonly Kaposi sarcoma and AIDS-related lymphoma. Infection by multiple organisms at multiple sites is the rule.

Primary infection with HIV causes only minor symptoms which may resemble infectious mononucleosis, or other viral syndrome, with fevers, myalgias, transient adenopathy and skin rash. This is the stage of active viral replication and dissemination. With development of the immune response, usually within 3 months, virus levels dramatically decrease and the patient enters a clinically "silent" period which often lasts many years. However, the CD4-receptor-coated T-lymphocytes, which are primarily responsible for cell-mediated immunity, gradually but progressively, decrease in number in the peripheral blood. A CD4 count below 200 cells/mm^3 (normal = 800–1000 cells/mm^3) is diagnostic of AIDS. Clinical immunodeficiency presents with signs and symptoms of impaired cellular immunity. Cellular immunity is primarily responsible for the body's defense against mycobacteria, fungi, parasites, certain viruses, and tumors. Because drug therapy has become more effective, AIDS patients live longer, develop a broader spectrum of OI, and have a greater risk of developing AIDS-related tumors. Malignancy, rather than infection, is now a major cause of death. Although AIDS-related diseases may affect all body systems and involve every region of the body, abdominal disease is increasingly common. Abdominal imaging studies are used to document the presence and severity of complications, and in some cases, to suggest the specific cause. Patients with abdominal disease and AIDS may present with dysphagia, abdominal pain, diarrhea, fever, or progressive weight loss with muscle wasting. Barium studies are being used with declining frequency because of the nonspecificity of most findings and the expanding clinical practice of treating AIDS symptomatically without identification of a specific GI pathogen. US and CT are the most useful modalities for evaluating the solid visceral organs, adenopathy, and the peritoneal cavity. MR has made no significant contribution to evaluating the abdomen in AIDS patients.

CD4 cell counts are correlated with high risk of specific pathogens in AIDS patients (24). Thrush and tuberculosis are seen most commonly in patients with CD4 counts of 250–500 cells/mm^3. *Pneumocystis carinii* pneumonia usually presents in patients with CD4 counts of less than 200 cells/mm^3. Kaposi sarcoma and AIDS-related lymphoma appear with counts in the range of 150–200 cells/mm^3. Counts of 75–125 cells/mm^3 are associated with esophageal candidiasis, and herpes simplex virus, toxoplasmosis, and cryptococcosis infection. Patients with CD4 counts below 50 cells/mm^3 have a median survival time of less than one year.

Opportunistic Infections are caused by organisms that are usually effectively controlled by normal cellular immunity. *Pneumocystis carinii* causes pneumonia in nearly 80% of AIDS patients. In patients treated with prophylactic aerolized pentamidine, extrapulmonary PC infection is common, affecting the liver, spleen, kidney, pancreas, and lymph nodes. *Mycobacterium avium-intracellulare* and *M. tuberculosis* are also frequent infections. MAI is a cause of bulky abdominal adenopathy, hepatosplenomegaly, and focal lesions in the liver and spleen. *Candida albicans* and cytomegalovirus are common causes of esophagitis as well as gastric antritis and duodenitis. *Cryptosporidium* and *Isospora belli* are protozoans, previously found only in animals, that infect the gastrointestinal tract and cause severe diarrhea.

Table 26.9. Abdominal Imaging Findings in AIDS

Adenopathy

Persistent generalized lymphadenopathy (reactive lymphoid hyperplasia)—mild retroperitoneal adenopathy (nodes <1 cm)—preceeds onset of AIDS

Lymph nodes >1.5 cm suggests ARL, KS, MTB, MAI

Liver

Hepatitis/cirrhosis due to HBV and HCV—especially in intravenous drug abusers

Hepatomegaly without focal lesions due to HCV, MAI, histoplasmosis

Hepatomegaly with focal lesions due to bacillary angiomatosis or ARL

Masses >5 cm due to ARL, KS, or amebic abscess

Masses (2–4 cm) due to ARL, hepatocellular carcinoma, metastatic disease

Microabscesses (<1 cm) due to MAI, MTB, *Candida*, histoplasmosis, coccidiomycosis

Biliary Tract

Acalculous cholecystitis due to CMV, *Cryptosporidium*

AIDS-related cholangitis—resembles sclerosing cholangitis—due to CMV, *Cryptosporidium, Microsporidium*

Papillary stenosis with dilated common bile duct

Long segment strictures of extrahepatic bile ducts

Spleen

Splenomegaly due to OI, ARL, and portal hypertension

Focal lesions >2 cm due to PC, MTB, ARL

Focal lesions <1 cm due to *Candida*, coccidiomycosis, KS, MAI, MTB, bacillary angiomatosis

Gastrointestinal tract

Esophagitis due to *Candida albicans*, CMV, MTB

Gastritis/antral narrowing due to CMV, Cryptosporidium, MTB, MAI, *Candida* or toxoplasmosis

Gastric nodules/mass due to KS or ARL

Duodenitis/small bowel thickened folds due to *Cryptosporidium, Isospora belli, Microsporidium, Giardia lamblia*, MTB. MAI

Colitis due to CMV, *Clostridium difficile, Salmonella, Campylobacter*

Acute proctitis/perirectal infiltrate in homosexual men due to sexual activity and *Neisseria gonorrhea, Chlamydia*, HSV, *Treponema pallidum*

Pancreas

Acute pancreatitis due to CMV, *Toxoplasma gondii, Cryptococcus neoformans, Candida*, and drug therapy

Irregular sclerosis with narrowing and focal dilatation of the pancreatic duct due to CMV, *Cryptosporidium, Microsporidium*

Solitary mass—ARL or MTB more likely cause than primary pancreatic neoplasm

Kidneys

Affected by OI, KS, ARL, polypharmacy, AIDS-related renal failure

Focal pylelonephritis due to MTB, MAI, aspergillosis, *Candida*

Parenchymal calcifications due to PC, MAI, CMV

Multiple parenchymal masses due to ARL

HIV nephropathy (10% of AIDS patients)—bilateral large echogenic kidneys/thick-walled collecting system due to multiple causes—predictive of early and progressive renal failure with early mortality

Bladder

Hemorrhagic cystitis/bladder wall thickening due to CMV, *Candida, Salmonella*, β-hemolytic streptococci

Kaposi's sarcoma

Bulky adenopathy (>1.5 cm) in retroperitoneum and mesentery

GI tract wall thickening, nodules, plaques, polypoid lesions, thickened folds

Focal lesions in liver and spleen

AIDS-related lymphoma

Bulky adenopathy (>1.5 cm)-mesentery, paraortic, pelvic

Hepatosplenomegaly

Focal lesions in liver, spleen, kidney

Focal masses/wall thickening GI tract, especially rectum and perianal area

***Mycobacterium avium-intracellulare* infection**

Bulky adenopathy (>1.5 cm)-retroperitoneal + mesenteric

Hepatosplenomegaly

Rare focal lesions, liver + spleen

***Pneumocystis carinii* infection**

Focal lesions in liver + spleen

Diffuse or punctate calcification liver, spleen, kidney, adrenal glands, lymph nodes

Abbreviations:			
AIDS	Acquired immunodeficiency syndrome	HIV	Human immunodeficiency virus
ARL	AIDS-related lymphoma	HSV	Herpes simplex virus
CMV	Cytomegalovirus	KS	Kaposi sarcoma
GI	Gastrointestinal	MAI	*Mycobacterium avium intracellulare*
HBV	Hepatitis B virus	MTB	*Mycobacterium tuberculosis*
HCV	Hepatitis C virus	OI	Opportunistic infections
		PC	*Pneumocystis carinii*

Cryptosporidium and cytomegalovirus are implicated as causes of AIDS-related cholangitis. Herpes virus, *Toxoplasma gondii, Entamoeba histolytica, Giardia lamblia*, and *Cryptococcus neoformans* are additional pathogens in AIDS patients.

Kaposi's Sarcoma is the most common malignancy associated with AIDS and is second only to PC pneumonia as the most common AIDS-defining illness (25). The tumor is always multicentric and arises from lymphatic epithelium found in all organs and tissues. The typical lesion is a vascular nodule on the skin or mucous membranes, in the GI tract, or in any solid visceral organ. AIDS-associated KS is divided into two clinical subtypes. Classic KS is a limited form of KS with lesions mostly confined to the face, extremities, and oral mucosa.

Classic KS may convert into epidemic KS at any time. Epidemic KS is disseminated, aggressive, and requires therapy. Lesions are found in lymph nodes, visceral organs, GI tract, and bone marrow. Most patients with internal involvement have multiple lesions on the skin. KS affects the GI tract in 40–50% of cases causing nodules, plaques, polypoid lesions, and thickened folds. Bulky adenopathy is sometimes present in the retroperitoneum and mesentery. Brightly enhancing lymphadenopathy is particularly suggestive of KS (79% positive predictive value)(26). In the liver, KS lesions appear as hyperechoic nodules on US, and as uniform-enhancing or ring-enhancing lesions on CT. AIDS-related KS is now believed to be caused by a herpes-type virus that is transmitted primarily by anal intercourse (27). KS is most common (90–95% of cases) in homosexual and bisexual men, and is uncommon in women and heterosexual men. The diagnosis should be confirmed with biopsy to avoid misdiagnosis

AIDS-Related Lymphomas are extremely aggressive neoplasms that respond poorly to therapy and commonly involve extra-nodal sites. Median survival is only 5–6 months (28). Extra-nodal involvement is found at presentation in 73–86% of patients, with the most common locations being the central nervous system (26%), bone marrow (22%), GI tract (17–54%), liver (12–29%), kidney (11%), and spleen (7%). Focal hepatic lesions are hypodense on contrast CT and vary from innumerable small lesions (~1 cm in size), to large solitary masses up to 15 cm in diameter. Hepatosplenomegaly is minimal or absent unless focal lesions are present. Spleen and renal lesions appear as hypodense nodules 1–3 cm in diameter. Evidence of GI tract involvement includes focal or diffuse wall thickening, which is often striking, and eccentric homogeneous masses. Rectal and perianal involvement is particularly common. Retroperitoneal or mesenteric lymph node enlargement is seen in only 64% of patients. Lymphoma may be the initial AIDS-defining illness.

More extensive descriptions of AIDS-related diseases affecting individual organs are provided in the appropriate chapters.

References

1. Meyers MA. Dynamic Radiology of the Abdomen: Normal and Pathological Anatomy. 3rd ed. New York: Springer-Verlag, 1988.
2. DeMeo JH, Fulcher AS, Austin RF, Jr. Anatomic CT demonstration of the peritoneal spaces, ligaments, and mesenteries: normal and pathologic processes. Radiographics 1995;15:755–770.
3. Arenas AP, Sanchez LV, Albillos JM, et al. Directs dissemination of pathological abdominal processes through perihepatic ligaments: identification with CT. Radiographics 1994;14:515–527.
4. Dodds WJ, Foley WD, Lawson TL, et al. Anatomy and imaging of the lesser peritoneal sac. AJR Am J Roentgenol 1985;141:567–575.
5. Sompayrac SW, Mindelzun RE, Silverman PM, Sze R. The greater omentum. AJR Am J Roentgenol 1997;168:683–687.
6. Korobkin M, Silverman PM, Quint LE, Francis IR. CT of the extraperitoneal space: normal anatomy and fluid collections. AJR Am J Roentgenol 1992;159:933–941.
7. Bechtold RE, Dyer Rb, Zagoria RJ, Chen MYM. The perirenal space: relationship of pathologic processes to normal retroperitoneal anatomy. Radiographics 1996;16:841–854.
8. Mastromatteo JF, Mindell HJ, Mastromatteo MF, et al. Communications of the pelvic extraperitoneal spaces and their relation to the abdominal extraperitoneal spaces: heli-

cal CT cadaver study with pelvic extraperitoneal injections. Radiology 1997;202:523–530.
9. Raptopoulos V, Kleinman PK, Marks S, Jr., et al. Renal fascial pathway: posterior extension of pancreatic effusions within the anterior perirenal space. Radiology 1986;158:367–374.
10. Walensky RP, Venbrux AC, Prescott CA, Osterman FA, Jr. Pseudomyxoma peritonei. AJR Am J Roentgenol 1996;167:471–474.
11. Levine MS, Scheiner JD, Rubesin SE, et al. Diagnosis of pneumoperitoneum on supine abdominal radiographs. AJR Am J Roentgenol 1991;156:713–735.
12. Puylaert JBCM, van der Zant FM, Rijke AM. Sonography and the acute abdomen: practical considerations. AJR Am J Roentgenol 1997;168:179–186.
13. Siewert B, Raptopoulus V. CT of the acute abdomen: findings and impact on diagnosis and treatment. AJR Am J Roentgenol 1994;163:1317–1324.
14. Maglinte DDT, Balthazar EJ, Kelvin FM, Megibow AJ. The role of radiology in the diagnosis of small-bowel obstruction. AJR Am J Roentgenol 1997;168:1171–1180.
15. Balthazar EJ. CT of small bowel obstruction. AJR Am J Roentgenol 1994;162:255–261.
16. Ha HK, Kim JS, Lee MS, et al. Differentiation of simple and strangulated small-bowel obstructions: usefulness of known CT criteria. Radiology 1997;204:507–512.
17. Hamrick-Turner JE, Chiechi MV, Abbitt PL, Ros PR. Neoplastic and inflammatory processes of the peritoneum, omentum, and mesentery: diagnosis with CT. Radiographics 1992;12:1051–1068.
18. Goerg C, Schwerk WB. Peritoneal carcinomatosis with ascites. AJR Am J Roentgenol 1991;156:1185–1187.
19. Einstein DM, Singer AA, Chilcote WA, Desai RK. Abdominal lymphadenopathy: spectrum of CT findings. Radiographics 1991;11:457–472.
20. Jackson F, Lalani Z. Ultrasound in the diagnosis of lymphoma: a review. J Clin Ultrasound 1989;17:145–171.
21. Weinshel EL, Peterson BA. Hodgkin's disease. CA-Cancer J Clin 1993;43:327–346.
22. Skarin AT, Dorfman DM. Non-Hodgkin's lymphomas: current classification and management. CA-Cancer J Clin 1997;47:351–372.
23. Amis ES, Jr. Retroperitoneal fibrosis. AJR Am J Roentgenol 1991;157:321–329.
24. Frank I, Fishman L. Epidemiology and clinical manifestations of human immunodeficiency virus infection. Semin Roentgen 1994;29:230–241.
25. Herndier BG, Friedman SL. Neoplasms of the gastrointestinal tract and hepatobiliary system in acquired immunodeficiency syndrome. Semin Liver Dis 1992;12:128–141.
26. Herts BR, Megibow AJ, Birnbaum BA, et al. High-attenuation lymphadenopathy in AIDS patients: significance of findings at CT. Radiology 1992;185:777–781.
27. Moore PS, Chang Y. Detection of herpes-virus-like DNA sequences in Kaposi's sarcoma in patients with and without HIV infection. N Engl J Med 1995;332:1181–1185.
28. Radin DR, Esplin JA, Levine AM, Ralls PW. AIDS-related non-Hodgkin's lymphoma: abdominal CT findings in 112 patients. AJR Am J Roentgenol 1993;160:1133–1139.

27
Liver, Biliary Tree, and Gallbladder

William E. Brant

short-time inversion-recovery, and fat-suppressed pulse sequences (7). Use of an expanding variety of contrast agents in MR improves characterization of tumors and detection of diffuse liver disease (8,9).

Radionuclide imaging of the liver is inferior to CT and MR for lesion detection but offers functional information in characterizing lesions such as focal nodular hyperplasia. Radionuclide blood pool imaging is very useful for definitive diagnosis of cavernous hemangioma. Fine-needle aspiration for cytology or core needle biopsy for histology, guided by US or CT, are popular and safe methods to obtain tissue diagnoses (10).

Anatomy

The vascular anatomy that defines the surgical approach to lesion resection is the anatomy most relevant to liver imaging (11–16). Hepatic vascular territories divide the liver into three lobes and four segments. The hepatic veins run in the *inter*lobar and *inter*segmental fissures, while the portal veins, hepatic arteries, and bile ducts run in the *intra*segmental parenchyma. Portal veins and hepatic arteries supply the parenchyma of the segments through which they course. Hepatic veins drain both segments bordering the fissures that the veins help define. The right and left lobes are separated by the major lobar fissure, defined by the middle hepatic vein. The right hepatic lobe is subdivided into anterior and posterior segments by the right intersegmental fissure, defined by the right hepatic vein. The left hepatic lobe is subdivided into medial and lateral segments by the left intersegmental fissure, defined by the left hepatic vein and by the fat-filled fissure of the ligamentum teres and falciform ligament. The caudate lobe lies between the fissure of the ligamentum venosum anteriorly and the inferior vena cava posteriorly (17). The caudate lobe is supplied by branches of both right and left hepatic arteries and portal veins. Hepatic venous drainage of the caudate lobe is by multiple small branches that enter the inferior vena cava directly. A numbering system developed by Couinaud (pronounced "kwee-NO") is commonly used internationally and provides further subdivision of hepatic segments (Table 27.1)(18,19).

The blood supply to the liver is approximately two-thirds via the portal vein and one-third via the hepatic artery. When intravenous contrast is administered as a bolus during rapid CT scanning, the maximum liver parenchymal enhancement will be delayed 1–2 minutes following initiation of injection. This delay reflects the transit time of contrast agent through the gastrointestinal tract before access to the liver through the portal vein. Tumors, which are supplied primarily by the hepatic artery, usually enhance maximally during the early hepatic arterial phase, while the liver parenchyma enhances maximally during the portal venous phase.

LIVER

Imaging Methods

CT, US, and MR all produce high-quality images of the liver parenchyma. Dynamic bolus contrast-enhanced spiral CT is the current method of choice for the bulk of hepatic imaging (1). Fast imaging techniques that control motion have increased the role of MR as a problem-solver and in some cases as the primary hepatic imaging modality. MR is preferred whenever iodinated contrast cannot be used. US is used as a screening method for patients with abdominal symptoms and suspected diffuse or focal liver disease. Color flow and spectral Doppler are used to assess hepatic vessels and tumor vascularity (2). Radionuclide imaging is used in the characterization of cavernous hemangiomas and focal nodular hyperplasia.

Spiral CT of the liver is performed using a biphasic technique. Intravenous contrast is administered rapidly by mechanical injector while scans are obtained initially during hepatic arterial phase and then during portal venous phase of hepatic enhancement (3,4). The most sensitive imaging technique for demonstration of focal liver lesions is CT combined with arterial portography. Contrast is delivered to the intrahepatic portal system by catheter injection of the splenic or superior mesenteric artery (5,6). Pseudolesions due to blood flow phenomena are common and complicate the interpretation of CT-arterial portography (4).

Hepatic MR imaging is performed with a bewildering array of fast spin-echo, breath-hold gradient recall,

Table 27.1. American and International Nomenclature for Anatomic Segments of the Liver

American	International	Number
Caudate lobe	Caudate lobe	I
Left lobe		
lateral segment	left lateral superior subsegment	II
	left lateral inferior subsegment	III
medial segment	left medial subsegment	IV
Right lobe		
anterior segment	right anterior inferior subsegment	V
	right anterior superior subsegment	VIII
posterior segment	right posterior inferior subsegment	VI
	right posterior anterior subsegment	VII

(Adapted from: Dodd GD. An American's guide to Couinaud's numbering system. AJR Am J Roentgenol 1993;161:574–575.)

Variations in hepatic arterial and portal venous blood supply to various areas of the liver cause defects in enhancement on both CT and MR contrast studies (4). These flow defects must be recognized to avoid mistaking them as mass lesions (20). The CT density of the normal liver is equal to or greater than the CT density of the normal spleen, both before and after intravenous contrast administration.

On US the normal liver is homogeneous with excellent visualization of small vascular structures within the parenchyma. The liver is isoechoic or slightly hyperechoic compared to the kidney, and is slightly hypoechoic compared to the spleen (see Fig. 36.4).

On MR T1WI, the normal liver is of slightly higher signal intensity than the spleen, and most focal lesions appear as low density masses. With T2WI, the normal liver is less than or equal to the spleen in signal strength, and most focal lesions appear as high intensity masses.

Diffuse Liver Disease

Hepatomegaly. Enlargement of the liver is usually judged subjectively on imaging studies. Rounding of the inferior border of the liver and extension of the right lobe of the liver inferior to the lower pole of the right kidney are evidence of hepatomegaly. A liver length of greater than 15.5 cm measured in the midclavicular line is considered enlarged. Reidel's lobe is a normal variant of hepatic shape found most often in women. It refers to an elongated inferior tip of the right lobe of the liver. The left lobe of the liver may, as a normal variant, be elongated and surround a portion of the spleen. Causes of hepatomegaly are listed in Table 27.2.

Fatty Infiltration is a common and nonspecific response of hepatocytes to injury and toxins (21). Hepatocytes become filled with cholesterol and triglycerides. Causes include alcoholism, obesity, malnutrition, hyperalimentation, steroid therapy, diabetes mellitus, pancreatitis, glycogen storage disease, and chemotherapy. Imaging is the best diagnostic method to document the condition since laboratory evaluation may be normal.

On CT, fat infiltration lowers the attention of the hepatic parenchyma and makes the liver appear less dense than the spleen. Differences in density between liver and spleen are most reliably judged on noncontrast images.

On post contrast images the spleen enhances maximally 1–2 minutes before maximal liver enhancement and is thus transiently brighter than the normal liver. On US, the liver parenchyma is increased in echogenicity in areas of fat infiltration. Conventional spin echo MR images show no significant abnormalities with fat infiltration (22). Gradient echo imaging with fat and water molecules in-phase and out-of-phase is the MR method most sensitive to fatty infiltration. On in-phase images, the signal from water and fat molecules are additive. On out-of-phase images, the signals from water and fat cancel out each other. A loss of signal intensity between in-phase and out-of-phase images is indicative of fatty infiltration. This is the same technique used to characterize benign adrenal adenomas (see Chapter 33).

Characteristic features of fatty infiltration include lack of mass effect (no bulging of liver contour or displacement of intrahepatic blood vessels), and angulated geometric boundaries between involved and uninvolved parenchyma. (23). Areas of fat infiltration may be multifocal with interdigitating fingers of normal and abnormal parenchyma. Fatty changes can develop within 3 weeks of hepatocyte insult and may resolve within 6 days of removing the insult. Patterns of fatty infiltration are strongly related to hepatic blood flow (4).

Diffuse uniform fatty infiltration with involvement of the entire liver is the most common pattern (Fig. 27.1). However, the degree of fat infiltration is commonly not uniform throughout the liver.

Focal fatty infiltration assumes a geographic or fan-shaped pattern with the same imaging features as diffuse infiltration. Vessels run their normal course through the area of involvement. Focal fatty infiltration may simulate a liver tumor, however, the area of involvement has a density characteristic of fat (24). Focal fatty infiltration is most common adjacent to the falciform ligament.

Focal sparing in a diffusely fatty infiltrated liver may be the most confusing pattern because spared areas of normal parenchyma may simulate a liver tumor (Fig. 27.2). The fat-spared area is most commonly in the medial segment of the left lobe (segment IV pseudotumor)(25). The fat-spared area is hypoechoic relative to

Table 27.2. Causes of Hepatomegaly

Vascular Congestion
Congestive heart failure
Hepatic vein thrombosis

Metabolic/Diffuse infiltration
Fatty infiltration
　alcohol
　drugs/chemotherapy
　hepatic toxins
　Gaucher's disease and lipidoses
Carbohydrate
　glycogen storage diseases
　diabetes mellitus
Iron
　hemochromatosis
Amyloid
　amyloidosis

Tumor/Cellular infiltrate
Diffuse metastases
Diffuse hepatocellular carcinoma
Lymphoma
Extramedullary hematopoiesis
Systemic mastocytosis

Cysts
Polycystic disease

Inflammation/Infection
Hepatitis
Sarcoidosis
Tuberculosis
Malaria

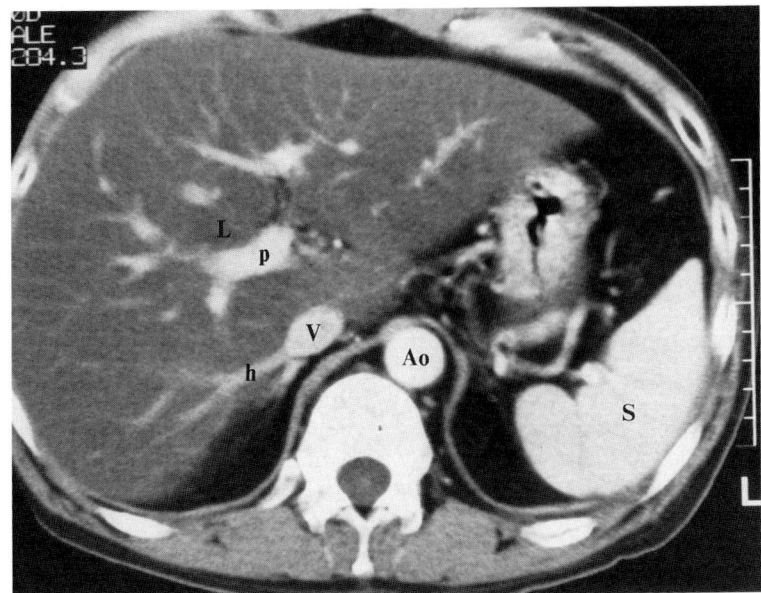

Figure 27.1. Diffuse Fatty Infiltration. CT reveals the density of the enhanced liver parenchyma (*L*) to be significantly less than the density of the enhanced splenic parenchyma (*S*). Portal (*p*) and hepatic (*h*) veins run their normal courses without displacement or distortion. *V*, inferior vena cava; *Ao*, aorta.

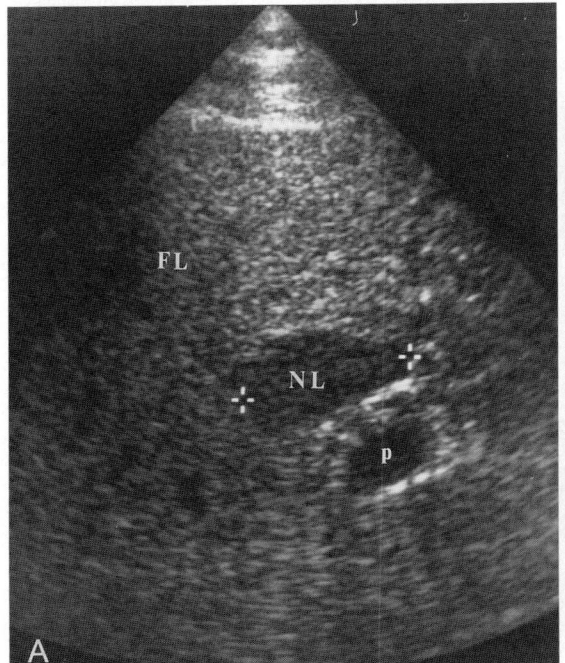

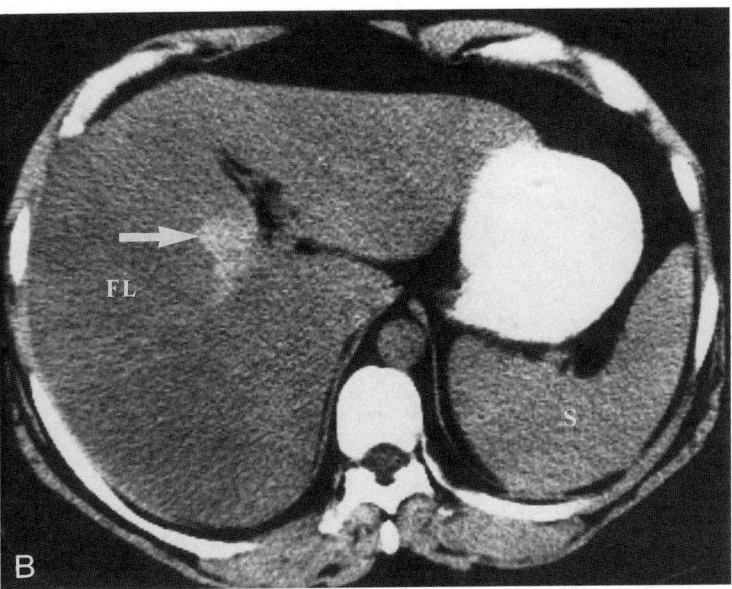

Figure 27.2. Fatty Infiltration with Focal Sparing. A. An US image demonstrates a focal hypoechoic area of normal liver (*NL*) near the portal vein (*p*) in a liver (*FL*) that is diffusely increased in echogenicity due to fatty infiltration. **B.** A CT image obtained without contrast enhancement demonstrates the spared area of normal liver (*arrow*) to be high density compared to the lower density of the fatty replaced liver (*FL*). Note the characteristic "flip-flop" appearance of fat density between CT and US. *S*, spleen.

the rest of the liver on US and is of higher density than the rest of the liver on CT. The remainder of the liver demonstrates features characteristic of diffuse fatty infiltration.

Acute Hepatitis most commonly causes no abnormalities on hepatic imaging. In some patients, diffuse edema lowers the parenchyma echogenicity and causes the portal venules to appear unusually bright on US. In acute fulminant hepatitis, areas of necrosis show as ill-defined areas of low density on CT (26).

Chronic Hepatitis is characterized pathologically by portal and perilobular inflammation and fibrosis. Imaging studies are insensitive to early pathologic changes. Fatty changes are minimal and the liver is usually not enlarged. US may show a subtle coarse increase in hepatic echogenicity. The primary role of imaging is to detect hepatocellular carcinoma.

Cirrhosis is characterized pathologically by diffuse parenchymal destruction, fibrosis with alteration of hepatic architecture, and innumerable regenerative nodules that replace normal liver parenchyma (27). Causes of cirrhosis include hepatic toxins (alcohol, drugs), infection (viral hepatitis B and C), biliary obstruction, and heredity (Wilson's disease). In the United States, 75% of patients with cirrhosis are chronic alcoholics. In Asia and Africa, most cases of cirrhosis are due to chronic active hepatitis. A variety of morphologic alterations are seen on imaging studies. These include hepatomegaly (early), hepatic atrophy (late), coarsening of hepatic parenchymal texture, irregularity (nodularity) of the liver surface, hypertrophy of the caudate lobe with shrinkage of the right lobe, and regenerating nodules. Extrahepatic signs of cirrhosis include evidence of portal hypertension, splenomegaly, and ascites. The pathological changes of cirrhosis are irreversible, but disease progression can be limited or stopped by eliminating the causative agent (stop drinking alcohol). Transjugular intrahepatic portosystemic shunts (TIPS) are effective treatment for por-

tal hypertension and long-term control of esophageal variceal bleeding. Liver transplantation is now established as effective treatment for end-stage liver disease.

US demonstrates heterogeneous parenchyma with coarse increase in echogenicity and decreased visualization of small portal triad structures. High frequency scanning of the liver surface reveals fine nodules. CT may be normal in the early stages, or reveal parenchymal inhomogeneity with patchy areas of increased and decreased attenuation. The liver surface is often nodular (Fig. 27.3). Areas of fatty replacement may be evident. MR spin echo imaging usually shows normal parenchymal signal intensity. Radionuclide scans demonstrate a shift of colloid activity to the bone marrow and spleen. The gross morphologic changes in the liver are usually evident. Hepatic activity is inhomogeneous.

Nodules are commonly present in the cirrhotic liver (Fig. 27.4)(Table 27.3)(28). A recurrent problem, not

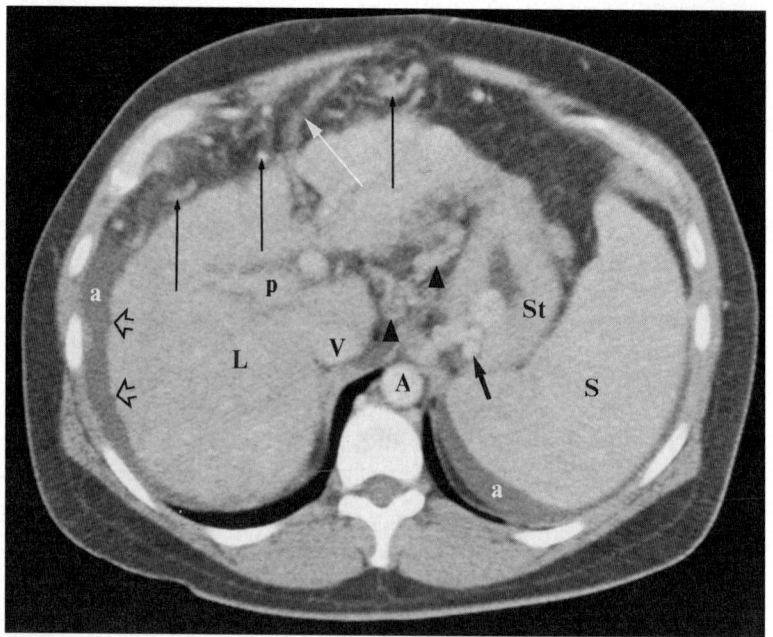

Figure 27.3. Cirrhosis and Portal Hypertension. A CT scan reveals atrophy of the liver (*L*) with diffuse nodularity of its surface (*open arrows*) and splenomegaly (*S*). Numerous enhancing portosystemic collateral vessels are evident including perihepatic (*long black arrows*), gastrohepatic (*arrowheads*), and gastric varices (*short arrow*). A dilated periumbilical vein (*white arrow*) is seen coursing out of the fissure of the ligamentum teres into the falciform ligament. Ascites (*a*) is also evident. *ST*, stomach; *V*, inferior vena cava; *A*, aorta.

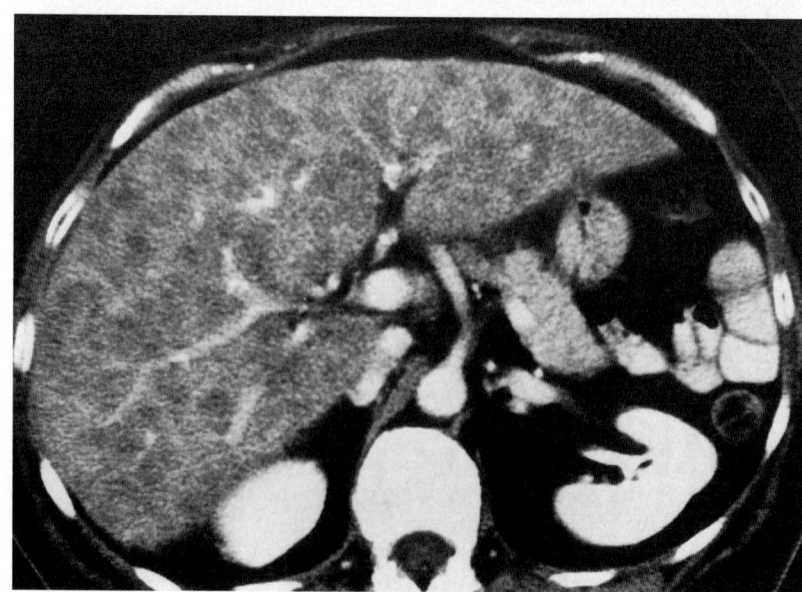

Figure 27.4. Regenerative Nodules in Cirrhosis. Innumerable low density nodules are evident throughout the liver in this patient with cirrhosis. Needle biopsy confirmed benign regenerative nodules.

yet solved, is detection of HCC and other malignancy in the cirrhotic liver and the differentiation of nodules of HCC from benign nodules (29,30). The most common nodules are *regenerative nodules*, which are a routine pathologic feature of cirrhosis due to attempted repair of hepatocyte injury. Regenerative nodules are composed primarily of hepatocytes that are surrounded by coarse fibrous septations. They have the same imaging characteristics as hepatic parenchyma but stand out as nodules because of their surrounding fibrous bands. Regenerative nodules are 3–10 mm in size. Small regenerative nodules cause the micronodular pattern of alcoholic cirrhosis. Iron deposits in regenerating nodules (siderotic nodules) causes slight increase in CT attenuation and mild hypointensity on T2WI on MR. *Adenomatous hyperplastic nodules* (dysplastic nodules) are proliferative precancerous lesions that may be found in conjunction with hepatocellular carcinoma. On CT and US, adenomatous hyperplastic nodules resemble regenerative nodules but are larger than 10 mm diameter. On MR, non-iron-containing adenomatous hyperplastic nodules are hyperintense on T1WI and hypointense to isointense on T2WI (31). High signal on T2WI is is indicative of foci of cellular atypia or malignancy (28). Small (<3 cm) *hepatocellular carcinomas* (HCCs) are homogeneous and hypoechoic with a thin peripheral hypoechoic halo on US. On CT, small HCCs appear as low density encapsulated masses that enhance rapidly

Table 27.3. Causes of Nodules in a Cirrhotic Liver

Regenerative nodules (nodules <10 mm)
Adenomatous hyperplastic nodules (nodules >10 mm)
Hepatocellular carcinoma
Confluent fibrosis
Focal fat infiltration
Focal fat sparing
Metastases

and quickly become hypodense with bolus contrast dynamic scanning (Fig. 27.5). Ringlike enhancement of the tumor capsule is characteristic. On MR, small HCCs are variable in signal intensity and show various combinations of hypointensity and hyperintensity on T1WI and T2WI (32). Hyperintensity on T2WI is suggestive of malignancy but some small HCC are hypointense on T2WI. A well-defined low intensity fibrous capsule may be evident on both T1WI and T2WI. *Confluent fibrosis* describes masslike areas of fibrosis found in livers with advanced cirrhosis (33,34). Extensive fibrosis produces wedge-shaped or radiating bandlike masses that are hypodense on noncontrast CT and may become hyperdense post-contrast administration. Volume loss of the affected portion of the liver is a key feature. A whole hepatic segment or lobe may be replaced by fibrosis. The areas of fibrosis are hypointense to liver parenchyma on T1WI and hyperintense on T2WI. As mentioned previously, *focal fat infiltration* or *focal fat sparing* may also produce nodules in the cirrhotic liver. *Metastases*, especially those due to breast carcinoma, may mimic the appearance of cirrhosis with regenerative nodules.

Portal Hypertension is a pathological increase in portal venous pressure that results in the formation of portosystemic collateral vessels that divert blood flow away from the liver and into the systemic circulation (35,36). Causes of portal hypertension include progressive vascular fibrosis associated with chronic liver disease, portal vein thrombosis or compression, and parasitic infections (schistosomiasis). Portal hypertension carries the risk of hemorrhage from varices and hepatic encephalopathy. The signs of portal hypertension include visualization of portosystemic collaterals (coronary, gastroesophageal, splenorenal, hemorrhoidal, and retroperitoneal) (Fig. 27.3), increased portal vein diameter (>13 mm), increased superior mesenteric and splenic vein diameters (>10 mm), portal vein thrombosis, splenomegaly due to vascular congestion, and ascites (37,38).

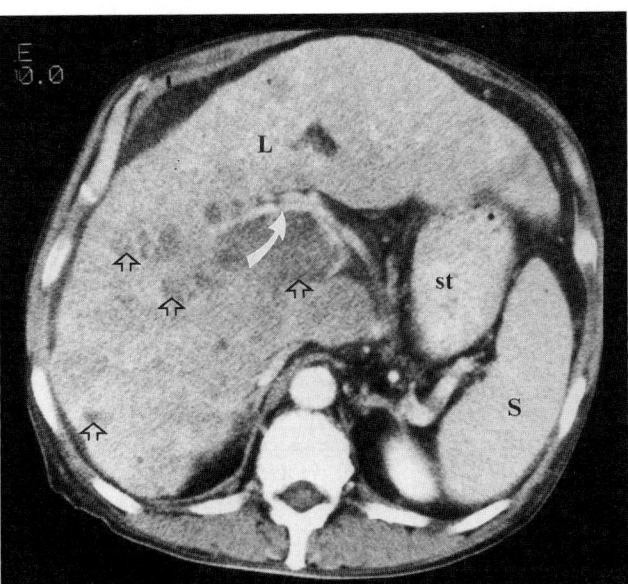

Figure 27.5. Hepatocellular Carcinoma. Contrast-enhanced CT demonstrates multiple hypodense nodules (*open arrows*) in the liver representing hepatocellular carcinoma. The portal vein (*curved arrow*) is compressed and distorted by tumor. *st*, stomach; *S*, spleen.

Portal Vein Thrombosis may occur as a complication of cirrhosis, or be caused by portal vein invasion or compression by tumor, hypercoagulable states, or inflammation (pancreatitis) (39). The cause is unknown is 8–15% of patients. On CT and US, the thrombus is seen as a hypodense plug within the portal vein. On MR, the thrombus is hyperintense on T1WI when acute and isointense when chronic. Signal is increased on T2WI. Portal hypertension is exacerbated, or may be caused, by portal vein thrombosis. *Cavernous transformation* of the portal vein develops when small collateral veins adjacent to the portal vein expand and replace the obliterated portal vein. These collateral veins appear as a tangle of small vessels surrounding the thrombosed portal vein.

Budd-Chiari Syndrome is caused by obstruction to hepatic venous outflow that may be due to obstruction of the suprahepatic IVC by a congenital membranous web (primary type) or by thrombosis of the hepatic veins caused by tumor, hypercoagulable states, or trauma (secondary type) (40).   Blood flow to the right and left hepatic lobes is severely impaired resulting in a characteristic "flip-flop" pattern on contrast-enhanced CT. On early images, the central liver enhances prominently while the peripheral liver enhances weakly. On delayed images, the periphery of the liver is enhanced, while contrast has washed out of the central liver. The caudate lobe is spared, due to its separate venous drainage to the IVC. The caudate lobe is characteristically enlarged and enhances normally. Thrombus may be seen in the hepatic veins, or they may be reduced in caliber and difficult to visualize. Comma shaped intrahepatic collateral vessels may be seen on CT or MR (the "comma sign").

Passive Hepatic Congestion is a common complication of congestive heart failure and constrictive pericarditis (41). Hepatic venous drainage is impaired and the liver becomes engorged and swollen. Findings include distention of the hepatic veins and IVC, reflux of intravenous contrast into the hepatic veins and IVC, increased pulsatility of the portal vein, and inhomogeneous contrast enhancement of the liver. Secondary findings commonly present include hepatomegaly, cardiomegaly, pleural effusions, and ascites.

Hemochromatosis may be primary (hereditary) or secondary due to excessive iron intake from either parenteral or dietary sources. In severe cases, CT demonstrates a diffuse increase in liver density to 75–130 H MR is more sensitive to hepatic iron overload and demonstrates marked diffuse loss of signal intensity on T2WI, and moderate loss of signal intensity on T1WI. Long-standing hemochromatosis places the patient at risk for cirrhosis and hepatocellular carcinoma (21).

Liver Masses

A major challenge of liver imaging is to differentiate common and benign liver masses such as cavernous hemangioma and simple hepatic cysts from malignant masses such as metastases and hepatoma (42). US can definitively characterize hepatic cysts; however, benign and malignant solid masses overlap in sonographic appearance. CT can characterize most cysts and cavernous hemangiomas but only with optimal technique and contrast administration. On MR, simple cysts and hemangiomas are hypointense on T1WI and extremely hyperintense on T2WI. These benign masses are typically homogeneous and have sharp outer margins. Malignant lesions on MR tend to be inhomogeneous with unsharp outer margins, peritumoral edema, and central necrosis. Most focal lesions are hypointense on T1WI and hyperintense on T2WI (43). Hyperintensity of focal lesions on T1WI may be due to the presence of fat, blood, proteinaceous material, or melanin in melanoma metastases (Table 27.4) (44). Diffuse hypointensity of liver, due to diffuse edema or iron overload, may make any lesion appear relatively hyperintense. Hypointensity on T2WI is commonly due to fibrosis (Table 27.5).

SOLID LIVER MASSES

Metastases are the most common malignant masses in the liver. Metastases are 20 times more common than primary liver malignancies. Of all patients who die of malignancy, 24–36% have liver involvement (45). Hepatic metastases most commonly originate from the gastrointestinal tract, breast, and lung. A wide spectrum of appearance of metastatic disease is seen on all imaging studies (Fig. 27.6). Metastases may be uniformly solid, necrotic, cystic, or calcified; they may be avascular or hypervascular. Most characteristic is band-like peripheral enhancement on arterial-phase images with rapid wash-out on delayed CT and MR images. Metastatic disease must be considered in the differential of virtually all hepatic masses (Table 27.6).

Table 27.4. Causes of Hyperintensity in Focal Liver Lesions on MR T1WI

Fat deposits	**Copper**
Focal fat infiltration	Intratumoral copper in
Fat deposition in tumor	hepatoma
Hepatoma	**Melanin**
Lipoma	Melanoma metastasis
Angiomyolipoma	**Contrast enhancement**
Hepatic adenoma	Gadolinium administration
Blood	Lipiodol administration
Hematoma	**Ghosting artifact**
Hemorrhage into tumor	Due to blood flow in adjacent
Proteinaceous material	vessels
Proteinaceous fluid in cysts	**Hypointensity of liver**
Necrosis/hemorrhage in	**parenchyma**
tumor	Edema due to passive
Abscess	hepatic congestion
Hematoma	Iron deposition in hepatocytes

Table 27.5. Causes of Hypointensity in Focal Liver Lesions on MR T2WI

Fibrous capsule	**Fibrous central scar**
Hepatoma (24–42% of HCC)	Fibrolamellar hepatocellular
Hepatic adenoma	carcinoma
Focal nodular hyperplasia (rare)	Focal nodular hyperplasia

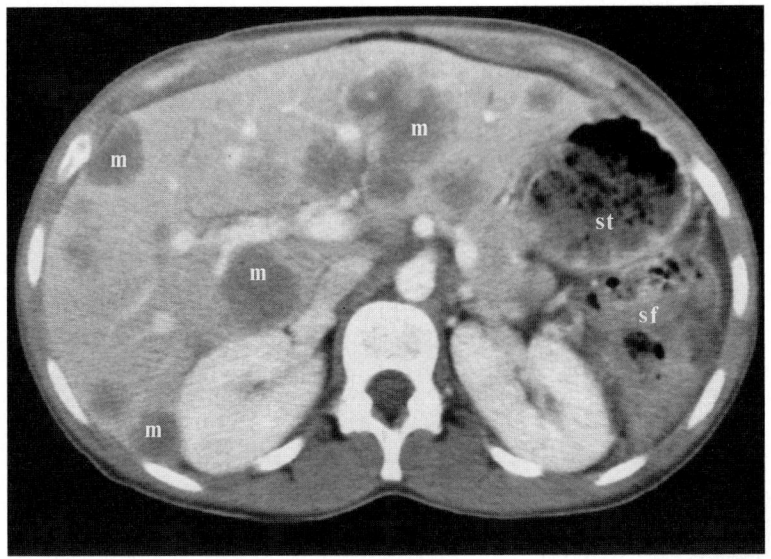

Figure 27.6. Metastases. CT of the liver demonstrates multiple low density solid masses (*m*) of varying size representing metastases from adenocarcinoma of the colon. *st*, stomach. *sf*, splenic flexure of the colon.

Table 27.6. Causes of Multiple Small (10 mm) Lesions in the Liver

Regenerative nodules in cirrhosis
Microabcesses (immunocompromised patient)
Multiple bacterial abscesses
Histoplasmosis
Lymphoma
Kaposi sarcoma (AIDS patient)
Hepatocellular carcinoma (multinodular form)
Sarcoidosis
Gamna-Gandy bodies (portal hypertension)
Metastases
  Breast carcinoma
  Lung carcinoma
  Ovarian carcinoma
  Gastric carcinoma
  Malignant melanoma
  Prostate carcinoma

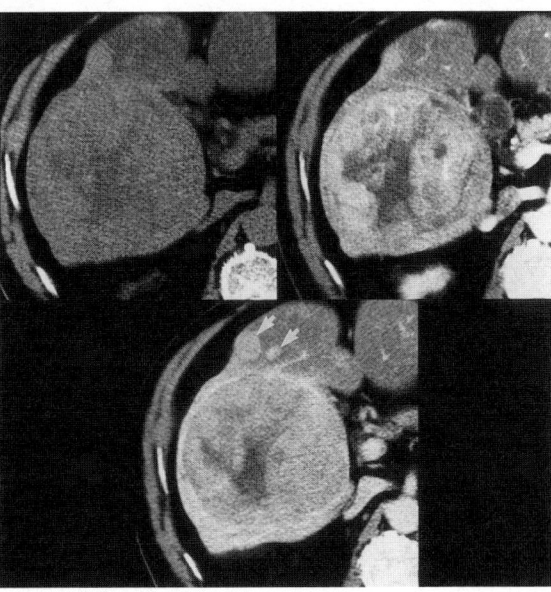

Figure 27.7. Hepatocellular Carcinoma. Three phase helical CT demonstrates the enhancement pattern of a larger hepatocellular carcinoma in the right lobe. The tumor is slightly hyperdense to parenchyma on the unenhanced scan (upper left) and shows intense enhancement on the early (arterial phase—upper right) scan and delayed (venous phase—lower) scan. The central low density is due to necrosis. Note the satellite lesions (*arrows*).

Hepatocellular Carcinoma is the most common primary malignancy of the liver. Risk factors include cirrhosis, chronic hepatitis, and a variety of carcinogens (sex hormones, aflatoxin, thorotrast). In the United States, most HCCs are found in patients with cirrhosis (usually due to alcohol abuse). In Asia, most HCCs are found in patients with chronic active hepatitis. Hepatomas demonstrate three major growth patterns that affect their imaging appearance: diffuse infiltrative, solitary massive (Fig. 27.7), and multinodular (Fig. 27.5). Detection of the diffuse pattern of tumor is particularly difficult, especially when the liver parenchyma is already altered by diffuse hepatic disease. Approximately 24% of tumors are surrounded by a fibrous capsule. This encapsulated HCC, a variant of the solitary form, is found more frequently in Asian populations and has a better prognosis. Intratumoral hemorrhage and necrosis are common due to a lack of stroma within the tumor (43,46). Calcifications (punctate, stippled, or rimlike) occur in approximately 10% of cases. Most lesions are hypervascular and demonstrate contrast enhancement on arterial-phase images that declines on delayed-phase images (Fig. 27.7). Detection of hepatoma on a background of cirrhosis and regenerative nodules is a major imaging challenge. Elevation in serum α-fetoprotein is found in 90% of patients and is strongly suggestive of hepatoma in patients with cirrhosis. The tumor metastasizes to lung, adrenal, lymph nodes, and bone.

Several imaging features are highly characteristic of HCC when present. Invasion of tumor into portal and hepatic veins occurs in up to 48% of cases (see Fig. 36.8). *Tumor thrombus* is visualized as a low density plug within an expanded vein. The intraluminal tumor enhances with contrast agent on CT and MR, and may demonstrate arterial signal with Doppler US. Portal vein thrombus is more common than hepatic vein thrombus. A *tumor capsule*, when present, is visualized as a sharply marginated rim of tissue that enhances in 90% of cases. The capsule has low signal intensity on both T1WI and T2WI and is hypoechoic on US. *Fatty metamorphosis* is a common histologic finding in HCC. However, imaging methods are insensitive to the presence of fat within the tumor. CT may demonstrate a focal area of tumor with attenuation values of fat. MR confirmation of fat is performed with chemical shift imaging (47). A *mosaic appearance* of the tumor is considered to be characteristic, but is found primarily in larger lesions (48). The mosaic pattern appears as multiple nodular areas of differing CT attenuation. The pattern is more obvious with enhancement of septations on post-contrast scans. *Arterioportal shunting* is seen as early or prolonged enhancement of the portal vein, or as a wedge-shaped area of parenchymal enhancement adjacent to the tumor (48). Abundant copper-binding protein in cancer cells may lead to *excessive copper accumulation* within the tumor. High copper concentration causes the tumor to appear hyperdense on noncontrast CT, and hyperdense (due to T1 shortening effect) on T1WI on MR (49,50).

Fibrolamellar Hepatocellular Carcinoma is a subtype of hepatocellular carcinoma found in younger patients (mean age, 23 years) with none of the risk factors for HCC, and non-elevated α-fetoprotein levels. The characteristic appearance is a large, lobulated hepatic mass with central scar and calcifications (Fig. 27.8). Although the tumor is less aggressive than HCC, stage at presentation tends to be advanced with malignant adenopathy present. Aggressive surgical management is indicated (51).

Cavernous Hemangioma is second only to metastases as the most common cause of a liver mass (52). It is the most common benign liver neoplasm, found in 7–20% of the population and more commonly in women. Up to 10% of patients have multiple lesions easily mistaken for metastases (Fig. 27.9). Many hemangiomas are discovered incidentally on hepatic imaging performed for other reasons. The tumor consists of large, thin-walled, blood-filled vascular spaces separated by fibrous septa. Blood flow through the maze of vascular spaces is extremely slow, resulting in characteristic imaging findings. Thrombosis within the vascular channels may result in central fibrosis and calcification. Most lesions are less than 5 cm in size, cause no symptoms, and are considered benign findings. Larger lesions occasionally cause symptoms by mass effect, hemorrhage, or arteriovenous shunting. The size of most cavernous hemangiomas is stable over time (53,54). Enlargement of a lesion is cause for reassessment.

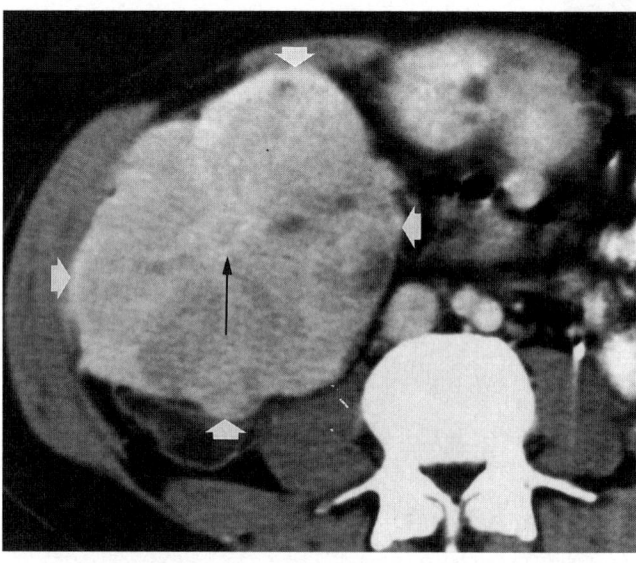

Figure 27.8. Fibrolamellar Hepatocellular Carcinoma. A CT scan demonstrates a large tumor (between *white arrows*) extending caudally from the right lobe of the liver. A characteristic stellate central scar (*black arrow*) is present.

Figure 27.9. Multiple Cavernous Hemangiomas. T2-weighted MR demonstrates multiple hyperintense cavernous hemangiomas (*h*) in the liver (*L*). These lesions were isointense with liver parenchyma on T1WI. *gb*, gallbladder; *rk*, top of right kidney; *lk*, left kidney.

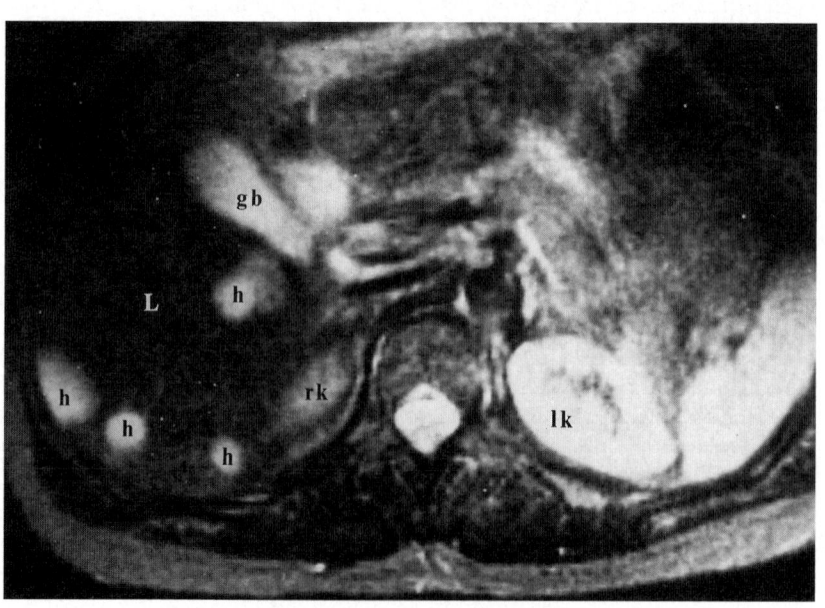

US demonstrates a well-defined, uniformly hyperechoic mass in 80% of patients. In a patient with no history of malignant disease and normal liver chemistries, only follow-up is generally recommended. No Doppler signal is obtained from most cavernous hemangiomas because the flow is too slow.

CT generally shows a well-defined, hypodense mass on unenhanced scans. The characteristic pattern of enhancement with bolus intravenous contrast is nodular enhancement from the periphery of the lesion that gradually becomes isodense or hyperdense compared to the liver parenchyma (Fig. 27.10). The contrast enhancement persists for 20–30 minutes following injection because of slow flow within the lesion.

Radionuclide scanning using technetium-labeled red blood cells as a blood pool agent is extremely accurate in the diagnosis of cavernous hemangioma. Hemangiomas are characterized by prolonged intense activity within the lesion on delayed images.

MR demonstrates a well-defined homogeneous mass that is hypointense or isotense on T1WI and brightens markedly with increasing amounts of T2-weighting (Fig. 27.9). Areas of fibrosis remain dark on all image sequences. However, the MR appearance of cavernous hemangioms overlaps that of cysts, abscesses, and hypervascular metastases (55). A more specific diagnosis can be made by administering intravenous gadolinium and observing early puddling peripheral enhancement in a pattern similar to contrast-enhanced CT.

Angiography has been the historical gold standard for hemangioma diagnosis. Normal-sized arteries feed an area of well-circumscribed vascular lakes with no neovascularity or arteriovenous shunting. Contrast remains pooled within the lesion late into the venous phase.

Biopsy may be required in atypical cases. Percutaneous biopsy can be safely performed using small needles (20-gauge and smaller). The characteristic finding is blood with normal epithelial cells and no malignant cells. Biopsy with large-bore needles has been associated with hemorrhage and death.

Focal Nodular Hyperplasia (FNH) forms a solid mass consisting of abnormally arranged hepatocytes, bile ducts, and Kupffer cells. Most lesions are less than 5 cm in diameter and are hypervascular with a central fibrous scar containing thick-walled blood vessels (56). Unlike hepatic adenoma, hemorrhage, necrosis, and infarction are extremely rare. Similar to hepatic adenoma, FNH is found most commonly in women, but is twice as common as hepatic adenoma and is not related to oral contraceptive use. Most tumors (80–95%) are solitary. Because of the presence of Kupffer cells, most (50–70%) FNH nodules will show normal or increased radionuclide activity on technetium sulfur colloid liver-spleen scans. This finding is highly suggestive of the diagnosis. On CT, MR, and US, most tumors appear homogeneous and solid with a central stellate fibrous scar. The typical finding on contrast enhanced CT and MR is brief (approximately 1 minute) and intense, uniform, tumor enhancement (42). On noncontrast CT, FNH is barely perceptible as an isodense or slightly hypointense focal lesion. On MR, FNH appears homogeneous and is nearly isointense to normal parenchyma on all imaging sequences. The central scar is hypointense on T1WI and hyperintense on T2WI. The margin of the mass is usually ill-defined, but

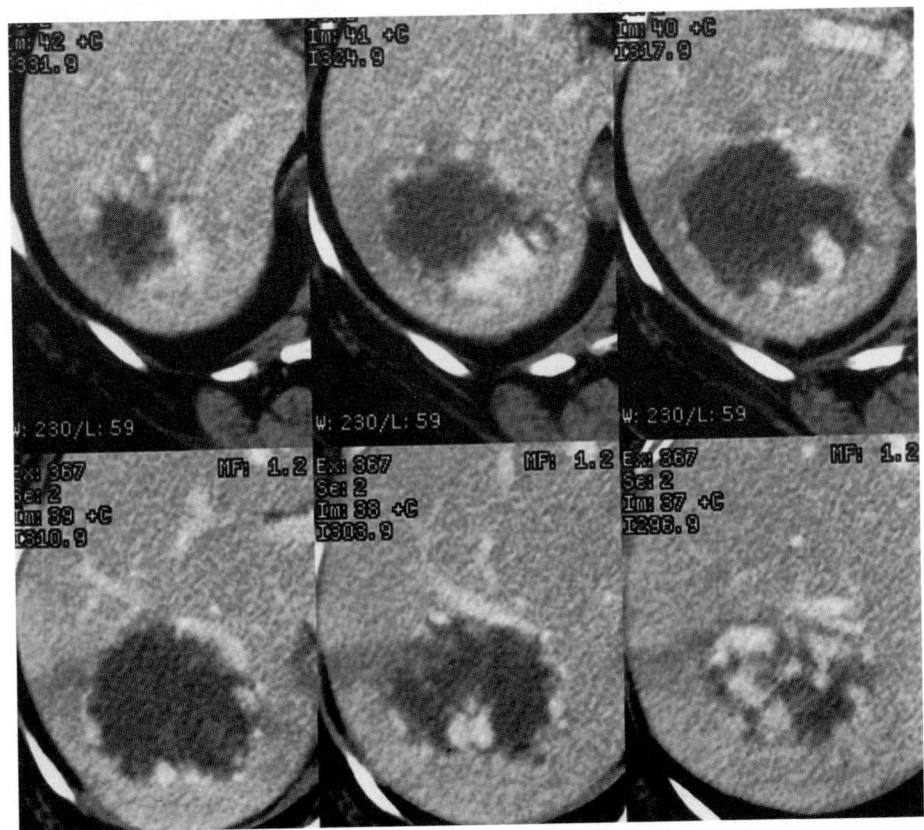

Figure 27.10. Cavernous Hemangioma. Images from a contrast-enhanced helical CT demonstrate the characteristic nodular pattern of enhancement from the periphery of the lesion.

occasionally shows a capsule-structure and mimics the appearance of HCC.

Hepatic Adenomas are rare, benign tumors that carry a risk of life-threatening hemorrhage and potential for malignant degeneration. Surgical removal of the tumor is advocated. They are found most commonly in women on long-term oral contraceptives. Additional risk factors include androgen steroid intake and glycogen storage disease. The tumor consists of sheets and cords of benign hepatocytes without a distinct acinar architecture. The hepatocytes occasionally contain abundant fat that may be demonstrated by MR (43). The tumor occurs as a solitary spherical mass up to 30 cm in diameter. Areas of necrosis, hemorrhage, and fibrosis are common. No imaging method can reliably differentiate hepatic adenoma from HCC. Common findings of MR include hyperintensity on T1WI due to fat or hemorrhage with a hypodense pseudocapsule due to compressed hepatic parenchyma. Prominent feeding vessels are commonly visualized around the periphery of the tumor. CT shows rapid and transient contrast enhancement (42).

Lymphoma involving the liver is usually diffusely infiltrative and undetectable by imaging methods. The multiple nodule pattern found in 10% of cases resembles metastatic disease. Some cases present as a large poorly defined hypodense mass with satellite nodules (57).

CYSTIC LIVER MASSES

Simple Hepatic Cyst is the second most common benign hepatic mass, found in up to 7% of the elderly population. Most are solitary, but they may be multiple, especially in patients with adult polycystic disease or tuberous sclerosis (Fig. 27.11). Cysts range in size from microscopic to 20 cm.

US is the best imaging modality to characterize hepatic cysts. Typical cysts are anechoic with thin walls and posterior acoustic enhancement. Occasionally, hepatic cysts may have internal debris and septa, especially if they have been infected.

When a cystic mass does not meet criteria for a simple cyst, the following lesions must be considered (58).

Pyogenic Abscess is usually caused by *Escherichia coli*, *Staphylcoccus aureus*, *Streptococcus*, or anaerobic bacteria. Patients present with fever and pain. Lesions may be solitary or a tight group of individual microabscesses (Fig. 27.12). Gas is present within the lesion in 20% of cases. Diagnosis is confirmed by percutaneous aspiration. Catheter or surgical drainage is indicated.

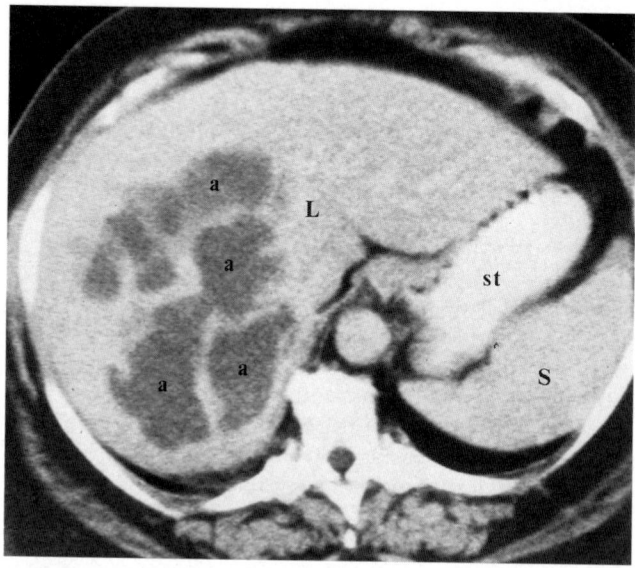

Figure 27.12. Pyogenic Abscess. A CT scan shows multiple low density areas (*a*) in the liver (*L*) representing a multiloculated pyogenic abcess. *st*, stomach; *S*, spleen.

Figure 27.11. Multiple Hepatic Cysts. Unenhanced CT scan of a patient with autosomal dominant polycystic disease shows multiple cysts (*c*) of varying size in the liver (*L*). Both right and left kidneys (*rk, lk*) are markedly enlarged, with parenchyma largely replaced by innumerable cysts.

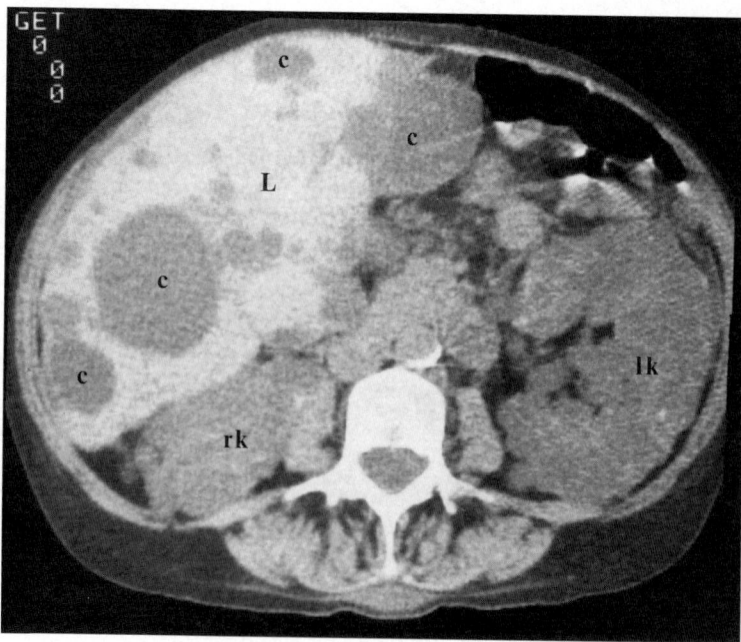

Amebic Abscess is usually solitary with thick nodular walls. The lesion may be indistinguishable from pyogenic abscess, however, the patient is usually not septic and has a history of travel to endemic areas. Amebic abscesses commonly occur in the right lobe of the liver (see Fig. 36.11), often cause elevation of the right hemidiaphragm, and may rupture through the diaphragm into the pleural space. In the United States, the diagnosis is typically confirmed by serology and the patient is treated with metronidazole. In endemic areas, the diagnosis is confirmed by aspiration of "anchovy paste" material and the patient is treated by repeated aspiration or catheter drainage.

Echinococcus Cyst is due to infestation with *Echinococcus* tapeworm. Single or multiple cystic masses usually have well-defined walls that commonly calcify. Daughter cysts may be visualized within the parent cyst (59). Diagnostic aspiration carries a risk of anaphylactic reaction. Treatment is albendazole or surgical excision.

Cystic/Necrotic Tumor must always be considered for atypical cystic masses. Metastases may be necrotic or predominantly cystic. Biliary cystadenoma and cystadenocarcinomas are rare primary tumors that resemble mucinous cystic tumors of the pancreas.

Liver Trauma

CT is the imaging method of choice for blunt abdominal trauma (60,61). The extent of liver injury can be classified as contusion, laceration, or intrahepatic or subcapsular hematoma. Contusions are seen as low-density areas in the liver without associated hemoperitoneum. Lacerations are shown as jagged linear or stellate lucencies in the liver associated with intrahepatic hematoma and hemoperitoneum (Fig. 27.13). Subcapsular hematomas cause lenticular-shaped low-density areas beneath the liver capsule that compress the hepatic parenchyma. CT helps determine therapy by accurate quantitation of the severity of injury and the volume of hemoperitoneum.

BILIARY TREE

Imaging Methods

Imaging of the biliary tree uses assorted techniques that differ in degrees of invasiveness (62). US and CT are highly sensitive in the detection of dilation of the bile ducts, though they are somewhat less effective in identifying its cause. US is the preferred screening method for biliary obstruction because of its low cost and convenience. Unenhanced helical CT has a reported sensitivity of 88% in detection of stones in the common bile duct (63). MR can also demonstrate biliary dilation, and may be more effective than CT or US in demonstrating associated tumors. Endoscopic retrograde cholangiography (ERCP) and percutaneous transhepatic cholangiography (PTC) supplement cross-sectional imaging methods by providing access to the biliary tree for contrast injection and subsequent catheter drainage. MR cholangiopancreatography (MRCP), performed using T2-weighted fast spin echo techniques, offers a non-invasive method of high resolution imaging of the biliary tree (64,65). Similar to contrast cholangiography, bile ducts demonstrate high signal intensity and stones are seen as hypodense filling defects (Table 27.7). Operative cholangiography is used to visualize nonpalpable bile duct stones at surgery, and T-tube cholangiography is used to visualize common duct stones following surgery. Radionuclide imaging, utilizing technetium-99m-imi-

Table 27.7. Causes of Filling Defects in the Bile Ducts

Biliary stones	Neoplasms	Parasites
Air bubbles	Cholangiocarcinoma	Ascaris lumbricoides
Blood clots	Ampullary carcinoma	Liver fluke
	Granular cell	
	myoblastoma	
	Mesenchymal tumor	

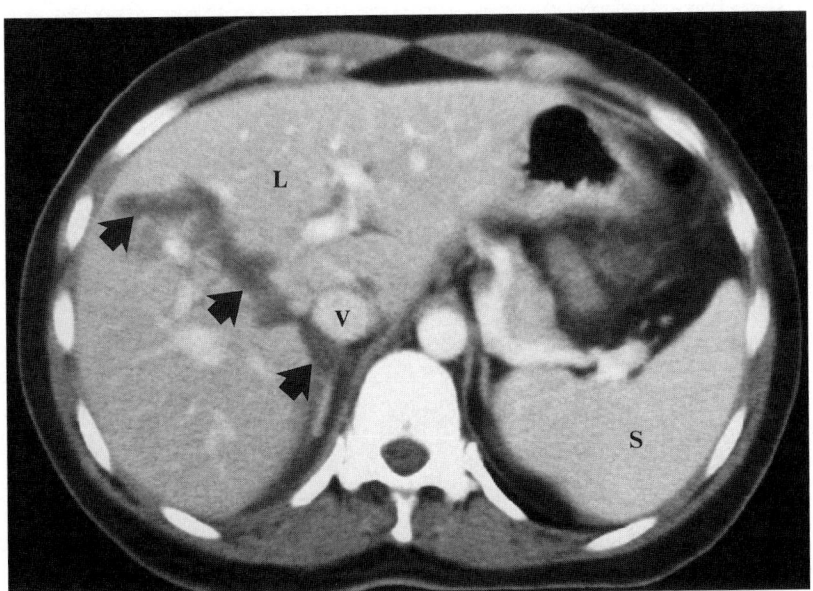

Figure 27.13. Liver Laceration. A CT scan of a patient injured in a motor vehicle accident demonstrates a jagged laceration (*arrows*) extending from posterior to the inferior vena cava (*V*) through the right lobe of the liver (*L*). Blood in the laceration is responsible for its low density. Hemoperitoneum was evident on lower CT slices (not shown). *S,* spleen.

nodiacetic acid, is useful for showing the patency of biliary-enteric anastomoses and for demonstrating bile leaks and fistulae. Scintigraphy has the greatest sensitivity for early obstruction. Intravenous cholangiography involved the use of highly toxic contrast agents and has been abandoned in favor of other techniques.

Anatomy

The bile ducts arise as bile capillaries between hepatocytes and join progressively larger branches until two main trunks are formed draining the right and left lobes of the liver. The ducts of the left hepatic lobe are more anterior than those of the right hepatic lobe. This relationship must be kept in mind when contrast cholangiography is performed. Contrast agents flow to the most dependent portions of the biliary tree and may not opacify nondependent ducts. Failure to fill ducts before gravitational repositioning must not be interpreted as evidence of obstruction (66).

The right and left hepatic ducts combine to form the *common hepatic duct* that courses with the portal vein and hepatic artery in the porta hepatis (67). The *cystic duct* courses posteriorly and inferiorly from the gallbladder to join the common hepatic duct and form the *common bile duct*. The common bile duct runs ventral to the portal vein and to the right of the hepatic artery, descending from the porta hepatis along the free right margin of the hepatoduodenal ligament to the duodenal bulb. The distal third of the common duct turns caudally and descends in the groove between the descending duodenum and the head of the pancreas just anterior to the inferior vena cava. The duct tapers distally as it ends in the sphincter of Oddi, which protrudes into the duodenum as the ampulla of Vater. The common bile duct and the pancreatic duct share a common orifice in 60% of individuals and have separate orifices in the remainder. However, because of their close proximity, tumors of the ampulla region generally obstruct both ducts.

Normal intrahepatic ducts are occasionally seen on US and on post-contrast helical CT with thin (5 mm) collimation (68). Normal intrahepatic bile ducts do not exceed 40% of the diameter of the adjacent portal vein, or 2 mm indiameter in the central liver, or 1.8 mm in diameter in the peripheral liver. The extrahepatic common duct is routinely visualized and does not exceed 6–7 mm in internal diameter. Normal ducts appear larger on contrast cholangiography studies because of distension and magnification. Slightly larger common ducts are also normal in elderly patients because of elastic tissue degeneration with aging. Cholecystectomy is not proven to alter normal common duct size. Care must be taken to differentiate an enlarged common duct from an enlarged hepatic artery. Color Doppler is useful to make this differentiation on US. Contrast enhancement of blood vessels makes differentiation easy on CT.

Biliary Dilatation

CT, US, and MR are highly effective at demonstrating the anatomic finding of biliary dilatation, which is usually equated with biliary obstruction (69). However, biliary obstruction may be present intermittently or in the early stage, without biliary dilation being present. Alternatively, biliary dilatation may be present without obstruction, such as after surgical decompression or bypass. Patients with clinical evidence of biliary obstruction (i.e., elevated alkaline phosphatase and direct hyperbilirubinemia) may not have biliary dilation. Hepatitis causes swelling of hepatocytes, which blocks biliary capillaries and causes intrahepatic cholestasis without surgical obstruction.

Signs of biliary dilation include (Fig. 27.14) the following: *a*) multiple branching tubular, round, or oval structures that course toward the porta hepatis, *b*) dilation of the common duct greater than 6 mm, and *c*) gallbladder diameter greater than 5 cm, when obstruction is distal to the cystic duct (69,70). Benign disease is responsible for

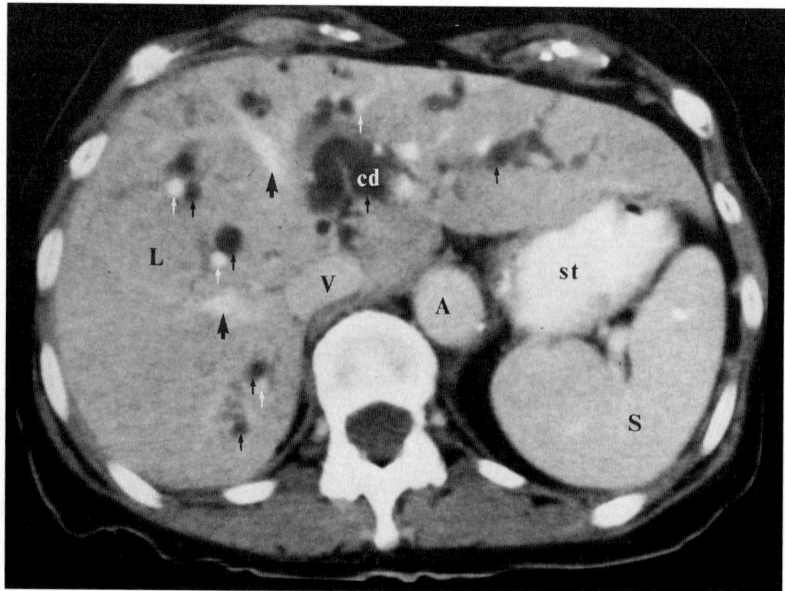

Figure 27.14. Biliary Dilation. A CT scan demonstrates dilated intrahepatic ducts (*small black arrows*) easily differentiated from portal veins (*small white arrows*) and hepatic veins (*black arrowheads*) by contrast enhancement of the blood vessels. The common hepatic duct (*cd*) is tortuous and dilated (12 mm diameter). Mild, diffuse, low density of the liver (*L*) compared to the spleen (*S*) indicates early diffuse fatty infiltration. *V*, inferior vena cava; *A*, aorta; *S*, stomach.

approximately 75% of cases of obstructive jaundice in the adult, while malignant disease causes the remainder. Gradual tapering of a dilated common duct suggests benign stricture. Gallstones may be identified in the bile duct surrounded by a crescent of bile. Abrupt termination of a dilated common duct is characteristic of a malignant process.

Infected bile is present in up to 10% of cases of complete biliary obstruction and 60% of cases of partial or intermittent biliary obstruction. Intravenous antibiotic therapy is warranted prior to biliary interventional procedures in the obstructed patient (71).

Causes of biliary dilation and obstruction (Table 27.8) include the following (69).

Table 27.8. Causes of Biliary Tract Obstruction

BENIGN—75%	MALIGNANT—25%
Benign stricture	Pancreatic carcinoma
Surgery/instrumentation	Ampullary/duodenal carcinoma
Trauma	Cholangiocarcinoma
Stone passage	Metastasis
Pancreatitis	
Cholangitis	
Choledochal cyst	
Stone impacted in duct	
Parasite (Ascariasis)	
Liver cyst	

Choledocholithiasis is responsible for approximately 20% of cases of obstructive jaundice in the adult (Fig. 27.15). Gallstones are present in the gallbladder in 10% of the population, but the presence of stones in the gallbladder does not necessarily mean that stones are the cause of ductal obstruction. In addition, 1–3% of patients with choledocholithiasis will have no stones in the gallbladder. Operative cholangiography is a routine component of cholecystectomy for gallstones. T-tube cholangiography is routinely performed in the postoperative period to look for residual stones. Patients with prior cholecystectomy are at high risk for common duct stones when they present with jaundice, or evidence of cholangitis. PTC and ERCP are the most efficacious examinations when common duct stones are highly suspected (Fig. 27.16).

Benign Stricture is the cause of 40–45% of obstructive jaundice in the adult. Causes of benign stricture include trauma, surgery, prior biliary interventional procedures, recurrent cholangitis, previous passage of stones through the bile ducts, radiation therapy, and perforated duodenal ulcer.

Pancreatitis is responsible for approximately 8% of cases of biliary obstruction.

Sclerosing Cholangitis is associated with a history of ulcerative colitis in 50% of cases. Sclerosing cholangitis is characterized by insidious onset of jaundice with progressive disease affecting both intrahepatic and extrahepatic bile ducts. Alternating dilation and stenosis pro-

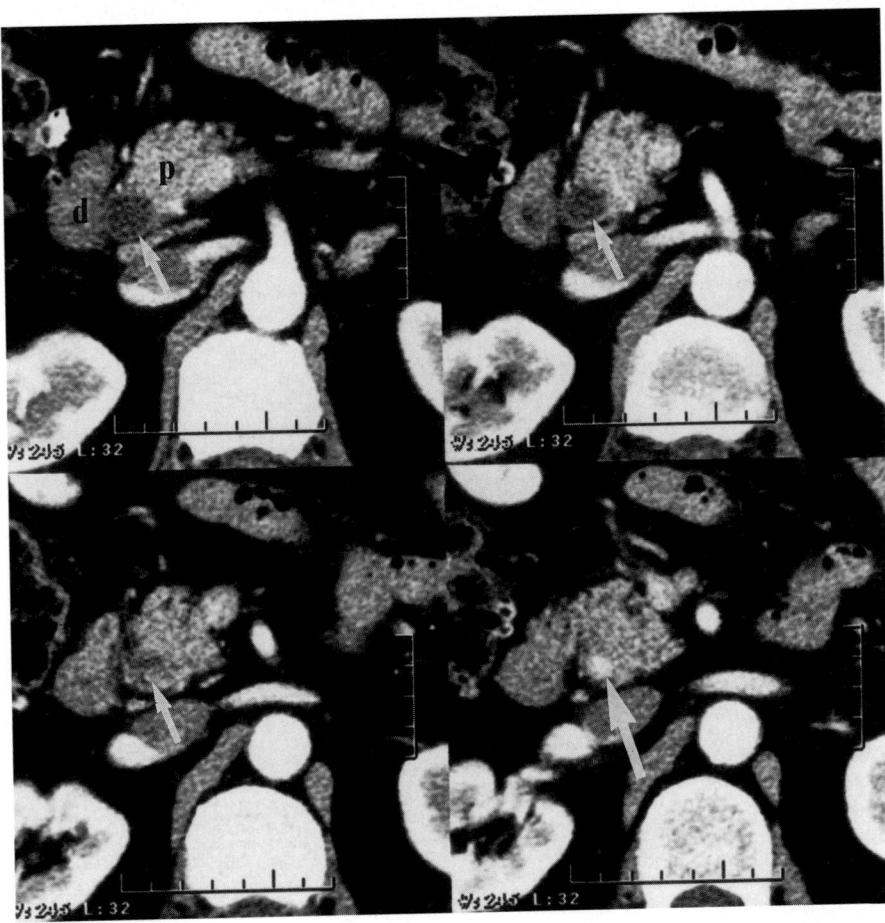

Figure 27.15. Obstructing Stone in Common Bile Duct. Serial CT images obtained from a jaundiced patient demonstrate dilatation of the common bile duct (*small arrows*) due to an obstructing high density gallstone (*large arrow*) impacted in the distal common bile duct. Note the course of the common bile duct in relationship to the head of the pancreas (*p*) and descending duodenum (*d*).

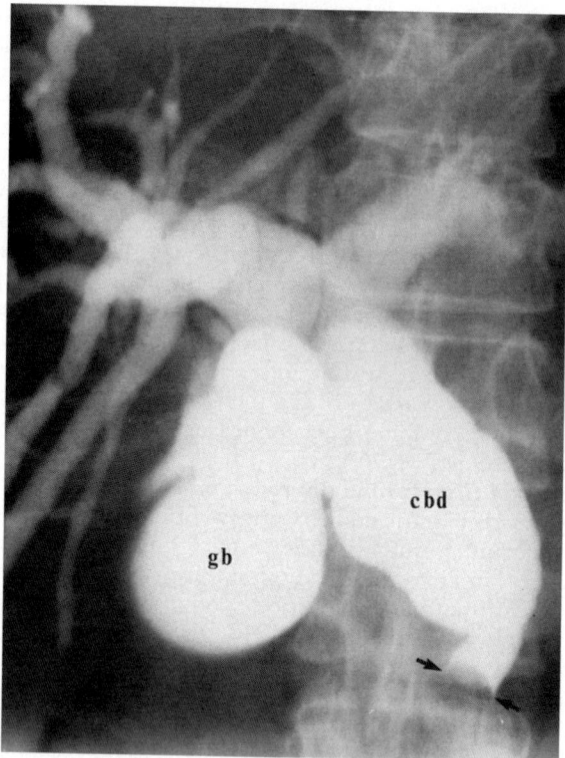

Figure 27.16. Choledocholithiasis. Percutaneous transhepatic cholangiogram demonstrates marked dilation of the common bile duct (*cbd*) and intrahepatic bile ducts. The gallbladder (*gb*) is filled with contrast and distended. The cause of obstruction and dilation is a radiolucent stone (*arrows*) impacted in the distal common bile duct. The proximal aspect of the stone is well-outlined by contrast.

duces a characteristic beaded pattern of intrahepatic ducts (72). Small saccular outpouching (duct divertic-ula), demonstrated on cholangiography, are considered to be pathognomonic.

AIDS-associated Cholangitis is characterized by thickening of the walls of the bile ducts and the gall-bladder due to inflammation and edema (73). Infection by opportunistic organisms, most commonly cyto-megalovirus and *Cryptosporidium*, as well as reaction to the human immunodeficiency virus itself, are implicated as the cause of observed disease. Bile ducts are com-monly dilated in association with stenosis at the am-pulla. Ulcers in the common duct, inflammatory changes in the duodenum, and additional evidence of infection with opportunistic organisms are commonly associated.

Oriental Cholangiohepatitis is an endemic disease in Southeast Asia characterized by recurrent attacks of jaundice, abdominal pain, fever, and chills (74). Intrahepatic and extrahepatic bile ducts are dilated and filled with soft pigmented stones and pus. The cause is uncertain but the disease is associated with parasitic in-festation (clonorchiasis, ascariasis) and nutritional defi-ciency. Findings include intraductal stones, severe extrahepatic biliary dilation, focal strictures, and straightening and rigidity of intrahepatic ducts.

Caroli's Disease is an uncommon congenital anomaly of the biliary tract characterized by saccular ec-tasia of the intrahepatic bile ducts without biliary ob-struction (75). The extrahepatic bile ducts are usually

spared. Only one hepatic lobe or segment may be af-fected, most commonly the left lobe. The cross-sectional imaging appearance is of diffusely scattered cysts that communicate with the bile ducts. The disease is associ-ated with medullary sponge kidney and autosomal re-cessive polycystic kidney disease. Complications include pyogenic cholangitis, liver abscess, and biliary stones. Cholangiocarcinoma develops in 7% of cases. Most cases present in childhood. Autosomal recessive inheritance is evident in some cases.

Choledochal Cysts are uncommon congenital anoma-lies of the biliary tree characterized by cystic dilation of the bile ducts (Fig. 27.17)(76,77). Most (60%) present in infancy or childhood. Some are discovered by fetal US. The condition is much more common in females (70–84% of cases). Patients present with abdominal pain, mass, and jaundice. The Todani classification of congenital bil-iary cysts is illustrated in Figure 27.18 (78).

Pancreatic and Ampullary Carcinomas are the cause of 20–25% of cases of biliary obstruction in the adult. Metastatic disease from lung, breast, gastroin-testinal tumors, and lymphoma account for 2% of cases.

Cholangiocarcinoma is the second most common ma-lignant primary hepatic tumor (79,80). The histology is usually adenocarcinoma. *Peripheral cholangiocarcinoma* (10%) presents as an intrahepatic hypodense mass with adjacent biliary dilatation present in only 25% of cases. Spiral CT demonstrates mild, thin, incomplete rim-like en-hancement with low tumoral attentuation in most cases (81). *Hilar cholangiocarcinoma* (Klastkin's tumor)(25%) oc-curs near the junction of the right and left bile ducts. The tumor is usually small, poorly differentiated, aggressive, and causes obstruction of both ductal systems.

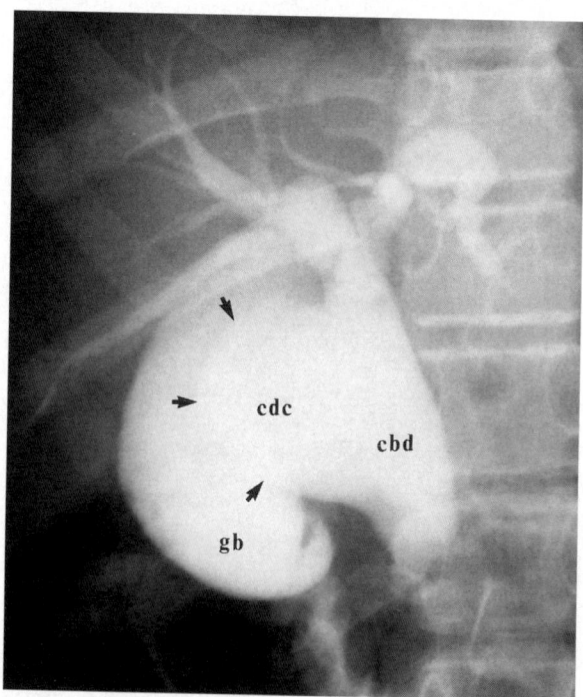

Figure 27.17. Choledochal Cyst. Endoscopic retrograde cholan-giography demonstrates cystic dilation (*cdc, arrows*) of the com-mon bile duct (*cbd*). The gallbladder (*gb*) and intrahepatic bile ducts are also opacified.

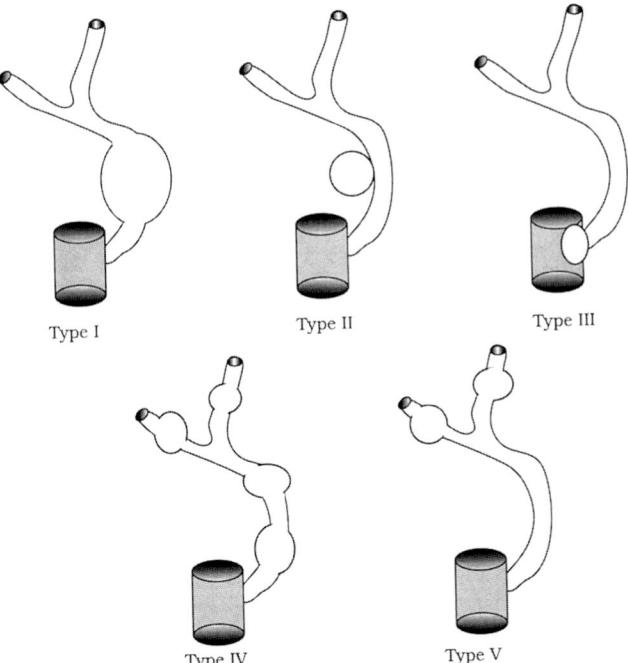

Type I   Type II   Type III

Type IV   Type V

Figure 27.18. Classification of Congenital Biliary Cysts. Type I choledochal cysts (80–90% of cases) are focal, saccular or fusiform, dilatations of the common bile duct. Type II cysts (2%) are true diverticuli of the common bile duct. Type III cysts (1.4–5%) are termed choledochoceles and are dilatations of the terminal intraduodenal portion of the common bile duct. Type IV cysts (19%) refers to multiple intrahepatic and extrahepatic bile duct cysts. Caroli's disease is classified Type V.

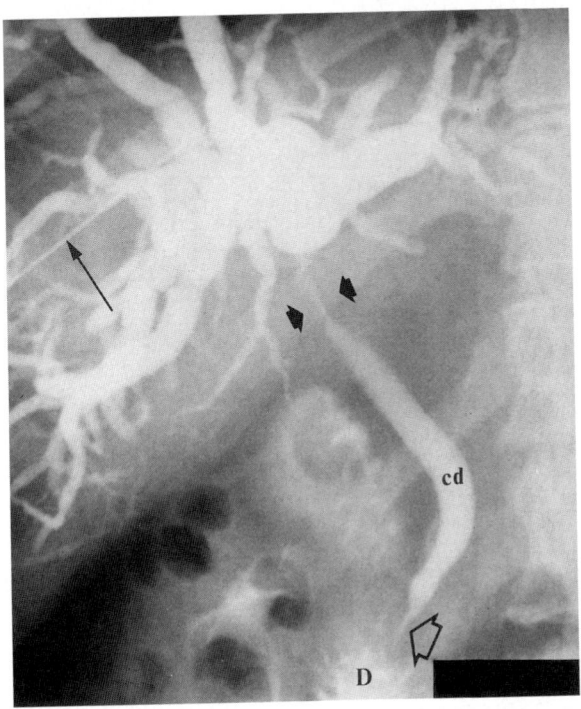

Figure 27.19. Cholangiocarcinoma. Percutaneous transhepatic cholangiogram (PTC) demonstrates abrupt focal narrowing (*short arrows*) of the proximal common bile duct (*cd*) near the bifurcation. The intrahepatic bile ducts are diffusely dilated. The common bile duct shows normal narrowing at the ampulla of Vater (*open arrow*). The PTC needle (*long arrow*) is evident. *D*, duodenum.

Extrahepatic cholangiocarcinoma (65%) causes stenosis or obstruction of the common bile duct in most (95%) cases (Fig. 27.19) and presents as an intraductal polypoid mass in 5%. Predisposing conditions include choledochal cyst, ulcerative colitis, Caroli's disease, *Clonorchis sinensis* infection, and primary sclerosing cholangitis. The tumor may be infiltrative, desmoplastic, and small, making imaging detection as well as needle biopsy difficult. Abrupt stricture with thickening of duct wall may be the only findings. Cross-sectional imaging is used to detect adenopathy and hepatic metastases. Prognosis is poor, with less than 20% of tumors resectable.

Gas in the Biliary Tract

Gas in the biliary tract is most commonly encountered in the patient with a surgically created biliary-enteric anastomosis, or who has had a sphincterotomy to facilitate stone passage (Table 27.9).

Cholecystoduodenal Fistula is most commonly due to erosion of a gallstone through the gallbladder and into the duodenum. When the gallstone is large, it may cause small bowel obstruction, i.e., "*gallstone ileus.*" The gallstone may also erode into the colon and pass spontaneously in the feces. Cholecystoduodenal fistula is most common in women because of the higher incidence of gallstones.

Choledochoduodenal Fistula is caused by a penetrating peptic ulcer eroding into the common bile duct (Fig. 27.20).

GALLBLADDER

Imaging Methods

US is the imaging method of choice for the gallbladder. It offers high anatomic detail, convenience, and cost efficiency. Gallbladder US is reviewed in detail in chapter 36. Cholescintigraphy utilizing technetium-99m-iminodiacetic acid has sensitivity and specificity comparable to US for the diagnosis of acute cholecystitis. Oral cholecystogram (OCG) remains useful in the diagnosis of cholelithiasis. Contrast agents taken orally are concentrated within the gallbladder and demonstrate gallstones as filling defects in the contrast pool. Plain films demonstrate calcified gallstones, porcelain gallbladder, and emphysematous cholecystitis. Gallstones and cholecystitis may be demonstrated by CT but the sensitivity is

Table 27.9. Causes of Gas in the Biliary Tract

Postsurgical
  Sphincterotomy
  Choledochoduodenostomy
  Choledochojejunostomy
Biliary-enteric fistula
  Cholecystoduodenal fistula (gallstone erodes into CBD)
  Choledochoduodenal fistula (ulcer penetrates CBD)
  Surgery/trauma
  Tumor erosion with fistula
Infection
  Emphysematous cholecystitis
  Pyogenic cholangitis

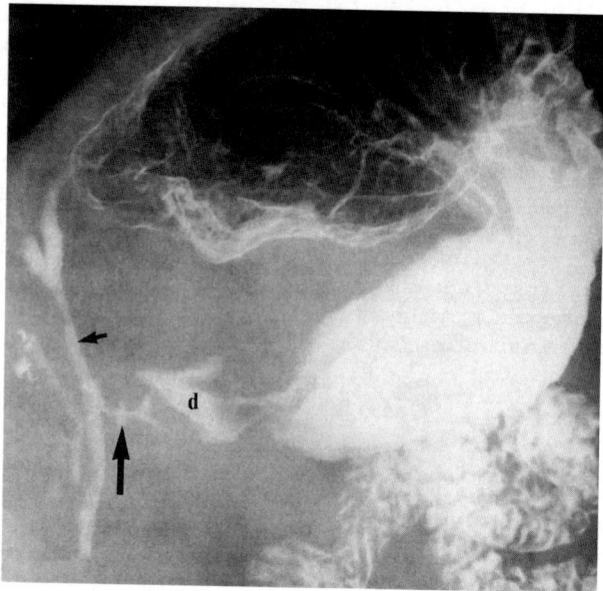

Figure 27.20. Choledochoduodenal Fistula. An upper gastrointestinal series demonstrates filling of the bile ducts due to a penetrating duodenal ulcer that created a fistula (*large arrow*) between the duodenum (*d*) and the bile ducts (*small arrow*).

low. CT is useful in the diagnosis and staging of gallbladder carcinoma. MR is occasionally used in the staging of gallbladder carcinoma.

Anatomy

The gallbladder lies on the underside of the liver in the fossa formed by the junction of the left and right lobes. While the position of the fundus is inconsistent, the neck of the gallbladder is invariably positioned in the porta hepatis and major interlobar fissure. The gallbladder fundus frequently causes a mass impression on the top of the duodenal bulb. Kinking and folding of the gallbladder is common and generally easily recognized by careful image analysis. The so-called phrygian cap, which is descriptive of folding of the gallbladder fundus, is a common normal variant (82). Septa within the gallbladder may be partial or complete. The spiral valves of Heister are small folds in the cystic duct.

The normal gallbladder is well-distended with bile and is easily visualized following a 4 hour fast. A gallbladder greater than 5 cm in diameter is considered enlarged (hydropic), while a gallbladder less than 2 cm in diameter is considered contracted. The normal gallbladder wall does not exceed 3 mm in thickness, measured from gallbladder lumen to liver parenchyma, when the gallbladder is distended. The normal gallbladder lumen is free of particulate debris and is fluid density on imaging studies.

Gallstones

Gallstones are present in 8% of the general population and 15% of the population aged 40–60. Approximately 85% of gallstones are predominantly cholesterol, while 15% are predominantly bilirubin and are related to hemolytic anemia. Approximately 10% of stones are suf-

ficiently radiopaque to be detected by plain film as laminated or faceted calcifications. Fissures within gallstones may contain nitrogen gas that appears on plain film as branching linear lucencies resembling a "crow's foot." Gallstones are most common in women (female:male = 4:1), and patients with hemolytic anemia, diseases of the ileum, cirrhosis, and diabetes mellitus.

US detects 95% of all gallstones whereas CT detects only 80–85%. Gallstones vary in CT attenuation from fat density to calcium density (83). Some gallstones are not visible because they are isodense with bile while some are missed because of their small size. Care must be taken to avoid interpreting contrast in adjacent bowel as cholelithiasis.

OCG demonstrates gallstones as filling defects within the contrast-filled gallbladder (Fig. 27.21) (84). Mobile gallstones will move with changes in patient position. OCG has a 10% false-negative rate for gallstones because they are obscured by stool, contrast, or air in overlying bowel. OCG can reliably be performed only in patients on normal fat-containing diets who have bilirubin levels below 2 mg/100 ml. Obstruction of the cystic duct, associated with chronic cholecystitis and stones, causes nonvisualization of the gallbladder on OCG. Additional causes of nonvisualization include poor intestinal absorption of contrast, prolonged fasting, and liver disease.

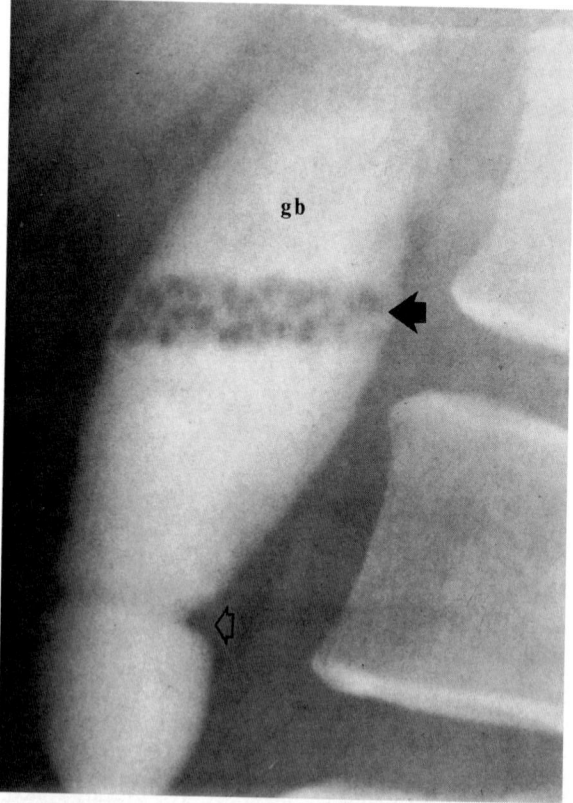

Figure 27.21. Gallstones. An upright film from an oral cholecystogram demonstrates multiple small gallstones (*closed arrow*) that float in contrast within the gallbladder lumen (*gb*). The high specific gravity of contrast causes some gallstones to float. A fold of mucosa (*open arrow*) produces partial septation of the gallbladder fundus. This is a normal variant.

US may clarify the cause of gallbladder nonvisualization by confirming gallbladder disease.

Differential considerations for lesions in the gallbladder that may be mistaken for gallstones include the following.

Sludge Balls or tumefactive biliary sludge result from biliary stasis. The bile thickens and forms mobile masses that move with changes in patient position.

Cholesterol Polyps are common benign, polypoid masses that result from accumulation of triglycerides and cholesterol in macrophages in the gallbladder wall. They are of no clinical significance. All are 10 mm or less in size (see Fig. 36.19).

Adenomyomatosis may be focal and present as a polypoid mass fixed to the gallbladder wall.

Adenomatous Polyps are small, usually flat masses fixed to the gallbladder wall.

Gallbladder Carcinoma may present as a polypoid mass. Most are 1 cm or more in size. Gallstones are usually present.

Acute Cholecystitis

Acute inflammation of the gallbladder is caused by gallstones obstructing the cystic duct in 90% of cases. Acalculous cholecystitis occurs nearly always in patients with predisposing conditions listed subsequently. Cholescintigraphy and sonography have comparable sensitivities and specificities in the diagnosis of acute cholecystitis.

Scintigraphic diagnosis of acute cholecystitis is based on obstruction of the cystic duct with nonvisualization of the gallbladder. The normal gallbladder demonstrates progressive accumulation of radionuclide activity over 30 minutes to 1 hour following injection of technetium-99m-iminodiacetic acid. Delayed visualization of the gallbladder may be seen in patients with biliary stasis due to fasting or hyperalimentation. Delayed images taken at 4 hours postradionuclide injection are needed to assess for this possibility. The test is considered positive if there is prompt tracer accumulation in the liver with excretion of tracer into the bowel and without gallbladder visualization at 4 hours. The test may be considered positive at 1 hour postradionuclide injection if the gallbladder does not visualize within 20 minutes of intravenous injection of morphine.

Confident US diagnosis of acute cholecystitis requires the presence of three findings: cholelithiasis, edema of the gallbladder wall seen as a band of echolucency in the wall, and a positive sonographic Murphy sign (see Fig. 36.20).

Although CT is not the imaging method of first choice for acute cholecystitis, findings that suggest the diagnosis include gallstones, distended gallbladder, thickened gallbladder wall, subserosal edema, high density bile, intraluminal sloughed membranes, pericholecystic stranding, and pericholecystic fluid (Fig. 27.22) (85).

Acalculous Cholecystitis causes special problems in diagnosis because the cystic duct is often not obstructed. Inflammation may be due to gallbladder wall ischemia or direct bacterial infection. Patients at risk for acalculous cholecystitis include those with biliary stasis due to lack of oral intake, posttrauma, postburn, postsurgery, or on total parenteral nutrition. Scintigraphy

usually demonstrates lack of gallbladder visualization. Although this finding is 90–95% sensitive for acalculous cholecystitis, it is only 38% specific. False-positive conditions for nonvisualization include hyperalimentation and prolonged severe illness, which are predisposing conditions for acalculous cholecystitis. US demonstrates a distended tender gallbladder with thickened wall but without stones (see Fig. 36.21). Many patients are too ill to elicit a reliable sonographic Murphy sign.

Sludge is a term used to describe the presence of thick particulate matter in highly concentrated bile. Calcium bilirubinate and cholesterol crystals precipitate in the bile when biliary stasis is prolonged because of a lack of oral intake, hyperalimentation, or biliary obstruction. Since sludge may be found in a fasting, but otherwise normal patient, its presence is not definitive evidence of gallbladder disease. Pus, blood, and milk of calcium are additional causes of dense bile.

Complications of acute cholecystitis include the following.

Gangrenous Cholecystitis indicates the presence of necrosis of the gallbladder wall (Fig. 27.22). The patient is at risk for gallbladder perforation. Findings include mucosal irregularity and asymmetric thickening of the gallbladder wall with multiple lucent layers, indicating mucosal ulceration and reactive edema.

Perforation of the Gallbladder is a life-threatening complication seen in 5–10% of cases. Perforation may occur adjacent to the liver resulting in pericholecystic abscess, into the peritoneal cavity resulting in generalized peritonitis, or into adjacent bowel resulting in biliary-enteric fistula. Overall mortality is as high as 24%. A focal pericholecystic fluid collection suggests pericholecystic abscess.

Emphysematous Cholecystitis results from infection of the gallbladder with gas-forming organisms, usually *E. coli* or *Clostridium perfringens*. Approximately 40% of

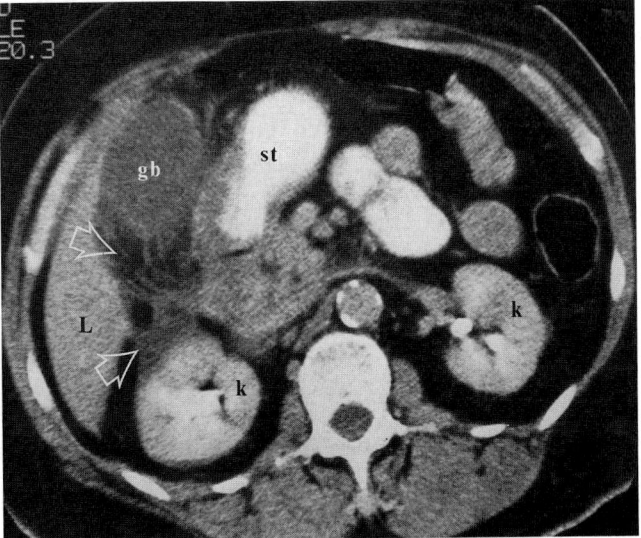

Figure 27.22. Gangrenous Cholecystitis. CT reveals a distended gallbladder (*gb*) with extensive pericholecystic inflammation manifest by globular and streaky soft tissue densities in the pericholecystic fat (*arrows*). *L*, liver; *k*, kidney; *s*, stomach.

patients are diabetic. Gallstones may or may not be present. Gas is demonstrated within the wall or within the lumen of the gallbladder by plain film or CT. On US, intramural gas has an arc-like configuration difficult to differentiate from calcification and porcelain gallbladder.

Mirizzi's Syndrome refers to the condition of biliary obstruction resulting from a gallstone in the cystic duct eroding into the adjacent common duct and causing an inflammatory mass that obstructs the common duct. Visualization of a stone at the junction of the cystic duct and the common hepatic duct in a patient with biliary obstruction and gallbladder inflammation suggests the diagnosis.

Chronic Cholecystitis

Chronic cholecystitis includes a spectrum of pathology that shares the presence of gallstones and chronic gallbladder inflammation. Patients with chronic cholecystitis complain of recurrent attacks of right upper quadrant pain and biliary colic. Imaging findings include gallstones, thickening of the gallbladder wall, contraction of the gallbladder lumen, delayed visualization of the gallbladder on cholescintigraphy, and poor contractility. Variants of chronic cholecystitis include the following.

Porcelain Gallbladder describes the presence of dystrophic calcification in the wall of an obstructed and chronically inflamed gallbladder (Fig. 27.23). The condi-

tion is associated with gallstones in 90% of cases. Porcelain gallbladder carries a 10–20% risk of gallbladder carcinoma. Cholecystectomy is usually indicated.

Milk of Calcium Bile, also called limy bile, is associated with an obstructed cystic duct, chronic cholecystitis, and gallstones. Particulate matter with a high concentration of calcium compounds is precipitated in the bile, making the bile radiopaque on plain films or CT. Dependent layering of bile can be demonstrated on plain film radiographs. The bile is extremely echogenic on US and gallstones may be visualized within it.

Thickening of the Gallbladder Wall

Thickening of the gallbladder wall is present when the wall thickness measured on the hepatic aspect of the gallbladder exceeds 3 mm in patients who have fasted at least 8 hours. Conditions associated with wall thickening include the following.

Acute and Chronic Cholecystitis. Wall thickening is a usual feature of acute cholecystitis and is present in 50% of cases of chronic cholecystitis.

Hepatitis causes reduction in bile flow, which results in reduced gallbladder volume and thickening of the gallbladder wall in approximately half of the patients.

Portal Venous Hypertension and Congestive Heart Failure may cause wall thickening by passive venous congestion.

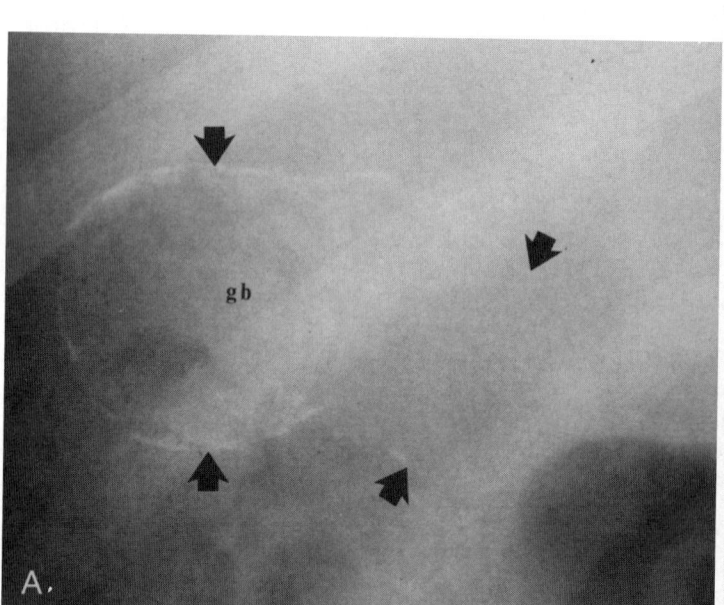

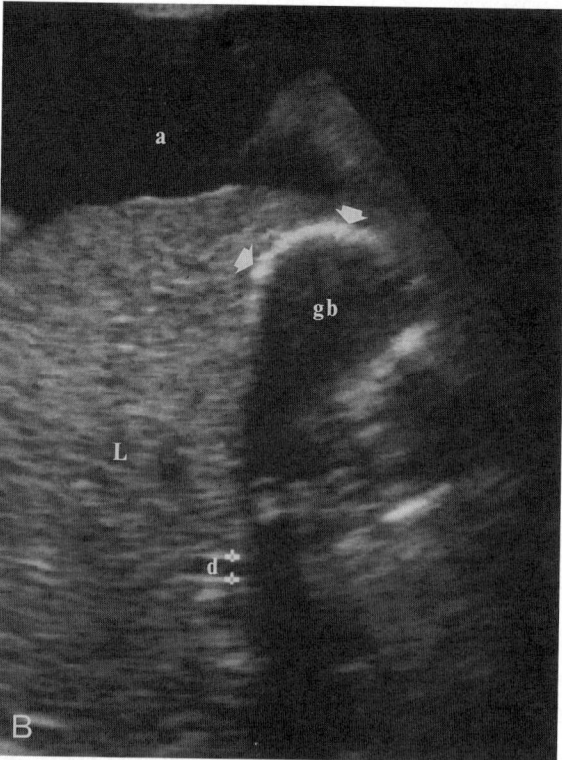

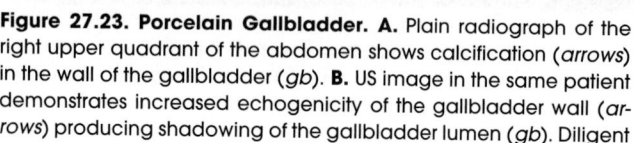

Figure 27.23. Porcelain Gallbladder. A. Plain radiograph of the right upper quadrant of the abdomen shows calcification (*arrows*) in the wall of the gallbladder (*gb*). **B.** US image in the same patient demonstrates increased echogenicity of the gallbladder wall (*arrows*) producing shadowing of the gallbladder lumen (*gb*). Diligent analysis with multiple views is needed to differentiate calcification in the gallbladder wall from large stones filling the gallbladder lumen. This patient also has cirrhosis with a shrunken nodular liver (*L*) and ascites (*a*). d, common bile duct.

AIDS is associated with thickening of the gallbladder wall and the the walls of the bile ducts (73). Opportunistic organisms are sometimes present.

Hypoalbuminemia is associated with thickened gallbladder wall in 60% of patients.

Gallbladder Carcinoma usually presents as a focal mass but may cause only focal wall thickening.

Adenomyomatosis is the most frequent benign condition of the gallbladder and is characterized by hyperplasia of the mucosa and smooth muscle. It is usually focal in the fundus, but may be diffuse throughout the gallbladder. Outpouchings of mucosa into or through the muscularis form characteristic Rokitansky-Aschoff sinuses (Fig. 27.24). The condition has no malignant potential. Coexisting gallstones are commonly present.

Gallbladder Carcinoma

Adenocarcinoma of the gallbladder is commonly overlooked or misdiagnosed preoperatively (86,87). The presence of gallstones in 70–80% of cases masks the findings of carcinoma, especially with US examination. Gallbladder carcinoma is a tumor of elderly women (>60 years, female:male = 4:1). Patients present with pain, anorexia, weight loss and jaundice. Calcification of the gallbladder wall (porcelain gallbladder) is a risk factor. Imaging findings include (see Fig. 36.22) the following: *a)* intraluminal soft tissue mass; *b)* focal or diffuse thickening of the gallbladder wall; *c)* soft tissue mass replacing the gallbladder; *d)* gallstones; *e)* extension of tumor into the liver, bile ducts, and adjacent bowel; *f)* di-

lated bile ducts; and *g)* metastases to regional lymph nodes and liver. Most tumors are unresectable at discovery.

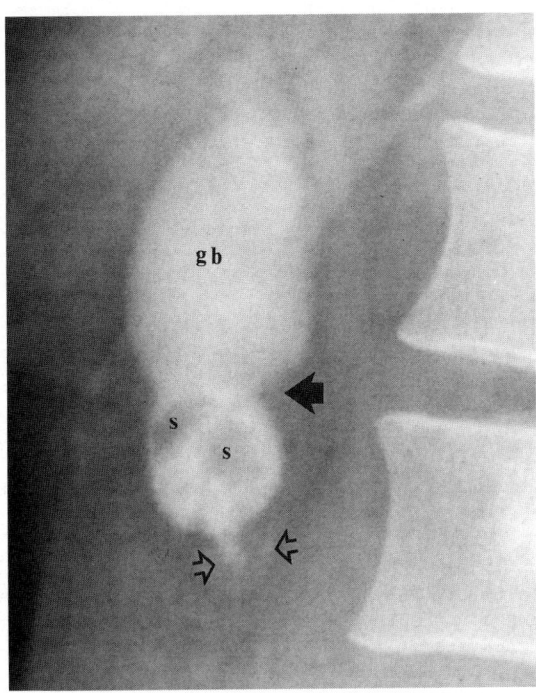

Figure 27.24. Adenomyomatosis. An oral cholecystogram reveals compartmentalization of the gallbladder (*gb*) fundus by a thick septa (*closed arrow*). Contrast extends into the thickened wall at the fundus filling Rokitansky-Aschoff sinuses (*open arrows*). Stones (*s*) in the fundus are seen as lucent filling defects.

References

1. Bluemke DA, Fishman EK. Spiral CT of the liver. AJR Am J Roentgenol 1993;160:787–792.
2. Grant EG, Schiller VL, Millener P, et al. Color Doppler imaging of the hepatic vasculature. AJR Am J Roentgenol 1992; 159:943–950.
3. Oliver JH III, Baron RL. Helical biphasic contrast-enhanced CT of the liver: technique, indications, interpretation, pitfalls. Radiology 1996;201:1–14.
4. Itai Y, Matsui O. Blood flow and liver imaging. Radiology 1997;202:306–314.
5. Lupetin AR, Cammisa BA, Beckman I, et al. Spiral CT during arterial portography. Radiographics 1996;16:723–743.
6. Nelson RC, Thompson GH, Chezmar JL, et al. CT during arterial portography: diagnostic pitfalls. Radiographics 1992; 12:705–718.
7. Soyer P, Bluemke DA, Rymer R. MR imaging of the liver. MRI Clin North Am 1997;5:205–221.
8. Van Beers BE, Gallez B, Pringot J. Contrast-enhanced MR imaging of the liver. Radiology 1997;203:297–306.
9. Ito K, Mitchell DG, Honjo K, et al. Biphasic contrast-enhanced multisection dynamic MR imaging of the liver: potential pitfalls. Radiographics 1997;17:693–705.
10. Dodd LG, Mooney EE, Layfield LJ, Nelson RC. Fine-needle aspiration of the liver and pancreas: a cytology primer for radiologists. Radiology 1997;203:1–9.
11. Mukai JK, Stack CM, Turner D, et al. Imaging of surgically relevant hepatic vascular and segmental anatomy. Part 1. Normal anatomy. AJR Am J Roentgenol 1987;149: 287–292.
12. Mukai JK, Stack CM, Turner DA, et al. Imaging of surgically relevant hepatic vascular and segmental anatomy. Part 2. Extent and resectability of hepatic neoplasms. AJR Am J Roentgenol 1987;149:293–297.
13. Winter TC III, Ngheim HV, Freeny PC, et al. Hepatic arterial anatomy: demonstration of normal supply and vascular variants with three-dimensional CT angiography. Radiographics 1995;15:771–780.
14. Soyer P, Bluemke DA, Bliss DF, et al. Surgical segmental anatomy of the liver: demonstration with spiral CT during arterial portography and mulitplanar reconstruction. AJR Am J Roentgenol 1994;163:99–103.
15. Gazelle GS, Haaga JR. Hepatic neoplasms: surgically relevant segmental anatomy and imaging techniques. AJR Am J Roentgenol 1992;158:1015–1018.
16. Sugarbaker PH. Surgical decision making for large bowel cancer metastatic to the liver. Radiology 1990;174: 621–626.
17. Dodds WJ, Erickson SJ, Taylor AJ, et al. Caudate lobe of the liver: anatomy, embryology, and pathology. AJR Am J Roentgenol 1990;154:87–93.
18. Dodd GD. An American's guide to Couinaud's numbering system. AJR Am J Roentgenol 1993;161:574–575.
19. Soyer P. Segmental anatomy of the liver: utility of a nomenclature accepted worldwide. AJR Am J Roentgenol 1993; 161:572–573.
20. Yu J-S, Kim KW, Sung KB, et al. Small arterial-portal venous shunts: a cause of pseudolesions at hepatic imaging. Radiology 1997;203:737–742.
21. Mergo PJ, Ros PR, Buetow PC, Buck JL. Diffuse disease of the liver: radiologic-pathologic correlation. Radiographics 1994;14:1291–1307.

22. Siegelman ES. MR imaging of diffuse liver disease—hepatic fat and iron. MRI Clin North Am 1997;5:347–365.

23. Itai Y, Murata S, Kurosaki Y. Straight border sign of the liver: spectrum of CT appearances and causes. Radiographics 1995;15:1089–1102.

24. Wang S-S, Chiang J-H, Tsai Y-T, et al. Focal hepatic fatty infiltration as a cause of pseudotumors: ultrasonographic patterns and clinical differentiation. J Clin Ultrasound 1990;18:401–409.

25. Kester NL, Elmore SG. Focal hypoechoic regions in the liver at the porta hepatis: prevalence in ambulatory patients. J Ultrasound Med 1995;14:649–652.

26. Itai Y, Sekiyama K, Ahmadi T, et al. Fulminant hepatic failure: observation with serial CT. Radiology 1997;202:379–382.

27. Brown JJ, Naylor MJ, Yagan N. Imaging of hepatic cirrhosis. Radiology 1997;202:1–16.

28. Taylor AJ, Carmody TJ, Quiroz FA, et al. Focal masses in cirrhotic liver: CT and MR imaging features. AJR Am J Roentgenol 1994;163:857–862.

29. Miller WJ, Baron RL, Dodd GD III, Federle MP. Malignancies in patients with cirrhosis: CT sensitivity and specificity in 200 consecutive transplant patients. Radiology 1994;193:645–650.

30. Dodd GD III, Miller WJ, Baron RL, et al. Detection of malignant tumors in end-stage cirrhotic livers: efficacy of sonography as a screening technique. AJR Am J Roentgenol 1992;159:727–733.

31. Choi BI, Takayasu K, Han MC. Small hepatocellular carcinomas and associated nodular lesions of the liver: pathology, pathogenesis, and imaging findings. AJR Am J Roentgenol 1993;160:1177–1187.

32. Earls JP, Theise ND, Weinreb JC, et al. Dysplastic nodules and hepatocellular carcinoma: thin-section MR imaging of explanted cirrhotic livers with pathologic correlation. Radiology 1996;201:207–211.

33. Ohtomo K, Baron RL, Dodd GD III, et al. Confluent hepatic fibrosis in advanced cirrhosis: appearance at CT. Radiology 1993;188:31–35.

34. Ohtomo K, Baron RL, Dodd GD III, et al. Confluent hepatic fibrosis in advanced cirrhosis: evaluation with MR imaging. Radiology 1993;189:871–874.

35. Bosch J, Pizcueta P, Feu F, et al. Pathophysiology of portal hypertension. Gastroenterology Clin N Am 1992;21:1–14.

36. Pieters PC, Miller WJ, DeMeo JH. Evaluation of the portal venous system: complementary roles of invasive and noninvasive imaging strategies. Radiographics 1997;17:879–895.

37. Cho KC, Patel YD, Wachsberg RH, Seeff J. Varices in portal hypertension: evaluation with CT. Radiographics 1995;15:609–622.

38. Subramanyam BR, Balthazar EJ, Madamba MR, et al. Sonography of portosystemic venous collaterals in portal hypertension. Radiology 1983;146:161–166.

39. Ito K, Higuchi M, Kada T, et al. CT of acquired abnormalities of the portal venous system. Radiographics 1997;17:897–917.

40. Cho K, Koo J-H, Kim Y-S, et al. Collateral pathways in Budd-Chiari syndrome: CT and venographic correlations. AJR Am J Roentgenol 1996;167:1163–1167.

41. Gore RM, Mathieu DG, White EM, et al. Passive hepatic congestion: cross-sectional imaging features. AJR Am J Roentgenol 1994;162:71–75.

42. Ito K, Honjo K, Fujita T, et al. Liver neoplasms: diagnostic pitfalls in cross-sectional imaging. Radiographics 1996;16:273–293.

43. Powers C, Ros PR, Stoupis C, et al. Primary liver neoplasms: MR imaging with pathologic correlation. Radiographics 1994;14:459–482.

44. Lee MJ, Hahn PF, Saini S, Mueller PR. Differential diagnosis of hyperintense liver lesions on T1-weighted MR images. AJR Am J Roentgenol 1992;159:1017–1020.

45. Baker ME, Pelley R. Hepatic metastases: basic principles and implications for radiologists. Radiology 1995;197:329–337.

46. Fujita T, Honjo K, Ito K, et al. High-resolution dynamic MR imaging of hepatocellular carcinoma with a phased-array body coil. Radiographics 1997;17:315–331.

47. Martin J, Sentis M, Zidan A, et al. Fatty metamorphosis of hepatocellular carcinoma: detection with chemical shift gradient-echo MR imaging. Radiology 1995;195:125–130.

48. Stevens WR, Johnson CD, Stephens DH, Batts KP. CT findings in hepatocellular carcinoma: correlation of tumor characteristics with causative factors, tumor size, and histologic tumor grade. Radiology 1994;191:531–537.

49. Ebara M, Watanabe S, Kita K, et al. MR imaging of small hepatocellular carcinoma: effect of intratumoral copper content on signal intensity. Radiology 1991;180:617–621.

50. Kitagawa K, Matsui O, Kadoya M, et al. Hepatocellular carcinomas with excessive copper accumulation: CT and MR findings. Radiology 1991;180:623–628.

51. Stevens WR, Johnson CD, Stephens DH, Nagorney DM. Fibrolamellar hepatocellular carcinoma: stage at presentation and results of aggressive surgical management. AJR Am J Roentgenol 1995;164:1153–1158.

52. Brant WE, Floyd JL, Jackson DE, Gilliland JD. The radiological evaluation of hepatic cavernous hemangioma. JAMA 1987;257:2471–2474.

53. Mungovan JA, Cronan JJ, Vacarro J. Hepatic cavernous hemangiomas: lack of enlargement over time. Radiology 1994;191:111–113.

54. Nghiem HV, Bogost GA, Ryan JA, et al. Cavernous hemangiomas of the liver: enlargement over time. AJR Am J Roentgenol 1997;169:137–140.

55. Semelka RC, Sofka CM. Hepatic hemangiomas. MRI Clin North Am 1997;5:241–253.

56. Beutow PC, Pantongrag-Brown L, Buck JL, et al. Focal nodular hyperplasia of the liver: radiologic pathologic correlation. Radiographics 1996;16:369–388.

57. Sanders LM, Botet JF, Straus DJ, et al. CT of primary lymphoma of the liver. AJR Am J Roentgenol 1989;152:973–976.

58. Murphy BJ, Casillas J, Ros PR, et al. The CT appearance of cystic masses of the liver. Radiographics 1989;9:307–322.

59. von Sinner W, te Strake L, Clark D, Sharif H. MR imaging of hydatid disease. AJR Am J Roentgenol 1991;157:741–745.

60. Wolfman NT, Bechtold RE, Scharling ES, Meredith JW. Blunt upper abdominal trauma: evaluation by CT. AJR Am J Roentgenol 1992;158:493–501.

61. Roberts JL, Dalen K, Bosanko CM, Jafir SZH. CT in abdominal and pelvic trauma. Radiographics 1993;13:735–752.

62. Burrell MI, Zeman RK, Simeone JF, et al. The biliary tract: imaging for the 1990s. AJR Am J Roentgenol 1991;157:223–233.

63. Neitlich JD, Topazian M, Smith RC, et al. Detection of choledocholithiasis: comparison of unenhanced helical CT and endoscopic retrograde cholangiopancreatography. Radiology 1997;203:753–757.

64. Reinhold C, Bret PM, Guibaud L, et al. MR cholangiopancreatography: potential clinical applications. Radiographics 1996;16:309–320.

65. Reinhold C, Bret PM. Current status of MR cholangiopancreatography. AJR Am J Roentgenol 1996;166:1285–1295.

66. Turner MA, Cho S-R, Messmer JM. Pitfalls in cholangiographic interpretation. Radiographics 1987;7:1067–1105.

67. Gazelle GS, Lee MJ, Mueller PR. Cholangiographic segmental anatomy of the liver. Radiographics 1994;14: 1005–1013.

68. Liddell RM, Baron RL, Ekstrom JE, et al. Normal intrahepatic bile ducts: CT depiction. Radiology 1990;176:633–635.

69. May GR, James EM, Bender CE, et al. Diagnosis and treatment of jaundice. Radiographics 1986;6:847–890.

70. Rosenthal SJ. Pitfalls and differential diagnosis in biliary sonography. Radiographics 1990;10:285–311.

71. Rege RV. Adverse effects of biliary obstruction: implications for treatment of patients with obstructive jaundice. AJR Am J Roentgenol 1995;164:287–293.

72. Majoie CMLM, Reeders JWAJ, Sanders JB, et al. Primary sclerosing cholangitis: a modified classification of cholangiographic findings. AJR Am J Roentgenol 1991;157: 495–497.

73. Miller FH, Gore RM, Nemcek AA Jr, Fitzgerald SW. Pancreaticobiliary manifestations of AIDS. AJR Am J Roentgenol 1996;166:1269–1274.

74. Lim JH. Oriental cholangiohepatitis: pathologic, clinical, and radiologic features. AJR Am J Roentgenol 1991;157: 1–8.

75. Miller WJ, Sechtin AG, Campbell WL, Pieters PC. Imaging findings in Caroli's disease. AJR Am J Roentgenol 1995; 165:333–337.

76. Kim OH, Chung HJ, Choi BG. Imaging of choledochal cyst. RadioGraphics 1995;15:69–88.

77. Savader SJ, Benenati JF, Venbrux AC, et al. Choledochal cysts: classification and cholangiographic appearance. AJR Am J Roentgenol 1991;156:327–331.

78. Todani T, Watanabe Y, Narusue M, et al. Congenital bile duct cysts: classification, operative procedure, and review of 37 cases, including cancer arising from choledochal cyst. Am J Surg 1977;134:263–269.

79. Soyer P, Bluemke DA, Reichle R, et al. Imaging of intrahepatic cholangiocarcinoma: 1. peripheral cholangiocarcinoma. AJR Am J Roentgenol 1995;165:1427–1431.

80. Soyer P, Bluemke DA, Reichle R, et al. Imaging of intrahepatic cholangiocarcinoma: 2. hilar cholangiocarcinoma. AJR Am J Roentgenol 1995;165:1433–1436.

81. Kim TK, Choi BI, Han JK, et al. Peripheral cholangiocarcinoma of the liver: two-phase spiral CT findings. Radiology 1997;204:539–543.

82. Meilstrup JW, Hopper KD, Thieme GA. Imaging of gallbladder variants. AJR Am J Roentgenol 1991;157:1205–1208.

83. Brink JA, Kammer B, Mueller PR, et al. Prediction of gallstone composition: synthesis of CT and radiographic features in vitro. Radiology 1994;190:69–75.

84. Maglinte DDT, Torres WE, Laufer I. Oral cholecystography in contemporary gallstone imaging: a review. Radiology 1991;178:49–58.

85. Fidler J, Paulson EK, Layfield L. CT evaluation of acute cholecystitis: findings and usefulness in diagnosis. AJR Am J Roentgenol 1996;166:1085–1088.

86. Lane J, Buck JL, Zeman RK. Primary carcinoma of the gallbladder: a pictorial essay. Radiographics 1989;9:209–228.

87. Rooholamini SA, Tehrani NS, Razavi MK, et al. Imaging of gallbladder carcinoma. Radiographics 1994;14:291–306.

28
Pancreas and Spleen

William E. Brant

PANCREAS

Imaging Techniques

CT and US provide high-quality images of the pancreatic parenchyma and are used as the primary imaging modalities for the pancreas (1). Helical CT technique optimizes contrast enhancement for detection of small tumors and provides the capability of CT angiography to detect vascular involvement by pancreatic tumor (2,3). Improved MR techniques and the use of gadolinium enhancement have increased its capability to detect and characterize pancreatic lesions (4). Endoscopic retrograde cholangiopancreatography (ERCP) provides excellent visualization of the lumen of the pancreatic duct, which is usually affected by any mass lesion of the pancreas (5,6). This procedure is performed by endoscopic cannulization of the bile and pancreatic ducts, followed by injection of a contrast agent and filming. Specialized MR techniques offer a noninvasive method of performing cholangiopancreatography (7,8). Arteriography is used in selected cases to define tumor vascularity. US- and CT-guided biopsy and drainage procedures play a major role in the diagnosis and treatment of pancreatic diseases (9,10).

Anatomy

The pancreas is a tongue-shaped organ, approximately 12–15 cm in length, that lies within the anterior pararenal compartment of the retroperitoneum (see Fig. 36.30). The pancreas is posterior to the left lobe of the liver, the stomach, and the lesser sac (Fig. 28.1). It is anterior to the spine, the inferior vena cava, and the aorta. Pancreatic tissue is best recognized by identification of the vessels around it. The neck, body, and tail of the pancreas lie ventral to the splenic vein, with the tail extending into the hilum of the spleen. The splenic vein and pancreas are anterior to the superior mesenteric artery. The head of the pancreas wraps around the junction of the superior mesenteric vein and the splenic vein, with the uncinate process of the pancreatic head extending under the superior mesenteric vein just anterior to the inferior vena cava. The splenic artery courses through the pancreatic bed in a tortuous course. Atherosclerotic splenic artery calcifications are easily mistaken for pancreatic calcifications. The lumen of the splenic artery may be mistaken for pancreatic cysts or a dilated pancreatic duct on CT without contrast or US.

Maximum dimensions for pancreatic size are a 3.0-cm diameter for the head, 2.5-cm diameter for the body, and 2.0-cm diameter for the tail. The gland is somewhat larger in young patients and progressively decreases in size with age. Because the gland is not encapsulated, fatty infiltration between the lobules in older patients gives the pancreas a delicate, feathery appearance on CT. The pancreatic duct is visualized with thin-slice (5 mm) CT and with US. It normally measures 3–4 mm in diameter in the head and tapers smoothly to the tail. Films from ERCP show the normal duct to be a bit larger owing to magnification effect and distension resulting from contrast injection (Fig. 28.2). The duodenum cradles the pancreatic head in the C-loop. Many pancreatic abnormalities show secondary effects on the duodenum (see Figs. 30.23, 30.24), and occasionally on the stomach and colon.

On MR, the pancreas is best seen on fat-suppressed T1WI (11). High protein content in the exocrine pancreas results in high signal of the pancreatic parenchyma. Tumors, pancreatitis, and atrophy decrease pancreas signal intensity on T1WI (12). On T2WI, pancreatic tissue is variable in signal intensity from as low as the liver is to as high as fat. Gadolinium will enhance the parenchyma, whereas adenocarcinoma enhances poorly and remains low density on T1WI.

Acute Pancreatitis

The diagnosis of acute pancreatitis is generally made clinically (10,13). The role of imaging is to clarify the diagnosis when the clinical picture is unclear, to assess the severity of the condition, to determine prognosis, and to detect complications. Inflammation of the pancreatic

Figure 28.1. Normal Pancreas CT. A Image through neck (*n*), body (*b*) and tail (*t*) of the pancreas. **B** Image through head (*h*) and uncinate process (*u*) of the pancreas. The majority of the pancreas lies anterior to the splenic vein (*s*) and its junction with the superior mesenteric vein (*v*) that forms the portal vein (*p*). The head and uncinate process lie caudal to the majority of the pancreas. The superior mesenteric artery (*a*) arises from the aorta posterior to the splenic vein and courses caudally just to the left of the superior mesenteric vein. The superior mesenteric artery is normally surrounded by a collar of clear fat.

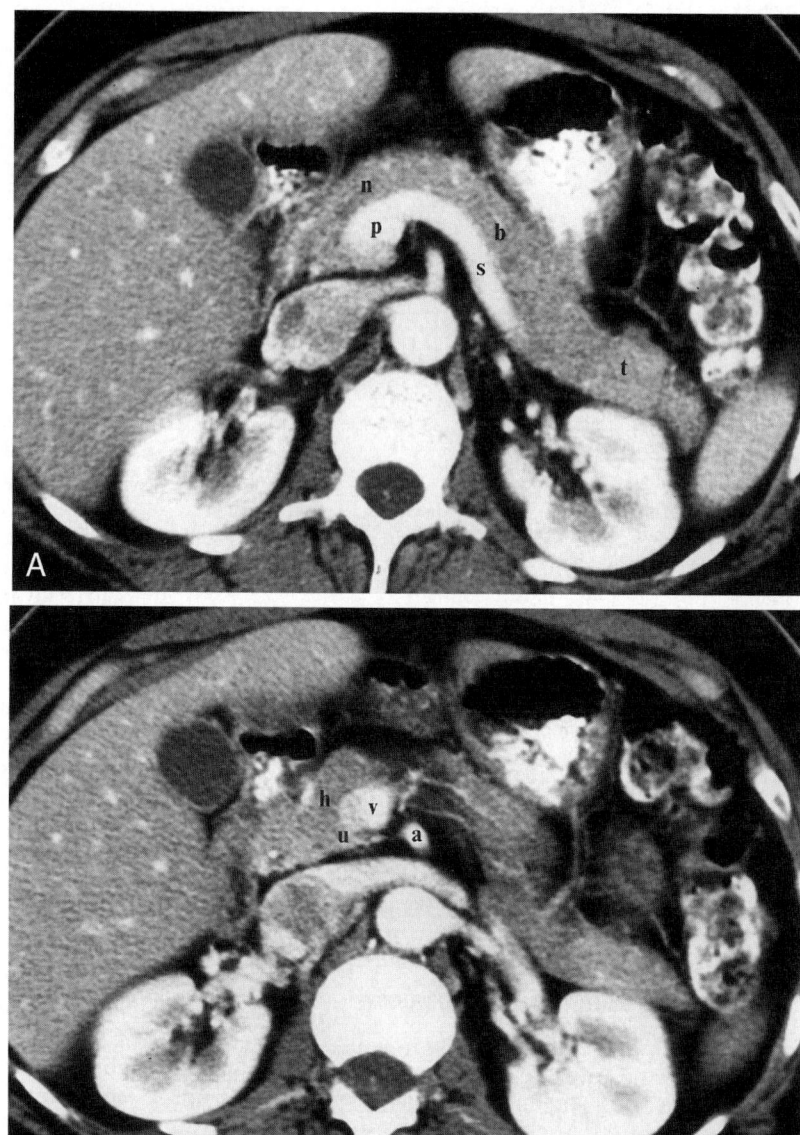

Figure 28.2. Normal Pancreatic Ducts. Radiograph from an ERCP demonstrates the main duct of Wirsung (*DW, black arrows*) and the accessory duct of Santorini (*DS, open arrow*). In this patient, the main duct drained separately into the major papilla (of Vater) with a different orifice for the common bile duct. The accessory duct drained into the minor papilla. Both ampullae were cannulated endoscopically and injected before this radiograph. A number of different variants of pancreatic duct anatomy exist. This variant is found in about 35% of individuals. Embryologically, the main duct is formed by the entire duct of the ventral pancreatic bud and the distal portion of the duct of the dorsal pancreatic bud. The main duct may join the common bile duct or have a separate orifice in the major papilla. The proximal portion of the duct of the dorsal pancreatic bud may be obliterated or persist as the accessory duct. *E*, endoscope.

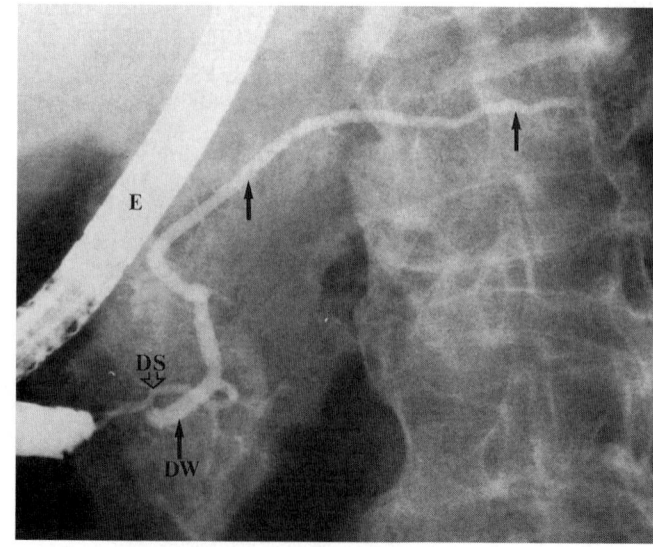

Table 28.1. Causes of Acute Pancreatitis

Alcohol abuse—most common cause of chronic pancreatitis
Gallstone passage/impaction—most common cause of acute pancreatitis
Metabolic disorders
    Hereditary pancreatitis—autosomal dominant
    Hypercalcemia
    Hyperlipidemia—types I and V
    Malnutrition
Trauma
    Blunt abdominal trauma
    Surgery
    ERCP
Penetrating ulcer
Malignancy
    Pancreatic adenocarcinoma
    Lymphoma
Drugs—steroids, tetracycline, furosemide, many others
Infection
    Viral—mumps, hepatitis, infectious mononucleosis, AIDS
    Parasitic—ascariasis, clonorchis
Structural
    Choledochocele
    Pancreas divisum
Idiopathic—20% of cases of acute pancreatitis

tissue leads to disruption of small pancreatic ducts, resulting in leakage of pancreatic secretions. Because the pancreas lacks a capsule, the pancreatic juices have ready access to surrounding tissues. Pancreatic enzymes digest fascial layers, spreading the inflammatory process to multiple anatomic compartments. Causes of acute pancreatitis are listed in Table 28.1.

Imaging studies of acute pancreatitis may be normal in mild cases. Dynamic contrast-enhanced CT provides the most comprehensive initial assessment; however, US is useful for follow-up of specific abnormalities, such as fluid collections. Abnormalities that may be seen in the pancreas include 1) focal or diffuse enlargement, 2) changes in density due to edema (see Fig. 36.31), and 3) indistinctness of the margins of the gland due to inflammation. Abnormalities in the peripancreatic tissues include stranding densities in the fat with indistinctness of the fat planes and thickening of affected fascial planes. Complications demonstrated by imaging are listed in Table 28.2 (Figs. 28.3,28.4,28.5; see 28.20) (10,13–15). Barium studies may demonstrate mass effect or inflammatory changes affecting adjacent bowel. US-directed or CT-directed aspiration biopsy may be needed to confirm the presence of pancreatic abscess. Image-directed catheter placement is an alternative to surgical drainage of pancreatic fluid collections.

Chronic Pancreatitis

Chronic pancreatitis is caused by recurrent and prolonged bouts of acute pancreatitis that cause parenchymal atrophy and progressive fibrosis. Both the exocrine and endocrine function of the pancreas may be impaired. The clinical diagnosis is often vague, so imaging is used both to confirm the diagnosis and to detect com-

plications. The morphologic changes of chronic pancreatitis include 1) dilation of the pancreatic duct, usually in a beaded pattern of alternating areas of dilation and constriction (Fig. 28.6); 2) decrease in visible pancreatic tissue because of atrophy (Fig. 28.7); 3) calcifications in the pancreatic parenchyma that vary from finely stippled to coarse, usually associated with alcoholic pancreatitis (Fig. 28.8); 4) fluid collections that are both intrapancreatic and extrapancreatic; 5) focal enlargement of the pancreas owing to benign inflammation and fibrosis; 6) dilation of the biliary duct because of fibrosis or mass in the pancreatic head; and 7) fascial thickening and chronic inflammatory changes in surrounding tissues (16). Differentiation between an inflammatory mass resulting from chronic pancreatitis and that of pancreatic carcinoma frequently requires image-directed biopsy.

Pancreatic Carcinoma

Ductal adenocarcinoma of the pancreas is a highly lethal tumor that is usually unresectable at presentation. The average survival time of a patient with this disease is only 5–8 months. It accounts for 3% of all cancers and is second only to colorectal cancer as the most common digestive tract malignancy. Radiographic assessment of resectability is critical because surgical resection offers the only hope of cure, yet the surgery itself carries a high morbidity. Scanning by CT should include rapid bolus contrast injection and thin slices (at least 5 mm). Adenocarcinoma appears as a hypodense mass distorting the contour of the gland (17). Associated find-

Table 28.2. Complications of Acute Pancreatitis

Pancreatic fluid collections—collections of enzyme-rich pancreatic juice.
    Acute—resolve spontaneously in 50% of cases. May be intrapancreatic, anterior pararenal space, lesser sac, or extend anywhere in the abdomen, into solid organs, or even into the chest.
    Pseudocyst—round or oval, encapsulated pancreatic fluid collection by encased by a fibrous capsule; require at least 4 weeks to develop. About 50% will spontaneously resolve; the remainder require catheter or surgical drainage.
Liquefactive necrosis of pancreatic parenchyma—seen as lack of parenchymal enhancement during bolus contrast administration on CT, often multifocal.
Phlegmon—focal mass attributable to fat necrosis, extravasated pancreatic fluid, inflammation, and edema
Infected necrosis—bacterial infection in necrotic tissue. Seen as an area of nonenhancing pancreatic tissue containing gas. Confirmed with needle aspiration. Infected necrosis generally requires surgical drainage.
Abscess—circumscribed collection of pus in area with little or no necrosis tissues. Seen as a fluid collection with a thick wall. Effectively treated with catheter drainage.
Hemorrhage—resulting from erosion of blood vessels and tissue necrosis. CT shows high-attenuation blood in the retroperitoneum
Pancreatic ascites—leakage of pancreatic secretions into peritoneal cavity.
Pseudoaneurysm—autodigestion of arterial walls by pancreatic enzymes results in pulsatile mass that is lined by fibrous tissue and maintains communication with parent artery.

Figure 28.3. Acute Necrotizing Pancreatitis. A CT scan performed with rapid bolus administration of intravenous contrast demonstrates enhancement of only the distal body of the pancreas (*p*). The pancreatic head and neck did not enhance and are lost in the fluid (*f*) extending from the pancreatic bed. This CT finding is indicative of pancreatic necrosis. *st*, stomach; *L*, liver; *ivc*, inferior vena cava; *ao*, aorta; *k*, kidney.

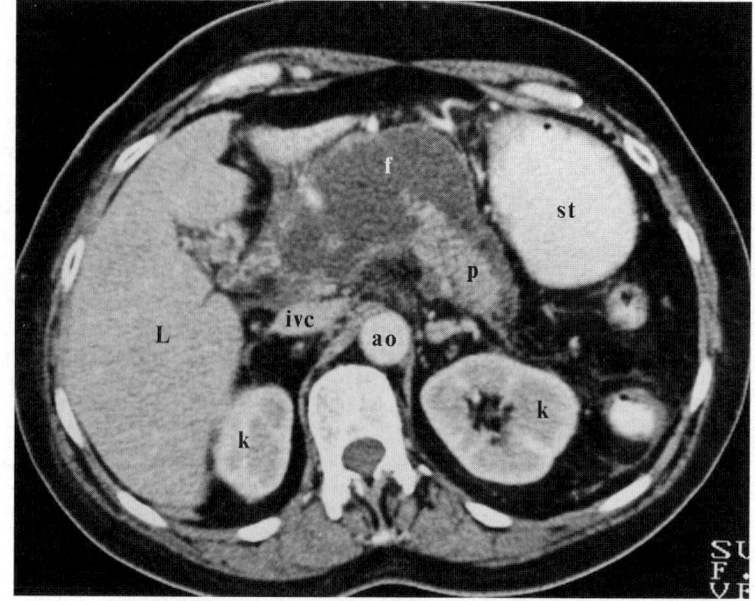

Figure 28.4. Pancreatic Abscess. Air (*A*) and fluid (*f*) extend from the bed of the pancreas (*p*) on this CT scan performed without intravenous contrast. Air in the pancreatic bed is indicative of abscess and/or fistulous communication with bowel. *st*, stomach; *l*, liver; *v*, inferior vena cava; *a*, aorta; *k*, kidney.

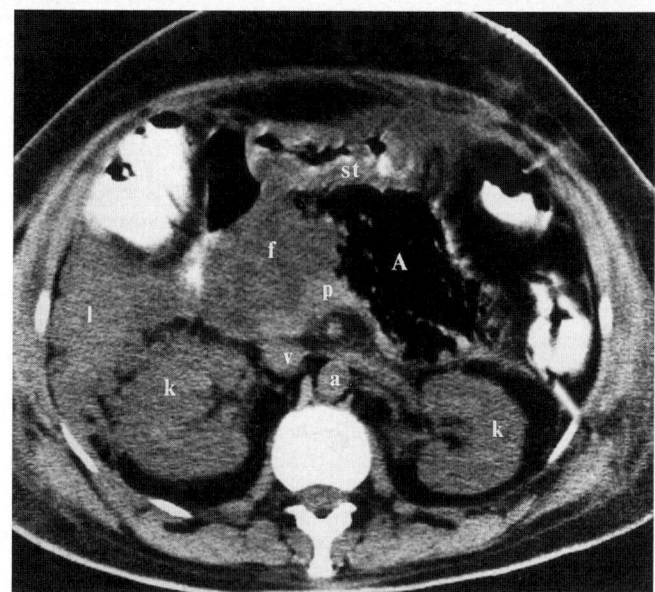

Figure 28.5. Pseudoaneurysm Caused by Acute Pancreatitis. Delayed CT image from a contrast-enhanced study shows central contrast enhancement (*arrow*) of a cystic lesion just inferior to the pancreas. Angiography subsequently confirmed a pseudoaneurysm arising from the splenic artery, caused by erosion of the artery by enzymes released by acute pancreatitis.

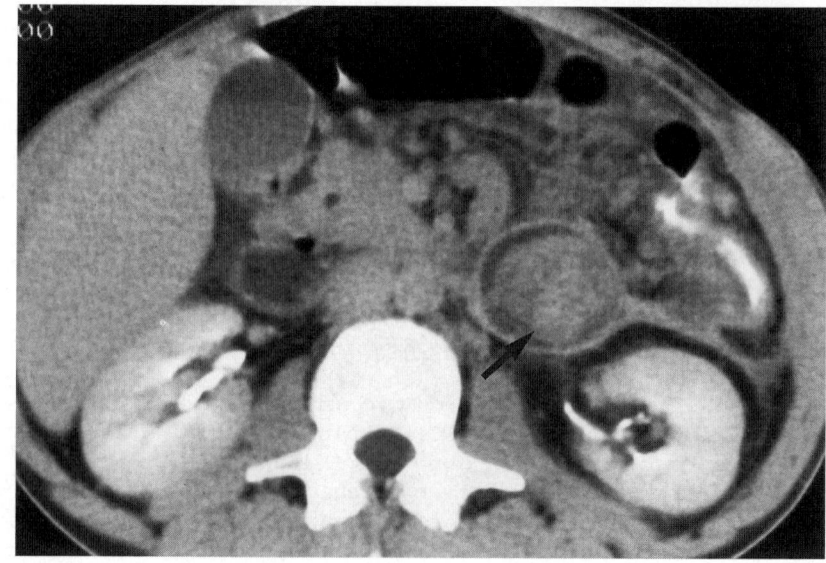

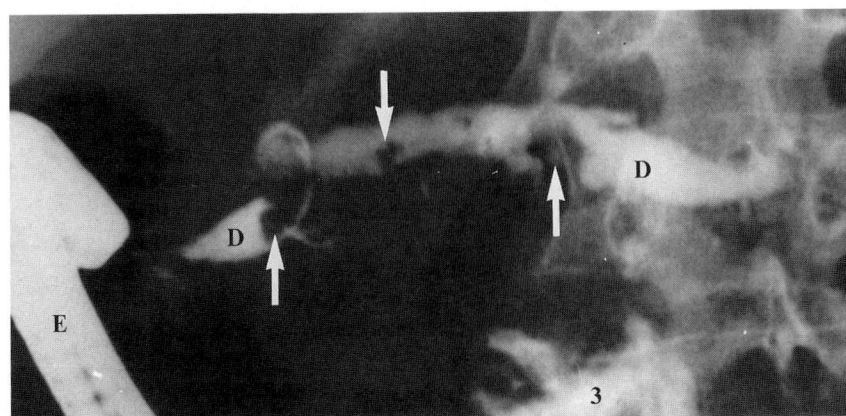

Figure 28.6. Chronic Pancreatitis. Radiograph from an ERCP after contrast injection into the pancreatic duct (*D*) demonstrates irregular dilation of the duct with multiple filling defects (*arrows*) as a result of stones and debris. Contrast is also present in the lumen of the third portion of the duodenum (3). *E*, endoscope.

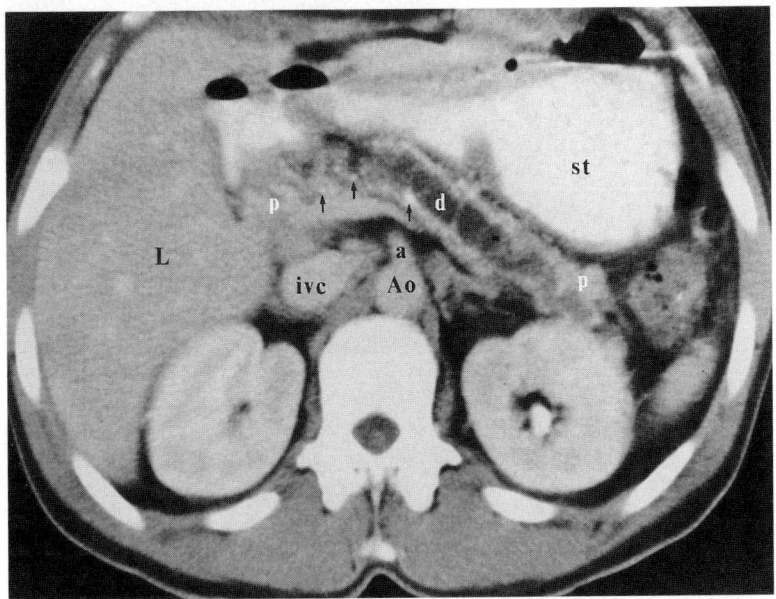

Figure 28.7. Chronic Pancreatitis. A CT scan with bolus intravenous contrast enhancement demonstrates marked dilation of the pancreatic duct (*d*) and atrophy of the pancreatic parenchyma (*p*). Punctate calcifications are also present (*arrows*). The aorta (*ao*) is seen at the origin of the superior mesenteric artery (*a*). *L*, liver; *st*, stomach; *ivc*, inferior vena cava.

ings include obstruction of the common bile duct (Fig. 28.9) and pancreatic duct and atrophy of pancreatic tissue beyond the tumor. Metastases commonly go to regional nodes, liver, and the peritoneal cavity. Signs of potential resectability include isolated pancreatic mass with or without dilation of the bile or pancreatic ducts (Fig. 28.10) or combined dilation of both the bile and pancreatic ducts without an identifiable pancreatic head mass. Signs of unresectability include the following: 1) extension of the tumor beyond the margins of the pancreas (Fig. 28.11), 2) tumor involvement of adjacent organs, 3) enlarged regional lymph nodes (>15 mm), 4) encasement or obstruction of peripancreatic arteries or veins (Fig. 28.12), 5) metastases in the liver, and 6) peritoneal carcinomatosis (3,17,18). Only 10–15% of patients have tumors that are potentially resectable using these criteria. Image-guided biopsy can confirm the diagnosis in patients whose tumors are deemed to be unresectable (Fig. 28.13). Tumor recurrence following the Whipple procedure is best detected with helical CT (19).

Islet Cell Tumors

Functioning islet cell tumors produce distinct clinical syndromes and usually present while the tumors are

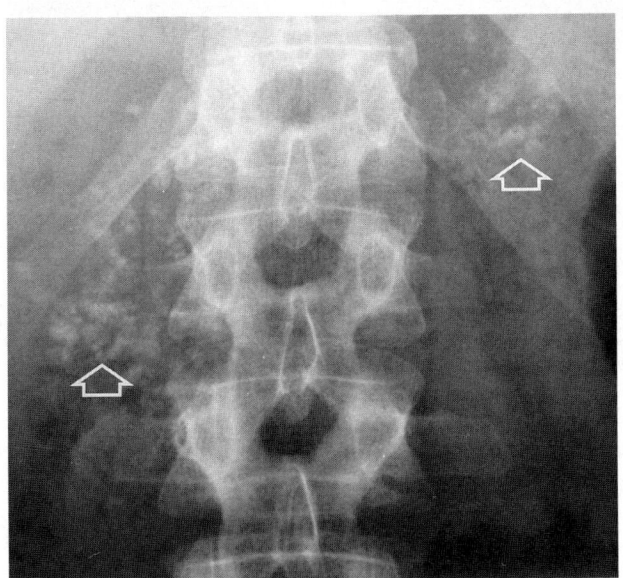

Figure 28.8. Pancreatic Calcifications. Plain radiograph of the upper abdomen demonstrates multiple calcifications (*arrows*) throughout the region of the pancreatic bed. Pancreatic calcifications of this type suggest chronic pancreatitis caused by alchol abuse or hereditary pancreatitis.

Figure 28.9. Pancreatic Carcinoma. Radiograph from an ERCP demonstrates a characteristic "rat-tail" appearance (*arrow*) of the dilated common bile duct (*CBD*) at the head of the pancreas due to pancreatic carcinoma. *E,* endoscope.

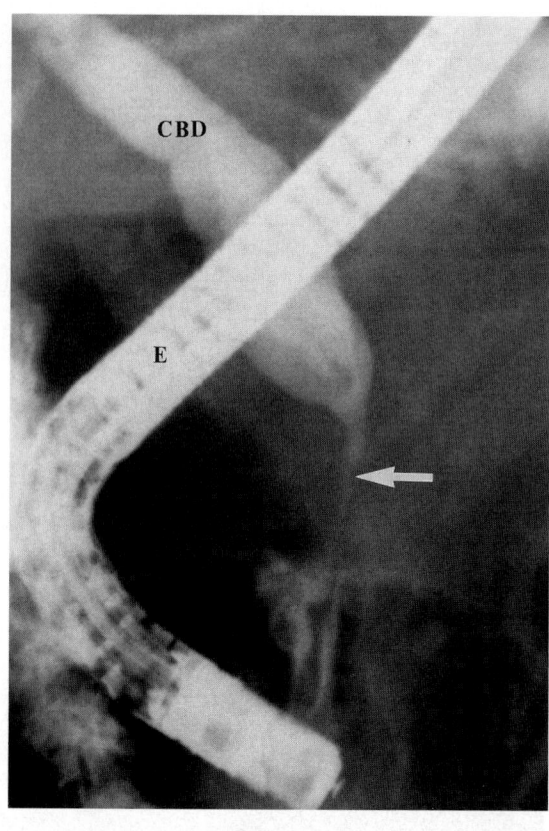

Figure 28.10. Potentially Resectable Pancreatic Carcinoma. CT demonstrates a small mass (*arrow*) in the neck of the pancreas that causes dilation of the pancreatic duct (*arrowhead*) and atrophy of the pancreatic body and tail. No metastases were seen in the liver, and regional lymph nodes were not enlarged. The patient underwent a successful Whipple procedure.

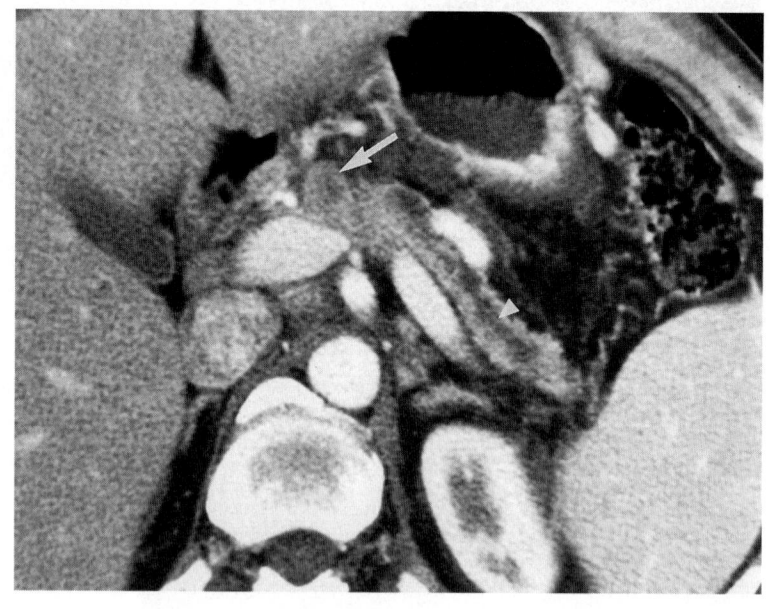

small (20). Insulinomas present with hypoglycemia, and gastrinomas present with peptic ulcers, diarrhea caused by gastric hypersecretion, or Zollinger-Ellison syndrome. Other islet cell tumors include glucagonoma (diabetes mellitus and painful glossitis), somatostatinoma (diabetes and steatorrhea), and vipoma (massive watery diarrhea). Nonfunctioning islet cell tumors are clinically silent until they present with symptoms of a growing, usually large, mass. Functioning tumors vary in malignant potential from 10% for insulinoma to 60% for gas-

trinoma and to 80% for glucagonoma. Up to 80% of nonfunctioning tumors are malignant.

Functioning islet cell tumors vary in size from 0.4 to 4.0 cm and require strict attention to technique for accurate preoperative identification. Most small islet cell tumors cannot be identified on precontrast CT. Because the lesions tend to be hypervascular, bolus contrast administration during rapid, thin-slice, helical CT scanning through the pancreatic bed offers the best chance of lesion visualization (21). The tumor stands out as an

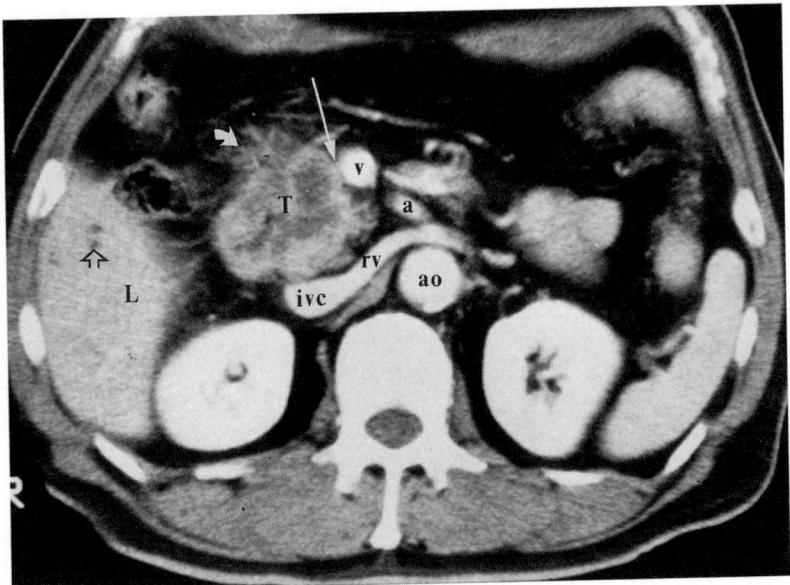

Figure 28.11. Unresectable Pancreatic Carcinoma. A CT with bolus intravenous contrast demonstrates an inhomogeneous necrotic tumor (*T*) in the head of the pancreas. The margins of the tumor are ill-defined (*curved arrow*), indicating invasion of peripancreatic tissues. The tumor extends (*long arrow*) to the superior mesenteric vein (*v*) but spares the superior mesenteric artery (*a*). Bile ducts (*open arrow*) in the liver (*L*) were dilated because of distal obstruction. *ivc*, inferior vena cava; *rv*, left renal vein; *ao*, aorta.

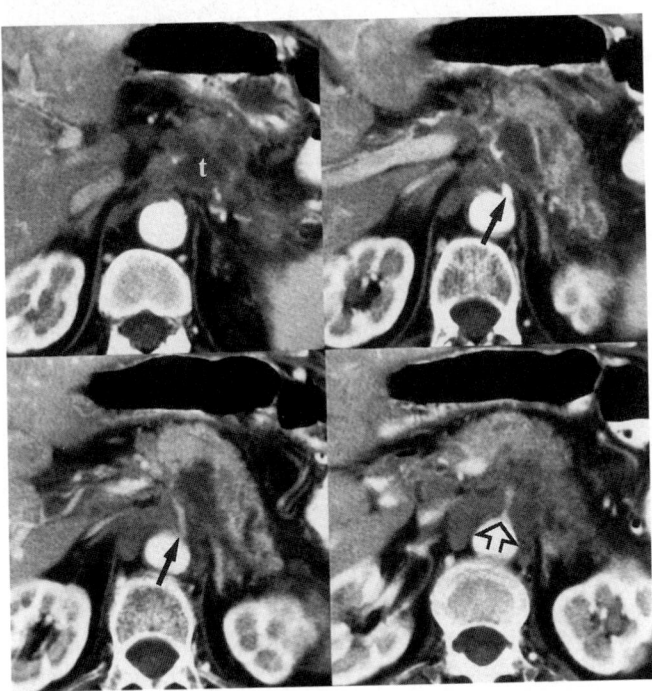

Figure 28.12. Unresectable Pancreatic Carcinoma. Four CT images demonstrate tumor encasement of the celiac axis (*closed arrows*) and superior mesenteric artery (*open arrow*). The periarterial fat is infiltrated and replaced with the soft tissue density of the tumor (*t*).

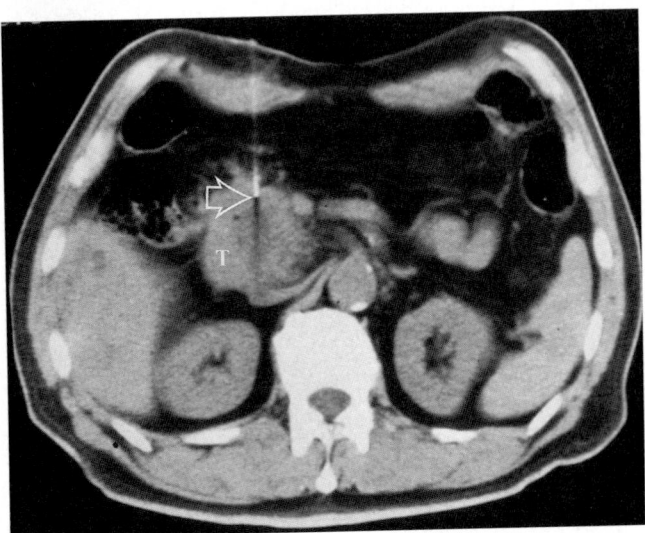

Figure 28.13. Percutaneous Pancreatic Biopsy. A CT is used to guide percutaneous biopsy of a pancreatic head tumor (*T*). A vertical needle course is selected to bring the needle tip (*arrow*) into the lesion. The *black streak* emanating from the needle indicates that the needle tip, not the needle shaft, is visualized. The biopsy confirmed pancreatic carcinoma.

Cystic Lesions

Pseudocysts resulting from pancreatitis are the most common pancreatic cystic lesions (22). They are of fluid density and have a definable fibrous wall that may be calcified. Internal septations and multiple loculations are common.

Abscess must be considered in any patient with a cystic pancreatic lesion and a fever. Most abscesses have indistinct walls and contain fluid and debris. The presence of gas bubbles within the cystic mass is good evidence for abscess. Image-directed aspiration confirms the diagnosis and may be followed by percutaneous catheter placement for treatment.

enhancing nodule within the pancreas. Sonography has proved extremely valuable for tumor localization during surgery. Islet cell tumors appear as hypoechoic masses within the pancreas. Octreotide is a somatostatin analogue that is used for scintographic detection of islet cell tumors.

Nonfunctioning islet cell tumors tend to be much larger, 6–20 cm diameter. Imaging findings include coarse calcifications, cystic degeneration, necrosis, local and vascular invasion, and metastases (Fig. 28.14) (20).

Figure 28.14. Nonfunctioning Malignant Islet Cell Tumor. The tumor (*t*) arising from the tail of the pancreas invaded the splenic artery and vein, causing a splenic infarction (*I*). Mass effect compresses and distorts the left kidney.

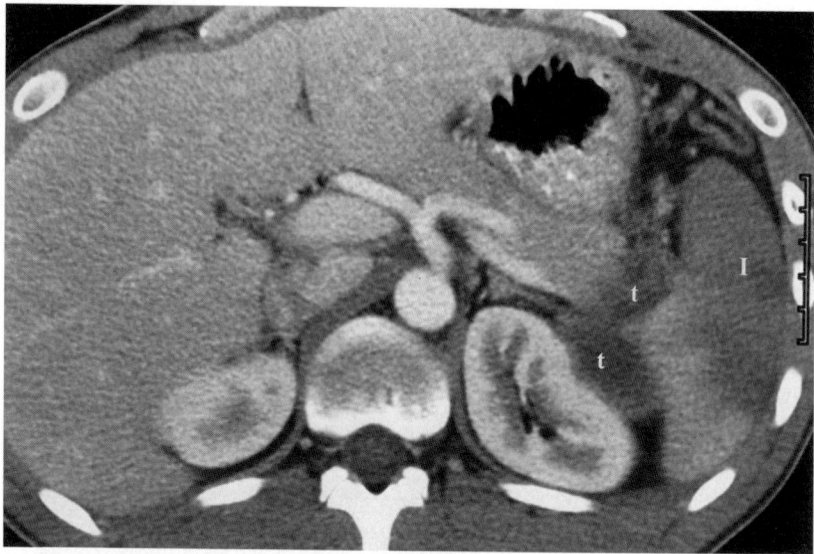

Figure 28.15. Mucinous Cystadenocarcinoma of the Pancreas. A CT demonstrates a multiloculated cystic tumor (*T, between arrows*) arising from the pancreas (*p*). No metastases in the liver (*L*) were evident. *v,* superior mesenteric vein; *a,* superior mesenteric artery; *ivc,* inferior vena cava; *ao,* aorta; *S,* spleen.

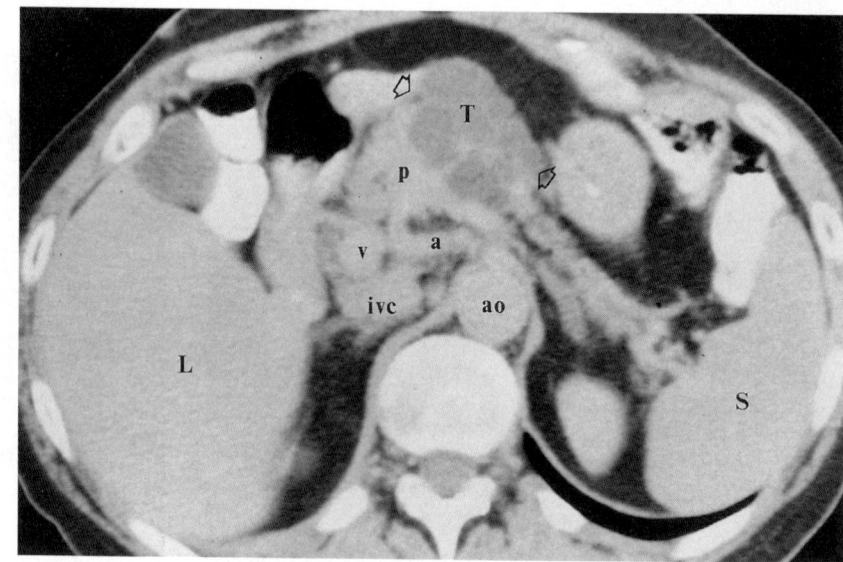

True Pancreatic Cysts, with epithelial lining, are found in 10% of patients with autosomal dominant polycystic disease, 30% of patients with von Hippel-Lindau syndrome, and some patients with cystic fibrosis. They appear as well-defined fluid-filled masses with walls of variable thickness. Patients with von Hippel-Lindau syndrome are prone to islet cell tumors and microcystic adenomas, in addition to multiple pancreatic cysts (23).

Cystic Tumors of the pancreas are uncommon (5–15% of pancreatic cysts). Islet cell tumors may appear cystic because of extensive necrosis. Cystic teratomas rarely arise in the pancreas and usually have characteristic hair, fat, calcifications, and cystic and solid components.

Microcystic Adenoma is a benign pancreatic tumor composed of innumerable small cysts 1 mm to 2 cm in size (24). The lining epithelial cells are rich in glycogen, resulting in the alternate name of glycogen-rich cystadenoma. The cysts may be so small that the tumor appears as a solid lesion on imaging studies. A characteristic feature is a central stellate fibrous scar that may be calcified. Approximately 80% of patients with this disease are aged 60 or older. This tumor also occurs in patients with von Hippel-Lindau syndrome. Base CT shows a well-defined mass with low attenuation near water density. Contrast enhancement is usually marked with demonstration of multiple internal septations in a honeycomb appearance. US commonly shows an echogenic mass with only a few of the larger cysts visible. Biopsy confirming the diagnosis will commonly allow surgery to be avoided.

Mucinous Cystic Tumors are all potentially malignant and require complete excision (25,26). The tumors produce large amounts of mucin and are predominantly cystic, with walls 1 to 2 mm thick with papillary projections of solid tissue. Large cysts are up to 5 cm in size. They are most commonly multilocular, but the occasional unilocular cyst will mimic a pancreatic pseudocyst (Fig. 28.15). Because of the high mucin production, branch or the main pancreatic ducts are commonly dilated. The tumors are hypovascular and enhance poorly. Thin section CT is needed to demonstrate the septations and dilation of small pancreatic ducts. Metastases to the liver tend to be cystic.

Pancreatic Trauma

The spectrum of traumatic pancreatic injuries includes pancreatitis, laceration, and transection. Pancreatic injuries are best documented by contrast-enhanced CT. Pancreatic lacerations appear as irregular lucent clefts in the pancreatic parenchyma, most commonly at the junction of the body and tail just to the left of midline (Fig. 28.16). Complete transection is rare.

SPLEEN

Imaging Techniques

CT and US remain the major techniques used to image the splenic parenchyma (27–34). Technetium sulfur colloid radionuclide scanning images both the liver and the spleen and can be used to confirm the presence of functioning splenic tissue. MR is somewhat disappointing in its ability to demonstrate splenic abnormalities because the signal intensity of the splenic parenchyma tends to parallel the signal intensity of pathologic lesions and shows insufficient contrast differentiation to identify the lesions (35). With the use of gadolinium enhancement, MR imaging of the spleen is improved (36,37).

Anatomy

The spleen is the body's largest lymphoid organ. Although it serves as a site of blood formation in the fetus, there is no hematopoetic activity in the normal adult spleen. The spleen sequesters abnormal and aged red and white blood cells and platelets and serves as a reservoir for red blood cells. The spleen occupies the left upper quadrant of the abdomen just below the diaphragm,

posterior and lateral to the stomach. Its diaphragmatic surface is smooth and convex, conforming to the shape of the diaphragm, whereas its visceral surface has concavities for the stomach, kidney, colon, and pancreas. Spleen size varies with age, nutrition, and hydration. The spleen is relatively large in children, reaching adult size by age 15. The average spleen dimensions in adults are 12 cm in length, 7 cm in width, and 3–4 cm in thickness. In older adults, the spleen progressively decreases in size with age. The splenic artery and vein course through the pancreas to the splenic hilum, where they divide into multiple branches. Splenic arteries are end arteries without anastomoses or collateral supply. Occlusion of the splenic artery or its branches produces infarction.

On all imaging studies, the spleen has a homogeneous appearance. On both CT and MR, lesions are best demonstrated on contrast-enhanced images. On CT, the normal spleen density is less than or equal to the density of normal liver on both noncontrast and contrast-enhanced images. On MR the spleen signal intensity is lower than hepatic parenchyma on T1WI images and higher than liver parenchyma on T2WI. US demonstrates a mid-level even echo pattern for the splenic parenchyma.

Transient pseudomasses are formed during rapid intravenous bolus administration of both CT and MR contrast agents due to variable rates of blood flow through the splenic parenchyma (36,38). Images taken during the arterial phase demonstrate irregular defects in parenchymal enhancement. One or two minutes later, the entire spleen is homogeneously enhanced on both CT and MR. Diffuse liver disease is associated with more prominent splenic pseudomasses during early enhancement.

Lobulations and clefts in the splenic contour are common and must not be mistaken for masses or splenic fractures.

Accessory spleens are found in approximately 10% of normal individuals. These appear as round masses, 1–3

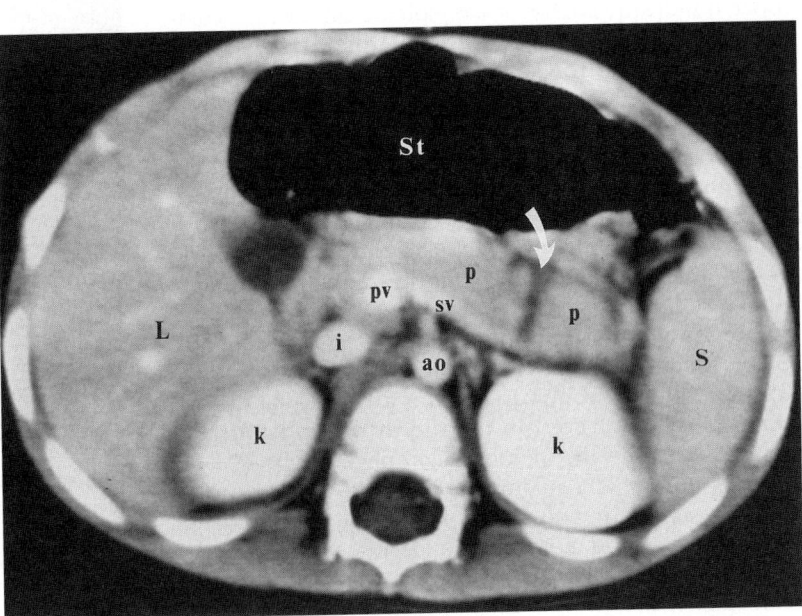

Figure 28.16. Transected Pancreas. Contrast-enhanced CT scan in a 2-year-old boy struck by an automobile demonstrates a lucent fissure (*arrow*) in the pancreas (*p*), indicating disruption of the parenchyma. The portal vein (*pv*) and splenic vein (*sv*) enhance normally. Surgery confirmed complete transection of the pancreas with an intact splenic vein and artery. *L*, liver; *S*, spleen; *St*, stomach; *i*, inferior vena cava; *ao*, aorta; *k*, kidney.

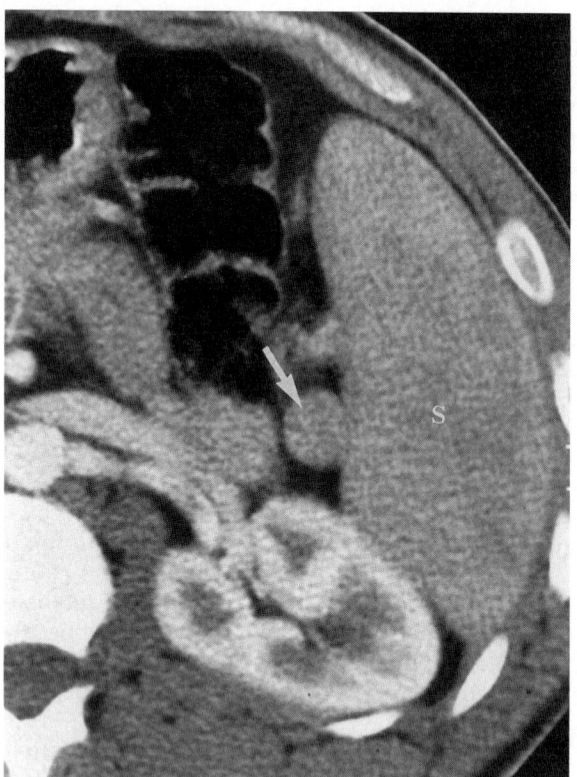

Figure 28.17. Accessory Spleen. An accessory spleen (*arrow*) is seen in the splenic hilum. Accessory spleens have the same imaging characteristics as the parent spleen (*S*).

cm in size, and of the same texture as normal splenic parenchyma (Fig 28.17) (28). They may be single or multiple and are usually located in the splenic hilum. Technetium sulfur colloid radionuclide scans can be used to confirm suspected accessory spleens as functioning splenic tissue.

Wandering Spleen is the term applied to a normal spleen positioned out of its normal location in the left upper quadrant. Laxity of the splenic ligaments, commonly found in association with abnormalities of intestinal rotation, allow the spleen to be positioned anywhere in the abdominal cavity (28). A wandering spleen may present as a palpable abdominal mass, although most cause no symptoms. The diagnosis is made by recognizing the normal shape and tissue texture of the spleen and the absence of normal spleen in the left upper abdomen and by identifying the blood supply from splenic vessels. Radionuclide scans confirm functioning splenic tissue.

Splenosis refers to multiple implants of ectopic splenic tissue that may occur after traumatic splenic rupture. Splenic tissue can implant anywhere in the abdominal cavity, or even in the thorax if the diaphragm has been ruptured. Splenosis complicates 40–60% of splenic injuries. The splenic implants are usually multiple and vary in size and shape. The tissue fragments enlarge over time and may simulate peritoneal metastases. Functioning splenic tissue is confirmed by radionuclide scanning.

Splenic Regeneration. After splenectomy, remaining accessory spleens, or splenules resulting from traumatic peritoneal seeding of splenic tissue may enlarge and resume the function of the resected spleen. When the spleen is removed, bits of nuclear material, called Howell-Jolly bodies, are routinely seen in red cells on peripheral blood smears. Disappearance of these Howell-Jolly bodies from peripheral blood is a clinical sign of splenic regeneration. Imaging studies demonstrate single or multiple spleenlike masses in the abdominal cavity in patients with a history of splenectomy.

Polysplenia is a rare congenital anomaly that features multiple small spleens, usually located in the right abdomen and associated with situs ambiguous (30). Both lungs are two-lobed. Most patients also have cardiovascular anomalies.

Asplenia (Ivemark's syndrome) is the congenital absence of the spleen, found in association with bilateral right-sidedness, midline liver, and bilateral three-lobed lungs (30). Major cardiac anomalies are present in 50% of cases. Most patients die before 1 year of age.

Splenomegaly

The diagnosis of splenic enlargement on imaging studies is usually made subjectively (Fig. 28.18). Although quantitative methods have been attempted, none have proved popular. Findings that suggest splenomegaly are any spleen dimension greater than 14 cm, projection of the spleen ventral to the anterior axillary line, inferior spleen tip extending more caudally than the inferior liver tip, or inferior spleen tip extending below the lower pole of the left kidney. Enlarged spleens frequently compress and displace adjacent organs, especially the left kidney.

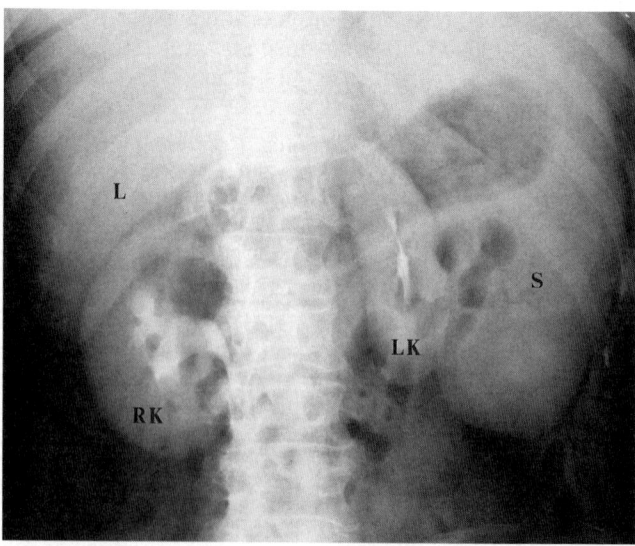

Figure 28.18. Splenomegaly. Radiograph from an excretory urogram demonstrates a massively enlarged spleen (*S*) in a patient with rheumatoid arthritis and Felty's syndrome. The left kidney (*LK*) is compressed and rotated by the large spleen. The inferior margin of the spleen extends well below the inferior margin of the liver (*L*). *RK*, right kidney.

Table 28.3. Causes of Splenomegaly

Congestive
Portal hypertension (50% of cases)
Portal vein thrombosis
Myeloproliferative disorders
Leukemia
Lymphoma (30% of cases)
Polycythemia vera
Idiopathic thrombocytopenia purpura
Sickle cell disease (in infants)
Thalasemia major
Hereditary spherocytosis
Myelofibrosis
Infection
Malaria (universal in endemic areas)
Schistosomiasis (endemic areas)
Infectious mononucleosis
Subacute bacterial endocarditis
AIDS
Intravenous drug abuse
Infiltrative
Systemic lupus erythematosus
Amyloidosis
Gaucher's disease

The causes of splenomegaly are exhaustive (Table 28.3). Most do not produce a change in spleen density, so differentiation is based upon associated imaging findings or on clinical evaluation (33). MR offers no significant benefit to the differential diagnosis of splenomegaly (35). Mild to moderate splenomegaly is seen with portal hypertension, AIDS, storage diseases, collagen vascular disorders, and infection. More marked splenomegaly is usually associated with lymphoma, leukemia, infectious mononucleosis, hemolytic anemia, and myelofibrosis.

Cystic Lesions

Posttraumatic Cysts are false cysts that lack an epithelial lining. They generally have thick walls and septations that commonly become calcified (30–40%) (Fig. 28.19) (34,39). The internal fluid may be complex owing to blood products, cholesterol crystals, or cellular debris. Posttraumatic cysts result from previous hemorrhage, infarction, or infection. They account for 80% of all splenic cysts.

Epidermoid Cysts are true epithelial-lined cysts that are probably developmental in origin. They have the same appearance as posttraumatic cysts but less frequently have calcification in their walls (5%).

Pancreatic Pseudocysts extend beneath the splenic capsule by tracking along the pancreatic tail to the splenic hilum (Fig. 28.20) (15). Splenic subcapsular pancreatic fluid collections develop in 1–5% of patients with pancreatitis. Internal debris and hemorrhage are commonly present. Imaging studies demonstrate associated findings of pancreatitis.

Bacterial Abscesses occur most commonly in spleens that are already diseased. They present with vague symptoms but have a high mortality when left untreated. They result from hematogenous spread of

infection (75%), trauma (15%), or infarction (10%). Abscesses appear as single or multiple low-density masses with ill-defined thick walls (30,34). US commonly demonstrates internal echoes resulting from inflammatory debris (see Fig. 36.27). Abscesses are low intensity on T1WI and high intensity on T2WI (35). They may contain gas or demonstrate air-fluid levels. Perisplenic fluid collections and left pleural effusions are common. Image-guided aspiration confirms the diagnosis. Treatment is by catheter drainage or splenectomy (40).

Microabscesses are found in patients with compromised immune systems attributable to AIDS, organ transplantation, lymphoma, or leukemia. The causes of microabscesses include fungi, tuberculosis, *Pneumocystis carinii*, histoplasmosis, and cytomegalovirus. Imaging studies demonstrate multiple small defects in the spleen, usually 5 to 10 mm, up to 20 mm, in size (Fig. 28.21) (32,41). The differential diagnosis of multiple small low density splenic defects is listed in Table 28.4.

Hydatid Cysts in the spleen are found in only 2% of patients with hydatid disease. Hydatid cysts are usually also present in the liver or lung. The lesions consist of spherical mother cysts that contain smaller daughter cysts and have internal septations and debris representing hydatid sand (42). Ringlike calcifications in the wall are usually prominent in the chronic stage.

Solid Lesions

Lymphoma is the most common malignant tumor involving the spleen. Commonly, the spleen involved with lymphoma, particularly Hodgkin's lymphoma, appears normal on all imaging studies. CT is only 65% sensitive in demonstrating splenic involvement with lymphoma (32). Patterns of involvement visible on imaging studies include diffuse splenomegaly, multiple masses of varying

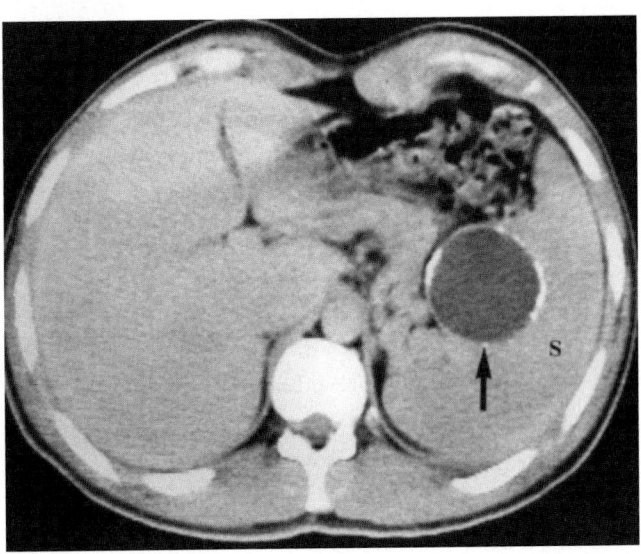

Figure 28.19. Posttraumatic Splenic Cyst. The well-defined cyst with calcified walls *(arrow)*, in the hilum of the spleen *(S)*, is the result of an old intrasplenic hemorrhage.

Figure 28.20. Pancreatic Pseudocysts in Spleen and Liver. Pancreatic fluid owing to acute pancreatitis tracts along blood vessels and fascial planes to form fluid collections (*arrows*) in the spleen (*S*), liver (*L*), and lesser sac (*LS*).

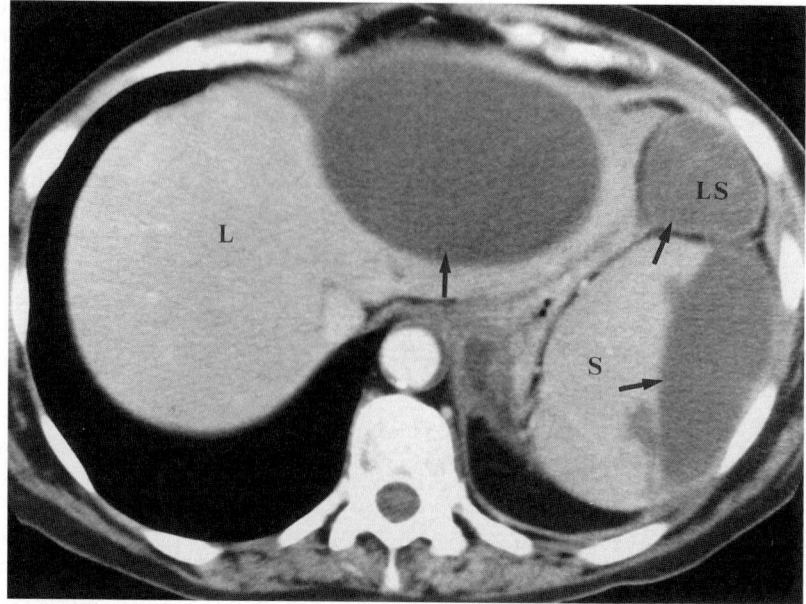

Figure 28.21. Microabscesses in the Spleen. Multiple lucent defects of varying size in the spleen (*S*) of this patient with AIDS are attributable to *Pneumocystis carnii* infection.

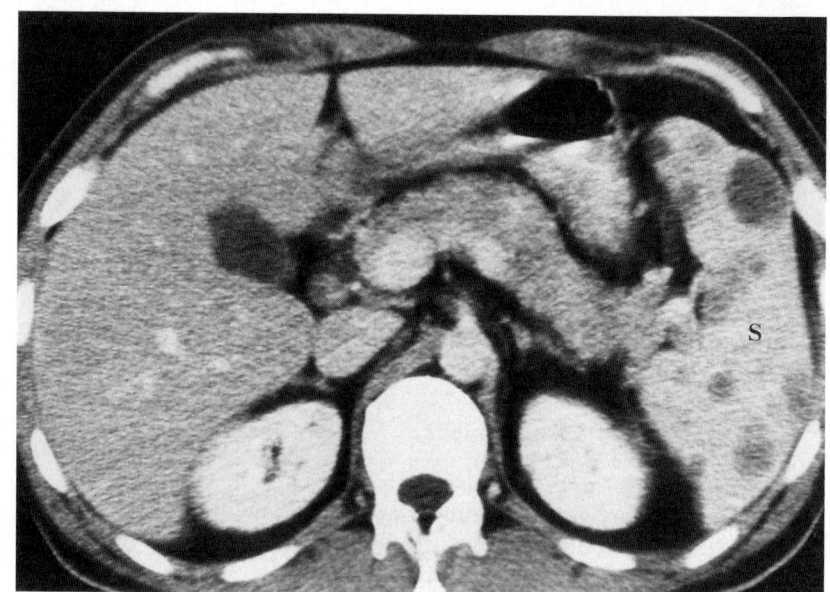

Table 28.4. Causes of Multiple Small (10 mm) Lesions in the Spleen

Microabcesses (immunocompromised patient)
Multiple bacterial abscesses
Histoplasmosis
Lymphoma
Kaposi sarcoma (AIDS patient)
Sarcoidosis
Gamna-Gandy bodies (portal hypertension)
Metastases
    Breast carcinoma
    Lung carcinoma
    Ovarian carcinoma
    Gastric carcinoma
    Malignant melanoma
    Prostate carcinoma

size, miliary nodules resembling microabscesses (Fig. 28.22), large solitary mass, and direct invasion from adjacent lymphomatous nodes. Adenopathy is frequently evident elsewhere in the abdomen when the spleen is involved with lymphoma. Lymphoma is a common predisposing condition for splenic infarction.

Metastases are found in the spleen on autopsy series in up to 7% of patients who die of cancer. Most splenic metastases are microscopic and are not detected by imaging studies. The most common tumors to metastasize to the spleen are malignant melanoma and lung, breast, ovary, prostate, and stomach carcinoma. Metastases appear as single or multiple low-density masses. On MR, metastases are low intensity on T1WI and high intensity on T2WI. The increased signal intensity of the lesions parallel the increased signal intensity

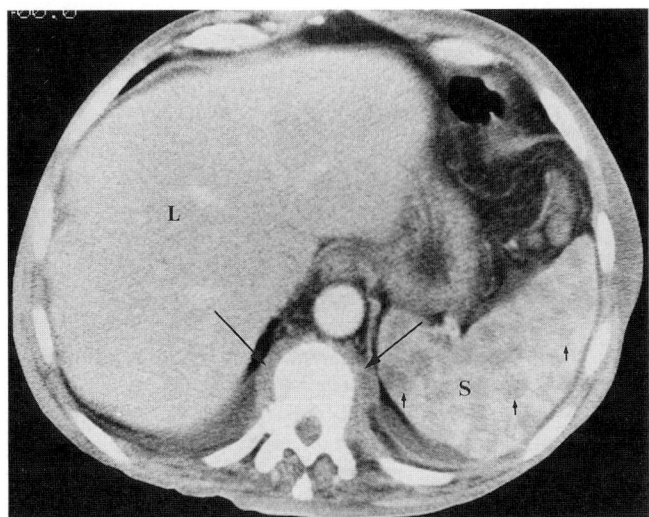

Figure 28.22. Lymphoma. Contrast-enhanced CT demonstrates inhomogeneous splenic parenchyma (*S*) with multiple focal masses (*small arrows*) of varying size. Confluent retrocrural adenopathy (*long arrows*) is also present. The liver (*L*) appears normal.

of the normal splenic parenchyma on T2WI, and the lesions may not be evident (35). Contrast enhancement is recommended for both CT and MR demonstration of metastases. Calcification is rare. Melanoma metastases commonly appear cystic.

Infarction is produced by occlusion of the main or branch splenic arteries. Causes of infarction include emboli (owing to endocarditis, atherosclerotic plaques, or cardiac valve thrombi), sickle cell disease, pancreatitis, pancreatic tumors, and arteritis. Additional predisposing conditions include myeloproliferative disorders, hemolytic anemias, and sepsis. Infarcts classically appear as wedge-shaped defects in the splenic parenchyma (Figs. 28.14,28.23). Multiple infarcts may fuse, however, and the wedge shape may be lost. The key finding is extension of a low-density area to an intact splenic capsule. Splenomegaly, especially due to lymphoma, is a predisposing condition. Complications of splenic infarctions include subcapsular hematomas, infection, and splenic rupture with hemoperitoneum (43).

Gamna-Gandy Bodies (also called siderotic nodules) are small hemorrhages in the spleen caused by portal hypertension. They are seen best on MR as multiple small low-intensity nodules on T1WI-weighted and T2*-weighted images. Signal intensity is low because of hemosiderin content (34). They do not enhance.

Hemangioma is the most common primary neoplasm of the spleen, found in 14% of patients on autopsy series. The tumor consists of vascular channels of varying size lined by a single layer of endothelium. Imaging studies demonstrate an appearance similar to hemangiomas in the liver. US shows a well-defined hyperechoic mass. On CT the lession may appear solid and may have central punctate or peripheral curvilinear calcification (29). On MR the lesion is low in signal intensity on T1WI and high in signal intensity on T2WI (44). The contrast enhancement pattern described for liver hemangiomas is seldom seen with splenic hemangiomas.

Angiosarcoma is a very rare malignancy arising in the spleen. The tumor is aggressive, usually presenting with widespread metastases, especially to the liver. Imaging studies demonstrate multiple well-defined enhancing nodules or diffuse spleen abnormality (30,32). Patients with thorotrast exposure are at increased risk.

AIDS

Splenomegaly associated with generalized lymphoid hyperplasia is the most common finding in patients with AIDS. Focal lesions in the spleen are usually caused by opportunistic infections such as pneumocytes, atypical mycobacterium, or Candida *Pneumocystis carinii*, atypical mycobacterium, or *Candida*. *Pneumocystis carinii* infection may cause multiple splenic calcifications (Table 28.5). AIDS-associated lymphoma and Kaposi sarcoma may also cause single or multiple solid-appearing lesions in the spleen.

Splenic Trauma

The spleen is the most commonly injured intra-abdominal organ following blunt trauma (39). Contrast-enhanced CT is the modality of choice to demonstrate the presence and extent of splenic injury.

Splenic lacerations are seen as irregular linear clefts through the splenic parenchyma (Fig. 28.24). Because the splenic capsule is disrupted, a perisplenic blood clot

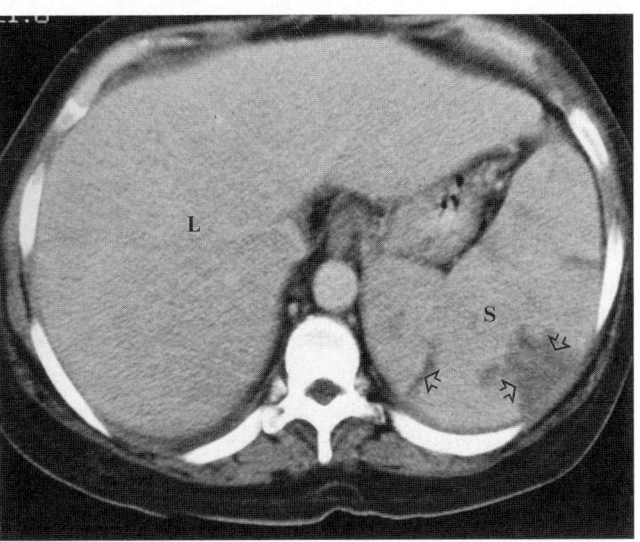

Figure 28.23. Splenic Infarction. A CT scan demonstrates wedge-shaped and linear areas of infarction (*arrows*) in the spleen (*S*) in this patient with splenomegaly of an unknown cause. Note that the infarctions extend to the splenic capsule. The liver (*L*) has a normal appearance.

Table 28.5. Causes of Multiple Splenic Calcifications

Histoplasmosis
Tuberculosis
Healed *Pneumocystis carinii* (AIDS patient)
Phleboliths
Hemangiomas

Figure 28.24. Multiple Splenic Lacerations. CT scan of a patient injured in an automobile accident reveals low-density jagged defects (*open arrow*) extending through the spleen (*S*), indicating multiple lacerations. A band of low density between liver and diaphragm (*closed arrow*) is evidence of hemoperitoneum.

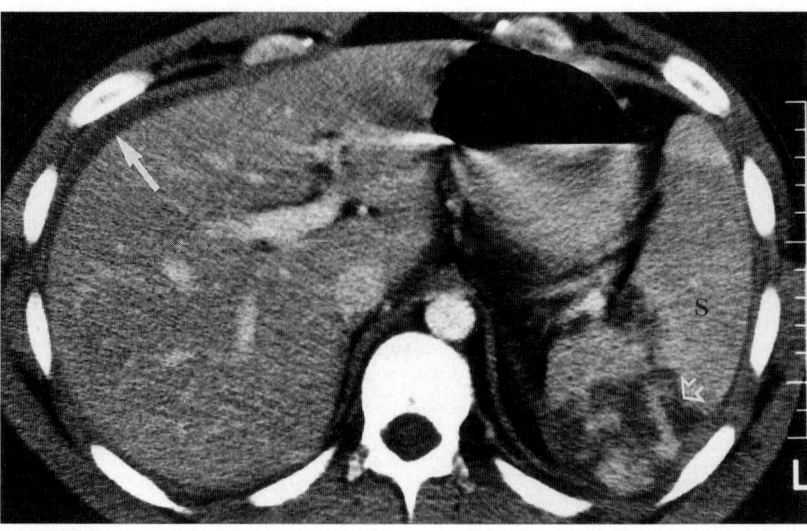

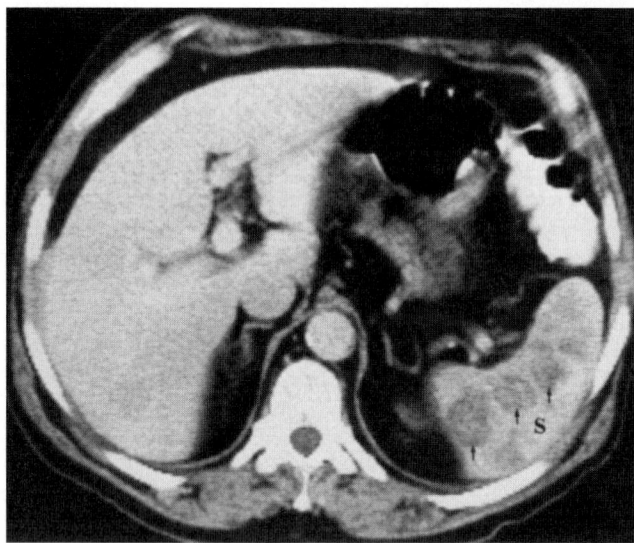

Figure 28.25. Intrasplenic Hematomas. A CT scan demonstrates multiple low-density foci (*arrows*) in the spleen (*S*), representing intrasplenic hematomas in this patient with blunt trauma to the left flank.

and intra-abdominal free blood are usually present. A shattered spleen describes multiple lacerations with disconnected portions of the splenic parenchyma.

Subcapsular hematoma produces a peripheral low-density lenticular shaped mass that flattens and displaces the splenic parenchyma inward and may bow the capsule outward. The splenic capsule may be thickened. The CT density and echogenicity of the hematoma changes with time.

Intrasplenic hematomas appear as irregular low-density areas within the parenchyma (Fig. 28.25). Hematomas may take up to 1 year to resolve. Some result in fibrous scars, calcifications, or posttraumatic splenic cysts.

References

1. Brant WE. Pancreas. In: Webb WR, Brant WE, Helms CA, eds. Fundamentals of Body CT. 2nd ed. Philadelphia: WB Saunders Co, 1998:223–233.

2. Fishman EK, Wyatt SH, Ney DR, et al. Spiral CT of the pancreas with multiplanar display. AJR Am J Roentgenol 1992;159:1209–1215.

3. Raptopoulos V, Steer ML, Sheiman RG, et al. The use of helical CT and CT angiography to predict vascular involvement from pancreatic cancer: correlation with findings at surgery. AJR Am J Roentgenol 1997;168:971–977.

4. Mergo PJ, Helmberger TK, Buetow PC, et al. Pancreatic neoplasms: MR imaging and pathologic correlation. Radiographics 1997;17:281–301.

5. Gulliver DJ, Cotton PB, Baillie J. Anatomic variants and artifacts in ERCP interpretation. AJR Am J Roentgenol 1991;156:975–980.

6. Slater GJ, Schapiro RH, O'Neill MJ, et al. Endoscopic retrograde pancreatography: imaging findings. AJR Am J Roentgenol 1995;165:1181–1186.

7. Reuther G, Kiefer B, Tuchmann A, et al. Imaging findings of pancreaticobiliary duct diseases with single-shot MR cholangiopancreatography. AJR Am J Roentgenol 1997;168:453–459.

8. Soto JA, Barish MA, Yucel EK, et al. MR cholangiopancreatography: findings on 3D fast spin-echo imaging. AJR Am J Roentgenol 1995;165:1397–1401.

9. Brandt KR, Charboneau JW, Stephens DH, et al. CT- and US-guided biopsy of the pancreas. Radiology 1993;187:99–104.

10. Balthazar EJ, Freeny PC, vanSonnenberg E. Imaging and intervention in acute pancreatitis. Radiology 1994;193:297–306.

11. Mitchell DG. MR imaging of the pancreas. Magn Reson Imaging Clin North Am 1995;3:51–71.

12. Mitchell DG, Shapiro M, Schuricht A, et al. Pancreatic disease: findings on state-of-the-art MR images. AJR Am J Roentgenol 1992;159:533–538.

13. Balthazar EJ, Robinson DL, Megibow AJ, et al. Acute pancreatitis: value of CT in establishing prognosis. Radiology 1990;174:331–336.

14. Johnson CD. CT of acute pancreatitis: correlation between lack of contrast enhancement and pancreatic necrosis. AJR Am J Roentgenol 1991;156:93–95.

15. Fishman EK, Soyer P, Bliss DF, et al. Splenic involvement in pancreatitis: spectrum of CT findings. AJR Am J Roentgenol 1995;164:631–635.

16. Luetmer PH, Stephens DH, Ward EM. Chronic pancreatitis: reassessment with current CT. Radiology 1989;171:353–357.

17. Megibow AJ. Pancreatic adenocarcinoma: designing the examination to evaluate the clinical questions. Radiology 1992;183:297–303.

18. Bluemke DA, Cameron JL, Hruban RH, et al. Potentially resectable pancreatic adenocarcinoma: spiral CT assessment with surgical and pathologic correlation. Radiology 1995; 197:381–385.

19. Bluemke DA, Abrams RA, Yeo CJ, et al. Recurrent pancreatic adenocarcinoma: spiral CT evaluation following the Whipple procedure. Radiographics 1997;17:303–313.

20. Buetow PC, Miller DL, Parrino TV, et al. Islet cell tumors of the pancreas: clinical, radiologic, and pathologic correlation in diagnosis and localization. Radiographics 1997;17: 453–472.

21. Buetow PC, Parrino TV, Buck JL, et al. Islet cell tumors of the pancreas: pathologic-imaging correlation among size, necrosis and cysts, calcification, malignant behavior, and functional status. AJR Am J Roentgenol 1995;165: 1175–1179.

22. Ros PR, Hamrick-Turner JE, Chiechi MV, et al. Cystic masses of the pancreas. Radiographics 1992;12:673–686.

23. Hough DM, Stephens DH, Johnson CD, et al. Pancreatic lesions in von Hippel-Lindau disease: prevalence, clinical significance, and CT findings. AJR Am J Roentgenol 1994; 162:1091–1094.

24. Buck JL, Hayes WS. Microcystic adenoma of the pancreas. Radiographics 1990;10:313–322.

25. Itoh S, Ishiguchi T, Ishigaki T, et al. Mucin-producing pancreatic tumor: CT findings and histopathologic correlation. Radiology 1992;183:81–86.

26. Procacci C, Graziani R, Bicego E, et al. Intraductal mucin-producing tumors of the pancreas: imaging findings. Radiology 1996;198:249–257.

27. Brant WE, Jain KA. Current imaging of the spleen. Radiologist 1996;3:185–192.

28. Dodds WJ, Taylor AJ, Erickson SJ, et al. Radiologic imaging of splenic anomalies. AJR Am J Roentgenol 1990;155: 805–810.

29. Ferrozzi F, Bova D, Draghi F, et al. CT findings in primary vascular tumors of the spleen. AJR Am J Roentgenol 1996; 166:1097–1101.

30. Freeman JL, Jafri SZH, Roberts JL, et al. CT of congenital and acquired abnormalities of the spleen. Radiographics 1993;13:597–610.

31. Görg C, Schwerk WB, Görg K. Sonography of focal lesions of the spleen. AJR Am J Roentgenol 1991;156:949–953.

32. Rabushka LS, Kawashima A, Fishman EK. Imaging of the spleen: CT with supplemental MR examination. Radiographics 1994;14:307–332.

33. Taylor AJ, Dodds WJ, Erickson SJ, et al. CT of acquired abnormalities of the spleen. AJR Am J Roentgenol 1991;157: 1213–1219.

34. Urrutia M, Mergo PJ, Ros LH, et al. Cystic masses of the spleen: radiologic-pathologic correlations. Radiographics 1996;16:107–129.

35. Torres GM, Terry NL, Mergo PJ, et al. MR imaging of the spleen. Magn Reson Imaging Clin North Am 1995;3:39–50.

36. Ito K, Mitchell DG, Honjo K, et al. Gadolinium-enhanced MR imaging of the spleen: artifacts and potential pitfalls. AJR Am J Roentgenol 1996;167:1147–1151.

37. Ito K, Mitchell DG, Honjo K, et al. MR imaging of acquired abnormalities of the spleen. 1997;168:697–702.

38. Miles KA, McPherson SJ, Hayball MP. Transient splenic inhomogeneity with contrast-enhanced CT: mechanism and effect of liver disease. Radiology 1995;194:91–95.

39. Do HM, Cronan JJ. CT appearance of splenic injuries managed nonoperatively. AJR Am J Roentgenol 1991;157: 757–760.

40. Schwerk WB, Görg C, Görg K, Restrepo I. Ultrasound-guided percutaneous drainage of pyogenic splenic abscesses. J Clin Ultrasound 1994;22:161–166.

41. Murray JG, Patel MD, Lee S, et al. Microabscesses of the liver and spleen in AIDS: detection with 5-MHz sonography. Radiology 1995;197:723–727.

42. Franquet T, Montes M, Lecumberri FJ, et al. Hydatid disease of the spleen: imaging findings in nine patients. AJR Am J Roentgenol 1990;154:525–528.

43. Görg C, Schwerk WB. Splenic infarction: sonographic patterns, diagnosis, follow-up, and complications. Radiology 1990;174:803–807.

44. Ramani M, Reinhold C, Semelka RC, et al. Splenic hemangiomas and hamartomas: MR imaging characteristics of 28 lesions. Radiology 1997;202:166–172.

29

Pharynx and Esophagus

William E. Brant

IMAGING METHODS

The upper gastrointestinal series (UGI), also called a barium meal, is a barium examination of the alimentary tract from the pharynx to the ligament of Treitz. A barium swallow or esophagram is a study more dedicated to evaluation of swallowing disorders and suspected lesions of the pharynx and esophagus. Barium sulfate preparations are ingested orally, and filming is performed during fluoroscopy. The fluoroscopic examination is commonly videotaped to allow for more detailed review of swallowing dynamics and motility (1). Double-contrast techniques using mucosal coating with barium combined with luminal distension are preferred for mucosal detail. Distension of the pharynx is provided by having the patient phonate (2). Distension of the esophagus is attained by having the patient ingest gas-producing crystals. Full-column, or single-contrast, technique uses barium suspension alone to fill and distend the esophagus. Mucosal relief views are collapsed views of the barium-coated esophagus.

Cross-sectional imaging techniques are used to stage malignancies of the pharynx and esophagus and to clarify findings seen with other imaging methods. CT complements barium studies and endoscopy of the esophagus by demonstrating the esophageal wall and adjacent structures to determine extent of disease. CT is poor at evaluating the mucosa and generally cannot differentiate inflammatory and neoplastic conditions. MR is preferred over CT for evaluation of the nasopharynx and is an alternative to CT for demonstrating the extent of esophageal disease. The clear depiction of blood vessels by MR is useful in confirming the presence of varices and in evaluating mediastinal vascular anatomy. Endoluminal sonography shows promise in the staging of esophageal tumors and in evaluation of the mediastinum.

This chapter reviews the pharynx as studied as part of a barium examination and for assessment of swallowing disorders. Cross-sectional imaging of the neck and pharynx is reviewed in chapter 9.

ANATOMY

The pharynx extends from the nasal cavity to the larynx and is arbitrarily divided into three compartments (Fig. 29.1) (3,4). The *nasopharynx* extends from the skull base to the soft palate. Its function is entirely respiratory, and the nasopharynx is not considered further in this chapter. The *oropharynx* is posterior to the oral cavity and extends from the soft palate to the hyoid bone. The *hypopharynx* (laryngopharynx) extends from the hyoid bone to the cricopharyngeus muscle. The base of the tongue forms the anterior boundary of the oropharynx (Fig. 29.1). The outline of the surface of the tongue is nodular because of the presence of lymphoid tissue forming the lingual tonsils and the circumvallate papillae, which contain taste buds (5). The lingual tonsils may hypertrophy and mimic a neoplasm. The epiglottis and aryepiglottic folds separate the larynx from the oropharynx and hypopharynx. The *valleculae* are two symmetrical pouches formed in the recess between the base of the tongue and the epiglottis. They are divided medially by the median glossoepiglottic fold and bounded laterally by the lateral glossoepiglottic folds. The *piriform sinuses* are deep, symmetrical, lateral recesses formed by the protrusion of the larynx into the hypopharynx.

The esophagus extends from the cricopharyngeus muscle at the level of C5–6 to the gastroesophageal junction (GEJ). The esophagus is a muscular tube formed by an outer longitudinal muscle layer and an inner circular muscle layer lined by stratified squamous epithelium. The esophagus lacks a serosal layer, which allows for rapid spread of tumor into adjacent tissues. The proximal one third of the esophagus is predominantly striated muscle, whereas the distal two-thirds, below the level of the aortic arch, is predominantly smooth muscle. Normal extrinsic impressions on the esophagus are made by the aortic arch, the left mainstem bronchus, and the left atrium. The normal esophageal mucosa is smooth and featureless when fully distended on air-contrast barium studies. With partial collapse, multiple longitudinal folds, 1–2 mm in thickness, become evident. Multiple regular, transverse folds, 1-mm thick, result from contraction of the longitudinal fibers in the muscularis mucosa. This pattern is called *feline esophagus* because it is typical of a normal esophagus in cats. In humans, it may be an early sign of dysmotility or esophagitis.

On cross-sectional imaging, the esophagus appears as an oval of soft tissue density usually surrounded by fat (6). The esophagus may contain air or contrast located

Figure 29.1. Double-contrast Pharyngogram.
Three radiographs of the pharynx coated with barium demonstrate normal anatomic structures: **(A)** nondistended lateral view; **(B)** distended lateral view, obtained by having the patient phonate "eee. . ."; and, **(C)** frontal (anteroposterior) view. The nasopharynx (*NP*) extends from the skull base to the soft palate (*sp*). The oropharynx (*OP*) spans from the soft palate to the hyoid bone (*HB*). The hypopharynx (*HP*) extends from the hyoid bone to the cricopharyngeus muscle (C5–6), which demarcates the pharynx and esophagus. The epiglottis (*e*) closes during swallowing to protect the larynx (*L*) from aspiration. The cricoid cartilage makes a prominent impression on the hypopharynx (*small white arrows*). The base of the tongue (*t*) has a normal lobulated appearance due to nodular lymphoid tissue. The valleculae (*v*) are recesses between the tongue and epiglottis, bordered by the median glossoepiglottic fold (*large black arrow*) and the lateral glossoepiglottic folds (*small black arrows*). The pyriform sinuses (*ps*) extend laterally and posterior to the larynx.

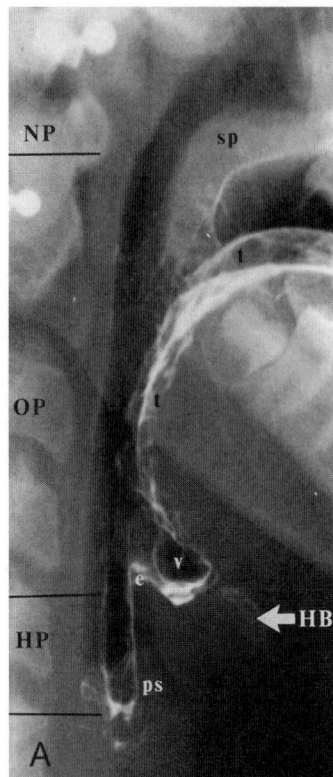
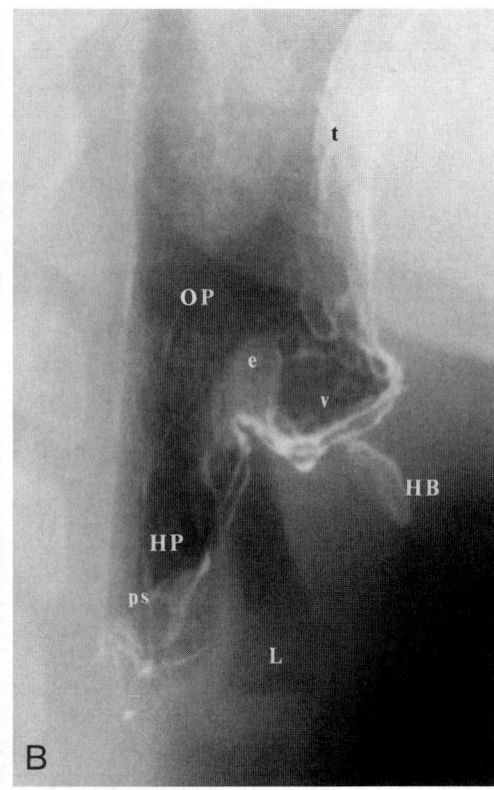
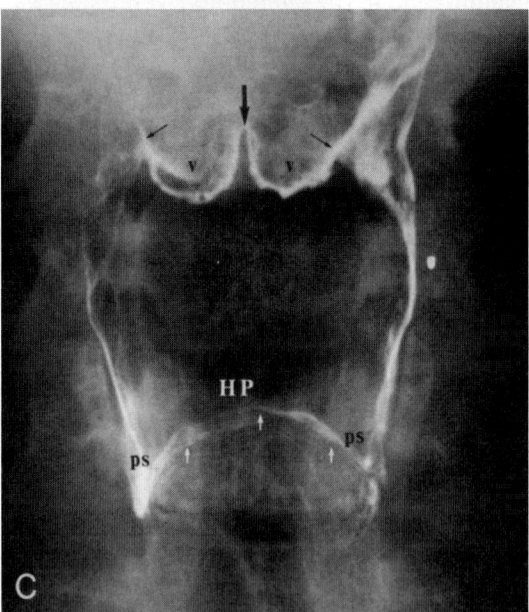

centrally within its lumen. Eccentric contrast or air should be considered abnormal. The wall of the distended esophagus should not exceed 3 mm in thickness.

Anatomy of the esophagogastric region is complex (7). The length of the esophagus is tubular, and its termination is saccular (Fig 29.2). The saccular termination is called the *esophageal vestibule*. The tubulovestibular junction is formed by a symmetrical muscular ring called the *A ring*. The *B ring* is an asymmetrical mucosal ring or notch that occurs at the junction of esophageal squamous epithelium with gastric columnar epithelium.

This squamocolumnar junction is also marked by the *Z line*, a thin ragged line of demarcation seen on double-contrast views of the lower esophagus. The B ring and the Z line are considered to be radiographic markers of the GEJ.

The esophageal hiatus is an angled opening in the diaphragm, formed by the edges of the diaphragmatic crura. On CT and MR, the crura appear as often prominent, teardrop-shaped structures of muscle density. With normal breathing, the proximal vestibule and A ring lie in the thorax. The midvestibule is in the esophageal hiatus, and the distal vestibule and B ring are in the abdomen. With swallowing, the vestibule opens and moves upward and the B ring may be seen 1 cm above the diaphragm.

NORMAL SWALLOWING AND MOTILITY

The normal process of swallowing can be divided into oral, pharyngeal, and esophageal phases (1–3,8,9). The oral stage involves the voluntary transport of a bolus from the oral cavity into the pharynx. The soft palate elevates and the tongue depresses to accommodate the bolus and channel it into the oropharynx. The oropharynx and hypopharynx receive the bolus and conduct it to the esophagus. Breathing is halted while the larynx elevates, the laryngeal vestibule closes, and the epiglottis and aryepiglottic folds close over the opening into the larynx and deflect the bolus through the lateral piriform sinuses.

The functional upper esophageal sphincter (UES), formed by the cricopharyngeus and other pharyngeal muscles, opens to receive the bolus. Peristalsis conveys ingested material through the tubular esophagus to the stomach. *Primary peristalsis* is composed of a rapid wave of inhibition that opens the sphincters, followed by a slow wave of contraction that moves the bolus. Normal peristalsis will clear the esophagus completely with each swallow. Radiographically, primary peristalsis appears as a stripping wave that traverses the entire esophagus from top to bottom. *Secondary peristalsis* is initiated by distension of the esophageal lumen. The peristaltic wave starts in the midesophagus and spreads simultaneously

up and down the esophagus to clear reflux or any part of a bolus left behind. Secondary waves have the same radiographic appearance as primary waves except that they start at the point of the retained barium bolus. *Tertiary waves* are nonproductive contractions associated with motility disorders. Irregular contractions follow one another at close intervals from the top to the bottom of the esophagus. These nonperistaltic contractions cause a corkscrew or beaded appearance of the esophageal barium column. The functional lower esophageal sphincter (LES) at the level of the esophageal vestibule relaxes and opens in response to swallowing, primary peristalsis, and proximal esophageal dilation.

Oral and pharyngeal swallowing are evaluated fluoroscopically with the patient in an upright position simulating normal eating. The lateral projection is most useful. Studies are videotaped for subsequent detailed study (1,9). Esophageal motility is evaluated by observing fluoroscopically at least five separate swallows of barium with the patient in a prone oblique position (10). The patient must be instructed to swallow only once, as continuous swallowing distends the esophagus and makes impossible the evaluation of primary peristalsis.

MOTILITY DISORDERS

Difficulty with swallowing has an increasingly high prevalence with age (11). Symptoms of abnormal oral or pharyngeal swallowing include difficulty initiating swallowing, globus sensation (lump in throat), cervical dysphagia, nasal regurgitation, hoarseness, coughing, or choking (9,11). Symptoms suggesting esophageal dys-

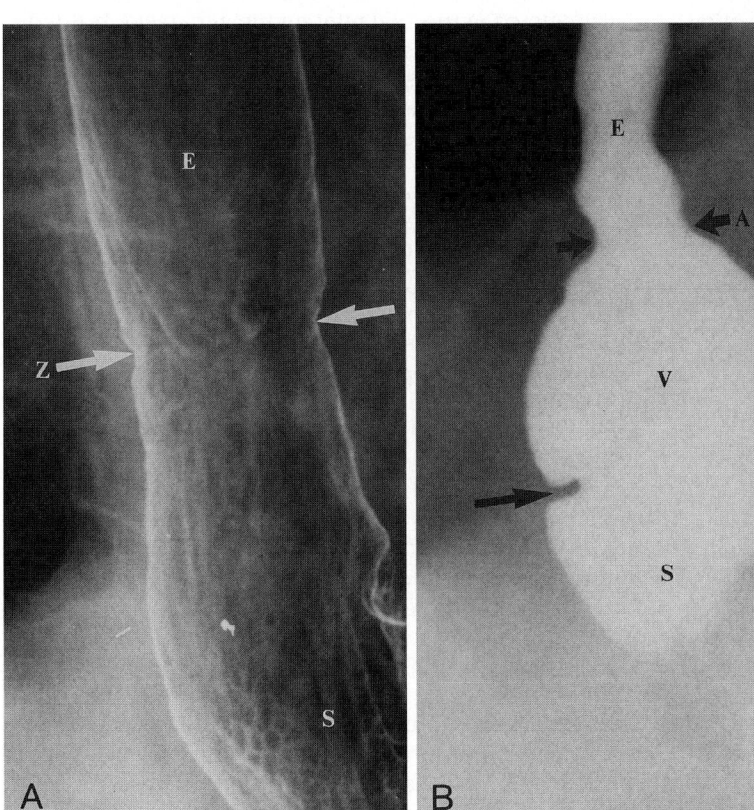

Figure 29.2. Anatomy of the Gastroesophageal Junction. Radiographs from a double-contrast barium study **(A)** and a single-contrast barium study **(B)** demonstrate the physiologic and anatomic landmarks of the gastroesophageal junction. The Z line (Z, *white arrows*), seen best on the double-contrast study, marks the junction of the squamous epithelium of the esophagus (*E*) and the columnar epithelium of the stomach (*S*). The single-contrast study demonstrates the esophageal vestibule (*V*) demarcated by the muscular A ring (*A, short black arrows*) and the mucosal fold of the B ring (*B, long black arrows*). The vestibule marks the location of the lower esophageal sphincter. The Z line and the B ring are markers of the gastroesophageal junction. Their location relative to the esophageal hiatus in the diaphragm varies with swallowing and other physiologic motions.

function include heartburn, dysphagia, "indigestion," and chest pain. Dysphagia is defined as the awareness of swallowing difficulty during the passage of solids or liquids from mouth to stomach. Patients complain of food "sticking in the throat" and of painful swallowing (odynophagia). These symptoms may be caused by anatomic abnormalities, tumors, or motility disorders. Subjective assessment of the location of the abnormality is not reliable. Detailed dynamic barium studies of the entire oropharyngeal–esophageal pathway with videofluoroscopy are needed for complete evaluation. Motility disorders that may cause dysphagia or aspiration are reviewed in this section. Radiographic findings of functional abnormalities of the pharynx and esophagus increase in prevalence with age, may not correlate with specific symptoms, and must be interpreted with caution (11).

Signs of Pharyngeal Dysfunction. *Pharyngeal stasis*, indicative of impaired pharyngeal transport, is seen as increased residual volume of swallowed material filling the valleculae and piriform sinuses. *Laryngeal penetration* is defined as entry of barium into the laryngeal vestibule without passage below the vocal cords. *Aspiration* implies barium passage below the vocal cords. Either finding may precipitate a cough. *Nasal regurgitation* occurs when the soft palate does not make a good seal against the posterior pharyngeal wall. Causes include neurologic impairment, muscular dystrophies, and structural defects in the palate. The major causes of pharyngeal dysfunction are listed in Table 29.1.

Cricopharyngeal achalasia is attributable to failure of complete relaxation of the UES, commonly resulting in dysphagia and aspiration. Barium swallow demonstrates a shelflike impression *(cricopharyngeal bar)* on the barium column at the pharyngoesophageal junction at the level of C5–6. The pharynx is distended, and bar-

Table 29.1. Causes of Pharyngeal Swallowing Dysfunction

Aging (primary presbyphagia)
Neurological disease
  Cerebrovascular accident
  Multiple sclerosis
  Movement disorders
  Neurodegenerative diseases
  Central nervous system infections
Muscle disease
  Muscular dystrophies
  Myasthenia gravis
Structural abnormalities
  Pharyngeal webs
  Zenker's diverticulum
  Tumors
Medications
Radiation
Gastroesophageal reflux
Zenker's diverticulum
Trauma
Postsurgical changes
Malignancy
  Oral cavity
  Pharynx
  Larynx

ium may overflow into the larynx and trachea. Because some normal individuals have a prominent cricopharyngeal impression, controversy exists as to how prominent the impression must be to be considered significant. Narrowing of the lumen greater than 50% is generally accepted as a definite cause of dysphagia (12). Cricopharyngeal dysfunction is commonly associated with neuromuscular disorders of the pharynx.

Esophageal achalasia is a disease of unknown etiology characterized by 1) absence of peristalsis in the body of the esophagus, 2) marked increase in resting pressure of the LES, and 3) failure of the LES to relax with swallowing. The abnormal peristalsis and LES spasm result in a failure of the esophagus to empty. Pathologically, cases show a deficiency of ganglion cells in the myenteric plexus (Auerbach's plexus) throughout the esophagus. The clinical presentation is insidious, usually at age 30–50 years, with dysphagia, regurgitation, foul breath, and aspiration. Radiographic signs include 1) uniform dilatation of the esophagus, usually with an air-fluid level present; 2) absence of peristalsis, with tertiary waves common in the early stages of the disease; 3) tapered "beak" deformity at the LES because of failure of relaxation (Fig. 29.3); and 4) increased incidence of epiphrenic diverticula and esophageal carcinoma. Treatment of achalasia is balloon dilation or Heller myotomy. Diseases that may mimic esophageal achalasia include the following.

Chagas' disease is caused by the destruction of ganglion cells of the esophagus due to a neurotoxin released by the protozoa, *Trypanosoma cruzi*, endemic to South America, especially eastern Brazil. The radiographic appearance of the esophagus is identical to achalasia. Associated abnormalities include cardiomyopathy, megaduodenum, megaureter, and megacolon.

Carcinoma of the GEJ may mimic achalasia, but tends to involve a longer segment of the distal esophagus, is rigid, and tends to show more irregular tapering of the distal esophagus and mass effect.

Peptic strictures are usually associated with normal primary peristalsis.

Diffuse esophageal spasm is a syndrome of unknown cause characterized by multiple tertiary esophageal contractions, thickened esophageal wall, and intermittent dysphagia and chest pain. Primary peristalsis is usually present, but the contractions are infrequent. Most patients are middle-aged.

Neuromuscular disorders are a common cause of abnormalities of the oral, pharyngeal, or esophageal phases of swallowing. The most common cause of neurologic dysfunction is cerebrovascular disease and stroke. Additional causes include parkinsonism, Alzheimer's disease, multiple sclerosis, neoplasms of the central nervous system, and posttraumatic central nervous system injury. Diseases of striated muscle, such as muscular dystrophy, myasthenia gravis, and dermatomyositis, predominantly affect the pharynx and proximal third of the esophagus.

Scleroderma is a systemic disease of unknown cause characterized by progressive atrophy of smooth muscle and progressive fibrosis of affected tissues. Women are most commonly affected, usually aged 20–40 years at the onset of disease. The esophagus is affected in

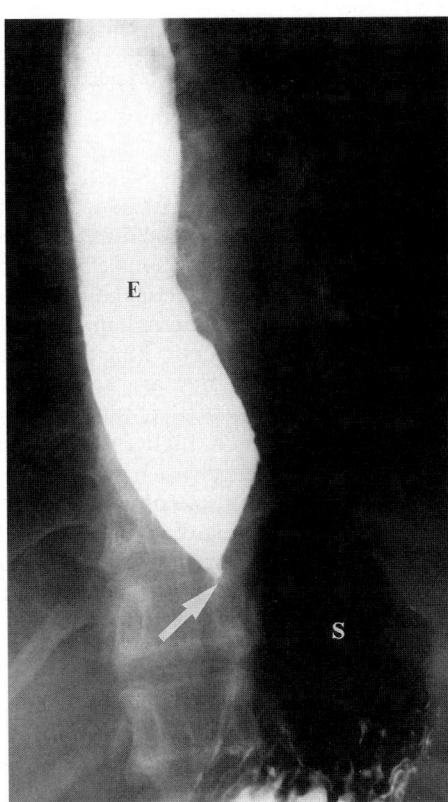

Figure 29.3. Esophageal Achalasia. Radiograph from a UGI series reveals uniform dilatation of the esophagus (*E*) to the level of the GEJ, where a beak (*arrow*) is formed by the barium column. Repeated observation by fluoroscopy confirmed failure of relaxation of the LES and prolonged retention of barium in the esophagus even in the upright position. *S*, stomach.

75–80% of patients. Radiographic findings (Fig. 29.4) include 1) weak to absent peristalsis in the distal two thirds (smooth muscle portion) of the esophagus, 2) delayed esophageal emptying, 3) a stiff dilated esophagus that does not collapse with emptying, and 4) wide gaping LES with free gastroesophageal reflux. Despite free reflux, tight strictures of the distal esophagus are uncommon.

Postoperative states, including surgery for malignancy of the tongue, larynx, and pharynx, commonly impair swallowing function as well as alter the morphology (9). Surgical resection is aimed at providing at least a 1-cm margin free of tumor and often results in removing large blocks of tissue and functionally altering the structures that remain.

Esophagitis frequently results in abnormal esophageal motility and visualization of tertiary esophageal contractions.

Gastroesophageal reflux (GER) occurs as a result of incompetence of the LES. The resting pressure of the LES is abnormally decreased and fails to increase with raised intra-abdominal pressure. As a result, increases in intra-abdominal pressure exceed LES pressure, and gastric contents are allowed to reflux into the esophagus. Symptoms of GER include substernal burning pain ("heartburn"), postural regurgitation (in supine posi-

tion), and development of reflux esophagitis, dysphagia, and odynophagia. Complications of GER include reflux esophagitis, stricture, and development of Barrett's esophagus.

The radiographic diagnosis of pathologic GER may be difficult because 20% of normal individuals show spontaneous reflux on UGI examination, and patients with pathologic GER may not demonstrate reflux without provocative tests (13). Monitoring of esophageal pH for 24 hours in an ambulatory patient is the most sensitive means of diagnosing abnormal GER.

Hiatus hernia has for years been considered synonymous with GER. There is, however, poor correlation between the presence of hiatus hernia and GER or reflux esophagitis. One area of controversy is the definition of hiatus hernia and the criteria used for diagnosis. The simplest definition is protrusion of any portion of the stomach into the thorax. Two major types of hernia are described. The most common is the *sliding hiatus hernia*, with the GEJ displaced more than 1 cm above the hiatus (Fig. 29.5). The esophageal hiatus is often abnormally widened to 3–4 cm. The upper limit of normal hiatal width is 15 mm, most easily measured by CT. The gastric fundus may be displaced above the diaphragm and present as a retrocardiac mass on a chest radiograph. The presence of an air-fluid level in the mass suggests the diagnosis. Small, sliding hiatus hernias commonly

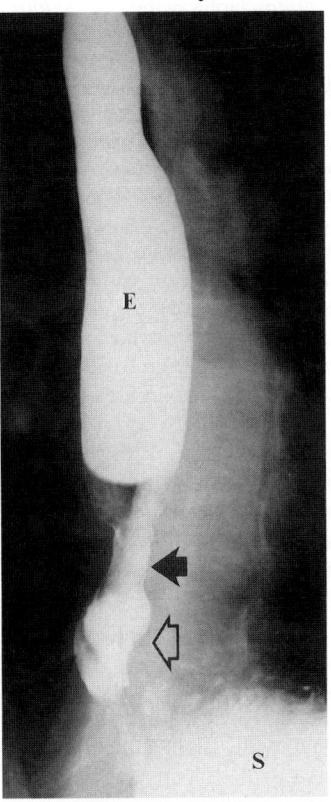

Figure 29.4. Scleroderma. Barium esophagram demonstrates the esophagus (*E*) to be dilated and lacking in peristaltic motion in its distal two-thirds on fluoroscopic observation. The GEJ (*open arrow*) is wide and is never observed to close. Reflux esophagitis causes stiffening and narrowing of the distal esophagus (*closed arrow*). *S*, stomach.

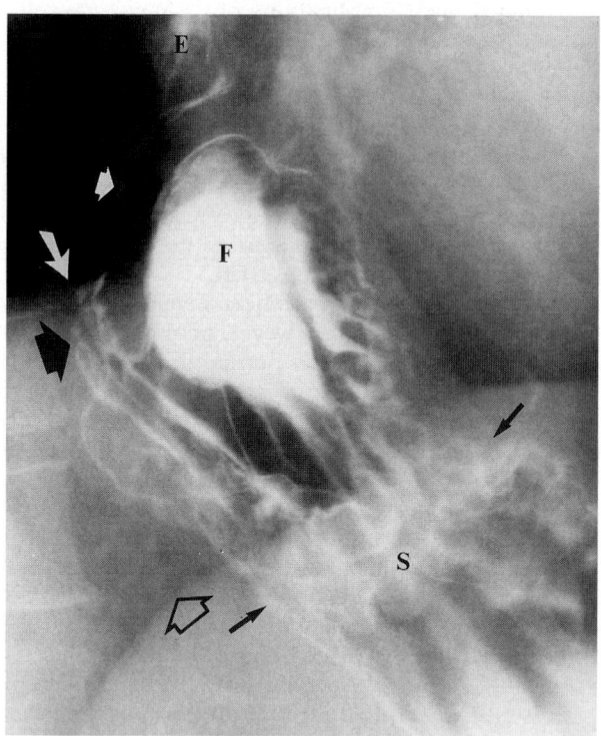

Figure 29.5. Hiatus Hernia. Left posterior oblique view from a UGI series demonstrates a large hiatus hernia. The fundus (*F*) of the stomach (*S*) extends well above the level of the left hemidiaphragm (*open arrow*). The widened (6 cm) esophageal hiatus makes an impression (*small black arrows*) on the body of the stomach. The GEJ (*fat black arrowhead*) is 5 cm above the left hemidiaphragm. The distal esophagus (*white arrowhead*) is bowed around the herniated stomach. The right hemidiaphragm (*white arrow*) projects well above the left hemidiaphragm on this view.

reduce in the upright position. Much less common (1% of the total) is the *paraesophageal hiatus hernia*, in which the GEJ remains in normal location, while a portion of the stomach, usually the fundus, herniates above the diaphragm. The mere presence of hiatus hernia is of limited clinical significance in most cases. The function of the LES and the presence of pathologic GER are the crucial factors in producing symptoms and causing complications. Large hiatus hernias, especially when the stomach is totally intrathoracic, are at risk for obstruction and volvulus.

OUTPOUCHINGS

Lateral pharyngeal diverticula are protrusions of pharyngeal mucosa through areas of weakness of the lateral pharyngeal wall, most common in the region of the tonsillar fossa and thyrohyoid membrane. They reflect increased intrapharyngeal pressure and are seen most commonly in wind instrument players.

Zenker's diverticulum arises in the hypopharynx just proximal to the UES. It is located in the posterior midline at the cleavage plane, known as Killian's dehiscence, between the circular and oblique fibers of the cricopharyngeus muscle (Fig. 29.6). The diverticulum

has a small neck that is higher than the sac, resulting in food and liquid being trapped within the sac. The distended sac may compress the cervical esophagus. Symptoms include dysphagia, halitosis, and regurgitation of food.

Midesophageal diverticula may be pulsion or traction diverticula. Pulsion diverticula occur as a result of disordered esophageal peristalsis. Traction diverticula occur because of fibrous inflammatory reactions of adjacent lymph nodes. Most midesophageal diverticula have large mouths, empty well, and are usually asymptomatic (Fig. 29.7).

Epiphrenic diverticula occur just above the LES, usually on the right side. They are rare and usually found in patients with esophageal motility disorders (Fig. 29.8). Because of a small neck, higher than the sac, they may trap food and liquids and cause symptoms.

Sacculations are small outpouchings of the esophagus that usually occur as a sequela of severe esophagitis (see Fig. 29.9). They are thought to result from the healing and scarring of ulcerations. Sacculations tend to change in size and shape during fluoroscopic observation.

ESOPHAGITIS

Esophagitis is a common disease with many causes. Radiologic evaluation will detect most cases of moderate

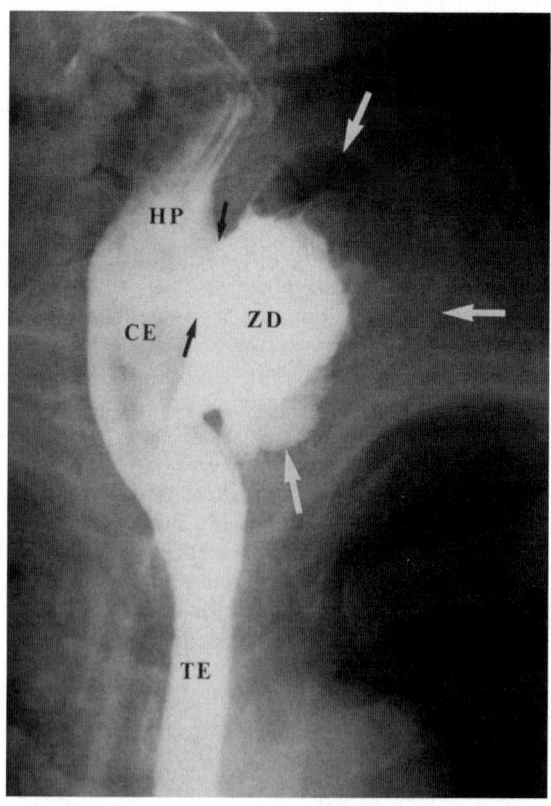

Figure 29.6. Zenker's Diverticulum. Barium swallow examination demonstrates a partially barium-filled outpouching (*ZD*) at the junction of the hypopharynx (*HP*) and cervical esophagus (*CE*). The full extent of the diverticulum is indicated by the *white arrows*. Note that the neck of the diverticulum (*black arrow*) is at a more cephalad location than its base, encouraging the trapping of food and liquid. *TE*, thoracic esophagus.

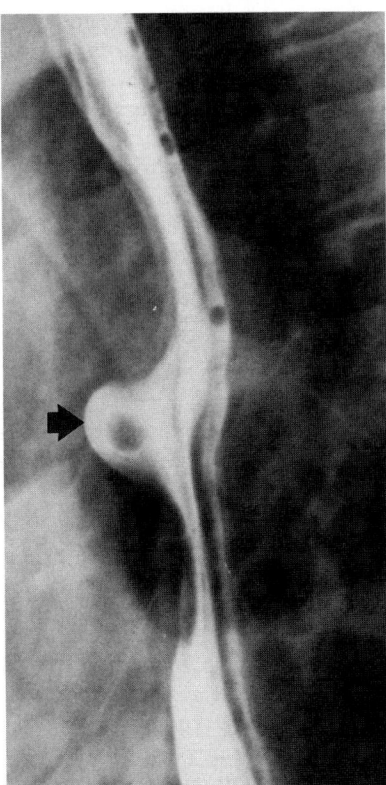

Figure 29.7. Pulsion Diverticulum. A barium swallow examination demonstrates a persistent mucosal outpouching (*arrow*) in the midesophagus. The patient was asymptomatic. Pulsion diverticula are formed when the mucosa and submucosa herniate through the muscularis.

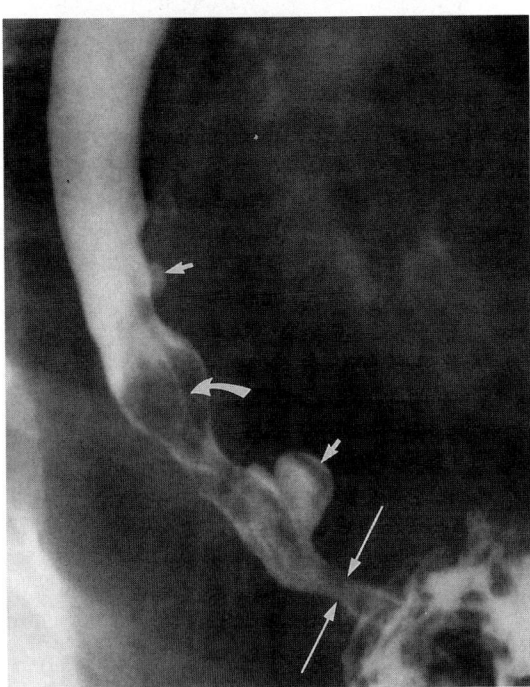

Figure 29.8. Epiphrenic Diverticula. A stricture (*long arrows*) of the distal esophagus has resulted in the formation of pulsion diverticula (*short arrows*). The filling defects (*curved arrow*) in the barium column are caused by retained boluses of meat proximal to the stricture.

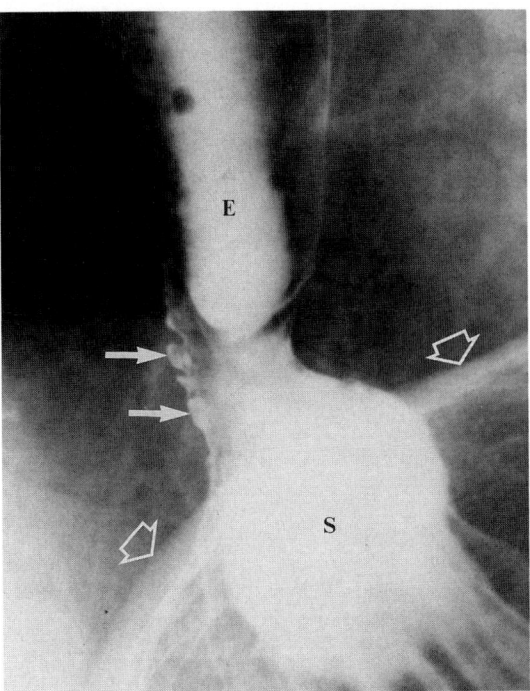

Figure 29.9. Reflux Esophagitis. A barium esophagram demonstrates stiffness and narrowing of the distal esophagus just above the level of the diaphragm (*open arrows*). Several prominent sacculations (*arrows*) are present, indicating long-standing and severe esophagitis. *E*, esophagus; *S*, stomach.

to severe esophagitis but will demonstrate less than half the cases of mild esophagitis. Attention to excellent technique and use of double-contrast studies are essential (14). Radiographic signs of esophagitis include *a*) thickened esophageal folds (>3 mm), *b*) limited esophageal distensibility (asymmetric flattening), *c*) abnormal motility, *d*) mucosal plaques and nodules, *e*) erosions and ulcerations, *f*) localized stricture, and *g*) intramural pseudodiverticulosis (barium filling of dilated 1–3 mm submucosal glands).

Reflux esophagitis (RE) is the result of esophageal mucosal injury owing to exposure to gastroduodenal secretions. The severity depends on the concentration of caustic agents including acid, pepsin, bile salts, caffeine, alcohol, and aspirin, as well as the duration of contact with the esophageal mucosa. The findings of reflux esophagitis are always most prominent in the distal esophagus and GEJ (Fig. 29.9). Early changes of reflux esophagitis include mucosal edema, which is manifest as a granular or nodular pattern of the distal esophagus. In contrast to the distinct borders of *Candida* plaques and nodules, reflux esophagitis nodules have poorly defined borders. Inflammatory exudates and pseudomembrane formation may mimic fulminant *Candida* esophagitis; however, the patient has symptoms of reflux rather than severe odynophagia.

Reflux esophagitis is the most common cause of esophageal ulcerations. The ulcers appear as discrete linear, punctate, or irregular collections of barium, usually surrounded by a radiolucent mound of edema. Distal prominence of the ulcerations is the key to differ-

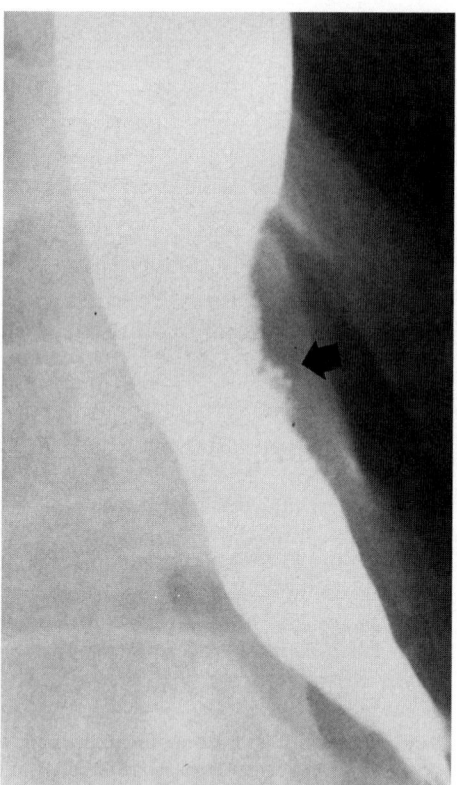

Figure 29.10. Candida Esophagitis. Barium esophagram in a patient with AIDS demonstrates "shaggy" esophageal mucosa (*arrow*) owing to multiple tiny plaques produced by *Candida albicans* esophagitis.

entiating RE ulcers from those of herpes esophagitis. Complications of RE include ulceration, bleeding, stricture, and Barrett's esophagus.

Barrett's esophagus is an acquired condition of progressive columnar metaplasia of the distal esophagus caused by chronic gastroesophageal reflux. Columnar rather than squamous epithelium lines the distal esophagus. The prevalence of Barrett's esophagus in patients with reflux esophagitis is about 10%, but may increase to 37% in patients with scleroderma. It is premalignant, with a 30–40 times increased risk of developing adenocarcinoma (see Fig. 29.20), resulting in a 15% prevalence of adenocarcinoma in patients with Barrett's esophagus. Clinical presentation is usually indistinguishable from reflux esophagitis. Adenocarcinoma may develop at any age. The characteristic radiographic appearance of Barrett's esophagus is a high (midesophageal) stricture or deep ulcer in a patient with GER (15). A reticular mucosal pattern of the esophageal mucosa, resembling areae gastricae of the stomach, is also suggestive. The diagnosis is confirmed by endoscopy and biopsy.

Infectious esophagitis is found most commonly in patients with compromised immune systems. It is increasingly common because of the use of steroids and cytotoxic drugs and because of the increasing prevalence of AIDS.

Candida albicans is the most common cause of infectious esophagitis and is highly prevalent in patients with AIDS. *Candida* of the oropharynx (thrush) is commonly

present and is usually diagnosed clinically. Odynophagia is a prominent symptom. Discrete plaquelike lesions demonstrated by double-contrast esophograms are most characteristic. The plaques appear as longitudinally oriented linear or irregular discrete filling defects etched in white with intervening normal-appearing mucosa. The lesions may be tiny and nodular, or giant and coalescent with pseudomembranes. Patients with AIDS tend to have more fulminant disease with a diffuse "shaggy" esophagus (Fig. 29.10).

Herpes simplex esophagitis begins as discrete vesicles that rupture to form discrete mucosal ulcers. The ulcers may be linear, punctate, or ringlike and have a characteristic radiolucent halo. Discrete ulcers on a background of normal mucosa involving the midesophagus is most characteristic of herpes. Nodules and plaques are usually absent.

Cytomegalovirus is a cause of fulminant esophagitis in patients with AIDS. Cytomegalovirus esophagitis is characteristically manifest as one or more large, flat mucosal ulcers (Fig. 29.11). Endoscopic biopsy or culture confirms the diagnosis.

Human Immunodeficiency Virus (HIV) esophagitis causes giant ulcers and severe odynophagia. Electron microscopy reveals HIV particles in the ulcers. The ulcers are large, flat, and usually in the midesophagus.

Tuberculosis. The esophagus is the least common portion of the gastrointestinal tract to be involved by tuberculosis. Manifestations include ulceration, stricture, sinus tract, and abscess formation (Fig. 29.12).

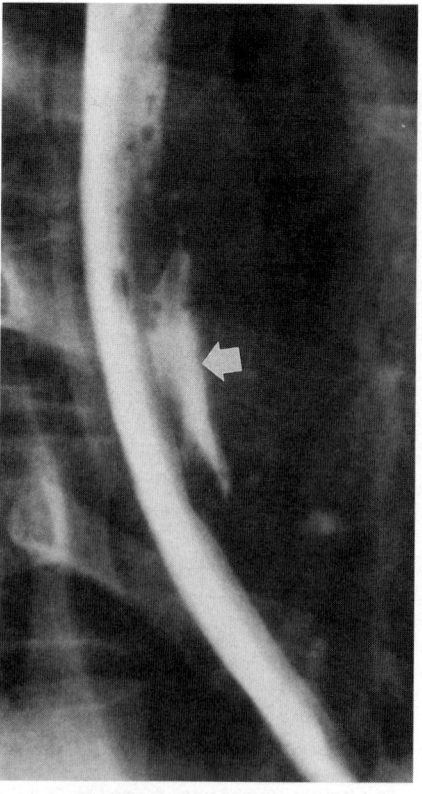

Figure 29.11. Cytomegalovirus Esophagitis. A large flat mucosal ulcer (*arrow*) in the distal esophagus is characteristic of cytomegalovirus esophagitis in a patient with AIDS.

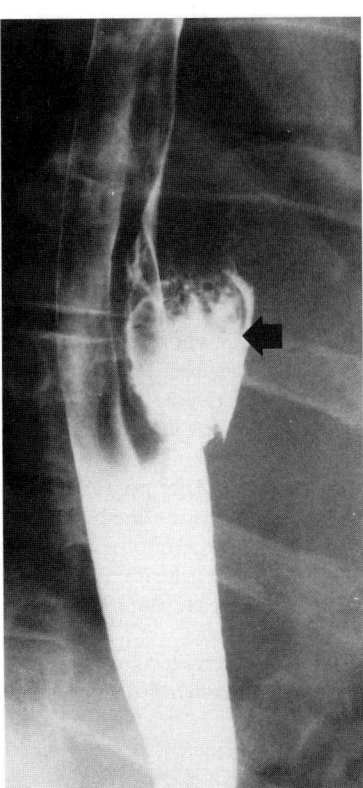

Figure 29.12. Tuberculous Esophagitis. Tuberculosis in an immunocompromised patient has ulcerated the esophagus and causes a periesophageal abscess (*arrow*).

Drug-induced esophagitis is the result of intake of oral medications that produce a focal inflammation in areas of contact with the mucosa. Drugs that cause this condition include tetracycline, doxycycline, quinidine, aspirin, indomethacin, ascorbic acid, potassium chloride, alprenolol chloride, and emepronium bromide. The radiographic appearance may be identical to herpes esophagitis, with discrete ulcers separated by normal mucosa in the midesophagus (Fig. 29.13). The diagnosis is suggested by a history of recent drug ingestion. Healing usually occurs within 7–10 days of discontinuing the offending medication.

Corrosive ingestion usually occurs as an accident in children or a suicide attempt in adults. Alkaline agents (liquid lye) produce deep (full-thickness) coagulation necrosis. Acid agents tend to produce more superficial injury. Ulceration, esophageal perforation, and mediastinitis may complicate the acute injury. Late complications are fibrosis and long or multiple strictures.

Crohn's disease may rarely manifest as discrete aphthous ulcers in the esophagus. Involvement of the small or large bowel by Crohn's disease is virtually always present. Crohn's disease of the esophagus should not be considered unless Crohn's disease of the bowel is already evident.

Radiation esophagitis occurs in patients with a history of thoracic radiation therapy for malignant disease. Acute radiation may cause shallow or deep ulcers in the area of involvement. With the development of fibrosis, the peristaltic wave is interrupted and a long smooth

stricture may develop within the radiotherapy field. Simultaneous radiotherapy and doxorubicin hydrochloride (Adriamycin) chemotherapy greatly accentuates esophageal inflammation.

ESOPHAGEAL STRICTURE

Strictures are defined as any persistent intrinsic narrowing of the esophagus (16). The most common causes are fibrosis induced by inflammation and neoplasm. Because radiographic findings are not reliable in differentiating benign from malignant strictures, all should be evaluated endoscopically.

Esophagitis. Chronic inflammation induces progressive fibrosis that eventually narrows the esophageal lumen. Acute and chronic findings of esophagitis commonly overlap.

Reflux esophagitis is the most common cause of esophageal stricture. Reflux strictures are usually confined to the distal esophagus (Figs. 29.14,29.15) and may be smooth and circumferential or asymmetric and irregular. Long-segment stricture may be induced by long-term nasogastric intubation. A *Schatzki ring* is a pathologic ringlike stricture at the level of the B ring, caused by reflux esophagitis.

Barrett's esophagus strictures tend to be high in the midesophagus and may be smooth and tapered or ringlike narrowings. The high position is because of a ten-

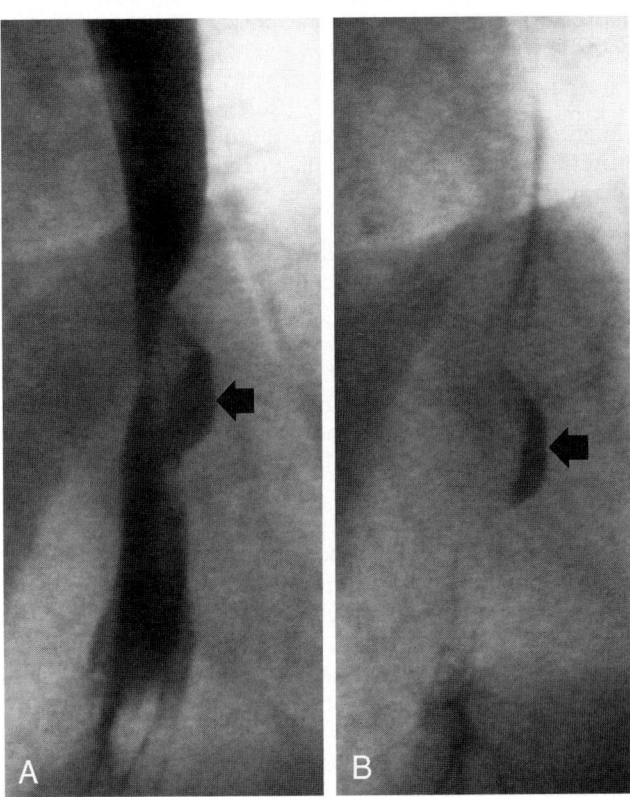

Figure 29.13. Drug-induced Esophagitis. A discrete ulcer of the distal esophagus is seen as a persistent collection of barium (*arrows*) on single contrast **(A)** and double contrast **(B)** views of the esophagus. The causative agent was indomethacin taken for severe ankylosing spondylitis.

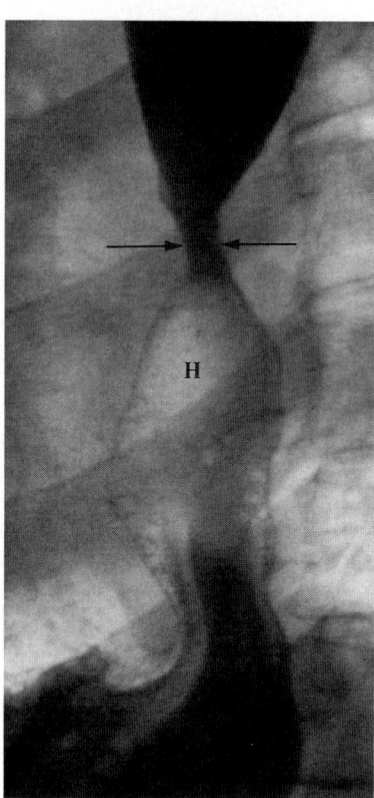

Figure 29.14. Short Stricture Resulting from Reflux Esophagitis. A short, narrowed area (*arrows*) of the distal esophagus extends to the top of a hiatus hernia (*H*) in this patient with chronic gastroesophageal reflux.

dency for strictures to occur at the squamocolumnar junction, which has been displaced to a position well above the GEJ.

Corrosives strictures are long and symmetrical. They commonly develop years after the initial injury.

Radiation strictures are confined to the radiotherapy field.

Neoplasm. An irregular, ulcerated, circumferential narrowing is most typical of malignant stricture (Fig. 29.16). Infiltrative tumors may cause smooth, rigid narrowing of the esophagus without a clear zone of transition. The mucosa may not be altered until tumor spread is substantial.

Webs are thin, delicate membranes that sweep partially across the lumen. They occur in both the pharynx and esophagus and are commonly multiple. Pharyngeal webs arise most commonly from the anterior wall of the hypopharynx. Esophageal webs may occur anywhere, but they are most common in the cervical esophagus just distal to the cricopharyngeus impression (Fig. 29.17). Most are incidental findings; however, they occasionally cause sufficient obstruction to result in dysphagia.

Extrinsic Compression. Malignancy or inflammation in the mediastinum may encase the esophagus and narrow its lumen. Causes include lung carcinoma, lymphoma, metastasis to mediastinal nodes, tuberculosis, and histoplasmosis.

ENLARGED ESOPHAGEAL FOLDS

Esophagitis. Thick folds occur most commonly with reflux esophagitis. Additional findings associated with esophagitis, such as ulcerations and nodules, are commonly present.

Varices appear as serpiginous filling defects (Fig. 29.18) that change in size with changes in intrathoracic pressure and that collapse with esophageal peristalsis and distension. They are best demonstrated on UGI with mucosal relief views. Spiral CT with bolus contrast enhancement demonstrates varices as enhancing vascular structures within and adjacent to esophageal wall near the GEJ. MR is also effective in demonstrating varices as vascular spaces, with signal void because of flowing blood.

Uphill varices refer to the portosystemic collateral veins that enlarge because of portal hypertension. Coronary vein collaterals connect with gastroesophageal varices that drain into the inferior vena cava via the azygos system. Uphill varices are usually only present in the distal esophagus.

Downhill varices are formed as a result of obstruction of the superior vena cava with drainage from the azygous

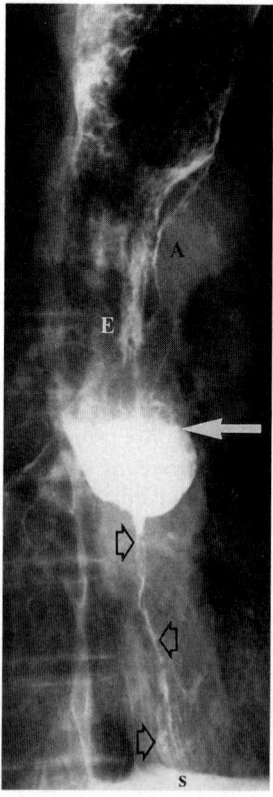

Figure 29.15. Long Stricture Resulting from Reflux Esophagitis. A long-segment stricture (*open arrows*) of the distal esophagus is apparent on this barium esophagram. The column of barium is abruptly narrowed to a thin irregular channel. Barium forms an air-fluid level (*white arrow*) on this upright view as it is retained in the esophagus before trickling through the stricture. Retained food particles and secretions cause a mottled appearance in the lumen of the proximal esophagus (*E*). The aorta (A) produces a normal impression on the left lateral aspect of the esophagus. *S*, stomach.

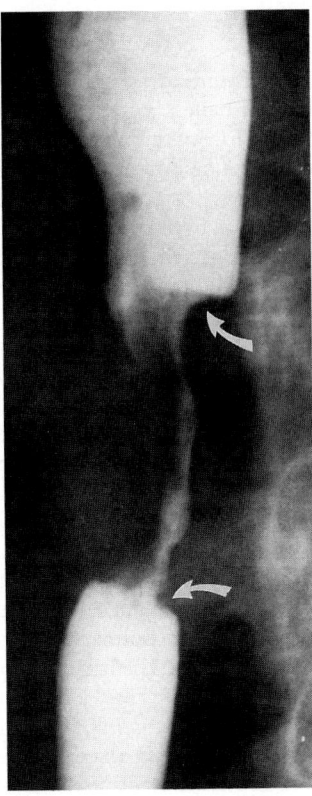

Figure 29.16. Stricture Caused by Carcinoma. A squamous cell carcinoma of the midesophagus causes an abrupt narrowing with irregular mucosa. The prominent shoulders (*arrows*) are characteristic of tumor.

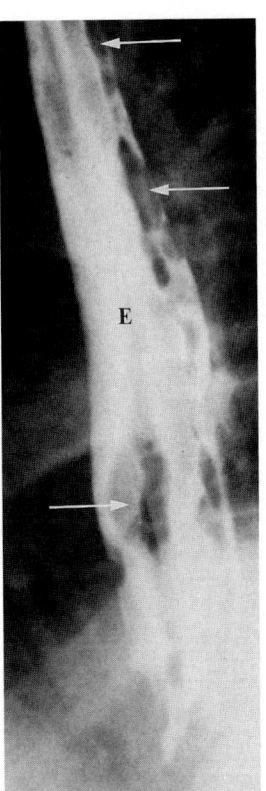

Figure 29.18. Varices. A single-contrast barium esophagram demonstrates sinuous tubular and nodular filling defects (*arrows*) in the esophagus (*E*). This patient has cirrhosis, portal hypertension, and a history of upper gastrointestinal bleeding.

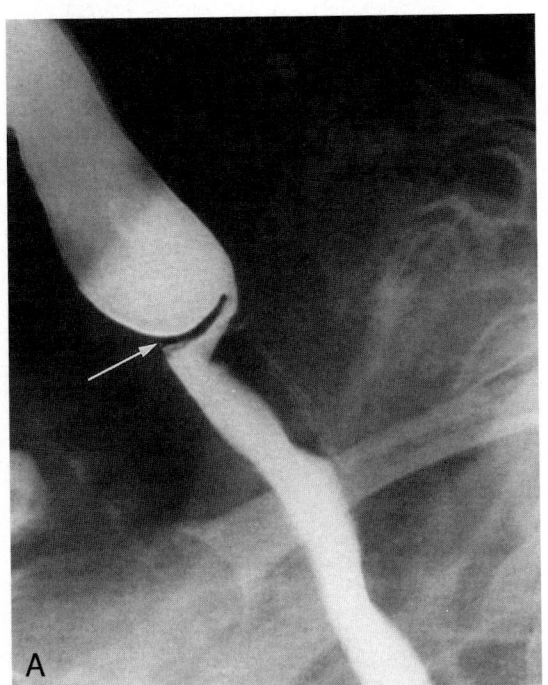

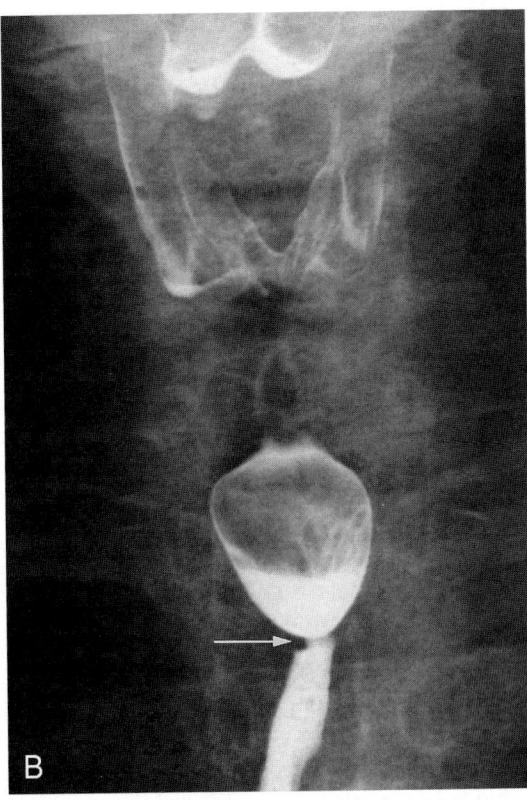

Figure 29.17. Esophageal Web. Lateral oblique **(A)** and frontal **(B)** views from a barium esophagram reveal a thin membrane (*arrows*) that extends across the lumen of the proximal esophagus, leaving only a narrow lumen for passage of food. The esophagus is dilated proximal to the web.

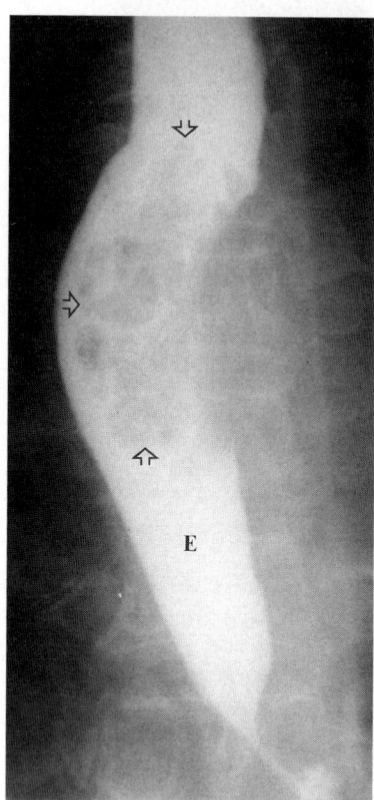

Figure 29.19. Squamous Cell Carcinoma. This squamous cell carcinoma appears as a polypoid mass (*arrows*) in the midesophagus (*E*) on this barium esophagram. Barium outlines the lobulations in the tumor.

Esophageal carcinoma is squamous cell carcinoma (Fig. 29.19) in 90% of cases, and the remainder are adenocarcinoma arising in Barrett's esophagus (Fig. 29.20), undifferentiated, or miscellaneous cell types. Because of rapid spread to adjacent structures, esophageal carcinoma is deadly, with a 5-year survival of only 5%. The tumor assumes four basic radiographic patterns. An annular constricting lesion, appearing as an irregular ulcerated stricture, is most common (Fig. 29.16). The polypoid pattern causes an intraluminal filling defect (Fig. 29.19). The infiltrative variety grows predominantly in the submucosa and may simulate a benign stricture. The least common pattern is that of an ulcerated mass. Predisposing conditions include cigarette and alcohol abuse, corrosive ingestion, and carcinoma of the head and neck. The typical patient is a 65-year-old man.

The tumor spreads quickly by direct invasion into adjacent tissues because of the lack of a serosal covering on the esophagus. Lymphatic spread may go to nodes in the neck, mediastinum, or below the diaphragm, depending on the location of the primary tumor in the esophagus. Hematogenous spread is to lung, liver, and adrenal gland.

CT, MR, or endoscopic US are used to define the extent of disease and determine surgical resectability (Table 29.2 and Fig. 29.21) (6,17,18). Findings include irregular thickening of the esophageal wall, eccentric narrowing of the lumen, dilation of the esophagus above the area of narrowing, invasion of periesophageal tissues, and metastases to

system through esophageal varices to the portal vein. Downhill varices usually predominate in the proximal esophagus.

Lymphoma may infiltrate the submucosa and thicken the folds. Lymphoma rarely involves the esophagus directly and is virtually never primary in the esophagus.

Varicoid carcinoma causes thick, tortuous, longitudinal folds that resemble varices but are rigid and persistent.

MASS LESIONS/FILLING DEFECTS

Pharyngeal carcinomas are well demonstrated by double-contrast pharyngography. Barium studies may detect tumors difficult to visualize endoscopically. Radiographic signs include *a)* intraluminal mass seen as a filling defect, abnormal luminal contour, or focal increased density; *b)* mucosal irregularity owing to ulceration or mucosal elevations, and *c)* asymmetrical distensibility due to infiltrating tumor or extrinsic nodal mass. Most pharyngeal tumors are squamous cell carcinomas that may arise on the base of the tongue, palatine tonsil, posterior pharyngeal wall, or the piriform sinus. Laryngeal tumors may impress on the pharynx or extend into it. Staging is best performed by CT or MR.

Lymphoma of the pharynx is usually manifest as a large, bulky tumor of the lingual or palatine tonsils. Lymphoma constitutes 15% of oropharyngeal tumors.

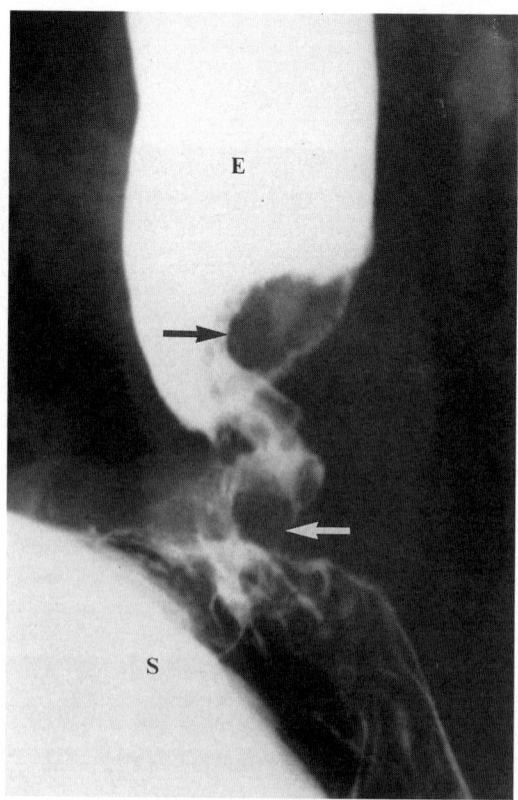

Figure 29.20. Adenocarcinoma in Barrett's Esophagus. A tumor in the distal esophagus (*E*) forms nodular (*arrows*) narrowing of the barium column. Endoscopy confirmed adenocarcinoma arising in Barrett's esophagus. *S*, stomach.

mediastinal lymph nodes and the liver. Obliteration of the fat space between the aorta, esophagus, and vertebral body is highly predictive of invasion of the aorta.

Gastric adenocarcinoma spreads from the fundus and GEJ into the distal esophagus. Adenocarcinoma of the distal esophagus may be either primary gastric or primary esophageal, arising in Barrett's esophagus.

Leiomyoma is the most common benign neoplasm of the esophagus. It is a firm, well-encapsulated tumor that arises in the wall. Ulceration is rare in the esophagus. Most are asymptomatic and discovered incidentally. Men

aged 25–35 years are affected most commonly (male-to-female ratio = 2 : 1). On UGI, most appear as smooth, well-defined wall lesions, although rarely they may be pedunculated or polypoid. Coarse calcifications are occasionally present and strongly indicative of leiomyoma. CT demonstrates a smooth, well-defined mass of uniform soft tissue density. The esophageal wall is eccentrically thickened. Leiomyosarcoma of the esophagus is exceedingly rare, accounting for less than 1% of esophageal malignancy.

Polyp. Fibroepithelial or fibrovascular polyps are a rare cause of esophageal filling defect. They appear as large ovoid or elongated intraluminal masses in the upper esophagus.

Extrinsic lesions may invade the esophagus or simulate an esophageal mass or filling defect. Causes include mediastinal adenopathy, lung carcinoma, and vascular structures.

Aberrant right subclavian artery arises from the aorta distal to the left subclavian artery. To reach its destination, it must cross the mediastinum behind the esophagus. It causes a characteristic upward-slanting linear filling defect on the posterior aspect of the esophagus (Fig. 29.22).

ESOPHAGEAL PERFORATION AND TRAUMA

Esophageal perforation is life-threatening event requiring prompt diagnosis and treatment. More than half the cases are related to esophageal instrumentation. Bleeding can be profuse, and infection is a great risk. Plain films demonstrate subcutaneous, cervical, or mediastinal emphysema within 1 hour of perforation. Chest radiographs may show a widened mediastinum and pleural effusion or hydropneumothorax. Contrast stud-

Table 29.2. Staging of Esophageal Carcinoma

Traditional Staging	TMN Staging[a]	Description
0	Tis	Carcinoma in situ
1	T1	Tumor invades lamina propria or submucosa
IIA	T2	Tumor invades muscularis propria
	T3	Tumor invades adventitia
IIB	T1, N1	Tumor invades lamina propria or submucosa + regional node metastases
	T2, N1	Tumor invades muscularis propria + regional node metastases
III	T3, N1	Tumor invades adventitia + regional node metastases
	T4	Tumor invades adjacent structures
IV	Any T, M1	Distant metastases
	N0	No regional node metastases
	N1	Regional node metastases
	M0	No distant metastases
	M1	Distant metastases

[a] American Joint Committee TNM Stating System for Esophageal Cancer (17).

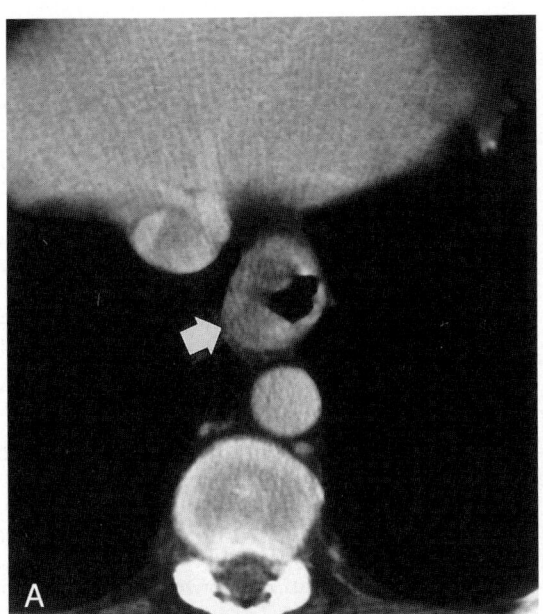
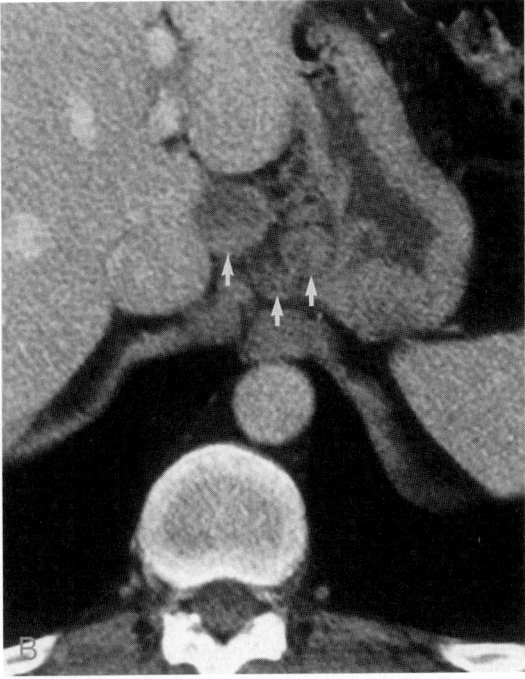

Figure 29.21. Esophageal Carcinoma. CT image of the distal esophagus **(A)** demonstrates eccentric thickening of the wall as a result of tumor. CT image just below the level of the gastroe-sophageal junction **(B)** in the same patient reveals enlarged lymph nodes in the gastrohepatic ligament because of metastases.

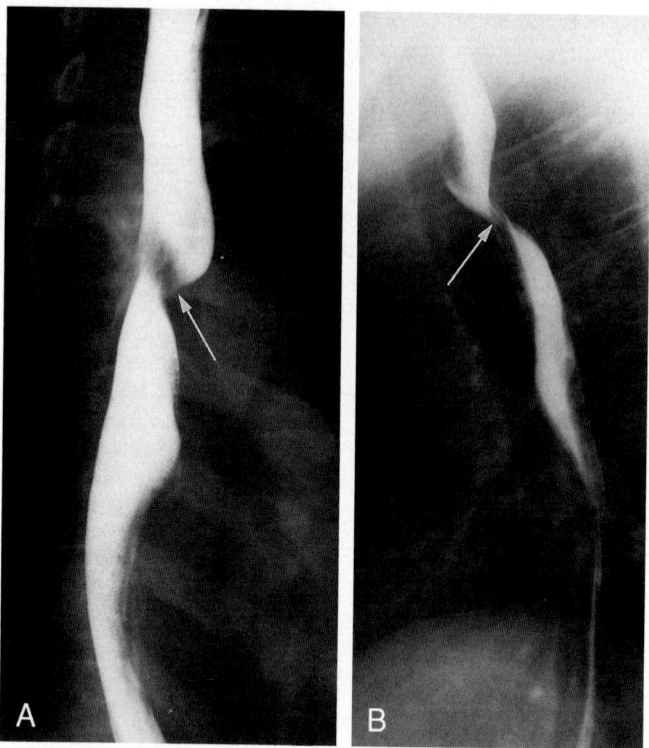

Figure 29.22. Aberrant Right Subclavian Artery. An aberrant right subclavian artery arising from the aortic arch distal to the left subclavian artery crosses behind the esophagus, causing a tubular extrinsic impression (*arrows*) on the esophagus. **A.** frontal view. **B.** lateral view.

ies should be performed with low-osmolar water-soluble agents to avoid the possibility of barium leakage into the mediastinum inciting an inflammatory reaction. The key finding is focal or diffuse extravasation of contrast outside the esophagus.

Trauma. Endoscopy, esophageal dilation procedures, or any type of instrumentation may perforate the esophageal wall. Knife and bullet wounds may perforate the esophagus. Blunt trauma may tear the esophagus by an explosive increase in intraesophageal pressure.

Boerhaave's syndrome refers to rupture of the esophageal wall as a result of forceful vomiting. The tear is virtually always in the left posterior wall near the left crus of the diaphragm. Esophageal contents usually escape into the left pleural space or into the potential space between the parietal pleura and left crus.

Mallory-Weiss tear involves only the mucosa and not the full thickness of the esophagus. The tears are usually caused by violent retching. Although endoscopy usually identifies the lesion, it is commonly missed on UGI. When seen, the tear appears as a longitudinally oriented barium collection, 1–4 cm in length, in the distal esophagus. It may be a cause of copious hematemesis.

Foreign body impaction in adults is usually attributable to bones or boluses of meat. Children may ingest any foreign object including toys, coins, and jewelry. Bones usually lodge in the pharynx, most often near the cricopharyngeus muscle. Meat impacts in the distal or midesophagus. Perforation occurs in only 1% of cases, but the risk increases if impaction persists more than 24 hours. Bones in the pharynx are difficult to differentiate from calcification of the thyroid and cricoid cartilages. Contrast studies show nonopaque foreign bodies as filling defects. Impacted foreign bodies may be removed by use of a Foley balloon catheter or wire basket or by gaseous distension of the esophagus with gas-producing crystals.

References

1. Ott DJ, Pikna LA. Clinical and videofluoroscopic evaluation of swallowing disorders. AJR Am J Roentgenol 1993;161: 507–513.
2. Rubesin SE, Jones B, Donner MW. Contrast pharyngography: the importance of phonation. AJR Am J Roentgenol 1987;148:269–272.
3. Donner MW, Bosma JF, Robertson DL. Anatomy and physiology of the pharynx. Gastrointest Radiol 1985;10: 196–212.
4. Rubesin SE, Rabischong P, Bilanuiuk LT, et al. Contrast examination of the soft palate with cross sectional correlation. Radiographics 1988;8:641–665.
5. Rubesin SE, Jessurun J, Robertson D, et al. Lines of the pharynx. Radiographics 1987;7:217–237.
6. Noh HM, Fishman EK, Forastiere AA, et al. CT of the esophagus: spectrum of disease with emphasis on esophageal carcinoma. Radiographics 1995;15:1113–1134.
7. Ott DJ, Gelfand DW, Wu WC, et al. Esophagogastric region and its rings. AJR Am J Roentgenol 1984;142:281–287.
8. Dodds WJ, Stewart ET, Longemann JA. Physiology and radiology of the normal oral and pharyngeal phases of swallowing. AJR Am J Roentgenol 1990;154:953–963.
9. Dodds WJ, Logemann JA, Stewart ET. Radiologic assessment of abnormal oral and pharyngeal phases of swallowing. AJR Am J Roentgenol 1990;154:965–974.

10. Ott DJ, Chen YM, Hewson EG, et al. Esophageal motility: assessment with synchronous video tape fluoroscopy and manometry. Radiology 1989;173:419–422.

11. Frederick MG, Ott DJ, Grishaw EK, et al. Functional abnormalities of the pharynx: a prospective analysis of radiographic abnormalities relative to age and symptoms. AJR Am J Roentgenol 1996;166:353–357.

12. Jones B, Donner MW. Examination of the patient with dysphagia. Radiology 1988;167:319–326.

13. Ott DJ. Gastroesophageal reflux: what is the role of barium studies? AJR Am J Roentgenol 1994;162:627–629.

14. Levine MS. Radiology of esophagitis: a pattern approach. Radiology 1991;179:1–7.

15. Levine MS. Barrett's esophagus: a radiologic diagnosis? AJR Am J Roentgenol 1988;151:433–438.

16. Karasick S, Lev-Toaff AS. Esophageal strictures: findings on barium radiographs. AJR Am J Roentgenol 1995;165:561–565.

17. American Joint Committee on Cancer. Manual for Staging of Cancer. 4th ed. Philadelphia: JB Lippincott Co, 1992.

18. Vilgrain V, Mompoint D, Palazzo L, et al. Staging of esophageal carcinoma: comparison of results with endoscopic sonography and CT. AJR Am J Roentgenol 1990;155:277–281.

30
Stomach and Duodenum

William E. Brant

Imaging Methods

The upper gastrointestinal (UGI) series is the standard radiographic method of examination of the stomach and duodenum. However, to attain a high sensitivity for the examination and to avoid missing significant pathology, multiple techniques must be used for the UGI (1). The single-contrast technique of filling and distending the stomach and duodenum with barium suspension is one such technique. It is usually supplemented by compression procedures effective in demonstrating abnormalities of the distal stomach and duodenum. Mucosal relief technique, which entails using small amounts of barium to coat the mucosa without distending the bowel, is useful in demonstrating abnormalities such as varices. Double-contrast technique, using high-density barium suspensions to coat the mucosa and ingestible effervescent granules to distend the organ, is optimal for demonstration of subtle features of the mucosal surface. As with any radiographic examination, attention to detail and tailoring the examination for the clinical problem is essential in producing good results.

CT, with use of spiral and air-contrast distention techniques, is a valuable adjunct to barium studies and endoscopy for abnormalities of the stomach wall and duodenum. CT can also help determine the extent of extraluminal disease (2). Optimal distension of the stomach and duodenum is mandatory for accurate CT interpretation. Gastric and duodenal distension may be attained by filling the organs with positive contrast agents or using effervescent granules to cause gaseous distension. The patient is positioned to optimize distension of the GI tract portion of greatest interest.

Anatomy

The GI tract is essentially a hollow tube consisting of four concentric layers of tissue (Fig. 30.1). The inner-most layer exposed to the lumen is the *mucosa*. The mucosa consists of epithelium supported by loose connective tissue of the lamina propria and a thin band of smooth muscle called the muscularis mucosae. The *submucosa* provides connective tissue support for the mucosa. The submucosa contains the primary vascular and lymphatic channels, lymphoid follicles, and autonomic nerve plexuses. The major muscular structure of the bowel wall is the *muscularis propria*, comprised of inner circular and outer longitudinal layers. The *serosa* or adventitia is the outer covering of the bowel. Lymphoid tissue in the GI tract is located in the mucosa (epithelium and lamina propria), the submucosa, and the mesenteric lymph nodes. As the major component of the mucosa-associated lymphoid tissue (MALT), lymphoid tissue plays a major role in host immune defenses and is a site of significant disease (3).

The appearance and position of the stomach and duodenum vary considerably from one individual to another. The terms used to describe the anatomic divisions of the stomach and duodenum are illustrated in Fig. 30.2. *Cardia* refers to the region of the gastroesophageal junction (GEJ). The *fundus* is that portion of the stomach above the level of the GEJ. The *body* of the stomach is the central two-thirds portion from the cardia to the *incisura angularis*. The incisura angularis is an acute angle formed on the lesser curvature that marks the boundary between the body and the antrum. The parietal cells, which produce hydrochloric acid, and the chief cells, which produce pepsin precursors, are located in the fundus and body. The *antrum* is the distal one-third of the stomach, and contains gastrin-producing cells but no acid-secreting cells.

The *pylorus* is the junction of the stomach with the duodenum, and the pyloric canal is the channel through the pylorus. The *duodenal bulb*, or cap, is the pyramidal first portion of the duodenum. The gallbladder frequently makes a prominant impression on the top of the bulb. The duodenum bulb, like the stomach, is covered on all surfaces by visceral peritoneum. The remainder of the duodenum is retroperitoneal and within the anterior pararenal compartment.

The second or descending portion of the duodenum is lateral to the head of the pancreas. The common bile duct and pancreatic duct pierce the medial aspect of the descending duodenum at the ampulla of Vater. The third or horizontal portion of the duodenum passes to the left between the superior mesenteric vessels and the inferior vena cava and aorta. The fourth or ascending portion of the duodenum ascends on the left side of the aorta to the level of L-2 and the ligament of Treitz, where its turns abruptly ventrally to form the duodenal-jejunal flexure.

The term "areae gastricae" refers to the detailed pattern of the gastric mucosa as demonstrated by double-

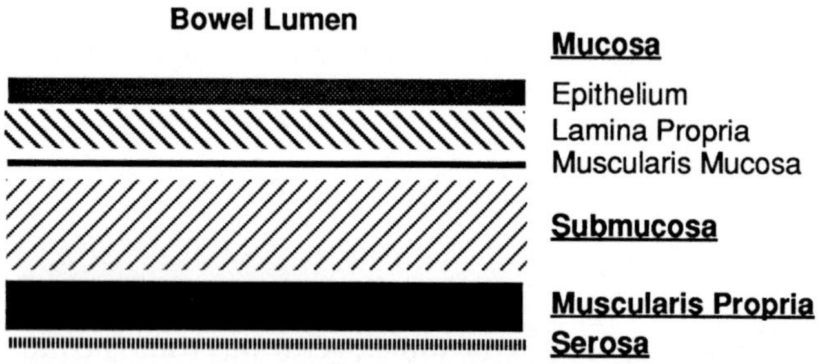

Bowel Lumen

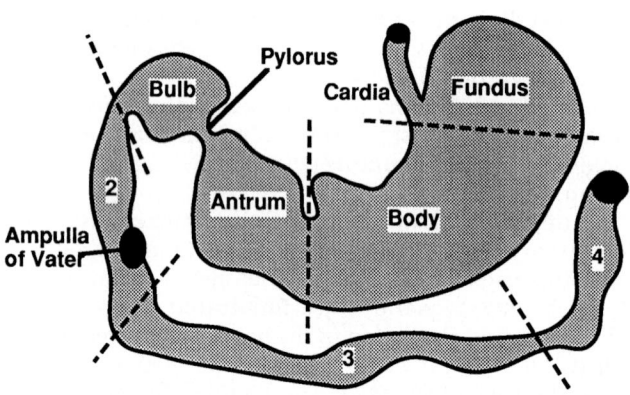

Figure 30.1. Layers of the Bowel Wall. The mucosa consists of three layers in close proximity to the bowel lumen. The submucosa consists of connective tissue, blood vessels, lymphatic channels and follicles, and autonomic nerve plexuses. The muscularis propria is the muscle layer responsible for peristalsis. The serosa is the outer covering layer.

Figure 30.2. Anatomy of UGI Tract. The stomach is divided anatomically into fundus, body, and antrum. The pylorus serves as a valve that separates the stomach and duodenum. The bile and pancreatic ducts empty into the duodenum at the ampulla of Vater. The duodenum is divided into bulb (or cap), descending (*2*), transverse (*3*), and ascending (*4*) portions.

contrast technique (Fig. 30.3). Normal areae gastricae varies from a fine reticular pattern to a course nodular pattern. The hallmark of normal is the regularity of the pattern in all areas in which it is visualized. The term "rugae" refers to the gastric mucosal folds that produce distinct radiolucent ridges when the stomach is partially distended. Rugae are composed of mucosa, the lamina propria, the muscularis mucosae, and portions of the submucosa. Disease in any of these structures may cause thickening of the gastric folds.

The lesser curvature of the stomach is attached to the liver by the lesser omentum. The greater omentum attaches to the greater curvature of the stomach. The lesser sac is the intraperitoneal space posterior to the stomach and anterior to the pancreas.

On CT the normal gastric wall does not exceed 5 mm thick, and the normal duodenal wall is less than 3 mm thick. Both organs must be fully distended to accurately assess wall thickness. A prominent pseudotumor, caused by inadequate distension, is often seen on CT near the GEJ (4).

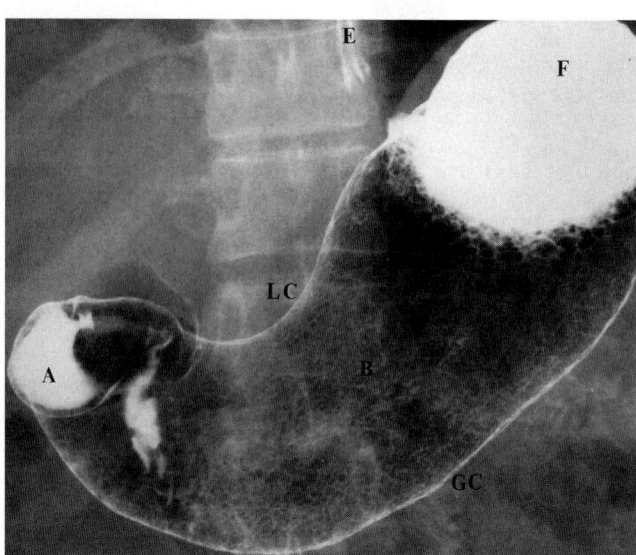

Figure 30.3. Normal Stomach. Double-contrast technique provides distension of the stomach with coating of its mucosa to demonstrate normal areae gastricae in the body (*B*) and antrum (*A*). *E*, esophagus. *F*, fundus. *LC*, lesser curvature. *GC*, greater curvature.

STOMACH

Helicobacter pylori Infection

In the past few years, *H. pylori* infection has been identified as the major cause of chronic gastritis, duodenitis, benign gastric and duodenal ulcers, gastric adenocarcinoma, and gastric lymphoma (5,6). *H. pylori* is a gram-negative spiral bacillus that colonizes the stomachs of as much as 80% of some populations. It will infect only gastric-like epithelium and is usually localized to the gastric antrum, living on surface epithelial cells beneath the mucous coat. It survives in gastric acid by using a powerful urease enzyme to break down urea into ammonia and bicarbonate, creating a more alkaline environment for itself. The prevalence of infection increases with age (>50% of Americans older than age 60) and in lower socioeconomic populations and in developing countries. Infection is chronic and causes a superficial gastritis, which is most commonly asymptomatic. Approximately 70% of peptic gastric ulcers, 95% of duodenal ulcers, and 50% of gastric adenocarcinoma are caused by this infection. Diagnosis of *H. pylori* infection is made by serology, urea breath tests, and endoscopic biopsy. Treatment is usually a combination of two to four drugs including one or more antibiotics (tetracycline, amoxicillin, metronidazole, clarithromycin), H$_2$ blockers to decrease acid secretion (omeprazole, lansoprazole, ranitidine), and occasionally a bismuth compound (Pepto-Bismol). Cure rates of 90% are reported although antibiotic resistance is emerging. Although spontaneous elimination of infection is rare, treatment of asymptomatic infected individuals is not currently recommended.

Gastric Filling Defects/Mass Lesions

Gastric Carcinoma is the third most common GI malignancy, following colon and pancreatic carcinoma. Most (95%) are adenocarcinomas; the remainder are diffuse anaplastic (signet-ring) carcinoma, squamous cell carcinoma, or rare cell types. Predisposing factors include smoking, pernicious anemia, atrophic gastritis, and gastrojejunostomy. *H. pylori* infection increases the risk of gastric carcinoma sixfold and is the cause of approximately half of gastric adenocarcinoma cases (7). Peak age is from 50–70 years with males predominating 2:1. The incidence of gastric carcinoma is as much as five times higher in Japan, Finland, Chile, and Iceland than in the United States. Mortality is high with a 5-year survival rate of 10–20%.

The tumor assumes four common morphologic growth patterns. One-third are polypoid masses that present as filling defects within the gastric lumen (Fig. 30.4). Many of these are broad-based and papillary in configuration. Another third are ulcerative masses presenting as malignant gastric ulcers. The remainder are infiltrating (Fig. 30.5), presenting as scirrhous carcinomas (15%), or superficial spreading, producing plaque-like tumors or bizarre thickened folds. Scirrhous carcinoma is characterized by diffuse infiltration of the gastric wall by poorly differentiated or undifferentiated carcinomatous cells (8). The wall of the stomach is thickened and rigid. The terms "linitis plastica" and "water-bottle stomach" may be applied to describe the resulting stiff narrowed stomach (Fig. 30.6). Additional causes of narrowed stomach are listed in Table 30.1.

Superficial spreading carcinoma spreads through the mucosa and submucosa producing nodular thickening or superficial mucosal ulceration. Intraluminal mass effect is minimal; however, the involved areas are thickened and rigid and involved rugae are thickened and distorted. Cancers are most common near the cardia (44%), in the antrum, and along the lesser curvature.

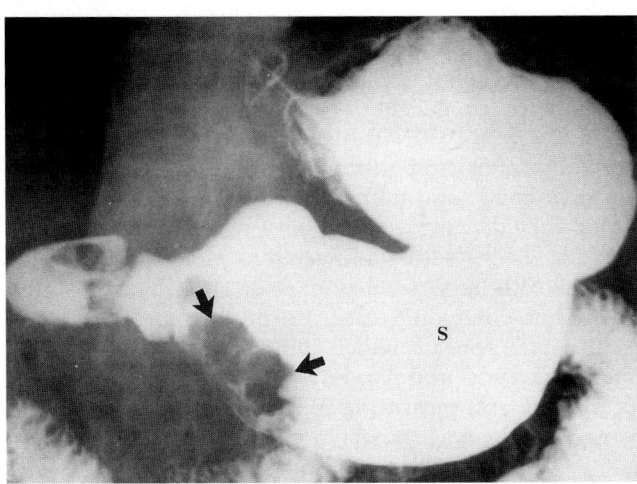

Figure 30.4. Polypoid Gastric Carcinoma. Single-contrast technique UGI series reveals a lobulated filling defect (*arrows*) in the antrum of the stomach (*S*).

Table 30.1. Narrowed Stomach

Neoplastic
Gastric adenocarcinoma (linitis plastica)
Lymphoma (antral narrowing + extension into duodenum)
Metastases (linitis plastica due to breast carcinoma)
Kaposi's sarcoma (AIDS)
Inflammatory
H. pylori gastritis (usually antral narrowing)
Corrosive ingestion (usually acid)
Radiotherapy (after 4500 rads)
AIDS (*Cryptosporidium* infection) (narrowed antrum + small bowel involvement)
Eosinophilic gastroenteritis (narrowing + wall thickening)
Infection (tuberculosis + syphilis—both rare)
Crohn's disease (rare)
Sarcoidosis (usually asymptomatic)
Extrinsic compression
Pancreatitis
Pancreatic carcinoma
Omental cake

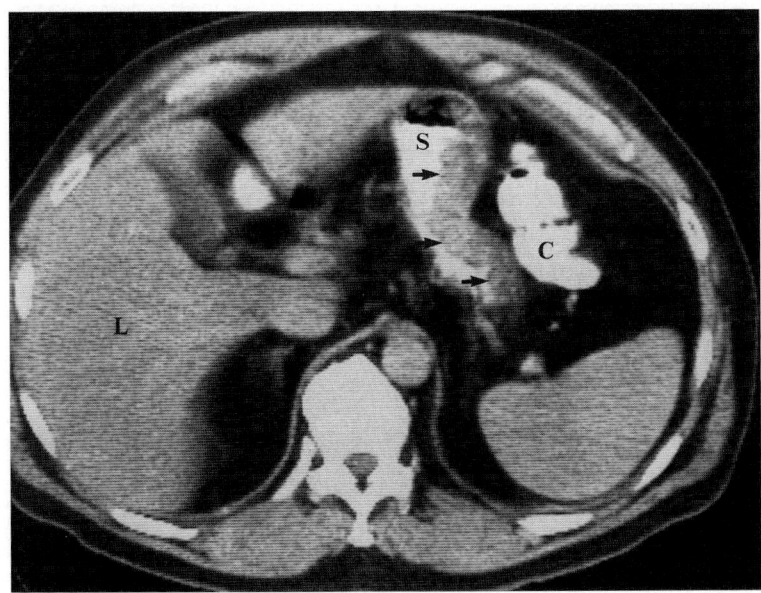

Figure 30.5. Scirrhous Carcinoma. CT demonstrates fixed nodular thickening (*arrows*) of the lateral wall of the stomach (*S*) caused by gastric adenocarcinoma. The outer margin of the stomach is well defined, giving evidence against extension of tumor through the wall. The CT also evaluates the liver (*L*) and regional lymph nodes for evidence of metastatic disease. *C*, splenic flexure of the colon.

The tumor spreads by direct invasion through the gastric wall to involve perigastric fat and adjacent organs, or it may seed the peritoneal cavity. Lymphatic spread is to regional lymph nodes including perigastric nodes along the lesser curvature, celiac axis, and hepatoduodenal, retropancreatic, mesenteric, and para-aortic nodes. Hematogenous metastases involve the liver, adrenal glands, ovaries, and, rarely, bone and lung. Intraperitoneal seeding presents as carcinomatosis or Kruckenberg ovarian tumors.

Early gastric cancers appear on barium studies as: *a)* gastric polyps with risk of malignancy increased for lesions larger than 1 cm (Fig. 30.4), *b)* superficial plaque-like lesions or nodular mucosa, and *c)* shallow, irregular ulcers with nodular adjacent mucosa. These lesions are most sensitively detected on double contrast studies (1).

CT is used to determine the extent of tumor to facilitate preoperative planning (Fig. 30.5). Transmural extension, intraperitoneal spread, or distant metastases limit treatment to palliative surgery or chemotherapy. Findings include *a)* focal, often irregular, wall thickening; *b)* diffuse wall thickening due to tumor infiltration (linitis plastica)(contrast enhancement is common); *c)* intraluminal soft tissue mass; *d)* bulky mass with ulceration; *e)* rare, large, exophytic tumor resembling leiomyosarcoma; *f)* extension of tumor into perigastric fat; *g)* regional lymphadenopathy; and *h)* metastases in the liver, adrenal, and peritoneal cavity. Mucinous adenocarcinomas frequently contain stippled calcifications.

Lymphoma accounts for 2% of gastric neoplasms. The stomach is the most common site of involvement of primary GI lymphoma, accounting for approximately 50% of cases (3). Most (80%) gastric lymphoma is non-Hodgkin's, currently classified as high-grade large cell or immunoblastic type. Chronic infection of the gastric epithelium with *H. pylori* is associated with risk of developing gastric lymphoma. Because lymphoma remains confined to the bowel wall for prolonged periods of time, it has a better prognosis than carcinoma with 5-year survival in the 62–90% range. Lymphoma demonstrates three morphologic patterns: polypoid solitary mass, ulcerative mass, and diffuse infiltration. UGI findings include the following: *a)* polypoid lesions (Fig. 30.7), *b)* irregular ulcers with nodular thickened folds, *c)* bulky tumors with large cavities, *d)* multiple submucosal nodules that commonly ulcerate and create a target or "bull's-eye" appearance, *e)* diffuse but pliable wall and fold thickening, and *f)* rarely, linitis plastica appearance of diffuse, stiff narrowing (9). Multiplicity of lesions favors lymphoma as the diagnosis.

CT findings that are helpful in differentiating gastric lymphoma from carcinoma include *a)* more marked thickening of the wall (may exceed 3 cm) (Fig. 30.8), *b)* in-

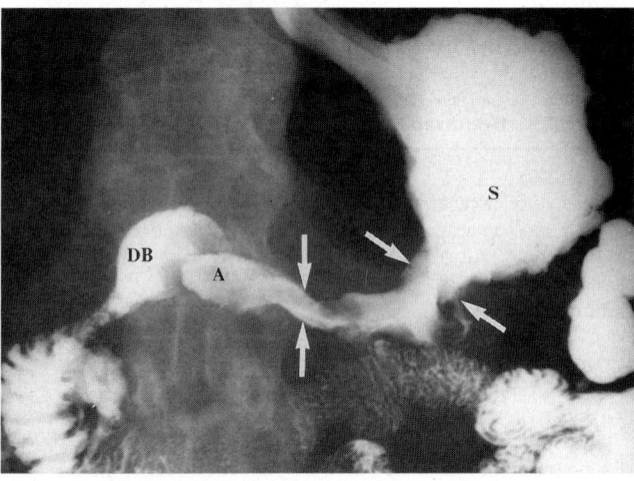

Figure 30.6. Linitis Plastica. Scirrhous gastric carcinoma causes fixed nodular narrowing (*arrows*) of the body and antrum (*A*) of the stomach (*S*). No peristalsis through this portion of the stomach was observed at fluoroscopy. Biopsy yielded undifferentiated adenocarcinoma. *DB*, duodenal bulb.

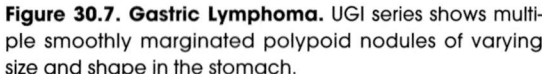

Figure 30.7. Gastric Lymphoma. UGI series shows multiple smoothly marginated polypoid nodules of varying size and shape in the stomach.

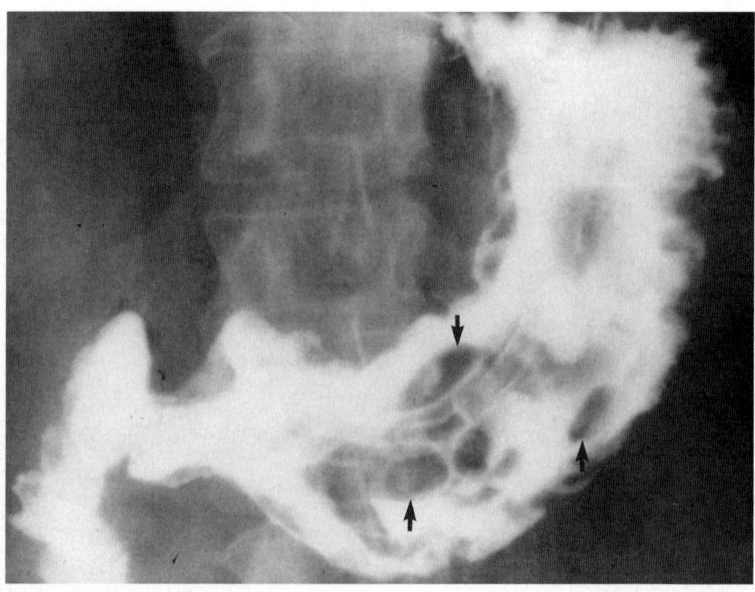

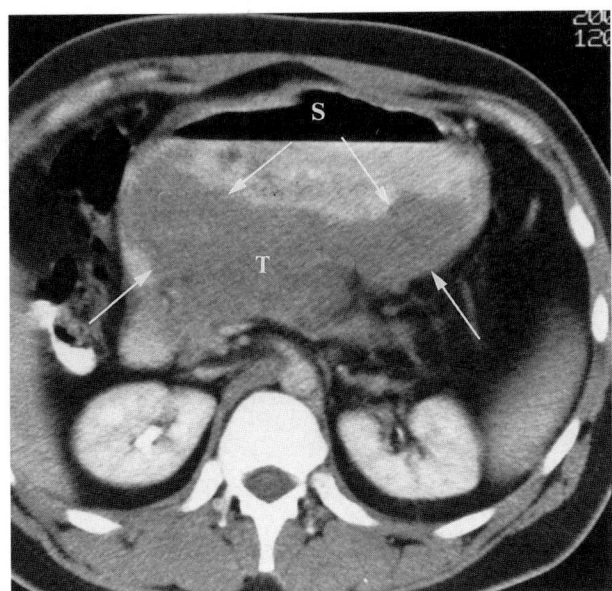

Figure 30.8. Gastric Lymphoma. CT demonstrates marked thickening (*arrows*) of the posterior gastric wall with a homogeneous tumor (*T*) extending into the lumen of the stomach (*S*). Endoscopic biopsy revealed large cell lymphoma.

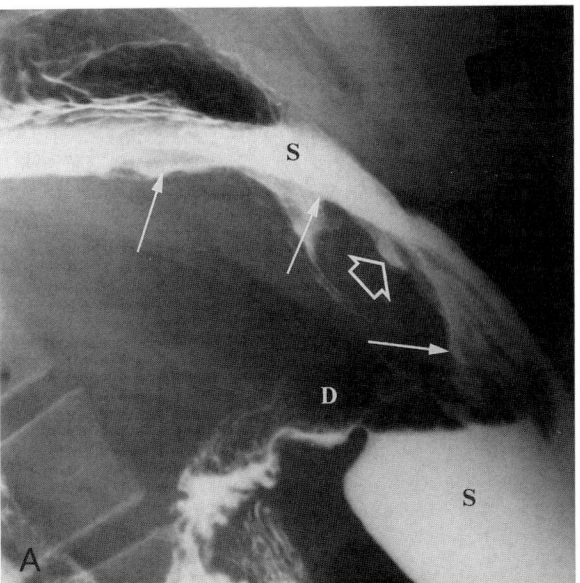

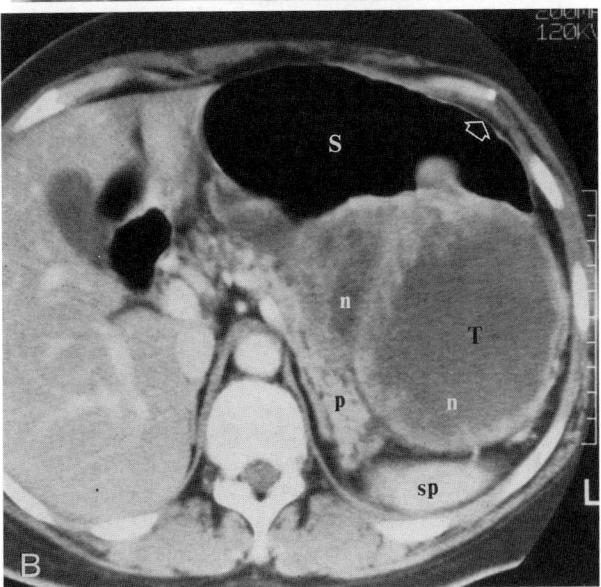

Figure 30.9. Gastric Leiomyosarcoma. A. Radiograph in lateral upright position demonstrates a huge posterior mass distorting the lumen (*arrows*) of the stomach (*S*). An ulcer (*open arrow*) is evident. *D*, duodenal bulb. **B.** CT of the same patient reveals the tumor (*T*) to be heterogeneous with large lucent areas representing necrosis (*n*). Note the thin, normal anterior wall (*open arrow*) of the stomach (*S*). The pancreas (*p*) is compressed against the spine by the mass. *sp*, spleen.

volvement of additional areas of the GI tract, *c*) absence of invasion of the perigastric fat, and *d*) more widespread and bulkier adenopathy.

Leiomyoma and Leiomyosarcoma arise from the smooth muscle of the gastric wall and grow as submucosal, subserosal, or exophytic tumors. Long-term silent growth to a large size is characteristic. The overlying mucosa is ulcerated in half of leiomyoma cases and the majority of leiomyosarcomas (Fig. 30.9). Dystrophic calcification is relatively common in both benign and malignant tumors and helps differentiate these lesions from other gastric tumors. Histologic differentiation of benign from malignant tumors is difficult; the differentiation is based upon size, gross appearance, and behavior of the tumor. On UGI, leiomyomas appear as submucosal nodules. Ulceration causes a bull's-eye appearance and may be responsible for significant bleeding. Leiomyosarcomas are larger submucosal lesions, commonly with single, multiple, or cavitary ulcerations.

CT is useful in characterizing the tumors because they are predominantly extraluminal. Benign tumors are smaller (4–5 cm, average size), are homogeneous in density, and show uniform diffuse enhancement. Malignant tumors tend to be larger (12 cm, average size) with central zones of low density caused by hemorrhage and necrosis (Fig. 30.9B) and show irregular patterns of enhancement.

Metastasis may present as submucosal nodules or ulcerated masses. They are commonly multiple. Common primary tumors are melanoma and breast and lung carcinoma. Breast cancer metastases cause linitis plastica.

Kaposi's Sarcoma, usually found in patients with AIDS, demonstrates a wide spectrum of appearances including polypoid mass, thickened folds, multiple submucosal masses, and linitis plastica.

Villous Tumors are adenomatous polypoid masses that produce multiple frond-like projections. Most are solitary and 3–9 cm in size although giant tumors may be as large as 15 cm. Malignant potential is high and varies with size of the lesion (50% for 2–4 cm lesions, 80% for lesions >4 cm). Barium trapped in the clefts between fronds produces a characteristic soap-bubble appearance. The tumors are mobile and deform with compression. All should be treated as malignant lesions.

Polyps are lesions that protrude into the lumen. Their appearance on double-contrast UGI series depends on whether they are on the dependent or nondependent surface. A polyp on the dependent surface appears as a radiolucent filling defect in the barium pool; a polyp on the nondependent surface is covered with a thin coat of barium (Fig. 30.10). The x-ray beam catches its margin in tangent, resulting in a lesion whose margins are etched in white. The *bowler hat sign* (see Fig. 32.5) is produced by the acute angle of attachment of the polyp to the mucosa. The *Mexican hat sign* consists of two concentric rings and is produced by visualizing a pedunculated polyp end-on.

Hyperplastic polyps account for 80% of gastric polyps. Most are less than 15 mm in diameter. They are not neoplasms, but rather hyperplastic responses to mucosal injury, especially gastritis. They may be located anywhere in the stomach, are frequently multiple (Table 30.2), but have no malignant potential.

Adenomatous polyps account for 15% of gastric polyps and are true neoplasms with malignant potential. Most are solitary, located in the antrum, and are larger than 2 cm in diameter. Polyps that are larger than 1 cm, lobulated, or pedunculated should have biopsies taken of them because of the risk of malignancy.

Hamartomatous polyps occur in Peutz-Jeghers syndrome. They have no malignant potential.

Ectopic Pancreas is a common intramural lesion, usually found in the antrum. Lobules of heterotopic pancreatic tissue, up to 5 cm in size, are covered by gastric mucosa. Most are nipple-shaped or cone-shaped with small central orifices.

Bezoar/Foreign Body. The term "bezoar" refers to an intraluminal gastric mass consisting of accumulated ingested material (Fig. 30.11). Bezoars may be composed of a wide variety of substances: trichobezoars are composed of hair; phytobezoars are composed of fruit or vegetable products. Any ingested foreign body may produce an intraluminal filling defect.

Extrinsic Impression. Masses adjacent to the stomach may produce filling defects. Extrinsic masses on the dependent surface produce ill-defined radiolucencies. The mucosa may be impressed upon by an extrinsic mass and be seen in profile as a white line. Pancreatic, splenic, hepatic, and retroperitoneal masses may impress upon the stomach. CT is excellent for demonstrating the nature of an extrinsic mass impression.

Thickened Gastric Folds/Thickened Wall

Gastric folds are usually considered to be thickened if they exceed 1 cm in the fundus and 5 mm in the antrum.

Normal Variant. Gastric folds are normally most prominent in the fundus and upper third of the greater curvature. Thickened folds, even those larger than 1 cm, in this region are often normal, but they require evaluation to exclude pathology.

Gastritis is a convenient label used to describe a wide variety of diseases affecting the gastric mucosa (10). Most of these diseases are inflammatory. The hallmarks of gastritis are thickened folds and superficial mucosal ulcerations (erosions). The thickened folds are usually caused by mucosal edema and superficial inflammatory infiltrate. *Erosions* are defined as defects in the mucosa that do not penetrate beyond the muscularis mucosae. *Aphthous ulcers* (also called varioliform erosions) are complete erosions that appear as tiny central flecks of barium surrounded by a radiolucent halo of edema (Fig. 30.12). Incomplete erosions appear as linear streaks and dots of barium. Erosions heal without scarring. Barium

Table 30.2. Multiple Gastric Filling Defects

Hyperplastic polyps
Adenomatous polyps (especially with polyposis syndromes)
Metastases
Lymphoma
Varices

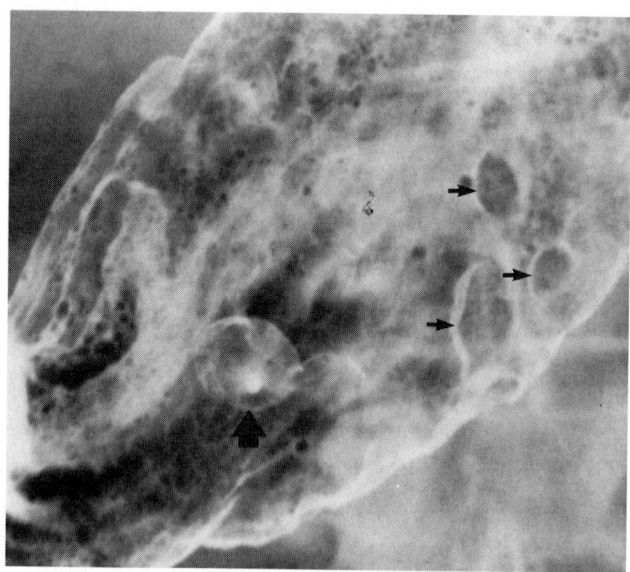

Figure 30.10. Benign Gastric Polyp. A polyp (*large arrow*) on the nondependent surface of the stomach is etched in white because it is coated with barium and suspended in the air-distended stomach. This polyp was benign at biopsy. Additional filling defects (*small arrows*) proved to be normal gastric folds.

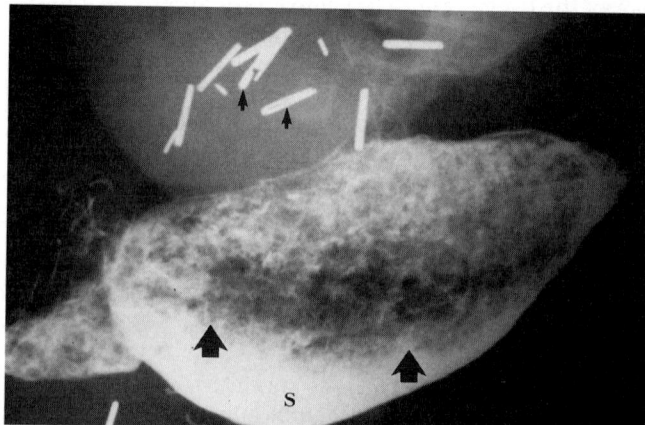

Figure 30.11. Bezoar. UGI series reveals an irregular mottled mass (*large arrows*) floating in the lumen of the stomach (*S*). The mass is composed of retained food fibers in this patient with poor gastric emptying due to scleroderma and multiple gastric surgeries. Numerous surgical clips (*small arrows*) are evident.

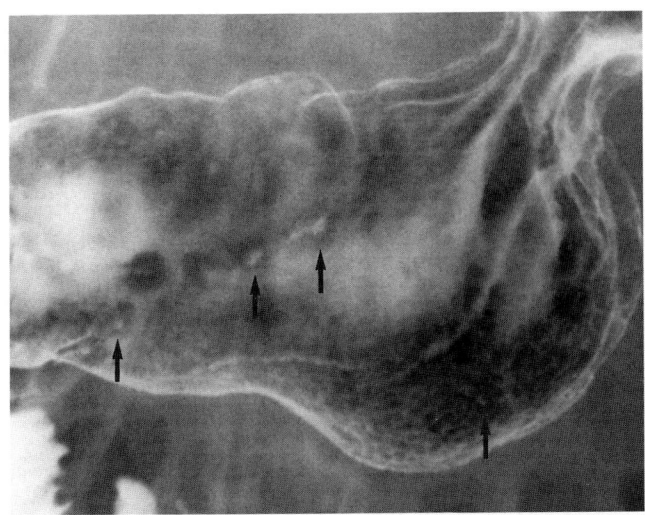

Figure 30.12. Erosions: Aphthous Ulcers. Film from an air-contrast UGI series demonstrates multiple aphthous ulcers seen as spots of dense barium surrounded by a lucent halo (*arrows*). Aphthous ulcers are superficial mucosal erosions that do not penetrate the muscularis mucosae. (Case courtesy of C. John Rosenquist, MD, University of California, Davis.)

precipitates may mimic erosions, appearing as distinct punctate barium spots but without the distinctive radiolucent halo of a true erosion.

Helicobacter pylori gastritis is the most common form of gastritis (5,6). Although most people who are infected with *H. pylori* are asymptomatic, most have gastritis endoscopically and pathologically. Almost all patients with benign gastric and duodenal ulcers have *H. pylori* gastritis. UGI findings of *H. pylori* gastritis include: *a)* thickening (<5 mm) of gastric folds, *b)* nodular folds, *c)* erosions, *d)* antral narrowing, *e)* inflammatory polyps, *f)* antral narrowing, and *g)* enlarged areae gastricae (11).

Acute erosive gastritis is caused by alcohol, aspirin and other nonsteroidal antiinflammatory agents, steroids, reflux of biliary or pancreatic secretions, and infection with herpes simplex, cytomegalovirus, or *Candida*. Double-contrast UGI findings include the following: *a)* erosions, *b)* thickened, nodular folds in the antrum, *c)* limited distensibility of the antrum, *d)* stiffness and limited peristalsis.

Crohn's gastritis characteristically involves the gastric antrum and proximal duodenum. Early stage disease manifests as apthous ulcers identical to those seen with erosive gastritis. More advanced disease shows antral narrowing, wall thickening, and fistulas.

Atrophic gastritis is a chronic autoimmune disease that destroys the fundic mucosa but spares the antral mucosa (10). Destruction of parietal cells results in decreased acid and intrinsic factor production that leads to vitamin B_{12} deficiency and pernicious anemia. Antibodies to parietal cells and intrinsic factors are found in peripheral blood samples. Characteristic UGI findings are as follows: *a)* decreased or absent folds in the fundus and body ("bald fundus"), *b)* narrowed, tube-shaped stomach (fundal diameter <8 cm), and *c)* small (1–2 mm) or absent areae gasricae.

Phlegmonous gastritis is an acute, often fatal, bacterial infection of the stomach. α-Hemolytic streptococci are the most common cause, but a variety of other bacteria have also been identified. It may arise as a complication of septicemia, gastric surgery, or gastric ulcers. Multiple abscesses are formed in the gastric wall, which is markedly thickened. The rugae are swollen. Barium may penetrate into abscess crypts in the gastric wall. Peritonitis develops in 70% of cases. Healing usually results in a severely contracted stomach.

Emphysematous gastritis is a form of phlegmonous gastritis caused by gas-producing organisms, usually *Escherichia coli* or *Clostridium welchii*. Most cases are caused by caustic ingestion, surgery, trauma, or ischemia. Multiple gas bubbles are apparent within the wall of the stomach.

Eosinophilic gastroenteritis is a diffuse infiltration of the wall of the stomach and small bowel by eosinophils. Any or all layers of the wall may be involved. The condition is associated with a peripheral eosinophilia as high as 60%. Initially, the folds are markedly thickened and nodular, especially in the antrum. When chronic, the antrum is narrowed with a nodular "cobblestone" mucosal pattern.

Ménétrier's disease, also called giant hypertrophic gastritis, is a rare condition characterized by excessive mucus production, giant mucosal hypertrophy, hypoproteinemia, and hypochlorhydria. UGI findings are as follows: *a)* markedly enlarged and tortuous but pliable folds in the fundus and body with antrum sparing (Fig. 30.13) and *b)* hypersecretion that has diluted the barium and impaired mucosal coating. CT exhibits wall thickening and nodular thick folds.

Varices appear as smooth, lobulated filling defects resembling thickened folds. They are most common in the fundus and usually accompany esophageal varices. Isolated gastric varices may occur with splenic vein occlusion.

CT with bolus contrast enhancement is an excellent method for confirming the presence of gastric varices (Fig. 30.14) as well as demonstrating their cause.

Neoplasm. Lymphoma and superfical spreading gastric carcinoma may produce distorted rigid gastric folds that are commonly ulcerated and appear nodular. The distal stomach is the most common location for neoplasms.

Gastric Ulcers

An ulcer is defined as a full-thickness defect in the mucosa. It frequently extends to the deeper layers of the stomach, including the submucosa and muscularis propria. About 95% of ulcerating gastric lesions are benign. All gastric ulcers should be examined endoscopically or be followed to complete radiographic healing.

Signs of an ulcer as demonstrated by a double-contrast UGI series include *a)* a barium-filled crater on the dependent wall (Fig. 30.15), *b)* a ring shadow due to barium coating the edge of the crater on the nondependent wall, *c)* a double ring shadow if the base of the ulcer is broader than the neck, and *d)* a crescentic or semilunar line when the ulcer is seen on tangent oblique view.

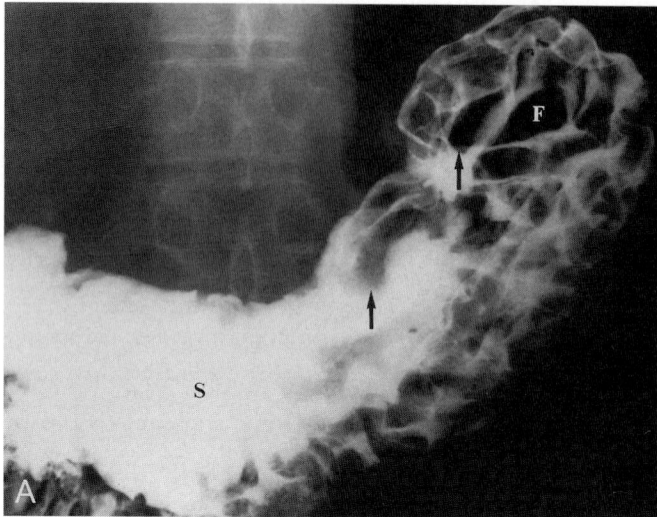

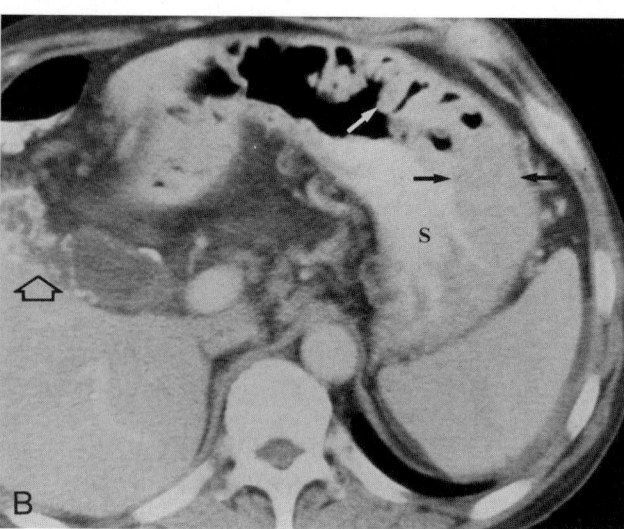

Figure 30.13. Ménétrièr's Disease. A. UGI series reveals marked thickening of the mucosal folds (*arrows*) in the fundus (*F*) and proximal body of the stomach (*S*). **B.** A CT scan of the same patient confirms the marked thickening of the folds (*arrows*) of the stomach (*S*). This patient also has calcification of the wall of the gallbladder (*open arrow*).

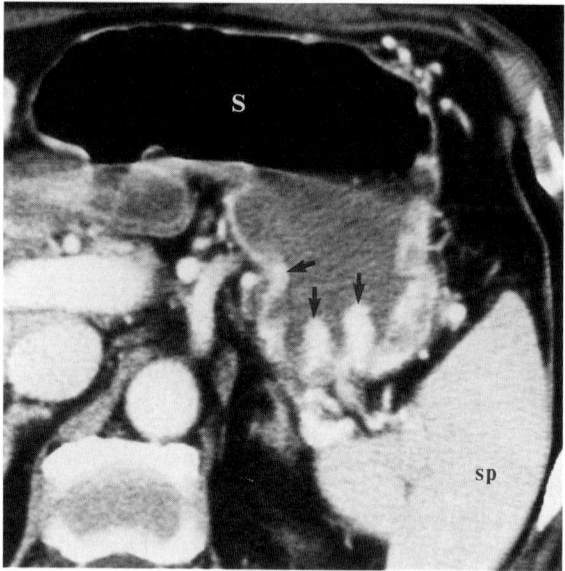

Figure 30.14. Gastric Varices. Helical CT with bolus intravenous contrast reveals markedly enhancing varices (*arrows*) protruding into the gastric lumen. *S*, stomach; *sp*, spleen.

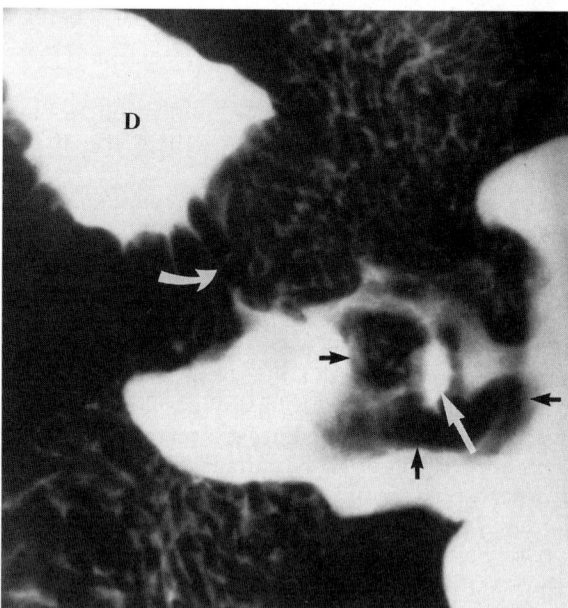

Figure 30.15. Benign Gastric Ulcer. Spot film from a UGI demonstrates a benign gastric ulcer (*straight white arrow*) in the antrum. Prominent, nodular folds (*black arrows*) surround the ulcer crater. The normal contracted pyloric channel (*curved white arrow*) is seen as a thin line of barium. *D*, normal distended duodenal bulb.

Some ulcers may be linear or rod-shaped. Ulcers are multiple in about 20% of patients.

Peptic Ulcer Disease. Benign gastric ulcers are caused by *H. pylori* infection (70%) and by nonsteroidal antiinflammatory medications (30%) (5). Duodenal ulcers are usually associated with increased production of acid although patients with gastric ulcers may have normal or even decreased acid levels. However, hydrochloric acid must be present for peptic ulceration to occur. Patients usually present with aching or burning pain within several hours after eating. Some patients with ulcers may be asymptomatic. The major complications of peptic ulcer disease are bleeding, obstruction, and per-

foration. Bleeding occurs in 15–20% of patients and is manifest by melena, hematemesis, or hematochezia. Gastric outlet obstruction complicates approximately 5% of cases. Ulcers may perforate into the free abdominal cavity or penetrate into adjacent organs. Free perforations usually present with an acute abdomen. Ulcer penetration into an adjacent organ is usually heralded by a marked increase in abdominal pain.

Benign Ulcers. The hallmark of benign ulcers and the basis for most radiographic signs of benignancy is mucosa that is intact to the very edge of an undermining ul-

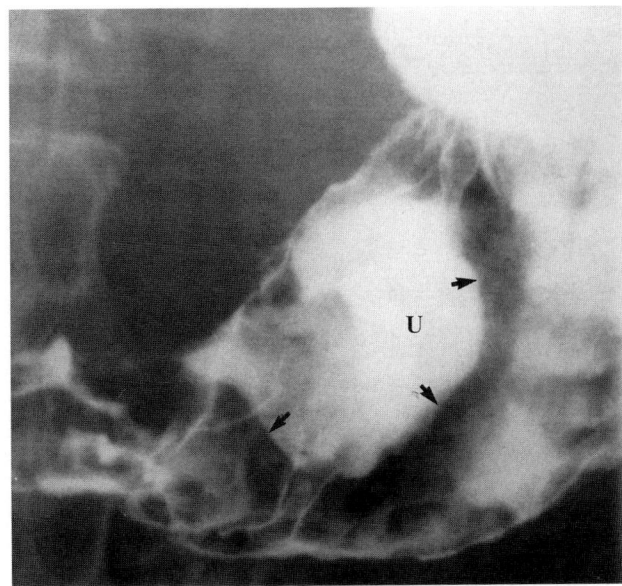

Figure 30.16. Carmen Meniscus Sign. A large, flat malignant ulcer (*U*) traps barium within its rounded edges, seen as a band of lucency (*arrows*) surrounding the barium collection. The barium collection is convex toward the gastric lumen.

cer crater. However, it should be recognized that even if the ulcers are radiographically "benign," as many as 3% will actually be malignant. Demonstration of complete and sustained healing is considered the only reliable radiographic evidence of benign ulcer. Signs of benignancy include *a*) a smooth ulcer mound with tapering edges, *b*) an edematous ulcer collar with overhanging mucosal edge, *c*) an ulcer projecting beyond the expected lumen, *d*) radiating folds extending into the crater, *e*) depth of ulcer greater than width, *f*) sharply marginated contour, and *g*) Hampton's line (a thin, sharp, lucent line that traverses the orifice of the ulcer). Hampton's line, best demonstrated on spot films obtained with compression, is caused by an overhanging gastric mucosa in an undermined ulcer.

The size, depth, and location of the ulcer, and the contour of the ulcer base are of no diagnostic value in differentiating benign from malignant ulcers. The differential diagnosis of "benign ulcer" includes *H. pylori* peptic disease, gastritis, hyperparathyroidism, radiotherapy, and Zollinger-Ellison syndrome.

Malignant Ulcers demonstrate signs that are the antithesis of benign ulcers. Evidence of irregular tumor mass or infiltration of the surrounding mucosa is evidence of malignancy. Signs of malignancy include *a*) an ulcer within the lumen of the stomach, *b*) an ulcer eccentrically located within the tumor mound, *c*) a shallow ulcer with a width greater than its depth, *d*) nodular, rolled, irregular, or shouldered edges, and *e*) Carmen meniscus sign (describes a large flat-based ulcer with heaped-up edges that fold inward to trap a lens-shaped barium collection that is convex toward the lumen) (Fig. 30.16). The differential diagnosis of "malignant ulcer" includes gastric adenocarcinoma, lymphoma, leiomyoma, and leiomyosarcoma.

CT is useful in demonstrating the extent of the tumor mass and the degree of involvement of the gastric wall.

DUODENUM

Duodenal Filling Defects/Mass Lesions

In the duodenal bulb, 90% of tumors are benign. In the second and third portions of the duodenum, tumors are 50% benign and 50% malignant. In the fourth portion of the duodenum, most tumors are malignant. Small, benign tumors of the duodenum usually present as smooth, polypoid filling defects. CT is helpful, but not specific, in predicting malignancy. Biopsy is usually required. Signs of malignancy include the following: *a*) central necrosis, *b*) ulceration or excavation, *c*) exophytic or intramural mass, and *d*) evidence of tumor beyond the duodenum (12).

Duodenal Adenocarcinoma, although being the most frequent malignant tumor of the duodenum, is a rare lesion. Malignant tumors are most common in the periampullary region and are rare in the bulb. Morphologic patterns include polypoid mass, ulcerative mass, and annular constricting lesion. Metastases to regional lymph nodes are present in two-thirds of patients at presentation. CT demonstrates the local extent of the tumor, as well as nodal and liver metastases.

Metastases to the duodenum may occur in the wall or subserosa of the duodenum. As the tumor grows, it may extend into the lumen and present as an intraluminal mass (Fig. 30.17) that may ulcerate. The most common primaries are breast, lung, and other GI malignancies. The duodenum may be invaded by tumors of adjacent organs including the pancreas and kidney.

Lymphoma in the duodenum usually presents as nodules with thickened folds. The nodules associated with lymphoma are distinctly larger than those seen with benign lymphoid hyperplasia.

Duodenal Adenoma presents as a polypoid lesion that may be pedunculated or sessile. Multiple adenomatous polyps are associated with polyposis syndromes. Villous adenomas have a high incidence of malignant degeneration and a characteristic "cauliflower" appearance on double-contrast UGI series.

Leiomyoma and Leiomyosarcoma present as an intramural, endoluminal, or exophytic mass (Fig. 30.18). Ulceration is common. Leiomyosarcoma ranges up to 20 cm size and is most common in the more distal duodenum. Leiomyosarcoma is the second most common primary malignant tumor of the duodenum.

Lipoma of the duodenum is a soft tumor that may grow to a large size. A definitive diagnosis can be made by CT demonstration of a uniform fat density mass.

Lymphoid Hyperplasia presents as small (1–3 mm) polypoid nodules diffusely throughout the duodenum. The condition is usually benign, especially in children. It is associated with immunodeficiency states in some adults. No evidence supports the concept that lymphoid hyperplasia is a precursor to lymphoma.

Gastric Mucosal Prolapse/Heterotopic Gastric Mucosa. Gastric mucosa may prolapse through the pylorus during peristalsis and cause a lobulated filling de-

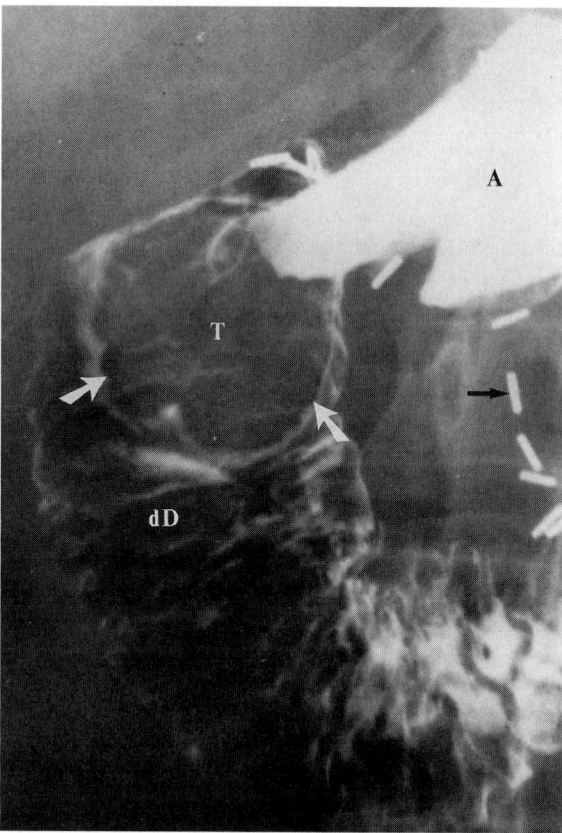

Figure 30.17. Metastasis to Duodenum. Double-contrast view demonstrates a lobulated tumor (*T, white arrows*) within the lumen of the descending duodenum (*dD*). Surgical biopsy revealed renal cell carcinoma metastatic to the duodenum. The surgical clips (*black arrow*) are from a radical left nephrectomy. *A*, antrum of the stomach.

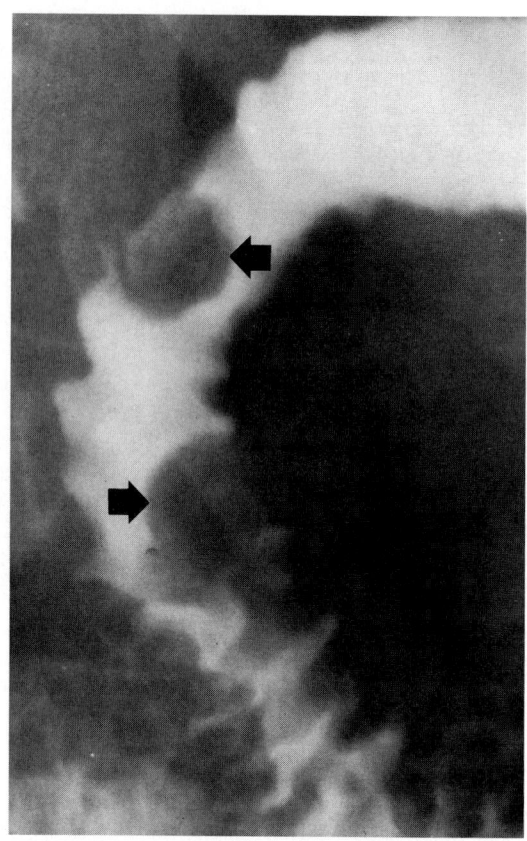

Figure 30.18. Duodenal Leiomyomas. Spot view from a UGI series shows two round, smooth filling defects (*arrows*) in the descending duodenum. Endoscopic biopsy confirmed two leiomyomas. The UGI appearance is nonspecific.

fect at the base of the duodenal bulb. The diagnosis is suggested by characteristic location and change in configuration with peristalsis.

Heterotopic gastric mucosa in the duodenal bulb is common on endoscopy (12%) but less frequently evident radiographically. The lesion has the appearance of areae gastricae in the duodenal bulb, or as clusters of 1–3 mm plaques on the smooth duodenal bulb mucosa (13). It may also appear as a solitary polyp that is indistinguishable from other polypoid lesions of the duodenum.

Brunner's Gland Hyperplasia/Adenoma. Brunner's glands are located in the submucosa of the proximal two-thirds of the duodenum and secrete an alkaline substance that buffers gastric acid. Diffuse nodular gland hyperplasia is a common cause of multiple filling defects and is associated with hyperacidity. Brunner's gland adenoma presents as a solitary filling defect and is identical in appearance to other benign duodenal nodules.

Ectopic Pancreas may also occur in the duodenum, most commonly in the proximal descending portion. A solitary mass with a central dimple is most characteristic.

Extrinsic Mass impressions on the duodenum may be made by the gallbladder; masses in the liver, pancreas, adrenal gland, kidney, or colon; pancreatic fluid collections; adenopathy; or aneurysms.

Thickened Duodenal Folds

The valvulae conniventes, or Kerckring's folds, of the small bowel begin in the second portion of the duodenum and continue throughout the remainder of the small bowel. The valvulae conniventes are permanent circular folds of mucosa supported by a core of fibrovascular submucosa. They are normally several millimeters wide and remain visible even with full distension of the duodenum. Folds greater than 2–3 mm wide are usually considered thickened.

Normal Variant. Thickened folds are a nonspecific radiographic finding that may be found in normal individuals. The radiographic diagnosis of a pathologic condition is more confident when there are additional findings.

Duodenitis refers to inflammation of the duodenum without discrete ulcer formation. The major cause of duodenitis is *H. pylori* infection. Alcohol and antiinflammatory medications cause a few cases. UGI findings include *a)* thickening (>4 mm) of the proximal duodenal folds, *b)* deformity of the duodenal bulb, and *c)* erosions.

Pancreatitis and Cholecystitis thicken the duodenal folds by paraduodenal inflammation. Both may also cause mass impressions on the duodenal lumen. CT or US demonstrate the extent and nature of the paraduodenal process.

Crohn's Disease of the duodenum usually involves the first and second portions and is almost always associated with contiguous involvement of the stomach. Duodenal involvement is manifest by thickened folds, aphthous ulcers, erosions, and single or multiple strictures.

Parasites. Giardiasis is caused by an overgrowth of the parasite *Giardia lamblia* in the duodenum and jejunum. Many patients are asymptomatic carriers, but patients with invasion of the gut wall have abdominal pain, diarrhea, and malabsorption. Giardiasis is a frequent cause of travelers diarrhea. Radiographic findings include *a)* distorted thickened folds in the duodenum and jejunum, *b)* hypermotility and spasm, and *c)* increased secretions.

Strongyloidiasis is caused by infection with the nematode, *Strongyloides stercoralis*, found in all areas of the world but most common in the warm, moist regions of the tropics. As with giardiasis, many patients are asymptomatic carriers. Invasion of the intestinal wall causes vomiting and malabsorption. The UGI findings include edematous folds, spasm, dilation of the proximal duodenum, and diffuse mucosal ulceration.

Lymphoma presents with nodular thickened folds.

Intramural Hemorrhage is caused by trauma, anticoagulation, and bleeding disorders. The regular pattern of thickened folds resembles a stack of coins. Partial or complete duodenal obstruction is usually present. The fixed retroperitoneal position of the third portion of the duodenum makes it susceptible to blunt abdominal trauma and compression against the lumbar spine.

Duodenal Ulcers and Diverticuli

Duodenal Ulcers are caused by *H. pyloris* infection in 95% of cases (5). Addition causes include antiinflammatory medications, Crohn's disease, Zollinger-Ellison syndrome, viral infections, or penetrating pancreatic cancer. Duodenal ulcers are associated with acid hypersecretion. Most (95%) are in the duodenal bulb with the anterior wall being most often involved. Radiographic diagnosis of a duodenal ulcer depends upon demonstration of the ulcer crater or niche. En face, the crater appears as a persistent collection of barium or air. In profile, ulcers project beyond the normal lumen (Fig. 30.19). Thickened folds often radiate toward the ulcer crater, which may be surrounded by a mound of edema. Although the shape is usually round or oval, linear ulcers also occur. Giant ulcers larger than 2 cm resemble diverticuli or a deformed bulb. Ulcer craters have no mucosal lining and therefore no mucosal relief pattern, and do not contract with peristalsis. Ulcer scarring may cause a pattern of radiating folds with a central barium collection that is indistinguishable from an acute ulcer. Endoscopy may be required to make the differentiation. Postbulbar ulcers represent about 5% of the total. Most involve the second and third portions of the duodenum, which are frequently narrowed.

Complications of duodenal ulcer disease include obstruction, bleeding, and perforation. Bleeding from a duodenal ulcer is most efficiently diagnosed endoscopi-

cally. Perforation may be manifest by pneumoperitoneum or a localized abnormal gas collection. Peptic duodenal ulcer is not a premalignant condition.

Zollinger-Ellison Syndrome is caused by a gastrin-secreting islet cell tumor (gastrinoma). Gastrinomas are found in the pancreas (75%), duodenum (15%), and in 10% in extraintestinal sites (liver, lymph nodes, and ovary). The islet cell tumor is malignant in 60% of cases. Gastrinomas also occur as part of the hereditary syndrome of multiple endocrine neoplasia, type I (MEN-I). Continuous gastrin secretion results in marked hyperacidity and multiple peptic ulcers in the duodenum, stomach, and jejunum. UGI studies show pathognomic findings of *a)* multiple peptic ulcers in the stomach, duodenal bulb, and, most characteristically, in the postbulbar duodenum; *b)* hypersecretion with high volume gastric fluid diluting the barium and impairing mucosal coating; and *c)* thick edematous folds in the stomach, duodenum, and proximal jejunum.

Flexural Pseudotumors are a common cause of a duodenal filling defect with a central barium collection, mimicking an ulcerated lesions. Appearing as rounded, swirled mucosal folds on the inner aspect of the flexure at the apex of the bulb, these tumors are redundant mucosa and have a variable appearance on different projections.

Duodenal Diverticula are common (5% of UGI series) and usually incidental findings. They may be multiple and may form in any portion of the duodenum, but are most common along the inner aspect of the descending duodenum (Fig 30.20). Diverticula are differentiated from ulcers on a UGI series by demonstration of mucosal folds entering the neck of the diverticulum and change in appearance with peristalsis. On plain abdominal radiographs, duodenal diverticuli may be seen as abnormal air collections. On CT they may be filled with fluid and mimic a pancreatic pseudocyst (Fig. 30.21), or they may contain air and fluid and mimic a pancreatic abscess (14). Rare complications include perforation and hemorrhage. Diverticuli adjacent to the ampulla of Vater

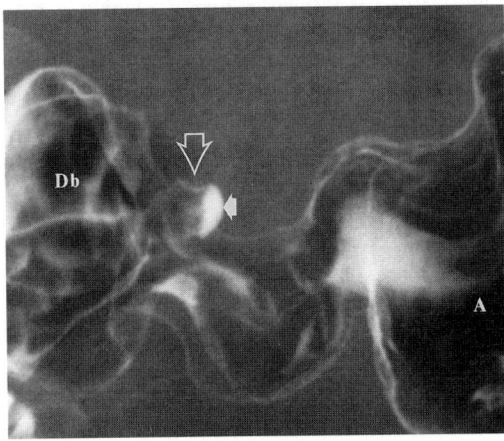

Figure 30.19. Peptic Ulcer. A UGI series demonstrates a persistent barium collection (*closed arrow*) that projects beyond the lumen of the base of the duodenal bulb (*Db*). A well-defined ulcer collar (*open arrow*) is present. *A*, gastric antrum.

may rarely obstruct the common bile duct or pancreatic duct.

Intraluminal Diverticula are caused by a thin, incomplete, congenital diaphragm that is stretched by moving intraluminal contents to form a "wind sock" configuration within the duodenum (Fig. 30.22).

Duodenal Narrowing

Annular Pancreas is the most common congenital anomaly of the pancreas. Pancreatic tissue encircles the descending duodenum and narrows its lumen (Fig. 30.23) (15). The abnormality occurs when the bilobed ventral component of the pancreas fuses with the dorsal pancreas on both sides of the duodenum. Although it often presents in childhood, especially in children with Down's syndrome, about half of the cases do not present until adulthood. Symptomatic adults present with nausea, vomiting, abdominal pain, and occasionally jaundice. The UGI series typically demonstrates eccentric or concentric narrowing of the descending duodenum. Annular pancreas is associated with a high incidence of postbulbar peptic ulceration in adults. CT confirms the diagnosis by demonstration of pancreatic tissue encircling the duodenum. Endoscopic retrograde cholan-

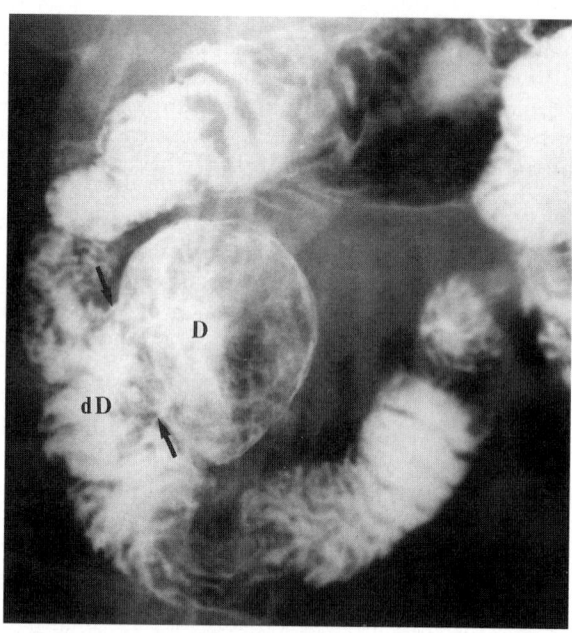

Figure 30.20. Duodenal Diverticulum. Radiograph from an UGI series demonstrates contrast and air filling a duodenal diverticulum (*D*) that originates from the medial aspect of the descending duodenum (*dD*). The neck of the duodenum is indicated by the *arrows*. (From Stone EE, Brant WE, Smith G. Computed tomography of duodenal diverticula. J Comput Assist Tomogr 1989;13:61–64.)

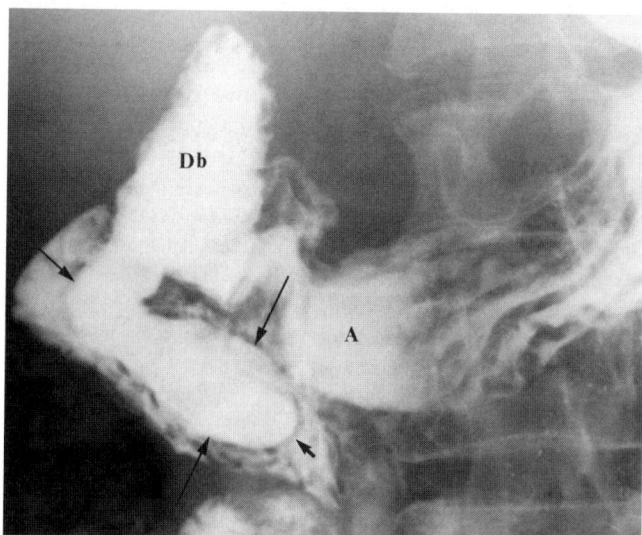

Figure 30.22. Intraluminal Diverticulum. A UGI series demonstrates a barium-filled "sock" (*long arrows*) within the lumen of the descending duodenum. The radiolucent wall of the diverticulum (*short arrow*) is outlined by barium, both within the diverticulum and within the lumen of the duodenum. *Db*, duodenal bulb. *A*, gastric antrum.

Figure 30.21. Duodenal Diverticulum. CT demonstrates a diverticulum (*D*) of the descending duodenum (*dD*) that is completely fluid-filled and extends to the pancreatic bed, mimicking a pancreatic pseudocyst. *S*, stomach. *sv*, splenic vein. (From Stone EE, Brant WE, Smith G. Computed tomography of duodenal diverticula. J Comput Assist Tomogr 1989; 13:61–64.)

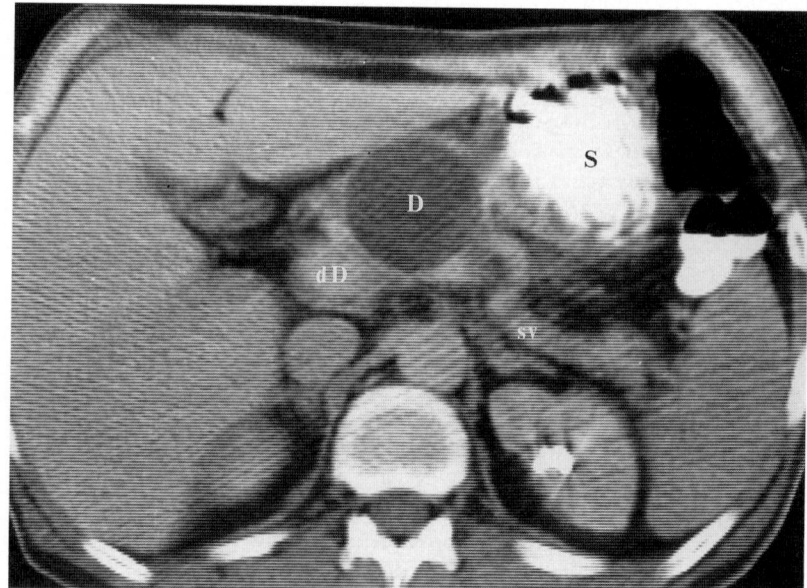

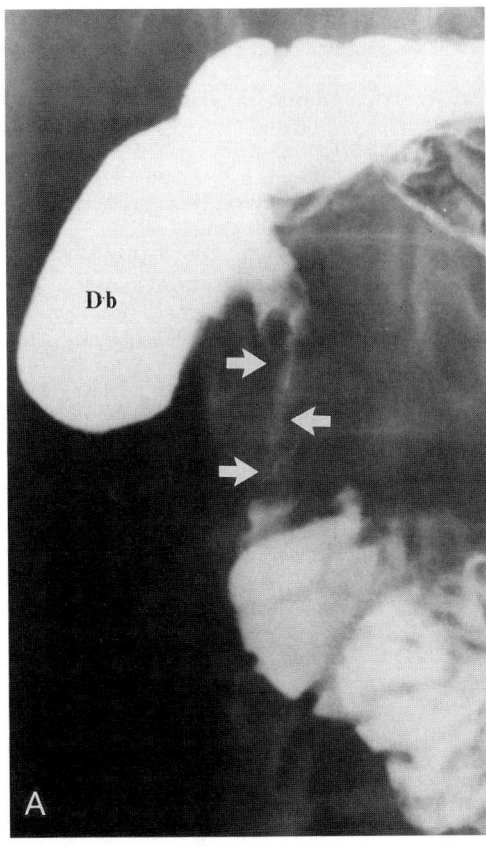

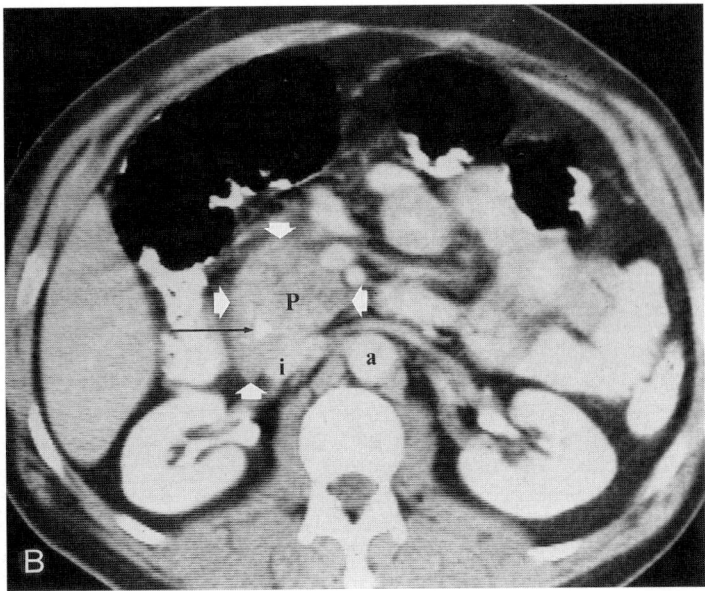

Figure 30.23. Annular Pancreas. A. UGI series demonstrates a 3-cm long circumferentially narrowed segment (*arrows*) of the descending duodenum. No ulceration was evident. *Db*, duodenal bulb. **B.** CT reveals normal pancreatic tissue (*P, white arrows*) encircling the narrowed descending duodenum (*black arrow*) confirming the diagnosis of annular pancreas. *i*, inferior vena cava. *a*, aorta.

giopancreatography demonstrates an annular pancreatic duct encircling the duodenum.

Duodenal Adenocarcinoma can present as a circumferential constricting lesion with tumor shoulders giving evidence of mass effect. Ulceration is common. CT demonstrates the extent of the lesion.

Lymphoma causes marked wall thickening and bulky paraduodenal lymphadenopathy that may narrow the lumen.

Postbulbar Ulcer is commonly associated with narrowing of the lumen of the second and third portions of the duodenum.

Extrinsic Compression, because of inflammation or tumor in adjacent organs, especially the pancreas (Fig. 30.24), may constrict the duodenal lumen.

Upper Gastrointestinal Hemorrhage

UGI hemorrhage refers to bleeding with the site of origin proximal to the ligament of Treitz. This hemorrhage has an average mortality of 8–10%. Causes in an approximate order of frequency are *a*) duodenal ulcer, *b*) esophageal varices, *c*) gastric ulcer, *d*) acute hemorrhagic gastritis, *e*) esophagitis, *f*) Mallory-Weiss tear, *g*) neoplasm, *h*) vascular malformation, and *i*) vascular enteric fistula.

Barium studies should be avoided in patients in the acute stages of UGI hemorrhage. Endoscopy is much more accurate than a UGI series in demonstrating the bleeding site (95% versus 45%). The UGI series may identify a lesion but does not indicate whether that le-

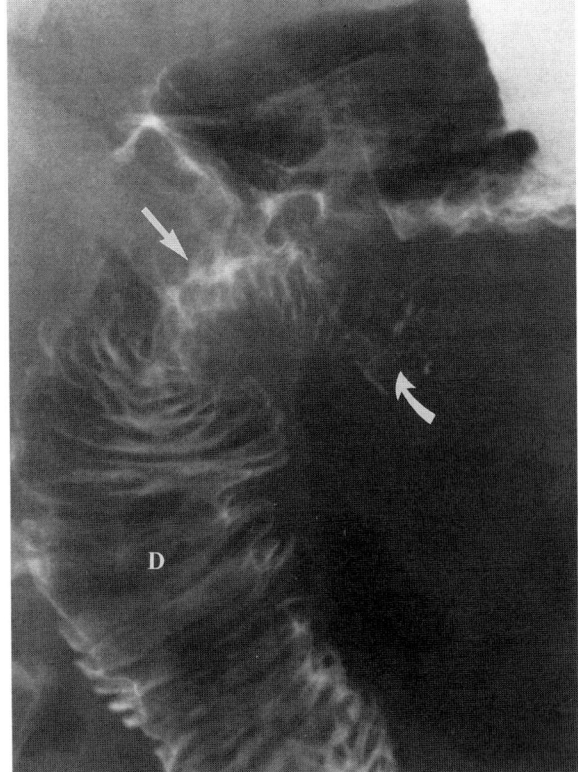

Figure 30.24. Pancreatic Carcinoma. Double-contrast UGI series reveals narrowing (*straight arrow*) of the proximal descending duodenum with ulceration that allows tracking of barium (*curved arrow*) into the pancreas. The cause was carcinoma of the pancreas. Normal folds and mucosal pattern are seen in the more distal descending duodenum (*D*).

sion is responsible for the bleeding. Also, retained barium in the GI tract following a UGI series will usually make performing angiography impossible. Helical CT angiography shows promise in identifying the bleeding site (16). Conventional angiography is used to localize active bleeding sites and provide therapy by infusion of vasoconstrictors or performance of transcatheter embolization.

References

1. Low VHS, Levine MS, Rubesin SE, et al. Diagnosis of gastric carcinoma: sensitivity of double-contrast barium studies. AJR Am J Roentgenol 1994;162:329–334.
2. Fishman EK, Urban BA, Hruban RH. CT of the stomach: spectrum of disease. Radiographics 1996;16:1035–1054.
3. Levine MS, Rubesin SE, Pantongrag-Brown L, et al. Non-Hodgkin's lymphoma of the gastrointestinal tract: radiographic findings. AJR Am J Roentgenol 1997;168:165–172.
4. Kaye MD, Young SW, Hayward R, Castellino RA. Gastric pseudotumor on CT scanning. AJR Am J Roentgenol 1980; 135:190–193.
5. Pattison CP, Combs MJ, Marshall BJ. *Helicobacter pylori* and peptic ulcer disease: evolution to revolution to resolution. AJR Am J Roentgenol 1997;168:1415–1420.
6. Cello JP. *Helicobacter pylori* and peptic ulcer disease. AJR Am J Roentgenol 1995;164:283–286.
7. Eurogast Study Group. An international association between *Helicobacter pylori* and gastric cancer. Lancet 1993; 341:1359–1362.
8. Levine MS, Kong V, Rubesin SE, et al. Scirrhous carcinoma of the stomach: radiologic and endoscopic diagnosis. Radiology 1990;175:151–154.
9. Levine MS, Pantongrag-Brown L, Aguilera NS, et al. Non-Hodgkin lymphoma of the stomach: a cause of linitis plastica. Radiology 1996;201:375–378.
10. Furth EE, Rubesin SE, Levine MS. Pathologic primer on gastritis: an illustrated sum and substance. Radiology 1995;197:693–698.
11. Sohn J, Levine MS, Furth EE, et al. Helicobacter pylori gastritis: radiographic findings. Radiology 1995;195:763–767.
12. Kazerooni EA, Quint LE, Francis IR. Duodenal neoplasms: predictive value of CT for determining malignancy and tumor resectability. AJR Am J Roentgenol 1992;159: 303–309.
13. Gore RM, Ghahremani GG, Miller FH. Mucosal features of the alimentary tract on double contrast barium studies. Radiologist 1995;2:283–295.
14. Stone EE, Brant WE, Smith G. Computed tomography of duodenal diverticula. Comput Assist Tomogr 1989;13: 61–64.
15. Pantoja E, Nagy F, Thomas HA, Jr, et al. Annular pancreas. Medical Radiography and Photography 1985;61:2–9.
16. Ettore GC, Francioso G, Garribba AP, et al. Helical CT angiography in gastrointestinal bleeding of obscure origin. AJR Am J Roentgenol 1997;168:727–730.

31
Mesenteric Small Bowel

William E. Brant

Imaging Methods

Disease of the mesenteric small intestine is relatively rare. Detailed radiographic study of the small bowel is justified only when clinical suspicion of small bowel disease is high. Small bowel disease is usually manifest by four major symptoms: colic, diarrhea, malabsorption, and bleeding (1,2). Colic is defined as recurrent and spasmodic abdominal pain with periods of relief every 2–3 minutes. Diarrhea caused by small bowel disease is less urgent than that caused by colon disease. Malabsorption is manifest by steatorrhea, foul-smelling stools, and weight loss. Bleeding from small bowel disease is usually occult and manifest by anemia. Because the majority of the mesenteric small intestine is out of reach of the endoscopist, diagnostic radiology has the primary responsibility for its evaluation.

The traditional method for radiographic examination of the small bowel is the small bowel follow-through examination (SBFT)(Fig. 31.1) tacked onto a standard upper gastrointestinal series (3). The patient is asked to continue drinking barium while a series of supine abdominal films are obtained until the terminal ileum and cecum are filled with barium. Fluoroscopic examination of the small bowel is then attempted. This study is notoriously insensitive. It is limited by overlap of bowel loops, poor distension, flocculation of barium, intermittent barium filling, and unpredictable transit time. Visualization of the distal ileum may be improved with double-contrast technique by insufflating the colon with air (SBFT with peroral pneumocolon).

Enteroclysis, or the small bowel enema, is the preferred method for detailed radiographic examination (Fig. 31.2)(4). This study provides more uniform distension of the bowel, even distribution of barium, superior anatomic detail, and shorter overall examination time. The study is performed by passing a specially designed 12-14 French enteroclysis catheter through the mouth or nose and into the distal duodenum or proximal jejunum. A guidewire is used for directional control of the

catheter during manipulation under fluoroscopy. The study may be performed single contrast using approximately 600 ml of barium or double contrast using 200 ml of barium followed by 1000 ml of methylcellulose to advance the barium and distend the bowel.

The small bowel lumen and mucosal surface are best demonstrated by barium studies. CT complements the barium examination by demonstrating the extraluminal component of bowel disease. In addition, CT evaluates the mesentery, adjacent solid organs, the peritoneal cavity, and the retroperitoneum. CT signs that aid in the differentiation of benign and malignant disease are listed in Table 31.1 (5,6).

US demonstrates the floating bowel loops in ascites and the dilated small bowel in ileus and small bowel obstruction. Real-time US may be used to evaluate peristalsis and help differentiate ileus and obstruction. Large small bowel masses and masses in the mesentery may be characterized by US.

Anatomy

The mesenteric small intestine is a tube approximately 7-m long that lies totally within the greater peritoneal cavity. The jejunum is arbitrarily defined as the proximal two-fifths of the mesenteric intestine, while the ileum is the distal three-fifths. The jejunum and ileum are suspended from the posterior abdominal wall by the small bowel mesentery. The small bowel mesentery is composed of connective tissue, blood vessels, and lymphatic vessels, and is covered by peritoneum, which reflects from the posterior parietal peritoneum. The root of the small bowel mesentery extends obliquely from the ligament of Treitz, just left of the L-2 vertebra, to the cecum, near the right sacroiliac joint. On CT the mesentery is defined by its normal vascular structures outlined by fat between loops of bowel. Normal mesenteric lymph nodes may be seen as soft tissue density nodules 5 mm or less in size. The concave border of the small bowel loops is the mesenteric border where the mesentery attaches. The convex border, facing away from the mesentery, is called the antimesenteric border. Identification of the border involved by disease can be of diagnostic value.

On CT and barium studies, the jejunum has a feathery mucosal pattern, more prominent valvulae conniventes, a wider lumen, and a thicker wall. The ileum has a less featured mucosal pattern, thinner, less frequent folds, narrower lumen, and a thinner wall. The transition between jejunum and ileum is gradual, and all loops are freely mobile. The general structure of the layers of the small bowel wall is shown in Figure 30.1. The

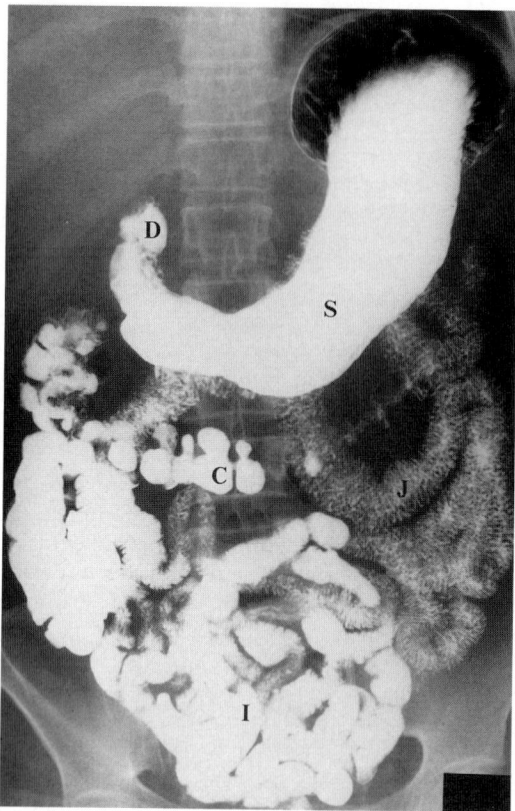

Figure 31.1. Normal Small Bowel Follow-through. The small bowel is demonstrated on an upper GI series by having the patient ingest additional barium and by taking additional radiographs to document passage of barium through the small bowel into the colon. The loops of jejunum (*J*) have a delicate feathery appearance in the left upper abdomen, whereas the loops of ileum (*I*) are coarse and featureless in the right lower abdomen. Barium has filled portions of the ascending and transverse colon (*C*), identified by its haustral folds. Colonic haustral folds extend only partway across the bowel lumen, and small bowel folds extend completely across the bowel lumen. *S*, stomach. *D*, duodenum.

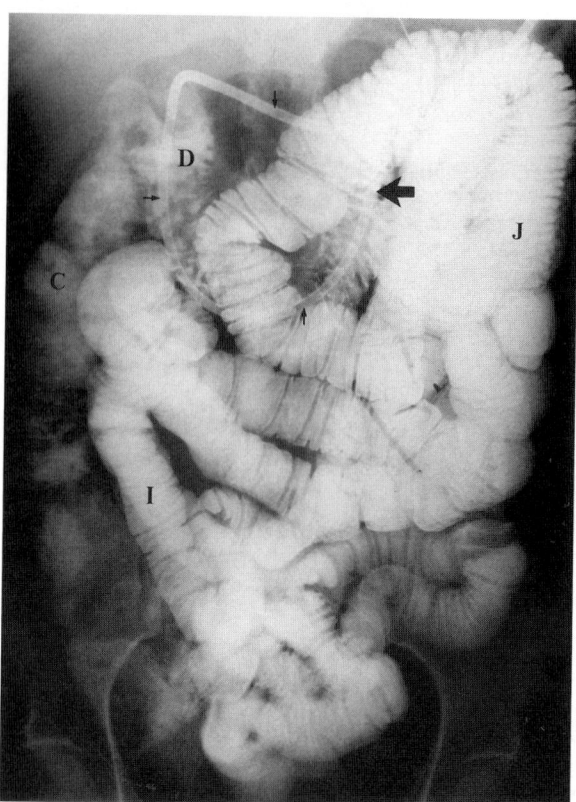

Figure 31.2. Normal Enteroclysis. The enteroclysis catheter (*small arrows*) has been passed through the C-loop of the duodenum to the location of the ligament of Treitz (*large arrow*), using fluoroscopy to guide catheter manipulation. The enteroclysis technique provides uniform distension of the jejunum (*J*) and ileum (*I*). Barium fills portions of the ascending colon (*C*). Note the small bowel folds crossing the entire diameter of the small bowel lumen. *D*, duodenum.

ileum has larger and more numerous lymphoid follicles in the submucosa. Villi are finger-like projections that extend from the entire mucosal surface of the small bowel. They are composed of loose connective tissue of the lamina propria. Tiny capillaries and lymphatic vessels (lacteals) extend to the submucosal vessels. The combination of valvulae conniventes and villi greatly expands the absorptive surface area of the small intestine. The caliber of the normal small bowel lumen is less than 3 cm with normal fold thickness of less than 3–4 mm and normal wall thickness of 2–3 mm. Normal lymph nodes seen in the mesentery are less than 3–4 mm in diameter.

Small Bowel Filling Defects/Mass Lesions

Neoplasms of the small intestine are rare accounting for only 2–3% of GI tumors. Benign neoplasms are about equal to malignant neoplasms in overall frequency. However, when the patient presents with symptoms, malignancy is three times more common. Presenting afflictions include obstruction, pain, weight loss, bleeding, and palpable mass.

Table 31.1. Diagnostic Findings of CT of the Gastrointestinal Tract

Benign Lesion	Neoplastic Lesion
Circumferential thickening	Eccentric thickening
Symmetrical thickening	Asymmetric thickening
Thickening <1 cm	Thickening >2 cm
Segmental or diffuse involvement	Focal soft tissue mass
Thickened mesenteric fat	Abrupt transition
Wall is homogeneous soft tissue density	Lobulated contour
"Double halo sign": dark inner ring/ bright outer ring	Spiculated outer contour
"Target sign": bright inner-dark, middle-bright outer (Fig. 31.13)	Luminal narrowing
	Regional adenopathy
	Liver metastases

Carcinoid tumors are the most common neoplasm of the small intestine, accounting for about one-third of all small bowel tumors (7). They are considered a low-grade malignancy that may recur locally or metastasize to the lymph nodes, liver, or lung. They arise from endocrine cells (enterochromaffin or Kulchitsky cells) deep in the mucosa. These cells produce vasoactive substances including serotonin and bradykinins. About 20% of all carcinoid tumors arise in the small bowel, most commonly in the ileum where 30% are multiple. Only 7%, those with liver metastases, present with carcinoid syndrome (cutaneous flushing, abdominal cramps and diarrhea) because the liver inactivates the vasoactive substances. The tumors grow slowly but cause a marked fibrotic response of the bowel wall and mesentery because the serotonin produced by the tumor induces an intense local desmoplastic reaction. Complications include stricture, obstruction, and bowel infarction induced by fibrosis of the mesenteric vessels. The tumors may be pedunculated and cause intussusception.

Radiographic signs of fibrosis and metastases resemble the findings of Crohn's disease and overshadow demonstration of the primary tumor (7). Barium studies show: *a)* luminal narrowing, *b)* thickened and spiculated folds, *c)* separation of bowel loops by mesenteric mass, or *d)* bowel loops drawn together by fibrosis, and *e)* primary lesion appearing as small (<1.5 cm) mural nodule or intraluminal polyp. CT findings that are pathognomonic of carcinoid tumor are: *a)* sunburst pattern of radiating soft tissue density in the mesenteric fat due to mesenteric fibrosis (Fig. 31.3), *b)* bowel wall thickening, *c)* primary lesion appearing as a small, lobulated soft tissue mass, occasionally with central calcification, usually in the distal ileum *d)* enlarged mesenteric nodes and liver masses due to metastatic disease.

Adenocarcinoma of the small bowel is about half as common as carcinoid tumor. It is most frequent in the duodenum and proximal jejunum, and is uncommon in the distal ileum, where carcinoid is most common. Most patients are symptomatic at presentation, and 30% have a palpable mass. Patients with adult celiac disease, Crohn's disease, and Peutz-Jeghers syndrome are at increased risk for small bowel carcinoma. Complications include bleeding, obstruction, and intussusception. Prognosis is poor, with a 5-year survival of 20%. Metastatic spread is by intraperitoneal seeding, lymphatic channels to regional nodes, and portal veins to the liver. Morphologically the tumor may be infiltrating, producing strictures; polypoid, producing filling defects; or ulcerating. Barium studies typically show a charac-

teristic "apple core" stricture of the small bowel (Fig. 31.4). CT demonstrates: *a)* solitary mass in the duodenum or jejunum (up to 8 cm diameter) or *b)* short segment asymmetric, irregular, circumferential thickening of the bowel wall (8).

Lymphoma is responsible for about 20% of all small bowel malignant tumors (9). The GI tract is the most common site for extranodal origin of lymphoma, and the small bowel is most commonly involved (10). Most cases are non-Hodgkin's lymphoma. Non-Hodgkin lymphoma clinically involves the GI tract in 30% of cases overall.

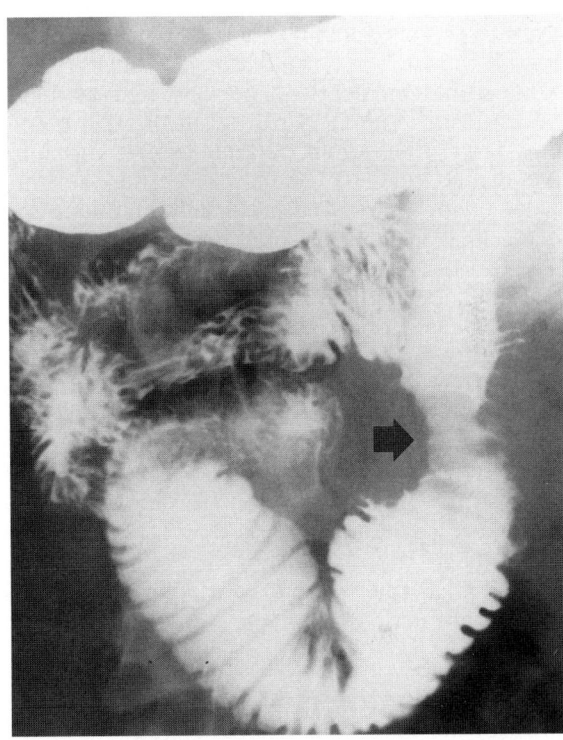

Figure 31.4. Adenocarcinoma Jejunum. Small bowel follow-through study demonstrates fixed constricting lesion of the jejunum. The folds in the involved area are thickened and effaced.

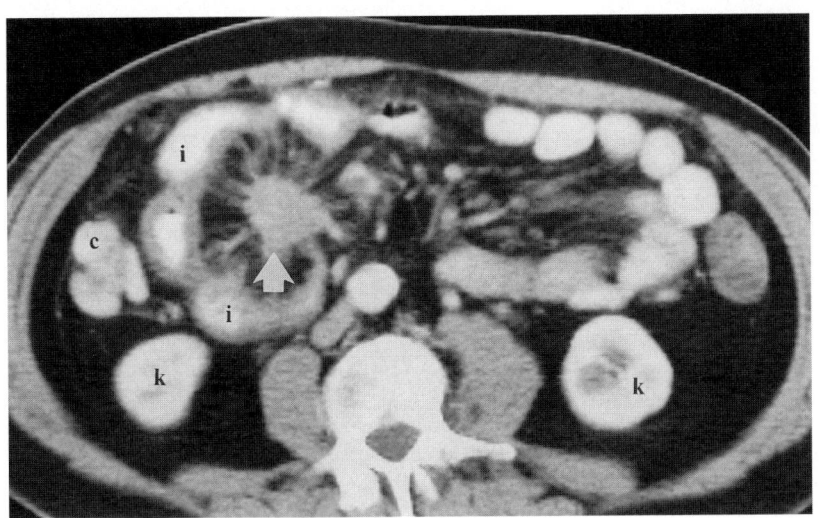

Figure 31.3. Carcinoid Tumor. CT scan shows classic "sunburst" appearance of radiating strands and mesenteric mass (*arrow*) due to carcinoid tumor arising in the ileum (*i*). *c*, ascending colon; *k*, kidney.

Lymphoma is most frequent in the distal ileum where the concentration of lymphoid tissue is the greatest. Morphologic patterns of involvement include diffuse infiltration, exophytic mass, polypoid mass, and multiple nodules. Multiple sites of involvement are seen in 10–25% of cases. Aneurysmal dilation of the lumen is a feature of lymphoma due to replacement of the muscularis and destruction of the autonomic plexus by tumor without inducing fibrosis. As a result, obstruction is uncommon.

Barium studies most commonly reveal: *a*) wall thickening with irregular, distorted folds due to submucosal infiltration of cells (Fig. 31.5); *b*) fold thickening may be smooth and regular in early stages due to lymphatic blockage in the mesentey; *c*) folds become effaced in later stages with greater cell infiltration into the bowel wall; *d*) narrowed, widened, or normal lumen; *e*) cavitary lesions containing fluid and debris; *f*) polypoid masses that may cause intussusception; *g*) rare multiple filling defects that are larger than 4 mm, variable in size, and nonuniform in distribution (10). Shallow ulceration is common.

CT demonstrates: *a*) circumferential wall thickening involving a long segment of small bowel, *b*) effacement of folds, *c*) mucosal nodularity, *d*) eccentric wall thickening (Fig. 31.5)(9). Exophytic lymphoma is generally of uniform soft tissue density and enhances little, if any with intravenous contrast administration. This is a differentiating finding in comparison with leiomyosarcoma and adenocarcinoma, which usually enhance prominently. CT readily demonstrates associated findings of lymphoma including mesenteric and retroperitoneal adenopathy and hepatosplenomegaly. The mesentery may show a large confluent mass encasing multiple bowel loops or enlarged individual nodes (Fig. 31.5). The "sandwich sign," characteristic of lymphoma, refers to sparing of rind of fat surrounding mesenteric vessels encased by lymphoma.

Burkitt's lymphoma in North America usually presents with intestinal involvement, especially of the ileocecal area in children and young adults. The malignancy is aggressive, with rapid doubling time and poor prognosis. Imaging studies show bulky tumors.

AIDS-related lymphoma is an aggressive high-grade non-Hodgkin's lymphoma with poor prognosis. Extranodal involvement, including small bowel lymphoma, is common. Adenopathy may be caused by lymphoma, Kaposi's sarcoma, or *Mycobacterium avium-intracellulare* infection. The radiographic findings are identical to those seen in immunocompetent patients (11).

Nodular Lymphoid Hyperplasia may involve the entire small bowel. The condition is differentiated from lymphoma by the uniform small size of the nodules (2–4 mm) and even distribution through the area of involvement (see Fig. 32.8). Lymphoid hyperplasia confined to the terminal ileum and proximal colon is usually considered incidental and may be related to recent viral infection. Diffuse lymphoid hyperplasia is associated with hypogammaglobulinemia, especially low IgA.

Metastases to the small bowel are common. The two most frequent routes are by peritoneal seeding, usually involving the mesenteric border, and by hematogenous spread, which usually implants on the antimesenteric border. Intraperitoneal implantation of the small bowel serosa is most commonly due to ovarian carcinoma in women, and colon, gastric, and pancreatic carcinoma in men. The mesenteric border of the small bowel is favored by the flow of fluid along the small bowel mesentery from the left upper to the right lower abdomen. Implantation is most common along the terminal ileum, cecum, and ascending colon. Peritoneal implants on the parietal peritoneum, and omentum (omental cake), as well as in

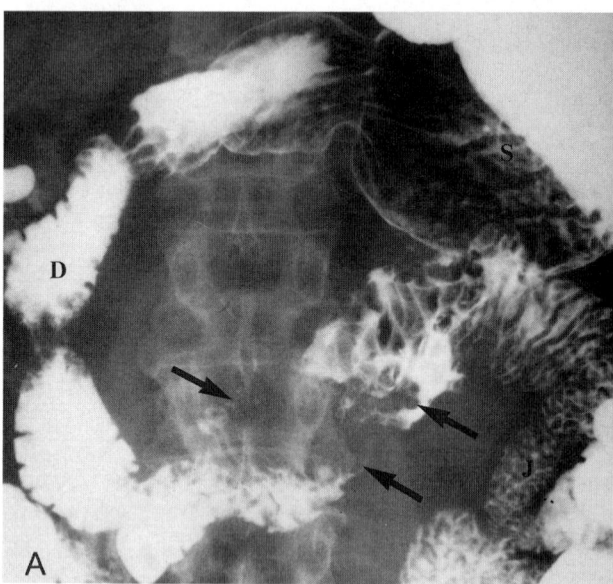

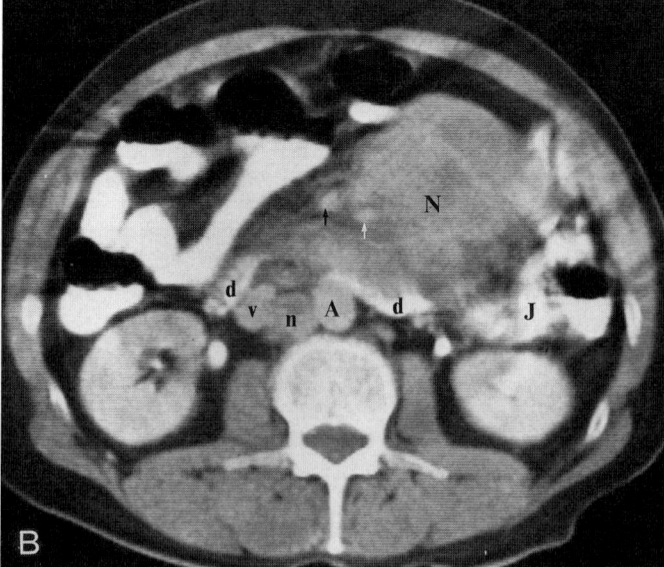

Figure 31.5. Non-Hodgkins Lymphoma. A. An UGI series demonstrates polypoid filling defects (*arrows*) in the third portion of the duodenum (*D*). The duodenal C-loop is widened and the jejunum (*J*) is displaced laterally. *S*, stomach. **B.** A CT scan of the same patient demonstrates the full extent of disease. A large mass of confluent enlarged lymph nodes (*N*) compresses and invades the duodenum (*d*), and displaces the jejunum (*J*). The adenopathy surrounds the superior mesenteric artery (*small white arrow*) and vein (*small black arrow*) creating a CT sandwich sign. An enlarged lymph node (*n*) is seen between the inferior vena cava (*v*) and the aorta (*A*).

the pouch of Douglas, are demonstrated by CT. Barium studies demonstrate nodules and tethering of folds due to mesenteric fibrosis.

Hematogenous metastases are deposited along the antimesenteric border where the submucosal blood vessels arborize. Common primary malignancies are melanoma, lung, breast, and colon carcinoma, and embryonal cell carcinoma of the testes. Barium studies demonstrate mural nodules of uniform or varying size anywhere in the small bowel. They may appear as target lesions, or ulcerate or cavitate (12).

Kaposi's Sarcoma in AIDS patients commonly involves the small intestine. About half of the patients with skin lesions have intestinal lesions as well. Barium studies demonstrate multiple mural nodules, often centrally umbilicated. CT demonstrates mesenteric, retroperitoneal, and pelvic adenopathy.

Leiomyoma and Leiomyosarcoma. Leiomyoma is the most frequent benign neoplasm of the mesenteric small bowel. Most (80%) occur in the jejunum and ileum with 20% in the duodenum. They are circumscribed, round, or lobulated tumors of the bowel wall. They may project into the lumen, be pedunculated or exophytic. The overlying mucosa may ulcerate and be a source of intestinal bleeding. CT shows a focal soft tissue mass. Homogeneous tissue density and uniform enhancement favor a benign tumor. Angiography demonstrates a hypervascular mass.

Leiomyosarcoma represents about 8% of small bowel malignant tumors. The tumor is more common in the ileum than the jejunum. Most are exophytic and grow to large size (11 cm), developing areas of necrosis and cystic changes. Ulceration and bleeding are common. They spread by direct extension to adjacent structures and by hematogenous routes to liver, lungs, and bone. Nodal metastases are uncommon. Like leiomyomatous tumors elsewhere, the malignant tumors are larger and more heterogeneous than benign tumors (Fig. 31.6). CT demonstrates ulceration and central tumor necrosis. Because the tumor is hypervascular, solid portions enhance avidly.

Adenoma accounts for about 20% of benign small bowel neoplasms. It is more common in the duodenum than in the mesenteric small intestine. The tumor is a benign proliferation of glandular epithelium, and has the potential for malignant degeneration. Barium studies demonstate an intraluminal polyp with a finely lobulated surface.

Lipoma is most common in the ileum. The tumor arises from the fat of the submucosa. Lipomas account for about 17% of benign small bowel tumors. Most are asymptomatic incidental findings, although some cause bleeding or intussusception. CT demonstration of a fat density (−50 to −100 H) tumor is diagnostic. Thin (5 mm) sections are recommended for the demonstration of fat density within small lesions.

Hemangioma is usually solitary and submucosal, projecting into the lumen as a polyp. These tumors are located predominantly in the jejunum. About two-thirds present with bleeding. Barium studies demonstrate a small polyp. The occasional presence of a calcified phlebolith suggests the diagnosis. They account for less than 10% of benign small bowel tumors.

Polyposis Syndromes cause multiple polypoid lesions of the small bowel. The differential diagnosis includes metastases, lymphoma, nodular lymphoid hyperplasia, Kaposi's sarcoma, and carcinoid tumors.

Peutz-Jeghers syndrome is an autosomal dominant inherited condition consisting of multiple hamartomatous polyps in the small intestine (most common), colon, and stomach associated with melanin freckles on the facial skin, palmar aspects of the fingers and toes, and mucous membranes (13). Hamartomatous polyps are a nonneoplastic, abnormal proliferation of all three layers of the mucosa, epithelium, lamina propria, and muscularis mucosae. The polyps are most common in the jejunum, are usually pedunculated, and are variable in size up to 4 cm. Patients are at increased risk for intussusception, GI tract adenocarcinoma, and extraintestinal malignancy (breast, pancreas, ovary). Barium studies demonstrates myriad polyps in involved areas of small intestine, separated by normal bowel segments.

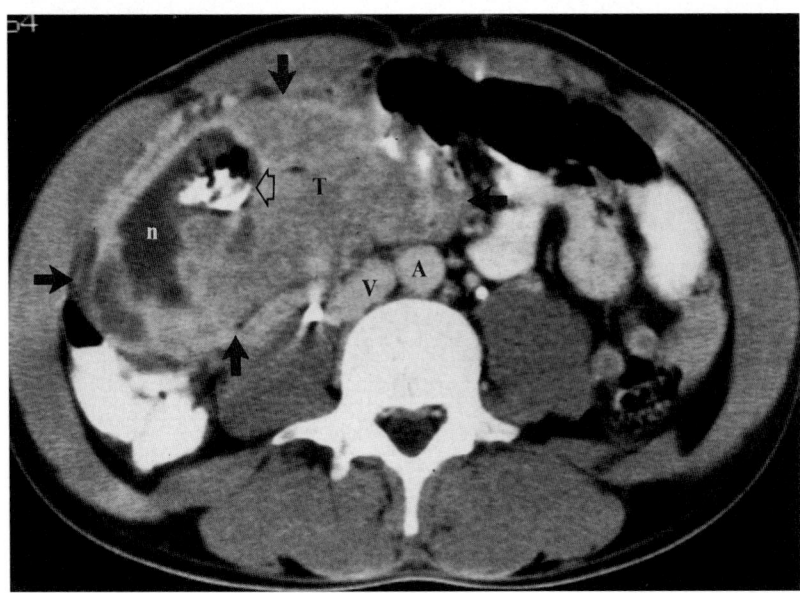

Figure 31.6. Leiomyosarcoma of the Ileum. Contrast-enhanced CT demonstrates a large tumor (*T*, between *closed arrows*) in the right abdomen encompassing a loop of ileum (*open arrow*). The tumor enhances with contrast (compare to muscle) and demonstrates low-density areas of necrosis (*n*). *V*, inferior vena cava. *A*, aorta.

Cronkhite-Canada syndrome involves the small bowel in about half the cases with multiple inflammatory polyps. The colon and stomach are always involved.

Gardner's syndrome of inherited adenomatous polyposis coli usually includes a few adenomatous polyps in the small bowel.

Juvenile GI polyposis is most common in the colon but occasionally involves the small bowel. Inflammatory polyps containing cysts filled with mucin develop secondary to chronic irritation. Most are round, smooth, and pedunculated.

Ascariasis is caused by infestation with the roundworm *Ascaris lumbricoides*. Ascariasis is found worldwide, but is most common in Asia and Africa. Endemic areas in the United States include rural southern Appalachia and the Gulf Coast states. Infestation is acquired by ingesting food or water contaminated with *Ascaris* eggs. The eggs hatch in the small bowel. Larvae penetrate the wall and migrate through the vascular system to the lungs, where they molt and grow before migrating up the bronchi and trachea to the larynx where they are again swallowed. Worms mature in the small bowel, especially in the jejunum, and may reach 15—35 cm in size. New generations of infective ova are excreted in feces. A large bolus of worms may obstruct the small bowel, especially in children, or cause intussusception. Worms can be identified on plain abdominal radiographs in 70% of cases (Fig. 31.7). Barium studies demonstrate worms as long linear filling defects. Barium ingested by the worms may be seen in their intestinal tract as a long, string-like white line.

Mesenteric Masses

Masses arising in the small bowel mesentery frequently present as a palpable abdominal mass. The mesenteric fat may be infiltrated by edema, hemorrhage, or inflammatory cells (14). The disorders may be diseases of the small intestine or be primary to the mesentery itself. CT, US, and MR provide the most diagnostic information. Carcinoid tumors, metastases, leiomyoma, and leiomyosarcoma may all have a prominent component of disease in the mesentery, and must also be considered.

Lymphoma causing bulky adenopathy is the most common solid mesenteric mass (Fig. 31.5).

Mesenteric Desmoid tumors are benign but locally aggressive, solid, fibrous, mesenteric tumors (15,16). They may be solitary (28%) or multiple (72%) and associated with Gardner's syndrome. US and CT demonstrate a heterogeneous solid mass with well-defined (68%) or infiltrative borders (Fig. 31.8).

Mesenteric Cysts are lymphangiomas that arise in the root of the small bowel mesentery (17). Most are thin-walled and multiloculated with internal fluid that may be chylous, serous, or bloody. US demonstrates a well-defined cyst with internal debris, and fluid-debris or fluid-

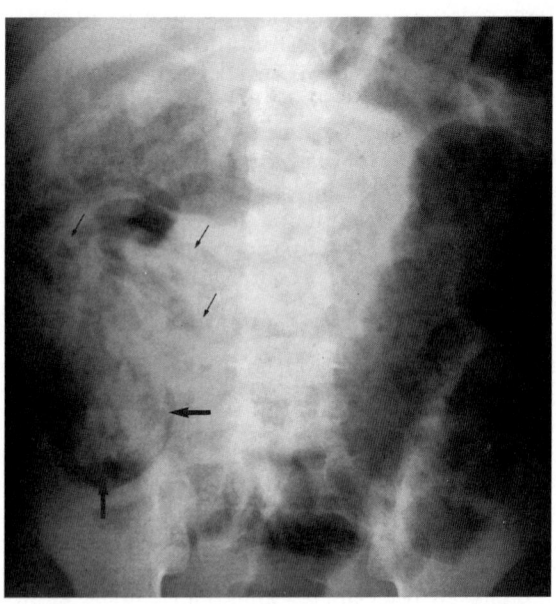

Figure 31.7. Ascaris Infestation. Plain radiograph demonstrates diffuse intestinal dilation. Roundworms in the ileum are seen as round and tubular soft tissue densities outlined by intestinal gas (*small arrows*). A large bolus of entangled worms (*large arrows*) plugged the distal ileum, causing small bowel obstruction.

Figure 31.8. Mesenteric Desmoid. A mesenteric desmoid tumor (*T*) arises in the small bowel mesentery and displaces bowel loops. Surgical biopsy confirmed the diagnosis, but the tumor could not be safely removed because of extensive involvement of bowel and mesenteric vessels.

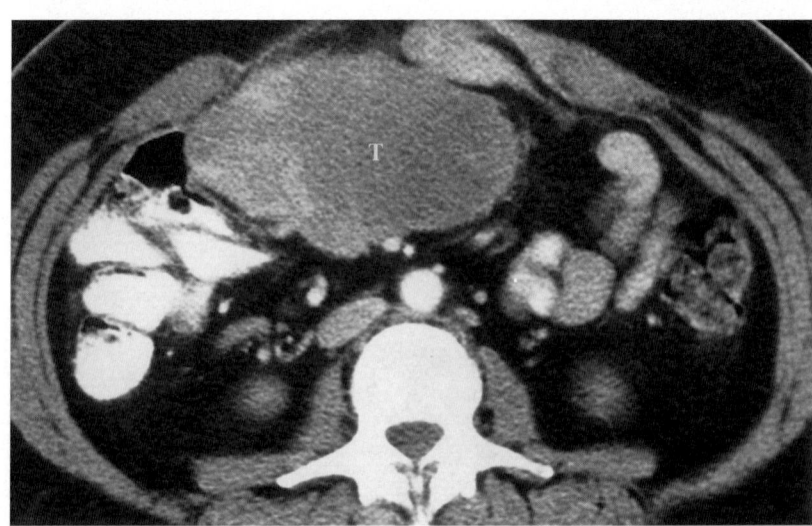

fat levels. CT shows a cystic mass, displacing loops of small bowel anteriorly and laterally. On MR, cyst contents are hyperintense on T2WI and hypointense on T1WI when serous, or hyperintense on T1WI when chylous or hemorrhagic.

GI Duplication Cyst is a congenital, partial, or complete replica of the small bowel. Most arise from the distal small bowel and may communicate with the normal intestinal lumen at one or both ends, or not at all. They are lined by intestinal epithelium. US,CT, and MR reveal a thick-walled cyst with usually serous contents (17).

Mesenteric Teratoma is heterogeneous with cystic and solid components (17). Demonstration of calcium or fat is a clue to radiographic diagnosis.

Diffuse Small Bowel Disease

Students of radiology dread learning about diseases of the small bowel because they are numerous, obscure, confusing, and lead to long lists of differential diagnosis (see Tables 31.3–31.5). A few common diseases cause the majority of small bowel abnormalities that most radiologists will encounter in routine practice. The rest of the list must be known to pass The Boards. Five rules, learned well, simplify the problem.

Rule #1. Dilatation of the small bowel lumen means small bowel obstruction or dysfunction of small bowel muscle.
Rule #2. Thickening of small bowel folds means infiltration of the submucosa.
Rule #3. Uniform, regular, straight thickening means infiltration by fluid (edema or blood).
Rule #4. Irregular, distorted, nodular thickening means infiltration by cells or nonfluid material.
Rule #5. The specific diagnosis requires matching the small bowel pattern with the clinical data.

The normal values for small bowel luminal diameter and fold anatomy is given in Table 31.2 (1,2,18,19).

Dilated Small Bowel Lumen (Table 31.3). The hallmark of mechanical bowel obstruction is a point of transition between dilated bowel and nondilated bowel at the site of obstruction. With muscle dysfunction, the small bowel dilatation is diffuse with no transition point. If no coexisting mucosal disease is present, the small bowel folds are straight and regular (Fig. 31.9). See chapter 26 for an expanded discussion of this topic.

Thickened Folds: Straight and Regular (Table 31.4). Infiltration of edema fluid or hemorrhage into the

Table 31.3. Dilated Small Bowel Lumen

Obstruction (has dilated/nondilated transition zone)
   Adhesions (75% of small bowel obstruction)
      Postsurgical
      Postperitonitis
   Incarcerated hernia
   Volvulus
   Extrinsic Tumor
   Congenital stenosis
   Intraluminal lesion
      Tumor: usually malignant
      Intussusception
      Foreign body
      Gallstone ileus
      Bezoar
      Ascaris (bolus of worms)
      Meconium
Muscle disfunction (no transition zone)
   Adynamic ileus
      Surgery
      Trauma
      Peritoneal inflammation
      Ischemia
      Drugs
         Opiates
         Barbiturates
         Anticholinergics
      Vagotomy
      Diabetic neuropathy
      Metabolic disorders
         Electrolyte imbalance
   Collagen diseases
      Scleroderma
      Dermatomyositis
   Malabsorption syndromes
      Celiac disease
   Chronic idiopathic pseudoobstruction

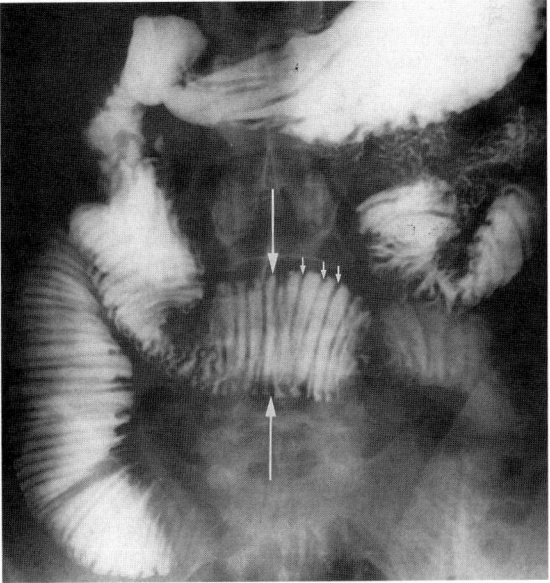

Figure 31.9. Dilated Small Bowel, Normal Folds. Small bowel follow-through examination reveals dilation of the small bowel lumen (>5 cm between *large arrows*) with normal thickness of well-defined folds (*small arrows*). The cause was small bowel obstruction caused by adhesions.

Table 31.2. Normal Small Bowel Measurements

Feature	Normal Values	
	Jejunum	Ileum
Diameter of lumen	3.0 cm	2.5 cm
Diameter of lumen during enteroclysis	4.5 cm	3.5 cm
Thickness of folds	2 mm	2 mm
Number of folds	4–7 per inch	2–4 per inch
Depth of folds	8 mm	8 mm

Table 31.4. Thickened Small Bowel Folds: Straight and Regular

Intestinal edema (diffuse)
    Hypoproteinemia
    Congestive heart failure
    Portal hypertension
    Lymphatic obstruction
        Tumor infiltration (lymphoma)
        Radiation
        Fibrosis of the mesentery
        Lymphangiectasis
    Zollinger-Ellison syndrome
    Lactase deficiency
Intestinal edema (short segment)
    Crohn's disease
    Eosinophilic gastroenteritis
Hemorrhage into bowel wall (long segment)
    Trauma
    Ischemia
    Anticoagulant therapy
    Bleeding disorders
    Vasculitis
        Henoch-Schönlein syndrome
        Connective tissue disease
        Radiation
        Thromboangiitis obliterans
Stomach and small bowel involved
    Ménétrier's disease
    Zollinger-Ellison syndrome
    Crohn's disease
    Lymphoma
    Eosinophilic gastroenteritis

Implies submucosal infiltration by fluid

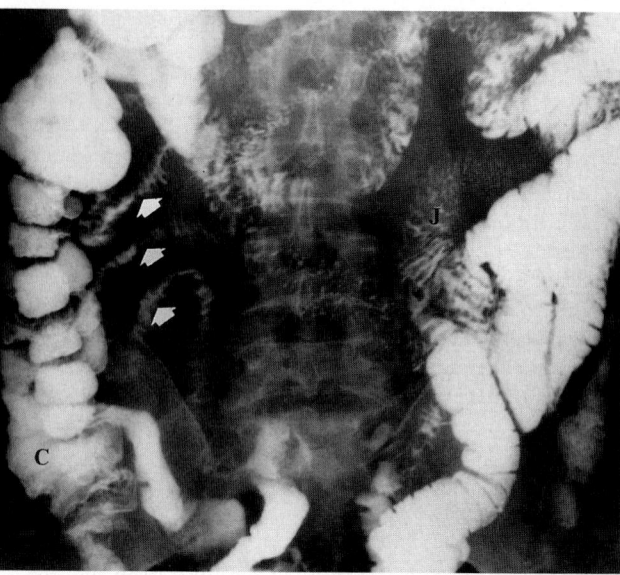

Figure 31.10. Thickened Folds—Regular—Intestinal Ischemia. Barium examination demonstrates a striking separation of multiple loops of ileum (*arrows*), indicating thickening of the bowel walls. The folds in involved loops are thickened and nodular due to edema and hemorrhage resulting from ischemia. A repeat study 1 month later documented complete resolution of all findings. *C*, colon. *J*, jejunum.

submucosa results in uniform straight thickening of the folds (Fig. 31.10). Hemorrhage usually causes thicker folds than edema and may result in scalloping or "thumbprinting" of some folds.

Thickened Folds: Irregular and Distorted (Table 31.5). This is the most difficult category of abnormality because many conditions are unusual. The distribution of fold abnormality helps to limit the differential diagnosis (Fig. 31.11).

Some conditions are included in several categories. Early Crohn's disease is characterized by edema and regular folds. More advanced Crohn's disease has inflammatory cell infiltrate and irregular folds. Lymphoma in the mesentery obstructs lymphatics and causes edema, and lymphoma in the bowel wall causes nodular, irregular folds. Lymphoma and Crohn's disease are the two most commonly encountered small bowel diseases.

Scleroderma produces atrophy of the muscularis of the small bowel by the process of progressive collagen deposition resulting in flaccid, atonic, dilated bowel. The valvulae conniventes are normal or thinned. A "hidebound" appearance of thinned folds tethered together is produced by contraction of the longitudinal muscle layer to a greater extent than the circular muscle layer. Excessive contraction of the mesenteric border of the small bowel results in formation of mucosal sacculations along the antimesenteric border. The jejunum and duodenum are more severly involved than the ileum. The di-

Table 31.5. Thickened Small Bowel Folds: Irregular and Distorted

Proximal (predominantly duodenum + jejunum)
    Giardiasis
    Strongyloides
    Whipple's disease
    Eosinophilic gastroenteritis
    Zollinger-Ellison syndrome
Distal (predominantly ileum)
    Lymphoma
    Crohn's disease
    Yersinia/Campylobacter
    Salmonella
    Tuberculosis
    Behçet's disease
    Cystic fibrosis
    AIDS-related infections
Diffuse
    Lymphoma
    Polyposis syndromes
    Amyloidosis
    Histoplasmosis
    Systemic mastocytosis
    Waldenström's macroglobulinemia
    Lymphoma
Stomach and small bowel involved
    Lymphoma
    Crohn's disease
    Eosinophilic gastroenteritis
    Whipple's disease
    Tuberculosis
    Mastocytosis

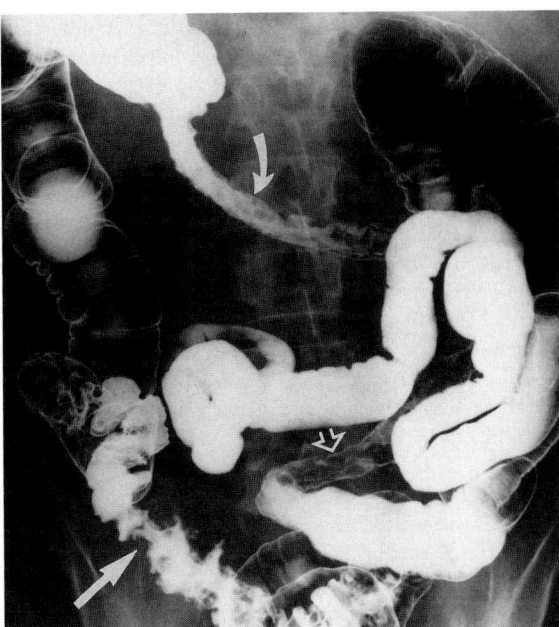

Figure 31.11. Thickened Folds—Irregular—Crohn's Disease. Crohn's disease of the ileum causes thickened folds (*straight arrow*) that are irregular and distorted. A more proximal segment of jejunum (*open arrow*) is effaced and narrowed. The transverse colon (*curved arrow*) is narrowed, stiffened, and has multiple inflammatory polyps producing filling defects. This is an excellent example of "skip lesions" characteristic of Crohn's disease.

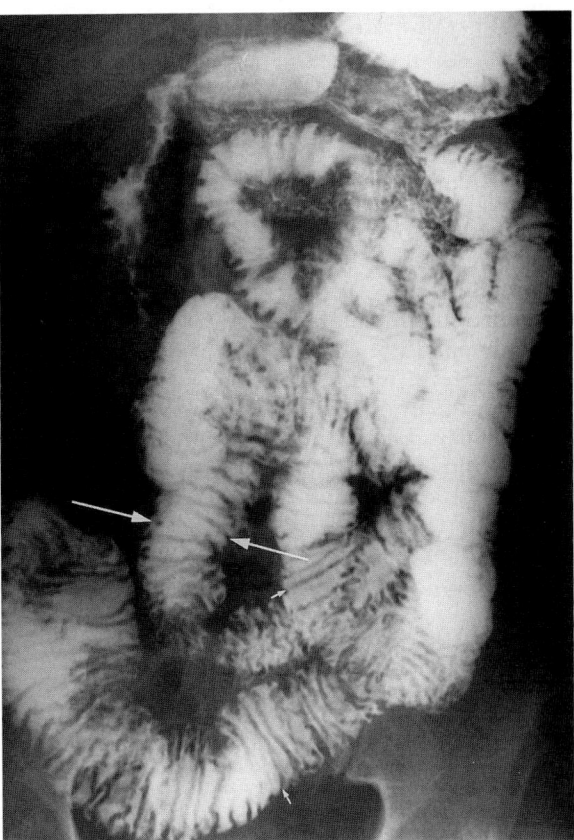

Figure 31.12. Adult Celiac Disease. Small bowel follow-through examination demonstrates dilation of the lumen of the small bowel (4 cm between *long arrows*). The folds are of normal thickness (*small arrows*), less than 3 mm. This patient with malabsorption became asymptomatic on a gluten-free diet.

agnosis is confirmed by skin changes and characteristic involvement of the esophagus. Malabsorption eventually occurs.

Adult Celiac Disease (nontropical sprue) presents with malabsorption, steatorrhea, and weight loss (20). Gluten, an insoluble protein found in wheat, rye, oats, and barley, acts as a toxic agent to the small bowel mucosa. The mucosa becomes flattened and absorptive cells decrease in number; villi disappear. The submucosa, muscularis, and serosa remain normal. Patients with long-term sprue have an increased risk of lymphoma and GI carcinoma. The classic radiographic findings are as follows: *a)* dilated small bowel, *b)* normal or thinned folds (Fig. 31.12) *c)* a decreased number of folds per inch in the jejunum (≤3) *d)* an increased number of folds per inch in the ileum (≥5). Findings are best demonstrated by enteroclysis. Five or more folds per inch in the jejunum makes the diagnosis unlikely. Fluid excess is often evident in the ileum. Transient intussusceptions may be observed.

Tropical Sprue has similar clinical and radiographic findings as nontropical sprue but is confined to India, the Far East, and Puerto Rico. The disease responds to administration of folate and antibiotics.

Lactase Deficiency. Lactase is required within the absorptive cells of the jejunum to properly digest disaccharides. Several population groups, including Chinese, Arabs, Bantu, and Eskimos, may become totally deficient in lactase during adult life. Secondary lactase deficiency may develop with alcoholism, Crohn's disease, and drugs such as neomycin. The nondigested lactose in

the small bowel causes increased intraluminal fluid and dilated small bowel with normal folds.

Intestinal Ischemia may result from embolism or thrombosis of the superior mesenteric artery or vein (21). Patients may present with an acute abdomen or vague symptoms. Arterial occlusion may be due to embolus, vasculitis, trauma, or adhesions. Venous thrombosis results from hypercoagulability states (neoplasms, oral contraceptives), inflammation (pancreatitis, peritonitis, abscess), or stasis (portal hypertension, congestive heart failure). Plain films demonstrate gaseous distention, thickened mucosal folds (thumbprinting), and, in some cases, intramural or portal venous gas. CT is preferred to barium studies to demonstrate characteristic abnormalities (Figs. 31.10,31.13): dilated lumen, thickened bowel wall, engorged mesenteric vessels, thrombus in the mesenteric arteries or veins, intramural or venous gas.

Radiation Enteritis occurs when large doses of radiation are given to adjacent organs. The small bowel is the most radiosensitive organ in the abdomen. Long segments of bowel may be involved, with thickening of folds and bowel wall. Peristalsis is impaired. Progressive fibrosis leads to tapered strictures commonly involving long segments. The bowel may be kinked and obstructed by adhesions. Fistulas to the vagina or other organs may also result. Computed tomography demonstrates wall thickening and increased density of the mesentery, and fixation of bowel loops.

Lymphangiectasia refers to gross dilation of the lymphatic vessels in the small bowel mucosa and submucosa. The primary form is a congenital lymphatic blockage, often associated with asymmetric edema of the extremities. Despite being congenital, symptoms often do not occur until young adulthood. Patients present with protein-losing enteropathy, diarrhea, steatorrhea, and recurrent infection. Secondary lymphangiectasia refers to lymphatic obstruction due to radiation, congestive heart failure, or mesenteric node involvement by malignancy or inflammation. The diagnosis is confirmed by jejunal biopsy. Barium study findings include diffuse fold thickening that is most pronounced in the jejunum, increased intraluminal fluid, and groups of tiny (1 mm) nodules due to distended villi. The pattern closely resembles Whipple's disease. CT helps the differentiation by revealing thickening of the bowel wall and mesenteric adenopathy in secondary lymphangiectasia.

Eosinophilic Gastroenteritis virtually always affects the gastric antrum, as well as all or part of the small bowel. Intense infiltration of eosinophils in the lamina propria causes thickening of the bowel wall and mucosal folds, often with luminal narrowing. Barium studies show thickened and straightened folds. Thickening of the bowel wall is evidenced by wide separation between bowel loops and is demonstrated by CT. Most patients have a history of allergic disorders. The disease is self-limited but recurrences are frequent.

Amyloidosis is a disease complex associated with extracellular infiltration of an amorphous protein material in body tissues (22). The disease may be primary or associated with multiple myeloma (10–15%), rheumatoid arthritis (20–25%), or tuberculosis (50%). Most cases are systemic but 10–20% are localized. The small bowel is the most common site of GI involvement. Amyloid deposits are seen throughout the wall of the small bowel, especially within the walls of small blood vessels resulting in ischemia and infarction. Deposits in the muscularis impair motility. Diffuse, irregular thickened folds may be seen throughout the small bowel. Nodules are sometimes present. Diagnosis is confirmed by biopsy.

Systemic Mastocytosis is a proliferation of mast cells in the skin, bones, lymph nodes, and GI tract. Urticaria pigmentosa is the characteristic skin manifestation. Osteoblastic bone changes are found in 70% of cases. Lymphadenopathy and hepatosplenomegaly are often present. The bowel wall and mucosal folds are thickened, and mucosal nodules up to 5 mm size are often evident (Table 31.6).

Whipple's Disease is an uncommon systemic disorder affecting the GI tract, joints, central nervous system, and lymph nodes. The disease is caused by Whipple's bacilli, Gram-positive, rod-shaped bacteria that are found within macrophages in many organs and tissues. Patients may present with arthritis, neurologic symptoms, or steatorrhea. Generalized lymphadenopathy is usually present. Enteroclysis demonstrates irregularly thickened folds most prominent in the jejunum. Demonstration of tiny (1 mm) sand-like nodules spread diffusely over the mucosa or in small groups is strong evidence of the disease. Increased luminal fluid is usual. CT reveals enlarged mesenteric lymph nodes that may have fat density.

AIDS Enteritis. In addition to lymphoma and Kaposi's sarcoma, AIDS patients are predisposed to multiple opportunistic infections of the GI tract (23). Infective agents usually occur in combination and in multiple GI sites.

Cryptosporidium and *Isospora belli* are protozoans that may infest the proximal intestine and cause a cholera-like diarrhea with life-threatening fluid loss. Barium studies show thickened folds and marked increased fluid.

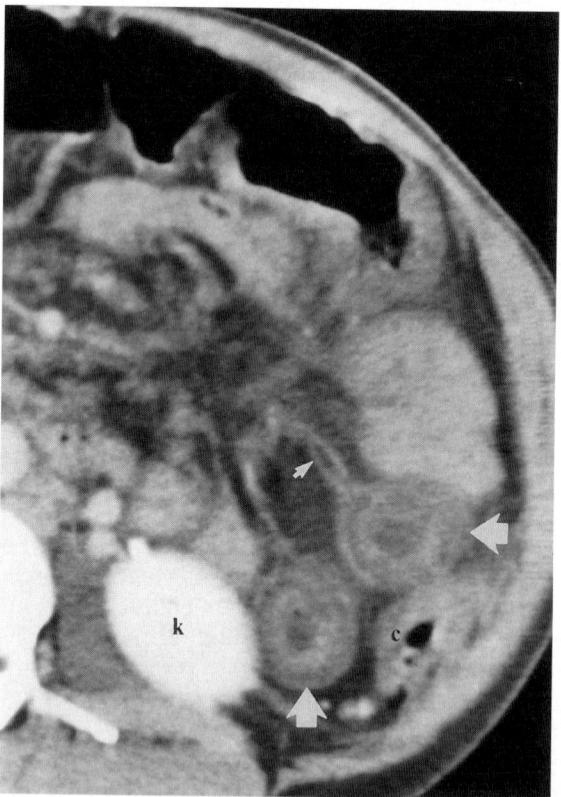

Figure 31.13. Intestinal Ischemia. CT demonstrates circumferential thickening of small bowel loops (*large arrows*) caused by intestinal ischemia due to portal vein thrombosis. A characteristic, benign, "target" appearance of bowel wall thickening is evident. The mesentery is edematous and congested (*small arrow*). *c*, descending colon; *k*, kidney.

Table 31.6. Tiny Small Bowel Nodules

Nodular lymphoid hyperplasia (2–4 mm)
Lymphoma (>4 mm)
Amyloidosis
Whipple's disease (1–2 mm)
Mycobacterium avium-intracellulare
Lymphangiectasia
Systemic mastocystosis (<5 mm)

Cytomegalovirus causes disease in the small bowel and colon as well as the lungs, liver, and spleen. Mucosal ulceration with bleeding and perforation are the major intestinal manifestations. Barium studies show thickened folds, loop separation, ulcers, and fistulae.

Mycobacterium avium-intracellulare is a common systemic infection in AIDS, involving lung, liver, spleen, bone marrow, lymph nodes, and intestinal tract. Barium studies show thickened, nodular folds with a sand-like mucosal pattern. CT demonstrates retroperitoneal and mesenteric adenopathy and focal lesions in the liver and spleen.

Candida, Amoeba histolytica, Giardia, Strongyloides, herpes simplex, and *Campylobacter* may also occur in AIDS patients.

Small Bowel Erosions and Ulcerations

Crohn's Disease is an inflammatory disease of uncertain etiology that may involve the GI tract from the esophagus to the anus (24,25). The disease is characterized by erosions, ulcerations, full-thickness bowel wall inflammation, and formation of noncaseating granulomas. Patients present, usually in their twenties and thirties, with diarrhea, abdominal pain, weight loss, and often fever. The typical course is one of remissions, relapse, and progression of disease. Patterns of GI involvement include colon and terminal ileum (55%), small bowel alone (30%), colon alone (15%), and proximal small bowel without terminal ileum (3%). Radiographic hallmarks of Crohn's disease are: *a*) aphthous erosions (see Fig. 30.12), *b*) confluent deep ulcerations, *c*) thickened and distorted folds (Fig. 31.11), *d*) fibrosis with thickened walls, contractures and stenosis, *e*) involvement of the mesentery, *f*) asymmetric involvement both longitudinally and around the lumen, *g*) skip areas of normal intervening bowel between disease segments (Fig. 31.11), and *h*) fistula and sinus tract formation. Aphthous ulcers are shallow, 1–2 mm depressions usually surrounded by a well-defined halo. Deep ulcerations are larger and often linear, forming fissures between nodules of elevated edematous mucosa ("cobblestone pattern")(Fig. 31.14). Fibrosis and progressive thickening of the bowel wall narrows the lumen, particularly of the terminal ileum, producing the "string sign" (Fig. 31.15). Mesenteric involvement is best demonstrated by CT. Ulceration along the mesenteric border may extend between the leaves of the mesentery. The mesenteric fat is infiltrated; the mesentery is thickened and retracted.

Complications of Crohn's disease are common and well shown by CT (see Fig. 32.14). Obstruction is usually partial and due to strictures or areas of severe ulceration and spasm. Fistulae are formed in 19% of patients with small bowel disease (Fig. 31.15). Fistulae are abnormal communications between two epithelial-lined organs. Most frequent are ileocolonic and ileocecal, but enterocutaneous, enterovesical, and colovesical fistulae are also common. Sinus tracts extend into inflammatory extraluminal masses from the bowel lumen (Fig. 31.15). Abscess and phlegmon formation in the mesentery, peritoneal cavity, retroperitoneum, and abdominal wall are common. Free perforation occurs in 3% of cases. Most

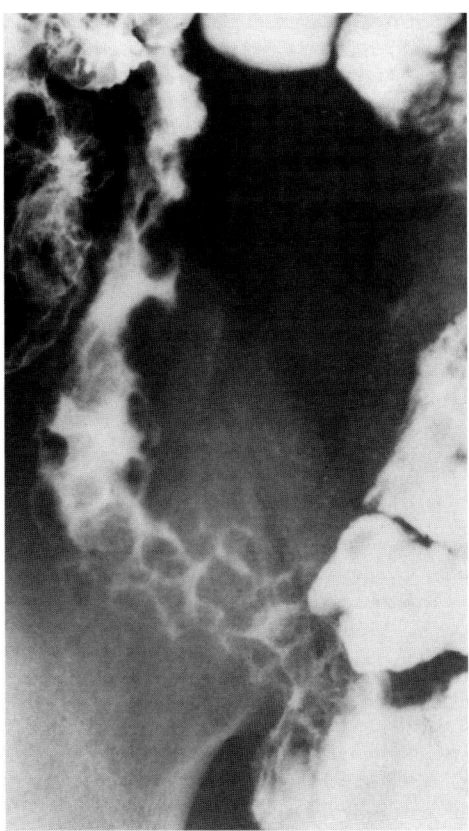

Figure 31.14. Crohn's Disease: Cobblestone Pattern. Coned-down view of the terminal ileum reveals cobblestone pattern of ulcerations and fissures between mounds of unaffected mucosa.

perforations are confined and form sinus tracts or fistulae. Carcinoma of the small and large bowel are increased in frequency with a prevalence of about 0.5% in Crohn's disease patients. Derangements of intestinal absorption cause megaloblastic anemia (vitamin B_{12} deficiency) and an increased incidence of gallstones and renal stones. Up to 20% of patients have arthritis or spondylitis that mimics ankylosing spondylitis.

Yersinia Enterocolitis is caused by infection with the Gram-positive bacilli, *Yersinia enterocolitica* or *Y. pseudotuberculosis*. Infection causes an acute enteritis with abdominal pain, fever, and often bloody diarrhea that mimics acute appendicitis or acute Crohn's disease. Children and young adults are most often affected. The infection runs a self-limited course of 8–12 weeks. Diagnosis is confirmed by stool culture. Radiographic findings are most pronounced in the last 20 cm of the ileum. They include aphthous ulcers, nodules up to 1 cm in size, wall thickening, and thickened folds that become effaced with increasing edema. Nodular lymphoid hyperplasia may appear during the resolution stage.

Campylobacter fetus subsp *jejuni* infection is clinically and radiographically similar to *Yersinia* enterocolitis. The disease usually lasts 1–2 weeks but relapses are common. Diagnosis is by stool culture.

Behçet's Disease is a multisystem disease due to a small vessel vasculitis that affects eyes, joints, skin, central nervous system, and the intestinal tract (26).

Figure 31.15. Crohn's Disease. A small bowel study in a patient with long-standing Crohn's disease demonstrates numerous sinus tracts and fistulas (*small arrows*) with extraluminal abscesses (*long arrows*). Fistulous connections extended between loops of small bowel as well as between ileum and the right ureter (not shown). The distal ileum (*i*) demonstrates irregular narrowing and separation from adjacent loops. Asymmetric involvement of a portion of the ileum has resulted in the formation of a sacculation (*large arrow*). The terminal ileum (*ti*) is narrowed and stiffened with a thick wall evidenced by separation from adjacent loops. *C*, cecum.

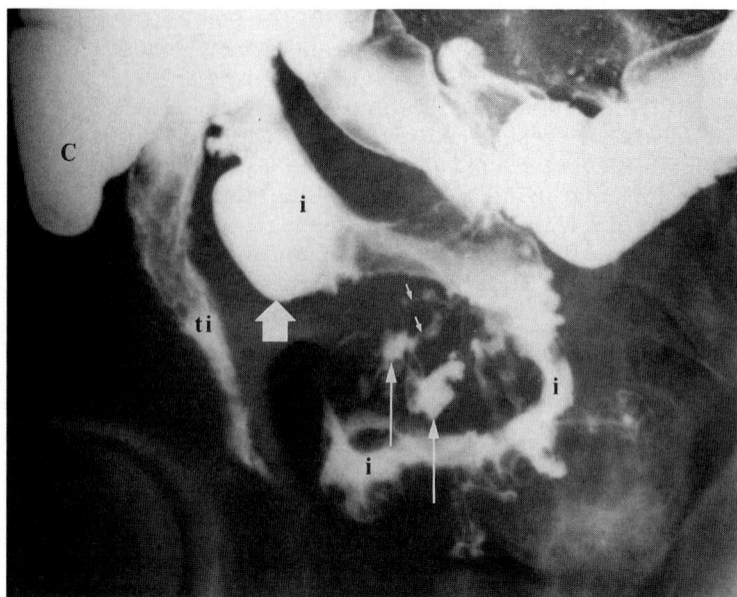

Prominent clinical features include relapsing iridocyclitis, mucocutaneous ulcerations, vesicles, pustules, and mild arthritis. Intestinal disease most commonly involves the ileocecal region, where Crohn's disease is closely mimicked with aphthous erosions, deep ulceration, stenosis, and fistula formation.

Tuberculosis presents as peritonitis or focal infection of the gut, most commonly involving the ileocecal area, closely mimicking Crohn's disease. Less than half of the patients have concurrent evidence of pulmonary tuberculosis. Barium studies demonstrate inflamed mucosa with transverse and stellate ulcers. The affected bowel becomes rigid and narrowed with nodular mucosa. The ileocecal valve is stiff and gaping with narrowed terminal ileum and cecum. CT shows characteristic findings of mesenteric adenopathy, high-density ascites, and peritoneal thickening accompanying the bowel wall thickening.

Small Bowel Diverticula

Small Bowel Diverticula are most common in the jejunum along the mesenteric border. They are outpouchings of mucosa through the bowel wall and between the leaves of the mesentery. They are commonly multiple and often asymptomatic. However, because of stasis of bowel contents within them, bacterial overgrowth may occur, resulting in deconjugation of bile salts and malabsorption. Vitamin B_{12} absorption may also be impaired, resulting in megaloblastic anemia. Additional complications include obstruction, acute diverticulitis, hemorrhage, and volvulus. Plain films may reveal featureless ovoid collections of air. Barium studies show the outpouchings, most with a neck smaller in diameter than the outpouching itself (Fig. 31.16). The diverticulum lacks mucosal folds and does not contract because of the lack of muscle within its wall. Diverticula are usually not recognized on CT.

Meckel's Diverticulum is the most common congenital anomaly of the GI tract, present in 2–3% of the population

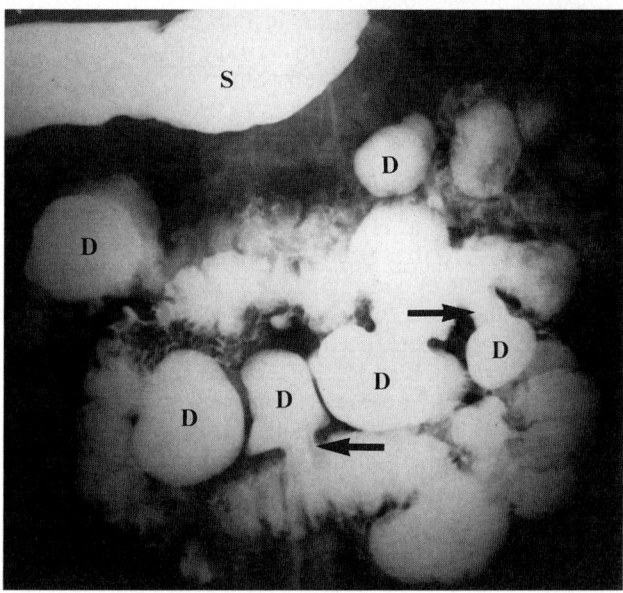

Figure 31.16. Small Bowel Diverticula. A small bowel series demonstrates numerous diverticula (*D*) extending from the duodenum and jejunum. The necks (*arrows*) of several diverticula are shown particularly well. *S*, stomach.

(27). The diverticulum varies from 2–8 cm in length, and is located on the antimesenteric border of the ileum up to 2 m from the ileocecal valve. The tip of the diverticulum may be attached to the umbilicus by a remnant of the vitelline duct. Ectopic gastric mucosa is present in up to 62% of cases. Peptic secretions may cause ulceration and bleeding. Other complications are intussusception, volvulus, and perforation. Radionuclide (Tc-99m-pertechnetate) scanning for ectopic gastric mucosa is the test of choice but is less reliable in adults than in children, and is negative when the diverticulum does not contain gastric mucosa. Enteroclysis is then the best method to demonstrate the diverticulum which appears as a blind sac attached to the antimesenteric border of the ileum.

Pseudodiverticula or sacculations are outpouchings along the antimesenteric border of the small bowel that result from disease of the small bowel. They occur most commonly in association with Crohn's disease (Fig. 31.14) or scleroderma. With fibrosis and contraction of the mesenteric border of the bowel, the unsupported antimesenteric border becomes pleated and forms sacculations.

References

1. Herlinger H, Maglinte D, eds. Clinical Radiology of the Small Intestine. Philadelphia: WB Saunders Company, 1989.
2. Rubesin SE, Rubin RA, Herlinger H. Small bowel malabsorption: clinical and radiologic perspectives—how we see it. Radiology 1992;184:297–305.
3. Trenkner SW, Hommeyer S. Practical imaging of the small bowel. Radiologist 1995;2:127–137.
4. Herlinger H. Barium examinations. In: Gore RM, Levine MS, Laufer I, eds. Textbook of Gastrointestinal Radiology. Philadelphia: WB Saunders, 1994:772–788.
5. Balthazar EJ. CT of the gastrointestinal tract: principles and interpretation. AJR Am J Roentgenol 1991;156:23–32.
6. Desai RK, Tagliabue JR, Wegryn SA, Einstein DM. CT evaluation of wall thickening in the alimentary tract. Radiographics 1991;11:771–783.
7. Buck JL, Sobin LH. Carcinoids of the gastrointestinal tract. Radiographics 1990;10:1081–1095.
8. Dudiak KM, Johnson CD, Stephens DH. Primary tumors of the small intestine: CT evaluation. AJR Am J Roentgenol 1989;152:995–998.
9. Rubesin SE, Gilchrist AM, Bronner M, et al. Non-Hodgkin lymphoma of the small intestine. Radiographics 1990;10:985—998.
10. Levine MS, Rubesin SE, Pantongrag-Brown L, et al. Non-Hodgkin's lymphoma of the gastrointestinal tract: radiographic findings. AJR Am J Roentgenol 1997;168:165–172.
11. Balthazar EJ, Noordhoorn M, Megibow AJ, Gordon RB. CT of small-bowel lymphoma in immunocompetent patients and patients with AIDS: comparison of findings. AJR Am J Roentgenol 1997;168:675–680.
12. McDermott VG, Low VHS, Keogan MT, et al. Malignant melanoma metastatic to the gastrointestinal tract. AJR Am J Roentgenol 1996;166:809–813.
13. Buck JL, Harned RK, Lichtenstein JE, Sobin LH. Peutz-Jeghers syndrome. Radiographics 1992;12:365–378.
14. Mindelzun RE, Jeffrey RB Jr, Lane MJ, Silverman PM. The misty mesentery on CT: differential diagnosis. AJR Am J Roentgenol 1997;167:61–65.
15. Eistein DM, Tagliabue JR, Desai RK. Abdominal desmoids: CT findings in 25 patients. AJR Am J Roentgenol 1991;157:275–279.
16. Forte MD, Brant WE. Spontaneous isolated mesenteric fibromatosis. Diseases Colon Rectum 1988;31:315–317.
17. Stoupis C, Ros PR, Abbitt PL, et al. Bubbles in the belly: imaging of cystic mesenteric or omental masses. Radiographics 1994;14:729–737.
18. Eisenberg RL. Gastrointestinal Radiology: A Pattern Approach. 2nd ed. Philadelphia: JB Lippincott, 1992.
19. Zalev AH. Radiographic diagnosis of diseases of the small intestine by pattern analysis. Applied Radiology 1994;(Oct.):20–26.
20. Rubesin SE, Grumbach K, Herlinger H, et al. Adult celiac disease and its complications. Radiographics 1989;9:1045–1066.
21. Lund EC, Han SY, Holley HC, Berland LL. Intestinal ischemia: comparison of plain radiographic and computed tomographic findings. Radiographics 1988;8:1083–1108.
22. Urban BA, Fishman EK, Goldman SM, et al. CT evaluation of amyloidosis: spectrum of disease. Radiographics 1993;13:1295–1308.
23. Feczko PJ. Gastrointestinal complications of immunodeficiency virus (HIV) infection. Semin Roentgen 1994;29:275–287.
24. Wills JS, Lobis IF, Denstman FJ. Crohn disease: state of the art. Radiology 1997;202:597–610.
25. Gore RM, Balthazar EJ, Ghahremani GG, Miller FH. CT features of ulcerative colitis and Crohn's disease. AJR Am J Roentgenol 1996;167:3–15.
26. Iida M, Kobayashi H, Matsumoto T, et al. Intestinal Behçet disease: serial changes at radiography. Radiology 1993;188:65–69.
27. Rossi P, Gourtsoyiannis N, Bezzi M, et al. Meckel's diverticulum: imaging diagnosis. AJR Am J Roentgenol 1996;166:567–573.

32
Colon and Appendix

William E. Brant

COLON

Imaging Methods

The primary imaging methods for detection of colon abnormalities are barium enemas. The single-contrast barium enema is generally favored for the evaluation of colonic obstruction, fistulas, and in old, seriously ill or debilitated patients. The double-contrast barium enema is favored for detection of small lesions (<1 cm), for documentation of inflammatory bowel disease, and for detailed imaging evaluation of the rectum (Fig. 32.1). Colonoscopy is a complementary procedure to barium studies that is limited by occasional failure to reach the right colon. Colonoscopy and proctoscopy are excellent for evaluating diagnostic problems posed by barium studies, and for biopsy of suspected neoplastic lesions.

As elsewhere in the GI tract, CT complements the barium examination by demonstrating intramural and extracolonic components of disease (1–3). It is excellent for demonstrating extrinsic inflammatory and neoplastic processes that affect the colon: abscesses, sinuses, and fistulas. A new investigational helical CT technique, called CT colography or virtual colonoscopy, utilizes reformatted two-dimensional and three-dimensional images to simulate endoscopic images and detect polyps and other mucosal abnormalities (4).

CT and MR images have been utilized for initial staging of colorectal carcinoma. However, both methods are limited in their ability to determine the extent of bowel wall tumor infiltration and involvement of regional lymph nodes. Transrectal US is more accurate than CT or MR in determining local tumor extent of rectal carcinomas, and is used in the evaluation of other rectal and perirectal disease (5,6). For the initial staging of colorectal carcinoma, CT and MR should be reserved for patients with suspected widespread local or disseminated disease. CT is useful in screening for recurrence of colorectal carcinoma because it can provide a comprehensive examination of the liver, abdominal cavity, and entire colon. MR is sensitive but nonspecific in the detection of local recurrence of rectal carcinoma.

Anatomy

The large intestine consists of the cecum and appendix, colon, rectum, and anal canal. It is approximately 1.5 m in length from the ileum to the anus. The large intestine is characterized by the *taenia coli*, three longitudinal bands of muscle that traverse the colon shortening it to form haustra, the sacculations created by puckering of the bowel wall. The major functions of the large intestine are the formation, transport, and evacuation of feces. These functions require mobility, absorption of water, and secretion of mucus. Infrequent peristalsis transports feces from the ascending and transverse colon to the sigmoid colon where fecal material is stored until defecation. The cecum and ascending colon absorb water from the highly liquid material received from the ileum. Mucus secreted by mucosal goblet cells protects the mucosa from injury, and is secreted in profuse amounts when the mucosa is irritated or injured.

The cecum is the large blind pouch that extends below the level of the ileocecal valve. The cecum generally lies in the right iliac fossa but may be quite mobile. It is usually covered on all sides by peritoneum (intraperitoneal), but may be fixed extraperitoneally, covered only on its ventral surface by peritoneum. The appendix is a long worm-like tube that hangs from near the apex of the cecum (Fig. 32.1). The ileocecal valve consists of two lips that project into the cecum forming a prominent mass. The ascending colon is extraperitoneal, lying in the anterior pararenal space, covered only on its ventral surface by peritoneum. The hepatic flexure forms two curves. The proximal, more posterior curve is closely related to the descending duodenum and right kidney. The more distal anterior curve is closely related to the gallbladder. The transverse colon is intraperitoneal and suspended from the transverse mesocolon that arises from the peritoneum covering the pancreas and sweeps transversely across the upper abdomen. The transverse mesocolon limits the superior extent of the small bowel loops. The splenic flexure is closely related to the tail of the pancreas and the caudal aspect of the spleen. The

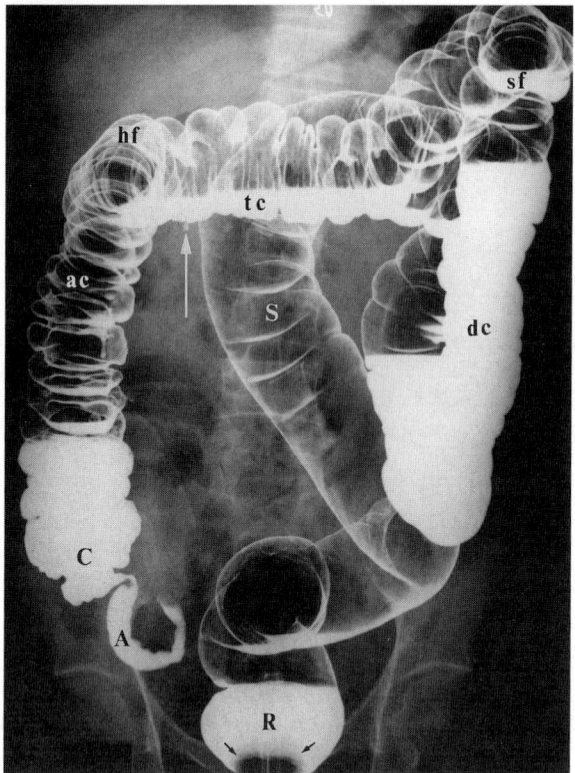

Figure 32.1. Double-Contrast Barium Enema. An upright radiograph from a double-contrast barium enema demonstrates normal colon anatomy. The appendix (*A*) extends from the cecum (*C*). The ascending colon (*ac*) extends to the hepatic flexure (*hf*), the coils of which must be examined by multiple oblique views. The transverse colon (*tc*) extends to the splenic flexure (*sf*), which continues as the descending colon (*dc*). This patient has a long sigmoid colon (*S*) that extends high into the abdomen. The transverse colon is relatively short. Patients with a short sigmoid colon usually have a long redundant transverse colon. The distended balloon at the tip of the enema catheter causes a lucent filling defect (*small arrows*) in the rectum (*R*). A tiny intramural diverticulum (*long arrow*) is seen in the proximal transverse colon.

splenic flexure is anchored to the diaphragm by the phrenicocolic ligament, which serves as a boundary between disease processes of the left subphrenic space and the left paracolic gutter.

The descending colon, like the ascending colon, is extraperitoneal within the anterior pararenal space and is covered by peritoneum only on its ventral surface. The sigmoid colon forms a redundant loop of variable length from the distal descending colon in the left iliac fossa to the rectum. The sigmoid colon is completely intraperitoneal and is suspended by the sigmoid mesocolon that allows considerable mobility. The sigmoid colon penetrates the peritoneum at the level of vertebrae S-2 to S-4 to continue as the extraperitoneal rectum. The rectum extends for approximately 12 cm in close relationship with the sacrum. Peritoneum forming the pouch of Douglas covers the ventral and lateral aspects of the rectum. The anal canal is 3–4 cm long and is invested by the sphincter ani and levator ani muscles. A series of vertical folds form the rectal columns of Morgagni, beneath which are the veins that when dilated, are hemorrhoids.

The colon can be recognized on CT and MR by its course, haustral markings, and fecal content. The thickness of the wall of the normal colon does not exceed 5 mm.

Colon Filling Defects/Mass Lesions

Filling Defect refers to a radiolucency in a barium pool caused by a protruding mass lesion. On barium enema examinations, filling defects may be polyps, tumors, plaques, air bubbles, feces, mucus, or foreign objects. Polyps are protrusions from the mucosa that produce filling defects in pools of barium or are etched in white when coated by barium and outlined by air on double-contrast studies. Polyps may be pedunculated on a stalk or sessile (Fig. 32.2). They may appear as "bowler hats" (Fig. 32.3) when viewed obliquely (7). The term "polyp" is generic for a protruding lesion and does not imply a histologic diagnosis. Air bubbles rise to the highest point of a contrast column (the "carpenter's level sign"), but fecal material usually remains dependent (8). Plaques are flat lesions that barely rise above the mucosal surface. An excellent pictorial glossary of findings on double contrast intestinal studies is provided by Rubesin and Laufer (9).

Colorectal Adenocarcinoma is the the most common malignancy of the GI tract and the second most common malignant tumor in the United States (10). Approximately 50% arise in the rectum and rectosigmoid area. Another 25% occur in the sigmoid colon, and the remaining 25% are evenly distributed throughout the remainder of the colon. Nearly all cancers of the colon are adenocarcinomas arising from preexisting adenomas. Most tumors are annular constricting lesions, 2–6 cm in diameter, with raised everted edges and ulcerated mucosa (Fig. 32.4). Polypoid tumors are less common, some

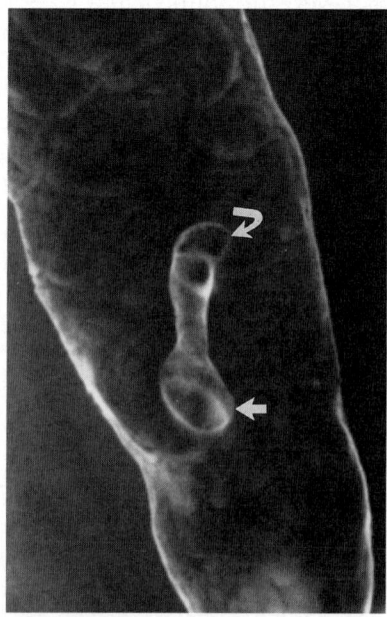

Figure 32.2. Pedunculated Polyp. Double-contrast barium enema demonstrates a long-stalked pedunculated polyp with a bulbous tip (*straight arrow*) arising (*curved arrow*) from the mucosa of the descending colon.

having the frond-like appearance of villous carcinoma. Infiltrating scirrhous tumors, so common in gastric carcinoma, are rare in the large intestine, unless the patient has ulcerative colitis. The tumor spreads by direct invasion through the bowel wall into pericolonic fat and adjacent organs (Figs. 32.5,32.6), lymphatic channels to regional nodes (11), and hematogenously through the

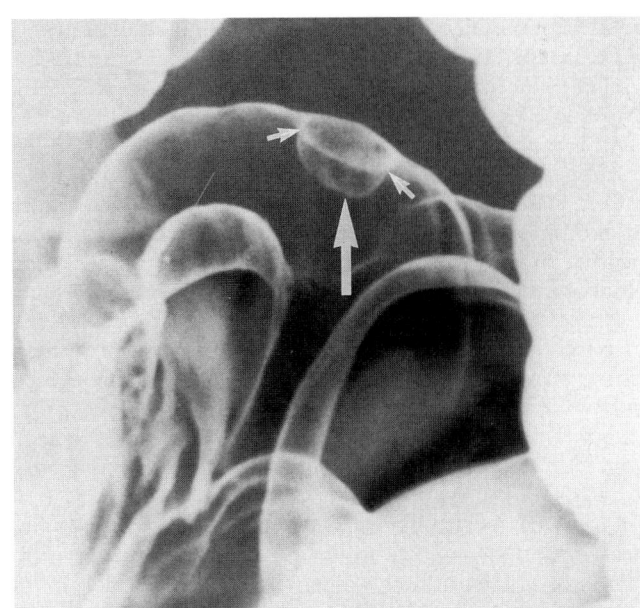

Figure 32.3. Bowler Hat Sign is produced by barium coating both the body of the polyp (*large arrow*) and the recesses (*small arrows*) between the base of the lesion and the normal colonic mucosa.

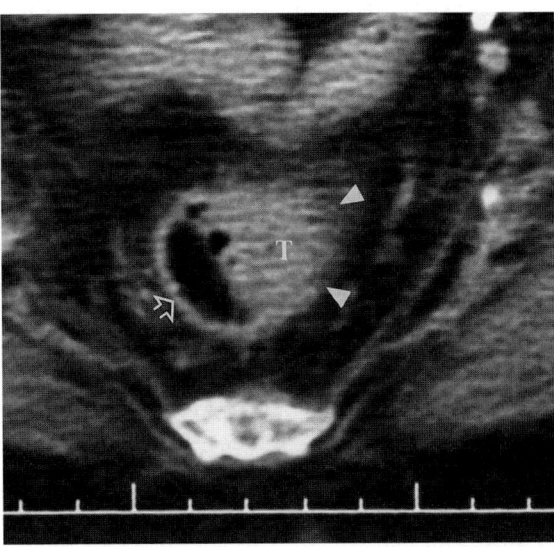

Figure 32.5. Rectal Carcinoma. CT demonstrates asymmetric thickening of the wall of the rectum (*T*) with soft tissue stranding densities (*arrowheads*) extending into the perirectal fat. Tumor invasion through the rectal wall was confirmed at surgery. Note the normal rectal wall on the opposite side (*open arrow*) with sharp definition of perirectal fat.

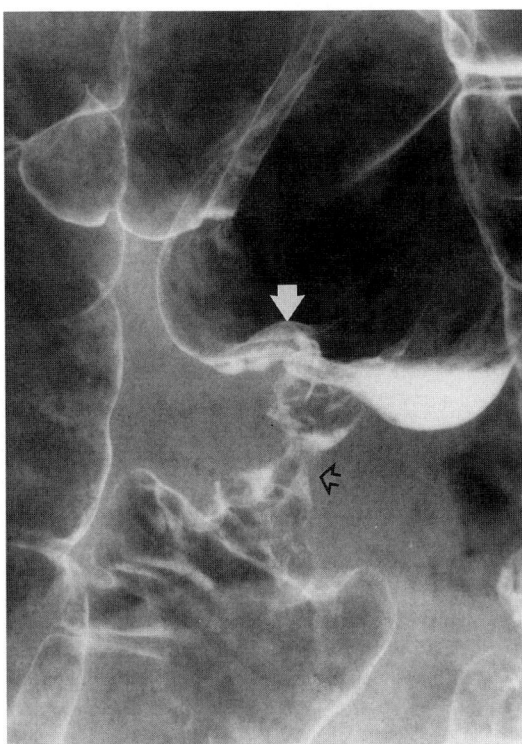

Figure 32.4. Colon Carcinoma. Radiograph of the sigmoid colon from a double-contrast barium enema demonstrates a characteristic "apple core" constricting lesion of colon carcinoma. The lumen is markedly narrowed (*open arrow*) and shoulders of the tumor cause a mass impression on the adjacent distended lumen (*solid arrow*).

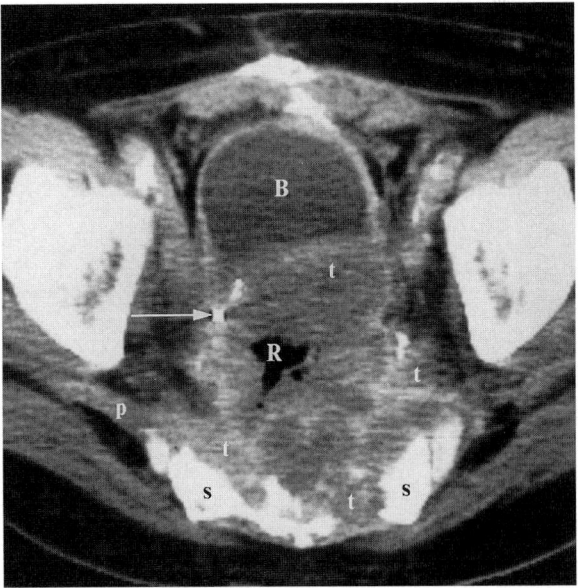

Figure 32.6. Advanced Rectal Carcinoma. A CT scan demonstrates carcinoma of the rectum (*R*) with widespread tumor extension (*t*) into the bladder (*B*), perirectal tissues, piriformis muscle (*p*), and sacrum (*s*). A stent (*arrow*) has been placed in the right ureter because of tumor obstruction at the ureteral vesical junction.

portal veins to the liver and systemic circulation (Table 32.1). Intraperitoneal seeding from a tumor that penetrates the colon wall may also occur. Obstruction is the most frequent complication. Other complications are uncommon but include perforation, intussusception, abscess, and fistula formation. Up to 20% of patients have a second tumor of the large bowel at diagnosis, usually an adenoma or another carcinoma. Approximately 5% of patients will have a second colorectal carcinoma either simultaneously or subsequently diagnosed. Patients with ulcerative colitis, Crohn's disease, familial adenomatous polyposis syndrome, and Peutz-Jeghers syndrome are at increased risk of colon carcinoma.

Local disease is best evaluated with transrectal or colonoscopic US. CT and MR are used for more advanced disease and to detect recurrence. Microscopic invasion through the bowel wall and tumor involvement of normal sized lymph nodes is not detected by CT or MR (12). A scheme for cross-sectional staging of colorectal carcinoma is given in Table 32.2.

Tumor recurrences are most common *a)* at the operative site, near the bowel anastomosis, *b)* in the peritoneal cavity, and *c)* in the liver and distant organs. Because the entire abdominal cavity must be surveyed to detect tumor recurrence, CT is the current method of choice.

Polyps. A polyp is defined as a localized mass that projects from the mucosa into the lumen. Because the majority of colorectal cancers are believed to arise from preexisting adenomatous polyps, the detection of colon polyps is a major indication for barium studies of the colon. The following "rules of thumb" can be applied. Polyps less than 5 mm are almost all hyperplastic, with a risk of malignancy less than 0.5%. Polyps 5–10 mm size are 90% adenomas, with a risk of malignancy of 1%. Polyps 10–20 mm in size are usually adenomas, with a risk of malignancy of 10%. Polyps larger than 20 mm are 50% malignant (13).

Hyperplastic polyps are non-neoplastic mucosal proliferations. They are round and sessile. Nearly all are less than 5 mm in size.

Adenomatous polyps are distinctly premalignant and a major risk for development of colorectal carcinoma. Adenomatous polyps are neoplasms with a core of connective tissue. Approximately 5–10% of the population older than 40 years have adenomatous polyps.

Hamartomatous polyps (juvenile polyps) represent approximately 1% of colon polyps. They are a common cause of rectal bleeding in children. The Peutz-Jeghers polyp is type of hamartomatous polyp.

Inflammatory polyps are usually multiple and associated with inflammatory bowel disease (14). They account for less than 0.5% of colorectal polyps.

Familial Adenomatous Polyposis Syndrome is approximately two-thirds inherited and one-third spontaneous. The inheritance pattern is autosomal dominant with high penetrance. The polyps are tubulovillous adenomas which usually are evident by age 20. Colorectal cancer will eventually develop in nearly all patients, so total colectomy with rectal mucosectomy and ileoanal pouch construction is the current recommended therapy. Polyps typically carpet the entire colon (Fig. 32.7).

Patients are at risk for numerous extracolonic manifestations including carcinomas of the small bowel, thy-

Table 32.1. Surgical-Pathologic Staging of Colorectal Carcinoma (Modified Dukes Classification)

Stage	Description
A	Limited to mucosa
B1	Extension into, but not through, muscularis propria
B2	Extension through muscularis propria; no nodes involved
C1	Limited to bowel wall; positive nodes
C2	Extension through bowel wall; positive nodes
D	Distant metastases

Table 32.2. Colorectal Carcinoma: CT and MR Staging

Stage	Description
I	Intraluminal mass without thickening of wall
II	Thickened wall or pelvic mass; no invasion or extension to side walls
IIIa	Thickened wall or pelvic mass with invasion of adjacent structures but not to pelvic side walls or abdominal wall
IIIb	Thickened wall or pelvic mass with extension to pelvic side walls and/or abdominal wall without distant metastases
IV	Distant mestastasis

(Adapted from Thoeni RF. Colorectal cancer: cross-sectional imaging for staging of primary tumor and detection of local recurrence. AJR Am J Roentgenol 1991;156:910.)

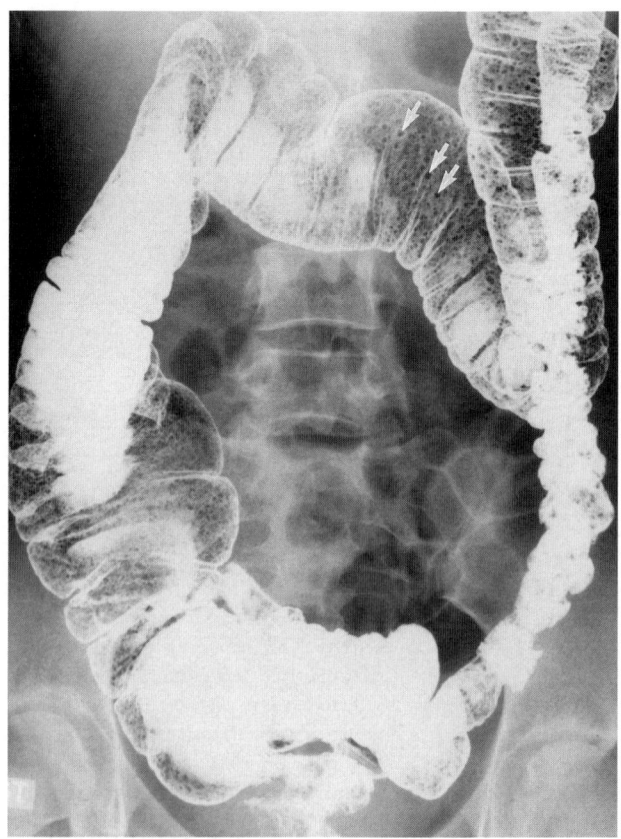

Figure 32.7. Familial Adenomatous Polyposis Syndrome. Double-contrast barium enema reveals the entire colonic mucosa to be carpeted with innumerable small polyps seen as tiny filling defects (*arrows*).

roid carcinoma, and mesenteric fibromatosis. Patients with associated bone and skin abnormalities including cortical thickening of the ribs and long bones, osteomas of the skull, supernumerary teeth, exostoses of the mandible, and dermal fibromas, desmoids, and epidermal inclusion cysts have been diagnosed as *Gardner's syndrome.* Those with associated tumors of the central nervous system have been grouped as *Turcot's syndrome.* These are variations of the same disease (15).

Hamartomatous Polyposis Syndromes. Hamartomatous polyps are non-neoplastic growths with a smooth muscle core covered by mature glandular epithelium. The hamartomatous polyps associated with the various syndromes have minor histologic differences. These lesions carry no risk of malignant transformation. However, patients with the hamartomatous polyposis syndromes may also develop adenomatous polyps which do carry a risk of malignancy. (16,17).

Peutz-Jeghers syndrome predominantly involves the small bowel, but most cases have gastric and colon polyps as well. The condition is autosomal dominant with incomplete penetrance. Dark pigmented spots on the skin and mucous membranes are characteristic. Risk of carcinoma arising from coexisting adenomatous polyps is 2–20%. Patients are at risk for breast cancer, uterine and ovarian cancer, and early age cancer of the pancreas.

Cowden's disease is a syndrome of multiple hamartomas including hamartomatous polyposis of the GI tract, with goiter and thyroid adenomas and increased risk of breast cancer and transitional cell carcinoma of the urinary tract. The syndrome is autosomal dominant and affects mainly Caucasians. All patients have mucocutaneous lesions with facial papules, oral papillomas, and palmoplantar keratoses.

Cronkhite-Canada syndrome is a disease of older patients with a mean age of onset of 60 years. Polyps are distributed throughout the stomach, small bowel, and colon. Associated skin findings include nail atrophy, brownish skin pigmentation, and alopecia. Patients present with watery diarrhea and protein-losing enteropathy.

Lymphoid Hyperplasia may involve the colon. The normal lymphoid follicular pattern of diffuse tiny nodules 1–3 mm in diameter with characteristic umbilication is most common in the terminal ileum and cecum but may involve any portion of the colon. The nodular lymphoid hyperplasia pattern of diffuse nodules larger than 4 mm (Fig. 32.8) is associated with allergic, infectious, and inflammatory disorders.

Lymphoma. The colon is less commonly involved with lymphoma than the stomach or small bowel (18). Involvement of the cecum or rectum is most common with anal and rectal lymphoma increasingly frequent in AIDS patients (Fig. 32.9). Morphologic patterns include

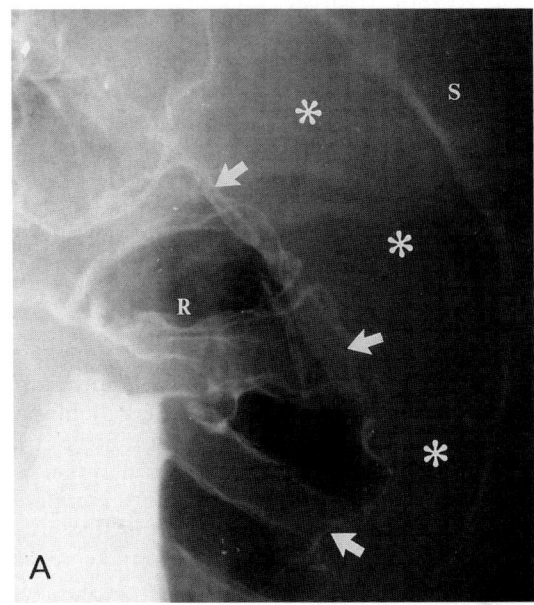

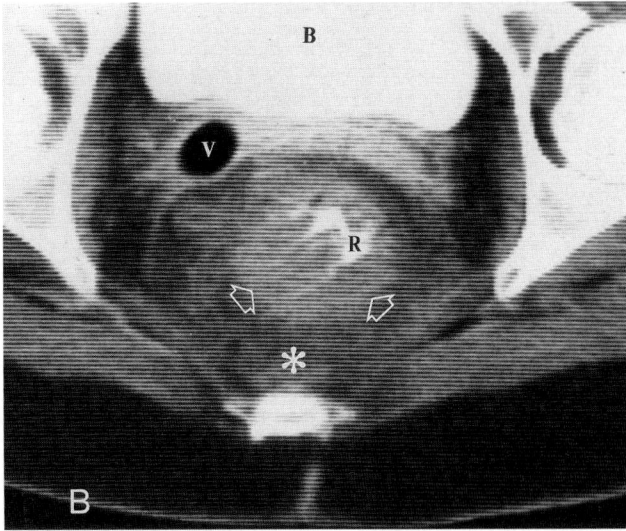

Figure 32.9. Rectal Lymphoma. A. Lateral view of the rectum from a double-contrast barium enema shows bizarre thickened folds (*arrows*) in the rectum (*R*) and marked widening of the presacral space (***). *S*, sacrum. **B.** A CT scan demonstrates irregular thickening of the wall (*arrows*) and distortion of the lumen of the rectum (*R*). The presacral space (***) is infiltrated with soft tissue density. *B*, bladder; *V*, vagina containing a tampon.

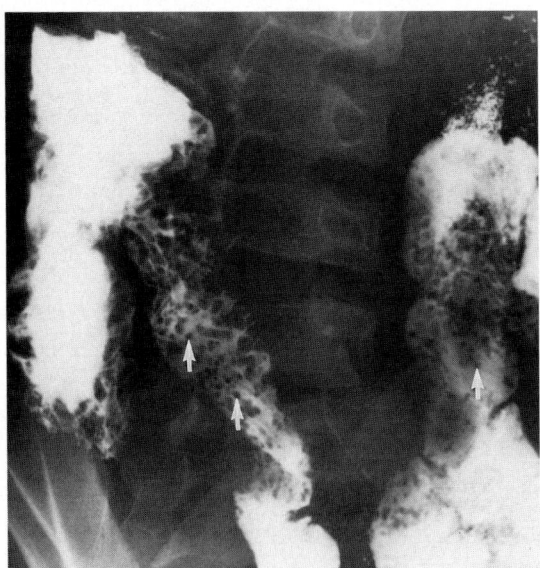

Figure 32.8. Nodular Lymphoid Hyperplasia. Single-contrast barium enema in a patient with hypogammaglobulinemia shows numerous small nodules (*arrows*) throughout the colon.

small to large nodules that may ulcerate, excavitate and perforate (Fig. 32.10), and diffuse infiltration of the bowel wall resulting in bulbous folds and thickened bowel wall. As in the small intestine, marked narrowing of the lumen is uncommon and aneurysmal dilation occurs when transmural disease destroys innervation. The diffuse multinodular form may be difficult to differentiate from nodular lymphoid hyperplasia. Lymphoma nodules vary is size although lymphoid hyperplasia nodules are uniform in size. Non-Hodgkin's lymphoma is most common.

Leiomyoma and Leiomyosarcoma of the colon account for less than 1% of GI tumors. They are more common in the stomach and small bowel than in the colon. As in the remainder of the GI tract, they may appear as exophytic, mural, or intraluminal masses (Fig. 32.11). Most are 25 mm or larger. Ulceration is relatively frequent.

Lipoma is the most common submucosal tumor of the colon. It is most frequent in the cecum and ascending colon (19). Nearly 40% present with intussusception. Barium studies demonstrate a smooth, well-defined elliptical filling defect, usually 1–3 cm in diameter. The tumors are soft and change shape with compression. CT demonstration of a fat-density tumor is definitive.

Extrinsic Masses commonly cause mass effect on the colon that may simulate intrinsic disease.

Endometriosis commonly implants on the sigmoid colon and rectum (20). Defects are frequently multiple and of variable size. Barium studies demonstrate sharply defined defects that compress but do not usually encircle the lumen. CT demonstrates complex cystic pelvic masses with high-density fluid components. Multiple pelvic organs may be incorporated into the mass. MR demonstrates masses with signal characteristics of hemorrhage.

Metastases may involve the colon by contiguous spread, spread along mesenteric fascial planes, by intraperitoneal seeding, through lymphatic channels, or by embolus through blood vessels. The involved colon demonstrates thickening of the wall, separation of folds, spiculation, angulations, narrowing, and serosal plaques (Fig. 32.12). Metastases often cannot be differ-

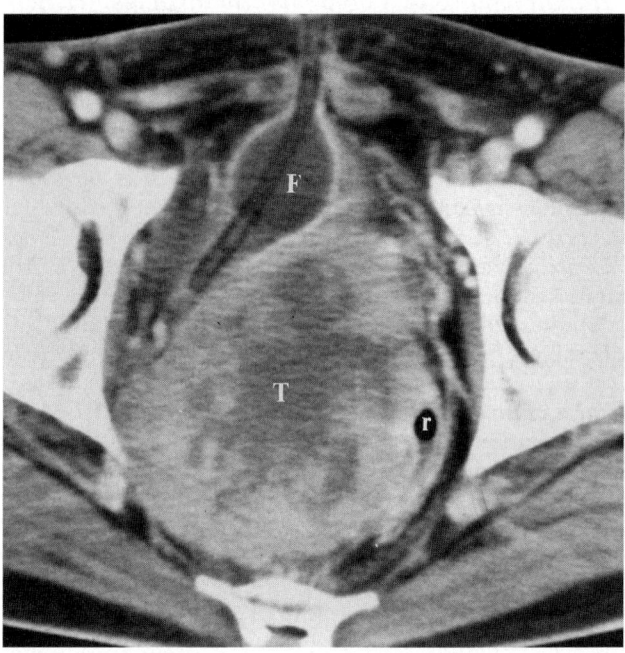

Figure 32.11. Leiomyosarcoma of the Rectum. A CT scan shows a large tumor (*T*) with an irregular low-density area of central necrosis arising exophytically from the wall of the rectum (*r*), which is displaced laterally and anteriorly. The tumor obstructed the bladder outlet, necessitating placement of a suprapubic Foley catheter (*F*).

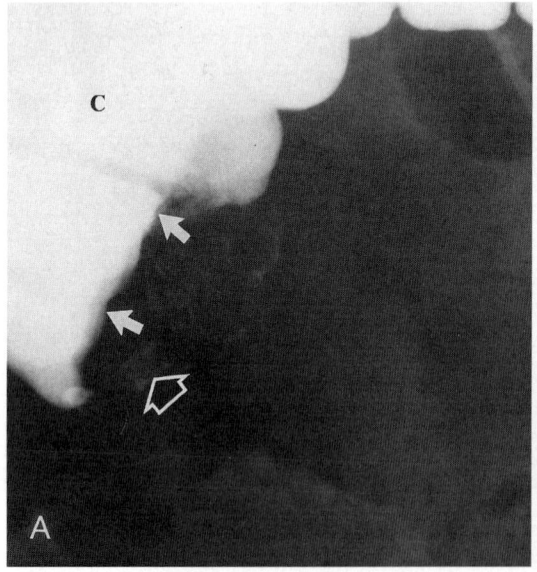
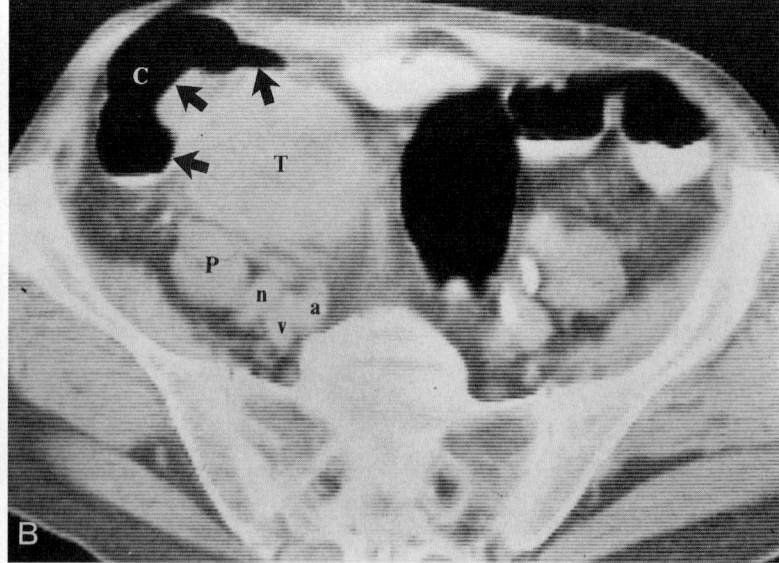

Figure 32.10. Cecal Lymphoma. A. Radiograph of the cecum from a single-contrast barium enema shows mass impression (*arrows*) on both the cecum (*C*) and appendix (*open arrow*). **B.** A CT scan demonstrates the full extent of the tumor mass (*T*) impressing (*arrows*) on the cecum (*C*). An enlarged node (*n*) is also seen adjacent to the common iliac artery (*a*) and vein (*v*). *P*, psoas muscle.

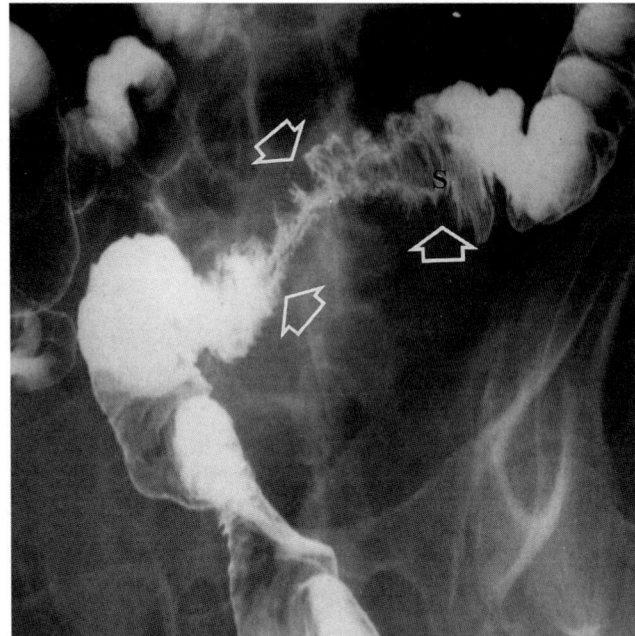

Figure 32.12. Serosal Metastases involving the Colon. Metastases from carcinosarcoma of the uterus implanted on the serosal surface of the sigmoid colon (*S*) cause narrowing and spiculation (*arrows*) of the lumen.

Table 32.3. Ulcerative Colitis vs. Crohn's Colitis

Ulcerative Colitis	Crohn's Colitis
Circumferential disease	Eccentric disease
Regional (continuous disease)	Skip lesions (discontinuous disease)
Predominantly left-sided	Predominantly right-sided
Rectum usually involved	Rectum normal in 50%
Confluent shallow ulcers	Confluent deep ulcers
No aphthous ulcers	Aphthous ulcers early
Collar button ulcers	Transverse and longitudinal ulcers
Terminal ileum usually normal	Terminal ileum usually diseased
Terminal ileum patulous	Terminal ileum narrowed
No pseudodiverticula	Pseudodiverticula
No fistula	Fistula common
High risk of cancer	Low risk of cancer
Risk of toxic megacolon	No toxic megacolon

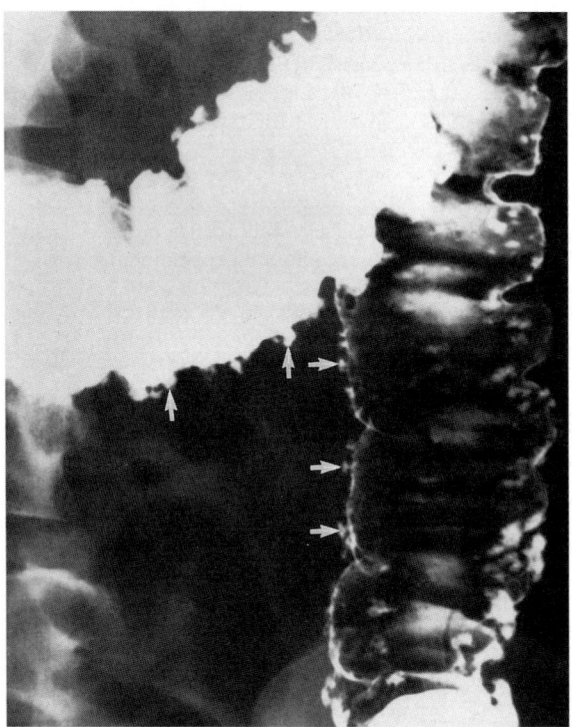

Figure 32.13. Ulcerative Colitis. Double-contrast barium enema shows a pattern of continuous involvement of the colon with innumerable submucosal collar button ulcers (*arrows*).

entiated from primary tumors by imaging methods. Crohn's disease and metastatic disease may also look exactly alike radiographically. CT or MR demonstrate contiguous involvement of the colon and rectum by pelvic tumors.

Extrinsic inflammatory processes, such as appendicitis, pelvic abscess, diverticular abscess, and pelvic inflammatory disease, cause mass effect, asymmetric tethering, and spiculation.

Colon Inflammatory Disease

Ulcerative Colitis is an uncommon idiopathic inflammatory disease involving primarily the mucosa and submucosa of the colon (21). The peak age for its appearance is 20–40 years, but onset of disease after age 50 is common. The disease consists of superficial ulcerations, edema, and hyperemia. The radiographic hallmarks of ulcerative colitis are granular mucosa, confluent shallow ulcerations, symmetry of disease around the lumen, and continuous confluent diffuse involvement (Table 32.3). An early fine, granular pattern is produced by mucosal hyperemia and edema that precedes ulceration. Superficial ulcers spread to cover the entire mucosal surface. The mucosa is stippled with barium adhering to the superficial ulcers. "Collar button ulcers" are deeper ulcerations of thickened edematous mucosa with crypt abscesses extending in the submucosa (Fig. 32.13). A coarse granular pattern is produced later by the replacement of diffusely ulcerated mucosa with granulation tissue. Late changes include a variety of polypoid lesions (14). Pseudopolyps are mucosal remnants in areas of extensive ulceration. Inflammatory polyps are small is-

lands of inflamed mucosa. Postinflammatory polyps are mucosal tags that are seen in quiescent phases of the disease. Hyperplastic polyps may occur during healing after mucosal injury. Involvement typically extends from the rectum proximally in a symmetric and continuous pattern. The terminal ileum is nearly always normal. Rare "backwash ileitis" may produce an ulcerated but patulous terminal ileum.

Complications of ulcerative colitis include *a*) strictures, usually 2–3 cm in length and commonly involving the transverse colon and rectum, *b*) colorectal adenocarcinoma, with an approximate risk of 1% per year of disease, *c*) toxic megacolon in 2–5% of cases (may be the initial manifestation), and *d*) massive hemorrhage.

Associated extraintestinal diseases include sacroiliitis mimicking ankylosing spondylitis in 20% of the cases, eye lesions including uveitis and iritis in 10% of the cases, cholangitis, and an increased incidence of thromboembolic disease.

Crohn's Disease involves the colon in two-thirds of all cases and is isolated to the colon in approximately one-third of all cases. Hallmarks of Crohn's colitis include early aphthous ulcers, later confluent deep ulcerations, predominant right colon disease, discontinuous involvement with intervening regions of normal bowel, asymmetric involvement of the bowel wall (Fig. 32.14A), strictures, fistulas, and sinus formation (Table 32.3). Pseudodiverticula of the colon are formed by asymmetric fibrosis on one side of the lumen, causing saccular outpouches on the other side. Involvement of the rectum is characterized by deep rectal ulcers and multiple fistulous tracts to the skin (Fig. 32.14B).

Pseudomembranous Colitis is an inflammatory disease of the colon, and occasionally the small bowel, characterized by the presence of a pseudomembrane of necrotic debris and overgrowth of *Clostridium difficile* (22). There are many contributing causes including antibiotics (clindamycin, streptomycin, lincomycin, any that change bowel flora), intestinal ischemia (especially following surgery), irradiation, long-term steroids, shock, and colonic obstruction. The disease presents as fulminant inflammatory bowel disease with diarrhea and foul stools. Plain radiographs reveal the following: *a)* dilated colon, *b)* nodular thickening of the haustra, and *c)* ascites. The colon may be greatly dilated, and toxic megacolon has been reported. Barium enema demonstrates an irregular lumen with thumbprint indentations similar to ischemic colitis. Superficial ulcers are common. Plaque-like defects on the mucosal surface are due to the pseudomembranes. The colitis is frequently patchy in distribution with sparing of the rectum. The condition is commonly first detected on CT which shows: *a)* marked wall thickening (average 15 mm) with halo or target appearance, *b)* characteristic stripes of intraluminal contrast media trapped between nodular areas of wall thickening (the accordion sign), *c)* mild pericolonic fat inflammation disproportionate with the marked colonic wall inflammation, and *d)* acites (35%).

Figure 32.14. Crohn's Colitis. A. A CT scan through the transverse colon (*T*) demonstrates asymmetric thickening of the colon wall characteristic of Crohn's colitis. The anterior wall (*open arrows*) is normal, although the posterior wall (*closed arrows*) is thickened and nodular. **B.** A more caudal CT scan in the same patient demonstrates numerous air-containing perirectal cutaneous fistulas (*f*). *r*, rectum.

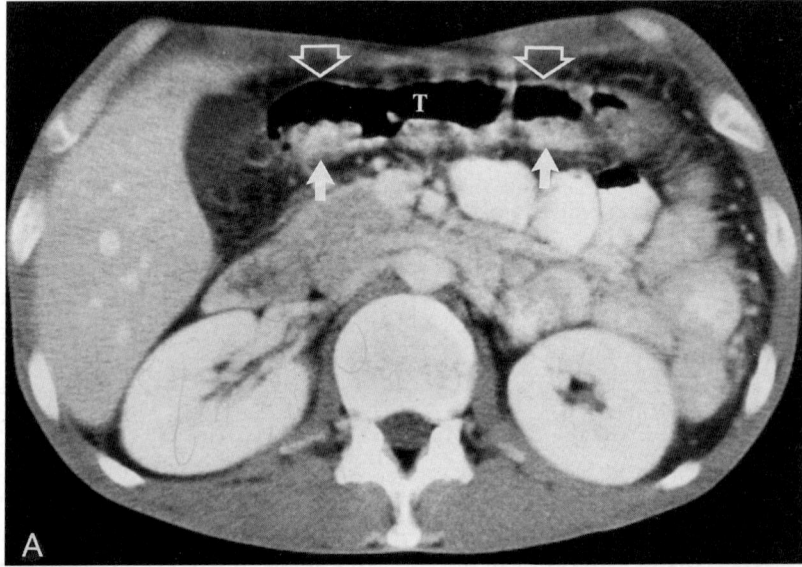

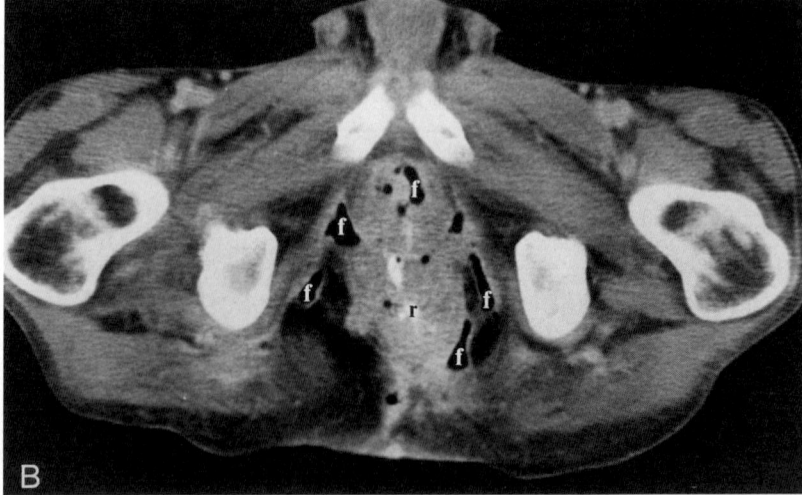

Amebiasis is an infection by the protozoan parasite *Entamoeba histolytica*. The disease is worldwide but particularly common in South Africa, Central and South America, and Asia. At least 5% of the population of the United States harbor amebae. Encysted amebae are ingested with contaminated food and water. The cyst capsule is dissolved in the small bowel, releasing trophozoites that migrate to the colon and burrow into the mucosa, forming small abscesses. The infection can spread throughout the body by hematogenous embolization or direct invasion. Amebic colitis produces dysentery with frequent bloody mucoid stools. Barium studies demonstrate a disease that closely mimics Crohn's colitis with aphthous ulcers, deep ulcers, asymmetric disease, and skip areas. The cecum and rectum are the primary sites of colonic disease. The terminal ileum is characteristically not involved. Complications include strictures, amebomas consisting of a hard fixed mass of granulation tissue that may simulate carcinoma, toxic megacolon, and fistulas, particularly following surgical intervention. Amebic liver abscess results from the spread of infection through the portal system and may be complicated by diaphragm perforation, pleural effusion, and thoracic disease.

Ischemic Colitis mimics ulcerative colitis and Crohn's colitis both clinically and radiographically. The causes of ischemic colitis include arterial occlusion due to arteriosclerosis, vasculitis, or arterial emboli; venous thrombosis due to neoplasm, oral contraceptives and other hypercoagulation conditions; and low flow states such as hypotension, congestive heart failure, and cardiac arrhythmias. The pattern of involvement generally follows the distribution of a major artery and is the clue to diagnosis. The superior mesenteric artery supplies the right colon from the cecum to the splenic flexure. The inferior mesenteric artery supplies the left colon from the splenic flexure to the rectum. The splenic flexure region and descending colon are the most susceptible areas to ischemic colitis. Early changes include thickening of the colon wall, spasm, and spiculation. As blood and edema accumulate within the bowel wall, multiple nodular defects are produced in a pattern called "thumbprinting" (Fig. 32.15). Progression of the disease results in ulcerations, perforation, scarring, and stricture. CT demonstrates symmetrical or lobulated thickening of the bowel wall with an irregular narrowed lumen. Submucosal edema may produce a low-density ring bordering on the lumen. Air in the bowel wall (pneumatosis) is highly suggestive of ischemia. Thrombus may occasionally be demonstrated within the superior mesenteric artery or vein.

AIDS-associated Colitis occurs most commonly in AIDS patients with CD4 lymphocyte counts below 200. Causative organisms are most commonly cytomegalovirus or cryptosporidiosis, although the human immunodeficiency virus itself may cause ulceration and colitis. Right colon disease is most common with wall thickening and ulceration (23).

Radiation Colitis may be indistinguishable radiographically from early ulcerative colitis. The diagnosis is made by confirmation of the involved colon being within an irradiation field. The rectosigmoid region is most commonly involved due to radiation of pelvic malignancy. Colitis is produced by a slowly progressive

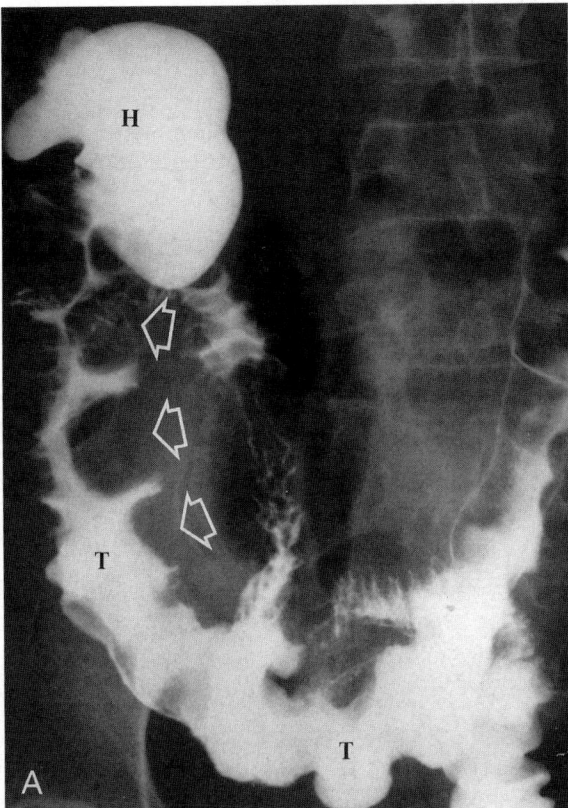

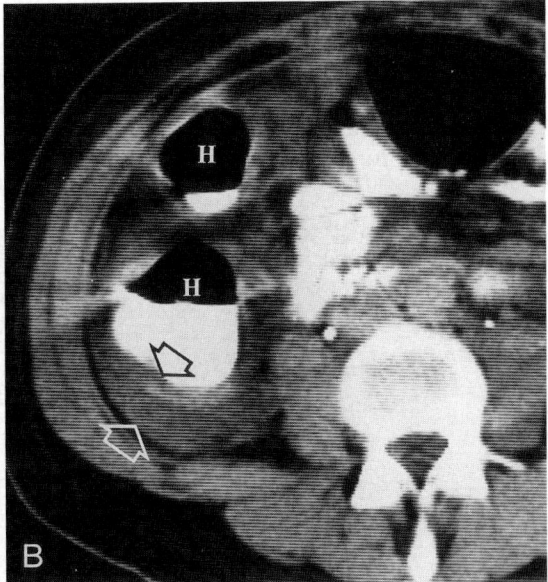

Figure 32.15. Ischemic Colitis. A. Double-contrast barium enema shows thumbprinting pattern (*arrows*) involving the proximal portion of a redundant transverse colon (*T*). *H*, hepatic flexure. **B.** A CT scan in the same patient reveals marked thickening (*arrows*) of the walls of the hepatic flexure (*H*). The patient presented clinically with abdominal pain and bloody stools.

endarteritis that causes ischemia and fibrosis. Radiographic findings include thickened folds, spiculation, ulceration, stricture, and occasionally fistula formation. Fibrosis results in a rigid, featureless bowel. Healing may include formation of pseudopolyps and postinflammatory polyps.

Cathartic Colon is due to chronic irritation of the mucosa by laxatives including castor oil, bisacodyl, and senna. The involved colon may be dilated and without haustra, or narrowed. The right colon is most commonly affected. Bizarre contractions are often observed. The diagnosis is made by clinical history.

Diverticular Disease

Colon Diverticulosis is an acquired condition in which the mucosa and muscularis muscosae herniate through the muscularis propria of the colon wall, producing a saccular outpouching (Fig. 32.16). Colon diverticula are classified as false diverticula because the sacs lack all of the elements of the normal colon wall. The condition is rare under age 25, but increases with age thereafter to affect 50% of the population over age 75. The major risk factor for diverticulosis is a low-residue diet. The condition is very uncommon in cultures where a high-residue diet is the norm, such as African native populations. The formation of diverticular sacs is usually associated with thickening of the muscularis propria, including both the circular muscle and the taenia coli. Severely affected portions of bowel are usually shortened in length, resulting in crowding of the thickened circular muscle bundles. Muscle dysfunction associated with diverticulosis may result in pain and tenderness without evidence of inflammation. Diverticulosis without diverticulitis is a cause of painless colonic bleeding that may be brisk and life-threatening.

Plain abdominal radiographs demonstrate diverticula as gas-filled sacs parallel to the lumen of the colon. Barium studies show diverticula as barium or gas-filled sacs outside the colon lumen. Sacs vary in size from tiny spikes to 2 cm in diameter. Most are 5–10 mm in diameter. They may occur anywhere in the colon but are most common and usually most numerous in the sigmoid colon. Some sacs are reducible and may disappear with complete filling of the lumen. Others may contain fecal residue. The associated muscle abnormality is seen as thickening and crowding of the circular muscle bands with spasm and spiked irregular outline of the lumen. CT demonstrates the muscle hypertrophy as a thickened colon wall and distorted luminal contour. The diverticula are shown as well-defined gas-filled or contrast-filled sacs outside the lumen (Fig. 32.16).

Diverticulitis is inflammation of diverticula, usually with perforation and intramural or localized pericolic abscess. Diverticulitis eventually complicates approximately 20% of the cases of diverticulosis. Clinical signs include painful mass, localized peritoneal inflammation, fever, and leukocytosis. Complications of diverticulitis include bowel obstruction, bleeding, peritonitis, and sinus tract and fistula formation. Diverticulitis is a less common cause of colon obstruction than is colon carcinoma. Obstruction due to diverticulitis is often temporarily relieved by smooth muscle relaxants such as glucagon. Colon bleeding is more often associated with diverticulosis than diverticulitis. Most diverticular abscesses are quickly walled off and confined, but free perforation with pus and air in the peritoneal cavity and diffuse peritonitis may occur. Sinus tracts may lead to larger abscess cavities in the peritoneal or retroperitoneal compartments. Fistulas are most common to the bladder (Fig 32.17), vagina, or skin, but may develop to any lower abdominal organ including fallopian tubes, small bowel, and other parts of the colon. Diverticulitis is efficiently diagnosed radiographically by barium enema or CT. Barium enema examination is considered safe except when signs of free intraperitoneal perforation or sepsis are present.

Hallmarks of diverticulitis on barium enema include deformed diverticular sacs, demonstration of abscess, and extravasation of barium outside the colon lumen.

Figure 32.16. Diverticulosis. A CT scan demonstrates air-filled and contrast-filled outpouchings (*arrows*) representing diverticuli in the transverse (*T*) and descending (*D*) colon.

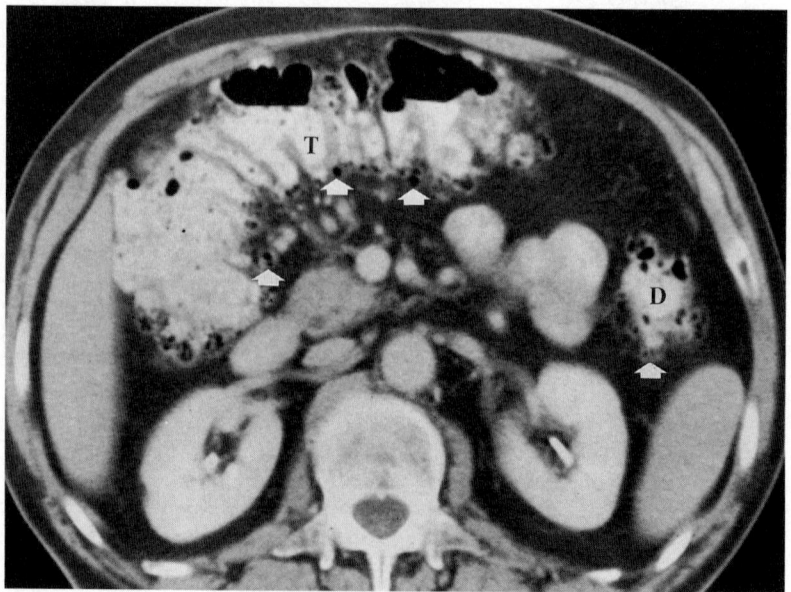

The smooth outline of the involved sacs are deformed by inflammation and perforation. The resulting abscess causes extrinsic mass effect on the adjacent colon (Fig. 32.18A). The colon lumen is narrowed but tapers at the margins of narrowing in distinction with the abrupt narrowing of carcinoma. Barium leaks into the abscess cavities, or forms tracks paralleling the colon lumen and often connecting multiple perforated sacs (the "double track sign"). CT excels at demonstrating the paracolic inflammation and abscess associated with diverticulitis, as well as complications such as colovesical fistula. CT findings are (Fig. 32.18B): *a)* localized wall thickening, *b)* inflammation of pericolonic fat, *c)* pericolonic abscess, *d)* diverticula at or near the site of inflammation.

Lower Gastrointestinal Hemorrhage

Although upper GI hemorrhage is usually readily diagnosed by gastric aspirate and endoscopy, lower GI hemorrhage is difficult to localize, even during surgery (24). The common causes of lower GI hemorrhage are listed in Table 32.4. Radionuclide imaging studies are usually selected as the screening examination of choice for confirming the presence of, and often localizing, lower GI bleeding. Technetium-99m-sulfur colloid or Tc-99m-red blood cell studies are capable of detecting bleeding at rates below 0.1 ml/min. A negative scintigraphic study

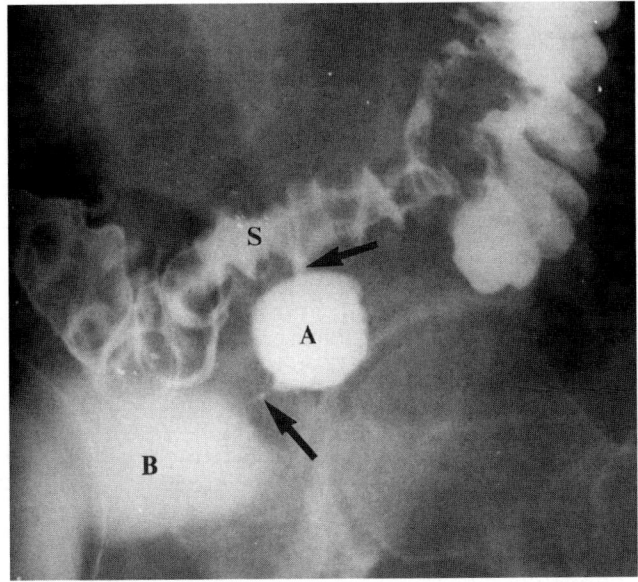

Figure 32.17. Diverticular Abscess and Colovesical Fistula. Single-contrast barium enema demonstrates barium filling a diverticular abscess (*A*) and opacifying the bladder (*B*). Thin columns of barium (*arrows*) outline fistulous tracts extending from the bowel lumen to abscess and from abscess to the bladder. The lumen of the sigmoid colon (*S*) is irregularly narrowed by the inflammatory process.

Table 32.4. Causes of Lower Gastrointestinal Hemorrhage

Cause	Percentage of Cases
Colon diverticula	40
Angiodysplasia	17–30
Colon carcinoma	7–16
Polyps	8
Rectal trauma/fissure/hemorrhoids	7
Duodenal ulcer	Rare
Meckel's diverticulum	Rare
Bowel ischemia	Rare

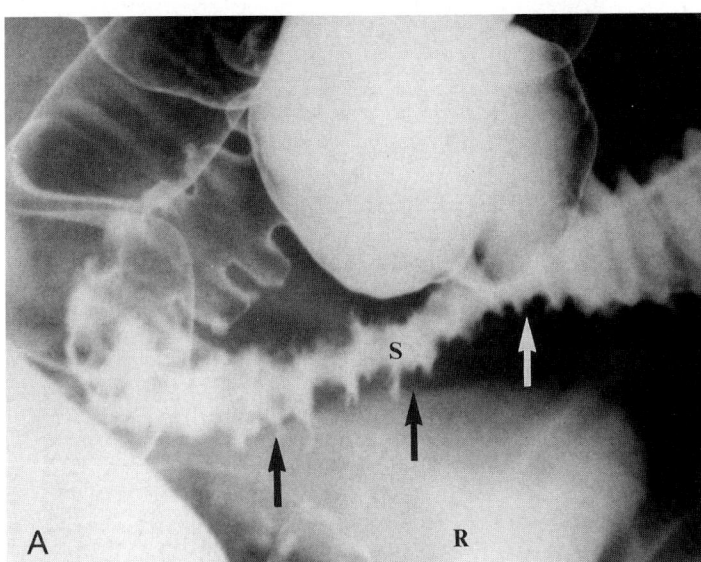
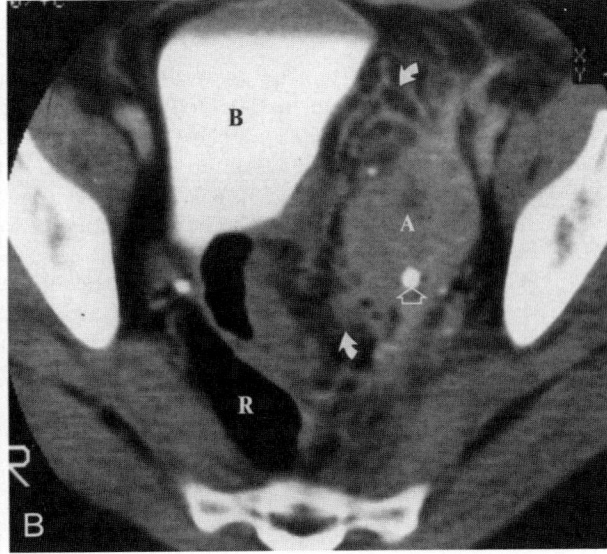

Figure 32.18. Diverticulitis. A. Barium enema shows a narrowed spiculated lumen (*arrows*) of a segment of the sigmoid colon (*S*). *R*, rectum. **B.** A CT scan demonstrates the extraluminal component of the disease. A large inflammatory mass (*A*) is seen in the soft tissues of the pelvis. Inflammatory reaction causes rounded and streaky soft tissue densities (*curved arrows*) in the adjacent fat. A drop of barium (*open arrow*) is seen in a diverticulum, encompassed within the inflammatory mass. The loop of involved sigmoid colon shown in **(A)** is just cephalad to the CT slice shown. *R*, rectum. *B*, bladder.

usually precludes the need for urgent angiography. Angiography requires bleeding rates of 0.5 ml/min or greater. However, angiography is more specific than scintigraphy in demonstrating the anatomic cause of bleeding and offers the possibility of nonoperative treatment by embolization or infusion of Pitressin. Colonoscopy is usually unrewarding because of the large quantities of sticky, melanotic stool. Barium enema is not used to evaluate acute hemorrhage because it usually cannot locate the source of bleeding and it will interfere with any subsequently needed angiographic procedure.

Angiodysplasia refers to ectasia and kinking of mucosal and submucosal veins of the colon wall. The condition results from a chronic intermittent obstruction of the veins where they penetrate the circular muscle layer. A maze of distorted, dilated vascular channels replaces the normal mucosal structures and are separated from the bowel lumen only by a layer of epithelium. Angiodysplasia is acquired, and probably related to aging. The average age of affected patients is 65 years. Bleeding is usually chronic, resulting in anemia, but may be acute and massive. Angiography demonstrates a tangle of ectatic vessels without an associated mass.

APPENDIX

Imaging Methods

Filling of the appendix is attained most reliably by single contrast barium enema examination. The appendix is also frequently visualized on abdominal films obtained 6 to 48 hours following oral administration of barium. Failure to fill the appendix with barium on barium enema examination is not definitive evidence of appendiceal disease. Both CT and US have proven extremely useful in the diagnosis of appendiceal disease, especially acute appendicitis.

Anatomy

The appendix arises from the posteromedial aspect of the cecum at the junction of the taenia coli, approximately 1–2 cm below the ileocecal valve. The appendix is a blind-ended tube that is 5–10 mm in diameter (on barium studies) (Fig. 32.1) and approximately 8 cm in length, although it may be up to 30 cm long. Its mucosa is heavily infiltrated with lymphoid tissue. The appendix is quite variable in position: it may be pelvic, retrocecal, or retrocolic, and intraperitoneal or extraperitoneal in location. The appendix always arises from the cecum on the same side as the ileocecal valve. A posterior position of the ileocecal valve indicates a posterior position of the appendix. On CT the normal appendix appears as a thin-walled tube less than 6 mm in diameter.

Acute Appendicitis

Acute appendicitis is the most common cause of acute abdomen. Frequently the clinical diagnosis is straightforward. However, patients with atypical presentations cause diagnostic problems. The most difficult patients are women of childbearing age, in whom ruptured ovar-

ian cysts and pelvic inflammatory disease may mimic acute appendicitis. Acute appendicitis results from obstruction of the appendiceal lumen. Continued mucosal secretions cause dilation and increased intraluminal pressure that impairs venous drainage and results in mucosal ulceration. Bacterial infection causes gangrene and perforation with abscess. Most periappendiceal abscesses are walled off, but free perforation and pneumoperitoneum occasionally occur.

Plain films will demonstrate an appendiceal calculus (appendicolith or fecalith) in approximately 14% of patients with acute appendicitis (Fig. 32.19). An appendicolith is formed by calcium deposition around a nidus of inspissated feces. The resultant calcification is usually laminated with a radiolucent center. Appendiceal abscess or periappendiceal inflammation may result in a visible soft tissue mass in the right lower quadrant (Fig. 32.20). The lumen of the cecum, as outlined by gas, will be deformed; localized ileus may be evident.

Barium enema examination is frequently nonspecific. Complete filling of the appendix to its bulbous tip is strong evidence against appendicitis. However, nonfilling of the appendix, as would be expected with luminal obstruction, has no diagnostic value of its own. Mass impression on the cecum has many causes besides appendicitis.

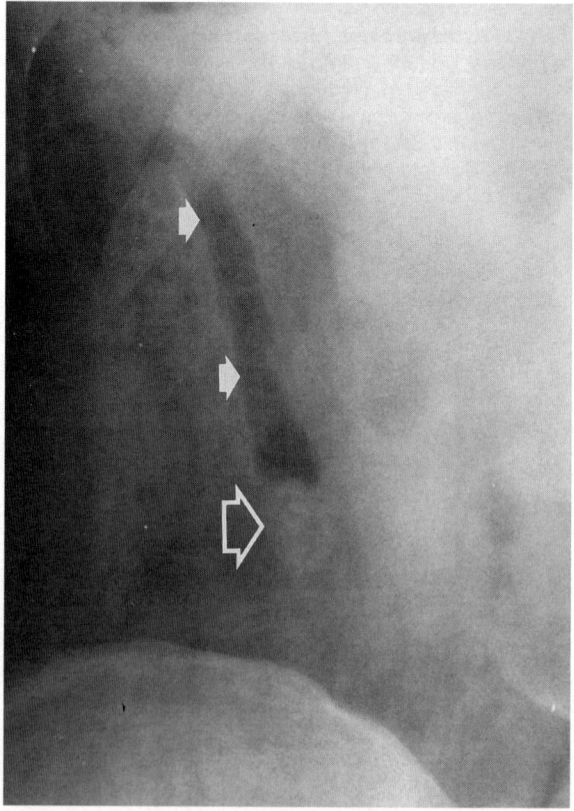

Figure 32.19. Appendicolith. Plain radiograph of the abdomen demonstrates a faintly calcified appendicolith (*open arrow*) that obstructed the appendiceal orifice. The lumen of the appendix (*closed arrows*) is dilated and air-filled because of stasis and bacterial overgrowth. Surgery confirmed acute appendicitis with a retrocecal appendix.

US, using the graded compression technique, is quite accurate in providing a definitive diagnosis (25). Slow graded compression is applied with a near-focus transducer to the area of maximum tenderness. The normal appendix has a diameter of less than 6 mm when compressed. US signs of acute appendicitis are: *a*) a noncompressible appendix larger than 6 mm in diameter, measured outer wall to outer wall (Fig. 32.21) and, *b*) visualization of a shadowing appendicolith. With perforation, sonography demonstrates a loculated pericecal fluid collection, a discontinuous wall of the appendix, and prominent pericecal fat. When the US examination is negative for appendicitis, an alternate diagnosis can frequently be suggested based on visualized abnormalities.

CT is the imaging method of choice when periappendiceal abscess is suspected (Fig. 32.22)(26). Definitive CT diagnosis of acute appendicitis is based on finding: *a*)

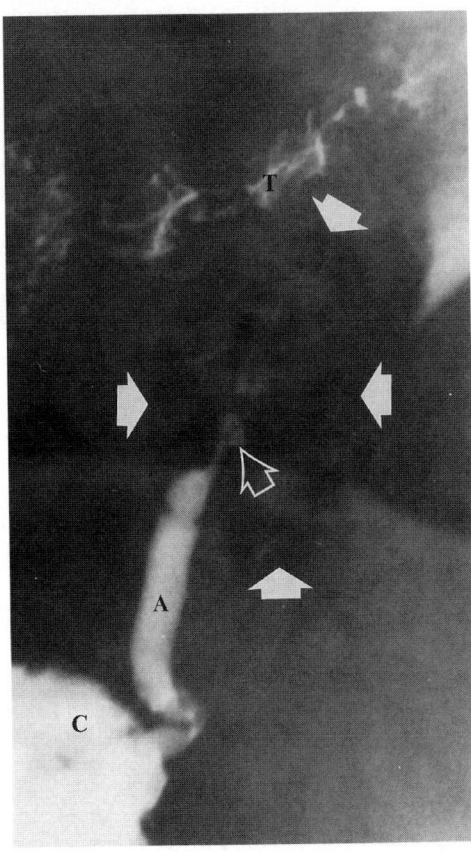

Figure 32.20. Appendiceal Abscess. Barium fills the lumen of the appendix (*A*) and extravasates from its tip (*open arrow*) into a large appendiceal abscess outlined by gas collections within it (*closed arrows*). *C*, cecum; *T*, transverse colon.

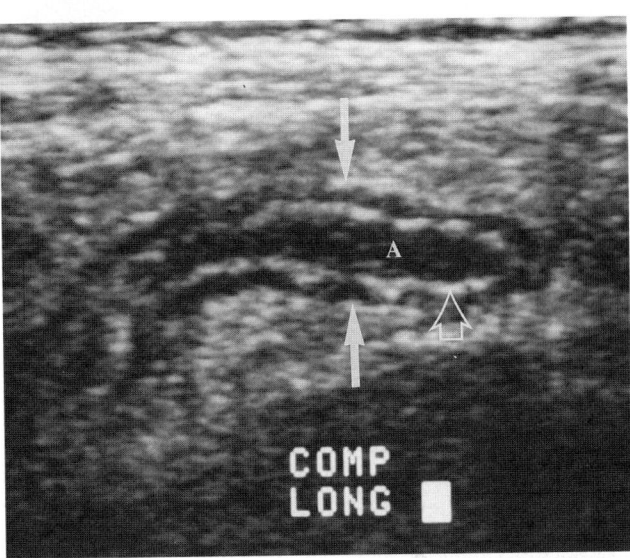

Figure 32.21. Acute Appendicitis. Graded compression US demonstrates a distended appendix (*A*) with a diameter (between *closed arrows*) of 10 mm. The mucosal interface produces a bright echogenic line (*open arrow*). Surgery confirmed an acutely inflamed and focally necrotic appendix. (Case courtesy of David A. Russell, MD, Cedar Rapids, Iowa.)

Figure 32.22. Periappendiceal Abscess. A CT scan demonstrates a dilated, fluid-filled cecum (*C*), an appendicolith (*open arrow*) obstructing the appendiceal orifice, and periappendiceal fluid and inflammation (*closed arrows*) resulting from appendiceal rupture.

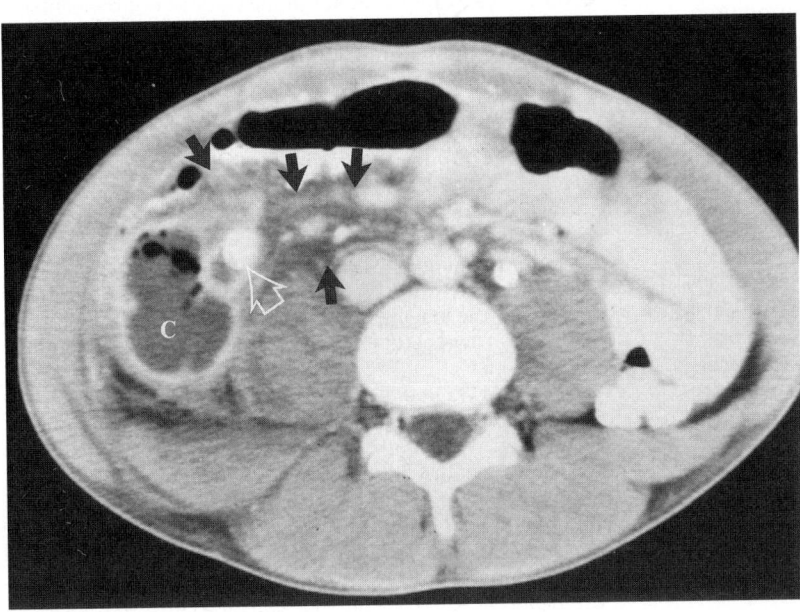

Figure 32.23. Appendiceal Mucocele. CT reveals a tubular cystic mass (*M*) with calcification in its wall (*arrow*) in the right lower quadrant of the abdomen.

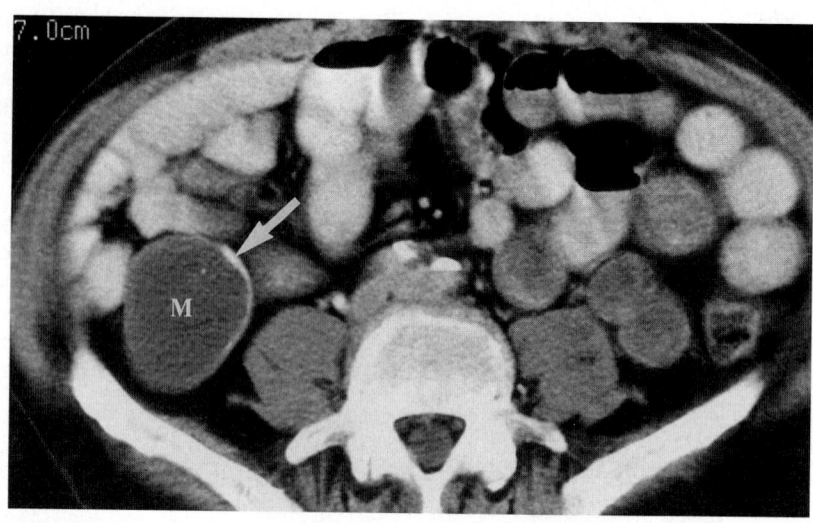

an abnormally dilated (>6 mm), enhancing appendix, *b*) enhancing appendix surrounded by inflammatory stranding, phlegmon or abscess, or *c*) pericecal abscess or phlegmon with a calcified appendicolith. Phlegmon is seen as an indurated soft tissue mass with a CT density greater than 20 H. A liquified mass less than 20 H in CT density is evidence of abscess. Abscesses larger than 3 cm generally require surgical or catheter drainage. Smaller abscesses or phlegmons commonly resolve on antibiotic treatment alone.

Mucocele of the Appendix

Mucocele refers to distension of all or a portion of the appendix with sterile mucus (27). The lumen is obstructed by appendicolith, foreign body, adhesions, or tumor. Some cases are due to mucinous cystadenomas or cystadenocarcinomas of the appendix. Continued secretion of mucus produces a large (up to 15 cm), well-defined cystic mass in the right lower quadrant (Fig. 32.23). Peripheral calcification may be present. Rupture of the mucocele may result in pseudomyxoma peritonei. Gelatinous implants spread throughout the peritoneal cavity, causing adhesions and mucinous ascites.

Appendiceal Tumors

Carcinoid is the most common tumor of the appendix, accounting for 85% of all tumors. The appendix is the most common location for carcinoid tumor, accounting for 60% of all carcinoids. Most occur near the tip and are round, nodular tumors up to 2.5 cm size. Most are solitary and have less tendency to metastasize than carcinoids elsewhere in the GI tract. Carcinoid syndrome is rare and the mesenteric reaction seen with small bowel carcinoid is usually absent.

Adenomas occur in the appendix usually in association with familial multiple polyposis. Isolated adenomas are usually mucinous cystadenomas associated with mucocele of the appendix.

Adenocarcinoma of the appendix is rare.

References

1. Balthazar EJ. CT of the gastrointestinal tract: principles and interpretation. AJR Am J Roentgenol 1991;156:23–32.
2. Desai RK, Tagliabue JR, Wegryn SA, Einstein DM. CT evaluation of wall thickening in the alimentary tract. Radiographics 1991;11:771–783.
3. Thoeni RF. Colorectal cancer: cross-sectional imaging for staging of primary tumor and detection of local recurrence. AJR Am J Roentgenol 1991;156:909–915.
4. Hara AK, Johnson CD, Reed JE. Colorectal lesion evaluation with CT colography. Radiographics 1997;17:1157–1167.
5. Kruskal JB, Kane RA, Sentovich SM, Longmaid HE. Pitfalls and sources of error in staging rectal cancer with endorectal US. Radiographics 1997;17:609–626.
6. St. Ville EW, Jafri SZH, Madrazo BL, et al. Endorectal sonography in the evaluation of rectal and perirectal disease. AJR Am J Roentgenol 1991;157:503–508.
7. Simms SM. Differential diagnosis of the bowler hat sign. AJR Am J Roentgenol 1985;144:585–587.
8. Mulloy JP, Scott RL. Differentiating colonic polyps from air bubbles on barium enema: the "carpenter's level sign." AJR Am J Roentgenol 1994;163:84–86.
9. Rubesin SE, Laufer I. Pictorial glossary of double contrast radiology. In: Gore RM, Levine MS, Laufer I, eds. Textbook of Gastrointestinal Radiology. Philadelphia: WB Saunders, 1994:50–80.
10. Buetow PC, Buck JL, Carr NJ, Pantongrag-Brown L. Colorectal adenocarcinoma: radiologic-pathologic correlation. RadioGraphics 1995;15:127–146.
11. McDaniel KP, Charnsangavej C, DuBrow RA, et al. Pathways of nodal metastases in carcinomas of the cecum, ascending colon, and transverse colon: CT demonstration. AJR Am J Roentgenol 1993;161:61–64.
12. Zerhouni EA, Rutter C, Hamilton SR, et al. CT and MR imaging in the staging of colorectal carcinoma: report of the Radiology Diagnostic Oncology Group II. Radiology 1996;200:443–451.
13. Olmstead WW, Ros PR, Sobin LH, Dachman AH. The solitary colonic polyp: radiologic-histologic differentiation and significance. Radiology 1986;160:9–16.
14. Buck JL, Dachman AH, Sobin LH. Polypoid and pseudopolypoid manifestations of inflammatory bowel disease. Radiographics 1991;11:293–304.
15. Harned RK, Buck JL, Olmsted WW, et al. Extracolonic manifestations of the familial adenomatous polyposis syndromes. AJR Am J Roentgenol 1991;156:481–485.

16. Harned RK, Buck JL, Sobin LH. The hamartomatous polyposis syndromes: clinical and radiologic features. AJR Am J Roentgenol 1995;164:565–571.

17. Cho GJ, Bergquist K, Schwartz AM. Peutz-Jeghers syndrome and the hamartomatous polyposis syndromes: radiologic-pathologic correlation. Radiographics 1997;17: 785–791.

18. Levine MS, Rubesin SE, Pantongrag-Brown L, et al. Non-Hodgkin's lymphoma of the gastrointestinal tract: radiographic findings. AJR Am J Roentgenol 1997;168:165–172.

19. Taylor AJ, Stewart ET, Dodds WJ. Gastrointestinal lipomas: a radiologic and pathologic review. AJR Am J Roentgenol 1990;155:1205–1210.

20. Szucs RA, Turner MA. Gastrointestinal tract involvement by gynecologic diseases. Radiographics 1996;16:1251–1270.

21. Gore RM, Balthazar EJ, Ghahremani GG, Miller FH. CT features of ulcerative colitis and Crohn's disease. AJR Am J Roentgenol 1996;167:3–15.

22. Ros PR, Buetow PC, Pantograg-Brown L, et al. Pseudomembranous colitis. Radiology 1996;198:1-9.

23. Murray JG, Evans SJJ, Jeffrey PB, Halvorsen RA Jr. Cytomegalovirus colitis in AIDS: CT features. AJR Am J Roentgenol 1995;165:67–71.

24. Zuckerman DA, Bocchini TP, Birnbaum EH. Massive hemorrhage in the lower gastrointestinal tract in adults: diagnostic imaging and intervention. AJR Am J Roentgenol 1993;161:703–711.

25. Jeffrey RB Jr, Jain KA, Nghiem HV. Sonographic diagnosis of acute appendicitis: interpretive pitfalls. AJR Am J Roentgenol 1994;162:55–59.

26. Curtin KR, Fitzgerald SW, Nemcek AA Jr, et al. CT diagnosis of acute appendicitis: imaging findings. AJR Am J Roentgenol 1995;164:905–909.

27. Madwed D, Mindelzun R, Jeffrey RB Jr. Mucocele of the appendix: imaging findings. AJR Am J Roentgenol 1992;159: 69–72.

Section VII GENITOURINARY TRACT

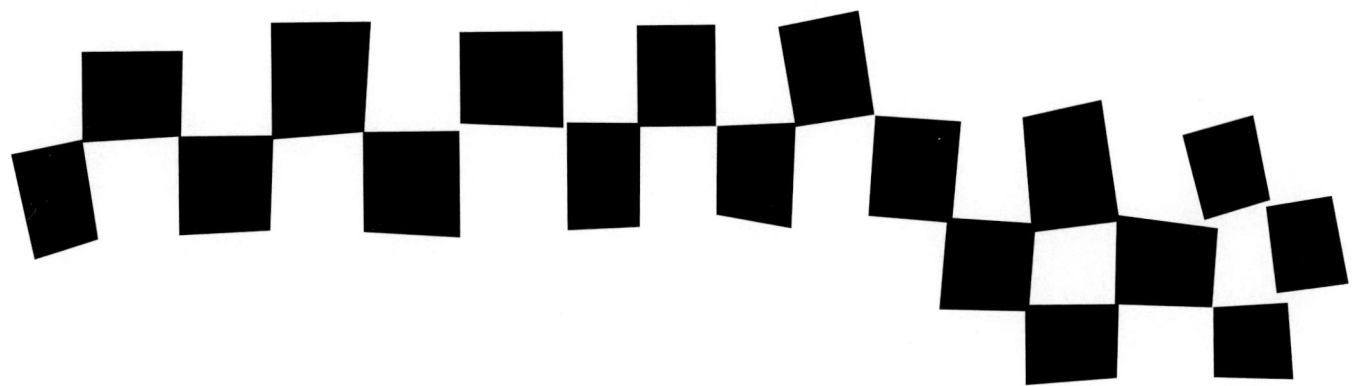

33
Adrenal Glands and Kidneys

William E. Brant

ADRENAL GLANDS

Imaging Methods

Challenges in adrenal imaging occur in three major clinical settings. First, a patient is referred for adrenal imaging because a hormonally active adrenal tumor is suspected on a clinical basis. The role of imaging is to locate and characterize the lesion. Second, adrenal imaging is requested to evaluate for metastatic disease. Third, an adrenal mass is incidentally detected on imaging studies performed for other indications. The significance of the finding must be assessed both radiographically and clinically.

CT is usually the adrenal imaging modality of choice in adults (1–5). US is excellent for screening the adrenal glands in infants and children, especially for detection of adrenal hemorrhage. MR can provide high-quality images of adrenal lesions and is useful in problem solving, especially with chemical-shift imaging to characterize benign adrenal adenomas. Arteriography, venography, venous sampling, radionuclide imaging, and percutaneous biopsy are reserved for selected problem cases.

Anatomy

The adrenal glands are composed of an outer cortex and an inner medulla that are functionally independent and distinct. The cortex secretes steroid hormones including cortisol, aldosterone, androgens, and estrogens. The medulla produces catecholamines.

The adrenal glands lie within the perirenal space surrounded by fat. The right adrenal gland is located posterior to the inferior vena cava (IVC) at the level where the IVC enters the liver. The right adrenal gland is between the right lobe of the liver and the right crus of the diaphragm just above the upper pole of the right kidney. The left adrenal gland lies just medial and anterior to the upper pole of the left kidney, posterior to the pancreas and splenic vessels, and lateral to the left crus of the diaphragm. On cross-sectional imaging, the adrenal glands appear triangular, linear, or inverted V- or Y-shaped. Each limb is smooth in outline and uniform in thickness with straight or concave borders. The limbs are 4–5 cm in length and 5–7 mm in thickness. The adrenal glands are of uniform soft-tissue density on CT and US. On MR, the normal adrenal is hypointense, about equal to striated muscle, on T1WI. On T2WI, the adrenals are isointense or slightly hypointense compared with the liver and hypointense compared with the spleen (6). MR may demonstrate corticomedullary differentiation in some normal patients and in most patients with adrenal hyperplasia. The cortex has higher signal intensity than the medulla.

Adjacent structures may cause major problems in adrenal imaging by mimicking adrenal masses. Tortuous splenic vessels, splenic lobulations, pancreatic projections, exophytic upper pole renal masses, portosystemic venous collaterals, retroperitoneal adenopathy, gastric diverticulum, and portions of the stomach may all cause adrenal pseudotumors. Judicious use of oral and intravenous contrast on CT, or supplemental US or MR studies, will reveal the true nature of these conditions.

Adrenal Hyperplasia

Half of the cases of biochemically hyperplastic glands will appear anatomically normal on CT and MR. In the remainder of cases, both glands will be diffusely enlarged but maintain their normal adrenal shape (Fig. 33.1). Uncommonly, hyperplasia may appear nodular and mimic solitary or multiple adenomas. In diffuse hyperplasia, the limbs of the adrenal glands are longer than 5 cm and exceed 10-mm thickness. Adrenal hyperplasia is present in 70% of the cases of Cushing's syndrome and 20% of the cases of Conn's syndrome. Adre-

Figure 33.1. Adrenal Hyperplasia. The limbs of both adrenal glands (*arrows*) are thickened and somewhat nodular. Differential considerations include hyperplasia, metastases, and granulomatous disease. Note the anatomic landmarks for the adrenal glands: *d*, crura of the diaphragm; *l*, right lobe of the liver; *i*, inferior vena cava; *a*, aorta.

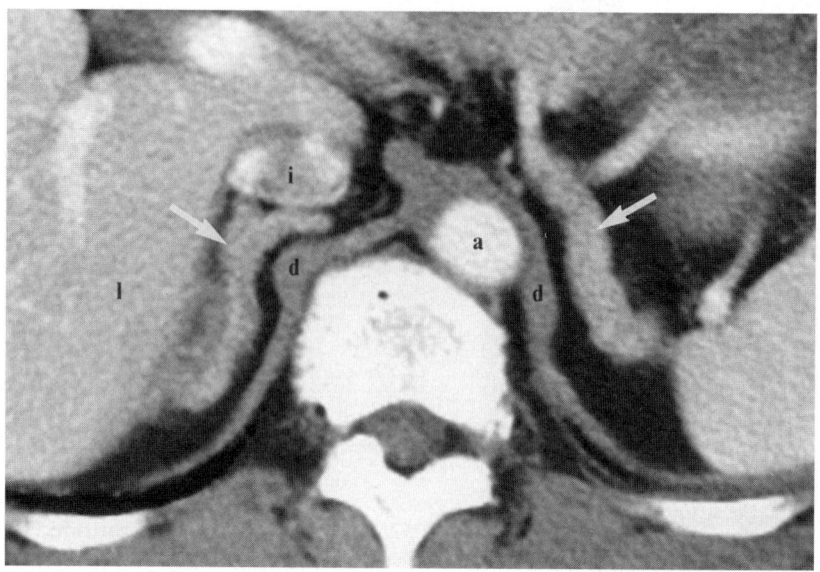

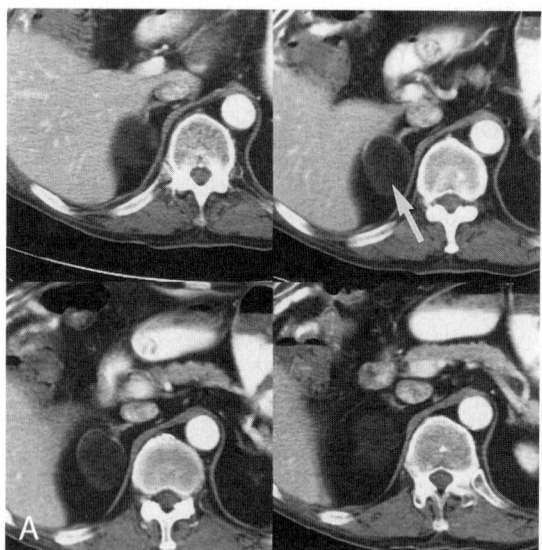

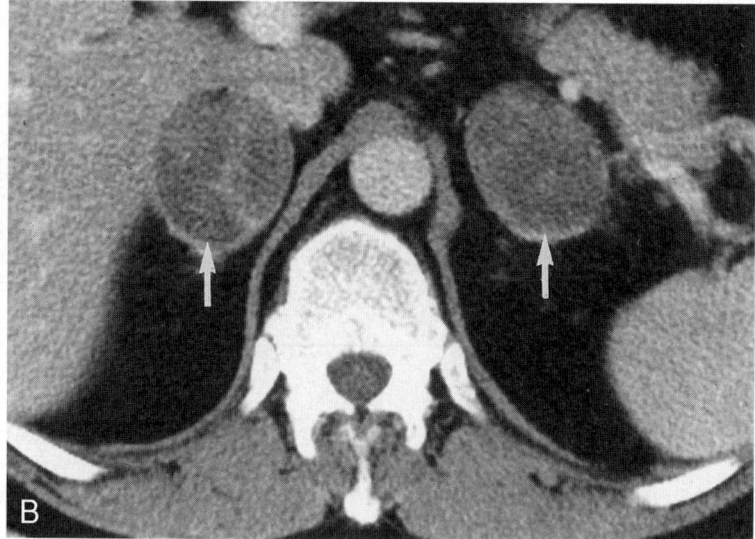

Figure 33.2. Benign and Malignant Adrenal Masses. A. Contrast enhanced CT: Low-density, well-defined mass extends from the right adrenal gland. Density measurement of −20 H confirms a benign lesion. **B.** Contrast-enhanced CT: Bilateral adrenal masses are inhomogeneous with attenuation values of 43–45 H, indicating high likelihood of malignancy. The lesions are metastases from lung carcinoma.

nal hyperplasia is important to differentiate from adrenal adenoma as a cause of endocrine syndromes. The syndrome is usually treated medically when hyperplasia is causative, whereas surgical removal of hyperfunctioning adrenal adenomas is usually curative. Metastatic disease, tuberculosis, and histoplasmosis may also cause diffuse adrenal enlargement and mimic the appearance of adrenal hyperplasia.

Adrenal Adenoma

Adrenal adenomas may secrete excessive hormone and cause one of the endocrine syndromes or be nonhyperfunctional and present as an unsuspected adrenal mass (1,3). Nonhyperfunctional adrenal adenomas are incidental findings in as much as 3–5% of the popula-

tion. Function of an adenoma cannot be determined by imaging appearance but is assessed clinically or, in problem cases, by venous sampling. Patients with hyperfunctioning adenomas are cured by surgical excision. The most likely cause of an incidentally discovered adrenal mass is a benign nonhyperfunctioning adenoma. These must be differentiated from an unsuspected metastasis or a rare, small, adrenal carcinoma. Incidental discovery of an adrenal metastasis as the first manifestation of an occult primary tumor is a rare event.

On CT, benign adenomas are typically small (<4 cm), well-defined, smooth, round, and homogeneous (3,7). Because benign adenomas are rich in lipids, they tend to be low in CT density (Fig. 33.2A) (8). On a nonenhanced CT scan, a measured CT density of less than 10 H (9,10) is strongly predictive of benign adenoma and virtually excludes a metastatic lesion. Benign adenomas enhance uniformly with intravenous contrast administration. Adrenal masses cannot be adequately characterized as benign by CT attenuation values on immediate postcontrast CT (10); however, CT scans repeated 1 hour after contrast administration may prove adequate. A study by Korobkin et al. (11) indicated that adrenal masses could be characterized as benign if they measured less than 30 H on scans obtained 1 hour after IV administration of 150 cc of contrast (11). Boland et al. (12) reported a 96% specificity for benign adrenal masses with a threshold value of 24 H or less, measured 12–18 minutes after contrast administration (Fig. 33.2B).

The US appearance parallels that of CT, with benign adenomas being small (<4 cm), well-defined, and homogeneous in echogenicity. Larger masses with heterogeneous echogenicity tend to be malignant.

On MR, T1WI show adenomas to be homogeneous and hypointense or isointense relative to the liver. On T2WI, benign adenomas are usually isointense or slightly hyperintense to liver (Fig. 33.3) (4). Some adenomas are substantially hyperintense to liver on T2WI and overlap with the appearance of adrenal metastases. Malignant lesions and pheochromocytoma tend to be very hyperintense to liver. Gadolinium administration shows mild enhancement and rapid washout in benign lesions and strong early enhancement with slow washout in malignant lesions.

Chemical-shift MR imaging is used to differentiate benign adenomas from metastases by demonstrating the higher fat content of benign adenomas (13–15). Two separate T1-weighted or gradient-echo pulse sequences are obtained, one with the water and fat resonant peaks aligned, and the other with them completely out of alignment (Fig. 33.4). A reduction in signal intensity on the out-of-phase image is evidence of fat in the tumor and confirms benign adenoma. Increased or unchanged signal on the out-of-phase image compared with the in-phase image indicates a nonfatty, probably malignant tumor. Occasional nonfatty adenomas will cause false-positive results.

In summary, adrenal adenomas may be characterized as benign by attenuation values of less than 10 H on unenhanced CT or less than 30 H on delayed images from enhanced CT, or by chemical-shift MR imaging showing reduced signal intensity on out-of-phase images. Percutaneous biopsy is reserved for tissue confirmation of suspected malignancy. Surgical excision is the treatment of choice for hyperfunctioning adenomas.

Adrenal Metastases

Adrenal metastases are exceedingly common, found in 27% of patients with malignant disease on autopsy series. The most common primary tumors are lung, breast, melanoma, gastrointestinal, and renal. Small lesions (<3–4 cm) tend to be homogeneous, well-defined, and difficult to distinguish from benign, nonhyperfunctioning adenomas. To complicate the issue, even in patients with known primary malignancy, up to 50% of small adrenal masses are benign adenomas and not metastases. Percutaneous biopsy will be needed in many cases to confirm the pathology (16).

Larger lesions (>4 cm) generally show features of malignancy, including inhomogeneous density, inhomogeneous enhancement, irregular outline, thick irregular rim, and invasion of adjacent structures. On CT, lesions with attenuation values of greater than 10 H on unenhanced scans or of greater than 30 H on delayed enhanced scans are possibly malignant (Fig. 33.2B) (11). MR demonstrates metastases to be hypointense relative to liver on T1WI and strongly hyperintense relative to the liver on T2WI. Gadolinium shows early enhancement and slow washout.

Adrenal Carcinoma

Adrenal carcinoma is an uncommon but lethal tumor. Most are large and invasive at presentation. About half

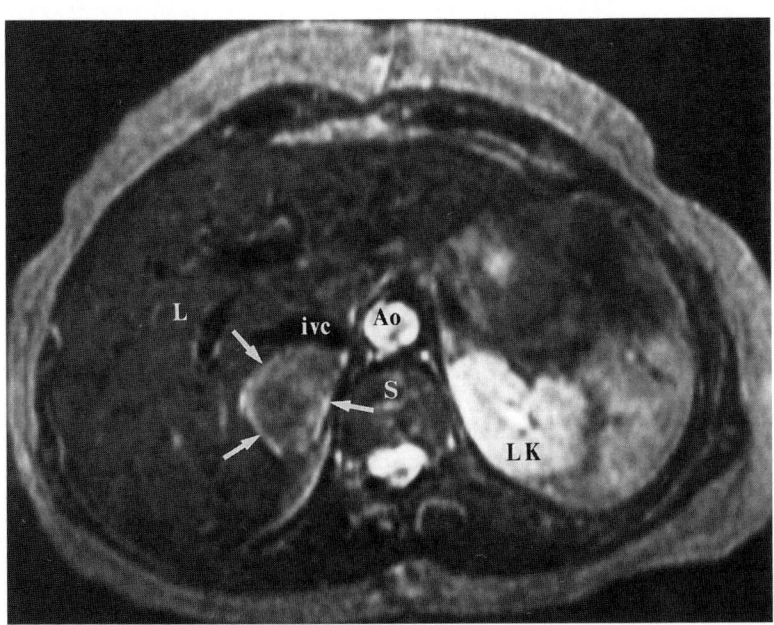

Figure 33.3. Benign Adrenal Adenoma. Axial plane T2-weighted MR image demonstrates a right adrenal mass (*arrows*) that proved to be a benign hyperfunctioning adenoma causing Conn's syndrome. *Ao,* aorta; *ivc,* inferior vena cava; *L,* liver; *LK,* left kidney; *S,* spine.

Figure 33.4. Chemical shift MR of Adrenal Mass.
A. In-phase gradient-echo image, with water and fat peaks aligned, shows a right adrenal mass (*arrow*) with signal intensity of 113. In-phase images appear gray and flat. **B.** Out-of-phase gradient-echo image, with water and fat peaks out of alignment, shows no significant change in signal intensity (115) of the right adrenal mass (*arrow*), indicating low fat content and high likelihood of malignancy. Out-of-phase images are more contrasty with prominent edge definition.

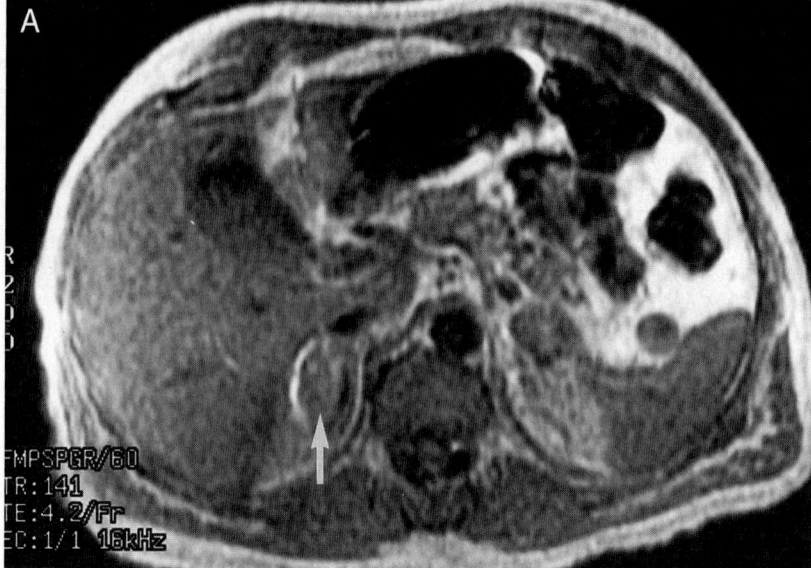

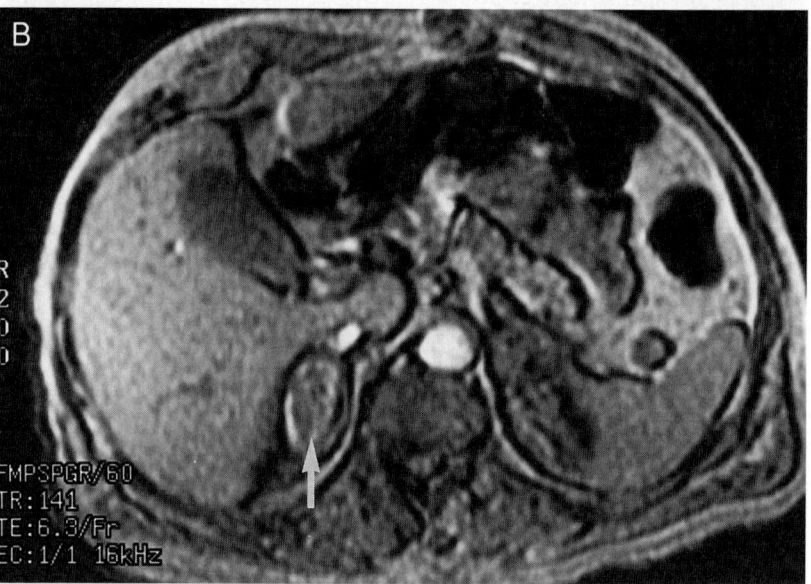

the carcinomas are hyperfunctioning and cause endocrine syndromes, most commonly Cushing's syndrome, virilization, or feminization.

The typical CT appearance is a large mass (4–20 cm), with areas of central necrosis and hemorrhage, and a pattern of irregular enhancement (1,3,7). Adrenal tumors larger than 4–5 cm in size should be removed because of the significant risk of carcinoma. Calcification is present in 30% of the tumors (Fig. 33.5). Hepatic and lymph node metastases are common. Tumor thrombus in the renal vein or IVC may be evident. Large tumors may be difficult to differentiate from hepatic masses.

On MR, T1WI demonstrate an inhomogeneous large mass, predominantly hypointense compared with liver. Signal intensity is increased on T2WI (Fig. 33.6) (4). Gadolinium enhancement or gradient echo imaging is useful to detect tumor thrombus. US with Doppler is also excellent for the evaluation of tumor thrombosis.

Cystic Adrenal Masses

Adrenal cysts are rare lesions that usually produce no symptoms and are discovered incidentally (17). True cysts are lined with endothelium or epithelium. Pseudocysts have a fibrous wall without lining cells and usually result from adrenal hemorrhage or infarction (Fig. 33.7). Parasitic cysts are usually echinococcal in origin. Adrenal cysts are more common in women and may be found at any age.

Cysts can be classified as uncomplicated and benign when they have thin walls (≥3 mm) with or without calcification, internal water density, do not exceed 5–6 cm in size, and do not enhance on CT. Calcification in cyst walls and septa is a common finding in all types of cysts (Fig. 33.7). Endothelial cysts tend to be multilocular with septal calcification. Hemorrhagic pseudocysts are usually unilocular with calcification in the wall. US demonstrates thin-walled anechoic cysts that may be septated.

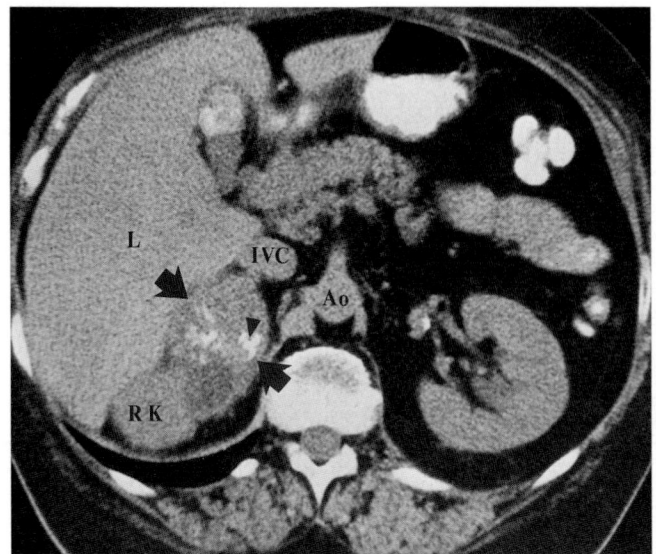

Figure 33.5. Adrenal Carcinoma. A CT scan of a patient with Cushing's syndrome demonstrates a 5-cm, irregularly marginated mass (*arrows*) with calcifications (*arrowhead*), replacing the right adrenal gland. *RK*, right kidney; *IVC*, inferior vena cava; *L*, liver; *Ao*, aorta.

Uncomplicated cysts are uniform low intensity on T1WI, uniform high intensity on T2WI, and do not enhance with gadolinium (6).

Cysts that are larger than 6 cm, have thick walls or solid components, show contrast enhancement on CT or MR, are inhomogeneous on MR, have echogenic fluid or internal debris on US, or produce symptoms should be considered for surgical removal. These lesions may be cysts complicated by hemorrhage or may be tumors with cystic degeneration, including metastases and pheochromocytoma. Percutaneous biopsy of the cyst wall is difficult, and percutaneous aspiration of cyst fluid may not be reliable to exclude malignancy.

On unenhanced CT, cysts may be difficult to differentiate from low-density benign adrenal adenomas. With intravenous contrast, adenomas generally demonstrate uniform enhancement, whereas uncomplicated cysts do not enhance.

Adrenal Myelolipoma

Myelolipomas are rare, nonfunctioning benign tumors arising from bone marrow elements in the adrenal gland. Identification of fat density within the tumor by CT or MR

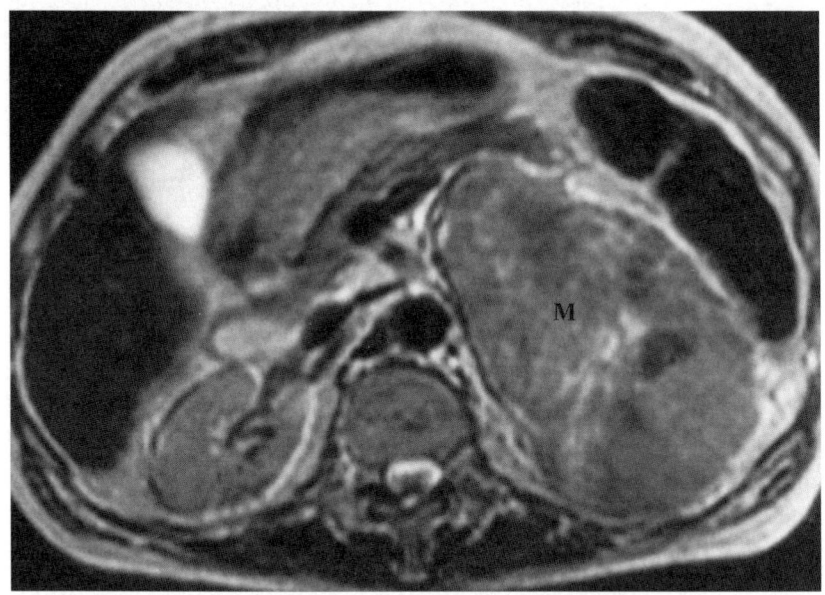

Figure 33.6. Adrenal Carcinoma. T2-weighted MR image shows huge inhomogeneous left adrenal mass (*M*). Areas of high and low signal intensity represent necrosis and hemorrhage.

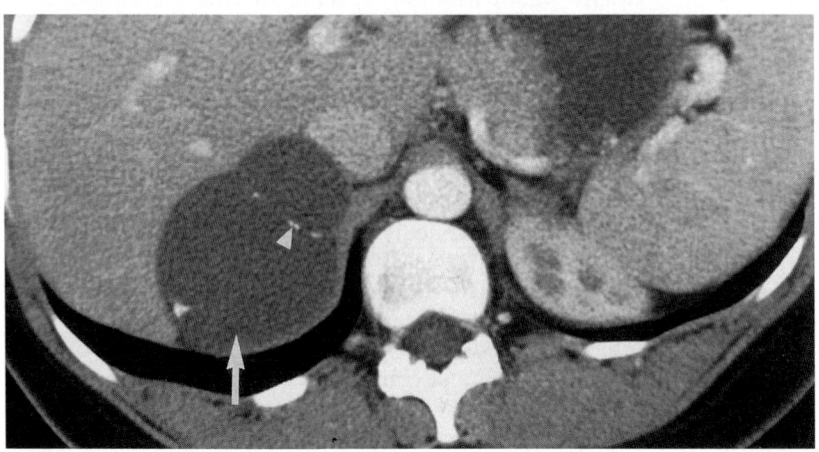

Figure 33.7. Posthemorrhagic Adrenal Cyst. CT shows a well-defined fluid-density lesion (*arrow*) of the right adrenal gland. Calcification (*arrowhead*) is evident in the wall and septation.

Figure 33.8. Adrenal Myelolipoma. Lesion (*between arrows*) of the left adrenal gland has large internal areas of fat density identical to surrounding retroperitoneal fat. Inhomogeneous attenuation is common.

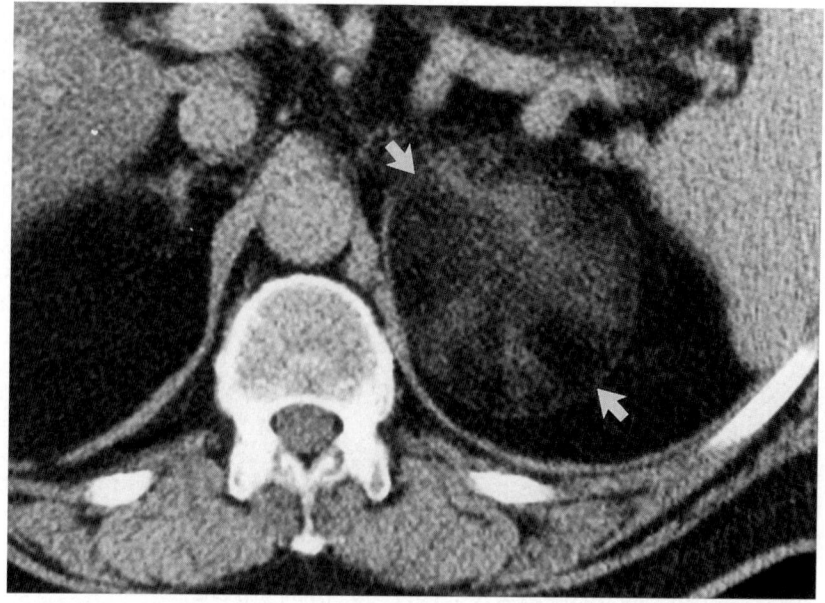

Figure 33.9. Adrenal Hemorrhage. Bilateral adrenal hemorrhage causes bilateral low-density adrenal masses (*arrows*). The hemorrhages followed severe trauma in an automobile accident.

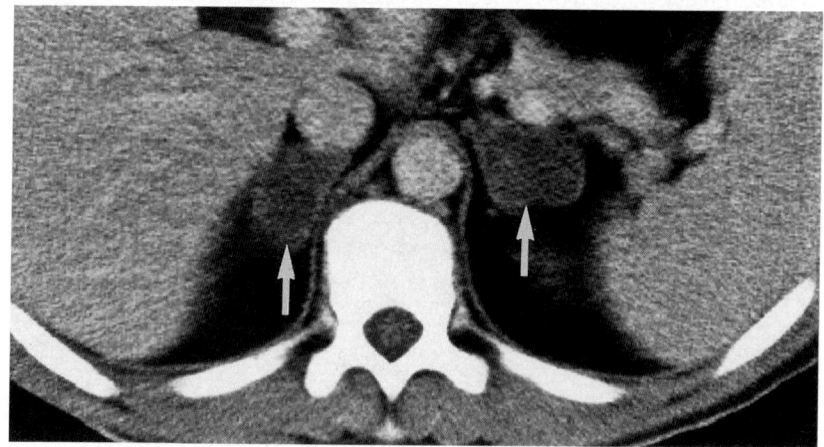

is definitive in making the diagnosis (Fig. 33.8) (18–20). Fat saturation pulse sequences confirm the diagnosis on MR (4). They have no malignant potential. These tumors range in size up to 30 cm and are frequently inhomogeneous because of their mixed components. Calcifications are present in 20%. On US, they may be extremely echogenic and blend in with retroperitoneal fat.

Adrenal Hemorrhage

Adrenal hemorrhage is most common in newborn infants, usually induced by episodes of hypoxia, birth trauma, or septicemia. Most cases are bilateral. In children, adrenal hemorrhage may be associated with child abuse (21). In adults, trauma and infection are the most common causes of adrenal hemorrhage. Unilateral hemorrhage is most common in adults, with the right adrenal most frequently affected. Bilateral hemorrhage may cause adrenal insufficiency.

Hemorrhage on CT is hypodense compared with the liver and spleen on contrast-enhanced studies (Fig. 33.9) (22). Stranding in the para-adrenal fat and thickening of the adjacent fascia are additional findings (23).

US demonstrates a hypoechoic mass that demonstrates the evolution over time that is characteristic of a hematoma.

MR demonstrates features of acute hemorrhage with short T1 and long T2 characteristics. T1WI show areas of signal intensity brighter than liver, whereas T2WI show bright signal intensity. Signal intensity changes with time and evolution of the hematoma.

Adrenal Calcification

Adrenal calcifications, in both children and adults, most commonly result from adrenal hemorrhage (Fig. 33.10). Tuberculosis and histoplasmosis may cause diffuse adrenal calcification associated with Addison's disease. Adrenal tumors that calcify include neuroblastoma and ganglioneuroma in children and adrenal carcinoma, pheochromocytoma, and ganglioneuroma in adults (24). Adrenal pseudocysts attributable to previous hemorrhage are the most common calcified adrenal masses in adults. Wolman's disease is a rare, autosomal recessive lipid disorder associated with enlarged calcified adrenal glands, hepatomegaly, and splenomegaly.

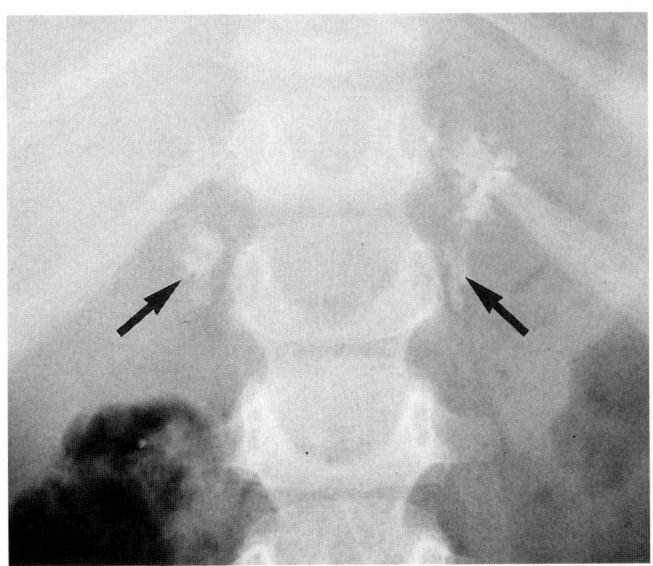

Figure 33.10. Adrenal Calcification. Plain radiograph of the abdomen in a 4-year-old child demonstrates calcification of both adrenal glands (*arrows*) resulting from bilateral adrenal hemorrhage as an infant.

Endocrine Syndromes

Cushing's syndrome is caused by excessive amounts of hydrocortisone and corticosterone released by the adrenal cortex. Clinical signs include truncal obesity, easy bruisability, generalized weakness, diabetes mellitus, and oligomenorrhea. Adrenal hyperplasia causes 70% of cases of noniatrogenic Cushing's syndrome. The hyperplasia is stimulated in 90% of cases by a pituitary microadenoma that produces adrenocorticotropic hormone (ACTH). MR of the sella is recommended for suspected pituitary adenomas. In 10% of cases, the source of ACTH is ectopic, usually from lung malignancies. Benign adrenal adenomas cause 20% of cases of Cushing's syndrome, and adrenal carcinoma causes the remaining 10% (see Fig. 33.5).

Conn's syndrome, produced by elevated levels of aldosterone, causes 1–2% of systemic hypertension. The clinical diagnosis is made by findings of persistent hypokalemia, increased serum and urine aldosterone, and decreased renin activity in the plasma. A solitary, benign, hyperfunctioning adrenal adenoma is the cause of 80% of cases, and adrenal hyperplasia is the cause of the remaining 20%. Adenomas are treated with surgical resection, whereas hyperplasia is treated medically. Adenomas that produce Conn's syndrome tend to be small (<2 cm); therefore, strict attention to excellent CT technique using thin (5 mm) slices is necessary for accurate localization (25). Adrenal venous sampling is used to confirm the site of excess aldosterone secretion and to differentiate adenoma from hyperplasia in problem cases (26).

Adrenogenital syndrome usually occurs in newborns and infants who have an enzyme deficiency (11β- or 22-hydroxylase) leading to deficient production of cortisol and aldosterone, and an excess of precursors, especially androgens. These infants have adrenal hyperplasia, which is usually well demonstrated by US (27). Both adrenal adenomas and carcinomas may be a cause of masculinizing or feminizing syndromes in older patients.

Pheochromocytoma is a rare tumor that causes hypertension, headaches, and tremors. Paroxysmal attacks are characteristic but not always present. Symptoms are produced by excessive secretion of catecholamines by the tumor. Pheochromocytoma is said to follow the "rule of tens": 10% are bilateral, 10% are extra-adrenal, 10% are malignant, and 10% are familial. Pheochromocytoma is associated with multiple endocrine neoplasia (MEN II), von Hippel-Lindau syndrome, and neurofibromatosis. Because 90% of pheochromocytomas arise in the adrenal medulla, the adrenal glands are usually scanned first.

CT is the usual imaging method of choice. The literature has traditionally advised against the use of intravenous contrast media in patients with pheochromocytoma because of a presumed risk of precipitating adrenergic crisis. More recent experience indicates a high level of safety with nonionic contrast media (28). Most tumors are larger than 2 cm in diameter. Tumors vary from purely solid to complex to predominantly cystic (Fig. 33.11) (29). Calcification is rare, but usually "eggshell" in configuration when present. If no lesion is found and clinical suspicion remains high, then scanning must be expanded to include the chest and remainder of the abdomen and pelvis. Extra-adrenal sites for pheochromocytoma include the organ of Zuckerkandl near the bifurcation of the aorta, the bladder (Fig. 33.12), and the para-aortic sympathetic chain.

MR may be the modality of choice to search for extra-adrenal pheochromocytoma (30). The tumor demonstrates very bright signal intensity on T2WI that makes it stand out from surrounding structures. Radionuclide scans using [131]I- or ^{123}I-metaiodobenzylquanidine (MIBG) are also effective in localizing pheochromocytoma; however, the agent is not widely available.

Addison's disease refers to primary adrenal insufficiency, which occurs only after 90% of the adrenal cortex is destroyed. The most common cause (60–70%) in the United States is idiopathic atrophy, which is probably an autoimmune disorder. The adrenal glands shrink and may not be detectable with imaging methods. Additional causes include tuberculosis, histoplasmosis, infarction, disseminated fungal infection, lymphoma, and metastatic tumor. Adrenal calcification suggests prior tuberculosis or histoplasmosis. Bilateral enlargement is seen with active infection. Lymphoma and metastases replace the glands with tumor.

KIDNEYS

Imaging Methods

Excretory urography (XU) has been the traditional method of imaging the kidneys; however, US, CT, and MR all provide better images of the renal parenchyma (31). Contrast-enhanced helical CT is the current best

Figure 33.11. Pheochromocytoma. CT in a patient presenting with severe hypertension reveals inhomogeneous mass (*arrow*) with areas of internal hemorrhage arising from the right adrenal gland.

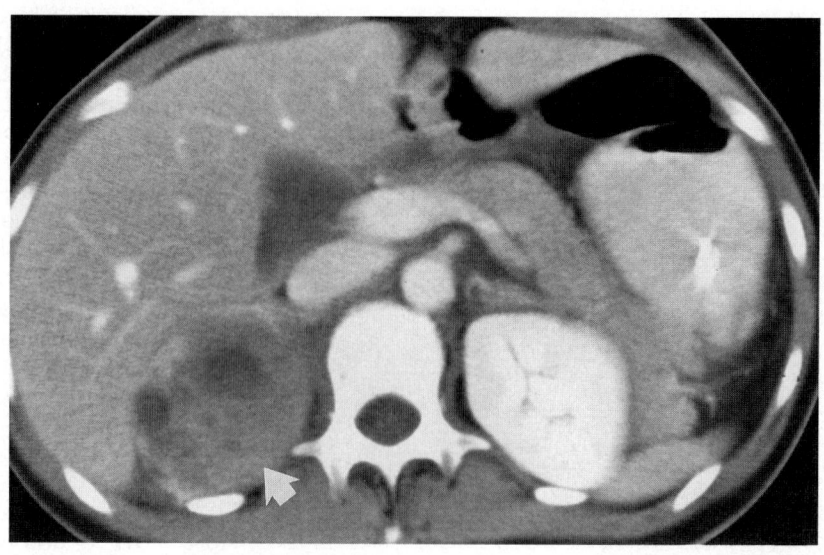

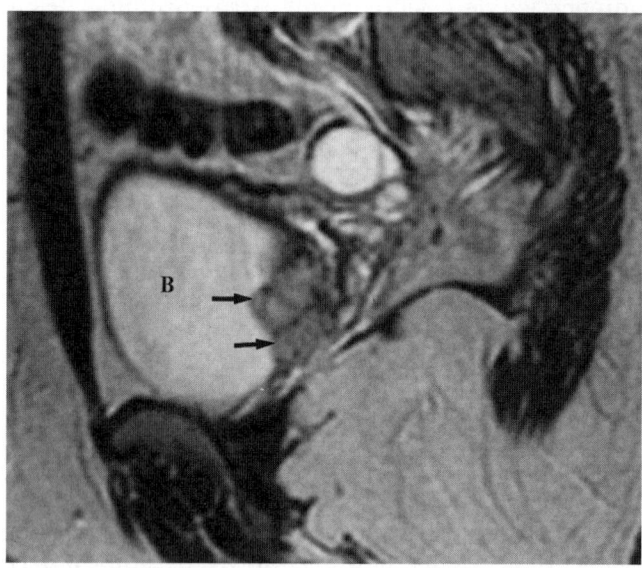

Figure 33.12. Pheochromocytoma in Bladder Wall. T2-weighted sagittal plane MR demonstrates a lobulated mass in the posterior wall of the bladder (*B*).

imaging study to detect and evaluate suspected renal tumors. Helical CT is usually performed as a three-stage study using 5-mm collimation with contiguous or overlapping slice reconstruction (see Fig. 33.16). Base scans are followed by corticomedullary phase scans at 30–40 seconds after onset of rapid contrast injection, followed by nephrogram phase scans at 120 seconds. US is used primarily to detect hydronephrosis and demonstrate kidney size. Renal masses may be discovered as an incidental finding on US of the abdomen. MR is a substitute for CT for patients in whom the use of intravenous iodinated contrast agents is contraindicated or whenever the CT study is equivocal. Color Doppler US is valuable in the assessment of venous involvement by renal tumors. Venography is useful whenever the question of venous involvement by tumor is not answered by CT, MR, or color Doppler US. Currently, arteriography is rarely used to diagnose or stage renal tumors, but may be required

for embolization procedures. Percutaneous biopsy, using US or CT for guidance, provides histologic confirmation of tumors that have already metastasized.

Anatomy

The kidneys are located within the cone of renal fascia (Gerota's fascia), surrounded by the fat of the perirenal space. The kidney is made up of lobes that consist of a pyramid-shaped medulla surrounded by cortex except at the apex of the pyramid. The cortex consists of all the glomeruli, proximal and distal convoluted tubules, and accompanying blood vessels. The peripheral cortex is immediately beneath the renal capsule, and the septal cortex extends down between the pyramids as the columns of Bertin. Prominent intrarenal cortex may simulate a renal mass (32). The medullary pyramids consist of the collecting tubules and the long, straight portions of the loops of Henle, as well as accompanying blood vessels. The apex of each pyramid is directed at the renal sinus and projects into a calyx. The term *papilla* refers to the innermost zone of the medulla, closest to the draining calyx. The kidneys gradually increase in size from birth to age 20. Renal length is relatively stable at 9–12 cm from ages 20 to 50 and gradually decreases thereafter.

Simple calyces are cup-shaped structures that drain one renal lobe (Fig. 33.13). Compound calyces drain several renal lobes and are more complex in shape. Compound calyces are more common at the poles of the kidney and are more prone to intrarenal reflux. The shape of each calyx is determined by the shape of the papilla. Disease of the papilla is reflected in the appearance of the calyx. The minor calyces join to form major calyces (infundibula), which drain into the renal pelvis. The appearance of the calyces and pelvis varies widely from patient to patient, and often from one kidney to another, even in the same patient. About 10% of the renal collecting systems are bifid or completely duplicated.

The main renal arteries originate laterally from the aorta, just below the origin of the superior mesenteric artery. The right renal artery courses posterior to the IVC, whereas the left renal artery courses posterior to

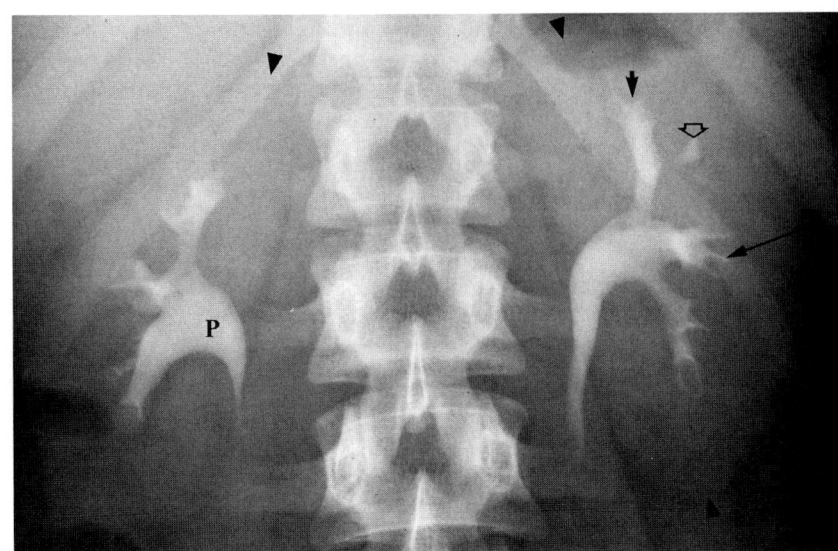

Figure 33.13. Normal Excretory Urogram. A radiograph of the kidneys taken 5 minutes after intravenous contrast injection demonstrates the enhanced renal parenchyma (*between arrowheads*) and the filled collecting system (*P*). The calyces (*long arrow*) are sharp and cup-shaped to accept the apex of the medullary pyramids. Upper pole calyces (*short arrow*) are usually compound because of drainage of multiple pyramids. Oblique views may be needed to confirm the normal appearance of calyces oriented anteriorly or posteriorly (*open arrow*). The normal kidney is equal in length to between three and four vertebral bodies.

the left renal vein. The main renal artery divides into ventral and dorsal branches as it enters the renal hilum. These branches divide into segmental arteries that supply separate portions of the kidney. Each is an end artery without anastomoses. Supplied segments of the kidney are therefore highly subject to infarction caused by emboli or occlusion. Interlobar arteries arise from segmental arteries and course in the columns of Bertin. Arcuate arteries are continuations of the interlobar arteries and course parallel to the renal capsule at the corticomedullary junction. Arcuate arteries give rise to intralobular arteries. Arterial divisions down to the level of the arcuate artery are demonstrable by color Doppler US.

The tight fibrous capsule that covers the kidney produces a sharp renal margin on CT. Perirenal fat continues into the renal sinus, outlining blood vessels and the collecting system. The renal fascia is commonly visualized on CT, especially when the fascia is thickened. Connective tissue septa extending between the renal capsule and the renal fascia subdivide the perirenal space into compartments and may be seen as linear strands in the perirenal fat.

On MR, T1WI demonstrate a high-density cortex and a lower density medulla. With T2WI, both the cortex and medulla brighten, but corticomedullary differentiation is often lost. The collecting systems may be difficult to visualize unless filled with urine.

Excretory urography will demonstrate corticomedullary differentiation when bolus contrast administration and rapid sequence filming are used. Because contrast agents are excreted by glomerular filtration, the cortex is opacified first, then the medulla is opacified as contrast passes into the collecting tubules. A tomogram late in the nephrogram phase will demonstrate uniform enhancement of the renal parenchyma. By 5 minutes postinjection, the collecting structures and ureters should be opacified (Fig. 33.13).

Because the kidneys actively concentrate contrast in the collecting tubules, renal masses seen on CT and XU will be hypodense compared with the enhanced renal parenchyma.

Congenital Renal Anomalies

Renal agenesis is associated with genital tract anomalies in the female. Ipsilateral adrenal agenesis is found in 10% of cases. In the remainder, the adrenal gland may appear enlarged. Compensatory hypertrophy of the opposite kidney is usually evident.

Horseshoe kidney is the most common renal fusion anomaly. The lower poles of the kidneys are joined across the midline by a fibrous or parenchymal band. As a result of fusion, the kidneys are malrotated, with the renal pelvises directed more anteriorly and the lower pole calyces directed medially (Fig. 33.14). The fused

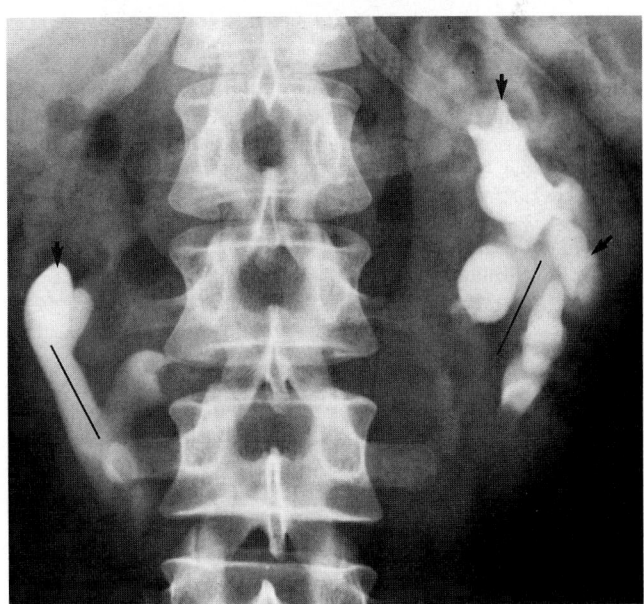

Figure 33.14. Horseshoe Kidney. Radiograph from an excretory urogram demonstrates the two kidneys extending across the spine and joined at their lower poles. Note the reversal of the long axis of each kidney (*black lines*) with the lower poles converging instead of diverging. The calyces (*arrows*) are blunted, reflecting urinary stasis created by the ureters having to cross anteriorly over the joined parenchyma.

kidney is low in position in the abdomen because normal ascent is prevented by renal tissue encountering the inferior mesenteric artery in the midline. Renal arteries are frequently multiple and ectopic in origin. Complications include increased susceptibility to trauma and urinary stasis leading to stones and infection. CT and US identify the midline isthmus of the kidney.

Crossed-fused renal ectopia may present as an abdominal mass because both kidneys are on the same side of the abdomen (Fig. 33.15). Renal arteries are invariably aberrant. The ureters insert in their normal locations in the bladder trigone.

Solid Renal Masses

NEOPLASTIC

Renal cell carcinoma (RCC) accounts for 85% of all renal neoplasms. It is most common in men (male-to-female ratio = 3:1), aged 50–70 years, and is bilateral in 2% (33). Because surgical resection provides the only chance for cure, early detection and accurate staging are critically important (34). Treatment is radical nephrectomy with removal of the renal fascia and its contents including the kidney, adrenal gland, perinephric fat, and hilar lymph nodes. Small RCC (<3 cm) have been treated with partial nephrectomy with good results.

Any solid renal mass should be considered suspect for renal cell carcinoma (Fig. 33.16). Hemorrhage and necrosis are common, and cystic and multicystic forms are also seen (5–10% of cases) (Fig. 33.17). Stippled central or peripheral calcifications are present in 10% of cases. The tumors are commonly hypervascular with numerous abnormal feeding vessels visualized. Tumor growth into the renal vein occurs in 30% of cases and extends into the IVC in 5–10%. Detection of venous invasion is critical to surgical planning. Metastases are present at diagnosis in 40% of cases. The tumor metastasizes most commonly to lung, local lymph nodes, liver, bone, adrenal glands, and the opposite kidney. Chest CT and radionuclide bone scans are effective in demonstrating distant metastases. Prognosis is directly related to the stage of the tumor at the time of diagnosis.

Contrast-enhanced CT (Fig. 33.16) is usually the tumor evaluation and staging method of choice (Table 33.1)(34). When intravenous contrast is contraindicated, however, MR is preferred. The tumor appears as a het-

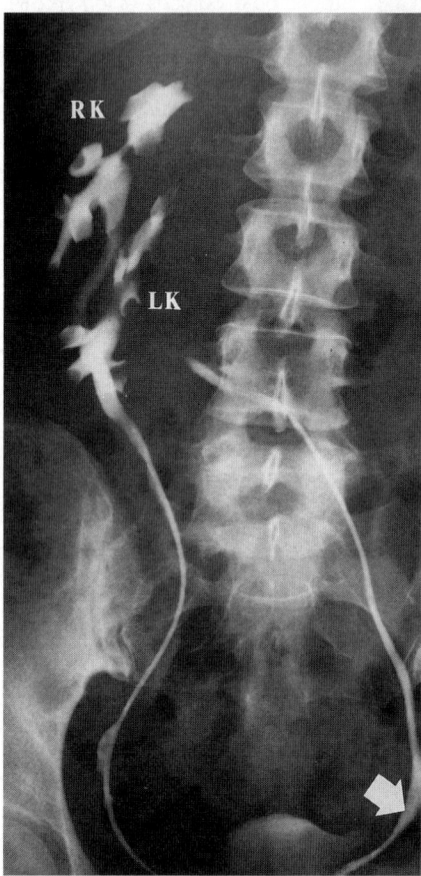

Figure 33.15. Crossed-fused Renal Ectopia. The left kidney (*LK*) is ectopic on the right side of the abdomen, and its parenchyma is fused to the parenchyma of the right kidney (*RK*). Note that the left ureter (*arrow*) inserts normally into the bladder.

Table 33.1. Staging of Renal Cell Carcinoma

Robson Stage	TMN Stage	Description	Imaging Findings
I	T1	Confined within renal capsule	Sharp renal margin
	T2	Tumor <2.5 cm	
		Tumor >2.5 cm	
II	T3a	Spread to perinephric fat but confined within the renal fascia	Poorly defined margin
			Discrete soft-tissue nodules in perirenal fat
III-A	T3b	Tumor thrombus in veins	Enlarged vessels + intraluminal mass
	T3c	Tumor in renal vein only	
	T4b	Tumor in IVC below diaphragm	
		Tumor in IVC above diaphragm	
III-B	N1–N3	Spread to local lymph nodes	Local lymph nodes >15 mm diameter
III-C		Tumor thrombus in vein and tumor spread to local lymph nodes	Enlarged vessels + intraluminal mass
			Local lymph nodes 15 mm diameter
IV-A	T4a	Direct invasion of adjacent organs	Tumor invasion of adjacent organs
IV-B	M1a–M1d, N4	Distant metastases	Distant metastases

(Adapted from Robson CJ, Churchill BM, Anderson W. The results of radical nephrectomy for renal cell carcinoma. J Urol 1969;101:297, and American Joint Committee on Cancer: Manual for staging of cancer. 3rd ed. 1998.)

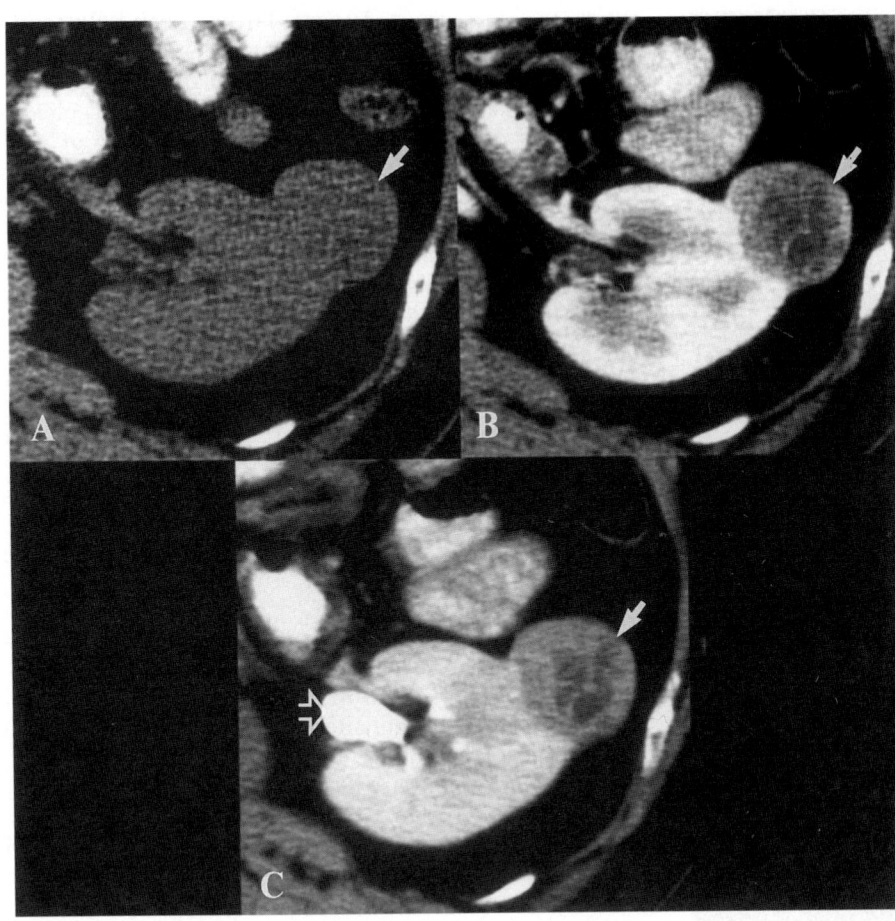

Figure 33.16. Renal Cell Carcinoma.
Three-phase helical CT demonstrates a solid mass (*arrows*) with internal necrosis arising from the left kidney. **A.** Base scan shows the mass is isodense with unenhanced renal parenchyma. **B.** Cortical nephrogram phase shows early enhancement of the mass. The renal cortex is enhanced, whereas the medullary pyramids have not yet received the contrast agent. **C.** Nephrogram (delayed) scan shows that the mass remains hypodense to the enhanced renal parenchyma. Contrast has now opacified the collecting system (*open arrow*).

erogeneous enhancing mass that is less dense than enhanced renal parenchyma. Low density areas within the tumor reflect hemorrhage and necrosis. CT is not accurate in the differentiation of stage I and stage II tumors, but this is of limited treatment significance. Stranding densities in the perirenal fat are usually attributable to edema or fibrosis from previous inflammation and are not a reliable sign of tumor spread. Discrete soft-tissue nodules in the perirenal fat are highly predictive of tumor spread into the fat. Preoperative percutaneous biopsy is indicated only when the tumor is believed to be metastatic on imaging studies. In this case, percutaneous biopsy of a metastatic lesion is usually more fruitful than biopsy of the renal tumor itself because well-differentiated RCC may be difficult to differentiate cytologically from normal renal cells. Venous tumor thrombus is seen as a low-density filling defect within a contrast-enhanced vein that is usually enlarged.

MR for tumor detection and staging usually includes T1WI before and after gadolinium injection, T2WI, and a fat suppression sequence if angiomyolipoma is suspected (35,36). RCC is isointense or hyperintense compared with renal parenchyma on T1WI and shows distinct enhancement with gadolinium administration. Hyperintensity on T1WI usually reflects tumoral hemorrhage, but fat suppression sequences should be used to ensure the high signal is not because of fat. Most RCCs are heterogeneous on T2WI, reflecting areas of tumor, necrosis, hemorrhage, and hemosiderin (Fig. 33.18). The staging accuracy of MR and CT is about equal.

US demonstrates solid renal cell carcinomas as a heterogeneous hypoechoic or mildly hyperechoic mass (see Fig. 36.54). Areas of hemorrhage and necrosis appear cystic. Doppler US of the renal vein and IVC shows tumor thrombus by demonstration of echogenic material in the vein associated with partial or complete absence of blood flow (37).

Excretory urography is insensitive to small tumors demonstrating only about half of the tumors 2-3 cm in size that are shown by CT. Larger tumors appear as contour bulges on the renal outline, defects in the nephrogram, areas of mottled enhancement, or by the presence of calcification.

Angiomyolipoma (AML) is an uncommon (1–3% of renal neoplasms) benign mesenchymal tumor composed of fat in varying amounts, smooth muscle, and abnormal blood vessels lacking elastic tissue (38). Most (80%) are solitary unilateral tumors discovered most commonly in middle-aged women. The remaining 20% are found in patients with tuberous sclerosis. These tumors are commonly multicentric and bilateral. Because of the abnormal thin-walled vessels, the tumors are prone to hemorrhage, which may be massive. Large solitary lesions are usually surgically removed. Follow-up of small lesions reveals slow growth (39). Imaging studies reflect the tissue composition of the tumor and can range from almost purely fat density to nearly homogeneously solid muscle density. Tumors may be as large as 20 cm and may be predominantly exophytic, mimicking nonrenal tumors.

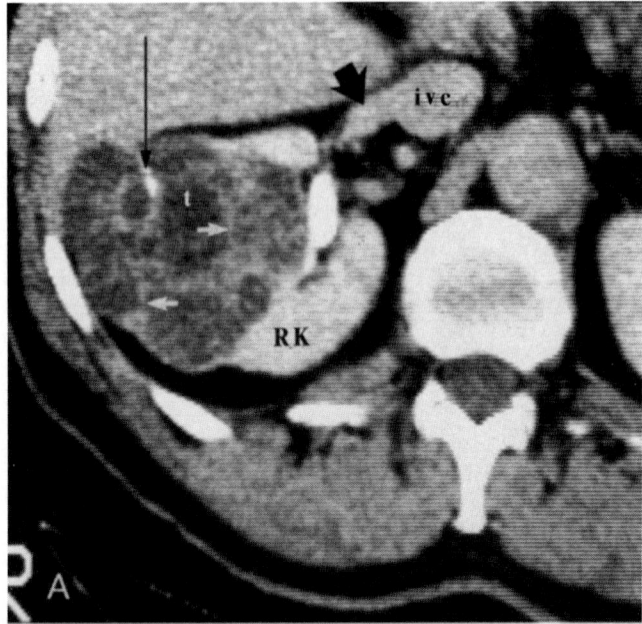

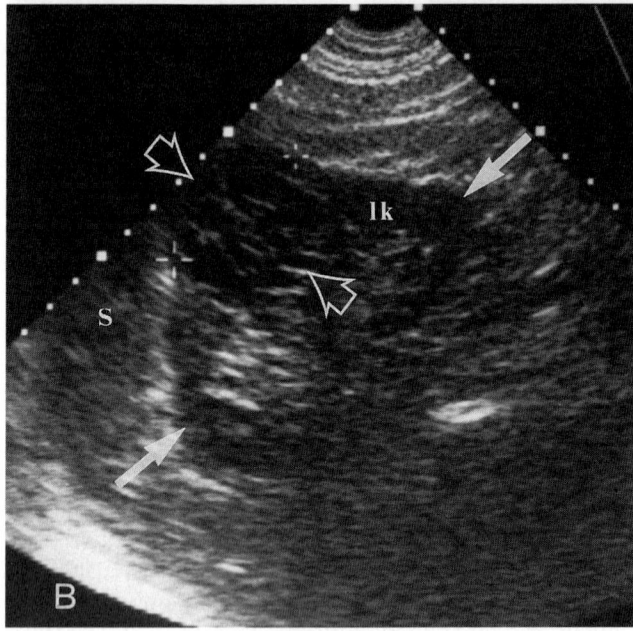

Figure 33.17. Renal Cell Carcinoma-Multicystic Appearance.
A. Contrast-enhanced CT scan reveals a lobulated tumor (*t*) in the right kidney (*RK*). Septations (*small arrows*) are evident between cystic areas. A focal calcification (*long black arrow*) is also present. The right renal vein (*black arrow*) and the inferior vena cava (*ivc*) are free of tumor thrombus. **B.** A US image in a different patient shows a multicystic mass (*between open arrows*) arising from the lateral aspect of the left kidney (*lk; between closed arrows*). The thin septations were lined by clear cells typical of renal carcinoma. *S*, spleen.

CT demonstration of even small quantities of fat density within the tumor is considered diagnostic of AML (Fig. 33.19). Thin-section (3-5 mm) CT is the preferred method to demonstrate fat in problem cases. Smooth muscle and vascular components of the tumor are seen as nodules and strands of soft tissue density. Vascular areas of the tumor may show striking contrast enhance-

ment. In a few reported cases, fat has been detected in association with calcification in a RCC. In these cases, the calcification was shown histologically to be ossification with associated marrow fat. Fat density in a solid renal tumor without calcification is diagnostic of AML (31,40).

US characteristically demonstrates a strikingly hyperechoic solid mass. Echogenicity of the tumor often exceeds renal sinus fat. Small tumors (<2 cm) are common incidental findings.

On MR, T1WI demonstrate the high-signal intensity of fat, which should be confirmed by fat-suppression technique. Coronal and sagittal MR is useful in confirming the renal origin of large masses.

Angiography classically demonstrates a hypervascular mass with enlarged feeding arteries and tortuous, dilated vessels with small aneurysms. Venous pooling is common, but there is no arteriovenous shunting. Angiography is useful for planning renal-sparing surgery.

Renal Adenoma. Controversy exists as to whether renal adenoma is a benign neoplasm or a small, well-differentiated renal cell carcinoma. By definition, adenomas are less than 3 cm in size, lack invasive features, and do not metastasize. Adenomas are indistinguishable from renal cell carcinoma by imaging methods.

Oncocytoma is a rare (3–6% of renal neoplasms) well-encapsulated, benign tumor composed of eosinophilic cells called oncocytes. Tumors may be large (up to 25 cm), but they average 5–8 cm. Hemorrhage and necrosis are rare. Most are solitary, but 6% are multiple or bilateral. Large tumors demonstrate a stellate central scar that is suggestive of the diagnosis. Angiography classically demonstrates a "spoke-wheel" configuration of radiating vessels. Most oncocytomas are indistinguishable from renal cell carcinoma by all imaging methods and must be surgically removed to confirm the diagnosis (41).

Lymphoma. Although primary renal lymphoma is rare, the kidney is commonly involved by metastatic lymphoma or by direct invasion. Most cases are non-

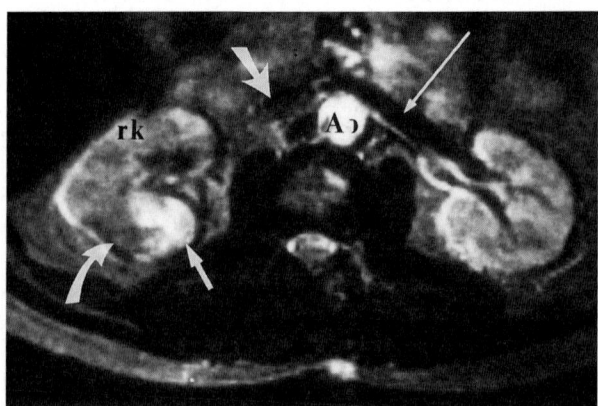

Figure 33.18. Renal Cell Carcinoma. T2-weighted MR image demonstrates inhomogeneous tumor in the right kidney with a bright cystic component (*small arrow*) and an isodense solid portion (*curved arrow*). The IVC (*large arrow*) is free of evidence of tumor thrombus. The left renal vein (*long arrow*) is well demonstrated. *Ao*, aorta.

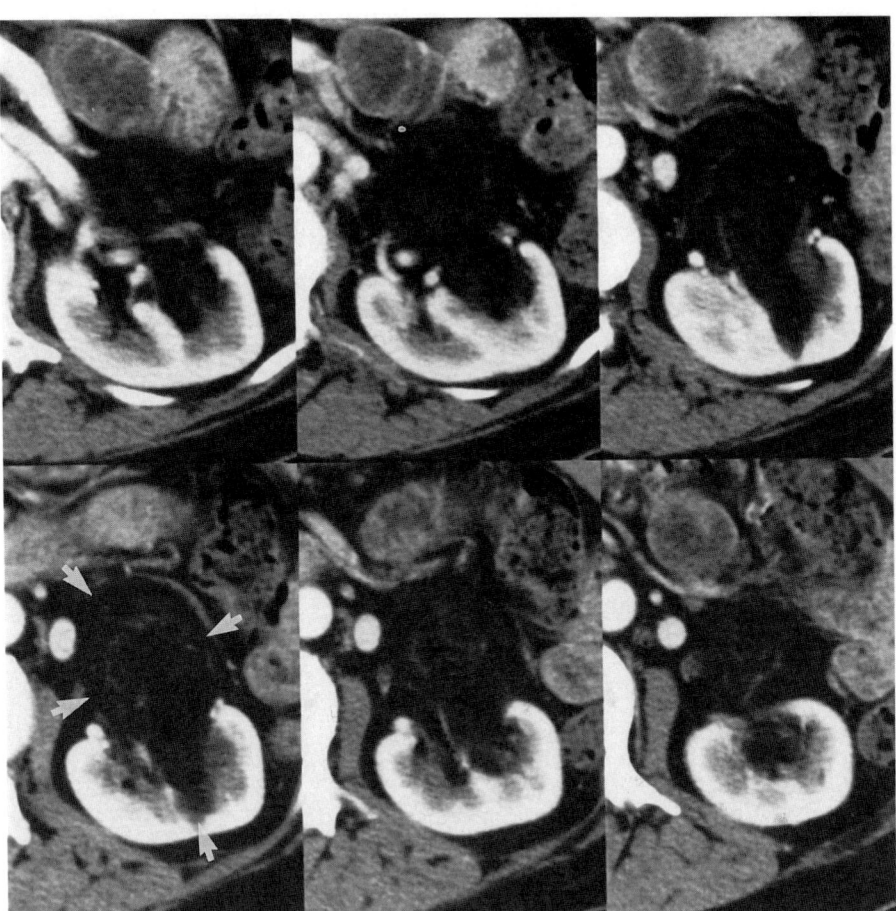

Figure 33.19. Angiomy
of helical CT images obtai
cortical phase of contrast er.
demonstrates a fat-density tumor
arrows) extending from the renal s.
the left kidney into the perirenal space.
density of the tumor is identical to perirene
fat.

Hodgkin's lymphoma. Patterns of renal involvement include diffuse disease enlarging the kidney, multiple bilateral solid renal masses (Fig. 33.20), solitary bulky tumor, and tumor invasion into the renal sinus.

CT shows lymphoma as a homogenous, round, poorly enhancing mass. Extensive retroperitoneal adenopathy favors the diagnosis.

Metastases. The kidneys are a frequent site of hematogeneous metastases; however, most are detected late in the course of malignancy (42). Most metastases appear as multiple, bilateral, small, irregular renal masses. Some are large, solitary, and not distinguishable from RCC. Common primary tumors include lung, breast, colon, and melanoma.

INFLAMMATORY

Xanthogranulomatous pyelonephritis is a rare inflammatory lesion that may diffusely involve an obstructed kidney or present as a focal renal mass (43). An obstructing stone, often a staghorn calculus, is usually present. The kidney is chronically infected, most commonly with *Proteus mirabilis*, and does not function in the affected areas. Renal parenchyma is destroyed and replaced by xanthoma cells, which are lipid-laden macrophages. CT and US demonstrate focal or diffuse hydronephrosis and a complex mass with areas of high and low density (see Fig. 36.61).

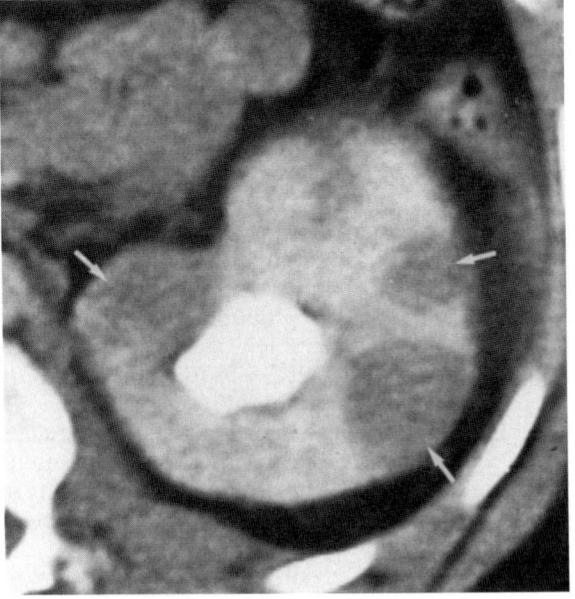

Figure 33.20. Renal Lymphoma. Non-Hodgkin's lymphoma manifests in this patient as multiple low-density solid masses (*arrows*) in the left kidney.

al Cyst. A large
the left kidney
features. The cyst is
has a sharp margin
nyma, and its wall is

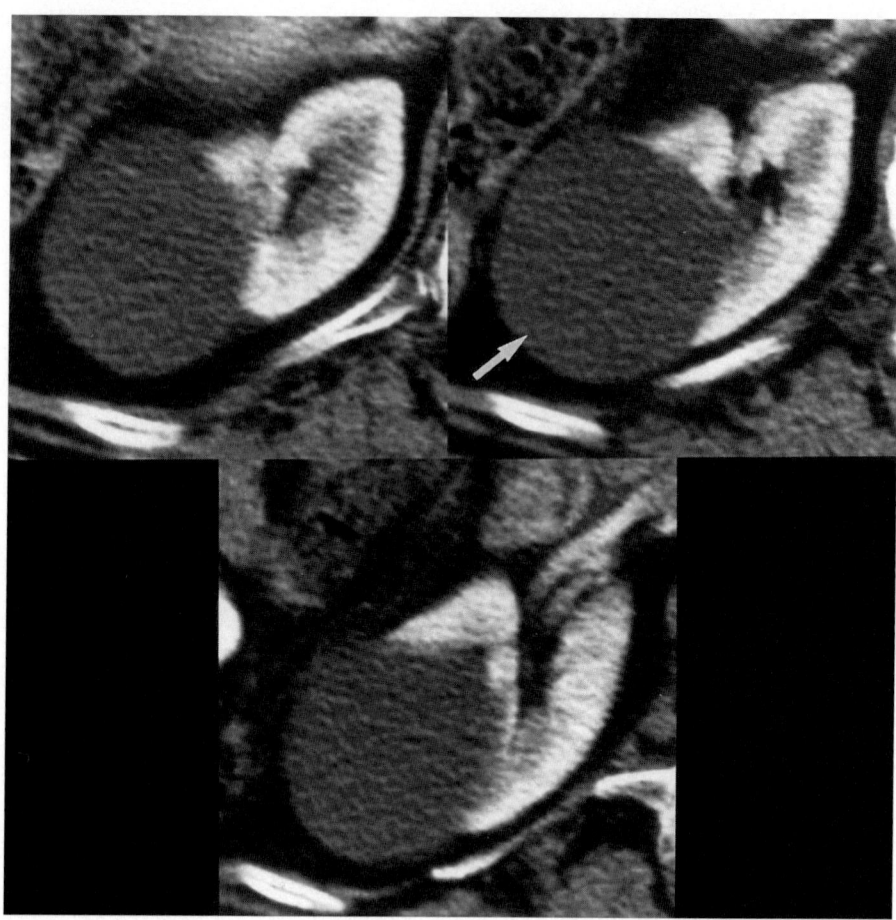

Cystic Renal Masses

Simple renal cyst is the most common renal mass. They are found in half the population older than age 55. Small cysts are asymptomatic. Large cysts (>4 cm) occasionally cause obstruction, pain, hematuria, or hypertension. Cysts are commonly multiple and bilateral. US, CT, and MR can each make a definitive diagnosis.

US criteria for simple renal cyst are *a)* round or oval anechoic mass, *b)* increased through transmission, *c)* sharply defined far wall, and *d)* thin or imperceptible cyst wall.

CT signs include *a)* sharp margination with the renal parenchyma, *b)* no perceptible wall, *c)* homogeneous attenuation near water density (−10 to +10 H), and *d)* absence of contrast enhancement (Fig. 33.21).

MR criteria include *a)* homogeneous, sharply defined round or oval mass, *b)* homogeneous low-signal intensity on T1WI, and *c)* homogeneous high-signal intensity similar to urine on T2WI. No enhancement should be seen after gadolinium administration.

XU shows cysts as lucent defects in the nephrogram with sharp round borders with the renal parenchyma. A beak or claw sign may be produced by the enhancing renal parenchyma. Findings on XU are not sufficiently specific to characterize renal masses as cysts. Sonography is the most cost-effective method to evaluate renal masses detected by XU (44).

Complicated Cyst. Simple renal cysts may be complicated by hemorrhage or infection. The resulting change in imaging characteristics may make differentiation from cystic renal tumors difficult. Bosniak (45) developed a classification system for cystic masses that helps to categorize these problematic lesions.

Category I lesions are simple cysts with the imaging findings just listed. US and CT are definitive when all characteristic findings are present.

Category II lesions are benign, with no further imaging or follow-up needed (see Fig. 33.24). Three types of cysts are in this category: *a)* cysts with delicate thin septations no more than 1-mm to 2-mm thick, *b)* cysts with delicate thin calcification in the wall or septum, and *c)* cysts that are hyperdense (60–100 H) on CT because of high concentration of protein or blood breakdown products and size of less than 3 cm. Larger lesions thought to be benign but with less characteristic findings are classified as category IIF lesions. Bosniak (46) recommends imaging follow-up of IIF lesions at 3, 6, and 12 months.

Category III lesions are indeterminate lesions that may be malignant. Most should be treated surgically. Findings include thick irregular calcification, irregular margins, thick or enhancing septa, areas of nodularity, thick walls, multilocular mass. Lesions in this category include hemorrhagic or infected simple cysts, multilocular cystic nephroma, multiloculated cysts, and cystic forms of RCC.

Category IV lesions are necrotic cystic neoplasms or tumors that arise in the wall of a cyst. Findings include irregular solid nodules, irregular thick shaggy walls, and septa with contrast enhancement of solid areas.

Small renal lesions may be particularly difficult to classify (31,47). Thin section CT (3- to 5-mm–thick slices) with bolus contrast enhancement and great attention to detail will assist in correct classification of lesions.

MR signal intensity depends on the amount of blood or proteinaceous material present within the cyst. Cyst fluid with signal characteristics similar to urine suggests a simple cyst. Higher signal intensity on T1WI suggests a complicated cyst, which may be indistinguishable from a solid mass.

Renal abscess usually results from pyelonephritis complicated by liquefactive necrosis. A focal renal mass with a thick wall is the most common appearance. Associated inflammatory changes include stranding densities in the perirenal space and thickening of the renal fascia. Renal abscesses may extend into the perirenal space and demonstrate an associated perirenal fluid collection (Fig. 33.22).

Renal cell carcinoma may appear as a predominantly cystic or multiloculated cystic mass (see Fig. 33.17) (48). Malignant tumor cells line the walls and septa. Thick walls, thick septations, and contrast enhancement are usually evident.

Multilocular cystic nephroma is an uncommon benign neoplasm consisting of a cluster of noncommunicating cysts of varying size separated by connective tissue septations (48,49). The tumor has a thick capsule with thin septations. They are discovered most commonly in male infants and children (<4 y) and middle-aged women (40–60 y). Surgical excision is usually recommended in adults to exclude renal cell carcinoma.

Renal Cystic Disease

MULTIPLE BILATERAL RENAL CYSTS

Autosomal dominant polycystic disease is transmitted by autosomal dominant inheritance but usually manifests clinically later in life. Renal parenchyma is progressively replaced by multiple noncommunicating cysts of varying size (Fig. 33.23). Renal volume increases with the number and size of the renal cysts. The cysts are commonly complicated by internal hemorrhage. The condition can be detected in neonates and children, but most patients present clinically between ages 30 and 50 years with hypertension and renal failure. Imaging diagnosis is confirmed by demonstration of cysts in the liver (60% of patients) and pancreas (10% of patients), and often in other organs. Extrarenal cysts seldom cause clinical problems. Associated cardiovascular abnormalities include intracranial berry aneurysms (20% of patients), mitral valve prolapse, bicuspid aortic valve, aortic aneurysms and dissections (50).

Multiple simple cysts must be differentiated from adult polycystic disease. Patients with multiple simple cysts are usually older, have fewer cysts, usually no renal failure, and no family history of renal cystic disease (Fig. 33.24). Cysts are not found in other organs.

von Hippel-Lindau disease is associated with multiple renal and pancreatic cysts, renal adenomas, and frequently multiple and bilateral renal cell carcinomas (24–45% of patients). Associated lesions include retinal angiomas and cerebellar hemangioblastomas. The disease is inherited with an autosomal dominant pattern that is not expressed in every individual with the gene (51,52).

Tuberous sclerosis combines multiple renal cysts (see Fig. 36.53) and multiple angiomyolipomas. Cutaneous, retinal, and cerebral hamartomas are associated. This condition also has an autosomal dominant inheritance pattern.

Acquired cystic kidney disease is the term applied to the development of multiple cysts in the native kidneys of patients on long-term hemodialysis. Affected kidneys are usually small, reflecting the chronic renal disease. Cysts are predominantly cortical and rarely exceed 2-cm size (Fig. 33.25). Solid renal adenomas and RCC (7%) also develop and are prone to spontaneous hemorrhage (53,54).

MEDULLARY CYSTIC DISEASE

Autosomal recessive polycystic kidney disease usually presents in the neonate and is detectable in the

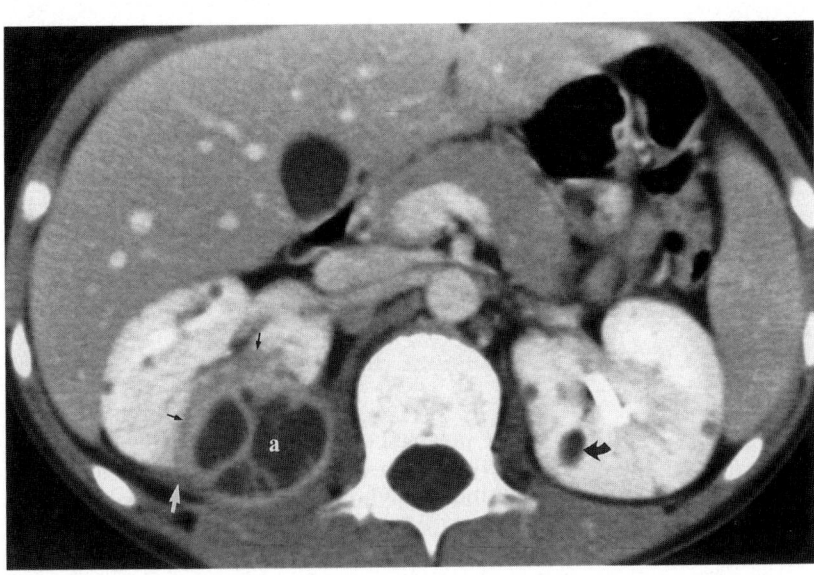

Figure 33.22. Renal Abscess. The right renal abscess (*a*) has characteristic thick walls and septations and internal fluid density. Edema reduces the CT density of the renal parenchyma adjacent to the mass (*small black arrows*) and infiltrates the perirenal space (*white arrow*). This patient also has multiple small renal cysts (*curved arrow*) due to autosomal dominant polycystic disease.

Figure 33.23. Adult Polycystic Disease. Contrast-enhanced CT demonstrates massive enlargement of both kidneys (*RK, LK*) and replacement of most of the renal parenchyma by multiple cysts (*c*). *p,* renal pelvis opacified with contrast.

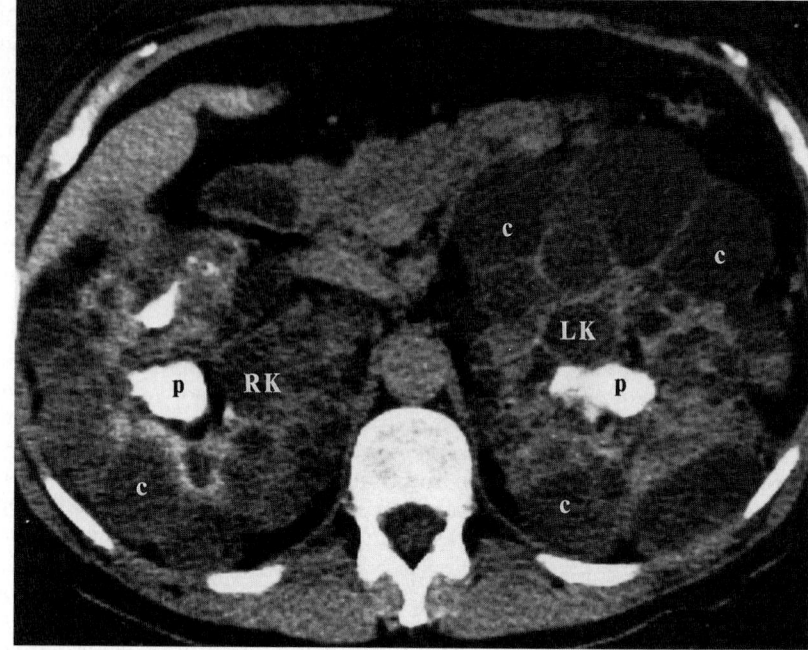

Figure 33.24. Multiple Renal Cysts. CT demonstrates multiple cysts (*open arrows*) in both kidneys. The right kidney has one cyst (*cc*) that does not meet criteria for a simple cyst because of visible thickening of its wall (*closed arrow*). The thick wall was the result of previous hemorrhage within the cyst. The renal veins (*rv, lv*) and inferior vena cava (*ivc*) are clearly seen. An enlarged retrocaval lymph node (*curved arrow*) is evident. *Ao,* aorta.

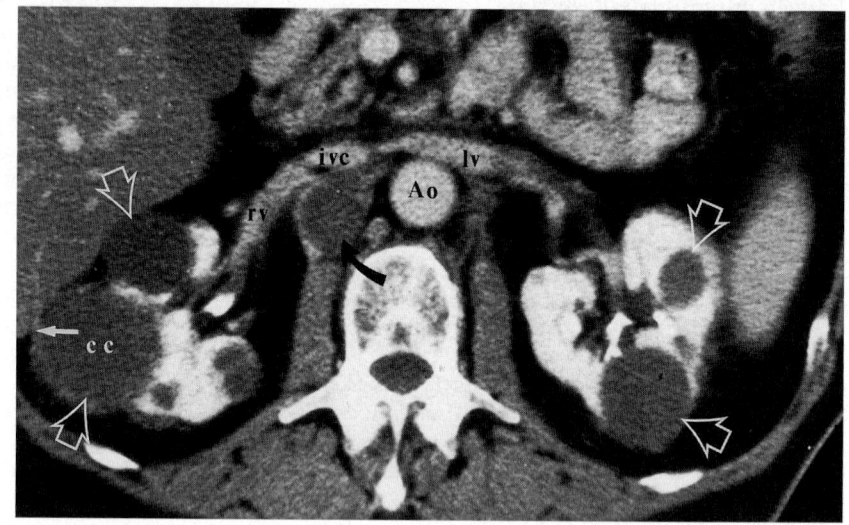

Figure 33.25. Acquired Cystic Kidney Disease. Noncontrast CT reveals both kidneys (*arrows*) are small and contain numerous small cysts. The patient has been on hemodialysis for 8 years.

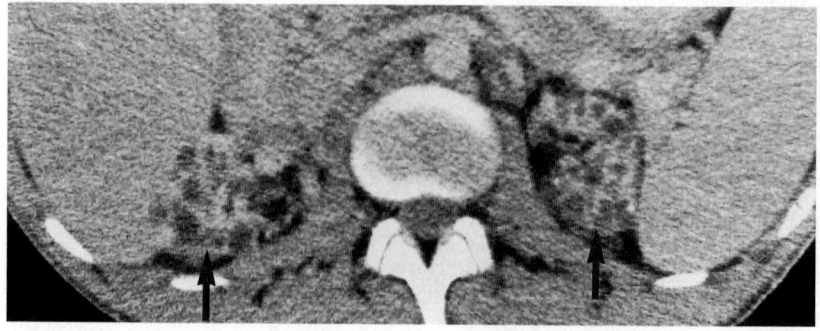

fetus. The condition is bilateral, relatively symmetrical, and characterized by marked enlargement of the kidneys and occasionally the liver. Affected patients have a combination of cystic renal disease and hepatic fibrosis. The disease runs a spectrum from severe renal disease at birth (infantile polycystic disease) to relatively mild renal disease with development of hepatic fibrosis and liver failure in childhood (juvenile polycystic disease) (55). The primary defect in the kidneys is diffuse dilatation of the collecting tubules (Fig. 33.26). The early prognosis depends on the number of abnormal nephrons. Most infants who present in renal failure die in the neonatal period. Infants with a larger number of normal nephrons have mild renal impairment and present at age 3–5 years with progressive liver failure and portal hypertension.

US is used to make the diagnosis in most cases (see Fig. 36.51). Both kidneys are large and echogenic centrally with a sonolucent rim of compressed cortex. Visualized cysts are generally small (<5 mm). Children with less severe renal disease develop larger cysts. US shows an enlarged echogenic liver with splenomegaly, dilated portal vein, and enlarged portosystemic collateral vessels in the older children who develop liver disease.

Medullary sponge kidney refers to dysplastic dilatation of the collecting tubules in the papilla. The dilatation is cylindrical or saccular in configuration. The condition causes urinary stasis in the papilla, which results in stone formation and occasionally infection (Fig. 33.27). Most patients are asymptomatic. There is no genetic predisposition and no risk of renal failure. The kidneys remain normal in size. The condition is usually bilateral and symmetrical but may be focal, unilateral, or asymmetrical. Striations or saccular contrast collections in the papilla on excretory urography are most characteristic. Stones in the papilla cause increased echogenicity in the medulla on US.

Uremic medullary cystic disease presents with renal failure, anemia, and salt wasting. The basic defect is progressive tubular atrophy with glomerular sclerosis and medullary cyst formation. The medullary cysts are generally too small to be visualized by current imaging methods. Kidney size is normal or small. Renal parenchymal echogenicity is usually increased.

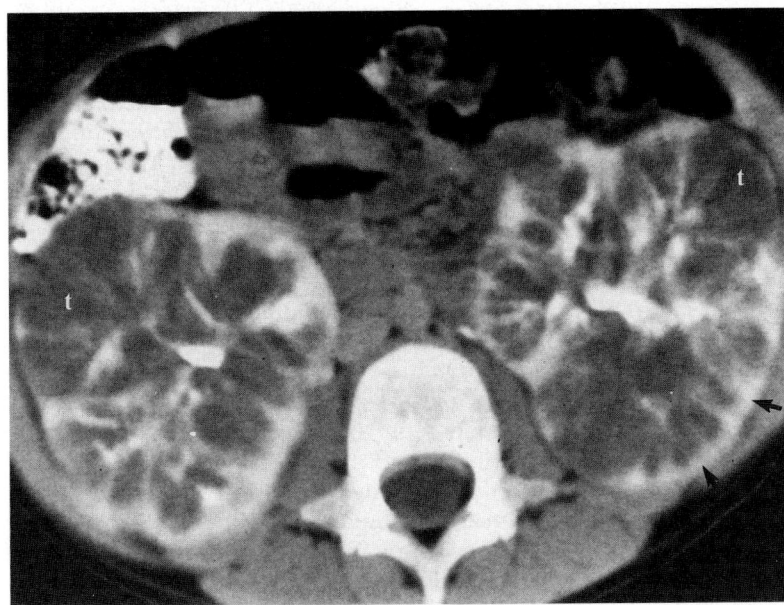

Figure 33.26. Autosomal Recessive Polycystic Disease. Contrast-enhanced CT in a 5-year-old child shows massive kidneys. The enhanced cortex (*arrows*) is thinned and nonenhanced collecting tubules (*t*) in the medulla are enlarged. No discrete cysts are evident.

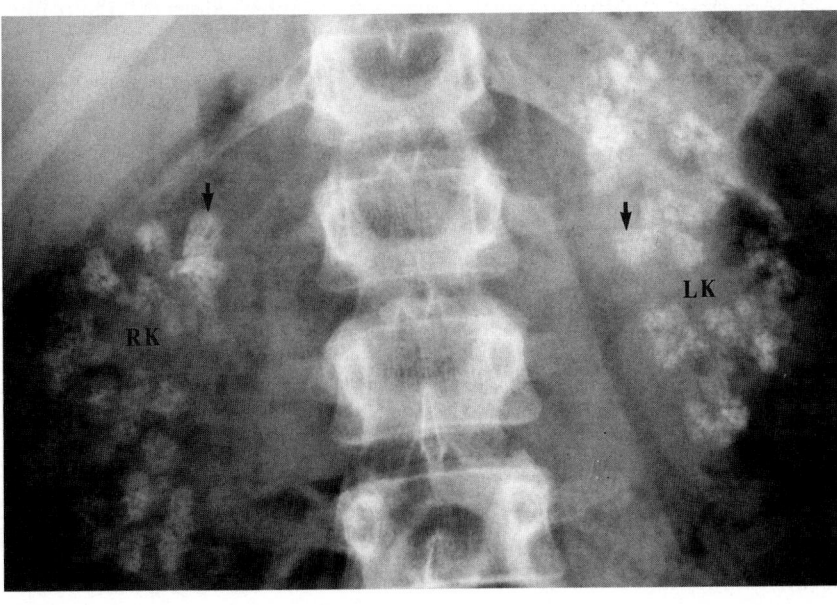

Figure 33.27. Medullary Sponge Kidney. Plain radiograph demonstrates innumerable calcifications (*arrows*) in the medullary regions of both right and left kidneys (*RK, LK*). The stones form in dilated collecting tubules in the medullary pyramids.

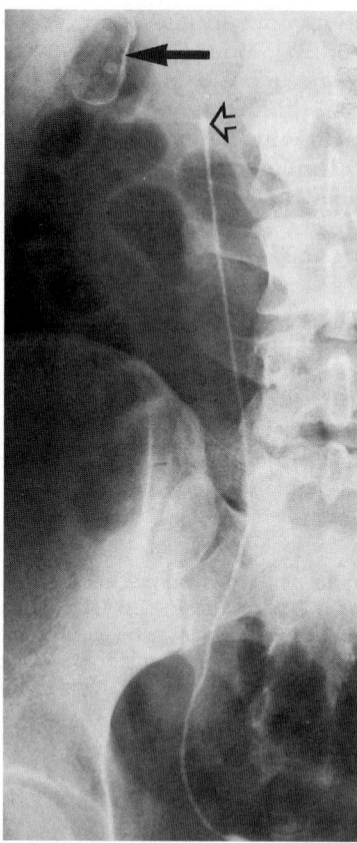

Figure 33.28. Multicystic Dysplastic Kidney. The dysplastic right kidney has shrunken to a small calcified mass (*closed arrow*) in this 25-year-old patient. Retrograde ureterogram shows an atretic ureter (*open arrow*) that terminates short of the kidney. Embryologic failure of union of the mesonephric blastema (which forms the renal parenchyma) and the ureteric bud (which forms the ureter and collecting system) is one cause of congenital cystic renal dysplasia.

MULTICYSTIC RENAL DISEASE

Multicystic dysplastic kidney is usually diagnosed in utero or at birth. The classic multicystic dysplastic kidney appears as a mass of noncommunicating cysts of varying size (see Fig. 36.52) (56). With time, the kidney progressively atrophies, so in the adult a nubbin of tissue, which is often calcified, is all that remains (Fig. 33.28). The ureter is commonly atretic.

Renal Infections

Acute pyelonephritis is usually the result of ascending urinary tract infection caused by Gram-negative organisms, especially *Escherichia coli* (57). Uncomplicated infection requires no imaging and often shows no imaging abnormalities (58). Imaging evaluation is indicated in patients who fail to respond to treatment or are severely ill. CT is more sensitive than US in demonstrating subtle changes in the renal parenchyma associated with uncomplicated pyelonephritis (Fig. 33.29). Complications such as renal or perirenal abscess are demonstrated by CT (Figs. 33.22, 33.30) or US (59). Predisposing factors include diabetes, obstruction, immune system compromise, drug abuse, chronic debilitating disease, and incomplete antibiotic treatment.

CT may be normal in some patients with mild uncomplicated pyelonephritis. In most patients, edema causes diffuse or focal swelling. Areas of high attenuation on precontrast scans suggest hemorrhagic inflammation. Contrast enhancement reveals streaks and wedges of low attenuation (Fig. 33.29) extending to the renal capsule, often associated with thickened septa in perinephric fat and thickening of Gerota's fascia. Inflammatory low-density masses may form in the renal parenchyma. A variety of confusing terms, including lobar nephronia and focal bacterial nephritis, have been applied to these masses. The Society of Uroradiology recommends abandoning these terms and using only the terms "acute pyelonephritis" with or without "focal, multifocal, or diffuse swelling" (57).

Emphysematous pyelonephritis is a form of acute pyelonephritis with air in the renal parenchyma. Most cases occur in patients with diabetes, obstruction, or immune compromise. The condition is rapidly progressive and often life threatening. Mixed flora infection with Gram-negative organisms is most common. Plain films

Figure 33.29. Acute Pyelonephritis. Edema and swelling associated with acute renal infection cause wedge-shaped defects (*arrows*) in the enhanced parenchyma of the right kidney. The left kidney is normal.

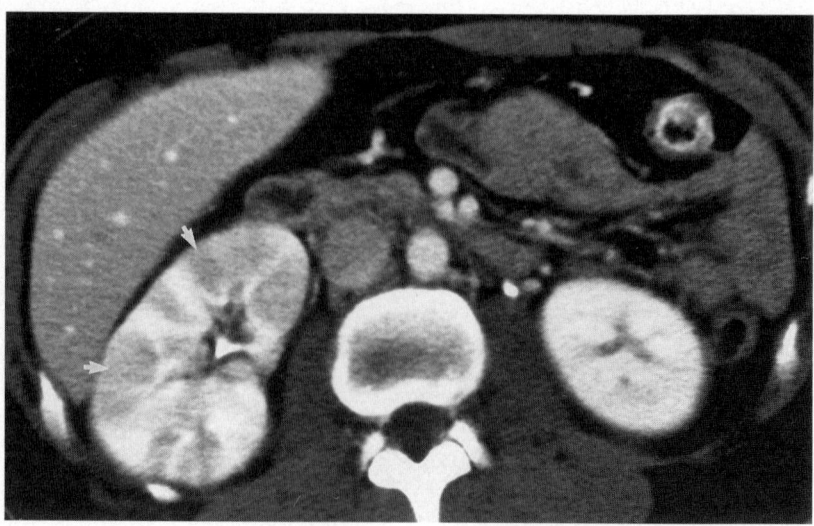

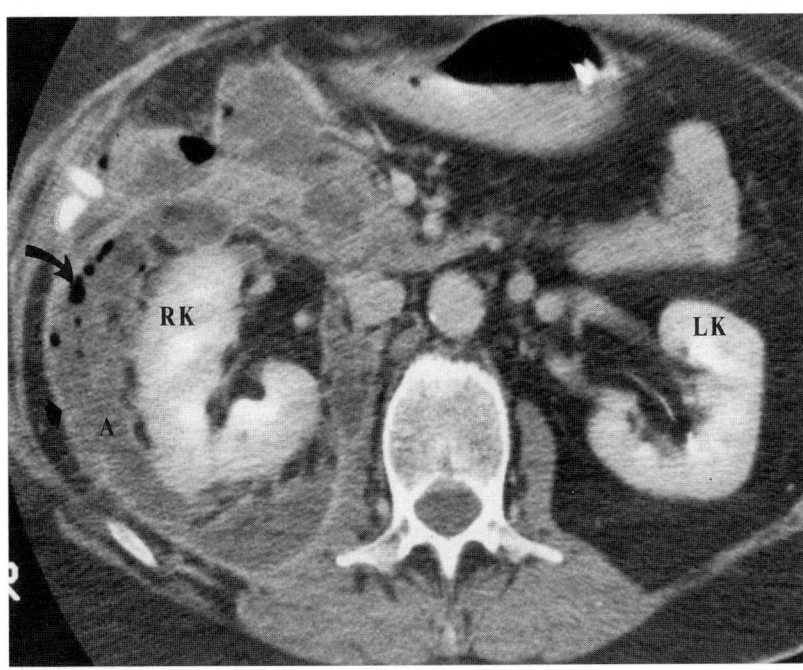

Figure 33.30. Perirenal Abscess. Contrast-enhanced CT scan discloses a low-density fluid collection (*A*) in the perirenal space between the right kidney (*RK*) and the thickened renal fascia (*arrowhead*). Gas bubbles (*curved arrow*) are seen within the perirenal abscess. *LK*, left kidney.

and CT demonstrate gas collections within the renal parenchyma (Fig. 33.31) (60).

Chronic Pyelonephritis and Reflux Nephropathy. Chronic pyelonephritis refers to chronic interstitial nephritis caused by infection (43). In children, vesicoureteral reflux of infected urine is the most common cause of chronic pyelonephritis. Intrarenal reflux, usually most prominent at the upper pole, damages the papilla, resulting in calyceal blunting with overlying cortical scarring. This process of progressive renal injury associated with reflux is referred to as *reflux nephropathy.* Adults may show stable residual findings of this childhood disease (Fig. 33.32). Chronic pyelonephritis in adults is most commonly associated with calculi and chronic obstruction. Neurogenic bladder, ileal conduits, and other causes of urinary stasis are predisposing conditions.

Both reflux nephropathy of childhood and chronic pyelonephritis in adults show similar imaging findings. The hallmark is a focal cortical scar that overlies a blunted calyx (Fig. 33.32). The disease is classically lobar, with normal lobes with normal calyces interposed between diseased lobes. These findings are best demonstrated on excretory urography but may also be evident on US and CT.

Renal tuberculosis may follow primary pulmonary tuberculosis by as much as 10–15 years. Active pulmonary tuberculosis is present in only 10% of cases of renal tuberculosis. Only 30% show any chest radiograph evidence of prior tuberculosis. Patients present with asymptomatic hematuria or sterile pyuria. Imaging studies often initially suggest the diagnosis when it is unsuspected clinically. CT is generally preferred over US and XU to demonstrate subtle findings.

The hallmarks of renal tuberculosis include parenchymal destruction and cavity formation eventually leading to parenchymal scarring, parenchymal masses owing to granuloma formation, fibrosis leading to strictures of the collecting system and ureters, and a wide variety of patterns of calcification. End-stage nonfunctional tuberculous kidneys may be hydronephrotic sacs or appear as atrophic and calcified masses in the renal bed (Fig. 33.33) (43).

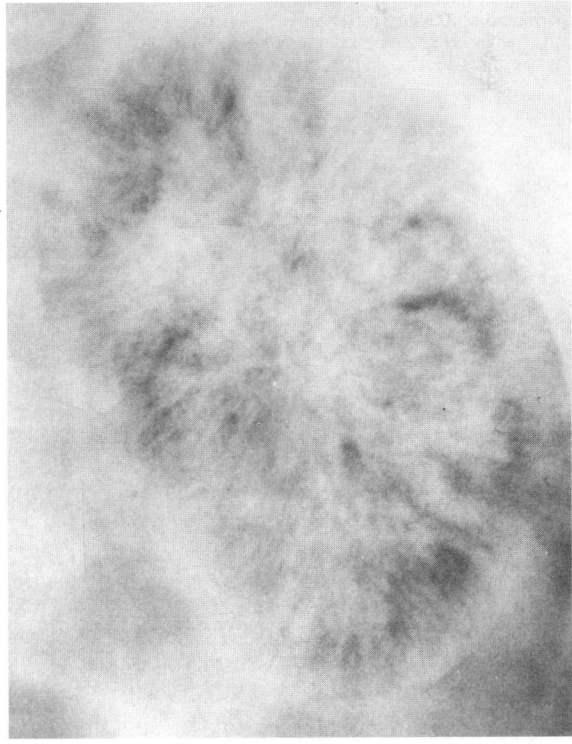

Figure 33.31. Emphysematous Pyelonephritis. Plain radiograph of the left kidney shows striations in the renal parenchyma caused by interstitial gas. This finding is indicative of life-threatening infection.

Figure 33.32. Reflux Nephropathy. Radiograph of the left kidney (*LK*) obtained as part of an excretory urogram demonstrates a blunted calyx (*arrow*) with an overlying cortical scar (*curved arrow*). These findings are indicative of reflux nephropathy.

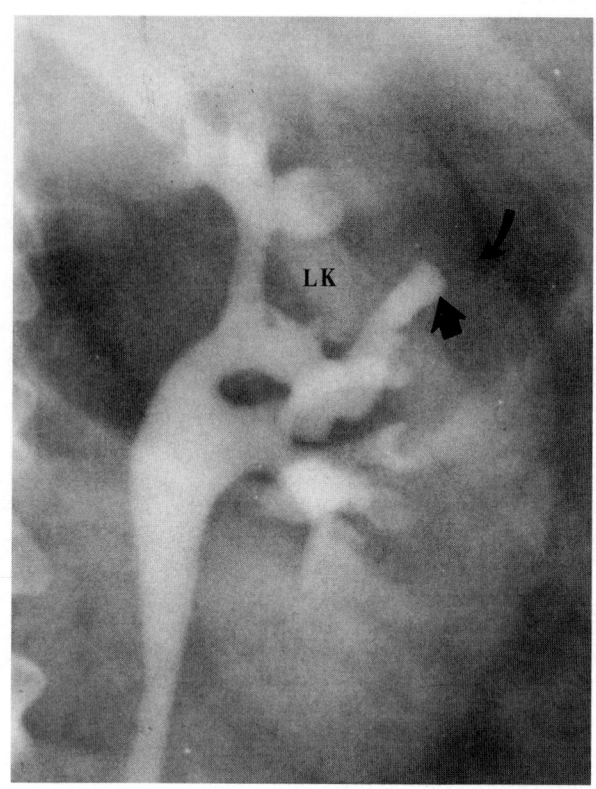

Figure 33.33. End-stage Renal Tuberculosis. The right kidney is small, nonfunctioning, and completely calcified because of chronic tuberculous infection. The left kidney is enlarged owing to compensatory hypertrophy resulting from long-standing reduced right renal function.

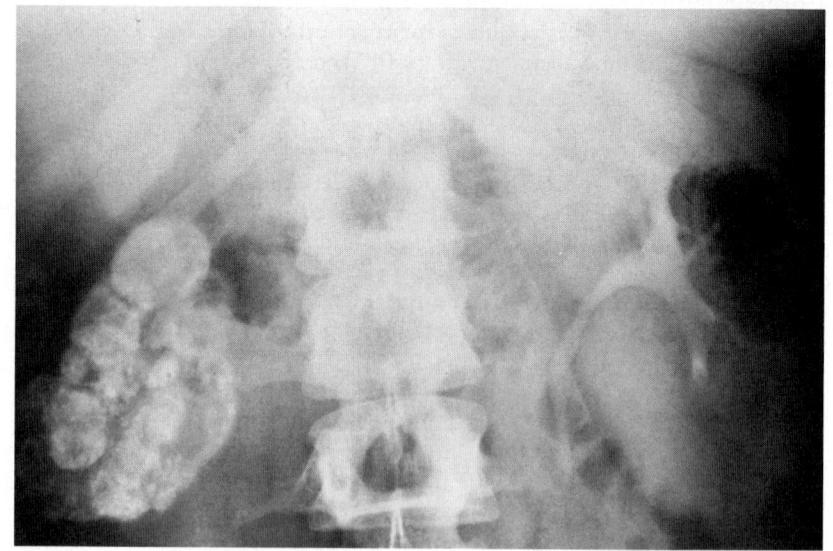

Renal Parenchymal Disease

Renal Failure. In patients with renal failure, US is usually requested to exclude hydronephrosis, assess renal size, and identify renal parenchymal disease. Bilateral hydronephrosis is a rare, but potentially reversible, cause of renal failure. Patients with acute renal failure and large (>12 cm) or normal-sized kidneys often require biopsy for definitive diagnosis of renal parenchymal disease. Patients with small (<9 cm) kidneys usually have irreversible end-stage renal disease and do not benefit from biopsy. Measurements of renal cortical thickness are unreliable in assessing residual renal function. Sonographic signs of renal parenchymal disease include a diffuse increase in parenchymal echogenicity often associated with loss of corticomedullary differentiation (see Fig. 36.47). Sonographic characterization of renal parenchymal changes correlated with renal size shortens the differential diagnosis of "medical renal disease" to a limited degree (Table 36.3).

Acquired Immunodeficiency Syndrome. Renal disease in AIDS encompasses a broad spectrum of abnormalities. AIDS-related nephropathy refers to focal and segmental glomerulosclerosis with associated tubular

Table 33.2. Causes of Bilateral Small Kidneys

Arterial hypotension (acute contrast reaction)
Generalized arteriosclerosis
Nephrosclerosis due to systemic hypertension
Chronic glomerulonephritis
Uremic medullary cystic disease

(Adapted from Davidson AJ. Radiology of the kidney. Philadelphia: WB Saunders, 1985:179.)

Table 33.3. Causes of Bilateral Large Kidneys

Proliferative disorders
    Acute glomerulonephritis
    Lupus nephritis
    Diabetic glomerulosclerosis
Parenchymal edema
    Acute tubular necrosis
    Acute cortical necrosis
    Acute bilateral pyelonephritis
Cell infiltration
    Lymphoma
    Leukemia
Protein deposition
    Multiple myeloma
    Amyloidosis
Urate deposition
    Urate nephropathy

(Adapted from Davidson AJ. Radiology of the kidney. Philadelphia: WB Saunders, 1985:221.)

Table 33.4. Causes of Unilateral Small Kidney

Renal artery stenosis
Global renal infarction
Radiation nephritis
Postobstructive atrophy
Postinflammatory atrophy
Congenital hypoplasia

(Adapted from Davidson AJ. Radiology of the kidney. Philadelphia: WB Saunders, 1985:151.)

abnormalities. Diffuse renal infection with associated calcification resulting from *Pneumocystis carinii, Mycobacterium avium intracellulare,* and *M. tuberculosis* have been reported. Patients with AIDS are exposed to nephrotoxic drugs such as pentamidine. Associated diseases such as lymphoma and dehydration caused by diarrhea and vomiting may contribute to renal injury. More than 50% of patients with AIDS demonstrate increased renal parenchymal echogenicity.

Bilateral small kidneys (<9 cm) imply a systemic disease process that injures both kidneys and usually reduces their function (Table 33.2). The conditions listed are generally indistinguishable by imaging methods.

Bilateral large kidneys (>12 cm) imply a systemic process that adds to renal size by deposition of protein, cells, or fluid (Table 33.3). Acute tubular necrosis is the most common cause of acute renal failure. Acute tubular necrosis is most commonly precipitated by renal is-

chemia or exposure to nephrotoxic substances including radiographic contrast agents.

Unilateral small kidney suggests global injury to the renal parenchyma as a result of a local unilateral rather than a systemic process (Table 33.4). Renal artery stenosis causes chronic renal ischemia and is a cause of systemic hypertension. The involved kidney is small and demonstrates a delayed nephrogram and a delay in the collecting system opacification on XU. Global renal infarction occurs as a result of sudden occlusion of a main renal artery due to embolus, thrombus, or trauma. Radiation nephritis results from inclusion of the kidney in a field of therapeutic radiation. Postobstructive atrophy may follow relief of chronic obstruction. Postinflammatory atrophy follows chronic infection. Congenital hypoplasia is an underdeveloped kidney with a reduced number of lobes (<5 lobes); the opposite kidney usually shows compensatory hypertrophy.

Unilateral Large Kidney. With the exception of a duplicated collecting system and compensatory hypertrophy, unilateral large kidneys are the result of acute local insults that affect only one kidney (Table 33.5). Renal vein thrombosis and renal artery infarction result in enlarged swollen kidneys in the acute state and small kidneys in the chronic state. Acute obstruction and acute pyelonephritis cause edematous swollen kidneys. Compensatory hypertrophy is usually associated with a small or poorly functioning opposite kidney (Fig. 33.33). Duplication of the collecting system is proved by excretory urography.

Nephrocalcinosis

Nephrocalcinosis is a broad term that refers to pathologic deposition of calcium in the renal parenchyma. Nephrocalcinosis is usually bilateral and the result of systemic disorders.

Cortical nephrocalcinosis is unusual, representing less than 5% of nephrocalcinosis. Causes include acute cortical necrosis precipitated by severe ischemia, chronic glomerulonephritis, and primary hyperoxaluria.

Medullary nephrocalcinosis is far more common and is usually related to hypercalcemic or hypercalciuric states (Table 33.6). Note that echogenic renal pyramids may result from medullary nephrocalcinosis, as well as other causes (see Fig. 33.27).

Renal Trauma

Contrast-enhanced CT provides the most comprehensive evaluation of renal trauma (61).

Table 33.5. Causes of Unilateral Large Kidney

Acute renal vein thrombosis
Acute arterial infarction
Obstructive uropathy
Acute pyelonephritis
Duplicated collecting system
Compensatory hypertrophy

(Adapted from Davidson AJ. Radiology of the kidney. Philadelphia, WB Saunders, 1985:255.)

Table 33.6. Causes of Medullary Nephrocalcinosis

Hyperparathyroidism
Medullary sponge kidney
Renal tubular acidosis (distal form)
Milk-alkali syndrome
Hypervitaminosis D
Hypercalcemic/hypercalciuric states

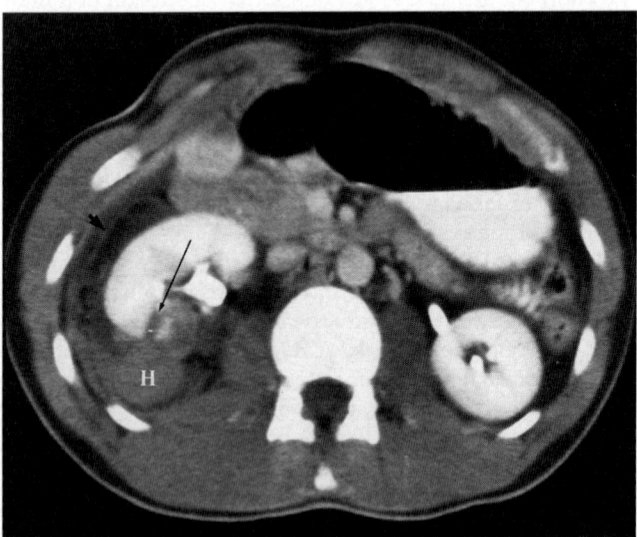

Figure 33.34. Renal Fracture. A postcontrast CT demonstrates a linear defect (*long arrow*) in the parenchyma of the right kidney, indicating a renal fracture. Blood has escaped from the kidney, resulting in a hematoma (*H*) in the perirenal space. The renal fascia (*short arrowhead*) is thickened.

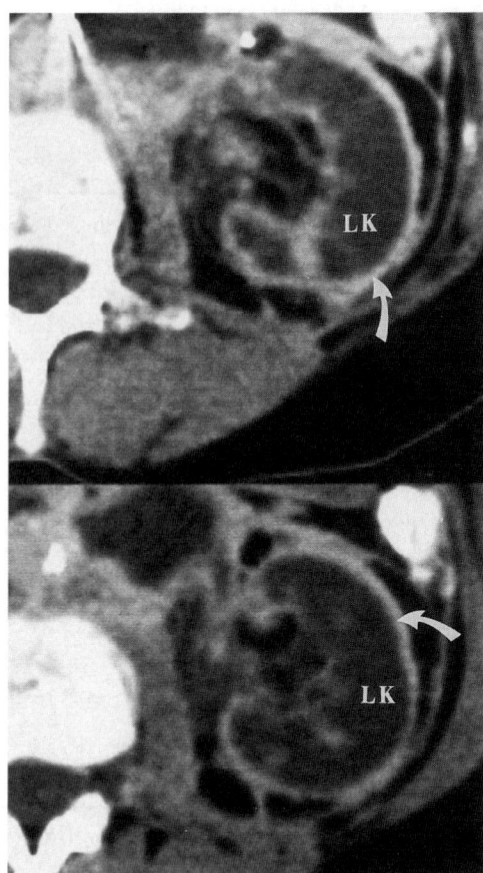

Figure 33.35. Acute Renal Artery Occlusion. Two images from a contrast-enhanced CT demonstrate the absence of enhancement of most of the parenchyma of the left kidney (*LK*), indicating occlusion of the main renal artery. Only a peripheral rim of the enhancement (the "cortical rim sign") (*arrow*), resulting from supply by capsular arteries, is present. In the setting of deceleration injuries, such as in motor vehicle accidents, a tear of the intima in the renal artery is the most likely cause.

Minor injuries constitute 75% of all renal injuries and require no specific treatment. The patient is usually observed for any complications. Renal *contusion* is a nonspecific term that refers to poorly defined areas of low attention that probably represent small intrarenal hematomas. The contused kidney functions poorly, and contrast filling of the collecting system is delayed. *Subcapsular hematoma* are confined between the tough renal capsule and the renal parenchyma. The hematoma usually causes a focal bulge in the renal contour. *Traumatic segmental infarctions* are caused by occlusion of an intrarenal artery. On CT, they appear as wedge-shaped, sharply marginated areas of low attenuation. They heal with a cortical scar. Small *lacerations* are small tears in the renal capsule (Fig. 33.34). Small collections of blood and urine are seen in perirenal space.

Intermediate injuries constitute 10–15% of renal injuries. Most are managed conservatively, but the risk for complication requiring surgery is increased. Large subcapsular hematomas are a risk for infection. Patients may develop fibrosis of the renal capsule, resulting in hypertension (Page kidney). Evacuation of the hematoma is performed in some cases. Large lacerations or *fractures* may include a tear in the collecting system, resulting in urinoma formation. The perirenal hematoma is large and commonly displaces the kidney. Bleeding is contained within Gerota's fascia. Most uroepithelial tears will heal spontaneously as long as no obstruction is present.

Major injuries account for 5–10% of the total. *Renovascular injury* is evidenced by failure of the kidney to enhance after intravenous contrast injection. Occlusion of the renal artery because of an intimal tear resulting in thrombosis should be suspected (Fig. 33.35). Arteriography may be required to identify the specific causative lesion. Immediate surgical repair is needed to preserve renal function. A *shattered kidney* refers to multiple lacerations resulting in devascularized fragments of parenchyma that fail to enhance on CT after intravenous contrast administration. The parenchyma is severely disrupted, and renal fragments may be widely displaced. Hemorrhage may be life threatening and require surgery to control.

References

1. Dunnick NR. Adrenal imaging: current status. AJR Am J Roentgenol 1990;154:927–936.

2. Francis IR, Gross MD, Shapiro B, et al. Integrated imaging of adrenal disease. Radiology 1992;184:1–13.

3. Dunnick NR, Korobkin M, Francis I. Adrenal radiology: distinguishing benign from malignant adrenal masses. AJR Am J Roentgenol 1996;167:861–867.

4. Lee MJ, Mayo-Smith WW, Hahn PF, et al. State-of-the-art MR imaging of the adrenal gland. Radiographics 1994;14:1015–1029.

5. Parsons R. The incidental adrenal lesion: an imaging update. Radiologist 1997;4:33–45.

6. Shady KL, Brown JJ. MR Imaging of the adrenal glands. Magn Reson Imaging Clin North Am 1995;3:73–85.

7. McLoughlin RF, Bilbery JH. Tumors of the adrenal gland: findings on CT and MR imaging. AJR Am J Roentgenol 1994;163:1413–1418.

8. Korobkin M, Giordano TJ, Brodeur FJ, et al. Adrenal adenomas: relationship between histologic lipid and CT and MR findings. Radiology 1996;200:743–747.

9. McNicholas MMJ, Lee MJ, Mayo-Smith WW, et al. An imaging algorithm for the differential diagnosis of adrenal adenomas and metastases. AJR Am J Roentgenol 1995;165:1453–1459.

10. Korobkin M, Brodeur FJ, Yutzy GG, et al. Differentiation of adrenal adenomas from nonadenomas using CT attenuation values. AJR Am J Roentgenol 1996;166:531–536.

11. Korobkin M, Brodeur FJ, Francis IR, et al. Delayed enhanced CT for differentiation of benign from malignant adrenal masses. Radiology 1996;200:737–742.

12. Boland GW, Hahn PF, Pètna C, Mueller PR. Adrenal masses: characterization with delayed contrast-enhanced CT. Radiology 1997;202:693–696.

13. Outwater EK, Siegelman ES, Radecki PD, et al. Distinction between benign and malignant adrenal masses: value of T1-weighted chemical-shift MR imaging. AJR Am J Roentgenol 1995;165:579–583.

14. Korobkin M, Lombardi TJ, Aisen AM, et al. Characterization of adrenal masses with chemical shift and gadolinium-enhanced MR imaging. Radiology 1995;197:411–418.

15. Outwater EK, Siegelman ES, Huang AB, Birnbaum BA. Adrenal masses: correlation between CT attenuation value and chemical shift ratio at MR imaging with in-phase and opposed-phase sequences. Radiology 1996;200:749–752.

16. Welch TJ, Sheedy PFI, Stephens DH, et al. Percutaneous adrenal biopsy: review of a 10-year experience. Radiology 1994;193:341–344.

17. Rozenblit A, Morehouse HT, Amis ES Jr. Cystic adrenal lesions: CT features. Radiology 1996;201:541–548.

18. Cyran KM, Kenney PJ, Memel DS, Yacoub I. Adrenal myelolipoma. Am J Roentgenol 1996;166:395–400.

19. Musante F, Derchi LE, Zappasodi F, et al. Myelolipoma of the adrenal gland: sonographic and CT features. AJR Am J Roentgenol 1988;151:961–964.

20. Rao P, Kenney PJ, Wagner BJ, Davidson AJ. Imaging and pathologic features of myelolipoma. Radiographics 1997;17:1373–1385.

21. Nimkin K, Teeger S, Wallach MT, et al. Adrenal hemorrhage in abused children: imaging and postmortem findings. AJR Am J Roentgenol 1994;162:661–663.

22. Sivit CJ, Ingram JD, Taylor GA, et al. Posttraumatic adrenal hemorrhage in children: CT findings in 34 patients. AJR Am J Roentgenol 1992;158:1299–1302.

23. Burks DW, Mirvis SE, Shanmuganathan K. Acute adrenal injury after blunt abdominal trauma: CT findings. AJR Am J Roentgenol 1992;158:503–507.

24. Kenney PJ, Stanley RJ. Calcified adrenal masses. Urol Radiol 1987;9:9–15.

25. Dunnick NR, G S Leight J, Roubidoux MA, et al. CT in the diagnosis of primary aldosteronism: sensitivity in 29 patients. AJR Am J Roentgenol 1993;160:321–324.

26. Doppman DL, Gill JR Jr. Hyperaldosteronism: sampling the adrenal veins. Radiology 1996;198:309–312.

27. Sivit CJ, Hung W, Taylor GA, et al. Sonography in neonatal adrenal hyperplasia. AJR Am J Roentgenol 1991;156:141–143.

28. Mukherjee JJ, Peppercorn PD, Reznek RH, et al. Pheochromocytoma: effect of nonionic contrast medium in CT on circulating catecholamine levels. Radiology 1997;202:227–231.

29. Schwerk WB, Gölorg C, Gölorg K, Restrepo IK. Adrenal pheochromocytomas: a broad spectrum of sonographic presentation. J Ultrasound Med 1994;13:517–521.

30. van Gils APG, Falke THM, van Erkel AR, et al. MR imaging and MIBG scintigraphy of pheochromocytomas and extra-adrenal functioning paragangliomas. Radiographics 1991;11:37–57.

31. Davidson AJ, Hartman DS, Choyke PL, Wagner BJ. Radiological assessment of renal masses: implications for patient care. Radiology 1997;202:297–305.

32. Yeh HC, Halton KP, Shapiro RS, et al. Junctional parenchyma: revised definition of hypertrophic column of Bertin. Radiology 1992;185:725–732.

33. Solokoff NH, deKernion JB, Figlin RA, Belldegrun A. Current management of renal cell carcinoma. CA Cancer J Clin 1996;46:284–302.

34. Zagoria RJ, Bechtold RE, Dyer RB. Staging of renal adenocarcinoma: role of various imaging procedures. AJR Am J Roentgenol 1995;164:363–370.

35. Choyke PL. Detection and staging of renal cancer. Magn Reson Imaging Clin North Am 1997;5:29–47.

36. Rominger MB, Kenney PJ, Morgan DE, et al. Gadolinium-enhanced MR imaging of renal masses. Radiographics 1992;12:1097–1116.

37. Habboub HK, Abu-Yousef MM, Williams RD, et al. Accuracy of color Doppler sonography in assessing venous thrombus extension in renal cell carcinoma. AJR Am J Roentgenol 1997;168:267–271.

38. Wagner BJ, Wong-You-Cheong JJ, Davis CJ, Jr. Adult renal hamartomas. Radiographics 1997;17:155–169.

39. Lemaitre L, Robert Y, Dubrulle F, et al. Renal angiomyolipoma: growth followed up with CT and/or US. Radiology 1995;197:598–602.

40. Hägelagenon O, Merran S, Paraf F, et al. Unusual fat-containing tumors of the kidney: a diagnostic dilemma. Radiographics 1997;17:129–144.

41. Davidson AJ, Hayes WS, Hartman DS, et al. Renal oncocytoma and carcinoma: failure of differentiation with CT. Radiology 1993;186:693–696.

42. Choyke PL, White EM, Zeman RK, et al. Renal metastases: clinicopathologic and radiologic correlation. Radiology 1987;162:359–363.

43. Kenney PJ. Imaging of chronic renal infections. AJR Am J Roentgenol 1990;155:485–494.

44. Einstein DM, Herts BR, Weaver R, et al. Evaluation of renal masses detected by excretory urography: cost-effectiveness of sonography versus CT. Am J Roentgenol 1995;164:371–375.

45. Bosniak MA. The small (<3.0 cm) renal parenchymal tumor: detection, diagnosis, and controversies. Radiology 1991;179:307–317.

46. Bosniak MA. Problems in the radiologic diagnosis of renal parenchymal tumors. Urol Clin North Am 1993;20:217–230.

47. Curry NS. Small renal masses (lesions smaller than 3 cm): imaging evaluation and management. AJR Am J Roentgenol 1995;164:355–362.

48. Hartman DS, Davis CJ, Sanders RC, et al. The multilocu-

lated renal mass: considerations and differential features. Radiographics 1987;7:29–52.

49. Agrons GA, Wagner BJ, Davidson AJ, Suarez ES. Multilocular cystic renal tumor in children: radiologic-pathologic correlation. Radiographics 1995;15:653–669.

50. Gabow PA. Autosomal dominant polycystic kidney disease: more than a renal disease. Am J Kidney Dis 1990;16: 403–413.

51. Choyke PL, Glenn GM, Walther MM, et al. von Hippel-Lindau disease: genetic, clinical, and imaging features. Radiology 1995;194:629–642.

52. Choyke PL, Filling-Katz MR, Shawker TH, et al. Von Hippel-Lindau disease: radiologic screening for visceral manifestations. Radiology 1990;174:815–820.

53. Heinz-Peer G, Schoder M, Rand T, et al. Prevalence of acquired cystic kidney disease and tumors in native kidneys of renal transplant recipients: a prospective US study. Radiology 1995;195:667–671.

54. Levine E, Slusher SL, Grantham JJ, Wetzel LH. Natural history of acquired renal cystic disease in dialysis patients: a prospective longitudinal CT study. AJR Am J Roentgenol 1991;156:501–506.

55. Blickman JG, Bramson RT, Herrin JT. Autosomal recessive polycystic kidney disease: long-term sonographic findings in patients surviving the neonatal period. AJR Am J Roentgenol 1995;164:1247–1250.

56. Strife JL, Souza AS, Kirks DR, et al. Multicystic dysplastic kidney in children: US follow-up. Radiology 1993;186: 785–788.

57. Talner LB, Davidson AJ, Lebowitz RL, et al. Acute pyelonephritis: can we agree on terminology? Radiology 1994;192:297–305.

58. Kawashima A, Sandler CM, Goldman SM, et al. CT of renal inflammatory disease. Radiographics 1997;17:851–866.

59. Lowe LH, Zagoria RJ, Baumgartner BR, Dyer RB. Role of imaging and intervention in complex infections of the urinary tract. AJR Am J Roentgenol 1994;163:363–367.

60. Joseph RC, Amendola MA, Artze ME, et al. Genitourinary tract gas: imaging evaluation. Radiographics 1996;16: 295–308.

61. Fanney DR, Casillas J, Murphy BJ. CT in the diagnosis of renal trauma. Radiographics 1990;10:29–40.

34

Pelvicalyceal System, Ureters, Bladder, and Urethra

William E. Brant

PELVICALYCEAL SYSTEM AND URETER

Imaging Methods

Excretory urography (XU) is the usual method used to demonstrate the pelvicalyceal system and ureter. High-grade urinary tract obstruction may preclude adequate visualization because of delayed renal function or poor concentration of contrast. Retrograde pyelography, performed by cystoscopic catheterization of the ureteral orifice followed by injection of contrast, is independent of renal function and provides high-quality images of the ureter and the collecting system. Similar images can be obtained by antegrade pyelography, performed via nephrostomy catheter; however, this procedure is more invasive. CT provides excellent images of the kidneys, collecting system, and ureter; it can demonstrate the extent of soft tissue lesions; and has the capability of differentiating tumor from stones and blood clots. US is the imaging method of choice for screening for hydronephrosis but is limited in its ability to demonstrate small uroepithelial tumors. Specialized MR techniques provide urographic images comparable to excretory urography (1,2).

Anatomy

The collecting tubules of a medullary pyramid coalesce into a variable number of papillary ducts that pierce the tip of the papilla and drain into the receptacle of the collecting system called a *minor calyx*. The projection of a papilla into the calyx produces a cup shape. The sharp-edged portion of the minor calyx projecting around the sides of a papilla is called the *fornix* of the calyx (see Fig. 33.13). Compound calyces, usually found at the poles of the kidney, are formed by the projection of two or more papilla into the calyx. *Infundibula* extend between minor calyces and the renal pelvis. The renal pelvis is triangular, with its base within the renal sinus. The apex of the pelvis extends downward to join the ureter. A so-called *extrarenal pelvis* (Fig. 34.1) is predominantly outside the renal sinus and is larger and more distensible than an intrarenal pelvis surrounded by renal sinus fat. An extrarenal pelvis should not be confused with hydronephrosis. There is endless variety in the size and arrangement of calyces and in the shape and appearance of the renal pelvis.

The ureters have an outer fibrous adventitia that is continuous with the renal capsule and with the adventitia of the bladder. The muscularis, responsible for ureteral peristalsis, consists of outer circular and inner longitudinal muscle bundles. The mucosa lining the entire pelvicalyceal system, ureters, and bladder is transitional epithelium. The ureters enter the bladder at an oblique angle. When the bladder wall contracts, the ureteral orifices are closed. The ureters propel urine by active peristalsis, which can be visualized fluoroscopically and by US. Jets of urine opacified by contrast are frequently seen within the bladder on XU and CT. Because of peristalsis, the diameter of the ureter at any particular instant is highly variable. Three main points of ureteral narrowing, where calculi are likely to become impacted, are *a)* the ureteropelvic junction, *b)* the site at which the ureter crosses the pelvic brim, and *c)* the ureterovesical junction.

Ureteral Duplication occurs in 1–2% of the population (Fig. 34.2) (3). Unilateral duplication is six times more common than bilateral duplication. The Weigert-Meyer rule states that with complete ureteral duplication, the ureter draining the upper pole passes through the bladder wall to insert inferior and medial to the ureter draining the lower pole. The upper pole ureter often ends as an ectopic ureterocele that is obstructed because of its ectopic insertion. The lower pole ureter inserts in, or near, the normal location in the bladder trigone and is subject to vesicoureteral reflux because of

Figure 34.1. Extrarenal Pelvis. The position of the left renal pelvis (*white arrow*) outside of the renal sinus enables the pelvis to distend with urine and to be larger than the normal right renal pelvis (*black arrow*). The extrarenal pelvis is a normal variant, not to be mistaken for hydronephrosis.

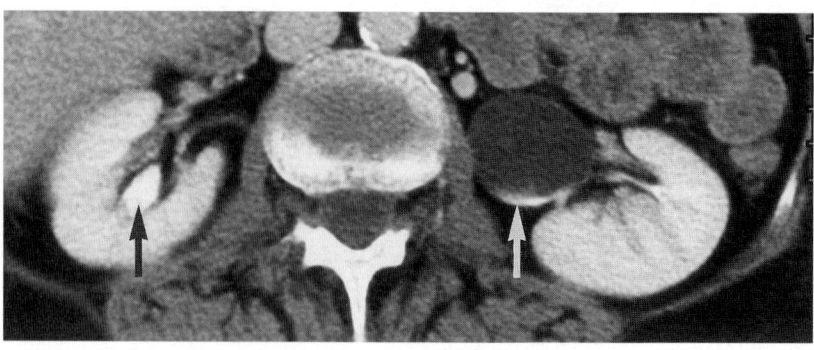

distortion of its passage through the bladder wall by the ectopic ureterocele. Complications of complete duplication include urinary tract infection, vesicoureteral reflux, and ureteropelvic junction obstruction of the lower pole system. Reflux into the lower pole collecting system in childhood may produce scarring and deformity of the lower pole of the kidney.

Excretory urography commonly demonstrates poor function or nonfunction of the obstructed upper pole system. The lower pole system is displaced inferiorly and commonly shows a "drooping lily" appearance. Reflux nephropathy of the lower pole system may be evident.

US, CT, or MR demonstrates cystic dilatation of the upper pole system, usually with marked parenchymal thinning. The upper pole ureter is commonly tortuous and dilated. The ectopic ureterocele and its associated dilated ureter may simulate a multiseptated cystic mass in the pelvis.

Bifid Renal Pelvis occurs in 10% of the population. Separate pelvices draining the upper and lower poles join at the ureteropelvic junction. This anomaly has no pathologic consequences.

Ureteropelvic Junction Obstruction is a common congenital anomaly that may go undiagnosed until adulthood. The amount of hydronephrosis and parenchymal atrophy present depends on the severity of obstruction. The condition is bilateral in 30% of cases but is often not symmetrical. Excretory urography and US demonstrate pelvicalyectasis with sharply defined narrowing at the ureteropelvic junction. The ureter is not dilated. In 15–20% of cases, an aberrant renal vessel causes the obstruction. Helical CT is effective in demonstrating the crossing vessel (4). In the majority of cases, the precise cause is unknown.

Retrocaval Ureter is a developmental variant in which the right ureter passes behind the inferior vena cava at the level of L3 or L4 vertebra (Fig. 34.3). The ureter exits anteriorly between the cava and the aorta to return to its normal position. The condition is associated with varying degrees of urinary stasis and proximal pyeloureterectasis. The anomaly is due to faulty embryogenesis of the inferior vena cava, with abnormal persistence of the right subcardinal vein anterior to the ureter instead of the right supracardinal vein posterior to the ureter.

Calculous Disease

Nephrolithiasis refers to the presence of calculi in the renal collecting system (5,6). Nearly 10% of the popula-

tion will form a renal stone in their lifetime. Sufficient calcium oxalate or calcium phosphate is present in 80% of renal calculi for them to be radiopaque on plain film. Struvite (magnesium ammonium phosphate) stones, formed in the presence of alkaline urine and infection, make up another 15% of renal calculi and are also radiopaque. Cystine stones comprise 1–2% of renal stone, are mildly radiopaque, and are found only in patients with congenital cystinuria. The remaining 3–4% of renal stones are composed of urate or xanthines and are radiolucent. *Milk of calcium* refers to a fine sediment-containing calcium that may be found in a calyceal divertic-

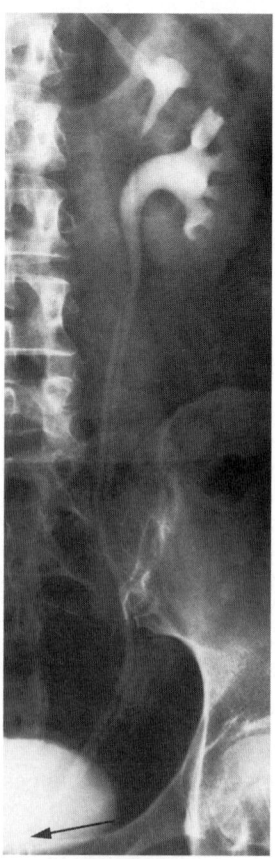

Figure 34.2. Ureteral Duplication. The left collecting system and ureter are completely duplicated. The ureter draining the upper pole of the left kidney inserts into the bladder inferior and medial (*arrow*) to the insertion of the ureter draining the lower pole collecting system.

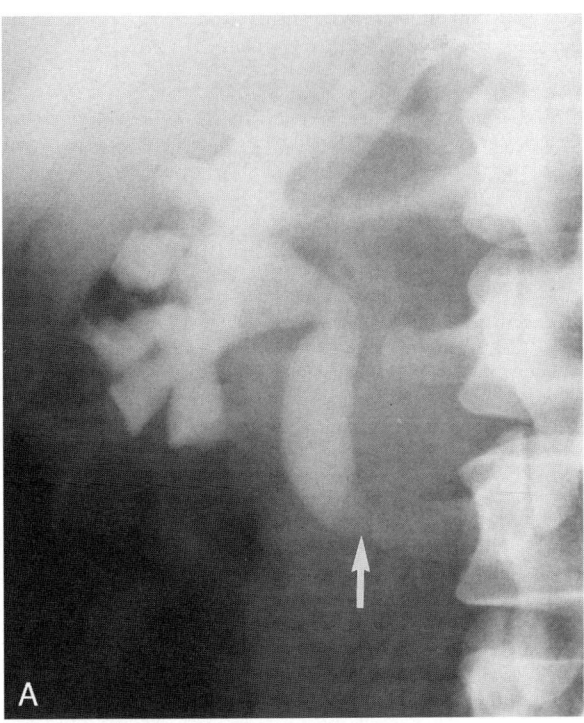
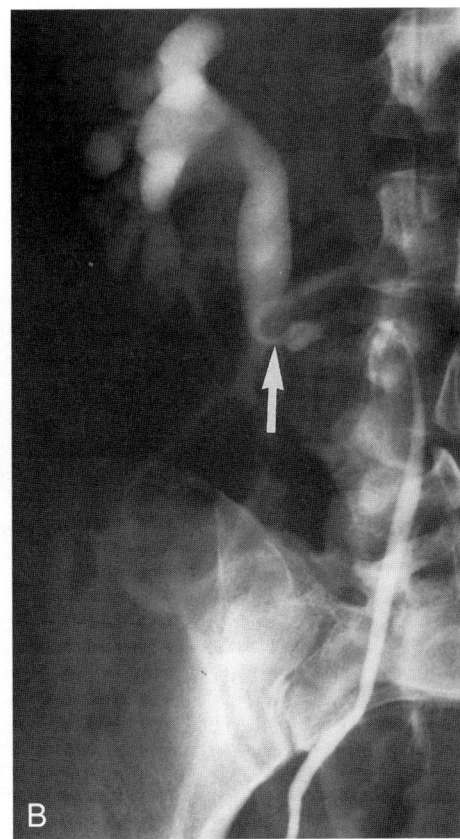

Figure 34.3. Retrocaval Ureter. A. The right renal collecting system and proximal right ureter are dilated. At the level of the transverse process of L3 vertebra, the ureter makes an abrupt turn to the left. The more distal ureter was poorly visualized but did not appear di- lated on this XU. **B.** Retrograde ureterogram documents the char- acteristic appearance of the ureter, which courses behind the infe- rior vena cava at the level of the sharp bend.

ulum or hydrocalyx that lacks drainage. Complications of renal calculi include obstruction, ureteral stricture, chronic renal infection, and loss of renal function. High-quality plain films to detect calculi and calcification are mandatory prior to contrast studies of the urinary tract.

Renal Calculi. Most renal calculi are demonstrated on plain films. Excretory urography demonstrates stones within the collecting system as filling defects within contrast-opacified urine. Staghorn calculi form casts of the pelvicalyceal system (see Fig. 26.15). Most are composed of struvite and are associated with chronic renal infection. US demonstrates both radiopaque and nonradiopaque stones as echodensities with acoustic shadowing (see Fig. 36.61). Large stones (>1.5 cm) are the easiest to identify with US. Small stones, which do not cast acoustic shadows, may blend in with renal si-nus fat and are often not detected by US. US is more sen-sitive than plain film for subtle calcification in the renal parenchyma (Fig. 36.46). All calculi appear dense on CT. Attenuation values > 100 H will differentiate a calculus from a tumor (20–50 H) or blood clot (<50 H). Calculi are best visualized on thin slice (5 mm) noncontrast CT.

Ureteral Calculi are a major cause of acute urinary tract obstruction and renal colic. Stones that form in the kidney are prone to pass into and obstruct the ureter (see Fig. 36.45). Stones less than 6 mm in size are likely to pass spontaneously through the ureter within 6 weeks. Stones

larger than 6 mm are likely to become lodged in the ureter and require intervention for removal. Calculi are most likely to be found at the three points of ureteral narrowing already described. Noncontrast CT is effectively used to detect ureteral calculi in patients with renal colic (Fig. 34.4) (7,8). The tissue rim sign, visualization of a rim of soft tissue surrounding a suspected ureteral calculus, is specific for ureterolithiasis and helps to differentiate stones in the ureter from extraurinary calcifications (9).

Hydronephrosis

Hydronephrosis is defined as dilatation of the upper urinary tract. Hydronephrosis is not synonymous with obstruction but has a number of causes that are de-scribed in this section. The terms *caliectasis, pyelecta-sis,* and *ureterectasis* are more precise in describing di-latation of portions of the urinary tract. US is an excellent screening modality for determining the pres-ence of urinary tract dilation.

Obstruction. The causes of obstruction include stone, stricture, tumor, and extrinsic compression. The degree of dilatation produced by obstruction is variable. In gen-eral, the more proximal and the more chronic the ob-struction, the greater is the degree of dilatation. Acute obstruction produced by an impacted stone often pro-duces minimal dilatation.

Figure 34.4. Ureteral Calculus on Noncontrast CT.
A. CT image through the kidneys in a patient with left flank pain demonstrates mild enlargement of the left renal pelvis (*arrow*). **B.** CT at the level of the seminal vesicles (*s*) shows a high-density stone in the distal left ureter. Note the "tissue rim sign." All urinary tract stones appear "white" on CT viewed at soft-tissue windows. **C.** More caudal image at the level of the base of the prostate (*P*) shows two phleboliths, not to be mistaken for ureteral stones. Their location is below the level of the distal ureter and they lack a tissue rim sign. *B*, bladder.

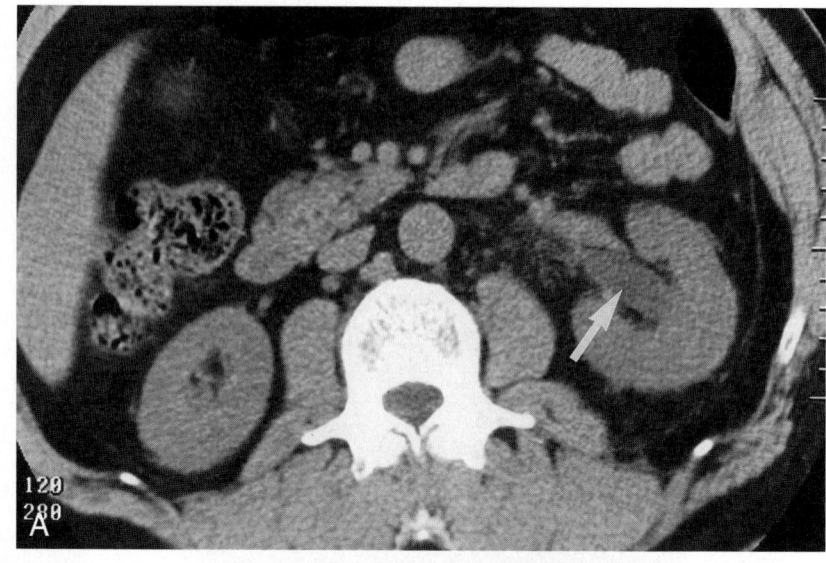

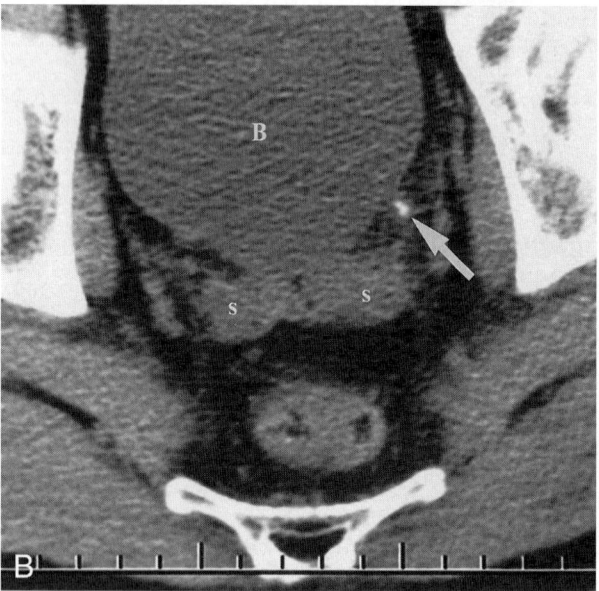

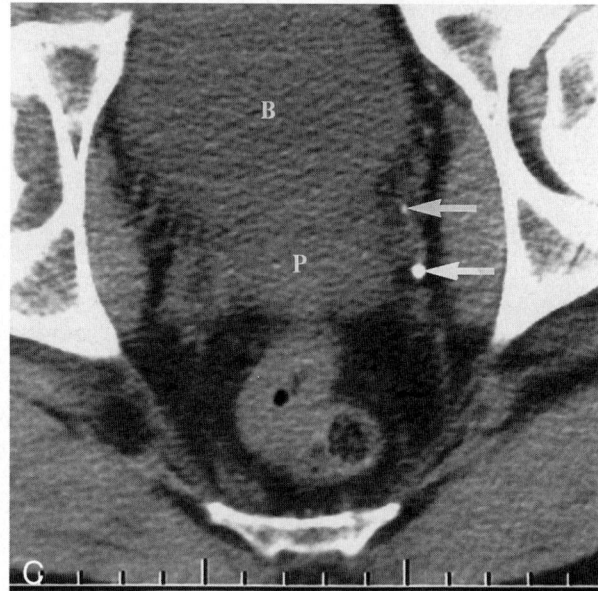

US demonstrates hydronephrosis as separation of normal sinus echogenicity by anechoic urine in the collecting system (see Fig. 36.43). The calyces become enlarged and blunted and are seen to connect with the dilated renal pelvis. Medullary pyramids may be hypoechoic, especially in children, and must be differentiated from dilated calyces. Pyramids are more peripheral, surrounded by more echogenic cortex, and do not connect with the renal pelvis. A peripelvic cyst can easily be mistaken for hydronephrosis on US (see Fig. 36.44).

XU signs of obstruction include *a)* increasingly dense nephrogram with time, *b)* delay in appearance of contrast in the collecting system, and *c)* dilated pelvicalyceal system and ureter to the point of obstruction (Fig. 34.5). ***Pyelosinus reflux*** may result from rupture of a fornix precipitated by contrast-induced diuresis superimposed on the increased hydrostatic pressure of an obstructed pelvicalyceal system. Urine and contrast extravasate into the renal sinus and perirenal space.

CT demonstrates dilatation of the collecting system, either with or without use of intravenous contrast. Delay in opacification of the obstructed kidney and dependent layering of unopacified urine over heavier contrast media may also be evident. The location and cause of obstruction can usually be identified (see Fig. 34.4).

Pyonephrosis refers to infection in an obstructed kidney. Pyonephrosis can result in rapid destruction of the renal parenchyma and must be treated promptly by relief of obstruction by ureteral stent or nephrostomy tube placement and antibiotics. US classically demonstrates a dilated collecting system filled with layering echogenic pus and debris. Shadowing calculi may also be evident. CT may be better than US in demonstrating the site and cause of obstruction. Excretory urography is usually not useful because the affected kidney functions poorly or not at all.

Vesicoureteral Reflux is a common cause of hydronephrosis in children. The basic defect is an abnormal ureteral tunnel at the ureterovesical junction and associated urinary tract infection. In adults, vesicoureteral reflux is usually associated with neurogenic bladder (Fig. 34.6) or bladder outlet obstruction. Chronic vesicoureteral reflux of infected urine causes reflux nephropathy. Vesicoureteral reflux is confirmed by demonstrating retrograde filling of the ureters on voiding cystourography or radionuclide cystography.

Congenital Megaureter is due to an aperistaltic segment of the lower ureter causing a functional obstruction and resulting in dilatation of the proximal ureter. The aperistaltic segment of the ureter demonstrates smoothly tapered narrowing without evidence of mechanical obstruction.

Prune Belly Syndrome, also called Eagle-Barrett syndrome, is a congenital disorder manifested by absence of the abdominal wall musculature, urinary tract anomalies, and cryptorchidism. The ureters are markedly dilated and tortuous, the bladder is large and distended, and the posterior urethra is dilated.

Polyuria, associated with acute diuresis and diabetes insipidus, may cause mild to severe hydronephrosis.

Filling Defect/Mass in Pelvicalyceal System or Ureter

Calculi are the most common cause of filling defects in the contrast-filled collecting system or ureter (Fig. 34.7). Most calculi (>85%) are radiopaque on plain radiographs. CT demonstrates all calculi as high-density objects with a CT density of >100 H. Stones in the ureter are differentiated from phleboliths on noncontrast CT by the presence of a soft-tissue rim surrounding the high-density stone (10).

Blood Clots cause nonradiopaque filling defects that can be differentiated from soft-tissue tumors by their change in appearance over time. Attenuation values on CT are usually < 50 H.

Transitional Cell Carcinoma (TCC) accounts for 85–90% of all uroepithelial tumors (11,12). Most (85%) have a papillary growth pattern that is exophytic, polypoid, and attached to the mucosa by a stalk. These le-

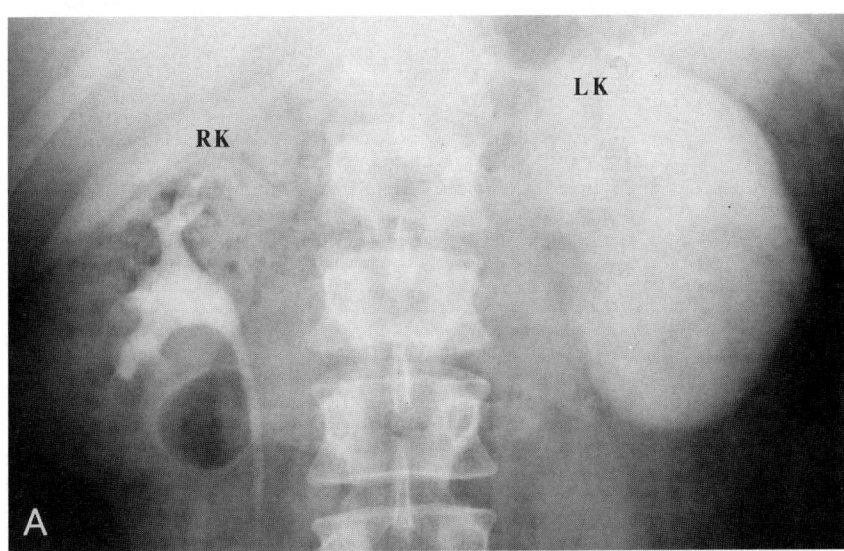

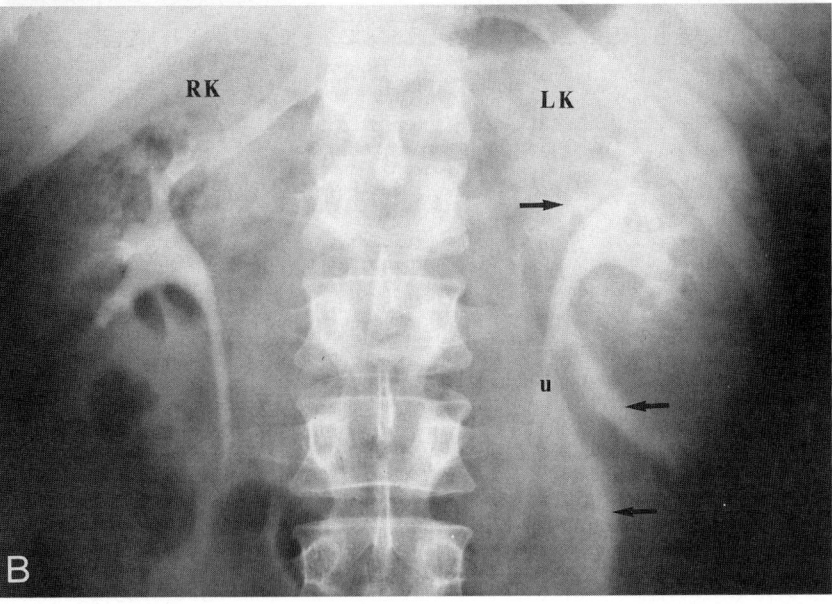

Figure 34.5. Obstruction with Pyelosinus Reflux. A. Radiograph taken at 10 minutes after intravenous injection of contrast demonstrates a persisting dense nephogram in the left kidney (*LK*) with delay of contrast excretion into the collecting system. The patient had an obstructing stone at the ureterovesical junction. The right kidney (*RK*) is normal. **B.** Radiograph obtained 2 hours after contrast injection reveals leakage of contrast (*arrows*) out of the left collecting system and into the renal sinus and the perirenal and periureteric spaces. Overdistension of the obstructed collecting system due to the diuretic effect of the contrast agent resulted in rupture of a calyceal fornix. *u,* left ureter.

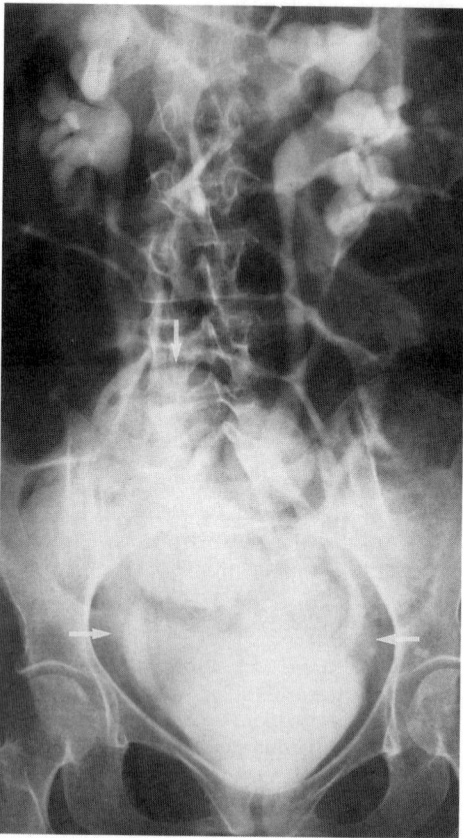

Figure 34.6. Vesicoureteral Reflux Due to Neurogenic Bladder. A cystogram demonstrates contrast filling the massively dilated bladder (*between arrows*) and refluxing into both ureters and pelvicalyceal systems.

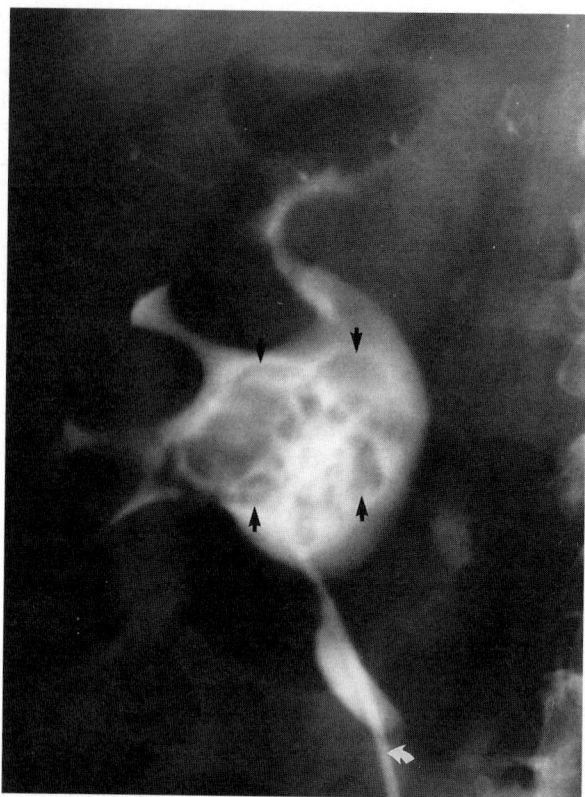

Figure 34.7. Multiple Calculi in the Renal Pelvis. A retrograde pyelogram demonstrates multiple filling defects (*arrows*) in the right renal pelvis that were proved to be radiolucent calculi. Contrast was injected into the renal pelvis via a catheter (*curved arrow*) in the right ureter that was inserted at cystoscopy.

sions cause a distinct filling defect in the collecting system or ureter (Figs. 34.8, 34.9). A stippled pattern of contrast material within the interstices of the papillary lesion is characteristic. Tumors in the ureter may demonstrate a "champagne glass" sign of ureteral dilatation distal to a filling defect (Fig. 34.9). This sign distinguishes tumor from a calculus that impacts in the ureter and causes distal spasm and narrowing. Nonpapillary tumors are nodular or flat and tend to be infiltrating and aggressive. They cause strictures of the collecting system or ureter rather than filling defects.

Most TCC occur in men (male-to-female ratio = 4:1) aged 60 and older. A variety of chemical agents used in the textile and plastic industries, drugs including cyclophosphamide and phenacetin, chronic urinary stasis (horseshoe kidney), and smoking play a role in the etiology of these tumors. The tumor metastasizes most commonly to regional lymph nodes, liver, lung, and bone.

TCC exhibits a strong tendency toward multiplicity. Patients with upper tract TCC have multicentric tumors in 20–44% of cases, and those with TCC of the ureter develop bladder TCC in 20–37% of cases. Careful evaluation of the entire urinary tract is warranted both at initial diagnosis and for follow-up. Standard treatment of TCC is total nephroureterectomy and excision of a cuff of the bladder surrounding the ureteral orifice.

CT demonstrates a mass within the collecting system

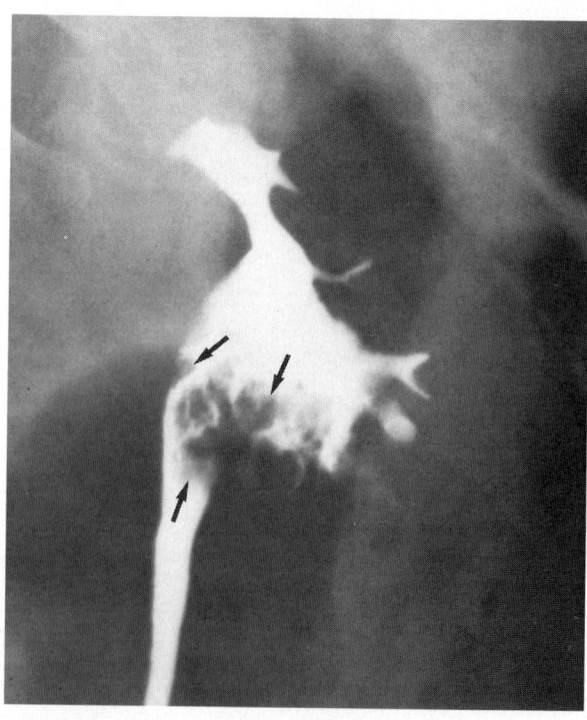

Figure 34.8. Transitional Cell Carcinoma. Radiograph from a retrograde pyelogram of the left kidney reveals a multilobulated filling defect (*arrows*) in the left renal pelvis. This was proved to be a TCC.

(Fig. 34.10) (13,14). Densities range from 8–30 H unenhanced and 18–55 H after contrast administration, enabling clear differentiation from calculi. CT demonstrates the extent of the tumor, including invasion of the kidney or surrounding structures, lymphadenopathy, and distant metastases (Table 34.1).

US demonstrates renal TCC as a discrete hypoechoic mass within the renal sinus (see Fig. 36.57). Small lesions may be subtle and easily missed. The absence of acoustic shadowing usually provides differentiation from calculi, although a few high-grade tumors have been reported to cast acoustic shadows.

Squamous Cell Carcinoma accounts for 10% of uroepithelial tumors. Chronic infection, calculi, and phenacetin abuse are major predisposing factors. Most tumors are infiltrating and superficially spreading, producing stricture or subtle filling defects.

Table 34.1. Staging of TCC in the Renal Pelvis and Ureter

Stage	Description
I	Tumor limited to uroepithelial mucosa and lamina propria
II	Tumor invades into, but not beyond, muscularis
III	Tumor invades beyond muscularis into periureteric or peripelvic fat or renal parenchyma
IV	Tumor invades adjacent organs or through the kidney into perinephric fat

(Adapted from American Joint Committee on Cancer. Manual for staging of cancer. 4th ed. Philadelphia: JB Lippincott Co, 1992:205–207.)

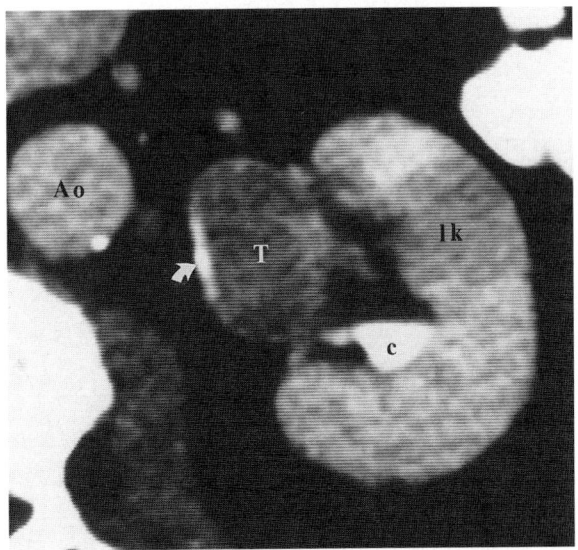

Figure 34.10. Transitional Cell Carcinoma. Contrast-enhanced CT reveals a tumor (*T*) in the enlarged pelvis of the left kidney (*lk*). A small amount of contrast (*arrow*) in the pelvis outlines the tumor. A calyx (*c*) proximal to the tumor is dilated due to obstruction. *Ao*, aorta.

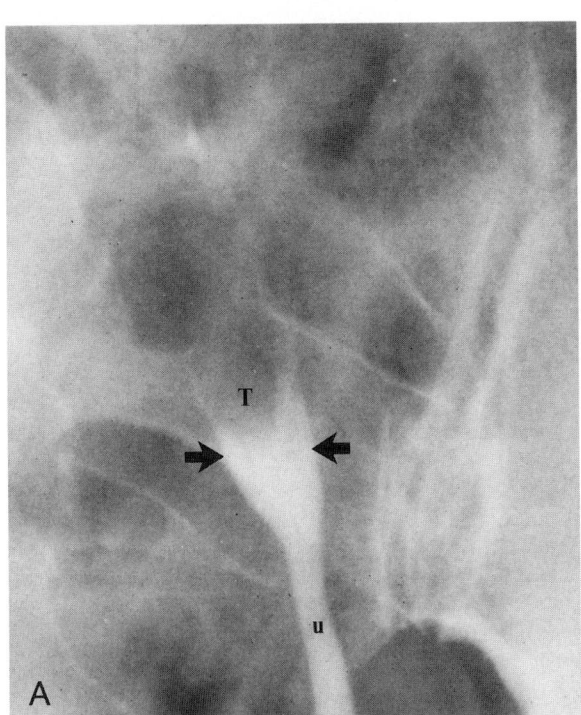

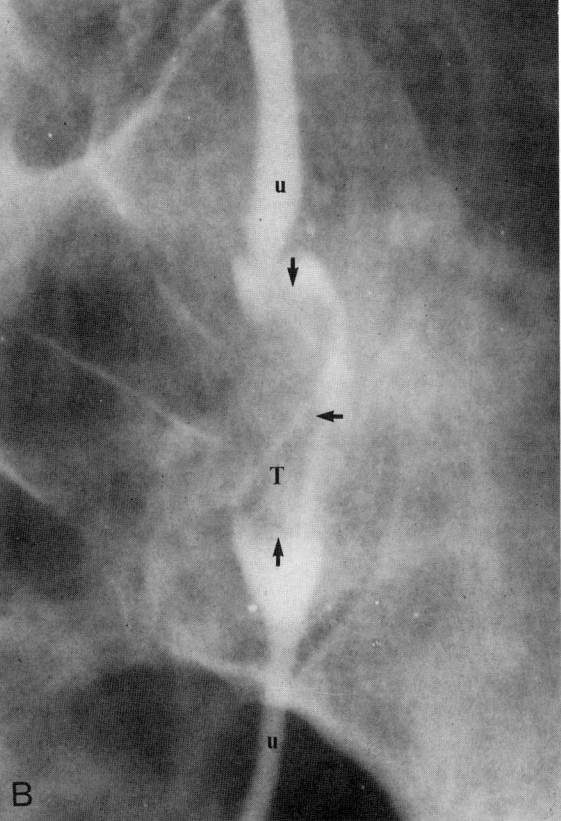

Figure 34.9. Transitional Cell Carcinoma. A. A retrograde ureterogram demonstrates widening of the ureter (*arrows*) distal to an obstructing tumor (*T*). The distal ureter assumes a champagne glass configuration because of the slow growth of the tumor. **B.** Additional contrast administration demonstrates the full extent of the tumor (*T, between arrows*). u, left ureter.

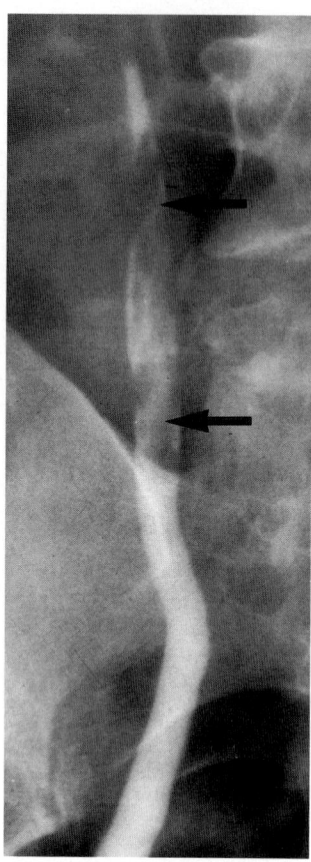

Figure 34.11. Fibroepithelial Polyp. The long sinuous filling defect (*arrows*) in the ureter is characteristic of fibroepithelial polyp.

Metastases are a rare cause of a filling defect. Common primary sites are the breast, melanoma, lung, stomach, and cervix.

Papillary Necrosis is ischemic necrosis of the tips of the medullary pyramids. Causes include infection, tuberculosis, sickle cell trait and disease, diabetes, and analgesic nephropathy. Necrotic papilla may remain in situ, slough into the collecting system causing a mobile filling defect, or disappear, resulting in a contrast collection in the papilla or a blunted calyx (see Fig. 34.17). Sloughed papilla may obstruct the ureter and cause renal colic.

Fibroepithelial Polyp is a benign fibrous polyp covered by transitional epithelium. It is most common in young adult men. The polyp is mobile and hangs from the mucosa by a long, thin stalk (Fig. 34.11).

Pyeloureteritis Cystica is a benign process of submucosal cyst formation associated with chronic urinary tract infection. Multiple, small (2–3 mm), smooth, round filling defects in the ureter are characteristic (Fig. 34.12). Cysts in renal pelvis tend to be larger, up to 2 cm.

Leukoplakia is a rare inflammatory condition of the uroepithelium related to chronic urinary tract infection and calculi. Squamous metaplasia with keratinization and desquamation results in irregular plaques in the renal pelvis, proximal ureter, and bladder. A key clinical feature is passage of flakes of desquamated epithelium in the urine. Leukoplakia is considered a premalignant condition in the bladder, but not in the ureter.

Malacoplakia is another rare inflammatory condition of the uroepithum caused by chronic infection, especially due to *Escherichia coli.* Smooth submucosal nodules composed of histiocytes produce multiple smooth filling defects in the distal ureter and bladder. This condition is not premalignant.

Stricture of Pelvicalyceal System or Ureter

A stricture is a fixed narrowing of the pelvicalyceal system or ureter. Strictures should be confirmed with multiple views taken in different projections. A diagnosis of ureteral stricture should never be made unless dilatation of the ureter or pelvis above the point of narrowing is present. Active peristalsis and the numerous normal kinks and bends in the ureter mimic strictures but lack the combination of fixed narrowing with proximal dilatation.

Inflammation from Stone. An impacted calculus may cause inflammation, which results in scarring and fibrosis producing a stricture.

Posttraumatic strictures result from surgery and instrumentation.

Uroepithelial Tumor. The infiltrating growth pattern of TCC characteristically causes strictures of the collecting system or ureters (Fig. 34.13). These account for 15%

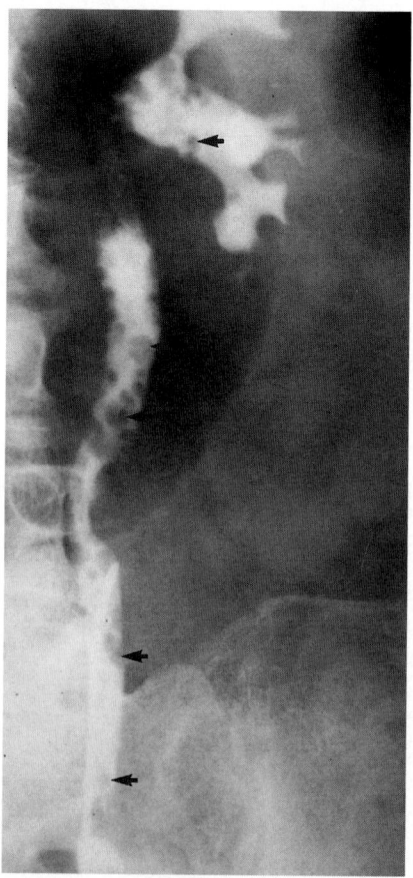

Figure 34.12. Pyeloureteritis Cystica. Retrograde pyeloureterogram demonstrates numerous well-defined, rounded filling defects (*arrows*) representing submucosal cysts in the left renal pelvis and ureter. The patient had a history of recurrent urinary tract infection.

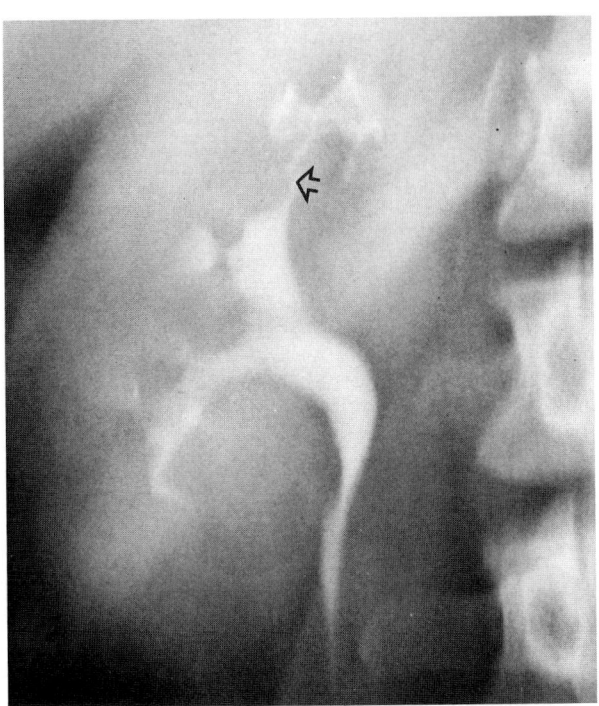

Figure 34.13. Transitional Cell Carcinoma. Radiograph from an excretory urogram demonstrates fixed narrowing (*arrow*) of the upper pole infundibulum. Compare with Figure 34.14.

of TCC. Squamous cell carcinoma is usually manifest as a stricture of the pelvis or ureter.

Tuberculosis and Schistosomiasis are two chronic inflammatory processes that are characterized by fibrosis and strictures. Differentiation from TCC may be difficult (Figs. 34.14, 34.15).

Extrinsic encasement by tumor or inflammatory processes is a common cause of stricture. Causes include lymphoma, cervical carcinoma, colon carcinoma, endometriosis, Crohn's disease, diverticulitis, and pelvic inflammatory disease.

Papillary Cavities

Calyceal Diverticuli are uroepithelium-lined cavities in the renal parenchyma that communicate via a narrow channel with the fornix of a nearby calyx (Fig. 34.16). They may be congenital, developing from a ureteral bud remnant, or acquired because of rupture of a cyst, infection, or reflux.

Papillary Necrosis may result in cavities at the papillary tips that fill with contrast on both antegrade and retrograde studies (Fig. 34.17). Larger cavities cause blunting of the calyces.

BLADDER

Imaging Methods

Evaluation of the bladder by standard excretory urography is usually sufficient to exclude most radiographically detectable bladder lesions. A cystogram, performed by instilling contrast agents directly into the bladder,

provides a more detailed examination. Fluoroscopic examination is performed during bladder filling to detect reflux. Films are obtained in frontal, lateral, and oblique positions. Films obtained during voiding demonstrate the bladder outlet and urethra. Postvoid films document residual urine. Although CT and MR play no significant role in bladder tumor detection, both are used to stage known bladder neoplasms. The urine-filled bladder is routinely used as a sonographic window to the pelvis. Intraluminal masses, calculi, bladder wall thickness, and bladder emptying can be reliably assessed by US (see chapter 37).

Anatomy

The normal filled urinary bladder is oval, with the floor parallel to, and 5–10 mm above, the superior aspect of the symphysis pubis. The size and shape of the bladder vary with the degree of bladder filling. The superior surface is covered by peritoneum, which extends to the side walls of the pelvis. The sigmoid colon and loops of small bowel, as well as the uterus in females, lie on top of the bladder and may cause mass impressions on the bladder dome. The inferior surface is extraperitoneal. Anteriorly, the bladder is separated from the symphysis pubis by fat in the extraperitoneal space of Retzius. Posteriorly, the bladder is separated from the uterus by the uterovesical peritoneal recess in females and from the rectum by the rectovesical peritoneal recess in males.

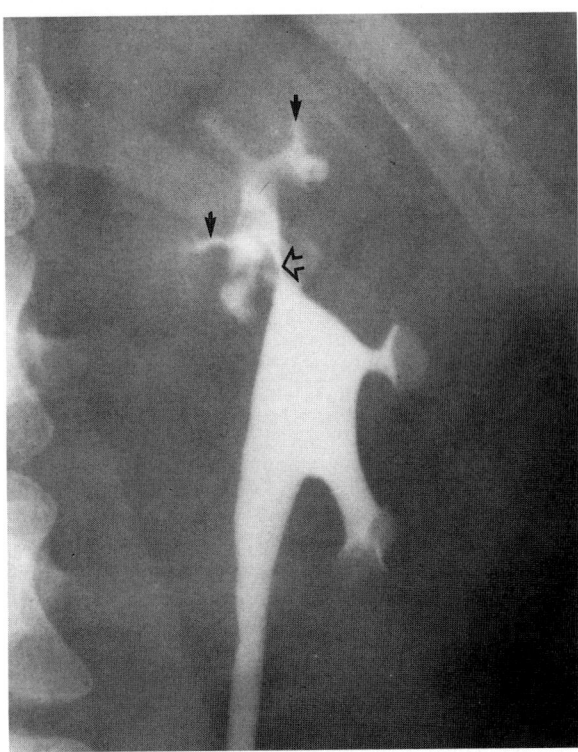

Figure 34.14. Tuberculosis. Active renal tuberculosis causes narrowing (*open arrow*) of the upper pole infundibulum of the left kidney, very similar to that seen with TCC in Figure 34.13. Note the additional areas of narrowing and irregularity (*arrowheads*) affecting upper pole collecting structures. The study is a retrograde ureterogram.

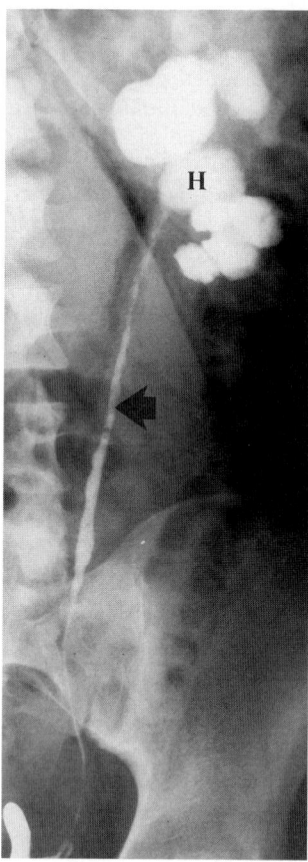

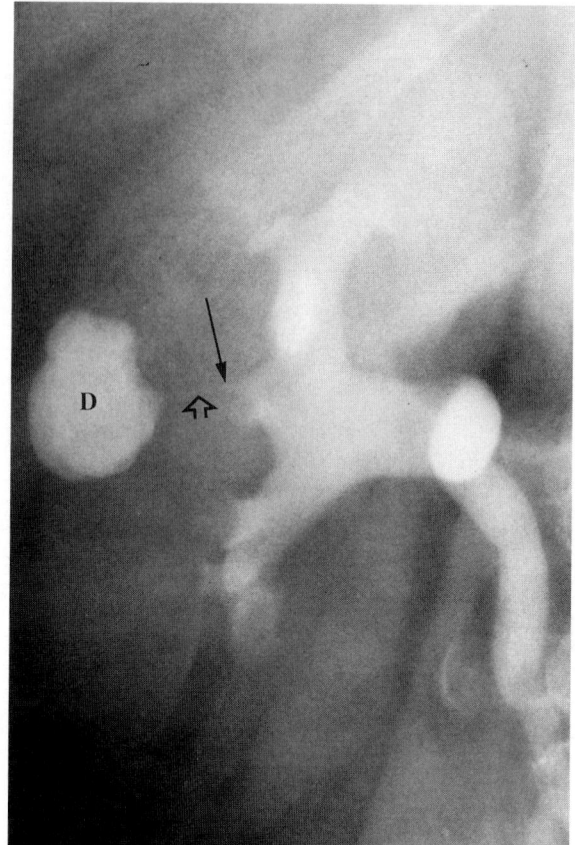

Figure 34.15. Tuberculosis. Retrograde contrast injection shows numerous filling defects, areas of narrowing, and mucosal irregularity involving the left ureter (*arrow*). A high-grade stricture at the ureteropelvic junction causes marked hydronephrosis (*H*).

Figure 34.16. Calyceal Diverticulum. An excretory urogram reveals a contrast-filled diverticulum (*D*) in the renal parenchyma. A tiny stream of contrast (*open arrow*) fills the tract, providing communication between the diverticulum and the calyceal fornix (*arrow*).

Figure 34.17. Papillary Necrosis. Multiple cavities (*arrows*) in the papilla fill with contrast during this excretory urogram in a patient with sickle cell trait. Most calyces are blunted. Low oxygen tension and high blood osmolality in the papillary tips predispose to sickling and ischemic injury.

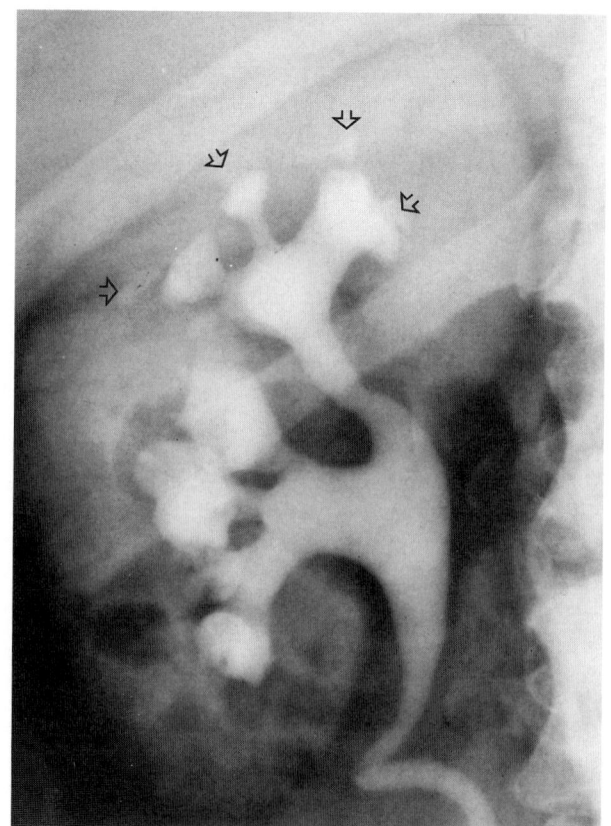

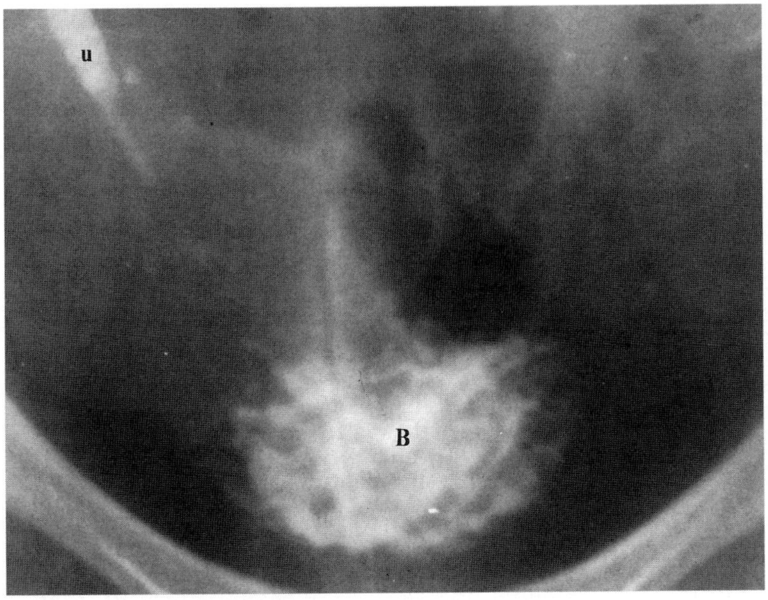

Figure 34.18. Normal Wrinkled Bladder Mucosa. Postvoid radiograph obtained as part of an XU demonstrates normal folds in the bladder mucosa with the bladder (*B*) near empty. The distal right ureter (*u*) is visualized.

The lining mucosa of the bladder is loosely attached to the muscular coat, so when the bladder is contracted, the mucosa appears wrinkled (Fig. 34.18). The bladder wall has four layers: an outer connective tissue adventitia, smooth muscle consisting of circular muscle fibers sandwiched between inner and outer layers of longitudinal fibers, submucosal connective tissue (the lamina propria), and the mucosa of transitional epithelium. The *trigone* is a triangle at the bladder floor formed by the two ureteral orifices and the internal urethral orifice. With voiding, the trigone descends 1–2 cm and transforms from a flat surface into a cone with the urethra at the apex.

On MR T1WI, the bladder wall is often indistinguishable from low-intensity urine (15). On T2WI the low-intensity bladder wall is well outlined by high-intensity urine and perivesical fat. Chemical shift artifact at water–fat interfaces may interfere with assessment of tumor invasion of the bladder wall.

Bladder Exstrophy results from a congenital deficiency in development of the lower anterior abdominal wall. The bladder is open, and its mucosa is continuous with the skin. Epispadias and wide diastasis of the symphysis pubis are associated. Ureteral obstruction, umbilical, and inguinal hernias are common. Management includes urinary diversion, bladder augmentation and skin grafting.

Thickened Bladder Wall/Small Bladder Capacity

The normal wall of a well-distended bladder should not exceed 5–6 mm in thickness (Fig. 34.19). The following conditions are associated with abnormal thickening of the bladder wall and, often, reduced bladder capacity.

Benign Prostatic Hypertrophy affects 50–75% of men older than age 50. Prostate enlargement projects into the base of the bladder, uplifting the bladder trigone and causing "J-hooking" of the distal ureters (Fig. 34.20). Chronic bladder outlet obstruction results in thickening and trabeculation of the bladder wall.

Prostate calcifications and bladder stones may be present. Prostate carcinoma must also be considered as a cause of prostate enlargement, although imaging methods cannot reliably differentiate benign enlargement from malignancy.

Urethral Stricture and Posterior Urethral Valves cause chronic obstruction to the outflow of urine from the bladder. The bladder wall thickens reflecting muscle hypertrophy in an attempt to overcome the obstruction. Voiding or retrograde urethrography demonstrates the urethral abnormality.

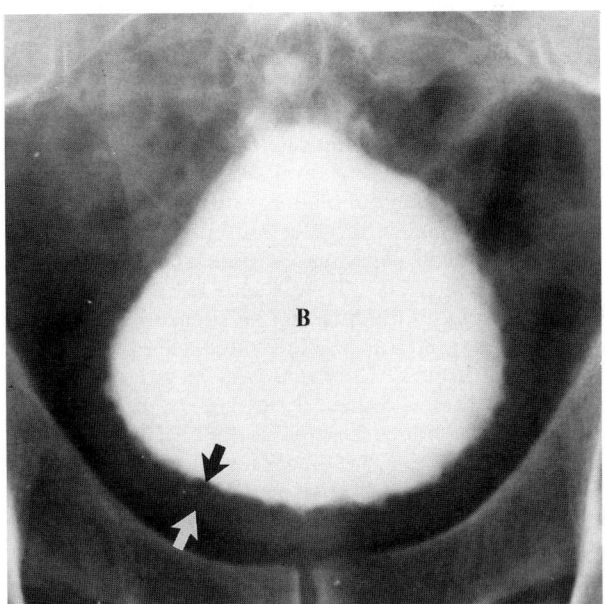

Figure 34.19. Bladder Wall Thickening. Radiograph from a cystogram in a patient with a neurogenic bladder and chronic urinary tract infections demonstrates a thickened bladder wall (*between arrows*) outlined by the contrast agent inside the bladder (*B*) and pelvic fat outside the bladder. Note the irregular contour of the bladder lumen caused by trabeculation of the muscle of the bladder wall.

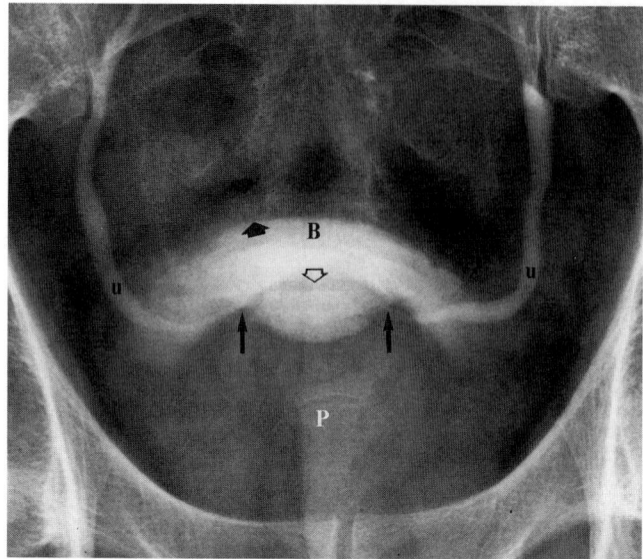

Figure 34.20. Benign Prostatic Hypertrophy. A radiograph from an excretory urogram shows marked uplifting of the bladder base because of massive enlargement of the prostate (*P*). The trigone (*open arrow*) and ureteral orifices (*black arrows*) are markedly elevated, resulting in a J-shaped appearance to the distal ureters (*u*). The bladder wall is thickened (*between black arrowheads*) and the bladder (*B*) mucosal pattern is prominent.

Neurogenic Bladder may be spastic or atonic. Causes include meningomyelocele, spinal trauma, diabetes mellitus, poliomyelitis, central nervous system tumor, and multiple sclerosis. Neurogenic bladders are prone to urinary stasis, chronic infection, and stone formation. Most neurogenic bladders eventually become trabeculated, thick-walled, and reduced in capacity (Fig. 34.19).

Cystitis. Inflammation of the bladder has many causes, including infection (bacteria, adenovirus, tuberculosis, schistosomiasis), drugs (cyclophosphamide), radiation, and autoimmune reaction.

MR demonstrates mucosal edema and inflammation as high-signal intensity on T2WI, easily differentiated from normal low-signal bladder wall.

Cystitis cystica is characterized by multiple fluid-filled submucosal cysts. Most cases are associated with bladder infection.

Cystitis glandularis is a further progression of cystitis cystica with proliferation of mucous secreting glands in the lamina propria. The cysts vary in size and may obstruct the ureteral orifice. Cystitis glandularis may be a precursor of adenocarcinoma of the bladder.

Bullous edema of the bladder wall is usually associated with chronic irritation from indwelling catheters. Grapelike cysts elevate the mucosa.

Interstitial cystitis is a chronic, idiopathic inflammation of the bladder found most often in women. The bladder capacity is progressively diminished, and the bladder wall thickens and becomes trabeculated and fibrotic.

Hemorrhagic cystitis is characterized by hemorrhage into the mucosa and submucosa. It is caused by bacterial or adenovirus infection.

Eosinophilic cystitis is an infiltration of the bladder wall by eosinophils. The cause is uncertain. The bladder wall is greatly thickened and frequently nodular.

Emphysematous cystitis is a form of bladder inflammation with gas within the bladder wall (Fig. 34.21). It is associated with poorly controlled diabetes mellitus, bladder outlet obstruction, and infection with *E. coli*, which ferment sugar in the urine to release carbon dioxide and hydrogen gasses. Gas within the bladder lumen is seen with emphysematous cystitis, instrumentation, and vesicocolic fistula.

Calcified Bladder Wall

Schistosomiasis of the urinary tract is caused by infestation with *Schistosoma haematobium*. The disease is most prevalent in North Africa, the Nile Valley, and Egypt. The larval cercariae of the blood fluke penetrate the skin of humans in infected water, enter the lymphatic vessels, and circulate eventually to the portal venous system, where the organism matures into adulthood. Adult females migrate to the vesical venous plexus and lay their eggs in the wall of the urinary bladder and ureter. The eggs incite a fibrosing granulomatous reaction that results in beaded stenosis and irregular dilatation of the ureters, and calcification of the walls of the distal ureters and bladder. The calcification is entirely the result of calcification of the eggs embedded within the wall (Fig. 34.22). The ureters become aperistaltic, resulting in vesicoureteral reflux. Eventually, the bladder may become shrunken, fibrotic, and contracted. Fistulas may develop in the perineum and scrotum. Renal disease develops slowly due to functional obstruction and reflux.

Tuberculosis affects the kidneys primarily and the ureters and bladder secondarily. Calcification affects the ureters proximally and may eventually extend into the distal ureters and bladder. Tuberculous infection of the bladder causes wall thickening and reduced capacity. Calcification of the bladder wall is uncommon and patchy.

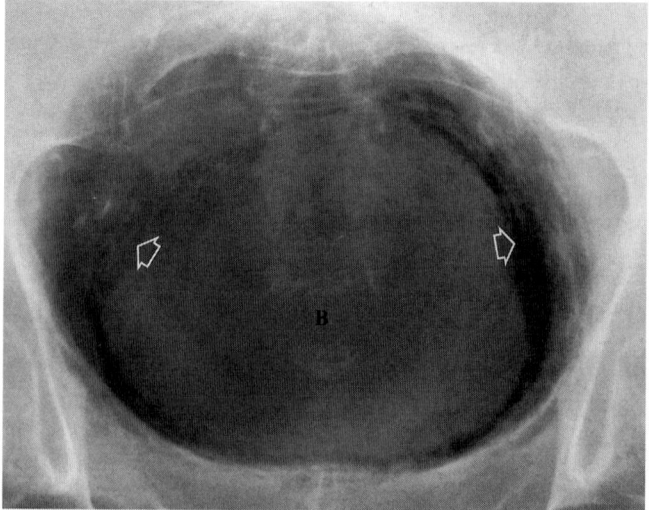

Figure 34.21. Emphysematous Cystitis. Air in the bladder wall is seen as a pattern of layering linear lucencies (*open arrows*) outlining the bladder (*B*) on this plain radiograph in a 67-year-old man with cystitis due to *Escherichia coli*.

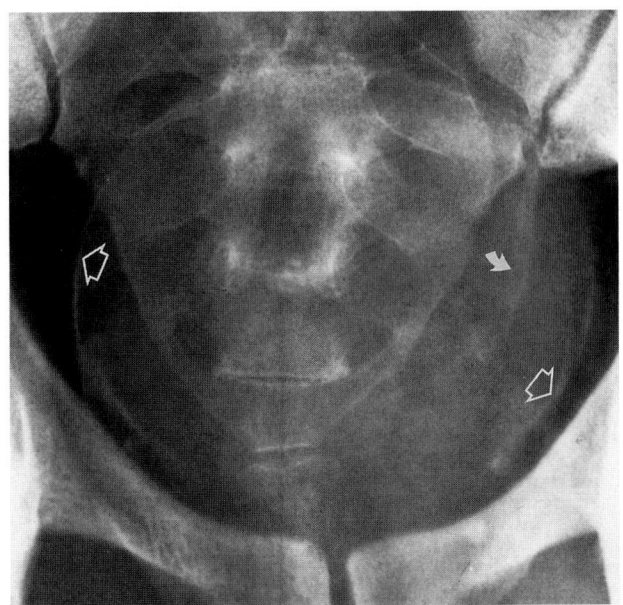

Figure 34.22. Schistosoma haematobium. Plain radiograph demonstrates calcification in the wall of the bladder (*open arrows*) and in the wall of the left ureter (*curved arrow*). The bladder is filled with urine. The patient is a 25-year-old Egyptian male.

Cystitis. Postirradiation cystitis, chronic infection, and cyclophosphamide-induced cystitis have been reported as causes of curvilinear or flocculent bladder wall calcification (16).

Neoplasm. Transitional cell and squamous cell carcinomas of the bladder may rarely calcify (1–7% incidence). Tumor calcification may be punctate or curvilinear and is best demonstrated by CT.

Bladder Wall Mass/Filling Defect

Simple Ureterocele is a congenital prolapse of the dilated distal ureter and orifice into the bladder lumen at the normal insertion site of the ureter into the trigone (17). It is usually an incidental finding in adults, although larger, simple ureteroceles may be associated with ureter obstruction, infection, and stone formation.

Excretory urography demonstrates a rounded filling defect in the bladder at the ureteral insertion. A "cobra head" or "spring onion" appearance is characteristic (Fig. 34.23). A radiolucent halo is produced by the wall of the ureter outlined both inside and outside by contrast.

US demonstrates a cystic mass at the ureteral orifice. Peristalsis of the ureter causes alternate filling and emptying of the ureterocele, as seen on real-time US.

Ectopic Ureterocele is usually associated with ureteral duplication (3). Females with ectopic ureters are prone to urinary incontinence because the ureter may insert distal to the external sphincter into the vestibule, uterus, or vagina. In males, the ectopic ureter usually inserts proximal to the external sphincter; no incontinence results. Insertion sites include the lower bladder, posterior urethra, seminal vesicles, vas deferens, and ejaculatory duct. Large ectopic ureteroceles may obstruct the opposite ureter or cause bladder outlet

obstruction because of their mass effect. The ectopic ureterocele appears as a cystic mass at the ectopic site of ureter insertion. The ureter is dilated and tortuous.

Transitional Cell Carcinoma of the bladder is the most common urinary tract neoplasm (18,19). TCC of the bladder is 50 times more common than TCC of the ureter. Although bladder tumors commonly develop in patients with primary TCC of the renal pelvis or ureter, only 2–4% of patients with bladder carcinoma have TCC of the ureter. Nonetheless, all patients with TCC deserve detailed screening of the entire uroepithelium.

Cross-sectional imaging is used to stage known bladder carcinoma (Table 34.2). Bladder carcinoma spreads by direct invasion through the bladder wall, by lymphatic spread to regional lymph nodes, and by hematogenous spread most commonly to bones, liver, and lung. Approximately 5% of patients have distant metastases at initial diagnosis.

XU plays a major role in screening the uroepithelium. Most bladder tumors appear as irregular filling defects (Fig. 34.24). Tumors larger than 1.5 cm are reliably detected by XU with inclusion of a postvoid film. The tumor may obstruct a ureteral orifice. Cystoscopic biopsy confirms the diagnosis.

MR is the imaging method of choice for staging bladder tumors (Table 34.2). On T1WI, tumor signal intensity is slightly higher than muscle but much lower than fat (15,19). On T2WI, the tumor appears brighter than bladder muscle, but not as bright as urine. MR is better than CT in predicting the depth of bladder wall invasion. T2WI demonstrate tumor invasion of the deep muscle layer as high-signal disruption of the normally low-signal bladder wall. Tumor extension into the perivesical fat is seen

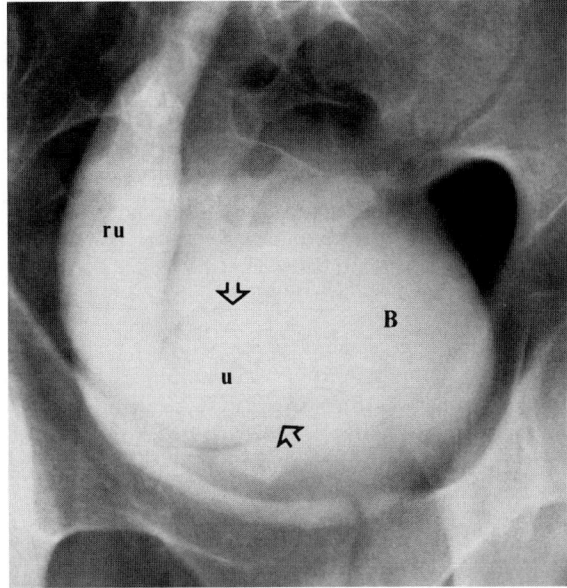

Figure 34.23. Simple Ureterocele. Oblique radiograph from an excretory urogram demonstrates dilation of the right ureter (*ru*) associated with a simple ureterocele (*u*) that protrudes into the lumen of the bladder (*B*). The radiolucent wall of the ureterocele (*arrows*) is outlined by contrast within the ureterocele and contrast within the bladder lumen. The wall of the ureterocele is made up of the wall of the ureter and the bladder mucosa.

Table 34.2. Staging of TCC in the Bladder

Jewett-Strong-Marshall System	TMN System	Description	MR Findings
O	Tis	Carcinoma in situ	Too small to be detected
O	Ta	Papillary tumor, confined to epithelium	Tumor confined to bladder wall; outer bladder wall seen as low-intensity band on T2WI
A	T1	Tumor invades lamina propria	Tumor confined to bladder wall; outer bladder wall seen as low-intensity band on T2WI
B1	T2	Tumor invades inner half of muscle layer	Tumor confined to bladder wall; outer bladder wall seen as low-intensity band on T2WI
B2	T3a	Tumor invades outer half of muscle layer	Tumor seen as high signal extending through the bladder wall but not into perivesical fat
C	T3b	Tumor invades perivesical fat	Tumor extension into perivesical fat seen on two planes
D1	T4a	Tumor invades surrounding organs	Tumor invades other pelvic organs
D1	T4b	Tumor invades pelvic or abdominal wall	Tumor invades pelvic side wall
D1	N1–3	Pelvic lymph node metastases	Pelvic nodes >1.0 cm
D2	M1	Distant metastases	Distant metastases
D2	N4	Lymph node metastases above aortic bifurcation	Abdominal nodes >1.0 cm

(Adapted from: Barentsz JO, Rujis SHJ, Strijk SP. The role of MR imaging in carcinoma of the urinary bladder. AJR Am J Roentgenol 1993;160:937–947; and Teeger S, Sica GT. MR imaging of bladder diseases. Magn Reson Imaging Clin North Am 1996;4:565–581.)

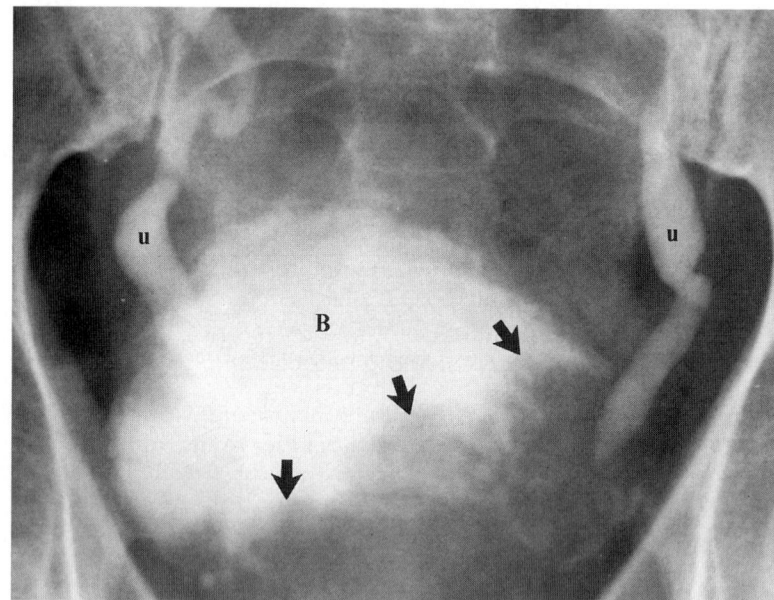

Figure 34.24. Transitional Cell Carcinoma. Radiograph from an excretory urogram reveals a lobulated mass (*arrows*) causing a large filling defect in the base of the bladder (*B*). Both ureters (*u*) are visualized.

on T1WI as low-signal tumor extending into high-signal fat. Pelvic lymph nodes are best visualized on T1WI. When larger than 1.0 cm, they are judged to be involved. MR cannot detect tumor involvement of smaller lymph nodes.

CT demonstrates TCC as a soft-tissue mass projecting into the bladder lumen or as a focal thickening of the bladder wall (Fig. 34.25). CT is poor at differentiating superficial noninvasive tumors from those that invade the bladder muscle and is therefore best used for staging advanced tumors. Perivesical spread is seen as soft-tissue density tumor in the perivesical fat. Like MR, CT detects lymph node involvement only by lymph node enlargement.

US demonstrates exophytic tumors as polypoid masses extending from the bladder wall. Infiltrating tumors may show as focal thickening of the bladder wall. Tumors may be difficult to recognize in the presence of diffuse bladder wall thickening and trabeculation. Transrectal and transurethral sonography may play a role in the staging of bladder tumors.

Squamous cell carcinoma accounts for 4% of bladder malignancy. It tends to develop in bladders chronically irritated by stones and infection.

Adenocarcinoma is rare, accounting for less than 1% of bladder malignancy. Most cases are associated with bladder extrophy or urachal remnants.

Benign bladder tumors include leiomyoma, hemangioma, pheochromocytoma, and neurofibroma. Most produce smooth filling defects.

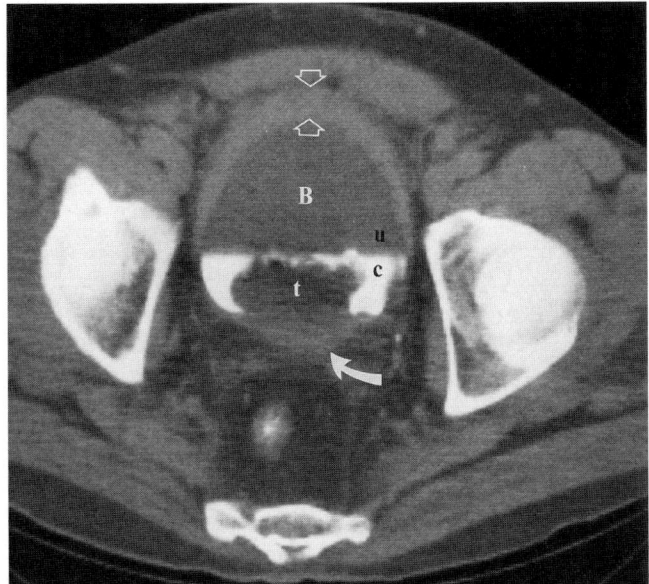

Figure 34.25. Transitional Cell Carcinoma. A CT scan demonstrates a large tumor (*t*) arising from the posterior wall of the bladder (*B*) and extending through the bladder wall into the perivesical fat (*curved arrow*). This tumor is stage III. The bladder wall is thickened (*arrows*) because of benign prostatic hypertrophy. Note that contrast (*c*) layers posteriorly while unopacified urine (*u*) layers anteriorly in this supine patient. On an excretory urogram, routine films of the bladder may miss lesions of the anterior bladder wall if all films are taken in the supine position.

Blood clots in the bladder are usually irregular in shape, move with changes in patient position, and change in size and appearance over time.

Bladder stones may migrate from the kidney or form primarily within the bladder because of urinary stasis or a foreign body (Fig. 34.26). Solitary stones are most common. Stones must be removed to cure chronic bladder infection. Chronic bladder stones increase the risk of developing bladder carcinoma.

Pear-shaped Bladder/Extrinsic Mass

Lymphadenopathy is a common cause of extrinsic mass impression on the bladder. Lymphoma and metastases from malignancy of pelvic organs are common causes.

Pelvic hemorrhage indents the bladder and displaces it to the opposite side. CT and MR confirm the presence of hematoma.

Pelvic lipomatosis refers to a condition of excessive perirectal and perivesical fat in the pelvis. The bladder is elongated and lifted up and out of the pelvis. Fat density is evident on CT and MR.

Iliac artery aneurysms tend to be clinically silent, but rupture is common and associated with high mortality. Calcification in the aneurysm may be apparent. Most iliac artery aneurysms are associated with aortic aneurysms.

Pelvic tumors may be manifest on plain film or excretory urography by mass impression on the bladder.

Psoas muscle hypertrophy may also cause a pear-shaped bladder (Fig. 34.27).

Bladder Outpouchings/Fistula

Bladder diverticula are herniations of the bladder mucosa between interlacing muscle bundles. Most are located posterolaterally near the ureterovesical junction (Fig. 34.28). Diverticula may contain stones or tumor and occasionally do not fill on cystograms. Complications of bladder diverticula include urinary stasis, infection, stone formation, vesicoureteral reflux, and bladder outlet obstruction (17).

Vesicocolonic fistula most commonly occurs as a complication of diverticulitis (see Fig. 32.17). Additional causes include colon or bladder carcinoma, ulcerative colitis, and Crohn's disease. The bladder is chronically infected, and the patient may complain of pneumaturia and fecaluria. The diagnosis is often made clinically. Barium enema and cystography detect only 35% of vesicocolonic fistulae. The fistulous tract is occasionally demonstrated by CT.

Vesicovaginal fistula is usually a complication of gynecologic surgery, especially for cervical carcinoma. Obstetric injury is an occasional cause.

Vesicoenteric fistula are almost always attributable to Crohn's disease.

Bladder Trauma

Susceptibility of the bladder to traumatic injury depends largely on the degree of bladder filling at the time of injury. A distended bladder is more prone to injury than a collapsed bladder.

Extraperitoneal bladder rupture (80% of bladder

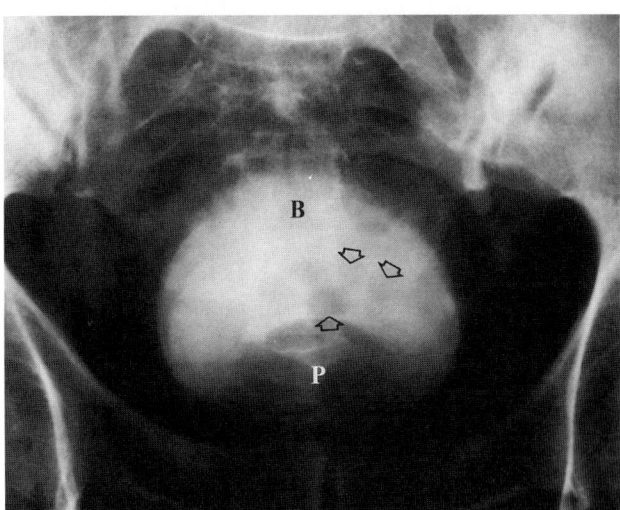

Figure 34.26. Bladder Stones. A radiograph of the bladder (*B*) taken as part of an excretory urogram demonstrates a prominent prostate (*P*) impression on the base of the bladder. Multiple radiolucent bladder stones (*arrows*) are seen within the contrast-filled bladder. Stones form as a result of stasis caused by chronic bladder outlet obstruction.

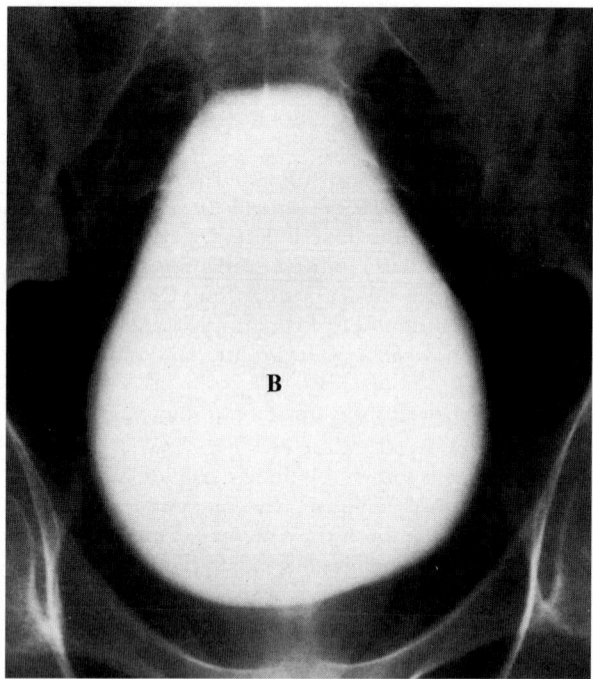

Figure 34.27. Pear-shaped Bladder. The bladder (*B*) on this excretory urogram is pear-shaped because of psoas muscle hypertrophy in this 16-year-old patient with muscular dystrophy.

ruptures) results from puncture of the bladder by a spicule of bone from a pelvic fracture. Contrast extravasation is into extraperitoneal compartments, most commonly the retropubic space of Retzius (Fig. 34.29). Contrast extravasation may extend into the anterior abdominal wall, thigh, and scrotum. XU is not an adequate screening method. Cystography or CT with distension of the bladder to at least 250 mL is required to exclude bladder rupture.

Intraperitoneal bladder rupture (20% of bladder ruptures) results from blunt trauma applied to a distended bladder. The sudden rise in intravesical pressure results in rupture of the bladder dome and extravasation into the peritoneal space. Contrast material flows into the paracolic gutters and outlines the loops of the bowel (Fig. 34.30). Intraperitoneal bladder rupture may clinically mimic acute renal failure. Urine output is decreased or absent, and serum creatinine is increased because of absorption of urine by the peritoneal surface.

URETHRA

Imaging Methods

The urethra is studied by retrograde and voiding urethrography (20,21). The retrograde urethrogram is a simple study of the anterior male urethra (Fig. 34.31). Contrast medium is injected into the anterior urethra by means of a syringe or catheter that occludes the meatal orifice. Films are exposed in the right posterior oblique projection. The anterior urethra normally distends fully because of resistance owing to the external sphincter at the level of the urogenital diaphragm. Complete filling of

the posterior urethra is not possible because contrast runs freely into the bladder. Voiding cystourethrography is performed by filling the bladder with contrast via a catheter. The catheter is removed, and films are obtained while the patient urinates into a basin on the fluoroscopy table. The voiding urethrogram demonstrates

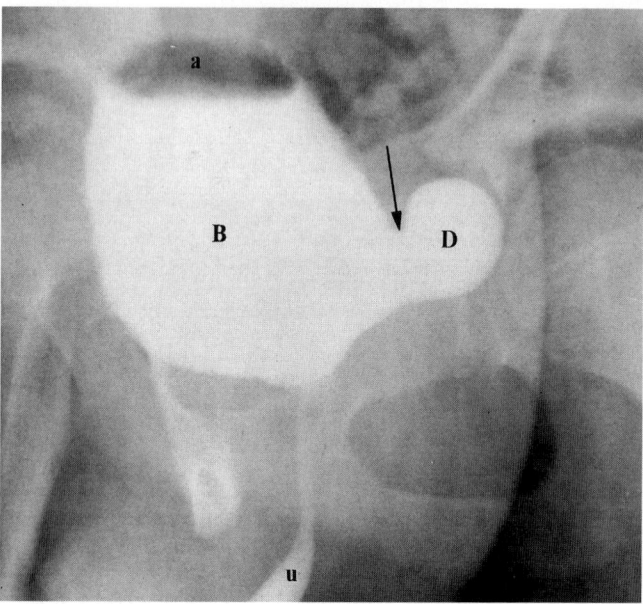

Figure 34.28. Bladder Diverticulum. A smooth-walled diverticulum (*D*) extends from the posterolateral aspect of the bladder (*B*) on this oblique radiograph from a cystogram. The diverticulum fills with contrast through a wide neck (*arrow*) that connects with the bladder lumen. Diverticula that arise in this location near the ureteral orifice may cause vesicoureteral reflux. Air (*a*) was introduced into the bladder by the catheter placed to instill contrast. Contrast is seen in the urethra (*u*) on this film taken during voiding.

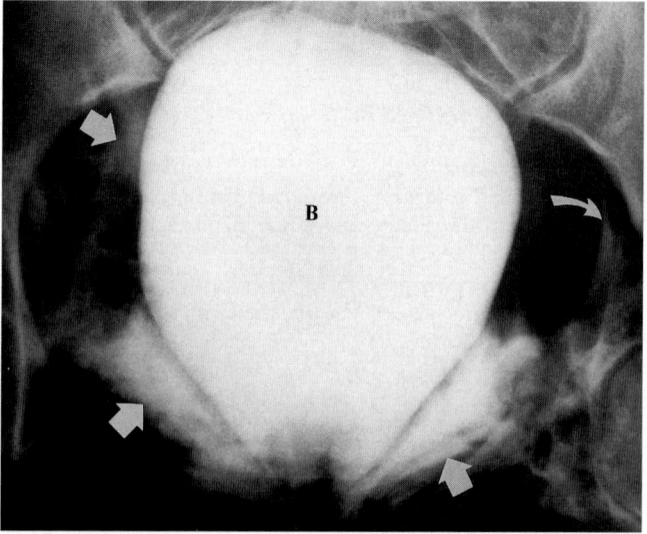

Figure 34.29. Extraperitoneal Bladder Rupture. Radiograph from a cystogram with the bladder (*B*) filled with contrast demonstrates extraperitoneal extravasation of contrast (*straight arrows*), characterized by its amorphous shape without distinct edges. A fracture of the acetabulum is evident (*curved arrow*).

distension of both the posterior and anterior urethra (Fig. 34.32).

Radiographic study of the female urethra may be conducted by voiding cystourethrogram or by retrograde urethrogram with a specially designed double-balloon catheter. The female urethra is also well studied by transrectal or perineal US and by MR (Fig. 34.33) (22–24).

Anatomy

The male urethra is divided into posterior and anterior portions by the inferior aspect of the urogenital di-

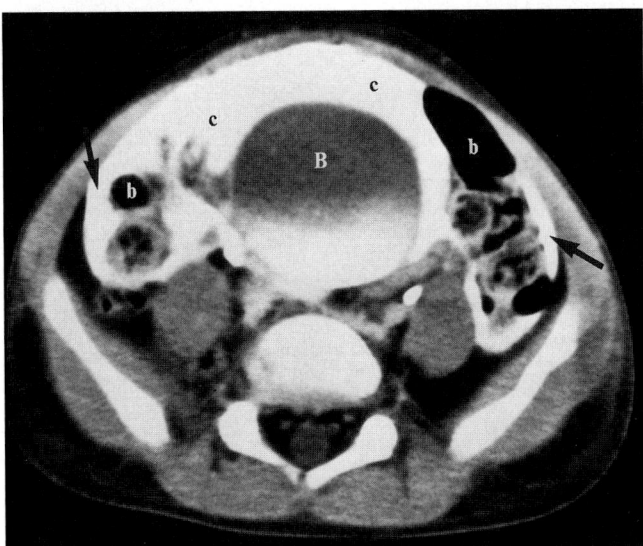

Figure 34.30. Intraperitoneal Bladder Rupture. A CT scan of a 5-year-old boy injured in a motor vehicle accident demonstrates contrast in the peritoneal cavity (*c, arrows*) surrounding loops of the bowel (*b*). The bladder (*B*) is distended with urine and layering contrast. The contrast agent in the peritoneal cavity strongly suggests bladder rupture. Perforated bowel may cause both air and oral contrast to be in the peritoneal cavity.

aphragm (see Figs. 34.31,34.32) (21,25). The posterior urethra consists of the *prostatic urethra* within the prostate gland, from the bladder neck to urogenital diaphragm, and the short *membranous urethra*, which is totally contained within the 1-cm thick urogenital diaphragm. The anterior urethra extends from the urogenital diaphragm to the external urethral meatus. It consists of the *bulbous urethra* extending from the urogenital diaphragm to the penoscrotal junction, and the *penile urethra* extending to the urethral meatus. The anterior urethra is entirely contained within the corpora-spongiosum penis except for the proximal 2 cm of the bulbous urethra, called the *pars nuda*.

The prostatic urethra runs vertically through the prostate over a length of 3–4 cm. An oval filling defect in the midportion of the posterior wall is the *verumontanum*. The ejaculatory ducts open into the urethra on either side of the verumontanum, and the prostatic glands empty into the urethra by multiple small openings that surround the verumontanum. The utricle, a müllerian remnant, is a small, saccular depression in the middle of the verumontanum.

The distal end of the verumontanum marks the beginning of the membranous urethra, which extends to the apex of the cone of the bulbous urethra. The voluntary external urethral sphincter within the urogenital diaphragm entirely surrounds the membranous urethra. Cowper's glands (Fig 34.34) are pea-sized accessory sex glands within the urogenital diaphragm on either side of the membranous urethra. Their ducts empty into the bulbous urethra 2 cm distally.

On retrograde urethrography, the bulbous urethra tapers to a cone shape as the urethra enters the external sphincter (see Fig. 34.31). The apex of the cone marks the division between the membranous and bulbous urethra. The penoscrotal junction that divides the bulbous and penile urethra is marked by the suspensory ligament of the penis, which causes a normal bend in the urethra. The entire anterior urethra is lined by the glands of Littré, whose secretions lubricate the urethra.

Figure 34.31. Retrograde Urethrogram. Contrast injected retrograde through the penile meatus demonstrates the penile (*pu*) and bulbous (*bu*) urethra demarcated by the suspensory ligament of the penis at the penoscrotal junction (*curved arrow*). The urethra tapers to a point at the urogenital diaphragm (*straight arrow*), marking the location of the membranous urethra. The verumontanum (*open arrow*) marks the location of the prostatic urethra.

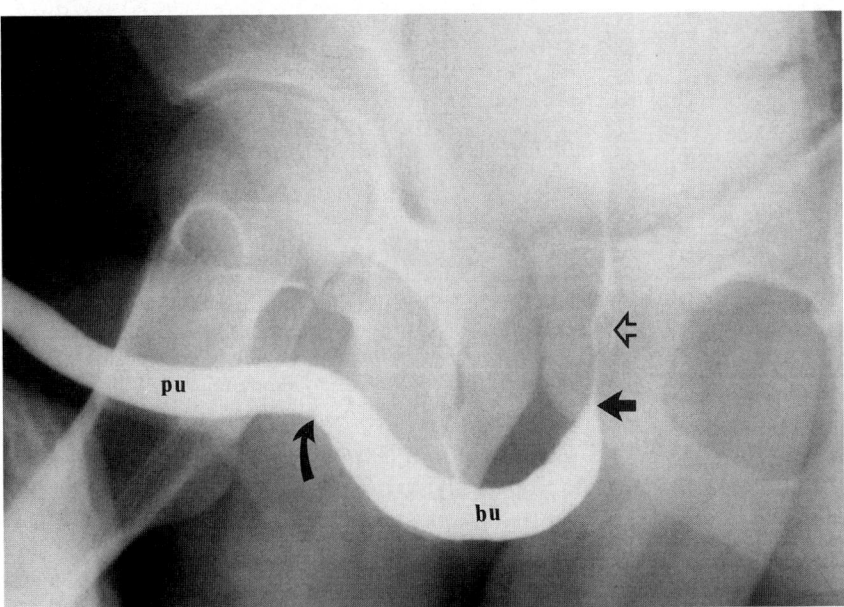

Figure 34.32. Voiding Cystourethrogram. Radiograph exposed while the patient is urinating demonstrates the entire urethra. The verumontanum (*open arrow*) is seen as an oval filling defect in the prostatic urethra. A slight constriction (*straight arrow*) at the lower edge of the verumontanum marks the location of the membranous urethra. The bulbous urethra (*bu*) extends to the penoscrotal junction (*curved arrow*). The penile urethra (*pu*) travels in the corpora spongiosum to the penile meatus. *B*, bladder.

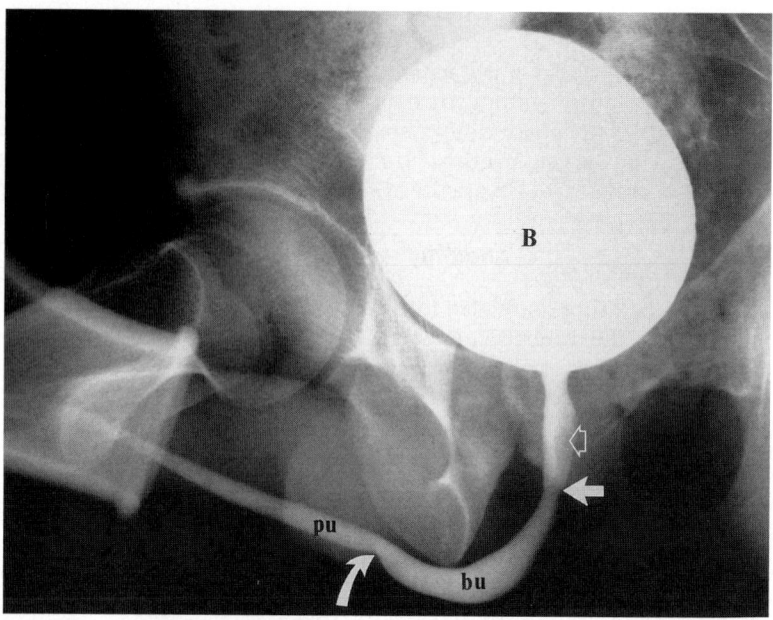

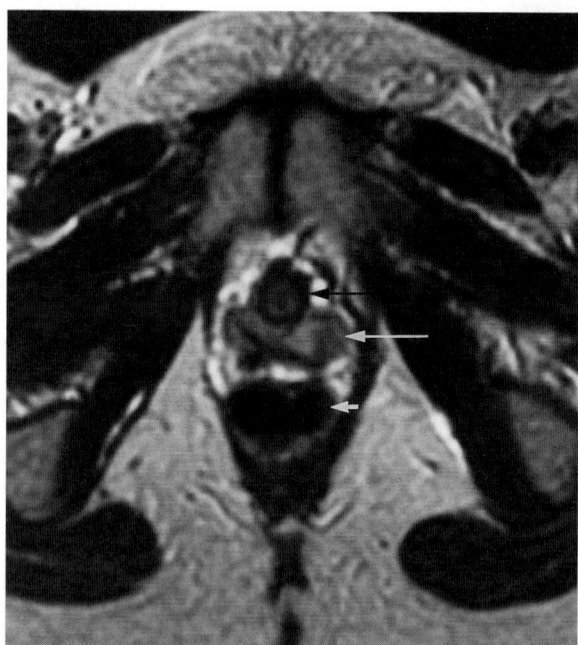

Figure 34.33. Female Urethra. T2-weighted MR demonstrates the zonal anatomy of the female urethra (*black arrow*) in the anterior wall of the vagina (*white arrow*). The outer smooth layer is low signal (*dark*), the submucosal layer is moderately bright, and the central mucosa is dark. The *arrowhead* indicates the rectum.

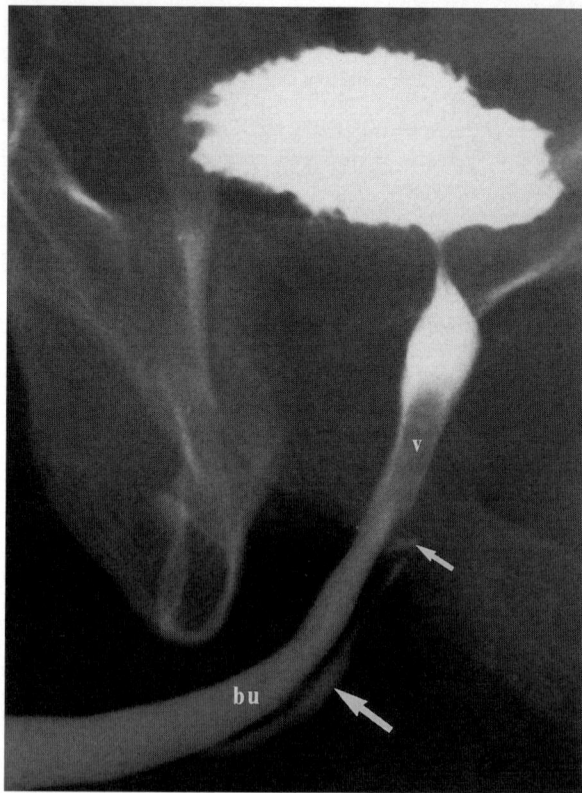

Figure 34.34. Cowper's glands. Voiding cystourethrogram shows filling of the ducts to Cowper's glands. The glands (*small arrow*) are in the urogenital diaphragm and their ducts (*large arrow*) drain into the bulbous urethra (*bu*). *v*, verumontanum.

Cowper's ducts and the utricle occasionally fill with contrast during urethrography in a normal patient. The filling of these structures with contrast occurs much more commonly in the presence of urethral strictures. Visualization of the glands of Littré is always abnormal and associated with chronic inflammation and urethral stricture (Fig. 34.35). Reflux of contrast into the prostatic ducts is also abnormal and is associated with prostatitis and distal urethral stricture (Fig. 34.36).

The female urethra varies in length from 2.5 to 4 cm.

The urethra is embedded in the anterior wall of the vagina and is lined throughout by periurethral glands. On MR, the urethra is isointense with the vaginal muscle on T1WI (23,24). On T2WI (Fig. 34.33), the normal urethra demonstrates a characteristic target appearance with dark inner and outer rings and a middle zone of high signal intensity. The middle zone corresponds to highly vascular submucosa and enhances markedly with gadopentetate administration. The dark inner zone is mucosa, and the dark outer zone is urethral smooth muscle.

Urethral Stricture

Urethral strictures are abnormal narrowings of the urethra resulting from fibrous scar tissue. They may involve the entire urethra or only a small portion. Abrupt, short-segment strictures are usually traumatic. Long-segment strictures may be either traumatic or inflammatory.

Causes of traumatic urethral strictures include instrumentation, indwelling catheters, prostatectomy procedures, chemical injury (podophyllin), saddle injuries (usually of the bulbous urethra), and pelvic fractures.

Most inflammatory strictures are attributable to gon-

orrhea. Bacteria become sequestered in the glands of Littré and incite the formation of granulation tissue and fibrosis. Additional etiologies include chlamydia, mycoplasma, tuberculosis, and schistosomiasis.

Complications of urethral strictures include the following:

- *Periurethral abscess* is usually on the ventral surface and may drain into the lumen or onto the skin, creating a periurethral fistula (Fig. 34.36).
- *False passage* is the most common complication of urethral stricture. It is usually iatrogenic because of attempted passage of catheters or instruments past the obstruction.
- *Stasis and infection* may cause disease of the upper urinary tracts including hydronephrosis, bladder hypertrophy, calculi, and chronic inflammation.
- *Carcinoma of the urethra* occurs as a complication of chronic urethritis and stricture. Carcinomas may appear as a filling defect in the urethra or as a change in

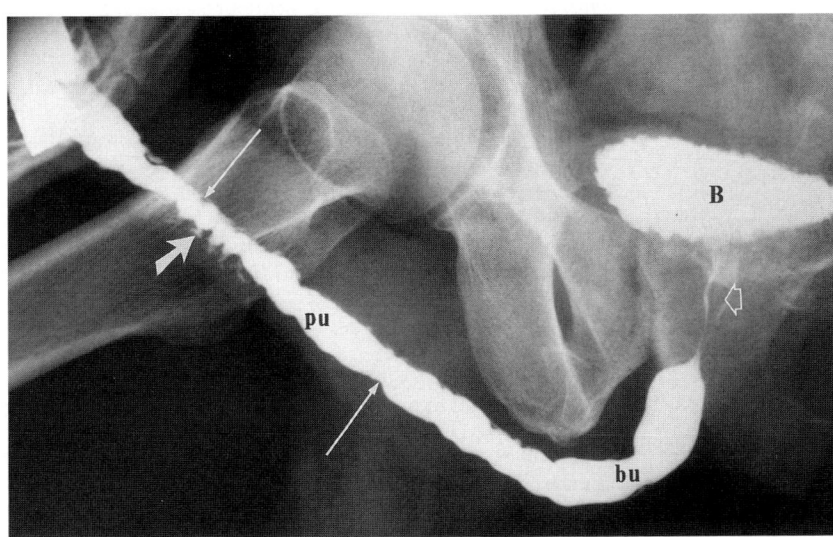

Figure 34.35. Urethral Strictures, Glands of Littré. Retrograde urethrogram demonstrates multiple strictures (*long arrows*) in the penile (*pu*) and bulbous (*bu*) urethra. Filling of the glands of Littré (*short arrow*) is evidence of urethritis. This patient had a history of multiple episodes of gonorrhea. The verumontanum (*open arrow*) marks the prostatic urethra. *B*, bladder.

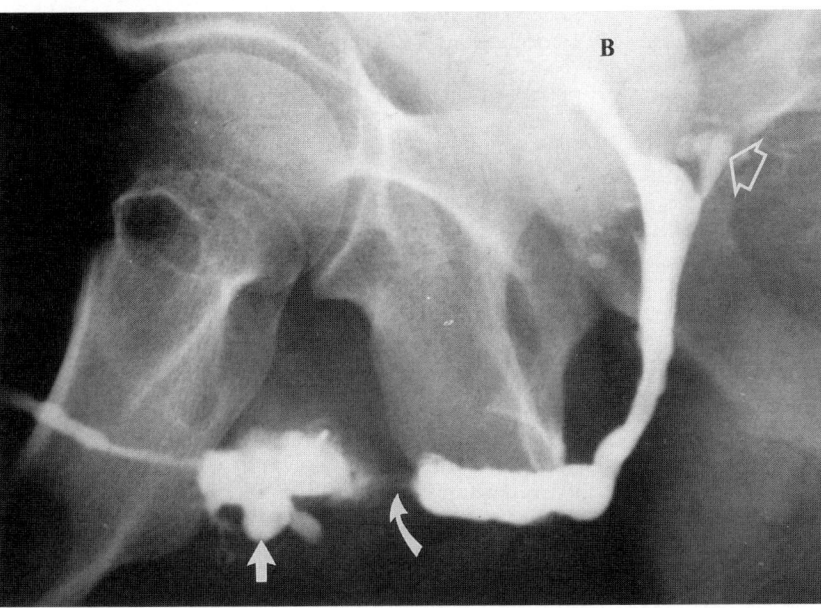

Figure 34.36. Periurethral Abscess and Fistula. Voiding cystourethrogram demonstrates a periurethral abscess (*arrow*) with a fistula into the scrotum. A stricture (*curved arrow*) is present, proximal to the abscess. Contrast is seen refluxing into the prostatic ducts (*open arrow*). *B*, bladder.

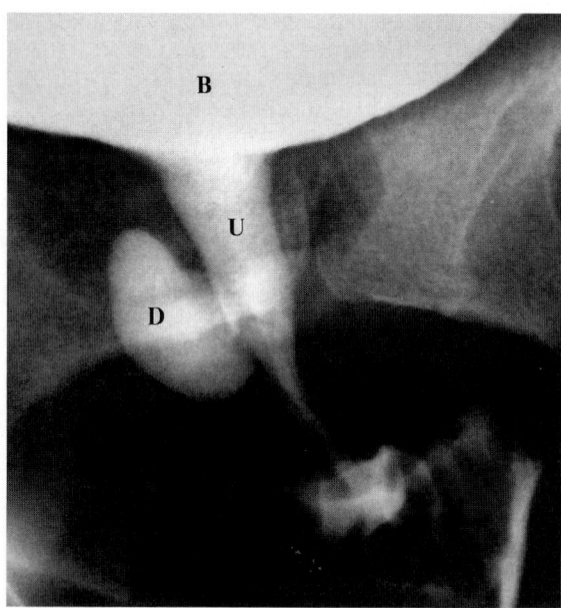

Figure 34.37. Urethral Diverticulum. Voiding cystourethrogram in a woman with recurrent urinary tract infections fills a urethral diverticulum (*D*). *B*, bladder; *U*, female urethra.

appearance of the stricture. Most are squamous cell carcinoma and most involve the anterior urethra (26). Rare tumors of the posterior urethra are usually TCC that occur as part of multiple uroepithelial neoplasia.

Urethral Diverticulum

Urethral diverticuli are smooth, saclike outpouchings of the urethra. They may be congenital or the result of infection or trauma. Because they serve as a site of urinary stasis, stone formation and recurrent infection are common complications. A diverticulum of the female urethra is an uncommon cause of recurrent urinary tract infection. It may be demonstrated by a postvoid film of an excretory urogram, voiding cystourethrogram (Fig. 34.37), transrectal or transperineal US, or MR.

Urethral Trauma

Traumatic injury to the posterior urethra occurs in about 10% of pelvic fractures. The junction between the prostatic and membranous urethra is the most common site of injury. Injury is suspected in patients with pelvic fractures or when blood is present at the urethral meatus. Retrograde urethrography should precede attempts at urethral catheterization. If a bladder catheter has already been inserted, the urethra can be studied by inserting a small (8F) pediatric feeding tube adjacent to the catheter and injecting contrast. The classification of posterior urethral injury is as follows:

Type 1 is a stretch injury due to pelvic hematoma.
Type 2 is a rupture of the membranous urethra at the apex of the prostate with extravasation above the urogenital diaphragm.
Type 3 is a rupture of both the membranous and bul-

bous urethra with disruption of the urogenital diaphragm and contrast extravasation both above and below the diaphragm.

A "straddle injury," falling astride a fixed object commonly injures the bulbous urethra. Instrumentation, foreign body insertion, or direct trauma to the penis may injure the penile urethra. Long-term bladder catheterization may injure any portion of the urethra. Autodigestion of the urethra because of drainage of pancreatic exocrine enzymes has been reported as a complication of pancreatic transplantation.

Complications of urethral injury are common and include stricture, incontinence, impotence, and pelvic and perineal sinus tracts and fistulas.

References

1. Rothpearl A, Frager D, Subraminian A, et al. MR urography: technique and application. Radiology 1995;194:125–130.
2. Tang Y, Yamashita Y, Namimoto T, et al. The value of MR urography that uses HASTE sequences to reveal urinary tract disorders. AJR Am J Roentgenol 1996;167:1497–1502.
3. Fernbach SK, Feinstein KA, Spencer K, et al. Ureteral duplication and its complications. Radiographics 1997;17:109–127.
4. Quillin SP, Brink JA, Heiken JP, et al. Helical (spiral) CT angiography for identification of crossing vessels at the ureteropelvic junction. AJR Am J Roentgenol 1996;166:1125–1130.
5. LeRoy AJ. Diagnosis and treatment of nephrolithiasis: current perspectives. AJR Am J Roentgenol 1994;163:1309–1313.
6. Bush WHJ. Radiologic aspects of urolithiasis. Radiologist 1994;1:31–43.
7. Sommer FG, Jeffrey RB Jr, Rubin GD, et al. Detection of ureteral calculi in patients with suspected renal colic: value of reformatted noncontrast CT. AJR Am J Roentgenol 1995;165:509–513.
8. Smith RC, Verga M, Dalrymple N, et al. Acute ureteral obstruction: value of secondary signs on helical unenhanced CT. AJR Am J Roentgenol 1996;167:1109–1113.
9. Kawashima A, Sandler CM, Boridy IC, et al. Unenhanced CT of ureterolithiasis: value of the tissue rim sign. AJR Am J Roentgenol 1997;168:997–1000.
10. Heneghan JP, Dalrymple NC, Verga M, et al. Soft-tissue "rim" sign in the diagnosis of ureteral calculi with use of unenhanced helical CT. Radiology 1997;202:709–711.
11. Winalski CS, Lipman JC, Tumeh SS. Ureteral neoplasms. Radiographics 1990;10:271–283.
12. Leder RA, Dunnick NR. Transitional cell carcinoma of the pelvicalices and ureter. AJR Am J Roentgenol 1990;155:713–722.
13. Urban BA, Buckley J, Soyer P, et al. CT appearance of transitional cell carcinoma of the renal pelvis: part 1. Early stage disease. AJR Am J Roentgenol 1997;169:157–161.
14. Urban BA, Buckley J, Soyer P, et al. CT appearance of transitional cell carcinoma of the renal pelvis: part 2. Advanced stage disease. AJR Am J Roentgenol 1997;169:163–168.
15. Teeger S, Sica GT. MR imaging of bladder diseases. Magn Reson Imaging Clin North Am 1996;4:565–581.
16. Pollack HM, Banner MP, Martinez LO, et al. Diagnostic considerations in urinary bladder wall calcification. AJR Am J Roentgenol 1981;136:791–797.
17. Fernbach SK, Feinstein KA. Abnormalities of the bladder in children: imaging findings. AJR Am J Roentgenol 1994;162:1143–1150.

18. Lamm DL, Torti FM. Bladder cancer, 1996. CA Cancer J Clin 1996;46:93–112.
19. Barentsz JO, Ruijs SHJ, Strijk S. The role of MR imaging in carcinoma of the urinary bladder. AJR Am J Roentgenol 1993;160:937–947.
20. Yoder IC, Papanicolaou N. Imaging the urethra in men and women. Urol Radiol 1992;14:24–28.
21. Amis ES Jr, Newhouse JH, Cronan JJ. Radiology of the male periurethral structures. AJR Am J Roentgenol 1988; 151:321–324.
22. Vargas-Serrano B, Cortina-Moreno B, Rodriguez-Romero R, et al. Transrectal ultrasonography in the diagnosis of ure-thral diverticula in women. J Clin Ultrasound 1997;25: 21–28.
23. Hricak H, Secaf E, Buckley DW, et al. Female urethra: MR imaging. Radiology 1991;178:527–535.
24. Siegelman ES, Banner MP, Ramchandani P, et al. Multicoil MR imaging of symptomatic female urethral and peri-urethral disease. Radiographics 1997;17:349–365.
25. McCallum RW. The adult male urethra: normal anatomy, pathology, and method of urethrography. Radiol Clin North Am 1979;17:227–244.
26. Mostofi FK, Davis CJ Jr, Sesterhenn IA. Carcinoma of the male and female urethra. Urol Clin North Am 1992;19:347–358.

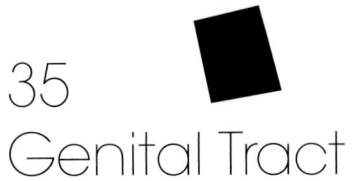

35
Genital Tract

William E. Brant

FEMALE GENITAL TRACT

The primary modality for imaging of the female genital tract is US using transabdominal and transvaginal techniques. MR and CT are used to stage and follow-up pelvic malignancies and to supplement US by providing additional characterization of lesions (1,2). In addition, many uterine and adnexal lesions may be discovered incidentally by pelvic CT or MR performed for other reasons (3). Hysterosalpingography (HSG) is combined with US, CT, and MR to diagnose congenital anomalies of the female genital tract and mechanical causes of infertility (4–6). The HSG is performed by cannulating the cervix and injecting a contrast agent into the lumina of the uterus and fallopian tubes. Free communication of these lumina with the peritoneal cavity should be evident. Hysterosonography is an alternative to HSG. Isotonic saline is injected into the uterine cavity while the pelvis is examined sonographically (7).

Anatomy

Normal MR Anatomy. The internal anatomy of the uterus is depicted best on T2WI (8). On T2WI, the endometrium appears as a high signal intensity central stripe surrounded by the low signal intensity junctional zone (Fig. 35.1). The bulk of the myometrium is intermediate signal intensity. The low signal intensity of inner junctional zone of the myometrium is due to lower water content. The entire uterus is low in signal intensity and the internal anatomy of the uterus is poorly seen on T1WIs. The cervix is largely composed of collagenous tissue that are low in signal intensity on both T1WI and T2WI, providing a dark background for visualization of hyperintense cervical carcinomas (see Fig. 35.11)(9). The endocervical epithelium and mucus is homogeneous high signal on T2WI. High-resolution MR using surface or intravaginal coils shows two zones in the cervical fi-bromuscular stroma, a darker inner zone contiguous with the uterine junctional zone and an intermediate signal outer zone distinctly darker than the myometrium (10). The parametrium is the fibrous tissue that separates the upper cervix from the bladder and extends laterally between the leaves of the broad ligament. Vaginal anatomy is also best seen on T2WI. The muscular vaginal wall is low in signal, but the central epithelium and mucus is high in signal.

The normal ovaries of fertile women are easily identified by the bright signal of the follicles demonstrated on T2WI. The follicles are low or intermediate in signal on T1WI. The cortex of the ovary in the premenopausal woman is darker in the signal than the medulla on T2WI (11). The postmenopausal ovary is more difficult to identify because of the absence of follicles and the cortex and medulla being nearly equal in signal on both T1WI and T2WI.

Normal CT Anatomy. The position of the uterus varies with the anatomy and size of the other pelvic organs, changing dramatically in position with filling of the bladder (12). Because CT is limited to axial slices, the outline of the uterus may appear lobulated or bulbus solely because of position. The uterus is uniform in soft-tissue density and its internal anatomy is not demonstrated by CT. Because the myometrium is highly vascular, the uterus enhances more than most other pelvic organs. Fluid in the uterine cavity is usually low density. The ovaries are easily mistaken for unopacified bowel loops in the pelvis. The vagina is seen in cross-section as a flattened ellipse of soft tissue density between the bladder and rectum. Normal fallopian tubes are not demonstrated by CT.

Hysterosalpingography is primarily used for the evaluation of infertility to demonstrate the morphology and patency of the uterine canal and fallopian tubes (Fig. 35.2)(5,6,13,14). Contrast injected into the uterine cavity outlines the endocervical canal, uterine cavity, and lumen of the fallopian tubes with free spill of contrast into the peritoneal cavity in the normal patient. The uterine cavity is sharply defined and triangular in shape with normal mild concavity in the fundal region. The size of the cavity varies with parity. The endocervical canal is cylindrical in shape, 3–4 cm in length and 1–3 cm in width. Folds in the endocervical mucosa form a normal serrated appearance. The normal fallopian tubes are 10–12 cm in length extending from the cornua of the uterus. The lumen is thread-like (1–2 mm) until it reaches the ampulla where it expands to 5–10 mm and rugal folds become visible. Patency of the tubes is confirmed by dispersal of contrast within the peritoneal cavity with outlining of bowel loops.

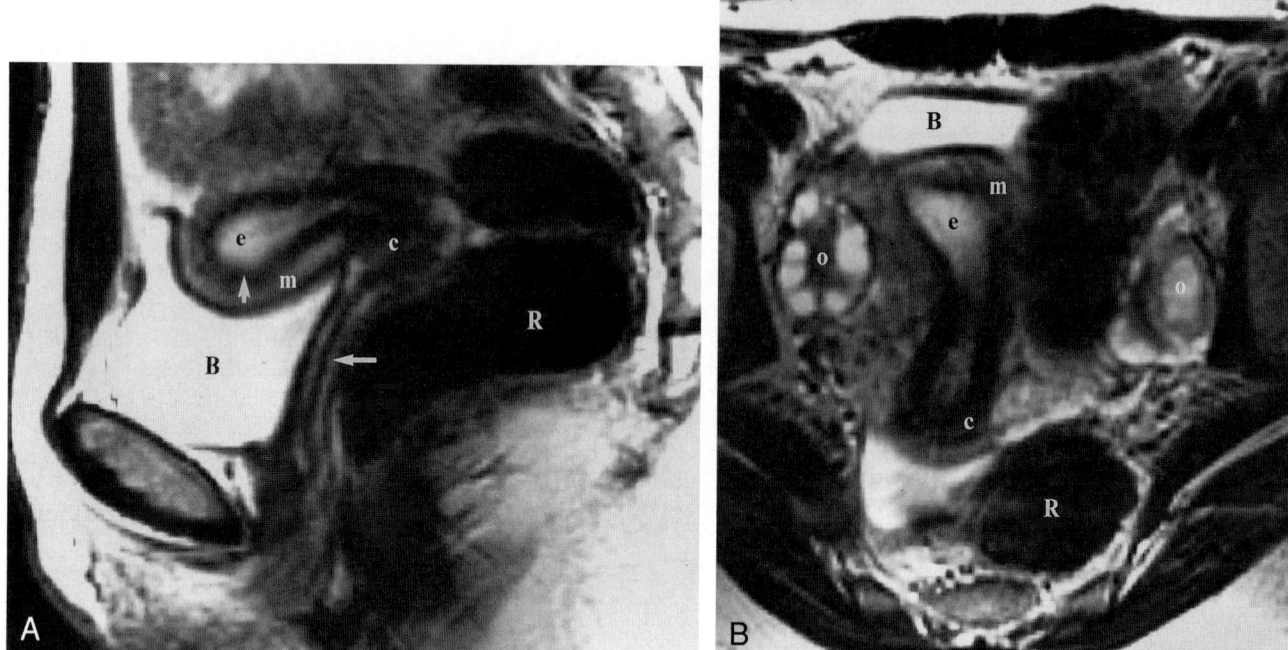

Figure 35.1. Normal MR Anatomy: Female. A. Sagittal midline T2WI. **B.** Axial T2WI. The uterus is in a normal anteverted position impressing on the bladder (*B*). The high signal intensity endometrium (*e*) is surrounded by the low signal intensity junctional zone (*arrowhead*) and the intermediate signal intensity myometrium (*m*). The cervix (*c*) is lower in signal intensity than the myometrium. Multiple follicles are seen on both ovaries (*o*). The vagina (*arrow*) has high intensity epithelium and low intensity muscular walls. *R*, rectum.

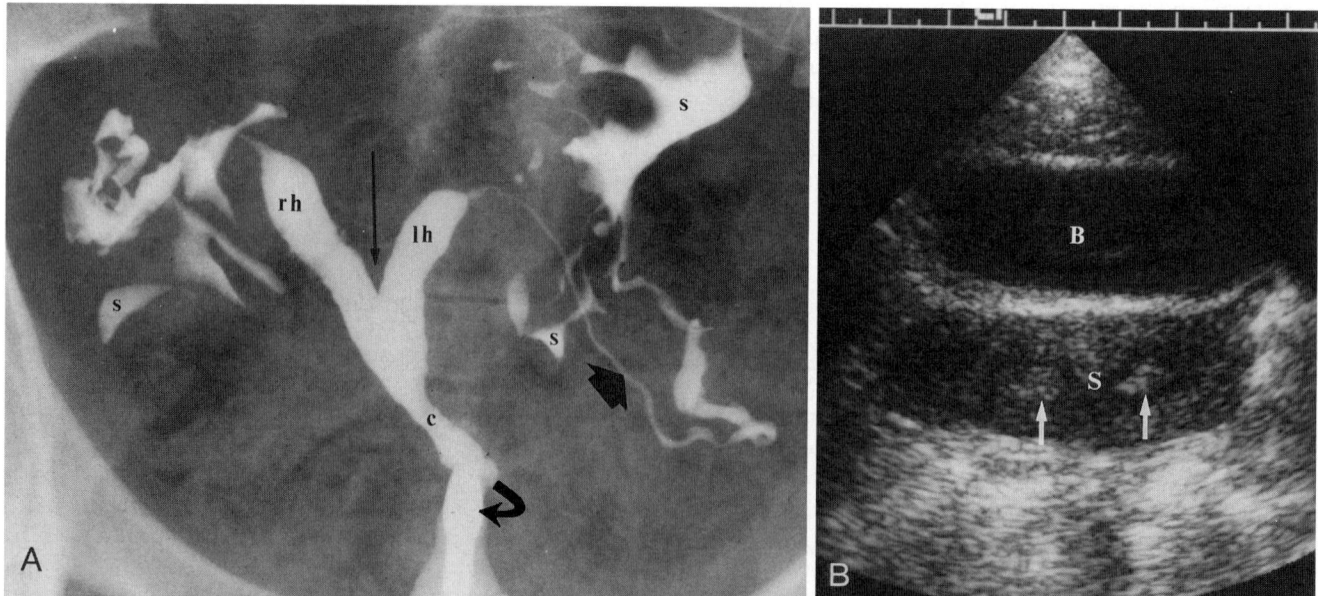

Figure 35.2. Septate Uterus. A. HSG demonstrates two horns of the uterine cavity (*rh, lh*) separated by a muscular septum (*long arrow*). The lumen of the left fallopian tube is well demonstrated (*arrowhead*), while the lumen of the right fallopian tube is obscured by the superimposed contrast. Free spill of contrast into the peritoneal cavity is evident (*s*), confirming the patency of both fallopian tubes. A contrast agent was injected into the uterus after placing a cannula (*curved arrow*) into the cervix (*c*). **B.** Axial plane US image of the uterus obtained through a filled bladder (*B*) demonstrates two separate uterine cavities (*arrows*) identified by their echogenic endometrium. The muscular septum (*S*) separating the uterine horns is evident.

Congenital Anomalies

Congenital anomalies of the female genital tract are a common cause of infertility, seen in up to 9% of women evaluated for infertility or repeated abortion. In addition, unrecognized anomalies may be mistaken for other types of pathology, such as leiomyoma.

Most anomalies result from arrested development or incomplete fusion of the paired müllerian duct that forms the uterus, cervix, and fallopian tubes. Urinary tract abnormalities are found in 20–50% of patients with uterine anomalies. Arrested müllerian duct development may result in uterine aplasia or unicornuate uterus with a single fallopian tube. Ipsilateral renal agenesis is found in 5–20% of patients with these anomalies. Failure of complete fusion of the müllerian duct results in varying degrees of duplication (Figs. 35.2, 35.3), from uterus didelphys, with two uteri, two cervices, and two vaginas; to bicornuate uterus with two uterine horns, one (unicollis) or two (bicollis) cervices, and one vagina; to a septate uterus with a midline septum dividing the uterus into two cavities. Uterine anomalies should be suspected when the uterus appears abnormal in size, contour, or position. The classification of the anomaly is made by a combination of physical examination, HSG to demonstrate the uterine cavity and fallopian tubes, and MR or US to define the contour of the uterus (Fig. 35.4)(4,15,16).

Gynecologic Malignancy

Ovarian Cancer represents 3% of all malignancy in women, but accounts for 15% of all cancer deaths. There are more than 20 histologic types of ovarian malignancy, however, epithelial (70%) and germ cell (15%) tumors account for the majority (17,18). Approximately 40% of ovarian tumors are malignant, two-thirds are cystic, and 25% are bilateral. The peak age of onset of ovarian cancer is 55–59. Ovarian malignancy has an insidious onset and a silent growth pattern that usually results in advanced disease at presentation in 70% of cases. CA-125 is a sero-

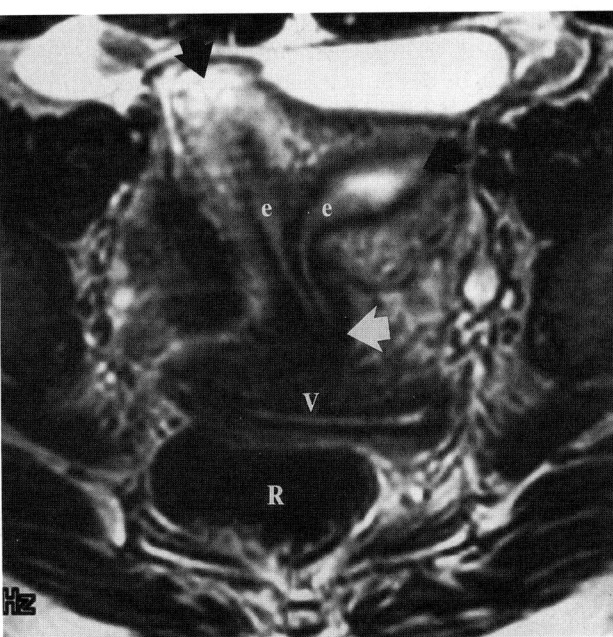

Figure 35.4. Bicornuate Unicollis Uterus. Axial plane T2-weighted MR image demonstrates two uterine horns (*black arrows*), each with a separate endometrial cavity (*e*) opening through a single cervix (*white arrow*). The high tissue differentiation and multiplanar capability of MR makes it ideal for defining congenital anomalies of the genital tract. *V*, vagina. *R*, rectum.

Table 35.1. Ovarian Cancer Staging (FIGO)

Stage	Description
I	**Tumor limited to ovaries**
Ia	Growth limited to one ovary
Ib	Growth limited to both ovaries
Ic	With malignant ascites or malignant peritoneal washings
II	**Tumor involves one or both ovaries with pelvic extension**
IIa	Extension to uterus and/or fallopian tubes
IIb	Extension to other pelvic tissues
IIc	With malignant ascites or malignant peritoneal washings
III	**Tumor involves one or both ovaries with peritoneal extension outside the pelvis and/or regional lymph node metastasis**
IIIa	Microscopic peritoneal metastasis beyond pelvis
IIIb	Macroscopic peritoneal metastasis beyond pelvis, 2 cm or less in greatest dimension, nodes are negative
IIIc	Peritoneal metastasis beyond pelvis more than 2 cm in greatest dimension and/or regional lymph node metastasis
IV	**Distant metastases**

FIGO = International Federation of Gynecology and Obstetrics
(Adapted from American Joint Committee on Cancer. Manual for Staging of Cancer. 4th ed. Philadelphia: JB Lippincott Company, 1992:167–169.)

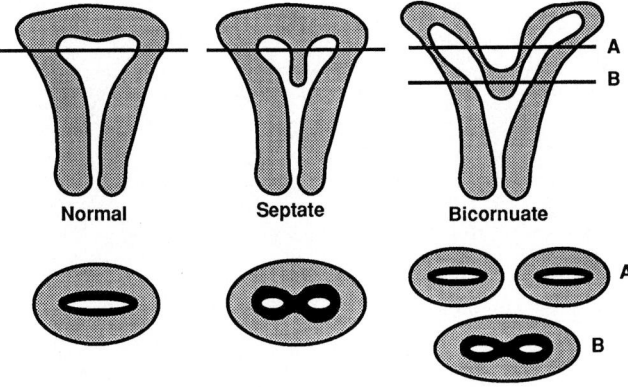

Figure 35.3. Uterine Anomalies. The normal uterus has a single oval endometrial cavity in axial plane images. The septate uterus has two endometrial cavities separated by a muscular septum. The fundus remains convex. The bicornuate uterus has two separate horns and a convex shape to the fundus. An axial plane image through the fundus (*A*) demonstrates no myometrial tissue between the two horns.

Normal   Septate   Bicornuate

logic marker for ovarian cancer found to be elevated in 80% of women with ovarian cancer. Unfortunately, it is more likely to be abnormal in advanced cancers and is elevated in only 25–50% of Stage I ovarian cancers. Survival correlates directly with the stage of disease which also determines treatment (Table 35.1)(19).

MR and CT signs of ovarian malignancy are similar to those listed for US in Chapter 37. Wall thickness greater than 3 mm, nodularity, vegetations, solid components, evidence of invasion of adjacent structures, ascites, contrast enhancement of the peritoneum and adenopathy are evidence of malignancy (Fig. 35.5).

Ovarian carcinoma spreads primarily by peritoneal seeding with small tumor nodules implanting on the peritoneum, mesentery, and omentum, and malignant ascites (Fig. 35.6). Secondary patterns of spread include direct extension to adjacent structures, lymphatic metastases to pelvic and retroperitoneal nodes, and late hematogenous spread to lung, liver, and bones. CT is used primarily for follow-up of known ovarian cancer (Fig. 35.7)(20). Because ovarian cancer is usually staged with surgical laparatomy, initial radiographic tumor staging is indicated only in clearly advanced cases. Initial treatment is total abdominal hysterectomy, bilateral salpingo-oophorectomy, omentectomy, and tumor debulking. Both CT and MR are poor in the detection of peritoneal metastases. Only tumor implants 2–3 cm in size in the absence of ascites and 0.5–1 cm in the presence of ascites are reliably detected. At the present time, MR is inferior to CT for ovarian cancer staging because of the difficulty differentiating tumor from bowel. No imaging method can reliably differentiate benign from malignant ovarian masses. This is not surprising because many cases are borderline malignant, even histologically.

Cervical Cancer is the most common gynecologic malignancy. Squamous carcinoma accounts for 95% and

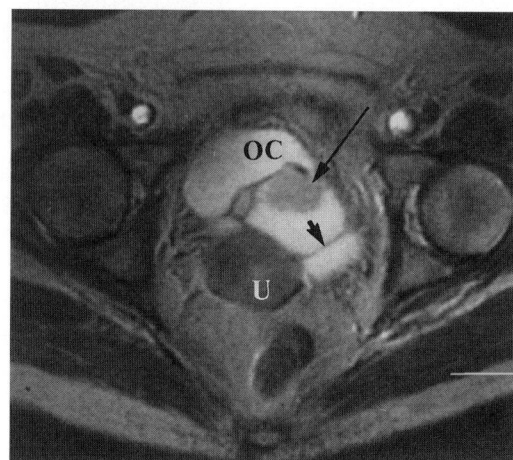
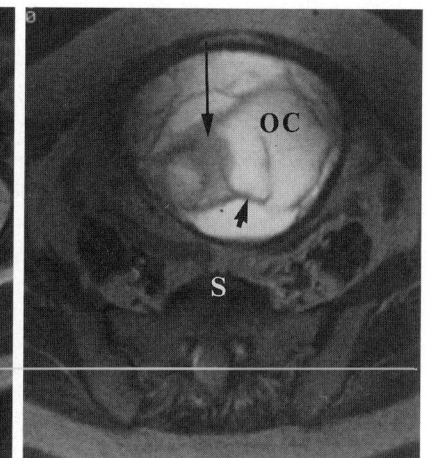

Figure 35.5. Ovarian Cystadenocarcinoma. Two axial plane, T2-weighted MR images demonstrated a complex pelvic mass (*OC*). The image on the left is at the level of the body of the uterus (*U*). The image on the right is 7 cm more superior, at the level of the sacral promontory (*S*). The fluid component of the mass was high intensity on both T1WI and T2WI, suggesting internal hemorrhage or proteinaceous fluid. Note the septations of varying thickness (*arrowheads*) and the solid nodular components (*arrows*).

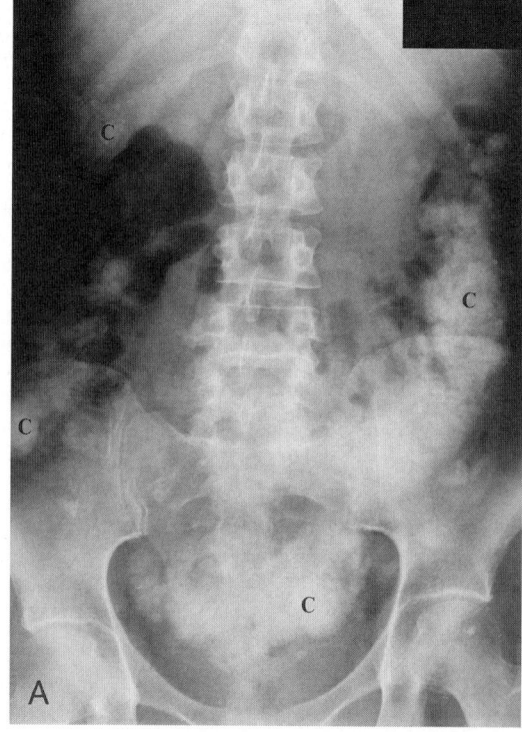
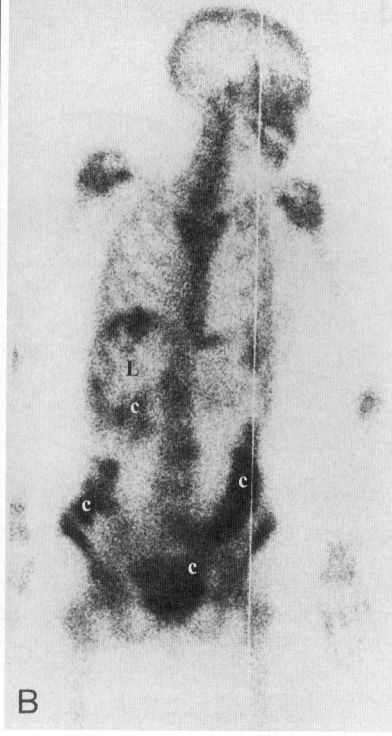

Figure 35.6. Metastatic Ovarian Carcinoma. A. A plain film radiograph of the abdomen demonstrates calcified implants of ovarian carcinoma (*C*) throughout the peritoneal cavity. **B.** A Tc-99m-MDP bone scan shows radionuclide uptake within the tumor nodules. Note the ghost of the liver (*L*) caused by tumor implantation on the peritoneal surface, rather than within, the liver. The pathologic diagnosis was metastatic papillary serous cystadenocarcinoma of the ovary.

adenocarcinoma for 5% of these cases. The peak age of onset is 45–55, but it is the second most common malignancy in women aged 15–34. Cervical cancer spreads predominantly by direct extension to involve the vagina, paracervical and parametrial tissues, and the bladder and rectum. Obstruction of the ureters is particularly common because of their proximity to the cervix. Lymphatic metastases to the pelvic, inguinal, and retroperitoneal nodes are common. Hematogenous metastases to the lung, bone, and brain occur only late in the course of the disease.

MR is usually preferred to CT for staging of proven disease (Table 35.2)(Fig. 35.8)(21). On T1WI, cervical carcinoma is isointense with the myometrium. On T2WI, the tumor is higher in signal compared with the lower signal in the normal tissue. A continuous rind of low signal cervical stroma surrounding the tumor is reliable evidence of the absence of parametrial invasion (9). Staging by CT requires excellent contrast enhancement to differentiate the tumor from normal tissue. Both MR and CT use node enlargement (>10 mm in short axis) as the primary criterion for involvement. This is inherently inaccurate because cervical cancer is known to involve nodes without enlarging them.

Endometrial Carcinoma is now the most common invasive gynecological malignancy. Histologically it is

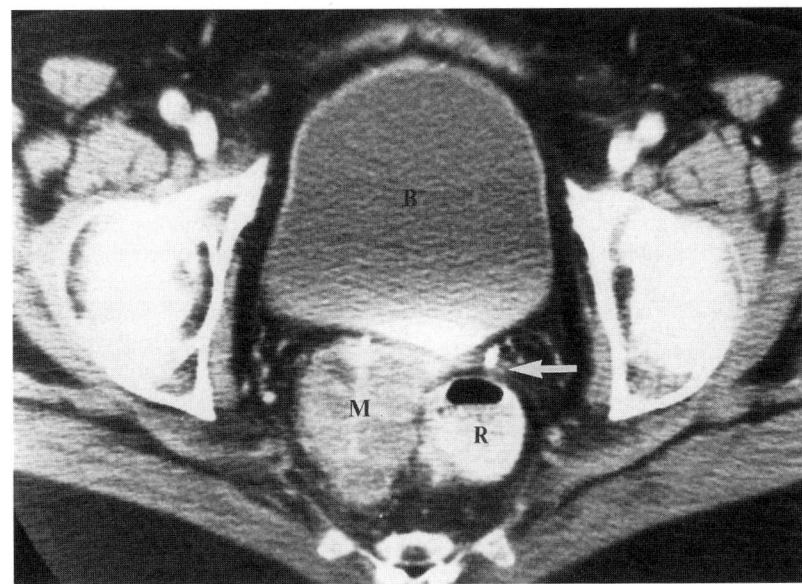

Figure 35.7. Recurrence of Ovarian Carcinoma. CT reveals an inhomogeneous solid mass (*M*) in the cul-de-sac in a patient who had undergone total hysterectomy and bilateral salpingo-oophorectomy for ovarian cancer. The top of the vaginal is marked by the *arrow*. This is a common location for ovarian tumor recurrence. *R*, rectum. *B*, bladder.

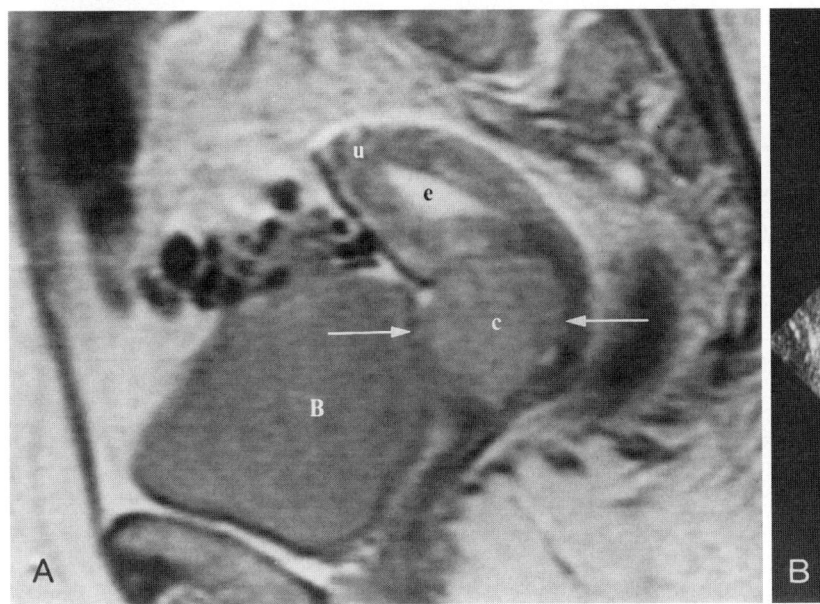

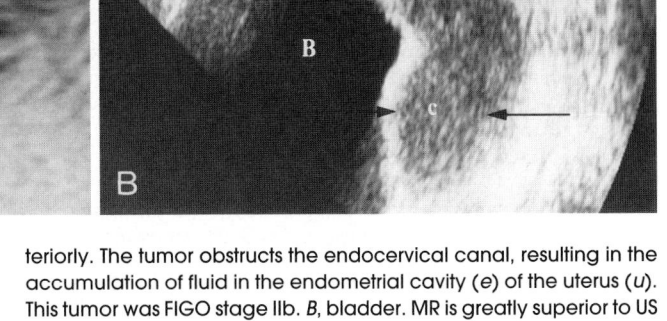

Figure 35.8. Cervical Carcinoma. Sagittal plane, proton density-weighted MR image **(A)**, and sagittal US image **(B)**, reoriented to match the MR, demonstrate a cervical carcinoma (*c*, between *arrows*) arising from the anterior lip of the cervix. The tumor invades the paracervical tissues anteriorly and the posterior lip of the cervix posteriorly. The tumor obstructs the endocervical canal, resulting in the accumulation of fluid in the endometrial cavity (*e*) of the uterus (*u*). This tumor was FIGO stage IIb. *B*, bladder. MR is greatly superior to US in revealing the extent of the tumor.

95% adenocarcinoma and 5% sarcoma. The peak age at onset is 55–62 years, with postmenopausal vaginal bleeding as the key symptom. The tumor spreads initially by invasion into the myometrium and cervix, followed by lymphatic spread to the pelvic and retroperitoneal nodes, then continued direct spread into the broad ligaments, parametrium, and ovaries. Peritoneal seeding will occur with penetration of the uterine serosa. Hematogenous spread to the lung, bone, liver, and brain occurs late in the course of the disease. Prognosis and treatment depend on stage of the disease (Table 35.3) with the most critical factors being the depth of myometrial invasion and the involvement of lymph nodes (22). Lymph node metastases are unlikely if myometrial invasion is less than 50% (23).

MR (Fig. 35.9) and transvaginal US have been used to stage the depth of myometrial invasion with accuracies for both reported in the 70–90% range (23–26). Gadolinium enhancement improves MR tumor staging (24,25). By MR. disease is considered confined to the en-dometrium (stage Ia) if the junction zone appears intact on T2WI. Invasion of the myometrium appears as high signal tumor invasion of the dark junctional zone or surrounding myometrium. Stage Ib and Ic are separated by measurement comparing tumor extension at its deepest point to the thickness of the myometrium. Transvaginal US staging is performed in a similar manner with the tumor appearing echogenic and the junctional zone myometrium appearing hypoechoic. CT and MR evidence of nodal metastases are lymph nodes larger than 10 mm in short axis.

Benign Conditions

Leiomyomas most commonly appear low-signal compared to myometrium on both T1WI and T2WI, although visualization is best on T2WI (Fig. 35.10)(8). Areas of degeneration and cystic change cause inhomogeneous high internal signal. The tumors are well-demarcated from adjacent myometrium by a discrete rim of low signal. Contrast enhancement does not improve leiomyoma detection or characterization (27).

On CT leiomyomas appear as homogeneous or heterogeneous masses that may be hypodense, isodense, or hyperdense relative to enhanced myometrium (28). Coarse calcifications within the mass are common and characteristic (Fig. 35.11). Cystic degeneration produces interior low density. Diffuse enlargement of the uterus and lobulation of its contour are common. Pedunculated leiomyomas may appear as adnexal rather than uterine masses.

Adenomyosis is best demonstrated on T2WI as focal or diffuse thickening of the junctional zone of the myometrium (>8 mm) with scattered foci of high signal in involved areas (8,29). Poor definition and ill-defined

Table 35.2. Cervical Cancer Staging (FIGO)

Stage		Description
0		**Carcinoma *in situ***
I		**Tumor confined to cervix**
	Ia	Preclinical invasive carcinoma diagnosed by microscopy only. Invasion no deeper than 5mm, no wider than 7mm
	Ib	Clinical lesions confined to cervix
II		**Tumor invades beyond cervix but not to pelvic wall or lower third of vagina**
	IIa	Without parametrial invasion
	IIb	With parametrial invasion
III		**Tumor extends to pelvic wall and/or involves lower third vagina and/or causes hydronephrosis**
	IIIa	No extension to pelvic side wall
	IIIb	Extension to pelvic widewall or hydronephrosis
IV	IVa	Tumor invades mucosa of bladder or rectum and/or extends to pelvic side walls
	IVb	Distant metastases

FIGO = International Federation of Gynecology and Obstetrics
(Adapted from American Joint Committee on Cancer. Manual for staging of cancer. 4th ed. Philadelphia: JB Lippincott Company, 1992:155–157.)

Table 35.3. Endometrial Cancer Staging (FIGO)

Stage		Description
0		Carcinoma *in situ*
I	Ia	Tumor limited to endometrium
	Ib	Tumor invasion of ≤50% thickness of myometrium
	Ic	Tumor invasion of >50% thickness of myometrium
II	IIa	Tumor invades cervical mucosa
	IIb	Tumor invades cervical mucosa and stroma
III		Tumor invades uterine serosa, parametrium, adnexa, or para-aortic lymph nodes
IV		Tumor invades mucosa of bladder or rectum and/or extends beyond the true pelvis or distant metastases

FIGO = International Federation of Gynecology and Obstetrics
(Adapted from Creasman WT. New Gynecologic Cancer Staging. Obstet Gynecol 1990;75:287–288.)

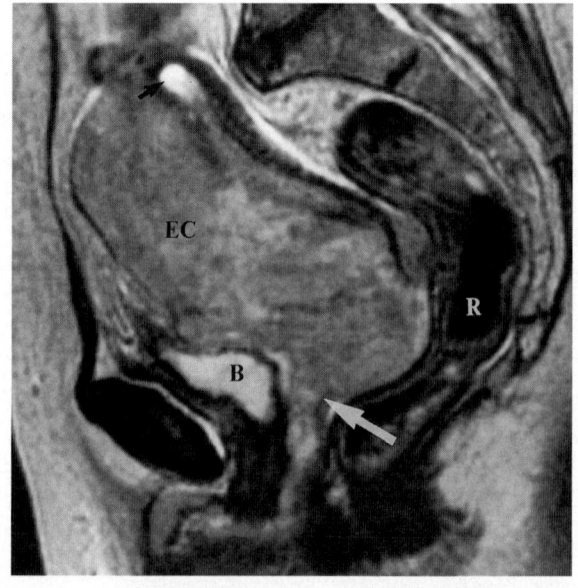

Figure 35.9. Endometrial Carcinoma. Midline sagittal plane T2-weighted MR shows extensive endometrial carcinoma (*EC*) invading and replacing the anterior myometrium and invading the upper vagina (*white arrow*), FIGO stage III. The anterior junctional zone is obliterated. Fluid (*black arrow*) is retained in the endometrial cavity in the uterine fundus. *R*, rectum. *B*, bladder.

margination differentiate adenomyosis from leiomyomas which are characteristically sharply circumscribed. Adenomyosis is not routinely evident on CT.

Nabothian cysts are retention cysts of the mucous-secreting glands of the cervical epithelium. They are common and are seen on MR as bright, round, well-defined structures in the cervix on T2WI (Fig. 35.12). On T1WI, they are isointense to urine or muscle.

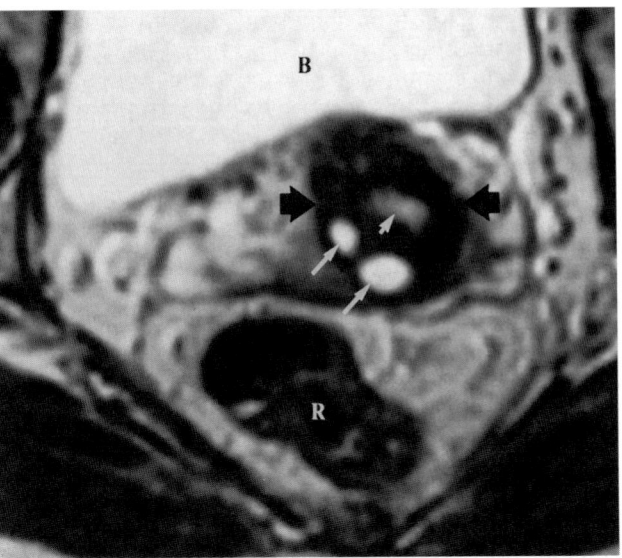

Figure 35.12. Nabothian Cysts. Axial T2WI demonstrates two nabothian cysts (*white arrows*) in the cervix (between *black arrows*). Note the normal low signal intensity of the cervix and the high signal of the endocervical canal (*white arrowhead*). *R*, rectum. *B*, bladder.

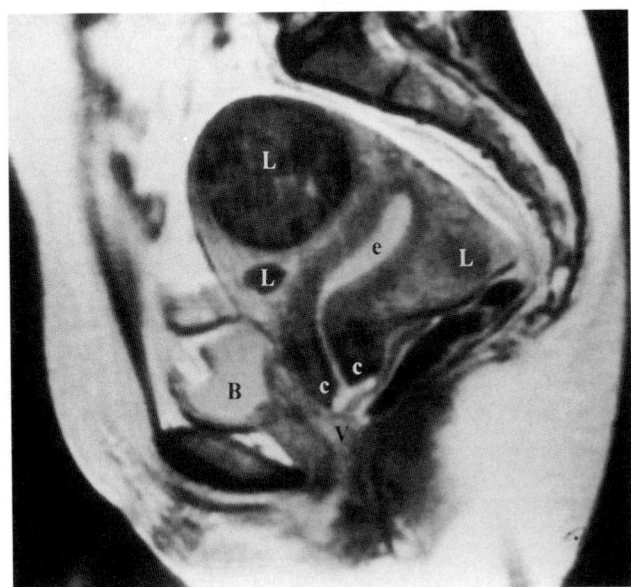

Figure 35.10. Multiple Leiomyomas. A midsagittal plane, T2-weighted MR image of the pelvis demonstrates multiple leiomyomas (*L*) which greatly enlarge and distort the uterus. The endometrial cavity (*e*) of the uterus and the cervix (*c*) are clearly demonstrated. *B*, bladder; *V*, vagina.

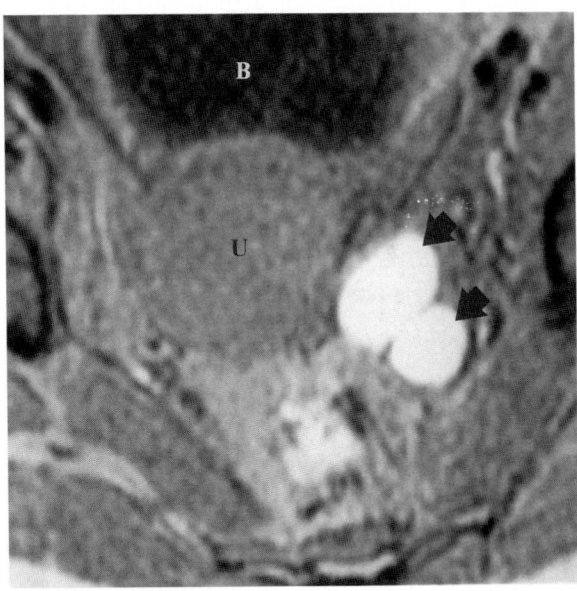

Figure 35.13. Hemorrhagic Follicular Cysts. Fat-suppressed T1WI shows high signal in two left ovarian cysts indicating internal hemorrhage. The cysts are well-defined, homogeneous, and lack any solid component. *U*, uterus. *B*, bladder.

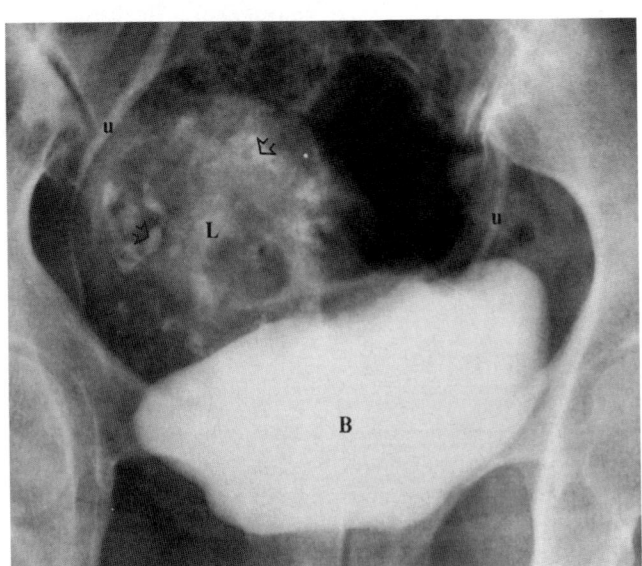

Figure 35.11. Leiomyoma Calcifications. A radiograph of the pelvis obtained as part of an excretory urogram demonstrates a leiomyoma (*L*) causing a mass impression on the bladder (*B*). Multiple characteristic "popcorn" calcifications (*open arrows*) are evident. *u*, ureters.

Physiological Ovarian Cysts contain simple fluid than is low signal on T1WI and high signal on T2WI (see Fig. 35.1)(30). A uniform, thin, dark wall is evident on T2WI. Gadolinium enhancement of the cyst wall is common but not constant. On CT they are well defined, thin walled, and have homogeneous internal density near water. Size less than 2.5 cm is indicative of physiological ovarian follicle.

Hemorrhagic Functional Ovarian Cysts appear high signal on T1WI if a large amount of methemoglobin is present (Fig. 35.13). If predominantly intact red blood cells are present, the cyst appear low signal on T2WI. Thus hemorrhagic cysts may be low signal on both T1WI and T2WI, high signal on T1WI and low signal on T2WI, or low signal on T1WI and high signal on T2WI (31,32). Layering of blood products may be present. The absence of gadolinium enhancement differentiates blood clot adherent to the cyst wall from a solid nodule. On CT, hemorrhagic cysts appear thin walled. Internal density may be near water or higher depending on the physical state of the blood products. Atypical cysts can be followed with US to determine if they resolve after one or two menstrual cycles.

Endometriomas are similar to hemorrhagic ovarian cysts in MR appearance (Fig. 35.14). Multiplicity, distorted shape, and shading favor endometriosis (31,32). Most hemorrhagic cysts are solitary and round. Most characteristic is high signal in multiple cysts on T1WI with low intensity "shading" on T2WI. Endometriomas commonly have a thick shaggy fibrotic wall containing hemosiderin-laden macrophages seen in a low-intensity rim on T2WI. Fat-saturation T1WI improves visualization of small implants on peritoneal surfaces (33).

On CT endometriomas appear as complex cystic pelvic masses, frequently with high density fluid components. Inflammation and fibrosis are prominent. Multiple pelvic organs may be incorporated into the mass.

Benign Cystic Teratoma characterization by MR depends on demonstration of fat by chemical shift artifact or fat-suppresion imaging (34). Fat or sebaceous material within the cyst follows the signal intensity of subcutaneous fat on all imaging sequences. Fat-fluid levels, layering of debris, dermoid plugs, and calcification are additional findings. A small percentage of cystic teratomas contain simple fluid showing low signal on T1WI and high signal on T2WI. These may be diagnosed as teratomas by demonstration of small deposits of fat in the walls (35). The presence of fat, teeth (Fig. 35.15), bone formation, hair, or fat-fluid levels allows definitive CT diagnosis in most cases (36).

Hydrosalpinx is a common finding on HSG performed for infertility (Fig. 35.16). Occlusion of the fallopian tube results in fluid accumulation and dilatation of the tube. The most common cause is pelvic infection.

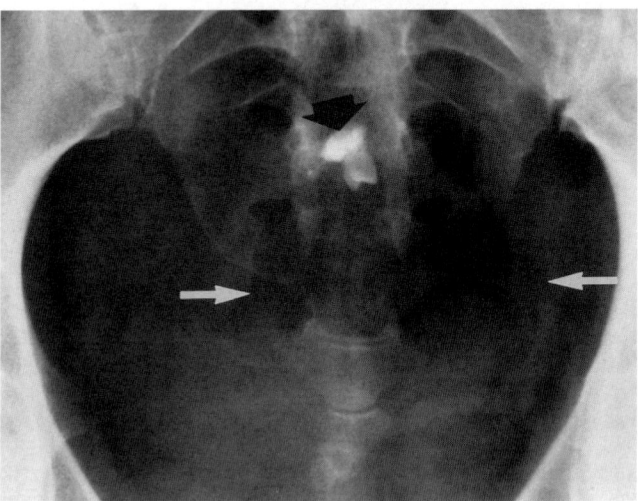

Figure 35.15. Benign Cystic Teratoma. A plain radiograph of the pelvis in a young woman demonstrates several well-formed teeth (*black arrow*). A subtle, well-defined mass of fat density is also present (*white arrows*). These findings are diagnostic of benign cystic teratoma.

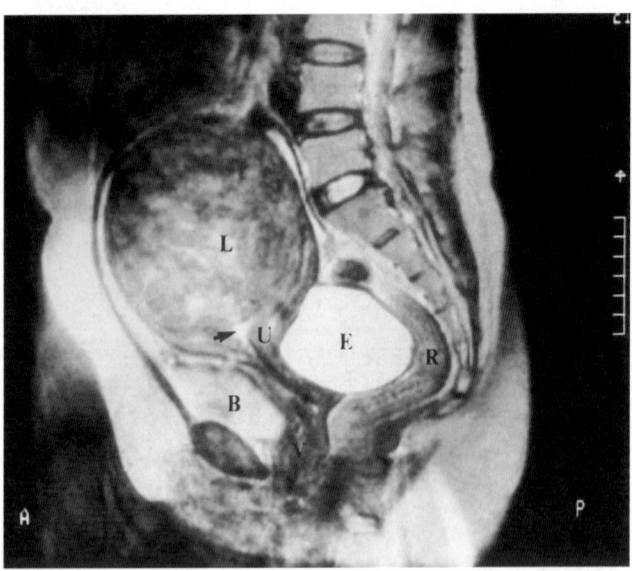

Figure 35.14. Endometrioma and Leiomyoma. A midsagittal plane, T2-weighted MR demonstrates a large leiomyoma (*L*) arising from the anterior aspect of the uterus (*U*) and a large endometrioma (*E*) in the cul-de-sac between uterus and rectum (*R*). The high-signal intensity of the endometrioma on a T2WI is nonspecific and compatible with any hemorrhagic cyst. The endometrial cavity of the uterus is indicated by the *arrowhead*. *B*, bladder; *V*, vagina. (Case courtesy of Roy A. Kottal, MD, Cedar Rapids, Iowa.)

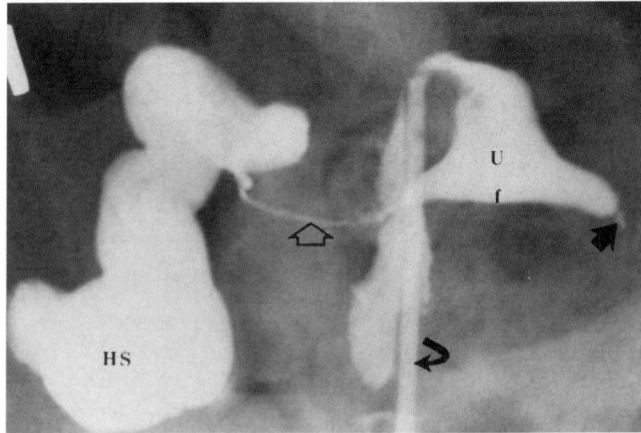

Figure 35.16. Hydrosalpinx. Hysterosalpingography demonstrates a retroflexed uterus (*U*) with the fundus (*f*) directed posteriorly and inferiorly. The left fallopian tube is occluded at the isthmus (*black arrow*). The right fallopian tube (*open arrow*) is massively dilated at its distal end, forming a hydrosalpinx (*HS*). Occlusion of the right fallopian tube is confirmed by the absence of peritoneal spill. The *curved arrow* indicates the cervical cannula.

MALE GENITAL TRACT

Testes and Scrotum

US, supplemented by color Doppler, is the imaging method of choice to demonstrate the testes and scrotal contents. MR using surface coils offers excellent spatial resolution, greater tissue contrast, and wider field of view, but has the disadvantages of greater cost and lesser availability. Radionuclide imaging provides useful information about perfusion, but with limited anatomic detail. CT is useful in the staging of testicular tumors and in locating undescended testes that are not found by US. US imaging of the testes and scrotum is covered in chapter 37.

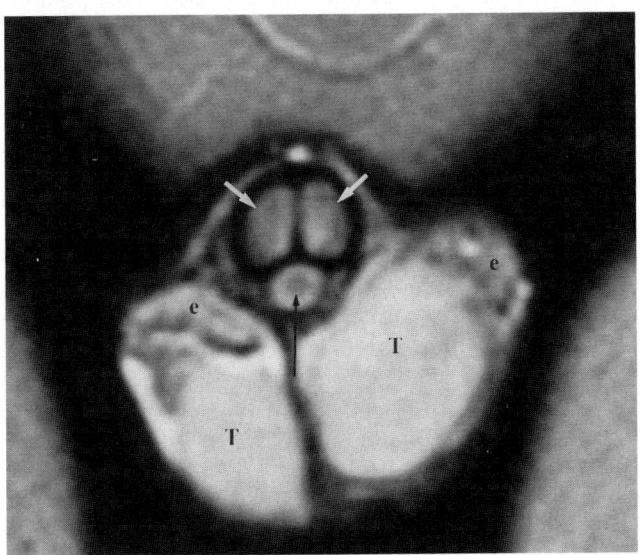

Figure 35.17. Normal MR Anatomy: Male. Coronal plane T2-weighted MR shows both testes (*T*) and the penis in cross-section. The testes are high in signal because of their high fluid content. The epididymis (*e*) is also high signal on T2WI but less than that of the testes. The paired corpora cavernosa (*white arrows*) are well demonstrated. The corpus spongiosum contains the urethra (*black arrow*).

Normal MR Anatomy. Because of its high fluid content, the testes are of uniform intermediate signal on T1WI and uniform high signal, slightly less than water, on T2WI (Fig. 35.17)(37,38). The tunica albuginea forms a well-defined 1 mm thick rim. Septations are often visualized radiating from the mediastinum to the tunica albuginea. A small amount of fluid is normally present in the scrotum between the layers of the tunica vaginalis. The epididymis is isointense to the testes on T1WI and brightens on T2WI, though to a lesser extent than the testis. The scrotum is intermediate signal reflecting the dartos muscle. The spermatic cord appears as numerous tubular structures representing the arteries and veins with MR signal determined by blood flow.

Undescended Testis. CT and MR are used to localize undescended testes not demonstrated by US to be within the inguinal canal. The testis, if present, will be seen between the lower pole of the kidney and the internal inguinal ring. In 3–5% of cases, the testis is congenitally absent. The undescended testis appears as an oval soft tissue mass up to 4 cm in size (Fig. 35.18). Because the undescended testis is usually atrophic, MR may show low or intermediate, instead of high signal, on T2WI.

Neoplasms. Germ cell tumors, stromal tumors, lymphoma and leukemia all appear on T2WI as low signal areas of tumor within the high signal normal testicular parenchyma (38). Normal parenchymal septations are disrupted by the tumor. High signal areas within tumors correspond to areas of hemorrhage. MR cannot reliably differentiate benign from malignant tumors.

CT and MR are used for staging of tumors. Lymphatic spread is most common with nodal involvement following an orderly ascending pattern. Inital spread is along gonadal lymphatics following testicular veins to renal hilar nodes. Alternatively, lymphatic metastases may follow the external iliac chain to the paraaortic nodes. Internal iliac and inguinal nodes are usually not involved. Lymphatic spread to the mediastinum and hematogenous spread to the lungs rarely occurs without

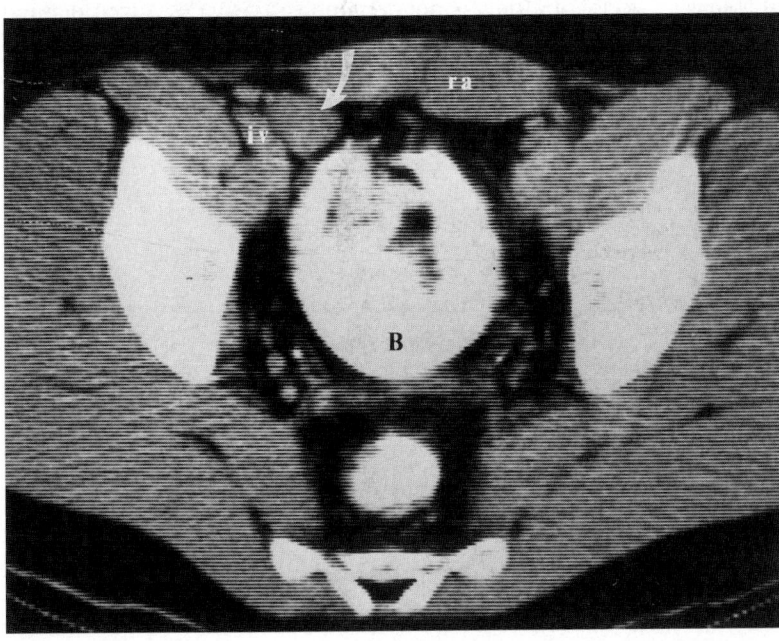

Figure 35.18. Undescended Testis. CT of a 25-year-old man demonstrates his right undescended testis (*arrow*) in the abdomen at the level of his right internal inguinal ring. The testis is similar to muscle in CT density. *B*, bladder; *iv*, external iliac vessels; *ra*, rectus abdominis muscle.

paraaortic disease, except for choriocarcinoma, which spreads hematogenously early.

Scrotal Fluid Collections. Simple hydroceles show signal characteristics of water, low signal on T1WI and high signal on T2WI. Hematoceles and pyoceles show high signal on T1WI, reflecting complex fluid or high protein content. Epididymal cysts show the signal of simple fluid. Spermatoceles commonly contain fat and high protein causing high signal on T1WI, and layering debris may be evident. Varicoceles appear as serpiginous tubular structures in the spermatic cord. Signal intensity corresponds to slow blood flow.

Epididymitis/Orchitis. Orchitis causes inhomogeneous signal on both T1WI and T2WI, indistinguishable from tumor. With epididymitis, the epididymis is enlarged but signal intensity on T2WI is unpredictable and may be increased, decreased, or normal. Dilated vessels in the spermatic cord reflect hypervascularity. Hydrocele is usually present.

Testicular Torsion is best evaluated with Doppler US or scintigraphy. With acute torsion, MR may demonstrate a characteristic twisted pattern of torsion of the spermatic cord with impaired blood flow evident. The testis appears heterogeneous on all image sequences (39).

Prostate and Seminal Vesicles

The role of imaging in prostate disease is heavily debated and has been the subject of numerous published studies (40). No imaging modality can reliably demonstrate the presence or absence of cancer in the prostate. That diagnosis relies on biopsy which is best performed using transrectal US for guidance (41). MR with endorectal coils and transrectal US offer (42–44)the best promise for staging of local disease. Either CT or MR may be used to demonstrate evidence of nodal and distant tumor spread.

Normal MR Anatomy. The prostate is divided into three glandular zones surrounding the urethra (Fig. 35.19)(45). The *peripheral zone* contains approximately 70% of prostate tissue and is draped around the remainder of the gland like a glove holding a baseball. Most prostate cancers (70%) arise in the peripheral zone. The *transitional zone* consists of two small areas of periurethral glandular tissue. Although it contains only 5% of prostatic tissue in the normal young man, it is the site of

benign prostatic hypertrophy and may enlarge greatly in the older man. The *central zone* consists of the glandular tissue at the base of the prostate through which course the ducts of the vas deferens and seminal vesicles and the ejaculatory ducts. Although the central zone makes up 25% of glandular tissue, only 10% of cancers arise there. The anterior portion of the prostate is occupied by nonglandular tissue called the anterior *fibromuscular stroma.* The *base* of the prostate is that portion adjacent to the base of the bladder and the seminal vesicles. The *apex* of the prostate rests on the urogenital diaphragm.

The seminal vesicles are symmetrically sized, lobulated, teardrop-shaped coiled ducts that occupy the groove between the base of the bladder and the base of the prostate posteriorly. Prominent veins are frequently visualized in the periprostatic tissues (46). Lymphatic drainage of the prostate goes to regional pelvic lymph nodes with channels to paraaortic and inguinal nodes. Periprostatic venous connections to vertebral veins offer a route for the hematogenous spread of tumor to the axial skeleton

On T1WI, the prostate gland is uniform low signal similar to skeletal muscle (47,48). The high signal periprostatic fat defines the margin of the prostate. Periprostatic veins and neurovascular bundles are low signal. On T2WI, the internal structure (zonal anatomy) of the prostate is demonstrated (Fig. 35.20). The peripheral zone is high in signal due to higher water content and looser acinar structure. The central zone is lower in signal due to more compact muscle fibers and acinar structure. The central and transitional zones become heterogeneous with age and development of benign prostatic hyperplasia. The anterior fibromuscular stroma is low in signal and has poorly defined margins. The seminal vesicles are low to intermediate signal on T1WI and brighten greatly on T2WI due to fluid within the tubules (49). The normal size of the seminal vesicles varies widely, and slight asymmetry is common.

Normal CT Anatomy. The prostate gland is seen at the base of the bladder as a homogeneous rounded soft tissue organ up to 4 cm in maximal diameter. Prostate zonal anatomy is not demonstrated by CT. A well-defined plane of fat separates the prostate from the obturator internus. The paired seminal vesicles produce a characteristic "bow-tie"-shaped soft tissue structure in the groove between the bladder base and the prostate.

Figure 35.19. Zonal Anatomy of the Prostate. The anatomy is illustrated in midsagittal plane (*left*) and axial plane (*right*) at the level of the vertical *dashed line* on the left.

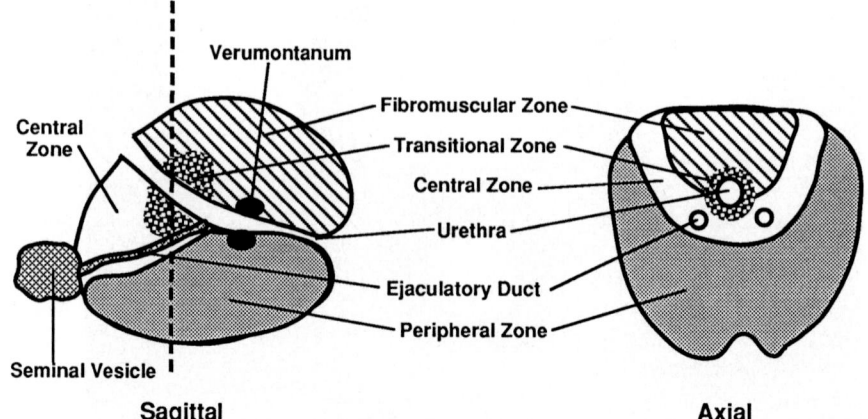

Verumontanum

Central Zone

Fibromuscular Zone

Transitional Zone

Central Zone

Urethra

Ejaculatory Duct

Peripheral Zone

Seminal Vesicle

Sagittal

Axial

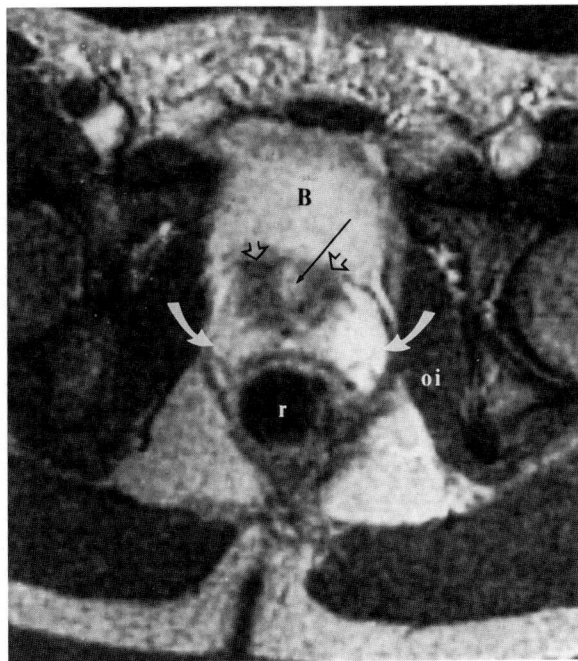

Figure 35.20. Normal Prostate by MR. Axial plane T2-weighted MR of a normal prostate obtained on a 1.5 tesla unit demonstrates the high-intensity peripheral zone (*curved arrows*), the urethra (*long arrow*), and the lower intensity transitional zone (*open arrows*). B, bladder; r, rectum; oi, obturator internus muscle.

Prostate Carcinoma. Prostate cancer is the third leading cause of cancer death in men. Approximately 10% of males over age 50 will develop clinical prostate carcinoma in their lifetime. Despite the high prevalence and importance of prostate disease, the diagnosis and treatment remain extremely controversial. One of the difficulties of dealing with prostate cancer is differentiating tumors with biological aggressiveness from those that are incidental findings. Nearly 50% of men older than 75 years of age will have prostate carcinoma on biopsy or autopsy. However, many of these cancers will not affect the patient's life span. The tumor is uncommon before age 50 and increases in incidence thereafter. The Gleason histologic grading system is used to assess the degree of differentiation of the tumor. A grade 1 is well differentiated, but a grade 5 is anaplastic. The Gleason score varies from 2–10 and adds the Gleason grade for the predominant and the secondary portions of the tumors. Tumor staging is by the American Urological Association system (Table 35.4). Most (95%) tumors are adenocarcinoma. Prostate cancer spreads by local extension, lymphatic vessels to regional nodes, and by hematogenous dissemination. Penetration of tumor through the capsule or into the seminal vesicles greatly worsens the prognosis (Fig. 35.21). Involvement of the axial skeleton by hematogenous metastases is common. Metastases to the lungs, liver, and kidneys occur in the terminal phases of the disease.

On MR T2WI, cancers appear as areas of low signal within the high signal peripheral zone (Fig. 35.21). Cancer is isointense with prostate tissue on T1WI, which are best used for assessing invasion of periprostatic fat and for detecting nodal involvement. Recent biopsy limits the specificity of MR because areas of hemorrhage may mimic tumor.

CT is limited to the demonstration of adenopathy and distant spread of tumor, because it cannot differentiate tumor from benign hyperplasia within the gland.

Benign Prostatic Hyperplasia begins at approximately age 40 and eventually occurs in all men. Hypertrophy and hyperplasia occur in glandular tissue in the transitional and periurethral zones accompanied by proliferation of supporting smooth muscle and stromal cells. The end result is focal or diffuse enlargement of the prostate. Pressure on the urethra obstructs bladder outflow and results in symptoms of hesitancy, decreased force and caliber of the urine stream, dribbling,

Table 35.4. Prostate Cancer Staging: 1992 Revision of TNM Classification

Stage	Description
Primary Tumor	
TX	**Not assessable**
T0	**Not evident**
T1	**Clinically apparent, not palpable or visible by imaging**
T1a	Found incidently in 5% or less of tissue resected
T1b	Found incidently in more than 5% of tissue resected
T1c	Identified by needle biopsy due to elevated PSA
T2	**Palpable or visible by imaging**
T2a	Involves half of one lobe or less
T2b	Involves more than half of one lobe, but not both lobes
T2c	Involves both lobes
T3	**Extends through prostate capsule**
T3a	Found unilaterally
T3b	Found bilaterally
T3c	Invades seminal vesicles
T4	**Fixed, or invades other structures**
T4a	Invades bladder neck, external sphincter, or rectum
T4b	Invades levator muscles or is fixed to pelvic wall
Regional Lymph Nodes	
NX	Regional lymph nodes cannot be assessed
N0	No regional lymph nodes metastases
N1	Metastases to single lymph node 2 cm or less in greatest dimension
N2	Metastases to single lymph node 2–5 cm in greatest dimension, or to multiple lymph nodes all less than 5 cm in greatest dimension
N3	Metastases to regional lymph node greater than 5 cm in greatest dimension
Distant Metastases	
MX	Metastases cannot be assessed
M0	No distant metastases
M1	Distant metastases present

(Adapted from Schroeder FH, Hermanek P, Denis L, et al. The TNM classification of prostate cancer. Prostate 1992;4(suppl):129–138.)

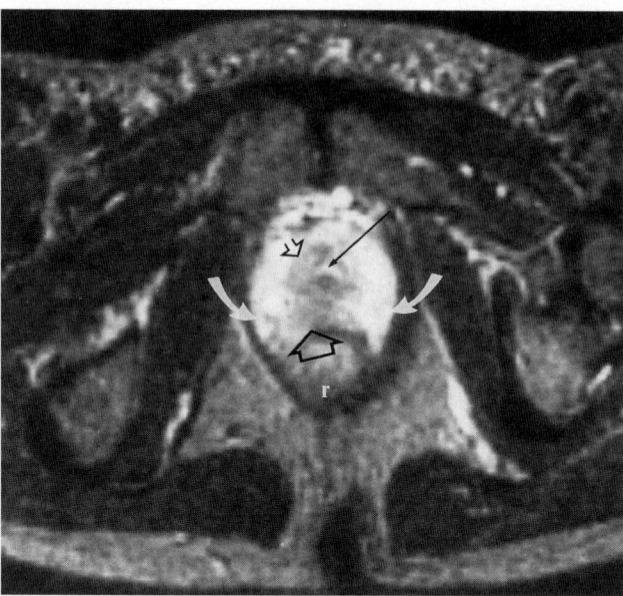

Figure 35.21. Prostate Carcinoma, Stage B2. Proton density-weighted, axial plane, 1.5 tesla MR image demonstates a low-intensity prostate carcinoma (*large open arrow*) in the peripheral zone (*curved arrows*). The tumor is confined to prostate gland and measures approximately 2 cm. The urethra (*long arrow*) and dark transitional zone (*small open arrow*) are evident. *r,* rectum.

frequency, nocturia, and postvoid residual. This progressive process is combatted by hypertrophy of the bladder wall musculature. Advanced symptoms require medical therapy (finasteride-Proscar, flutamide, casodex, etc.) balloon dilatation, stents, or transurethral resection (TURP)(50).

CT findings include the following: *a)* enlargement of the prostate, commonly with lobulated contour and visible high and low density nodules; *b)* coarse calcifications; *c)* cystic degeneration; *d)* bladder wall thickening and trabecuation.

MR shows prostate enlargement with heterogeneous central gland on T2WI. Areas of cystic degeneration are low signal on T1WI and high signal on T2WI.

References

1. Outwater EK, Dunton CJ. Imaging of the ovary and adnexa: clinical issues and applications of MR imaging. Radiology 1995;194:1–18.
2. Olson MC, Posniak HV, Tempany CM, Dudiak CM. MR imaging of the female pelvic region. RadioGraphics 1992; 12:445–465.
3. Slanetz PJ, Hahn PF, Hall DA, Mueller PR. The frequency and significance of adnexal lesions incidentally revealed by CT. AJR Am J Roentgenol 1997;168:647–650.
4. Pellerito JS, McCarthy SM, Doyle MB, et al. Diagnosis of uterine anomalies: relative accuracy of MR imaging, endovaginal sonography, and hysterosalpingography. Radiology 1992;183:795–800.
5. Yoder IC, Hall DA. Hysterosalpingography in the 1990s. AJR Am J Roentgenol 1991;157:675–683.
6. Krysiewicz S. Infertility in women: diagnostic evaluation with hysterosalpingography and other imaging techniques. AJR Am J Roentgenol 1992;159:253–261.
7. Hoetzinger H. Hysterosonography and hysterography in benign and malignant diseases of the uterus—a comparative in vitro study. J Ultrasound Med 1991;10:259–263.
8. Kier R. Magnetic resonance imaging of the uterus. MRI Clin North Am 1994;2:189–210.
9. Mezrich R. Magnetic resonance imaging applications in uterine cervical cancer. MRI Clin North Am 1994; 2:211–243.
10. deSouza NM, Hawley IC, Schwieso JE, et al. The uterine cervix on in vitro and in vivo MR images: a study of zonal anatomy and vascularity using an enveloping cervical coil. AJR Am J Roentgenol 1994;163:607–612.
11. Outwater EK, Talerman A, Dunton C. Normal adnexa uteri specimens: anatomic basis of MR imaging features. Radiology 1996;201:751–755.
12. Foshager MC, Walsh JW. CT anatomy of the female pelvis: a second look. RadioGraphics 1994;14:51–66.
13. Ott DJ, Fayez JA. Hysterosalpingography: A Text and Atlas. Baltimore: Urban & Schwarzenberg, 1991.
14. Karasick S, Lev-Toaff AS, Toaff MEA. Imaging of uterine leiomyomas. AJR Am J Roentgenol 1992;158:799–805.
15. Fielding JR. MR imaging of Müllerian anomalies: impact on therapy. AJR Am J Roentgenol 1996;167:1491–1495.
16. Woodward PJ, Wagner BJ, Farley TE. MR imaging in the evaluation of female infertility. RadioGraphics 1993;13: 293–310.
17. Wagner BJ, Buck JL, Seidman JD, McCabe KM. Ovarian epithelial neoplasms: radiologic-pathologic correlation. RadioGraphics 1994;14:1351–1374.
18. Brammer HM III, Buck JL, Hayes WS, et al. Malignant germ cell tumors of the ovary: radiologic-pathologic correlation. RadioGraphics 1990;10:715–724.
19. Qazi F, McGuire WP. The treatment of epithelial ovarian cancer. CA Cancer J Clin 1995;45:88–101.
20. Forstner R, Hricak H, Occhipinti K, et al. Ovarian cancer: staging with CT and MR imaging. Radiology 1995;197: 619–626.
21. Hricak H, Yu KK. Radiology in invasive cervical cancer. AJR Am J Roentgenol 1996;167:1101–1108.
22. Creasman WT. New gynecologic cancer staging. Obstet Gynecol 1990;75.
23. Scoutt LM, McCarthy SM, Flynn SD, et al. Clinical stage I endometrial carcinoma: pitfalls in preoperative assessment with MR imaging. Radiology 1995;194:567–572.
24. Yamashita Y, Harada M, Sawada T, et al. Normal uterus and FIGO stage I endometrial carcinoma: dynamic gadolinium-enhanced MR imaging. Radiology 1993;186: 495–501.
25. Yamashita Y, Mizutani H, Torashima M, et al. Assessment of myometrial invasion by endometrial carcinoma: transvaginal sonography vs contrast-enhanced MR imaging. AJR Am J Roentgenol 1993;161:595–599.
26. DelMaschio A, Vanzulli A, Sironi S, et al. Estimating the depth of myometrial involvement by endometrial carcinoma: efficacy of transvaginal sonography vs MR imaging. AJR Am J Roentgenol 1993;160:533–538.
27. Hricak H, Finck S, Honda G, Göranson H. MR imaging in the evaluation of benign uterine masses: value of gadopentetate dimeglumine-enhanced T1-weighted images. AJR Am J Roentgenol 1992;158:1043–1050.
28. Casillas J, Joseph RC, Guerra JJ Jr. CT appearance of uterine leiomyomas. Radiographics 1990;10:999–1007.
29. Kang S, Turner DA, Foster GS, et al. Adenomyosis: specificity of 5 mm as the maximum normal uterine junctional zone thickness in MR images. AJR Am J Roentgenol 1996; 166:1145–1150.

30. Outwater EK, Mitchell DG. Normal ovaries and functional cysts: MR appearance. Radiology 1996;198:397–402.

31. Jain KA, Jeffrey RB Jr. Evaluation of pelvic masses with magnetic resonance imaging and ultrasonography. J Ultrasound Med 1994;13:845–853.

32. Jain KA. Prospective evaluation of adnexal masses with endovaginal gray-scale and duplex and color Doppler US: correlation with pathologic findings. Radiology 1994;191:63–67.

33. Ha HK, Lim YT, Kim HS, et al. Diagnosis of pelvic endometriosis: fat-suppressed T1-weighted vs. conventional MR images. AJR Am J Roentgenol 1994;163:127–131.

34. Stevens SK, Hricak H, Campos Z. Teratomas versus cystic hemorrhagic adnexal lesions: differentiation with proton-selective fat-saturation MR imaging. Radiology 1993;186:481–488.

35. Yamashita Y, Hatanaka Y, Torashima M, et al. Mature cystic teratomas of the ovary without fat in the cystic cavity: MR features in 12 cases. AJR Am J Roentgenol 1994;163:613–616.

36. Dodd GD III, Budzik RF Jr. Lipomatous tumors of pelvis in women: spectrum of imaging findings. AJR Am J Roentgenol 1990;155:317–322.

37. Baker LL, Hajek PC, Burkhard TK, et al. MR imaging of the scrotum: normal anatomy. Radiology 1987;163:89–92.

38. Cramer BM, Schlegel EA, Thueroff JW. MR imaging in the differential diagnosis of scrotal and testicular disease. RadioGraphics 1991;11:9–21.

39. Mattrey RF. Magnetic resonance imaging of the scrotum. Semin Ultrasound CT MR 1991;12:95–108.

40. D'Amico AV. The role of MR imaging in the selection of therapy for prostate cancer. MRI Clin North Am 1996;4:471–479.

41. Melchior SW, Brawer MK. Role of transrectal ultrasound and prostate biopsy. J Clin Ultrasound 1996;24:463–471.

42. Harris RD, Schned AR, Heaney JA. Staging of prostate cancer with endorectal MR imaging: lessons from a learning curve. RadioGraphics 1995;15:813–829.

43. Jager GJ, Ruijter ETG, van de Kaa CA, et al. Local staging of prostate cancer with endorectal MR imaging: correlation with histopathology. AJR Am J Roentgenol 1996;166:845–852.

44. Presti JC Jr., Hricak H, Narayan PA, et al. Local staging of prostatic carcinoma: comparison of transrectal sonography and endorectal MR imaging. AJR Am J Roentgenol 1996;166:103–108.

45. Hardt NS, Kaude JV, Li KC, et al. Sonography of the prostate: in vitro correlation of sonographic and anatomic findings in normal glands. AJR Am J Roentgenol 1988;151:955–959.

46. Neumaier CE, Martinoli C, Derchi LE, et al. Normal prostate gland: examination with color Doppler US. Radiology 1995;196:453–457.

47. White Nunes L, Schiebler MS, Rauschning W, et al. The normal prostate and periprostatic structures: correlation between MR images made with and endorectal coil and cadaveric microtome sections. AJR Am J Roentgenol 1995;164:923–927.

48. Banson ML. Normal MR anatomy and techniques for imaging of the male pelvis. MRI Clin North Am 1996;4:481–496.

49. Secaf E, Nuruddin RN, Hricak H, et al. MR imaging of the seminal vesicles. AJR Am J Roentgenol 1991;156:989–994.

50. Keetch DW, Andriole GL. Medical therapy for benign prostatic hypertrophy. AJR Am J Roentgenol 1995;164:11–15.

Section VIII ULTRASOUND

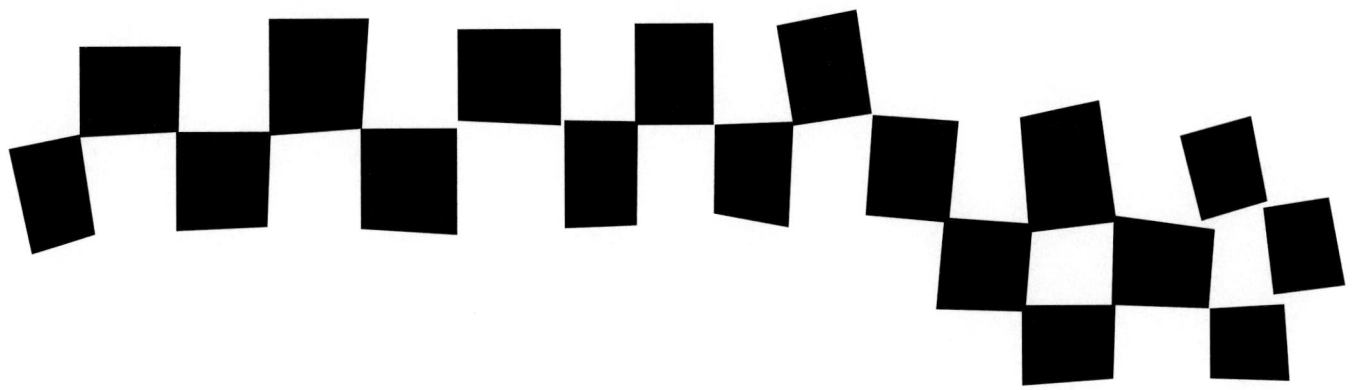

36
Abdomen Ultrasound

William E. Brant

Ultrasound (US) is firmly established as a primary imaging modality for comprehensive evaluation of the abdomen including the abdominal organs, the peritoneal cavity, and the retroperitoneum. Its role includes screening for disease, evaluation and follow-up of known abnormalities, and guidance of biopsy, aspiration, and catheter drainage procedures. Comprehensive examination commonly includes the use of Doppler and color flow imaging, as well as specialized techniques of transvaginal or transrectal US to demonstrate pelvic extension of disease. This chapter provides the basics for understanding effective use of US in examining the abdomen.

PERITONEAL CAVITY

Normal US Anatomy. The normal peritoneal cavity is a potential space best appreciated when fluid is present. The peritoneal membrane lines the abdominal cavity and covers, in whole or in part, the intraabdominal organs. Numerous peritoneal ligaments, folds, and recesses are visualized when outlined by fluid within the peritoneal cavity. US examination for the presence of fluid includes inspection of the subdiaphragmatic and subhepatic regions, the pericolic gutters and the pelvic cul-de-sac. Tiny volumes of intraperitoneal fluid are best detected by transvaginal US. Firm transducer pressure and changes in patient position are needed to inspect between bowel loops for fluid collections. Solid organs and fluid serve as sonographic windows to the abdomen and gas in bowel, the ribs, spine, and bony pelvis serve as obstacles.

Intraperitoneal Fluid. Fluid within the peritoneal cavity flows, under the effect of gravity, along peritoneal reflections to peritoneal recesses. The hepatorenal recess (Morison's pouch) and the pelvic cul-de-sac are the two most dependent recesses in the supine patient. They connect via the paracolic gutters. Fluid outlining intraperitoneal organs provides an opportunity to evaluate organ surface abnormalities, such the fine nodularity of cirrhosis. Transudative ascites, urine, and bile are anechoic (Fig. 36.1). Fluid with echogenic particles, layering debris, or septations may be hemorrhage, pus, malignant ascites, or spilled gastrointestinal contents.

Free intraperitoneal fluid outlines recesses and compartments which retain their normal shape. Loops of bowel float and sway freely within free fluid. Loculated fluid collections, abscesses, and cystic masses create their own space, displace bowel and adjacent organs, and are usually more round and tense.

Intraperitoneal Abscess. Although CT is commonly preferred for detection of small intraperitoneal abscesses, US readily demonstrates most abscesses. Because abscesses most commonly form in the dependent recesses, the pelvis must be included in every examination. Abscesses appear as loculated collections of fluid (Fig. 36.2) that may be anechoic to densely echogenic. Fluid levels, internal debris, septations, thick walls, and gas within the abscess are common. Gas is brightly echogenic and associated with reverberation artifact and acoustic shadowing. An abscess containing extensive gas may be mistaken for gas-filled bowel and overlooked. Some abscesses appear solid. Changes in patient position show shifting of the particle pattern when liquid. Doppler and color flow US show the presence or absence of internal blood vessels. Abscesses have mass effect and displace adjacent structures.

Intraperitoneal Tumor. Metastases are the most common tumor of the peritoneal surface. Fluid and gravity distribute malignant cells throughout the peritoneal cavity where they implant upon visceral or parietal peritoneal surfaces. The greater omentum is fertile ground and thickens with tumor implantation to form "omental cake," a layer of solid tissue separating bowel from con-

Figure 36.1. Ascites. Longitudinal US image shows anechoic ascites (*a*) surrounding the spleen (*S*). Fluid outlines the gastrosplenic ligament (*white arrow*). Note the small bare area of the spleen (*black arrow*) where reflections of the peritoneum from the spleen to the diaphragm prevent access of intraperitoneal fluid. A right pleural effusion (*e*) is seen above the diaphragm (*curved arrow*).

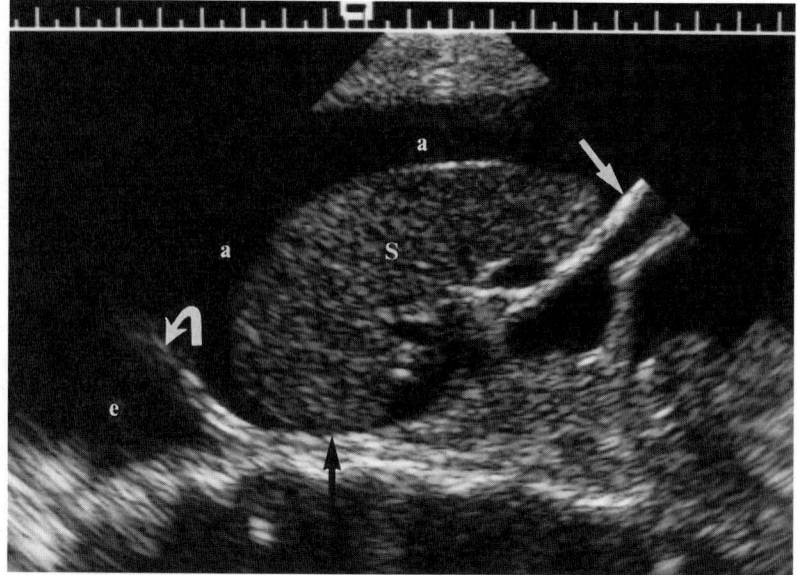

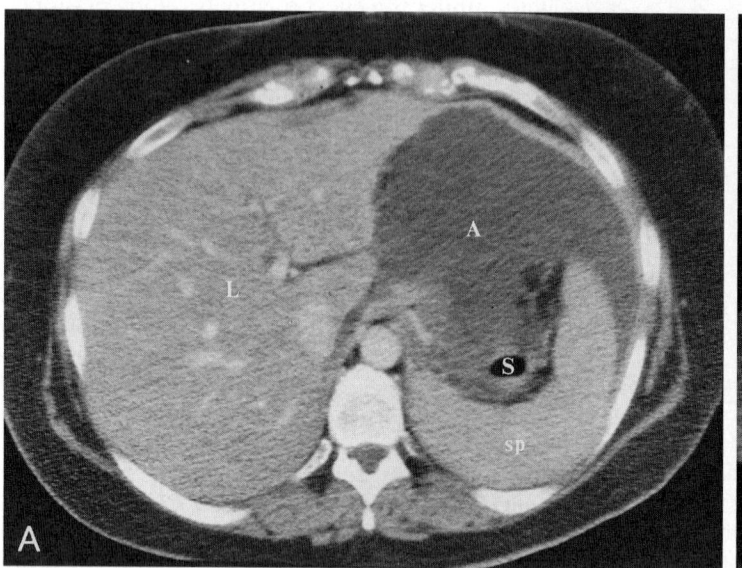

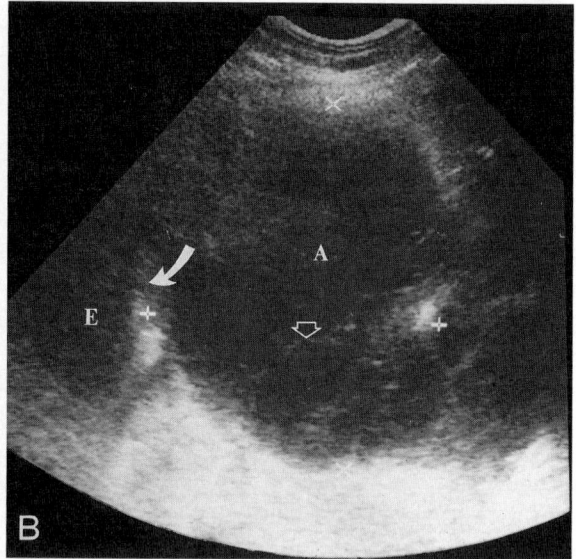

Figure 36.2. Left Subphrenic Abscess. A. A CT scan demonstrates a loculated fluid collection (*A*) in the left subphrenic space following gastric bypass surgery. The stomach (*S*) is displaced posteriorly. *L*, liver; *sp*, spleen. **B.** US in the same patient demonstrates internal sep- tations (*open arrow*) within the fluid collection (*A*, between cursors) that are not apparent on the CT study. A pleural effusion (*E*) is seen above the diaphragm (*curved arrow*). The abscess contained gram-negative organisms.

tact with the anterior abdominal wall. Metastatic implants appear as hypoechoic solid masses of varying size on peritoneal surfaces. Ascites is usually present, with echogenic debris and septations common. The most common tumors of origin are ovarian, colon, pancreas, and gastric carcinoma.

Primary peritoneal tumors include mesothelioma, desmoids, carcinoids, and lymphoma. These appear as predominantly hypoechoic solid masses. Acoustic shadows may arise from dense fibrous tissue or calcifications.

RETROPERITONEUM

Normal US Anatomy. The retroperitoneum is that portion of the abdomen behind the posterior parietal peritoneum. The anatomy of its three compartments is described in chapter 26. Its organs are discussed separately. US of the abdominal aorta and inferior vena cava are discussed in chapter 40. The crura of the diaphragm must not be mistaken for adenopathy. Both are hypoechoic linear bands of muscle. The right crus is larger, more lobular, and inserts lower, extending to L3 vertebral body. The left crus is more uniform in thickness inserting on L1 and L2 vertebral bodies. The crura serve as landmarks for identification of the adrenal gland. The psoas and quadratus lumborum muscles show the typical hypoechoic pattern of muscle with longitudinally oriented echogenic fibrous strands dividing muscle bundles. Echogenic retroperitoneal fat surrounds and defines organs, vessels, and other structures.

Retroperitoneal Adenopathy. Enlarged lymph nodes are homogeneous, hypoechoic, and round or oval (Fig. 36.3). Accentuated sound transmission may be present, and some enlarged solid nodes are so hypoechoic they appear cystic. A solitary node larger than 1.5 cm in short axis diameter, or multiple nodes larger than 1.0 cm, are considered to be pathologically enlarged. Lymphoma is characterized by confluence of enlarged nodes to form a solid mass which surrounds vessels and organs. Causes of retroperitoneal adenopathy are lymphoma (most common), tumor metastastases (testicular, renal, pelvic, gastrointestinal malignancies, and melanoma), and infection, especially in AIDS patients.

Retroperitoneal Tumors are most commonly of mesenchymal origin and include liposarcoma, leiomyosarcoma, and malignant fibrous histiocytoma. These are aggressive tumors that invade organs and muscles and are difficult to remove surgically. Most are large, heterogenous, and partially cystic. Benign lipomas consist of fat identical in appearance with normal retroperitoneal fat. Germ cell tumors in the retroperitoneum may be primary or secondary, and benign or malignant.

Retroperitoneal Fluid Collections include hemorrhage, infection, urinoma, pancreatic fluid collections, and cystic masses (lymphoceles, lymphangiomas, renal cysts, and teratomas). Porto-systemic collaterals and other enlarged blood vessels are differentiated by Doppler US. As within the peritoneal cavity, retroperitoneal fluid may be anechoic or echogenic, with particulate cellular debris and layering fluid levels. Echogenic clotted blood may appear as a solid mass. Absence of internal vascularity on Doppler examination and change in appearance with time are distinguishing features.

LIVER

US is an efficient imaging method to screen patients for diffuse and focal hepatic disease. For focal liver metastases, its sensitivity is near that of CT and MR; however its images are more difficult to reproduce for follow-up comparisons, and benign and malignant nodules cannot usually be distinguished. Color Doppler US is valuable in the assessment of liver vasculature, the diagnosis of portal and hepatic vein thrombosis and portal hypertension, and in evaluating the vascularity of liver tumors (1).

Normal US Anatomy. The echogenicity of the liver parenchyma is homogeneous and equal to or slightly greater than that of the kidney (Fig. 36.4). The surface of the liver is normally smooth and the inferior margin of the liver is sharp-edged. The lobar and segmental anatomy of the liver is described and illustrated in chapter 27 (2). The hepatic veins are seen as echolucent tubes with thin walls that converge into the inferior vena cava. The portal veins, hepatic arteries, and bile ducts, encompassed by fibrofatty tissue, form the portal triads which are normally visualized as echogenic spots throughout the liver. Doppler US is used to differentiate blood vessels from bile ducts and small hepatic cysts and to confirm blood flow (1).

Diffuse Liver Disease

Fatty Infiltration causes an increase in echogenicity of the liver making affected areas distinctly more echogenic than normal renal parenchyma. Fatty infiltration also increases the attenuation of the US beam diminishing visualization of the diaphragm and commonly requiring a lower frequency transducer to examine deep portions of the liver (Fig. 36.5). The hepatic echotexture appears coarsened and visualization of the portal triads is decreased. The various patterns of fatty infiltration are reviewed in chapter 27. The "flip-flop" pattern of fatty infiltration as seen on US compared with CT is useful in confirming the diagnosis of focal fatty infiltration and focal fat sparing (see Fig. 27.2). Fat infiltrated areas are

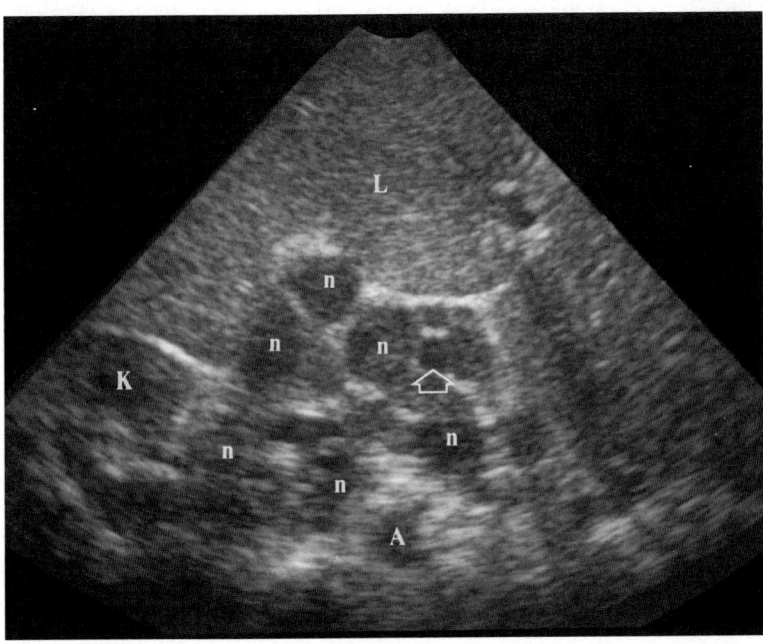

Figure 36.3. Lymphoma. An axial plane US demonstrates multiple enlarged hypoechoic lymph nodes (*n*) surrounding and displacing the aorta (*A*) and celiac axis (*open arrow*). The adenopathy extends into the hilum of the right kidney (*K*). *L*, liver.

Figure 36.4. Normal Liver. Longitudinal US image demonstrates normal liver (*L*) and right kidney (*K*). The liver parenchyma is of uniform echogenicity, approximately equal to the parenchymal echogenicity of the kidney. The liver is well-visualized to the level of the diaphragm (*curved arrow*). Small portal triad structures (*straight arrow*) are seen throughout the liver parenchyma.

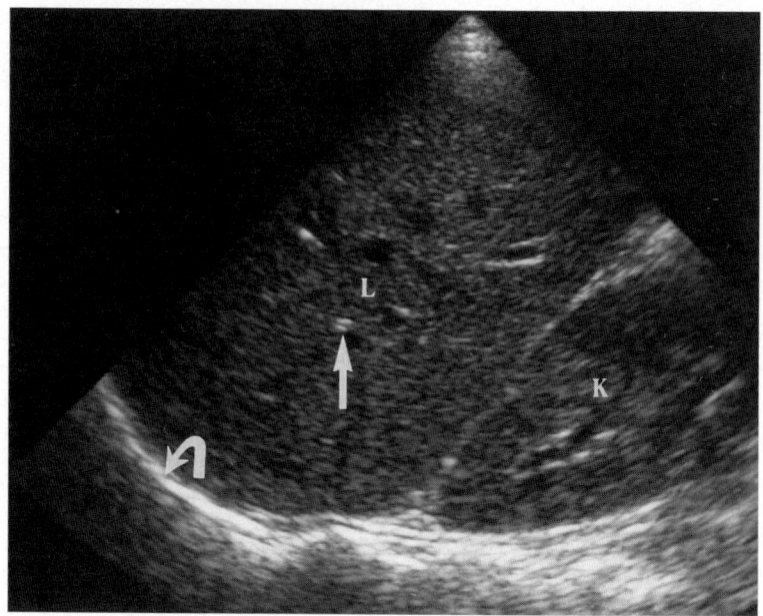

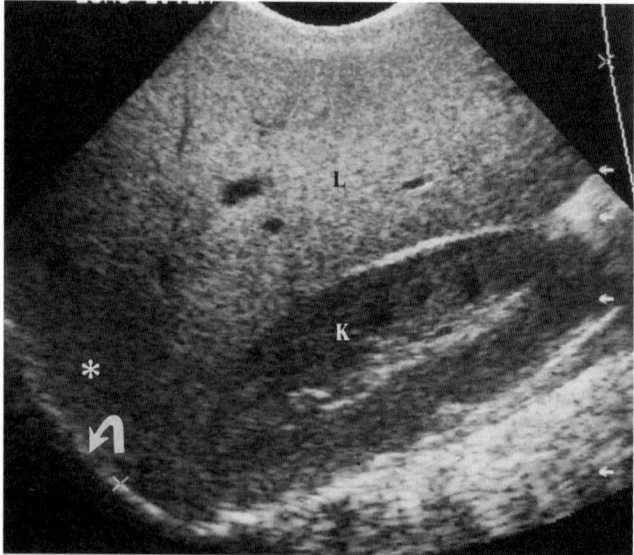

Figure 36.5. Diffuse Fatty Infiltration. Longitudinal image demonstrates the liver parenchyma (*L*) to be coarsened and significantly more echogenic than the parenchyma of the right kidney (*K*). Decreased sound wave penetration is evidenced by decreased echo intensity (***) near the diaphragm (*curved arrow*). Visualization of small portal triad structures is lost.

bright on US and dark on CT. Focally sparred areas within diffuse fatty infiltration are dark on US and bright on CT.

Acute Hepatitis results in diffuse hepatic edema which reduces the echogenicity of the liver, resulting in a "*starry sky*" appearance. The portal triads appear unusually bright on the darkened background of edematous parenchyma. The starry sky appearance has also been described with diffuse leukemic or lymphomatous infiltrate, toxic shock syndrome, and diffuse decrease in glycogen stores in the liver (3).

Passive Hepatic Congestion refers to stasis of blood in the liver due to congestive heart failure (4). US findings include hepatomegaly, distention of the inferior vena cava and hepatic veins, and pulsatile portal vein flow seen on Doppler due to transmission of right atrial activity through congested sinusoids. Ascites, pleural effusion, and pericardial effusion are often present.

Cirrhosis. US reflects the morphological changes in the liver associated with cirrhosis (5). Hepatic echotexture is usually coarsened and heterogeneous with multiple vague nodules commonly evident. The surface of the liver examined with high frequency transducers shows fine or coarse nodularity. Echogenicity is increased in proportion to the degree of fatty infiltration. With alcoholic cirrhosis the right lobe is shrunken, and the left lobe and caudate lobe are enlarged. Advanced cirrhosis results in a small liver. The normal triphasic Doppler waveform of the hepatic veins is flattened in cirrhosis with loss of the reverse flow component caused by atrial systole (6). US is insensitive (<45%) to detection of malignancy in cirrhotic livers, however US demonstration of a discrete focal mass is highly predictive of malignancy (7).

Portal Hypertension. US evidence of portal hypertension includes demonstration of portosystemic collateral vessels (Fig. 36.6), dilatation of the portal vein (>13 mm), dilatation of the splenic and superior mesenteric veins (>10 mm), splenomegaly, and ascites (8). The hepatic artery may be enlarged and tortuous. Doppler demonstration of reversed (hepatofugal) flow in the portal vein is diagnostic of portal hypertension (Fig. 36.7). Flow in a dilated paraumbilical vein traversing the falciform ligament and anterior abdominal wall is also highly specific for portal hypertension. Color Doppler is very useful in the detection of splenorenal, retroperitoneal, and coronary vein collaterals.

Portal Vein Thrombosis is evidenced by the presence of echogenic clot within an enlarged portal vein (9). Color Doppler confirms complete occlusion or demonstrates

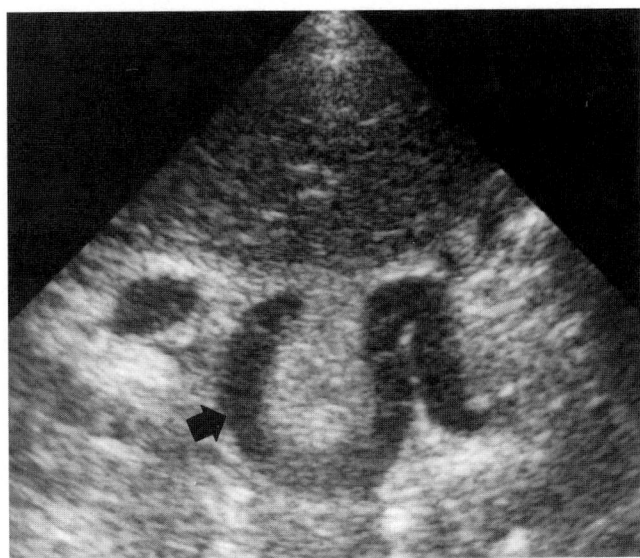

Figure 36.6. Portosystemic Collaterals. A tortuous collateral vessel (*arrow*) is seen in the splenic hilum in a patient with advanced portal hypertension.

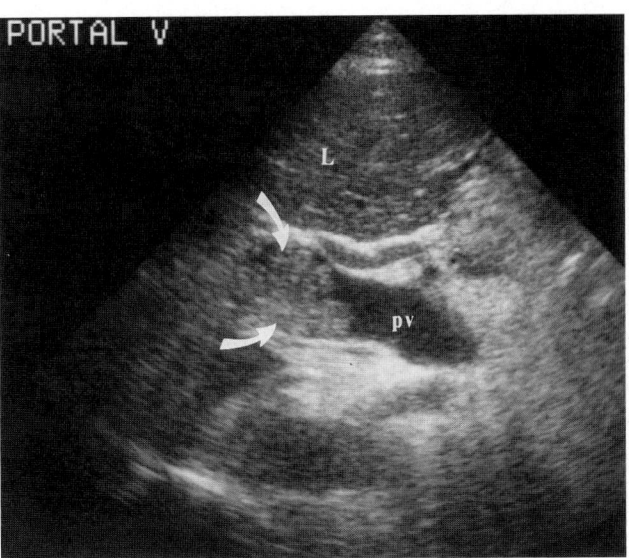

Figure 36.8. Portal Vein Invasion. The portal vein (*pv*) is enlarged and partially filled with tumor thrombus (*arrows*) from hepatocellular carcinoma. *L*, liver.

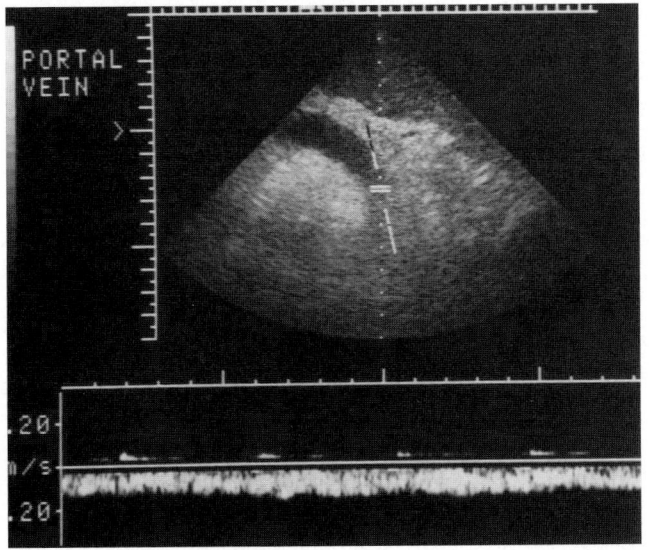

Figure 36.7. Reversed Flow in the Portal Vein. The spectral waveform below the baseline indicates venous flow away from the transducer. The anatomic image confirms that this flow direction is out of, instead of into, the liver indicating advanced portal hypertension.

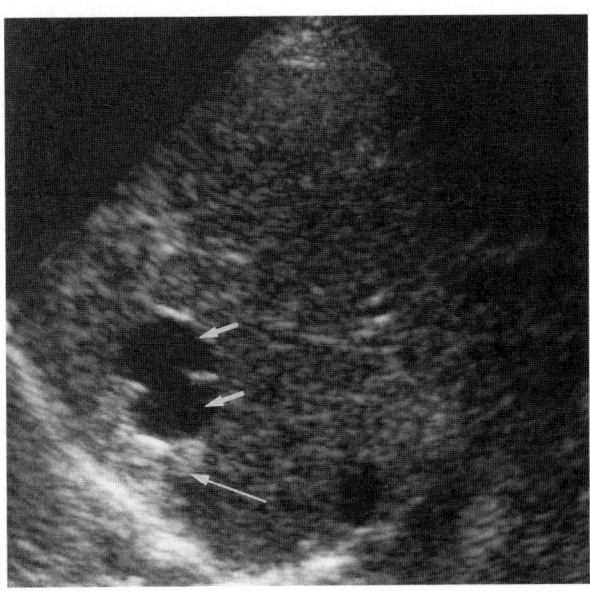

Figure 36.9. Simple Hepatic Cysts. Two simple cysts (*short arrows*) appear as well defined anechoic masses with accentuated sound transmission (*long arrow*).

residual flow around the thrombus. The thrombus itself varies in appearance from anechoic to hyperechoic, depending upon the age of the thrombus. Tumor thrombus from invasion of the portal vein by hepatoma (Fig. 36.8) is confirmed by spectral Doppler demonstration of arterial waveforms in the thrombus within the portal vein.

Liver Masses

Cysts are common and easily identified and characterized by US. Simple hepatic cysts contain anechoic fluid, have thin walls, and demonstrate posterior acous-

tic enhancement (Fig. 36.9). Most are septated and have a lobulated, rather than spherical, contour. They vary in size from tiny to huge and are commonly multiple. Small cysts may mimic vessels on quick inspection. Doppler is useful to confirm their avascular nature.

Cavernous Hemangiomas are commonly identified on hepatic sonograms. The classic US appearance is a well-defined homogeneous hyperechoic mass (Fig. 36.10). Doppler usually shows no internal blood flow although on occasion with slow flow, high sensitivity settings, very low velocity flow is detected. Large lesions may contain hypoechoic thrombosis, fibrosis, and calci-

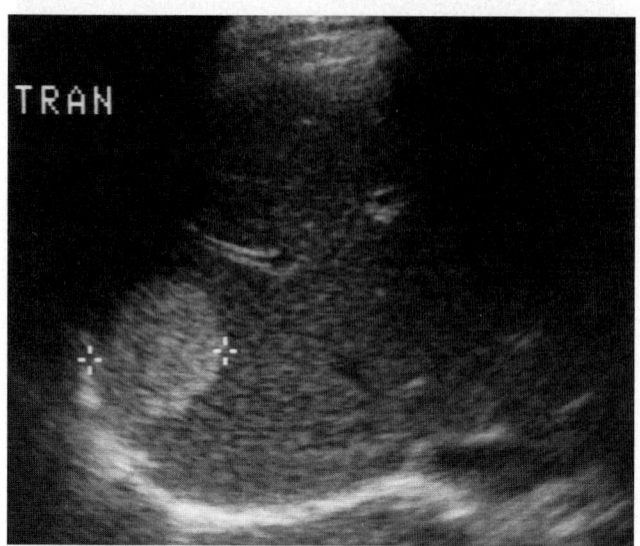

Figure 36.10. Cavernous Hemangioma. US defines a homogeneous, sharply marginated, hyperechoic mass (between cursors (+)) in the right lobe of the liver. This appearance is classic for cavernous hemangioma.

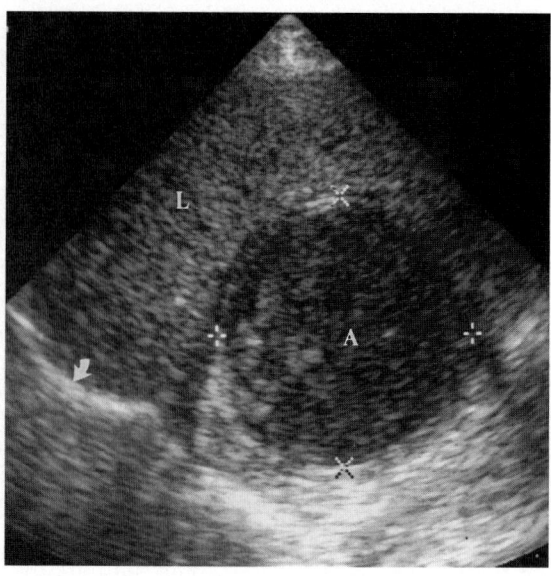

Figure 36.11. Amebic Abscess. A well-defined hypodense mass (*A*, between calipers) is seen in the right lobe of the liver (*L*). Note the proximity to the right hemidiaphragm (*arrow*). Amebic abscesses in the liver may rupture through the diaphragm into the right pleural space.

fication. Most lesions remain stable in size over time, but about 2% show enlargement. Classic appearing lesions in patients with normal liver function tests usually require no followup. Atypical lesions should be have a 6-month follow-up US or be confirmed with other imaging modalities as discussed in Chapter 27.

Metastases vary greatly in appearance from hypoechoic to hyperechoic and from homogeneous to heterogeneous to calcified. Metastatic disease must be considered in the differential diagnosis of all solid and atypical cystic lesions in the liver.

Hepatocellular Carcinoma may be solitary, multifocal, or diffuse. Detection in the diseased liver is commonly difficult with US. Most are hypervascular with prominent vascularity shown by color Doppler. Tumor invasion of the portal and hepatic veins is common (Fig. 36.8). Tumors may be hyperechoic with internal fat to hypoechoic and heterogeneous due to nonliquefactive necrosis. Any solid mass detected by US in a diseased liver is suspicious for hepatocellular carcinoma.

Abscesses usually appear as complex fluid collections (Fig. 36.11) containing echogenic fluid, fluid-fluid layers, or gas. Healed abscesses commonly calcify.

Microabscesses occur most commonly in immunocompromised patients with fungal or parasitic septicemia. Target lesions with central echogenic spot and peripheral hypoechoic halo are common. The differential diagnosis of multiple small (<10 mm) lesions in the liver is given in Table 27.6.

Other Masses, including hepatic adenoma, focal nodular hyperplasia, sarcoma, and peripheral cholangiocarcinoma, have a varied and nonspecific sonographic appearance. They range from hypoechoic to hyperechoic and may contain areas of internal hemorrhage, necrosis, fibrosis, or calcification. Characterization of these non-specific masses is often best performed with three-phase contrast-enhanced helical CT. The final diagnosis often depends on percutaneous biopsy.

BILE DUCTS

Normal US Anatomy. Intrahepatic bile ducts run in the portal triads in the company of the portal veins and hepatic arteries. Normal intrahepatic ducts may be visualized with high resolution US. Intrahepatic ducts normally do not exceed 2 mm in diameter in the central liver or 40% of the diameter of the adjacent portal vein. The junction of the right and left lobe bile ducts to form the common hepatic duct marks the division between the intrahepatic and extrahepatic portions of the biliary tree. The junction of the cystic duct with the common hepatic duct marks the commencement of the common bile duct. Because this junction is seldom visualized with US, the generic term "common duct" is used to identify the duct in the porta hepatis. The common duct courses anterior to the main portal vein, the right portal vein and the right hepatic artery in the portal region. The hepatic artery is commonly tortuous in the porta hepatis, but the common duct runs a straight course parallel to the portal vein. This straight portion of the common duct is routinely measured, with normal values in adults of 4–6 mm diameter from inner wall to inner wall. After age 60, an additional millimeter per decade is added to the normal range, so a 70-year-old patient may have a normal common duct as large as 7 mm.

As the portal triad structures course through the free edge of the hepatoduodenal ligament, a "Mickey Mouse" configuration is formed with the common duct forming Mickey's right ear (Fig. 36.12). The normal common bile duct can be traced descending adjacent to the pancreatic

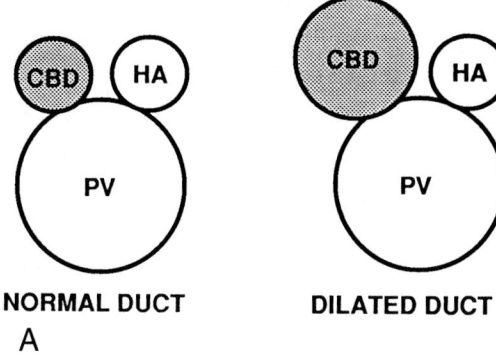

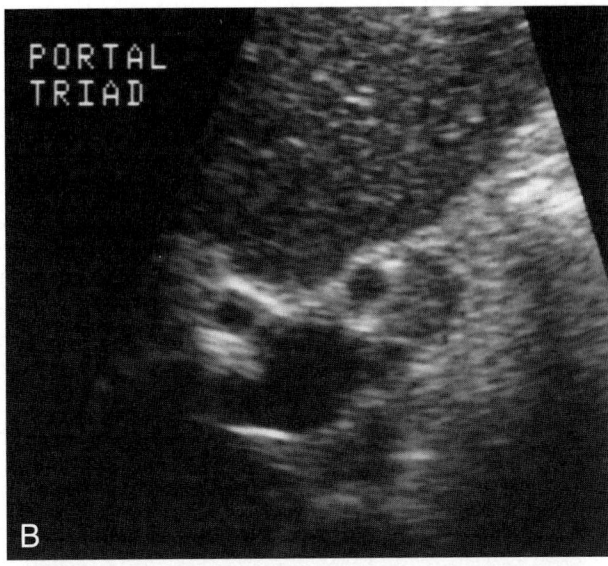

Figure 36.12. "Mickey Mouse" Configuration of the Portal Triad. A. Anatomic drawing demonstrates the anatomic relationships of the common bile duct (*CBD*), hepatic artery (*HA*), and portal vein (*PV*). Dilation of the common bile duct enlarges Mickey's right ear. **B.** US image of Mickey Mouse.

head to its insertion at the Ampulla of Vater. Normal variants that may cause confusion include a "replaced" right hepatic artery arising from the superior mesenteric artery and coursing between the portal vein and inferior vena cava to the porta hepatis. An elongated gallbladder neck may be mistaken for a dilated common duct. Low insertion of the cystic duct causes the appearance of two common ducts. Doppler identification of vascular structures is helpful in confusing cases.

Dilatation of the Biliary Tree

Dilated intrahepatic ducts are tortuous like the branches of an oak tree, exceed 40% of the diameter of the adjacent portal vein, and are visualized in the periphery of the liver. Gray-scale US shows "too many tubes" in the liver (Fig. 36.13), but color Doppler US offers rapid differentiation of patent blood vessels and dilated bile ducts. Dilated extrahepatic ducts exceed 6–7 mm in diameter, and appear as enlargement of Mickey's right ear in the hepatoduodenal ligament. The dilated duct should be followed to the level of obstruction, where careful evaluation will demonstrate the cause of obstruction in 80% of patients.

Choledocholithiasis. Stones in the bile ducts appear as echogenic objects within the lumen of the duct (Fig. 36.14). Unfortunately, not all intraluminal stones will cast a distinct acoustic shadow. Technique must be optimized to demonstrate shadowing. Nonetheless, US detection of obstructing common duct stones is only about 75% sensitive. Abrupt termination of a dilated common duct is an indication for contrast cholangiography. Calcification in the hepatic artery may mimic the appearance of stones in the biliary tree.

Gas in the Biliary Tree is most commonly the result of surgical procedures, such as choledochoenterostomy or sphincterotomy (see Table 27.9). Additional causes include gas-producing infection, fistulous connection with the intestinal tract (gallstone ileus, perforation duodenal ulcer), and trauma. Air in bile ducts causes bright linear or globular reflections with shadowing and ring-down ar-

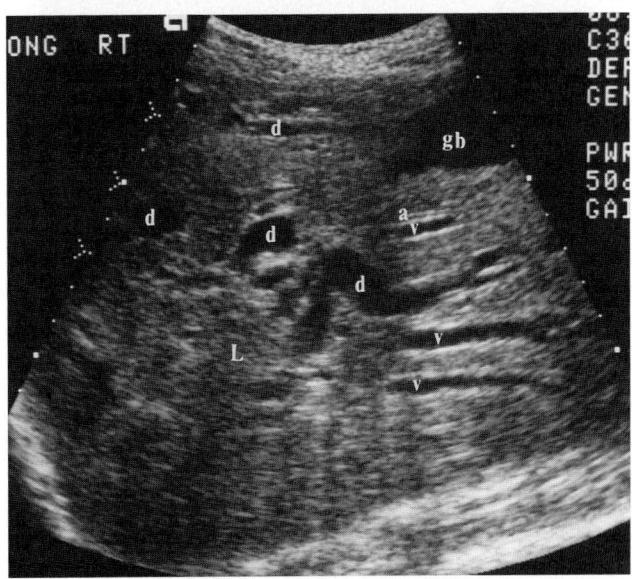

Figure 36.13. Bile Duct Dilation. Longitudinal US image demonstrates "too many tubes" in the liver (*L*). Dilated bile ducts (*d*), veins (*v*), and arteries (*a*) are most easily distinguished by use of spectral or color Doppler. Dilated bile ducts tend to be more tortuous and less uniform in diameter than arteries or veins. *gb*, gallbladder.

tifacts. Air will move in the biliary tree with changes in patient positioning. Ducts are usually dilated when air is present.

Cholangiocarcinoma. Hilar cholangiocarcinoma (Klatskin tumor) and extrahepatic cholangiocarcinoma tend to be small (<3 cm) when they present with biliary obstruction. US demonstrates the tumor as a focal mass at the point of obstruction (Fig. 36.15), nodular thickening of the bile duct wall, or polypoid intraluminal mass (10,11). The visualized mass is most commonly isoechoic with the liver parenchyma but may be hypoechoic or hyperechoic. Abrupt termination of a dilated duct without a mass being seen may be the only finding. Adjacent portal veins may be invaded and obstructed by tumor.

Oriental Cholangiohepatitis. US reveals bile ducts that are focally dilated or stenotic (12). Multiple stones with and without shadowing are evident in the bile ducts. Debris, "biliary mud," may fill and layer within dilated ducts. Most patients originate from Southeast Asian countries.

AIDS-related Cholangitis features dilated intra- and extrahepatic bile ducts with thickening of the walls of the bile ducts and gallbladder (13). Sludge is commonly seen, but stones are usually not present. A unique finding is an echogenic nodule representing edema of the papilla of Vater at the termination of the dilated common bile duct (14).

Biliary Ascariasis. Worms that colonize the intestinal tract may find their way into the biliary tree and gallbladder. Living worms may obstruct the biliary tree and gallbladder and cause cholangitis, cholecystitis, and pancreatitis with a high associated mortality. Worms are seen by US as moving tubular echogenic structures with an echolucent core (15).

Congenital Biliary Cysts. The classification of congenital biliary cysts is illustrated in Figure 27.18. US is excellent in demonstrating the morphology of cystic masses and their relationship to the biliary tree.

GALLBLADDER

Normal US Anatomy. The gallbladder is found on the undersurface of the liver with the gallbladder neck positioned in the interlobar fissure. Normal bile is anechoic. The normal wall does not exceed 3 mm in thickness. The mucosa is echogenic and the smooth muscle layer of the wall is hypoechoic. The diameter of the gallbladder is less than 4 cm in 96% of normals. Most patients are examined after an overnight fast although a 4-hour fast is usually sufficient to ensure gallbladder distension. Patients are examined in multiple positions to displace gallstones and demonstrate their mobility. The neck region should be carefully examined to avoid overlooking impacted stones. Normal folds in the gallbladder neck and cystic duct may cause acoustic shadows and mimic gallstones.

Echogenic Bile. Bile becomes echogenic when it is highly concentrated and cholesterol crystals and calcium bilirubinate granules precipitate as *sludge*. Sludge commonly layers in the gallbladder (Fig. 36.16) and may become quite viscous and form "sludge balls" or tumefactive sludge. Sludge balls usually move within the gallbladder but do not cast acoustic shadows. Floating cholesterol crystals are seen as bright reflectors with short comet tail artifacts. Air in bile has a similar appearance. Sludge is not definitive evidence of gallbladder disease but is indicative of prolonged lack of bile turnover in the gallbladder. Prolonged fasting is the most common cause, but sludge is usually present with gall-

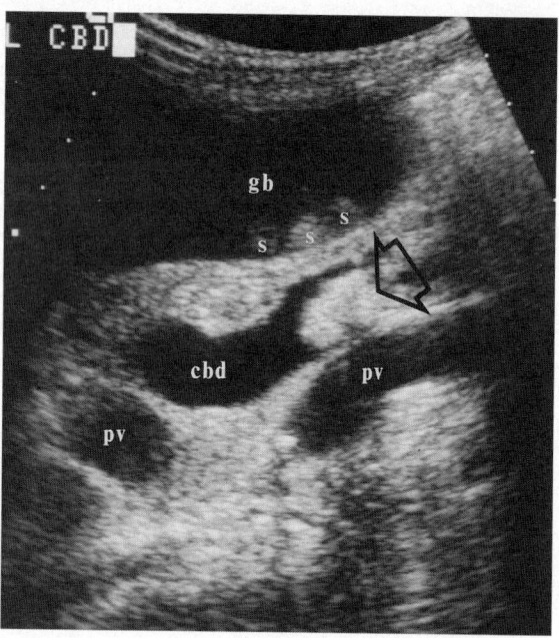

Figure 36.14. Choledocholithiasis. US image of the porta hepatis demonstrates a large stone (*arrow*) obstructing the common bile duct (*cbd*) and resulting in its dilation (13 mm diameter). The gallbladder (*gb*) is dilated and contains several nonshadowing sludge balls (*s*) formed as a result of biliary stasis. *pv*, portal vein.

Figure 36.15. Cholangiocarcinoma. Tumor (*arrow*) obstructs and dilates the common bile duct (*d*) in the porta hepatis. *v*, portal vein; *a*, hepatic artery.

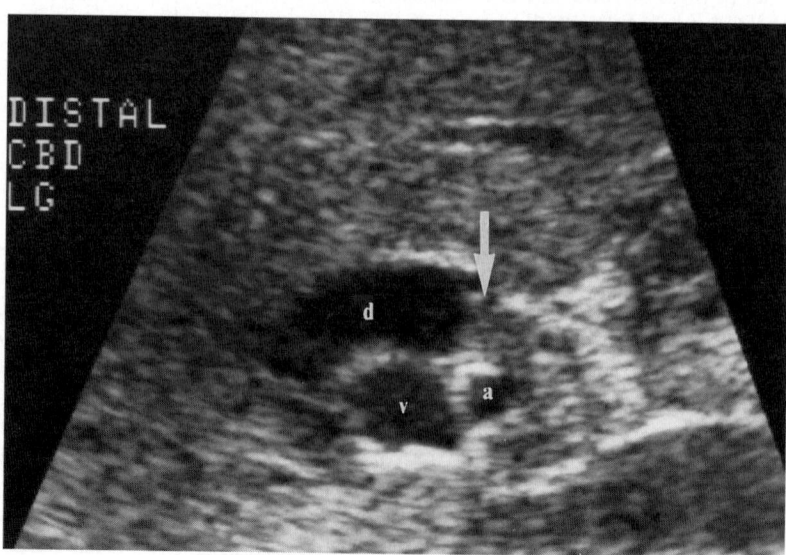

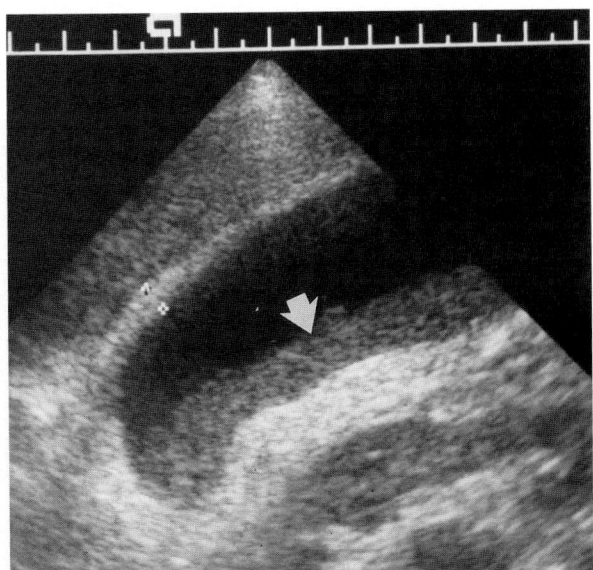

Figure 36.16. Echogenic Bile. Highly concentrated echogenic bile (*arrow*) layers dependently within the gallbladder. The gallbladder wall is thickened (between cursors) to 6 mm in this patient with acute cholecystitis.

Table 36.1. Causes of Gallbladder Wall Thickening

Contracted gallbladder after eating
Gallbladder disease
   Acute cholecystitis
   Chronic cholecystitis
   Adenomyomatosis
   Gallbladder carcinoma
   AIDS cholangiopathy
   Sclerosing cholangitis
Nonbiliary disease
   Hypoproteinemia
   Ascites
   Edema due to congestive heart failure
   Hepatitis
   Portal hypertension
   Portal lymph node obstruction
   Cirrhosis

bladder and biliary obstruction. Sludge is not produced by routine overnight fasting in preparation for gallbladder examination. Additional causes of echogenic bile are blood, pus, and parasites.

Thickened Gallbladder Wall. The gallbladder wall is considered thickened when it exceeds 3 mm as measured between the gallbladder lumen and the liver parenchyma (Fig. 36.16). Causes of thickening include gallbladder disease and nonbiliary processes (Table 36.1). The most common causes are ascites, hypoproteinemia, and cholecystitis.

Gallstones

US is the imaging method of choice for detection of gallstones with a sensitivity of greater than 90%.

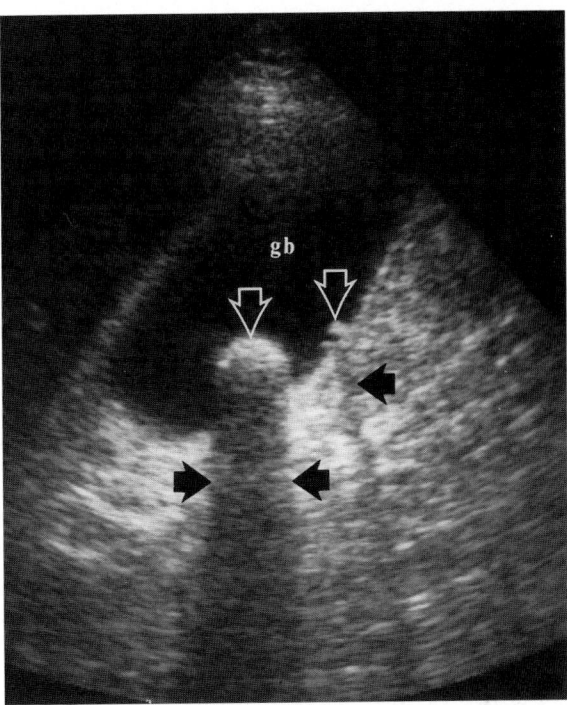

Figure 36.17. Gallstones. US demonstrates focal echodensities of varying size (*open arrows*) within the gallbladder lumen (*gb*). Acoustic shadows (*closed arrows*) extend from the echodensities. Moving the patient into the upright position resulted in a change in position of the gallstones.

Gallstones appear within the gallbladder lumen as echogenic objects which cast acoustic shadows and move with changes in patient position (Fig. 36.17). When these finding are present, specificity for gallstones is 100%. However, the demonstration of acoustic shadowing is strongly dependent on technique. When shadows are not evident with a suspected gallstone, a switch to a higher frequency transducer with focal zone adjusted at the depth of the stone will commonly demonstrate the elusive shadow.

Gallstones may be nonmobile due to adhesion to the gallbladder wall, but acoustic shadowing should be demonstrable. Cholesterol polyps and adenomatous polyps are nonmobile, non-shadowing, soft tissue nodules attached to the gallbladder wall. Sludge balls appear as echogenic foci that move, or are adherent to the wall, but do not shadow.

Wall-Echo-Shadow (WES) Sign. When the gallbladder is completely filled with gallstones, a confident diagnosis becomes more difficult because the gallbladder resembles an air-filled loop of bowel. The WES sign is definitive evidence of a stone-filled gallbladder (Fig. 36.18). Gallstones produce a "clean" dark shadow, and air in bowel produces a "dirty" brighter shadow (16).

Polyps appear as echogenic non-shadowing nodules that extend from the gallbladder wall (Fig. 36.19). Most are cholesterol polyps which are smaller than 1 cm and are commonly multiple. Adenomatous polyps are rare and indistinguishable from cholesterol polyps. Polyps larger than 1 cm may be malignant.

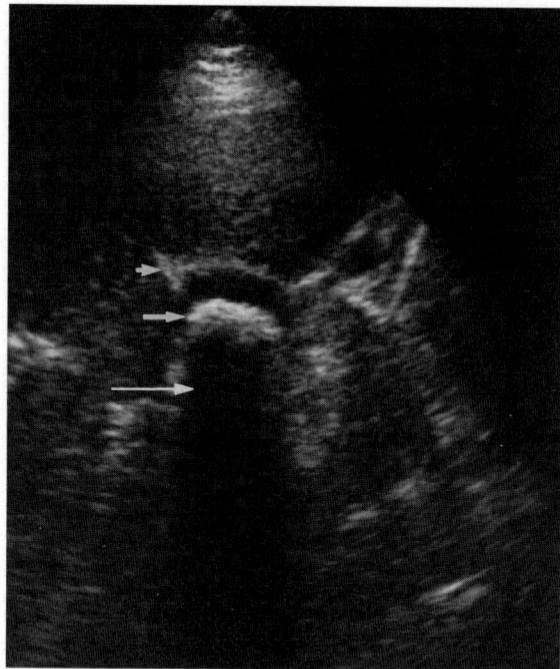

Figure 36.18. Wall-Echo-Shadow Sign. A thin layer of bile separates the gallbladder wall (*arrowhead*) from the bright echo (*short arrow*) of gallstones which cast a dense acoustic shadow (*long arrow*). This appearance has also been called the "double arc shadow sign."

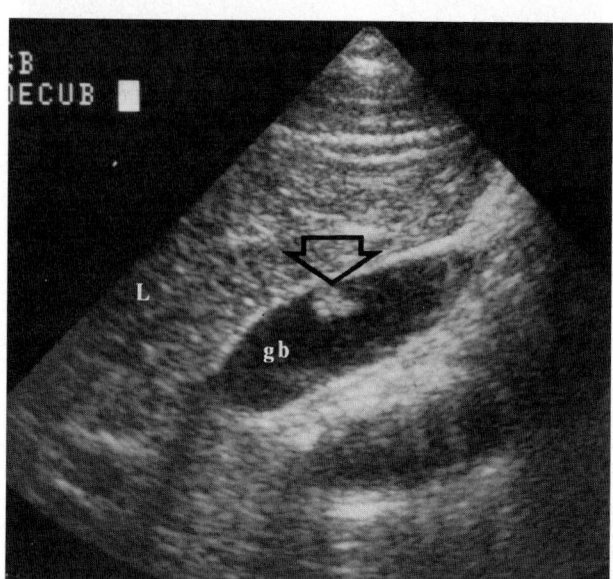

Figure 36.19. Cholesterol Polyp. An echogenic nodule (*arrow*) extends from the nondependent wall of the gallbladder into the lumen (*gb*). The lesion does not cause acoustic shadowing. *L*, liver.

Acute Cholecystitis

US is commonly performed in patients who present with acute right upper quadrant pain (16). US evidence of acute cholecystitis includes (Fig. 36.20) the following: *a)* gallstones, *b)* thickened gallbladder wall, *c)* focal gallbladder tenderness elicited by transducer pressure directly over the gallbladder (positive Murphy sign), *d)* pericholecystic fluid, *e)* dilated gallbladder, and *f)* power Doppler evidence of wall hyperemia (17). An unequivocally positive Murphy sign is highly predictive of acute cholecystitis (92%). A negative or equivocal Murphy sign is evidence against acute cholecystitis. A striated appearance of a thickened gallbladder wall is evidence of gangrenous cholecystitis (18). Pericholecystic fluid collections larger than 1 cm are evidence of gallbladder perforation. The absence of gallstones is not evidence against cholecystitis in patients who are at risk for acalculous cholecystitis (Fig. 36.21). These patients usually have a prolonged illness associated with major surgery, trauma, burns, prolonged hospitalization, parenteral nutrition, and sepsis.

Emphysematous Cholecystitis is usually due to ischemia in elderly male diabetics. Gas develops in the gallbladder wall and lumen in association with gas-producing bacterial infection of the gallbladder. Perforation occurs commonly and mortality is high. The diagnosis is suggested on US by bright reflections in the gallbladder wall associated with ring-down artifact (19). Gas bubbles in the lumen move and produce comet-tail artifacts. Air may be present in the bile ducts. The diagnosis is confirmed by CT or plain film confirmation of air in the gallbladder. Immediate surgery is indicated.

Gallbladder Carcinoma

Because gallstones are usually present, the signs of gallbladder carcinoma may be overlooked during US examination. Three major patterns of disease have been described (20). A mass replacing the gallbladder is the most common appearance (40–65% of cases). A normal gallbladder is not evident. The mass is strikingly heterogeneous due to enveloped gallstones, tumor, and necrotic debris. Diffuse or focal thickening of the gallbladder wall is the second pattern seen in 20–30% of cases. The wall is thicker and more irregular than walls thickened by other causes. The least common pattern (5–10%) is a soft tissue mass within the gallbladder lumen (Fig. 36.22). An intraluminal mass larger than 10 mm is suspicious for cancer. Cholesterol polyps are usually less than 5 mm in size. Benign adenomatous polyps uncommonly exceed 10 mm diameter. Additional findings associated with gallbladder cancer include biliary obstruction, adenopathy, liver metastases, and invasion of adjacent structures.

Porcelain Gallbladder refers to calcification of the gallbladder wall complicating chronic cholecystitis. US demonstrates a highly echogenic wall with acoustic shadowing. Porcelain gallbladder is a predisposing condition to gallbladder carcinoma.

Adenomyomatosis appears on US as focal or diffuse thickening of the gallbladder wall. The gallbladder fundus is nearly always involved. Rokitansky-Aschoff sinuses are a characteristic morphologic feature. These are pockets of mucosa within the hypertrophied smooth muscle wall. These pockets commonly contain precipitated cholesterol crystals which are very echogenic and produce comet-tail artifacts (Fig. 36.23). This benign

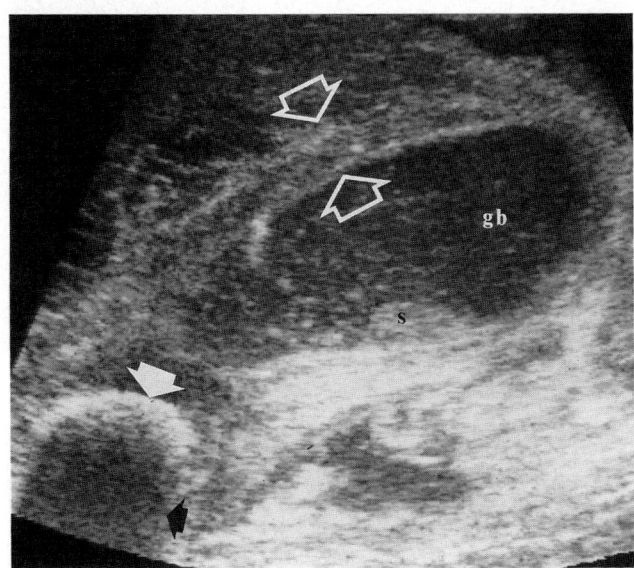

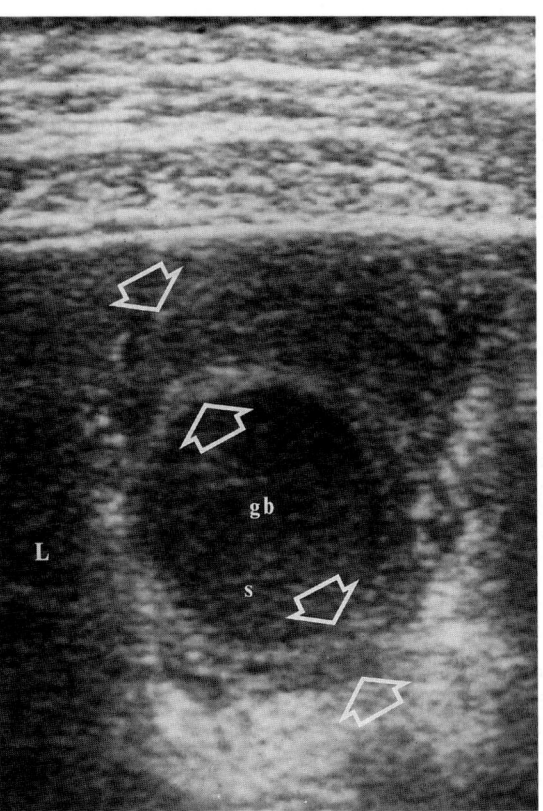

Figure 36.20. Acute Cholecystitis. US image through the long axis of the gallbladder (*gb*) demonstrates a large gallstone (*closed white arrow*) impacted in the neck of the gallbladder and casting an acoustic shadow (*black arrow*). The gallbladder wall is thickened (*open arrows*) and edematous. Echogenic sludge (*s*) is seen within the gallbladder lumen, giving evidence of bile stasis. A sonographic Murphy sign was present.

Figure 36.21. Acalculous Cholecystitis. Transverse image of the gallbladder (*gb*) demonstrates marked thickening and edema of the wall (*arrows*) and echogenic sludge (*s*) in the lumen. A sonographic Murphy sign was elicited. No gallstones were present. *L,* liver.

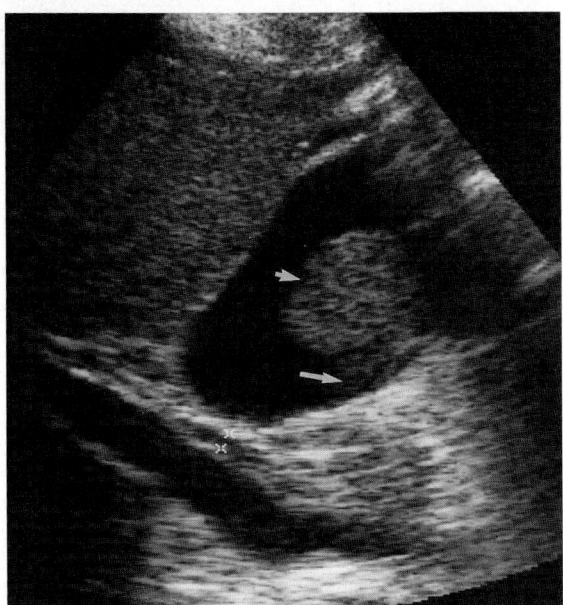

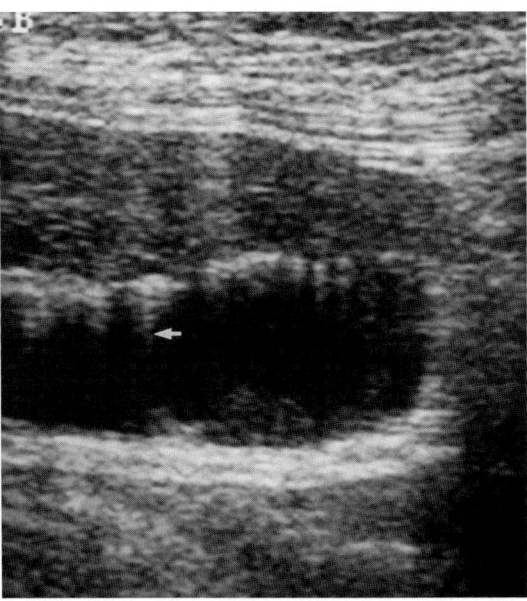

Figure 36.22. Gallbladder Carcinoma. A soft tissue mass (*arrowhead*) extends into the gallbladder lumen from an area of focally thickened gallbladder wall (*arrow*).

Figure 36.23. Adenomyomatosis. V-shaped comet-tail artifacts (*arrow*) extend from the gallbladder wall thickened due to adenomyomatosis. The comet-tail reverberation artifacts are due to cholesterol crystals within Rokitansky-Aschoff sinuses.

Figure 36.24. Accessory Spleen. A well-defined nodule with the same echotexture as the splenic parenchyma is seen in the splenic hilum. The spleen has a normal US appearance.

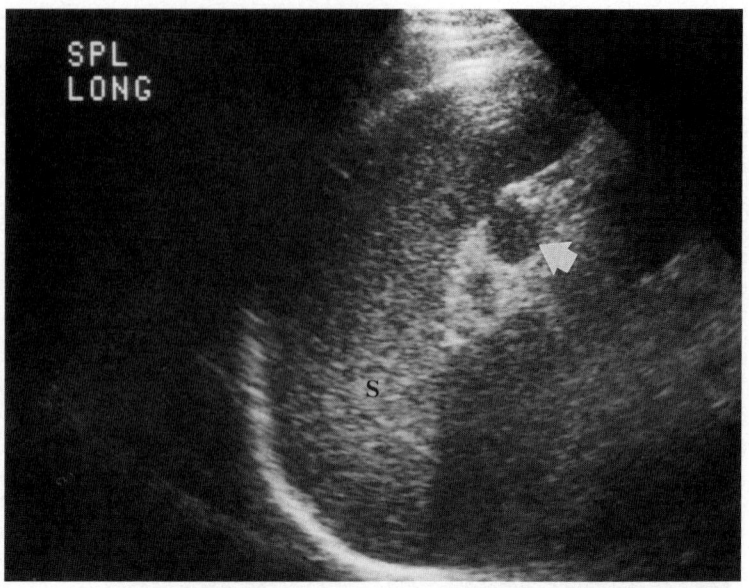

condition has no malignant potential, but may mimic gallbladder carcinoma on US studies.

SPLEEN

Normal US Anatomy. The spleen is best visualized with US with a posterolateral intercostal approach with the patient supine (Fig. 36.24). With the patient in a right lateral decubitus position, the spleen may be difficult to visualize because of expansion of the left lung. When the spleen is large an anterior subcostal approach with the patient in deep inspiration is also useful. The splenic parenchyma is homogeneous and normally more echogenic than the liver. Its borders are smooth, sharply defined, and commonly lobulated. Doppler demonstrates the splenic artery and vein in the splenic hilum and their branches within the spleen.

Accessory Spleens appear as rounded, well-defined masses, in or near the splenic hilum (Fig. 36.24). They are homogeneous and isoechoic with spleen parenchyma. Blood supply by branches of the splenic artery or vein is diagnostic (21).

Splenomegaly is evidenced by splenic length >12 cm or thickness >6 cm. The parenchyma usually remains homogeneous and normal in appearance no matter what the cause of splenic enlargement (Fig. 36.25)(see Table 28.3).

Cystic Lesions

Post-traumatic Cysts account for 80% of cystic lesions of the spleen (22). Most are well-defined, anechoic, with accentuated through-transmission. Thick walls with ringlike calcification are common.

True Epithelial Cysts are indistinguishable from post-traumatic cysts although calcification in the wall is less common.

Pancreatic Fluid Collections are nearly always subcapsular in location (Fig. 36.26). Associated findings of pancreatitis confirm the diagnosis.

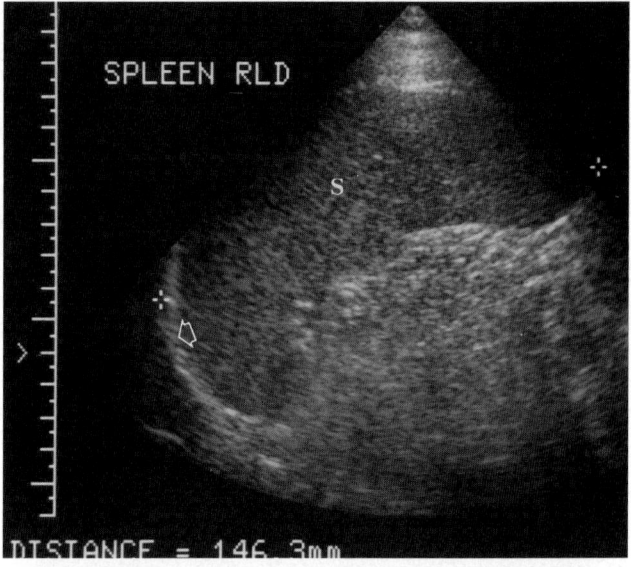

Figure 36.25. Splenomegaly. US image in coronal plane from the left side demonstrates enlargement of the spleen (*S*, between *calipers*). The spleen parenchyma is of homogeneous normal echogenicity. The diaphragmatic surface of the spleen conforms to the shape of the diaphragm (*arrow*).

Aneurysms of the Splenic Artery are common and present as a hypoechoic mass in the region of the splenic hilum. Atherosclerotic calcification in the aneurysm wall is usually present. Doppler reveals arterial blood flow. Rupture causes a high mortality. Pseudoaneurysms of the splenic artery are usually caused by pancreatitis. Real-time scanning reveals a fluid collection with thin, noncalcified walls. Doppler demonstrates internal arterial flow and communication with the splenic artery.

Abscesses usually demonstrate echogenic fluid, layering debris, and air (Fig. 36.27) although some contain anechoic fluid (23). US-guided percutaneous aspiration

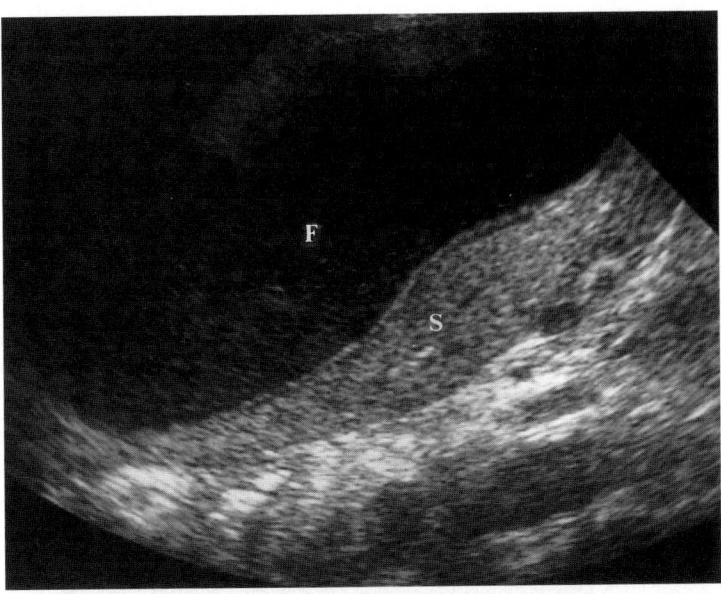

Figure 36.26. Subcapsular Pancreatic Fluid Collection in the Spleen. Pancreatic fluid (*F*) due to acute pancreatitis has tracked beneath the splenic capsule and compressed the splenic parenchyma (*S*).

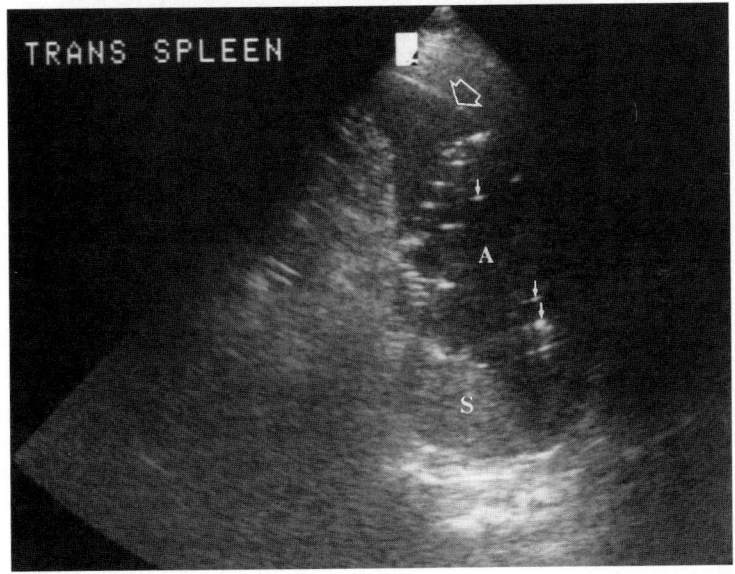

Figure 36.27. Splenic Abscess. Coronal plane US image demonstrates extensive destruction of the splenic parenchyma by a large abscess (*A*) containing air bubbles seen as mobile echogenic foci distributed through the fluid of the abscess (*small arrows*). Only a small remnant of normal splenic parenchyma (*S*) remains. The *open arrow* indicates the left hemidiaphragm.

for diagnosis and catheter placement for treatment are safe procedures (24).

Microabscesses are most common in immunocompromised patients. High frequency transducers reveal multiple tiny hypoechoic lesions (25). Common causes are *Mycobacterium tuberculosis*, *M. avium intracellulare*, *Candida*, and *Pneumocystis carinii*. The differential diagnosis is listed in Table 28.4.

Solid Lesions

Lymphoma. Hypoechoic lesions in the spleen in patients with lymphoma are very likely to be foci of lymphoma. Lesions range from numerous and small to solitary and large. However, the spleen may be enlarged without lymphoma involvement or appear normal and still be diffusely infiltrated.

Infarctions appear hypoechoic or anechoic and are usually wedge-shaped and extend to the splenic capsule (Fig. 36.28)(26). Parenchymal borders may be sharply defined or irregular. Hemorrhage associated with infarction may dissect beneath the capsule or the capsule may rupture resulting in hemoperitoneum. Most patients with infarction have a predisposing cause.

Hemangiomas are usually homogeneous and hyperechoic, but have a much more variable appearance than they have in the liver. A complex mass appearance with multiple cystic areas has been described (27). Calcifications occur in areas of fibrosis.

Metastases are non-specific in appearance, usually hypoechoic and multiple.

Hematoma. Sonography is now commonly used to screen for free intraperitoneal blood in patients with blunt abdominal trauma. Splenic lacerations, subcapsular and intraparenchymal hematomas are commonly demonstrated. The US appearance of the hematoma varies with age and composition (Fig. 36.29). Most are well-defined and hypoechoic.

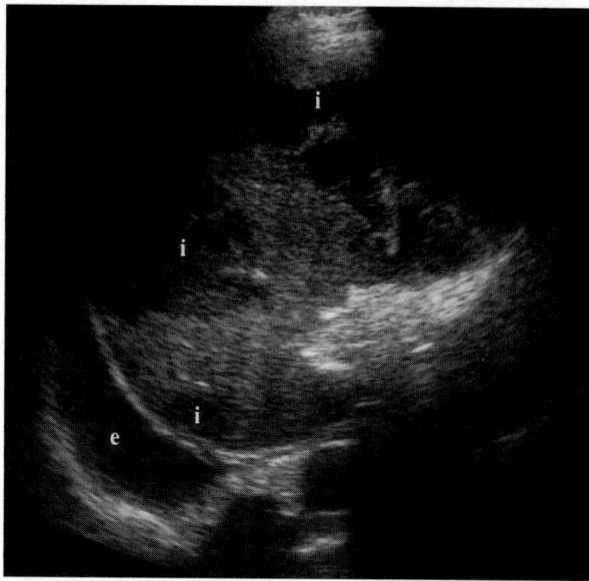

Figure 36.28. Splenic Infarctions. Acute splenic infarctions (*i*) appear as irregular and wedge-shaped, peripheral, hypoechoic regions in the spleen. An associated pleural effusion (*e*) is also evident.

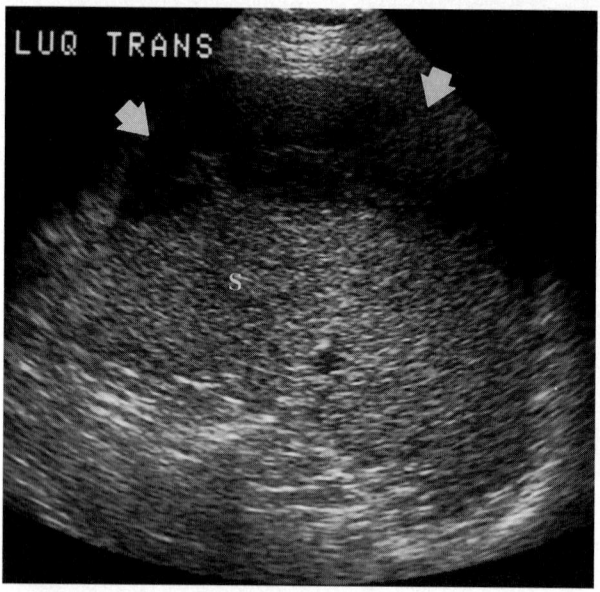

Figure 36.29. Subcapsular Splenic Hematoma. US demonstrates a heterogeneous low-density fluid collection (*arrows*) beneath the splenic capsule flattening the splenic parenchyma (*S*).

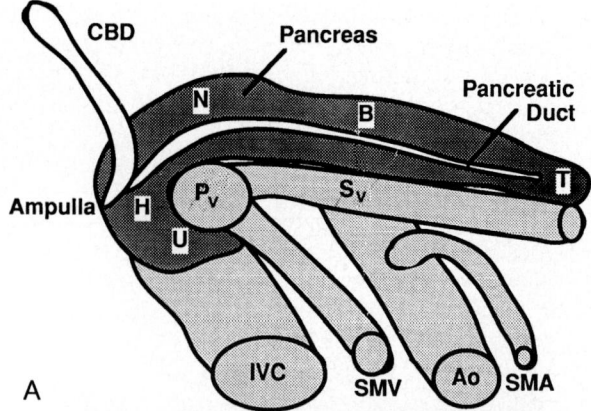

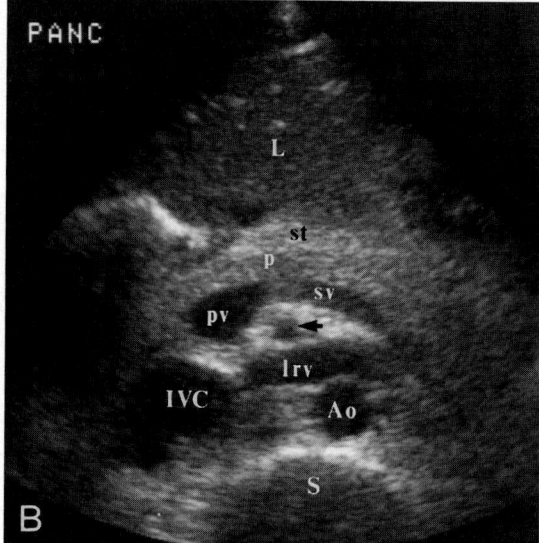

Figure 36.30. Normal Pancreas Anatomy. A diagram **(A)** and an US in transverse plane **(B)** demonstrate the normal anatomy of the pancreas. The majority of the pancreas lies anterior to the splenic vein (*sv*) and its junction with the superior mesenteric vein (*SMV*) forming the portal vein (*pv*). The head (*H*) and uncinate process (*U*) of the pancreas cradle the origin of the portal vein. The pancreatic neck (*N*) is anterior to the SV-SMV confluence, and the uncinate process and inferior vena cava (*IVC*) are posterior to the confluence. The superior mesenteric artery (*SMA, arrow*) arises from the aorta (*Ao*) dorsal to the splenic vein. The left renal vein (*lrv*) passes between the SMA and aorta to the inferior vena cava. The left lobe of the liver (*L*) offers a good sonographic window to the pancreas. The stomach (*st*) and lesser sac (collapsed) are anterior to the pancreas. *CBD,* common bile duct; *S,* spine; *B,* body of the pancreas; *T,* tail of the pancreas; *p,* pancreas.

PANCREAS

Normal US Anatomy. The pancreas may be a difficult organ to image with US. Vascular landmarks are the key to its identification (Fig. 36.30). The body and tail of the pancreas are immediately anterior to the splenic vein as it courses from the splenic hilum toward the liver. The neck of the pancreas is anterior to the junction of the splenic vein with the superior mesenteric vein that marks the commencement of the portal vein. The head of the pancreas envelops this confluence and lies anterior to the inferior vena cava. It is important to remember that a portion of the pancreatic head, the uncinate process lies caudal to the splenic vein, between the superior mesenteric vein and the inferior vena cava.

The echogenicity of the pancreas depends upon the amount of fatty infiltration. In children and young adults, the pancreas is about equal in echogenicity to the liver. In older adults, the pancreas becomes more echogenic with progressive fat infiltration. The pancreatic duct may be seen in a large number of normal individuals. The normal duct does not exceed 3 mm in diameter and tapers progressively toward the tail.

The left lobe of the liver serves as the best sonographic window to the pancreas. The distal stomach lies between the liver and the pancreas. The hypoechoic muscular wall of the stomach should not be mistaken for the pancreatic duct. Gas in the stomach, or more often in the transverse colon, commonly prevents visualization of the pancreas, especially if the left lobe of the liver is small. Progressive transducer pressure is most effective in displacing gas to visualize the pancreas. The tail of the pancreas can be visualized through the spleen concentrating on the region of the splenic hilum.

Pancreatitis

Acute Pancreatitis. US findings include: diffuse glandular enlargement, decrease in echogenicity due to edema, and poorly defined gland margins (Fig. 36.31). In mild cases, the US examination may be normal. Focal pancreatitis most commonly involves the pancreatic head. US examination should include documentation of the presence of gallstones and dilatation of the biliary tree. The ampullary region should be carefully examined for an impacted gallstone. US is excellent for detection and follow-up of fluid collections (Figs. 36.32, 36.33). Fluid accumulates most commonly around the pancreas, in the lesser sac, and in the splenic hilum. Examination should be extended into the pelvis, especially if fluid is seen tracking caudal to the pancreas. Discrete cystic collections should be examined with Doppler to detect pseudoaneurysms. The splenic, portal,

and superior mesenteric veins are examined for evidence of thrombosis.

Chronic Pancreatitis. Because of fibrosis and diffuse glandular atrophy, the pancreas is reduced in size and increased in echogenicity making its identification with US more difficult. Calcifications produce focal echodensities and, often, acoustic shadowing. The pancreatic duct shows a pattern of alternating dilatation and constriction. Calcifications are commonly seen within the

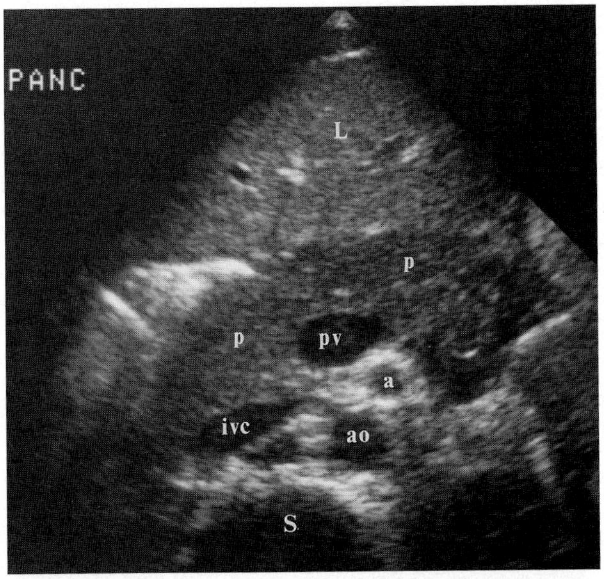

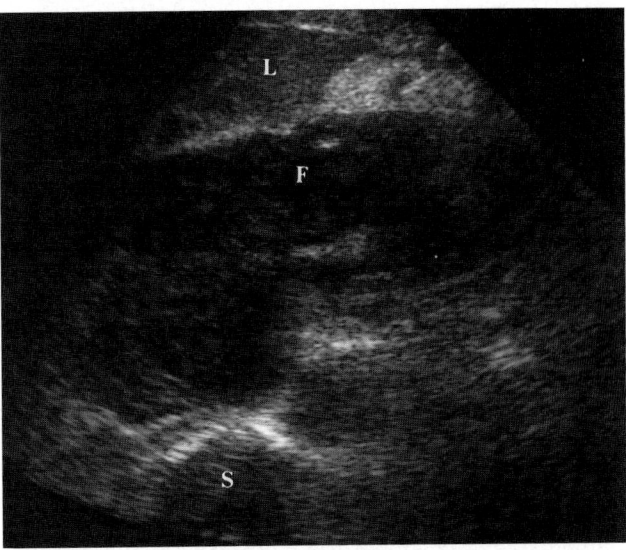

Figure 36.32. Necrotizing Pancreatitis. The anatomic landmarks for the pancreas are obliterated and replaced by heterogeneous fluid (*F*) in this patient with acute severe necrotizing pancreatitis. *S,* spine; *L,* liver.

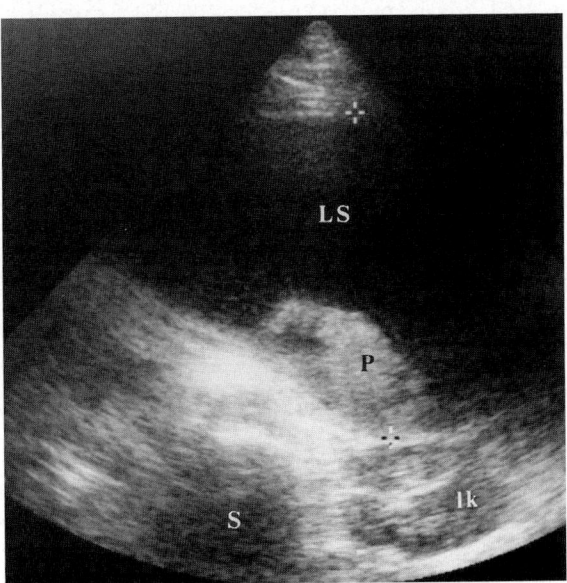

Figure 36.31. Acute Pancreatitis. Axial plane US image reveals a diffuse decrease in the echogenicity of the pancreatic parenchyma (*p*) compared to the liver (*L*) because of diffuse edema of acute inflammation. The normal pancreas is more echogenic than the normal liver (Fig. 36.30B). No discrete fluid collections were evident. *pv,* portal vein; *a,* superior mesenteric artery; *ivc,* inferior vena cava; *ao,* aorta; *S,* spine.

Figure 36.33. Pancreatic Fluid Collection in Lesser Sac. US scan in axial plane shows a large collection of fluid (*LS*) in the lesser sac anterior to the pancreas (*P*). US is excellent for following the evolution of pancreatic fluid collections. *S,* spine; *lk,* left kidney.

duct (Fig. 36.34). Signs of acute pancreatitis are commonly superimposed on chronic pancreatitis.

Solid Pancreas Masses

Adenocarcinoma appears as a hypoechoic mass (Fig. 36.35) or as a subtle alteration of acoustic texture in the pancreas. Biliary and pancreatic ductal obstruction is easily identified. Sudden termination of dilated ducts in a hypoechoic mass is a characteristic appearance. Doppler is used to detect the vascular encasement or invasion that commonly makes the tumor non-resectable (28). The liver and retroperitoneum should be carefully examined for metastatic nodules and adenopathy.

Chronic Pancreatitis. A mass of solid fibrinous tissue caused by chronic pancreatitis may be indistinguishable from adenocarcinoma. Ductal dilatation may be present. A major use of US is to guide percutaneous biopsy to provide pathological differentiation of this common clinical problem.

Islet Cell Tumors are predominantly hypoechoic compared to pancreatic paremchyma (29). Cystic degeneration, hemorrhage, fibrosis, and calcification cause a wide variety in appearance. Transabdominal US detects 20–75% of insulinomas and only 20–30% of gastrinomas. Endoscopic US improves detection to 77–94% range. Intraoperative US demonstrates 75–100% of small tumors and serves as a major aid to the surgeon having difficulty identifying the tumor.

Metastases, especially from colon carcinoma, may mimic pancreatic adenocarcinoma (30).

Lymphoma commonly involves the peripancreatic lymph nodes causing multiple or confluent hypoechoic masses.

Cystic Pancreas Masses

Pseudocysts appear as well-defined, smooth-walled, anechoic masses. Multiple loculations and internal septations are common. Internal debris and fluid-fluid levels are indicative of hemorrhage or infection. US is an excellent way to provide imaging follow-up of pseudocysts to confirm resolution or determine the need for drainage.

Abscess. US demonstrates a fluid collection that is usually ill-defined and contains echogenic fluid. Gas bubbles that move, shadow, and cause comet-tail artifacts are strong evidence of infection. US is used to guide aspiration and catheter drainage.

Multiple Pancreatic Cysts are seen in patients with autosomal dominant polycystic disease and those with von Hippel-Lindau syndrome (31). Solitary true epithelial-lined cysts are rare.

Pseudoaneurysms develop in the peripancreatic region most commonly as a complication of pancreatitis with enzyme erosion of arterial walls. US demonstrates a discrete cystic mass in close proximity to an artery. Doppler US confirms arterial flow within the lumen of the pseudoaneurysm. A small neck of connection with the parent artery can be identified by flow jets.

Microcystic Adenoma, although composed of innumerable small cysts, commonly appears as a solid lesion on US (32). A few larger cysts may be demonstrated. An echogenic central stellate scar with calcification is characteristic. CT should be performed to demonstrate distinctive enhancement of honeycomb septations.

Mucinous Cystic Tumors demonstrate cysts 2 cm or larger in size (Fig. 36.36). Internal septations and papil-

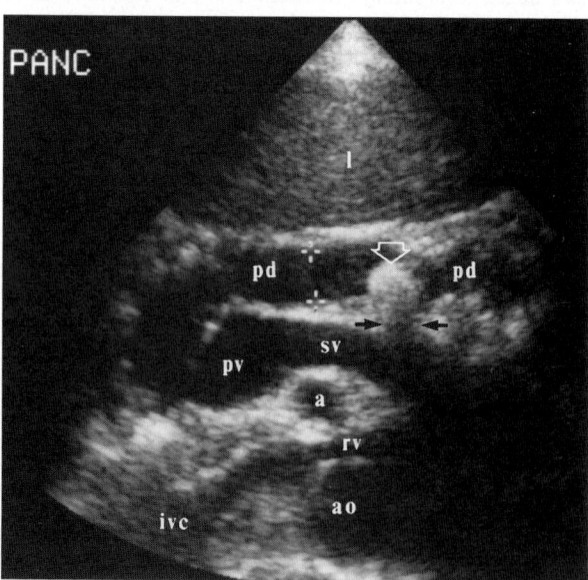

Figure 36.34. Chronic Pancreatitis. US in axial plane demonstrates a calculus (*open arrow*) in the markedly dilated pancreatic duct (*pd*). The calculus is seen as an echogenic focus with acoustic shadowing (*black arrows*). The pancreatic parenchyma is atrophic, consistent with chronic pancreatitis. The pancreatic duct measures 8.7 mm in diameter (*calipers*). A detailed knowledge of anatomy is needed to correctly identify all structures visualized. Doppler US is helpful in confirming vascular structures. *ao*, aorta; *a*, superior mesenteric artery; *ivc*, inferior vena cava; *rv*, left renal vein; *sv*, splenic vein; *pv*, portal vein; *l*, liver.

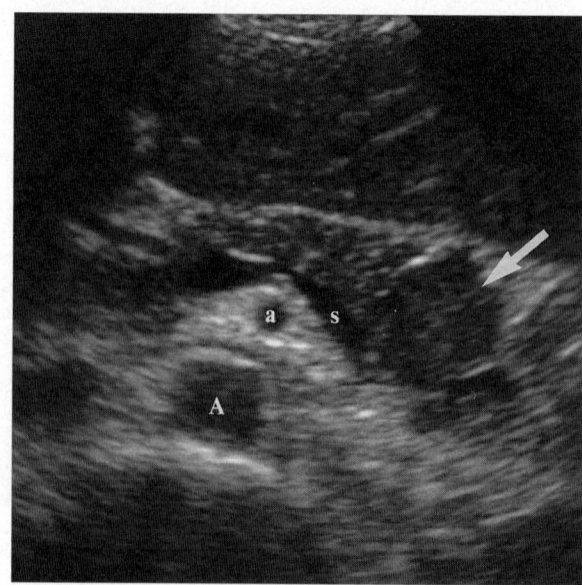

Figure 36.35. Adenocarcinoma of the Pancreas. The tumor is seen as a subtle hypoechoic mass (*arrow*) causing a focal bulge in the contour of the tail of the pancreas. *A*, aorta; *a*, superior mesenteric artery; *s*, splenic vein.

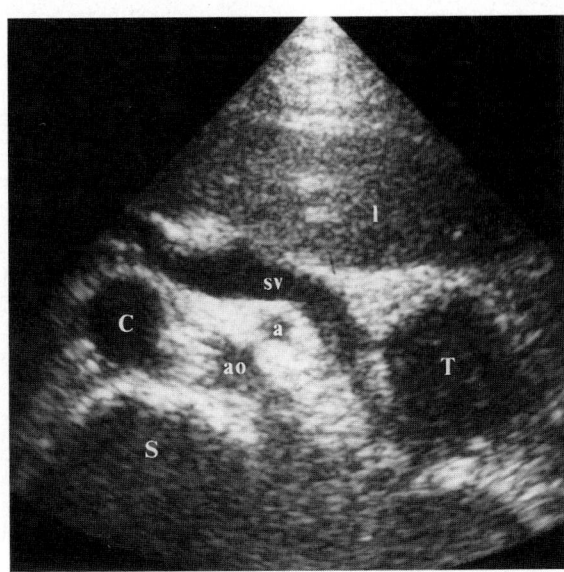

Figure 36.36. Mucinous Cystadenocarcinoma of the Pancreas. Axial plane US demonstrates a unilocular cystic tumor (*T*) arising from the tail of the pancreas. A cyst (*C*) was present on the right kidney. The inferior vena cava was not distended when this image was taken. *S*, spine; *ao*, aorta; *a*, superior mesenteric artery; *sv*, splenic vein; *l*, liver.

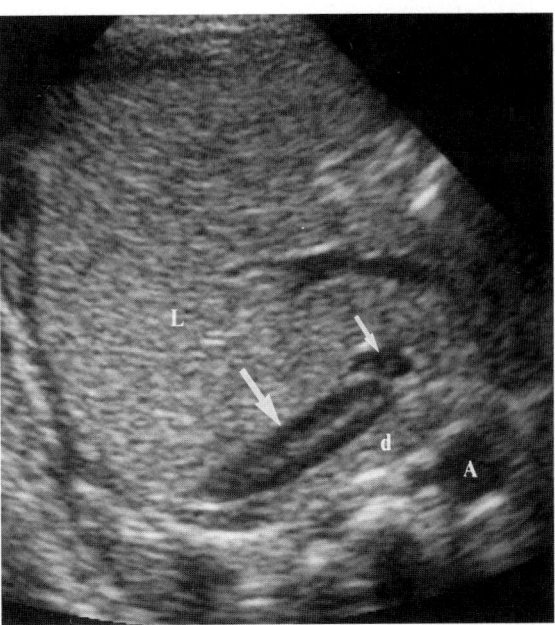

Figure 36.37. Normal Adrenal Gland. Transverse US image in an infant demonstrates the normal anatomic landmarks for identification of the right adrenal gland (*large arrow*), found posterior to the inferior vena cava (*small arrow*), between the right lobe of the liver (*L*) and the right crus (*d*) of the diaphragm. *A*, aorta.

lary projections from 1–2 mm thick walls are demonstrated. Dilatation of the pancreatic ducts accompany tumors that produce large volumes of mucin (33,34). Bengin and malignant tumors cannot be differentiated.

ADRENAL GLANDS

Normal US Anatomy. The normal adrenal glands may be difficult to visualize sonographically in the adult, but are usually quite prominent in the newborn (Fig. 36.37). The right adrenal gland is best seen on a transverse image just above the upper pole of the right kidney. The Y- or V-shaped adrenal gland is seen just posterior to the inferior vena cava as the IVC enters the liver. The right adrenal is visualized between the right lobe of the liver and the right crus of the diaphragm. The left adrenal is best seen between the upper pole of the left kidney and the aorta on an angled coronal plane. The adrenals are hypoechoic compared to retroperitoneal fat and isoechoic compared to the crura of the diaphragm. The medulla is seen as a thin echogenic line surrounded by the hypoechoic cortex. The limbs of the normal adult adrenal gland are 4–5 cm in length and 5–7 mm in width. In infants the adrenal glands normally appear large due to persistence of the "fetal" portion of the gland (35). The fetal cortex rapidly involutes in the first 3 weeks of life (36).

Although CT is more sensitive than US for detection of small adrenal masses, US is useful for: characterizing adrenal masses as cystic, followup of presumed benign adrenal masses, and confirming the origin of large retroperitoneal masses (37).

Adrenal Hyperplasia appears as bilateral diffuse enlargement or as multiple bilateral small nodules (35).

Hyperplastic glands are seen with the adrenal endocrine syndromes. The differential diagnosis of bilateral enlarged adrenal glands includes infection (especially tuberculosis, histoplasmosis, and cytomegalovirus), metastatic disease, and lymphoma. Patients with AIDS may have adrenal enlargement due to mycobacterial, fungal, or viral infection.

Adrenal Adenomas appear as solid, homogeneous, adrenal masses with echogenicity similar to renal parenchyma (Fig. 36.38). US offers no specific findings that differentiate benign from malignant masses. Masses larger than 4 cm should be considered suspicious for malignancy.

Adrenal Carcinomas are indistinguishable from adenomas when the tumor is small (<4 cm). Larger carcinomas are inhomogeneous with areas of necrosis, hemorrhage, and calcification. Real-time imaging and Doppler are useful to detect tumor invasion of adrenal or renal veins and the inferior vena cava.

Pheochromocytoma arising in the adrenal gland can usually be demonstrated by US, because most are large (5–6 cm)(Fig. 36.39). Most are sharply marginated and predominantly solid with cystic areas of necrosis and hemorrhage commonly present (38). Predominantly cystic pheochromocytomas are less common.

Adrenal Myelolipoma appears as a highly echogenic mass in the adrenal bed (39, 40). They may be easily overlooked. Mixed hyperechoic and hypoechoic areas correspond to fatty and myeloid elements within the tumor. The diagnosis is confirmed by demonstration of internal fat density by CT. Other echogenic masses in the adrenal region include renal angiomyolipoma, teratoma, lipoma, and liposarcoma.

Figure 36.38. Benign Adrenal Adenoma. Longitudinal US demonstrates a homogeneous 3.5 cm mass (*A*, between *arrows*) arising from the right adrenal gland. The mass is outlined by echogenic fat. This is a nonhyperfunctioning adrenal adenoma that was discovered incidentally. *L*, liver; *RK*, right kidney.

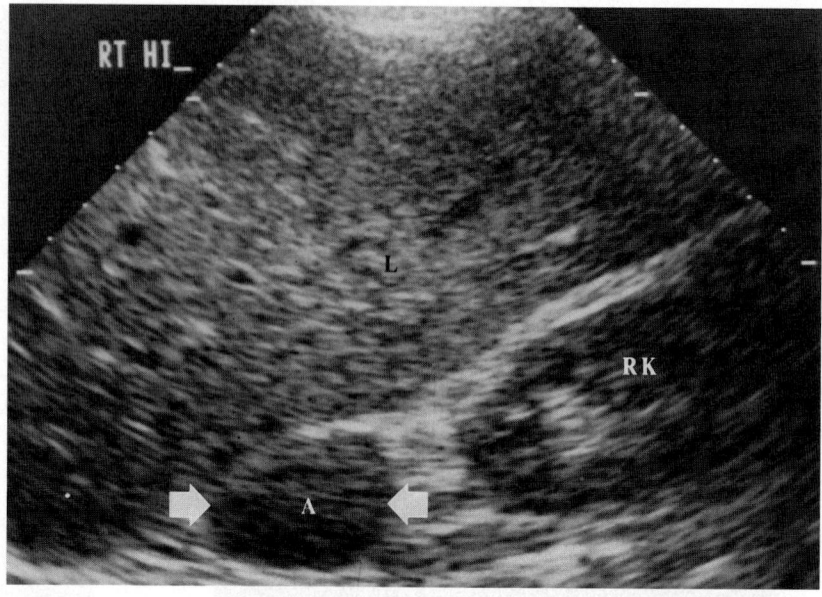

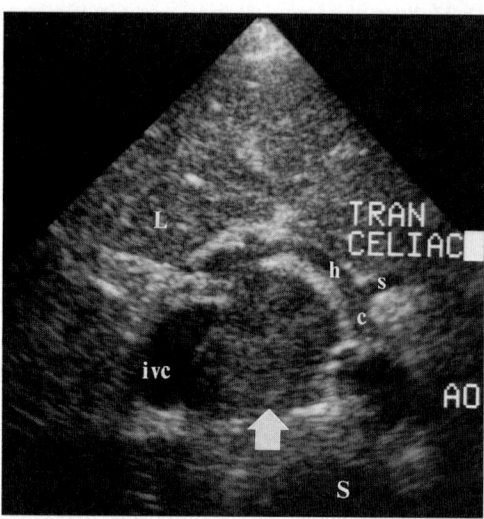

Figure 36.39. Pheochromocytoma. Axial plane US demonstrates the adrenal tumor extending between the inferior vena cava (*ivc*) and aorta (*AO*). The origin of the celiac axis (*c*) from the aorta and its branches, the common hepatic artery (*h*) and the splenic artery (*s*) are clearly seen. *L*, liver; *S*, spine.

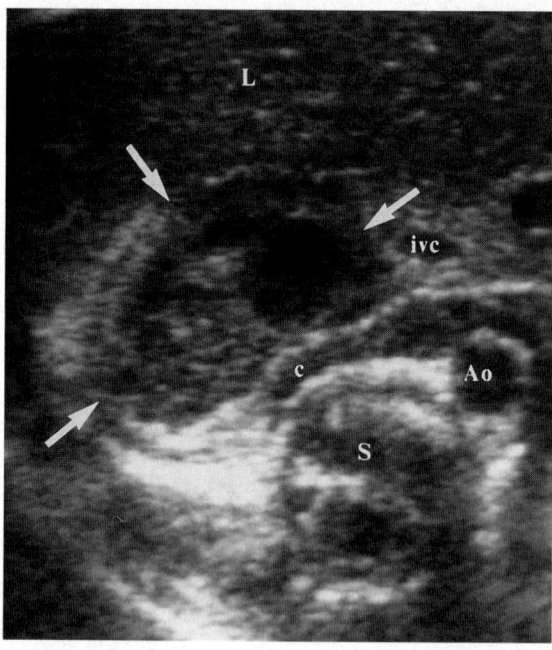

Figure 36.40. Adrenal Hemorrhage. The adrenal gland in a 2-week old infant is identified by its location between liver (*L*), inferior vena cava (*ivc*), and right crus of the diaphragm (*c*). *Ao*, aorta; *S*, spine.

Adrenal Cysts. US may be utilized to differentiate benign cysts from cystic tumors. Uncomplicated benign cysts have thin walls and septa (<3 mm), anechoic internal fluid, and demonstrate accentuated through-transmission (41). Calcification in walls and septa is common in all types of benign cysts. Echogenic internal fluid or debris, thick walls, solid components, and large size (>6 cm) suggest possible malignancy.

Adrenal Hemorrhage. US initially demonstrates hyperechoic, mass-like enlargement of the adrenal gland (Fig. 36.40). With time, the adrenal mass rapidly becomes hypoechoic and progressively decreases in size. The gland may return entirely to normal or evolve into a pseudocyst that commonly develops calcifications in its walls within 2—4 weeks of the hemorrhage. Eventual collapse of the pseudocyst results in coarsely calcified adrenal glands. In the neonate, adrenal hemorrhage is usually bilateral and due to hypoxic stress. In the adult, adrenal hemorrhage is usually unilateral and right-sided (85%).

KIDNEYS

Normal US Anatomy. US demonstrates the complex internal anatomy of the kidney with a wide range of normal variation in appearance (Fig. 36.41). The renal cortex is isoechoic or slightly hypoechoic compared to the liver and distinctly hypoechoic compared to the spleen. The medullary pyramids are visualized as hypoechoic cone-shaped structures surrounded by the more echogenic cortex. This corticomedullary differentiation is striking in the newborn and becomes less noticeable with age (Fig. 36.42). Lucent pyramids should not be mistaken for hydronephrosis. The central sinus contains fat, blood vessels, the collecting system, and lymphatics. Central sinus echogenicity is the same as perirenal fat. Blood vessels appear as lucent tubular structures

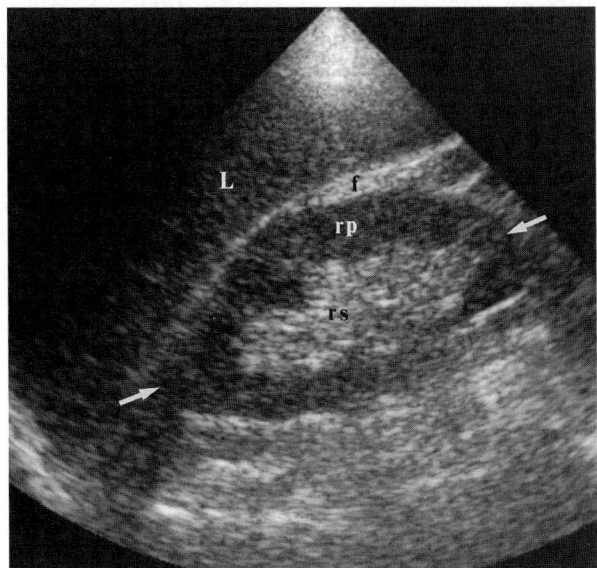

Figure 36.41. Normal Kidney. A long axis US view of the right kidney (between *arrows*) obtained through the liver (*L*) demonstrates echogenicity of the normal renal parenchyma approximately equal to the echogenicity of the normal liver. The renal sinus (*rs*), containing vessels, the collecting system, and fat, is hyperechoic compared to the renal parenchyma (*rp*). The margins of the kidney are outlined by echogenic perirenal fat (*f*). Morison's pouch is a recess of the peritoneal cavity between the kidney and the liver that usually fills with fluid when ascites is present.

with flow demonstrated by Doppler. In well hydrated patients, minimally dilated collecting structures may be normally visualized. The contour of the kidney is smooth and may be lobulated by the normal renal lobes. Adult kidneys range from 9 to 13 cm in length. The *junctional parenchymal defect* is a normal anatomic variant caused by incomplete fusion of the upper and lower poles of the kidney. Sonography demonstrates a wedge-shaped echogenic defect in the renal parenchyma at the junction of the upper and middle thirds of the kidney.

Obstruction. US is commonly the imaging method of first choice for the diagnosis of urinary obstruction. Beware, there are numerous pitfalls in using US to make this diagnosis. The key US finding in obstruction is hydronephrosis. Hydronephrosis is recognized as fluid distension of the collecting system with communication between round fluid-filled calyces and the dilated renal pelvis (Fig. 36.43). A dilated ureter appears as a fluid-filled tube extending from the renal pelvis. However, in acute obstruction such as from a stone impacted in the ureter, the degree of collecting system dilatation may be slight even though the obstruction is severe. Moreover, the presence of hydronephrosis does not always mean obstruction. Additional causes of pelvicalyectasis are listed in Table 36.2. Structures that may mimic hydronephrosis include peripelvic cysts (Fig. 36.44), multiple simple cysts in the renal sinus, and an extrarenal pelvis. An *extrarenal pelvis* is one that extends outside the renal sinus. This type of pelvis is commonly fluid-filled but is a normal variant not associated with dilated calyces or ureter. Comparison with previous studies may help in making the correct diagnosis. The ureterovesical junction should be examined with color Doppler to detect the presence or absence of a ureteral jet. Doppler evaluation of the renal arteries may also be helpful. A resistance index greater than 0.70 in the arcuate artery suggests suggests obstruction (42).

Stones. All renal stones, regardless of composition, appear on US as bright echogenic foci (Fig. 36.45)(43). Stones as small as 5 mm may be identified if they cast

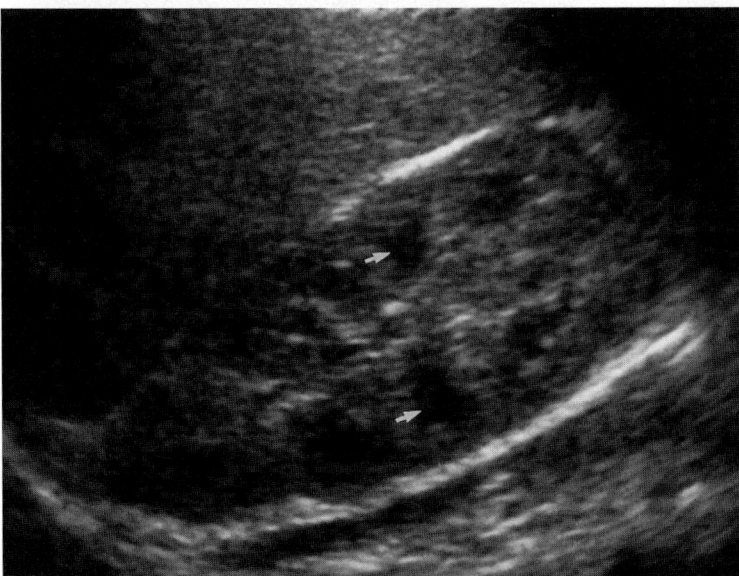

Figure 36.42. Normal Infant Kidney. In newborns and infants, the renal cortex is more echogenic than in older children and adults, causing the medullary pyramids (*arrows*) to appear more lucent and resemble hydronephrosis. Note that the lucent pyramids correspond anatomically to the location of the renal medulla, that the pyramids do not interconnect, and that the renal pelvis is not dilated.

an acoustic shadow (44). However, when acoustic shadowing is not evident, often due to technical factors, small stones may be overlooked because they blend in with echogenic renal sinus fat. Technical factors that improve the capability to demonstrate shadowing include: imaging the stone in the focal zone of the transducer, center-

ing the stone within the US beam, and using high frequency transducers.

Nephrocalcinosis refers to calcification in the renal medullary pyramids which appear echogenic rather than echolucent (Fig. 36.46). US is highly sensitive to even faint calcification that may not be visible on plain radiographs. Acoustic shadowing is present only when calcification is dense. Common causes include furosemide therapy in the newborn, hypercalciuric states such as hyperparathyroidism, medullary sponge kidney, and renal tubular acidosis.

Diffuse Renal Parenchymal Disease. US is commonly used to evaluate patients with acute and chronic renal failure. Rarely (<5% of cases), bilateral renal obstruction will be a cause of acute renal failure. Causes of bilateral obstruction include leaking abdominal aortic aneurysm, tumor (especially cervical carcinoma), and retroperitoneal fibrosis. These rare cases will benefit from relief of obstruction. In the remainder of patients, US reveals the size and morphology of the kidneys. End-stage renal disease is associated with small echogenic, often difficult to visualize, kidneys (Fig. 36.47)(Table 36.3). When the kidneys are smaller than 9 cm in adults, reversible renal disease is unlikely and renal biopsy is

Figure 36.43. Hydronephrosis due to Ureteropelvic Junction Calculus. Coronal plane US of the right kidney (*RK*) reveals mild dilation of the calyces (*long white arrows*) and renal pelvis (*p*) due to an impacted stone (*s, between open arrows*) at the ureteropelvic junction. Note the dark acoustic shadow (between *short white arrows*) cast by the calculus.

Table 36.2. Causes of Hydronephrosis

Obstruction
Vesicoureteral reflux
Distended bladder
Relieved obstruction with persistent dilatation
Pregnancy
Diabetes insipidus
Active diuresis

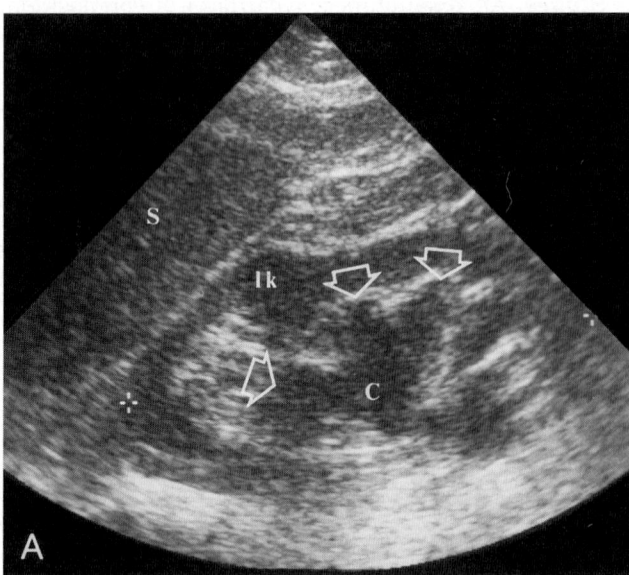
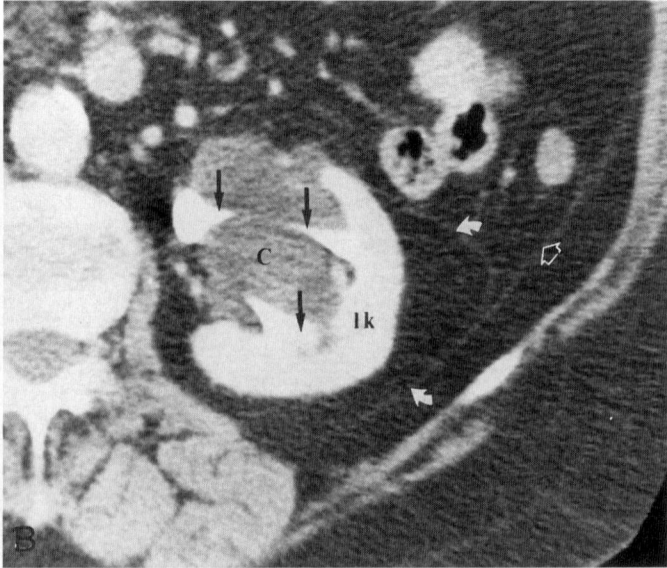

Figure 36.44. Peripelvic Cyst. A. Long axis US image of the left kidney (*lk*) reveals a fluid-filled structure (*C*) in the renal sinus. Lobulations (*arrows*) of the cystic mass resemble dilated calyces. *S*, spleen. **B.** A CT image of the left kidney (*lk*) reveals the calyces and pelvis (*black arrows*) to be stretched around the peripelvic cyst (*C*).

Cysts that arise in the renal sinus assume the shape of the sinus as they slowly enlarge, mimicking hydronephrosis. Note the visualization of the renal fascia (*curved arrows*) and lateroconal fascia (*open arrow*) in this patient.

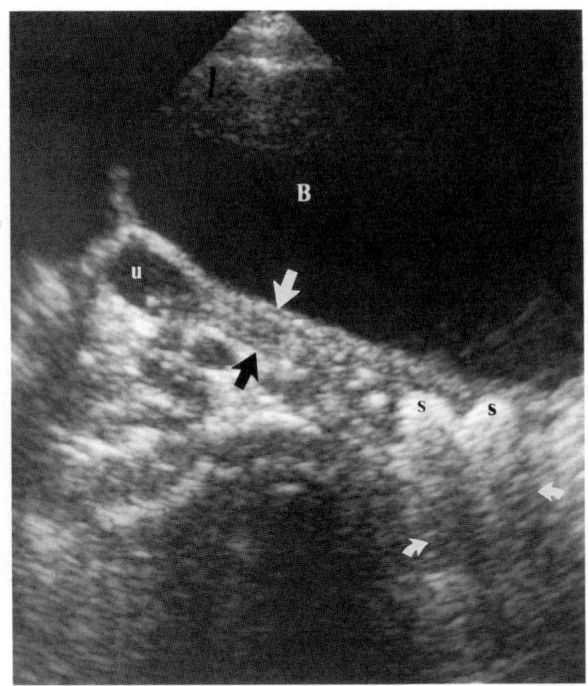

Figure 36.45. Calculi in Distal Ureter. Sagittal plane US image of the distal right ureter (*u*) demonstrates two stones (*s*) impacted at the ureterovesical junction. Faint acoustic shadows (*curved arrows*) are cast by the stones. Just proximal to the stones the ureter is filled with echogenic debris (*arrows*) due to infection developing as a result of urinary stasis. *B*, bladder.

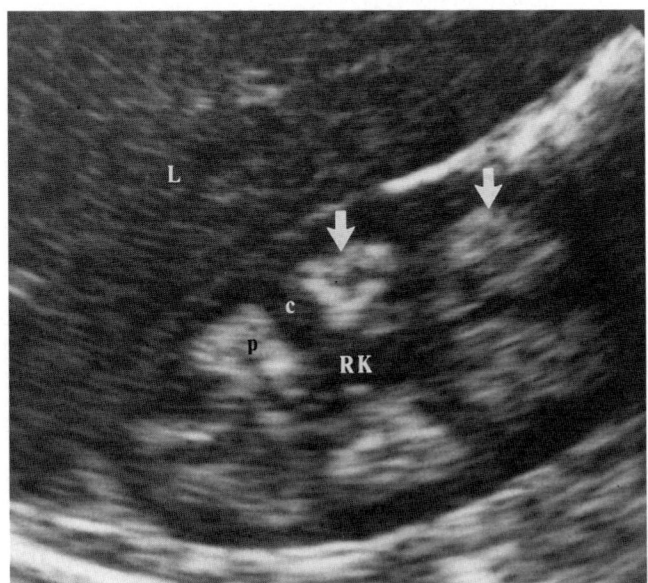

Figure 36.46. Medullary Nephrocalcinosis. Longitudinal US of the right kidney (*RK*) demonstrates abnormal increased echogencity of the medullary pyramids (*p, arrows*). Compare to Figures 36.41 and 36.42. The echogenicity of the intrarenal cortex (*c*)(columns of Bertin) is normal. *L*, liver

seldom justified. Diffuse and focal renal parenchymal thinning and scarring provide rough estimates of renal parenchymal loss. Enlarged kidneys (>12 cm) suggest an infiltrative process such as acute glomerulonephritis, leukemia, lymphoma, or renal vein thrombosis (edema). AIDS nephropathy is characterized by an enlarged diffusely echogenic kidney (Fig. 36.48). Enlarged kidneys are an indication for Doppler examination of the renal veins, and may warrant a renal biopsy to detect a treatable condition. US may demonstrate an unsuspected condition such as a form of renal cystic disease.

Renal Masses

Sonography plays a significant role in both the detection and characterization of renal masses. Real-time gray-scale US is used to determine if a mass is a simple cyst, a complicated cyst, a complex mass, or an entirely solid mass. Doppler is used to demonstrate the internal vascularity to characterize a neoplasm.

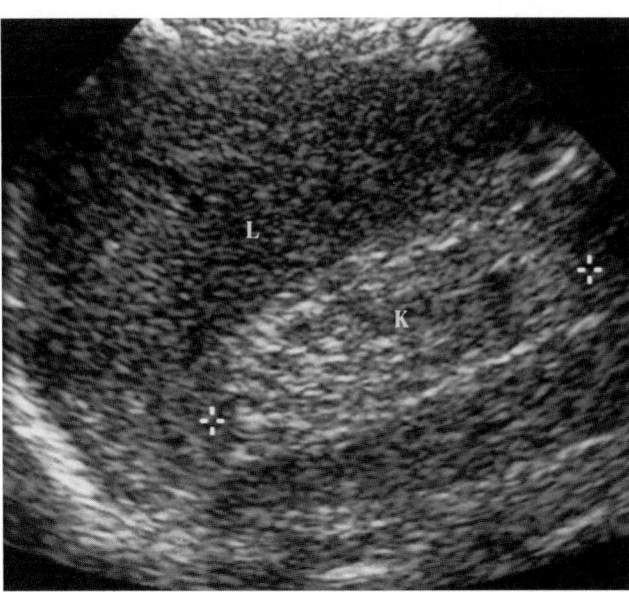

Figure 36.47. End-Stage Kidney. In this patient with advanced renal failure, both kidneys (*K*) were small (between *cursors* (+))(6–7 cm in length), diffusely echogenic, and difficult to visualize due to loss of normal renal morphology. The echogenicity of the renal parenchyma exceeds the echogenicity of the liver parenchyma (*L*).

Table 36.3. Medical Renal Diseases with Echogenic Renal Parenchyma in Adults

Acute glomerulonephritis
Chronic glomerulonephritis
Hypertensive nephrosclerosis
Diabetic glomerulosclerosis
Lupus nephritis
Lymphoma
AIDS
Amyloidosis

Figure 36.48. AIDS Nephropathy. Both kidneys in this patients with AIDS and impaired renal function were diffusely enlarged (>14 cm) and diffusely increased in echogenicity. Compare the right kidney parenchyma (*K*) to the liver parenchyma (*L*).

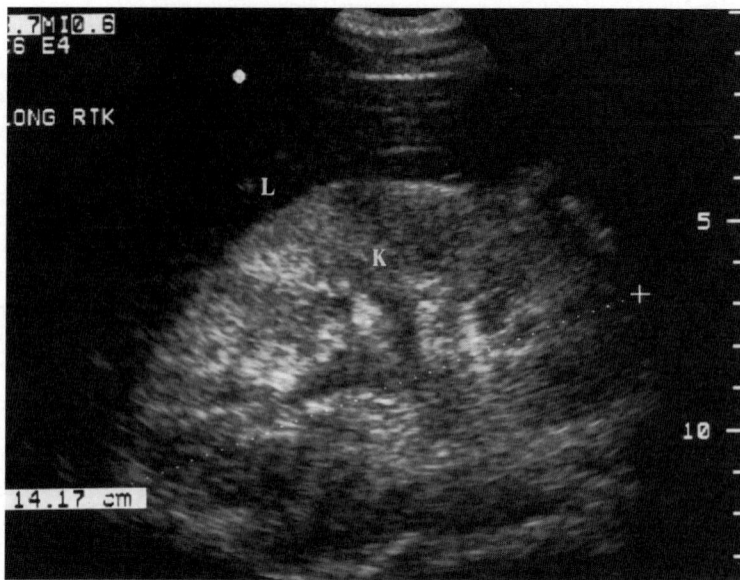

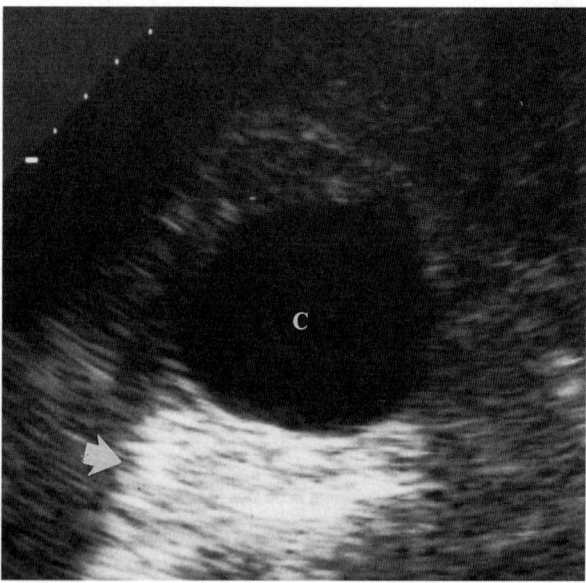

Figure 36.49. Simple Renal Cyst. Transverse image of the kidney shows a simple renal cyst (*C*) with imperceptibly thin walls, anechoic internal fluid, and accentuated sound transmission (*arrow*).

Simple Cysts are diagnosed accurately and easily by US. Characteristic findings are (Fig. 36.49) the following: *a*) anechoic contents, *b*) well-defined far wall, *c*) acoustic enhancement deep to the lesion, *d*) imperceptibly thin walls. Small cysts may have artifactual internal echoes due to slice thickness limitations. Acoustic enhancement may depend upon optimizing technique. All cysts should have a sharply defined back wall. Cysts with thin septations or thin peripheral curvilinear calcifications still qualify as benign cysts.

Complicated Cysts have any of the following findings which disqualify their characterization as a simple cyst: internal debris, echogenic clot, fluid-debris levels, thick septations, thick walls, blood vessels in septations, thick or coarse calcification (see Figure 33.17). Differential di-

agnosis of a complicated cystic mass includes: hemorrhage or infection in simple cyst, cystic tumor, abscess, obstructed upper pole duplication, calyceal diverticulum, lymphoma, aneurysm, and pseudoaneurysm.

Peripelvic Cysts form in the renal sinus, are multilobed, and may closely resemble hydronephrosis (Fig. 36.44). Peripelvic cysts are differentiated from hydronephrosis by demonstration of lack of communication with each other or dilated renal pelvis, echogenic fat between the tip of the medullary pyramid and the cyst, and lack of a dilated ureter. Problem cases require excretory urography or CT.

Renal Cystic Disease is discussed in detail in chapter 33. US is a reliable, safe, and accurate method to demonstrate size, number, and character of cysts in the kidney as well as other organs (Figs. 36.50–36.53).

Renal Cell Carcinoma (RCC) is, by far, the most common solid renal mass in adults. On US, 50% are hyperechoic compared to renal parenchyma (Fig. 36.54), 30% are isoechoic, 10% are hypoechoic and 5–10% are predominantly cystic, 20–30% have coarse, punctate, central calcification. Highly echoic RCC may be confused with angiomyolipoma (AML) although RCC tends to be more heterogeneous and may have cystic components (45). CT or MR may be needed to demonstrate fat in the tumor. Isoechoic tumors are detected when they distort the renal contour. Tumors become cystic because of necrosis and internal hemorrhage. Doppler demonstration of internal vascularity is strong evidence of RCC.

With detection of a solid renal mass the US examination should be extended to detect tumor invasion of the renal vein and inferior vena cava. Signs of tumor thrombus include (Fig. 36.55): echogenic mass in vein, enlarged vein, enlarged collateral vein, lack of or displacement of venous flow on color Doppler, and arterial Doppler signal within the vein due to tumor neovascularity.

Angiomyolipoma. The classic US appearance, seen in 80% of cases, is a uniformly hyperechoic renal mass with sharp borders (Fig. 36.56)(46). The echogenicity of the

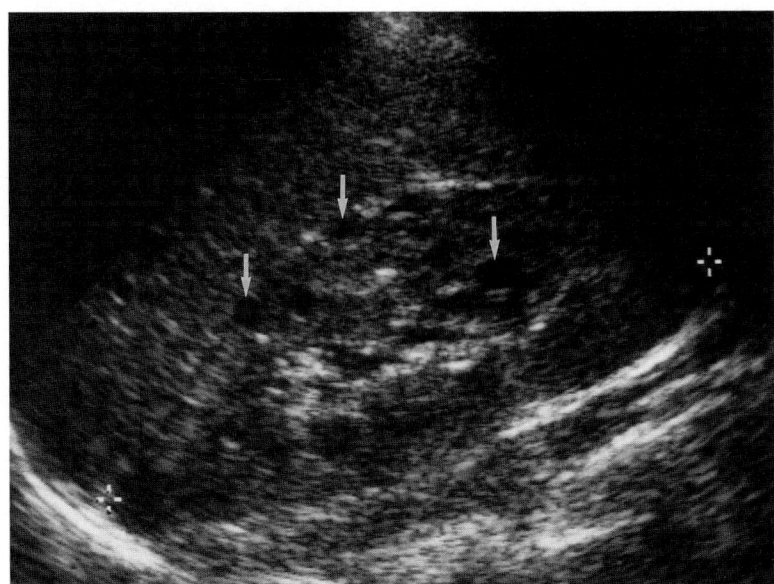

Figure 36.50. Autosomal Dominant Polycystic Disease. The kidney of a 21-year-old patient with a family history of cystic renal disease shows multiple small cysts (*arrows*) and mild enlargement. These findings are an early manifestation of autosomal dominant polycystic disease.

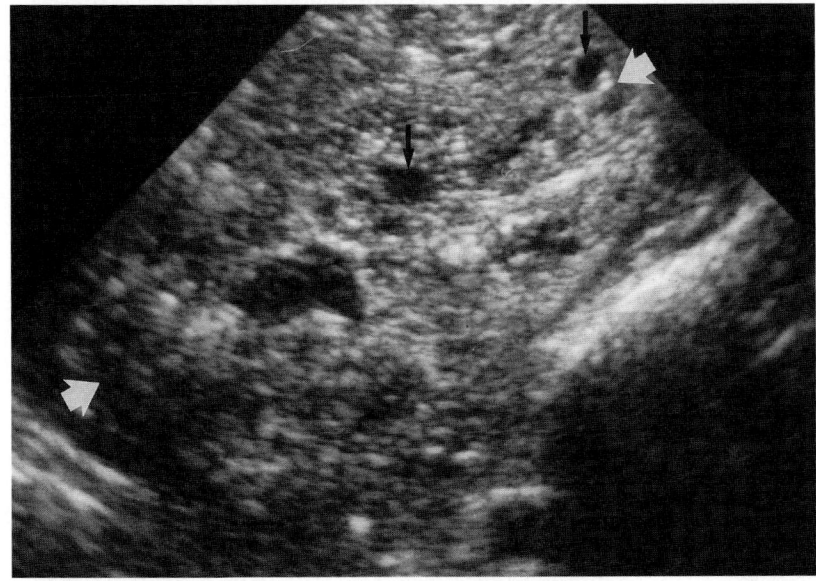

Figure 36.51. Autosomal Recessive Polycystic Disease. The kidney (between *white arrows*) of a 5-year-old with impaired renal and hepatic function shows mottled increased echogenicity and several small parenchymal cysts (*black arrows*).

mass is at least equal to that of renal sinus fat. Tumors which lack substantial fat are often indistinguishable from other renal tumors. Weak acoustic shadowing in the absence of calcification is seen with AML but not with RCC. Angiomyolipoma is typically hypervascular but rarely has any cystic components. Definitive diagnosis is made by CT or MR demonstration of fat within the tumor. Calcification in the tumor is extremely rare.

Transitional Cell Carcinoma (TCC) is commonly overlooked by US. Tumors may be small, infiltrative, or stenosing. A solid mass within or arising from the central renal sinus is suspicious (Fig. 36.57). US is best used to differentiate a solid mass in the renal sinus from a peripelvic cyst. Focal hydronephrosis may be caused by a small TCC, or TCC may appear as soft tissue nodule within a dilated pelvis.

Lymphoma typically produces multiple hypoechoic masses, each of which has a uniform pattern of fine low-level echoes reflecting the homogeneous cellular structure. Doppler demonstration of internal vessels differentiates lymphoma from cysts containing echogenic fluid. Growth patterns include single dominant mass, multiple masses, diffuse infiltration causing renal enlargement, and invasion of the renal sinus from confluent retroperitoneal adenopathy.

Renal Infection

Acute Pyelonephritis frequently produces no US abnormalities. Severe cases alter the echogenicity of the renal parenchyma due to edema, local inflammation, and focal bleeding (Fig. 36.58). Masslike areas of focal inflammation have been called lobar nephronia, focal nephritis, and a variety of other names that mostly cause confusion. These finding should be viewed as US evidence of severe pyelonephritis and probably nothing

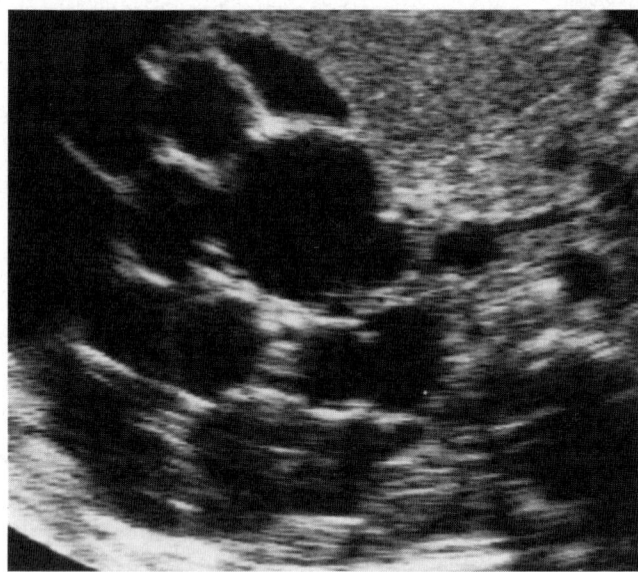

Figure 36.52. Multicystic Dysplastic Kidney. The right kidney is totally replaced by cysts of varying size, the classic appearance of multicystic dysplastic kidney. The left kidney appeared normal. A radionuclide scan demonstrated absent function on the right and normal function on the left.

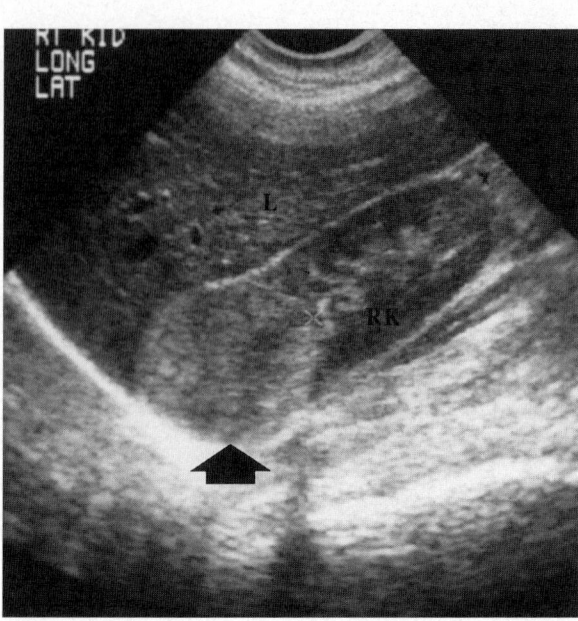

Figure 36.54. Renal Cell Carcinoma. An US image in the long axis of the right kidney (*RK*) reveals a solid, hyperechoic mass (*arrow*) at the upper pole. *L*, liver.

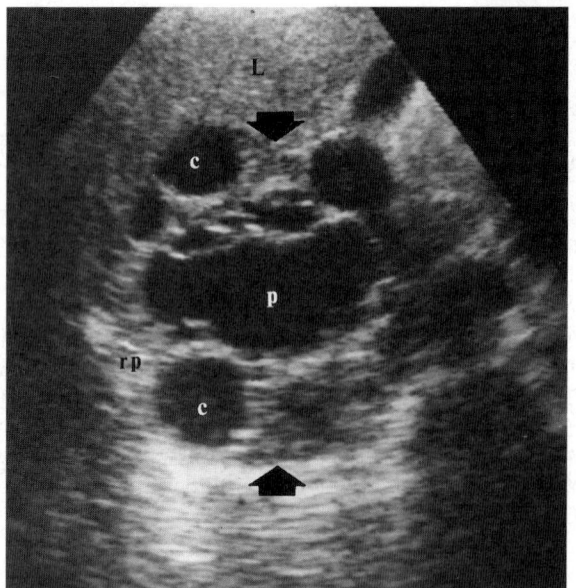

Figure 36.53. Tuberous Sclerosis. Transverse US view of the right kidney (between *arrowheads*) reveals multiple simple cysts (*c*) of varying size in the renal parenchyma (*rp*). The renal pelvis (*p*) is dilated because of mass effect and partial obstruction caused by the renal cysts. *L*, liver.

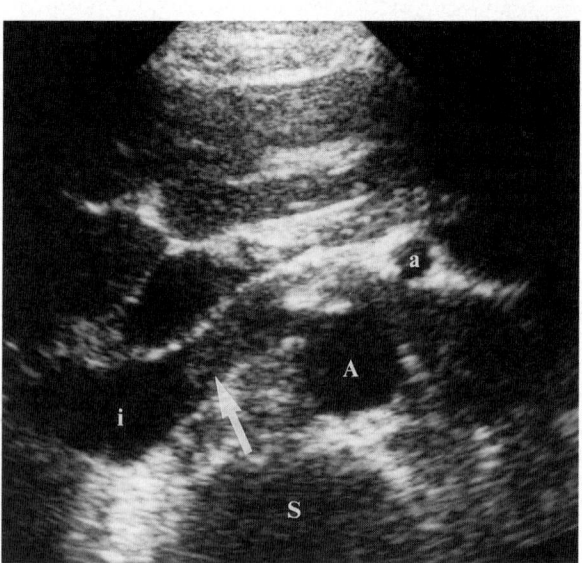

Figure 36.55. Extension of Renal Cell Carcinoma into Renal Vein. Transverse image reveals an enlarged left renal vein with intraluminal soft tissue (*arrow*) extending to its junction with the inferior vena cava (*i*) in patient with renal cell carcinoma in the left kidney. *A*, aorta; *a*, superior mesenteric artery; *S*, spine.

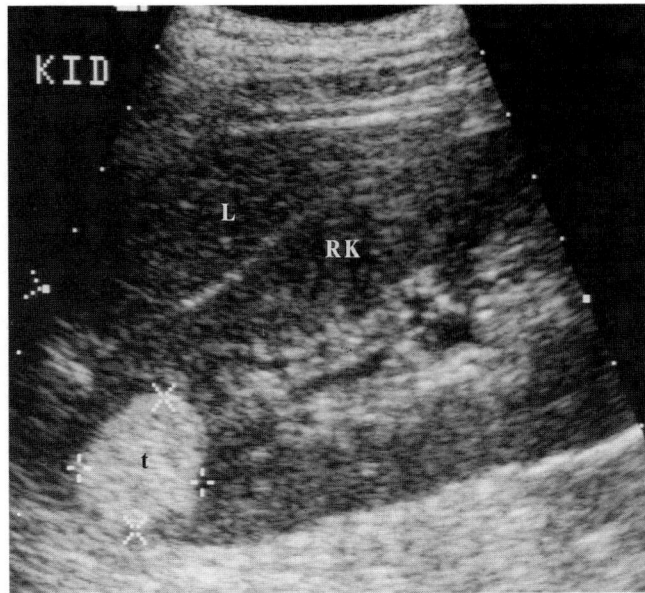

Figure 36.56. Angiomyolipoma. An US image through the long axis of the right kidney (*RK*) demonstrates a well-defined, uniformly hyperechoic tumor (*t*) in the upper pole. This appearance is strongly suggestive of angiomyolipoma. *L*, liver.

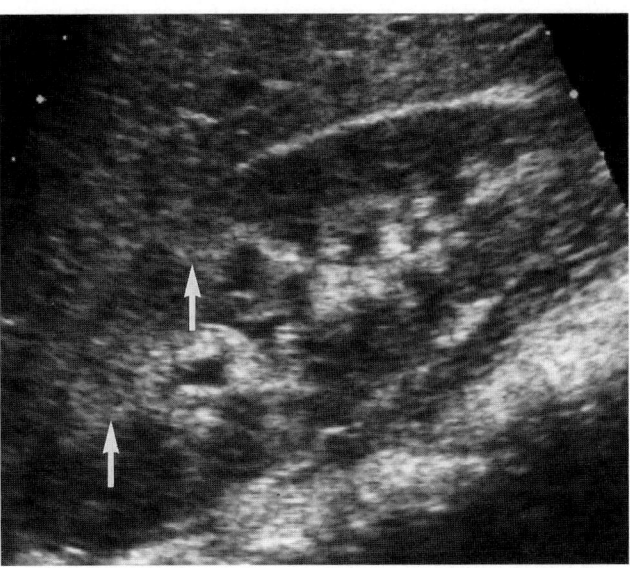

Figure 36.58. Acute Pyelonephritis. Focal areas of increased echogenicity (*arrows*) indicate inflammation and hemorrhage due to acute bacterial infection.

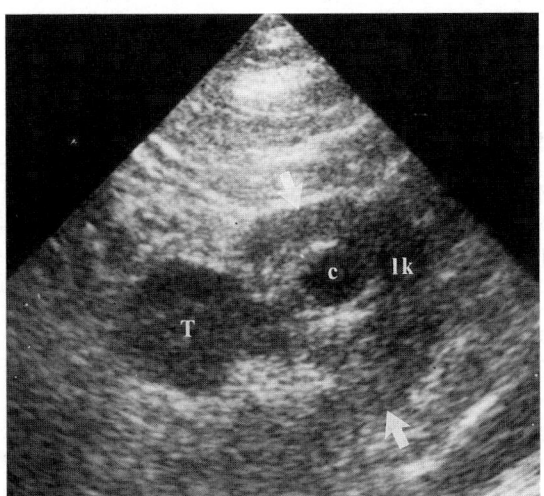

Figure 36.57. Transitional Cell Carcinoma. An US image of the left kidney (*lk*, between *arrows*) in transverse plane shows the tumor (*T*) as a hypoechoic mass. The echogenicity of the mass is only slightly greater than that of a dilated calyx (*c*).

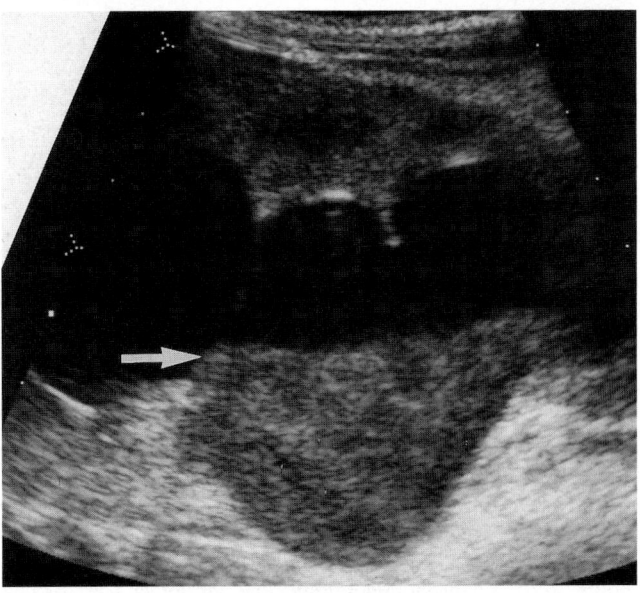

Figure 36.59. Pyonephrosis. US view of the left kidney with the patient in right lateral decubitus position reveals layering pus (*arrow*) in a dilated, obstructed collecting system.

more (47). US is performed in patients with urinary tract infection to detect hydronephrosis, renal abscess, or perirenal abscess.

Pyonephrosis refers to infection within a dilated and obstructed renal collecting system. Echogenic debris, often with a shifting urine-debris level, is seen within a dilated pelvicalyceal system in an infected patient (Fig. 36.59). Gas in the collecting system produces shifting echogenic foci with shadowing and reverberation arti-

fact. About 10% of cases of pyonephrosis are indistinguishable from uncomplicated hydronephrosis, so guided aspiration for diagnosis is indicated in clinically suspicious cases. Pyonephrosis is an indication for urgent percutaneous or surgical drainage.

Renal Abscess appears as a poorly marginated intrarenal cystic mass containing echogenic fluid (Fig. 36.60). The appearance may change rapidly over a few days with extension of infection into and beyond the

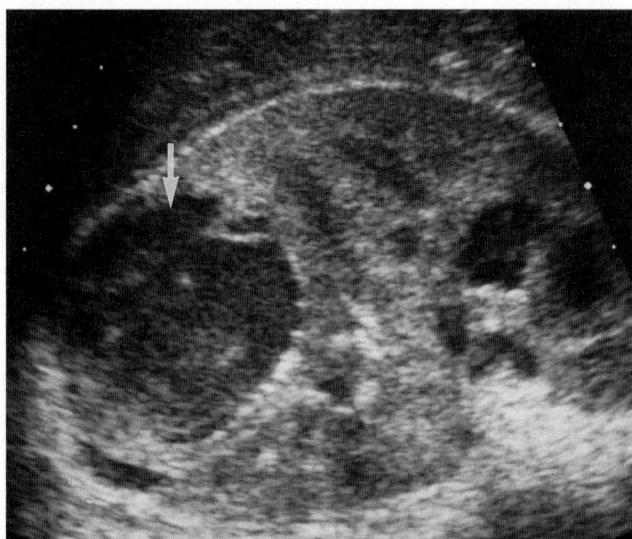

Figure 36.60. Renal Abscess. A cystic mass (*arrow*) in the upper pole of the kidney contains heterogeneous echogenic fluid. US-guided aspiration yielded coliform bacteria.

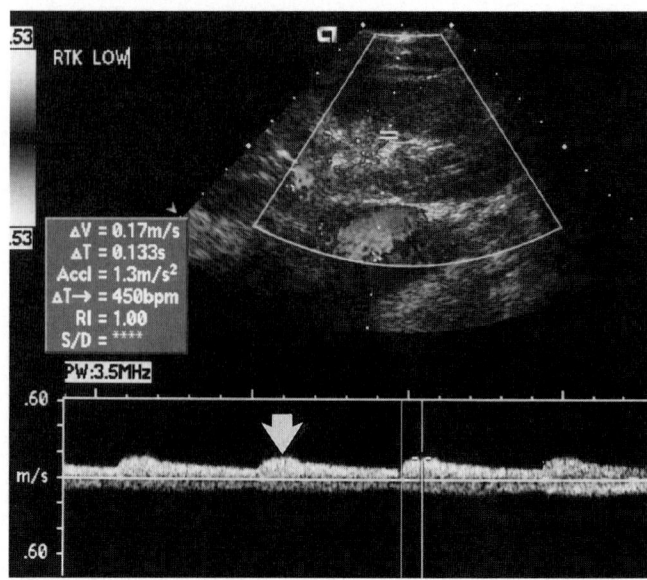

Figure 36.62. Renal Artery Stenosis. Doppler spectrum obtained from an intrarenal artery reveals tardus-parvus waveform with delayed and stunted peak systolic velocities (*arrow*).

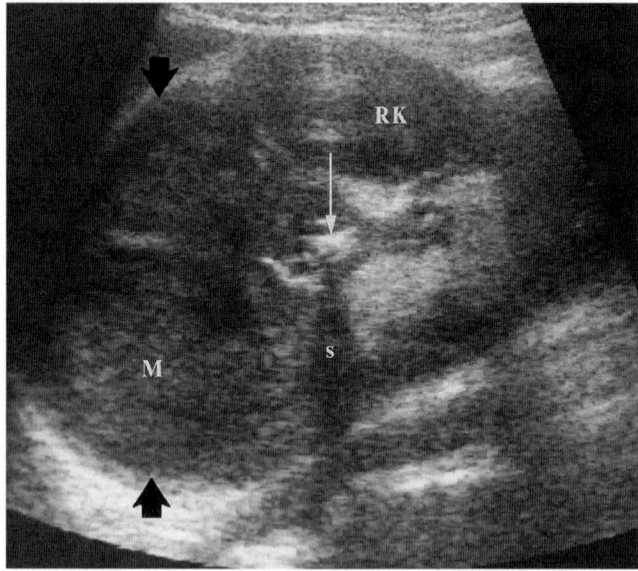

Figure 36.61. Xanthogranulomatous Pyelonephritis. Long axis US of the right kidney (*RK*) reveals a hypoechoic mass (*M*, between *arrows*) enlarging the upper pole. An obstructing stone (*long white arrow*) casting an acoustic shadow (*s*) is seen in the renal sinus The kidney was chronically infected and was surgically removed, confirming xanthogranulomatous pyelonephritis.

perirenal space. Small abscesses may be effectively treated with antibiotics, but larger abscesses (>2 cm) may require percutaneous drainage. Extensive perirenal abscess usually requires surgical drainage.

Renal Tuberculosis is characterized by the multiplicity of findings present including parenchymal scarring, calcification, intraparenchymal cavities with echogenic contents, and dilated calyces without accompanying di-

latation of the renal pelvis. US findings are seldom specific.

Xanthogranulomatous Pyelonephritis is suggested by US demonstration of a shadowing stone in the renal pelvis, dilated collecting structure commonly filled with echogenic debris, mass-like distortion and enlargement of the kidney, and extension of disease into the perirenal space. The renal parenchyma is frequency hypoechoic reflecting edema and inflammation (Fig. 36.61).

Reflux Nephropathy is suggested by US findings of focal renal parenchyma thinning with an underlying echogenic scar extending from the renal sinus toward the periphery, or a dilated calyx beneath the parenchymal thinning. The process is distinctly focal with the remainder of the kidney usually appearing normal.

Renal Doppler

Renal Artery Stenosis is commonly a difficult US diagnosis due to limited visualization of the renal arteries in large patients and the frequency of accessory renal arteries which may be stenosed and cause hypertension but are not detected with US (48). Significant renal artery stenosis is evidenced by parvus-tardus spectral waveforms in intrarenal arteries (see chapter 40). Normal intrarenal artery spectral waveforms demonstrate a near vertical early systolic upstroke. Parvus-tardus waveforms show a diminished peak systolic velocity (parvus) and a delayed time to peak systole (tardus)(Fig. 36.62)(49). Systolic acceleration values less than 300 cm/sec^2 are abnormal. Additional signs of renal artery stenosis are main renal artery peak systolic velocity greater than 100 cm/sec and renal artery to aortic peak systolic velocity ratio of greater than 3.5.

Renal Vein Thrombosis occurs in clinical settings of nephrotic syndrome, dehydration, trauma, coagulopathy, or thrombosis of the inferior vena cava. Acute complete thrombosis causes an enlarged, hypoechoic, edematous kidney without detectable blood flow in the renal vein by spectral or color Doppler. Waveforms in the renal artery are diminished in velocity and show a high resistance pattern with diminished diastolic forward flow. Incomplete venous thrombosis usually does not enlarge the kidney. Clot may be seen in the renal vein with flow on color Doppler diverted around the thrombus. Enlarged venous collateral vessels may be visualized.

Renal Transplant Evaluation includes detailed US imaging and Doppler examination. Visualization of small fluid-filled collecting structures is common and normal. Serial US examinations, or radionuclide renograms, are often needed to confirm that hydronephrosis is due to obstruction. Perirenal fluid collections are common and include: hematoma, seroma, urinoma, lymphocele, and abscess. US-guided aspiration is used to obtain fluid for laboratory differentiation. Doppler US is used to visualize and confirm patency of the entire length of the renal artery and vein. Doppler waveforms and resistive indices are not useful in differentiating acute rejection from acute tubular necrosis from acute drug reaction in the setting of acute transplant dysfunction. US-guided parenchymal biopsy is commonly used to make the diagnosis histologically.

References

1. Grant EG, Schiller VL, Millener P, et al. Color Doppler imaging of the hepatic vasculature. AJR Am J Roentgenol 1992; 159:943–950.
2. Lafortune M, Madore F, Patriquin H, Breton G. Segmental anatomy of the liver: a sonographic approach to the Couinard nomenclature. Radiology 1991;181:443–448.
3. Cazier PR, Sponaugle DW. "Starry sky" liver with fasting: variations in glycogen stores? J Ultrasound Med 1996;15: 405–407.
4. Gore RM, Mathieu DG, White EM, et al. Passive hepatic congestion: cross-sectional imaging features. AJR Am J Roentgenol 1994;162:71–75.
5. Brown JJ, Naylor MJ, Yagan N. Imaging of hepatic cirrhosis. Radiology 1997;202:1–16.
6. Colli A, Cocciolo M, Riva C, et al. Abnormalities of Doppler waveform of the hepatic veins in patients with chronic liver disease: correlation with histologic findings. AJR Am J Roentgenol 1994;162:833–837.
7. Dodd GD III, Miller WJ, Baron RL, et al. Detection of malignant tumors in end-stage cirrhotic livers: efficacy of sonography as a screening technique. AJR Am J Roentgenol 1992;159:727–733.
8. Subramanyam BR, Balthazar EJ, Madamba MR, et al. Sonography of portosystemic venous collaterals in portal hypertension. Radiology 1983;146:161–166.
9. Parvey HR, Raval B, Sandler CM. Portal vein thrombosis: imaging findings. AJR Am J Roentgenol 1994;162:77–81.
10. Hann LE, Greatrex KV, Bach AM, et al. Cholangiocarcinoma at the hepatic hilus: sonographic findings. AJR Am J Roentgenol 1997;168:985–989.
11. Robledo R, Muro A, Prieto ML. Extrahepatic bile duct carcinoma: US characteristics and accuracy in demonstration of tumors. Radiology 1996;198:869–873.
12. Lim JH. Oriental cholangiohepatitis: pathologic, clinical, and radiologic features. AJR Am J Roentgenol 1991;157: 1–8.
13. Miller FH, Gore RM, Nemcek AA, Jr,, Fitzgerald SW. Pancreaticobiliary manifestations of AIDS. AJR Am J Roentgenol 1996;166:1269–1274.
14. Da Silva F, Boudghene F, Lecomte I, et al. Sonography in AIDS-related cholangitis: prevalence and cause of an echogenic nodule in the distal end of the common bile duct. AJR Am J Roentgenol 1993;160:1205–1207.
15. Ali M, Khan AN. Sonography of hepatobiliary ascariasis. J Clin Ultrasound 1996;24:235–241.
16. Rosenthal SJ. Pitfalls and differential diagnosis in biliary sonography. Radiographics 1990;10:285–311.
17. Uggowitzer M, Kugler C, Schramayer G, et al. Sonography of acute cholecystitis: comparison of color and power Doppler sonography in detecting hypervascularized gallbladder wall. AJR Am J Roentgenol 1997;168:707–712.
18. Teefey SA, Baron RL, Bigler SA. Sonography of the gallbladder: significance of striated (layered) thickening of the gallbladder wall. AJR Am J Roentgenol 1991;156:945–947.
19. Bloom RA, Libson E, Lebensart PD, et al. The ultrasound spectrum of emphysematous cholecystitis. J Clin Ultrasound 1989;17:251–256.
20. Rooholamini SA, Tehrani NS, Razavi MK, et al. Imaging of gallbladder carcinoma. Radiographics 1994;14:291–306.
21. Subramanyam BR, Balthazar EJ, Horii SC. Sonography of the accessory spleen. AJR Am J Roentgenol 1984;143: 47–49.
22. Urrutia M, Mergo PJ, Ros LH, et al. Cystic masses of the spleen: radiologic-pathologic correlations. Radiographics 1996;16:107–129.
23. Görg C, Schwerk WB, Görg K. Sonography of focal lesions of the spleen. AJR Am J Roentgenol 1991;156:949–953.
24. Schwerk WB, Görg C, Görg K, Restrepo I. Ultrasound-guided percutaneous drainage of pyogenic splenic abscesses. J Clin Ultrasound 1994;22:161–166.
25. Murray JG, Patel MD, Lee S, et al. Microabscesses of the liver and spleen in AIDS: detection with 5-MHz sonography. Radiology 1995;197:723–727.
26. Goerg C, Schwerk WB. Splenic infarction: sonographic patterns, diagnosis, follow-up, and complications. Radiology 1990;174:803–807.
27. Ros PR, Moser RP, Jr., Dachman AH, et al. Hemangioma of the spleen: radiologic-pathologic correlation in ten cases. Radiology 1987;162:73–77.
28. Ralls PW, Wren SM, Radin R, et al. Color flow sonography in evaluating the resectability of periampullary and pancreatic tumors. J Ultrasound Med 1997;16:131–140.
29. Buetow PC, Miller DL, Parrino TV, Buck JL. Islet cell tumors of the pancreas: clinical, radiologic, and pathologic correlation in diagnosis and localization. Radiographics 1997;17:453–472.
30. Charnsangavej C, Whitley NO. Metastases to the pancreas and peripancreatic lymph nodes from carcinoma of the right side of the colon: CT findings in 12 patients. AJR Am J Roentgenol 1993;160:49–52.
31. Hough DM, Stephens DH, Johnson CD, Binkovitz LA. Pancreatic lesions in von Hippel-Lindau disease: prevalence, clinical significance, and CT findings. AJR Am J Roentgenol 1994;162:1091–1094.
32. Buck JL, Hayes WS. Microcystic adenoma of the pancreas. Radiographics 1990;10:313–322.
33. Itoh S, Ishiguchi T, Ishigaki T, et al. Mucin-producing pancreatic tumor: CT findings and histopathologic correlation. Radiology 1992;183:81–86.
34. Procacci C, Graziani R, Bicego E, et al. Intraductal mucin-producing tumors of the pancreas: imaging findings. Radiology 1996;198:249–257.
35. Sivit CJ, Hung W, Taylor GA, et al. Sonography in neonatal adrenal hyperplasia. AJR Am J Roentgenol 1991;156: 141–143.

36. Scott EM, Thomas A, McGarrigle HHG, Lachelin GCL. Serial adrenal ultrasonography in normal neonates. J Ultrasound Med 1990;9:279–283.

37. Westra SJ, Zaninovic AC, Hall TR, et al. Imaging of the adrenal gland in children. Radiographics 1994;14: 1323–1340.

38. Schwerk WB, Görg C, Görg K, Restrepo IK. Adrenal pheochromocytomas: a broad spectrum of sonographic presentation. J Ultrasound Med 1994;13:517–521.

39. Musante F, Derchi LE, Zappasodi F, et al. Myelolipoma of the adrenal gland: sonographic and CT features. AJR Am J Roentgenol 1988;151:961–964.

40. Cyran KM, Kenney PJ, Memel DS, Yacoub I. Adrenal myelolipoma. AJR Am J Roentgenol 1996;166:395–400.

41. Rozenblit A, Morehouse HT, Amis ES, Jr. Cystic adrenal lesions: CT features. Radiology 1996;201:541–548.

42. Platt JF, Rubin JM, Ellis JH. Acute renal obstruction: evaluation with intrarenal duplex Doppler and conventional US. Radiology 1993;186:685–688.

43. LeRoy AJ. Diagnosis and treatment of nephrolithiasis: current perspectives. AJR Am J Roentgenol 1994;163: 1309–1313.

44. Middleton WD, Dodds WJ, Lawson TL, Foley WD. Renal calculi: sensitivity for detection with ultrasound. Radiology 1988;167:239–244.

45. Siegel CL, Middleton WD, Teefey SA, McClennan BL. Angiomyolipoma and renal cell carcinoma: US differentiation. Radiology 1996;198:789–793.

46. Wagner BJ, Wong-You-Cheong JJ, Davis CJ, Jr. Adult renal hamartomas. Radiographics 1997;17:155–169.

47. Talner LB, Davidson AJ, Lebowitz RL, et al. Acute pyelonephritis: can we agree on terminology? Radiology 1994;192:297–305.

48. Hèlènon O, Rody FE, Correas J-M, et al. Color Doppler US of renovascular disease in native kidneys. Radiographics 1995;15:833–854.

49. Halpern EJ, Needleman L, Nack TL, East SA. Renal artery stenosis: should we study the main renal artery or segmental vessels? Radiology 1995;195:799–804.

37
Genital Tract and Bladder Ultrasound

William E. Brant

BLADDER

The full bladder is used as an acoustic window to the pelvis for evaluation of the genital tract. Abnormalities of the bladder may be mistaken for abnormalities of other organs of the pelvis. Alternatively, large cystic masses may be mistaken for the bladder. Ultrasound (US) is valuable for evaluation of bladder wall, distal ureters, intravesical, and extravesical masses.

Normal US Anatomy. The urine-filled bladder is thin-walled and contains anechoic urine. The normal wall measures 3 mm when the bladder is distended and 5 mm when collapsed. The volume of bladder contents may be calculated by the standard formula for volume of a prolate ellipse (length × width × height × 0.52). US measurements may be used to calculate postvoid urine residual and overdistended bladder volumes when the bladder is neurogenic. Ureteral jets are spurts of urine into the bladder due to ureteral peristalsis. They are best visualized by color Doppler but are occasionally seen on gray-scale US as swirling microbubbles. Visualization of ureteral jets confirms patency of the ureter (1,2). In males the prostate is seen as a hypoechoic soft tissue mass at the bladder base (Fig. 37.1). With enlargement the prostate elevates the bladder base. The urethral orifice makes a V-shaped depression in the prostate.

Bladder Masses

Bladder Diverticula appear as fluid-filled sacs that project from the bladder wall (Fig. 37.2)(3). Bladder mucosa herniates through a defect in the bladder wall producing a fluid-filled mass that communicates with the main bladder lumen through a small orifice. The wall of the diverticulum lacks a muscle layer and is thinner than the bladder wall. The orifice may be inconspicuous and require a diligent search to detect. Color Doppler may be used to detect a jet of urine flow through the diverticular orifice when pressure is applied to the lower abdomen. Diverticula may not empty completely with voiding and serve as a site of urine stasis predisposing to infection and stone formation. US may demonstrate floating and layering debris in the urine with infection and shadowing stones within the diverticulum or bladder. The presence of a soft tissue mass within the diverticulum suggests a complicating carcinoma.

Simple Ureteroceles produce small oval fluid-filled masses projecting into the bladder lumen. The size of the ureterocele changes as it fills and empties with ureteral peristalsis. The location at the ureterovesical junction may be confirmed by observing ureteral jets originate from the ureterocele.

Ectopic Ureteroceles are found with ureteral duplication and produce variable sized fluid-filled masses in the bladder lumen (Fig. 37.3). The ureterocele commonly remains unchanged in size after voiding. The distal ureter is dilated and tortuous.

Bladder Carcinoma may appear as a polypoid mass, focal, or multifocal thickening of the bladder wall (4). Irregular papillary surface to the tumor may be evident. Tumors may be single or multiple, and occur with increased incidence within diverticula. Tumor can be differentiated from blood clot by Doppler demonstration of blood vessels within the mass.

Bladder Stones appear as brightly echogenic objects that cast acoustic shadows. Most stones will move with changes in patient position but some are adherent to the bladder wall. Stones may also be seen in the distal ureter, in ureteroceles, and in diverticula.

Foreign Bodies are usually echogenic and linear, angulated, or geographic in appearance, rather than round or oval like stones. Many will cast acoustic shadows and move within the bladder.

Blood Clots may produce layering fluid-debris levels when small or heterogeneous masses when large. Doppler shows no internal vascularity. Clots change in appearance and size with time.

Thickened Bladder Wall

Bladder Outlet Obstruction causes muscle hypertrophy and trabeculation of the bladder wall. US demonstrates thickening of the wall and marked irregularity of its luminal surface (Fig. 37.4). Causes include prostate enlargement, neurogenic bladder, urethral stricture, ectopic ureterocele, tumors, and blood clots.

Cystitis due to any cause may produce focal or diffuse thickening of the bladder wall, often associated with layering or mass-like echogenic debris within the urine (5). The mucosa may be raised and echolucent due to edema. Air within the bladder wall or lumen produces bright echoes with acoustic shadowing or ring-down artifact.

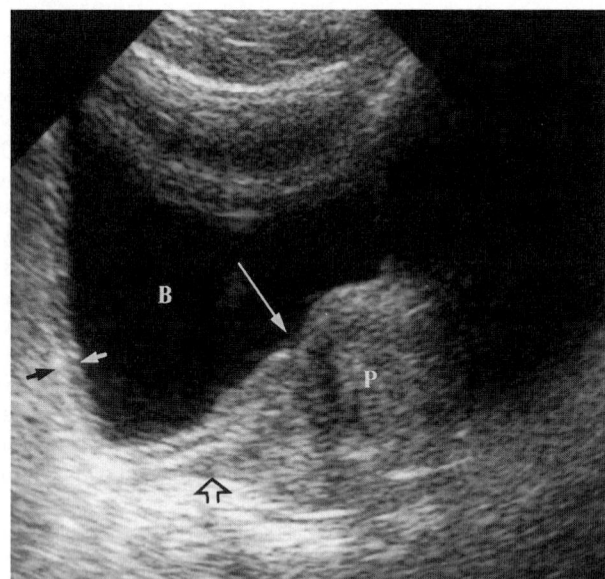

Figure 37.1. Enlarged Prostate. Midline sagittal US image shows an enlarged prostate (*P*) protruding into and elevating the base of the bladder (*B*). The urethral orifice (*long arrow*) forms a V-shaped depression in the prostate. The seminal vesicles (*open arrow*) are also seen. The bladder wall is mildly thickened (between *short arrows*).

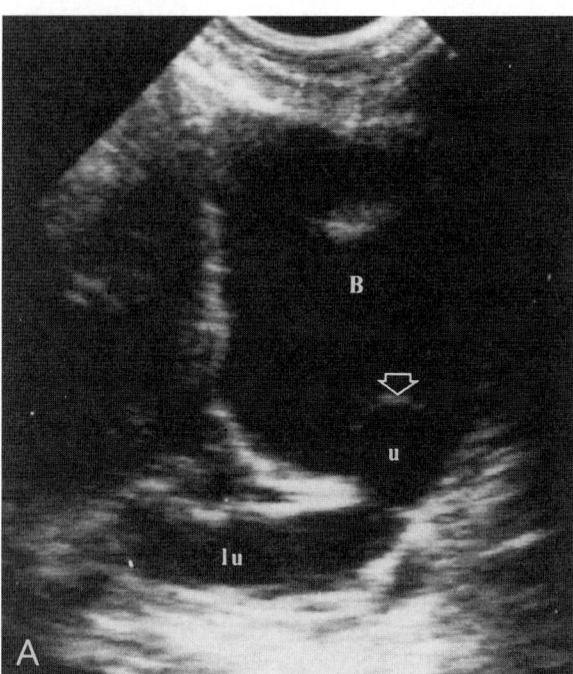

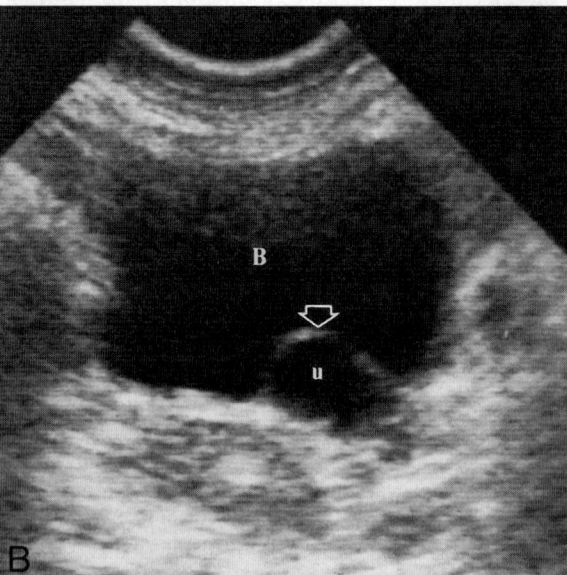

Figure 37.3. Ectopic Ureterocele. US images in left sagittal **(A)** and transverse **(B)** planes demonstrate an ectopic ureterocele (*u*) of the left upper pole ureter (*lu*) protruding into the lumen of the bladder base. The upper pole collecting system was hydronephrotic, but the lower pole collecting system was normal. The wall of the ureterocele (*arrows*) is clearly seen. The ureterocele changes in size with peristalsis of the ureter. *B*, bladder.

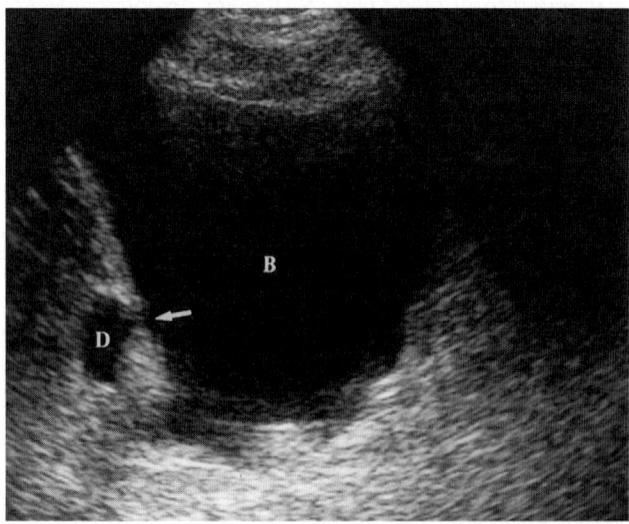

Figure 37.2. Bladder Diverticulum. Axial plane image shows a urine-filled diverticulum (*D*) projecting through a defect (*arrow*) in the bladder wall. *B*, bladder.

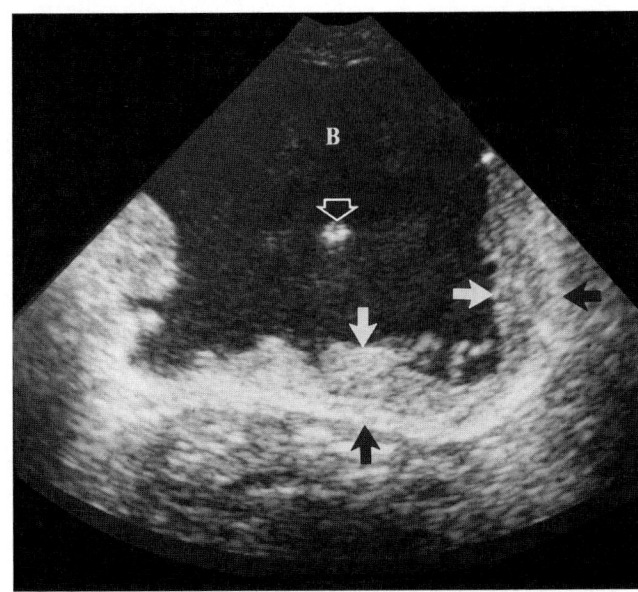

Figure 37.4. Thickened Bladder Wall. Axial US of a neurogenic bladder (*B*) demonstrates marked thickening (*arrows*) of the bladder wall with trabeculation. The patient had an indwelling foley catheter, the tip of which is evident (*open arrow*).

Bladder Carcinoma is difficult to differentiate from benign bladder wall thickening unless a polypoid mass is present. Early stage tumors are usually not demonstrated with US.

FEMALE GENITAL TRACT

US is the primary imaging modality for evaluation of the female genital tract and pelvis. The utility and accuracy of ultrasound have been dramatically increased by the development of transvaginal tranducers and color Doppler imaging (6–8). US is used as an adjunct to physical examination to confirm the presence of a pelvic mass, and to evaluate its size, contour, and character, determine the organ of origin, evaluate for involvement of other organs, and detect the presence of ascites, hydronephrosis, and metastases. The US examination is initiated transabdominally using the distended urinary bladder as a window to the pelvis. The transvaginal approach is used to improve visualization of all lesions and to overcome the limitations of limited bladder filling and obesity. Color flow US is used to identify pelvic blood vessels, identify vascular lesions of the pelvis, and detect neovascularity of tumors.

Uterus

Normal US Anatomy. The uterus in the postpubertal woman is smoothly contoured and pear-shaped (Fig. 37.5). The myometrium is uniform mid-level echogenicity with the endometrium distinctly more echogenic. The thickness of the endometrial echo varies with stage of the menstrual cycle. The innermost myometrium, called the *junctional zone*, may appear as a thin hypoechoic layer adjacent to the echogenic endometrial stripe.

Normal uterine dimensions in the adult woman are 6–8 cm in length, 4–6 cm in width, and 3–4 cm in anteroposterior diameter. Following menopause, the uterus atrophies to approximately 6 × 2 × 2 cm. The prepubertal, infantile, uterus is cigar-shaped. The cervix makes up about one-third the length of the uterus in the adult woman and about two-thirds of the length of the uterus in the prepubertal girl. Normal uterine positions in the pelvis include tilted forward (anteverted—most common), tilted backward toward the sacrum (retroverted), or folded anteriorly (anteflexed) or posteriorly (retroflexed)(Fig. 37.6). The normal uterus may also be tilted right or left toward the pelvic side walls. The position of the uterus is altered by the degree of bladder filling. The retroverted or retroflexed uterus appears more globular on transabdominal scanning. The normal vagina appears as a flattened muscular tube with echogenic mucosa (Fig. 37.6).

The US examination must always be correlated with the stage of the menstrual cycle which affects the normal brightness and thickness of the endometrial stripe (9). At the end of menstruation, the endometrial stripe is thin (2–3 mm) and discrete. During the *proliferative phase* the stripe thickens to 8 mm and remains brightly echogenic and distinct. From ovulation to menstruation through the *secretory phase* (Fig. 37.7) the endometrium progressively thickens to 15 mm and becomes less well defined. The junction zone appears as a hypoechoic halo surrounding the bright endometrium. In the normal postmenopausal woman, the echogenic endometrial stripe does not exceed 5–7 mm in thickness. During the normal fertile years, pregnancy must always be considered. Abnormalities of the first trimester of pregnancy are reviewed in chapter 38.

Congenital Anomalies are best defined by correlation of physical examination, US or MR imaging, and hysterosalpingography. US may define two uterine horns, two distinct endometrial cavities, and an abnormal shape of the uterus (see Figs. 35.2, 35.3). The kidneys should be examined for associated anomalies such as renal agenesis.

Leiomyomas (fibroids) are exceeding common benign smooth muscle tumors of the myometrium that can develop in all women of all ages. They are suspected when the uterus is enlarged or altered in contour. Leiomyomas are virtually always multiple. They may be completely within the myometrium, subserosal or submucosal in location. Leiomyomas may also be pedunculated and predominantly extrauterine, simulating an adnexal mass (10). Color flow US demonstration of vascular supply contiguous with the myometrium is definitive in confirming uterine origin of these exophytic leiomyomas. Uncomplicated leiomyomas may be isoechoic, hypoechoic, or hyperechoic compared to normal myometrium (Fig. 37.8). Leiomyomas may undergo atrophy, internal hemorrhage, cystic degeneration, fibrosis, and calcification (11,12). A "popcorn" pattern of calcification is characteristic and definitive on plain film radiographs (see Fig. 35.11). On US they are typically heterogeneous and vary from hypoechoic to hyperechoic, sometimes causing acoustic shadowing. No imaging modality can reliably differentiate benign leiomyoma from the rare leiomyosarcoma.

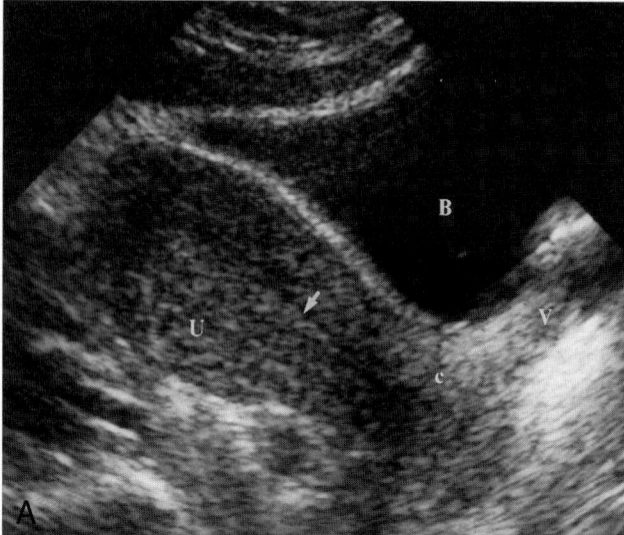
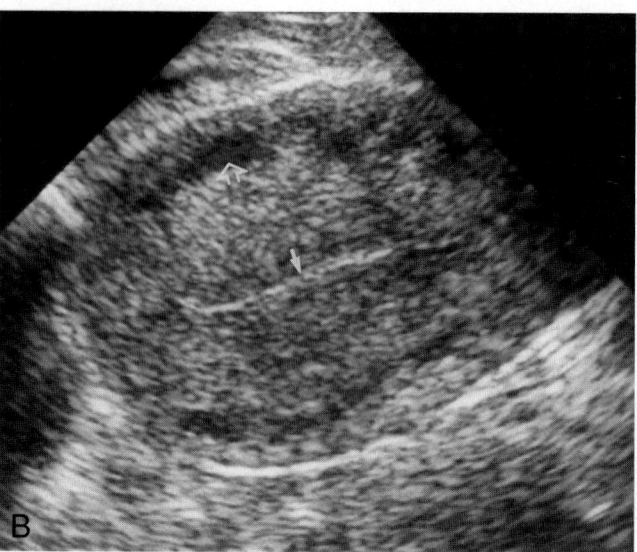

Figure 37.5. Normal Uterus. A. Transabdominal sagittal plane image through the urine-filled bladder (*B*) demonstrates the smooth contour and pear-shape of the normal uterus (*U*). The endometrial stripe (*arrow*) is more echogenic than the surrounding myometrium. The cervix (*c*) protrudes into the upper vagina (*V*) at the intersection between the long axis of the uterus and the axis of the vagina.

B. Transvaginal sagittal plane image of the uterus demonstrates the improved resolution of this technique. The endometrial stripe (*arrow*) is more sharply defined and the myometrium is more clearly evaluated. Lucencies (*open arrow*) in the peripheral myometrium are due to normal blood vessels, as confirmed by Doppler.

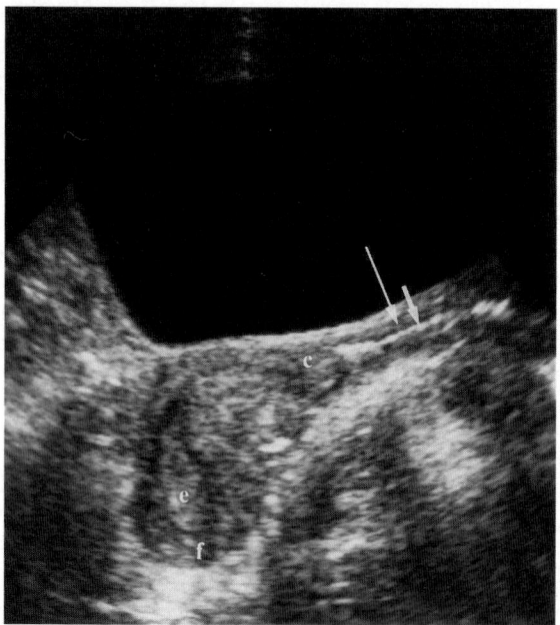

Figure 37.6. Retroflexed Uterus. The uterus is flexed with the fundus (*f*) directed posteriorly toward the sacrum on this sagittal midline transbladder image. A retroflexed or retroverted uterus may be mistaken for a pelvic mass on both physical examination and US. The vagina is well seen with its hypoechoic muscular walls (*long arrow*) and echogenic mucosa (*short arrow*). *c*, cervix. *e*, endometrium.

Retroposition of the uterus and uterine anomalies, such as a bicornuate uterus, must be differentiated from leiomyoma. Leiomyomas may cause menorrhagia or vaginal bleeding unrelated to menstrual cycles. Exophytic tumors may torse and be a cause of acute pelvic pain. The

tumors are responsive to female hormones and commonly accelerate in growth during pregnancy. Correspondingly, they involute with menopause.

Arcuate Artery Calcifications are seen as discrete echogenic foci in the outer third of the myometrium of postmenopausal women (6). They are seen more commonly in women who are diabetic or hypertensive.

Thickened Endometrial Stripe. The thickness of the endometrial stripe must always be correlated with age, menstrual history, and stage of the menstrual cycle (6). The full thickness of the echogenic endometrium, including both anterior and posterior walls, is measured perpendicular to the long axis of the uterus (Fig. 37.9)(13). In women having active menstrual cycles, the endometrial stripe may measure up to 14 mm during the secretory phase. However, in postmenopausal women the endometrium normally does not exceed 5–7 mm in thickness. Hormone replacement therapy thickens the endometrium in postmenopausal women by 1–3 mm (14). In women with abnormal vaginal bleeding, US demonstration of abnormal endometrial thickness is an indication for endometrial biopsy. A normal endometrial thickness measurement averts the need for biopsy (15). The causes of thickening of the endometrium include (16):

Endometrial carcinoma. Thickness of the stripe may be uneven with an ill-defined irregular contour. This cancer is most common in women over age 50. Postmenopausal vaginal bleeding is a common presentation.

Endometrial hyperplasia is caused by unopposed or prolonged estrogen stimulation and is most common in perimenopausal and postmenopausal women. The endometrium is thickened and inhomogeneous with small cysts commonly present.

Endometrial polyps are result from focal hyperplasia or

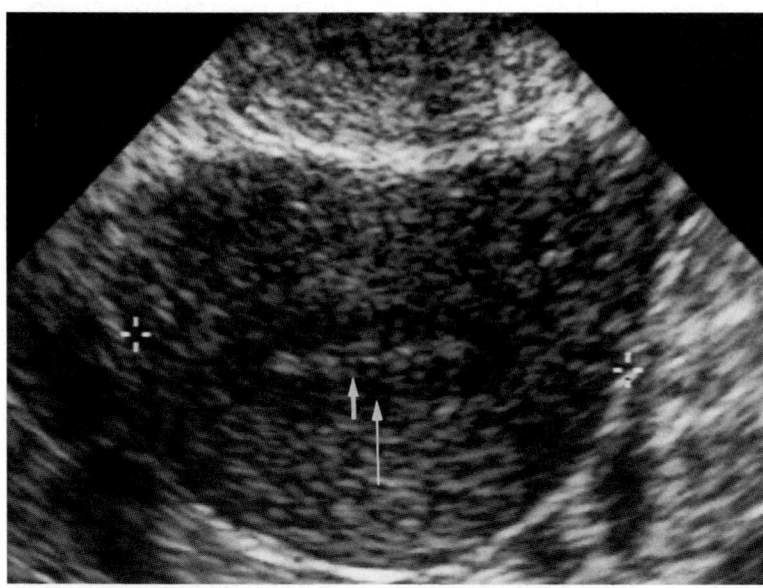

Figure 37.7. Secretory Phase Endometrium. Coronal transvaginal image of the uterus (between *calipers*) shows thickening of the endometrium (*short arrow*) and the hypoechoic halo of the surrounding junctional zone (*long arrow*) of the myometrium in a patient in second half of her menstrual cycle.

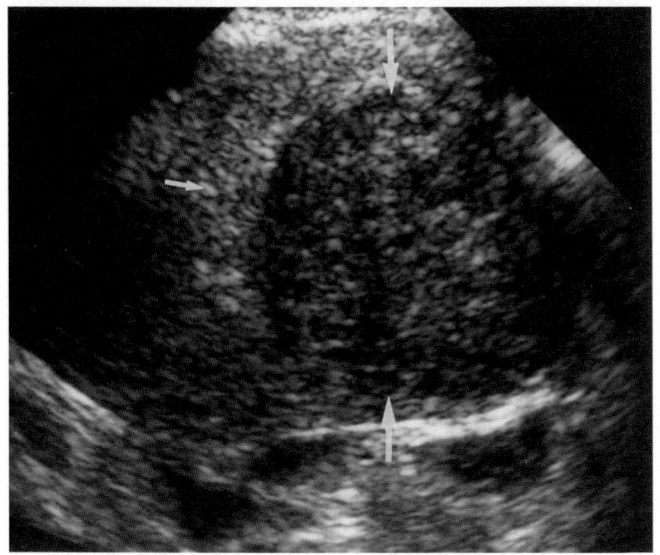

Figure 37.8. Leiomyoma. Transvaginal image of the uterus shows a hypoechoic leiomyoma (between *large arrows*) displacing the endometrial stripe (*small arrow*).

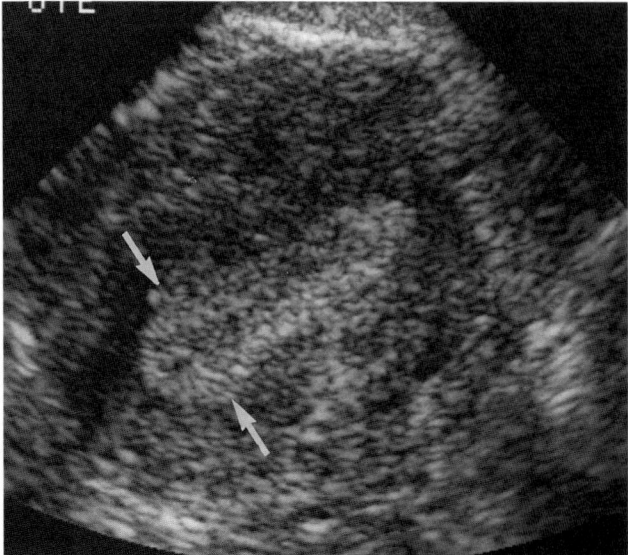

Figure 37.9. Thickened Endometrial Stripe. Transvaginal US demonstrates thickening of the endometrial stripe to 15 mm (measured between arrows) in a postmenopausal woman with vaginal bleeding. Subsequent endometrial biopsy showed endometrial hyperplasia.

adenomatous neoplasia of the endometrium. They are most common between ages 30 and 60. Malignant transformation is reported in 1–4%. About 20% are multiple. US demonstrates a focal echogenic polypoid mass in the endometrium or diffuse endometrial thickening.

Endometritis may be a complication of instrumentation, the postpartum state, or be associated with pelvic inflammatory disease. The endometrium appears thickened and irregular. Fluid may be seen in the endometrium. Gas echoes in the endometrial cavity are the most specific finding.

Other, less common, causes include tamoxifen therapy, incomplete abortion, metastatic carcinoma, and submucosal leiomyoma. Pregnancy must never be forgotten as a possibility.

Fluid in the Endometrial Cavity. The fluid may be blood, mucus, or purulent material. Hematometrium refers to blood in the endometrial cavity and hematocolpos describes blood filling the vagina.

In postmenopausal women causes include: cervical stenosis, cervical carcinoma, endometrial carcinoma, endometrial polyps, and pyometrium (see Fig. 35.8)(17).

In the premenopausal women causes include: congenital obstruction due to imperforate hymen, vaginal septum, vaginal or cervical atresia; acquired cervical obstruction due to instrumentation, radiation, or carcinoma; menorrhagia; and pregnancy.

Adenomyosis is the condition of focal or diffuse invasion of the myometrium by benign endometrium ("internal endometriosis"). It is found commonly in multiparous women over age 30 (9–30% incidence on hysterectomy specimens) (18,19). The islands of endometrium within the myometrium appear as echogenic or hypoechoic ill-defined nodules, diffuse heterogeneous echotexture of the myometrium, or focal asymmetric thickening of the myometrium. The uterus is usually enlarged. Findings are best demonstrated by transvaginal US.

Nabothian Cysts result from obstruction of the ducts of mucous-secreting glands of the epithelial lining of cervix and are commonly visualized on tranvaginal US. They are anechoic, frequently multiple and vary in size 2–3 mm up to 4 cm.

Ovaries and Adnexa

Normal US Anatomy. The adnexa contains the ovaries, fallopian tubes, broad ligament, and ovarian and uterine vessels, all of which may be involved in pathological conditions. US demonstrates the ovaries as oval soft tissue structures with multiple small cystic follicles (Fig. 37.10). The ovaries average $4 \times 3 \times 2$ cm in size, with a maximum of 5 cm in any one dimension. The maximum ovarian volume for an adult woman, calculated by the standard formula (length $\times$ width $\times$ height $\times$ 0.52), is 15 cc. The ovaries show characteristic morphological changes with the menstrual cycle (20). Following menstruation, the ovaries are at their smallest with the follicles measuring less than 5 mm. During the estrogen phase, follicles enlarge to 10–15 mm size with one dominant follicle attaining 20–25 mm size by midcycle. Rupture of the dominant follicle releases the ovum and the corpus luteum forms at the site of the dominant follicle. Ovulation releases fluid which pools in the cul-de-sac. All remaining follicles normally involute following ovulation. Hemorrhage into the corpus luteum or any follicle produces a *hemorrhagic functional cyst*.

The ovaries vary widely in location, but usually lie in a shallow ovarian fossa in the angle between the external iliac vessels anteriorly and the ureter posteriorly with the fallopian tubes draped over and around them. The fallopian tubes are not visualized unless enlarged, however the broad ligament is clearly seen when it is outlined by fluid in the pelvis. Transvaginal US is the most effective way to evaluate the ovaries.

Postmenopausal Ovaries are atrophic, lack follicles, and are often difficult to visualize. Mean ovarian volume decreases from 8 cc at age 40–44 to less than 1.0 cc at age 70. Estrogen replacement therapy maintains ovarian size at near premenopausal volumes. Development of follicles, up to 3–4 cm size occurs normally in up to one-third of postmenopausal women (21). These have the appearance of simple cysts with thin walls and no internal echoes. Most will disappear on follow-up examination.

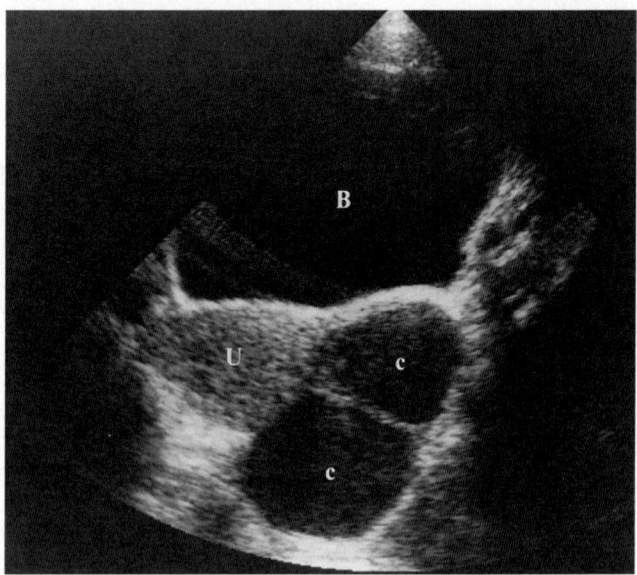

Figure 37.11. Hemorrhagic Follicular Cysts. An US image in a transverse plane through the full bladder (*B*) reveals two cystic masses (*c*) in the left adnexa. Note the low level internal echoes due to hemorrhage in these surgically confirmed follicular cysts. *U*, uterus.

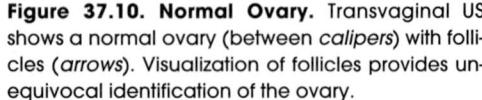

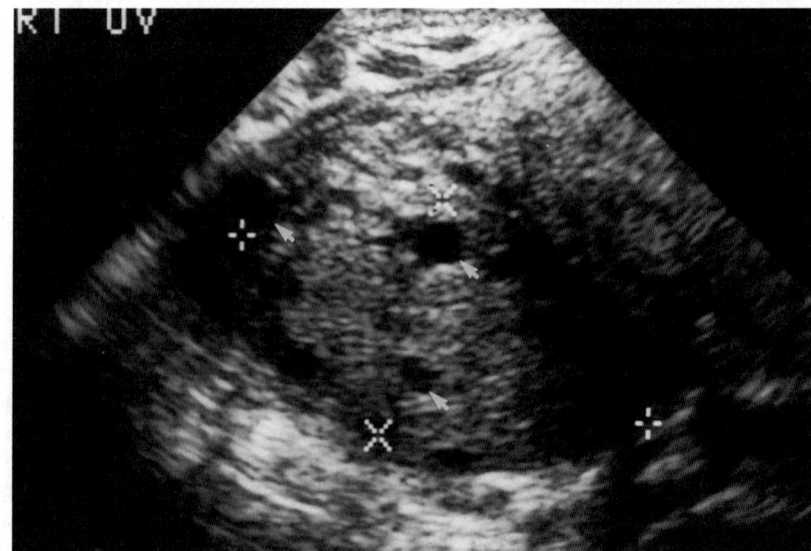

Figure 37.10. Normal Ovary. Transvaginal US shows a normal ovary (between *calipers*) with follicles (*arrows*). Visualization of follicles provides unequivocal identification of the ovary.

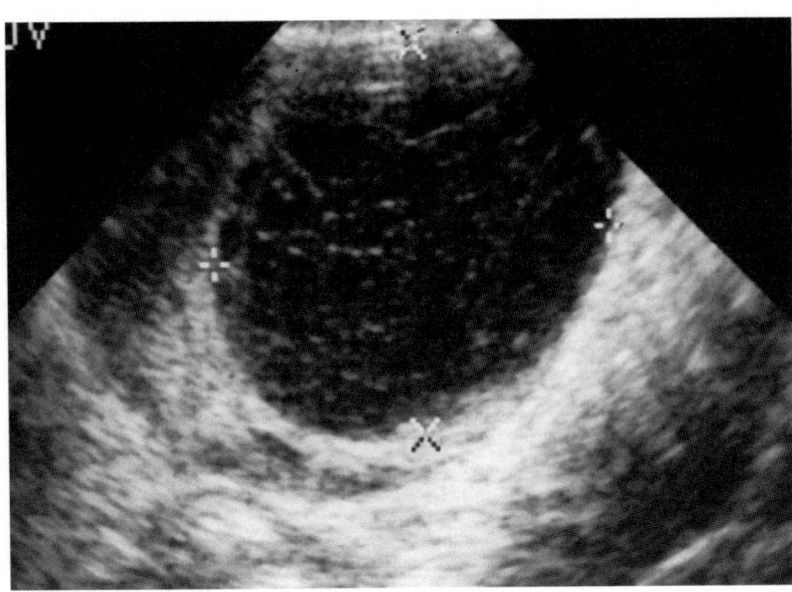

Figure 37.12. Hemorrhagic Functional Cyst. Transvaginal US shows the complex internal echogenicity of a hemorrhagic functional cyst (between *calipers*) which resolved on follow-up US examination 2 months later.

ADNEXAL MASSES

Functional Ovarian Cysts are the most common ovarian masses. Small cysts, up to 2.5 cm, should generally be considered to be normal follicles. Pathologic *follicular cysts* up to 20 cm may result from excessive accumulation of fluid or internal hemorrhage (Fig. 37.11). *Corpus luteal cysts* result from hemorrhage into a physiologic corpus luteum. Functional cysts may rupture or undergo torsion. Diagnosis is made by the demonstration of a round, smooth, usually unilocular ovarian cyst that resolves on follow-up examination after one or two menstrual cycles. Hemorrhage into the cyst may cause a complex internal echogenicity with septal strands, echogenic fluid, and layering (Fig. 37.12)(22).

Pelvic Inflammatory Disease and Endometriosis have a very similar appearance on all imaging studies and are considered together. Both cause masses which are predominantly cystic with complex internal fluid and adhesions that may encompass adjacent structures such as the ovary or bowel into a complex mass (Fig. 37.13). Differentiation is made primarily by clinical history.

Pelvic inflammatory disease is the term applied to acute or chronic inflammation of the tubes, ovaries, and pelvic peritoneum. Patients are usually in their teens and 20s and present with pain, fever, and vaginal discharge. Causes of the disease include gonococcus, chlamydia, anaerobic bacteria, and tuberculosis. The disease runs a spectrum from endometritis to salpingitis to hydrosalpinx (see Fig. 35.16) and tubo-ovarian abscess. US demonstrates a complex ill-defined adnexal mass that often includes a dilated, pus-filled fallopian tube, swollen ovary, and adhesions to adjacent structures. Fluid is usually present in the cul-de-sac (23).

Endometriosis is the occurrence of aberrant endometrial tissue outside the uterus. Patients are commonly in their 20s and 30s, and present with infertility, dysmenorrhea, and dyspareunia. Many cases involve small implants on the peritoneum that are not visualized by US.

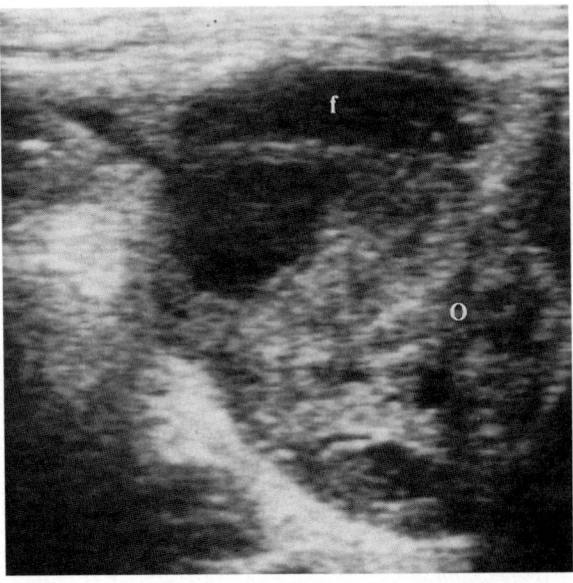

Figure 37.13. Tubo-ovarian Abscess. US of the left adnexa reveals a complex mass with fluid enveloping the left ovary. Physical examination reveals marked pelvic tenderness with fixation of the pelvic organs.

Transvaginal US distinctly improves detection (24,25). Larger deposits may form cystic masses filled with old blood, a condition termed the "chocolate cyst" (Fig. 37.14).

Ovarian Tumors, whether benign or malignant, are predominantly cystic. The tumors most commonly encountered are the epithelial tumors, serous and mucinous cystadenoma and cystadenocarcinoma, and benign cystic teratoma. US is used to differentiate functional ovarian cysts from ovarian tumors, and to provide findings used to assess the risk of malignancy.

Benign Cystic Teratomas, also called dermoid cysts, are benign germ cell tumors usually discovered in patients aged 10–30. They are the most common ovarian

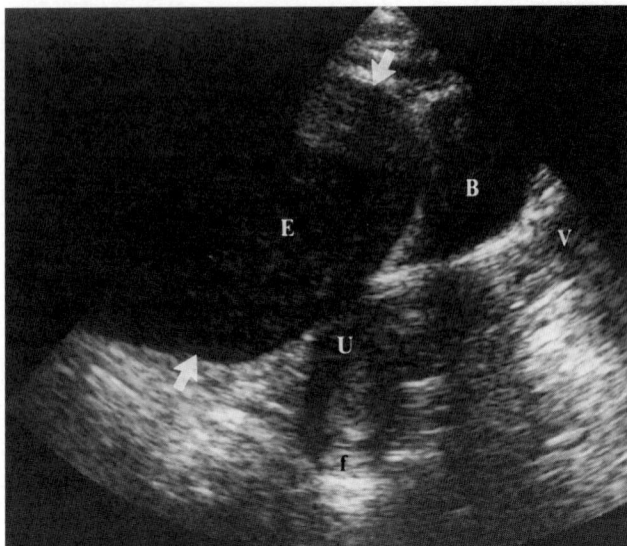

Figure 37.14. Endometrioma. A large endometrioma (*E*, between *arrows*) causes a mass impression on the bladder (*B*). The uterus (*U*) is retroflexed with the fundus (*f*) directed posteriorly. *V*, vagina.

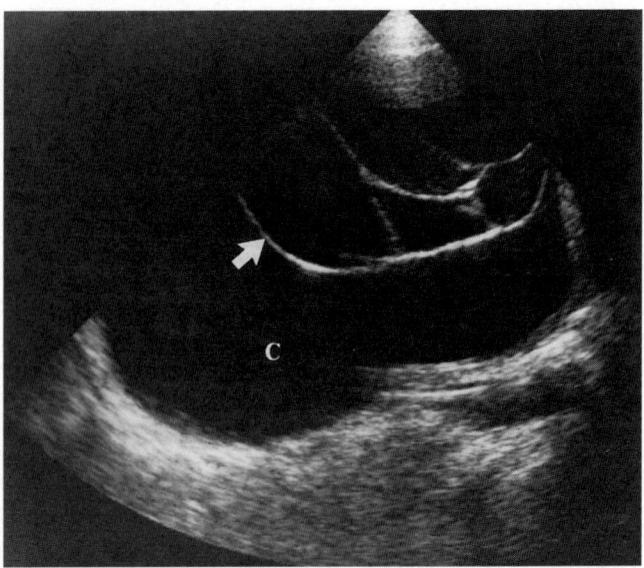

Figure 37.16. Benign Mucinous Cystadenoma. This ovarian tumor caused a huge mass, filling the pelvis and lower abdomen. An US confirmed a cystic mass (*C*) with a network of fine septations (*arrow*). The absence of detectable solid components suggests a benign tumor.

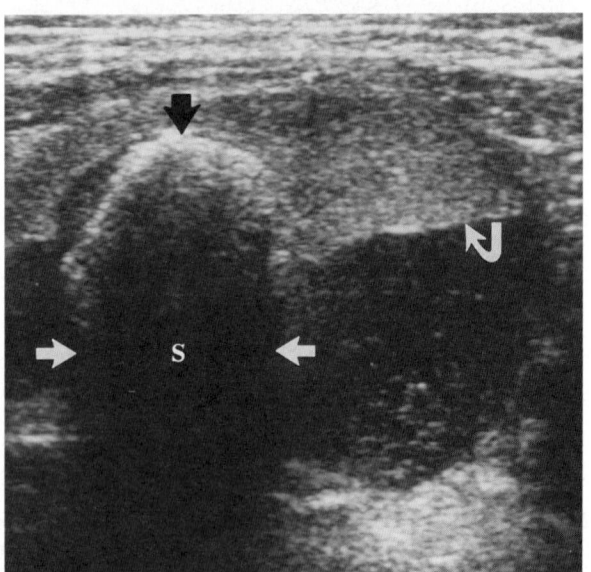

Figure 37.15. Benign Cystic Teratoma. An US of a pelvic mass demonstrates a fluid-fluid layer (*curved arrow*) and a large area of calcification (*black arrow*) with acoustic shadowing (*S*, between *white arrows*). Surgery confirmed a benign cystic teratoma containing teeth (the calcified portion), fat and hair (the fluid-fluid layer). (Case courtesy of Roy A. Kottal, MD, Cedar Rapids, Iowa.)

neoplasm. They are bilateral in 15–25% of cases. Although predominantly cystic, the presence of mature ectodermal elements such as bone, teeth, and hair give them a complex and varied appearance (Fig. 37.15)(26). The most characteristic appearance is a cystic mass with complex fluid and a mural nodule, the "dermoid plug." Fluid-fluid levels are common. Another classic appearance is the "tip of the iceberg" sign of an echogenic mass

that fades into acoustic shadowing due to sound absorption. The diagnosis can often be confirmed by a plain film radiograph that demonstrates teeth or bone (see Fig. 35.15).

Epithelial Tumors arise from the epithelial covering of the ovary. As a group they account for 65–75% of all ovarian neoplasms. Most present as predominantly cystic masses. Pathological differentiation of benign and malignant forms is sometimes difficult resulting in some being classified as "borderline" malignant. Bilateral tumors are common and more frequent with malignant types (27,28).

Serous cystadenoma and cystadenocarcinoma comprise 30% of all ovarian neoplasms and 40% of all ovarian malignancies. Serous cystadenomas are thin-walled usually unilocular cysts with anechoic fluid. Serous cystadenocarcinomas are multiloculated with thick walls, thick septa, and papillary projections into fluid that may be echogenic.

Mucinous cystadenoma and cystadenocarcinoma comprise 20% of ovarian neoplasms. About 85% are benign. Mucinous tumors may be huge filling the pelvis and extending high into the abdomen. Most have multiple septations (Fig. 37.16) and their fluid is echogenic due to the presence of mucin. Rupture spreads mucin-secreting cells throughout the peritoneal cavity and may result in pseudomyxoma peritonei.

Endometrioid tumors are nearly always malignant. Most are cystic masses with papillary projections.

Other epithelial cell types include clear cell carcinoma (unilocular cyst with a mural nodule), Brenner tumor (solid, benign), and undifferentiated epithelial tumor (aggressive, ill-defined, cystic or solid).

Germ Cell Tumors include the benign cystic teratoma previously described, struma ovarii in which thyroid tissue predominates, dysgerminomas which consist of undifferentiated germ cells, yolk sac (endodermal sinus) tumor, and immature teratoma (29,30). The latter tumors are predominantly solid with small areas of hemorrhage or necrosis.

Stromal Tumors include Sertoli-Leydig cell tumors (10–20% malignant) which may cause masculinization, thecoma (produces estrogen) and fibromas (associated with ascites and pleural effusions—Meigs syndrome).

Metastases to the Ovary occur most commonly with gastrointestinal and breast carcinomas. A *Krukenberg tumor* is a metastasis to the ovary from a mucin-producing tumor of the gastrointestinal tract (31). Most metastases to the ovary are bilateral and solid. Cystic metastases may be indistinguishable from a primary ovarian tumor.

Signs of Malignancy. Since most pelvic masses are discovered, or initially evaluated, by US, every effort should be made to assess the risk of malignancy. Transvaginal US aids substantially in the evaluation. The following signs correlate with an increased risk of malignancy (32–34):

1. Solid consistency—the more solid tissue present the greater the risk of malignancy. Solid tissue includes thick walls, thick septations, and papillary projections (Fig. 37.17). Unilocular cysts or cysts with thin septations are likely to be benign (Fig. 37.16). Thick-walled, multilocular, masses with solid nodules are likely to be malignant. Echogenic masses, or portions of masses, that transmit sound poorly are likely to be malignant.

2. Size greater than 10 cm correlates with a 64% risk of malignancy in postmenopausal women (35). Masses less than 5 cm are more likely to be benign.
3. Color flow US demonstration of blood vessels within septations is strong evidence of neoplasm. Hemorrhagic functional cysts may be complex in appearance but lack internal vascularity.
4. High velocity flow during diastole on spectral Doppler of arteries supplying the mass is strong evidence of neovascularity. A resistance index less than 0.4, or a pulsatility index less than 1.0 suggests malignancy. This finding is not specific. Benign lesions may show "malignant" index values and malignant lesions may have "benign" index values (Fig. 37.18).
5. Age—The risk of malignancy of an ovarian mass increases with the patient's age from 24% at age 50–60 to 60% above age 80 (35).
6. Extension of tumor outside the ovary to the uterus, broad ligament, or other pelvic organs is strong evidence of malignancy. However, inflammatory processes such as tubo-ovarian abscess and endometriosis, may produce similar extension of disease.
7. Ascites, even in absence of visualized tumor implants, is an ominous finding in the presence of an adnexal mass. Peritoneal implants from ovarian carcinoma are commonly minute and may not be detected by US or other imaging methods.
8. Evidence of metastatic spread including tumor implants on peritoneal surfaces, omental cake, and enlarged lymph nodes are clear signs of malignancy (Fig. 37.19).

Ovarian Torsion is a result of axial rotation of the ovary about its vascular pedicle causing acute severe pelvic pain due to arterial occlusion and venous stasis (36). The torsed ovary become swollen, hemorrhagic, and often necrotic depending on the severity of torsion. An ovarian mass may serve as the lead point. The fallopian tube is commonly torsed as well adding to the complexity of the adnexal mass. US reveals a swollen hemorrhagic edematous mass with peripheral follicles. Free fluid is frequently present in the cul-de-sac. Differentiation from other complex masses is often not possible. Doppler evaluation is not always reliable due to normal variations in adnexal flow. Reduced or absent arterial flow to the involved ovary suggests the diagnosis. The presence of central venous flow is indicative of ovarian viability (36).

Polycystic Ovary Disease is technically a clinical and biochemical diagnosis based on findings of hirsutism, amenorrhea, infertility, and obesity. Both ovaries maintain a normal appearance but are enlarged (in 70% of cases) and contain multiple follicles (>5 per ovary). In 30% of cases the ovaries are normal in size, and functionally normal ovaries with multiple follicles may simulate polycystic ovaries (37).

Nonovarian Cysts in the pelvis include abscess from appendicitis or diverticulitis, urachal cysts in the midline above the bladder, lymphocele in patients with prior pelvic node dissection, and paraovarian cysts in the mesosalpinx arising from wolffian duct remnants

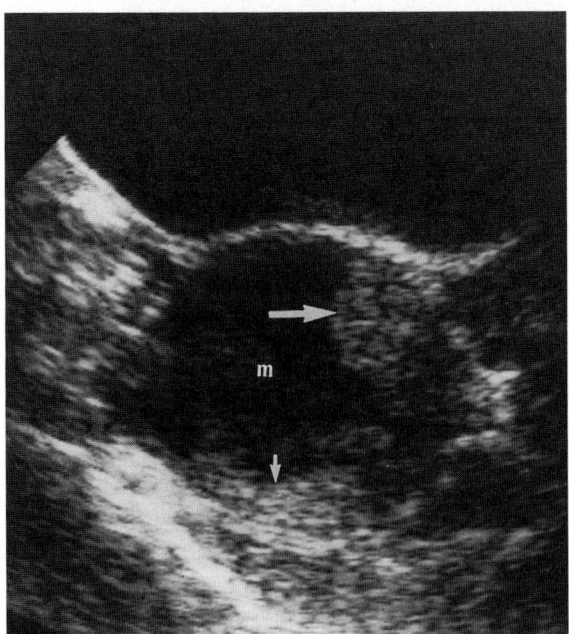

Figure 37.17. Ovarian Carcinoma. US of an adnexal mass (*m*) shows it to be predominantly cystic but with a thick wall (*small arrow*) and a prominent solid nodule (*large arrow*) projecting from its wall. Doppler demonstration of vascularity within the solid nodule confirms neoplastic tissue.

Figure 37.18. Doppler of Ovarian Mass. The spectral Doppler sample volume (*long arrow*) is placed in a blood vessel identified by color Doppler in the wall of an ovarian mass. The Doppler spectrum shows an intermediate resistance pattern with a resistance index (RI) of 0.50 favoring benignancy. The mass proved to be a hemorrhagic follicular cyst. The resistance index is calculated by measuring the peak systolic velocity (*open arrow*) and the end diastolic velocity and using the formula for resistance index (see Table 40.2). The velocity measurements are not angle corrected.

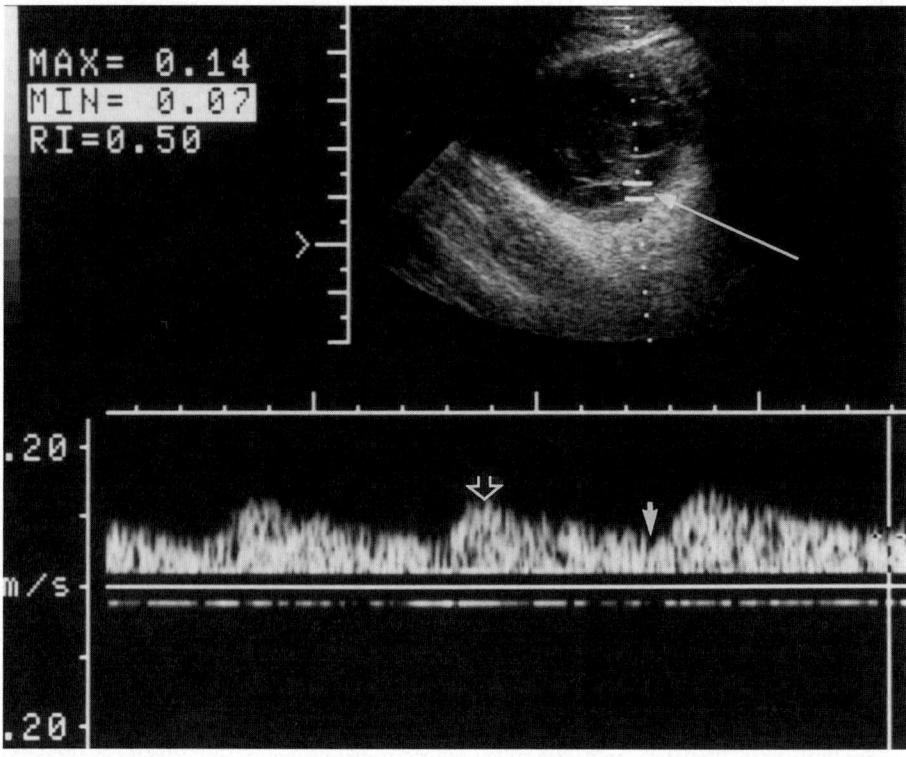

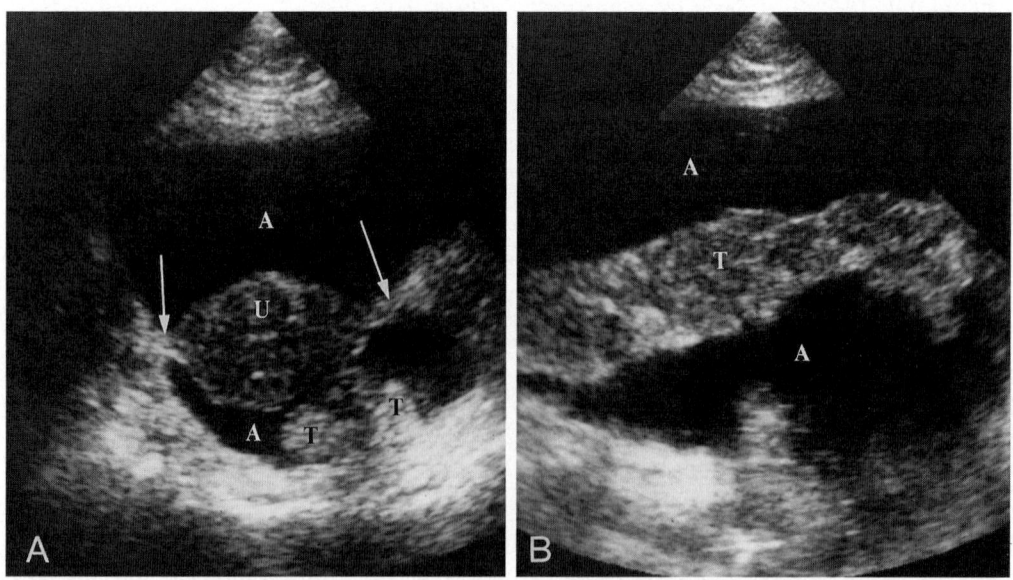

Figure 37.19. Metastatic Ovarian Carcinoma. A. An US image of the pelvis in a 68-year-old woman presenting with sudden onset of ascites confirmed ascites (*A*) with tumor implants (*T*) on the peritoneal surfaces. The uterus (*U*) is seen in transverse section, with the broad ligaments (*arrows*) outlined by fluid. **B.** A sagittal US image from the upper abdomen demonstrates tumor implantation (*T*) on the greater omentum outlined by fluid (*A*). This appearance has been called "omental cake."

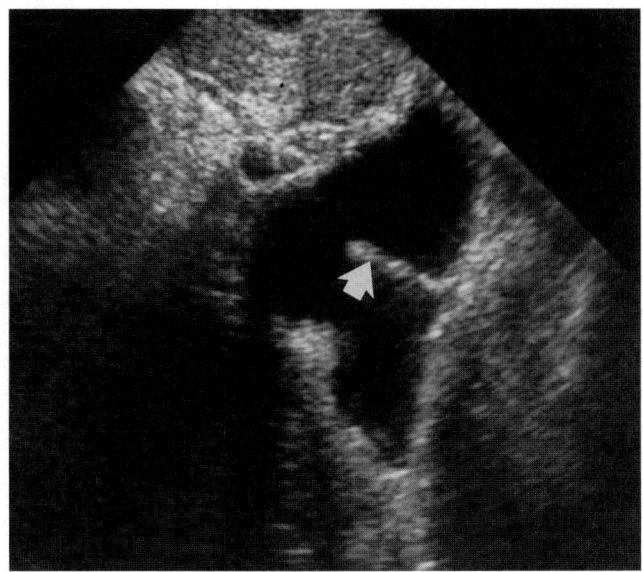

Figure 37.20. Hydrosalpinx. Transvaginal US demonstrates the tubular nature of an adnexal mass confirming hydrosalpinx. Folds (*arrow*) are commonly visualized in a dilated fallopian tube.

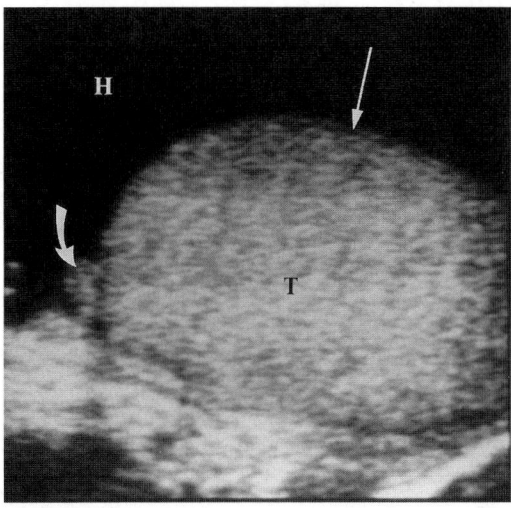

Figure 37.21. Normal Testis, Large Hydrocele. An US image through the long axis of the testis (*T*) demonstrates its homogeneous midlevel echogenicity. The head of the epididymis is seen as a small nodular structure (*curved arrow*) at the superior aspect of the testis. The tunica albuginea (*straight arrow*) is the tough fibrous capsule that covers the testis. The hydrocele (*H*) surrounds all portions of the testis except its posterior portion, where the testis is attached to the scrotal wall.

(38,39). Sonographic demonstration of a separate ovary on the same side as the adnexal mass suggests the diagnosis of nonovarian mass.

Hydrosalpinx can produce a large complex cystic mass. Folds in the dilated fallopian tube may simulate septa in an ovarian tumor (Fig. 37.20). Fluid within the mass is commonly echogenic. Transvaginal US is best for demonstrating the tubular nature of the mass. Other findings of pelvic inflammatory disease may be present.

MALE GENITAL TRACT

Testes and Scrotum

Normal US Anatomy. The normal testis is ovoid and smooth, measuring approximately 3.5 cm in length and 2.0–3.0 cm in diameter (Fig. 37.21)(40). It is covered by a dense fibrous capsule called the tunica albuginea. The testis consists of 250 lobules made up of seminiferous tubules that are the site of spermatozoa development. The seminiferous tubules unite to form the tubuli recti, rete testes, and finally efferent ductules, which exit the testis at the mediastinum. The mediastinum is an invagination of the tunica albuginea on the posterior surface of the testes that provides access for the testicular vessels and exit for efferent ductules (Fig. 37.22). The efferent ductules carry seminal fluid to the epididymis. The epididymis is a highly convoluted tubule that is tightly applied to the posterior aspect of the testis (41). The head of the epididymis (globus major) is the enlarged (7–8 mm diameter) superior portion of the epididymis adjacent to the superior pole of the testes. The body of the epididymis is 1–2 mm in diameter and courses caudally along the posterior-lateral testis. The tail (globus minor) is the pointed lower extremity of the epididymis at the lower pole of the testis. The ductus deferens is the continuation of the epididymis that ascends along the

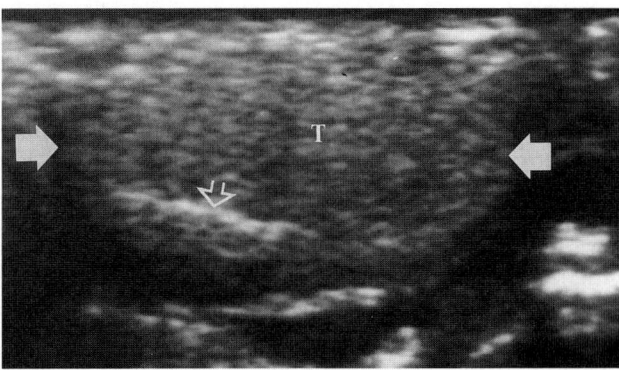

Figure 37.22. Mediastinum of the Testis. The normal mediastinum testis is seen as an echogenic linear stucture (*open arrow*) paralleling the long axis of the testis (*T*, between *arrows*). Testicular vessels and ducts enter and exit the testis through the mediastinum.

posterior-medial aspect of the testis to become a component of the spermatic cord and traverse the inguinal canal. The appendix testis is a müllerian duct remnant seen as a small, oval structure just beneath the head of the epididymis. The appendix epididymis is a small, stalked appendage of the epididymal head. Torsion of the appendix testis or appendix epididymis may clinically mimic testicular torsion.

The scrotum consists of many layers of different tissue (Fig. 37.23). The thickness of the scrotal skin is usually 3–6 mm, with a maximum of 8 mm. The tunica vaginalis is a peritoneal membrane that forms a closed serous sac that covers the medial, anterior, and lateral aspects of the testis and the lateral aspect of the epididymis. This space normally contains 1–2 ml of fluid. Excessive fluid in this space is termed a hydrocele. The tunica vaginalis

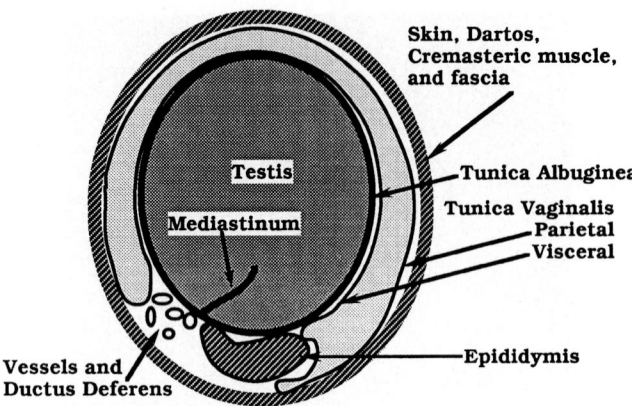

Figure 37.23. Normal Scrotal Anatomy. Drawing of a cross-section of the scrotum demonstrates the testis encapsulated by the tunica albuginea and largely surrounded by the potential space lined by the tunica vaginalis. The testis is attached to the scrotal wall posteriorly, where the testicular blood vessels, ductus deferens, and epididymis reside.

leaves a bare area posteriorly that anchors the testis to the scrotal wall. A midline septum divides the scrotum into two separate compartments.

The spermatic cord is formed at the internal inguinal ring, courses through the inguinal canal and abdominal wall, and suspends the testes in the scrotum. The spermatic cord consists of the ductus deferens; the testicular, deferential, and external spermatic arteries; the pampiniform plexus of veins; lymphatic vessels, and the covering cremaster muscle. Enlargement of the pampiniform plexus of veins is termed a varicocele. Color flow and power Doppler US can evaluate arterial flow in the spermatic cord and testes (42,43). After entering the testis, the testicular artery forms the capsular arteries which course just beneath the tunica albuginea. The capsular arteries give rise to the centripetal branches which flow toward the mediastinum through the testicular parenchyma. Color flow images of one testes should always be compared to color flow images of the opposite testis.

US demonstrates the testes to be homogeneous in echogenicity with an echotexture similar to the thyroid (Fig. 37.21). The mediastinum is seen as a prominent echogenic line along the posterior aspect of the testis. Fluid in the space formed by the tunica vaginalis provides the best visualization of the components of the epididymis. The epididymis has a coarser, more heterogeneous appearance than the testis.

Undescended Testis. About 3% of full-term newborns have an undescended testis. Most of these testes will spontaneously descend by 1 year of age, leaving 1% with cryptorchidism. Spontaneous descent after 1 year of age is unlikely. To preserve fertility, orchipexy is recommended by 2 years of age. Long-term retention of an undescended testis is associated with a dramatically increased risk of testicular neoplasm, especially seminoma. The undescended testis may be located anywhere along the course of descent, from the lower pole of the kidney to the superficial inguinal ring. Most

(70–80%) are identified by US in the inguinal canal. The remainder, located in the abdomen, are best demonstrated by CT or MR (44). The inguinal canal runs an oblique, medially directed course through the flat muscles of the abdominal wall between the deep and superficial inguinal rings. The deep inguinal ring is located midway between the anterior superior iliac spine and the symphysis pubis. The superficial inguinal ring is located just above the pubic crest. Most undescended testes are atrophic, as small as 1 cm in size, and appear hypoechoic compared to normal testis. The bulbous termination of the gubernaculum, called the pars infravaginalis gubernaculi, must not be mistaken for the undescended testis (45). The gubernaculum is a cord-like structure that guides the testes into the scrotum during descent. The gubernaculum atrophies after normal testicular descent, but when descent is incomplete the pars infravaginalis gubernaculi persists as a fibrous or gelatinous mass. Correct identification of the testis is assured by demonstration of the testicular mediastinum.

ACUTE SCROTAL PAIN

Doppler US has largely replaced radionuclide studies as the imaging method of first choice for patients with acute scrotal pain. Doppler US is essential in the differentiation of torsion and infection (46–48)(Table 37.1).

Testicular Torsion results from anomalous suspension of the testis by a long spermatic cord with associated complete investment of the testis and epididymis by the tunica vaginalis resulting in the testis being not securely anchored to the scrotum. This anatomic variant is usually bilateral and has been termed the "bell and clapper" deformity. Surgical correction within 6 hours of torsion will usually preserve testicular function. Delay of surgery for 12 hours or more results in a salvage rate under 20%. The peak ages for testis torsion are the newborn period and ages 13–16 years.

US findings of acute torsion include enlargement of the testis and epididymis with a diffuse but sometimes heterogeneous decrease in echogenicity due to edema. The spermatic cord is enlarged and the Doppler signal from the spermatic cord is decreased or lost. Demonstration of normal flow on one side and absent or decreased flow on the symptomatic side provide the most reliable evidence of torsion and testicular ischemia. Spontaneous detorsion may result in reactive hyperemia which mimics epididymo-orchitis. A clinical history of decreasing pain prior to sonography suggests the possibility of detorsion.

Table 37.1. Causes of Acute Painful Scrotum

Common
Acute epididymitis/orchitis
Acute testicular torsion
Uncommon
Torsion of appendix epididymis
Torsion of appendix testis
Incarcerated inguinal hernia
Hemorrhage into a testicular tumor

Radionuclide perfusion studies utilizing technetium-99m pertechnetate demonstrate decreased vascular flow with a rounded cold area in the location of the affected testis. When torsion is present for more than 24 hours, the "doughnut sign" may appear. This is seen as a central cold area representing the underperfused testis surrounded by a rim of increased radionuclide activity due to dartos hyperemia.

Acute Epididymo-orchitis. Although testicular torsion is most common in patients under 20 years, acute epididymitis is most common after age 20. The onset of pain and swelling is more gradual with epididymitis. Pyuria is commonly present. *Escherichia coli, Staphylcoccus aureus*, gonococcus, and tuberculosis are the most common causative organisms.

US demonstrates thickening and enlargement of the epididymis. Color Doppler demonstrates diffuse increased blood flow on the affected side as compared to the opposite side. Hypervascularity may be confined to the epididymis or the testis, or involve both. Hydrocele is common. Inflammatory changes in the testis occur in 20% of cases (Fig. 37.24).

Radionuclide perfusion imaging shows increased vascular flow in the spermatic cord on the affected side. Radionuclide activity in the affected hemiscrotum may also be increased because of reactive hyperemia.

Torsion of the Appendix Testis or Appendix Epididymis is a common cause of acute scrotal pain in children (49,50). Presentation mimics testicular torsion. US demonstrates enlarged hypoechoic masses medial or posterior to the epididymal head associated with hydrocele, thickening of the scrotal wall, and normal testes. Treatment is symptomatic with spontaneous resolution expected.

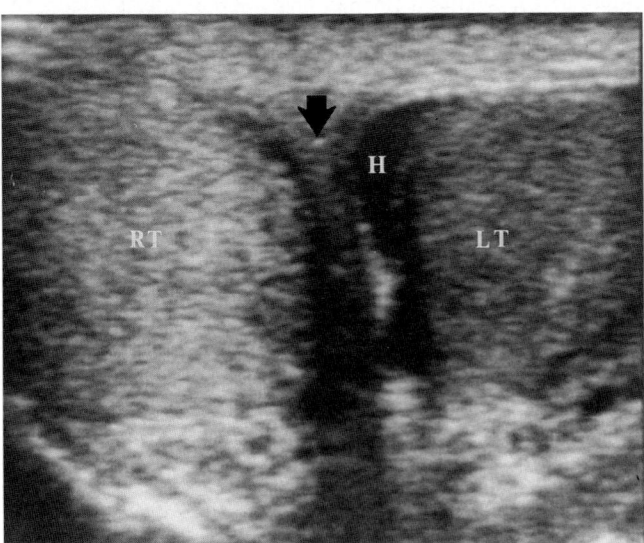

Figure 37.24. Acute Orchitis. Transverse US view of the scrotum demonstrates the left testis (*LT*) to be diffusely hypoechoic compared to the right testis (*RT*). A small hydrocele (*H*) is seen in the left hemiscrotum. The midline septum (*arrow*) dividing the scrotum into two separate compartments is evident.

SCROTAL MASSES

US is 80–95% accurate in differentiating intratesticular from extratesticular masses. The majority of intratesticular masses are malignant (Table 37.2). Every intratesticular lesion should be considered to be potentially malignant until it is proven to be benign. Most extratesticular lesions are benign and are caused by inflammation or trauma (51,52)(Table 37.3).

Table 37.2. Differential Diagnosis of Intratesticular Lesions

Malignant
Primary germ cell tumor
  Seminoma
  Nonseminoma
  Embryonal cell carcinoma
  Teratoma
  Choriocarcinoma
  Mixed cell tumor
Secondary malignancy
  Leukemia and lymphoma
  Metastasis
Benign
Inflammatory
  Orchitis
  Epididymo-orchitis
  Mumps
  Abscess
Torsion/infarction
Gonadal stromal tumor
  Leydig cell tumor
  Sertoli cell tumor
Cysts
  Cyst of the tunica albuginea
  Benign testicular cyst
Trauma/hemorrhage

Table 37.3. Differential Diagnosis of Extratesticular Lesions

Extrinsic to epididymis
Scrotal fluid collections
  Hydrocele
  Hematocele
  Pyocele
Varicocele
Scrotal hernia
Epididymal lesions
Cystic
  Spermatocele
  Epididymal cyst
  Abscess
Solid
  Sperm granuloma
  Epididymitis
  Sarcoidosis
  Adenomatoid tumor

Intratesticular Lesions

Primary Testicular Neoplasms constitute 4–6% of all male genitourinary tumors and 1% of all male malignancies. Most (95%) are germ cell tumors. These occur most commonly in the 25–35-year-old age group and present as a unilateral painless mass (53,54).

Seminomas constitute 50% of germ cell tumors. They are less aggressive and are sensitive to radiation therapy. Seminomas are histologically monotonous, consisting of sheets of uniform cells intermixed with fibrous strands. Reflecting the histology, US demonstrates the tumor to be homogeneous and hypoechoic (Fig. 37.25).

Nonseminomatous Tumors. The remainder of germ cell malignancies can be grouped as nonseminomatous tumors. As a group they are more aggressive and resistant to radiation therapy. Cell types include embryonal cell carcinoma (20–25%), teratoma (5–10%), and choriocarcinoma (1–3%). The remainder are of mixed cell type. All tend to be heterogeneous because of mixed cellularity as well as the presence of hemorrhage and necrosis. US demonstrates the heterogeneity and shows irregular areas of high and low density, cystic areas, and calcification (Fig. 37.26). A hydrocele is present in 15% of patients with germ cell tumors.

Lymphatic spread of tumor is most common, with a usual pattern of orderly ascending nodal involvement. Initial spread is along gonadal lymphatic vessels following the testicular veins to renal hilar nodes. Lymphatic metastases may also follow the external iliac chain to the paraaortic nodes. The internal iliac and inguinal nodes are rarely involved. Extensive metastatic involvement of the lymph nodes mimics lymphoma in young males. The primary tumor in the testis may be clinically occult, yet is effectively demonstrated by ultrasound. Hematogenous spread to the lungs usually follows lymphatic spread, except in choriocarcinoma, which spreads hematogenously early. Both CT and MR are excellent methods for initial tumor staging and follow-up.

Lymphoma, Leukemia, and Metastases from other primary tumors are more common than germ cell tumors in patients over age 50. The testis serves as a sanctuary for disease because of ineffective access of chemotherapy. Involvement of the testis may be diffuse or focal. Tumors are usually of lower echogenicity than normal parenchyma (Fig. 37.27)(55). Careful comparison with the opposite testis may be necessary for detection of lesions. Renal cell and prostate carcinoma are the most common tumors to metastasize to the testis.

Testicular Microlithiasis appears on US as diffuse, punctate, nonshadowing, hyperechoic foci throughout the testicular parenchyma (Fig. 37.28)(56,57). It is a benign condition of microcalcifications within the seminiferous tubules, but is associated with an incidence of testicular carcinoma as high as 40%. Nearly all cases are

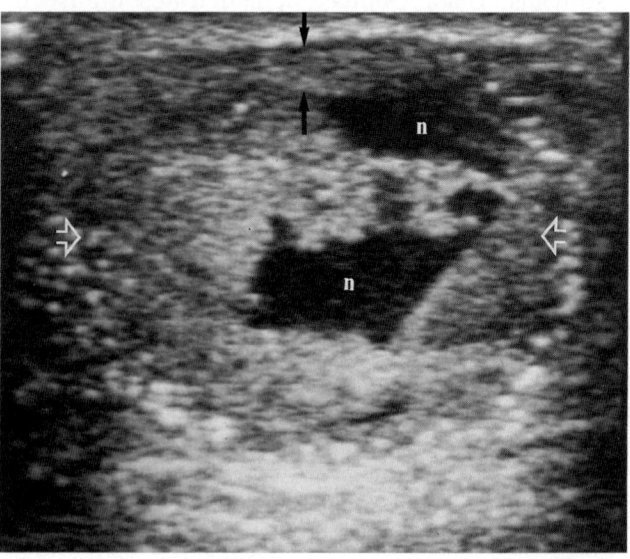

Figure 37.26. Choriocarcinoma. An US view of a testis in long axis demonstrates a large tumor (between *open arrows*) replacing the testicular parenchyma. Note the marked inhomogeneity of the tumor with large areas of necrosis (*n*). The residual testicular parenchyma is indicated by the *black arrows*.

Figure 37.25. Seminoma. Longitudinal US demonstrates near-complete replacement of the testes (between *arrowheads*) by a homogeneous hypoechoic mass (*S*) that proved to be seminoma. Only a thin rim of normal testicular parenchyma remains (between *arrows*).

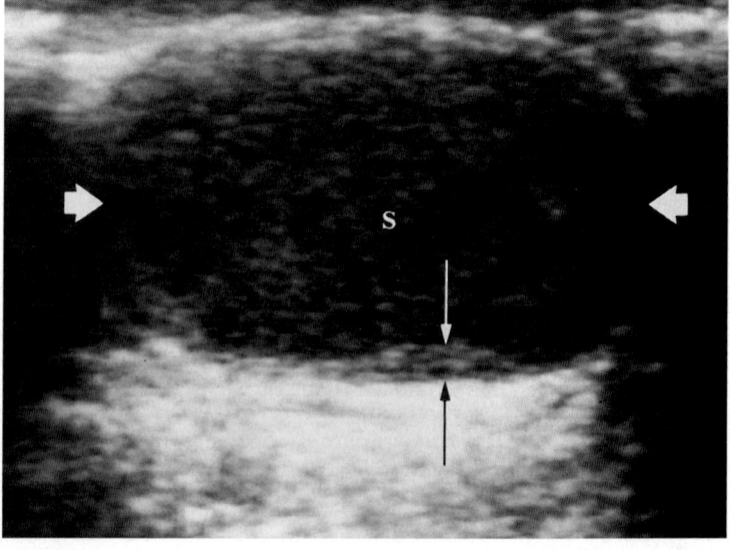

bilateral. Additional associations include cryptorchidism and infertility.

Orchitis and Abscess. Most inflammations of the testis are associated with epididymitis. Mumps is an additional cause of orchitis. The testis with orchitis is enlarged with edematous areas that may be irregular in outline (Fig. 37.24). A fluid-filled mass suggests abscess formation. Testicular abscess may rupture through the tunica albuginea and result in a pyocele.

Infarction. Testis infarction may result from torsion or trauma. The infarct may appear as a focal low-density area or diffuse low density of the entire testis. With time, the testis shrinks and becomes fibrotic.

Gonadal Stromal Tumors. Leydig and Sertoli cell tumors account for 3–6% of all testicular tumors; 3% are

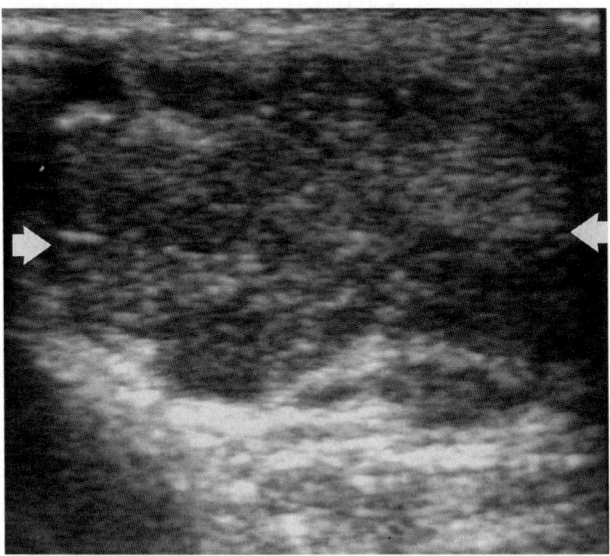

Figure 37.27. Malignant Melanoma Metastasis. Long axis view of the testis reveals complete replacement of parenchyma by an inhomogeneous, predominantly hypoechoic tumor (between *arrowheads*). No recognizable normal parenchyma remains.

bilateral; up to 15% are malignant. They appear as small, solid masses.

Cysts. Benign testicular cysts are incidental findings in 8–10% of males (Fig. 37.29). Cysts of the tunica albuginea are well defined, small (2–5 mm in diameter), and peripheral (58,59). Both types are filled with serous fluid.

Dilated Rete Testis may mimic a complex intratesticular mass (60,61). US demonstrates multiple small spherical or tubular cystic structures in the region of the mediastinum of the testis (Fig. 37.30). Nearly all cases are associated with abnormalities of the epididymis including spermatocele, epididymal cysts, or history of epididymitis or vasectomy.

Trauma/Hemorrhage. In the setting of trauma, the role of imaging is to detect a ruptured testis. Most (90%) ruptured testes can be salvaged by surgery performed in the first 72 hours following trauma. Intratesticular hematoma and hematocele are the major indicators of testis rupture. Discrete fractures are identified in a minority of cases. Color Doppler US is useful in detecting intratesticular vascular disruption and in avoiding mistaking a normal vascular cleft for a fracture.

Extratesticular Lesions

Scrotal Fluid Collections. A hydrocele is the accumulation of serous fluid between the visceral and parietal layers of the tunica vaginalis (Figs. 37.21, 37.23). It is the most common cause of painless scrotal swelling. Although many cases are idiopathic, hydrocele may accompany malignant tumors, torsion, and inflammation. Hematoceles result from trauma or surgery. Pyoceles usually result from rupture of an abscess into the space between the layers of the tunica vaginalis. Internal septations and loculations are common with hematoceles and pyoceles.

Varicoceles are dilated serpiginous veins of the pampiniform plexus (Fig. 37.31). They occur in 15–20% of males and are the most common correctable cause of

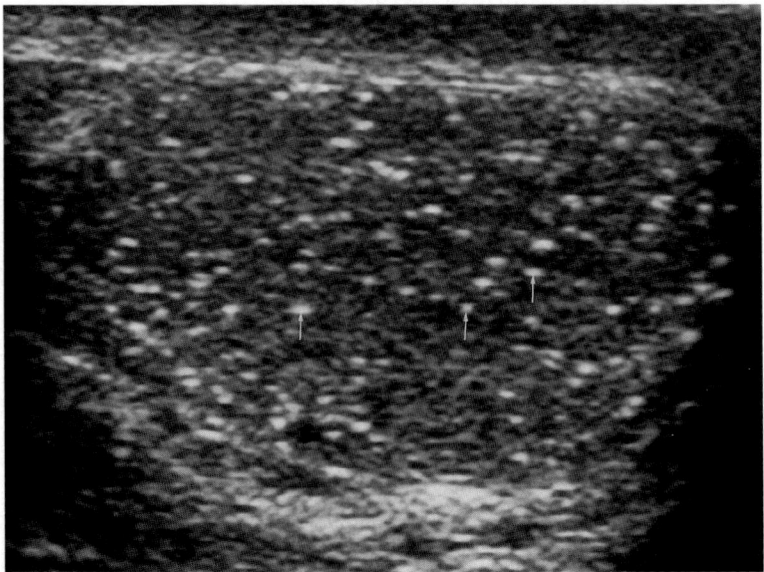

Figure 37.28. Testicular Microlithiasis. Innumerable tiny echogenic spots (*arrows*) are evident throughout the testicular parenchyma. This benign condition carries a high risk of associated testicular carcinoma.

male infertility. Acute onset of a varicocele in an adult male aged 40 or older may be a sign of neoplastic obstruction of the ipsilateral gonadal or renal vein.

Scrotal Hernias may contain omentum, small bowel, or colon. The herniated mass extends through the inguinal canal to the scrotum (Fig. 37.32).

Cystic Epididymal Lesions. *Spermatoceles* are cysts of the epididymal head that contain sperm and cellular debris (Fig. 37.33). *Epididymal cysts* contain clear serous fluid and may occur anywhere along the course of the epididymis. Loculations and septations within the cysts are common. Spermatoceles range in size up to several centimeters (62).

Solid Epididymal Lesions. *Sperm granuloma* form when sperm extravasate into the soft tissues surrounding the epididymis. *Chronic epididymitis*, resulting from incompletely resolved acute epididymitis, causes an ir-

regular, hard, tender mass (Fig. 37.34). *Sarcoidosis* may cause a painless, solid epididymal mass and involve the testis. *Adenomatoid tumors* are benign, slow-growing epididymal neoplasms.

Prostate

The major indication for transrectal US of the prostate gland is to guide needle biopsy for diagnosis of prostate cancer (63). Early enthusiasm for use of transrectal US as a screening examination for prostate cancer has been dampened by well-documented sensitivity of only 60% for US examination alone. Additional indications include detection of abscess, infertility with suspicion of ob-

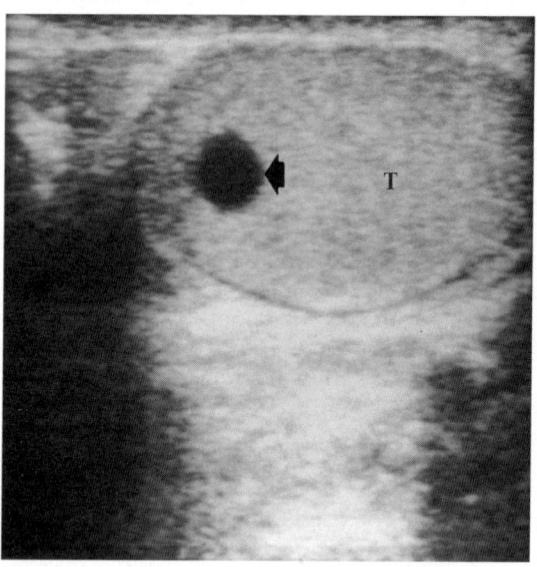

Figure 37.29. Testicular Cyst. A benign testicular cyst is viewed as a well-defined, spherical, uniformly anechoic mass (*arrow*) within the testis (*T*). Care must be taken to differentiate simple testicular cysts from cystic necrosis within testicular tumors.

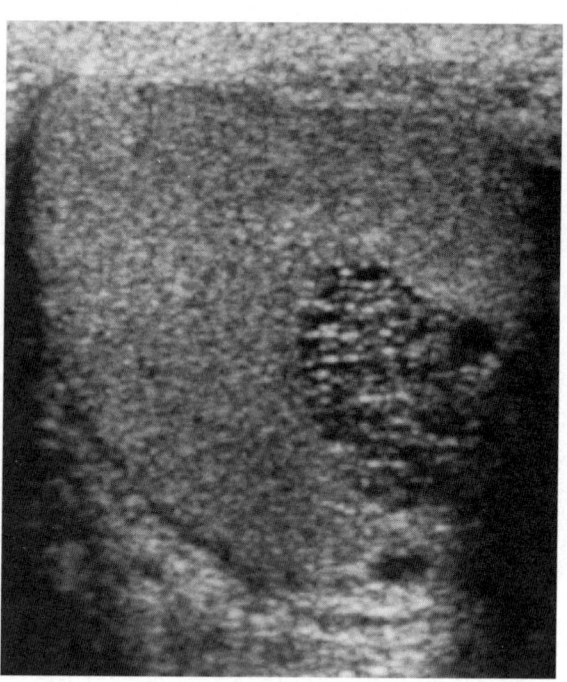

Figure 37.30. Dilated Rete Testis. A complex appearing mass (*arrow*) is made up of numerous tiny cystic tubular structure and is located in the mediastinum of the testis.

Figure 37.31. Varicocele. Sagittal view of the scrotum demonstrates a network of curving tubular structures (*arrows*) at the superior pole of the testis (*T*). Color Doppler US confirmed slow venous flow within these dilated vessels.

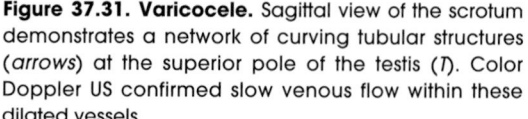

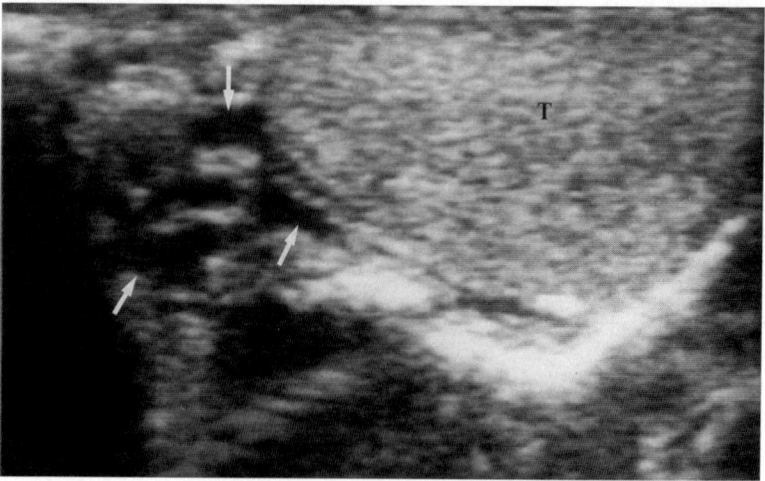

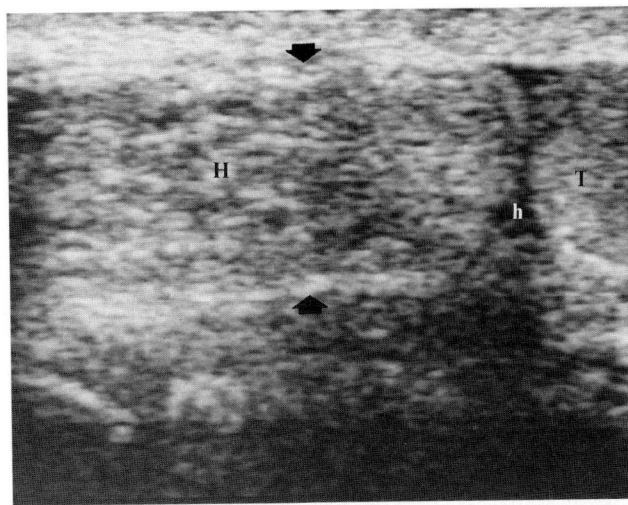

Figure 37.32. Inguinal Hernia. Sagittal plane image reveals a moderately echogenic mass in the inguinal canal (*H*, between *arrowheads*). With straining, the mass approached the superior pole of the testis (*T*). With relaxation in the supine position the hernia was reduced. A small hydrocele (*h*) was also present. Surgery confirmed a small inguinal hernia with omentum extending through the inguinal canal into the superior aspect of the scrotum.

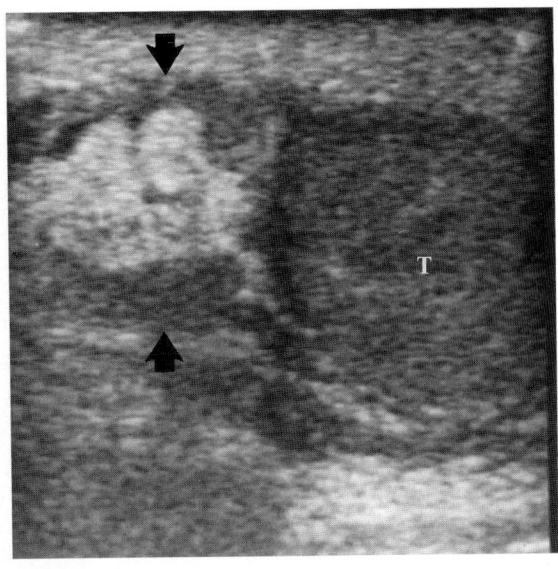

Figure 37.34. Chronic Epididymitis. The epididymis (*arrows*) is grossly enlarged and has a large central echogenic area, representing fibrosis and chronic inflammation. The testis (*T*) is diffusely hypoechoic because of diffuse orchitis.

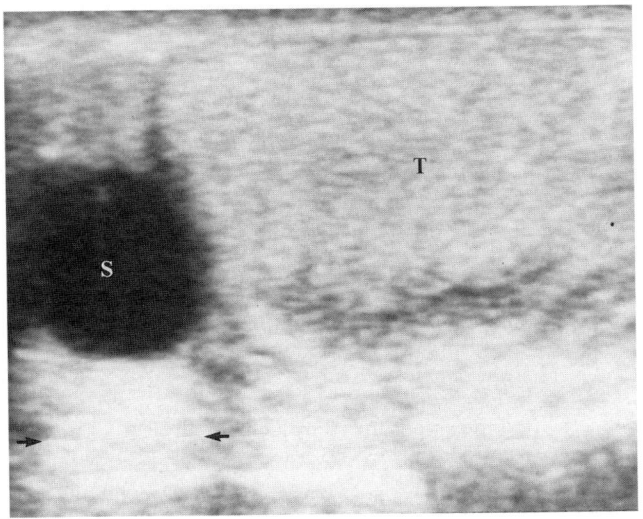

Figure 37.33. Spermatocele. Long axis US image of the testis displays a well-defined extratesticular cyst (*S*) at the superior pole of the testicle (*T*). Debris within the spermatocele produces floating particles within the fluid. Acoustic enhancement (*arrows*) is evident deep to the spermatocele.

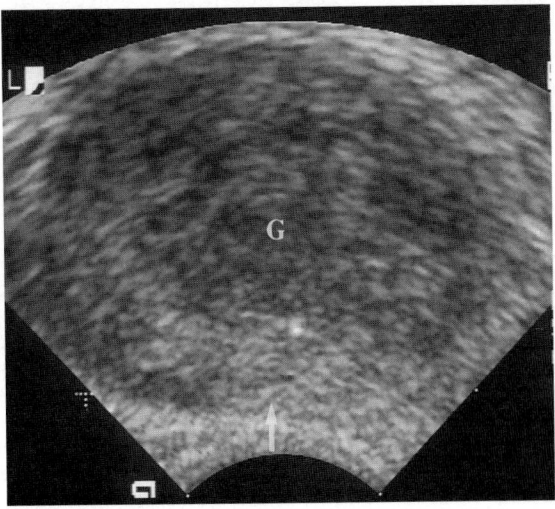

Figure 37.35. Prostate Anatomy. Transrectal US images of the prostate are routinely viewed inverted. The transducer is at the bottom, rather than the top of the image. This sagittal image shows the normal peripheral zone (*arrow* near the transducer) to be slightly echogenic compared to the hypoechoic, more heterogeneous central gland (*G*).

struction of the ejaculatory ducts or atresia of the seminal vesicles and for examination of the posterior urethra.

Normal US Anatomy. On transabdominal US the prostate is seen as a rounded organ at the base of the bladder (Fig. 37.1). Enlargement of the prostate elevates the base of the bladder. The urethral orifice can usually be identified as a V-shaped indentation in the prostate. The zonal anatomy of the prostate is described in chapter 35. On transrectal US, the central and peripheral zones are nearly equal in echogenicity and are usually

distinguished mainly by position (Fig. 37.35). It is useful to describe the gland on ultrasound as having a *peripheral zone* and an *inner gland* comprising the central and transitional zones and their pathologic alterations. The anterior fibromuscular stroma is seen as a hypoechoic area at the anterior superior aspect of the gland. US can be used to calculate the volume of the prostate gland using the formula width × height × length × 0.52. Larger than 30 cc (or 30 gm) is considered enlarged.

The seminal vesicles are seen as hypoechoic, lobu-

Figure 37.36. Normal Seminal Vesicles. Transrectal US image shows the normal hypoechoic convoluted tubular appearance of the seminal vesicle (*arrow*). *B,* bladder.

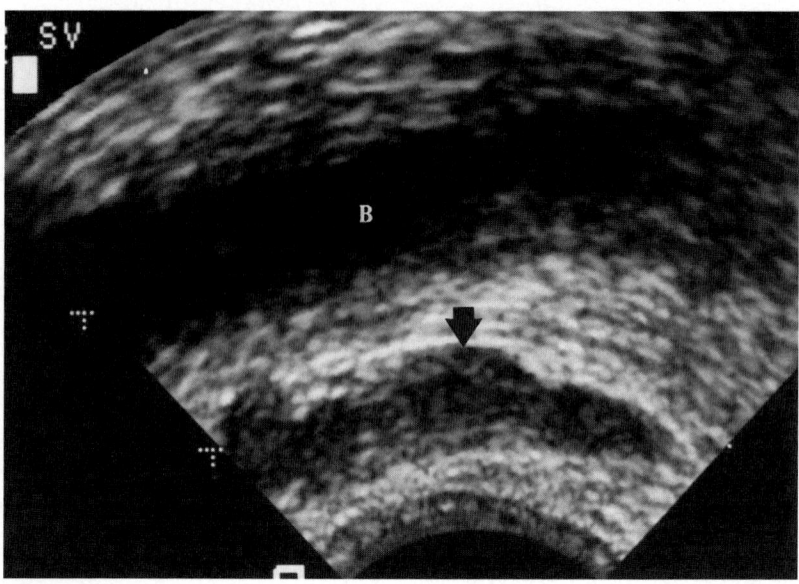

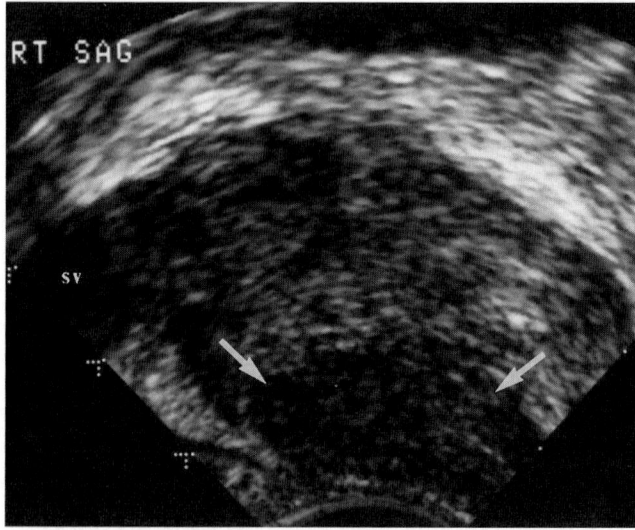

Figure 37.37. Prostate Cancer. Right sagittal transrectal US image shows a distinct hypoechoic nodule (*arrows*) in the peripheral zone. US-guided transrectal needle biopsy confirmed prostate carcinoma. *sv,* seminal vesicle.

Table 37.4. Causes of Peripheral Hypoechoic Nodule in the Prostate

Carcinoma
Benign prostatic hypertrophy
Prostatitis
Infarction
Fibromuscular hyperplasia

Table 37.5. Cystic Lesions in the Prostate

Müllerian duct cyst (midline)
Utricle cyst (midline)
Prostate retention cyst (associated with BPH)
Seminal vesicle cyst
Ejaculatory duct cyst

lated, tubular structures in the groove between the base of the bladder and the base of the prostrate (Fig. 37.36).

Prostate Carcinoma. Screening for prostate carcinoma currently includes digital rectal examination and serum prostate-specific antigen (PSA) testing (64). Prostate-specific antigen is a glycoprotein produced only by the prostate gland. Elevated PSA levels suggest the presence of cancer with the risk of malignancy increasing with the PSA value. The normal serum PSA level is 0–4 ng/ml. False positive elevation of PSA levels is generally due to benign prostate hyperplasia (BPH). For this reason some centers use a PSA-density calculation of PSA value divided by size of the prostate estimated clinically or measured by transabdominal or transrectal US.

US signs of prostate cancer are *a)* distinct hypoechoic nodule (Fig. 37.37), *b)* poorly marginated hypoechoic area in the peripheral zone, *c)* mass effect on surrounding tissues, *d)* asymmetric enlargement of the prostate, *e)* deformation of prostatic contour and, *f)* heterogeneous area in the homogeneous gland, and *g)* focal increased vascularity in the peripheral zone with color flow US (65). All findings are nonspecific (Table 37.4), and random biopsies of the prostate yield carcinoma as commonly as 20% of cases. Sonographic guidance provides a safe and accurate method to obtain tissue from specific areas of the prostate gland. Indications for US-guided needle biopsy include: suspicious palpable nodule, suspicious nodule visualized by US, or elevated prostate

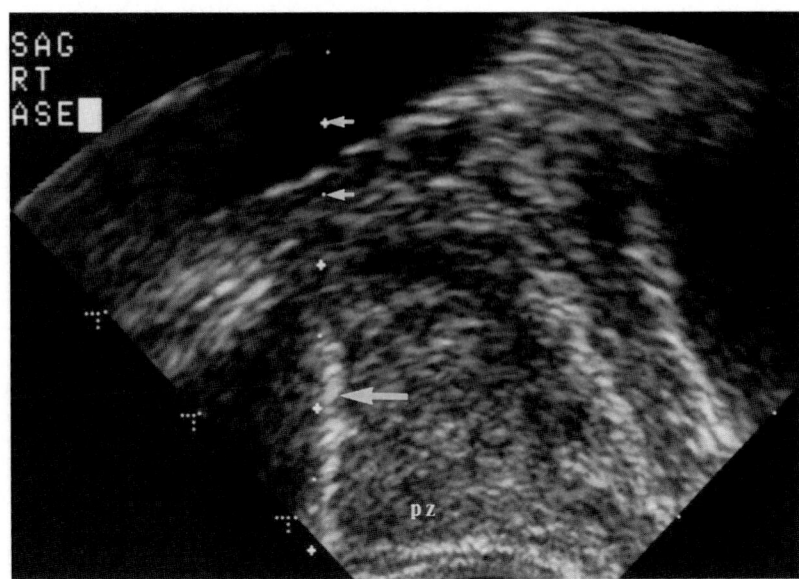

Figure 37.38. US-guided Prostate Biopsy. The dotted line (*small arrows*) indicates the expected needle tract when biopsy needle is passed through a needle guide attached to the US transducer. The operator aims at the target lesion, advances the needle just into the peripheral zone (*pz*), and fires the spring-loaded core-biopsy needle to obtain a tissue specimen for histology. The needle tract (*large arrow*) is shown in this image obtained during the needle firing.

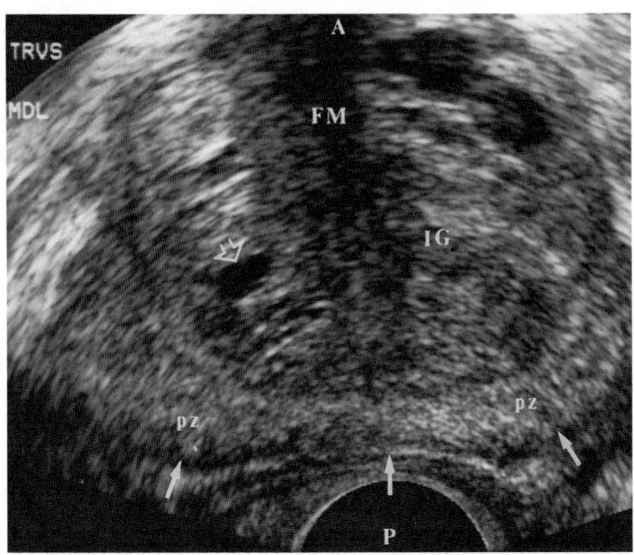

Figure 37.39. Benign Prostatic Hypertrophy. Transrectal axial US view through the midprostate demonstrates excellent differentiation of a normal peripheral zone (*pz, solid arrows*). The inner gland (*IG*) demonstrates mild enlargement and heterogeneity that is characteristic of benign prostatic hypertrophy. A small prostatic cyst is evident (*open arrow*). The hypoechoic fibromuscular zone (*FM*) is anterior. *A*, anterior; *P*, posterior.

specific antigen (Fig. 37.38). Both transrectal and transperineal routes are used for prostate biopsy. The transperineal route is more painful, and the transrectal route requires preprocedure antibiotics. Our practice had been to routinely obtain a total of 6-10 18-gauge core biopsy specimens from different areas of gland, always including all four quadrants.

Benign Prostatic Hyperplasia is a nodular hypertrophy of the glandular tissue of the transitional zone, usually beginning in the 5th decade of life. The transitional zone becomes enlarged and heterogeneous and com-

presses the urethra and the central zone (Fig. 37.39). Discrete nodules, some with cystic changes, may be visualized. The enlargement is often marginated circumferentially by a pseudocapsule. The size of the prostate exceeds 30 gm (ml). The prostatic urethra becomes elongated, tortuous, and compressed, causing bladder outlet obstruction. Stasis of urine may lead to the formation of bladder stones. The bladder base is commonly elevated and the bladder wall may be thickened.

Acute Prostatitis is usually caused by *E. coli* infection. The gland is swollen and edematous. Prostatic abscess is demonstrated by US as a focal collection of echogenic fluid within the gland (Fig. 37.40). Septations may be present. Transrectal US may be used to direct needle aspiration of a suspected abscess.

Chronic Prostatitis results from incompletely resolved acute prostatitis. Large prostatic calculi are common and serve as a reservoir for persistent and relapsing infection.

Prostatic Calculi form spontaneously or result from chronic inflammation. Most calculi are periurethral and form from the corpora amylacea, a proteinaceous material formed in the prostate gland. On US calculi are brightly echogenic and commonly produce acoustic shadows. Although they may be found in areas of cancer, they are not a sign of cancer and do not develop from the malignant process.

Prostatic Cysts are relatively common findings on prostate imaging examinations. Cystic lesions of the prostate are listed in Table 37.5 (66,67).

Ejaculatory Duct Obstruction is an uncommon but treatable cause of male infertility (68). Causes include congenital obstruction, urethritis, and instrumentation. The normal ejaculatory ducts are not commonly visible on transrectal US. Obstruction of the ducts is suggested by presence of a cyst posterior to the prostatic urethra, commonly associated with dilatation of the seminal vesicles. Needle aspiration or surgical resection of the obstructing cyst is frequently curative.

Figure 37.40. Prostate Abscess. Transverse transrectal US reveals an abscess (*arrows*) in the right side of the prostate gland in a patient with fever, pelvic pain, and pyuria. The abscess contained purulent debris seen on US as floating particulate matter.

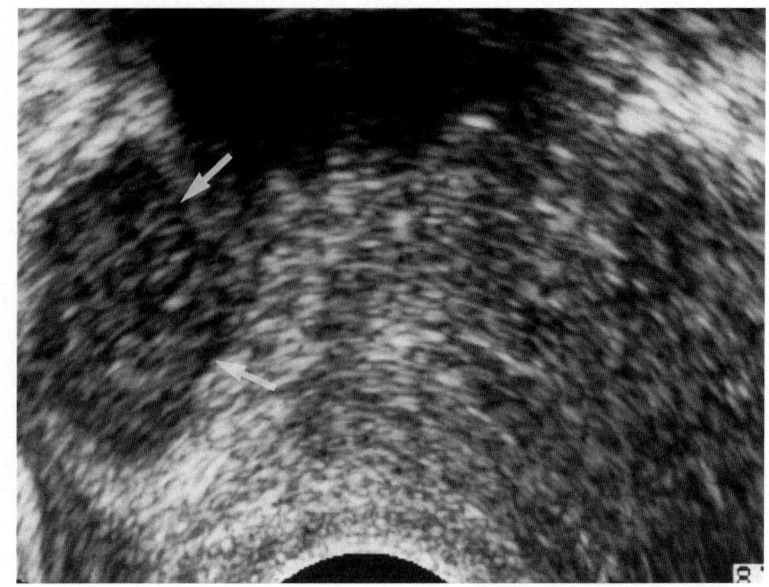

References

1. Abulafia O, Sherer DM, Lee PS. Postoperative color Doppler flow ultrasonographic assessment of ureteral patency in gynecologic oncology patients. J Ultrasound Med 1997;16:125–129.
2. Burge HJ, Middleton WD, McClennan BL, Hildebolt CF. Ureteral jets in healthy subjects and patients with unilateral ureteral calculi: comparison with color Doppler ultrasound. Radiology 1991;180:437–440.
3. Maynor CH, Kliewer MA, Hertzberg BS, et al. Urinary bladder diverticula: sonographic diagnosis and interpretive pitfalls. J Ultrasound Med 1996;16:189–194.
4. Abu-Yousef MM. Ultrasound of bladder tumors. Semin Ultrasound CT MR 1986;7:275–286.
5. Gooding GAW. Ultrasound of the bladder. The Radiologist 1996;3:311–317.
6. Mogavero G, Sheth S, Hamper UM. Endovaginal sonography of the nongravid uterus. RadioGraphics 1993;13:969–981.
7. Fleishcher AC, Kepple DM. Transvaginal color duplex sonography: clinical potentials and limitations. Semin Ultrasound CT MR 1992;13:69–80.
8. Chang TS, Böhm-Vélez M, Mendelson EB. Nongynecologic applications of transvaginal sonography. AJR Am J Roentgenol 1993;160:87–93.
9. Santolaya-Forgas J. Physiology of the menstrual cycle by ultrasonography. J Ultrasound Med 1992;11:139–142.
10. Baltarowich OH, Kurtz AB, Pennell RG, et al. Pitfalls in the sonographic diagnosis of uterine fibroids. AJR Am J Roentgenol 1988;151:725–728.
11. Karasick S, Lev-Toaff AS, Toaff MEA. Imaging of uterine leiomyomas. AJR Am J Roentgenol 1992;158:799–805.
12. Cohen JR, Luxman D, Sagi J, et al. Ultrasonic "honeycomb" appearance of uterine submucous fibroids undergoing cystic degeneration. J Clin Ultrasound 1995;23:293–296.
13. Atri M, Nazarnia S, Aldis AE, et al. Transvaginal US appearance of endometrial abnormalities. RadioGraphics 1994;14:483–492.
14. Zalud I, Conway C, Schulman H, Trinca D. Endometrial and myometrial thickness and uterine blood flow in postmenopausal women: the influence of hormonal replacement therapy and age. J Ultrasound Med 1993;12:737–741.
15. Aleem F, Predanic M, Calame R, et al. Transvaginal color and pulsed Doppler sonography of the endometrium: a possible role in reducing the number of dilatation and curettage procedures. J Ultrasound Med 1995;14:139–145.
16. Hulka CA, Hall DA, McCarthy K, Simeone JF. Endometrial polyps, hyperplasia, and carcinoma in postmenopausal women: differentiation with endovaginal sonography. Radiology 1994;191:755–758.
17. Zalel Y, Tepper R, Cohen I, et al. Clinical significance of endometrial fluid collections in asymptomatic postmenopausal women. J Ultrasound Med 1996;15:513–515.
18. Reinhold C, Atri M, Mehio A, et al. Diffuse uterine adenomyosis: morphologic criteria and diagnostic accuracy of endovaginal sonography. Radiology 1995;197:609–614.
19. Reinhold C, McCarthy S, Bret PM, et al. Diffuse adenomyosis: comparison of endovaginal US and MR imaging with histopatholoic correlation. Radiology 1996;199:151–158.
20. Ritchie WG. Sonographic evaluation of normal and induced ovulation. Radiology 1986;161:1–10.
21. Levine D, Gosink BB, Wolf SI, et al. Simple adnexal cysts: the natural history in postmenopausal women. Radiology 1992;184:653–659.
22. Fried AM, Kenney CM III, Stigers KB, et al. Benign pelvic masses: sonographic spectrum. RadioGraphics 1996;16:321–334.
23. Bulas DI, Ahlstrom PA, Sivit CJ, et al. Pelvic inflammatory disease in the adolescent: comparison of transabdominal and transvaginal sonographic evaluation. Radiology 1992;183:435–439.
24. Volpi E, De Grandis T, Zuccaro G, et al. Role of transvaginal sonography in the detection of endometriomata. J Clin Ultrasound 1995;23:163–167.
25. Kupfer MC, Schwimer SR, Lebovic J. Transvaginal sonographic appearance of endometrioma: spectrum of findings. J Ultrasound Med 1992;11:129–133.
26. Hertzberg BS, Kliewer MA. Sonography of benign cystic teratoma of the ovary: pitfalls in diagnosis. AJR Am J Roentgenol 1996;167:1127–1133.
27. Wagner BJ, Buck JL, Seidman JD, McCabe KM. Ovarian epithelial neoplasms: radiologic-pathologic correlation. RadioGraphics 1994;14:1351–1374.
28. Buy J-N, Ghossain MA, Sciot C, et al. Epithelial tumors of the ovary: CT findings and correlation with US. Radiology 1991;178:811–818.

29. Brammer HM III, Buck JL, Hayes WS, et al. Malignant germ cell tumors of the ovary: radiologic-pathologic correlation. RadioGraphics 1990;10:715–724.

30. Surratt JT, Siegel MJ. Imaging of pediatric ovarian masses. RadioGraphics 1991;11:533–548.

31. Shimizu H, Yamasaki M, Ohama K, et al. Characteristic ultrasonographic appearance of the Krukenberg tumor. J Clin Ultrasound 1990;18:697–703.

32. Buy J-N, Ghossain MA, Hugol D, et al. Characterization of adnexal masses: combination of color Doppler and conventional sonography compared with spectral Doppler analysis alone and conventional sonography alone. AJR Am J Roentgenol 1996;166:385–393.

33. Stein SM, Laifer-Narin S, Johnson MB, et al. Differentiation of benign and malignant adnexal masses: relative value of gray-scale, color Doppler, and spectral Doppler sonography. AJR Am J Roentgenol 1995;164:381–386.

34. Jain KA. Prospective evaluation of adnexal masses with endovaginal gray-scale and duplex and color Doppler US: correlation with pathologic findings. Radiology 1994;191:63–67.

35. Rulin MC, Preston AL. Adnexal masses in postmenopausal women. Obstet Gynecol 1987;70:578–581.

36. Fleischer AC, Stein SM, Cullinan JA, Warner MA. Color Doppler sonography of adnexal torsion. J Ultrasound Med 1995;14:523–528.

37. Pache TD, Wladimiroff JW, Hop WCJ, Fauser BCJM. How to discriminate between normal and polycystic ovaries: transvaginal US study. Radiology 1992;183:421–423.

38. Barloon TJ, Brown BP, Abu-Yousef MM, Warnock NG. Paraovarian and paratubal cysts: preoperative diagnosis using transabdominal and transvaginal sonography. J Clin Ultrasound 1996;24:117–122.

39. Kim JS, Woo SK, Suh SJ, Morettin LB. Sonographic diagnosis of paraovarian cysts: value of detecting a separate ipsilateral ovary. AJR Am J Roentgenol 1995;164:1441–1444.

40. Older RA, Watson LR. Ultrasound anatomy of the normal male reproductive tract. J Clin Ultrasound 1996;24:389–404.

41. Black JAR, Patel A. Sonography of the normal extratesticular space. AJR Am J Roentgenol 1996;167:503–506.

42. Gooding GA. Sonography of the spermatic cord. AJR Am J Roentgenol 1988;151:721–724.

43. Horstman WG, Middleton WD, Melson GL, Siegel BA. Color Doppler US of the scrotum. RadioGraphics 1991;11:941–957.

44. Friedland GW, Chang P. The role of imaging in the management of the impalpable undescended testis. AJR Am J Roentgenol 1988;151:1107–1111.

45. Rosenfield AT, Blair DN, McCarthy S, et al. The pars infravaginalis gubernaculi: importance in identification of the undescended testis. AJR Am J Roentgenol 1989;153:775–778.

46. Burks DD, Markey BJ, Burkhard TK, et al. Suspected testicular torsion and ischemia: evaluation with color Doppler sonography. Radiology 1990;175:815–821.

47. Berman JM, Beidle TR, Kunberger LE, Letourneau JG. Sonographic evaluation of acute intrascrotal pathology. AJR Am J Roentgenol 1996;166:857–861.

48. Herbener TE. Ultrasound in the assessment of the acute scrotum. J Clin Ultrasound 1996;24:405–421.

49. Cohen HL, Shapiro MA, Haller JO, Glassberg K. Torsion of the testicular appendage—sonographic diagnosis. J Ultrasound Med 1992;11:81–83.

50. Strauss S, Faingold R, Manor H. Torsion of the testicular appendages: sonographic appearance. J Ultrasound Med 1997;16:189–192.

51. Doherty FJ. Ultrasound of the nonacute scrotum. Semin Ultrasound CT MR 1991;12:131–156.

52. Gerscovich EO. High-resolution ultrasonography in the diagnosis of scrotal pathology: I. normal scrotum and benign disease. J Clin Ultrasound 1993;21:355–373.

53. Tessler RN, Tublin ME, Rifkin MD. Ultrasound assessment of testicular and paratesticular masses. J Clin Ultrasound 1996;24:423–436.

54. Gerscovich EO. High-resolution ultrasonography in the diagnosis of scrotal pathology: II. tumors. J Clin Ultrasound 1993;21:375–386.

55. Mazzu D, Jeffrey RB Jr, Ralls PW. Lymphoma and leukemia involving the testicles: findings on gray-scale and color Doppler sonography. AJR Am J Roentgenol 1995;164:645–647.

56. Miller RL, Wissman R, White S, Ragosin R. Testicular microlithiasis: a benign condition with a malignant association. J Clin Ultrasound 1996;24:197–202.

57. Backus ML, Mack LA, Middleton WD, et al. Testicular microlithiasis: imaging appearances and pathologic correlation. Radiology 1994;192:781–785.

58. Gooding GAW, Leonhardt W, Stein R. Testicular cysts: US findings. Radiology 1987;163:537–538.

59. Hamm B, Fobbe F, Loy V. Testicular cysts: differentiation with US and clinical findings. Radiology 1988;168:19–23.

60. Brown D, Benson CB, Doherty FJ, et al. Cystic testicular mass caused by dilated rete testis: sonographic findings in 31 cases. AJR Am J Roentgenol 1992;158:1257–1259.

61. Weingarten BJ, Kellman GM, Middleton WD, Gross ML. Tubular ectasia within the mediastinum testis. J Ultrasound Med 1992;11:349–353.

62. Black JAR, Patel A. Sonography of the abnormal extratesticular space. AJR Am J Roentgenol 1996;167:507–511.

63. Smith JA Jr. Transrectal ultrasonography for the detection and staging of carcinoma of the prostate. J Clin Ultrasound 1996;24:455–461.

64. Brawer MK. How to use prostate-specific antigen in the early detection or screening for prostatic carcinoma. CA Cancer J Clin 1995;45:148–164.

65. Newman JS, Bree RL, Rubin JM. Prostate cancer: diagnosis with color Doppler sonography with histologic correlation of each biopsy site. Radiology 1995;195:86–90.

66. Jarow JP. Transrectal ultrasonography of infertile men. Fertil Steril 1993;60:1035–1039.

67. Hamper UM, Epstein JI, Sheth S, et al. Cystic lesions of the prostate gland—a sonographic—pathologic correlation. J Ultrasound Med 1990;9:395–402.

68. Meacham RB, Townsend RR, Drose JA. Ejaculatory duct obstruction: diagnosis and treatment with transrectal sonography. AJR Am J Roentgenol 1995;165:1463–1466.

38
Obstetric Ultrasound

William E. Brant

IMAGING METHODS

Ultrasound is the imaging method of choice for dating the pregnancy, monitoring fetal growth, assessing fetal well-being, and evaluating fetal anatomy and maternal pelvic organs. Transvaginal sonography is particularly useful in the assessment of first-trimester pregnancy and in the demonstration of fetal anatomic structures deep in the pelvis. Modern US offers superb anatomic detail in real time, keeping up with the frequently vigorous motion of the fetus. MR is used occasionally as a supplement to US imaging when the US examination is equivocal (1). MR offers excellent detail of maternal pelvic organs, unobscured by bone, gas, or fat. Demonstration of fetal anatomy is limited by fetal motion but may be overcome by fetal sedation and fast scan techniques (2). CT is the method of choice for pelvimetry (3).

THE ULTRASOUND EXAMINATION

An obstetric US examination consists of a survey of the uterus and maternal pelvic organs, measurements of the fetus to date the pregnancy and assess fetal growth, and a survey of fetal anatomy. Standards for the performance of obstetric ultrasound examinations have been published by the American Institute of Ultrasound in Medicine (4). In the first trimester, the location and appearance of the gestational sac is documented. The embryo is identified, crown–rump length measured, and fetal cardiac activity confirmed. Fetal number is documented, and the uterus and adnexa are examined. Second- and third-trimester sonography includes assessment of fetal life and number, fetal position, amount of amniotic fluid, placental location and appearance, fetal measurements (biparietal diameter, head circumference, abdominal circumference, femur length), and evaluation of the uterus and adnexa. Assessment of fetal anatomy includes the cerebral ventricles, a four-chamber view of the heart, and images of the spine, stomach, bladder, umbilical cord insertion site, and renal regions. The literature refers to "Level I" obstetric ultrasounds as routine or standard examinations and "Level II" examinations as targeted to scrutinize fetal anatomy and detect anomalies.

FIRST TRIMESTER

The first trimester covers the period from conception to the end of the 13th menstrual week. This includes the entire embryonic period (0–10 wk) and is a time of dynamic growth and the differentiation and development of most organ systems. The embryo and fetus have the greatest risk of maldevelopment, injury, and death during this period because of external factors (infection, drugs, radiation) or chromosome abnormalities. About 40% of implanted zygotes are menstrually aborted, and another 25–35% of surviving embryos will threaten to abort during the first trimester.

Normal Gestation

The presence of a pregnancy is confirmed by a positive serum β-human chorionic gonadotropin (β-hCG)test or by a positive enzyme linked immunoassay (ELIZA) urinary pregnancy test. Radioimmunoassay for serum β-hCG allows pregnancy to be detected within 2 weeks of conception (as early as 23 menstrual days) and before a normal gestational sac can be detected by either transabdominal or transvaginal US. The early gestational sac can generally be seen by transvaginal sonography at 3.5–4.5 menstrual weeks as a tiny cystic structure implanted within the echogenic decidua, the *intradecidual sign* (Fig. 38.1). This sign is not specific for early intrauterine pregnancy and may be mimicked by fluid collections or endometrial cysts in the presence of ectopic

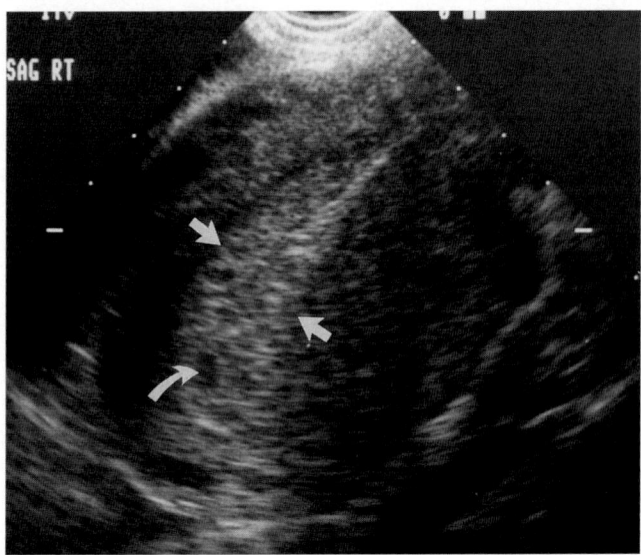

Figure 38.1. Intradecidual Sign. Transvaginal US image of the uterus in a sagittal plane demonstrates thickening of the endometrial stripe (*arrows*) due to decidual reaction. A tiny (6 mm) gestational sac (*curved arrow*) is implanted within the thickened decidua near the uterine fundus. The size of the sac corresponds to a pregnancy of approximately 4 weeks' menstrual age.

Table 38.1. US Characteristics of a Normal Gestational Sac[a]

Intradecidual sign—before 5 weeks' GA
Double decidual sac sign—after 5 weeks' GA (>98% of IUP)
Well-defined round/or oval anechoic sac
Echogenic decidua >2 mm thick
Position in upper uterine body midway between uterine walls
Growth in MSD >1.2 mm/day
Yolk sac 2–6 mm in diameter:
   Always present when MSD ≥ 20 mm on transabdominal US
   Always present when MSD ≥ 8 mm on transvaginal US
Embryo:
   Always present when MSD ≥25 mm on transabdominal US
   Always present when MSD ≥16 mm on transvaginal US

[a] The gestational sac diameter is measured in three orthogonal planes, and the measurements are averaged to calculate the mean sac diameter (MSD). (Adapted from Nyberg DA, Laing FC, Filly RA, et al. Ultrasonographic differentiation of the gestational sac of early intrauterine pregnancy from the pseudogestational sac of ectopic pregnancy. Radiology 1983;146:755–759; and from Levi CS, Lyons EA, Lindsay DJ. Early diagnosis of nonviable pregnancy with endovaginal. US Radiology 1988;167:383–385.)

pregnancy (5). A normal gestational sac is often visualized by the transabdominal approach by 5 menstrual weeks. The normal gestational sac appears on US as a smoothly contoured, round or oval, fluid-containing structure positioned in the endometrial cavity near the fundus of the uterus (Table 38.1)(6). The normal sac has an echogenic border greater than 2-mm thick, which represents the choriodecidual reaction. A *double decidual sac sign* (Fig. 38.2) is evident in about 85% of normal pregnancies. The double sac sign is produced by visualization of three layers of decidual reaction early in pregnancy (7). The term *decidua* refers to the endometrium of the pregnant uterus. The decidua vera lines the en-

dometrial cavity, and the decidua capsularis covers the gestational sac. The decidua basalis contributes to the formation of the placenta at the site of implantation. A small amount of fluid in the endometrial cavity separates the decidua vera from the decidua capsularis, enabling visualization of the "double sac." The free margin of the gestational sac consists of chorion and decidua capsularis and is normally at least 2-mm thick. The double sac is not complete because of placental attachment to the uterine wall. A well-visualized double sac is excellent evidence of intrauterine pregnancy. An absent double sac sign is evidence of an abnormal intrauterine pregnancy or an ectopic pregnancy.

The yolk sac (Fig. 38.3) is a 2- to 6-mm diameter, spherical, cystic structure that is connected to the midgut of the embryo by a thin stalk, the vitelline duct. The yolk sac is the earliest site of blood cell formation in the embryo. It floats freely in fluid between the amniotic and chorionic membranes. It is generally the earliest structure visualized within the gestational sac and serves as definitive evidence of early pregnancy. The yolk sac should always be visualized in normal pregnancy in gestational sacs of 20-mm mean sac diameter by transabdominal sonography or 8-mm mean sac diameter by transvaginal sonography.

The earliest demonstration of the embryo is the *double bleb sign* (Fig. 38.4), produced by the amniotic sac and the yolk sac with the embryonic disc between them (8). Embryos as small as 2-mm long can be detected by transvaginal sonography. The earliest embryonic cardiac

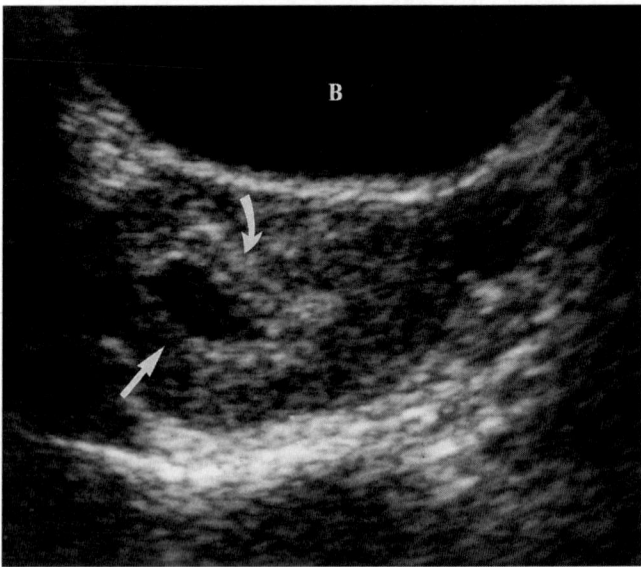

Figure 38.2. Double Decidual Sac Sign. A transverse image of the uterus obtained transabdominally through a filled bladder (*B*) demonstrates a gestational sac with two decidual layers in the endometrial cavity. The two echogenic lines (*curved arrow*) are formed by the decidua vera lining the endometrial cavity and the decidua capsularis covering the gestational sac. The placental implantation site on the posterior aspect of the uterus (*straight arrow*) has a single echogenic stripe due to the decidua basalis.

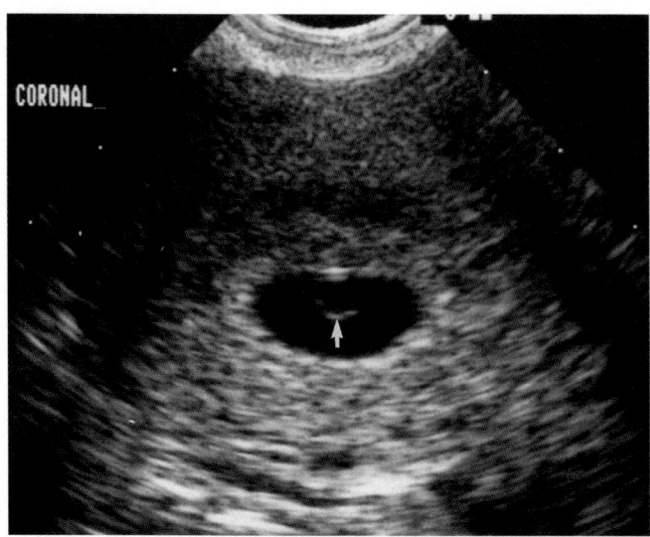

Figure 38.3. Yolk Sac. The yolk sac (*arrow*) is seen within the gestational sac by transvaginal US in a coronal plane. The normal yolk sac is less than 6 mm in diameter, spherical, and fluid filled with a thin wall. Demonstration of the yolk sac within the uterus confirms intrauterine pregnancy.

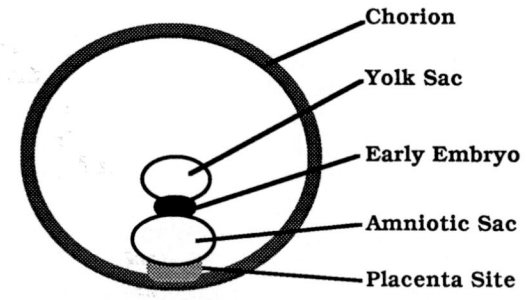

Figure 38.4. Double Bleb Sign. The double bleb is formed by the yolk sac and the amniotic sac suspended in the fluid of the early chorionic sac. The embryo is seen as a tiny disclike structure between the two blebs. Early cardiac activity can frequently be observed in the embryonic disc.

activity can be detected by careful inspection of the embryonic disc by real-time US. Transvaginal sonography may demonstrate tiny normal embryos in which cardiac activity cannot be confirmed. Cardiac activity should always be seen transvaginally in embryos that can be visualized by transabdominal US.

Gestational age in the first trimester is estimated by measuring the mean diameter of the gestational sac (MSD, or mean sac diameter) or the crown–rump length of the embryo or fetus. A normal gestational sac grows at a rate of approximately 1.2 mm/day MSD.

Patients who present with vaginal bleeding and pelvic pain during the first trimester are commonly referred for US examination. The differential diagnosis is listed in Table 38.2.

Table 38.2. Vaginal Bleeding in the First Trimester

Differential Diagnosis
Spontaneous abortion
Anembryonic pregnancy
Embryonic demise
Demise of a twin
Ectopic pregnancy
Subchorionic hemorrhage
Implantation bleed
Gestational trophoblastic disease

Spontaneous Abortion

Abortion is the termination of pregnancy before 20 weeks' gestational age. *Spontaneous abortion* is the termination of pregnancy by natural causes. Approximately 10–15% of all known pregnancies end in spontaneous abortion. Up to 60% of spontaneous abortions have chromosomal abnormalities. A number of clinical terms are used to describe abortion. *Threatened abortion* refers to the occurrence of vaginal bleeding and uterine cramping with a closed cervical os in early pregnancy. Threatened abortion complicates roughly 25% of all pregnancies. *Inevitable abortion* presents with cervical dilation and fetal or placental tissues within the cervical os. With *complete abortion*, all uterine contents have been expelled. *Incomplete abortion* refers to the presence of residual products of conception within the uterus. In *missed abortion*, the fetus has died but remains within the uterus. *Habitual abortion* is defined as three or more successive spontaneous abortions. *Anembryonic pregnancy* or *blighted ovum* is a pregnancy in which the embryo has died and is no longer visible or never developed.

"Empty" Gestational Sac. A gestational sac without an embryo demonstrated by US is compatible with a very early intrauterine pregnancy or a nonviable intrauterine pregnancy (blighted ovum) (Fig 38.5). An empty gestational sac must be differentiated from a pseudogestational sac associated with ectopic pregnancy (Fig. 38.6). A gestational sac is considered to be abnormal if it demonstrates the following features (Table 38.3): large size without an embryo or yolk sac, distorted shape, irregular contour, thin or weak choriodecidual reaction, absence of a double decidual sac, or abnormal position. Any one of the major criteria or three of the minor criteria are considered diagnostic. Large sac size without visualized yolk sac or embryo and a distorted sac contour have a reported 100% specificity and positive predictive value for identification of nonviable pregnancy (6). The original criteria reported by Nyberg et al. (6,7) have been refined by the use of transvaginal transducers, which improve visualization of anatomic detail (9). Most authors recommend allowing a 1–2 mm margin of error and repeating any equivocal scans in several days (10). Growth of the gestational sac by less than 1 mm/day MSD is strong evidence of abnormal sac development (11).

Embryonic or Fetal Demise is diagnosed by US confirmation of the absence of cardiac activity. Absence of

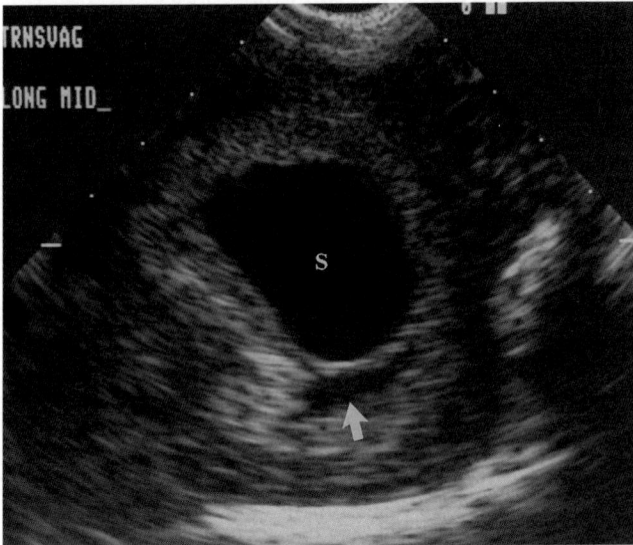

Figure 38.5. Anembryonic Pregnancy. An empty gestational sac (*S*) measuring 28 mm in MSD is demonstrated within the uterus by transvaginal US. Blood (*arrow*) is present in the endometrial cavity. In a normal intrauterine pregnancy, an embryo should always be demonstrable by transvaginal US when the MSD exceeds 16 mm.

Table 38.3. Ultrasound Characteristic of an Abnormal Gestational Sac[a]

Major criteria
  Absence of yolk sac when:
    MSD ≥20 mm on transabdominal US
    MSD ≥8 mm on transvaginal US
  Absence of embryo when:
    MSD ≥25 mm on transabdominal US
    MSD ≥16 mm on transvaginal US
  Distorted sac shape
  Growth <1 mm MSD/day
Minor criteria
  Irregular sac contour
  Thin decidual reaction ≦2 mm
  Weak decidual echo amplitude
  Absent double decidual sac sign
  Sac positioned low in the uterus

[a] The gestational sac diameter is measured in three orthogonal planes, and the measurements are averaged to calculate the mean sac diameter (MSD).
(Adapted from: Nyberg DA, Laing FC, Filly RA, et al. Ultrasonographic differentiation of the gestational sac of early intrauterine pregnancy from the pseudogestational sac of ectopic pregnancy. Radiology 1983;146:755–759; and from Levi CS, Lyons EA, Lindsay DJ. Early diagnosis of nonviable pregnancy with endovaginal US. Radiology 1988;167:383–385.)

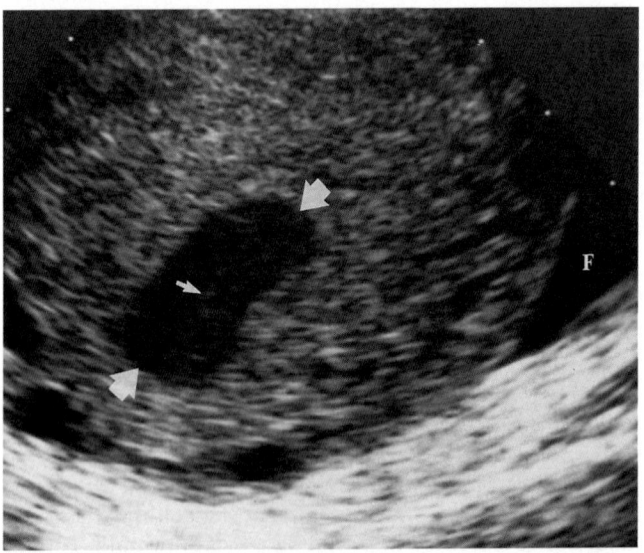

Figure 38.6. Pseudogestational Sac. Fluid within the endometrial cavity (*large arrows*) in a patient with an ectopic pregnancy mimics an intrauterine gestational sac. Echogenic material due to blood (*small arrow*) within the fluid cavity may mimic an embryo. The uterus is imaged in the sagittal plane with an intravaginal transducer. Fluid (*F*) is seen in the cul-de-sac.

cardiac activity in a fetus or an embryo large enough to be visualized by transabdominal US is definitive evidence of death. Because of the increased sensitivity of transvaginal US in demonstrating cardiac activity, all cases of suspected demise of small embryos should be confirmed by transvaginal US, which may demonstrate cardiac activity even in embryos as small as 1.5 mm

crown–rump length (CRL). Transvaginal US may also visualize small, normal, living embryos (<5 mm CRL) without demonstrating cardiac activity. Absence of cardiac activity in embryos larger than 5 mm on transvaginal US is considered diagnostic of embryonic demise (missed abortion) (12). Embryos smaller than 5 mm without cardiac activity should be rescanned in a few days to confirm demise (13).

Quantitative serum β-hCG levels have been correlated with US findings to assist in the identification of abnormal pregnancies. Great caution is advised, however, because of differences in the way that individual laboratories report serum β-hCG results and in the wide variation in values obtained by different laboratories. In summary, discriminatory levels will vary with the resolution of the US scanner used and the laboratory reporting the hormonal assay.

Ectopic Pregnancy

Ectopic pregnancy occurs in only 1.4% of all pregnancies, but it is the major cause of pregnancy-related deaths. Misdiagnosis of ectopic pregnancy remains one of the most common areas for medical malpractice litigation. Patients at high risk for ectopic pregnancy include those with a history of pelvic inflammatory disease, tubal surgery, endometriosis, ovulation induction, previous ectopic pregnancy, or use of intrauterine device for contraception. Ninety-five percent of ectopic pregnancies occur in the fallopian tube, most commonly in the isthmic portion. Interstitial ectopic pregnancies, developing in the portion of the tube passing through the uterine wall, may grow to large size before rupture, resulting in catastrophic hemorrhage (14). Additional sites for ectopic implantation include the abdominal cavity, ovary, and cervix. All patients with a positive pregnancy test (serum β-hCG), and vaginal bleeding, pelvic pain, or adnexal mass must be considered at risk for ectopic pregnancy.

A completely confident diagnosis of ectopic pregnancy can be made sonographically only when a living embryo is positively demonstrated to be in a position outside of the uterus. This occurs in only 5–10% of ectopic pregnancies. Transvaginal sonography increases the possibility of demonstrating a live ectopic pregnancy. In any other circumstance, we are dealing with a situation of relative risk (Table 38.4) (15). When an intrauterine pregnancy is documented by US, the risk of coexisting ectopic pregnancy is extremely low, estimated at 1 in 30,000. Concurrent intrauterine and extrauterine pregnancies do occur, however, especially in patients taking ovulation-inducing drugs. When an adnexal mass other than a simple corpus luteal cyst is demonstrated, or a moderate or large amount of fluid is present in the pelvis, the risk of ectopic pregnancy is high. Even when the US examination is entirely normal, a patient with a positive pregnancy test remains at risk for ectopic pregnancy.

Table 38.4. Risk of Ectopic Pregnancy as Determined by Ultrasound Findings

Ultrasound Finding	Approximate Risk
IUP Confirmed	
General population	1 in 30,000
Patient taking ovulation-inducing drugs	1 in 6000–7000
IUP not confirmed	43%
Living ectopic fetus	100%
Adnexal mass	83%
Moderate/large fluid	83%
Adnexal mass + pelvic fluid	94%
Normal pelvic sonogram	8%

(Adapted from Mahony BS, Filly RA, Nyberg, DA, Callen PW. Sonographic evaluation of ectopic pregnancy. J Ultrasound Med 1985;4:221–228.)

The role of US, then, is to demonstrate findings that determine relative risk. This assessment, in conjunction with clinical history and physical examination, determines the next step in the patient's evaluation.

US findings in ectopic pregnancy include demonstration of an extrauterine gestational sac appearing as a fluid-containing structure with an echogenic ring, the *tubal ring sign* (Fig. 38.7) (16,17). A living or dead embryo might or might not be evident. The ectopic gestational sac must be differentiated from a corpus luteal cyst, which develops on the ovary at the site of ovulation. The corpus luteal cyst appears as a thin-walled cyst projecting eccentrically from the ovary. Clotted blood from hemorrhage within a corpus luteal cyst may simulate an embryo. A key differentiating finding is whether the cystic mass arises from the ovary. Most ectopic pregnancies implant in the fallopian tube and are separate from the ovary. Implantation of ectopic pregnancy on the ovary is a rare event. Corpus luteal cysts always arise from the ovary. Hematosalpinx or ruptured ectopic pregnancy may appear as an amorphous solid or complex adnexal mass lacking an embryo or sac (18). Blood in the cul-de-sac usually appears as echogenic fluid but may be entirely echolucent if liquid, or echogenic and solid-appearing if clotted (19). Stimulation of the endometrium by the hormones associated with the ectopic pregnancy causes thickening of the central stripe of the uterus. Blood in the endometrial cavity causes a *pseudogestational sac* (Fig. 38.6) in up to 20% of ectopic pregnancies. A true gestational sac is differentiated from "pseudosac" by the presence of a yolk sac or embryo. A double decidual sac sign suggests a true gestational sac, but is not totally reliable because some pseudosacs may also show a double decidual sac sign. Doppler studies demonstrate absent or minimal peritrophoblastic flow with pseudosacs and high-velocity, low impedance flow with true gestational sacs (20).

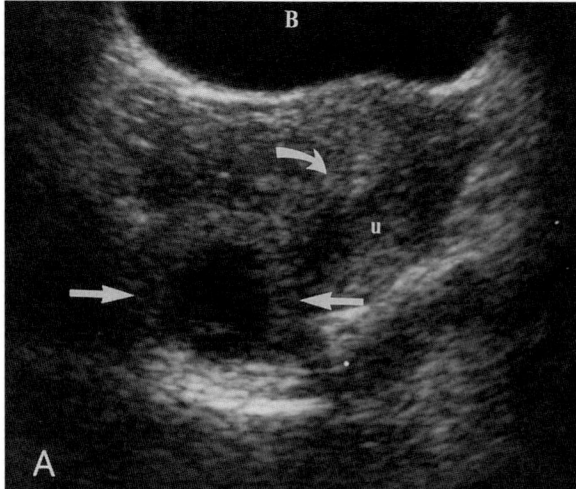

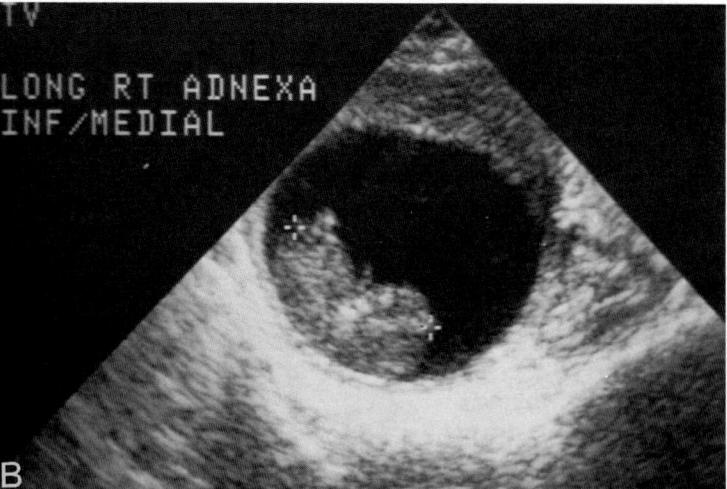

Figure 38.7. Ectopic pregnancy. A. Transabdominal US in a transverse plane through the bladder B demonstrates a cystic mass (*arrows*) with a thick echogenic wall in the right adnexa. The uterus (*u*) is empty but has a thickened endometrial stripe (*curved arrow*) resulting from decidual reaction. **B.** Transvaginal examination in the same patient demonstrates a 20-mm embryo (between *caliper marks* (+)) in the extrauterine sac. No cardiac activity was present.

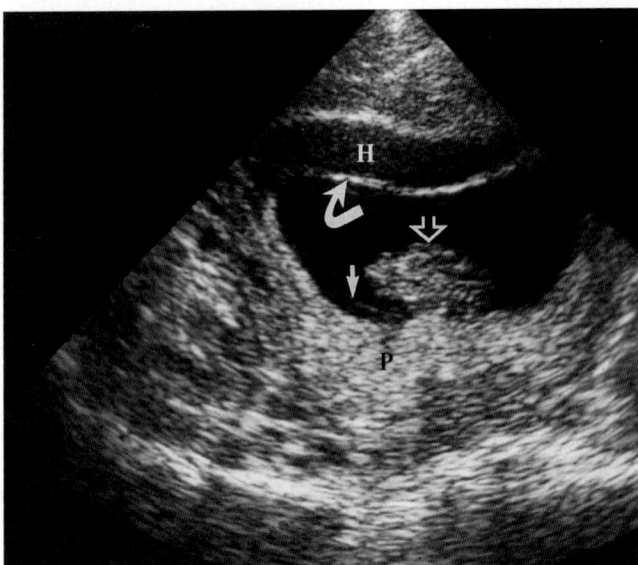

Figure 38.8. Subchorionic Hemorrhage. Hemorrhage (*H*) extends beneath the chorion (*curved arrow*) from the edge of the placenta (*P*). A living 11-week fetus (*open arrow*) was present. Note the normal separation of the thin amniotic membrane (*straight arrow*) from the surface of the placenta.

Subchorionic Hemorrhage

Subchorionic hemorrhage (Fig. 38.8) is a common finding in the bleeding patient before 20 weeks' gestational age (21). All cases are believed to develop because of venous bleeding from separation of the margin of the placenta. The hematoma collects preferentially beneath the chorion because the chorion is more easily separated from the myometrium than is the placenta. Patients may be asymptomatic if the hematoma remains confined or may present with vaginal bleeding if the hematoma leaks through the cervix. In most patients, a subchorionic hematoma is an innocent finding; however, an increased rate of spontaneous abortion has been reported in some series associated with large hematomas (>60 mL), advanced maternal age (>35 y), and early gestational age (<8 wk).

The US appearance of the hemorrhage varies with age. Acute bleeding is anechoic to hypoechoic. With clotting, it becomes hyperechoic and heterogeneous. With lysis, the hematoma reverts to being hypoechoic to anechoic.

Implantation Bleeding is a nonspecific term that refers to small collections of blood at the site of attachment of the chorion to the endometrium. These are in essence small areas of subchorionic bleeding that occur early in pregnancy. Sonographic follow-up is warranted to assess for progression.

Gestational Trophoblastic Disease

Gestational trophoblastic disease is a group of neoplasms that range from benign to highly malignant (22,23). All are derived from abnormal placental tissues and occur as sequelae to pregnancy. Both benign and malignant tumors produce human chorionic go-

nadotropin. Marked elevation of β-hCG levels is characteristic and serial measurement is a sensitive and reliable indicator of tumor activity. Gestational trophoblastic disease complicates about one in 1000–2000 pregnancies in the United States but has a much higher incidence in the Far East and in Latin America.

Hydatidiform Mole is the most common (80%) and most benign form of the disease but maintains a potential for malignant sequelae. The placenta demonstrates edema and proliferation of trophoblasts. The villi become swollen and vesicular, resembling a bunch of grapes. Patients present with hyperemesis, pregnancy-induced hypertension, or vaginal bleeding. The uterus may be enlarged (50%), normal (35%), or small (15%) for dates. Two types of hydatidiform mole exist. *Complete mole* (70%) involves the entire placenta, lacks a fetus, and is diploid in karyotype. *Partial mole* (30%) involves only a portion of the placenta, is usually associated with a fetus, and is triploid in karyotype (due to fertilization of an ovum by two sperm). This condition is lethal to the fetus. Rarely, a normal fetus may coexist with a complete mole in a twin pregnancy. Prognosis for the fetus in these cases is grim because of maternal complications of the mole.

US in complete mole classically demonstrates the uterus to be filled with innumerable tiny cysts, often described as a "snowstorm" appearance because of the multiple echogenic foci (Fig. 38.9). Most vesicles are 1–2 mm in size but range up to 30-mm size. Partial mole demonstrates changes in only a portion of the placenta. The associated fetus usually has multiple anomalies. Early in the first trimester, the classic appearance may not be evident. Molar pregnancy may appear as an ane-

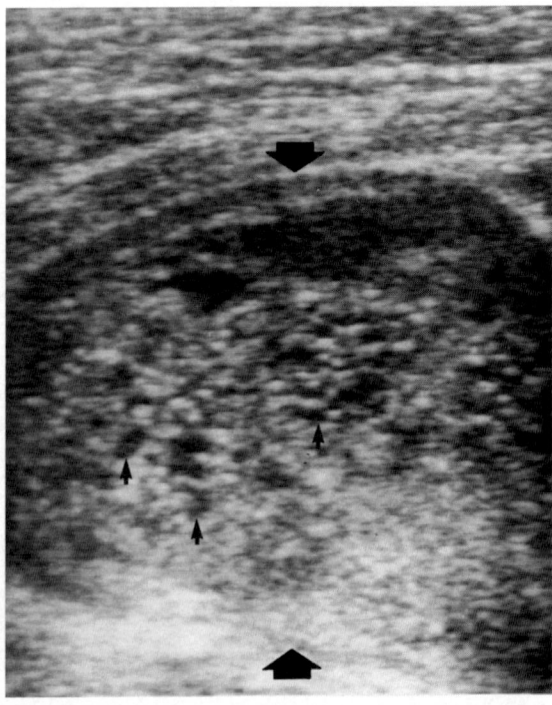

Figure 38.9. Hydatidiform Mole. The uterus (between *large arrowheads*) is filled with echogenic material interspersed with numerous tiny cysts (*small arrows*), representing swollen chorionic villi.

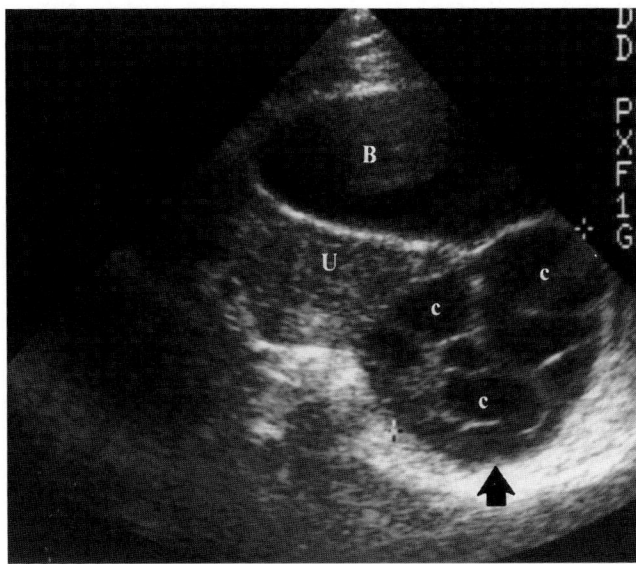

Figure 38.10. Theca Lutein Cysts. Transabdominal image in a transverse plane demonstrates the left ovary (*arrow*) to be greatly enlarged by numerous cysts (*c*) in this patient with persistent gestational trophoblastic disease. The uterus (*U*) is normal in size. *B*, bladder.

choic fluid collection that mimics anembryonic pregnancy or appears echogenic and solid. Transvaginal US helps to demonstrate the characteristic vesicles. Theca lutein cysts are seen as large, septated, bilateral cysts massively enlarging the ovaries in up to 50% of cases (Fig. 38.10). Theca lutein cysts result from ovarian hyperstimulation resulting from high circulating levels of β-hCG.

Invasive Mole (chorioadenoma destruens) refers to invasion of molar tissue into, but usually not beyond, the myometrium. It is seen in about 10% of patients, usually evident after treatment for hydatidiform mole.

Choriocarcinoma is a highly aggressive malignancy that forms only trophoblasts without any villous structure. Choriocarcinoma is locally invasive, spreads into the myometrium and parametrium, and hematogenously metastasizes to any site in the body. The β-hCG levels that rise or plateau in the 8–10 weeks following evacuation of molar pregnancy suggest invasive or metastatic gestational trophoblastic disease.

US is relatively insensitive in demonstrating a locally invasive mole. Nodules in the myometrium are suggestive, but the sonographic appearance overlaps that of degenerating fibroids and ovarian dysgerminomas. CT and MR demonstrate uterine enlargement, focal myometrial masses, dilated vessels, and areas of hemorrhage and necrosis within highly vascular tumor. Metastases may be found in any organ.

FETAL MEASUREMENTS AND GROWTH

Dating the pregnancy and determining the appropriateness of fetal growth are essential to obstetric care. Clinical dating is based on history of the mother's last menstrual period (LMP) and bimanual assessment of uterine size. Sonographic dating is based on measurements of the gestational sac and the embryo or fetus. Serial measurements of fetal parameters are used to document growth. By convention, pregnancies are dated from the first day of the LMP. The terms *gestational age* (GA), which is the clinical standard, and *menstrual age* are usually considered to be synonymous terms and are based on the average 28-day menstrual cycle. Conception is assumed to occur 14 days following the LMP. Term is 40 weeks, with an acceptable range of 37–42 weeks.

Gestational Sac Size is used in the first trimester to estimate GA when no embryo is visualized. The gestational sac diameter is measured in three orthogonal planes, and the results are averaged. The MSD is accurate to within approximately 1 week's menstrual age.

Crown–Rump Length (CRL) is measured from the top of the head to the bottom of the torso of the visualized embryo or fetus (Fig. 38.7B). The CRL is useful until about 10–12 weeks' GA, when other fetal measurements become more accurate. Charts provide GA estimations accurate to approximately 0.5 week's menstrual age.

Biparietal Diameter (BPD) is measured on an axial image of the fetal head at the level of the third ventricle and thalamus (Fig. 38.11). By convention, the measurement is made from the outer table of the near cranium to the inner table of the far cranium. The measurement is affected by head shape and provides an inaccurate estimate of GA if significant dolichocephaly (elongated skull) or brachycephaly (round skull) is present.

Head Circumference (HC) is the outer perimeter of the fetal cranium measured in the same plane as the BPD. The HC measurement is relatively independent of head shape.

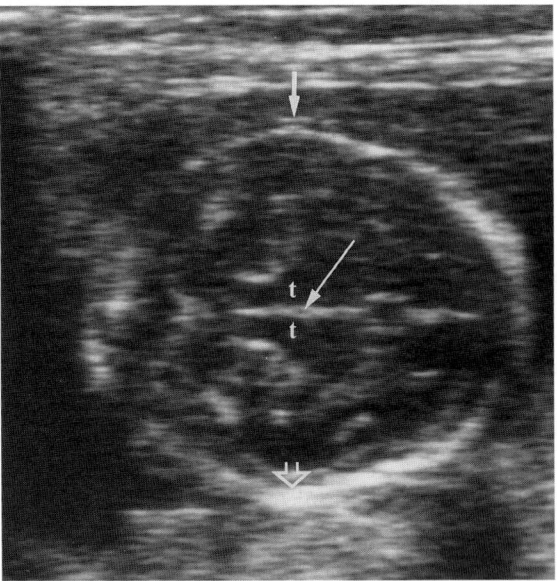

Figure 38.11. Transthalamic (BPD/HC) Plane. Axial image of the fetal cranium demonstrates the paired thalami (*t*) on either side of the midline third ventricle (*long arrow*). The BPD is measured in this plane from the outer surface of the near cranium (*closed arrow*) to the inner surface of the far cranium (*open arrow*). The head circumference is measured in this same plane.

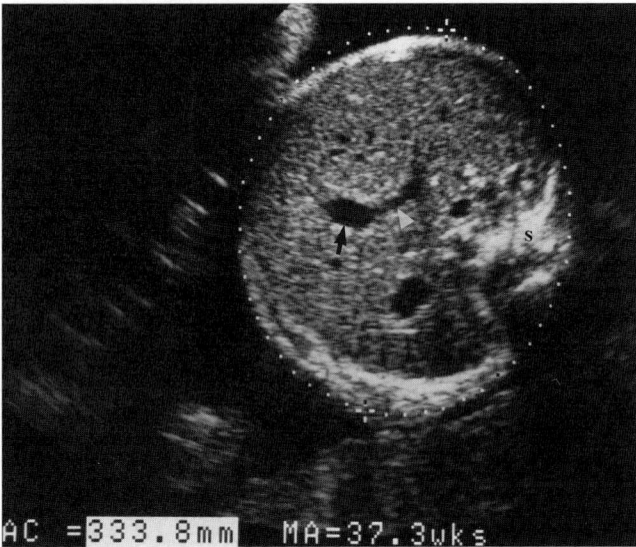

AC =333.8mm   MA=37.3wks

Figure 38.12. Abdominal Circumference. The correct plane of measurement of the abdominal circumference is an axial plane showing a round abdomen at the level of the umbilical vein (*black arrow*) junction with the left portal vein (*white arrowhead*). The umbilical vein appears oval and is seen in the midline at about one-third the anteroposterior diameter of the abdomen. The spine (*s*) casts an acoustic shadow.

Abdominal Circumference (AC) is the outer perimeter of the fetal abdomen measured on an axial plane image at the level of the intrahepatic portion of the umbilical vein (Fig. 38.12).

Femur Length (FL) is the measurement of the ossified portion of the femoral diaphysis. The entire femur must be imaged, and the femoral shaft must be centered in the beam so that it casts an acoustic shadow.

Gestational age estimates are most accurate in early pregnancy and become progressively less accurate as the pregnancy advances. The composite age, calculated by averaging the GA estimates of multiple parameters, is more accurate than any single parameter. Fetal anomalies may make individual parameters inaccurate for estimation of GA. Body parts with structural anomalies should be excluded from the composite GA estimation. The composite of BPD, HC, AC, and FL measurements predicts GA accurate to about 1.2 weeks at 12–18 weeks, but the composite age is accurate to only about 3.1 weeks at 36–42 weeks. Gestational age is assigned at the time of the first US and is not changed thereafter. All subsequent US examinations are compared with the first examination to assess fetal growth.

Intrauterine Growth Retardation

Fetuses with impaired intrauterine growth retardation (IUGR) have an increased risk of intrauterine demise and a perinatal mortality four to eight times greater than normal-sized fetuses. Half the survivors have significant morbidity, including intrapartum fetal distress, hypoglycemia, hypocalcemia, meconium aspiration pneumonia, impaired immune function, retarded neurologic development, and learning disabilities (24). A fetus or newborn is

considered *small for gestational age* if its weight is below the 10th percentile for GA. This definition will encompass normal infants who are constitutionally small and infants with IUGR who are pathologically small. The challenge is to separate the growth-restricted fetuses from those who are normal. Impaired growth may be caused by factors that are intrinsic to the fetus or related to a hostile fetal environment (Table 38.5). Fetuses with intrinsic insults have fixed defects and will not benefit from early delivery. The pattern of growth impairment tends to occur early in the second trimester and tends to be *symmetrical* in that the head, abdomen, and femur are all proportionally small. Fetuses exposed to an extrinsically impaired growth environment will usually benefit from therapy that commonly includes early delivery. Growth impairment occurs in the late second and third trimesters and tends to be *asymmetrical* in that the fetal abdomen is disproportionally small relative to the head and femur. The AC is small because of diminished glycogen stores in the fetal liver and decreased subcutaneous fat.

Many US criteria have been proposed to diagnose IUGR, but none individually is highly accurate. A multiparameter approach using estimated fetal weight (EFW), amniotic fluid volume, and the presence or absence of maternal hypertension has the greatest accuracy for diagnosis (24). The first step in diagnosis is to establish an accurate GA. An early US provides assignment of GA, which should not be changed on subsequent examinations. When the first US is obtained in the third trimester, GA is assigned on the basis of BPD, HC, and FL measurements, recognizing the increasing imprecision of GA estimations in the third trimester. Estimated fetal weight is determined from established charts by measurement of AC and BPD, or AC and FL. The error range of these weight predictions is large: 15–18% for 95% of cases and even greater for 5% of cases. IUGR is diagnosed confidently when the EFW is below the 6th percentile for GA and is excluded when the EFW is above the 20th percentile for GA. When the EFW is between the 6th and 20th percentile, IUGR is diagnosed if oligohydramnios or maternal hypertension is present, and it is likely not present if the amniotic fluid volume is normal or elevated and the mother is normotensive. US follow-up of fetuses with IUGR should be performed weekly or biweekly and include measurement of growth parameters, assessment of amniotic fluid volume, biophysical profile score, and spectral Doppler. Normal fetal weight

Table 38.5. Causes of Intrauterine Growth Retardation

Intrinsic causes
   Chromosome abnormalities (trisomy, triploidy)
   Intrauterine infection (rubella, CMV, toxoplasmosis)
   Structural abnormalities (congenital heart disease)
   Teratogen exposure
Extrinsic causes
   Primary placental insufficiency
   Maternal hypertension
   Chronic maternal diseases (anemia, renal failure)
   Maternal malnutrition
   Maternal smoking, alcohol, and drug abuse
   Multiple gestation

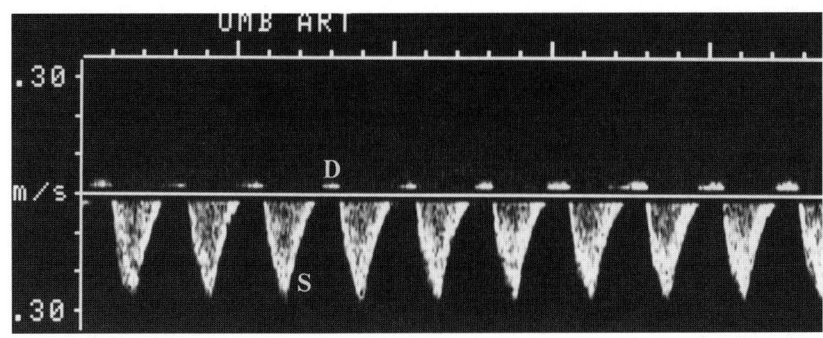

Figure 38.13. Umbilical Artery Doppler. Spectral Doppler tracing from an umbilical artery shows a high vascular resistance pattern with flow toward the placenta during systole (*S*) and reversal of blood flow direction in diastole (*D*). This finding is highly indicative of severe fetal distress. The fetus died 4 days after this examination.

gain in the third trimester is 100–200 g/wk. An amniotic fluid index of 5 cm or less is strongly predictive of poor outcome (25).

Biophysical Profile is a test to identify compromised fetuses. Four parameters assess for acute hypoxia: reactive fetal heart rate (nonstress test), respiratory activity, gross motor movements, and fetal tone. One parameter evaluates chronic hypoxia, the amniotic fluid volume. A variety of different techniques are used for assessment and scoring (26). A score of 2 is given for a normal response, and 0 is given for an abnormal response. The fetus is at extreme risk for fetal demise within 1 week with a score of 0 or 2, and it is at no immediate risk with a score of 8 or 10.

Umbilical Cord Doppler US is not accurate in the diagnosis of IUGR but is valuable for monitoring the pregnancy and detecting fetal compromise (24,25). Spectral Doppler tracings are obtained from the umbilical artery in a free-floating loop of umbilical cord. A systolic-to-diastolic ratio (see chapter 40) of 4.0 or greater, or the absence of forward flow in diastole, is strongly predictive of severe fetal compromise. Reversal of flow in diastole is a particularly ominous finding indicative of high risk for fetal demise within 1–7 days if the fetus is left in utero (Fig. 38.13).

Fetal Macrosomia

Fetal macrosomia is defined as estimated fetal weight above the 90th percentile for GA or a fetal weight above 4000 g. Risk factors include maternal diabetes, maternal obesity, previous history of macrosomic infant, and excessive weight gain during pregnancy. Complications of macrosomia are manifest at delivery and include shoulder dystocia, traumatic delivery, fractures, brachial plexus injury, perinatal asphyxia, neonatal hypoglycemia, and meconium aspiration.

THE FETAL ENVIRONMENT

Uterus and Adnexa in Pregnancy

Uterine Leiomyomas are the most common solid pelvic masses encountered during pregnancy (27). Fibroids commonly enlarge and undergo cystic degeneration as the pregnancy advances. They are associated with bleeding, premature uterine contractions, malpresentation, and obstruction during labor. Leiomyomas must be differentiated from uterine contractions.

Contractions are transient, although they may persist up to an hour. They typically appear homogeneous and isoechoic with the myometrium. They bulge the inner, but generally not the outer, margin of the uterine wall. Leiomyomas are persistent, more heterogeneous, may have calcifications, and typically bulge the outer margin of the uterine wall. Doppler US demonstrates splaying of myometrial vessels around leiomyomas but no vessel displacement in areas of myometrial contraction (28).

Corpus Luteal Cysts are the most common cystic pelvic masses found in pregnancy. Internal hemorrhage causes enlargement up to 10–15 cm size, internal echoes, and septations. Most of these cysts regress by 16–18 weeks' GA. Differential diagnosis includes benign cystic teratoma, cystadenoma, hydrosalpinx, and para-ovarian cyst.

Theca Lutein Cysts form due to an exaggerated corpus luteum response to high levels of hCG. They appear as bilateral multicystic enlargement of the ovaries (Fig. 38.10). They occur most commonly with gestational trophoblastic disease, pregnancy with more than one fetus, and the use of ovulation-inducing drugs.

Cervical Incompetence may be congenital or result from cervical lacerations, excessive cervical dilation, or therapeutic abortion. The incompetent cervix is incapable of retaining a pregnancy to term. Preterm delivery is the single most common cause of a poor neonatal outcome. An obstetric history of recurrent loss of pregnancy in the second trimester establishes the diagnosis. US is used to measure and follow cervical length and appearance (Fig. 38.14). Scans are best performed transvaginally or translabially from the introitus with the bladder empty (29). A full urinary bladder compresses the lower uterus and falsely elongates the length of the cervix. The normal cervical length is 2.5–4 cm throughout gestation. Cervical length is measured in sagittal plane between the internal os marked by a V-shaped notch and the external os marked by a triangular echodensity. The endocervical canal is seen as a thin hypoechoic or hyperechoic line. The relative risk of preterm delivery increases as cervical length decreases, with the greatest risk for cervical lengths of less than 3.0 cm (30). Cervical dilation is measured between the anterior and posterior surface of the cervical canal. Dilation of the cervical canal > 8 mm is indicative of cervical incompetence. Membranes may be seen bulging into the cervical canal. Sutures associated with cervical cerclage are seen on US as echogenic linear structures with acoustic shadowing.

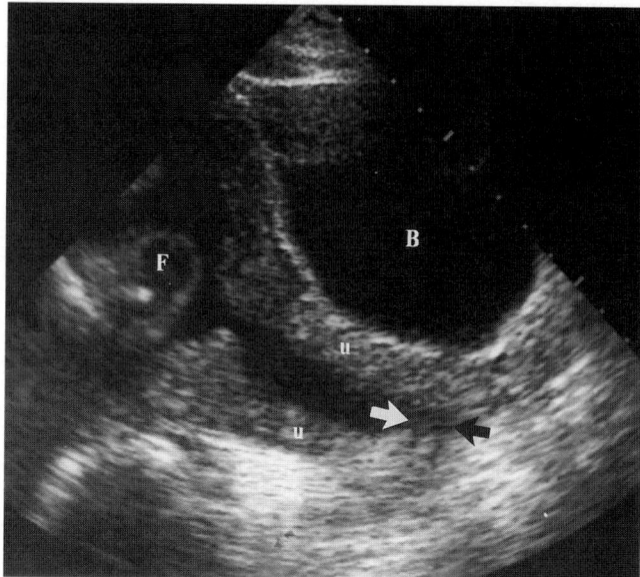

Figure 38.14. Cervical Incompetence. The cervix, measured between the internal os (*white arrow*) and the external os (*black arrow*), is shortened to 9 mm in this patient with a history of multiple spontaneous abortions in the second trimester. An overdistended bladder (*B*) may compress the anterior and posterior walls of the lower uterine segment (*u*) together and mimic the cervix. The fetus (*F*) was 23 weeks' GA.

Placenta and Membranes

Normal Placenta is first apparent on US at about 8 weeks as a focal thickening at the periphery of the gestational sac (31). The disclike shape of the placenta becomes evident by 12 weeks, and by 18 weeks the placenta is finely granular and homogeneous with a smooth covering chorionic membrane along its fetal surface. The retroplacental complex of decidual and myometrial veins forms a prominent sonographic landmark (Fig. 38.15). As the gestation advances, the placenta becomes more heterogeneous, with focal echolucencies owing to venous lakes and areas of fibrin deposition. Septations become prominent sonographic features throughout the placenta and cause undulations of the placental surface. Calcifications occur along the septations and are dispersed randomly throughout the placenta. These are normal changes of aging and should not be interpreted as indicators of disease. The normal placenta has a maximum thickness of 4 cm and a minimal thickness of 1 cm (32). Thick placentas are associated with maternal diabetes, maternal anemia, hydrops from immune and nonimmune causes, and chronic uterine infections. Thin placentas are associated with pre-eclampsia, placental insufficiency, IUGR, and trisomy 13 and 18.

Placenta Previa is present when part or all of the placenta covers the internal cervical os (Fig. 38.16). Placenta previa is present at term in 0.3–0.6% of live births. Placenta previa is suggested by US in as many as 45% of pregnancies examined in the first and second trimesters. These cases are the result of low implantation of the placenta and filling of the bladder, distorting the lower uterine segment and cervix. As the pregnancy

progresses, the muscular portion of the cervix elongates and increases the distance from the margin of the placenta to the cervical os. Risk factors for placenta previa include previous cesarean section, previous placenta previa, lower uterine surgical scars, and multiple previous pregnancies. Patients usually present with painless vaginal bleeding in the third trimester. Bleeding is initiated by the effacement of the cervix and dilation of the cervical os, which disrupts the vascular bed of the placenta. US confirmation of placenta previa should be performed transperineally, with the bladder empty to allow optimal identification of both the edge of the placenta and the internal os of the cervix (33). When the placenta covers the entire cervical os, the previa is complete. When an edge of the placenta covers a portion of the cervical os, the previa is partial or marginal.

Placental Abruption is defined as the premature separation of a normally positioned placenta from the myometrium (34). Separation is associated with hemorrhage from the maternal vessels at the base of the placenta. Abruption complicates 0.5–1.3% of pregnancies and is implicated in 15–25% of perinatal deaths. Risk factors include maternal hypertension, smoking, cocaine abuse, and previous history of abruption. *Subchorionic hemorrhage* (marginal abruption) occurs because of a separation at the edge of the placenta (see Fig. 38.8). Bleeding is usually venous and preferentially accumulates beneath the chorionic membrane adjacent to the placenta. *Retroplacental hemorrhage* occurs with more central abruption. Bleeding is usually arterial and accumulates beneath the placenta as an anechoic or mixed hypoechoic mass (Fig. 38.17). The hemorrhage may be isoechoic and difficult to differentiate from the

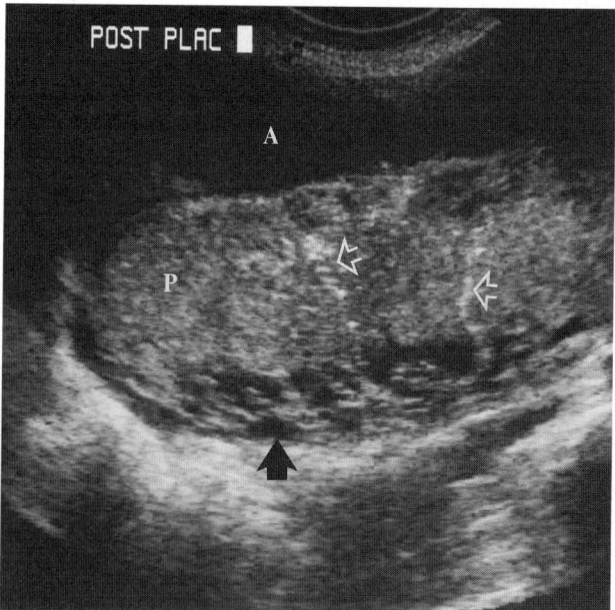

Figure 38.15. Normal Placenta. A transabdominal scan at 33 weeks' GA demonstrates a normal placenta (*P*) with calcified septations (*open arrows*). The retroplacental complex of veins (*black arrow*) appears as a network of tubular lucencies beneath the placenta. *A*, amniotic cavity.

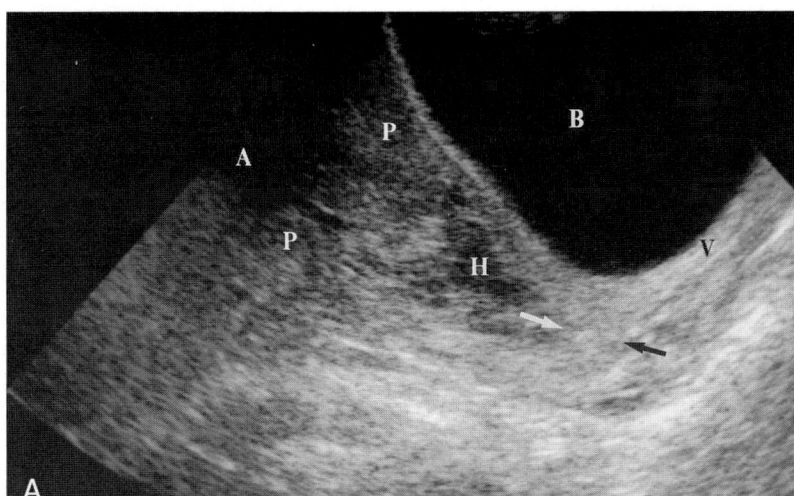

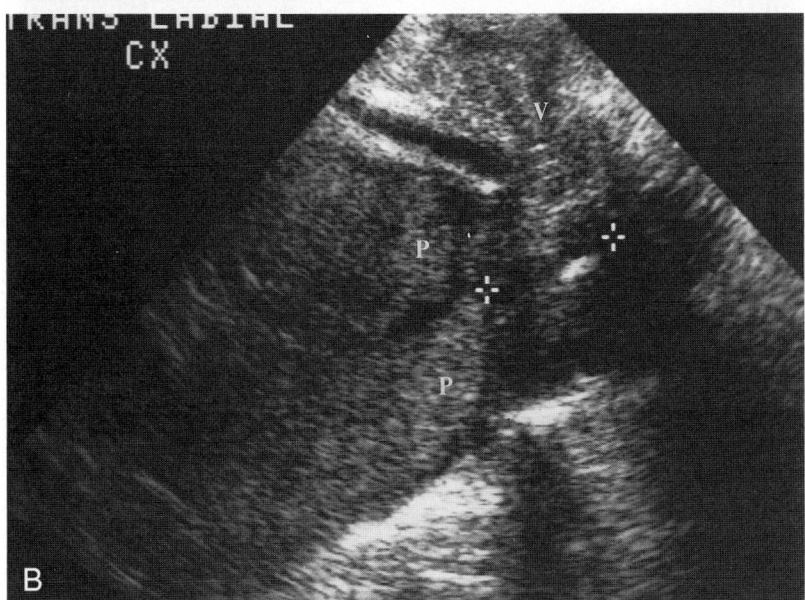

Figure 38.16. Placenta Previa. A. Transabdominal US shows a shortened cervix (between *arrows*) measuring 18 mm. The placenta (*P*) covers the internal os (*white arrow*). A small hematoma (*H*) is seen between the placenta and the cervix. *A,* amniotic cavity; *B,* bladder; *V,* vagina. **B.** Translabial US, in a different patient, shows complete placenta previa (*P*). On translabial scanning, US beam is parallel to the vagina (*V*) and perpendicular to the cervix (between *cursors*), making the cervix easier to visualize.

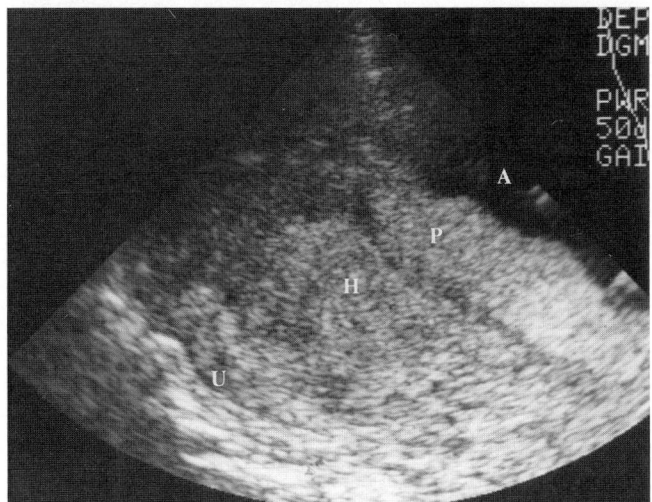

Figure 38.17. Placental Abruption. The placenta (*P*) is displaced away from the wall of the uterus (*U*) by an echogenic hematoma (*H*). Note the absence of visualization of the retroplacental complex of veins. *A,* amniotic cavity.

placental tissue. The diagnosis is suggested by demonstrating disruption of the retroplacental complex of veins and thickening of the placenta (>4 cm).

Placenta Accreta is an abnormal adherence of the placenta to the uterine wall. Invasion of the uterine wall by the placenta is referred to as *placenta increta* and penetration of the uterine wall is *placenta percreta*. The decidua basalis and retroplacental complex of veins are completely or partially absent. Failure of the abnormally adherent placenta to separate completely from the myometrium during labor results in hemorrhage. Risk factors include prior cesarean section, prior placenta accreta, and prior placenta previa. Scarring of the uterus results in the defective formation of decidua. US findings include absence of vascular channels in the retroplacental region, increased echogenicity of tissues deep to the placenta, and visualization of retroplacental vessels within the bladder lumen (35). Placenta previa is usually also present.

Chorioangioma is a benign vascular placental mass supplied by the fetal circulation. It appears on US as a solid hypoechoic, sometimes septated, mass in the placenta, usually close to the chorionic surface. Doppler demonstration of arterial waveforms at the fetal heart rate in vessels supplying the tumor is diagnostic. Vascular shunting may cause fetal high-output cardiac failure and fetal hydrops.

Umbilical Cord. The normal umbilical cord consists of two arteries and one vein surrounded by Wharton's jelly (36). It has a normal diameter of 1–2 cm. A single-artery umbilical cord is found in about 1% of pregnancies and has a 10–20% association with congenital malformations. Associated anomalies include cardiac, urinary tract, and central nervous system malformations, omphalocele, trisomy 13, and trisomy 18 (37). Masses in the umbilical cord include allantoic cysts, hematomas, hemangiomas, and teratomas.

Placental Membranes consist of an outer layer (*chorion*) and an inner layer (*amnion*). These membranes commonly remain separated by a layer of fluid (Fig. 38.18) until 14–16 weeks' GA when the two membranes fuse. The amnion is visualized on US as a thin membrane floating in fluid. Occasional persistence of chorioamniotic separation into the third trimester is believed to be of no clinical significance.

Amniotic Band Syndrome is caused by the disruption of the amnion, enabling the fetus to enter the chorionic cavity (38). The fetus becomes entangled in fibrous bands that cross the chorionic cavity (Fig. 38.19). Entrapment of fetal parts results in amputation deformities that range from mild to incompatible with life. Typical abnormalities include asymmetrical absence of the cranium resembling anencephaly, encephaloceles, gastroschisis and truncal defects, spinal deformities, and extremity amputations. The amniotic bands trapping the fetus may be visualized.

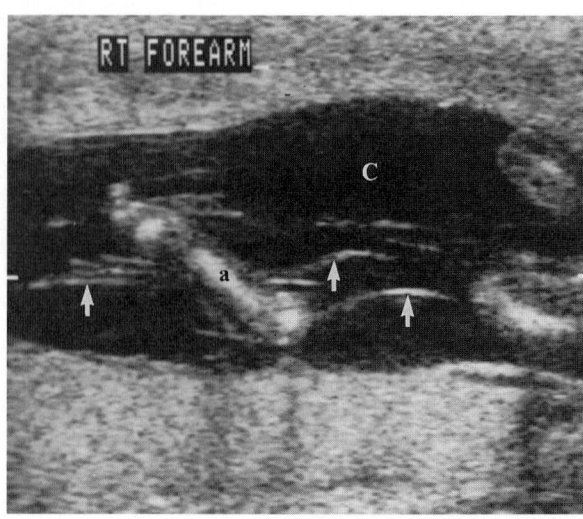

Figure 38.19. Amniotic Band Syndrome. The forearm (*a*) of a fetus at 15 weeks' GA is entangled within fibrous bands (*arrows*) that extend across the chorionic cavity (*C*).

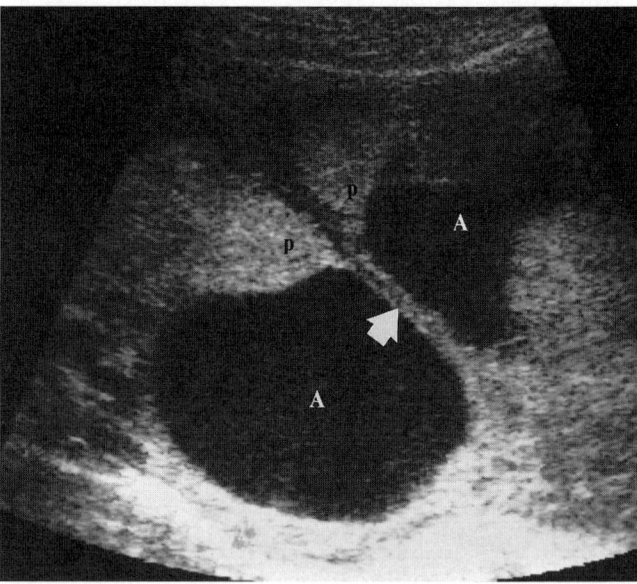

Figure 38.20. Amniotic Sheet. A fibrous band covered by chorioamniotic membranes (*arrow*) extends from the placenta (*p*) across the amniotic cavity (*A*). The uterine synechia forms a shelf-like structure that partially compartmentalizes the uterine cavity. The fetus has free access to both compartments.

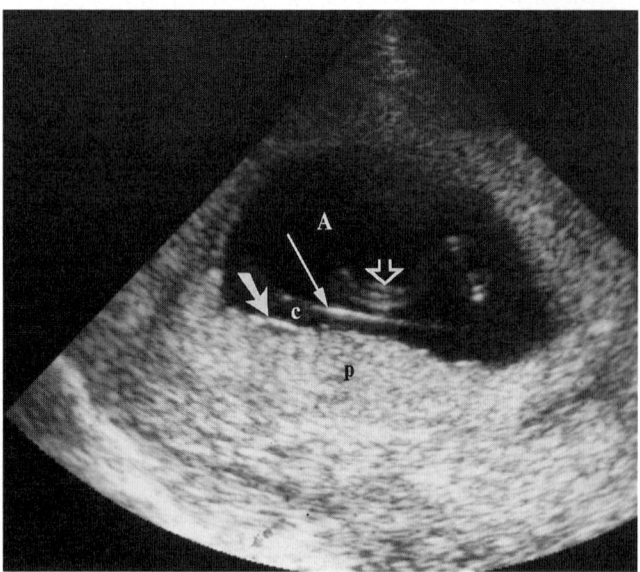

Figure 38.18. Normal Chorioamniotic Separation. The thin amniotic membrane (*long arrow*) is separated from the chorionic membrane (*short arrow*) covering the placenta (*p*) by fluid within the chorionic sac (*c*). The umbilical cord (*open arrow*) floats in the fluid of the amniotic sac (*A*).

Amniotic Sheets (uterine synechia) are membranous structures that project into the uterine cavity (39,40). They demonstrate a characteristic appearance with a bulbous-free edge, thinner midportion, and a thickened base (Fig. 38.20). The fetus is able to move freely about the sheet of tissue. No fetal deformities are associated with this condition, which makes it distinct from the amniotic band syndrome. The amniotic sheets arise from folding of the chorioamniotic membranes over an intrauterine adhesion. Patients at increased risk for amniotic sheets include those with prior history of dilation and curettage or therapeutic abortion. An increased rate of cesarean section because fetal malpresentation has been reported.

Amniotic Fluid

Normal Amniotic Fluid is essentially a dialysate of maternal serum in early pregnancy. As the pregnancy advances, fetal urine becomes the major source of amniotic fluid. The composition of amniotic fluid is dynamic, with turnover of the entire volume every 3 hours. The fetus swallows amniotic fluid at a rate up to 450 mL per 24 hours. Transudate from the fetal lungs contribute a small volume. Water crosses placental membranes in response to osmotic gradients. Amniotic fluid is essential in promoting normal development and maturation of the fetal lungs. Suspended particles in amniotic fluid visualized by US are attributable to normal vernix (desquamated fetal skin), blood, or meconium.

Amniotic Fluid Index is a rough US measurement of amniotic fluid volume obtained by measuring the deepest pockets of four quadrants of the uterus and adding these values together. Pockets are selected that do not include fetal parts or umbilical cord. Normal values are 5–20 cm.

Polyhydramnios is an excessive amount of amniotic fluid, traditionally defined as greater than 2 L of fluid at delivery. US is used to confirm excessive fluid any time in pregnancy. Because amniotic fluid volume is difficult to measure; the diagnosis is usually made subjectively by visual inspection. The visual proportion of fluid relative to the size of the fetus is greatest early in the second trimester and decreases progressively to term. Polyhydramnios is suggested by large pockets of fluid relative to the age of the pregnancy. An amniotic fluid index greater than 20 cm or a single fluid pocket greater than 8 cm deep is strongly suggestive of polyhydramnios. Another clue is failure of the fetal abdomen to be in contact with both anterior and posterior uterine wall after 24 weeks' GA. Excessive fluid is associated with preterm labor, premature rupture of membranes, and substantial maternal discomfort. About 60% of cases are idiopathic, 15–20% are related to maternal disease (diabetes mellitus, preeclampsia, anemia, obesity), and 20–25% are associated with fetal anomalies. About half of all fetuses with anomalies will have polyhydramnios. Gross polyhydramnios has a higher association with fetal anomalies than mild polyhydramnios. Associated anomalies include anencephaly, encephalocele, gastrointestinal obstructions, abdominal wall defects, achondroplasia, and hydrops (isoimmunization).

Oligohydramnios refers to an abnormally low amniotic fluid volume. Fluid pockets are small, fetal parts are crowded, fetal surface features such as the face are difficult to visualize, and the amniotic fluid index measures less than 5 cm. Measurement of the largest fluid pocket in the vertical direction of less than 1 cm is indicative of severe oligohydramnios. Causes of oligohydramnios include premature rupture of membranes, IUGR, renal anomalies (lack of urine output), fetal death, eclampsia, and postdate pregnancies. A major complication of severe oligohydramnios is fetal lung immaturity.

Multiple Pregnancy

Twins occur in 1 of every 90 births (41). Morbidity and mortality are significantly increased in twin pregnancy compared with singleton pregnancy. Twins account for 12–13% of all neonatal deaths. Twin morbidity includes prematurity, polyhydramnios, increased incidence of congenital anomalies, discordant growth, and cord accidents. Relative risk is increased if the fetuses share a placenta (monochorionic, 20%) as opposed to each fetus having its own placenta (dichorionic, 80%) (42). Twins that share a single amniotic cavity (monoamniotic) have the highest risk for morbidity, including conjoined twinning and intertwining of the umbilical cords. Visualization of two separate placentas, or determination that the twins are of different sex, is definitive proof of lower risk dichorionic twinning. Unfortunately, about half of dichorionic twins will have a fused placenta. Visualization of a membrane separating the twins confirms diamniotic twins. Monochorionic twins usually have vascular anastomoses at the placental level, making them at risk for twin transfusion syndrome and twin embolization syndrome.

Twin Transfusion Syndrome results from shunting of blood from one twin to the other through vascular connections in the placenta (43). The abnormality ranges in severity from minor discordance in growth to severe IUGR in one twin, with hydropic fluid overload in the other twin. Severe disparity in amniotic fluid volume may be present, with one twin experiencing polyhydramnios while the other twin is virtually anhydramniotic ("a stuck twin"). The mortality rate may be as high as 70%.

Twin Embolization Syndrome is an uncommon complication of the death of one twin in utero (42). Blood products from the dead twin are shunted through placental interconnections to the live twin, resulting in disseminated intravascular coagulopathy and multifocal tissue infarction.

FETAL ANOMALIES

General

Fetal Hydrops refers to the pathologic accumulation of fluid in body cavities and tissues. US demonstrates ascites, pleural and pericardial effusions, and subcutaneous edema (Fig. 38.21). *Immune hydrops* is caused by blood group incompatibility between mother and fetus. Modern treatment, including fetal transfusion, is highly successful. *Nonimmune hydrops* is caused by a host of conditions including cardiac disorders, infections, chromosomal anomalies, twin pregnancy, urinary obstruction, and umbilical cord complications. The cause of many cases is not identified. The prognosis for nonimmune hydrops remains poor.

α-Fetoprotein (AFP) and Triple Marker Screening. AFP is a protein produced by the fetal liver. Concentrations of AFP are highest in the fetal serum, with small amounts present in the amniotic fluid (AF-AFP) and minute amounts detectable in maternal serum (MS-AFP). Open neural tube and other skin defects allow AFP to leak into the amniotic fluid and maternal serum in abnormally large quantities. Routine MS-AFP screen-

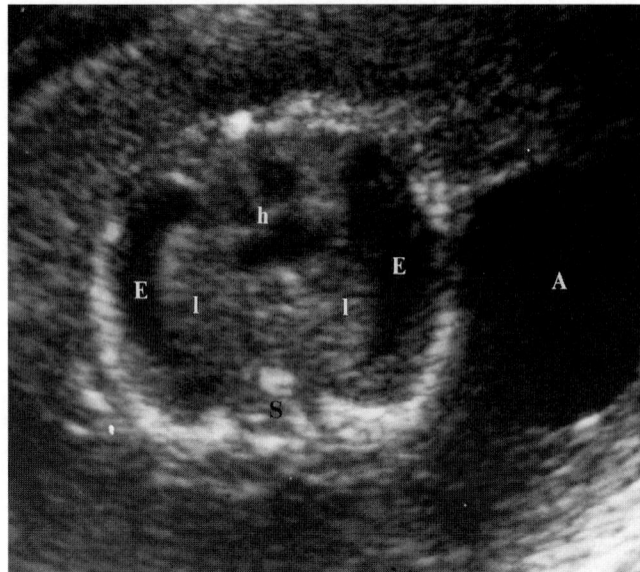

Figure 38.21. Fetal Hydrops. A transverse image through the fetal thorax at the level of the heart (*h*) demonstrates bilateral pleural effusions (*E*) outlining the lungs (*l*). The fetal chest is viewed from above, with the spine (*S*) posterior. This fetus also had ascites. A pocket of amniotic fluid (*A*) is seen adjacent to the right side of the fetus.

Table 38.6. Causes of Elevated MS-AFP

Erroneous gestational dating
Multiple pregnancy
Fetal demise
Neural tube defects
   Anencephaly
   Spina bifida
   Encephaloceles
Abdominal wall defects
   Gastroschesis
   Omphalocele
   Amniotic band syndrome
Cystic hygroma
Placental abnormalities
   Subchorionic hemorrhage
   Chorioangioma
Unexplained—fetus at high risk for:
   IUGR
   Fetal death
   Preterm delivery
   Preeclampsia
   Oligohydramnios

The MS-AFP, or triple marker screening, is performed at 16–18 weeks' GA as determined by menstrual history. The normal values for MS-AFP vary with GA, reaching maximum values at 30–32 weeks' gestation. Patients with abnormal MS-AFP or triple marker screening are routinely referred for US dating, fetal examination, and consideration of amniocentesis for karyotyping. The

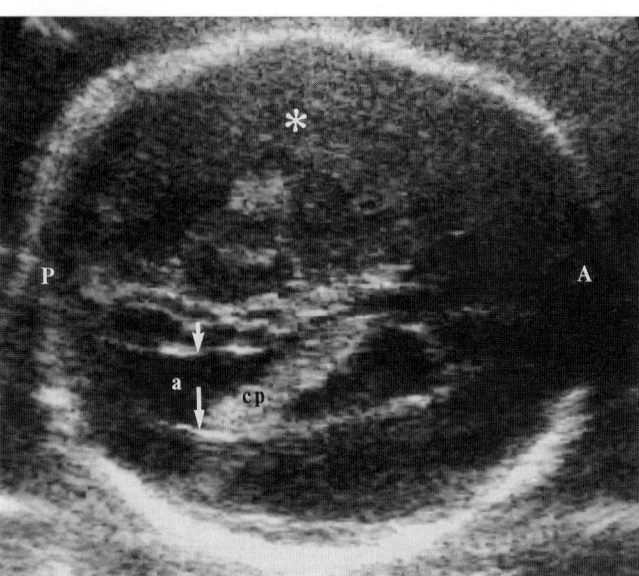

Figure 38.22. Transventricular Plane. The choroid plexus (*cp*) hangs dependently in the atria (*a*) of the lateral ventricle marking the lateral ventricular wall (*long arrow*). The ventricular atrium is measured from its medial wall (*short arrow*) to its lateral wall. The normal ventricular atrium does not exceed 10 mm in width at anytime during pregnancy. The near hemisphere (***) is obscured by reverberation artifact from the near skull. *A*, anterior; *P*, posterior.

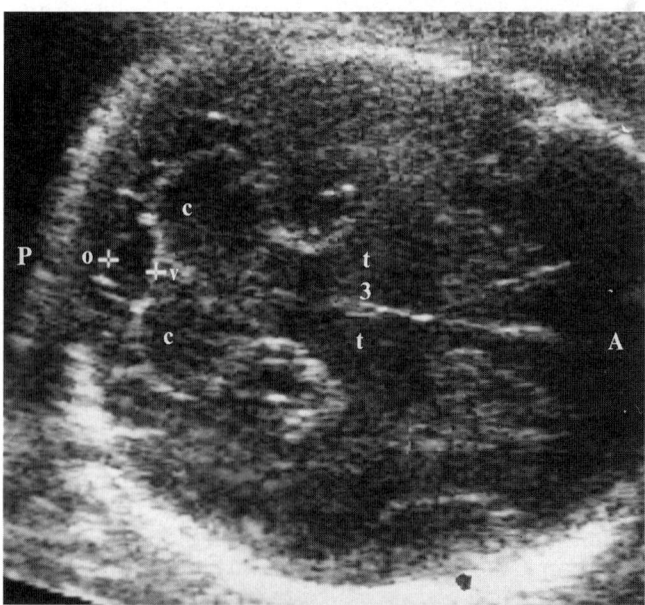

Figure 38.23. Transcerebellar Plane. Landmarks for the transcerebellar plane are the thalami (*t*), third ventricle (*3*), and cerebellar hemispheres (*c*). The cisterna magna (between *cursors* (+)) is measured from the vermis (*v*) to the occiput (*o*). The normal cisterna magna measures 2–11 mm throughout pregnancy. *A*, anterior; *P*, posterior.

ing is performed in Great Britain, California, and elsewhere to aid in detection of neural tube defects and other fetal anomalies. Triple marker screening refers to expanded maternal serum screening programs that have added β-hCG and unconjugated estriol (uE3) determinations to MS-AFP screening. Results are reported as multiples of the median (MOM) values. AFP is considered elevated when *greater than* 2.50 MOM. Low values for the triple marker screen are correlated with maternal age to yield a risk for chromosome abnormalities, especially trisomy 21 and trisomy 18.

Table 38.7. Algorithm for Diagnosis of Congenital Brain Abnormalities

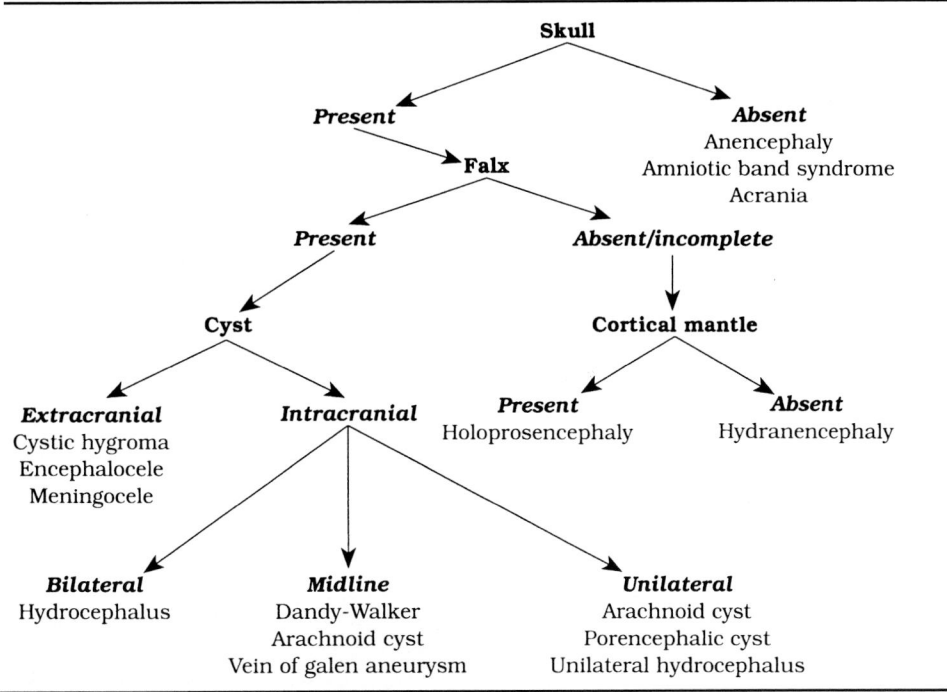

(From Carrasco CR, Stierman ED, Hornsberger HR, Lee TG. An algorithm for prenatal ultrasound diagnosis of congenital CNS abnormalities. J Ultrasound Med 1985;4:163–168.)

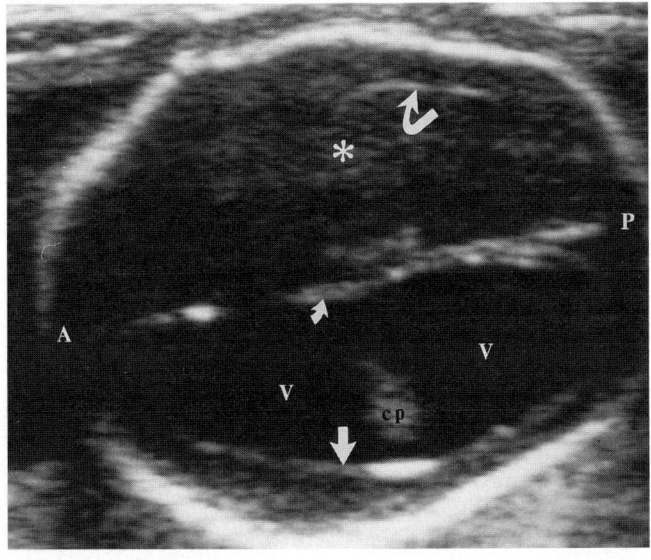

Figure 38.24. Ventriculomegaly. An axial image in the transventricular plane of a fetus with aqueduct stenosis demonstrates massive enlargement of the lateral ventricles (*V*). The choroid plexus (*cp*) dangles dependently from its medial attachment, marking the location of the lateral ventricular wall (*arrow*). The falx (*small curved arrow*) is seen as an echogenic stripe in the midline. The near hemisphere (*) is obscured by reverberation artifact from the near skull, but the lateral ventricular wall (*large curved arrow*) remains evident. *A*, anterior; *P*, posterior.

differential diagnosis for elevated AFP is listed in Table 38.6.

Chromosome Abnormalities may be suspected when multiple or major fetal anomalies are detected by US. Advanced maternal age (>35 y at delivery) or a parent or previous child with aneuploidy or chromosomal translocation anomalies are risk factors for fetal chromosome abnormalities. Fetuses with structural anomalies detected on US have an 11–35% risk of associated chromosome abnormality. Fetal conditions with significant high risk of chromosome abnormality include holoprosencephaly, Dandy-Walker syndrome, cystic hygroma, cardiac malformations, omphalocele, duodenal atresia, facial anomalies, and early symmetric IUGR. Chromosome analysis is performed on samples obtained by amniocentesis or chorionic villous sampling.

Trisomy 21, Down's syndrome, is the most common chromosome abnormality, occurring in 1 of 660 births (44). Although women older than age 35 have a 1 in 250 risk of carrying a fetus with trisomy 21, 80% of fetuses with Down's syndrome are born to younger women. Triple marker serum screening will detect about 60% of affected fetuses. A variety of US findings serve as markers for the condition. Major structural defects found in Down's fetuses include congenital heart disease (endocardial cushion defects), duodenal atresia, and hydrocephalus. Nuchal fold thickening greater than 6 mm in the second trimester is strongly associated. The skinfold is measured from the occipital bone to the external skin surface on the transcerebellar plane view. If two or more of the following findings are present, trisomy 21 is likely: short femur, short humerus, echogenic bowel, mild fetal renal pyelectasis, intracardiac echogenic focus, hypoplastic middle phalanx of 5th finger.

Trisomy 18 is the second most common chromosome anomaly, occurring in 1 of 3000 births. A large number of structural abnormalities may occur, but the most common identified by US are IUGR, complex congenital heart disease, congenital diaphragmatic hernia, omphalocele, neural tube defects, Dandy-Walker complex, clenched hands, and single umbilical artery.

Central Nervous System, Face, and Neck

Anomalies of the CNS occur in 1 of 1000 live births. Survivors are often severely handicapped and require long-term care. Effective US screening for CNS anomalies can be performed by examination of three crucial axial planes through the fetal brain (45). The *transthalamic plane* is used to measure the BPD and HC (see Fig. 38.11). Abnormalities of head shape, microcephaly, macrocephaly, and major structural abnormalities are evident in this plane. The third ventricle varies in appearance from a single echogenic line to a slitlike structure less than 3.5 mm in width (46). The *transventricular plane* is an axial plane at the level of the ventricular atria (Fig. 38.22). The dominant landmark is the echogenic choroid plexus, which normally fills the atrium nearly completely. Measurements of atrial diameter made perpendicular to the walls do not normally exceed 10 mm (47,48). The *transcerebellar plane* is an axial scan in ap-

proximately 10–15° of inclination from the canthomeatal line. The anatomic landmarks include the inferior portion of the third ventricle and the cerebellar hemispheres outlined by fluid in the cisterna magna (Fig. 38.23). The normal cisterna magna measures 2–11 mm in width. A small cisterna magna (<2 mm) suggests a Chiari II malformation, but may also be seen with massive ventriculomegaly. A large cisterna magna (>11 mm) may be a normal variant (mega-cisterna magna) or Dandy-Walker malformation, arachnoid cyst, or cerebellar hypoplasia. When these three planes are anatomically normal, the risk of CNS anomaly is approximately 0.005%. An algorithm for sorting out fetal CNS anomalies is given in Table 38.7 (49).

Ventriculomegaly is an anatomic finding with many causes that can be grouped into the categories of obstructive hydrocephalus (obstruction to flow of cerebrospinal fluid), cerebral atrophy (ex vacuo), and maldevelopment (such as agenesis of the corpus callosum).

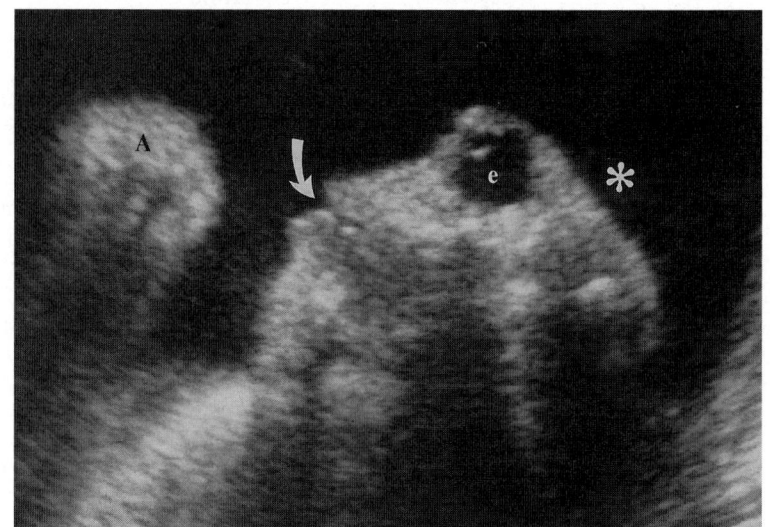

Figure 38.25. Anencephaly. A sagittal image through the head of a fetus demonstrates absence of the cranial vault (*) above the level of the eye (*e*). The mouth and lips are evident (*arrow*). *A*, fetal arm.

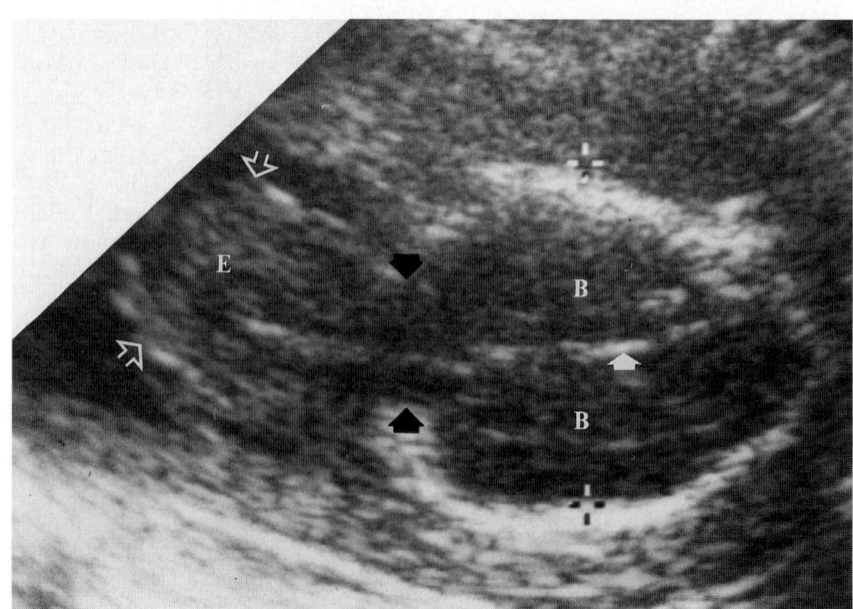

Figure 38.26. Encephalocele. Axial US image through the fetal skull demonstrates herniation of brain tissue (*B*) through a large defect in the skull (*black arrows*), forming an occipital encephalocele (*E*, between *open arrows*). The falx (*white arrow*) is seen as an echogenic midline stripe.

Ventriculomegaly detected in utero carries a poor prognosis. Up to 80% of fetuses with ventriculomegaly have associated anomalies. The US signs of ventriculomegaly include diameter of ventricular atrium >10 mm, separation of choroid plexus from the ventricular wall by >3 mm, and a "dangling choroid" (47,48,50). The choroid plexus hangs dependently in the ventricle and marks the position of the lateral ventricular wall (Fig. 38.24). The most common causes of ventriculomegaly seen in the fetus include Chiari II malformation and aqueductal stenosis.

Anencephaly is the most common neural tube defect. US findings include absence of the cranial vault and cerebral hemispheres above the level of the orbits (Fig. 38.25). The cerebral hemispheres may be replaced by an amorphous neurovascular mass (area cerebrovasculosa) (51,52). The condition is inevitably fatal.

Cephaloceles are brain and/or fluid-filled sacs that protrude through a defect in the bony calvarium (53). They are found in the occipital (75%), frontoethmoid (13%), and parietal (12%) regions. Meningoceles contain only cerebrospinal fluid, whereas encephaloceles contain brain tissue (Fig. 38.26).

Spina Bifida refers to a spectrum of spinal abnormalities resulting from failure of the complete closure of the neural tube. The condition ranges from simple nonfusion of the vertebral arches with intact skin (spina bifida occulta), to protruding sacs containing cerebrospinal fluid, spinal cord, or nerve roots (myelomeningocele), to a totally open spinal defect (myeloschisis). Spina bifida may occur anywhere in the spine but most often occurs in the lumbosacral region. US findings include outward splaying rather than inward convergence of the laminae, defect in the soft tissues overlying the bony abnormality, and a protruding sac containing fluid and often neural tissues (Fig. 38.27) (54,55). The associated functional neuromuscular defect often results in club foot deformities and dislocated hips. Associated cranial abnormalities of the Chiari II malformation provide clues to the presence of the spinal defect. Ventriculomegaly is present in 75% of cases. The "lemon sign" refers to bossing of the frontal bones, causing a lemon-shaped appearance to the head in the axial plane (Fig. 38.28A). The "banana sign" is produced by compression of the cerebellar hemispheres into a banana shape. The cisterna magna is small or obliterated (Fig. 38.28B).

Chiari II Malformations are associated with 95% of myelomeningoceles. The cranial abnormality consists of caudal displacement of the cerebellar tonsils, pons, and medulla. The fourth ventricle is elongated, the posterior fossa is small, and the cisterna magna is obliterated.

Holoprosencephaly refers to a spectrum of disorders characterized by a failure of the prosencephalon to divide and form separate right and left hemispheres and thalami. Associated facial anomalies including hypotelorism, cyclopia, and proboscis are common (Fig. 38.29) (56). Alobar holoprosencephaly is the most severe form and demonstrates absence of the falx and interhemispheric fissure with a single midline ventricle. The semilobar and lobar forms demonstrate greater degrees of midline separation.

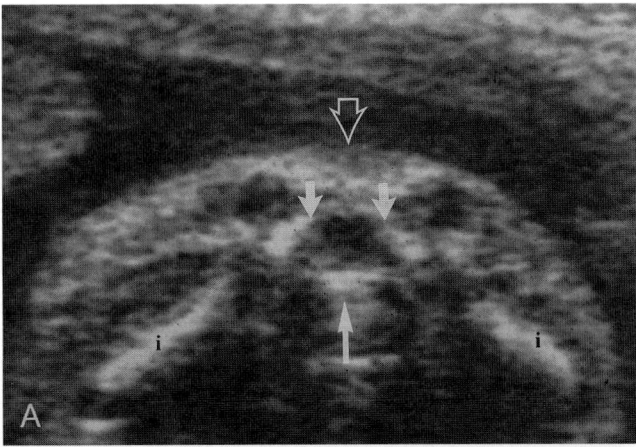

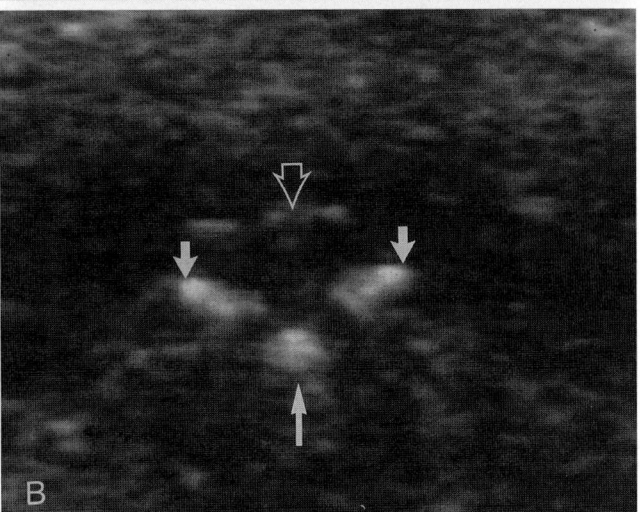

Figure 38.27. Normal Spine and Meningomyelocele. A. Normal spine. Posterior transverse image through a normal fetal spine at the L4–5 level demonstrates the ossified portion of the vertebral body (*long arrow*) anteriorly and the converging ossified portions of the lamina (*short arrows*) posteriorly. The skin overlying the posterior aspect of the vertebra is intact (*open arrow*). *i*, iliac crest. **B.** Meningomyelocele. Posterior transverse image through a spina bifida defect demonstrates the ossified portion of the vertebral body (*long arrow*) anteriorly and the diverging ossified portions of the lamina (*short arrows*) posteriorly. A small fluid-containing sac (*open arrow*) protrudes through the defect.

Hydranencephaly refers to total destruction of the cerebral cortex, believed to be caused by the occlusion of the internal carotid arteries. The cranial vault contains fluid, but no cortical mantle is visible. The falx may be present but is usually incomplete. The brainstem and structures supplied by the vertebral arteries appear normal.

Dandy-Walker Malformation results from the maldevelopment of the roof of the fourth ventricle. The cisterna magna is enlarged and communicates directly with the fourth ventricle through its absent roof. The posterior fossa is enlarged, and the tentorium is elevated (Fig. 38.30). The cerebellar hemispheres are usually hypoplastic. Hydrocephalus is usually present. The condition varies in severity across a broad spectrum. Less severe abnormalities are usually called Dandy-Walker

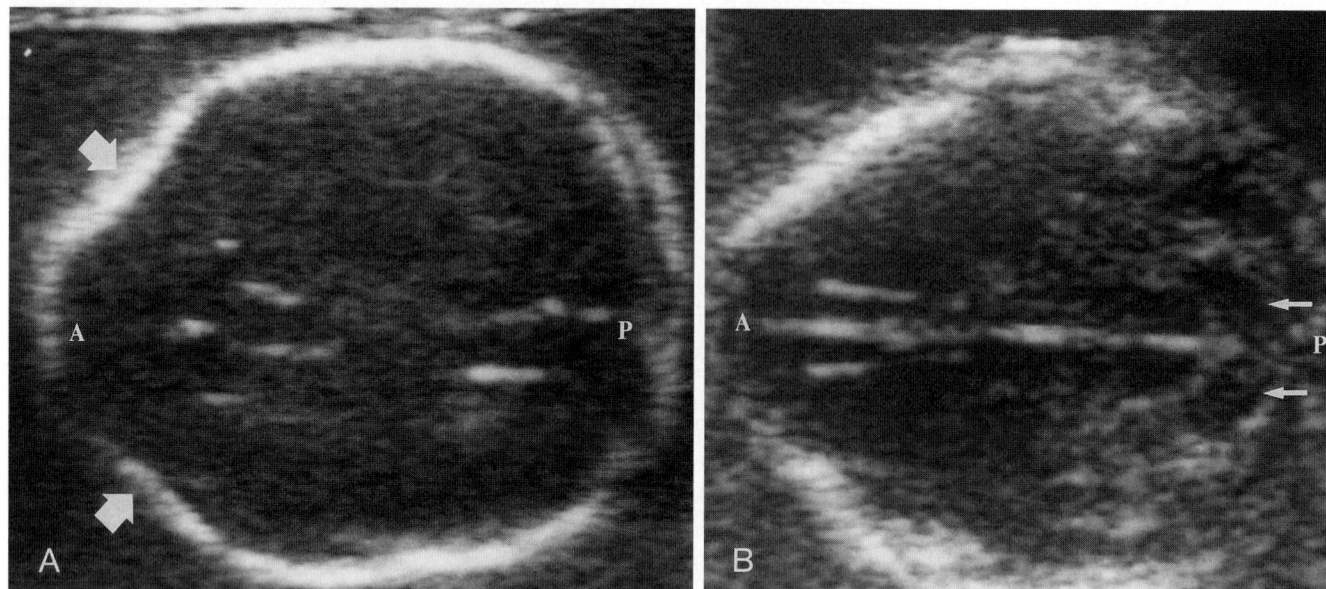

Figure 38.28. Lemon and Banana Signs. A. Lemon sign. Concavity of the frontal bones (*arrows*) causes a "lemon" shape to the fetal skull in axial plane images. This appearance suggests a possible spina bifida defect. **B.** Banana sign. Compression of the cerebellar hemispheres associated with downward herniation of the brainstem and the Chiari II malformation results in an hypoechoic "banana" (*arrows*) in the posterior aspect of the fetal skull in axial plane. *A*, anterior; *P*, posterior.

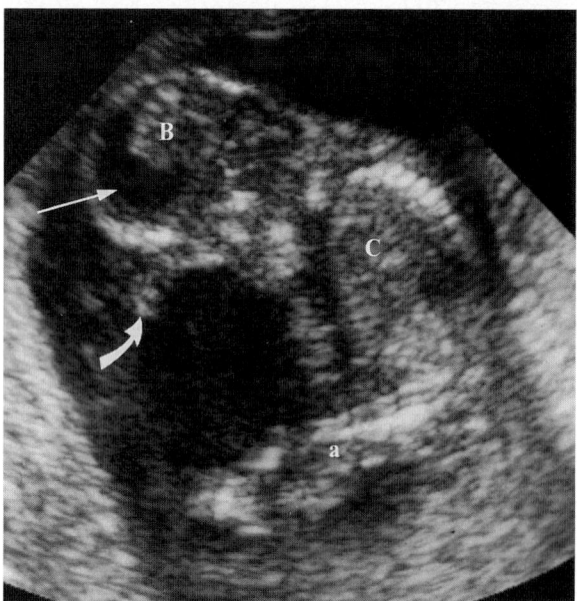

Figure 38.29. Holoprosencephaly. Sagittal plane transvaginal image of a 12-week fetus demonstrates a proboscis (*curved arrow*) protruding from the midface and the enlarged fused ventricles (*straight arrow*) of alobar holoprosencephaly. *B*, brain; *C*, chest; *a*, arm.

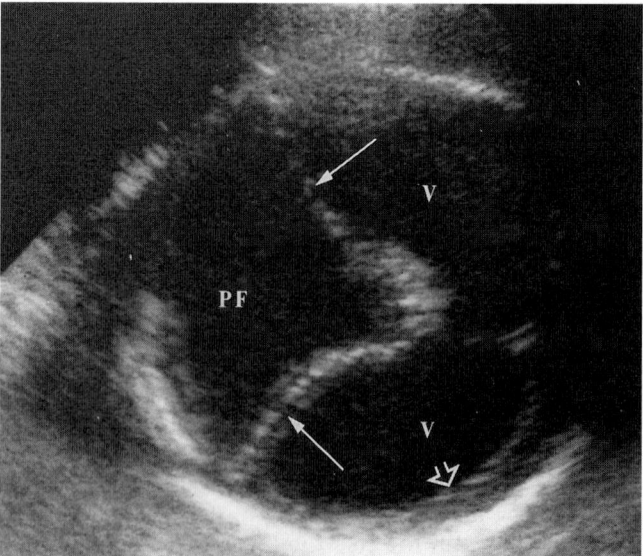

Figure 38.30. Dandy-Walker Malformation. Low axial plane image demonstrates cystic enlargement of the posterior fossa (*PF*) demarcated by the elevated tentorium (*arrows*). The lateral ventricles (*V*) are markedly enlarged and the cortical mantle (*open arrow*) is thinned.

variants (57). Arachnoid cysts and large cisterna magna are differentiated by their lack of communication with the fourth ventricle.

Choroid Plexus Cysts are found in 1–3% of normal fetuses during the second trimester. The cysts themselves cause no clinical problem and nearly always resolve. Because they are present in 30% of fetuses with trisomy 18, their discovery causes concern for the presence of chromosome abnormality. In most cases, detailed US examination, which includes echocardiography and examination of the fetal hands, will demonstrate additional structural abnormalities that justify amniocentesis for

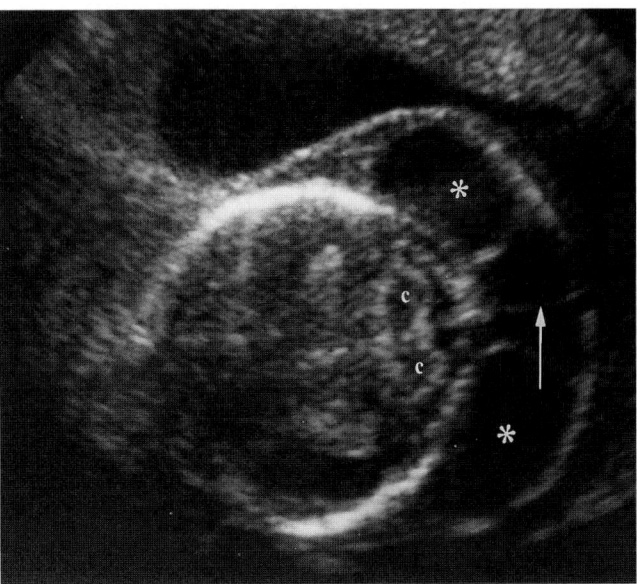

Figure 38.33. Cystic Hygroma. A multiseptated cystic mass (*) extends over the occipital region of the fetal skull. Cystic hygroma is differentiated from occipital cephalocele by demonstration of the midline septum (*arrow*) due to the nuchal ligament and by absence of a bony defect in the skull.

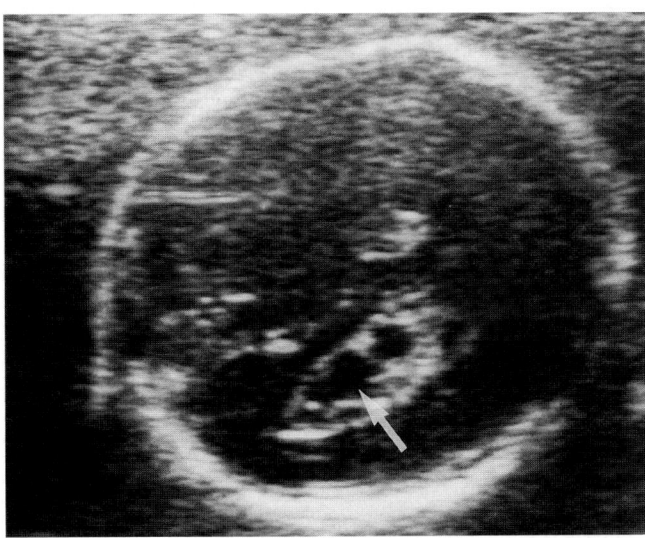

Figure 38.31. Choroid Plexus Cyst. A multiloculated cyst (*arrow*) is seen in the choroid plexus of the lateral ventricle.

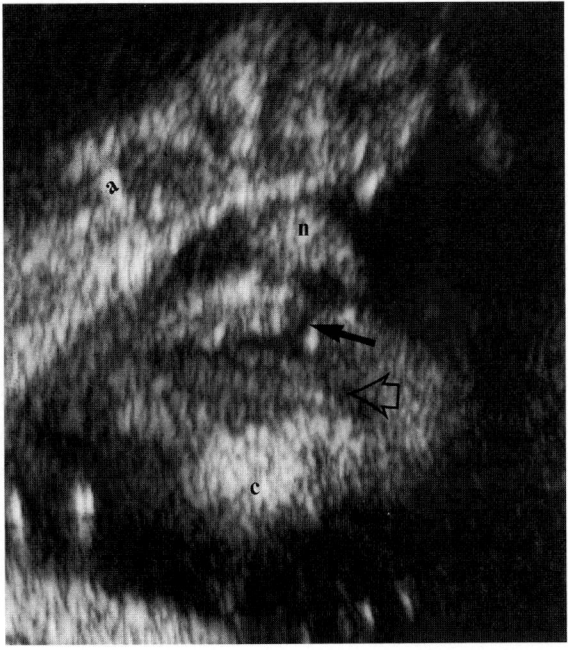

Figure 38.32. Cleft Lip. Coronal view of the fetal face reveals a cleft (*arrow*) in the left lip extending into the left nares. The mouth (*open arrow*), nose (*n*), and chin (*c*) are evident. An arm (*a*) extends across the forehead.

karyotyping. Controversy exists as to whether amniocentesis is warranted when choroid plexus cysts are an isolated finding. Size, bilaterality, and appearance of the cysts are not distinguishing features (Fig. 38.31). The preponderance of data suggests that amniocentesis is not necessary if thorough US examination is negative for additional abnormalities (58).

Cleft Lip and Cleft Palate account for 13% of all congenital anomalies found in the United States. Lateral clefting involves both lip and palate in 50% of cases, the lip alone in 25%, and the palate alone in 25%. The condition is bilateral in 20–25% of cases. Up to 60% of affected fetuses have additional anomalies including polydactyly, congenital heart disease, and trisomy 21. US diagnosis is made on demonstration of a groove extending from one of the nostrils through the lip (Fig. 38.32) (59). Median cleft lip is a completely different entity associated with holoprosencephaly and accounting for less than 0.7% of all cases of cleft lip. A coronal plane sonogram of the face demonstrates a wide central defect in the upper lip and palate.

Cystic Hygroma is a fluid collection in the fetal neck caused by failure of the lymphatic system to develop normal connections with the venous system in the neck (60). US demonstrates a bilateral nuchal cystic mass with a prominent midline septum representing the nuchal ligament (Fig. 38.33) (59). Up to 70% have abnormal karyotypes including Turner's syndrome and Down's syndrome. Generalized lymphangiectasia and fetal hydrops may occur and are always fatal when they do.

Chest and Heart

Congenital Diaphragmatic Hernia is a disorder in which abdominal contents protrude into the thorax

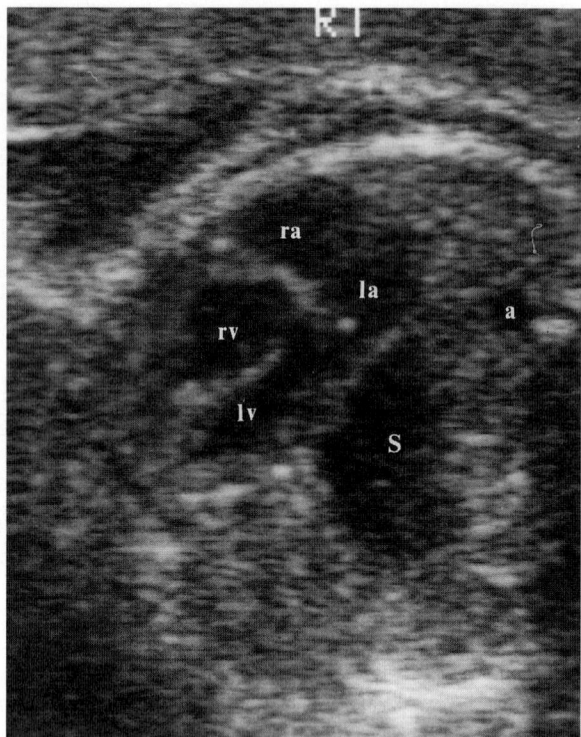

Figure 38.34. Congenital Diaphragmatic Hernia. Axial plane image of the fetal thorax viewed from above. Herniation of the stomach (*S*) into the left thorax displaces the heart into the right thorax. The heart is seen in four-chamber view. *ra*, right atrium; *rv*, right ventricle; *la*, left atrium; *lv*, left ventricle; *a*, descending aorta.

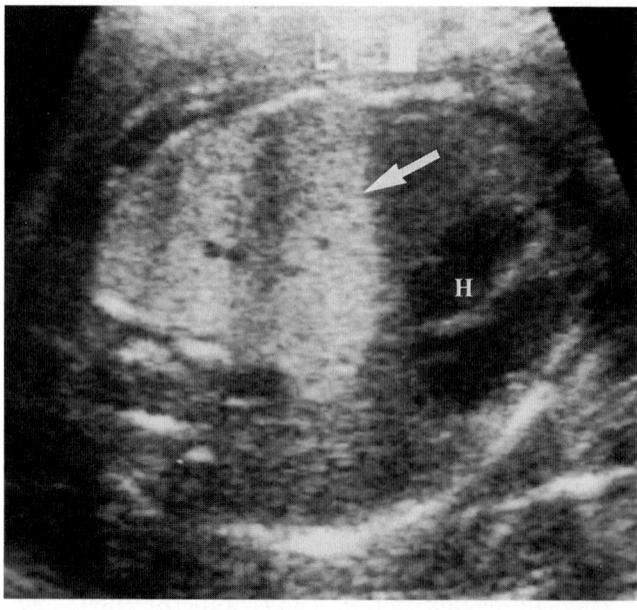

Figure 38.35. Cystic Adenomatoid Malformation. An echogenic solid-appearing mass (*arrow*) is seen in the thorax displacing the heart (*H*). The appearance is characteristic of type III, cystic adenomatoid malformation.

through defects in the diaphragm. The most common type involves the foramen of Bochdalek at the posterolateral aspect of the diaphragm. The majority (75%) occur on the left side (Fig. 38.34). Anteromedial defects at the foramen of Morgagni also occur. US findings include

displacement of the heart and mediastinum; fluid-filled, solid, or multicystic mass in the chest; absence of the stomach in the abdomen; and polyhydramnios (61). Associated defects, especially cardiac and CNS, are common. Mortality is high (50–80%) because of pulmonary hypoplasia.

Cystic Adenomatoid Malformation is a congenital hamartomatous lesion of the lung, usually affecting one lobe (62). The lesion consists of single or multiple cysts that vary in size from microscopic to larger than 2 cm size. Type I lesions appear on US as single or multiple cysts larger than 2 cm size. Type II lesions consist of multiple smaller cysts of uniform size less than 2 cm. Type III lesions appear as echogenic solid masses because the cysts are microscopic (Fig. 38.35). Polyhydramnios and fetal hydrops may occur.

Pulmonary Sequestration is a mass of lung tissue supplied by systemic arteries and separated from its normal bronchial and pulmonary vascular connections (63,64). *Intralobar sequestrations* (75–85%) are contained within the pleural covering of an otherwise normal lobe of the lung. Pulmonary venous drainage is maintained. Most present in adults. US detection in the fetus is rare. *Extralobar sequestrations*, though less common (15–25%), are much more frequently evident on fetal US. These are accessory lobes, contained within their own pleura, and supplied by both systemic arteries and veins. US demonstrates a homogeneous echogenic solid lung mass that displaces the mediastinum. Color Doppler is used to demonstrate the systemic supplying artery arising from the thoracic aorta. Hydrops may occur.

Fetal Heart Anomalies. Congenital heart disease is a major cause of neonatal morbidity and mortality. Precise

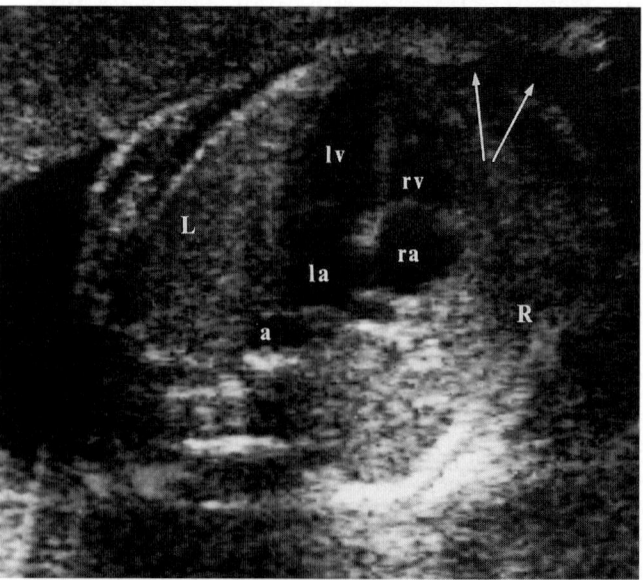

Figure 38.36. Four-Chamber View of the Heart. Axial plane image of the fetal thorax viewed from above demonstrates a normal four-chamber view of the heart. Note the orientation of the axis of the heart relative to the midline of the chest (*arrows*). *la*, left atrium; *lv*, left ventricle; *ra*, right atrium; *rv*, right ventricle; *a*, descending aorta; *L*, left thorax; *R*, right thorax.

US diagnosis of fetal heart abnormalities often requires specialized equipment and a high level of expertise. The presence of many major structural abnormalities of the fetal heart can be recognized on the four-chamber heart view (65–67). The four-chamber view is obtained on an axial scan through the fetal chest just above the diaphragm (Fig. 38.36). The apex of the heart is directed at the left anterior chest wall at a 45° angle on the same side as the fetal stomach. Deviation from this position suggests a cardiac malformation or a thoracic mass (see Figs. 38.34, 38.35). Pericardial effusions appear as an anechoic band surrounding the myocardium. The ventricles are approximately equal in size and slightly smaller than their corresponding atria. Motion of the atrioventricular valves is observed in this plane. Papillary muscles in the ventricles may be echogenic and prominent. Discrepancies in chamber size or valve motion suggest cardiac malformations and the necessity to perform a more detailed examination.

Abdomen

Normal Fetal Abdomen. The abdomen of the fetus is significantly different from the abdomen of the older child or adult. The fetal abdomen is large relative to body length compared with the adult. The liver is large, and the left lobe is larger than the right lobe. The umbilical vein is an important US landmark. Half the blood it carries goes directly to inferior vena cava via the ductus venosus. The remainder perfuses the liver via the left portal vein. The adrenal glands are up to 20 times larger in relative size because of the presence of the "fetal zone." The pelvis is relatively small, and pelvic organs extend into the lower abdomen. Swallowing begins at 11–12 weeks' GA. The fetal stomach should be fluid filled by 18 weeks' GA (68,69). The small bowel is moderately echogenic, centrally located, and blends with the liver (70). By the third trimester, peristalsis in small bowel loops can be observed. The visualized small bowel loops are normally less than 6-mm in diameter and less than 15 mm in length. The colon is visualized after 20 weeks as a tubular structure around the periphery of the abdomen The colon progressively fills with meconium but does not exceed 23 mm in diameter. Normal fetal kidneys are seen as paired, slightly hypoechoic structures adjacent to the spine. The renal sinus appears as an echogenic stripe. Fetal lobulation causes an undulating contour of the kidneys. The length of normal fetal kidneys in millimeters is approximately equal to GA in weeks. The bladder should be observed to fill and empty. Because amniotic fluid is predominantly urine, a normal amniotic fluid volume implies at least one functioning kidney.

Absent Stomach. Failure to visualize the fetal stomach by 18 weeks' GA is a significant abnormality in about half the cases. Causes include obstruction (esophageal atresia, chest mass), impaired swallowing (facial clefts and neuromuscular disorders), low amniotic fluid volume, and ectopic stomach (diaphragmatic hernia). In the remaining cases, absence of fluid in the stomach is a normal variant, probably representing recent gastric emptying. Follow-up US is warranted to detect delayed filling.

Double Bubble is descriptive of fluid distension of the stomach and proximal duodenum (Fig. 38.37). Fluid dilatation of the duodenum is abnormal and indicative of duodenal atresia or stenosis, annular pancreas, or volvulus. Down's syndrome should be considered. Half the cases have additional anomalies.

Bowel Obstruction is suggested by dilation of the small bowel of greater than 6 mm. Causes include jejunal or ileal atresia or stenosis, volvulus, meconium ileus, and enteric duplication. A dilated and tortuous ureter should not be misinterpreted as dilated bowel.

Meconium ileus causes small bowel obstruction by impaction of abnormally thick meconium in the distal ileum. Meconium ileus is nearly always associated with cystic fibrosis. The combination of dilated bowel with echogenic meconium suggests the diagnosis.

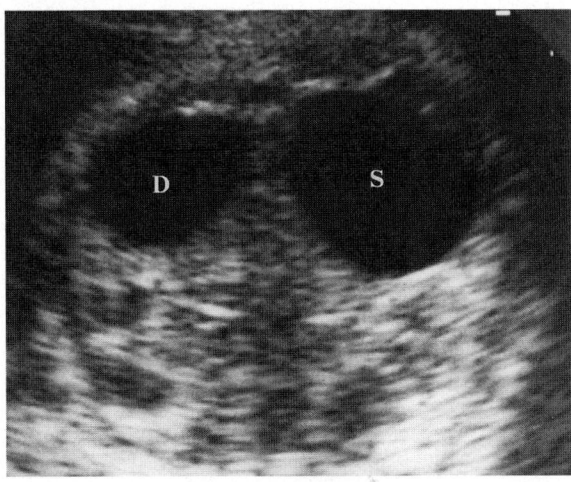

Figure 38.37. "Double Bubble." Fluid distension of the stomach (*S*) and duodenal bulb (*D*) is caused by obstruction at the level of the descending duodenum.

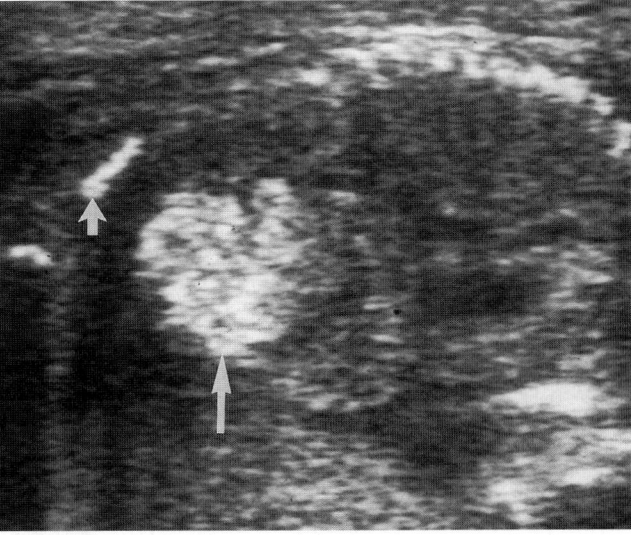

Figure 38.38. Echogenic Bowel. Abnormally echogenic bowel (*long arrow*) creates an echogenic mass in the lower fetal abdomen. The echogenicity of the mass of bowel is equal to that of the iliac wing (*short arrow*).

Meconium Peritonitis results from perforation of a bowel segment. Spillage of meconium into the peritoneal cavity causes a sterile peritonitis that results in calcifications in the peritoneal cavity, meconium pseudocysts, ascites, bowel dilatation, and polyhydramnios. The cause is commonly not identified and may be due to vascular insult to small bowel. Identified causes include meconium ileus (cystic fibrosis), bowel atresia, and volvulus.

Echogenic Bowel. Meconium, consisting of desquamated cells, proteins, and bile pigments, fills the distal small bowel by 15–16 weeks. Its US appearance ranges from echolucent to moderately echogenic. Small bowel is considered abnormally echogenic when its echogenicity is equal to or greater than that of adjacent bone (Fig. 38.38). This finding is normal in half the cases, but serves as a marker of significant abnormality in the other half. Associations include cystic fibrosis, chromosome abnormalities (trisomy 21, trisomy 18), small bowel atresia, volvulus, and fetal viral infection (cytomegalovirus) (71).

Urinary Obstruction. The most common causes of hydronephrosis in the fetus are ureteropelvic junction obstruction, ectopic ureterocele, and posterior urethral valves. Dilation of the renal pelvis greater than 10-mm AP diameter or greater than 50% of the AP diameter of the kidney in axial section (Fig. 38.39), or unequivocal calyectasis are definitive evidence of significant hydronephrosis. Assessment of bladder filling and amniotic fluid volume is necessary to determine the severity of obstruction.

Minimal dilatation of the renal pelvis presents a clinical problem. Up to 20% of fetuses show a dilated renal pelvis greater or equal to 3 mm, and another 40% show detectable (1–2 mm) fluid distension of the pelvis. This mild dilatation is most often due to physiologic reflux that is normal in the second and third trimesters. Some significant obstruction may show only mild dilatation in the second trimester; follow-up US in the third trimester is warranted to detect development of calyectasis or progression of pyelectasis (72). Elective postnatal examinations of equivocal cases should be performed at 1–2 weeks of age to avoid underestimation of hydronephrosis due to early postnatal oliguria.

Renal Cystic Disease is commonly detected in utero. Multicystic dysplastic kidney appears as multiple noncommunicating cysts of varying size (Fig. 38.40). Because affected kidneys do not function, bilateral multicystic dysplastic kidney is associated with oligohydramnios and is not compatible with life. Massive enlargement of both kidneys associated with oligohydramnios suggests autosomal recessive polycystic dis-

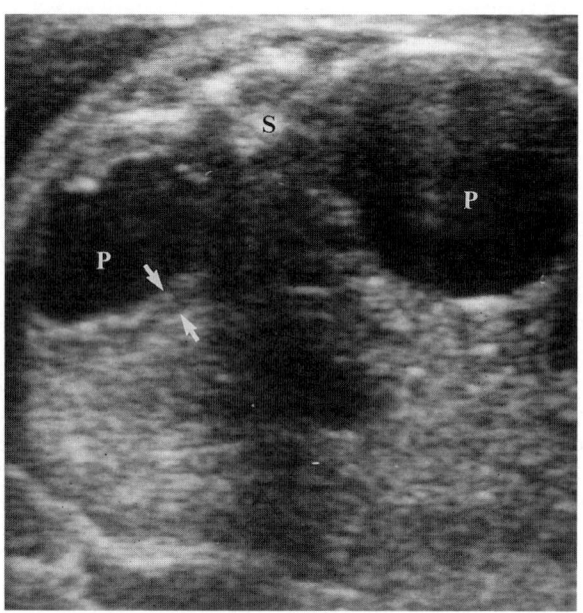

Figure 38.39. Hydronephrosis. Posterior axial plane US of the abdomen demonstrates marked bilateral enlargement of the renal pelves (*P*) in a male fetus with posterior urethral valves. The renal cortex is markedly thinned (*arrows*). *S*, spine.

Figure 38.40. Multicystic Dysplastic Kidney. The kidney (*outlined by arrows*) is largely replaced by multiple noncommunicating cysts (*c*).

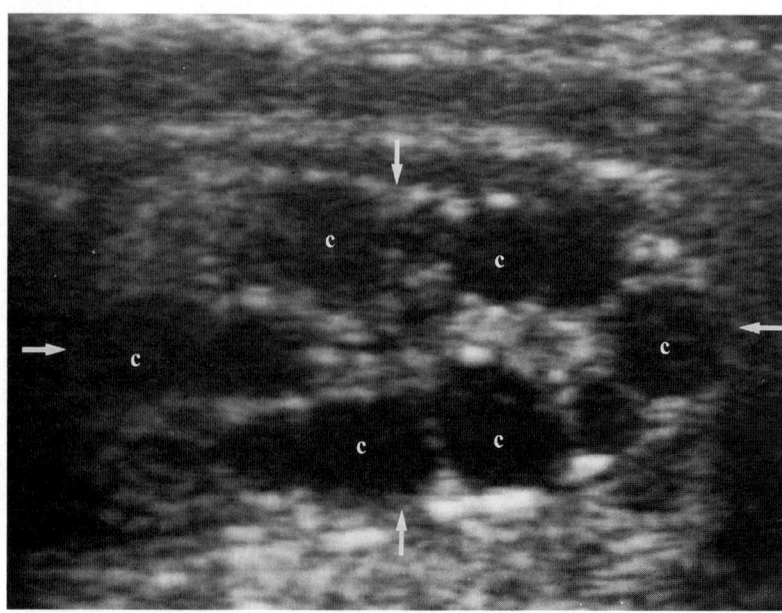

ease. The kidneys are predominantly echogenic with a sonolucent rim. Discrete cysts are not evident. Autosomal dominant polycystic kidney disease is occasionally detected in utero. The kidneys are enlarged but lack the sonolucent rim of infantile polycystic kidney disease. Occasional discrete cysts are visualized. Obstructive uropathy such as posterior urethral valves may result in cystic renal dysplasia. Affected kidneys are hydronephrotic, with increased parenchymal echogenicity and cysts of varying size. The kidneys may be dysplastic without cysts being visualized by US.

Gastroschisis results from a defect in the anterior abdominal wall on the right side of the umbilicus (Fig. 38.41) (73,74). The defect is usually 2–5 cm in size. Bowel herniates through the defect and floats freely in the amniotic fluid with no covering membrane. Small defects may be associated with bowel ischemia, resulting in thickening of the wall of the herniated bowel. The cord insertion site is normal. Gastroschisis is most commonly an isolated defect without chromosomal anomaly or recurrence risk. Postnatal repair is usually successful, so the prognosis is excellent.

Omphalocele is a more serious abdominal wall defect that is about equal in frequency to gastroschisis (73,74). The defect is midline at the umbilicus with herniation of abdominal contents into the base of the umbilical cord. Both liver and bowel are commonly present in the herniation. A membrane consisting of peritoneum and amnion covers the omphalocele. The umbilical cord inserts through the membrane (Fig. 38.42). Associated anomalies are common (67–88%), including cardiac, CNS, urinary tract, and gastrointestinal malformations. Chromosome anomalies are found in up to 40% of cases. The ventral wall defect may include the heart (ectopia cordis).

Skeleton

Skeletal Dysplasias are a heterogeneous group of disorders of skeletal growth resulting in bones of abnormal size and shape (Fig 38.43). US findings that are highly associated with the presence of a generalized skeletal dysplasia include shortening of extremity bones, fractures, bowing of long bones, demineralization, and a small thorax (75). Finding of short femur length mandates detailed bone examination with measurement of additional long bones. A ratio of femur length to foot length of less than 0.9 suggests a skeletal dysplasia, whereas a ratio greater than 0.9 is usually associated with a constitutionally small or growth-retarded fetus. Additional findings that help categorize the skeletal dys-

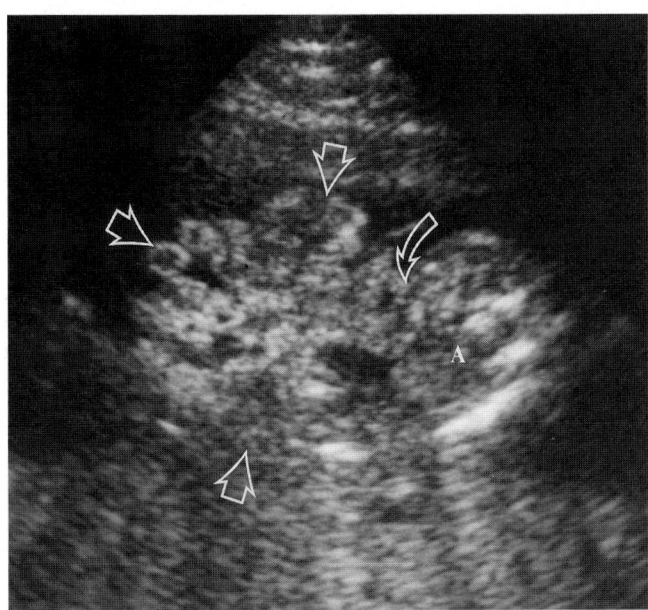

Figure 38.41. Gastroschisis. Transverse plane US through the fetal abdomen demonstrates herniation of multiple bowel loops (*arrows*) through a defect in the anterior abdominal wall (*curved arrow*). The bowel loops float freely in amniotic fluid and are not confined within a membrane. *A*, fetal abdomen.

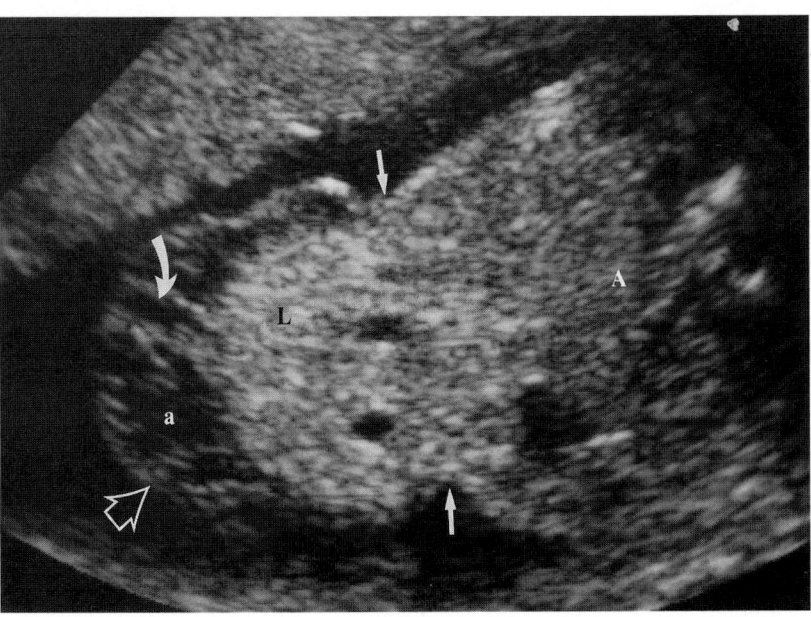

Figure 38.42. Omphalocele. The liver (*L*) herniates through a large defect (*small arrows*) in the anterior abdominal wall in this fetus with omphalocele. The umbilical vein (*curved arrow*) is included within the herniation. The herniated abdominal contents are confined within a membrane (*open arrow*). Ascites (*a*) is present within the omphalocele and within the fetal abdomen (*A*).

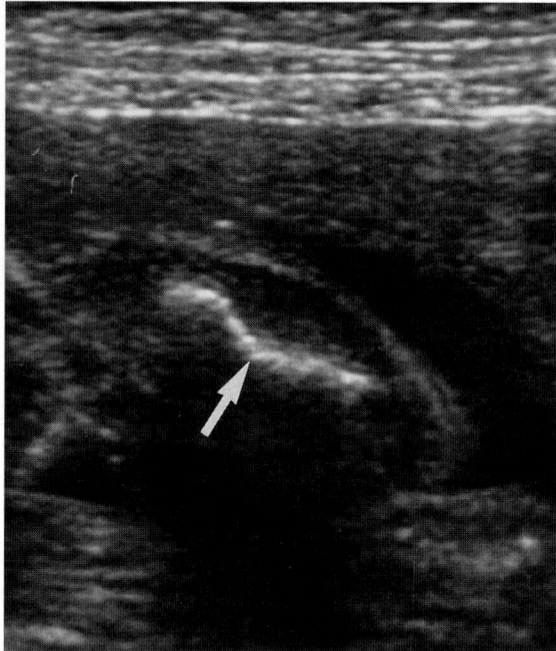

Figure 38.43. Osteogenesis Imperfecta. A longitudinal image of the femur demonstrates poor mineralization and central bowing due to a fracture (*arrow*).

plasia include polydactyly, abnormal head shape, spine anomalies, midface hypoplasia, abnormal bone configuration, ventriculomegaly, polyhydramnios, and hydrops. Precise diagnosis of a skeletal dysplasia may be difficult unless there is a family history. An algorithmic approach is then recommended (76).

Thanatophoric dwarfism is the most common lethal skeletal dysplasia. Distinguishing features include small thorax, cloverleaf skull, large head, hydrocephalus, and polyhydramnios. *Achondroplastic dysplasia* is an autosomal dominant trait that is lethal in homozygous form and nonlethal in heterozygous form. Because at least one parent must have the condition, the US diagnosis is made on the basis of proximal limb shortening. *Osteogenesis imperfecta* is a heterogenous group of disorders with both autosomal dominant and recessive inheritance patterns. The hallmark of the disease is osteoporosis that may manifest on US as diminished bone brightness. Additional features include bone thickening with fractures and callus formation, bone bowing, a small chest, and protuberant abdomen.

Examination of the fetal hands and feet may yield characteristic findings that suggest a variety of syndromes and chromosome abnormalities (77). Clenched hands with overlapping index fingers suggests trisomy 18. Polydactyly with polycystic kidneys suggests Meckel-Gruber syndrome. Hypoplasia of the middle phalanx of the fifth digit in association with femur and humerus shortening suggests Down's syndrome.

References

1. Angtuaco TL, Shah HR, Mattison DR, et al. MR imaging in high-risk obstetric patients: a valuable complement to US. Radiographics 1992;12:91–109.

2. Levine D, Hatabu H, Gaa J, et al. Fetal anatomy revealed with fast MR sequences. AJR Am J Roentgenol 1996;167:905–908.

3. Federle MP, Cohen HA, Rosenwein MF, et al. Pelvimetry by digital radiography: a low-dose examination. Radiology 1982;143:733–735.

4. American Institute of Ultrasound in Medicine. Guidelines for performance of the antepartum obstetrical ultrasound examination. Rockville, MD: American Institute of Ultrasound in Medicine, 1991.

5. Laing FC, Brown DL, Price JF, et al. Intradecidual sign: is it effective in diagnosis of an early intrauterine pregnancy? Radiology 1997;204:655–660.

6. Nyberg DA, Laing FC, Filly RA. Threatened abortion: sonographic distinction of normal and abnormal gestation sacs. Radiology 1986;158:397–400.

7. Nyberg DA, Laing FC, Filly RA, et al. Ultrasonographic differentiation of the gestational sac of early intrauterine pregnancy from the pseudogestational sac of ectopic pregnancy. Radiology 1983;146:755–759.

8. Yeh H-C, Rabinowitz JG. Amniotic sac development: ultrasound features of early pregnancy–the double bleb sign. Radiology 1988;166:97–103.

9. Levi CS, Lyons EA, Lindsay DJ. Early diagnosis of nonviable pregnancy with endovaginal US. Radiology 1988;167:383–385.

10. Rowling SE, Coleman BG, Langer JE, et al. First-trimester US parameters of failed pregnancy. Radiology 1997;203:211–217.

11. Nyberg DA, Mack LA, Laing FC, et al. Distinguishing normal from abnormal gestational sac growth in early pregnancy. J Ultrasound Med 1987;6:23–27.

12. Pennell RG, Needleman L, Pajak T, et al. Prospective comparison of vaginal and abdominal sonography in normal early pregnancy. J Ultrasound Med 1991;10:63–67.

13. Brown DL, Emerson DS, Felker RE, et al. Diagnosis of early embryonic demise by endovaginal sonography. J Ultrasound Med 1990;9:631–636.

14. Chen G-D, Lin M-T, Lee M-S. Diagnosis of interstitial pregnancy with sonography. J Clin Ultrasound 1994;22:439–442.

15. Russell SA, Filly RA, Damato N. Sonographic diagnosis of ectopic pregnancy with endovaginal probes: what really has changed? J Ultrasound Med 1993;3:145–151.

16. Fleischer AC, Pennell RG, McKee MS, et al. Ectopic pregnancy: features at transvaginal sonography. Radiology 1990;174:375–378.

17. Brown DL, Doubilet PM. Transvaginal sonography for diagnosing ectopic pregnancy: positivity criteria and performance characteristics. J Ultrasound Med 1994;13:259–266.

18. Frates MC, Brown DL, Doubliet PM, et al. Tubal rupture in patients with ectopic pregnancy: diagnosis with transvaginal US. Radiology 1994;191:769–772.

19. Nyberg DA, Hughes MP, Mack LA, et al. Extrauterine findings of ectopic pregnancy at transvaginal US: importance of echogenic fluid. Radiology 1991;178:823–826.

20. Dillon EH, Feyock AL, Taylor KJW. Pseudogestational sacs: Doppler US differentiation from normal or abnormal intrauterine pregnancy. Radiology 1990;176:359–364.

21. Bennett GL, Bromley B, Lieberman E, et al. Subchorionic hemorrhage in first-trimester pregnancies: prediction of pregnancy outcome with sonography. Radiology 1996;200:803–806.

22. Wagner BJ, Woodward PJ, Dickey GE. Gestational trophoblastic disease: radiologic-pathologic correlation. Radiographics 1996;16:131–148.

23. Green CL, Angtuaco TL, Shah HR, et al. Gestational tro-

phoblastic disease: a spectrum of radiologic diagnosis. Radiographics 1996;16:1371–1384.

24. Doubilet PM, Benson CB. Sonographic evaluation of intrauterine growth retardation. AJR Am J Roentgenol 1995; 164:709–717.

25. Dubinsky T, Lau M, Powell F, et al. Predicting poor neonatal outcome: a comparative study of noninvasive antenatal testing methods. AJR Am J Roentgenol 1997;168:827–831.

26. Finberg HJ, Kurtz AB, Johnson RL, et al. The biophysical profile: a literature review and reassessment of its usefulness in the evaluation of fetal well-being. J Ultrasound Med 1990;9:583–591.

27. Strobelt N, Ghidini A, Cavallone M, et al. Natural history of uterine leiomyomas in pregnancy. J Ultrasound Med 1994; 13:399–401.

28. Kessler A, Mitchell DG, Kuhlman K, et al. Myoma vs. contraction in pregnancy: differentiation with color Doppler imaging. J Clin Ultrasound 1993;21:241–244.

29. Hertzberg BS, Bowie JD, Weber TM, et al. Sonography of the cervix during the third trimester of pregnancy: value of the transperineal approach. AJR Am J Roentgenol 1991; 157:73–76.

30. Iams JD, Goldenberg RL, Meis PJ, et al. The length of the cervix and the risk of spontaneous premature delivery. N Engl J Med 1996;334:567–572.

31. Brant WE. Ultrasonography of the placenta. Perspect Radiol 1989;2:157–170.

32. Harris HD, Barth RA. Sonography of the gravid uterus and placenta: current concepts. AJR Am J Roentgenol 1993; 160:455–465.

33. Hertzberg BS, Bowie JD, Carroll BA, et al. Diagnosis of placenta previa during the third trimester: role of transperineal sonography. AJR Am J Roentgenol 1992;159:83–87.

34. Nyberg DA, Mack LA, Benedetti TJ, et al. Placental abruption and placental hemorrhage: correlation of sonographic findings with fetal outcome. Radiology 1987;164:357–361.

35. Finberg HJ, Williams JW. Placenta accreta: prospective sonographic diagnosis in patients with placenta previa and prior Cesarean section. J Ultrasound Med 1992;11: 333–343.

36. Dudiak CM, Salomon CG, Posniak HV, et al. Sonography of the umbilical cord. Radiographics 1995;15:1035–1050.

37. Nyberg DA, Mahony BS, Luthy D, et al. Single umbilical artery—prenatal detection of concurrent abnormalities. J Ultrasound Med 1991;10:247–253.

38. Burton DJ, Filly RA. Sonographic diagnosis of the amniotic band syndrome. 1991;156:555–558.

39. Randel SB, Filly RA, Callen PW, et al. Amniotic sheets. Radiology 1988;166:633–636.

40. Finberg HJ. Uterine synechiae in pregnancy: expanded criteria for recognition and clinical significance in 28 cases. J Ultrasound Med 1991;10:547–555.

41. Benson CB, Doubilet PM. Sonography in multiple gestations. Radiologist 1994;1:147–154.

42. Filly RA, Goldstein RB, Callen PW. Monochorionic twinning: sonographic assessment. AJR Am J Roentgenol 1990; 154:459–469.

43. Brown DL, Benson CB, Driscoll SG, et al. Twin–twin transfusion syndrome: sonographic findings. Radiology 1989; 170:61–63.

44. Benacereff BR. Use of sonographic markers to determine the risk of Down syndrome in second-trimester fetuses. Radiology 1996;201:619–620.

45. Filly RA, Cardoza JD, Goldstein RB, et al. Detection of fetal central nervous system anomalies: a practical level of effort for a routine sonogram. Radiology 1989;172:403–408.

46. Hertzberg BS, Kliewer MA, Freed KS, et al. Third ventricle: size and appearance in normal fetuses through gestation. Radiology 1997;203:641–644.

47. Farrell TA, Hertzberg BS, Kliewer MA, et al. Fetal lateral ventricles: reassessment of normal values for atrial diameter. Radiology 1994;193:409–411.

48. Alagappan R, Browning PD, Laorr A, et al. Distal lateral ventricular atrium: reevaluation of normal range. Radiology 1994;193:405–408.

49. Carrasco CR, Stierman ED, Harnsberger HR, et al. An algorithm for prenatal ultrasound diagnosis of congenital CNS abnormalities. J Ultrasound Med 1985;4:163–168.

50. Hertberg BS, Lile R, Foosaner DE, et al. Choroid plexus-ventricular wall separation in fetuses with normal-sized cerebral ventricles at sonography: postnatal outcome. AJR Am J Roentgenol 1994;163:405–410.

51. Goldstein RB, Filly RA. Prenatal diagnosis of anencephaly: spectrum of sonographic appearances and distinction from the amniotic band syndrome. AJR Am J Roentgenol 1988; 151:547–550.

52. Goldstein RB, Filly RA, Callen PW. Sonography of anencephaly: pitfalls in early diagnosis. J Clin Ultrasound 1989; 17:397–402.

53. Goldstein RB, LaPidus AS, Filly RA. Fetal cephaloceles: diagnosis with US. Radiology 1991;180:803–808.

54. Budorick NE, Pretorius DH, Nelson TR. Sonography of the fetal spine: technique, imaging findings, and clinical implications. AJR Am J Roentgenol 1995;164:421–428.

55. Filly RA, Simpson GF, Linkowski G. Fetal spine morphology and maturation during the second trimester-sonographic evaluation. J Ultrasound Med 1987;6:631–636.

56. McGahan JP, Nyberg DA, Mack LA. Sonography of facial features of alobar and semilobar holoprosencephaly. AJR Am J Roentgenol 1990;154:143–148.

57. Estroff JA, Scott MR, Benacerraf BR. Dandy-Walker variant: prenatal sonographic features and clinical outcome. Radiology 1992;185:755–758.

58. Nadel AS, Bromley BS, Frigoletto Jr. FD, et al. Isolated choroid plexus cysts in the second-trimester fetus: is amniocentesis really indicated? Radiology 1992;185:545–548.

59. Brant WE. Ultrasound of the fetal face and neck. Radiologist 1994;1:235–244.

60. Zadvinskis DP, Benson MT, Kerr HH, et al. Congenital malformations of the cervico-thoracic lymphatic system: embryology and pathogenesis. Radiographics 1992;12: 1175–1189.

61. Guibaud L, Filiatrault D, Garel L, et al. Fetal congenital diaphragmatic hernia: accuracy of sonography in the diagnosis and prediction of outcome after birth. AJR Am J Roentgenol 1996;166:1195–1202.

62. Rosado-de-Christenson ML, Stocker JT. Congenital cystic adenomatoid malformation. Radiographics 1991;11: 865–886.

63. Bromley B, Parad R, Estroff JA, et al. Fetal lung mass: prenatal course and outcome. J Ultrasound Med 1995;14: 927–936.

64. Rosado-de-Christenson ML, Frazier AA, Stocker JT, et al. Extralobar sequestration: radiologic-pathologic correlation. Radiographics 1993;13:425–441.

65. McGahan JP. Sonography of the fetal heart: findings on the four chamber view. AJR Am J Roentgenol 1991;156: 547–553.

66. Brown DL, DiSalvo DN, Frates MC, et al. Sonography of the fetal heart: normal variants and pitfalls. AJR Am J Roentgenol 1993;160:1251–1255.

67. Benacerraf BR. Sonographic detection of fetal anomalies of the aortic and pulmonary arteries: value of the four-chamber view vs direct images. AJR Am J Roentgenol 1994;163: 1483–1489.

68. Hertzberg BS, Kliewer MA. Ultrasound of the fetal gastrointestinal tract. Radiologist 1996;3:123–129.

69. Hertzbeg BS. Sonography of the fetal gastrointestinal tract: anatomic variants, diagnostic pitfalls, and abnormalities. AJR Am J Roentgenol 1994;162:1175–1182.

70. Parulekar SG. Sonography of normal fetal bowel. J Ultrasound Med 1991;10:211–220.

71. Rypens FF, Avni EF, Abehsera MM, et al. Areas of increased echogenicity in the fetal abdomen: diagnosis and significance. Radiographics 1995;15:1329–1344.

72. Anderson N, Clautice-Engle T, Allan R, et al. Detection of obstructive uropathy in the fetus: predictive value of sonographic measurements of renal pelvic diameter at various gestational ages. AJR Am J Roentgenol 1995;164:719–723.

73. Brant WE. Sonographic evaluation of the fetal abdominal wall. Radiologist 1995;2:149–161.

74. Emanuel PG, Garcia GI, Angtuaco TL. Prenatal detection of anterior abdominal wall defects with US. Radiographics 1995;15:517–530.

75. Bowerman RA. Anomalies of the fetal skeleton: sonographic findings. AJR Am J Roentgenol 1995;164:973–979.

76. Spirt BA, Oliphant M, Gottlieb RH, et al. Prenatal sonographic evaluation of short limbed dwarfism: an algorithmic approach. Radiographics 1990;10:217–236.

77. Bromley B, Benacerraf B. Abnormalities of the hands and feet in the fetus: sonographic findings. AJR Am J Roentgenol 1995;165:1239–1243.

39

Chest, Thyroid, Parathyroid, and Neonatal Brain Ultrasound

William E. Brant

CHEST

Ultrasound is an excellent supplement to plain film radiography and computed tomography for the problem-solving evaluation of the chest and to guide interventional procedures in the thorax (1,2). US can image into and through pleural effusions and lung consolidation to evaluate the thorax opacified on plain films. Its portability allows evaluation of critically ill patients who are impractical to move for a CT. US examination of the chest must always be correlated with preliminary chest radiography.

Pleural Space

Normal US Anatomy. Air in the lungs completely reflects the US beam and prohibits examination deeper into the chest. However, when pleural fluid displaces air-filled lungs away from the chest wall, disease in the pleural space can be optimally evaluated with US. The pleural space is examined by a direct intercostal approach with the US transducer applied directly to the chest, or by an abdominal approach imaging through the diaphragm from the abdomen. The ribs are used as sonographic landmarks for direct chest imaging (Fig. 39.1). A linear array transducer applied to the chest wall shows the ribs as curving echoes that cast acoustic shadows. The visceral pleura-air filled lung interface is seen within 1 cm of the rib echo as a bright echogenic surface that moves with respiration (the "gliding" sign). The moving lung surface is well visualized when the transducer is turned to parallel the intercostal space. Fluid in the pleural space is seen just superficial to the gliding pleura. From the abdomen, the diaphragm is seen as a bright curving interface due to intense sound reflection from the air-filled lung above it. Organs beneath the diaphragm (liver, spleen) are artifactually reproduced above the diaphragm due to multi-path sound reflection (the "mirror-image" artifact)(Fig. 39.2).

Pleural Fluid displaces the lung away from the chest wall allowing visualization of the pleural space (Fig. 39.1C). Most pleural fluid is anechoic, or hypoechoic with floating particulate matter (3). The fluid separates the visceral and parietal pleural surfaces. From an abdominal approach (Fig. 39.2B), hypoechoic fluid is seen above the diaphragm, the inside of the thorax is visualized, and the mirror image artifact is not present. Septations not evident on CT are commonly visualized (Fig. 39.3). Collapsed or consolidated lung moves with respiration within the fluid in the pleural space. Fluid that is echogenic, contains floating particles or layering debris, or is septated is an exudate (4). Fluid that is anechoic may be an transudate, exudate, or even empyema. Loculations of pleural fluid and suspected empyemas can be localized and evaluated with US visualization used to guide needle aspiration and drainage catheter placement (5).

Pleural Thickening complicates inflammatory and malignant disease of the thorax. US demonstrates uniform, undulating, or plaque-like thickening of the pleura (Fig. 39.3). The visceral pleura is easily evaluated. The parietal pleura is partially obscured by reverberation artifact in the near field.

Pleural Masses. Pleural metastases or tumors such as mesotheliomas are seen as nodular pleural thickening or hypoechoic soft tissue masses in the pleural space projecting from the pleural surface (6).

Lung Parenchyma

Normal US Anatomy. The air-filled lung with its covering visceral pleura completely blocks transmission of US into the thorax (Fig. 39.1A,B). The gliding visceral surface of the lung is easily seen, but reverberation artifact is displayed deep to that surface. However, consolidation, atelectasis, or tumor that extends to the visceral pleural surface produces a window for US examination.

Consolidation refers to filling of the air spaces of the lung with fluid and inflammatory cells. This process "solidifies" the lung and provides a medium for sound transmission (7). The consolidated lung appears solid and hypoechoic with echogenicity similar to liver. Sonographic air bronchograms and air alveolograms may be seen within the consolidated lung. Air-filled

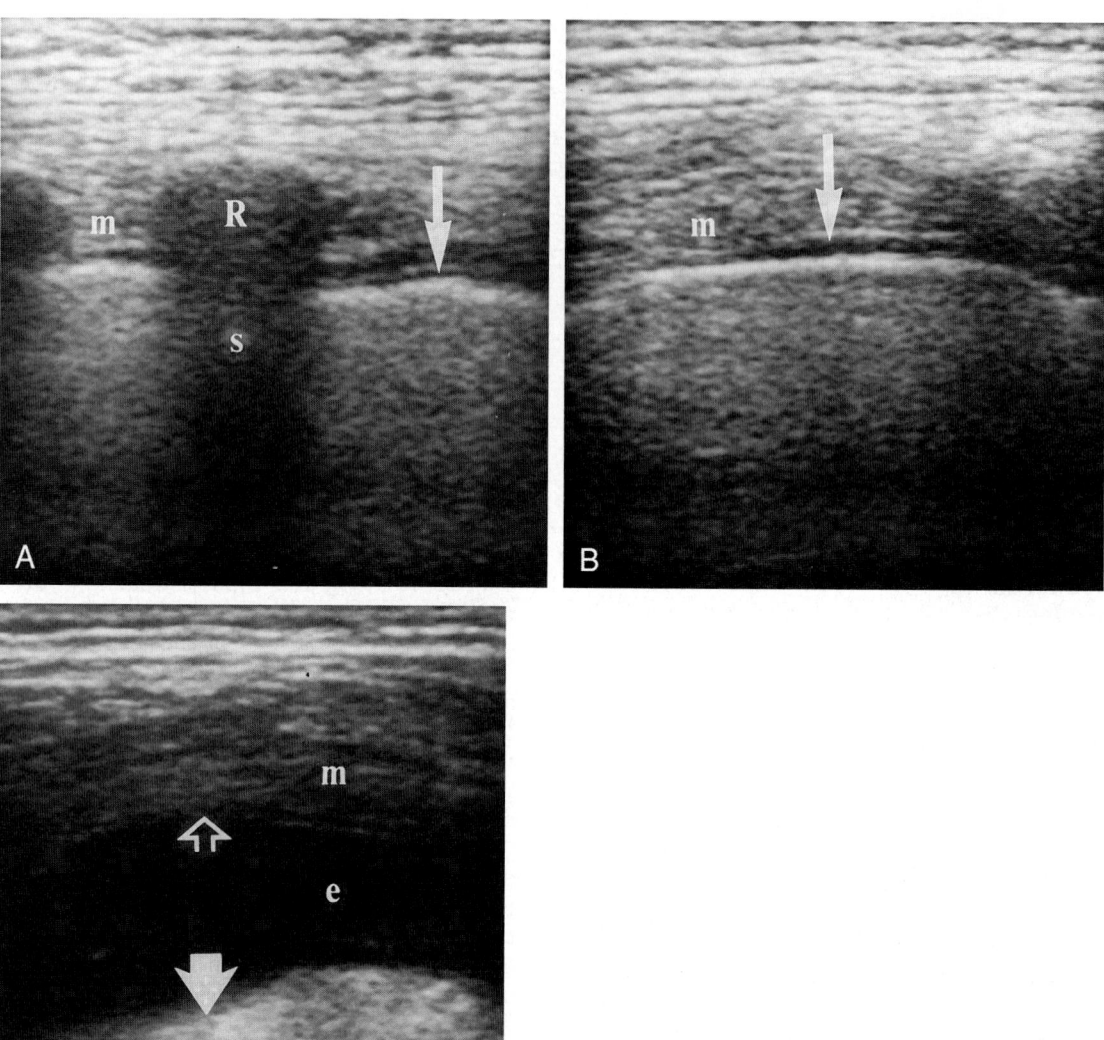

Figure 39.1. Pleural Space: Intercostal Approach. A. Longitudinal US image of the chest shows a rib (*R*) and its acoustic shadow (*s*). The pleural space is approximately 1 cm deep to the surface of the rib. The visceral pleura–air filled lung interface (*arrow*) is identified by its movement with respiration. Intercostal muscle (*m*) is seen between the ribs. **B.** Aligning the transducer parallel to the ribs in the intercostal space enables improved visualization of the pleural space (*arrow*). *m*, intercostal muscle. **C.** A pleural effusion (*e*) separates the visceral pleura (*closed arrow*) from the parietal pleura (*open arrow*). *m*, intercostal muscle.

bronchi produce bright linear reflections. Air trapped in alveoli surrounded by consolidated lung produces globular bright echoes with comet-tail artifacts. Sonographic fluid bronchograms appear as anechoic fluid-filled tubes extending from the hilum of the lung. Color flow US demonstrates pulmonary vessels extending through the consolidated lung.

Atelectasis. Collapse of the air spaces with absorption of air also results in solidification of the lung (Fig. 39.4). With atelectasis the lung volume is decreased and bronchi and pulmonary blood vessels are crowded together. Collapsed lung always accompanies large pleural effusions. The atelectatic lung is wedge-shaped and sharply defined by its covering pleura.

Lung Masses surrounded by air-filled lung are not visualized by US, but those that extend to the visceral pleura or are accompanied by peripheral consolidation or atelectasis may be seen and evaluated. US guidance may be effectively used to aspirate or biopsy lung masses in areas difficult to access with fluoroscopy or CT. Central tumor necrosis, hemorrhage within tumors, and lung abscesses are effectively evaluated (8).

Pulmonary Sequestration is a congenital partition of lung tissue that does not communicate with the bronchial tree. Most occur at the lung base. Intralobar sequestrations are within the visceral pleura. Extralobar sequestrations are invested by their own separate pleura. US is used to confirm the diagnosis by demon-

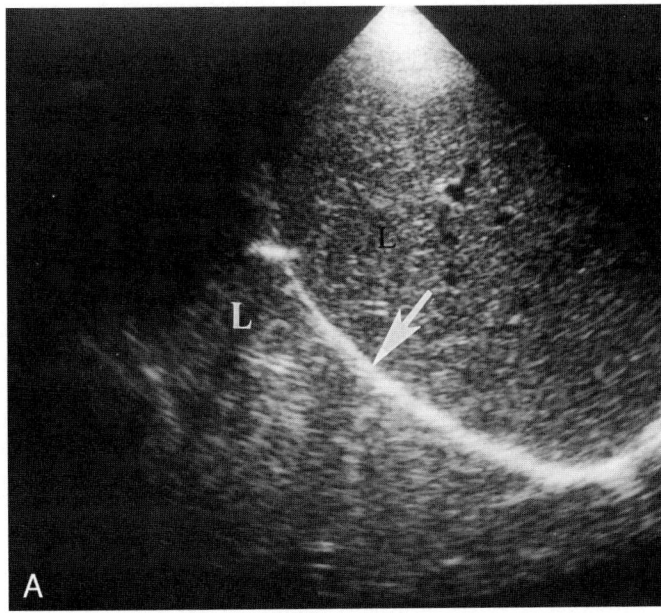

Figure 39.2. Pleural Space: Abdominal Approach. A. Examination of the chest may be performed from an abdominal approach using the liver (*L*) as a sonographic window. The diaphragm is seen as a bright curving line. Normal air-filled lung causes the liver (*black L*) to be reproduced as a mirror-image artifact (*white L*) above the diaphragm. **B.** A pleural effusion (*e*) eliminates the mirror-image artifact and allows visualization of the chest wall (*arrow*) through the diaphragm and pleural space. Note the rib shadows (*s*).

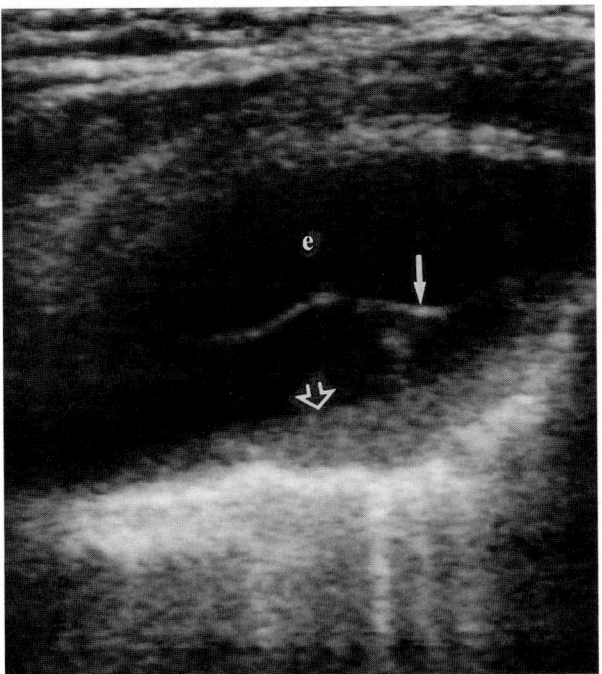

Figure 39.3. Pleural Thickening. Intercostal US image demonstrates a small pleural effusion (*e*) with septation (*closed arrow*). The visceral pleura (*open arrow*) is thickened.

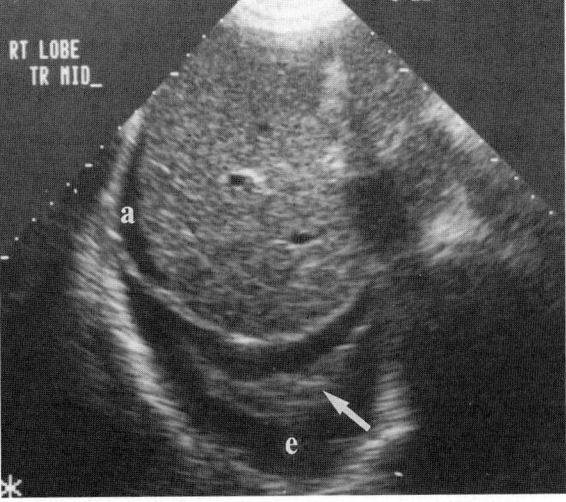

Figure 39.4. Atelectasis. A transverse image through the liver reveals a pleural effusion (*e*) surrounding a tongue of collapsed lung (*arrow*). The patient also has ascites (*a*).

Mediastinum

Normal US Anatomy. The superior and anterior mediastinum are effectively evaluated with US using a parasternal or supramanubrial approach (9). The posterior mediastinum is less accessible because of spine and lung. Large lesions create sonographic windows to the mediastinum. Imaging downward into the superior mediastinum from just above the sternal manubrium demonstrates the innominate veins and the arteries arising from the aortic arch. Doppler US assists in the identification of vessels.

stration of a feeding artery arising from the aorta. Extralobar sequestration drain via a systemic vein, whereas intralobar sequestrations connect to the pulmonary veins.

Vascular Lesions. Elongation and tortuosity of the brachiocephalic artery is a common cause of mediastinal widening in older adults. This diagnosis is easily confirmed by US which can also exclude other masses of the superior mediastinum.

Mediastinal Masses. Thymic masses, substernal extension of thyroid enlargement, adenopathy, and other mediastinal masses are effectively demonstrated by US which can confirm their cystic or solid nature and vascularity. Lesions that can be visualized by US can usually have biopsies done on them using US guidance to avoid critical structures (10). Continuation of thyroid tissue into the mediastinum is a straight-forward diagnosis. Enlarged lymph nodes are usually homogeneous and hypoechoic. Confluent adenopathy due to lymphoma produces a solid, homogeneous, hypoechoic mass that encompasses and displaces blood vessels.

THYROID

Imaging of the thyroid gland is a controversial topic. Thyroid nodules are exceedingly common although thyroid cancer is uncommon and death from thyroid malignancy is rare (11–13). High resolution US is extremely sensitive in detecting thyroid nodules, however, imaging signs to differentiate benign from malignant lesions are nonspecific and unreliable. This creates a recurring clinical problem of what to do with the many nodules detected sonographically. Because of this difficulty, the indications for US of the thyroid are debated. US is used to precisely guide percutaneous biopsy of thyroid nodules, to screen patients at high risk for thyroid cancer, to identify recurrent disease in patients with known thyroid cancer, and to determine if palpable nodules arise from the thyroid gland. CT and MR supplement US by staging of invasive thyroid cancers, evaluating for postoperative recurrence of thyroid cancer, and demonstrating extension of goiter into the thorax. Radionuclide imaging, discussed in chapter 58, evaluates the physiological function of the gland and determines the activity of nodules.

Normal US Anatomy. The thyroid gland consists of paired lobes of near-equal size (5 × 2 × 2 cm) connected across the trachea by a thin thyroid isthmus (see Fig. 58.1). The thyroid parenchyma is homogeneous with fine medium-level echogenicity greater than muscle (Fig. 39.5). Anatomic landmarks include the midline air-filled trachea which casts an air shadow, the common carotid artery and internal jugular vein which parallel the lateral edge of the thyroid lobes, the longus colli muscles posteriorly, and the sternohyoid, sternothyroid, and sternocleidomastoid muscles anteriorly. Small pools of colloid (colloid cysts) are routinely visualized within the normal gland (Fig. 39.6). The thyroid lobes are often mildly asymmetric in size. The esophagus may protrude from behind the trachea on the left side and must not be mistaken for a thyroid or parathyroid mass or lymph node. The superior thyroid artery and vein are imaged between the upper pole of the thyroid and the longus colli. The recurrent laryngeal nerve and inferior thyroid artery and vein are seen posterior to the lower poles. The thyroid is easily imaged with the patient in a supine position with the neck extended by placement of a pillow beneath the shoulders.

Thyroid Nodules

The Problem. Thyroid nodules can be palpated in 4–7% of the general population and are found at autopsy in 50% of thyroid glands that are normal to palpation (14). High resolution US demonstrates thyroid nodules in 35–45% of asymptomatic adults, with a higher incidence of nodules in women (15–17). Thyroid cancer, on the other hand, affects only 0.1% of the population. Thyroid cancer is less than 1% of all cancer and is the cause of less than 0.5% of all cancer deaths. The ratio of benign thyroid nodules to thyroid cancer can be estimated at 500:1. The challenge of imaging studies and clinical evaluation is to establish the liklihood of malignancy and to select out for surgery only those patients with thyroid malignancy.

US is highly sensitive for the detection of thyroid nodules, however, its specificity for determining malignancy

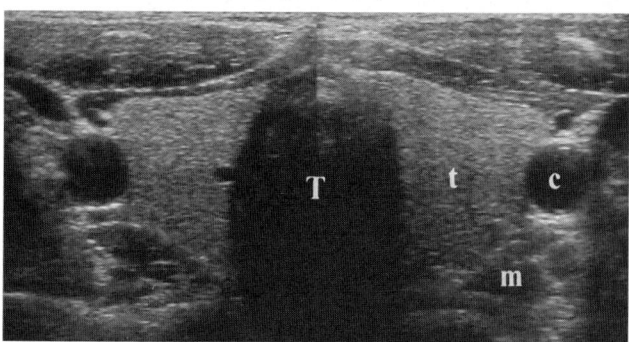

Figure 39.5. Normal Thyroid. Symmetric lobes of homogeneous thyroid tissue (*t*) are seen on either side of the trachea (*T*) on this transverse image. Anatomic landmarks include the carotid arteries (*c*) and longus colli muscle (*m*).

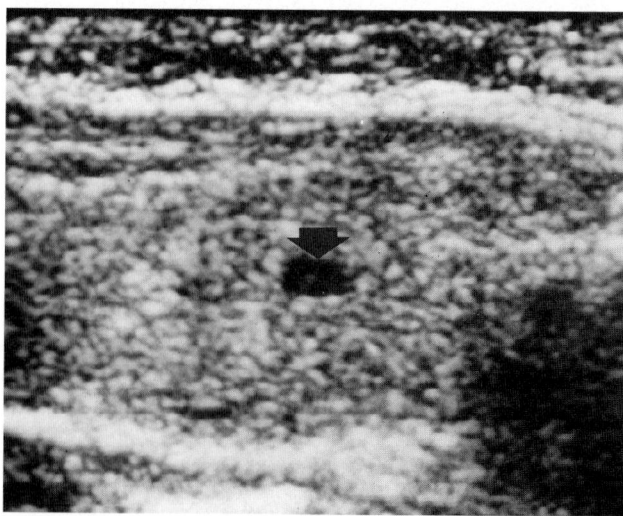

Figure 39.6. Colloid Cyst. Longitudinal US shows a colloid cyst (*arrow*) in the right lobe of the thyroid. Colloid cysts are small (<5 mm), well-defined, and of no clinical significance.

Table 39.1. Differentiation of Benign and Malignant Thyroid Nodules

Evidence Favoring Benign Nodule	Evidence Favoring Malignant Nodule	Indeterminate Evidence Found with Both Benign and Malignant Nodules
Extensive cystic component	Irregular contour	Hypoechoic nodule
Sharply defined margin	Poor margination	Isoechoic nodule
Peripheral calcification	Microcalcifications (25)	Solid nodule
Homogeneously hyperechoic	Size >4–5 cm	Amorphous dense calcification
Comet tail artifacts (26)	Single cold nodule on radionuclide scan (15% malignant)	Echolucent halo
Multiple nodules on radionuclide scan	Age <20 years	Multiple nodules on US
Hot on radionuclide scan	History of neck irradiation, especially in childhood	Increased flow on color Doppler US
	Family history of thyroid malignancy, especially medullary carcinoma	
	Male	

Table 39.2. Causes of Multiple Thyroid Nodules on US

Common
- Multinodular goiter
- Multiple benign adenomas
- Hashimoto thyroiditis (micronodules)(31)
- Subacute thyroiditis
- Chronic thyroiditis

Uncommon
- Carcinoma + benign adenomas
- Anaplastic carcinoma
- Lymphoma
- Acute thyroiditis

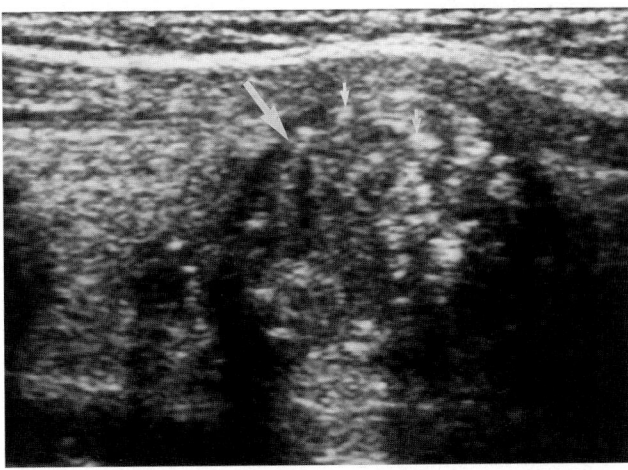

Figure 39.7. Papillary Carcinoma of the Thyroid. Longitudinal image reveals a solid nodule (*large arrow*) containing numerous microcalcifications (*small arrows*). The presence of microcalcifications in a thyroid nodule is highly indicative of malignancy. Biopsy proved papillary carcinoma.

is low. Neither MR nor CT can improve that specificity. This is not surprising because the histologic differentiation of benign follicular adenoma from well differentiated follicular carcinoma is based solely on identification of vascular invasion. Radionuclide imaging is far less sensitive than US in the demonstration of thyroid nodules. Although no signs are specific, multiple parameters can be used together to make a clinical judgement regarding risk of thyroid malignancy (Table 39.1). Nodules considered suspicious for malignancy should undergo fine needle aspiration biopsy (FNA) for diagnosis. US is a precise imaging method to guide FNA (18–20).

Although true thyroid cysts are extremely rare, many benign nodules demonstrate cystic degeneration. An extensive cystic component is strong evidence of benignancy. Most of these benign cystic lesions demonstrate internal debris and some degree of wall irregularity and solid components. This finding is not specific however. Although most thyroid cancers are solid masses, some have cystic areas within them. Radionuclide scans classify nodules as hypofunctioning ("cold")(see Fig. 58.4), hyperfunctioning ("hot")(see Fig. 58.5), or indeterminate. Single cold nodules have a 15% incidence of malignancy, and malignancy is exceedingly rare in hot nodules. If a radionuclide scan demonstrates multiple nodules, the risk of malignancy is about 1%. However, demonstration of multiple nodules by US is *not* a sign of benignancy (Table 39.2)(21). Papillary thyroid cancer is multicentric in 20% of cases, and benign nodules are found to coexist with thyroid cancer in 33% of cases undergoing

surgery (22). Most benign nodules and most thyroid cancers are hypoechoic relative to normal thyroid parenchyma. However, a nodule that is predominantly hyperechoic is very likely to be benign (23). Benign nodules tend to be well marginated and smooth in contour. Malignancies are usually poorly marginated and irregular in contour. However, many thyroid nodules violate these trends. An echolucent rim (see Fig. 58.4) is a sign of a slow growing nodule, but may be found with both benign and malignant nodules. Up to 20% of malignant nodules have a sonolucent peripheral halo (24). Calcifications are common in all thyroid nodules. Peripheral or eggshell calcification is highly characteristic of benign lesions whereas microcalcifications (small echodense particles usually without acoustic shadows)(Fig. 39.7) are strongly indicative of malignancy (25). Amorphous dense calcifications are found with both benign and malignant nodules. Comet tail artifacts, which arise from inspissated colloid, are a strong sign of a benign nodule (26). A history of neck irradiation, particularly in childhood, increases the risk of malignancy by 5–10 fold. Regression of nodule size following thyroid hormone therapy is a sign of a benign nodule. Color flow

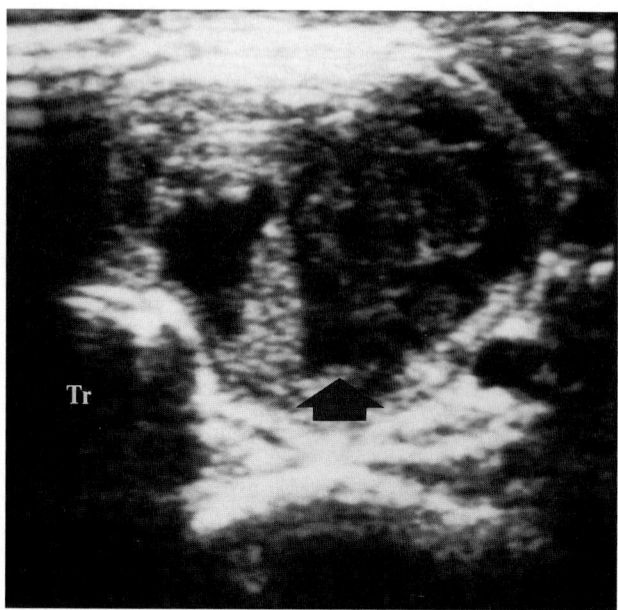

Figure 39.8. Degenerated Follicular Adenoma. Transverse US of the left lobe of the thyroid shows a well defined mass (*arrow*) with large irregular areas of cystic degeneration. Regressive changes are common in follicular adenomas and adenomatous nodules. *Tr*, trachea.

US is not helpful in the differentiation of benign and malignant thyroid nodules (27,28). Biopsy is indicated for all nodules with malignant features, and for nodules larger than 15 mm with indeterminate features. Nodules smaller than 15 mm can be followed by physical examination for evidence of enlargement.

BENIGN THYROID NODULES

Adenomatous Nodules, also called colloid nodules, are the most common thyroid nodule. They are not neoplasms but benign growths resulting from cycles of hyperplasia and involution of thyroid tissue. They are usually multiple, and associated with diffuse enlargement of the thyroid gland. Individual nodules are isoechoic or hypoechoic to thyroid parenchyma, and commonly show degenerative changes with prominent cystic components, necrosis, hemorrhage, and calcification.

Follicular Adenoma is the most common benign neoplasm. Autonomous hyperfunctioning adenomas are a cause of hyperthyroidism, but most adenomas cause no alteration of overall thyroid function. Most are solitary, solid, and well encapsulated. They may be hypoechoic, hyperechoic, or isoechoic to thyroid parenchyma. Hyperfunctioning adenomas are commonly strikingly hypervascular on color flow US. Degenerative changes (Fig. 39.8) include focal necrosis, hemorrhage, edema, infarction, fibrosis, and calcification.

Thyroid Cysts are extremely rare, epithelial-lined, simple cysts. Most cystic nodules found in the thyroid are actually cystic degeneration of an adenomatous nodule or a follicular adenoma.

Hemorrhage may occur into an adenomatous nodule or a follicular adenoma, or spontaneously into normal parenchyma. Patients present with sudden neck pain and subsequent swelling. US reveals a hypoechoic nodule with internal debris.

MALIGNANT THYROID NODULES

Papillary Thyroid Carcinoma (75% of thyroid cancer) is one of the least aggressive cancers in humans (29). Most patients are female (4:1). Nodules are hypoechoic and commonly multiple. Punctate internal calcification is common and highly indicative of malignancy (Fig. 39.7). Involved cervical nodes may contain similar calcifications. The tumor spreads commonly to regional nodes, but rarely (2–3% of cases) to lung and bone. Five-year survival is 95–99%.

Follicular Thyroid Carcinoma (10–15%) is also a slow growing malignancy, but invasion of blood vessels is characteristic with common hematogenous spread to lung and bone. Lymphatic spread to cervical nodes is uncommon. Most tumors are solitary, isoechoic, and ill-defined. Cystic areas, hemorrhage, and necrosis are common. Five-year survival is about 65%.

Medullary Thyroid Carcinoma (5%) is a neuroendocrine malignancy that arises from parafollicular C-cells that secrete calcitonin, which serves as a tumor marker. About 20% of cases are familial and associated with multiple endocrine neoplasia (MEN II). US appearance is similar to papillary carcinoma with coarse internal calcifications common (80%). Five-year survival is 65%.

Anaplastic Thyroid Carcinoma (<5%) is a lethal malignancy of the elderly (29). The tumor grows rapidly and metastasizes widely. US shows a ill-defined, inhomogenous, hypoechoic, solid mass. Five-year survival is less than 4%.

When using US, CT, or MR for initial staging of thyroid malignancy or follow-up for recurrence, one must consider the common routes of spread of the specific type of malignancy to optimally plan the imaging study. The impressive contrast resolution of MR makes it excellent for determining involvement of muscles, larynx, esophagus and other cervical structures by large invasive tumors. Recurrence of tumor may be demonstrated by MR. On T2WI, tumor has high signal intensity, brighter than muscle, and fibrosis in the thyroid bed has low signal intensity, less than or equal to muscle. Lymph node involvement is determined primarily by size criteria. Normal lymph nodes in the neck are less than 10 mm in diameter.

Lymphoma accounts for 4% of thyroid malignancy and is most common in elderly women (30). Most is of the non-Hodgkin's type. A solitary strikingly hypoechoic mass is most common although some cases demonstrate multiple nodules. Associated enlarged cervical nodes are common. Nearly all patients with primary thyroid lymphoma also have Hashimoto thyroiditis.

Metastasis. Metastatic disease to the thyroid gland is rare. The most common primary tumors to metastasize to the thyroid are breast, lung, kidney, and malignant melanoma.

Diffuse Thyroid Disease

The diagnosis of most diffuse diseases of the thyroid is made clinically and US is seldom indicated. US can be helpful when thyroid enlargement is asymmetric and a neoplasm is suspected.

Goiter is a general term that means diffuse thyroid enlargement. Goiter may be associated with increased, decreased, or normal thyroid function. The range of normal thyroid size is great. Thyroid enlargement is best judged subjectively. Helpful US signs of thyroid enlargement are thickening of the isthmus greater than 3 mm (Fig. 39.9) and outward bulge of the anterior surface of the gland. US measurement is useful in assessing and following thyroid gland size in determining response to therapy.

Nontoxic Goiter is caused by iodine deficiency, goitrogens in the diet, or deficiency of thyroid enzymes. US shows an enlarged gland with homogeneous parenchyma.

Adenomatous Goiter, also called multinodular goiter, affects about 5% of the population of the United States. Adenomatous hyperplasia is the cause of 80% of thyroid nodules. Adenomatous goiter refers to the generalized enlargement of the thyroid that occurs when multiple hyperplastic nodules are present. US shows coarsening and heterogeniety of the thyroid parenchyma with coarse calcifications commonly present. Each nodule must be individually evaluated for signs of malignancy.

Hashimoto Thyroiditis (chronic lymphocytic thyroiditis) is an autoimmune disease that affects primarily women. About 10–15% of patients are clinically hypothyroid. It is the most common cause of hypothyroidism and goiter in adults in the United States. Circulating antithyroid antibody is associated with diffuse lymphomatous infiltration of the gland. US demonstrates diffuse thyroid enlargement with inhomogeneous low density parenchyma (Fig. 39.10). No normal parenchyma is present. A pattern of multiple tiny nodules, 1–6 mm size, is highly indicative of the disease (31). Patients are at risk for development of lymphoma. Large hypoechoic nodules should be considered for biopsy (32).

Graves' Disease is the most common cause of hyperthyroidism. The gland is usually enlarged twofold to threefold, homogeneous, and without nodules (Fig. 51.3). Color Doppler US demonstrates striking diffuse increased vascularity with multiple small areas of intrathyroid flow, the "thyroid inferno" (33).

Subacute (Viral) Thyroiditis, also called De Quervain or granulomatous thyroiditis, presents with thyroid pain and hyperthyroidism following an upper respiratory infection. Iodine uptake is usually decreased or absent in the acute stages. The disease runs a subacute course of a few weeks to a few months. Affected portions of the gland are swollen, edematous, and hypoechoic on US (34).

Acute Suppurative Thyroiditis is rare bacterial infection of the thyroid gland. Often only a portion of the gland is involved. US is helpful in the detection and aspiration of abscesses.

Riedel's Thyroiditis is a rare inflammatory disease of progressive fibrosis that eventually destroys the thyroid

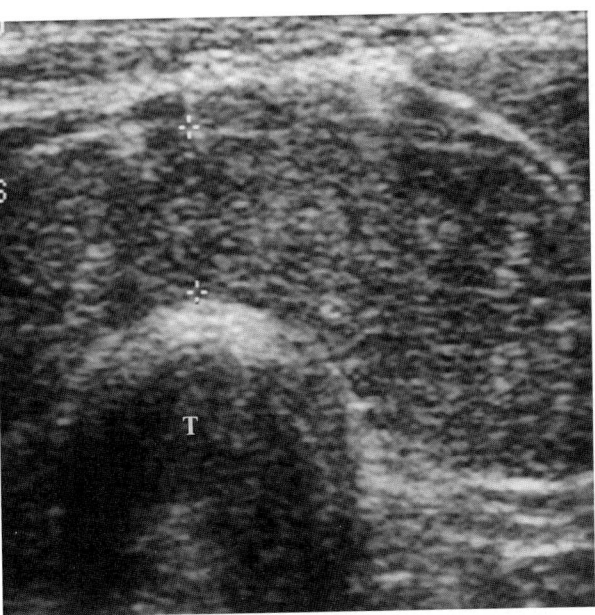

Figure 39.9. Goiter. Transverse image shows thickening of the thyroid isthmus to 12 mm (between *cursors*). *T,* trachea.

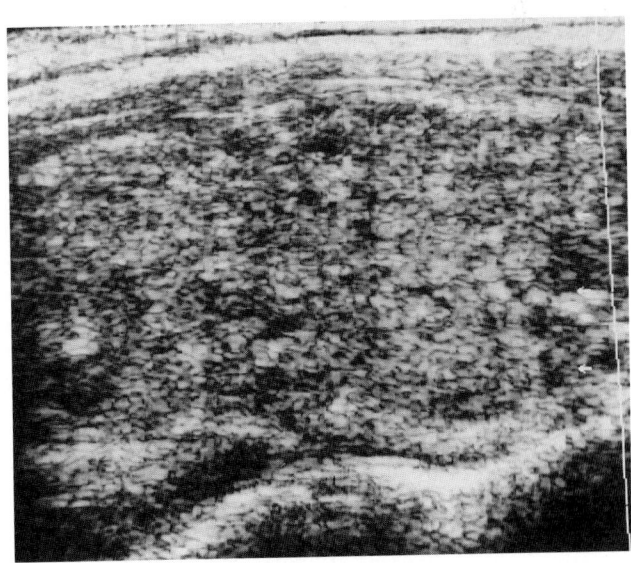

Figure 39.10. Hashimoto Thyroiditis. Longitudinal image through one lobe of the thyroid shows heterogeneous parenchyma without discrete nodules.

gland and commonly extends into the neck. The gland is diffusely enlarged and inhomogeneous. US is used to show extension into the neck with encasement of cervical blood vessels.

PARATHYROID

Imaging of the parathyroid glands is another controversial topic (35). The primary indication is preoperative localization of parathyroid adenomas or hyperplastic parathyroid glands in the setting of clinically diagnosed

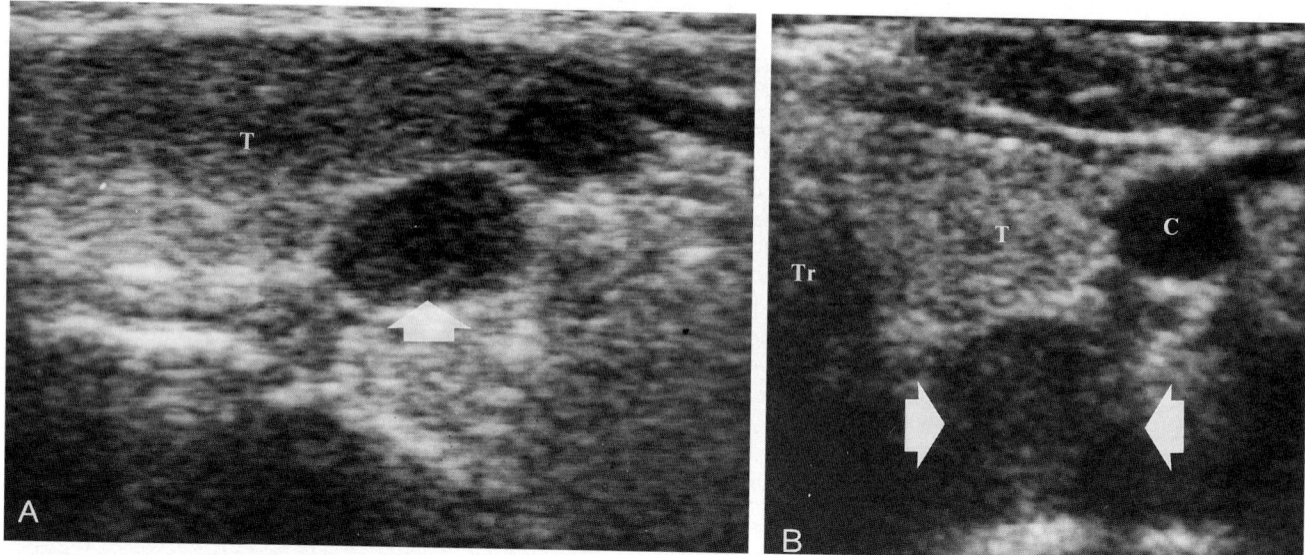

Figure 39.11. Parathyroid Adenoma. Longitudinal **(A)** and transverse **(B)** US images demonstrate a parathyroid adenoma (*arrows*) at the lower pole of the left thyroid lobe. *T*, thyroid; *Tr*, trachea; *C*, common carotid artery.

hyperparathyroidism. Preoperative localization makes resection easier and reduces surgical morbidity. Preoperative imaging is particularly useful in patients with previous neck surgery. US, CT, MR, and radionuclide imaging have all been used in this setting. Of these, radionuclide imaging is the most sensitive and accurate (see chapter 58)(36). However, because 80–85% of abnormal parathyroid glands are located in the neck, US is able to demonstrate the majority. Imaging has no role in hypoparathyroidism.

Normal US Anatomy. Normal parathyroid glands measure only 5 × 3 × 1 mm in size, and are not usually demonstrated by any imaging method. Most enlarged glands are found beneath the thyroid lobes between the trachea and carotid sheath (see Fig. 58.1). Ectopic glands may be found between the upper pole of the thyroid and the thymus.

Hyperparathyroidism

Primary hyperparathyroidism is a common disease that affects women two to three times more commonly than men. More than half the patients are above age 50. A single benign hyperfunctioning adenoma is the cause in 85% of cases (see Table 58.4). Multiple gland enlargement is responsible for 14% and parathyroid carcinoma is the cause of 1%. Most cases of hyperplasia involve all glands, although usually asymmetrically. The diagnosis is suspected on the basis of unexplained hypercalcemia and is confirmed by elevated serum parathyroid hormone level. In secondary and tertiary hyperparathyroidism, elevated parathormone levels are caused by diffuse or nodular glandular hyperplasia. Secondary hyperparathyroidism occurs as a result of chronic hypocalcemia in patients with chronic renal failure. The parathyroid glands are overstimulated and become hyperplastic. When the chonically overstimulated glands become autonomous, the term tertiary hyperparathyroidism is used. Parathormone may also be produced by non-endocrine tumors such as renal cell and bronchogenic carcinoma.

Parathyroid Adenomas appear as homogeneous, hypoechoic, solid, oval, and well-defined masses, 8–15 mm in size (Fig. 39.11). Color Doppler demonstrates hypervascularity. On MR T1WI, adenomas show low intensity similar to muscle. On T2WI, the adenomas showed high intensity similar to or greater than fat. Because adenomas may be isointense with fat, T2WI alone provide an incomplete examination. CT is best performed with intravenous contrast to demonstrate the contrast enhancing parathyroid nodules.

Rarely, parathyroid adenomas may show cystic degeneration or calcification. Thyroid nodules may appear similar to parathyroid adenomas on US although degenerated parathyroid adenomas may mimic cystic thyroid masses. US may be used to guide needle biopsy. Cells of parathyroid origin can be readily differentiated from thyroid cells cytologically although fluid aspirated from degenerated parathyroid nodules have high parathyroid hormone levels (37).

Parathyroid Hyperplasia affects all the parathyroid glands but the degree of enlargement is frequently asymmetric. Hyperplastic glands have the same imaging characteristics as parathyroid adenomas.

Parathyroid Carcinoma is distinguished by larger size (>20 mm) than parathyroid adenomas. Tumors are usually more heterogenous with cystic degeneration and occasional calcification. The contour is lobulated or ill-defined. Color flow US is useful to demonstration invasion of adjacent vessels or muscle. The diagnosis is most commonly confirmed at surgical resection.

Ectopic Parathyroids are best localized by radionuclide imaging. CT (Fig. 39.12) or MR is usually needed to show the anatomic relationships when they are located in the mediastinum.

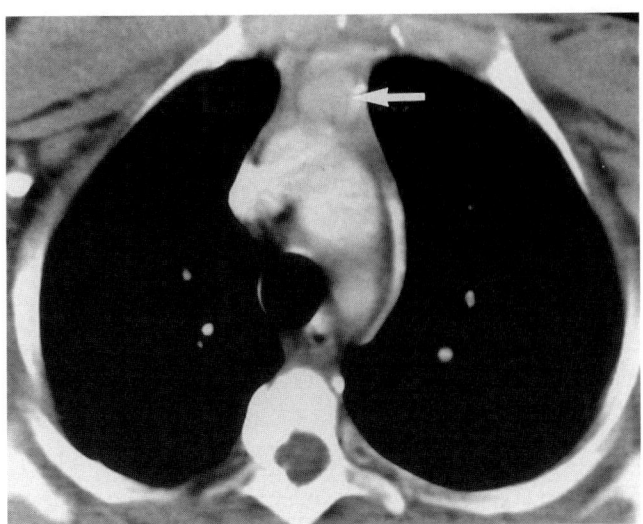

Figure 39.12. Ectopic Parathyroid Adenoma. Contrast-enhanced CT of the chest confirms the presence of an ectopic parathyroid adenoma (*arrow*) in the mediastinum just anterior to the top of the aortic arch.

NEONATAL BRAIN

Sonography of the neonatal brain has become an integral part of the care of the neonate, allowing detailed evaluation of intracranial structures to be performed at the infant's bedside. The standard examination is relatively simple to perform, takes only a few minutes, and requires no sedation. The fact that the examination can be performed portably in the nursery where the infant can be kept warm and well-monitored offers great advantage over CT and MR brain imaging. Indications for neonatal head US include: detection and confirmation of congenital brain abnormalities, detection and follow-up of hydrocephalus and other sequelae of infection, and evaluation for brain injury due to hypoxia.

Normal US Anatomy. Routine cranial sonograms are performed through the anterior fontanelle. The anterior fontanelle remains open until about 2 years of age, but examinations may be difficult after 12–14 months of age because of its smaller size. Standard views are taken in coronal and sagittal planes, and are frequently supplemented by views in the axial plane, or through the posterior fontanelle, open sutures, or the foramen magnum.

Examinations are performed at bedside keeping the infant warm, covered and monitored in the isolette. The infant is positioned to optimize access to the anterior fontanelle. High frequency 5 and 7.5 MHz sector transducers with a wide angle of view are preferred. The transducer is thoroughly cleansed with alcohol between each patient. In coronal plane the brain is examined from anterior to the frontal horns to the occipital cortex. Standard views are recorded through the frontal horns, third ventricle, and trigone (Fig. 39.13). Sagittal views include midline and parasagittal scans obtained 10° laterally through the frontal horns and bodies of the lateral ventricles and 20° laterally through the temporal horns (Fig. 39.14). Axial views (Fig. 39.15) through the thin squama of the temporal bone provide excellent demonstration of the third ventricle, the cortex abutting the inside of the cranium, and the circle of Willis for Doppler studies. Key anatomic landmarks to be indentified on every cranial US include: the lateral, third, and fourth ventricles; cavum septum pellucidum/cavum vergae; corpus callosum; choroid plexus in the temporal horn, atrium, and body of the lateral ventricles and in the roof of the third ventricle; cerebellar vermis; caudate nucleus, thalamus and caudothalamic groove. These structures are illustrated in Figures 39.13 to 39.15. The posterior fontanelle and foramen magnum can be effectively used as windows to the posterior fossa.

Congenital Brain Abnormalities

Congenital brain abnormalities are among the most common human malformations. Obstetric US has progressed to the point that most brain abnormalities can be detected or suspected in utero. Anomalies of the face, head, or other organ systems in the newborn suggest possible brain anomalies. Cranial US in the neonate can be used in these settings to confirm suspected abnormalities. Discussions of the classifications and findings of various brain malformations are provided in chapters 8 and 38.

Infection

Meningitis occurs as a result of hematogenous spread of bacteria from respiratory infections, or direct spread from ear or sinus infections. *Hemophilus influenza*, *Escherichia coli*, and group B streptococcus are the most common causative organisms. Bacteria in the subarachnoid space cause inflammation of the pia and arachnoid. US findings (Fig. 39.16) in meningitis include: *a*) echogenic sulci; *b*) echogenic debris in the ventricles; *c*) enlarged ventricles, often due to obstruction by inflammatory exudate; *d*) increased echogenicity and shaggy thickening of the ependyma; and *e*) transient extraaxial fluid collections. US may be used to detect complications including persistent hydrocephalus, abnormal parenchymal echogenicity representing infarction or cerebritis, and brain abscess.

TORCH organisms cause congenital infections affecting the central nervous system. TORCH refers to **T**oxoplasma gondii, **o**ther conditions including syphilis, **r**ubella, **c**ytomegalovirus (CMV), and **h**erpes simplex type 2. Congenital CMV infection is the most common and may cause severe brain destruction. Necrotizing periventricular infection causes periventricular calcification, subependymal cysts, and microcephaly. Toxoplasmosis causes scattered brain calcifications especially in the basal ganglia, multicystic encephalopathy, and porencephaly. Herpes causes cystic periventricular encephalomalacia, hemorrhagic infarction, and scattered brain calcifications, as well as retinal dysplasia. Rubella uncommonly causes recognizable brain injury, but microcephaly, vasculopathy, and massive calcification have been reported.

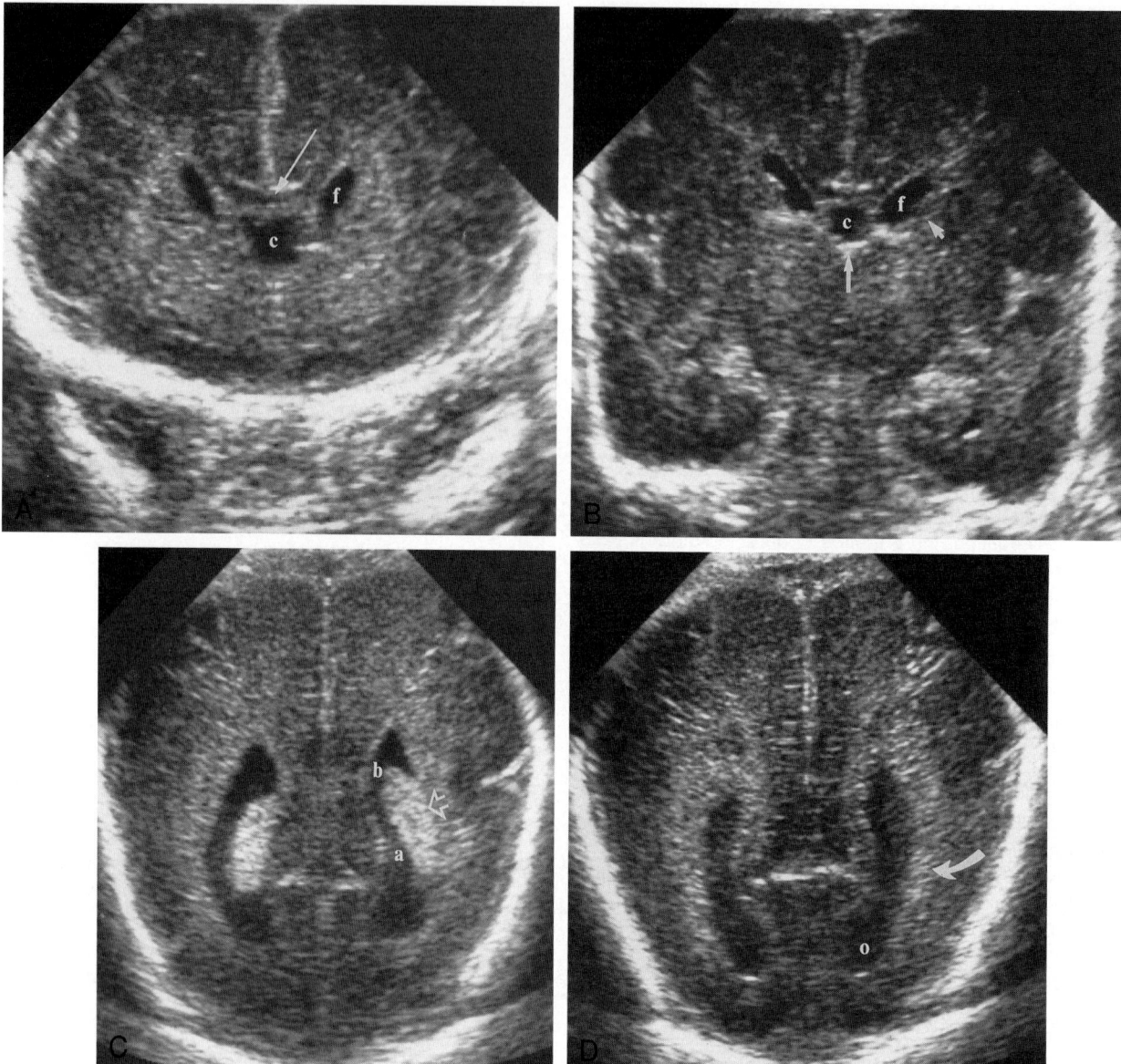

Figure 39.13. Normal Cranial US: Coronal Plane. The normal brain of a 29-week premature infant is imaged through the anterior fontanelle. **A.** Anterior image shows frontal horns of the lateral ventricles (*f*), cavum septum pellucidum (*c*), and corpus callosum (*long arrow*). **B.** Midline image shows choroid plexus in the roof of the 3rd ventricle (*short arrow*), cavum septum pellucidum (*c*), frontal horns of the lateral ventricle (*f*), and caudate nucleus (*arrowhead*).

C. Posterior image through the body (*b*) and atria (*a*) (trigone) of the lateral ventricles demonstrates the choroid plexus (*open arrow*) which lays dependently against the down (left) side of the ventricles. **D.** More posteriorly angled image shows the occipital horns (*o*) of the lateral ventricles and the moderately echogenic normal periventricular white matter (*curved arrow*).

Ischemic Brain Injury

Premature infants, born at less than 34 weeks gestational age or with birth weight less than 1500 grams, are extremely susceptible to ischemic brain injury. Subependymal hemorrage in the residual germinal matrix and periventricular leukomalacia are the two most common forms of hypoxic brain injury in premature infants (38). They are responsible for a 5–15% incidence of cerebral palsy (spastic motor deficits) and a 25–50% incidence of cognitive disabilities in surviving premature infants. Cranial sonograms are routinely performed on premature infants to detect these brain injuries and to monitor for treatable complications.

Germinal Matrix is a fragile gelatinous mass of tissue found in the fetal brain between the ependyma lining the ventricles and the caudate nucleus. The germinal matrix is highly vascular and is a major source of hemorrhage when it becomes ischemic. The germinal matrix is the source of neuroblasts and spongioblasts which migrate to the brain surface to form the glial cells of the cortex. The germinal matrix involutes by 32 weeks of gestational

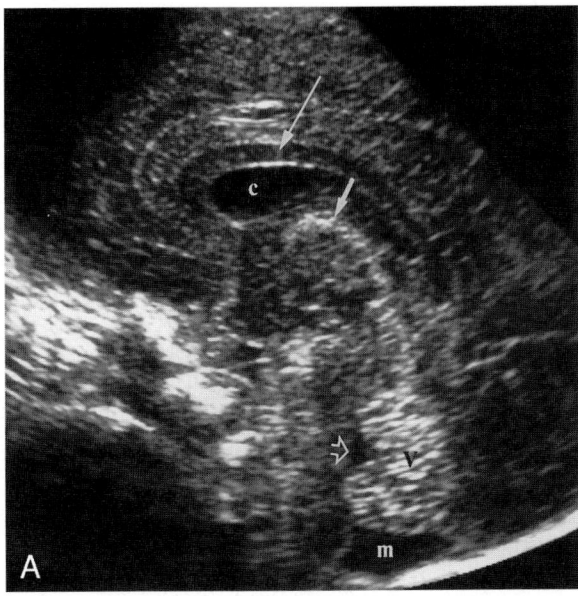
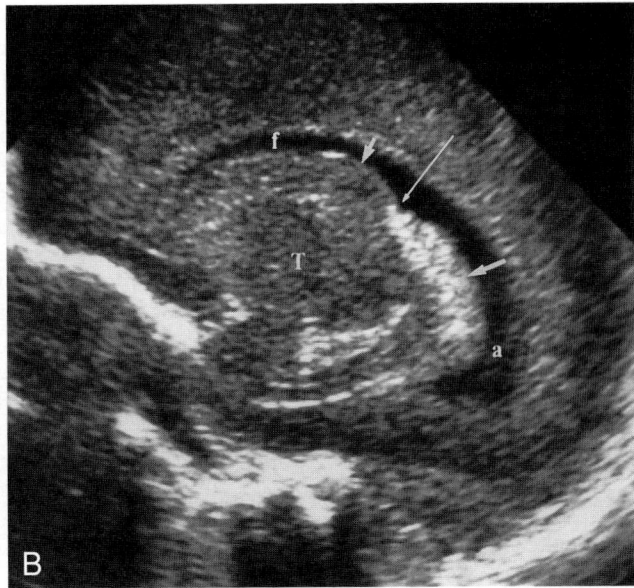

Figure 39.14. Normal Cranial US: Sagittal Plane. A. Midline image shows the corpus callosum (*long arrow*), cavum septum pellucidum (*c*), echogenic choroid plexus in the roof of the 3rd ventricle (*short arrow*), echogenic cerebellar vermis (*V*), the 4th ventricle (*open ar-* row), and the cisterna magna (*m*). **B.** Laterally angled image shows the frontal horn (*f*) and atrium (*a*) of the lateral ventricle, the caudate nucleus (*arrowhead*), caudothalamic groove (*long arrow*), choroid plexus (*short arrow*) and thalamus (*T*).

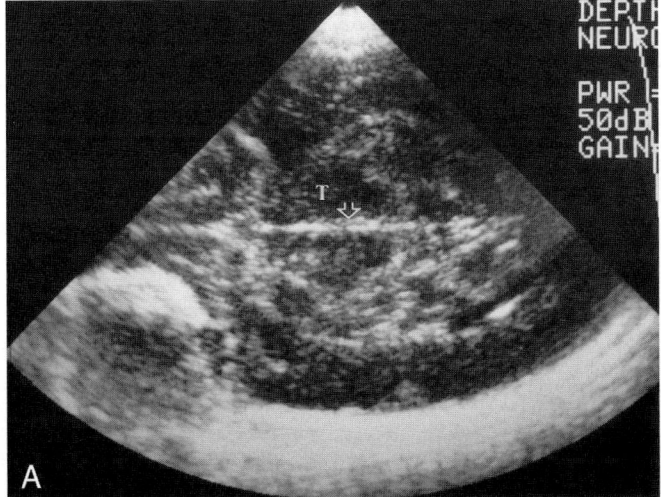
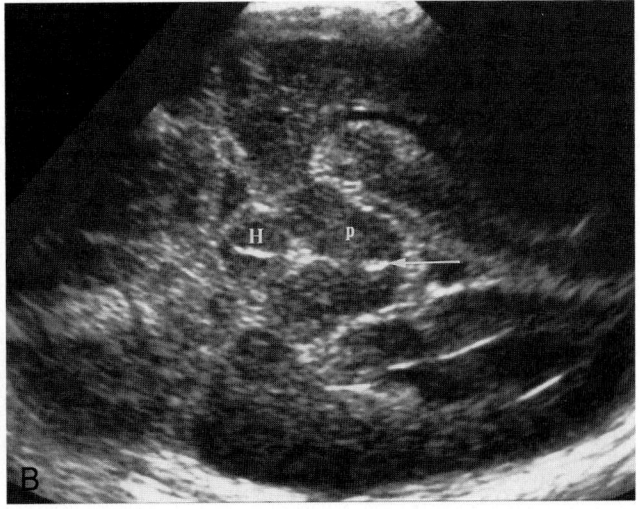

Figure 39.15. Normal Cranial US: Axial Plane. A. Image shows the walnut-shaped thalamus (*T*) which contains the 3rd ventricle (*open arrow*). **B.** Image at a slightly lower level shows the hypothalamus (*H*) and heart-shaped cerebral peduncles (*p*). The aqueduct of Sylvius is seen as an echogenic dot (*arrow*) posteriorly. The circle of Willis surrounds the hypothalamus in the suprasellar cistern.

age, so only premature infants are susceptible to germinal matrix hemorrage.

Germinal Matrix Hemorrhage (GMH), also called subenpendymal or intraventricular hemorrhage, occurs in the residual germinal matrix overlying the frontal horn and body of the lateral ventricles. The incidence is reported at 30–55% in infants born at 24–32 weeks gestation. Most hemorrhages originate in the region of the caudothalamic groove (Fig. 39.17) where the germinal matrix is most prominent in the premature infant. The hemorrhage may remain confined but commonly rup- tures into the ventricle resulting in intraventricular hemorrhage, ependymitis, and hydrocephalus. Most (97%) GMH occurs in the first week after birth. Ventriculomegaly develops in the first two weeks after hemorrhage and may persist for 3–6 months.

US demonstrates confined subependymal hemorrhage as a focus of bright echogenicity anterior to caudothalamic groove (Fig. 39.17). On coronal views the echogenic clot is at the floor of the frontal horn, obscuring the caudate nucleus. Hemorrhage into the ventricle is seen as echogenic clots in an enlarging ventricle. Hemorrhage frequently has the same echogenicity as the choroid plexus. Hemorrhage is differentiated from choroid plexus by location and appearance. Because no choroid plexus is present in the frontal and occipital horns of the lateral ventricles, any echogenic foci in these locations likely represent hemorrhage. Asymmetric enlargement of the choroid plexus is suspicious for hemorrhage. Parenchymal hematomas (Fig. 39.18) result from hemorrhagic infarction caused by obstruction of the

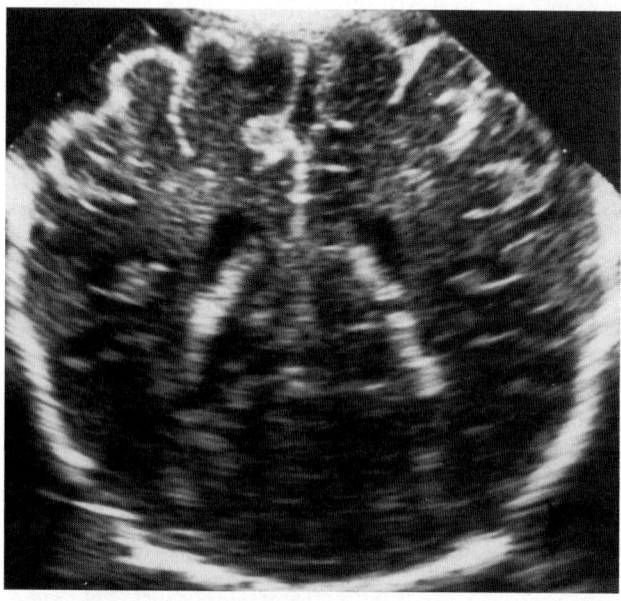

Figure 39.16. Meningitis. Coronal plane US shows marked increased echogenicity of the gyri and sulci associated with diffuse brain atrophy and increased extraaxial fluid space.

medullary veins by the germinal matrix hemorrhage. A commonly used grading system for classifying the severity of hemorrhage is described in Table 39.3. The sonographic appearance of hematomas follows a predictable evolution. The hematoma is initially densely echogenic, then becomes progressively echolucent centrally as it shrinks. Clots in the ventricles characteristically maintain an echogenic rim. Eventually the clots resolve completely. Cellular debris from the hemorrhage is seen as echogenic material floating within the intraventricular cerebrospinal fluid.

Hydrocephalus is a common sequelae of GMH. Hydrocephalus may result from obstruction of cerebrospinal fluid pathways by clot, organizing ependimitis, or arachnoid granulation obstruction. Spastic paralysis results from injury to the corticospinal tracts as they course in close proximity to the site of hemorrhage. Cognitive defects and learning disorders may also result from the brain injury.

Periventricular Leukomalacia refers to lesions caused by hypoxic injury in the periventricular white matter. The periventricular white matter, at the angles of the lateral ventricles, is in a watershed zone between the arterial blood supply of the basal ganglia and the immature arterial supply to the cerebral cortex. After 34 weeks gestational age, maturation of cerebral arterial supply moves the watershed zones from the periventricular area to the cortex between cerebral arteries territories. Hypoxia in the premature infant may cause infarction of the periventricular white matter, followed by necrosis, cyst formation, and gliosis. This injury results from arterial infarction, whereas the parenchymal injury from GMH results from venous infarction. The initial injury is usually not detected by US unless the damaged area of brain becomes echogenic due to hemorrhage. In this

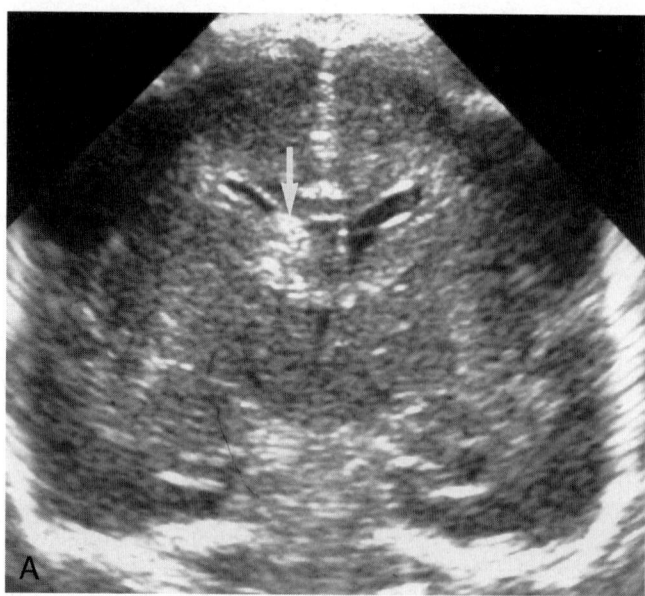
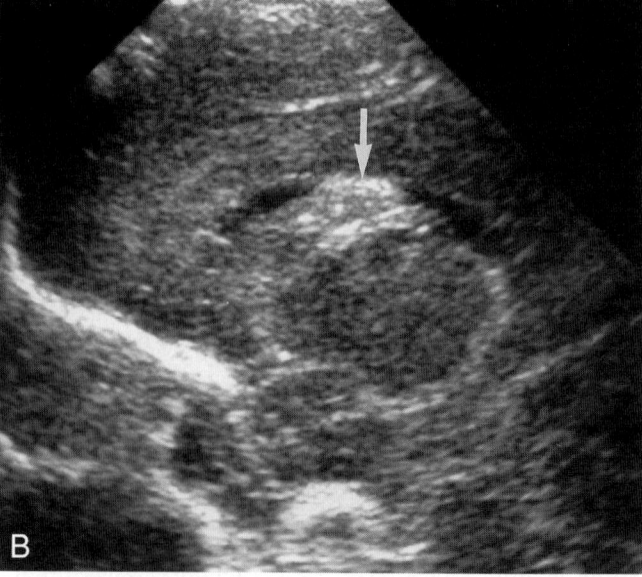

Figure 39.17. Grade I Germinal Matrix Hemorrhage. Coronal **(A)** and angled sagittal **(B)** plane images show abnormal echogenicity (*arrows*) overlying the caudate nucleus indicating germinal matrix hemorrhage.

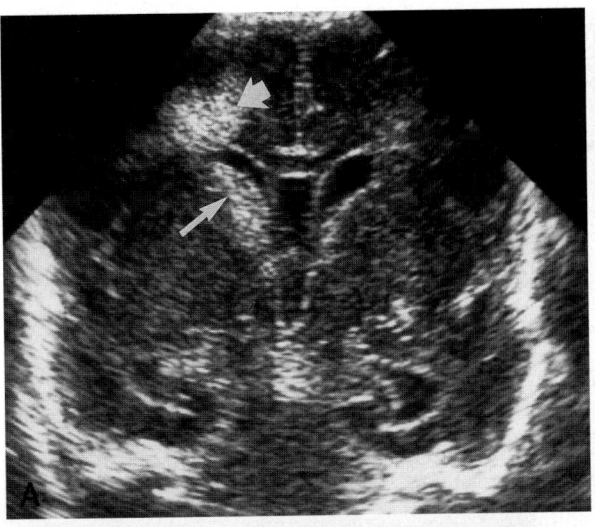

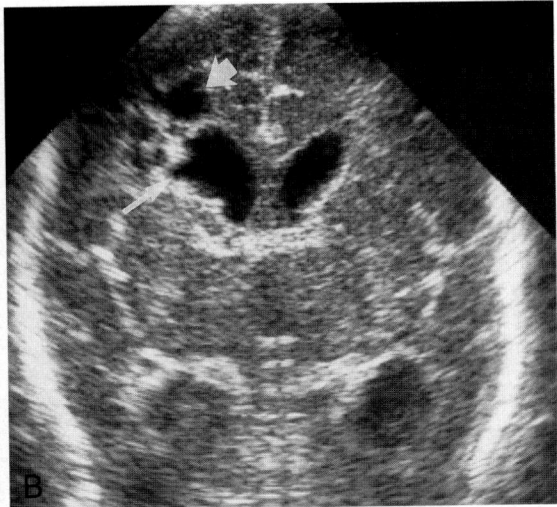

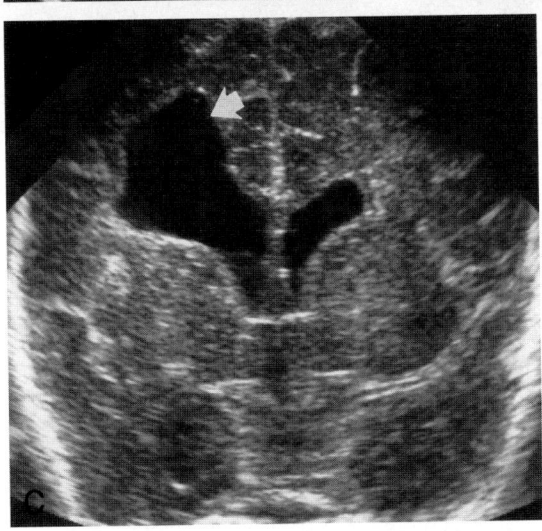

Figure 39.18. Grade 4 Germinal Matrix Hemorrhage Resulting in Porencephaly. A. Coronal brain image on the second day of life for a premature infant shows hemorrhage in the caudate nucleus (*long arrow*) and in the periventricular brain parenchyma (*short arrow*). **B.** Image obtained one month later shows small area of porencephaly extending into the caudate nucleus (*long arrow*) and focus of cystic encephalomalacia in the brain parenchyma (*short arrow*). The ventricles are enlarged. **C.** Follow-up image obtained at 15 weeks of age shows large area of brain destruction resulting in porencephaly (*short arrow*).

Table 39.3. Classification of Germinal Matrix Hemorrhage

Grade	Description
1	Small hemorrhage confined to germinal matrix.
2	Small hemorrhage with extension into lateral ventricles. Ventricles may dilate transiently but are not filled with blood.
3	Large hemorrhage that fills and dilates the ventricles with blood.
4	Intraparenchymal hemorrhagic venous infarction caused by obstruction of the medullary veins draining the periventricular white matter.

case, US (Fig. 39.19) demonstrates foci of increased echogenicity in the periventricular white matter at the lateral angles of the lateral ventricles. This finding resolves in 2–4 weeks when periventricular cysts may be visualized. Within 2–4 months, these cysts may enlarge, coalesce and form porencephalic cysts, resolve completely, or result in ventriculomegaly due to brain atrophy.

Diffuse Cerebral Edema may result from profound cerebral ischemia in premature or full-term infants. US signs of diffuse cerebral edema include: decreased visibility of the sulci and gyri, slit-like ventricles, and diffuse increased parenchymal echogenicity. Severe hypoxia may cause cystic areas of brain destruction and diffuse brain atrophy resulting in microcephaly, and severe motor and mental impairment. Slit-like lateral ventricles as an isolated finding is a common normal variant in premature infants (39). Other, often subtle, signs of cerebral edema must be present before the diagnosis can be made sonographically. CT and MR are more sensitive than US for evidence of diffuse hypoxic injury in infants.

Neurodevelopmental Deficits are caused by the brain parenchymal injury due to GMH, PVL, or diffuse hypoxia. Spastic diplegia or quadriplegia are caused by injury to the corticospinal tracts. Developmental delay, learning disabilities and mild mental retardation also occur. Severe mental retardation is uncommon. More severe long-term prognosis is associated with Grade 3 and Grade 4 GMH, persistence of ventriculomegaly, large parenchymal cysts and brain atrophy (40).

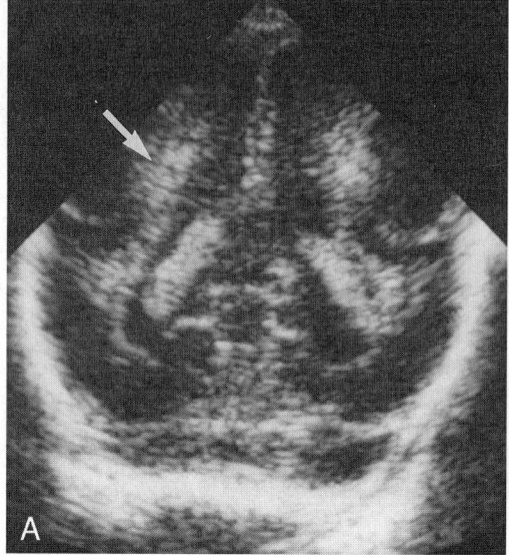
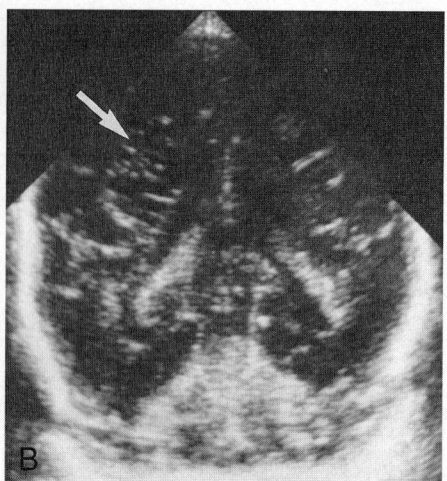

Figure 39.19. Periventricular Leukomalacia. A. US obtained a few hours after an episode of severe hypoxia in a premature infant shows increased echogenicity (*arrow*) in the periventricular white matter bilaterally. **B.** Follow-up US one month later shows the characteristic periventricular cysts (*arrow*) resulting from white matter necrosis.

References

1. Brant WE. The Thorax. In: Rumack CM, Wilson SR, Charboneau JW, eds. Diagnostic Ultrasound. 2nd ed. St. Louis: Mosby, 1998:575–597.
2. Brant WE. Chest. In: McGahan JP, Goldberg BB, eds. Diagnostic Ultrasound—A Logical Approach. Philadelphia: Lippincott-Raven, 1998:1063–1086.
3. Wernecke K. Sonographic features of pleural disease. AJR Am J Roentgenol 1997;168:1061–1066.
4. Yang PC, Luh KT, Chang DB, et al. Value of sonography in determining the nature of pleural effusion: analysis of 320 cases. AJR Am J Roentgenol 1992;159:29–33.
5. Klein JS, Schultz S, Heffner JE. Interventional radiology of the chest: image-guided percutaneous drainage of pleural effusions, lung abscesses, and pneumothorax. AJR Am J Roentgenol 1995;164:581–588.
6. Görg C, Schwerk WB, Görg K, Walters E. Pleural effusion: an "acoustic window" for sonography of pleural metastases. J Clin Ultrasound 1991;19:93–97.
7. Targhetta R, Chavagneux R, Bourgeois JM, et al. Sonographic approach to diagnosing pulmonary consolidation. J Ultrasound Med 1992;11:667–672.
8. Targhetta R, Bourgeois JM, Marty-Double C, et al. Peripheral pulmonary lesions: ultrasonic features and ultrasonically guided fine needle aspiration biopsy. J Ultrasound Med 1993;12:369–374.
9. Wernecke K, Pötter R, Peters PE, et al. Parasternal mediastinal sonography: sensitivity in the detection of anterior mediastinal and subcarinal tumors. AJR Am J Roentgenol 1988;150:1021–1026.
10. Rubens DJ, Strang JG, Fultz PJ, Gottlieb RH. Sonographic guidance of mediastinal biopsy: an effective alternative to CT guidance. AJR Am J Roentgenol 1997;169:1605–1610.
11. Brander A, Viikinkoski P, Nickels J, Kivisaari L. Thyroid gland: US screening in a random adult population. Radiology 1991;181:683–687.
12. Gagel RF, Goepfert H, Callender DL. Changing concepts in the pathogenesis and management of thyroid carcinoma. CA Cancer J Clin 1996;46:261–283.
13. Brander A, Viikinkoski P, Tuuhea J, et al. Clinical versus ultrasound examination of the thyroid gland in common clinical practice. J Clin Ultrasound 1992;20:37–42.
14. Rojeski MT, Gharib H. Nodular thyroid disease. N Engl J Med 1985;313:428–436.
15. James EM, Charboneau JW. High frequency (10 MHz) thyroid ultrasonography. Semin US CT MR 1985;6:294–304.
16. Brander A, Viikinkoski P, Nickels J, Kivisaari L. Thyroid gland: US screening in middle-aged women with no previous thyroid disease. Radiology 1989;173:507–510.
17. Bruneton JN, Balu-Maestro C, Marcy PY, et al. Very high frequency (13 MHz) ultrasonographic examination of the normal neck: detection of normal lymph nodes and thyroid nodules. J Ultrasound Med 1994;13:87–90.
18. Takashima S, Fukuda H, Kobayashi T. Thyroid nodules: clinical effect of ultrasound-guided fine-needle aspiration biopsy. J Clin Ultrasound 1994;22:535–542.
19. Lin J-D, Huang B-Y, Weng H-F, et al. Thyroid ultrasonography with fine-needle aspiration cytology for the diagnosis of thyroid cancer. J Clin Ultrasound 1997;25:111–118.
20. Boland GW, Lee MJ, Mueller PR, et al. Efficacy of sonographically guided biopsy of thyroid masses and cervical lymph nodes. AJR Am J Roentgenol 1993;161:1053–1056.
21. Brkljacic B, Cuk V, Tomic-Brzac H, et al. Ultrasonic evaluation of benign and malignant nodules in echographically multinodular thyroids. J Clin Ultrasound 1994;22:71–76.
22. Hay ID. Papillary thyroid carcinoma. Endocrinol Metab Clin North Am 1990;19:545–576.
23. Solbiati L, Voterrani L, Rizzatto G, et al. The thyroid gland with low uptake lesions: evaluation by ultrasound. Radiology 1985;155:187–191.
24. Propper RA, Skolnick ML, Weinstein BJ, et al. The nonspecificity of the thyroid halo sign. J Clin Ultrasound 1980; 8:129–132.
25. Takashima S, Fukuda H, Nomura N, et al. Thyroid nodules: re-evaluation with ultrasound. J Clin Ultrasound 1995;23: 179–184.
26. Ahuja A, King W, Metreweli C. Clinical significance of the comet-tail artifact in thyroid ultrasound. J Clin Ultrasound 1996;24:129–133.

27. Clark KJ, Cronan JJ, Scola FH. Color Doppler sonography: anatomic and physiologic assessment of the thyroid. J Clin Ultrasound 1995;23:215–223.

28. Shimamoto K, Endo T, Ishigaki T, et al. Thyroid nodules: evaluation with color Doppler ultrasonography. J Ultrasound Med 1993;12:673–678.

29. Wells SA Jr. Recent advances in the treatment of thyroid carcinoma. CA Cancer J Clin 1996;46:258–260.

30. Takashima S, Morimoto S, Ikezoe J, et al. Primary thyroid lymphoma: comparison of CT and US assessment. Radiology 1989;171:439–443.

31. Yeh H-C, Futterweit W, Gilbert P. Micronodulaton: ultrasonographic sign of Hashimoto thyroiditis. J Ultrasound Med 1996;15:813–819.

32. Takashima S, Matsuzuka F, Nagareda T, et al. Thyroid nodules associated with Hashimoto thyroiditis: assessment with US. Radiology 1992;185:125–130.

33. Ralls PW, Mayekawa DS, Lee KP, et al. Color-flow Doppler sonography in Graves disease: "thyroid inferno." AJR Am J Roentgenol 1988;150:781–784.

34. Tokuda Y, Kasagi K, Iida Y, et al. Sonography of subacute thyroiditis: changes in the findings during the course of the disease. J Clin Ultrasound 1990;18:21–26.

35. Udelsman R. Parathyroid imaging: the myth and the reality. Radiology 1996;201:317–318.

36. Gordon BM, Gordon L, Hoang K, Spicer KM. Parathyroid imaging with 99m-Tc-sestamibi. AJR Am J Roentgenol 1996;167:1563–1568.

37. Sacks BA, Pallotta JA, Cole A, Hurwitz J. Diagnosis of parathyroid adenomas: efficacy of measuring parathormone levels in needle aspirates of cervical masses. AJR Am J Roentgenol 1994;163:1223–1226.

38. Volpe JJ. Current concepts of brain injury in the premature infant. AJR Am J Roentgenol 1989;153:243–251.

39. Patel MD, Cheng AG, Callen PW. Lateral ventricular effacement as an isolated sonographic finding in premature infants: prevalence and significance. AJR Am J Roentgenol 1995;165:155–159.

40. Roth SC, Baudin J, McCormick DC, et al. Relation between ultrasound appearance of the brain of very preterm infants and neurodevelopmental impairment at eight years. Developmental Medicine and Child Neurology 1993;35:755–768.

40
Vascular Ultrasound

Raymond S. Dougherty
William E. Brant

Spectral Doppler US and color flow vascular imaging supplement gray-scale US by identifying blood vessels, confirming the presence of blood flow and its direction, detecting vessel stenosis and occlusion, assessing the perfusion of organs and tumors, and characterizing blood flow dynamics to detect physiological abnormalities (1). This chapter reviews the basics of vascular US examination and Doppler interpretation.

DOPPLER BASICS

Understanding the Doppler Spectrum

Doppler Effect refers to the change in the frequency of sound waves that occurs because of motion of a sound source, a sound reflector, or a sound receiver (2–5). Johann Doppler of Salzburg, Austria described this phenomenon in 1842. In medical diagnosis, the Doppler effect is used to confirm blood flow by detecting the change in frequency of US waves that occurs when sound is reflected from moving clumps of red blood cells (RBCs). The echoes reflected from RBCs are very weak, having a signal intensity up to 10,000 times less than that of contiguous soft tissue; thus, Doppler US instruments require a high sensitivity to weak signals and instrument settings must be routinely optimized.

Doppler Shift is the change in frequency between the US waves emitted by the transducer and the US waves returning to the transducer after reflection from moving RBCs (Fig. 40.1). This shift in sound frequency results from the Doppler effect. The reflected sound frequency increases when blood flow direction is toward the Doppler signal and decreases when the direction is away from the Doppler signal. An increase in frequency is termed a positive Doppler shift; the sound waves are compressed by encountering RBCs moving toward the sound source. A decrease in frequency is termed a negative Doppler shift as the reflected sound waves are stretched by RBCs moving away from the sound source. The presence of a Doppler shift within a blood vessel confirms the presence of blood flow. The direction of the Doppler shift toward a higher or lower frequency indicates the direction of blood flow. Doppler shift frequencies are within the range of human hearing and produce distinctive audible sound patterns that characterize normal and abnormal arterial and venous blood flow.

Doppler Equation. The Doppler equation describes, in mathematical form, the relationship between the Doppler frequency shift (ΔF) and the velocity (V) of the moving RBCs that produce the shift.
where

$$\Delta F = (Fr - Ft) = \frac{2(V)(Ft)(\cos\theta)}{(C)}$$

$\Delta F = (Fr-Ft)$ = the Doppler frequency shift
Ft = frequency of the transmitted Doppler US beam (the transducer frequency)
Fr = frequency of the reflected US beam (shifted by RBC motion)
V = RBC velocity (blood flow velocity)
θ = the Doppler angle = the angle between the direction of blood flow and the direction of the Doppler US beam
C = speed of sound in tissue (assumed to be constant at 1540 m/sec)

The frequency shift (ΔF) is proportional to the following: 1) the velocity (V) of the moving RBCs; 2) the frequency of the transmitted Doppler US beam (Ft); and 3) the cosine of the angle between the incident Doppler US beam and the direction of blood flow. This angle is called the Doppler angle and is symbolized by the Greek letter theta (θ). The direction of blood flow is assumed to be parallel to the walls of the visualized blood vessel being interrogated (Fig. 40.2). The Doppler US beam can be steered by controls on the US unit. The direction of the

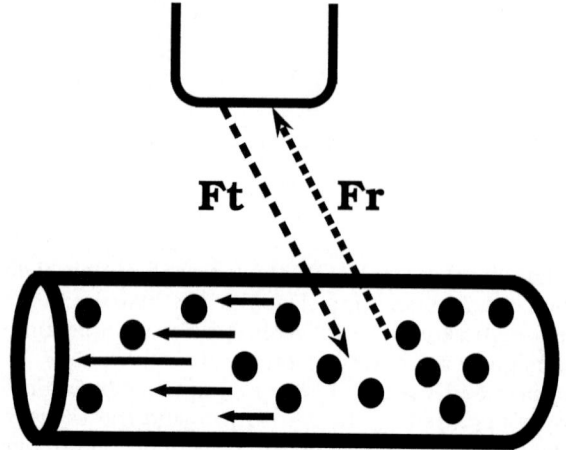

Figure 40.1. Doppler Frequency Shift. The transmitted Doppler US beam (*Ft*) encounters red blood cells moving toward it within a visualized blood vessel. The RBC motion causes an increase in frequency of the returning echo (*Fr*) due to the Doppler effect. The US instrument detects and measures the frequency of the returning Doppler signal confirming the presence of blood flow and its direction by the presence and direction of the Doppler frequency shift.

Table 40.1. Cosine Values

Angle	Cosine
0°	1
10°	0.98
20°	0.93
30°	0.87
40°	0.77
50°	0.64
60°	0.50
70°	0.34
80°	0.17
90°	0

Doppler beam is indicated on the US image by a dotted or dashed line.

The Doppler frequency shift's direct proportionality to the *cosine* of the Doppler angle has important implications (Table 40.1). First, the largest frequency shift—that is, the largest Doppler signal—will be obtained when the Doppler US beam is directed straight down the barrel of the vessel ($\theta = 0°$, cosine 0° = 1). Second, no Doppler shift will occur when the Doppler US beam is directly perpendicular to blood flow ($\theta = 90°$, cosine 90° = 0). Small errors in Doppler angle estimation cause only small errors in velocity calculations at small Doppler angles, but small errors in Doppler angle estimation cause large errors in velocity calculations at angles close to 90°. **As a general rule, Doppler scanning should be performed keeping Doppler angles at 60° or less.**

By algebraic manipulation we can rewrite the Doppler equation as follows:

$$V = \frac{(\Delta F)(C)}{2(Ft)(\cos\theta)}$$

The US unit detects and measures the frequency of the

Doppler beam reflected from moving RBCs (Fr) and calculates the Doppler frequency shift ($\Delta F = Ft - Fr$). The transmission frequency (Ft) is determined by the transducer used in the examination. The speed of sound in human tissue is assumed to be constant (C). The operator communicates the Doppler angle to the US unit by aligning the Doppler angle "wings" to be parallel with the walls of the vessels examined (Figs. 40.2, 40.3).

Because depth of a structure in an US image is measured by the time delay between transmission of the US into tissue and return of the echo from the structure, we can limit Doppler information to a selected Doppler "sample volume" by use of a "time window." The length of the time window determines the size of the sample volume and the time delay of the time window determines its depth. Thus, we can restrict Doppler information to a small portion of a single visualized vessel. On most Doppler US units the relative size and location of the Doppler sample volume is indicated by two short parallel lines along the Doppler beam indicator line (Figs. 40.2, 40.3). Simultaneous gray scale imaging and Doppler scanning is called duplex US. Both spectral and color Doppler imaging are examples of duplex imaging.

Doppler Spectral Display. Returning Doppler signals are processed using a fast Fourier transform spectrum analyzer, which sorts the range and mixture of Doppler frequency shifts into individual components and displays them as a function of time on a velocity (or frequency shift) scale (Fig. 40.3). Analysis is performed rapidly enough to be displayed in real time. The horizontal scale (x-axis) of the Doppler spectrum represents time in seconds. The vertical scale (y-axis) represents blood flow velocity in m/sec or cm/sec. Because velocity and Doppler frequency shift are directly related mathematically, Doppler frequency shift may alternatively be used on the vertical scale without changing the appearance of the

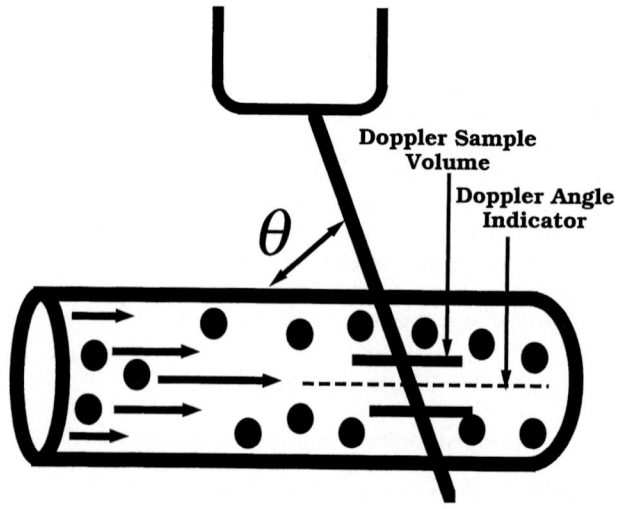

Figure 40.2. Doppler Angle. The Doppler angle, θ, is defined as the angle between the Doppler US beam and the direction of blood flow, which is assumed to be parallel to the walls of the blood vessel. The Doppler sample volume is indicated by two parallel lines. The Doppler angle indicator is displayed as a dashed line within the sample volume. The US unit has a control knob that is used to align the Doppler angle indicator with the blood vessel walls.

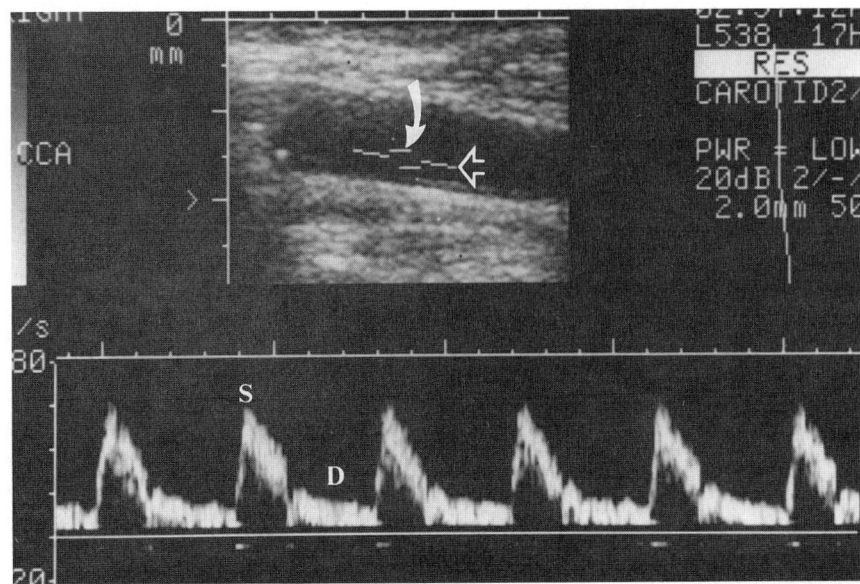

Figure 40.3. Duplex Doppler US. US image shows the Doppler spectrum of the common carotid artery. The vertical scale shows blood flow velocity in meters per second. The horizontal scale shows time in seconds. The Doppler trace demonstrates peak velocities in systole (*S*) and low flow velocities in diastole (*D*). A 2-mm Doppler sample volume (*curved arrow*) is placed by the sonographer in the midportion of the artery visualized by real-time US. Only Doppler shifts originating from this sample volume are analyzed for display. An estimated Doppler angle of 50° is communicated to the US unit computer by aligning the angle indicator (*open arrow*) parallel to the vessel walls.

Doppler spectrum. Because blood flow velocity provides the most diagnostically useful information, velocity is the usual choice for the vertical axis. Each pixel (bright dot) in the spectral display represents a group of RBCs moving at a specific velocity at a given moment in time. The more RBCs moving at that specific velocity and time, the brighter the pixel. Flow toward the Doppler beam (positive frequency shift) is displayed above the zero baseline, and flow away from the Doppler beam (negative frequency shift) is displayed below the zero baseline. Peaks of higher velocity occur during ventricular systole, and periods of lower velocity represent ventricular diastole.

Spectral Waveforms. Different blood vessels have unique flow characteristics that can be recognized by the Doppler spectral waveform (Doppler "signature") they produce (6,7). Factors that affect the appearance of the spectral waveform include the following: cardiac contraction, vessel compliance, and downstream vascular resistance. Cardiac arrhythmias are reflected in the periodicity of the systolic peaks and the velocities reached during each cardiac contraction. A major determinant of a spectral waveform's appearance is the resistance to blood flow offered by the vascular bed supplied by the artery being studied. Vessels can be categorized as high-resistance or low-resistance based on their Doppler spectral waveform. **High-resistance** spectral waveforms are characterized by velocities that increase sharply with systole, decrease rapidly with cessation of ventricular contraction, and show little or no forward flow during diastole (Fig. 40.4). Blood flow direction may reverse briefly during early diastole, producing a triphasic waveform. Blood flow in high-resistance arteries is always under considerable pressure and encounters constricted arterioles that impede forward blood flow. Pulse pressures traveling down the arterial tree are highly reflected, which results in minimal flow to the capillary bed during diastole. Diastolic flow velocity is low, absent, or reversed, and pulse pressure is high. The ratio of systolic velocity to diastolic velocity (pulsatility) is high. Vessels normally showing a high-resistance pattern Doppler

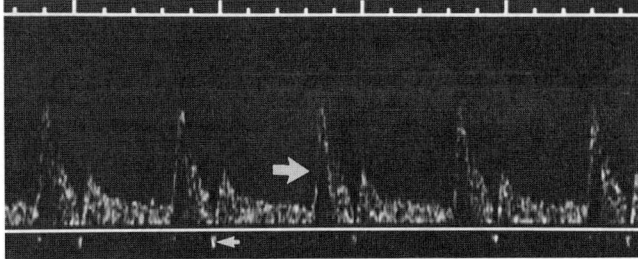

Figure 40.4. High-Resistance Doppler Spectrum. A high-resistance waveform is characterized by rapid systolic upstroke (*arrow*), low flow velocities during diastole, and, commonly, reversal of flow direction (*arrowhead*) in early diastole.

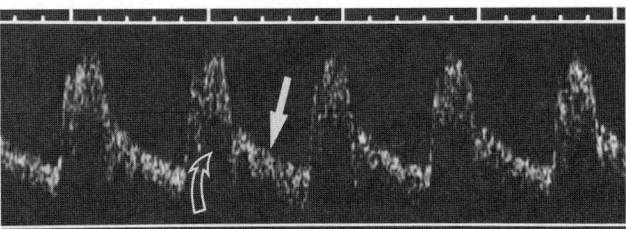

Figure 40.5. Low-Resistance Doppler Spectrum. A low-resistance waveform is characterized by relatively high-flow velocities throughout diastole (*arrow*). The narrow spectrum and clean systolic window (*open arrow*) is characteristic of laminar blood flow.

waveform include arteries that supply primarily skeletal muscle at rest including the iliac, femoral, popliteal, subclavian, and brachial arteries. The external carotid artery waveform is relatively high-resistance in appearance. **Low-resistance** spectral waveforms are characterized by a slower increase in flow velocity with onset of systole and a gradual decrease in velocity during diastole with continued forward flow throughout the cardiac cycle (Fig. 40.5). Arteries that supply vital organs characteristically have a low resistance waveform; they include

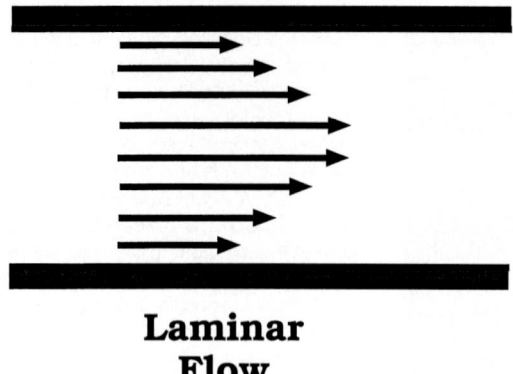

Laminar Flow

Figure 40.6. Laminar Blood Flow. Blood flow in most normal arteries is arranged in an orderly layering pattern with the highest velocity in the midstream and the lowest velocity near the vessel wall.

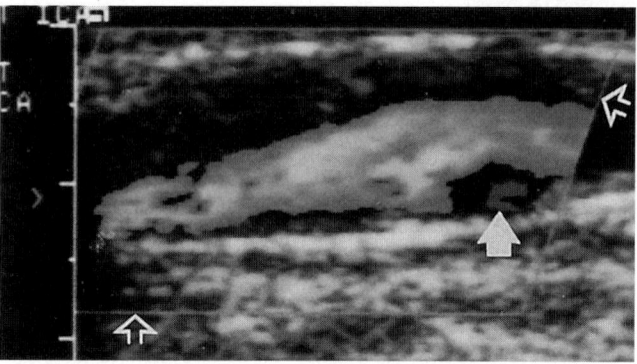

Figure 40.7. (Color Plates) Normal Flow Reversal at Bifurcation. Flow in the internal carotid artery is shown in red with areas of higher flow velocity shown in yellow. A normal area of blood flow reversal (*closed arrow*) is seen in the carotid bulb. Note how the true color change is outlined in black. The color Doppler interrogation area is marked on the image by the box outlined in white (*open arrows*).

the internal carotid, hepatic, and renal arteries. The superior mesenteric artery waveform has a high-resistance pattern during fasting and a low-resistance pattern after eating, thus reflecting opening of intestinal tract arterioles and increased blood flow. The common carotid artery, with 70% of its blood flow going to the internal carotid artery, has a low-resistance spectral waveform.

Laminar Blood Flow. Most normal arteries and large veins have a laminar pattern of blood flow. Blood flow velocity is highest at the center of the vessel and progressively diminishes closer to the vessel wall (Fig. 40.6). The Doppler waveform of laminar flow is characterized by a "narrow spectrum"—a narrow band of blood flow velocities throughout the cardiac cycle with a "window" beneath the spectral trace in systole (Fig. 40.4). Large arteries such as the aorta have "plug" flow characterized by uniform flow velocities extending from the center to near the vessel wall. At vessel bifurcations, the division of blood flow results in a small area of reversed blood flow near the vessel wall opposite the flow divider (Fig. 40.7).

Tortuous blood vessels demonstrate normal slowing of blood flow on the inner aspect of the curve with acceleration of blood flow on the outer aspect of the curve. The highest velocities are seen at the outer aspect of the vessel rather than at midlumen. Blood flow velocity returns to a laminar distribution a short distance downstream from the curve.

Disturbed Blood Flow. Turbulent and disturbed spectral waveforms are usually—but not always—indicative of pathological changes in blood flow. Disturbed blood flow is a loss of the normal orderly laminar flow pattern. Characteristic spectral signs of disturbed blood flow are as follows: increased velocity, spectral broadening, simultaneous forward and reverse flow, and fluctuations of flow velocity over time (5). Peak systolic velocity increases with severity of vessel stenosis. *Spectral broadening* is widening of the spectral waveform that reflects a broader range of flow velocities within the Doppler sample volume. Spectral broadening increases with the severity of flow disturbance. However, normal spectral broadening occurs when the size of the Doppler sample volume is large compared to the size of the vessel or when the sample volume is placed near the vessel wall instead of midlumen. Flow velocity fluctuation and simultaneous forward and reverse flow characterize turbulence. Turbulence is most pronounced downstream from a severe vessel stenosis where eddy currents are produced as the high velocity flow slows and occupies a larger vessel area.

Velocity Ratios. Blood flow velocity calculations depend on accurate estimation of the Doppler angle. When the Doppler angle cannot be determined because of poor visualization of the interrogated blood vessel or the vessel's tortuosity (as with the umbilical artery in the cord), velocity cannot be accurately calculated. When the Doppler angle indicator is not displayed, the US instrument calculates Doppler velocities by assuming the Doppler angle is 0° (cosine 0° = 1). Velocity ratios can be calculated from the spectral waveform and used to estimate vascular resistance and hemodynamics. The ratios are independent of absolute velocity measurements. Velocity ratios in common use are listed in Table 40.2.

Assessing Arterial Stenosis. Acute narrowing of the blood vessel lumen disturbs laminar flow. Doppler characterization of vessel stenosis is based upon changes in blood flow pattern and velocity. To assess the degree of stenosis, Doppler spectra are routinely obtained in three areas of the vessel lumen (Fig. 40.8): 1) proximal to stenosis, 2) at the point of maximal stenosis, and 3) 1–2 cm downstream from the stenosis. Laminar flow is generally present proximal to the stenosis. Within the

Table 40.2. Doppler Velocity Ratios

A/B Ratio (Systolic/Diastolic Ratio)	$= \dfrac{\text{Peak Systolic Velocity}}{\text{End Diastolic Velocity}}$
Resistance Index (RI) (Pourcelot Index (PoI))	$= \dfrac{\text{Peak Systolic Velocity} - \text{End Diastolic Velocity}}{\text{Peak Systolic Velocity}}$
Pulsatility Index (PI)	$= \dfrac{\text{Peak Systolic Velocity} - \text{End Diastolic Velocity}}{\text{Temporal Mean Velocity}}$

stenotic zone, velocity is increased but usually remains laminar. The severity of stenosis correlates best with the highest blood flow velocity during peak systole. The highest velocity may be in a very small region, and a careful search of the vessel is needed. In the poststenotic zone, flow spreads out, causing turbulence and eddy currents to occur and produce broadening of the Doppler spectrum. Downstream from severe stenosis (>50%), the Doppler signals are dampened producing the **parvus-tardus** waveform. Flow velocities are low (parvus) with a slow systolic upstroke (tardus)(see Fig. 40.22)(8,9).

Color Flow US

Currently, three different techniques are used to produce color flow US images. **Color Doppler imaging** (CDI) superimposes Doppler flow information on a standard gray-scale B-mode real-time US image (10,11). The B-mode image is displayed in shades of gray, and

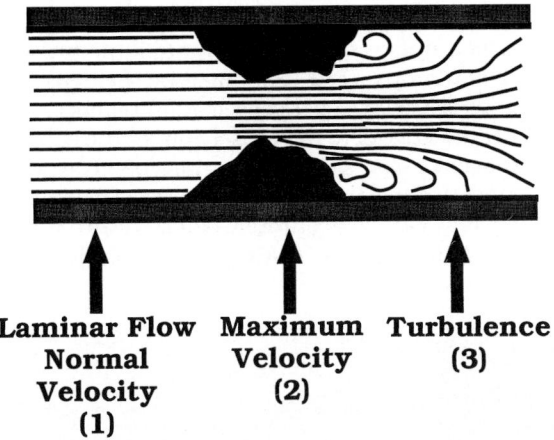

Figure 40.8. Assessing Arterial Stenosis. To assess a vessel plaque for stenosis, Doppler spectra are obtained: *1)* proximal to the plaque where blood flow velocity is normal and flow is laminar; *2)* in the area of the plaque where flow usually remain laminar but where flow velocity is at maximum; and *3)* downstream from the plaque where turbulence and eddy currents are detected.

the Doppler flow information is displayed on the same image in color (Fig. 40.9). Most of the same principles and limitations of spectral Doppler apply to color Doppler imaging. **Color Doppler energy** (CDE) displays color flow information obtained from integration of the power of the Doppler signal, rather than the Doppler frequency shift (1,12–14). Another name for this technique is Power Doppler. Color Doppler energy displays information more directly related to the number of moving RBCs than to their velocity (Fig. 40.10). CDE is relatively angle-independent and is more sensitive to slow flow than is CDI. The third method of color flow imaging is called **color velocity imaging** (CVI)(15). Color velocity imaging is not a Doppler technique. CVI tracks the movement of structure in the US image from one moment to the next. In effect, CVI images blood like a soft tissue and stores a unique texture pattern for comparison with a subsequent image. Movement of the blood flow speckle pattern is displayed as a color flow image.

On the color Doppler image flow directed toward the transducer is usually colored red whereas flow away from the transducer is usually colored blue. The operator may arbitrarily change the coloring of the Doppler information. The color map used is displayed as part of the color US image. Faster blood flow velocities are colored in lighter shades while slower blood flow is colored in darker shades. Color shading is dependent on mean velocities, not peak velocities. Thus, peak velocities cannot be estimated from the color image alone and must be determined from spectral Doppler. A normal laminar flow pattern will demonstrate lighter shades in the midstream and darker shades near the vessel walls, reflecting rapid flow in the middle of the vessel and slower flow near its walls. Disturbed flow, such as turbulence, is indicated by a wide range of colors without a discernible pattern.

Changes in color within a blood vessel on a color flow US image may be caused by: a) change in the Doppler angle, b) change in blood flow velocity, or c) aliasing. A change in Doppler angle causes a change in Doppler frequency shift which, on a color flow image, produces a change in the color displayed. Variations in the Doppler

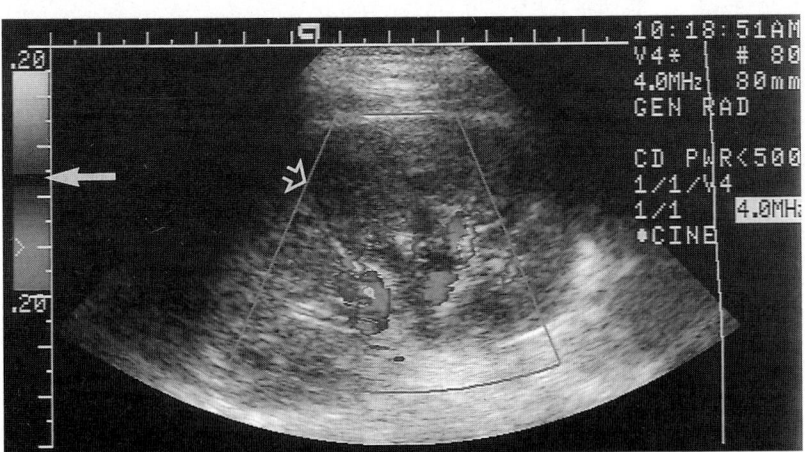

Figure 40.9. (Color Plates) Color Doppler Image. This color Doppler image of blood flow in the kidney displays arteries entering the kidney in red/yellow and veins leaving the kidney in blue/green. The color Doppler area of interrogation (sample volume) is etched by thin white lines (*open arrow*). Any detected Doppler shift within this area is displayed in color. The kidney and surrounding tissue are displayed in gray scale. The color Doppler map on the left is set to show blood flow toward the Doppler beam in red/yellow at the top of the scale and blood flow away from the Doppler beam in blue/green at the bottom of the scale. The zero flow baseline is represented by the black bar (*arrow*) in the center of the color map.

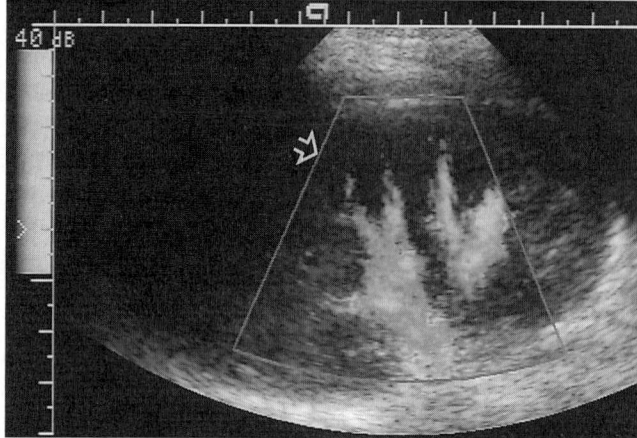

Figure 40.10. (Color Plates) Color Doppler Energy (Power Doppler) Image. Color Doppler energy image of the same kidney as displayed in Fig. 40.9 shows the increased sensitivity of CDE. Blood vessels are detected more peripherally in the kidney. However, CDE lacks the capability to show blood flow direction. Arteries and veins are displayed in the same color shades. The CDE area of interrogation is indicated by the white box (*open arrow*).

angle may be caused by diverging US beams from sector or curved array transducers, a blood vessel curving through the color image, or a combination of both. Color flow images are used to detect changes in blood flow velocity for further analysis by spectral Doppler. To interpret a color flow image, inspect the color map for color display orientation; then analyze the image for variations in Doppler angle and blood flow velocity.

Doppler Limitations and Artifacts

Aliasing is a limitation of pulsed Doppler US that occurs with both spectral and color flow Doppler (11,16). Aliasing happens with high-velocity blood flow and improper velocity scale and baseline settings. Aliasing on spectral displays is seen as a wraparound" of peak velocities to the opposite end of the scale (Fig. 40.11). The highest velocities are cut off one side of the scale and artifactually displayed on the opposite side of the scale. Aliasing on CDI "wraps around" high velocities onto the opposite color scale (Fig. 40.12). For example, velocities too high for the red-scale setting are artifactually displayed as shades of blue. Color aliasing must be distinguished from true color changes caused by flow reversal or change in the Doppler angle. True color changes are always surrounded by a black border whereas CDI aliasing color shifts lack this black border.

Aliasing occurs when the pulse Doppler sampling rate is too low for a given Doppler signal frequency, thus resulting in an inaccurate frequency measurement. The US instrument measures the frequency of returning Doppler signal piece by piece by a series of pulses. The rate at which pulses can be transmitted (the **pulse repetition frequency** or PRF) is limited by the depth of the vessel interrogated. Deeper vessels require more time for the US beam to travel to the vessel and for the echo to return. To avoid aliasing, the PRF must be at least twice the frequency of the signal to be detected. The maximum frequency that can be accurately detected without aliasing is called the **Nyquist limit** and is equal to one-half

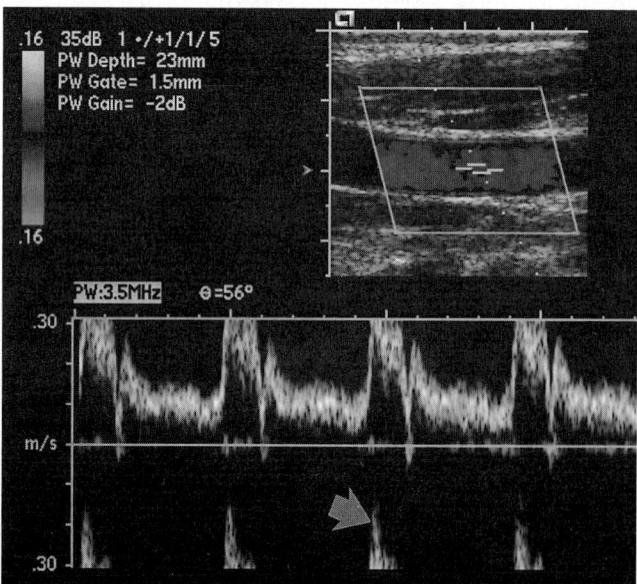

Figure 40.11. (Color Plates) Aliasing on Spectral Doppler. The high velocity peaks (*arrow*) of the spectral Doppler display are cut off at the top, "wrapped around," and displayed at the bottom of the spectral display. The spectral Doppler scale on the left is set with a Nyquist limit of 0.30 m/sec, too low for the peak velocities encountered within the interrogated blood vessel.

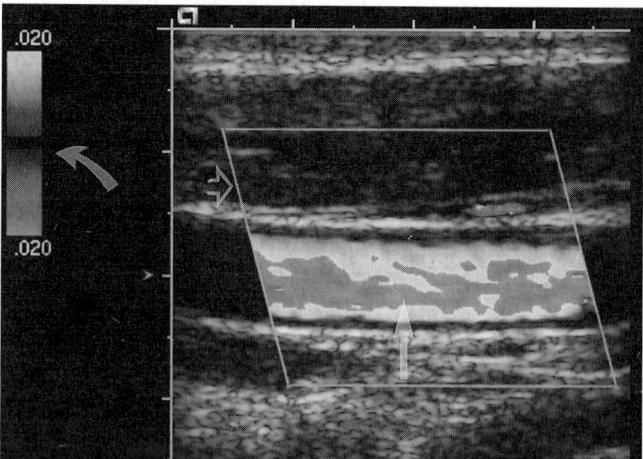

Figure 40.12. (Color Plates) Aliasing on Color Doppler Imaging. The color map (*curved arrow*) is set for red/yellow color at the top of the scale to indicate flow toward the Doppler beam and for blue/green color at the bottom of the scale to indicate flow away from the Doppler beam. The direction of the Doppler beam is indicated by the parallel sides (*open arrow*) of the color Doppler sample volume box shown in white. The dominant color within the visualized blood vessel is red/yellow indicating the direction of blood flow is from right to left. The higher velocity of blood flow in the center of the blood vessel exceeds the low velocity scale setting (Nyquist limit =0.020 m/sec) and is displayed in green, the high velocity color on the opposite end of the color scale. The lack of a black border around the color shift is a sign of aliasing.

the PRF. The Nyquist limit is displayed at the top and bottom of the spectral Doppler scale and the color map. In CDI, aliasing may be helpful and serve as a tag for high velocities associated with significant stenosis. Aliasing may be eliminated by proper adjustment of the Doppler scale and baseline settings, by using a lower-frequency Doppler transducer or increasing the Doppler angle.

Incorrect Doppler Gain. When the Doppler gain is set too low, Doppler information may be lost and blood flow may not be detected. The CDI image with too high gain demonstrates color in nonflow areas and random color noise. Correct gain settings are attained by turning up the gain setting until noise appears on the image then slightly lowering the setting.

Velocity Scale Errors. Velocity range settings that are too high may obscure low velocity flow. Vessels that are patent with slow flow may be considered thrombosed. When velocity scale settings are too low, aliasing occurs; such aliasing is corrected by adjusting scale and baseline settings.

Color Flash. Any motion of a reflector relative to the transducer produces a Doppler shift. Rapid movement of the transducer itself may produce a Doppler shift and a flash of color projected over the gray scale image. Most instruments incorporate motion discriminators that suppress color flash in hyperechoic but not in hypo-echoic areas. Color flash is accentuated in cysts, the gallbladder, other hypoechoic nonvascular structures, and also by high color sensitivity settings.

Tissue Vibration Artifact. Tissue vibration may produce color display in perivascular tissues indicating flow where none is present. Tissue vibration artifact is produced in nonflow areas by bruits, arteriovenous fistulas, and shunts.

Fluid Motion. Color signal can be produced during CDI by motion of fluids other than blood. Motion of fluid within cysts and the bowel may be misinterpreted as blood flow. Ureteral peristalsis produces a jet of color in the bladder that confirms patency of the ureter.

CAROTID ULTRASOUND

Stroke

Approximately 500,000 strokes occur in the United States each year, resulting in 150,000 deaths. The public health cost for the disabilities of stroke exceed $15 billion per year. Atherosclerotic lesions of the extracranial vessels are estimated to cause 75% of strokes having either a thrombotic or embolic cause (17).

During the last decade, the management of atherosclerotic carotid disease has changed significantly. In 1991, two randomized prospective multicenter studies, the North American Symptomatic Carotid Endarterectomy Trial (NASCET) (18) and the European Carotid Stenosis Trial (ECST) (19) demonstrated a clear benefit of carotid endarterectomy in patients with an internal carotid artery (ICA) stenosis ≥70% of the diameter as defined by conventional angiography. An important difference between the NASCET and ECST studies is the method of measuring the stenosis (Fig. 40.13). NASCET measured the degree of narrowing as the ratio of the diameter of the stenosis to the diameter of the normal ICA distal to the stenosis on catheter angiography. The ECST measured carotid stenosis in a more traditional fashion, comparing the residual lumen diameter to an approximation of the original vessel diameter. A 70% ECST stenosis is approximately equal to a 50% NASCET stenosis.

NASCET found an unequivocal difference between the risk of stroke in patients receiving the best medical care alone and those undergoing endarterectomy. The risk of ipsilateral stroke after two years is 26% for those treated medically and 9% for those treated surgically. Similarly, the ECST found a sixfold decrease in stroke in endarterectomy patients. If the stenoses had been measured as in the NASCET study, this decrease may have been more significant. Most investigators regard the NASCET study as the gold standard that makes carotid endarterectomy the standard of care for symptomatic carotid stenosis ≥70% of the diameter. The ECST confirmed that patients with stenoses <30% of the diameter are best managed medically. The NASCET subgroup of patients with stenosis 30–69% of the diameter did not benefit from endarterectomy. However, this group contained both hemodynamically significant (>50% of the diameter) and insignificant lesions. Reliable data do not exist for the 30–69% subgroup, but clinical trials are ongoing.

The Asymptomatic Carotid Atherosclerosis Study (ACAS) (20) demonstrated a 53% aggregate stroke risk reduction with carotid endarterectomy for stenosis ≥60% of the diameter in asymptomatic individuals. In men, the risk reduction is 66%; in women, 17%. A second trial in asymptomatic patients conducted by the Veterans Administration (21) showed a substantial reduction in transient ischemic attacks (TIA) in patients with stenosis ≥50% of the diameter but no stroke re-

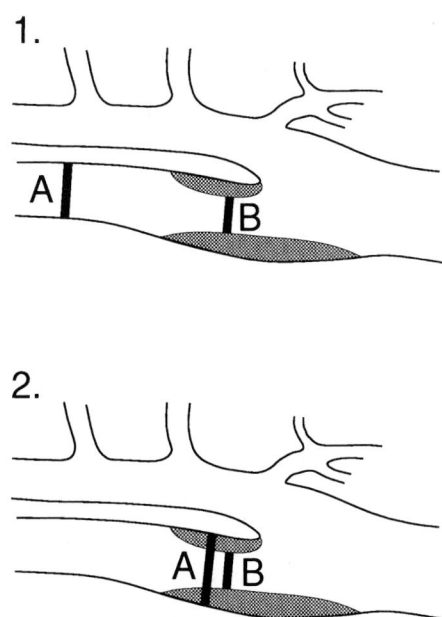

Figure 40.13. Percent Carotid Stenosis. Carotid % Stenosis: (A-B)/A ×100% **1.** NASCET **2.** ECST (traditional). See text.

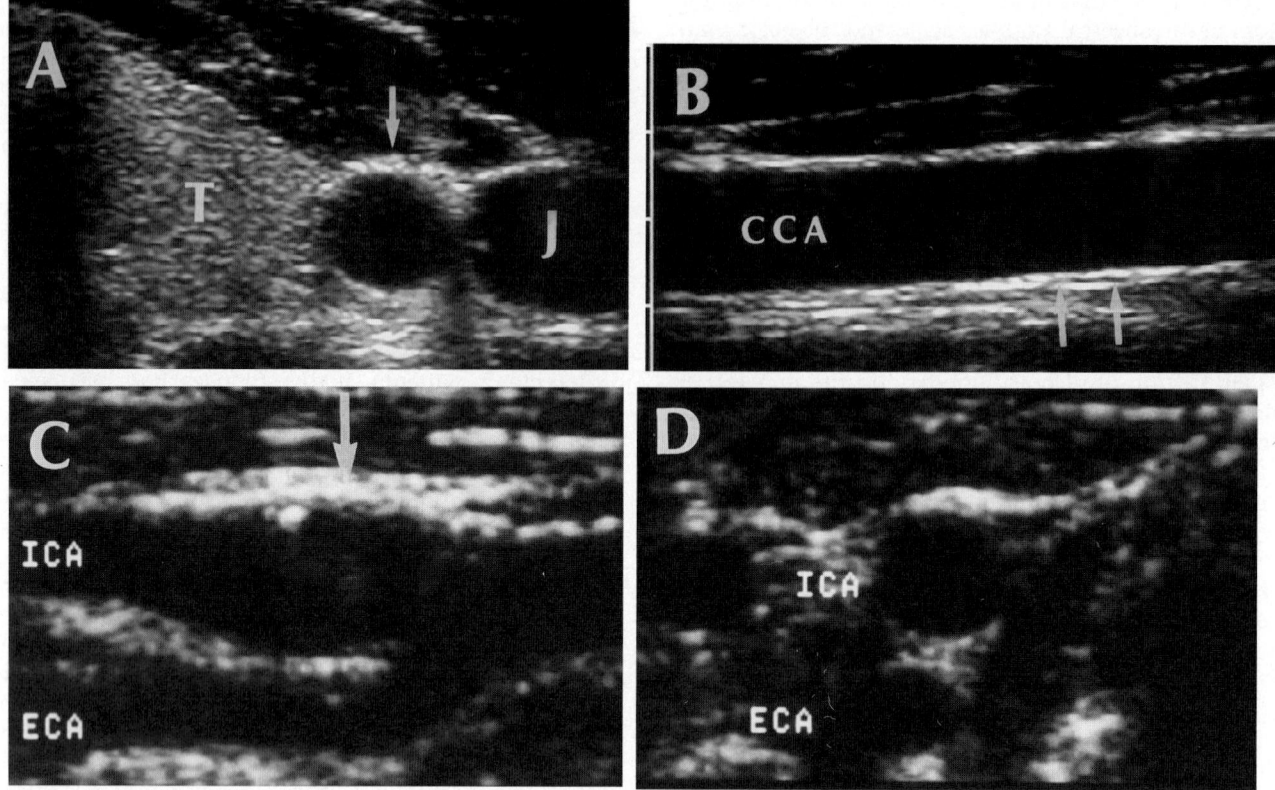

Figure 40.14. Carotid Anatomy. A. Transverse gray scale US image of the left common carotid artery (*arrow*) at the level of the thyroid (*T*). The CCA is positioned medial to the jugular vein (*J*) and lateral to the thyroid. **B.** Longitudinal image of the right CCA. Normal intima-media complex (*arrows*). **C.** Longitudinal image of the carotid bifurcation and carotid bulb (*arrow*). **D.** Transverse image of the carotid bifurcation. *CCA,* common carotid artery; *ICA,* internal carotid artery; *ECA,* external carotid artery.

duction. These studies are not perfect in design, and have been criticized. The management of the asymptomatic stenosis remains controversial.

Anatomy and Technique

Anatomy. The right common carotid artery (CCA) arises from the bifurcation of the inominate artery. The left CCA arises from the aortic arch. The CCAs ascend anterolaterally up the neck, medial to the jugular vein, and lateral to the thyroid. Each artery measures 6–8mm in diameter. US evaluation of the CCA often shows the three layers of the normal vessel wall— the echogenic intima, hypoechoic media, and echogenic adventitia. The distance between these two echogenic lines (intima-media complex) is normally less than 1.2mm. The CCA dilates in the common carotid bulb and bifurcates into the internal (ICA) and external (ECA) carotid arteries at the C-3/4 level. The bifurcation may occur anywhere from the C-1 to T-2 level. The ECA assumes an antero-*medial* course off the carotid bulb 70% of the time. It is intermediate (overlaps ICA) in 20% of patients and reversed (lateral) in 10% of patients. The ECA has branch vessels that supply the head and face, and it measures 3–4mm in diameter. The ICA assumes a postero*lateral* course off the carotid bulb, supplies the brain, and measures 5–6 mm in diameter. The portion of the arterial

Table 40.3. ICA versus ECA

Internal Carotid Artery	External Carotid Artery
Larger (6 mm)	Smaller (3–4 mm)
No branches	Branch vessels
Usually posterolateral	Usually anteromedial
Courses posteriorly to mastoid	Courses anteriorly to face
Low-resistance flow pattern	High-resistance flow pattern
Carotid bulb at origin	"Temporal tap" maneuver

wall between the ICA and ECA at their origin is called the *flow divider.* The vertebral arteries are the first branches of the subclavian arteries with the left the same size or larger than the right in 75% of cases. They ascend in the transverse foramen of C-2 to C-6. Normal carotid anatomy is illustrated in Figure 40.14. Sonographic characteristics that aid in the differentiation of the ICA and ECA are shown in Figures 40.15, 40.16, and Table 40.3.

Technique. Duplex US of the carotid arteries is performed using a linear 5–10 MHz transducer with the patient in the supine position. The patient's head is rotated away from the side being examined. The cervical carotid arteries are evaluated in the longitudinal plane using gray scale, color flow, and spectral Doppler imaging. Findings are confirmed in the transverse plane.

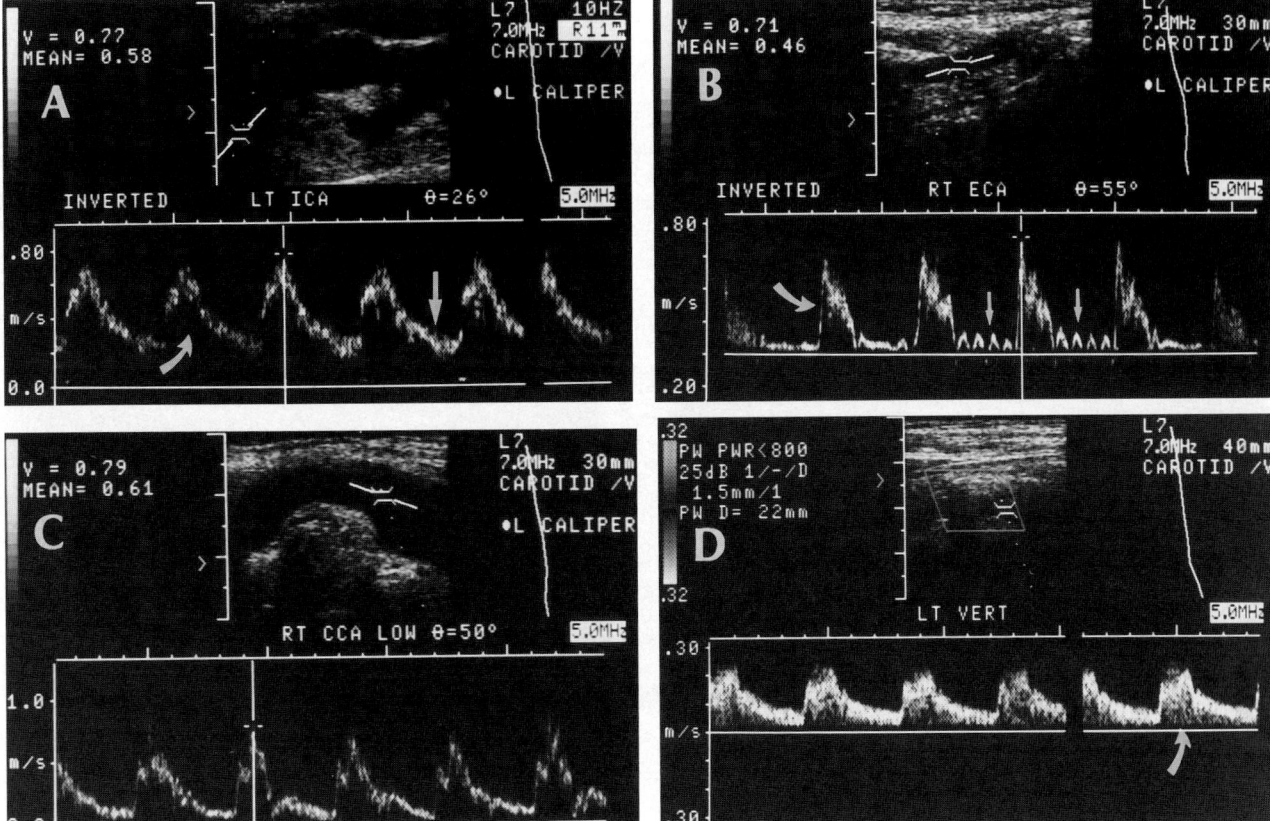

Figure 40.15. Normal Carotid Spectral Waveforms. A. Internal carotid artery (*ICA*)—low-resistance waveform. Note the prominent diastolic flow (*arrow*) and clean systolic window (*curved arrow*). **B.** External carotid artery (*ECA*)—high-resistance waveform. The rapid systolic upstroke is characteristic (*curved arrow*). The "sawtooth" pattern (*arrows*) is the result of the temporal tap. The sonographer palpates the pulse and then digitally taps either the superficial temporal or preauricular branch of the ECA. The tapping is transmitted back to the ECA as the "sawtooth" pattern on the spectral display. This maneuver helps distinguish the ECA from the ICA (no "sawtooth") in difficult cases. **C.** Common carotid artery (*CCA*)—hybrid waveform. The CCA typically is more ICA-like since 70% of its blood flows into the ICA. **D.** Vertebral Artery (*VA*)—low-resistance waveform. The VA often demonstrates spectral broadening caused by its small size and location (poor visualization). Note the filling in of the systolic window with spectral broadening (*curved arrow*).

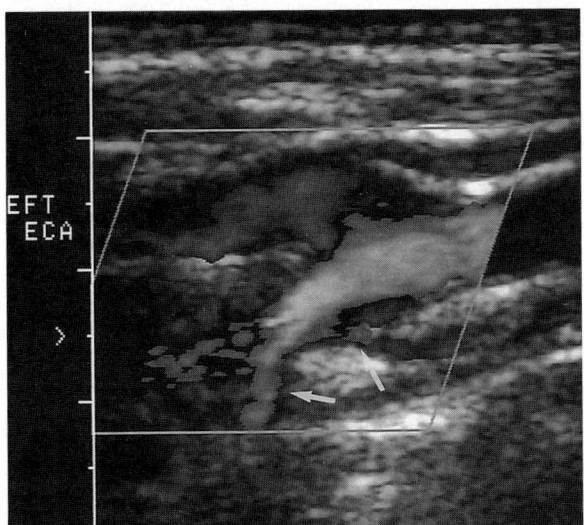

Figure 40.16. (Color Plates) External Carotid Artery. Note vessel branches (*arrows*).

Plaque Evaluation

Intimal Hyperplasia. Diffuse thickening (>1.2mm) of the intima-media complex of the CCA has been linked to an increased risk of atherosclerotic vascular disease including TIA, stroke, and coronary artery disease (22–24). Serial wall thickness measurements have been used to monitor the clinical response to specific treatments for atherosclerosis. Measurable decreases in the CCA wall thickness have occurred with Lovastatin use and dietary therapy for hypercholesterolemia (25).

Plaque Formation. Carotid plaques are most commonly found within 2cm of the bifurcation. Injury to the vascular endothelium results in the deposition of a fatty streak in the wall of the artery. Plaque growth results from progressive deposition of lipids, proliferation of smooth muscle cells, and migration of fibrocytes. The plaque contains a lipid core with a variable fibrous cap. As the plaque increases in size, the shearing forces of blood flow to which it is subjected cause repeated episodes of fissuring and intraplaque hemorrhage with

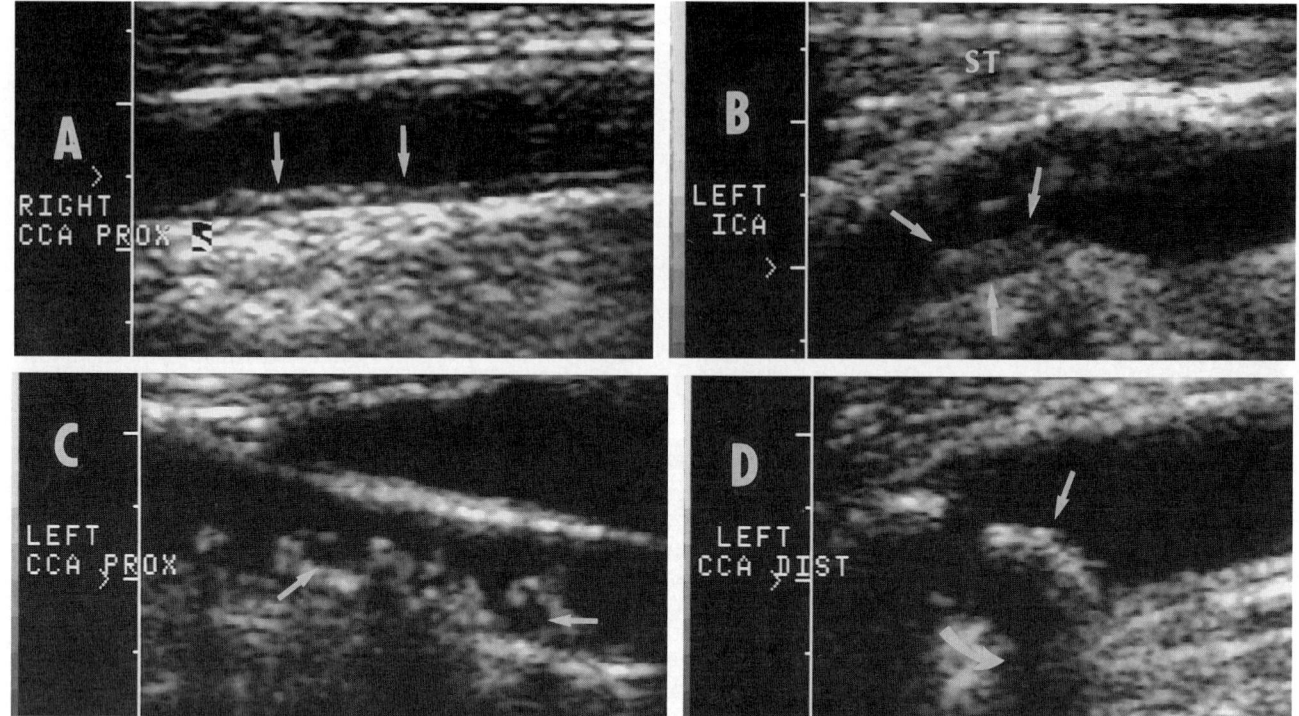

Figure 40.17. Plaque. A. Intimal hyperplasia (*arrows*). **B.** Predominantly homogeneous plaque (*arrows*) demonstrates echotexture similar to the surrounding soft tissue (*ST*). **C.** Heterogeneous plaque with sonolucent areas representing intraplaque hemorrhage (*arrows*). **D.** Calcified plaque (*arrow*) with distal acoustic shadowing (*curved arrow*).

interval healing. During this process, the plaque can rupture and cause cerebral emboli (26).

Plaque Characterization. No universal system exists to characterize plaque. Plaque is usually described by surface characteristics, density, and texture (Figs. 40.17, 40.18) (22,26–28).

Surface characteristics consist of smooth, irregular, and ulcerated. Having approximately a 60% sensitivity and specificity, US is unreliable in the diagnosis of plaque ulceration. Gray scale US findings suggestive of ulceration include undercutting of the plaque margin, a sonolucent area that extends to the surface of the plaque, and a divot or crater on the surface of the plaque. Color Doppler may demonstrate flow into the crater with flow reversal.

Hypoechoic, isoechoic, and hyperechoic are the terms used to describe plaque density. The more hypoechoic (or anechoic) the higher the lipid content of the plaque. Isoechoic plaques contain more smooth muscle and hyperechoic plaques contain a large amount of fibrous tissue. Color Doppler is useful to help identify areas of anechoic plaque not seen in the vessel lumen because they are isoechoic with blood.

Plaque texture is either homogeneous or heterogeneous. Because of its high content of fibrous tissue, homogeneous plaque is smooth and similar in echotexture to the surrounding soft tissues. Heterogeneous plaque is complex and has at least one focal area of sonolucency representing intraplaque hemorrhage. Intraplaque hemorrhage is identified on sonography, which has approximately a 90% sensitivity and 85% specificity. Heter-

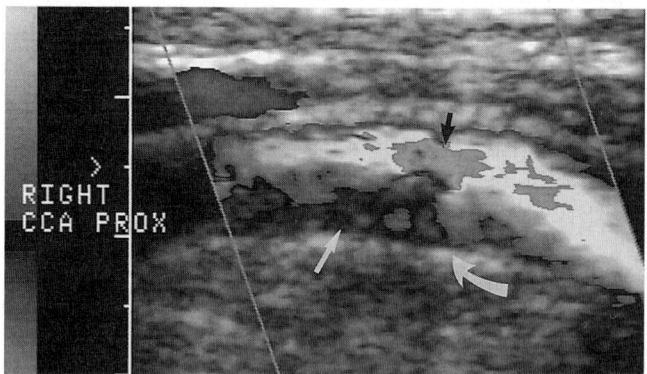

Figure 40.18. (Color Plates) Ulcerated Plaque. Color Doppler demonstrates a heterogeneous plaque (*white arrow*) with a vortex of color (flow reversal) extending into the plaque. This represents an angiographically proven ulcer crater (*curved arrow*). Area of green color shift (*black arrow*) represents aliasing because of increased flow velocity caused by stenosis.

ogeneous plaque can have either a smooth or irregular surface. All ulcerated plaques are heterogeneous but not all heterogeneous plaques ulcerate. Plaque calcification is a nonspecific finding and is seen in both homogeneous and heterogeneous plaque.

Plaque Significance. Heterogeneous plaque is accepted as a risk factor for a subsequent neurologic event. However, many asymptomatic individuals have heterogeneous plaque. How many of these individuals have a subsequent TIA or stroke remains controversial. No study to date demonstrates a definite stroke reduction from endarterectomy or medical management based on the US characteristics of plaque. Polak (29) found that the severity of ICA stenosis more closely predicts stroke or TIA than plaque characterization. In the authors' opinion, until conclusive evidence exists that plaque morphology can predict stroke, spectral Doppler (velocity parameters) remains the most important factor in carotid duplex interpretation. Color Doppler and gray scale imaging are complementary.

Stenosis

Duplex US is well established in screening for carotid stenosis. Properly performed, duplex US has sensitivity and specificity exceeding 90%. However, many studies, including NASCET, have shown marginal diagnostic accuracy (sensitivity, 67%; specificity, 78%). Most investigators believe the poor statistics are caused by suboptimal quality control and no standardization of the duplex scans by the institutions involved in the study. The cost-effectiveness of duplex sonography is well-recognized when symptomatic individuals are screened. The rate of positive angiograms (>50% stenosis) increases from 30% to more than 70%, thus decreasing the number of unnecessary angiograms and their associated risk (30).

Internal Carotid Artery. Numerous velocity criteria exist for grading ICA stenosis. The most common velocity parameters include the following: peak systolic velocity (PSV), end-diastolic velocity (EDV), peak systolic velocity ICA to CCA ratio, and the diastolic velocity ICA to CCA ratio. Color Doppler and gray scale images are used to facilitate interpretation, particularly when the velocity parameters are discordant. Color Doppler mapping of the ICA also helps in identifying areas of suspected high flow (aliasing), thus significantly shortening the examination time (Fig. 40.19).

PSV is the most accurate parameter for stenoses greater than 50% and less than 90%. A stenosis less than 50% is more accurately graded with gray scale and color flow imaging in the transverse plane. For a stenosis approximately 50% of the diameter, spectral broadening of the ICA waveform and a mild increase in PSV are noted. For a stenosis greater than 90–95%, the PSV falls as stenosis approaches occlusion. The ICA/CCA ratio is most helpful when the CCA velocities are abnormal (Table 40.4). The diastolic velocity (>100cm/sec) and diastolic velocity ratios help in distinguishing high-grade (>80% diameter) stenosis from lesser degrees. Polak (26) states that individuals with an EDV>140cm/sec are a subset of patients at high risk for stroke.

Since the NASCET study, many investigators have published revised criteria for grading ICA stenosis (Table 40.5)(31–40). These studies demonstrate the wide variability between vascular laboratories. Examples of the pre-NASCET criteria are shown in Table 40.6. Each vascular US laboratory must develop

Table 40.4. Abnormal Common Carotid Artery (CCA) Velocities

Symmetric CCA Velocities	
Bilateral Low < 50 cm/sec	Bilateral High > 100 cm/sec
Low cardiac output	High cardiac output
CHF	hypertension
cardiomyopathy	hyperthyroid
pericardial effusion	bradycardia
Wide diameter arteries	Narrow diameter arteries

Asymmetric CCA Velocities	
Unilateral Low < 50 cm/sec	Unilateral High > 100 cm/sec
Severe proximal stenosis	Technical (i.e Tortuous)
Severe distal stenosis or occlusion	CCA stenosis
Wide diameter CCA	Narrow diameter CCA
Long segment stenosis	Contralateral severe stenosis

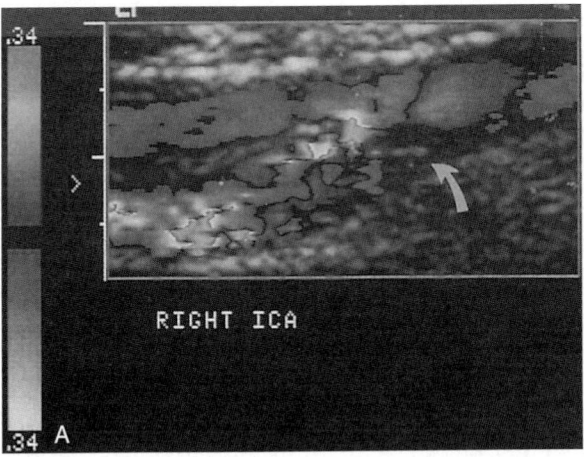

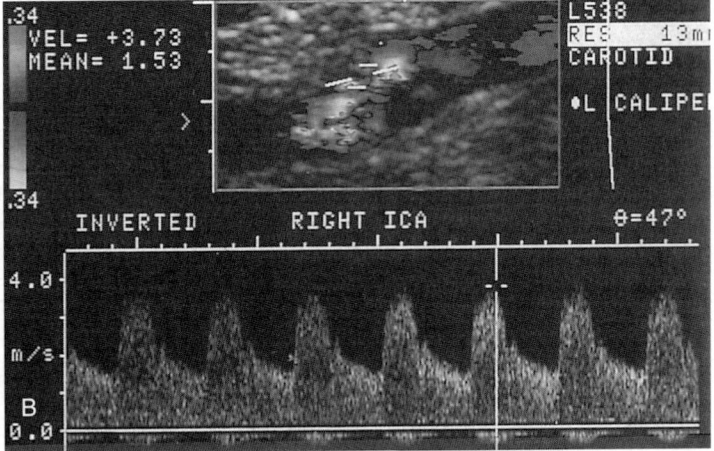

Figure 40.19. (Color Plates) Internal Carotid Artery Stenosis. A. Longitudinal color Doppler image of the carotid bifurcation demonstrates an eccentric atherosclerotic plaque (*arrow*) at the origin of the ICA. The markedly heterogeneous color display distal to the plaque is indicative of severe turbulence due to significant stenosis. **B.** The color Doppler image is used to direct placement of the spectral Doppler sample volume in the area of maximum flow velocity. Spectral Doppler waveform shows measurement of peak systolic flow velocity at 3.73 m/sec (*upper left*), indicating critical stenosis. Note the "filling in" of the Doppler waveform, known as spectral broadening, indicative of turbulence.

Table 40.5. New Doppler Criteria Based on NASCET

Author	Cut-Off (%Stenosis)	Parameter	Value
Hunink et al. (1993) (31)	70	PSV	>230 cm/s
Moneta et al. (1993) (32)	70	SVR	>4.0
Neale et al. (1994) (33)	70	PSV	>270 cm/s
		EDV	>110 cm/s
Faught et al. (1994)(34)	70	PSV	>130 cm/s
Hood et al. (1996) (37)		EDV	>100 cm/s
Carpenter et al. (1995) (35)	60	PSV	>170 cm/s
		EDV	>40 cm/s
		SVR	>2.0
		DVR	>2.4
Moneta et al. (1995) (36)	60	PSV	>290 cm/s
		EDV	>80 cm/s
Browman et al. (1995) (39)	70	PSV	>175 cm/s
		PSV	<40 cm/s
Carpenter et al. (1996) (38)	70	PSV	>210 cm/s
		EDV	>70 cm/s
		SVR	>3.0
		DVR	>3.3
Lefsrud et al. (1997) (40)	70	PSV	>230 cm/s
		EDV	>70 cm/s
		SVR	>3.2

PSV = peak systolic velocity
EDV = end diastolic velocity
SVR = peak systolic velocity ratio (ICA/CCA)
DVR = end diastolic velocity ratio (ICA/CCA)
cm/s = centimeters/second

Table 40.6. Pre-NASCET Doppler Criteria

Diameter Stenosis (%)	PSV (cm/sec)	EDV (cm/sec)	SVR (ICA/CCA)	DVR (ICA/CCA)
1–39%				
Bluth et al.	<110	<40	<1.8	<2.6
Carroll	<110 >25		<1.5	<2.6
40–59%				
Bluth et al.	<130	<40	<1.8	<2.6
Carroll	>120	<40	<1.8	<2.6
60–79%				
Bluth et al.	>130	>40	>1.8	>2.6
Carroll	>130	>40	>1.8	>2.6
80–99%				
Bluth et al.	>250	>100		
100 >3.7	>5.5			
80–90%				
Carroll	>250 <25	>80–135	>3.7	>5.5

PSV = peak systolic velocity
EDV = end diastolic velocity
SVR = peak systolic velocity ratio (ICA/CCA)
DVR = end diastolic velocity ratio (ICA/CCA)
(Modified from Bluth E, et al. Radiographics 1988;8:487–516; Carroll BA. Radiology 1991;178:303–313.)

Table 40.7 Peak Systolic Velocity Ratio (SVR) and % Stenosis

Velocity Ratio	Diameter Stenosis
2:1	50%
3.5:1	75%
7:1	90%

its own criteria or pick an existing table that accurately correlates with conventional angiography, clinical outcomes data, and the desired sensitivity and specificity at their institution.

Common Carotid Artery. The normal velocity in the CCA is 50–100 cm/sec in the population older than age 50. No velocity tables exist for grading CCA stenosis. However, some vascular labs use ICA parameters. Along with gray scale and color flow imaging, a PSV ratio can be used to estimate the percent of the stenosis. The velocity at the stenosis is divided by the velocity proximal to the stenosis (Table 40.7, Fig. 40.20). If a significant stenosis exists in the extreme proximal portion of the CCA or at its origin, the CCA may have a parvus-tardus waveform (Fig 40.21).

External Carotid Artery. Because the ECA predominantly supplies the face, the degree of stenosis (or occlusion) does not affect clinical management or stroke reduction. However, a significant ECA stenosis can alter the waveform of the CCA and cause elevated flow velocities in the ICA. A high ECA stenosis may cause a neck bruit.

Vertebral Artery. No well-established velocity parameters exist for determination of vertebral artery stenosis. Because treatment is limited and the vertebral artery origin and size is so variable, the detection of stenosis and occlusion is not clinically useful. Analysis is usually limited to confirming the presence and normal direction of blood flow.

Occlusion

Common Carotid Artery occlusion is easily identified by duplex scanning. No spectral waveform or color flow can be elicited. Echogenic clot can often be seen filling the CCA lumen. Antegrade flow is usually present in the ipsilateral ICA secondary to retrograde flow through the ECA to the carotid bifurcation and into the ICA. Spectral analysis in this situation demonstrates reversed flow in the ECA (Fig. 40.22).

Internal Carotid Artery occlusion is suggested when no flow is identified in the vessel with spectral analysis and color flow imaging. On gray scale imaging, the ICA diameter may be small and filled with echogenic thrombus. A brief systolic pulse (followed by a flow reversal) is usually present at the proximal end of the obstruction caused by "thumping" of blood against the occlusion. The CCA waveform has a high-resistance flow pattern with decreased diastolic flow velocities more characteristic of the ECA. This pattern is often called "externalization of the CCA" (Fig. 40.23). If the patient has well-developed ipsilateral ECA to ICA collateral flow intracranially, the CCA may not be externalized. In this circumstance, the ECA waveform becomes more low resistance or ICA-like, often called "internalization of the ECA" because it then supplies brain parenchyma (Fig. 40.24).

The distinction between total occlusion of the ICA and trickle flow is of critical importance. Patients with trickle flow are candidates for carotid endarterectomy and those with total occlusions are not (Fig. 40.25). Despite advances in duplex US, 5–7% of trickle flows are not detected on gray scale, spectral Doppler, or color Doppler imaging. Power Doppler may improve the detection rate. MR angiography (MRA) has an accuracy similar to duplex US. Therefore, catheter angiography is still recommended to exclude a "string sign" when the Doppler suggests occlusion.

Inominate/Subclavian Artery. Occlusion of the inominate artery or left subclavian artery proximal to the origin of the vertebral artery results in the *subclavian steal syndrome.* In this circumstance, the upper extremity receives blood from the CCA through the circle of Willis and down the vertebral artery. Spectral Doppler demonstrates reversed flow in the vertebral artery. Partial subclavian steal results in reversed flow during systole and antegrade flow during diastole in the vertebral artery because of a severe stenosis of the inominate or left subclavian artery (Fig. 40.26).

Common Pitfalls

Angle of Insonation. Ensure that the angle of insonation is between 30°–60°. Spectral analysis with angles of interrogation >60° may cause large errors in velocity.

Tortuous and Narrow Vessels. The laminar flow pattern is disrupted as blood flows through a sharp bend. Reporting of the higher velocity at the outer bend in a tortuous vessel may overestimate the degree of stenosis or falsely suggest a stenosis when none is present (Fig 40.27).

Carotid Bulb. Normal flow reversal is usually noted in the carotid bulb opposite the flow divider (Fig. 40.7) and should not be mistaken for pathologic flow.

Calcified Plaque. Dense calcification can make obtaining velocities in portions of the ICA impossible because of acoustic shadowing. As a result, a significant stenosis may not be detected. Color flow imaging is helpful in this situation. If the color flow into and out from behind the plaque is homogeneous, the presence of a significant stenosis is unlikely. However, if flow proximal to the plaque is homogeneous and flow distal to the plaque heterogeneous, a significant stenosis should be suspected (Fig. 40.28).

Contralateral High-grade Carotid Stenosis. With unilateral ICA occlusion or high-grade stenosis, flow ve-

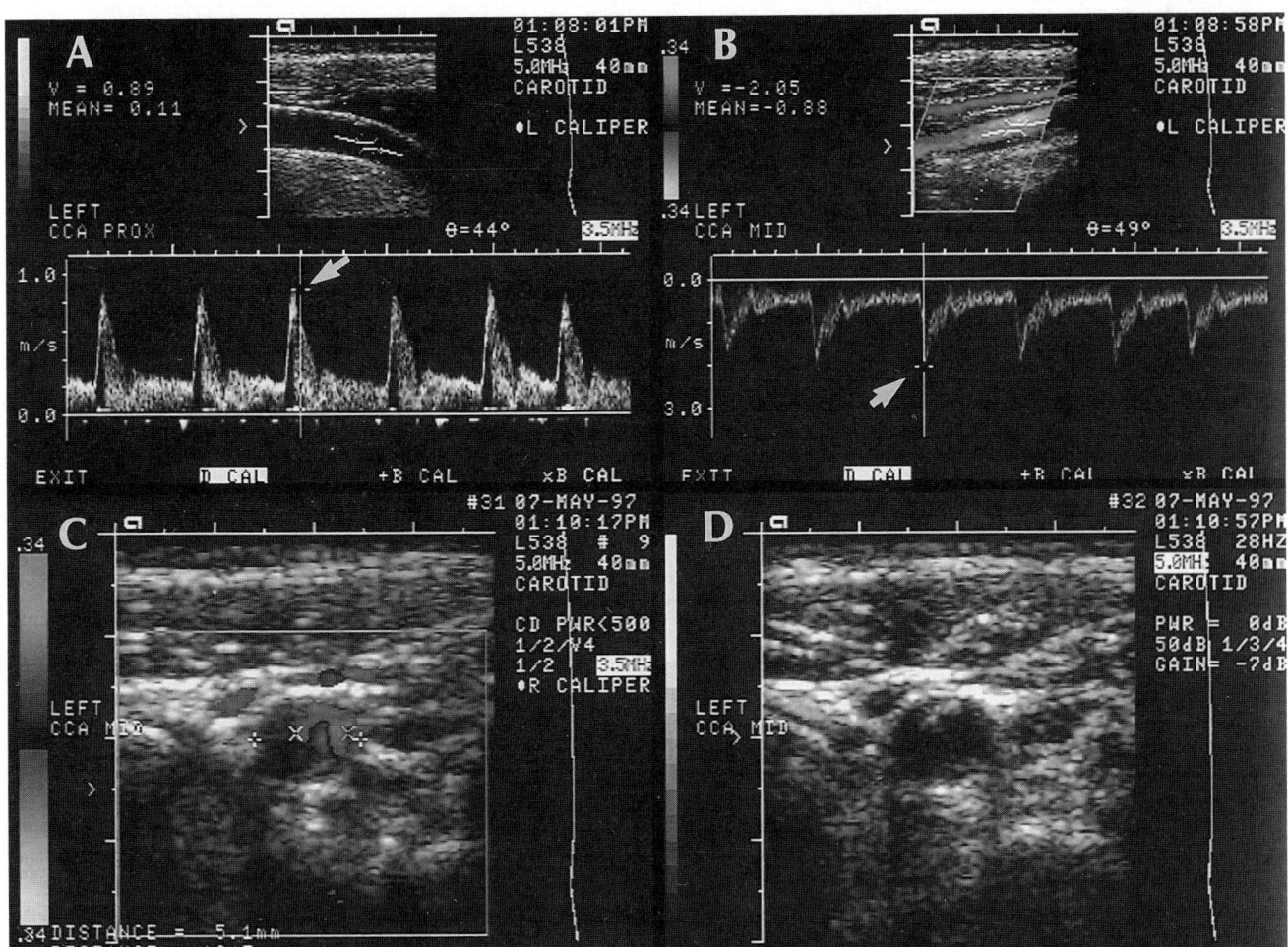

Figure 40.20. (Color Plates) Common Carotid Artery Stenosis. A. Proximal left CCA peak systolic velocity is 0.89 m/sec (*arrow*). **B.** Mid–left CCA peak systolic velocity is 2.05 m/sec (*arrow*). The velocity ratio (mid/proximal) is 2.3 indicating ≥.50% diameter left CCA stenosis (Table 40.7). Transverse color Doppler **(C)** and gray scale **(D)** images confirm the degree of stenosis secondary to mildly heterogeneous plaque. MR angiography graded the stenosis at 60% diameter.

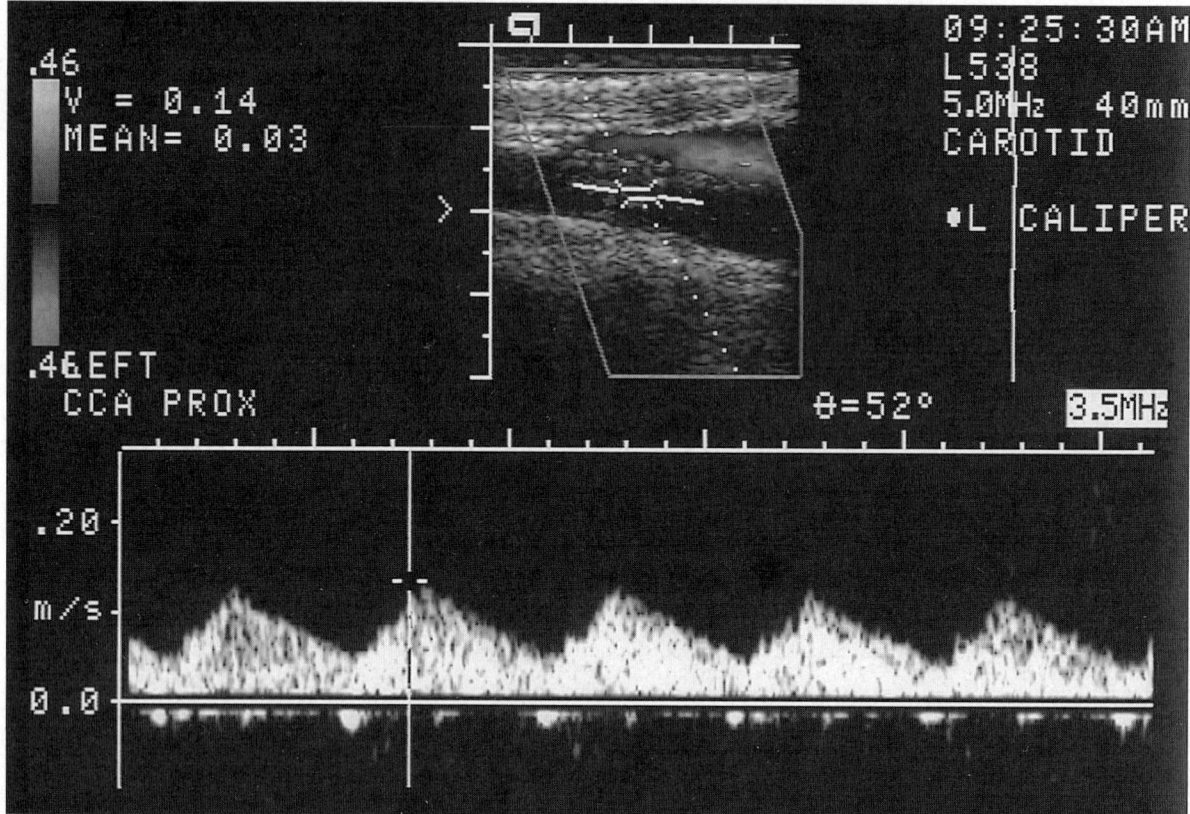

Figure 40.21. (Color Plates) Common Carotid Artery Origin Stenosis. A parvus-tardus waveform is shown in the left proximal CCA with a low peak systolic velocity of 0.14 m/sec (*upper left*) cor-responding to an angiographically proven severe origin stenosis of the left CCA.

locity in the contralateral CCA and ICA may be elevated to maintain cerebral perfusion pressure.

Bilateral ICA Disease causes physiologic flow alterations that complicate determining which side represents the more significant disease.

Tandem Lesions. The presence of more than one high-grade stenotic lesion can lead to interpretation errors. A significant intracranial ICA lesion causes a reduction in PSV with absence of diastolic flow in the cervical portion of the ICA. Alternately, a significant proximal CCA lesion lowers the PSV and increases the diastolic flow. In either circumstance, a stenosis in the cervical ICA may be underestimated.

Mistaking ECA for ICA When ICA Is Occluded. Remember that the ECA waveform may be internalized because of collateral flow. Use the temporal tap and look for branch vessels to identify the ECA (Figs. 40.16, 40.24).

Near Occlusion of the ICA. As the ICA approaches occlusion, the PSV and EDV may approach normal. The severity of the stenosis can be grossly underestimated if gray scale and color flow imaging are not performed.

Postendarterectomy. Following endarterectomy, the vein or polytetrafluoroethylene patch (PFTE) sutures may remain visible along the arterial wall (Fig. 40.29). A patulous carotid artery at the operative site is common. Complications include restenosis (~10–15% within the first year due to intimal hyperplasia), intimal flaps, and clamp strictures. Intraoperative US can help the assessment of surgical result prior to closure. The postendarterectomy waveform often has a high-resistance flow pattern similar to the ECA. Turbulent flow is often caused by the absence of the smooth endothelial lining.

Nonatherosclerotic Carotid Disease. Remember that not all carotid disease is atherosclerotic. Takayasu's arteritis and radiation fibrosis cause diffuse concentric wall thickening and narrowing of the lumen. Fibromuscular dysplasia in the cervical CCA produces irregular intimal thickening over the full length of the artery. Carotid dissection can be traumatic, inflammatory, degenerative, or spontaneous. Systolic flow reversal and intimal flaps can be seen. Carotid body tumors or vascular invasion from metastases can be visualized using duplex scanning.

Valvular Heart Disease. Significant aortic stenosis produces a bilateral parvus-tardus waveform, and aortic insufficiency demonstrates a bisiferous pulse with the second systolic peak higher than the first.

A simplified approach to carotid duplex interpretation is provided in Table 40.8 . The ideal carotid imaging algorithm is at best controversial, and a detailed discussion is beyond the scope of this chapter. For both medical and economic reasons, a combination of noninvasive studies—MRA and duplex US—has replaced catheter angiography in most patients. In our institutions, duplex US is used to screen patients. Therefore, we use sensitive but less specific velocity parameters. If a significant

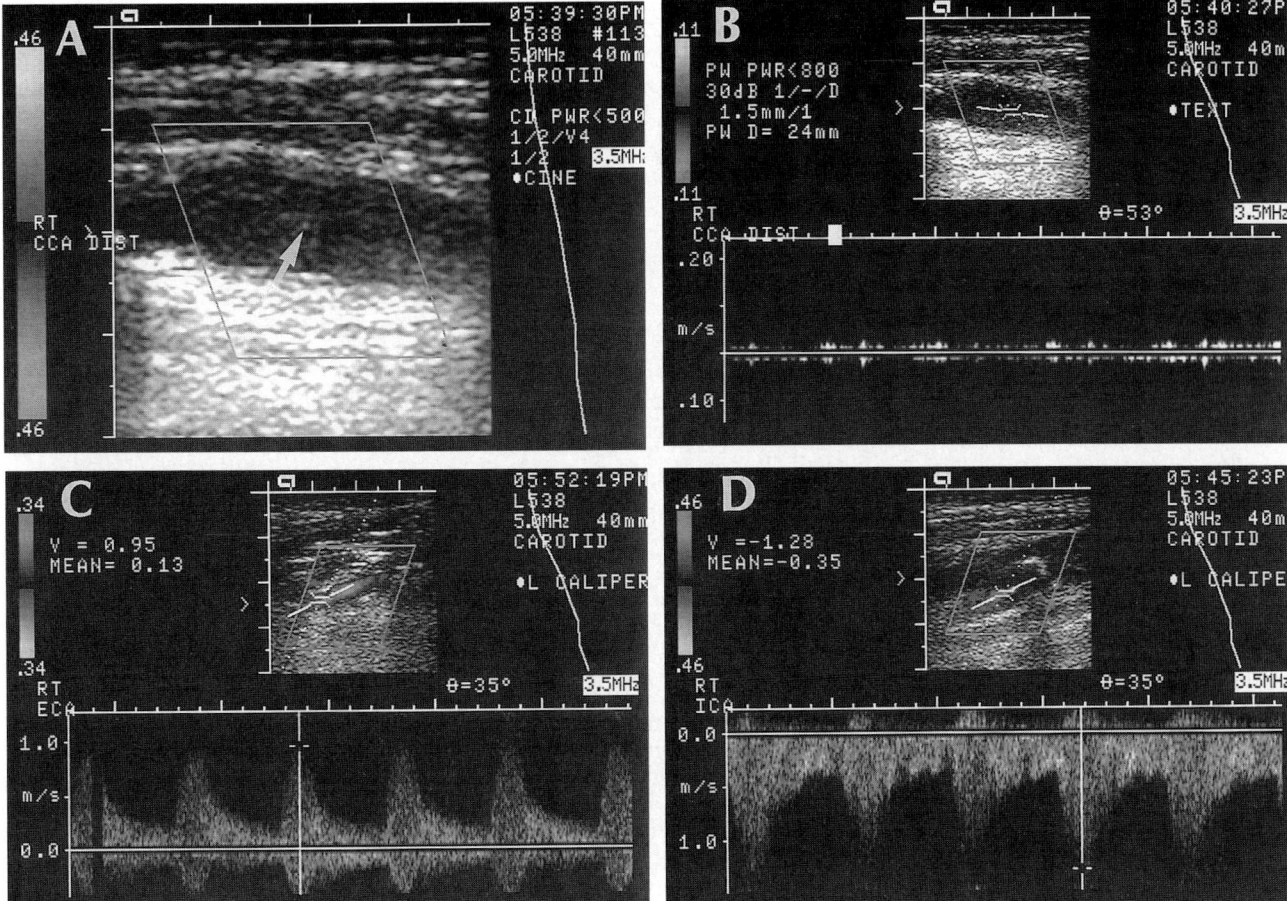

Figure 40.22. (Color Plates) Common Carotid Artery Occlusion. A. Longitudinal color Doppler image of the right CCA shows echogenic thrombus (arrow) with absence of color indicating no blood flow. **B.** Spectral Doppler confirms no CCA flow. The irregular signal near the baseline is due to noise. **C.** Spectral Doppler of the right ECA demonstrates retrograde flow (toward the heart). **D.** Spectral Doppler of the right ICA shows antegrade flow (toward the head). See text for explanation.

Table 40.8. Carotid Duplex Interpretation—Checklist

1. Keep angle of insonation <60°
2. Is the CCA flow normal? (50–100 cm/sec)
3. If CCA velocities are normal and symmetric
   —use the PSV to grade stenosis
4. If CCA velocities abnormal or asymmetric
   —use ICA/CCA ratio and search for cause.
5. Use the EDV to help identify very high grade stenosis
   —>100cm/s suggests >80% diameter stenosis
6. Confirm all findings on gray scale and color Doppler
7. Assess direction of flow in vertebral arteries

CCA = common carotid artery
PSV = peak systolic velocity
EDV = end diastolic velocity
ICA/CCA = ICA peak systolic velocity/CCA peak systolic velocity

stenosis is suspected, an MRA is performed for confirmation. Catheter angiography is reserved for difficult cases and confirmation of carotid occlusion. Asymptomatic stenoses >70% of the diameter receive endarterectomy. Because management is controversial, Asymptomatic patients with stenoses >60% of the diameter are evaluated on an individualized basis.

ABDOMINAL VESSELS

Anatomy

Abdominal Aorta. The abdominal aorta enters the abdomen through the aortic hiatus of the diaphragm and descends just to the left of midline and anterior to the spine. It bifurcates into the bilateral common iliac arteries at approximately the level of L4. The aorta has five main branches. Three originate from the ventral aorta: the celiac axis, the superior mesenteric artery, and the inferior mesenteric artery. The left and right renal arteries originate laterally from the aorta. The proximal aorta measures 2.5 cm and tapers distally to measure approximately 1.5–2.0 cm at the bifurcation (see Fig. 24.14). Spectral analysis demonstrates a triphasic waveform. Color Doppler is useful to identify thrombus.

Inferior Vena Cava. The IVC courses toward the heart just to the right of midline and to the right of the aorta. As it reaches the liver, the IVC is contained in a deep groove on the liver's posterior surface. It traverses the liver and diaphragm and empties into the right atrium. The sonographically detectable branches include the hepatic and renal veins. The renal veins are anterior to their corre-

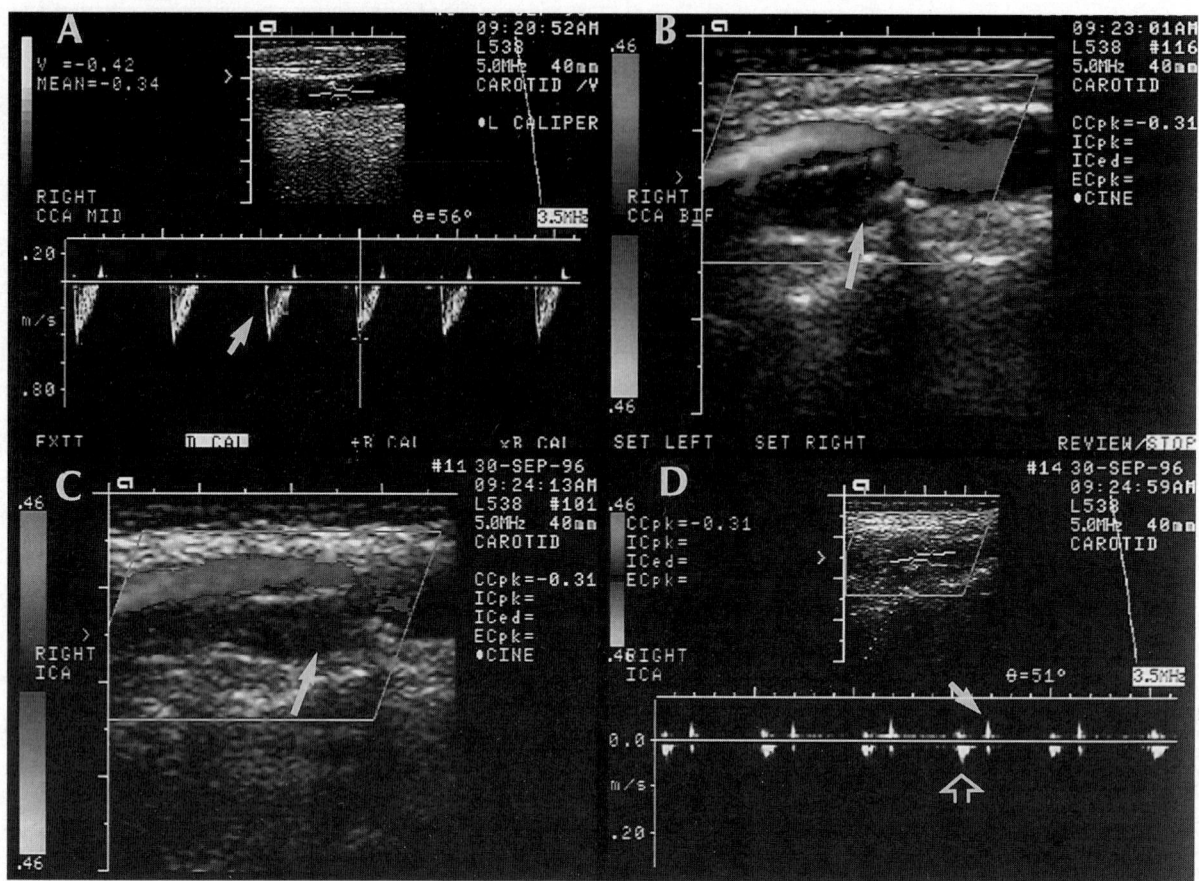

Figure 40.23. (Color Plates) Internal Carotid Artery Occlusion. A. Spectral Doppler waveform in the right mid CCA illustrates "externalization" of the CCA (*arrow*). The CCA waveform resembles the high resistance ECA waveform. Longitudinal color Doppler images of the right carotid bifurcation **(B)** and right ICA **(C)** demonstrates echogenic thrombus and the absence of color flow (*arrow*) in the ICA. Color Doppler flow (*red*) is present in the ECA. **D.** Spectral Doppler interrogation of the ICA at the proximal end of the occlusion shows the typical bi-directional flow. Antegrade flow (*open arrow*) slams into the occlusion resulting in flow reversal (*arrow*). During scanning an audible carotid "thump" can be heard.

Figure 40.24. (Color Plates) Internal Carotid Occlusion. Color image and spectral Doppler demonstrate "internalization" of the ECA waveform due to ICA occlusion with intracranial ECA collateral flow to the ICA system. The temporal tap (*arrows*) confirms that the artery visualized is the ECA.

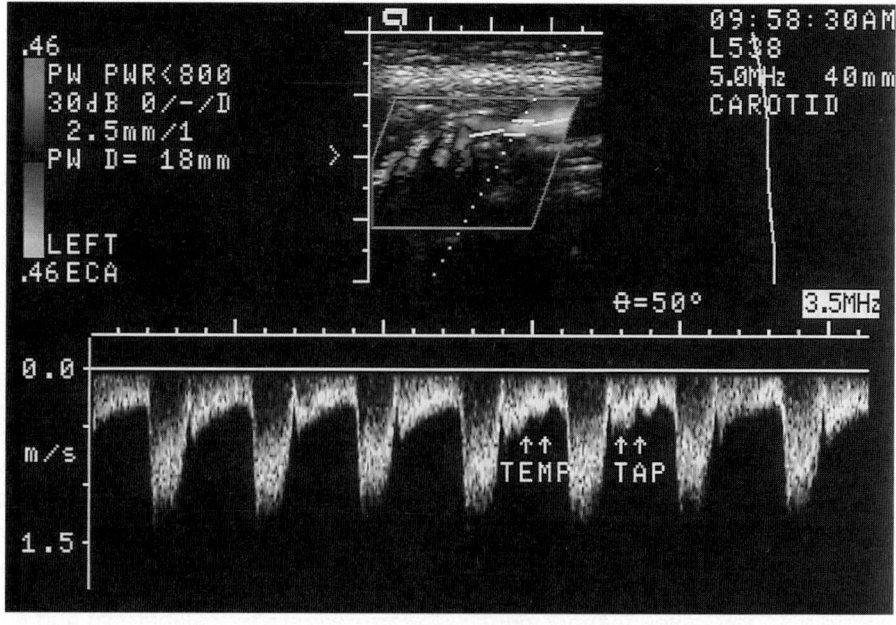

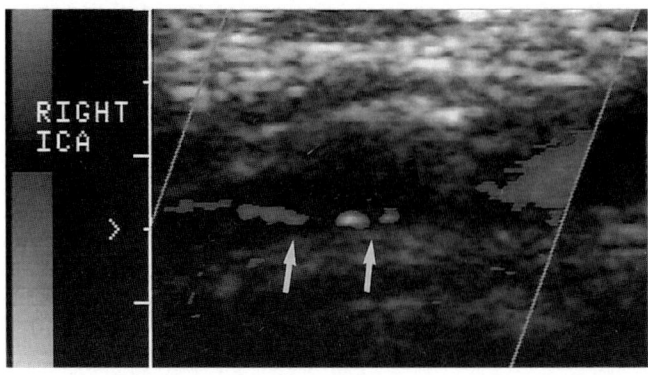

Figure 40.25. (Color Plates) String Sign. Near occlusion of the right ICA demonstrates "trickle flow" (*arrows*).

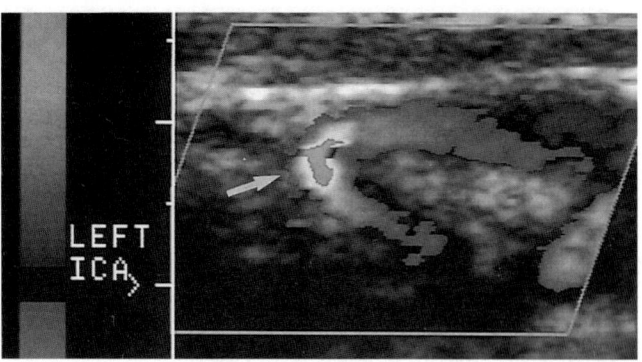

Figure 40.27. (Color Plates) Tortuous Vessel. Color Doppler image of ICA shows a sharp turn. Aliasing and turbulence (*arrow*) indicate the disruption in laminar flow as blood flows around a bend.

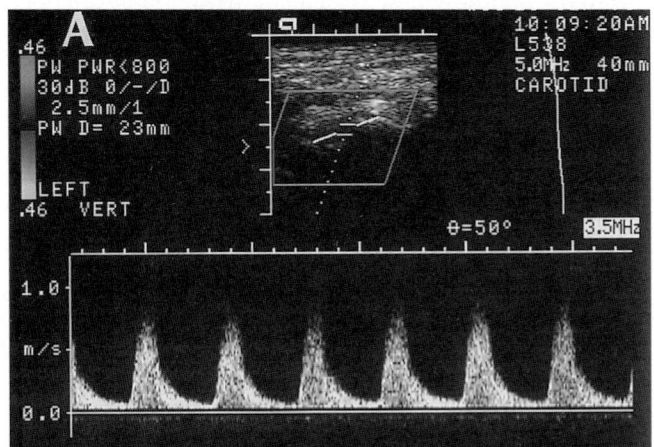

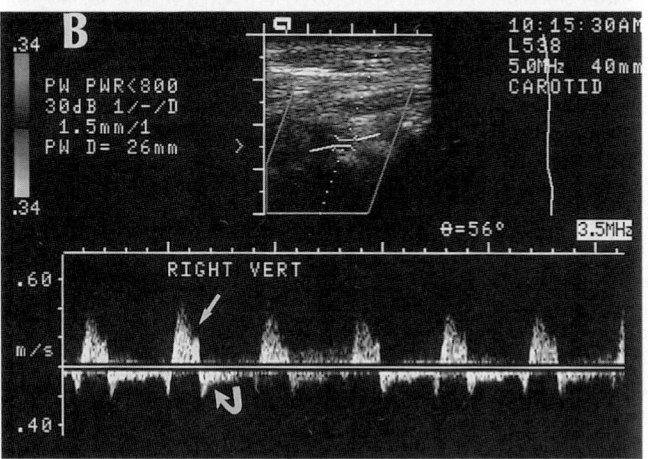

Figure 40.26. Subclavian Steal. A. Flow is reversed in the left vertebral artery (flow is away from the brain). **B.** Partial subclavian steal. In another patient, results in reversed flow during systole (*arrow*) and antegrade flow during diastole (*curved arrow*).

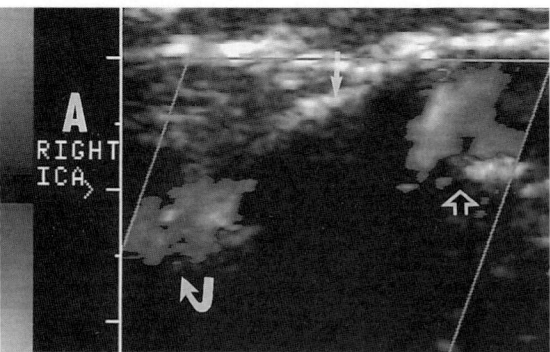

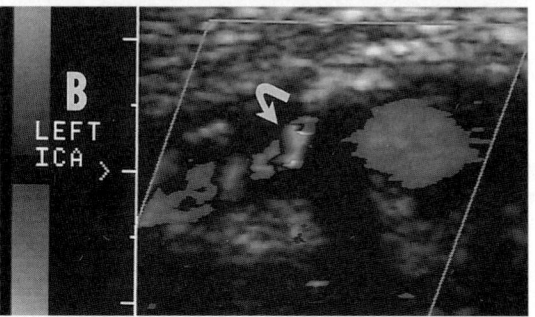

Figure 40.28. (Color Plates) Calcified Plaques. A. Longitudinal color Doppler image of a right ICA. Visualization of the lumen is limited behind a calcified plaque (*arrow*) due to sound absorption/shadowing. However, the flow is homogeneous (*red*) both entering (*open arrow*) and exiting (*curved arrow*) from behind the plaque. The absence of turbulent flow after the plaque bodes against a significant stenosis. **B.** In contrast, this longitudinal color Doppler image demonstrates heterogeneous or turbulent flow (aliasing) exiting from behind the calcified plaque (*curved arrow*). This patient had a severe stenosis at angiography despite only mild to moderate velocity elevation.

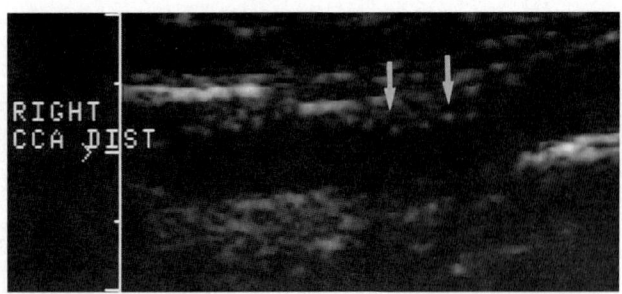

Figure 40.29. Postendarterectomy. Note the typical "dot-dash" pattern of the synthetic PFTE sutures (*arrows*).

Table 40.9. Aortic Aneurysm Rupture

Size	Rupture Rate
> 4 cm	10%
4–7 cm	25%
7–10 cm	45%
>10 cm	60%

sponding arteries and enter the IVC at right angles. The left renal vein is three times longer than the right. The hepatic veins enter the IVC from the posterior surface of the liver. Many embryologic variations of the IVC exist, including an interrupted IVC that does not extend above the renal arteries, a left-sided IVC, and a duplicated IVC. The left renal vein can be retroaortic or circumaortic.

Aneurysm

Abdominal Aorta. More than 90% of abdominal aortic aneurysms (AAA) involve the infrarenal aorta. Most are fusiform and enlarge at the rate of 2–4mm per year. Surgery is recommended for aneurysms >5cm. This recommendation stems from Darling's autopsy data of aneurysm rupture rates shown in Table 40.9 (41). The rupture rate for an aneurysm >5cm is currently estimated at about 8% per year with lifetime risks of 25–49% (42); thus, surgery is reasonable but not universally accepted. Some surgeons operate on smaller aneurysms (42,43). Some use rapid expansion rates (>1cm per year) as an additional criteria for elective surgery for aneurysms <6cm (44). Currently, no definitive patient selection process exists for elective aneurysm repair. Aneurysm size, clinical risk factors, and operative mortality rates (1–3% in experienced centers) are important factors.

Duplex US has a diagnostic accuracy of almost 100%, is readily available, and is cost-effective. Therefore, it has become the imaging modality of choice for diagnosing and following asymptomatic AAAs. The aorta is imaged from the diaphragm to the iliac bifurcation using a linear 3.5–5.0MHz transducer in both the longitudinal and transverse planes. Limitations include patient obesity, bowel gas, and difficulty identifying the origins of the renal arteries. An AAA is defined as a focal enlargement of the aorta greater than 3cm in the anteroposterior (AP) diameter. The AP dimension of the aorta should be measured in both the transverse and longitudinal plane to ensure accuracy. Many atherosclerotic aortas are tortuous, and if measured obliquely, measurement errors occur. The AP dimension can be overestimated in the transverse plane and underestimated in the longitudinal plane. The authors report the longitudinal measurement provided it is concordant with the transverse measurement. The aorta normally tapers from proximal to distal. If it enlarges distally, it is technically considered aneurysmal regardless of the absolute measurement (Fig. 40.30).

Figure 40.30. Abdominal Aortic Aneurysm (AAA). A. Longitudinal image of a distal AAA measuring 5.1cm in the AP dimension (*cursors*). **B.** Longitudinal image shows extension of the aneurysm into the right common iliac artery (*cursors*). **C.** The maximum dimension of the aneurysm is confirmed in the transverse plane. **D.** Longitudinal image showing the fusiform nature of the AAA.

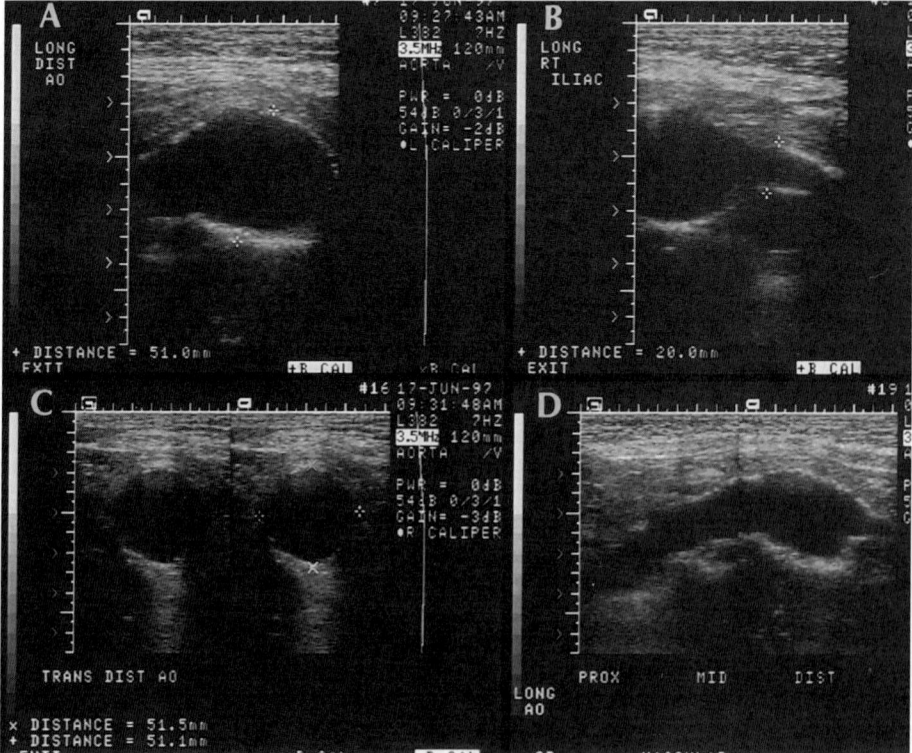

In addition to sizing the aneurysm, US can identify intraluminal thrombus, which generally appears hypoechoic. Thrombus can be isoechoic to blood within the aorta making it invisible on gray scale imaging; therefore, color Doppler is useful in this situation. Inflammatory aneurysms have a hypoechoic ring surrounding the aorta corresponding to the perianeurysmal fibrosis. Aortic rupture can be diagnosed with US if a retroperitoneal hematoma is present. CT is the diagnostic modality of choice for suspected leaking aneurysm, rupture, inflammatory aneurysm, and for defining the aneurysm's relationship to the surrounding retroperitoneal structures.

Following AAA repair, the aortic graft demonstrates discrete echogenic walls. US is used to confirm patency of the graft, to assess for perigraft fluid collections, and to evaluate for anastomotic stenosis or aneurysm. Perigraft fluid collections seen more than three months after surgery may indicate hemorrhage or infection. Anastomotic aneurysms typically occur at the iliac anastomosis. They appear as focal circumscribed bulges off the distal end of the graft.

Abdominal aortic dissection can be diagnosed when US discloses an intimal flap or color flow US identifies flow in the false lumen (Fig. 40.31). Chronic dissection is difficult to identify because the false lumen is often filled with clot. CT and MR remain the preferred diagnostic modalities.

Iliac Arteries. Approximately two-thirds of AAAs extend into the common iliac arteries; however, extension into the external iliac artery is uncommon. The normal common iliac arteries measure <15 mm in the AP dimension. Isolated iliac artery aneurysms are rare. Common iliac artery aneurysms can rupture or erode into the adjacent iliac vein, colon, or ureter.

Thrombosis

Inferior Vena Cava. The IVC is examined in sagittal, coronal, and transverse planes using a linear 3.5–5.0 MHz transducer. The renal and hepatic vein communications with the IVC are usually seen. The characteristic waveform in the IVC results from transmission of right atrial pulsations. The tracing is similar to that of the hepatic veins. Patency is confirmed by color flow and a normal spectral tracing.

IVC thrombosis usually extends from the peripheral veins. Bilateral lower extremity edema is present, and if acute, patients typically experience severe pain. Other clinical symptoms and signs are related to organ involvement (renal failure, bowel ischemia, etc.). Gray scale imaging demonstrates intraluminal clot (Fig 40.32) that often expands the IVC. Remember that congestive heart failure also distends the hepatic veins and IVC. With the current high-resolution transducers, the slow-flowing blood can be mistaken for a clot. Doppler demonstrates the absence of flow in complete occlusion and diverted flow with partial obstruction. In partial thrombosis, the spectral waveform is usually blunted with loss of the transmitted cardiac pulsation and respiratory phasicity.

Tumor extension into the IVC causes a tumor throm-

bosis (Fig. 40.32), which appears similar to bland thrombus. If arterial flow is identified in the IVC lumen within the mass, the diagnosis of tumor thrombus can be made confidently. The most common tumor to extend into the IVC is renal cell carcinoma. Less common tumors include hepatoma, adrenal cell carcinoma, pheochromocytoma, and lymphoma. Benign tumors that rarely invade the IVC include angiomyolipoma and atrial myxoma. Leiomyosarcoma is the most common primary tumor of the IVC.

Extrinsic compression from any intraperitoneal or retroperitoneal process such as lymphadenopathy, hepatomegaly, retroperitoneal fibrosis, or hematoma can cause obstruction and thrombosis of the IVC.

Budd-Chiari syndrome (segmental obstruction of the hepatic veins) can involve the IVC. Causes include hypercoagulable states, trauma, tumor invasion, and membranous obstruction of the suprahepatic IVC (web or diaphragm). US demonstrates echogenic thrombus within, reduced caliber of, or nonvisualization of the hepatic veins. The spectral waveform is often monophasic.

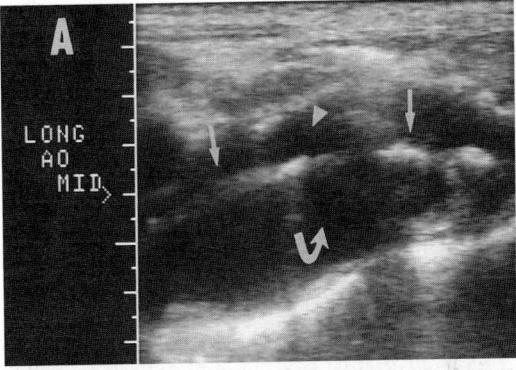

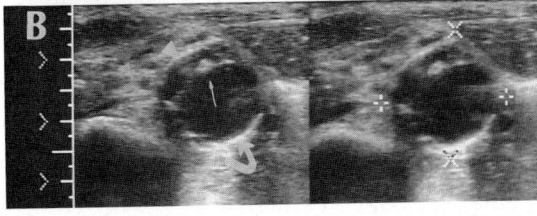

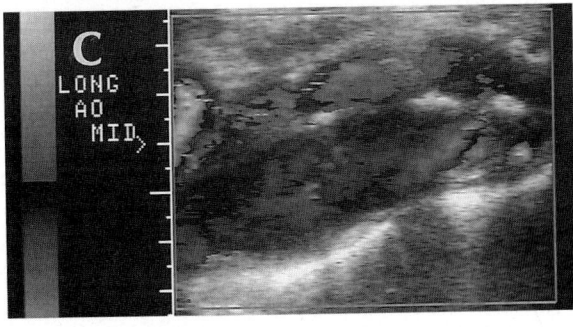

Figure 40.31. (Color Plates) Aortic Dissection. Longitudinal **(A)** and transverse **(B)** images of a 4.2 cm aortic aneurysm with a dissection. An echogenic intimal flap is identified (*arrows*) separating the true (*arrowhead*) from false (*curved arrow*) lumen. **C.** Longitudinal color Doppler image demonstrates antegrade flow in the smaller true lumen (*red*) and retrograde flow in the larger false lumen (*blue*).

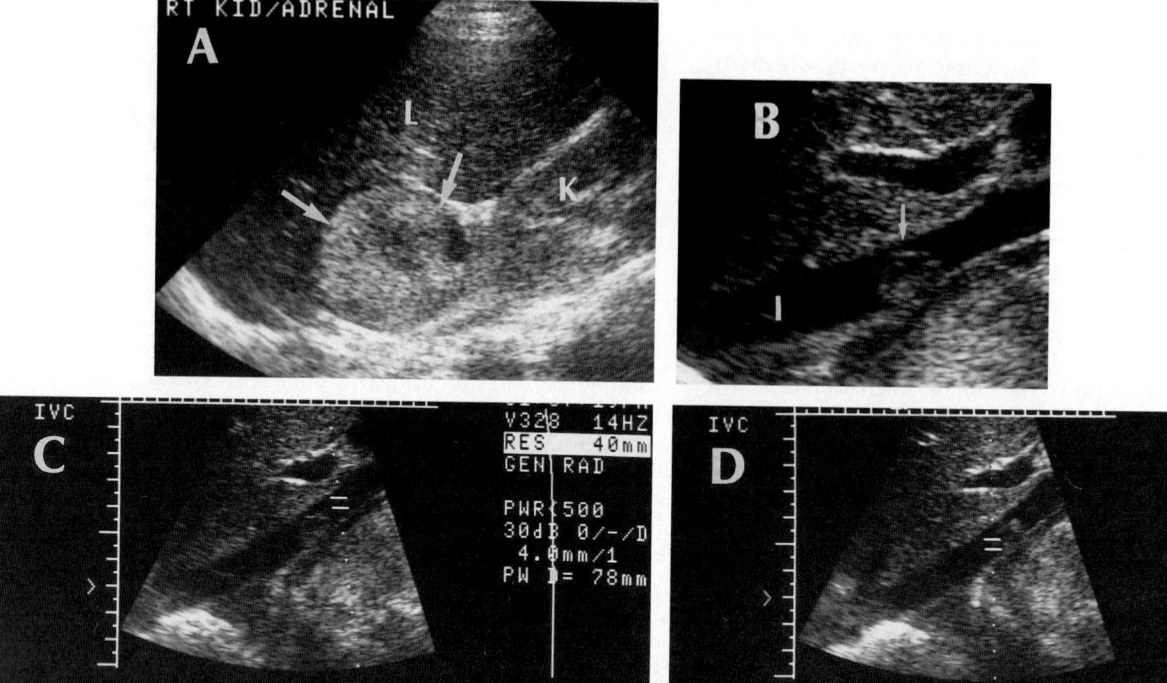

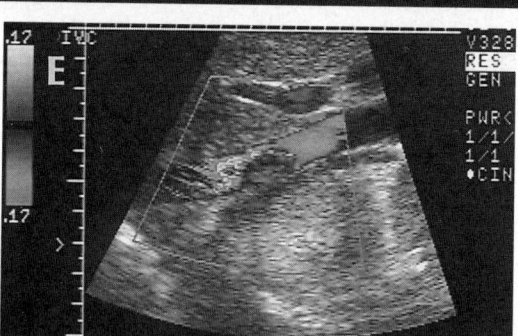

Figure 40.32. (Color Plates) IVC Tumor Thrombus. A. Longitudinal image shows an echogenic right suprarenal mass (*arrows*). *L*, liver; *K*, kidney. **B.** Longitudinal image of the IVC (*I*) showing an echogenic intraluminal mass (*arrow*). Spectral analysis demonstrates mild blunting of the IVC waveform caudad to the mass **(C)** and the normal waveform cephalad to the mass **(D). E.** Color Doppler image shows flow around the intraluminal mass. **Diagnosis:** pheochromocytoma with tumor extension into the IVC.

Aortic Thrombosis. Gray scale imaging of the abdominal aorta may appear normal when aortic thrombosis is present because it can occur in the absence of an aneurysm and the clot can be echolucent. Spectral and color Doppler imaging confirm the presence of a thrombosis.

TIPS Evaluation

Transjugular intrahepatic portosystemic shunt (TIPS) has become commonplace in the treatment of life-threatening portal venous hypertension with variceal bleeding refractory to sclerotherapy and intractable ascites. The TIPS procedure involves creating a tract between a hepatic and portal vein, most commonly the right hepatic vein to the right portal vein. Because early shunt malfunction is often asymptomatic, the ability to predict shunt failure is of prime importance. If diagnosed, rein-

tervention can be performed in a timely fashion to prevent a catastrophic variceal bleed and to increase the longevity of the stent.

Technique. The patient is imaged using 2.5–3.5 MHz curvilinear or sector transducer. A common protocol for monitoring a TIPS calls for a pre-TIPS US, a US within 24 hours following the procedure, at three months after TIPS, and then at 6-month intervals. Additional interval US is performed if the clinical situation suggests shunt malfunction (e.g., recurrent bleeding or ascites). Transjugular portal venograms are routinely performed at six months, one year following the procedure, and then annually (45).

The pre-TIPS US defines the anatomy and establishes the patient's baseline hemodynamics prior to the procedure (46). Gray scale US evaluates the size and echotexture of the hepatic and splenic parenchyma. Spectral and color Doppler establish the patency and direction of flow in the main, right, and left portal veins; the hepatic veins; and IVC. Velocity measurements can be obtained in the main portal vein and hepatic arteries. Enlarged collateral vessels (patent umbilical vein, etc.) are documented and the amount of ascites is noted. The right internal jugular vein is assessed for patency.

After the TIPS procedure, the shunt is easily visualized on US as an echogenic tubular structure coursing from a portal vein to a hepatic vein. The anatomic survey is repeated as per the pre-TIPS protocol. In addition, duplex interrogation of the stent is performed. The angle-corrected peak systolic velocities at the portal vein end of the stent, the middle of the stent, and the hepatic vein end of the stent are obtained. Normal postshunt velocities range from 100–200 cm/sec. Following shunting, the collateral vessels disappear and ascites resolves in many patients. In two-thirds of patients, blood flow in the right and left portal vein reverses (becomes hep-

atofugal) secondary to diversion through the stent. The immediate post-TIPS US establishes a new baseline and looks for immediate thrombosis of the stent as well as hemorrhagic complications (Fig. 40.33) (45–47).

Shunt Malfunction usually results from thrombosis or pseudointimal hyperplasia of the stent. The latter can occur within a few weeks after TIPS, and significant stenoses are often detected within six months. Stenosis is usually focal and can occur anywhere in the stent but is more common in the hepatic vein end. Diffuse pseudointimal hyperplasia occurs less commonly.

Nearly all shunt stenoses manifest as decreased velocity within the stent because of preferential shunting through the lower resistance collateral venous pathways present in portal hypertension. However, several recent articles have shown high-velocity stenosis within the TIPS stent (47). Duplex US is nearly 100% accurate in detecting shunt occlusion. No spectral waveform or color

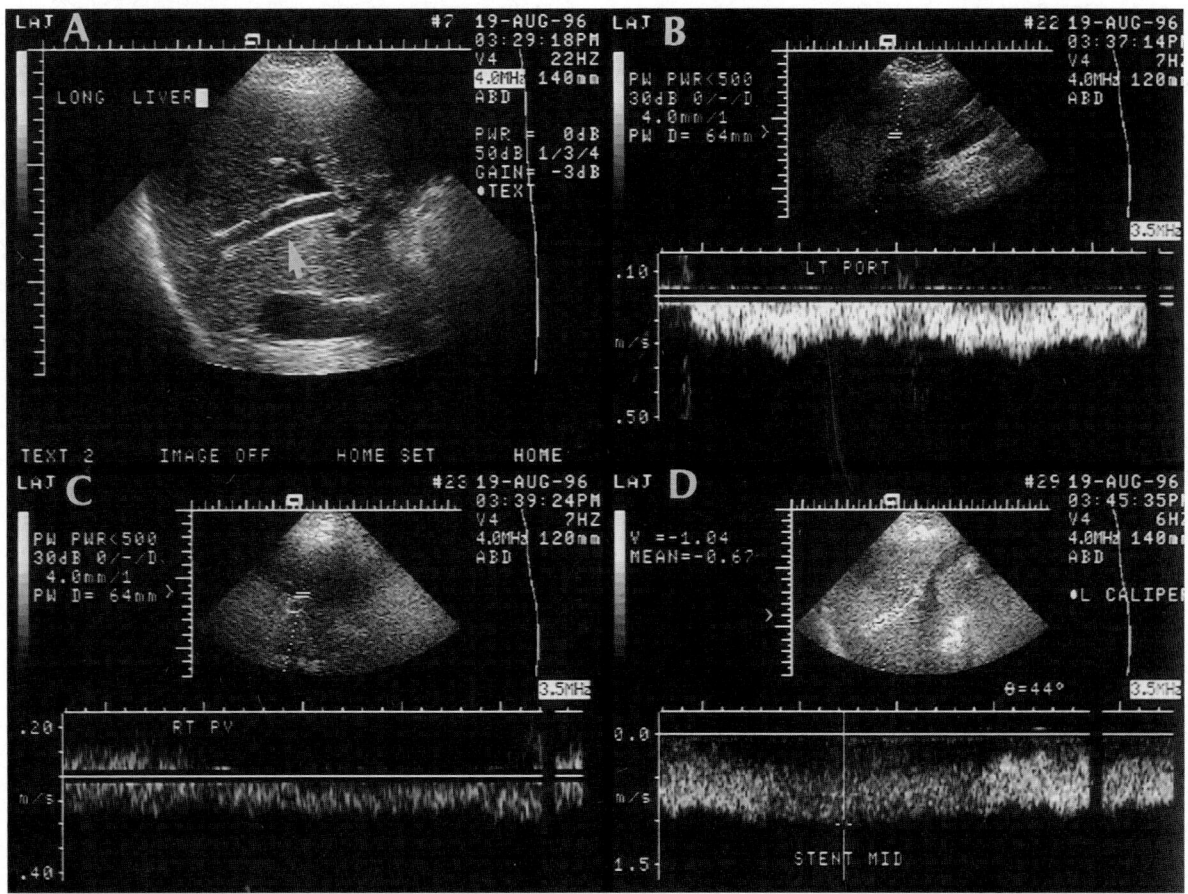

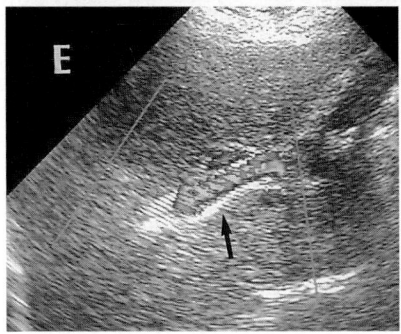

Figure 40.33. (Color Plates) TIPS US. A. Longitudinal gray scale image shows the TIPS stent (arrow). Spectral Doppler interrogation of the left portal vein **B** and anterior branch of the right portal vein **C** shows the "normal" hepatofugal flow seen in about two-thirds of patients following TIPS. The Doppler tracings are below the baseline indicating flow away from the transducer. **D.** Normal midstent velocity of 1.04 m/sec. **E.** Color Doppler image demonstrates a patent TIPS stent (arrow).

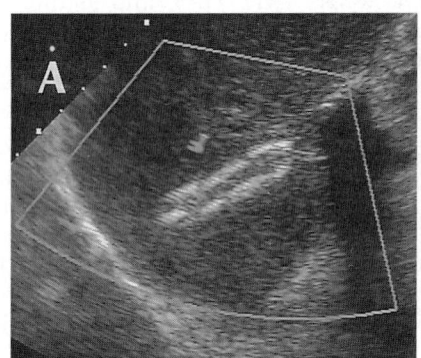
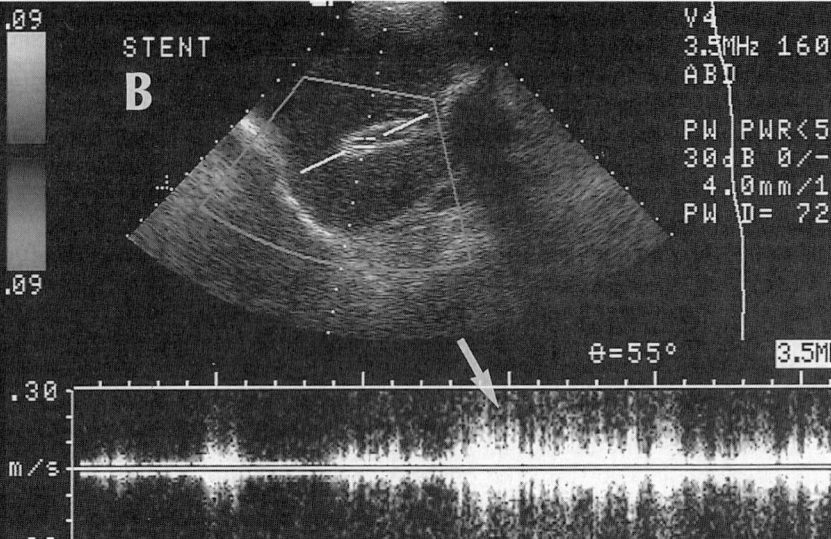

Figure 40.34. TIPS Occlusion. Color Doppler **(A)** and spectral Doppler **(B)** show an occluded TIPS shunt. Echogenic thrombus is seen in the stent with the absence of flow on color flow imaging. The pulsed wave Doppler shows artifact (*arrow*) but no flow.

Table 40.10. Duplex Evaluation of TIPS Malfunction

Criteria (45–53)	Parameter
	Change from Baseline:
Collaterals	Recurrent, new or increased
Ascites	Recurrent, new or increased
Right/Left Portal Vein Flow	Hepatofugal to Hepatopetal
Draining Hepatic Vein Flow	Reversed
Shunt Velocity:	**Abnormal if:**
Kanterman et al. (47)	Peak <90 or ≥ 190 cm/sec
	Distal <90 or ≥ 220 cm/sec
Feldstein et al. (45)	Peak <50 cm/sec
Chong et al. (48)	Peak <50 cm/sec
Foshager et al. (46)	Peak <60 cm/sec
Peak Shunt velocity change:	**Change from Baseline:**
Kanterman et al. (47)	Decrease >40 cm/sec
	Increase >60 cm/sec
Dodd et al. (49)	Decrease >50 cm/sec
	Increase >50 cm/sec
Main portal vein velocity:	**Abnormal if:**
Kanterman et al. (47),	<30 cm/sec
Suratt et al. (52),	
Longo et al. (53)	

flow is identified within the shunt (Fig. 40.34). Parameters for the early detection of shunt malfunction are shown in Table 40.10 (45–53). The methodology, parameters, location of velocity measurements within the stent, small patient numbers, and individual patient manifestations of portal hypertension have made establishing universally accepted criteria for shunt malfunction difficult.

US is a screening test used to decide when transjugular portography should be performed. The absolute or temporal change in PSV within the shunt is a sensitive indicator of malfunction. Measuring the PSV in more than one region within the stent increases the chance of finding an early focal stenosis. A peak shunt velocity of <50cm/sec portends a bad prognosis. Velocities between 50–100cm/sec remain equivocal and should be individualized to each patient and compared to the baseline post-TIPS study. A stent velocity decrease of more than 50 cm/sec from baseline indicates a potential shunt malfunction; thus, portography is warranted. Shunt velocities >200 cm/sec suggest shunt stenosis particularly if the velocity has increased >50 cm/sec above the established baseline. Because velocity in the main portal vein increases after shunting, a MPV velocity <30 cm/sec indicates possible shunt stenosis. Recurrence of ascites, recanalization of collateral pathways, and return of hepatopetal flow in the right and left portal veins predict early shunt malfunction. In the authors' institution, if any of the above changes occur, the patient is referred for transjugular portography and potential shunt revision (Fig. 40.35).

PERIPHERAL ARTERIES

In the lower extremity, duplex US is the diagnostic modality of choice for evaluating the complications of arterial puncture and monitoring arterial bypass grafts. This noninvasive technique is also evolving as an important adjunct in the evaluation of atherosclerotic peripheral vascular disease (ASPVD). In the upper extremity, ASPVD is uncommon distal to the subclavian arteries. Therefore, US is limited to evaluation of thoracic outlet syndrome (discussed under venous US) and dialysis grafts.

Anatomy

In the lower extremity (Fig 24.15), the femoral and popliteal arteries travel with an accompanying vein. The patient is imaged supine using a 5–10 MHz linear transducer. The common femoral artery arises at the inguinal ligament and quickly bifurcates into the profunda femoris and superficial femoral artery (SFA). The SFA travels along the anteromedial thigh, through the adductor (Hunter's) canal, and becomes the popliteal artery. Below the knee the popliteal artery branches into the anterior tibial artery and a short tibioperoneal trunk that quickly bifurcates into the peroneal and posterior tibial arteries. The anterior tibial artery descends anteriorly and terminates in the dorsalis pedis artery. The peroneal artery terminates above the ankle; the posterior tibial artery continues behind the medial malleolus supplying the plantar surface of the foot. The normal Doppler waveform is a high-resistance, triphasic pattern. Peak systolic velocity decreases from proximal to distal, averaging 110 cm/sec in the femoral artery and 70 cm/sec in the popliteal artery.

In the upper extremity, the right subclavian artery arises from the inominate artery and the left originates from the aortic arch. Their origins can usually be identified from a supraclavicular approach. The subclavian arteries lie superficial to the veins. The distal subclavian artery is difficult to visualize due to the clavicle and is generally better imaged from an infraclavicular approach. The subclavian artery continues as the axillary artery, and the axillary artery becomes the brachial artery, which courses along the medial aspect of the arm. At the elbow, the brachial artery branches into the ulnar and radial arteries, which continue into the hand and form the palmar arches. Like the leg, the Doppler waveforms, at rest, are high-resistance and triphasic. Peak systolic velocity is 110 cm/sec in the proximal subclavian artery and decreases to approximately 85 cm/sec in the axillary artery.

Arterial Puncture Complications

Pseudoaneurysm is a contained rupture of an artery wall with a persistent connection (neck) to the artery that results in a pulsatile mass (54–57). Most are seen in the common femoral artery as a complication of arterial catheterization. Other causes are surgery or trauma. The recent use of larger bore catheters for procedures such

as coronary angioplasty have increased the incidence of pseudoaneurysm to as high as 6%.

US reliably differentiates pseudoaneurysms from other groin masses. Gray scale imaging demonstrates a predominantly echolucent mass, sometimes multilocular, that may contain internal echoes or mural thrombus. The mass is located immediately adjacent to the artery. Color Doppler shows the connection to the artery and documents flow within the mass in the typical "yin-yang" pattern. Interrogation over the neck shows the characteristic "to and fro" spectral waveform (Figs. 40.36, 40.37).

US guided compression is a safe, successful, and cost-effective method of treating postcatheterization pseudoaneurysms. Informed consent is obtained from the patient because pain, distal embolization, rupture and thrombosis of the femoral artery, deep venous thrombosis, and technical failures are potential problems. Patients receive pain medications and local anesthesia upon request. Contraindications include infection, large hematoma, and femoral artery puncture above the inguinal ligament. A contraindication or technically inadequate compression occurs in approximately 10–15% of patients.

The neck of the pseudoaneurysm is compressed using direct pressure from the US transducer during color flow sonography. Enough pressure is applied to obliterate flow in the pseudoaneurysm while maintaining flow in the common femoral artery. Distal pulses are monitored, and compression is held for 20–30 minutes and then slowly released. If flow to the pseudoaneurysm is detected, compression is immediately resumed. This cycle is continued until no extraluminal flow is seen and the pseudoaneurysm is completely thrombosed (Fig. 40.36D). If operator or patient fatigue occurs (usually after 1–2 hours) before complete thrombosis, the process can be repeated the following day. The authors have had several cases of apparent failure that on 24-hour follow-up had spontaneously thrombosed. If successful, standard post–femoral artery catheterization orders are followed including bedrest for six hours. A follow-up scan is obtained within the next 2–3 days to ensure closure. In the rare circumstance of a recurrent pseudoaneurysm, recom-

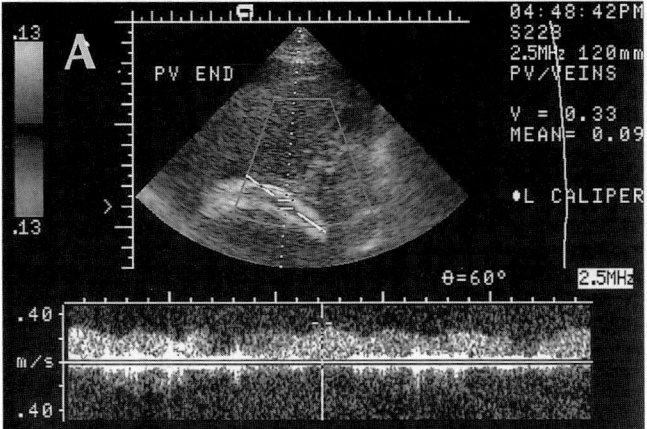
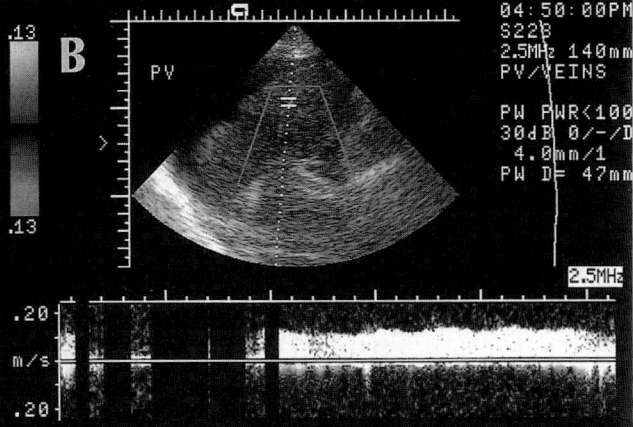

Figure 40.35. TIPS Malfunction. Same patient as Figure 40.34 on follow-up US shows a decreased velocity within the stent of 0.33 m/sec **(A)** and hepatopetal flow (above the baseline) in the right portal vein **(B)** indicating shunt stenosis. The patient underwent successful shunt revision.

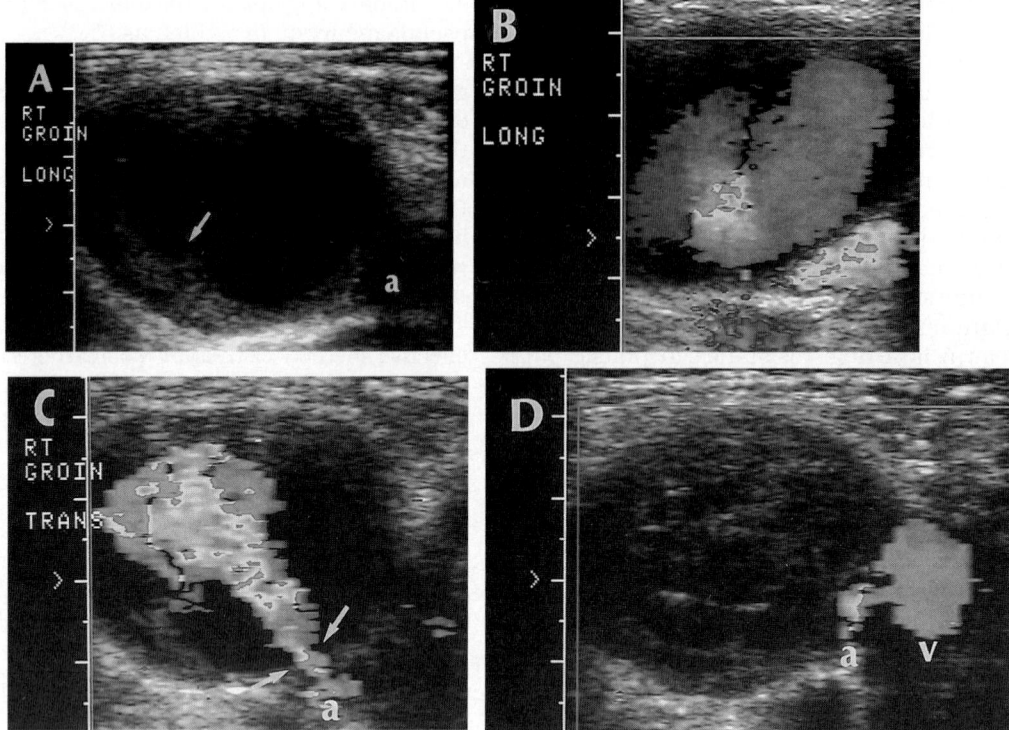

Figure 40.36. (Color Plates) Pseudoaneurysm. A. An echolucent mass with thrombus (*arrow*) is seen adjacent to the common femoral artery (*a*). **B.** Color Doppler image demonstrates the characteristic swirling or "yin-yang" flow. **C.** Transverse color Doppler image demonstrates the neck of the pseudoaneurysm with a "jet" (*arrows*) of blood flow into the mass. **D.** Following successful compression, no flow is seen within the thrombosed pseudoaneurysm. *a*, common femoral artery; *v*, common femoral vein.

Figure 40.37. (Color Plates) Pseudoaneurysm. Spectral Doppler tracing over the neck of a pseudoaneurysm showing the characteristic "to and fro" waveform. During systole, blood flows into the pseudoaneurysm (*arrow*); during diastole (*curved arrow*), blood flows out of the pseudoaneurysm.

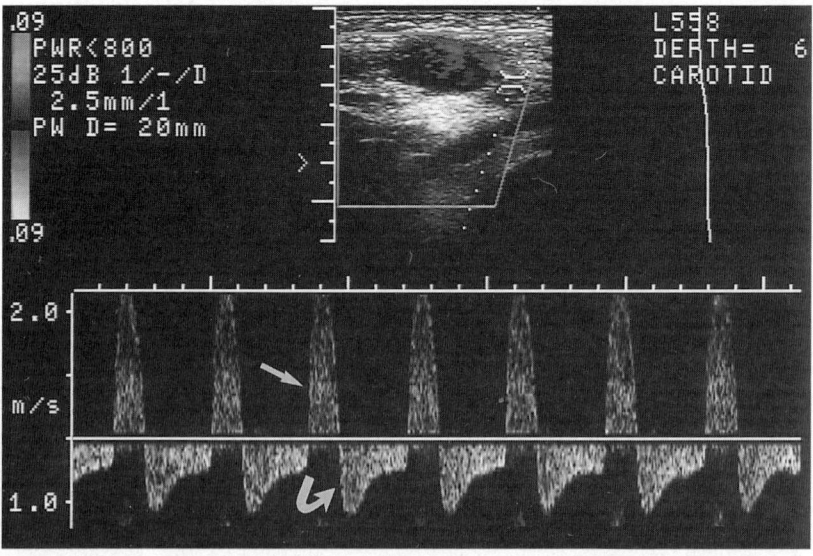

pression is almost always successful. Although the compression technique is usually performed in the groin, it is applicable to pseudoaneurysms resulting from brachial or axillary artery procedures.

Successful occlusion of pseudoaneurysms amenable to compression is achieved in 80–90% of patients. A slightly higher success rate is noted for pseudo-aneurysms <4 cm. Masses with long necks are easier to compress. Anticoagulation decreases the success rate, but compression is still successful in about two-thirds of patients. If medically feasible, anticoagulation is discontinued prior to the compression. Surprisingly, the success rate of compression is not altered by the duration of the pseudoaneurysm (57).

Arteriovenous Fistula (AVF) generally result from simultaneous puncture of the artery and vein. Less common than pseudoaneurysms, AVFs are often small and resolve spontaneously. In a large AVF, the feeding artery has a low resistance waveform with increased diastolic flow, atypical for an extremity artery. The draining vein is distended and demonstrates high velocity pulsatile flow. These characteristic findings are usually only present within several centimeters of the fistula (Fig. 40.38). With a small AVF, duplex imaging may be normal. Color flow imaging guides the placement of the Doppler gate. Color Doppler shows a heterogeneous and markedly disorganized color pattern overlying the fistula caused by soft tissue vibration. This appearance is sometimes called a color Doppler bruit. With appropriate technical adjustments, the fistulous tract often can be seen (54,55).

Hematoma. Perivascular masses immediately following arterial puncture are most commonly hematomas. Sonographically, hematomas range from anechoic to hypoechoic with a complex echo pattern. No internal flow can be demonstrated. Hematomas cannot be distinguished from thrombosed pseudoaneurysms, seromas, or abscesses.

Aneurysm

The popliteal arteries are the most common site of aneurysm in the peripheral vascular system. The popliteal artery is considered aneurysmal when it measures greater than 2 cm. Unlike aneurysms in the abdominal aorta, popliteal aneurysms are unlikely to rupture. Mural thrombus within the aneurysms may cause distal embolization and potential limb loss.

Stenosis and Occlusion

In most circumstances, the diagnosis of significant peripheral arterial occlusive disease is made on clinical grounds based on the symptom of claudication and physical exam findings. Noninvasive testing is primarily used to confirm the diagnosis prior to angiography. The primary noninvasive techniques include continuous wave Doppler, plethysmography, the ankle-brachial index, segmental pressure measurements and pulse volume recordings. Discussion of these modalities is beyond the scope of this chapter. Evaluation with duplex sonography (55,58,59) continues to evolve for diagnosing peripheral vascular stenosis in the native arterial

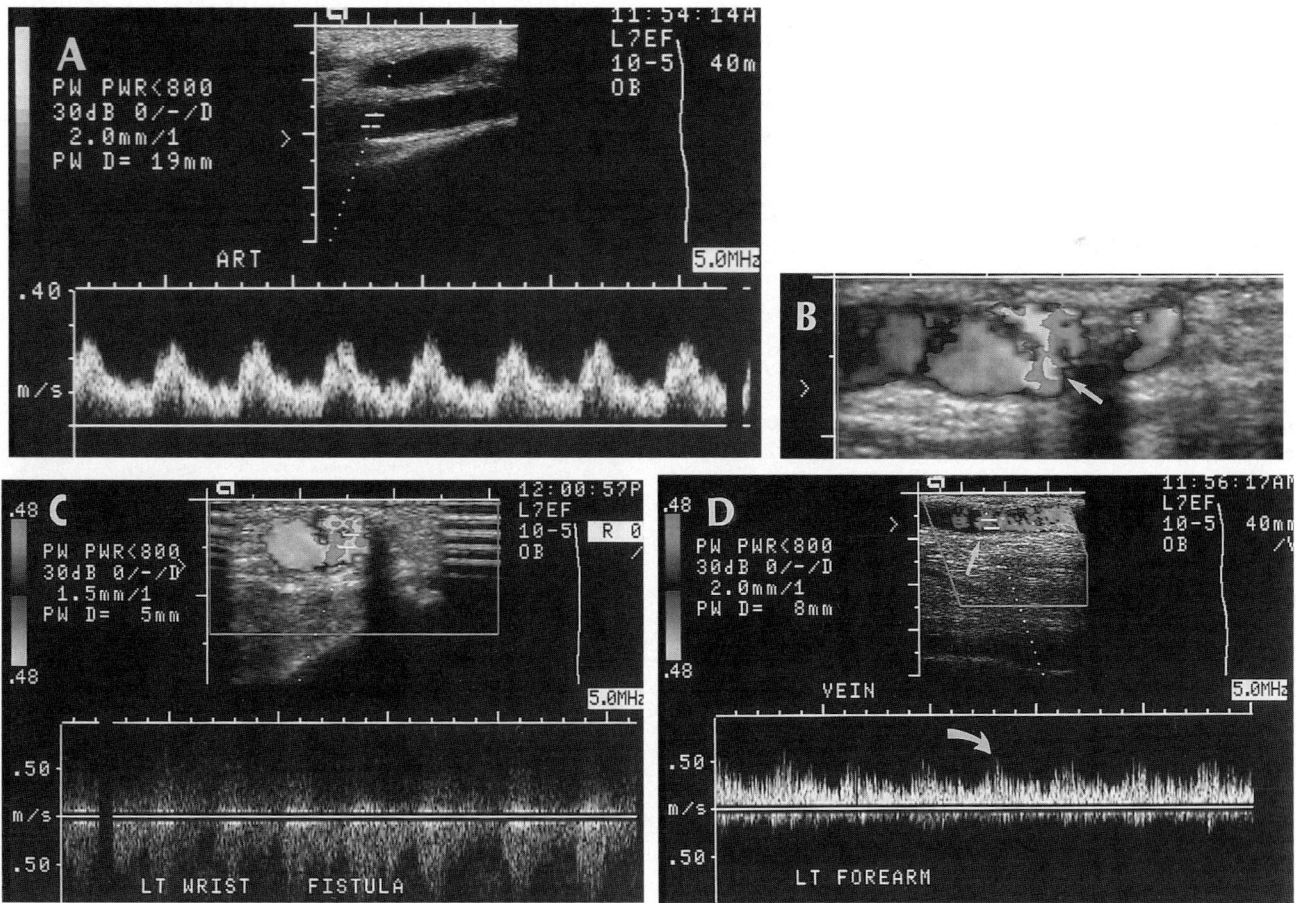

Figure 40.38. (Color Plates) Arteriovenous Fistula—Left Wrist. A. The feeding artery demonstrates a low-resistance waveform uncharacteristic of an extremity artery. **B.** Color Doppler image demonstrates the typical heterogeneous, turbulent flow pattern (*arrow*) at the level of the fistula. **C.** Pulsed wave Doppler tracing showing a pulsatile, turbulent (spectral broadening) waveform with bi-directional flow at the level of the fistula. **D.** The draining vein is dilated (*arrow*) and exhibits a pulsatile (arterialized) waveform (*curved arrow*).

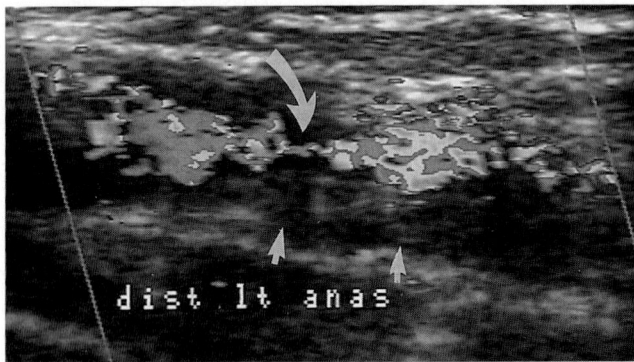

Figure 40.39. (Color Plates) Synthetic Graft Anastomotic Stenosis. Longitudinal color Doppler image at the left distal anastomosis of an aorto-bi-iliac graft. Predominantly homogeneous fibrointimal hyperplasia (*arrows*) and a significant stenosis (*curved arrow*) is evident. The velocity proximal in the graft is approximately 0.53 m/sec and at the anastomosis 1.80 m/sec. Using Table 40.7, this represents about a 75% diameter stenosis (confirmed angiographically).

system. Currently, it remains complementary to the clinical evaluation but may have a role in selecting patients for percutaneous intervention rather than surgery. Vascular surgeons require either catheter or MR angiography for an arterial road map preoperatively and typically do not operate solely on the basis of the US findings. In addition, the definitive treatments—angioplasty or stent placement—can often be performed at the time of the diagnostic study.

The transducer typically used for peripheral arterial mapping is a linear 5–7.5 MHz transducer. Gray scale imaging locates the vessels and evaluates plaque. Color Doppler mapping has drastically decreased imaging time by identifying areas of narrowing and turbulent flow where spectral tracings are then obtained.

The previously described waveform changes before, at, and after a stenosis apply in the peripheral arterial system. Proximal to a significant stenosis, the waveform may be normal or demonstrate a monophasic waveform, decreased PSV, and no diastolic flow. A high-velocity jet is usually at (or just after) the stenosis. Distal to a significant stenosis, the parvus-tardus waveform may be seen. The waveforms can be markedly different for the same degree of stenosis in different individuals. This difference is influenced by the blood inflow, runoff, collateral flow, and medications.

Because of the wide range of normal velocities, the PSV has not been reliable in grading stenosis. Instead velocity ratios are more predictive. The high velocity in the stenosis is divided by the "normal" velocity proximal to the stenosis. Although the numbers vary among investigators, the percent stenosis using velocity ratios can be estimated using the values shown in Table 40.7. Properly performed, sensitivities for detecting stenosis in the femoral-popliteal arteries are 85–90%.

Duplex US has a sensitivity greater than 90% in diagnosing occlusion in the lower extremity. Most errors in diagnosis are technical; most commonly, "trickle" flow is overlooked.

Graft Surveillance

In contrast to native vessels, sonography has established itself as the noninvasive modality of choice in monitoring peripheral bypass grafts (55,58,60).

Synthetic Grafts. Dacron grafts typically give a corrugated appearance, and PTFE grafts typically show two parallel echogenic lines. Synthetic grafts are rarely used for grafting below the knee. Graft failure usually results from a complication at the anastomotic connections to the native artery (Fig. 40.39) such as stenosis or pseudoaneurysm. Anastomotic pseudoaneurysms may not have the typical appearance described previously in this chapter because the communication between the pseudoaneurysm and the bypass graft anastomosis is almost always larger than those acquired following arterial puncture. Occasionally, a patulous anastomosis can mimic a pseudoaneurysm (Fig. 40.40). Such complications typically occur within the first two years following surgery. Progressive disease in the native arteries causes graft failure due to poor inflow or outflow. Fibrointimal hyperplasia within the graft lumen is a late complication, usually 5–10 years following surgery. No good data exist using velocity criteria for evaluation of synthetic graft failure, but velocity ratios are commonly used.

Autologous Vein Grafts. Of two techniques typically performed, the most common is the reversed saphenous vein graft; the second is the in situ graft. In the former, the vein is removed from its normal location, reversed, and anastomosed to the proximal and distal artery. For the in situ graft, only the proximal and distal ends of the saphenous vein are mobilized and anastomosed to the proximal and distal artery. In this type of graft, the venous valves are lysed to allow flow down the extremity.

During the first month following surgery, Doppler is used to assess the technical success of the operation. Perivascular fluid collections, anastomotic failure, poor vein selection, AVF, and residual valves are detected. Most important, Doppler confirms patency of the graft.

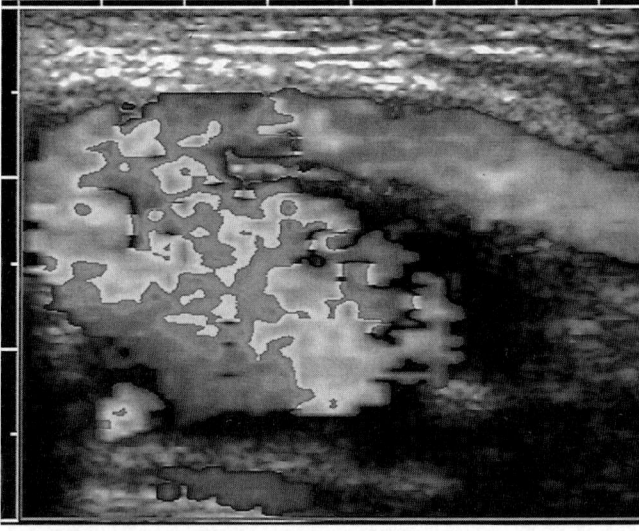

Figure 40.40. (Color Plates) Graft Anastomosis. Color Doppler image shows heterogeneous flow pattern at a patulous proximal femoral-popliteal graft anastomosis. A graft anastomotic pseudoaneurysm has a similar appearance.

Between 1 month and 2 years following surgery, intimal hyperplasia causes a focal stenosis in approximately 20% of patients. The hyperplasia usually occurs at the site of venous valves. Gray scale and color flow is used to identify areas of potential stenosis. A doubling of velocity within the graft is considered to be a 50% diameter or significant stenosis. The velocity obtained at the suspected stenosis is divided by the velocity in the graft 2–4 cm more proximal. The protocol is slightly modified at the anastomoses: the velocity at the proximal anastomosis is divided by the velocity 4–6cm distally into the graft. At the distal anastomosis, the velocity is divided by the velocity in the native artery in a "normal" segment distal to the graft. It is not uncommon for the velocity ratio at the distal anastomosis to be 2 because the distal native arteries are usually smaller than the graft. A velocity in the graft less than 45 cm/sec usually indicates impending graft failure. This protocol has proven more sensitive to early graft abnormalities than clinical symptoms or ABI measurements. The reported accuracy approaches 95%, but Doppler can overestimate the stenosis. Intervention is usually considered for a stenotic lesion when the velocity triples (Figs. 40.41 and 40.42).

Graft failures longer than two years after surgery are usually due to progression of native atherosclerotic vascular disease.

Dialysis Grafts. Dialysis grafts are typically inserted into the forearm with a side to side, end to side, or loop anastomosis. Such a graft can be either a synthetic or an autologous vein. The primary indication for Doppler evaluation is patency. Complications include anastomotic pseudoaneurysms, aneurysms, or stenoses. Accuracy of Doppler US for the detection of stenosis approaches 90%.

VENOUS ULTRASOUND

Lower Extremity

Duplex US is clearly recognized as the diagnostic modality of choice in evaluating lower extremity swelling for deep venous thrombosis (DVT) (26,61–63). Cronan et al. pooled data from multiple studies and found a sensitivity of 95% and a specificity of 98% for duplex US. Other modalities such as MR venography and contrast venography are reserved for instances when duplex is

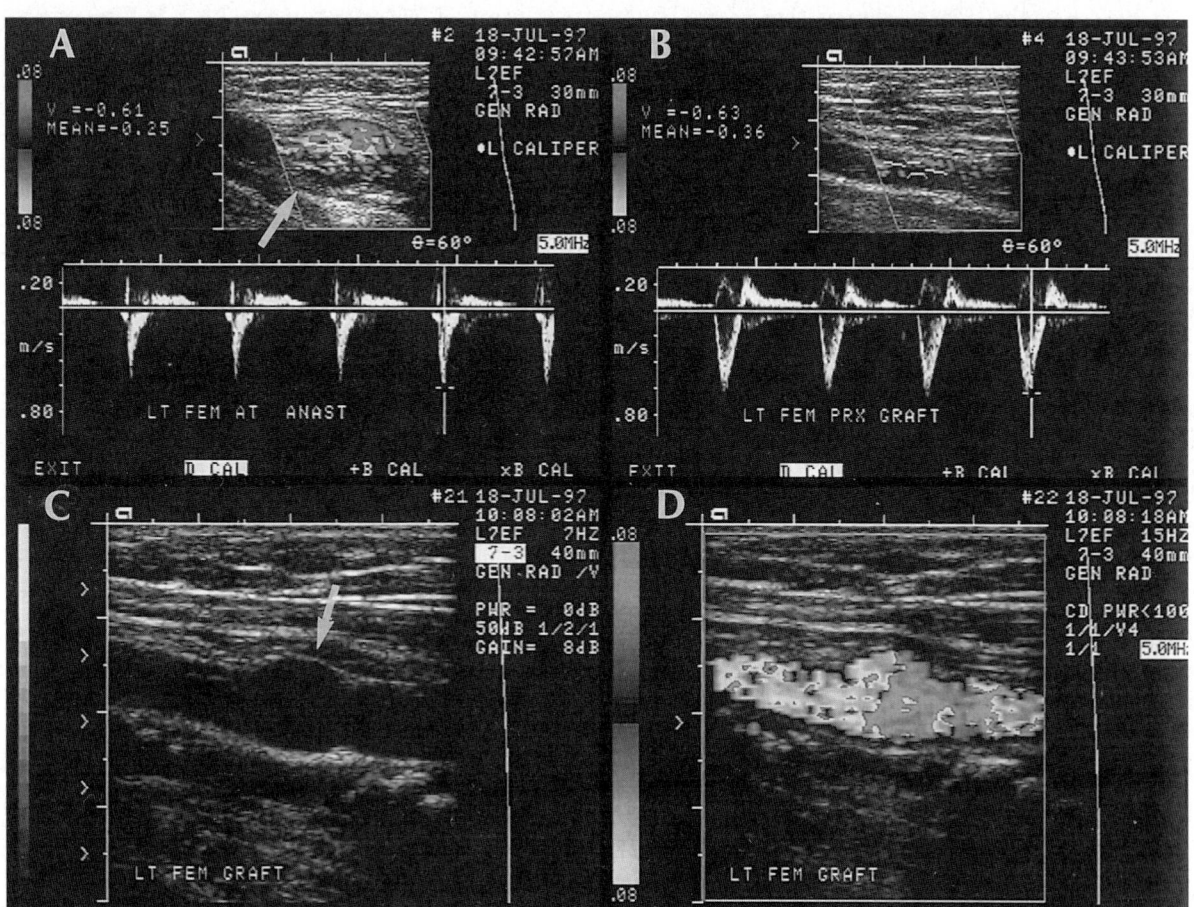

Figure 40.41. (Color Plates) Reversed Saphenous Vein Graft. A. Spectral Doppler tracing at the proximal anastomosis of a left femoral-popliteal vein graft has a velocity of 0.61 m/sec. Mild aneurysmal dilatation and heterogeneous flow (*arrow*) is not uncommon. **B.** Velocity obtained 4–6cm into the graft is nearly identical (0.63 m/sec) indicating no significant anastomotic stenosis. **C.** Mild saccular dilatation within the graft (*arrow*) corresponds to the location of a saphenous vein valve. **D.** Longitudinal color Doppler image confirms patency at the valve. Stenoses most commonly occur at the location of the valves.

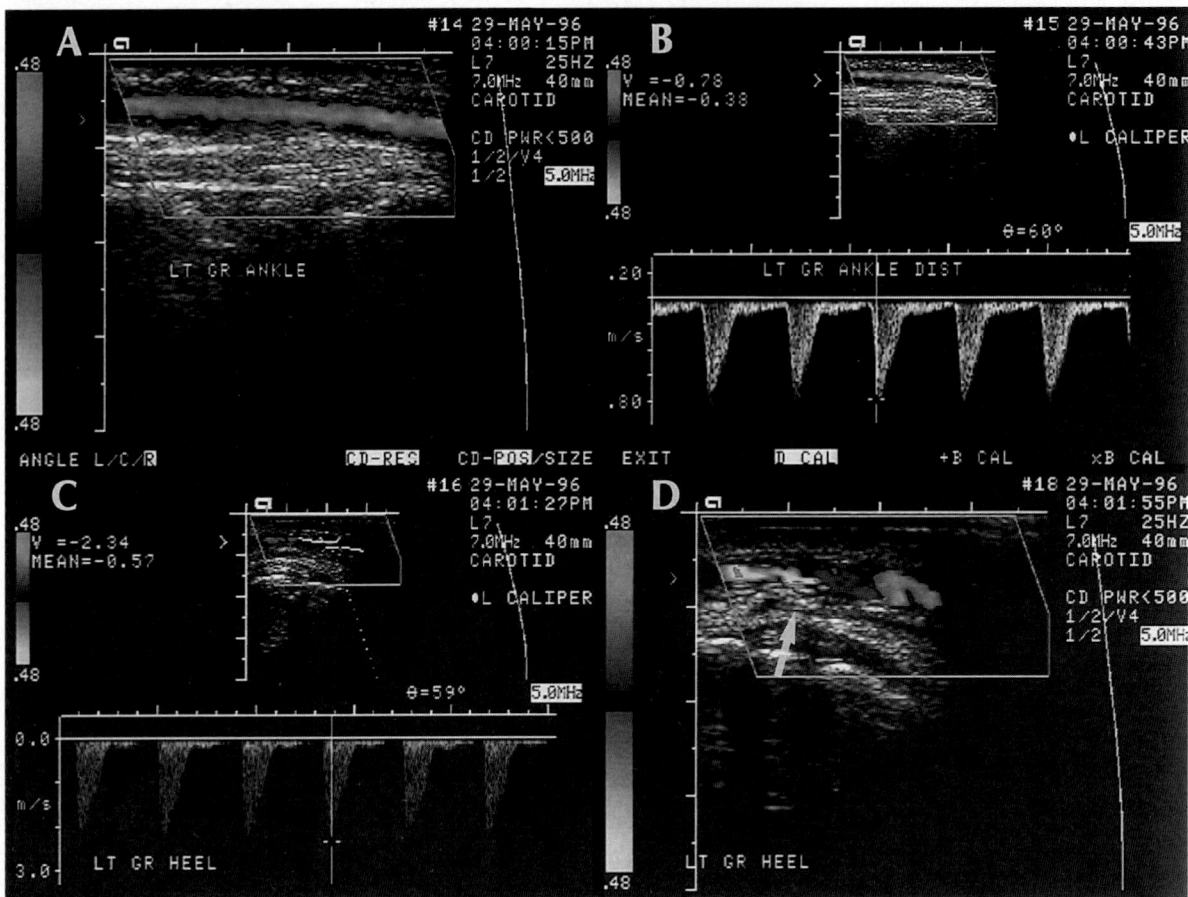

Figure 40.42. (Color Plates) Popliteal to Plantar Artery Vein Graft Stenosis. Color Doppler **(A)** and spectral tracing **(B)** within the vein graft demonstrates homogenous color flow (*red*) and a velocity of 0.78 m/sec. More distally within the graft the velocity has increased to 2.34 m/sec **(C)** and heterogeneous, turbulent flow (*arrow*) is noted on color Doppler **(D)**. Using Table 40.7, this tripling of the velocity corresponds to approximately a 75% stenosis. This patient had a nonhealing foot ulcer that responded to surgical revascularization.

nondiagnostic, when pelvic or IVC clot is suspected, or if calf clot will be treated.

Anatomy. The deep venous system of the lower extremity consists of veins that parallel the arteries both anatomically and in name (Fig. 40.43). In the calf, the anterior tibial, posterior tibial, and peroneal veins converge just below the knee to form the popliteal vein. The popliteal vein continues into the thigh through the adductor canal as the superficial femoral vein (SFV). Near the groin, the profunda femoris vein joins the SFV to form the common femoral vein (CFV). The popliteal and SFV are partially or completely duplicated in approximately 25% of patients. The calf veins have many normal variations.

The greater and lesser saphenous veins comprise the superficial venous system of the lower extremity (Fig. 40.43). The greater saphenous vein originates on the medial side of the ankle, ascends anteromedially along the thigh, and empties into the CFV at the inguinal ligament. The lesser saphenous vein originates laterally at the ankle, ascends posteriorly along the calf, and empties into either the popliteal or greater saphenous vein. Small perforating veins containing valves connect the superficial to the deep system in the calf and lower thigh. Flow is directed from the superficial to the deep system.

The CFV ascends medial to the artery into the pelvis and becomes the external iliac vein. The internal iliac vein joins the external iliac vein to become the common iliac vein over the sacrum. The common iliac veins join to form the IVC.

Technique. The deep veins of the lower extremity are examined from the inguinal ligament (junction of greater saphenous with CFV) through the popliteal fossa. Examination of the CFV/SFV is performed in the supine position with a linear 5–7.5 MHz transducer in a slight reverse trendelenberg position. In the transverse plane, compression and release of the veins are performed every 1 cm to the popliteal fossa. Behind the knee, the popliteal vein is examined in a similar fashion with the patient prone and knee flexed 15°. If a thrombus is present, longitudinal views are performed to determine its extent. Doppler interrogation demonstrates respiratory phasicity and flow augmentation is created by squeezing the calf or having the patient plantar flex the foot (Fig. 40.44). Color Doppler evaluation of the deep venous system confirms patency and unidirectional flow and is par-

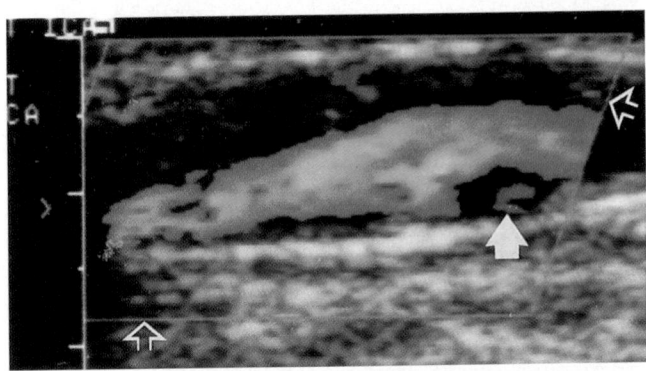

Figure 40.7. Normal Flow Reversal at Bifurcation.

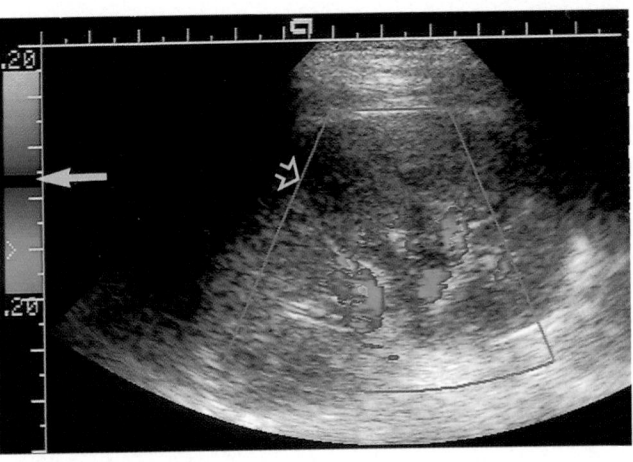

Figure 40.9. Color Doppler Image.

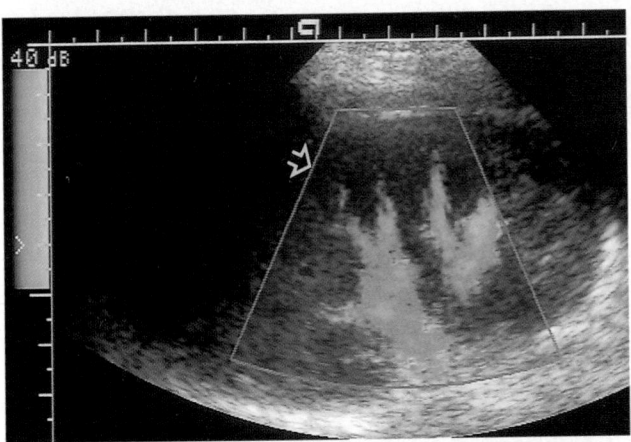

Figure 40.10. Color Doppler Energy (Power Doppler) Image.

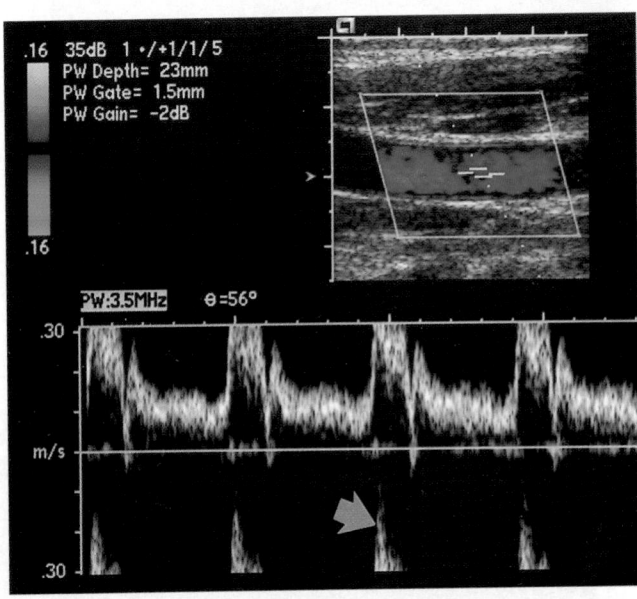

Figure 40.11. Aliasing on Spectral Doppler.

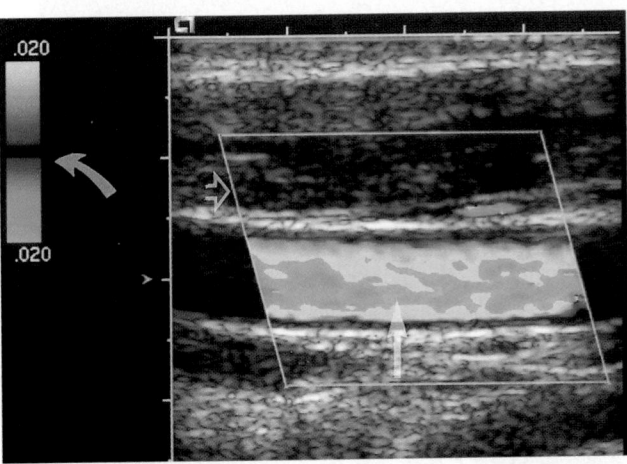

Figure 40.12. Aliasing on Color Doppler Imaging.

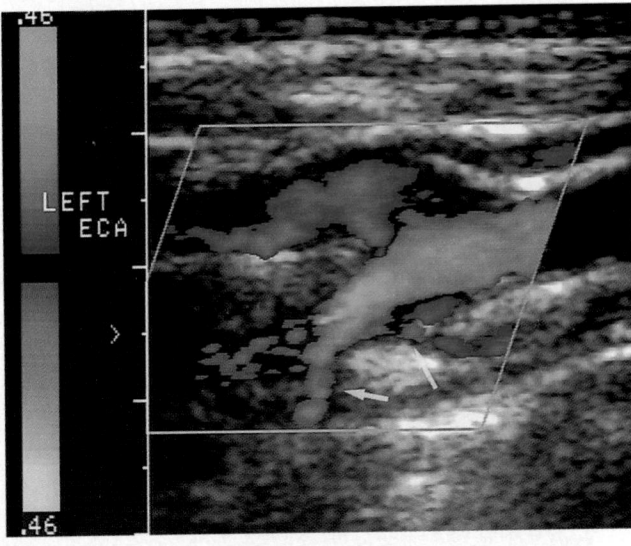

Figure 40.16. External Carotid Artery.

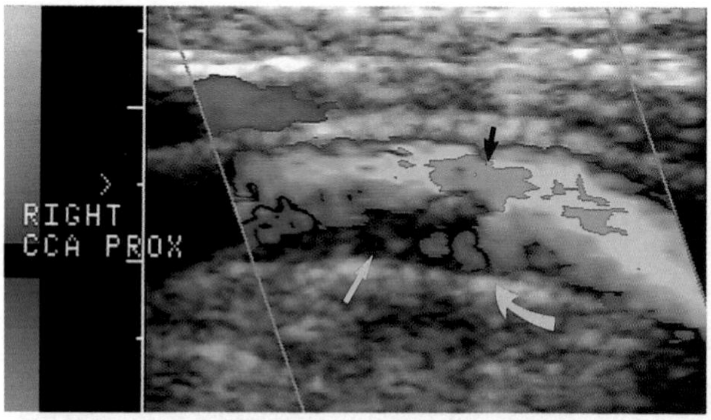

Figure 40.18. Ulcerated Plaque.

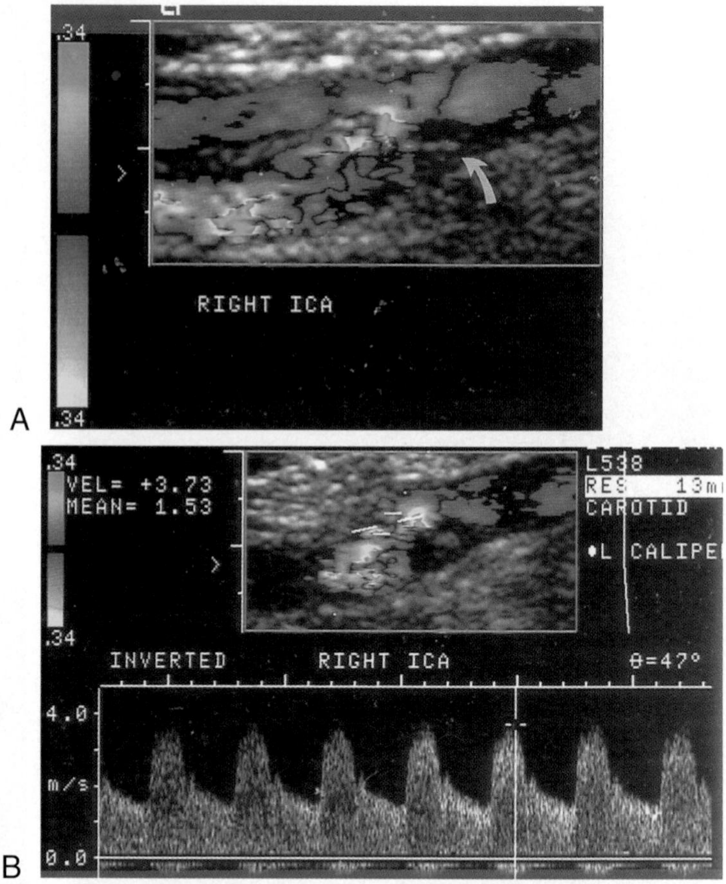

Figure 40.19. Internal Carotid Artery Stenosis.

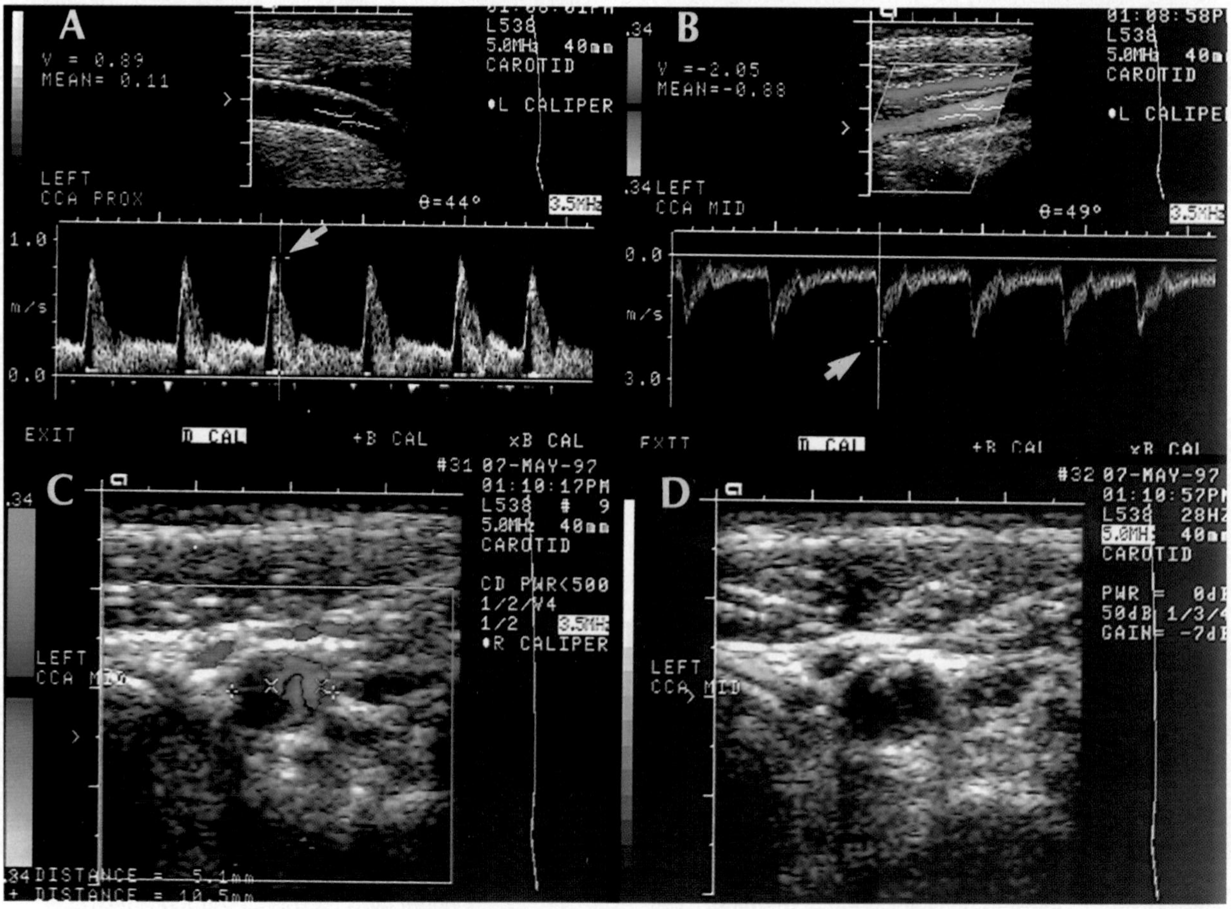

Figure 40.20. Common Artery Stenosis.

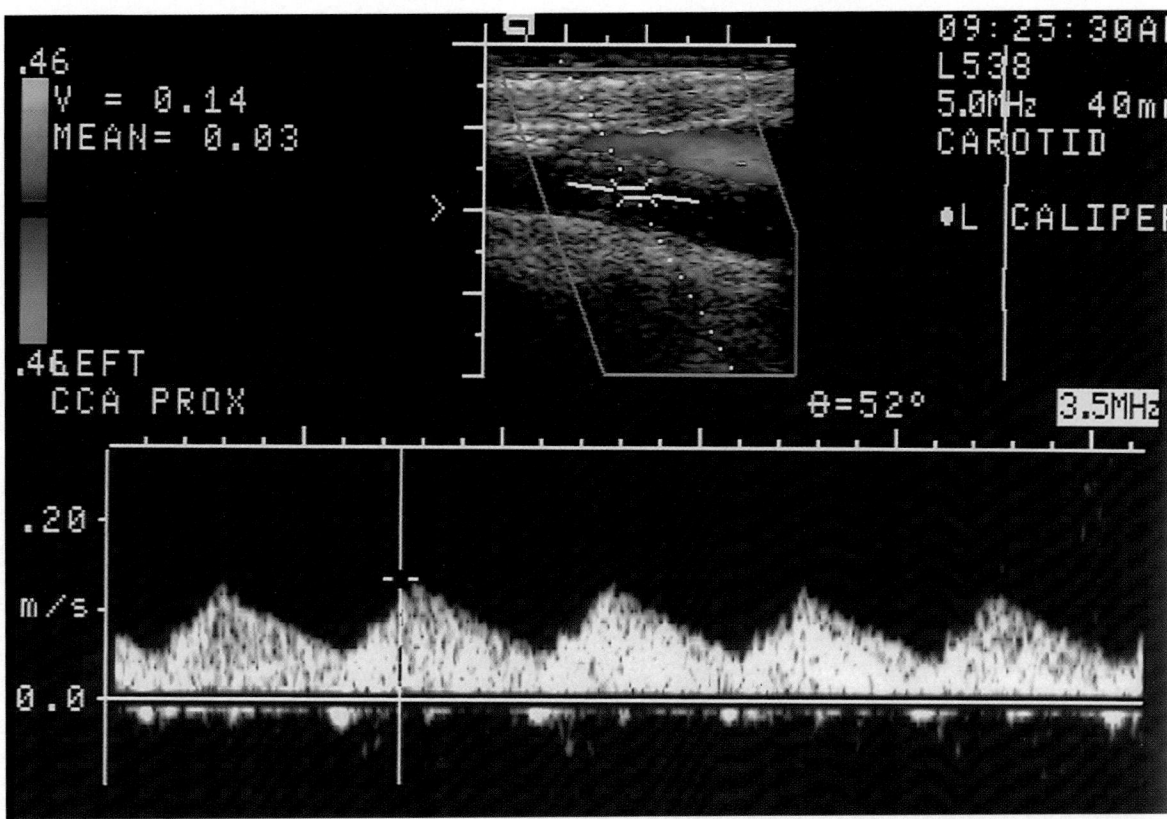

Figure 40.21. Common Carotid Artery Origin Stenosis.

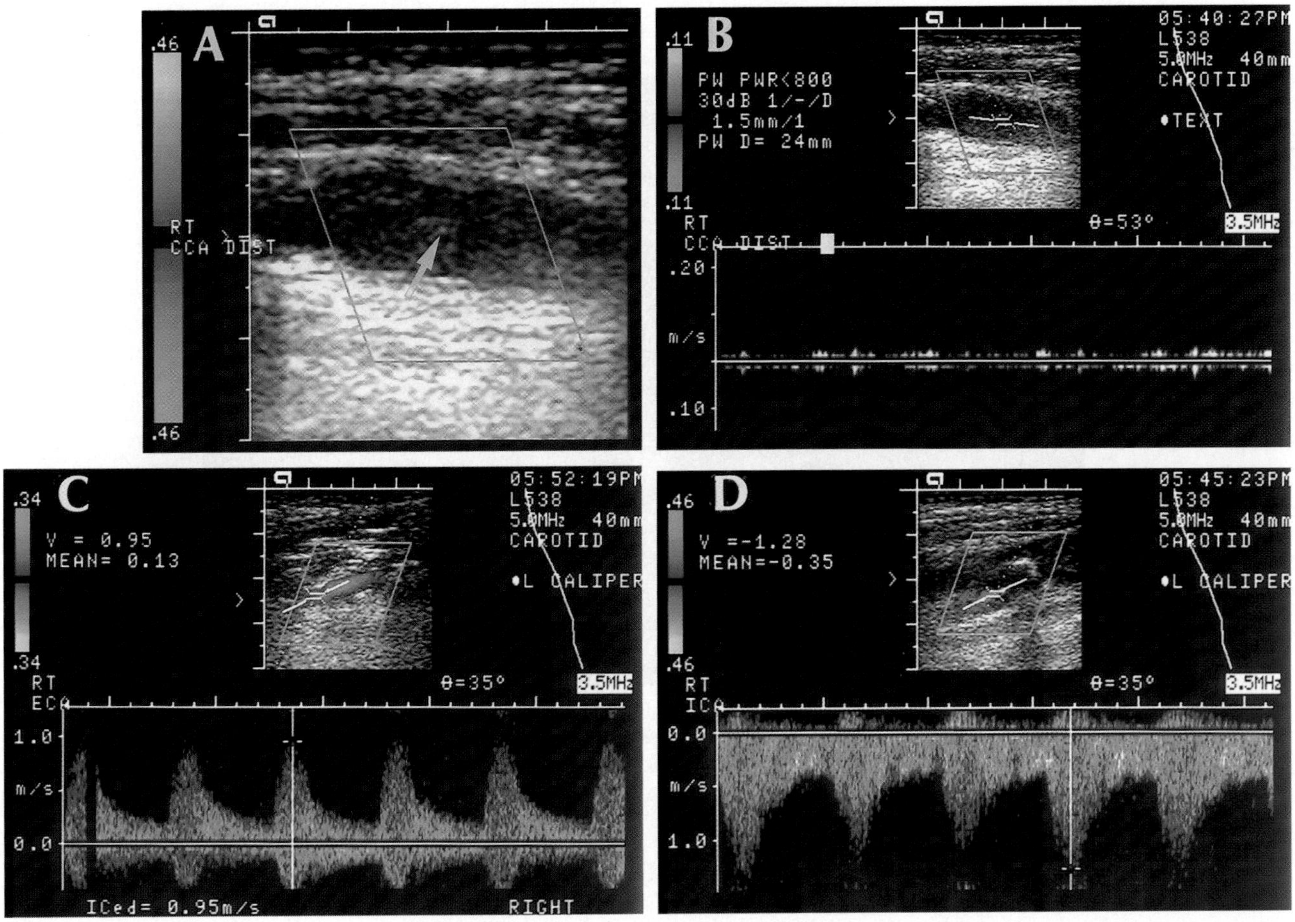

Figure 40.22. Common Carotid Artery Occlusion.

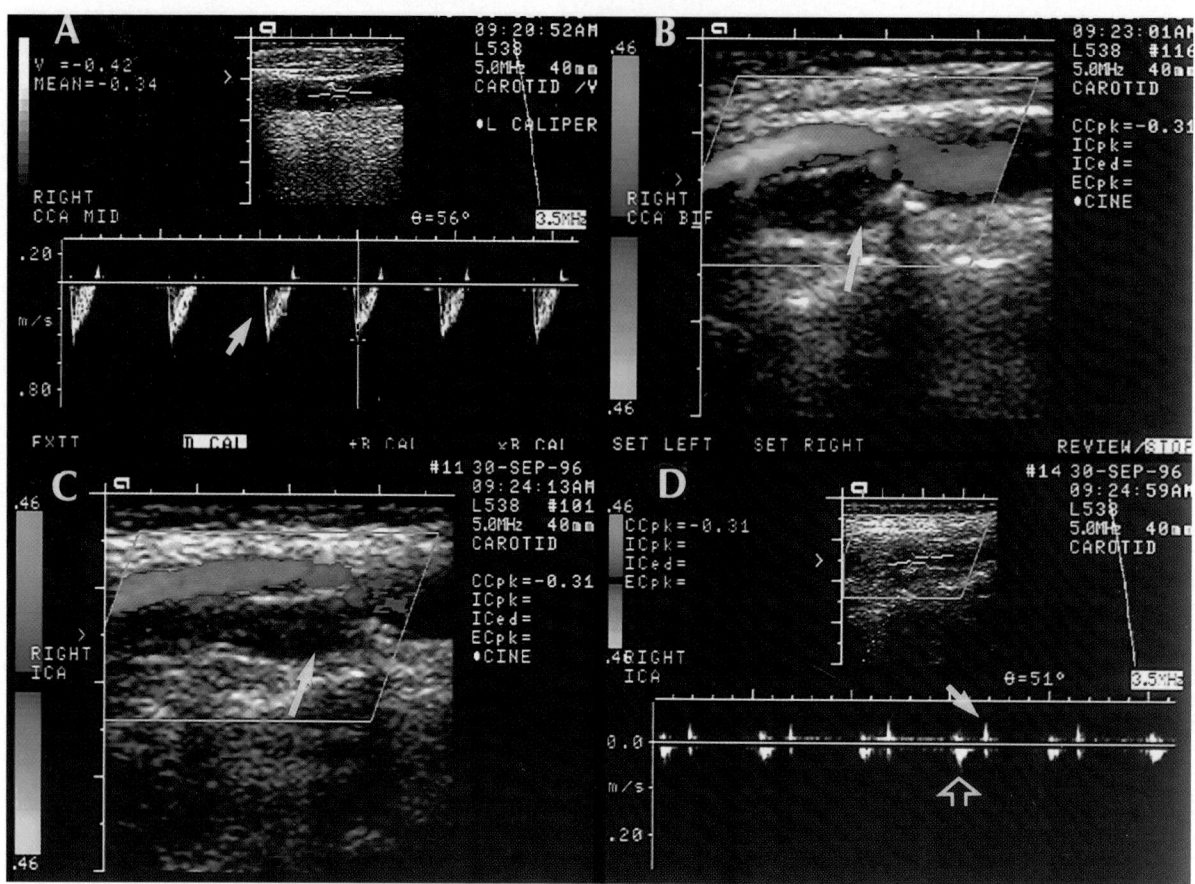

Figure 40.23. Internal Carotid Artery Occlusion.

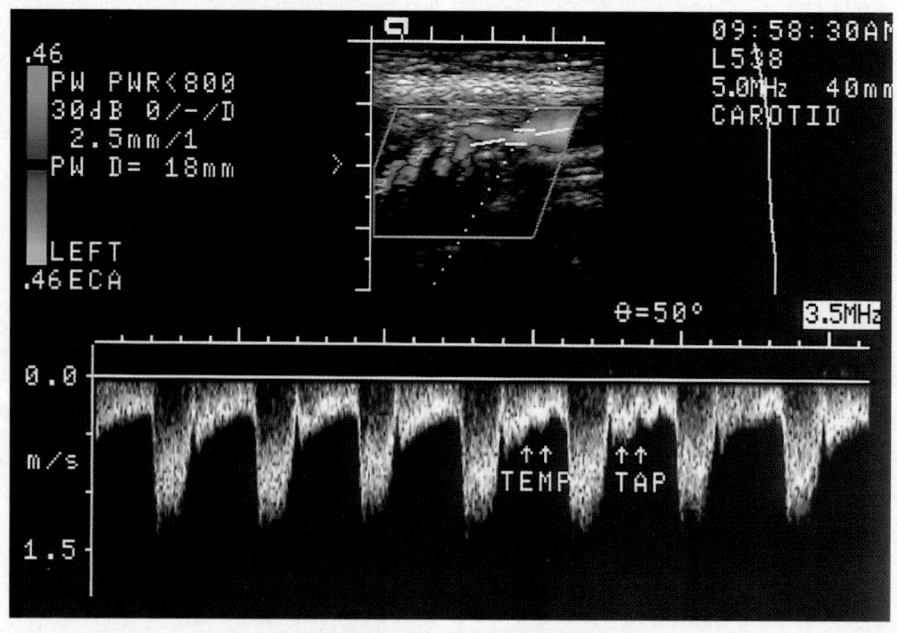

Figure 40.24. Internal Carotid Occlusion.

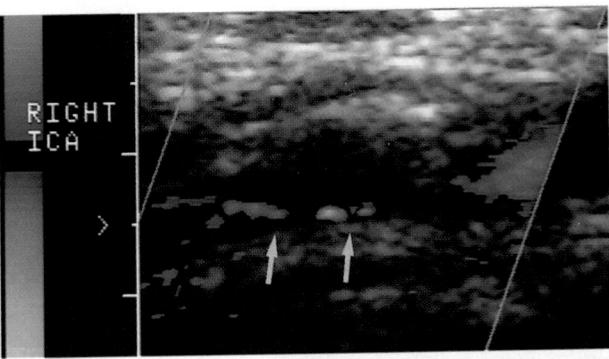

Figure 40.25. String Sign.

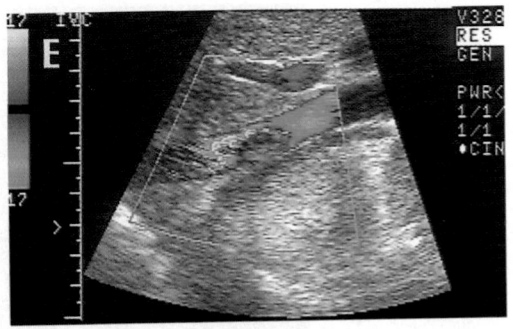

Figure 40.32E. IVC Tumor Thrombus.

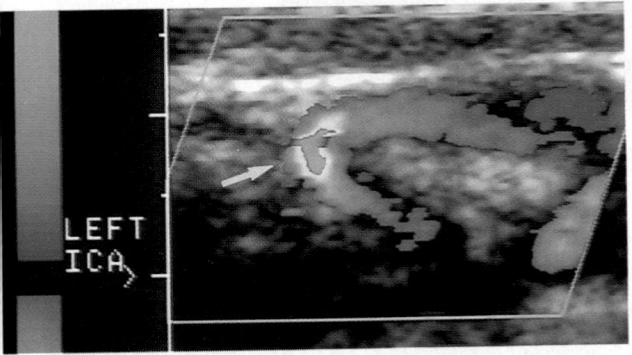

Figure 40.27. Tortuous Vessel.

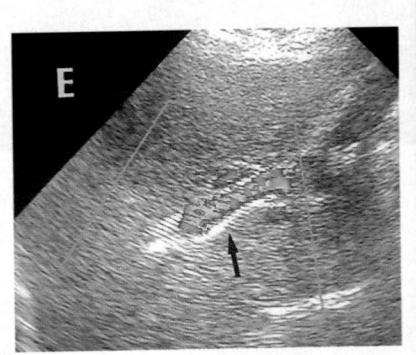

Figure 40.33E. TIPS US.

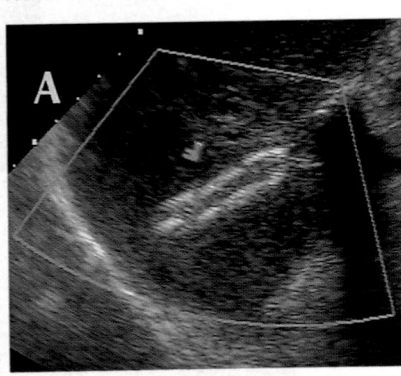

Figure 40.34A. TIPS Occlusion.

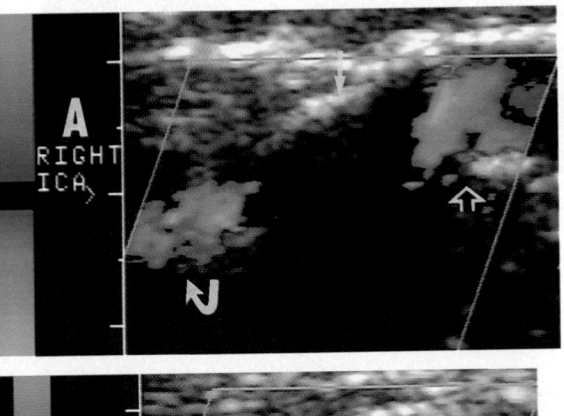

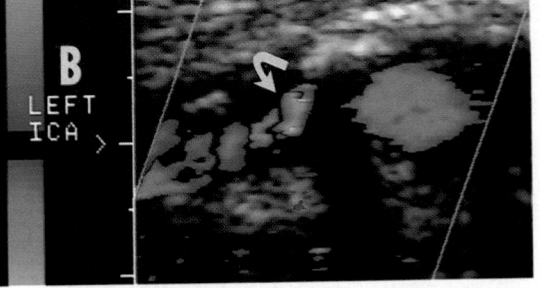

Figure 40.28. Calcified Plaques.

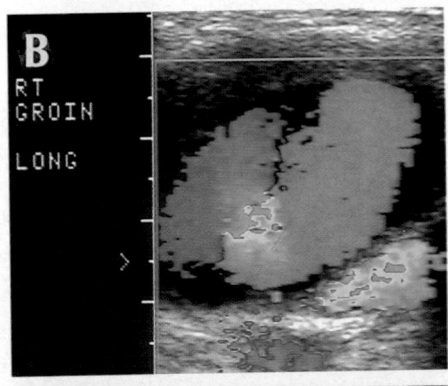

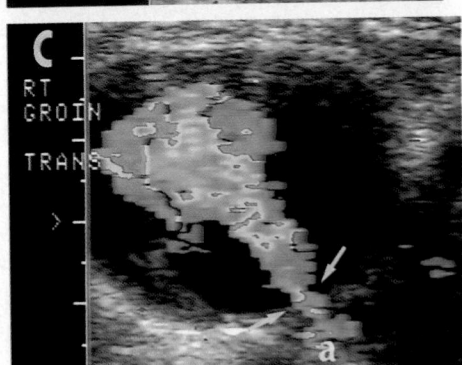

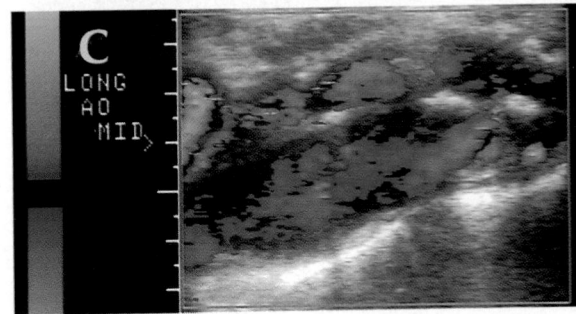

Figure 40.31C. Aortic Dissection.

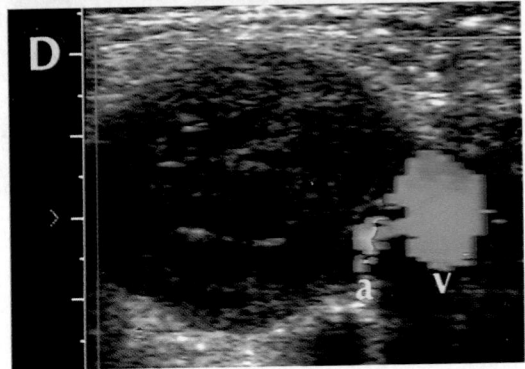

Figure 40.36. Pseudoaneurysm.

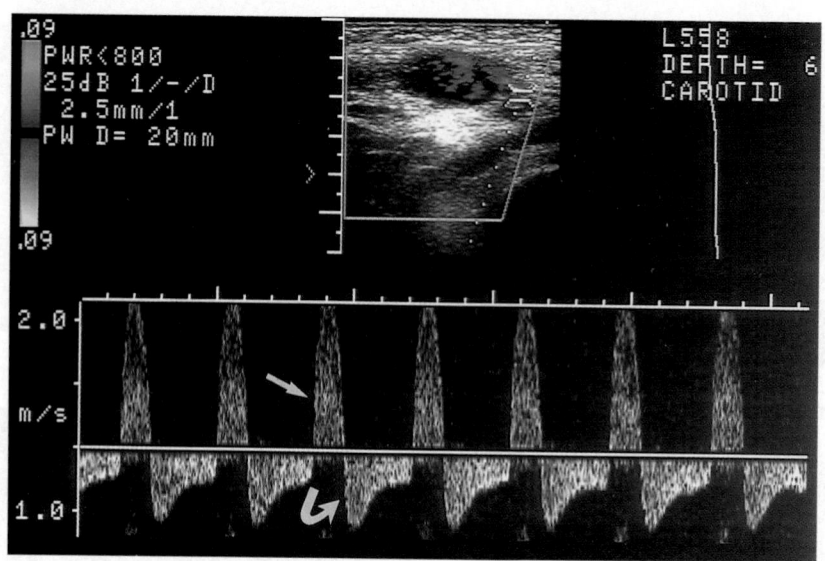

Figure 40.37. Pseudoaneurysm.

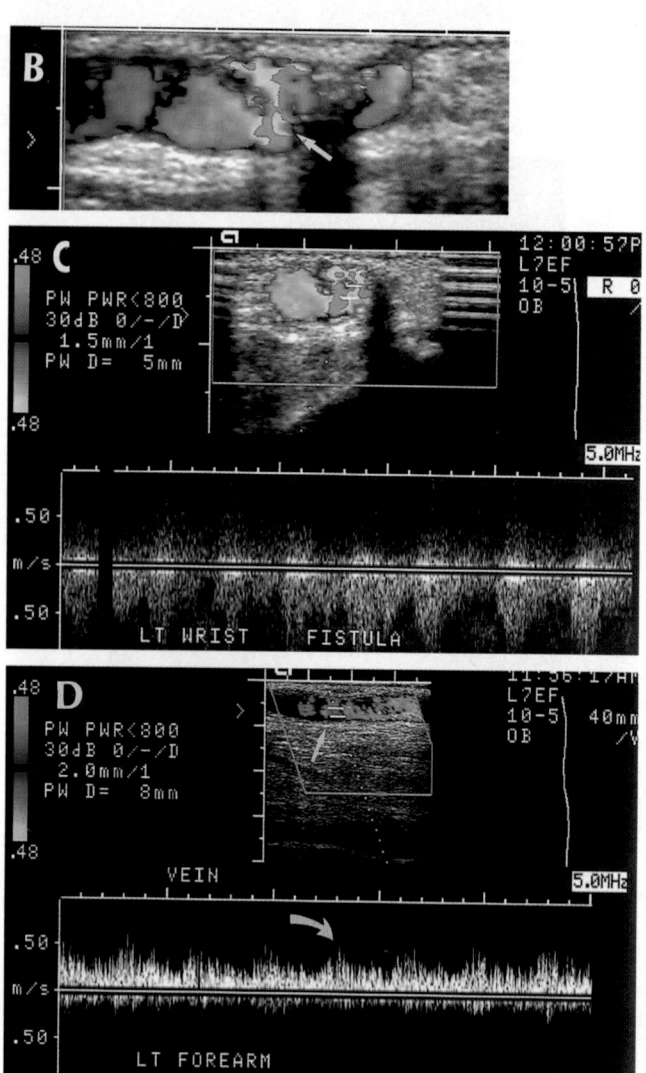

Figure 40.38. Arterio venous Fistula—Left Wrist.

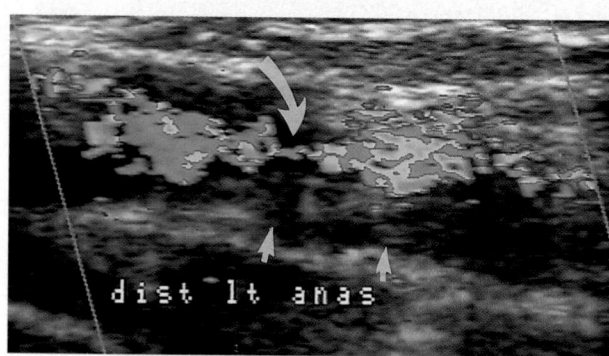

Figure 40.39. Synthetic Graft Anastomatic Stenosis.

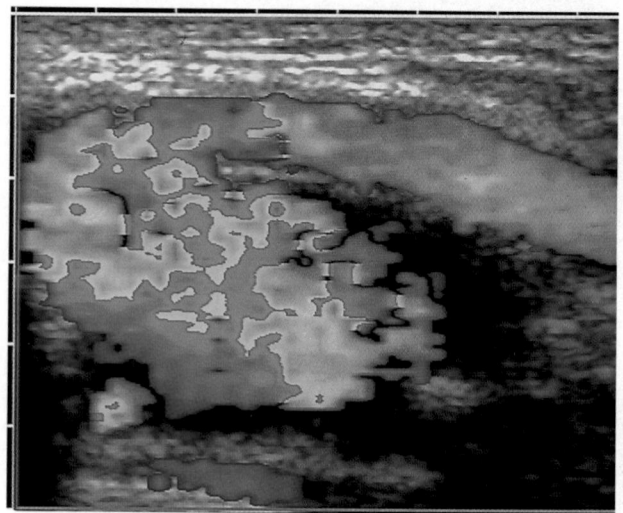

Figure 40.40. Graft Anastomosis.

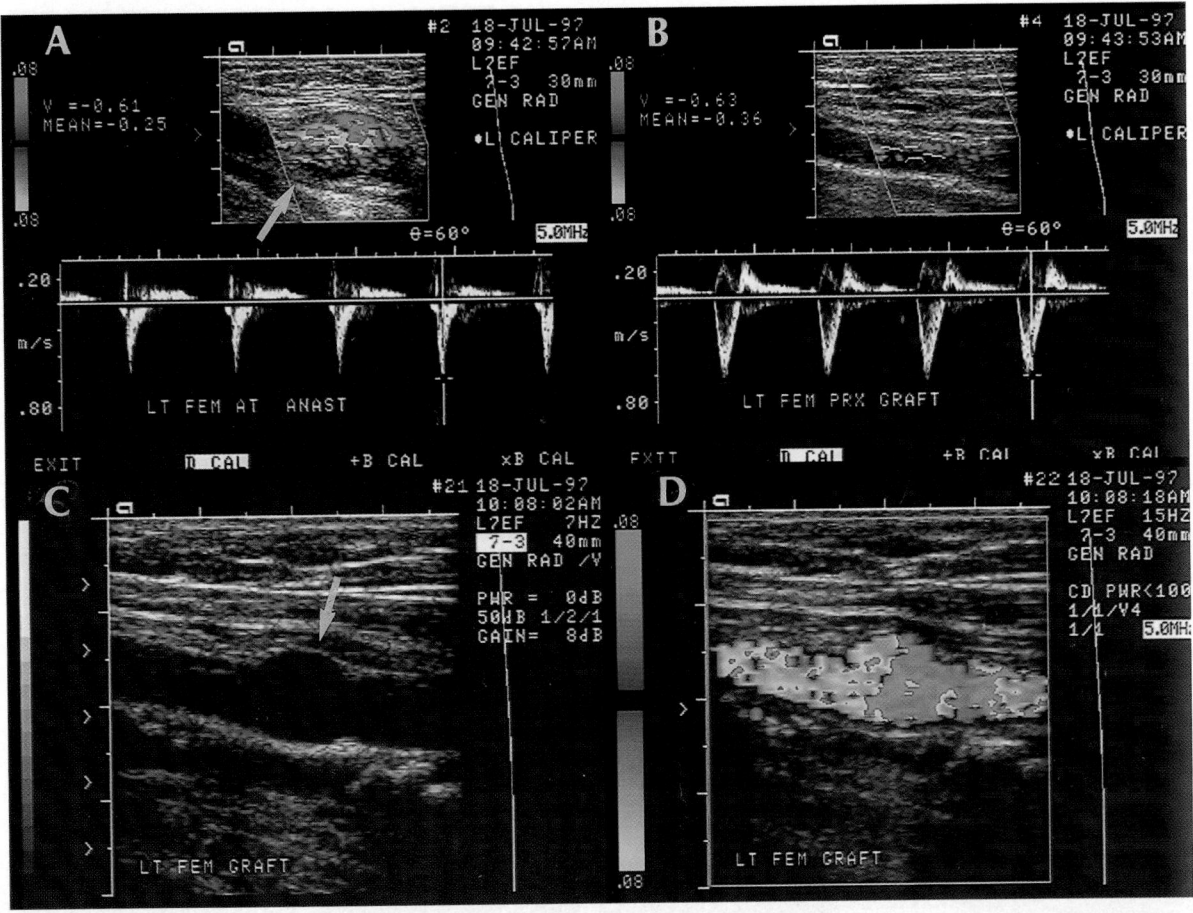

Figure 40.41. Reversed Saphenous Vein Graft.

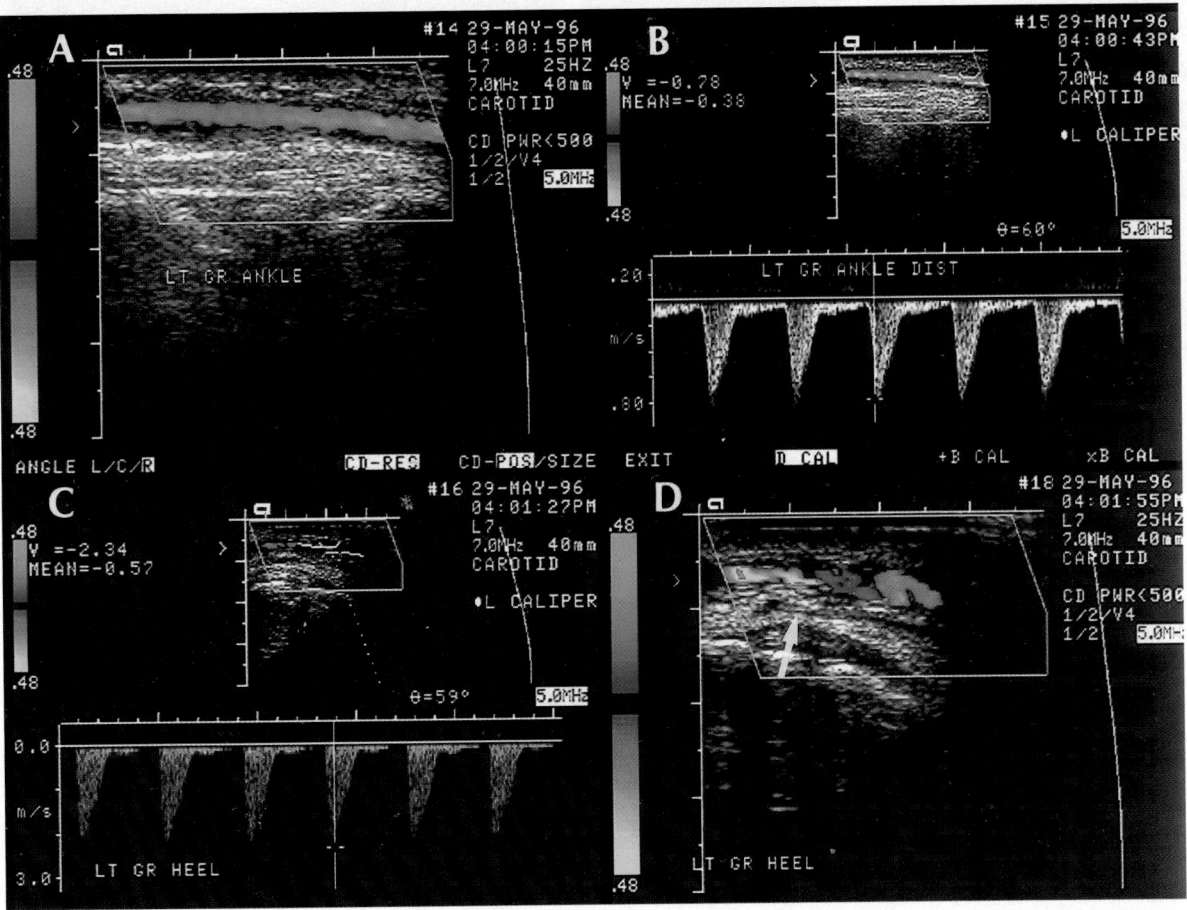

Figure 40.42. Popliteal to Plantar Artery Vein Graft Stenosis.

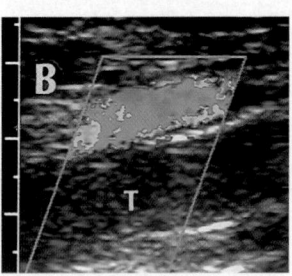

Figure 40.45B. Deep Vein Thrombosis.

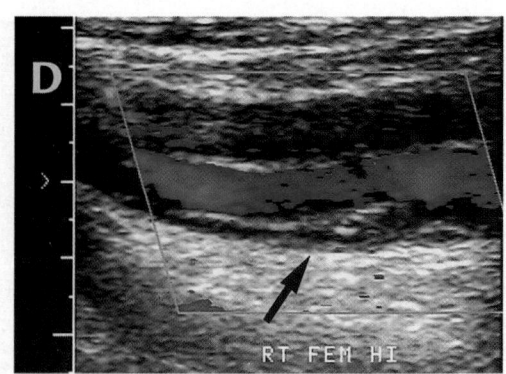

Figure 40.46D. Chronic Deep Venous Thrombosis.

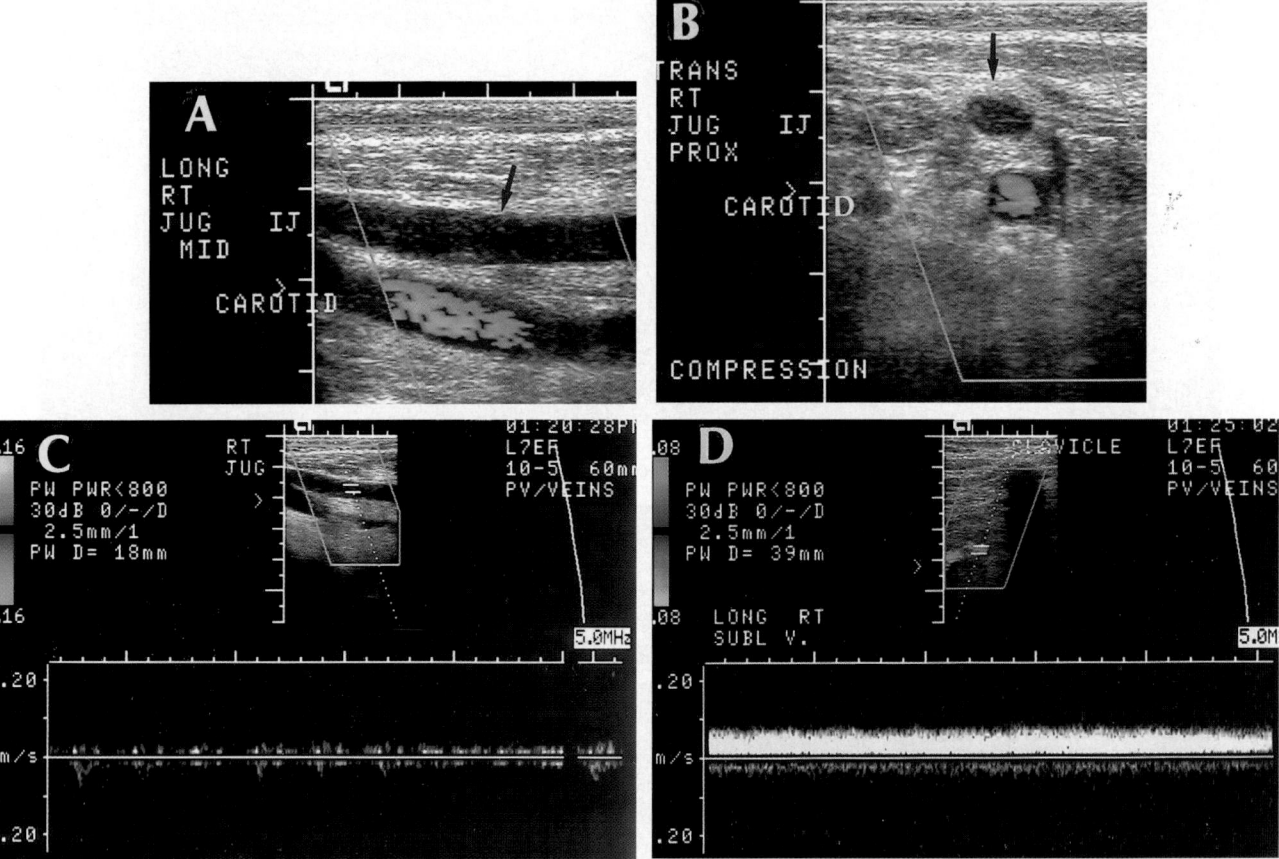

Figure 40.49. Internal Jugular Vein Thrombosis.

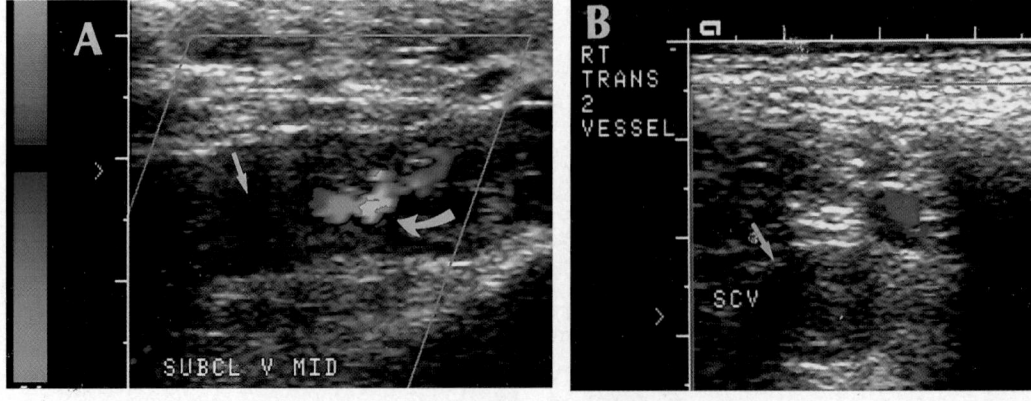

Figure 40.50. Subclavian Vein Thrombosis.

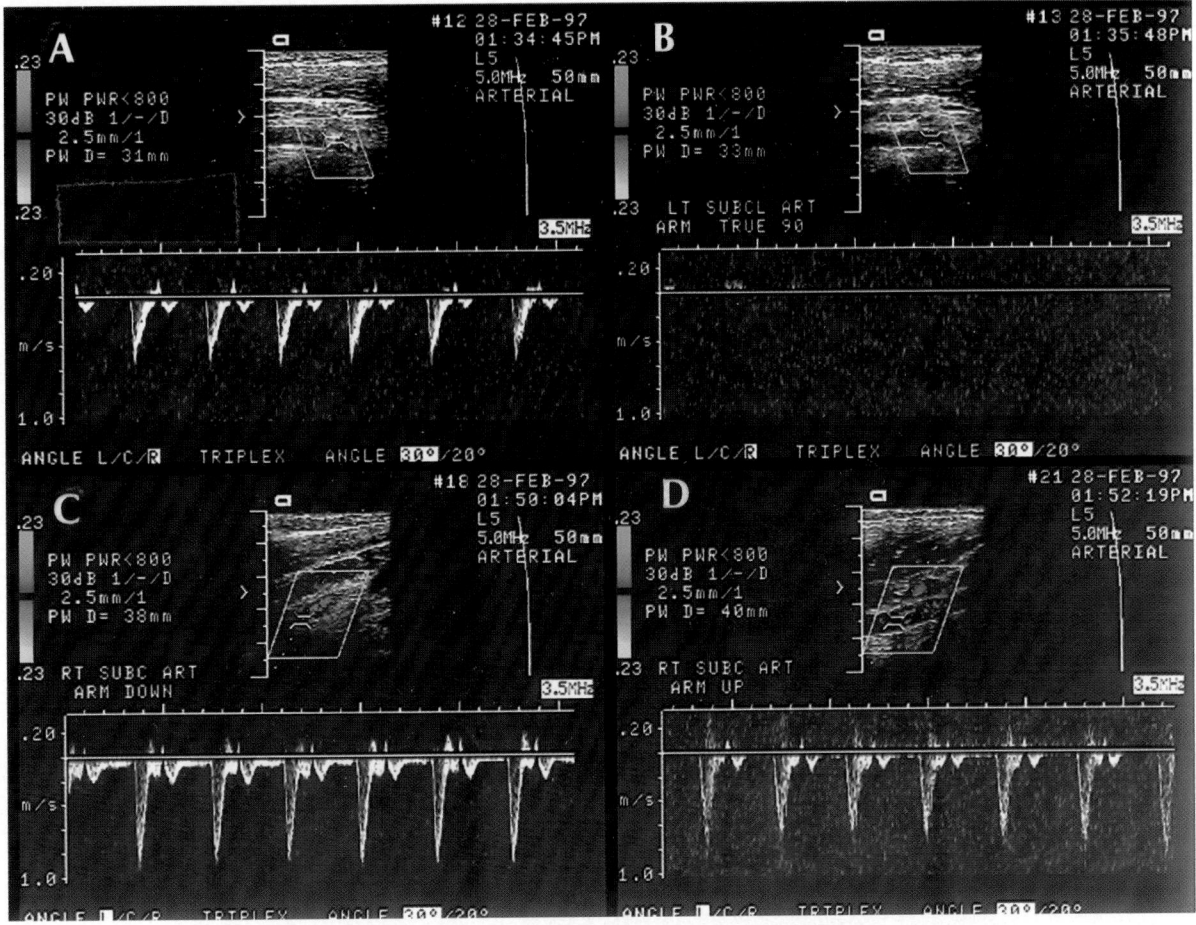

Figure 40.52. Thoracic Outlet Syndrome: Arterial.

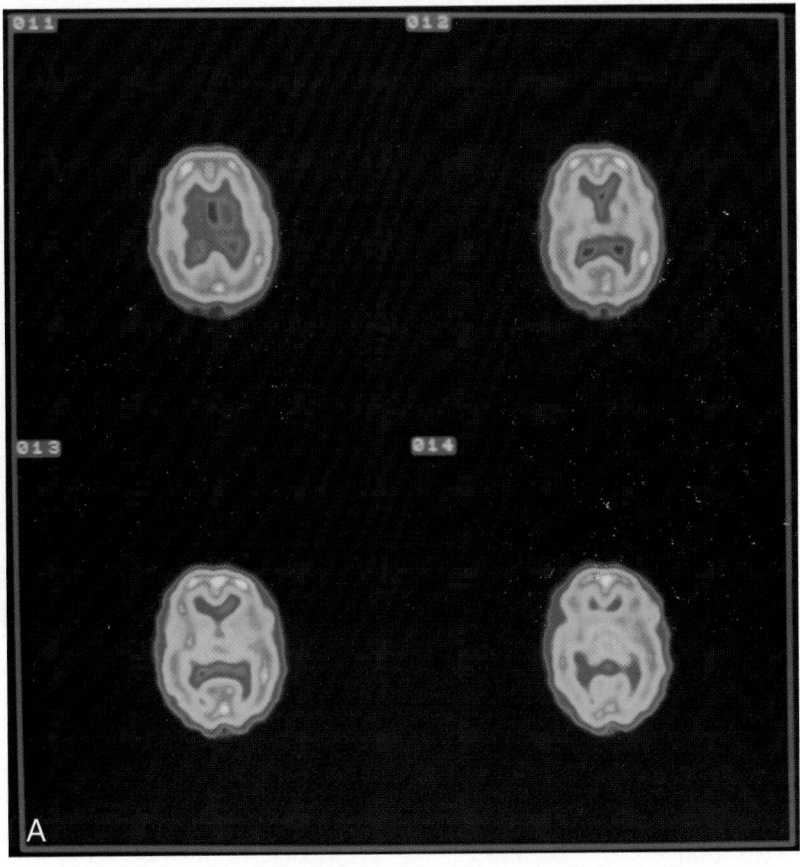

Figure 63.1A. Normal Study.

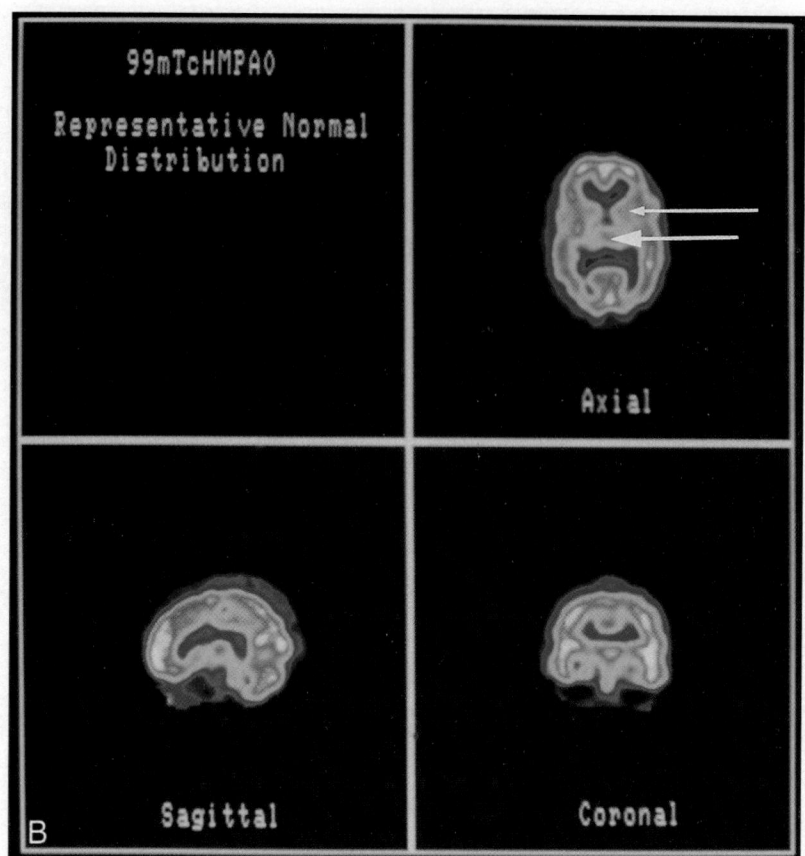

Figure 63.1B. Normal Study.

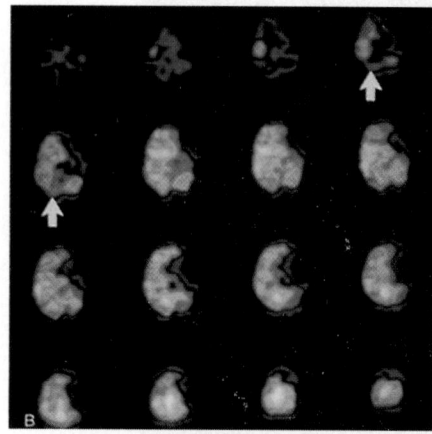

Figure 63.2. Cerebral Infarction.

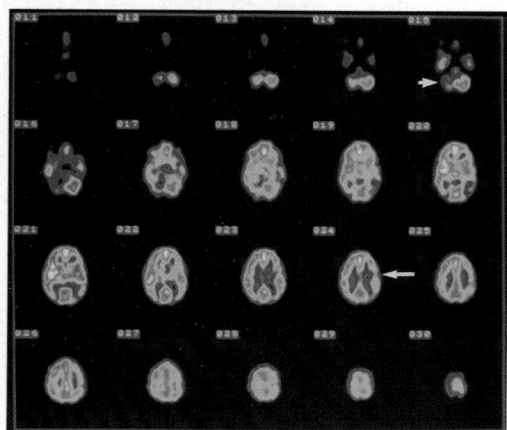

Figure 63.3. Crossed Cerebral Diaschisis.

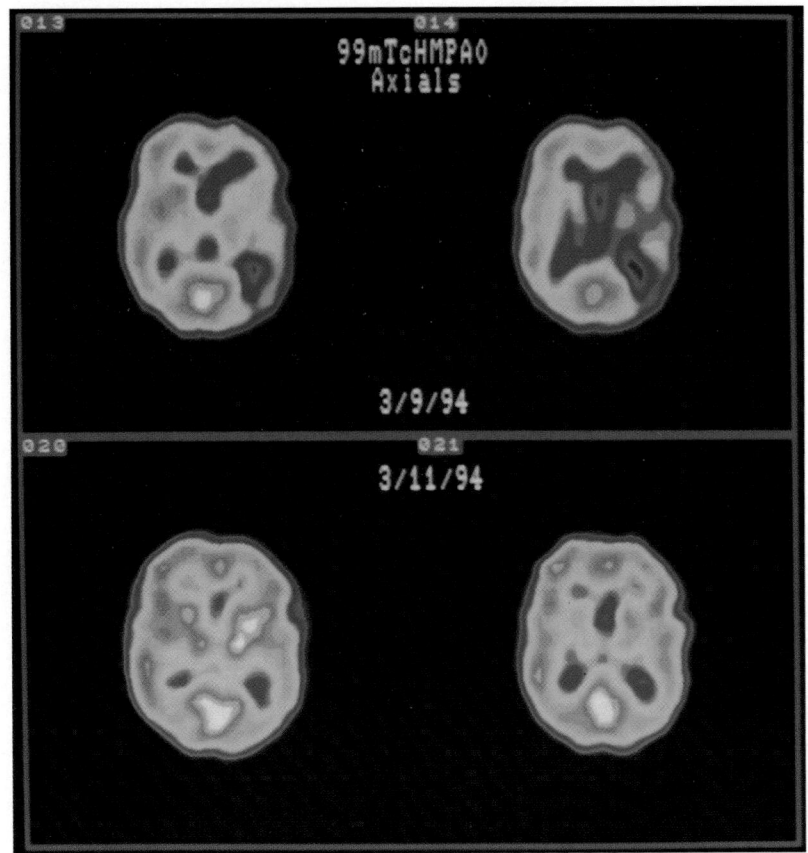

Figure 63.4. Positive Balloon Occlusion Study.

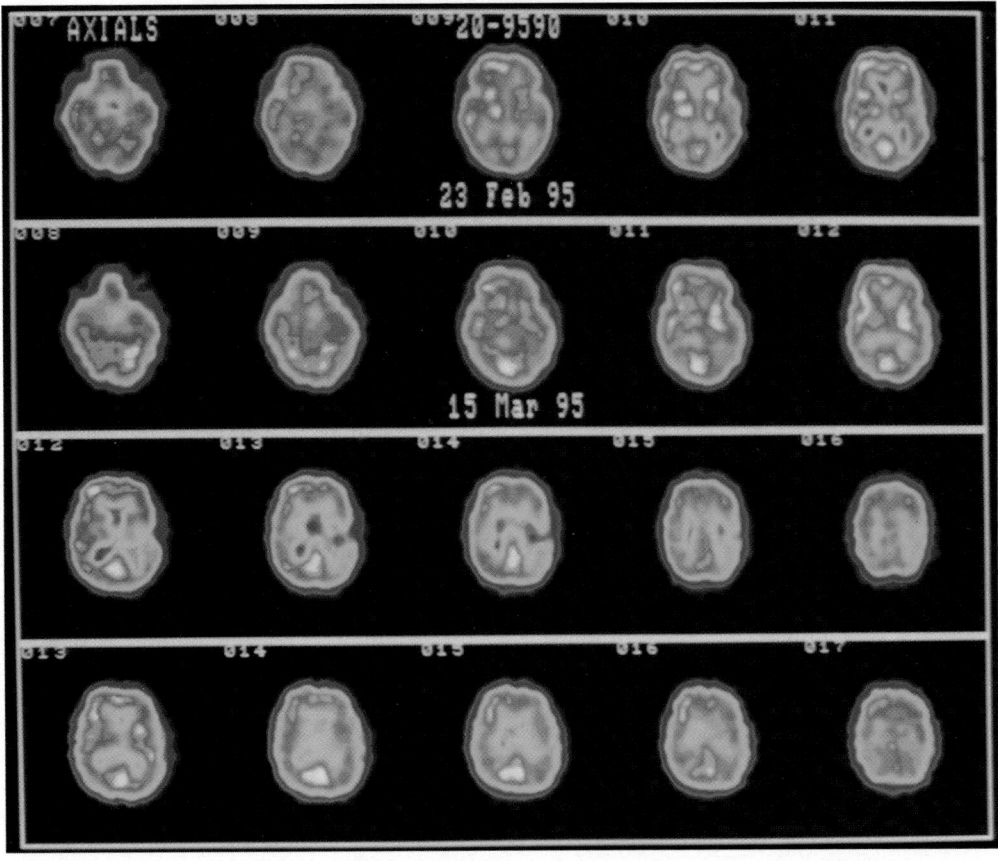

Figure 63.5. Catheter-induced Resolving Ischemic Neurologic Deficit (RIND).

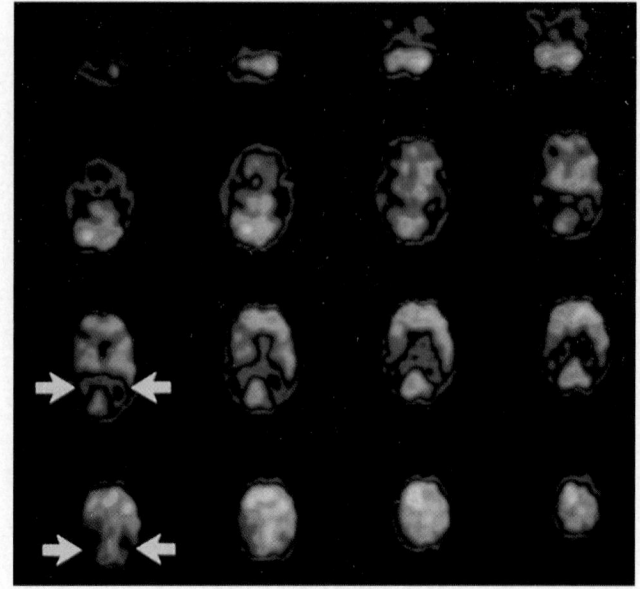

Figure 63.6. Alzheimer's Dementia.

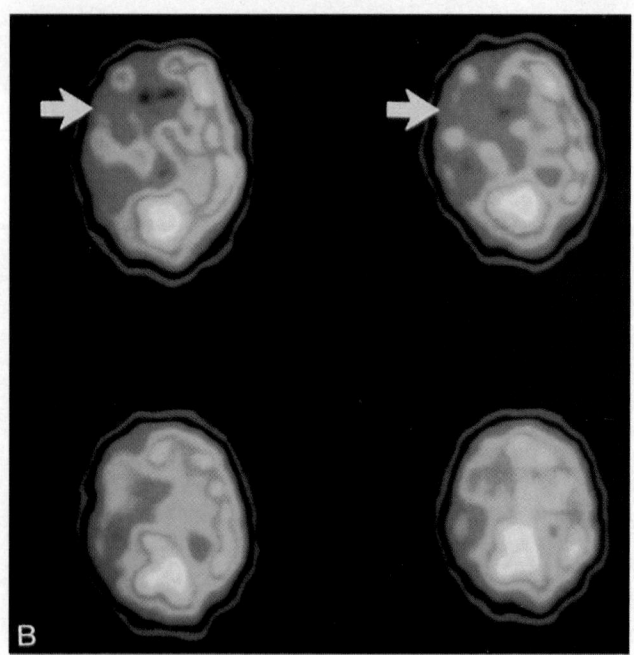

Figure 63.7B. Seizure Focus.

ticularly useful in areas or patients difficult to examine (e.g., the adductor canal and obese patents). Power Doppler's increased sensitivity occasionally augments the color Doppler examination.

Because of the many anatomic variations and duplication of the calf veins, duplex US is time-consuming and probably does not have the diagnostic accuracy

needed to exclude a small thrombus. Most clinicians do not anticoagulate an isolated calf DVT because it is not a cause of pulmonary emboli and often spontaneously resolves. For these reasons, the authors do not routinely perform duplex US of the calf veins. Up to 20% of calf vein DVTs propagate to the popliteal or SFV. To diagnose clot propagation and prevent pulmonary embolus,

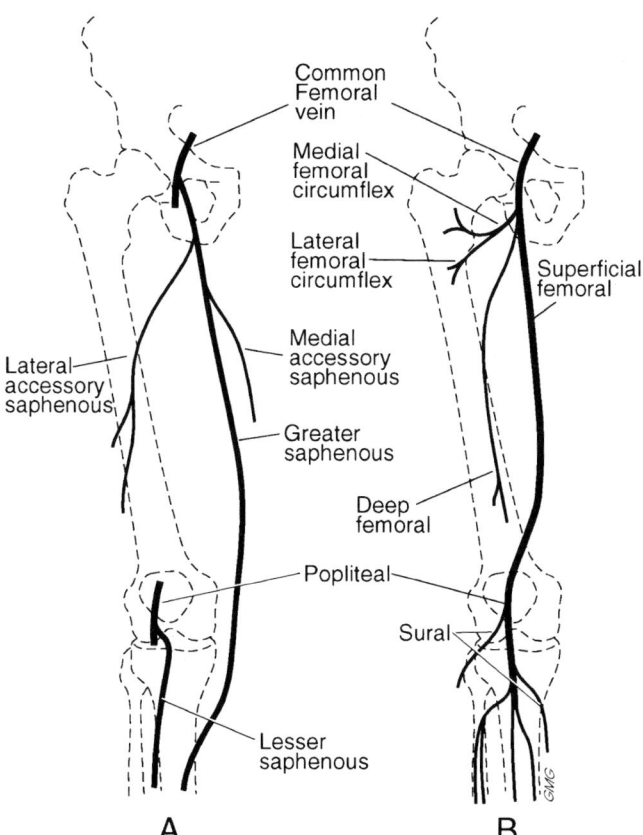

Figure 40.43. Lower Extremity Venous Anatomy. A. Superficial system. **B.** Deep system.

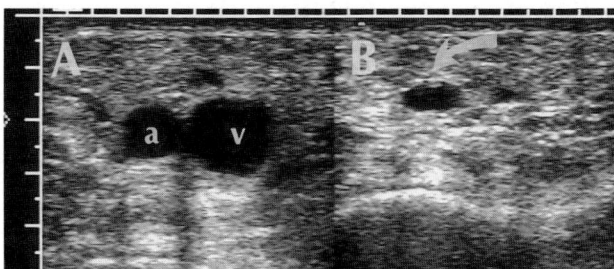

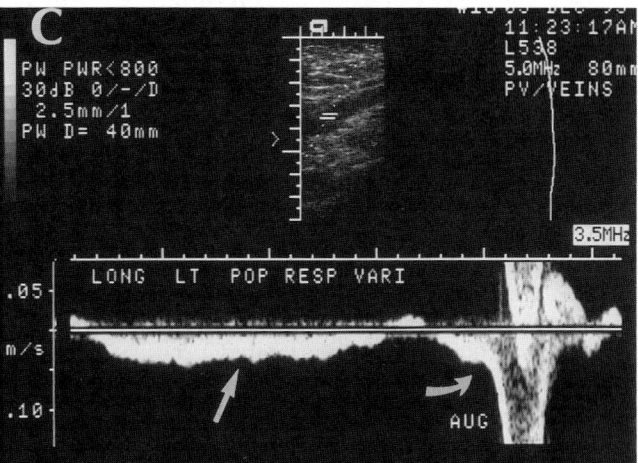

Figure 40.44. Normal Venous Compressibility, Respiratory Phasicity, and Augmentation. A. Transverse gray scale imaging demonstrates the normal common femoral artery (*a*) and vein (*v*). **B.** With compression, the normal vein is obliterated and the arterial lumen (*curved arrow*) persists. Enough compression has been ap-

plied to deform the arterial lumen (making it more oval) but not obliterate it. **C.** Spectral Doppler shows the normal respiratory phasicity (*arrow*) and augmentation from squeezing the calf (*curved arrow*) in the normal popliteal vein.

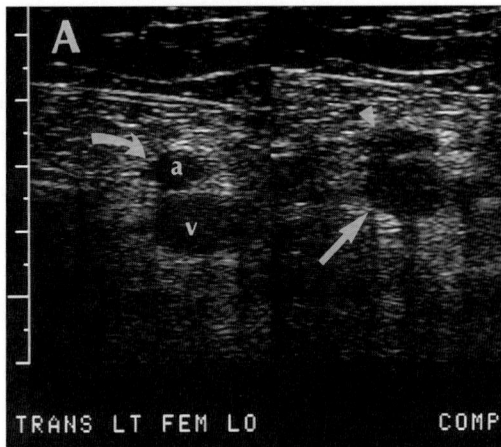

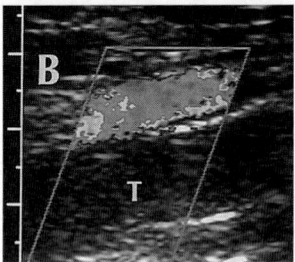

Figure 40.45. (Color Plates) Deep Venous Thrombosis. A. Transverse images without (*left*) and with (*right*) compression demonstrates a noncompressible, distended superficial femoral vein (*v, arrow*) diagnostic of a DVT. Note enough pressure has been applied to deform the artery (*a, arrowhead*) when compared to the adjacent image without compression (*curved arrow*). **B.** Longitudinal color Doppler image of the superficial femoral vein demonstrates echogenic thrombus (*T*) and no color flow. Flow is present in the superficial femoral artery anteriorly.

serial evaluation every 3–5 days is therefore important in patients who remain symptomatic after conservative therapy.

Deep Venous Thrombosis. Risk factors for developing DVT include prolonged immobilization, age, pregnancy, use of oral contraceptives, surgery, trauma, myocardial infarction, congestive heart failure, malignancy, polycythemia, prior DVT, or any other hypercoagulable state. The clinical presentation and physical examination findings are unreliable in making the diagnosis. Differential diagnoses include Baker's cyst, cellulitis, popliteal artery aneurysm, edema from multiple causes (CHF, lymphatic, renal failure, etc.), chronic venous insufficiency, extrinsic venous compression, superficial thrombophlebitis, and hematoma. The importance of making the diagnosis cannot be underestimated because 90% of pulmonary emboli arise in the lower extremities and untreated DVT results in pulmonary embolus in as many as 50% of cases.

The most accurate US criterion for the diagnosis of DVT is loss of compressibility of the vein. The veins of the deep venous system are easily compressible with light pressure. The maximum pressure required to obliterate a normal vein in any patient is less than that required to deform the shape of the adjacent artery. Other findings

include distention of the vein and visualization of intraluminal thrombus (Fig. 40.45). Because a significant number of clots are isoechoic to flowing blood, the latter finding is less reliable. Color Doppler demonstrates an intraluminal defect or color void. CDI may be as accurate as compression US. Spectral Doppler exhibits a lack of augmentation of signal when the clot is between the point of interrogation and foot. Doppler may also show a loss of respiratory phasicity caudad to the clot. If the respiratory phasicity is lost in the CFV, an iliac or IVC clot should be suspected. Loss of augmentation of signal in the CFV with release of valsalva is also suggestive of a more cephalad obstruction. A complete evaluation uses all these techniques.

It is important to realize the limitations of US diagnosis. The iliac and pelvic veins are not adequately evaluated in most patients. Obesity and severe edema can cause technically inadequate examinations. The adductor canal can be difficult to visualize even in thin patients. The saphenous vein or collaterals can be mistaken for the SFV. Duplications of the deep venous system can lead to diagnostic error, particularly if one system is clotted and the other is patent. Extrinsic venous compression by nodes or tumor can cause loss of respiratory phasicity and augmentation.

The distinction between ***acute*** and ***chronic*** DVT is difficult on all imaging modalities including contrast venography. Six months following a DVT, 50% of patients have persistent abnormalities on US. Typically, chronic clot does not expand the lumen of the vein and appears more echogenic than an acute clot. Echogenic strands are often noted in the lumen. The walls of the vein also appear thickened, irregular, and echogenic, and the vein is incompletely compressible (Fig. 40.46). Color Doppler evaluation often demonstrates collateral vessels. We obtain a baseline duplex US just prior to discontinuing anticoagulation therapy to help distinguish acute versus chronic changes in the future. Otherwise, with recurrent symptoms, a chronic DVT may be inadvertently diagnosed as an acute or recurrent DVT subjecting the patient to life-long anticoagulation. If a clot appears chronic and unchanged from baseline, an interval follow-up US in 2–3 days is performed to assess change. Acute clot superimposed on chronic changes remains a difficult US diagnosis. Venography may be required.

Chronic Venous Insufficiency occurs in approximately 40% of individuals following an episode of acute DVT. Venous insufficiency results when the lower extremity venous valves are destroyed or become incompetent. CDI detects valvular insufficiency by demonstrating flow reversal for more than 1 second during valsalva. Compressing the thigh muscle while interrogating the venous system more distally demonstrates reversed flow or augmentation. Both the deep system cephalad to the popliteal vein and the saphenous system can be evaluated with this technique. Reversal of flow from the deep to the superficial system through the perforating veins can often be documented. Many variations of thigh and calf compression techniques are reported in the literature.

Upper Extremity

Although not as well-studied, duplex US has become a useful screening modality for the venous evaluation of the upper extremity, particularly for DVT and symptoms suggestive of thoracic outlet syndrome (26,64).

Anatomy. The superficial venous system is the primary drainage pathway for the upper extremity. The basilic vein courses along the ulnar side of the forearm and medial upper arm and continues as the axillary vein. The cephalic vein ascends on the radial aspect of the forearm and continues laterally to the shoulder.

The cephalic vein joins the axillary vein just below the clavicle. The axillary vein continues as the subclavian vein at the lateral border of the first rib (Fig. 40.47). After it receives the internal jugular vein, it continues as the brachiocephalic vein to the superior vena cava. The deep system consists of small, paired brachial veins that course with the artery and empty into the basilic vein.

Technique. A complete evaluation of the upper extremity includes the bilateral evaluation of the axillary, subclavian, and internal jugular veins. The same technique used for the lower extremity can be applied

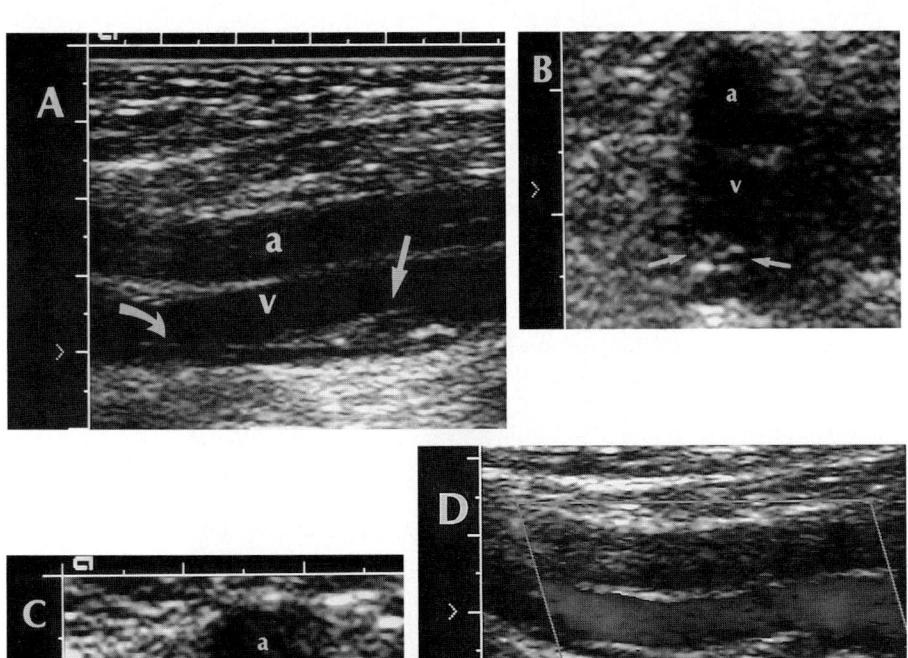

Figure 40.46. (Color Plates) Chronic Deep Venous Thrombosis A. Longitudinal image of the right SFV (*v*) and the SFA (*a*) in a patient with a prior DVT. The wall of the vein appears thickened and irregular with areas of increased echogenicity (*arrow*). An echogenic strand is seen within the lumen (*curved arrow*). **B.** Transverse image through the SFV without compression shows the thickened irregular wall inferiorly (*arrows*). The vein is not distended. **C.** Transverse image shows complete compression except for the thickened wall (*arrows*). **D.** Longitudinal Color Doppler image confirms the gray scale findings (*arrow*) showing patency of the residual lumen (*blue*). Serial examinations were unchanged.

Figure 40.47. Upper Extremity Venous Anatomy.

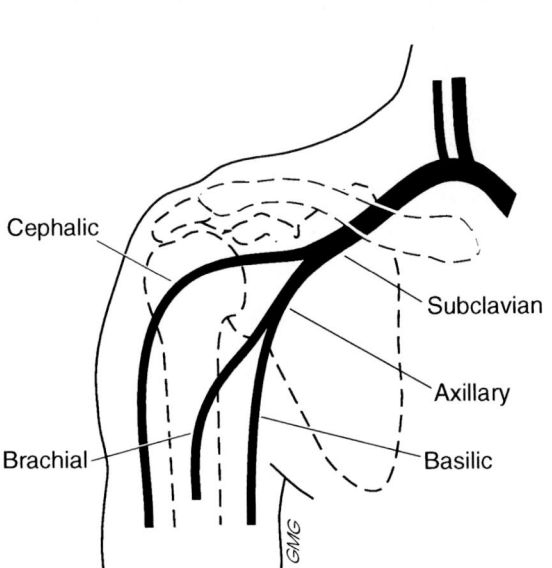

Figure 40.48. Normal Subclavian Vein Waveform. Normal venous waveform demonstrates respiratory phasicity and transmitted cardiac pulsations.

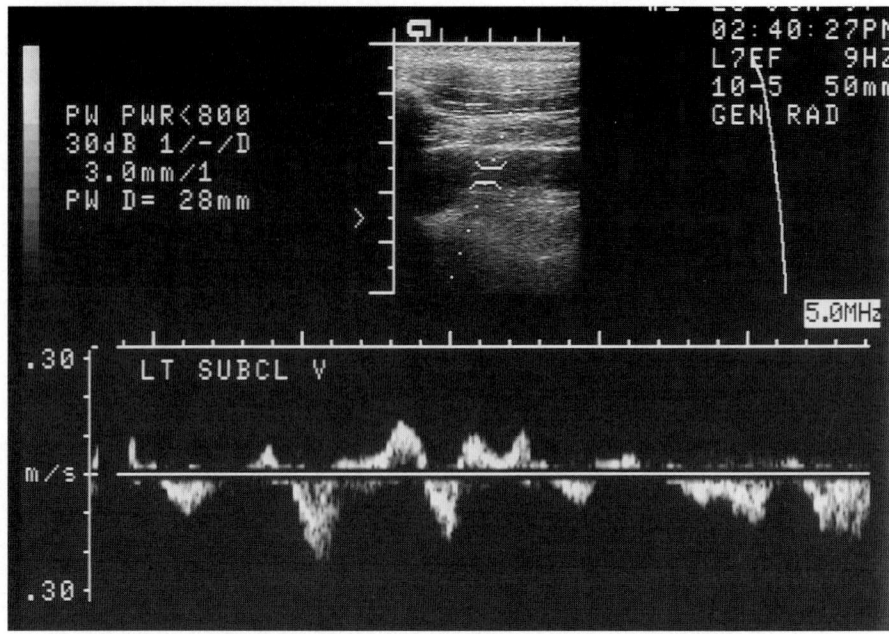

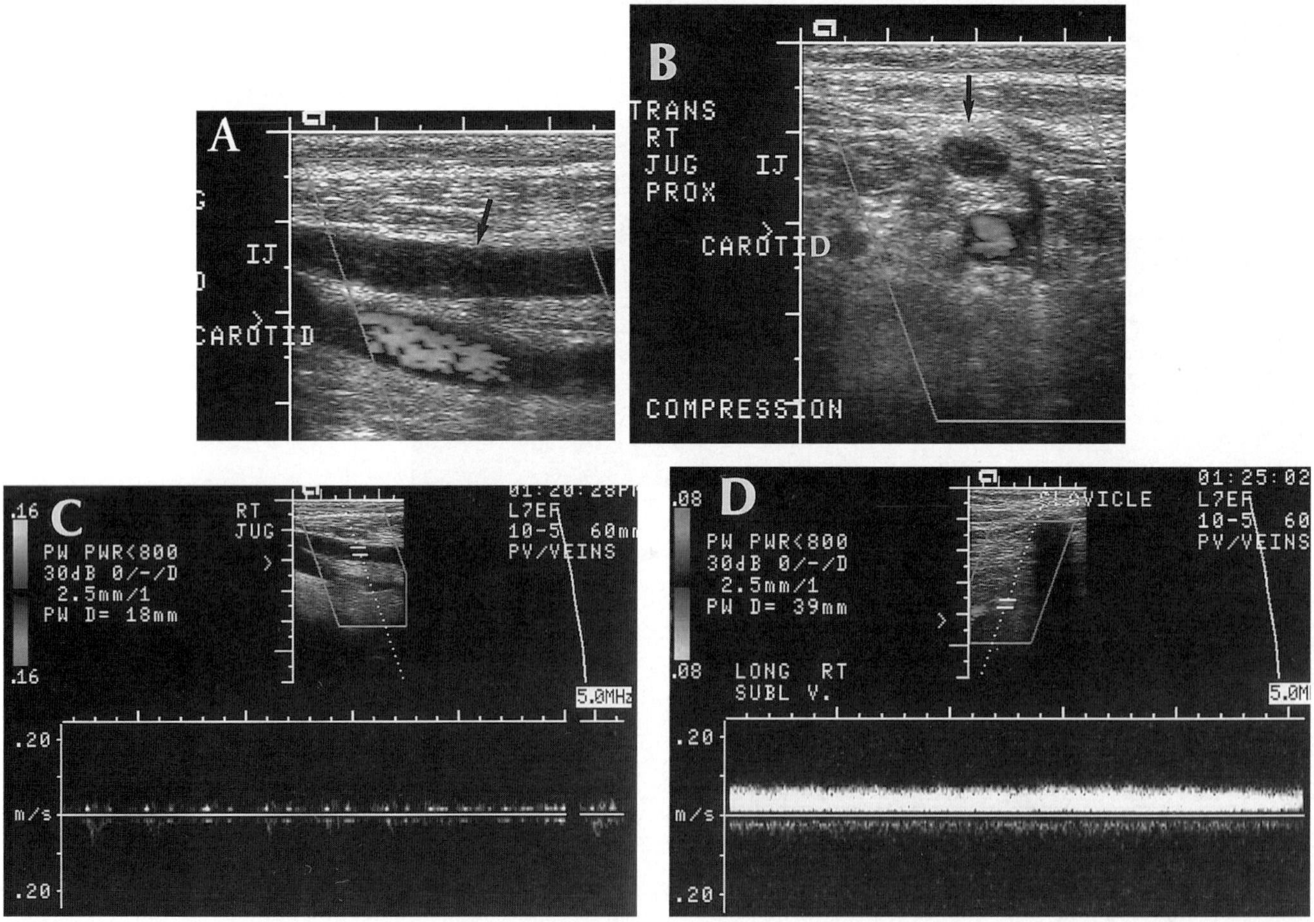

Figure 40.49. (Color Plates) Internal Jugular Vein Thrombosis. Longitudinal **(A)** and transverse **(B)** color Doppler images of the right internal jugular (*IJ*) vein shows noncompressible echogenic thrombus (*arrows*). Color flow (*red*) is seen in the right common carotid artery and no flow in the IJ. **C.** Spectral Doppler confirms no flow in the right IJ. **D.** The proximal right subclavian vein has a blunted, monophasic waveform suggesting a central obstruction.

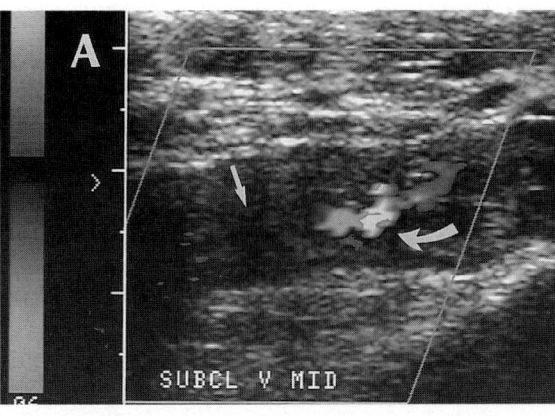
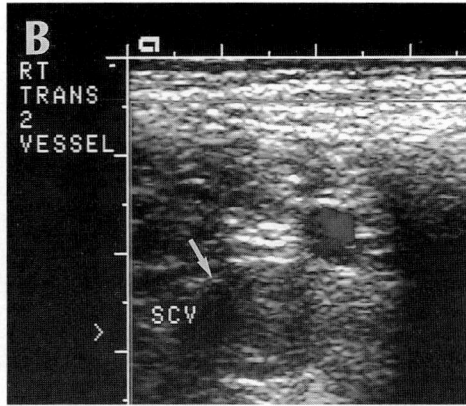

Figure 40.50. (Color Plates) Subclavian Vein Thrombosis. Longitudinal **(A)** and transverse **(B)** color Doppler images of the right subclavian vein (*SCV*). The distended vein is filled with echogenic thrombus (*arrows*). The longitudinal image demonstrates some residual patent lumen (*curved arrow*).

in the upper extremity above the elbow. Evaluation of the central veins, especially the subclavian, is limited because the overlying clavicle limits visualization; thus, the compression technique cannot be used. Color Doppler is the mainstay of evaluation of the central veins.

In lieu of compression, the "sniff" test is useful in the subclavian vein. With sniffing, the diameter of the subclavian vein will decrease and often completely collapse. With valsalva, the vein will increase in diameter. These maneuvers are performed bilaterally, and the response is compared.

Duplex evaluation of the venous waveforms reveal normal respiratory phasicity and transmitted cardiac pulsations (Fig. 40.48) in the central veins. The further from the thoracic inlet, the more monophasic the waveform. Loss of the normal pulsatility (monophasic waveform) centrally when compared to the contralateral side suggests a proximal central obstruction (Fig. 40.49).

Deep Venous Thrombosis. Upper extremity DVT is usually the result of a current or previous indwelling catheter. A coexistent ipsilateral internal jugular vein clot is often present (Fig. 40.49). Venous stasis in the upper extremity due to extrinsic compression or thoracic outlet syndrome is less common. In contrast to the lower extremity, upper extremity DVT is associated with pulmonary embolism in only 12% of cases. The diagnosis of DVT employs the same principles as for the lower extremity in addition to the techniques described above (Fig. 40.50). Although no large studies have compared duplex US to contrast venography, most consider US as the initial imaging modality. Contrast venography, CT, and MR venography are reserved for patients with a high clinical probability of DVT despite a negative duplex examination.

Thoracic Outlet Syndrome. The most common presentation for a patient with thoracic outlet syndrome is pain due to compression of the brachial plexus. Venous obstruction resulting in arm swelling is more common than arterial obstruction. Venous compression occurs on the subclavian vein as it passes between the first rib and scalene muscles at the thoracic inlet. Intermittent arm swelling, effort thrombosis, and pain are the usual

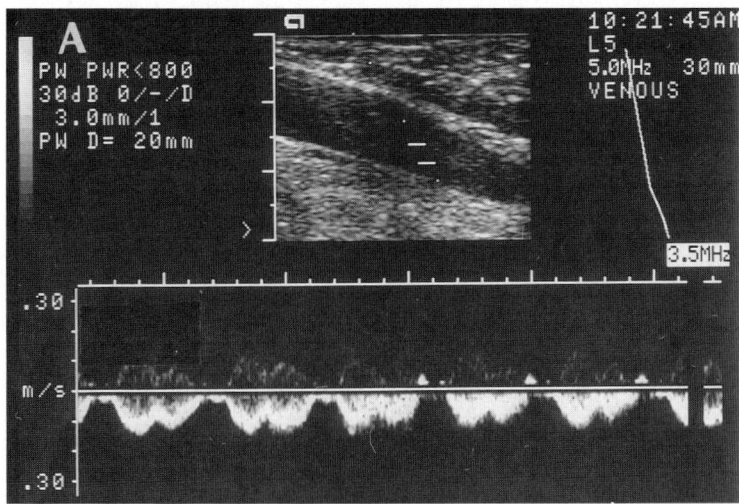

Figure 40.51. Thoracic Outlet Syndrome: Venous. A. Normal subclavian vein waveform with the arm at the patient's side. *(Continued)*

Figure 40.51. *(Continued).* **B.** With the arm abducted the Doppler tracing is blunted (more monophasic). The contralateral side demonstrated no blunting of the waveform with abduction.

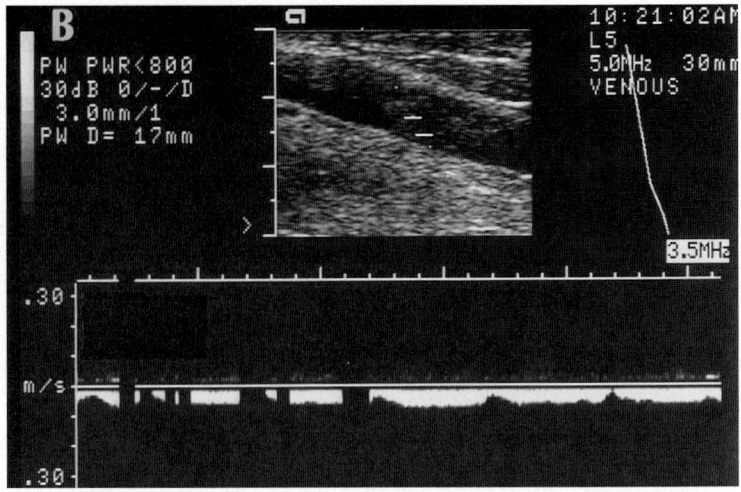

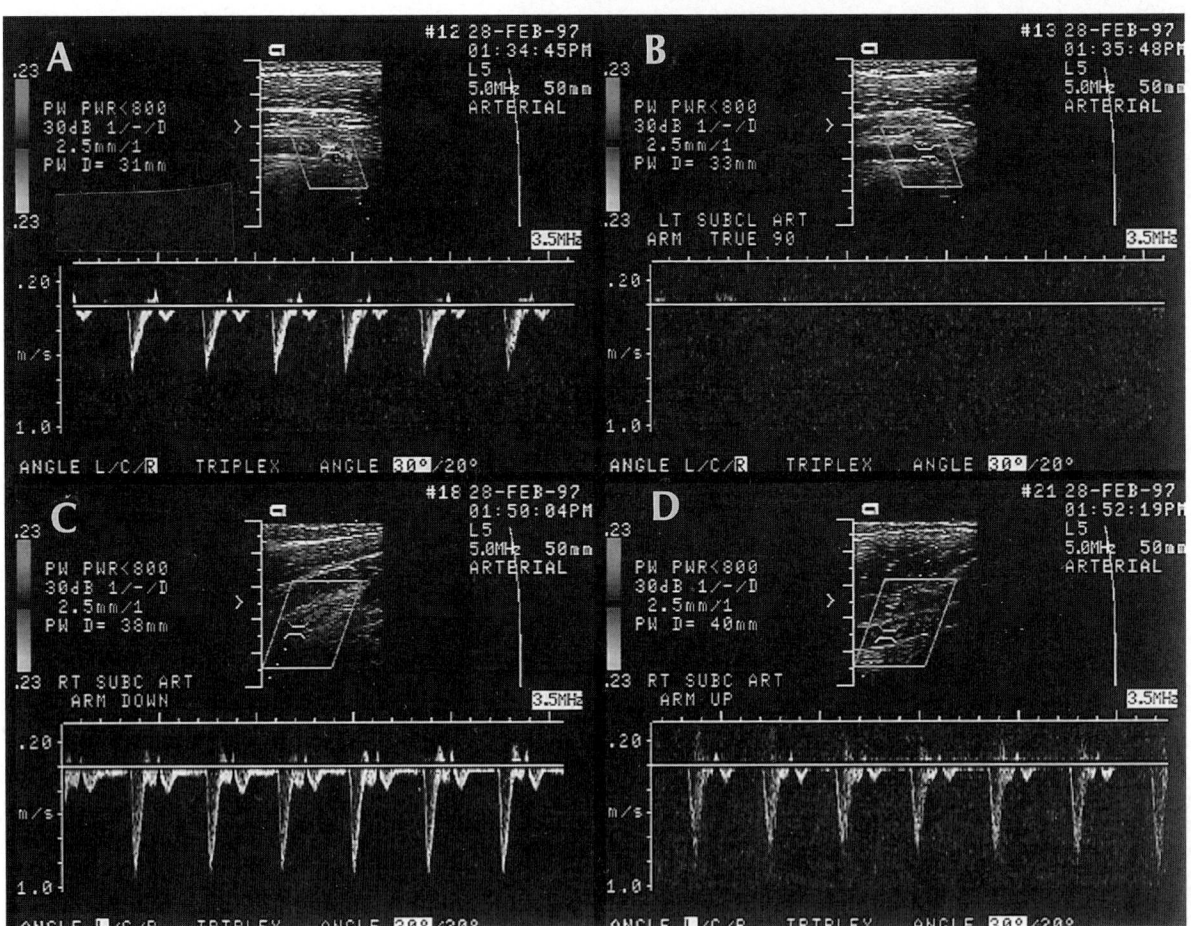

Figure 40.52. (Color Plates) Thoracic Outlet Syndrome: Arterial. A. Normal triphasic, high resistance waveform in the left subclavian artery with the arm at the patient's side. **B.** Abduction of the left arm causes obliteration of the left radial pulse on physical exam. The Doppler tracing confirms the clinical finding demonstrating complete occlusion of the left subclavian artery. **C, D.** The right subclavian artery has normal triphasic, high resistance flow with the arm at the patient's side and in abduction (no thoracic outlet syndrome).

symptoms. If frank clot is not identified, the patient should be examined with the arm at the side and at various degrees of abduction. With use of pulse wave and color Doppler imaging, compression is likely if flow ceases or a dampening of the waveform occurs. No dampening is seen on the unaffected side. Similarly, a blunted arterial waveform or absent flow is seen if the subclavian artery is affected (Figs. 40.51, 40.52).

References

1. Newman JS, Adler RS, Bude RO, et al. Detection of soft-tissue hyperemia: value of power Doppler sonography. AJR Am J Roentgenol 1994;163:385–389.

2. Nelson TR, Pretorius DH. The Doppler signal: where does it come from and what does it mean? AJR Am J Roentgenol 1988;151:439–447.

3. Merritt CRB. Doppler US: the basics. Radiographics 1991; 11:109–119.

4. Rubin JM. Spectral Doppler ultrasound. Radiographics 1994;14:139–150.

5. Burns PN. The physical principles of Doppler and spectral analysis. J Clin Ultrasound 1987;15:567–590.

6. Zwiebel WJ, Fruechte D. Basics of abdominal and pelvic duplex: instrumentation, anatomy, and vascular Doppler signatures. Semin Ultrasound CT MR 1992;13:3–21.

7. Maulik D. Hemodynamic interpretation of the arterial Doppler waveform. Ultrasound Obstet Gynecol 1993; 3:219–227.

8. Kotval PS. Doppler waveform parvus and tardus—a sign of proximal flow obstruction. J Ultrasound Med 1989; 8:435–440.

9. Bude RO, Rubin JM, Platt JF, et al. Pulsus tardus: its cause and potential limitations in detection of arterial stenosis. Radiology 1994;190:779–784.

10. Powis RL. Color flow imaging. Radiographics 1994;14: 415–428.

11. Mitchell DG. Color Doppler imaging: principles, limitations, artifacts. Radiology 1990;177:1–10.

12. Weskott HP. Amplitude Doppler US: slow blood flow detection tested with a flow phantom. Radiology 1997;202:125–130.

13. Bude RO, Rubin JM. Power Doppler sonography. Radiology 1996;200:21–23.

14. Rubin JM, Bude RO, Carson PL, et al. Power Doppler US: a potentially useful alternative to mean frequency-based color Doppler US. Radiology 1994;190:853–856.

15. Bohs LN, Friemel BH, McDermott BA, et al. Real-time system for angle-independent US of blood flow in two dimensions: initial results. Radiology 1993;186:259–261.

16. Pellerito JS, Troiano RN, Quedens-Case C, et al. Common pitfalls of endovaginal color Doppler flow imaging. Radiographics 1995; 15:37–47.

17. Santilli JD, Santilli SM, Rodnick JE. Prevention of stroke caused by carotid bifurcation stenosis. Am Fam Phys 1996; 53:549–556.

18. North American Symptomatic Carotid Endarterectomy Trial Collaborators. Beneficial effect of carotid endarterectomy in symptomatic patients with high-grade carotid stenosis. N Engl J Med 1991;325:445–453.

19. European Carotid Surgery Trialist's Collaborative Group. MRC European carotid surgery trial: interim results for symptomatic patients with severe (70–99%) or with mild (0–29%) carotid stenosis. Lancet 1991;337:1235–1243.

20. Executive Committee for the Asymptomatic Carotid Atherosclerosis Study. Endarterectomy for asymptomatic carotid artery stenosis. JAMA 1995;273:1421–1428.

21. Hobson RW, Weiss DG, Fields WS, et al. Efficacy of carotid endarterectomy for asymptomatic carotid stenosis. N Engl J Med 1993;328:221–227.

22. Carroll BA. Carotid sonography. Radiology 1991;178: 303–313.

23. O'Leary DH, Polak JF, Krommal RA, et al. Thickening of the carotid wall. A marker for atherosclerosis in the elderly? Stroke 1996;27:224–231.

24. Burke GL, Evans GW, Riley WA, et al. Arterial wall thickness is associated with prevalent cardiovascular disease in middle-aged adults. The Atherosclerosis Risk In Communities (ARIC) Study. Stroke 1995;26:386–391.

25. Hodis H, Mack W, Labrec L, et al. Reduction in carotid arterial wall thickness using lovastatin and dietary therapy. A randomized, controlled trial. Ann Intern Med 1996;124: 548–556.

26. Polak JF. Peripheral Vascular Sonography: A Practical Guide. Baltimore: Williams & Wilkins, 1992.

27. Bluth EI, Stavros AT, Marich KW, et al. Carotid duplex sonography: a multicenter recommendation for standardized imaging and Doppler criteria. Radiographics 1988; 8:487–506.

28. Polak JF. Sonographic evaluation of the carotid arteries in patients with transient ischemic attacks, strokes, or carotid bruits. RSNA Special Course in US 1996:91–97.

29. Polak JF, O'Leary DH, Kronmal RA, et al. Sonographic evaluation of carotid artery atherosclerosis the elderly: relationship of disease severity to stroke and transient ischemic attack. Radiology 1993;188:363–370.

30. O'Leary DH, Clouse ME, Potter JE, et al. The influence of noninvasive tests on the selection of patients for carotid angiography. Stroke 1995;16:264–267.

31. Hunink MG, Polak JF, Barlan MM, et al. Detection and quantification of carotid artery stenosis: efficacy of various Doppler velocity parameters. AJR 1993; 160:619–625.

32. Moneta GL, Edwards JM, Chitwood RW, et al. Correlation with North American Symptomatic Carotid Endarterectomy Trial (NASCET) angiographic definition of 70% to 99% internal carotid artery stenosis with duplex scanning. J Vasc Surg 1993;17:152–157.

33. Neale ML, Chambers JL, Kelly AT, et al. Reappraisal of duplex criteria to assess significant carotid stenosis with special reference to reports from the North American Symptomatic Carotid Endarterectomy Trial and the European Carotid Surgery Trial. Stroke 1994;20:642–649.

34. Faught WE, Mattos MA, van Bemmelen PS, et al. Color-flow duplex scanning of carotid arteries: new velocity criteria based on receiver operator characteristic analysis for threshold stenoses used in the symptomatic and asymptomatic carotid trials. J Vasc Surg 1994;19:818–828.

35. Carpenter JP, Lexa FJ, Davis JT. Determination of sixty percent or greater carotid artery stenosis by duplex Doppler ultrasonography. J Vasc Surg 1995;22:697–705.

36. Moneta JL, Edwards JM, Papanicolaou G, et al. Screening for asymptomatic internal carotid artery stenosis: duplex criteria for discriminating 60% to 99% stenosis. J Vasc Surg 1995;21:989–994.

37. Hood DB, Mattos MA, Mansour A, et al. Prospective evaluation of new duplex criteria to identify 70% internal carotid artery stenosis. J Vasc Surg 1996;23:254–261.

38. Carpenter JP, Lexa FJ, Davis JT. Determination of duplex Doppler US criteria appropriate to the North American Symptomatic Carotid Endarterectomy Trial. Stroke 1996; 27:695–699.

39. Browman MW, Cooperberg PL, Harrison PB, et al. Duplex ultrasonography criteria for internal carotid stenosis of more than 70% diameter: angiographic correlation and receiver operating characteristic curve analysis. Canad Assoc Radiol J 1995;46:291–295.

40. Lefsrud RD, James ME, Huston J. Redefined duplex US criteria for diagnosis of carotid stenosis. Scientific Paper Presentation, American Roentgen Ray Society, Boston, MA, 1997.

41. Darling RC, Messina CR, Brewster DC, et al. Autopsy study of unoperated abdominal aortic aneurysms. Circulation 1977;56:161–164.

42. Geroulakis G, Nicolaides A. Infrarenal abdominal aortic aneurysms. Eur J Vasc Surg 1992;6:616–622.

43. Ernst CB. Abdominal aortic aneurysm. N Engl J Med 1993; 16:1167–1172.

44. Scott RAP, Wilson NM, Ashton HA, et al. Is surgery necessary for abdominal aortic aneurysm less than 6 cm in diameter? Lancet 1993;342:1395–1396.

45. Feldstein VA, Patel MD, LaBerge JM. Transjugular intrahepatic portosystemic shunts: accuracy of Doppler US in determination of patency and detection of stenosis. Radiology 1996;201:141–147.

46. Foshager MC, Ferral H, Finlay DE, et al. Color Doppler sonography of transjugular intrahepatic portosystemic shunts (TIPS). AJR Am J Roentgenol 1994;163:105–111.

47. Kanterman RY, Darcy MD, Middleton WD, et al. Doppler sonography findings associated with transjugular intrahepatic portosystemic shunt malfunction. AJR Am J Roentgenol 1997;168:567–572.

48. Chong WK, Malisch TA, Mazer MJ, et al. Transjugular intrahepatic portosystemic shunt: US assessment with maximum flow velocity. Radiology 1993;189:789–793.

49. Dodd GD, Zajko AB, Orons PD, et al. Detection of transjugular intrahepatic portosystemic shunt dysfunction: Value of duplex Doppler sonography. AJR Am J Roentgenol 1995;164:1119–1124.

50. Feldstein VA, LaBerge JM. Hepatic vein flow reversal at duplex sonography: a sign of transjugular intrahepatic portosystemic shunt dysfunction. AJR Am J Roentgenol 1994;162:839–841.

51. Foshager MC, Ferral H, Nazarian GK, et al. Duplex sonography after transjugular intrahepatic portosystemic shunts (TIPS): normal hemodynamic findings and efficacy in predicting shunt patency and stenosis. AJR Am J Roentgenol 1995;165:1–7.

52. Suratt RS, Middleton WD, Darcy MD, et al. Morphologic and hemodynamic findings a sonography before and after creation of a transjugular intrahepatic portosystemic shunt. AJR Am J Roentgenol 1993;160:627–630.

53. Longo JM, Bilbao JI, Rousseau HP, et al. Transjugular intrahepatic portosystemic shunt: evaluation with Doppler sonography. Radiology 1993;186:529–534.

54. Carrol BA. Pulsatile groin mass in the postcatheterization patient. RSNA Special Course in US 1996:107–115.

55. Polak JF. Peripheral arterial disease: evaluation with color flow and duplex sonography. Radiol Clin North Am 1995;33:71–89.

56. Foshager MC, Finlay DE, Longley DG, et al. Duplex and color Doppler sonography of complications after percutaneous interventional vascular procedures. Radiographics 1994;14:239–253.

57. Coley BD, Roberts AC, Fellmeth BD, et al. Postangiographic femoral artery pseudoaneurysms: further experience with US-guided compression repair. Radiology 1995;194:307–311.

58. Zwiebel WJ. Painful legs after walking. RSNA Special Course in US 1996:133–141.

59. Polak JF. Arterial sonography: efficacy for the diagnosis of arterial disease of the lower extremity. AJR Am J Roentgenol 1993;161:235–243.

60. Beidle TR, Brom-Ferral R, Letourneau JG. Surveillance of infrainguinal vein grafts with duplex sonography. AJR Am J Roentgenol 1994;162:443–448.

61. Dorfman GS, Cronan JJ. Venous ultrasonography. Radiol Clin North Am 1992;30:879–893.

62. Cronan JJ. Venous thromboembolic disease: The role of US. Radiology 1993;186:619–630.

63. Bluth EI. Leg swelling with pain or edema. RSNA Special Course in US 1996:99–105.

64. Beidle TR, Letourneau JG. Arm swelling. RSNA Special Course in US 1996:125–132.

Section IX   BONES AND JOINTS

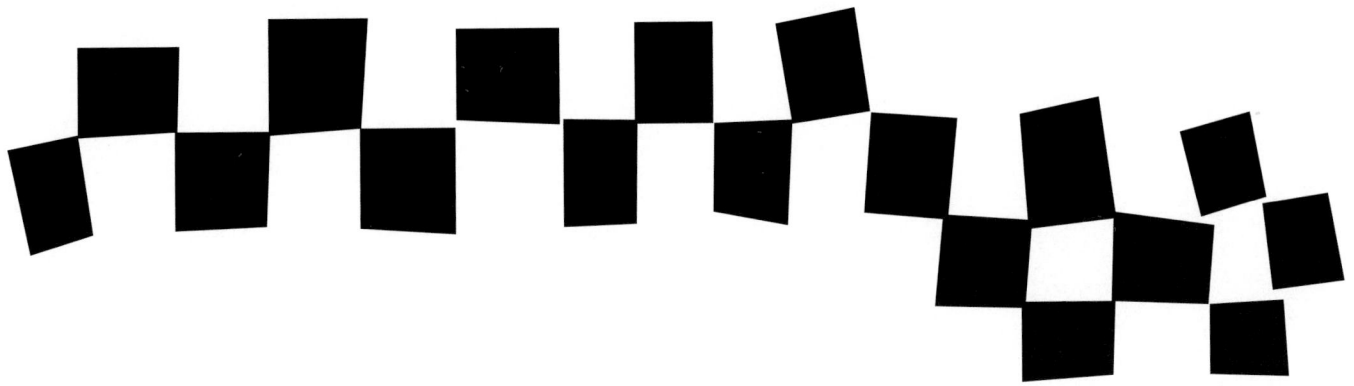

41
Benign Cystic Bone Lesions

Clyde A. Helms

A benign, bubbly, cystic lesion of bone is one of the more common skeletal lesions a radiologist encounters. The differential diagnosis can be quite lengthy and is usually structured on how the lesion looks to the radiologist, using his or her experience as a guide. This method, called pattern identification, certainly has merit, but it can lead to a very long differential diagnosis and many erroneous conclusions if not tempered with some logic.

In general, if a differential diagnosis will yield the correct diagnosis 95% of the time, most would consider it a useful differential list; however, it would not be appropriate to accept a 1-in-20 miss rate for fractures and dislocations. In general, the shorter the differential diagnosis list, the more helpful it is to clinicians and the easier it is to remember. A shorter differential list will usually have a lower accuracy rate than a long list; however, many times the longer lists contain such rare entities that the accuracy does not really increase substantially. For most of the entities in bone radiology, a 95% accurate differential is acceptable. If one wants to be more accurate than that, simply add more diagnoses to the list of differential possibilities.

When the differential diagnosis is long, as in the differential for bubbly, cystic lesions of bone, it can be difficult to recall all of the entities that should be mentioned. A mnemonic can be helpful in recalling long lists of information and is recommended.

FEGNOMASHIC

FEGNOMASHIC is a mnemonic that serves as a nice starting point for discussing possibilities that appear as benign, cystic lesions in bone. This mnemonic has been in general use for many years. By itself, it is merely a long list–14 entities–and needs to be coupled with other criteria to shorten the list into manageable form for each particular case. For instance, the age of the patient will help add or eliminate many of the possibilities. If multiple lesions are present, only half a dozen entities need to be discussed. Methods of narrowing the differential are discussed later in this chapter.

The first step in approaching a benign, cystic bone lesion is to be certain it is really benign. The criteria for differentiating benign from malignant are covered in chapter 42. Once it is established that the lesion is truly a benign, cystic lesion, FEGNOMASHIC will enable a differential diagnosis that is at least 95% accurate. Memorizing the 14 entities in this differential is easily done (Table 41.1).

The next step after learning the names of all of the lesions is getting some idea of each lesion's radiographic appearance. This is when experience becomes a factor. For the medical student or first-year resident, it is difficult to go beyond saying that they *all* look cystic, bubbly, and benign. The third-year resident should have no trouble differentiating between a unicameral bone cyst and a giant cell tumor because he or she has seen examples of each many times before and knows their appearance.

After getting a feel for what each lesion looks like radiographically and overcoming the frustration that builds when one realizes that many of them look alike, one should try to learn ways to differentiate each lesion from the others. I have developed a number of keys that I call discriminators, which will help to differentiate each lesion. These discriminators are 90–95% useful (I will mention when they are more or less accurate, in my experience) and are by no means intended to be absolutes or dogma. They are guidelines but have a high accuracy rate.

Textbooks rarely state that a finding "always" or "never" occurs. They temper descriptions with "virtually always," "invariably," "usually," or "characteristically." I have tried to pick out findings that come as close to "always" as I can, realizing that I will only be approximately 95% accurate. That is good enough for most radiologists.

The following is only a brief description of each entity, as more complete descriptions are readily available in any skeletal radiology text. What is emphasized here are the points that are unique for each entity, thereby en-

Table 41.1 Discriminators for Benign Lytic Bone Lesions – Mnemonic: FEGNOMASHIC

Letter	Represents	Characteristics
F	*Fibrous dysplasia*	No Periosteal reaction
E	*Enchondroma*	1. Calcification present (except in phalanges).
		2. Painless (no periostitis).
	Eosinophilic granuloma	Younger than age 30
G	*Giant cell tumor*	1. Epiphyses closed.
		2. Abuts the articular surface (in long bones).
		3. Well defined with a nonsclerotic margin (in long bones).
		4. Eccentric.
N	*Nonossifying fibroma*	1. Younger than age 30.
		2. Painless (no periostitis).
		3. Cortically based.
O	*Osteoblastoma*	Mentioned when ABC is mentioned (especially in the posterior elements of the spine).
M	*Metastatic diseases and myeloma*	Older than age 40.
A	*Aneurysmal bone cyst*	1. Expansile.
		2. Younger than age 30.
S	*Solitary bone cyst*	1. Central.
		2. Younger than age 30.
H	*Hyperparathyroidism (brown tumor)*	Must have other evidence of HPT.
I	*Infection*	Always mention.
C	*Chondroblastoma*	1. Younger than age 30.
		2. Epiphyseal.
	Chondromyxoid	No calcified matrix.

abling differentiation from the others. Table 41.1 is a synopsis of these discriminators.

FIBROUS DYSPLASIA

Fibrous dysplasia is a benign congenital process that can be seen in a patient of any age and can look like almost any pathologic process radiographically. It can be wild-looking, a discrete lucency, patchy, sclerotic, expansile, multiple, and many other descriptions. It is, therefore, difficult to look at a bubbly lytic lesion and unequivocally say it is or is not fibrous dysplasia. It would be better if the FEGNOMASHIC differential started on a positive note, say, with giant cell tumor or chondroblastoma, for which there are some definite criteria. Because fibrous dysplasia is first on the list, we might as well deal with it.

How do you know whether to include or exclude fibrous dysplasia if it can look like almost anything? Experience is the best guideline. In other words, look in a few texts and find as many different examples as possible; get a feeling for what fibrous dysplasia looks like.

Fibrous dysplasia will not have periostitis associated with it; therefore, if periostitis is present, one may safely exclude fibrous dysplasia. Fibrous dysplasia virtually never undergoes malignant degeneration and should not

Figure 41.1. Fibrous Dysplasia. This patient has polyostotic fibrous dysplasia with diffuse involvement of the pelvis as well as the proximal right femur. When the pelvis is involved with fibrous dysplasia, the ipsilateral femur on the affected side is invariably also involved.

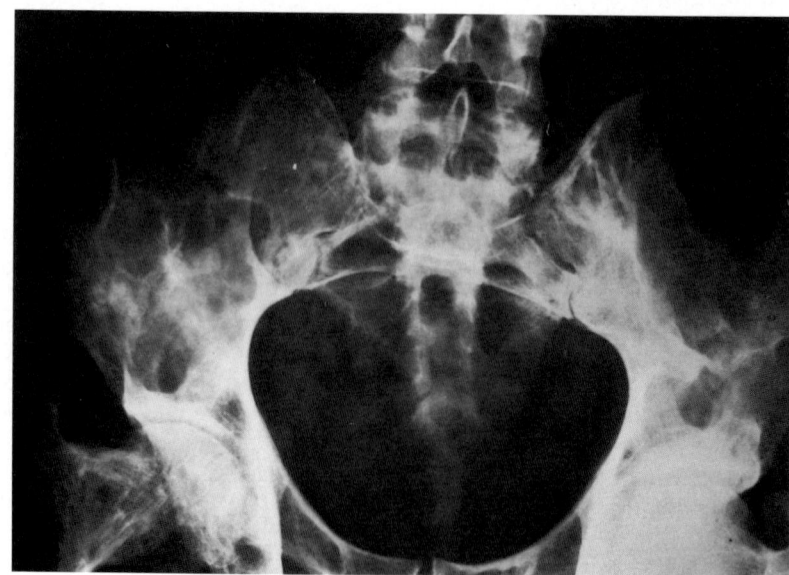

be a painful lesion unless there is a fracture. An occult fracture often occurs in long bones with fibrous dysplasia; therefore, it is not unusual to have it present with pain and no obvious fracture seen in a long bone. Pain in a flat bone, such as the ribs or pelvis (non–weight-bearing bones), should not occur with fibrous dysplasia.

Fibrous dysplasia can be either monostotic (most commonly) or polyostotic and has a predilection for the pelvis, proximal femur, ribs, and skull. When it is present in the pelvis, it is invariably present in the ipsilateral proximal femur (Fig. 41.1). I have seen only one case in which the pelvis was involved with fibrous dysplasia and the proximal femur was spared. The proximal femur, however, may be affected alone, without involvement in the pelvis (Fig. 41.2).

Fibrous dysplasia often involves the ribs. It typically has an expansile, lytic appearance in the posterior ribs (Fig. 41.3) and a sclerotic appearance in the anterior ribs.

The classic description of fibrous dysplasia is that it has a ground-glass or smoky matrix. This description confuses people as often as it helps them, and I do not recommend using ground-glass appearance as a buzz word for fibrous dysplasia. Fibrous dysplasia is often purely lytic and becomes hazy or takes on a ground-glass look as the matrix calcifies (Fig. 41.4). It can go on to calcify significantly, and then it presents as a sclerotic lesion (Fig. 41.5). Also, I often see lytic lesions with a pathologic diagnosis other than fibrous dysplasia that

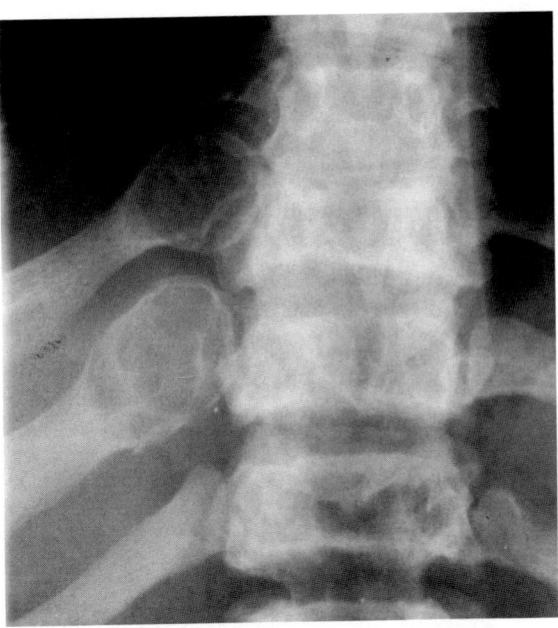

Figure 41.3. Fibrous Dysplasia. When fibrous dysplasia affects the ribs, the posterior ribs often demonstrate a lytic expansile appearance, as in this example. When the anterior ribs are involved, they are most often sclerotic in appearance. Note also the involvement of the thoracic spine.

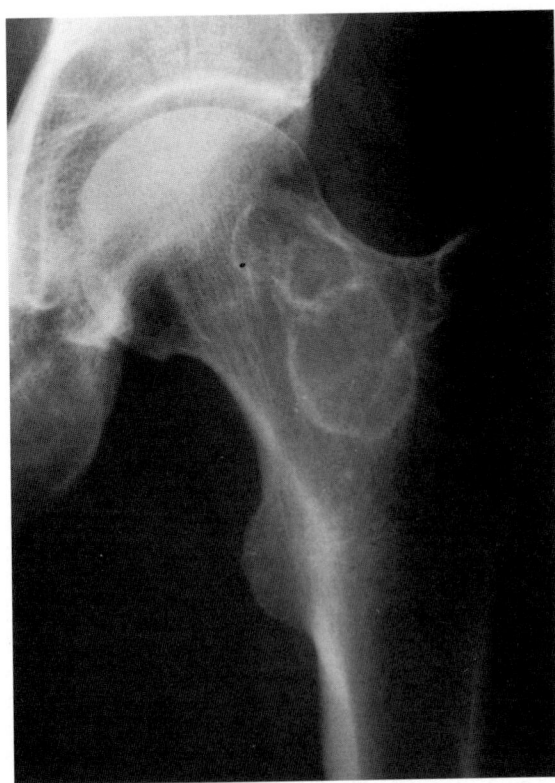

Figure 41.2. Fibrous Dysplasia. This patient has a well-defined lytic lesion with a hazy, ground-glass appearance in the neck of the left femur. The pelvis was uninvolved. It is not unusual for monostotic fibrous dysplasia to involve the proximal femur and spare the pelvis.

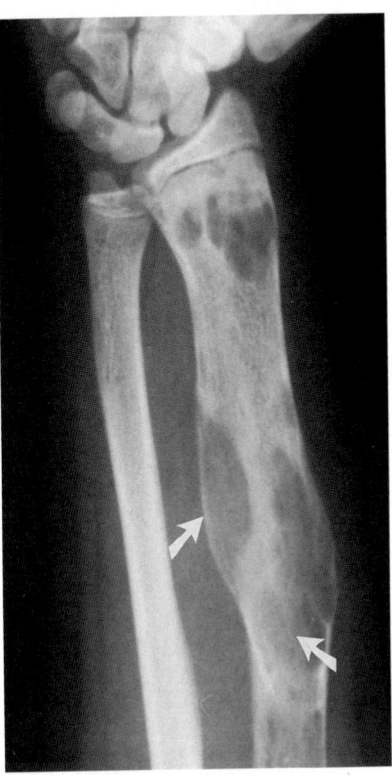

Figure 41.4. Fibrous Dysplasia. Polyostotic fibrous dysplasia is seen in the radius in this child. Parts of this lesion have a hazy, ground-glass appearance (*arrows*), whereas others are more lytic appearing. A hazy, ground-glass appearance is often present in fibrous dysplasia, but just as often, the appearance can be purely lytic or even sclerotic.

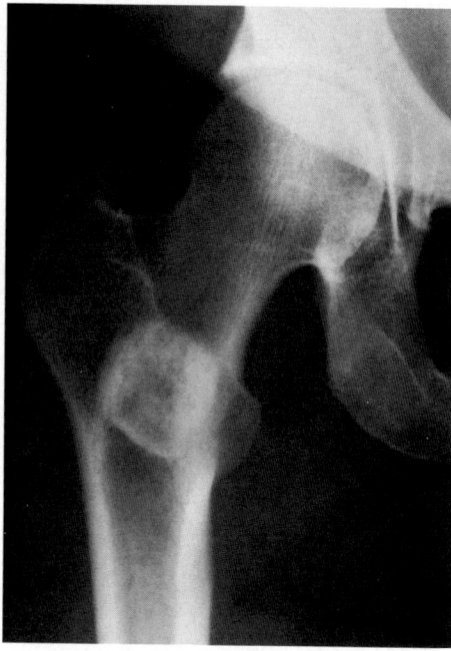

Figure 41.5. Fibrous Dysplasia. This predominantly sclerotic lesion in the intertrochanteric region of the right hip is a characteristic appearance for monostotic fibrous dysplasia in this location.

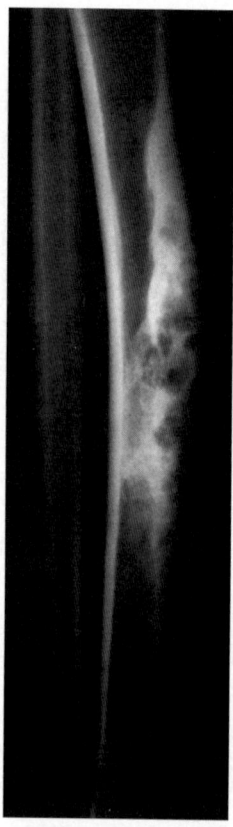

Figure 41.6. Adamantinoma. This expansile, mixed lytic and sclerotic process in the midshaft of the tibia is characteristic for fibrous dysplasia. An adamantinoma has an identical appearance and should be considered in any tibial lesion that resembles fibrous dysplasia. Biopsy showed this to be an adamantinoma.

have a distinct ground-glass appearance; therefore, the ground-glass quality can be misleading.

Adamantinoma. When a lesion is encountered in the tibia that resembles fibrous dysplasia, an adamantinoma should also be mentioned. An adamantinoma is a malignant tumor that radiographically and histologically resembles fibrous dysplasia (Fig. 41.6). It occurs almost exclusively in the tibia and the jaw (for unknown reasons) and is rare. Because it is rare, one may choose not to include it in the differential—a misdiagnosis will not occur more than once or twice in a lifetime.

McCune-Albright Syndrome. Polyostotic fibrous dysplasia occasionally occurs in association with café au lait spots on the skin (dark-pigmented, frecklelike lesions) and precocious puberty. This complex is called McCune-Albright syndrome. The bony lesions in this syndrome, and even in the simple polyostotic form, often occur unilaterally, that is, throughout one half of the body. This does not happen often enough to be of any diagnostic use in differentiating fibrous dysplasia from other lesions.

The presence of multiple lesions of fibrous dysplasia in the jaw has been termed cherubism. This is from the physical appearance of the child with puffed-out cheeks having an angelic look. The jaw lesions in cherubism regress in adulthood.

Discriminator. No periosteal reaction.

ENCHONDROMA AND EOSINOPHILIC GRANULOMA

Enchondroma

Enchondromas occur in any bone formed from cartilage and may be central, eccentric, expansile, or nonexpansile. They invariably contain calcified chondroid matrix except when in the phalanges. An enchondroma is the most common benign cystic lesion in the phalanges (Fig. 41.7). If a cystic lesion is present without calcified chondroid matrix anywhere except in the phalanges, I do not include enchondroma in my differential.

Often it is difficult to differentiate between an enchondroma and a bone infarct. An infarct usually has a well-defined, densely sclerotic, serpiginous border (Fig. 41.8), whereas an enchondroma does not (Fig. 41.9). An enchondroma often causes endosteal scalloping, whereas a bone infarct will not. Although these criteria are helpful in separating an infarct from an enchondroma, they are not foolproof.

It is difficult, if not impossible, to differentiate an enchondroma from a chondrosarcoma. Clinical findings (primarily pain) serve as a better indicator than radiographic findings, and indeed pain in an apparent enchondroma should warrant surgical investigation. Periostitis should not be seen in an enchondroma either. Trying to differentiate histologically an enchondroma from a chondrosarcoma is also difficult, if not impossible, at times. Biopsy of an apparent enchondroma should not be performed routinely for histologic differentiation.

Multiple enchondromas occur on occasion; this condition has been termed Ollier's disease (Fig. 41.10). It is not hereditary and does not have an increased rate of malignant degeneration. The presence of multiple en-

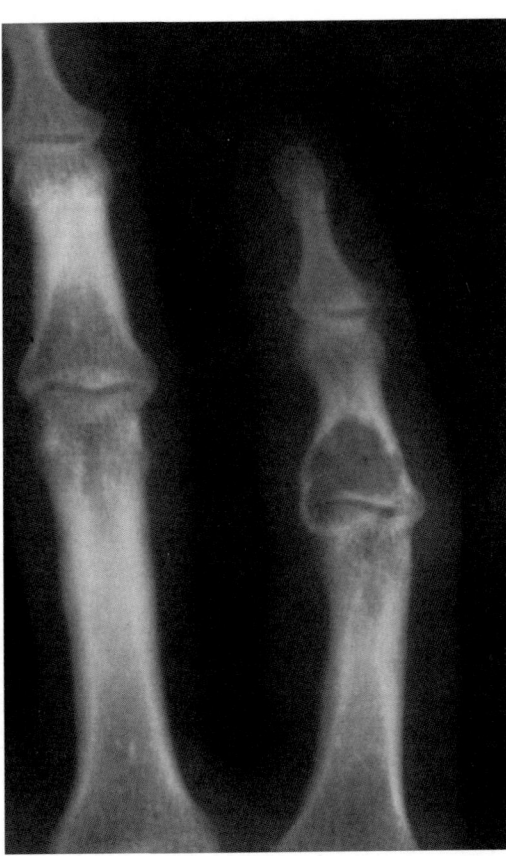

Figure 41.7. Enchondroma. A lytic lesion in the phalanges is most commonly an enchondroma. This is the only location in the skeleton where an enchondroma does not contain calcified chondroid matrix. These most often present with pathologic fractures, as in this example.

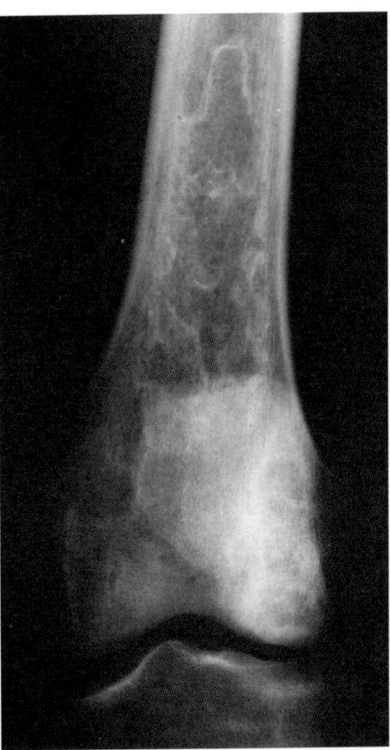

Figure 41.8. Bone Infarct. This lytic lesion in the distal femur with a calcified, serpiginous border is typical for a bone infarct. Occasionally, the differential between a bone infarct and an enchondroma can be difficult on plain films; however, in this example, an infarct is easily diagnosed.

chondromas associated with soft-tissue hemangiomas is known as Maffucci's syndrome (Fig. 41.11). This syndrome also is not hereditary; however, it does have an increased incidence of malignant degeneration of the enchondromas.

Discriminators. 1. Must have calcification (except in phalanges). 2. No periostitis or pain.

Eosinophilic Granuloma

Eosinophilic granuloma is a form of histiocytosis X, the other forms being Letterer-Siwe disease and Hand-Schüller-Christian disease. Although these forms may be merely different phases of the same disease, most investigators categorize them separately. The bony manifestations of all three disorders are similar and are discussed in this review simply as EG.

Eosinophilic granuloma, unfortunately for radiologists, has many appearances (1). It can be lytic or sclerotic; it may be well defined or ill defined; it might or might not have a sclerotic border; and it might or might not elicit a periosteal response. The periostitis, when present, is typically benign in appearance (thick, uniform, wavy) but can be lamellated or amorphous. Eosinophilic granuloma can mimic Ewing's sarcoma and present as a permeative (multiple small holes) lesion.

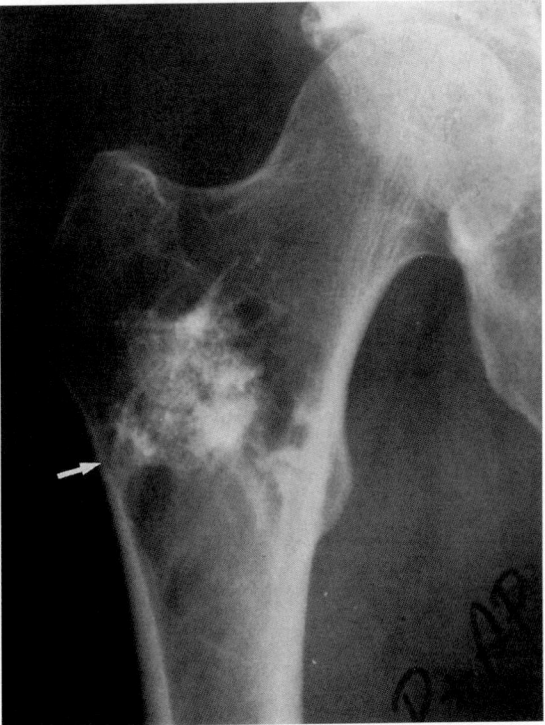

Figure 41.9. Enchondroma. This mixed lytic, sclerotic lesion in the intertrochanteric region of the right femur shows the stippled punctate calcification typical for chondroid matrix seen in an enchondroma. Some endosteal scalloping is seen on the lateral cortex (*arrow*), but this is subtle.

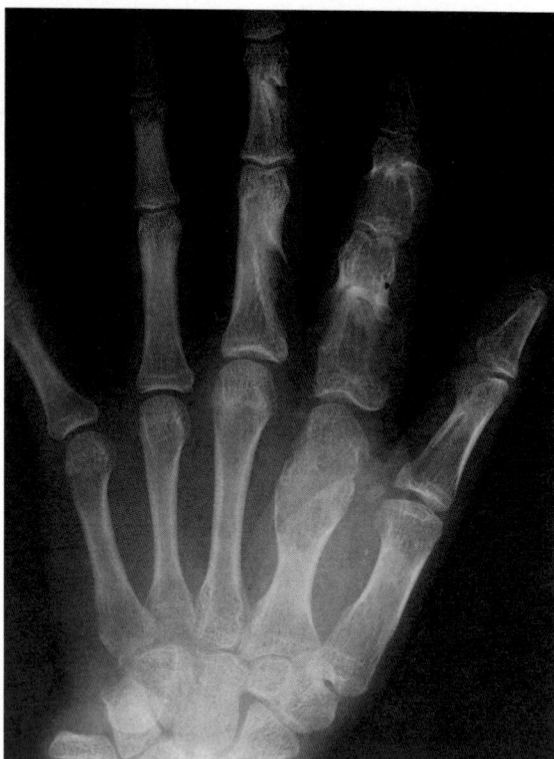

Figure 41.10. Ollier's Disease. Multiple enchondromas are present throughout the hand. This is a typical example of Ollier's disease.

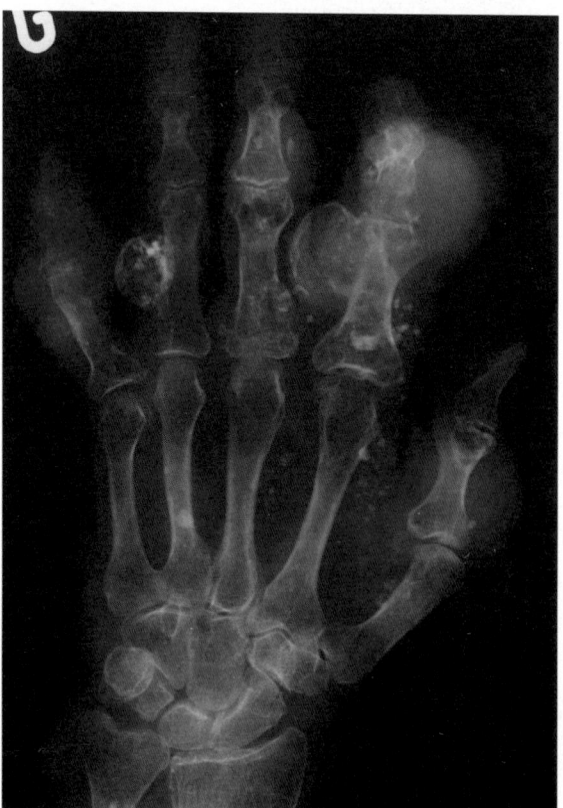

Figure 41.11. Maffucci's Syndrome. Multiple enchondromas associated with phleboliths are present in the phalanges. This combination of findings invariably represents hemangiomas and enchondromas in Maffucci's syndrome.

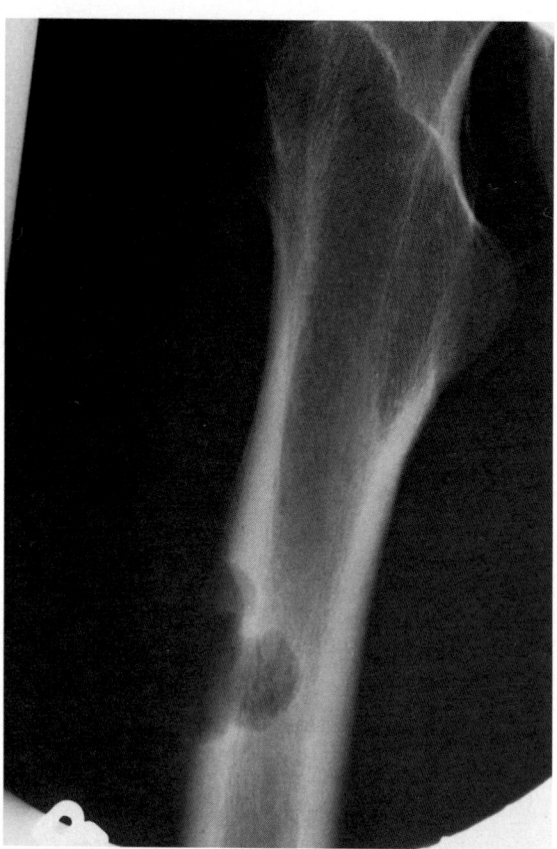

Figure 41.12. Eosinophilic Granuloma. A well-defined lytic lesion is seen involving the cortex of the proximal femur in this 20-year-old patient. Biopsy showed this to be EG.

How, then, can one distinguish EG from any of the other lytic lesions in this differential? Remember that it is difficult to exclude EG from almost any differential of a bony lesion, be it benign or malignant. Eosinophilic granuloma occurs almost exclusively in patients less than the age of 30 years (usually <20 y); therefore, the patient's age is the best criterion. I recommend mentioning EG as a differential possibility for *any* lesion in a patient less than the age of 30. Because EG can look like anything, so long as the radiograph is not of an arthritide or trauma, EG can be mentioned without even looking at the film!

Eosinophilic granuloma is most often monostotic (Fig. 41.12), but it can be polyostotic (Fig. 41.13) and, thus, has to be included whenever multiple lesions are present in a patient younger than the age of 30 years.

Eosinophilic granuloma might or might not have a soft-tissue mass associated, so the presence or absence of a soft-tissue mass will not help in the differential diagnosis. I know of no entity in which presence or absence of an associated soft-tissue mass will warrant inclusion or exclusion of the process from a differential. It is important to note the presence of a soft-tissue mass (or its absence), but it will do little to narrow the differential diagnosis.

Most radiologists are inept at evaluating the soft tissues because they are difficult to see, and computed tomography and magnetic resonance imaging have made it un-

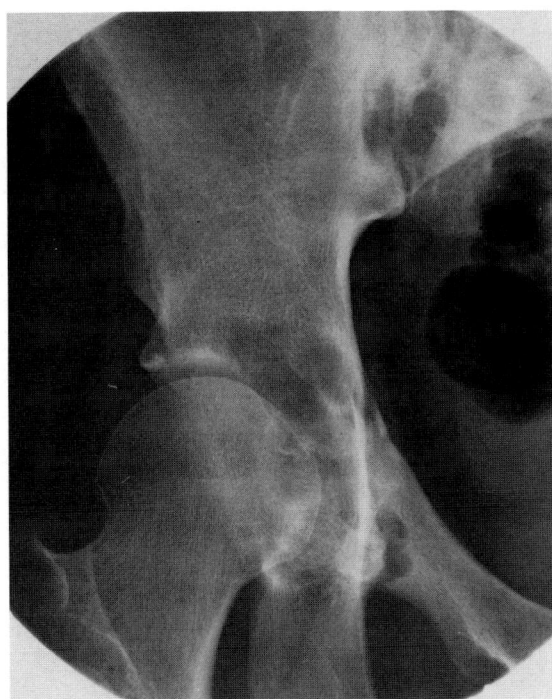

Figure 41.13. Eosinophilic Granuloma. Well-defined lytic lesions are present throughout the pelvis in this 24-year-old patient. In addition to the lesion around the right hip, a lesion is seen at the right sacroiliac joint. Biopsy showed this to be EG.

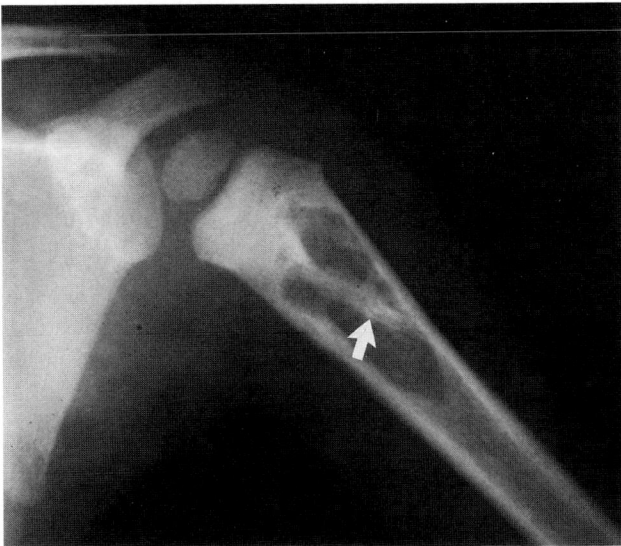

Figure 41.14. Eosinophilic Granuloma. This well-defined lytic lesion contains a bony sequestrum (*arrow*), which is typical for osteomyelitis or EG. Biopsy revealed this to be EG.

necessary in most cases to rely on plain films for the soft tissues. Fortunately, in most cases, the presence or absence of a soft-tissue mass will not alter the differential diagnosis. The treating physician will undoubtedly want to know whether the soft tissues are involved and to what extent; this can be satisfactorily demonstrated with MR.

Eosinophilic granuloma occasionally has a bony sequestrum (Fig. 41.14). Only a few other entities have been described that on occasion have bony sequestra:

osteomyelitis, lymphoma, and fibrosarcoma; therefore, when a sequestrum is identified, EG, osteomyelitis, lymphoma, and fibrosarcoma should be considered. As discussed in chapter 40, an osteoid osteoma will often give an appearance of a sequestration when the nidus is partially calcified.

Clinically, EG might or might not be associated with pain; therefore, clinical history is noncontributory for the most part.

Discriminator. Must be less than age 30 years.

GIANT CELL TUMOR

Giant cell tumor is an uncommon, somewhat controversial lesion with several schools of thought as to its radiographic appearance. I subscribe to the most widely used approach, as do the majority of radiologists and pathologists (2).

First, it is important to realize that one is unable to tell whether a giant cell tumor is benign or malignant, regardless of its radiographic appearance. Histologically, a giant cell tumor cannot be divided into either a benign or a malignant category. Most surgeons curettage and pack the lesions and consider them benign unless they recur. Even then, they can still be benign and recur a second or third time. About 15% of giant cell tumors are thought to be malignant on the basis of their recurrence rate. When malignant, they can metastasize to the lungs, but they do so infrequently.

Four classic radiographic criteria for diagnosing giant cell tumors exist. If any of these criteria are not met when looking at a lesion, giant cell tumor can be eliminated from the differential diagnosis.

1. Giant cell tumor occurs only in patients with closed epiphyses; this is valid at least 98–99% of the time and is extremely useful. I will not entertain the diagnosis of giant cell tumor in a patient with open epiphyses.
2. The lesion must be epiphyseal and abut the articular surface (Fig. 41.15). There is disagreement as to whether giant cell tumors begin in the epiphyses or metaphyses or from the physeal plate itself; however, except for rare cases, when radiologists see the lesions, they are epiphyseal and are flush against the articular surface. The metaphysis also has some of the tumor in it because the lesions are generally very large. When one sees a giant cell tumor, it will be epiphyseal. Perhaps more importantly, it should be flush against the articular surface of the joint. This occurs in 98–99% of giant cell tumors; therefore, if I have a lesion that is separated from the articular surface by a definite margin of normal bone, I will not include giant cell tumor in the diagnosis. This rule does not apply in flat bones, such as in the pelvis or in the apophyses, which have no articular surfaces (Fig. 41.16).
3. Giant cell tumors are said to be eccentrically located in the bone, as opposed to being centrally placed in the medullary cavity. When a bony lesion is quite large, it can be difficult to tell whether it is central or eccentric. I do not find this to be a terribly useful description, but it is one of the classic "rules" of a giant cell tumor.

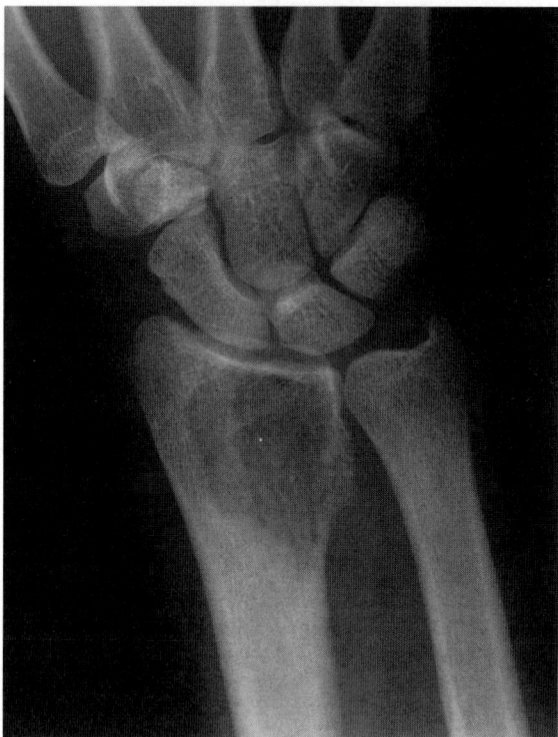

Figure 41.15. Giant Cell Tumor. A well-defined lytic lesion without a sclerotic margin is seen abutting the articular surface of the distal radius in a patient who has closed epiphyses. These are all characteristics of a giant cell tumor.

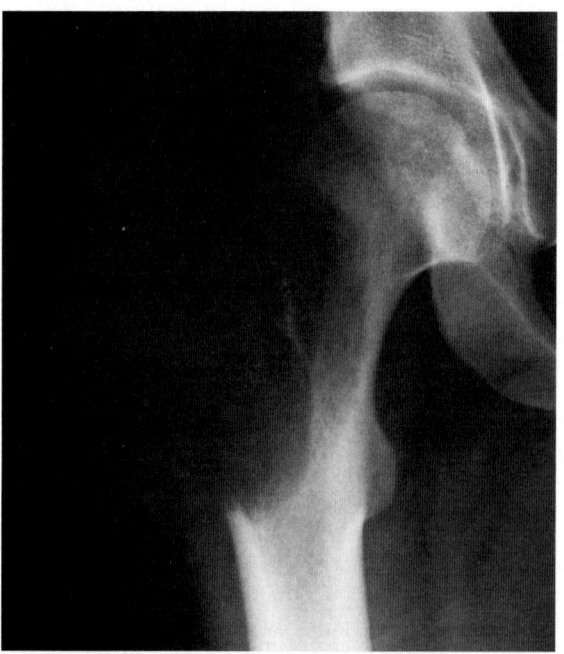

Figure 41.16. Giant Cell Tumor. This well-defined lytic lesion that does not have a sclerotic margin completely involves the greater trochanter. The apophyses have the same differential diagnosis as lesions in the epiphyses, which makes giant cell tumor a strong possibility in this example. Biopsy showed this to be a giant cell tumor.

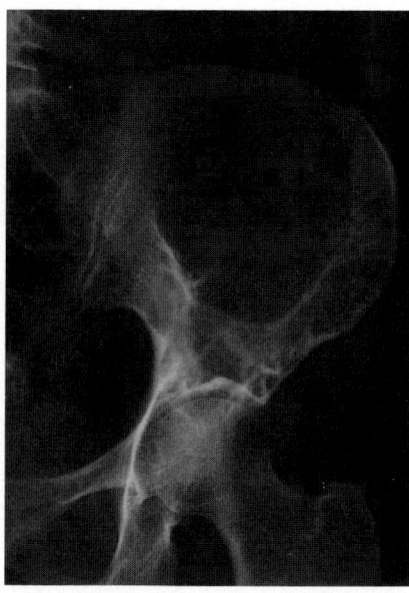

Figure 41.17. Giant Cell Tumor. A large, well-defined lytic lesion in the iliac wing is seen, which does contain a sclerotic margin and does not appear to abut any articular surface. The pelvis is a good location for giant cell tumor, which this proved to be at biopsy. The usual rules for giant cell tumors such as presence of a nonsclerotic margin do not apply in flat bones.

4. The lesion must have a sharply defined zone of transition (border) that is not sclerotic. This is a very helpful finding in giant cell tumor. The only places this does not apply is in flat bones, such as the pelvis (Fig. 41.17), and the calcaneus.

It is important to realize that the four criteria for a giant cell tumor apply only to giant cell tumors and not to any other lesion. For instance, I know of no other lesion that depends on whether the epiphyses are open or closed. No other lesion in any of my lists use as a diagnostic factor whether the zone of transition is sclerotic or not (many lesions, such as nonossifying fibromas, will usually have a sclerotic margin, but it does not occur enough to include as a discriminator). No other lesion must always abut the articular surface, and no other lesion has the classic description of being eccentrically placed (although several lesions, including nonossifying fibroma and chondromyxoid fibroma, are eccentric most of the time).

Although these four criteria apply well for giant cell tumor, they do not apply at all for any other lesions. Residents have a tendency to apply these criteria to every lytic lesion encountered for the simple reason that they have learned the four criteria.

Once one of the criteria is violated, the remainder do not even have to be used to eliminate a giant cell tumor. For instance, if a lytic lesion is found in the middiaphysis of a bone, giant cell tumor can be excluded. There is no need to check further to see whether it is eccentric, whether it has a nonsclerotic margin, or whether the epiphyses are closed.

Again, these rules will be greater than 95% effective

and, in my experience, close to 99% effective. If one or two cases are found that do not fit the criteria, another pathologist should review the slides. Many pathologists refer to aneurysmal bone cysts as giant cell tumors; hence, they have giant cell tumors that do not obey any of the criteria. These pathologists may be correct, but they are not in the mainstream of what most people use for giant cell tumor criteria, both radiographically and histologically.

Discriminators. 1. Epiphyses must be closed. 2. Must abut the articular surface. 3. Must be well defined with a nonsclerotic margin. 4. Must be eccentric.

NONOSSIFYING FIBROMA

A nonossifying fibroma (NOF) is probably the most common bone lesion encountered by radiologists. It reportedly occurs in up to 20% of children and usually spontaneously regresses so as to be seen only rarely after the age of 30. "Fibrous cortical defect" is a common synonym, although some people divide the two lesions on the basis of size, with a fibrous cortical defect being smaller than 2 cm in length (Fig. 41.18) and an NOF being larger than 2 cm (Fig. 41.19). Histologically, these lesions are identical; therefore, it seems appropriate to refer to them all as NOFs rather than to subdivide them by their size.

Nonossifying fibromas are benign, asymptomatic lesions that typically occur in the metaphysis of a long bone, emanating from the cortex. They classically have a thin, sclerotic border that is scalloped and slightly expansile (Fig. 41.20); however, this is a general descrip-

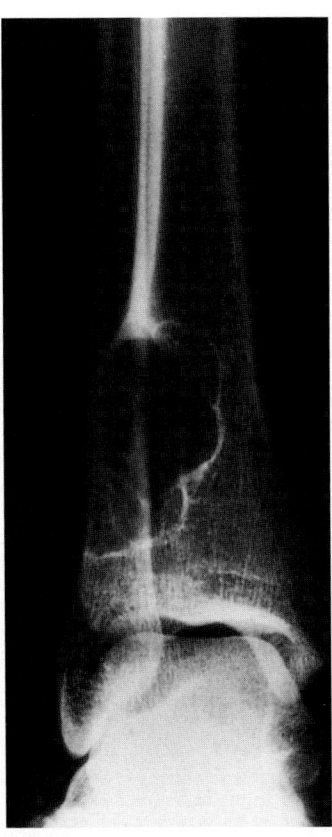

Figure 41.19. Nonossifying Fibroma. A large, well-defined lytic lesion, which is slightly expansile with scalloped sclerotic margins, is seen in the distal tibia in this young patient. This is a characteristic appearance of an NOF. The examination was obtained for a sprained ankle and not for this asymptomatic lesion.

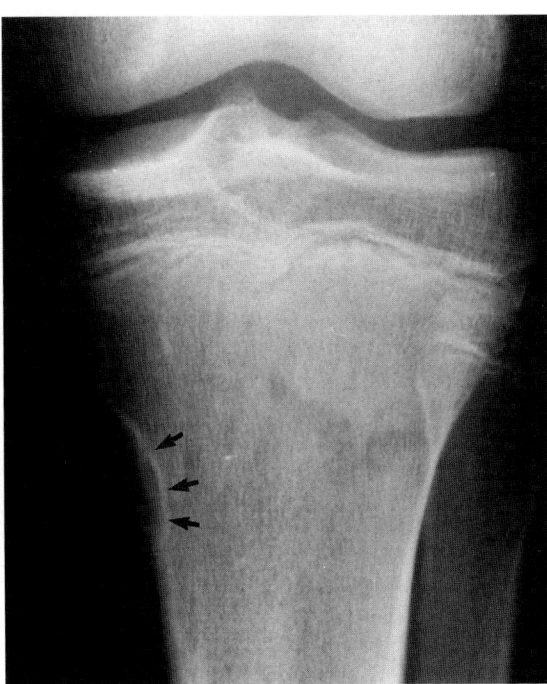

Figure 41.18. Fibrous Cortical Defect. A well-defined lytic lesion is seen in the medial metaphysis of this tibia (*arrows*), which is typical for a fibrous cortical defect.

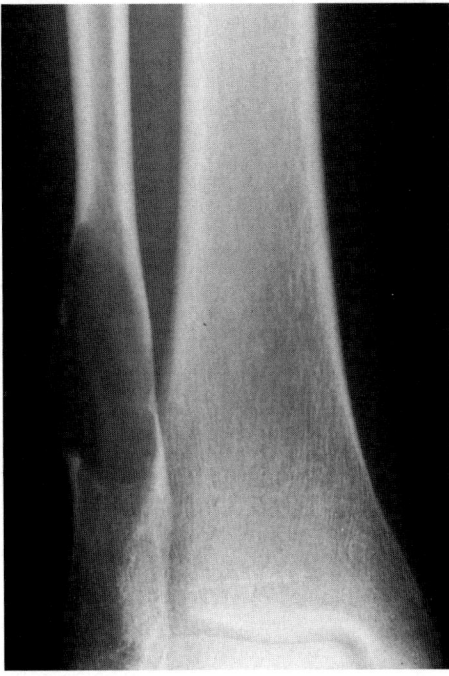

Figure 41.20. Nonossifying Fibroma. A well-defined, expansile lytic lesion in the distal fibula is noted in this asymptomatic patient, which is characteristic for an NOF.

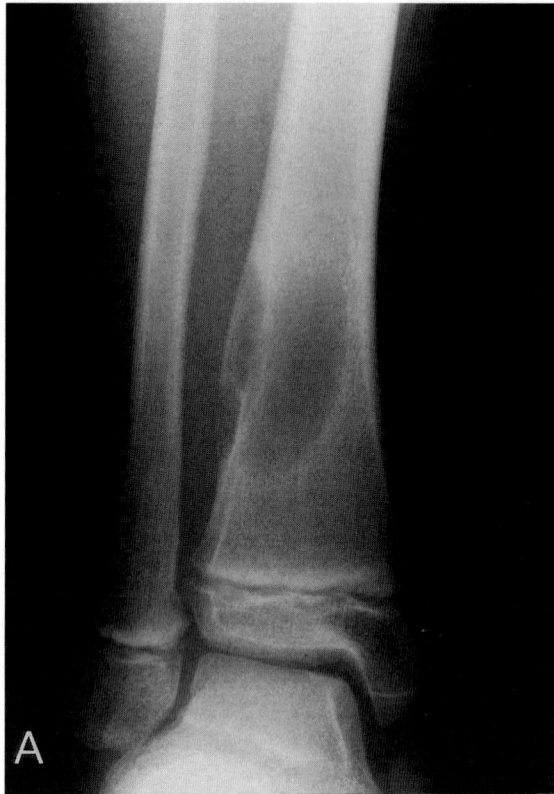

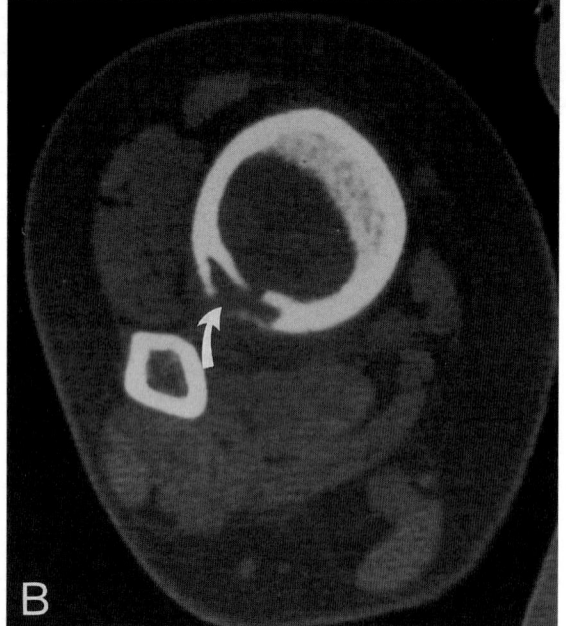

Figure 41.21. Nonossifying Fibroma. A. A well-defined, lytic lesion that is minimally expansile is seen in the distal tibia in this child who was examined for a sprained ankle. **B.** A CT examination showed apparent cortical destruction (*arrow*), which was believed to be suggestive of an aggressive lesion. Biopsy showed this to be a nonossifying fibroma. Both CT and MR will often show apparent cortical destruction, which is merely cortical replacement by benign fibrous tissue.

tion that probably applies to only 75% of the lesions and could equally apply to most of the lesions in FEGNO-MASHIC. They do not have to have expansion or a scalloped or sclerotic border, and are not limited to the metaphyses. Then how are they best recognized? The best way is to familiarize oneself with their general appearance by looking at examples in textbooks. That can be done in 15 minutes. It is important to recognize these lesions because they are what I call "don't touch" lesions (see chapter 39); that is, the radiologist's diagnosis should be the final word and thereby supplant a biopsy. These lesions are so characteristic that no differential diagnosis should be entertained, although a few entities can indeed occasionally simulate them.

If a CT or MR is obtained of an NOF, there will often appear to be interruption of the cortex, which can be misinterpreted as cortical destruction (Fig. 41.21). This merely represents cortical replacement by benign fibrous tissue and should not warrant further investigation.

If the patient is older than 30 years of age, NOF should not be included in the differential diagnosis. Nonossifying fibromas must be asymptomatic and exhibit no periostitis, unless there is an antecedent history of trauma. They routinely "heal" with sclerosis and eventually disappear (Fig. 41.22), usually around the ages of 20–30 years. During this healing period, they can appear hot on a radionuclide bone scan because there is osteoblastic activity. These lesions can occasionally get quite large (Fig. 41.23); therefore, growth or change in size should not alter the diagnosis. They are most commonly seen about the knee but can occur in any long bone. Occasionally, multiple NOFs are seen about the knee, each of which is characteristic in appearance.

Discriminators. 1. Must be younger than age 30 years. 2. No periostitis or pain. 3. Cortically based.

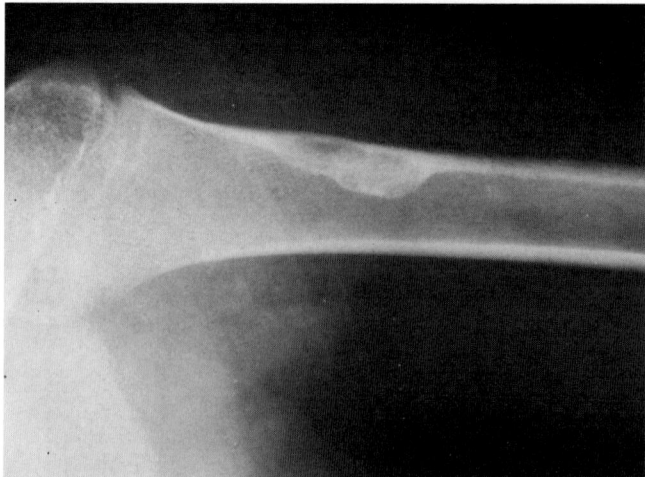

Figure 41.22. Healing Nonossifying Fibroma. A predominantly sclerotic lesion, which is minimally expansile and well defined, is seen in the proximal humerus in this child who is asymptomatic. This is a typical appearance of a disappearing or healing, NOF. With time, this lesion will melt into the normal bone and essentially disappear.

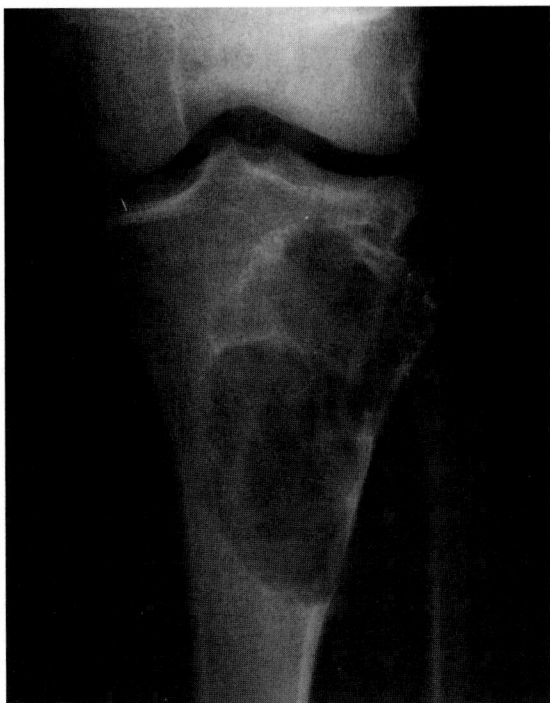

Figure 41.23. Nonossifying Fibroma. This large, well-defined lytic lesion with faint sclerotic margins is seen in the proximal tibia. It has a very typical appearance for a giant cell tumor; however, it has sclerotic margins and does not abut the articular surface. The lesion underwent biopsy and was found to be an NOF. (Case courtesy of Larry Yeager, MD, Redwood City, California.)

OSTEOBLASTOMA

Osteoblastomas are rare lesions that could justifiably be excluded from this differential without the fear of missing a diagnosis more than once in a lifetime. Why, then, include them? The mnemonic FEGNOMASHIC would not have nearly the same ring without the extra vowel, so osteoblastoma remains.

Osteoblastomas have two appearances: 1) They look like large osteoid osteomas, and are often called giant osteoid osteomas. Because osteoid osteomas are sclerotic lesions and do not resemble bubbly lytic lesions, this is not the type of osteoblastoma we are concerned with in this differential. 2) They simulate aneurysmal bone cysts (ABCs). They are expansile, often having a soap bubble appearance. If an ABC is being considered, so should an osteoblastoma. Osteoblastomas commonly occur in the posterior elements of the vertebral bodies, and about half of the cases demonstrate speckled calcifications (Fig. 41.24). A classic radiology differential is that of an expansile lytic lesion of the posterior elements of the spine, which includes osteoblastoma, ABC, and tuberculosis.

Discriminator. Mentioned when ABC is mentioned (especially in the posterior elements of the spine).

METASTATIC DISEASE AND MYELOMA

Metastatic disease should be considered for any lytic lesion—benign or aggressive in appearance—in a patient more than 40 years of age. Metastatic disease can appear perfectly benign radiographically (Fig. 41.25), so it is not valid to say, "Because this lesion looks benign, it should not be a metastasis." Most metastatic disease

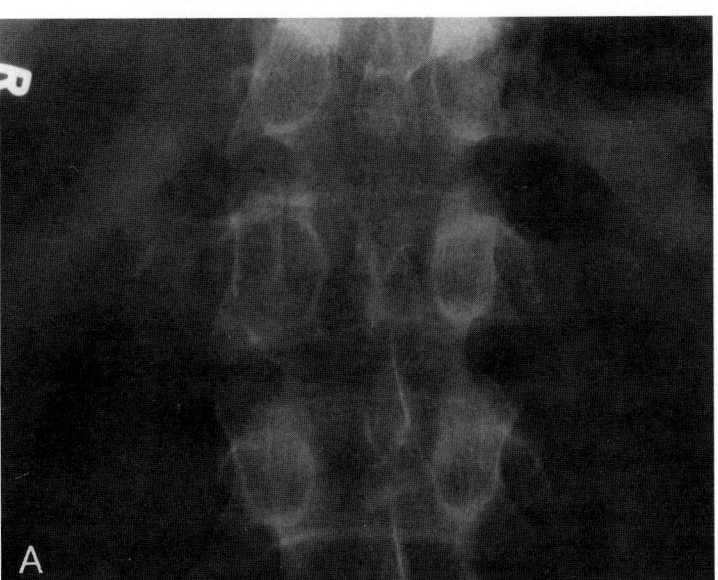

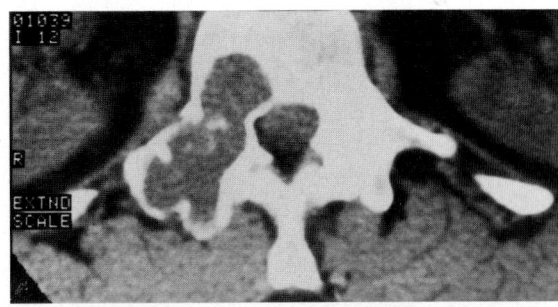

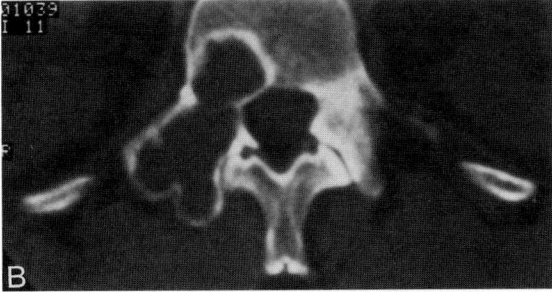

Figure 41.24. Osteoblastoma. A lytic expansile lesion involving the right T-12 pedicle and transverse process is seen on this anteroposterior plain film in **(A)** which is seen on the CT scan **(B)** to extend into the vertebral body. It has intact cortices and contains some calcified matrix. This is a classic example of an osteoblastoma of the spine.

has an aggressive appearance and will not be in the FEGNOMASHIC differential, but a significant number appear benign. In fact, metastases can have any radiographic appearance; therefore, any bone lesion in a patient older than the age of 40 should have metastatic disease as a consideration, unless trauma or arthritis is the primary concern.

For statistical purposes, I do not mention metastatic disease in a patient younger than the age of 40. I will be correct more than 99% of the time using 40 as a cut-off age. Otherwise, metastatic diseases would have to be mentioned in every single case of a lytic lesion, and I prefer to limit the list of differential possibilities. I am not claiming that metastatic disease does not occur in patients younger than the age of 40, only that I consider it acceptable to miss it (unless given a history of a known primary neoplasm).

Although myeloma most commonly presents as a diffuse permeative process in the skeleton (Fig. 41.26), it can present as either a solitary lesion (Fig. 41.27) or as multiple lytic lesions. Bubbly, lytic bone lesions of myeloma are more correctly called plasmacytomas. I mention plasmacytoma separately from metastatic disease because it can occur in a slightly younger population (age greater than 35 years is my cut-off) and can precede clinical or hematologic evidence of myeloma by 3 to 5 years. In general, there is no harm in lumping all metastatic disease, including myeloma, into one group and using greater than age 40 as the limiting factor.

Virtually any metastatic process can present as a lytic, benign-appearing lesion; therefore, it serves no purpose to try to guess the source of the metastatic disease from its appearance. In general, lytic expansile metastatic diseases tend to come from thyroid and renal tumors (Fig. 41.28). The only metastatic lesion that is said to *always* be lytic is renal cell carcinoma.

Discriminator. Must be older than age 40 years.

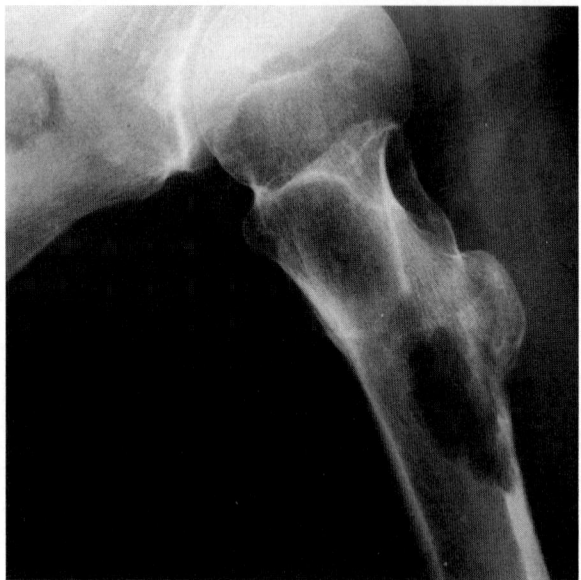

Figure 41.25. Metastatic Disease. A well-defined lytic lesion is seen in the proximal femur in this 50-year-old patient who has pain associated with this lesion. Biopsy showed this to be a renal metastasis. A significant number of metastatic lesions can have a completely benign appearance, as in this example.

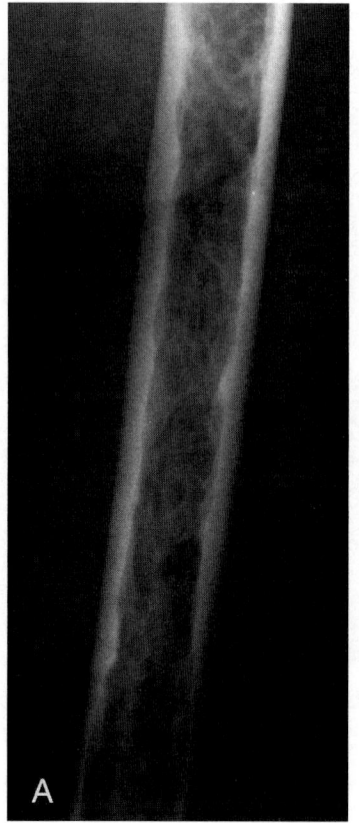

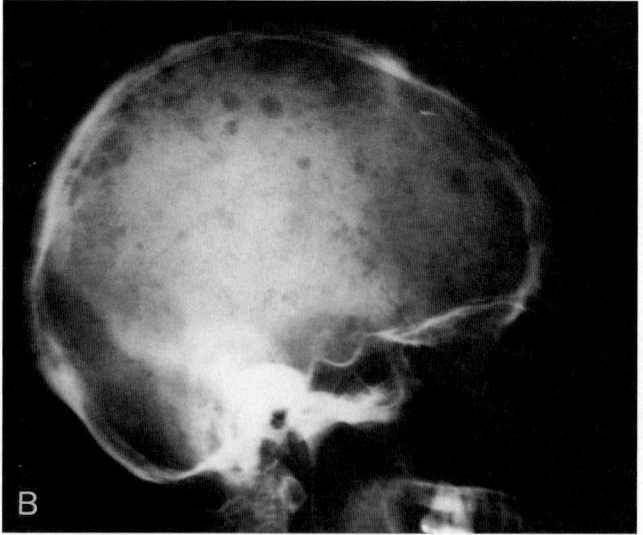

Figure 41.26. Multiple Myeloma. A. A diffuse permeative pattern is present throughout the femur in this patient with multiple myeloma. **B.** A lateral skull film shows a typical presentation of multiple myeloma in the skull with multiple small holes throughout the calvarium, which are well defined.

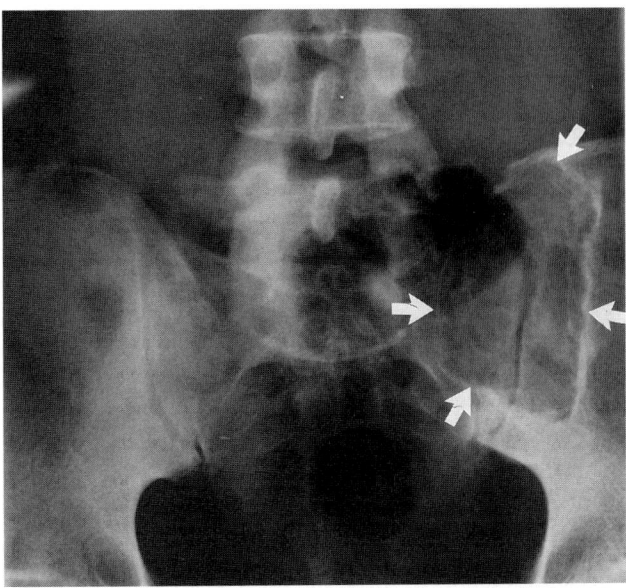

Figure 41.27. Plasmacytoma. A large, well-defined lytic lesion is seen in the left ilium (*arrows*) in this patient with multiple myeloma. This is a common location for a plasmacytoma. Like metastases, plasmacytomas often have a completely benign appearance.

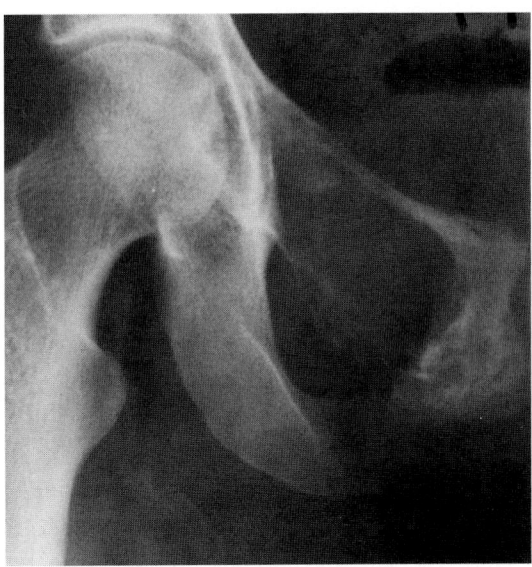

Figure 41.29. Aneurysmal Bone Cyst. An expansile lytic lesion is present in the superior pubic ramus in this 20-year-old patient who presents with pain. This is a fairly typical appearance for an ABC.

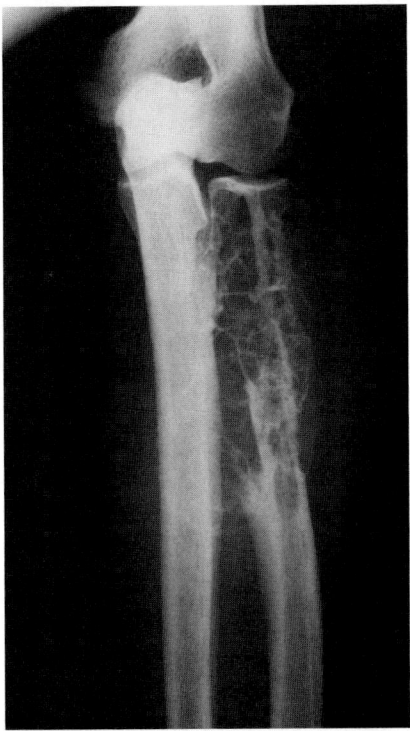

Figure 41.28. Metastatic Disease. An expansile lesion with a soap-bubble appearance is present in the proximal radius in a patient with renal cell carcinoma. An expansile lytic lesion is a common finding with renal or thyroid metastatic disease.

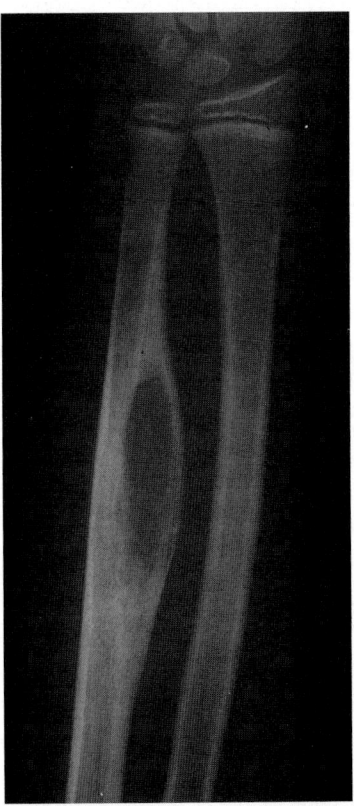

Figure 41.30. Aneurysmal Bone Cyst. A well-defined expansile lesion is seen in the midshaft of the ulna in a child who presents with pain in this region. This is a characteristic appearance for an ABC.

ANEURYSMAL BONE CYST

Aneurysmal bone cysts are the only lesions I know of that are named for their radiographic appearance. They are virtually always aneurysmal or expansile (Figs. 41.29, 41.30). Rarely, an ABC will present before it is ex-

pansile, but that is unusual enough not to worry about. Aneurysmal bone cysts primarily occur in patients who are less than the age of 30, although occasionally one will be encountered in older patients. I use bony expansion and age of less than 30 years as fairly rigid guidelines and seldom miss the diagnosis of ABC.

Aneurysmal bone cysts are, like giant cell tumors, somewhat controversial. There are apparently two types of ABCs: a primary type and a secondary type. The secondary type occurs in conjunction with another lesion or from trauma, whereas a primary ABC has no known cause or association with other lesions. Secondary ABCs have been said to occur with giant cell tumors, osteosarcomas, and almost any other lesion. I have seen dozens of ABCs and have seen only one in association with another lesion, so I doubt that this occurs very often. As to occurring after trauma, I do not understand why they would be age-limited if trauma were causative. Also, malignant tumors were once thought to occur after trauma because of the frequent association of a history of antecedent trauma with malignant bone tumors. This is not seriously considered today and is thought to be coincidental. I suspect that ABCs and trauma are also coincidental, but this is mere speculation.

Aneurysmal bone cysts typically present because of pain. They can occur anywhere in the skeleton, and there is no location that would make them more highly ranked in the differential diagnosis. As with osteoblastoma, they often occur in the posterior elements of the spine.

Discriminators. 1. Must be expansile. 2. Must be younger than age 30 years.

SOLITARY BONE CYST

Solitary bone cysts are also called simple bone cysts or unicameral bone cysts. They are not necessarily unicameral (one compartment), however. This is the only lesion in FEGNOMASHIC that is always central in location (Fig. 41.31). Many of the other lesions may be central, but a solitary bone cyst can be excluded if it is not. It is one of the few lesions that does not occur most commonly around the knees. Two thirds to three fourths of these lesions occur in the proximal humerus (Fig. 41.32) and proximal femur (Fig. 41.33). Applying this rule by itself is not that helpful, or one third to one fourth of the lesions would be missed.

Solitary bone cysts are usually asymptomatic unless fractured, which is a common occurrence. Even when pathologic fractures occur, they rarely form periostitis. A classic radiographic finding for a solitary bone cyst is the fallen fragment sign (see Fig. 41.32). This occurs when a piece of cortex breaks off after a fracture in a solitary bone cyst, and the piece of cortical bone sinks to the gravity-dependent portion of the lesion. This has not been described in any other lesion and indicates a fluid-filled cystic lesion, rather than a lesion filled with matrix.

Solitary bone cysts occur almost exclusively in young patients (less than 30 years of age). Although long bones are most commonly involved, solitary bone cysts have been described in almost every bone in the body. They begin at the physeal plate in long bones and grow into the shaft of the bone; therefore, they are not epiphyseal lesions. They can, however, extend up into an epiphysis after the plate closes, but this is unusual. A fairly common location is in the calcaneus, where they have a characteristic location adjacent to the inferior surface of the calcaneus (Fig. 41.34).

Discriminators. 1. Must be central. 2. Must be younger than age 30 years. 3. No periostitis.

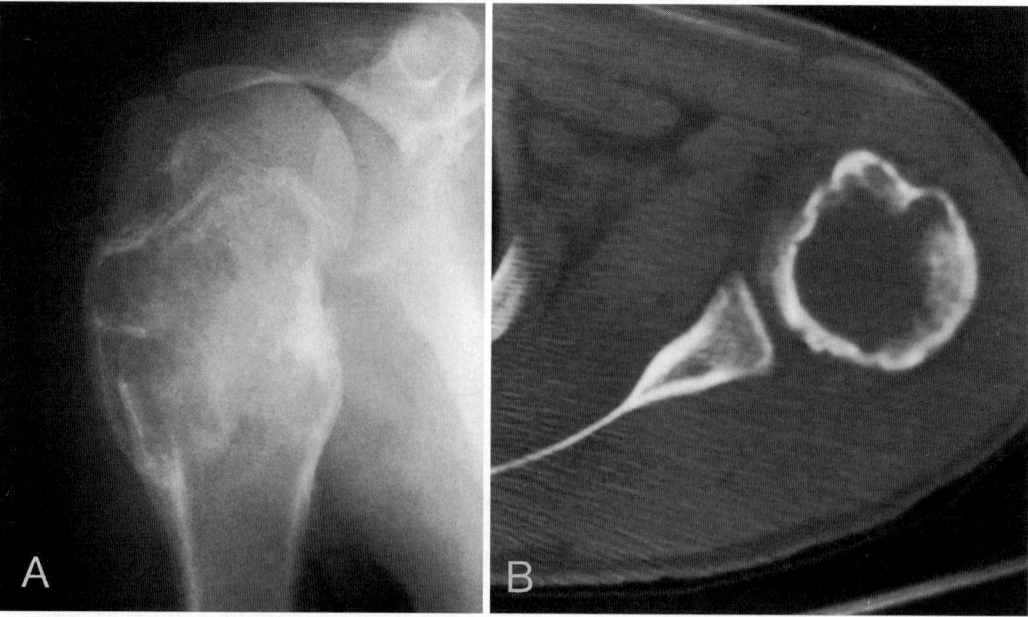

Figure 41.31. Solitary Bone Cyst. A plain film **(A)** and a CT scan **(B)** of the proximal humerus show a central, well-defined lytic lesion in this young person, which is typical in location and appearance for a solitary bone cyst. Note on the CT the central location of this lesion, which is characteristic.

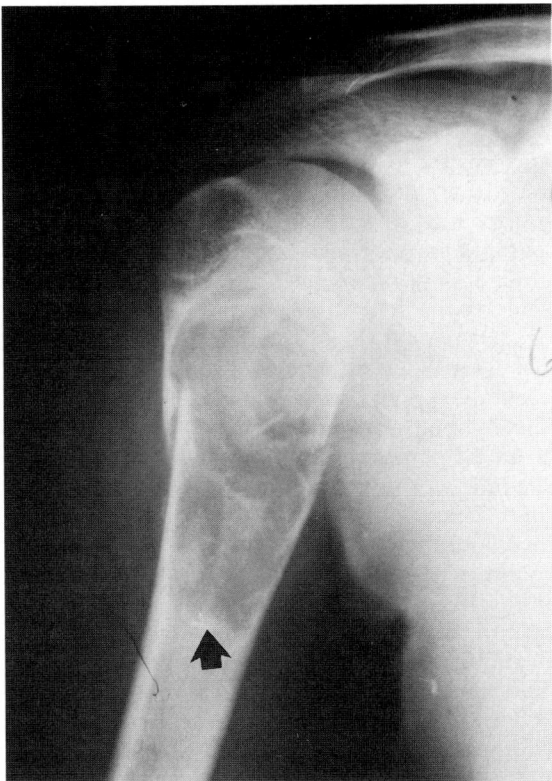

Figure 41.32. Solitary Bone Cyst. A well-defined lytic lesion is present in the proximal humerus in this child who suffered a fracture through the lesion. The location and central appearance, as well as the age of the patient, are characteristic for a solitary bone cyst. A piece of cortical bone has broken off and descended through the serous fluid contained within the lesion and can be seen in the dependent portion of the lesion (*arrow*) as a fallen fragment sign. A fallen fragment sign is said to be pathognomonic for a unicameral bone cyst.

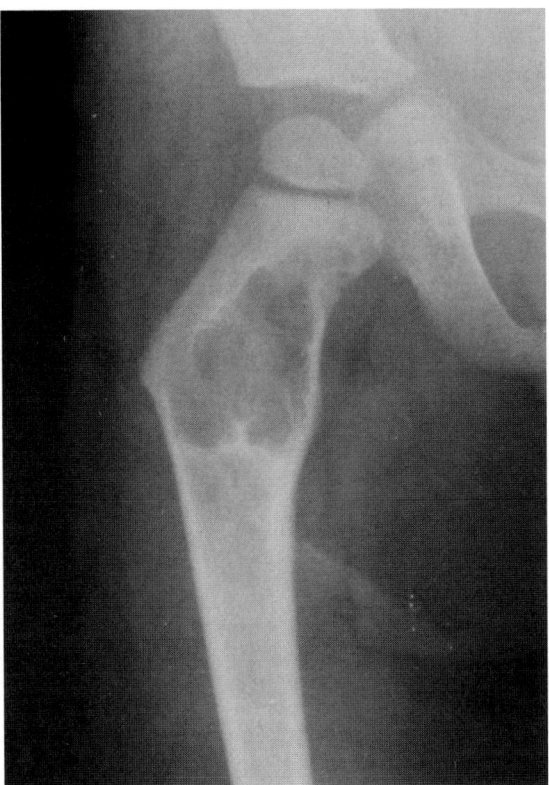

Figure 41.33. Solitary Bone Cyst. A well-defined lytic lesion, which is central in location, is seen in the proximal femur in this child. This is characteristic for a solitary bone cyst.

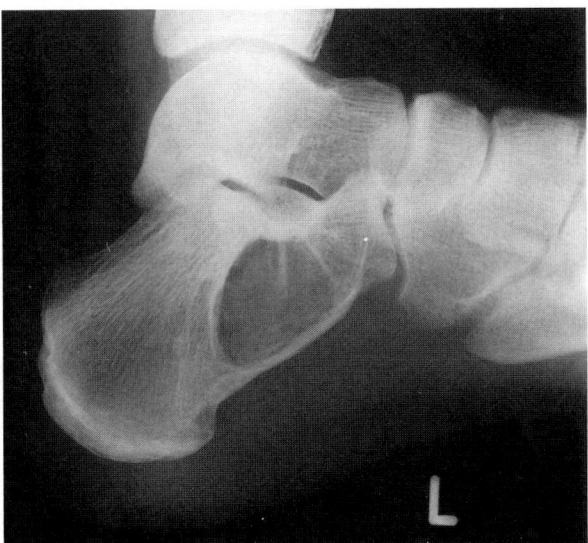

Figure 41.34. Solitary Bone Cyst. A well-defined lytic lesion is seen in the calcaneus abutting the inferior surface, which is typical in location and appearance for a solitary bone cyst. A solitary bone cyst in the calcaneus occurs almost exclusively in this location and is not subject to pathologic fracture as readily as when one occurs in the proximal femur and humerus.

HYPERPARATHYROIDISM (BROWN TUMORS)

Brown tumors of hyperparathyroidism (HPT) can have almost any appearance, from a purely lytic lesion (Fig. 41.35) to a sclerotic process. Generally, when the patient's HPT is treated, the brown tumor undergoes sclerosis and will eventually disappear. If a brown tumor is going to be considered in the differential diagnosis, additional radiographic findings of HPT should be seen. Subperiosteal bone resorption is pathognomonic for HPT and should be searched for in the phalanges (particularly in the radial aspect of the middle phalanges) (Fig. 41.35), distal clavicles (resorption), medial aspect of the proximal tibias, and sacroiliac joints. If the physes are open they should have a frayed, ragged appearance, as in rickets, owing to the effect of parathormone. Osteoporosis or osteosclerosis might suggest that renal osteodystrophy with secondary HPT is present, but subperiosteal resorption must be present, or brown tumor can be safely excluded from the differential.

Most authorities believe that brown tumors occur most commonly in primary HPT; however, because we see so many more patients with secondary HPT, more

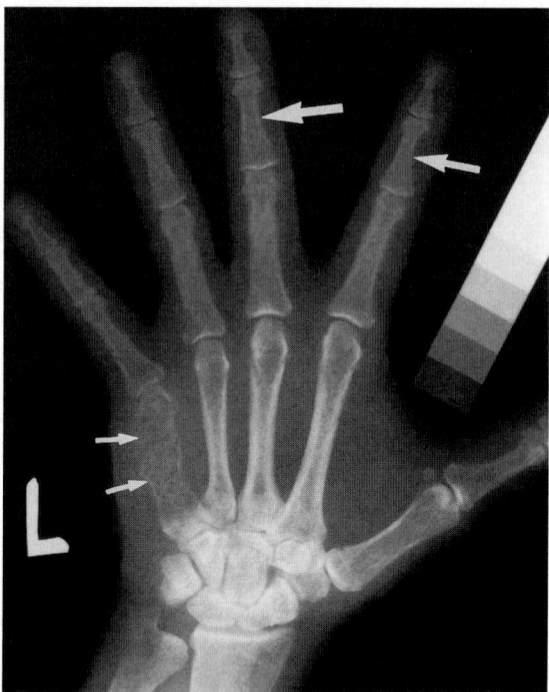

Figure 41.35. Brown Tumor. An expansile lytic lesion is seen in the fifth metacarpal (*small arrows*), and a second, smaller lytic lesion is seen in the proximal portion of the fourth proximal phalanx. This patient can be noted to have subperiosteal bone resorption, best seen in the radial aspect of the middle phalanges (*large arrows*), which makes the diagnosis of hyperparathyroidism with multiple brown tumors most likely.

brown tumors are seen in patients with secondary rather than primary HPT.

Discriminator. Must have other evidence of HPT.

INFECTION

Unfortunately, there is no reliable way radiographically to exclude a focus of osteomyelitis. It has a protean radiographic appearance and can occur at any location and in a patient of any age. It might or might not be expansile, have a sclerotic or nonsclerotic border, or have associated periostitis (3). Therefore, infection will be in almost every differential diagnosis of a lytic lesion, which is acceptable, as it is one of the most common lesions encountered. Soft-tissue findings such as obliteration of adjacent fat planes are notoriously unreliable and even misleading, as tumors and EG can do the same thing.

When osteomyelitis occurs near a joint, if the articular surface is abutted, invariably the joint will be involved and show either cartilage loss or an effusion (Fig. 41.36), or both. This finding is not particularly helpful, as any lesion can cause an effusion, but it is occasionally useful in ruling out osteomyelitis when no effusion is present and the lesion abuts the articular surface.

If a bony sequestrum is present, osteomyelitis should be strongly considered (Fig. 41.37). As mentioned previously, the only lesions described that demonstrate sequestra are infection, EG, lymphoma, and fibrosarcoma, with osteoid osteoma sometimes mimicking a sequestrum. The finding of a sequestrum in osteomyelitis can be significant for treatment in that it usually requires surgical removal rather than antibiotics alone because a sequestrum is a focus of devitalized bone that does not have a blood supply and will not be effectively treated with parenteral medication.

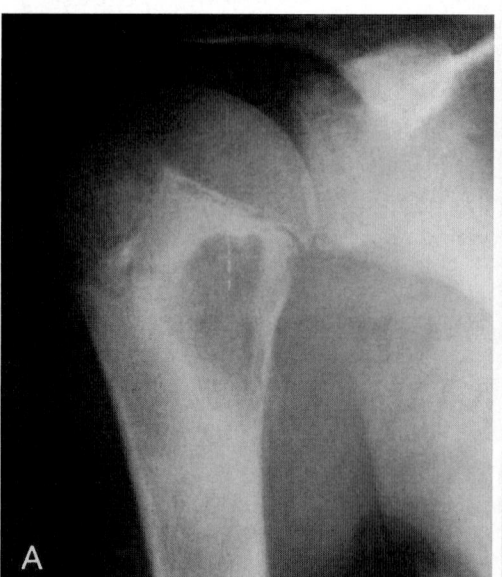
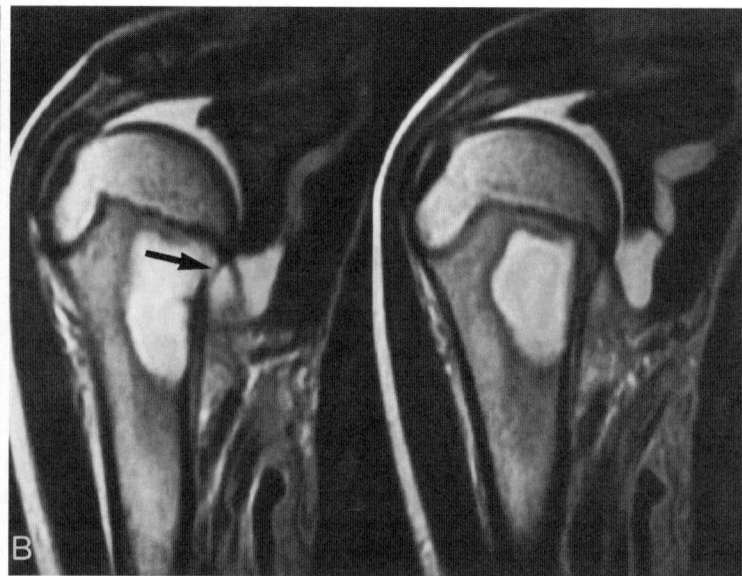

Figure 41.36. Brodie's Abscess. A. A plain film of the proximal humerus in this child with shoulder pain reveals a well-defined lytic lesion in the medial metaphysis. **B.** A T2-weighted MR of the humerus shows the lesion to have high signal and an associated joint effusion. The probable site of connection to the joint can be seen (*arrow*), which likely represents a draining abscess. Aspiration of the joint fluid revealed pus. This is a large focus of osteomyelitis or Brodie's abscess. (Case courtesy of Rick Harnsberger, MD, Salt Lake City, Utah.)

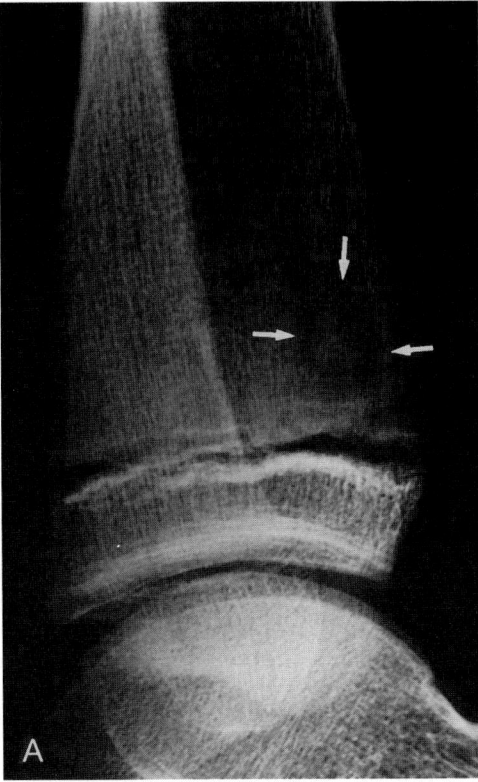
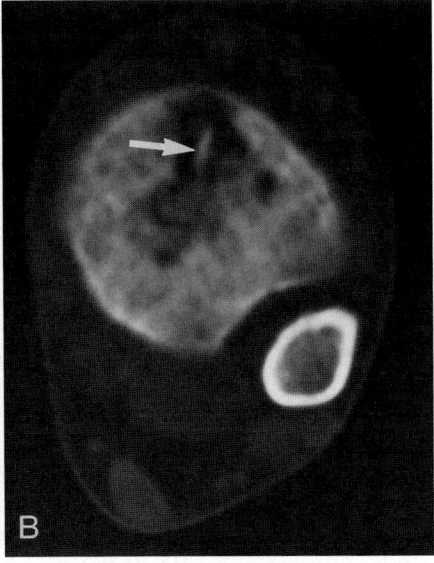

Figure 41.37. Osteomyelitis. A. A lytic lesion is present in the distal tibia, which is only faintly seen on the plain film (*arrows*). **B.** A CT scan through this area reveals a lytic lesion that contains a calcific density within (*arrow*), which is a bony sequestrum. In retrospect, the sequestrum can be faintly seen on the original plain film. This is an area of osteomyelitis with a bony sequestration.

For this reason, CT is routinely recommended when osteomyelitis is considered.

Discriminator. None.

CHONDROBLASTOMA

Chondroblastomas are rare lesions but are among the easiest lesions for radiologists to deal with because they occur only in the epiphyses (Fig. 41.38) (a handful of cases have been reported in the metaphyses but this is rare) and they occur almost exclusively in patients younger than the age of 30 years. From 40% to 60% demonstrate calcification, so absence of calcification is not helpful. Presence of calcification is helpful as long as it is certain that it is not detritus or sequestra from infection or EG, both of which can occur in the epiphyses.

The differential diagnosis of a lytic lesion in the epiphysis of a patient less than 30 years of age is simple: *1)* infection (most common), *2)* chondroblastoma, and *3)* giant cell tumor (it has its own diagnostic criteria, so it can usually be definitely ruled out or in). This is an old, classic differential and probably encompasses 98% of epiphyseal lesions.

A caveat on epiphyseal lesions is to consider always the possibility of a subchondral cyst or geode (Fig. 41.39), which has been described in four disease processes: *1)* degenerative joint disease (must have joint space narrowing, sclerosis, and osteophytes), *2)* rheumatoid arthritis, *3)* calcium pyrophosphate dihy-

drate crystal disposition disease or pseudogout, and *4)* avascular necrosis. Be certain no joint pathology that might indicate one of these processes is present, or an unnecessary biopsy of a geode might be performed on the basis of the differential of an epiphyseal lesion.

Apophyses are identical to epiphyses as far as the differential diagnosis of lytic lesions, with the exception of geodes, which only occur adjacent to articular surfaces. The carpal bones, the tarsal bones, and the patella have a tendency to behave like epiphyses in their differential diagnosis of lesions. Therefore, a lytic lesion in these areas has a similar differential diagnosis as an epiphyseal lesion.

Discriminator. 1. Must be less than 30 years of age. 2. Must be epiphyseal.

CHONDROMYXOID FIBROMA

Like the osteoblastoma, the chondromyxoid fibroma is such a rare lesion that failure to mention it is probably not going to result in missing more than one in a lifetime. Why include it then? I recommend not including it, but it is part of the classic FEGNOMASHIC differential. If it is mentioned, at least know what it looks like. Basically, chondromyxoid fibromas resemble NOFs. Unlike NOFs, however, they can be seen in a patient of any age. Chondromyxoid fibromas often extend into the epiphyses (Fig. 41.40), whereas NOFs rarely do. They can present with pain, also, which will not occur with an NOF. They have been reported to progress from a benign pro-

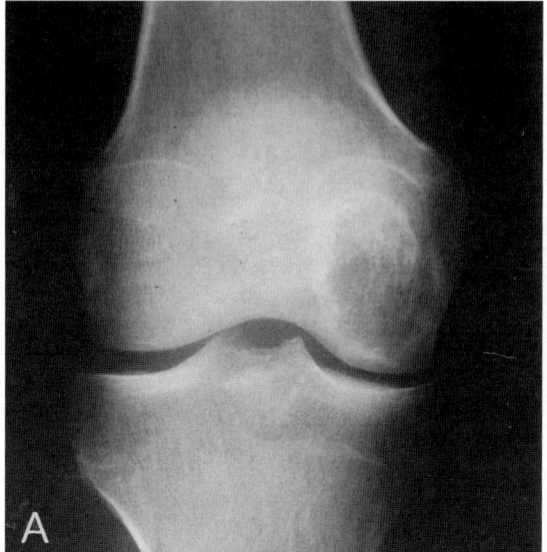

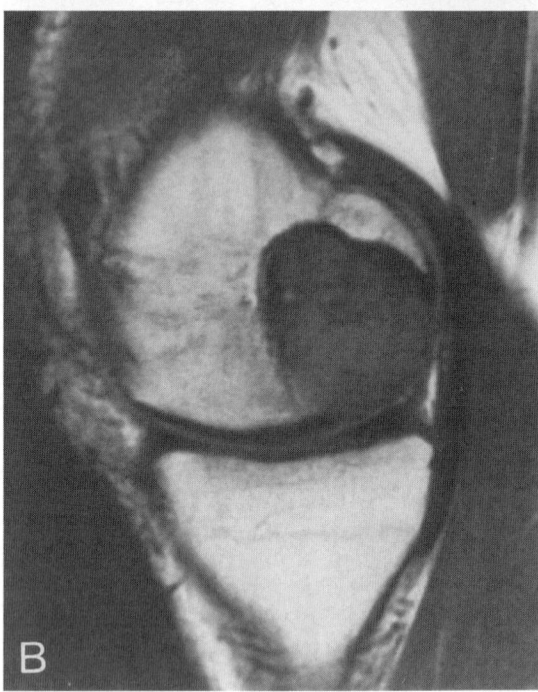

Figure 41.38. Chondroblastoma. A. A plain film in this young patient shows a well-defined lytic lesion in the medial femoral condyle. **B.** A sagittal T1-weighted MR through the medial knee joint reveals a fairly homogeneous lesion that abuts the articular surface. Biopsy showed this to be a chondroblastoma.

cess to an aggressive and even malignant lesion, but this is extremely rare. Even though chondromyxoid fibromas are cartilaginous lesions, calcified cartilage matrix is virtually never seen radiographically.

Discriminator. 1. Mention when an NOF is mentioned. 2. No calcified matrix.

SUMMARY

That, in essence, is the differential diagnosis for a benign cystic lesion of bone. It is probably 98% accurate,

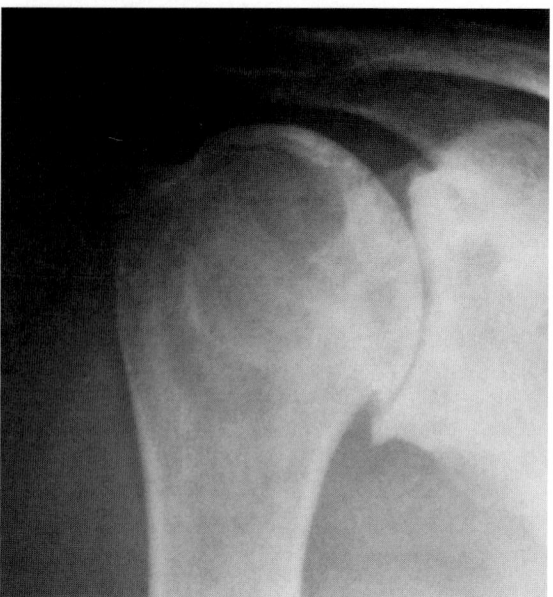

Figure 41.39. Geode. A large, well-defined lytic lesion in the proximal humerus is present, which is associated with marked degenerative disease of the glenohumeral joint. When definite degenerative joint disease is present and associated with a lytic lesion, the lytic lesion should be considered to be a geode. A biopsy was performed, which confirmed this to be a geode, or subchondral cyst; however, the biopsy could have been avoided.

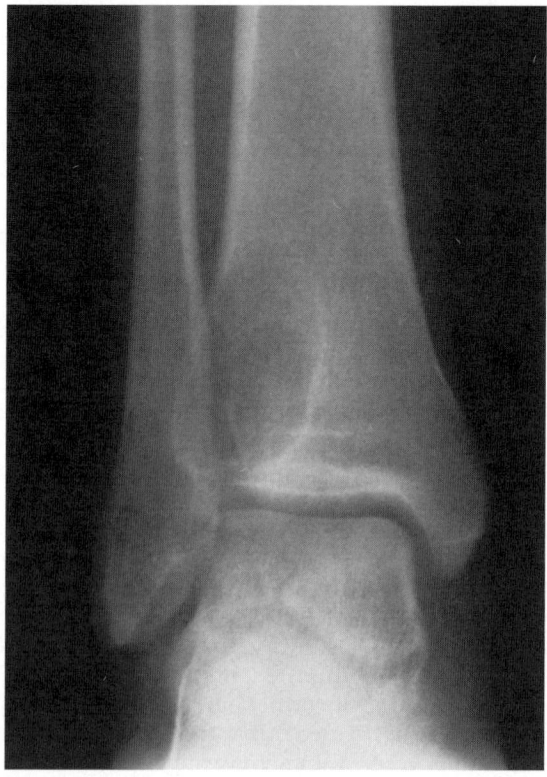

Figure 41.40. Chondromyxoid Fibroma. A well-defined lytic lesion in the distal tibia that extends slightly into the epiphysis is noted on this anteroposterior plain film. A nonossifying fibroma could certainly have this appearance; however, this underwent biopsy and was found to be a chondromyxoid fibroma. Chondromyxoid fibromas often will extend into the epiphysis, as in this example, whereas NOFs usually will not.

which is good enough for most radiologists. To increase the accuracy to 99%, it would be necessary to add many uncommon or rare lesions, and the whole process would become too confusing for most radiologists to learn and apply. If there is a favorite lesion that is not on this list, by all means add it. Likewise, if the list is already too cumbersome, forget about osteoblastoma and chondromyxoid fibroma. I am unable to make it much simpler than that and still be reasonably accurate.

Some of the lesions I have purposefully omitted are intraosseous ganglion, pseudotumor of hemophilia, hemangioendothelioma, ossifying fibroma, intraosseous lipoma, glomus tumor, neurofibroma, plasma cell granuloma, and schwannoma. Others could be added to this list, of course, but are best left to the pathologist–not the radiologist–for the diagnosis.

There are several features that are somewhat useful in separating the various lesions in FEGNOMASHIC. For instance, if the patient is younger than the age of 30 years, be sure to consider *EG, chondroblastoma, NOF, solitary bone cyst*, and *ABC* (Table 41.2). If the patient is more than 30 years of age, those five lesions can be excluded. Note that this is not a differential diagnosis for lesions in patients less than the age of 30; it simply means these entities should not be mentioned in older patients. For those younger than the age of 30, other lesions such as fibrous dysplasia and infection must also be mentioned.

There are a few lytic lesions that have no good discriminators other than age and, therefore, must be mentioned routinely. I call these lesions "automatics" because one should automatically mention them regardless of the location or appearance of the lesion. *Infection* and *EG* must be mentioned for those younger than the age of 30 years, whereas *metastatic disease* and *infection* must be included in any differential in a patient older than the age of 40 years (Table 41.3). These lesions have a protean radiographic appearance and should be mentioned not only in the benign, cystic differential, but also for an aggressive lesion.

If periostitis or pain is present (assuming no trauma, which can be a foolhardy assumption), you can exclude *fibrous dysplasia, solitary bone cyst, NOF*, and *enchon-*

droma (Table 41.4). If the lesion is epiphyseal, the differential is *infection, giant cell tumor, chondroblastoma* (and do not forget *geodes*) (Table 41.5). If the patient is more than 40 years of age, add metastatic disease and myeloma and remove chondroblastoma from the epiphyseal list.

The epiphyseal differential tends to apply also to the tarsal bones (especially the calcaneus), the carpal bones, and the patella. In the calcaneus, a unicameral bone cyst should also be considered and has a characteristic appearance and location (see Fig. 41.34). Apophyses are "epiphyseal equivalents" and have the same differential as epiphyses. The difference between an epiphysis and an apophysis is that epiphyses contribute to the length of a bone, whereas apophyses serve as ligamentous attachments.

A classic differential for benign, cystic rib lesions is the mnemonic FAME, in which F = *fibrous dysplasia*, A = *ABC*, M = *metastatic diseases* and *myeloma*, and E = *enchondroma* and *EG* (Table 41.6).

If there are multiple lytic lesions present, FEEMHI is a useful mnemonic of the lesions in FEGNOMASHIC, which can be multiple. F = *fibrous dysplasia*, E = *enchondroma*, E = *EG*, M = *metastatic disease* and *myeloma*, H = *hyperparathyroidism* (brown tumor), and I = *infection* (Table 41.7).

A few findings that just do not seem to narrow the differential diagnosis are presence or absence of a soft-tis-

Table 41.2. Lesions in Patients Younger Than 30 Years of Age

EG
ABC
NCF
Chondroblastoma
Solitary bone cyst

Table 41.3. "Automatics"

Younger than age 30
  Infection
  EG
Older than age 40
  Infection
  Metastatic disease and myeloma

Table 41.4. Lesions That Have No Pain or Periostitis

Fibrous dysplasia
Enchondroma
NOF
Solitary bone cyst

Table 41.5. Epiphyseal Lesions

Infection
Giant cell tumor
Chondroblastoma
Geode

Table 41.6. Differential for Rib Lesions

Fibrous dysplasia
ABC
Metastatic disease and myeloma
Enchondroma and EG

Table 41.7. Multiple Lesions (FEEMHI)

Fibrous dysplasia
EG
Enchondroma
Metastatic disease and myeloma
Hyperparathyroidism (brown tumors)
Infection

sue mass, expansion of the bone (except it must be present in an ABC), a sclerotic or nonsclerotic border (except it must be nonsclerotic in giant cell tumor), presence or absence of bony struts or compartments in the lesion, and size of the lesion.

If calcified matrix is identified in a lesion, it is tempting to narrow the differential to either the osteoid series or the chondroid series of lesions, depending on the character of the matrix. Be careful of this. Very few radiologists can reliably differentiate chondroid from osteoid matrix. Routine calcification of a lesion or debris, detritus, or sequestrations in osteomyelitis can mimic chondroid or osteoid calcification and be misleading. The only lesion that must exhibit calcified matrix is the enchondroma (except in the phalanges). Chondroblastomas and osteoblastomas demonstrate calcified matrix about half the time, and chondromyxoid fibromas never have radiographically demonstrable calcified matrix.

DIFFERENTIAL DIAGNOSIS OF A SCLEROTIC LESION

Many lytic lesions spontaneously regress and are not usually seen in patients more than 30 years of age. When these lesions regress, they often fill in with new bone and have a sclerotic or blastic appearance. Therefore, when a sclerotic focus is identified in a 20- to 40-year-old patient, especially if it is an asymptomatic, incidental finding, the following lesions should be considered: NOF (Fig. 41.41), EG, aneurysmal bone cyst, solitary bone cyst, and chondroblastoma. Several other lesions should be included that can also appear sclerotic: fibrous dysplasia, osteoid osteoma, infection, brown tumor (healing), and perhaps a giant bone island (Fig. 41.42). In any patient older than the age of 40 years, the number one possibility should be metastatic disease.

References

1. David R, Oria R, Kumar R, et al. Radiologic features of eosinophilic granuloma of bone. Pictorial essay. AJR Am J Roentgenol 1989;153:1021–1026.
2. Dahlin D. Giant cell tumor of bone: highlights of 407 cases. AJR Am J Roentgenol 1985;144:955–960.
3. Gold R, Hawkins R, Katz R. Pictorial essay. Bacterial osteomyelitis: findings on plain radiography, CT, MR, and scintigraphy. AJR Am J Roentgenol 1991;157:365–370.

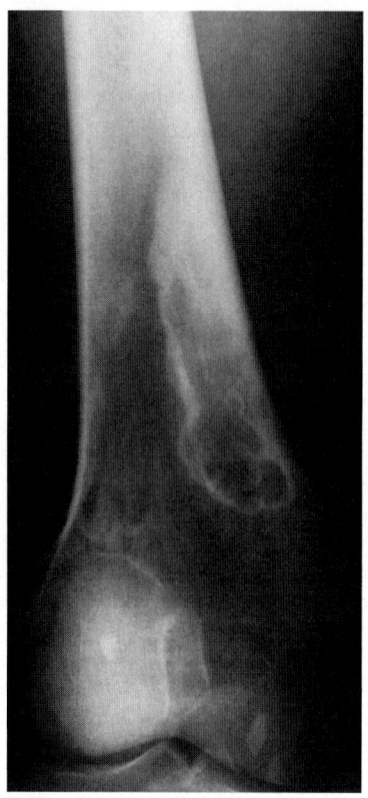

Figure 41.41. Healing Nonossifying Fibroma. A plain film of the femur in this 15-year-old patient reveals several mixed lytic, sclerotic lesions in the diametaphyseal region, which are well defined. The large lesion has diffuse sclerosis in its proximal two-thirds. These represent NOFs that are starting to sclerose and disappear.

Figure 41.42. Giant Bone Island. A large sclerotic lesion is present in the right supra-acetabular region of the ilium, which represents a giant bone island. The slightly feathered margins of the trabeculae blending in with the normal bone, and the long axis of the lesion being in the direction of primary weight bearing, are characteristic for a bone island.

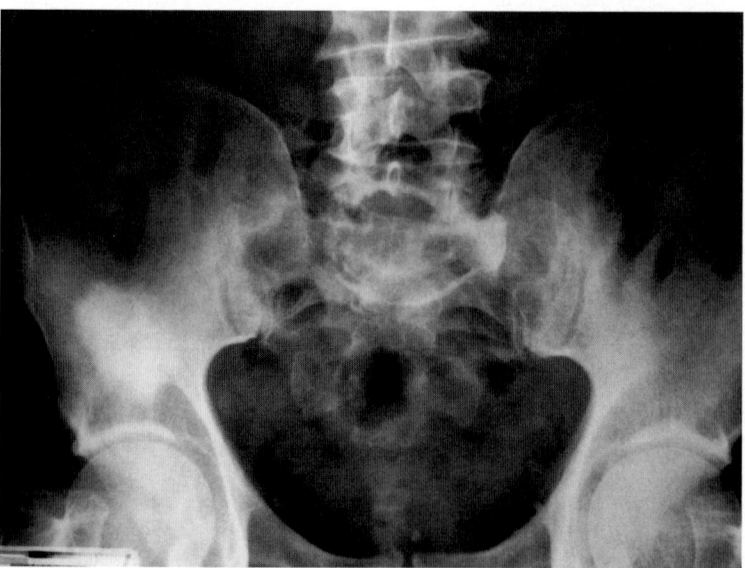

42

Malignant Bone and Soft-Tissue Tumors

Clyde A. Helms

RADIOGRAPHIC FINDINGS

Malignant bone tumors, thankfully, are not very common. Nevertheless, every radiologist should be able to recognize them and give a useful differential diagnosis. First, how does one recognize a malignant tumor and differentiate if from a benign process? This can be difficult and often impossible. Recognizing that it is *aggressive* is usually easy, but stating that it is *malignant* is another matter altogether. Processes such as infection and eosinophilic granuloma can mimic malignant tumors and are, of course, benign. They will often be included in the differential diagnosis of an aggressive lesion along with malignant tumors. What radiologic plain film criteria are useful for determining malignant versus benign? Standard textbooks give four aspects of a lesion to be examined: 1) cortical destruction, 2) periostitis, 3) orientation or axis of the lesion, and 4) zone of transition. Let me discuss each of these criteria and show why only the last one–the zone of transition–is accurate to a 90% plus rate. It is important to recognize that these are plain film criteria and do not apply to CT or MR imaging in many instances.

Cortical Destruction

Benign fibro-osseous lesions and cartilaginous lesions often have part of their noncalcified matrix (fibrous matrix or chondroid matrix, both of which are radiolucent on plain films) replacing cortical bone, which can give the false impression of cortical destruction on plain films (Fig. 42.1) or CT. Also, benign processes such as infection and eosinophilic granuloma can cause extensive cortical destruction and mimic a malignant tumor. It is well known that aneurysmal bone cysts cause such thinning of the cortex as to make the cortex radiographically undetectable (Fig. 42.2). For these reasons, cortical destruction can occasionally be misleading. Cortical destruction always makes one think of a malignant lesion when using the "gestalt approach," but the lesion must also have other criteria for a malignant process, such as a wide zone of transition.

Periostitis

Periosteal reaction occurs in a nonspecific manner whenever the periosteum is irritated, whether it is irritated by a malignant tumor, a benign tumor, infection, or trauma. Callus formation in a fracture is actually just periosteal reaction of the most benign type. Periosteal reaction occurs in two types: benign or aggressive, based more on the timing of the irritation than on whether it is a malignant or benign process causing the periostitis. For example, a slow-growing benign tumor will cause thick, wavy, uniform or dense periostitis (Fig. 42.3A) because it is a low-grade chronic irritation that gives the periosteum time to lay down thick new bone and remodel into more normal cortex. A malignant tumor causes a periosteal reaction that is high-grade and more acute; hence, the periosteum does not have time to consolidate. It appears lamellated (onion-skinned) (Fig. 42.3B) or amorphous or even sunburstlike. If the irritation stops or diminishes, the aggressive periostitis will solidify and appear benign. Therefore, when periostitis is seen, the radiologist should try to characterize it into either a benign (thick, dense, wavy) type or an aggressive (lamellated, amorphous, sunburst) type. Unfortunately, judging the lesion by its periostitis can be very misleading. First, it takes considerable experience to characterize periostitis accurately because many times the reaction is not clearly benign or aggressive. Second, many benign lesions cause aggressive periostitis, such as infection, eosinophilic granuloma, aneurysmal bone cysts, osteoid osteomas, and even trauma. Seeing *benign* periostitis, however, can be very helpful because malignant lesions will not cause benign periostitis. Some investigators with great experience in dealing with malignant bone tumors state that the only way benign periostitis can occur in a malignant lesion is if there is a concomitant fracture or infection. Exceptions to this are extremely uncommon.

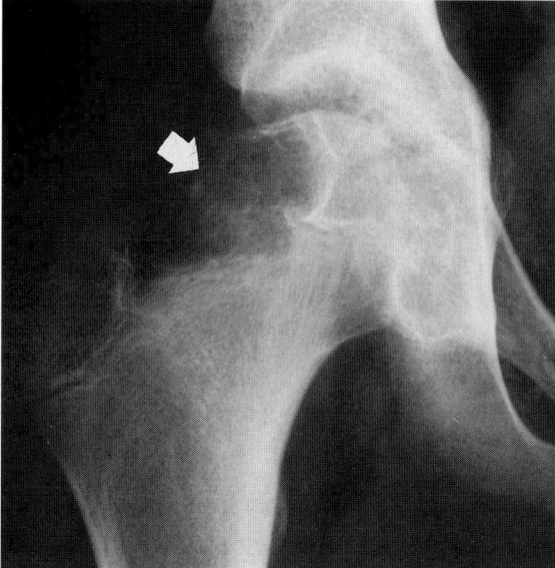

Figure 42.1. Apparent Cortical Destruction. This benign chondroblastoma has noncalcified chondroid tissue replacing cortical bone in the proximal femur (*arrow*), which gives this lesion a destructive appearance. This is an example of cortical replacement, rather than cortical destruction, which can be very confusing if one uses cortical destruction as an aggressive or malignant key. Note in this example that the zone of transition is narrow, as one would expect in a benign lesion such as this.

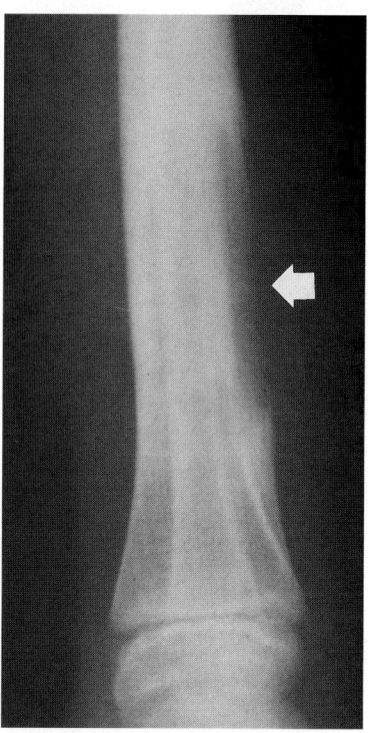

Figure 42.2. Aneurysmal Bone Cyst. This benign lesion has thinned the cortex to such a degree as to make it imperceptible (*arrow*). As in Figure 42.1, this could be misconstrued as cortical destruction, giving the false impression of a malignant or very aggressive lesion.

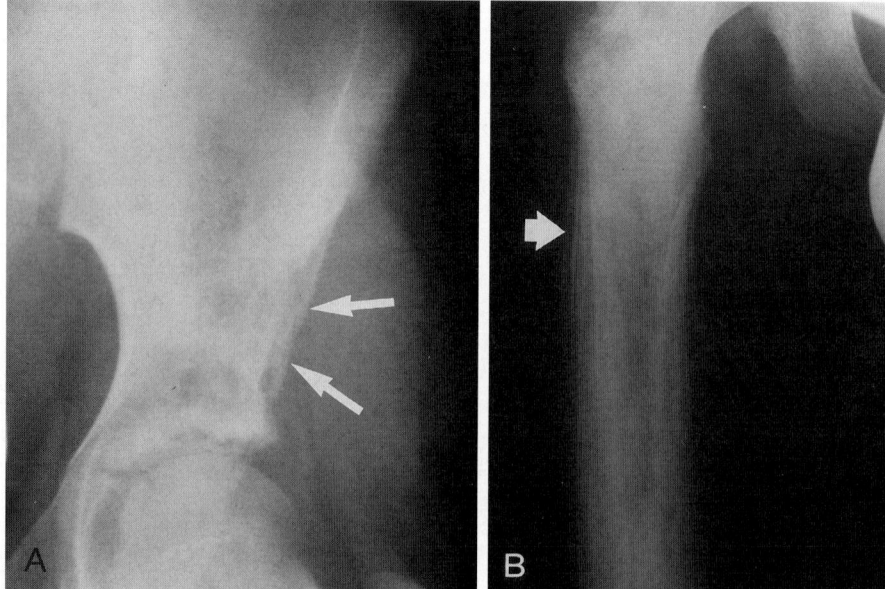

Figure 42.3. Periostitis. A. Benign periostitis. Thick, wavy periostitis (*arrows*) along the ilium in a child with a permeative lesion in the pelvis is characteristic for infection or eosinophilic granuloma. Ewing's sarcoma was initially considered in the differential; however, the benign periostitis would make a malignant lesion very unlikely. Biopsy showed this lesion to be eosinophilic granuloma.

B. Aggressive periostitis. Lamellated or onion-skin periostitis (*arrow*) is characteristic of an aggressive process such as in this patient with Ewing's sarcoma of the femur. Again, this aggressive type of periostitis could conceivably occur in a benign process such as infection or eosinophilic granuloma.

Orientation or Axis of the Lesion

This is a very poor determinant of benign versus aggressive lesions and rarely helps determine into which category the lesion should be placed. It has been said that if a lesion grows in the long axis of a long bone, rather than being circular, it is benign. There are simply too many exceptions for this to be helpful. For example, Ewing's sarcoma, an extremely malignant lesion, usually has its axis along the shaft of a long bone. Conversely, many fibrous cortical defects are circular, yet totally benign. Thus, the axis of the lesion is not helpful in assessing benignity versus malignancy.

Zone of Transition

This is without question the most reliable plain film indicator for benign versus malignant lesions. Unfortunately, it also has some drawbacks. The zone of transition is the border of the lesion with the normal bone. It is said to be "narrow" if it is so well defined that it can be drawn with a fine-point pen (Fig. 42.4). If it is imperceptible and cannot be clearly drawn at all, it is said to be "wide" (Fig. 42.5). Obviously, all shades of gray lie in between, but most lesions can be characterized as having either a narrow or wide zone of transition. If the lesion has a sclerotic border, it, of course, has a narrow zone of transition. If a lesion has a narrow zone of tran-

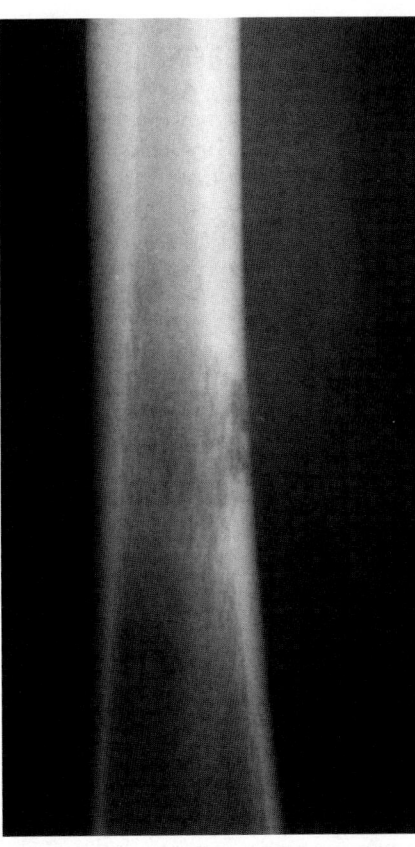

Figure 42.5. Wide Zone of Transition. A lytic, permeative process is seen in the midshaft of the femur in this patient that on biopsy was found to be a malignant fibrous histiocytoma. The zone of transition in this lesion is said to be wide, as it cannot be easily drawn with a fine-point pen. A permeative lesion such as this, by definition, has a wide zone of transition.

sition, a benign process should be considered as the most likely possibility.

The exceptions to this are rare. If a lesion has a wide zone of transition, it is aggressive, although not necessarily malignant. As with aggressive periostitis, many benign lesions as well as malignant lesions can cause a wide zone of transition. A few of the same processes that can cause aggressive periostitis and thereby mimic a malignant tumor can have a wide zone of transition (i.e., infection and eosinophilic granuloma). They are aggressive in their radiographic appearance because they are usually fast-acting, aggressive lesions. The zone of transition is usually easier to characterize than the periostitis, plus it is always present to evaluate; whereas, many lesions, benign or malignant, have no periostitis. For these reasons, the zone of transition is the most useful indicator of whether a lesion is benign or malignant.

A lesion consisting of multiple small holes is said to be "permeative" (see chapter 45 for discussion of the difference between a permeative and a pseudopermeative lesion). It has no perceptible border and therefore has a wide zone of transition. Round cell tumors such as multiple myeloma, reticulum cell sarcoma (primary lymphoma of bone), and Ewing's sarcoma are typical of this type of lesion. Infection and eosinophilic granuloma also can have this same appearance.

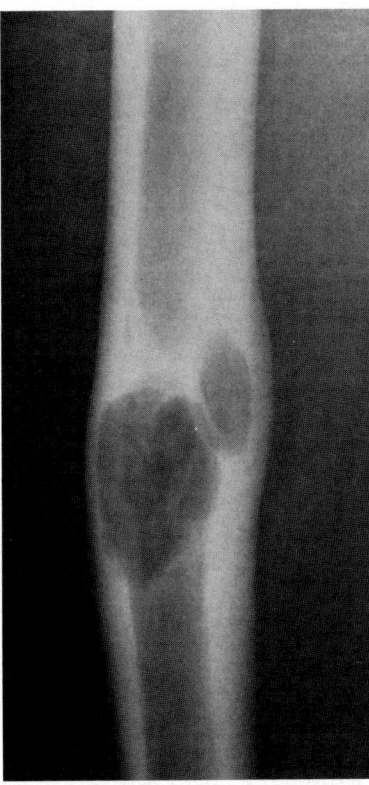

Figure 42.4. Narrow Zone of Transition. When the margins of a lesion can be drawn with a fine-point pen, as in this example, it is said to be a narrow zone of transition, which is characteristic of a benign lesion. A narrow zone of transition might or might not have a sclerotic border. This is a nonossifying fibroma.

Once it is decided that a particular lesion is most likely malignant, the differential is fairly straightforward. First, the list of malignant tumors is relatively short, and, second, most tumors follow somewhat strict age groupings. Jack Edeiken (1), one of the preeminent bone radiologists of our era, evaluated 4000 malignant bone tumors and found that they could be diagnosed correctly 80% of the time just by using the patient's age. He basically divides the tumors into decades of when they usually affect a patient. For example, osteosarcoma and Ewing's sarcoma are the only childhood primary malignant tumors of bone, and after the age of 40, only metastatic disease, myeloma, and chondrosarcoma are common (Table 42.1). Although there are certainly outliers that are uncommon, these age guidelines are extremely useful. It is inappropriate to mention Ewing's sarcoma in a 40-year-old patient or metastatic disease in a 15-year-old patient, unless there is a known primary tumor. In fact, *any* bone lesion, regardless of its appearance, could be a metastatic lesion and would be suspicious in a patient with a known primary tumor.

Table 42.1. Age of Patients with Malignant Tumors

1–30	Ewing's sarcoma, ostogenic sarcoma
30–40	Giant cell tumor, parosteal sarcoma, fibrosarcoma, malignant fibrous histiocytoma, reticulum cell sarcoma
Over 40	Chondrosarcoma, metastatic disease, myeloma

Magnetic Resonance Imaging

Although plain films are the best modality for characterizing a bony lesion, that is, being able to distinguish benign from malignant and generating a differential diagnosis, MR is without question the imaging procedure of choice for determining the extent of a lesion, both in the skeleton and in the soft tissues. For this reason, if resection of a tumor is contemplated, MR should be performed.

In assessing benignity versus malignancy, MR is somewhat controversial (2). Benign lesions tend to be well marginated, to have uniform and homogeneous signal, not to encase neurovascular structures, and not to invade bone. Malignant lesions tend to have irregular margins, inhomogeneous signal, and may encase neurovascular structures or invade bone.

Although almost all tumors will have low signal on T1-weighted images, which become very high in signal intensity with T2 weighting (as will fluid collections), there are a few exceptions. Fibrosarcomas, malignant fibrous histiocytomas, and desmoid tumors can occasionally demonstrate low signal on both T1-weighted and T2-weighted sequences. Any tumor with calcification will be low in signal on both T1 and T2 sequences.

In some instances, MR will characterize the lesion better than plain films and enable a specific diagnosis to be made. Lipomas are easily diagnosed with MR by their homogeneous high signal on T1-weighted images and

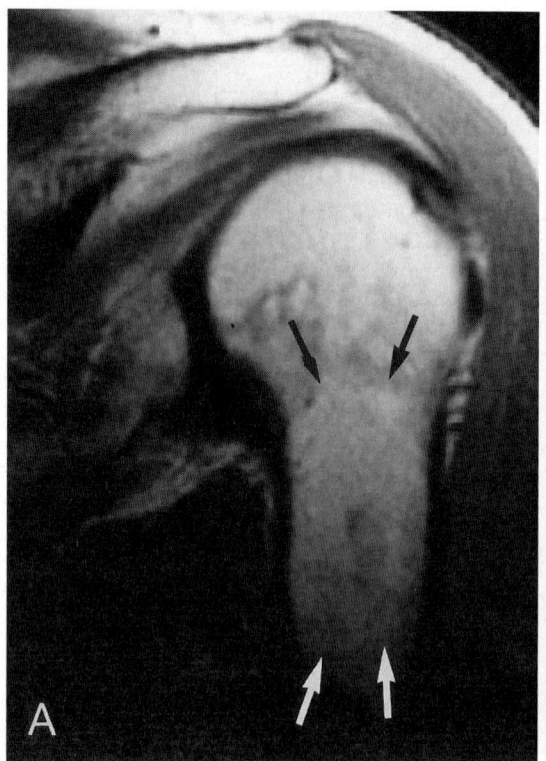
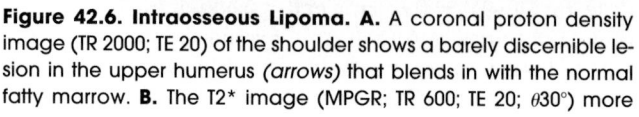
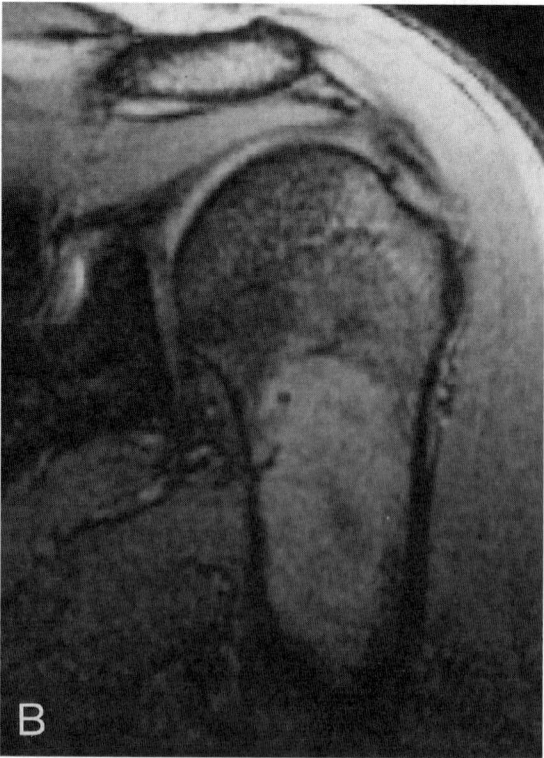

Figure 42.6. Intraosseous Lipoma. A. A coronal proton density image (TR 2000; TE 20) of the shoulder shows a barely discernible lesion in the upper humerus *(arrows)* that blends in with the normal fatty marrow. **B.** The T2* image (MPGR; TR 600; TE 20; $\theta 30°$) more readily reveals the lesion and again shows it having signal characteristics similar to that of the subcutaneous fat. This is virtually pathognomonic for a fatty lesion; in this case, an intraosseous lipoma.

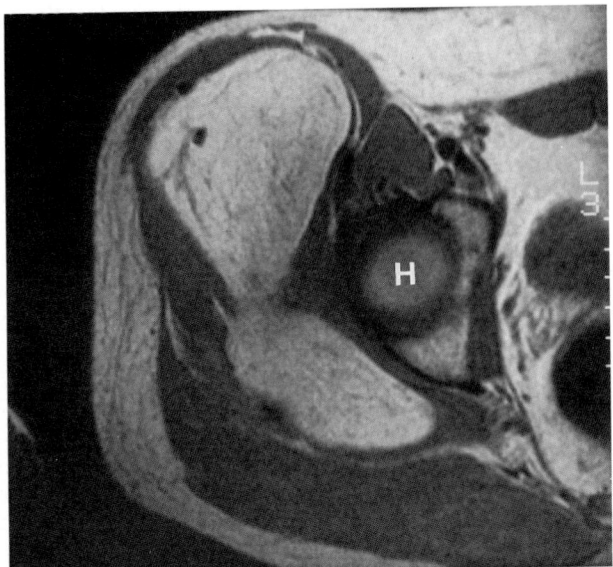

Figure 42.7. Lipoma. This axial proton-density image (TR 2000; TE 20) through the pelvis shows a large bilobed lesion lateral to the hip (H), which has sharp margins and signal characteristics similar to the subcutaneous fat. This is a lipoma. Lipomas will usually contain a small amount of low signal linear tissue, as in this example, which should not be cause to consider this lesion malignant.

sharp margins whether they are intraosseous (Fig. 42.6) or in the soft tissues (Fig. 42.7). Hemangiomas and arteriovenous malformations most commonly have mixed high and low signal on both sequences because of the combination of fatty elements and blood (Fig. 42.8). They characteristically have low-signal serpiginous vessels visible.

The finding of a low signal mass on T1-weighted images that is high in signal on T2-weighted images is sus-

picious for a tumor, but this is a very nonspecific finding and needs to be correlated clinically. Intramuscular injection sites can mimic soft-tissue tumors (Fig. 42.9), as can any area of soft-tissue trauma. Many malignant tumors exhibit high signal radiating from involved bone, which is soft-tissue edema and virtually indistinguishable from tumor spread.

TUMORS

Osteosarcoma

The most common malignant primary bone tumor is an osteosarcoma. These occur almost exclusively in children and young adults (< 30 years old). Some texts describe a second peak of osteosarcoma around the sixth decade, but this is probably because of secondary osteosarcoma in Paget's disease and because of prior radiation. Although osteosarcoma typically occurs toward the end of a long bone, it may occur anywhere in the skeleton with enough frequency that location is not a helpful discriminator. These lesions are usually destructive, with obvious sclerosis present from either tumor new bone formation or reactive sclerosis (Fig. 42.10); however, on occasion an osteosarcoma can be entirely lytic. These are usually telangiectatic osteosarcomas. There are many different types and classifications of osteosarcomas, but it serves little purpose for the radiologist to try to distinguish between most of them. Magnetic resonance imaging of an osteosarcoma generally reveals a large soft-tissue component with heterogeneous high and low signal on both T1WIs and T2WIs (Fig. 42.11).

Parosteal Osteosarcoma

A type of osteosarcoma that should be distinguished from the central osteosarcoma is the parosteal osteosar-

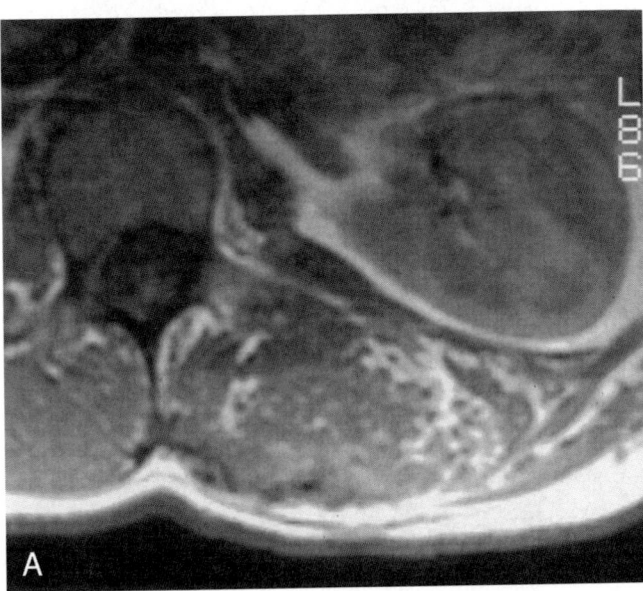

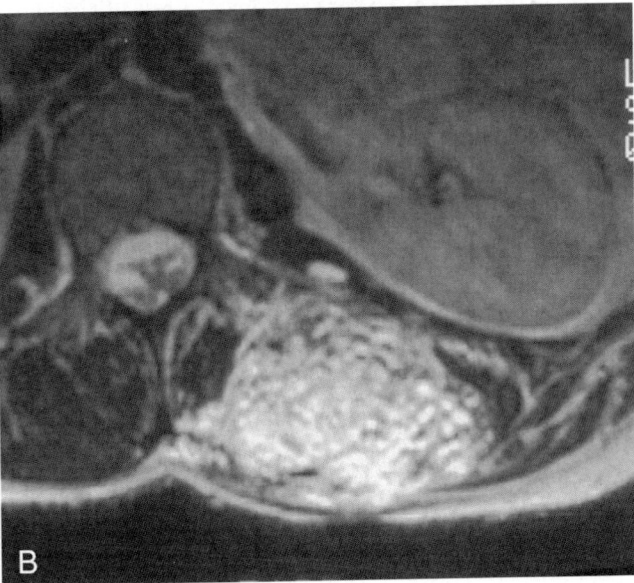

Figure 42.8. Hemangioma. A. A T1-weighted axial image (TR600; TE 11) through the midback in a 30-year-old patient with a mass shows a predominantly low signal mass with stippled areas of high signal representing fat around numerous vessels. **B.** A FSE T2-weighted axial image (TR 3700; TE 102) reveals inhomogeneous high signal with punctate areas of very bright signal representing vessels. Hemangiomas typically have mixed fatty and vascular tissue, which gives high signal on both T1 and T2 sequences.

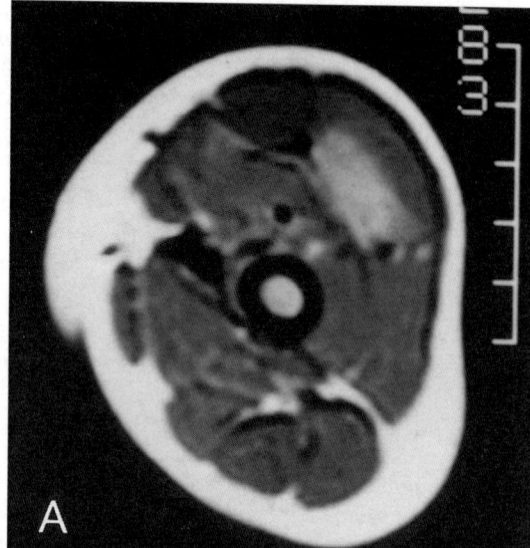

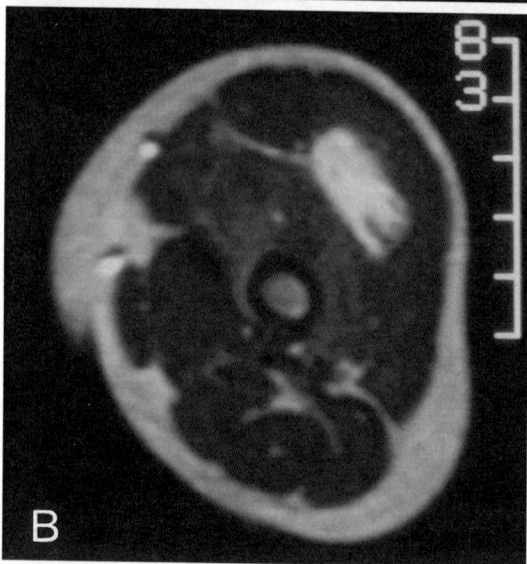

Figure 42.9. Intramuscular Injection Sites. Proton density **(A)** (TR 2000; TE 20) and T2-weighted **(B)** (TR 2000; TE 70) axial images through the left thigh of a child show a mass in the anterior thigh that resembles a typical soft-tissue tumor. This, however, is an intramuscular injection site.

coma. A parosteal osteosarcoma originates from the periosteum of the bone and grows outside the bone (Fig. 42.12). It often wraps around the diaphysis without breaking through the cortex at all. It occurs in an older age group than the central osteosarcomas and is not as aggressive or as deadly as long as it has not extended into the medullary portion of the bone. Treatment used to consist of merely shaving the tumor off the bone from which it was arising; however, recurrence rates were so high that now wide-bloc excisions are performed. Once a parosteal osteosarcoma violates the cortex of the adjacent bone, it is considered to be as aggressive as a central osteosarcoma and is treated in a similar fashion, that is, by amputation or radical excision. The radiologist needs to evaluate the lesion for invasion of the adjacent cortex to help determine treatment and prognosis.

This is best done with CT or MR (Fig. 42.12B,D). A common location from which parosteal osteosarcomas arise is the posterior femur, near the knee.

A lesion that can mimic an early parosteal osteosarcoma in this location is a cortical desmoid tumor. A cortical desmoid tumor is an avulsion injury that is totally benign but can appear somewhat aggressive. Unfortunately, it can appear malignant histologically, so biopsy can lead to disastrous consequences. Amputations for benign cortical desmoid tumors that were confused with malignancies have occurred.

Another lesion that can be confused with a parosteal osteosarcoma is an area of myositis ossificans. Like cortical desmoid tumors, areas of myositis ossificans can be histologically confused for malignancies with disastrous consequences. Differentiation is, of course, vital. Fortunately, differentiation between parosteal osteosarcoma and myositis ossificans is usually easily done radiographically. (See chapter 39 for discussion of differential points between parosteal osteosarcoma and myositis ossificans, and cortical desmoid tumors.)

Ewing's Sarcoma

The classic Ewing's sarcoma is a permeative (multiple small holes) lesion in the diaphysis of a long bone in a child (see Fig. 42.3B). Only about 40% of these tumors occur in the diaphysis, however, with the remainder be-

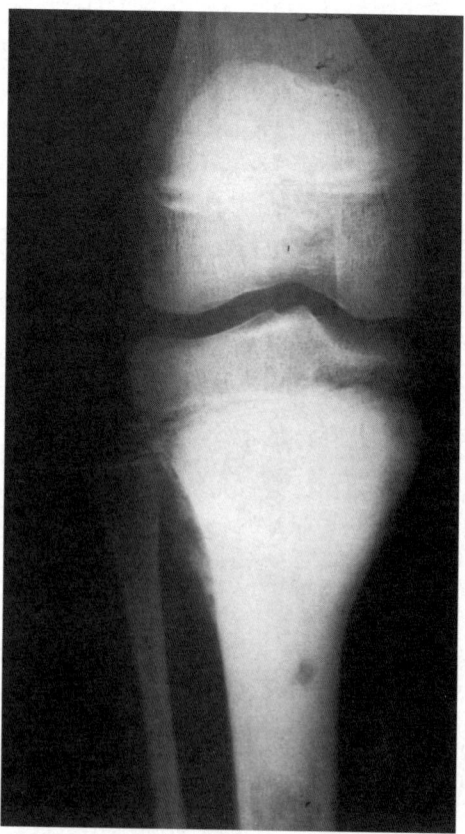

Figure 42.10. Osteosarcoma. A densely sclerotic lesion in the proximal tibia of a child is noted, which is characteristic for an osteogenic sarcoma.

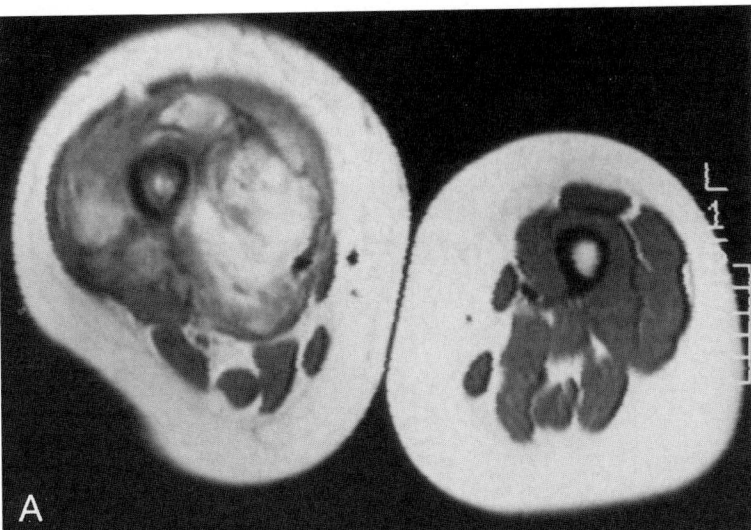

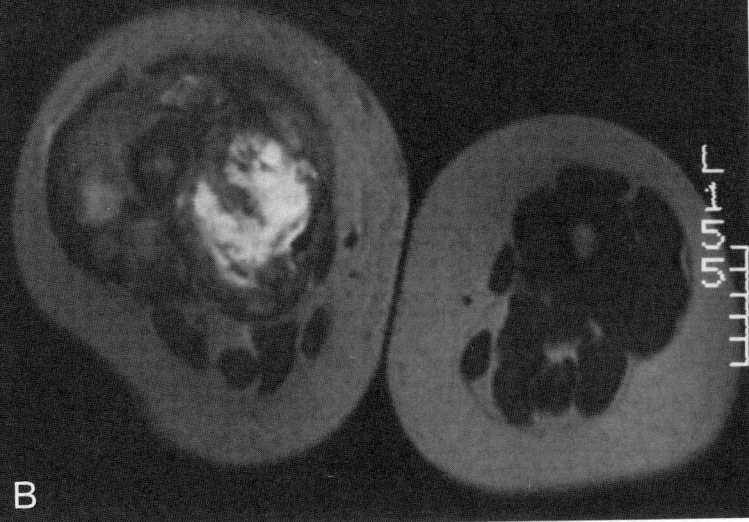

Figure 42.11. Osteosarcoma. A proton density **(A)** (TR 2000; TE 20) and T2-weighted **(B)** (TR 2000; TE 60) image of the thighs in this teenager shows a lesion in the right femur, which is surrounded by a huge soft-tissue mass. The soft-tissue mass has mixed high and low signal on both imaging sequences and is very inhomogeneous. A biopsy revealed this to be an osteosarcoma.

ing metaphyseal, diametaphyseal, and in flat bones. They do tend to be primarily in children and adolescents, although a significant number occur in patients in their 20s, especially in flat bones. Although most often permeative in appearance, they can elicit reactive new bone that can give the lesion a partially sclerotic or "patchy" appearance. Ewing's sarcomas often have an onion-skin type of periostitis, but they can also have periostitis that is sunburst or amorphous in character (Fig. 42.13). Rarely, if ever, will a Ewing's sarcoma have benign-appearing periostitis (thick, uniform, or wavy).

If benign periostitis is present, other lesions should be considered instead, such as infection and eosinophilic granuloma. The classic differential diagnosis for a permeative lesion in a child is Ewing's sarcoma, infection, and eosinophilic granuloma. These three entities can appear radiologically identical. Ewing's sarcoma should be removed from the differential diagnosis if definite benign periostitis or a sequestration is present. The presence or absence of a soft-tissue mass is not helpful in distinguishing between these three lesions. The presence of symptoms is not helpful, as all three entities can be symptomatic.

Chondrosarcoma

Chondrosarcomas have a protean appearance that makes it difficult, at times, to make the diagnosis with any assurance. They most commonly occur in patients older than the age of 40 years. Chondrosarcoma rarely occurs in children, although occasionally one will be encountered from malignant degeneration of an osteochondroma (3). It can be extremely difficult to differentiate histologically a low-grade chondrosarcoma from an enchondroma (3). The diagnosis of chondrosarcoma usually initiates radical excision and therapy, although it is debatable (and somewhat controversial) whether a low-grade chondrosarcoma is even a malignant tumor. For these reasons, the diagnosis of "possible chondrosarcoma" should be reserved for those lesions that are painful (Fig. 42.14) or that show definite aggressive characteristics, such as periostitis and destruction. The truth of the matter is neither radiologists nor pathologists can reliably distinguish between enchondromas and low-grade chondrosarcomas.

Chondrosarcoma should be considered in the diagnosis any time there is a bony or soft-tissue mass with

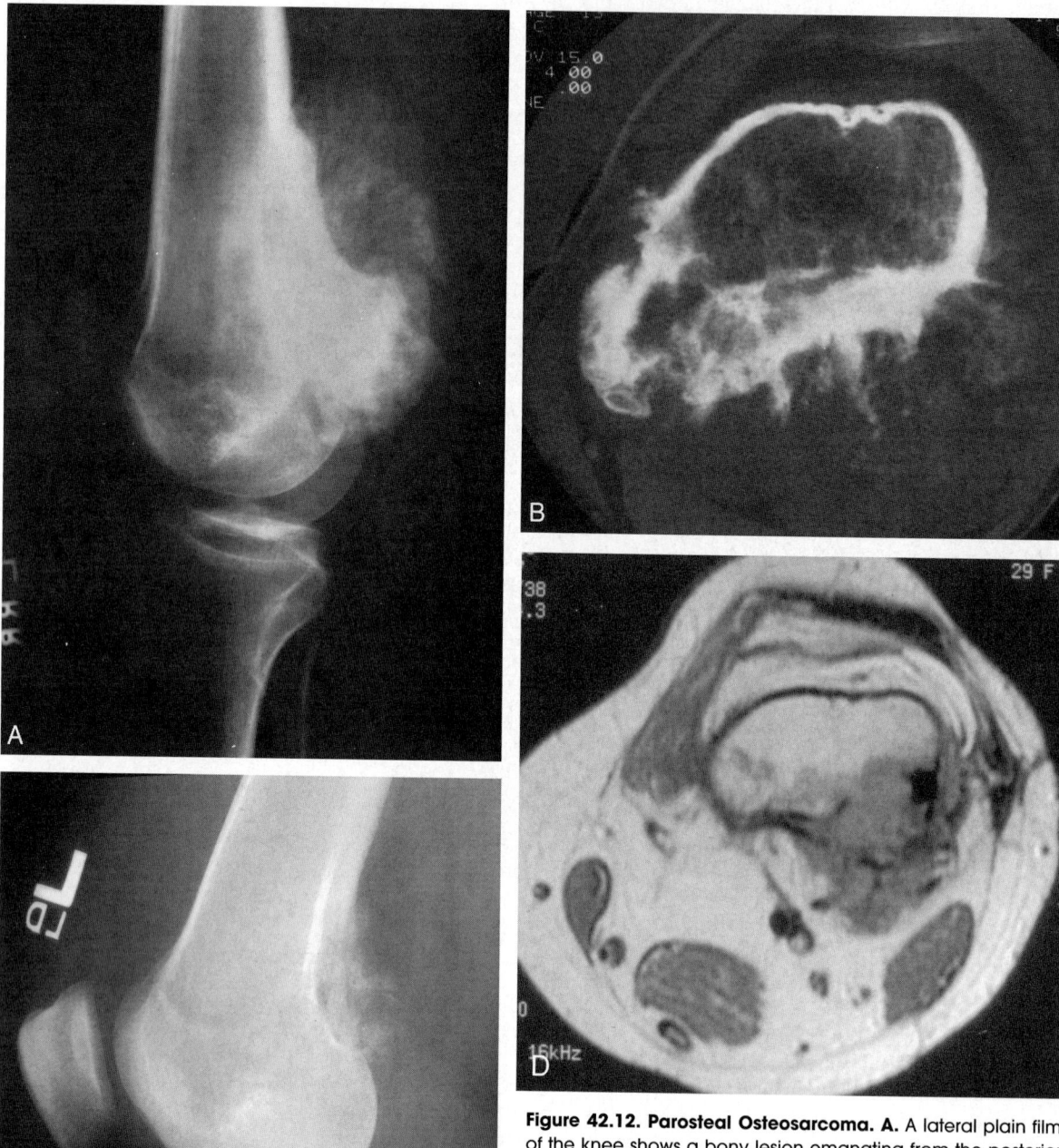

Figure 42.12. Parosteal Osteosarcoma. A. A lateral plain film of the knee shows a bony lesion emanating from the posterior cortex of the distal femur with a large, calcified soft-tissue mass. Note that the densest calcification is central and the periphery is only faintly calcified, characteristics that are typical for a parosteal osteosarcoma. **B.** A CT through the lesion reveals the tumor to be invading the medullary portion of the bone. This is a poor prognostic sign and is essential information to the surgeon. **C.** A lateral plain film in a different patient with a parosteal os-teosarcoma shows soft-tissue calcification extending from the posterior femur. **D.** A proton-density axial image (TR 200; TE 20) reveals considerable bony involvement. It also shows the vas-cular structures to be uninvolved with the soft-tissue component.

amorphous, snowflake calcification in an older patient (>40 years) (Fig. 42.15). Without the presence of calcified chondroid matrix, the lesion is indistinguishable from any other aggressive lytic lesion, such as metastatic disease, plasmacytoma, fibrosarcoma, malignant fibrous histocytoma, or infection. Usually the radiologist can only give a long differential diagnosis such as this, which is entirely acceptable. The lesion will have to undergo biopsy at any rate, so it is not necessary for the radiologist to make the diagnosis. This is the case for most malignant tumors.

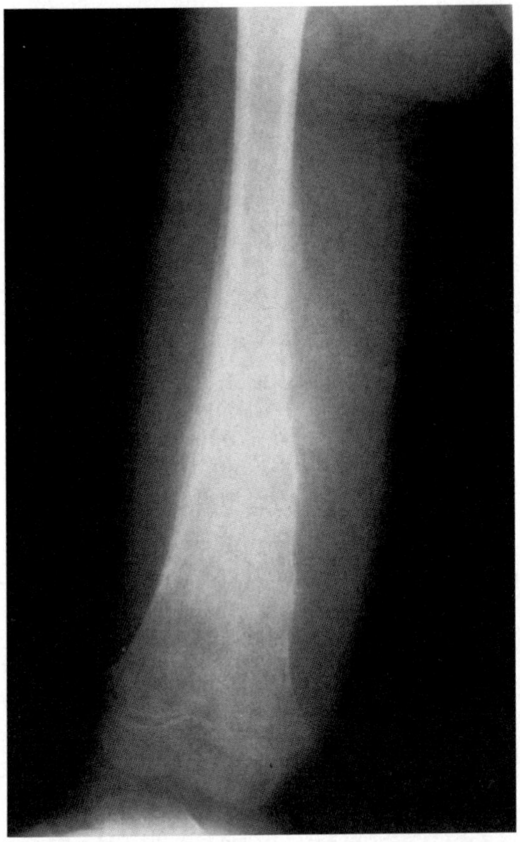

Malignant Giant Cell Tumor

Approximately 20% of giant cell tumors are malignant. Unfortunately, there does not seem to be any way to predict which giant cell tumor will become malignant. Radiologically, the benign and malignant giant cell tumors appear identical. Histologically, the benign and

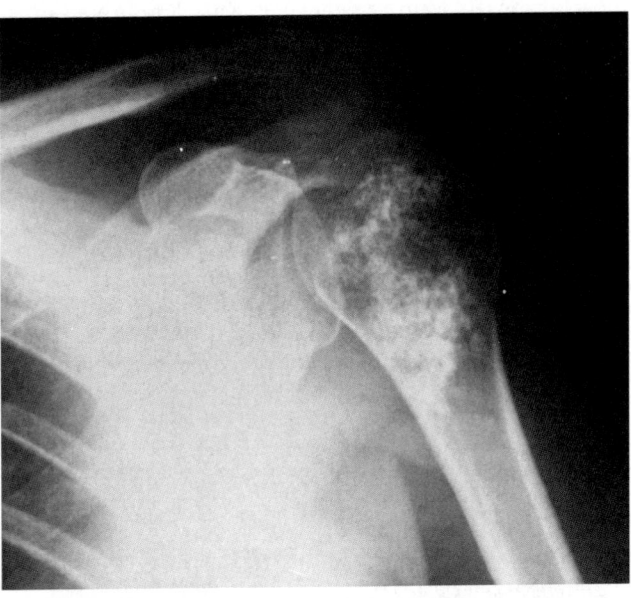

Figure 42.14. Chondrosarcoma. Typical snowflake, or popcornlike, amorphous calcification in the proximal humerus is seen, which is typical of an enchondroma. This patient, however, had pain associated with this lesion, and on biopsy, this was found to be a chondrosarcoma. (Case courtesy of Dr. Tomas Jimenez-Robinson, Rio Piedras, Puerto Rico.)

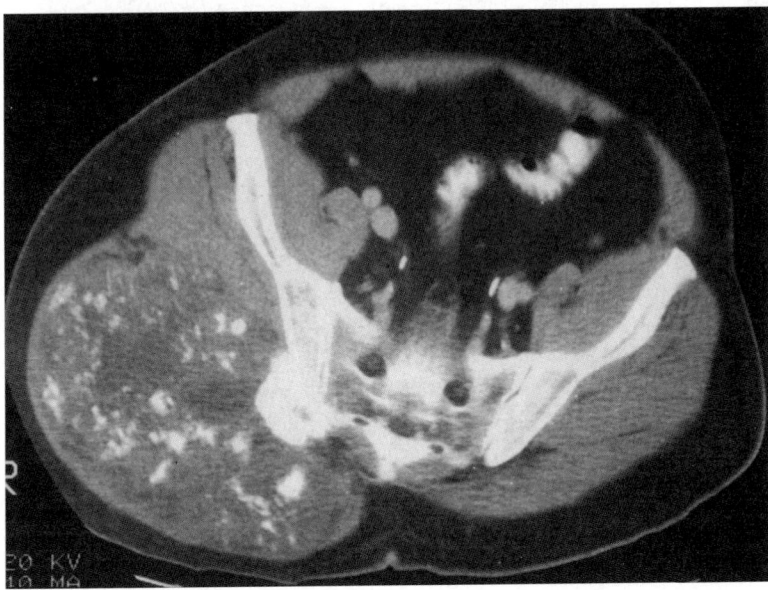

Figure 42.13. Ewing's Sarcoma. An anteroposterior plain film of the femur of a child shows a predominantly sclerotic process with large amounts of sunburst periostitis in the diaphysis, which on biopsy was found to be Ewing's sarcoma.

Figure 42.15. Chondrosarcoma. A large soft-tissue mass with amorphous, irregular calcification is seen in a lesion arising from the ilium on this CT of the pelvis. This is typical for a chondrosarcoma.

malignant giant cell tumors are the same. If metastases (usually to the lung) occur, or if a previously resected giant cell tumor recurs, the tumor is considered by most oncologists to be malignant. Malignant giant cell tumors tend to occur primarily in the fourth decade of life.

Fibrosarcoma

Fibrosarcomas are lytic malignant tumors that do not produce osteoid or chondroid matrix. True fibrosarcomas are today considered to be very uncommon lesions with most of what were once called fibrosarcomas actually being malignant fibrous histiocytomas. They usually do not cause reactive new bone and, therefore, are almost always lytic in appearance. This lytic appearance may take any form, from permeative (Fig. 42.16) to moth-eaten to a fairly well-defined area of lysis (Fig. 42.17). The age range for fibrosarcoma is quite broad, but they tend to predominate in the fourth decade. This is one of the few malignant tumors that can, on occasion, have a bony sequestrum.

Malignant Fibrous Histiocytoma

These tumors were originally classified as fibrosarcomas by most pathologists but have come into their own grouping in the past few decades. MFH is one of the most

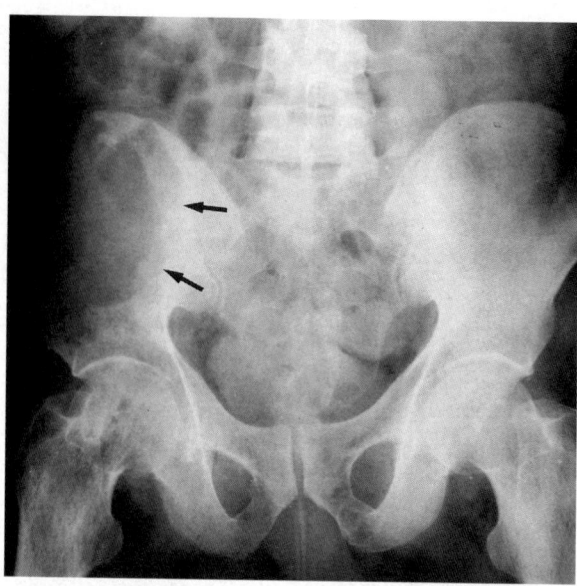

Figure 42.17. Fibrosarcoma. A large, lytic, destructive process of the entire right iliac wing (*arrows*) is noted, which is fairly well defined. On biopsy, this was shown to be a fibrosarcoma. Fibrosarcomas can be very slow growing and will occasionally have a narrow zone of transition such as this.

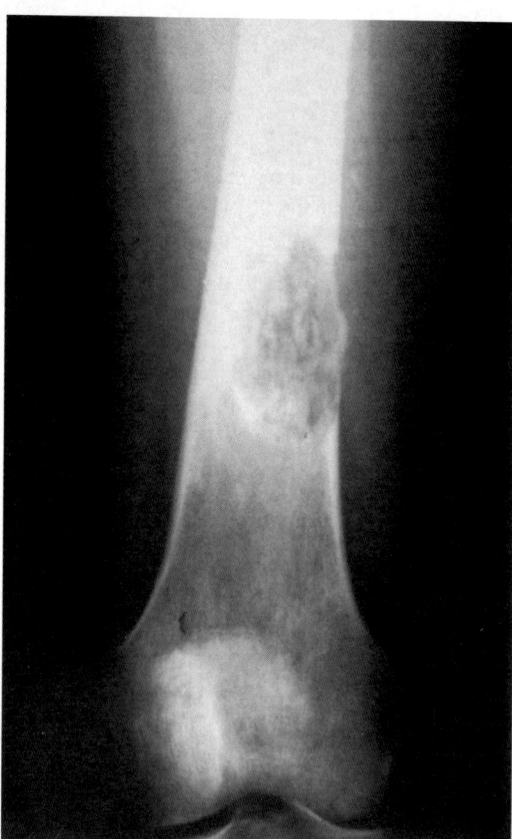

Figure 42.16. Fibrosarcoma. An ill-defined lytic lesion that is permeative or moth-eaten in appearance is seen in the diaphysis of the femur that on biopsy was shown to be a fibrosarcoma.

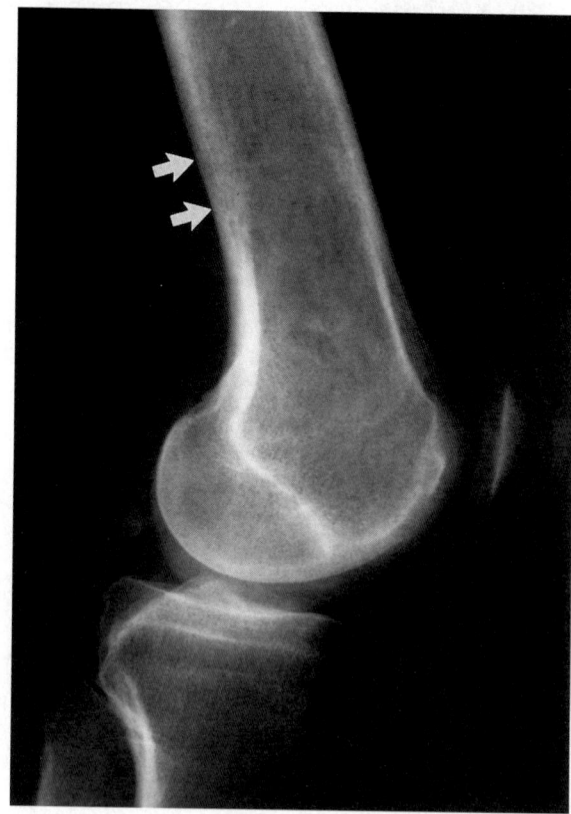

Figure 42.18. Malignant Fibrous Histiocytoma. A moth-eaten or permeative process in the distal femur, with some involvement of the posterior cortex (*arrows*), is seen on this lateral radiograph. In a patient less than the age of 30 years, a Ewing's sarcoma, eosinophilic granuloma, or infection would be the differential diagnosis. In a patient more than the age of 30, infection and malignant fibrous histiocytoma would be more common. A reticulum cell sarcoma could have a similar appearance.

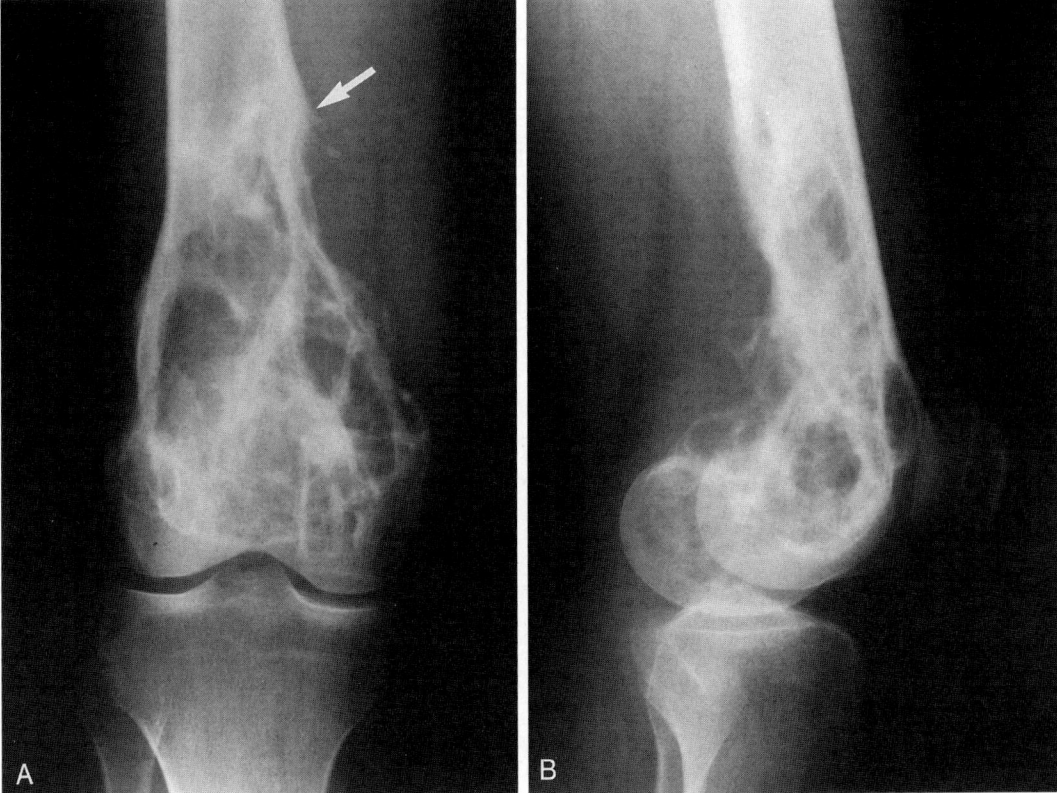

Figure 42.19. Desmoid Tumor. A multilocular, heavily septated, destructive, lytic lesion of the distal femur is noted in these anteroposterior **(A)** and lateral **(B)** plain films of the femur, which is fairly characteristic for a desmoid tumor. The thick septa and narrow zone of transition are characteristic of a benign process, whereas the Codman's triangle (*arrow*) and large amount of bony destruction indicate an aggressive process.

common bone and soft-tissue tumors, with true fibrosarcomas, as mentioned earlier, being uncommon. Radiologically, they appear identical to fibrosarcomas: lytic lesions with variations extending from permeative (Fig. 42.18) to fairly well defined. Like fibrosarcomas, they may, on occasion, have a bony sequestrum.

Desmoid Tumor

A desmoid tumor (not to be confused with a cortical desmoid; see chapter 39) is a half-grade fibrosarcoma. It has also been called a desmoplastic fibroma or aggressive fibromatosis. These lesions, like fibrosarcoma, are lytic, but are usually fairly well defined because of their slow growth. They often have benign periostitis present that has thick spicules or "spikes." They usually have a multilocular appearance with thick bony septa (Fig. 42.19). They are slow growing and do not metastasize, but they can exhibit inexorable tumor extension into surrounding soft tissues with devastating results. Like fibrosarcoma and malignant fibrous histiocytomas, these lesions can exhibit a bony sequestrum.

Reticulum Cell Sarcoma (Primary Lymphoma of Bone)

This is a rare neoplasm that has a radiologic appearance identical to Ewing's sarcoma, that is, a permeative or moth-eaten pattern (Fig. 42.20). Primary lymphoma of bone tends to occur in an older age group than Ewing's sarcoma, and, whereas Ewing's sarcomas are typically systemically symptomatic, patients with primary lymphoma of bone are often asymptomatic. It is said to be the only malignant tumor that can involve a large amount of bone while the patient is asymptomatic.

Metastatic Disease

Metastatic lesions must be included in *any* differential diagnosis of a bone lesion in a patient greater than the age of 40 years. They can have virtually any appearance. They can mimic a benign lesion or an aggressive primary bone tumor. It can be difficult, if not impossible, to judge the origin of the tumor from the appearance of the metastatic focus, although some appearances are fairly characteristic. For instance, multiple sclerotic foci in a man are most likely prostatic metastases (Fig. 42.21), although lung, bowel, or almost any other metastatic tumor could present like this. In a woman, the same picture would most likely be from breast metastases. Although nearly every metastatic bone lesion can be either lytic or blastic, the only primary tumor that virtually never presents with blastic metastatic disease is renal cell carcinoma. The classic differential diagnosis for an expansile, lytic metastasis is renal cell or thyroid carcinoma (Fig. 42.22).

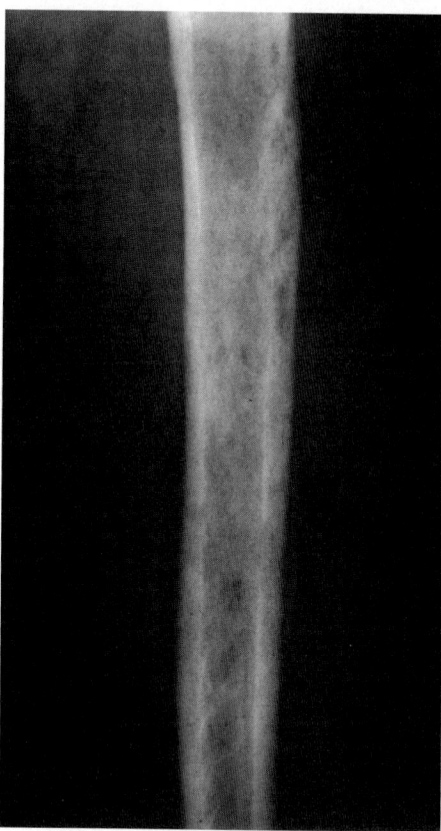

Figure 42.20. Primary Lymphoma of Bone. A diffuse permeative pattern is seen throughout the humerus in this 35-year-old patient that is characteristic of primary lymphoma of bone.

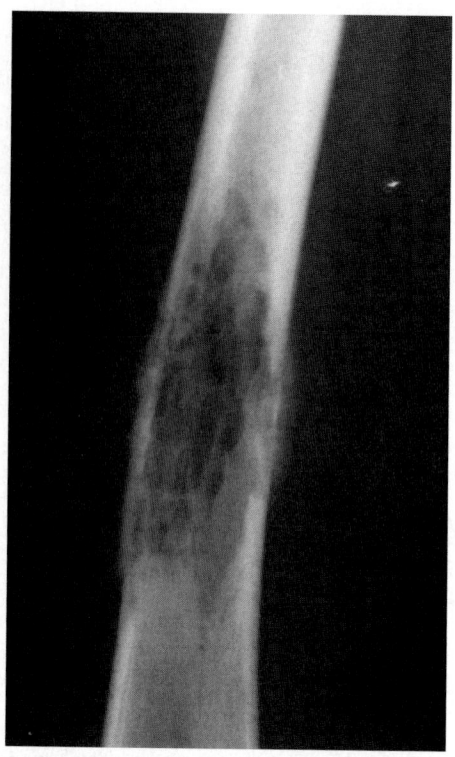

Figure 42.22. Metastatic Renal Cell Carcinoma. A lytic lesion in the diaphysis of the femur is noted, which is typical for renal cell carcinoma. As many as one-third of renal cell carcinomas present initially with a bony metastasis. Renal cell carcinoma virtually never presents with a blastic metastatic focus.

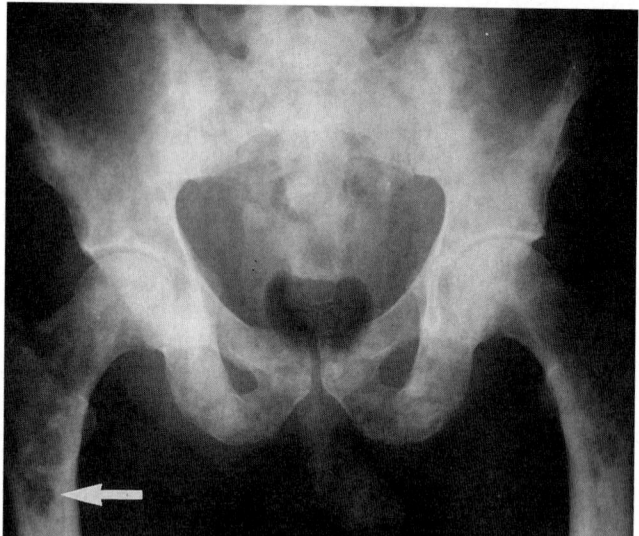

Figure 42.21. Metastatic Prostate Carcinoma. Diffuse blastic metastases are seen throughout the pelvis and proximal femurs with a lytic, destructive lesion seen in the right proximal femur (*arrow*). Prostate metastases tend to be blastic but can occasionally be lytic.

Myeloma

Like metastases, myeloma should only be considered in a patient older than the age of 40 years, although some radiologists use age 35 for the lower limits of myeloma. Myeloma typically has a diffuse permeative appearance (Fig. 42.23) that can mimic a Ewing's sarcoma or primary lymphoma of bone. Because of the age criteria, Ewing's sarcoma and myeloma are not in the same differential, however. Myeloma frequently involves the calvarium (Fig. 42.24). Rarely, myeloma can present with multiple sclerotic foci resembling diffuse metastatic disease. Myeloma is one of the only lesions that is not characteristically hot on a radionuclide bone scan; therefore, radiologic "bone surveys" are performed in place of radionuclide bone scans when evidence of myeloma is found clinically. Occasionally, myeloma will present with a lytic bone lesion called a plasmacytoma. This lesion can mimic any lytic bone lesion, benign or aggressive, in its appearance; it can precede other evidence of myeloma by up to 3 years.

Soft-Tissue Tumors

There is no concise, useful differential diagnosis for soft-tissue tumors, whether or not there is calcification, bony destruction, fat plane involvement, and so forth. The two most common soft-tissue tumors, ***malignant fi-***

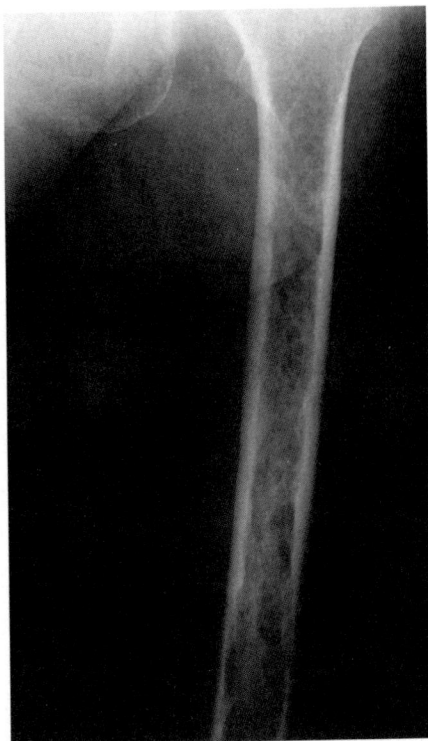

Figure 42.23. Multiple Myeloma. A diffuse, moth-eaten pattern is seen throughout the diaphysis of the femur in this 45-year-old patient that is characteristic for myeloma. Primary lymphoma of bone could have a similar appearance.

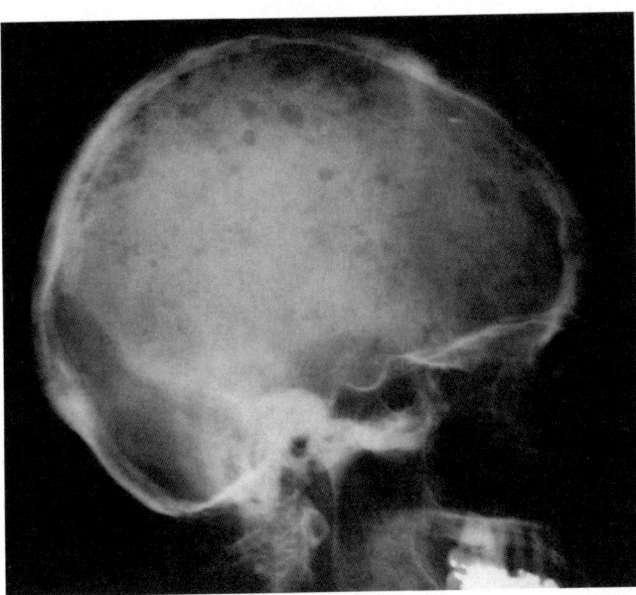

Figure 42.24. Multiple Myeloma. A lateral view of the skull shows multiple lytic lesions in the calvarium, which is a characteristic appearance of multiple myeloma.

fat present. There are at least three subtypes of liposarcomas, two of which have only small amounts of fat present. Therefore, one is generally left to giving descriptions of size and extent of the tumor and letting the pathologist determine the diagnosis.

Synovial sarcomas, or synoviomas, only rarely originate in a joint. They are often adjacent to joints but probably arise from synovial tissue in tendon sheaths rather than in joints themselves. There are no malignant tumors that routinely need to be considered in the differential diagnosis of joint lesions.

Synovial osteochondromatosis is a benign joint lesion that probably occurs from metaplasia of the synovium and leads to multiple calcific loose bodies in a joint. This can histologically mimic a chondrosarcoma, and therefore is best diagnosed radiographically, as it has a pathognomonic radiographic appearance (Fig. 42.25). Up to 30% of the time, the loose bodies do not calcify, however, and the osteochondromatosis then can mimic pigmented villonodular synovitis.

Pigmented villonodular synovitis is a benign synovial soft-tissue process that causes joint swelling and pain and, occasionally, joint erosions (Fig. 42.26). It virtually never has calcifications associated with it. The MR appearance of PVNS is characteristic. Marked low signal lining the synovium is seen on T1- and T2-weighted images because of the hemosiderin deposits (Fig. 42.27).

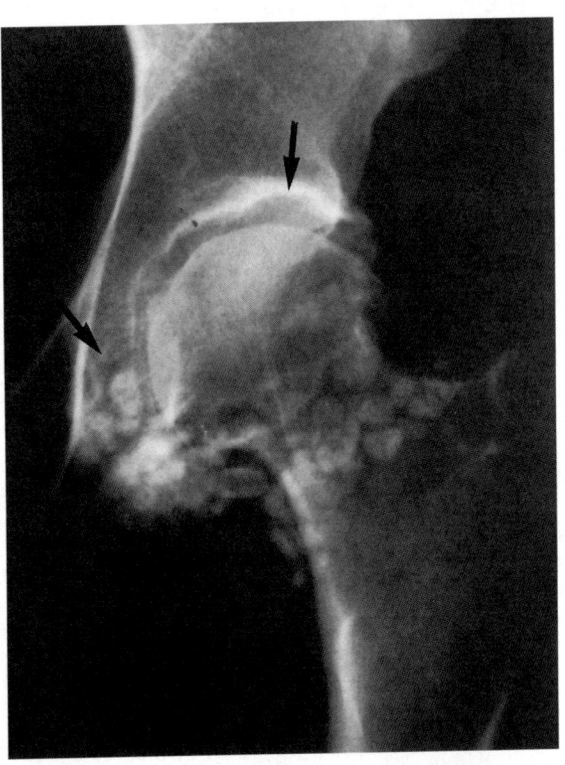

Figure 42.25. Synovial Osteochondromatosis. Multiple calcific loose bodies in a hip joint, as in this example, are virtually pathognomonic for synovial osteochondromatosis. Notice the erosions in the acetabulum (*arrows*). In up to 30% of cases, the loose bodies are nonossified; in such cases, this process is indistinguishable from PVNS.

brous histiocytoma and **liposarcoma**, should be mentioned as the most likely possibilities for any soft-tissue tumor, but any cell type can produce a benign or malignant tumor and mimic any other soft-tissue tumor. A lipoma, obviously, can be separated out by the appearance of fat, but a liposarcoma might or might not have

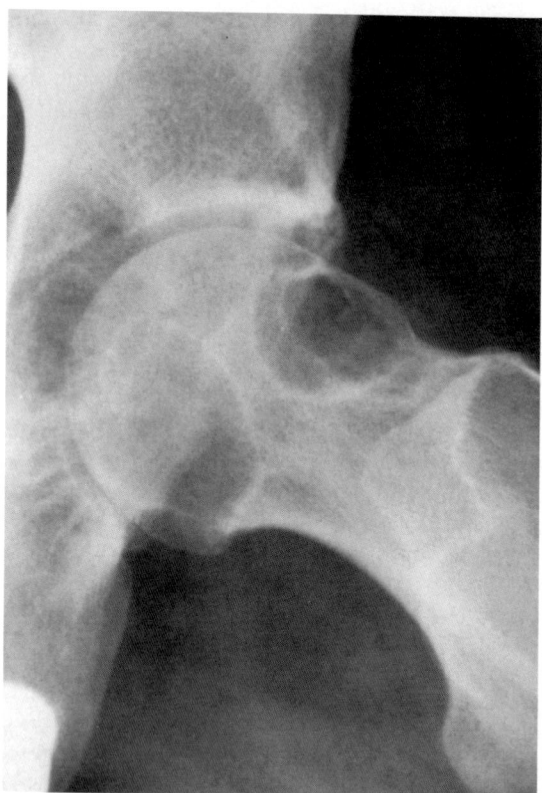

Figure 42.26. Pigmented Villondular Synovitis. Large erosions in the femoral head and acetabulum are characteristic for PVNS; however, nonossified synovial osteochondromatosis could present, such as in this example.

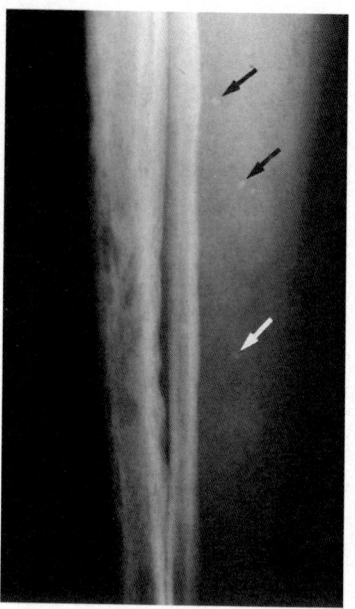

Figure 42.28. Hemangioma. Multiple irregular lytic lesions, predominantly cortical in nature, are seen in the tibia in this patient with a soft-tissue mass. Cortical holes such as this occur almost exclusively in radiation and soft-tissue hemangioma. Note the phleboliths in the posterior soft-tissues (*arrows*) that are often seen in hemangioma and make this an easy diagnosis.

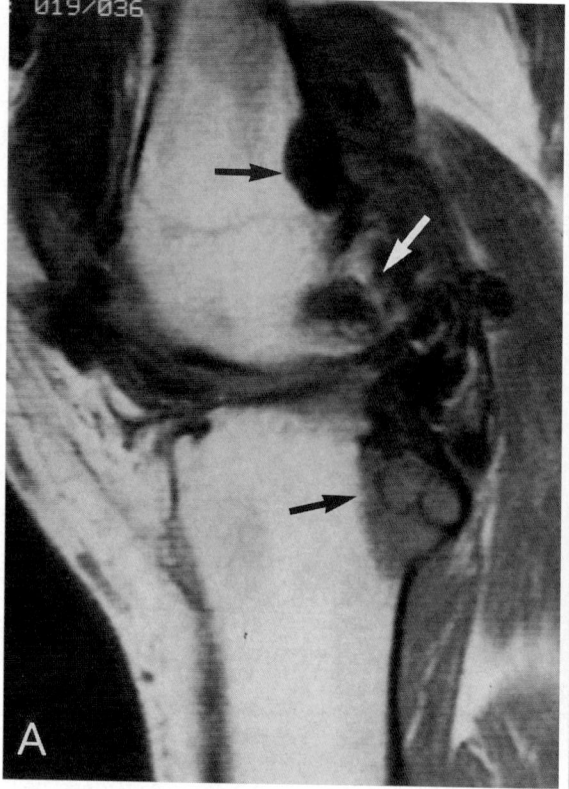

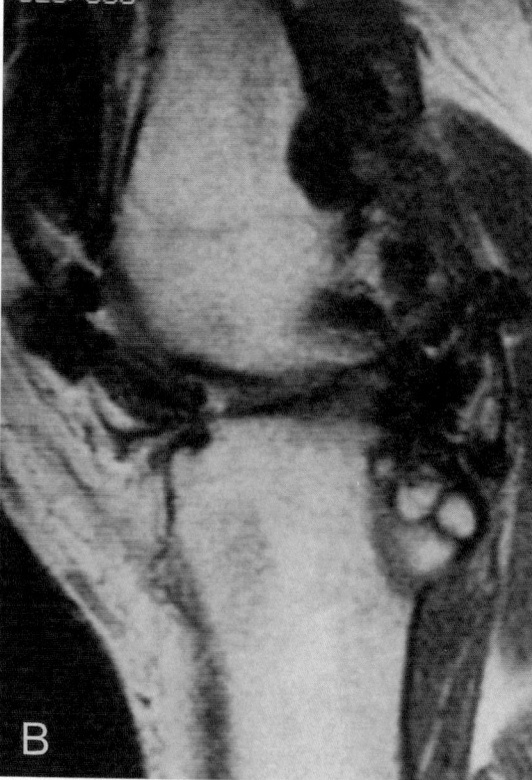

Figure 42.27. Pigmented Villondular Synovitis. Proton-density **(A)** (TR 1500; TE 20) and T2-weighted **(B)** (TR 1500; TE 60) sagittal images of the knee in this patient with painful swelling show diffuse low signal throughout the synovium and eroding into the bone (*arrows*). The low signal on both T1-weighted and T2-weighted images is typical for hemosiderin deposits in PVNS.

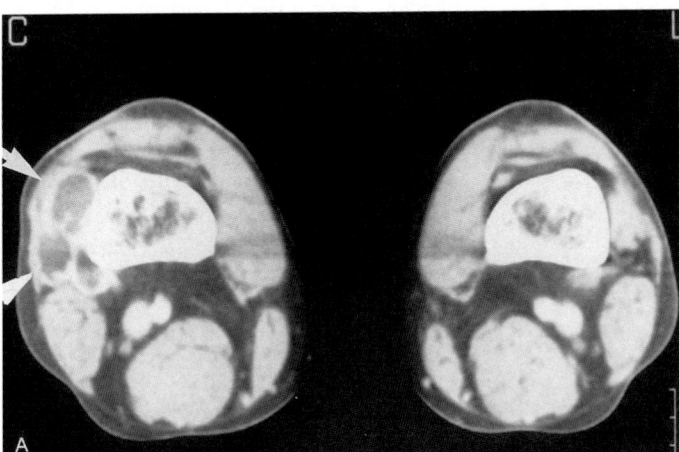

Figure 42.29. Atypical Synovial Cyst. A. A CT scan through the distal femurs in a patient with a soft-tissue mass around the right knee shows a multilocular soft-tissue mass adjacent to the distal right femur (*arrows*). **B.** A proton-density MR (TR 2000; TE 20) through the same area shows intermediate intensity signal in a homogeneous multilocular soft-tissue mass (*arrows*). **C.** A T2-weighted image (TR 2000; TE 60) shows high-intensity signal in the lesion, which is typical for fluid, although a tumor could have these signal characteristics This was an atypical synovial cyst arising from the knee joint.

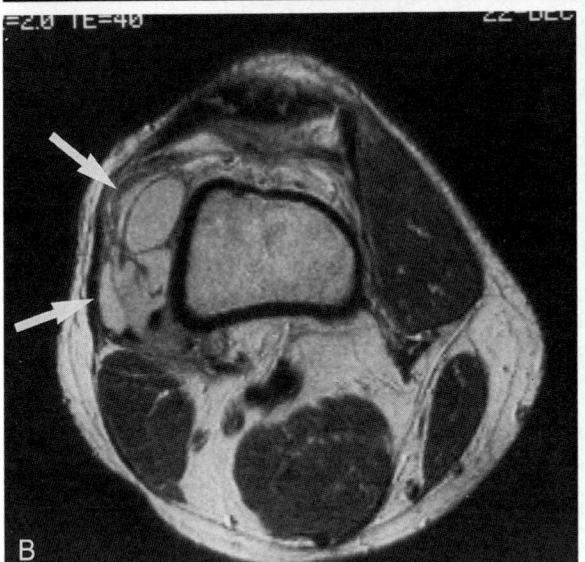
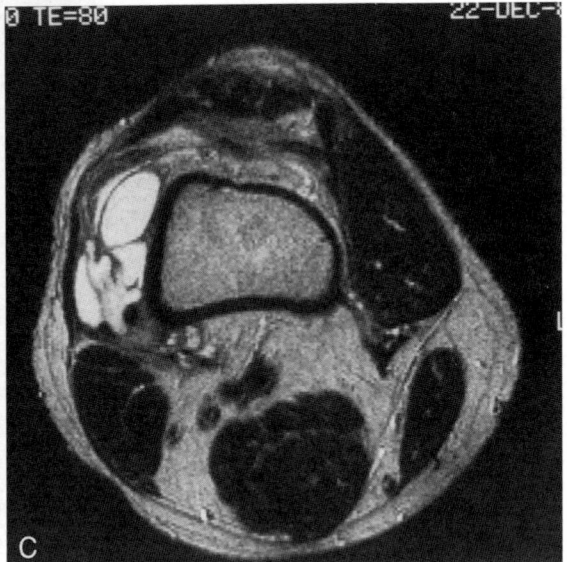

Chronic bleeding into a joint, so-called hemosiderotic arthritis, could have a similar appearance, but is even more rare than PVNS.

Hemangiomas will often have phleboliths associated with them and often cause cortical holes in adjacent bone that can mimic a permeative or moth-eaten pattern (Fig. 42.28), a pseudopermeative pattern. The true permeative pattern of round cell lesions occurs in the intramedullary or endosteal part of the bone and can be differentiated from a pseudopermeative pattern by the intact cortex.

Atypical synovial cysts, such as Baker's cysts around the knee, can present as a soft-tissue mass and result in an unnecessary biopsy. On CT, these lesions may not be appreciated as fluid-filled lesions and their association with a joint can be easily overlooked.

Magnetic resonance imaging will demonstrate a very high signal intensity with T2 weighting that is very homogeneous and often septated (Fig. 42.29).

References

1. Edeiken J. Roentgen Diagnosis of Diseases of Bone. 3rd ed. Baltimore: Williams & Wilkins, 1981.
2. Berquist T, Ehman R, King B, Hodgman C, et al. Value of MR imaging in differentiating benign from malignant soft-tissue masses: study of 95 lesions. Am J Roentgenol 1990;155:1251–1255.
3. Brien EW, Mirra JM, Kerr R. Benign and malignant cartilage tumors of bone and joint—their anatomic and theoretical basis with an emphasis on radiology, pathology and clinical biology. 1. The intramedullary cartilage tumors [review]. Skeletal Radiol 1997;26(6):325–353.

43
Skeletal Trauma

Clyde A. Helms

SPINE
HAND AND WRIST
ARM
PELVIS
LEG

Most of the differential diagnoses in skeletal radiology that I use are geared to be 95% inclusive; that is, the correct diagnosis will be mentioned 95% of the time. The yield can be increased by lengthening the list, but if the list gets too long, it can be unwieldy and less useful for the clinician. In trauma cases, however, being right 95% of the time is not good enough. Missing the correct diagnosis 5% of the time is unacceptable. Fractures simply should not be missed.

Before starting with specific examples, a few key points should be kept in mind concerning radiology of trauma. First, have a high index of suspicion. Every radiologist in the world has missed fractures on radiographs because they were not sufficiently attuned to the possible presence of a fracture. Often, the history is either nonexistent or misleading, and the anatomic area of concern is therefore overlooked. When in doubt, examine the patient. Orthopaedic surgeons rarely miss seeing fractures on radiographs because they have examined the patient, they know where the patient hurts, and they have a high index of suspicion. Second, always get two radiographs at 90° to each other in every trauma case. A high percentage of fractures are seen only on one view (the anteroposterior or the lateral) and will therefore be missed unless two views are routinely obtained. Third, once a fracture is identified, do not forget to look at the rest of the film. About 10% of all cases have a second finding that often is as significant or even more so than the initial finding. Many fractures have associated dislocation, foreign bodies, or additional fractures, so be sure to examine the entire film.

Finally, do not hesitate to obtain a CT scan or an MR study if the plain films fail to confirm what is believed to be present clinically. MR imaging is being used more frequently as a primary imaging tool for trauma, replacing CT or radionuclide studies in cases in which the plain films are negative or equivocal. Make sure that an expensive examination such as CT or MR is truly going to affect patient care rather than just show an abnormality and then have the same treatment whether positive or negative. For example, there is no reason to do a CT scan or an MR study to find a subtle or occult fracture of the radial head in the elbow because the patient is going to

have a posterior splint regardless of the results of the advanced study (assuming the patient had trauma to the elbow, has pain, and the plain film shows a displaced posterior fat pad indicative of fluid in the joint). On the other hand, an elderly patient who has hip pain after a fall and has a negative plain film would benefit from an MR study because his treatment will depend on whether or not an occult fracture is present.

SPINE

The cervical spine is one of the most commonly filmed parts of the body in a busy emergency department and can be one of the most difficult examinations to interpret. One of the most important pieces of information for the radiologist to have is the clinical history. If the patient has been involved in an automobile accident and has no neck pain, it is extremely unlikely that a fracture is present. So-called precautionary radiographs are not justified. On the other hand, if the plain films are negative in a trauma victim who has neck pain or neurologic deficits, obtain a CT scan (1).

Usually, a cross-table lateral view of the C-spine is obtained first in order to avoid unduly moving the patient who might have a cervical fracture. If the lateral C-spine appears normal, the remainder of the C-spine series, including flexion and extension views (if the patient can cooperate) is obtained.

What does one look for on the lateral C-spine? First, make certain that all seven cervical vertebral bodies can be visualized. A large number of fractures are missed because the shoulders obscure the lower C-spine levels (Fig. 43.1). If the entire cervical spine is not visualized, repeat the film with the shoulders lowered.

Next, evaluate five parallel (more or less) lines for step-offs or discontinuity as follows (Fig. 43.2):

Line 1 is the prevertebral soft tissue and extends down the posterior aspect of the airway; it should be several millimeters from the first three or four vertebral bodies and then moves further away at the laryngeal cartilage. It should be less than one vertebral body width from the anterior vertebral bodies from C3 or C4 to C7, and it should be smooth in its contour.

Line 2 follows the anterior vertebral bodies and should be smooth and uninterrupted. Anterior osteophytes can encroach on this line and extend beyond it and should therefore be ignored in drawing this line. Interruption of the anterior vertebral body line is a sign of a serious injury (Fig. 43.1B).

Line 3 is similar to the anterior vertebral body line (line 2) except that it connects the posterior vertebral bodies.

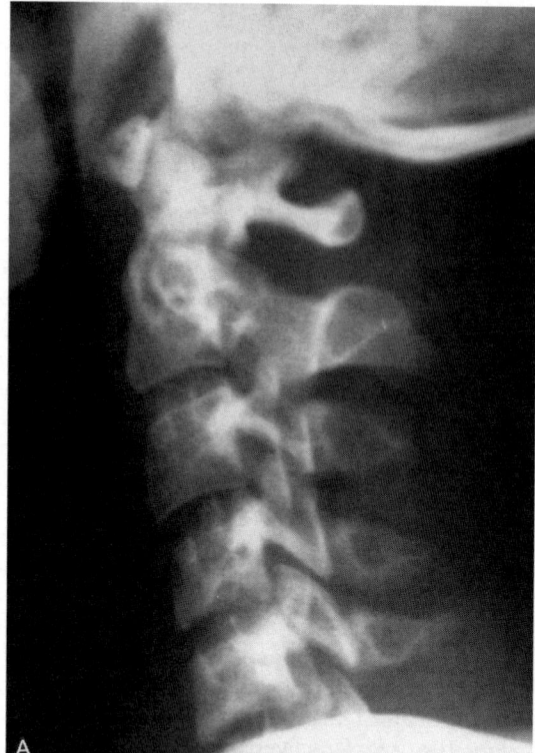

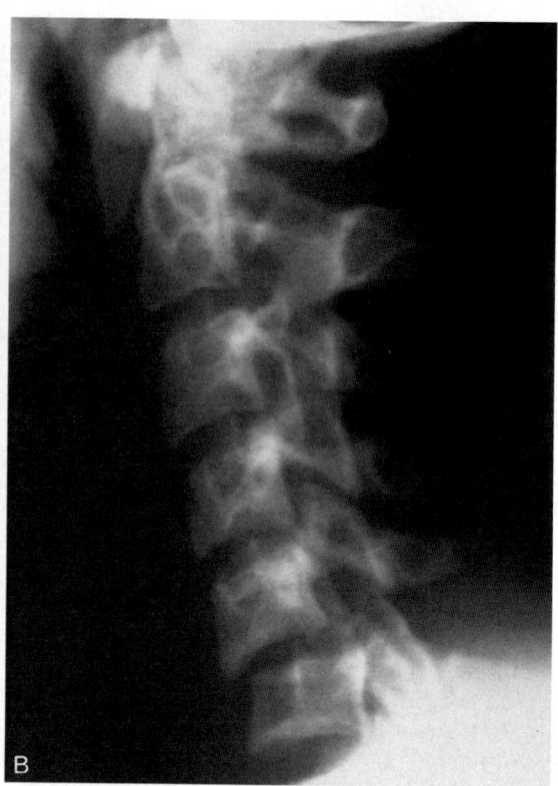

Figure 43.1. Shoulders Obscuring C5–6 Dislocation. This patient presented to the emergency department after an injury suffered while diving into a shallow swimming pool. He had neck pain but no neurologic deficits. **A.** The initial radiograph obtained of the C-spine was interpreted as within normal limits. Only five cervical vertebrae are visible, however, because of high-riding shoulders. **B.** A repeat examination with the shoulders lowered reveals a dislocation of C5 on C6. To visualize C7, the shoulders were lowered even further. The C7 vertebral body must be visualized on every lateral C-spine examination in a trauma setting.

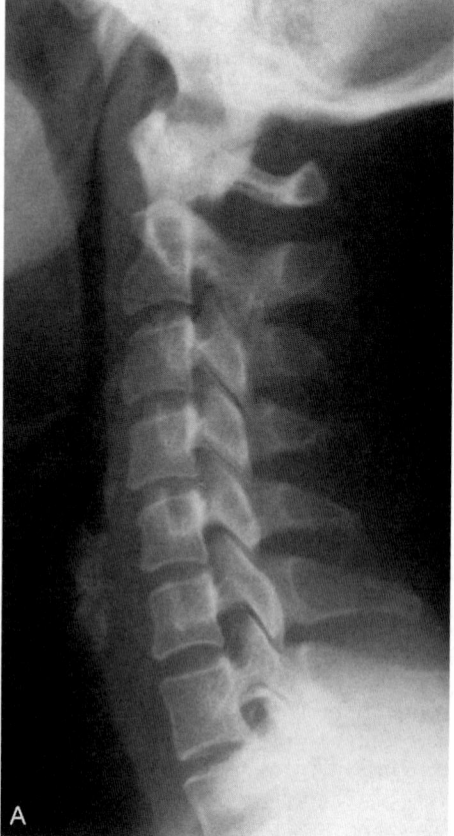

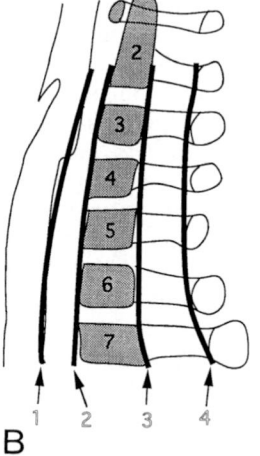

Figure 43.2. Normal Lateral Cervical Spine. A. Lateral radiograph of a normal cervical spine. **B.** Diagrammatic representation of a lateral C-spine showing four parallel lines that should be observed in every lateral C-spine examination. Line 1 is the soft-tissue line that is closely applied to the posterior border of the airway through the first four or five vertebral body segments and then widens around the laryngeal cartilage and runs parallel to the remainder of the cervical vertebrae. Line 2 demarcates the anterior border of the cervical vertebral bodies. Line 3 is the posterior border of the cervical vertebral bodies. Line 4 is drawn by connecting the junction of the lamina at the spinous process, which is called the spinolaminal line. It represents the posterior extent of the central canal that contains the spinal cord itself. These lines should be generally smooth and parallel with no abrupt step-offs.

Like line 2, it should be smooth and uninterrupted, and any disruption signifies a serious injury.

Line 4 connects the posterior junction of the lamina with the spinous processes and is called the spinolaminal line. The spinal cord lies between lines 3 and 4; therefore, any offset of either of these lines could mean a bony structure is impinging the cord. It takes very little force against the cord to cause severe neurologic deficits, and any bony structure lying on the cord must be recognized as soon as possible.

Line 5 is not really a line so much as a collection of points—the tips of the spinous processes. They are quite variable in their size and appearance, although C7 is consistently the largest. A fracture of one of the spinous processes, by itself, is not a serious injury, but it occasionally heralds other, more serious injuries.

After visually inspecting these five lines on the lateral C-spine, then inspect the C1–2 area a little more closely. Make certain that the anterior arch of C1 is no greater then 2.5 mm from the dens (Fig. 43.3). Any greater separation than this (except in children, for whom up to 5.0 mm can be normal) is suspicious for disruption of the transverse ligament between C1 and C2 (Fig. 43.4).

The disc spaces are examined next to see that there is no inordinate widening or narrowing, either of which could indicate an acute traumatic injury. If a disc space is narrowed, it will usually be secondary to degenerative disease, but make certain that associated osteophytosis and sclerosis are present before diagnosing degenerative disease.

The examination of the lateral C-spine as described here can be done in less than 1 minute. If it is normal, then the remainder of the examination can be completed, including flexion and extension views. It is imperative that the patient initiate the flexion and extension without help from the technician or anyone else. A patient, if conscious and semialert, will not injure himself or herself with voluntary flexion and extension and will have muscle guarding preventing motion if there is an injury present. Even gentle pressure to aid in flexion or extension can cause severe injury if a fracture or dislocation is present.

A few examples of fractures, dislocations, and other abnormalities are illustrated in the following paragraphs.

Jefferson Fracture. A blow to the top of the head, such as when an object falls directly on the apex of the skull, can cause the lateral masses of C1 to slide apart, splitting the bony ring of C1. This is called a Jefferson fracture (Fig. 43.5). It nicely illustrates how a bony ring will not break in just one place, but must break in several places. This is a rule that is seldom violated. All the vertebral rings, when fractured, must fracture in two or more places. The bony rings of the pelvis behave similarly.

Computed tomography is excellent at demonstrating the complete bony ring of C1 and shows the fractures, as well as any associated soft-tissue mass, much better than plain films do. In diagnosing a Jefferson fracture on plain film, the lateral masses of C1 must extend beyond the margins of the C2 body (Fig. 43.5A). Just seeing asymmetry of the spaces on either side of the dens is not enough to make the diagnosis, as this can be normally asymmetrical with rotation or with rotatory fixation of the atlantoaxial joint.

Rotatory Fixation of the Atlantoaxial Joint is a somewhat controversial, little understood process in which the atlantoaxial joint becomes fixed and the C1–C2 bodies move en mass instead of rotating on one another. It is easily diagnosed with open-mouth odontoid views. In the normal odontoid view, the spaces lateral to the dens (odontoid) are equal. With rotation of the head to the left the space on the left widens, and with rotation to the right the space on the right widens. With rotatory fixation, one of the spaces is wider than the other and stays wider even with rotation of the head to the opposite side (Fig. 43.6). This is a relatively innocuous malady that by itself is usually treated with a soft cervical collar, gentle traction, or both. It is rarely associated with disruption of the transverse ligaments at C1–2 (di-

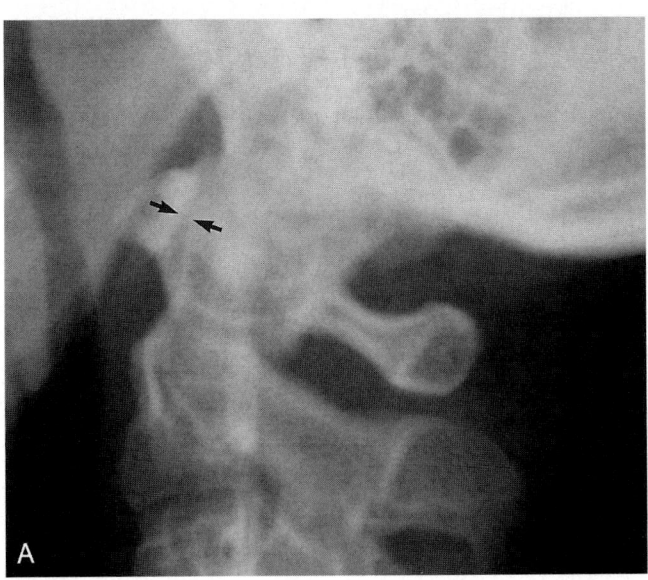

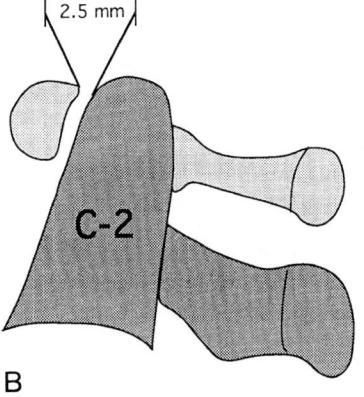

Figure 43.3. Normal C1 and C2. A lateral radiograph **(A)** and drawing **(B)** of the upper cervical spine showing the normal distance of the anterior arch of C1 less than 2.5 mm in distance from the odontoid process (dens) of C2 (*arrows*).

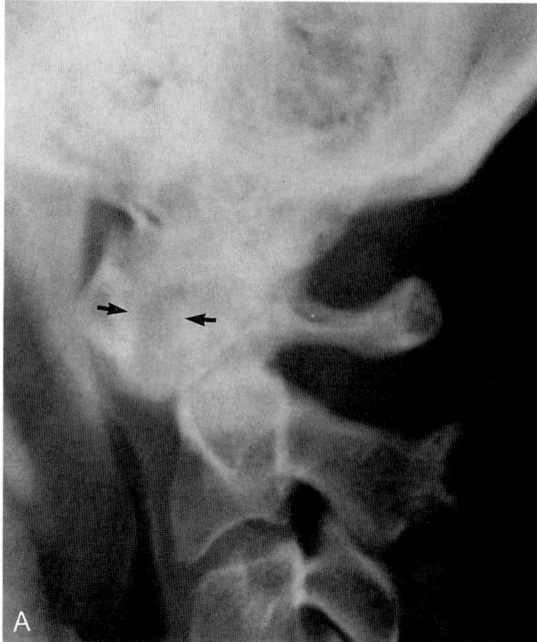

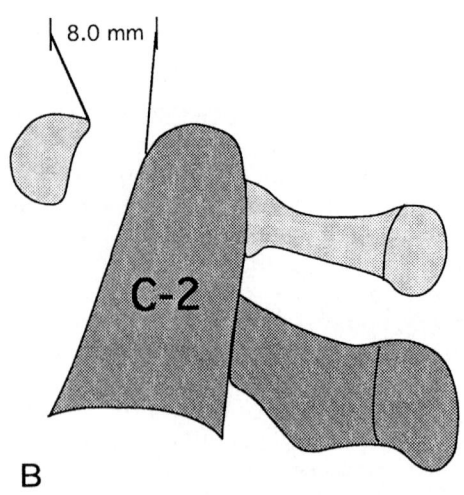

Figure 43.4. C1–2 Dislocation. A lateral radiograph **(A)** and drawing **(B)** of the upper cervical spine in a patient who suffered trauma to the neck shows the anterior arch of C1 is 9 mm anterior to the odontoid process of C2 (*arrows*). This is diagnostic of a dislocation of C1 on C2 and indicates rupture of the transverse ligaments that normally hold these vertebral segments together.

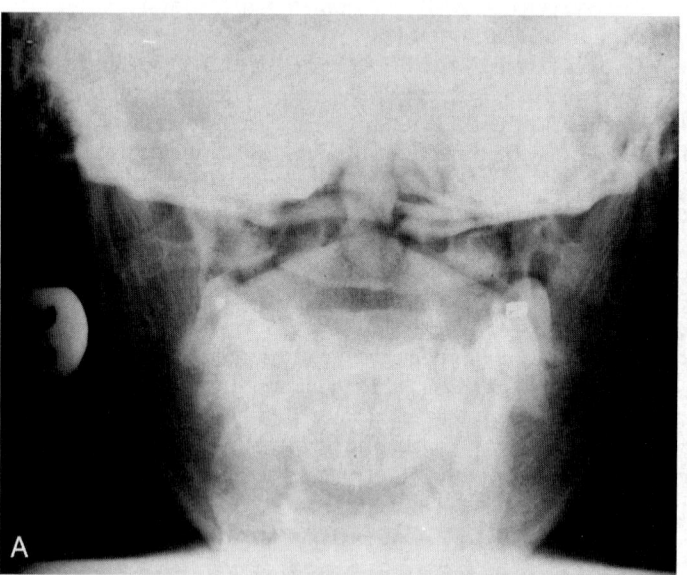

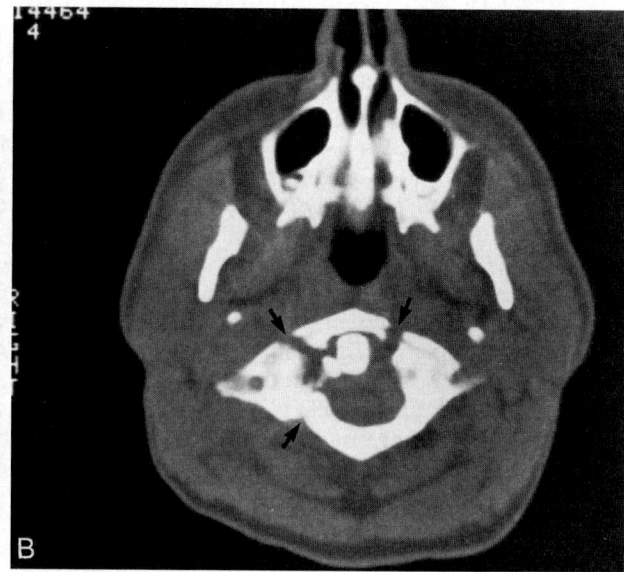

Figure 43.5. Jefferson Fracture. A. An AP open-mouth odontoid view is suspicious for the lateral masses of C1 being laterally displaced on the body of C2. Because of overlying structures, however, this is difficult to appreciate. **B.** A CT examination was obtained and shows multiple fracture sites in the C1 ring (*arrows*). This is called a Jefferson fracture. Computed tomography should be routinely used in spinal trauma because of frequent shortcomings of plain films.

agnosed by an increase of greater than 2.5 mm in the space between the anterior arch of C1 and the dens), however, and when it is, it is then a serious problem. It usually presents spontaneously or after very mild trauma such as an unusual sleeping position.

"Clay-Shoveler's" Fracture. Another relatively innocuous injury is a fracture of the C6 or C7 spinous process called a "clay-shoveler's" fracture. Supposedly, workers shoveling sticky clay would toss the shovel full of clay over their shoulders; once in a while, the clay would stick to the shovel, causing the ligaments attached to the spinous processes (supraspinous liga-

ments) to undergo a tremendous force, pulling on the spinous process and avulsing it. This can occur at any of the lower cervical spinous processes (Fig. 43.7).

"Hangman's" Fracture. A "hangman's" fracture is an unstable, serious fracture of the upper cervical spine that is caused by hyperextension and distraction (such as hitting one's head on a dashboard). This is a fracture of the posterior elements of C2 and, usually, displacement of the C2 body anterior to C3 (Fig. 43.8). These patients actually do better than one might think. They often escape neurologic impairment because of the fractured posterior elements of C2 that, in effect,

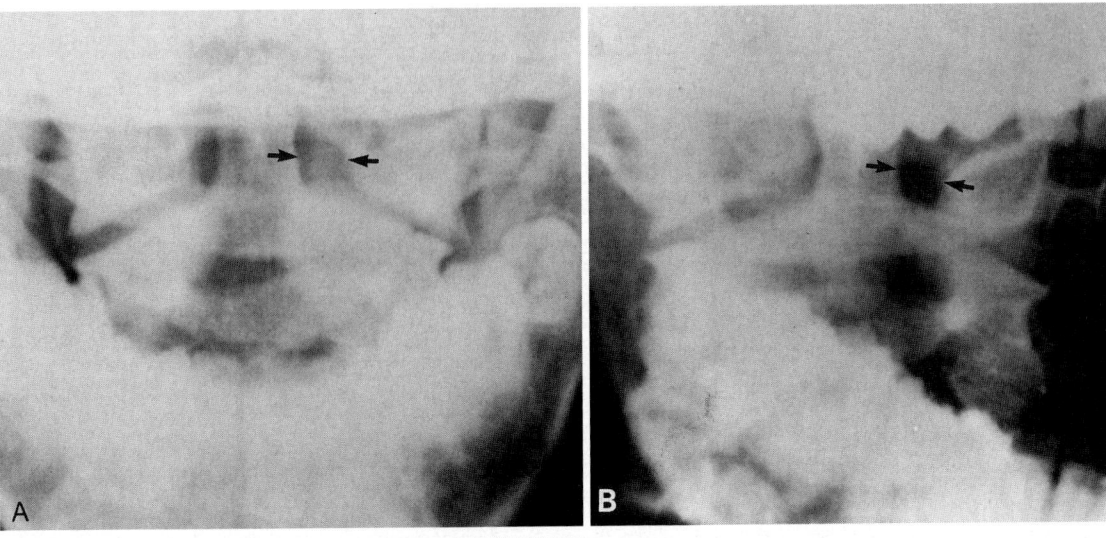

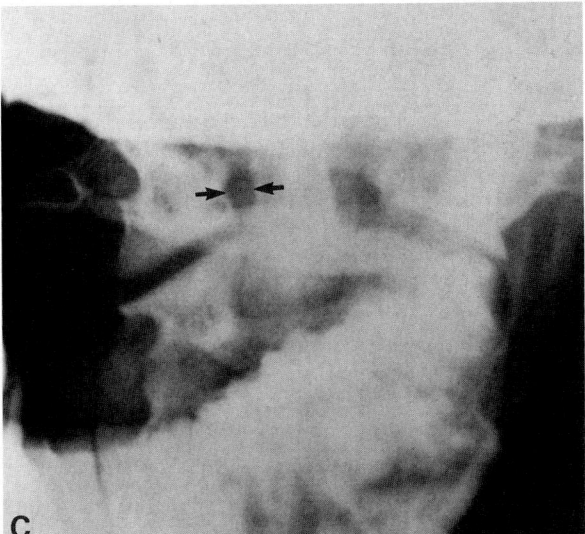

Figure 43.6. Rotary Fixation of the Atlantoaxial Joint. This patient presented to the emergency department with pain and decreased motion in the cervical spine. **A.** An AP open-mouth odontoid view shows the space on the left side of the odontoid between the odontoid and the lateral mass of C1 (*arrows*) is wider than the corresponding space on the right side. This is often the result of rotation. Therefore, open-mouth odontoid views with right and left obliquities were obtained. **B.** This view shows rotation of the patient's head to the left, which causes the space on the left side of the odontoid process (*arrows*) to be wider than that on the right, which is appropriate. **C.** This view, however, shows that when the patient turns the head to the right, the space on the right (*arrows*) does not get wider than the space on the left. This is diagnostic of rotary fixation of the atlantoaxial joint.

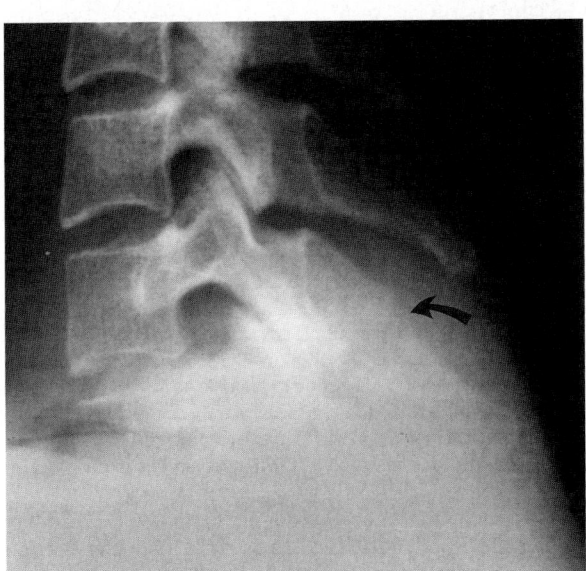

Figure 43.7. Clay Shoveler's Fracture. A nondisplaced fracture of the C7 spinous process (*arrow*) is noted that is diagnostic of a clay shoveler's fracture.

causes a decompression and takes pressure off the injured area.

Flexion-Teardrop Fracture. Severe flexion of the cervical spine can cause a disruption of the posterior ligaments with anterior compression of a vertebral body. This is called a flexion "teardrop" fracture (Fig. 43.9). A teardrop fracture is usually associated with spinal cord injury, often from the posterior portion of the vertebral body being displaced into the central canal.

Unilateral Locked Facets. Severe flexion associated with some rotation can result in rupture of the apophyseal joint ligaments and facet joint dislocation. This can result in locking of the facets in an overriding position that, in effect, causes some stabilization to protect against further injury. This is called unilateral locked facets (Fig. 43.10). It occasionally occurs bilaterally.

"Seatbelt Injury." "Seatbelt injury" is seen secondary to hyperflexion at the waist (as occurs in an automobile accident while restrained by a lap belt). This causes distraction of the posterior elements and ligaments and anterior compression of the vertebral body. It usually involves the T12, L1, or L2 level. Several variations of this

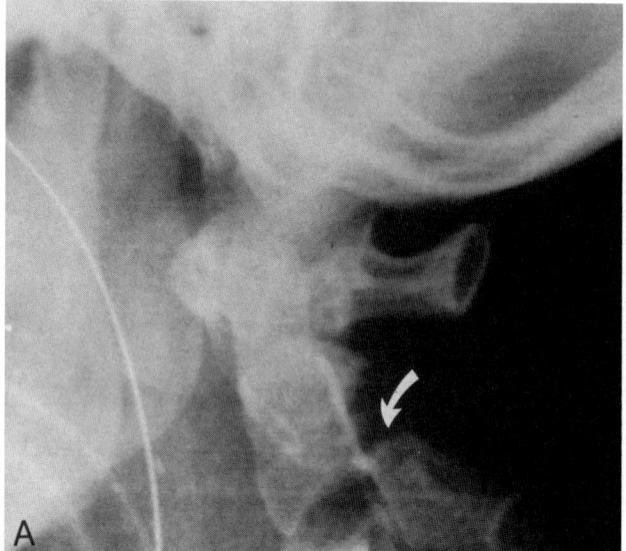

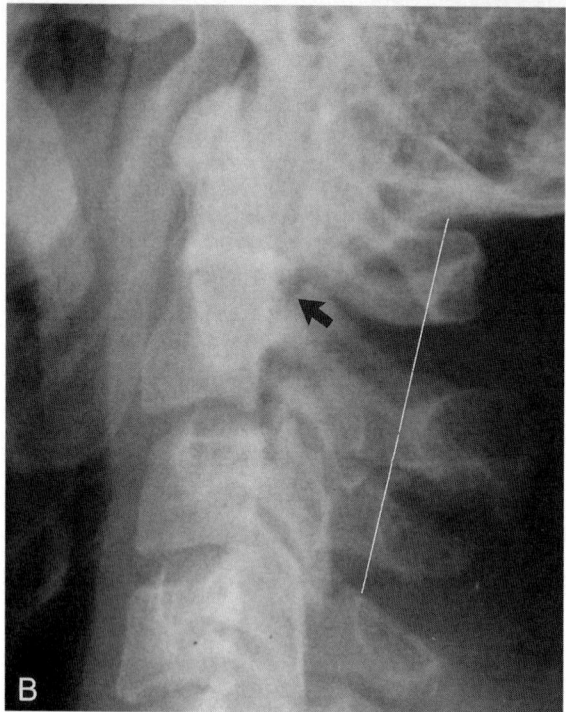

Figure 43.8. Hangman's Fracture. A. Lateral films of a patient with a hangman's fracture shows an obvious example of the posterior elements of the CT vertebral body fractured and displaced inferiorly (*arrow*). **B.** This view shows a very subtle fracture through the posterior elements of C2 (*arrow*) in another patient. A line drawn through the spinolaminal lines of the posterior elements shows the C2 spinolaminal line to be offset posteriorly in this example.

injury can occur: a fracture of the posterior body is called a Smith fracture and a fracture through the spinous process is called a Chance fracture. Horizontal fractures of the pedicles, laminae, and transverse processes can also occur (Fig. 43.11).

Spondylolysis. A somewhat controversial spinal abnormality that might or might not be caused by trauma is spondylolysis. Spondylolysis is a break or defect in the pars interarticularis portion of the lamina (Fig. 43.12). On oblique views, the posterior elements form the figure

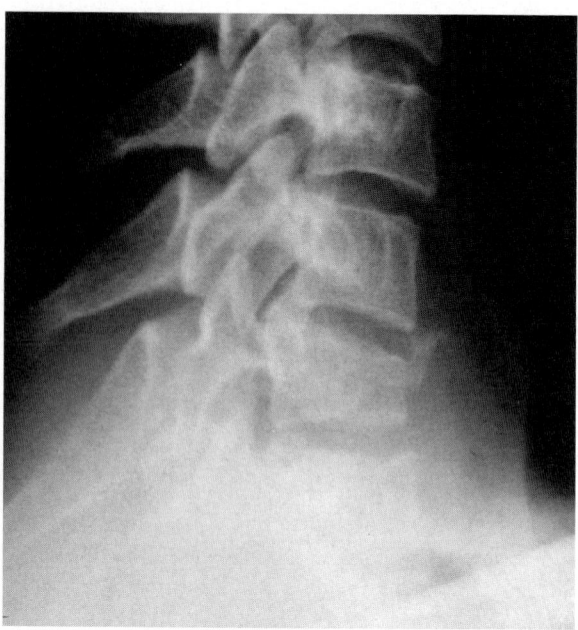

Figure 43.9. Flexion Teardrop Fracture. This patient suffered a hyperflexion injury in an automobile accident and presented to the emergency department with severe neurologic deficits. A lateral x(ib)-ray of the lower cervical spine shows wedging anteriorly of the C7 vertebral body with some displacement of the posterior vertebral line at C7 into the central canal. A small avulsion fracture off the anterior body is also noted.

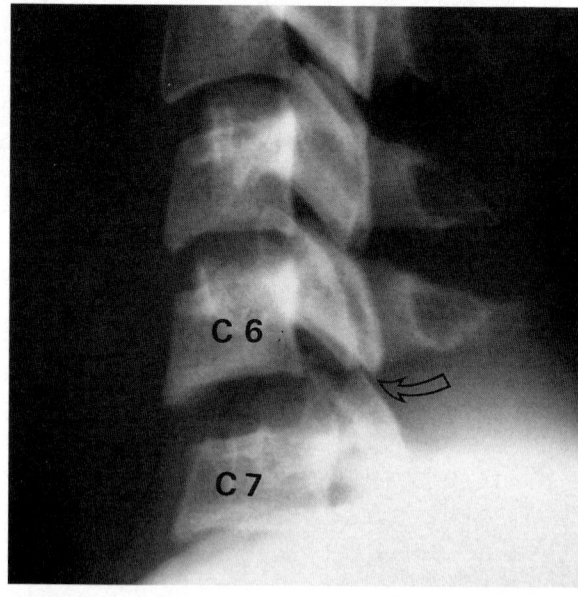

Figure 43.10. Unilateral locked facets. The C6–7 disc space is abnormally widened, and the C7 vertebra is posteriorly located in relation to C6. Also note the C-7 facets, which are dislocated and locked on the C6 facets (*arrow*). When the facets are perched in this manner, it is termed locked facets, which are unilateral in this example.

of a "Scottie dog," with the transverse process being the nose, the pedicle forming the eye, the inferior articular facet being the front leg, the superior articular facet representing the ear, and the pars interarticularis (the portion of the lamina that lies between the facets) equivalent

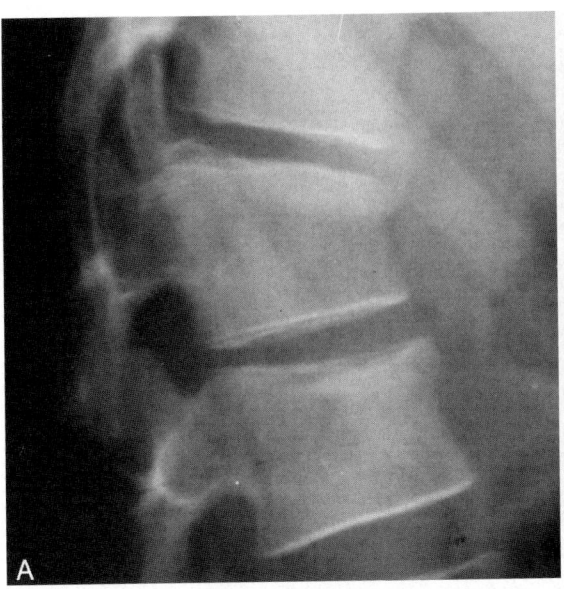 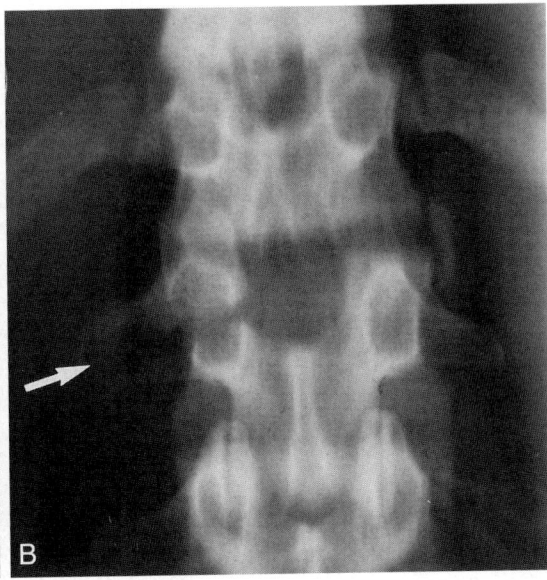

Figure 43.11. Seatbelt Fracture. Hyperflexion at the waist can cause anterior wedging of the vertebral body in the lower thoracic or upper lumbar region as shown in **(A).** By itself, although painful, it is somewhat innocuous; however, **(B)** shows a horizontal fracture through the right transverse process and pedicle (*arrow*) because of extreme traction during the flexion injury. When fracture of the posterior elements occurs, this injury is considered to be unstable and potentially debilitating. Any anterior wedging injury to a vertebral body should have the posterior elements of that level closely inspected.

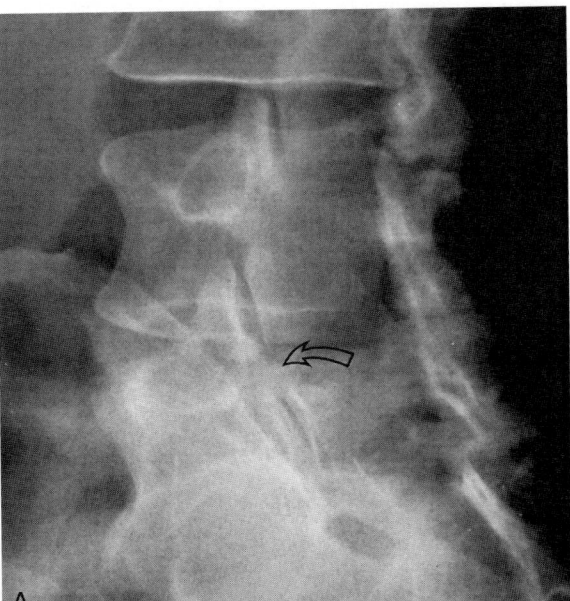

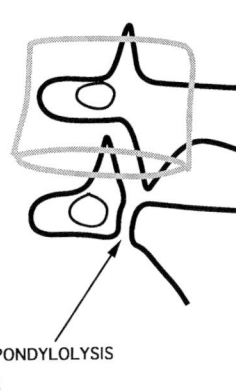

SPONDYLOLYSIS

B

Figure 43.12. Spondylolysis. A. An oblique plain film of the lumbar spine shows a defect in the neck of the "Scottie dog" at L5 (*arrow*), which is diagnostic of a spondylolysis. **B.** A drawing of an oblique view of the lumbar spine shows how a spondylolysis appears as a "collar" around the Scottie dog's neck.

to the neck of the dog. If a spondylolysis is present, the pars interarticularis, or the neck of the dog, will have a defect or break. It often looks as if the Scottie dog has a collar around the neck.

The cause of a spondylolysis is controversial but thought to be congenital and or posttraumatic. Many believe this is a stress-related injury from infancy that develops when toddlers try to walk and repeatedly fall on their buttocks, sending stress to their lower lumbar spine. The significance of spondylolysis is just as controversial as its etiology. More and more clinicians are coming to the viewpoint that a spondylolysis is an inci-

dental finding with no clinical significance in most cases. Certainly some patients have pain related to a spondylolysis and get relief after surgical stabilization. It is important to identify spondylolysis preoperatively in patients undergoing lumbar discectomy so that the possibility of clinical symptoms from the spondylolysis that can mimic disc symptoms can be evaluated. Although plain films can usually show spondylolysis, CT will show it to better advantage, as well as demonstrate any associated disc disease. Magnetic resonance will show spondylolysis, but it can be difficult to see and is easily overlooked with this method.

Figure 43.13. Spondylolisthesis. A. A lateral plain film of the lumbar spine shows that the L5 vertebral body is slightly anteriorly offset on the S1 body as noted by the posterior margins *(arrows)*. **B.** The drawing illustrates this more clearly. Because this offset is less than 25% as measured by the length of the S1 endplate, it is termed a grade 1 spondylolisthesis. A grade 2 offset is more than 25% but less than 50% of the length of the S1 endplate.

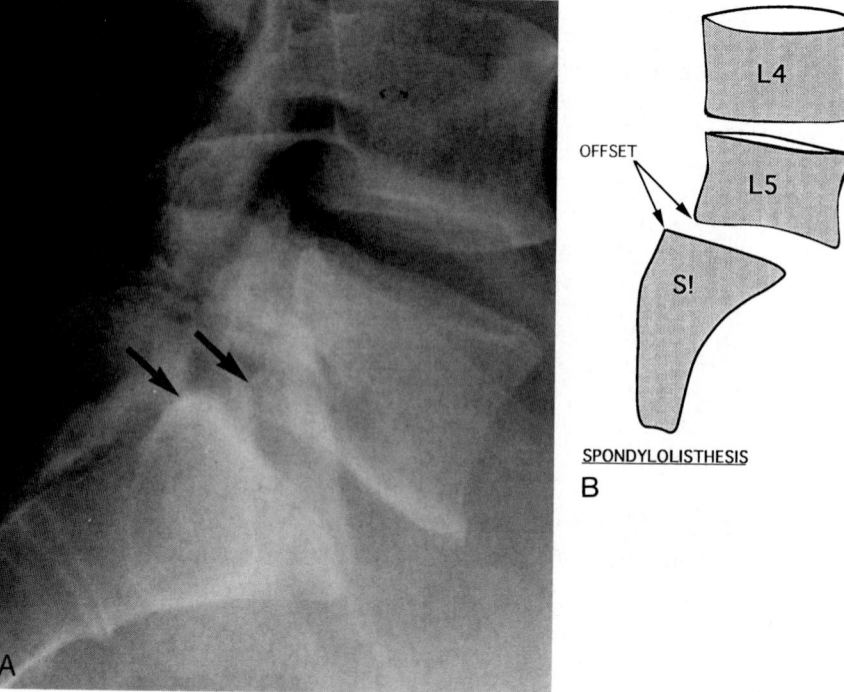

If spondylolysis is bilateral and the vertebral body in the more cephalad position slips forward on the more caudal body, spondylolisthesis is said to be present (Fig. 43.13). Spondylolisthesis might or might not be symptomatic and by itself has no clinical significance. If severe, it can cause neuroforaminal stenosis and can impinge on the nerve roots in the central spinal canal. If it is symptomatic, it can be stabilized surgically.

HAND AND WRIST

Several seemingly innocuous fractures in the hand require surgical fixation rather than just casting and, therefore, should be recognized by the radiologist as serious injuries.

Bennett's Fracture. One such fracture is a fracture at the base of the thumb into the carpometacarpal joint, a Bennett's fracture (Fig. 43.14). Because of the insertion of the strong thumb adductors at the base of the thumb, it is almost impossible to keep the metacarpal from sliding off its proper alignment. It almost always requires internal fixation. The radiologist occasionally has to remind a nonorthopaedic practitioner of this, as well as closely examine the alignment of a Bennett's fracture in plaster that has not been internally fixed with wires.

A comminuted fracture of the base of the thumb that extends into the joint has been termed a Rolando fracture (Fig. 43.15), and a fracture of the base of the thumb that does not involve the joint has been called a pseudo-Bennett's fracture.

Mallet Finger or Baseball Finger is an avulsion injury at the base of the distal phalanx (Fig. 43.16) where the extensor digitorum tendon inserts. With the extensor tendon inoperative, the distal phalanx flexes without opposition, which can result in a flexion deformity and in-

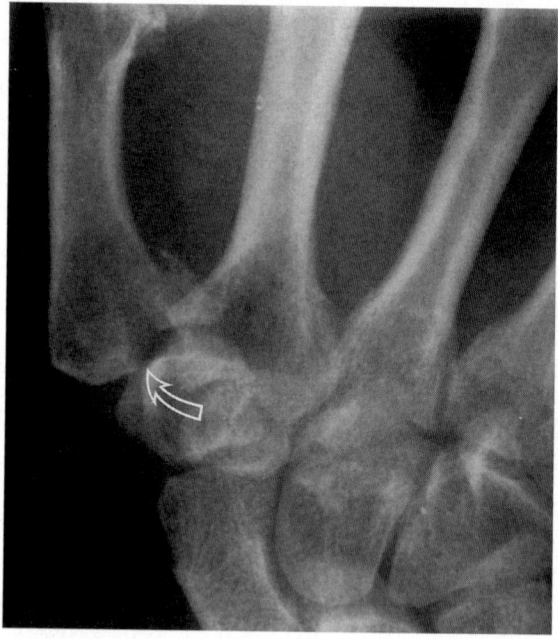

Figure 43.14. Bennett's Fracture. A small corner fracture of the base of the thumb is noted that involves the articular surface of the base of the thumb *(arrow)*; this is a serious injury that almost always requires internal fixation.

ability to extend the distal phalanx if not properly treated.

A fracture at the volar aspect of the base of the interphalangeal and metacarpophalangeal joints from an avulsion of the volar plate can appear innocent but often requires surgical intervention. The volar plate is a dense fibrocartilaginous band that covers the joint on the volar aspect and can get interposed in the joint once it is torn, often requiring surgical removal.

"Gamekeeper's Thumb." Another innocent-appearing fracture that often requires internal fixation is an avulsion on the ulnar aspect of the first metacarpophalangeal joint (Fig. 43.17); this is where the ulnar collateral ligament of the thumb inserts. If the ulnar collateral ligament is torn, normal function of the thumb can be impaired, and this can have a serious result if not properly treated. This injury is called a "gamekeeper's thumb" because of the propensity of English game wardens to acquire it from breaking rabbits' necks between their thumb and forefinger. A more current scenario is falling on a ski pole and having the pole jam into the webbing between the thumb and index finger. This avulsion injury usually requires pinning to fix the ligament securely.

Lunate/Perilunate Dislocation. A fall on the outstretched arm can result in any number of wrist fractures and dislocations. One serious such injury is the lunate/perilunate dislocation. This occurs when the ligaments between the capitate and the lunate are disrupted, allowing the capitate to dislocate from the cup-shaped articulation of the lunate. This is best seen on lateral views. Ordinarily, on the lateral view the capitate should be seen seated in the cup-shaped lunate (Figs. 43.18, 43.19A). In a dorsal dislocation (the capitate occasionally dislocates volarly, but this is uncommon), the capitate and all of its surrounding bones, including the metacarpals, come to lie dorsal to a line drawn through the radius and the lunate (Figs. 43.19B, 43.20). If the capitate then pushes the lunate volarly and tips it over, the line drawn up through the radius shows the lunate volarly displaced and the line goes through the capitate. This has been termed a lunate dislocation (Figs. 43.19C, 43.21). Failure to diagnose and treat this disorder can result in permanent median nerve impairment, as it can get impinged by the volarly displaced lunate.

A lunate or perilunate dislocation can be diagnosed on an AP view of the wrist by noting a triangular or pie-shaped lunate (Fig. 43.21B). Ordinarily, the lunate has a rhomboid shape on the AP view, with the upper and lower borders parallel.

Several fractures are known to be associated with a perilunate dislocation, the most common of which is a transscaphoid fracture. The capitate, radial styloid, and triquetrum are also known to fracture frequently when a perilunate dislocation occurs.

Hook of the Hamate Fracture. One of the most difficult wrist fractures to identify radiologically is a fracture of the hook of the hamate. A special view, the carpal tunnel view, should be obtained when trying to see the hook of the hamate. This view is obtained with the wrist (palm down) flat on an x-ray plate and the fingers pulled dorsally. The x-ray beam is angled about 45°, parallel to the palm of the hand so that the carpal tunnel is in profile. The hook of the hamate is seen as a bony protuberance off the hamate on the ulnar aspect of the carpal tunnel. A fractured hook of the hamate is often identified with the carpal tunnel view (Fig. 43.22) but can occasionally be very difficult to visualize. A CT scan will often show an obvious fracture that the plain film does not (Fig. 43.23) and should be considered in any possible carpal fracture when plain films are not diagnostic.

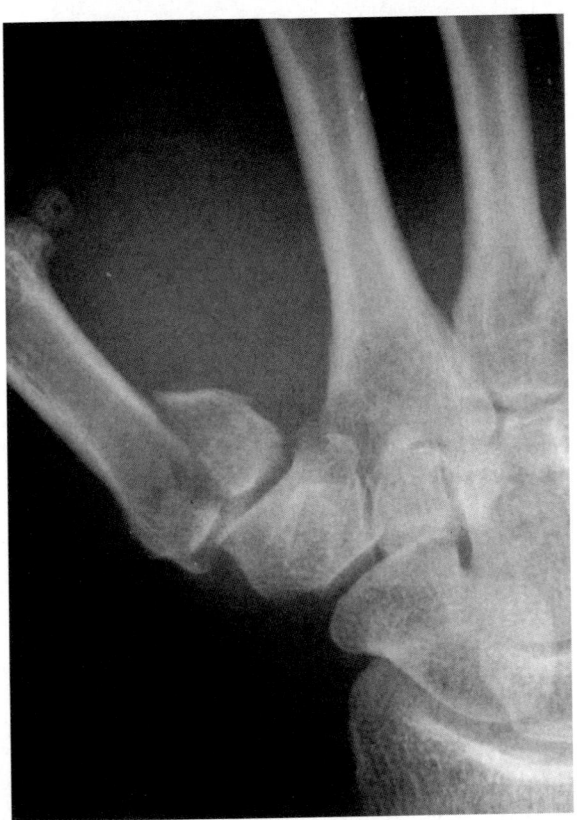

Figure 43.15. Rolando Fracture. A comminuted fracture of the base of the thumb that extends into the articular surface is a more serious type of Bennett's fracture, which has been termed a Rolando fracture.

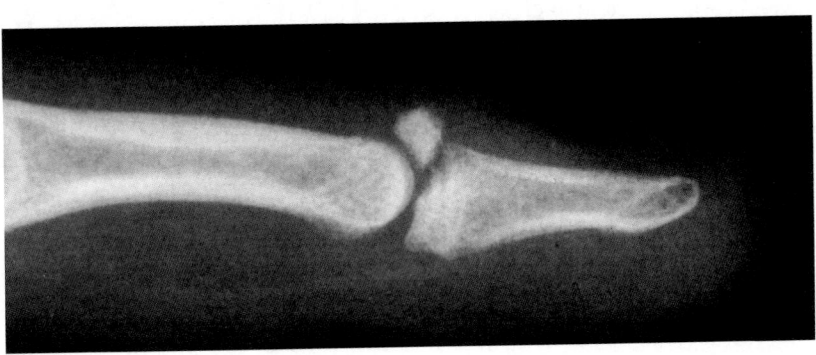

Figure 43.16. Mallet Finger. A small avulsion injury is noted at the base of the distal phalanx, which is where the extensor digitorum tendon inserts. This is termed a mallet finger or baseball finger because it is often caused by a baseball striking the distal phalanx and causing the avulsion.

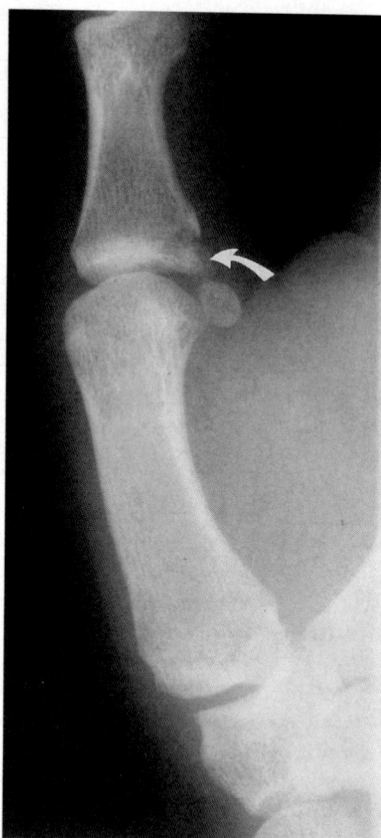

Figure 43.17. Gamekeeper's Thumb. A small avulsion injury on the ulnar aspect of the first metacarpophalangeal joint (*arrow*) is diagnostic of a gamekeeper's thumb. This is the insertion site for the ulnar collateral ligament and usually requires internal fixation.

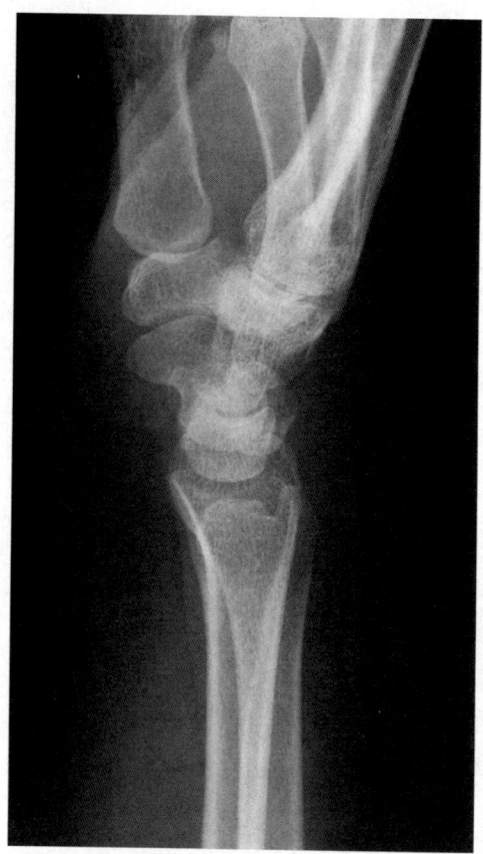

Figure 43.18. Normal Lateral Radiograph of the Wrist. The normal lateral view should show the lunate seated in the distal radius and the capitate seated in the lunate. A line drawn up through the radius should connect all three structures. Compare this radiograph with the drawing in Figure 43.19A.

A fracture of the hook of the hamate most commonly occurs from a fall on the outstretched hand. A clinical setting that has gained attention in sports-medicine circles is that of a professional athlete who participates in an activity in which the butt of a club, bat, or racket is held in the palm of the hand. Overswinging can result in the butt of the club levering off the hook of the hamate. This has been seen in professional baseball players, tennis players, and golfers. It is not seen in amateurs because they usually are not strong enough to exert enough force to lever the hook off and, if they do, will usually terminate that activity, allowing healing, whereas a professional will continue participation, which can lead to a nonunion of the fracture.

Rotary subluxation of the navicular is another wrist injury seen after a fall onto the outstretched hand. This results from rupture of the scapholunate ligament, which allows the scaphoid (navicular) to rotate dorsally. On an AP wrist plain film, a space is seen between the navicular and the lunate (Fig. 43.24) where ordinarily they are closely opposed. This has been called the "Terry Thomas" sign after the famous British actor with a gap between his two front teeth.

Navicular Fracture. A fracture of the navicular is a potentially serious injury because of the high rate of avascular necrosis that occurs with this injury. When avascular necrosis occurs, it usually requires surgical

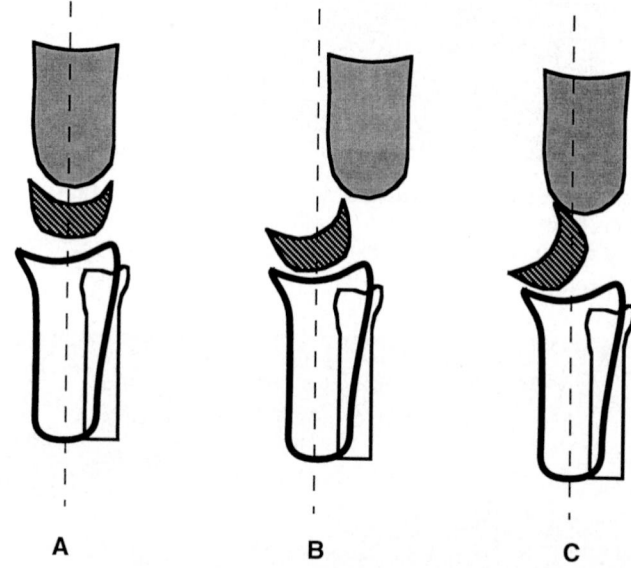

A   B   C

Figure 43.19. Perilunate and Lunate Dislocations. Schematic depiction of normal lateral wrist **(A)**, perilunate dislocation **(B)**, and lunate dislocation **(C)**. (Dorsal is to the right.)

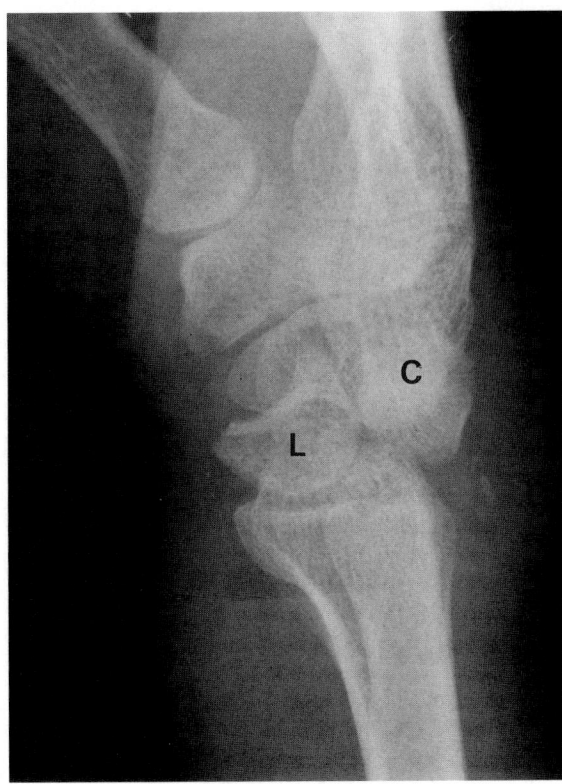

Figure 43.20. Perilunate Dislocation. Although the lunate (*L*) is normal in relation to the distal radius, the capitate (*C*) and the remainder of the wrist are dorsally displaced in relation to the lunate. Compare this radiograph with the drawing in Figure 43.19B.

intervention with bone grafting to obtain healing. This fracture can be very difficult to detect initially; therefore, whenever a fracture of the navicular is clinically suspect (trauma with pain over the snuffbox of the wrist), the wrist should be casted and repeat radiographs obtained in 1 week. Often, the fracture is then visualized because of the disuse osteoporosis and hyperemia around the fracture site.

If avascular necrosis of the navicular develops, it is the proximal fragment that undergoes necrosis because the blood supply to the navicular begins distally and runs proximally. A fracture with disruption of the blood supply thus leaves the proximal pole without a vascular supply; hence, it dies. Avascular necrosis is diagnosed by noting increased density of the proximal pole of the navicular compared with the remainder of the carpal bones (Fig. 43.25).

Avascular necrosis can occur in other carpal bones, most commonly the lunate. This is called Kienböck's malacia and is most often caused by trauma; however, it is also thought to be idiopathic. It is diagnosed by noting the increased density to the lunate bone, which might or might not go on to collapse and fragmentation (Fig. 43.26). It often requires surgical bone grafting and occasionally, removal or proximal carpal row fusion. It has a high association with a discrepancy between the length of the radius and the ulna as seen at the radiocarpal joint. If the ulna is shorter than the radius, it is termed negative ulnar variance and there is an increased incidence of Kienböck's malacia (Fig. 43.26). If the ulna is longer than the radius, it is termed positive ulnar variance and there is an increased incidence of triangular fibrocartilage tears.

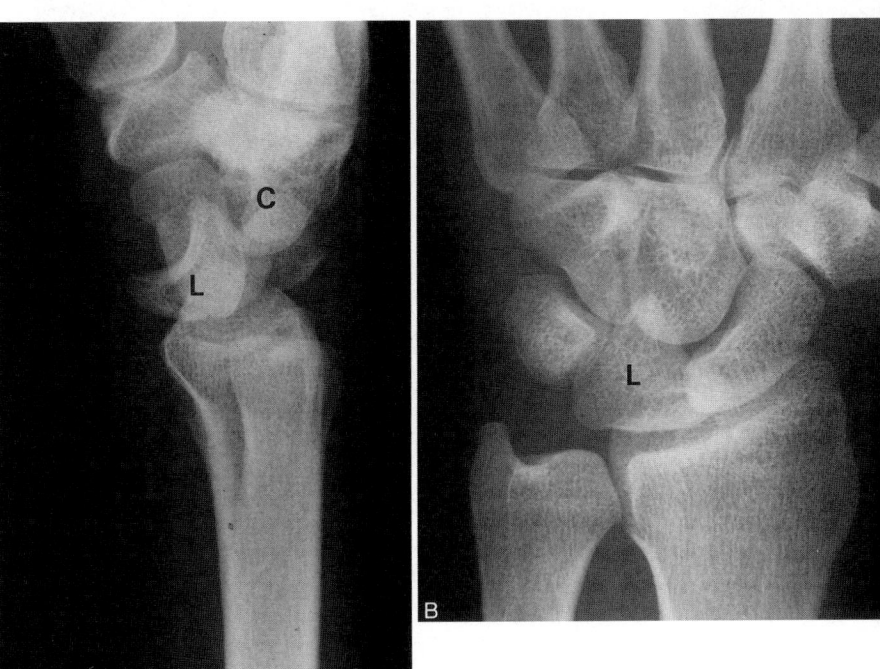

Figure 43.21. Lunate Dislocation. A. The lateral radiograph of the wrist shows the lunate (*L*) tipped off of the distal radius, whereas the capitate (*C*) seems to be normally aligned in relation to the radius, yet is dislocated from the lunate. Compare this with the drawing in Figure 43.19C. The AP view shows a pie-shaped lunate **(B)** (*L*) rather than a lunate with a more rhomboid shape. A pie-shaped lunate on the AP view is diagnostic of a perilunate or lunate dislocation.

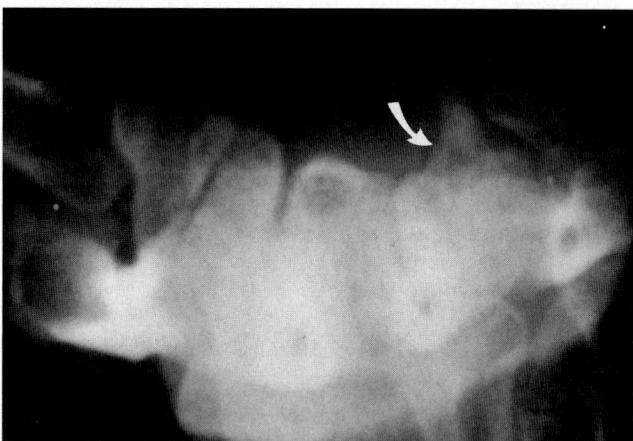

Figure 43.22. Fracture of the Hook of the Hamate. The hook of the hamate is seen on a carpal tunnel view in this patient and has an area of sclerosis with a faint cortical break (*arrow*). This represents a fracture at the base of the hook of the hamate.

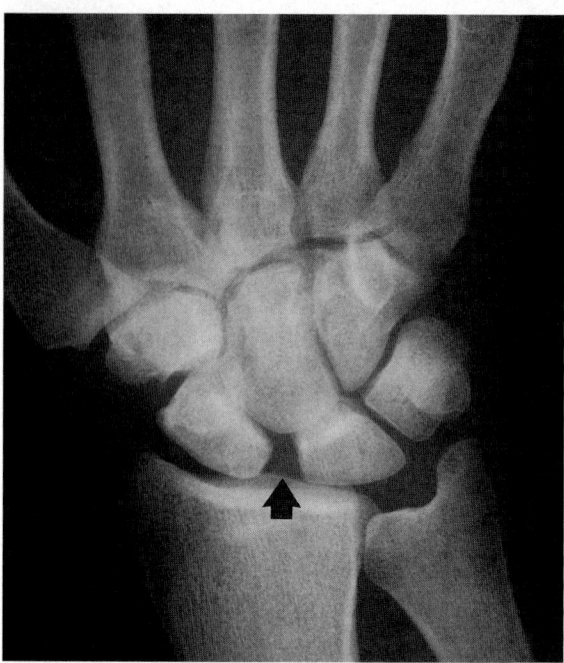

Figure 43.24. Rotatory Subluxation of the Navicular. An AP view of the wrist shows a gap or space between the navicular and the lunate (*arrow*). This is abnormal and represents the "Terry Thomas" sign, which means the scapholunate ligament is ruptured. This is diagnostic of a rotatory subluxation of the navicular.

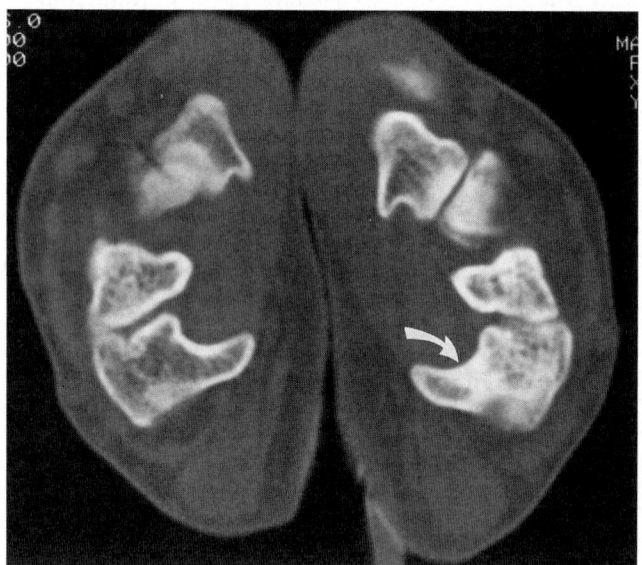

Figure 43.23. A CT of a Fractured Hamate. A CT scan through the wrist in this patient shows a faint lucency surrounded by sclerosis in the left hamate (*arrow*), which represents a fracture through the base of the hook of the hamate with moderate reactive sclerosis. This could not be seen in the plain films, even in retrospect.

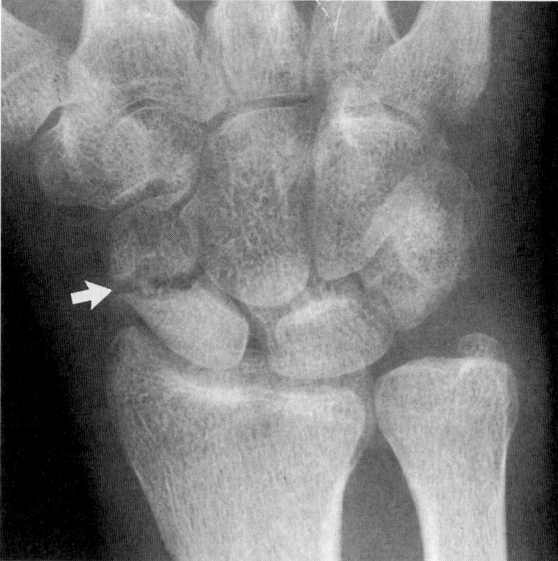

Figure 43.25. Avascular Necrosis of the Navicular. An AP view of the wrist shows a fracture through the waist of the navicular (*arrow*). The proximal half of the navicular is slightly sclerotic in relation to the remainder of the carpal bones, which indicates avascular necrosis of the proximal half.

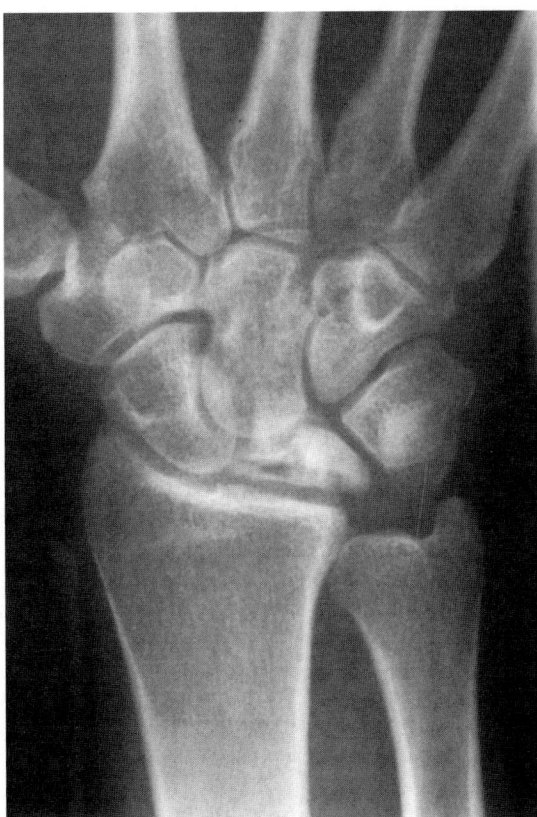

Figure 43.26. Kienböck's Malacia. An AP view of the wrist reveals the lunate to be sclerotic and abnormal in shape. The lunate has collapsed because of aseptic necrosis. This is known as Keinböck's malacia. Note that the ulna is shorter than the radius, this is termed negative ulnar variance, which is often associated with Kienböck's malacia.

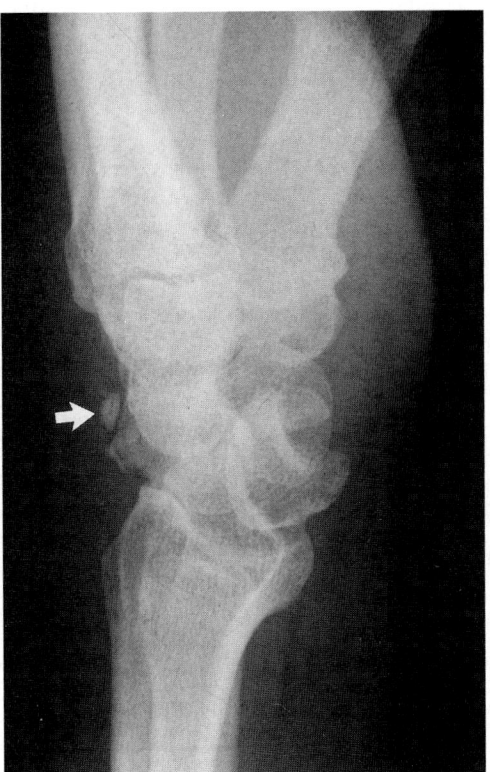

Figure 43.27. Triquetral Fracture and Perilunate Dislocation. A perilunate or lunate dislocation is present (it is difficult to classify exactly which has occurred because both the lunate and the capitate are out of their normal position). A small avulsion is seen on the dorsum of the wrist (*arrow*), which is virtually diagnostic of an avulsion off the triquetrum. It is often associated with a lunate or perilunate dislocation.

A common avulsion fracture in the wrist is a triquetral fracture. It is best seen on a lateral film, which shows a small chip of bone off the dorsum of the wrist (Fig. 43.27). This is virtually pathognomonic of an avulsion from the triquetrum.

ARM

Colles' Fracture. One of the most common fractures of the forearm is a fracture of the distal radius and ulna after a fall on an outstretched arm. This results in a dorsal angulation of the distal forearm and wrist and is called a Colles' fracture (Fig. 43.28). When the fracture angulates volarly, it is called a Smith's fracture (Fig. 43.29). A Smith's fracture is a much less common occurrence than a Colles' fracture. Sometimes the radius and ulna suffer a traumatic insult, and the force on the bones causes bending instead of a frank fracture. This has been termed a plastic bowing deformity of the forearm (Fig. 43.30) and is often treated by breaking the bones while the patient has undergone anesthesia and resetting them. Left untreated, a plastic bowing deformity can result in reduced supination and pronation.

Monteggia Fracture. The forearm is a two-bone system that has some of the same properties as a ring bone. As mentioned previously, a solid ring cannot break in

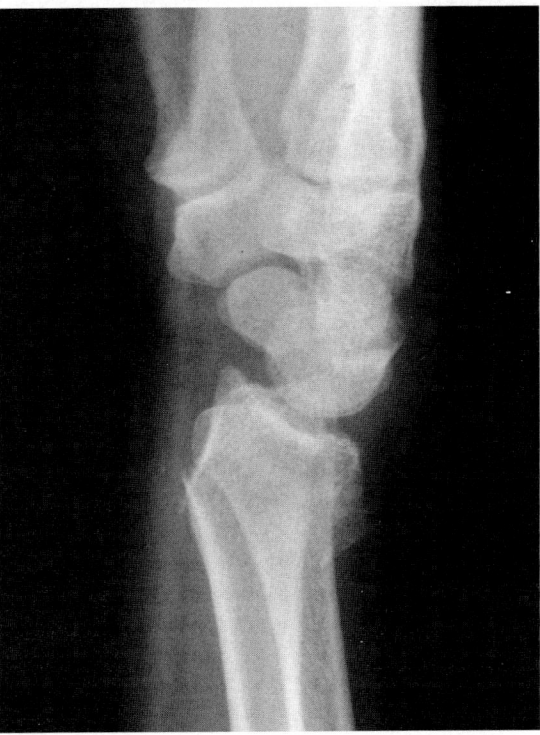

Figure 43.28. Colles' Fracture. A fracture of the distal radius with dorsal angulation is noted, which has been termed a Colles' fracture.

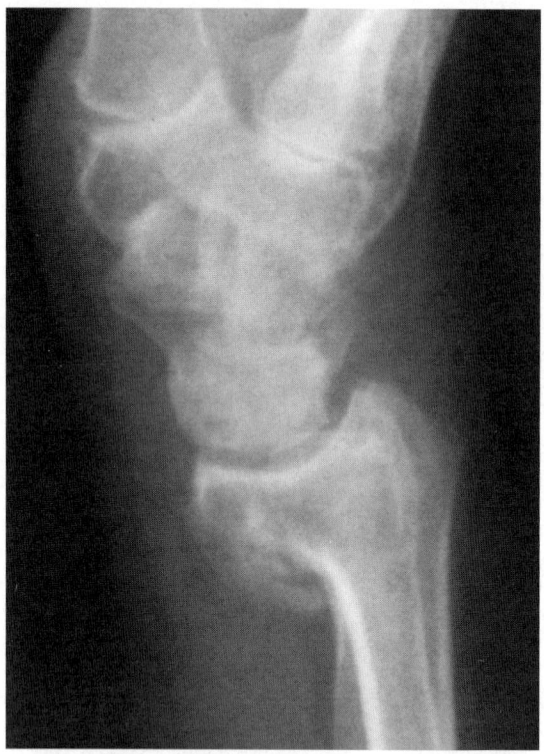

Figure 43.29. Smith's Fracture. A fracture of the distal radius with volar angulation such as this is called a Smith's fracture. This is a much less common injury than the Colles' fracture, shown in Figure 43.28.

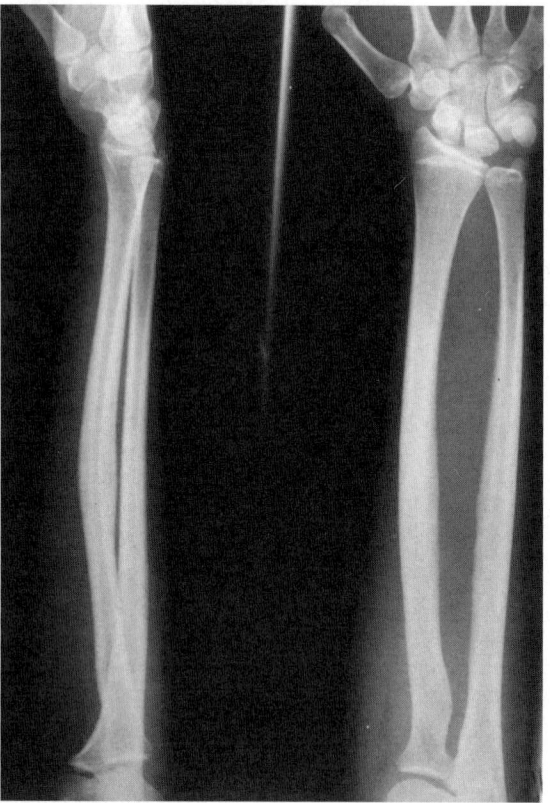

Figure 43.30. Plastic Bowing Deformity of the Forearm. These AP and lateral views of the forearm of a child show the radius to be abnormally bowed anteriorly. This has been termed a plastic bowing deformity of the forearm and occurs only in children.

only a single place, it must break in at least two points. In the forearm, a fracture of one bone should be accompanied by a fracture of the other. If the second fracture is not present, a dislocation of the nonfractured bone usually occurs. The most common example of this is a fracture of the ulna with a dislocation of the proximal radius (Fig. 43.31). This is called a Monteggia fracture. It has also been termed a nightstick injury, from a police officer hitting someone with a nightstick. The person being hit instinctively raises the arm for protection and the nightstick falls on the ulna, fracturing it and dislocating the radial head. The dislocated radial head can be missed clinically and develop into aseptic necrosis with subsequent elbow dysfunction. Whenever the forearm is fractured, the elbow must be examined to exclude a dislocation.

Galeazzi Fracture. A fracture of the radius with dislocation of the distal ulna is called a Galeazzi fracture (Fig. 43.32). This is much less common than a Monteggia fracture, and because the deformity of the dislocated ulna is usually obvious, it is rarely missed clinically.

A helpful indicator of a fracture about the elbow is a displaced posterior fat pad. Ordinarily, the posterior fat pad is not visible on a lateral view of the elbow because it is tucked away in the olecranon fossa of the distal humerus. When the joint becomes distended with blood

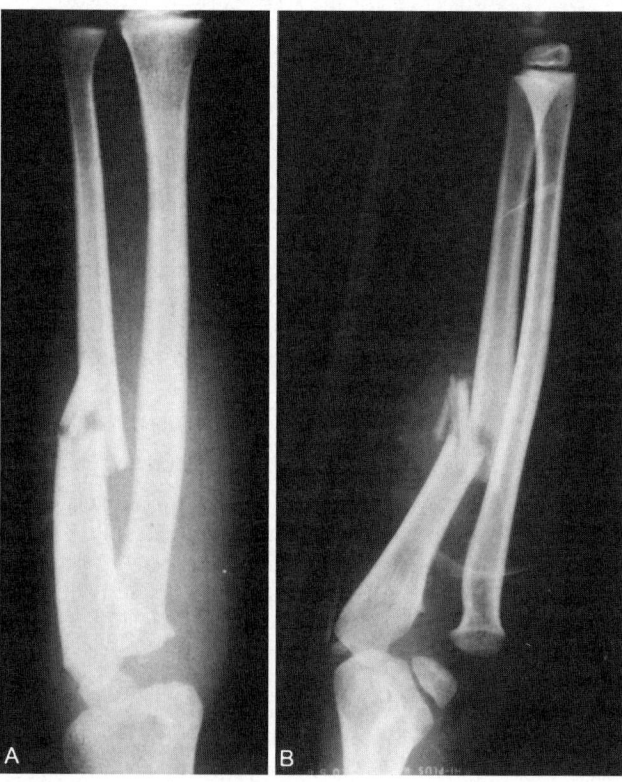

Figure 43.31. Monteggia Fracture. A blow to the forearm such as with a policeperson's nightstick can result in a fracture of the ulna **(A)**. Although the head of the radius appears normally placed in **(A)** the lateral examination shown in **(B)** reveals the head of the radius to be displaced. Failure to recognize this abnormality can result in death of the radial head, with subsequent elbow dysfunction. This illustrates the importance of always obtaining two views of a bone after trauma.

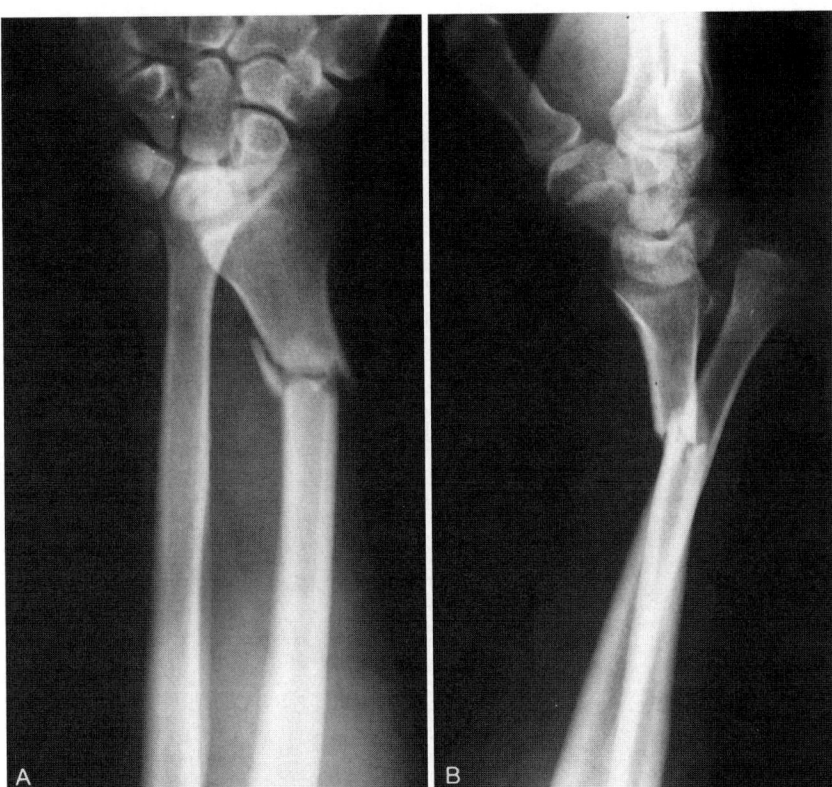

Figure 43.32. Galeazzi Fracture. A. A fracture of the distal radius in this patient is seen on the AP view without a definite fracture of the ulna. **B.** This view shows an obvious dislocation of the distal ulna, which would almost certainly not be missed clinically. This has been termed a Galeazzi fracture and is much less common than the Monteggia fractures.

secondary to a fracture, the posterior fat pad is displaced out of the olecranon fossa and is visible on the lateral view (Fig. 43.33A). Therefore, in the setting of trauma, a visible posterior fat pad indicates a fracture. In an adult (epiphyses closed), the fracture site is almost always the radial head (Fig. 43.33B). In a child (epiphyses open), it is usually indicative of a supracondylar fracture (Fig. 43.34).

Often, the fracture itself is not visualized, and extraordinary steps are taken by clinicians and radiologists alike to demonstrate the fracture. These steps include oblique views, special radial head views, tomograms, and even CT scans or MR studies. These are absurd attempts to document pathology that will be treated identically whether or not it is radiographically recorded. As long as there is no obvious deformity or loose body, it does not matter whether the fracture is definitely identified or not in a patient with a posttraumatic painful elbow and a visible posterior fat pad. An infection, an arthritide, or any elbow effusion could cause a joint effusion and a displaced posterior fat pad, but the clinical setting would not be to rule out a fracture.

The anterior fat pad also gets displaced with a joint effusion. Ordinarily it is visible as a small triangle just anterior to the distal humeral diaphysis on a lateral film (Fig. 43.35). With an effusion, it gets displaced superiorly and outward from the humerus and has been called a "sail sign" because it resembles a spinnaker sail (see Figs. 43.33, 43.34).

Shoulder Dislocations are generally easily diagnosed, both clinically and radiographically. The most common shoulder dislocation is the anterior dislocation. It is at least 10 times more common than a posterior dis-

location. For all practical purposes, anterior and posterior dislocations are the only two types of shoulder dislocations about which to be concerned.

An anterior dislocation occurs when the arm is forcibly externally rotated and abducted. This is commonly seen when football players "arm tackle," when kayakers "brace" with the paddle above their heads and allow their arms to get too far posterior, when skiers plant their uphill pole and get it stuck, and from other similar athletic positions. Radiographically, the diagnosis is easily made on an AP shoulder film: the humeral head is seen to lie inferiorly and medial to the glenoid (Fig. 43.36). The humeral head often impacts on the inferior lip of the glenoid causing an indentation on the posterosuperior portion of the humeral head; this is called a Hill-Sachs deformity. The presence of a Hill-Sachs deformity is said to indicate a greater likelihood of recurrent dislocation, and some surgeons use it as an indicator to intervene surgically to prevent a recurrence. A bony irregularity or fragment off the inferior glenoid, which occurs from the same mechanism as the Hill-Sachs deformity, is called a Bankart deformity. It is not seen radiographically as often as the Hill-Sachs deformity.

A posterior dislocation can be a difficult diagnosis to make, both clinically and radiographically. An AP view may look completely normal, or nearly so. On the AP view of a normal shoulder, the humeral head should slightly overlap the glenoid (Fig. 43.37), forming what has been called a "crescent sign." In a patient with a posterior dislocation, this crescent of bony overlap is usually absent and a small space is seen between the glenoid and the humeral head (Fig. 43.38).

The best way to diagnose unequivocally a dislocated

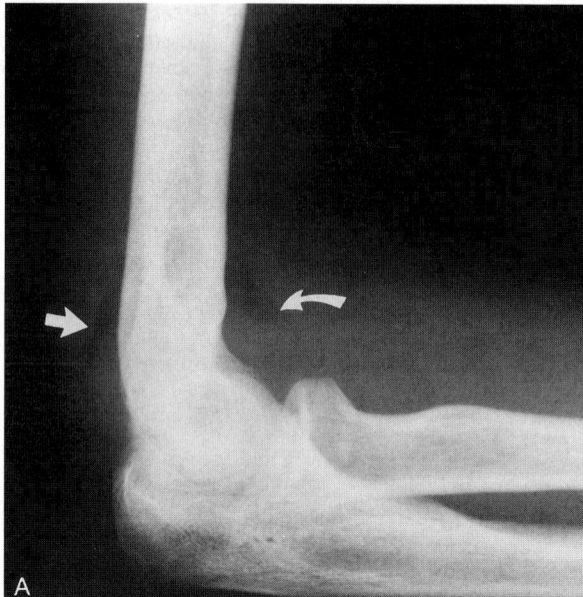

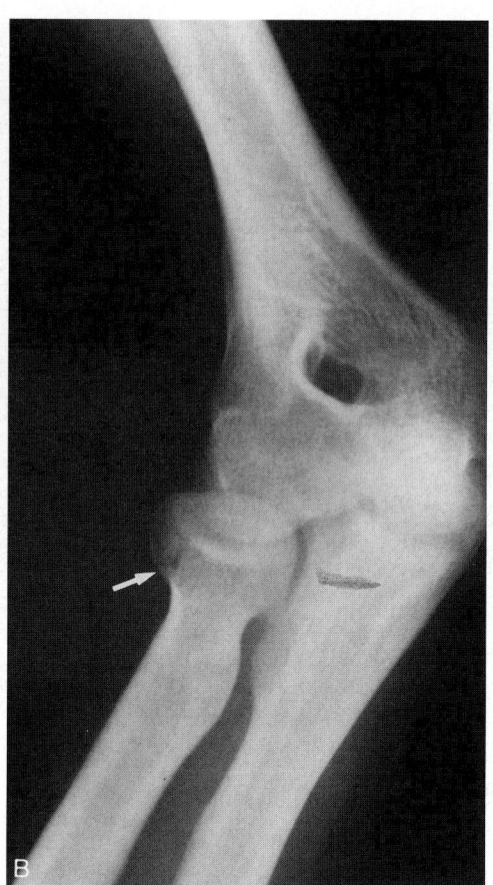

Figure 43.33. Displaced Elbow Fat Pads. A. On the lateral view of this elbow, the posterior fat pad is faintly visible (*arrow*) and the anterior fat pad is elevated and anteriorly displaced (*curved arrow*). These findings indicate a fracture about the elbow that in an adult should be in the radial head. **B.** An oblique view shows the fracture of the radial head (*arrow*). Even without seeing the fracture on the radiographs, it should be surmised to be present when the posterior fat pad is visualized in the setting of trauma. The elevated and displaced anterior fat pad has been termed a sail sign.

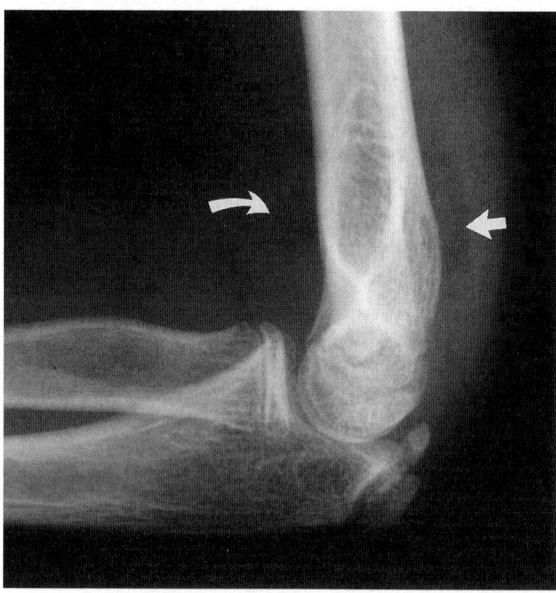

Figure 43.34. Displaced Elbow Fat Pads. A lateral view of the elbow in this child shows a posterior fat pad (*arrow*) and a sail sign anteriorly (*curved arrow*). This is indicative of a fracture about the elbow, which in a child (epiphyses are open) usually means a supracondylar fracture.

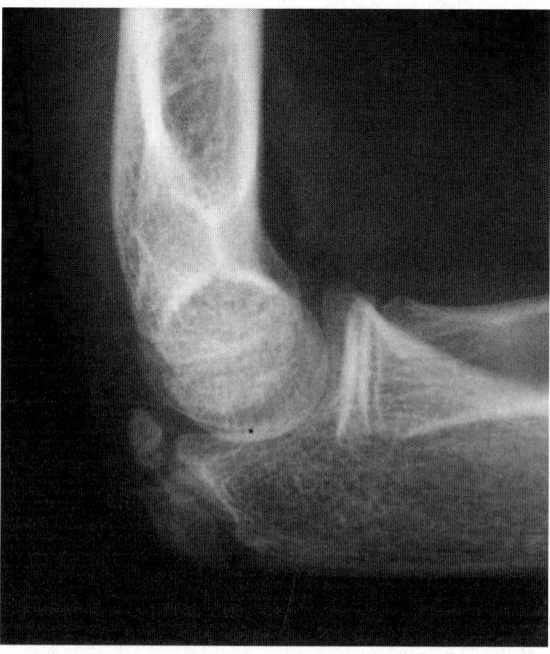

Figure 43.35. Normal Anterior Fat Pad of the Elbow. Note the lucency just anterior to the humerus of this normal elbow and compare this with the sail sign of the anterior fat pads in Figures 43.33 and 43.34.

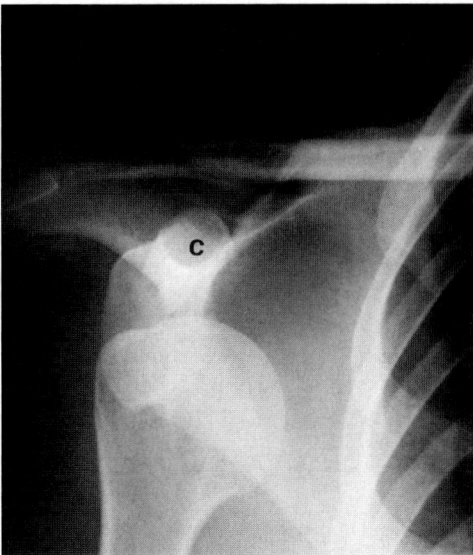

Figure 43.36. Anterior Shoulder Dislocation. An AP view of the right shoulder shows the humeral head to lie medial to the glenoid and inferior to the coracoid process (*C*). This is diagnostic of an anterior dislocation of the shoulder.

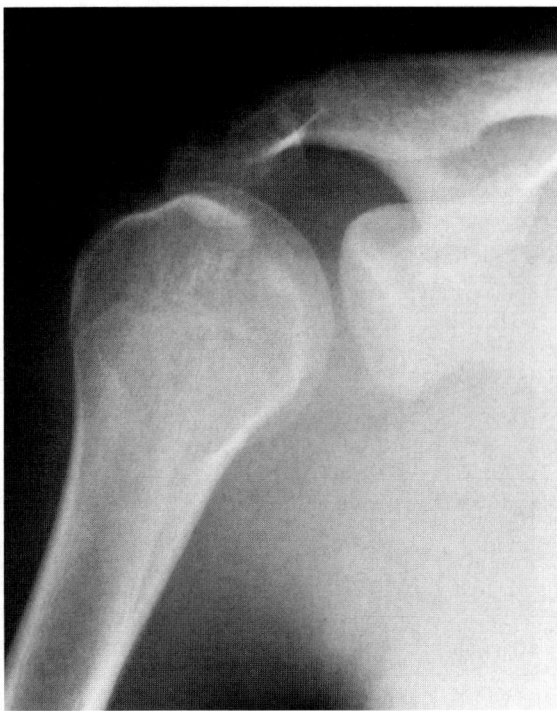

Figure 43.38. Posterior Shoulder Dislocation. Note that the humeral head in this patient is slightly displaced from the glenoid on the AP view. This is termed absence of the crescent sign and is often seen with a posterior dislocation. Compare this with the normal shoulder in Figure 43.37.

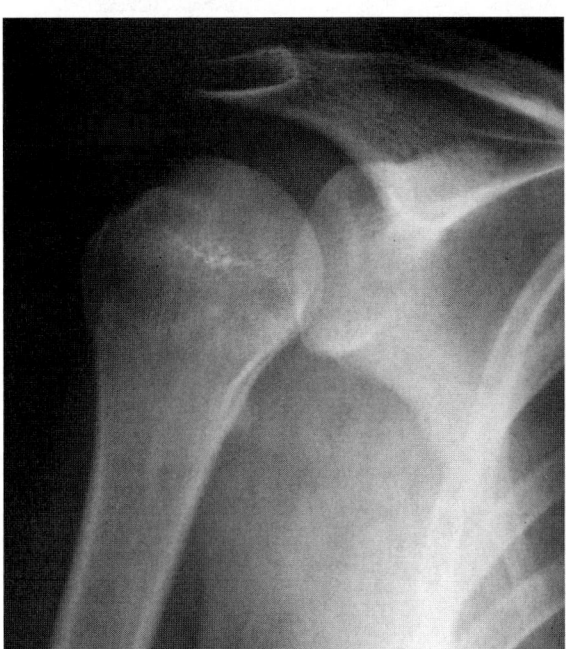

Figure 43.37. Normal AP View of the Shoulder. Note in this example of a normal shoulder that the humeral head slightly overlaps the glenoid, which has been termed the crescent sign.

shoulder is to obtain a transscapular view. An axillary view will show basically the same thing but requires the patient to move the arm and shoulder, which can be painful and may even redislocate the shoulder if it has spontaneously reduced itself. The transscapular view is obtained by angling the x-ray beam across the shoulder in the same plane as the blade of the scapula. This gives an en face view of the glenoid, and the humeral head can easily be related to it as either normal, anterior (Fig. 43.39), or posterior. Because of frequently overlapping

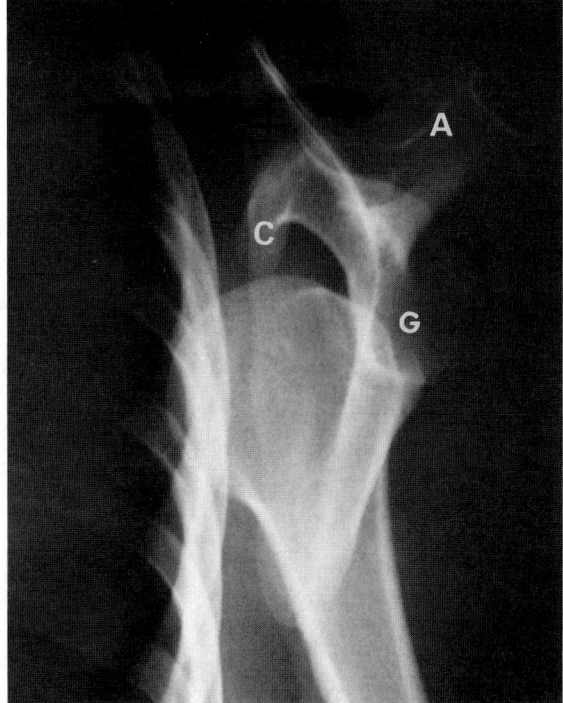

Figure 43.39. Transscapular View of an Anterior Dislocation. This transscapular view of the shoulder is obtained by aiming the x-ray beam parallel to the shoulder blade. The coracoid process (*C*) can be seen anteriorly and the spine of the acromion (*A*) can be seen posteriorly. Both of these structures extend inwardly and meet at the glenoid (*G*). The humeral head is seen in this example to lie anterior to the glenoid.

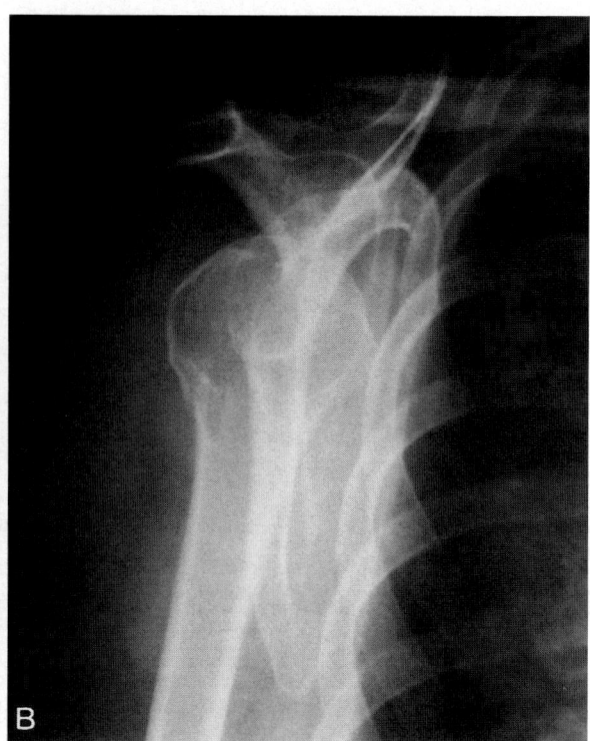

Figure 43.40. Pseudodislocation of the Shoulder. A. An AP view of the shoulder in this patient who had trauma to the shoulder shows the humeral head to be inferiorly placed in relation to the glenoid with absence of the normal crescent sign. A dislocation was suspected. **B.** The transscapular lateral film, however, reveals the humeral head to be normally placed over the glenoid. This is a pseudodislocation owing to a hemarthrosis. A search for an occult fracture should be made. In this case, a fracture can be seen in **(A)** (*arrow*), which caused bleeding into the joint.

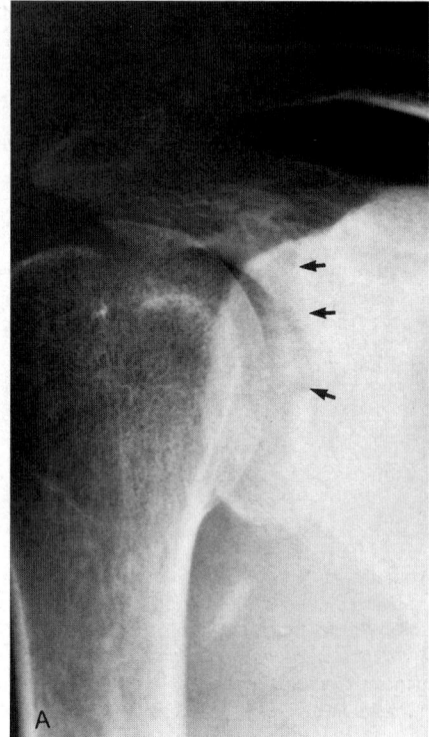

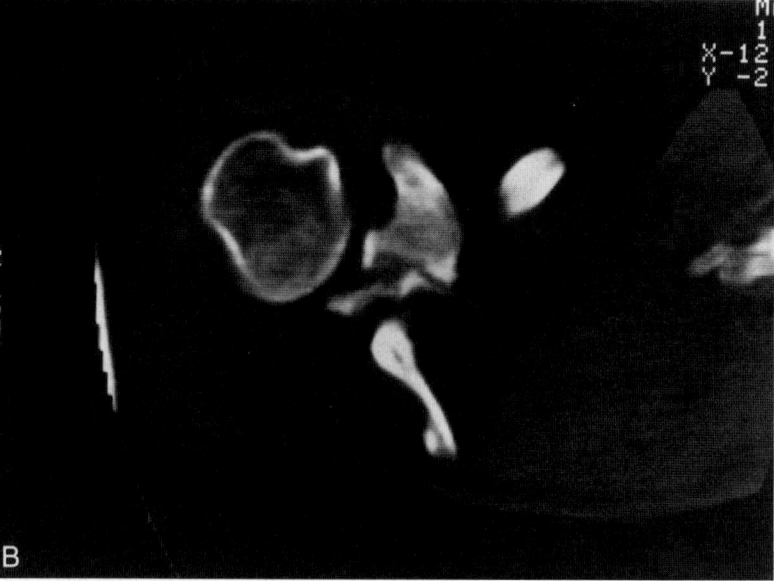

Figure 43.41. Fracture of the Glenoid. A. An AP view of the shoulder demonstrates a faint lucency indicative of a fracture of the glenoid (*arrows*) with a fragment of bone seen inferior to the joint. **B.** The full extent of the fracture cannot be appreciated until the CT is examined. On the CT scan, the fracture can be seen to extend fully through the scapula and is seen to be slightly displaced in the articular portion.

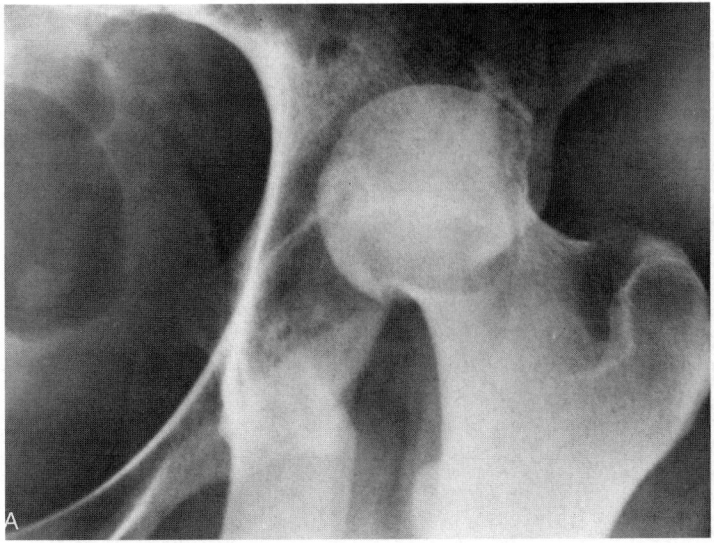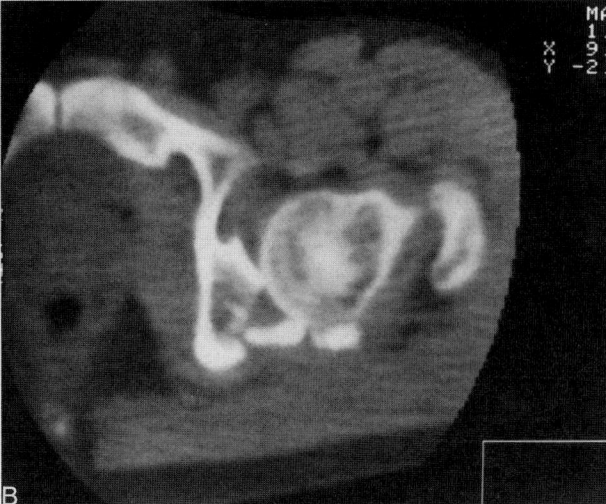

Figure 43.42. Dislocation of the Hip. A. An AP plain film of the left hip shows dislocation of the femoral head, which lies slightly superior to the acetabulum. **B.** Fractures are easily identified on the CT scan. A cortical break through the articular surface of the posterior acetabulum as well as the dislocation is identified.

ribs and clavicles, the exact anatomy is often difficult to discern on the transscapular view. To find the glenoid, one has to find the coracoid, the spine of the acromion, and the blade of the scapula. These three structures all lead to the glenoid and form a "Y" around it. All that is necessary to find the center of the glenoid is to find two of those bony landmarks, usually the coracoid and the blade of the scapula. The humeral head can then be found and its position determined.

An entity that can be mistaken for a dislocated shoulder is a traumatic hemarthrosis, which displaces the humeral head inferolaterally on the AP film (Fig. 43.40). Because the anterior dislocation displaces inferomedially, it should not be confused with this. The posterior dislocation will easily be excluded by looking at a transscapular view. This has been termed a pseudodislocation. It should be recognized so that attempts to "reduce" the "dislocation" are not made. Also, it can predict a subtle or occult humeral head fracture.

If a fracture is suspected about the shoulder and the plain films are negative or equivocal, a CT scan should be performed. A complex joint such as the shoulder or hip is best examined with CT scanning when the full extent of the fracture needs to be identified (Fig. 43.41).

PELVIS

Fractures of the Pelvis, and especially those involving the acetabulum, can be difficult to evaluate completely with plain films alone. Computed tomography scanning should be considered in almost all acetabular fractures because of the possibility of free fragments and subtle fractures that plain films do not show (Fig. 43.42).

Sacral Fractures are said to occur in half the cases that have pelvic fractures. They can be difficult to see on even the best of films because the sacrum is often hidden by bowel gas. In looking for sacral fractures, one should examine the arcuate lines of the sacrum bilater-

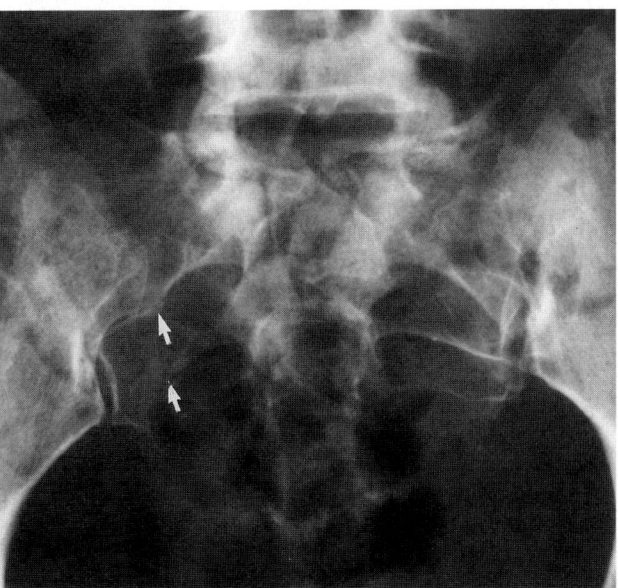

Figure 43.43. Fracture of the Sacrum. An AP view of the sacrum in this patient shows normal arcuate lines on the left side of the sacrum that are interrupted on the right side (*arrows*). Interruption of these lines indicates a fracture through this portion of the sacrum.

ally to see whether they are intact. Fractures often interrupt these lines and, because of the side-to-side asymmetry, can therefore be easily identified (Fig. 43.43).

Sacral Stress Fractures in patients who are osteoporotic or who have undergone radiation therapy can present as patchy or linear sclerosis on the sacral ala that might or might not show cortical disruption on plain films (Fig. 43.44A). These should be differentiated from metastatic disease because of their characteristic location, appearance, and history of prior radiation and by seeing a cortical break. Computed tomography will usually, but not always, demonstrate cortical disruption

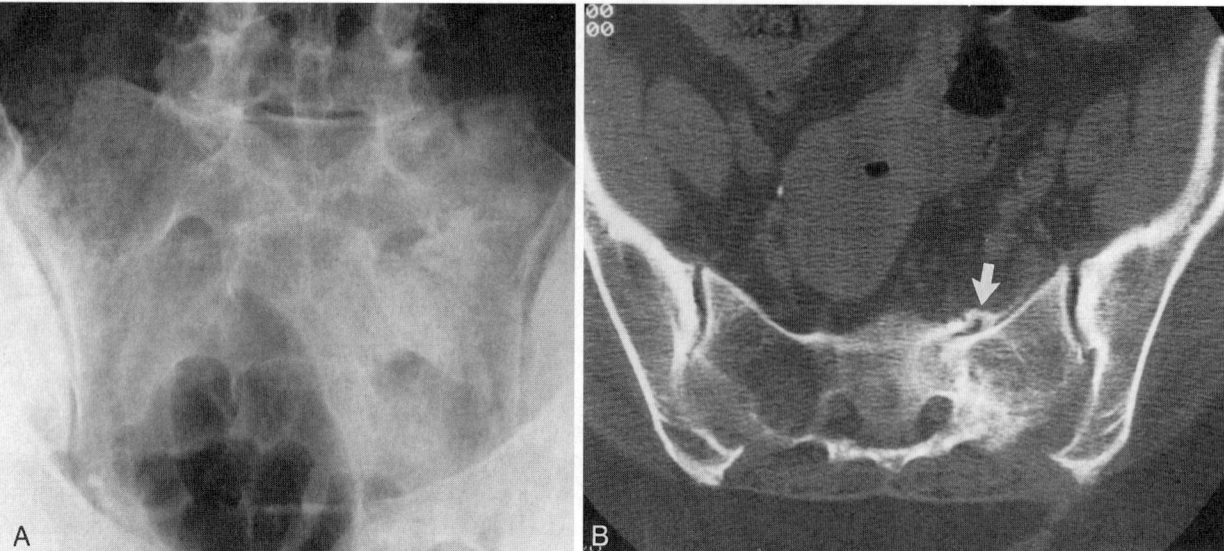

Figure 43.44. Sacral Stress Fracture. A. Faint sclerosis is noted in the left part of the sacrum as compared with the right in this patient complaining of pelvic pain. A radionuclide bone scan showed increased isotope uptake on the left half of the sacrum, and metastatic disease was postulated. **B.** A CT scan through this region that demonstrates a cortical disruption (*arrow*) indicative of a fracture. This is a characteristic plain film and CT appearance of a stress fracture of the sacrum.

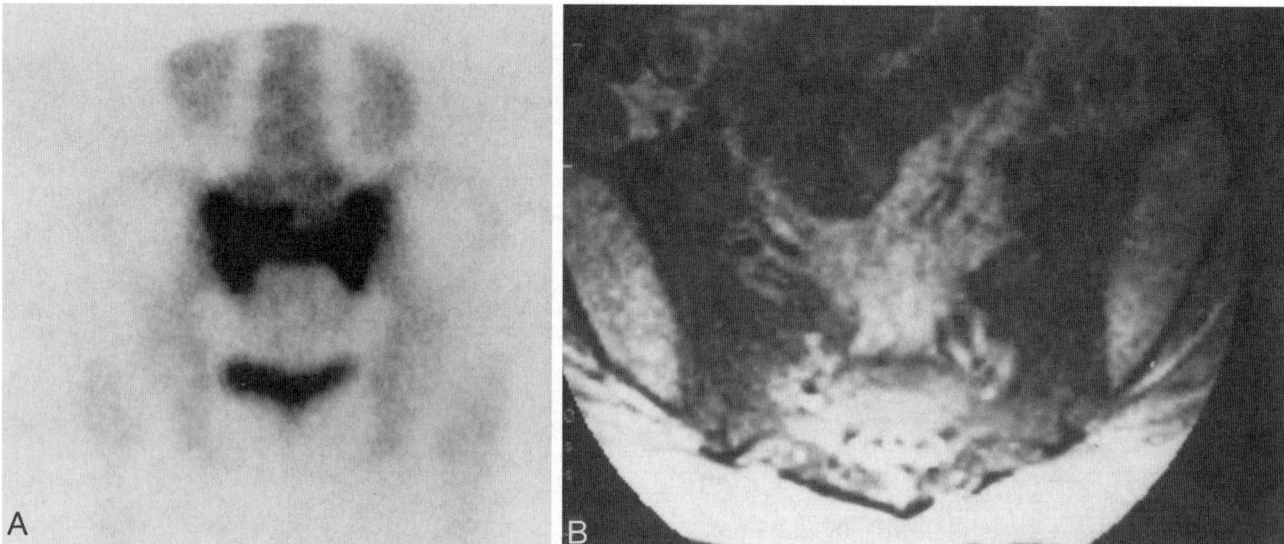

Figure 43.45. Sacral Stress Fracture. A. A radionuclide bone scan in an osteoporotic patient with pelvic pain shows a classic "Honda sign" seen with bilateral sacral stress fractures. **B.** A T1-weighted coronal MR in this patient shows diffuse low signal throughout the sacrum adjacent to the sacroiliac joints bilaterally. This represents edema and hemorrhage in the fractures and corresponds to the bone scan Honda sign.

(Fig. 43.44B). These fractures have a characteristic appearance on radionuclide bone scans (Fig. 43.45A), which is termed the Honda sign because of its appearance to the logo of the car. The Honda sign is seen only with bilateral stress fractures; unilateral fractures will have increased radionuclide uptake throughout one sacral ala. Magnetic resonance imaging will demonstrate an area of diffuse low signal on T1WIs corresponding to the area of involvement (Fig. 43.45B). Sacral stress fractures have also been termed insufficiency fractures, indicating that the underlying bone is abnormal, similar to a pathologic fracture.

Avulsion Injuries affect the pelvis quite often and should be easily recognized by radiologists. On occasion, an avulsion injury can have an aggressive appearance and, if not diagnosed radiographically, a biopsy might be performed. This can be calamitous as avulsion injuries have been known to mimic malignant lesions histologically, with a misdiagnosis leading to radical treatment (Fig. 43.46). Therefore, when an avulsion injury is a consideration, it becomes a "do not touch" lesion (see chapter 39). Common sites for pelvic avulsions include the ischium, the superior and inferior anterior iliac spines (Fig. 43.47), and the iliac crest. These injuries are said to

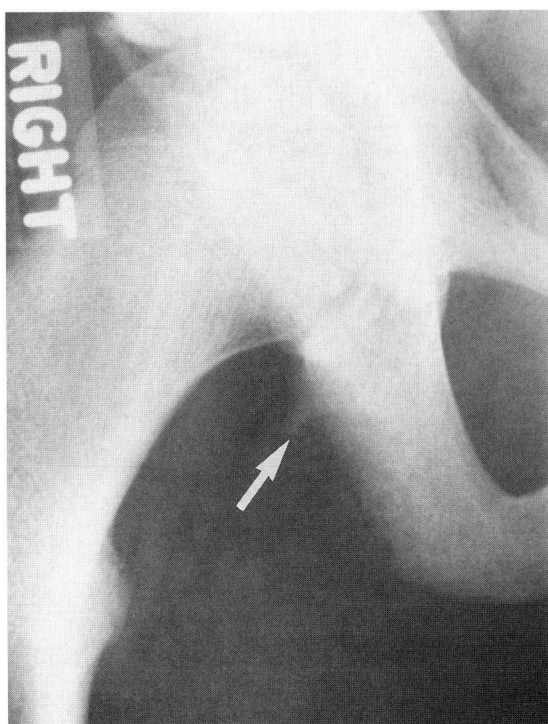

Figure 43.46. Avulsion off the Ischium. An AP view of the pelvis shows an area of cortical disruption and periostitis at the right ischium (*arrow*) in a patient complaining of pain at this site. These findings are characteristic for an ischial avulsion and should not undergo biopsy.

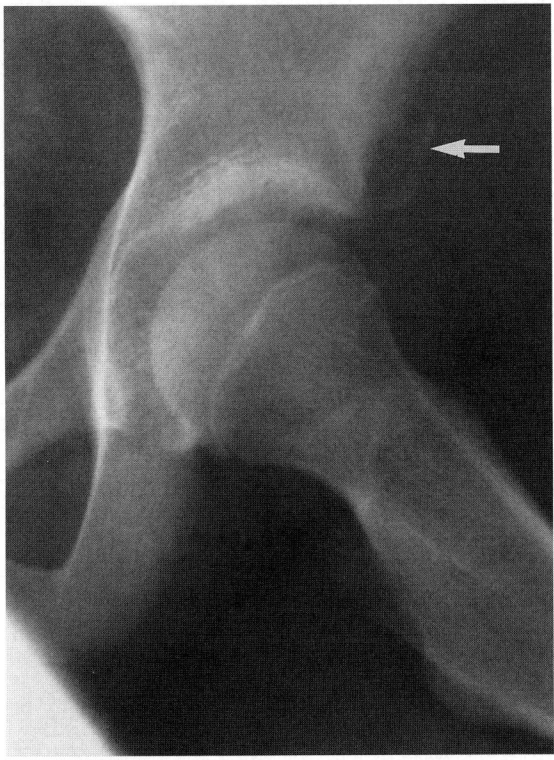

Figure 43.47. Rectus Femoris Avulsion. An AP plain film of the left hip shows a faint calcific density superior to the acetabulum (*arrow*), which is characteristic for an avulsion of the rectus femoris muscle from the anterior inferior iliac spine.

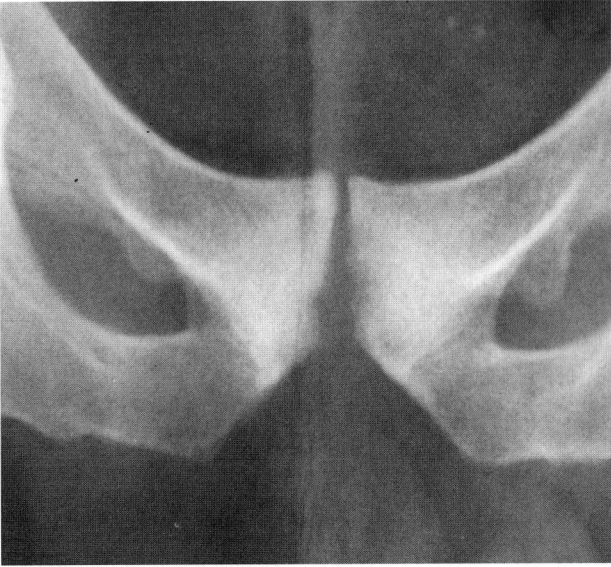

Figure 43.48. Osteoarthritis of the Symphysis Pubis. Sclerosis with erosion is noted at the symphysis in this ultramarathoner complaining of severe pubic pain. This is characteristic of DJD or osteoarthritis at this site in such an overuse setting. Erosions are ordinarily not seen in DJD, except in certain joints such as the symphysis pubis, sacroiliac, and the acromioclavicular.

be fairly common in long jumpers, sprinters, hurdlers, gymnasts, and cheerleaders.

Another area in the pelvis that can demonstrate radiologic findings as a result of stress is the symphysis pubis. In ultramarathoners, cross-country skiers, soccer players, and other athletes the symphysis can be affected by degenerative joint disease or osteoarthritis. (Fig. 43.48). The hallmarks of DJD are sclerosis, joint space narrowing, and osteophytosis. In certain joints, however, erosions can occur as a result of DJD. These joints include the temporomandibular joint, the acromioclavicular joint, the symphysis pubis, and the sacroiliac joint.

When the sacroiliac joints are involved with DJD, this can closely resemble an HLA-B27 spondyloarthropathy (Fig. 43.49) and lead to erroneous diagnosis and treatment. Large osteophytes can develop across the sacroiliac joints and mimic sclerosis or even a tumor (Fig. 43.50).

LEG

Overt fractures in the femur and lower leg are, for the most part, straightforward and deserve no special radiologic treatment for fear of missing subtle abnormalities.

Stress Fractures, however, need to be considered in anyone with hip or leg pain, as overlooking the diagnosis can lead to a complete fracture. The most serious stress fracture, and fortunately, one of the rarest, is the femoral neck stress fracture (Fig. 43.51). Many of these progress to complete fractures (Fig. 43.52) that, with continued weight bearing, can displace; these are very serious lesions.

Stress fractures also occur in the distal diaphysis of the femur and in the proximal, middle, and distal thirds

Figure 43.49. Osteoarthritis of the Sacroiliac Joint. Sclerosis and erosions (*arrow*) are seen in the left sacroiliac joint in this young, professional dancer. Although this has the appearance of an inflammatory arthritis, this is also seen in DJD or osteoarthritis secondary to overuse.

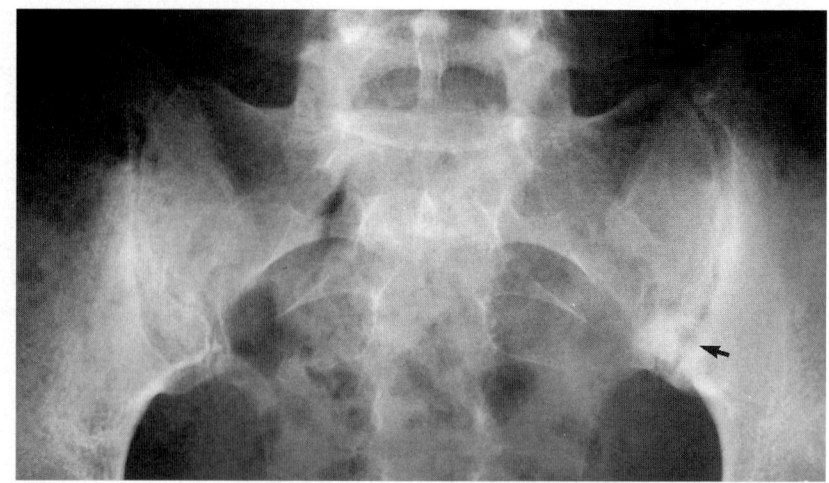

Figure 43.50. Sacroiliac Osteophytes. A. An AP view of the pelvis in this marathoner shows dense sclerosis over both sacroiliac joints. **B.** A CT through this area demonstrates dense, bridging osteophytes, characteristic of DJD.

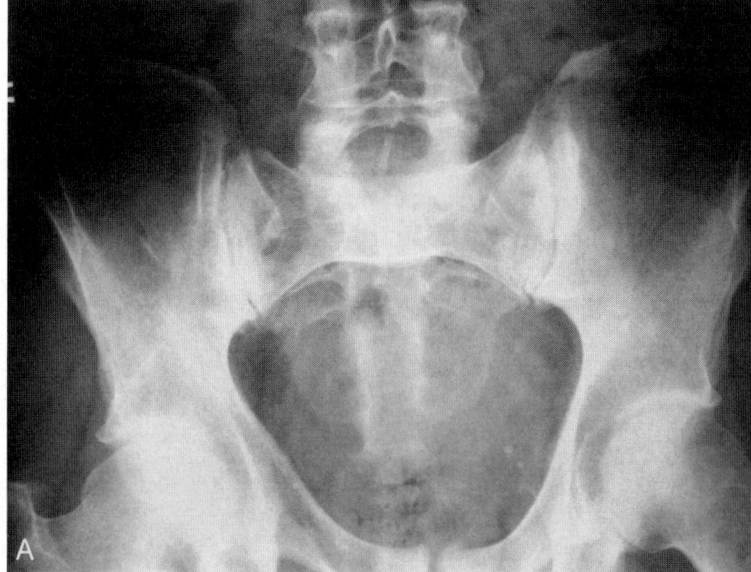

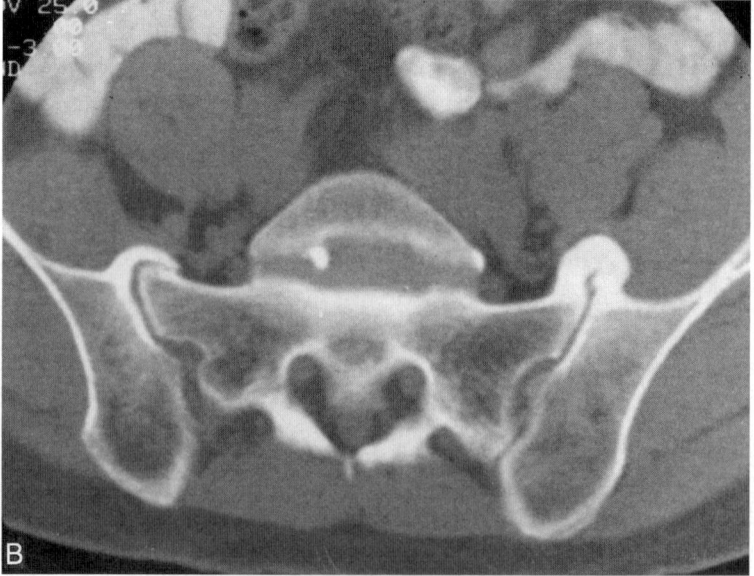

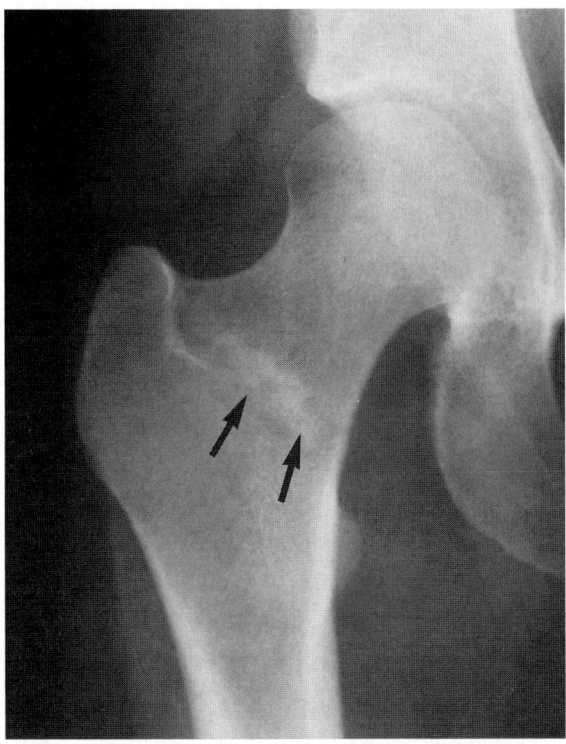

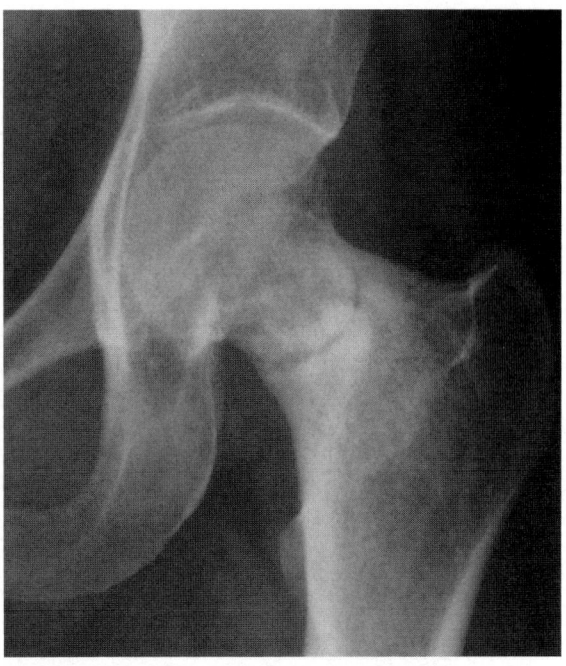

Figure 43.52. Stress Fracture of the Femoral Neck. A linear lucency with surrounding sclerosis is seen in the femoral neck in this jogger with hip pain. This is a severe femoral neck stress fracture.

Figure 43.51. Femoral Stress Fracture. An area of linear sclerosis (*arrows*) is seen at the base of the femoral neck in a runner with hip pain. This is diagnostic of a stress fracture of the femur. (Case courtesy of Dr. David Simms, Wichita, Kansas.)

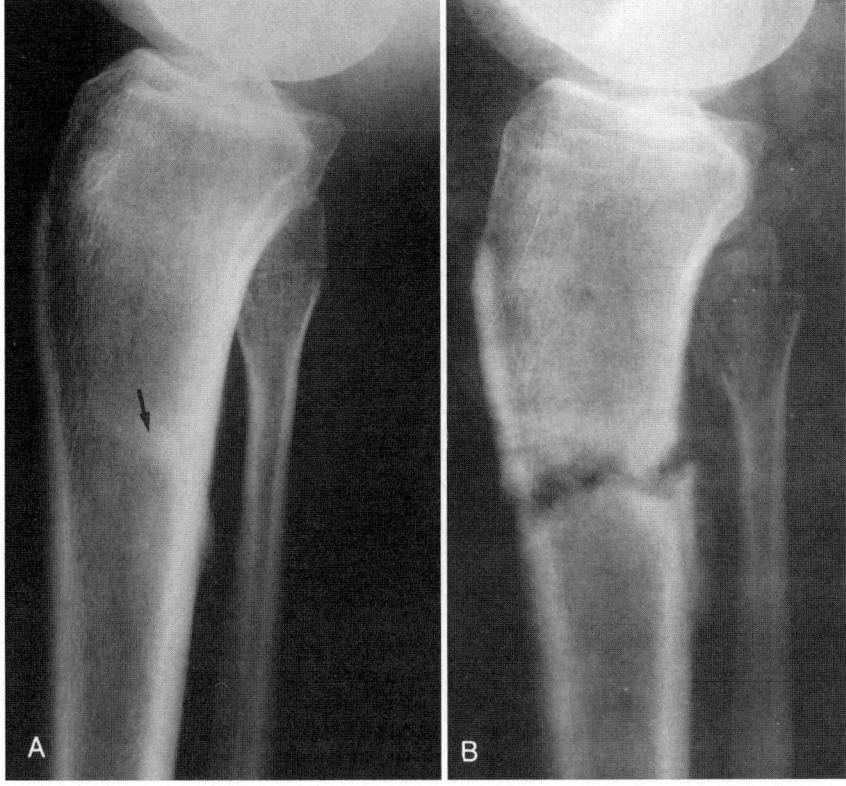

Figure 43.53. Stress Fracture of the Proximal Tibia. A. A faint linear sclerotic area (*arrow*) is seen, which is characteristic for a stress fracture of the proximal tibia. **B.** This view shows the result of continued exercise in this patient: a complete fracture of the tibia and of the proximal fibula.

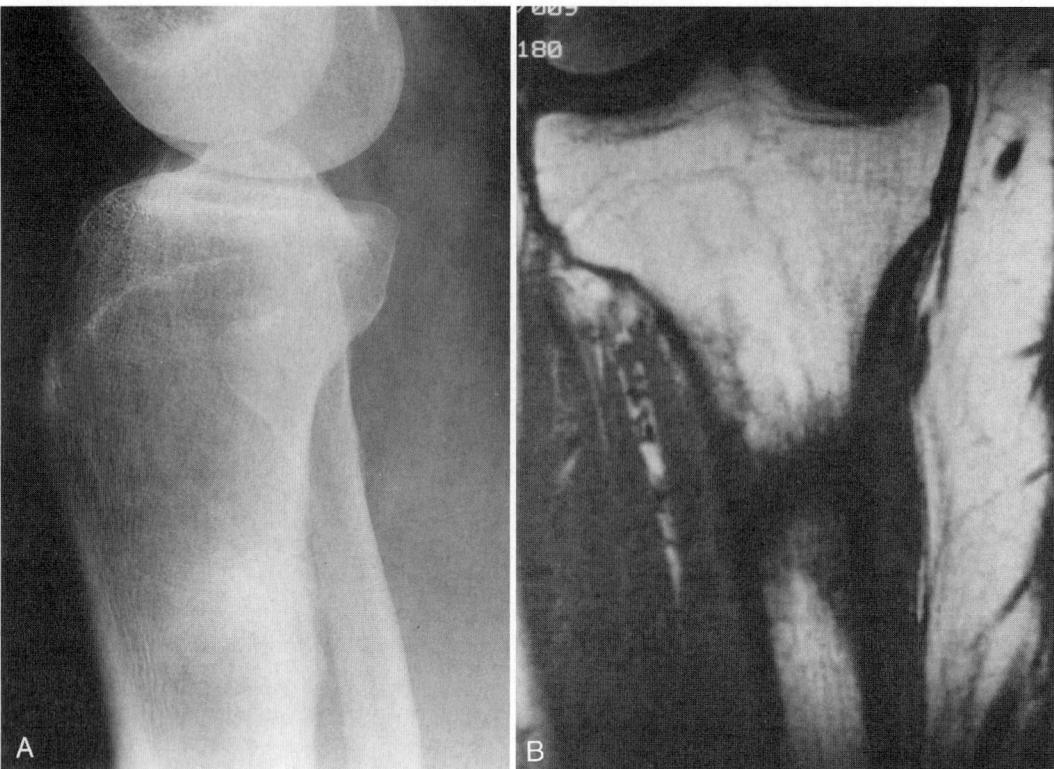

Figure 43.54. Stress Fracture of the Tibia. A. An irregular focus of sclerosis is seen in the posterior proximal tibia with adjacent periostitis. There was concern that this might represent a primary bone tumor, and the surgeons recommended a biopsy. **B.** An MR scan was performed, however, which shows a linear low signal area running obliquely across the tibia on this T1-weighted coronal image, which is characteristic for a stress fracture. No significant soft-tissue mass was found. The patient's recent history included an increase in his jogging. A stress fracture was diagnosed on the basis of these images.

of the tibia. All of these stress fractures need to be treated with the utmost caution because complete fractures are not uncommon with continued stress (Fig. 43.53). Sclerosis in a weight-bearing bone that has a horizontal or oblique linear pattern should be considered a stress fracture until proved otherwise. A history of repetitive stress is not always obtained, so the diagnosis should not depend solely on the history.

A stress fracture occasionally will appear somewhat aggressive, with aggressive periostitis and no definite linearity to the sclerosis (Fig. 43.54A). If this is mistaken for a tumor and undergoes biopsy, it can be confused with a malignancy, with subsequent radical therapy. These should, therefore, not undergo biopsy under any circumstance. If the clinical presentation is unusual for a stress fracture and the plain films are not diagnostic, take additional films 1 or 2 weeks later. Computed tomography and MR sometimes will better delineate the lesion (Fig. 43.54B) and should show normal soft tissues. Stress fractures can be difficult to diagnose radiologically early on but should be straightforward after several weeks.

One final stress fracture that deserves mention because it is frequently misdiagnosed clinically and overlooked radiographically is the calcaneal stress fracture (Fig. 43.55). It is often clinically misdiagnosed as a "heel spur" or plantar fasciitis and can be a somewhat subtle radiographic finding.

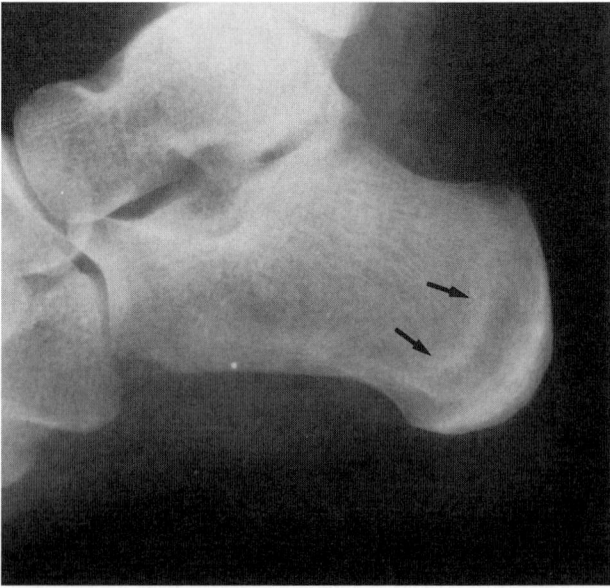

Figure 43.55. Calcaneal Stress Fracture. A linear band of sclerosis is seen in the posterior calcaneus (*arrows*), which is diagnostic for a stress fracture of the calcaneus.

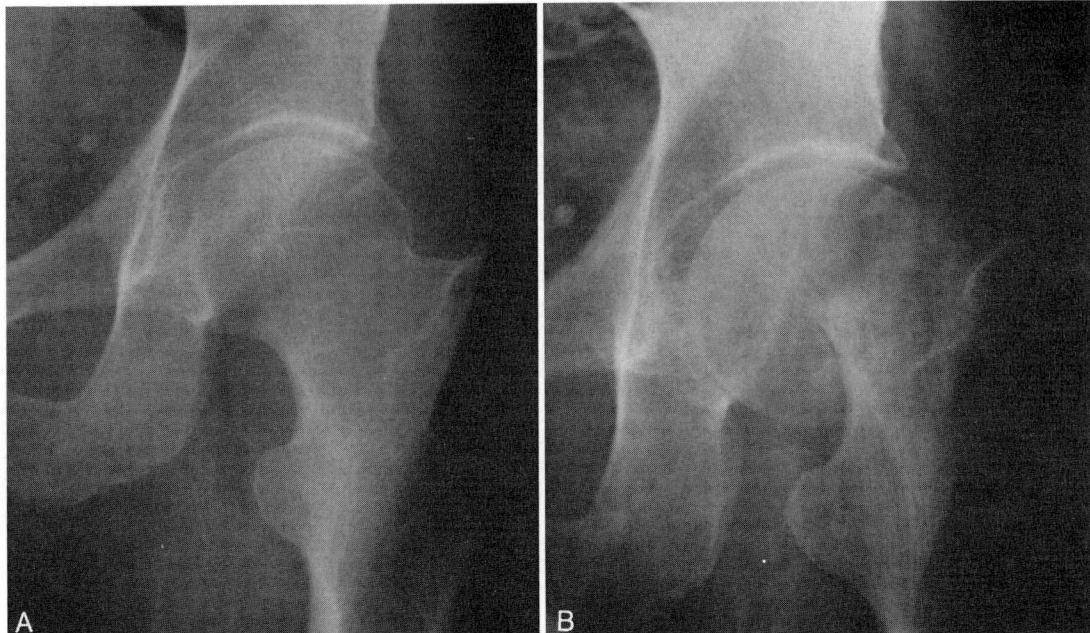

Figure 43.56. Fracture of the Hip. A. An AP view of the hip was obtained in an elderly man following a fall. It was interpreted as normal, and the patient was dismissed from the emergency department. Two weeks later, the patient returned to the emergency department unable to walk and another radiograph **(B)** was obtained. It shows a complete fracture through the femoral neck. In retrospect, the fracture can be faintly seen in **(A)** and should have been picked up initially. Fractures of the hip in the elderly can be very difficult to see and should be diligently searched for with additional views when the clinical setting is appropriate.

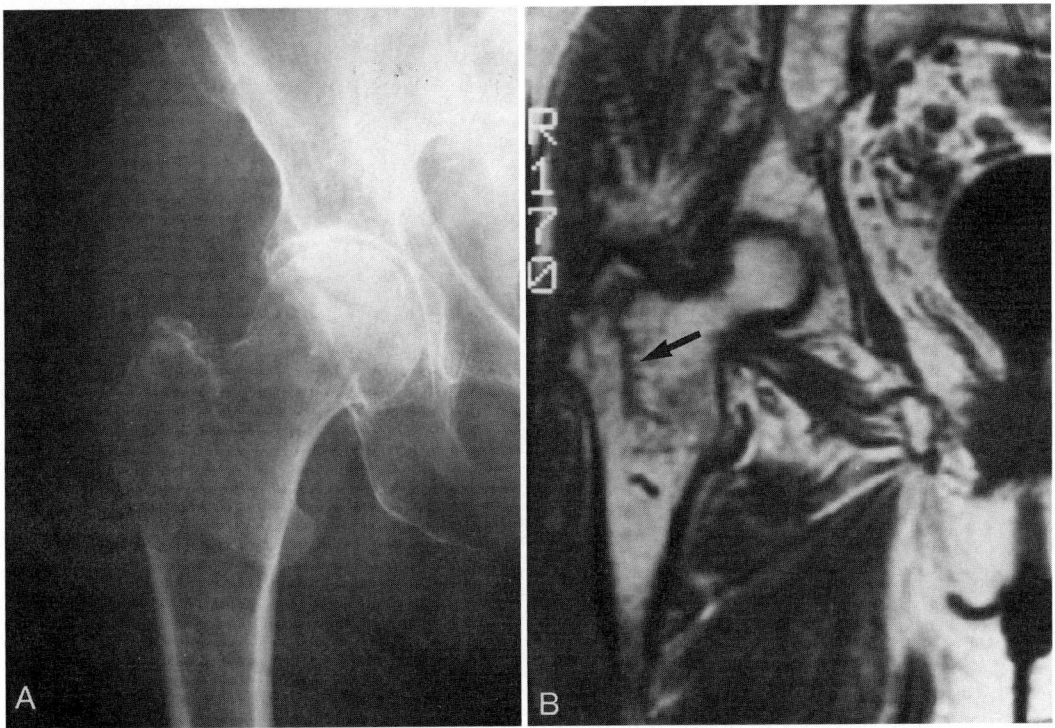

Figure 43.57. Occult Fracture of the Hip. A. An AP plain film in an elderly patient with hip pain after a fall appears normal. **B.** A coronal T1-weighted MR was obtained because of the clinical suspicion of a fracture and shows linear low signal in the intertrochanteric region (*arrow*), confirming the fracture.

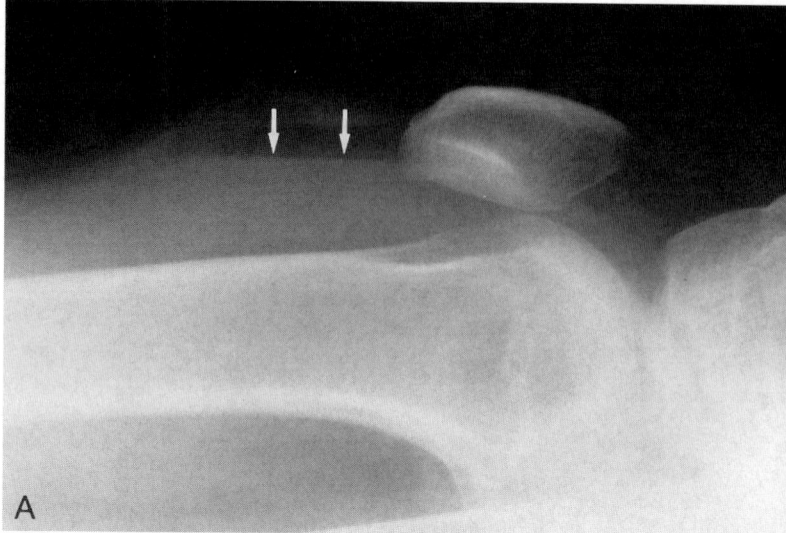

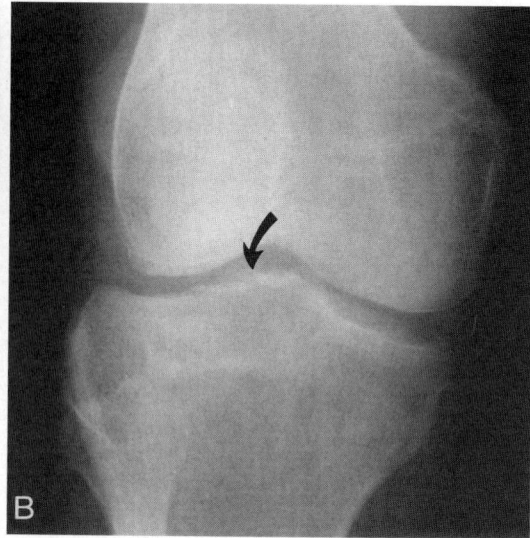

Figure 43.58. Tibial Plateau Fracture. A. A cross-table lateral plain film of the knee reveals a fat-fluid level (*arrows*), which indicates a fracture with fatty marrow leaking into the joint. **B.** An AP view shows a barely discernible fracture (*arrow*) near the tibial spines, indicative of a tibial plateau fracture.

Hip Fracture. Overt fractures in the lower extremity are uncommonly missed on radiographs; however, a few exceptions should be noted. Hip fractures in the elderly population can be very difficult to detect (Fig. 43.56), and a high index of suspicion should be maintained. A negative plain film in an elderly patient with hip pain after trauma (even relatively mild trauma) does not exclude a femoral neck fracture. Magnetic resonance imaging has been shown to be very useful in demonstrating femoral neck fractures that are occult (Fig. 43.57).

Tibial Plateau Fracture. Another fracture that can be difficult to exclude on routine plain films is a tibial plateau fracture. A cross-table lateral plain film should be obtained in cases of knee trauma to look for a fat-fluid level (Fig. 43.58); this indicates a fracture that allows fatty marrow to leak into the knee joint. In the appropriate clinical setting, tomograms or CT may be necessary to make the diagnosis.

Lisfranc Fracture. A serious fracture in the foot that can be missed radiographically when little or no displacement occurs is the so-called Lisfranc fracture (Fig. 43.59). It is named after a surgeon in Napoleon's army who would do forefoot amputations in patients with gangrenous toes as a result of frostbite. The Lisfranc fracture is a fracture-dislocation of the tarsometatarsals. If the dislocation is slight, it can be easily overlooked. A key to normal alignment is that the medial border of the second metatarsal should always line up with the medial border of the second cuneiform. If it does not, a Lisfranc fracture-dislocation should be suspected. This fracture is seen most commonly in patients who catch the forefoot in something such as a hole in the ground, or a horseback rider falling and hanging by the forefoot in the stirrups. It is commonly seen as a neurotrophic or Charcot joint in diabetics.

Fracture of the Calcaneus can be difficult to appreciate on routine radiographs. Böhler's angle is a

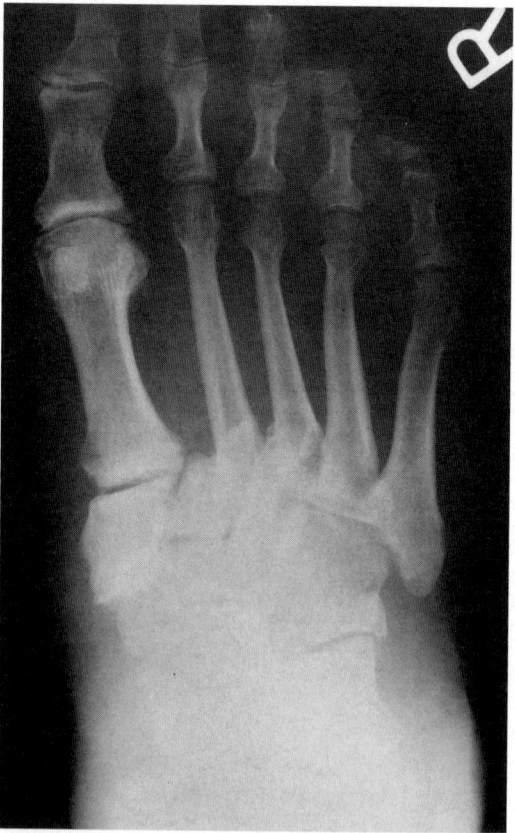

Figure 43.59. Lisfranc Fracture. An AP view of the foot in this patient shows a space between the first and second metatarsals with the base of the second metatarsal displaced off the second cuneiform. This is indicative of a Lisfranc fracture dislocation.

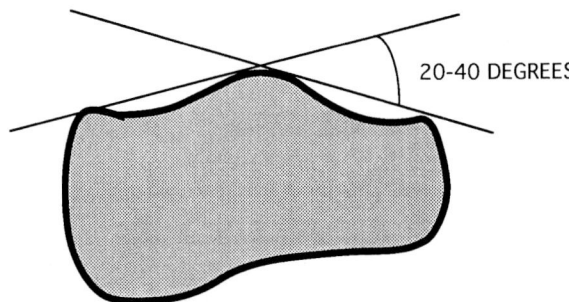

Figure 43.60. Böhler's Angle in a Normal Calcaneus. This drawing depicts the normal calcaneus with a line across the anterior process extending to the apex of the calcaneus intersecting with a line from the posterior portion of the calcaneus to the apex. This is termed Böhler's angle, and when it becomes flattened or less than 20°, a calcaneal fracture should be diagnosed.

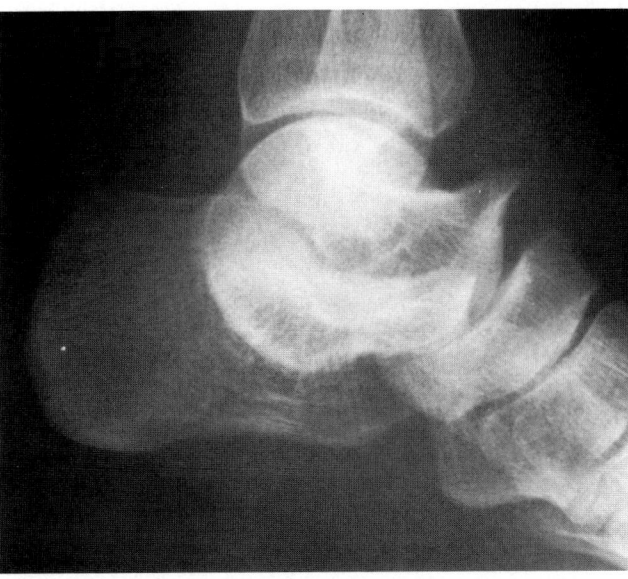

Figure 43.61. Calcaneal Fracture. Böhler's angle in this calcaneus is less than 20°, which is indicative of a fracture of the calcaneus.

normal anatomic landmark that should be looked for in every foot film when trauma has occurred (Fig. 43.60). If this angle is narrower than 20° it indicates a compression of the calcaneus, as seen in jumping injuries (Fig. 43.61).

This is a fairly simplified overview of some commonly overlooked fractures and dislocations and should not be interpreted as a substitute for the more complete texts listed in the references (2,3).

References

1. Vandemark R. Radiology of the cervical spine in trauma patients: practice pitfalls and recommendations for improving efficiency and communication. AJR Am J Roentgenol 1990; 155:465–472.
2. Rogers LF. Radiology of Skeletal Trauma. New York: Churchill Livingstone, 1982.
3. Rockwood CA Jr, Green DP, Bucholz RW. Fractures in adults. 3rd ed. Philadelphia: JB Lippincott, 1991.

44
Arthritis

Clyde A. Helms

OSTEOARTHRITIS

Osteoarthritis, or degenerative joint disease (DJD), is the most common arthritide. It is believed to be caused by trauma—either overt or as an accumulation of microtrauma for the years, although there is also an hereditary form called primary osteoarthritis that occurs primarily in middle-aged women. The hallmarks of DJD are *joint space narrowing, sclerosis,* and *osteophytosis* (Table 44.1 and Fig. 44.1). If all three of these findings are not present on the radiograph, another diagnosis should be considered. Joint space narrowing is the least specific finding of the three, yet it is virtually always present in DJD. Unfortunately, it is also seen in almost every other joint abnormality.

Sclerosis should be present in varying amounts in all cases of DJD unless severe osteoporosis is present. Osteoporosis will cause the sclerosis to be diminished. For instance, in long-standing rheumatoid arthritis in which the cartilage has been destroyed, DJD often occurs with very little sclerosis. Osteophytosis will be diminished in the setting of osteoporosis also. Otherwise, sclerosis and osteophytosis should be prominent in DJD.

The only disorder that will cause osteophytes without sclerosis or joint space narrowing is diffuse idiopathic skeletal hyperostosis (1). This is a common bone-forming disorder that at first glance resembles DJD, except that there is no joint space narrowing (or disc space narrowing in the spine) and there is no sclerosis (Fig. 44.2). Diffuse idiopathic skeletal hyperostosis is not believed to be caused by trauma or stress as is DJD and is not painful or disabling as DJD can be. Millions of dollars per year are awarded to federal employees at retirement, representing "disability" payments for supposed DJD acquired during their employment, when in fact, these retirees have diffuse idiopathic skeletal hyperostosis and have been misdiagnosed.

Osteoarthritis is divided into two types: primary and secondary. Secondary osteoarthritis is what radiologists refer to when speaking of DJD. It is, as mentioned, secondary to trauma of some sort. It can occur in any joint in the body but is particularly common in the hands, knees, hips, and spine.

Primary osteoarthritis is a familial arthritis that affects middle-aged women almost exclusively and is seen only in the hands. It affects the distal interphalangeal joints, the proximal interphalangeal joints, and the base of the thumb in a bilaterally symmetrical fashion (Fig. 44.3). If it is not bilaterally symmetrical, the diagnosis of primary osteoarthritis should be questioned.

A type of primary osteoarthritis that can be very painful and debilitating is erosive osteoarthritis. It has the identical distribution mentioned for primary osteoarthritis but is associated with severe osteoporosis of the hands, as well as erosions. It is uncommon, and radiologists generally see little of this disorder. It is also called Kellgren's arthritis.

There are a few exceptions to the classic triad of findings seen in DJD (sclerosis, narrowing, and osteophytes). Several joints also exhibit erosions as a manifestation of DJD: the *temporomandibular joint*, the *acromioclavicular joint*, the *sacroiliac joints*, and the *symphysis pubis* (Table 44.2). When erosions are seen in one of these joints, DJD must be considered or inappropriate treatment may be instituted (Fig. 44.4).

A subchondral cyst, or geode (taken from the geologic term used when a volcanic rock has a gas pocket that leaves a large cavity in the rock), is often found in joints affected with DJD. Geodes are cystic formations that occur around joints in a variety of disorders (including, in addition to **DJD, rheumatoid arthritis, calcium pyrophosphate dihydrate crystal deposition disease,** and **avascular necrosis** (Table 44.3)(2). Presumably, one method of geode formation is that synovial fluid is forced into the subchondral bone, causing a cystic collection of joint fluid. Another etiology is following a bone contusion in which the contused bone forms a cyst. They rarely cause problems by themselves but are often misdiagnosed as something more sinister (Fig. 44.5).

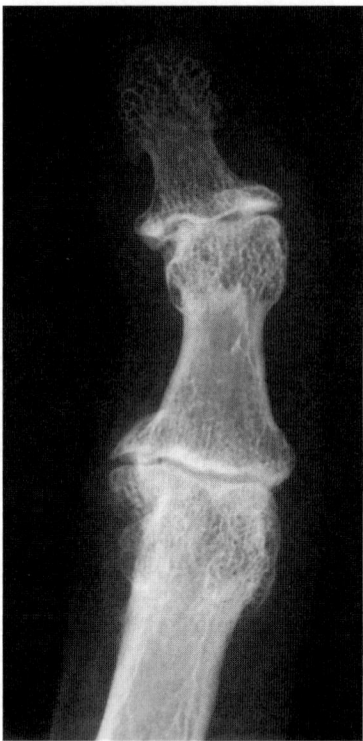

Figure 44.1. Osteoarthritis (DJD). A plain film of a finger with osteoarthritis (DJD) of the distal and proximal interphalangeal joints. Both joints demonstrate joint space narrowing, subchondral sclerosis, and osteophytosis, which are hallmarks of degenerative joint disease.

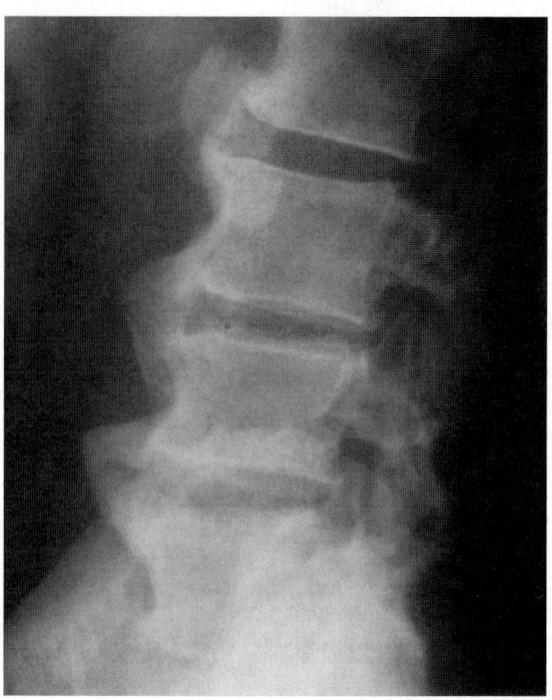

Figure 44.2. Diffuse Idiopathic Skeletal Hyperostosis. A lateral view of the lumbar spine shows extensive osteophytosis without significant disc space narrowing or sclerosis. This is a classic picture for diffuse idiopathic skeletal hyperostosis.

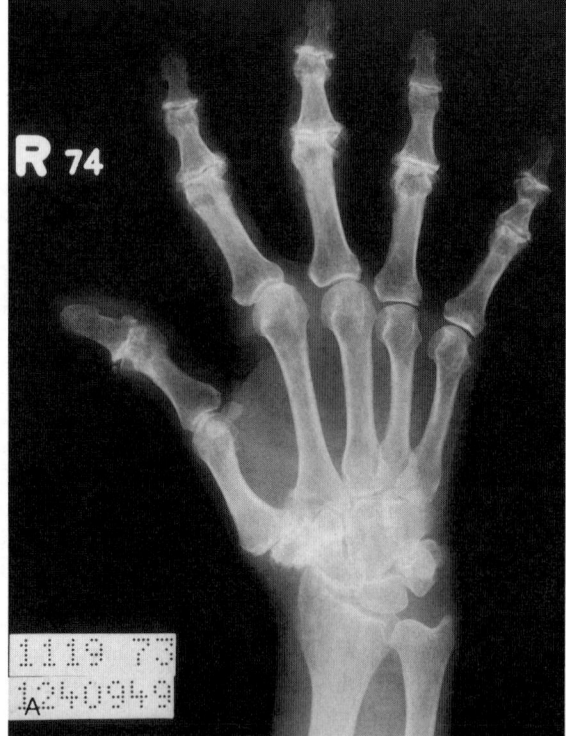

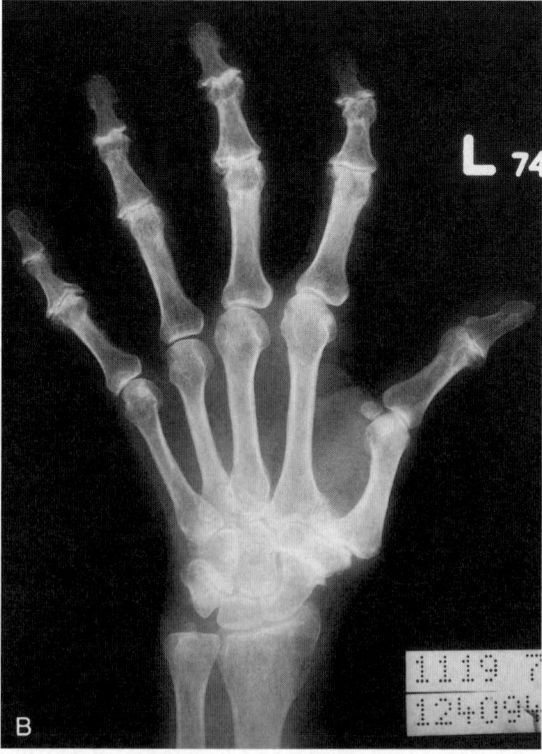

Figure 44.3. Primary Osteoarthritis. Bilateral hand films **(A,B)** in a patient with primary osteoarthritis. Present are classic findings of osteophytosis, joint space narrowing, and sclerosis at the distal interphalangeal joints, the proximal interphalangeal joints, and at the base of the thumb. This is bilaterally symmetrical, which is typical for primary osteoarthritis.

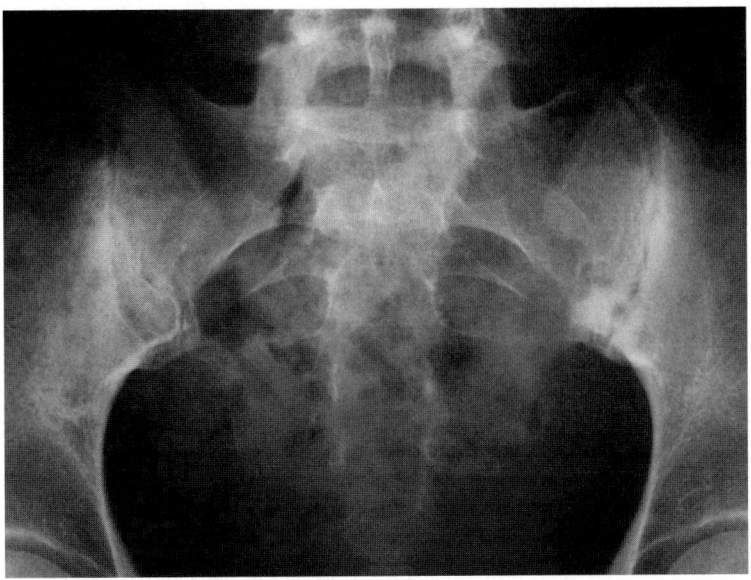

Figure 44.4. Osteoarthritis of the SI Joint. A young woman who is a professional dancer complained of left-sided hip pain. An AP film of the pelvis demonstrated left SI joint sclerosis, joint irregularity, and erosions. A complete workup to rule out an HLA B-27 spondyloarthropathy was negative, and no laboratory or clinical evidence for infection was found. Her clinical history pointed to this being completely occupation-related, and an aspiration biopsy to rule out infection was therefore not performed. This is not an unusual appearance for DJD of the SI joints.

Table 44.1 Hallmarks of DJD

Joint space narrowing
Sclerosis
Osteophytes

Table 44.2 Joints That Have Erosions As a Feature of DJD

Sacroiliac
Acromioclavicular
Temporomandibular
Symphysis pubis

Table 44.3 Diseases in Which Geodes Are Found

DJD
Rheumatoid arthritis
CPPD
AVN

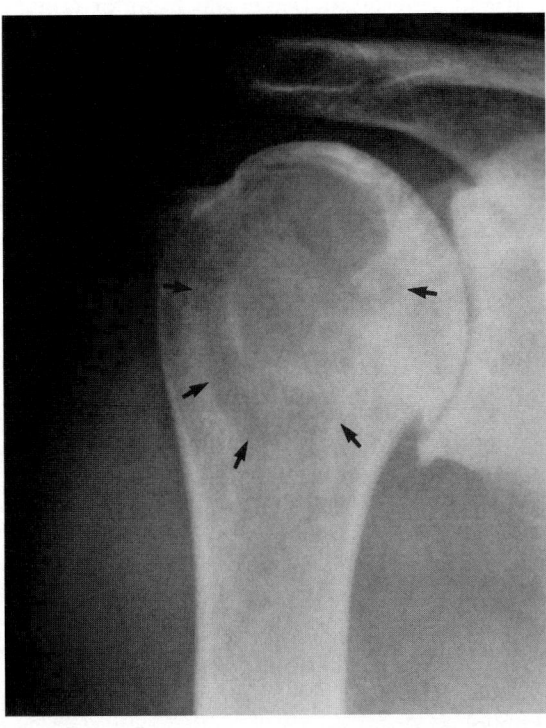

Figure 44.5. Subchondral Cyst or Geode of the Shoulder. This patient has marked DJD of the shoulder with joint space narrowing, sclerosis, and osteophytosis. A large lytic process (*arrows*) is seen in the humeral head, which is a subchondral cyst or geode often seen in association with DJD. Because of the DJD in the shoulder, a biopsy to rule out a more sinister lesion in the humeral head should be avoided.

RHEUMATOID ARTHRITIS

Rheumatoid arthritis is a connective tissue disorder of unknown etiology that can affect any synovial joint in the body. The radiographic hallmarks are **soft-tissue swelling**, **osteoporosis**, **joint space** narrowing, and **marginal erosions**. In the hands, it is classically a **proximal** process that is **bilaterally symmetrical** (Table 44.4 and Fig. 44.6). There are so many exceptions to these rules, however, that I have come to regard them as no better than 80% accurate. Rheumatoid arthritis has a large variety of appearances, and from its radiographic appearance alone, it can be very difficult to diagnose with any degree of assurance.

Rheumatoid arthritis in large joints is fairly characteristic in that it causes marked joint space narrowing and is associated with osteoporosis. Erosions might or might not be present and tend to be marginal, that is, away from the weight-bearing portion of the joint. In the hip, the femoral head tends to migrate axially, whereas in osteoarthritis, it tends to migrate superolaterally (Figs. 44.7, 44.8). In the shoulder, the humeral head tends to be "high-riding" (Fig. 44.9). Other things to think of when confronted with a high-riding shoulder are a torn rotator cuff and CPPD (Table 44.5).

When rheumatoid arthritis is long-standing, it is not unusual for secondary DJD to superimpose itself on the findings one would expect with rheumatoid arthritis. This picture of DJD differs somewhat from that usually seen, in that the sclerosis and osteophytes are considerably diminished in severity as compared with the joint space narrowing (Fig. 44.10).

HLA-B27 SPONDYLOARTHROPATHIES

A group of diseases that was formerly known as rheumatoid variants is now known as the seronegative, HLA-B27-positive spondyloarthropathies. These disorders are all linked to the HLA-B27 histocompatibility antigen. Included in this group of diseases are ankylosing spondylitis, inflammatory bowel disease, psoriatic arthritis, and Reiter's syndrome. They are characterized by bony ankylosis, proliferative new-bone formation, and predominantly axial (spinal) involvement.

One of the more characteristic findings in these disorders is that of syndesmophytes in the spine. A syndesmophyte is a paravertebral ossification that resembles an osteophyte, except that it runs vertically, whereas an osteophyte has its orientation in a horizontal axis. Sometimes it can be difficult to decide whether a particular paravertebral ossification is an osteophyte or a syndesmophyte based on its orientation alone (Fig. 44.11). Bridging osteophytes and large syndesmophytes can have a similar appearance, with both having an orientation halfway between vertical and horizontal. How should one evaluate those cases? Look at the other vertebral bodies and use the ossifications on them to determine whether they are osteophytes or syndesmophytes. If no other level is involved, one might not be able to tell one from the other.

Syndesmophytes are classified as to whether they are marginal and symmetrical or nonmarginal and asymmetrical. A marginal syndesmophyte has its origin at the edge or margin of a vertebral body and extends to the margin of the adjacent vertebral body. They are invariably bilaterally symmetrical as viewed on an AP spine film. Ankylosing spondylitis classically has marginal, symmetrical syndesmophytes (Fig. 44.12). Inflammatory bowel disease has an identical appearance when the spine is involved. Nonmarginal, asymmetrical syndesmophytes are generally large and bulky. They emanate from the vertebral body away from the endplate or margin and are unilateral or asymmetrical as viewed on an AP spine film (Figs. 44.11, 44.13). Psoriatic arthritis and Reiter's syndrome classically have this type of syndesmophyte.

Table 44.4 Hallmarks of Rheumatoid Arthritis

Soft-tissue swelling
Osteoporosis
Joint space narrowing
Marginal erosions
Proximal distribution (hands)
Bilaterally symmetric

Table 44.5 Causes of High-riding Shoulder

Rheumatoid arthritis
CPPD
Torn rotator cuff

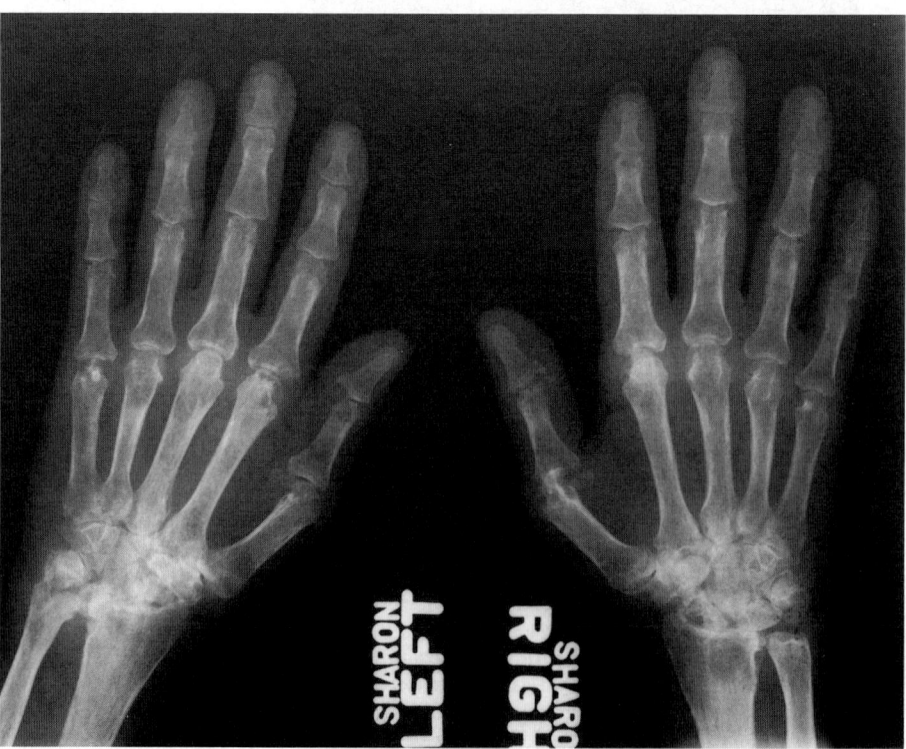

Figure 44.6. Rheumatoid Arthritis. An erosive arthritis affecting primarily the carpal bones and the metacarpophalangeal joints is seen that has associated osteoporosis and soft-tissue swelling (note the soft-tissue over the ulnar styloid processes). It is a bilaterally symmetrical process in this patient, which is classic.

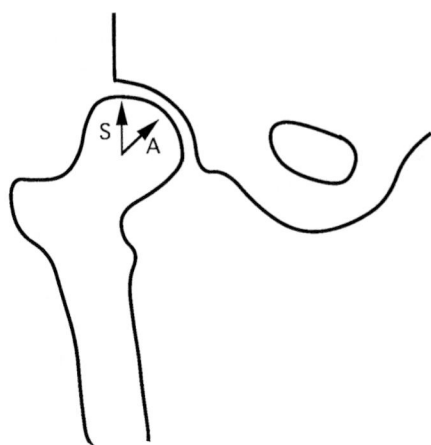

Figure 44.7. Migration of the Femoral Head. A drawing of the hip showing routes of migration of the femoral head. Osteoarthritis of the hip tends to cause superior (S) migration of the femoral head in relation to the acetabulum, whereas rheumatoid arthritis tends to cause axial (A) migration of the femoral head in relation to the acetabulum.

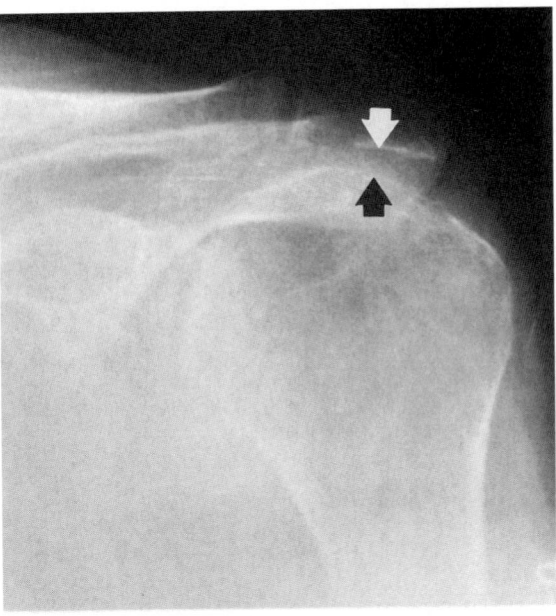

Figure 44.9. Rheumatoid Arthritis in the Shoulder. An AP view of the shoulder in this patient with rheumatoid arthritis shows that the distance between the acromion and the humeral head is diminished (*arrows*). Ordinarily, this space is about 1 cm in width to allow the rotator cuff to pass freely beneath the acromion. This is a common finding in rheumatoid arthritis as well as in CPPD.

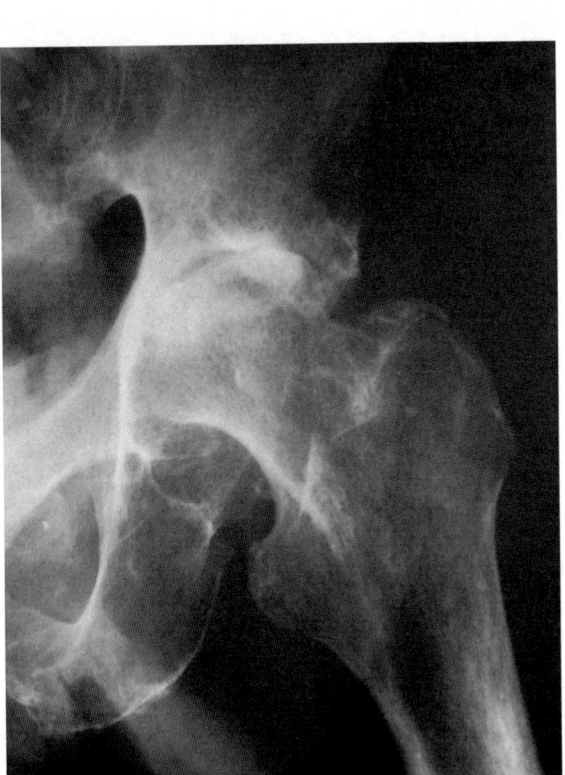

Figure 44.8. Rheumatoid Arthritis of the Hip. Note the severe joint space narrowing in this patient with rheumatoid arthritis. The femoral head has migrated in an axial direction with fairly concentric joint space narrowing. Minimal secondary degenerative changes have occurred as noted by the sclerosis in the superior portion of the joint; however, these have been diminished somewhat by the osteoporosis that usually accompanies rheumatoid arthritis.

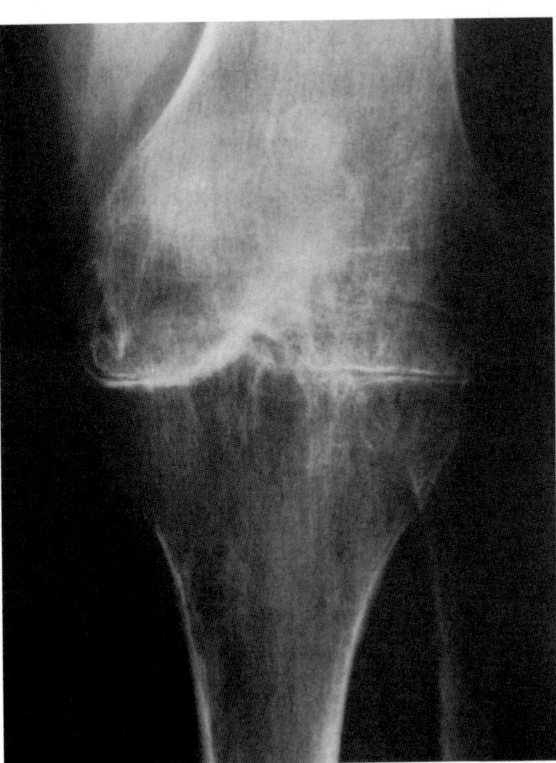

Figure 44.10. Secondary Degenerative Disease in the Knee in a patient with Rheumatoid Arthritis. This patient has a history of long-standing rheumatoid arthritis. An AP view of the knee shows severe osteoporosis and joint space narrowing. Secondary DJD is occurring, as evidenced by the sclerosis and osteophytosis; however, these findings are out of proportion to the severe joint space narrowing. When DJD narrows a joint to this extent, the osteophytosis and sclerosis are invariably much more pronounced.

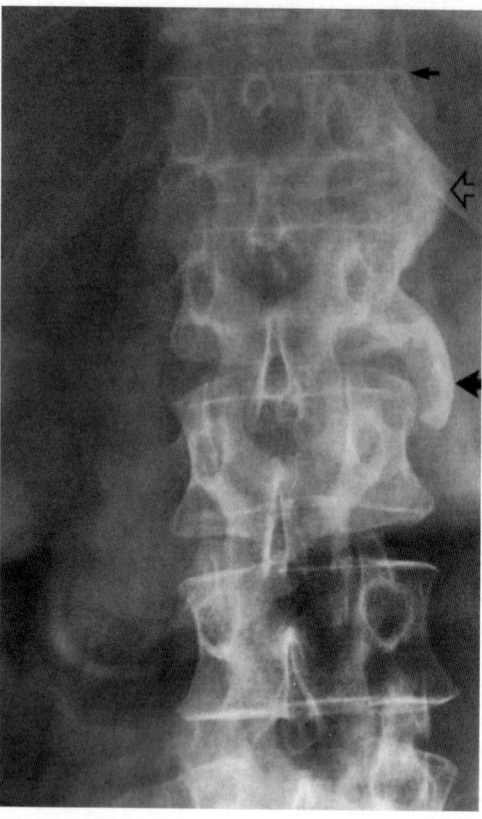

Figure 44.11. Psoriasis with Syndesmophytes. The large paravertebral ossification on the left side of the T12–L1 disc space (*open arrow*) is difficult to differentiate between an osteophyte and a syndesmophyte. Either could have this appearance. The paravertebral ossification at the left L1–2 disc space (*large solid arrow*) definitely has a vertical rather than a horizontal orientation, , however, as does the faint ossification seen at the T11–12 disc space (*small solid arrow*). These definitely represent syndesmophytes. It makes sense, therefore, to assume logically that the ossification at the T12–L1 disc space is almost certainly a syndesmophyte as well. This patient has large nonmarginal, asymmetrical syndesmophytes, which are typical of psoriatic arthritis or Reiter's disease. This patient has psoriasis.

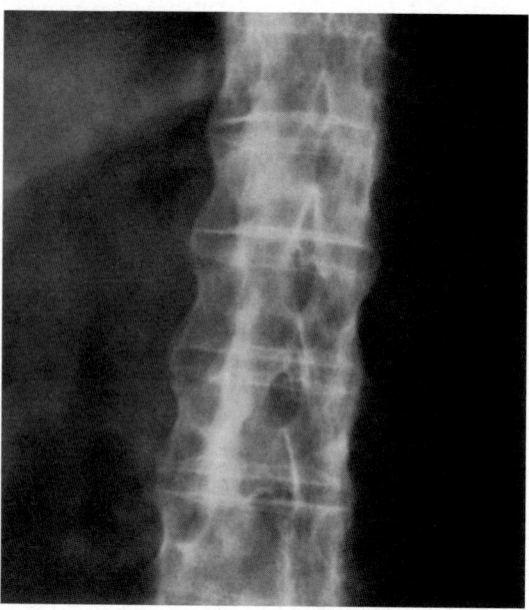

Figure 44.12. Marginal, Symmetrical Syndesmophytes in Ankylosing Spondylitis. Bilateral marginal syndesmophytes are seen bridging the disc spaces throughout the lumbar spine in this patient. This is a so-called bamboo spine and is classic for ankylosing spondylitis and inflammatory bowel disease.

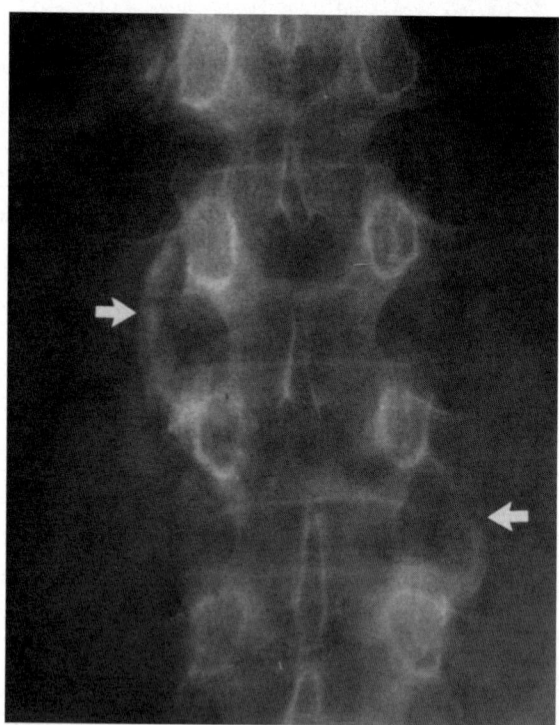

Figure 44.13. Syndesmophytes in Psoriatic Arthritis. Large, bulky, nonmarginal, asymmetrical syndesmophytes (*arrows*) are seen in this patient with psoriatic arthritis.

Involvement of the sacroiliac (S-I) joints is common in the HLA-B27 spondyloarthropathies. The patterns of involvement, like the patterns of involvement of the spine, are somewhat typical for each disorder. Ankylosing spondylitis and inflammatory bowel disease typically cause bilaterally symmetrical SI joint disease, which is initially erosive in nature and progresses to sclerosis and fusion (Figs. 44.14, 44.15). It is extremely unusual to have asymmetrical or unilateral SI joint disease in these two disorders.

Reiter's syndrome and psoriatic arthritis can exhibit unilateral or bilateral SI joint involvement. It seems that it is bilateral about 50% of the time. It is often asymmetrical when it is bilateral, but exact symmetry can be difficult to assess; therefore, when it is definitely bilateral and not clearly asymmetrical, consider the SI joints to be in the bilateral symmetrical category. This means that if there is bilateral, symmetrical SI joint disease, it could be caused by any of the four HLA-B27 spondyloarthropathies. If there is unilateral (or clearly asymmetrical) SI joint involvement, one can exclude ankylosing spondylitis and inflammatory bowel disease and consider Reiter's syndrome or psoriatic disease. In this latter example, one would also have to consider infection and DJD (remember that DJD can cause erosions in the SI joints). Although seen less commonly, gout can also affect the SI joints unilaterally (Table 44.6 and Figs. 44.4, 44.16).

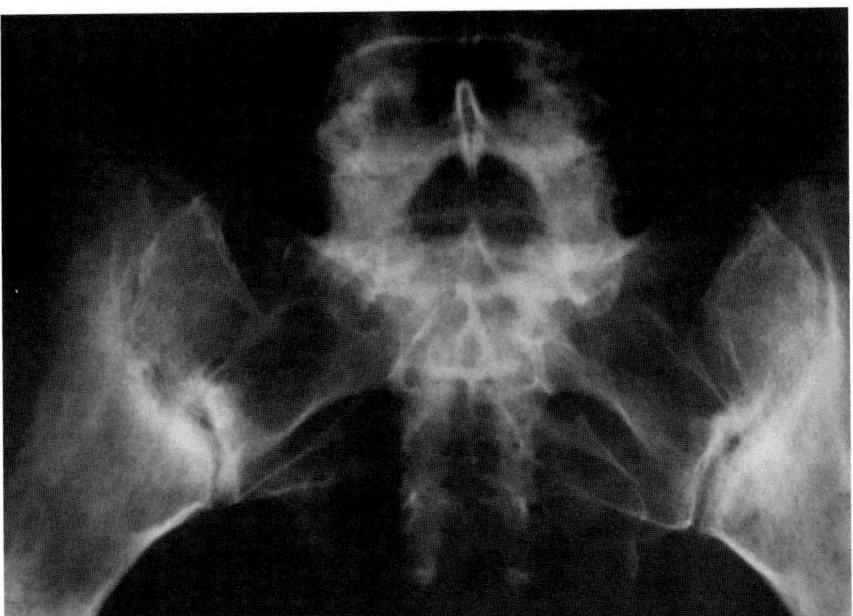

Figure 44.14. Ankylosing Spondylitis. Bilateral symmetrical, SI joint sclerosis and erosions are seen in this patient with ankylosing spondylitis. Inflammatory bowel disease could have a similar appearance. Although this is classic for these two disorders, it would not be that unusual for psoriatic disease or Reiter's syndrome also to have this appearance. Although less likely, it would be possible for infection and even DJD to be bilateral in this fashion.

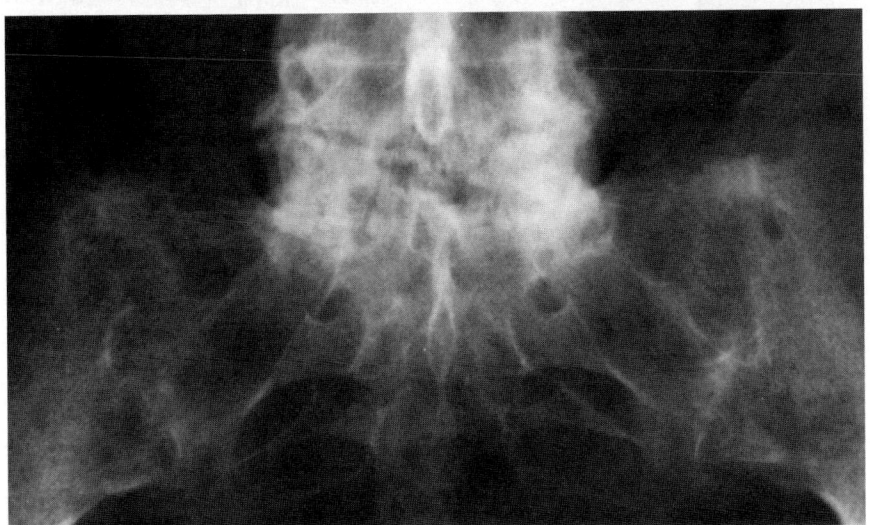

Figure 44.15. Fusion of the SI Joints in Ankylosing Spondylitis. Bilateral complete fusion of the SI joints in this patient with ankylosing spondylitis makes the SI joints totally indistinguishable. Inflammatory bowel disease could have a similar appearance.

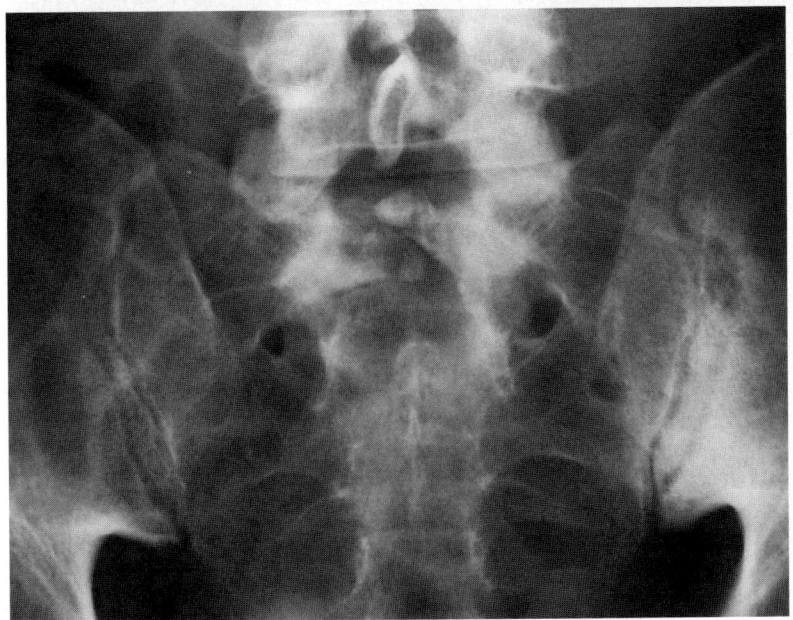

Figure 44.16. Psoriasis with SI Joint Disease. Unilateral SI sclerosis and erosions are seen in this patient with psoriasis. Ankylosing spondylitis and inflammatory bowel disease virtually never have this appearance.

Table 44.6 Causes of Sacroiliac Joint Disease

Ankylosing spondylitis
Inflammatory bowel disease
Psoriasis
Reiter's syndrome
Infection
DJD
Gout

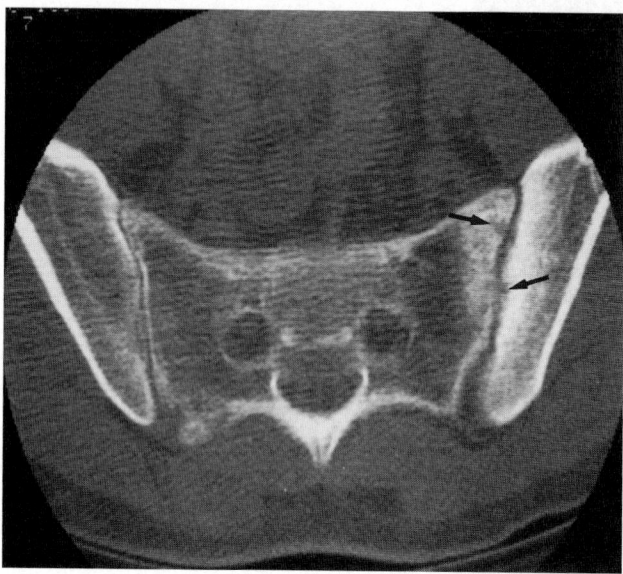

Figure 44.17. CT of the SI Joints in Psoriasis. A computed tomography scan through the SI joints in this patient with psoriasis shows unilateral SI joint sclerosis and erosions (*arrows*), typical for psoriasis or Reiter's disease.

Computed tomography can be very helpful in examining the SI joints and is considered by many to be the diagnostic procedure of choice because of the unobstructed view of the entire joint (Fig. 44.17).

Large-joint involvement with the HLA-B27 spondyloarthropathies is uncommon (except for ankylosing spondylitis), but when it does occur, the arthropathy will resemble rheumatoid arthritis (Fig. 44.18). The hips are involved in up to 50% of the patients with ankylosing spondylitis.

Small-joint involvement, specifically in the hands and feet, is not common in ankylosing spondylitis and inflammatory bowel disease. Psoriasis causes a distinctive arthropathy that is characterized by its distal predominance, proliferative erosions, soft-tissue swelling, and periostitis. Proliferative erosions are different from the clean-cut, sharply marginated erosions seen in all other erosive arthritides in that they have fuzzy margins with wisps of periostitis emanating from them (Fig. 44.19A). The severe forms are often associated with bony ankylosis across joints (Fig. 44.19) and arthritis mutilans deformities. A fairly common finding is a calcaneal heel spur that has fuzzy margins as opposed to the well-corticated heel spur seen in DJD or posttrauma (Fig. 44.20).

Reiter's syndrome causes identical changes in every respect to psoriasis, with the exception that the hands are not as commonly involved as the feet. The interphalangeal joint of the great toe is a commonly affected location in Reiter's disease (Fig. 44.21).

CRYSTAL-INDUCED ARTHRITIS

The crystal-induced arthritides include primarily gout and pseudogout (CPPD). Ochronosis and Wilson's disease are so rare that they are not covered in this chapter.

Figure 44.18. Ankylosing Spondylitis with Hip Disease. An AP view of the pelvis in this patient with ankylosing spondylitis shows bilateral complete fusion of the SI joints. Concentric left hip joint narrowing is present with axial migration of the femoral head. This would be a typical finding in rheumatoid arthritis or, as in this example, in ankylosing spondylitis. Note the secondary DJD changes in the left hip as well.

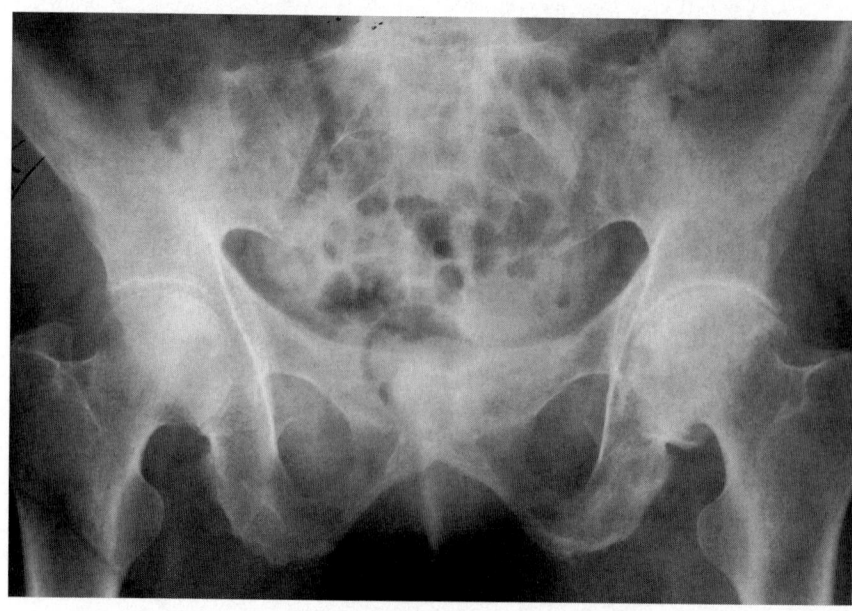

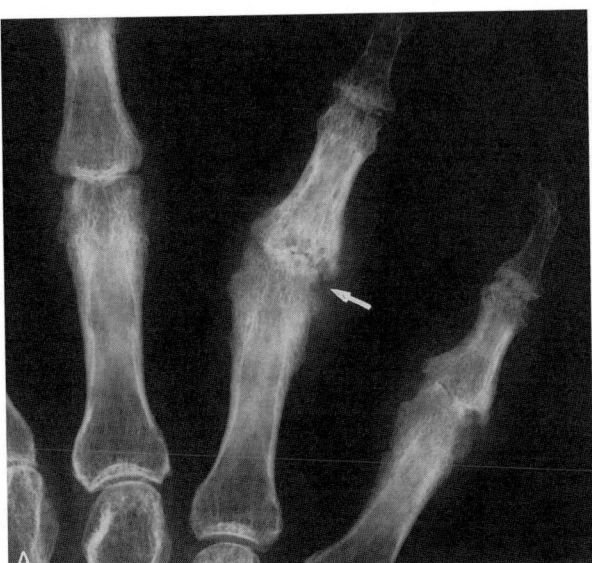
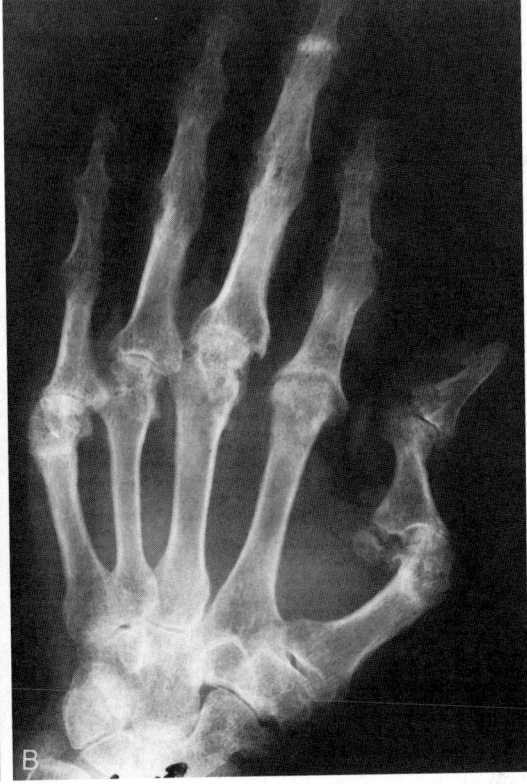

Figure 44.19. Psoriatic Arthritis. A. Cartilage loss at the proximal interphalangeal joints of the third, fourth, and fifth digits in this hand is apparent, with erosions noted most prominently in the third digit (*arrow*). These erosions are not sharply demarcated but are covered with fluffy new bone. These are termed proliferative erosions. Note also the periostitis along the shafts of each of the proximal phalanges. **B.** Advanced psoriatic arthritis. Fusion or ankylosis is apparent across the proximal interphalangeal joints of the second through the fifth digits. Several of the distal interphalangeal joints are also ankylosed. Severe joint space narrowing at the metacarpophalangeal joints is noted. This distal arthridite is typical for psoriatic arthritis in advanced stages.

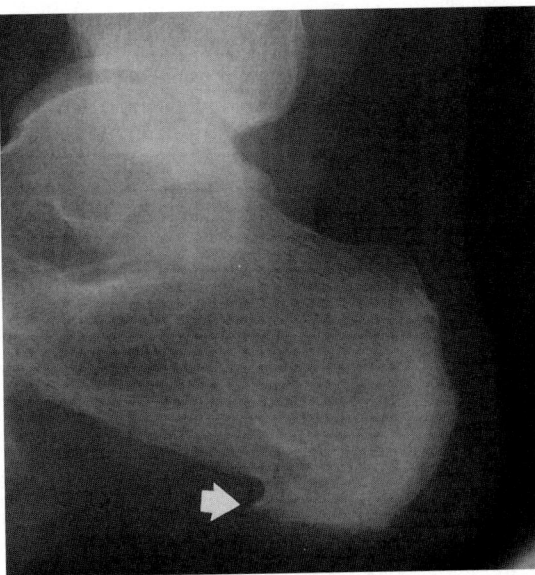

Figure 44.20. Reiter's Syndrome. A lateral view of a calcaneus in a patient with Reiter's syndrome shows poorly defined new bone on the posteroinferior margin of the calcaneus with a calcaneal spur (*arrow*), which is also poorly defined. This is typical of psoriatic or Reiter's disease as opposed to the well-formed calcaneal spur in DJD.

Gout

Gout is a metabolic disorder that results in hyperuricemia and leads to monosodium urate crystals being deposited in various sites in the body, especially joint cartilage. The actual causes of the hyperuricemia are myriad and include heredity.

The arthropathy caused by gout is very characteristic radiographically. It takes 4–6 years for gout to cause radiographically evident disease, and most patients are treated successfully long before the destructive arthropathy occurs; therefore, gouty arthritis is not commonly encountered.

The classic radiographic findings in gout are ***well-defined erosions***, often with sclerotic borders or overhanging edges; ***soft-tissue nodules*** that calcify in the presence of renal failure; and a ***random distribution*** in the hands ***without marked osteoporosis*** (Table 44.7 and Fig. 44.22). Even though erosions with overhanging edges occur with gout, they can occur in other disorders as well and are by no means pathognomonic. The sclerotic margins of the erosions are rarely seen in any other arthridite; therefore, this is a very useful differential point. Gout typically affects the metatarsophalangeal joint of the great toe (Fig. 44.23). In the advanced stages,

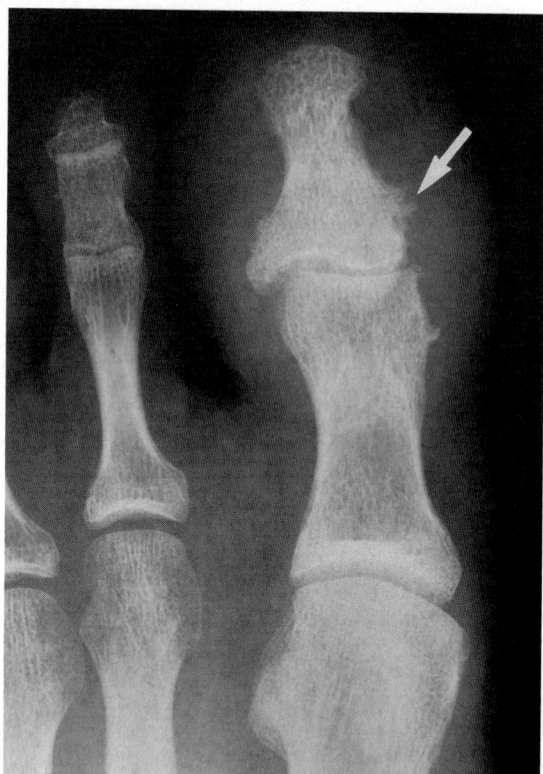

Figure 44.21. Reiter's Syndrome. An AP view of the large toe in a patient with Reiter's disease shows fluffy periostitis (*arrow*) in the erosions adjacent to the interphalangeal joint of the great toe. Marked soft-tissue swelling is also present throughout the great toe. These changes are typical in appearance and location for Reiter's disease or psoriasis.

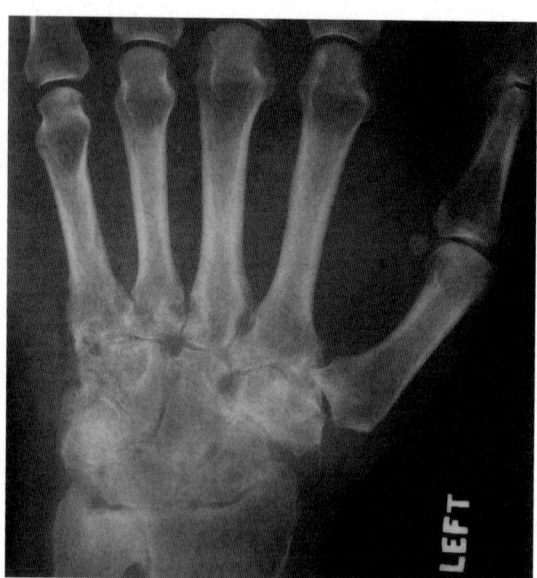

Figure 44.22. Gout. Sharply marginated erosions, some with a sclerotic margin, are noted throughout the carpus and proximal metacarpals. These erosions are classic in gout. Note the absence of marked demineralization.

Table 44.7 Hallmarks of Gout

Well-defined erosions (sclerotic margins)
Soft-tissue nodules
Random distribution
No osteoporosis

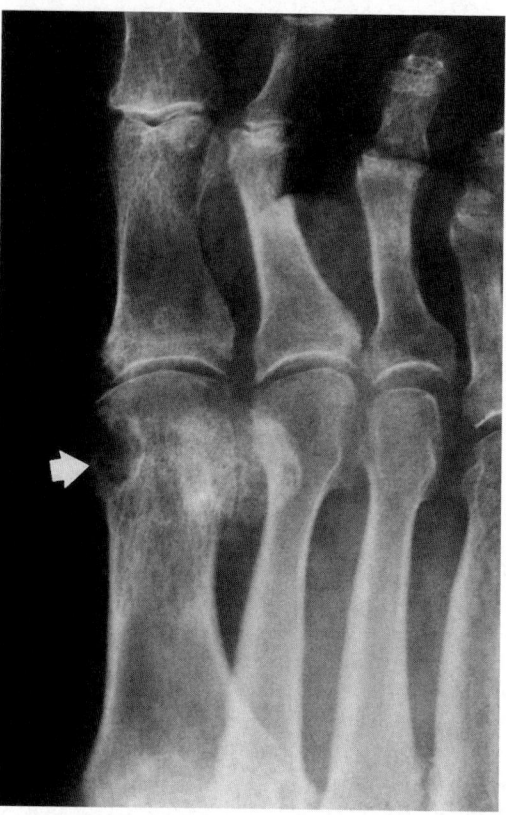

Figure 44.23. Gout. A sharply marginated erosion with an overhanging edge (*arrow*) and a sclerotic margin is seen in the metatarsophalangeal in the great toe in this patient with gout. This appearance and location are classic for gout, whereas psoriasis and Reiter's disease usually involve the interphalangeal joint and do not have erosions that are this sharply marginated.

it can be very deforming (Fig. 44.24). Patients with gout often have chondrocalcinosis because they have a predisposition for pseudogout (CPPD). As many as 40% of patients with gout concomitantly have CPPD.

Pseudogout (Calcium Pyrophosphate Dihydrate Crystal Deposition Disease)

Calcium pyrophosphate dihydrate crystal deposition disease has a classic triad: pain, cartilage calcification, and joint destruction. The patient may have any combination of one or more of this triad at any one time. Each of these is addressed individually in some detail in this chapter, but note that two of the three are radiographic findings. This is a disorder that is best diagnosed radiographically.

The pain of CPPD is nonspecific. It can mimic that of gout (hence the term "pseudogout") or infection or just

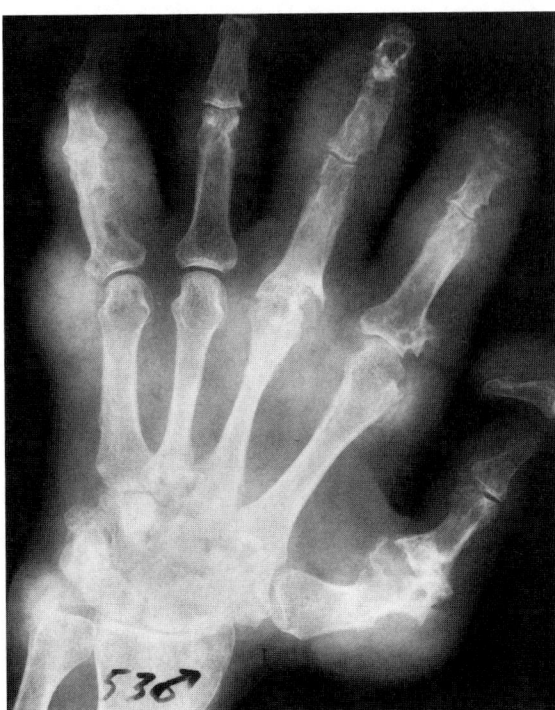

Figure 44.24. Advanced Gout. Marked diffuse and focal soft-tissue swelling is present throughout the hand and wrist in this patient with long-standing gout. Destructive, large, well-marginated erosions, some with overhanging edges, are noted near multiple joints. The focal areas of soft-tissue swelling are called tophi, some of which are calcified. These only calcify with coexistent renal disease.

about any arthritis. It typically is intermittent for a large number of years until DJD occurs and becomes the main cause of pain.

Cartilage calcification, known as chondrocalcinosis, can occur in any joint but tends to affect a few select sites in most patients. These are the medial and lateral compartments of the **knee** (Fig. 44.25), **the triangular fibrocartilage of the wrist** (Fig. 44.26), and the **symphysis pubis** (Table 44.8). Chondrocalcinosis in these areas is virtually diagnostic of CPPD (3). When CPPD crystals occur in the soft tissues, such as in the rotator cuff of the shoulder, a radiograph cannot differentiate between CPPD and calcium hydroxyapatite, which occurs in calcific tendinitis. Calcium hydroxyapatite does not occur in the joint cartilage except in extremely unusual cases; therefore, all chondrocalcinosis can be considered to be secondary to CPPD.

The joint destruction or arthropathy is virtually indistinguishable from DJD. In fact, it *is* DJD. It is caused by CPPD crystals eroding the cartilage. There are a few features of the DJD caused by CPPD that will help distinguish it from DJD caused by trauma or overuse, however. The main difference is one of location. The CPPD has a proclivity for the **shoulder**, the **elbow** (Fig. 44.27), the **radiocarpal joint** in the wrist (Fig. 44.28), and the **patellofemoral joint** of the knee (Table 44.9). These are areas not normally involved by DJD of wear and tear (such as in the distal interphalangeal joints of the hand, the hip, and the medial compartment of the knee). When

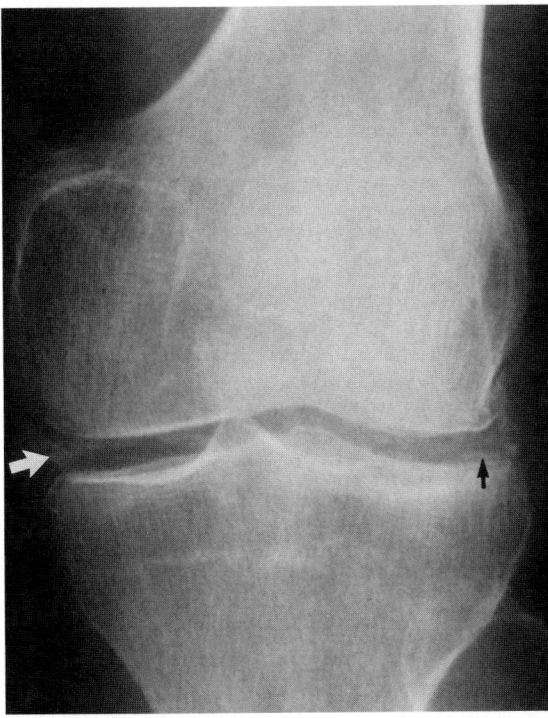

Figure 44.25. Chondrocalcinosis in the Knee. Cartilage calcification known as chondrocalcinosis is seen in the fibrocartilage (*white arrow*) and in the hyaline articular cartilage (*black arrow*) in this patient with CPPD.

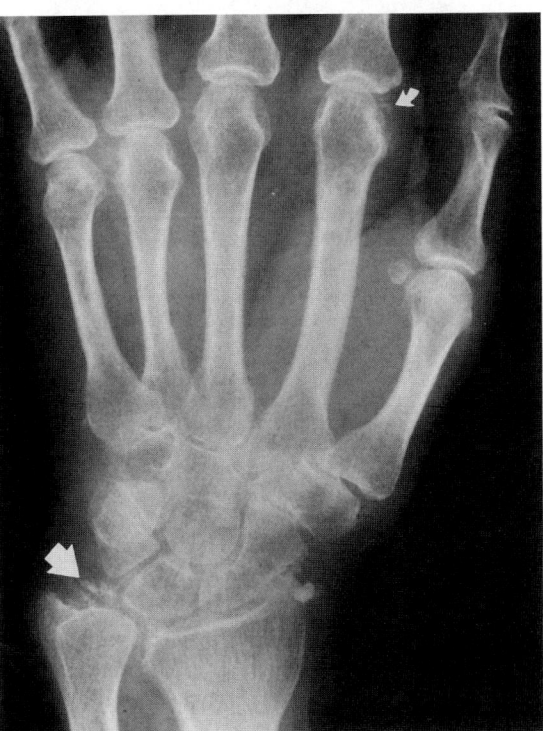

Figure 44.26. Chondrocalcinosis in the Wrist. This patient with CPPD exhibits chondrocalcinosis in the triangular fibrocartilage of the wrist (*large arrow*). A small amount of chondrocalcinosis is also seen in the second metacarpophalangeal (*small arrow*). Triangular ligament calcification is one of the more common locations for chondrocalcinosis to occur.

Table 44.8 Most Common Location of Chondrocalcinosis in CPPD

Knee
Triangular fibrocartilage of wrist
Symphysis pubis

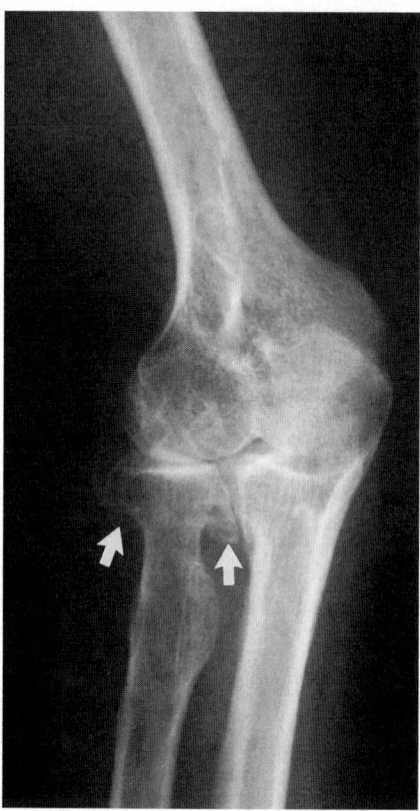

Figure 44.27. Calcium Pyrophosphate Dihydrate Deposition Disease Arthropathy. Degenerative joint disease of the elbow is seen in this patient with CPPD. Note the joint space narrowing with minimal sclerosis and large osteophytes (*arrows*). Osteophytes of this nature are termed drooping osteophytes and are often seen in CPPD. The elbow is an unusual place for DJD to occur except in the setting of CPPD.

DJD is seen in the joints that CPPD tends to involve, a search for chondrocalcinosis should be made. If necessary, a joint aspiration for CPPD crystals may be required to confirm the diagnosis.

Occasionally, the arthropathy of CPPD causes such severe destruction that a neuropathic or Charcot joint is mimicked on the radiograph. This has been termed a pseudo-Charcot joint. It is not a true Charcot joint because of the presence of sensation (4).

There are three diseases that have a high degree of association with CPPD. These are **primary hyperparathyroidism**, **gout**, and **hemochromatosis** (Table 44.10). This is not a differential diagnosis for chondrocalcinosis. These are diseases that tend to occur at the same time that CPPD occurs. If the patient has one of these three disorders, he or she is more likely to have CPPD than is a nonaffected person. There is probably no good reason to work up every patient with chondrocalci-

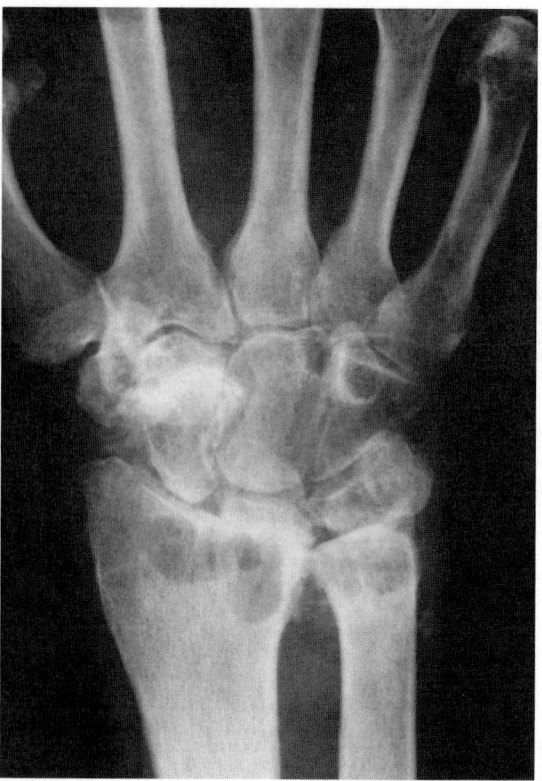

Figure 44.28. Calcium Pyrophosphate Dihydrate Crystal Deposition Disease Arthropathy. Marked DJD at the radiocarpal joint is seen in this patient with CPPD. Severe joint space narrowing and sclerosis with large subchondral cysts or geodes are all hallmarks of DJD. This is an unusual location for DJD except in the setting of CPPD.

Table 44.9 Most Common Location of Arthropathy in CPPD

Shoulder
Radiocarpal joint
Patellofemoral joint
Elbow

Table 44.10 Disease with High Association with CPPD

Primary hyperparathyroidism
Gout
Hemochromatosis

nosis for one of the three associated diseases because they are so uncommon and CPPD is extremely common.

COLLAGEN-VASCULAR DISEASES

Scleroderma, systemic lupus erythematosus, dermatomyositis, and mixed connective tissue disease are all grouped together as collagen-vascular diseases. The striking abnormality in the hands in each of these disorders is osteoporosis and soft-tissue wasting. Systemic lupus erythematosus characteristically has severe ulnar

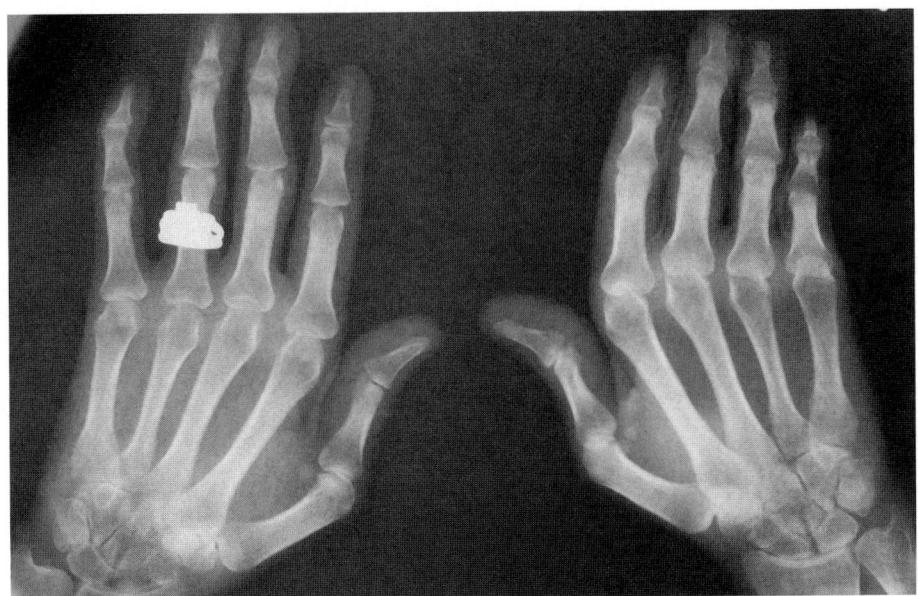

Figure 44.29. Systemic Lupus Erythematosus. Marked soft-tissue wasting, as noted by the concavity in the hypothenar eminence, with ulnar deviation of the phalanges, seen primarily in the right hand, are hallmarks of systemic lupus erythematosus.

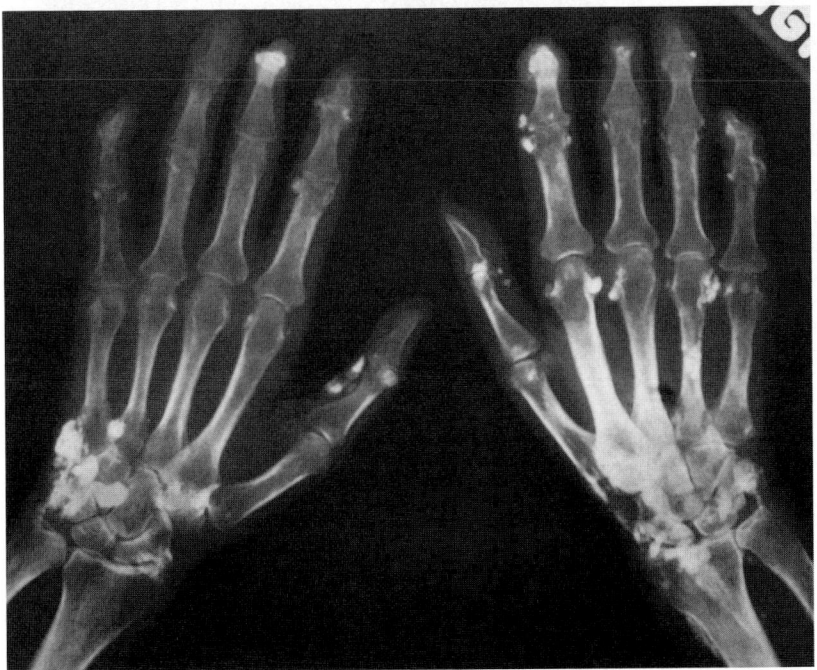

Figure 44.30. Scleroderma. Diffuse subcutaneous soft-tissue calcification is seen throughout the hands and wrists in this patient with scleroderma. Soft-tissue wasting and osteoporosis are also present, as well as bone loss in multiple distal phalanges secondary to the vascular abnormalities often present in this disease.

deviation of the phalanges (Fig. 44.29). Erosions are generally not a feature of these disorders. Soft-tissue calcifications are typically present in scleroderma (Fig. 44.30) and dermatomyositis. The calcifications in scleroderma are typically subcutaneous, whereas in dermatomyositis they are intramuscular in location. Mixed connective tissue disease is an overlap of scleroderma, systemic lupus erythematosus, polymyositis, and rheumatoid arthritis. It has a myriad of radiographic findings.

SARCOID

Sarcoidosis is a disease that causes deposition of granulomatous tissue in the body, primarily in the lungs, but also in the bones. In the skeletal system, it

has a predilection for the hands, where it causes lytic destructive lesions in the cortex. These often have a so-called lace-like appearance, which is characteristic (Fig. 44.31). It can have associated skin nodules in the hands.

HEMOCHROMATOSIS

Hemochromatosis is a disease of excess iron deposition in tissues throughout the body leading to fibrosis and eventual organ failure. Twenty to fifty percent of patients with hemochromatosis have a characteristic arthropathy in the hands that should suggest the diagnosis. The classic radiographic changes are essentially DJD, which involves the second through the fourth metacarpophalangeal joints (Fig. 44.32). Up to 50% of

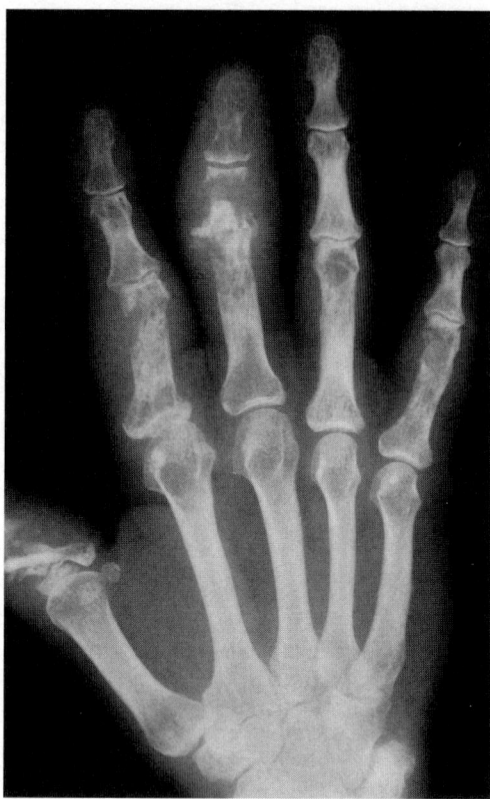

Figure 44.31. Sarcoid. An AP view of the hand in this patient with sarcoid demonstrates classic changes of bony involvement with this granulomatous process. Note the lacelike pattern of destruction seen most prominently in the proximal phalanges and in the distal third phalanx. Soft-tissue swelling and some areas of severe bony dissolution are also noted, which occur in more advanced patterns of sarcoid. These changes are typically limited to the hands but can rarely occur in other parts of the skeleton.

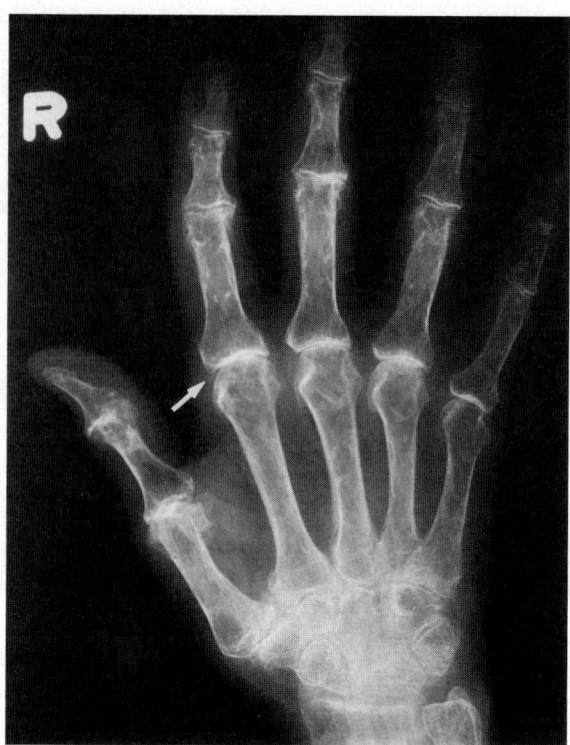

Figure 44.32. Hemochromatosis. An AP view of the hand in this patient with hemochromatosis shows severe joint space narrowing throughout the hand, which is most marked at the metacarpophalangeal joints. Associated sclerosis at the metacarpophalangeal joints with large osteophytes seen off the metacarpal heads suggests DJD. These are very unusual joints for DJD to occur in, yet this is the classic appearance of hemochromatosis. No chondrocalcinosis is seen in the triangular cartilage in this patient; however, a small amount of chondrocalcinosis can be seen at the second metacarpophalangeal (*arrow*). Fifty percent of patients with hemochromatosis also have CPPD.

the patients with hemochromatosis also have CPPD; therefore, a search should be made for chondrocalcinosis. Another finding that is often seen in hemochromatosis is called squaring of the metacarpal heads. They appear enlarged and blocklike as a result of the large osteophytes commonly seen in this disorder. The osteophytes are often said to be "drooping" because of the unusual way they hang off the joint margin.

MULTICENTRIC RETICULOHISTIOCYTOSIS

Multicentric reticulohistiocytosis is a very rare disorder that is also called lipoid dermatoarthritis. It is a disease of cutaneous xanthomas that are associated with a mutilating arthritis of the hands, which is very characteristic (5). Multiple erosions, predominantly in the phalanges, are found that are strikingly bilaterally symmetrical and not associated with osteoporosis (Fig. 44.33). Rheumatoid arthritis usually is mentioned in the differential diagnosis because of the erosions and bilateral symmetry; however, the distal distribution and lack of osteoporosis are against rheumatoid. Multicentric reticulohistiocytosis can proceed to an arthritis mutilans or can spontaneously arrest.

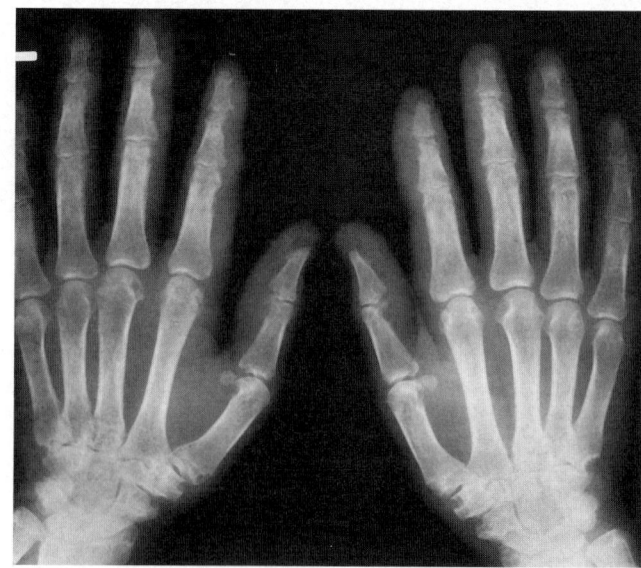

Figure 44.33. Multicentric Reticulohistiocytosis. An AP view of the hand in this patient reveals multiple soft-tissue nodules seen best in the second digits bilaterally with diffuse erosions that are sharply demarcated and strikingly bilaterally symmetrical. There is little or no osteoporosis. These changes are classic for multicentric reticulohistiocytosis.

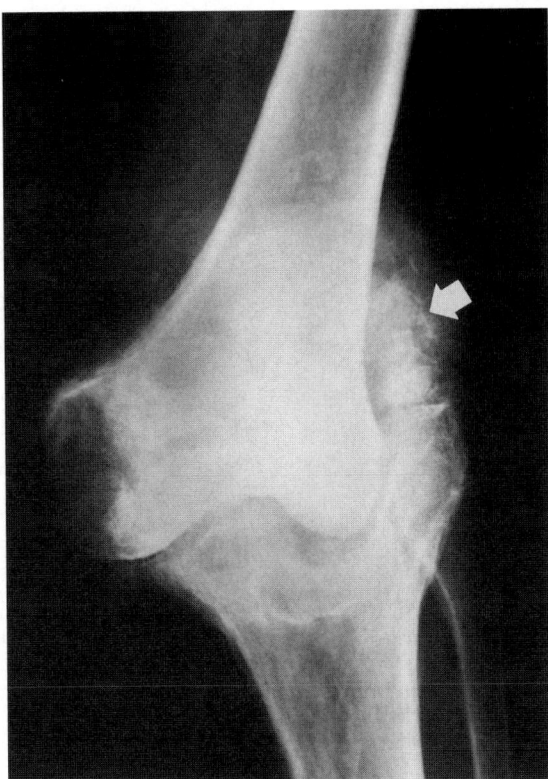

Figure 44.34. Charcot Joint. An AP view of the knee in this patient with tabes dorsalis shows the classic changes of a neuropathic or Charcot joint. Note the severe joint destruction, the subluxation, and the heterotopic new bone (*arrow*).

**Table 44.11 Hallmarks of a
Neuropathic Joint**

Joint destruction
Dislocation
Heterotopic new bone formation

NEUROPATHIC OR CHARCOT JOINT

The radiographic findings for a Charcot joint are characteristic and almost pathognomonic. A classic triad has been described that consists of *joint destruction*, *dislocation*, and *heterotopic new bone* (Table 44.11 and Fig. 44.34).

Joint destruction is seen in every type of arthritis and therefore seems very nonspecific; however, nothing causes as severe destruction in a joint as a Charcot joint. Progressive joint destruction occurs in a neuropathic joint because the joint is rendered unstable by inaccurate muscle action and is unprotected by intact nerve reflexes. Early in the development of a Charcot joint, the joint destruction may merely appear to be joint space narrowing. It is extremely difficult to make the diagnosis this early. In the spine, instead of joint space destruction, there is disc space destruction (Fig. 44.35).

Dislocation, like joint destruction, can be present in varying degrees. Early on the joint may have subluxation instead of dislocation.

Heterotopic new bone has also been termed debris or detritus and consists of soft-tissue calcification or

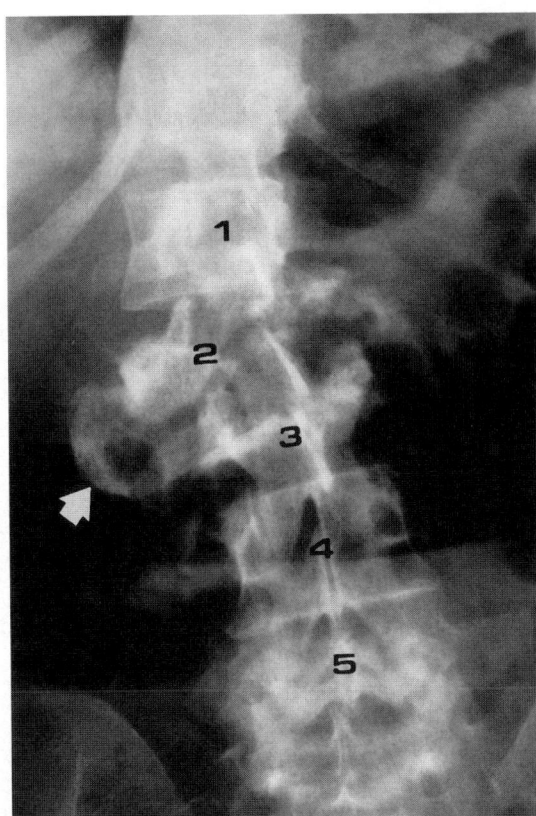

Figure 44.35. Charcot Spine. An AP view of the spine in this paraplegic patient shows severe destruction of the L2 and L3 vertebral bodies and the intervening disc space, heterotopic new bone (*arrow*), and malalignment or dislocaton. *Numbers* indicate lumbar vertebrae.

clumps of ossification adjacent to the joint. It too can be present in varying amounts.

The most commonly seen Charcot joint today is in the foot of a diabetic. The disease typically affects the first and second tarsometatarsal joints in a fashion similar to a Lisfranc fracture (Fig. 44.36).

Tabes dorsalis from syphilis is rarely seen today. More commonly seen is a Charcot joint in a patient with paralysis who continues to use the affected limb for support. A Charcot joint that is also seen on occasion is the so-called pseudo-Charcot joint in CPPD.

HEMOPHILIA, JUVENILE RHEUMATOID ARTHRITIS, AND PARALYSIS

Why would clinically disparate entities like paralysis, juvenile rheumatoid arthritis, and hemophilia be covered in the same section? Because they are usually radiographically indistinguishable.

The classic findings for JRA and hemophilia are *overgrowth of the ends of the bones* (epiphyseal enlargement) associated with *gracile diaphyses* (Fig. 44.37). Joint destruction might or might not be present. A finding that is purported to be classic for JRA and hemophilia is widening of the intercondylar notch of the knee. This sign can be quite variable and difficult to use. It is rarely present when the other classic signs are not also present and obvious.

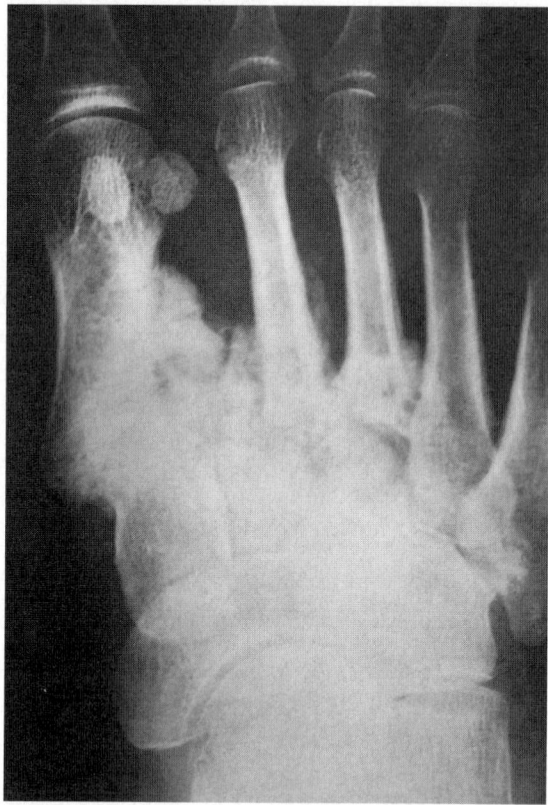

Figure 44.36. Lisfranc Charcot Joint. Dislocation of the second and third metatarsals along with joint destruction and large amounts of heterotopic new bone are present in the foot of this diabetic patient. These findings are classic for a Charcot joint, which has been termed a Lisfranc fracture-dislocation. It is most commonly seen secondary to trauma rather than as a Charcot joint but is the most common neuropathic joint seen today.

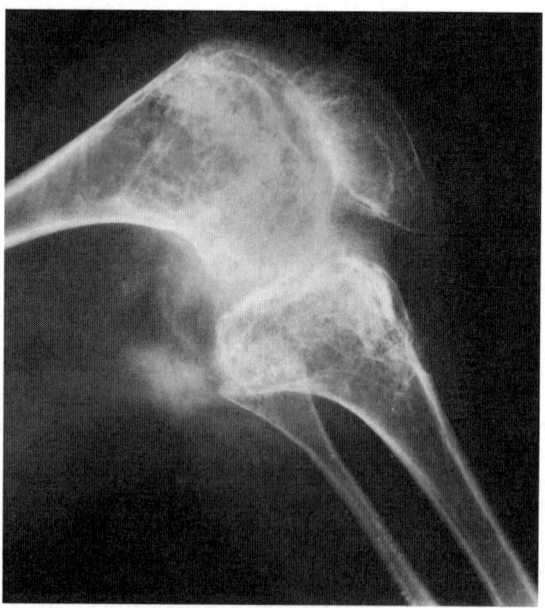

Figure 44.37. Juvenile Rheumatoid Arthritis. A lateral view of the knee in this patient with JRA shows the classic findings of overgrowth of the ends of the bones and associated gracile diaphyses. These changes can also be seen in patients with hemophilia or paralysis.

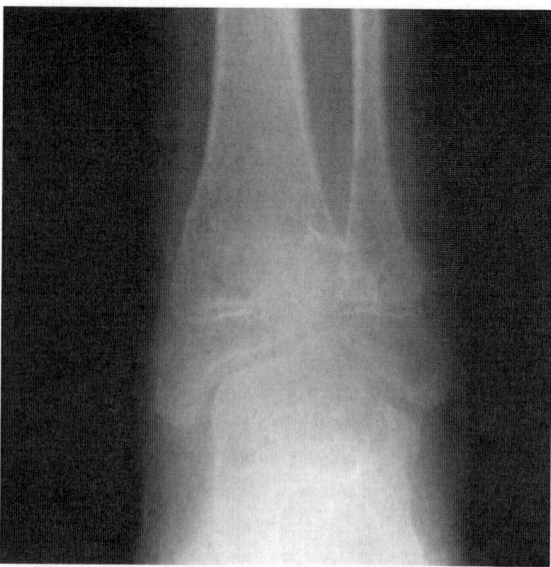

Figure 44.38. Muscular Dystrophy Simulating JRA or Hemophilia. An AP view of the ankle in this patient with muscular dystrophy shows subtle changes of overgrowth of the distal tibia and fibular epiphyses. Marked tibiotalar slant, which can also be present in JRA or hemophilia, is also present.

Another process that can mimic the findings in JRA and hemophilia is a joint that has undergone disuse from paralysis (Fig. 44.38). It has always been said that the reason the epiphyses are overgrown in JRA and hemophilia is because of the hyperemia; however, many other things cause hyperemia without affecting the size of the epiphyses (such as rheumatoid arthritis and infection). The common denominator shared by JRA, hemophilia, and paralysis is disuse. This is most likely what causes the overgrowth of the ends of the bones seen in all three of these disorders.

SYNOVIAL OSTEOCHONDROMATOSIS

Synovial osteochondromatosis is a relatively common disorder caused by a metaplasia of the synovium, resulting in deposition of foci of cartilage in the joint. Most of the time, these cartilaginous deposits calcify and are readily seen on a radiograph (Fig. 44.39). It is most commonly seen in the knee, hip, and elbow. Up to 30% of the time, the cartilaginous deposits do not calcify. In these cases, all that is seen on the radiograph is a joint effusion, unless erosions or joint destruction occur (Fig. 44.40).

The calcifications begin in the synovium and then tend to shed into the joint, where they can cause symptoms of free fragments or "joint mice." They then embed into the synovium and tend not to be free in the joint after a while. It is usually necessary to perform a complete synovectomy to relieve the symptoms.

PIGMENTED VILLONODULAR SYNOVITIS

Pigmented villonodular synovitis is a rare, chronic, inflammatory process of the synovium that causes synovial proliferation. A swollen joint with lobular masses

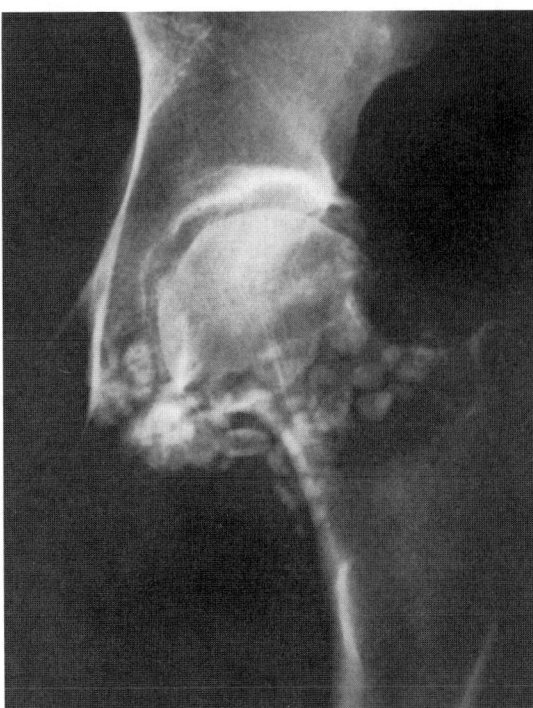

Figure 44.39. Synovial Osteochondromatosis. An AP view of the hip in this patient with left hip pain shows multiple calcified loose bodies in the hip joint, which is virtually diagnostic of synovial osteochondromatosis.

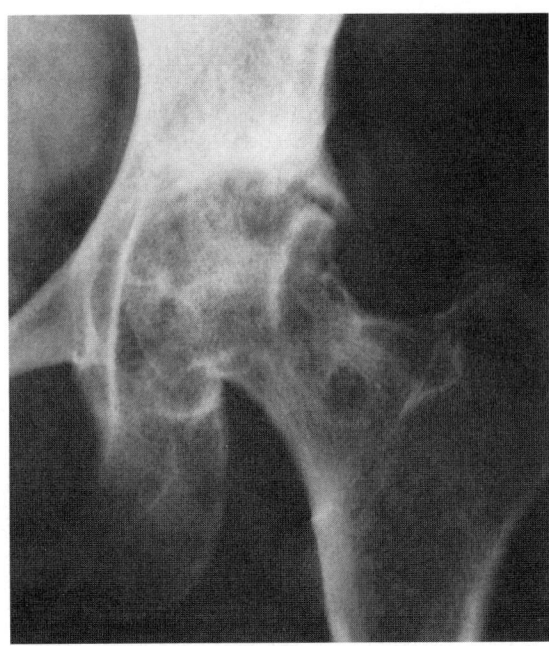

Figure 44.41. Pigmented Villonodular Synovitis. An AP view of the hip in this patient shows joint space destruction and bony erosions throughout the femoral head and neck. Pigmented villonodular synovitis or synovial chondromatosis could have this appearance.

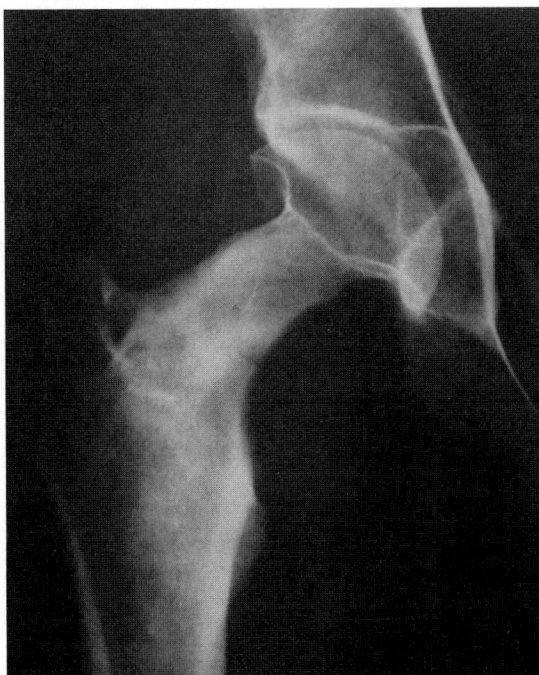

Figure 44.40. Synovial Osteochondromatosis without Calcification. An AP view of the hip in this patient shows the femoral neck to be eroded, with the femoral head having an "apple core" appearance. This has occurred from the pressure erosion of multiple nonossified loose bodies in the joint. This is nonossified synovial osteochondromatosis (which is probably more properly termed synovial chondromatosis). It usually does not cause this degree of bony erosion and is indistinguishable from pigmented villonodular synovitis.

of synovium occurs and causes pain and joint destruction (Fig. 44.41). It rarely, if ever, calcifies. It has been termed giant cell tumor of tendon sheath and tendon sheath xanthoma when it occurs in a tendon sheath, which is not unusual. Joints with PVNS look radiographically identical to noncalcified synovial osteochondromatosis, yet they are much less common. Therefore, whenever pigmented villonodular synovitis is a consideration, synovial osteochondromatosis (noncalcified) should be mentioned. Pigmented villonodular synovitis has a characteristic appearance on magnetic resonance imaging with low-signal hemosiderin seen lining the synovium on both T1- and T2-weighted images (Fig. 44.42).

SUDECK'S ATROPHY

Also known as shoulder-hand syndrome and reflex sympathetic dystrophy, Sudeck's atrophy is a poorly understood joint affliction that typically occurs after minor trauma to an extremity, resulting in pain, swelling, and dysfunction. Severe, patchy osteoporosis and soft-tissue swelling are seen radiographically (Fig. 44.43). It typically affects the distal part of an extremity such as a hand or foot, yet intermediate joints such as the knee and hip are believed by some to be occasionally involved. The pain usually subsides, but the osteoporosis may persist. The swelling, with time, will subside and the skin may become atrophic. It is important for the radiologist to recognize the aggressive osteoporosis in this disorder and differentiate it from disuse osteoporosis so that the treating physician can begin aggressive physical therapy.

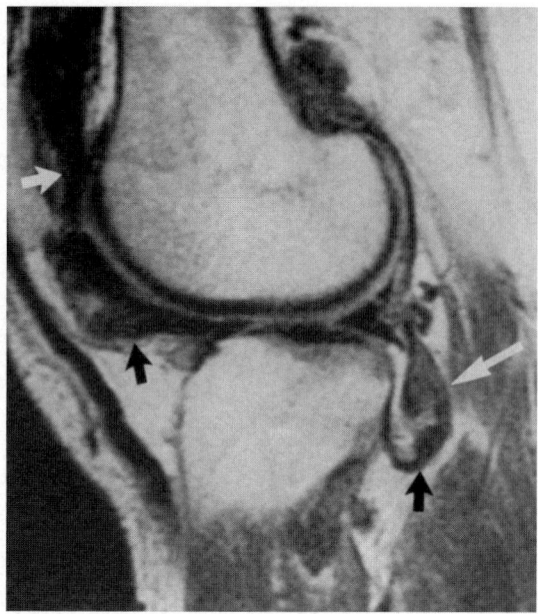

Figure 44.42. Pigmented Villonodular Synovitis. A sagittal T2-weighted MR (TR 1500; TE 60) in a knee with pigmented villonodular synovitis shows low signal masses of tissue in the joint (*arrows*) with only a small amount of high signal joint fluid visible. This is a characteristic appearance of pigmented villonodular synovitis with MR.

JOINT EFFUSIONS

Most joint effusions are clinically obvious and do not require radiographic validation. The elbow is an exception. In the setting of trauma to the elbow, an effusion indicates a fracture. The radiographic signs of an elbow effusion are generally clearly seen (displaced fat pads, as described in chapter 36) and have proved to be valid. Clinical determination of an elbow effusion can be difficult; therefore, the radiologist can be very helpful in this area.

Clinical determination of a hip effusion is also very difficult. The presence of a hip effusion can be valuable in certain clinical settings. For instance, a patient with pain in the hip and an effusion should have the joint aspirated to rule out an infection. If only pain were present, an aspiration would probably not be performed. The radiology literature mentions displacement of the fat stripes about the hip as being an indicator for an effusion, but this has been proved to be unfounded. The only fat pad around the hip that gets displaced with an effusion is the obturator internus, and it is uncommonly seen.

The radiographic sign for a knee effusion that seems to be the most reliable is the measurement of the distance between the suprapatellar fat pad and the anterior femoral fat pad (Fig. 44.44). A distance between these two fat pads of more than 10 mm is definite evidence for an effusion. A distance of less than 5 mm is normal. A distance of 5–10 mm is equivocal. It does not make any difference if there is an effusion in the knee–the patient gets treated the same, regardless. If it were vital to the patient, one could aspirate the joint or perform an MR study to find out. I should point out that an MR should

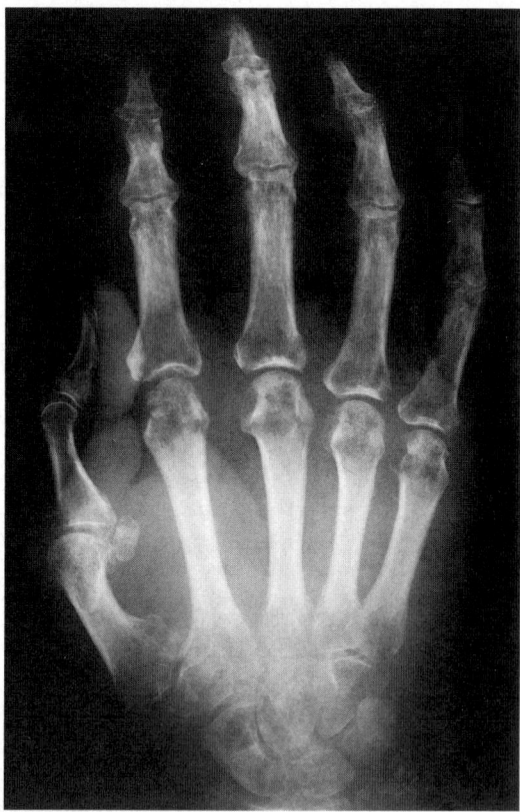

Figure 44.43. Sudeck's Atrophy. Diffuse soft-tissue swelling and marked osteoporosis that is so aggressive it has a spotty or permeative appearance is noted around all of the joints in the hand. This patient has severe hand pain and dysfunction following minor trauma. This is characteristic of Sudeck's atrophy.

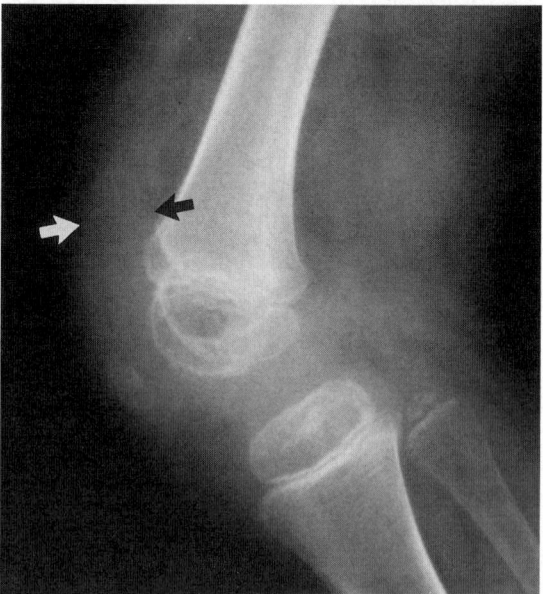

Figure 44.44. Knee Joint Effusion. This patient has joint fluid in the knee, with widely displaced fat pads. The suprapatellar fat pad (*white arrow*) is more than 5 mm from the anterior suprafemoral fat pad (*black arrow*), which indicates a joint effusion. The suprapatellar fat pad is difficult to see in this example.

never be performed just to see whether there is fluid in the joint.

Shoulder effusions are very difficult to detect unless they are massive enough to displace the humeral head inferiorly, as with a fracture and hemarthrosis (see chapter 36). Fortunately, as with most other joints, treatment is not based solely on the presence or absence of an effusion, so it hardly matters. The same is true in the ankle, wrist, and smaller joints.

AVASCULAR NECROSIS

Avascular necrosis, or aseptic necrosis, can occur around almost any joint for a host of reasons including steroids, trauma, a variety of underlying disease states, and even idiopathically. It is often seen in renal transplant patients.

The hallmark of AVN is increased bone density at an otherwise normal joint. Increased density at a narrowed joint usually indicates DJD; however, if either osteophytes or joint space narrowing are absent, another disorder should be considered.

The earliest sign of AVN is a joint effusion. This often is not visible radiographically or is so nonspecific that it does not help with the diagnosis unless the clinical setting had already raised suspicion for AVN. The next sign for AVN is a patchy or mottled density (Fig. 44.45). In the knee, this density increase can occur throughout an entire condyle, whereas in the hip, it often involves the entire femoral head. Next, a subchondral lucency develops

that forms a thin line along the articular surface (Fig. 44.46). This lucent line has been described as being an early indicator for AVN, whereas, in fact, it is a late finding. Also, the lucent line stage is often not present in the evolution of AVN. Therefore, using the lucent line as one of the main criteria for AVN can lead to missing early findings in some cases and missing the diagnosis completely in others.

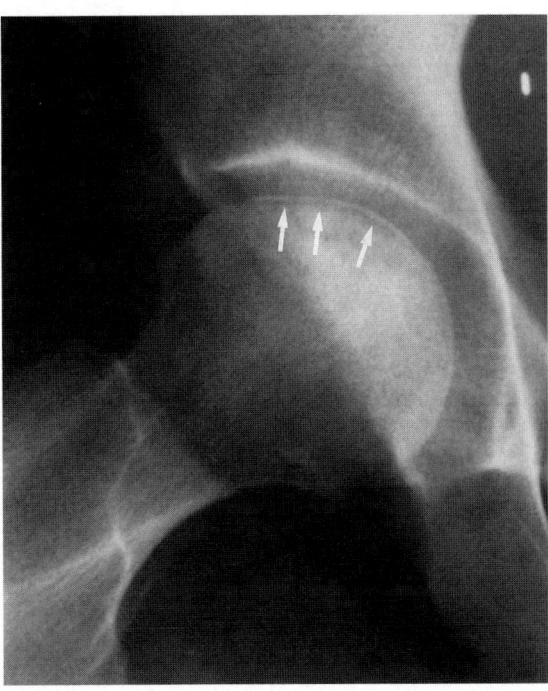

Figure 44.46. Avascular Necrosis of the Hip. A definite subchondral lucency (*arrows*) is seen in the weight-bearing portion of this hip with AVN. Patchy sclerosis throughout the femoral head is also noted.

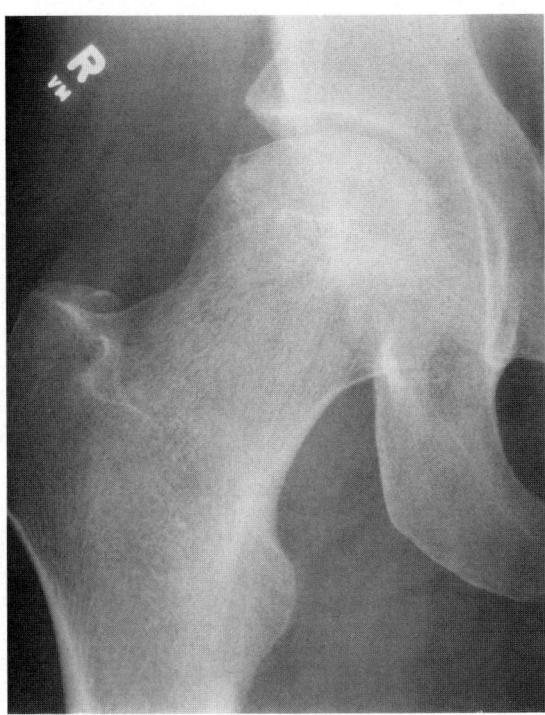

Figure 44.45. Early Avascular Necrosis of the Hip. Patchy sclerosis is present in the femoral head in this patient with a renal transplant and avascular necrosis of the right hip. No subchondral lucency or articular surface irregularity in the weight-bearing region is yet present, with the exception of a small cortical irregularity seen laterally.

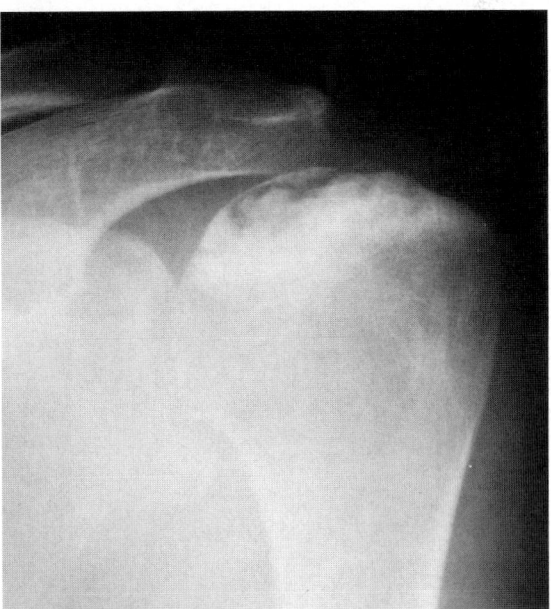

Figure 44.47. Avascular Necrosis of the Shoulder. Articular surface collapse is present in this shoulder with long-standing AVN. Dense bony sclerosis is also present.

Figure 44.48. Avascular Necrosis of the Hip.
An axial T1WI (TR 600; TE 20) of the hips shows
a focal area of abnormality in the left femoral
head (*arrow*), which is characteristic for AVN.
The low signal serpigenous border is a typical
finding, as is the anterior location.

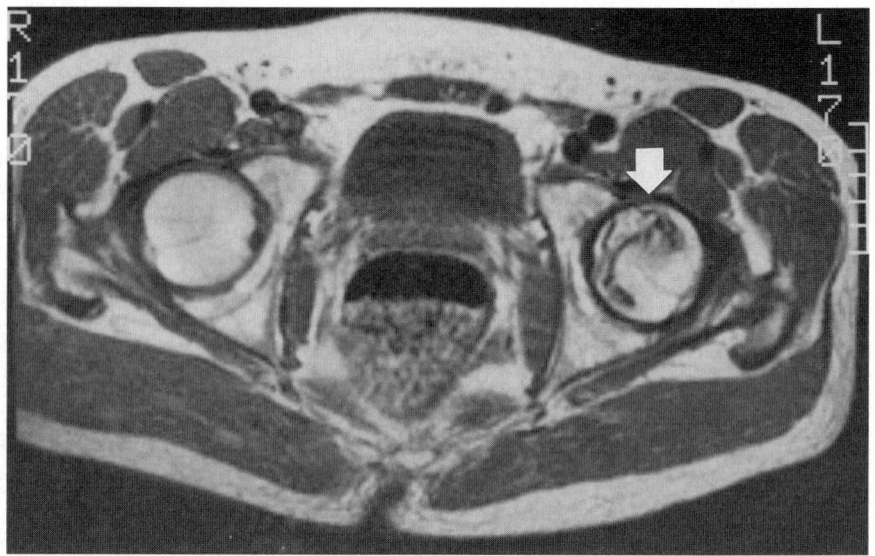

Figure 44.49. Early Avascular Necrosis of the Hip.
A coronal T1WI **(A)** (TR 600; TE 20) and a coronal
GRASS image **(B)** (TR 500; TE 15; θ15°) show bilateral
AVN that is more advanced in the left hip. The T1 WI
(A) shows diffuse low signal intensity in the femoral
necks that increases on the GRASS T2* image **(B)**.
This is typical for edema or hyperemia seen in AVN.
Note the bilateral joint effusions seen as high signal
on the T2* image **(B)**.

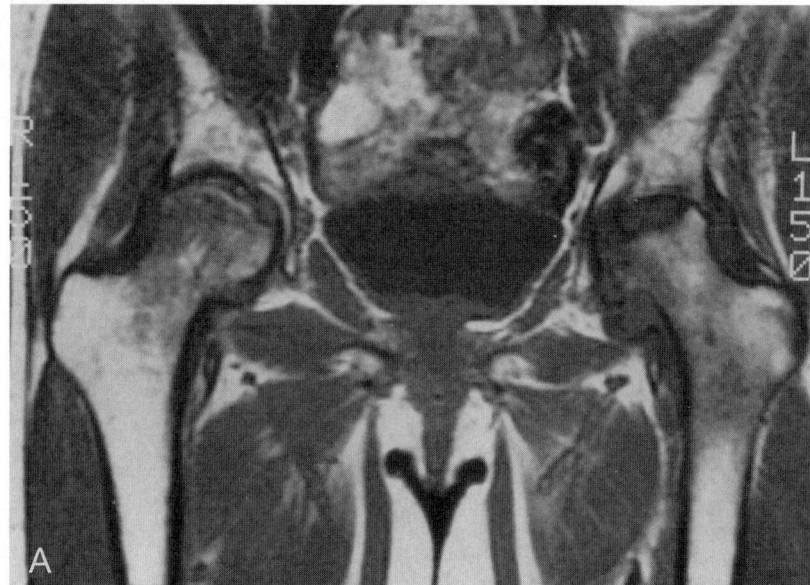

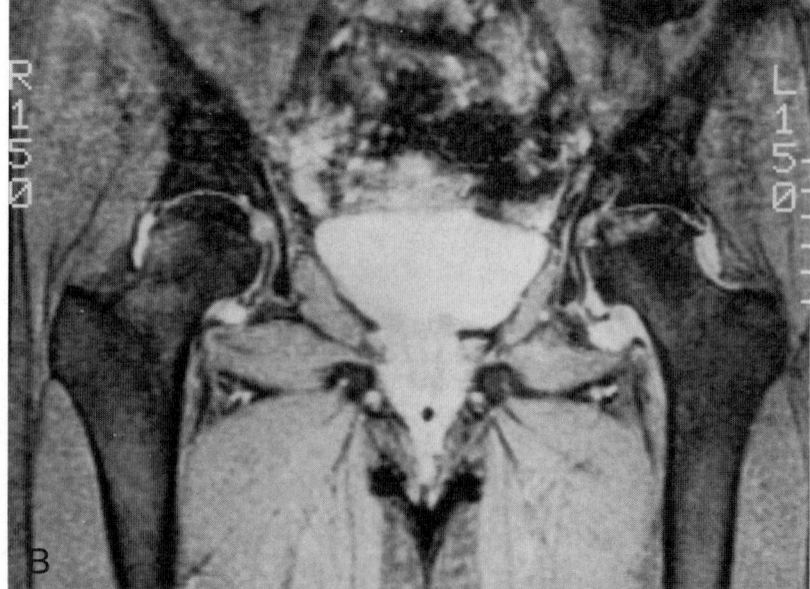

The final sign in AVN is collapse of the articular surface and joint fragmentation (Fig. 44.47). I must stress that these changes all occur on only one side of a joint, which makes for an easy diagnosis because almost everything else around joints involves both sides of the joint.

Magnetic resonance imaging is extremely useful in evaluating AVN. It is the most sensitive imaging study available, often showing AVN when plain films or radionuclide scans are normal (6). In the hip, AVN typically has an area of low or mixed signal on T1-weighted images that is located in the anterosuperior portion of the femoral head (Figs. 44.48, 44.49). If the anterior portion of the femoral head is not involved, the diagnosis of AVN should be questioned, as it is uncommon to present otherwise. Posterior femoral head AVN can occasionally be found after posterior dislocation of the hip because of impaction of the femoral head on the posterior column of the acetabulum.

A form of AVN that is smaller and more focal than that just described is osteochondritis dissecans. It is most likely caused by trauma; however, this is controversial, with one school of thought believing the cause is idiopathic. It occurs most often in the knee at the medial epicondyle (Fig. 44.50). It also is frequently seen in the dome of the talus (Fig. 44.51) and occasionally in the capitellum (Fig. 44.52). Osteochondritis dissecans frequently leads to a small fragment of bone being sloughed off and becoming a free fragment in the joint, a "joint mouse" (see Fig. 44.50).

Avascular necrosis is one of the disorders around joints in which subchondral cysts or geodes can occur.

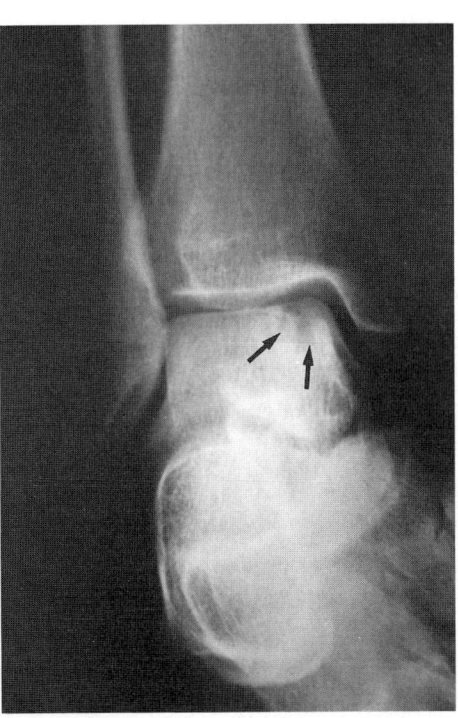

Figure 44.51. Osteochondritis Dissecans of the Talus. A focal area of AVN in the talus as seen here (*arrows*) is called osteochondritis dissecans. The talus is the second most common site after the knee and, as in the knee, can cause a joint mouse, or loose body in the joint.

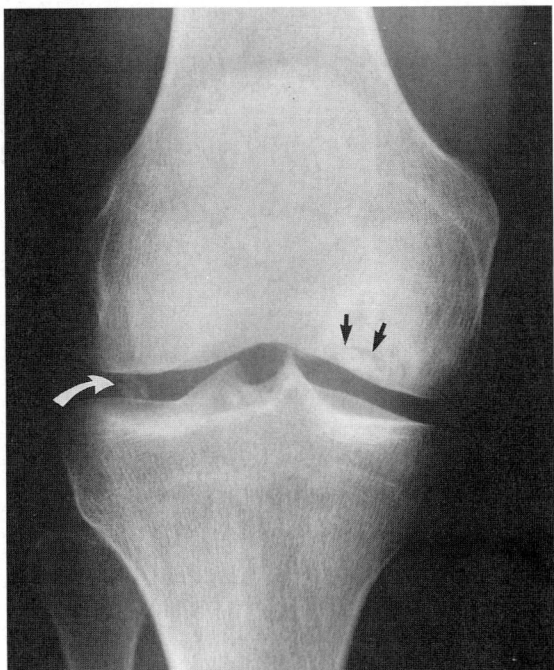

Figure 44.50. Osteochondritis Dissecans. A small focal area of avascular necrosis in the medial epicondyle of the femur (*black arrows*) is present, which is an area of osteochondritis dissecans. Part of the area of AVN has shed a bony fragment (*white arrow*) that is loose in the joint, which is known as a joint mouse.

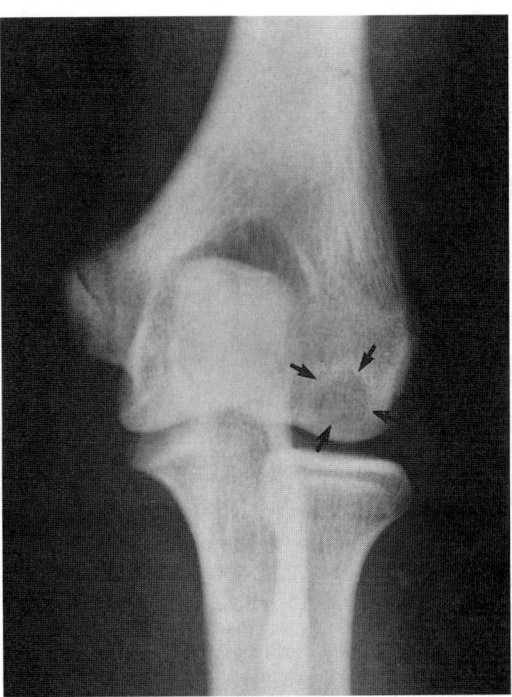

Figure 44.52. Osteochondritis Dissecans of the Elbow. The third most common site for osteochondritis dissecans is in the capitellum of the elbow. The faint lucency seen in this capitellum (*arrows*) was at first believed to be a chondroblastoma or an area of infection.

It is the only one of the four disorders (rheumatoid arthritis, DJD, and CPPD being the others) that can have an essentially normal joint and have a geode (Fig. 44.53). The other abnormalities will have any or a combination of joint space narrowing, osteophytes, osteoporosis, chondrocalcinosis, or other findings.

A host of names have been ascribed to epiphyseal avascular necrosis, usually with the eponym being the first person to describe the disorder. These are believed to be idiopathic for the most part but can also occur secondary to trauma. A few of the more common epiphyses involved are the following: the carpal lunate, Kienböck's

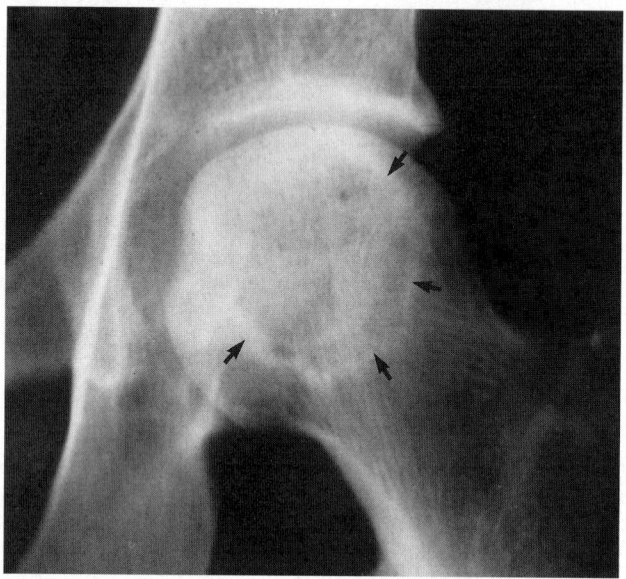

Figure 44.53. Geode in the Hip. A large cystic lesion (*arrows*) is seen in this patient with AVN of the hip. Note the adjacent patchy sclerosis, indicative of avascular necrosis. A subchondral cyst or geode should be considered any time a lytic lesion is found around a joint.

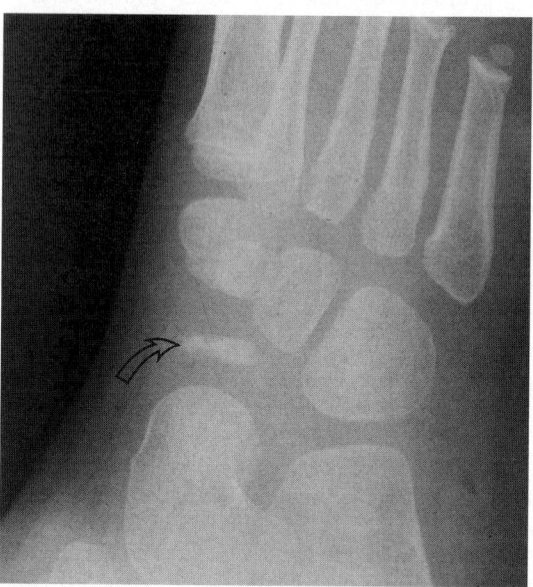

Figure 44.55. Köhler's Disease. Flattening and sclerosis of the tarsal navicular (*arrow*) in children is thought by many to be AVN and is called Köhler's disease. Others have found this to be an asymptomatic normal variant and believe that it is an incidental finding.

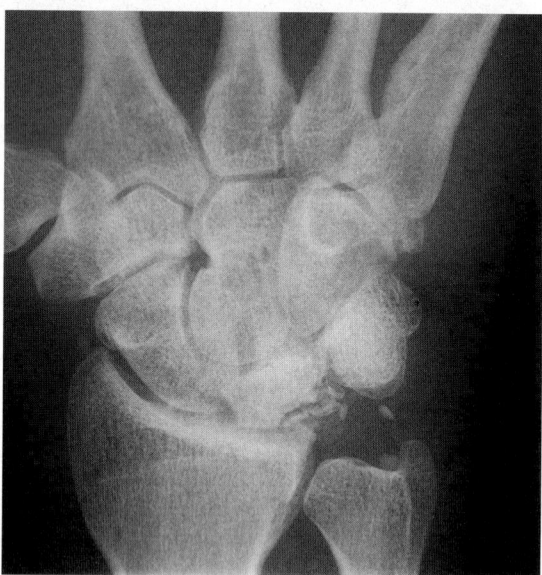

Figure 44.54. Kienböck's Malacia. Avascular necrosis of the lunate, Kienböck's malacia, is demonstrated in this patient's wrist. The increased density and partial fragmentation of the lunate are characteristic for AVN. Also, note the slightly shortened ulna (in comparison with the radius), which is called negative ulnar variance. Negative ulnar variance is said to have a high association with Kienböck's malacia.

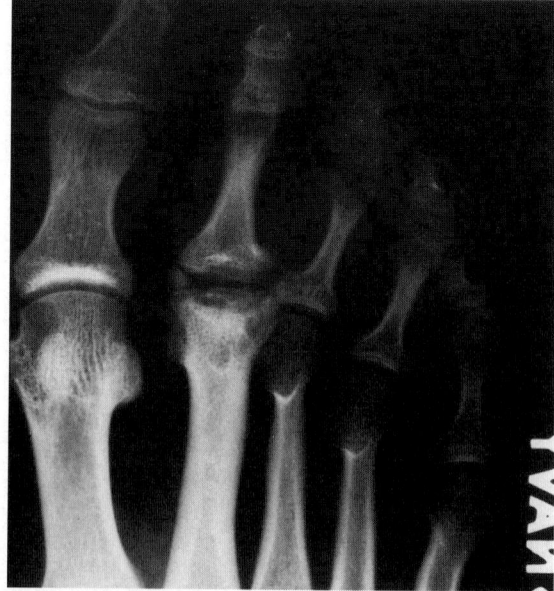

Figure 44.56. Freiberg's Infraction. Flattening, collapse, and sclerosis of the second metatarsal head, as seen in this patient, is typical of AVN or Freiberg's infraction. It can also involve the second, third, or fourth metatarsal heads. Note the compensatory hypertrophy of the cortex of the second metatarsal, which is invariably found with this disorder.

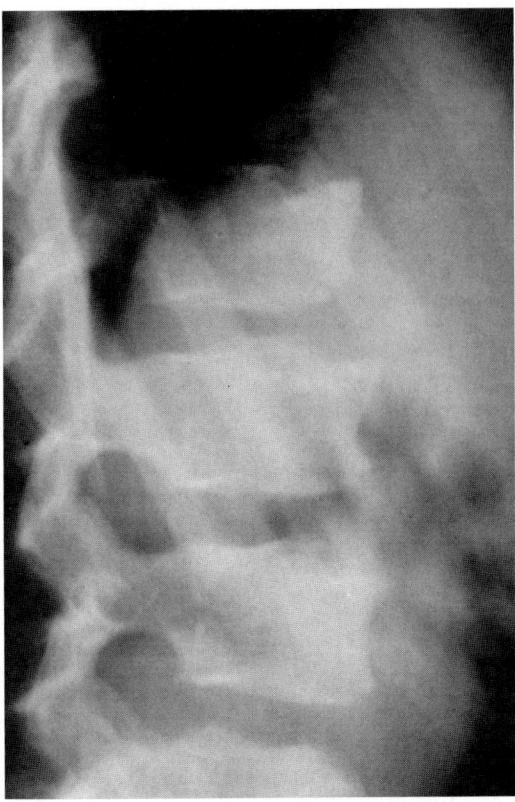

Figure 44.57. Scheuermann's Disease. Avascular necrosis of the apophyseal rings of the vertebral bodies is called Scheuermann's disease. He originally described a painful kyphosis with multiple vertebral bodies involved. It is most commonly seen without kyphosis or pain and with only a few vertebral bodies involved.

malacia (Fig. 44.54); the tarsal navicular, Köhler's disease (Fig. 44.55); the metatarsal heads, Freiberg's infraction (Fig. 44.56); the femoral head, Legg-Perthes disease; the ring epiphyses of the spine, Scheuermann's disease (Fig. 44.57); and the tibial tubercle, Osgood-Schlatter disease, also called surfer's knees. Magnetic resonance imaging can be very useful in identifying AVN in these sites. It shows diffuse low signal on T1-weighted images that involves the entire area of avascular necrosis (Fig. 44.58).

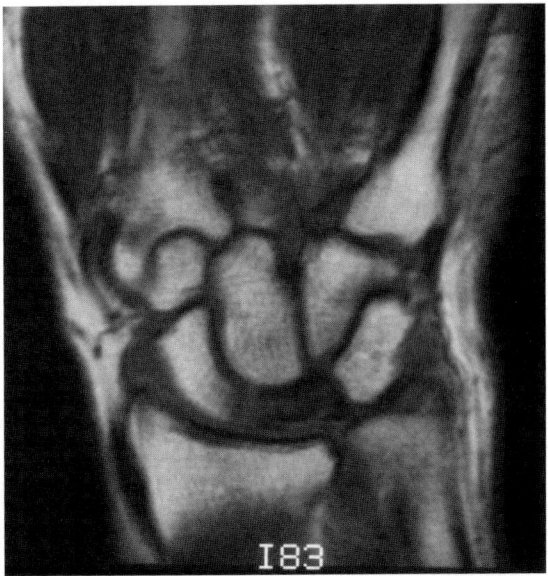

Figure 44.58. Kienböck's Malacia. A T1-weighted (TR 600; TE 20) coronal MR of the wrist shows low signal throughout the lunate, which is characteristic for AVN of the lunate, Kienböck's malacia.

References

1. Resnick D, Shaul S, Robins J. Diffuse idiopathic skeletal hyperostosis with extraspinal manifestations. Radiology 1975; 115:513–524.
2. Resnick D, Niwayama G, Coutts R. Subchondral cysts (geodes) in arthritic disorders: pathologic and radiographic appearance of the hip joint. AJR Am J Roentgenol 1977;128: 799–806.
3. Resnick D, Niwayama G, Goergen T, et al. Clinical, radiographic and pathologic abnormalities in calcium pyrophosphate dihydrate deposition disease (CPPD): pseudogout. Radiology 1977;122:1–15.
4. Helms CA, Chapman GS, Wild JH. Charcot-like joints in calcium pyrophosphate dihydrate deposition disease. Skeletal Radiol 1981;7:55–58.
5. Gold R, Metzger A, Mirra J, et al. Multicentric reticulohistiocytosis (lipoid dermatoarthritis). An erosive polyarthritis with distinctive clinical, roentgenographic, and pathologic features. AJR Am J Roentgenol 1975;124:610–624.
6. Mitchell D, Kressel H, Arger P, et al. Avascular necrosis of the femoral head: morphologic assessment by MR imaging, with CT correlation. Radiology 1986;161:739–742.

45
Metabolic Bone Disease

Clyde A. Helms

OSTEOPOROSIS

Osteoporosis is defined as diminished bone *quantity* in which the bone is otherwise normal. This contrasts to osteomalacia in which the bone quantity is normal but the *quality* of the bone is abnormal in that it is not normally mineralized. Osteomalacia results in excess nonmineralized osteoid. It is not possible in most cases to distinguish between osteoporosis and osteomalacia on plain films; hence, many prefer the term "osteopenia" for the plain film finding of diminished mineralization.

There are myriad causes of osteoporosis, the most common of which is primary osteoporosis (so-called senile osteoporosis or osteoporosis of aging). This is seen most commonly in postmenopausal women and is a major health concern because of the increase of vertebral body and hip fractures in this patient population.

Secondary osteoporosis implies that an underlying disorder, such as thyrotoxicosis or renal disease, has caused the osteoporosis. Only about 5% of the cases of osteoporosis are of the secondary type. The differential diagnosis for secondary osteoporosis is quite long and probably should not be memorized. One cannot even be sure whether it is osteoporosis or osteomalacia on the basis of the plain films; therefore, the differential for presumed osteoporosis would have to include the causes of osteomalacia.

The main radiographic finding in osteoporosis is thinning of the cortex. Although this can be seen in any bone, it is most reliably demonstrated in the second metacarpal at the middiaphysis. The normal metacarpal cortical thickening should be approximately one-fourth to one-third the thickness of the metacarpal (Fig. 45.1). In osteoporosis, this cortical thickness is decreased (Fig. 45.2). The metacarpal cortex (and all bony cortices, for that matter) decreases in thickness normally with age and is thinner in females than in males of the same age. Several tables have been published that give the normal metacarpal cortical measurement that have age and sex adjustments to allow the determination of normal. Unfortunately, these only determine the mineralization of the peripheral skeleton and do not seem to relate to whether vertebral body or hip fractures will occur.

Measurement of the bone mineral content in the axial skeleton can be done by one of several methods that use computed tomography to assess the bone quantity in the spine. There is much debate about which method is superior and even about whether knowing the bone mineral content is clinically more helpful than just knowing the age and sex of the patient, which is fairly accurate for predicting the bone-mass quantity. Most agree that knowing the axial bone mineral measurement does not help predict which patients are at risk for vertebral body and hip fractures.

Exercise and proper diet seem to help delay the onset of primary osteoporosis.Calcium additives have not been shown to reverse the process of primary osteoporosis. Estrogen clearly plays a role in alleviating postmenopausal osteoporosis, yet its use in a widespread manner is somewhat controversial.

A type of osteoporosis that can be seen in a patient of any age is disuse osteoporosis. It results from immobilization from any cause, most commonly following treatment of a fracture. The radiographic appearance of disuse osteoporosis is different from primary osteoporosis in that it occurs somewhat more rapidly and gives the bone a patchy appearance (Fig. 45.3). This is from osteoclastic resorption in the cortex causing intracortical holes. If allowed to continue with disuse, the bone would resemble any bone with marked osteoporosis, that is, severe cortical thinning.

Occasionally, aggressive osteoporosis from disuse can mimic a permeative lesion such as a Ewing's sarcoma or multiple myeloma because of the multiple cortical holes that project over the medullary space, thus resembling a medullary permeative process (Fig. 45.4). The way to dif-

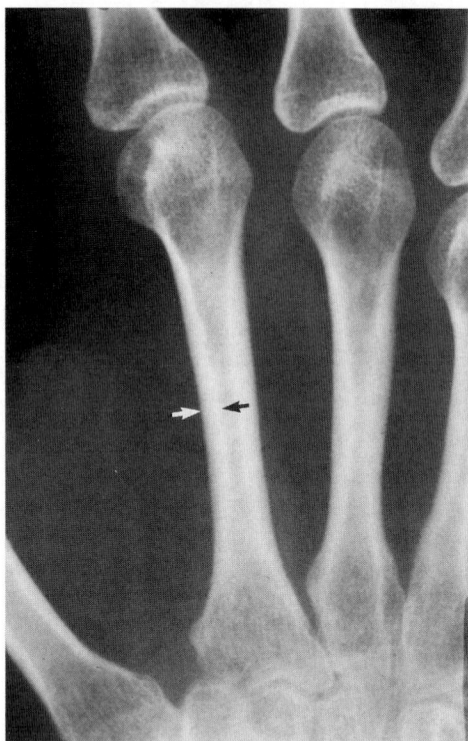

Figure 45.1. Normal Mineralization. The cortical width (*arrows*) at the midsecond metacarpal in this patient with normal mineralization is greater than one third of the total width of the metacarpal.

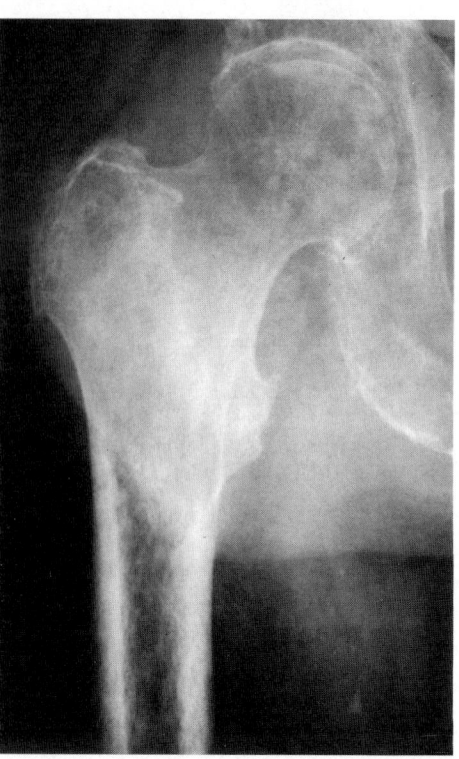

Figure 45.3. Disuse Osteoporosis. A mottled, patchy appearance is present in the proximal right femur in this patient with aggressive disuse osteoporosis secondary to an amputation. Note the mottled, irregular cortex seen in the femoral shaft, which is representative of cortical holes that can be seen in aggressive osteoporosis.

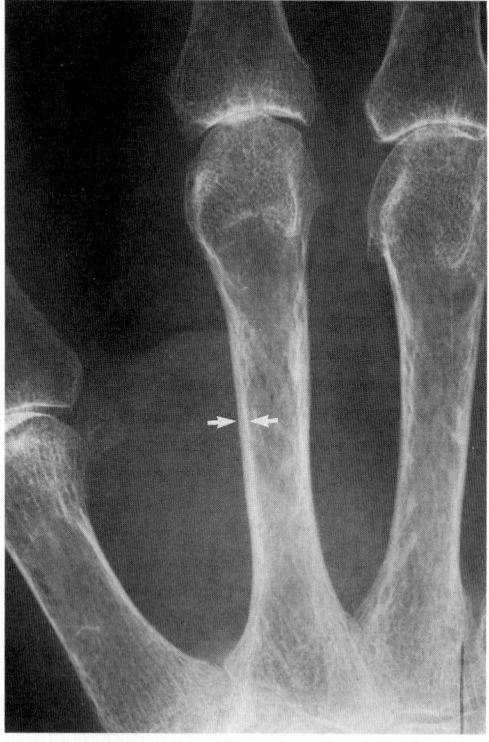

Figure 45.2. Osteoporosis. Severe cortical narrowing (*arrows*) at the midsecond metacarpal cortex is seen in this patient with severe osteoporosis. Note the intracortical tunneling that occurs in more aggressive forms of osteoporosis.

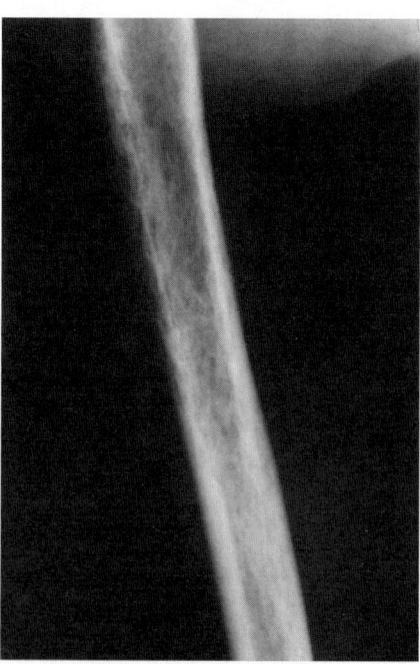

Figure 45.4. Aggressive Osteoporosis. Multiple small holes are seen in the cortex and overlying the medullary space in the proximal humerus of this patient who has suffered a stroke. This represents aggressive osteoporosis from disuse and is mimicking an aggressive permeative process. These holes are, however, almost entirely within the cortex of the bone.

ferentiate a true intramedullary permeative process from an intracortical process such as osteoporosis is to observe the cortex and see whether it is solid or riddled with holes (Fig. 45.5). If the cortex is solid, one can assume the permeative process is emanating from the medullary space (Fig. 45.6); if the cortex has multiple small holes, assume the permeative pattern is from the cortical process. I call a permeative appearance that is secondary to cortical holes a "pseudopermeative" process to distinguish it from a true permeative process (1).

Other causes for a pseudopermeative process include hemangioma and radiation. A hemangioma can cause cortical holes in two ways: from focal hyperemia causing focal osteoporosis or by the blood vessels themselves tunneling through the cortex (Fig. 45.7). Radiation can cause cortical holes in bone and mimic a permeative pattern because of the death of cortical osteocytes, which can result in large lacunae in the cortex (Fig. 45.8). The cortical holes from radiation can be large, in which case they would not be confused with a true permeative process, but they can also be small and resemble an aggressive lesion.

If a permeative lesion is found, the differential diagnosis is usually an aggressive process such as Ewing's sarcoma, infection, or eosinophilic granuloma in a young person (< age 30 y) or multiple myeloma, metastatic car-

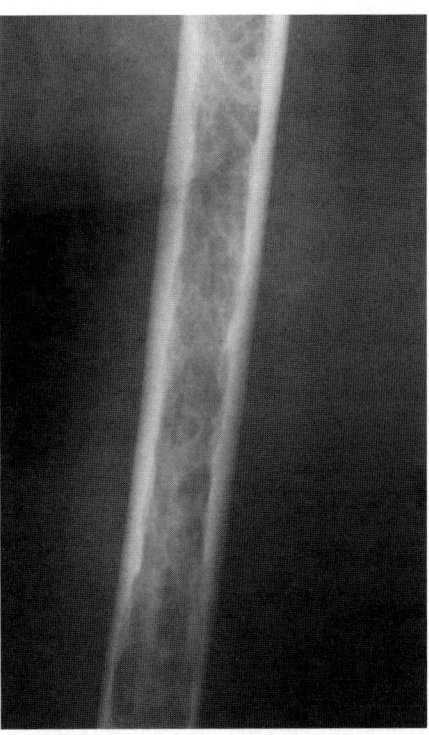

Figure 45.6. Myeloma Causing a Permeative Process. A diffuse permeative process throughout the femur is seen in this patient with myeloma. Note that the cortex is solid, although the endosteum has some scalloping. This is a true permeative process.

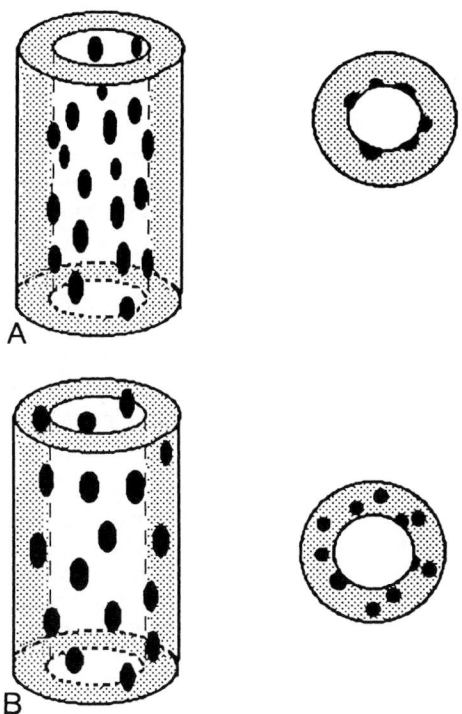

B) PSEUDOPERMEATIVE

Figure 45.5. Differentiation of Permeative Process. A. Schematic of a permeative lesion. A true permeative process has multiple small holes secondary to endosteal involvement with sparing of the cortex. This represents a marrow process. **B.** Schematic of a pseudopermeative process. A pseudopermeative process such as osteoporosis has multiple small cortical holes that are then superimposed over the marrow, giving a similar appearance to a permeative process.

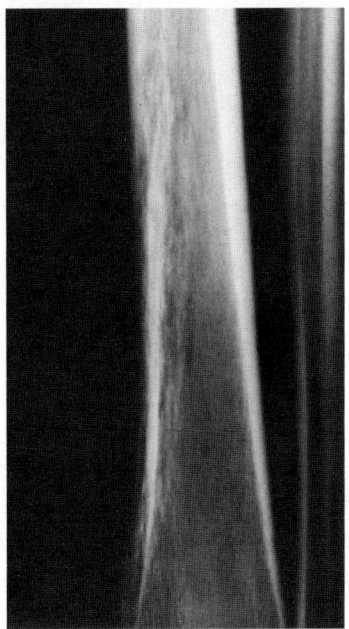

Figure 45.7. Pseudopermeative Process Secondary to Hemangioma. A permeative pattern is seen in the distal tibia in this patient with pain and swelling. It was thought to represent a Ewing's sarcoma, and a biopsy was performed with subsequent heavy loss of blood. This was found to be a hemangioma. An examination of the cortex demonstrates that the medial aspect is diffusely riddled with cortical holes, compared with the lateral aspect. The endosteum laterally also is completely spared, making a marrow process very unlikely. Hemangioma, radiation, and osteoporosis can cause a pseudopermeative process, although in this example, osteoporosis and radiation would be unlikely because of its focal nature.

cinomatosis, or primary lymphoma of bone in an older patient. If, however, the permeative pattern is a result of cortical holes, that is, a pseudopermeative pattern, the differential diagnosis is considerably less sinister: *aggressive osteoporosis, hemangioma,* or *radiation changes*. This differential diagnosis does not arise often but is very useful when it does (Table 45.1).

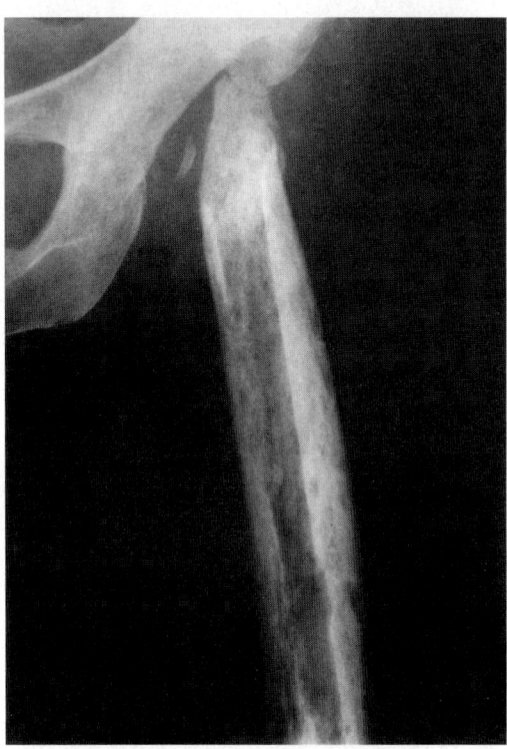

Figure 45.8. Pseudopermeative Pattern Secondary to Radiation. This patient had a fibrosarcoma treated with excision of the femoral head and subsequent radiation. A follow-up film shows a diffuse permeative pattern throughout the proximal femur. Because the cortex is riddled with holes, it was thought that this was secondary to radiation rather than tumor recurrence. This is a pseudopermeative appearance secondary to radiation.

Table 45.1. Differential Diagnosis of Pseudopermeative Pattern

Aggressive osteoporosis(st)
Hemangioma(st)
Radiation

OSTEOMALACIA

Osteomalacia is the result of too much nonmineralized osteoid. The most common cause is renal osteodystrophy. The radiographic findings are almost identical to those of osteoporosis, and, for the most part, the two disorders are indistinguishable. The only findings that are pathognomonic for osteomalacia are Looser's fractures, which are fractures through large osteoid seams (Fig. 45.9). They are extremely uncommon but tend to occur in the femur, pelvis, and scapula.

In children, osteomalacia is called rickets. It causes the epiphyses to become flared and irregular and the long bones to undergo bending from the bone softening (Fig. 45.10). As in adults, the most common cause is renal disease, although other causes such as biliary disease and dietary insufficiencies are occasionally seen.

HYPERPARATHYROIDISM

Hyperparathyroidism occurs from excess parathyroid hormone. Parathyroid hormone causes osteoclastic resorption in bone, which leads to osteoporosis and osteomalacia. Primary HPT is caused by parathyroid adenomas and hyperplasia. Up to 40% of patients with primary HPT will demonstrate skeletal abnormalities radiographically. The most common cause of HPT is from renal disease, which leads to secondary HPT. Secondary HPT is the result of the parathyroids secreting excess PTH in response to the hypocalcemia that occurs.

The radiographic sign that is pathognomonic for HPT is subperiosteal bone resorption. It is seen most commonly on the radial aspect of the middle phalanges of the hand (Fig. 45.11), but it can be seen in any long bone in the body. It is commonly seen on the medial aspect of the

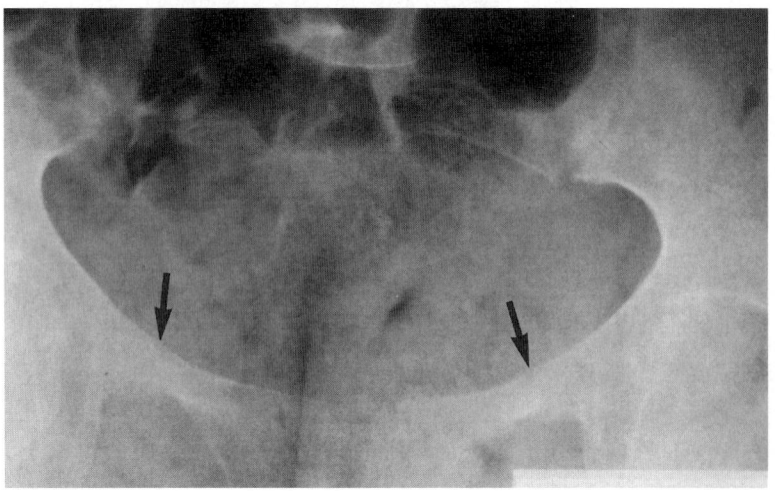

Figure 45.9. Looser's Fractures in Osteomalacia. Bilateral pubic rami fractures (*arrows*) are faintly identified in this patient with osteomalacia secondary to phenytoin (Dilantin) therapy. These are called Looser's fractures and are pathognomonic for osteomalacia, although they are uncommonly seen.

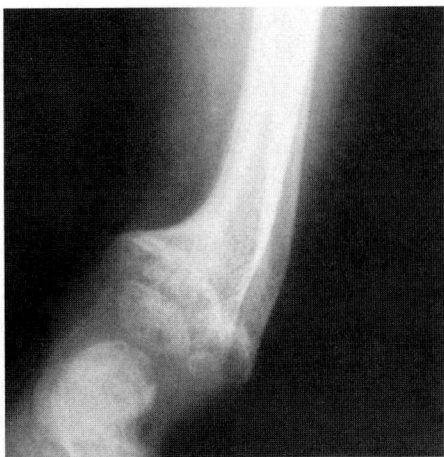

Figure 45.10. Rickets. Osteomalacia in children is called rickets and is identified by fraying and splaying of the epiphyses as well as bending of the bone secondary to softening. This patient had renal osteodystrophy.

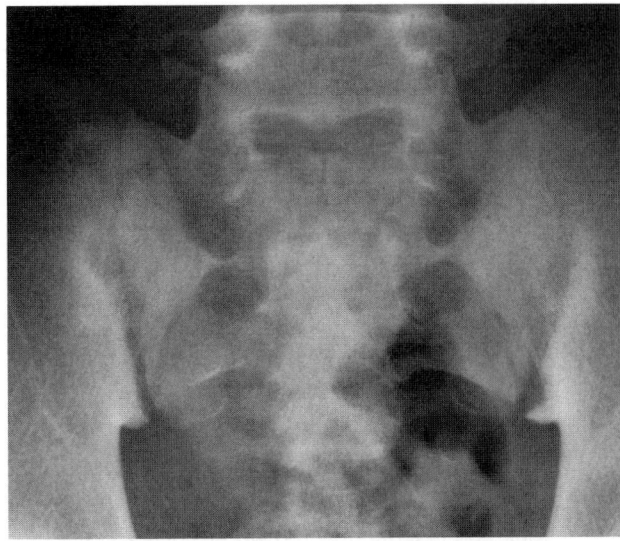

Figure 45.12. Hyperparathyroidism. Bilateral sacroiliac joint erosive changes with sclerosis are present in this patient with renal osteodystrophy and secondary hyperparathyroidism. Bilateral sacroiliac joint changes such as this are often seen with HPT.

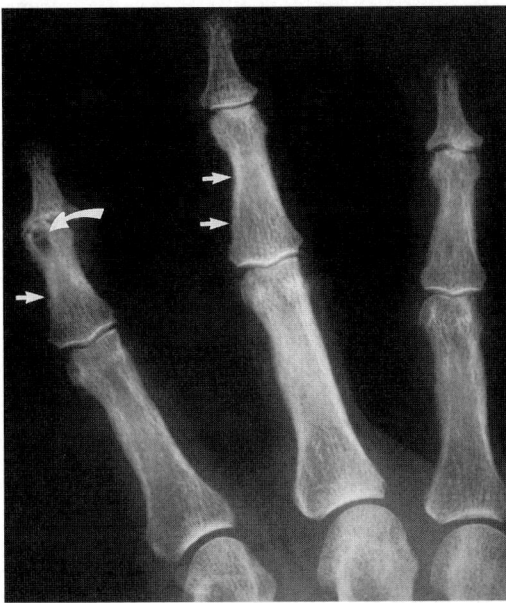

Figure 45.11. Hyperparathyroidism. Subperiosteal bone resorption can be seen at the radial aspect of the middle phalanges (*straight arrows*), which is pathognomonic for HPT. The lytic lesion seen in the distal middle phalanx (*curved arrow*) may be a small brown tumor.

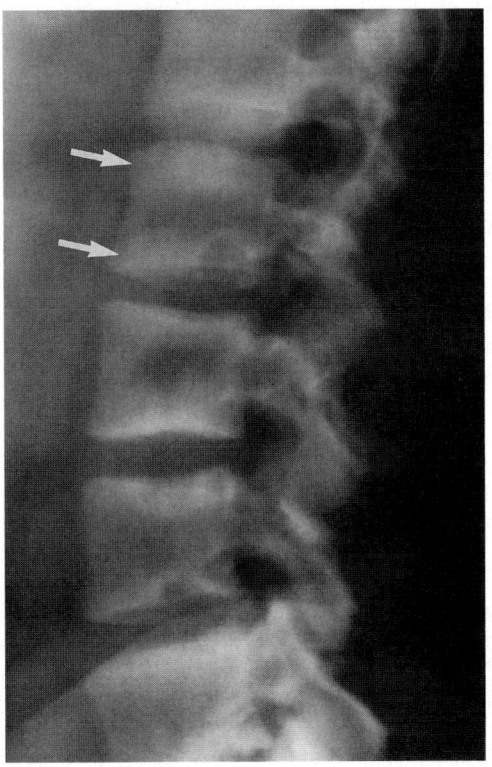

Figure 45.13. Hyperparathyroidism. Sclerotic bands present at the vertebral body endplates (*arrows*) are characteristic of a rugger jersey spine. This is seen in HPT.

proximal tibia, at the sacroiliac joints (Fig. 45.12), and in the distal clavicle.

Other radiographic findings include osteosclerosis, usually diffuse, but often involving the spine in a manner resembling the stripes on rugby jerseys, hence, the name "rugger jersey spine" (Fig. 45.13). Brown tumors are cystic lesions that are often expansile and aggressive in appearance (Fig. 45.14). They were once said to be more common in primary HPT but are seen more commonly associated with secondary HPT today because of the overwhelming preponderance of patients with secondary disease compared with primary disease. A brown tumor can have a variety of appearances, so the only thing char-

acteristic about it is that it is associated with subperiosteal bone resorption. If the underlying HPT is treated, the subperiosteal resorption may disappear before the brown tumor does. This is not commonly seen, however.

Metabolic bone surveys (plain films of the hands, spine, and long bones) were once routinely obtained in

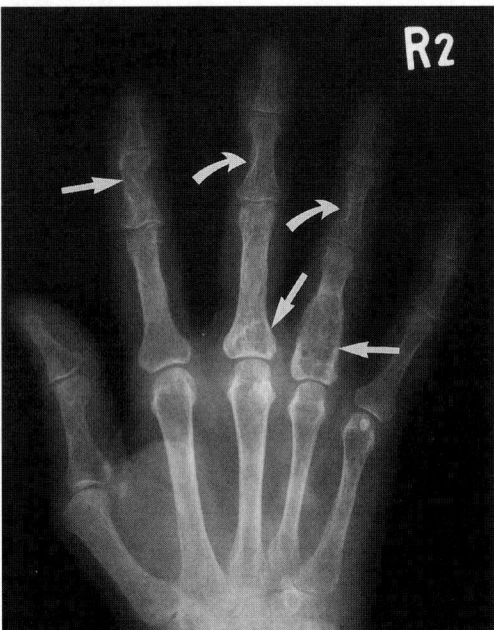

Figure 45.14. Brown Tumors in HPT. Several lytic lesions are present in the phalanges (*straight arrows*) in this patient with HPT; these are brown tumors. Note the subperiosteal bone resorption in the radial aspect of the middle phalanges (*curved arrows*), which is pathognomonic for HPT.

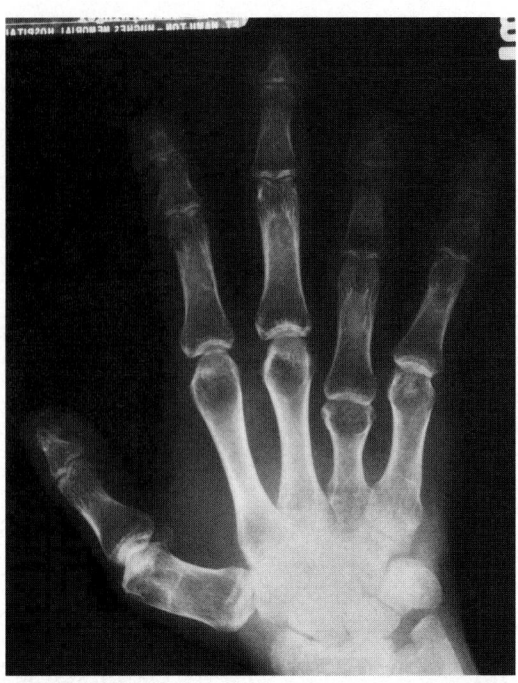

Figure 45.15. Pseudohypoparathyroidism. Brachydactyly is present in several of the metacarpals in this patient with pseudohypoparathyroidism. A short fourth metacarpal as seen here is a frequent finding in this entity.

patients to look for subperiosteal bone resorption, brown tumors, osteosclerosis, calcifications, and Looser's fractures. They are no longer recommended, however, as the yield of positive findings is extremely low and rarely will a positive finding affect treatment. In place of the metabolic bone survey, it is now recommended that plain films of the hands be obtained to look for subperiosteal resorption (2). A radionuclide bone scan can be obtained in selected cases, which will show increased radionuclide uptake by brown tumors and Looser's fractures. Also, investigation of causes of hypercalcemia, which can be caused by metastatic disease or metabolic bone disease, should include a bone scan (3).

HYPOPARATHYROIDISM

Hypoparathyroidism occurs because of a deficiency of the parathyroid glands to secrete normal amounts of PTH. Few skeletal changes occur in hypoparathyroidism. The calvarium on occasion will show thickening, and calcification in the basal ganglia of the brain has been described.

PSEUDOHYPOPARATHYROIDISM AND PSEUDOPSEUDOHYPOPARATHYROIDISM

Pseudohypoparathyroidism is caused by a congenital failure of tissues to respond to PTH. The parathyroid glands are normal in these cases. Treating these patients with PTH is of no help because the problem lies in the end organs, not the parathyroid glands. A characteristic appearance is seen in these patients: obesity, round facies, short stature, and brachydactyly (Fig. 45.15). The

tubular bones of the hands and feet are often all short. In pseudopseudohypoparathyroidism, there is no parathyroid abnormality and no end-organ problem; these patients merely resemble patients with pseudohypoparathyroidism. In summary, hypoparathyroidism is a parathyroid gland problem, pseudohypoparathyroidism is an end-organ problem, and pseudopseudohypoparathyroidism is a mimicker of pseudohypoparathyroidism morphologically.

PITUITARY GLAND HYPERFUNCTION

A secreting adenoma or hyperplasia of the anterior lobe of the pituitary gland will result in accelerated bone growth. If it occurs before the epiphyses close, it causes giantism. If it occurs after the epiphyses are closed, the result is acromegaly.

Acromegaly has several characteristic radiographic features in the skeletal system. The skull film invariably shows calvarial thickening, enlarged sinuses, and an enlarged sella turcica. The jaw is prognathic. The terminal tufts of the distal phalanges become hypertrophied and have a so-called spade appearance (an appearance not unlike a spade or shovel) (Fig. 45.16). The joint spaces are occasionally minimally enlarged because of hypertrophy of the hyaline articular cartilage. Early degenerative joint disease ensues because the cartilage itself is abnormal. The soft tissues also hypertrophy, with various measurements of soft-tissue thickening used by some as an indicator for acromegaly. For instance, thickening of the heel pad adjacent to the calcaneus has been used as a sign of acromegaly.

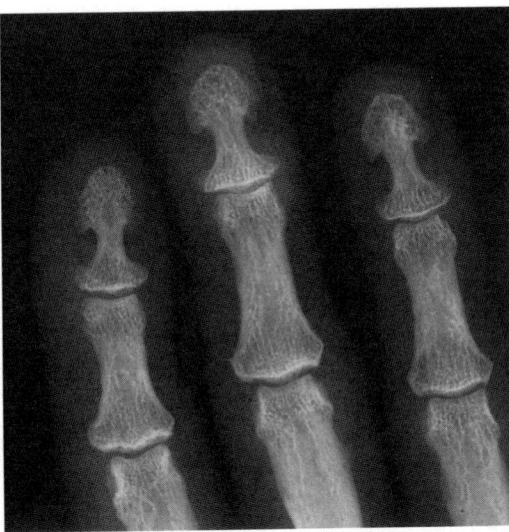

Figure 45.16. Acromegaly. Enlargement of the distal tufts in the phalanges (so-called spade tufts) are characteristic for acromegaly.

THYROID GLAND HYPERFUNCTION

In children, hyperthyroidism can result in increased skeletal maturation; however, this is seldom marked. A rare manifestation of hyperthyroidism in adults is thyroid acropachy. This occurs only after prior thyroidectomy and the cause is unknown. A characteristic-appearing periostitis occurs in the metacarpals and phalanges of the hands and feet (Fig. 45.17). It invariably involves the ulnar aspect of the fifth metacarpal, a useful differential point that can be used to tell thyroid acropachy from other causes of diffuse periostitis such as hypertrophic pulmonary osteoarthropathy and pachydermal periostitis, a rare form of idiopathic periostitis and skin thickening.

THYROID GLAND HYPOFUNCTION

Decreased thyroid secretion, or cretinism, results in delayed skeletal maturation in children. Delay in ossification of epiphyseal centers with occasional appearance of "stippled" epiphyses is seen. A delay in epiphyseal closure also occurs, in some instances with failure of epiphyseal closure noted in the third and fourth decade.

OSTEOSCLEROSIS

The radiographic finding of diffuse increased bone density, osteosclerosis, is somewhat uncommon, yet every radiologist must have a differential diagnosis for this process. Fortunately, it is a rather short differential and there are criteria to narrow down the list of possibilities.

The list of diseases that can cause diffuse osteosclerosis is quite long, but a list that includes 95–98% of the pathologic processes is all that is really necessary. The entities I include in the differential diagnosis of diffuse osteosclerosis are listed in Table 45.2.

The mnemonic I use to remember them is "*Regular Sex Makes Occasional Perversions Much More Pleasurable*

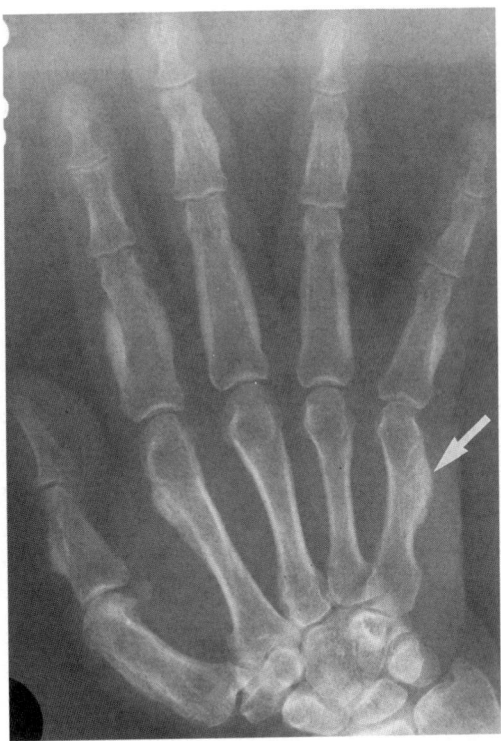

Figure 45.17. Thyroid Acropachy. Extensive periostitis is noted in the metacarpals and phalanges in this patient with thyroid acropachy. It is characteristic to have marked involvement of the ulnar aspect of the fifth metacarpal (*arrow*) in this entity.

Table 45.2. Differential Diagnosis of Diffuse Bony Sclerosis (Dense Bones)

Renal osteodystrophy(st)
Sickle cell disease(st)
Myelofibrosis(st)
Osteopetrosis(st)
Pyknodysostosis(st)
Metastatic carcinoma(st)
Mastocytosis(st)
Paget's disease(st)
Athletes(st)
Fluorosis

And Fantastic." I will cover each of these topics in generalities, trying to point out the features of each that should be looked for to allow inclusion or exclusion from the differential.

Renal Osteodystrophy

Anything that causes HPT can cause osteosclerosis, but renal disease is by far the most common disease in which osteosclerosis is seen. Although the most common presentation of renal osteodystrophy is osteopenia, about 10–20% of the patients with renal osteodystrophy will exhibit osteosclerosis, and the reasons for it are unknown. As mentioned previously, the sine qua non of renal osteodystrophy is subperiosteal bone resorption, seen earliest and most reliably at the radial aspect of the

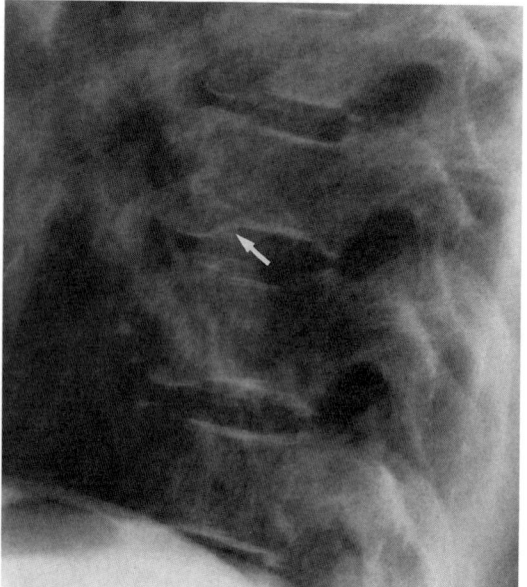

Figure 45.18. Sickle Cell Disease. Step-off deformities (*arrow*) are seen in the endplates of several vertebral bodies in this patient with sickle cell disease. They are also called fish vertebrae.

middle phalanges of the hands. Without this finding, osteosclerosis caused by renal disease should not be entertained.

Sickle Cell Disease

Like renal osteodystrophy, the underlying cause of dense bones in sickle cell disease is unknown. It only occurs in a small percentage of patients. Additional signs to look for are bone infarcts and step-off deformities of the vertebral body endplates (Fig. 45.18). These are also called "fish" vertebrae after their appearance like the vertebrae found in fish. Avascular necrosis of the hip is frequently an accompanying finding.

Myelofibrosis

Also called agnogenic myeloid metaplasia, myelofibrosis is a disease caused by progressive fibrosis of the marrow in patients older than 50 years of age. It leads to anemia with marked splenomegaly and extramedullary hematopoiesis. Whenever osteosclerosis is seen in a patient older than 50 years of age, a search should be made for a large spleen and extramedullary hematopoiesis (Fig. 45.19).

Osteopetrosis

This is a hereditary abnormality that results in extremely dense bones throughout the skeleton (Fig. 45.20). There are congenita and tarda forms, with different degrees of severity in each. The congenita form occurs at birth and can be lethal. Anemia, jaundice, hepatosplenomegaly, and infections are often present in this form. The tarda form is seen in older children and adults and has milder clinical problems. The tarda form may be so mild that it has no clinical findings. Although uncom-

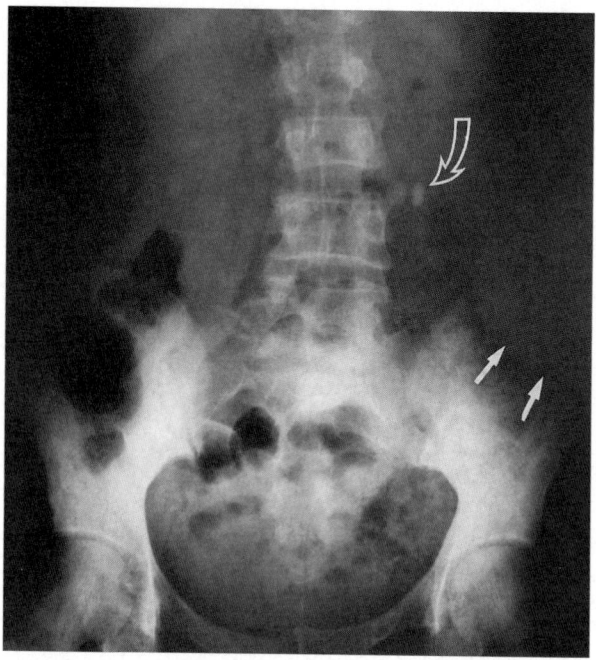

Figure 45.19. Myelofibrosis. Diffuse increased bone density is seen throughout the pelvis and spine in this patient with myelofibrosis. The spleen is markedly enlarged (*straight arrows*), and opaque iron tablets (*curved arrow*) can be seen, which were taken for the anemia that is often found in this disorder.

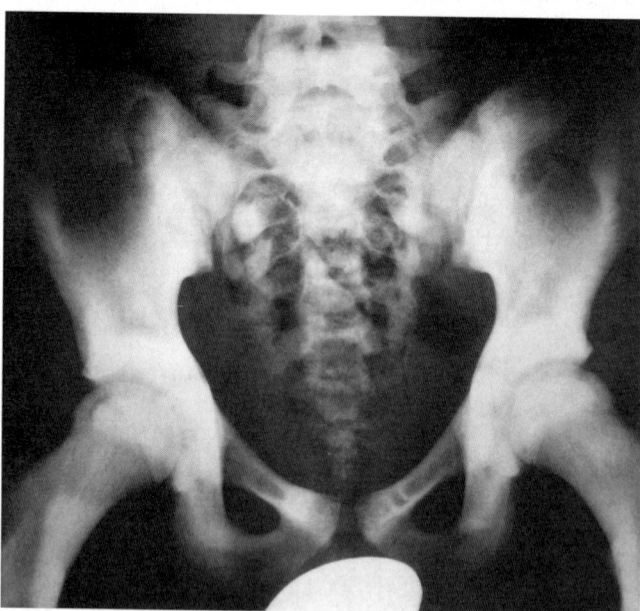

Figure 45.20. Osteopetrosis. Marked, diffuse bony sclerosis is seen throughout the skeleton in this patient with osteopetrosis.

mon, it is not so rare that one will never see a case; therefore, it should be included in this differential diagnosis. A characteristic finding is the so-called bone-in-bone appearance often seen in the vertebral bodies in which the vertebrae have a small replica of the vertebral body inside the normal one. Also characteristic are the "sandwich vertebrae" in which the endplates are densely sclerotic, giving the appearance of a sandwich (Fig.

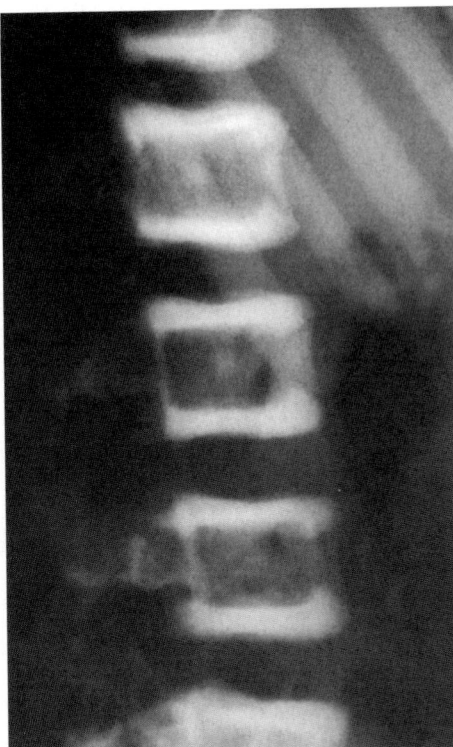

Figure 45.21. Sandwich Vertebrae. Dense bands of sclerosis parallel to the endplates are seen in this patient with osteopetrosis. These are called sandwich vertebrae, which are much more distinct than the dense bands of sclerosis seen in a rugger jersey spine (see Fig. 45.13).

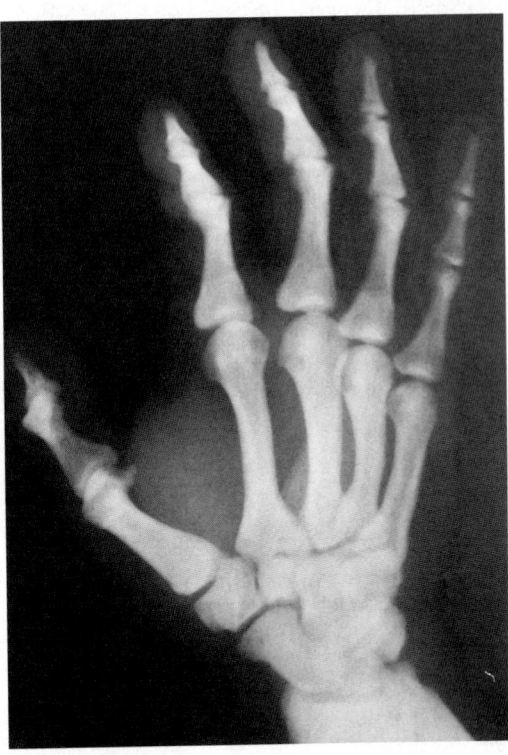

Figure 45.22. Pyknodysostosis. Diffuse, dense sclerosis is seen throughout the hand and wrist in this patient with pyknodysostosis. Note the absent distal phalangeal tufts that appear pointed and sclerotic, which is virtually pathognomonic for pyknodysostosis.

45.21). The sandwich vertebrae appearance resembles a rugger jersey spine but can be differentiated by being much denser and more sharply defined.

Pyknodysostosis

This is the other congenital abnormality with dense bones that should be considered in the differential diagnosis of osteosclerosis. It is seen less commonly than osteopetrosis. These patients are typically short and have hypoplastic mandibles. The distinguishing radiographic finding that is essentially pathognomonic is acro-osteolysis with sclerosis. The distal phalanges often have the appearance of chalk that has been put into a pencil sharpener: they are pointed and dense (Fig. 45.22). No other disease process has this appearance. Another name for this disorder is Toulouse-Lautrec syndrome, named for the famous artist who was afflicted with pyknodysostosis.

Metastatic Carcinoma

Only rarely will diffuse metastatic carcinoma cause a problem in diagnosis. I have seen only a handful of cases in which diffuse metastatic carcinoma mimicked diffuse osteosclerosis, and in every case, the primary tumor was either prostate or breast carcinoma. If cortical destruction or a lytic component is present, it simplifies the differential diagnosis, so a search should be made for these.

Mastocytosis

This is another rare disorder that can cause uniform increased bone density. Unfortunately, there are no other plain film findings that might help with the diagnosis. Patients with this disease have thickened small bowel folds with nodules, but, of course, to see them, an upper gastrointestinal contrast study must be performed (Fig. 45.23). Urticaria pigmentosa is a characteristic skin lesion found in these patients.

Paget's Disease

Diffuse Paget's disease that could be confused with one of the other diseases in the differential diagnosis of generalized osteosclerosis is very rare. Paget's disease classically causes bony enlargement (Fig. 45.24), but this is not always present. It occurs most commonly in the pelvis (Fig. 45.25), where it has been said the iliopectineal line on the pelvic brim must be thickened if Paget's disease is present. In fact, the iliopectineal line is usually, but not always, thickened. Paget's disease can occur in any bone in the body, including the smaller bones of the hands and feet.

Paget's disease has three distinct phases visible radiographically: a lytic phase, a sclerotic phase, and a mixed lytic–sclerotic phase. The lytic phase often has a sharp leading edge called a flame-shaped or blade-of-grass leading edge (Fig. 45.26). In a long bone, with the sole exception being the tibia, Paget's disease always starts at

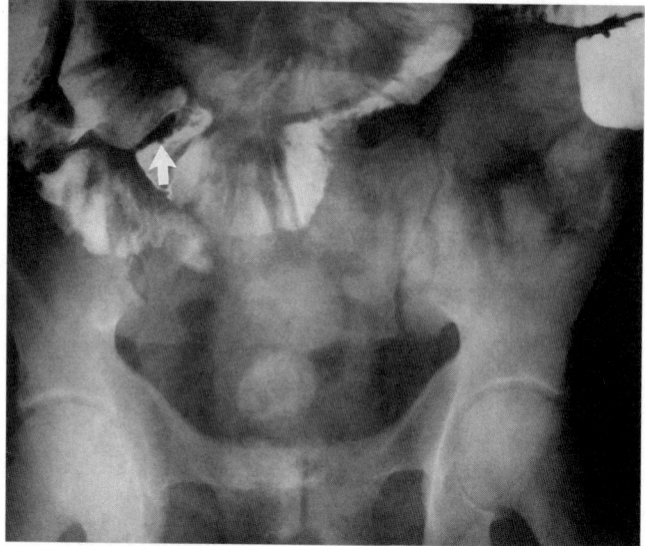

Figure 45.23. Mastocytosis. Uniform increased bone density is seen throughout the pelvis in this patient with mastocytosis. Small bowel thickened folds with nodules (*arrow*) can be seen in this barium study; these are often found in mastocytosis.

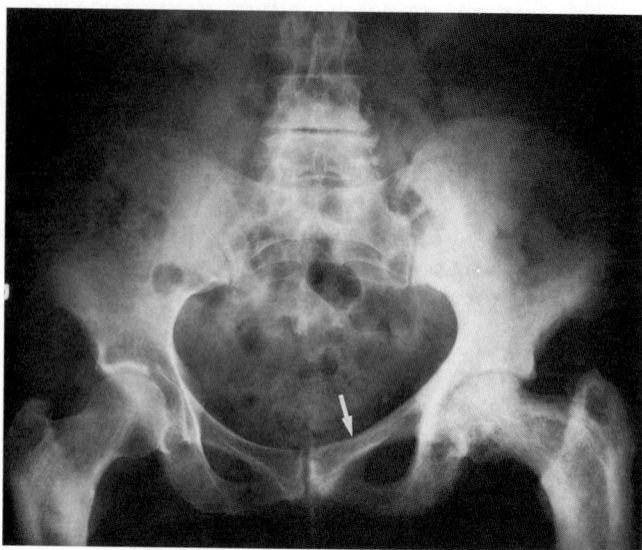

Figure 45.25. Paget's Disease. Bony sclerosis with some bony enlargement is seen in the left pelvis and proximal femur of this patient and is characteristic of Paget's disease. Note the cortical thickening of the left superior pubic ramus (*arrow*), which is called thickening of the iliopectineal line and is commonly seen in Paget's disease.

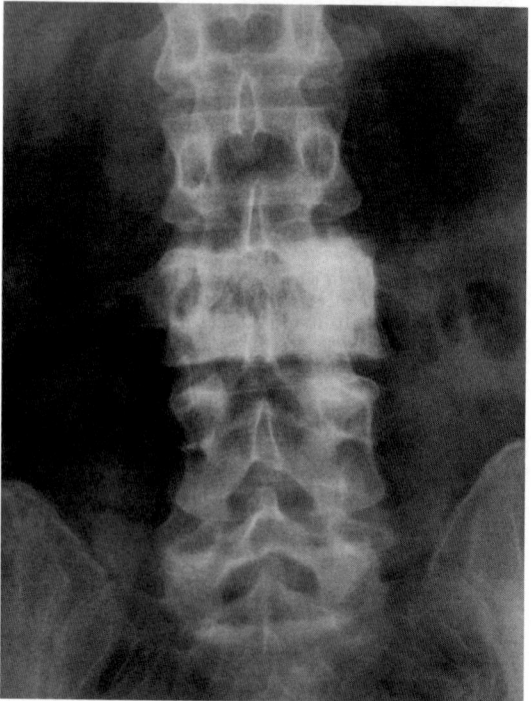

Figure 45.24. Paget's Disease. Dense, bony sclerosis with overgrowth of the vertebral body is seen at the L3 vertebra in this patient with Paget's disease. The left L3 pedicle is markedly dense and enlarged.

the end of the bone; therefore, if a lesion is present in the middle of a long bone and does not extend to either end, one can safely exclude Paget's disease.

Athletes

Plain film radiographs of professional athletes quite often demonstrate increased cortical thickness and appar-

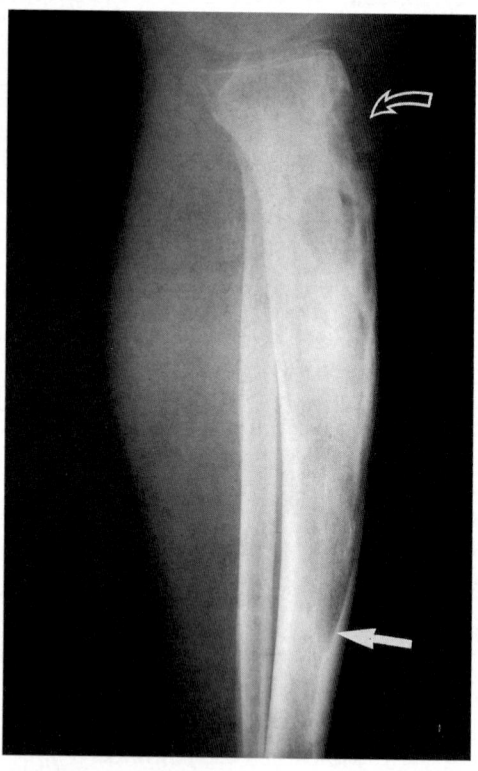

Figure 45.26. Paget's Disease. A lytic process involving the proximal two-thirds of the tibia is noted and has a blade of grass or flame-shaped leading edge (*straight arrow*), which is characteristic for Paget's disease. This represents the lytic phase of Paget's disease. The sclerotic phase of Paget's disease can be seen in the midportion of this lesion, and an area of probable sarcomatous degeneration can be seen in the proximal tibia (*curved arrow*), where apparent cortical destruction is noted. This represents all three phases or stages of Paget's disease.

ent diffuse osteosclerosis to the point of appearing pathologic. Undoubtedly, increased stress causes hypertrophy of bone as well as muscle. The increased density in these otherwise normal subjects is occasionally misinterpreted as abnormal, with extensive workups and even bone biopsy resulting.

Fluorosis

This is a rare disorder that is usually a result of chronic intake of fluoride in certain geographic areas where large amounts of fluoride are present in the drinking water. It can also be a result of long-term therapy with sodium fluoride for osteoporosis.

A radiographic finding that patients with fluorosis often have is ligamentous calcification. Calcification of the sacrotuberous ligament is said to be characteristic for fluorosis.

SUMMARY

There are other categories of disease that could be covered in a chapter on metabolic bone disease, but most of the remaining disorders are exceedingly rare and not likely to be seen by most radiologists on a routine basis.

References

1. Helms C, Munk P. Pseudopermeative skeletal lesions. Br J Radiol 1990;63:461–467.
2. Cooper KL. Radiology of metabolic bone disease. Endocrinol Metab Clin North Am 1989;18:955–976.
3. McAfee JG. Radionuclide imaging in metabolic and systemic skeletal diseases. Semin Nucl Med 1987;17:334–349.

46
Skeletal "Don't Touch" Lesions

Clyde A. Helms

POSTTRAUMATIC LESIONS
NORMAL VARIANTS
OBVIOUSLY BENIGN LESIONS
CONCLUSION

Skeletal "don't touch" lesions are those processes that are so radiographically characteristic that a biopsy or additional diagnostic tests are unnecessary. Not only does the biopsy result in unnecessary morbidity and cost, but in some instances, as is discussed in this chapter, a biopsy can also be frankly misleading and lead to additional unnecessary surgery.

Most radiology training stresses giving a differential diagnosis of a lesion, leaving it up to the clinician to decide between the various entities. For the "don't touch" lesions, however, a differential list is inappropriate as that often makes the next step in the decision-making process a biopsy. Because these lesions do not need to undergo biopsy for a final diagnosis, a radiologic diagnosis should be made without a list of differential possibilities. These lesions can be classified into three categories: 1) posttraumatic lesions, 2) normal variants, and 3) lesions that are real but obviously benign.

POSTTRAUMATIC LESIONS

Myositis ossificans. is an example of a lesion that should not undergo biopsy because its aggressive histologic appearance can often mimic a sarcoma (1). Unfortunately, radical surgery has been performed based on the histologic appearance of myositis ossificans when the radiologic appearance was diagnostic. The typical radiologic appearance of myositis ossificans is circumferential calcification with a lucent center (Fig. 46.1). This is often best appreciated on a computed tomography scan. (Fig. 46.2). A malignant tumor that mimics myositis ossificans has an ill-defined periphery and a calcified or ossific center (Fig. 46.3). Periosteal reaction can be seen with myositis ossificans or with a tumor. Occasionally, the peripheral calcification of myositis ossificans can be too faint to appreciate; in these cases, a computed tomography scan should help, or delayed films 1 or 2 weeks later are recommended. Biopsy should be avoided when myositis ossificans is a clinical consideration.

Avulsion Injury. Another posttraumatic entity in which a biopsy can be misleading is any avulsion injury (2,3). These injuries can have an aggressive radiographic appearance, but because of their characteristic location at ligament and tendon insertion sites (e.g., an-terior-inferior iliac spine or ischial tuberosity), they should be recognized as benign. (Figs. 46.4, 46.5). As with myositis ossificans, delayed films of several weeks will usually allow the problem case to become more radiographically clear. Biopsy can lead to the mistaken diagnosis of a sarcoma and should therefore be avoided. Any area undergoing healing can have a high nuclear-to-chromatin ratio and a high mitotic figure count, thereby occasionally simulating a malignancy histologically.

Cortical Desmoid is a process on the medial supracondylar ridge of the distal femur that is considered by many to be the result of an avulsion of the adductor magnus muscle. It occasionally simulates an aggressive lesion radiographically, and histologically, it can look malignant (4). In many instances, biopsy has led to amputation for this benign, radiographically characteristic lesion (Fig 46.6, 46.7). Cortical desmoids occur only on the posteromedial epicondyle of the femur. They might or might not be associated with pain and can have increased radionuclide uptake on a bone scan. They might or might not exhibit periosteal new bone and usually occur in young people. Biopsy should be avoided in all cases. Painful cortical desmoids should become asymptomatic with rest.

Trauma can lead to large, cystic geodes or subchondral cysts near joints and can be mistaken for other lesions, resulting in a biopsy being ordered. Although the biopsy specimen is not likely to mimic a malignant process, it is nevertheless avoidable. Because geodes from degenerative disease almost always are associated with additional findings such as joint space narrowing, sclerosis, and osteophytes, a diagnosis should be made radiographically (Fig. 46.8). On occasion, however, the additional findings are subtle and can be missed (Fig. 46.9). Geodes can also occur in the setting of calcium pyrophosphate dihydrate crystal disease, CPPD, rheumatoid arthritis, and avascular necrosis (5,6).

Discogenic Vertebral Sclerosis. An entity that is often confused for metastatic disease to the spine is discogenic vertebral disease. It can mimic metastatic disease very closely, and unless the radiologist is familiar with this process, it can lead to an unnecessary biopsy (7). Discogenic vertebral disease most often is sclerotic and focal (Fig. 46.10). It is always adjacent to the endplate, and the associated disc space should be narrow. Osteophytosis is invariably present. It really is a variant of a Schmorl's node and should not be confused with a metastatic focus. On occasion it can be lytic or even mixed lytic–sclerotic. The typical clinical setting is a middle-aged woman with chronic low back pain. Old films often confirm the benign nature of this process. In the setting of disc space narrowing and osteophytosis, focal

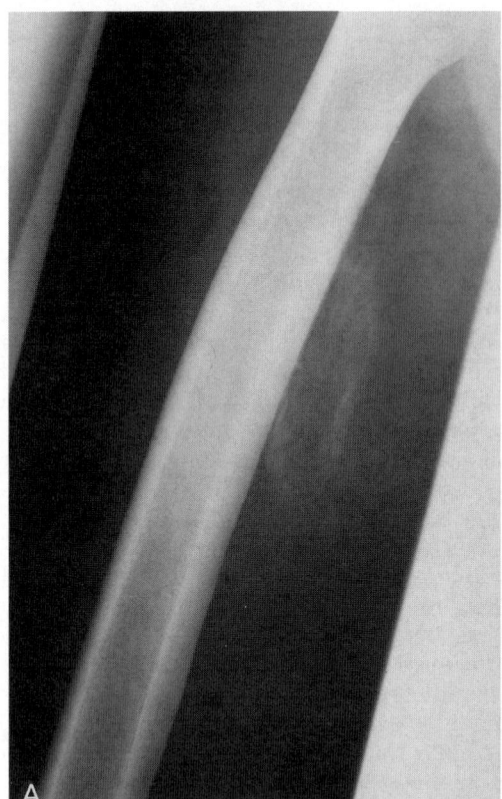

Figure 46.1. Myositis Ossificans. A. A plain film of the femur in this patient who presented with a soft-tissue mass shows a calcific density adjacent to the posterior cortex of the femur, which is calcified primarily in its periphery. If it is difficult on the plain film alone to state definitely that this is peripheral, circumferential calcification, a computed tomographic scan, as shown in **(B),** can be helpful in showing that the calcification is unequivocally peripheral in nature. This is virtually diagnostic of myositis ossificans.

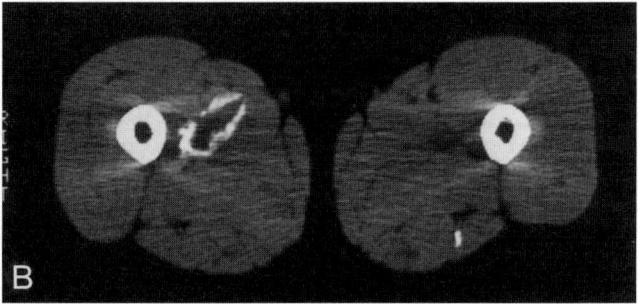

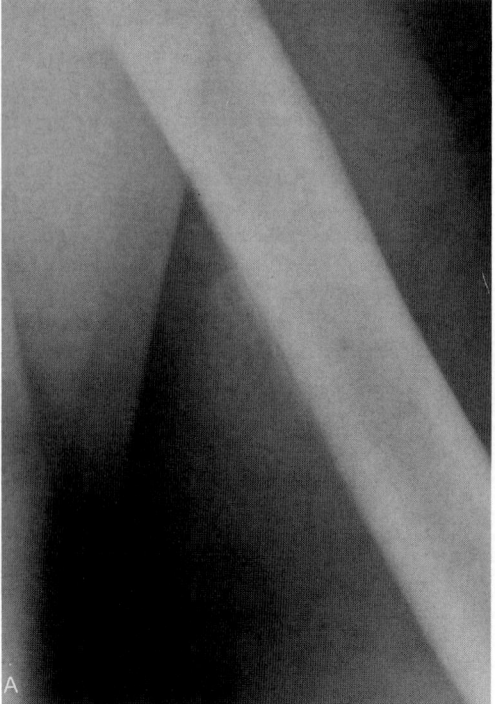

Figure 46.2. Myositis Ossificans. A. Hazy calcification is seen adjacent to the humeral shaft with underlying periosteal reaction noted. It is difficult to ascertain whether the calcification is circumferential. **B.** A CT scan through this mass shows that the calcification is unequivocally circumferential in nature, making the diagnosis of myositis ossificans a certainty.

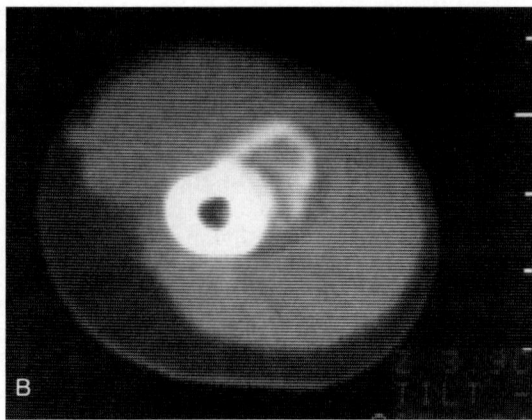

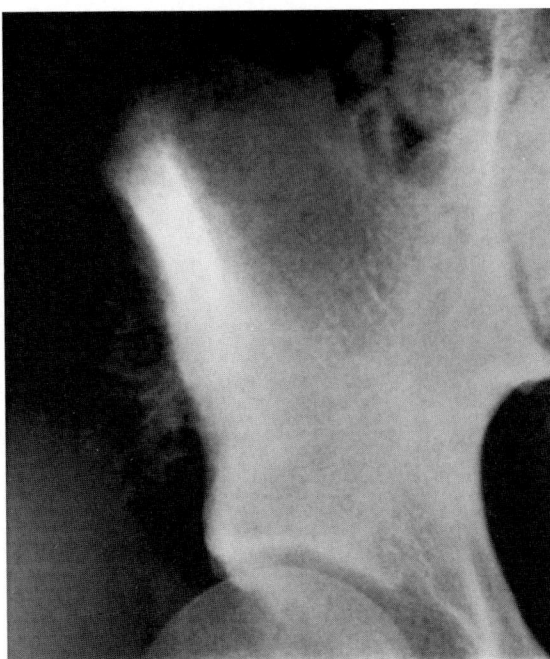

Figure 46.3. Osteogenic Sarcoma. Hazy, ill-defined calcification is seen adjacent to the iliac wing in this patient, which can be ascertained from the plain film as definitely not being circumferential in nature. Even though a prior history of trauma was obtained in this case, myositis ossificans is not a consideration with this appearance of calcification. Biopsy showed this to be an osteogenic sarcoma.

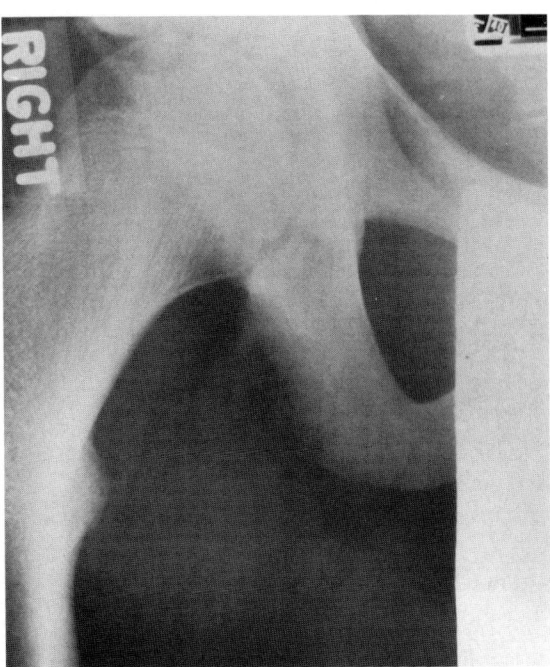

Figure 46.5. Avulsion Injury. Cortical irregularity with a Codman's triangle of periostitis is seen along the ischial tuberosity that was at first thought to represent a malignancy. Because of the characteristic location, an avulsion injury was considered and the lesion was observed. It healed without sequelae. (Case courtesy Dr. John Wilson, San Francisco, California.)

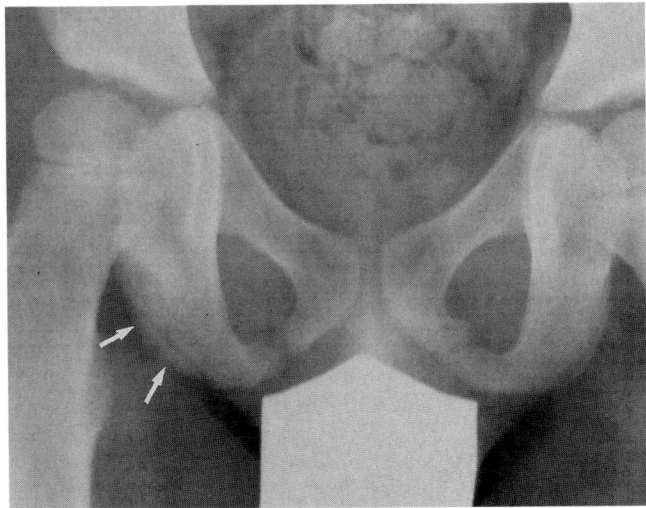

Figure 46.4. Avulsion Injury. Cortical irregularity (*arrows*) at the ischial tuberosity in this patient with pain over this region raises the question of possible tumor. This is a classic appearance, however, for an avulsion injury from this region, and a biopsy should be avoided.

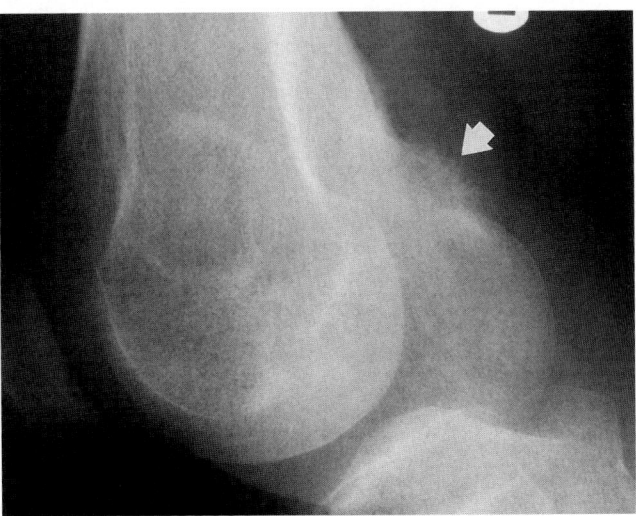

Figure 46.6. Cortical Desmoid. A focal cortical irregularity in this patient is seen in the posterior aspect of the femur (*arrow*) with adjacent periostitis noted. Although a tumor such as an early parosteal osteosarcoma could perhaps have this appearance, this is a characteristic location and appearance for a cortical desmoid and should not undergo biopsy. Pain will disappear with rest.

sclerosis adjacent to an endplate should not undergo biopsy.

Fracture. Occasionally, a fracture will be the cause of extensive osteosclerosis and periostitis, which can mimic a primary bone tumor (Fig. 46.11). Lack of immobilization can result in exuberant callus, which can be misinterpreted as aggressive periostitis or even new tumor

bone. Results of a biopsy in such a case might resemble a malignant lesion; therefore, any case associated with trauma should be carefully reviewed for a fracture.

Pseudodislocation of the Humerus. Another traumatic process that can be misdiagnosed radiologically, leading to inappropriate treatment and morbidity, is a pseudodislocation of the humerus (Fig. 46.12). This re-

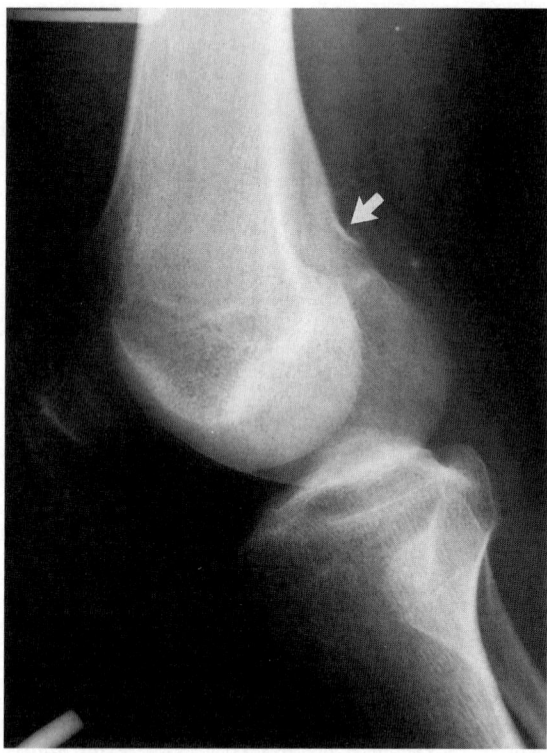

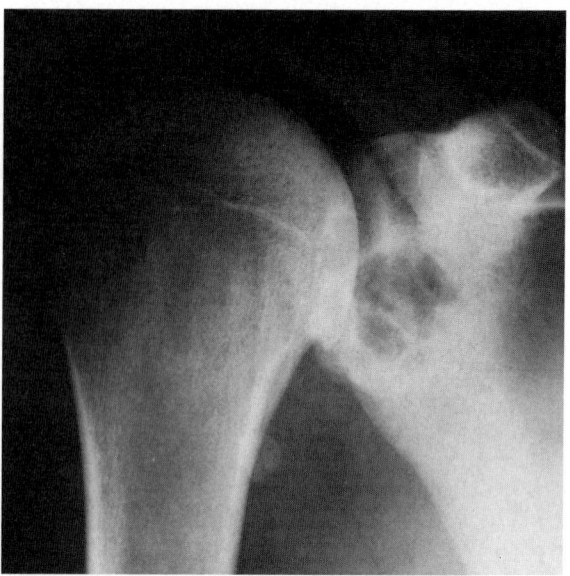

Figure 46.8. Geode. A large cystic lesion was found in the shoulder in this middle-aged weight lifter, and the possibility of a metastatic process was considered. Because the humeral head has sclerosis and osteophytosis as well as a loose body in the joint, degenerative disease of the shoulder was diagnosed; this makes the cystic lesion almost certainly a geode or subchondral cyst.

Figure 46.7. Cortical Desmoid. A well-defined cortical defect is seen in the posterior distal femur (*arrow*), which is a common appearance for a fairly well-healed cortical desmoid.

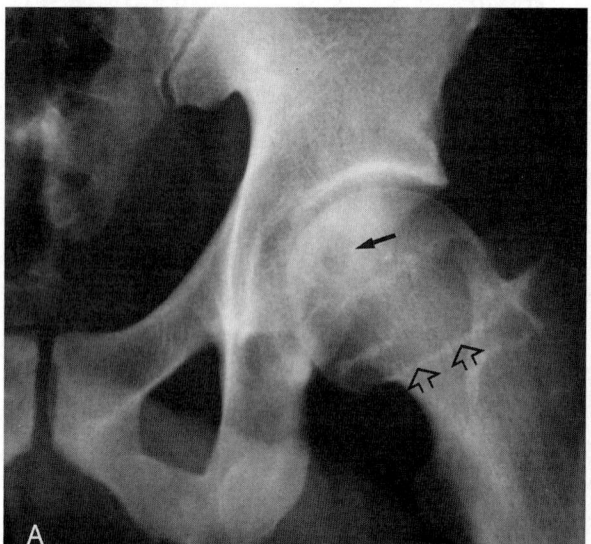

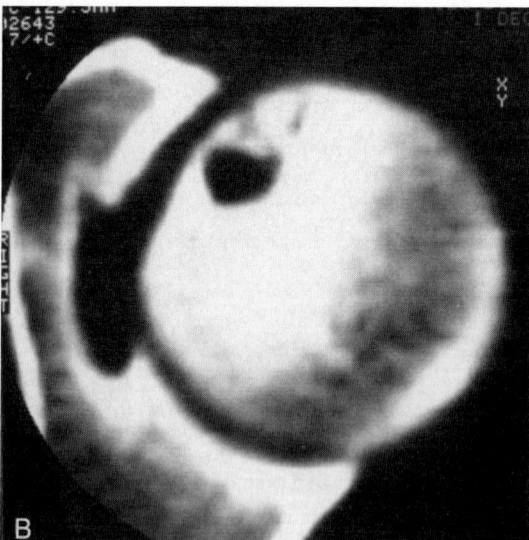

Figure 46.9. Geode. A. A cystic lesion was noted in the femoral head (*arrows*) of a young man with a painful hip. **B.** A computed tomography scan through this area shows the subarticular nature and adjacent sclerosis. The differential diagnosis of infection, eosinophilic granuloma, and chondroblastoma was given. A ring of osteophytes (*open arrowheads*) was noted in retrospect on the plain film **(A)** in the subcapital region, which indicates degenera- tive disease of the hip. Degenerative joint disease is extremely un- usual in a 20-year-old healthy man; however, it makes the lytic le- sion in the femoral head almost certainly a subchondral cyst or geode. This was an active soccer player who had been playing with pain in his hip for several years following an injury that had caused the degenerative disease. Unfortunately, a biopsy was performed anyway and a subchondral cyst or geode was confirmed.

Figure 46.10. Discogenic Vertebral Sclerosis. This patient has sclerosis on the inferior portion of the L4 vertebral body associated with minimal osteophytosis and joint space narrowing at the adjacent disc space. This is the classic appearance for discogenic vertebral sclerosis, and a biopsy to rule out metastatic disease should not be performed.

sults from a fracture with hemarthrosis, which causes distension of the joint and migration of the humeral head inferiorly (8). An axial or transscapular view shows it is not anteriorly or posteriorly dislocated (the usual forms of shoulder dislocation) but merely inferiorly subluxated. On an anteroposterior view, it can mimic a posterior dislocation in that the normal superimposition of the humeral head and the glenoid is missing. Often, attempts are made to "relocate" the humeral head, which, of course, are both fruitless (because it is not dislocated) and painful. A fracture is invariably present, and if not seen on the initial films, it should be sought after with additional views. The transscapular or the axial view is the key to making the diagnosis of a pseudodislocation. If necessary, the joint can be aspirated to confirm the presence of a bloody effusion and to show the normal position of the humeral head when fluid has been removed from the joint.

NORMAL VARIANTS

Dorsal Defect of the Patella. A normal variant that has been described in the patella that can be mistaken for a pathologic process is a lytic defect in the upper, outer quadrant called a dorsal defect of the patella (Fig. 46.13) (9). It can mimic a focus of infection, osteochondritis dissecans, or a chondroblastoma. It is a normal developmental anomaly, however, and because of its characteristic location, it should not undergo biopsy. On magnetic resonance imaging, it will have an appearance similar to many other bony lesions, that is, low signal on

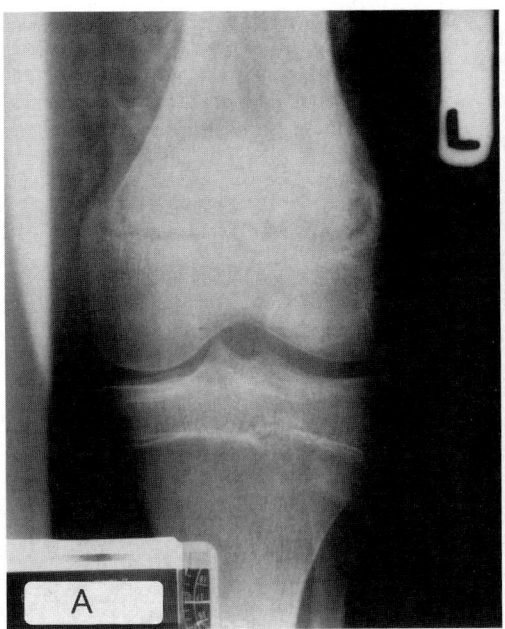
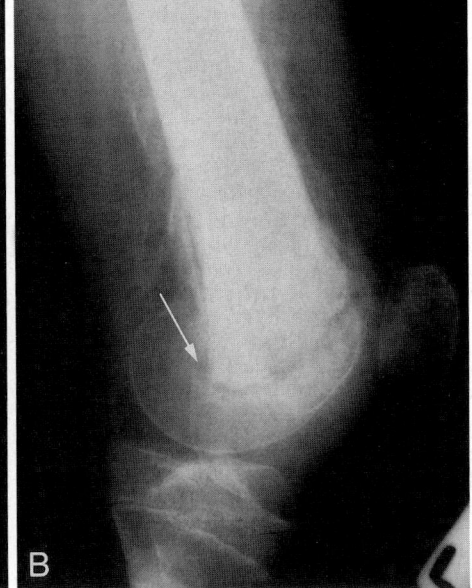

Figure 46.11. Fracture Mimicking Osteosarcoma. A. This 16-year-old patient had experienced pain around the knee for 2 weeks before these radiographs. The knee films showed diffuse sclerosis and extensive periostitis about the distal femur, which is thought to be characteristic for an osteogenic sarcoma. The periosteal reaction, however, was thought to be much too thick, dense, and wavy to represent malignant type of periostitis. **B.** A small offset of the epi-physis can be seen (*arrow*), which indicates an epiphyseal slippage consistent with a Salter epiphyseal fracture. This teenager had fallen off a bicycle and fractured the femur, yet continued to be active. The lack of immobility caused exuberant periostitis or callus with a large amount of reactive sclerosis, all of which mimicked an osteogenic sarcoma.

T1-weighted images and high signal on T2-weighted images (Fig. 46.14).

Pseudocyst of the Humerus. Another entity often confused for a lytic pathologic lesion is a pseudocyst of the humerus (Fig. 46.15). This is merely an anatomic variant caused by the increased cancellous bone in the region of the greater tuberosity of the humerus that gives this region a more lucent appearance on radiographs (10,11). With hyperemia and disuse caused by rotator cuff problems or any other shoulder disorder, this area of lucency may appear strikingly more lucent and mimic

a lytic lesion. Many of these have mistakenly undergone biopsy, and several have even had repeat biopsies after the initial pathology report stated "normal bone, no lesion in specimen." Because of the associated hyperemia from the shoulder disorder (be it rotator cuff injury or whatever), a bone scan can show increased radionuclide

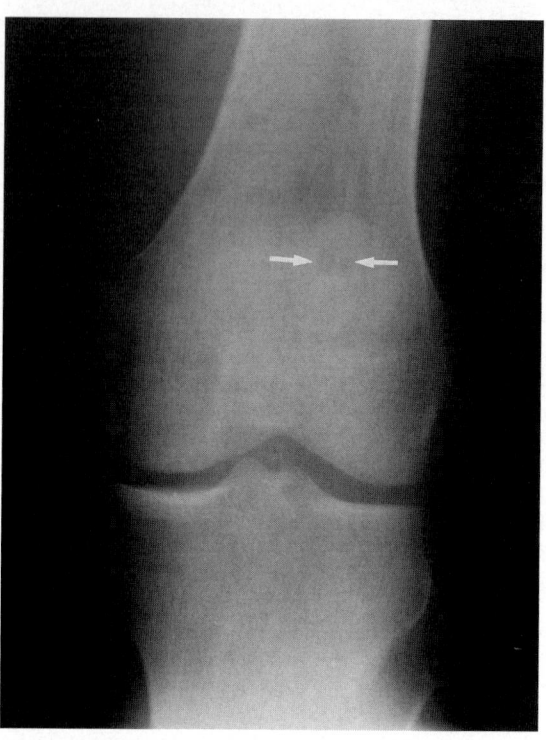

Figure 46.13. Dorsal Defect of the Patella. A lytic defect in the upper outer quadrant of the patella was seen in this patient (*arrows*), which is characteristic for a normal variant called dorsal defect of the patella. It occurs only in the upper outer quadrant and should be asymptomatic.

Figure 46.12. Pseudodislocation of the Shoulder. The humeral head in this patient is inferiorly placed in relation to the glenoid, which is the characteristic location when a hemarthrosis is present. A minimally displaced fracture of the neck of the humerus with avulsion of the greater tuberosity has occurred (*arrow*), causing the hemarthrosis.

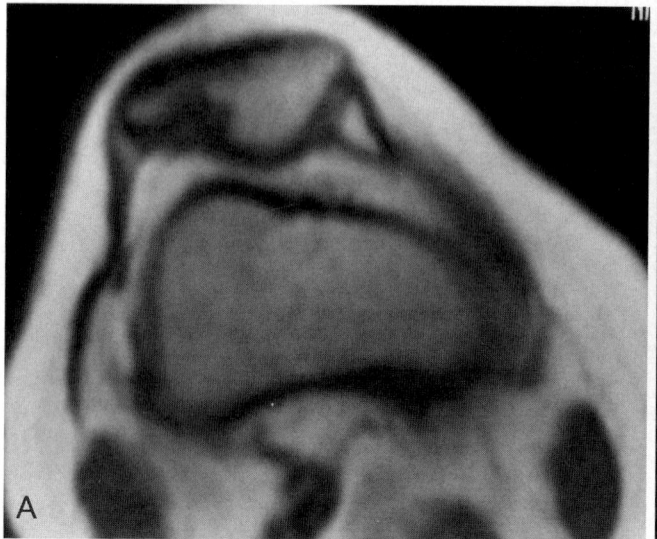

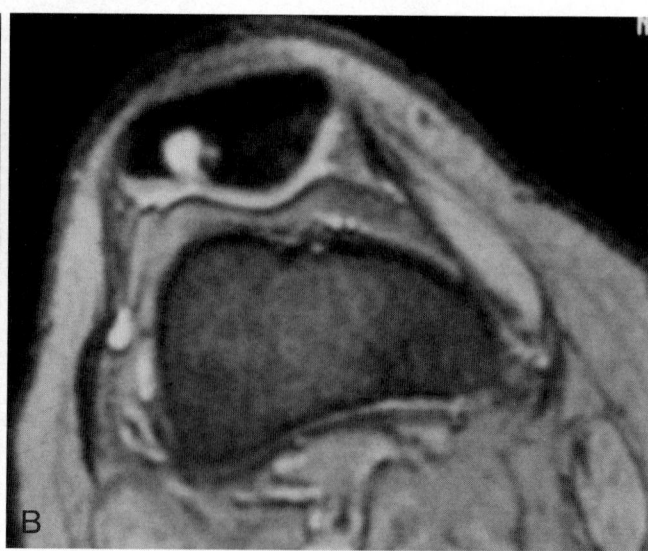

Figure 46.14. Dorsal Defect of the Patella. A. An axial T1-weighted MR shows a focal area of low signal in the patella in a subarticular location in the lateral facet of the patella. **B.** The axial T2-weighted image shows high signal in the lesion. This is typical in location and appearance for a dorsal defect of the patella.

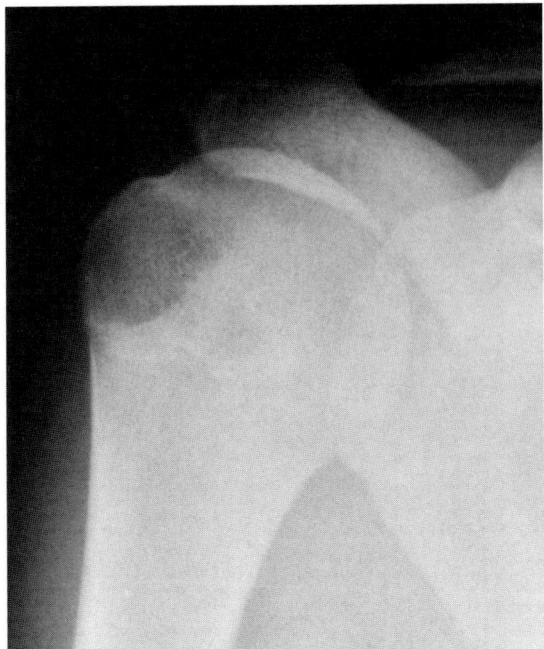

Figure 46.15. Pseudocyst of the Humerus. A well-defined lytic process is seen in the greater tuberosity, which was thought to represent a lytic lesion. This patient was symptomatic and had increased radionuclide uptake on isotope bone scan. This is a characteristic location and appearance, however, for a pseudocyst of the humerus, which merely represents decreased cortical bone in this region. This becomes more pronounced when pain in the shoulder is present and hyperemia or disuse osteoporosis occurs.

uptake and thus sway the surgeon to perform a biopsy of this normal variant. It is radiographically characteristic in its location and appearance and should not undergo biopsy. Although other lesions, such as a chondroblastoma, infection, or even a metastatic focus, could occur in a similar location, they do not have quite the same appearance as a pseudocyst of the humerus.

Os Odontoideum. A normal variant of the cervical spine that may, in fact, be posttraumatic is an os odontoideum (12). It is an unfused dens that may move anterior to the C2 body with flexion and can mimic a fractured dens (Fig. 46.16). Many of these require surgical fixation; some surgeons fuse every case, believing that they are all unstable. Radiologists should recognize that this process is not acute and, thus, save the patient halo fixation and possible immediate surgical intervention. Most of these cases are seen after trauma, and if no neurologic deficits are present, these patients can be seen electively and spared the horrors associated with treatment of the acutely fractured cervical spine. The radiologic signs for recognizing an os odontoideum are the smooth, often well-corticated, inferior border of the dens and the hypertrophied, densely corticated anterior arch of C1 (13). This latter finding presumably represents compensatory hypertrophy and indicates a long-standing condition.

OBVIOUSLY BENIGN LESIONS

Multiple real lesions exist that should be recognized radiographically as benign and left alone. These are lesions that should be diagnosed by the radiologist, not

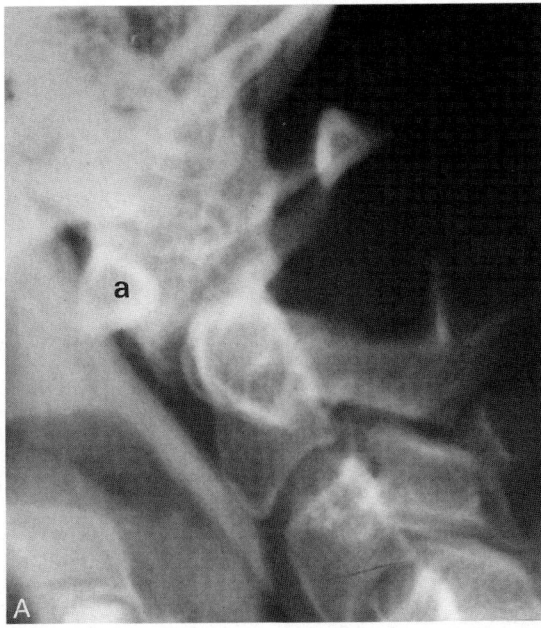
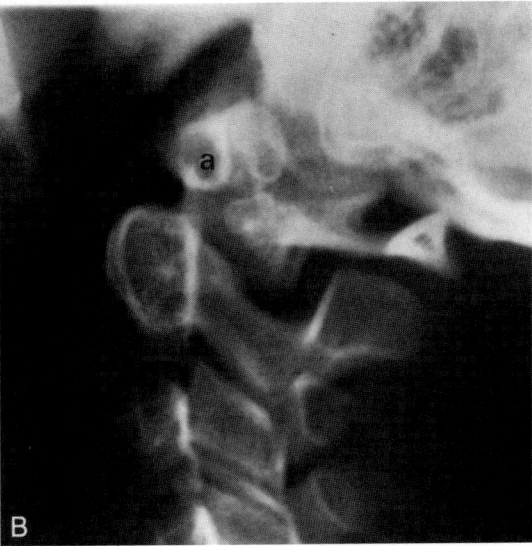

Figure 46.16. Os Odontoideum. Flexion **(A)** and extension **(B)** views show the anterior arch (a) of the C1 vertebrae has moved markedly anterior in relation to the body of C2 in flexion. The odontoid or dens is difficult to see but appears to be separated from the body of C2. Because of the smooth borders of the separated dens and because of the cortical hypertrophy of the anterior arch of C1, this can safely be called an os odontoideum, which is a congenital or long-standing posttraumatic abnormality rather than an acute fracture. Obviously, patients with this condition should have no neurologic problems, yet in many instances are still believed to be unstable and undergo surgically fusion. This, however, can be done on an elective basis.

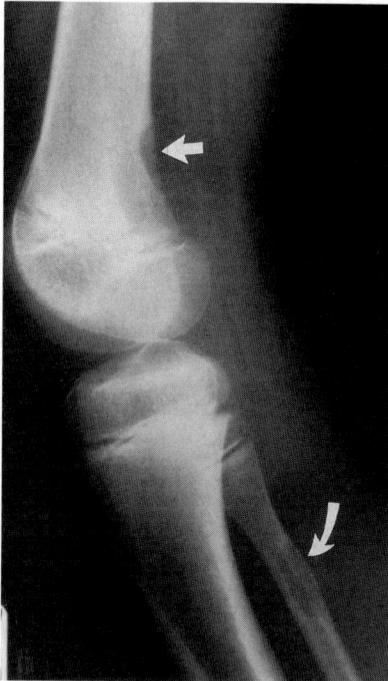

Figure 46.17. Nonossifying Fibroma. A well-defined, slightly expansile, lytic lesion is seen in the fibula (*curved arrow*); this is characteristic for a nonossifying fibroma. A second lytic lesion is seen in the posterior distal femur (*straight arrow*), which is also typical in appearance for a nonossifying fibroma.

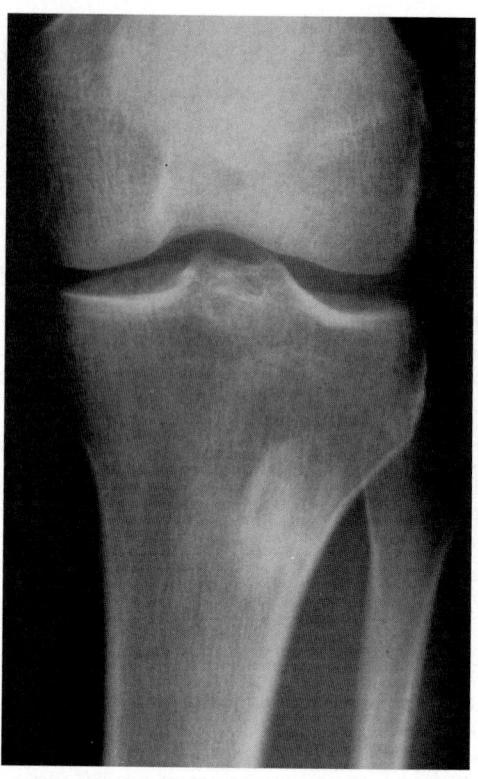

Figure 46.18. Healing Nonossifying Fibroma. A minimally sclerotic process is seen in the proximal tibia, which was thought by the surgeons to represent a focus of infection or an osteoid osteoma, even though the patient was asymptomatic. This is a characteristic appearance for a disappearing or healing nonossifying fibroma and should not undergo biopsy.

Figure 46.19. Nonossifying Fibroma. AP **(A)** and lateral **(B)** films of the tibia show a large, well-defined, minimally expansile lytic lesion of the proximal tibia, which is characteristic for a nonossifying fibroma. Even though the patient was asymptomatic, biopsy was performed and the diagnosis confirmed. (Case courtesy Dr. Larry Yeager, Redwood City, California.)

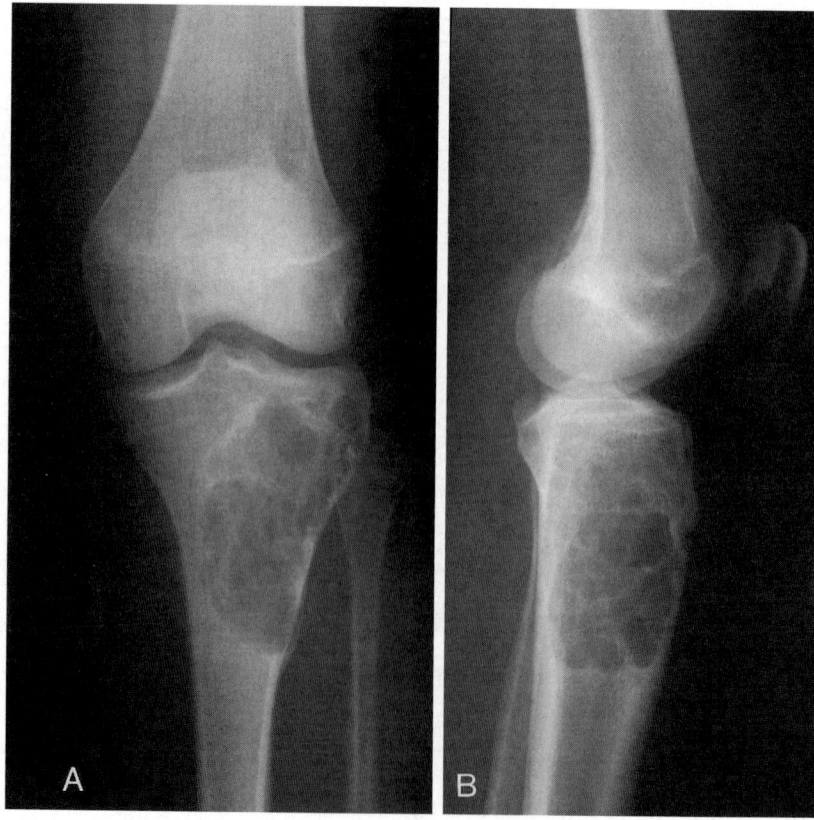

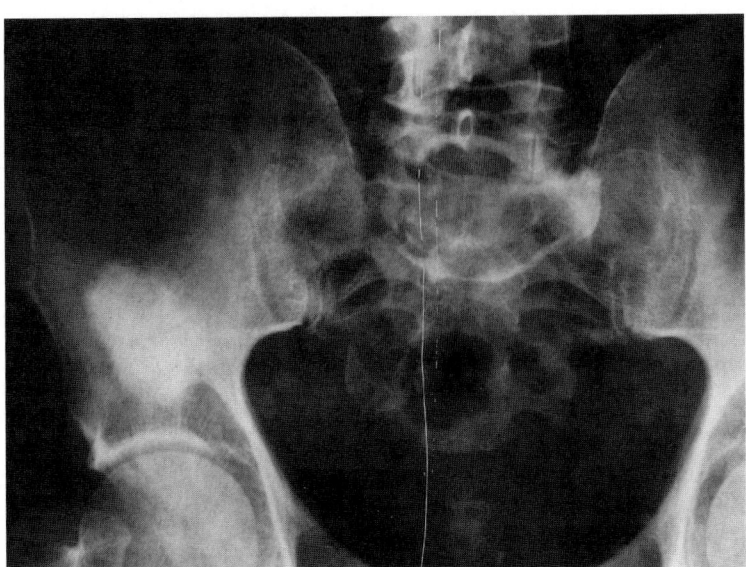

Figure 46.20. Giant Bone Island. A large sclerotic focus is seen in the right iliac wing. Note how the lesion is somewhat spherical or oblong in the lines of trabecular stress, which is characteristic for a bone island. This patient was asymptomatic and had no evidence of a primary carcinoma.

the pathologist. Listing a differential in these cases often spurs the surgeon to a biopsy, when, in fact, no biopsy should be necessary.

Nonossifying Fibroma. Perhaps the most often encountered lesion in this category is the nonossifying fibroma. Nonossifying fibroma is identical to a fibrous cortical defect, but the term is usually reserved for defects larger than 2 cm. They are, classically, lytic lesions located in the cortex of the metaphysis of a long bone and have a well-defined, often sclerotic, scalloped border with slight cortical expansion (Fig. 46.17). They are almost exclusively found in patients younger than the age of 30 years; hence, the natural history of the lesion is involution. As they involute, they fill in with new bone, giving it a sclerotic appearance (Fig. 46.18); thus, they can have some increased radionuclide activity on bone scans. They are most often mistaken for an area of infection, eosinophilic granuloma, fibrous dysplasia, or aneurysmal bone cyst. They are asymptomatic and have never been reported to be associated with malignant degeneration. On occasion, a pathologic fracture can occur through these lesions, but most surgeons do not advocate prophylactic curettage to prevent fracture, as with unicameral bone cysts. Nonossifying fibromas can be quite large but invariably have a benign appearance (Fig. 46.19), and biopsy should be avoided. The asymptomatic nature should help differentiate them from most of the other lesions in the differential diagnosis and thereby preclude even giving a differential diagnosis. On occasion, they are found to be multiple, yet each lesion is so characteristic that they should be easily diagnosed.

Bone Islands are not a radiographic dilemma when they are 1 cm or less in size. Occasionally, however, they grow to golf ball size or larger and mimic sclerotic metastases (Fig. 46.20). They are always asymptomatic. Radiographically, two signs can be found to help distinguish giant bone islands from metastases. First, bone islands usually are oblong, with their long axis in the axis of stress on the bone, for example, in a long bone they align themselves along the axis of the diaphysis. Second,

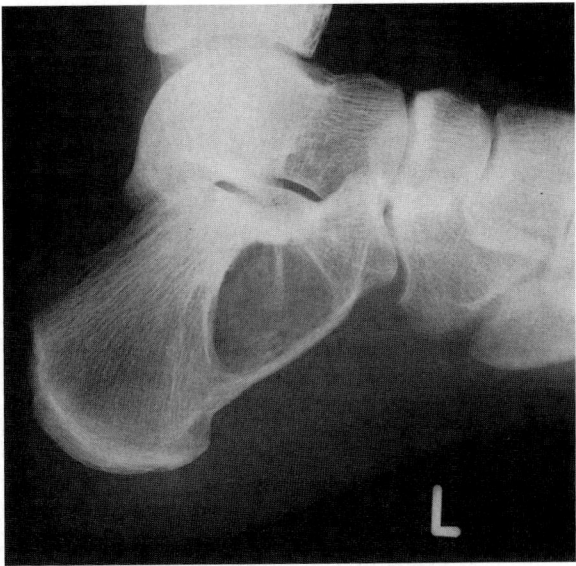

Figure 46.21. Unicameral Bone Cyst. A well-defined lytic lesion on the anterior-inferior portion on the calcaneus, as in this example, is virtually pathognomonic for a unicameral bone cyst or simple bone cyst. Because this is an area of diminished stress, it is thought not to be necessary to curettage and pack this lesion prophylactically in an effort to avoid a pathologic bone fracture, which is often done in the femur and humerus with unicameral bone cysts.

the margins of a bone island, if examined closely, will show bony trabeculae extending from the lesion into the normal bone in a spiculated fashion (14). This is characteristic of a bone island and helpful in differentiating it from a more aggressive process.

Unicameral Bone Cysts are often prophylactically curettaged and packed so as to prevent fracture with subsequent deformity. When these cysts occur in the calcaneus, however, they should be left alone. They always occur in the anterior-inferior portion of the calcaneus (Fig. 46.21), an area that does not receive undue

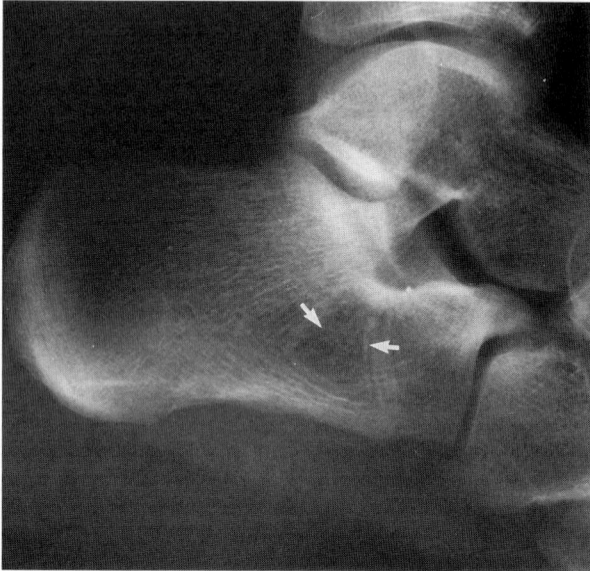

Figure 46.22. Pseudocyst of the Calcaneus. An area of radiolucency is seen on the anterior-inferior portion of the calcaneus (*arrows*) similar to the example in Figure 46.21, but not as well defined. This is a pseudocyst similar to the pseudocyst of the humerus that results from diminished stress through this region.

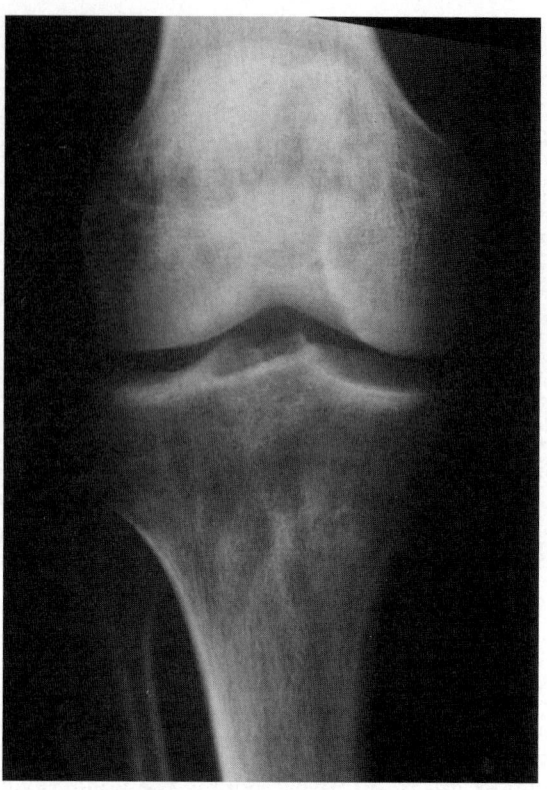

Figure 46.23. Early Bone Infarct. Patchy demineralization is seen in the distal femur and proximal tibia in this patient with systemic lupus erythematosus. The opposite leg was similarly involved. This is characteristic for early bone infarcts and should not be confused with infection or metastatic disease.

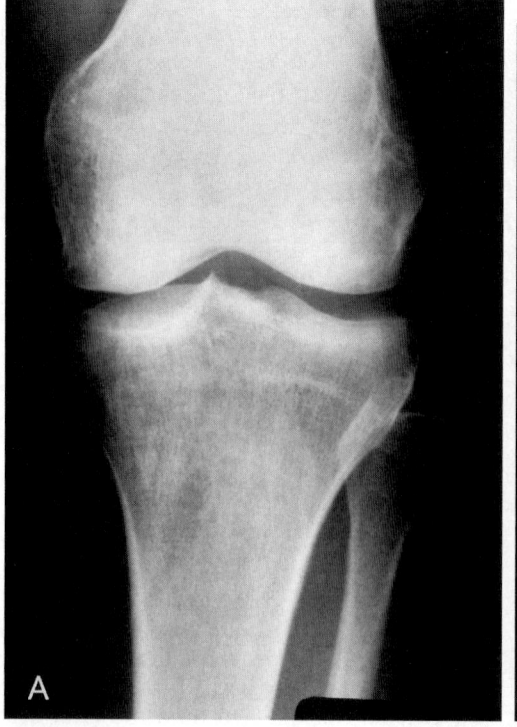

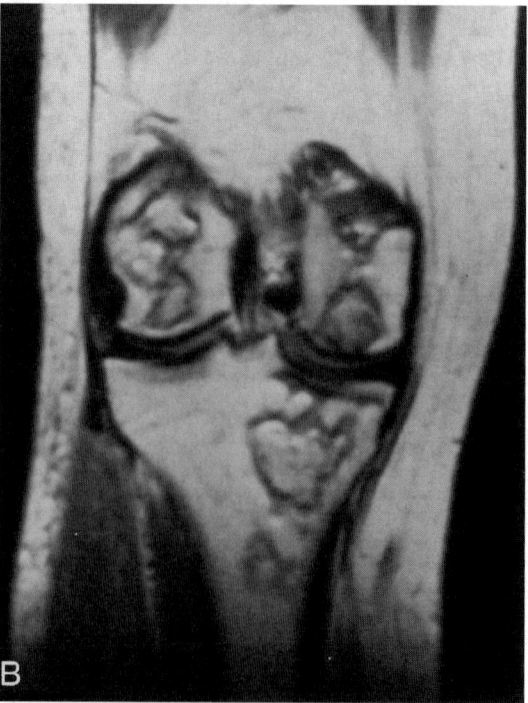

Figure 46.24. Bone Infarct. A. A plain film of the knee shows a permeative pattern in the proximal tibia, which was at first thought to be infection or a primary tumor. **B.** A T1-weighted coronal MR shows the characteristic serpiginous border seen with bone infarct in the tibia and in the femur. Magnetic resonance imaging can on occasion better characterize the ill-defined early bone infarct, as in this example. This patient has systemic lupus erythematosus.

stress. In fact, a pseudotumor of the calcaneus is seen in the identical position because of the absence of stress and resulting atrophy of bony trabeculae (Fig. 46.22). These lesions are asymptomatic, only rarely fracture, and should not suffer the same fate as their counterparts in long bones, that is, surgical removal.

Bone Infarction. Early in the course of its development, a bone infarct can have a patchy or a mixed lytic–sclerotic pattern or even resemble a permeative process (Fig. 46.23) (15). In a patient with bone pain and a permeative bone lesion, many aggressive disorders head the differential list and a biopsy soon ensues. If this process can be noted to be multiple and in the diametaphyseal region of a long bone, especially if the patient has an underlying disorder such as sickle cell anemia or systemic lupus erythematosus, areas of early bone infarction should be considered. In some cases, the characteristic MR appearance of an infarct may save a patient from biopsy when the plain films are equivocal (Fig. 46.24).

CONCLUSION

These are but a few of the many examples of circumstances in skeletal radiology in which the well-trained radiologist can be of invaluable assistance to the clinician and the patient by helping avert a needless biopsy. Dozens of other examples are nicely shown in normal variant textbooks, which are widely available. Because of the potential harm in performing a needless biopsy, the examples described in this chapter are stressed. When these lesions are encountered by the radiologist, a differential diagnosis should not be offered, as it will often lead the surgeon to a biopsy in an attempt to get a diagnosis. A biopsy in many of these entities is not only unnecessary but can be misleading.

References

1. Murray R, Jacobson H. The Radiology of Skeletal Disorders. 2nd ed. New York: Churchill Livingstone, 1977:603.
2. Wootton J, Cross M, Holt K. Avulsion of the ischial apophysis. J Bone Joint Surg 1990;72B:625–627.
3. Schneider R, Kaye J, Ghelman B. Adductor avulsive injuries near the symphysis pubis. Radiology 1976;120:567–569.
4. Barnes G, Gwinn J. Distal irregularities of the femur simulating malignancy. AJR Am J Roentgenol 1974;122:180–185.
5. Ostiere S, Seeger L, Eckardt J. Subchondral cysts of the tibia secondary to osteoarthritis of the knee. Skeletal Radiol 1990;19:287–289.
6. Resnick D, Niwayama G, Coutts R. Subchondral cysts (geodes) in arthritic disorders: pathologic and radiographic appearance of the hip joint. AJR Am J Roentgenol 1977;128:799–806.
7. Martel W, Seeger J, Wicks J, et al. Traumatic lesions of the discovertebral junction in the lumbar spine. AJR Am J Roentgenol 1976;127:457–464.
8. Helms C, Richmond B, Sims R. Pseudodislocation of the shoulder: a sign of an occult fracture. Emerg Med 1986;18:237–241.
9. Johnson JF, Brogdon BG. Dorsal effect of the patella: incidence and distribution. AJR Am J Roentgenol 1982;139:339–340.
10. Helms C. Pseudocyst of the humerus. AJR Am J Roentgenol 1979;131:287–292.
11. Resnick D, Cone R. The nature of humeral pseudocysts. Radiology 1984;150:27–28.
12. Minderhoud J, Braakman R, Penning L. Os odontoideum: clinical, radiological, and therapeutic aspects. J Neurol Sci 1969;8:521–544.
13. Holt RG, Helms CA, Munk PL, et al. Hypertrophy of C-1 anterior arch: useful sign to distinguish os odontoideum from acute dens fracture. Radiology 1989;173:207–209.
14. Onitsuka H. Roentgenologic aspects of bone islands. Radiology 1977;124:607–612.
15. Munk PL, Helms CA, Holt RG. Immature bone infarcts: findings on plain radiographs and MR scans. AJR Am J Roentgenol 1989;152:547–549.

47
Miscellaneous Bone Lesions

Clyde A. Helms

There are a host of bony conditions, diseases, and syndromes that do not fit conveniently into any of the preceding chapters, yet should be given some mention in an attempted overview of musculoskeletal radiology. These are listed alphabetically for lack of a more scientific basis.

ACHONDROPLASIA

The most common cause of dwarfism is achondroplasia, a congenital, hereditary disease of failure of endochondral bone formation. The femurs and humeri are more profoundly affected than the other long bones, although the entire skeleton is abnormal. A characteristic finding is that the spine typically has narrowing of the interpedicular distances in a caudal direction (Fig. 47.1), the opposite of normal, in which the interpedicular distances get progressively wider as one proceeds down the spine. The long bones are short but have normal width, giving them a thick appearance.

AVASCULAR NECROSIS

The term "avascular necrosis" (AVN) refers to the lack of blood supply with subsequent bone death and ensuing bony collapse in an articular surface. The etiology of AVN is an extensive differential that most commonly includes *trauma, steroids, aspirin, renal disease, collagen vascular diseases, alcoholism,* and *idiopathic* causes (Table 47.1) (1). The radiographic appearance ranges from patchy sclerosis (Fig. 47.2A) to articular surface collapse and fragmentation (Fig. 47.3). Just before collapse, a subchondral lucency is occasionally seen (Fig. 47.4); however, this is a late and inconstant sign of AVN. Magnetic resonance imaging is extremely valuable in demonstrating the presence and extent of AVN (Fig. 47.2B,C), even when plain films are apparently normal. Magnetic resonance imaging is currently considered to be the most efficacious way to evaluate a joint for AVN (2). It is useful not only in AVN of the hip but also in the knee, wrist, foot, and ankle.

HYPERTROPHIC PULMONARY OSTEOARTHROPATHY

Hypertrophic pulmonary osteoarthropathy is manifested by clubbing of the fingers and periostitis, usually in the upper and lower extremities (Fig. 47.5), which might or might not be associated with bone pain. It is most commonly seen in patients with lung cancer, but many other etiologies have been reported, including bronchiectasis, gastrointestinal disorders, and liver disease. The actual mechanism of formation of periostitis secondary to a distant malignancy or other process is unknown. The differential diagnosis for periostitis in a long bone without an underlying bony abnormality would include *hypertrophic pulmonary osteoarthropathy, venous stasis, thyroid acropachy, pachydermoperiostosis,* and *trauma* (Table 47.2).

MELORHEOSTOSIS

Melorheostosis is a rare, idiopathic disorder characterized by thickened cortical new bone that accumulates near the ends of long bones, usually only on one side of the bone, and has an appearance likened to "dripping candle wax" (Fig. 47.6). It can affect several adjacent bones and can be symptomatic.

MUCOPOLYSACCHARIDOSES (MORQUIO'S, HURLER'S, AND HUNTER'S SYNDROMES)

The mucopolysaccharidoses are a group of inherited diseases characterized by abnormal storage and excretion in the urine of various mucopolysaccharidoses such as keratin sulfate (Morquio's) and heparan sulfate (Hurler's). These patients have short stature, primarily from shortened spines, and characteristic plain film findings. In the spine, patients with Morquio's have platyspondyly (generalized flattening of the vertebral bodies) with a central anterior projection or "beak" off the vertebral body, as viewed on a lateral plain film (Fig. 47.7). Hurler's and Hunter's show platyspondyly with a beak that is anteroinferiorly positioned (Fig. 47.8). The pelvis in these disorders is similar in appearance to that of achondroplasts, with wide, flared iliac wings and broad femoral necks. A characteristic finding in the hands is a pointed proximal fifth metacarpal base that has a notch appearance to the ulnar aspect (Fig. 47.9).

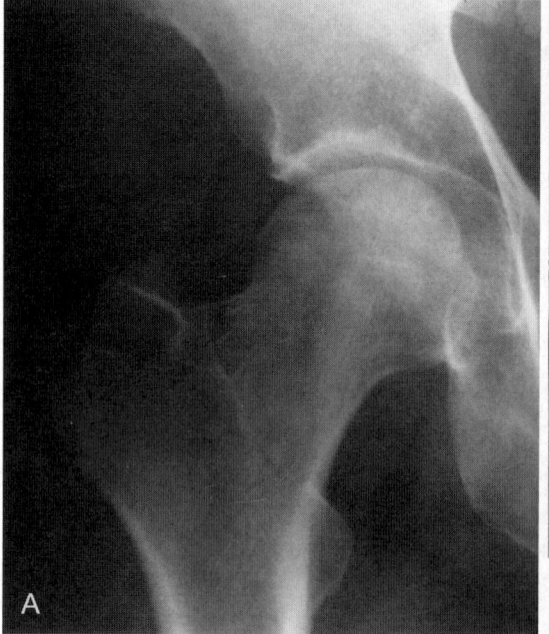

Figure 47.1. Achondroplasia. An anteroposterior plain film of the spine in this patient with achondroplasia demonstrates narrowing of the interpedicular distance (*arrows*) in a caudal direction, which is characteristic of this disorder. Ordinarily, the interpedicular distance widens in each vertebra in a caudal direction.

MULTIPLE HEREDITARY EXOSTOSIS

Also known as diaphyseal aclasia, this is a not uncommon hereditary disorder that seems to affect multiple members of a family with multiple osteochondromas, or exostoses. An osteochondroma is a cartilage-capped bone outgrowth that may be pedunculated or sessile in appearance. In the multiple hereditary form, the knees are virtually always involved (Fig. 47.10). Undertubulation (a widened diameter of the bone) is invariably present at the site of the exostosis. The incidence of malignant degeneration in this population has been reported to be as high as 20%. As with solitary osteochondromas, the more axially situated lesions are more prone to undergo malignant degeneration, whereas the more peripheral lesions are less likely to do so. The proximal femurs are frequently involved and have a characteristic appearance (Fig. 47.11).

Table 47.1. Common Causes of AVN

Trauma
Steroids
Renal disease
Collagen vascular diseases
Alcoholism
Idiopathic causes

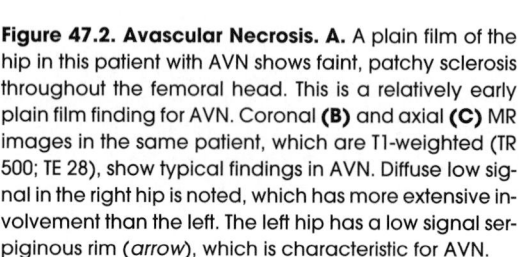

Figure 47.2. Avascular Necrosis. A. A plain film of the hip in this patient with AVN shows faint, patchy sclerosis throughout the femoral head. This is a relatively early plain film finding for AVN. Coronal **(B)** and axial **(C)** MR images in the same patient, which are T1-weighted (TR 500; TE 28), show typical findings in AVN. Diffuse low signal in the right hip is noted, which has more extensive involvement than the left. The left hip has a low signal serpiginous rim (*arrow*), which is characteristic for AVN.

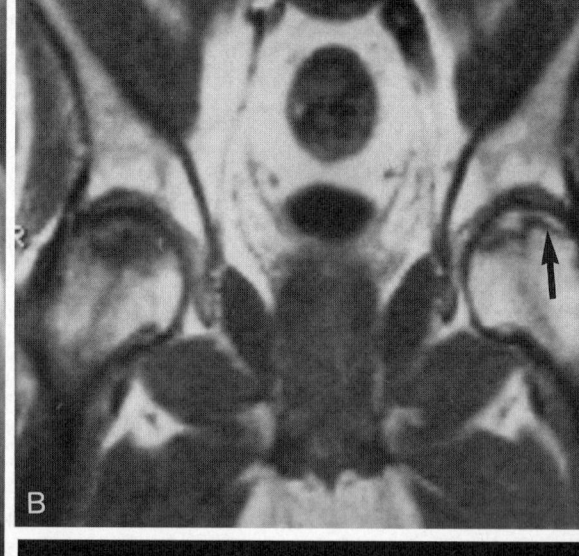

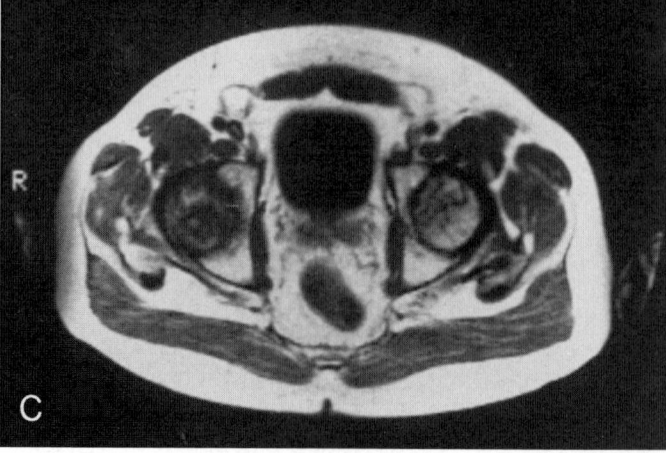

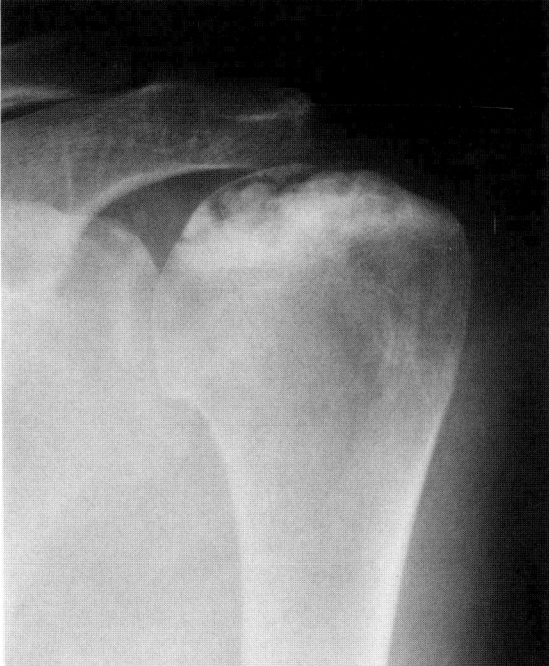

Figure 47.3. Avascular Necrosis. An anteroposterior plain film of the shoulder reveals articular surface collapse in this patient who was treated with steroids for systemic lupus erythematosus. This is an advanced stage of AVN.

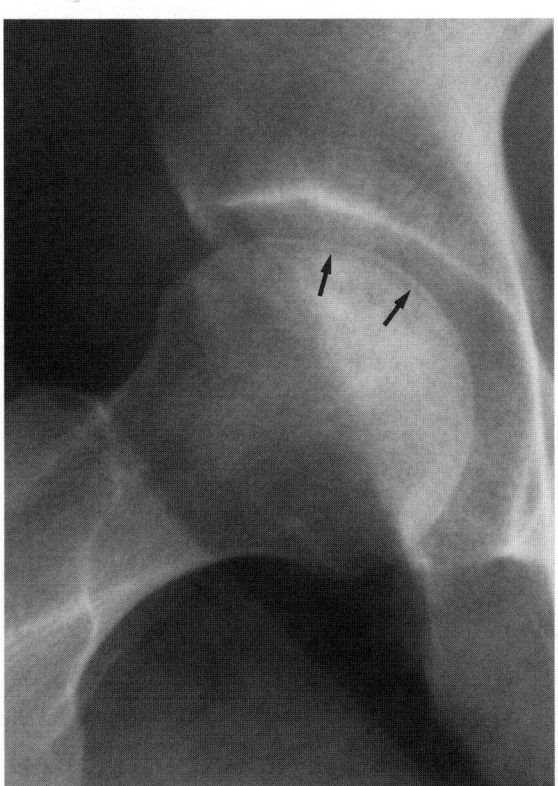

Figure 47.4. Avascular Necrosis. An anteroposterior frog-leg lateral view of the hip in this patient with sickle cell disease shows a sub-chondral lucency (*arrows*) and patchy sclerosis in the femoral head, indicative of AVN. This is a relatively advanced stage of AVN. The subchondral lucency is often better demonstrated with the frog-leg lateral view.

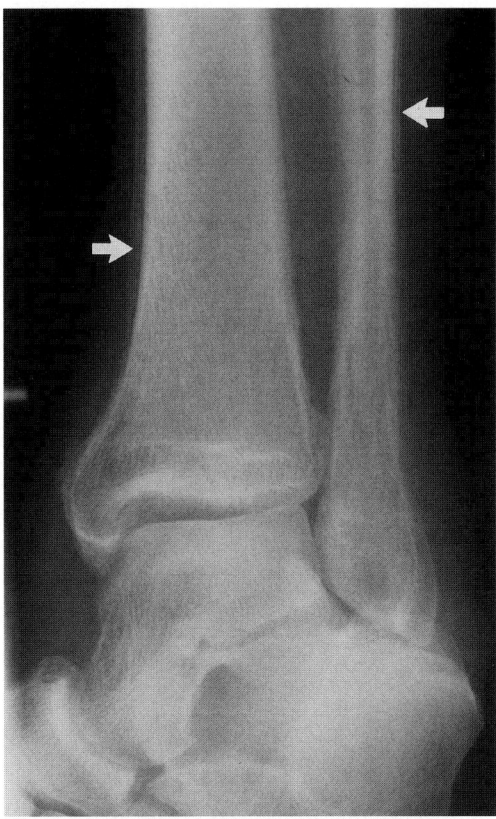

Figure 47.5. Hypertrophic Pulmonary Osteoarthrosis. Periostitis can be seen along the shafts of the distal tibia and fibula (*arrows*) in this patient with bronchogenic carcinoma and leg pain. This is characteristic for hypertrophic pulmonary osteoarthrosis.

Table 47.2. Periostitis without Underlying Bony Lesions

Trauma
Hypertrophic pulmonary osteoarthropathy
Venous stasis
Thyroid acropachy
Pachydermoperiostosis

OSTEOID OSTEOMA

The etiology of osteoid osteoma is unknown. It may be an infection (bacterial or viral) or a slow-growing tumor, but nobody knows. It is a painful lesion that occurs almost exclusively in patients less than 30 years of age and is treated successfully with surgical excision.

Radiographically, an osteoid osteoma is said to have a classic appearance, but it has many different appearances, which can make diagnosis difficult (3). The classically described radiographic appearance is a cortically based sclerotic lesion in a long bone that has a small lucency within it that is called the nidus (Fig. 47.12A). It is the nidus that causes the pain and the surrounding reactive sclerosis. If the nidus is surgically removed, complete cessation of pain is the rule. Computed tomography is often very helpful in demonstrating the exact location of the nidus (Fig. 47.12B).

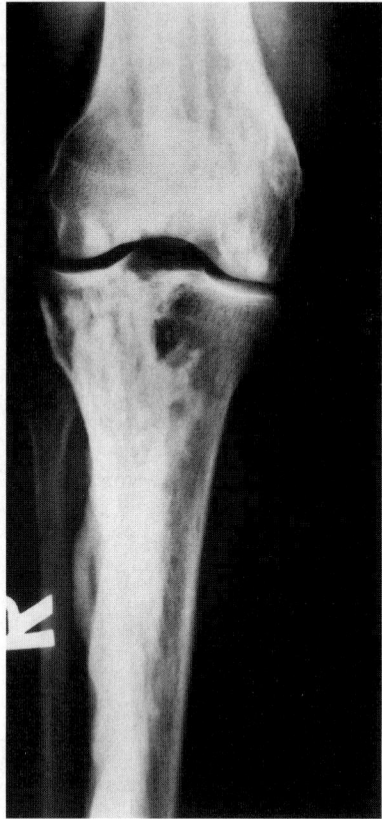

Figure 47.6. Melorheostosis. Dense, wavy, new bone is seen adjacent to the lateral tibial cortex, which has a dripping candle wax appearance, which is classic for melorheostosis. A similar pattern can be seen in the medial aspect of the distal femur.

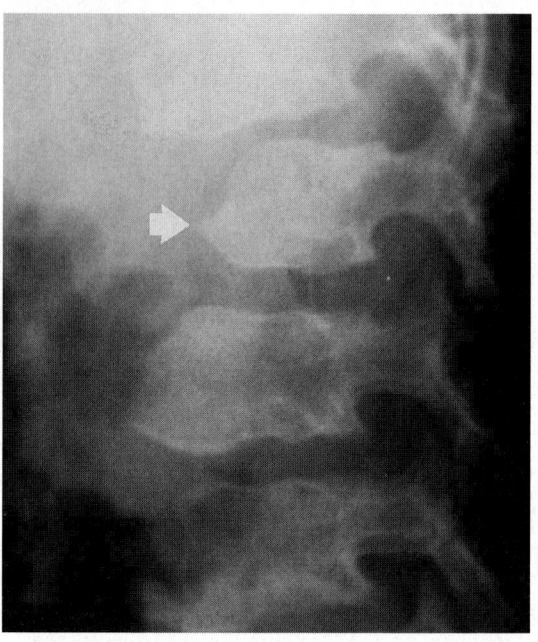

Figure 47.8. Hurler's Syndrome. A lateral plain film of the spine in this patient with Hurler's syndrome shows an inferiorly placed bony projection extending anteriorly off the vertebral bodies (*arrow*).

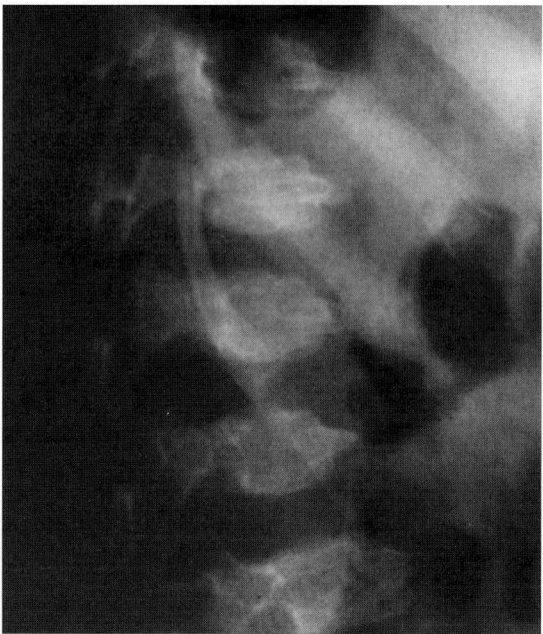

Figure 47.7. Morquio's Syndrome. A lateral plain film of the spine reveals a central beak or anterior bony projection off the vertebral bodies in this patient with Morquio's syndrome.

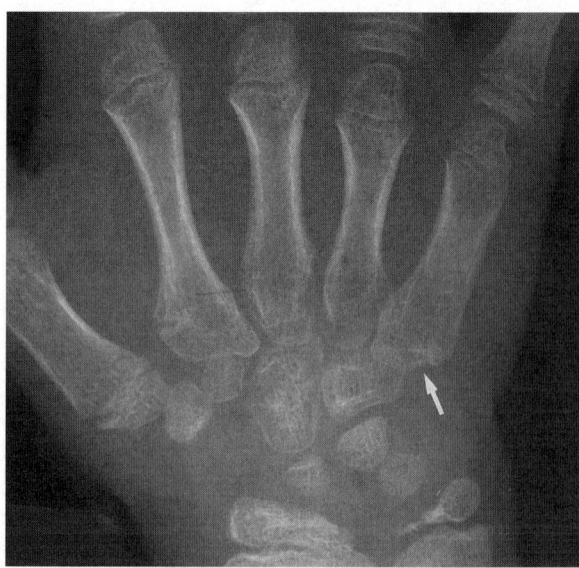

Figure 47.9. Hurler's Syndrome. An anteroposterior plain film of the hand in this patient with Hurler's syndrome shows a notch (*arrow*) at the base of the fifth metacarpal, which is a characteristic finding in all of the mucopolysaccharidoses.

If the nidus of an osteoid osteoma is located in the medullary rather than the cortical portion of a bone, or if it is located in a joint, there is much less reactive sclerosis present. This gives the lesion a different overall appearance than the more common cortical lesion in that it does not appear as sclerotic. Up to 80% of osteoid osteomas are located intracortically, with the remainder being in the intramedullary part of a bone. Rarely, an osteoid osteoma will present in the periosteum, causing exuberant periostitis.

The nidus itself is usually lucent but often develops some calcification within it. It then has the appearance

of a sequestrum, as is seen in osteomyelitis. If the nidus calcifies completely, it blends in with the surrounding sclerosis and cannot be seen on most radiographs. Therefore, the diagnosis of an osteoid osteoma in no way depends on seeing a nidus.

Because an osteoid osteoma resembles osteomyelitis, regardless of the appearance of the nidus, it can be difficult to differentiate the two radiographically. It cannot be reliably done with plain films, computed tomography, or MR. However, because the nidus is extremely vascular, it avidly accumulates radiopharmaceutical bone-scanning agents. An osteoid osteoma will have an area of increased uptake corresponding to the area of reactive sclerosis but, in addition, will demonstrate a second area of increased uptake corresponding to the nidus (Fig. 47.13). This has been termed the double-density sign (4). In contrast, osteomyelitis has a photopenic area corresponding to the plain film lucency that represents an avascular focus of purulent material. The natural history of an osteoid osteoma is presumed to be spontaneous regression, as they are rarely seen in patients older than the age of 30.

OSTEOPATHIA STRIATA

Also known as Voorhoeve's disease, this disorder is manifested by multiple 2- to 3-mm–thick linear bands of sclerotic bone aligned parallel to the long axis of a bone (Fig. 47.14). It usually affects multiple long bones and is asymptomatic; hence, it is usually an incidental finding.

OSTEOPOIKILOSIS

Osteopoikilosis is an hereditary, asymptomatic disorder that is usually an incidental finding of multiple small (3–10 mm) sclerotic bony densities affecting primarily the ends of long bones and the pelvis (Fig. 47.15). It has no clinical significance other than that it can be confused for diffuse osteoblastic metastases.

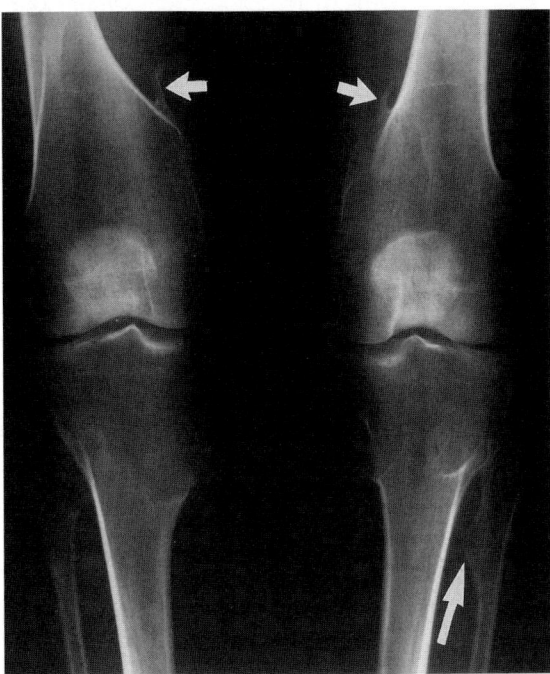

Figure 47.10. Multiple Hereditary Exostosis. The knees are involved in virtually every case of multiple hereditary exostosis. They typically show not only multiple exostoses (*arrows*) but marked undertubulation in the metaphyses.

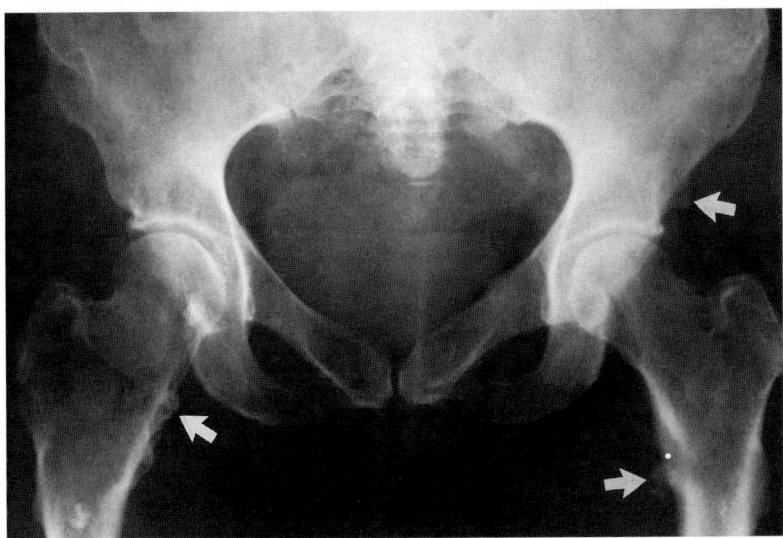

Figure 47.11. Multiple Hereditary Exostosis. The femoral necks are often involved in multiple hereditary exostosis. They will show undertubulation, as in this example, and usually have one or more exostoses (*arrows*).

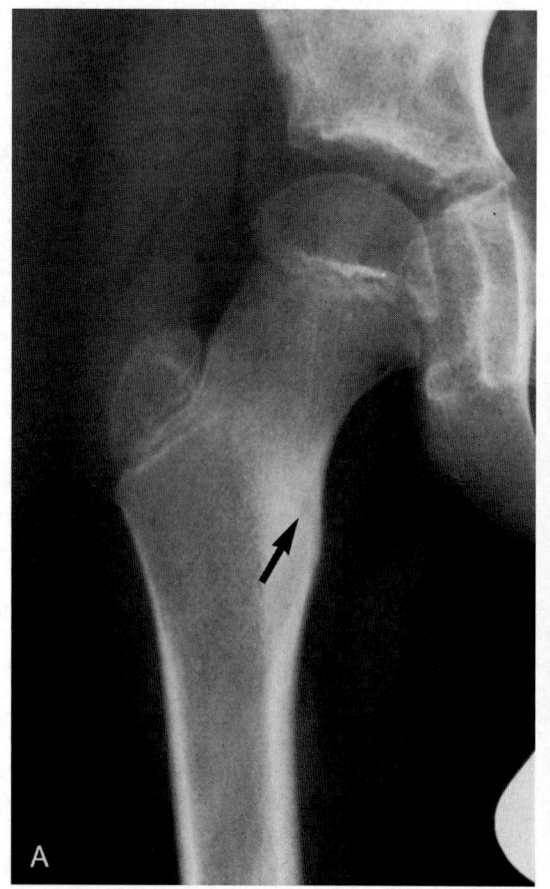

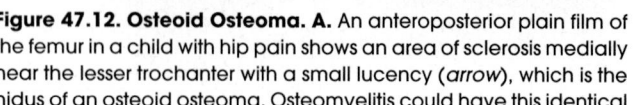

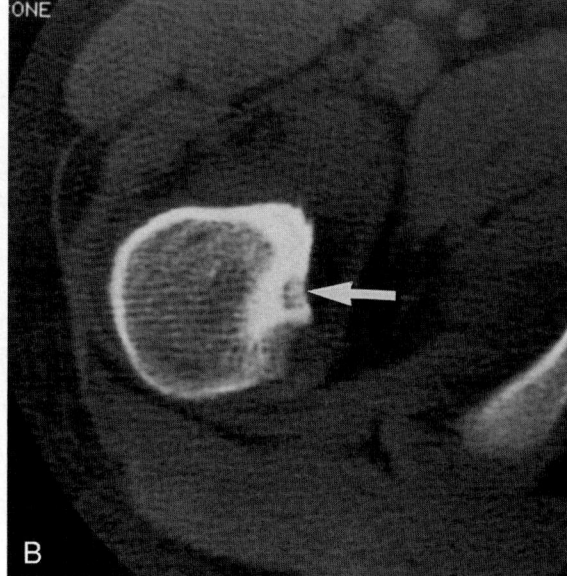

Figure 47.12. Osteoid Osteoma. A. An anteroposterior plain film of the femur in a child with hip pain shows an area of sclerosis medially near the lesser trochanter with a small lucency (*arrow*), which is the nidus of an osteoid osteoma. Osteomyelitis could have this identical appearance. **B.** A computed tomographic scan of the femur shows the sclerosis medially and the lucent nidus (*arrow*) to better advantage. The CT scan gives the surgeon a more precise anatomic location of the nidus than the plain film.

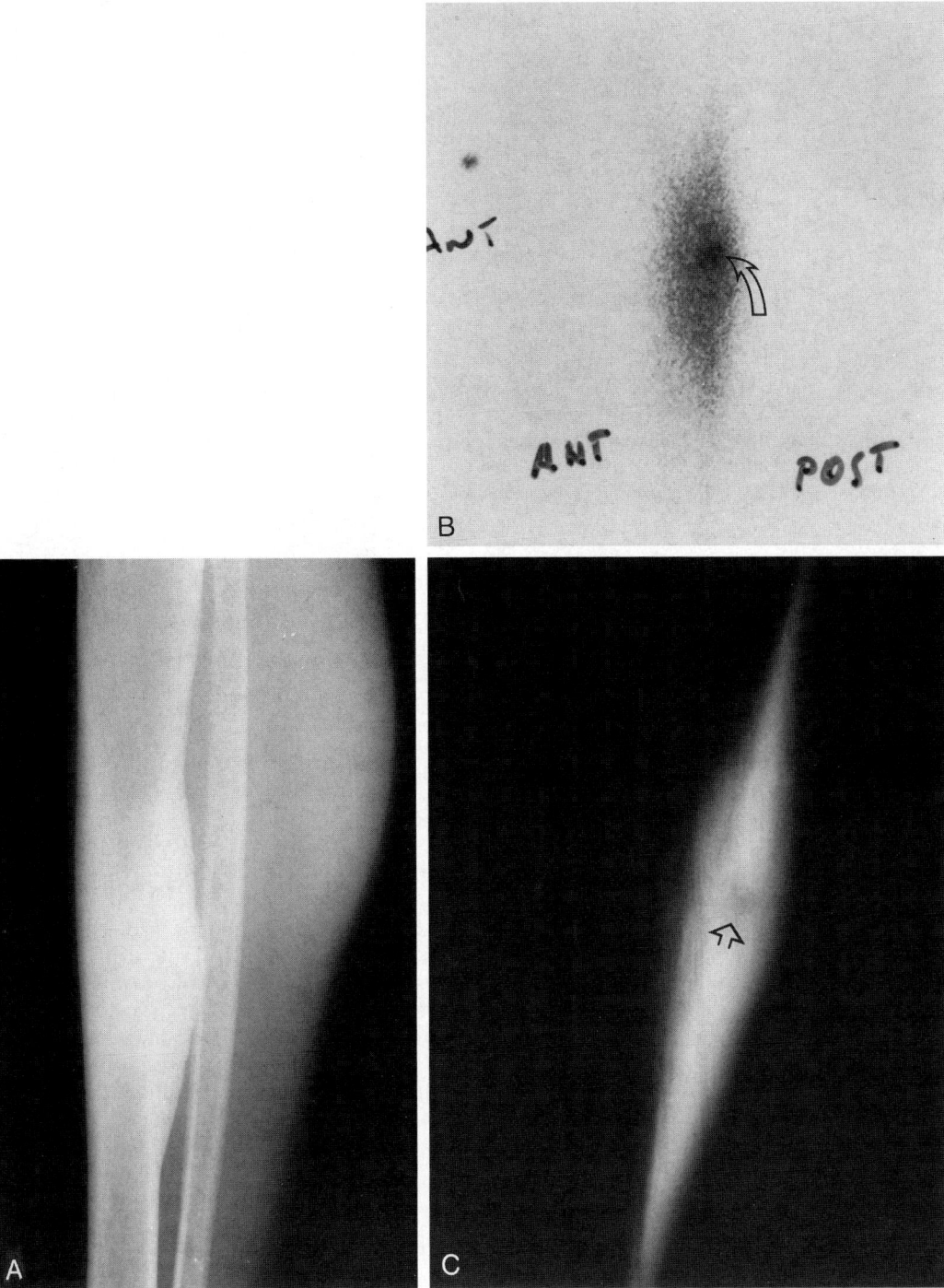

Figure 47.13. Osteoid Osteoma. A. A lateral plain film of the tibia in this child with leg pain shows cortical thickening in the posterior diaphysis. No lucency in the sclerotic area could be identified. **B.** A radionuclide bone scan reveals uptake corresponding to the area of sclerosis in the tibia, with a more marked area of uptake centrally (*arrow*), which is the double-density sign of an osteoid osteoma. **C.** The surgical specimen shows the nidus (*arrow*) as a faint lucency within the sclerotic bone.

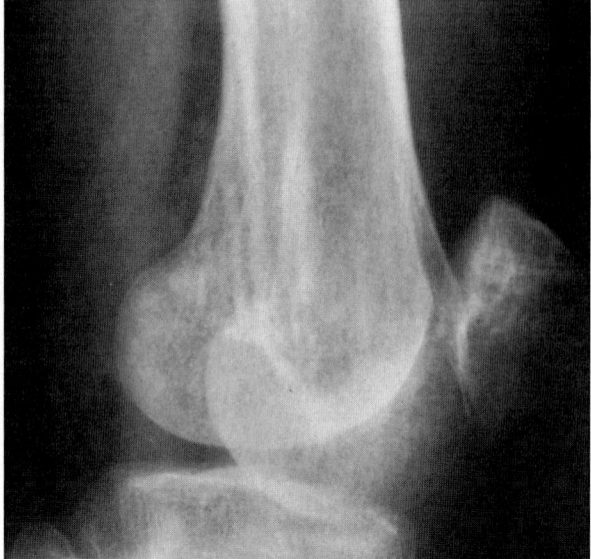

Figure 47.14. Osteopathia Striata. Multiple linear dense streaks are seen in the distal femur, which are characteristic of osteopathia striata.

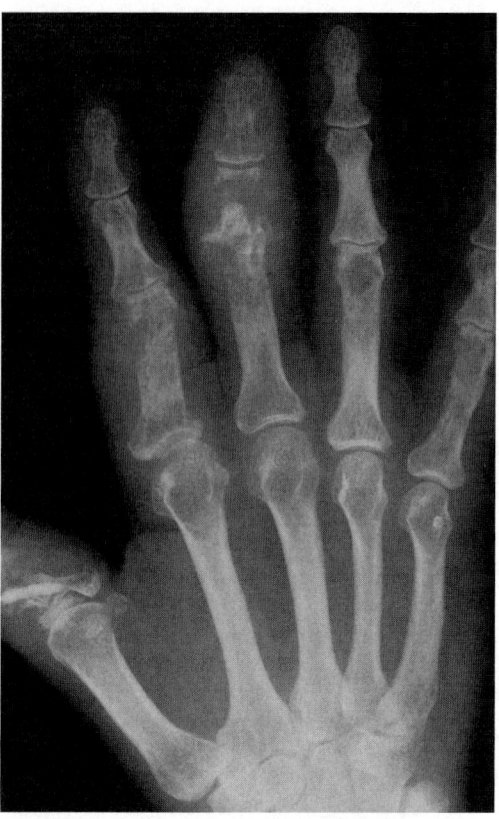

Figure 47.16. Sarcoid. An anteroposterior plain film of the hands in a patient with sarcoidosis shows multiple lytic lesions, many of which demonstrate a lacelike pattern.

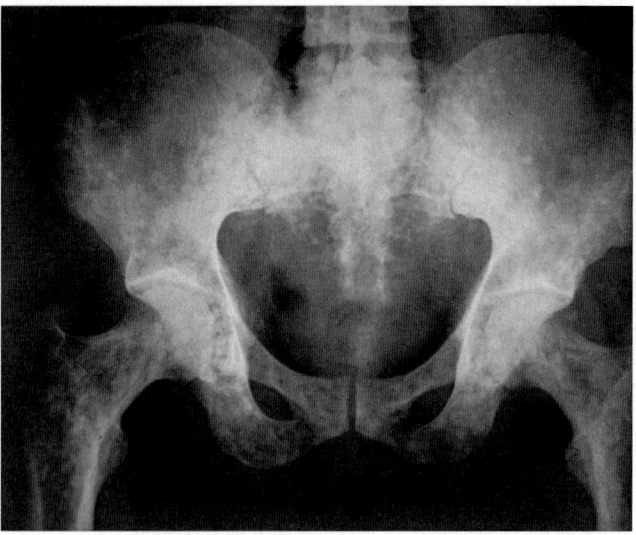

Figure 47.15. Osteopoikilosis. An anteroposterior view of the pelvis reveals multiple small, round sclerotic foci throughout the pelvis and femurs. This is diagnostic of osteopoikilosis. This is occasionally mistaken for metastatic disease.

SARCOIDOSIS

Sarcoidosis is a noncaseating granulomatous disease that primarily affects the lungs. When the musculoskeletal system is involved, the hands are mainly affected, with the spine and long bones only infrequently involved. Sarcoid causes a characteristic lacelike pattern of bony destruction in the hands (Fig. 47.16). Multiple phalanges are typically affected in either one or both hands. It is so radiographically characteristic that there is almost no differential diagnosis for this pattern.

TRANSIENT OSTEOPOROSIS OF THE HIP

This poorly understood disorder is an idiopathic process that begins with a painful hip with no underlying disorder or other findings other than osteoporosis, which is limited to the painful hip. Some believe it is early AVN; however, this has not been proved. Its appearance on MR is similar to early AVN (5) in that low signal on T1-weighted images is seen throughout the femoral head and neck (Fig. 47.17). Transient osteoporosis of the hip invariably is self-limited with full resolution. It tends to occur more often in males.

PACHYDERMOPERIOSTOSIS

Pachydermoperiostosis is a rare, familial disease that is manifested by thickening of the skin of the extremities and face, clubbing of the fingers, and widespread periostitis. It seems to be more common in black patients. The periosteal reaction is similar to that of hypertrophic pulmonary osteoarthropathy, but pachydermoperiostosis is rarely painful.

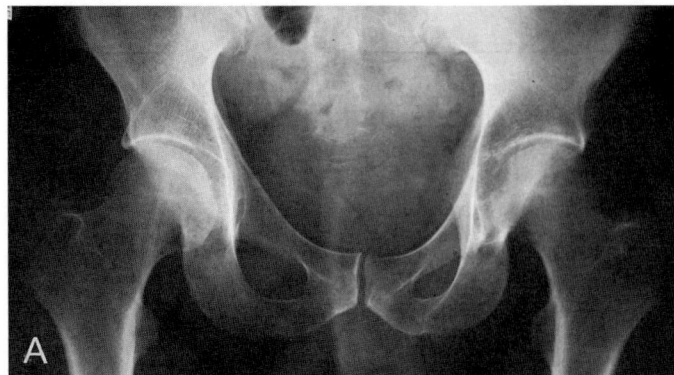

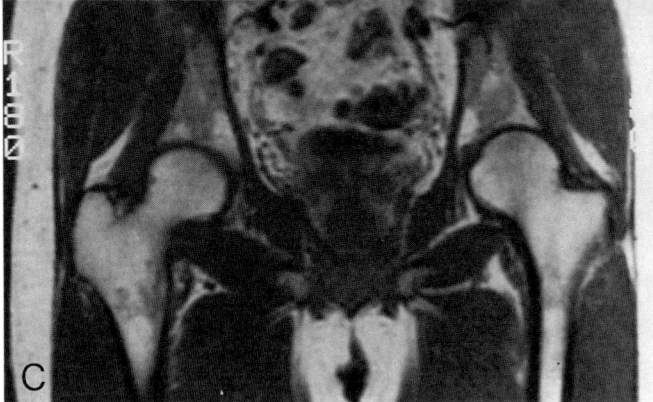

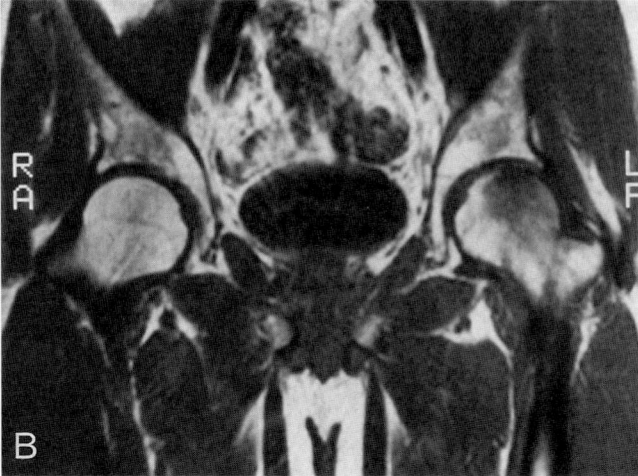

Figure 47.17. Idiopathic Transient Osteoporosis of the Hip. A. A plain film of a 40-year-old man with left hip pain shows osteoporosis involving the left hip, with no other abnormalities seen. **B.** A T1-weighted (TR 700; TE 12) coronal MR done at the same time as the plain film shows low signal in the superior portion of the left femoral head. This is a characteristic appearance for AVN but is a nonspecific finding. Clinically, this patient had no underlying causes for AVN, and he was treated conservatively. **C.** Seven months later, after near total cessation of the hip pain, a repeat MR (TR 600; TE 20) shows no abnormality in the hip. This is consistent with idiopathic transient osteoporosis of the hip.

References

1. Mankin H. Nontraumatic necrosis of bone (osteonecrosis). N Engl J Med 1992;326:1473–1479.
2. Mitchell D, Kressel H, Arger P, et al. Avascular necrosis of the femoral head: morphologic assessment by MR imaging, with CT correlation. Radiology 1986;161:739–742.
3. Marcove R, Heelan R, Huvos A, et al. Osteoid osteoma. Diagnosis, localization, and treatment. Clin Orthop 1991; 267:197–201.
4. Helms CA, Hattner RS, Vogler JB III. Osteoid osteoma: radionuclide diagnosis. Radiology 1984;151:779–784.
5. Takatori Y, Kokubo T, Ninomiya S, et al. Transient osteoporosis of the hip. Magnetic resonance imaging. Clin Orthop 1991;271:190–194.

48

Magnetic Resonance Imaging of the Knee

Clyde A. Helms

TECHNIQUE
MENISCI
CRUCIATE LIGAMENTS
COLLATERAL LIGAMENTS
PATELLA
BONY ABNORMALITIES

MR of the knee has developed into one of the most frequently requested examinations in radiology. This is because of its inherent accuracy in depicting internal derangements and its ability to allow orthopaedic surgeons to use the study as a road map for subsequent therapeutic arthroscopic procedures. Also, MR has a very high negative predictive value; therefore, a normal MR knee examination is highly accurate in excluding an internal derangement (1,2).

TECHNIQUE

The proper imaging protocol is essential for a high diagnostic accuracy rate. If the appropriate sequences are obtained, an accuracy of 90–95% can be expected. A sagittal T1-weighted (or proton-density) sequence is essential for examining the menisci, and 4-mm or 5-mm thick slices with a relatively small field of view and at least a 192 matrix are recommended. The knee should be imaged using a dedicated knee coil and externally rotated about 5–10° (do not exceed 10°) to put the anterior cruciate ligament in the plane of imaging. T2 spin-echo or T2* GRASS (gradient recalled acquisition in the steady state) sagittal images are obtained primarily to examine the cruciate ligaments. With T2-weighted spin-echo images, meniscal tears may be difficult to see; however, they will be picked up on the proton-density images.

Fast spin echo (FSE) sequences are particularly poor for examining the menisci. Even when performed as fast proton-density images with a short echo train length, they have too much blurring to allow for accurate demonstration of meniscal tears.

Coronal images are obtained to examine the collateral ligaments and to look for meniscocapsular separations. These abnormalities can generally only be seen with T2WIs. T1-weighted coronal images are therefore a waste of time because nothing can be seen on these images that cannot seen eqaully as well on the sagittal images or the T2 or T2* coronal images. T2* GRASS coronal images or repeating the sagittal spin-echo sequences in the coronal plane are imperative. The coronal images are rarely useful for seeing a meniscal tear that cannot be appreciated on the sagittal images.

Axial images are obtained for use by technicians as a scout view and can also be used for viewing the patellofemoral cartilage and for examining a medial patellar plica. As in the coronal images, to afford an opportunity to see any pathology, T1WIs or T2WIs must be obtained.

MENISCI

The normal meniscus is a fibrocartilagenous, C-shaped structure that is uniformly low in signal on both T1-weighted and T2-weighted sequences. Many centers have found that the menisci are more easily examined if they fat-suppress the T1 or proton-density sequences (Fig. 48.1). With T2* sequences, the menisci will usually demonstrate some internal signal. With T1WIs, any signal within the meniscus is abnormal, except in children, where some signal is normal and represents normal vascularity.

Meniscal Degeneration. Meniscal signal that does not disrupt an articular surface is representative of intrasubstance degeneration (Fig. 48.2), which is myxoid degeneration of the fibrocartilage. It most likely represents aging and normal wear and tear. It is not thought to be symptomatic, and cannot be diagnosed clinically or with arthroscopy. Some choose, therefore, not to mention intrasubstance degeneration in the radiology interpretation. A grading scale for meniscal signal that is widely used is the following (Fig. 48.3): grade 1, rounded or amorphous signal that does *not* disrupt an articular surface; grade 2, linear signal that does *not* disrupt an articular surface; and grade 3, rounded or linear signal that disrupts an articular surface (Fig. 48.4). Grades 1 and 2 are intrasubtance degeneration and should not be reported as "grade 1 or 2 tears." The term "tear" often leads to an unnecessary arthroscopy (arthroscopy is not indicated for intrasubstance degeneration). Grade 3 is a meniscal tear.

Mensical Tear. When high signal in a meniscus disrupts the superior or inferior articular surface, a meniscal tear is diagnosed (Fig. 48.4). Meniscal tears have many different configurations and locations; an oblique tear extending to the inferior surface of the posterior horn of the medial meniscus is the most common type. In a small but significant percentage of cases, it can be virtually impossible to be certain if meniscal high signal disrupts an articular surface. In these cases it is recommended that the surgeon be advised that it is too close to call. The surgeon can then rely on his or her clinical expertise to decide if arthroscopy is warranted, and if it is, the MR will guide the surgeon to the location of the questionable tear. If these equivocal cases are excluded, the remaining cases will have an extremely high accuracy rate.

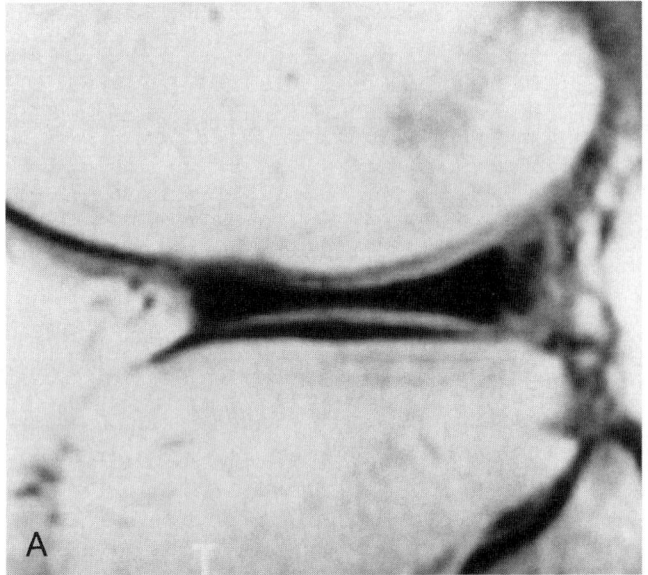

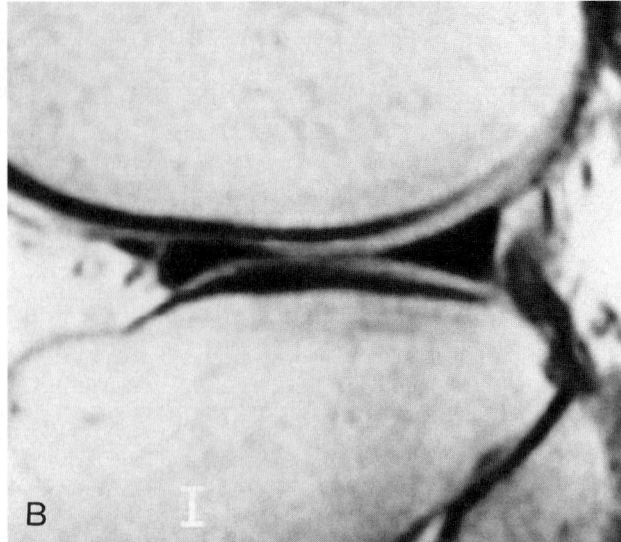

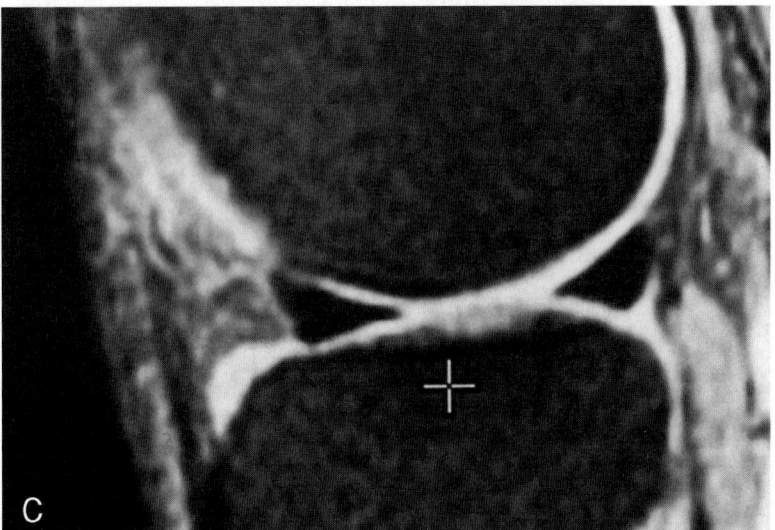

Figure 48.1. Normal Meniscus. A. A T1-weighted sagittal image (TR 600; TE 30) through a normal lateral meniscus demonstrates uniform low signal in the meniscus. This is a section through the body of the meniscus as it has a bow-tie configuration. Two sections of the body should be seen in each meniscus with 4-mm or 5-mm thick slices. **B.** In the same T1-weighted sequence, this sagittal image demonstrates uniform low signal in the anterior and posterior horns of this normal lateral meniscus. **C.** This sagittal proton density image (TR 2000; TE 20) shows how fat suppression accentuates the menisci.

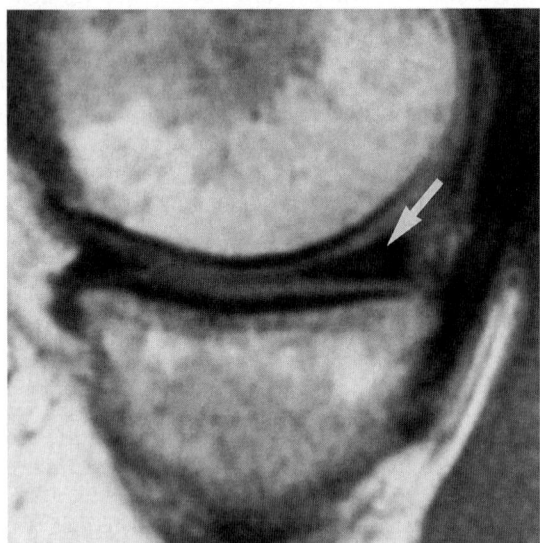

Figure 48.2. Intrasubstance Degeneration. Faint intermediate signal can be seen in the posterior horn of this meniscus (*arrow*) that does not disrupt the articular surface of the meniscus. This is intrasubstance degeneration.

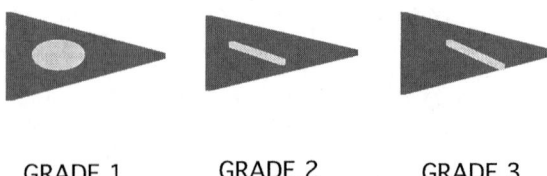

GRADE 1   GRADE 2   GRADE 3

Figure 48.3. Grading Scale for Menisci. A schematic of the MR grading scale for meniscal abnormalities. Grade 1 is rounded or amorphous signal in the meniscus that does not disrupt an articular surface. Grade 2 is linear signal that does not disrupt an articular surface. Grades 1 and 2 represent intrasubstance degeneration. Grade 3 is signal that does disrupt an articular surface and indicates a meniscal tear.

It has been shown that MR imaging sensitivity for meniscal tears decreases significantly when the anterior cruciate ligament (ACL) is torn (3). These frequently overlooked tears occur in the periphery of the meniscus and in the posterior horn of the lateral meniscus. Hence, great care must be used in examining these areas of the menisci in patients with ACL tears.

Bucket-handle Tear. Another very common meniscal tear is a bucket-handle tear. This is a vertical longitudinal tear that can result in the inner free edge of the meniscus becoming displaced into the intercondylar

notch (Fig. 48.5). It is most easily recognized by observing on the sagittal images that only one image is present that has the bow-tie appearance of the body segment of the meniscus (Fig. 48.6). Normally, two contiguous sagittal images with a bow-tie shape are seen because the normal meniscus is 10–12 mm in width and the sagittal images are 4–5 mm in thickness. On the coronal images, a bucket-handle tear may reveal the meniscus to be shortened and truncated; however, the torn meniscus often remodels and truncation cannot be appreciated. The displaced inner edge of the meniscus (the "handle" of the bucket) is often seen in the intercondylar notch on sagittal or coronal views (Fig. 48.7); however, it can occasionally be difficult to find the displaced meniscal fragment.

Discoid Meniscus. A discoid meniscus is a large meniscus that can have many different shapes—lens-shaped, wedged, flat, and others. Whether it is congenital or acquired is not known, but most are found in children or young adults. It is seen laterally in up to 3% of

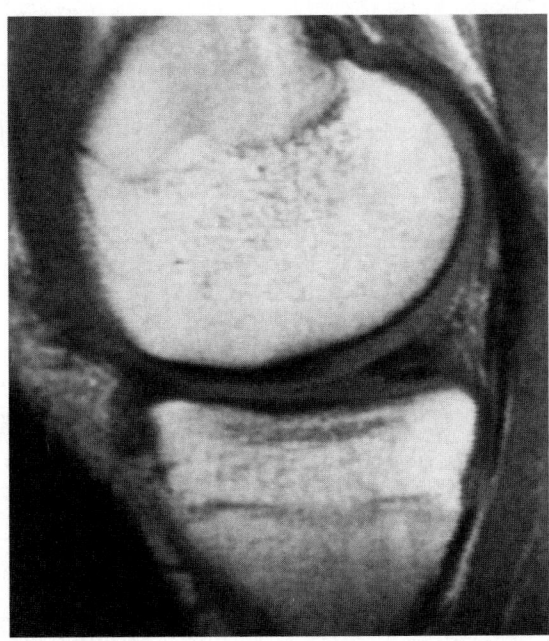

Figure 48.4. Meniscal Tear. This T1-weighted sagittal image (TR 600; TE 30) shows linear high signal in the posterior horn of the meniscus that disrupts the inferior articular surface. This is the appearance of a meniscal tear.

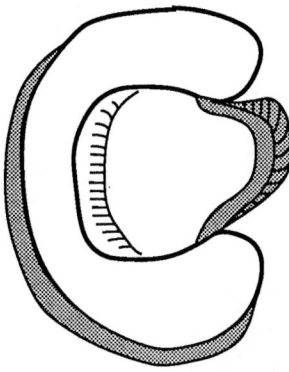

Figure 48.5. Bucket-handle Tear. This drawing illustrates a bucket-handle tear with the torn free edge of the meniscus displaced as the handle of the bucket.

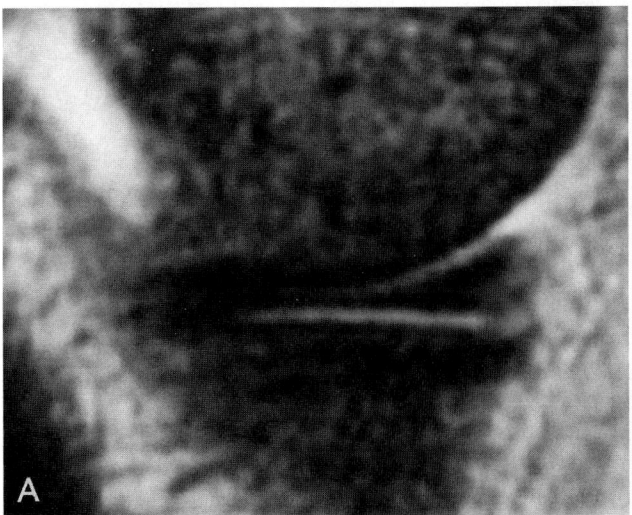
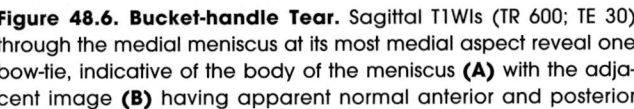
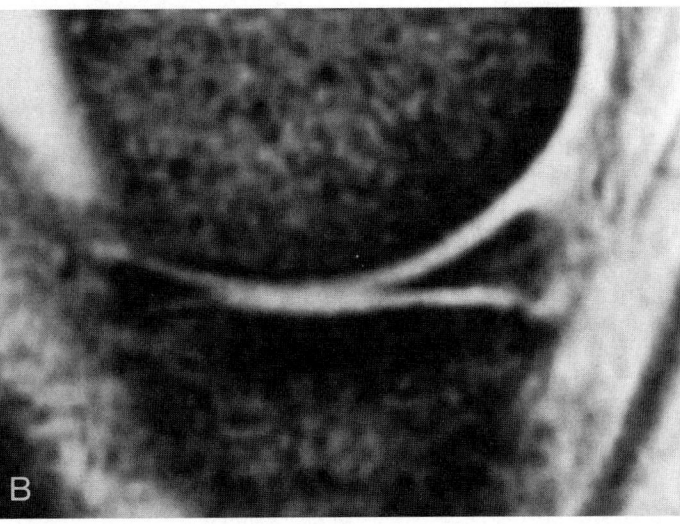

Figure 48.6. Bucket-handle Tear. Sagittal T1WIs (TR 600; TE 30) through the medial meniscus at its most medial aspect reveal one bow-tie, indicative of the body of the meniscus **(A)** with the adjacent image **(B)** having apparent normal anterior and posterior

horns. However, since there should be two consecutive sagittal images with a bow-tie configuration, this indicates a bucket-handle tear.

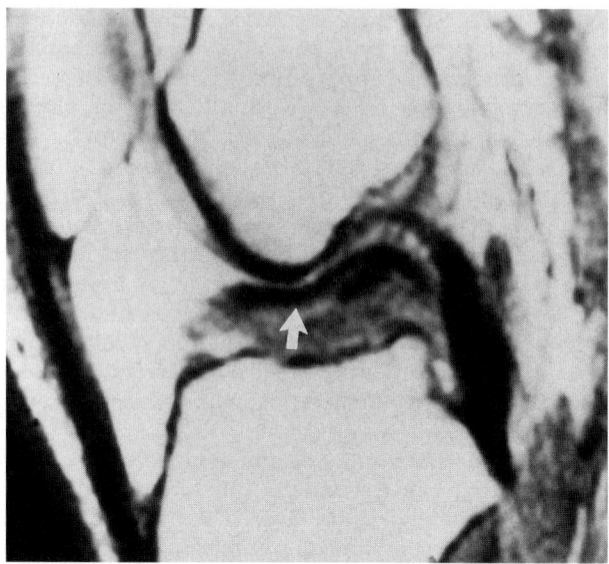

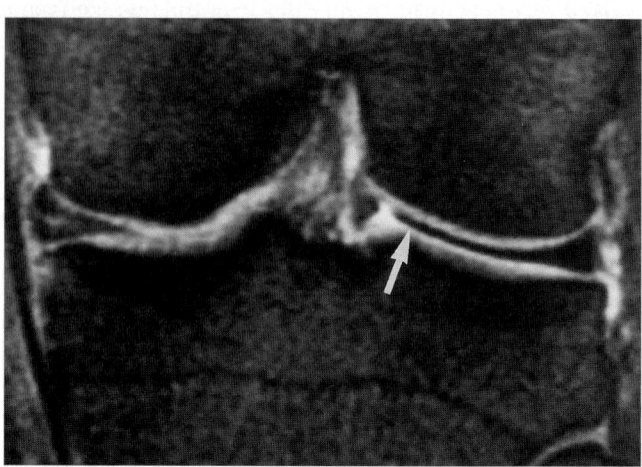

Figure 48.7. Displaced Fragment in Bucket-handle Tear. A sagittal T1WI (TR 600; TE 30) through the intercondylar notch in a patient with a bucket-handle tear reveals the displaced free fragment or handle (*arrow*) just anterior to the PCL.

Figure 48.8. Discoid Lateral Meniscus. A coronal GRASS image (TR 500; TE 30; θ, 30°) through the intercondylar notch shows a large lateral meniscus with meniscal tissue extending into the notch medially (*arrow*).

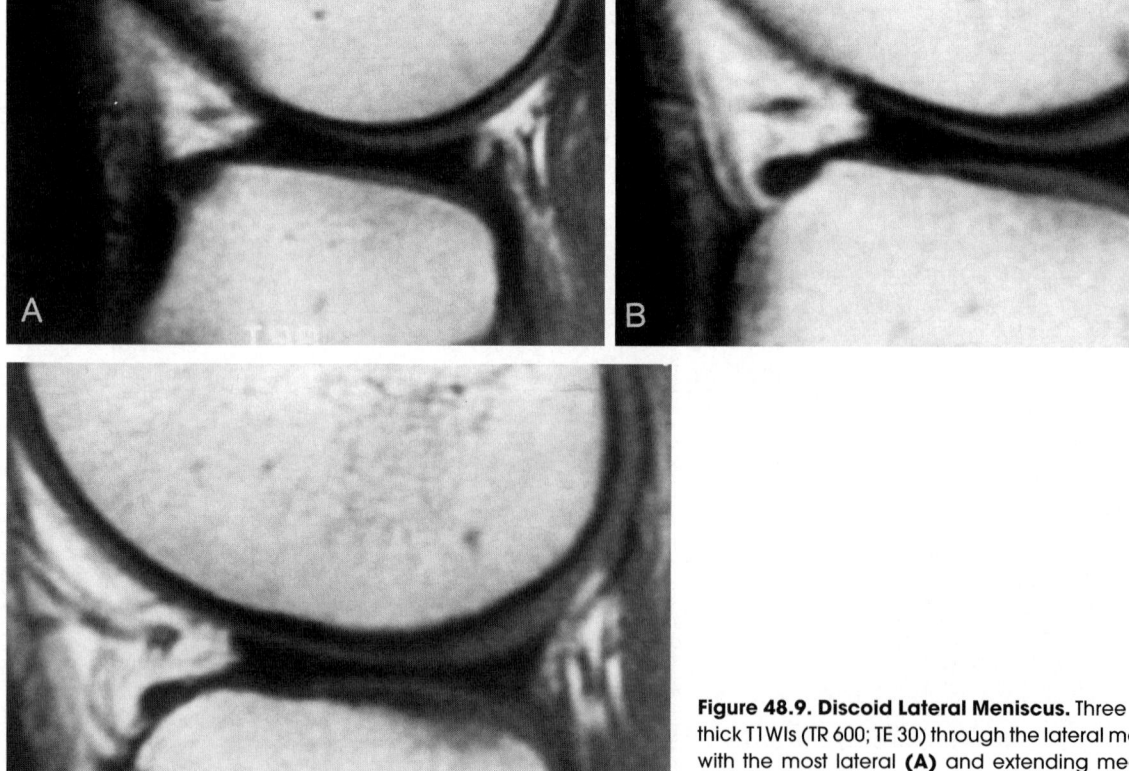

Figure 48.9. Discoid Lateral Meniscus. Three consecutive 5-mm thick T1WIs (TR 600; TE 30) through the lateral meniscus, beginning with the most lateral **(A)** and extending medially **(B,C)**, each show the meniscus to have a bow-tie configuration. As only two images should have a bow-tie shape, indicative of the body of the meniscus, this is diagnostic of a discoid lateral meniscus. (Fig. 48.8 is a coronal GRASS image of the same knee.)

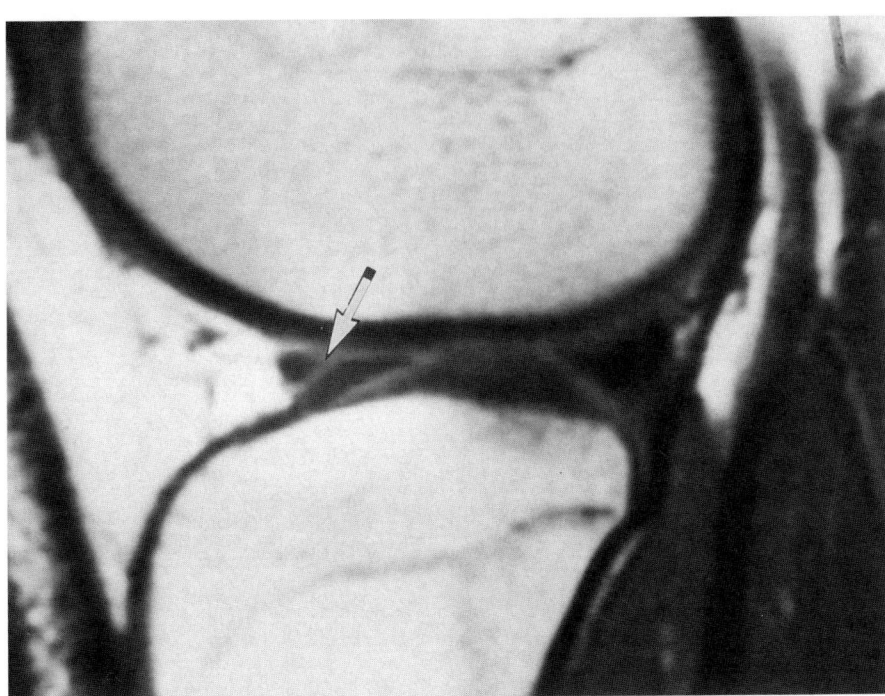

Figure 48.10. Pseudotear from a Transverse Ligament. A sagittal T1WI (TR 600; TE 30) through the lateral meniscus shows linear high signal through the upper anterior horn (*arrow*), which resembles a tear. This is the insertion of the transverse ligament onto the meniscus.

the population, with a discoid medial meniscus being much less common. A discoid meniscus is thought to be more prone to tear than a normal meniscus, and it can be symptomatic even without being torn. Although they are easily identified on coronal images by noting meniscal tissue extending into the tibial spines at the intercondylar notch (Fig. 48.8), they are most reliably diagnosed by noting more than two consecutive sagittal images that show the meniscus with a bow-tie appearance (Fig. 48.9)(4).

Transverse Ligament. The lateral meniscus often has what appears to be a tear on the anterior horn near its upper margin, which is a pseudotear from the insertion of the transverse ligament (Fig. 48.10). This can easily be differentiated from a real tear by following it medially across the knee in Hoffa's fat pad where it inserts into the anterior horn of the medial meniscus. The function of the transverse ligament is unknown.

CRUCIATE LIGAMENTS

Anterior Cruciate Ligament. The normal anterior cruciate ligament (ACL) is seen in the intercondylar notch as a linear, predominantly low signal structure on T1WIs; it often shows some linear striations near its insertion onto the medial tibial spine when viewed on sagittal images (Fig. 48.11). When torn, the ACL is most often simply not visualized although sometimes the actual disruption will be seen (Fig. 48.12). T2WI or T2WI are imperative for obtaining the highest accuracy in diagnosing ACL tears because fluid and hemorrhage will often obscure the ligament on T1WI. Partial tears or sprains of the ACL are manifested by high signal within an otherwise intact ligament.

Posterior Cruciate Ligament. The normal posterior cruciate ligament (PCL) is a gently curved, homoge-

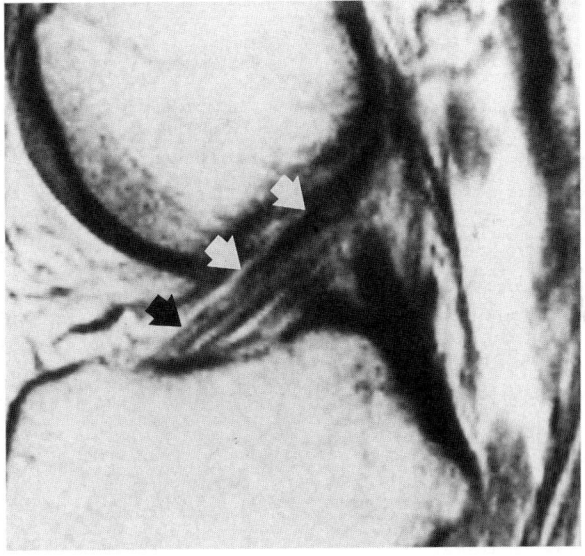

Figure 48.11. Normal ACL. A sagittal T1WI (TR 600; TE 30) through the intercondylar notch shows the normal appearance of the ACL (*arrows*).

neously low signal structure (Fig. 48.13) that is infrequently torn and even less frequently repaired by surgeons. When torn, it takes on diffuse intermediate signal throughout (Fig. 48.14). This increased signal usually does not get brighter with T2WI and is therefore often overlooked. Most orthopaedic surgeons do not even inspect the PCL at arthroscopy and do not repair it when torn because it rarely is a cause of instability.

Meniscofemoral Ligament. A low signal, round structure is often seen just anterior or posterior to the PCL, as seen in the sagittal views. A loose body or a free fragment of a piece of torn meniscus can have this ap-

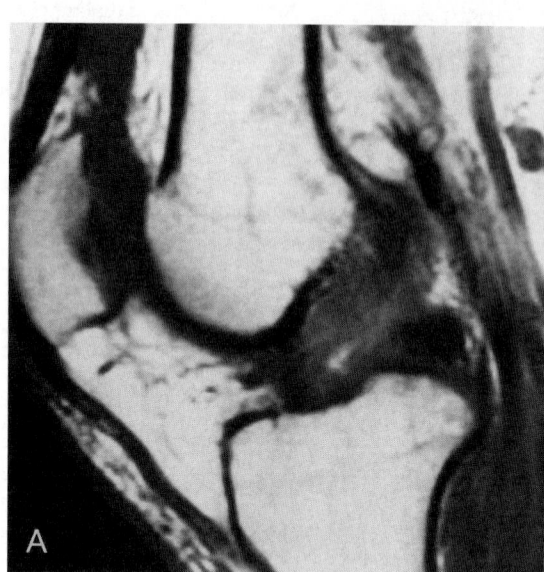

Figure 48.12. Torn ACL. A. A sagittal T1WI (TR 600; TE 30) through the intercondylar notch does not reveal any structure that resembles a normal ACL. This is a common MR appearance of a torn ACL. **B.** A sagittal GRASS image (TR 500; TE 30; θ 30°) in the same knee shows fibers of the torn ACL that are disrupted centrally (*arrow*).

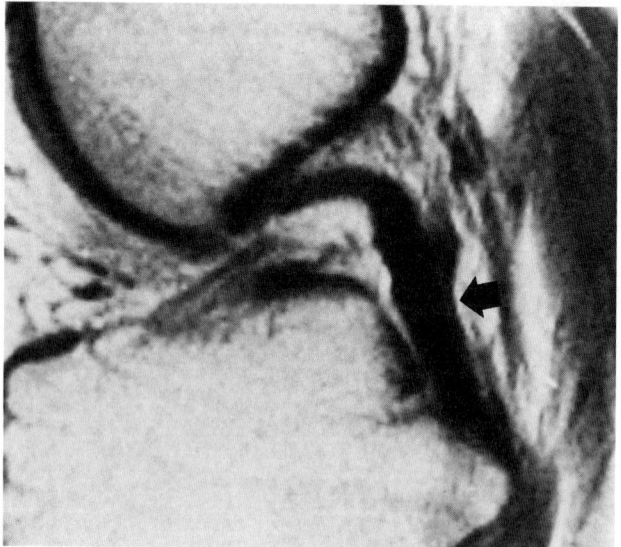

Figure 48.13. Normal PCL. A sagittal T1WI (TR 600; TE 30) through the intercondylar notch shows the appearance of the normal PCL with its characteristic uniform low signal (*arrow*).

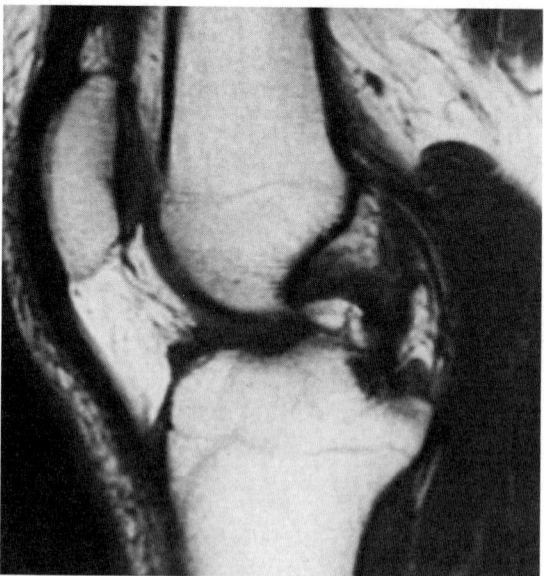

Figure 48.14. Torn PCL. A sagittal T1WI (TR 600; TE 30) through the intercondylar notch reveals the PCL to have diffuse intermediate signal throughout. This is typical for a torn PCL.

pearance (Fig. 48.15), but it is most commonly caused by a meniscofemoral ligament that extends obliquely across the knee from the medial femoral condyle to the posterior horn of the lateral meniscus. If it passes in front of the PCL, it is called the ligament of Humphry, and if it passes behind the PCL, it is called the ligament of Wrisberg (Fig. 48.16). One or the other of these ligaments is present in up to 72% of all knees.

The insertion of the ligament of Humphry or Wrisberg onto the lateral meniscus can produce a pseudotear sim-

ilar to that caused by the transverse ligament on the anterior horn of the lateral meniscus (Fig. 48.17). Prior to calling a tear on the upper aspect of the posterior horn of the lateral meniscus, care must be taken to look for a meniscofemoral ligament to be certain it is not a pseudotear from the ligament's insertion. Similarly, prior to calling a loose body in front of or behind the PCL, care must be taken to try to follow the structure across to the lateral meniscus to determine if it is a meniscofemoral ligament.

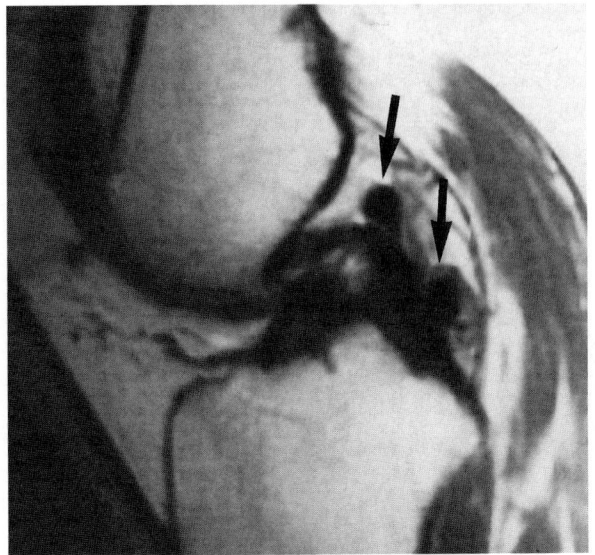

Figure 48.15. Free Fragment of a Torn Meniscus. A sagittal T1WI (TR 600; TE 30) through the intercondylar notch in this patient with a torn meniscus shows two rounded low signal structures (*arrows*) that are free fragments of meniscal tissue. A meniscofemoral ligament of Wrisberg could have the appearance of either of these loose bodies.

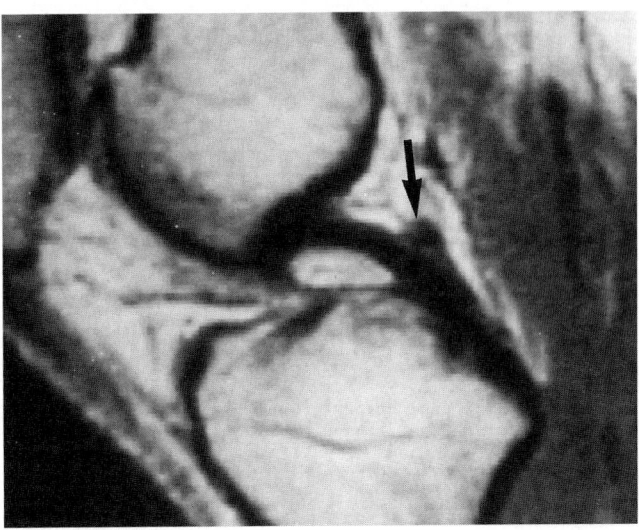

Figure 48.16. Ligament of Wrisberg. A sagittal T1WI (TR 600; TE 30) through the intercondylar notch shows a rounded low signal structure posterior to the PCL, which is the meniscofemoral ligament of Wrisberg (*arrow*).

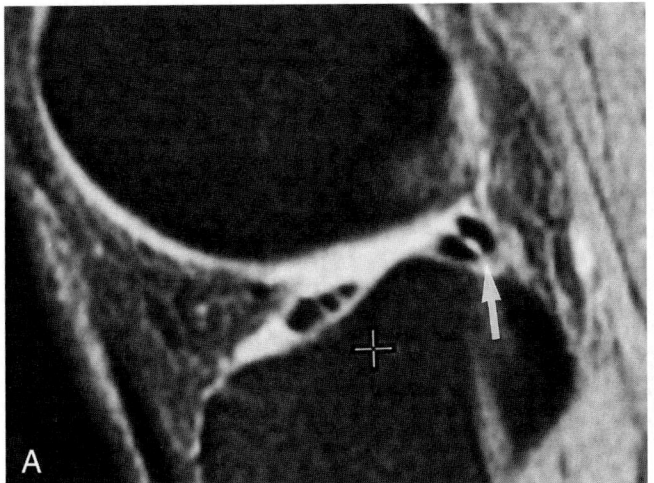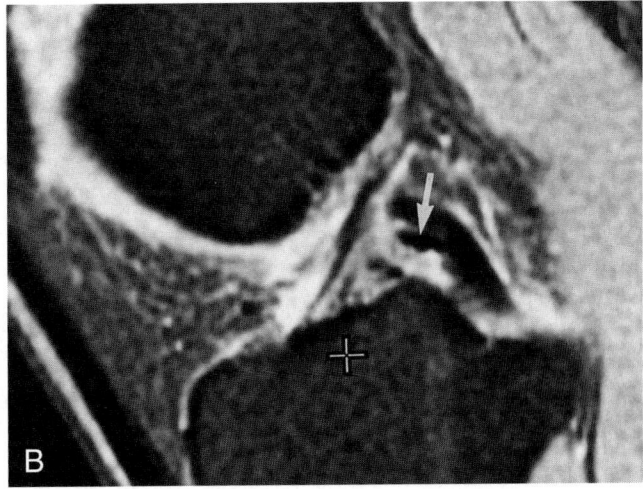

Figure 48.17. Pseudotear from Ligament of Humphry insertion. A. A sagittal proton density fat suppressed image (TR 2000; TE 20) through the lateral meniscus reveals an apparent tear of the posterior horn (*arrow*). (The "speckled" appearance in the anterior horn of the lateral meniscus is a frequently seen normal variant and should not be confused for a torn meniscus.) **B.** On the image thru the intercondylar notch a ligament of Humphry (*arrow*) is seen anterior to the PCL. The ligament of Humphry could be followed on adjacent images from anterior to the PCL to its insertion on the posterior horn of the lateral meniscus.

COLLATERAL LIGAMENTS

Medial Collateral Ligament. The medial collateral ligament (MCL) originates on the medial femoral condyle and inserts on the tibia. It is closely applied to the joint and is intimately associated with the medial joint capsule and the medial meniscus. The MCL is uniformly low in signal on T1 and T2 or T2* sequences. Injuries to the MCL usually occur from a valgus stress to the lateral part of the knee (such as a "clipping" injury in football).

A grade 1 injury represents a mild sprain and is diagnosed on MR by noting fluid or hemorrhage in the soft tissues medial to the MCL. The ligament is otherwise normal. A grade 2 injury is a partial tear and is seen as high signal in and around the MCL on T2 or T2* coronal sequences. The ligament is intact, although the deep or superficial fibers may show minimal disruption (Fig. 48.18). A grade 3 injury is a complete disruption of the MCL. It can be best appreciated on T2 or T2* images (Fig. 48.19).

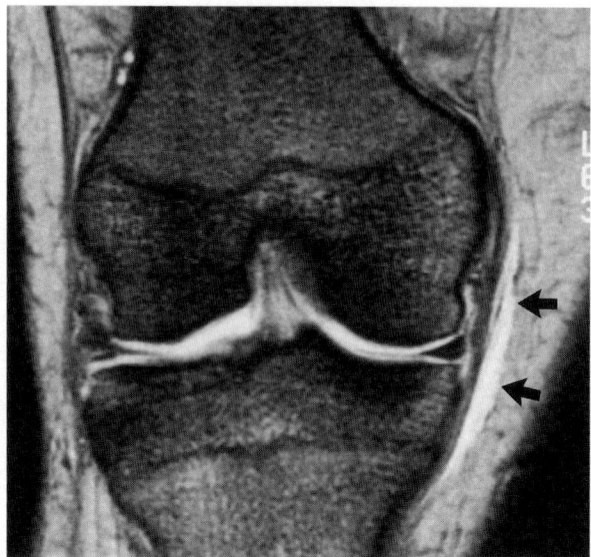

Figure 48.18. Partial Tear of the MCL. A GRASS coronal image (TR 500; TE 15; θ 30°) reveals high signal adjacent to the MCL (*arrows*), which represents edema and hemorrhage from a partial tear or sprain of the MCL. The MCL is clearly intact; hence, a complete tear is easily excluded.

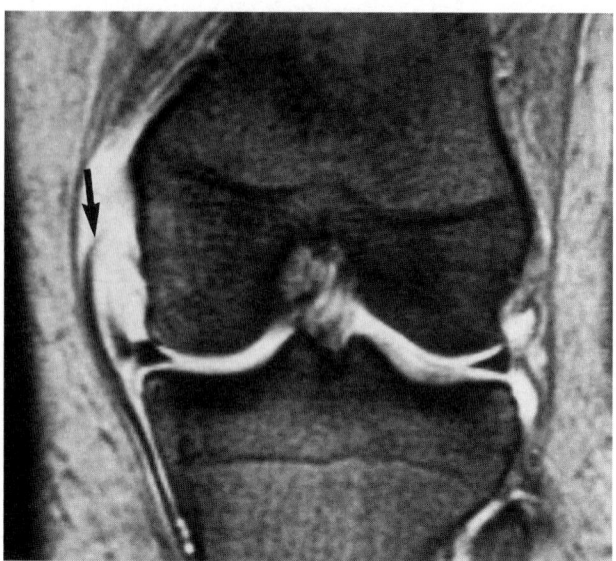

Figure 48.19. Torn MCL. A coronal GRASS image (TR 500; TE 15, θ 30°) shows a large joint effusion with the MCL disrupted proximally (*arrow*). In addition, joint fluid can be seen extending between the medial meniscus and the MCL, which indicates a meniscocapsular separation. Neither of these diagnoses could be made on the T1-weighted coronal images.

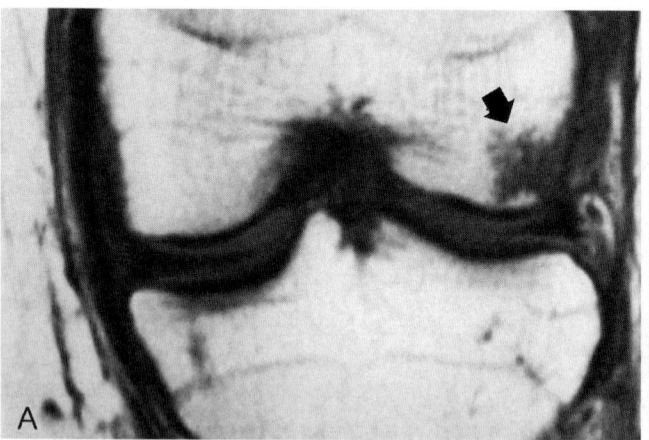

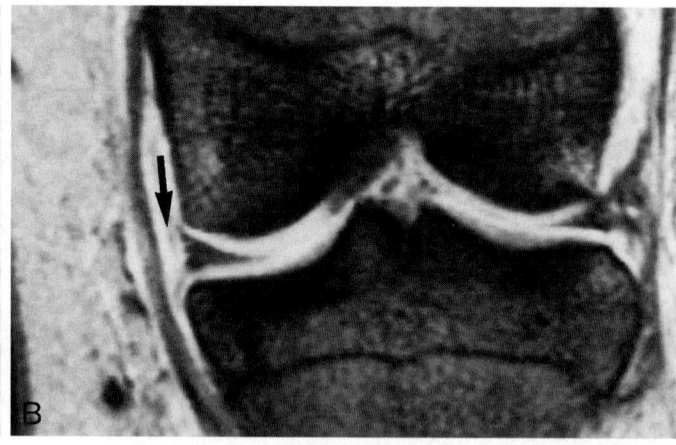

Figure 48.20. Meniscocapsular Separation. A. A T1-weighted coronal image (TR 600; TE 30) reveals a contusion of the lateral femoral condyle (*arrow*), indicative of a valgus strain, which is often associated with a MCL tear. The MCL appears normal on this image; however, the linear low signal in the soft tissues just adjacent to the MCL is suggestive of fluid. This would indicate a partial tear or sprain of the MCL. **B.** A coronal GRASS image (TR 500; TE 15; θ 30°) in the same knee reveals fluid between the medial meniscus and the MCL (*arrow*), which is diagnostic for a meniscocapsular separation. Faint high signal in the MCL and adjacent to it indicates a partial tear. A T2 or T2* sequence in the coronal plane is necessary to see these abnormalities.

A meniscocapsular separation occurs when the medial meniscus is torn from its attachment to the joint capsule. It occurs most commonly at the site of the MCL and often occurs concomitantly with an MCL injury. It is easily recognized on a T2 or T2* coronal image by noting joint fluid extending between the medial meniscus and the capsule (Fig. 48.20). It is essential to use T2 or T2* sequences as a T1WI will not detect the fluid between the meniscus and the capsule.

Lateral Collateral Ligament. The lateral collateral ligament consists of three parts. The most posterior structure is the tendon of the biceps femoris, which inserts onto the head of the fibula. Next, anterior to the biceps is the true lateral collateral ligament, also called the fibulocollateral ligament, which extends from the lateral femoral condyle to the head of the fibula. The biceps and the fibulocollateral ligament usually join and insert onto the head of the fibula in a conjoined fashion. Anterior to the fibulocollateral ligament is the iliotibial band, which extends into the fascia more anteriorly and blends into the lateral retinaculum on the patella. The lateral collateral ligament is infrequently torn.

PATELLA

Chondromalacia Patella. The patellar cartilage commonly undergoes degeneration, causing exquisite pain

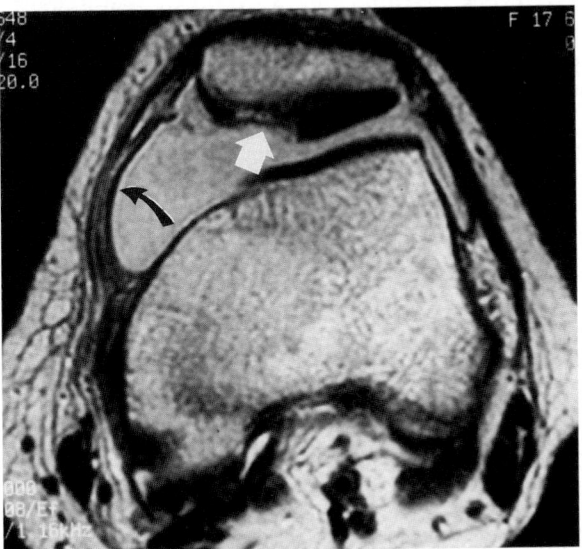

Figure 48.21. Chondral Defect in Patella. An axial FSE T2WI (TR 3000; TE 108) through the patella shows a large cartilage defect on the apex and medial facet of the patella (*arrow*) in this patient who suffered a dislocated patella. Note the high signal throughout the medial retinaculum (*curved arrow*), a frequent finding after a patella dislocation.

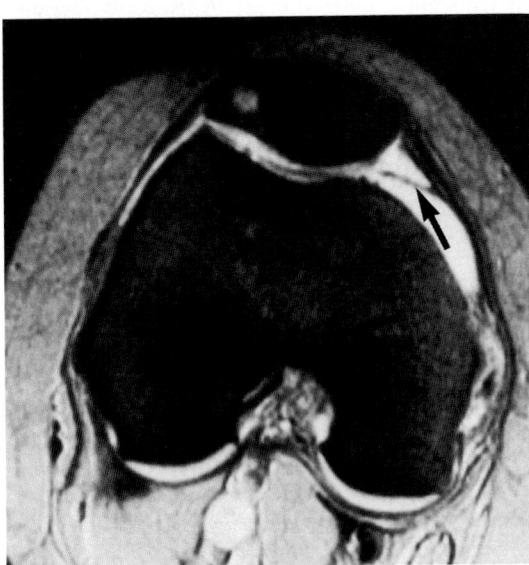

Figure 48.22. Plica. An axial GRASS image (TR 500; TE 15; θ 30°) through the patella shows a low signal linear structure (*arrow*) extending from the medial capsule toward the medial facet of the patella. This is a medial patellar plica that is not abnormally thickened. Without the joint effusion or the T2WI, the plica would not be visualized.

and tenderness. This is called chondromalacia patella. It can be diagnosed on sagittal images but is more easily identified on axial images. Because hyaline articular cartilage has the same signal intensity as joint fluid on T1-weighted sequences, T2 or T2* sequences are necessary to diagnose chondromalacia patella in most instances.

Chondromalacia patella begins with focal swelling and degeneration of the cartilage. This can be seen as low or high signal foci in the cartilage. Its progression causes thinning and irregularity of the articular surface of the cartilage, and finally underlying bone is exposed. This final stage occurs more commonly from trauma than from wear and tear. A frequent cause of a patellar cartilage defect is dislocation of the patella in which the patella strikes the lateral femoral condyle and displaces a piece of patella articular cartilage (Fig. 48.21).

Patellar Plica. A normal structure seen in over half of the population is the medial patellar plica. It is an embryologic remnant from when the knee was divided into three compartments. It is a thin, fibrous band that extends from the medial capsule toward the medial facet of the patella (Fig. 48.22). A suprapatellar and infrapatellar plica also exist. The medial patellar plica can, on rare occasions, thicken and cause clinical symptoms indistinguishable from a torn meniscus; this has been termed "plica syndrome." An abnormal plica can be easily removed arthroscopically.

BONY ABNORMALITIES

Contusions. The most frequently encountered bony abnormality seen with MR is a contusion. A contusion represents microfractures from trauma (5). They are also called bone bruises. They are easily identified on T1-weighted sequences as subarticular areas of inhomogeneous low signal (Fig. 48.23). With T2 weighting, a con-

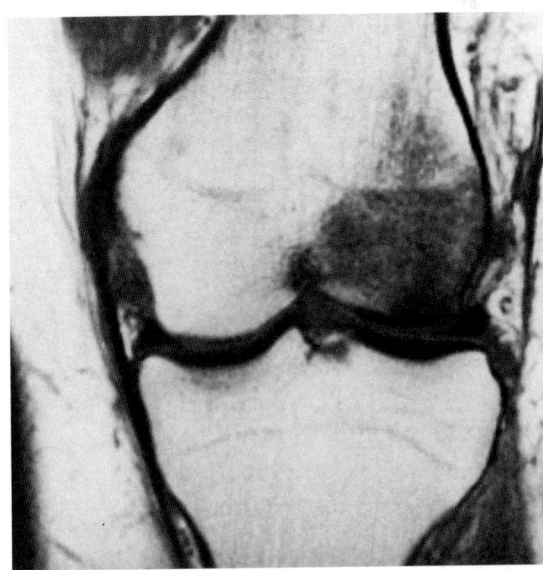

Figure 48.23. Contusion. A coronal T1WI (TR 600; TE 30) shows a focus of low signal in the lateral femoral condyle, which is subarticular. This is a characteristic appearance for a severe bone contusion.

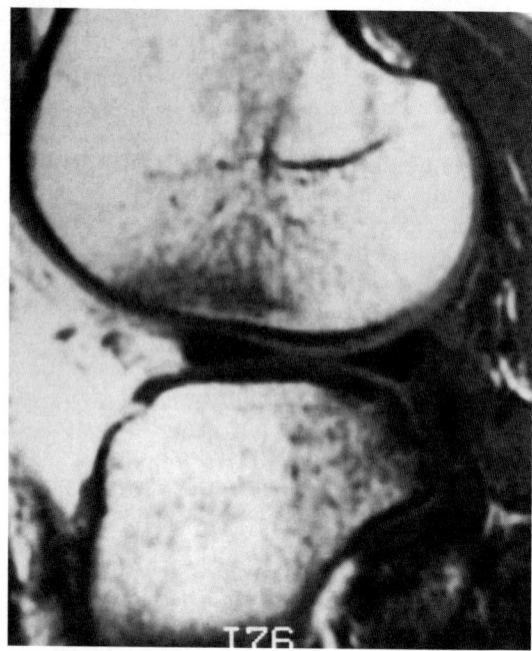

Figure 48.24. Contusion. A sagittal T1WI through the lateral compartment shows irregular low signal in a subarticular location of the posterior tibial plateau and in the anterior part of the lateral femoral condyle. These findings are characteristic for bone contusions. This distribution of contusions in the posterior lateral tibial plateau and anterior in the lateral femoral condyle is almost always associated with a torn ACL.

tusion will show increased signal for several weeks, depending on its severity. Seeing increased signal with T2* images can be difficult because of the susceptibility artifacts of the bone seen with T2* images. Contusions can progress to osteochondritis dissecans if they are not

treated with diminished weight bearing; hence, an isolated bone contusion, with no other internal derangement, is a serious finding that requires protection.

A commonly seen contusion is one that occurs on the posterior part of the lateral tibial plateau (Fig. 48.24). It is invariably associated with a torn ACL. Acute ACL tears have been reported to have this type of contusion in over 90% of cases (6).

Fractures. MR imaging is useful in examining fractures about the knee. Tibial plateau fractures can be imaged precisely with computed tomography; however, MR allows the soft tissues to be seen in addition to any bony abnormalities. A fracture that occurs which is almost always associated with an internal derangement is the Segond fracture. A small, bony fragment pulled off the posterior lateral tibial joint line by an avulsion of the lateral joint capsule, it is almost always associated with an ACL tear.

References

1. Crues JI, Mink J, Levy T, et al. Meniscal tears of the knee: accuracy of MR imaging. Radiology 1987;164:445–448.
2. Mink JH, Deutsch AL. Magnetic resonance imaging of the knee. Clin Orthop 1989;244:29–47.
3. De Smet A, Graf B. Meniscal tears missed on MR imaging: relationship to meniscal tear patterns and anterior cruciate ligament tears. AJR 1994;162:905–911.
4. Silverman J, Mink J, Deutsch A. Discoid menisci of the knee: MR imaging appearance. Radiology 1989;173:351–354.
5. Mink JH, Deutsch AL. Occult cartilage and bone injuries of the knee: detection, classification, and assessment with MR imaging. Radiology 1989;170:823–829.
6. Murphy B, Smith R, Uribe J, et al. Bone signal abnormalities in the posterolateral tibia and lateral femoral condyle in complete tears of the anterior cruciate ligament: a specific sign? Radiology 1992;182:221–224.

49
Magnetic Resonance Imaging of the Shoulder

Clyde A. Helms

ANATOMY
ROTATOR CUFF
BONY ABNORMALITIES
GLENOID LABRUM
BICEPS TENDON
SUPRASCAPULAR NERVE ENTRAPMENT

MR of the shoulder is well accepted for its diagnostic utility for abnormalities of the rotator cuff and the glenoid labrum. It has been shown by some investigators to have a high degree of accuracy (1–4), while others report a barely acceptable rate of accuracy. MR of the shoulder has nevertheless replaced standard arthrography and computed tomographic arthrography for examining the rotator cuff and the glenoid labrum in the vast majority of diagnostic imaging centers.

ANATOMY

The rotator cuff is comprised of the tendons of four muscles that converge on the greater and lesser tuberosities of the humerus: the supraspinatus, infraspinatus, subscapularis, and teres minor (Fig. 49.1). Of these, the supraspinatus most commonly causes clinically significant problems, and is the one that is most commonly surgically treated. The supraspinatus tendon lies just superior to the scapula and inferior to the acromioclavicular (AC) joint and acromion. It inserts onto the greater tuberosity of the humerus. Two to three centimeters proximal to its insertion is a section of the tendon called the "critical zone." This area is reported to have decreased vascularity and is therefore less likely to heal following trauma. The critical zone of the supraspinatus tendon is where most rotator cuff tears occur.

The glenoid labrum is a fibrocartilaginous ring that surrounds the periphery of the bony glenoid of the scapula. It serves as an attachment site for the capsule and broadens the base of the glenohumeral joint to allow increased stability. Tears or detachments of the glenoid labrum most commonly occur from, and result in, dislocations or instability of the humerus.

ROTATOR CUFF

The rotator cuff commonly suffers from what has been termed "impingement syndrome." Impingement of the critical zone of the supraspinatus tendon occurs from abduction of the humerus, which allows the tendon to be impinged between the anterior acromion and the greater tuberosity. The tendon can also be impinged by the undersurface of the AC joint if downward-pointing osteophytes or a thickened capsule is present. Other theories exist for impingement syndrome, including natural degeneration from aging and a predisposition for the critical zone to undergo degeneration due to decreased blood supply. Most investigators agree that whatever the cause, the natural course of impingement syndrome is a complete, or full-thickness, tear of the rotator cuff.

The rotator cuff is best seen on oblique coronal images that are aligned parallel to the supraspinatus muscle (Fig. 49.2). Both T1- (or proton density) and T2-weighted sequences are typically performed, although little diagnostic information is present on the T1WIs and they are not obtained by many radiologists. Multiple acceptable variations of imaging sequences are available to demonstrate the normal and abnormal structures that can be seen in the oblique coronal plane. The most commonly employed protocol is a spin-echo proton-density and T2-weighted sequence. Some prefer to use a spin-echo T1WI in conjunction with a GRASS or other type of T2* sequence. A fat suppressed fast spin echo (FSE) T2-weighted oblique coronal is gaining popularity as the primary sequence for imaging the rotator cuff in many imaging centers. The slice thickness should be no greater than 5 mm, and 3 mm is preferable. As with most joint imaging, a small field of view (16–20 cm) is recommended. A dedicated shoulder coil or a surface coil placed anteriorly over the shoulder is necessary, although no particular type of shoulder coil appears to be clearly superior.

In examining the rotator cuff, the most anterior oblique coronal images will show the critical zone of the supraspinatus tendon. A useful landmark for noting the supraspinatus tendon is the AC joint, which is an anterior structure and usually easily located. The infraspinatus tendon is seen on the more posterior images and can easily be mistaken for the tendon of the supraspinatus. The supraspinatus tendon can be differentiated from that of the infraspinatus by noting the more horizontal course of the supraspinatus as compared with the infraspinatus, which runs obliquely inferiorly to superiorly.

The normal supraspinatus tendon is said to be uniformly low in signal on all pulse sequences (Fig. 49.3). Unfortunately, this is not always the case. In fact, it usually has some intermediate-to-high signal in the critical zone, which causes much confusion. If the signal in the critical zone gets brighter on the T2WIs, it is abnormal and represents either tendinitis (many investigators prefer the term "tendinosis" or "tendonopathy" over tendinitis, as no inflammatory cells are found histologically) or

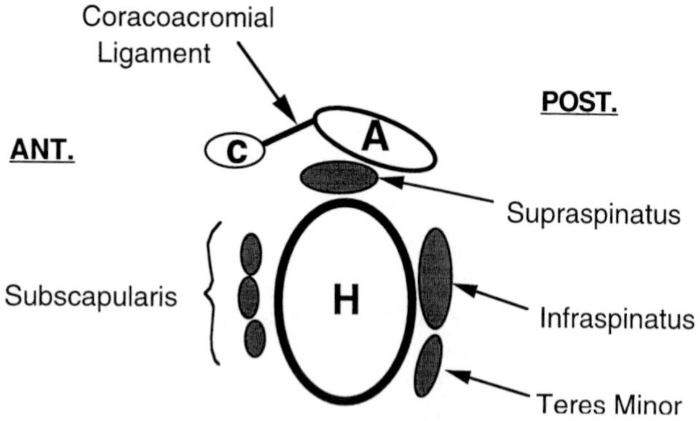

Coracoacromial
Ligament

POST.

ANT.

C   A

H

Supraspinatus

Subscapularis

Infraspinatus

Teres Minor

Figure 49.1. Schematic of Shoulder Anatomy. This drawing shows the rotator cuff muscles in a sagittal plane (anterior is on the left). *C,* coracoid; *A,* acromion; *H,* humeral head.

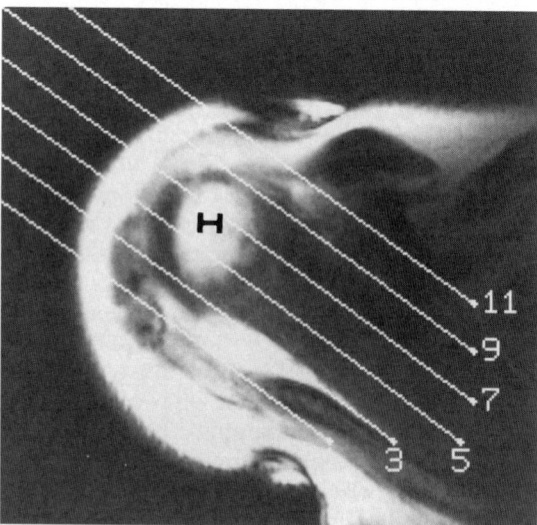

Figure 49.2. Scout View for Oblique Coronal Images. This axial image through the supraspinatus shows the cursors angled along the plane of the supraspinatus muscle (anterior on top) *H,* humeral head.

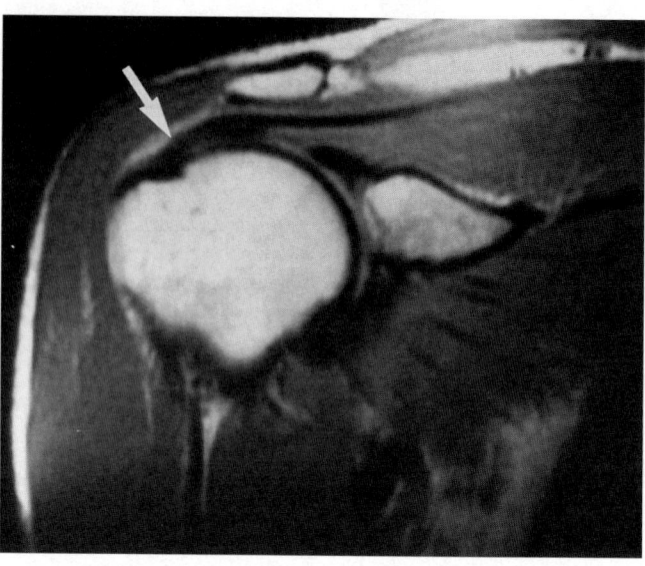

Figure 49.3. Normal Supraspinatus Tendon. A T1-weighted (TR 600; TE 30) oblique coronal image shows a normal supraspinatus tendon (*arrow*) with uninterrupted low signal extending from the musculo-tendinous junction to the insertion on the greater tuberosity.

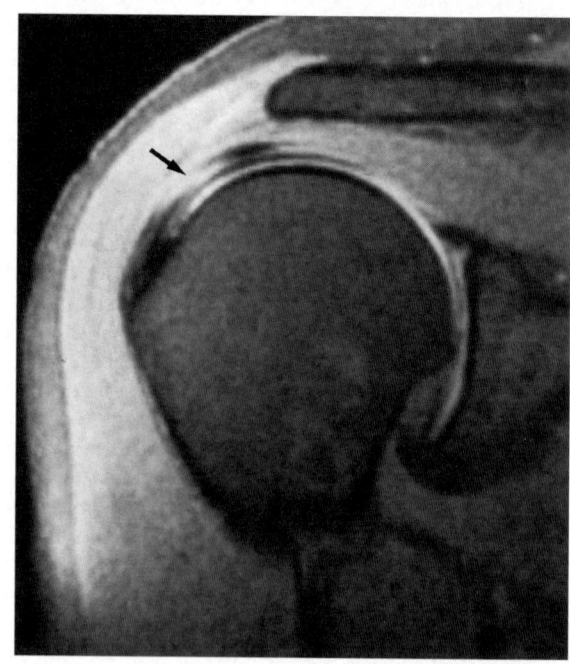

Figure 49.4. Partial Tear of the Supraspinatus Tendon. A T1-weighted (TR 700; TE 20) oblique coronal image with fat saturation shows high signal in the critical zone of the supraspinatus tendon (*arrow*) with the tendon appearing very irregular. A small amount of fluid is seen in the subacromial bursa. Arthroscopy confirmed a partial tear on the bursal side of the supraspinatus tendon.

a partial tear (severe tendinitis) (Fig. 49.4). However, if it disappears or has the same signal intensity as the adjacent muscle on T2-weighted sequences, it may represent one of many different processes:

1. Partial volume averaging of peritendinous fat can cause some high signal in the supraspinatous tendon on the oblique coronal images; this does not get brighter on T2WIs.

2. If the plane of the oblique coronal images is slightly off of the plane of the tendon, muscle slips can be partially volume averaged, which may appear as relatively high signal on T1WIs but will not get brighter with T2WIs.

3. The so-called "magic angle" effect can cause apparent high signal in a tendon that lies at 55° to the bore of the magnet (as does the critical zone of the supraspinatus tendon)(5). This high signal will not be seen on T2WIs (or any sequence with a long TE). This is believed to be a common cause of high signal in the critical zone on T1WIs.

4. Myxoid and fibrillar degeneration of the supraspinatus tendon are commonly found in autopsy specimens in older patients. The majority of asymptomatic shoulders in patients over the age of 50 are believed to have some tendon degeneration in the supraspinatus; this has been termed "tendonopathy." This is seen as high signal in the critical zone on T1WIs that

does not increase with T2 weighting (6). It has not been determined if this can be symptomatic.

Because high signal can be seen in the critical zone of the supraspinatus in a variety of normal situations, how can one differentiate the normal from the abnormal? As long as the T2WIs do not show the signal getting brighter, it probably does not matter. Tendon degeneration (tendonopathy) can be seen in asymptomatic shoulders of all ages; hence, it needs to be correlated with the clinical picture. If the signal gets brighter on T2WIs it must be considered pathologic–either tendinitis or a partial tear. If, in addition, fluid is present in the subacromial bursa, a small full-thickness tear should be mentioned as a possibility even if a definite tendon disruption cannot be seen. A small amount of fluid can be seen in the subacromial bursa because of a partial tear, but if a substantial amount of fluid is found, suspicion for a full-thickness tear should be high. It should be noted that fluid in the subacromial bursa can also occur from isolated subacromial bursitis or for several days following a therapeutic injection into the bursa.

If disruption of the supraspinatus tendon is seen, obviously a full-thickness tear is present. In these cases fluid is invariably present in the subacromial bursa (Fig. 49.5). Care should be made to look for retraction of the supraspinatus muscle, as marked retraction will obviate some types of surgery.

Thus, three categories exist for the appearance of the supraspinatus tendon. a) High signal on T1WIs that does not get brighter on T2WIs. This can represent one of several processes in a normal tendon or myxoid degeneration, also called tendonopathy. This should basically be considered "normal" as it has not been proved that tendonopathy is symptomatic. b) High signal on T1WIs that gets brighter on T2-weighted sequences. Little or no fluid is present in the subacromial bursa. This represents tendinitis or a partial tear. c) If tendon disruption and/or a large amount of fluid is present in the subacromial bursa with high signal in the critical zone on T1WIs and T2WIs, a full-thickness tear should be diagnosed.

BONY ABNORMALITIES

The undersurface of the anterior acromion and the AC joint should be examined for osteophytes or irregularities that can be responsible for impingement syndrome (Fig. 49.6). In the proper clinical setting an anterior acromioplasty will relieve the symptoms of impingement syndrome and prevent a more serious full-thickness rotator cuff tear. It is imperative that the surgeon also remove any AC joint undersurface irregularity, if present, or failed surgery can occur.

Abnormalities of the humeral head include sclerosis and cystic changes about the greater tuberosity, which are commonly present in patients with impingement syndrome and rotator cuff tears. Bony impaction on the posterosuperior aspect of the humeral head can be seen in patients with anterior instability of the humeral head. This is called a Hill-Sachs lesion and is best identified on the superior-most two or three axial images (Fig. 49.7). The normal humeral head should be round on the superior slices; any irregularity seen posteriorly is abnormal.

GLENOID LABRUM

Tears of the glenoid labrum cause glenohumeral joint instability. They are commonly caused by dislocations, but less traumatic episodes, such as repeated trauma from throwing, can result in labral tears. Torn or detached labra are often repaired arthroscopically with good results.

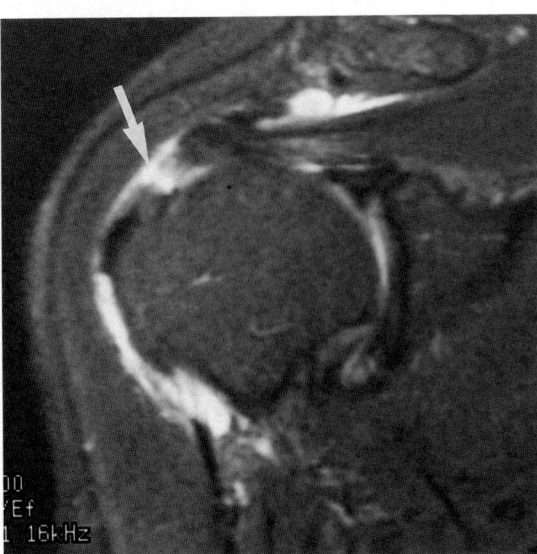

Figure 49.5. Torn Supraspinatus Tendon. An oblique coronal FSE T2 image (TR 3000; TE 60) with fat suppression shows disruption of the supraspinatus tendon (*arrow*) and fluid in the torn tendon.

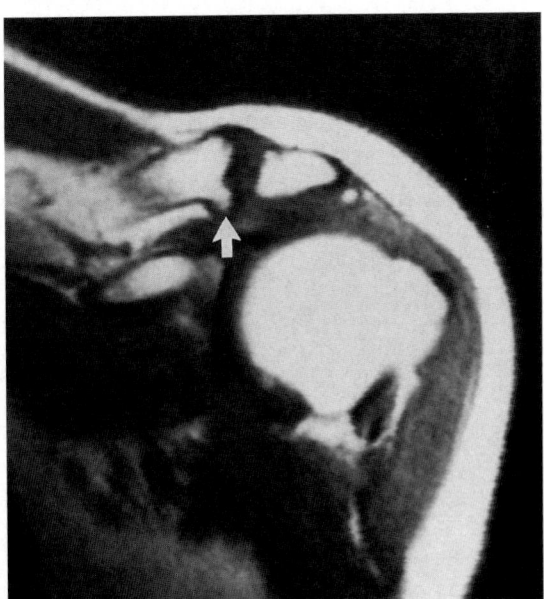

Figure 49.6. Acromioclavicular Joint Osteophytes. An oblique coronal T1WI (TR 600; TE 30) reveals osteophytes extending inferiorly off the AC joint (*arrow*). This is a common source of impingement on the supraspinatus tendon.

The glenoid labrum is best imaged on axial T2-weighted or T2*-WIs. T1-weighted axial images are not necessary to diagnose labral abnormalities and can be omitted from the shoulder protocol. Fluid in the joint makes for easier assessment of the labrum, hence MR arthrography has evolved into a routine exam in many centers. It is performed by injecting a 1:200 dilution of Gd-DTPA with saline into the joint using fluoroscopic guidance.

The normal labrum is a triangular-shaped low-signal structure as viewed on an axial image, with the anterior labrum usually larger than the posterior labrum (Fig. 49.8). The anterior labrum is much more commonly involved with tears than the posterior, and the superior labrum is even less commonly involved. The superior labrum is evaluated on the oblique coronal views.

If no joint effusion is present, a labral tear can be difficult to see unless it is quite severe. If joint fluid extends between the bony glenoid and the base of the labrum, a detached labrum is present. Tears in the body of the labrum are diagnosed by noting fluid extending into the labrum or by truncation of the labrum (Fig. 49.9). Superior labral tears are called SLAP lesions (**S**uperior **L**abrum **A**nterior to **P**osterior)(Fig. 49.10). They are seen most frequently in throwing athletes secondary to the pull of the long head of the biceps which inserts on the superior labrum. They are also seen in older patients in association with cuff tears.

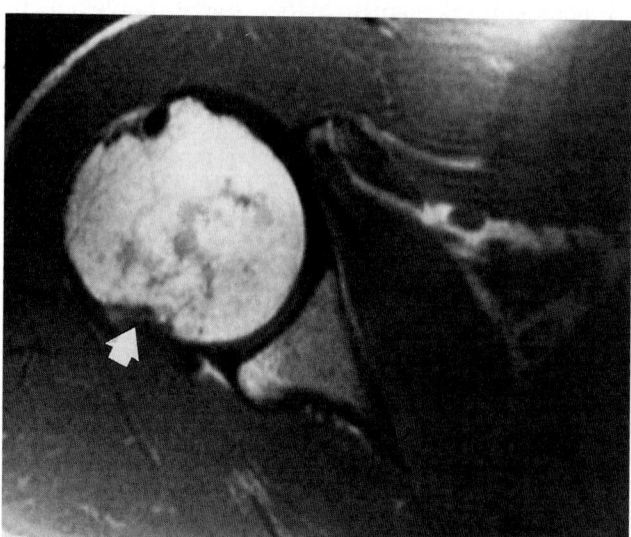

Figure 49.7. Hill-Sachs Lesion. An axial T1WI (TR 600; TE 30) through the superior portion of the humeral head shows a posterior impaction (*arrow*) caused by the glenoid labrum during an anterior dislocation of the humerus. This has been termed a Hill-Sachs lesion.

Figure 49.8. Normal Labrum. An axial T2* GRASS image (TR 600; TE 30; θ 20°) shows a normal anterior (*black arrow*) and posterior (*white arrow*) glenoid labrum. The anterior labrum is usually larger than the posterior labrum.

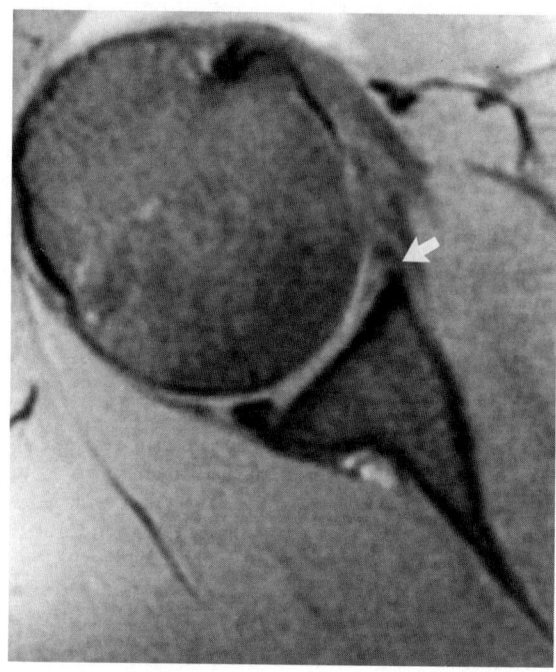

Figure 49.9. Torn Labrum. An axial T2* GRASS image (TR 500; TE 9; θ 20°) shows disruption of the anterior labrum (*arrow*). Note the normal posterior labrum for comparison.

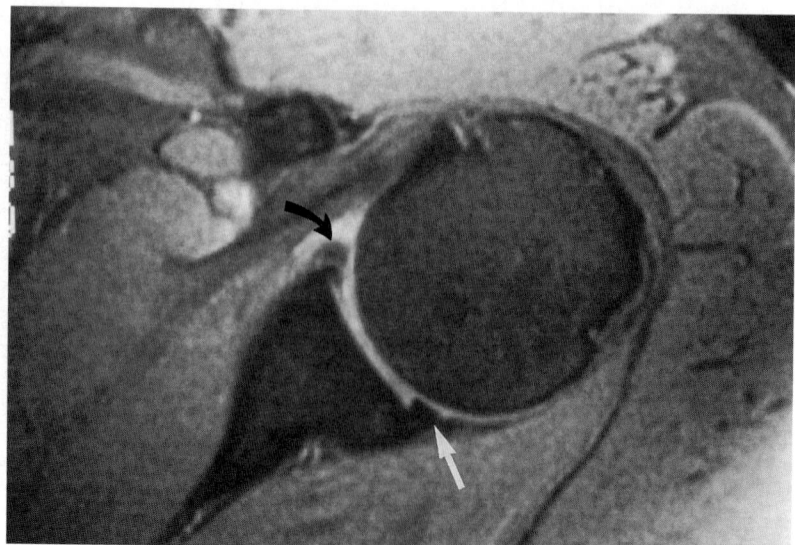

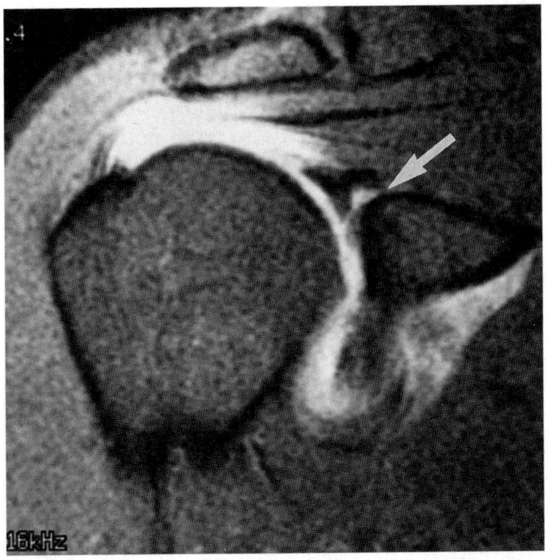

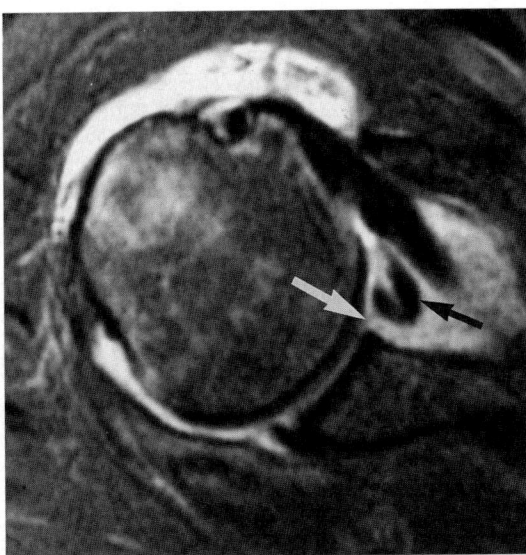

Figure 49.10. SLAP Lesion. An oblique coronal T1-weighted (TR 500; TE 19) image with fat suppression following a Gd-DTPA arthrogram shows a detached superior labrum (*arrow*). The rotator cuff is also shown to be torn.

Figure 49.11. Insertion of Glenohumeral Ligament and a Sublabral Foramen. This axial FSE T2WI (TR 3500; TE 54) with fat suppression reveals linear intermediate signal extending obliquely across the anterior labrum, which simulates a tear. This is the insertion of the middle glenohumeral ligament (*black arrow*) onto the labrum. The labrum also appears to be detached from the bony glenoid (*white arrow*), however, this is a sublabral foramen which is a normal variant seen only in the anterosuperior labrum.

The attachment of the glenohumeral ligaments to the labrum can cause a linear high signal that can mimic a tear (Fig. 49.11), so care must be taken to be certain high signal fluid is actually present in the tear (7).

Two normal variants in the anterior labrum which can mimic a torn or detached labrum have been described, They both occur solely in the anterosuperior portion of the labrum, an area where tears are uncommon. The first is a sublabral foramen which is an opening beneath the anterosuperior labrum and the bony glenoid which mimics a detachment (Fig. 49.11). This is seen in up to 20% of the population. A second variant is called a Buford complex. It consists of an absent anterosuperior labrum in association with a thickened "cord-like" middle glenohumeral ligament. This is seen in about 3% of the population.

BICEPS TENDON

The long head of the biceps tendon runs in the bicipital groove between the greater and lesser tuberosities and inserts onto the superior labrum. It can be impinged by an abnormal acromion in the same way the supraspinatus tendon is impinged, resulting in tenosynovitis or tendinitis. In tenosynovitis, fluid can be seen in the tendon sheath surrounding an otherwise normal tendon. Because fluid in the glenohumeral joint can normally fill the biceps tendon sheath, this diagnosis is difficult to make with MR alone. If the tendon is enlarged and/or has signal within it, tendinitis is present (Fig. 49.12). If the tendon is not seen on one or more of the axial images, it is disrupted or dislocated. Dislocation is uncommon, but when it occurs the tendon can be seen to lie anteromedial to the joint.

SUPRASCAPULAR NERVE ENTRAPMENT

The suprascapular nerve is made up of branches from the C-4, C-5, and C-6 roots of the brachial plexus. It

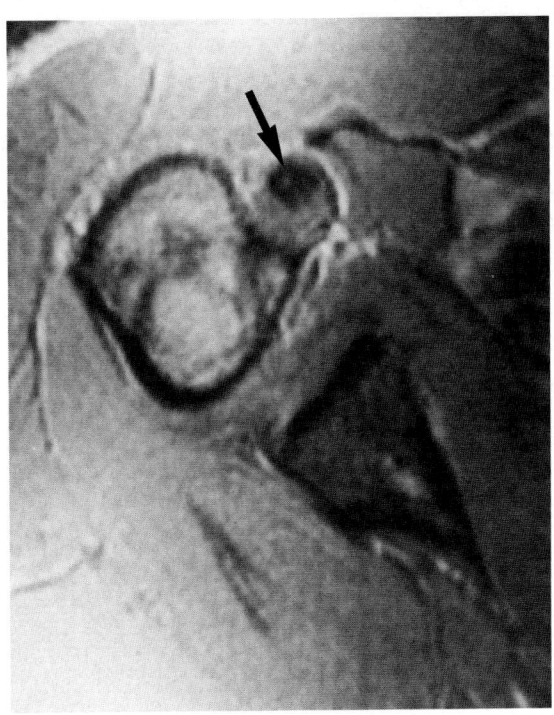

Figure 49.12. Biceps Tendinitis. An axial T2* GRASS image (TR 600; TE 30; θ 30°) shows the biceps tendon (*arrow*) to be swollen and filled with high signal, indicating tendinitis.

runs superior to the scapula, from anterior to posterior, just medial to the coracoid process. It gives off a branch that innervates the supraspinatus muscle as it courses

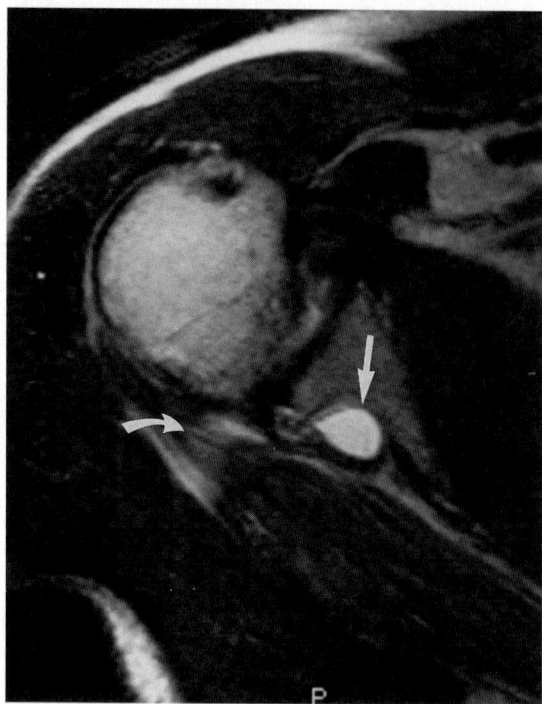

Figure 49.13. Ganglion in Spinoglenoid Notch. An axial T2 image (TR 1850; TE 80) reveals a large high-signal mass posterior to the scapula in the spinoglenoid notch (*arrow*). This is a ganglion that has impressed the suprascapular nerve, causing shoulder pain and atrophy of the infraspinatus muscle. Note the high signal in the infraspinatus muscle (*curved arrow*), which indicates fatty infiltration from atrophy.

posteriorly in the suprascapular notch, and then innervates the infraspinatus muscle after it runs through the spinoglenoid notch in the posterior scapula. It can easily be entrapped by a tumor or a ganglion as it runs above the scapula because it is bounded superiorly by a transverse ligament both anteriorly and posteriorly. A fairly common finding is a ganglion in the spinoglenoid notch that impresses the infraspinatus portion of the nerve with resultant pain and atrophy of the infraspinatus muscle (Fig. 49.13). This is most commonly seen in males who are athletic, particularly weight lifters. The ganglion can be percutaneously drained with CT guidance or surgically removed. They can also spontaneously rupture, which results in cessation of symptoms (8). There is a near 100% association of a torn posterior labrum with these cysts.

References

1. Palmer W, Brown J, Rosenthal D. Rotator cuff: evaluation with fat-suppressed MR arthrography. Radiology 1993;188: 683–688.
2. Singson RD, Hoang T, Dan S, Friedman M. Mr evaluation of rotator cuff pathology using T2-weighted fast spin-echo technique with and without fat suppression. AJR Am J Roentgenol 1996;166(5):1061–1065.
3. Rafii M, Firooznia H, Sherman O, et al. Rotator cuff lesions: signal patterns at MR imaging. Radiology 1990;177(3): 817–823.
4. Zlatkin MB, Iannotti JP, Roberts MC, et al. Rotator cuff tears: diagnostic performance of MR imaging. Radiology 1989;172: 223–229.
5. Erickson S, Cox I, Hyde J, et al. Effect of tendon orientation on MR imaging signal intensity: a manifestation of the "magic angle" phenomenon. Radiology 1991;181:389–392.
6. Kjellin I, Ho CP, Cervilla V, et al. Alterations in the supraspinatus tendon at MR imaging: correlation with histopathologic findings in cadavers. Radiology 1991;181: 837–841.
7. Kaplan P, Bryans K, Davick J, Otte M, Stinson W, Dussault R. MR imaging of the normal shoulder: variants and pitfalls. Radiology 1992;184:519–524.
8. Fritz R, Helms C, Steinbach L, Genant H. Suprascapular nerve entrapment: evaluation with MR imaging. Radiology 1992;182:437–444.

50
Magnetic Resonance Imaging of the Foot and Ankle

Clyde A. Helms

Magnetic resonance imaging (MR) is playing an increasingly important role in the examination of the foot and ankle (1). Orthopaedic surgeons and podiatrists are learning that critical diagnostic information can be obtained in no other way and are relying on MR for many therapeutic decisions.

TENDONS

One of the more common reasons to perform MR of the foot and ankle is to examine the tendons. Although multiple tendons course through the ankle, only a few are routinely affected pathologically. These are primarily the flexor tendons, located posteriorly in the ankle. The extensor tendons, located anteriorly, are rarely abnormal. Only those tendons that are more commonly seen to be abnormal will be discussed in detail.

Tendons can be directly traumatized or be injured from overuse. Either etiology can result in a) *tenosynovitis*, which is seen on MR as fluid in the tendon sheath with the underlying tendon appearing normal; b) *tendinitis* or a partial tear, which is seen as focal or fusiform swelling of the tendon with signal within the tendon that gets bright on T2-weighted images or T2*-weighted images; thinning or attenuation of the tendon is a more severe form of tendinitis that can be recognized on MR; and c) *tendon rupture*, which is best identified on axial images by noting the absence of a tendon on one or more images. Complete tendon disruption can be difficult to see on sagittal or coronal images because of the tendency for tendons to run oblique to the plane of imaging. An exception to this is the Achilles tendon, which is usually best seen on a sagittal image (2).

It is important to distinguish between tendinitis and a complete disruption because surgical repair is often warranted for the latter and not for the former. Making the distinction clinically is often difficult.

Achilles Tendon

The Achilles tendon does not have a sheath associated with it; therefore, tenosynovitis does not occur. Tendinitis is commonly seen in the Achilles tendon; however, it is such an easy clinical diagnosis that MR is usually not necessary. Complete disruption is commonly seen in athletes and in males who are approximately 40 years of age. It is also commonly associated with other systemic disorders that cause tendon weakening, such as rheumatoid arthritis, collagen vascular diseases, crystal deposition diseases, and hyperparathyroidism.

Achilles tendon disruption can be treated surgically or by placing the patient in a cast with equinus positioning (marked plantar flexion) for several months. Which treatment is superior is a controversial issue, with both methods of treatment seemingly working well. MR is being used by many surgeons to help decide if surgery should be performed. If a large gap is present (Fig. 50.1), some surgeons feel surgery should be performed for reapposition of the torn ends of the tendon; on the other hand, if the ends of the tendon are not retracted, nonsurgical treatment is preferred. No published papers have shown that this is, in fact, scientifically valid.

Posterior Tibial Tendon

The posterior tibial tendon is the most medial and the largest, except for the Achilles, of the flexor tendons (Fig. 50.2). The flexor tendons are easily remembered and identified by using the mnemonic "Tom, Dick, and Harry," with Tom representing the posterior tibial tendon, Dick the flexor digitorum longus tendon, and Harry the flexor hallucis longus tendon. The posterior tibial tendon inserts onto the navicular, second to fourth cuneiforms, and the bases of the second to fourth metatarsals. As it sweeps under the foot, it provides some support for the longitudinal arch; hence, problems in the arch or plantar fascia can sometimes lead to stress on the posterior tibial tendon with resulting tendinitis or even rupture. Posterior tibial tendinitis and rupture are commonly encountered in patients with rheumatoid arthritis.

Differentiation of tendinitis from tendon rupture can be difficult, and MR has become very valuable for making this distinction (3). Most surgeons will operate on a disrupted posterior tibial tendon; however, nonoperative therapy is usually preferred for tendinitis.

Posterior tibial tendinitis is seen on axial T1WI as swelling and/or signal within the normally low signal tendon on one or more images (Fig. 50.3). T2WI or T2*-

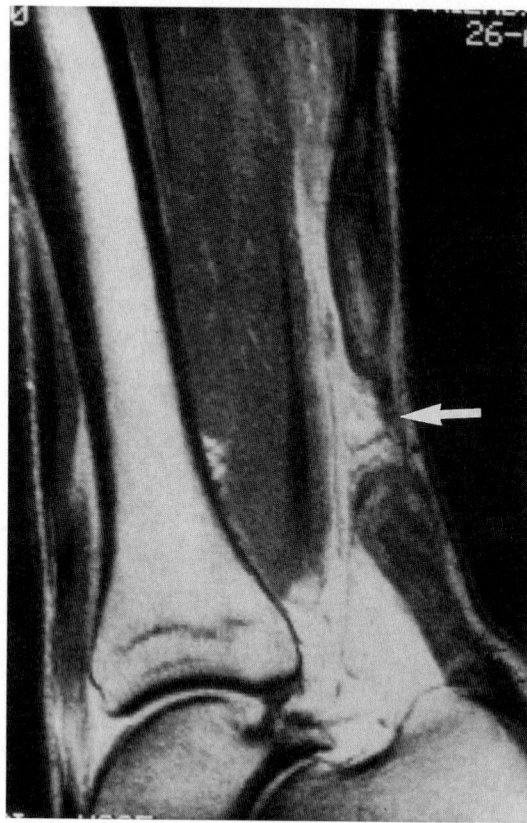

Figure 50.1. Torn Achilles Tendon. A sagittal T1WI (TR 600; TE 30) reveals the Achilles tendon to be torn with a 2-cm gap. Only a thin remnant of the tendon remains intact across the gap (*arrow*). Note the high signal in the swollen ends of the separated tendon, indicative of hemorrhage and edema.

weighted images show the signal in the tendon getting brighter. Tendon disruption is diagnosed by noting the absence of the tendon on one or more axial images. This typically occurs just at or above the level of the tibiotalar joint.

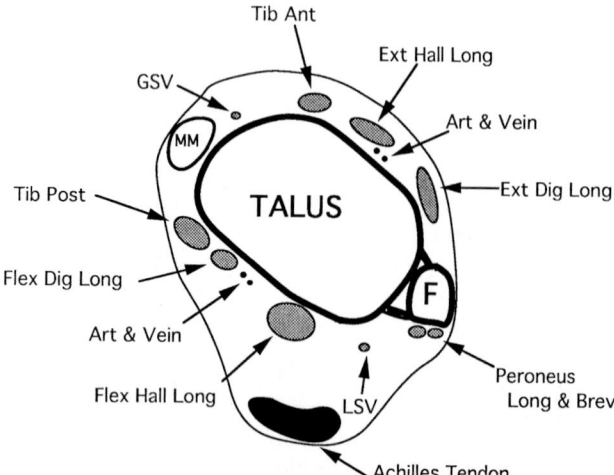

Figure 50.2. Schematic of Axial Ankle Anatomy. This drawing of the tendons around the ankle at the level of the tibiotalar joint shows the relationship of the flexor tendons posteriorly and the extensor tendons anteriorly. *F*, fibula; *MM*, medial malleolus; *GSV*, greater saphenous vein; *LSV*, lesser saphenous vein.

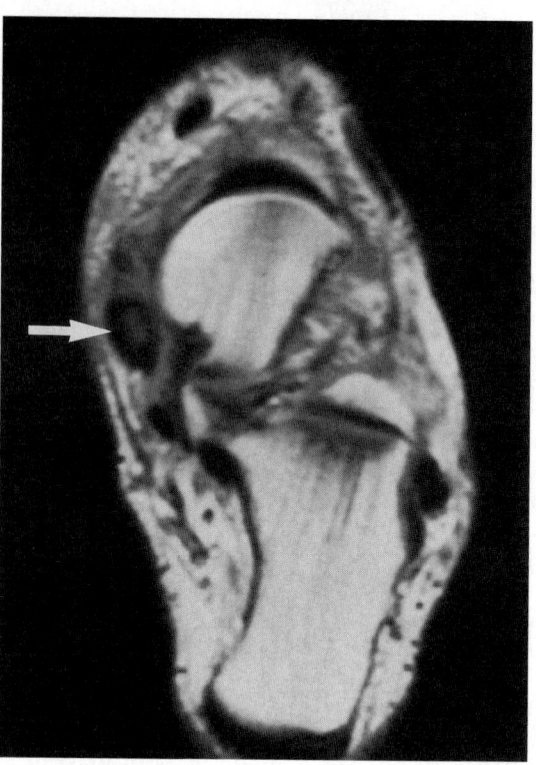

Figure 50.3. Posterior Tibial Tendon Tendinitis. A proton-density (TR 2000; TE 20) axial image through the ankle at the level of the mid-calcaneus shows the posterior tibial tendon (*arrow*) swollen and containing high signal. This is the appearance of marked tendinitis.

Flexor Hallucis Longus Tendon

The flexor hallucis longus (FHL) tendon is easily identified near the tibiotalar joint because it is usually the only tendon at that distal level that has muscle still attached. In the foot the FHL can be seen beneath the sus-

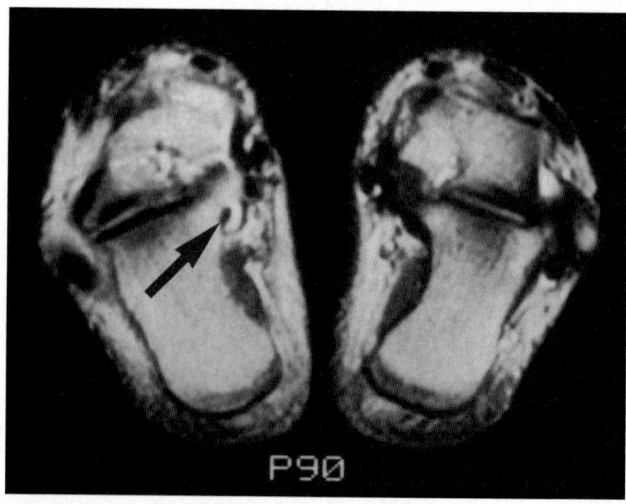

Figure 50.4. Flexor Hallucis Longus Tenosynovitis. A T2-weighted (TR 2000; TE 80) axial image of both ankles in this ballet dancer with a painful right ankle reveals fluid in the tendon sheath around the flexor hallucis longus tendon (*arrow*). This needs to be correlated with the clinical examination as fluid can normally extend into the tendon sheath of the flexor hallucis longus tendon from the tibiotalar joint in up to 20% of normal patients

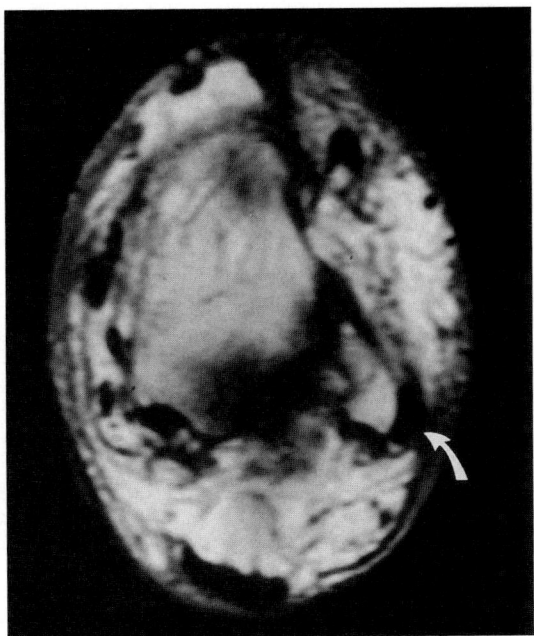

Figure 50.5. Dislocated Peroneus Longus Tendon. An axial T1WI (TR 600; TE 30) in this skier who injured the ankle in a fall shows a low signal rounded structure (*arrow*) lateral to the lateral malleolus. This is a dislocated peroneus longus tendon.

tentaculum talus, which it uses as a pulley to plantar flex the foot.

The FHL is known as the Achilles tendon of the foot in ballet dancers because of the extreme flexion positions they employ. Ballet dancers often will have tenosynovitis of the FHL, seen on MR as fluid in the sheath surrounding the tendon (Fig. 50.4). Care must be taken to have clinical correlation because fluid can be seen in the FHL tendon sheath from a connection to the ankle joint, which has an effusion in as many as 20% of normal patients. Rupture of the FHL is rare.

Peroneus Tendons

The peroneus longus and peroneus brevis tendons can be seen posterior to the distal fibula, to which they are bound by a thin fibrous structure, the superior retinaculum. The fibula serves as a pulley for the tendons to work as the principal everter of the foot. The tendons course close together adjacent to the lateral aspect of the calcaneus until a few centimeters below the lateral malleolus where they separate, with the peroneus brevis tendon inserting onto the base of the fifth metatarsal and the peroneus longus tendon crossing under the foot to the base of the first metatarsal. Avulsion of the base of the fifth metatarsal from a pull by the peroneus brevis tendon is known as a "dancer's fracture" or a Jones fracture.

Disruption of the superior retinaculum, often seen in skiing accidents (4), can result in displacement of the peroneus tendons (Fig. 50.5) and must be surgically corrected. It often occurs with a small bony avulsion, called a flake fracture, off the fibula.

Entrapment of the peroneus tendons in a fractured calcaneus or fibula can occur, and is easily diagnosed with MR. This can be a difficult diagnosis to make clinically. Complete disruption of the peroneal tendons is uncommon but is easily noted with MR.

AVASCULAR NECROSIS

Avascular necrosis commonly occurs in the foot and ankle. The talar dome is the second most common location of osteochondritis dissecans (the knee is the most common site). Magnetic resonance is useful in identifying and staging osteochondritis dissecans. Even when not apparent on plain films, magnetic resonance imaging can show osteochondritis dissecans as a focal area of low signal in the subarticular portion of the talar dome on T1WI. On T2WI or T2*-weighted images, if high signal is seen surrounding the dissecans fragment in the bone at the bed of the fragment or throughout the fragment (Fig. 50.6), the fragment is most likely unstable. If the

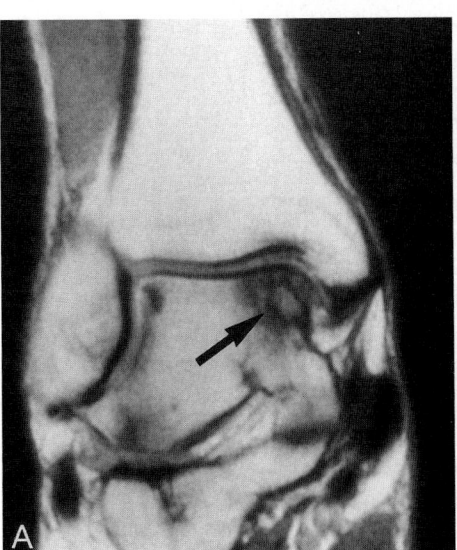
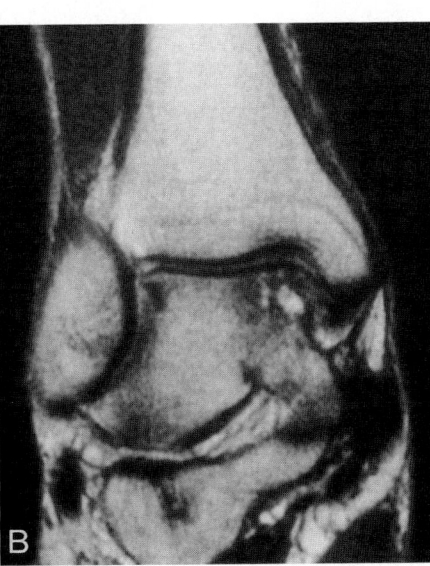

Figure 50.6. Unstable Osteochondritis Dissecans of the Talus. A. A proton-density (TR 2000; TE 20) coronal image through the talus shows a focus of low signal in the medial subarticular part of the talus (*arrow*). This is a characteristic appearance for osteochondritis dissecans. **B.** A T2-weighted (TR 2000; TE 80) image shows high signal throughout the focus of osteochondritis dissecans, which indicates an unstable fragment.

Figure 50.7. Avascular Necrosis of the Tarsal Navicular. A T1-weighted (TR 600; TE 30) sagittal image of the ankle in this patient with pain on the dorsum of the foot shows diffuse low signal throughout the tarsal navicular. This is a characteristic appearance for avascular necrosis and will often precede any plain film findings.

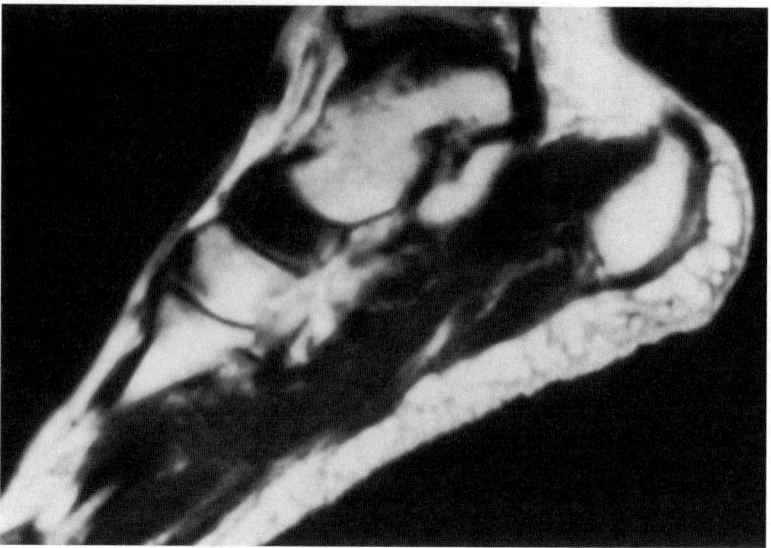

fragment has become displaced and lies in the joint as a loose body, MR can sometimes be useful to localize it; however, loose bodies in any joint can be exceedingly difficult to find.

Diffuse low signal throughout a tarsal bone on T1WI is typical for avascular necrosis. This occasionally occurs in the tarsal navicular (Fig. 50.7). MR can be useful in making this diagnosis when plain films are normal or equivocal.

TUMORS

A few tumors have a predilection for the foot and ankle (5). Up to 16% of synovial sarcomas occur in the foot.

Desmoid tumors are commonly seen in the foot. Giant cell tumors of tendon sheath (also called xanthomas and pigmented villonodular synovitis) are often found in the tendon sheaths of the foot and ankle (Fig. 50.8). They are characterized by marked low signal in the synovial lining and in the tendons on T1WI and T2WI, just as pigmented villonodular synovitis appears in a joint.

The differential diagnosis for calcaneal tumors is similar to that of the epiphyses—giant cell tumor, chondroblastoma, and infection—with a unicameral bone cyst added.

Soft-tissue tumors in the medial aspect of the foot and ankle can press on the posterior tibial nerve, resulting in tarsal tunnel syndrome (6). Clinically, patients with

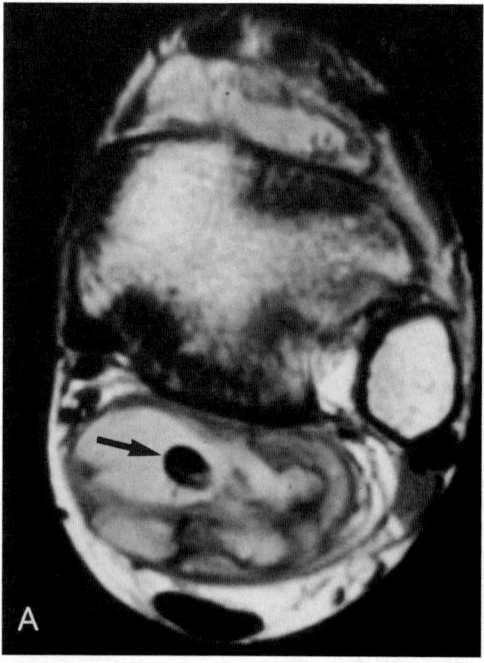

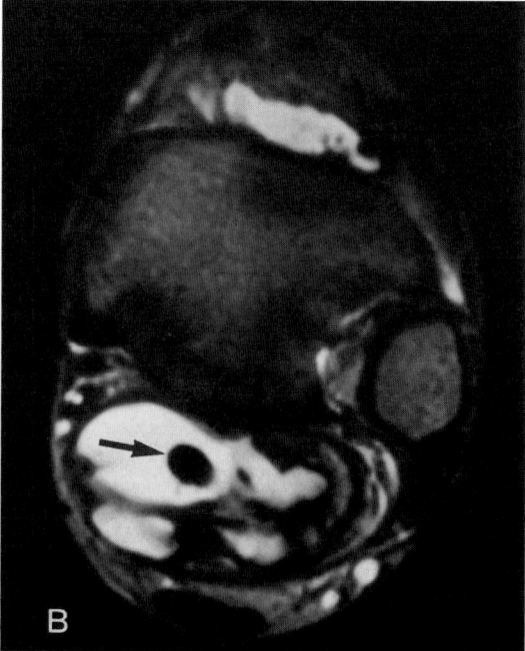

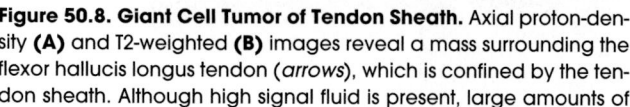

Figure 50.8. Giant Cell Tumor of Tendon Sheath. Axial proton-density **(A)** and T2-weighted **(B)** images reveal a mass surrounding the flexor hallucis longus tendon (*arrows*), which is confined by the tendon sheath. Although high signal fluid is present, large amounts of low signal material is lining the distended tendon sheath. This low signal is hemosiderin, which is typically found in a giant cell tendon of tendon sheath. Pigmented villonodular synovitis in a joint has an identical appearance.

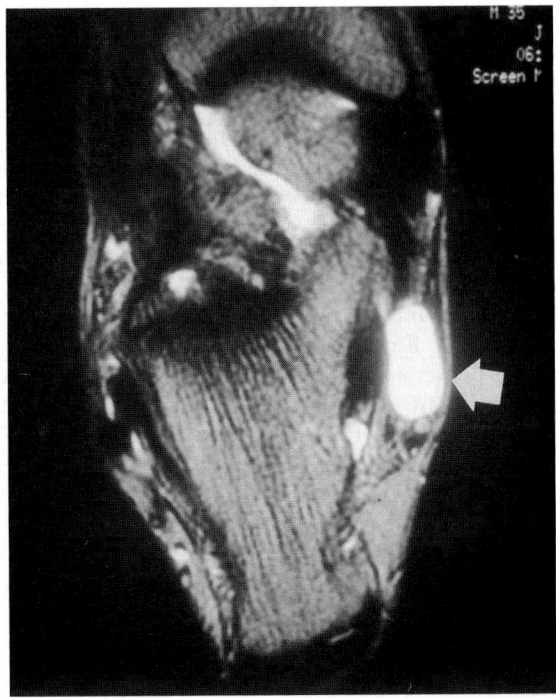

Figure 50.9. Ganglion Causing Tarsal Tunnel Syndrome. A FSE T2-weighted axial image of the ankle in a patient complaining of pain and paresthesia on the plantar aspect of the foot shows a homogeneous high signal mass (*arrow*) lying adjacent to the flexor hallucis longus tendon. This is the position of tarsal tunnel which contains the tibial nerve that can be impinged by a mass, such as in this case, resulting in tarsal tunnel syndrome. This was a ganglion.

tarsal tunnel syndrome present with pain and paresthesia in the plantar aspect of the foot. In the aforementioned mnemonic, "Tom, Dick, and Harry," the "and" is for artery, nerve, and vein. It is the position of the posterior tibial nerve. The nerve is easily compressed in the tarsal tunnel, which is bounded medially by the flexor retinaculum, a strong fibrous band that extends across the medial ankle joint for approximately 5–7 cm in a superior-to-inferior direction. Ganglions and neural tumors, both of which can look similar on T1WI and T2WI, often lie in the tarsal tunnel (Fig. 50.9) and compress the posterior tibial nerve, resulting in pain and paresthesia on the plantar aspect of the foot extending into the toes. Tarsal tunnel syndrome often occurs secondary to trauma or fibrosis, or it can occur idiopathically. Regardless, this syndrome may not respond to surgical intervention; hence, MR is valuable in delineating a treatable lesion in many cases.

Anomalous muscles in the foot or ankle are reported to be present in up to 6% of the population. These can be mistaken for a tumor and biopsy may be performed unnecessarily. MR will show these "tumors" to have imaging characteristics identical to normal muscle (Fig. 50.10) and to be sharply circumscribed. Accessory soleus and peroneus brevis muscles are the most common accessory muscles encountered around the foot and ankle.

LIGAMENTS

MR is not the best way to diagnose acute ankle ligament abnormalities. The clinical evaluation is usually

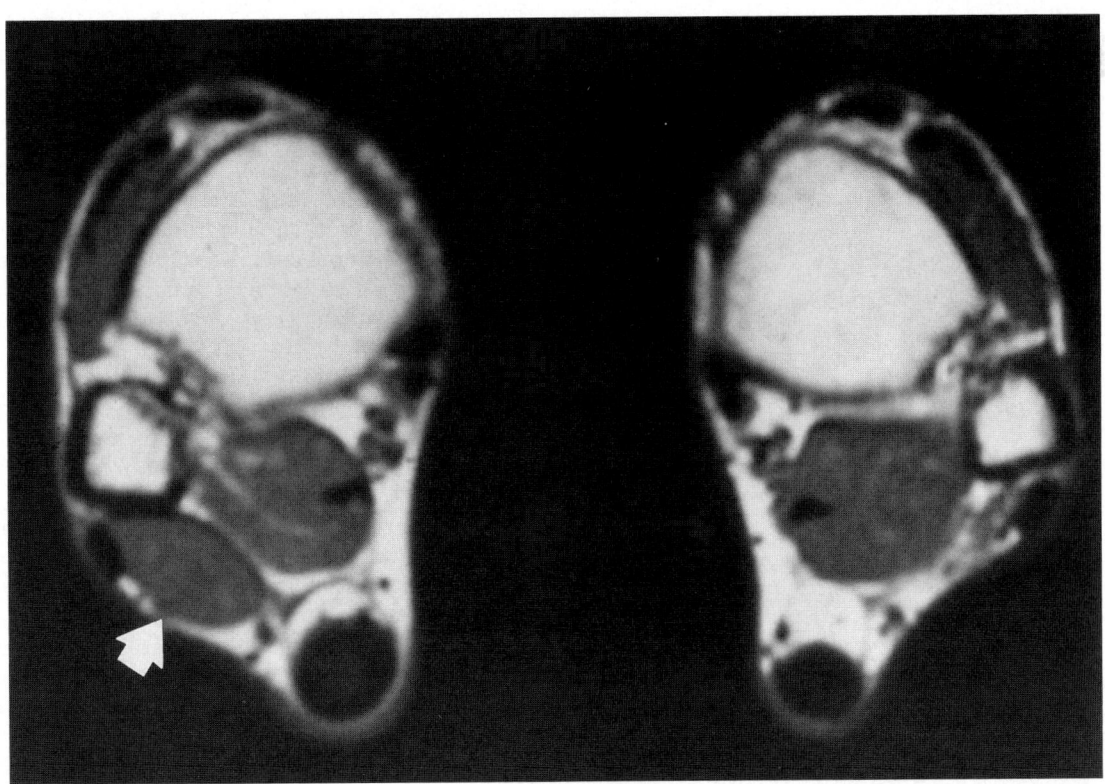

Figure 50.10. Anomalous Muscle. An axial T1WI of both ankles in this patient complaining of a mass in the right ankle shows an anomalous muscle (*arrow*) lateral to the flexor hallucis longus muscle that is responsible for the mass the patient feels.

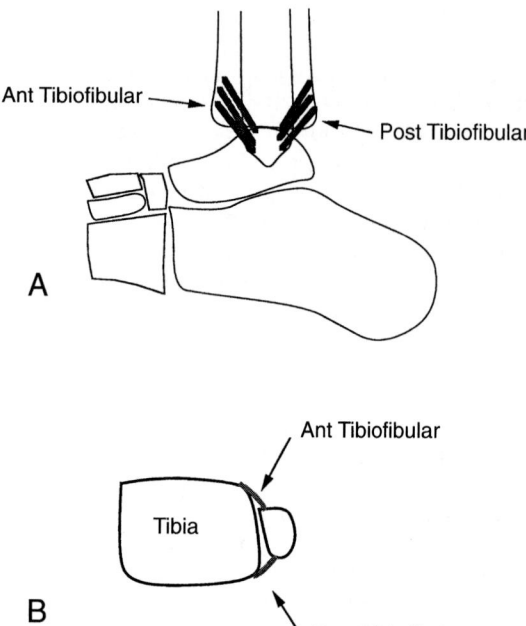

Figure 50.11. Schematic of Lateral Collateral Ligaments. A. This drawing of the ankle in a lateral view shows how the anterior and posterior tibiofibular (*tib-fib*) ligaments extend off the fibula and course superiorly to the tibia. **B.** A drawing in the axial plane shows that the fibula has a flat or convex surface at the origin of these ligaments.

straightforward and no diagnostic imaging of any type is necessary. Nevertheless, in clinically equivocal cases or when the examination is ordered for other reasons, the ligaments can be clearly evaluated with high-quality MR in most instances (7).

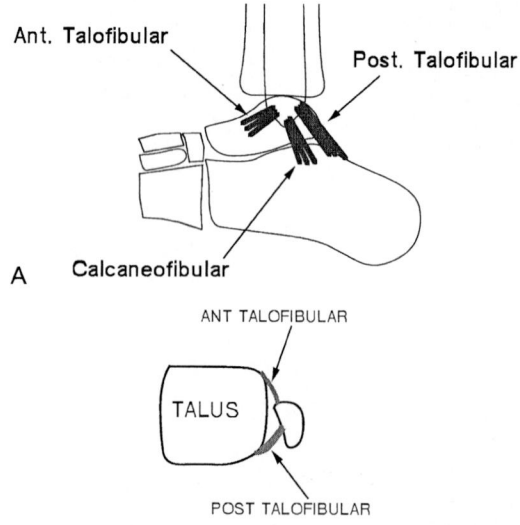

Figure 50.12. Schematic of Lateral Collateral Ligaments. A. This drawing of the ankle in a lateral view shows how the anterior and posterior talofibular ligaments, and the calcaneofibular ligament extend off the fibula and course inferiorly. These ligaments arise off of the fibula more distally than the anterior and posterior tibiofibular ligaments. **B.** A drawing in the axial plane shows that the anterior and posterior talofibular ligaments arise from the level of the distal fibula, which has a concave medial surface, the malleolar fossa.

The deltoid ligament lies medially as a broad band beneath the tendons. Although often seen on coronal images deep to the posterior tibial tendon, it has a variable anatomic appearance. Injury to the deltoid ligament accounts for only 5–10% of ankle ligament sprains.

The lateral ligaments are injured in over 90% of ankle sprains. The lateral complex is made up of two parts: a superior group, the anterior and posterior tibiofibular ligaments that make up part of the syndesmosis (Fig. 50.11), and an inferior group, the anterior and posterior talofibular ligaments and the calcaneofibular ligament (Fig. 50.12). The anterior and posterior tibiofibular ligaments can be seen on axial images at or slightly below the tibiotalar joint. The anterior and posterior talofibular ligaments are seen on the axial images just below the tibiotalar joint and emanate from a concavity in the distal fibula called the malleolar fossa (Fig. 50.12B). The most commonly torn ankle ligament is the anterior talofibular ligament. It is easily identified when a joint effusion is present because it makes up the anterior capsule of the joint (Fig. 50.13). The anterior talofibular ligament is usually torn without other ligaments being involved; however, if the injury is severe enough, the next ligament to tear is the calcaneofibular ligament. Finally, with very severe trauma, the posterior talofibular ligament will tear.

On sagittal T2WI or T2*-weighted images, the posterior tibiofibular ligament can mimic a loose body in the joint (Fig. 50.14). This pitfall is very common and is clinically significant: unnecessary surgery for a presumed loose body can occur because of failure to recognize the normal anatomy.

Several entities have a high association with chronic tears of the lateral ligaments. These include chronic lateral ankle instability, sinus tarsi syndrome, and anterolateral impingement syndrome.

Patients with sinus tarsi syndrome present with lateral ankle pain and tenderness and a perception of hindfoot instability. The sinus tarsi is the cone-shaped space between the talus and the calcaneus that opens up laterally. It is a fat-filled space through which traverse several important ligaments that provide subtalar stability. In sinus tarsi syndrome these ligaments are torn and the fat is replaced with granulation tissue or scar tissue. Hence, on T2WI there may be high (granulation tissue) or low (scar) signal, but on T1WI there is low signal in the sinus tarsi (Fig. 50.15). In the acutely sprained ankle, the sinus tarsi may have replacement of the fat due to hemorrhage and edema, which will resolve.

Anterolateral impingement syndrome results from hypertrophy and scarring of the synovium in the lateral gutter of the ankle. The lateral gutter is the space between the tibia and fibula and is bound by the lateral ankle ligaments. Patients with anterolateral impingement syndrome present with lateral ankle pain and inability to dorsiflex normally. They often have a click on dorsiflexion. Arthroscopic resection of the scar tissue has been reported with good results. MR images show low-signal tissue in the lateral gutter on T2WI (Fig. 50.16). The anterior talofibular ligament is commonly torn or fibrosed in this condition.

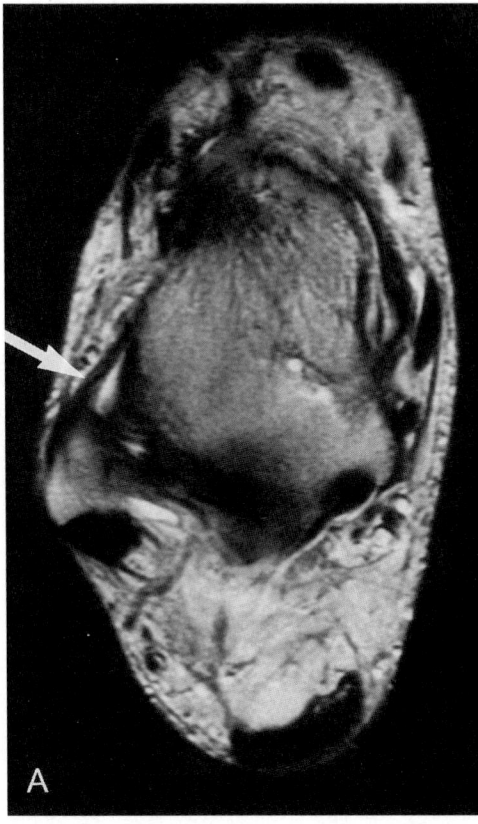

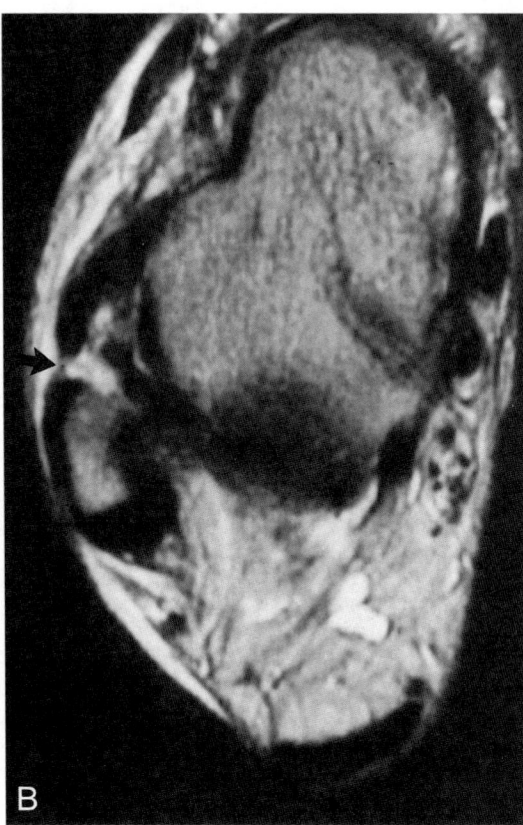

Figure 50.13. Anterior Talofibular Ligament. A. An axial T2WI (TR 4000; TE 76) through the distal fibula at the level of the malleolar fossa (the concave medial surface of the fibula) shows an intact anterior talofibular ligament (*arrow*) that makes up part of the joint capsule at this level. Note the high signal joint fluid adjacent to the ligament. **B.** This axial T2WI (TR 3200; TE 100) at the level of the malleolar fossa reveals a thickened anterior talofibular ligament that has a disruption (*arrow*). The marked thickening of the ligament indicates a chronic process. (Case courtesy of Dr. Jerrold Mink, Los Angeles, CA.)

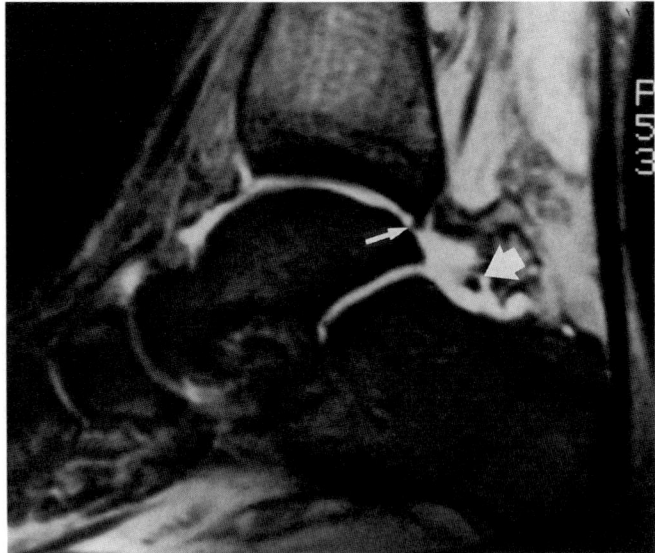

Figure 50.14. Posterior Tibiofibular Ligament and Loose Body. A sagittal T2* GRASS image (TR 500; TE 15; Θ 30°) through the midankle in a patient with occasional locking and a plain film (not shown) that demonstrates a calcified loose body near the posterior talus reveals two apparent loose bodies. The more posterior one (*large arrow*) matches the calcified loose body on the plain film. The other one (*small arrow*) is not a loose body but is the posterior tibiofibular ligament, which often resembles a loose body on sagittal T2WI.

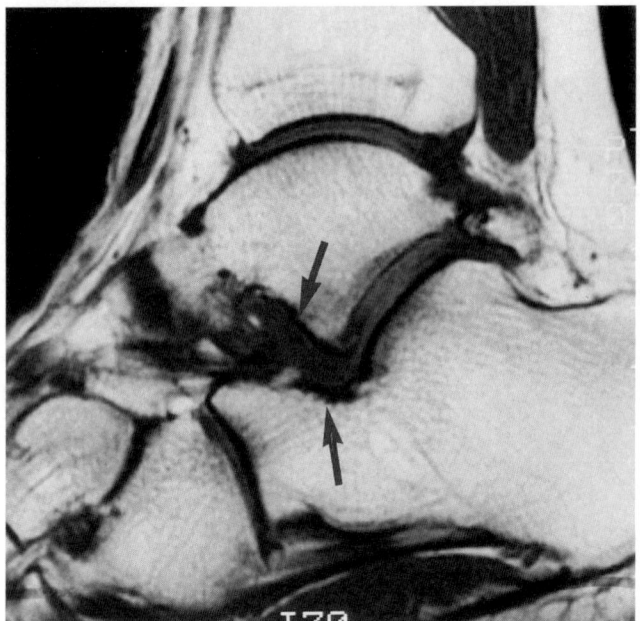

Figure 50.15. Sinus Tarsi Syndrome. A sagittal T1-weighted image in a patient with chronic lateral ankle pain shows absence of the normal fat in the sinus tarsi (*arrows*). This is virtually diagnostic of sinus tarsi syndrome except in the setting of an acute ankle sprain.

BONY ABNORMALITIES

Tarsal coalition is a common cause of a painful flatfoot. It occurs most commonly at the calcaneonavicular joint and the middle facet of the talocalcaneal joint (Fig. 50.17). Up to 80% of patients with tarsal coalition have bilateral coalition. It can be difficult (or impossible) to see the coalition on plain films; however, CT and MR will show bony coalition with a high degree of accuracy. The coalition can also be fibrous or cartilaginous. In these cases, secondary findings, such as joint space irregularity at the affected joint or degenerative joint disease at nearby joints that are subjected to accentuated stress, can be seen. For now, MR is not superior to CT for tarsal coalition.

Fractures of the foot and ankle are usually well documented with plain films. Stress fractures, however, can be difficult to radiographically or clinically diagnose, and they can mimic more sinister abnormalities. MR will show stress fractures as linear low signal on T1WI with high signal on T2 weighting (Fig. 50.18).

MR has had mixed reviews when used for diagnosing osteomyelitis in the foot. In diabetic patients with foot infections, diagnosing osteomyelitis is important because the treatment is often much more aggressive—including amputation—than if the bone is not involved. Unfortunately, MR is not highly accurate in this regard. If

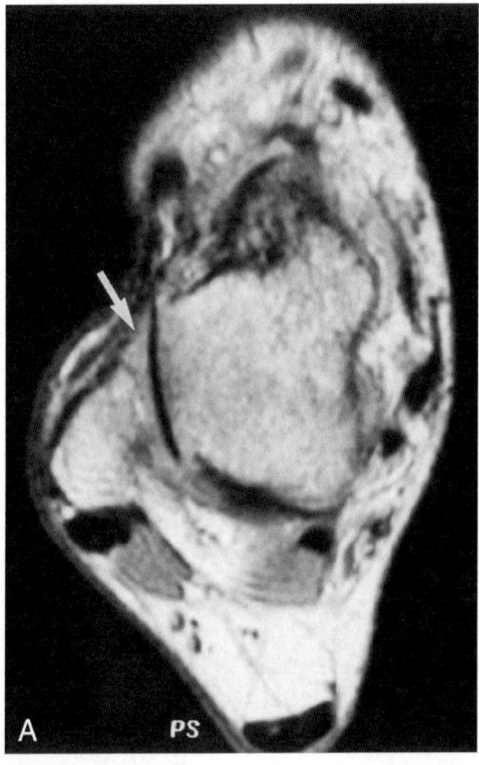

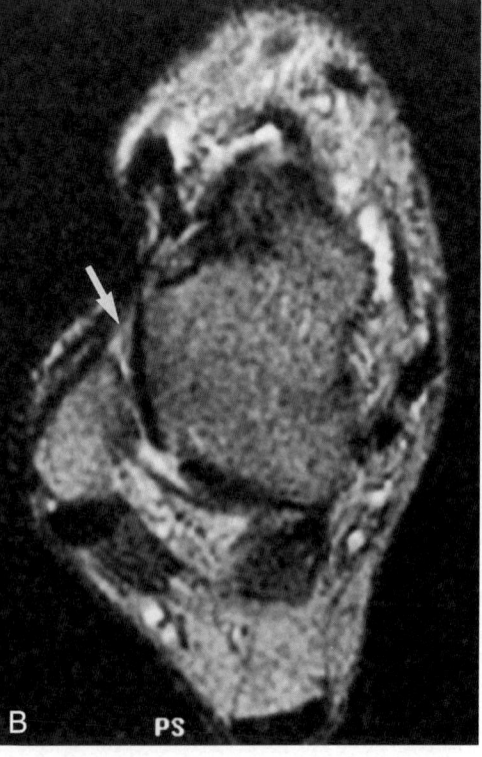

Figure 50.16. Anterolateral Impingement Syndrome. Axial images through the ankle in a patient with chronic lateral pain, and inability to fully dorsiflex show intermediate signal in the lateral gutter (*arrow*) on proton density **(A)** which remains intermediate in intensity on the T2WI **(B)**. This is scar tissue and hypertrophied synovium, which is typical for anterolateral impingement syndrome.

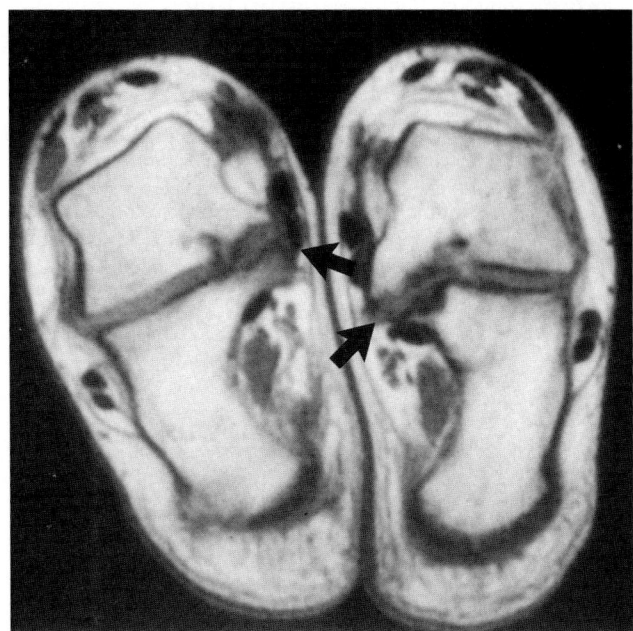

Figure 50.17. Tarsal Coalition. An axial T1WI in a patient with painful flat feet shows bilateral talocalcaneal coalition (*arrows*), which is primarily fibrous. The normal joint space is irregular and widened bilaterally. In cases of suspected coalition, both ankles should be imaged as coalition often occurs bilaterally.

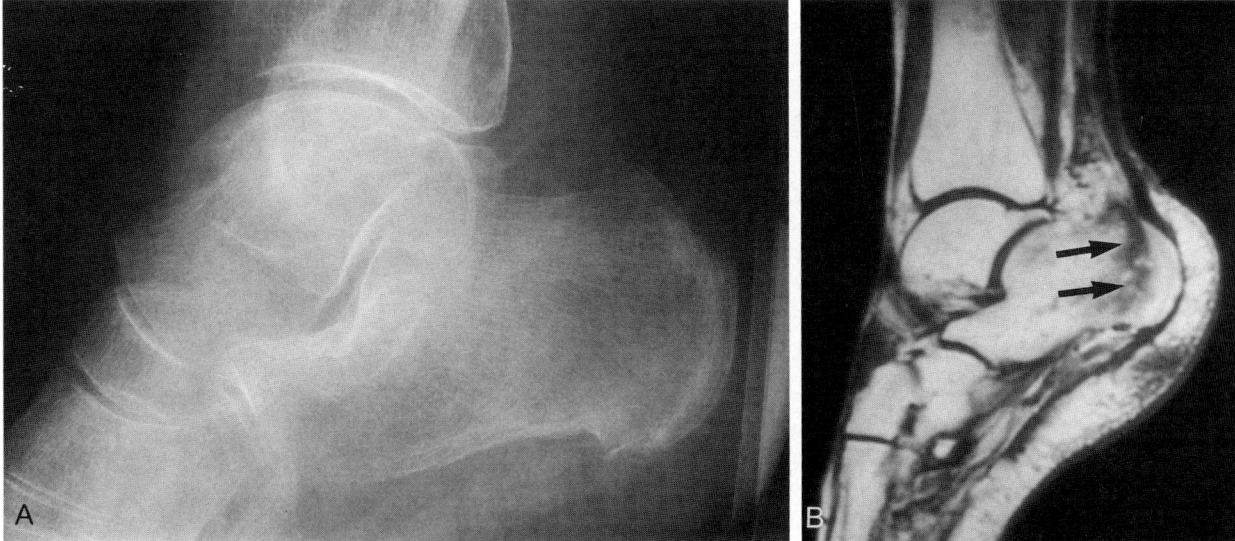

Figure 50.18. Calcaneal Stress Fracture. A 70-year-old patient with a prior history of lung cancer presented with heel pain and a normal plain film **(A)**. A bone scan showed diffuse increased radionuclide uptake throughout the posterior calcaneus. A sagittal T1-weighted MR **(B)** revealed a linear area of low signal (*arrows*), which is characteristic for a stress fracture. Metastatic disease would not have this appearance.

the marrow appears normal, MR is highly accurate in predicting no osteomyelitis; however, if low signal is present in the marrow around a joint, osteomyelitis may or may not be present. Low signal can be caused by edema or hyperemia without infection. MR is therefore very sensitive but not very specific in diagnosing osteomyelitis in the foot and ankle (8).

References

1. Kneeland J, Macrandar S, Middleton W, et al MR imaging of the normal ankle: correlation with anatomic sections. AJR Am J Roentgenol 1988;151:117–126.
2. Quinn S, Murray W, Clark R, Cochran C. Achilles tendon: MR imaging at 1.5 T. Radiology 1987;164:767–770.
3. Rosenberg Z, Cheung Y, Jahss M, et al. Rupture of posterior tibial tendons: CT and MR imaging with surgical correlation. Radiology 1988;169:229–236.
4. Oden R. Tendon injuries about the ankle resulting from skiing. Clin Orthop 1987;216:63–69.
5. Keigley B, Haggar A, Gaba A, et al. Primary tumors of the foot: MR imaging. Radiology 1989;171:755–759.
6. Erickson S, Quinn S, Kneeland J, et al. MR imaging of the tarsal tunnel and related spaces: normal and abnormal findings with anatomic correlation. AJR Am J Roentgenol 1990; 155:323–328.
7. Erickson S, Smith J, Ruiz M, et al. MR imaging of the lateral collateral ligament of the ankle. AJR Am J Roentgenol 1991; 156:131–136.
8. Erdman W, Tamburro F, Jayson H, et al. Osteomyelitis: characteristics and pitfalls of diagnosis with MR imaging. Radiology 1991;180:533–539.

Section X PEDIATRIC RADIOLOGY

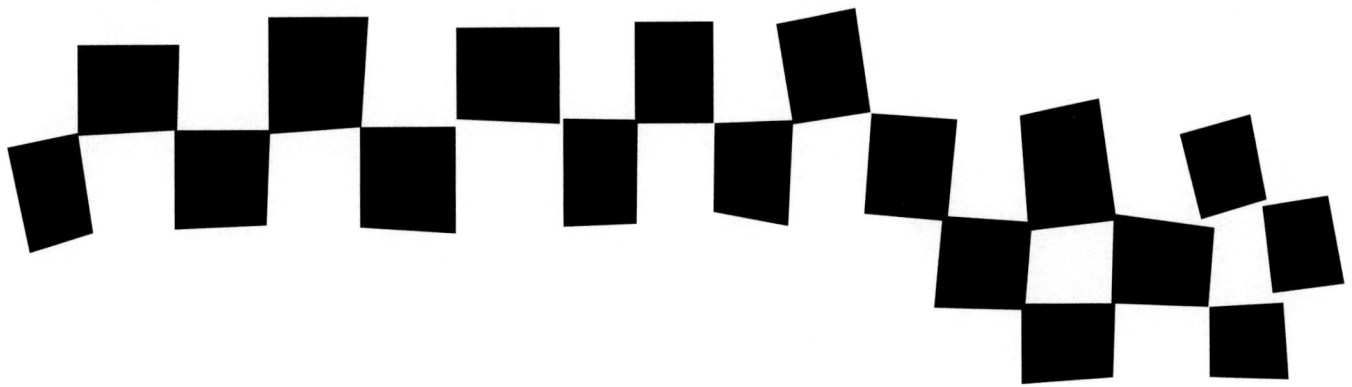

Susan D. John
Leonard E. Swischuk

PULMONARY INFILTRATIVE PATTERNS

Pulmonary infiltrates in children are classified in the same way as in adults as being either primarily alveolar or interstitial. It should also be noted whether the infiltrates are focal or diffuse and unilateral or bilateral. Some infiltrates occur in a central or parahilar distribution, whereas others are predominantly peripheral or basal in location. Mixed patterns also occur. An understanding of the causes of these various patterns is necessary to provide a useful interpretation of lung infiltrates in children.

Alveolar Patterns

Alveolar Consolidation occurs when the alveoli are filled with some substance, usually fluid. When such a consolidation is focal, the fluid most often is exudate resulting from bacterial pneumonia (Fig. 51.1) (Table 51.1). The most common organism varies with the age of the child: *Haemophilus influenzae* is most common before 2 years of age and *Streptococcus pneumoniae* is most common in older children. Currently, staphylococcal infections are not particularly common, and mycoplasma infections occasionally produce focal consolidating pneumonias.

Consolidations with viral infections are not particularly common but can occur with more serious viral infection such as adenovirus, influenza, parainfluenza, and respiratory syncytial virus. There is some question as to whether these consolidations represent true air-space consolidations. It is likely that they represent intense interstitial disease causing compression of the alveoli and mimicking the findings of air-space consolidations. The same may be true of mycoplasma infections.

Gram-negative infections are not very common in children, and primary tuberculosis should be considered, particularly when the infiltrate is accompanied by hilar lymphadenopathy. Other causes of focal lung consolidations in children include fungal infection, pulmonary infarction, lung contusion, and focal pulmonary hemorrhage.

Atelectasis. An important observation when faced with a focal lung density is whether it is associated with volume loss. If volume loss is present, the problem is most likely attributable to atelectasis: a very common occurrence with childhood viral respiratory tract infections. Generally, volume loss will not be seen with a bacterial pneumonia until it begins to resolve. Atelectasis is also very common in patients with acute asthma (Fig. 51.2). The clinical presentation in such patients is often very helpful. Solid infiltrates in a patient with acute asthma are much more likely to be the result of atelectasis. Pneumonia in a patient with asthma does not result in an asthma attack, but rather has the same clinical symptoms as in any other child (i.e., high fever, cough, chest pain).

Multiple Patchy Lung Opacities can be seen with a wide variety of conditions (Table 51.2). Once again, these opacities reflect filling of the alveolar space with exudate, edema, or blood. If patchy infiltrates are confined to one lobe, a bacterial or *Mycoplasma* infection is the most likely cause. Multiple bilateral alveolar infiltrates suggest bacterial infection (most commonly, *Staphylococcus*) (Fig. 51.3) or fungal disease. Opportunistic infections in immunocompromised patients are much more likely to be multiple and bilateral. Pneumonias caused by aspiration tend to present with multiple patchy pulmonary opacities. The pneumonitis associated with hydrocarbon ingestion typically occurs in the medial portions of the lung bases (Fig. 51.4). Other less common causes of patchy alveolar opacities include milk allergy, hypersensitivity pneumonitis, uremic lung disease, near drowning, and pulmonary hemorrhage (i.e., idiopathic pulmonary hemosiderosis).

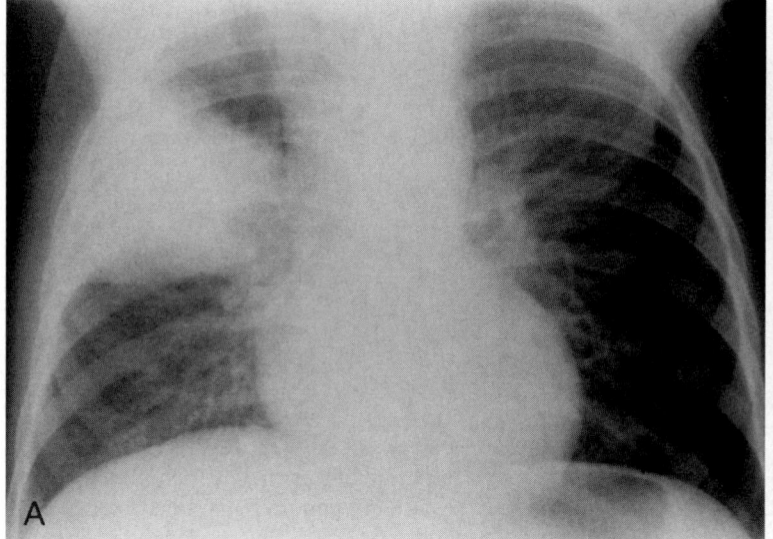

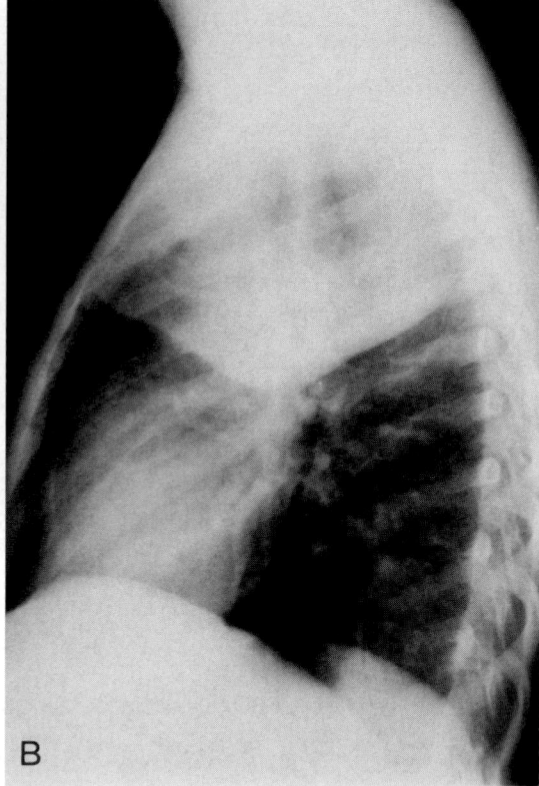

Figure 51.1. Bacterial Pneumonia. A. Frontal view. **B.** Lateral view. Typical alveolar consolidation is seen in the right upper lobe. Note that the fissures are not displaced, indicating that there is little volume loss.

Table 51.1. Focal Alveolar Consolidation

Bacterial pneumonia
  <2 years of age
    H. influenzae
  >2 years or age
    S. pneumoniae
    M. pneumoniae
    Staphylococcus
Nonbacterial infection
  Tuberculosis
  Actinomycosis
Pulmonary infarction
Pulmonary contusion

Table 51.2. Multiple Patchy Lung Opacities

Infection
  Staphylococcus
  Mycoplasma
  Fungal
  Opportunistic organisms
Aspiration
  Hydrocarbon ingestion
  Near drowning
Immune-mediated pneumonitis
  Milk allergy
  Hypersensitivity pneumonitis
Pulmonary hemorrhage
Pulmonary edema

Interstitial Patterns

Pulmonary Infections that primarily involve the bronchi and peribronchial interstitium (e.g., viruses, *Mycoplasma pneumoniae*, pertussis, *Chlamydia*) are often associated with areas of segmental or subsegmental atelectasis that can also appear as patchy pulmonary opacities. These are often clustered around the lung hila, unlike bacterial infections, which tend to lie more peripherally. Nevertheless, atelectasis and patchy pneumonia may be indistinguishable unless the atelectasis is seen to resolve rapidly on a repeat chest radiograph.

Parahilar Peribronchial Opacity due to bronchial and peribronchial inflammation and edema occurs commonly in children because of conditions associated with bronchitis and peribronchitis (Table 51.3). This pattern

Table 51.3. Parahilar Peribronchial Opacity

Acute (Infection)
  Viral
  Mycoplasma
  Chlamydia
  Pertussis
Chronic
  Asthma
  Cystic fibrosis
  Immunologic deficiency disease
  Chronic aspiration

appears as ill-defined increased soft-tissue densities in the parahilar regions that radiate outward along the bronchovascular tracts. This can lead to the "shaggy heart" appearance (Fig. 51.5) and is most often seen with viral infections (1–3). Bilateral hilar adenopathy and scattered areas of subsegmental atelectasis are common associated findings (Fig. 51.6). This pattern is very different from the more peripheral alveolar opacification that is most often seen with bacterial pneumonias. A superimposed consolidating bacterial pneumonia can develop later in the course of a viral lower respiratory tract infection. *Mycoplasma pneumoniae* and pertussis infections also commonly produce this pattern (4). *Chlamydia trachomatis* infection has a similar appearance and usually occurs just after the newborn period (Fig. 51.7). When chronic, one should consider asthma, cystic fibro-

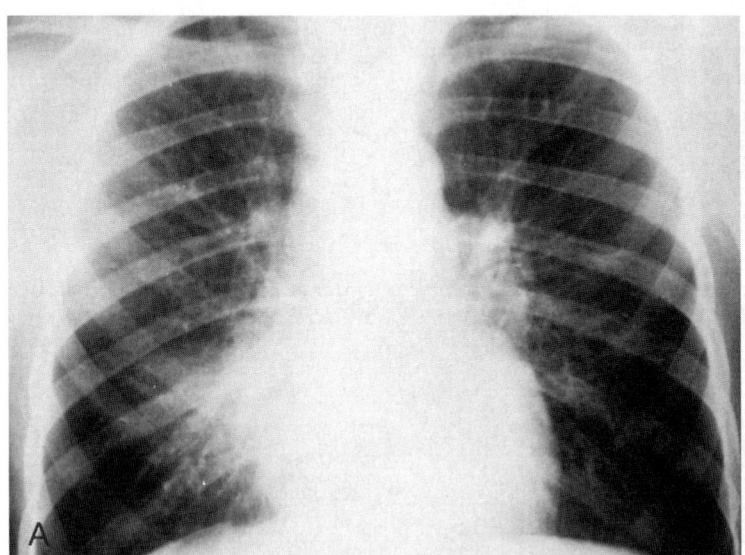

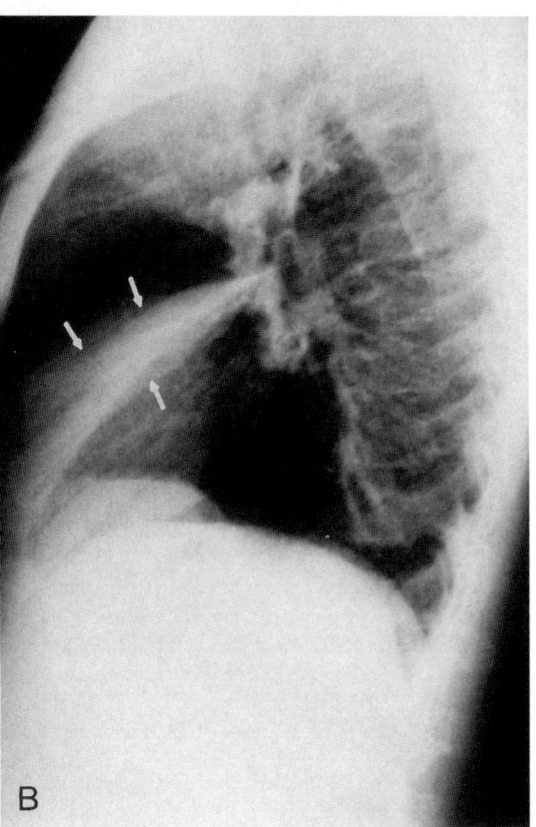

Figure 51.2. Acute Asthma. A. Opacity silhouettes the right heart border on the frontal view. **B.** Lateral view shows displacement of the horizontal and oblique fissures (*arrows*) indicating right middle lobe atelectasis.

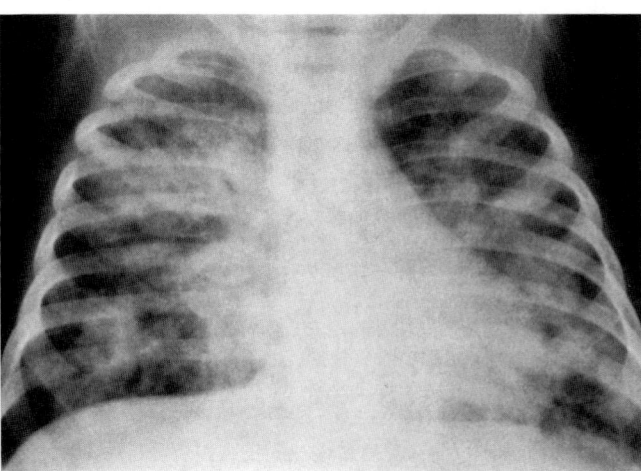

Figure 51.3. Staphylococcal Pneumonia. Multiple, bilateral alveolar opacities are typical of bacterial pneumonia.

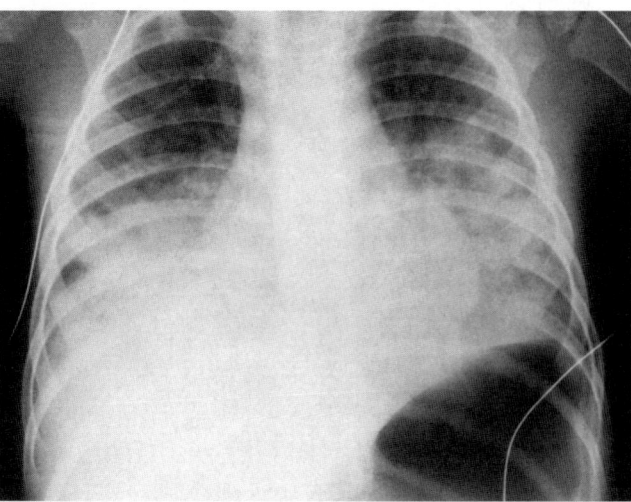

Figure 51.4. Hydrocarbon Aspiration. Bilateral patchy alveolar opacities are seen in the lung bases in this child who ingested kerosene.

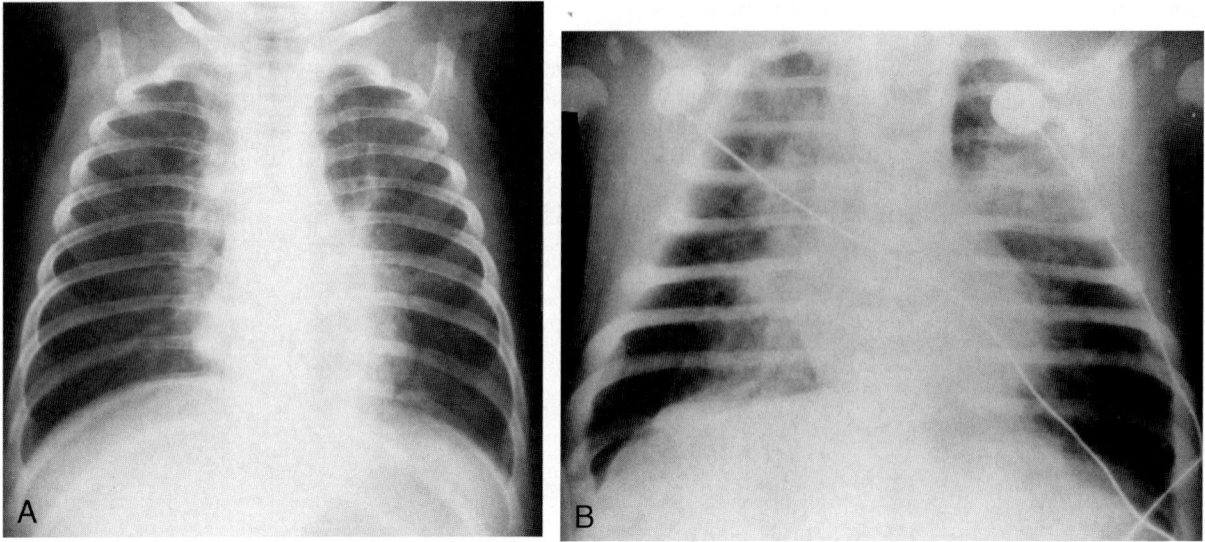

Figure 51.5. Viral Infection. A. Bilateral parahilar peribronchial infiltrates are typical of viral lower respiratory tract infections. **B.** More pronounced inflammatory edema produces dense parahilar regions leading to the "shaggy heart" appearance.

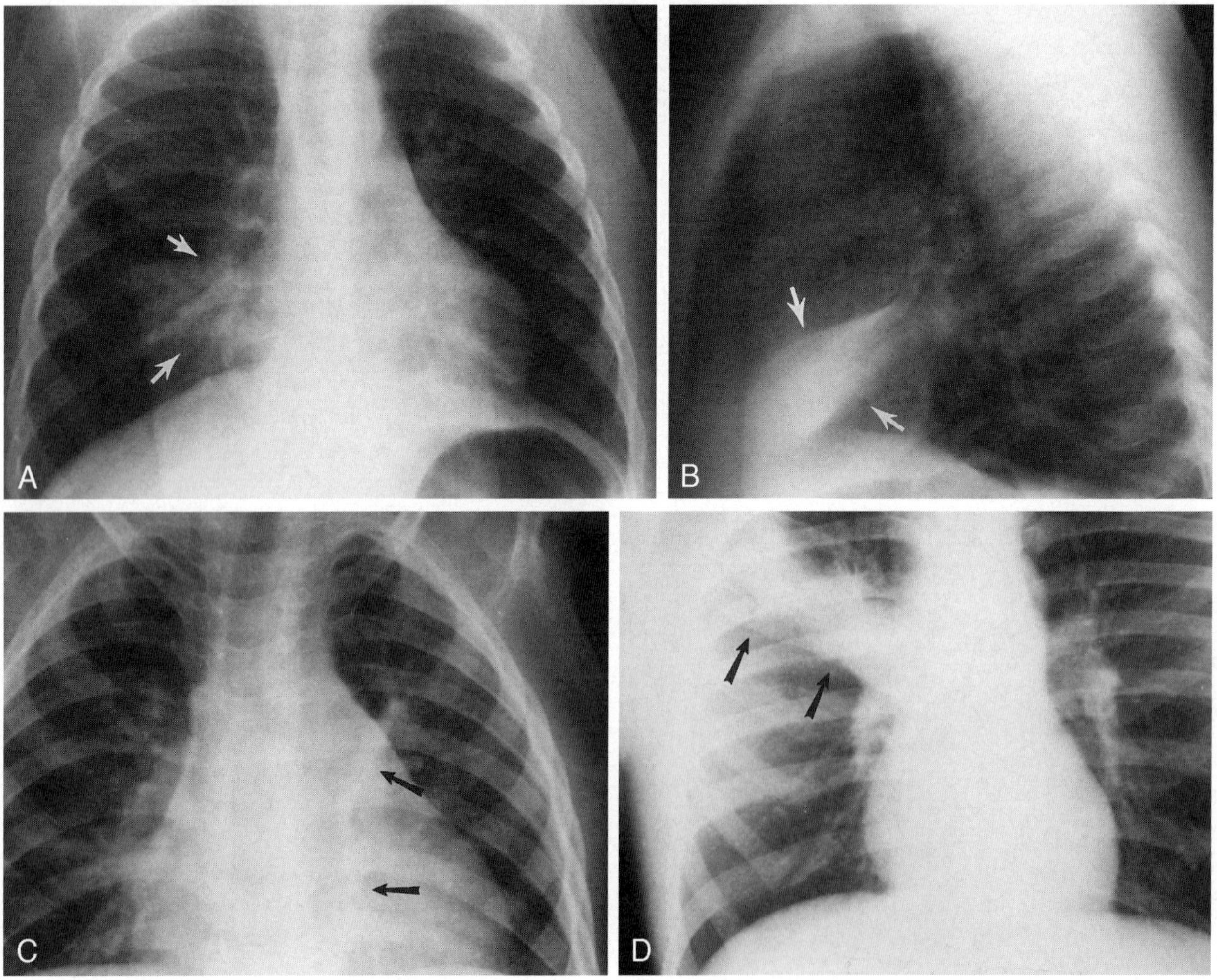

Figure 51.6. Viral Lower Respiratory Tract Infection with Atelectasis. A, B. The typical parahilar peribronchial infiltrates are accompanied by right middle lobe atelectasis (*arrows*). **C.** Note linear segmental atelectasis (*arrows*). **D.** Classic right upper lobe atelectasis (*arrows*).

sis (5)(see Fig. 51.18), immunologic deficiency diseases, and chronic aspiration.

Hazy, Reticular, or Reticulonodular Opacities that occur diffusely in the lungs indicate interstitial lung pathology caused by the same conditions that cause parahilar peribronchial infiltrates (Table 51.4). The most common cause of an interstitial pattern in the lungs of a child is either a viral or *Mycoplasma* infection (Fig. 51.8). In general, bacterial infections of the lung do not have this appearance, except in the newborn period when bacterial pneumonia can present as diffuse haziness or reticulonodularity. Fungal infections, such as *Histoplasma capsulatum* and *Coccidioides immitis*, can also occasionally result in an interstitial pattern.

Pulmonary edema, when it is confined to the interstitial space, also can produce hazy lungs, but more often creates a reticular pattern in the lungs. Cardiogenic pulmonary edema occurs when the pulmonary venous

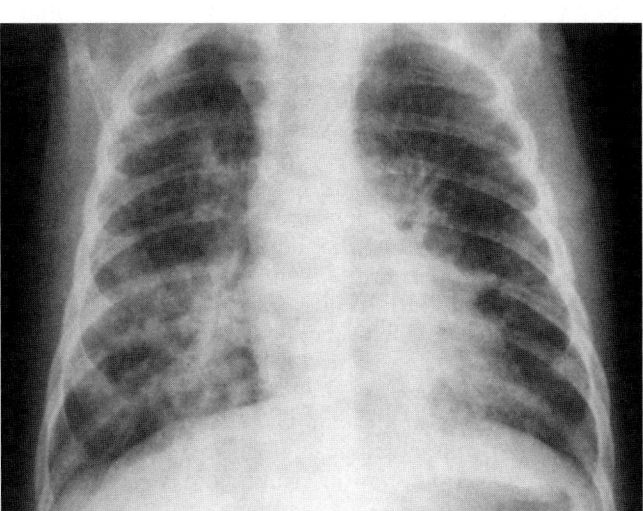

Figure 51.7. Chlamydia Pneumonitis. Prominent parahilar peribronchial infiltrates with slight nodularity are seen in the lung bases. The appearance is similar to that seen with viral infections.

Table 51.4. Hazy, Reticular, or Reticulonodular Patterns

Infection
  Viral
  Mycoplasma
  Fungal
Pulmonary edema
  Heart disease
  Acute renal failure
  Near drowning
  Increased intracranial pressure
  Inhalation injury
  Drug overdose
  ''Adult'' respiratory distress syndrome
Pulmonary lymphangiectasia/hemangiomatosis
Idiopathic pulmonary hemosiderosis
Interstitial pneumatosis
Histiocytosis X
Tuberous sclerosis
Connective tissue diseases
Malignancy
  Leukemia/lymphoma
  Lymphangitic metastasis

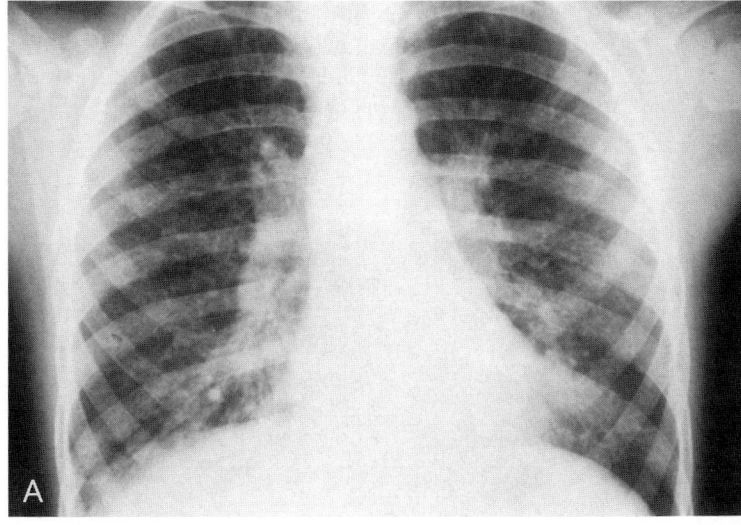
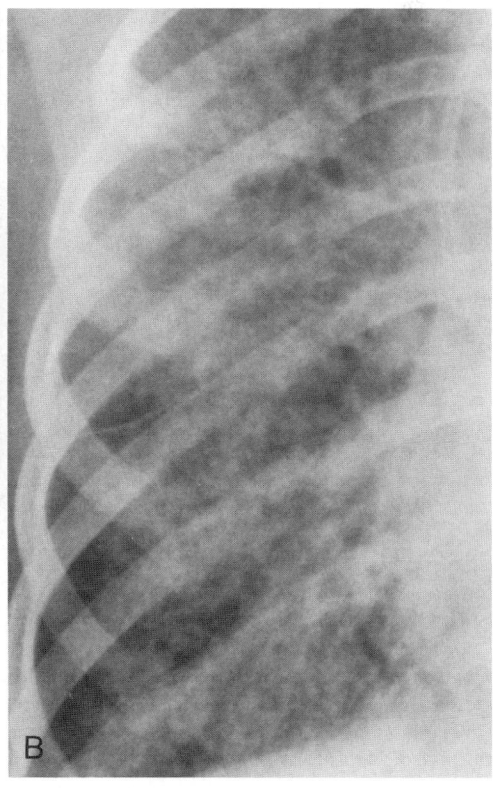

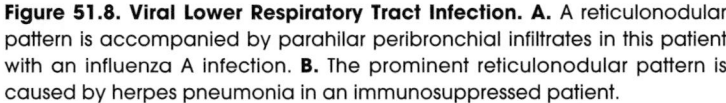

Figure 51.8. Viral Lower Respiratory Tract Infection. A. A reticulonodular pattern is accompanied by parahilar peribronchial infiltrates in this patient with an influenza A infection. **B.** The prominent reticulonodular pattern is caused by herpes pneumonia in an immunosuppressed patient.

pressures are elevated because of left-sided myocardial failure or congenital lesions that impede blood flow through the left side of the heart (e.g., pulmonary vein atresia, cor triatriatum, hypoplastic left heart syndrome). Noncardiogenic causes of pulmonary edema are probably more common in children. One of the most common causes of pulmonary edema in children is acute glomerulonephritis (Fig. 51.9). Sodium and fluid retention leads to hypervolemia, which can then result in cardiomegaly and pulmonary vascular congestion with edema. The radiographic appearance can be indistinguishable from edema caused by cardiac failure. Other noncardiogenic causes of pulmonary edema in children include near drowning, increased intracranial pressure, inhalation injuries, drug overdose, and adult respiratory distress syndrome.

Pulmonary lymphangiectasia is a rare condition that consists of dilated lymphatic channels secondary to ei-

ther abnormal embryonic development of the lymphatic system or obstruction of lymphatic drainage. The dilated lymphatics result in a coarsely nodular or reticular pattern in the lungs, usually seen in newborns (Fig. 51.10). Pulmonary hemangiomatosis is a similar rare condition. Recurrent hemorrhage into the lungs in patients with idiopathic pulmonary hemosiderosis eventually leads to a chronic diffuse haziness or reticularity of the lungs. The reticuloendothelioses cause an interstitial pattern that often is more prominent in the upper lung zones. The lung volumes are normal or increased, which differs from fibrotic conditions in which the lung volumes tend to be decreased.

Interstitial lung disease that predominates in the lower lobes can be seen with tuberous sclerosis, connective tissue diseases, and primary interstitial pneumonitides (e.g., desquamative, lymphocytic). Leukemia, lymphoma, and lymphatic metastases to the lungs can also cause a reticular or reticulonodular infiltrative pattern. Mycoplasmal pneumonitis sometimes presents as a unilobar reticular pattern (Fig. 51.11).

Miliary Nodules. Occasionally, interstitial disease results in tiny nodules (<5 mm in diameter), known as a miliary pattern (Table 51.5). This pattern in children is most often the result of hematogenous dissemination of tuberculosis or histoplasmosis (Fig. 51.12), although viral pneumonitis, idiopathic pulmonary hemosiderosis, and metastatic disease can also have this appearance.

HIV Infection. Patients with HIV infection are prone to be infected by opportunistic organisms. The patterns of infiltration are varied and include consolidations, reticulonodular infiltrates, and miliary infiltrates. Consolidations usually are seen with bacterial and fungal infections and only occasionally with viral infections. Reticulonodular infiltrates generally are seen with viral infections and tuberculosis. Miliary infiltrates occur with viral infections and tuberculosis. Patients with HIV infection are still infected with common organisms, except that infections occur unexpectedly or may be more pronounced.

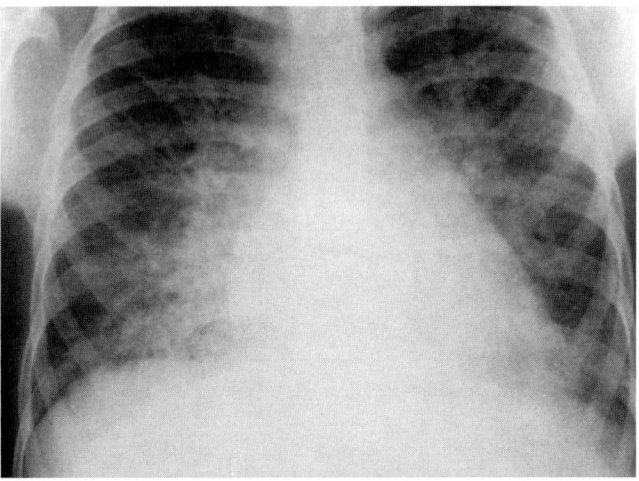

Figure 51.9. Acute Glomerulonephritis. Marked bilateral passive congestion is associated with mild cardiomegaly.

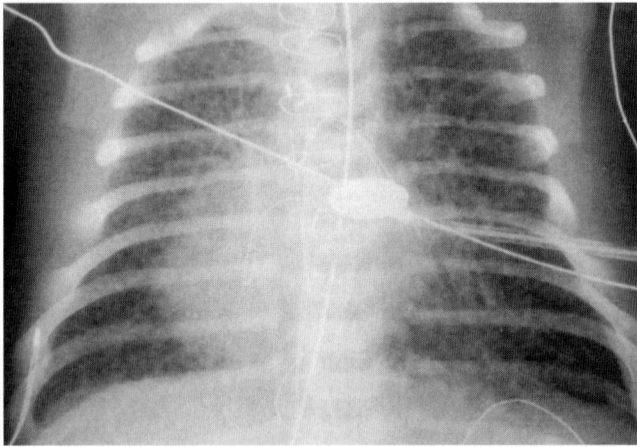

Figure 51.10. Pulmonary Lymphangiectasia. The diffuse reticulonodular pattern throughout both lungs is due to dilated lymphatics in the interstitium. Dextrocardia is also present. The patient underwent surgical repair of total anomalous pulmonary venous return, type I.

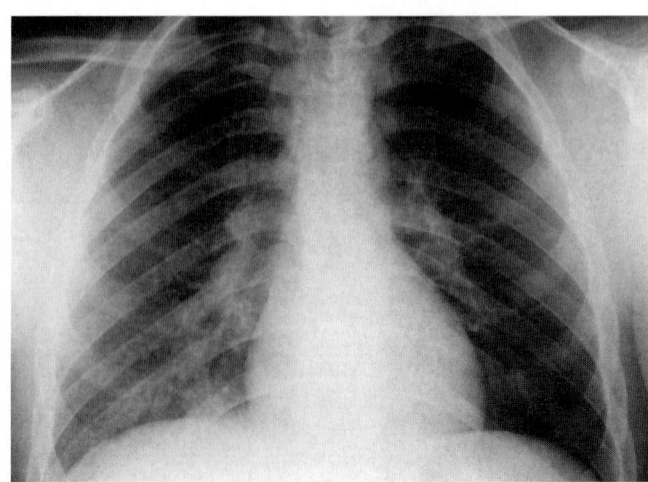

Figure 51.11. Mycoplasma Pneumonia. Reticulonodular and hazy infiltrates involve only the right lower lobe. The left lung is normal.

Table 51.5. Miliary Nodules

Infection
  Tuberculosis
  Histoplasmosis
  Viral
Idiopathic pulmonary hemosiderosis
Metastatic disease

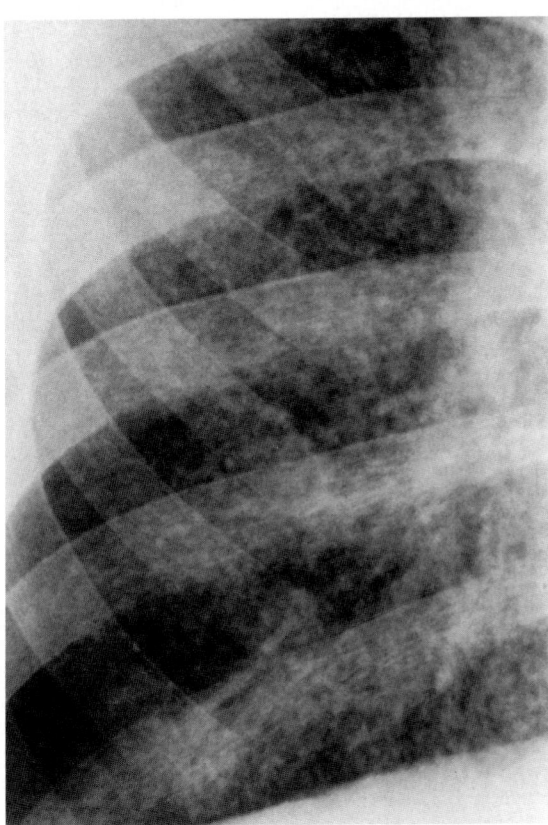

Figure 51.12. Miliary Tuberculosis. The numerous tiny nodules in the lungs of this immunosuppressed patient represent hematogenous dissemination of tuberculosis.

ABNORMALITIES OF AERATION

Pulmonary aeration abnormalities are best evaluated on the chest radiograph by observing the following criteria: *a)* the relative size of a lung or hemithorax, *b)* the degree of radiolucency of the lung, and *c)* the pulmonary vascularity or blood flow to the lung. Bilateral smallness of the lungs is commonly because of less than complete inspiration. The technical difficulties of obtaining good inspiratory chest films in children are significant. The lungs may appear small if the diaphragm is elevated either because of neuromuscular abnormality or the presence of large masses or fluid collections in the abdomen. Infrequently, inspiratory obstruction of the trachea can lead to bilateral underaeration of the lungs. Such obstruction is attributable to intratracheal masses, foreign bodies, or extrinsic compression of the trachea by anomalous vascular structures. A hyperlucent but small

hemithorax usually signifies some degree of pulmonary hypoplasia, either congenital or acquired.

Pulmonary Hypoplasia

Congenital Pulmonary Hypoplasia is associated with hypoplasia or the absence of the ipsilateral pulmonary artery; the pulmonary vessel branches will be diminished in size on the radiographs. Congenital lung hypoplasia is sometimes associated with congenital heart disease, most often tetralogy of Fallot or persistent truncus arteriosus. In cases of tetralogy of Fallot, the left lung is hypoplastic. In other patients, congenital lung hypoplasia is asymptomatic and may not be noted until later in life.

Pulmonary hypoplasia in the neonate can be unilateral or bilateral. Bilateral pulmonary hypoplasia is most often the result of compression of the lungs during fetal development. Congenital dysplasias and syndromes associated with short ribs and a small thoracic cage (asphyxiating thoracic dystrophy, thanatophoric dwarfism, Ellis-van Creveld syndrome) compress the lungs and cause hypoplastic lungs (Fig. 51.13). The degree of hypoplasia is often severe and leads to the demise of these infants. Chromosomal abnormalities such as the trisomies are associated with hypoplastic lungs, and,in some infants, hypoplasia is "primary" and unexplained (6).

The most common cause of intrathoracic compression of the fetal lungs is congenital diaphragmatic hernia. Although the hernia itself is most often unilateral, the increased volume of the thorax on the side of the hernia causes compression of the contralateral lung, resulting in bilateral and asymmetrical lung hypoplasia (Fig. 51.14). The degree of hypoplasia varies in severity; the earlier in gestation that the hernia occurs, the more severe the lung hypoplasia. Pulmonary insufficiency is the most significant cause of morbidity and mortality in

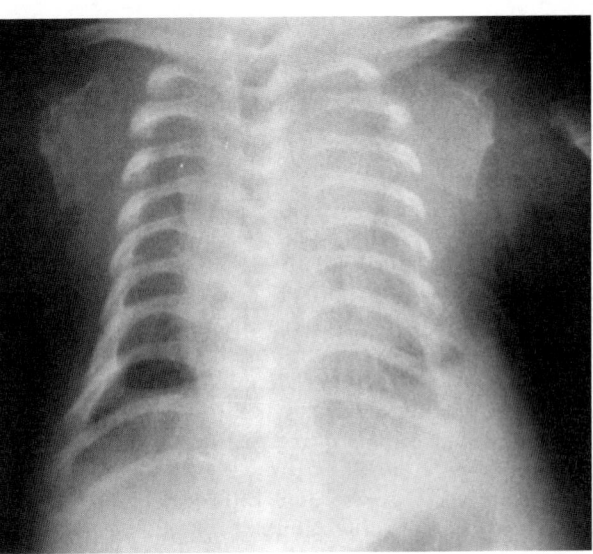

Figure 51.13. Lung Hypoplasia. The very small thoracic cage caused by rib shortening in this thanatophoric dwarf is associated with marked lung hypoplasia.

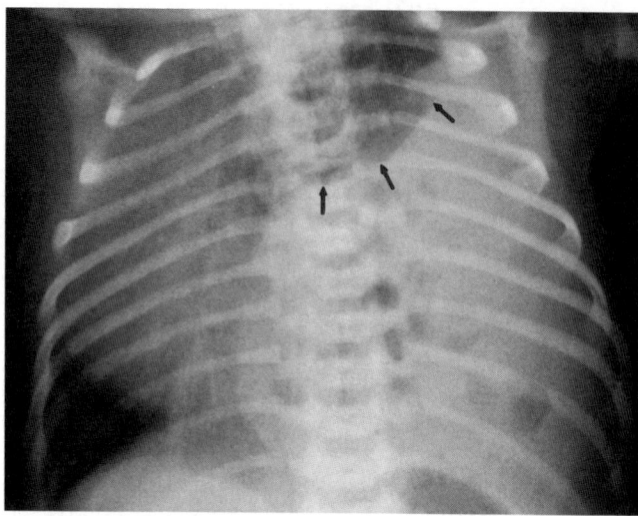

Figure 51.14. Congenital Diaphragmatic Hernia. Multiple air-filled and fluid-filled loops of bowel in the left hemithorax displace the mediastinum into the right hemithorax. Note the small, hypoplastic left lung (*arrows*).

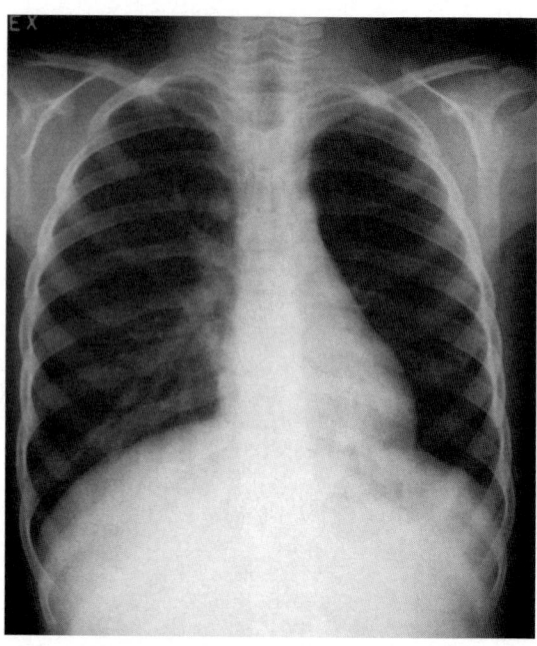

Figure 51.16. Swyer-James Lung. The left lung is small and relatively hyperlucent when compared with the right lung. The left pulmonary vascularity is decreased.

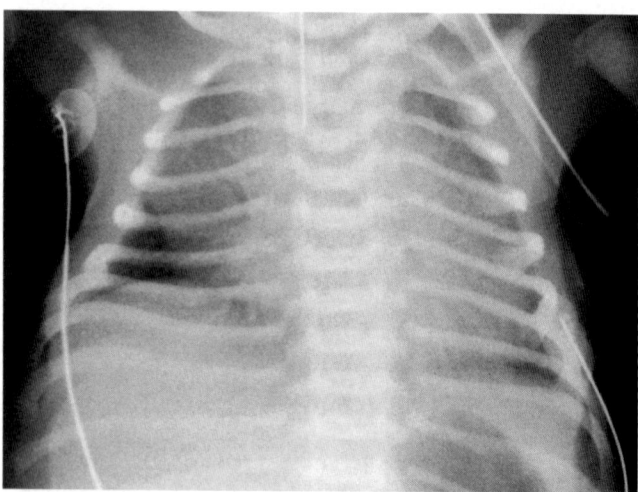

Figure 51.15. Lung Hypoplasia. Bilateral hypoplastic lungs in this newborn infant were the result of oligohydramnios due to leaking amniotic membranes.

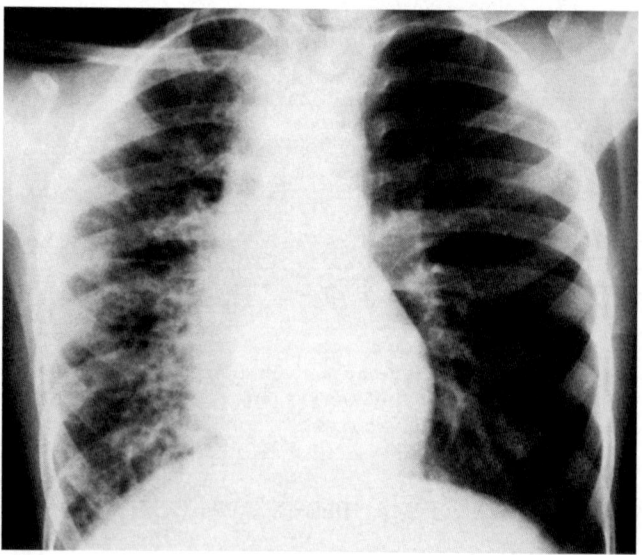

Figure 51.17. Unilateral Pulmonary Vein Atresia. The right lung is small with a diffuse reticularity that is very likely due to fibrosis from prolonged pulmonary edema and/or infection in this patient with pulmonary vein atresia on the right.

these infants. Infants with less severely hypoplastic lungs can be supported with artificial ventilation or extracorporeal membranous oxygenation (ECMO) until their lungs develop enough to permit survival. Other causes of intrathoracic compression leading to bilateral pulmonary hypoplasia include bilateral hydro-chylothorax, large intrathoracic cysts or tumors (neuroblastoma, teratoma, cystic adenomatoid malformation), or marked cardiomegaly.

Extrathoracic compression of the fetal lungs is most often because of oligohydramnios, which results from fetal urinary tract abnormalities, or abnormal amniotic fluid production or leakage (Fig. 51.15). Potter's syndrome due to bilateral renal agenesis, congenital renal cystic disease, and obstructive uropathy (posterior urethral valves, prune belly syndrome) commonly result in hypoplastic lungs. Additional causes include neuromuscular abnormalities with persistent elevation of the diaphragm or prolonged distension of the abdomen by large abdominal masses or ascites.

Swyer-James Syndrome is an acquired hypoplastic lung that develops after severe obliterative bronchiolitis with bronchiolar obstruction, bronchiectasis, and distal air-space destruction (Fig. 51.16). Air enters the lung by air-drift phenomenon but becomes trapped because of the bronchiolar obstruction. Air trapping results in a lung that changes very little in size between inspiration and expiration. This important feature distinguishes the hypoplastic Swyer-James lung from the congenitally hypoplastic lung, although it is not present in all cases. Radionuclide ventilation-perfusion studies can be used to verify the expiratory airway obstruction as well as the diminished perfusion of the hypoplastic lung. Although the Swyer-James lung is classically clear and hyperlucent, some patients show a fibrotic reticular pattern in the hypoplastic lung. Other causes of a unilateral small reticular lung include acquired hypoplasia because of radiation therapy or unilateral pulmonary vein atresia or stenosis (Fig. 51.17). The reticularity of the lung in pulmonary vein atresia results from a combination of interstitial pulmonary edema, fibrosis, and dilated interstitial lymphatics.

Table 51.6. Bilateral Lung Hyperinflation

Diffuse peripheral obstruction
  Viral bronchitis/bronchiolitis
  Asthma
  Cystic fibrosis
  Immunologic deficiency diseases
  Chronic aspiration
  Graft vs. host disease
Central obstruction
  Extrinsic
    Vascular anomalies
    Mediastinal masses
  Intrinsic
    Tracheal foreign body
    Tracheal neoplasm/granuloma

Bilateral Lung Hyperinflation

Bilateral overaeration of the lungs is most often caused by airway obstruction that can be central or diffuse and peripheral (Table 51.6).

Small Airway Obstruction. Obstructive emphysema due to widespread small airway obstruction is common and attributable to viral bronchitis and bronchiolitis, asthma, and cystic fibrosis. Acute bronchiolitis in infants often is accompanied by severe air trapping and overinflation of the lungs with little or no other visible pulmonary abnormality. Infants with cystic fibrosis can present with an appearance identical to bronchiolitis (3). Cystic fibrosis should be considered in any infant who presents with multiple episodes of bronchiolitis (Fig. 51.18). Hyperinflation tends to be less severe in older children with viral lower respiratory tract infections, but the mechanism (mucosal edema and bronchospasm secondary to inflammation) is the same. Peripheral small airway obstruction with parahilar peribronchial infiltrates is seen with certain immunologic deficiency diseases, chronic aspiration, and graft versus host disease.

Central Airway Obstruction leading to bilateral overaeration of the lungs is less common than peripheral obstruction. Intratracheal foreign bodies, neoplasms, granulomas, and intrinsic stenoses of the trachea are all rather rare. More commonly, tracheal obstruction is caused by extrinsic compression by cysts, neoplasms, adenopathy, or congenital vascular abnormalities.

A right-sided aortic arch is the key radiographic clue to the presence of a vascular lesions (Fig. 51.19). Most cases of double aortic arch consist of a large posterior, right-sided arch and a small anterior, left-sided arch that encircle the esophagus and trachea. The diagnosis may be verified by barium esophagram, which shows a reverse S-shaped indentation of the esophagus (Fig. 51.20). Lateral radiographs demonstrate the tracheal

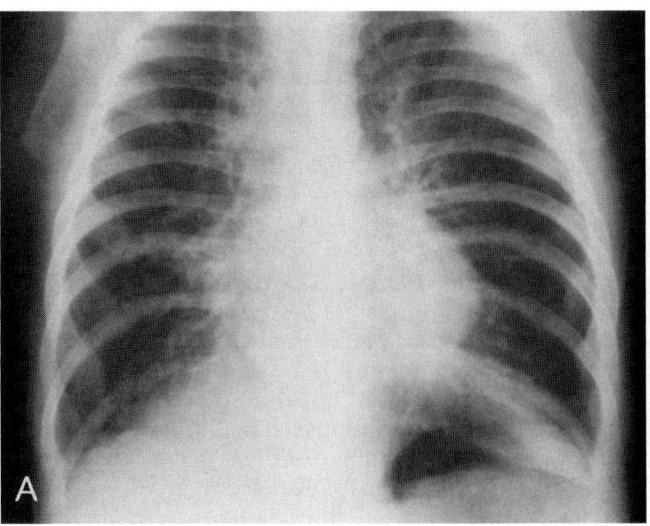
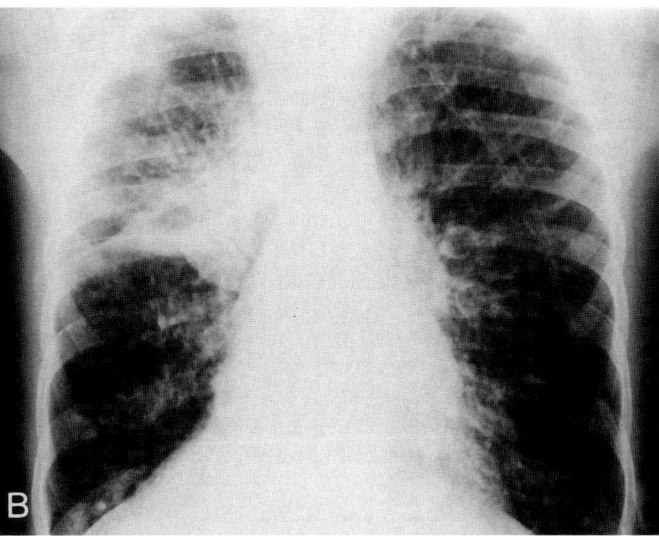

Figure 51.18. Cystic Fibrosis. A. The early stages of cystic fibrosis are often manifest only by parahilar peribronchial infiltrates and hyperinflation of the lungs. This appearance resembles that seen with viral lower respiratory tract infections or bronchiolitis. **B.** Later, the characteristic changes of end-stage cystic fibrosis are seen, including bronchial wall thickening, bronchiectasis, and persistent atelectasis.

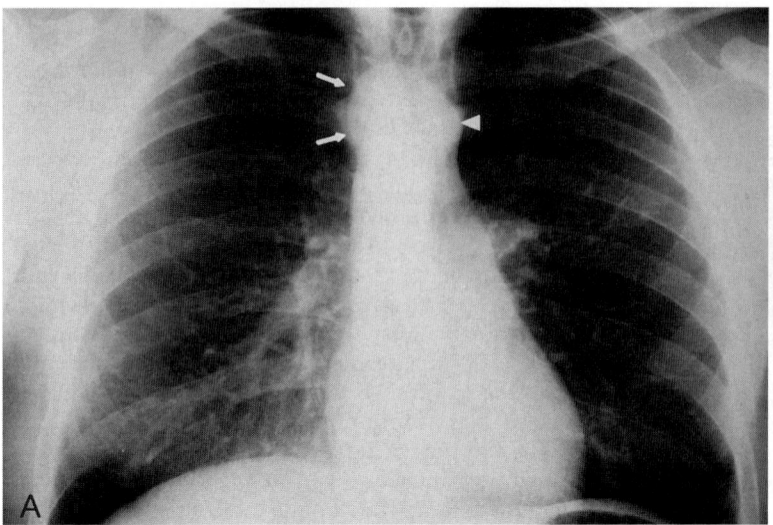

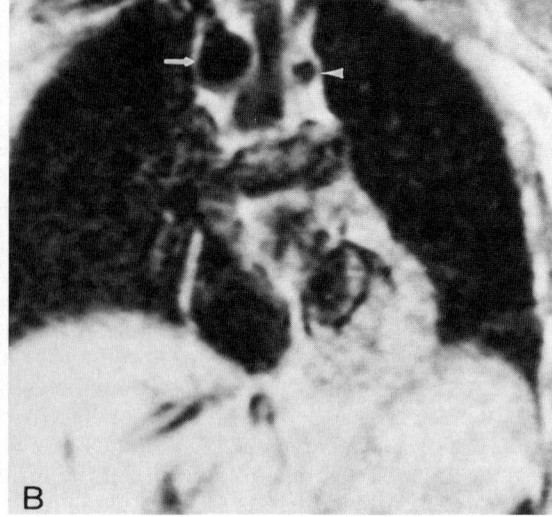

Figure 51.19. Double Aortic Arch. A. A right-sided aortic arch displaces the trachea to the left (*arrows*). A smaller nodular opacity seen to the left of the trachea is the left aortic arch (*arrowhead*).

B. Coronal MR clearly defines the large right aortic (*arrow*) and the smaller left arch (*arrowhead*), which encircle and compress the trachea.

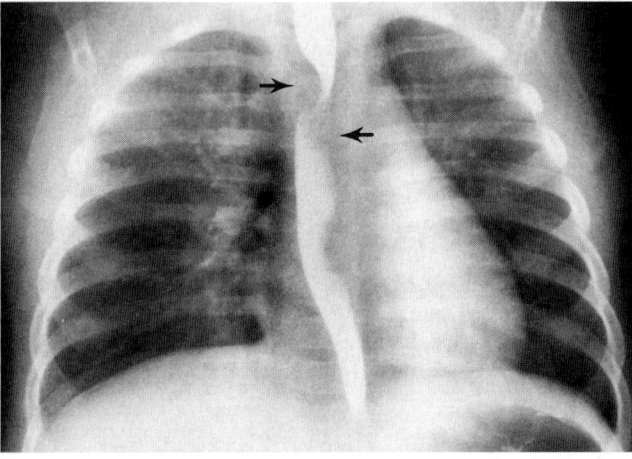

Figure 51.20. Double Aortic Arch. The encircling aortic arches compress the esophagus, creating a reverse-S configuration (*arrows*) on the barium esophogram. Note that the right arch is higher and more prominent than the left.

narrowing and posterior compression. Final diagnosis may be made with MR (Fig. 51.19).

Similar radiographic abnormalities are seen when the ring consists of a right ascending aortic arch, an aberrant left subclavian artery that passes posterior to the esophagus, and a ligamentum arteriosum or persistent ductus arteriosus stretching from the left subclavian artery to the pulmonary artery anterior to the trachea. The precise anatomy can be beautifully demonstrated by MR (Fig. 51.19)(7).

The pulmonary sling anomaly is a rare condition that may also result in tracheal compression and bilateral hyperaeration of the lungs. The left pulmonary artery arises from the right pulmonary artery, and as it courses to the left lung, it passes between the trachea and esophagus and compresses the trachea posteriorly (Fig.

51.21). The right lung may be either underaerated or overaerated.

Asymmetrical or Unilateral Aeration Abnormalities

Pulmonary aeration abnormalities are frequently asymmetrical or unilateral. A large, hyperlucent hemithorax most often indicates overinflation of an entire lobe or lung. This hyperaeration may be due to obstructive emphysema (Table 51.7) or compensatory overinflation resulting from decreased volume of the contralateral lung. The pulmonary vascularity is the key to differentiation. Obstructive emphysema generally results in diminished size of the pulmonary vessels because of compression and hypoxia-induced reflex arterial spasm (Fig. 51.22). With compensatory hyperinflation, the pulmonary vessels are normal or even increased in size. If doubt remains, inspiratory and expiratory frontal views of the chest, or fluoroscopy, can be helpful. The general rule is that the lung that does not change or changes the least in volume is the abnormal lung (Fig. 51.23). This holds true whether the lung is obstructed and overinflated or it is small because of atelectasis or hypoplasia. The only exception is mild congenital pulmonary hypoplasia, which is associated with relatively normal lung dynamics.

Congenital Lobar Emphysema consists of obstructive emphysema of a single lobe of the lung, most commonly the left upper, right upper, and right middle lobes, in this order. Usually emphysema is the result of segmental bronchial cartilage underdevelopment, which leads to expiratory airway collapse and a ball-valve type of obstruction. Early in the newborn period, the obstructed lobe may be opaque because of delayed clearance of fluid distal to the obstruction. Gradually, the fluid clears and the involved lobe becomes air-filled and overinflated (Fig. 51.24). A severely enlarged emphysematous lobe can occupy the entire hemithorax and erro-

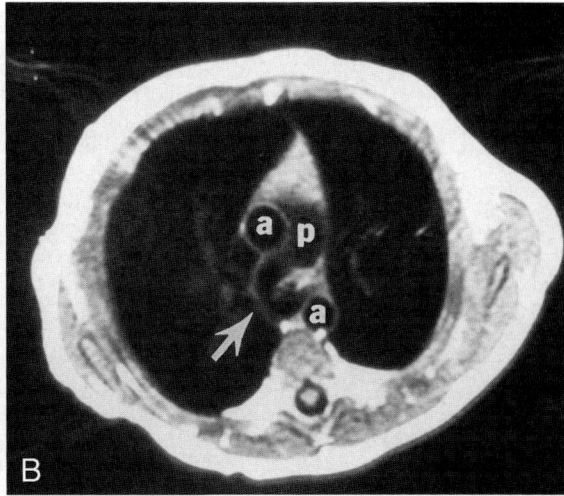

Figure 51.21. Aberrant Left Pulmonary Artery: Pulmonary Sling. A. The right lung is slightly small compared to the left. **B.** MR demonstrates the typical course of the aberrant left pulmonary artery (*arrow*). *a*; ascending and descending aorta. *p*; pulmonary artery. (From Swischuk LE. Imaging of the Newborn, Infant, and Young Child. 4th Ed. Williams & Wilkins, Baltimore, 1996.)

Table 51.7. Unilateral Obstructive Emphysema

Bronchial foreign body
Mucous plug
Congenital lobar emphysema
Bronchial stenosis/atresia
Tuberculosis
Vascular anomalies
Mediastinal masses

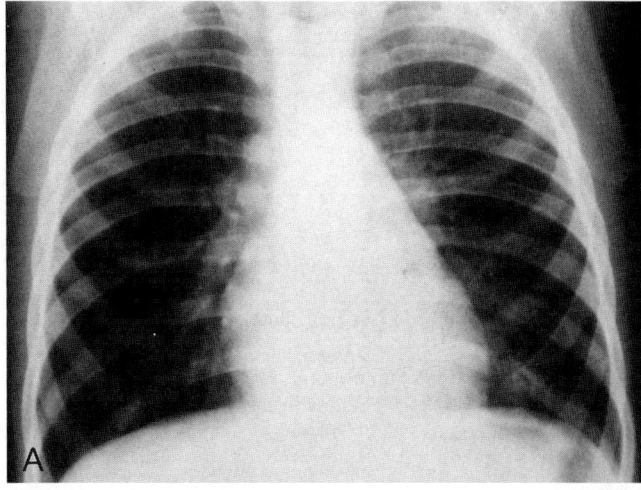

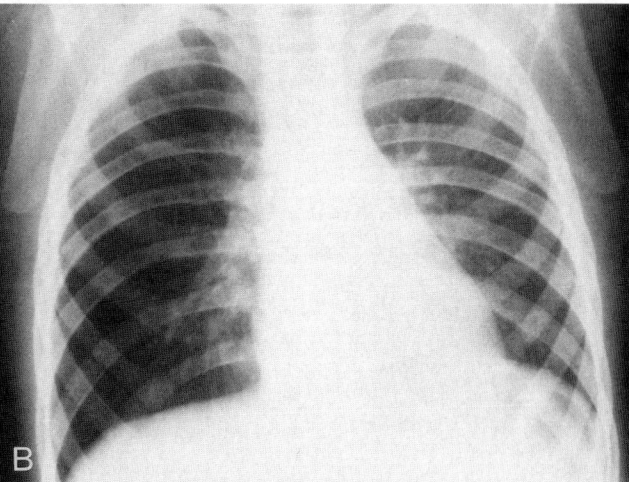

Figure 51.23. Bronchial Foreign Bodies. A. On inspiration, the right lung is slightly larger and more radiolucent than the left. **B.** With expiration, the left lung decreases in size, but the right lung remains overinflated. This indicates obstructive emphysema on the right, in this case due to pieces of walnut in the right mainstem bronchus.

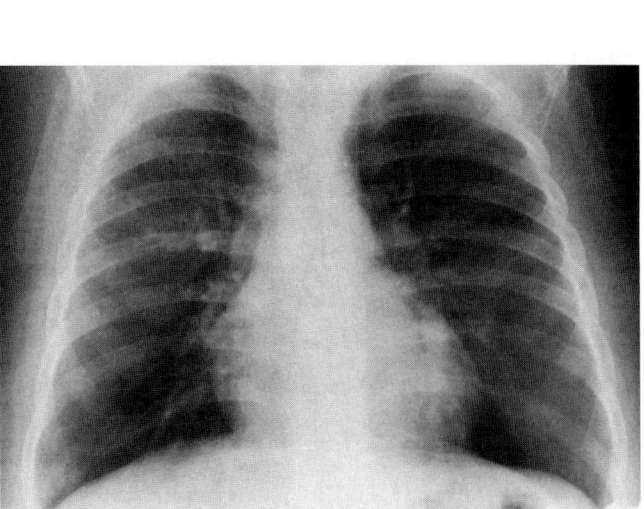

Figure 51.22. Obstructive Emphysema. The pulmonary vessels on the left are small when compared with those on the right. Bronchial obstruction was due to a mucous plug in this patient with viral bronchitis.

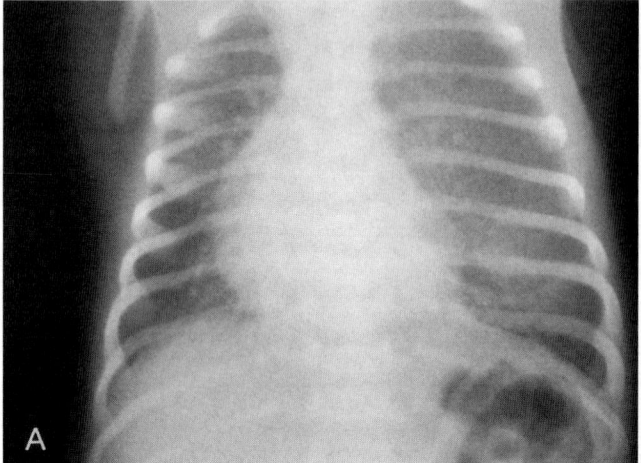

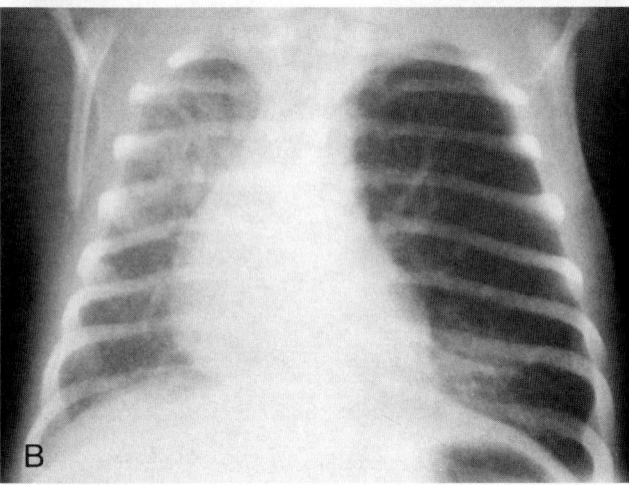

Figure 51.24. Congenital Lobar Emphysema. A. On the initial newborn film, the left upper lobe appears large and hazy because of fluid trapped in the obstructed lung. **B.** A later film shows that the fluid has cleared, leaving a typical overinflated left upper lobe with compressive atelectasis of the left lower lobe.

neously appear as a pneumothorax or of emphysema of the entire lung. Careful inspection reveals the collapsed, compressed adjacent lobes of the lung, confirming the diagnosis (Fig. 51.25). A similar appearance can occur in the rare case of bronchial stenosis or atresia. Classically, an oval opacity is seen adjacent to the overinflated lung near the hilum, representing a collection of mucus (mucocele) within the obstructed bronchus.

Endobronchial Lesions. In older infants and children, obstructive emphysema is most often the result of an endobronchial foreign body or a mucous plug (see Fig. 51.21). Mucous plugs occur most often in asthmatics and in children with viral lower respiratory tract infections. Other less common causes of unilateral obstructive emphysema include endobronchial masses

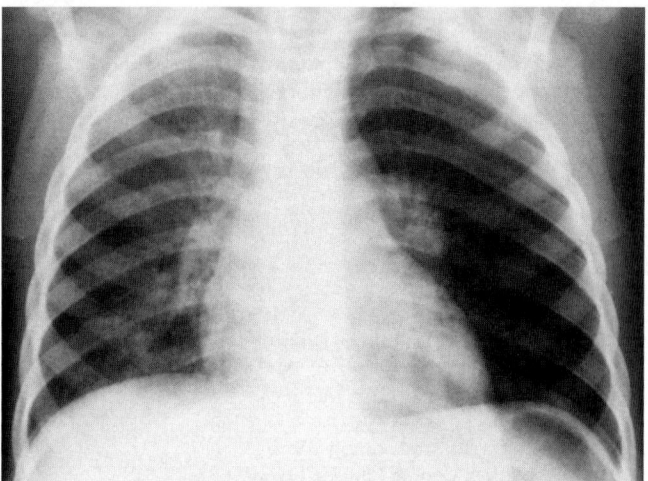

Figure 51.26. Primary Tuberculosis. Left hilar adenopathy and tuberculous granulomas of the left main bronchus cause obstructive emphysema of the left lung.

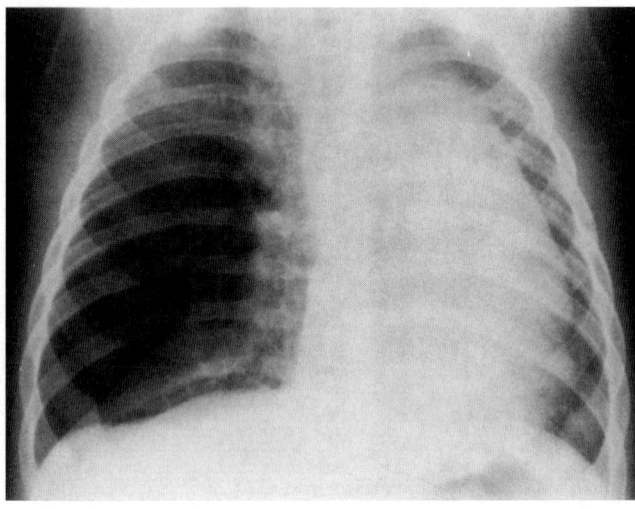

Figure 51.25. Congenital Lobar Emphysema. The right middle lobe is overinflated causing compression of the right upper and lower lobes and shift of the mediastinum to the left.

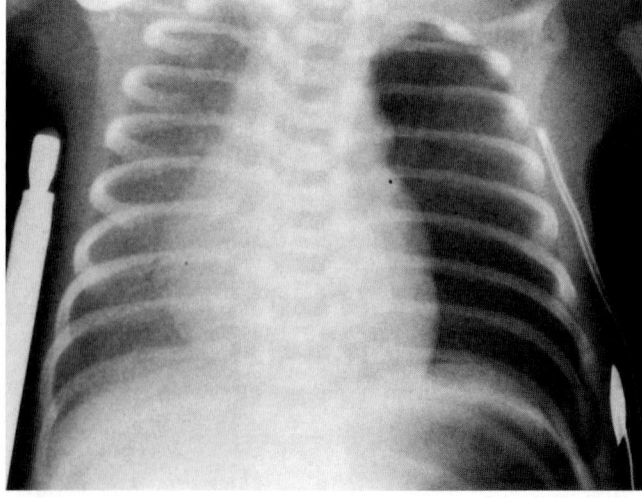

Figure 51.27. Pneumothorax in a Neonate. A left anterior pneumothorax causes increased radiolucency of the left lung and increased sharpness of the left heart border. Because the infant is supine, the free air lies anteriorly and a lateral lung edge is not visualized.

such as tuberculous granulomas (Fig. 51.26) and extrinsic compressing lesions such as anomalous blood vessels and mediastinal tumors and cysts. Pneumothorax may cause a large hyperlucent hemithorax that mimics obstructive emphysema. In supine patients, the pleural air may lie entirely along the anterior surface of the lung and no free lung edge will be visible. Clues to the presence of an anterior pneumothorax include increased radiolucency of the hemithorax with increased sharpness of the mediastinal border (Fig. 51.27). In newborns, a pneumothorax can compress the normal thymus gland, creating a mediastinal "pseudomass." Rarely, an air-filled lung cyst, or pneumatocele, or a markedly dilated stomach in a diaphragmatic hernia can occupy an entire hemithorax, rendering it hyperlucent.

PULMONARY CAVITIES

Cavities in the lungs of children are most often inflammatory or postinflammatory.

Lung Abscesses usually are a complication of a bacterial pneumonia and are frequently multiple. The wall of an abscess is thick and irregular, and some contain air-fluid levels (Fig. 51.28). An abscess may form distal to a bronchial obstruction, which in children is often due to a retained foreign body. Cavitary tuberculosis is rare in childhood and echinococcal cysts are rare outside of endemic areas.

Pneumatoceles are thin-walled lung cavities which most commonly result from pulmonary infections. Staphylococcal pneumonia is classically associated with pneumatocele formation, although they can occur with other infections, including tuberculosis (Fig. 51.29). Pneumatoceles develop from a bronchial obstruction that leads to air trapping and alveolar rupture. Pneumatoceles can become large and cause significant mass effect. More often the pneumatoceles remain relatively small and resolve spontaneously. Occasionally, pneumatoceles rupture, leading to pneumothorax or pneumomediastinum. Other causes of pneumatoceles in children include blunt chest trauma (Fig. 51.30), hydrocarbon pneumonitis, and Langerhans' cell histiocytosis.

Congenital Lung Cysts are uncommon, usually thin-walled and more commonly occur in the lower lobes. Most are asymptomatic unless they become infected or undergo rapid expansion with the development of a tension phenomenon.

Cystic Adenomatoid Malformation is a rare congenital lesion of the lung characterized by abnormal lung tissue containing dysplastic adenomatous tissue within communicating cysts of variable sizes. The radiographic appearance can vary from a predominantly solid lesion with multiple tiny cysts to multiple large thin-walled cysts that mimic congenital lobar emphysema (Fig. 51.31)(8). In the newborn period, the cysts usually are fluid-filled and the lesion has the appearance of a solid mass. With time, air replaces the fluid and small cysts become apparent. The cysts gradually enlarge and can cause enough mass effect to lead to respiratory distress. The malformation is usually unilateral and can affect any portion of the lung.

Congenital Diaphragmatic Hernia. Air-filled loops

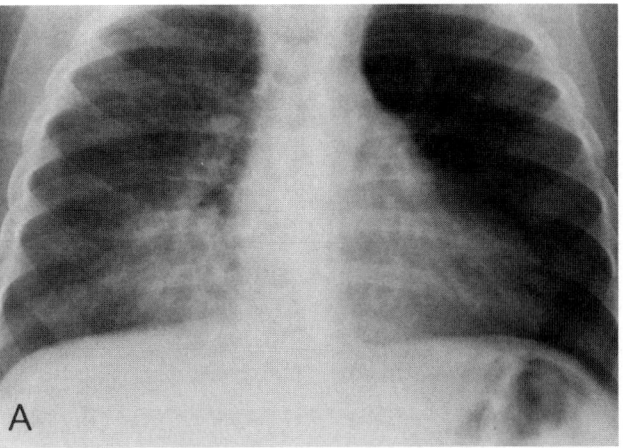

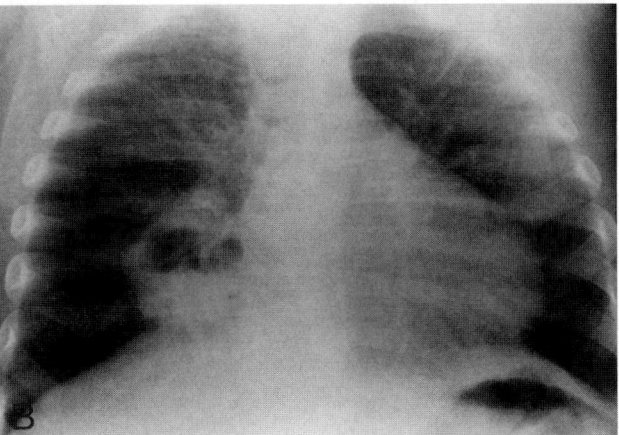

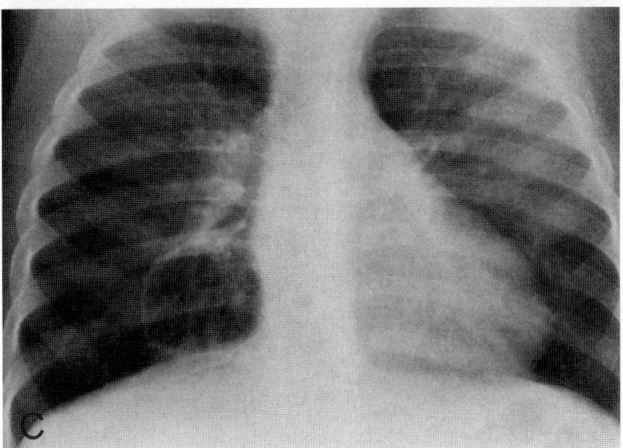

Figure 51.28. Pulmonary Abscess. A. A typical bacterial pneumonia is seen in the right middle lobe. **B.** Later, cavitation has developed in the central portion of the pneumonia and an air-fluid level is evident. This is a typical appearance for a lung abscess. **C.** With healing, the thick walls of the abscess become thin.

of bowel in a congenital diaphragmatic hernia can resemble the multiple cysts of cystic adenomatoid malformation. An important clue to the correct diagnosis of diaphragmatic hernia is the absence or paucity of gas-filled bowel loops within the abdomen (Fig. 51.32). Congenital diaphragmatic hernias most often occur through the foramen of Bochdalek, which lies posteriorly and laterally in each hemidiaphragm. Left-sided hernias

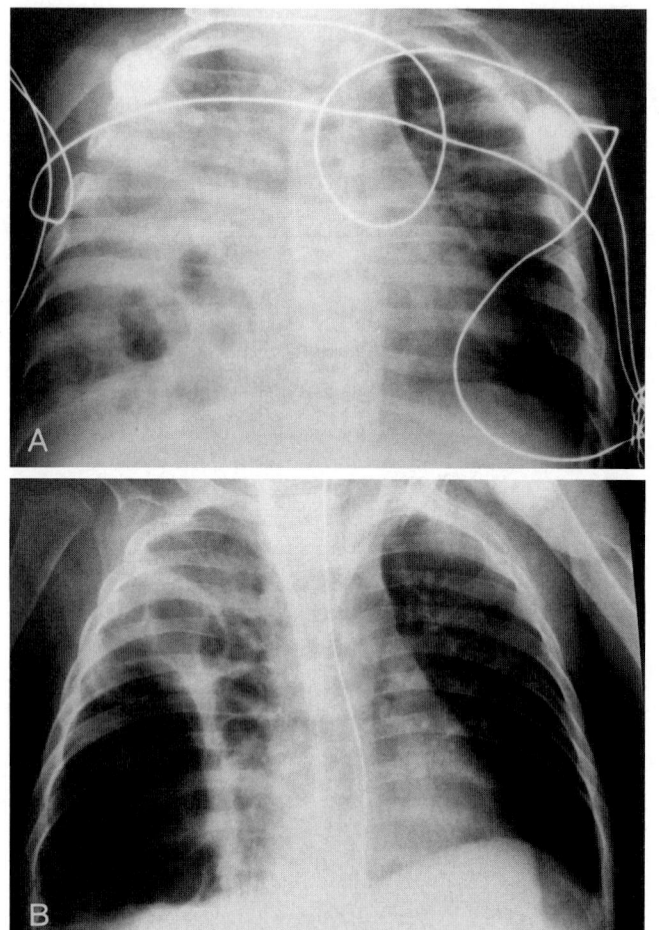

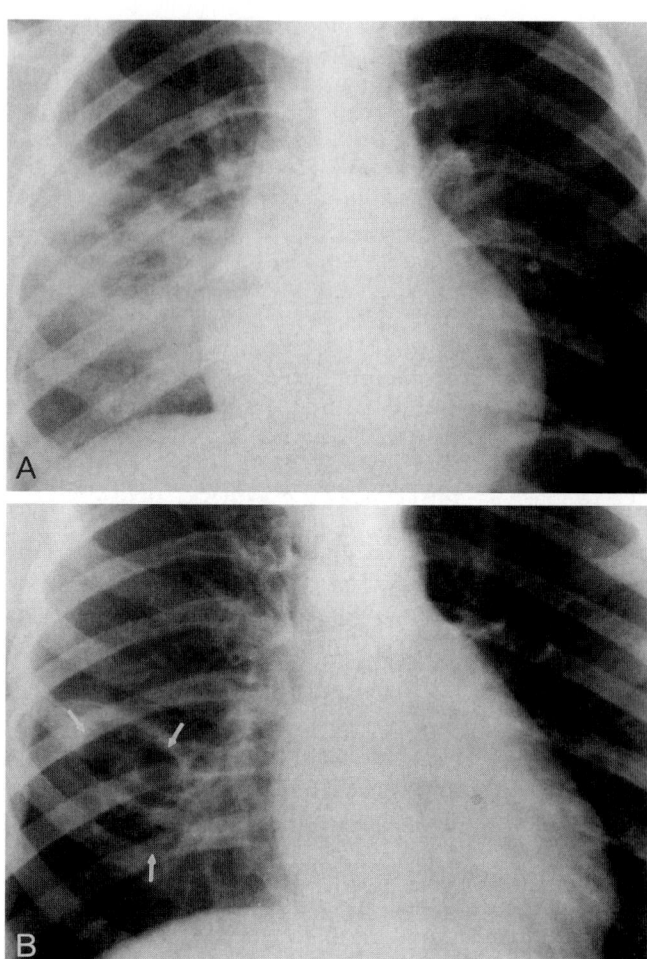

Figure 51.29. Postinflammatory Pneumatocele. A. Large air spaces are developing within consolidated right lung due to progressive primary tuberculosis. **B.** A later radiograph shows marked enlargement of the pneumatoceles.

Figure 51.30. Posttraumatic Pneumatocele. A. A motor vehicle accident resulted in a right lung contusion. **B.** After the contusion resolves, a thin-walled pneumatocele remains (*arrows*).

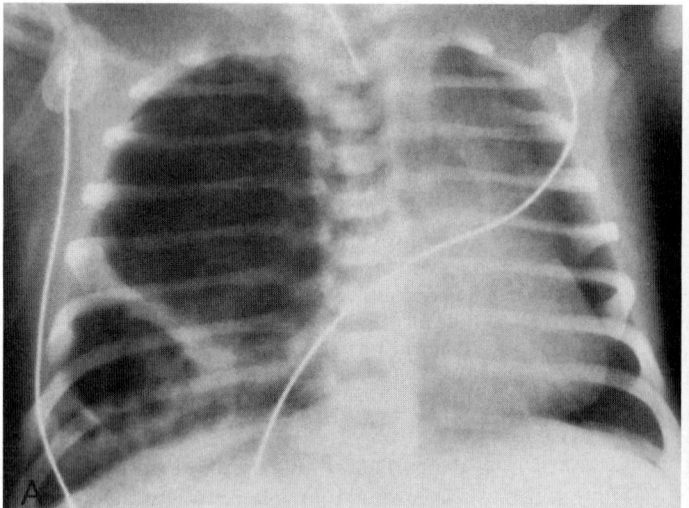

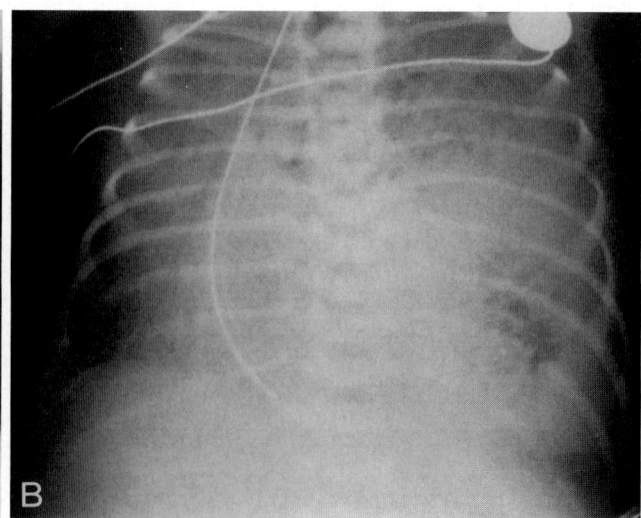

Figure 51.31. Cystic Adenomatoid Malformation. A. Multiple air-filled cysts of widely variable size expand the right lung and shift the mediastinum to the left. **B.** In another patient, the congenital mal-formation is predominantly solid or fluid-filled, with multiple, small air-filled cysts of varying sizes. Note that the mass in the left lung displaces the mediastinum and nasogastric tube to the right.

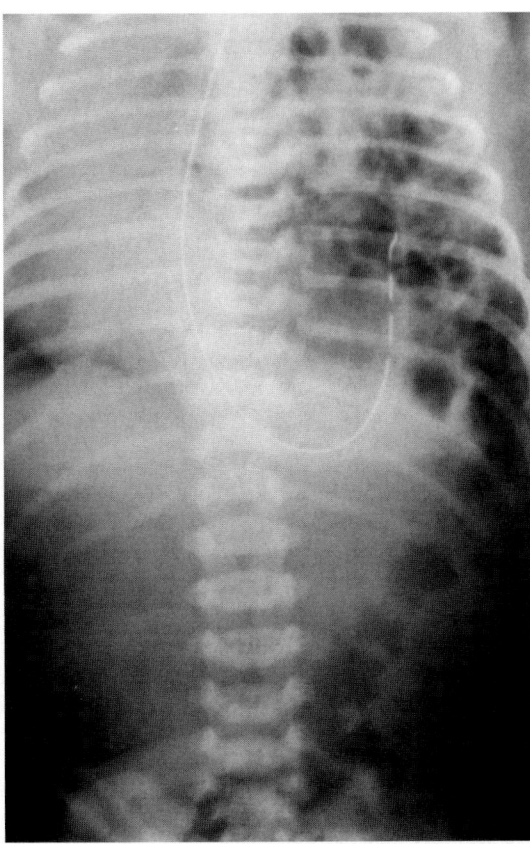

Figure 51.32. Congenital Diaphragmatic Hernia. The left hemithorax is filled with multiple air-filled loops of bowel, displacing the mediastinum to the right. The course of the nasogastric tube and the absence of normal bowel loops are clues to the diagnosis.

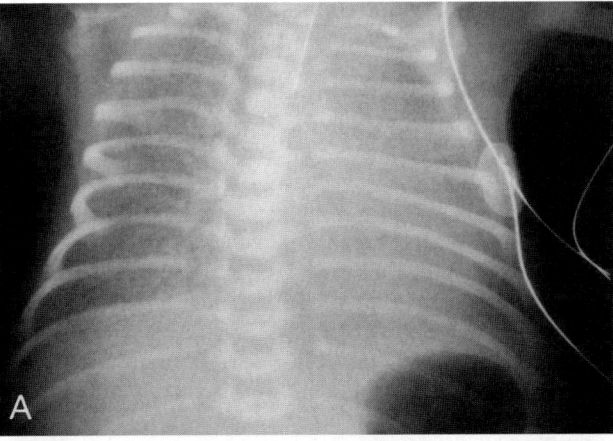

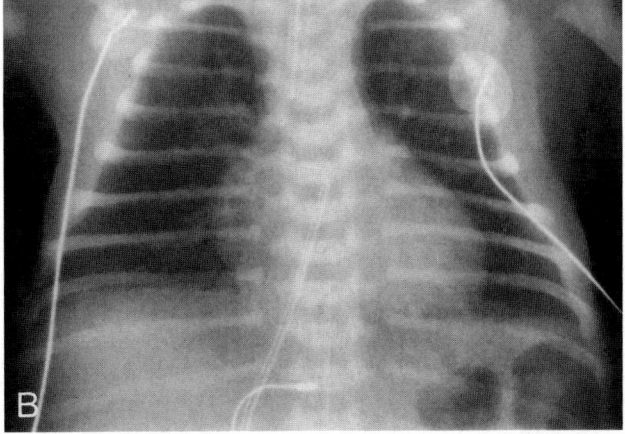

Figure 51.33. Surfactant Deficiency Disease. A. Shortly after birth, the lungs are small and diffusely opaque with air bronchograms that extend into the periphery of the lung. This is a typical appearance for surfactant deficiency disease. **B.** After treatment with endotracheal surfactant, the lung volumes have dramatically improved and lung opacity has virtually disappeared.

are much more common. Hernias through the foramen of Morgagni, which lies anteriorly, are less common and usually are less severe. Infants with large diaphragmatic hernias usually present with severe respiratory distress immediately after birth. Compression of the ipsilateral lung in utero causes it to be hypoplastic, and often the contralateral lung is also small. The patients are profoundly hypoxic, and persistent fetal circulation due to hypoxia-induced pulmonary hypertension usually further compromises the infant's condition. Even with early diagnosis and surgery, the mortality of this condition remains high. ECMO has been helpful in some patients by circumventing the problem of pulmonary hypertension and the right-to-left shunting of blood away from the lungs. Congenital diaphragmatic hernia may present later in life more frequently than generally appreciated (9–11).

LUNG DISEASE IN THE NEONATE

The conditions leading to respiratory distress in the newborn infant are numerous and can be divided into those treated medically and those requiring surgical intervention. Surgical conditions consist primarily of congenital and developmental abnormalities that result in a space-occupying lesion within the chest (diaphragmatic hernia, congenital lobar emphysema, chylothorax, pneu-

mothorax, cystic adenomatoid malformation). This section will deal with pulmonary parenchymal disease of the newborn.

Surfactant Deficiency Disease (hyaline membrane disease) is one of the most common causes of respiratory distress in the newborn (12,13). It is most common in premature infants, however, it occasionally occurs in term infants of diabetic mothers. In both cases, lung immaturity is the main predisposing factor. The primary abnormality is a lack of surfactant normally produced by the type II alveolar cells. This substance is responsible for decreasing the surface tension of the alveoli. When absent, the alveoli are poorly distensible and remain collapsed. A cycle of hypoxia, acidosis, and diminished perfusion results. Clinically, these infants present with respiratory distress within the first few hours after birth. The classic radiographic findings of surfactant deficiency disease consist of lungs that are small in volume and have a finely granular pattern with air bronchograms that extend into the lung periphery (Fig. 51.33). The granular pattern reflects the histologic findings of distended alveolar ducts and terminal bronchioles superimposed over generalized alveolar collapse. When the alveolar and terminal bronchials overdistend, small, round, 1–2 mm bubbles result. During expiration, the air bronchograms and granular pattern disappear and the lungs become totally opaque. Currently, with surfactant therapy, these changes are very transient (Fig. 51.33).

Similar lung opacities can be seen with neonatal pneumonia, pulmonary lymphangiectasia, neonatal-retained fluid syndrome, and congenital heart abnormalities associated with severe pulmonary venous obstruction. However, unlike patients with hyaline membrane disease, the lung volumes in these conditions are normal to increased (Fig. 51.34). In a few cases of neonatal pneumonia, the lung pattern is indistinguishable from respiratory distress syndrome. Until recently, the primary form of therapy of this condition consisted of positive pressure-assisted ventilation, which attempts to force

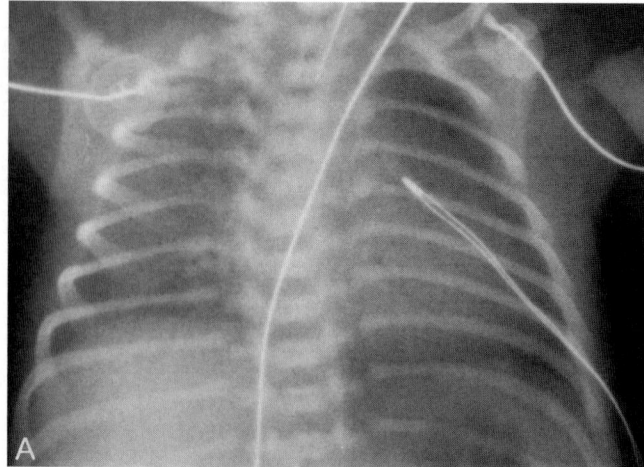

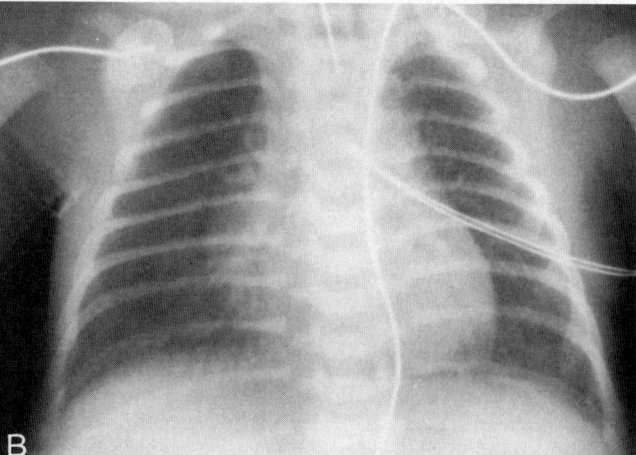

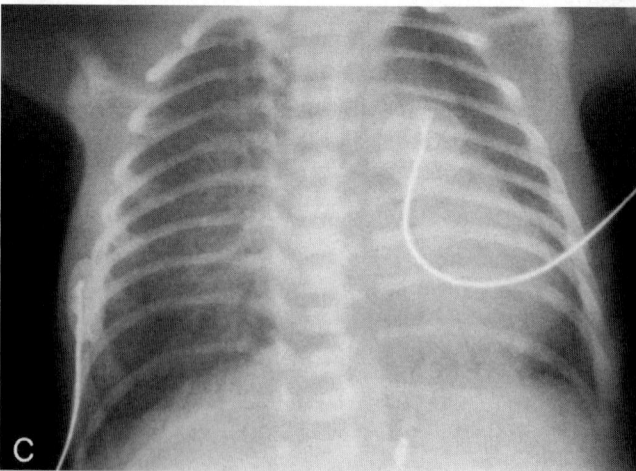

Figure 51.36. Patent Ductus Arteriosus in Surfactant Deficiency Disease. A. Newborn films showed typical small granular lungs due to hyaline membrane disease. **B.** Following surfactant therapy, the lungs increased in volume and became clear. **C.** A few days later, the heart has enlarged and, although the lungs have increased in volume, they have also become more opaque. The lung opacity represents pulmonary edema due to the development of a patent ductus arteriosus.

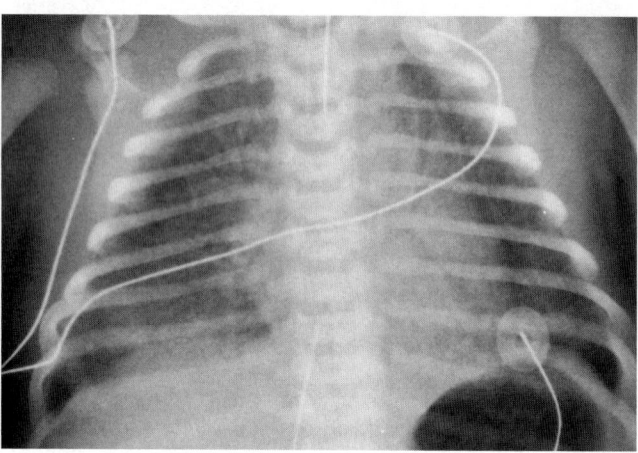

Figure 51.34. Neonatal Pneumonia. The lungs are diffusely hazy with a granular appearance that is similar to that seen with surfactant deficiency disease. Note, however, that the lungs are normal in volume.

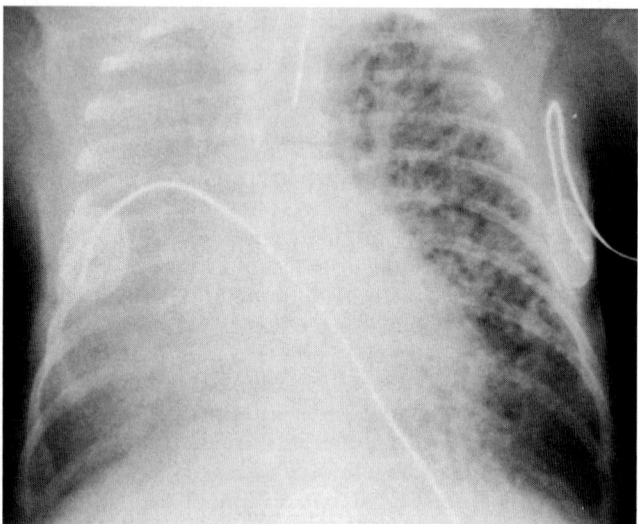

Figure 51.35. Pulmonary Interstitial Emphysema. Serpiginous bubbles of interstitial air extend to the periphery of the left lung. The interstitial air causes the lung to be stiff and hyperexpanded, even during expiration.

air deeper into the respiratory tree and alveoli. Although in some patients the use of assisted ventilation significantly improves oxygenation, in others, the elevated airway pressures result in complications due to air leakage from the distended terminal airways. Air dissects through the interstitium and lymphatics (pulmonary interstitial emphysema), creating a radiographic pattern of serpiginous bubbles that extends all the way to the lung periphery (Fig. 51.35). Unlike the air bronchograms of uncomplicated hyaline membrane disease, the bubbles of pulmonary interstitial emphysema do not collapse upon expiration. Pneumomediastinum and pneumothorax are other common complications of positive pressure ventilation. Air also can dissect into the pericardium and peritoneum, and occasionally air embolism can develop with devastating consequences. All complications are now much less commonly encountered because of the advent of surfactant therapy.

The hypoxemia associated with the respiratory distress syndrome sometimes leads to persistent patency of the ductus arteriosus. Often radiographic changes are the first clue to this complication. Suggestive findings include lungs that are large and increasingly opaque with loss of the granular pattern, cardiomegaly, and pulmonary vascular congestion (Fig. 51.36). The increased lung opacity is due to pulmonary edema. Neurogenic pulmonary edema, due to cerebral hypoxic injury and hemorrhage, is a common noncardiac cause of pulmonary edema in the premature infant.

Bronchopulmonary Dysplasia. Continued use of positive pressure-assisted ventilation and high oxygen concentration damages the lung parenchyma and results in the condition known as bronchopulmonary dysplasia (BPD). Initially described in four stages, now most authors recognize an edematous phase and a bubbly phase. The initial edematous phase results from oxygen toxicity and hypoxia. Damage to the basement membrane of the capillaries causes them to leak fluid into the interstitium of the lungs. The lungs become hazy and in some cases even reticular. The hazy pattern is most common currently encountered in premature infants.

Because there is no dysplasia in this phase, it has been suggested that this phase be termed the "**leaky lung syndrome**" (12,13). Pathophysiologically this phase of the disease resembles the acquired respiratory distress syndrome (ARDS).

The leaky lung syndrome can occur in conjunction with the bubbly phase of BPD (Fig. 51.37). However, in most cases the conditions are somewhat separated. The bubbly phase results from the overdistention of some alveolar groups while others remain atelectatic. Originally believed to be exclusively a late stage, it is now known that bubbly lungs can occur early, even within days after birth (14). The problem even can be seen in patients who are born with clear lungs and who do not have surfactant deficiency disease. These patients resemble those with the Wilson-Mikity syndrome. Possibly, both conditions result the same phenomenon of overdistention of certain alveolar groups with remaining atelectasis in other alveolar groups. Why this occurs is not known but it is related to structural pulmonary immaturity of the lungs and both result in chronic pulmonary disease.

The edematous phase of BPD is treated with fluid restriction, diuretics and, in advanced cases, the administration of steroids. The latter heals the basement membrane of the capillaries and stops the oozing of fluid into the interstitium. The bubbly phase is treated by decreasing positive pressures on the airway.

The radiographic findings of BPD consist of overaerated lungs with bubbles of varying size (Fig. 51.38). The findings are similar in the Wilson-Mikity syndrome except that in the early stages, with rapid onset, the bubbles tend to be smaller. In other cases, the bubbly pattern is less pronounced, but pulmonary fibrosis and scattered areas of segmental atelectasis are seen.

Retained Lung Fluid is also known as wet lung disease, transient tachypnea of the newborn, and transient respiratory distress of the newborn. However, the problem is simply retained lung fluid. In some cases the lungs are reticular in appearance while in others they are diffusely hazy. Other conditions can produce these

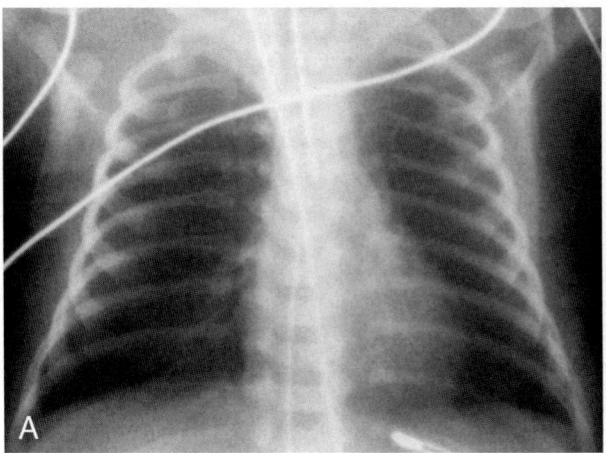
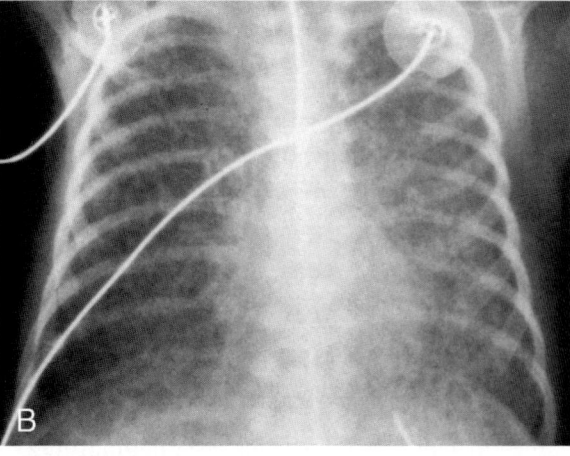

Figure 51.37. Leaky Lung Syndrome. A. A premature infant is born with clear lungs. **B.** A few days later, the lungs, although well expanded, are hazy to opaque. This is due to pulmonary edema as seen in the leaky lung syndrome. Early bubble formation, characteristic of bronchopulmonary dysplasia, is also present.

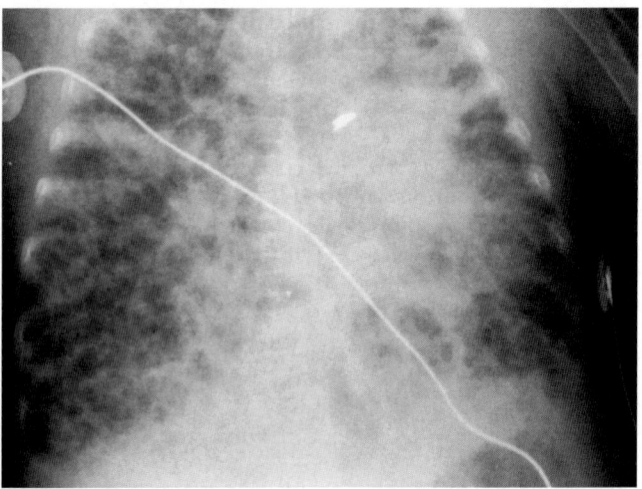

Figure 51.38. Bronchopulmonary Dysplasia. Bubbly appearance, with bubbles of various sizes, is typical of advanced bronchopulmonary dysplasia.

Table 51.8. Diffusely Hazy or Reticular Lungs (Neonate)

Decreased lung volumes
  Poor inspiration
  Hyaline membrane disease
Normal-to-increased lung volumes
  Retained fluid
  Aspiration (amniotic fluid/meconium)
  Pneumonia
  Pulmonary edema
  Pulmonary lymphangiectasia

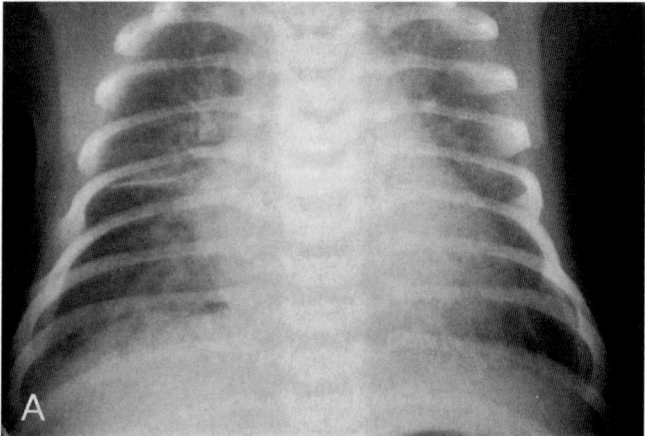

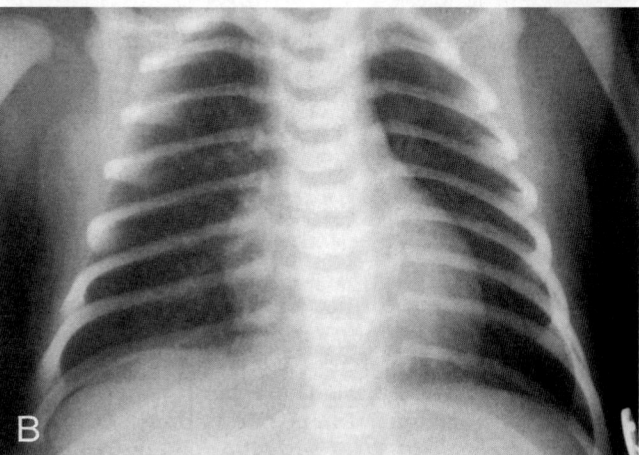

Figure 51.39. Retained Fluid Syndrome. A. On the first day of life, the chest radiograph of this term newborn shows diffuse lung haziness, streaky parahilar opacities, and bilateral pleural effusions. **B.** The following day, all of these abnormalities have resolved. This is the typical sequence of events in an infant with retained lung fluid.

patterns (Table 51.8), but the most common is the retained fluid syndrome. It occurs in otherwise normal, term infants and is especially common in infants delivered by cesarean section, due to the lack of squeezing of the chest as it passes through the vaginal canal.

In some cases the streaky parahilar opacities resembles pneumonia, while in other cases granularity of the lungs, resembles surfactant deficiency disease. In all cases the lungs are overaerated and the findings are bilateral. The findings are transient and disappear in 24-48 hours (Figs. 51.39, 51.40).

Meconium Aspiration. Intrauterine fetal distress can lead to the passage of meconium which can be aspirated into the tracheobronchial tree. Aspirated meconium particles cause obstruction of small peripheral bronchioles, resulting in unevenly distributed areas of subsegmental atelectasis with alternating areas of overdistension. This creates a coarsely reticulonodular or nodular appearance of the lungs (Fig. 51.41). In some infants, mostly fluid is aspirated resulting in rapid radiographic clearing with little residual air trapping. In severe cases, air trapping results in complications such as pneumothorax and pneumomediastinum. Because of the resulting hypoxia, persistent fetal circulation is also a common complication (see "Patent Ductus Artesiosus"). Treatment

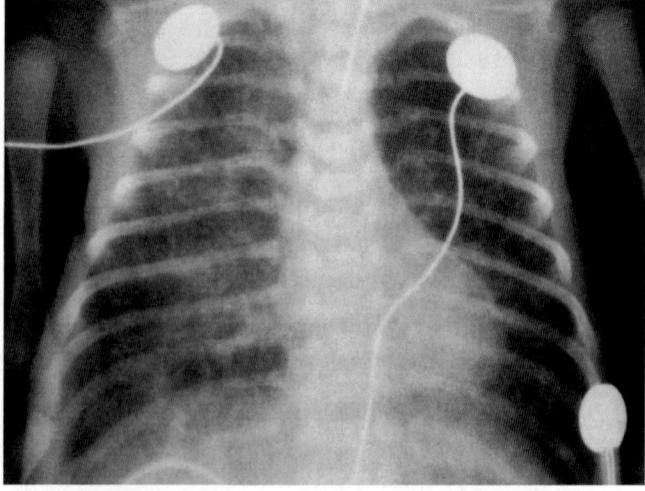

Figure 51.40. Neonatal Pneumonia. In this patient with neonatal pneumonia, the diffuse reticular pattern in both lungs resembles retained fluid. Early alveolar changes are present in the central regions of the right lung.

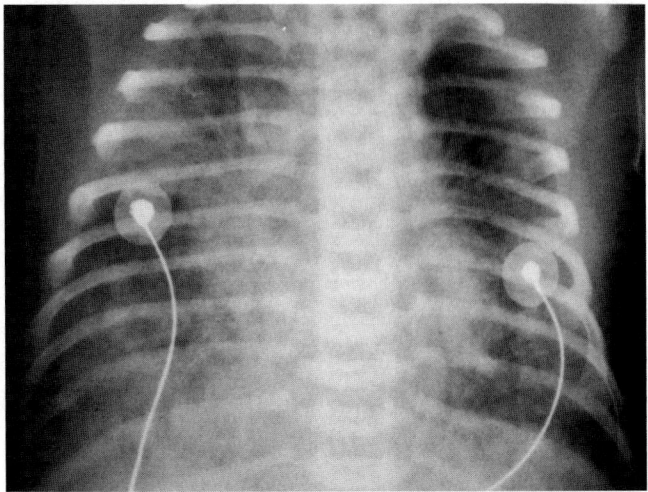

Figure 51.41. Meconium Aspiration. A coarse, reticulonodular pattern throughout both lungs is typical of meconium aspiration.

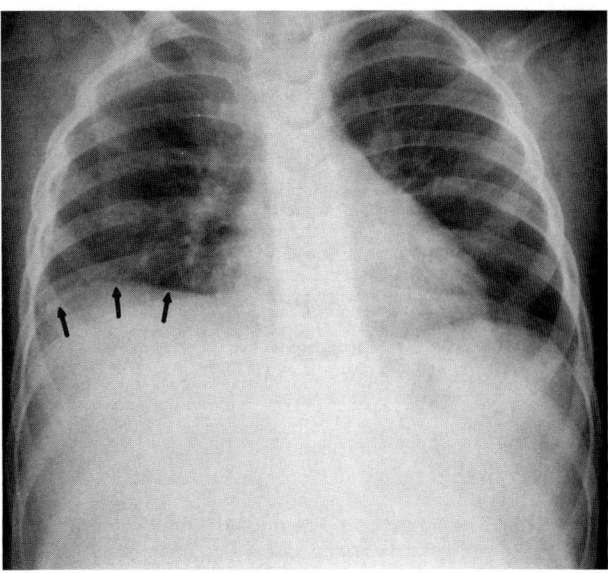

Figure 51.42. Right Pleural Effusion. Flattening and lateral displacement of curvature of the right hemidiaphragm (*arrows*), indicates the presence of subpulmonic pleural fluid.

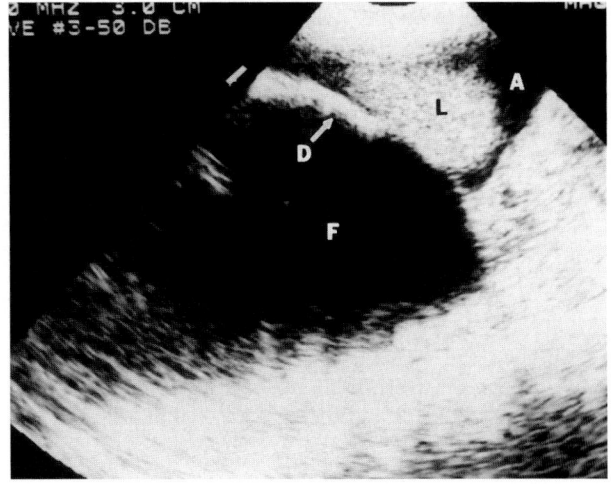

Figure 51.43. Chylothorax. US identifies fluid in the pleural space (*F*) as well as ascites (*A*) surrounding the liver (*L*). D, diaphragm.

consists of endotracheal suctioning and the administration of humidified oxygen.

Pulmonary Lymphangiectasia is a rare condition that can occur as an isolated abnormality or be associated with congenital heart disease or generalized lymphangiectasia (see Fig. 51.10). The isolated form results from abnormal pulmonary lymphatic development with dilated and obstructed lymphatic channels. The lungs often are hyperinflated and pleural effusions may also occur. Lymphangiectasia associated with congenital heart disease usually is seen with conditions leading to severe pulmonary venous obstruction (i.e., hypoplastic left heart syndrome, total anomalous pulmonary venous return type III, or pulmonary vein atresia).

ECMO is becoming more widely used for the support of infants with life-threatening respiratory disease. The technique consists of a bypass of the pulmonary blood flow through a semipermeable silicon membrane. The procedure interrupts the cycle of pulmonary hypertension and persistent fetal circulation (right-to-left shunting) and diminishes the damaging effect of high oxygen concentrations and barotrauma to the lungs. ECMO is commonly used in patients with congenital diaphragmatic hernia, surfactant deficiency disease, meconium aspiration syndrome, neonatal sepsis and pneumonia. While on the extracorporeal circuit, the lungs invariably become completely opaque because the lungs collapse (15). Occasionally, pleural effusions will also be present but are obscured on chest radiographs by the opacity of the lungs. In such cases, the lungs often fail to re-expand despite increasing ventilator pressures. US can be used to identify the pleural fluid.

PLEURAL THICKENING AND EFFUSIONS

Generalized thickening of the pleural space because of the accumulation of fluid has the same configurations in children as in adults. The most easily recognized pattern is thickening along the lateral and apical portions of the lung. Subpulmonic collections can mimic an elevated diaphragm, but characteristic flattening and laterally displaced curvature of the dome are clues to the presence of subpulmonic pleural fluid (Fig. 51.42). A totally opaque hemithorax of normal or increased volume is nearly always due to a large collection of pleural fluid. Opacification of an entire lung by pneumonia is very unusual in children. However, occasionally a large cyst or intrathoracic mass can occupy most of the hemithorax. In such cases one should look for residual radiolucency in the costophrenic angle, which is not present when pleural fluid is the cause of total opacification of a hemithorax. The presence of pleural fluid is easily verified by US (Fig. 51.43). The type of fluid in the pleural space (serous effusion, inflammatory exudate, chyle, or blood) cannot be determined radiographically.

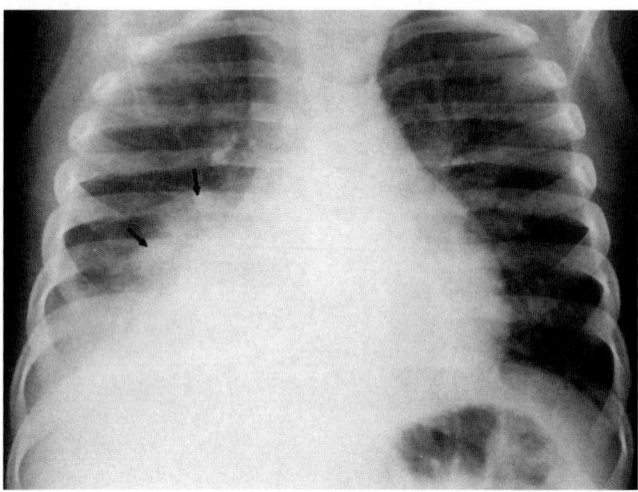

Figure 51.44 Pneumococcal Pneumonia with Pleural Effusion. A right pleural effusion partially obscures the consolidating pneumonia of the right middle lobe (*arrows*). The right hemidiaphragm is obscured by the effusion.

Table 51.9. Pleural Effusions

Unilateral
  Pneumonia/empyema
  Chylothorax
  Iatrogenic
  Trauma
  Intraabdominal inflammation
  Intrathoracic neoplasm
  Ruptured aneurysm of ductus arteriosus
Bilateral
  Renal disease
  Lymphoma
  Neuroblastoma
  Congestive heart failure
  Collagen vascular diseases
  Fluid overload

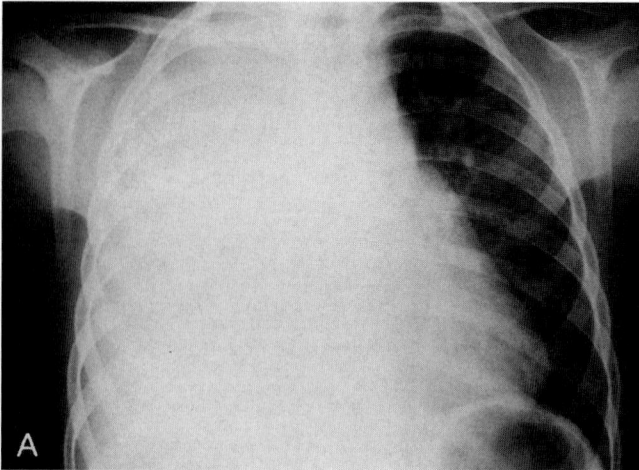

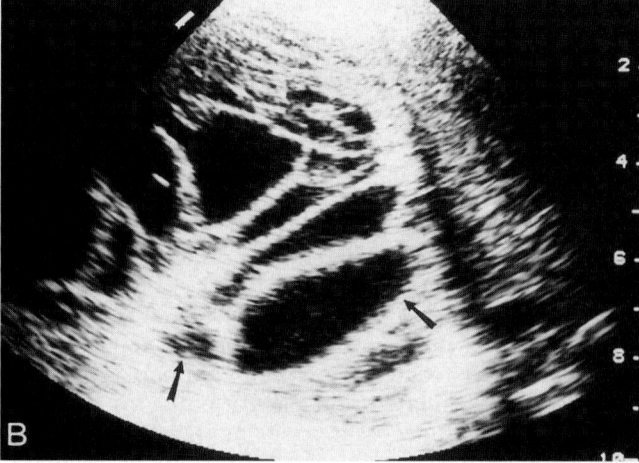

Figure 51.45. Empyema. A. The entire right hemithorax is opacified with shift of the mediastinum to the left. **B.** US confirms a large collection of fluid (pus) in the right pleural space with multiple thick septations (*arrows*).

Unilateral Pleural Effusions are most commonly associated with pneumonia in the ipsilateral lung (Fig. 51.44 and Table 51.9). Such effusions are often transudates, but empyema is likely if the collection is large (Fig. 51.45). Empyemas most often occur with staphylococcal, *Haemophilus*, and pneumococcal pneumonias. Serous effusions may be seen with a variety of infections, including mycoplasma. Inflammation below the diaphragm, particularly abscesses or pancreatitis can also result in pleural effusions. Rarely, a unilateral effusion will accompany an intrathoracic tumor that involves the pleura (Fig. 51.46).

Bilateral Serous Pleural Effusions are most commonly seen in patients with renal diseases such as acute glomerulonephritis or nephrotic syndrome, lymphoma (usually non-Hodgkin's) (Fig. 51.47), or neuroblastoma. Congestive heart failure, collagen vascular diseases, and fluid overload may also result in pleural effusions.

Hemothorax is usually the result of trauma, either direct chest wall trauma with or without rib fractures, or aortic rupture from deceleration injury. Occasionally, bleeding disorders can also result in hemothorax. Rarely, an aneurysm of the ductus arteriosus can rupture and bleed into the pleural space.

Chylothorax is the most common cause of massive pleural effusion in the neonate. Chylous effusions are usually unilateral and right-sided (Fig. 51.48). The cause of chylothorax is uncertain but likely possibilities are traumatic tear or congenital defect of the thoracic duct. Chylous effusions that occasionally result from superior vena cava thrombosis are more difficult to manage. Pulmonary lymphangiectasia is a rare cause of chylothorax. Most chylothoraces resolve following thoracentesis, although occasionally chest tube drainage is required.

Complications of Indwelling Catheters in thoracic vessels are a relatively common and iatrogenic cause of pleural fluid (16,17).

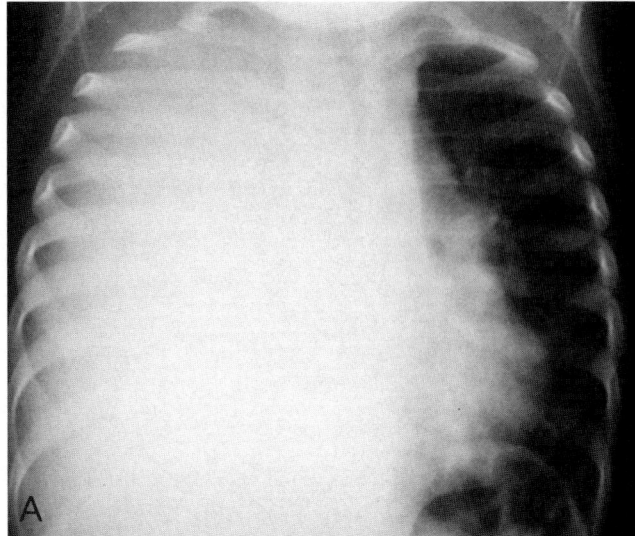

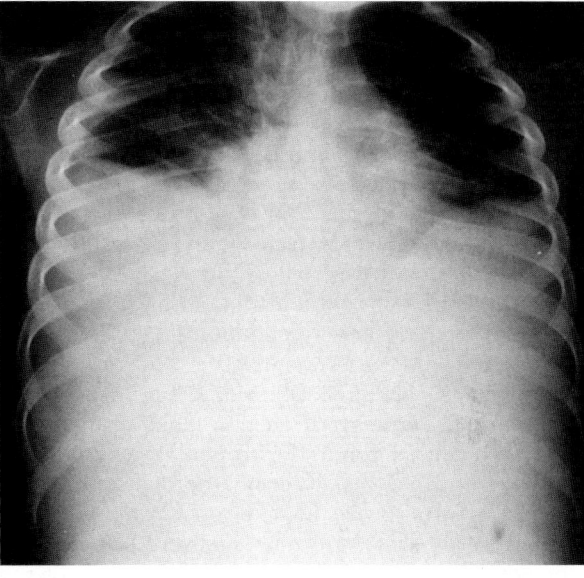

Figure 51.46. Pleural Effusion Associated with a Thoracic Neoplasm. A. Pleural fluid causes complete opacification of the right hemithorax and shift of the mediastinum to the left. **B.** On drainage of the effusion, a large right intrathoracic mass (teratoma) becomes apparent.

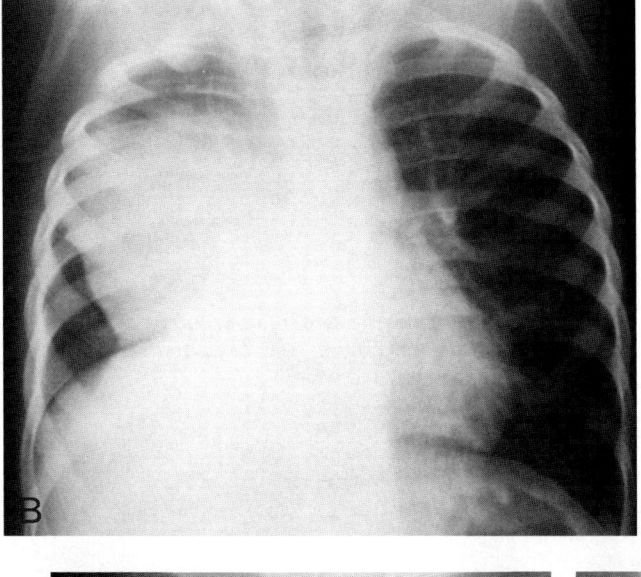

Figure 51.47. Bilateral Pleural Effusions–Lymphoma. Large bilateral subpulmonic pleural effusions are evident in a patient with abdominal non-Hodgkin's lymphoma.

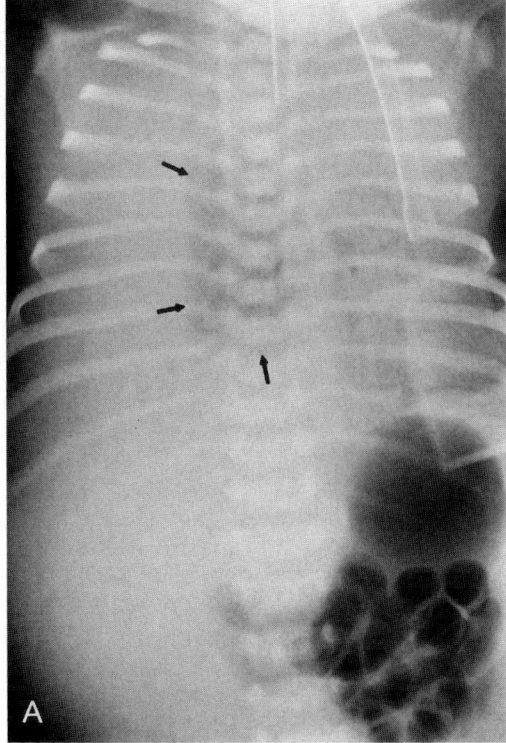

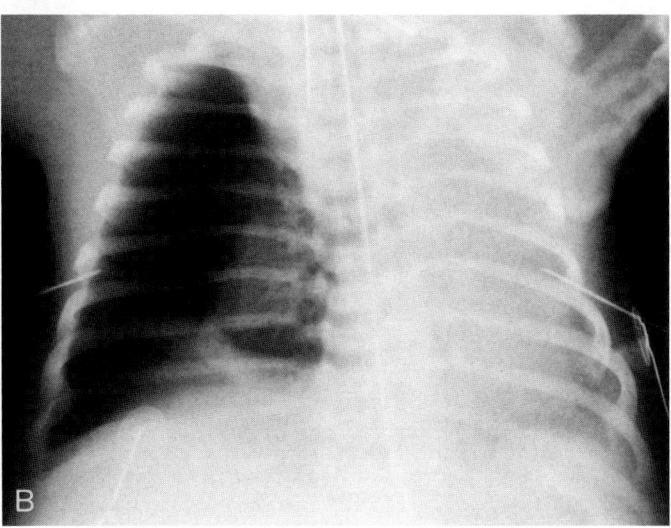

Figure 51.48. Neonatal chylothorax. A. The right hemithorax is opaque and the mediastinum is shifted into the left chest. Note the small right lung (*arrows*). **B.** After the chylous effusion is drained, the hypoplastic right lung becomes more clearly visible.

LUNG MASSES

The most common pulmonary "mass" in children is a pseudomass caused by a spherical pneumonia (Fig. 51.49). Such an appearance is not uncommon at certain stages of pneumonia in children. Pulmonary abscess have a mass-like appearance, usually with central cavitation. Postinflammatory granulomas due to tuberculosis or fungal infections are the most common true lung mass. Such granulomas are usually small and are very often calcified (Fig. 51.50). Plasma cell granuloma, or postinflammatory pseudotumor, is a reactive lesion that develops from a healing pneumonia. Calcification is uncommon and the lesion gradually resolves over a period of years. Nodules have also been reported following atypical measles pneumonia.

Bronchogenic Cysts are lined with respiratory epithelium and filled with mucoid liquid. They occur in the lung parenchyma or in the mediastinum (Fig. 51.51). A subcarinal location is very common (Fig. 51.52). Some are connected to the bronchial tree and are air-filled. They are readily demonstrable with CT or MR.

Pulmonary Sequestration is a mass of lung tissue that lacks a connection to the bronchial tree and is supplied by abnormal vessels from the descending aorta (18). Sequestrations are divided into *extralobar* (covered by their own pleura) or *intralobar* (covered by the pleura of the adjacent normal lung). Most appear as a triangu-

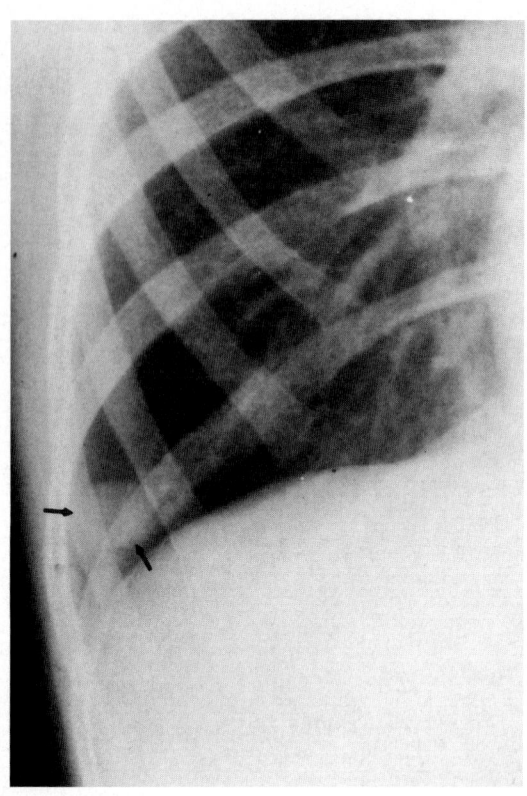

Figure 51.50. Histoplasma Granuloma. The small, round, well-defined mass in the right costophrenic angle (*arrows*) proved to be a granuloma due to histoplamosis.

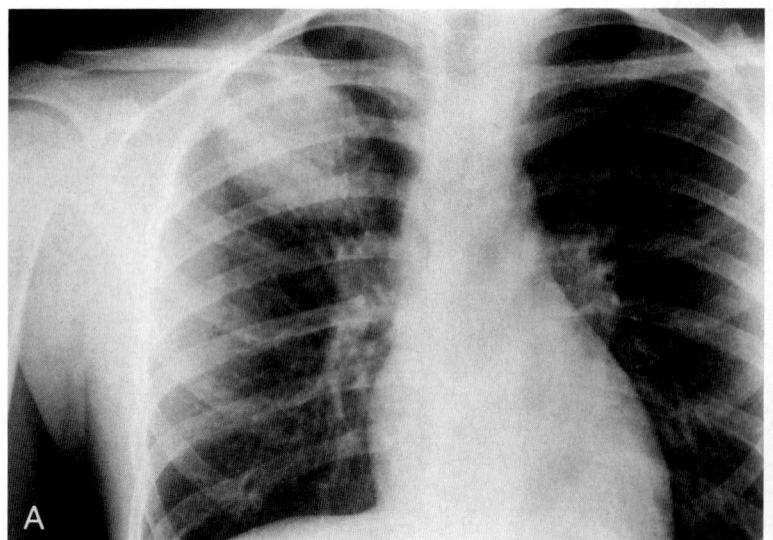

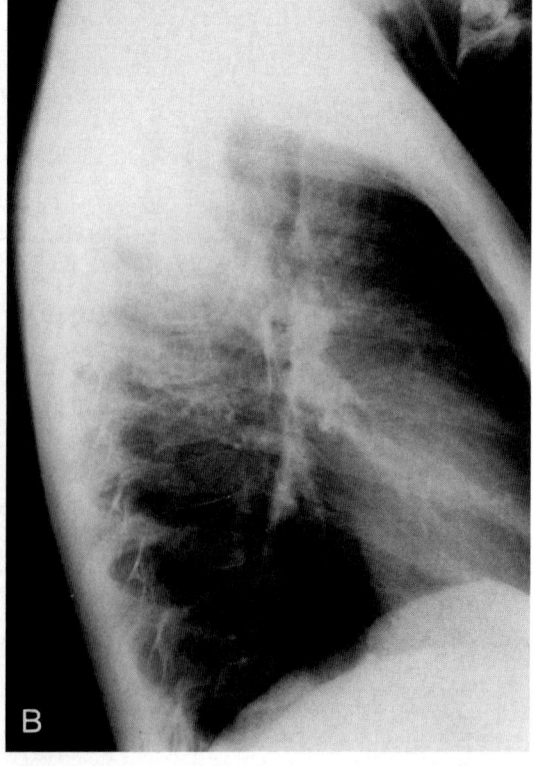

Figure 51.49. Round Pneumonia. A,B. This pneumonia of the right upper lobe has a round, mass-like configuration on both views.

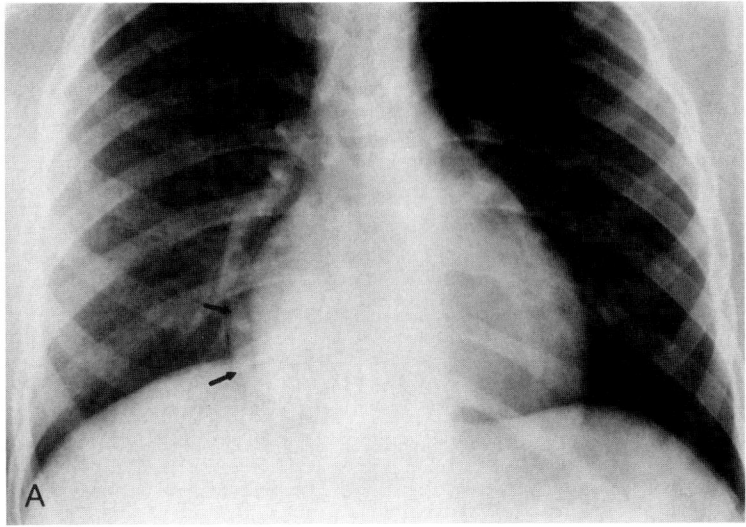

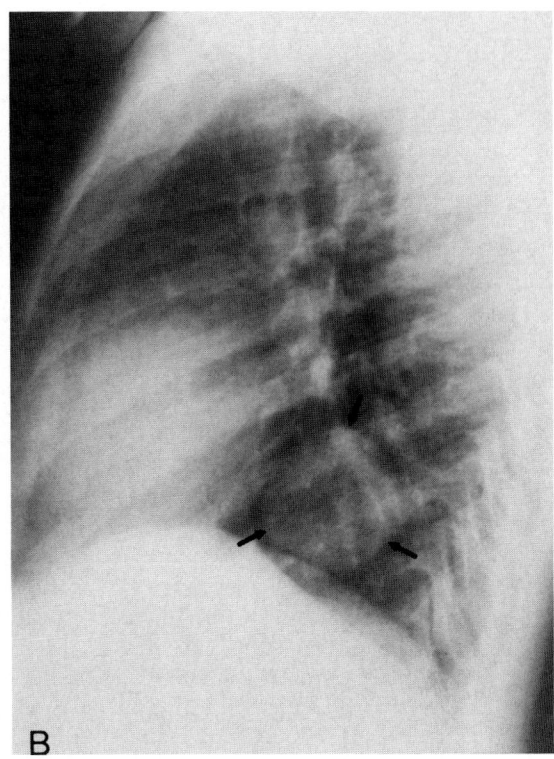

Figure 51.51. Bronchogenic Cyst. A. A rounded opacity peeks out from behind the right heart border (*arrows*). **B.** A lateral view more clearly shows the round, well-defined cyst (*arrows*) in the right lower lobe.

lar or oval-shaped mass in the medial and basal portion of a lung, more commonly on the left (Fig. 51.53A). Air is sometimes present within sequestrations because of collateral air drift. Most are clinically silent until they become infected and present as recurrent pneumonia. The diagnosis is made by demonstrating the abnormal blood supply by US, CT, or MR angiography (Fig. 51.53B,C)(19).

Rare Pulmonary Masses. Other rare causes of a pulmonary mass usually have few distinguishing features. A mass connected to an unusually large vessel is likely a pulmonary arteriovenous malformation. A central, oval-shaped nodule associated with overaeration of the involved lobe suggests the diagnosis of a mucocele in a patient with bronchial atresia. Primary lung tumors are rare and the majority are benign. Pulmonary hamartoma is a benign congenital tumor that occasionally contains characteristic flocculent calcifications. Rarely, laryngeal papillomas can spread into the trachea and the lungs. Primary pulmonary malignancies are very rare and include sarcomas, primitive neuroectodermal tumors, and squamous cell carcinoma. Pulmonary blastoma is a rare neoplasm composed of both epithelial and mesenchymal elements. These tumors can be either solid or cystic.

Metastases. By far the most common malignant neoplasm in the lung during childhood is mestastasis, whether single or multiple. The most common childhood tumors to metastasize to the lungs are Wilms' tumor, Ewing's sarcoma, osteosarcoma, and rhabdomyosar-

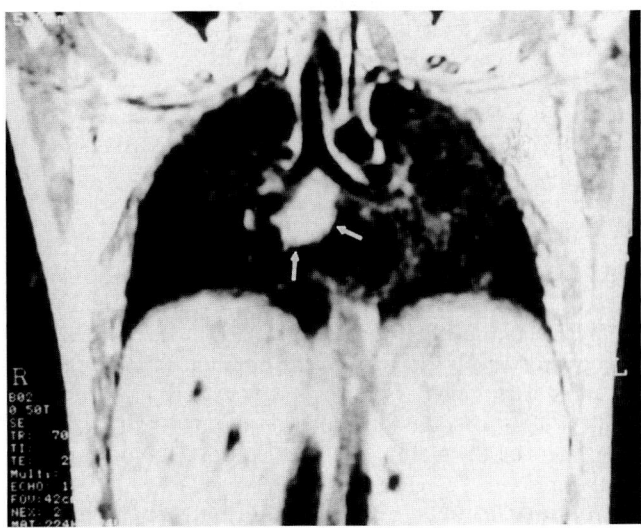

Figure 51.52. Brochogenic cyst. A coronal MR demonstrates a high intensity, fluid-filled cyst in a characteristic subcarinal location (*arrows*).

coma. Other masses and nodules that can be multiple include granulomas (most often fungal), abscesses, hemangiomas, and Wegener's granulomatosis. Cavitary nodules are characteristic of septic emboli, Wegener's granulomatosis, laryngeal papillomatosis, sarcoidosis, and metastases.

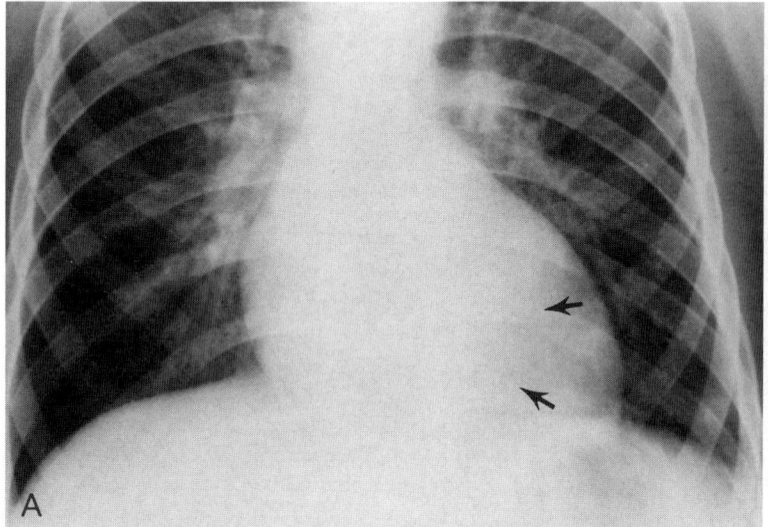

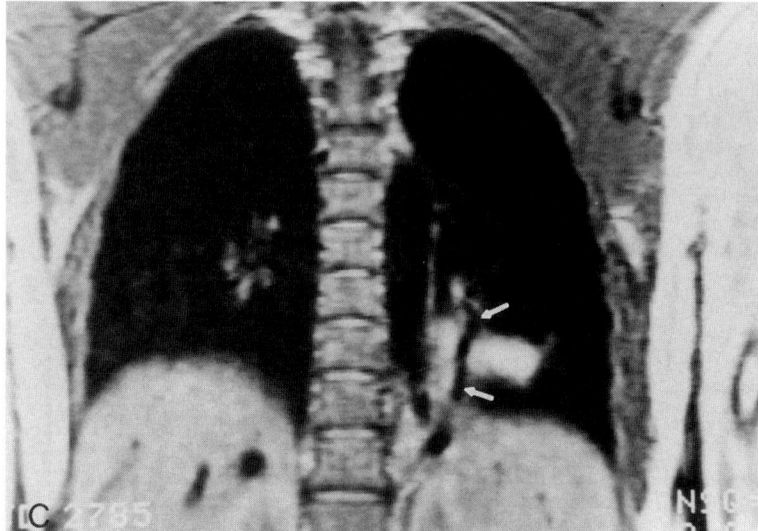

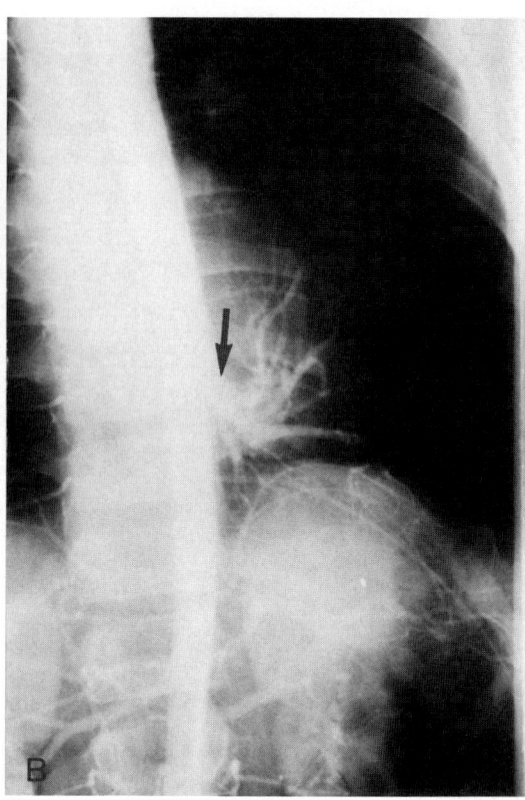

Figure 51.53. Pulmonary Sequestration. A. A poorly defined opacity is seen through the cardiac silhouette on the left (*arrows*). **B.** Angiography demonstrates the abnormal vessels (*arrow*) arising from the descending aorta that supply the sequestrated lung tissue. **C.** Coronal MR image in another patient shows a left lower lobe sequestration that appears as a high-intensity mass associated with a large abnormal vessel (*arrows*).

MEDIASTINAL AND HILAR MASSES

The division of the mediastinum into anterior, middle, and posterior compartments is the most useful scheme for categorizing mediastinal masses in both children and adults. This discussion will use an arbitrary system based on the division of the chest into roughly thirds on the lateral view.

Thymus Gland is the primary normal structure in the anterior mediastinum and is also the most common cause of an apparent anterior mediastinal mass. The normal thymus gland varies widely in its appearance sometimes causing considerable confusion in interpreting an infant or young child's chest radiograph. The gland is commonly very prominent at birth, remains easily visible up to approximately 2 years of age, and may be seen in an older child. On posteroanterior chest radiographs, the thymus gland causes smooth bilateral widening of the superior mediastinum. The gland overlies and silhouettes the upper cardiac borders, although sometimes a small notch is visible at the junction between the thymus and the heart (Fig. 51.54A,B). The border of the thymus gland may have a wavy contour

due to compression by the overlying ribs (Fig. 51.54C). One thymic lobe may appear more prominent than the other and have a triangular configuration called the "sail" sign (Fig. 51.54D). This appearance is more commonly seen on the right and may be mistaken for lung pathology lobar consolidation), particularly if the patient is in slightly right-sided rotated position. On the lateral view of the chest, the thymus lies over the anterosuperior portion of the cardiac silhouette in the retrosternal space (Fig. 51.54E). The normal thymus gland can have more unusual configurations, such as extensions high into the superior mediastinum, the lower neck, or posteriorly between the innominate and left brachiocephalic arteries. Only rarely do these atypical positions result in symptoms.

Stress atrophy of the thymus is an interesting phenomenon that occurs secondary to almost any type of illness or to the use of steroids. The thymus rapidly shrinks in size during illness, only to return to normal size after the infant has recovered. Occasionally, rebound hypertrophy follows stress atrophy. When stress atrophy is severe, the mediastinum appears very narrow suggesting absence or hypoplasia of the thymus gland

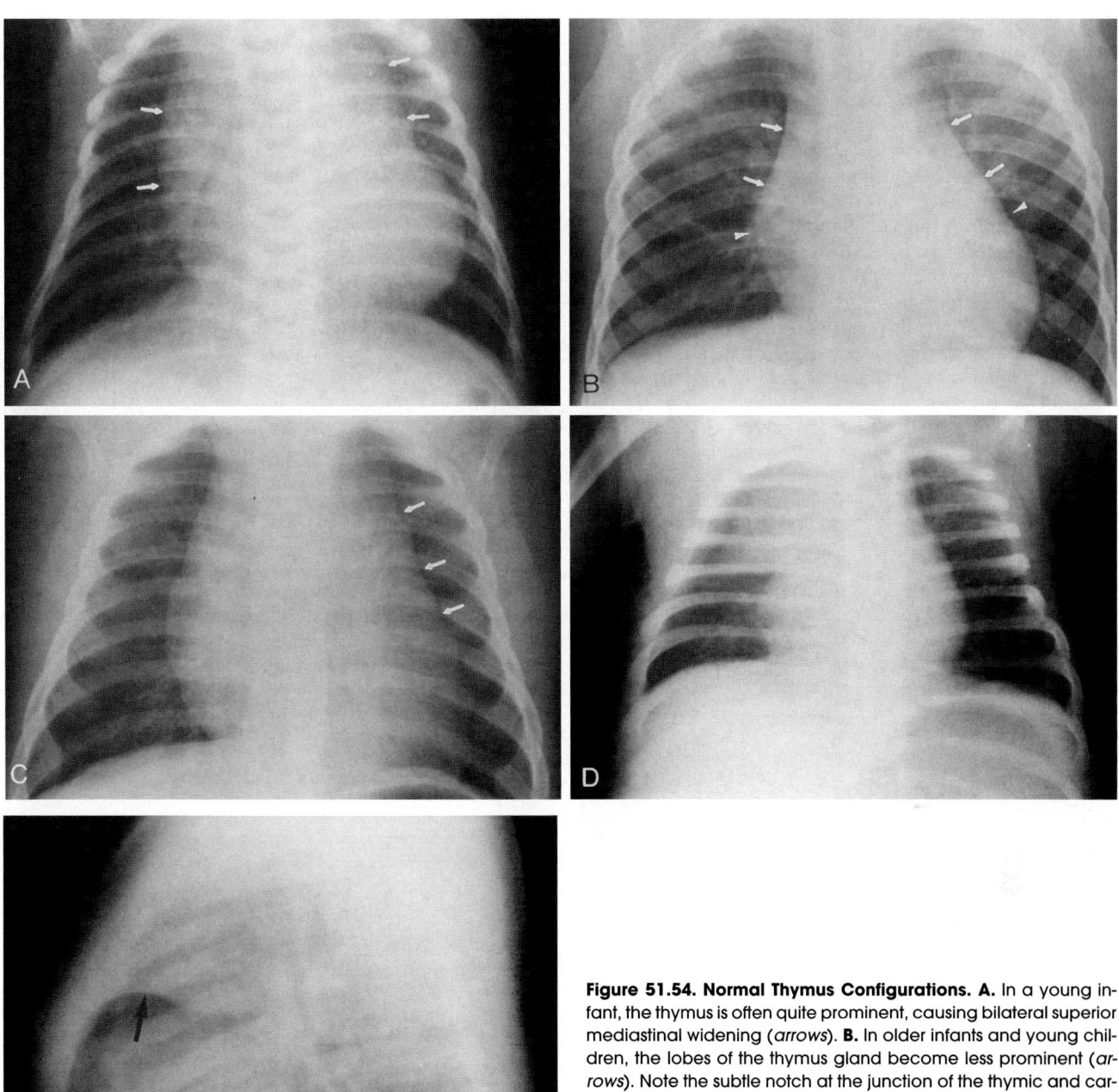

Figure 51.54. Normal Thymus Configurations. A. In a young infant, the thymus is often quite prominent, causing bilateral superior mediastinal widening (*arrows*). **B.** In older infants and young children, the lobes of the thymus gland become less prominent (*arrows*). Note the subtle notch at the junction of the thymic and cardiac shadows (*arrowheads*). **C.** The wavy thymic contour on the left is due to compression by the ribs (*arrows*). **D.** The right thymic lobe is prominent with a configuration that has been likened to a sail. **E.** The thymus gland has a straight inferior border (*arrow*) seen in the retrosternal space on the lateral view.

(Fig. 51.55). The distinction between thymic atrophy and aplasia becomes important in infants who are suspected of having certain immunologic disorders. The best known of these is the DiGeorge syndrome, which consists of thymic aplasia, absence of the parathyroid glands, cardiovascular, and a variety of other, congenital anomalies. This syndrome is caused by the faulty development of the third and fourth pharyngeal pouches. US is helpful in identifying a small thymus gland that is not apparent radiographically (20).

A large thymus gland is nearly always a normal gland in an infant. Leukemia or lymphoma can infiltrate the thymus gland, sometimes causing massive enlargement

(Fig. 51.56). Thymic cysts are uncommon developmental lesions that are best seen with US as well-defined, round, lesions that are anechoic unless complicated by hemorrhage or infection. Spontaneous hemorrhage into the thymus gland has been described in newborn infants. When pneumothorax is present in a neonate, the thymus gland can become compressed and elevated by the free air, creating a pseudomass in the superior mediastinum (Fig. 51.57). This mass-like compression of the thymus gland may be a clue to a subtle anterior pneumothorax.

On cross-sectional imaging, the thymic lobes have a smooth, somewhat triangular shape with homogeneous texture (Fig. 51.58) (21). Bulging or convexity of the borders of the thymus gland suggests pathologic enlargement, particularly if the trachea or the great vessels are displaced or compressed. Primary neoplasms and cysts produce focal alterations of attenuation or signal intensity, whereas infiltration by leukemia or lymphoma or hemorrhage results in a more diffuse and heterogenous parenchymal pattern. Overall, MR probably is best in defining whether a thymus gland is normal or abnormal.

Anterior Mediastinal Masses. The majority of masses in the anterior mediastinum in children are tumors, most commonly dermoids and teratomas. Dermoids are benign tumors comprised only of ectodermal elements, whereas teratomas contain elements from all dermal layers. Teratomas commonly contain calcifications that are best demonstrated by CT (Fig. 51.59). Other neoplasms in the anterior mediastinum include thyroid tumors, hemangiomas, and cystic hygromas (usually extending from the neck). US is an excellent means of evaluating an enlarged thyroid gland and easily differentiates cysts from neoplasms (Fig. 51.60). Cystic hygroma is a congenital malformation of lymphatic origin. US shows a multiloculated cystic mass (Fig. 51.61) (22). Hemangiomas tend to be echogenic

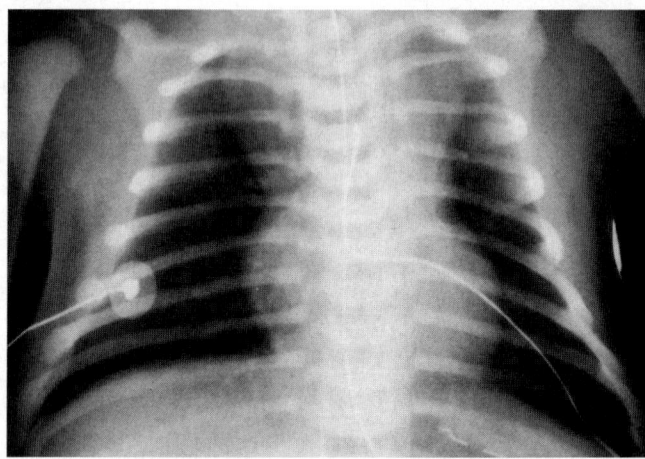

Figure 51.57. Thymic Pseudomass. The thymus gland is elevated and compressed by the bilateral anterior pneumothoraces, creating the appearance of a superior mediastinal mass.

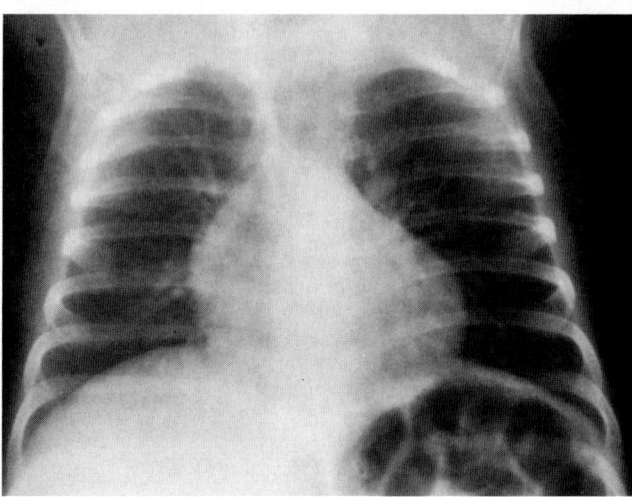

Figure 51.55. Stress Atrophy of the Thymus. The superior mediastinum is narrow due to absence of a thymic shadow in this infant suffering from failure to thrive.

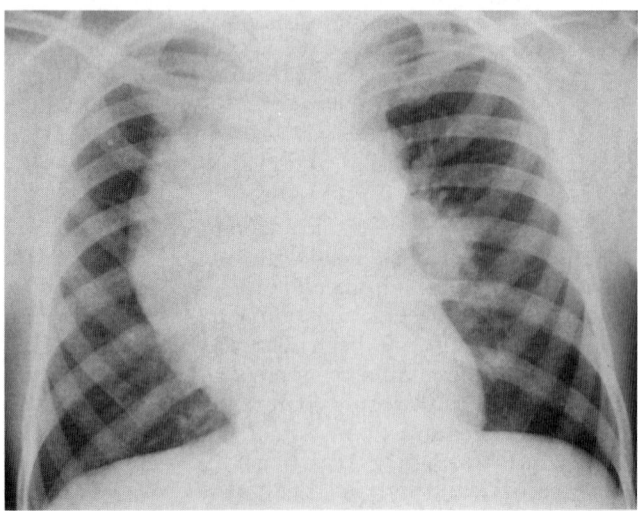

Figure 51.56. Hodgkin's Lymphoma. The thymus is massively enlarged due to lymphomatous involvement.

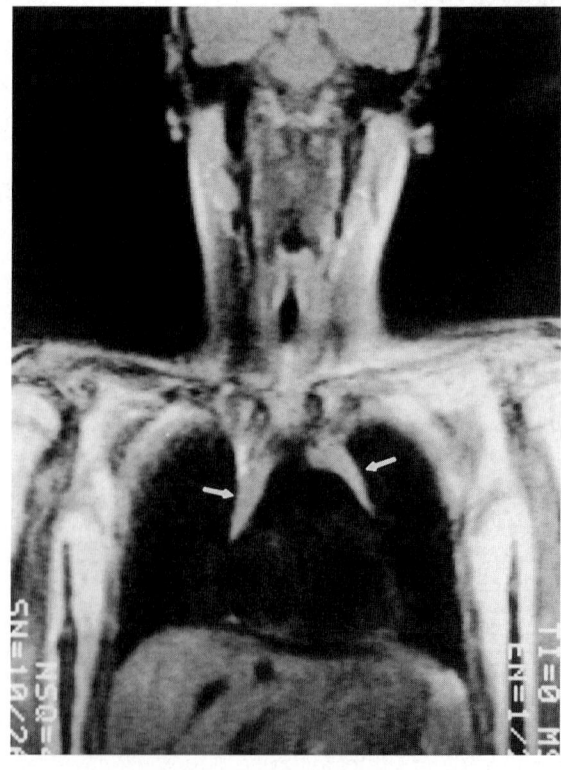

Figure 51.58. Normal Thymus Gland: MR. The normal thymus gland is elegantly demonstrated on this coronal MR image in an older child (*arrows*).

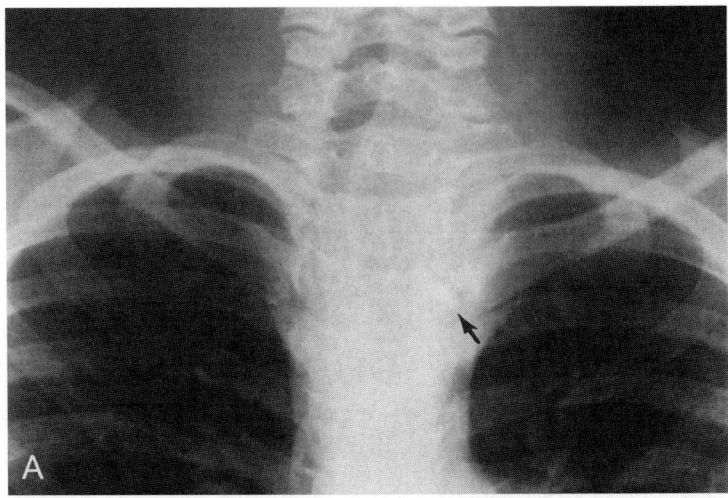

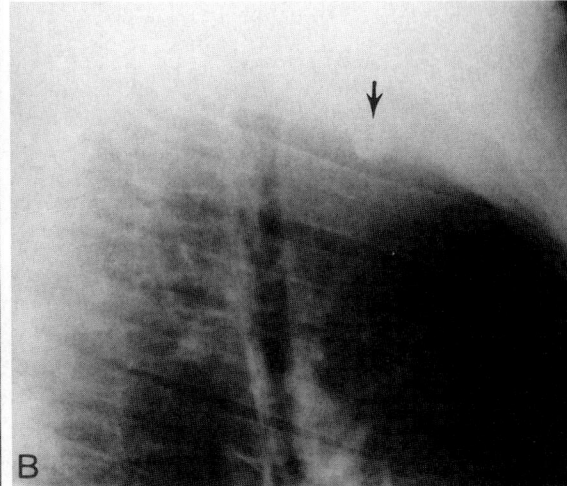

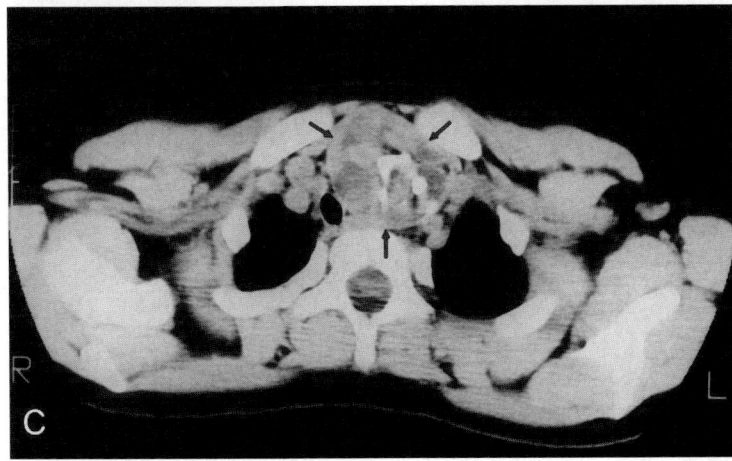

Figure 51.59. Mediastinal Teratoma. A. A superior mediastinal mass displaces the trachea to the right. A tooth-like calcification is seen within the mass (*arrow*). **B.** Lateral view shows the anterior location of the mass and the calcification (*arrow*). **C.** A CT scan reveals the heterogenous nature of this teratoma (*arrows*), which contains dense calcifications and hypodense areas representing fat.

with small cystic areas representing vascular lakes in the cavernous type of hemangioma. Blood flow is demonstrable with color Doppler imaging.

Middle Mediastinal Masses. Normal structures in the middle mediastinum from which masses can arise include lymph nodes, the airway, the esophagus, and the heart and great vessels.

Lymphadenopathy is by far the most common middle mediastinal mass. Inflammatory lymphadenopathy is much more common than neoplastic disease, but when massive adenopathy is seen, lymphoma or leukemia should be given primary consideration (Fig. 51.62). Hilar lymph node enlargement may accompany mediastinal adenopathy or may occur alone. Bilateral hilar adenopathy most commonly is the result of viral lower respiratory tract infections in children. Mycoplasmal, fungal, and tuberculous infections must also be considered (Fig. 51.63). Other causes of adenopathy include histiocytosis X, metastatic disease, sarcoidosis and Wegener's granulomatosis.

Unilateral lymphadenopathy is the most common radiographic finding of primary tuberculosis in children and is often associated with an area of opacity in the ipsilateral lung (the Ghon complex)(Fig. 51.64)(23). The lung opacity can be atelectasis or alveolar infiltrate. Unilateral lymphadenopathy is seen frequently with mycoplasma or fungal infections of the lung and occa-

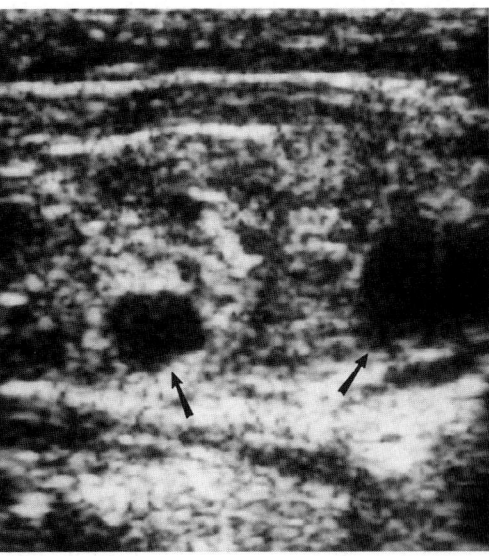

Figure 51.60. Thyroid Enlargement. US demonstrates colloid cysts (*arrows*) in an enlarged thyroid gland of a patient with multinodular goiter due to congenital dyshormonogenesis. Note the inhomogenous texture of the gland, a common finding in diffuse thyroid disease.

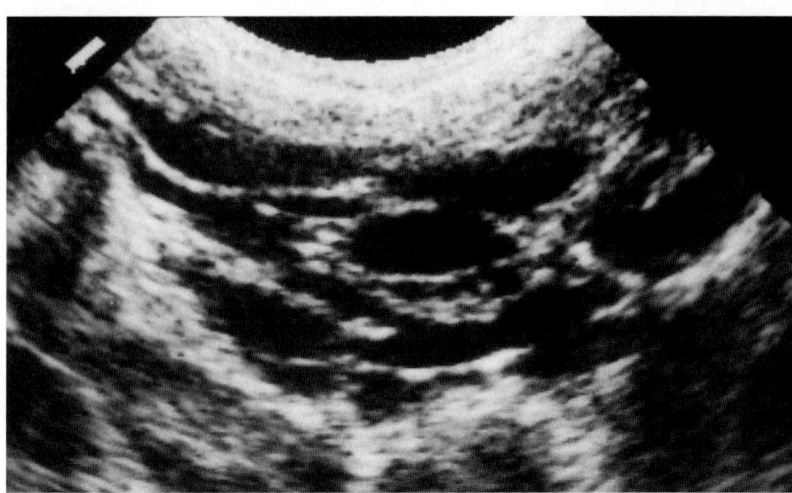

Figure 51.61. Lymphangioma. US shows the characteristic multicystic appearance of a lymphangioma.

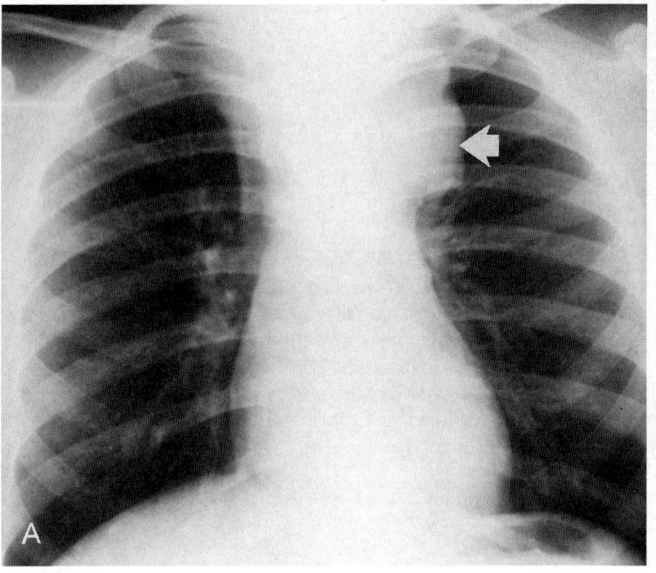

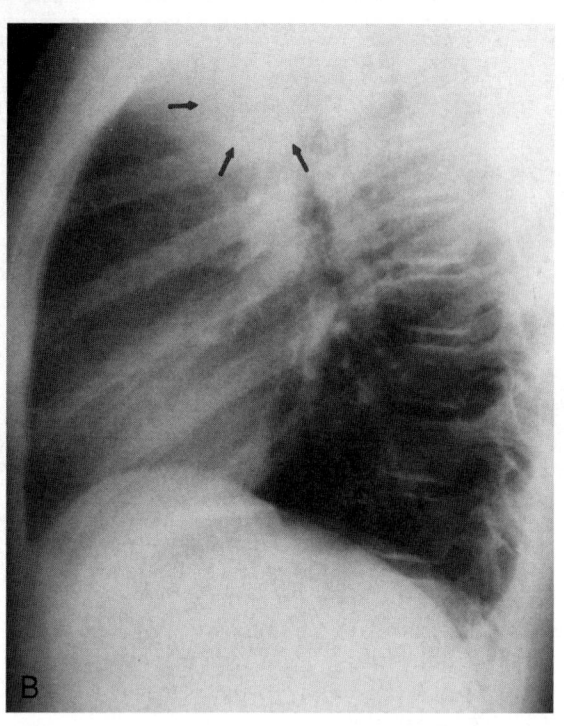

Figure 51.62. Histocytic Lymphoma. A. The large left paratracheal mass (*arrow*) represents lymphadenopathy due to lymphoma. **B.** Lateral view shows the middle mediastinal location of this mass (*arrows*).

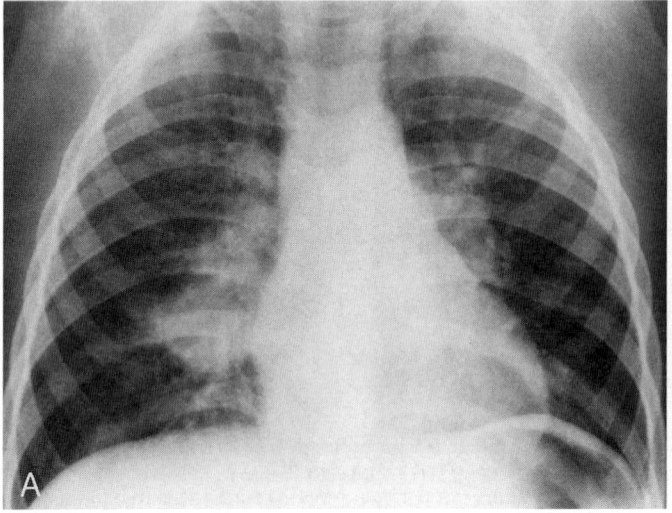

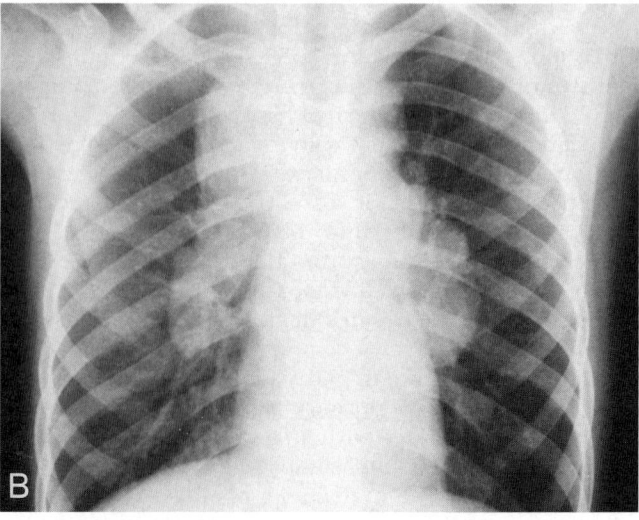

Figure 51.63. Bilateral Hilar Adenopathy. A. Prominent nodular, hilar opacities represent lymph nodes in this patient with primary tuberculosis. **B.** The bilateral hilar and paratracheal masses represent lymphadenopathy due to Hodgkin's lymphoma.

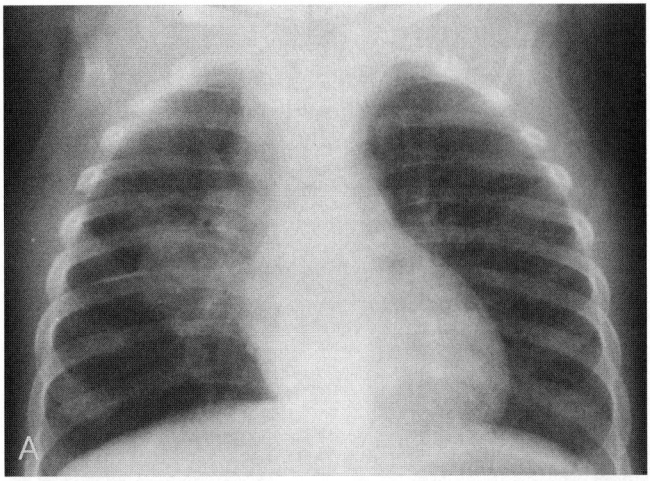

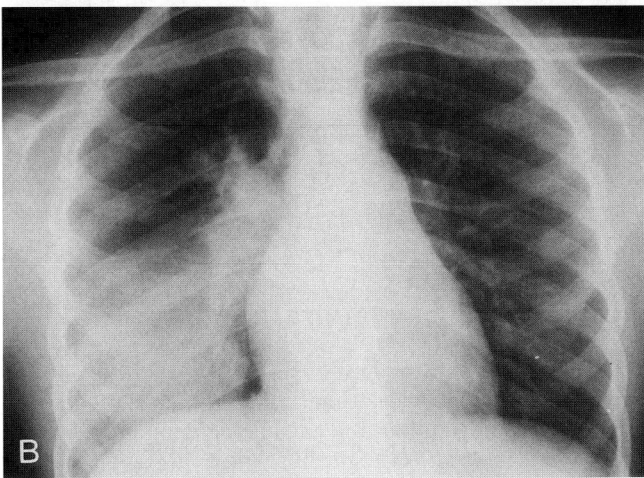

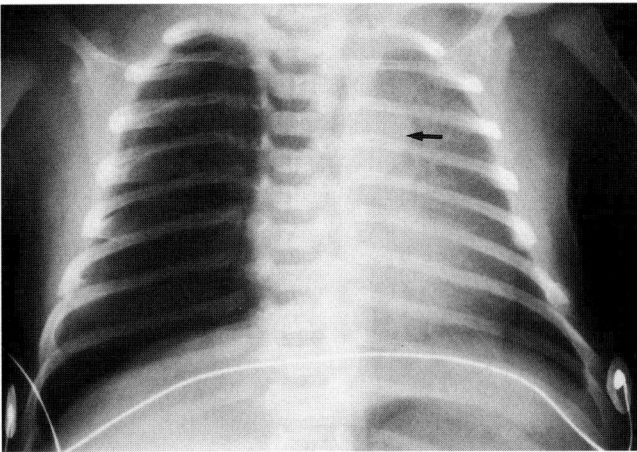

Figure 51.65. Ductus Bump. The prominent "bump" (*arrow*) that is seen along the upper descending aorta represents the dilated infundibulum of the ductus arteriosus in this newborn infant.

Figure 51.64. Unilateral Hilar Adenopathy. A. Right hilar adenopathy and adjacent parenchymal opacity comprise the typical Ghon complex of primary tuberculosis. **B.** Right hilar adenopathy is associated with a bacterial pneumonia.

sionally with a bacterial pneumonia. Unilateral lymphadenopathy associated with a viral infection is uncommon. Neoplastic lymph node enlargement can be unilateral or bilateral.

Cystic masses in the middle mediastinum can be associated with the airway or the esophagus. Bronchogenic cysts have a smooth, round appearance and commonly occur around the carina (see Fig. 51.52)(24). Esophageal duplication cysts are developmental abnormalities due to abnormal division of the neurenteric complex. These cysts usually do not communicate with the esophagus but displace and compress the esophagus on contrast studies. In some cases, gastric mucosa will be present in the cyst lining leading to ulceration and hemorrhage.

Enlarged vascular structures may present as a middle mediastinal mass. Aortic aneurysms are rare in childhood, except for those associated with trauma or with connective tissue disorders such as the Marfan or Ehler-Danlos syndromes. In the newborn infant, a small bump along the upper descending aorta is caused by a dilated infundibulum of the ductus arteriosus after closure (Fig. 51.65). Normally this "ductus bump" disappears in the

first weeks of life. Enlargement or persistence of this bump in later infancy suggests an aneurysm of the ductus arteriosus. Enlargement of the aorta and the main pulmonary artery will be addressed later in this chapter.

A mass along the upper left cardiac border can be caused by herniation of the left atrial appendage through a partial pericardial defect, or by a coronary artery aneurysm. Coronary artery aneurysms occur in children with periarteritis nodosa or the mucocutaneous lymph node syndrome. Enlargement of the azygos vein presents as a mass in the right paratracheal region. In children, this most often occurs with total anomalous pulmonary venous return to the azygos vein or absence of the inferior vena cava with azygos continuation.

Posterior Mediastinal Masses are largely of neurogenic origin. Close inspection of the vertebra and posterior ribs may reveal pedicle erosion, interpedicular or rib space widening, or bone erosions which are clues to a mass extending into the spinal canal. In such cases, the mass is most often a neoplasm of the neuroblastoma-ganglioneuroma group (Fig. 51.66). These tumors are probably congenital in origin and arise in paraspinal sympathetic nerve tissue. Primary thoracic neuroblastoma has a more favorable prognosis than neuroblastoma which originates in the abdomen. Ganglioneuroma is the benign counterpart of neuroblastoma and the two lesions cannot be reliably distinguished from one another radiographically. Calcifications may be seen in both lesions, and it is believed that some neuroblastomas can mature to ganglioneuromas.

Neurofibromas also occur in the posterior mediastinum and cause widening of intervertebral foramina (Fig. 51.67). These tumors can be solitary but more often occur with the neurofibromatosis syndrome. Anterior thoracic meningoceles also occur in patients with neurofibromatosis and have a similar radiographic appearance. Neurenteric cysts are a form of enteric duplication cysts that communicate with the spinal canal. The cysts lie in the posterior mediastinum and are almost always associated with vertebral anomalies. Spinal cord anomalies may also be present. MR is the procedure of choice

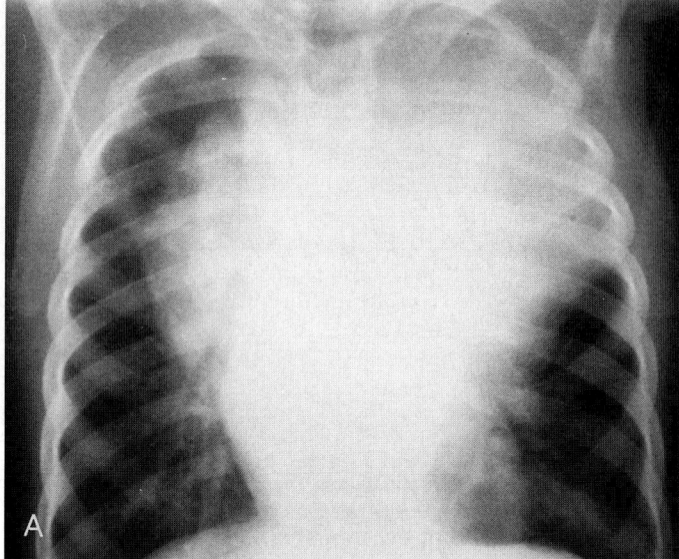

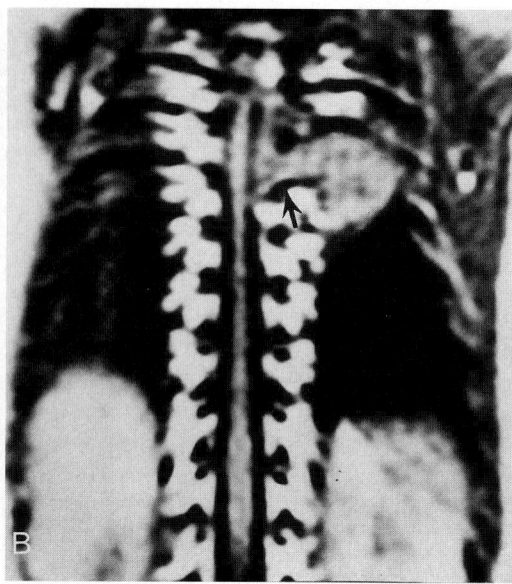

Figure 51.66. Thoracic Neuroblastoma. A. A large mediastinal mass is associated with thinning of the posterior and medial portion of the left second rib and widening of the T2-3 rib space localizing the mass to the posterior mediastinum and suggesting intraspinal extension. **B.** Coronal MR of a different patient demonstrates extension of a left posterior mediastinal tumor into the spinal canal (*arrow*).

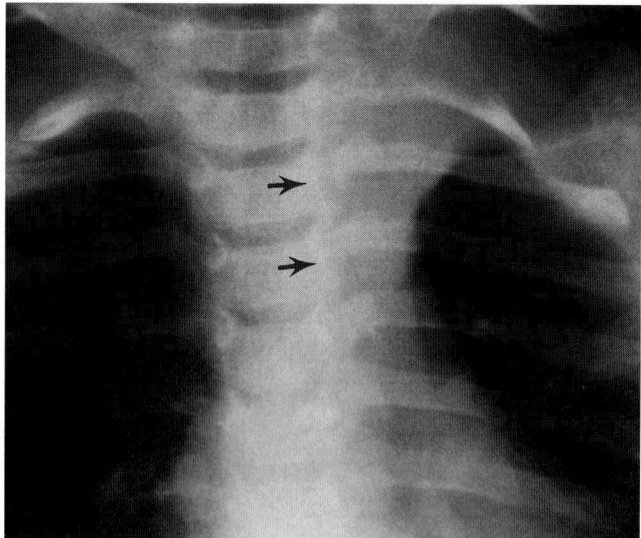

Figure 51.67. Neurofibromatosis. The soft-tissue mass in the superior and posterior mediastinum on the left deforms the left pedicles (*arrows*) of several of the upper thoracic vertebrae, suggestig neurogenic origin of the mass.

for evaluating this condition. A posterior mediastinal inflammatory mass occasionally accompanies inflammatory conditions of the spine. Rare causes of a posterior mediastinal mass include lymphangioma, teratoma, lymphoma, and sarcoma. Diaphragmatic hernias through the foramen of Bochdalek and pulmonary sequestration often present as masses in the inferior portion of the posterior mediastinum adjacent to the diaphragm.

CONGENITAL HEART DISEASE

A wide variety of imaging modalities are now available for diagnosing and evaluating congenital heart disease in children. Many congenital cardiac abnormalities that previously required angiocardiography can now be diagnosed noninvasively by echocardiography and MR (25). Perhaps the radiologist's most important role is the identification and classification of cardiovascular abnormalities by plain radiography. Although the specific diagnosis often will not be apparent on the plain films, a systematic approach to plain film interpretation will allow catagorization into one of several groups of lesions. This section will provide a framework for an organized scheme for radiographic evaluation of congenital heart disease.

Assessment begins with the pulmonary vascularity (26). Vascular patterns are placed in one of three broad groups: *increased* (congested), *decreased*, and *normal* (Fig. 51.68 and Table 51.10). If the vascularity is increased, one should attempt to distinguish active congestion from passive congestion.

Active Congestion occurs whenever the amount of blood flowing through the pulmonary vasculature has increased. This occurs in conditions with left-to-right shunts and with preferential blood flow into the lower pressure pulmonary circulation. Left-to-right shunts do not become radiographically apparent until the output of the right ventricle (RV) is approximately two and a half times greater than that of the left ventricle (LV). At this point, the pulmonary vessels become increased in diameter and are visible farther than usual into the periphery of the lungs (Fig. 51.68A). The vessels may appear tortuous but the margins remain relatively distinct. In borderline cases, if the diameter of the right descending pulmonary artery (PA) is less than that of the trachea, a left-to-right shunt is unlikely.

Passive Congestion reflects elevation of the pulmonary venous pressure, which can result from obstruction or dysfunction of the left side of the heart. As venous pressure increases and the veins dilate, edema fluid leaks into the perivascular interstitial tissues, causing the margins of the vessels to become less distinct on the chest radiograph (Fig. 51.69B). As pulmonary venous hypertension increases, alveolar pulmonary edema and pleural effusions develop. In patients with large left-to-right shunts and left heart failure, a mixed pattern of passive and active congestion occurs.

Decreased Pulmonary Vascularity indicates diminished blood flow to the lungs, most often due to obstruction of the right ventricular outflow tract and associated right-to-left shunts. Oligemia causes the lungs to appear more radiolucent and the vessels to appear uniformly thin and wispy (Fig. 51.68C). A diminished caliber of the peripheral two-thirds of the pulmonary arteries com-

bined with prominence of the central pulmonary arteries is characteristic of pulmonary arterial hypertension due to increased pulmonary vascular resistance.

Normal Pulmonary Vascularity is usually seen in patients with uncomplicated valvular disease, coarctation of the aorta, and mild forms of cardiomyopathy. The vessels retain a normal contour and diameter until congestive heart failure develops.

Asymmetry of Pulmonary Blood Flow is most commonly seen in tetralogy of Fallot, persistent truncus arteriosus, and valvular pulmonic stenosis. In tetralogy of Fallot, the blood flow to the left lung tends to be diminished. Blood flow to either lung, or occasionally only one lobe, can be decreased in persistent truncus arteriosus. In valvular pulmonic stenosis, the abnormal valve tends to direct the blood flow preferentially into the left pulmonary arterial system, although an enlarged left PA and increased blood flow to the left lung is seldom apparent on the radiographs of children. Alteration of the pulmonary vasculature due to aeration abnormalities of one lung has been discussed previously.

The next step in radiographic interpretation of con-

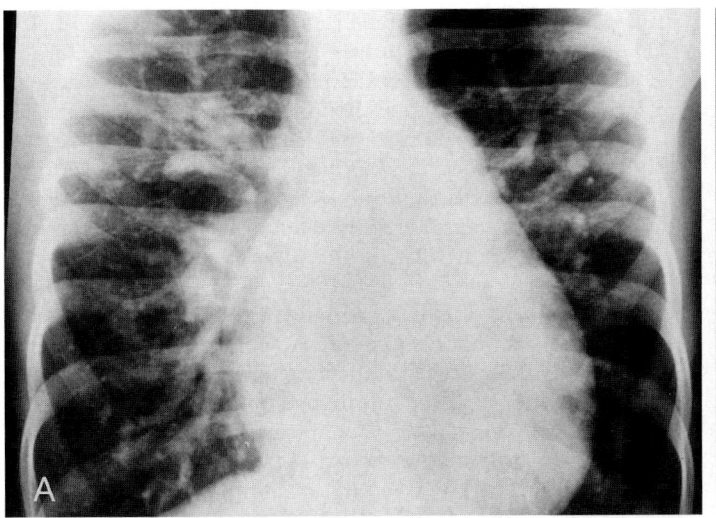

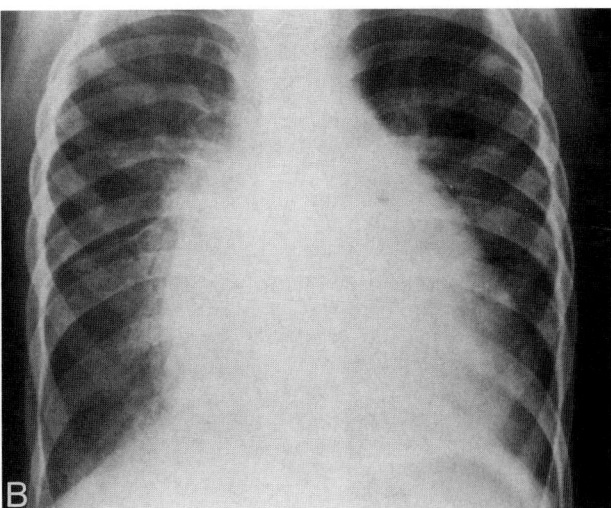

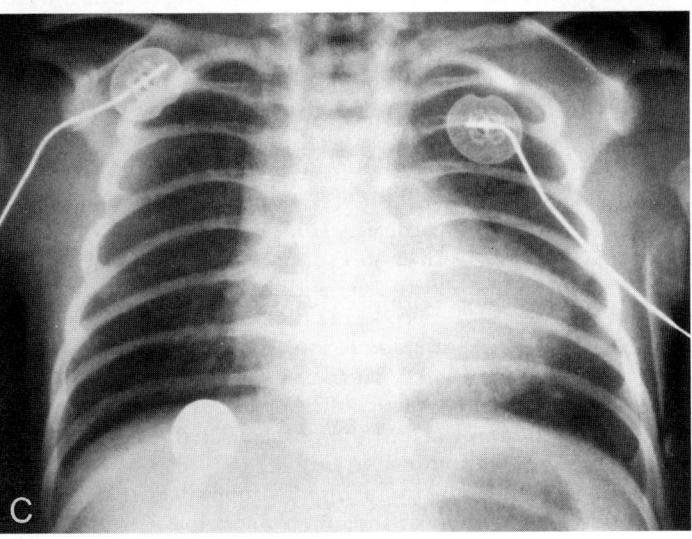

Figure 51.68. Pulmonary Vascular Patterns. A. *Active congestion.* Note the large but distinct pulmonary vessels extending into the periphery of the lung due to left-to-right shunting in a patient with a large VSD. **B. *Passive congestion.*** Indistinctness of the pulmonary vascular markings due to mitral insufficiency indicates passive vascular congestion. **C. *Decreased vascularity.*** A paucity of vessels in both lungs is due to tetralogy of Fallot. Note the right aortic arch and the charactertistic "boot" cardiac configuration due to right ventricular hypertrophy.

Table 51.10. Pulmonary Vascular Patterns

Increased vascularity (active) without cyanosis
ASD
VSD
PDA
Aortic-pulmonary window
Ruptured aneurysm of sinus of Valsalva
Coronary artery fistula
Partial anomalous pulmonary venous return
Increased vascularity (active) with cyanosis
Total anomalous pulmonary venous return (types I, II)
Persistent truncus arteriosus
Complete endocardial cushion defect
Transposition of the great vessels complex
Single ventricle (without pulmonary stenosis)
Increased vascularity (passive)
Total anomalous pulmonary venous return (type III)
Pulmonary vein atresia
Hypoplastic left heart syndrome (in failure)
Cor triatriatum
Decreased vascularity
Tetralogy of Fallot
Pseudotruncus arteriosus
Hypoplastic right heart syndrome (right-to-left shunt)
Tricuspid atresia
Pulmonary atresia
Tricuspid stenosis
Hypoplastic right ventricle
Ebstein's anomaly
Uhl's anomaly
Trilogy of Fallot
Single ventricle or transposition of great vessels with pulmonary stenosis or atresia
Tricuspid or pulmonary insufficiency with right-to-left shunt
Normal vascularity
Left heart lesions
Coarctation of the aorta
Interrupted aortic arch
Hypoplastic left heart syndrome (before failure develops)
Endocardial fibroelastosis
Cardiomyopathy
Aberrant left coronary artery
Mitral stenosis and insufficiency
Aortic stenosis and insufficiency
Cor triatriatum
Right heart lesions (without right-to-left shunt)
Pulmonary stenosis or insufficiency
Tricuspid insufficiency

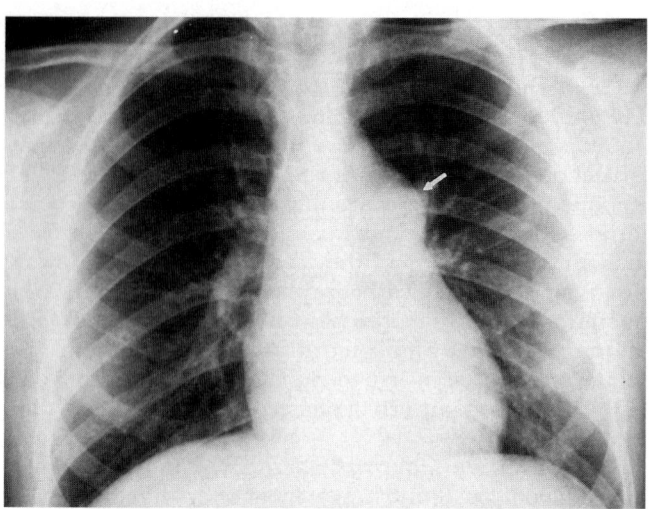

Figure 51.69. Pulmonary Artery Enlargement. Poststenotic dilation of the pulmonary artery is seen in this patient with valvular pulmonic stenosis (*arrow*).

genital heart disease is assessment of the main pulmonary artery and aorta.

Pulmonary Artery. An enlarged PA is seen with generalized increased pulmonary blood flow, in valvular pulmonic stenosis due to poststenotic dilation (Fig. 51.69), and in pulmonary valve insufficiency due to increased right ventricular output. An enlarged PA will often be higher in position than a normal pulmonary artery and can be mistaken for a large aortic knob. A small or absent PA shadow occurs with decreased blood flow due to pulmonary outflow obstruction or with an abnormal position of the PA such as with persistent truncus arteriosus or transposition of the great vessels.

Aorta. Evaluation of the aorta includes estimation of size, position, and contour abnormalities. The size of the aorta is assessed in the region of the aortic knob. The aorta may appear small because of hypoplasia, (in hypoplastic left heart syndrome), and with certain left-to-right shunts (atrial septal defect [ASD], ventricular septal defect [VSD]). Since the aorta in children is normally small relative to adults and a truly small aorta may be difficult to recognize. Enlargement of the ascending aorta and the aortic knob is most often poststenotic dilation due to valvular aortic stenosis, or increased aortic blood flow seen with aortic valve insufficiency, left-to-right shunting at the great vessels level (patent ductus arteriosus, persistent truncus arteriosus), and severe tetralogy of Fallot. Generalized aortic enlargement can occur with systemic hypertension. The most common abnormality of the contour of the aorta is the notching that occurs at the site of coarctation of aorta. Dilation of the aorta proximal and distal to the coarctation results in the characteristic "figure-3" sign (Fig. 51.70).

Right-sided Aortic Arch is most often an isolated anomaly. However, it can also accompany congenital heart disease, especially persistent truncus arteriosus or tetralogy of Fallot. A right aortic arch is seen as a bulge or fullness in the right paratracheal region, slightly above the usual level of a left-sided aortic arch. The trachea will be displaced to the left by a right aortic arch (Fig. 51.71). In addition, a right descending aorta can be visualized just to the right of the spine in many cases (Fig. 51.71B). A barium esophagram confirms the diagnosis by demonstrating a right-sided indentation. A right-sided aortic arch may be a clue to the presence of a vascular ring such as a double aortic arch or aberrant left subclavian artery with an encircling ligamentum arteriosum. In such cases, the barium swallow reveals opposing indentations in the barium-filled esophagus in a "reverse-S" configuration (see Fig. 51.20).

Cardiomegaly is an important indicator of cardiac disease in children and often accompanies congenital heart disease. Unfortunately, the estimation of cardiac

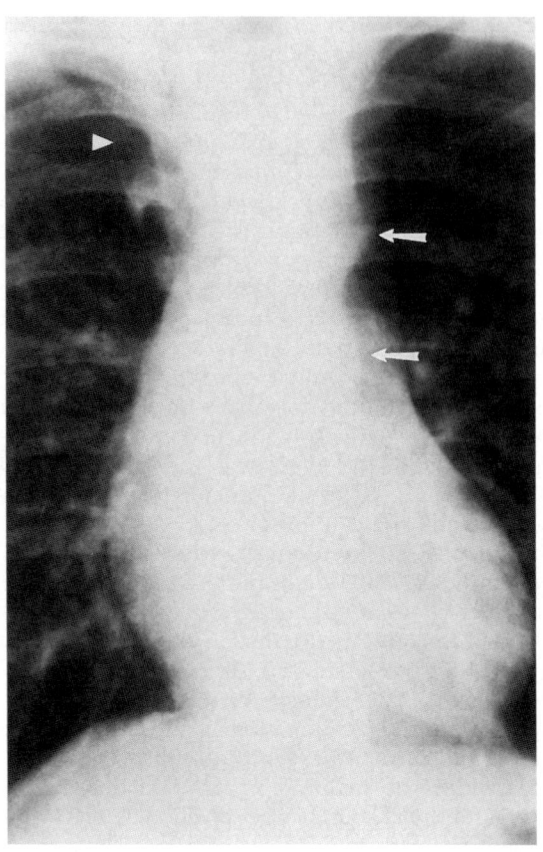

Figure 51.70. Coarctation of the Aorta. Pre- and poststenotic dilation of the aorta creates the characteristic "figure-3" sign (*arrows*). The patient also has an azygous fissure (*arrowhead*).

enlargement in children is somewhat subjective and measurements such as the cardiothoracic ratio are usually not helpful. Beware of the normally prominent thymus gland overlying the heart and of films taken in a poor degree of inspiration that can erroneously suggest cardiac enlargement. The configurations of enlargement of specific cardiac chambers are the same as those seen in adults. Generalized cardiomegaly with a globular appearance suggests pericardial fluid which can easily be confirmed with US (Fig. 51.72). Pericardial effusions in children commonly accompany viral infections or rheumatic fever. Other causes include acute or chronic renal failure, collagen vascular diseases, bacterial infections, and, rarely, tuberculosis, fungal infections, and pericardial metastases. Blood in the pericardial space is usually the result of trauma. Generalized cardiac enlargement also occurs with conditions causing increased blood volume and elevated cardiac outputs, including renal diseases, inappropriate secretion of antidiuretic hormone, large arteriovenous fistulae, chronic anemias (especially sickle cell disease and thalassemia), and hyperthyroidism.

Acyanotic Heart Disease with Increased Pulmonary Vascularity

Actively increased pulmonary vascularity in the absence of cyanosis most often occurs when a defect allows oxygenated blood from the left side of the heart or the aorta to be shunted back to the right side of the heart or the pulmonary circulation. Because no desaturated blood is shunted into the systemic circulation, cyanosis

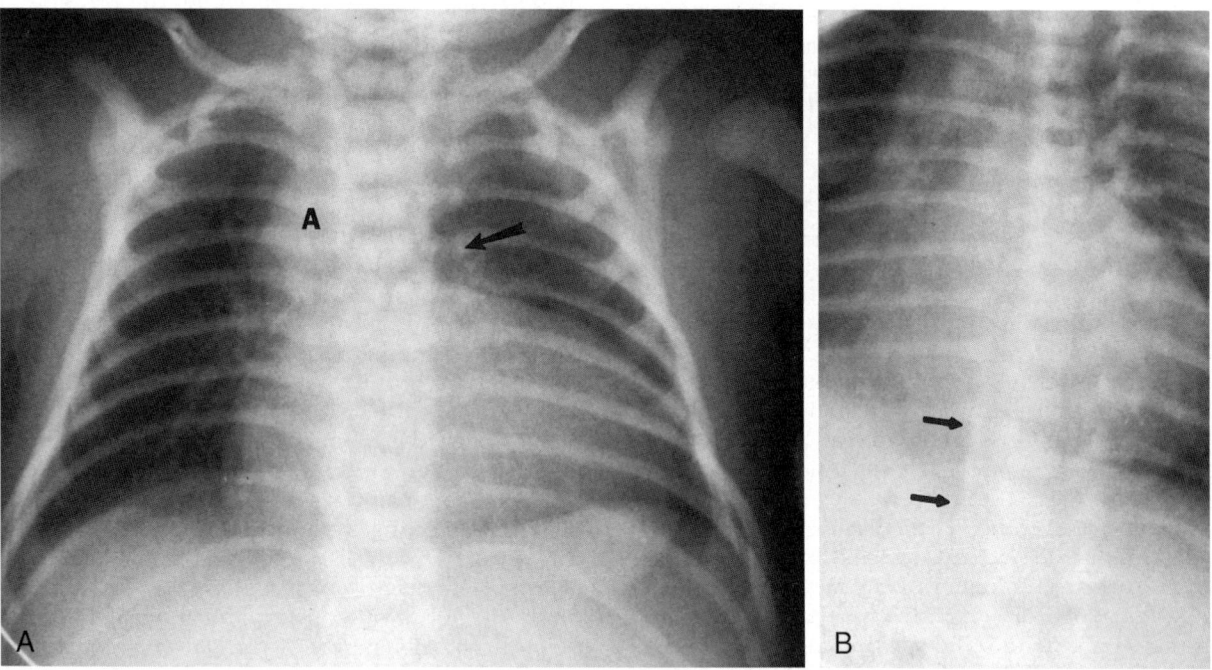

Figure 51.71. Right Aortic Arch. A. The right aortic arch (*A*), boot-shaped heart, and concave pulmonary artery segment (*arrow*) are characteristis of tetralogy of Fallot. **B.** With slight obliquity to the right, the descending right aorta is seen (*arrows*), just to the right of the spine.

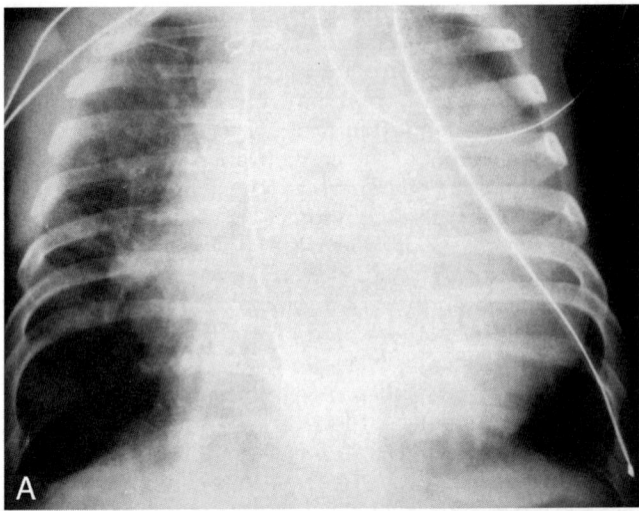

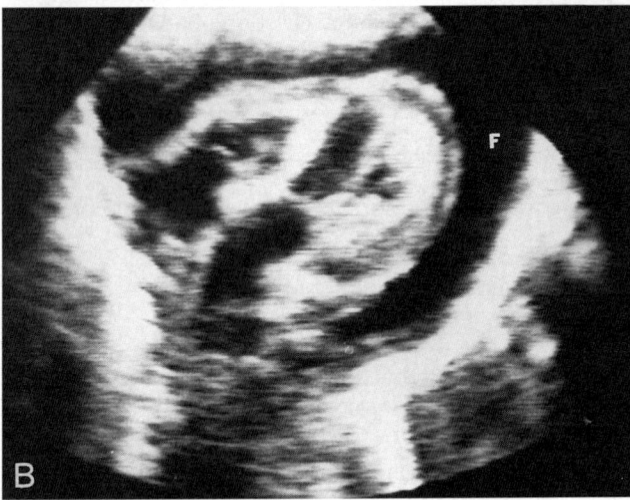

Figure 51.72. Pericardial Effusion. A. The cardiac silhouette is markedly enlarged and has a rounded, globular appearance due to a pericardial effusion that developed following open heart surgery. **B.** US is the best method for verifying pericardial fluid (*F*).

does not occur. The increased blood volumes recirculating through the right heart and pulmonary circulation results in cardiac enlargement and increased size of the pulmonary vessels. The most common conditions in this category are VSD, ASD, and patent ductus arteriosus (PDA).

Ventricular Septal Defect is the most common congenital heart abnormality after bicuspid aortic valve. VSD occurs frequently as an isolated anomaly, although it may accompany many of the cyanotic forms of congenital heart disease. The defect is categorized according to its location within the ventricular septum. Most are perimembranous defects in the membranous portion of the septum near the fusion of the membranous and muscular portions. Defects in the muscular septum are less common and tend to be smaller and less hemodynamically significant than the perimembranous defect. The third type of defect is uncommon and develops high in the membranous septum because of abnormal development of the conus portion of the truncus arteriosus.

This type is most often seen with persistent truncus arteriosus or tetralogy of Fallot.

Newborns with VSD are usually asymptomatic. A murmur will often not be detected until after the newborn period. This delay in manifestation of left-to-right shunting is the result of the normal phenomenon of postnatal pulmonary vascular involution. In the fetus, the walls of the pulmonary arteries are thicker than in postnatal life, resulting in increased pulmonary vascular resistance and relative right ventricular hypertrophy. Elevated pulmonary vascular pressure inhibits blood flow through the lungs and through the septal defect. During the early postnatal period, the pulmonary vascular resistance diminishes, allowing left-to-right shunting through the septal defect. In patients with moderate-to-large VSDs, symptoms usually develop within the first 2 years of life. Small defects can close spontaneously.

The characteristic findings in VSD are PA enlargement, increased pulmonary vascularity, and cardiomegaly that is predominantly left-sided (Fig. 51.73). Increased pulmonary venous return results in volume overload of the left atrium and ventricle, leading to their dilation. LV dilation causes a "drooping" shape of the left cardiac border. LA enlargement is best seen on the lateral or left anterior oblique view as a bulge along the upper posterior cardiac border that causes posterior displacement of the esophagus and the left mainstem bronchus. If the shunt is large, biventricular dilation enlargement occurs.

Atrial Septal Defect is much less common than VSD. The most common type of ASD occurs centrally at the fossa ovalis, the ostium secundum defect. Because the shunt is low-pressure, these children seldom develop symptoms in infancy or early childhood. If the shunt persists as the child grows older, the risk of developing pulmonary hypertension increases. As the pressure in the right side of the heart rises, the shunt becomes balanced and eventually reverses to a right-to-left shunt. This phenomenon is referred to as Eisenmenger's physiology, and can be seen with any left-to-right shunt.

The LA is not enlarged with ASD because of rapid shunting of blood away from the left atrium into the right side of the heart. Typically, the RA is enlarged, causing prominence of the right cardiac border on the frontal view (Fig. 51.74). On the lateral view, RV enlargement produces fullness in the retrosternal space. In both ASD and VSD, the aorta is rather small, as the shunt is below the level of the great vessels.

The ostium primum type of ASD (endocardial cushion defect) is caused by abnormal development of the primitive endocardial cushions that form the interatrial and interventricular septa and atrioventricular valves. This condition commonly occurs in trisomy 21. The specific malformation ranges from two separate atrioventricular valves with a low ASD and a VSD to the complete form with a common atrioventricular ring and a five-leaflet valve. The mitral valve is cleft and abnormally positioned resulting in elongation of the left ventricular outflow tract, creating a "goose neck" appearance on angiography (Fig. 51.75). The partial form behaves hemodynamically as a simple atrial left-to-right shunt with only mild degrees of mitral or tricuspid insufficiency. The clinical

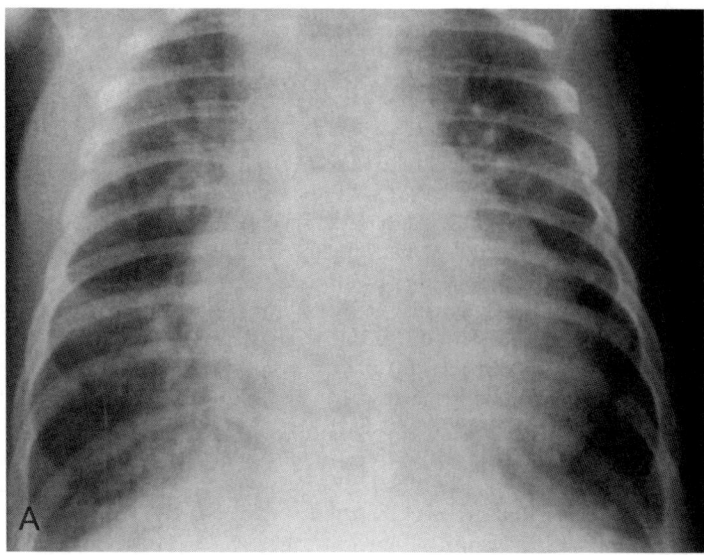

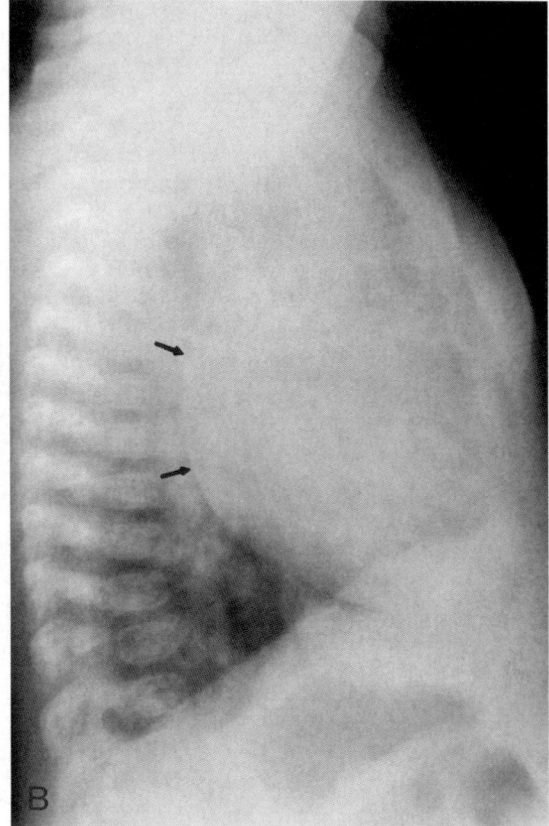

Figure 51.73. Ventricular Septal Defect. A. Increased pulmonary vascularity and cardiac enlargement that is predominantly left-sided are characteristic of VSD. **B.** Lateral view demonstrates left atrial enlargement (*arrows*).

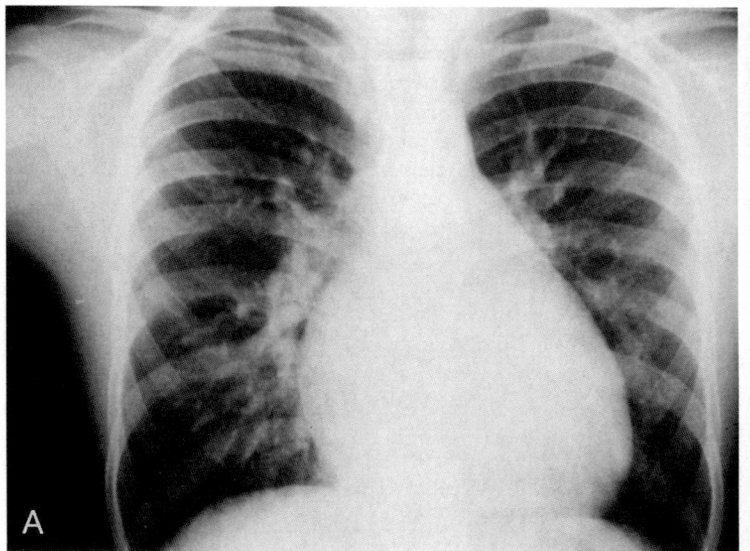

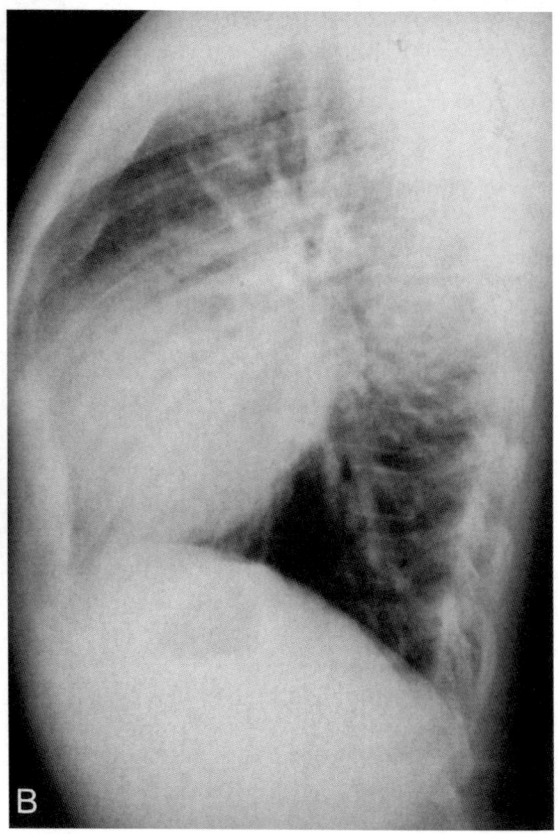

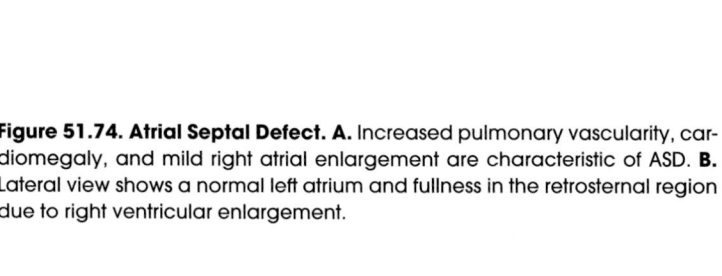

Figure 51.74. Atrial Septal Defect. A. Increased pulmonary vascularity, cardiomegaly, and mild right atrial enlargement are characteristic of ASD. **B.** Lateral view shows a normal left atrium and fullness in the retrosternal region due to right ventricular enlargement.

course of the complete form is much more severe. The shunts are large and usually bi-directional because of the abnormal valve development. The patients are cyanotic and tend to develop pulmonary hypertension and congestive heart failure early. Radiographically, these patients present with marked cardiomegaly with right atrial and right ventricular predominance and pulmonary vascular engorgement (Fig. 51.76).

Patent Ductus Arteriosus. The ductus arteriosus connects the pulmonary artery and aorta in fetal life. Normally, this structure begins to close immediately after birth, but in some infants closure is delayed. Prolonged patency is a common complication of hypoxia in the premature infant. In many infants, the cause of persistent patency is unknown, Symptoms develop within the first 2 years of life. Blood is shunted from the

aorta through the ductus to the PA, resulting in increased blood volumes flowing through the left side of the heart. Consequently, the LA, LV, and PA become dilated with active pulmonary vascular engorgement. An enlarged proximal aorta differs from the small aorta that is seen with ASD and VSD (Fig. 51.77). In young infants with large shunts, cardiomegaly tends to be more generalized and the size of the aorta is difficult to evaluate because of overlying thymus. PDA is easily diagnosed by angiography and echocardiography.

Aortic Pulmonary Window is a rare condition that is very similar to PDA both hemodynamically and radiographically. The abnormality results from failure of complete division of the primitive truncus arteriosus which leaves a communication between the aorta and the PA just above the valves. Other rare conditions that result in shunting of blood from the aorta to the PA include rupture of an aneurysm of the sinus of Valsalva and fistulas between the coronary arteries and the coronary sinus, pulmonary artery, or right cardiac chambers.

Cyanotic Heart Disease with Increased Pulmonary Vascularity

This category consists of a group of complex heart abnormalities whose common feature is the admixture of oxygenated and deoxygenated blood that is circulated systemically, resulting in cyanosis.

Transposition anomalies of the great vessels are lesions with abnormal anterior-to-posterior positioning of the aorta and PA and with abnormalities of the relationship between the atria and ventricles and their connections to the great vessels.

Complete Transposition of the Great Vessels is the most common form of cyanotic congenital heart disease with increased pulmonary blood flow. In this condition, the position of the aorta and PA are reversed. The ven-

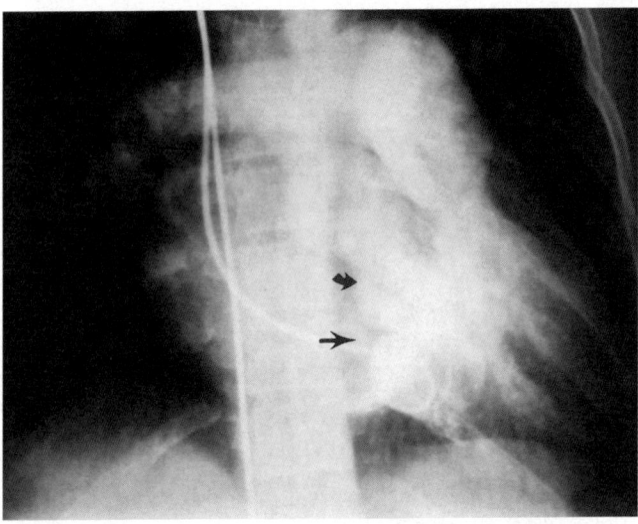

Figure 51.75. Endocardial Cushion Defect. Angiocardiography demonstrates the cleft mitral valve (*arrow*) and the elongated left ventricular outflow tract (*curved arrow*), the "goose-neck deformity."

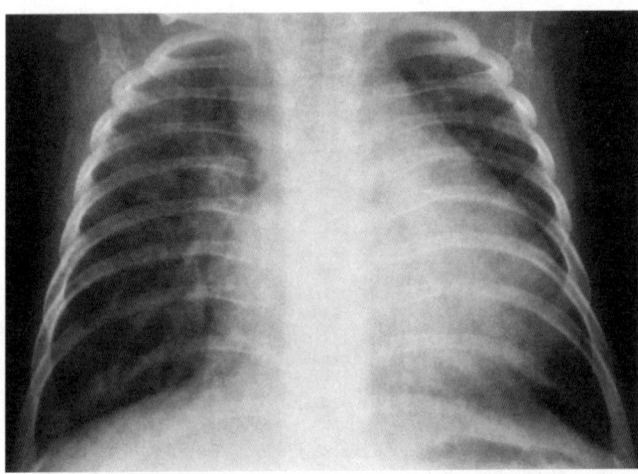

Figure 51.76. Endocardial Cushion Defect. Increased pulmonary vascularity with marked cardiomegaly and right atrial enlargement are typical of endocardial cushion defect.

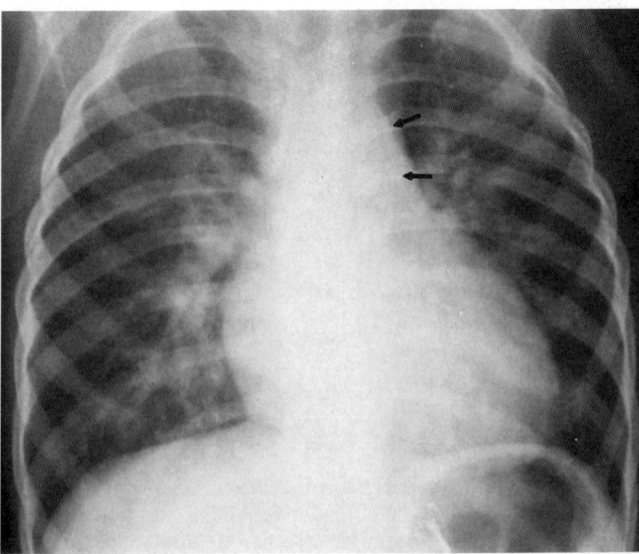

Figure 51.77 Patent Ductus Arteriosus. The heart is enlarged with left-sided prominence, increased pulmonary vascularity, and prominent aorta (*arrows*).

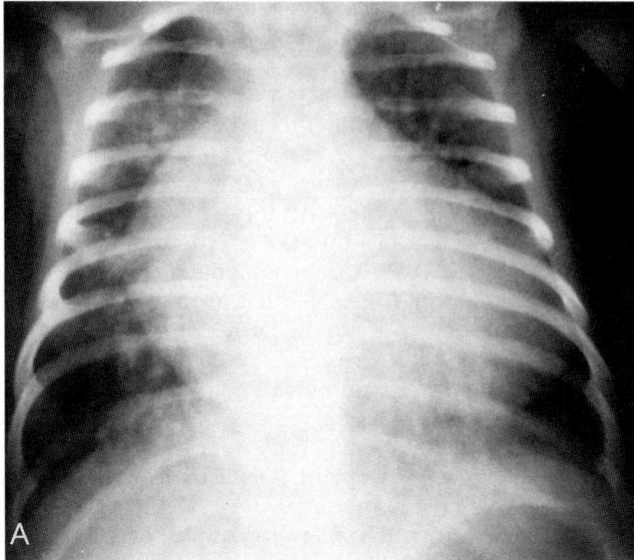

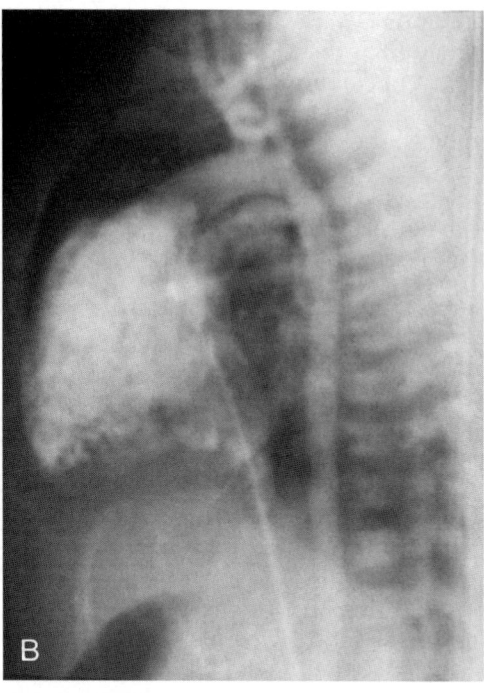

Figure 51.78. Transposition of the Great Vessels. A. The heart is enlarged with a typical "egg" shape. The superior mediastinum is narrow and the pulmonary vascularity is increased. **B.** Angiocardiography (in lateral view) shows the aorta arising anteriorly from the right ventricle.

tricles lie in their normal position with aorta arising anteriorly from the RV and the PA arising posteriorly from the LV. This results in two separate circulations, one through the pulmonary circulation and the other systemic. Communications that allow the infant to survive are most commonly a VSD, ASD, or PDA. Bidirectional shunting through these communications allows adequate mixing of the blood if the shunts are large enough. If pulmonary stenosis is not present, blood flows preferentially into the low-resistance pulmonary circulation resulting in increased pulmonary venous return and pronounced volume overloading. Congestive heart failure develops in the first weeks of life. The prognosis is more favorable with associated pulmonary stenosis.

Cardiomegaly with an oval configuration develops in the first few days of life (Fig. 51.78). The superior mediastinum and base of the heart are narrow because of thymic atrophy and the abnormal alignment of the aorta and PA. Both active and passive pulmonary vascular congestion can be seen. On lateral views of the chest, the anteriorly placed aorta causes increased opacity in the retrosternal region. Angiocardiography establishes the diagnosis (Fig. 51.78). Currently, these patients are sent so rapidly to surgery for the so-called "great vessel switch" procedure, that the classic radiographic findings may not develop.

Corrected Transposition of the Great Vessels. In corrected transposition, ventricular inversion (left-to-right reversal) accompanies the transposed positions of the aorta and PA resulting in functional correction of the transposition. Blood circulates through the heart RA to LV to PA to the pulmonary circulation, and LA to RV to aorta to the systemic circulation. The anatomic right ventricle functions as a left ventricle and vice versa.

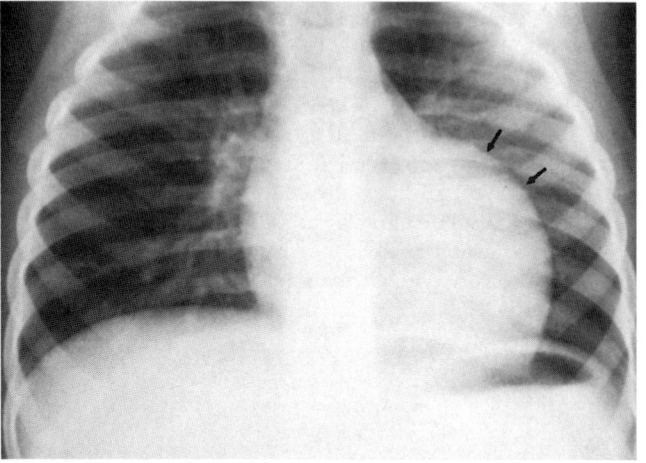

Figure 51.79. Congenitally Corrected Transposition. The transposed aorta arising from the inverted right ventricle on the left causes characteristic prominence along the upper left cardiac border (*arrows*).

Because the aorta lies anteriorly and to the left, this condition is often called L-transposition, while complete transposition is called D-transposition. Patients with the simple form of corrected transposition tend to be asymptomatic, but patients with coexisting cardiac defects (VSD, pulmonary stenosis, conduction defects) have an unfavorable prognosis. The diagnosis is suggested radiographically by a characteristic prominence along the upper left cardiac border that is due to the right ventricular outflow tract and the left-sided aorta (Fig. 51.79).

Double-outlet Right Ventricle is characterized by an aorta that is anterior and arises from the right ventricle. The PA, however, also empties the right ventricle, originating entirely from the right ventricle (type I), or overriding a high VSD and draining both the left and right ventricles (type II or the Taussig-Bing anomaly). The hemodynamics are similar to complete transposition of the great vessels. Radiographic findings are also similar. However, because the aorta and PA are oriented in a more side-to-side fashion, the cardiac waist is usually of normal or even increased width, unlike the narrow waist seen in transposition.

Total Anomalous Pulmonary Venous Return (TAPVR) is a condition in which the pulmonary veins, instead of emptying into the LA, return blood to the right side of the heart via the RA, coronary sinus, or a systemic vein. This anomaly can occur in conjunction with other major cardiac defects, but this discussion will refer only to the isolated form. The best-known classification of the types of TAPVR was described by Darling et al. In all types, the pulmonary veins converge into a single common vein before emptying into the anomalous site. In type I TAPVR, the most common form, the abnormal vein empties into a large supracardiac vein (a persistent left superior vena cava, the left brachiocephalic vein, the right superior vena cava, or the azygos vein). In the type II anomaly, the common vein drains into the coronary sinus or directly into the RA. In the type III anomaly, the common vein travels through the esophageal hiatus to empty into the portal vein or, less commonly, an abdominal systemic vein. TAPVR types I and II overload the right side of the heart, causing dilation of the RA, RV, and PA and engorgement of the pulmonary vessels. Communication with the left side of the heart is mandatory for survival and usually occurs as an ASD or patent foramen ovale. The classic radiographic configuration of the type I anomaly is the "snowman" heart, so named because of prominence of the superior mediastinum due to

a large, inverted U-shaped vessel that empties into the superior vena cava (Fig. 51.80). This configuration is only present when the abnormal common pulmonary vein enters the persistent left superior vena cava or vertical vein. In the other forms of the type I anomaly and in the type II anomaly, the cardiac configuration is less specific. Type II findings resemble those of the transposition complex of lesions. In the type I anomaly, if the abnormal vein empties into the azygos vein, it will be dilated.

Type III TAPVR is hemodynamically and radiographically distinct from the other forms. Although blood is directed incorrectly to the right side of the heart, the length and small caliber of the common vein increases the resistance to flow and creates pulmonary venous obstruction. The pulmonary vessels appear thin with hazy margins caused by pulmonary interstitial edema and passive vascular engorgement (Fig. 51.81). The heart does not enlarge. The differential diagnosis includes hypoplastic left heart syndrome and pulmonary vein atresia.

Persistent Truncus Arteriosus occurs when the primitive truncus arteriosus fails to divide normally into the aorta and pulmonary arteries. Both vessels are fed by a single vessel that overrides a high VSD. The Collete-Edwards classification is based on the site of origin of the pulmonary artery (Fig. 51.82). The degree of cyanosis is variable and symptoms depend largely on the amount of pulmonary blood flow. Most often the chest radiograph shows cardiomegaly and active pulmonary vascular congestion. In most forms of persistent truncus, concavity is seen at the usual site of the main PA and strongly suggests the diagnosis. A right aortic arch is present in 30% of the cases (Fig. 51.83). The aorta (truncus) is often dilated with a high arch and an elevated left PA.

Single Ventricle refers to a group of anomalies in which one ventricle is rudimentary, leaving the other large ventricle as the only functional ventricle. An underdeveloped right ventricle is most common. The connections between ventricles and the atrioventricular

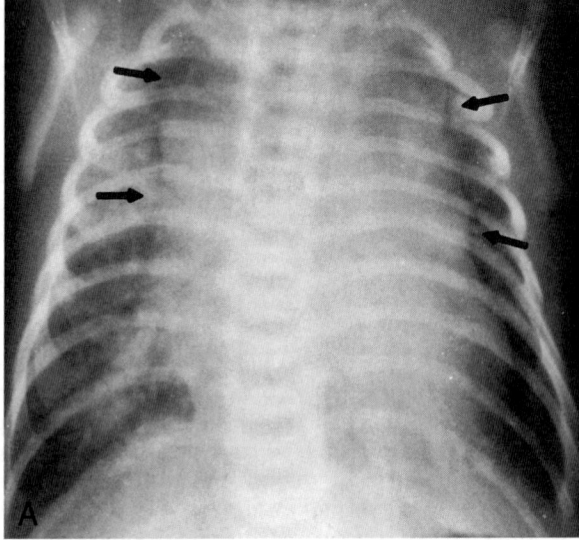
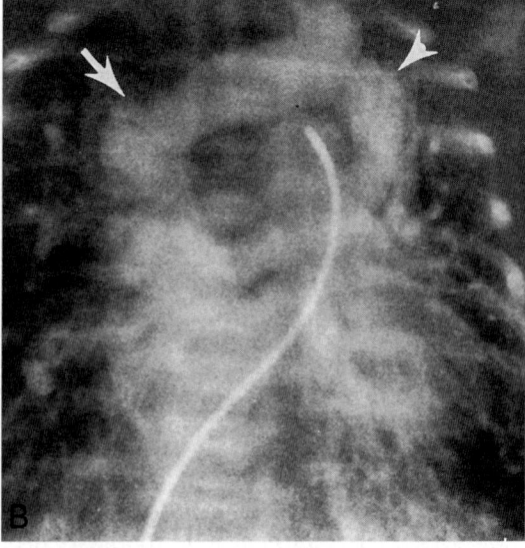

Figure 51.80. Total Anomalous Pulmonary Venous Return: Type I. A. The characteristic "snowman" (*arrows*) or "figure-8" configuration results from cardiomegaly combined with prominence of the supe-

rior mediastinum due to the anomalous pulmonary vein. **B.** Cardioangiogram demonstrate the inverted-U shaped vessel (*arrows*) which constitutes the upper portion of the snowman.

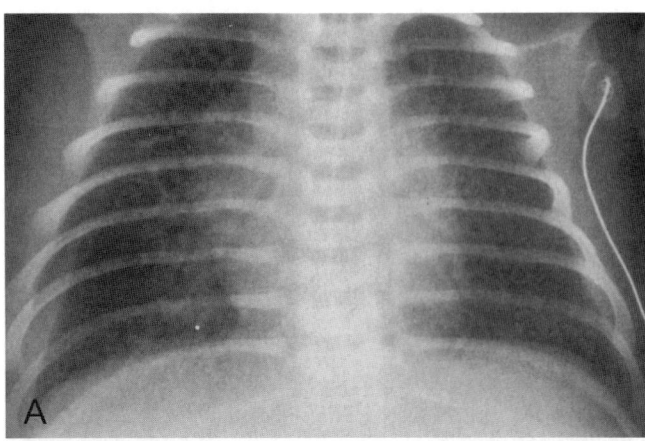

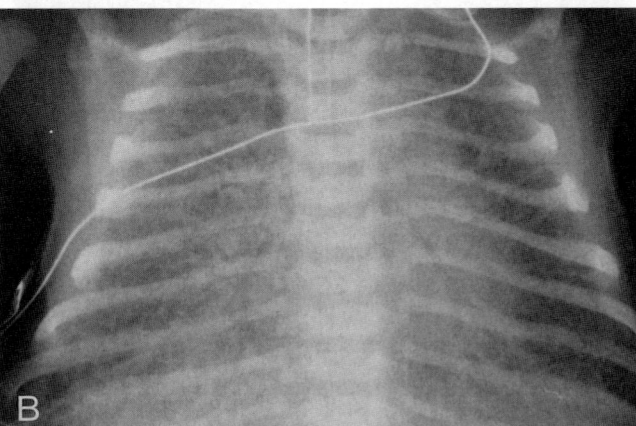

Figure 51.81. Total Anomalous Pulmonary Venous Return: Type III. A. The heart is normal in size with thin and somewhat indistinct pulmonary vessels due to passive vascular congestion. A prominent interstitial pattern in the lungs represents pulmonary edema. Bilateral pleural effusions are present. **B.** Another patient has more severe pulmonary edema. Once again, note the normal heart size.

valves, aorta, and PA are variable. Associated lesions include pulmonary valve stenosis, PA atresia, and transposition of the great vessels. If pulmonary stenosis is not present, mixing of saturated and unsaturated blood occurs in the single chamber, and the radiographs show cardiomegaly and pulmonary vascular engorgement. When pulmonary stenosis is present, blood flow to the lungs is diminished and cyanosis is more severe. Echocardiography is usually diagnostic, however, angiocardiography or MR is sometimes needed for complete demonstration of the anatomy.

Decreased Pulmonary Vascularity

A decreased pulmonary vascular pattern usually indicates a condition in which the flow through the right side of the heart is obstructed. This obstruction can occur anywhere from the tricuspid valve to the pulmonary arteries. Often an intracardiac right-to-left shunt, which varies with the severity of right ventricular outflow obstruction, is also present.

Tetralogy of Fallot is the most common anomaly to cause diminished pulmonary vascularity and is the most common cause of cyanotic congenital heart disease. The

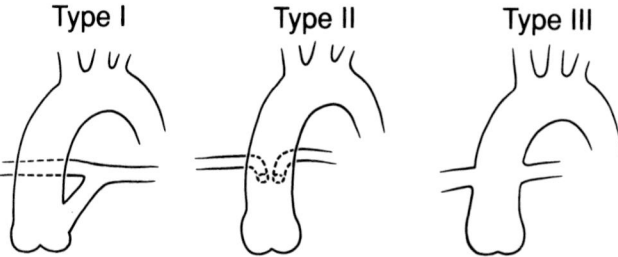

Figure 51.82. Persistent Truncus Arteriosus Classification. These diagrams illustrate the basic forms of the original Collett-Edwards classification of persistent truncus arteriosus.

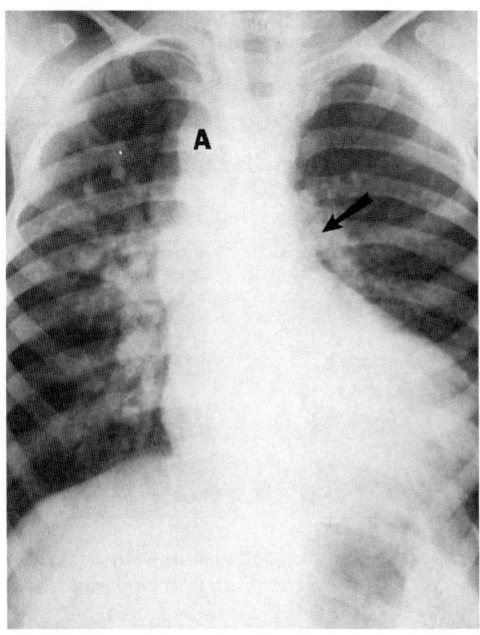

Figure 51.83. Persistent Truncus Arteriosus. Note oval cardiomegaly, increased pulmonary vascularity, a concave pulmonary artery segment (*arrow*) and a right aortic arch (*A*).

classic components are *a*) a high VSD, *b*) pulmonary stenosis (usually infundibular, with or without valvular stenosis), *c*) right ventricular hypertrophy, and *d*) an aorta that overrides the VSD. A right aortic arch occurs in 25% of cases and PA coarctation, hypoplasia, or absence are common.

The degree of pulmonary stenosis is the most critical component of this anomaly. Severe stenosis leads to marked right-to-left shunting and aortic enlargement, causing greater overriding (Fig. 51.84). Greater right-to-left shunting results in more severe cyanosis. Patients with mild pulmonary stenosis are usually acyanotic and asymptomatic ("pink" or "balanced" tetralogy of Fallot).

Patients with moderate-to-severe forms of tetrology have a characteristic radiographic appearance. The pulmonary vascularity is decreased with a shallow or concave PA shadow. Right ventricular hypertrophy causes lateral and superior displacement of the cardiac apex without overall enlargement of the cardiac silhouette, creating the classic "boot-shaped" heart (Fig. 51.85). Unequal pulmonary blood flow due to PA hypoplasia or

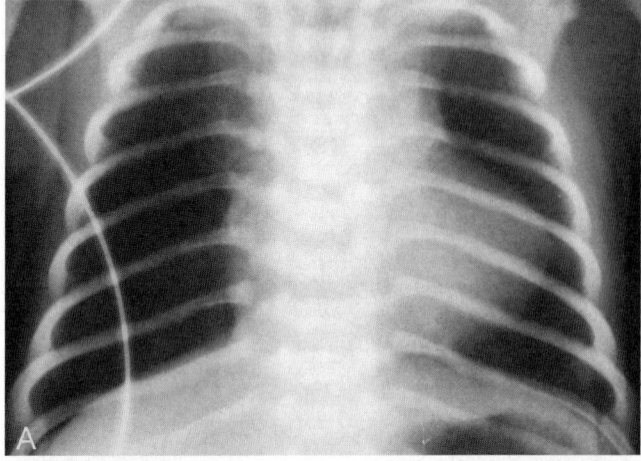

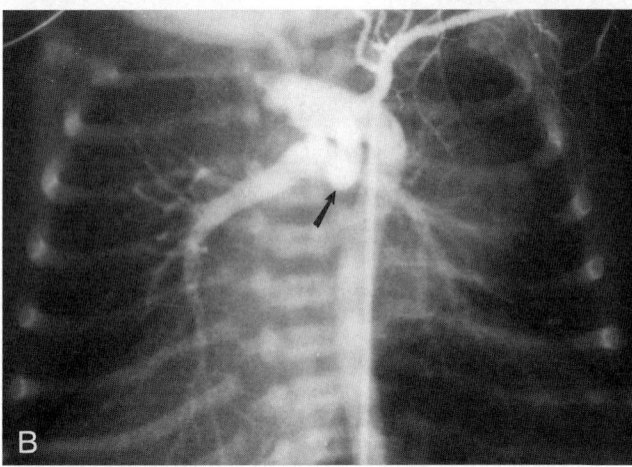

Figure 51.84. Tetralogy of Fallot with Pulmonary Atresia. A. Pulmonary vascularity is diminished, and the heart is enlarged. **B.** Aortogram identifies the patent ductus arteriosus (*arrow*), which supplies blood from the aorta to the pulmonary arterial system in this patient with pulmonary atresia.

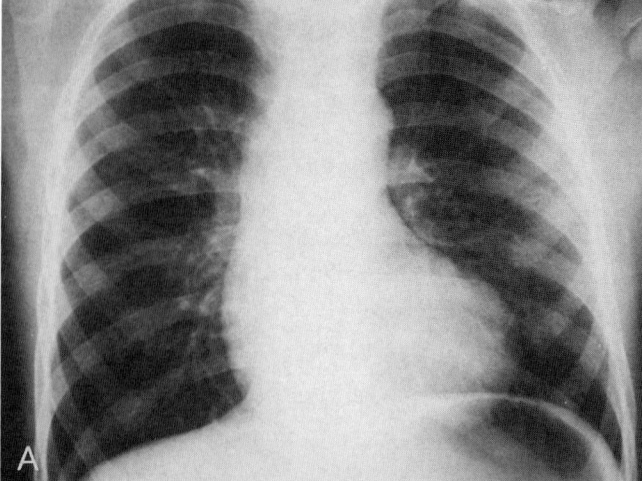

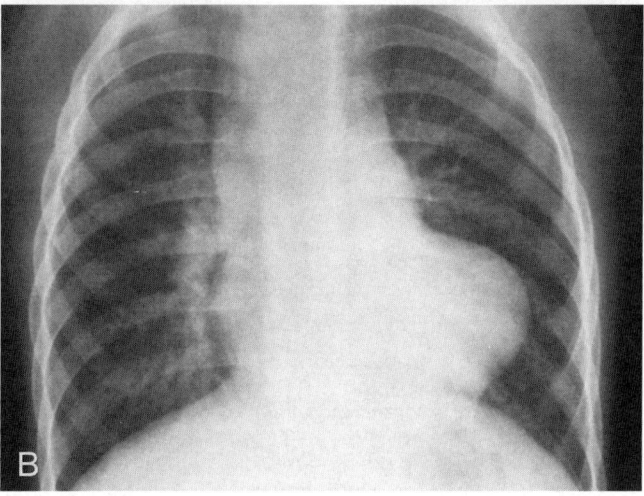

Figure 51.85. Tetralogy of Fallot. A. A boot-shaped appearance to the heart is created by an upwardly displaced cardiac apex due to right ventricular hypertrophy and a concave pulmonary artery shadow. **B.** Another patient with a boot-shaped heart and right aortic arch.

atresia (usually the left) is a common finding. The combination of a right aortic arch and decreased pulmonary vascularity is highly suggestive of tetralogy of Fallot or persistent truncus arteriosus.

Hypoplastic Right Heart syndrome consists of tricuspid atresia usually with pulmonary atresia or stenosis and an underdeveloped right ventricle. Isolated hypoplasia of the right ventricle is rare. The common features are a small right ventricle with right-to-left shunting through an ASD, resulting in cyanosis. A VSD or PDA can also be present. Nonspecific cardiomegaly and diminished pulmonary vascularity are seen radiographically. The PA shadow is flat or concave and the RA is enlarged (Fig. 51.86). The smaller the ASD, the larger is the size of the RA. tricuspid atresia may be accompanied by transposition of the great vessels. When this occurs, the PA drains the LV and, if no pulmonary stenosis is present, the pulmonary vascularity is engorged.

Pulmonary Atresia is considered a part of the hypoplastic right heart syndrome when accompanied by an intact ventricular septum. In most cases, the pulmonary valve is atretic and the RV and tricuspid valve

are hypoplastic. Less commonly, the RV and tricuspid valve are near normal and blood that enters the RV is regurgitated back into the RA, resulting in marked RA enlargement (Fig. 51.87). In either case, survival requires a PDA to shunt blood into the pulmonary circulation. Prostaglandin E_1 is used to help maintain ductal patency until surgery can be performed.

In patients with pulmonary atresia with a VSD, the RV is not hypoplastic. This situation occurs in severe tetralogy of Fallot and in pulmonary atresia with VSD and systemic collaterals (the old Collete-Edwards type IV truncus arteriosus). The most significant difference between these two conditions is the derivation of pulmonary blood flow. In severe tetralogy of Fallot, blood reaches the lungs through a long, tortuous, "wandering" PDA. The other form of pulmonary atresia with VSD relies on primitive systemic collaterals that transport blood from the aorta to the PA branches.

Ebstein's Anomaly consists of a malformed, enlarged tricuspid valve that is displaced downward, resulting in

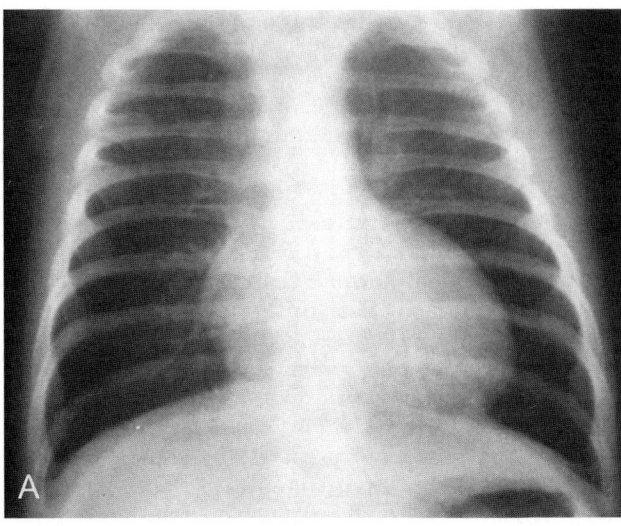
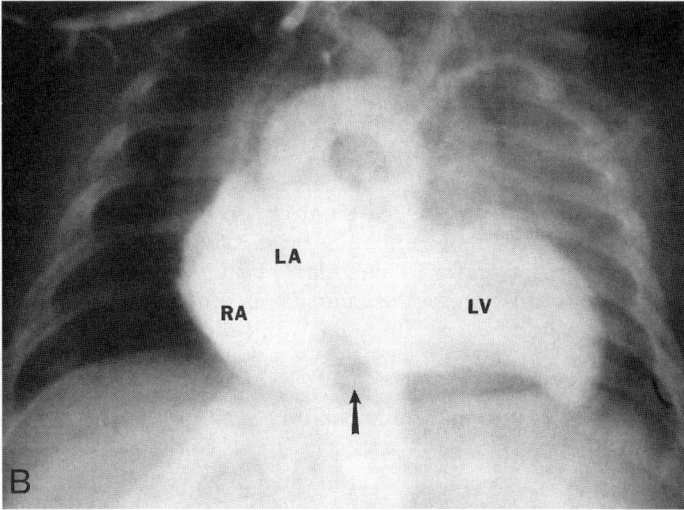

Figure 51.86. Tricuspid Atresia. A. Pulmonary vascularity is decreased with a concave pulmonary artery segment, and the right atrium and left ventricle are enlarged. **B.** Angiocardiography shows contrast in the right atrium (*RA*), left atrium (*LA*), and enlarged left ventricle (*LV*). A bare area is seen due to lack of filling of the right ventricle (*arrow*).

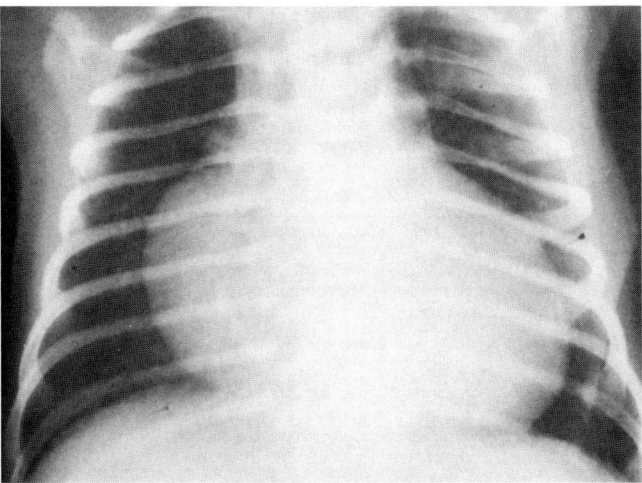

Figure 51.87. Pulmonary Atresia with Intact Ventricular Septum. Marked right atrial enlargement is present due to regurgitation of blood from the right ventricle with an atretic outflow tract and intact ventricular septum. Right ventricular size is near normal.

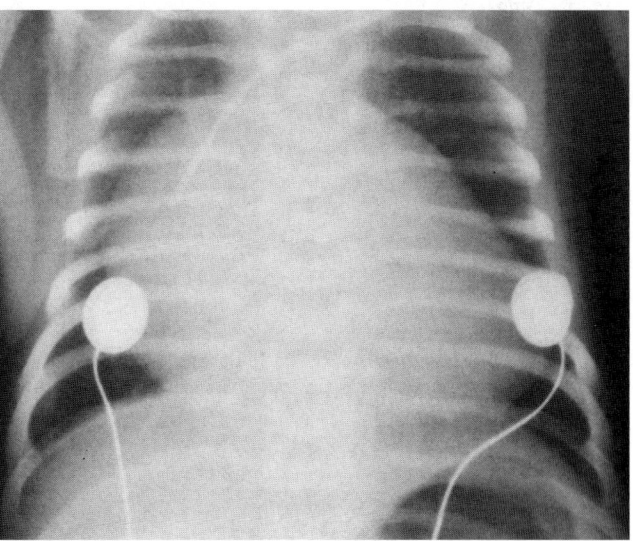

Figure 51.88. Ebstein's Anomaly. Severe cardiomegaly with marked right atrial enlargement and decreased pulmonary vascularity is typical for Ebstein's anomaly.

atrialization of a large portion of the RV. The remaining RV is very small. The atrialized portion has abnormal musculature, contracts ineffectively, and causes functional obstruction of RA emptying. Atrial right-to-left shunting results in cyanosis in the more severely affected patients. Clinical symptoms and radiographic findings depend on the degree of downward displacement of the tricuspid valve. Cardiomegaly is mainly right-sided with decreased pulmonary vascularity and a flattened PA shadow (Fig. 51.88). Occasionally, the small displaced RV is seen as a bulge along the upper left cardiac border, causing a squared cardiac appearance.

Uhl's anomaly is rare and consists of focal or complete absence of the RV myocardium. The very thin, poorly contractile RV functionally impairs the flow of blood through the right side of the heart. The clinical and radiographic findings are similar to those of Epstein's anomaly.

Normal Pulmonary Vascularity

Congenital cardiac anomalies with normal pulmonary vascularity are predominantly abnormalities of the cardiac valves and great vessels. Most have left-sided obstruction. When a concomitant left-to-right shunt is present, cardiac failure develops early the pulmonary vascularity becomes congested. In the absence of a left-to-right shunt, patients can go for many years without left ventricular failure.

Congenital Valve Stenosis most commonly affects the aortic or pulmonary valves. The radiographic findings in children are similar to those seen in adults, and consist of hypertrophy of the ventricle that ejects blood through the stenotic valve and poststenotic dilation of the affected artery (Fig. 51.89). Ventricular hypertrophy alters the shape of the heart with little change in the size of the heart. LV hypertrophy causes a more rounded appearance of the left cardiac border. RV hypertrophy produces fullness in the retrosternal region on the lateral view and lateral displacement of the cardiac apex on the posteroanterior view. In valvular pulmonic stenosis, poststenotic dilation of the main PA is often accompanied by prominence of the left PA and increased blood flow to the left lung. This finding is less commonly seen in children than in adults.

Aortic and pulmonary stenosis may also occur above or below the valve. Subvalvular is more common than supravalvular aortic stenosis. The subvalvular narrowing is due either to a discrete diaphragm or to disproportionate hypertrophy of the subaortic intraventricular septum. Supravalvular aortic stenosis is most often associated with Williams syndrome (idiopathic hypercalcemia of infancy) (Fig. 51.90) The features of this syndrome include supravalvular aortic stenosis and other systemic and pulmonary vascular stenoses, facial dysmorphism, mental and growth retardation, and hypercalcemia due to abnormal regulation of vitamin D metabolism. Subvalvular (infundibular) pulmonary stenosis is most often seen in tetralogy of Fallot. Supravalvular pulmonary stenosis usually consists of multiple areas of narrowing in the peripheral PA. The subvalvular and supravalvular forms are usually not associated with poststenotic great vessel dilation.

Congenital Valve Insufficiency is very rarely isolated, but sometimes accompanies other cardiac anomalies. In general, valvular insufficiency causes dilation of the cardiac chambers or vessels on both sides of the involved valve (Fig. 51.91). The resulting cardiac configurations are the same as those seen in adults with valvular insufficiency.

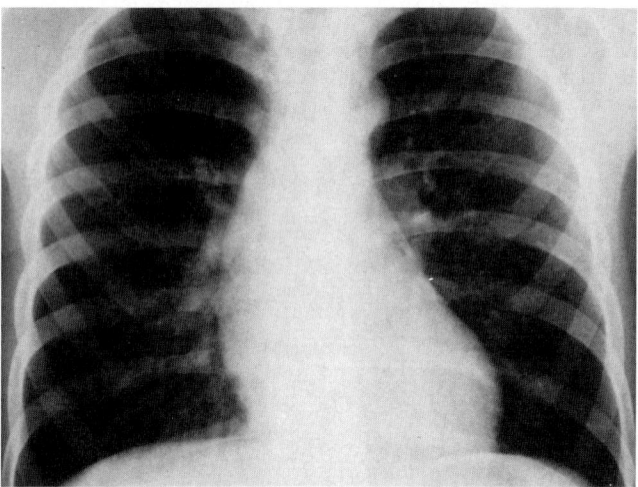

Figure 51.89. Aortic Valve Stenosis. The ascending aorta and aortic arch are prominent in this 5-year-old child with congenital aortic stenosis.

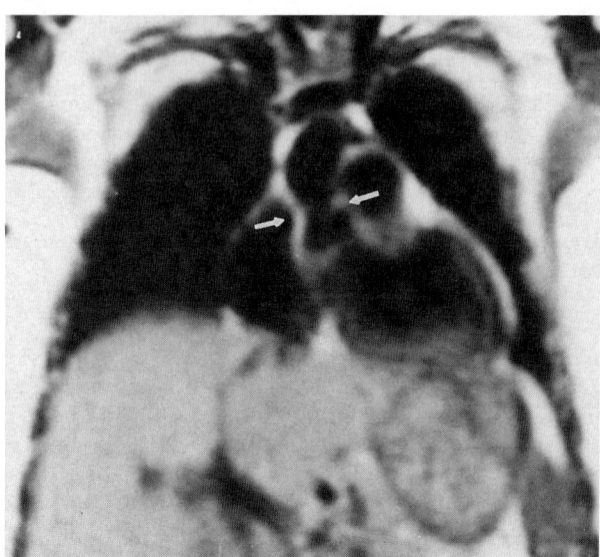

Figure 51.90. Supravalvular Aortic Stenosis (Williams Syndrome). Coronal MR demonstrates the short-segment narrowing of the aorta just above the sinus of Valsalva (*arrows*).

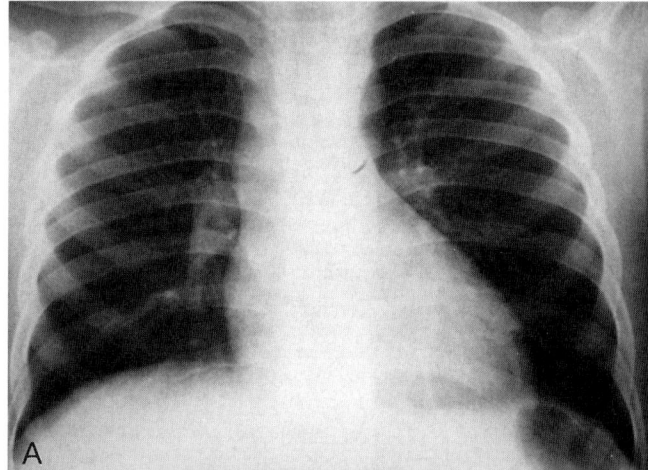

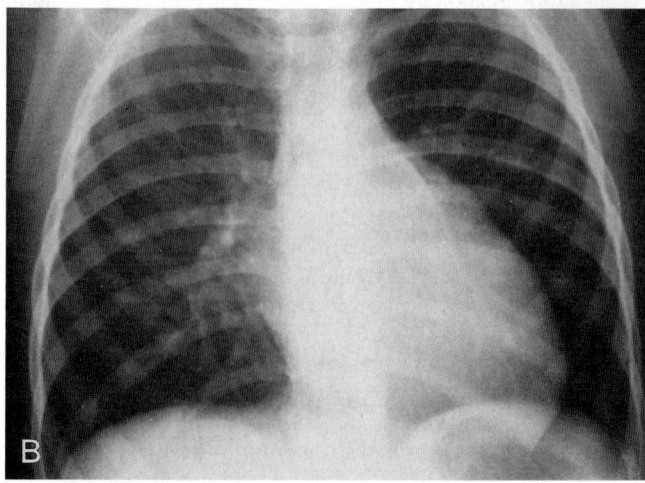

Figure 51.91. Congenital Valvular Insufficiency. A. The dilation of the left ventricle and the ascending aorta are characteristic of aortic valve insufficiency. **B.** Left atrial and left ventricular dilation, in another patient, are found with congenital mitral insufficiency.

Coarctation of the Aorta occurs in two distinct forms: the juxtaductal (adult) type, which lies at or just distal to the ductus arteriosus, and the rarer preductal (infantile) form, which is a long-segment narrowing. Coarctation of the aorta often is commonly associated with bicuspid aortic valve, PDA, or VSD. Patients with the preductal form undergo a more severe clinical course, frequently developing congestive heart failure during the first month of life. Patients with the juxtaductal form usually remain asymptomatic until later in childhood, except in those cases with a left-to-right shunt. Older children present with hypertension, discrepancies in the blood pressure between the upper and lower extremities, and a heart murmur. In juxtaductal coarctation, the aortic narrowing leads to pressure overloading and hypertrophy of the LV. The heart is usually normal in size but eventually develops rounding and prominence of the left cardiac border. Pre- and post-stenotic dilation of the aorta causes the "figure-3" sign (Fig. 51.92A). In some cases, poststenotic dilation extends along the entire descending thoracic aorta. Collateral circulation develops, usually involving the in-

tercostal arteries causing notching along the inferior edge of the posterior ribs from T-4 to T-8 (Fig. 51.92B). This finding usually is not visible until the patient is 7 or 8 years of age. Coarctation of the aorta is frequently di-

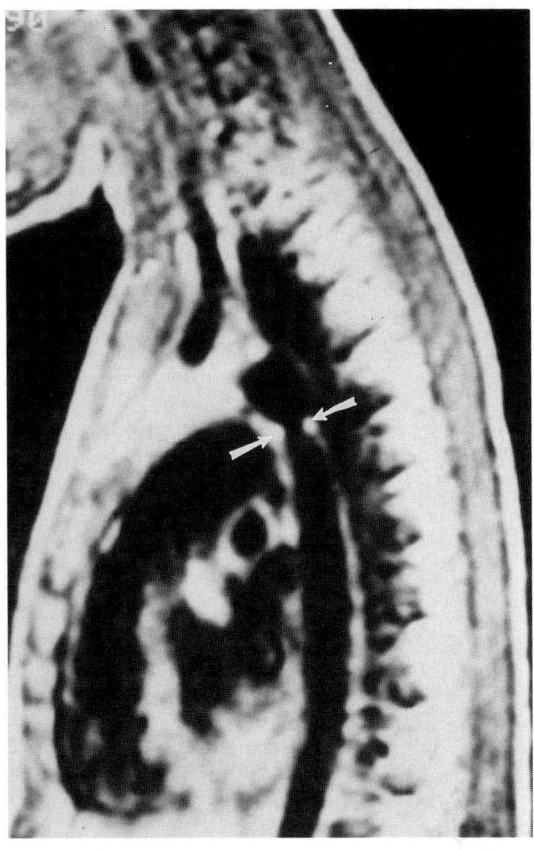

Figure 51.93. Coarctation of the Aorta. A slightly oblique sagittal MR image clearly shows the area of coarctation (*arrows*).

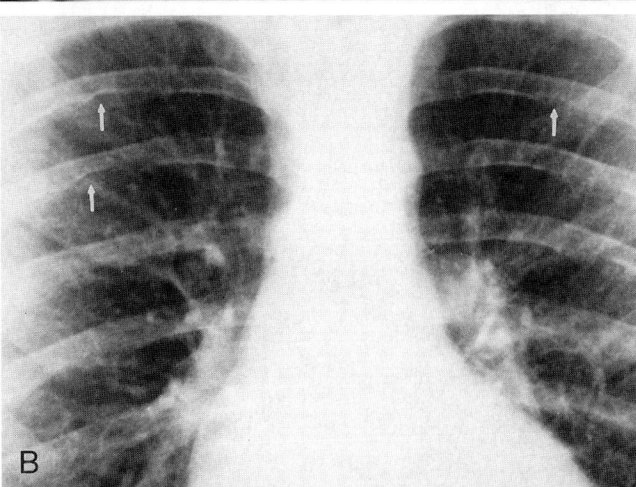

Figure 51.92. Coarctation of the Aorta. A. The rounded prominence of the left cardiac border is due to left ventricular hypertrophy. The figure-3 sign is difficult to see in this patient. **B.** The small notches along the inferior edges of the upper ribs bilaterally (*arrows*) are indicative of collateral circulation.

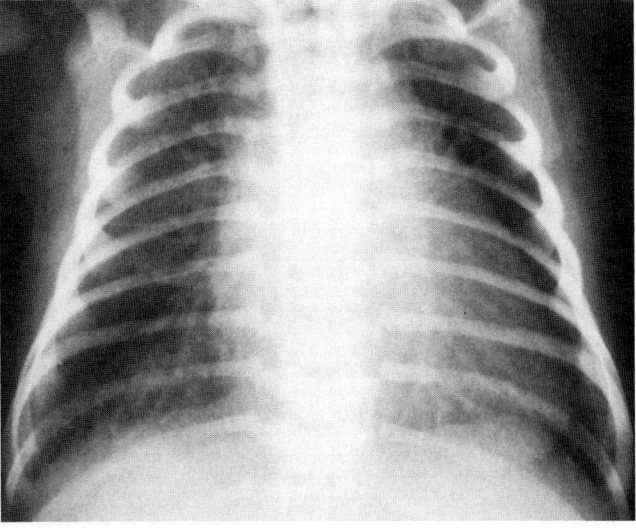

Figure 51.94. Hypoplastic Left Heart Syndome. The cardiomegaly and passive pulmonary vascular congestion usually develop within the first few days of life.

agnosed by echocardiography with further definition of anatomy by MR (Fig. 51.93).

Hypoplastic Left Heart Syndrome consists of lesions characterized by underdevelopment of the left side of the heart. The anomalies range from isolated atresia of the ascending aorta or aortic or mitral valves, to aortic and mitral valve atresia combined with marked hypoplasia of the LA, LV, and ascending aorta. In all cases blood flow through the left heart is severely impaired and a PDA is necessary to allow blood to reach the systemic circulation. Although the heart size and pulmonary vascularity can appear normal in the first few hours of life, cardiomegaly and congestive heart failure usually develop within the first 2 days. The pulmonary vasculature becomes passively congested and a diffusely hazy or reticular pattern develops in the lungs due to interstitial

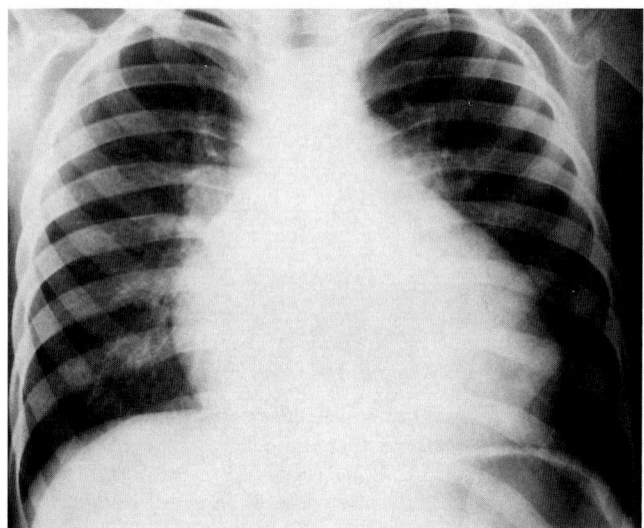

Figure 51.95. Cardiomyopathy. Marked cardiomegaly with left-sided predominence and early passive vascular congestion is seen in this child with idiopathic cardiomyopathy.

pulmonary edema (Fig. 51.94). The diagnosis is usually made by echocardiography.

Cor Triatriatum is a rare anomaly that presents in early infancy with pulmonary venous obstruction. In this anomaly the pulmonary veins empty into a common vein, which is abnormally incorporated into the LA. A partial membrane creates an extra chamber along the superior and dorsal aspect of the LA and variably obstructs venous emptying into the LA. The usual radiographic findings are cardiomegaly and passive venous congestion without evidence of LA enlargement.

Cardiomyopathies can also present with a normal pulmonary vascular pattern. Cardiomyopathies may accompany a variety of conditions in children including bacterial or viral infections, autoimmune diseases, toxic insults, and hereditary neuromuscular diseases. Asymmetrical septal hypertrophy is an unusual form of cardiomyopathy associated with subvalvular hypertrophic aortic stenosis. Radiographic findings of cardiomyopathy include cardiomegaly that may be generalized or predominantly left-sided (Fig. 51.95). The pulmonary vascularity remains normal until congestive heart failure develops. Endocardial fibroelastosis is a condition in which the left ventricular myocardium becomes markedly thickened with increased amounts of elastic and fibrous tissue. This results in marked LV and LA enlargement. The heart has a rounded configuration because of the thickened myocardium (Fig. 51.96). The enlarged LV often encroaches on the RV and impairs RV function. The LV can cause left lower lobe atelectasis by compression of the left lower lobe bronchus. Congestive heart failure usually occurs early in infancy.

Cardiac Malpositions

Cardiac malpositions are a confusing group of abnormalities and a detailed description of these conditions will not be attempted here. Nevertheless, mastery of the

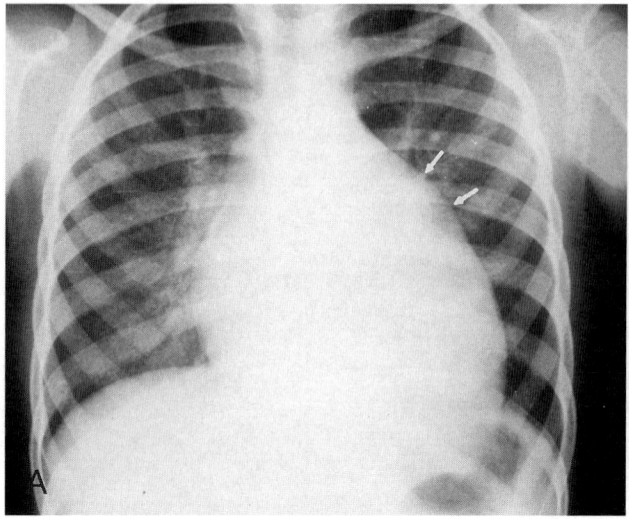

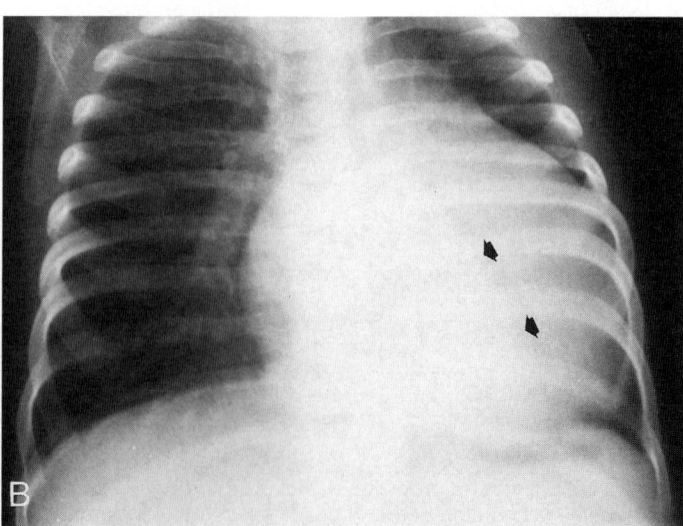

Figure 51.96. Endocardial Fibroelastosis. A. Note enlargement of the left atrium (*arrows*) and left ventricle. **B.** Another patient has a markedly enlarged left ventricle that has resulted in left lower lobe atelectasis (*arrows*).

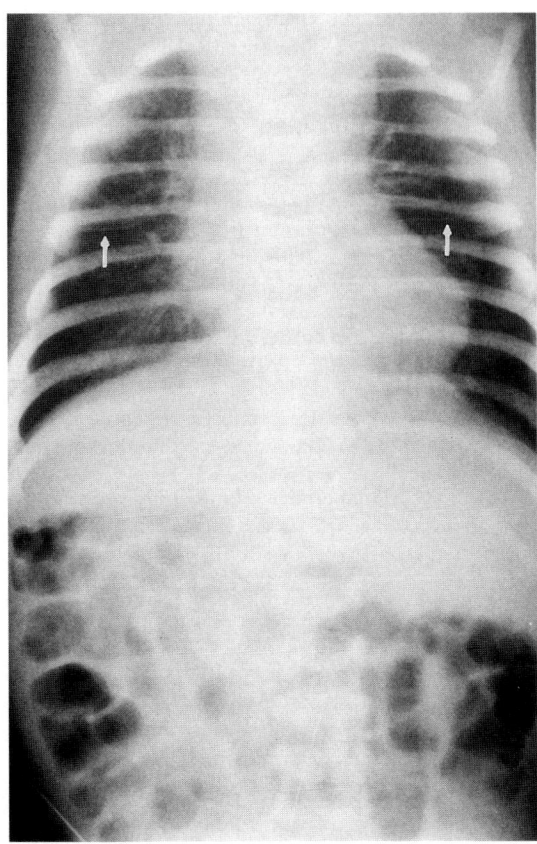

Figure 51.97. Asplenia Syndrome. Bilateral horizontal lung fissures (*arrows*) are indicative of bilateral right-sidedness. The liver has a midline configuration.

terminology used to describe these conditions can help provide a basic understanding of the anatomy involved. *Dextrocardia* implies a heart that lies to the right of the spine because of primary malpositioning during development. *Levocardia* is the normal position of the heart, to the left of the spine. When faced with cardiac malpositioning, one must then determine the position of the abdominal organs (i.e., the abdominal situs). In general, the RA will lie on the same side as the liver and the LA will lie on the side opposite the liver. *Situs solitus* refers to the normal position of the viscera with the liver on the right and the stomach on the left. The reversed position is referred to as *visceral situs inversus*.

Inversion refers to reverse positioning of anatomic structures, usually from right-to-left and vice versa, and thus a dextroposed heart can be either inverted or noninverted. The atria and ventricles can be inverted simultaneously or separately, and are referred to as *concordant* if they remain normally related to each other (i.e., the LA connected to the LV and the RA to the RV). If the LA is connected to the RV, the condition is referred to atrioventricular *discordance*.

Mirror-image Dextrocardia is the most common type of cardiac malposition. The cardiac chambers are completely inverted and the cardiac apex points to the right. Normal anteroposterior chamber relationships are preserved and there is no discordance. Visceral situs inver-

sus is present and the incidence of congenital heart disease is increased only slightly.

Dextroversion refers to right-sided rotation of the cardiac position so that the RA and RV are more posterior and the LA and LV lie anterior. Chamber inversion does not occur. Visceral situs solitus or inversus can be present, and in either case congenital cyanotic heart disease is frequent. Other variations of dextroposition are relatively rare.

Asplenia-Polysplenia Syndromes. Visceral heterotaxia and congenital heart disease are common components of the cardiosplenic (asplenia-polysplenia) syndromes. The asplenia (Ivemark's) syndrome is associated with more severe forms of congenital heart disease than the polysplenia syndrome. The liver often lies in the midline and intestinal malrotation is common. The asplenia syndrome can be thought of as bilateral right-sidedness (absent spleen, bilateral three-lobed lung, bilateral superior vena cava) (Fig. 51.97). Polysplenia resembles bilateral left-sidedness (multiple spleens, bilateral bilobed lungs, interrupted inferior vena cava with azygous continuation, biliary atresia). Situs inversus with levocardia is a rare situation. Systemic venous abnormalities and congenital heart disease with RV outflow track obstruction are common associated abnormalities.

References

1. Swischuk LE, Hayden CK Jr. Lower respiratory tract infection in children (Is roentgenographic differentiation possible?). Pediatr Radiol 1986;16:278–284.
2. Khamapirad RT, Glezen WP. Clinical and radiographic assessment of acute lower respiratory tract disease in infants and children. Semin Respir Infect 1987;2:130–151.
3. Wildin SR, Chonmaitree T, Swischuk LE. Roentgenographic features of common pediatric viral respiratory tract infections. Am J Dis Child 1988;142:43–46.
4. Guckel C, Benz-Bohm G, Widemann B. Mycoplasmal pneumonias in childhood: roentgen features, differential diagnosis and review of the literature. Pediatr Radiol 1989;19:499–503.
5. Amodio JB, Berdon WE, Abramson SJ. Cystic fibrosis in childhood: pulmonary, paranasal sinus, and skeletal manifestations. Semin Roentgenol 1987;22:125–135.
6. Lowe GM, Donaldson JS, Backer CL. Vascular rings: 10-year review of imaging. Radiographics 1991;11:637–646.
7. Swischuk LE, Richardson CJ, Nichols MM, et al. Primary pulmonary hypoplasia in the neonate. J Pediatr 1979;95:573–577.
8. Rosado-de-Christenson ML, Stocker JT. From the archives of the AFIP congenital cystic adenomatoid malformation. Radiographics 1991;11:865–886.
9. Byard RW, Bohn DJ, Wilson G, et al. Unsuspected diaphragmatic hernia: a potential cause of sudden and unexpected death in infancy and early childhood. J Pediatr Surg 1990;25:1166–1168.
10. Manning PB, Murphy JP, Rayunor, SC, et al. Congenital diaphragmatic hernia presenting due to gastrointestinal complications. J Pediatr Surg 1992;27:1225–1228.
11. Swischuk, LE. Vomiting blood for three days. Pediatr Emerg Care 1994;10:241–243.
12. Swischuk LE, Shetty B, John SD. The lungs in immature infants; how important is surfactant therapy in preventing chronic lung problems? Pediatr Radiol 1996;26:508–511.
13. Swischuk LE, John S D. Immature lung problems: can our

nomenclature be more specific? AJR Am J Roentgenol 1996;166:917–918.

14. Fitzgerald P, Donoghue V, Gorman W. Bronchopulmonary dysplasia: a radiographic and clinical review of 20 patients. Br J Radiol 1990;63:514–517.

15. Gross GW, Cullen J, Kornhauser MS. Thoracic complications of extracorporeal membrane oxygenation: findings on chest radiographs and sonograms. AJR Am J Roentgenol 1992;158:353–358.

16. Amodio JB, Abramson SJ, Berdon WE, et al. Iatrogenic causes of large pleural fluid collections in the premature infant: ultrasonic and radiographic findings. Pediatr Radiol 1987;17:104–108.

17. Goutail-Flaud MF, Sfez M, Berg A, et al. Central venous catheter-related complications in newborns and infants: a 587-case survey. J Pediatr Surg 1991;26:645–650.

18. John PF, Beasley SW, Mayne V. Pulmonary sequestration and related congenital disorders: a clinico-radiological review of 41 cases. Pediatr Radiol 1989;20:4–9.

19. West MS, Donaldson JS, Shkolnik A. Pulmonary sequestration: diagnosis by ultrasound. J Ultrasound Med 1989; 8:125–130.

20. Han BK, Babcock DS, Oestreich AE. Normal thymus in infancy: sonographic characteristics. Radiology 1989;170: 471–474.

21. Siegel MJ, Glazer HS, Wiener JI, Molina PL. Normal and abnormal thymus in childhood: MR imaging. Radiology 1989; 172:367–371.

22. Liu P, Daneman A, Stringer DA. Real-time sonography of mediastinal and juxtamediastinal masses in infants and children. J Can Assoc Radiol 1988;39:190–202.22.

23. Leung AN, Müller NL, Pineda PR, FitzGerald JM. Primary tuberculosis in childhood: radiographic manifestations. Radiology 1992;182:87–91.

24. DuMontier CM, Graviss ER, Siberstein MJ, McAllister WH. Bronchogenic cysts in children. Clin Radiol 1985;36: 431–436.

25. Bisset GS, III. Magnetic resonance imaging of congenital heart disease in the pediatric patient. Radiol Clin North Am 1991;29:279–291.

26. Swischuk LE, Stansberry SD. Pulmonary vascularity in pediatric heart disease. J Thorac Imag 1989;4:1–6.

52
Pediatric Abdomen and Pelvis

Susan D. John
Leonard E. Swischuk

GASTROINTESTINAL TRACT

Gastrointestinal Obstruction

Gastrointestinal (GI) obstruction is a more common problem in infants and children than in adults, and must be distinguished from numerous other causes of vomiting and abdominal distension. For the most part, congenital obstructions present early in life, usually in the first 30 days. We have found it helpful to consider the various causes of obstruction under four age-group categories, for the most likely causes shift in importance according to a child's age (Table 52.1). The basic job of the imager is to determine the location or level of obstruction and, if possible, the cause. Even in this day of sophisticated imaging it is the plain abdominal film, with decubitus or upright augmentation, that provides the most information. Determination of the site of obstruction depends upon noting the most distal extent of the air-filled, abnormally distended portion of the GI tract. Where the abnormally distended air column ends is the most likely level of obstruction.

Hypopharyngeal/Upper Esophageal Obstruction is most commonly caused in children by a spastic cricopharyngeus muscle. However, this condition is not very common and there is debate as to whether a prominent cricopharyngeus muscle indentation alone is always symptomatic. The cause of symptomatic spasm is often underlying brain stem disease, but in many cases the spasm is idiopathic. In refractory cases, surgical division of the muscle may be required.

Difficulties with swallowing also can occur with inflammatory processes such as epiglottitis, retropharyngeal abscess, tonsillar abscess, or a number of tumors or cysts that occur in this area. A large pharyngeal diverticulum may produce obstruction. These diverticula can be congenital or iatrogenic due to perforation of the hypopharynx during intubation. They are best demonstrated with barium swallow.

ESOPHAGEAL OBSTRUCTIONS

Esophageal Atresia and Tracheoesophageal Fistula. The most common congenital obstruction of the esophagus is esophageal atresia (Table 52.2). The site of obstruction is usually in the upper third of the esophagus. An air-filled upper esophageal pouch is classic (Fig. 52.1). The pouch may be chronically distended in utero due to swallowed amniotic fluid, causing pressure on the trachea that results in focal tracheomalacia. When severe, respiratory difficulty can persist even after repair of the esophageal obstruction.

Esophageal atresia is frequently associated with tracheoesophageal fistula. Most commonly, the fistula extends from the trachea, just above the carina, to the distal esophageal pouch. The fistula allows air to enter the stomach and intestines, in some cases in large volumes. Air in the stomach differentiates esophageal atresia without fistula from esophageal atresia with fistula. Without a fistula there is no way for air to get into the stomach or intestines. The proximal, obstructed esophageal pouch is often distended with air (Fig. 52.1). If necessary, the pouch can be demonstrated with barium, but only a small amount should be administered through a nasoesophageal tube, to prevent aspiration. Fistulae to the upper pouch also occur but are rare.

Esophageal atresia is more common in trisomy 21 and is associated with vertebral anomalies, duodenal atresia, and imperforate anus. Esophageal atresia results from faulty separation of the GI tract from the neurenteric tube with subsequent faulty canalization of the esophagus. A variety of communications may exist between the esophageal pouch and the spine, ranging from fibrous bands to actual fistulae. If the communication involutes at both ends and only the central portion remains, a neurenteric cyst results. Conversely, if an esophageal communication persists, a diverticulum is formed and a spinal communication leads to a meningocele. Faulty separation of the trachea and esophagus may also result in fistulae, fibrous bands, or diverticula. Tracheoesophageal fistula located high in the esophagus without esophageal atresia is the third most common abnormality in this group of lesions, following esophageal atresia with a distal tracheoesophageal fistula, and isolated esophageal atresia. The fistula is usually identified with barium swallow (Fig. 52.2).

Table 52.1. Most Common Causes of GI Tract Obstruction by Age

Age	Cause of Obstruction
0–1 Month	Congenital anomalies
	Atresia/stenosis
	Malrotation/volvulus
	Hirschsprung's disease
	Meconium plug/small left colon syndrome
	Meconium ileus
1–6 Months	Hernias
6 Months–3 years	Intussusception
3 Years and older	Perforated appendicitis
	Adhesions
	Regional enteritis

Table 52.2. Causes of Esophageal Obstruction

Congenital atresia/stenosis
Web/diverticulum
Foreign body
Stricture (peptic, caustic)
Extrinsic compression (cysts, neoplasms, vascular)
Achalasia

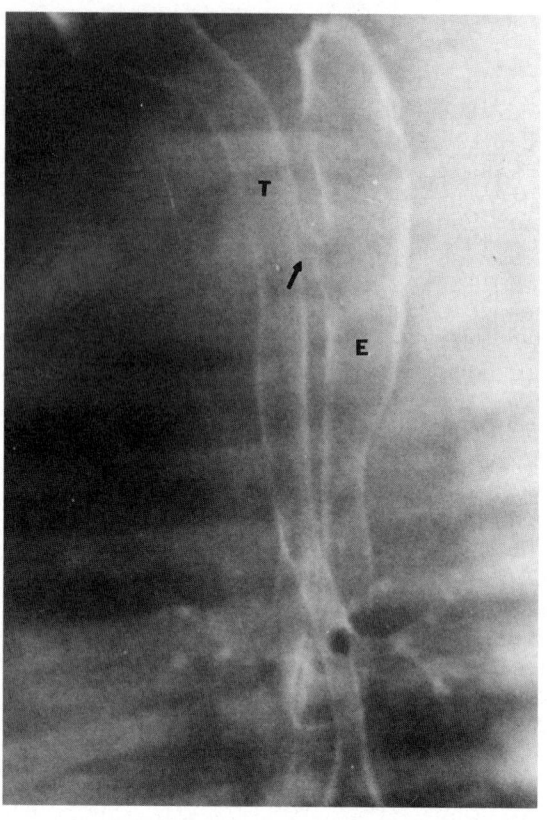

Figure 52.2. Tracheoesophageal Fistula. The trachea (*T*) and esophagus (*E*) are connected by a fistula (*arrow*).

Figure 52.1. Esophageal Atresia. A. Frontal view demonstrates the blind, air-filled upper esophageal pouch (*arrows*). Note the gas within the stomach and intestines which indicates the presence of an associated lower tracheoesophageal fistula. **B.** Lateral view in another patient demonstrates the typical air-filled pouch (*arrows*). A catheter is present in the pouch. The trachea is compressed and displaced by the pouch.

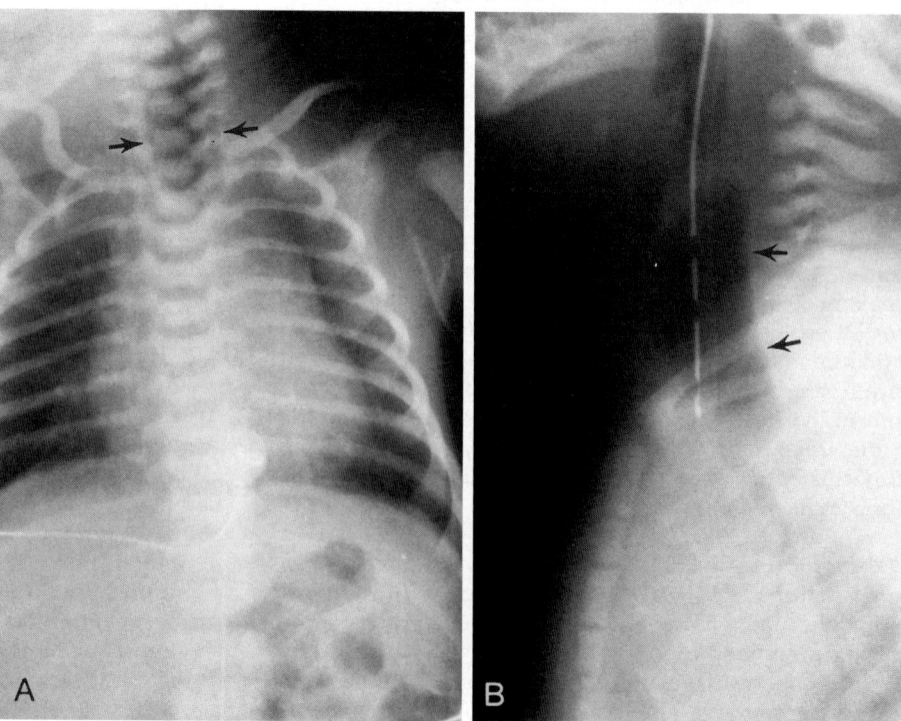

Congenital Esophageal Stenosis is a far less common cause of congenital esophageal obstruction. As in esophageal atresia, esophageal stenosis arises from faulty tracheal and esophageal separation where tracheobronchial cartilage remnants remain in the wall of the esophagus. On barium swallow, small diverticula (mucous glands) can be seen in the areas of stenosis.

Congenitally Short Esophagus with intrathoracic stomach is not truly a congenital lesion. Even though seen at birth, this condition more likely represents the aftermath of chronic prenatal hiatal hernia with gastroesophageal reflux and subsequent peptic esophageal stricture (Fig. 52.3).

Other uncommon congenital causes of esophageal obstruction include esophageal webs and diverticula.

Esophageal obstruction can also result from a variety of extrinsic lesions that produce pressure on the esophagus. Acquired esophageal obstructive lesions are primarily strictures or foreign bodies. Esophageal neoplasms are extremely rare in infants and children and malignant neoplasms are virtually nonexistent.

Peptic Esophagitis is associated with gastroesophageal reflux (GER) and can be seen with or without hiatus hernia. Although GER is very common in infants, peptic esophagitis with stricture is a relatively uncommon complication. GER may be primary (chalasia), due to a lax gastroesophageal sphincter, or secondary to a gastric outlet obstruction. The cause of gastric obstruction (pylorospasm, pyloric stenosis, gastric diaphragm, gastric ulcer disease) must be identified and treated for reflux to stop. GER is most reliably identified with 24-hour pH monitoring, but this procedure is cumbersome. Nuclear scintigraphy, the barium upper gastrointestinal (UGI) series, and US with color Doppler can be quite sensitive (Fig. 52.4)(1).

Peptic esophageal strictures usually are short and located in the distal third of the esophagus. The occasional case of Barrett esophagus with a high stricture can also be encountered. Peptic strictures may be irregular or surprisingly smooth mimicking the findings of achalasia (Fig. 52.5). Achalasia is uncommon as a cause of esophageal obstruction in children.

Caustic Esophagitis with stricture usually results from accidental ingestion of alkaline substances such as sodium hydroxide, potassium hydroxide (lye), or alkaline disk batteries. Disk batteries can become lodged in the esophagus and leak their alkaline contents, producing deep burns of the mucosa and submucosa. All alkaline burns cause deep penetrating injury that commonly results in stricture. Acids, even swallowed in significant quantities, produce more superficial burns. Although mucosal injury may be extensive, deep mural injury with fibrotic stricture is less common. Lye strictures lead to long areas of irregular narrowing (Fig. 52.6). Burns due to an ingested battery or medication (aspirin, tetracycline, Clinitest tablets) are more focal with stricture.

Epidermolysis Bullosa is an hereditary condition characterized by inflammatory skin and mucosal lesions that can heal with fibrosis resulting in esophageal stricture.

Acute Esophagitis. Esophageal obstruction due to acute inflammatory disease without stricture can also be seen. Acute inflammation with spasm occurs with monilial, herpetic, or peptic esophagitis. Monilial and herpetic esophagitis are a common problem with AIDS patients.

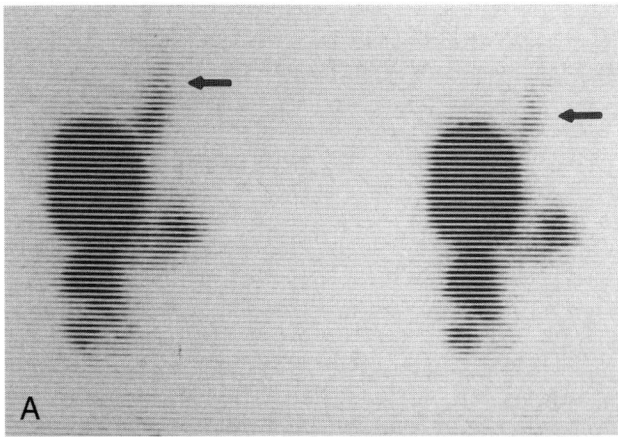

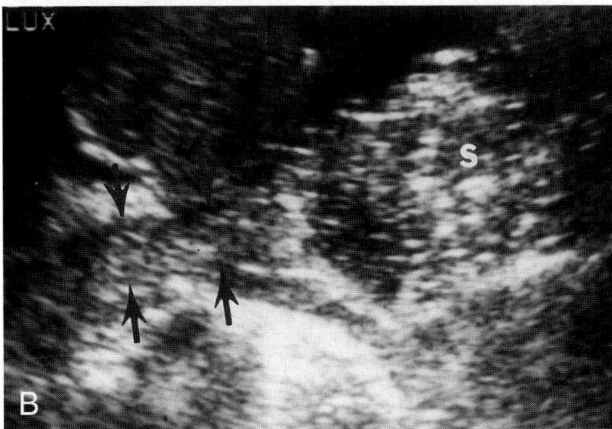

Figure 52.4. Gastroesophageal Reflux. A. Nuclear scintigraphy reveals reflux into the esophagus (*arrows*). **B.** US demonstrates fluid refluxing from the stomach (S) into the esophagus (*arrows*). This finding is more apparant in real-time.

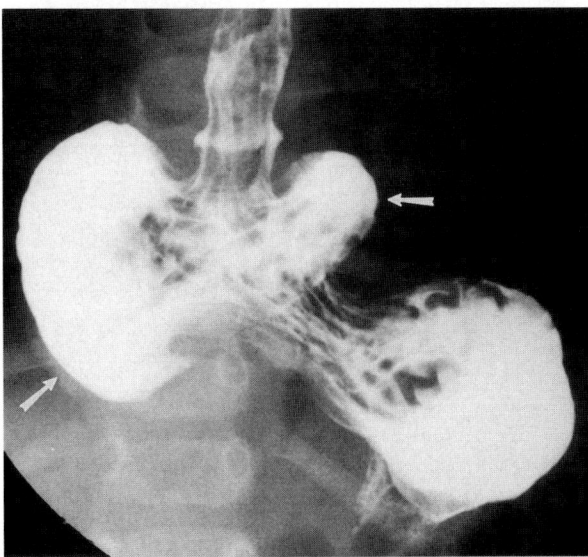

Figure 52.3. Intrathoracic Stomach. A large portion of the stomach (*arrows*) is above the diaphragm.

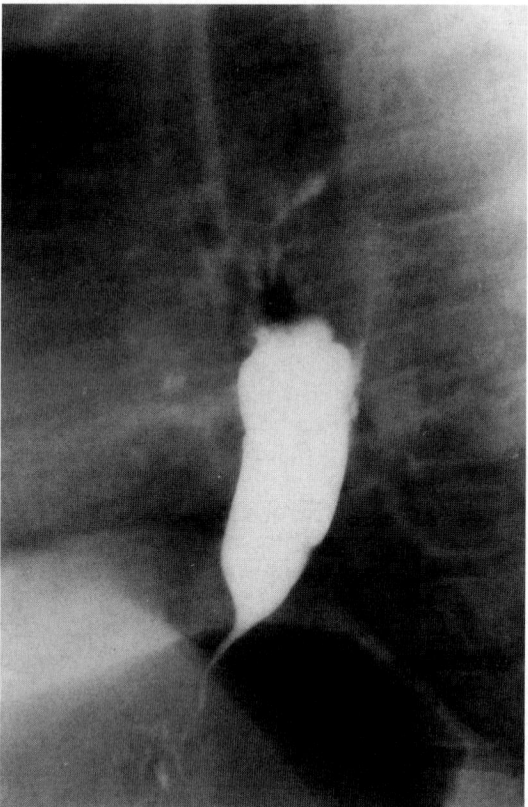

Figure 52.5. Peptic Stricture. The beak-like narrowing of the distal esophagus (*arrow*) mimics achalasia.

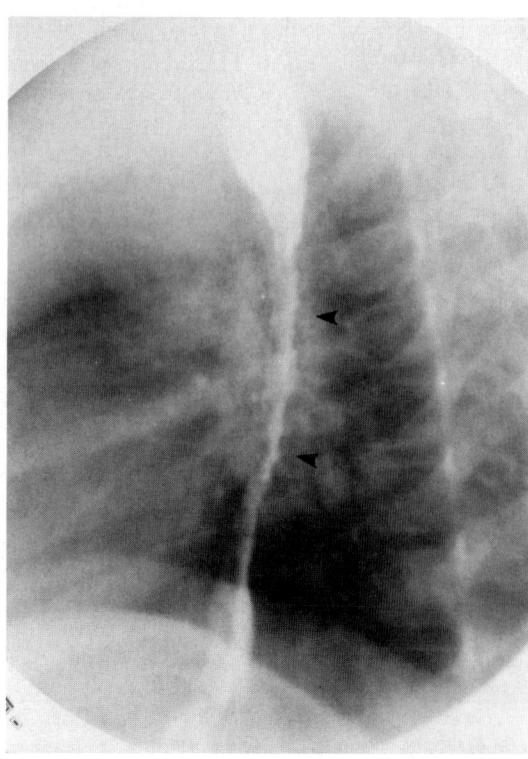

Figure 52.6. Caustic (Lye) Stricture. Note the characteristic long segment irregular configuration of the stricture (*arrows*).

GASTRIC OBSTRUCTION

Congenital obstructing lesions of the stomach are far less common than congenital obstructing lesions elsewhere in the GI tract (Table 52.3). Gastric distension on radiographs does not always indicate ostruction in infants. A large gas-filled stomach is occasionally found in normal infants, and persistent asymptomatic gastric distension occurs in infants receiving prostaglandins for ductal-dependent congenital heart disease (2).

Gastric Atresia is believed to result from a vascular insult to the stomach in utero. In the newborn infant if obstruction of the stomach is complete, radiographs show no air distal to the stomach (Fig. 52.7). Usually no further studies are required. In some cases, atresia takes the form of a gastric diaphragm or membrane which, if incomplete, will allow some gas distal to the obstructing web. US or a UGI series can be used to identify the incomplete diaphragm.

Gastric atresia may occur with congenital epidermolysis bullosa with stricturing due to inflammatory insult to the mucosa. *Microgastria* occurs with other GI atresias or VATER syndrome and is commonly associated with the polysplenia/asplenia syndromes.

Gastric Duplications must be critically located in the antrum or be very large to result in obstruction. They are best demonstrated with US where they appear sonolu-

Table 52.3. Causes of Gastric Obstruction

Atresia/antral diaphragm	Gastritis/ulcer disease
Duplication cyst	Volvulus
Pylorospasm	Microgastria
Hypertrophic pyloric stenosis	

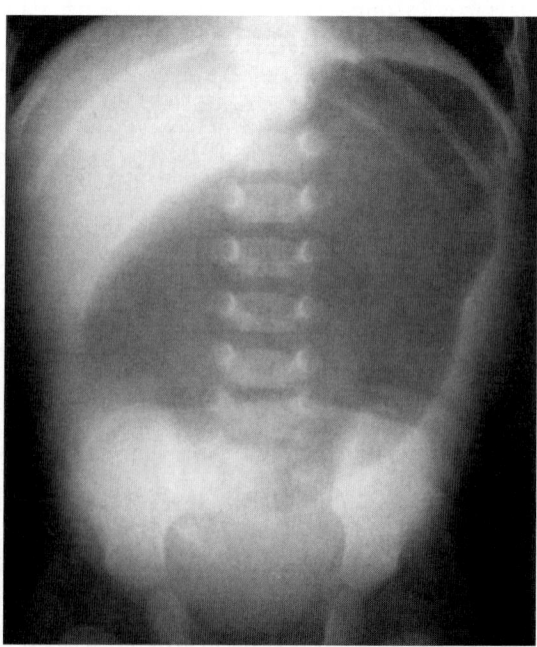

Figure 52.7. Gastric Atresia. Typical findings consist of a dilated air-filled stomach, with no air distal to the pylorus.

cent with a wall that demonstrates both mucosal and muscular layers (see Fig. 52.76).

Gastric Volvulus is an uncommon cause of gastric obstruction

Pylorospasm is a reactive problem due to insult to the gastric mucosa or muscle contraction from some other cause of stress. Mucosal inflammation may be due to milk allergy or peptic disease with ulceration. Most cases are due to simple spasm of the pyloric muscle. Real-time US demonstrates persistent contraction of the antropyloric region and poor emptying of liquids from the stomach. Occasionally minimal (less than 3 mm) thickening of the outer circular muscle can be seen (Fig 52.8). Intermittently, the antropylorus opens and gastric contents pass into the duodenum. The findings also can be demonstrated with UGI series, but US usually suffices. Antispasmodic therapy can be helpful in simple cases without predisposing cause.

Hypertrophic Pyloric Stenosis is now usually considered to be an acquired condition that, in some cases, may be related to prolonged pylorospasm. It most often develops between 2 and 8 weeks of age and is characterized by hypertrophy of the pyloric muscle. US is the preferred examination because of its ability to directly assess the thickness of the pyloric muscle and to provide real-time evaluation of contraction of the pyloric canal (3). The pyloric muscle measures 3 mm or more in thickness whereas the pyloric canal is elongated beyond 14 mm (Fig. 52.9) The pylorus is in fixed spasm and very little fluid passes through it. In atypical cases the pyloric canal is fixed in spasm, but the muscle measures 2–3 mm in thickness, whereas normal muscle measures no more than 1.5 mm in thickness. These patients may be

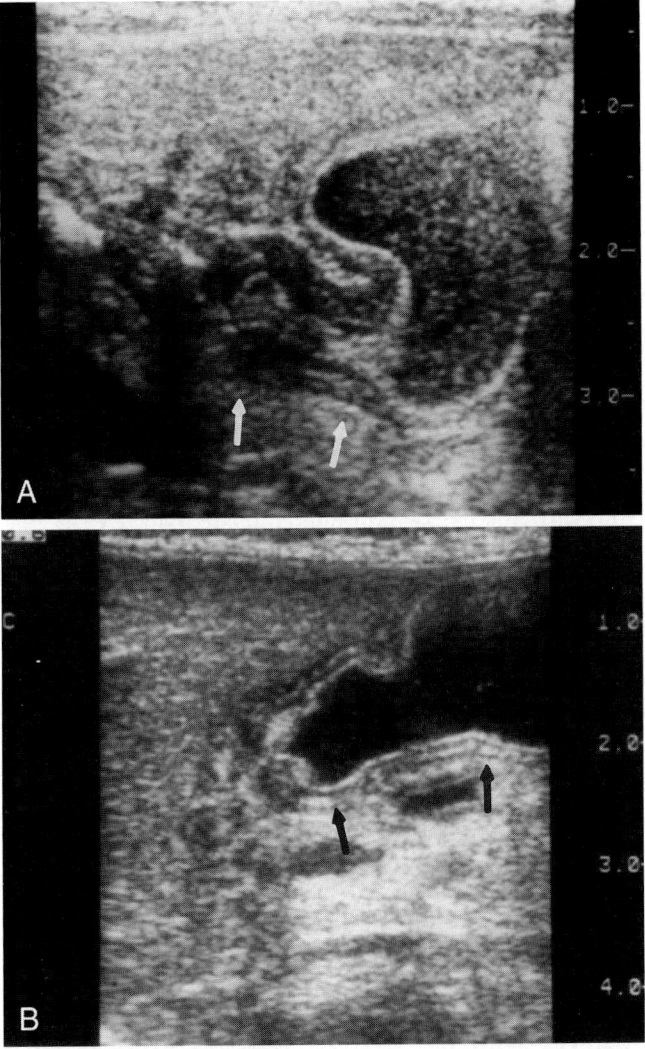

Figure 52.8. Pylorospasm US Features. A. The antrum is contracted. The muscle is slightly thickened but measures less than 3mm (*arrows*). **B.** After treatment with antispasm medication, the antrum opens, peristaltic activity is present, and the muscle has returned to normal thickness (*arrows*).

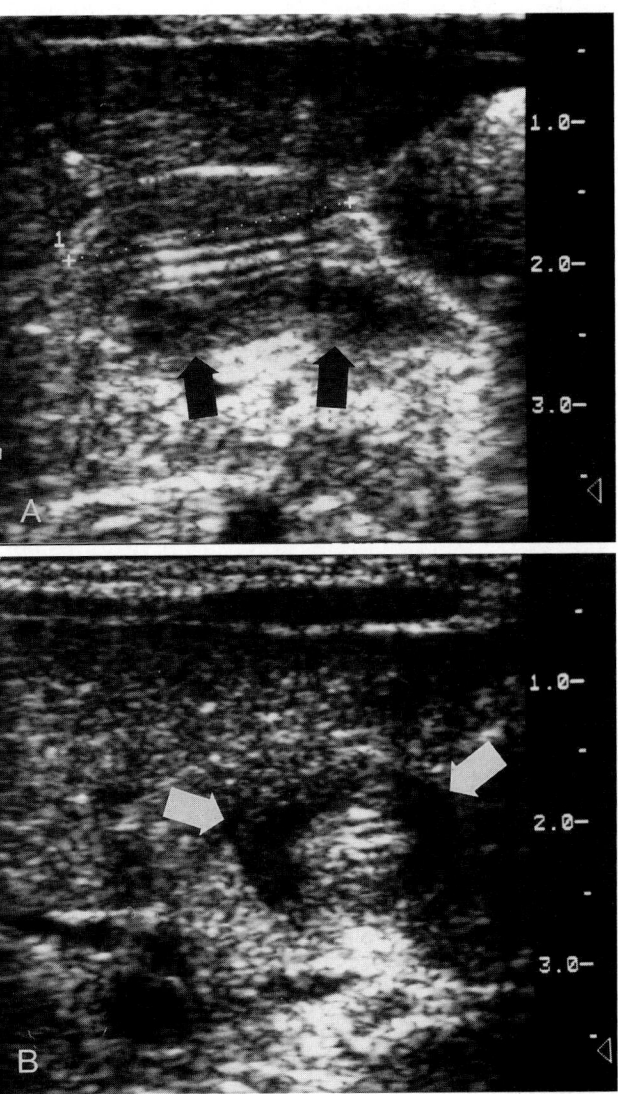

Figure 52.9. Pyloric Stenosis. A. Longitudinal view through the pylorus demonstrates the classic elongated pyloric canal (*arrows*) with thick outer hypoechoic muscle measuring nearly 5 mm in thickness. Note the echogenic layers of mucosa and the linear collections of fluid in the lumen. The canal measures 2.04 cm in length (*between cursors*). **B.** Cross-sectional view demonstrates the typical sonolucent donut configuration (*arrows*).

treated medically but should be followed closely, as some may progress to classic pyloric stenosis.

Tangential imaging of the normal, but contracted, pyloric canal may result in an erroneous impression of muscle thickening (Fig. 52.10). Furthermore, it has been demonstrated in pyloric stenosis that at the 6 o'clock and 12 o'clock positions, the pyloric muscle may not be as hypoechoic as it is at the 3 o'clock and 9 o'clock positions. As the circular muscle passes over the 6 and 12 o'clock positions, more acoustic interfaces are encountered and more echogenicity results. Finally, if the stomach is overfilled, the pyloric muscle mass can assume a posterior, upwardly curving position, making it more difficult to identify. With overdistention the stomach appears squared off at the antrum (Fig. 52.11). It may be necessary to empty the stomach with a nasogastric tube to allow the antropyloric canal to come into the viewing field (4).

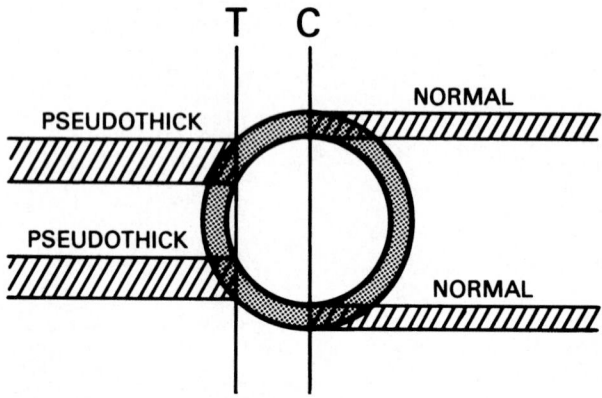

Figure 52.10. Tangenital Imaging Error. If the US beam traverses the center (*C*) of the pylorus, individual tissue layers will be imaged in a plane that allows a true measurement. With tangenital imaging (*T*), pseudothickening results. (From Hayden CK Jr, Swischuk LE, Rytting JE, et al. Gastric ulcer disease in infants: US findings. Radiology 1987; 164:131–134.)

Gastric Ulcer Disease is another acquired cause of acquired cause obstruction discussed later in this chapter. It is also best identified with US.

Gastric Tumors are quite uncommon, but produce the same findings as in adults. Gastric teratomas can occur in the neonate and can be quite large at presentation.

Gastric Bezoars are less common than in previous years. Bezoars may consist of hair (trichobezoar), milk products (lactobezoar), vegetable material (phytobezoar), or cloth that is chronically chewed and swallowed, especially by retarded children. Air or barium outlining the bezoar is diagnostic (Fig. 52.12). On US, an echogenic arc over the bezoar is characteristic. The arc is caused by echoes from the layer of air trapped between the bezoar and the gastric wall.

DUODENAL OBSTRUCTION

Congenital duodenal obstructions are more common than acquired obstructions in pediatric patients (Table 52.4). Plain films localize the level of obstruction that determines whether further imaging is required.

Duodenal Atresia/Annular Pancreas. When the stomach and duodenal bulb are distended ("double bubble" sign) and no gas is present distally (Fig. 52.13), the best diagnostic possibilities are duodenal atresia or annular pancreas. No further imaging is required. Occasionally, a small amount of air may be seen in the distal GI tract in duodenal atresia with an anomalous Y configuration of the hepatopancreatic duct. The upper limb connects to the pre-atretic duodenum, and the lower limb connects to the postatretic duodenum allowing air to pass into the distal small bowel. Air distal to a double-bubble obstructive pattern also can be seen with duodenal stenosis or incomplete duodenal web. Contrast studies are indicated in these cases to distinguish them from volvulus. US can demonstrate the dilated duodenal bulb with any cause of duodenal obstruction.

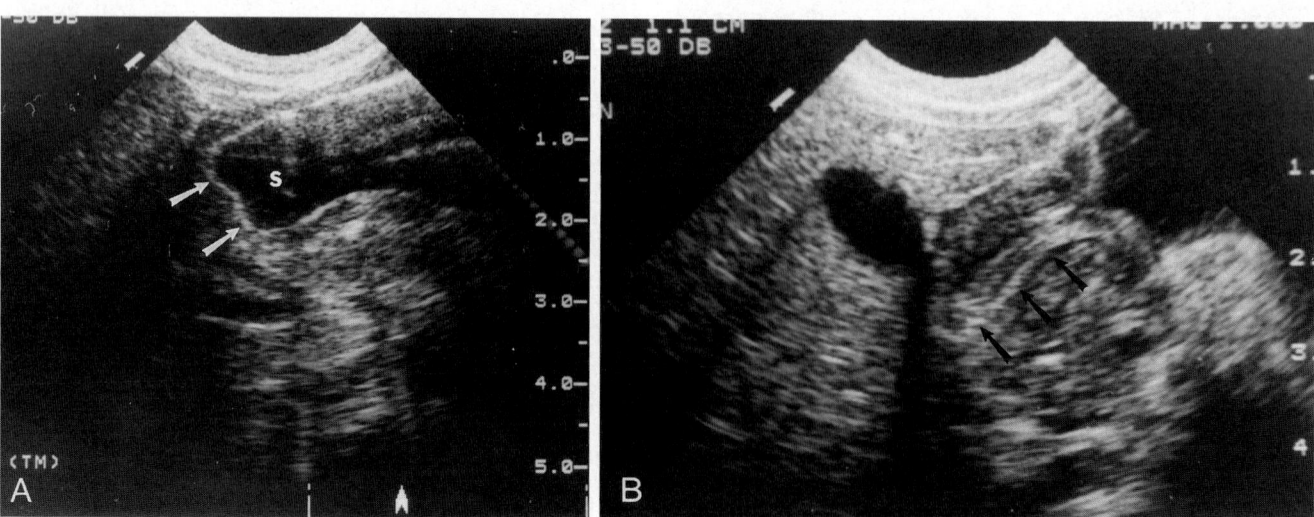

Figure 52.11. Overdistended Stomach. A. The fluid-filled stomach (*S*) is overdistended causing a squared-off appearance of the antrum (*arrows*). The pyloric channel is not visualized because it is posteriorly directed. **B.** With partial emptying of the stomach, the pylorus (arrows) has now come into view.

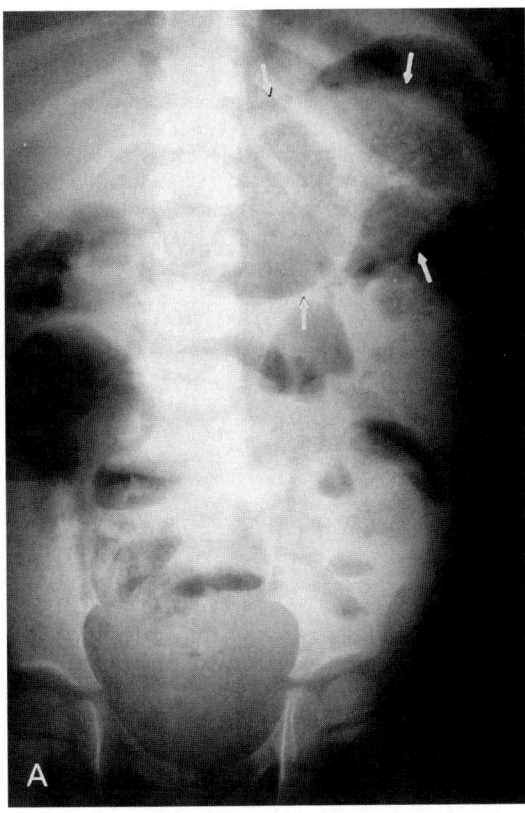

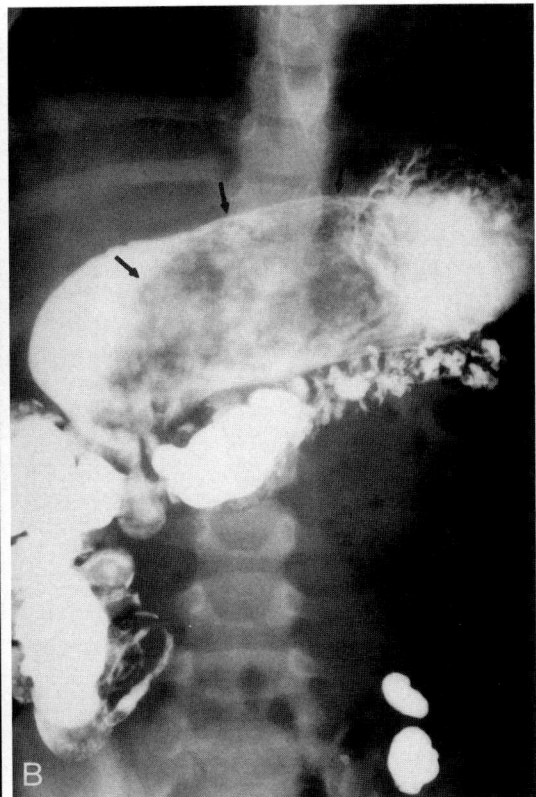

Figure 52.12. Bezoar. A. A filling defect (*arrows*) is seen in the stomach. **B.** UGI series demonstrates barium in the interstices of the intra-luminal mass (*arrows*), characteristic of a bezoar.

Table 52.4.   Causes of Duodenal Obstruction

Atresia/stenosis/diaphragm	Hematoma
Annular pancreas	Neoplasm (duodenum, pancreas,
Duodenal band	liver)
Midgut volvulus	Peptic ulcer disease

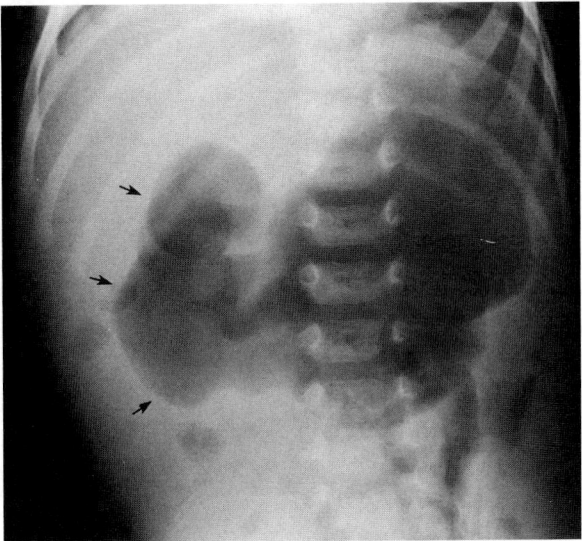

Figure 52.14. Midgut Volvulus. The stomach, duodenal bulb, and descending duodenum (*arrows*) are distended, but the remainder of the intestine shows sparse gas.

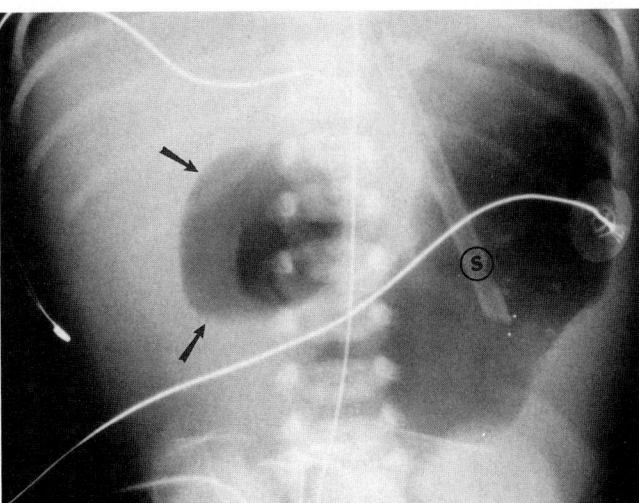

Figure 52.13. Duodenal Atresia. The classic double-bubble sign consists of a distended duodenal bulb (*arrows*) and a distended stomach (*S*).

Midgut Volvulus. When the obstruction of the duodenum is located at the third or fourth portions of the duodenum, the most likely causes are duodenal diaphragm or intestinal malrotation with an obstructing peritoneal band (midgut volvulus). The stomach and duodenum are dilated on radiographs, with gas usually present in the distal bowel (Fig. 52.14). In the supine position, the dis-

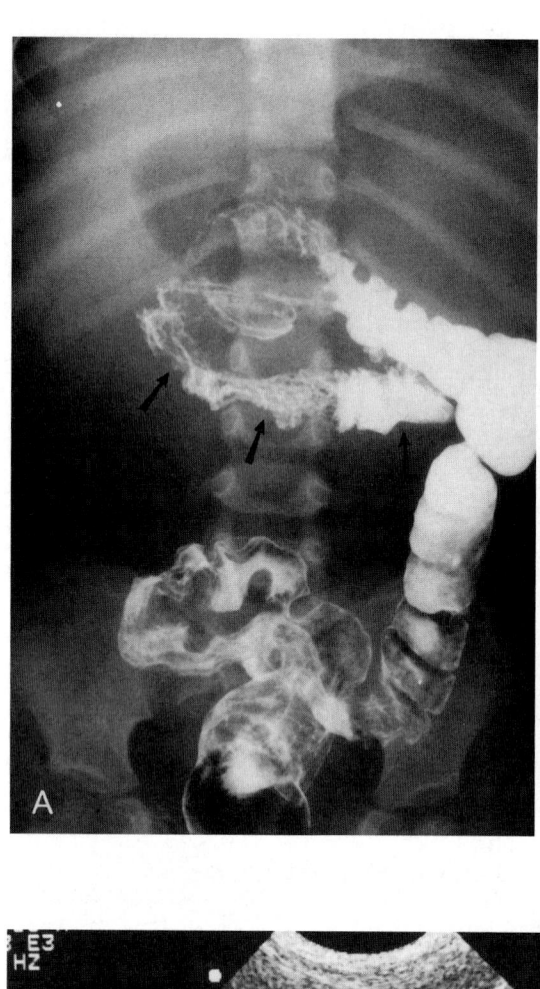

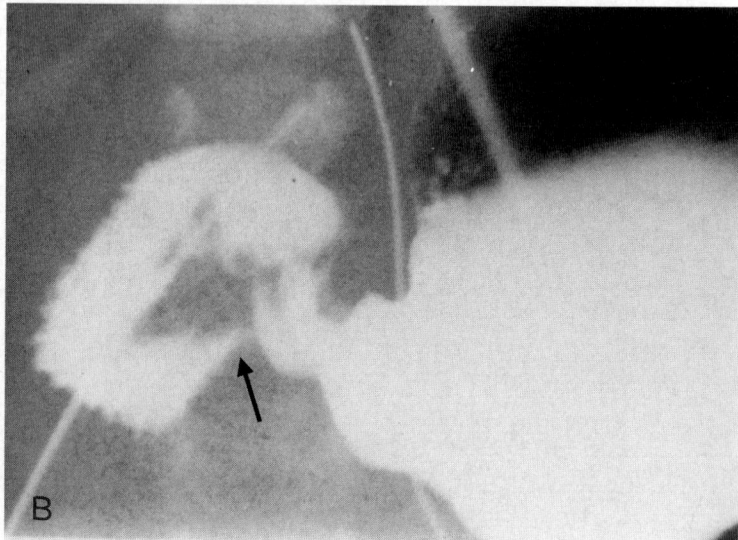

Figure 52.15. Midgut Volvulus. A. Barium enema demonstrates the typical high medial position of the ascending colon and cecum (*arrows*) with a twisted loop of hepatic flexure. **B.** UGI series demonstrates the typical beak-like obstruction (*arrows*) of the third portion of the duodenum, secondary to volvulus. The beak characteristically lies at or just to the right of the spine. **C.** US demonstrates the superior mesenteric vein (*SMV*) in an abnormal position to the left of the superior mesenteric artery (*SMA*). **D.** UGI series demonstrates typical spiraling of the small bowel (*arrows*). *D*, descending duodenum; *S*, stomach.

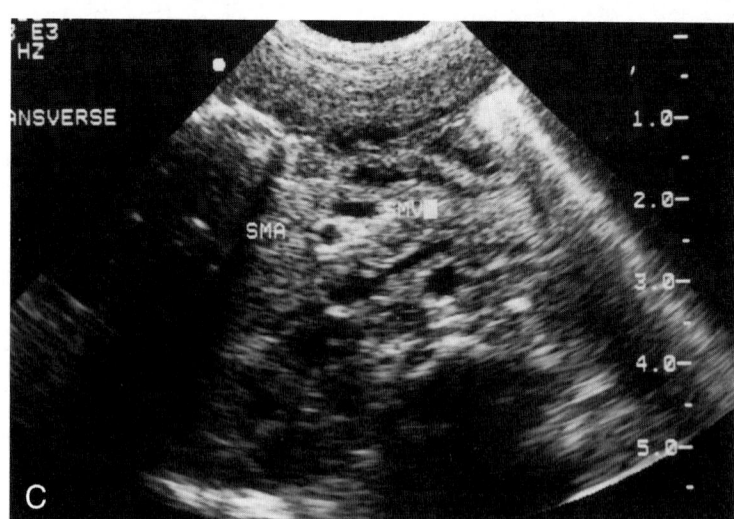

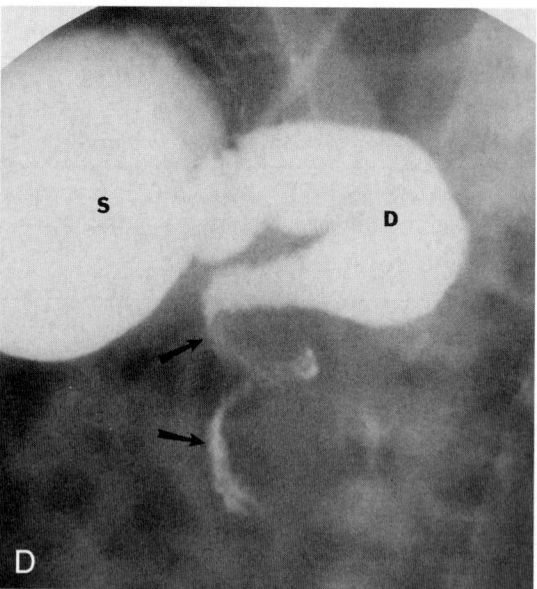

tended duodenum may contain fluid rather than air, erroneously suggesting a gastric obstruction. A contrast study is mandatory to determine whether volvulus is present. In the past, the barium enema was commonly used to show the cecum displaced high into the mid abdomen, just under the transverse colon (Fig. 52.15A). However, because the cecum tends to be mobile in normal infants, any position lower than the transverse colon cannot be interpreted as representative of midgut volvulus. The UGI series is now more commonly used to directly demonstrate obstruction of the duodenum. If

midgut volvulus is present, a characteristic beak deformity is seen at the point of obstruction, usually just before the duodenum crosses the midline (Fig. 52.15B). US demonstrates these findings along with reversal of the position of the superior mesenteric artery and vein which is indicative of intestinal malrotation (Fig. 52.15C). Normally the superior mesenteric vein lies to the right of the artery, but with malrotation the vein sits anterior or to the left of the artery.

Total obstruction at this site also can be seen with the peritoneal band (Ladd's bands) that frequently accom-

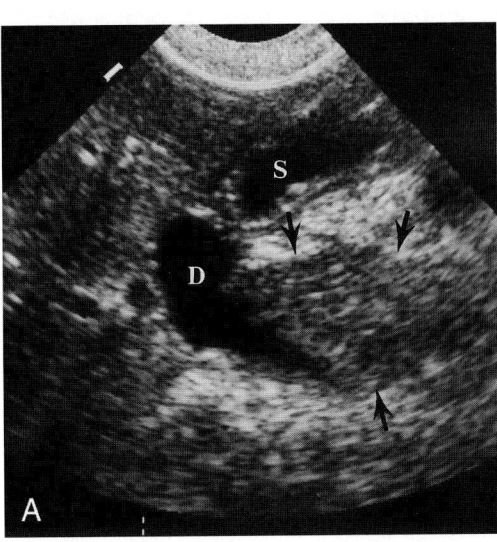 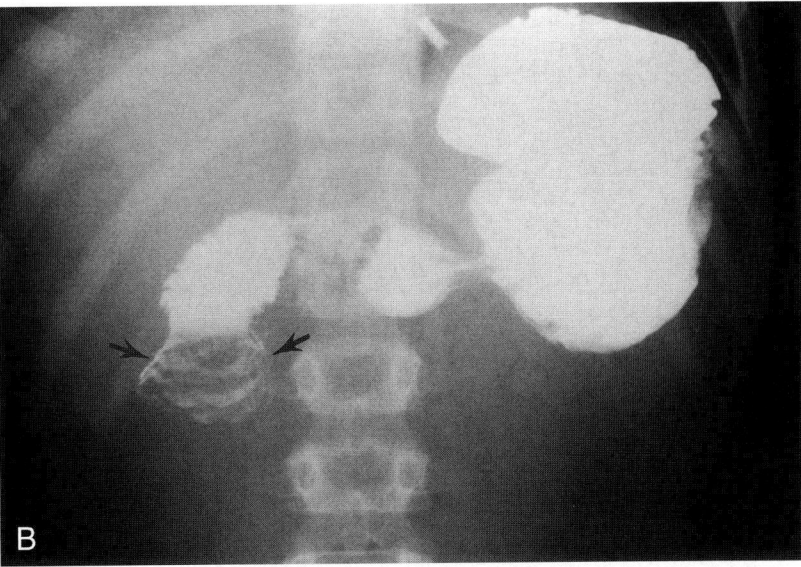

Figure 52.16. Duodenal Hematoma. A. US demonstrates an echogenic hematoma (*arrows*) causing obstruction of the duode- num (*D*). *S*, stomach. **B.** UGI series in another patient demonstrates the typical intramural filling defect of the hematoma (*arrows*).

pany rotational abnormality of the intestines. The defor- mity due to these bands appears as an oblique indenta- tion of the third or fourth portion of the duodenum. With a little time (5–10 minutes) some barium will pass through the obstruction and outline a corkscrew ap- pearance of the small bowel when volvulus is present (Fig. 52.15D). The small bowel is malpositioned in the right or midabdomen rather than in its usual left upper quadrant position. Bowel edema due to venous stasis may also be encountered.

Occasionally midgut volvulus is intermittent and gas is seen throughout the GI tract. Generalized intestinal dilatation is usually present. Most cases demonstrate obstruction of the third or fourth portions of the duode- num and midgut volvulus should be presumed present until proven otherwise. Other congenital abnormalities leading to obstruction at this level are duodenal webs and diaphragms, enteric duplication cyst and, rarely, a preduodenal portal vein.

Duodenal Hematoma is perhaps the most common acquired cause of duodenal obstruction. Hematomas usually result from blunt abdominal trauma and can be detected with US or UGI series (Fig. 52.16). The com- monest cause of duodenal hematoma in childhood is the battered child syndrome. These patients also may sus- tain trauma to the pancreas resulting in pancreatitis.

Obstruction of the duodenum secondary to peptic ul- cer disease is not nearly as common in children as it is in adults. Tumors of any type arising within or adjacent to the duodenum are rare, but can produce obstruction. The findings in these patients are no different from those seen in adults.

SMALL INTESTINAL OBSTRUCTION

Small intestinal obstruction in the neonate and young infant is more likely to be congenital whereas, in the

Table 52.5. Causes of Small Intestinal Obstruction

Atresia/stenosis	Perforated appendicitis
Meconium ileus	Regional enteritis
Incarcerated hernia	Posttraumatic hematoma/stricture
Intussusception	

older child, acquired problems are more common (Table 52.5). Congenital small bowel obstructions occur more commonly in the distal small bowel. In the neonate it is difficult to distinguish distal small bowel obstruction from colonic obstruction on plain radiographs. Obstruc- tion anywhere between the ileum and the rectum can produce a similar pattern of numerous dilated loops of intestine. A contrast enema must be performed to better localize the cause of obstruction.

Jejunal Atresia. With proximal obstruction one is dealing with jejunal atresia. Plain films demonstrate a variable number of distended loops of jejunum (Fig. 52.17). Often no further contrast studies are required. A variation of intestinal atresia, described as *apple peel small bowel*, consists of diffuse atresia of the small bowel with multiple sites of severe stenosis and a spiral config- uration of the atretic segment. This condition tends to be familial. Segmental volvulus of the small bowel can oc- cur anywhere along its length, but is uncommon. Simi- larly, internal hernias are rare.

Ileal Atresia and Meconium Ileus are the most com- mon causes of distal small bowel obstruction in the neonate. In both conditions, contrast studies reveal a characteristic generalized microcolon, indicating that meconium has not passed normally into the colon dur- ing fetal life. Meconium ileus is usually the earliest man- ifestation of cystic fibrosis. It results from abnormally thick meconium that forms plugs that cannot pass

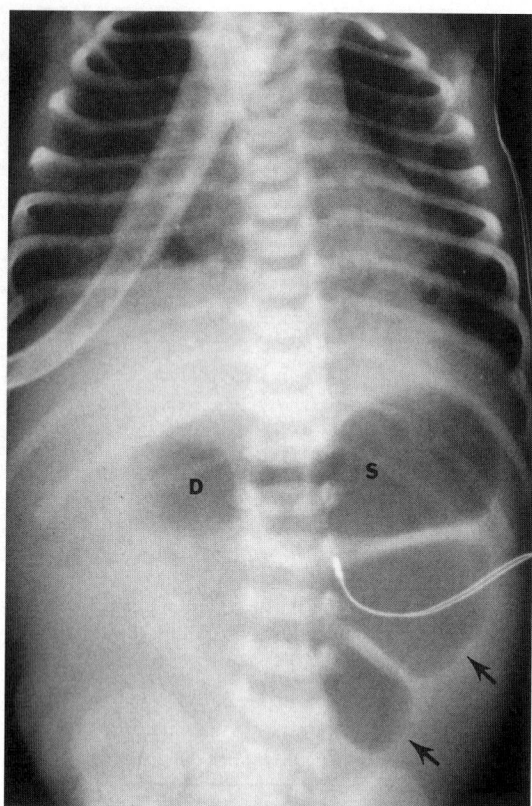

Figure 52.17. Jejunal Atresia. Plain film shows distention of the stomach (*S*), duodenum (*D*), and loops of the upper intestine (*arrows*). No air is present distal to the proximal jejunum.

through the ileocecal valve (Fig. 52.18). Plain radiographs demonstrate grossly distended loops of intestine with bubbly intestinal contents. When air-fluid levels are present, ileal atresia is the more likely diagnosis. It is important to distinguish between the two conditions, for ileal atresia is corrected surgically although meconium ileus is often treated with water soluble contrast enema. When performing such an enema, contrast material should reflux into the terminal illeum to outline, as well as lubricate, the inspissated meconium plugs. This procedure should be performed carefully because of the increased risk of perforation of a microcolon. If contrast does not reflux into the terminal ileum, surgery is required for definitive diagnosis as well as treatment.

Meconium Plug Syndrome is a misleading name for a condition due to functional immaturity and abnormal peristalsis of the distal colon. Also known as the *small left colon syndrome*, this condition should not be confused with meconium ileus. With the meconium plug syndrome, a dilated colon full of meconium with an empty distal descending colonic segment is characteristic (Fig. 52.19). This condition is more common in normal large infants and infants of diabetic mothers. The condition is transient and can often be treated by rectal stimulation or saline enemas. In more persistent cases, an enema using contrast that contains the detergent Tween 80 (such as Gastrografin) can be used to irritate the colon and stimulate defecation. Normal ganglion cells are present.

Hirschsprung Disease is differentiated from meconium plug syndrome by biopsy or follow-up. In Hirschsprung disease, functional colonic obstruction is due to congenital absence of ganglion cells in the distal colon resulting in abnormal peristalsis. The rectum is always involved but the extent of proximal involvement varies. Barium enema findings can be confusing in the neonatal period, for although the aganglionic segment is characteristically contracted, a well-defined change in caliber at the zone of transition is frequently not present. Tortuosity or corrugation of the narrowed aganglionic segment of the colon is commonly seen (Fig. 52.20). Barium evacuation is delayed usually well beyond 24 hours. This finding helps differentiate Hirschsprung disease from meconium plug syndrome, which usually resolves quickly after the enema examination. Diagnosis of Hirschsprung disease is definitively made with rectal biopsy. Necrotizing enterocolitis is an uncommon but serious complication of Hirschsprung disease due to stasis colitis.

Incarcerated Inguinal Hernia is the most common cause of low intestinal obstruction after 6 months of age. The findings of intestinal obstruction on plain films are characteristic, and the key to radiologic diagnosis is visualization of a unilaterally prominent inguinal fold or loops of air-filled bowel in the scrotum (Fig. 52.21). US can identify the incarcerated intestine in the inguinal canal or scrotum and can differentiate a hernia from other causes of scrotal swelling.

Intussusception. After 6 months of age, intussusception becomes an increasingly important acquired cause of intestinal obstruction. In young children, most intussusceptions are ileocolic and the cause is idiopathic. Redundant, inflamed mucosa or lymph nodes may act as the lead point. Definable lead points such as diverticula, polyps, or tumors are more commonly encountered in neonates and in older children.

Abdominal radiographs may be normal or may demonstrate intestinal obstruction. In approximately half the cases, the head of the intussusceptum is seen on plain films (Fig. 52.22A). US is a very effective and reliable imaging modality for the demonstration of intussusception (5,6). Characteristically, an oval mass is seen in the longitudinal section and a round mass is seen in cross-section. The outer ring is sonolucent with variably echogenic concentric inner rings (Fig. 52.22B). The findings result from indrawing of a portion of bowel into the more distal bowel (usually ileum into colon). The concentric rings represent layers of edematous intestine alternating with layers of mesentery (7). Often anechoic fluid, echogenic mesentery, and small lymph nodes can be identified in the center of the intussusceptum (Fig. 52.22C). Color Doppler US has been used to determine viability of the involved intestine (8,9). Nonsurgical reduction should be attempted in any case with no evidence of free air or peritonitis (Fig. 52.22D). Small amounts of free fluid are commonly seen with US and do not necessarily indicate perforation.

Barium was almost exclusively used for hydrostatic reduction in the past. The main disadvantage of barium is that if perforation occurs, barium leaks into the peritoneal cavity, and peritonitis results. We have used

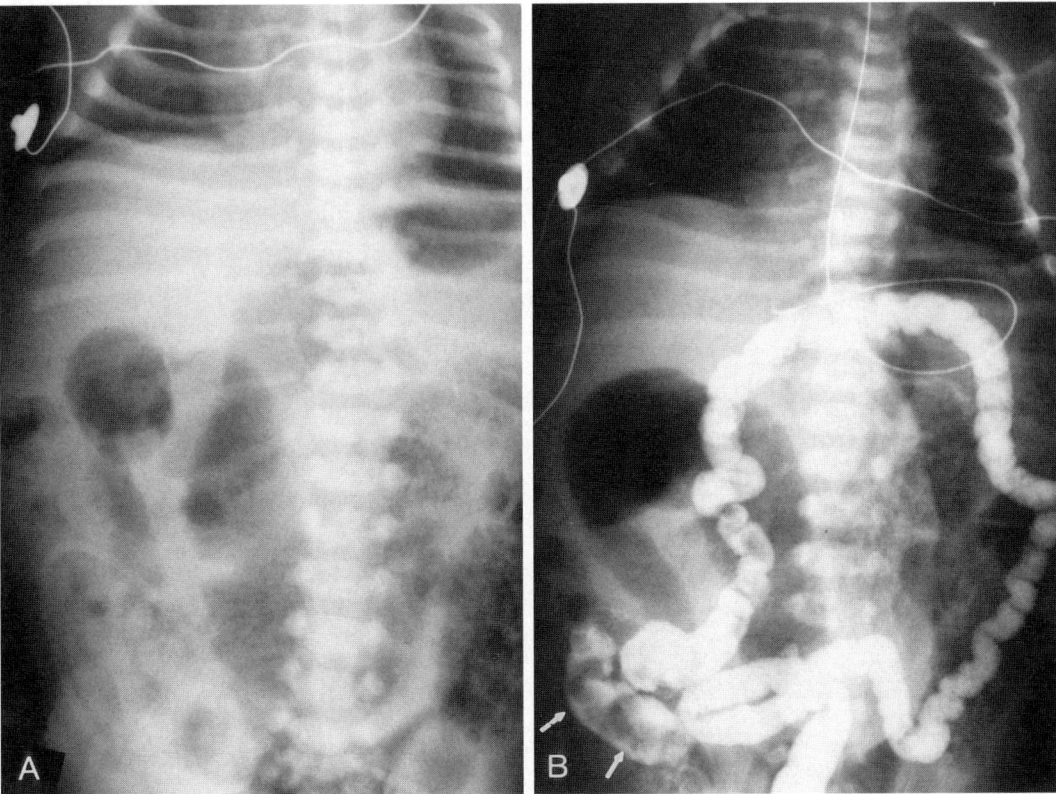

Figure 52.18. Meconium Ileus. A. Plain film shows the "soap-bubble" effect of air mixed with meconium in the numerous distended loops of intestine. **B.** Contrast enema demonstrates a typical micro-colon with reflux into the terminal ileum which is filled with pellets of meconium (*arrows*).

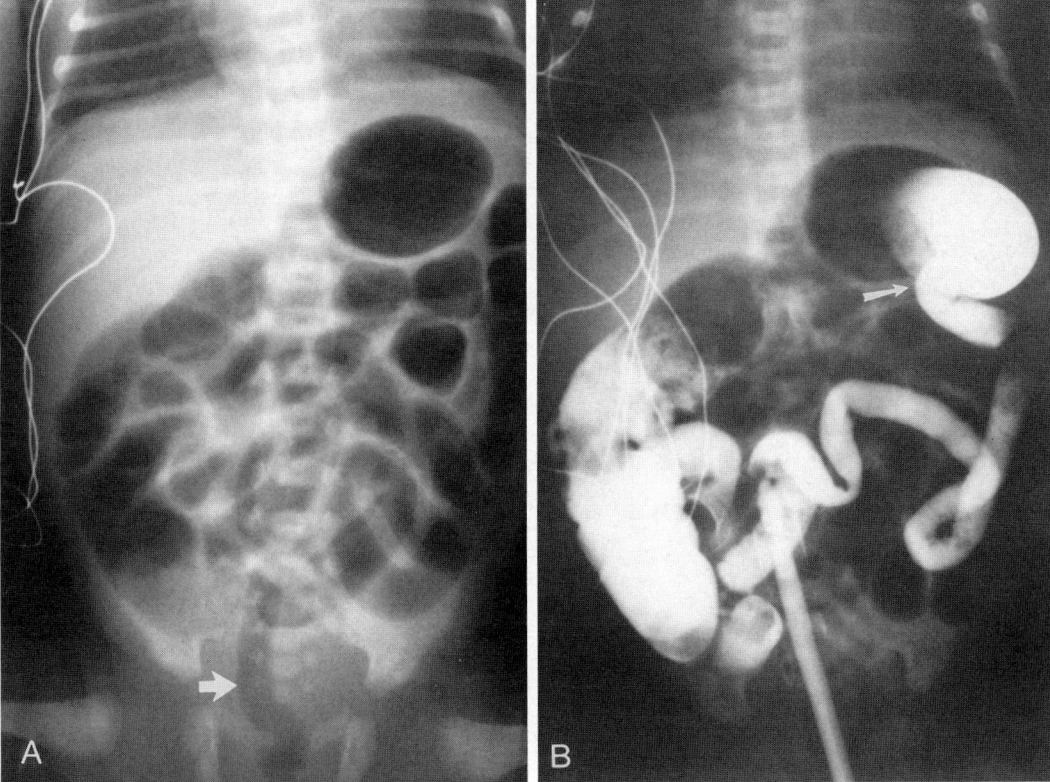

Figure 52.19. Meconium Plug Syndrome (Small Left Colon Syndrome). A. Numerous loops of intestine are distended with air. Also, note air in the relatively narrow rectosigmoid colon (*arrow*). **B.** Contrast enema demonstrates a small left colon with the characteristic transition zone (*arrow*). These findings mimic those of Hirschsprung's disease.

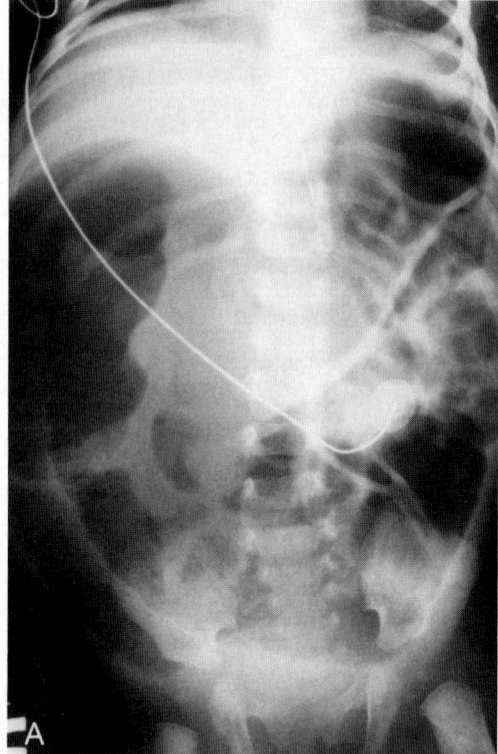

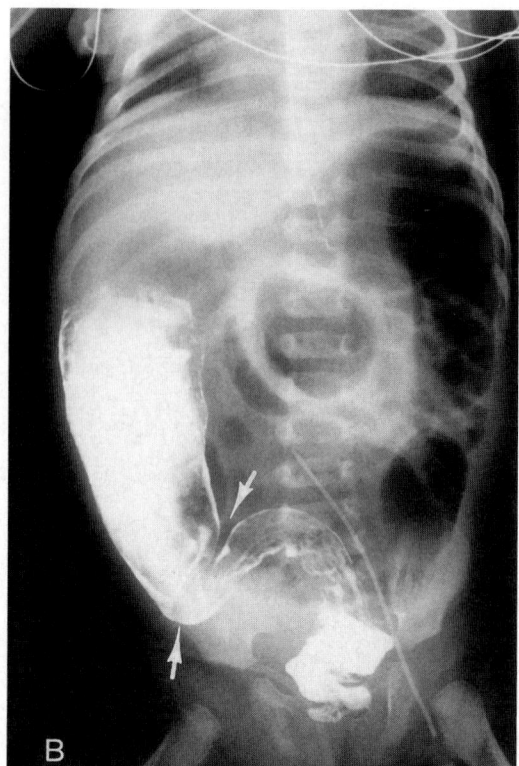

Figure 52.20. Hirschsprung Disease. A. Plain film demonstrates an enormously distended colon. No gas is present in the rectum. **B.** Contrast study demonstrates a narrowed rectum and sigmoid, with a classic transition zone (*arrows*). The colon above this area is dilated. It is not unusual for the sigmoid colon to flop over to the right side in infants. **C.** Another infant has spasms and irregularity of the aganglionic segment.

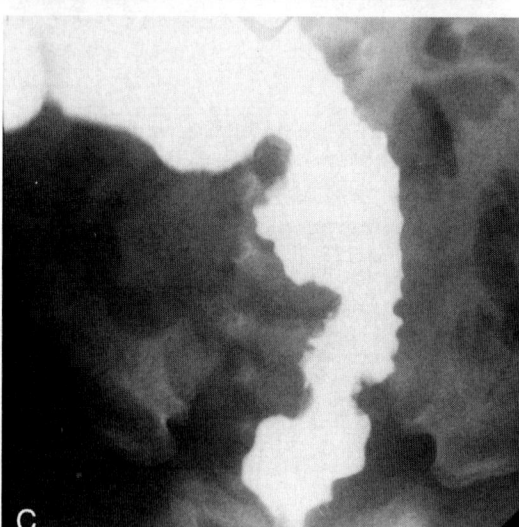

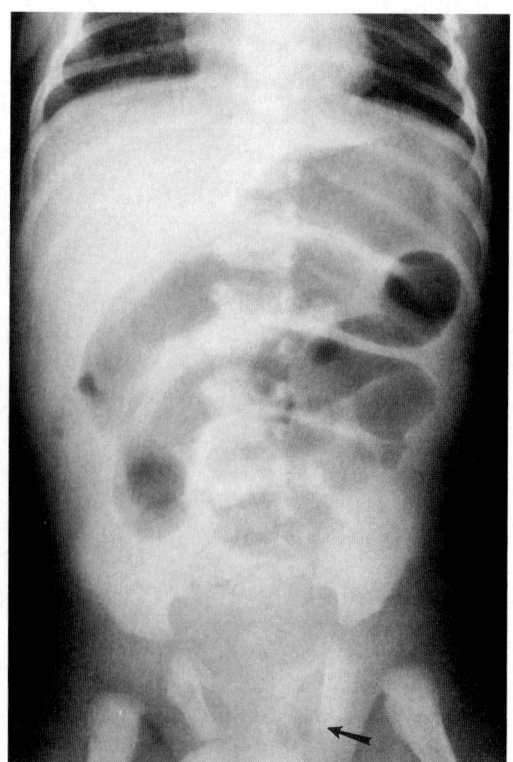

Figure 52.21. Inguinal Hernia. Numerous loops of intestine are distended signifying the presence of intestinal obstruction. Air is seen in the hernia in the left inguinal region (*arrow*).

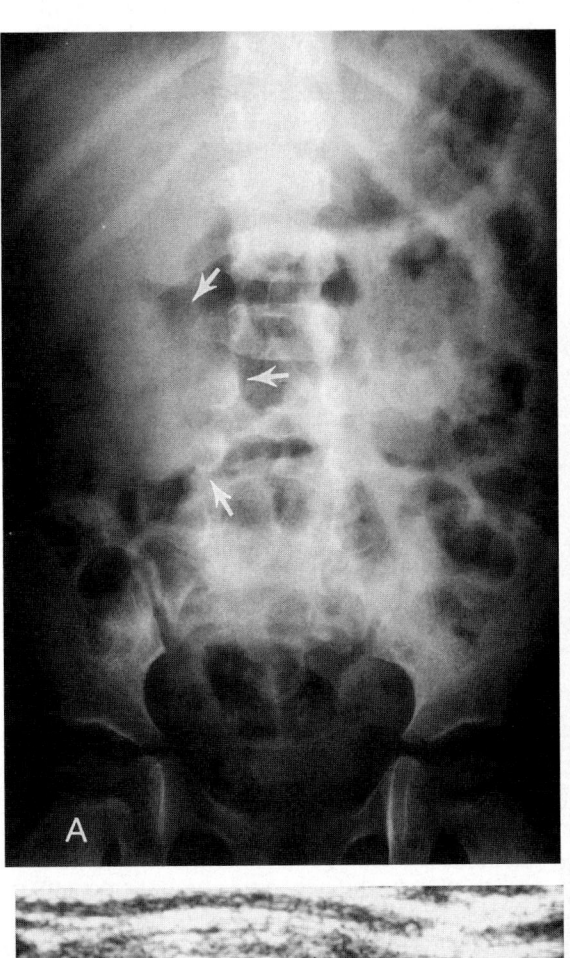

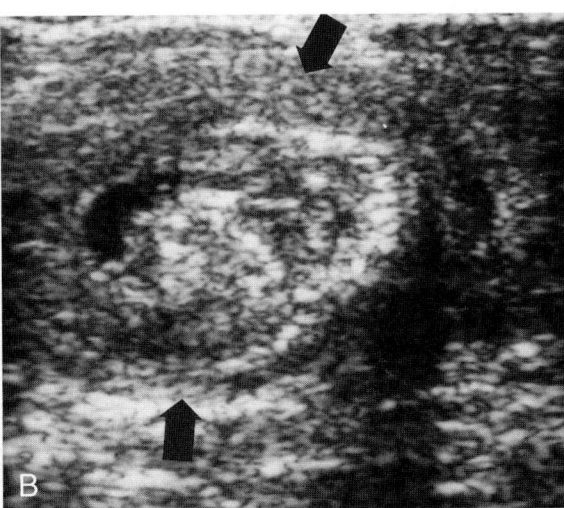

Figure 52.22. Intussusception. A. Plain film suggests a soft-tissue mass in the right upper quadrant (*arrows*). **B.** Transverse US through the intussusception demonstrates the typical donut configuration (*arrows*) with a small crescent of trapped fluid. **C.** Intussusception in another patient shows a concentric ring configuration. A mesenteric lymph node (*arrow*) is included with the intussuscepting bowel segment. **D.** Contrast enema demonstrates the typical appearance of the intussusception (*arrows*).

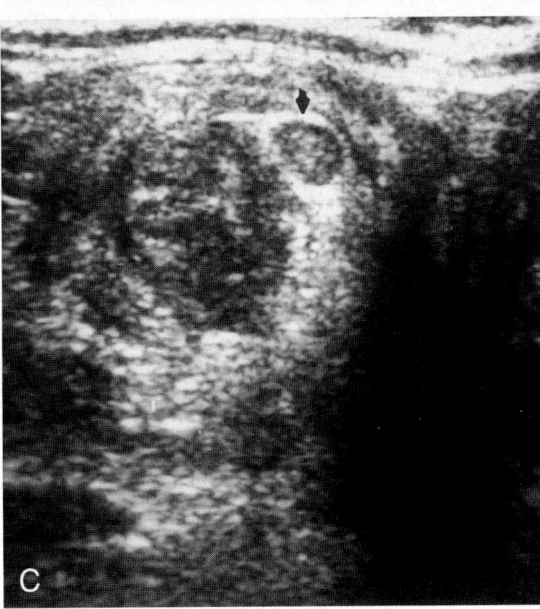

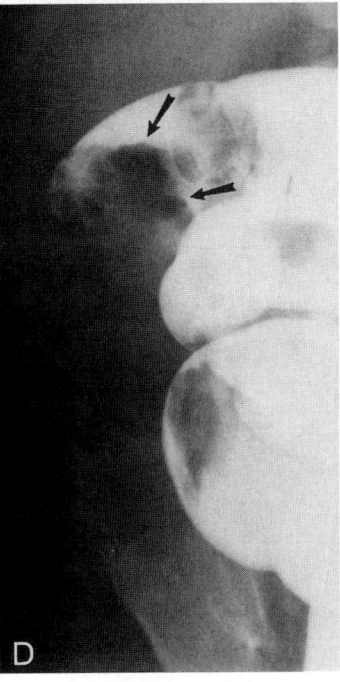

Gastrografin diluted 5:1 for years and have found it satisfactory (10,11). However with air reduction, the greater pressures that can be generated in the colon improve the rate of successful reduction. A water-soluble contrast column needs to be elevated to a height of 4–5 feet to equal the 120 mm Hg pressure generated with air pumps. With this pressure, reduction rates are 80–90%. US-guided hydrostatic reduction is advocated by some but has not gained wide acceptance (12–15).

When intussusception is initially refractory to reduction, repeated attempts are often helpful. Avoiding the use of sedation improves reduction rates by permitting the patients to increase intraabdominal pressure via Valsalva maneuver (16). The only contraindication to nonsurgical reduction of intussusception is the presence of free air or signs and symptoms of peritonitis. The duration of symptoms and the presence of small bowel obstruction are not usually considered deterrents. Recurrent intussusception occurs in approximately 5–10% of cases.

Appendicitis. After approximately 2 years of age, perforated appendicitis becomes an increasingly common cause of intestinal obstruction. No obstruction occurs with acute, nonperforated appendicitis. Once the appendix perforates, obstruction gradually develops because of a combination of functional obstruction and abscess formation (Fig. 52.23). Symptoms may initially improve once perforation occurs. Nevertheless, radio-

graphic evidence of low intestinal obstruction in the older child should be considered to be caused by perforated appendicitis until proven otherwise. Plain films may show a right lower quadrant mass, but free air is usually not seen. Abscesses can be demonstrated with US or CT. Barium enema demonstrates the abscess adhering to various portions of the GI tract.

Regional Enteritis patients clinically mimic those with chronic appendiceal abscess. US shows the thickened wall of the involved small bowel, but contrast studies better evaluate the extent of involvement and provide the definitive findings. Other diseases, such as tuberculosis, lymphoma, and *Yersinia* colitis, are much less common but produce findings that may be difficult to differentiate from regional enteritis.

COLONIC OBSTRUCTION

Congenital obstructions of the colon are more common than acquired obstructions (Table 52.6).

Hirshsprung Disease is less difficult to diagnose in later infancy and childhood than in the neonatal period. A narrowed distal aganglionic segment is visualized leading to a zone of transition beyond which the proximal colon is dilated (Fig. 52.24).

Functional Megacolon is a common condition in childhood that is associated with spasm of the puborectalis muscle. In many instances, the muscle spasm is secondary to anal fissures; in other cases it is idiopathic and probably multifactorial. Prominence of the puborectalis sling provides the major clue to diagnosis (Fig. 52.25) . These patients can hold considerable volumes of stool in their colon.

Imperforate or Ectopic Anus is a common cause of obstruction in the neonate. Anatomic deficits range from simple membranous anal atresia to arrest of the colon as it descends through the puborectalis sling, with fistula formation from the blind-ending rectal pouch to some part of the genital or urinary tract (Fig. 52.26). In females, the fistula may empty into the bladder, uterus, or vagina. In males, it tends to enter into the urethra or bladder. In both sexes it can enter the perineum. Sacral and urinary tract anomalies, hydrometrocolpos, and persistent cloaca are associated. When sacral abnormalities are present, the spinal cord and canal should be screened with US for abnormalities such as tethering or masses (17). Virtually all of these patients have neurogenic bladder dysfunction (18).

All associated anomalies should be demonstrated along with the location of the fistula. US demonstrates the end of the pouch. The fistula may be injected directly or may opacify during retrograde voiding cystourethrog-

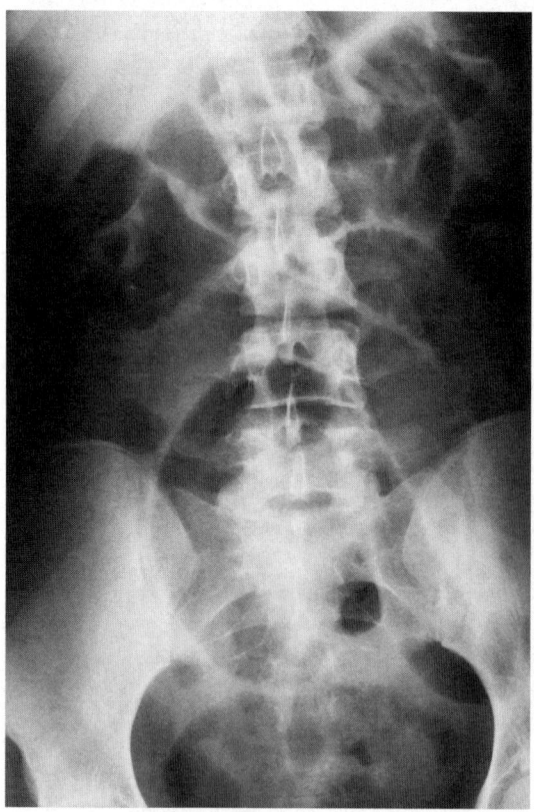

Figure 52.23. Perforated Appendicitis. Numerous loops of distended small bowel are seen with a paucity of gas in the right lower quadrant. A mild scoliosis with concavity to the right is present. A functional small bowel obstruction is present.

Table 52.6. Causes of Colonic Obstruction

Meconium plug syndrome (small left colon)	Colon atresia/stenosis
Hirschsprung disease	Inflammatory stricture
Functional megacolon	Volvulus
Ectopic (imperforate) anus	Trauma
	Neoplasm

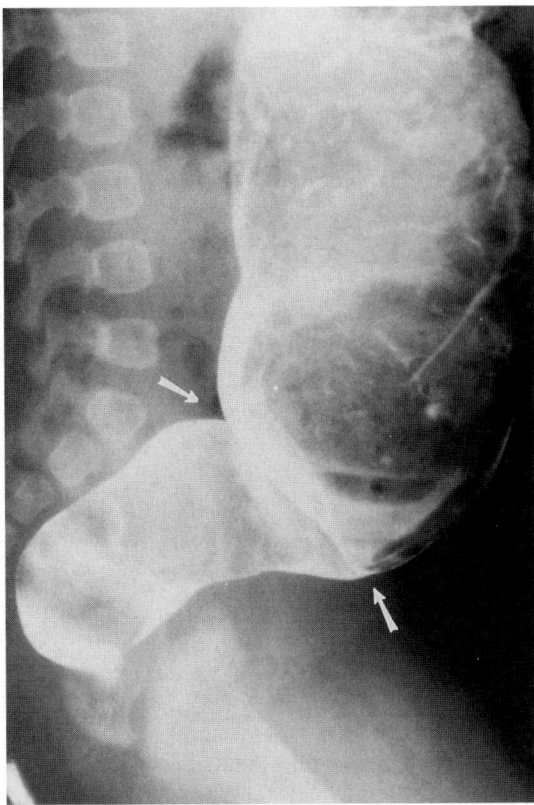

Figure 52.24. Hirschsprung Disease (Older Child). A characteristic transition zone (*arrows*) is seen between the dilated feces-filled colon above and the relatively narrowed rectum below.

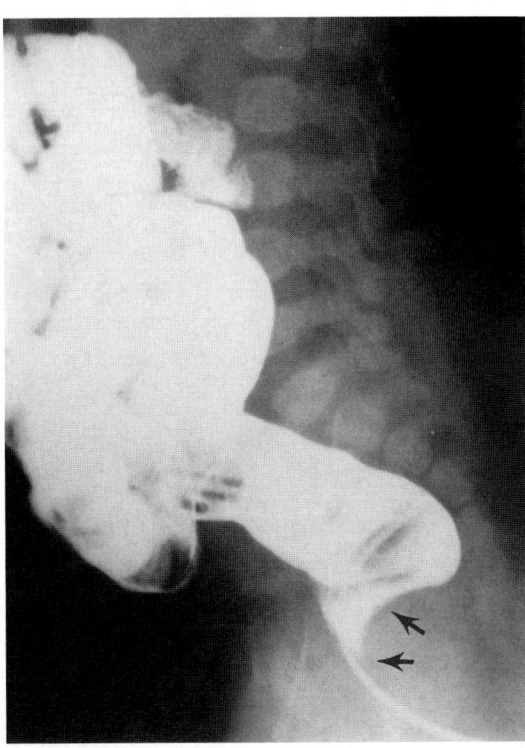

Figure 52.25. Functional Megacolon. The pronounced indentation of the posterior rectum (*arrows*) is typical of a prominent puborectalis sling.

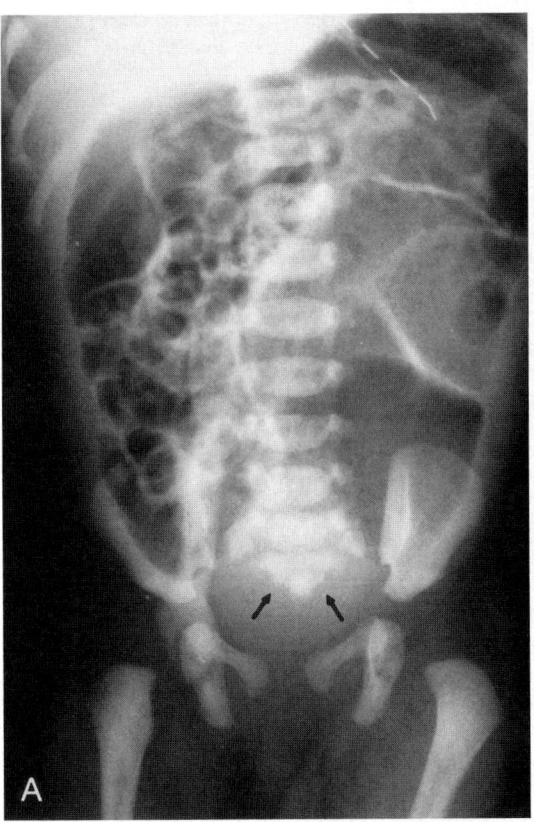

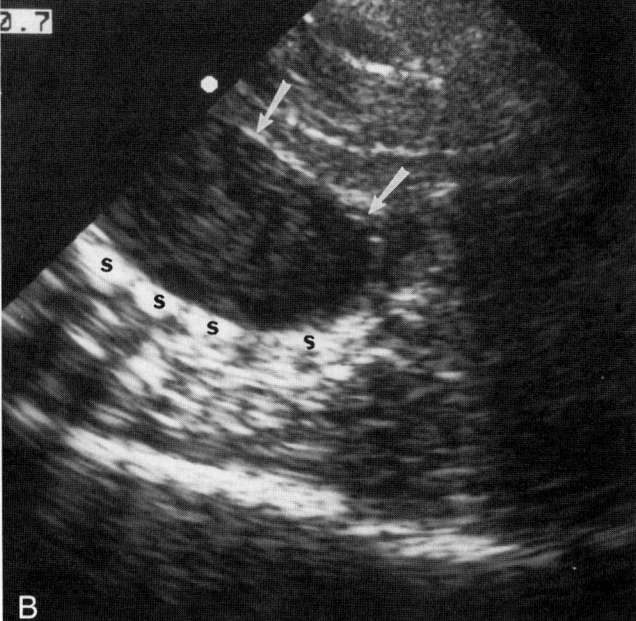

Figure 52.26. Imperforate Anus. A. Loops of colon are distended in the upper abdomen with gas evident in the small bowel. The rectum is not visualized. The sacrum (*arrows*) is underdeveloped. **B.** Sagittal US in another infant demonstrates the distended distal pouch (*arrows*) that overlies the sacral segments (*S*). The pouch ends at the lowermost sacral segment.

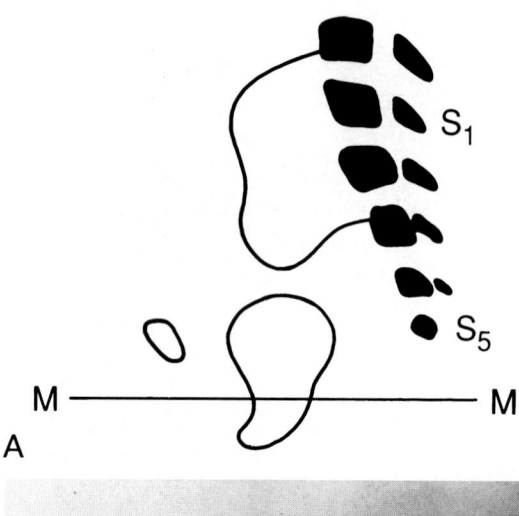

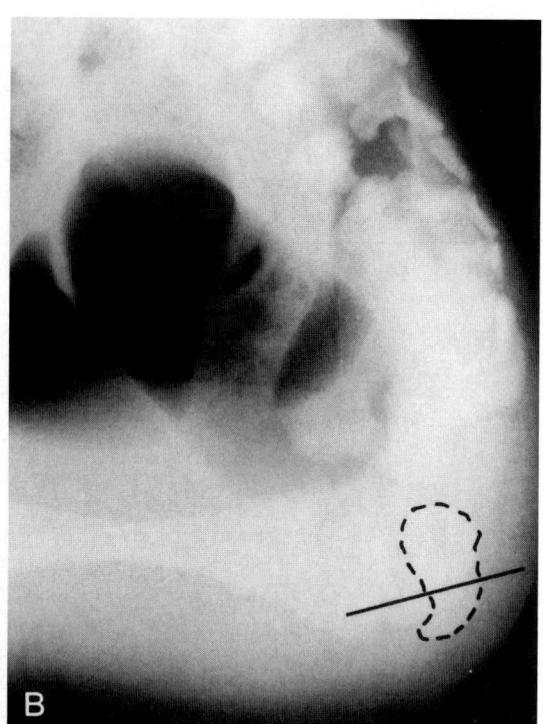

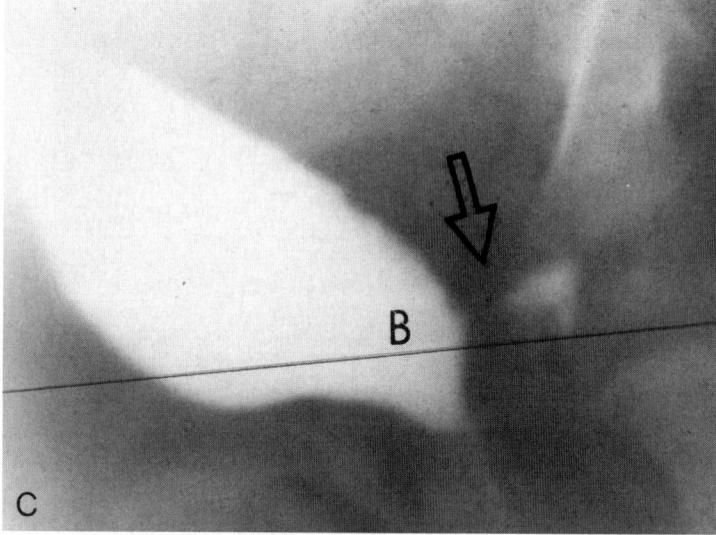

Figure 52.27. Imperforate Anus: Cremin's M Line. A. The M line is drawn horizontally through the junction of the middle and lower thirds of the ischium (*M*). The line demarcates the level of the puborectalis sling. S_1, S_5, sacral segments. **B.** Cross-table lateral film with the buttocks elevated in another infant demonstrates the distal air-filled pouch or the hindgut. Note the position of the M line. The pouch ends well above the M line, indicating a high imperforate anus. **C.** The same patient demonstrates a fistula (*arrow*) from the bladder (*B*) to the rectum. Cremin's line is drawn on the image.

raphy. In females, flush retrograde vaginography may be required. If the fistula empties above the puborectalis sling, it can be presumed that the puborectalis muscle is hypoplastic and that continence will be difficult to accomplish with any surgical procedure. If the fistula empties below the puborectalis sling, the puborectalis muscle is usually more developed and achieving continence is more likely. The "M" line of Cremin has been used to determine the level at which the blind pouch ends (Fig. 52.27). This line is drawn perpendicular to the long axis of the ischia on lateral view, and passes through the junction between the middle and lower third of the ischia. If the blind pouch and fistula end above the line, the fistula is considered high. If they end below the line, it is considered low, and if they end at the line, it is considered intermediate. Intermediate fistulae usually pose the same problems as high fistulae.

Colon Atresia is relatively rare and is evident in the neonatal period. Massive distension of the colon is seen proximal to the area of atresia or stenosis (Fig. 52.28).

Acquired Causes of colonic obstruction are relatively uncommon except for perforated appendicitis and regional enteritis. Inflammatory strictures associated with ulcerative colitis and necrotizing enterocolitis tend to be smooth and appear similar to those in adults. They may be single or multiple. Colonic strictures can also be found in children with cystic fibrosis (19). Tumors of the colon are uncommon and the findings are similar to those seen in adults. Trauma to the colon, producing obstruction, is seen with motor vehicle accidents or, more commonly, the battered child syndrome. Sigmoid and cecal volvulus are much less common in children than in adults, but the findings are the same. Volvulus occurs more frequently in bedridden patients and in retarded children.

Inflammation and Infection

GASTROINTESTINAL TRACT

Esophagitis in children is caused by peptic disease, caustic ingestion, viral and monilial infection. Peptic esophagitis tends to involve the lower third of the esophagus but, with severe reflux, may involve the entire esophagus. Findings consist of thickening of the esophageal wall, stiffening of the esophagus, lack of normal peristaltic activity, and ulcers which may be deep (Fig. 52.29). Nonfibrotic narrowing occurs in the early stages but later fibrotic stricturing results. With caustic

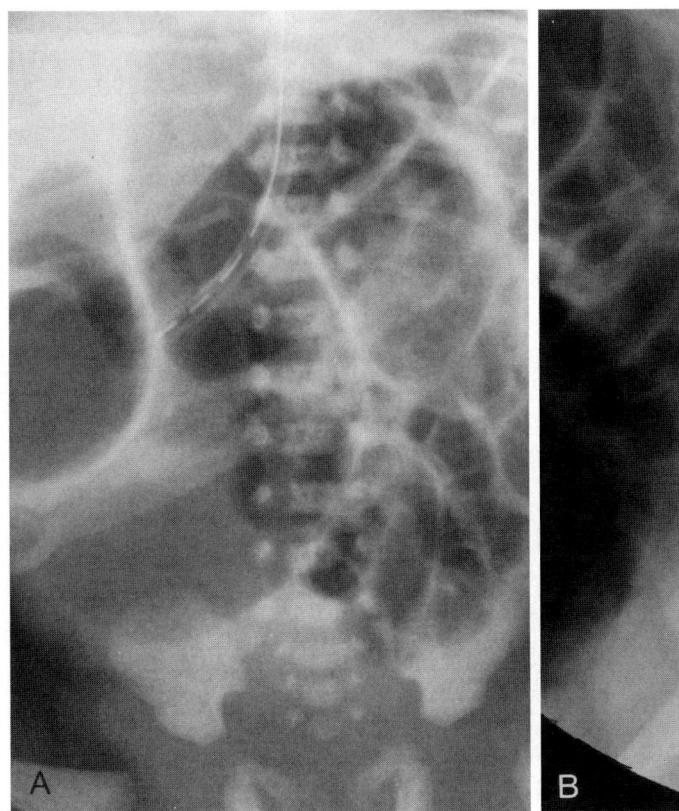

Figure 52.28. Colon Atresia. A. Plain film demonstrates numerous loops of distended intestine. **B.** Retrograde contrast study demon-strates the blind-ending microcolon (*arrow*). The proximal colon is air-filled and distended.

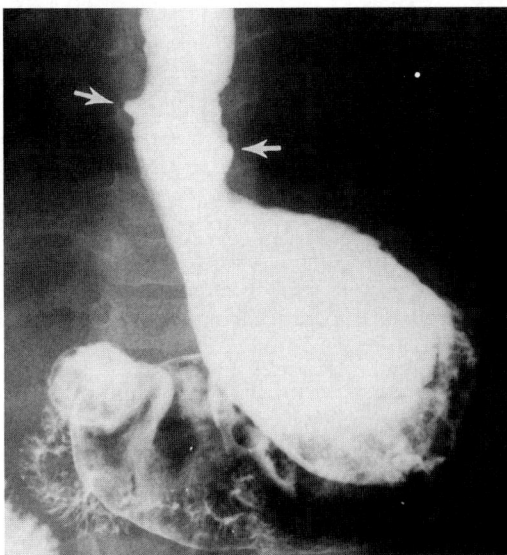

Figure 52.29. Peptic Esophagitis. Inflammation of the distal esoph-agus causes narrowing, mucosal irregularity, and ulcers (*arrows*).

ingestion, extensive esophageal burns are the rule. Perforation into the mediastinum can occur. Contrast studies are usually performed only in the late stages to demonstrate strictures (see Fig. 52.6). Viral (usually her-pes) esophagitis causes small superficial ulcers, best demonstrated with double contrast studies. The ulcers can be diffuse or focal and may result in intense spasm with severe dysphagia. Monilial esophagitis causes mu-cosal irregularities with intense spasm of the esophagus leading to pseudodiverticuli.

Gastritis is usually due to peptic disease in infants and young children. The findings resemble those seen in adults; superficial ulcerations and delicate, edematous, cobblestoned appearance of the mucosa. Milk allergy commonly causes gastritis in infants leading to vomiting and bleeding. On UGI series these patients demonstrate intense antropyloric spasm. With US, thickening of the mucosa can be detected. Ingestion of acidic caustic sub-stances is more likely to result in gastritis than esophagitis, especially when large volumes of high-spe-cific gravity acids are ingested.

Duodenitis is usually caused by peptic disease which is more common in children than usually believed. Ulcer craters are sometimes visualized. Children present with bleeding more often than adults.

Viral Gastroenteritis is the most common inflamma-tory condition of the small bowel. US shows dilated fluid-filled loops with thickened mucosa. Plain abdominal films may show extensive gas within the GI tract that may, at first, erroneously suggest mechanical obstruc-tion.

Regional Enteritis affects the terminal ileum as the primary site of involvement. Regional enteritis of the proximal small bowel, stomach, or esophagus is rather rare. The radiographic findings are identical to those in adults and consist of a variable lengths of narrowed ir-regular terminal ileum, with or without linear ulcers and sinus tracts (Fig. 52.30). The transmural bowel wall

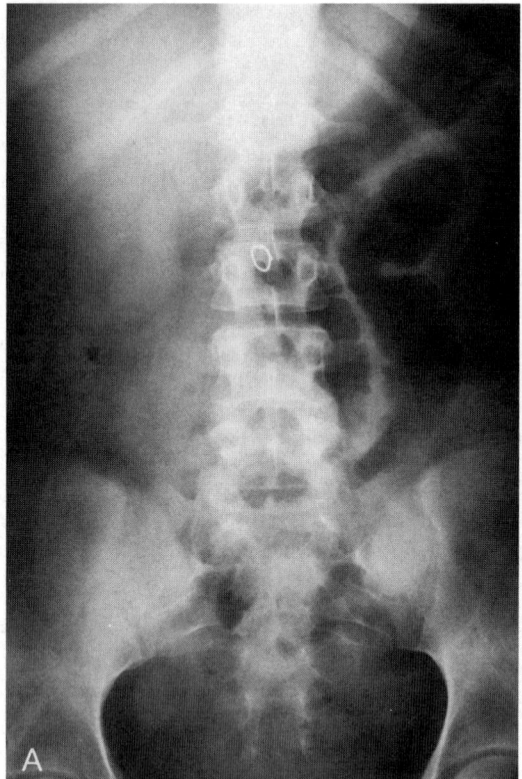

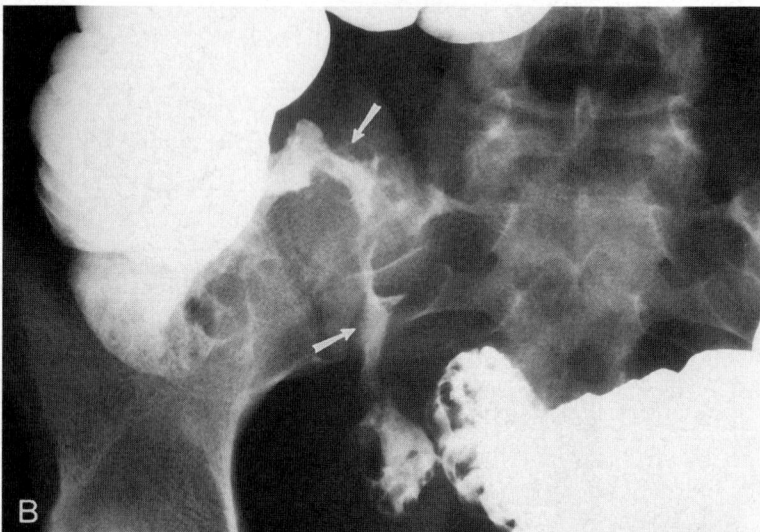

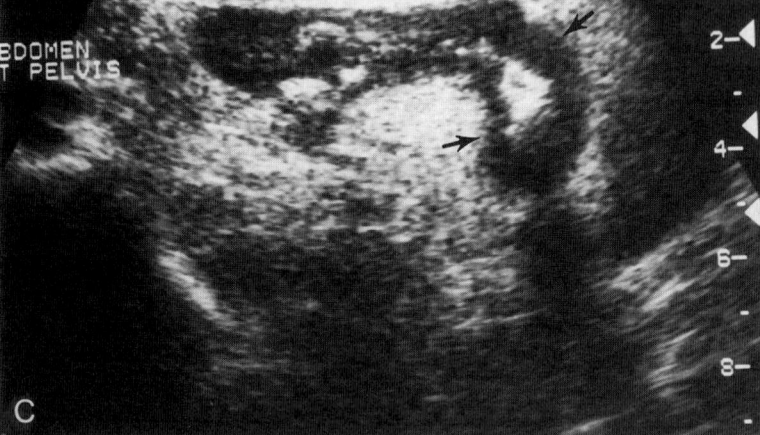

Figure 52.30. Regional Enteritis. A. Plain radiograph shows two dilated, obstructed small bowel loops with a paucity of gas in the right side of the abdomen. **B.** Barium enema demonstrates the markedly narrowed and irregular terminal ileum (*arrows*). Note that the tip of the cecum is also involved. **C.** US reveals transmural hypoechoic thickening of the wall of the terminal ileum (*arrows*).

thickening common in these patients is readily demonstrable with US (20).

Colitis. Almost every condition that produces colitis in the adult can produce colitis in infants and children. Almost any form of colitis manifests thickening of the colonic wall or mucosa on US.

Necrotizing Enterocolitis (NEC), on the other hand, is almost exclusively a pediatric problem most commonly seen in premature infants. Its etiology is hypoperfusion and hypoxia of the gut and the clinical findings tend to mimic those of sepsis. However, the passage of blood per rectum is more common with NEC. Initial radiographs demonstrate only dilated loops of small bowel and colon. The hallmark of the disease is pneumatosis cystoides intestinalis (Fig. 52.31A,B). Pneumatosis results from destruction of the mucosa with passage of gas produced by bacteria (*Escherichia coli*) into the bowel wall and, in

some cases, into the portal venous system (Fig. 52.31C). Pneumatosis cystoides intestinalis appears as linear, curvilinear, or bubbly-to-granular collections of air. Small bubbles of portal vein gas that are not visible radiographically can be detected with US as echogenic intravascular foci in the liver. The presence of portal vein gas has been considered a dire prognostic sign, but with aggressive treatment, it is of less concern. Many patients develop strictures, most commonly in the colon. NEC is treated by withholding feedings, administering antibiotics, and blood transfusions. Surgical intervention is necessary when perforation or peritonitis occurs. Free air, indicating intestinal perforation, is best demonstrated with cross-table lateral or left lateral decubitus views of the abdomen. Fixed dilated bowel loops are presumed to be ischemic and nonviable and an indication for surgical intervention.

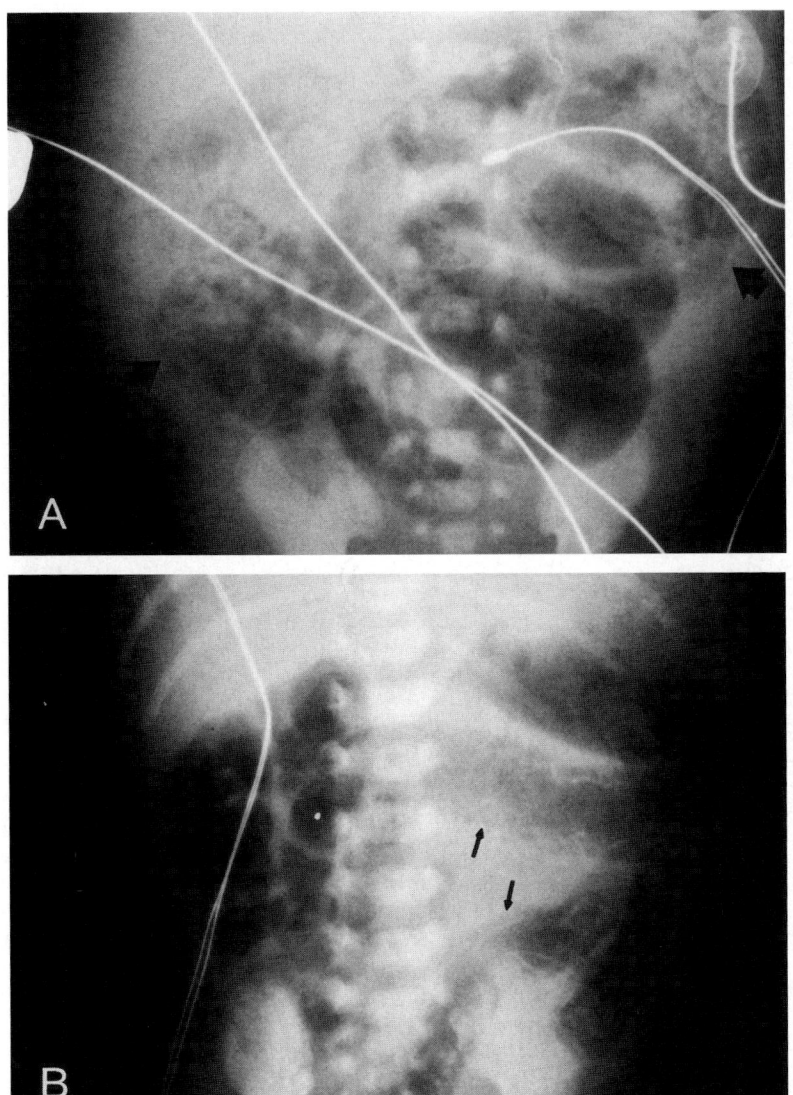

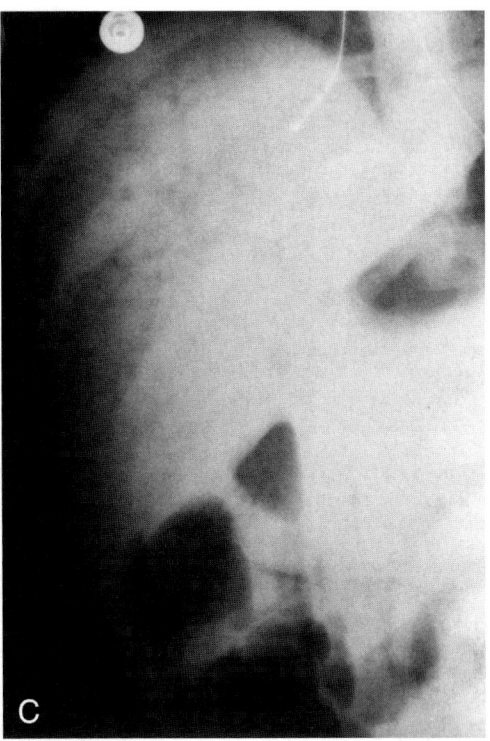

Figure 52.31. Necrotizing Enterocolitis. A. Multiple loops of distended bowel have bubbly and linear radiolucencies in the bowel wall representing pneumatosis intestinalis (*arrows*). **B.** Another patient with marked pneumatosis of the wall of the colon (*arrows*). **C.** The branching radiolucencies in the liver represent air within the portal venous system .

Typhlitis (neutropenic colitis) is a localized necrotizing colitis, usually involving the cecum, that develops in patients with leukemia when they are severely neutropenic. Findings mimic those of acute appendicitis or acute regional enteritis. The clinical setting suggests the correct diagnosis. On US the affected bowel wall is echogenic and thickened (21)(Fig. 52.32). Barium enema shows cecal abnormalities including thumb printing, spasm, and mucosal irregularity (Fig. 52.33). Hemolytic-uremic syndrome caused by *E. coli* can be preceded by a hemorrhagic colitis that has similar findings (22).

Appendicitis. In nonperforated appendicitis the abdomen often is relatively airless with one or two loops of air-filled small bowel or cecum in the right lower quadrant. Scoliosis with concavity to the right frequently is associated with spasm and indistinctness of the lateral edge of the right psoas muscle. Fecaliths, seen in 50% of cases, are strong presumptive evidence of appendicitis in a patient with an acute abdomen. When fecaliths are found in asymptomatic patients, some advocate elective prophylactic appendectomy.

US demonstrates a fluid-filled, swollen appendix with destruction of the mucosa (Fig. 52.34). The abnormal appendix measures greater than 6 mm in diameter and is tender and noncompressible (23–25). When perforation occurs, the appendix decompresses and is more difficult to detect with US (26). Color Doppler may show hyperemic periappendiceal soft tissues or fluid collections (27,28). Fecaliths are readily demonstrated with US.

With perforation of the appendix, clinical findings improve but never become normal. The radiograph, however, usually becomes distinctly abnormal, as the generalized inflammatory process in the area of perforation causes functional obstruction of the small bowel (see Fig. 52.23). Abscesses are best detected with US or CT. On US appendiceal abscesses vary from anechoic to solid in appearance (Fig. 52.35). Barium enema demonstrates plastering of the inflammatory process to portions of the colon and small bowel.

Mesenteric Adenitis clinically mimics appendicitis but is a self-limiting condition with no complications. US demonstrates enlarged lymph nodes in the right lower quadrant (Fig. 52.36) and a normal appendix. The enlarged nodes show increased blood flow with color

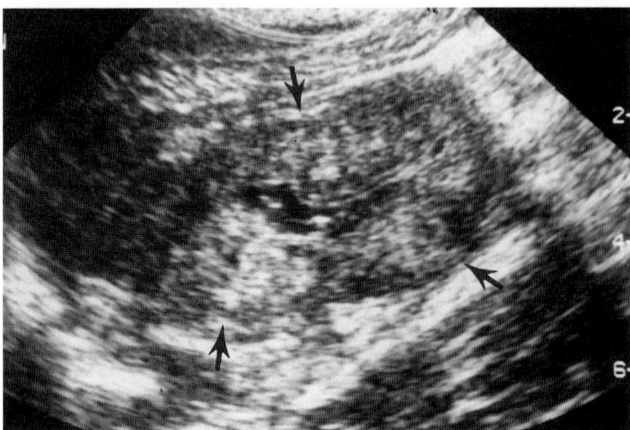

Figure 52.32. Typhilitis. US demonstrates marked echogenic thickening of the cecal wall (*arrows*).

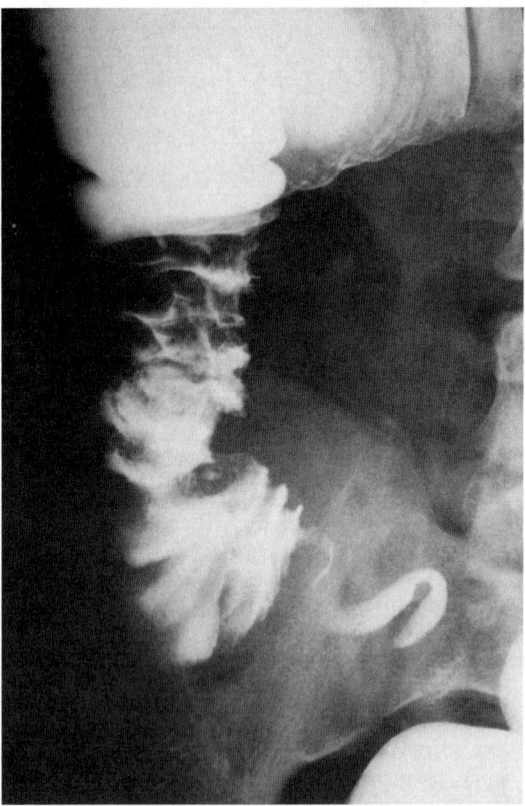

Figure 52.33. Typhilitis. Note the spasm, thumbprinting, and mucosal thickening involving the cecum.

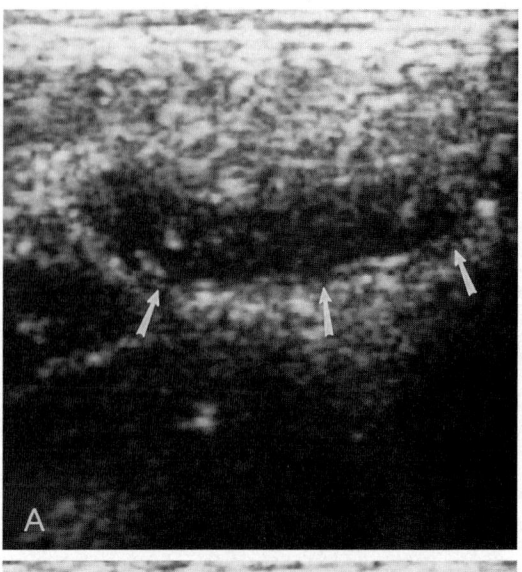

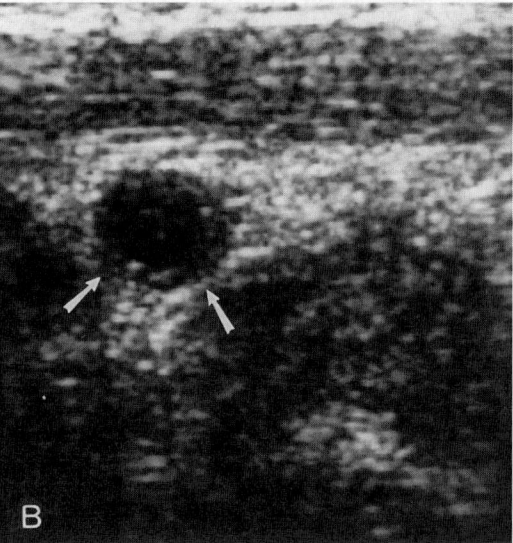

Figure 52.34. Acute Appendicitis. A. A longitudinal US image of the appendix demonstrating a fluid-filled lumen (*arrows*), which could not be compressed. **B.** The appendix in cross-section. Note the areas of decreased echogenicity of the mucosal lining of the appendix (*arrows*).

Doppler US. Giant mesenteric adenitis can produce a mass-like lesion in the right lower quadrant with considerable distortion of the terminal ileum and cecum.

Bacterial Peritonitis in children is caused by perforated appendicitis and generalized sepsis. Children with nephrotic syndrome are more prone to develop generalized bacterial peritonitis. Free fluid in the abdomen is the main imaging finding.

Meconium Peritonitis results from intrauterine intestinal perforation that occurs as a result of a fetal bowel obstruction or ischemia with bowel necrosis. In some patients, active perforation remains after birth and the patient presents with a clinical picture of peritonitis. In other cases, the perforation seals off in utero, and the extruded meconium is palpated as an abdominal mass. This meconium sometimes calcifies and is identified on plain films. Calcified meconium appears as scattered amorphous or curvilinear calcifications throughout the peritoneal cavity (Fig. 52.37A). Free meconium may enter the scrotum through a patent processus vaginalis. Residual masses of meconium can be identified sonographically (Fig. 52.37B). Calcifications create multiple scattered, bright echoes that have been likened to a "snowstorm." Infants with calcifications but no evidence of obstruction or active peritonitis can be managed nonsurgically. The calcifications slowly disappear. Some patients may develop bowel obstruction later in childhood due to adhesions.

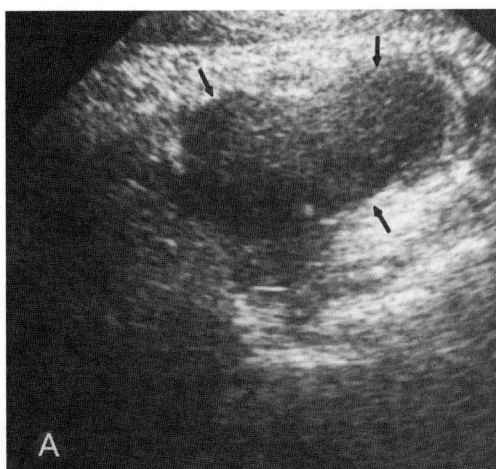

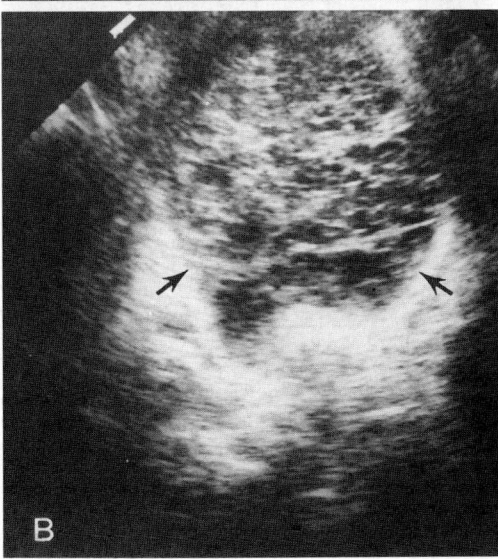

Figure 52.35. Abscesses Secondary to Perforated Appendicitis. A. US shows a complex oval fluid collection (*arrows*) in the right lower quadrant. **B.** This abscess developed postappendectomy and demonstrates a large amount of echogenic debris within the abscess fluid (*arrows*).

HEPATOBILIARY

Cholecystitis is more common than usually believed in the pediatric population. The findings are the same as in adults. The inflamed gallbladder is distended, shows a thickened wall, and may show surrounding edema (29). Cholecystitis occurs in otherwise healthy children but is also seen in patients who are HIV-positive. Gallstones also are more common than previously appreciated in infants and children. Many gallstones are due to the presence of a hemolytic anemia.

Ascending Cholangitis can occur at any age with the same findings as in adults. Ascending cholangitis, due to abnormal pancreatic duct insertion into the common bile duct, has been considered a strong etiologic factor in the development of choledochal cysts in infancy.

Hepatitis is not uncommon in children, but there are few imaging findings. If the liver is very edematous, it may appear hypoechoic on US.

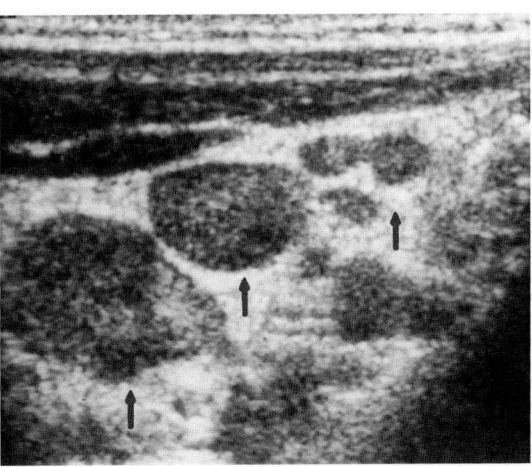

Figure 52.36. Mesenteric Adenitis. Multiple enlarged, hypoechoic lymph nodes (*arrows*) are seen on US of the right lower quadrant.

Biliary Atresia and Neonatal Hepatitis account for most cases of cholestatic jaundice in the neonate. Hepatitis in the newborn can be related to infection with a specific virus (hepatitis B virus, cytomegalovirus) or associated with familial or metabolic conditions that result in cholestatic jaundice (alpha-1-antitrypsin deficiency, Byler disease). Diffuse extrahepatic bile duct atresia is believed to result from chronic viral cholangiohepatitis. Less common are intrahepatic ductal atresia and focal atresia of the bile ducts, which is presumably caused by an intrauterine vascular insult.

Neonatal hepatitis is treated medically although extrahepatic bile duct atresia requires prompt surgical correction. US alone usually does not adequately distinguish between the two conditions (Fig. 52.38) and is used primarily to exclude other causes of obstructive jaundice such as choledochal cysts, inspissated bile syndrome, or obstructing masses or gallstones. The gallbladder is small or absent in most patients with extrahepatic biliary atresia, although in 20% a normal gallbladder is seen. In extrahepatic biliary atresia, hepatobiliary scintigraphy shows normal hepatic tracer uptake but no excretion into the bile ducts or GI tract (30,31). Tracer activity within the GI tract strongly supports the diagnosis of neonatal hepatitis and virtually excludes extrahepatic biliary atresia. Phenobarbital is sometimes administered prior to the examination to enhance the biliary excretion of the isotope and improve the discriminatory value of the examination. The definitive diagnosis of biliary atresia is made by liver biopsy and intraoperative cholangiography.

Pancreatitis in childhood is usually caused by blunt trauma, especially child abuse. On US, the pancreas may appear entirely normal or enlarged and hypoechoic. The gold standard for diagnosis of acute pancreatitis is the serum amylase level. In severe cases, peripancreatic extravasation of lipase causes lipolysis and increased echogenicity of otherwise undetectable fat. Because infants and children have little intraabdominal fat, the demonstration of peripancreatic echogenic fat strongly suggests the diagnosis of acute pancreatitis (Fig. 52.39). US is useful for detection and follow-up of peripancreatic

Figure 52.37. Meconium Peritonitis. A. Numerous amorphous calcifications are seen scattered throughout the peritoneal cavity. **B.** US revealed a hypoechoic mass (*M*), representing residual meconium in the peritoneal cavity. Note the scattered echogenic calcifications adjacent to the mass (*arrows*).

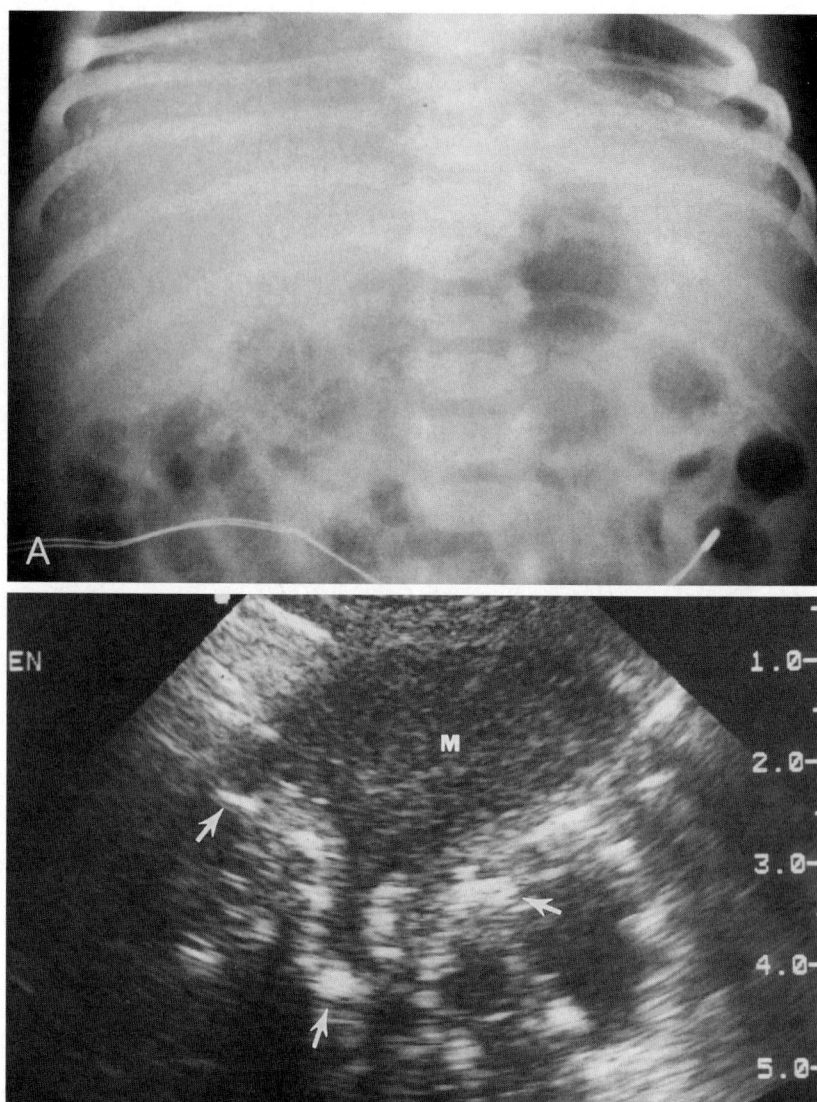

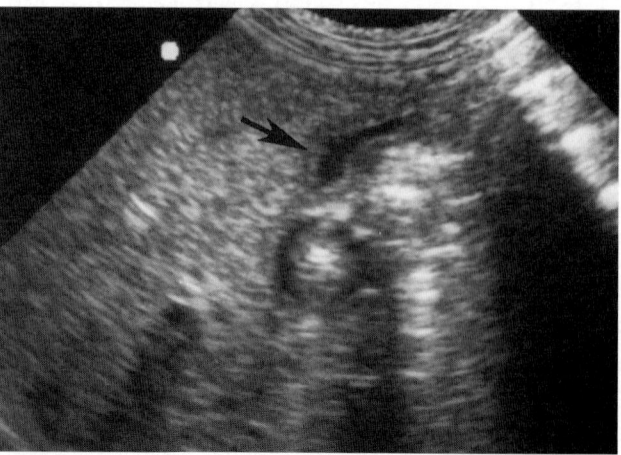

Figure 52.38. Neonatal Hepatitis. US identifies a small gallbladder (*arrow*) and no evidence of dilated bile ducts.

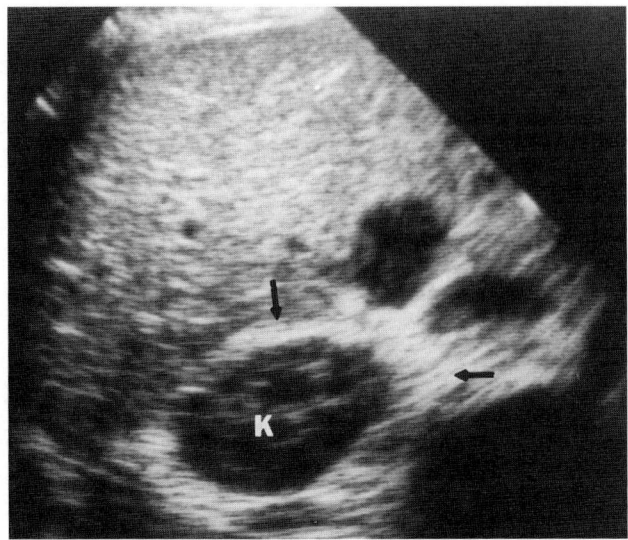

Figure 52.39. Pancreatitis. The perirenal fat (*arrows*) shows prominent increased echogenicity. *K*, kidney.

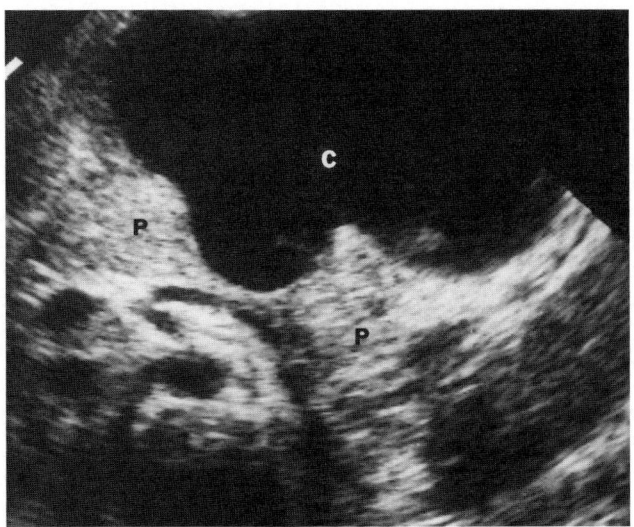

Figure 52.40. Pancreatic Pseudocyst. Posttraumatic pancreatitis in a battered child was complicated by the development of a large lobulated pseudocyst (*C*). *P*, pancreas.

fluid collections which usually resolve spontaneously in children (Fig. 52.40)(32).

Gastrointestinal Bleeding

The causes of GI bleeding in patients in the pediatric age group are numerous and depend upon the age of the patient (Table 52.7).

In the neonate, common causes include necrotizing enterocolitis, milk allergy, and the enterocolitis that sometime accompanies Hirschsprung disease. Ulcer disease and hemorrhagic gastritis are often associated with hypoxia or sepsis. Anal fissures are a common cause of rectal bleeding.

In older infants and children, peptic ulcer disease is an important cause of UGI tract bleeding. Coagulopathies

Table 52.7. Causes of GI Bleeding

Peptic ulcer disease	Anal fissures
Enterocolitis	Bleeding disorders
Necrotizing enterocolitis	Henoch-Schönlein purpura
Milk allergy	Hemolytic uremic syndrome
Hirschsprung disease	Juvenile polyps
Regional enteritis	Meckel's diverticulum
Ulcerative colitis	Intussusception
Hemorrhagic gastritis of the	Portal vein thrombosis
newborn	

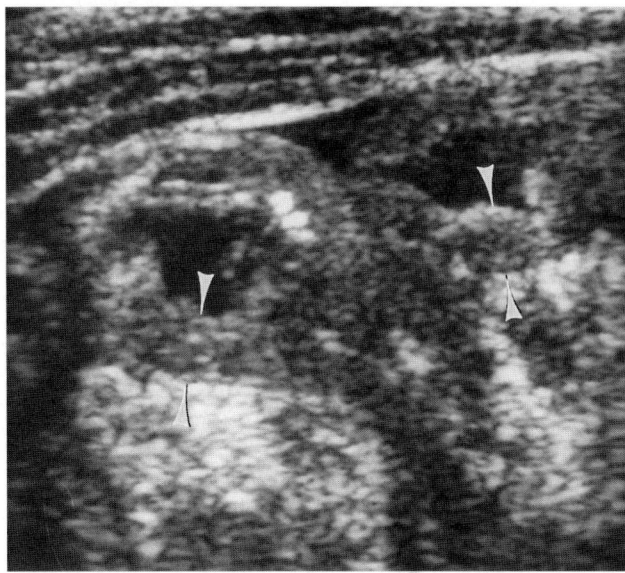

Figure 52.41. Henoch-Schönlein Purpura. The bowel wall (*arrows*) is echogenic and thickened due to mucosal and submucosal edema and hemorrhage.

can result in intestinal hematomas. Bloody diarrhea is a common component of *E. coli*-associated hemolytic uremic syndrome in young children. GI bleeding may be the presenting symptom of unsuspected portal vein thrombosis. Henoch-Schönlein purpura is a vasculitis of unknown etiology that affects the skin, GI tract, joints, and kidneys. In half of the cases, crampy abdominal pain and intestinal bleeding occur. US demonstrates segmental and circumferential echogenic thickening of the bowel wall (Fig. 52.41)(33). Abdominal symptoms may precede the characteristic skin rash.

Rectal bleeding in older children is most often caused by juvenile polyps, which are most common in the sigmoid and rectum. Painless, sometimes profuse, rectal bleeding may occur with Meckel's diverticulum. Meckel's diverticulum arises from the ileum approximately 80 centimeters from the ileocecal valve. Ectopic gastric or pancreatic tissue, found in 20–30% of Meckel's diverticula, is a site for ulceration, hemorrhage, and perforation. The best initial examination to identify a bleeding Meckel's diverticulum is a Tc-99m-pertechnate scan (see chapter 59). The tracer localizes in the ectopic gastric mucosa (Fig. 52.42). Diverticula without gastric mucosa

Figure 52.42. Meckel's Diverticulum. A scan performed with Tc-99m-pertechnate shows an abnormal collection of tracer in the right lower quadrant (*arrow*), the intensity of which parallels that of the stomach (*S*). Gastric mucosa within the diverticulum is responsible for the tracer localization. *B*, bladder.

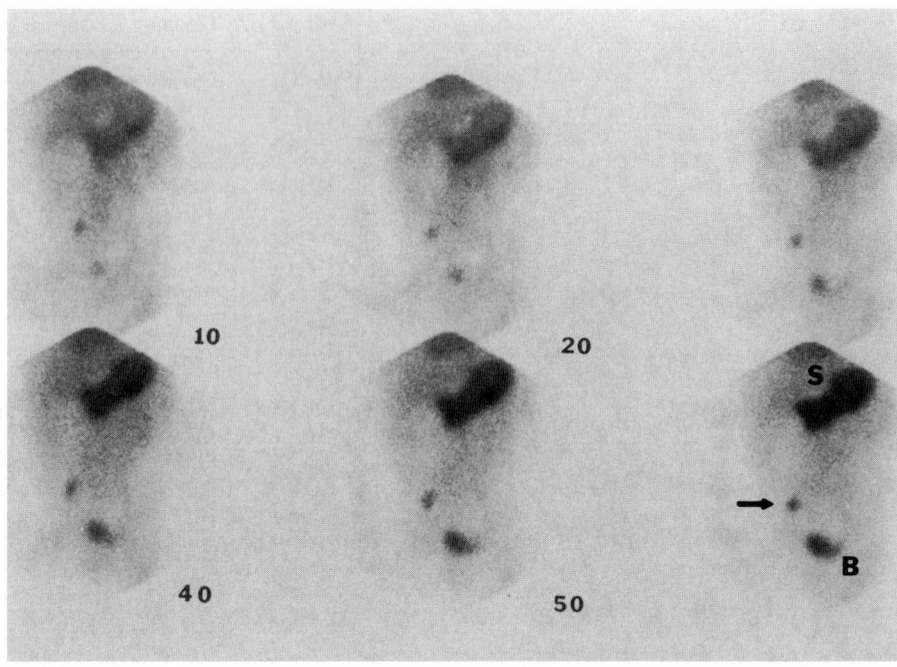

are missed. Intussusception is an important cause of painful hematochezia in young children.

GENITOURINARY TRACT

Normal Anatomy

Neonatal kidneys are proportionately larger and more lobulated than kidneys in older children and adults. On US, the renal cortex in infants under two or three months of age is normally echogenic although the medullary pyramids are quite hypoechoic and should not be mistaken for hydronephrosis or renal cysts (Fig. 52.43). Newborn female infants have a prominent uterus due to stimulation by maternal estrogen (Fig. 52.44). The uterus remains enlarged for 2 or 3 months and then involutes and remains small until puberty. In males, the epididymis in neonates and young infants is larger than in older children and adults (Fig. 52.45).

Renal Abnormalities

Urinary Tract Infection is a common problem in infants and children,especially in females. Ascending infection, originating in the lower urinary tract, can lead to chronic reflux, scarring, and growth impairment of the kidneys. In neonates, urinary tract infection is usually hematogenous and accompanies generalized sepsis. Obstructive uropathy can lead to urinary tract infection. Isolated cystitis may be bacterial or viral and is manifest by thickening of the mucosa of the bladder, demonstrated by US or cystourethrography (Fig. 52.46).

Renal Abscess is uncommon in children but is very adequately demonstrated with US and CT (Fig. 52.47) as a round or oval cystic-like structure that may contain debris. Multiple renal abscesses are usually seen in im-

munocompromised patients. These patients also are prone to fungal infection which can cause complete impaction of the calyces, pelvis, and ureter and result in anuria. Hydropyonephrosis is seen with US as dilated renal pelvis and calyces containing abundant debris.

Reflux Nephropathy. Primary vesicoureteral reflux, frequently accompanied by infection, leads to renal growth impairment, scarring, and atrophy. Primary reflux is due to abnormal insertion of the ureter into the bladder, resulting in a "golf hole orifice." The normal ureter inserts at a slant and, as the bladder distends and its wall stretches, a valve-like mechanism compresses the ureter and prevents reflux. With the congenital golf hole orifice, the ureter enters more horizontally (Fig. 52.48) and the valve-like closure is lost. Because this abnormality is frequently familial, asymptomatic siblings should probably also be evaluated for reflux.

Reflux can also occur as a secondary phenomenon in children with lower urinary tract infection. Bladder wall thickening accompanying cystitis can alter the ureteral insertion allowing reflux to occur. The Hutch diverticulum, a periureteral bladder diverticulum also alters the ureteral insertion resulting in vesicoureteral reflux and infection.

Reflux is evaluated with voiding cystourethrography and nuclear scintigraphy (see chapter 60)(34,35). The latter is more sensitive, but provides poor anatomic detail, whereas the former provides precise definition of the urethral, bladder, and ureteropelvic anatomy. Scintigraphy is often favored in females, because evaluation of the urethra is not usually important. In males, cystourethrography is the initial study of choice to detect obstructing lesions such as posterior urethral valves.

Reflux is graded from I through V (Fig. 52.49). Grade I reflux occurs only into the distal ureter and is of questionable significance. Grade II reflux reaches the kidney,

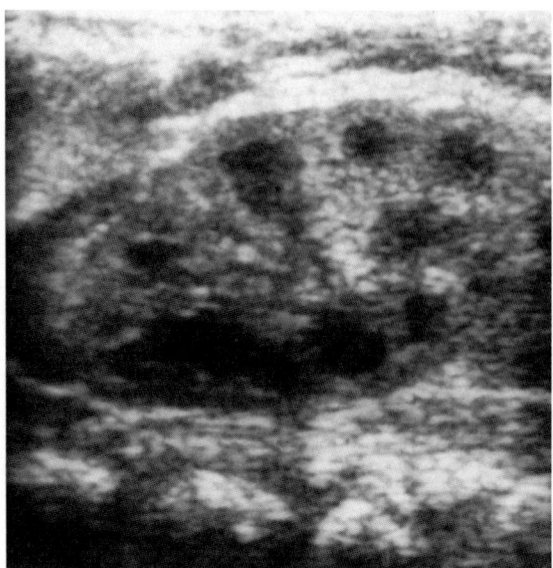

Figure 52.43. Normal Neonatal Kidney. Note the lobulated appearance of the kidney and the sonolucent medullary pyramids, which are often misinterpreted for cysts. Echogenicity of the cortex is similar to that of the liver and is normal.

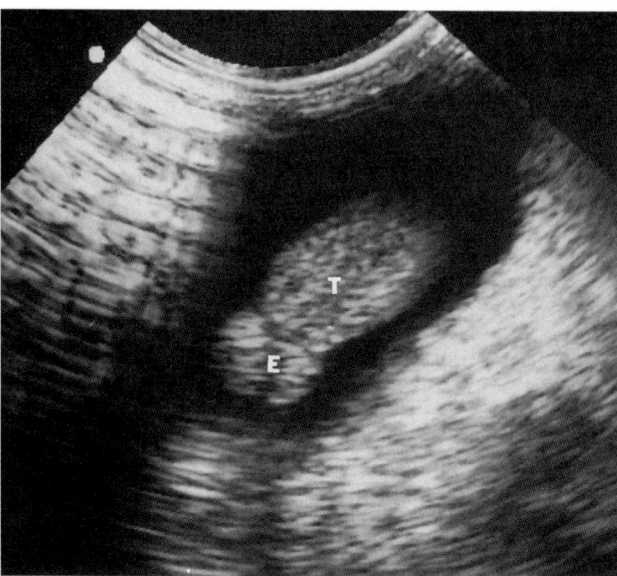

Figure 52.45. Prominent Epididymis in a Newborn. The testicle (*T*) and prominent epididymis (*E*) are surrounded by a hydrocele.

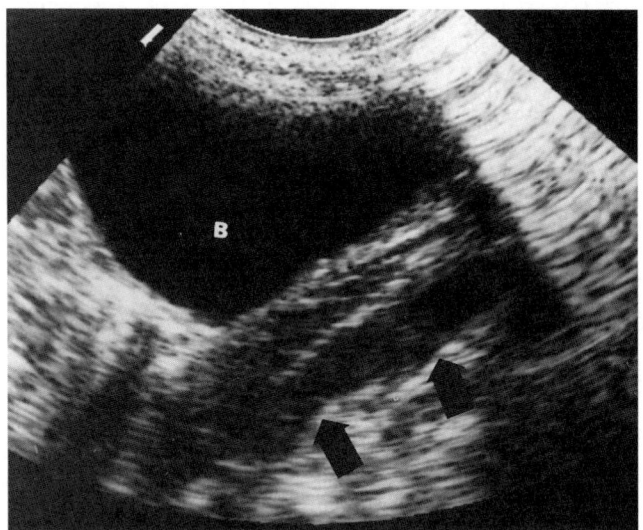

Figure 52.44. Prominent Uterus in a Newborn. US shows a normally enlarged uterus (*arrows*) in a newborn female infant. *B*, bladder.

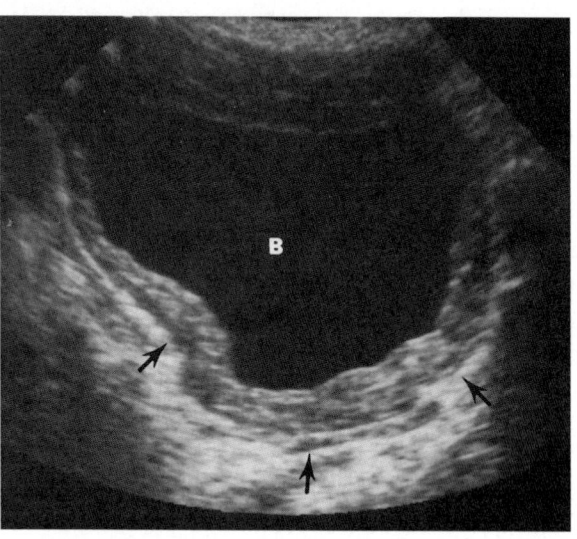

Figure 52.46. Cystitis. The bladder wall is thickened (*arrows*) due to infection.

but without dilation of the collecting system. Grade III reflux reached the kidney and the collecting system is mildly dilated whereas grade IV reflux is characterized by gross dilation of the renal pelvis, calyces and ureter. Marked tortuosity of the ureter with gross hydroureter and hydronephrosis indicate grade V reflux. Grades I through III reflux patterns are usually treated medically with prolonged prophylactic antibiotics. Grades IV and V reflux usually require surgical correction with reimplantation of the ureter.

Renal Parenchymal Disease. Nearly all types of chronic renal parenchymal disease lead to increased

echogenicity of the renal parencyma (Fig. 52.50). Eventually renal biopsy is required for diagnosis. In acute glomerulonephritis and nephrotic syndrome renal echogenicity is normal, but the kidneys may appear plump and swollen. In the neonate, acute tubular necrosis can transiently produce marked echogenicity of the kidneys. The condition is self-limiting and may involve either the cortex or the medulla or both (Fig. 52.50C). Echogenic renal pyramids may be seen transiently in the normal neonate as well as associated with a variety of conditions including hypercalciuric states, storage diseases, and protein deposition (Table 52.8)(36–38).

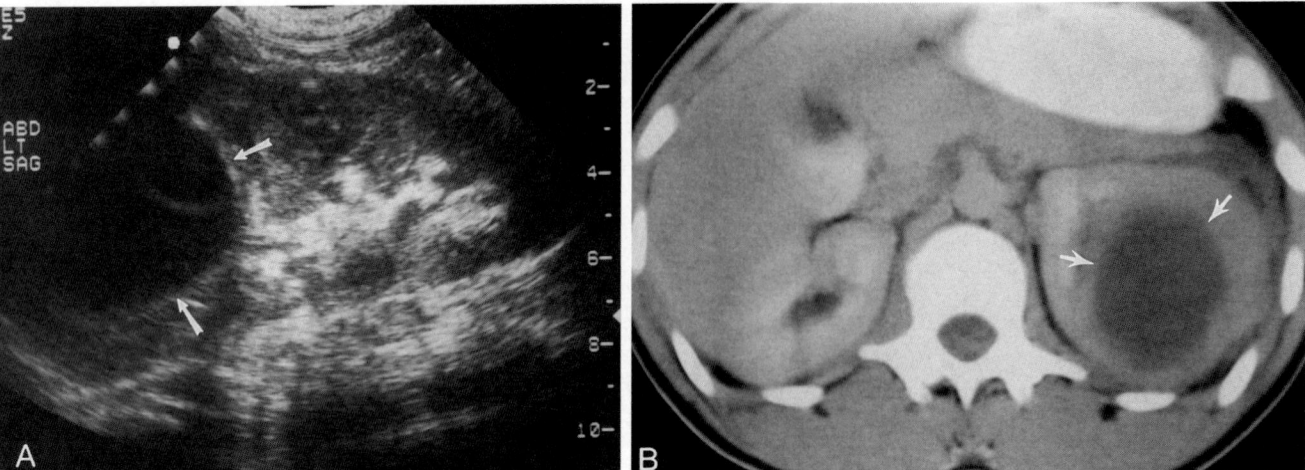

Figure 52.47. Renal Abscess. A. US shows an anechoic abscess (*arrows*) in the upper pole of the left kidney. **B.** A CT study with contrast enhancement also demonstrates the abscess (*arrows*) in the enlarged left kidney. Compare with the normal right kidney.

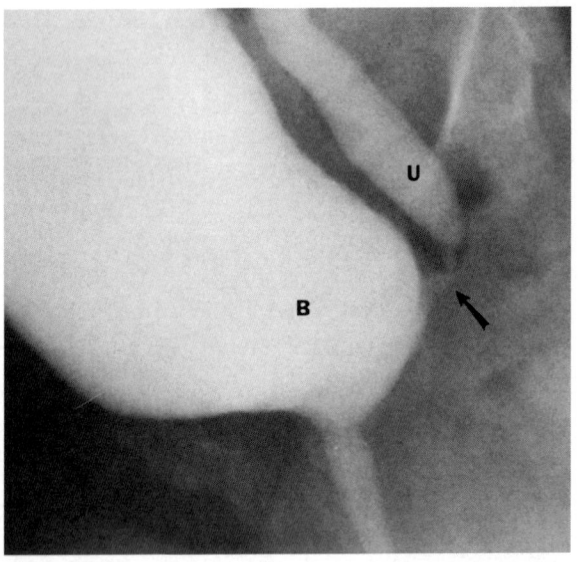

Figure 52.48. Horizontal Ureteral Insertion with Reflux. Reflux of contrast from the bladder (*B*) opacifies and dilates the left ureter (*U*). Note the horizontal orientation of the distal ureter (*arrow*).

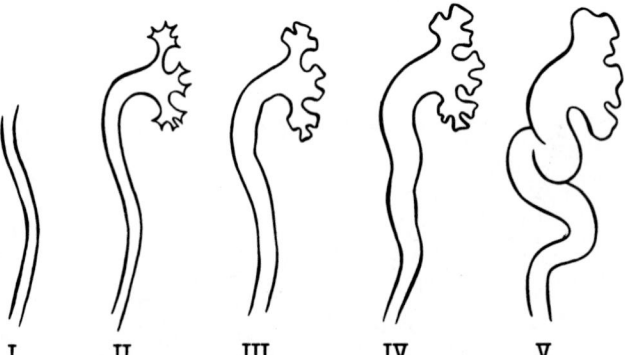

Figure 52.49. Classification of Reflux. Reflux into the distal ureter is Grade I. Reflux into the upper collecting system with no dilation of the upper tract is Grade III. Grade III reflux shows similar findings, but with mild blunting of the calyces. All of these findings are exaggerated in Grade IV reflux with marked hydroureter and calyceal dilatation. When the ureter is massively dilated and tortuous and the upper tract are markedly dilated, Grade V reflux is present. (International classification modified after Levit SB. Medical versus surgical treatment of primary vesicoureteral reflux: report of the International Reflux Study Committee. Pediatrics 1981;67:392–400.)

Hydronephrosis can result from obstructive uropathy, vesicoureteral reflux, or simple volume overload of the collecting system. The latter is rare and occurs with Bartter's syndrome, diabetes insipidus, and psychogenic water drinking. Urinary tract obstruction can be located anywhere from the renal pelvis to the urethra with the most common site at the ureteropelvic junction. Ureteropelvic junction obstruction is congenital and results from a short segment stenosis just at the ureteropelvic junction. It is believed to result from an intrauterine vascular insult, and may be bilateral or unilateral. The calyces and pelvis are dilated with no dilation of the ureter (Fig. 52.51A). The degree of obstruction can be assessed with furosemide washout nuclear scintigraphy (Fig. 52.51B–D), and Doppler resistive index (39).

Stenosis of the more distal ureter is uncommon. Total megaureter usually results from stenosis of the distal ureter as it enters the bladder or from gross vesicoureteral reflux. With gross reflux, the distal ureter is widely patent, but with primary megaureter it is narrowed (Fig. 52.52) and dysfunctional. Hydronephrosis secondary to lower urinary tract problems will be discussed later in this chapter.

Duplication and Ectopic Ureterocele. Incomplete duplication and positional abnormalities of the kidneys, such as ectopic and horseshoe kidney, appear no different than they do in adults. One condition that presents commonly in infancy is complete duplication of kidney and ureter with an ectopic and dilated ureter from the upper pole (ectopic ureterocele). Ectopic ureterocele is

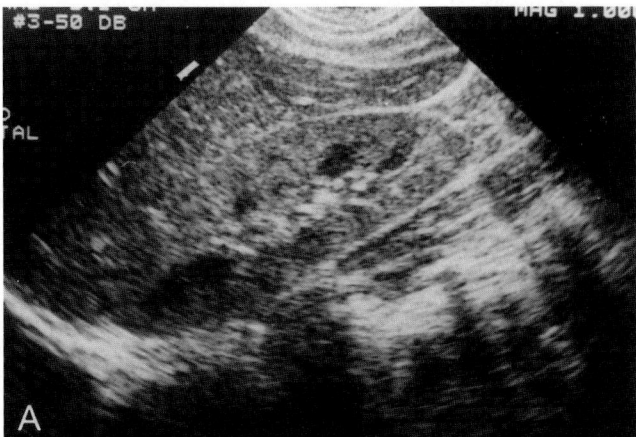

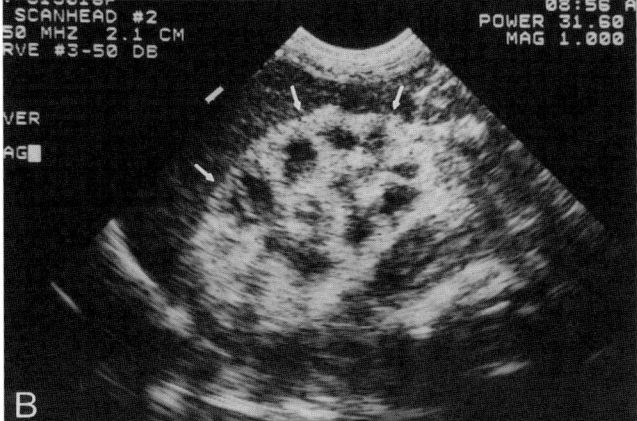

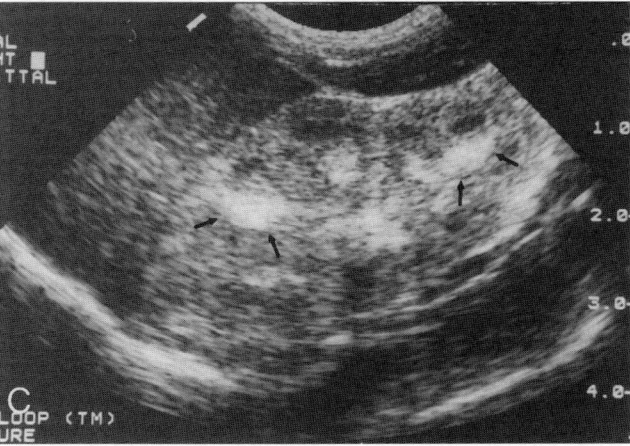

Figure 52.50. Diffuse Renal Parenchymal Disease. A. Increased echogenicity of the renal cortex (*arrows*) is seen in a patient with hemolytic uremic syndrome. **B.** Marked increased echogenicity of a neonatal kidney (*arrows*) due to acute tubular necrosis. Note the sonolucent medullary pyramids. **C.** In this neonate, increased echogenicity of the tips of the medullary pyramids (*arrows*) was a transient finding that could be considered normal.

Table 52.8. Echogenic Renal Pyramids

Normal neonate
Tamm-Horsfall proteinuria
Sickle-cell disease
Hypercalciuria
    Renal tubular acidosis
    Medullary sponge kidney
    Hyperparathyroidism
    Drugs (furosemide, steroids, vitamin D)
    Prolonged immobilization
    Bartter syndrome
    Williams syndrome
Autosomal recessive polycystic kidney disease
Storage diseases
    Glycogen storage disease IA
    Hurler's mucopolysaccharidosis
    Lesch-Nyhan syndrome
    Oxalosis

modality of choice for demonstration of the ureterocele, but cystourethrography and retrograde pyelography are used to evaluate the ureters. Reflux into the lower pole ureter may be seen (Fig. 52.53C). The obstructed ectopic ureter is dilated and tortuous and inserts into the bladder (most common), urethra, or even the vagina, leading to chronic dribbling.

Renal Vein Thrombosis is the result of dehydration and sepsis and is most common in the neonatal period. It also commonly occur with the nephrotic syndrome due to the hypercoagulable state. The findings are enlargement of the kidney, loss of its normal architecture, and visualization of thrombus in the renal veins and inferior vena cava. Color Doppler US usually provides the diagnosis.

Bilateral Renal Agenesis. Decreased output of urine with oligohydramnios and fetal compression leads to hypoplastic lungs and the characteristic deformities of Potter syndrome. Because the lungs are severely hypoplastic, the condition is usually lethal. At birth, the infant has severe respiratory distress and refractory pneumothoraces. The adrenal glands appear large, lose their usual triangular shape, and may be mistaken for kidneys (Fig. 52.54).

Renal Atrophy usually results from long-standing urinary tract infection and reflux. The greatest risk exists when reflux occurs under the age of 2 years. Less renal damage occurs with reflux and infection occurring later in childhood. Atrophy can also result from a vascular insult to the kidney.

Renal Cystic Disease is reviewed in detail in chapter 33. US is the imaging modality of choice in infants and children, and its common use has led to the realization that simple renal cysts are more common in infancy and childhood than previously suspected (Table 52.9) (40–42).

Renal Calculi are more common in infants and children than originally believed. In the past it was believed that an underlying metabolic abnormality had to be present before renal stones would develop. This has been proven to be untrue and many children have renal cal-

more common in females. The upper kidney may be hydronephrotic (Fig. 52.53A) or atrophic and difficult to visualize. The round, oval, or lobulated ureterocele is classic (Fig. 52.53B). The ureterocele may be flaccid and can be made to disappear with the pressures generated during voiding cystourethrography. Therefore, US is the

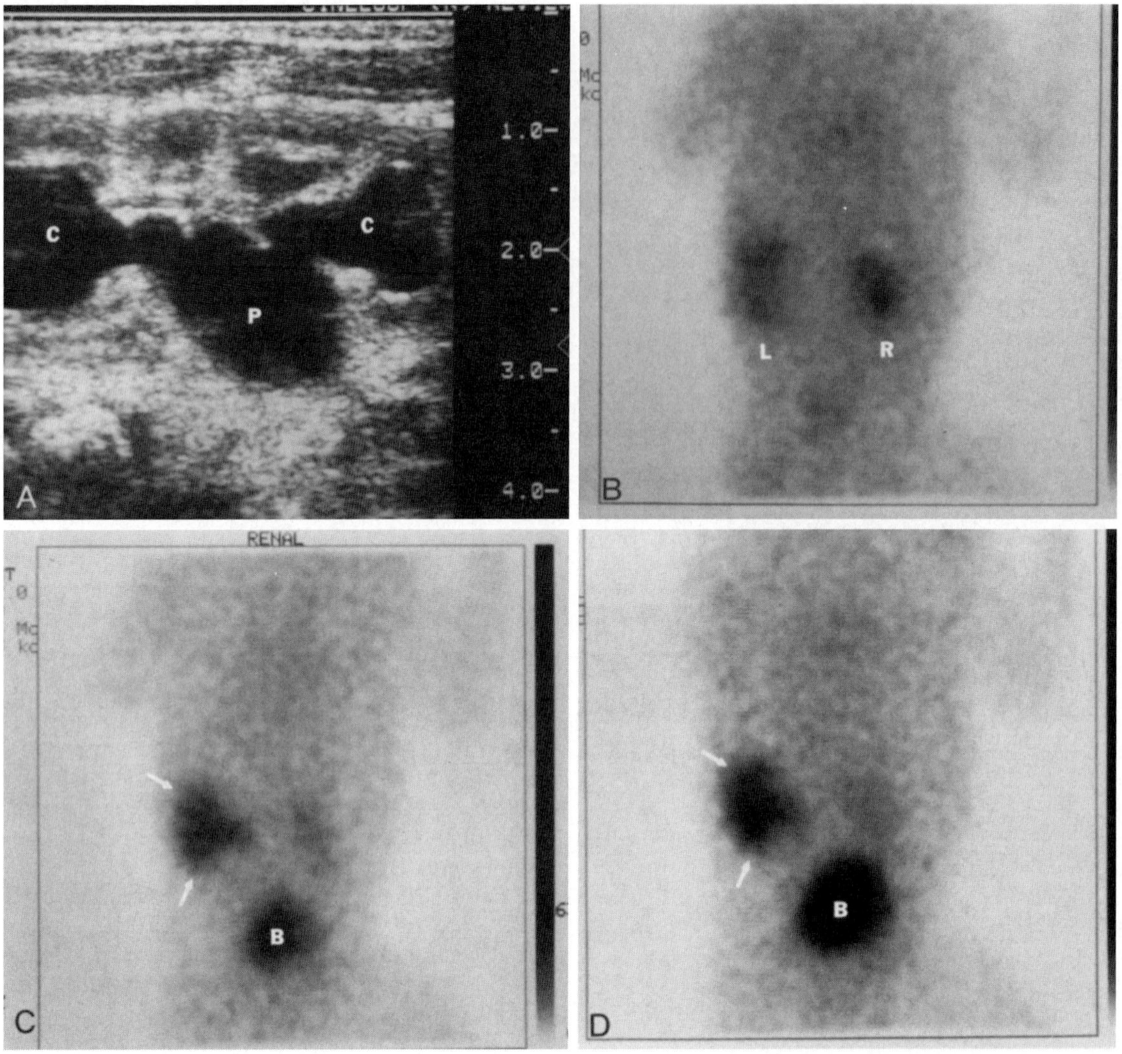

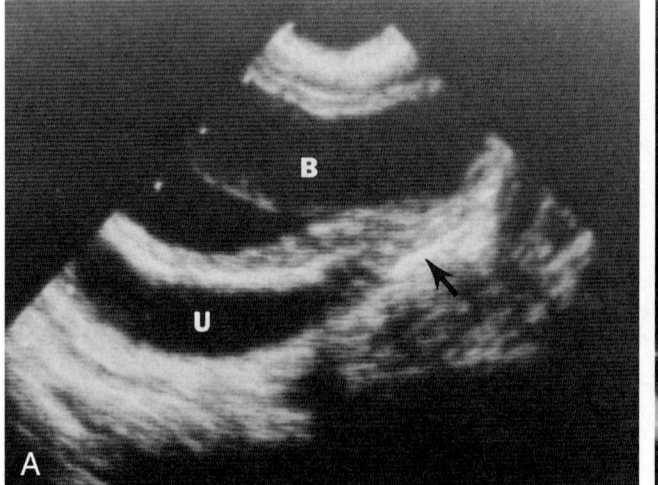

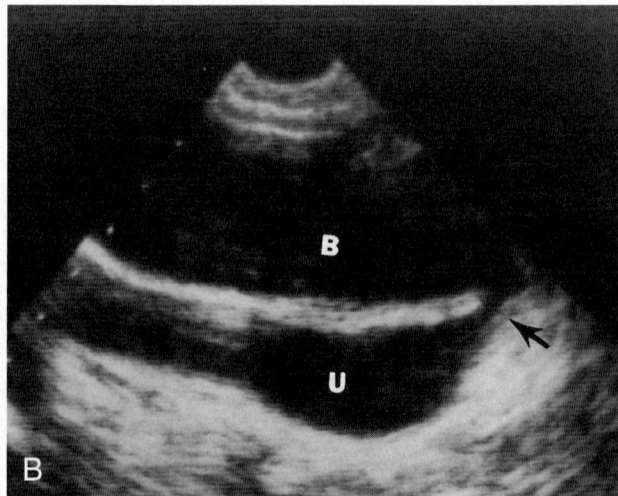

Figure 52.51. Ureteropelvic Junction Obstruction. A. Sonogram demonstrates a dilated renal pelvis (*P*) and markedly dilated renal calyces (*C*). **B.** Nuclear scintigraphy, early phase, demonstrates activity in both the right (*R*) and left (*L*) kidneys. Note that less activity is seen in the left kidney. **C.** Fifteen minutes later, there is marked accumulation of radioactive tracer in the left kidney (*arrows*); some is now accumulating in the bladder (*B*). The right kidney has emptied and is normal. **D.** After the administration of furosemide no activity is seen in the right kidney, increased activity is seen in the bladder (*B*), and marked activity has persisted in the obstructed left kidney (*arrow*).

Figure 52.52. Megaureter. A. Primary megaureter is diagnosed when the dilated ureter (*U*) demonstrates a persistently spastic distal segment (*arrow*). *B*, urinary bladder. **B.** Refluxing ureter (*U*) demonstrates similar dilation, but the distal end is open (*arrow*). *B*, urinary bladder. (From Hayden CK Jr, Swischuk LE. Pediatric ultrasonography, 2nd ed. Baltimore: Williams & Wilkins, 1992.)

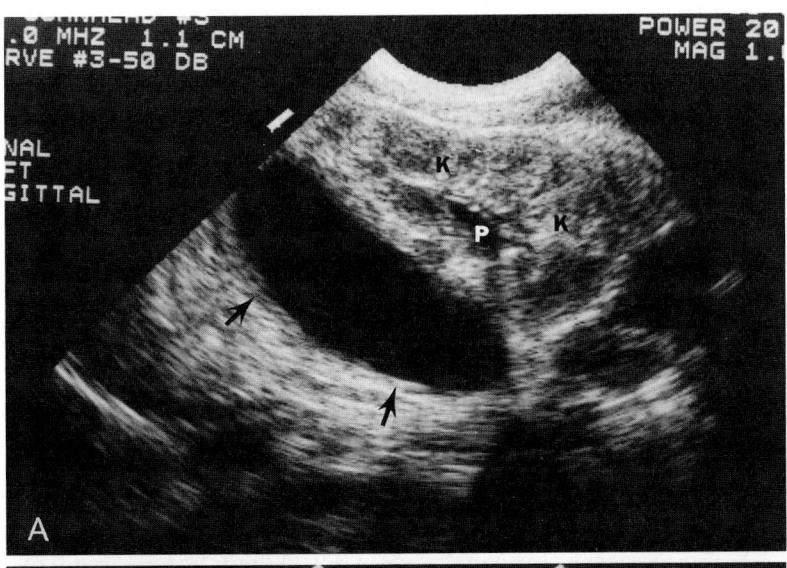

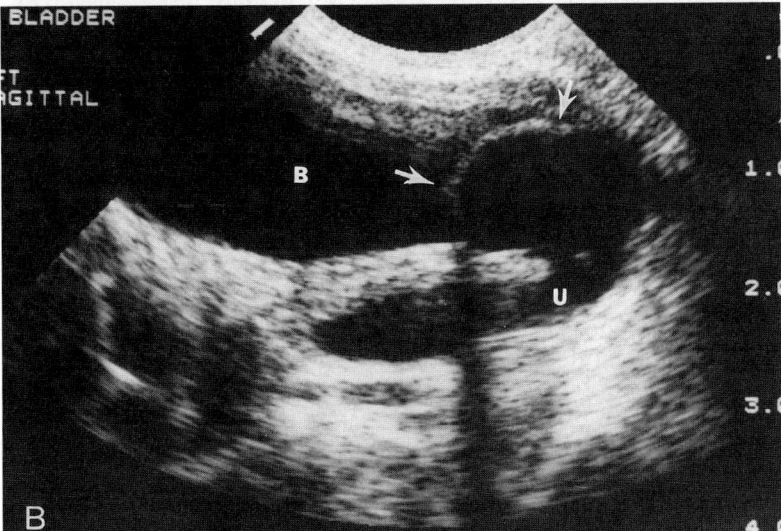

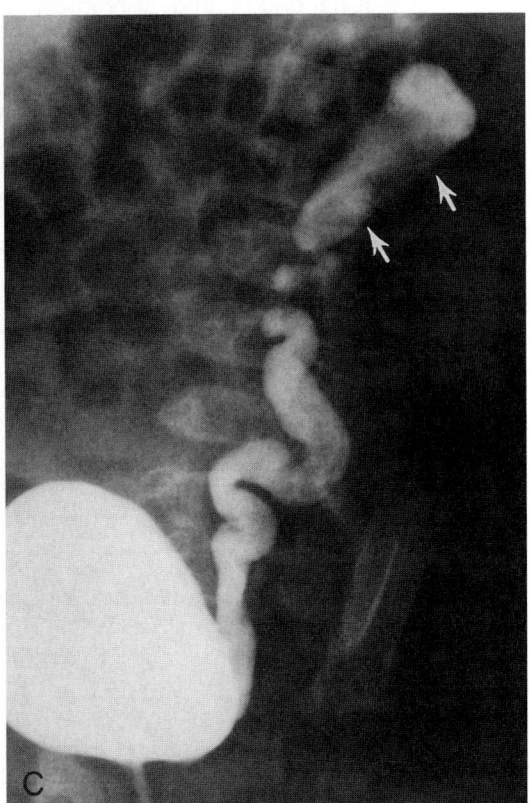

Figure 52.53. Ectopic Ureterocele. A. Sagittal US of the left kidney demonstrates a hydronephrotic upper pole (*arrows*) and a compressed lower renal segment (*K*). *P*, renal pelvis. **B.** Sagittal sonogram through the urinary bladder (*B*) demonstrates the distended ureterocele (*arrows*) projecting into the bladder base. The distal ureter (*U*) is dilated as it inserts into the ureterocele. **C.** Cystogram confirms reflux into the tortuous ureter, and dilated upper segment (*arrows*). This is the same segment as demonstrated in the upper pole of the kidney in **(A).**

culi without underlying metabolic disease. Diffuse nephrocalcinosis is seen with renal tubular acidosis (distal tubules), chronic glomerulonephritis, oxalosis, or with any cause of hypercalcemia. Nephrocalcinosis can appear smooth and homogenous throughout the parenchyma or be more punctate.

Large Kidneys. Unilateral enlargement of a kidney results from hydronephrosis, multicystic dysplastic kidney, renal vein thrombosis, or renal tumors. Bilateral renal enlargement can be seen with hydronephrosis, polycystic kidney disease, storage diseases, and glomerulonephropathies, including the nephrotic syndrome. Bilateral renal enlargement due to neoplasms is less common, although leukemia or lymphoma may infiltrate the renal parenchyma bilaterally.

Nephroblastomatosis. Small islands of primitive metanephric blastema, which are thought to be a precursor of Wilm's tumor, commonly exist in the kidneys of the normal newborn infant. These primitive cells usually spontaneously regress by 4 months of age. A diffuse and proliferative form of persistent renal blastema is referred to as nephroblastomatosis. The abnormal tissue can

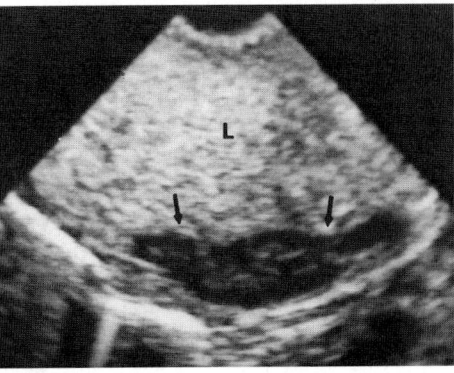

Figure 52.54. Renal Agenesis. In this patient with bilateral renal agenesis (Potter syndrome), the large but normal adrenal gland (*arrows*) may erronously suggest the presence of a kidney. *L*, liver.

form as multiple discrete nodules within the renal parenchyma or may completely replace the renal cortex. Nephroblastomatosis appears on CT or intravenous pyelogram as bilateral lobulated and enlarged kidneys with marked compression, stretching, and distortion of the pelvicalyceal structures (Fig. 52.55). On US, the kidneys are enlarged, lobular, and echogenic, or enlarged with diffuse hypoechoic thickening of the cortex. Small, focal metanephric rests are often difficult to visualize by US and are better evaluated with contrast-enhanced CT (43). Because of its malignant potential, nephroblastomatosis is usually treated with chemotherapy.

Bladder and Urethral Abnormalities

Rhabdomyosarcoma is the most common tumor to affect the lower urinary tract in children. This tumor arises from the prostate gland in males and from the vagina in females. It is usually quite large and detected early in infancy. Findings include a grapelike tumor mass with elevation of the bladder base and obstruction of the bladder neck.

Table 52.9. Renal Cysts

Single
  Simple cyst
  Calyceal diverticulum
  Abscess
  Multilocular cystic nephroma
Multiple
  Multicystic dysplastic kidney
  Polycystic kidney disease
  Glomerulo cystic disease
  Medullary cystic disease (juvenile nephronophthesis)
  Tuberous sclerosis
  Turner syndrome
  von Hippel-Lindau disease
  Zellweger syndrome
  Beckwith-Wiedemann syndrome
  Meckel-Gruber syndrome

Diverticula of the bladder may be due to chronic obstruction or neurogenic bladder. The congenital Hutch diverticulum occurs at the ureterovesicle junction and is associated with reflux. Bladder diverticula are a common feature of the cutis laxa syndrome. Urachal remnants may appear as a diverticulum or cyst in the midline at the dome of the bladder

Extrophy of the bladder is readily recognized clinically. Radiographic findings include widening of the symphysis pubis with splaying of the pelvic bones.

Prune Belly Syndrome occurs almost exclusively in male infants and demonstrates absence of the abdominal musculature with a large, patulous bladder. It is unknown whether the muscular abnormality is secondary to chronic intrauterine abdominal distension or is a primary abnormality. The enlarged bladder is associated with marked vesicoureteral reflux and hydronephrosis. Cystography demonstrates the large, floppy bladder and massively dilated ureters (Fig. 52.56). Urachal remnants are common.

Posterior Urethral Valve is the most common cause of urethral obstruction in infants, and also occurs almost exclusively in male infants. The type I valve (most common) obstructs below the verumontanum. Abnormal migration and insertion of the urethrovaginal folds result in a sail-like valve that causes antigrade obstruction with marked dilation of the posterior urethra, bladder hypertrophy and trabeculation, and vesicoureteral reflux (Fig. 52.57A). The type II valve is a nonobstructive mucosal fold extending from the verumontanum to the bladder neck. The type III valve is a transverse diaphragm located below the verumontanum (Fig. 52.57B).

Neurogenic Bladder causes functional lower urinary tract obstruction. The bladder may appear large and atonic, or small, spastic, and contracted with marked trabeculation and thickening of the bladder wall.

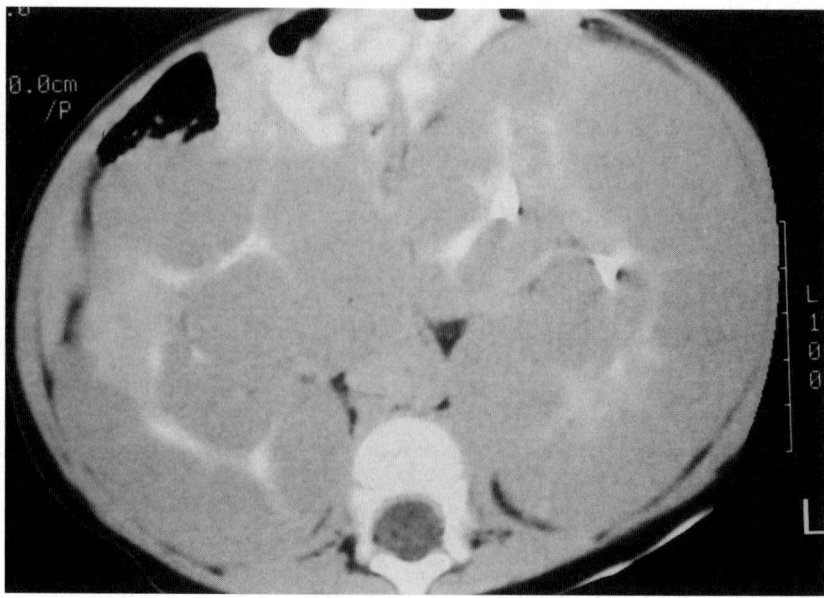

Figure 52.55. Nephroblastomatosis. The kidneys are massively enlarged with lobulated thickening of the parenchyma and stretching and compression of the collecting structures.

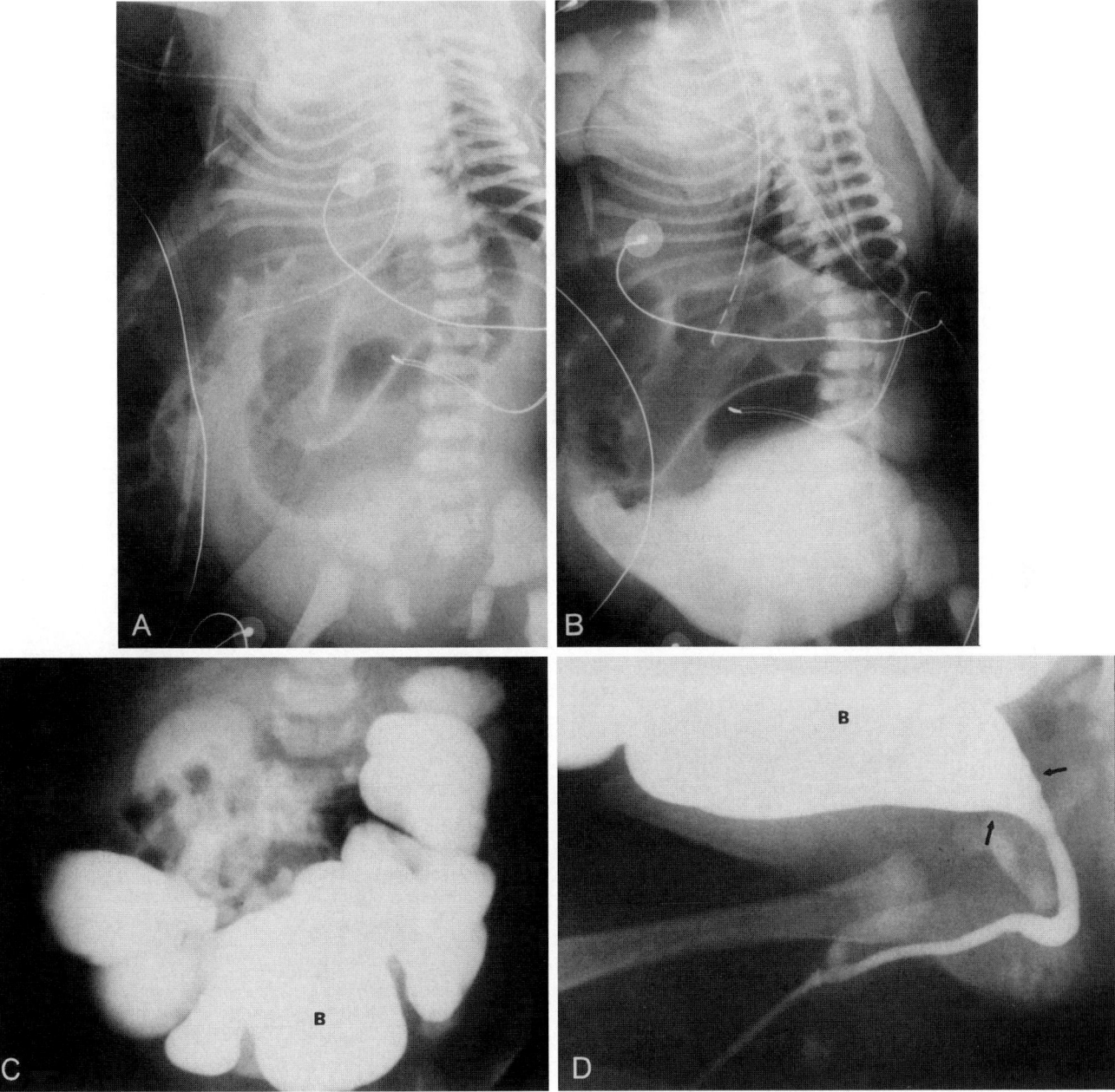

Figure 52.56. Prune Belly Syndrome (Eagle-Barrett Syndrome). A. Plain film demonstrates the large sagging abdomen. **B.** Retrograde cystogram shows the large floppy urinary bladder in the lower abdomen. **C.** Another patient with a large bladder (*B*) and massive re-flux into grossly dilated ureters and upper collecting systems on both sides. **D.** Lateral view of the bladder (*B*) demonstrates the characteristic cone-shaped posterior urethra-bladder neck region (*arrows*).

Genital Abnormalities

Ambiguous Genitalia result from a number of congenital abnormalities. Imaging is used to demonstrate the presence or absence of a vagina and uterus to aid with gender assignment. This is best accomplished with US, although retrograde vaginography may be required in some cases. In complex cases, every orifice on the perineum is injected with contrast. When a urogenital sinus is present, both the urethra and vagina empty into it (Fig. 52.58). The length of the sinus determines the type of surgical repair (44). A common cause of ambiguous genitalia is congenital adrenal hyperplasia which causes masculinization of the external genitalia of a normal female. The clitoris is enlarged but a normal vagina and uterus are present.

Testicular Abnormalities are reviewed in chapters 35 and 37.

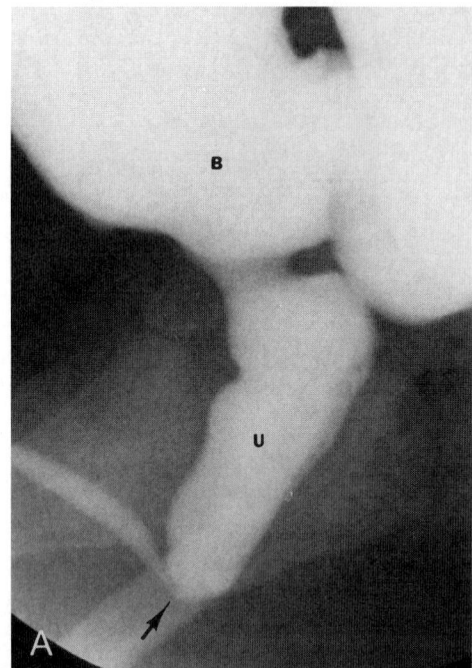

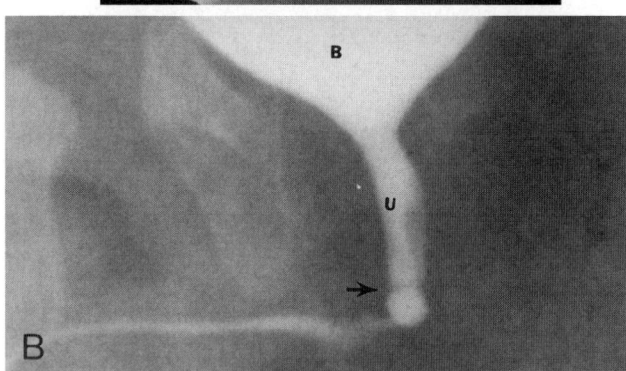

Figure 52.57. Posterior Urethral Valve. A. Typical type I valve, produces obstruction of the distal posterior urethra (*arrow*). The valve itself is seldom visualized. *U*, dilated posterior urethra; *B*, urinary bladder. Massive reflux into dilated ureters is evident posterior to the bladder. **B.** The thin diaphram (*arrow*) in the distal posterior urethra is characteristic of type III valve. *U*, urethra; *B*, bladder.

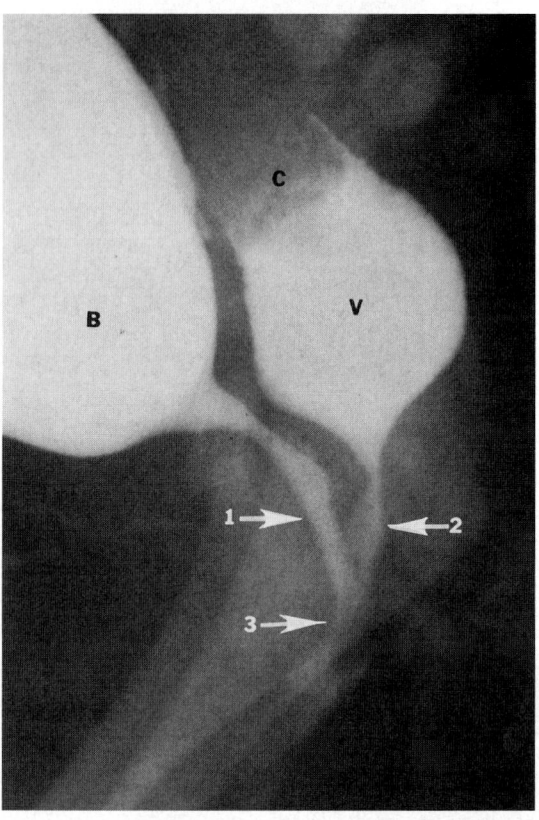

Figure 52.58. Urogenital Sinus. A short urogenital sinus (*3*) receives drainage from vagina (*V*) via a fistula (*2*) and from the urinary bladder (*B*) via the urethra (*1*). The cervix (*C*) is seen as a filling defect in the contrast-filled vagina.

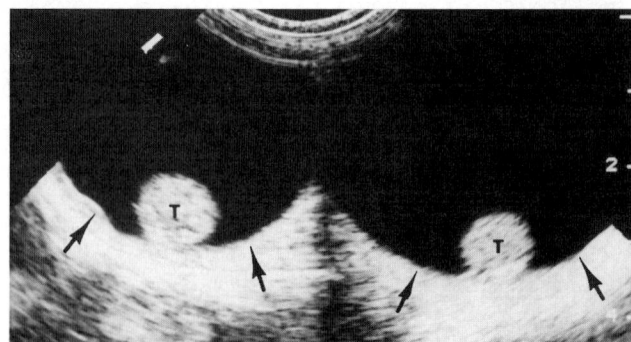

Figure 52.59. Hydrocele. Transverse US demonstrates bilateral hydroceles (*arrows*) which partially surround the testicles(*T*) anchored to the posterior scrotal wall.

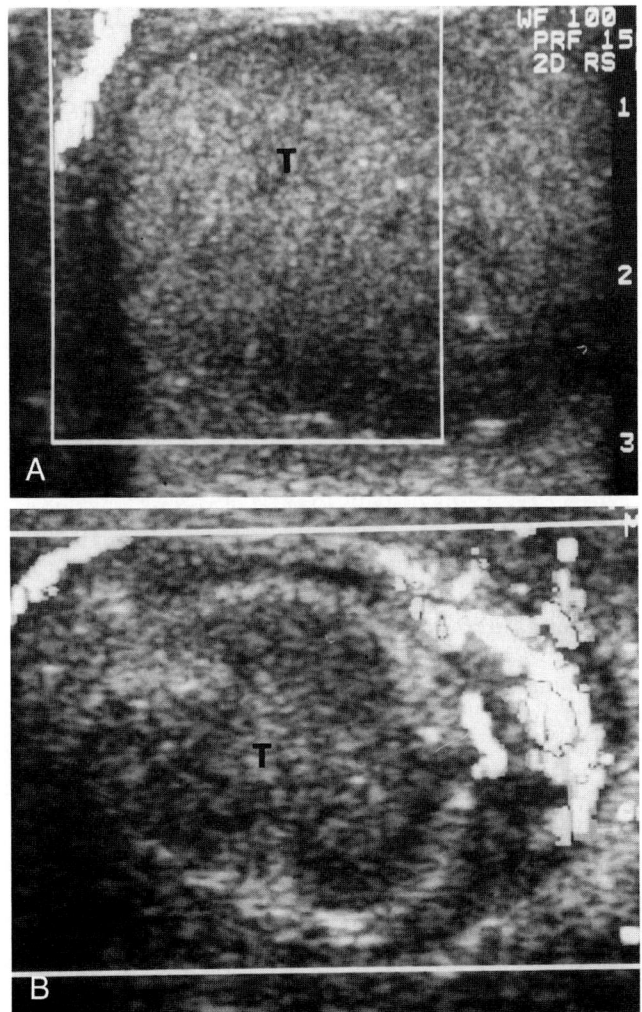

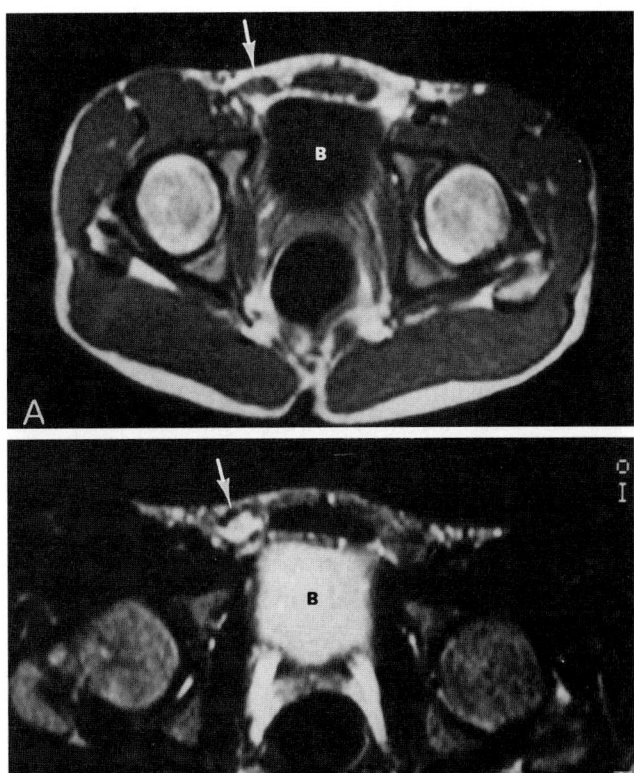

Figure 52.61. Ectopic Testicle. A. T1-weighted axial view of the inguinal region demonstrates the low-signal testicle (*arrow*) in the inguinal canal. **B.** T2WI demonstrates the testicle to be of high signal intensity (*arrow*). *B*, urinary bladder.

Figure 52.60. Testicular Torsion. A. Acute torsion is accompanied by slightly decreased echogenicity of the testis (*T*) and absence of flow with color Doppler (area within the white box). **B.** Another patient who presented after 3 days of pain has a heterogeneous and hypoechoic testis (*T*). Increased flow is seen surrounding the testis, but no intratesticular flow is present.

The most common cause of a scrotal mass in childhood is hydrocele (Fig. 52.59). Hydroceles may be congenital or develop in association with testicular inflammation, trauma, or torsion. The identification of blood flow helps to differentiate orchitis from acute testicular torsion. With torsion, blood flow is decreased within the testis (Fig. 52.60), but with orchitis, blood flow is increased within the testis (45,46). A nonpalpable testis usually indicates an undescended testis. Most undescended testes can be found in the inguinal region (Fig. 52.61) and are easily identified by US. MR is well suited for detection of testes that reside in the pelvis (47). Testicular tumors are uncommon in childhood. The most common neoplasm is the infantile embryonal (yolk-sac) carcinoma. US verifies the solid nature of a testicular mass, but cannot differentiate the type of tumor (48). Multiple hypoechoic masses can occur with congenital adrenal hyperplasia due to small adrenal rests within the testes (49).

ABDOMINAL MASSES

Abdominal masses are common in infants and children, and imaging plays an important role in their diagnosis and management. Plain radiographs provide clues to the location of the mass and the presence of calcifications. US is usually the most valuable procedure for the initial evaluation. US differentiates cystic from solid masses, indicates the organ of origin, and commonly suggests the diagnosis. CT or MR may be needed when the mass is large, poorly defined or obscured by bowel gas.

Pseudomasses may be caused on abdominal radiographs by a fluid-filled stomach, urinary bladder, or a loop of intestine. Structures outside the abdomen, such as large skin lesions, umbilical hernias, and meningomyelocele, can also mimic an abdominal mass.

Renal and Adrenal Masses

The most common abdominal masses in infants and children are enlarged kidneys due to hydronephrosis or cystic renal disease (50).

Wilms Tumor is the most common renal neoplasm of childhood. It arises from the primitive metanephric epithelium and demonstrates varied histologies classified into favorable and unfavorable groups. The prognosis is dependent on tumor histology and resectability, with survival of greater than 90% for tumors with favorable histology (51). Wilms tumor presents as a nontender, rapidly growing, unilateral abdominal mass in a young child. The mean age of presentation is three years. Bilateral tumors are found in 10% of patients, more commonly in children with associated congenital anomalies or nephroblastomatosis.

On US, Wilms tumor characteristically is a well-defined, predominantly solid mass arising from the kidney (Fig. 52.62A). Hypoechoic or anechoic areas within the tumor are due to necrosis. Hydronephrosis is commonly present. Wilms tumor has a propensity to extend into the renal vein, inferior vena cava, and even the right atrium. All of these structures must be evaluated preoperatively (Fig. 52.62B). CT is used to evaluate large tumors and the lungs which are a common site of metastasis (52). Either CT or MR can be used to exclude small masses in the contralateral kidney, which can be difficult to identify with US (Fig. 52.62B,C). Calcification is uncommon in Wilms tumor.

Renal Cell Carcinoma is very rare in young children, but it sometimes occurs in older children and adolescents. Like Wilms tumor, renal cell carcinoma usually presents as an asymptomatic abdominal mass, although hematuria is sometimes present. Hypertension is less common with renal cell carcinoma than with Wilms tumor. The imaging characteristics of renal cell carcinoma are indistinguishable from Wilms tumor.

Other Malignant Tumors are rare in children. Clear-cell sarcoma and rhabdoid tumor of the kidney were once considered variants of Wilms tumor. They are distinguished by a very poor prognosis and different metastatic patterns. The primary tumors have an identical imaging appearance to Wilms tumor, but bone metastases are common in clear-cell sarcoma, and rhabdoid tumor is associated with brain metastases and second intracranial primaries. Metastatic disease to the kidneys is uncommon. The kidneys may be infiltrated by leukemia or lymphoma.

Mesoblastic Nephroma is the most common renal tumor of the neonate. Like Wilms tumor, mesoblastic nephroma arises from the metanephric blastema. These tumors are indistinguishable on US. Although mesoblastic nephroma is usually considered to be benign, cases of metastasis to the brain have been reported (53,54).

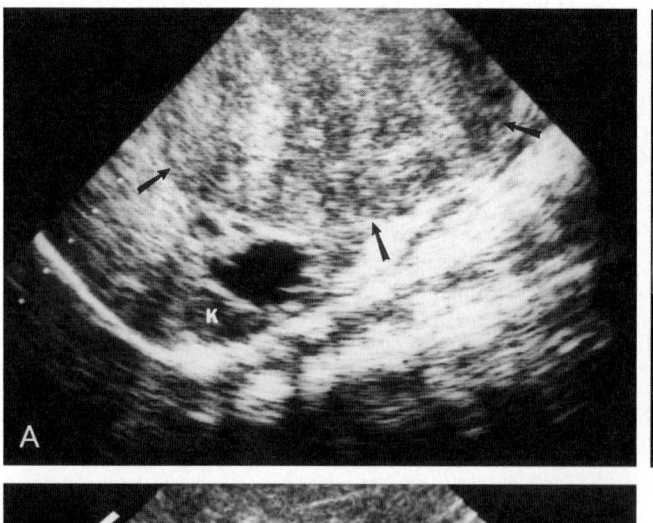

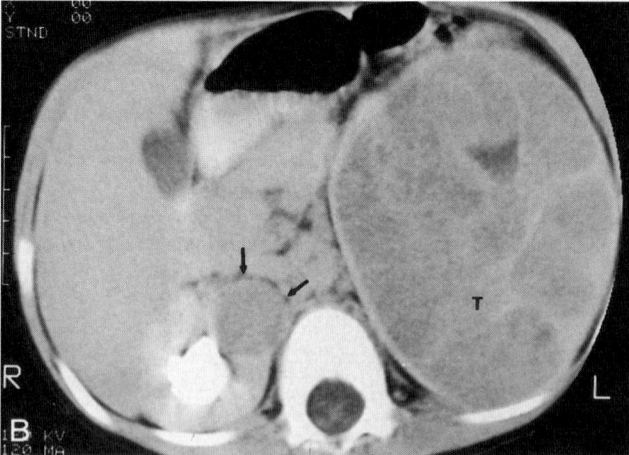

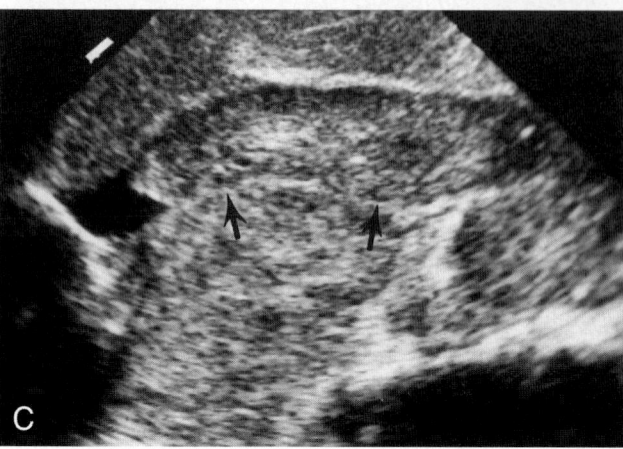

Figure 52.62. Wilms Tumor. A. US demonstrates a large mass (*arrows*) with a heterogenous echotexture arising from the kidney (*K*). Note the hydronephrosis of the involved kidney. **B.** CT scan shows the large, partially cystic Wilms tumor (*T*) on the left, and identifies a smaller tumor mass in the contralateral kidney (*arrows*). **C.** Tumor extension into the inferior vena cava (*arrow*) in another patient is seen with US.

Adrenal Hemorrhage. Suprarenal masses characteristically cause downward and outward displacement of the kidney. In the newborn, the most common cause of adrenal enlargement is adrenal hemorrhage. Predisposing factors include large babies, obstetric trauma, neonatal sepsis, and hypoxia. The infants usually present with an abdominal mass, jaundice, and anemia, but small hemorrhages may go unnoticed. Hemorrhage occurs more frequently on the right and is occasionally bilateral. Older children develop adrenal hemorrhage due to trauma, meningococcemia, or anticoagulant therapy.

US is an ideal modality for evaluating adrenal hemorrhage (55). The normal adrenal gland in the newborn is larger and more easily visualized than that of the adult. The gland appears as an inverted V-shaped structure with an echogenic central region and a peripheral hypoechoic zone (Fig. 52.63). Hemorrhage enlarges the gland and causes loss of the V shape. Initially, the hematoma resembles a solid, highly echogenic mass (Fig. 52.64). As the hemorrhage resolves, it becomes increasingly hypoechoic, starting in the central region and progressing peripherally. The hematoma decreases in size within the 1st week and sometimes calcifies. The calcifications begin around the rim of the gland, but eventually a small, completely calcified gland remains. Adrenal insufficiency rarely develops. Adrenal hemorrhage may be complicated by compression of the kidney, renal vein thrombosis, or infection.

Neuroblastoma belongs to a group of neural crest origin tumors that range from the benign ganglioneuroma to the malignant neuroblastoma (56,57). Neuroblastoma arises from the adrenal gland or from sympathetic ganglia in the retroperitoneum, posterior mediastinum,

neck, or pelvis. It is a neoplasm of early childhood presenting in children less than 5 years of age. Most children present with advanced disease and large abdominal masses. Symptoms are often related to bone metastases or intraspinal extension. In contrast to Wilms tumor, neuroblastomas are poorly marginated masses that frequently extend across the midline and into the chest. The kidney may be invaded and the tumor mistaken for an intrarenal mass. Calcifications are much more common in neuroblastoma than in Wilms tumor, with an incidence as high as 50–75% (Fig. 52.65A).

Most neuroblastomas appear echogenic and heterogeneous. In some cases, a characteristic echogenic nodule can be identified within the larger part of the tumor mass (Fig. 52.65B). CT and MR can be used to better define the extent of involvement of large tumors and to detect metastatic deposits (Fig. 52.65C). Neuroblastoma metastasizes to the liver, lymph nodes and bone marrow (58). MR demonstrates intraspinal extension (Fig. 52.65D) bone marrow infiltration and encasement of blood vessels without using intravenous contrast. Skeletal metastases are shown with bone scintigraphy. I-131-meta-iodobenzylguanidine resembles norepinephrine and is metabolized by neuroblastoma, pheo-

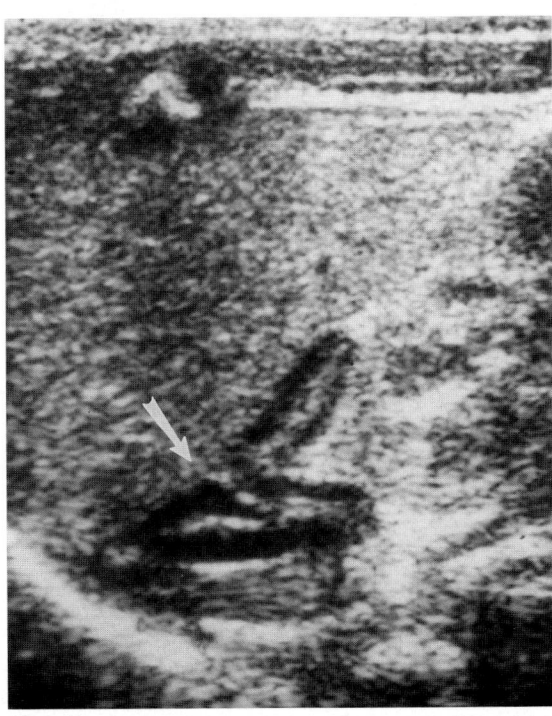

Figure 52.63. Normal Adrenal Gland. Note the characteristic "Y" shape (*arrow*) of the normal adrenal gland sitting astride the kidney.

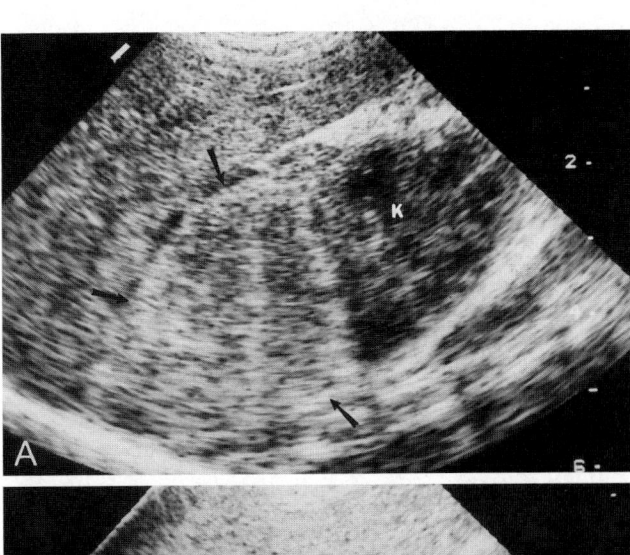

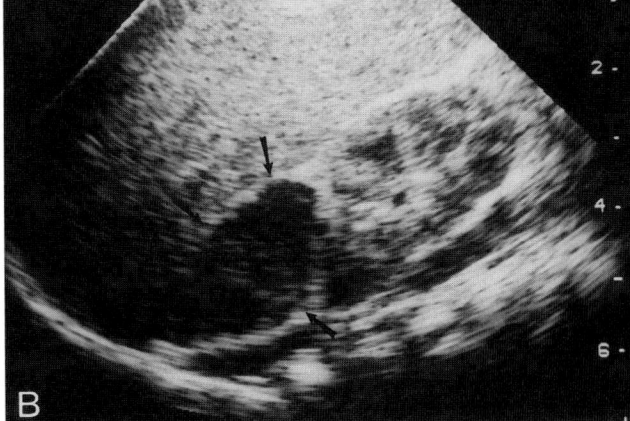

Figure 52.64. Adrenal Hemorrhage. A. In the early stages, hemorrhage into the adrenal gland presents as an echogenic suprarenal mass (*arrows*) that displaces the kidney inferiorly (*K*). **B.** As the hemorrhage resolves, the clot becomes smaller and more hypoechoic (*arrows*).

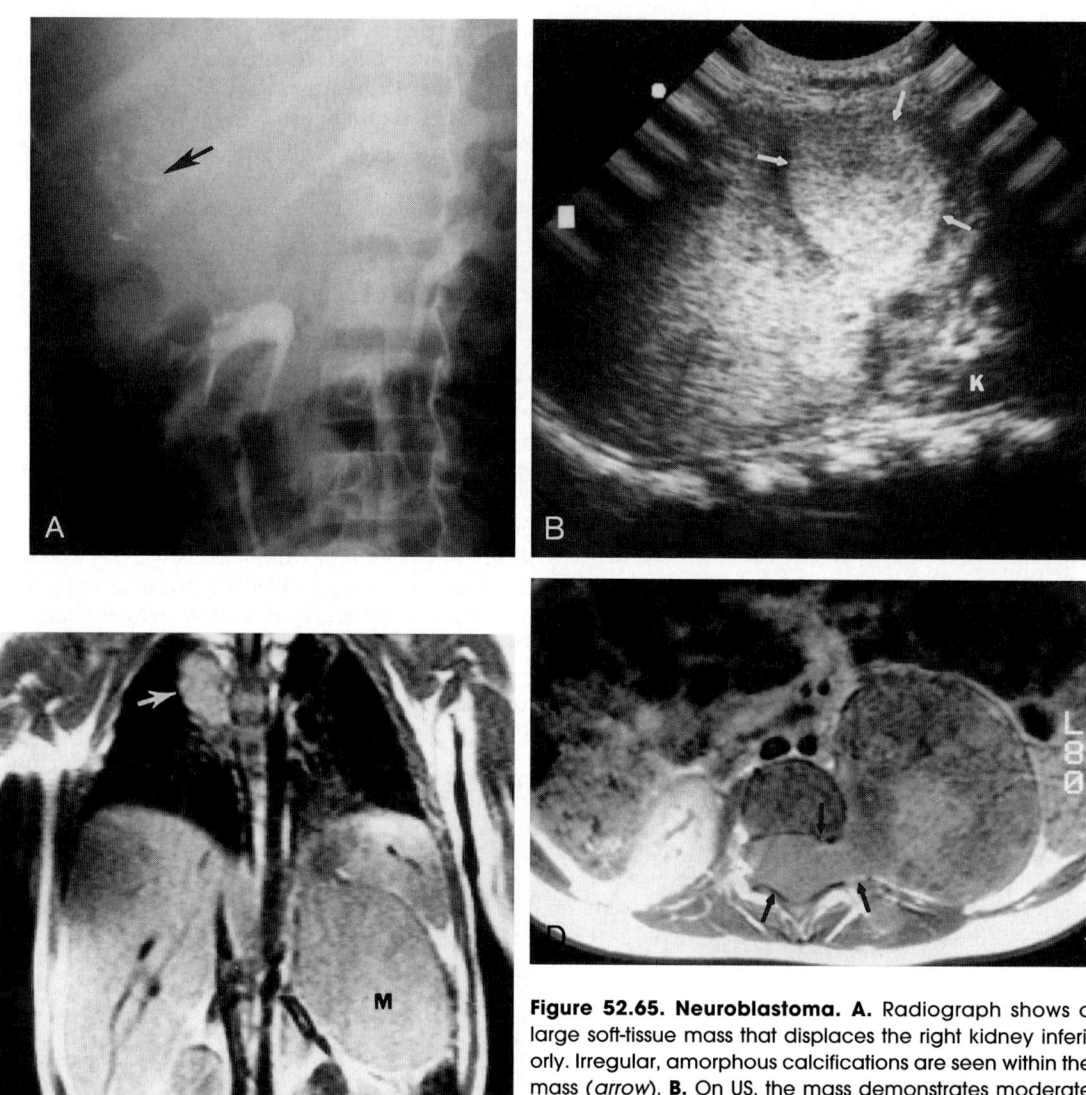

Figure 52.65. Neuroblastoma. A. Radiograph shows a large soft-tissue mass that displaces the right kidney inferiorly. Irregular, amorphous calcifications are seen within the mass (*arrow*). **B.** On US, the mass demonstrates moderate echogenicity. Note the characteristic echogenic nodule within the mass (*arrows*). *K*, kidney. **C.** MR, in a different patient, shows a large mass (*M*), displacing the left kidney. A second tumor mass is identified adjacent to the spine in the right upper hemithorax (*arrow*). **D.** Axial T1WI in another patient clearly shows tumor extension into the spinal canal (*arrows*).

chromocytoma, and other catecholamine producing tumors. This tracer is taken up by the primary tumor and metastases, and has been used to stage and monitor the therapy of neuroblastoma (59–61).

Other tumors of the adrenal gland are quite rare in children. Adrenocortical carcinoma is highly malignant and locally invasive with CT and US characteristics similar to neuroblastoma. Benign adenomas, pheochromocytomas, and congenital adrenal cysts are very rare in children.

Diffuse Adrenal Enlargement occurs with adrenocortical hyperplasia which causes the adrenogenital syndrome. The enlarged adrenals may have an undulating configuration described as cerebriform (Fig. 52.66)(62). Marked, reversible, adrenal enlargement is seen in in-

fants treated with ACTH (adrenocorticotropic hormone) for infantile spasm (63).

Wolman's Disease is a rare lipidosis that results in enlarged, densely calcified adrenal glands. Plain films are usually diagnostic. Wolman's disease is usually fatal at an early age.

Hepatobiliary Masses

A variety of cystic and solid masses may arise from the liver and biliary tract in children (Table 52.10). Most conditions can be differentiated with US.

Acute Hydrops of the Gallbladder is a poorly understood condition probably caused by transient obstruction of the cystic duct. It has been associated with the

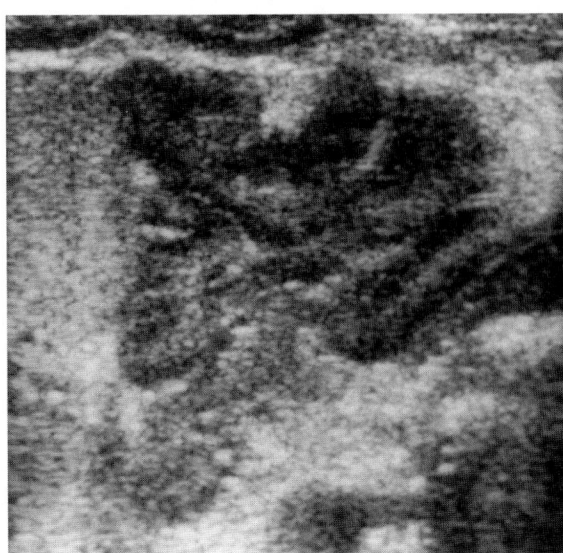

Figure 52.66. Congenital Adrenal Hyperplasia. Note the undulating configuration of the enlarged adrenal gland.

Table 52.10. Cystic Abdominal Masses

Renal cysts (see Table 52.9)	Pancreatic pseudocyst
Enteric duplication cyst	Cerebrospinal fluid pseudocyst
Mesenteric cyst	Abscess/parasitic cyst
Hydrops of the gallbladder	Lymphangioma
Choledochal cyst	Teratoma/dermoid cyst
Ovarian cyst	Tumor (necrotic)
Urachal cyst	Adrenal hemorrhage (resolving)

mucocutaneous lymph node syndrome, although in many cases the cause is unknown. US shows a markedly enlarged, tender gallbladder with a thin wall. A similar appearance can be seen with acute acalculous cholecystitis, although the gallbladder distension is less pronounced and gallbladder wall thickening is present. Transient distension of the gallbladder sometimes occurs in the neonate, particularly in premature infants. Prolonged total parental nutrition and sepsis have been implicated as possible etiologic factors.

Choledochal Cyst. Jaundice, pain, and a right upper quadrant mass comprise the classic triad of findings seen with a choledochal cyst. Young infants more commonly present with fluctuating jaundice, pain, and fever. The most common type of choledochal cyst is a localized, fusiform dilation of the common bile duct below the cystic duct. Choledochal cysts are usually diagnosed by US, appearing as a cystic mass in the porta hepatis, separate from the gallbladder and associated with dilated intrahepatic ducts (Fig. 52.67). Hepatobiliary scintigraphy confirms that the cyst communicates with the biliary tract, aiding in differentiation from other cystic abdominal masses (see Table 52.8).

Hepatic Cysts are less common in infants and children than in adults. Solitary congenital cysts of the liver are usually encountered as an incidental finding at US or CT. US shows a sharply defined anechoic masses in the hepatic parenchyma. Some cysts are very large and pedunculated, and their hepatic origin may be difficult to ascertain.

Multiple hepatic cysts occur in patients with the autosomal dominant polycystic disease. Acquired hepatic cysts may be solitary or multiple and are most commonly of infectious origin (Fig. 52.68). Resolving hematoma of the liver may also appear as a well-defined cystic lesion.

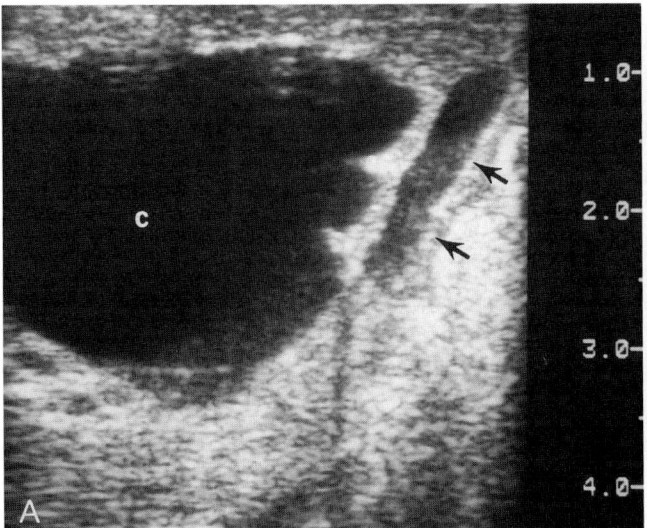
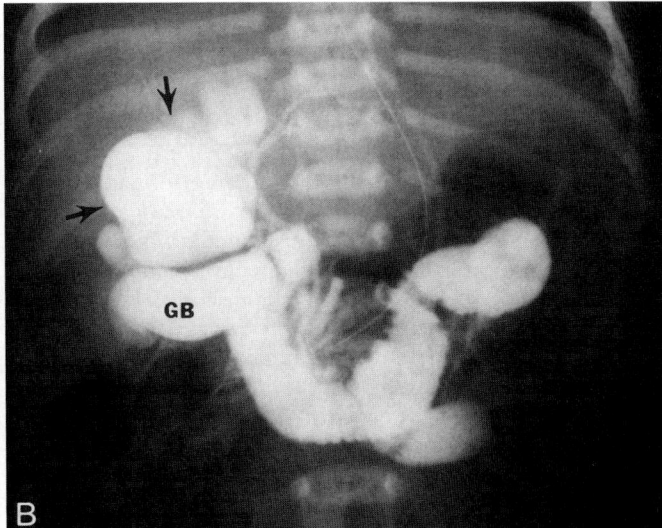

Figure 52.67. Choledochal Cyst. A. US shows a large, multilobulated anechoic cyst (*C*) that is adjacent to, but separate from, the gallbladder (*arrows*). **B.** Cholangiography confirms the presence of a large intrahepatic choledochal cyst (*arrows*) involving the right hepatic duct. *GB*, gallbladder.

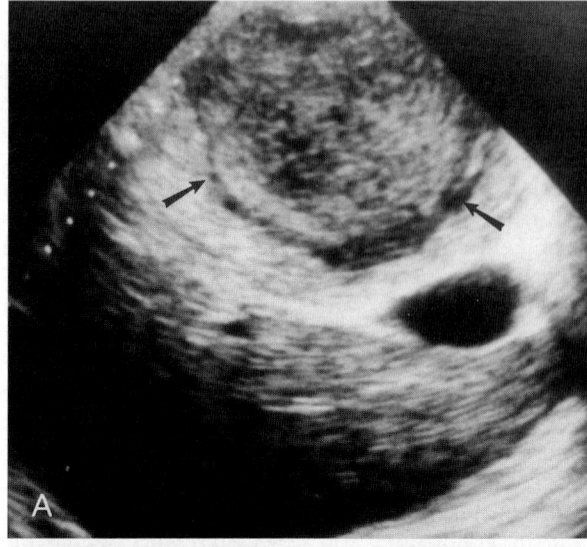

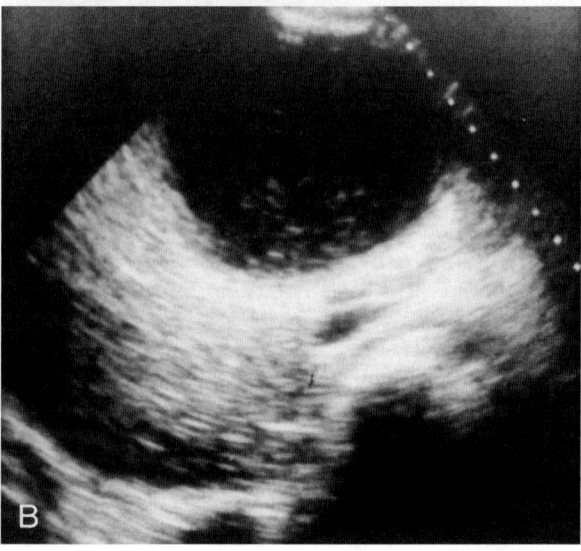

Figure 52.68. Amebic Abscess of the Liver. A. The initial US revealed a large complex mass (*arrows*) within the liver. The mass is well defined with a sonolucent rim. **B.** With therapy, the abscess becomes hypoechoic with a few floating echodensities in the dependent portion of the cyst.

Hemangioendothelioma may be solitary or multiple and is associated with with cutaneous hemangiomas in 40% of cases. It is the most common benign liver tumor encountered in infancy. This tumor may be complicated by high-output cardiac failure, hemorrhage, hemolytic anemia, or thrombocytopenia due to sequestration of platelets within the tumor. The typical sonographic appearance is a complex mass containing large anechoic sinusoids and associated with large draining vessels (Fig. 52.69). Doppler US demonstrates the vascular nature of these tumors. The lesions concentrate the tracer used for scintigraphic blood pool imaging. On CT and MR, the lesion has an appearance similar to that seen with cavernous hemangiomas in adults.

Mesenchymal Hamartoma is an uncommon benign tumor seen most often in infants and young children. Hamartomas are usually solitary and predominantly cystic with multiple thin septa and intervening nodules of solid tissue. The CT shows multiple areas of low attenuation within the tumor mass.

Hepatic Adenomas are rare in childhood but have been reported in association with Fanconi's anemia or glycogen storage disease type I.

Focal Nodular Hyperplasia presents as a mass-like lesion that can be confused with hepatic adenoma. Scintigraphy using sulfur colloid demonstrates normal-to-increased tracer uptake in many cases, differentiating it from adenomas that do not concentrate the tracer.

Metastatic Disease. Neuroblastoma is the most common childhood tumor to metastatize to the liver, followed by lymphoma, leukemia, and Wilms tumor. Metastatic lesions are usually multiple, and their imaging appearance is usually nonspecific.

Hepatoblastoma is a tumor of early childhood, presenting before 3 years of age. **Hepatocellular carcinoma** is more commonly seen in older children and adolescents. Sonographically, these tumors appear as single or multiple hyperechoic lesions, sometimes containing hypoechoic or anechoic areas due to hemorrhage or necrosis. Invasion of the hepatic or portal veins may be identified. On CT, the tumors appear as lesions of low attenuation with variable contrast enhancement (Fig. 52.70). MR is comparable with CT for the initial diagnosis of these tumors, however, MR is more sensitive in the detection of postoperative tumor recurrence (64).

Other less common primary malignant tumors in children include undifferentiated (embryonal) sarcoma and embryonal rhabdomyosarcoma of the biliary ducts. The latter tumor typically occurs in children between 2–5 years of age. When the tumor originates in a major bile duct, patient present with jaundice. Those tumors that originate within the intrahepatic ducts cannot be differentiated from other primary malignancies of the liver.

Splenic Lesions

Splenomegaly is a relatively common cause of a left upper quadrant mass in children. Splenic enlargement is most often secondary to a systemic illness. Common causes include hematologic diseases, infections, portal hypertension, and infiltrative diseases (mucopolysaccharidoses, reticuloendothelioses, leukemia, and lymphoma). The imaging characteristics are usually nonspecific and insufficient for diagnosing the cause of splenomegaly.

In the newborn and young infant, splenomegaly most often occurs because of bacterial sepsis and infection. Hepatomegaly is usually also present. In older children, infections such as infectious mononucleosis, typhoid fever, and cat-scratch fever are more common. Splenic abscess is uncommon in children and is most often associated with an impaired immune system. US shows splenic abscesses appear as multiple small, poorly defined and hypoechoic lesions (Fig. 52.71).

Cystic Masses of the spleen are uncommon and include congenital epidermoid cysts, posttraumatic pseudocysts, and echinococcal cysts (see chapter 28). Cystic lymphangiomatosis is a benign lymphatic malformation with a characteristic, multiloculated cystic appearance.

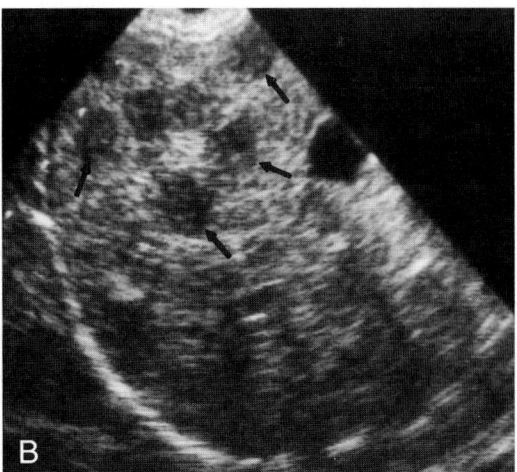

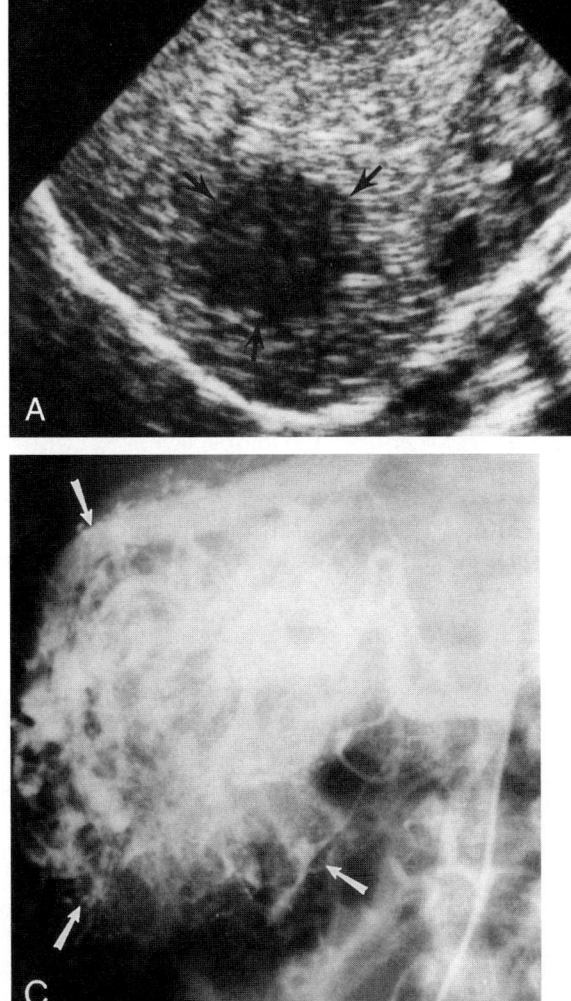

Figure 52.69. Vascular Neoplasms of the Liver. A. Hemangioma. US demonstrates a round, sonolucent mass (*arrows*) within the right lobe of the liver. This was a solitary hemangioma. **B.** Multiple sonolucent liver masses (*arrows*) represent hemangioendotheliomatosis. **C.** Arteriography demonstrates the marked vascularity (*arrows*) of an hemangiomendothelioma. (Fig. 52.69A courtesy of C. Keith Hayden, Jr. MD, Fort Worth, TX.)

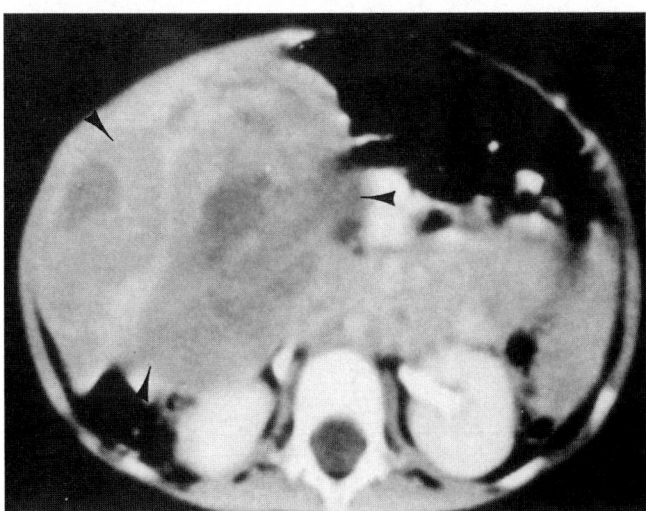

Figure 52.70. Hepatoblastoma. A CT scan demonstrates a large inhomogeneous tumor within the right lobe of the liver (*arrows*).

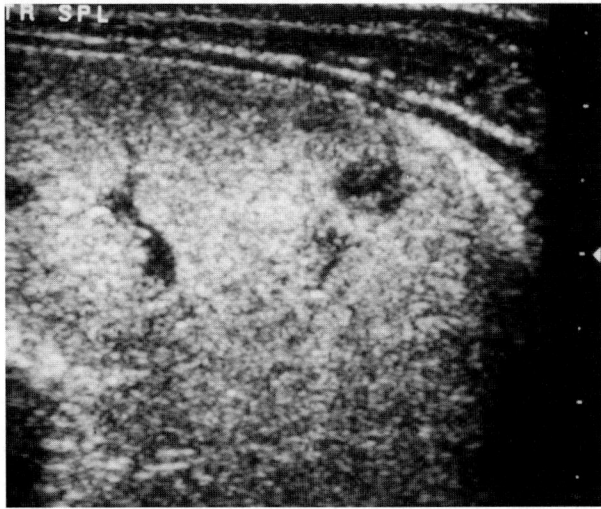

Figure 52.71. Cat Scratch Disease. US demonstrates multiple hypoechoic nodules in the spleen, characteristic of this infection.

Splenic Neoplasms. Primary neoplasms of the spleen (hemangioma, hamartoma, angiosarcoma) are rare. Lymphoma and leukemia commonly involve the spleen. However, splenic involvement with lymphoma does not necessarily result in splenic enlargement. Conversely, children with leukemia or lymphoma may have an enlarged spleen without neoplastic involvement.

Splenic Infarction. In children, infarction of the spleen occurs as a complication of sickle cell anemia, leukemia, or cardiac valvular disease. Acute splenic infarction results in decreased echogenicity on US and diminished contrast enhancement on CT. A rare cause of splenic infarction in children is torsion of a wandering spleen (Fig. 52.72).

Gastrointestinal and Pancreatic Masses

Enteric Duplication Cysts. A majority of abdominal masses that arise from the GI tract or pancreas are cystic. Enteric duplication cysts are most common in the small bowel (specifically ileum). Most are asymptomatic, but those that contain ectopic gastric or pancreatic tissue may ulcerate or hemorrhage. The cyst can act as a lead point for intussusception or volvulus. Diagnosis is usually best accomplished by US. The cysts appear as simple anechoic round to oval masses with characteristic two-layered wall (65). The inner wall is echogenic mucosa and the thin outer wall is hypoechoic muscle (Fig. 52.73). Because most enteric duplication cysts do not communicate with the intestinal lumen, GI contrast studies are of little value. Cysts that contain gastric mucosa are detectable by scintigraphy using technetium-99m-pertechnate.

Mesenteric and Omental Cysts are occasionally seen in the first decade of life and are considered to be a form of lymphangioma. These cysts are thin-walled with multiple internal septations. The wall of the cyst has a single layer rather than the double layer seen with duplication cysts.

Acquired Cysts are often a complication of ventriculoperitoneal shunts used for the treatment of hydrocephalus. The cysts are located near the tip of the shunt tubing (Fig. 52.74).

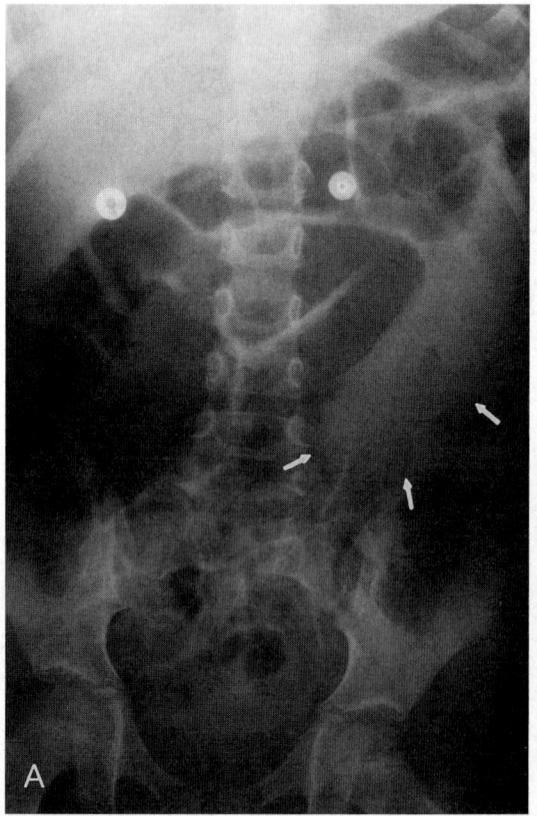

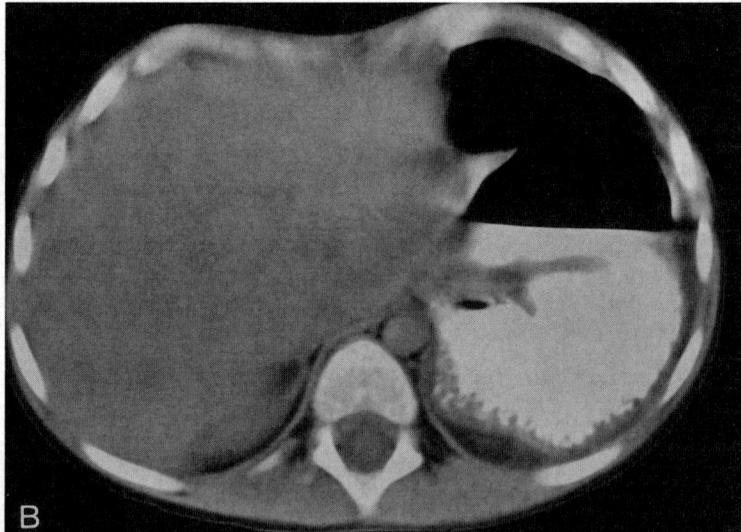

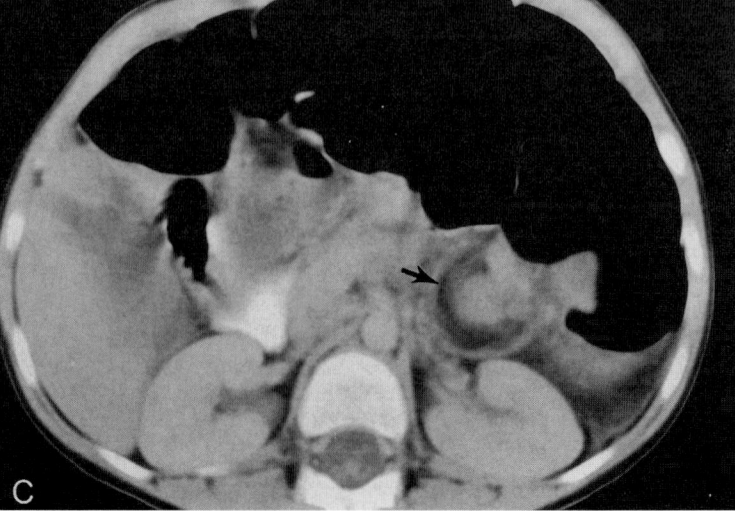

Figure 52.72. Splenic Torsion. A. Plain radiograph shows a soft-tissue mass in the left abdomen (*arrows*). A normal splenic shadow is not seen. **B.** A CT scan confirms absence of the spleen in the usual location in the left upper quadrant. **C.** A more caudal image demonstrates a donut appearance that represents the torsed splenic pedicle (*arrow*).

Pancreatic Cysts. The most common cystic mass of pancreas is a pseudocyst secondary to pancreatitis. True congenital cysts of the pancreas are rare and occur chiefly in association with autosomal dominant polycystic kidney disease or von Hippel-Lindau syndrome.

Pancreatic Neoplasms are rare in children. The most common is the benign islet cell adenoma (insulinoma), which is usually small and difficult to demonstrate. Papillary-cystic neoplasm of the pancreas is an uncommon tumor that contains variable amounts of cystic and solid tissue. Rare pancreatic neoplasms include adenocarcinoma, hamartoma, lymphangioma, pancreatoblastoma, and cystadenoma.

Tumors of the GI Tract are uncommon in infants and children. Lymphoma is the most common malignant tumors of the small intestine. Inflammatory polyps or polyps associated with one of the colonic polyposis syndromes are the most common colon lesions. Colon tumors in infancy are likely to be a leiomyoma, leiomyosarcoma, or lymphoma. Tumors of the mesentery and omentum are primarily Burkitt's lymphoma or metastases.

Pseudomasses of the GI tract are primarily inflammatory in nature; the most common of these is the appendiceal abscess (Fig. 52.75). Other intestinal pseudomasses include bowel thickening due to inflammatory bowel disease and intussusception.

Masses of the Reproductive Organs

Abdominal and pelvic masses that arise from the reproductive system are very common in young females.

Ovarian Cysts in children and adolescents are usually simple follicular or corpus luteum cysts (66,67). These cysts are common in neonates because of maternal hormonal stimulation. Most remain asymptomatic and spontaneously resolve without surgical intervention. Those cysts that are very large (>5 cm) or that are complicated by hemorrhage or torsion require aspiration or removal. Simple ovarian cysts appear on US as round or oval anechoic masses with a thin rim (Fig. 52.76A). In adolescents, hemorrhage into ovarian cysts is a cause of pain. When this occurs, the cyst appears more complex (Fig. 52.76B,C).

Complex Adnexal Masses must usually be differentiated on clinical grounds rather than imaging characteristics. Infection and abscess due to pelvic inflammatory disease is common in adolescents. Ectopic pregnancy must always be considered in postmenarchal females. The most common ovarian tumor is the benign teratoma. On US, teratomas vary from an entirely cystic mass to a predominantly solid mass with internal cystic components (Fig. 52.77A,B). A recognizable tooth within the mass is a pathognomonic finding (Fig. 52.77C). Malignant teratomas are accompanied by ascites, evidence of intraperitoneal spread, and metastasis to the liver. The

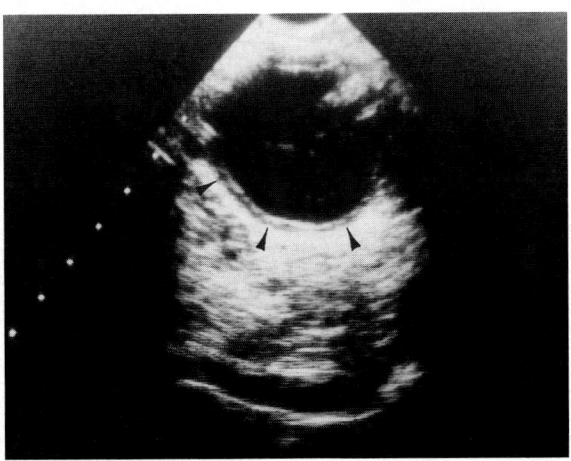

Figure 52.73. Enteric Duplication Cyst. US reveals an anechoic cyst with a well-defined 2-layered wall that consists of an inner echogenic mucosal layer and a thin outer muscular layer (*arrows*).

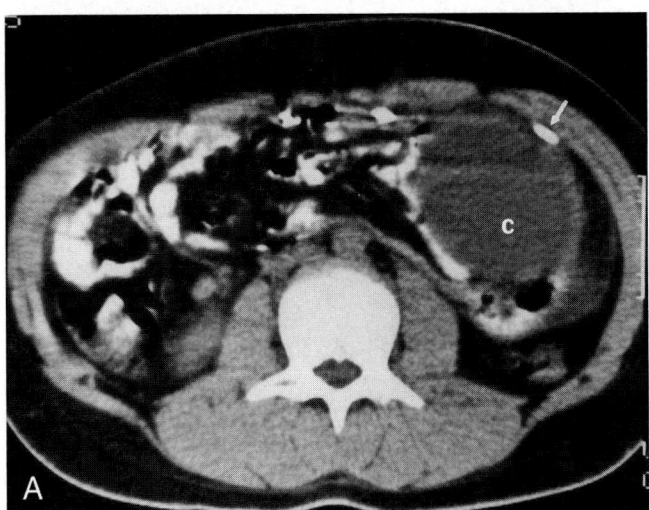
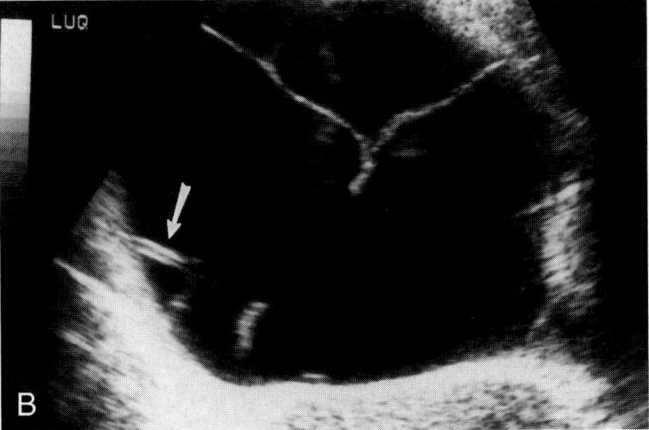

Figure 52.74. Cerebrospinal Fluid Pseudocyst. A. A CT scan demonstrates a loculated collection of fluid (*C*) in the left abdomen. The tip of the ventriculoperitoneal shunt lies adjacent to this fluid collection (*arrow*). **B.** US identifies the shunt tip (*arrow*) surrounded by a loculated pseudocyst, in another patient.

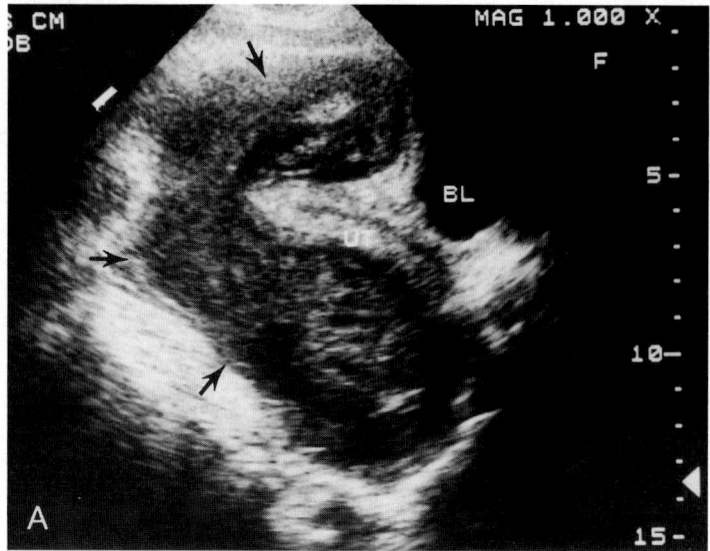

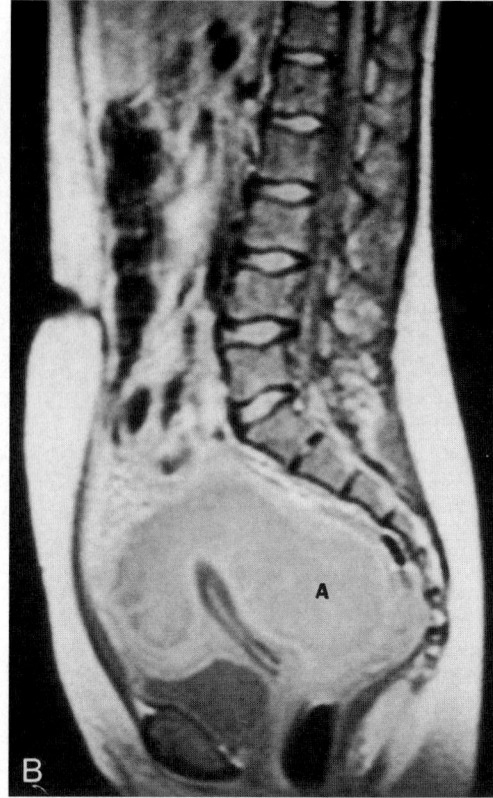

Figure 52.75. Appendiceal Abscess. A. US reveals a large, elongated complex mass (*arrows*) that extends from the pouch of Douglas over the uterine fundus. *UT*, uterus; *BL*, bladder. **B.** MR confirmed the presence of a large, high intensity abscess (*A*). This patient was only mildly symptomatic and was referred for evaluation of an "ovarian cyst."

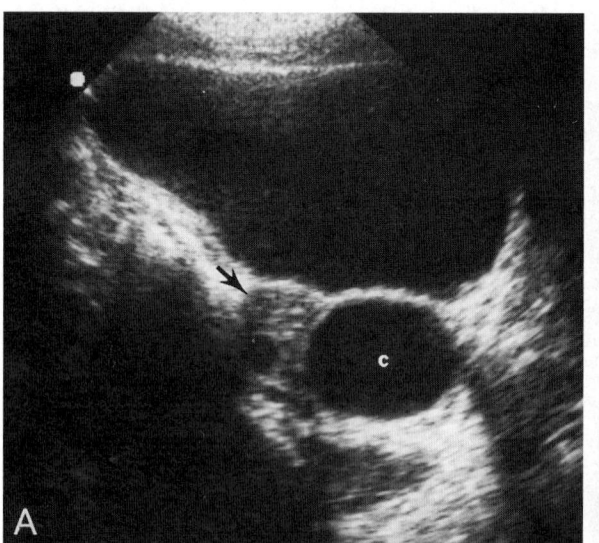

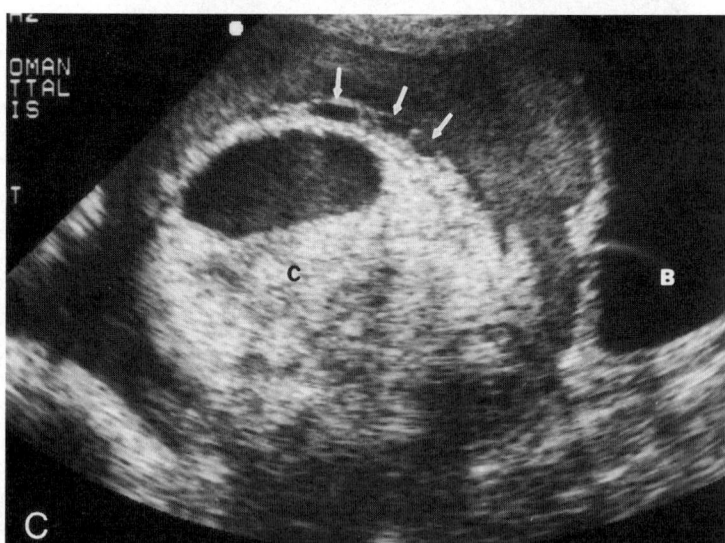

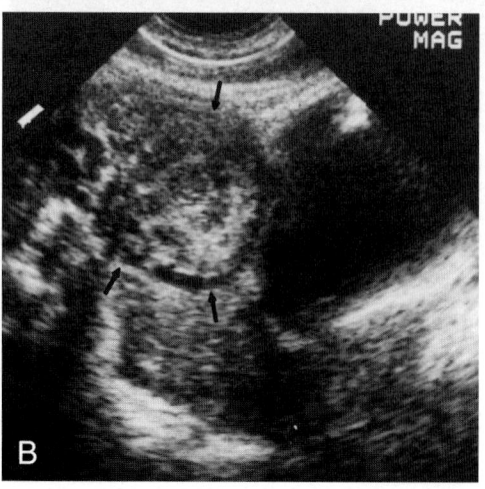

Figure 52.76. Ovarian Cyst. A. US shows a round, anechoic cyst (*C*) with a thin wall extending from the ovary (*arrow*). This appearance is characteristic of a simple follicular or corpus luteum cyst. **B.** Heterogeneous and echogenic clot is seen within an ovarian cyst that has undergone hemorrhage (*arrows*). **C.** A large hemorrhagic corpus luteum cyst (*C*) is seen in a patient on coumadin. Note the blood-fluid level within the cyst and several small follicles within the compressed and displaced ovary (*arrows*).

larger the component of solid tissue, the more likely is the tumor to be malignant. Less common ovarian neoplasms of childhood include dysgerminoma, cystadenoma and cystadenocarcinoma, and granulosa cell tumor.

Enlarged Uterus is sometimes the cause of a palpable abdominal mass. Pregnancy must be considered in adolescents. Congenital vaginal obstruction with hydrometrocolpos presents in the newborn period or at puberty. In most cases, US identifies the enlarged uterus filled with anechoic fluid in the newborn, or echogenic blood in the adolescent (Fig. 52.78A,B)(68). MR is useful for classifying the vaginal abnormality in older patients (Fig. 52.78C).

Rhabdomyosarcoma arises from the anterior wall of the vagina, or in the male from the prostate or bladder trigone (69). Because rhabdomyosarcoma frequently infiltrates the pelvic floor and surrounding structures, CT or MR are usually preferable to US for determining the extent of the disease.

Presacral Masses

Sacrococcygeal Teratoma. In the newborn and young infant, the most common presacral mass is a sacrococcygeal teratoma. These teratomas are frequently calcified and sometimes contain teeth. The presence of calcium and fat within a presacral lesion virtually assures the diagnosis (Fig. 52.79A).

Neuroblastoma can also develop as a primary tumor in the presacral space (Fig. 52.79B,C). Amorphous irregular calcifications are common and characteristic. Presacral neuroblastomas carry better prognosis than those that arise in the upper abdomen.

Sacral Chordoma is an uncommon neoplasm. Plain radiographs demonstrate destruction and expansion of the sacrum. Typical flocculant cartilaginous calcifications are often present.

Anterior Sacral Meningoceles are presacral masses that are associated with deformity of the sacrum. This deformity consists of a crescent-shaped sacrum due to a

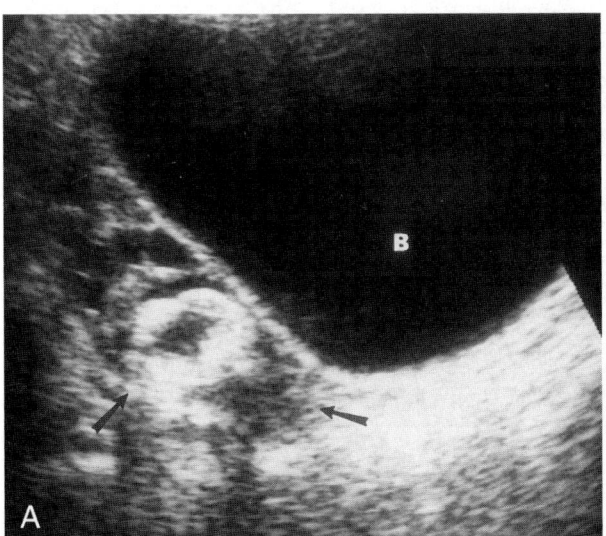

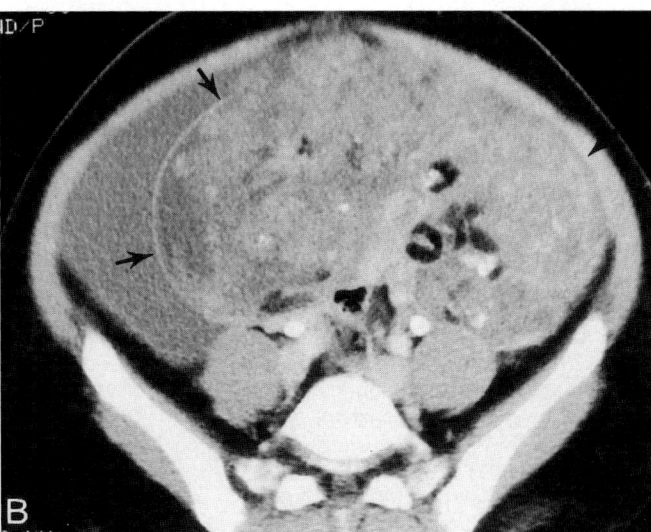

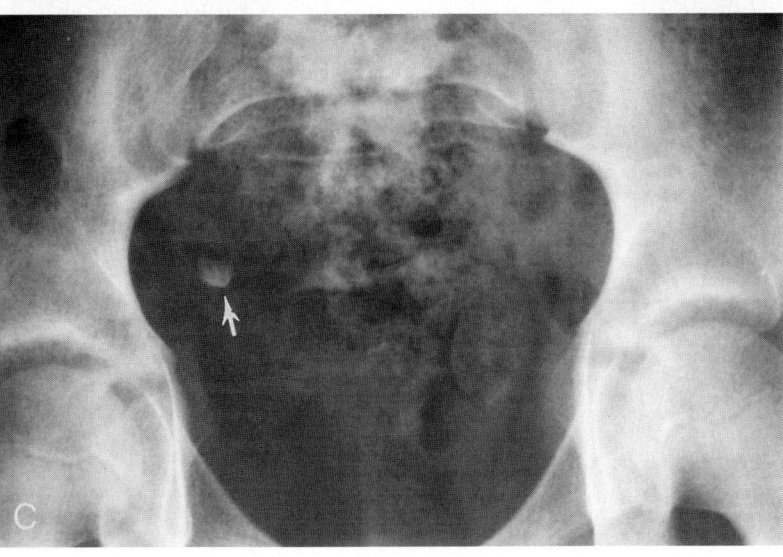

Figure 52.77. Ovarian Teratoma. A. US demonstrates a complex adnexal mass that contains both cystic and solid components as well as intensely echogenic areas of calcium and fat (*arrows*). *B*, bladder. **B.** A CT scan of a different patient shows a very large ovarian teratoma. The mass (*arrows*) is heterogenous with scattered calcifications and areas of fat density. **C.** Plain film of the pelvis reveals a formed calcification that closely resembles a tooth (*arrow*).

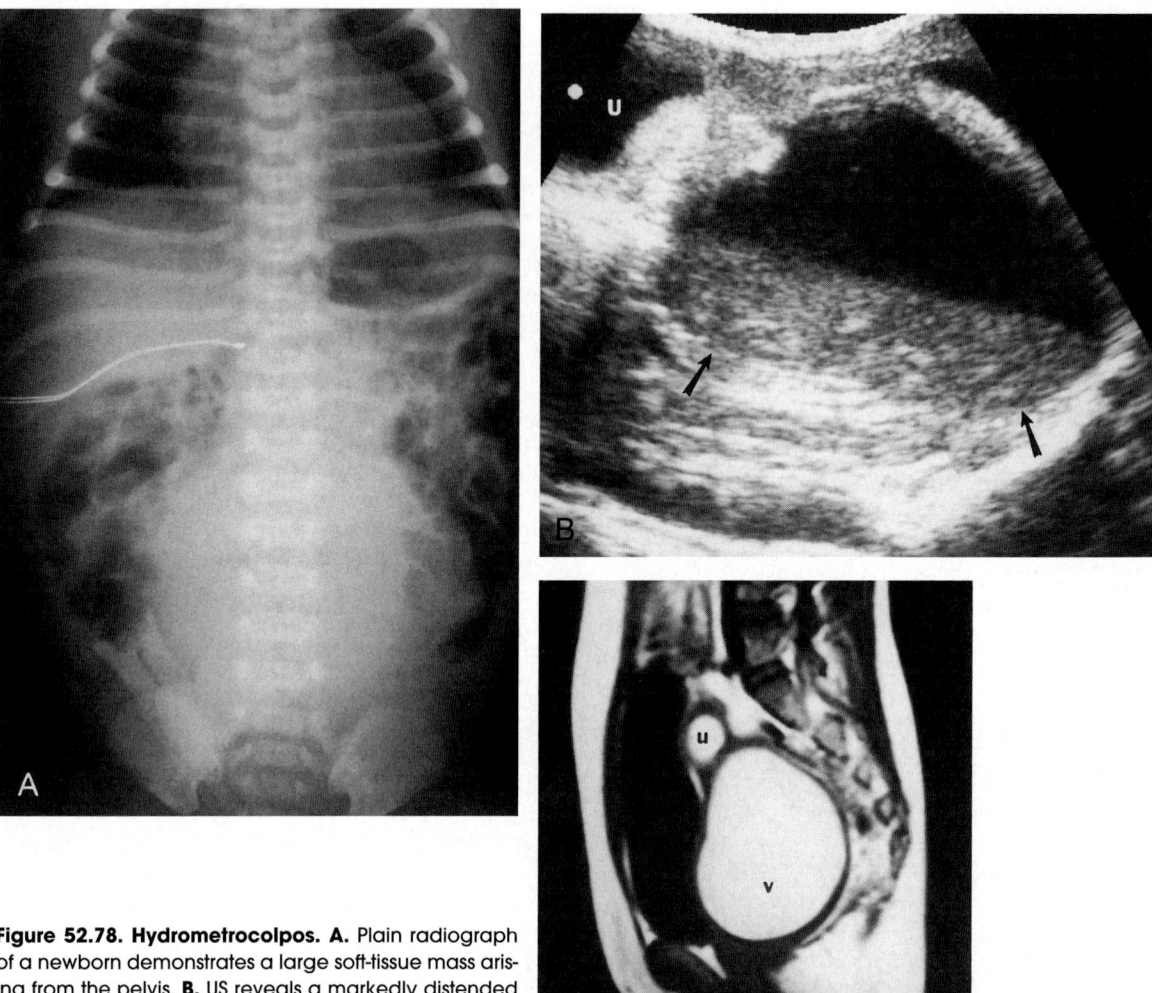

Figure 52.78. Hydrometrocolpos. A. Plain radiograph of a newborn demonstrates a large soft-tissue mass arising from the pelvis. **B.** US reveals a markedly distended upper vagina containing both fluid and debris (*arrows*). A smaller amount of fluid is seen in the uterus (*U*) superiorly. **C.** In an older girl, MR shows a markedly distended vagina (*V*) filled with high-intensity blood proximal to the vaginal membrane. *U*, uterus.

concave lateral defect through which the meningocele extends. Anterior sacral meningocele is commonly seen with anorectal abnormalities and in patients with neurofibromatosis.

Neuroenteric cysts are also occasionally seen in the presacral space and can also be associated with anterior sacral defects.

References

1. Hirsch W, Kedar R, Preiss U. Color Doppler in the diagnosis of the gastroesophageal reflux in children: comparison with pH measurements and B-mode ultrasound. Pediatr Radiol 1996;26:232,235.
2. Kriss WM. Desai NS. Relation of gastric distention to prostaglandin therapy in neonates. Radiology 1997;203:219–221.
3. Hernanz-Schulman M, Sells LL, Ambrosino MM, et al. Hypertrophic pyloric stenosis in the infant without a palpable olive: accuracy of sonographic diagnosis. Radiology 1994;193,771–776.
4. Swischuk LE, Hayden CK Jr, Stansberry SD. Sonographic pitfalls in imaging of the antropyloric region in infants. Radiographics 1989;9:437–447.
5. Bhisitkul DM, Listernick R, Shkolnik A, et al. Clinical application of ultrasonography in the diagnosis of intussusception. J Pediatr 1992;121:182–186.
6. Verschelden P, Filiatrault D, Garel L, et al. Intussusception in children: Reliability of US in diagnosis—a prospective study. Radiology 1992;184:741–744.
7. del-Pozo G, Albillos JC, Tejedor D. Intussusception: US findings with pathologic correlation-the crescent-in-doughnut sign. Radiology 1996;199:688–692.
8. Lam AH, Firman K. Value of sonography including color Doppler in the diagnosis and management of long standing intussusception. Pediatr Radiol 1992;22:112–114.
9. Kong M-S, Wong H-F, Lin S-L, et al. Factors related to detection of blood flow by color Doppler ultrasonography in intussusception. J Ultrasound Med 1997;16:141–144.
10. Shiels WE II, Maves CK, Hedlung GL, Kirks DR. Air enema for diagnosis and reduction of intussusception: clinical experience and pressure correlates. Radiology 1991;181:169–172.

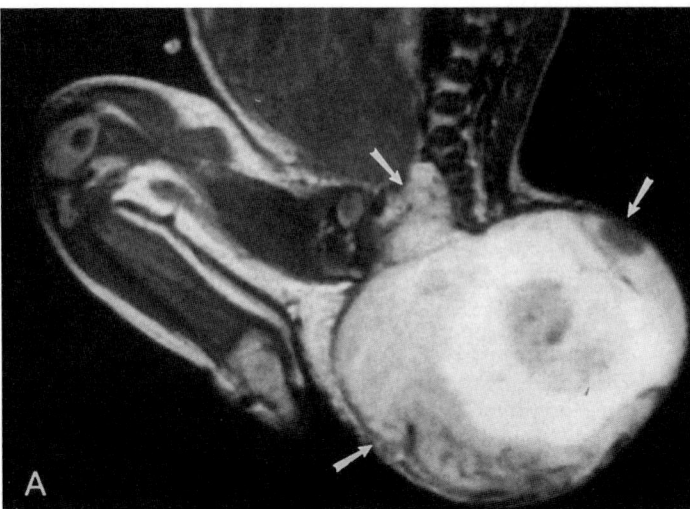

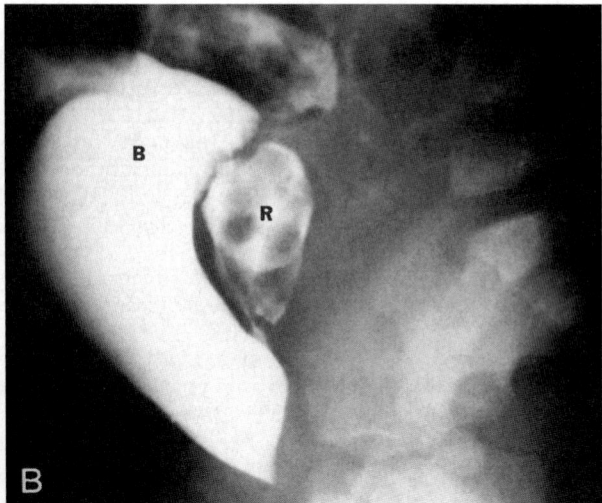

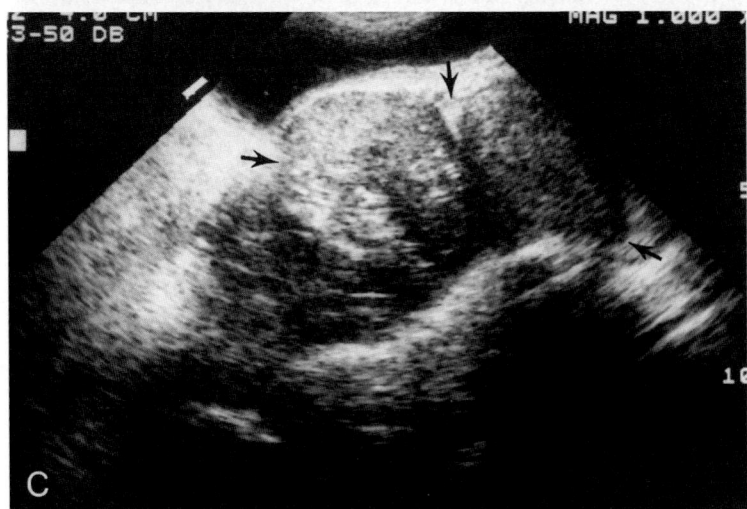

Figure 52.79. Presacral Masses. A. A large complex mass (*arrows*) extending from the presacral region is a sacrococcygeal teratoma. **B.** A neuroblastoma in the presacral space displaces the bladder (*B*) and rectum (*R*) anteriorly. **C.** US shows a homogeneous, moderately echogenic mass in the presacral space (*arrows*) caused by neuroblastoma. (Fig. 52.79A courtesy of Tom Boulden, MD, Memphis, TN.)

11. Stein M, Alton DJ, Daneman A. Pneumatic reduction of intussusception: 5-year experience. Radiology 1992;183:681–684.
12. Wood SK, Kim JS, Suh SJ, et al. Childhood inutssusception: US-guided hydrostatic reduction. Radiology 1992;182:77–80.
13. Riebel TW, Nasir R, Weber K. US-guided hydrostatic reduction of intussusception in children. Radiology 1993;188:513–516.
14. Rohrschneider WK, Troger J. Hydrostatic reduction of intussusception under US guidance. Pediatr Radiol 1995;25:530–534.
15. Peh WC, Khong P, Chan KL, et al Sonographically guided hydrostatic reduction of childhood intussusception using Hartmann's solution. AJR Am J Roentgenol 1996;167:1237–1241.
16. Shiels WE II, Kirks DR, Keller GL, et al. Colonic perforation by air and liquid enemas: Comparison study in young pigs. AJR 1993;160:931–935.
17. Tsakayannis DE, Shamberger RC. Association of imperforate anus with occult spinal dysraphism. J Pediatr Surg 1995;30:1010–1012.
18. Boemers TM, Beek FJ, van Gool JD, et al. Urologic problems in anorectal malformations. Part 1. Urodynamic findings and significance of sacral anomalies. J Pediatr Surg 1996;31:407–410.
19. Zerin JM, Kuhn-Fulton J, White SJ, et al. Colonic strictures in children with cystic fibrosis. Radiology 1995;194:223–226.
20. Sarrazin J, Wilson SR. Manifestations of Crohn disease at US. Radiographics 1996;16:499–520.
21. Alexander JE, Williamson SL, Seibert JJ, et al. The ultrasonographic diagnosis of typhlitis (neutropenic colitis). Pediatr Radiol 1988;18:200–204.
22. Friedland JA, Herman TE, Siegel MJ. *Escherichia coli* 0157:H7-associated hemolytic-uremic syndrome: value of colonic color Doppler sonography. Pediatr Radiol 1995;25(Suppl1):65–67.
23. Kao SC, Smith WL, Abu-Yousef MM, et al. Acute appendicitis in children: sonographic findings. AJR Am J Roentgenol 1989;153:375–379.
24. Sivit CJ, Newman KD, Boenning DA, et al. Appendicitis: usefulness of US in diagnosis in a pediatric population. Radiology 1992;185:549–552.
25. Quillin SP, Siegel MJ. Appendicitis in children: color Doppler sonography. Radiology 1992;184:745–747.
26. Hayden CK Jr, Kuchelmeister J, Lipscomb TS. Sonography of acute appendicitis in childhood: perforation versus nonperforation. J Ultrasound Med 1992;11:209–216.
27. Quillin SP, Siegel MJ. Diagnosis of appendiceal abscess in children with acute appendicitis: value of color Doppler sonography. AJR Am J Roentgenol 1995;164:1251–1254.

28. Patriquin HB, Garcier J-M, Lafortune M, et al. Appendicitis in children and young adults: Doppler sonographic-pathologic correlation. AJR Am J Roentgenol 1996:166;629–633.

29. Haller JO. Sonography of the biliary tract in infants and children. AJR Am J Roentgenol 1991;157:1051–1058.

30. Abramson SJ, Treves S, Teele RL. The infant with possible biliary atresia: evaluation by ultrasound and nuclear medicine. Pediatr Radiol 1982;12:1–5.

31. Majd M. ^{99m}Tc-IDA scintigraphy in the evaluation of neonatal jaundice. Radiographics 1983;3:88–99.

32. King LR, Siegel MJ, Balfe DM. Acute pancreatitis in children: CT findings of intra- and extrapancreatic fluid collections. Radiology 1995;195:196–200.

33. Couture A, Veyrac C, Baud C, et al. Evaluation of abdominal pain in Henoch-Schönlein syndrome by high frequency ultrasound. Pediatr Radiol 1992;22:12–17.

34. Hayden CK Jr, Swischuk LE, Fawcett HD, et al. Urinary tract infections in childhood: a current imaging approach. Radiographics 1986;6:1023–1038.

35. Berdon WE. Contemporary imaging approach to pediatric urologic problems. Radiol Clin North Am 1991;29:605–618.

36. Starinsky R, Vardi O, Batasch D, Goldberg M. Increased renal medullary echogenicity in neonates. Pediatr Radiol 1995;25:43–45.

37. Shultz PK, Strife JL, Strife CF, McDaniel JD. Hyperechoic renal medullary pyramids in infants and children. Radiology 1991;181:163–167.

38. Riebel TW, Abraham K, Wartner R, Muller R. Transient renal medullary hyperechogenicity in ultrasound studies of neonates: Is it a normal phenomenon and what are the causes? J Clin Ultrasound 1993;21:225–231.

39. Kessler RM, Ouevedo H, Lankau CA, et al. Obstructive vs nonobstructive dilatation of the renal collecting system in chidren: Distinction with Duplex sonography. AJR Am J Roentgenol 1993;160:353–357.

40. Hayden CK Jr, Swischuk LE. Renal cystic disease. Semin Ultrasound CT MR 1991;12:361–373.

41. Strife JL, Souza AS, Kirks DR, et al. Multicystic dysplastic kidney in children: US follow-up. Radiology 1993;186:785–788.

42. Karmazyn B, Zerin JM. Lower urinary tract abnormalities in children with multicystic dysplastic kidney. Radiology 1997;203:223–226.

43. White KS, Kirks DR, Bove KE. Imaging of nephroblastomatosis: an overview. Radiology 1992;182:1–5.

44. Gambino J, Caldwell B, Dietrich R, et al. Congenital disorders of sexual differentiation: MR findings. AJR Am J Roentgenol 1992;158:363–367.

45. Burks DD, Markey BJ, Burkhard TK, et al. Suspected testicular torsion and ischemia: evaluation with color Doppler sonography. Radiology 1990;175:815–821.

46. Atkinson GO Jr, Patrick LE, Ball TI Jr, Stephenson CA, et al. The normal and abnormal scrotum in children: evaluation with color Doppler sonography. AJR Am J Roentgenol 1992;158:613–617.

47. Kier R, McCarthy S, Rosenfield AT, et al. Nonpalpable testes in young boys: evaluation with MR imaging. Radiology 1988;169:429–433.

48. Aragona F, Pescatori E, Talenti E, et al. Painless scrotal masses in the pediatric population: prevalence and age distribution of different pathologic conditions—a 10-year retrospective multicenter study. J Urol 1996;155:1424–1426.

49. Avila NA, Premkumar A, Shawker TH, et al. Testicular

adrenal rest tissue in congenital adrenal hyperplasia: Findings at Gray-scale and color Doppler US. Radiology 1996;198:99–104.

50. McHugh K, Stringer DA, Hebert D, Babiak CA. Simple renal cysts in children: diagnosis and follow-up with US. Radiology 1991;178:383–385.

51. D'Angio GJ, Breslow N, Beckwith JB, et al. Cancer 1989;64; 349–360.

52. Cohen MD. Commentary: Imaging and staging of Wilms tumors: problems and controversies. Pediatr Radiol 1996;26: 307–311.

53. Heidelberger KP, Ritchey ML, Dauser RC, et al. Congenital mesoblastic nephroma metastatic to the brain. Cancer 1993;72:2499–2502.

54. Schlesinger AE, Rosenfield NS, Castle VP, Jasty R. Congenital mesoblastic nephroma metastatic to the brain: a report of two cases. Pediatr Radiol 1995;25:Suppl 1:S73–S75.

55. Heij HA, Taets van Amerongen AH, Ekkelkamp S, Vos A. Diagnosis and management of neonatal adrenal haemorrhage. Pediatr Radiol 1989;19:391–394.

56. David R, Lamki N, Fan S, et al. Many faces of neuroblastoma. Radiographics 1989;9:859–882.

57. Forman HP, Leonidas JC, Berdon WE, et al. Congenital neuroblastoma: evaluation with multimodality imaging. Radiology 1990;175:365–368.

58. Ruzal-Shapiro C, Berdon WE, Cohen MD, Abramson SJ. MR imaging of diffuse bone marrow replacement in pediatric patients with cancer. Radiology 1991;181:587–589.

59. Hibi S, Todo S, Imashuku S, Miyazaki T. ^{131}I-Meta-iodobenzylguanidine scintigraphy in patients with neuroblastoma. Pediatr Radiol 1987;17:308–313.

60. Paltiel HJ, Gelfand J, Elgazzar AH, et al. Neural crest tumors: I-1213 MIBG imaging in children. Radiology 1994; 190:117–121.

61. Suc A, Lumbroso J, Rubie H, et al. Metastatic neuroblastoma in children older than one year: prognostic significance of the initial metaiodobenzylguanidine scan and proposal for a scoring system. Cancer 1996;77:805–811.

62. Avni EF, Rypens F, Smet MH, Galetty E. Sonographic demonstration of congenital adrenal hyperplasia in the neonate: the cerebriform pattern. Pediatr Radiol 1993;23: 88–90.

63. Liebling MS, Starc TJ, McAlister WH, et al. ACTH induced adrenal enlargement in infants treated for infantile spasms and acute cerebellar encephalopathy. Pediatr Radiol 1993; 23:454–456.

64. Boechat MI, Kangarloo H, Ortega J, et al. Primary liver tumors in children: comparison of CT and MR imaging. Radiology 1988;169:727–732.

65. Barr LL, Hayden CK Jr, Stansberry SD, Swischuk LE. Enteric duplication cysts in children: are their ultrasonographic wall characteristics diagnostic? Pediatr Radiol 1990;20:326–328.

66. Siegel MJ. Pediatric gynecologic sonography. Radiology 1991;179:593–600.

67. Surratt JT, Siegel MJ. Imaging of pediatric ovarian masses. Radiographics 1991;11:533–548.

68. Blask AR, Sanders RC, Gearhart JP. Obstructed uterovaginal anomalies: demonstration with sonography: Part I. Neonates and infants. Radiology 1991;179:79–83.

69. Agrons GA, Wagner BJ, Lonergan G, et al. Genitourinary rhabdomyosarcoma in children: Radiologic-pathologic correlation. Radiographics 1997;17:919–937.

Section XI NUCLEAR RADIOLOGY

Section Editors:

John M. Bauman
Frederic A. Conte

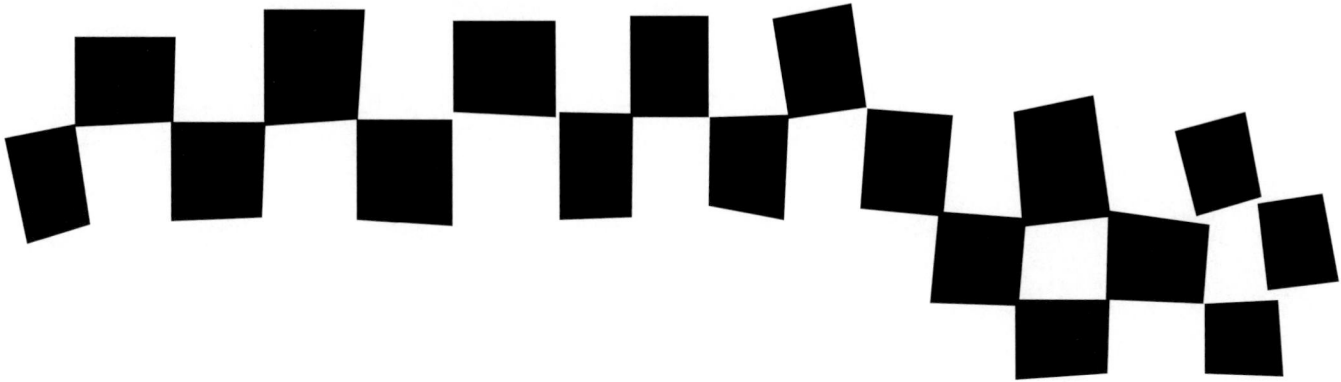

53
Introduction to Nuclear Medicine

John M. Bauman

INTRODUCTION
IMAGING PRINCIPLES
AN APPROACH TO IMAGE INTERPRETATION
SECTION OVERVIEW

INTRODUCTION

Nuclear radiology encompasses both therapeutic and diagnostic modalities that support practically every field of medical endeavor. Radiographic, ultrasonographic, and MR studies provide important anatomic or structural information from which pathologic processes are inferred. On the other hand, nuclear medicine studies sacrifice the high resolution of the other imaging techniques but provide physiologic and functional information not otherwise available. Despite changes in referral patterns and the advent of managed care, nuclear medicine studies remain among the most cost-effective for the diagnosis and management of a variety of diseases.

The material in this section is intended to provide an overview of the specialty and at the same time serve as the basis of review for those residents preparing for board examinations. The information should also be useful to those who may not practice nuclear radiology regularly or may not have done so recently.

IMAGING PRINCIPLES

The basic principles of diagnostic nuclear radiology are simple to grasp, yet somehow seem to elude first-year residents as they are overwhelmed with information at the outset of their training. The concept of nuclear imaging is based on the external detection and mapping (image formation) of the biodistribution of radioactivity that has been previously administered to a patient. The knowledge of the normal patterns of uptake, distribution, and in some cases excretion or lack thereof permit us to make decisions concerning the presence or absence of disease.

Sometimes a radioisotope of a naturally occurring element essential to normal biologic function (e.g., Iodine-123) or an analog (e.g., Technetium-99m Pertechnetate, Tc-99m-O_4) is used without additional chemical alteration. More commonly a radioactive isotope is combined with a physiologically "active" compound in vitro and administered intravenously or orally. Thus Tc-99m-O_4 may be combined with a diphosphonate compound for skeletal imaging. If the same radioactive compound is com-

bined with an iminodiacetic acid derivative, the biologic distribution reflected by the images will be that of a biliary scan. This simple concept is the foundation for imaging the biodistribution of radiolabeled blood cells, monoclonal antibodies and peptides, and energy substrates such as glucose and fatty acids. If this unifying principle can be kept in mind while reading the various sections on nuclear imaging, the diverse number and types of studies may seem somewhat less bewildering.

One problem frequently encountered among junior residents is failure to develop an approach to interpretation of nuclear medicine images. Radiology residents who have no difficulty devising a standard approach to the interpretation of chest radiographs or CT of the brain seem at a loss when viewing nuclear medicine studies. As with everything else in medicine, an orderly approach is best.

AN APPROACH TO IMAGE INTERPRETATION

Obviously a basic fund of anatomic, physiologic, and nuclear imaging knowledge is necessary in order to make intelligent differential diagnoses based on nuclear medicine images. The suggested approach to image interpretation provided here will make more sense after reading the remainder of the nuclear medicine section, and for the resident, will be of greater value after the second or third nuclear medicine rotation.

The initial portion of this discussion will be most helpful to those preparing to take case formally at the radiology board examination or in a conference setting. However, the basic principles may be applied whenever one is presented with an unknown case and expected to wax eloquent. The contribution to accurate diagnosis of a logical, comfortable, habitual approach to image interpretation cannot be emphasized enough, particularly to those facing the stress of oral examination.

When presented with a nuclear medicine study it is essential first to determine the radiopharmaceutical that was used to create the images. Obviously for a clinical case this information may already be known and in the board examination setting the examiner typically provides the information. Nonetheless, it is a good exercise to discern this information oneself if possible and thereby sharpen one's analytical and case-taking skills. It also indicates to the examiner that the candidate is using a rational and logical approach to interpretation and some latitude or good will may result as a consequence.

Determining the radiopharmaceutical and therefore the type of study may be as simple as reviewing the film margins for textual information. It is poor form to ask, "What type of study is this?" when the information is readily at hand. At the same time one may also glean important information about the age and sex of the patient, the site of injection, the temporal sequence when multiple images are present, the type of images (planar or tomographic, static, or dynamic), and patient orientation during imaging (right/left, oblique, posterior, upright/supine, etc.).

If the radiopharmaceutical information is not provided, then the first step in analysis is based on determining the relative count density of the images. Typically, images of Tc-99m-O_4 labeled radiopharmaceuticals have relatively high count density. Medium and higher energy isotopes (Indium-111, Gallium-67, Iodine-131, etc.) have lower count density based on lower administered dose and poor imaging characteristics—they produce relatively noisy images. A notable exception to this generalization is arterial flow studies performed with Tc-99m labeled radiopharmaceuticals. Because these studies are performed as dynamic acquisitions at a typical rate of 1–5 seconds/frame, they too will have a low count density.

Thus, the number and type of images presented should be noted. If a series of frames is provided, the study is either a dynamic acquisition with the typical timing of seconds or minutes per frame, or possibly a series of SPECT image slices that will usually have more counts and appear somewhat smoothed because of the processing algorithms employed.

Next study the biodistribution of activity in the images: Is there evidence of cardiac or great vessel blood pool activity? Is skeletal activity present? If so, is it marrow or cortical activity? What organs or structures are visualized? From a knowledge of the biodistribution evident on the images and a reasonable assumption about the likely radioisotope, one may make some conjecture as to the most likely radiopharmaceutical in use.

It may still be impossible to determine the exact radiopharmaceutical and study or even recognize specific anatomy depending on the experience of the individual and the rarity of the case. However the analysis provides a context for indirectly posing questions to the person presenting the case: "I can see from the relatively poor count density that this study was most likely performed with a high energy isotope such as Iodine-131 . . . I see hepatic, renal, and bladder activity on these anterior images as well as foci of increased activity in a pattern suggestive of large bowel . . . if this is Iodine-131, I suspect that this may be part of a whole body study in search of thyroid carcinoma metastasis . . . if so additional imaging of the thyroid bed with pinhole magnification is indicated and it would be important to review the entire study . . . if not, I would also consider the possibility that this could be a Gallium-67 study although it would have to be within 24 hours or so of the injection as that is when renal excretion chiefly occurs."

The ellipses (. . .) above represent short pauses that give the person presenting the case a chance to provide feedback as to the accuracy of your comments. This technique informs the presenter that while you may not be certain of the case immediately, you do in fact have some experience and knowledge as well as a logical approach to image interpretation. If the examiner does not offer comments after your initial attempt at analysis, it is

entirely appropriate to state that without further information concerning the type of study, it would be difficult if not impossible to continue. This approach is always better than blunt interrogation of the presenter. In fact it is not uncommon that when residents with a good approach do miss the actual diagnosis, their performance appears much better than others who may "get the case" but without a clear and logical style.

After determining the type of study, proceeding with the rest of the analysis is fairly straightforward. Again, a basic knowledge of the normal biodistribution of the radiopharmaceutical and the usual indications for performing the study is required. Given these plus a relatively rudimentary understanding of anatomy and physiology one can "make the finding(s)" with relative certainty. A word of caution is in order. There are two common errors that continue to cause problems for each new generation of residents. First, it is extremely difficult to "see what is not there." Always "take attendance" and be certain that all organs and structures that should be "present" on a given study are visualized with their normal pattern and relative uptake of radiopharmaceutical. Next, frequently more than one finding of importance will exist. It is easy to suffer from search satisfaction and quit looking for additional abnormalities after one is found. A rigid approach to image analysis is required to prevent both of these errors.

When studying dynamic series such as arterial flow studies, Tc-99m labeled red blood cell studies for GI hemorrhage localization, renal function images, and so forth, it is important to note the time per frame because you will need to make comments concerning the timing of the arrival of the radiopharmaceutical in various structures. This information may be critical to image interpretation and is frequently overlooked by the neophytes. Identifying changes from one frame to the next may be difficult. One approach to enhance and speed detection of abnormalities and asymmetries is to study the first frame or two relatively closely and then move directly to the last frame. Direct comparison of early and late images will demonstrate changes between the two most dramatically and will allow you to direct your attention to the appropriate areas on the intervening images and define the correct timing of events. It is helpful to "back through" the images from last to first after identifying any abnormalities on the later images. This approach will rapidly identify with great temporal and anatomic accuracy the exact time of appearance and location of GI hemorrhage, for example.

An orderly approach to image analysis for static images is also required, but will vary based on the type of study in question. Here are specific techniques for some common studies that may be helpful.

Skeletal Imaging. Review the images provided with a "top-down" approach, first addressing skeletal structures. Note areas of increased or decreased activity without attaching strong clinical significance to them initially. Always comment on the renal activity that should normally be present and use this as a reminder to evaluate soft tissue activity for abnormal increases, decreases, and asymmetry.

SPECT Myocardial Perfusion Imaging. Always view

the raw data images first, if available, and evaluate for quality control issues, artifacts, and ancillary and incidental findings (breast attenuation, motion, pacemaker artifact, pulmonary uptake, breast tumor, etc.). Always review the exercise data to confirm adequacy of stress or determine what—if any—pharmacologic agent was employed. Next review the short axis slices, then the vertical long axis slices, and finally the horizontal long axis slices. Note the presence or absence of areas of increased or decreased perfusion and whether they appear fixed or seem to change. Note chamber size and whether or not it changes. Attempt to confirm the presence of any defects in two planes. Formulate a working hypothesis to explain the constellation of findings present.

Ventilation-Perfusion Imaging for Pulmonary Embolus. Always review a chest radiograph first, if provided. If not initially provided, comment that review of the radiograph is essential prior to making a definitive statement about the likelihood of pulmonary embolus. Review the perfusion study in its entirety first. Note the presence of any defects, their relative sizes (lobar, segmental, subsegmental), and their locations. Attempt to confirm the findings in more than one view. Once the number and location of the defects are known, attempt to match these defects in the corresponding areas on the ventilation study. Summarize the findings verbally reciting the number and size of matched and mismatched defects. Offer a probability of pulmonary embolus based on the findings.

Hepatobiliary Imaging. For this and any other study where flow studies and dynamic imaging are performed, studying the images in the order in which they were acquired is best: flow study first, then dynamic images using the approach outlined previously, and finally static images (right lateral or left anterior oblique views would be typical) if any. Note the temporal sequence of the arrival of the arterial bolus in the kidneys, spleen, and finally liver if an arterial flow study of the abdomen is provided. With approximately 80% of hepatic blood flow arriving courtesy of the portal system, the liver should appear later than the other organs—if it does not, portal hypertension may be present. Early flow to the gallbladder fossa implies significant inflammation. On the dynamic series, note the appearance of the early images, then study the later images: Are gallbladder activity and bowel activity present? If so, "back through" the images and note their first appearance. Is activity visualized in the normal sequence of intrahepatic ducts, common hepatic duct, gallbladder, common bile duct, and duodenum? Is there activity in any areas other than expected—stomach, esophagus, or free spill into the peritoneum? Are there any focal accumulations of labeled bile in the liver, gallbladder fossa, or elsewhere?

When taking a case it is best to follow your initial comments concerning the findings with a final image review as you verbally summarize what you believe to be pertinent to diagnosis. It is not uncommon to realize only as the summary is presented aloud that a specific diagnosis is indicated or that the findings significantly limit the differential diagnosis.

For a situation in which a finding has been made but no explanation is readily apparent based on one's experience or study, it is helpful to contemplate the finding while considering a standard list of generic causes as well as mechanisms that might lead to the finding.

One sample generic list uses the mnemonic, VINDICATE as follows: Vascular (any cause of increased/decreased blood flow, collagen vascular diseases); Infectious (always include TB, Fungal, HIV); Neoplastic (benign or malignant, primary or metastatic); Drug-induced (radiopharmaceutical preparation and QC, recent prior radiopharmaceutical administration or contrast study, thyroid hormone ingestion), Idiopathic (sarcoidosis, amyloidosis); Congenital, Artifact (related to patient, clothing, imaging equipment, computer processing, or film processing or exposure); Trauma; Endocrine/metabolic (Paget's disease, hyperparathyroidism, etc.).

If the physiologic mechanisms of radiopharmaceutical localization are understood, then mechanistic explanations for findings allow another route to a solution. Thus, from a mechanistic standpoint, increased activity on a bone scan is caused by either increased delivery of radiopharmaceutical to the bone or increased incorporation due to either increased osteoblastic activity or increased dwell time for extraction by normally functioning osteoblasts. Reasons for increased delivery include the following: arterial injection, localized inflammation due to trauma, infection or tumor, arteriovenous malformation, increased use of a limb, neurologic reflex increased flow, and apparent increased uptake with actual reduced uptake in the contralateral body part. Reasons for increased osteoblastic activity include the following: normal growth in epiphyseal bone and enhanced repair in response to fracture, infection, and benign or malignant tumors. Increased dwell time may be caused by constricting clothing, tourniquets, venous obstruction, and lymphatic obstruction.

As a demonstration of this approach, note the two images in Figure 53.1. Using the techniques previously described, can you make the diagnosis? First of all, what is the most likely isotope? Are these static images or dynamic images? Planar or SPECT? What structures do you recognize? Given that the isotope is Tc-99m and that structures visualized include liver, spleen, cardiac blood pool, lungs, marrow, and vessels, can you suggest what the radiopharmaceutical might be? With significant blood pool activity, one should consider early imaging with almost any Tc-99m labeled pharmaceutical, but the count density is too high for those simple molecules that wash out rapidly. This suggests that labeled cells or possibly proteins or antibodies might be in use. If the latter, the imaging was performed early while the radiopharmaceutical was still circulating. If labeled red cells were used, should not the heart and great vessels demonstrate much greater activity relative to the marrow? What about labeled white blood cells?

Given that the study is a Tc-99m-HMPAO labeled white blood cell study, what are the findings? Note that splenic uptake is much greater than liver, more so than usual. Note that the liver is separated from the right ribcage by a few centimeters. This latter finding implies ascites, and the entire pattern suggests significant hepatocellular disease such as cirrhosis. Now what of the focus of increased activity superimposed on the left

Figure 53.1. Unknown study.

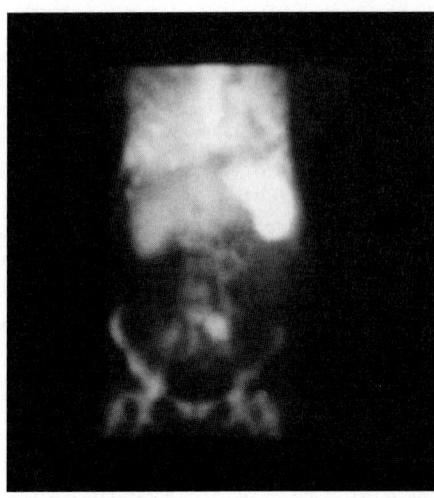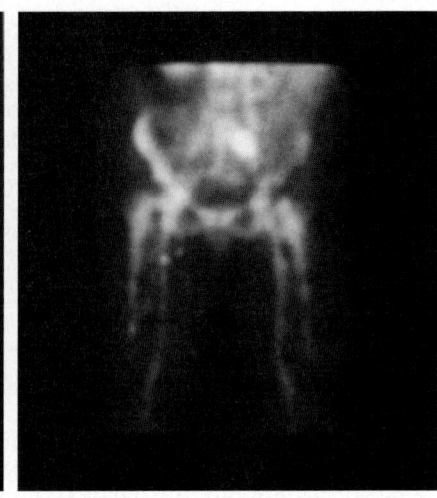

sacroiliac joint? We cannot ascertain whether this activity is superficial or deep or somewhere in-between without at least a posterior image, if not a left lateral view or an oblique. Is this an abscess in a cirrhotic patient or maybe a decubitus ulcer posterior to the left sacroiliac joint? Perhaps not. Note the fine serpiginous areas of increased activity stranding away from the large egg-shaped focus and consider mechanisms of localization: chemotaxis to sites of inflammation, and anything that causes increased flow and therefore delivery of the labeled cells. Final differential diagnosis (without any other image or clinical information): possible left lower quadrant or decubitus abscess in a cirrhotic patient with ascites versus caput medusa with varices containing circulating labeled cells.

Oblique and lateral imaging confirmed the location of the white cell collection in the anterior abdominal wall. Physical examination of the patient in the nuclear medicine clinic revealed no decubitus and a soft, compressible, palpable, noninflamed mass in the anterior abdominal wall. Correlation with a CT study demonstrated a giant varix in the expected location.

The foregoing discussion is not meant to be all-encompassing and does not do justice to the entire spectrum of studies and diseases that will be encountered. However, it should provide a starting point for development of one's own approach to image analysis and case-taking skills. Consider using the images in each of the subsequent chapters as sample unknown cases and attempt to analyze them before reading the captions. This sort of practice will undoubtedly enhance one's ability to take unknown cases with greater confidence and accuracy.

SECTION OVERVIEW

For this edition of the text, the nuclear radiology section has been thoroughly revised and updated with multiple new images and current references. The nuclear cardiology section in particular has been expanded and modernized to reflect current thinking concerning myocardial viability determination. A separate chapter on the rapidly expanding area of nuclear oncology has been added. In every case, the authors have attempted to provide clear, concise, current, and useful information. I have no doubt that you will find that they have succeeded.

54

Essential Science of Nuclear Medicine

Frederic A. Conte
Jerrold T. Bushberg

DEFINITIONS

Difference Between γ-rays (Gamma) and X-rays

The electromagnetic spectrum of radiation can be divided into non-ionizing and ionizing radiation. Non-ionizing radiation includes commonly encountered forms of electromagnetic radiation such as visible light, microwave, and radiofrequencies (used in radio transmissions and in MR). The ionizing radiation includes x-rays and γ-rays used in diagnostic medical imaging. The primary difference between x-rays and γ-rays lies in their origin. X-rays are extranuclear in origin and can be produced from the interaction of bombarding photons or electrons with an atom; γ-rays are produced from within the atomic nucleus as unstable nuclei transition to a more stable state. The source of x-rays for diagnostic radiology is the x-ray tube, which produces x-rays with energies below 100 keV. The source of γ-rays is the radioactive or unstable nuclide, i.e., radionuclide which typically produce photons with energies higher than 100 keV (Table 54.1). The production of images from these two sources is different and has a direct effect on the radiation dose delivered to a person. Diagnostic x-ray imaging is "transmission" imaging in which the x-ray photons from an external source traverse tissue where some are absorbed and some emerge to form the image. Each additional x-ray image requires an additional radiation exposure raising the dose to the patient. Nuclear medicine imaging with γ-rays is "emission" imaging in which the source resides within the patient and the photons are emitted and subsequently detected by the gamma camera imaging system. This emission imaging only requires additional acquisition time to obtain more images (views).

Ionizing radiation can also come in a particulate form. The particle of medical interest is the β-particle, which is an electron that has its origin within the unstable nucleus. As opposed to x-rays and γ-rays, β-particles interact quite easily with matter, traveling only a few millimeters in tissue as they transfer their energy to the surrounding tissue. Although not of imaging importance, it is this energy transferring property that produces a high dose within a short range and provides a therapeutic usefulness in such entities as Graves' disease and thyroid cancer with Iodine-131.

Units

Various units to describe radiation and its effects have been established. Because the scientific community is in transition between conventional units and the Système Internationale (SI), a table of both units with their conversion factors is provided in Table 54.2. *Activity* is used to describe the quantity of the radionuclide being administered and represents the rate of nuclear transformations, denoted by **Curies** (Ci) in conventional units and **Becquerels** (Bq) in SI units. The **Roentgen** is the unit utilized to express radiation exposure and is a measure of the ability of x-rays and γ-rays to produce a given amount of ionization in a given volume of air. From a biologic point of view, the important consideration is how much of the radiation exposure is deposited in an individual at a particular location. *Absorbed dose* is the amount of energy deposited by ionizing radiation per unit mass in joules/kg; the conventional unit is the radiation absorbed dose (**rad**) and the SI unit is the **Gray** (Gy). Because certain types of radiation are more biolog-

Table 54.1. Radionuclides

Radionuclide (symbol)	Method of Production	Mode of Decay (%)	Principal Imaging Photons keV (abundance)	$T_p1/2$	Comments
Chromium-51 (Cr-51)	Nuclear Reactor (Neutron Activation)	EC (100)	320 (9)	27.8 d	Used for in vivo red cell mass determinations, not for imaging; samples counted in sodium iodide well counter.
Cobalt-57 (Co-57)	Cyclotron	EC (100)	122 (86) 136 (11)	271 d	Primarily used as a uniform flood field source for gamma camera quality control.
Fluorine-18 (F-18)	Cyclotron	β^+ (97) EC (3)	511 (AR)	110 m	This radionuclide accounts for more than 80% of all clinical PET use; typically formulated as fluorodeoxyglucose (FDG).
Gallium-67 (Ga-67)	Cyclotron	EC (100)	93 (40) 184 (20) 300 (17) 393 (4)	78 h	In practice, the 93, 184, and 300 keV photons are used for imaging.
Indium-111 (In-111)	Cyclotron	EC (100)	171 (900) 245 (94)	2.8 d (67.2 h)	Principally utilized when optimal imaging occurs more than 24 hrs after injection; both photons used in imaging.
Iodine-123 (I-123)	Cyclotron	EC (100)	159 (83)	13.2 h	Replaced I-131 for most diagnostic imaging application to reduce radiation dose.
Iodine-125 (I-125)	Nuclear Reactor (Neutron Activation)	EC (100)	35 (6) 27 (39) 28 (76) 31 (20)	60.2 d	Used as I-125 Albumin for in vivo blood/plasma volume determinations; not utilized for imaging, samples counted in well-counter.
Iodine-131 (I-131)	Nuclear Reactor (U-235 Fission)	β^- (100)	284 (6) 364 (81) 637 (7)	8.0 d	Typical use now reserved for therapeutic applications; imaging is limited by high energy photon (364 keV) and high patient dosimetry mostly from β^- particles.
Krypton-81m (Kr-81m)	Generator Product	IT (100)	190 (67)	13 s	Ultrashort lived parent (Rb-81, 4.6 h) and high expense limit the use of this agent.
Molybdenum-99 (Mo-99)	Nuclear Reactor (U-235 Fission)	β^- (100)	181 (16) 740 (12) 780 (4)	67 h	The source (parent) for Mo/Tc generators; not used directly; 740 and 780 keV photons used to identify contamination of Tc-99m elution as ``moly breakthrough.''
Phosphorus-32 (P-32)	Nuclear Reactor (Neutron Activation)	β^- (100)		14.3 d	Used in treatment of polycythemia vera, metastatic bone disease, and serous effusions.
Samarium-153 (Sm-153)	Nuclear Reactor (U-235 Fission)	β^- (100)	103 (28)	46 h	Used for palliative treatment of metastatic bone pain.
Strontium-89 (Sr-89)	Nuclear Reactor (U-235 Fission)	β^- (100)	910 (.02)	50.5 d	Used for palliative treatment of metastatic bone pain.
Technetium-99m (Tc-99m)	Generator Product	IT (100)	140 (90)	6.02 h	This radionuclide, typically in kit form, accounts for more than 70% of all imaging studies.
Thallium-201 (Tl-201)	Cyclotron	EC (100)	69–80 (94) 167 (10)	73.1 h	Majority of photons are low energy x-rays (69–80 keV) from Mercury 201 (Hg-201), the daughter of Tl-201.
Xenon-133 (Xe-133)	Nuclear Reactor (U-235 Fission)	β^- (100)	81 (37)	5.3 d	Xe-133 is a heavier than air gas; low abundance and energy of photon reduces image resolution.

Legend: s, sec; h, hours; EC, Electron Capture; β^-, Beta Minus Decay; d, day; β^+, Beta Plus Decay; IT, Isomeric Transition (i.e. gamma ray emission); AR, Annihilation Radiation

ically damaging than others, a radiation weighting factor (also called quality factor) is multiplied by the absorbed dose to yield the *dose-equivalent*, which is measured in **rem** (roentgen equivalent man) in conventional units and the **Sievert** (Sv) in SI units. The dose-equivalent unit allows comparison between the various ionizing radiation sources (photons, β-particles, α-particles). Because the quality factor is equal to one for photons and electrons, one roentgen approximately equals 1 rad in the diagnostic energy range for soft tissue, which ap-

proximately equals 1 rem (Fig. 54.1). That is, 1 R ≈ 1 rad (.01 Gy) ≈ 1 rem (.01 Sv).

Radiation Exposure

To the Worker. The total average exposure for an x-ray technician results in an annual dose equivalent of only 100–150 mrem while for the nuclear medicine technician it is 200–300 mrem. The majority of whole body radiation to a nuclear medicine worker comes from ex-

Table 54.2. Conventional and SI Radiologic Units and Conversion Factors

| Quantity | Conventional Units | | Multiply by the conventional units to obtain SI units | SI Units | | |
	Name	Symbol		Name	Symbol	Example
Activity	Curie	Ci	3.7×10^{10}	Becquerel[b]	Bq	10 mCi = 370 MBq
Exposure	Roentgen	R	2.58×10^{-4}	Coulomb per Kilogram	C/Kg	
Absorbed dose	Radiation Absorbed Dose	rad[a] (acronym)	10^{-2}	Gray[c]	Gy	100 rad = 1 Gy
Dose Equivalent	Roentgen-Equivalent Man	rem (acronym)	10^{-2}	Sievert	Sv	100 rem = 1 Sv

[a] 1 rad = .01 joule/kg
[b] 1 Bq = 1 disintegration/sec
[c] 1 Gray = 1 joule/kg

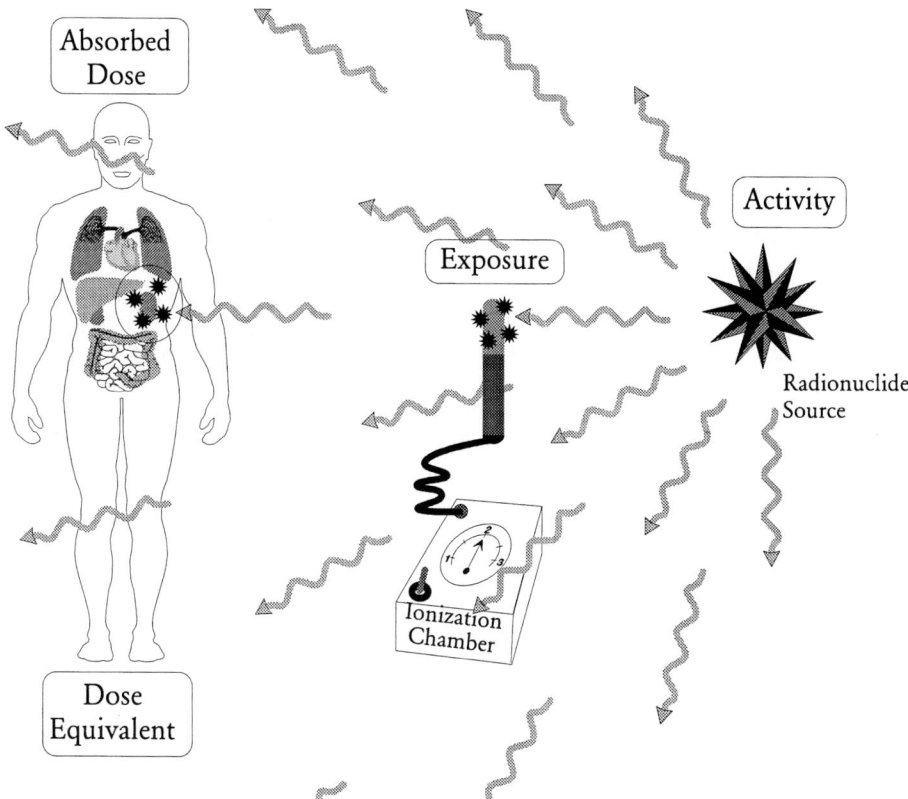

Figure 54.1. Graphical Representation of Radiation Units. The unit of measurement that is used to measure radioactivity is determined by where radioactivity is measured. **Activity** (curie/becquerel), whether occurring outside the body or inside, is measured at the source. **Exposure** (roentgen/coulomb per Kg) is measured by an ionization chamber the radioactivity as it transits air. **Absorbed Dose** (rad/gray) is a measure of radioactivity that has interacted with the tissue where it deposits its energy. **Dose Equivalent** (rem/Sievert) compares the effects on tissue by different types of radioactivity: α-particles, β-particles, and photons. The particles deposit more energy to the tissue than photons.

posure to the dosed patient during imaging. Localized extremity exposure doses from radiopharmaceutical preparation and injection can be higher.

The NRC occupational limits for radiation exposure are 5000 mrem/yr for workers and 100 mrem/yr for the public (not a patient).

The primary risk from any increased radiation exposure is an increased risk for cancer. For each additional rem, the lifetime increased risk of cancer is approximately 5×10^{-4} (5% per Sievert). With the cancer incidence risk in the general population at 33%, each additional rem will increase the risk by .05%. Therefore, an occupational whole body dose of 1 rem (e.g., 100 mrem/yr $\times$ 10 rem) will increase the risk of developing cancer from 33 to 33.05%. With these numbers, several caveats to radiation exposure need to be remembered: any increased risk is spread over a lifetime; increased risks from exposure is additive; and the minimum latency of cancer is 5–8 years with the mean for solid tissue tumors being closer to 20–25 years.

Because contamination in the workplace also increases radiation exposure to the worker, several guidelines can be followed to minimize contamination: follow universal precautions; wear protective clothing; use plastic-backed absorbent to restrict any spills; wash hands frequently; use covers over collimators that can be discarded if contaminated; monitor and wipe test frequently (see below); and avoid smoking, eating, or drinking when handling radioactivity.

To the Patient. The average total annual radiation dose to the population in the United States is 370 mrem/yr. Natural background radiation from atmospheric and terrestrial sources contributes 300 mrem/yr (80%) while man-made sources, primarily from medical procedures, provide the other 70 mrem/yr (20%).

Because nuclear medicine procedures involve radionuclides and radiopharmaceuticals that are variably transient in the human body, dosimetric considerations include not only the initial activity administered but the biodistribution, the physical and biologic half-lives, as well as possible pathologic processes. On a relative scale, the dose to the whole body of most nuclear medicine diagnostic procedures is equivalent to one-third to four times the average annual dose-equivalent from natural background. That is, whole body dose for nuclear medicine examinations range from 100 mrem for a bone scan to 1.3 rem for a Ga-67 procedure. An additional dosimetry term that relates directly to the patient is the concept of "critical organ." The critical organ is identified as the organ or tissue in a radiopharmaceutical procedure that receives the largest dose of radiation or that has the highest radiosensitivity. The dose to the critical organ depends on the radionuclide concentration by the organ, geometric factors, the effective retention in that organ, and the relative radiosensitivity of the organ. Interestingly, in many cases the dose to any organ (the target organ) comes as much from the organ itself as it does from the surrounding tissue (the source).

The pregnant patient faced with a nuclear medicine procedure is a common problem. There are no absolute contraindications regardless of the nuclear medicine exam being considered. Risk-versus-benefit evaluation determines the indication for the exam. If the radionuclide exam is indicated and cannot be postponed until after term, measures to minimize the dose can be employed such as halving the adult dose (and doubling the imaging time) and increasing hydration to enhance excretion.

A lactating female who is administered a radiopharmaceutical requires counseling to proscribe feeding her infant for a specified length of time. The guidelines for these lengths of time are based on the physical and biologic half-lives of the radionuclides (called effective half-lives), which, in turn, predict when the breast milk is safe to drink. The recommended times for successions of feeding are listed in Table 54.3. If the breast milk is measured, use the concentration values in the table to resume feeding; otherwise use the recommended times. For a quick, but very conservative method to arrive at the time for cessation of breast feeding, a good rule of thumb is to use eight physical half-lives of the radionuclide which will leave less than 1% of the radioactivity by the time breast feeding is resumed. Using this rule for Tc-99m agents, two days would be recommended for cessation.

Radiation Safety in the Workplace

General Guidelines. The common goals of radiation safety are to minimize exposure to radiation, whether to the worker, patient, or public and to be as cost-effective per dose as possible. Individuals exposed to radiation can delimit their exposure by observing three very basic principles: time, distance, and shielding. Specifically, *a)* limit the time, which, for the worker, can translate into being familiar enough with procedures that it is per-

Table 54.3. Recommendations for Cessation of Breast Feeding After Administration of Radiopharmaceuticals to Mothers

Radiopharmaceuticals	Administered Activity	Imaging Procedure	Safe Breast Milk Concentration (μCi/ml)	Cessation of Breast Feeding until Breast Milk is Safe
Tc-99m Sodium Pertechnetate	10 mCi	Thyroid Scan & Meckel's Scan	8.2×10^{-2}	24 hrs
Tc-99m kits (general rule)	5 to 25 mCi	All	8.2×10^{-2}	24 hrs
Tc-99m DTPA	10 to 15 mCi	Renal Scan	1.2×10^{-1}	16.8 hrs
Tc-99m MAA	3 to 5 mCi	Lung Perfusion Scan	1.2×10^{-1}	9.6 hrs
Tc-99m SC	5 mCi	Liver Spleen Scan	1.6×10^{-1}	14.4 hrs
Tc-99m MDP	15 to 25 mCi	Bone Scan	2.1×10^{-1}	16.8 hrs
Ga-67 Citrate	6 to 10 mCi	Infection & Tumor Scans	2.1×10^{-3}	4 wks
Tl-201 Chloride	3 mCi	Myocardial Perfusion	2.4×10^{-3}	3 wks
Sodium I-123	30 μCi	Thyroid Uptake	1.2×10^{-4}	3 days
Sodium I-123	200 to 400 μCi	Thyroid Scan	"	5 days
Sodium I-131	5 μCi	Thyroid Uptake	4.1×10^{-7}	68 days
Sodium I-131	10 μCi	Thyroid Cancer Metascan or Graves Therapy	"	(155 days) Discontinue[1]
Sodium I-131	29.9 μCi	Outpatient Therapy for Hyper-Functioning Nodule	"	(168 days) Discontinue[1]
Sodium I-131	100 μCi or more	Thyroid Cancer Treatment (Ablation)	"	(170 days) Discontinue[1]

DTPA. diethylenetriaminopentaacetic acid; MAA, macroaggregated albumin; SC, sulphur colloid; MDP. methylene diphosphonate
[1] Discontinuance is based not only on the excessive time recommended for cessation of breast feeding but also on the high dose the breast themselves would receive during the radiopharmaceutical breast transit.

formed efficiently thus minimizing exposure; *b)* maximize the distance, observing the inverse square law where radiation exposure, like heat from a candle flame, drops off very rapidly as the intensity decreases with the square of the distance from the source; and *c)* use shielding when possible. Shielding with thin lead aprons in diagnostic radiology is quite effective in stopping the low-energy scatter photons. In nuclear medicine, because of the higher energy photons, shielding is confined to containers for the source activity, such as in preparation vials and syringes.

Regulations. The Nuclear Regulatory Commission (NRC) governs nuclear material and its by-products. By-products include reactor-produced radionuclides, such as Molybdenum-99 and I-131. The NRC does not regulate accelerator-produced radioactive material; individual states govern their possession and use of these. The NRC licenses users (individuals or institutions) and governs many nuclear medicine proceedings including the standards for protection against radiation (radiation protection program), waste disposal, granting licenses, surveys, instrumentation, and training requirements. Many states, after accepting the responsibility to regulate radioactive materials, become "agreement states" and license users and enforce regulations compatible with that of the NRC.

The central goal of a radiation protection program is called ALARA, which promotes efforts to keep radiation exposures *as low as reasonably achievable.* As a requirement of the NRC, ALARA represents an administrative philosophy to encourage, enforce, teach, and observe all possible ways to minimize radiation doses and exposure. The ALARA program extends into personnel exposure (worker), misadministrations (patient), and environmental releases (general public) to achieve this dose minimization goal.

The NRC regulations that cover nuclear medicine are covered in the Code of Federal Regulations parts 19, 20, and 35. Part 19 covers the rights and responsibilities of workers to maintain a safe environment, and employers to educate their workers. Part 20 covers regulations of radiation protection for facilities to include dose limits for personnel and environment. Part 35 focuses on medical utilization of radiation sources, listing misadministration definitions and training requirement for authorized users. Board certification in diagnostic radiology or nuclear medicine suffices to qualify the individual as an authorized user in most states.

Safety Instruments

Two radiation detectors have a place in the radiation safety of a department. The Geiger-Müller (GM) detector is a gas-filled survey meter that measures counts per minute. The GM meter is a very sensitive radiation detector that is useful for localizing very small quantities of activity, but will not accurately quantify it. Its primary use, therefore, is as a lab survey instrument looking for contamination. The ion chamber, another gas-filled detector, is used to accurately measure radiation exposure, especially at high levels. The ion chamber has several uses, including to quantify exposure levels, to assay

doses prior to administration (dose calibrator, see later discussion), and to check packages for compliance with transportation regulations.

Radiopharmaceutical Possession and Handling

In general, compliance regulations require "cradle to grave" documentation of all radioactive substances. These requirements begin with an authorized individual ordering the radiopharmaceuticals, then setting standards for packaging and shipping, followed by procedures for the receipt of the package, and finally demonstrating documentation of its use (patient or research) and disposal. Meticulous records of each step are imperative for adequate documentation of the "life" of a radioactive substance.

Radiation Monitoring

In a personnel monitoring program, all workers exposed to radiation wear either a thermoluminescent dosimeter or, more commonly, a film badge. For the film badge, the film is processed and the optical density is related to the radiation exposure. Depending on the relative risk of exposure, reporting programs for personnel dosimeters can be established on a monthly (e.g., nuclear medicine technologists and angiographers) or a quarterly (e.g., mammography) basis.

The nuclear medicine workplace requires frequent monitoring for contamination. A typical monitoring program is as follows:

Daily. A GM survey meter is used to check over all work surfaces and trash. If any reading is 2 times background, then decontaminate (wash area) and resample until background reading, or less than twice background in an unrestricted area (general public area). Dose rates in unrestricted areas must be less than 2 mrem/hr and less than 100 mrem/week; however, all potential exposures should be kept ALARA. Label all contaminated trash as radioactive and store for decay (10 physical half-lives).

Weekly. Perform a radiation field survey using an ion chamber to survey controlled areas of workplace.

Weekly. Wipe test multiple sample areas of the workplace. Count in a multichannel analyzer attached to a multisample well counter using a wide energy window for 1 minute. Acceptable threshold is 200 disintegrations per minute per 100 cm^2 of surface area. If exceeded, then decontaminate and resample until within limits.

RADIOPHARMACEUTICALS

Functional Imaging

The major difference between images from radionuclides and those from x-ray sources is their greater functional information content. Most x-ray images carry a predominance of anatomic information; this is less true for Doppler US images and MR dynamic flow images. For nuclear medicine images, anatomic information is primarily inferred from the functional image. This functional image reflects not only the physiologic biodistribution (function) of the labeled tracer, but also the anatomic, pathologic, and artifact overlays present at the time of imaging. Recalling that the administered radiopharmaceuticals are delivered in tracer quantities to limit the patient absorbed dose, imaging is necessarily longer than for corresponding x-ray images.

Mechanism of Localization of Radiopharmaceuticals

A radiopharmaceutical is a compound to which a radionuclide is attached. The compound, sometimes in concert with the radionuclide, dictates the biodistribution of the radiopharmaceutical. Many radiopharmaceuticals act like analogs of natural biologic compounds, and thus localize via one of several methods. For example, Tc-99m-pertechnetate is analogous to the iodide molecule and distributes to the thyroid, salivary glands, stomach, and kidneys. Technetium-99m sulfur colloid acts like a colloid particle of approximately 1 micron and distributes throughout the reticuloendothelial system (liver, spleen, and bone marrow). Substituted iminodiacetic acid Tc-99m agents are analogous to bilirubin and are actively transported into hepatocytes and excreted into the biliary tree. See Table 54.4 for other examples.

Moly Generator

Nuclear medicine procedures are best served by a radionuclide that has a physical half-life long enough to allow for imaging in a reasonable amount of time, but not so long as to continue to radiate the patient much beyond that imaging. To provide for short-lived radionuclides, generators containing the parent material are constructed to provide an extended source of the daughter.

The most common radionuclide in nuclear medicine procedures, Tc-99m, comes from a generator, named for this parent-daughter relationship, the Mo-99 (Molybdenum)-Tc-99m generator (also known as the Moly generator). Molybdenum-99 decays with a physical T(1/2) of 67 hours, while Tc-99m decays with a 6 hour T(1/2)(Fig. 54.2). The Mo-99 is adsorbed to an alumina column. As the Tc-99m evolves on the column, it is easily removed by elution, as needed, by passing normal saline over the column, exchanging chloride for Tc-99m, in the form of sodium pertechnetate (Na Tc-99m O_4). Two types of Moly generators are commercially available (Fig. 54.3). The wet generator has a large reservoir of saline attached to

Table 54.4. Biodistribution: Mechanism of Localization of Radiopharmaceuticals

Imaging Procedure	Radiopharmaceuticals	Mechanism of Localization	Closest Biochemical Analog	Critical Organ (rad/mCi)
Lung Perfusion Scan	Tc-99m Macroaggregated albumin (MAA)	Capillary blockade	Thromboembolus	Lungs (0.15–0.48)
Lung Ventilation Scan	Xe-133 gas	Compartment localization	Air	Trachea (0.64)
Bone Scan	Tc-99m methylene diphosphonate	Chem-adsorption onto bone crystal	Phosphate	Bladder (0.1–0.2)
Hepatobiliary Scan	Tc-99m Iminodiacetic Acid (IDA)	Active hepatocyte cellular transport	Bilirubin	Gallbladder (0.12–0.18)
Myocardial Perfusion Scan	Tl-201 Chloride	ATP transport system	Potassium	Kidneys (0.4–0.9)
Labeled WBC Scan	In-111 WBC Tc-99m HMPAO	Active migration of leukocyte to site of infection or inflammation after binding of radionuclide to intracellular component	Migratory Leukocyte	Spleen (8.4–18.0) (0.79)
Renal Scan	Tc-99m DTPA Tc-99m MAG3 (mertiatide)	Glomerular filtration Glomerular filtration and Tubular secretion	Inulin p-Aminohippurate (PAH)	Bladder (0.07–0.6)
Thyroid	I-123	Active transport	Iodine	Thyroid (11.0–20.0)
Brain Scan	Tc-99m HMPAO (hexametazime)	Lipophilic passive transport	Fatty Acid	Lachyrmal Gland (5.16)
Gated Equilibrium Blood Pool Scan	Tc-99m Labeled RBCs	Compartment Localization of RBC after Tc-99m binds to intracellular hemoglobin	RBC	Spleen (2.2)
Tumor Imaging	Ga-67 Citrate	Unknown; iron receptor theory	Ferric ion	Colon (0.6–0.9)
	In-111 Oncoscint Monoclonal Antibody (Satumomab Pendetide)	Antibody-Antigen Complex	Antibody	Spleen (3.2)
Meckel's Scan	Tc-99m Pertechnetate	Active ion transport	Iodide	Thyroid (0.12–0.18)
Liver Spleen Scan	Tc-99m colloid	Reticuloendothelial phagocytosis	Colloid particle	Liver (0.2–0.4)

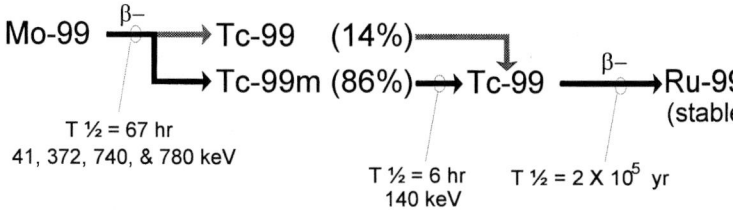

Figure 54.2. Mo-99/Tc-99m Decay Scheme. The Mo-99 decays with both high-energy photons and β-particles (electrons). Fourteen percent of Mo-99 decays directly to Tc-99, while the other 86% it produces metastable Tc-99m. Tc-99m gives up its 140 keV photon and reaches Tc-99.

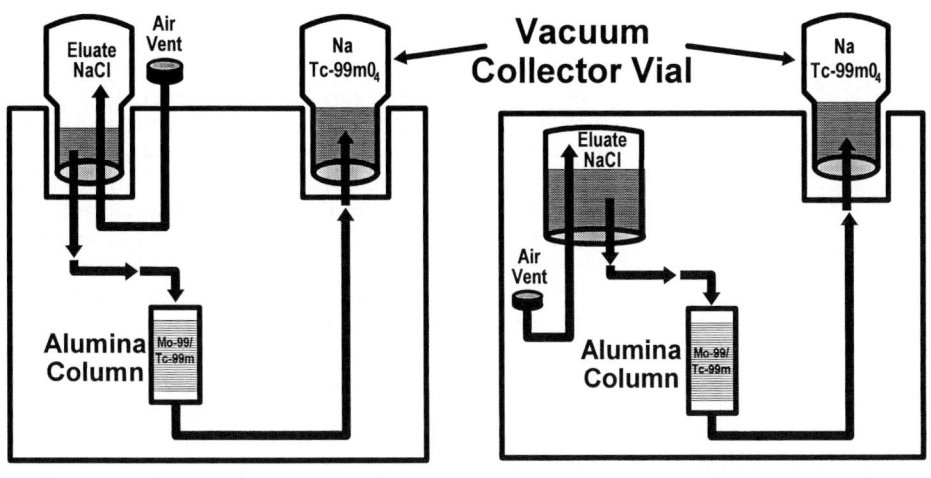

Figure 54.3. Wet/Dry Generators. Both dry and wet generators use a vacuum collection vial; the difference is in the source of the NaCl eluate. The dry generator has a replaceable vial while the wet generator has a fixed one. Both types of generators use the alumina column and are, therefore, susceptible to aluminum and Mo-99 (Moly) breakthrough. The end product is also the same: Sodium Pertechnetate (Na Tc-99mO₄).

one end of the column with which a vacuum bottle, attached to the other end, can extract the Tc-99m pertechnetate. The column is always "wet." The dry generator requires that a small saline vial be attached to one end, and the vacuum extraction vial to the other. The column is left "dry" after the elution.

After eluting (also know as milking) the Moly generator, the shorter-lived daughter, Tc-99m, begins immediately to re-accumulate on the column. This regrowth occurs at a predictable rate and dictates the yield at the subsequent elution (Fig. 54.4). The key times for regrowth and their yields include: 6 hrs, 50% of activity; 23 hrs, maximum activity. It can be readily appreciated from an inspection of the generator elution curve that eluting every 24 hours is both convenient and efficacious with respect to yield.

The quality control for the Moly generator consists of checking every elution for Mo-99 and aluminum breakthrough, that is, escape from the column. Although uncommon, the consequences of Moly breakthrough are important enough to mandate this quality control procedure for each elution. The assay for Moly breakthrough looks for the very high-energy photons, 740 and 780 keV, emitted by Mo-99. The entire eluate is placed in a lead container, called a Moly Pig, that absorbs the majority of the 140 keV Tc-99m photons, but allows the higher energy Mo-99 photons to pass. This pig is then assayed in a dose calibrator with the Mo-99 button selected. The NRC limits are 0.15 microcuries of Mo-99 per millicurie of Tc-99m at the time of administration.

Aluminum breakthrough will cause Tc-99m kits to flocculate. These colloid particles will cause increased

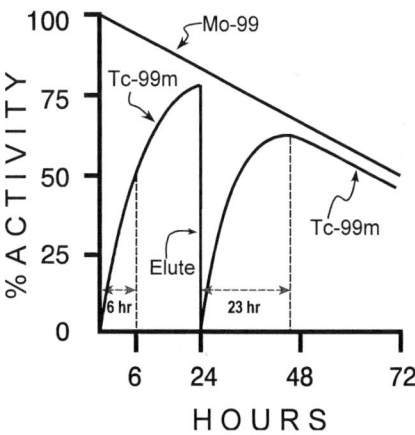

Figure 54.4. Mo-99/Tc-99m Generator Elution Curves. The regrowth of the daughter (Tc-99m) on the column takes a predictable course after each elution. Inspection of the curves reveals that approximately 50% of the activity will be present 6 hours after an elution and that maximum activity is achieved at 23 hours after elution. This is convenient for a daily morning-scheduled elution and allows for an unplanned elution by midday if needed.

lung uptake on a sulfur colloid liver spleen scan and increased liver uptake on a bone scan. The quality control procedure to check for aluminum breakthrough is the colorimetric spot test where a drop of eluate is placed on the colorimetric paper and compared with a standard. The maximum permissible amount of aluminum is 10 micrograms/ml of eluate.

Radiochemical Purity

Many of the Tc-99m based radiopharmaceuticals are produced by adding the generator elute, the "free" or unbound Tc-99m pertechnetate (TcO₄), to a "cold" kit containing the chelate (e.g., MDP, DTPA, DISIDA) and a reducing agent, usually stannous chloride. The reducing agent enables the stable Tc-99m with a valence of +7 to react with the chelate. Occasionally, a kit will require heat, such as sulfur colloid and MAG3, to allow for the chelation to occur. Aside from the desired Tc-99m chelate, several radiochemical impurities can occur as a result of the introduction of either air or water into the kit vial. Air, which can be inadvertently introduced at the time of kit preparation, causes the oxidation of stannous chloride (Sn^{+2} to Sn^{+4}). This inhibits the reduction of Tc-99m, thus interfering with the complexation of the radiopharmaceutical. Water, which can be introduced prior to kit preparation, will hydrolyze stannous chloride to stannous hydroxide, a colloid. Another impurity, formed after kit preparation, is the production of hydrolyzed reduced Tc-99m, also know as Tc-99m dioxide.

Radiochemical purity is defined as the percentage of the total radioactivity in a source that is present in the form of the desired chemical (i.e., the radiopharmaceutical). The Food and Drug Administration mandates testing of radiopharmaceuticals for radiochemical purity. Currently, radiochemical purity testing is required for HM-PAO, teboroxime, sestamibi, and MAG3. The procedure to test for impurities involves separating the different species based on solubility using appropriate solvents. Various solvents and media are used in the separation method but the most common method is thin-layer chromatography, which consists of glass fiber strips impregnated with silica gel. After placing a drop of the radiopharmaceutical on the end (origin) of a thin-layer chromatography strip, the strip is placed, origin end down, in a shallow pool of solvent until the solvent front reaches the top. Because free Tc-99m is soluble in acetone and saline, it migrates with the solvent front, leaving behind the insoluble species for that particular solvent. In saline, both Tc-99m dioxide and Tc-99m tin colloid are insoluble and remain at the origin while the Tc-99m radiopharmaceutical migrates with any free Tc-99m to the top. In acetone, only the free Tc-99m migrates to the top, leaving behind all other species. By cutting the strips into an origin half and a solvent front half, each part of the total strip can be counted in a sodium iodide well counter. The total value of radiochemical impurities is calculated by subtracting from 100% the sum of the percentage of the various impurities present (free Tc-99m, Tc-99m tin colloid and Tc-99m dioxide). No NRC limits are set for radiochemical purity, but the United States Pharmacopoeia (USP), which sets standards for pharmacies, has defined the lower limits of acceptability for purity at 95% for free Tc-99m, 92% for Tc-99m sulfur colloid, and 90% for all other Tc-99m radiopharmaceuticals.

Misadministrations

Misadministration of a radiopharmaceutical is a regulatory (NRC) definition. Misadministrations can be divided into those occurring during a diagnostic procedure and those occurring during a therapeutic procedure. Because of the inherent dosimetric potential, the radioiodines, I-123 and I-131, are identified specifically in the definition of misadministrations. The current NRC definition of misadministration is as follows:

1. For the radioiodines, I-123 and I-131, for dosages greater than 30 microcurie, a diagnostic or therapeutic misadministration occurs when: *a*) the dose is given to the wrong patient or the patient receives the wrong pharmaceutical, *b*) the administered dose differs from the prescribed dose by more than 20% and that difference is greater than 30 microcurie.
2. For all other radiopharmaceuticals other than the radioiodines, a diagnostic misadministration occurs when both: *a*) the radiopharmaceutical is given to the wrong patient, or when the wrong radiopharmaceutical, wrong route of administration or wrong dose (other than is prescribed-no percentage specified) is given to a patient and *b*) the dose to the patient exceeds 5 rems or the dose to any organ exceeds 50 rems.
3. For all other radiopharmaceuticals other than the radioiodines, a therapeutic misadministration occurs when either: *a*) the radiopharmaceutical is given to the wrong patient, or when the wrong radiopharmaceutical is given, or the wrong route of administration is used, or *b*) the administered dose differs from that prescribed by more than 20%.

Federal law requires that misadministrations of radiopharmaceuticals be reported to the NRC no later than the next calendar day after the discovery of the misadministration. This must be followed by a written report within 15 days that details a number of items including the cause of the misadministration and proposed corrective actions.

IMAGING AND DETECTORS OF RADIATION

Image Content

Almost all nuclear medicine procedures that produce images are accomplished with the gamma camera (also known as a scintillation camera). Because nuclear medicine images reflect the biodistribution of the radiopharmaceutical, interpretation of gamma camera images must be tempered with a knowledge of not only the patterns of the normal and pathologic processes, but also with a knowledge of the influence of the individual patient's physiology, habitus, and positioning, as well as with the technical aspects of the exam. In nuclear medicine technical aspects may take an overriding, and sometimes dangerously subtle, dominance in their contribution to the final image output. A mastery of the basic details of image acquisition combined with a awareness of the artifactual patterns, will enable the interpreting physician to avoid erroneous conclusions caused by the myriad interplay of physiologic, anatomic, and technical factors.

Gamma Camera

The essential components in the construction of a gamma camera, as we follow a photon out of the patient, include the collimator, the sodium iodide crystal, the photomultiplier (PM) tubes, electronic positioning and correction circuitry, electronic pulse height analyzer (PHA), and output device (CRT, Film, computer). Because photons emanate omnidirectionally from the patient, the lead collimator serves to select photons from a single projection, reducing the detection of scatter and other low energy emissions. The γ-photons interact with the sodium iodide crystal, converting to a light flash that is proportional to its initial energy. To assess the amount of energy in the light flash, a bank of photomultiplier tubes juxtaposed to the crystal converts the light to a summed voltage (pulse) that, after massage by the electronic positioning and correction circuitry, is screened by the pulse height analyzer (PHA) for acceptance. The PHA is set by the console operator based on the administered radionuclide and its appropriate photon energy (ies). For those photons accepted by the PHA, a position indicator is output to the CRT, film, and/or computer matrix. This entire process, called an event, can take place in as little as 10 seconds.

Prior to the PHA analysis, but after the positioning circuitry, the voltage event is subjected to various correction matrices. These are camera- and manufacturer-specific, but in essence are attempts to correct for slight variations in PM tube sensitivities and variations in crystal properties that, together, can cause inaccuracies in PM voltage response and, subsequently, event positioning on the crystal. One or more correction matrices can be present in a camera. Some of the more commonly found matrices include uniformity, energy, and linearity.

Over the past five years the electronics of the gamma camera head has become digital. Only the initial voltage from the photomultipler tube has remained analog. Digitization of the detector head improves energy resolution, count rate performance, and multiple-window spatial registration. These heads are more reliable and offer greater stability for tomographic imaging.

Photopeak

Although each radionuclide has one or more imaging photon energies (Table 54.1), interactions between the original photon and the patient and camera produce a wide range of energies that are all detected by the gamma camera. These various energies can be displayed by most gamma cameras using the multichannel analyzers, which plots frequency of event against photon energy. The desired photon energy is called the photopeak. The energies outside the photopeak are undesirable because they do not represent the true source of the radionuclide. This latter fact is caused by scatter, and is the major source for decreased image quality. Comparing the photospectrum curves of the radionuclide by itself with that of the patient demonstrates dramatically the ability of the patient to contribute to scatter and, thereby, to image degradation (Fig. 54.5). Furthermore, the larger the patient and the greater the gamma camera distance to the patient, the greater the scatter, attenuation, and image degradation. As stated earlier, the PHA is used to select the desired photon energy by placing a "window" of acceptance of plus and minus 10% around

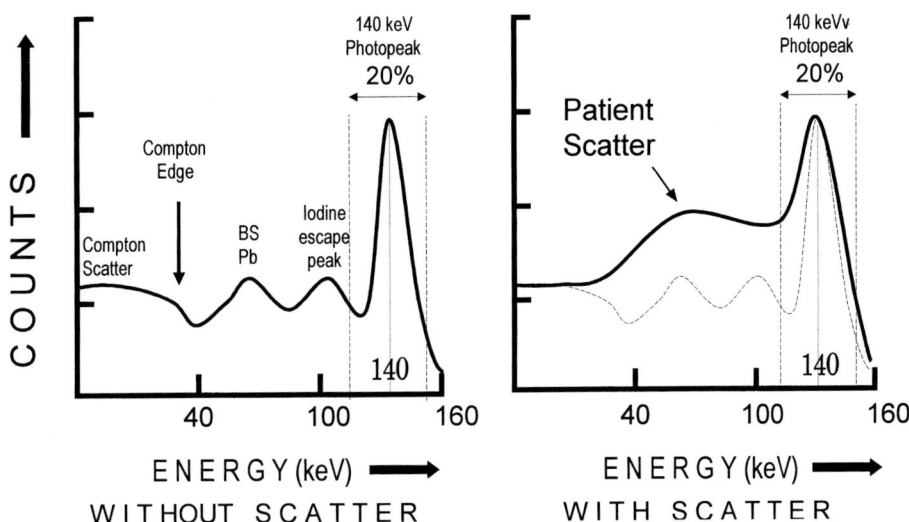

Figure 54.5. Tc-99m Photospectrums. The left photospectrum describes the energies present from the radionuclide imaged by itself (without scatter), while the right photospectrum is from the radionuclide imaged from inside a patient (with scatter). The primary energies of the curve include the following: *a)* Compton Scatter (0–50 keV); *b)* Compton Edge at 50 keV—note that in the patient, scatter contributes to a broad increase in the 90–140 keV level; *c)* Backscatter (*BS*)—primary gamma undergoes 180° scatter from behind the crystal and upon reentering the crystal they are completely absorbed; *d)* Lead X-ray Peak (*Pb*)—photoelectric absorption in lead shielding of camera housing causes 75–90 keV x-ray photons; *e)* Iodine Escape Peak (112 keV)—Iodine K-shell electrons escape the sodium iodide crystal with an energy of 28 keV, therefore an incoming gamma of say 140 keV would lose this much energy before it was registered by the PM tubes (140-28 = 112 keV); and *f)* Photopeak—for imaging purposes, a 20% window over the 140 keV photopeak defines the limits of acceptance of detected energies. Note that some of the scatter photons from the patient are accepted, contributing to decreased image quality (loss of resolution).

the photopeak, thereby limiting the contribution of scatter to the image. Multiple windows can be simultaneously acquired in this manner as would be needed, for example, by Gallium-67 (93, 184, and 300 keV) and Indium-111 (172 and 245 keV).

Quality Control of the Gamma Camera

The quality control program of a nuclear medicine department must cover instrumentation (Table 54.5) as well as radiopharmaceutical preparation. The goal of the QC of a gamma camera is to assure both the uniform response of the detectors (PM tubes) and the correct location of the scintillation events occurring in the crystal.

The quickest and easiest check of a gamma camera is by the daily acquisition of an intrinsic (no collimator) flood image. An intrinsic flood field image is obtained by exposing the entire crystal to either a uniform source of radioactivity, typically from a point source, Tc-99m, or a commercially prepared sheet source, Co-57. Regardless of source used, it must deliver count rates with less than 1% variation across the surface of the crystal. This is accomplished by positioning the point source at least 4 collimator crystal widths from the detector; the sheet source which is placed on the detector face during the acquisition of the flood, is purchased with the manufacturer's guarantee that there is less than 1% inherent variation. A visual inspection of the flood will give an adequate qualitative assessment of nonuniformities. The human eye can detect significant nonuniformities of 5% or more. Results from quantitative analysis, performed by flood field-specific software, along with the flood image itself, can be logged into a computer-based database for detection of subtle changes over time. If the pattern is abnormal, remedies include reloading correction matrices, replacing PM tubes, and addressing other electronic or mechanical problems (Fig. 54.6).

In a similar vein, a quantitative value of general camera performance can be obtained by comparing the uniformity flood field image acquired with and without the uniformity correction. This difference value, termed "data loss," represents additional processing time imposed by the correction circuits to reach a set number of counts. Using a 1 to 2 million count flood, the data loss can be calculated as the percentage difference between the time required to obtain an intrinsic flood with and without the uniformity correction turned on. Typically, differences under 15% are normal for most recent gamma camera systems. Greater differences significantly prolong imaging times and require either a reacquisition of the uniformity or other correction matrix or implicate a hardware electronic problem requiring a service call.

Two basic QC procedures performed to assure correct positioning of events are spatial resolution and linearity (Fig. 54.7). These are generally performed weekly by acquiring a flood with a specially designed phantom sandwiched between a Co-57 sheet source and the camera, with or without the collimator. Alternatively, a Tc-99m point source at 4-collimator distance can be substituted for the sheet source. Several commercial bar phantoms, such as PLES (parallel lines equally spaced) and four quadrant, are available to assess spatial resolution using a series of equally spaced lead bars. Linearity can also be assessed by visual inspection of any of these straight bar phantoms, or can be individually assessed by a dedicated phantom such as an orthogonal (perpendicular to crystal) holed phantom. Generally, inspection of these types of floods will reveal any linearity distortion such as pincushion or barreling.

Collimators

The collimator is composed of perforated lead or tungsten and is positioned on the face of the aluminum-encased sodium iodide crystal detector. Its purpose is to reduce both scatter and obliquely angled photons, allowing only those photons that pass through the collimator holes to be detected (Fig. 54.8). There are two basic collimator designs, pinhole and multihole (Fig. 54.9).

The pinhole collimator is a single-holed collimator that allows only photons within the angle subtended by the pinhole to reach the detector. The geometry inverts the image and, depending on its distance from the aperture, distorts it through magnification. Magnification translates into high-resolution images, but the small aperture

---

Table 54.5. Planar and SPECT Camera Recommended Quality Control Procedures

Procedure	Frequency	Camera System	Comment
Flood Field	Daily	Planar	Intrinsically or extrinsically; intrinsic flood is acquired for 1 to 2 million counts with and without uniformity correction; percent difference should be less than 15% for most systems.
Sensitivity	Weekly	Planar	Intrinsically or extrinsically; result is in counts per minute per μCi
Spatial Resolution	Weekly	Planar	Intrinsic or extrinsic; use bar phantom
Linearity	Weekly	Planar	Bar phantom or multi-holed phantom
High Count Collimator Flood	Weekly	SPECT	30 million counts for 64 × 64 matrix; 90 million counts for 128 × 128 matrix
Center of Rotation (COR)	Weekly	SPECT	Corrected to less than 0.5 pixel for 64 × 64 matrix; to less than 1.0 pixel for 128 × 128 matrix
Pixel Calibration	Monthly	SPECT	Measurement of pixel size in both X and Y direction; used for attenuation correction
Jaszczak or Carlson Phantom	Quarterly	SPECT	Commercially available phantoms that test total system performance

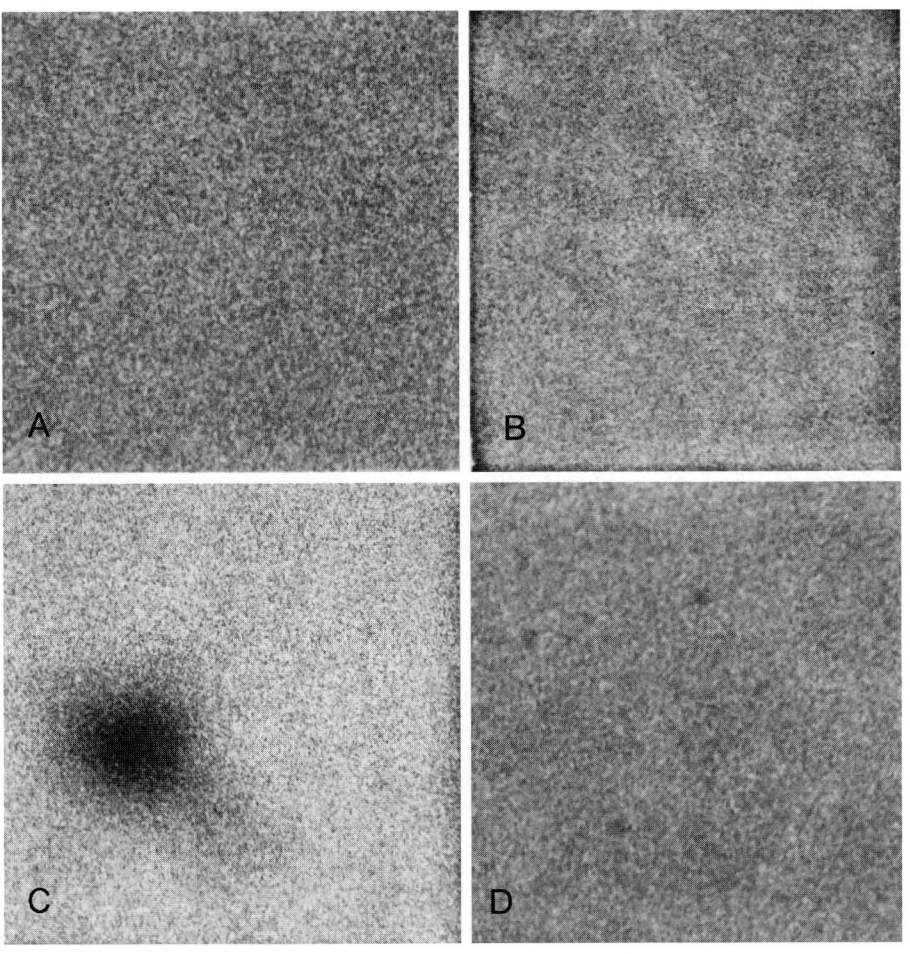

Figure 54.6. Intrinsic Floods. A. Normal uniform flood, with correction matrices applied. **B.** Same camera as in **(A)**, but with the correction matrices turned off. The correction matrices are able to compensate sometimes for striking nonuniformities in the flood field. These corrections are acceptable as long as they do not represent too great a data loss and prolong imaging times. **C.** Uncorrectable off-peak PM tube. The photopeak for this PM tube had drifted down and was accepting more counts than its neighboring PM tubes. **D.** Uncorrectable crystal hydration ("measles"). The dark spots are areas in the crystal where water has breached the manufacturer's watertight seal to gain access to a hygroscopic sodium iodide crystal. The expensive crystal had to be replaced.

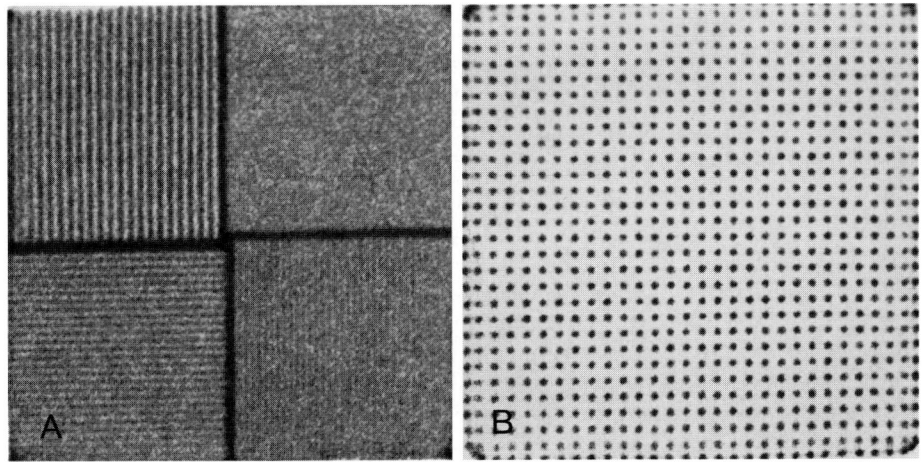

Figure 54.7. Spatial Resolution and Linearity of a Gamma Camera. Both of these floods were acquired without the collimator using a Co-57 sheet source over the phantom. **A.** Four quadrant bar phantom. Distance between bars is equal within a quadrant, but progressively diminishes between quadrants. This bar flood demonstrates lack of visibility of the bars in the quadrant with the narrowest bars. Rotating the bars 90° will allow the entire crystal to checked. Linearity can also be assessed with this phantom. **B.** Orthogonal holed phantom. Pincushion (inward) and barrel (outward) distortion can easily be evaluated by visual inspection of this flood. Both are absent here.

lowers sensitivity and imposes long acquisition times to achieve adequate image photon statistics. The large cone of lead renders the pinhole collimator applicable across a large range of photon energies from 140 keV (Tc-99m) to 364 keV (I-131). The pinhole collimator finds its major clinical use in imaging the thyroid and focal areas of the skeleton in a bone scan.

Multiholed collimators are classified as parallel, diverging, converging, or fan-beam. By far the most common of the multiholed collimators is the parallel collimator, which produces an image without distortion in a one-to-one correspondence with the source. The long axis of the holes of the collimator are perpendicular to the face of the crystal and parallel to each other, separated by lead septa of varying thickness. The physical design of the holes and septa dictates the sensitivity, energy range, and resolution of the parallel collimator. Thicker septa are used with higher energy photons to

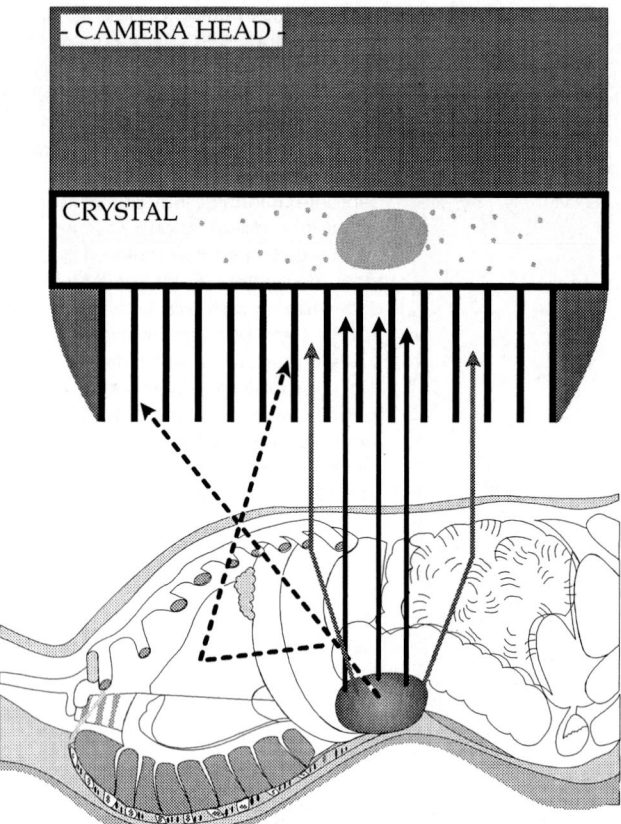

Figure 54.8. Function of a Collimator. The function of a collimator is to reduce scatter and correctly localize the source of the radionuclide in the patient. For example, a Tc-99m radiopharmaceutical localized primarily in the kidney will radiate 140 keV photons omnidirectionally. Those perpendicular to a parallel collimator will be detected at their corresponding anatomic location on the crystal. Because of the 20% window around the Tc-99m photopeak, some scatter photons (*solid gray lines*) will still be accepted and cause a slight degradation of image quality. But the majority of scatter, falling below the acceptance window (see photospectrums in Fig. 54.5), will be rejected due to either their low energy (not represented) or to their oblique incidence of the collimator (*dashed lines*).

prevent septal penetration, but result in decreased sensitivity due to reduction of the crystal surface area exposed to holes. Deeper holes increase resolution by narrowing the field of view, but also decrease sensitivity by excluding more aberrant photons. Differences in septal and hole design create a functional classification, i.e., high-resolution collimator for bone scans, high-sensitivity/low-resolution collimator for flow imaging, and high-energy collimator for Ga-67/I-131 images. Most planar imaging (two-dimensional imaging as opposed to three-dimensional as in single-photon emission computed tomography (SPECT)) is accomplished with parallel hole collimators, which includes bone, renal, hepatobiliary and myocardial imaging. Fan-beam collimators have higher sensitivity for a given resolution and are used for brain and myocardial SPECT imaging. To gain additional sensitivity in SPECT imaging, multihead gamma camera systems have been designed and are commercially available from most vendors.

The quality control for collimators is directed at assessing the integrity of the collimator. Imperfections from damaged septa in the collimator will introduce nonuniformities causing image degradation. Aside from the visual inspection of the actual collimator, a high-count extrinsic flood, performed on an annual basis, may reveal more subtle defects.

Dose Calibrator

As a mandatory requirement by the NRC, all diagnostic and therapeutic doses must be calibrated prior to administration. (See "Misadministrations" for prescription limits.) The dose calibrator is an ionization chamber, not a sodium iodide crystal. It is a cylinder that holds a defined volume of inert gas and a cylindrical collecting electrode (Fig. 54.10). A voltage applied across the electrodes will not pass current until the gas is ionized by radiation emitted from a radiopharmaceutical in the well. The measurement of the current is proportional to the activity for a given radionuclide. By calibrating to known radionuclides and known amounts of activity, the current can be equated to dose activity. A series of buttons imprinted with the radionuclide names resides on the face of the unit. A calibration factor is assigned to each button, unique for that particular radionuclide, to adjust the correct proportionality between current and activity. The dose calibrator will read activity with any button selected, but it is only accurate for the isotope for which the button has been calibrated. As opposed to the well-counter which measures only in the microcurie range, the dose calibrator is capable of measuring quantities in the curie, millicurie, and microcurie ranges. The well-counter, therefore, cannot act as a substitute for a dose calibration.

The quality control for the dose calibrator consists of periodic checks on its performance. Constancy, performed daily, measures the activity of long-lived reference sources to look for deviations from expected values. Using long physical T (1/2) isotopes such as Co-57 (120 keV) in the Tc-99m channel, and Cs-137 (662 keV) in the Molybdenum-99 (Mo-99) channel, the measured activity must agree with calculated activity ±5%. Linearity, performed quarterly, assesses the accuracy of measurements over a wide range of activity, usually from 10 microcuries to the maximum administered dose, which in most labs is around 200 millicuries. With a high activity Tc-99m source, a series of measurements is collected either over a 48 hours period of time, or by using commercially available simulated decay (leaded) cylinders. These measurements are compared with calculated (using decay factors) measurements should agree within ±10%. Accuracy, performed annually, measures certified sources of different photon energies, typically Co-57 and Cs-137, obtained from the National Institute of Standards and Technology (formerly the National Bureau of Standards). Their measurements must agree with known source measurements within ±10%. At installation and after repairs, geometry, is evaluated to compensate for measurements made of sources in different volume dilutions or in different containers. Glass and plastic

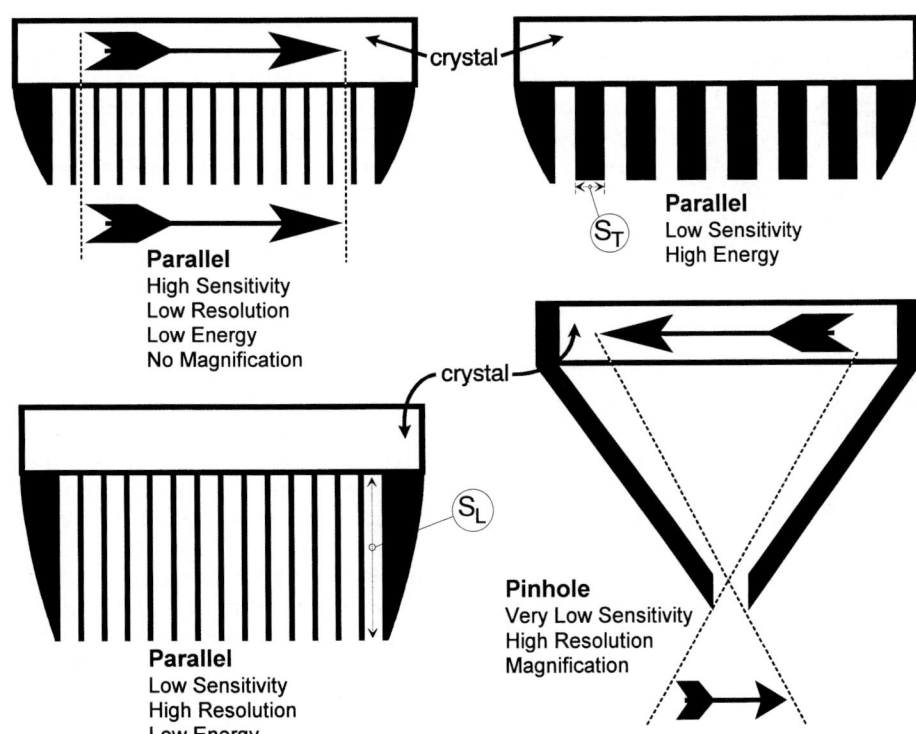

Parallel
High Sensitivity
Low Resolution
Low Energy
No Magnification

Parallel
Low Sensitivity
High Energy

Parallel
Low Sensitivity
High Resolution
Low Energy

Pinhole
Very Low Sensitivity
High Resolution
Magnification

Figure 54.9. Collimator Types. Parallel multiholed collimators are the principle lead collimator used in nuclear medicine imaging. The septa (lead walls between the holes) confer the properties of resolution, energy, and sensitivity. The longer the septa, the higher the resolution. The wider the septa (S_T), the higher the energy which can be imaged without septal penetration of unwanted photons. The shorter the septa (S_L), the higher the sensitivity. The count rate is inversely proportional to the square of the septal length (S_L). Note the lack of magnification and distortion with parallel collimators as opposed to the pinhole collimator.

Figure 54.10. Dose Calibrator.

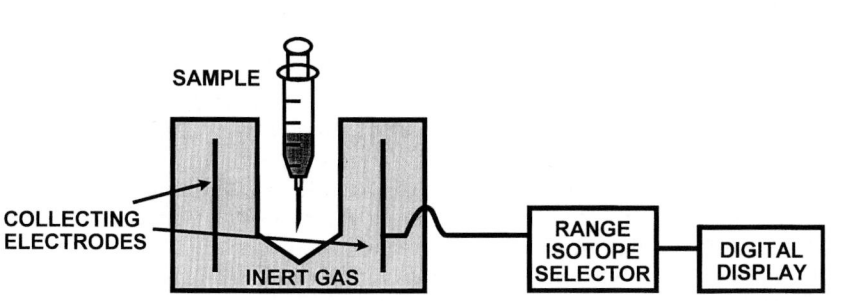

syringes can affect readings significantly. The operator applies these calculated correction factors to activity measurements, e.g., 2% is added for volumes greater than 20 ml.

Sodium Iodide Well Counter

The sodium iodide well counter is used to quantify small amounts of activity in examinations such as an in vitro Schilling test or survey wipe tests. Constructed of a sodium iodide cylinder with a hole drilled in it, sitting on a single photomultiplier tube, and surrounded by lead on all sides, the design provides for good geometric and detection efficiency (Fig. 54.11).

The quality control for the sodium iodide well counter consists of daily assessment of the high voltage and sensitivity. Additionally, resolution, chi-square, and linearity are checked quarterly.

Thyroid Uptake Probe

The thyroid uptake probe is used to quantitate the percentage of radioactive iodine taken up by the thyroid and to survey workers (called bioassay) for possible radioio-

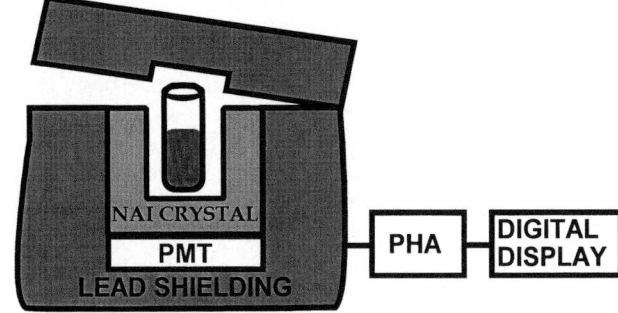

Figure 54.11. Sodium Iodide Well Counter.

dine contamination, most notably after radioiodine therapeutic administrations that may have resulted in some of the radioiodine entering the body (called internal contamination). Constructed of a single 2-inch or 3-inch thick sodium iodide crystal, 5 cm in diameter, juxtaposed to a single photomultiplier, the field of view is defined by a cone shaped flat-field collimator (Fig. 54.12). No imaging is performed with this probe, only quantitative count measurements that are performed at a fixed

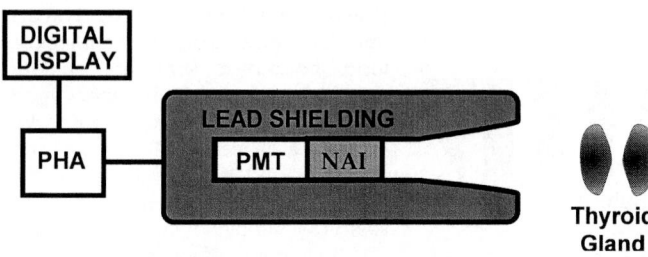

Figure 54.12. Thyroid Uptake Probe.

crystal-to-patient distance. The quality control for the thyroid uptake probe is identical to that of the sodium iodide well counter.

SINGLE-PHOTON EMISSION COMPUTED TOMOGRAPHY IMAGING

Concept

In diagnostic radiology, computed tomography is achieved by the calculation (reconstruction) of a three dimensional image from multiple x-ray transmissions through the body. To accomplish computed tomography in nuclear medicine, the three-dimensional image representing the volume of distribution of the administered radiopharmaceuticals is reconstructed from detection of multiple emissions from the body. This form of CT is termed "single-photon emission computed tomography," or SPECT. Unlike x-ray CT where one slice may be acquired at a time, SPECT simultaneously acquires multislice raw data in the form of two-dimensional planar images.

There are two major advantages of SPECT over planar imaging: a) image contrast is improved by minimizing the superimposition of activity present in a planar two-dimensional image, and b) improved three-dimensional localization of radiopharmaceutical results from the cross-sectional display of activity. Additionally, there is the theoretical advantage of being able to quantify the distribution of a radiopharmaceutical in the body. One disadvantage to SPECT needs to be noted. Because of the average increased detector-to-patient distance from the rotating camera head, spatial resolution is actually less in the tomographic images when compared to planar images.

Instrumentation of Rotational SPECT

SPECT can be accomplished by limited angle tomography, but rotational tomography is the dominant modality in the current clinical setting. In its elementary design, rotational tomography consists of a conventional gamma camera that is capable of orbiting the patient who lies on a table positioned on the axis of rotation. There is a commercial tendency to attach the camera to a gantry, as in most x-ray CT units, and to increase the number of camera heads from one to two or three. Rotating ring detectors can also be used in dedicated SPECT systems. All of these design modifications tend to optimize image quality.

Acquisition and Orbits. Camera head orbits can be up to 360° and, depending on the manufacturer, can be circular, elliptical or body contouring. These noncircular orbits decrease the camera to patient distance and increase spatial resolution (Fig. 54.13). As the detector traverses its orbit, a series of planar images, referred to as projections or views, is acquired either continuously or at discrete angular intervals. These are the raw data used by the computer to reconstruct the tomographic images. Acquisition parameters are changed to tailor image acquisition to the patient and the clinical question to be addressed. Parameters under user control include the number of views, the time for each view, and the computer matrix size. Because of the low number of photons available for each projection during the SPECT acquisitions, a 64 × 64 matrix is usually optimal. 128 × 128 matrices are usually reserved for very high photon flux scans, such as bone scans, or for multiheaded SPECT systems.

The sum of the number of views, the time for each view, and the time for gantry movement is the total acquisition time. Most patients can tolerate acquisition times of 30–45 minutes. The greater the number of views, the better the image resolution and quality, provided each view has acquired enough counts to minimize statistical artifacts. Sixty views over 360° will produce an adequate SPECT image. Once the number of stops has been chosen, the ability of the patient to lie still will dictate the time per view. As an example: 60 stops over 360° at 30 seconds a stop with 5 seconds per gantry movement will require approximately 33 minutes to complete. Acquisition parameters must be selected to balance image quality with patient comfort. When choosing acquisition parameters, any patient motion will significantly degrade the reconstructed image.

Reconstruction. High-speed computers accomplish the mathematical reconstruction from the raw planar data sets to the tomographic images. The quickest method of reconstruction is the filtered backprojection. This method generates the three-dimensional volume from the planar data and then uses digital filters to alter noise and smooth or sharpen the images. The reconstruction method and choice of filters that is generally vendor-specific must be optimized for each particular camera/computer combination. A second reconstruction method called iterative has gained favor as computer systems have become faster and cheaper. The iterative method applies multiple error corrections to the planar data sets to achieve a less noisy, more precise, tomographic image volume.

Scatter and Attenuation Correction. The goal of attenuation and scatter correction is to improve image quality and accurately describe the tomographic distribution of radioactivity in the patient-source. As can be deduced from Figure 54.5, a large percentage of patient counts come from scatter sources. Additionally, attenuation by the patient biases the planar images to superficial body parts.

The most accurate method of correcting attenuation artifacts is to apply attenuation correction matrices to the planar raw data that are derived from simultaneous emission-transmission imaging. The patient is the emis-

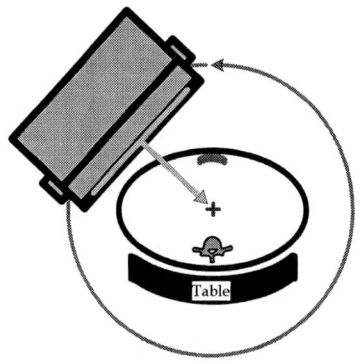 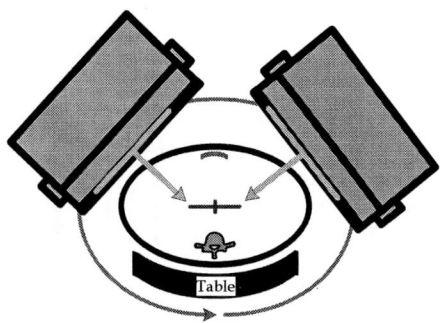

CIRCULAR   ELLIPTICAL

sion source and an external scanning or fixed line source is the transmission source. This fix requires a multihead camera system and can be used for the heart, thorax and abdomen.

Scatter correction is accomplished in one of several ways and is applied to routine planar images as well as to planar raw images used for tomography. A very simple method uses an asymmetric energy window to limit the scattered events that are accepted. A more sophisticated method employs multiple-energy windows during the acquisition. Between 16 to 64 windows span the photopeak and Compton scatter region of the energy spectrum. The true photopeak is estimated and only counts that fit the photopeak profile are accepted.

Display. Immediately after the acquisition of the raw data, but before the reconstruction, a cine display of the raw data should be performed to detect any unsuspected patient motion that might prevent a valid SPECT reconstruction. The reconstructed image can be displayed in classical tomographic planes: transaxial, coronal, and sagittal. Cinematic display of the rotating three-dimensional images and volume rendering are display options that have been used to enhance localization of abnormal activity. EKG-gating of the planar images can be performed during tomographic myocardial acquisitions. The display then allows for 'beating' tomographic slices of the heart to interrogate for wall-motion abnormalities.

Quality Control of SPECT Systems

Gamma Camera. The most important component of a SPECT system is the planar gamma camera. Any deficiencies in the planar capabilities of a SPECT system are amplified during the reconstruction process of the tomographic images. For example, an uncorrected flood-field nonuniformity defect or an off-peaked PM tube will produce subtle ring or blur artifacts in the three-dimensional images. In addition to the routine planar camera quality control, several SPECT-specific quality control procedures are necessary to minimize artifact formations (Table 54.5). Collimator imperfections will manifest as nonuniformities on the SPECT raw data. The effect of these collimator imperfections can be minimized by mathematically applying a statistically high-count extrinsic collimator flood to each individual raw planar im-

age prior to reconstruction. This extrinsic collimator flood is computer acquired using a Co-57 sheet source, for 30 million counts when using a 64 × 64 matrix and for 90 million when using a 128 × 128 matrix.

COR. The camera's mechanical center of rotation (COR) must be calibrated with the center of the computer's matrix as it is projected from the face of the crystal (Fig. 54.14). For various mechanical and electronic reasons these are not perfectly aligned. An offset greater than half a pixel for a 64 × 64 matrix will result in loss of contrast and resolution, and distortion in the tomographic images. The COR calibration is performed by imaging a point or line source at multiple opposing intervals over 360°. The COR is then calculated by averaging the difference in the sets of offset of the source from the matrix center as seen by the opposing pairs of images. The COR value is stored by the computer for use during the ensuing reconstruction of the three-dimensional images. When this calibration factor is applied during reconstruction, the matrix centers are shifted to align with the mechanical rotational center. This COR calibration must be performed for each collimator, zoom factor and matrix size used for SPECT acquisitions.

Pixel Size Calibration. Attenuation correction refers to attempts to compensate for the loss of photons due to absorption as they traverse tissue. Photons arising from deeper tissue have greater attenuation. Attenuation correction compensates for these losses by adding counts back into the reconstructed slices. Attenuation correction for SPECT images is usually only performed for solid body parts such as the abdomen, pelvis, and head. Pixel size calibration prior to attenuation correction is a necessary quality control procedure to match the matrix size with the physical dimensions of the body part being imaged. Pixel calibration is easily performed by acquiring two point or line sources separated by a known distance; the computer calculates and stores the pixels per millimeter calibration factor for subsequent attenuation corrections.

Phantoms. As a general assessment of the total performance of a SPECT system, commercially available phantoms can be imaged. Fluid-filled phantoms are designed so that after Tc-99m is added to the fluid, areas of cold and hot activity are present in varying dimensions. A subsequent SPECT acquisition, reconstruction,

Figure 54.14. Center of Rotation (COR). This illustration is diagrammatically exaggerated for teaching purposes. The COR represents the difference between mechanical center of rotation (*black dashed arrow/black dot*) and the center of the projected image matrix (*gray dashed arrow/black circle*). This difference must be adjusted to less than a half pixel for a 64 × 64 matrix, and one pixel for 128 × 128 matrix, to avoid SPECT reconstruction defects.

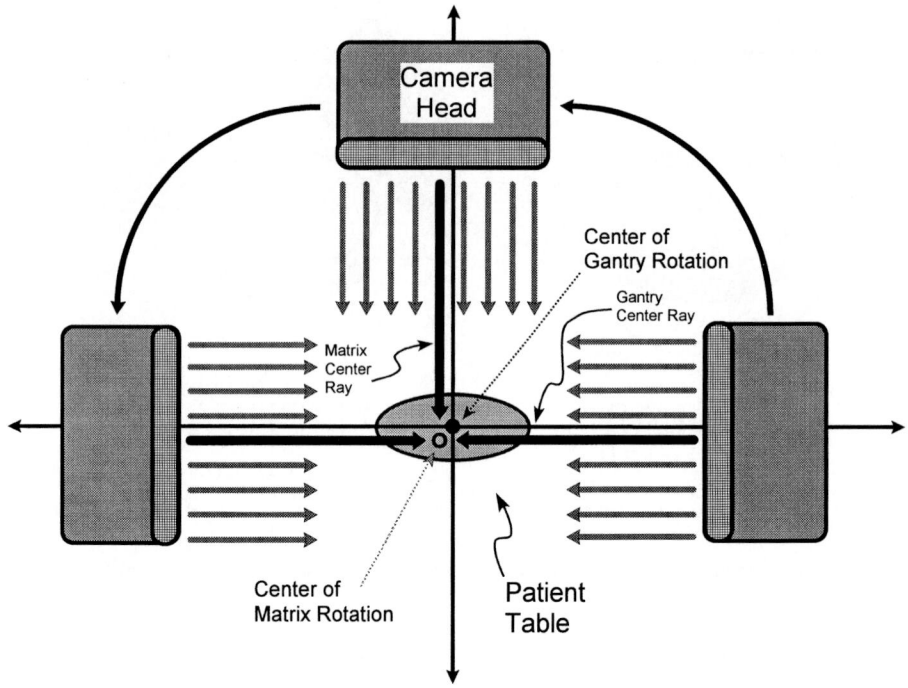

and display of the phantom will test the SPECT system's contrast, resolution, field uniformity, and attenuation correction.

POSITRON EMISSION TOMOGRAPHY

Concept and Instrumentation

Whereas SPECT is typically designed for the detection and tomographic imaging of single-photon emitting radionuclides, PET deals with the detection and tomographic imaging of dual-photon positron-emitting (positive electron) radionuclides. These proton rich radionuclides, such as carbon-11, nitrogen-13, oxygen-15 and fluorine-18, are short-lived, cyclotron-produced isotopes which decay by releasing a positron from the nucleus. Once released, the positron travels only a few millimeters in tissue before combining with a negative electron and converting to annihilation radiation composed of two photons of 511 keV each (energy equivalent of an electron's mass) that are emitted in 180° opposite directions. In a dedicated PET scanner, these annihilation photons are detected by a pair of opposed ring detectors and are accurately localized by high-speed coincident circuitry along a line. From these lines, and using filters and computer reconstruction techniques, tomographic images of the distribution of the positron radionuclide can be calculated and displayed.

Positron Emission Tomography–Enabled Gamma Camera Systems

Two approaches to imaging PET agents have been devised using the conventional gamma camera. The first approach employs 511-keV collimators that typically weigh up to 400 lb. each. Gantry design, extra shielding of the detector head, and the collimator changer all have

to be designed or modified to accommodate these heavy collimators. The acquisition follows the typical SPECT protocols and orbits. Despite a system sensitivity of only 20% compared to Tc-99m, clinical results of PET agents using SPECT have proven equivalent to dedicated PET scanners for the heart and for tumors greater than 2 cm in diameter.

The second approach takes advantage of the electronic evolution of the digital detector head. The digital detector head provides for very high-count rates that are critical to PET imaging within an acceptable patient-comfort time. By removing the collimators and employing coincidence circuitry in opposed dual-head gamma cameras, high-resolution SPECT acquisition of PET agents can be accomplished in less than an hour with a resultant image quality similar to that of dedicated PET scanners (Fig. 54.15).

Advantages. Positrons have been successfully labeled into compounds that have produced PET images demonstrating physiologic and biochemical processes. This has been particularly true in the fields of cerebral, cardiac, and oncologic metabolism. These functional images have till recently enjoyed higher resolutions than SPECT, due in large measure to the higher energy photons, efficient suppression of scattered radiation, and dedicated detector systems (Table 54.6). The recent introduction of PET-enabled mutlihead gamma camera systems has expanded the capability of PET imaging to sites outside dedicated PET centers.

Disadvantages. The high initial costs of a dedicated PET scanner, as well as the moderate investment in personnel necessary to operate the unit, have limited the proliferation of dedicated PET scanners. Additionally, some of the very short-lived positron radionuclides require an on-site cyclotron for their production.

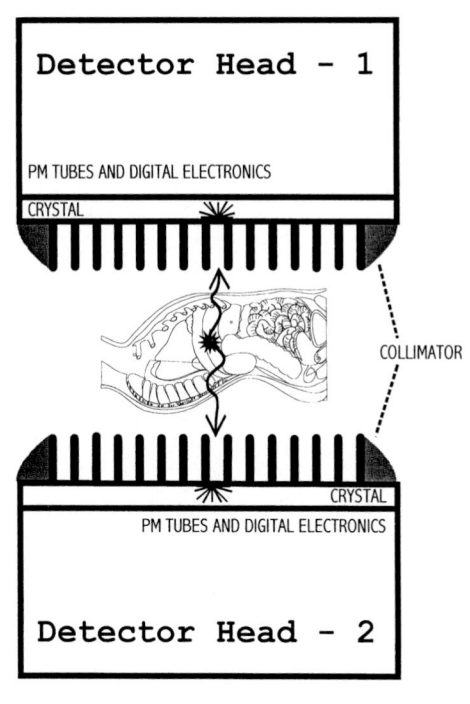

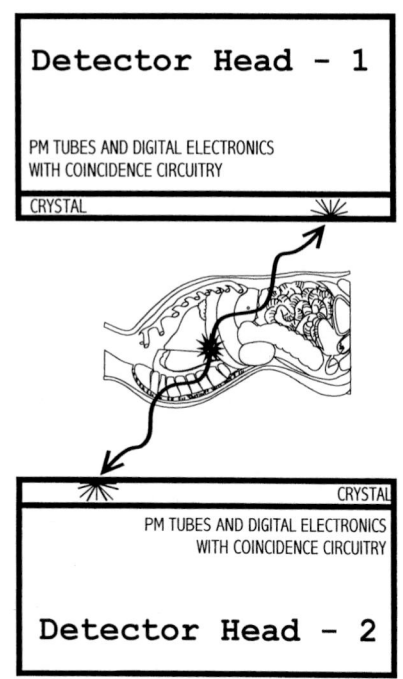

A   **B**

Figure 54.15. PET-Enabled Gamma Camera Systems. A. PET imaging can be accomplished with 511 keV collimators in either a single or, as depicted here, dual-headed configuration. The gamma cameras rotate around the patient and reconstruction is similar to SPECT acquisitions. **B.** Alternatively, a dual-opposed gamma camera system with coincidence circuitry can be used to image PET agents. Although more costly than typical gamma camera, the resultant image quality approaches that of dedicated PET scanners.

Table 54.6. Comparison of SPECT and PET

	SPECT	PET
Principle of raw image formation	Collimation	Annihilation coincidence detection
Transverse slice reconstruction	Filter backprojection	Filter backprojection
Radionuclides	Tc-99m and other single photon emitting radionuclides	Positron emitters
Spatial resolution	12 mm (1 head) 7 mm (3 heads)	5 mm
Attenuation correction	Crude	Accurate (with a transmission source)
Scatter rejection	Good	Excellent
Cost	$400,000 (1 head) $700,000 (3 heads)	$2,000,000 (plus need for on-site cyclotron if nuclides other than F-18 and Rb-82 are to be used)

Suggested Readings

Alazraki NP, Mishkin FS. Fundamentals of Nuclear Medicine. 2nd ed. New York: The Society of Nuclear Medicine, 1988: 3–20.

Brown ML, David Collier B, eds. Syllabus: A Categorical Course in Nuclear Medicine. Oak Brook: SNA Publications, 1996.

Bushberg JT, Seibert JA, Leidholdt EM, Boone JM. The Essential Physics of Medical Imaging. Baltimore: Williams & Wilkins, 1994.

English RJ, Brown SE. SPECT Single-Photon Emission Computed Tomography: A Primer. 2nd ed. New York: The Society of Nuclear Medicine, 1990.

Graham LS. Quality assurance for SPECT. In: Freeman LM, Weissmann HS, eds. Nuclear Medicine Annual 1989. New York: Raven Press, 1989:81–108.

Kowalsky RJ, Perry JR. Radiopharmaceuticals in Nuclear Medicine Practice. Norwalk, CT: Appleton & Lange, 1987.

Mettler FA, Guiberteau MJ. Essentials of Nuclear Medicine Imaging. 3rd ed. Philadelphia: WB Saunders Co., 1991.

Romney, BM, Nickloff, EL, Esser, PD, et al. Radionuclide Administration to nursing mothers: mathematically derived guidelines. Radiology 1986;160:549–554.

Simmons GH, ed. The Scintillation Camera. New York: The Society of Nuclear Medicine, 1988.

Sorensen JA, Phelps ME. Physics in Nuclear Medicine. 2nd ed. Philadelphia: WB Saunders Co., 1987.

U.S. National Academy of Sciences (1989). Report by the Committee on the Biological Effects of Ionizing Radiations ("BEIR-V"). National Academy of Sciences/National Research Council, Washington, DC.

55
Skeletal System Scintigraphy

Robert J. Telepak
Philip W. Wiest
Michael F. Hartshorne

PHYSIOLOGY AND TECHNICAL
INTERPRETATION

Musculoskeletal imaging studies performed with gamma cameras and Technetium-99m (Tc-99m) labeled diphosphonates are a staple of nuclear medicine. Bone scans are performed to assist in the medical care of tens of thousands of patients each week in the United States. The bone scan is a map of osteoblastic activity that occurs in response to a variety of benign and malignant conditions. It is an excellent complement to anatomic studies of the skeletal system. After injection, blood flow is required to deliver the radiopharmaceutical to the extracellular space around functioning osteoblasts. Within minutes, they begin to assemble labeled diphosphonates into the hydration shell of hydroxyapatite crystals as they are formed and modified. Osteoclastic function is not measured by this technique.

PHYSIOLOGY AND TECHNICAL

Skeletal scintigraphy has a resolution of about 5 mm in the best conditions. Adult intravenous doses of 20 mCi (740 mBq) or more Tc-99m diphosphonates are adequate for static imaging 3 to 4 hours after injection. Vigorous osteoblastic activity in juvenile skeletons, healing fractures, pathologic conditions stimulating skeletal blood flow, and bone repair increase the bone labeling. The Tc-99m diphosphonates are excreted by glomerular filtration by the kidneys. In a normal subject, 50% is excreted by 4 hours, and up to 80% of the injected diphosphonate will be excreted by 24 hours. Normal renal function clears soft-tissue activity, which improves the quality of bone images because of improved target to background ratios. Even though radioactivity is falling, the ratio improves and the resulting images become sharper. Decreased renal function for any reason degrades image quality. Waiting 3–4 hours before imaging is a compromise between remaining radioactivity and reduction of background around the skeleton. "Spot-view," "whole-body," and SPECT imaging technology may be used. High-resolution, low-energy collimation is most commonly used for good quality images. Ultra-high-resolution collimation will produce a minor improvement in image quality at the price of a geometric increase in imaging time. For the very patient imager, a pinhole collimator produces exquisite images of limited areas of the skeleton. The bone scan should be tailored as necessary to answer the clinical question for which the scan was ordered.

INTERPRETATION

Trauma to the skeleton may be undetectable on standard radiographic examinations. The classic insufficiency (stress) fracture may be caused by overuse of the normal skeleton or normal use of weakened bone. Radiographically demonstrated trauma precedes scintigraphically detectable fracture healing by approximately 10 days. Decreased or normal osteoblastic activity is seen at the fracture site in this first phase of repair. The subsequent osteoblastic activity then shows as a "hot spot" weeks before the calcified callus appears on a radiograph (Figs. 55.1, 55.2). In an uncomplicated fracture, repaired bone returns to normal appearance as the callus at the fracture site remodels over a period of months (Fig. 55.3). A complicated fracture in a weight-bearing bone healing with angulation may take many years to return to normal bone scan activity. Some fractures show remodeling on bone scans for life.

Prosthetic Joint Replacements may loosen and/or become infected. For about 6 months after hip replacement surgery the bone around the prosthesis is expected to have increased osteoblastic activity. Thereafter, increased labeling correlates with infection, loosening, and heterotopic bone formation, depending upon the pattern of localization. Radiographs and occasionally radiolabeled white blood cell scans are required to evaluate abnormal findings (Fig. 55.4).

Arthropathies and Arthridities. Inflammation of a joint creates increased blood flow and increases radiopharmaceutical supplied to those portions of the bone bounded by the synovial capsule. Increased bone labeling is seen in toxic synovitis, septic joints, inflammation associated with early degenerative conditions, and connective tissue arthropathies. In early osteoarthropathy, high-resolution bone scan images detect increased subchondral bone labeling long before there are radiographic findings. Intense, abnormal labeling also is seen in neuropathic joints long before the abnormality is detected by radiographs (Fig. 55.5).

Osteomyelitis. In a large bone such as a tibia, acute hematogenous infection of bone that precedes radiographic abnormality can be sensitively and specifically diagnosed by three-phase bone scans. Early arterial flow seen seconds after injection (first phase), increased blood pool seen for a few minutes before bone labeling begins (second phase), and intense delayed labeling 3 or

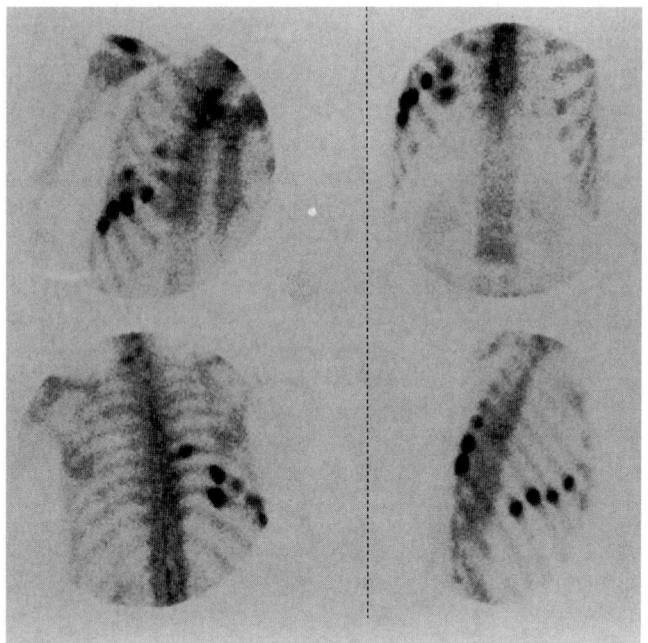

Figure 55.1. Multiple Rib Fractures. Vigorous osteoblastic repair activity is seen in two rows of fractures which were not visible on radiographs. Note the difference in lesion distribution from the metastases in scans of Figures 55.13 and 55.14.

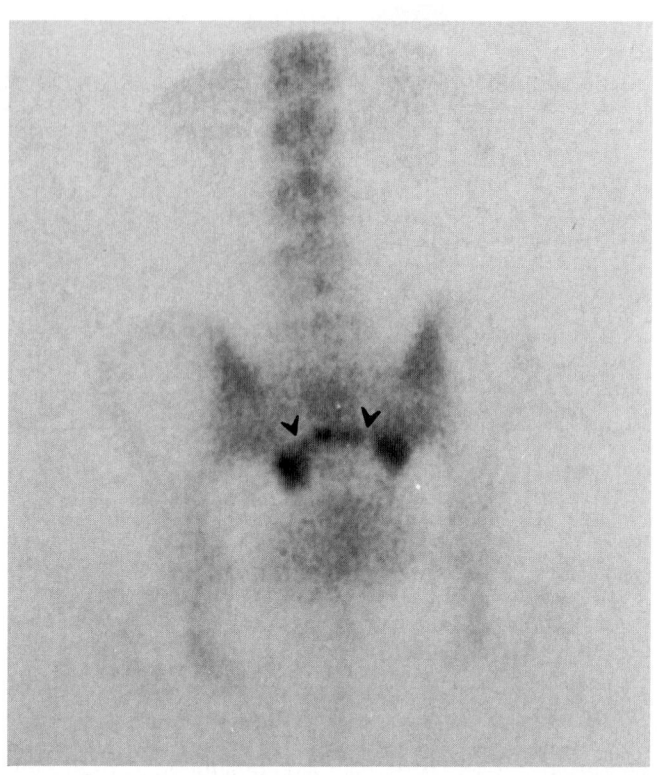

Figure 55.2. Occult Sacral Fracture. A posterior image of the pelvis shows a horizontal line of increased uptake (*arrowheads*) across the sacrum, which marks healing along a painful fracture that is invisible on radiographs.

Figure 55.3. Fracture Healing. Serial bone scans of the lower thoracic and lumbar spine at intervals of months show a normal spine followed by a compression fracture of L-1 which gradually heals only to be replaced by new fractures at T-9 and T-12. Note the horizontal, linear pattern of a simple vertebral compression fracture.

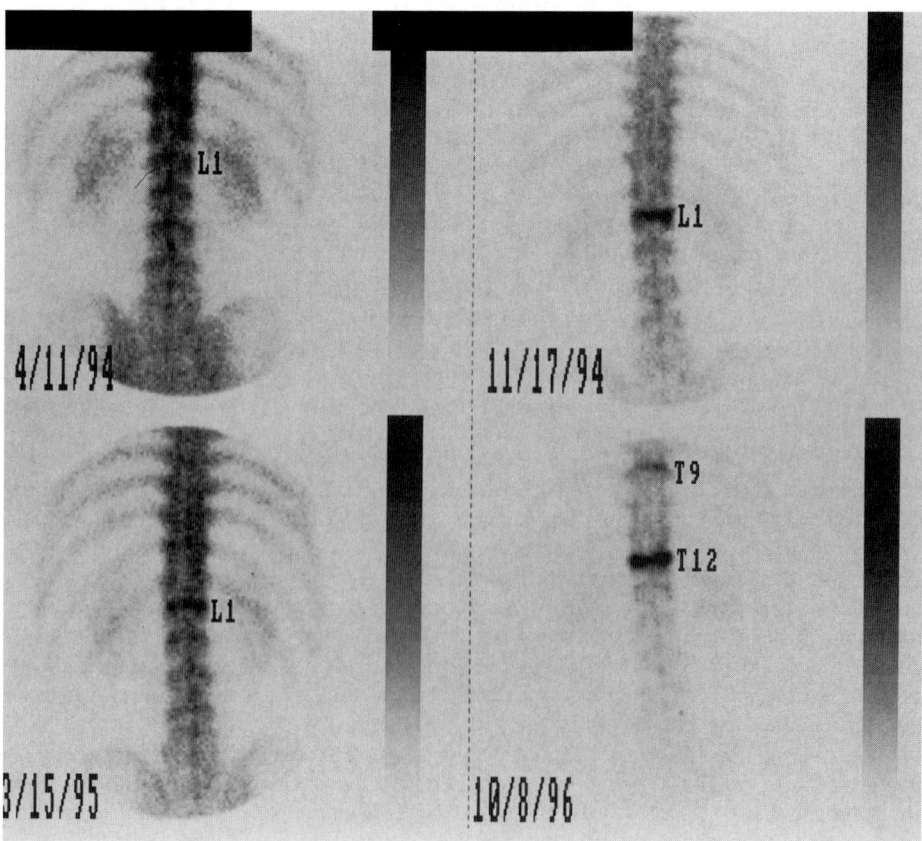

Figure 55.4. Hip Prosthesis Loosening. Anterior images of the pelvis, hips, and femurs show intense labeling around the femoral (*arrows*) and acetabular (*arrowheads*) components of a 2-year-old total hip arthroplasty. Both had loosened without infection.

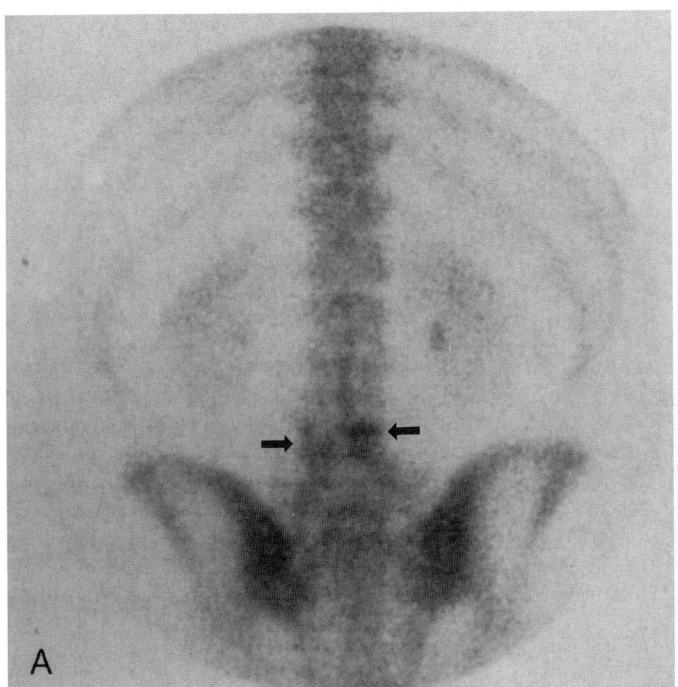

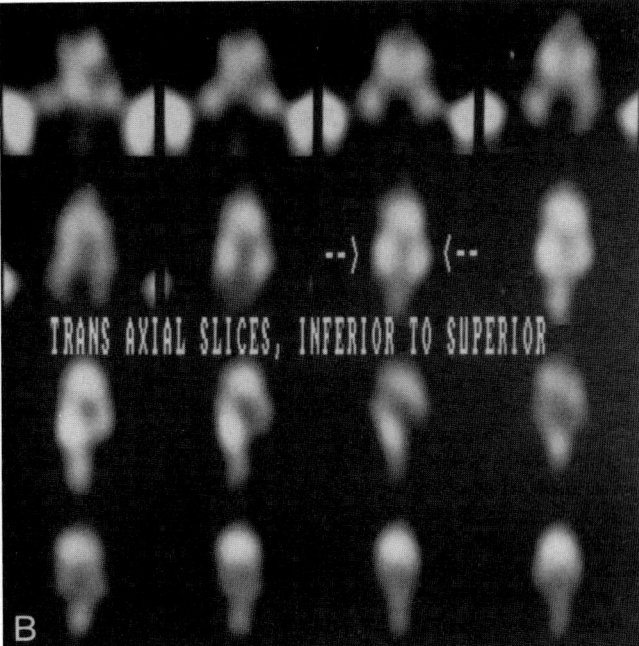

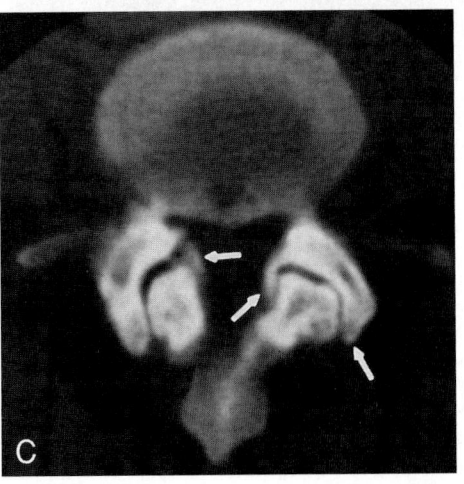

Figure 55.5. L4–5 Facet Degenerative Arthropathy. A. A planar, posterior image of the lumbar spine shows small areas of increased activity (*arrows*) in the lower lumbar spine in a patient with chronic low back pain. **B.** Transaxial SPECT images of the same lumbar spine start at the L5–S1 facet joint level and continue up to the L3–4 level. Note the conspicuity of the abnormality. Areas of increased bone labeling at the L4–5 facet joints are marked by *arrows*. **C.** The CT of the same level shows hypertrophic spurs (*arrows*) embracing the facet joints.

more hours after injection (third phase) is characteristic of early infection. This phenomena requires several days of symptoms before it develops. Radiographic changes may not be seen for 10–14 days. The scan is more difficult to read and not as specific when the target is small (like the bones of the foot) in comparison with the resolving power of the camera (Figs. 55.6, 55.7). False-negative examinations are reported in children when the duration of clinical illness is brief.

A cellulitis adjacent to bone is seen as soft tissue areas of increased activity on the arterial and immediate blood pool phases with little or no increased activity in the bone on the third phase. In the peripheral skeleton where bones are small, it is frequently impossible to tell the difference between an infection adjacent to a bone with increased soft tissue and increased periosteal labeling from an infection within the bone. Even in images of large bones, it may be necessary to use very high resolution systems to separate enhanced periosteal osteoblastic labeling from osteoblastic activity inside the infected cortex. Bone scans may take months to normalize after infections of bone are sterilized. Images of chronic osteomyelitis of bone are not distinguishable from normal healing after infection.

Vascular Phenomena. There is a strong vascular influence on the labeling of bones. Increased blood flow stimulates increased osteoblastic *and* osteoclastic activity. The bone scan reflects the former effect. Common pathologic conditions, such as tumor and trauma, cause hyperemia and increased blood pooling with increased delivery of radiopharmaceuticals to the bone's osteoblasts. This is an appropriate response to injury. Reflex sympathetic dystrophy is an example of an inappropriate, increased vascular response to little or no injury. The release of sympathetic vascular tone causes arteries to dilate (Fig. 55.8). A bone scan is a simple test of the vascular status of a bone or bone graft. If osteoblasts are labeled, the blood supply must be intact. Acute avascular necrosis shows no labeling of the affected bone. Bone subjected to radiation therapy may lose blood supply and osteoblastic activity. Square-edged radiation portals produce typical areas of decreased labeling (Fig. 55.9).

Heterotopic Bone. Repair of soft-tissue injuries sometimes leads to the formation of heterotopic bone. Histologically, normal bone may form from differentiating fibroblasts after trauma. Muscle crush injuries healing with the formation of heterotopic bone (myositis os-

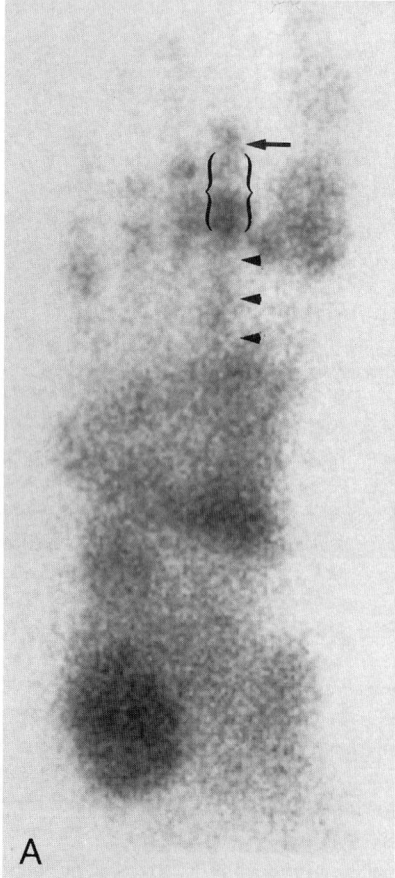
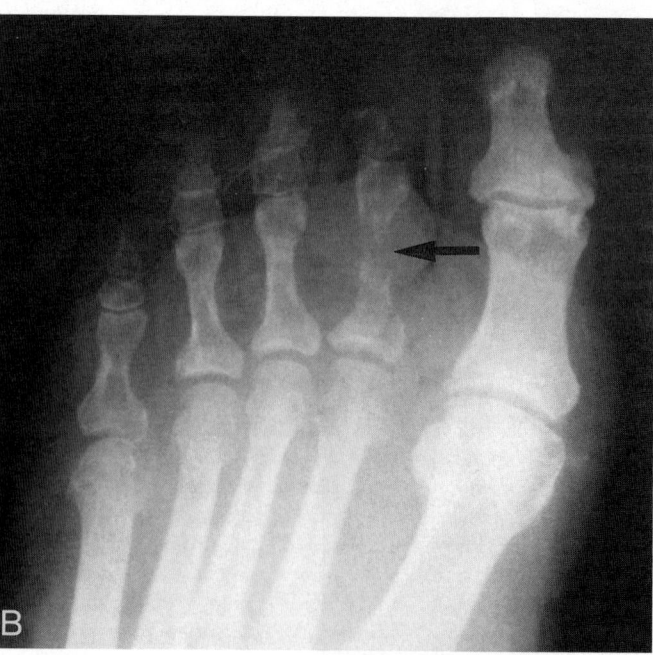

Figure 55.6. Osteomyelitis of the Second Toe and Metatarsal and Septic Second Metatarsal Phalangeal Joint. A. A plantar bone scan shows increased activity in the second proximal phalanx (*arrow*), metatarsal phalangeal joint (*brackets*), and second metatarsal (*arrowheads*) indicating reactive bone stimulated by the infection. Decreased activity distal to that point corresponds with necrotic tissue. **B.** A radiograph shows destructive changes in the second proximal phalanx (*arrow*), but appears normal in the second metatarsal phalangeal joint and metatarsal phalangeal shaft.

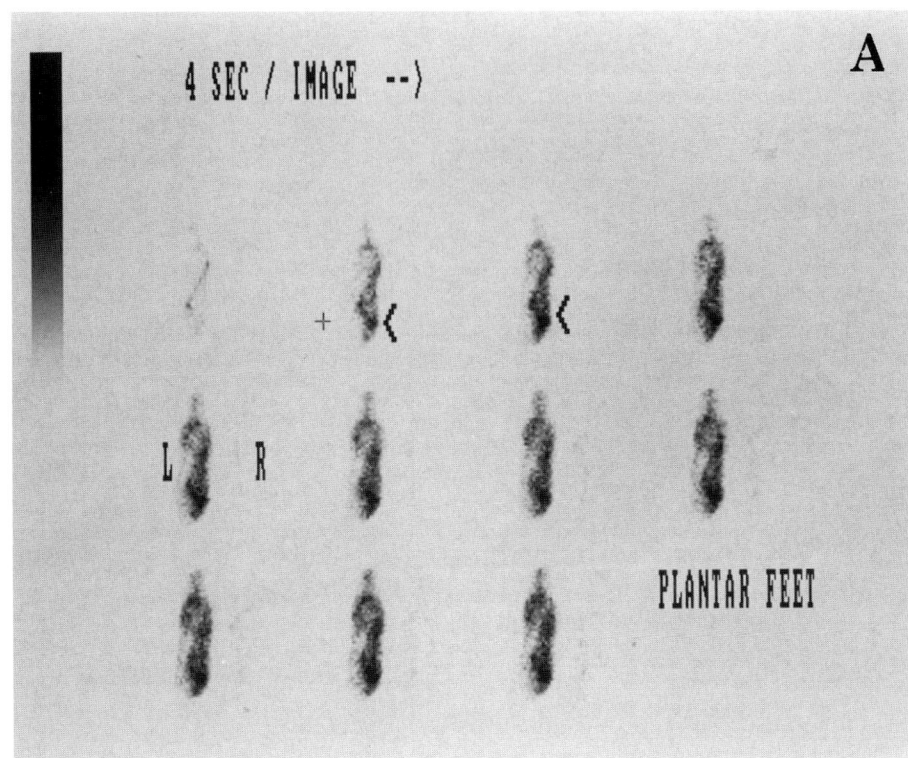

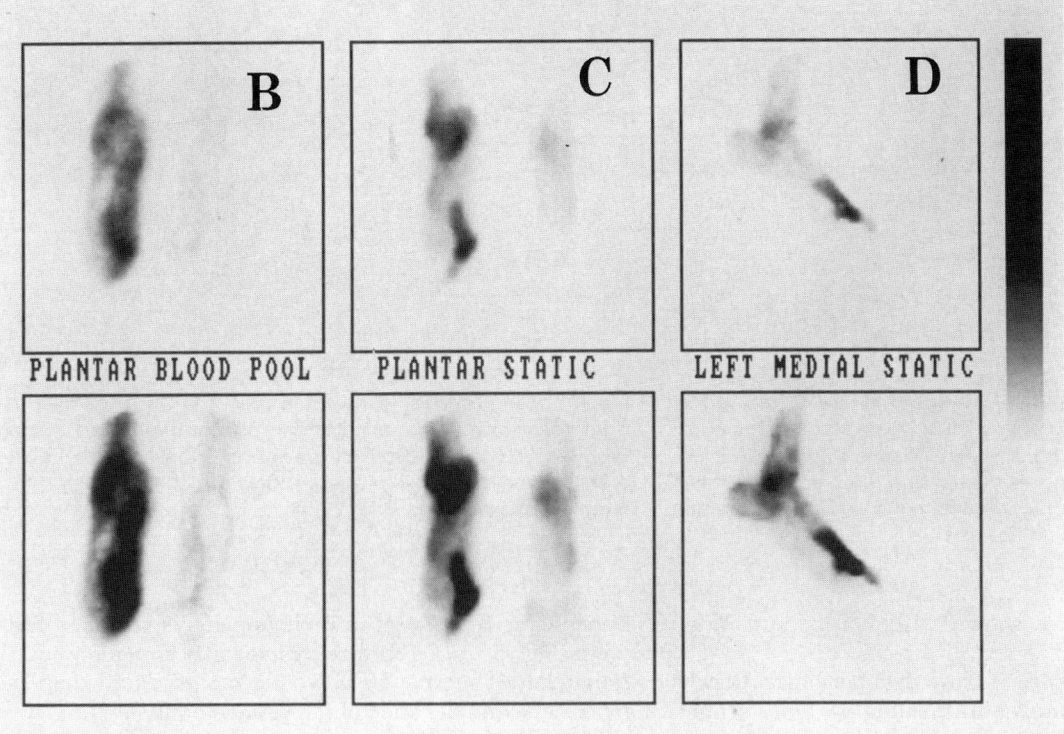

Figure 55.7. First Metatarsal Osteomyelitis and Septic First Metatarsal Phalangeal Joint. The plantar flow study **(A)** shows intense, early flow to the left foot and first metatarsal head (*arrowheads*). The immediate plantar blood pool images **(B)** show diffuse increased blood pooling in the same areas. The plantar **(C)** and left medial **(D)** views of the static bone scan show intense osteoblastic activity in the entire first metatarsal and in the first metatarsal joint.

sificans) are readily labeled on bone scans weeks before the plain film shows signs of calcification. Soft tissues around joint prostheses, in paralyzed limbs, and in burn injuries are common sites of heterotopic bone formation.

Metabolic Conditions. Increased parathormone levels (or the presence of tumor-produced parathormone-like substances) simultaneously increase serum calcium and phosphate. Calcium/phosphate complexes precipitate in the thyroid gland, lungs, and stomach. This "metastatic calcification" is rarely seen on radiographs but is routinely visible on bone scans. Other generalized skeletal abnormalities such as tumoral calcinosis, hypertrophic osteoarthropathy, systemic mastocytosis, and many other diseases with calcification or ossifica-

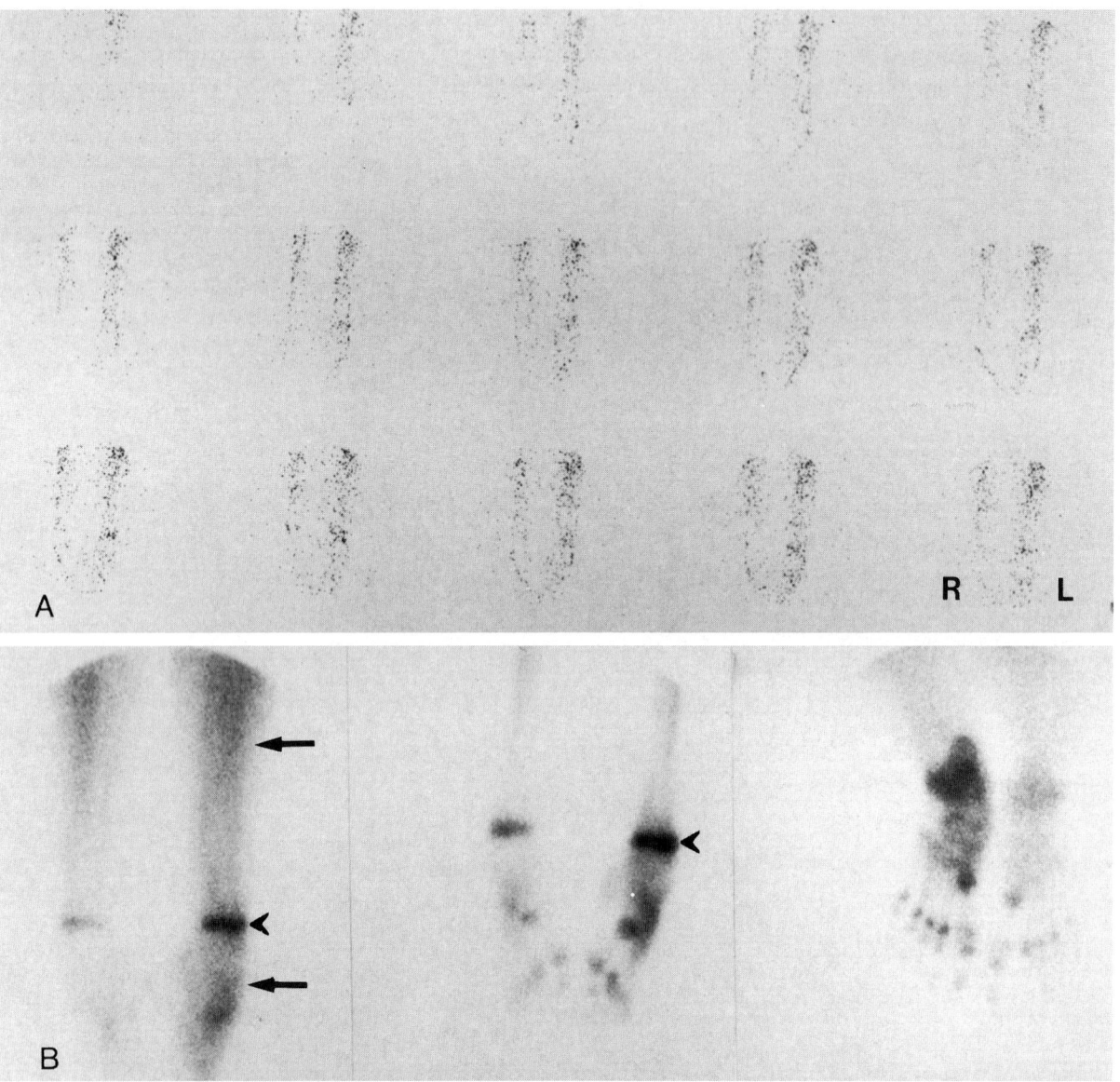

Figure 55.8. Reflex Sympathetic Dystrophy. Three phase bone scan in a 13-year-old with a painful left ankle and foot. **A.** The initial bolus, filmed at 1 second per frame in the anterior projection with heels together, arrives in the left foot (*L*) and ankle earlier than the right foot (*R*). **B.** The early blood pool image (*left*) shows greater blood pooling (*arrows*) in the same area. The 3-hour delayed images (*center* and *right*, anterior and plantar projections, respectively) show a generalized increase in bone labeling. Note the preferential labeling of the physeal plates, which is expected in a juvenile patient.

tion of tissues may be shown with bone scans (Fig. 55.10).

Bone Dysplasias. Benign bone dysplasias frequently show the expected increase in labeling on bone scans. Paget's disease of bone, fibrous dysplasia, enchondromas, exostoses, and many other benign conditions of bone are detected by bone scan. Comparison with skeletal radiographs will clarify these multicentric diagnoses. An efficient way to screen the whole skeleton is the bone scan. In the osteolytic phase of Paget's disease of bone, the radiographic changes are accompanied by marked increases in bone labeling. This repair continues with increased labeling during the radiographic stage of sclerotic, expansile pagetic bone. The increased activity on bone scans may eventually disappear as repair is complete (Fig. 55.11). Fibrous dysplasia is a benign condition of bone that may be polyostotic. It is readily detected by bone scans because of its intense bone labeling.

Primary Bone Tumors. There are two principle ways in which bone tumors are detected by bone scans. Osteosarcomas and chondrosarcomas may have abnormal osteoblastic or chondroblastic activity associated with the production of abnormal tumor calcification. This is a malignant process with the tumor itself being "hot" (Figs. 55.12, 55.13). Metastases from calcifying or ossifying primary tumors to other nonskeletal sites may also take up Tc-99m diphosphonates directly, making them readily detected by scintigraphy. The Tc-99m

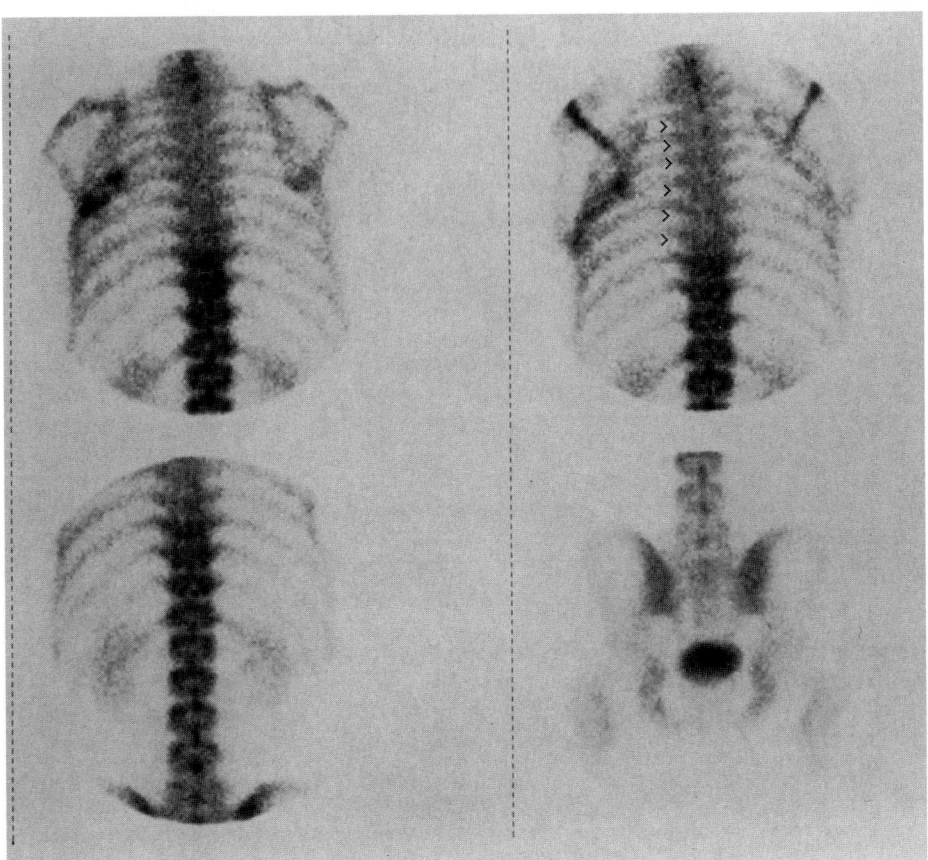

Figure 55.9. Radiation Therapy Changes. Decreased uptake is seen in the thoracic spine (*arrowheads*) within the radiotherapy portal. Note reactive changes in the lateral left ribs where a lateral thoracotomy was performed in this patient with bronchogenic carcinoma of the lung.

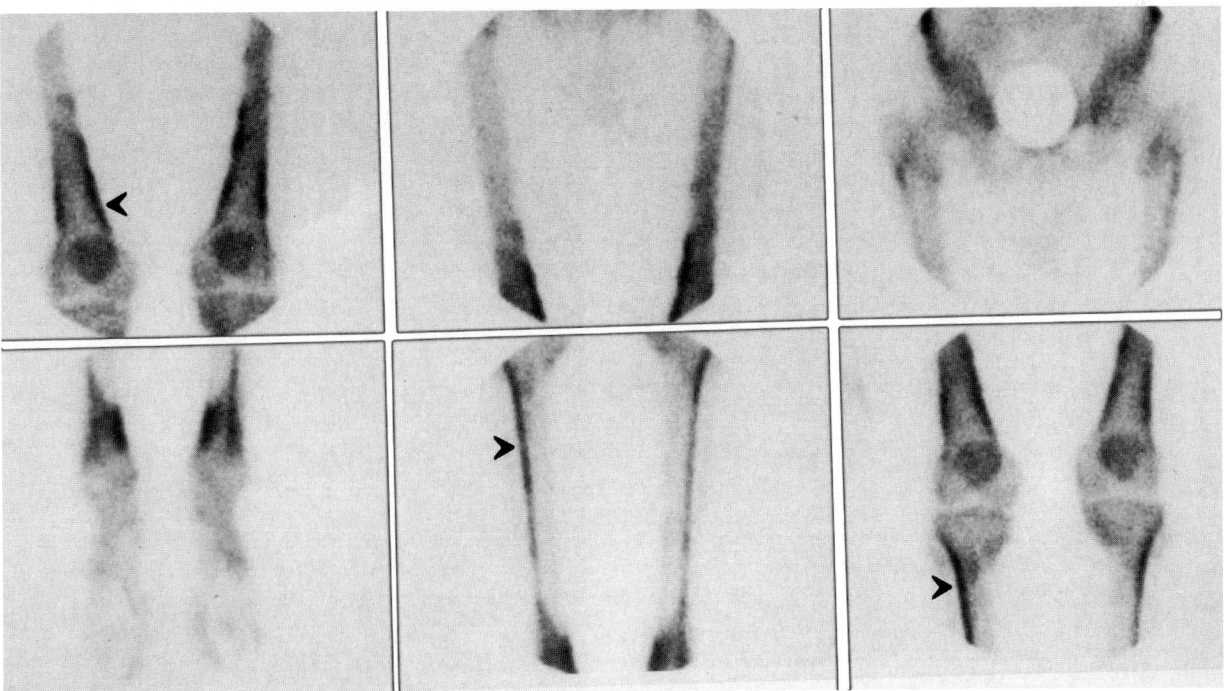

Figure 55.10. Hypertrophic Osteoarthropathy. A scan done to evaluate for metastases in a patient with carcinoma of the lung shows increased periosteal labeling (*arrowheads*), principally in the metaphyses of the lower extremity. The patient does not have metastases.

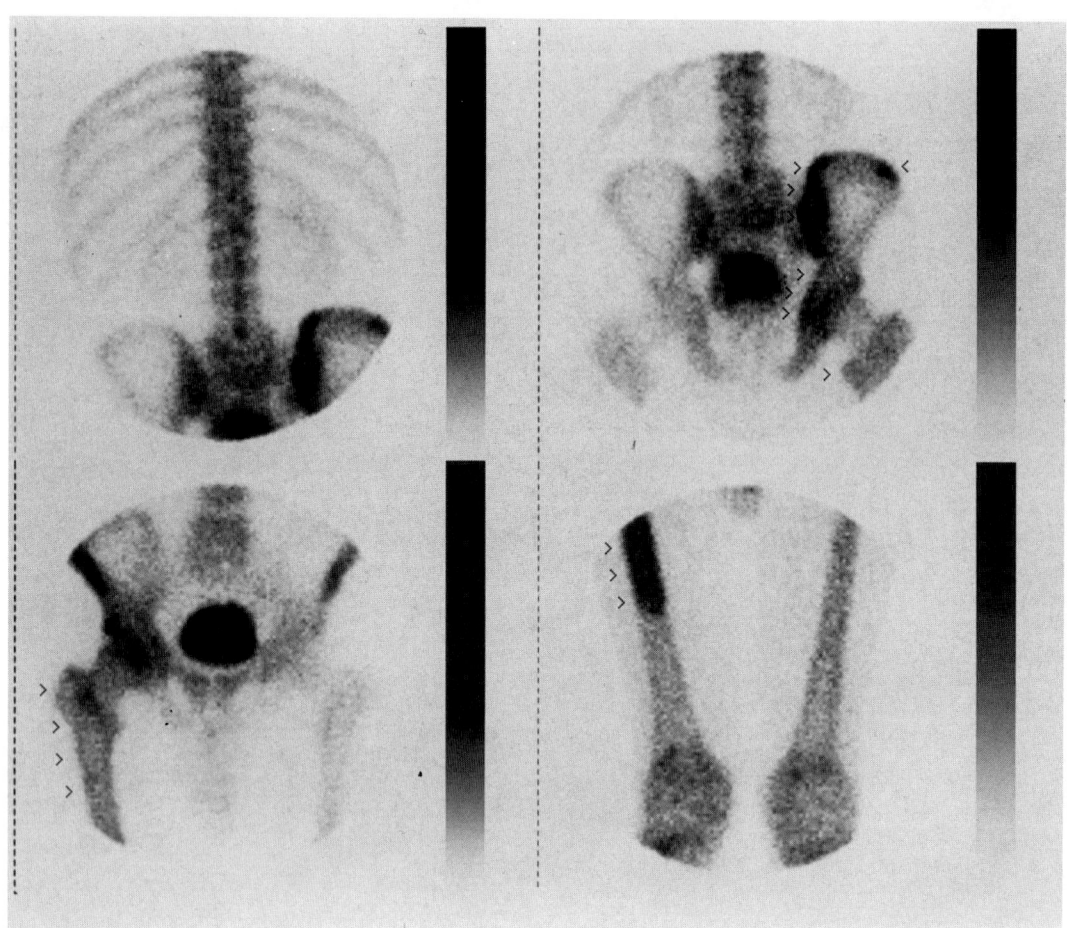

Figure 55.11. Paget's Disease of Bone. Image of the pelvis and femurs of a 60-year-old man with carcinoma of the prostate. There is abnormal, increased uptake in the right hemipelvis and proximal right femur (*arrowheads*), which is characteristic of pagetic bone. Note the distal "flame edge" of the pagetic portion of the femur. The patient does not have metastatic cancer.

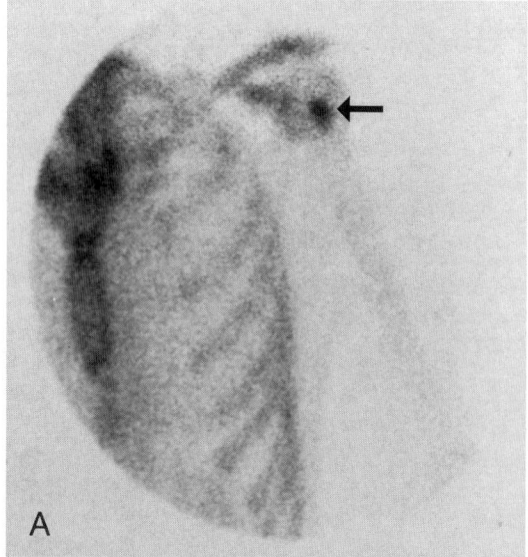

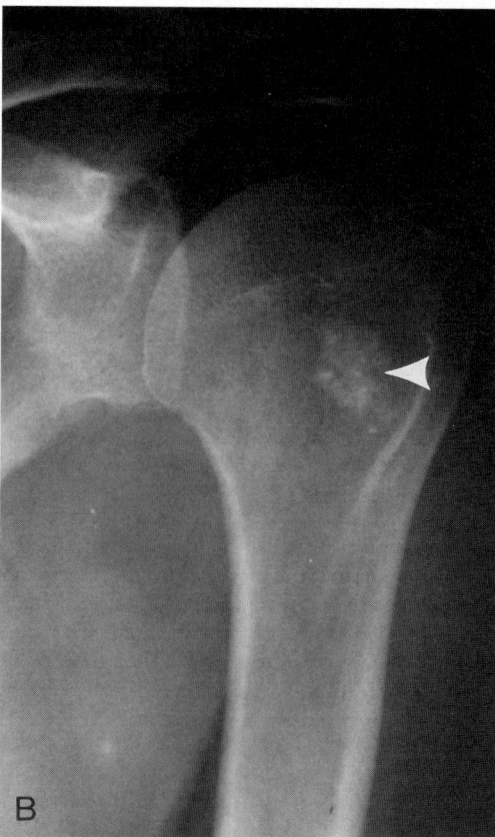

Figure 55.12. Low-grade Chondrosarcoma. A. An area of reactive bone (*arrow*) is seen in the proximal left humeral metaphysis. **B.** A radiograph shows the calcified cartilaginous matrix (*arrowhead*) of this tumor.

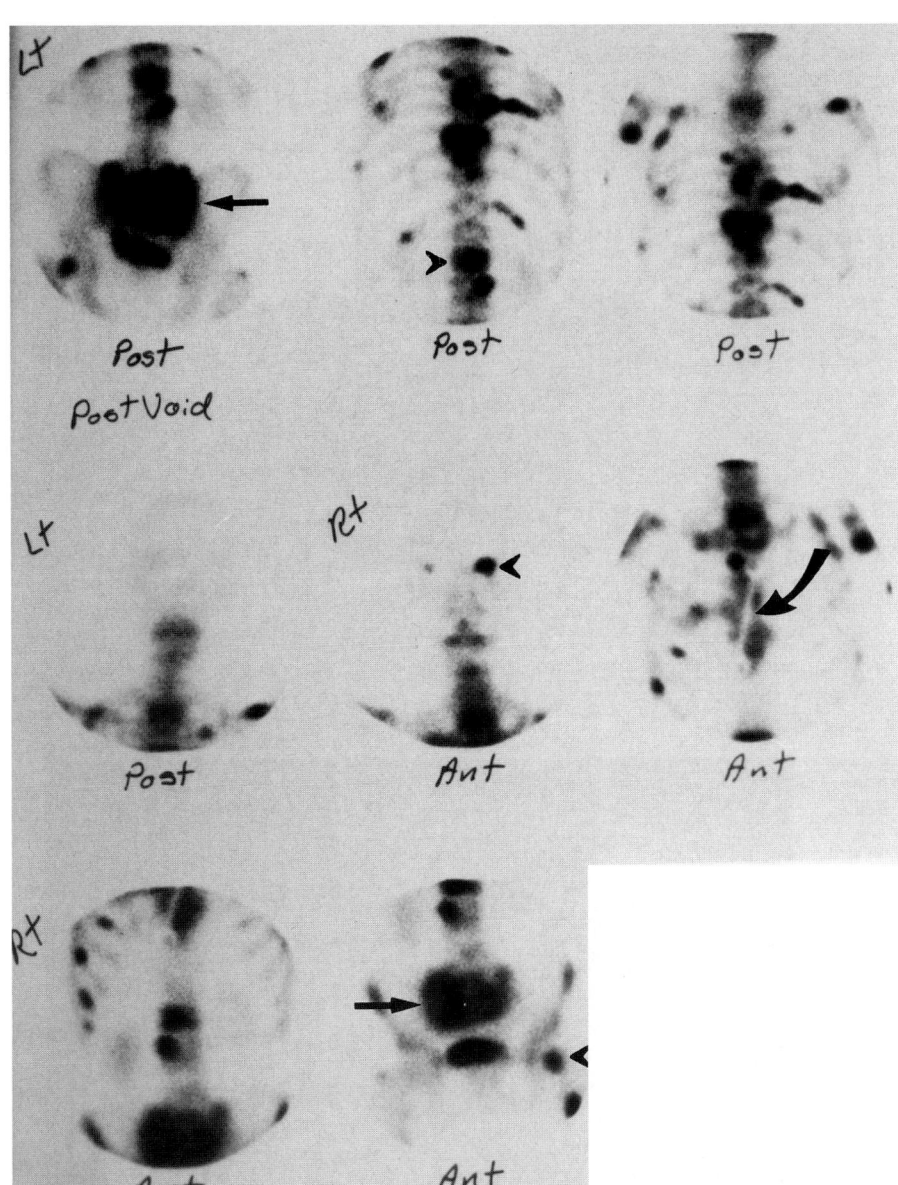

Figure 55.13. Osteogenic Sarcoma and Metastases. A 65-year-old man with a bone marrow burden of plutonium. A large primary tumor replaced the sacrum (*arrows*) and is seen as the most intense area of uptake. The balance of the skeleton shows multiple metastases (*arrowheads*), which have similarly intense labeling. There is a wrench (*curved arrow*) projecting over the sternum. The patient kept it to adjust a mechanical collar he wore for the last 6 months of his life because of extensive cervical vertebral metastases that threatened quadriplegia.

diphosphonate may also be avidly concentrated by the normal osteoblasts reacting to the destructive presence of the primary tumor. This common process makes the bone adjacent to tumors much more intense than the surrounding bone. Some malignancies may arise in the soft tissues adjacent to bone and invade through periosteum into the bone. In either case, the resulting reactive osteoblastic changes show the extent of invasion without showing the tumor itself. An extremely destructive bone tumor may destroy bone more quickly than repair can be effected. Thus, a "cold" defect in a bone with a primary malignancy is an indication of an aggressive tumor. High-grade sarcomas may show this phenomenon.

Metastatic Malignancy. The most common use of the bone scan is for the detection and monitoring of metastatic tumor involving the skeleton. The tumors monitored include prostate, lung, breast, thyroid, and renal carcinoma among many others. The majority of metastases afflict the axial skeleton in a pattern that re-

flects the distribution of the erythropoietic marrow. The likelihood of a metastasis peripheral to erythropoietic marrow is low. Most metastases are multiple at the time of discovery. Comparison bone scans at intervals of 3–6 months allow an accurate assessment of tumor spread (Fig. 55.14).

A knowledge of a given primary tumor's propensity to metastasize to the skeleton is helpful for scan interpretation. Confusion arises if an inexperienced observer cannot distinguish between common degenerative or post-traumatic changes and metastases. Merely counting the hot spots is of little value in the management of oncologic problems. Experience is necessary to judge metastatic disease in the skeleton. As metastases progress and regress, increases in labeling reflect the status of repair bone, not the status of the metastases. Increased numbers and size of individual lesions usually indicates that the tumor load of the skeleton is expanding. Increased *intensity* of the individual lesions (in the absence of new le-

Figure 55.14. Superscan. Numerous prostate cancer metastases produce "hot" spots of intense isotope accumulation that leave little or none of the radiopharmaceutical for renal excretion.

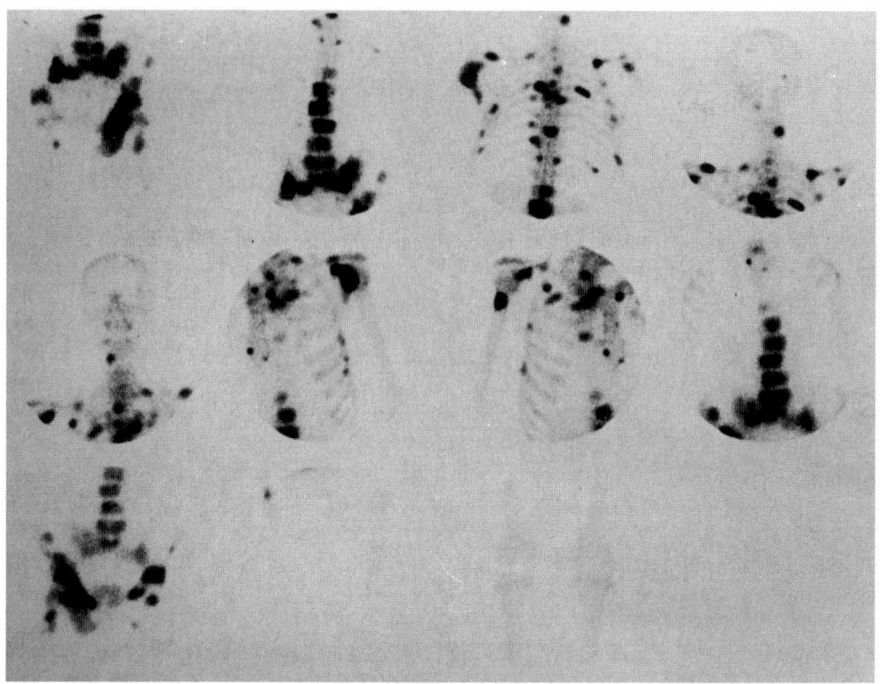

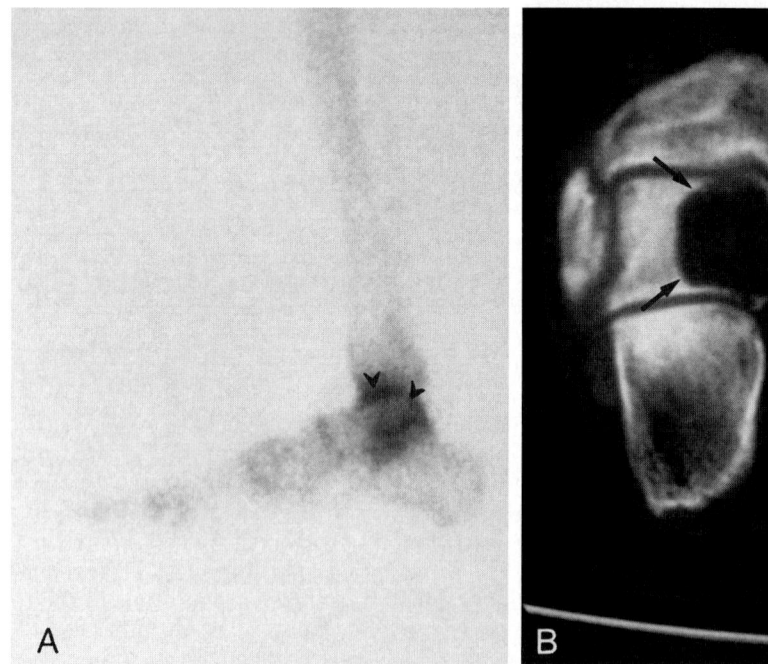

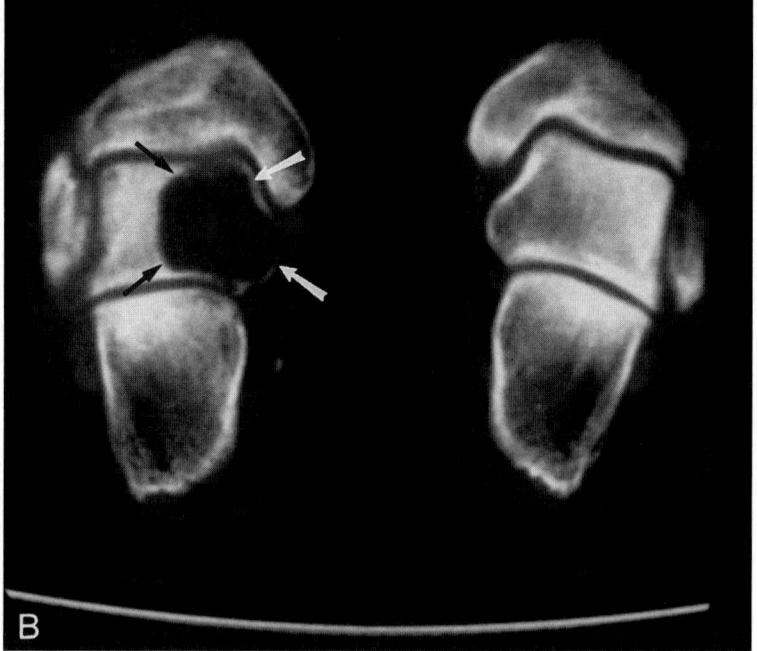

Figure 55.15. Aggressive Metastasis. A. A medial projection bone scan of the ankle and foot of a patient with renal cell carcinoma shows a halo of increased activity (*arrowheads*) around the ankle joint. **B.** A CT scan of the ankles shows a scooped out lesion (*arrows*) of the right talus where the metastasis has destroyed bone so fast that repair bone has no chance to form. The talus does not show a hot spot. The bone scan is abnormal because of hemarthrosis irritation of the synovium. Increased blood supplied to the inflamed synovium brings with it increased radiopharmaceutical, which labels all of the bones of the joint.

sions) frequently means that the tumor has become static and that the osteoblasts around it are engaged in vigorous repair. This "flare" response is usually a good indicator that a tumor has been checked by therapy.

Aggressive metastases may destroy bone so quickly that there is no repair (Fig. 55.15). Special attention should also be paid to those metastases in a critical, weight-bearing bone such as the femur. Early detection and treatment can prevent pathologic fractures that add to the suffering of a terminal illness. The bone scan can guide biopsy in cases where pathologic diagnosis of a bone lesion is required (Fig. 55.16).

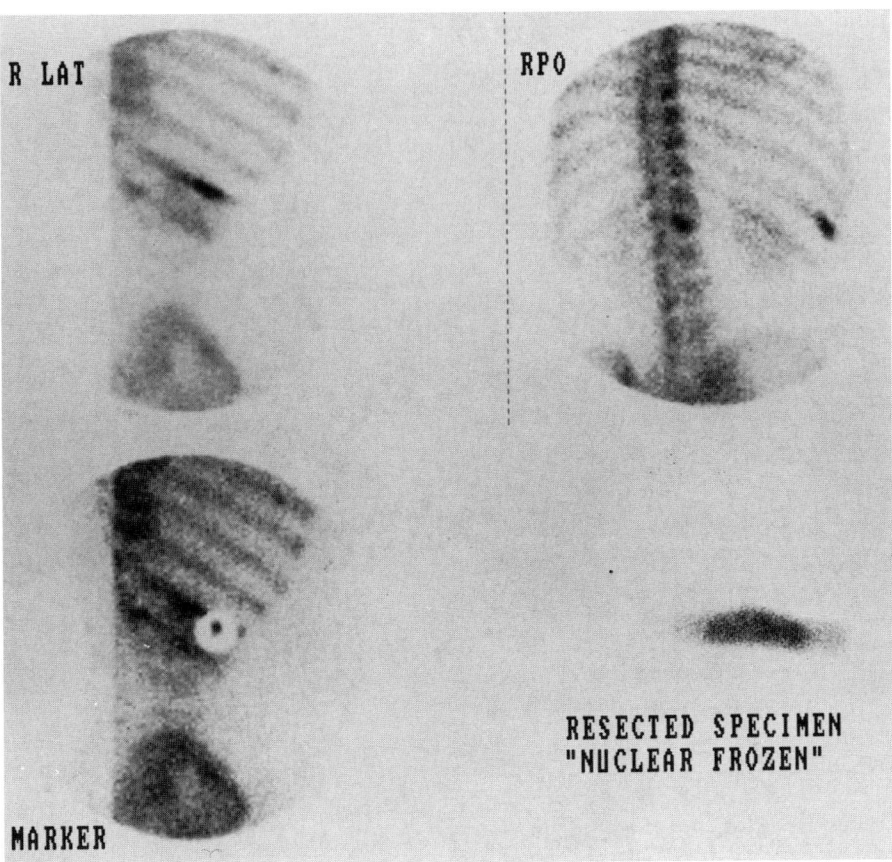

Figure 55.16. Resection of a Solitary Metastasis. A solitary metastasis from an adenocarcinoma of unknown origin is located with a "cold" lead ring maneuvered over the right lateral rib lesion before surgery to locate the correct rib for resection. On the way to the surgical pathologist, the resected rib was imaged to confirm that the correct rib had been resected.

Suggested Readings

Collier BD, Hellman RS, Krasnow AZ. Bone SPECT. Semin Nucl Med 1987;17:247–266.

Drane WE. Myositis ossificans and the three-phase bone scan. AJR Am J Roentgenol 1984;142:179–180.

Kozin F, Soin JS, Ryan LM, et al. Bone scintigraphy in the reflex sympathetic dystrophy syndrome. Radiology 1981;138:437–443.

Matin P. Bone scintigraphy in the diagnosis and management of traumatic injury. Semin Nucl Med 1983;8:108–122.

Maurer AH, Chen DCP, Carmago EE, et al. Utility of three-phase skeletal scintigraphy in suspected osteomyelitis: concise communication. J Nucl Med 1981;22:941–949.

Merkow RL, Jane JM. Current concepts of Paget's disease of bone. Orthop Clin North Am 1984;15:747–763.

McNeil BJ. Value of bone scanning in neoplastic disease. Semin Nucl Med 1984;14:277–286.

Orzel JA, Rudd TG. Heterotopic bone formation: clinical laboratory and imaging correlation. J Nucl Med 1985;26:125–132.

Rosenthal DI, Chandler HC, Azizi R, et al. Uptake of bone agents by diffuse pulmonary metastatic calcifications. AJR Am J Roentgenol 1977;129:871–874.

Schauwecker DS. The scintigraphic diagnosis of osteomyelitis. AJR Am J Roentgenol 1992;158:9–18.

Schuster HL, Sadowski D, Friedman JM. Radionuclide bone imaging as an aid in the diagnosis of fibrous dysplasia. J Oral Surg 1979;37:267–270.

Stevenson JS, Bright RW, Dunson GL, et al. Technetium-99m phosphate bone imaging: a method for assessing bone graft healing. Radiology 1974;110:391–396.

Subramanian G, McAfee JG, Blair RJ, et al. Technetium-99m-methylene diphosphonate-a superior agent for skeletal imaging: comparison with other technetium complexes. J Nucl Med 1975;18:744–755.

Sullivan DC, Rosenfield NS, Ogden J, Gottschalk A. Problems in the scintigraphic detection of osteomyelitis in children. Radiology 1980;135:731–736.

Tyler JL, Derbekyan V, Lisbona R. Early diagnosis of myositis ossificans with Technetium-99m diphosphonate imaging. Clin Nucl Med 1984;9:256–258.

Wellman H, Schauwecker D, Robb JA, et al. Skeletal scinti-imaging and radiography in the diagnosis and management of Paget's disease. Clin Orthop 1977;127:55–62.

Weiss PE, Mall JC, Hoffer PB, et al. 99m Tc-methylene diphosphonate bone imaging in the evaluation of total hip prosthesis. Radiology 1979;133:727–729.

Williamson BR, McLaughlin RE, Wang GJ, et al. Radionuclide bone imaging as a means of differentiating loosening and infection in patients with a painful total hip prosthesis. Radiology 1979;133:723–725.

56
Pulmonary Scintigraphy

Rhonda A. Wyatt

A scintigraphic lung scan is a physiologic map that evaluates the primary functions of the lung, pulmonary vasculature perfusion, and segmental bronchioalveolar tree ventilation. Most commonly, ventilation-perfusion (V/Q) scans are used to evaluate patients suspected of having pulmonary thromboembolism (PE). Although the techniques for performing V/Q scans have not changed much since their introduction in the 1960s, in an attempt to provide more accurate results, the criteria for interpreting the studies have been constantly revised. Different schema that compare defects present on the perfusion scan with those found on the ventilation scan and/or chest x-ray (CXR) have been developed in order to estimate the probability of PE. This chapter describes radiopharmaceuticals used, examination technique, imaging protocols, and criteria for the interpretation of V/Q scans.

ANATOMY AND PHYSIOLOGY

Understanding the segmental anatomy of the lungs (Fig. 56.1) is vital to the interpretation of lung scans. The three-dimensional location of ventilation or perfusion defects must be individually determined and correlated with the segmental or subsegmental anatomy of the lung. Pulmonary embolism will have a segmental or subsegmental distribution pattern. This visual pattern is the fundamental diagnostic feature of pulmonary embolism.

Although pulmonary ventilation occurs primarily via the branching bronchial system, other pathways exist by which distal alveoli can be aerated. The pores of Kohn connect adjacent alveoli, and the canals of Lambert connect alveoli with respiratory, terminal, and preterminal bronchioles. These canals and pores permit collateral ventilation of alveoli whose conducting airways have become blocked. Collateral air drift is dynamic and is mediated by neurohormonal control that can be altered by pathologic events, atmospheric/alveolar gas tension, and drugs.

Ventilation and pulmonary blood flow both demonstrate marked gravity effects. When a patient is in an upright posture, the gradient for blood flow is from the apices to the lung bases; the apex receives only one-third of the blood volume that the base receives. A corresponding ventilation gradient exists when the patient sits upright. Since the intrapleural pressure is less at the bases, the differential negative intrapleural pressure at the apices causes alveoli there to remain more open at expiration than basilar alveoli. Therefore, basilar alveoli undergo greater respiratory cycle changes in size. This results in greater gas exchange occurring in the base compared to the apex. On average, ventilation at the base is 1.5–2 times that of the apex. When a patient is supine, the ventilation gradient shifts from superioinferior to anteroposterior, and perfusion is increased to the dependent posterior portions of the lungs (1).

Normally, capillary perfusion and alveolar ventilation are matched in order to maximize gas exchange. Diseases that produce localized hypoxia invoke autoregulatory mechanisms that divert blood flow away from the hypoxemic pulmonary segments. These dynamic changes prevent nonventilated lung segments from being perfused. Conversely, localized hypoperfusion rarely induces localized bronchoconstriction. Thus, primary vascular disorders such as pulmonary embolism, if unassociated with parenchymal consolidation or pulmonary infarction, usually have normal ventilation (1).

VENTILATION LUNG SCAN

Radiopharmaceuticals

Xenon-133. Xe-133 is a radioisotope widely used to perform ventilation lung scans. A noble gas produced by fission of U-235 in a nuclear reactor, Xe-133 has a half-life of 5.3 days, and it decays by beta minus emission. The emitted beta-particle (374 keV) is responsible for most of the radiation dose delivered to the lungs. The principle photon energy is 81 keV. Xe-133 ventilation scans should be performed before perfusion lung scans because Compton scatter from the higher energy Tc-99m macroaggregated albumin (MAA) downscatters into the

Figure 56.1. Pulmonary Segment Anatomy. Broncho-pulmonary segments of the right lung: *1)* apical; *2)* posterior; *3)* anterior; *4)* lateral; *5)* medial; *6)* superior; *7)* medial basal; *8)* posterior basal; *9)* lateral basal; *10)* anterior basal. Bronchopulmonary segments of the left lung; *11)* apical posterior; *12)* anterior; *13)* superior lingual; *14)* inferior lingual; *15)* superior; *16)* anterior medial; *17)* lateral basal; *18)* posterior basal. *LPO,* left posterior oblique; *POST,* posterior; *RPO,* right posterior oblique; *RAO,* right anterior oblique, *ANT,* anterior; *LAO,* left anterior oblique; *RLAT,* right lateral; *LLAT,* left lateral. (Adapted with minor modifications from Sostman HD, Gottschalk A. Diagnostic nuclear medicine. 2nd ed. Baltimore: Williams & Wilkins, 1988:513.)

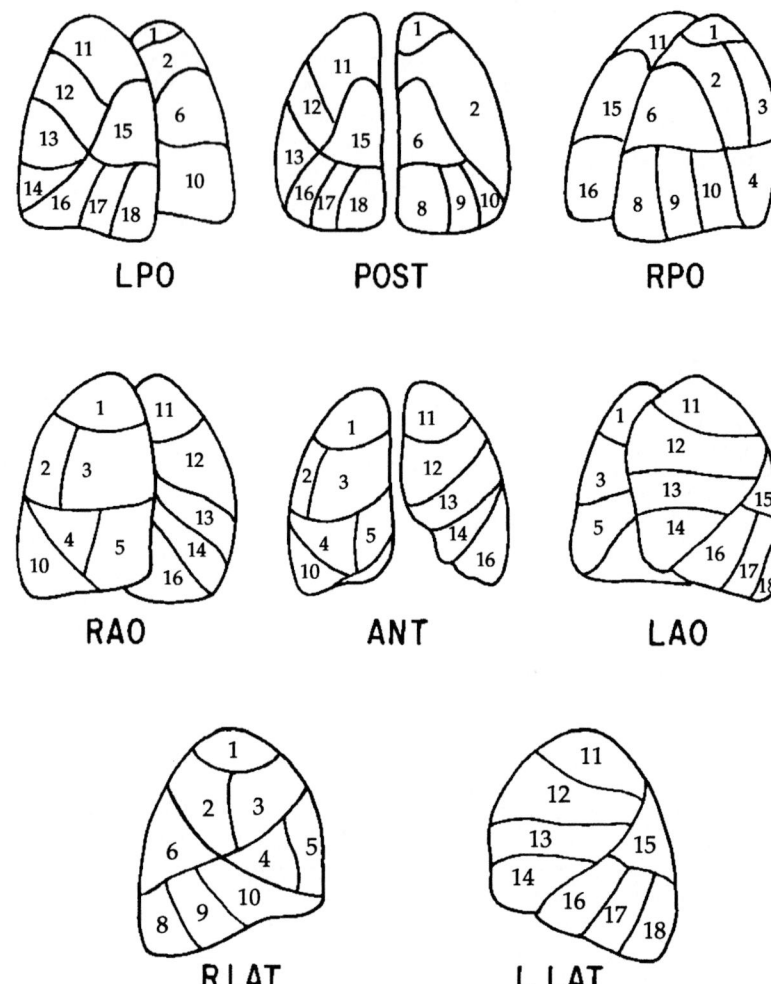

region of the 81 keV photopeak of the Xe-133 and would thus interfere with ventilation images. Soft tissue attenuation of the low-energy 81 keV photons is significant, yielding relatively poor resolution images. The usual adult dose of Xe-133 for a ventilation scan is 10–20 mCi (370–540 MBq).

Xenon-127. Xe-127 is a cyclotron-produced isotope with a physical half-life of 36.4 days. It decays by electron capture with principle photon energies of 203 keV (65%), 172 keV (22%), and 365 keV (18%). Because it has energy photons, Xe-127 ventilation scans can be performed after the perfusion scan, since downscatter image deterioration is not a significant problem. If the perfusion scan is normal, a ventilation scan is not necessary. Conversely, if the perfusion scan is abnormal, the Xe-127 scan can be performed in the projection that best demonstrates segments corresponding to perfusion defects. Unfortunately, because Xe-127 is cyclotron-produced, it is both expensive and of limited availability. The usual adult dose is 8–15 mCi (296–555 MBq). The higher energy of Xe-127 necessitates the use of a medium-energy collimator and requires that more shielding be used. Because of its longer half-life, the gas must be stored much longer prior to disposal.

Krypton-81m. Kr-81m is the other noble gas used for ventilation scans. Having an extremely short half-life of only 13 seconds, Kr-81m is produced from a Rb-81-Kr-81m generator. Kr-81m decays by isomeric transition and has a 191 keV photon energy. The Rb-81 parent has a half-life of only 4.7 hours, and the Rb-81-Kr-81m generator also has a short life span of approximately 1 day. Rubidium-81 is cyclotron-produced; therefore, the generator is expensive and of limited availability. As a result, using Kr-81m is only practical at institutions that conduct a high volume of lung scans. The short half-life of Kr-81m eliminates the need for storage and disposal of radioactive gas. It can be directly vented into the room as long as the room has good air circulation. The usual adult dose is 10–20 mCi (370–740 MBq).

Technetium-99m Aerosols. Ventilation scans can be performed using aerosolized rather than gaseous agents. Radioisotope-labeled aerosols are produced by nebulizing radiopharmaceuticals into a fine mist that is inhaled. Tc-99m diethylenetriaminepentaacetic acid (DTPA) is the most commonly used radioaerosol. Historically, In-111 or In-113m DTPA and colloids have also been used for this purpose. The advantages of Tc-99m aerosols are that they are widely available, inexpensive, and most importantly have a 140 keV photopeak ideal for gamma camera imaging. Shielded nebulizers produce a fine mist when air or oxygen is forced through a reservoir holding the radioisotope. The mist is passed through a settling bag, which traps larger particles. The mist is delivered to the patient via a nonrebreathing valve and is inhaled. The process is inefficient; only 2–10% of the aerosolized radioisotope is deposited within the lungs. Of 30 mCi of nebulized Tc-99m DTPA, only 1–2 mCi actually are deposited within the lungs.

The site of deposition of the aerosolized particles depends on the size of the inhaled particle. The larger the particle, the greater the gravitational effect and the more central the site of deposition. Particles larger than 2 microns localize in the trachea and pharynx. Current aerosol nebulizers can produce microaerosols of less than 0.5 microns. Thus, microaerosol particles are small enough to reach the distal portions of the tracheobrochial tree. Microaerosol localization reflects regional ventilation. Localized airway turbulence owing to airway narrowing affects deposition of aerosol particles. The greater the turbulence, the higher the likelihood of particles impacting the walls of an airway and depositing there. Patients with narrowed airways caused by asthma, bronchitis, or chronic obstructive pulmonary disease (COPD) have more central deposition of the particles than normal patients. This results in poor visualization of the peripheral lung fields. The clearance half-life of Tc-99m aerosols from the lungs is 60–90 minutes. The half-life is approximately 20 minutes shorter in tobacco smokers, owing to their increased alveolar permeability.

Dosimetry. The critical organ for Xe-133 is the trachea, which receives a dose of 0.64 rad/mCi. The lung dose is 0.01–0.04 rad/mCi whereas the whole-body absorbed dose is 0.001 rad/mCi. Xenon-127 has no particulate emission, and its higher energy photons are absorbed less by soft tissues than Xe-133. As a result, the total dose to the lungs from Xe-127 is approximately one-third that of Xe-133.

The lungs are the critical organ for Kr-81m ventilation scans, having an absorbed dose of 0.05 rad per 20 mCi/min whereas the whole-body absorbed dose is 0.001 rad per 20 mCi/min.

The lungs are also the critical organ for ventilation scans using Tc-99m aerosols. The lungs receive an absorbed dose of 0.1 rad/mCi, the bladder wall a dose of 0.18 rad/mCi, and the entire body a dose of 0.01 rad/mCi.

Ventilation Scan Technique

Ventilation scanning using radioactive gases requires special equipment to prevent leakage of the gas into the imaging room. Gas delivery systems consist of a shielded spirometer, oxygen delivery system, and a xenon charcoal trap. The room in which ventilation scans are performed should be well ventilated and have negative pressure flow. Because xenon is heavier than air, it pools at floor level.

Xenon-133 Ventilation Scanning. The patient is initially fitted with an air-tight face mask. While he or she takes a maximal inspiration, Xe-133 is injected into the mask intake tubing and exhaled xenon is vented to the xenon trap. The patient is instructed to hold his or her breath as long as possible. A posterior projection 100,000 count first-breath image of the lungs is then obtained. The ventilation system is switched so that the patient rebreathes the air–Xe-133 mixture. After 5 minutes of rebreathing, a posterior 100,000 count equilibrium image is obtained. The distribution of Xe-133 activity on the equilibrium image represents aerated lung volume. The ventilation system is readjusted so that the patient breathes in fresh air and exhales the Xe-133 mixture into a trap. Serial posterior 30-second washout images are obtained over a 5-minute interval. The Xe-133 normally washes out of the lungs within 3–4 minutes (2). Because the lung bases are better ventilated than the apices, the Xe-133 washes out of the bases faster than the apices in a normal patient. If possible, all images should be performed with the patient in an upright position.

Xenon-127 Ventilation Scanning is performed in the same manner as Xe-133 ventilation lung scans. The Xe-127 ventilation scan need be performed only if the perfusion scan is abnormal.

Krypton-81m Ventilation Scanning. The high-photon energy of Kr-81m allows ventilation scans to follow perfusion scans. Kr-81m images are matched to each perfusion scan image. Immediately after each perfusion image and without moving, the patient inhales Kr-81m and the corresponding ventilation image is obtained. This process is repeated until ventilation and perfusion images are obtained in all six positions. Because of its very short half-life, Kr-81m activity in the lungs is proportional to regional ventilation and images are equivalent to single-breath Xe-133 images. Krypton-81m decays before equilibrium occurs; therefore, equilibrium and washout images are not possible. However, repeat images can be obtained as needed.

Technetium-99m Aerosol Ventilation Scanning. The patient inhales the nebulized aerosol while in the supine position to avoid the normal apex to base gravity gradient. After inhaling the Tc-99m aerosol for 3–5 minutes, the patient sits upright and is imaged in the same positions as for the perfusion lung scan. Because the Tc-99m aerosol remains fixed in the lungs for several minutes after deposition, obtaining ventilation images in different positions is possible. The exhaled aerosol is trapped in a filter that is stored until decay is sufficient for safe disposal. Because breath-holding and deep-breathing maneuvers are not needed, the aerosol ventilation scan requires little active patient cooperation and is much easier to perform in critically ill patients.

A Tc-99m aerosol ventilation lung scan can be performed either before or after the perfusion lung scan. If the perfusion scan is performed first, a small dose (0.5 mCi) of Tc-99m MAA is used with a large dose (30 mCi) of Tc-99m DTPA. If the ventilation scan is performed first, 5–10 mCi of Tc-99m DTPA and 5 mCi of Tc-99m MAA are administered.

PERFUSION LUNG SCAN

Radiopharmaceuticals

Perfusion lung scanning is based on the principal of capillary blockade. Particles slightly larger than the pulmonary capillaries (>8 microns) are injected intravenously and travel to the right heart where venous blood is uniformly mixed. Radiolabeled particles in the pulmonary arterial blood pass into the distal pulmonary circulation. Because the radioactive particles are larger than the capillaries, they lodge in the precapillary arterioles. Their distribution in the lung reflects the relative blood flow to pulmonary segments. Pulmonary segments with decreased or absent blood flow show diminished radioactivity.

Tc-99m-MAA is the radiopharmaceutical used to perform most perfusion lung scans. MAA is prepared by heat denaturation of human serum albumin. The MAA particles are irregularly shaped molecules with size range and the number of particles in commercially available kits tightly controlled. Most particles are in the 20–40 micron size range with 90% of the particles between 10–90 microns. Particles larger than 150 microns should not be injected because they can obstruct arterioles. The size and number of particles in a kit are checked by counting a sample volume in a light microscopy hemocytometer. Tc-99m-MAA is prepared by adding Tc-99m-pertechnetate (Tc-99mO_4) to the MAA kit. The volume and activity of the Tc-99mO_4 determines the number of particles per mCi (MBq) in the Tc-99m-MAA solution. The biological half-life of MAA particles in the lung is 2–9 hours. The MAA leaves the lungs by breaking down into smaller particles that pass through the alveolar capillaries into the systemic circulation where they are removed by the reticuloendothelial system. The physical half-life of Tc-99m-MAA is 6 hours.

A minimum of 60,000 Tc-99m MAA particles must be injected to ensure reliable count statistics. Insufficient particles result in an inhomogeneous distribution that can result in false-positive scans. Typically 200,000–500,000 particles are injected. In the average human lung, approximately 280 million pulmonary arterioles/capillaries are present. Thus, about 1 vessel in 1000 is occluded in the perfusion scan. In most patients this large safety margin precludes any significant alteration of pulmonary hemodynamics. However, several types of patients should receive a reduced number of particles during a perfusion scan. Patients with pulmonary hypertension can destabilize with occlusion of even a small number of arterioles and should be given only 100,000 particles. Patients with right-to-left shunts should also be administered fewer particles because the shunt allows particles to bypass the lungs, become lodged in systemic peripheral vascular beds, and cause capillary blockade in the heart, kidneys, and brain. Because they have fewer pulmonary arterioles than adults, children should also be injected with only 100,000 particles. To perform reduced count imaging, each perfusion view is imaged for a longer time interval allowing for nearly equivalent count statistics.

Alternatively, the kit can be reconstituted with higher than usual Tc-99m activity per particle. The normal 5 mCi dose can be administered, but with fewer particles. The kit manufacturer usually provides instructions regarding altering the number of injected particles. Contraindications to perfusion lung scanning include severe pulmonary hypertension and allergy to human serum albumin products.

Human Albumin Microspheres **(HAM)** have previously been used for perfusion lung scans. However, a significant number of allergic reactions to HAM particles has been reported and HAM is no longer commercially available in the United States.

Dosimetry. The normal adult dose is 3–5 mCi (111–185 MBq). The lung is the critical organ and receives an absorbed dose of 0.15–0.5 rad/mCi. The whole body and gonadal absorbed dose are 0.15 rad/mCi.

Perfusion Scan Technique

The syringe containing the Tc-99m MAA should be gently agitated prior to injection to resuspend all particles. The patient is injected in the supine position while taking slow, deep breaths to minimize the pulmonary perfusion gravitational gradient (2). Blood should not be drawn into the syringe because aspirated blood may form clots, which become labeled by the Tc-99m MAA. Injection of clumped Tc-99m MAA particles or labeled clot can result in multiple focal hot spots scattered through the lungs. If this occurs, the remainder of the lung is poorly visualized and significant findings may be obscured.

The patient is imaged after the injection is completed using a large field of view, high-resolution gamma camera. If the patient's condition permits, he or she is imaged in the upright sitting position. The upright position provides the best lung expansion and improves visualization of small defects—especially at the lung bases. Images (500,000 count) are obtained in the anterior, posterior, right lateral, left lateral, right posterior oblique, and left posterior oblique positions. Supplemental anterior oblique and decubitus views can be added to clarify findings on the standard views.

V/Q SCANS

Indications. The most common indication for V/Q scans is diagnosis of suspected PE. This examination has also been used to monitor pulmonary function of lung transplants, to provide preoperative estimates of lung function in lung carcinoma patients in whom pneumonectomy is planned (split lung function study), to evaluate right to left shunts, and to conduct serial assessment of inflammatory lung disease. The CXR should be evaluated prior to obtaining a V/Q scan. Infiltrates, effusions, pulmonary edema, or pneumothorax may explain sudden respiratory deterioration and eliminate the need for a V/Q scan.

Normal Ventilation Scans (Fig. 56.2A) have homogeneous radiopharmaceutical distribution throughout all lung fields on all three phases of the scan. A subtle base-to-apex gradient may be seen because more lung parenchyma is located at the base than the apex. The first-breath Xe-133 image is often grainy because it has relatively poor count statistics. However, it still reflects regional lung volume. The equilibrium images look similar to first-breath images but have greater activity. The washout phase of the study demonstrates rapid clearance of the Xe-133 from the lungs. Normal half-time for xenon washout is less than 1 minute. Washout is complete within 3 minutes. Retention (trapping) of xenon in the lungs in a focal or diffuse pattern is an indication of obstructive lung disease (Fig. 56.3).

Xe-127 scans are similar to Xe-133 scans except that the image borders are more sharply defined. The higher photon energy of Xe-127 is less attenuated by the soft tissues. Krypton-81m scans are first-breath images because of the ultrashort half-life of Kr-81m. Kr-81m images appear similar to Xe-133 images except faint tracer activity can be visualized within the trachea on Kr-81m scans.

Tc-99m DTPA aerosol scans resemble Tc-99m MAA perfusion scans. However, activity is normally also present within the trachea and mainstem bronchi. Central deposition of the Tc-99m aerosol may occur as a variant in smokers. Swallowed Tc-99m DTPA aerosol is sometimes seen within the esophagus and stomach.

Normal Perfusion Scans show well-defined margins of both lungs on all views with sharply defined costophrenic angles. A mild apex to base count activity gradient is present due to the physical difference in lung thickness of the base compared to the apex. Tracer distribution should otherwise be homogeneous (Fig. 56.2B).

The heart causes a smoothly defined defect along the left medial lung border that is curvilinear in all projections. A prominent, focal triangular margin suggests the presence of a perfusion defect abutting the heart. The hila are prominent even in normal patients. Focal asymmetric hilar perfusion defects are abnormal. Cardiomegaly, tortuosity of the aorta, and mediastinal or hilar enlargement cause defects along the medial border of the lung associated with less well defined corresponding defects on the ventilation scan. The size and shape of any mediastinal structure on the V/Q scan should match its appearance on the CXR.

Abnormal Scans. Focal defects or inhomogeneous tracer distribution are abnormal on either ventilation or perfusion scans. Focal perfusion defects should be compared with corresponding areas on the ventilation scan and vice versa. The relative size and shape of V/Q defects should then be correlated with corresponding areas on a recent CXR. The CXR should be obtained with the same patient position as the V/Q images; i.e., upright V/Q images should be compared to upright CXR. Ideally, the correlative CXR should have been performed no more than 6–12 hours prior to the V-Q scan. CXR findings may change rapidly in patients with deteriorating respiratory status.

Ventilation scans are abnormal if areas of delayed xenon wash-in or washout are present. Defects on the single-breath image may disappear on the equilibrium images when xenon bypasses obstructed pulmonary bronchioles through the pores of Kohn and canals of Lambert. Air drift through these alternate pathways permits the xenon to enter and leave the alveoli distal to obstruction. Movement by collateral air drift proceeds more

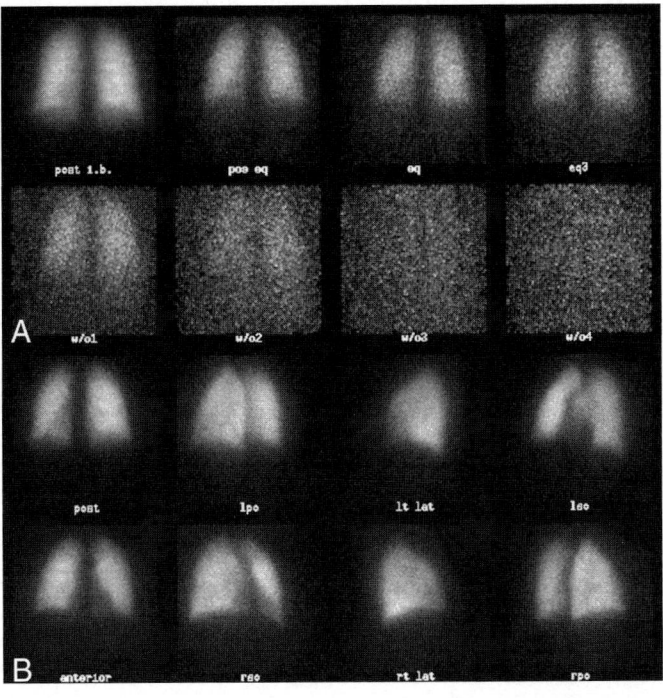

Figure 56.2. Normal V/Q Scan. A. Normal Xe-133 ventilation lung scan, top two rows. *post ib,* posterior initial breath; *pos eq,* posterior equilibrium; *eq,* equilibrium; *eq3,* equilibrium after 3 minutes; *wo/1,* 1 minute after start of washout; *wo/2,* 2-minute washout; *wo/3,* 3-minute washout; *wo/4,* 4-minute washout. **B. Normal Tc-99m MAA perfusion lung scan,** bottom two rows. *post,* posterior; *lpo,* left posterior oblique; *lt lat,* left lateral; *lao,* left anterior oblique; bottom row anterior; *rao,* right anterior oblique; *rt lat,* right lateral; *rpo,* right posterior oblique.

Figure 56.3. Chronic Obstructive Pulmonary Disease. A. Ventilation scan, posterior projection, top two rows. Obstructive changes in middle and upper lobes cause retention of Xe-133 on 4-minute washout image (*post wo/4*). *post ib,* posterior initial breath; *post eq,* posterior equilibrium; *lpo eq,* left posterior oblique equilibrium; *rpo eq,* right posterior oblique equilibruim; second row, post washout images 1–4 minutes. **B. Tc-99m MAA perfusion scan,** bottom two rows, labeling same as in Figure 56.2. Patchy, inhomogeneous uptake is seen primarily in middle and upper lung zones. Perfusion defects match those seen on initial breath image of the ventilation scan.

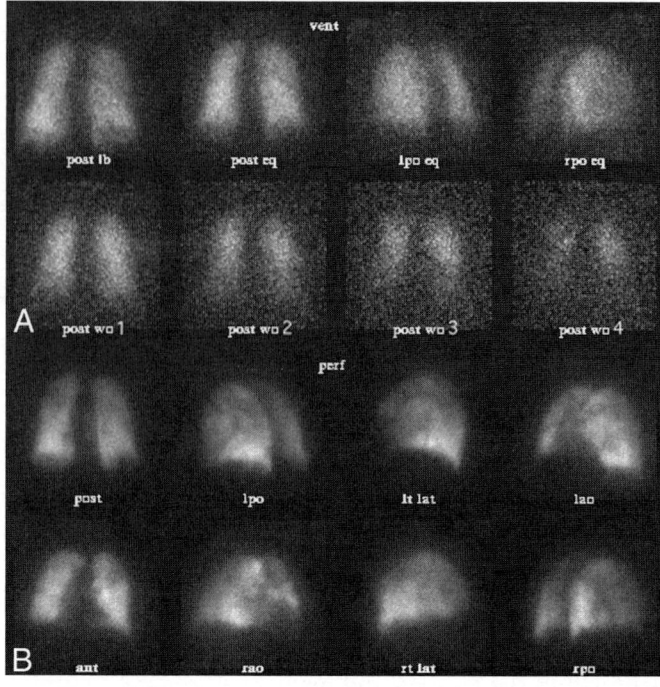

slowly than through the bronchioles, resulting in delayed wash-in and washout. Focal areas of abnormal retention therefore suggest focal obstructive lung disease (Fig. 56.3).

PULMONARY EMBOLISM

Pulmonary embolism is one of the common causes of death in the United States. Dahlen and Alpert (3) estimated that 30% of untreated patients with pulmonary embolism die as a consequence of their emboli, in comparison to 10–16% mortality for patients treated with anticoagulant therapy. Anticoagulants are, however, not a benign form of therapy. Anticoagulants place patients at significant risk for life-threatening bleeding and should not be prescribed without high probability for the diagnosis of thrombosis.

Pulmonary emboli originate from thrombi within the deep venous system of the legs and pelvis. Predisposing factors include prolonged immobilization, surgery (particularly intrapelvic or hip surgery), history of prior PE, preexisting cardiac disease, estrogen therapy (particularly in smokers), hypercoagualable states such as cancer, and congenital defects of thrombolysis.

PE is a very difficult to diagnose clinically. In 70% of patients who survive pulmonary emboli, the emboli may not be clinically suspected (4). The classic triad of dyspnea, hemoptysis, and pleuritic chest pain occurs in less than 20% of patients with pulmonary emboli. Larger emboli increase the likelihood of symptoms (5,6). Symptoms associated with PE, however, are nonspecific. Pulmonary or cardiac infection or inflammation, cancer, and pneumothorax produce similar symptoms. An electrocardiogram should be performed in patients sus-

pected of having PE to detect cardiac causes for chest pain or dyspnea. If a patient develops acute cor pulmonale because of pulmonary emboli, the electrocardiogram will show signs of right heart strain.

Radiographic Findings of PE. The CXR is normal in 12% of patients with PE. The classic findings are a wedge-shaped, pleural-based infarct (Hampton's hump), or a wedge-shaped area of oligemia (Westermark's sign). The most common CXR finding of patients with PE is atelectasis or opacities in the region with emboli (7).

Recently, spiral CT and MR have been used to diagnose pulmonary emboli. The sensitivity of spiral CT is 73–95 % with a specificity of 87–97% (8,9). Spiral CT and MR accurately detect emboli in the segmental or larger pulmonary arteries but may not display more peripheral emboli (10).

Scintigraphic Findings of DVT. A radionuclide venogram may be performed in conjunction with a perfusion lung scan. Tc-99m MAA is divided between two syringes and injected into the veins on the dorsum of the feet instead of into the arm. The nuclear venogram is most sensitive for thrombi occurring above the knees. Deep venous thrombi are indicated by obstruction of the veins that show cutoff of activity and multiple collateral vessels.

Preliminary studies using Tc-99m- and In-111-labeled antifibrin monoclonal antibodies (11,12) and Tc-99m labeled peptides (13) indicate high sensitivity and specificity for detecting deep venous thrombi. Acute thrombi demonstrate focal areas of asymmetric uptake within the deep venous system. Heparin reduces the intensity of uptake of the antifibrin monoclonal antibodies. These techniques are helpful in differentiating chronic and recurrent acute DVT.

V/Q SCAN INTERPRETATION

Multiple, bilateral perfusion defects with a normal ventilation scan are the classic diagnostic findings of pulmonary embolism (Fig. 56.4). Pulmonary emboli that completely occlude pulmonary arteries produce segmental perfusion defects that extend to the pleural surface. However, nonembolic processes that fill, destroy, or replace lung parenchyma also produce marked perfusion defects. In addition, tumors, pneumonia, and COPD cause perfusion defects. The ventilation scan is performed to improve the low specificity of the perfusion scan. The bronchial tree is unaffected by vascular embolization; thus, ventilation of the embolized region remains normal. Most nonembolic lung diseases have both abnormal ventilation and perfusion, which are typically matched defects. Pulmonary emboli are more common in the lower lobes because more pulmonary blood flow goes to the basilar pulmonary segments.

Criteria categorize V/Q scan findings according to the likelihood that emboli will be demonstrated on pulmonary angiography. All interpretation schema are based on carefully analyzing perfusion scan defects to determine if they correspond to anatomic segments or subsegments of the lung. An understanding of the segmental anatomy of the lung is essential. The shape, location, and size of any defect is analyzed for fit to a specific pulmonary segment on all views. The use of a segmental anatomy chart increases reading consistency and intraobserver agreement.

Size of segmental defect must be assessed. By definition, a defect of less than 25% of a pulmonary segment is a small defect, 25–75% a moderate defect, and greater than 75% a large defect. Subsegmental defects are summed to constitute full segment equivalents. Two moderate or four small perfusion defects are equivalent to a full segment defect. Even experienced readers tend to underestimate the size of segmental defects (14).

Interpretation schemes compare defects visualized on the perfusion scan with corresponding regions of the ventilation scan and CXR. A perfusion defect that demonstrates normal ventilation is termed a *mismatched defect*. A perfusion defect the same size and location as a ventilation defect is called a *matched defect*. Perfusion defects that match ventilation and CXR abnormalities in size and location are called *triple match defects*. The size and number of matched and/or mismatched segmental defects are used to estimate the likelihood that the defects represent pulmonary emboli.

Nonsegmental defects should be compared to CXRs to determine if a mass, effusion, mediastinal or hilar structure is responsible for the perfusion scan finding. Non–wedge-shaped defects, or wedge-shaped defects that do not correspond to segmental anatomy, are usually not due to pulmonary emboli. Common nonsegmental defects include cardiomegaly, pleural effusions (Fig. 56.5), adenopathy, hilar and parenchymal masses, cardiac pacemakers (Fig 56.6), pneumonia, large bullae, atelectasis, pulmonary hemorrhage, and aortic aneurysm or tortuosity.

Diagnostic Criteria. Biello criteria (15) originally categorizes V/Q scans as normal, low probability, intermediate, or high probability. The PIOPED study used a modified Biello schema with more detailed categorizations of V/Q scan patterns (6). The PIOPED classification has undergone several revisions after retrospective analysis of the data pointed out subcatagories of incorrectly classified scan patterns (7,16–20). The amended PIOPED criteria are listed in Table 56.1 (Figs 56.2, 56.5–56.7).

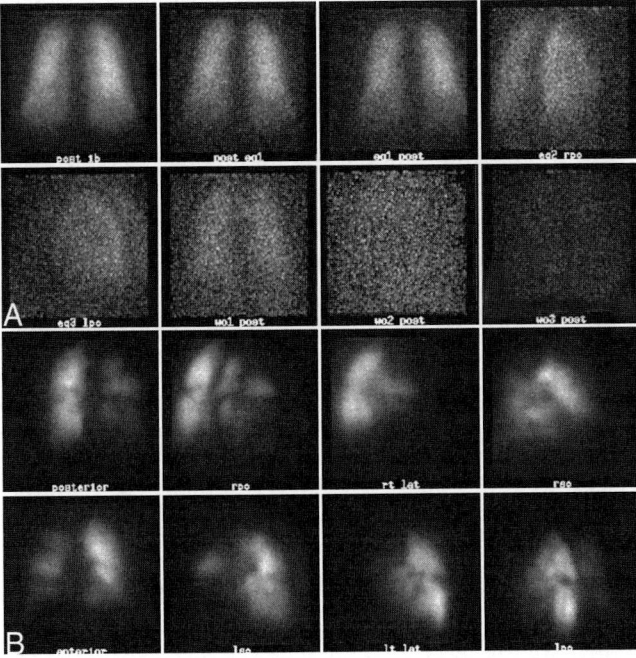

Figure 56.4. High probability V/Q scan. A. Xe-133 ventilation scan (top two rows) is normal. **B. Tc-99m MAA Perfusion scan** (bottom two rows). Perfusion scan demonstrates absence of perfusion to most segments of the right lung with multiple subsegmental defects in the left lung. Labeling is the same as in Figure 56.2.

Stripe and Fissure Signs. Two types of perfusion defects not listed in either the original PIOPED or Biello criteria have been found to strongly correlate with a normal pulmonary angiogram. Central perfusion defects that have a rim or stripe of increased activity around them have a less than 10% probability of being due to PE (21,22). The defect should be seen in different views to *not* extend to the pleural surface. The surrounding stripe of perfused lung is called the *stripe sign*. Pulmonary emboli perfusion defects extend to the pleural surface and have no intervening stripe of perfused lung.

Perfusion defects that match the location and shape of the major or minor fissures of the lung usually represent pleural effusions tracking up the fissures (Fig. 56.5)(23). When this defect is seen, the lateral view can be repeated with the patient in the supine or decubitus position to demonstrate layering of the fluid. The *fissure sign* correlates with the presence of a pleural effusion on CXR.

PIOPED Findings. The PIOPED study was designed to evaluate the usefulness of V/Q scans for diagnosing acute PE. In the original study 13% of patients had high probability V/Q scans, 39% intermediate, 34% low, and 14% normal or near normal scans. The interobserver agreement in classifying scans was very good (92–95%) for normal/near normal scans and high probability scans, but was significantly worse for low and intermediate scans (25–30%)(6). The prevalence of thromboembolism in patients who underwent angiography was 33%. The sensitivity of a high probability scan was 41% with a specificity of 97%.

The positive predictive value for a high probability scan was 91% in patients with no prior history of PE but fell to 74% in those who had previously documented pulmonary emboli. Prior PE may leave residual perfusion defects that cannot be distinguished from acute emboli. Use of 2 segmental equivalents as the criteria for high probability yielded a likelihood for PE of 71%. Use of 2.5 segmental equivalent mismatched defects was 100% predictive of PE (17).

The negative predictive value of a normal/near normal scan was 91–96% while that of a low probability scan was 84–88%. Patients with normal or nearly normal V/Q scans are unlikely to have clinically significant PE (24).

Clinical Assessment and V/Q Scan Interpretation. The V/Q scan should not be interpreted in a clinical vacuum. The PIOPED study demonstrated that adding the clinical assessment to V/Q scan interpretation improved the chance of correctly evaluating the patient's risk of having PE. Of patients with high-probability scans and a high clinical suspicion, 96% had emboli on pulmonary angiography. Of patients with low probability scans and low clinical suspicion, 96% had no evidence of PE on angiography. Patients with high-probability scans but intermediate clinical suspicion had an 88% positive PE rate while those with high-probability scans and low clinical suspicion had a 56% positive PE rate. Patients with high probability scans and high or intermediate clinical suspicion have a high risk of having pulmonary emboli that justifies treatment with anticoagulants. Patients with low-probability scans and low clinical suspicion have very low chance of having PE.

V/Q Scans and Pulmonary Angiography. Patients with intermediate probability scans have a significant risk of having PE. However, the V/Q scan alone is insufficient in determining that of these require anticoagulation therapy. Patients with intermediate probability scans (Fig. 56.8) and multiple risk factors or clinical findings suggestive of DVT should undergo another ex-

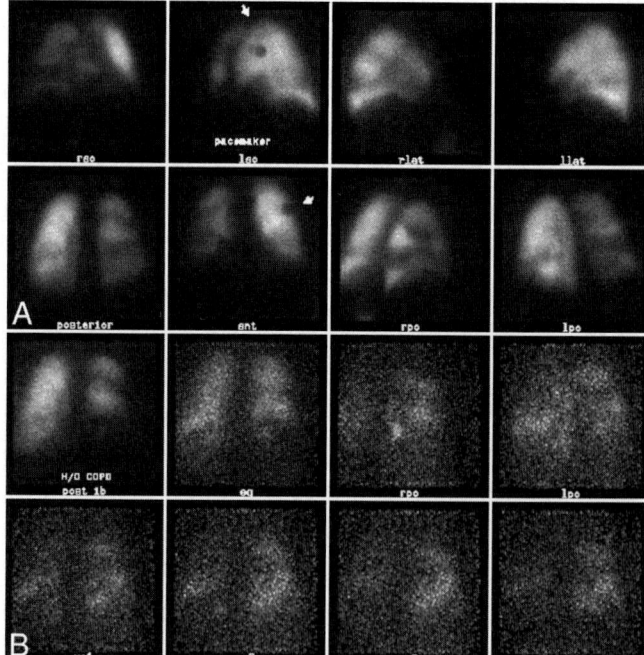

Figure 56.6. Chronic Obstructive Pulmonary Disease. A. Tc-99m MAA perfusion (top two rows). Moderate to large bilateral perfusion defects match the ventilation scan defects. A nonsegmental defect is also present over the left upper lobe representing an artifact secondary to a cardiac pacemaker (*arrow*). **B. Xe-133 Ventilation Scan** (bottom two rows). Patchy defects are seen in the mid and lower lung zones on the right on the initial breath image (*post ib*). The defects partially fill in on the equilibrium images (*eq, rpo, lpo*). Persistent retention of Xe-133 is seen in these same regions on the washout images (*wo/1, wo/2, wo/3, wo/4*). Labeling is the same as in Figure 56.2.

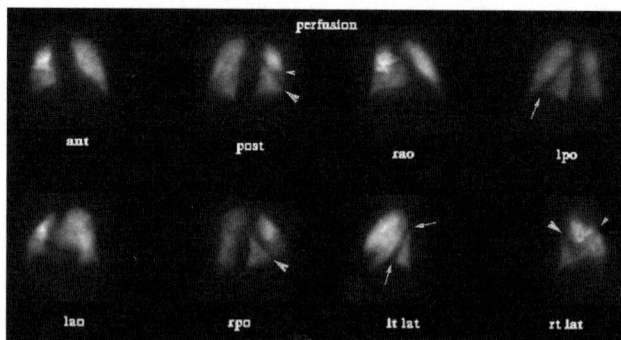

Figure 56.5. Low Probability Perfusion Scan with Bilateral Pleural Effusions. Scan demonstrates bilateral wedge shaped defects that correspond to pleural effusions within the major fissures bilaterally (*open arrows*) and the minor fissure on the right (*closed arrow*).

Table 56.1. Amended PIOPED Criteria

V/Q Scan Category	Criteria	Likelihood of PE	Prevalence of PE

High	2 or more mismatched perfusion segments or segmental equivalents without corresponding ventilation or CXR abnormalities:
	  a. ≥2 large segmental perfusion defects
	  b. 1 large and 2 moderate segmental defects
	  c. ≥4 moderate segmental defects
		≥80%	87%

Intermediate	1. 1 moderate to ≤2 large mismatched segments or segmental equivalents without corresponding ventilation or CXR abnormalities 2. Triple matched defects in the lower lung zone 3. Single moderate matched V/Q defects with normal CXR 4. Corresponding V/Q defects and small pleural effusion 5. Findings difficult to classify as normal, high, or low	20–79%	35%
Low	1. Multiple matched V/Q defects with a normal CXR 2. Corresponding V/Q defects and CXR opacities (triple matched defects) in the middle or upper lung zones. 3. Corresponding V/Q defects and large pleural effusions (>⅓ of the hemithorax) 4. Any perfusion defect with substantially larger CXR abnormality 5. Any defect with a rim of surrounding normally perfused lung (stripe sign) 6. >3 small perfusion defects with normal CXR 7. Nonsegmental perfusion defects	≤19%	12%
Very Low	<3 small perfusion defects with a normal CXR		2.5%
Normal	No defects present on the perfusion scan or they exactly match the shape of the lungs on CXR		0

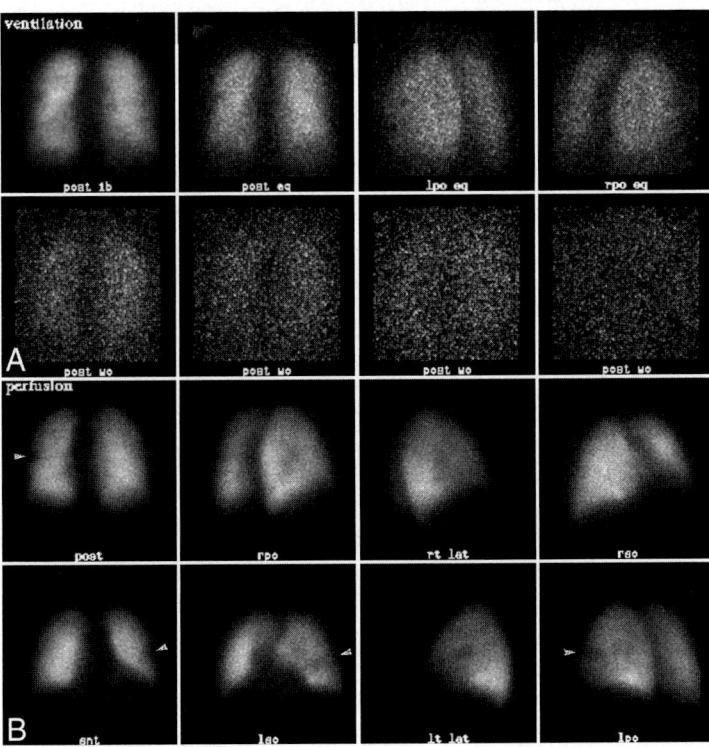

Figure 56.7. Intermediate Probability V/Q Scan. A. Xe-133 ventilation scan (top two rows) demonstrates a moderate sized defect in the anterior medial basal segment of the left lower lobe (*open arrow*). **B. Tc-99m MAA perfusion lung scan** (bottom two rows). A single, moderate sized matched perfusion defect is seen in the anterior medial basal segment of the left lower lobe (*arrows*).

amination such as Doppler US. If DVT is diagnosed, the patient can be placed on anticoagulants that would treat the DVT and serendipitously treat any PE. If the noninvasive search for DVT is negative, then pulmonary angiography should be performed. The location of mismatched defects on the perfusion scan would be the most likely sites for PE. The perfusion scan thus could be used to direct the pulmonary angiogram, allowing for a more selective examination. Pulmonary angiograms should also be strongly considered to confirm the diagnosis of PE in patients with high-probability scans when anticoagulation is risky. It also may be indicated in patients with low-probability scans but high clinical suspicion for having PE (25).

Follow-up V/Q Scans Post Anticoagulation. Most patients with PE show a gradual reduction in the size of perfusion defects with normalization of their scans within 3 months. Defects still present after 3 months of anticoagulation will usually remain as permanent abnormalities. The larger the initial defect, the less likely it is to completely resolve. The older the patient, the slower the rate of defect resolution and the less likely the scan will return to normal.

Follow-up scans done within 2 weeks of the initiation of anticoagulation therapy may show new defects that do not represent recurrent emboli. Large central thrombi may fragment and produce small distal thrombi. Thus emboli that were previously nonocclusive may become obstructive and show as new defects. The diagnosis of recurrent PE is more likely if multiple new large or moderate defects are present in areas that were previously normal (Fig. 56.9).

False-positive V/Q Scans. Mismatched perfusion defects can represent chronic pulmonary emboli in patients with a remote history of PE. Follow-up V/Q scans after patients have been placed on oral anticoagulants are useful as baselines in this patient population. If no old scans are available, it is impossible to determine which emboli are old and which are new. Patients with a history of PE are at higher risk of having a PE than patients without such a history. Mismatched perfusion defects can also be produced by extrinsic compression of the pulmonary vessels. Mass lesions in the mediastinum, hila, or pulmonary parenchyma may compress the pliable pulmonary vessels, particularly the veins. Adenopathy can impinge on the pulmonary vessels. Aneurysmal dilation of the thoracic aorta or congenital vascular abnormalities may rarely compress the pulmonary vascularity. The pulmonary vessels may also become entrapped and obstructed by mediastinal fibrosis. Pulmonary vessels can be obstructed by nonthrombotic intraluminal processes. Malignancies such as renal cell carcinoma may grow intravascularly or embolize to the pulmonary vessels. Sarcomas of the pulmonary arteries and lymphatic carcinomatosis have produced false-positive V/Q scans. Vasculitis, with obliterative lesions in the pulmonary vessel, such as Takayasu's arteritis and systemic lupus erythematosus can cause false-positive scans. Radiation therapy produces mismatched perfusion defects due to vasculitis or fibrosis. These are often geometric rather than segmental in shape.

False-negative V/Q Scans. V/Q scans may be falsely negative if the emboli are only partially occlusive. Very small emboli may produce perfusion defects too small to be visualized on a perfusion scan.

Figure 56.8. Intermediate Probability V/Q Scan. Tc-99m MAA perfusion scan demonstrates multiple bilateral small and moderate defects (*arrows*). The Xe-133 ventilation scan was normal.

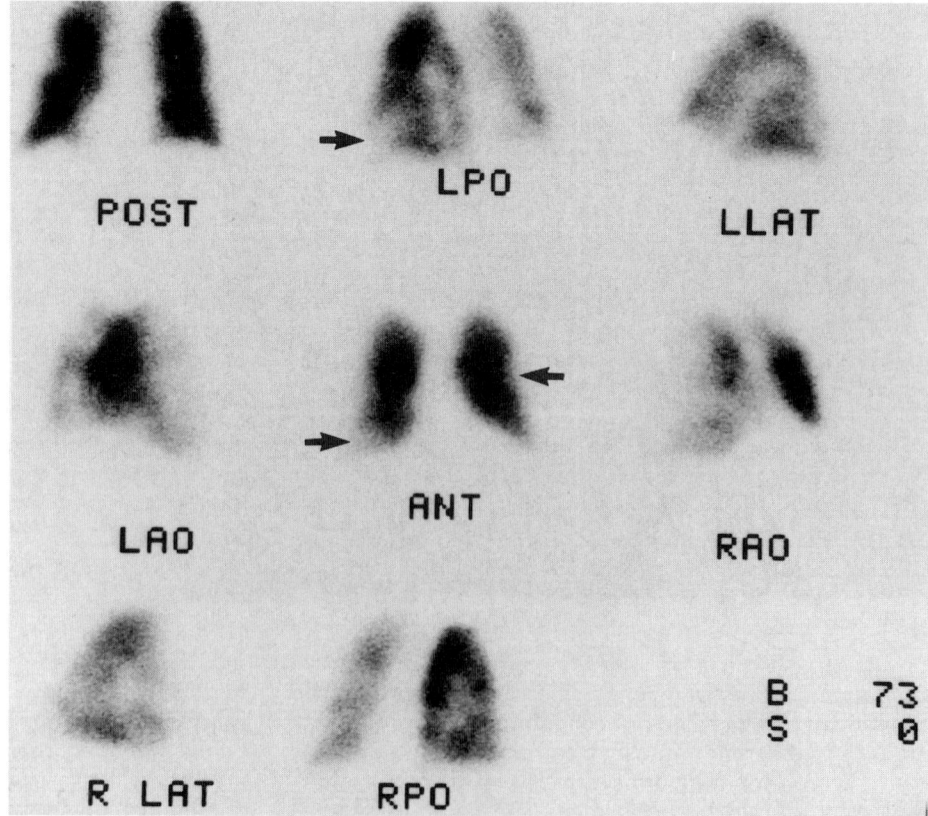

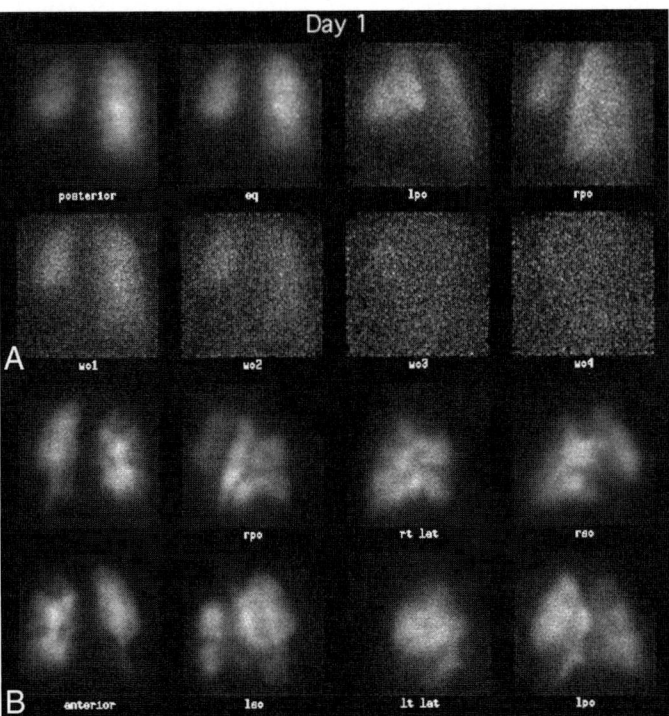

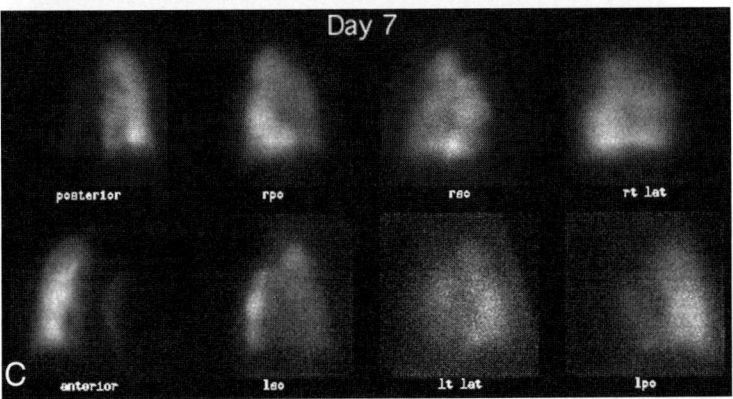

Figure 56.9. Recurrent Pulmonary Emboli. A. Xe-133 ventilation scan (top two rows) demonstrates lack of ventilation of most of the left lower lobe due to a pleural effusion. **B. Tc-99m MAA perfusion scan** (third and fourth rows) demonstrates multiple moderate and large mismatched perfusion defects in the right lung. **C.** Repeat Tc-99m MAA perfusion scan was performed one week later. Patient had recurrent symptoms while being treated with heparin. Marked improvement is seen in the perfusion defects previously noted in the right lung indicates resolution of some of the emboli with therapy. The left lung on the new scan shows almost complete abscence of perfusion indicative of new emboli to the lungs despite anticoagulation.

NONTHROMBOEMBOLIC PULMONARY DISEASE

Asthma produces bronchospastic narrowing of the airways resulting in decreased ventilation. Focal segmental or subsegmental ventilation defects are present on the first-breath image during an acute asthma attack. These defects may wash in later on the equilibrium images. Defects associated with mucus plugs may persist. Bronchospasm induces localized hypoxia, which in turn produces localized vasoconstriction and perfusion scan defects that match the ventilation defects. The V/Q scan of an asthma patient successfully treated with bronchodilators shows improvement compared with scans performed during the attack. The transient nature of the V/Q defects caused by asthma helps distinguish them from the fixed defects due to COPD. Most V/Q defects caused by asthma will resolve with 24 hours of bronchodilator therapy.

Lung Neoplasms produce V/Q scan abnormalities. The location and size of the tumor determine the findings on the lung scan, not the tumor type. Benign tumors cannot be distinguished from malignant ones on V/Q scans. Focal parenchymal masses and extrinsic mediastinal or chest wall tumors that displace lung parenchyma tend to produce matching V/Q defects which correspond to the size and shape of the mass on CXR.

The V/Q defects do not correspond to segmental anatomy unless the mass has invaded or compressed a local branch of the bronchovascular tree. The compliant pulmonary vessels are more easily compressed than the cartilage-reinforced bronchi. A common V/Q pattern seen with a lung tumor is a wedge-shaped area of reduced or absent perfusion with either normal ventilation or a ventilation defect matching the mass itself. When a small perihilar lung carcinoma obstructs the pulmonary

Figure 56.10. Quantitative Tc-99m MAA Perfusion Scan. The percentage of the pulmonary perfusion to each lung is calculated based on the relative counts over each lung on the posterior image.

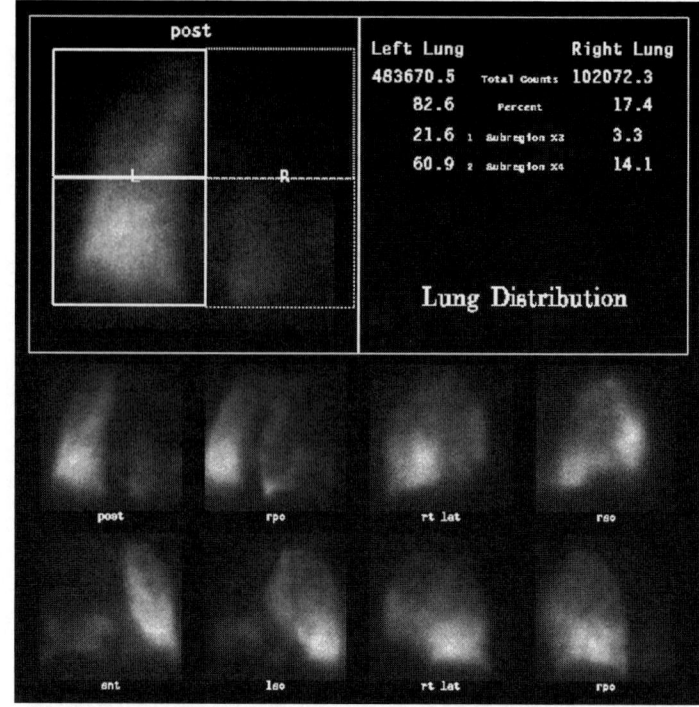

vessels but not the bronchi, a mismatched segmental or subsegmental perfusion defect occurs, mimicking pulmonary embolism. If the carcinoma obstructs the adjacent bronchus or bronchiole as well as the pulmonary vessels, then the ventilation defect may match the perfusion defect.

Quantitative Perfusion Lung Scan. Perfusion lung scans are useful in preoperatively estimating a lung carcinoma patient's postsurgical pulmonary function. The quantitative perfusion scan is performed in the same manner as a regular perfusion lung scan except that a single posterior image is obtained for a specified time interval or fixed number of counts. Regions of interest are drawn around each lung and the counts over each lung are obtained. The percentage of the total count that each lung contributes is calculated (Fig. 56.10). The postoperative FEV1 (forced expiratory volume in 1 second) is estimated by multiplying the preoperative FEV1 by the percent perfusion going to the lung that will remain after pneumonectomy. A patient needs to have a postoperative FEV1 of 800–1000 ml to have adequate lung function.

Chronic Obstructive Pulmonary Disease. The narrowed airways associated with COPD reduce ventilation. Xenon scans demonstrate delayed wash-in and delayed washout. First-breath images may have defects that gradually fill in on the equilibrium phase. Xenon washes out of the affected area more slowly than the rest of the lung and may still be visible on images more than 3 minutes after the patient was switched to breathing room air.

Perfusion lung scans are also frequently abnormal. Localized hypoxia in the lung induces localized vasoconstriction. Destruction of lung and inflammatory narrowing of blood vessels produces areas of reduced perfusion.

Regions of the lung that demonstrate obstructive changes on the ventilation scan usually have corresponding abnormalities on the perfusion scan (Figs. 56.3, 56.6). When the ventilatory changes are widespread, the perfusion scan has a mottled appearance (20). Perfusion scans may be normal if the ventilatory obstructive changes produce little hypoxia or vascular damage. Since COPD tends to affect the lung apices more than the bases, V/Q abnormalities are usually more pronounced at the apices. However, alpha-1-antitrypsin deficiency produces more pronounced emphysematous changes in the lower lobes, which are reflected on the V/Q scan.

Inflammatory/Infectious Disease of the Lung. Areas of consolidation on CXR will be abnormal on a V/Q scan. Consolidated airways do not ventilate and produce defects on xenon scans. The resulting local hypoxia produces reflex vasoconstriction which causes perfusion defects in the consolidated region. Perfusion defects are often smaller than the consolidated region on CXR. If the perfusion defect appears larger than the CXR abnormality, pulmonary emboli may be present as well as the infiltrate.

Tc-99m aerosols have also been used to evaluate inflammatory diseases of the lung (26,27). Normals have a Tc-99m aerosol clearance half-life of approximately 60 minutes. Increased permeability of inflamed pulmonary epithelium shortens the clearance time. Alveolitis and adult respiratory distress syndrome have rapid Tc-99m aerosol clearance. Smokers also have faster than normal aerosol clearance. Conversely, processes that thicken the alveolar membranes or cause fibrosis will have prolonged Tc-99m aerosol clearance. Abnormal aerosol clearance is a very sensitive, but nonspecific indicator of inflammation.

Smoke Inhalation. Many patients with serious burns also have inhalation injury of the lungs. Of patients admitted to a hospital for burns, 20–30% develop pulmonary complications and 70–75% of these patients die (1). Smoke consists of a mixture of toxic gases and particles. Inhalation of these toxins combine with thermal injury to produce severe pulmonary damage. A CXR is insensitive in detecting early inhalation injury with a lag period of 12–48 hours before the x-ray becomes abnormal (1). Xenon in saline ventilation scans have proven useful in detecting inhalation lung injury (28). Xenon-133 under pressure will dissolve in saline. When injected intravenously, the xenon remains in solution until it reaches the lungs. In the alveolar capillaries, the xenon diffuses across the capillary membrane into the alveoli and is exhaled. Normally, the xenon washes out of the lungs in less than 2 minutes. Areas of inhalational injury demonstrate retention of xenon. The xenon in saline study is 92% accurate in detecting lung injury.

References

1. Fraser RG, Paré JA, Paré PD, et al. Diagnosis of Diseases of the Chest. 3rd ed. Philadelphia: WB Saunders, 1988: 3–35,53–64,71–82,127–137.
2. Parker JA, Coleman RE, Siegel BA, et al. Procedure guideline for lung scintigraphy: 1.0. J Nucl Med 1996;37: 1906–1910.
3. Dahlen JE, Alpert JS. Natural history of pulmonary embolism. Prog Cardiovasc Dis 1975;17:259–270.
4. Palevsky HI. The problems of the clinical and laboratory diagnosis of pulmonary embolism. Semin Nucl Med 1991;21: 276–280.
5. Bell WR, Simon TL, DeMets DL. The clinical features of submassive and massive pulmonary emboli. Am J Med 1977; 62:355–360.
6. The PIOPED Investigators. Value of the ventilation/perfusion scan in acute pulmonary embolism. Results of the Prospective Investigation of Pulmonary Embolism Diagnosis (PIOPED). JAMA 1990;263:2753–2759.
7. Worsley DF, Alavi A. Comprehensive analysis of the results of the PIOPED study. J Nucl Med 1995;36:2380–2387.
8. vanRossum AB, Treurniet FE, Kieft GJ, et al. Role of spiral volumetric computed tomographic scanning in the assessment of patients with clinical suspicion of pulmonary embolism and an abnormal ventilation/perfusion scan. Thorax 1996;51:23–28.
9. Sostman HD, Layish DT, Tapson VF, et al. Prospective comparison of helical CT and MR imaging in clinically suspected acute pulmonary embolism. J Magn Reson Imaging 1996; 6:275–281.
10. Robinson PJ. Ventilation-perfusion lung scanning and spiral computed tomography of the lungs: competing or complementary modalities? Eur J Nucl Med 1996;193: 1547–1553.
11. Schaible TF, Alavi A. Antifibrin scintigraphy in the diagnostic evaluation of acute deep venous thrombosis. Semin Nucl Med 1991; 21:313–324.
12. DeFaucal P, Peltier P, Planchon B, et al. Evaluation of indium-111-labeled antifibrin monoclonal antibody for the diagnosis of venous thrombotic disease. J Nucl Med 1991; 32:785–791.
13. Muto P, Lastoria S, Varrella P, et al. Detecting deep venous thrombosis with technetium-99m-labeled synthetic peptide P280. J Nucl Med 1995;36:1384–1391.
14. Morrell NW, Nijran KS, Jones BE, et al. The underestimation of segmental defect size in radionuclide lung scanning. J Nucl Med 1993;34:370–374.
15. Biello DR, Mattar AG, McKnight RC, et al. Ventilation-perfusion studies in suspected pulmonary embolism. AJR Am J Roentgenol 1979;133:1033–1037.
16. Sostman HD, Coleman RE, DeLong DM, et al. Evaluation of revised criteria for ventilation-perfusion scintigraphy in patients with suspected pulmonary embolism. Radiology 1994;193:103–107.
17. Gottschalk A, Sostman HD, Coleman RE, et al. Ventilation-perfusion scintigraphy in the PIOPED study. Part II. Evaluation of the scintigraphic criteria and interpretations. J Nucl Med 1993;34:1119–1126.
18. Henry JW, Stein PD, Gottschalk A, et al. Pulmonary embolism among patients with a nearly normal ventilation/perfusion lung scan. Chest 1996;110:395–398.
19. Gottschalk A, Stein PD, Henry JW, et al. Matched ventilation, perfusion and chest radiographic abnormalities in acute pulmonary embolism. J Nucl Med 1996;37: 1636–1638.
20. Elgazzar AH, Silberstein EB, Hughes J. Perfusion and ventilation scans in patients with extensive obstructive airways disease: utility of single-breath (washin) xenon-133. J Nucl Med 1995;36:64–67.
21. Sostman HD, Gottschalk A. The stripe sign: a new sign for diagnosis of nonembolic defects on pulmonary perfusion scintigraphy. Radiology 1982;142:737–741.
22. Sostman HD, Gottschalk A. Prospective validation of the stripe sign in ventilation-perfusion scintigraphy. Radiology 1992;184:455–459.
23. Goldberg SN, Richardson DD, Palmer EL, et al. Pleural effusion and ventilation/perfusion scan interpretation for acute pulmonary embolus. J Nucl Med 1996;37: 1310–1313.
24. Kipper MS, Moser KM, Kortman KE, et al. Long term follow-up of patients with suspected pulmonary embolism and a normal lung scan. Chest 1982;82:411–415.
25. Juni JE, Alavi A. Lung scanning in the diagnosis of pulmonary embolism: the emperor redressed. Semin Nucl Med 1991;21:281–296.
26. Susskind H. Technetium-99m-DTPA aerosol to measure alveolar-capillary membrane permeability. J Nucl Med 1994;35:207–209.
27. Line BR. Scintigraphic studies of inflammation in diffuse lung disease. Radiol Clin North Am 1991;29:1095–1114.
28. Lull RJ, Anderson JH, Telepak RJ, et al. Radionuclide imaging in the assessment of lung injury. Semin Nucl Med 1980;10:302–310.

57

Cardiovascular System Scintigraphy

Robert J. Telepak
Philip W. Wiest
Michael F. Hartshorne

Nuclear medicine applications in the cardiovascular system include maps of myocardial perfusion, gated ventricular function studies of the blood pool in the ventricles, and detection and quantitation of intracardiac shunts.

MYOCARDIAL PERFUSION SCANS

Technique

Each of the perfusion agents may be imaged with planar techniques or with SPECT. Meticulous quality control of the stress and rest images is essential. The comparison of images between stress and rest requires identical repositioning so that the same areas of myocardium are visualized. Poor positioning will lead to false-positive interpretations of ischemia and infarct.

The three principle coronary artery distributions of the left ventricle (LV) are the left anterior descending artery (LAD), the left circumflex artery (LCX), and the posterior descending artery (PDA). Each artery normally provides an equal intensity of myocardial labeling at any given level of cardiac work. Perfusion of the thinner right ventricular wall is considerably less than that of the LV, but can be imaged using the same techniques (Figs. 57.1–57.3).

Exercise on a treadmill, or simulation of exercise by infusion of dipyridamole or adenosine, is used in conjunction with perfusion agents to increase radionuclide delivery to the normal myocardium. Step-wise increases in physical exercise are monitored by sequential electrocardiogram (ECG), blood pressure, and pulse measurements, while the patient is queried for symptoms of angina. The radiopharmaceutical is injected under conditions of maximal exercise, which should be continued for 30–60 seconds after injection to obtain optimal mapping of stress perfusion. Adequacy of the exercise challenge can be estimated simply from a calculation of the "double product" (DP) (systolic pressure × heart rate = DP). The DP correlates with an individual's myocardial work performed; the duration of exercise and heart rate alone may not. For exercise to be judged as adequate, the DP should double, or preferably triple, from rest to peak exercise, and should rise to above 20,000.

For those patients who cannot perform physical exercise, coronary vasodilatation can be pharmacologically forced. Intravenous dipyridamole or adenosine vasodilate normal coronary arteries, but do not effectively increase flow through vessels that are stenosed. Those areas which cannot dilate normally will appear to have a scan defect compared with the rest of the myocardium.

In the late 1980s, most Nuclear Medicine clinics shifted to SPECT imaging for myocardial perfusion studies. Planar images are not quite as sensitive or specific in the detection of myocardial infarction and ischemia as SPECT and are infrequently performed currently. Different strategies are used in myocardial perfusion studies. Some are dictated by the equipment available in a given clinic. Each has its own strengths and weaknesses.

Radiopharmaceuticals

Three gamma-emitting radiopharmaceuticals are readily available for mapping the flow of blood to the myocardium.

Thallium-201 (Tl-201), an analog of the potassium ion (K$^+$), is delivered to capillary beds by regional blood flow and is actively pumped into viable cells by the sodium/potassium (Na$^+$/K$^+$) adenosine triphosphatase pump. Cyclotron production at a remote site (requiring shipping), a long physical half-life (73 hours), low energy, poorly penetrating photons (mostly 69-83 keV γ-rays), and a relatively high absorbed dose (0.24 rad/mCi whole body at the usual dose of 2-5 mCi) combine to make Tl-201 a less than ideal agent for imaging. However, because of its active transport into cells, it is a more physiologic radionuclide than the technetium-99m (Tc-99m)-labeled agents.

A widely used technique utilizes Tl-201 with exercise stress or a dipyridamole challenge. Images are usually acquired as soon after injection as possible. However, some authors advocate waiting for 5–10 minutes to allow the exercised patient to stop breathing heavily so that movement of the heart heaving up and down with the diaphragm will be minimzed. Delayed imaging also limits an artifact caused by the "upward creep" of the heart. As the lungs decrease in volume slowly after exercise, the average level of the diaphragm is raised shifting the

Figure 57.1. Normal Exercise/Rest Planar Tc-99m Sestamibi Myocardial Scan. Anterior (*Ant*), left anterior oblique (*LAO 40, LAO 70*), and left lateral (*L LAT*) planar views of a 380-pound patient, with the upper row representing stress and the lower row representing rest injections of the radiopharmaceutical. Note the superb image quality in spite of the patient's large size.

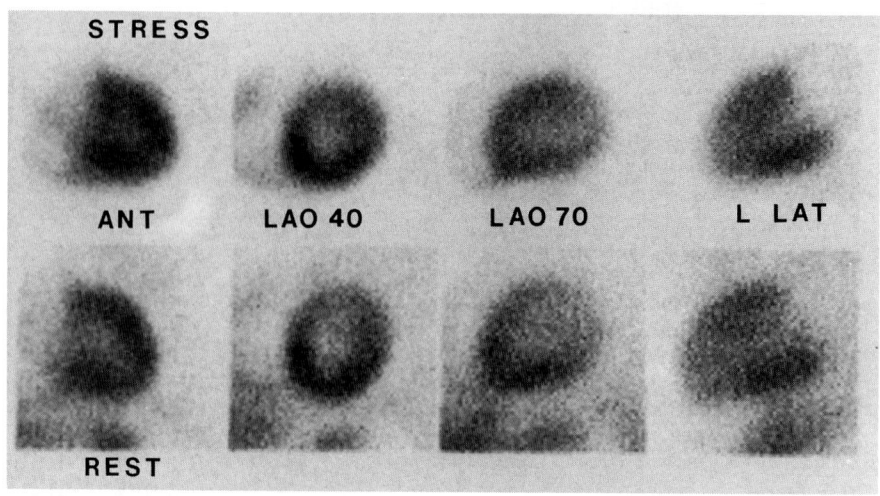

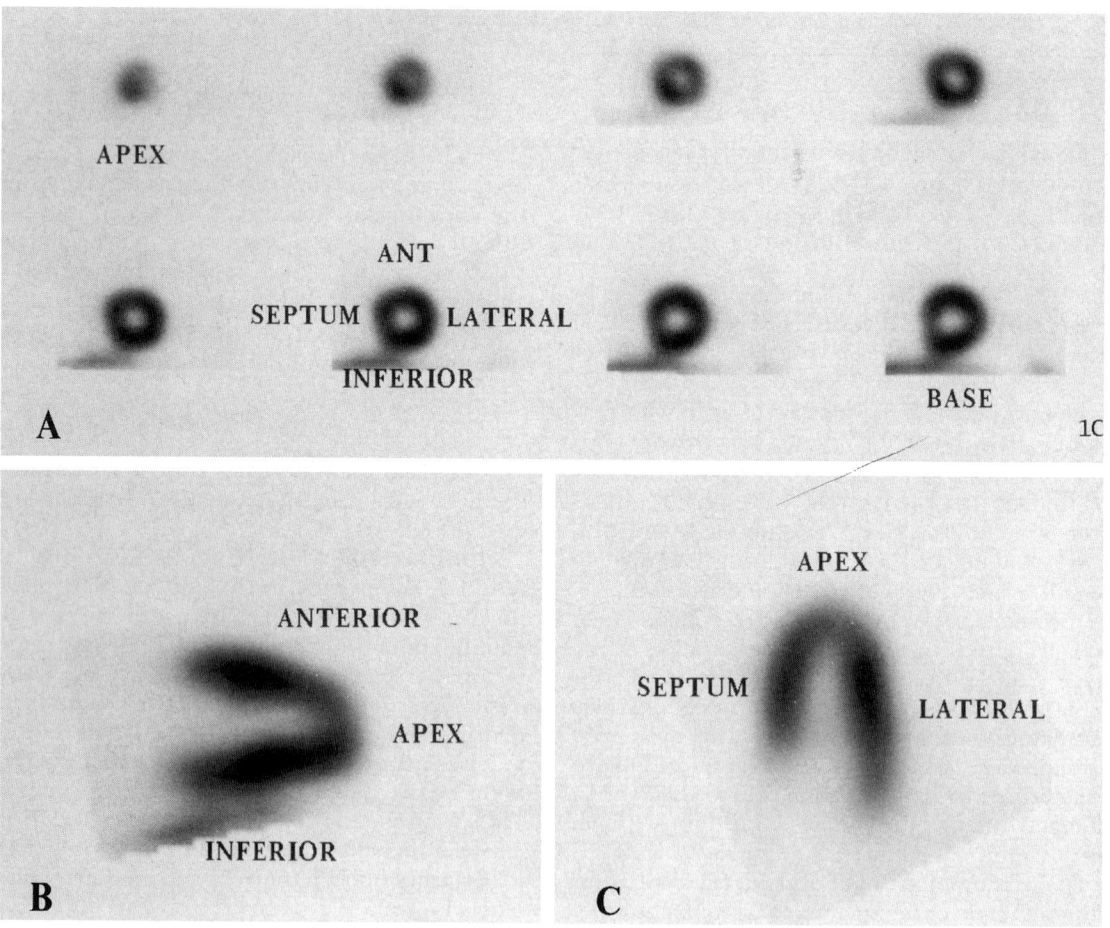

Figure 57.2. Normal SPECT Projections. Short axis **(A)**, vertical long axis **(B)**, and horizontal long axis **(C)** images in standard projections show the walls of left ventricle. In the short axis images an apical "button" starts the series which extends back to the base of the ventricle. The names of the walls for the short axis images are best given by the diagram in Figure 57.3. In the vertical long axis images the anterior and inferior (or posterior) walls are seen. In the horizontal long axis images the short septum and long lateral or "free" walls are well seen. The long axis images also show the apex very well.

CARDIAC CIRCULATION

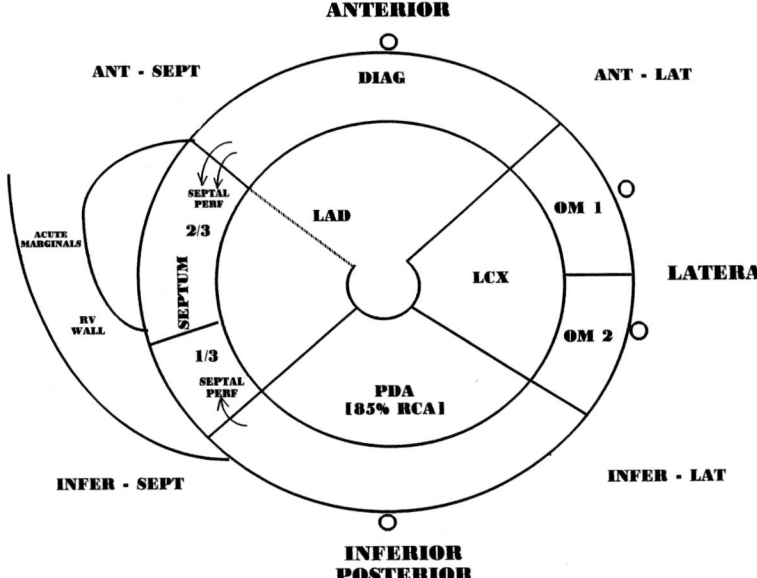

Figure 57.3. LV Short Axis Vascular Distributions and Wall Names. The schematic diagram locates the expected position of the principle coronary arteries. The left anterior descending artery (*LAD*) usually serves the apex. The names of the wall segments are listed in a clockwise fashion as *Anterior, Anterior-Lateral, Lateral, Inferior-Lateral, Inferior, Inferior-Septal, Septal,* and *Anterior-Septal.* The LAD sends diagonal vessels (numbered with digits in the order with which they leave the LAD . . . e.g., D1, D2, etc.) onto the Anterior and Anterior-Lateral walls and Septal Perforators down into the septum. The Left Circumflex (*LCX*) sends obtuse marginal (*OM*) branches along the free wall numbered in their sequence (*OM1, OM2,* etc.) The posterior descending artery (*PDA*), which arises from the right coronary artery (*RCA*) 85% of the time and serves the inferior wall and the inferior-septal wall. If you do not know these names and locations by heart you cannot speak with a cardiologist.

heart upward. This shift in location of the heart produces an artifactual shift in radionuclide activity that may be misinterpreted as ischemia.

The effective half-life (T1/2), or 50% washout, of Tl-201 from the normal myocardium is about 4 hours. A complex "redistribution" of the isotope within the myocardium is governed by rates of washout from myocardial cells, renal excretion, and shifts of the isotope between muscle, visceral, and other compartments. Rest imaging is usually done 3–4 hours after injection. With quantitative software packages regional washout of Tl-201 can be measured. Low rates of Tl-201 washout are a good marker of ischemia. In addition to clinical data (ECG, angina, etc.), the initial Tl-201 images of the chest and heart may help assess the heart's performance. High lung activity immediately after exercise usually indicates that left ventricular failure occurred during exercise. Dilation of the heart with exercise is another indicator of failure. Both phenomena have a severe prognosis for subsequent cardiac events (angina, infarction, arrhythmia, and sudden death) (Fig. 57.4). A nonquantitative strategy for improving the visual detection of ischemic myocardium by Tl-201 scintigraphy calls for a "reinjection" of 1 millicurie of Tl-201 just before delayed, rest imaging. Even with planar techniques the correct detection of ischemia is increased. Also, fewer areas of infarction will be misdiagnosed.

Technetium-99m is used to label two myocardial perfusion agents.

Tc-99m Sestamibi (trade name Cardiolite), is taken up by the perfused myocardium by passive diffusion and is bound in the myocyte, mostly within myocardial mitochondria. There is no significant redistribution effect with this agent. Washout is negligible. Imaging of the 15–20 mCi dose is delayed for 30 minutes to 1 hour after stress (or dipyridamole challenge) to allow for biliary clearance (which reduces liver background activity near the heart). Because there is no redistribution nor

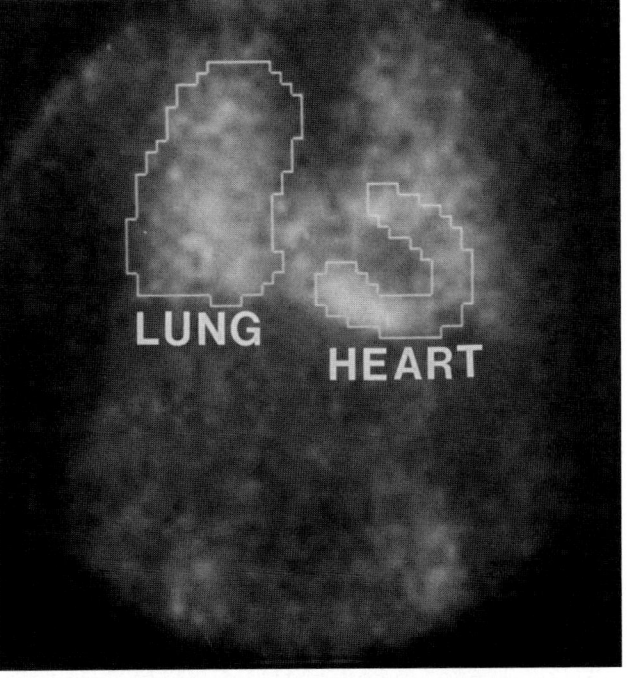

Figure 57.4. Abnormal Tl-201 Lung/Heart Ratio. This frame is an anterior projection acquired immediately after the start of a stress SPECT study. The lung:heart ratio of 0.77 is markedly elevated, indicating that the patient experienced heart failure during exercise.

significant washout of Tc-99m Sestamibi, a repeat injection of 15–20 mCi for resting images is commonly performed on a different day. Either stress or rest imaging can be done first. An alternative approach uses a small dose (8 mCi) for the initial scan (rest or exercise) and a larger dose (22 mCi) one hour later (exercise or rest). This strategy leaves open a question about polluting the second scan with radiopharmaceutical left over from the first scan.

Tc-99m Tetrofosmin (trade name Myoview), is rapidly extracted from the blood by perfused myocardium in a fashion that resembles Tc-99m Sestamibi. The manufacturer claims that it has less liver background than Tc-99m Sestamibi. The user should make up his or her own mind about this claim and check the prices of these two competing products.

Both of the Tc-99m-labeled agents are prepared from Tc-99m pertechnetate and stocked pharmaceutical kits. Studies may be performed on an as-needed basis. Both are easy to image radiopharmaceuticals with good soft-tissue penetration (140 keV gamma energy) and a high photon flux from typical doses of 8–22 mCi. In addition the Tc-99m agents also provide an opportunity with the same injection to perform gated first pass or gated SPECT studies which can be used to estimate left ventricular functional parameters such as left ventricular ejection fraction (LVEF) which are discussed later in this chapter.

Dual Isotope Myocardial Scans. An innovative way to maximize the logistical throughput of a clinic performing myocardial perfusion scans involves the use of a Tl-201 and a Tc-99m agent for sequential scans. Perhaps the most widely used dual isotope scan technique uses a resting Tl-201 scan done at the convenience of the Nuclear Medicine clinic's schedule followed by a Tc-99m (Sestamibi or Tetrofosmin) scan scheduled at the convenience of the cardiologist or other provider performing the stress or pharmacological challenge. Because the energy and photon flux of the Tc-99m scan is higher than the Tl-201 scan there is no problem with cross talk between the rest and stress images. Excellent scan quality can be combined with one day convenience.

Interpretation

Myocardical Ischemia. Interpretation of myocardial perfusion scans is difficult but important. Subtle abnormalities can signal serious coronary artery disease. Observer experience is essential for an accurate diagnosis. Parametric methods of perfusion image analysis have been employed in attempts to standardize diagnosis. Circumferential profiles of isotope distribution and analyses of regional rates of Tl-201 washout, compared with normal data bases, make interpretation more sensitive in the detection of ischemia. Displayed as graphic data, "bull's-eye" maps of SPECT images, and three-dimensional reconstruction of SPECT data, these aids in interpretation may be overly sensitive. If an abnormality is truly present, it should also be visible in the planar or SPECT images. Depending on the statistical assumptions used and the population studied the sensitivity

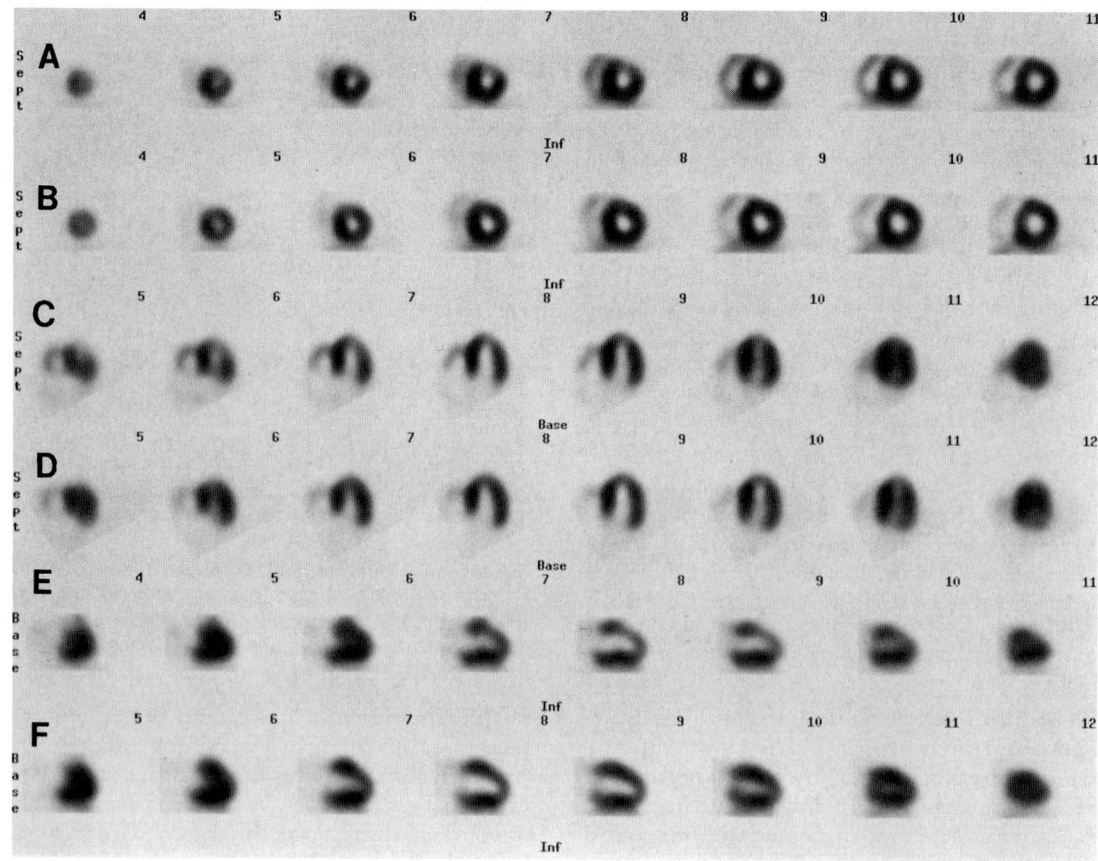

Figure 57.5. SPECT of LAD Reversible Ischemia. The row of short axis stress images **(A)** has a perfusion defect in the anterior wall (*arrows*) which perfuses normally in the rest of short axis images **(B)**. This is also visible in the horizontal long axis stress **(C)** and vertical long axis stress images **(E)** which have the same perfusion defect (*arrows*). At rest the matched images **(D,E,F)** show normal perfusion.

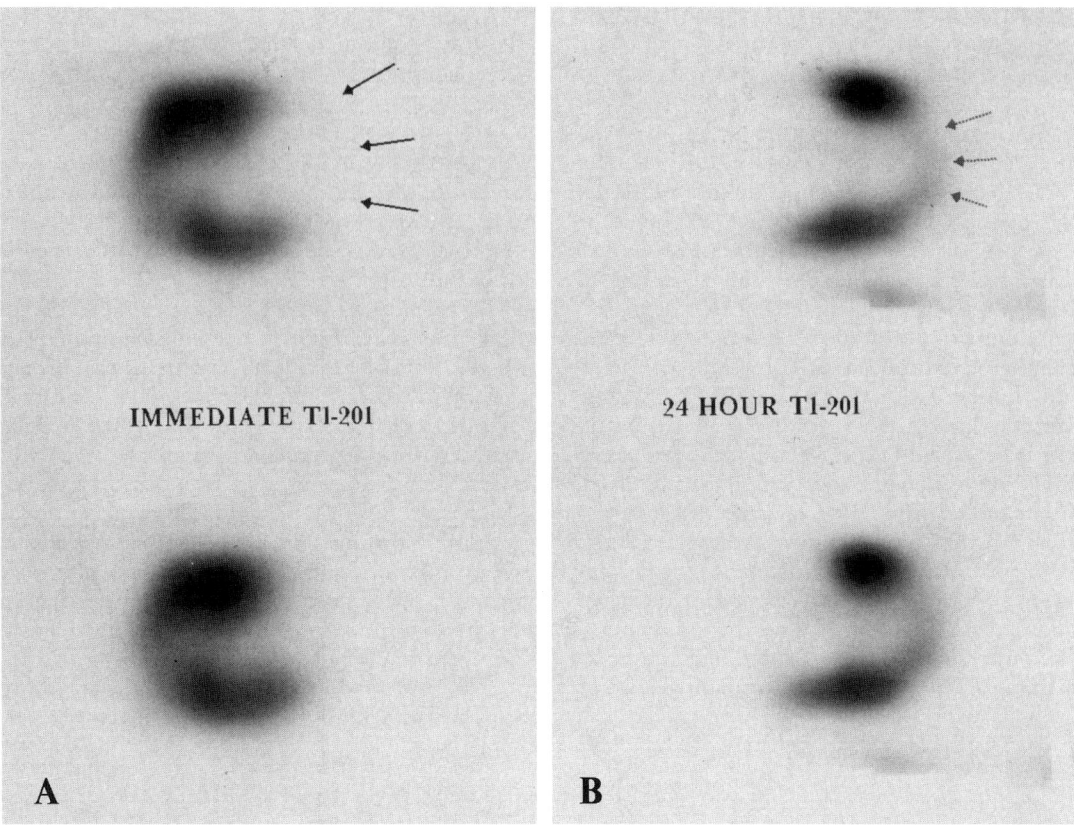

Figure 57.6. Hibernating Myocardium. Two vertical long axis Tl-201 images at rest **(A)** are compared with matched images at 24 hours **(B)**. The large anteroapical defect (*arrows*) partly fills in over time in-dicating that some hibernating (viable) myocardium is present in the midst of what looked initially to be infarcted tissue.

and specificity for detecting myocardial ischemia are in the percent range of the high 80s or low 90s. The myocardial perfusion scan also detects other causes of ischemia (including left bundle branch block, coronary vasculitis, and small vessel disease) which cannot be seen on coronary arteriography and thereby reduce its apparent specificity. In addition to detecting significant coronary artery atherosclerotic disease, the presence and severity of ischemic myocardium correlates strongly with the prognosis for adverse cardiac events including angina and cardiac death (Fig. 57.5).

Images of the heart map relative regional perfusion. Areas of myocardium with poor blood supply, usually because of atherosclerosis, fail to increase labeling by the perfusion agent during exercise. The most important feature of the myocardial perfusion test is comparison of the stress and rest images to detect areas of ischemia that are inadequately perfused at exercise yet viable. These areas are redundantly called "*reversibly ischemic.*" Ischemia detected by either exercise or pharmacological dilation of normal vessels usually corresponds with angiographic abnormalities in coronary arteries. Correction of the anatomic abnormality by angioplasty, laser atherectomy, or coronary artery bypass surgery is expected to relieve the ischemia. A frequent location of ischemic tissue is immediately adjacent to an area of infarct. This is called *peri-infarct ischemia* and may overlie or surround an infarct.

Some arterial distributions have naturally recruited collaterals or bypass grafts that produce apparent discrepancies between angiographic and scintigraphic studies. Abnormal anatomy in a coronary artery may not produce hemodynamically significant changes in blood flow to the myocardium. Not all ischemia is produced by large vessel atherosclerosis. Capillary disease in diabetics, left bundle branch block, vasospasm, vasculitis, or cardiomyopathy (dilated or hypertrophic) may produce ischemic myocardium even with normal arteries.

Hibernating Myocardium. Severe ischemia may be so slow to "reverse" on Tl-201 imaging that it will not be detected by rest images at 3–4 hours after exercise. Imaging at 24 hours, or a Tl-201 second injection rest study, may be required to detect extreme ischemia. The Tc-99m-labeled agents are routinely given as two separate injections, but evidence suggests that rest-injected Tl-201 studies may be best for detecting the severe ischemia that leads to a phenomenon known as "hibernating myocardium." Hibernating myocardium is important to diagnose as it simulates infarction by not contracting at rest. It remains viable, however, and will return to normal function after revascularization (Fig. 57.6). Ischemia may not be detected if there is inadequate exercise, inadequate pharmacological challenge, or balanced triple vessel disease. Fortunately, it is uncommon for all three coronary arteries to be hemodynamically compromised equally.

Myocardial Infarction produces layers of nonperfused scar tissue that are detected as areas of thin myocardium with decreased labeling at *both* exercise (or pharmacological dilation of coronary arteries) *and* rest. The extent of an infarct, from subendocardial to transmural, is reflected by the size and degree of the perfusion defect (Fig. 57.7). Technical artifacts from attenuation of the perfusion agent's radiation may be produced by SPECT tables, breast tissue, and subdiaphragmatic structures. These may appear as fixed defects superimposed on planar or SPECT images. This may lead to a false-positive reading of infarction. A false-positive interpretation of ischemia should not occur as long as the artifact does not change between stress and rest imaging.

Three techniques are in use to reduce the artifactual appearance of fixed defects seen with myocardial perfusion scanning. The simplest relies on scanning of the patient in the prone position. This changes the position of the heart, diaphragm and the subdiaphragmatic organs and reduces the appearance of inferior wall fixed defects which are misinterpreted as posterior descending artery distribution infarctions. Unfortunately, obese patients in whom there is plenty of subdiaphragmatic attenuation, may not be able to lay prone for this scan (Fig. 57.8).

Another technique that avoids misinterpretation of fixed artifactual defects as infarctions relies on gating the acquisition. This is best done with the Tc-99m labeled agents. It is a very simple technique with planar scans and somewhat more involved with SPECT scans. A cine replay of the gated study allows assessment of wall motion. The normal wall moves inward during systole, thickens as it contracts, and becomes brighter on the display. A wall that looks thin but moves well is probably not infarcted.

The elegant solution to the problem of artifactual defects has only recently become available. This relies on the simultaneous SPECT acquisition of an emission *and* a transmission scan performed with a radioactive source of a different energy than that used for the emission scan. With a transmission scan allowance for the emission photons lost due to attenuation can be made and the resulting SPECT scans are surprisingly artifact free. A related improvement on this scheme incorporates correction for photons scattered from the emission source but still accepted by the imaging system. A combination of attenuation and scatter correction promises truly quantitative imaging in the future (Fig. 57.9).

Stunned Myocardium. A single myocardial perfusion scan cannot determine the age of an infarct. Acute in-

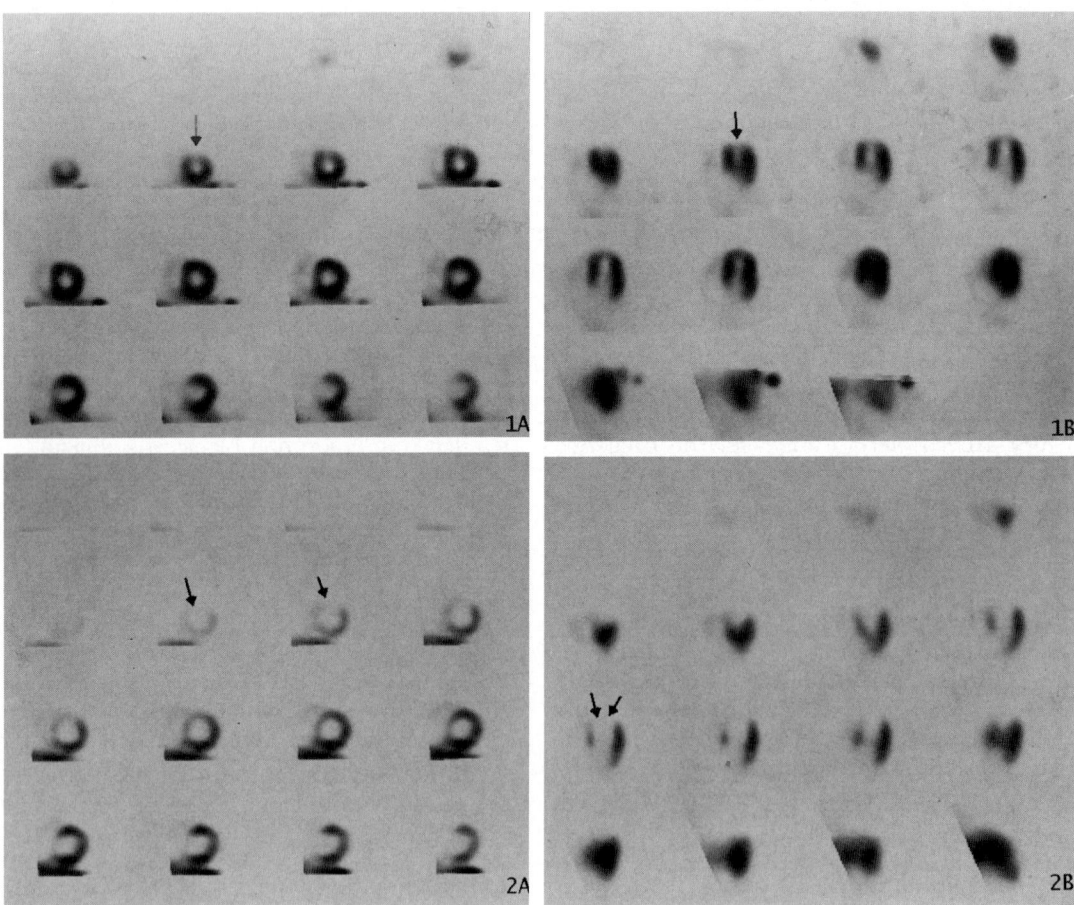

Figure 57.7. Resting Images of Infarcts of the LAD. Short axis **(1A)** and horizontal long axis **(1B)** SPECT images show a small anterior LAD infarct (*arrows*). This is compared with another patient who has a much larger LAD infarct **(2A,2B)** in the same vascular distribution (*arrows*). Note that the second patient's infarct extends from the anterolateral wall to and includes the septum. The ventricle is also dilated at rest.

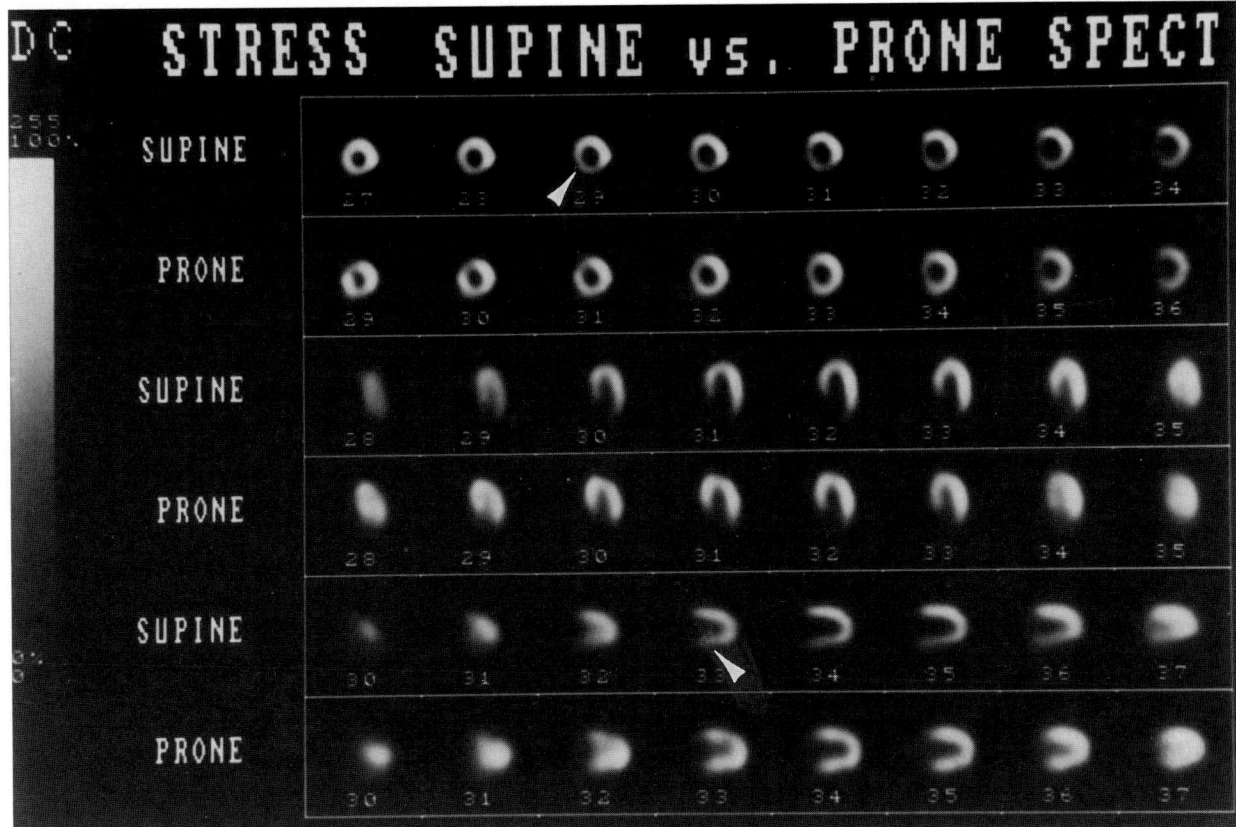

Figure 57.8. Stress versus Prone Imaging. Tc-99m Sestamibi imaging with a single headed SPECT camera shows a defect in the inferior wall during stress imaging (*arrowheads*) which is not present when the patient is reimaged in the prone position.

farcts usually appear larger than old infarcts when imaged with Tl-201. Temporarily damaged cells around infarcted cells, "stunned myocardium," will neither contract nor take up Tl-201 for a few days. As repair occurs, the apparent perfusion defect shrinks.

Infarct Avid Scans. Acute infarcts may also be detected with Tc-99m pyrophosphate labeling. Ionized calcium released from myocytes forms dystrophic calcifications with phosphates and a "hot spot" is formed adjacent to infarcted tissue. Antimyosin antibodies labeled with Tc-99m or indium-111 (In-111) also localize on the fringes of acute infarctions. The need for imaging of acute infarction is clinically infrequent, usually when the patient has left bundle branch block. Contused myocardium is also detected with these techniques.

GATED BLOOD POOL SCANS

The radionuclide ventriculogram (RVG) is a study that uses circulating, Tc-99m-labeled red blood cells to evaluate the size, wall motion, and functional parameters of the left ventricle. Right ventricle (RV) evaluation is better accomplished by the first pass study, to be discussed later.

Technique

A simple method to label red blood cells begins with an intravenous (IV) injection of a tin (Sn)-pyrophosphate compound. This is used to prepare the patient's red blood cells for labeling by a subsequent IV injection of 99m-technetium. Doses of up to 30 mCi are commonly used for typical adult patients. Electrocardiographic leads on the limbs or chest are used to obtain a suitable gating signal (the R wave) for the computer. Using the ECG as a measure of the cardiac cycle's length, the cardiac cycle is divided into a minimum of 16 frames for analysis of systolic function. Higher temporal resolution of 32 frames per cardiac cycle is required for measurement of diastolic function. The result of this acquisition is a composite, "averaged" series of images representing the patient's cardiac cycle. Data from a sufficient number of cardiac cycles (several hundred) must be obtained to make the images statistically significant for analysis. Typical acquisition time is 5–20 minutes per view (Fig. 57.10).

Analysis of the functional parameters of the LV, including the LV ejection fraction (LVEF) and first derivative (dV/DT; where V is LV volume and T is time) of the LV volume curve, is most accurate from images obtained in the "best septal" left anterior oblique view. This view produces the greatest separation of the activity of the LV from that of the RV. A zoomed acquisition of the RV and LV is recommended rather than images of the entire chest.

Computer processing of the image data by spatial and temporal smoothing algorithms improves both the visual analysis of wall motion and the accuracy and precision

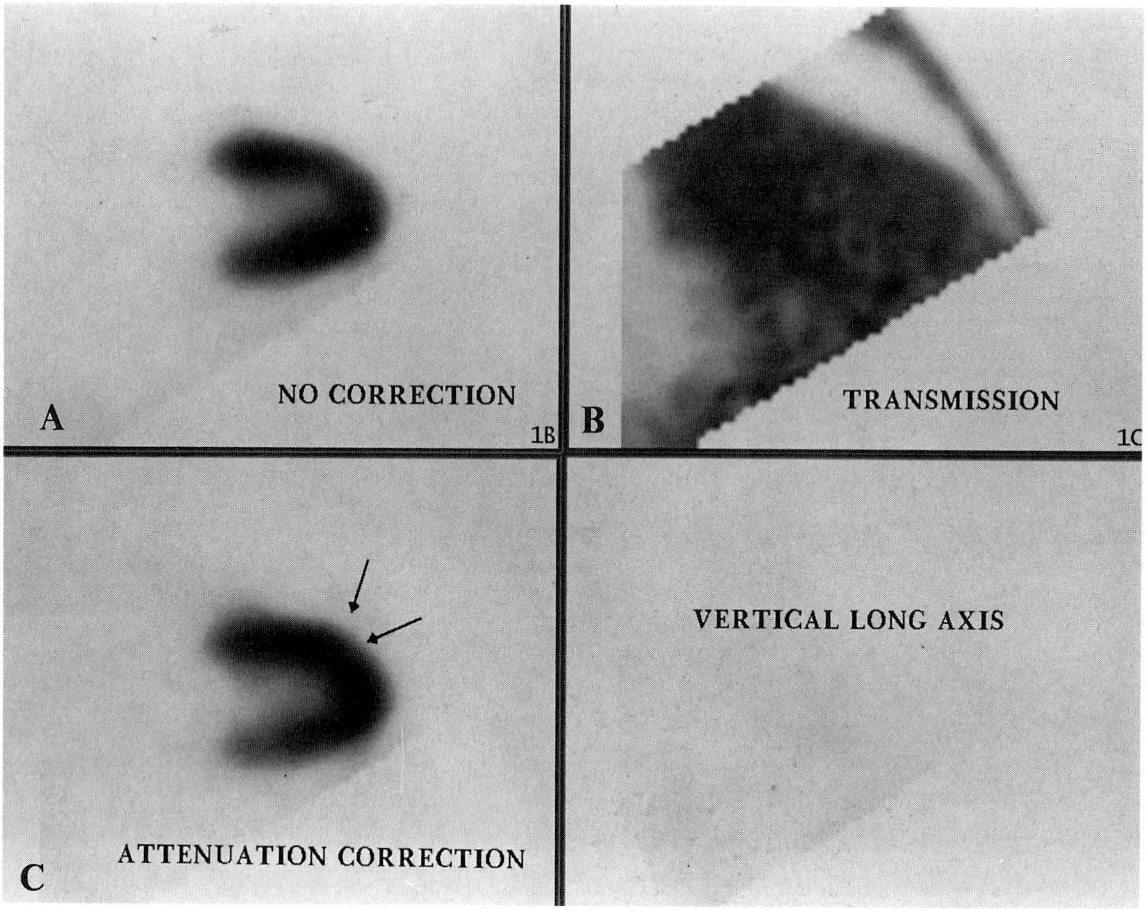

Figure 57.9. Attenuation Correction. An anterior wall defect caused by large breasts is corrected by simultaneous transmission and emission scans. A noncorrected vertical long axis scan **(A)** shows an apparent anterior wall defect which disappears when the transmission scan **(B)** is used to correct for the assymetric attenuation **(C)**. The anterior wall (*arrows*) is normal.

of the derived functional parameters. Outlining the edge of the ventricular blood pool in each frame of the study with second derivative edge detection methods is superior to threshold detection or manually drawn regions of interest. The volume curve is generated by plotting the number of counts in the ventricle versus time during the cardiac cycle. This curve generates the LVEF, which measures the change in volume between end diastole and end systole. The LVEF is the single best parameter of LV function (Fig. 57.11).

Arrhythmias such as frequent premature beats and atrial fibrillation tend to falsely lower the LVEF. The R-R (R-wave) interval histogram from the ECG can demonstrate the presence of arrhythmias. Most nuclear medicine computer systems allow analysis of selected populations of beats of the same R-R interval to yield a more accurate LVEF.

Additional functional parameters are easily obtained. The dV/DT of the LV volume curve gives important information on the rates (average or maximal) of systolic emptying and diastolic filling.

Cardiac Output (CO) in liters per minute may be calculated if the heart rate, the LVEF and the left ventricular end diastolic volume (LVEDV) are known. The product of all three is the CO. The first two are easy to obtain.

The LVEDV can be measured by comparing the count rate of a blood sample of known volume with the count rate of the ventricle at end diastole and end systole. This requires attenuation correction of the image data to allow for radioactivity absorbed by the chest wall.

Another, simpler method to measure the CO uses a "count-based ratio method." The ratio of the total counts to the maximum counts in the diastolic frame is entered into an equation that also requires a calibration of the voxel size for the acquisition and depends on constants derived from the formula for a sphere. The resulting measurement of the LVEDV has about the same error as more complicated methods and allows a rapid estimate of the CO (Fig. 57.12).

The exact range of normal for functional parameters of the RVG will depend on multiple factors. These include the camera used, the field of view (degree of zoom), number of frames acquired, counts within each image, method of computer filtering of the data, and methods of background correction and edge detection. Each laboratory should establish its own normal range. In the authors' clinic the clinically established normal resting LVEF is approx 65%, with a standard deviation of 5%. (The normal range of 2 standard deviations is 55–75%.)

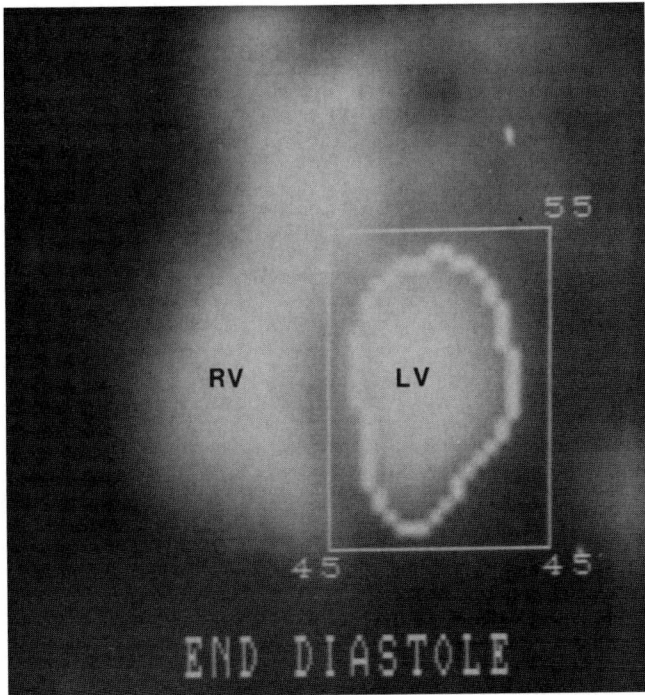

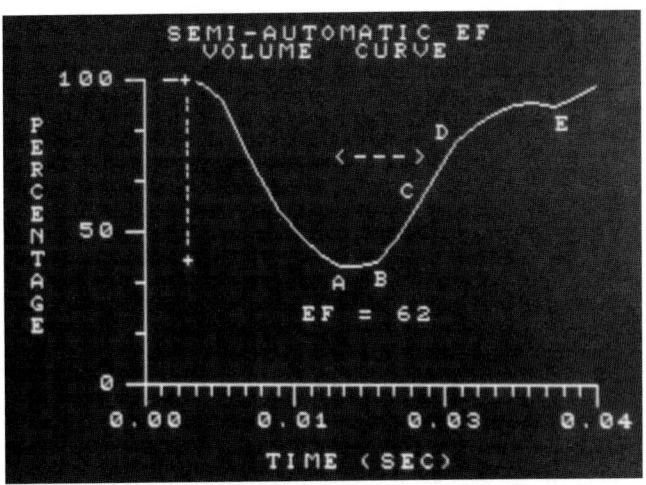

Figure 57.10. Normal Gated Blood Pool Image. An end-diastolic image is shown with a computer-generated region of interest around the left ventricle (*LV*) blood pool. The right ventricle (*RV*) is adjacent.

Figure 57.11. Left Ventricular Time Activity Curve. The graph shows this curve (from the patient in Fig. 57.10) that displays the ventricles relative volume during the cardiac cycle. *The vertical dashed line* represents the relative stroke volume expressed as an ejection fraction of 62%. The curve begins at end diastole, *A* marks end systole, *B* marks the start of diastolic filling, *C* marks the peak filling rate, *D* the end of rapid filling, and *E* the beginning of the atrial "kick." The *horizontal dashed line* shows the interval of the first third of diastole during which more than half of the stroke volume is recovered.

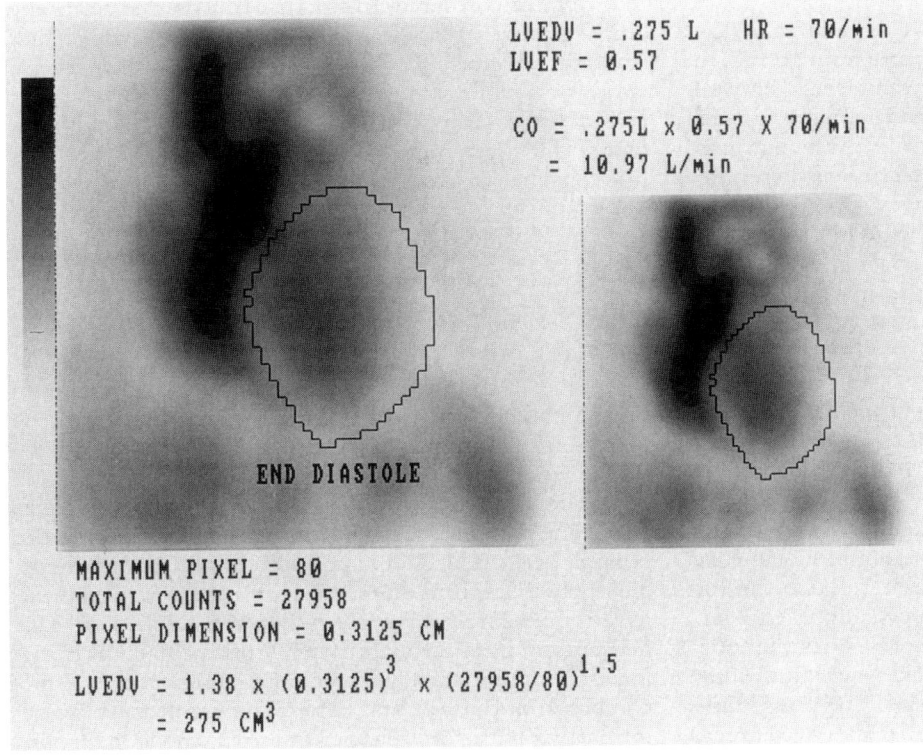

Figure 57.12. Sample Calculations of Cardiac Output (CO). The LVEDV calculation uses the count based ratio method which requires measurement of the total counts in the end diastolic ROI, the maximum pixel counts in the same ROI, and measurements of the size of a pixel in centimeters. In this case the dilated LV has a LVEDV of 275 cubic centimeters. Multiplying the LVEDV by the LVEF and heart rate gives a global CO of 10.97 L/min.

Interpretation

Left Ventricular Ejection Fraction. The most common causes of elevated LVEF values include mitral or aortic valvular regurgitation, hypertrophic cardiomyopathy, and high cardiac output states such as those found in hyperthyroidism.

Low LVEF values are usually seen in patients with prior myocardial infarction, ischemia (with congestive heart failure), and cardiomyopathy of any cause. A common application of the RVG is monitoring for the development of cardiotoxicity from chemotherapeutic drugs. The dV/DT curve is a somewhat more sensitive measure of the systolic and diastolic dysfunction that accompanies the progression of dilated and hypertrophic cardiomyopathy.

End-diastolic Volume. The relative end-diastolic size and shape of the RV and LV chambers (RVEDV and LVEDV) should be always noted. Though they appear roughly equal in a normal best-septal left anterior oblique view, the RVEDV is normally greater than the LVEDV. If no intracardiac shunts are present, the stroke volumes of the ventricles are equal because the RV ejection fraction is smaller than the LVEF. As the LV fails for any reason, it dilates and usually becomes rounder in shape. (See figure 57.12 for an example of a dilated left ventricle.)

Wall Motion of various regions of the LV can be assessed from an overlay of end-diastolic and end-systolic edge images. This is best evaluated by visually observing a cine display of the beating heart in two orthogonal views. The left posterior oblique view of the LV is imaged at a right angle to the best septal view. There is limited utility of anterior and other views done in oblique projections.

As the ventricular wall is damaged or infarcted, the progression of wall motion abnormality is from normal to hypokinetic to akinetic. If an aneurysm forms, the wall will become dyskinetic. To determine the degree of abnormality, it is important to concentrate on the margins of the LV chamber, which is the interface of the endocardial surface and blood. The observer should attempt to correlate a suspicion of abnormal wall motion in one view with this same area on the orthogonal view. Color computer displays that enhance the margins of the chambers may make subtle wall motion abnormalities more detectable.

It is very important to correlate RVG wall motion abnormalities whenever possible with myocardial perfusion images. Areas of myocardial infarction will usually be seen to have some degree of abnormal wall motion on the RVG study.

Fourier phase analysis provides powerful additional information on the amount of motion (amplitude) of various LV wall segments and also their relative timing (phase). The amplitude image is especially useful for confirming areas suspected to be hypokinetic or akinetic on the cine display. Damaged areas of myocardium contract with less vigor than normal areas. The phase display may help detect such areas because damaged areas contract slowly (tardykinesis). Dyskinetic aneurysmal areas are dramatically displayed using Fourier amplitude and phase images. There is wall motion of the segment displayed on the amplitude image but it is opposite (180° out of phase) compared with undamaged areas (Figs. 57.13, 57.14).

Valvular Regurgitation. Another use of fourier amplitude images is in the calculation of valvular regurgitation. Each pixel in an amplitude image is coded with a number proportional to the blood volume change under that pixel during the cardiac cycle. A simple total of the pixel values in all the LV and RV pixels outlined with region-of-interest markers will produce a ratio of the LV to RV stroke volume. The ratio can be used to calculate the regurgitant fraction. This method works only when there are regurgitant valves on one side of the septum. It cannot tell aortic regurgitation from mitral regurgition, however (Fig 57.15).

The RVG studies can be easily performed in an intensive care setting with a mobile gamma camera and computer system. They are also valuable to serially assess the effect of therapeutic measures.

Exercise RVG. The RVG study can also be done repeatedly while the patient is exercising on a bicycle ergometer at various work load levels. This is an excellent method to monitor cardiac functional response to exercise. The exercise RVG study is technically much more difficult to accomplish than resting study. The patient must be cooperative and capable of exercising. The 2–3 minute periods for each exercise level usually supply a minimally acceptable amount of statistical counts in the gated images. Finally, a large amount of data must be processed and reviewed because each stage of the study is comparable with a resting study (Table 57.1).

Normal patients increase their LVEF and dV/DT significantly while decreasing their LV end-systolic volume. The relative cardiac output can be measured from one stage to another and rises with increasing work load. Abnormal exercise RVG response can be seen in several ways, such as an increase of LVEDV more than 10%, lack of increase or even a fall in LVEF with greater work loads, and development of wall motion abnormalities due to ischemia brought on by the exercise.

RIGHT VENTRICULAR STUDIES

First Pass Function Studies

Right ventricular function is more difficult to assess by the RVG study than is LV function. This is because labeled activity in the RV cannot be isolated as well from other chambers as can LV activity. RV function is best assessed by analyzing images from the first pass of a radionuclide bolus through the right-sided chambers and lungs before the overlapping left-sided chambers are seen. The patient is usually imaged in the right anterior oblique projection. A bolus of up to 30 mCi of high specific-activity isotope must be very rapidly injected followed immediately by a nonradioactive flush dose. This activity will pass through the RV in three to eight heartbeats. Some systems allow acquisition as a gated study composed of these beats. Others allow retrospective reformatting of the first pass data into a cine loop display. These techniques yield a small amount of data compared with the many hundreds of beats in a resting RVG study.

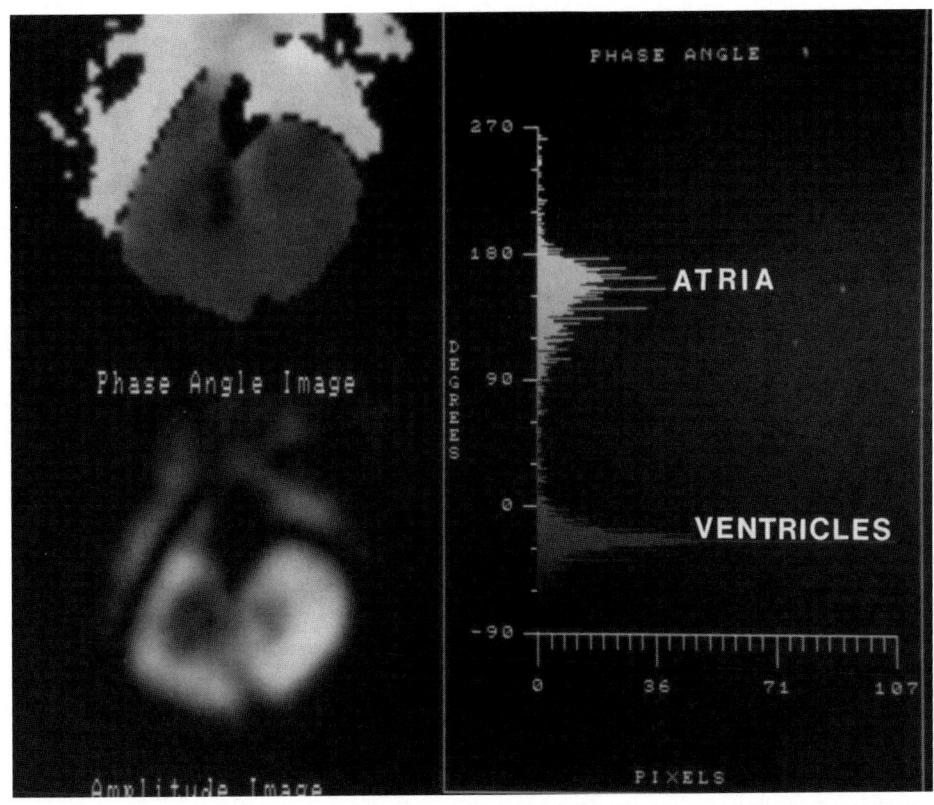

Figure 57.13. Normal Fourier Phase and Amplitude Images from the Same Patient in Figures 57.10 and 57.11. The lower (*Amplitude*) image shows the relative displacement of blood in each chamber of the heart. The pixel brightness depicts the relative degree of motion. The upper (*Phase*) image shows the relative timing of contraction of each chamber. The histogram summarizes the number of pixels with a given phase angle. The cardiac cycle is represented on an arbitrary scale of −90° to 270°. Note that the *gray pixels* representing ventricular motion are tightly grouped around −30°, indicating synchronous contraction. Approximately 180° up the time scale, there is a cluster of *white* pixels corresponding to atrial motion.

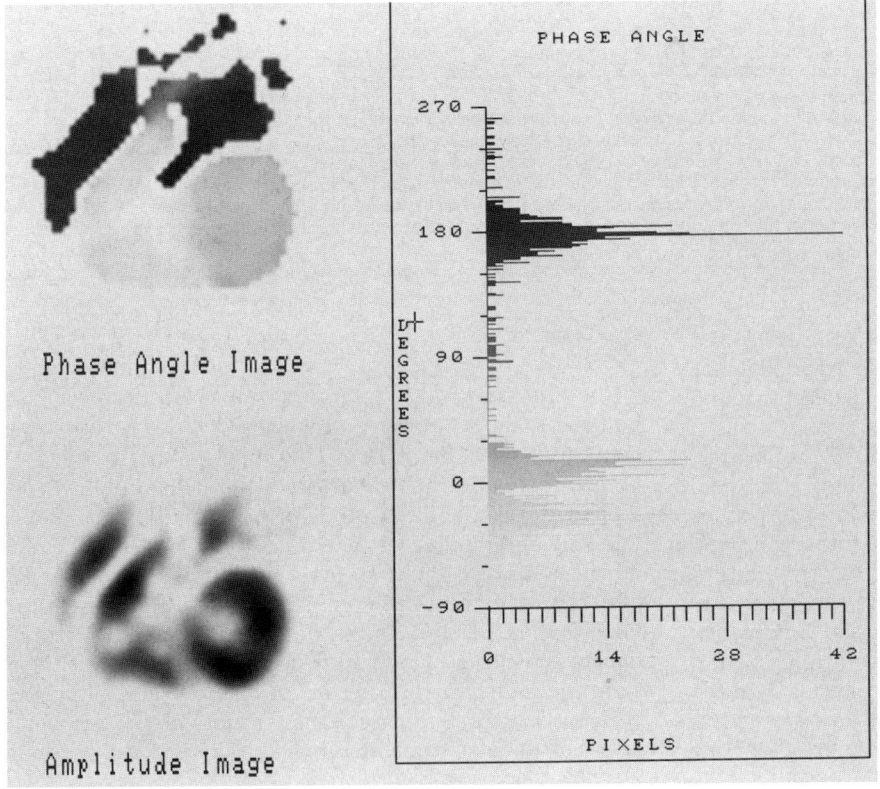

Figure 57.14. Fourier Phase and Amplitude in Left Bundle Branch Block (LBBB). Two separate populations of phase values are seen in the RV and LV. The lighter colored RV contracts before the darker colored LV. This is much easier to see in color!

Figure 57.15. Mitral Regurgitation Calculated from a Fourier Amplitude Image. The total counts in the LV and RV ROIs yield a 1.5-1 LV/RV stroke ratio with a 0.33 regurgitant fraction. This is the same patient used for Figure 57.12. The global CO of 10.97 is multiplied by the complement of the regurgitant fraction (0.67) to generate a forward CO of 7.35 L/min.

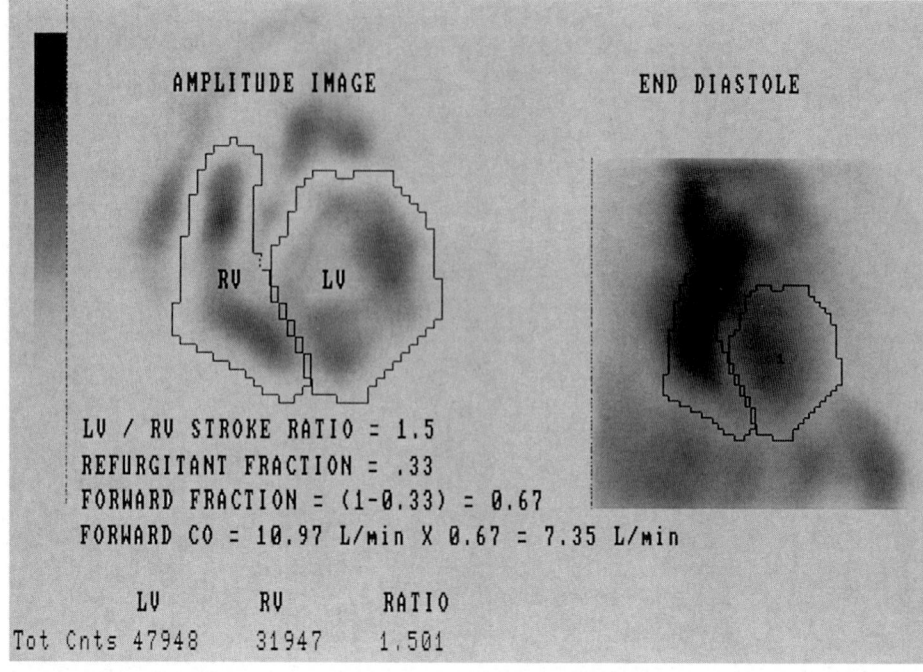

AMPLITUDE IMAGE   END DIASTOLE

RV   LV

LV / RV STROKE RATIO = 1.5
REFURGITANT FRACTION = .33
FORWARD FRACTION = (1-0.33) = 0.67
FORWARD CO = 10.97 L/min X 0.67 = 7.35 L/min

	LV	RV	RATIO
Tot Cnts	47948	31947	1.501

Table 57.1. Poor Diastolic Function

Exercise Radionucldie Ventriculogram-Relative Volumes and Cardiac Output								
Level	HR	BP	DP(k)	LVEF	rLVEDV	rLVESV	rLVSV	rCO
Rest	78	150	11.7	0.56	1.00	1.00	1.00	1.00
EX1	101	152	15.4	0.60	0.83	0.76	0.89	1.16
EX2	102	158	16.1	0.64	0.90	0.74	1.03	1.35
EX3	106	158	16.7	0.64	0.96	0.79	1.10	1.50
EX4	115	170	19.6	0.68	0.91	0.66	1.11	1.63
EX5	133	190	25.3	0.72	0.77	0.49	1.00	1.70
EX6	153	192	29.4	0.71	0.59	0.39	0.75	1.47
Post-EX	162	162	26.2	0.70	0.69	0.47	0.86	1.79

This exercise radionuclide ventriculogram shows that the patient worked hard during six levels of bicycle exercise as the heart rate (*HR*) rose from 78 to 153, while systolic blood pressure (*BP*) rose from 150 to 192 with a resultant rise in double product (*DP*) from 11.7 to 29.4 K. The left ventricular ejection fraction (*LVEF*) rises appropriately from 0.56 to 0.71 at peak exercise. However, the ventricle fills poorly during exercise as relative end-systolic volume (*rLVESV*) goes progressively down (normal) *but* relative end-diastolic volume (*rLVEDV*) goes down (abnormal). The stroke volume (*rLVSV*) changes little and the only improvement in relative cardiac output (*rCO*) is the result of increased heart rate. Poor diastolic function (poor compliance) limits exercise endurance in this otherwise healthy individual. This is a superb example of the quantitative data inherent in nuclear medicine images.

A region of interest is established around the RV and a time activity curve allows an RV ejection fraction to be measured for each beat. An average RV ejection fraction is calculated (Fig. 57.16).

There is a good RVEF technique that is not widely available. It uses Xenon-133 in saline solution for injection. During a slow venous infusion the Xe-133 passes through the right side of the heart and into the lungs, where it immediately fills the alveoli and is exhaled. In this way, overlapping activity never enters the left side of the heart. A gated study over many seconds is possible. Data from many beats can be collected and processed in a manner identical to the standard RVG of the LV. In the authors' clinics the mean Xe-133 RVEF is 42% with a standard deviation of 5% with a normal range of 32-52% (Fig. 57.17).

First Pass Flow Studies

The first pass study in an anterior projection can also be used to detect abnormalities of blood flow to one lung compared with the other. The effect of extrinsic compression on a pulmonary artery by a mediastinal or hilar mass can be easily detected, especially if Fourier phase analysis and display of the data is used. Abnormal blood flow to a lung segment such as is seen in pulmonary sequestration can be detected. The first pass study can be used to measure the transit time of an injected bolus between ventricles. There is a delay in passage of blood from the right ventricle to the left ventricle which typifies congestive heart failure. Obstruction of the superior vena cava is also easily diagnosed in a matter of seconds (Fig. 57.18).

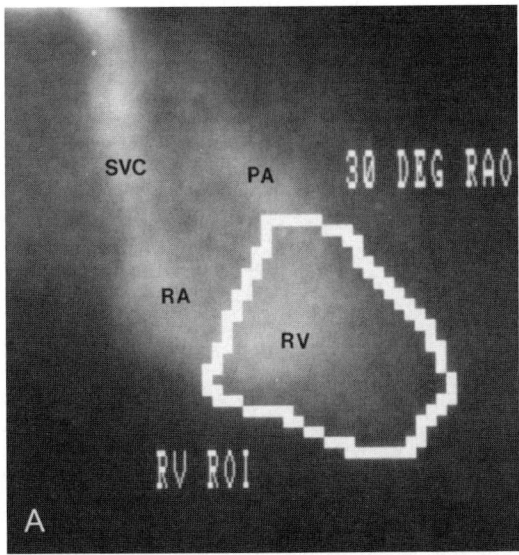
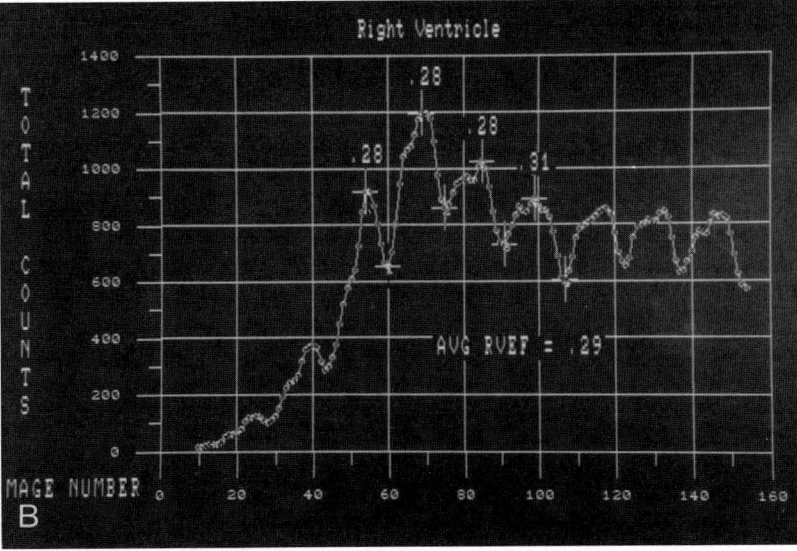

Figure 57.16. Right Ventricular First Pass Function Study. A. Fast dynamic right ventricular ejection fraction by first pass. The acquisition totaled 512 frames taken at 40 millisecond intervals in the right anterior oblique (*RAO*) projection as a radioactive bolus traversed the right atrium (*RA*) and ventricle (*RV*). An image of the *RV* is made by summing dozens of individual frames. A fixed region of interest (*ROI*) is drawn around the RV. *SVC*, superior vena cava; *PA*, pulmonary artery. **B.** A time activity curve from the ROI in **(A)** shows the relative volume of the ventricle rising and falling with diastole and systole. Peaks and valleys in the curve are flagged and beat by beat ejection fractions are averaged.

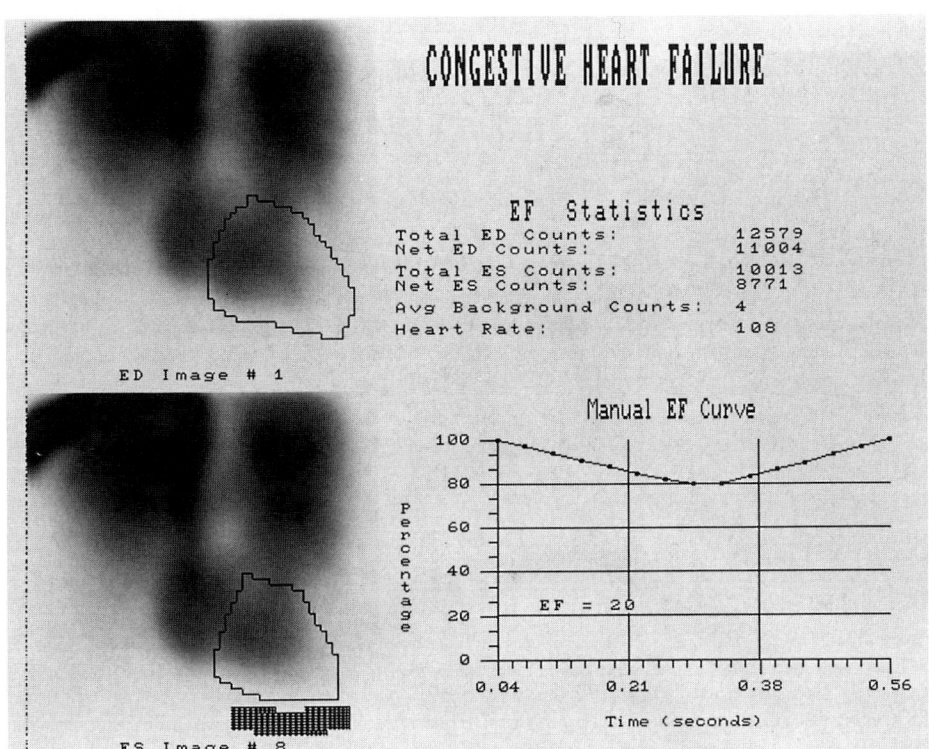

Figure 57.17. Xe-133 Right Heart Gated First Pass Study. Xe-133 in saline is slowly infused for a gated first pass study. It is shown with RAO end diastolic and end systolic frames and their respective ROIs around the RV blood pool. The RVEF in this patient with congestive heart failure is only 20%.

Figure 57.18. Superior Vena Cava (SVC) Obstruction. A first pass study with one second frames is shown in the anterior porjection after injection in the right antecubital vein. Serpiginous collateral veins on the chest wall probably communicate with the intercostal and azygous veins. Very little flow courses through the SVC into the right atrium and ventricle (*arrow*). The patient required stenting of the SVC to relieve obstruction caused by encircling tumor.

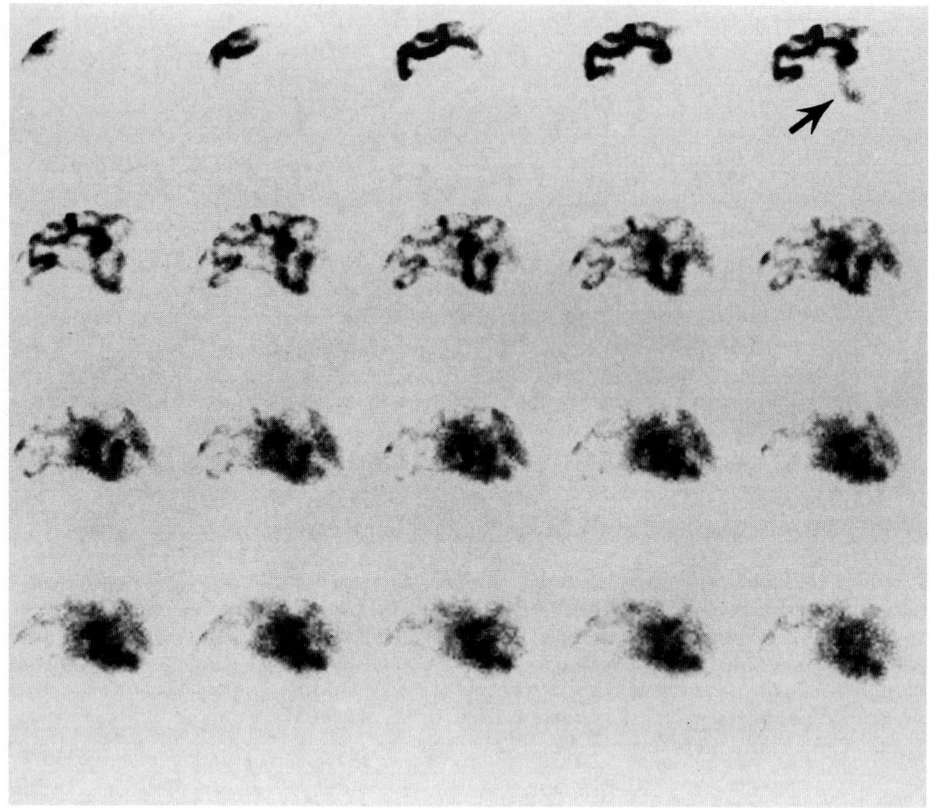

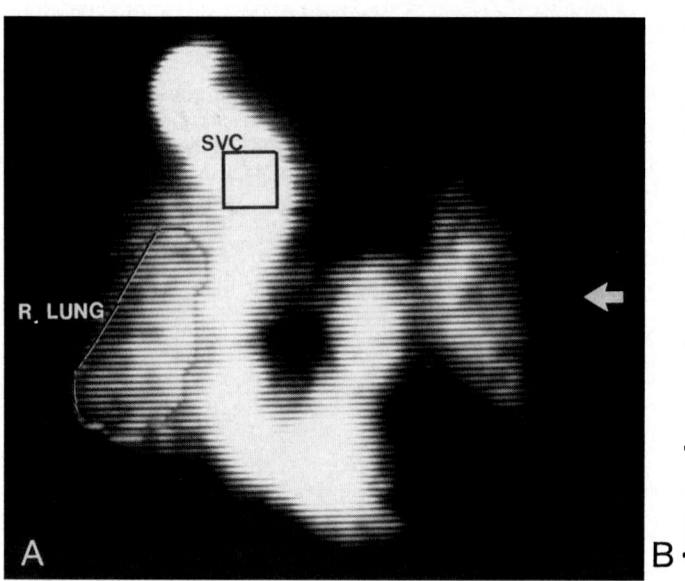

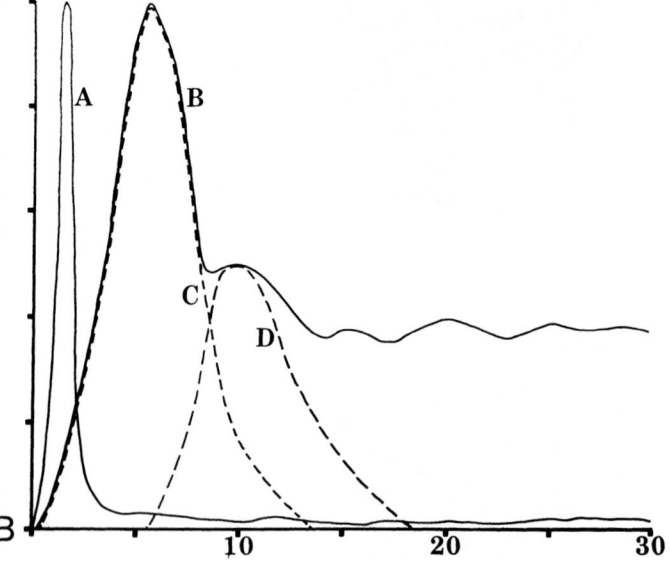

Figure 57.19. Abnormal Left-to-right Shunt Study. A. Regions of interest are drawn around the superior vena cava (*SVC, square box*) and the right lung (*R lung*) on image data from a first pass flow study. Note lack of activity in the *LV* (*arrow*) in this summary of images from the dextrophase of the flow. **B.** Graph showing time activity curve of the activity within the two regions shown in **(A)**. *A* is the sharp bolus injection passing through the superior vena cava. *B* is the right lung time activity curve, which rises exponentially but does not follow the fitted gamma variate curve (*C*) on the way down. This indicates early recirculation due to a left to right shunt. The shunt is quantified by comparing the area under *C* with the area under the fitted recirculation gamma variate (*D*).

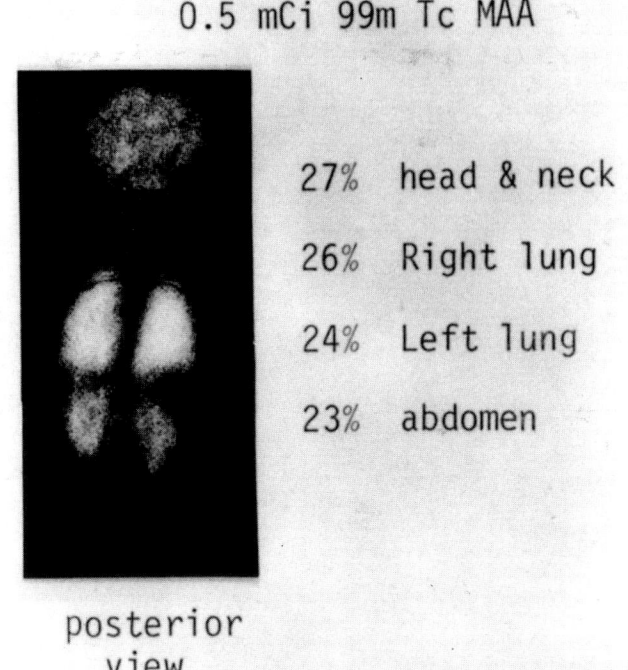

0.5 mCi 99m Tc MAA

27%   head & neck

26%   Right lung

24%   Left lung

23%   abdomen

posterior
view

Figure 57.20. Abnormal Right-to-Left Shunt Study. A significant portion of the injected Tc-99m macroaggregated albumin (*MAA*) particles are seen in capillary beds outside the lungs in the brain and kidneys. This indicates and measures the amount of shunted blood.

Left-to-right Intracardiac Shunts can be detected and quantified using a first pass imaging technique. Instead of using a region of interest over the RV for analysis, an area of lung is used. In a normal person, the bolus of activity passes into and out of the lung exponentially in a way that can be mathematically described by a gamma function. If a left-to-right shunt is present, some blood that has gone through the lungs to the left side of the heart reenters the right side of the heart and is pumped back into the lungs. This causes a prolonga-

tion of the washout of activity from the lung region of interest. A gamma-variate curve fitting method can be used to detect and quantify the amount of the left-to-right shunt. The method is sensitive to detect shunts with a ratio as low as 1.2:1, far below the 2:1 shunt that can be detected by chest radiograph (Fig. 57.19).

Right-to-left Shunts can be detected by using an IV injection of macroaggregated albumin particles. In a normal person, less than 10% of the injected dose should pass through normal arteriovenous shunts in the lungs and be found in the systemic circulation. After injection, static images of the patient's whole body are performed. Regions of interest are taken over the lungs, head, neck, abdomen, and extremities. In this way, the amount of radioactivity outside the lungs in the systemic circulation can be quantified. The study can be repeated at a later date to check progression (Fig. 57.20).

Suggested Reading

Bacharach SL, Green MV, Borer JS. Instrumentation and data processing in cardiovascular nuclear medicine: evaluation of ventricular function. Semin Nucl 1979;9:257–274.

Berman DS, Hosen K, Van Train K, et al. Technetium 99m sestamibi in the assessment of chronic coronary artery disease. Semin Nucl Med 1991;21:190–212.

Bonow RO, Dilszian V. T1-201 for assessment of myocardial viability. Semin Nucl Med 1991;21:230–241.

Green MV, Bacharach SL. Functional imaging of the heart: methods, limitations, and examples from gated blood pool scintigraphy. Progr Cardiovasc Dis 1986;28:319–348.

Jones RH. Use of radionuclide measurements of left ventricular function for prognosis in patients with coronary artery disease. Semin Nucl Med 1987;17:95–103.

Parker DA, Karvelis KC, Thrall JH, Froelich JW. Radionuclide ventriculography: methods. In: Gerson MC, ed. Cardiac Nuclear Medicine. New York: McGraw Hill, 1991:81–125.

Rozanski A, Berman DS. The efficacy of cardiovascular nuclear medicine exercise studies. Semin Nucl Med 1987;17:104–120.

Treves S, Parker JA. Detection and quantification of intracardiac shunts. In: Strauss HW, Pitt B, eds. Cardiovascular Nuclear Medicine. St Louis; CV Mosby, 1979:148–161.

58
Endocrine Gland Scintigraphy

Marc G. Cote
John M. Bauman

THYROID

Imaging Methods

Diagnosis and treatment of thyroid disease require the evaluation of thyroid function, anatomy including palpatory findings, and tissue characterization of thyroid lesions (1,2). Radionuclide scintigraphy and measurement of radioiodine uptake form the basis of functional assessment of the thyroid.

Radionuclide scintigraphy is used to assess the physiologic function of the gland and to determine the presence or functional status of nodules. Thyroid imaging is most commonly indicated to evaluate hyperthyroidism. Solitary palpable thyroid nodules are best evaluated initially with fine needle aspiration (FNA).

Normal thyroid parenchyma appears relatively homogeneous with technetium-99m-pertechnetate (Tc-99m-O_4) or Iodine-123 (I-123) scintigraphy. Iodine is trapped via active transport and organified onto the tyrosine contained in intrathyroidal thyroglobulin within thyroid follicles. Tc-99m-O_4 is only trapped and will subsequently wash out of the gland because it is not organified. I-123 is the agent of choice for thyroid imaging especially when imaging nodules (Table 58.1). Tc-99m-O_4 is best reserved for imaging hyperthyroid patients in conjunction with a Iodine-131 (I-131) radioactive iodine uptake (RAIU—the percentage of the administered dose present in the thyroid gland at a specific time after oral administration, usually 24 hours).

The functional status of a thyroid nodule may be categorized as hyperfunctioning ("hot"), hypofunctioning ("cold"), or indeterminate (sometimes called "warm") relative to the normal parenchymal uptake of radioiodine. Hot nodules usually represent hyperfunctioning adenomatous tissue and are rarely malignant. Although solitary cold nodules are hypofunctioning adenomatous tissue in approximately 40% of cases, they may harbor malignancy in up to 15% of cases (3). Indeterminate nodules have the same significance as cold nodules. The term "warm" should be avoided because it is easily misunderstood by the referring physician to have the same clinical significance as a "hot" nodule. Indeterminate nodules are due to normal activity overlying or surrounding a hypofunctioning cold nodule.

Tc-99m-O_4 is inexpensive but has the disadvantage of a lower target-to-background ratio. Also, if a nodule is hot with Tc-99m-O_4, an additional I-123 study must be performed to exclude a discordant nodule. A discordant nodule demonstrates increased Tc-99m-O_4 uptake but decreased I-123 uptake, thus potentially harboring malignancy. Discordant nodules still have the ability to trap Tc-99m-O_4 but have lost their ability to organify iodine. Because pertechnetate imaging is performed 4-6 hours after administration, initial trapping of the radiopharmaceutical may reveal uptake that is isointense or increased relative to normal parenchyma. Imaging of I-123 is performed at 18–24 hours after administration so any Iodine which may have been trapped has time to wash out of the gland prior to imaging, thus revealing the true nature of the nodule.

It is possible to detect nonpalpable abnormalities using a gamma camera with a pinhole collimator. Abnormalities smaller than 1 cm cannot be reliably resolved because of the inherent limitations of the Anger camera.

Historically, the RAIU served as a measure of thyroid function for many years prior to the development of laboratory assays. The development of accurate serological methods of measuring serum levels of thyroid hormones and ultra-sensitive 3rd and 4th generation thyroid-stimulating hormone (TSH) assays (4) provides a superior method of evaluating thyroid function. Serum TSH is the single best test for screening thyroid function. Only in cases of suspected pituitary or hypothalamic disease is the TSH alone insufficient for screening thyroid functional status. Measurement of the RAIU is usually indicated for one of three reasons: *a)* differentiating Graves' disease (uptake high, usually >35% at 24 hrs) from subacute or factitious hyperthyroidism (uptake usually <2%), *b)* assisting in the calculation of radioactive iodine dose for treatment of Graves' disease, and *c)* assessing suspected toxic multinodular goiters.

If the 24 hour RAIU is to be performed with I-131, 5–10 uCi is administered orally. No imaging is possible with this dose of this agent. I-123 administered orally may be used to perform both the imaging and uptake studies in

Table 58.1. Radiopharmaceuticals Used for Thyroid Imaging

Isotope	Half-life	Principal Gamma Ray (keV)	Advantages	Disadvantages	Comments
I-123	13 hours	159	Physiologic Good organ-to-background ratio Same dose can be used for imaging and uptake	Expensive Image 4 hours after administration	
I-131	8 days	364	Inexpensive Widely available Long half-life	High radiation dose per mCi High-energy photon Unsuitable for gamma camera imaging	Whole-body scans used for evaluation of residual thyroid and metastatic disease in patients with thyroid cancer
Tc-99m	6 hours	140	Inexpensive Excellent imaging qualities	Requires separate dose of I-123 or I-131 for uptake measurements Must repeat imaging with I-123 if hot nodule found	

doses of 200–400 uCi. For the uptake, a nonimaging uptake probe is used to obtain counts in a neck phantom standard. At 24 hours counts are obtained of the patient's neck, thigh, and of the background activity. Some laboratories also count the patient at 4–6 hours so that rapid turnover patients are not missed. Rapid turnover patients show a markedly elevated 4–6 hour RAIU (25–50%) but a lower if not normal 24 hour RAIU. Rapid turnover is seen in the setting of Graves' disease when the small dose of radioactive iodine is rapidly organified and released into the blood stream as thyroid hormone and subtracted with the thigh background counts.

$$\% \text{ Uptake} = \frac{\text{Neck} - \text{thigh cpm} \times 100}{\text{Standard} - \text{background cpm}}$$

where cpm = counts per minute.

Normal = 10–30% at 24 hours (highly dependent on iodine intake).

Anatomy, Physiology, and Embryology

The thyroid is located in the lower part of the neck. It consists of two lobes of approximately equal size (5 × 2 cm) positioned on either side of the trachea and connected across the midline by the thin thyroid isthmus inferiorly (Fig. 58.1). A mild degree of asymmetry in size of the lobes is common. The lobes of the thyroid lie between the carotid artery and jugular vein laterally and the trachea medially. They rest on the longus colli muscles posteriorly and are covered by the sternohyoid, sternothyroid, and prominent sternocleidomastoid muscles anteriorly. A pyramidal lobe (normal variant) extends upward from the isthmus or most commonly from the left lobe in as many as 40% of individuals and represents a lower thyroglossal duct remnant. Histologically, the thyroid gland is composed of thyroid hormone secreting follicular cells arranged in acini, with central collections of colloid. Embryologically, follicular cells originate from endoderm at the base of the tongue that descend to their usual position in the neck. Failure of the thyroid to descend may result in a lingual thyroid. Lingual thyroid pediatric patients are at high risk of developing hypothyroidism.

Thyroglossal duct persistence beyond the second gestational month of the thyroid's descent tract may occur and result in a persistent thyroglossal duct. Perifollicular cells ("C cells"), which produce calcitonin, comprise a small proportion of the cell population. Embryologically, perifollicular C cells are of ectodermal origin from the fourth pharyngeal pouch and descendants of the amine precursor uptake and decarboxylation (APUD) system.

The role of the thyroid gland is the production, storage, and release of thyroid hormones. TSH, produced by the anterior portion of the pituitary gland, regulates the production and release of thyroid hormones. TSH secretion is regulated by hypothalamic thyrotropin-releasing hormone (TRH) and suppressed by circulating thyroxine (T4) and triiodothyronine (T3). Dietary iodine is absorbed in the stomach and upper small bowel where it is rapidly reduced to iodide. It is trapped by active transport from the blood stream by the follicular cells of the thyroid where it is incorporated (organified) onto the tyrosine contained in the intrathyroidal thyroglobulin in the production of T4 and T3. Depending on the dietary content, about 25% of ingested iodine is taken up by the thyroid and 75% is excreted in the urine. Recommended daily adult allowance for iodine is 100–150 mg. This is greatly exceeded in most developed countries such as the United States. The daily intake of iodine in the United States may be as much as 500 mg from some of the rich sources in the North American diet: commercial breads, seafood, and dairy products. However iodine deficiency is still endemic in certain parts of the world, particularly the Andes, Himalayas, and inland areas of Europe and Africa. Iodine uptake competes with the monovalent anion of pertechnetate, perchlorate, and thiocyanates. Thiocyanates are found in vegetables such as cabbage and turnips.

Hypothyroidism

In endemic areas, hypothyroidism is usually caused by dietary iodine deficiency (with a goiter [enlarged gland] present) although in iodine-replete areas, the commonest noniatrogenic cause is chronic thyroiditis (Hashimoto's disease), in which a goiter is also usually present. Prior treatment of hyperthyroidism with ra-

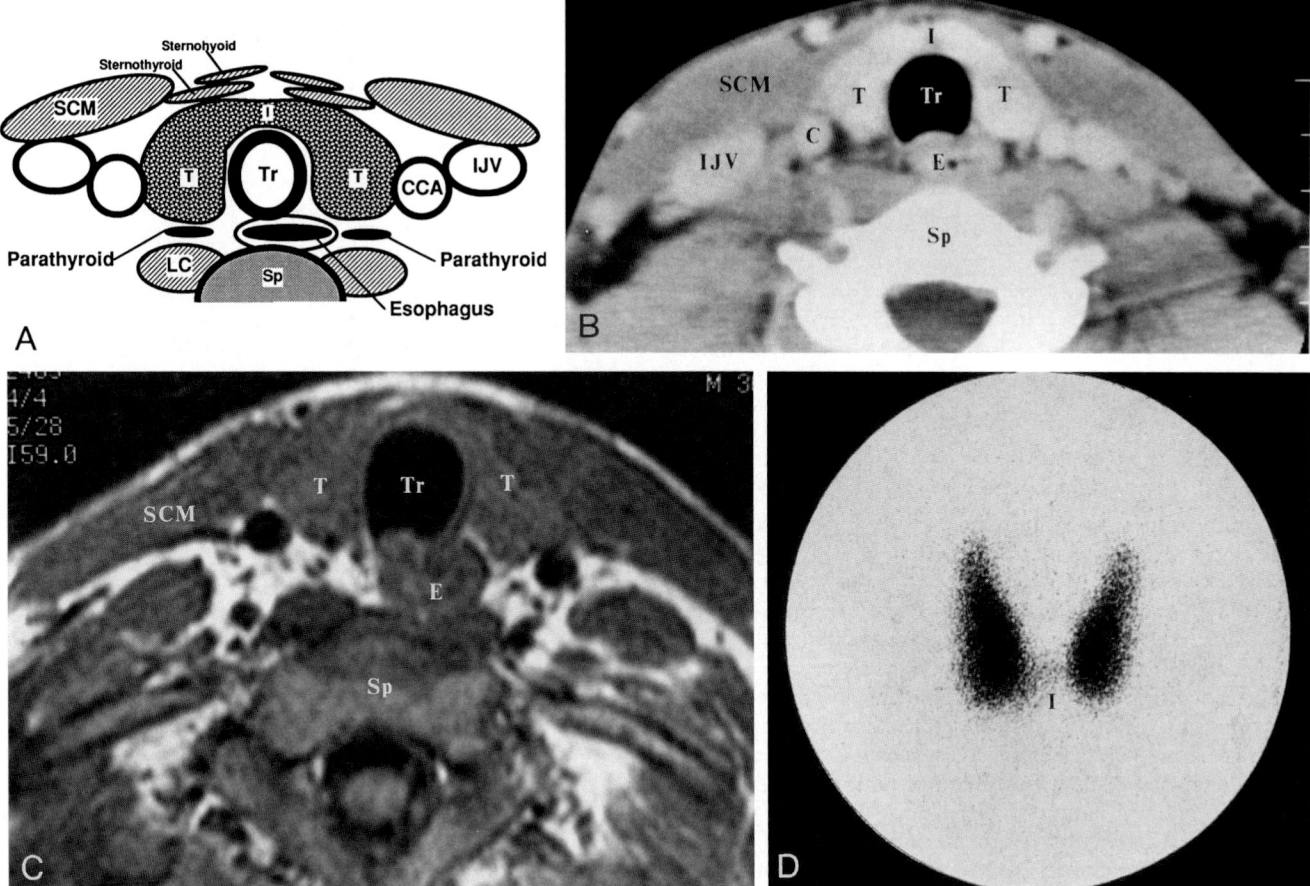

Figure 58.1. Normal Thyroid. Diagram **(A)**, CT image **(B)**, and T1-weighted MR image **(C)** of the thyroid gland in cross-section. **D.** Normal I-123 thyroid scan. *T*, thyroid gland; *I*, isthmus of thyroid gland; *Tr*, trachea; *CCA*, common carotid artery; *IJV*, internal jugular vein; *E*, esophagus; *SCM*, sternocleidomastoid muscle; *LC*, longus colli muscle; *Sp*, spine.

dioactive iodine is another common cause (no goiter). Neonatal hypothyroidism is caused by thyroid dysgenesis (agenesis, hypoplasia, or ectopia). Pediatric lingual thyroid has a 30% chance of developing hypothyroidism. Hypothyroidism's usual clinical features include weight gain, cold intolerance, sluggishness, fatigue, and dry skin. Laboratory findings include elevated serum TSH and low serum T4.

Hyperthyroidism

Graves' disease (diffuse toxic goiter) is the most common cause of hyperthyroidism. Other causes include subacute or painless thyroiditis, toxic nodular goiter and factitious hyperthyroidism due to ingestion of thyroid hormone tablets. Hyperthyroidism's clinical features include weight loss, increased appetite, tremor, heat intolerance, palpitations, muscle weakness, goiter, exophthalmus, and mood changes or irritability. Laboratory findings include a markedly decreased (suppressed) serum TSH and an elevated serum T4.

Goiter

Goiter refers to the clinical finding of generalized thyroid enlargement. Goiter may be associated with increased, decreased, or normal thyroid hormonal function. Thyroid enlargement may be suspected by physical examination and its accurate extent determined by a variety of imaging techniques. Goiters extending into the thorax may be imaged with the use of I-123. Tc-99m-O₄ is not particularly useful with substernal goiter because of the large amount of blood pool activity within the chest.

Multinodular Goiter is a commonly used clinical term for adenomatous hyperplasia. Imaging studies reveal a diffusely abnormal enlarged nodular gland with heterogeneous uptake of the radiopharmaceutical or a pattern of multiple discrete hot nodules on a background of normal or "cool" parenchyma. Photopenic regions should be palpated and dominant palpable nodules should be marked to assure that they do not represent a dominant cold nodule. A recent study reported a 4.1% rate of malignancy in patients with a dominant palpable cold nodule in the setting of multinodular goiter. The hot nodules represent autonomously functioning thyroid adenomas which are usually benign (5) (Fig. 58.2)

Nontoxic Goiter may be related to iodine deficiency, goitrogens in the diet, medications, or a thyroid enzymes deficiency. The gland is usually soft and symmetric, but may appear multinodular with age.

Thyroiditis. All types of thyroiditis are characterized by rapid asymmetric glandular enlargement, with or

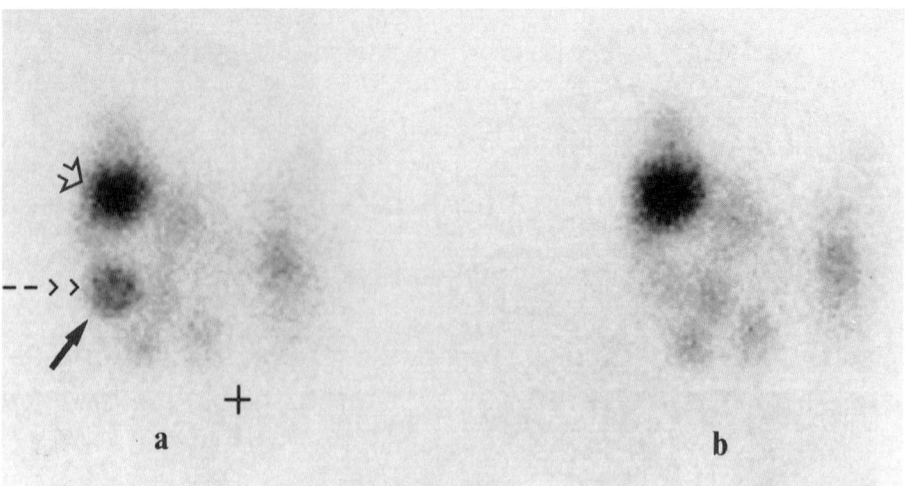

Figure 58.2. Thyroid Nodules. Two images from an I-123 Thyroid scan. A radioactive marker (*closed arrow*) was placed over a 2 cm palpable nodule in the right thyroid lobe for the image on the left (*a*). The image on the right (*b*), without the marker, demonstrates the palpable nodule to be cold. A second palpable nodule in the right upper lobe (*open arrow*) is shown to be hot. Biopsy confirmed a papillary thyroid cancer with multinodular goiter. This case illustrates the importance of palpating and marking nodules.

without nodularity. Inflammatory changes may fixate the gland to adjacent structures and simulate malignancy. Infection of the thyroid gland may be acute and suppurative due to gram-positive bacteria or subacute due to viral infection which may often involve only a portion of the gland. Immunocompromised patients such as diabetics with multinodular goiters have a greater risk of developing suppurative infections. Suppurative infection is associated with hemorrhage, necrosis, and abscess formation. Subacute viral infection usually causes focal edematous enlargement of the gland. Subacute viral infection may have a protean presentation that mimics some of the clinical features of Graves' disease due to release of all preformed thyroid hormone as a response to the inflammation. The RAIU allows for differentiation of this syndrome from Graves' disease. Unlike Graves' disease with its high RAIU and intense thyroid scan appearance, subacute viral patients have a very low RAIU such that scintigraphy of the thyroid gland is rarely indicated. The majority of patients with subacute thyroiditis will resolve and return to a euthyroid state after a transient period of hypothyroidism and elevation of RAIU as the gland returns to normal.

Graves' Disease is the most common cause of hyperthyroidism. It is an autoimmune disorder in which thyroid-stimulating antibodies cause hyperplasia and hyperfunction of the thyroid gland. The gland is usually enlarged twofold to threefold, homogeneous on thyroid scan, and without palpable nodules (Fig. 58.3). The treatment of choice for non-pregnant, non-breast feeding adults with Graves' disease is oral I-131 in conjunction with beta blockers such as propranolol to control symptoms during therapy. Treatment options include subtotal thyroidectomy or antithyroid drugs such as propylthiouracil, methimazole, and carbimazole.

Iodine-131 in the form of sodium iodide has been in use for many years. It is given by mouth either as a capsule or as a liquid. After uptake by the gland the high energy beta particles (mean energy of 0.19 MeV) deliver an average of one rad per microcurie (1000 rads per millicurie) to the thyroid cells. There is very little radiation dose to structures outside the thyroid gland because the average range of the beta particles is 0.8–1.0 mm in soft tissue. Most patients will become euthyroid or hypothyroid after a single dose. Of all patients, 10–20% require

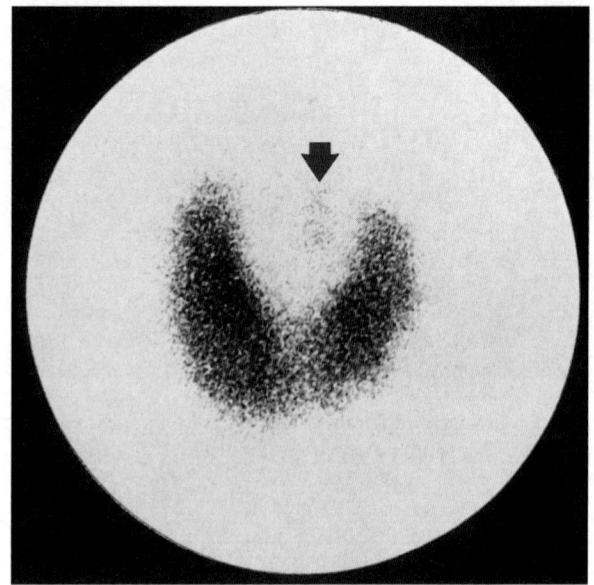

Figure 58.3. Graves' Disease. This I-123 scan demonstrates diffuse thyroid enlargement without nodules. A pyramidal lobe is visualized (*arrow*).

a second or third dose. Patients generally become euthyroid by 10–12 weeks after therapy and frequently become hypothyroid by 6–12 months. Estimation of the dose of I-131 is empiric. A commonly used formula is:

$$\text{Dose in mCi} = \frac{100 - 150 \text{ Ci/g} \times \text{wt of the gland in g}}{\text{RAIU \% uptake} \times 1000}$$

resulting in a typically administered oral dose of approximately 5–15 mCi of I-131. The higher the dose, the quicker the response and the sooner the patient becomes hypothyroid. The smaller the dose, the longer it takes to become euthyroid and the later the development of hypothyroidism. However, it appears that hypothyroidism cannot be avoided, merely delayed by using small doses of I-131. Therefore it has become a common policy in many centers to give larger doses of I-131 in the range of 15–25 mCi with the understanding that hypothyroidism is inevitable and is easily treated with daily replacement levothyroxine. It is important to document with laboratory testing that females of childbearing age are not pregnant prior to treatment with radioactive iodine because iodine crosses the placental barrier and will damage the fetal thyroid.

Complications are uncommon. Transient worsening of thyrotoxicosis is however fairly common. It occurs a few days to 2–3 weeks after treatment and is due to the release of preformed thyroid hormone from disrupted follicles. Occasionally patients develop symptoms of subacute thyroiditis, with pain and tenderness in the thyroid, often radiating to the ears or jaw. Temporary hypoparathyroidism and recurrent laryngeal nerve damage have been reported after radioactive iodine treatment but both are exceedingly rare. Though serious and life-threatening, thyroid storm is a very rare complication, more often seen after surgery in inadequately prepared patients. The patient's risk of genetic damage is no greater than their baseline pre-treatment risk provided they wait 6 months prior to conception. Carcinogenesis is not statistically increased over baseline (6).

Thyroiditis

All forms of thyroiditis may be mistaken for tumor because of rapid asymmetric enlargement and nodularity.

Subacute (Viral) Thyroiditis, has many eponyms but is commonly known as de Quervain's or granulomatous thyroiditis. Subacute thyroiditis presents with thyroid pain and hyperthyroidism following an upper respiratory infection as the gland is disrupted and releases its thyroid hormone into the blood stream. Iodine uptake is usually decreased or absent in the acute stages. The disease runs a subacute course of a few weeks to a few months before healing and returning back to a euthyroid state.

Hashimoto's Thyroiditis is the most common cause of goiter and primary hypothyroidism in adults in developed countries. It is an autoimmune disorder with circulating antithyroid antibody. Histology demonstrates diffuse lymphocytic infiltration of the gland. The thyroid is diffusely enlarged with a rubbery palpable texture. Its early phase is a hyperthyroid-like picture that subsequently evolves into its final hypothyroid sine qua non.

Riedel's Thyroiditis is a rare inflammatory fibrosing process that involves the thyroid and commonly extends into the neck. Radionuclide uptake is absent (cold) in the involved areas.

Secondary Hyperthyroidism may develop in patients with hydatidiform moles or choriocarcinoma. A subunit of the hCG produced by these conditions demonstrates considerable similarity to TSH thereby directly stimulating the thyroid. Clinical history and serum determination of HCG should be performed if this is a consideration.

Thyroid Nodules

Thyroid nodules are extremely common, although thyroid cancer is relatively rare (7,8). Nodules can be palpated in 4–7% of American adults who are asymptomatic for thyroid disease. Autopsy studies demonstrate thyroid nodules in 50% of patients with clinically normal thyroid glands (9). US studies can detect thyroid nodules in 36–41% of middle-aged adults (10) with some studies reporting even higher rates (11) of 67%. Thyroid cancer, on the other hand affects only 0.1% of the population. The incidence of thyroid cancer is approximately 12,000 new cases each year (12). Thyroid cancer represents less than 1% of all cancer and is responsible for less than 0.5% of all cancer death. The challenge of clinical evaluation and imaging studies is to establish the likelihood of malignancy and to select for surgery only those patients at high risk for thyroid malignancy.

US should not be used as a screening tool because it is highly sensitive for the detection of thyroid nodules but its specificity for determining malignancy is low. Recent consensus panels have discouraged the routine use of US for screening. Neither MR nor CT improve specificity. This is not surprising because the histologic differentiation of benign follicular adenoma from well-differentiated follicular carcinoma is based solely on identification of vascular invasion.

On the basis of radioiodine or technetium pertechnetate uptake during imaging, nodules may be classified as hypofunctioning (cold) (Fig. 58.4), relative to the rest of the gland, hyperfunctioning (hot) (Fig. 58.5), or indeterminate. In a patient with a nodular goiter the main concern is whether or not thyroid carcinoma is present. Single cold nodules have a 10–15% incidence of malignancy, although malignancy is exceedingly rare in hot nodules. A multinodular gland with one or more cold nodules may harbor cancer in up to 5% of patients. If Tc-99m-O_4 is used for imaging and a hot nodule is discovered, imaging must be repeated with I-123 as thyroid carcinoma may occasionally trap Tc-99m-O_4, resulting in a hot nodule. This nodule would be cold with I-123.

The differential diagnosis of thyroid nodules is as follows:

Follicular Adenoma is the most common benign neoplasm of the thyroid and represents about 20% of thyroid nodules. There are many subtypes based on histologic criteria, including Hürthle cell adenoma, colloid adenoma, and others. Most are solitary, round or oval, and well encapsulated. Regressive changes are extremely common and greatly affect a nodule's imaging appearance. These include focal necrosis, hemorrhage, edema, infarction, fibrosis, and calcification

Adenomatous Hyperplasia is responsible for up to 50% of thyroid nodules. Adenomatous nodules, also called colloid nodules, are not true neoplasms but are the result of cycles of hyperplasia and involution of a thyroid lobule. They are frequently multiple, but one nodule may be dominant. Regressive changes are common including necrosis, hemorrhage, cystic degeneration, and calcification.

Thyroid Cysts are extremely rare. Most cystic nodules found in the thyroid are actually cystic degeneration of an adenomatous nodule or a follicular adenoma. The incidence of malignancy within a thyroid cyst (13) is reported to be in the range of 0.5% to 3.0%. Therefore fluid should be submitted for cytology and the area aspirated should have adequate sampling.

Hemorrhagic Cysts also usually represent hemorrhage into an adenomatous nodule or a follicular adenoma. Hemorrhage into normal parenchyma also may produce a hemorrhagic cyst.

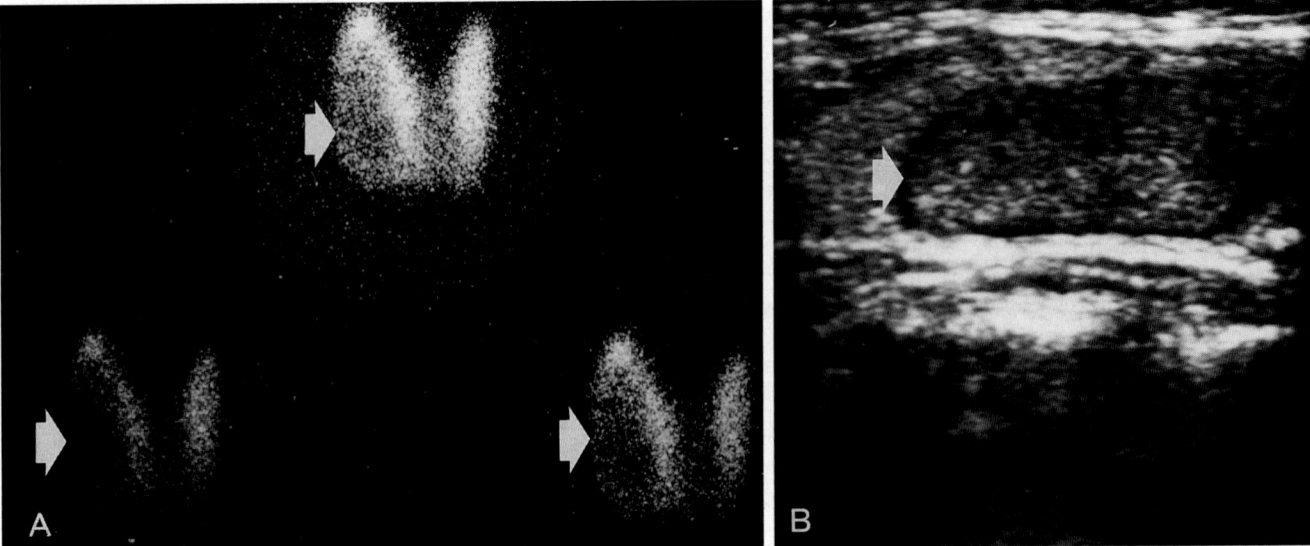

Figure 58.4. Cold Nodule: Follicular Adenoma. A. An I-123 scan photographed at three different intensities demonstrates a large hypofunctioning nodule (*arrows*) in the right thyroid lobe. **B.** Longitudinal US image of the right thyroid lobe reveals a well-defined solid nodule (*arrow*) with a hypoechoic rim.

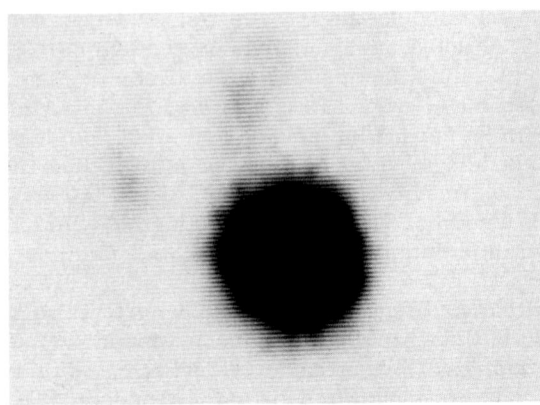

Figure 58.5. Hot Nodule. A hyperfunctioning adenoma demonstrates intense radionuclide activity with suppression of function of the remainder of the gland.

Table 58.2. Signs Suggesting Benign Etiology

Extensive cystic component
Multiple nodules
Hot on radionuclide scan
Peripheral calcification
Shrinkage in size following LT4 suppression hormone therapy
Sudden onset
Female gender
Older patient

Table 58.3 Signs Suggesting Malignancy

Imaging
  Solid nodule
  Cold on radionuclide scan
  Irregular contour
  Poor margination
  Size >4–5 cm
Clinical
  Hard on palpation
  History of neck irradiation
  Age <20 years
  Male
  Familial history of thyroid cancer

Thyroid Cancer. It is estimated that 14,000 new thyroid cancer cases occur each year resulting in more than 1,000 deaths per year (14) in the U.S. Thyroid cancer's annual incidence is approximately 4 per 100,000 population (15). Malignant nodules cannot be reliably differentiated from benign nodules by any imaging method. Fine-needle aspiration with good sampling technique and good cytological support is essential in every suspicious case. However, a number of criteria can be used to assess the relative risk of malignancy (Tables 58.2, 58.3). Every assessment of thyroid nodules must consider all clinical and imaging features. A nodule that is hot on radioiodine scan is extremely unlikely to be malignant. A nodule that is solitary and cold on scintigraphy has a 6% to 10% chance of being malignant (16). A history of neck irradiation, particularly in childhood, increases the risk of malignancy by fivefold to tenfold (0.3 to 12.5 per 10,000 person-years) (17–19). Nodules with extensive cystic component (>50% cystic), or well-defined peripheral calcification as seen at US are unlikely to be malignant. Regression of nodule size following thyroid hormone therapy is a sign of a benign nodule. Large, predominantly solid nodules with irregular contour and poor margination on ultrasound examination are likely to be malignant. Five year survival rates with treatment (20,21) are approximately 90–95%. The histologic types of thyroid malignancy are as follows:

Papillary Carcinoma is the most common type, and is responsible for 75% of cases. Patients are predominantly female (female:male = 4:1) with an average age of 45. The major route of spread is lymphatic to regional nodes, followed by hematogenous dissemination to lungs and bone (Fig 58.6).

Follicular Carcinoma represents 15% of cases, and is also more common in females. The primary route of spread is hematogenous to lung and bone. Prognosis is not as good as for papillary carcinoma.

Medullary Carcinoma arises from perifollicular cells (C cells) and is associated with multiple endocrine neoplasia (MEN II) in some cases. Calcitonin is a useful tumor marker. The prognosis is worse than for papillary or follicular carcinoma. The tumor spreads by both lymphatic and hematogenous routes. Although the tumor does not concentrate I-131 metastases can be detected by thallium-201 (Tl-201), Tc-99m(V) DMSA (dimercaptosuccinic acid, pentavalent form) and I-123/131-MIBG (metaiodobenzylguanidine). I-131-MIBG has also been used for treatment.

Anaplastic Carcinoma is an extremely lethal malignancy with no effective treatment and a 5-year survival rate of less than 4%. The tumor invades locally very aggressively and spreads early to distant sites, generally occurs in an older population.

The initial post-thyroidectomy I-131 whole body scan with its 72-hour RAIU, the surgical pathology report of the thyroid tumor, its size, presence of contralateral lobe involvement or noninvolvement, and lymph node status determination allow for initial staging of the tumor and treatment planning. One must consider the common routes of spread for the specific type of malignancy to optimally plan the imaging study and subsequent treatment. For non-iodine avid tumors, lymph node involvement is determined primarily by size criteria with subsequent pathological confirmation. Normal lymph nodes in the neck are less than 10 mm in diameter. Som (22) provides an excellent review of the anatomy and description of cervical lymph nodes.

Whole-body radionuclide scans using I-131 are effective in demonstrating thyroid metastases and tumor recurrence following thyroidectomy for papillary carcinoma (Fig. 58.7). However, radionuclide whole-body scans are ineffective in medullary and anaplastic carcinoma because of the lack of iodine uptake by the tumor.

Radioiodine (I-131) scans of the whole body, neck, and chest are performed to determine the completeness of surgery and to evaluate the response to treatment. Uptake of I-131 in the thyroid bed frequently represents residual thyroid tissue. Salivary, stomach, bowel, and bladder activity represents physiologic traces of iodine distribution. Focal activity in the lungs, skeleton, or in the neck remote from the thyroid bed is pathologic. Nasal secretions may contain radioiodine. A contaminated pocket handkerchief should not be mistaken for a metastasis. Similarly some breast uptake may occur. This should not be confused with lung metastasis. Unfortunately, some patients may have non-I-131-avid thyroid tumor but demonstrate persistent disease as noted by elevated serum thyroglobulin. Tl-201 (23,24) and more recently Tc-99m-Sestamibi (25) and Tc-99m-tetrofosmin (26) have shown some utility in imaging non-I-131-avid thyroid tumor.

Radioiodine Therapy. Most authorities agree with post thyroidectomy ablation in primary thyroid tumors greater than 1.5 cm. Some disagreement now exits in the literature on the treatment of patients with I-131 if primary tumor size is less than 1 cm.

According to the Nuclear Regulatory Commission regulations, patients receiving 30 mCi or more of I-131 require hospitalization until the residual amount of I-131 falls below 30 mCi or a rate meter reading of less than 5 mrad per hour at one meter (27). Doses close to 30 mCi are frequently used on an outpatient basis to ablate residual thyroid following thyroidectomy. Some authors advocate larger doses on the grounds that 30 mCi is inadequate to ablate thyroid cancer and may cause a stun-

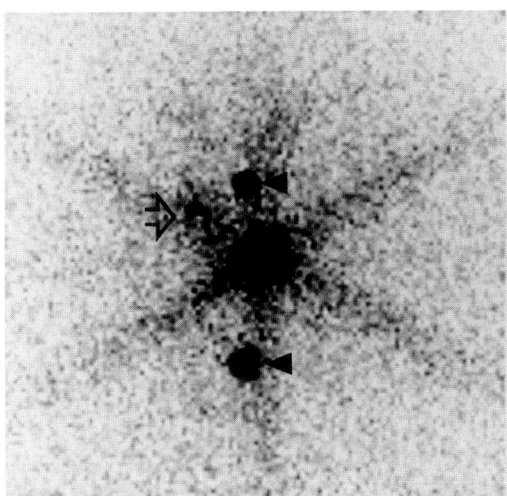
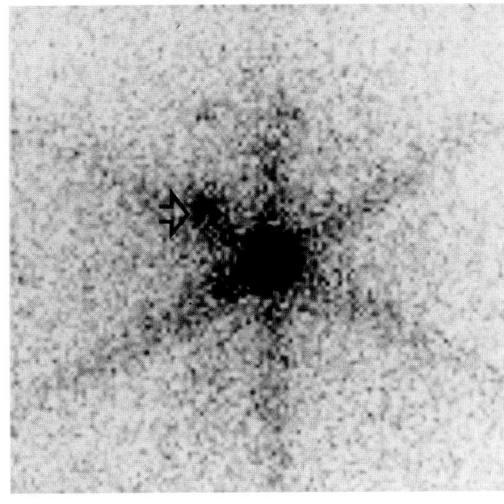

Figure 58.6. Thyroid Cancer Metastasis. I-131 scan of the neck in patient who has undergone near total thyroidectomy for thyroid cancer. *Arrowheads* indicate radioactive markers of the chin and suprasternal notch. The large star artifact is due to septal penetration of the collimator. The center of the star represents the original thyroid bed. A lymph node metastasis is evident in the right upper neck (*open arrows*).

ning effect that makes the thyroid more radioresistant on subsequent treatment. Doses of 100–200 mCi are frequently used depending on the tumor cytology, its size, and the presence of capsular, vascular, or lymph node involvement.

The patient should be hypothyroid with a serum TSH greater than 40 IU/ml prior to whole body I-131 imaging or ablation because elevated TSH is the strongest determinant in activating active transport of the iodine into the thyroid cell. This is to ensure maximal stimulation of residual thyroid and/or thyroid cancer and thereby promote appropriate localization of the radioiodine. Iodine-rich foods such as shellfish, bread, and kelp should be avoided at least 1 week prior to therapy. Dairy products should also be limited because these are also a rich source of "cold" iodine, which can inhibit uptake of the I-131. A radiographic study with iodinated contrast will delay therapy by at least two to 3 months unless clinical maneuvers to deplete the patient of the exogenous iodine is performed.

The frequency of side effects varies directly with the dose of radioiodine administered. Doses greater than 100 mCi may cause sialoadenitis which may lead to permanent xerostomia. For this reason patients should be strongly encouraged to drink copious amounts of water and suck on sialogogues such as lemon drops or sour candy for 3–7 days post therapy. Pulmonary fibrosis has been reported in patients who have had multiple doses of radioiodine therapy for extensive pulmonary disease. Leukemia has been reported in patients who have received cumulative doses in excess of 600–800 mCi (28,29).

Metastases to the thyroid gland are rare. The most common primary tumors which metastasize to the thyroid are breast, lung, kidney, malignant melanoma, and lymphoma.

PARATHYROID

Parathyroid disorders are classified in terms of function: excessive parathyroid hormone (PTH) production or hyperparathyroidism, and insufficient PTH production or hypoparathyroidism. Imaging studies of the parathyroid glands are performed to localize parathyroid abnormalities in patients with hyperparathyroidism that has been confirmed clinically. There is no role for imaging in hypoparathyroidism. The causes of hyperparathyroidism are listed in Table 58.4.

Imaging Methods

Approximately 80–85% of abnormal parathyroid glands are located near the thyroid. Ectopic locations for abnormal parathyroid tissue include: thymus (10–15%), posterior mediastinum (5%), retroesophageal (1%), within the carotid sheath (1%), and parapharyngeal (0.5%). US, scintigraphy with Tl-201, Tc-99m-Sestamibi (Tc-99m-MIBI), CT or MR have various sensitivities and specificities that depend on whether the patient has had prior surgery (30). At centers with very experienced surgeons, surgery is curative in 92–98% of patients with previously unoperated hyperparathyroidism (31), but re-operation success decreases to 62% in patients that require a repeat surgery. Localization procedures are indicated in patients who are surgical failures requiring a second surgery and may be helpful prior to a first operation when the local surgical experience is limited (32).

Tc-99mO₄/Tl-201 Radionuclide Subtraction Imaging has been used to detect parathyroid adenomas with a sensitivity of about 75% and a specificity of 90% (33).

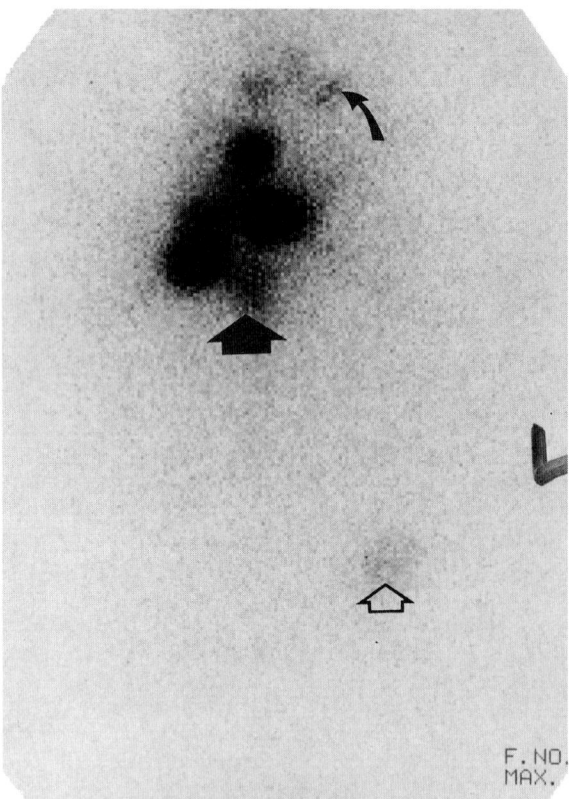

Figure 58.7. Lymph Node Metastases. I-131 whole body scan post thyroidectomy shows intense radionuclide activity in papillary carcinoma lymph node metastases in the neck (*solid arrow*). Normal activity is present in the stomach (*open arrow*) and submandibular salivary glands (*curved arrow*).

Table 58.4. Causes of Hyperparathyroidism

Primary Hyperparathyroidism
    Solitary parathyroid adenoma, 85%
    Parathyroid hyperplasia, 10%
    Multiple parathyroid adenomas, 4%
    Parathyroid carcinoma, 1%
Secondary Hyperparathyroidism
    Diffuse or adenomatous parathyroid hyperplasia due to calcium-losing renal disease
Tertiary Hyperparathyroidism
    Autonomous parathyroid function resulting from long-standing secondary hyperparathyroidism
Paraneoplastic Syndromes
    Ectopic parathormone production
    Bronchogenic carcinoma
    Renal cell carcinoma

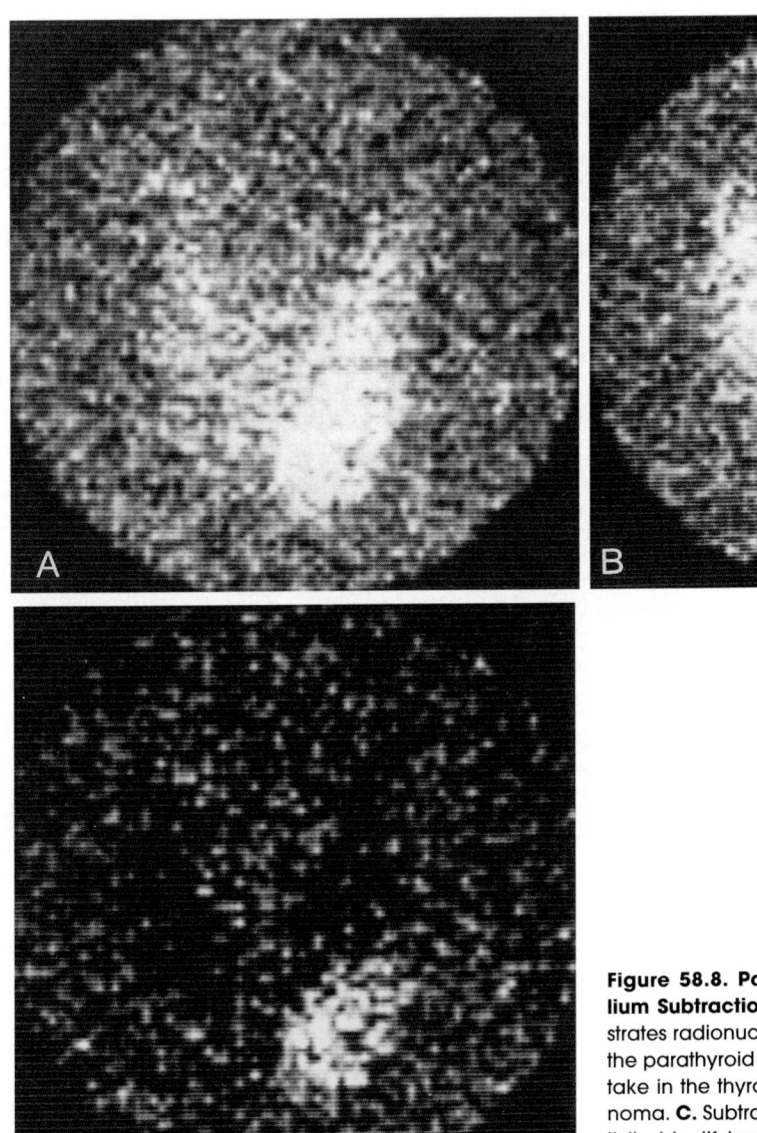

Figure 58.8. Parathyroid Adenoma: Technetium-Thallium Subtraction Technique. A. Thallium image demonstrates radionuclide activity in both the thyroid gland and the parathyroid adenoma. **B.** Tc-99m-O₄ image shows uptake in the thyroid gland but not in the parathyroid adenoma. **C.** Subtraction image shows a residual focus of activity, identifying a parathyroid adenoma at the lower pole of the left thyroid lobe.

Thyroid tissue concentrates both Tc-99mO$_4$ and Tl-201 (Fig. 58.8). Parathyroid adenomas Take up Tl-201 but not Tc-99mO$_4$. This is the basis for dual isotope imaging. First the Tl-201 images are acquired and then without moving the patient, Tc-99mO$_4$ is administered and imaging at the technetium peak is performed. The Tc-99mO$_4$ images are subsequently subtracted from the Tl-201 images. A residual focus of activity indicates the presence of a parathyroid adenoma (Fig. 58.8). It is vital that the patient does not move at all, otherwise erroneous results will be obtained. False-positive results can be seen with Tl-201 uptake in thyroid nodules, sarcoid containing lymph nodes, or metastases to the neck as the technique is predicated on the presence of an underlying normal thyroid gland.

Sestamibi and Tetrofosmin Imaging. Recently Tc-99m-MIBI and Tc-99m-tetrofosmin (Tc-99m-Tfos) have virtually replaced Tc-99mO$_4$/Tl-201 subtraction imaging at most centers. Both of these agents have similar sensitivities and specificities to other imaging methods (30,34). When Tc-99m-MIBI or Tc-99m-Tfos are used for parathyroid imaging, immediate and delayed images of the neck and mediastinum are performed. Parathyroid adenomas may or may not be visualized on initial imaging, but tend to retain the radiopharmaceutical on delayed (1–2 hour) images while the normal thyroid gland washes out (Fig. 58.9). Retention occurs in the mitochondria-rich cells of the adenoma. False negatives may be seen in clear cell adenomas which histologically contain a paucity of mitochondria.

Anatomy

Most people (80%) have four parathyroid glands, two superior and two inferior. However, autopsy studies have demonstrated that 20% of individuals have three, five, or six parathyroid glands. The superior parathyroid glands arise from the fourth branchial pouch along with the thyroid gland and are seldom ectopic (35). The inferior parathyroid glands arise from the third branchial

Figure 58.9. Parathyroid Adenoma: Technetium Sestamibi Scan. *Arrows* indicate focus of radionuclide activity in the lower pole of the right lobe of the thyroid. Surgery confirmed a parathyroid adenoma.

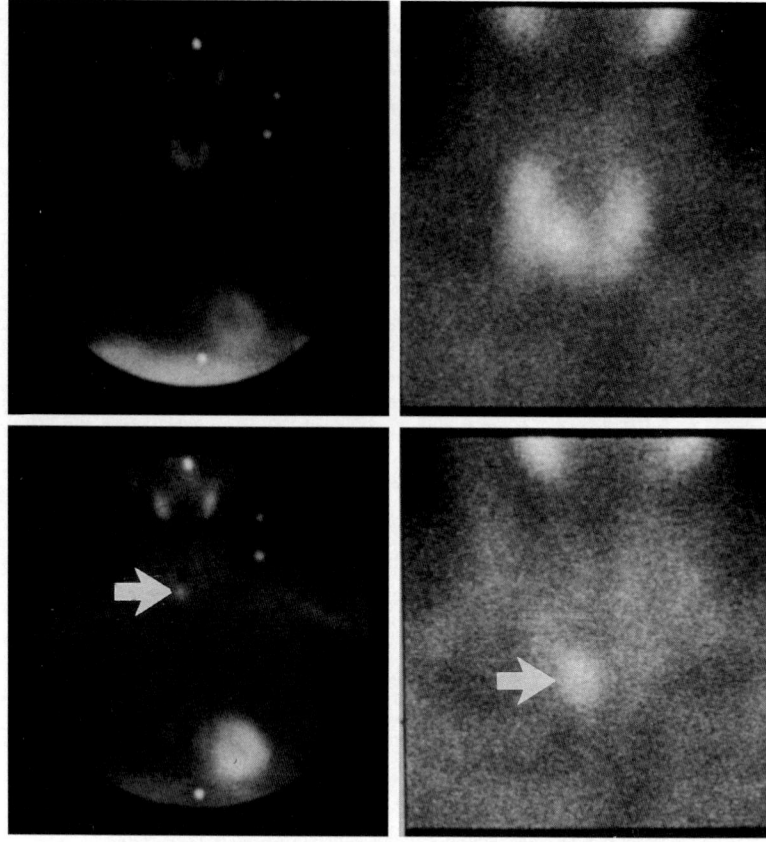

pouch along with the thymus and are more commonly ectopic, usually in the mediastinum. Normal glands measure $5 \times 3 \times 1$ mm in size and average 10–80 mg. Because they are so small and flat, normal glands are not usually demonstrated by any imaging method. The normally located parathyroid glands are found posterior to the thyroid lobes superficial to the longus colli muscles (see Fig. 58.1), and between the trachea and carotid sheath.

Parathyroid Adenoma

Parathyroid adenomas are characteristically oval in shape and 8–15 mm in greatest diameter. Their cellularity is homogeneous, giving a uniform internal appearance on all imaging modalities.

Multiple Gland Disease

Parathyroid hyperplasia cannot be differentiated from multiple parathyroid adenomas by imaging methods. Hyperplasia affects all of the parathyroid glands but is frequently asymmetric. The individual glands have the same imaging appearance as parathyroid adenomas.

Parathyroid Carcinoma

Carcinomas are usually larger than adenomas (at least 2 cm in size). The internal architecture is much more heterogeneous, with cystic degeneration more common. Invasion of adjacent muscle or vessels may be demon-

strated. The differentiation of parathyroid carcinoma from a large adenoma can usually be made only histologically.

Ectopic Parathyroid

Ectopic parathyroids are most common in the anterosuperior mediastinum or low in the neck. Immediate and delayed imaging of the neck and mediastinum with Tc-99m-MIBI or Tc-99m-Tfos have a diagnostic sensitivity of 75% (34). Tc-99m-MIBI or Tc-99m-Tfos imaging currently seems the modality of choice for identifying ectopic parathyroids in view of the improved target to background visualization when compared to Tl-201. CT, MR and scintigraphy all have reported sensitivities of approximately 75%.

ADRENAL

High-resolution anatomic imaging of the adrenal glands is performed by CT, MR, or US and is discussed in chapter 33. Functional imaging of hyperplastic or neoplastic adrenal disorders can be performed with the following radiopharmaceuticals I-131-6-iodomethyl-19-norcholesterol (NP59), or I-131-MIBG (meta-iodo-benzyl-guanidine). NP59, a cholesterol analog, is taken up by adrenal cortical tissue. Cholesterol is a common precursor of mineralocorticoids, glucocorticoids and androgens. MIBG is taken up by cells of adrenal medullary origin such as pheochromocytoma. In addition tumors of neural crest origin such as neuroblastoma and medullary thyroid cancer often concentrate MIBG. MIBG detects neuroblastomas and their metastases in >90% of cases (36). Note that NP59 is available only for investigational use in the U.S., although it is available commercially in many other countries.

Indium-111 Pentetreotide is a synthetic somatostatin analogue but with a longer plasma half life than native somatostatin. This radiopharmaceutical is showing promise in imaging a wide variety of neuroendocrine tumors. Sensitivities vary according to tumor type with carcinoid and paraganglioma having fairly high sensitivities (37).

References

1. McDougall IR. Thyroid Diseases in Clinical Practice. New York: Oxford University Press, 1992.

2. Sandler MP, Patton JA, Gross MD, et al. Endocrine Imaging. Norwalk, CT: Appleton & Lange, 1992.

3. Belfiore A, LaRose GL, LaPorta GA, et al. Cancer risk in patients with cold thyroid nodules: Relevance of iodine intake, sex, age, and multinodularity. Am J Med 1992;93:363–369.

4. Spencer CA, Schwartzbein D, Guttler RB, et al. Thyrotropin (TSH)-releasing hormone stimulation test responses employing third and fourth generation TSH assays. J Clin Endocrinol Metab 1993;76:494–498.

5. Meier DA, Dworkin HJ, eds. The autonomously functioning thyroid nodule. J Nucl Med 1991;32:30.

6. Hall P, Holm LE, Lundell G, et al. Cancer risks in thyroid cancer patients. Br J Cancer 1991;64:159–163.

7. Rojeski MT, Gharib H. Nodular thyroid disease: evaluation and management. N Engl J Med 1985;313:428–436.

8. James EM, Charboneau JW, Hay ID. The thyroid. In: Rumack CM, Wilson SR, Charboneau JW, eds. Diagnostic Ultrasound. St. Louis: Mosby Year Book, 1991:507–523.

9. Mortenson JD, Woolner LB, Bennett WA. Gross and microscopic findings in clinically normal thyroid glands. Clin Endocrinol Metab 1955;15:1270–1280.

10. Brander A, Viikinkoski P, Nickels J, et al. Thyroid gland: US screening in a random adult population. Radiology 1991;181:683–687.

11. Ezzat S, Sarti DA, Cain DR, et al. Thyroid incidentalomas: prevalence by palpation and ultrasonography. Arch Intern Med 1994;154:1838–1840.

12. Silverberg E, Boring CC, Squires TS. Cancer statistics 1990. Ca Cancer J Clin 1990;40:9–26.

13. Meier DA, Dworkin HJ, eds. The autonomously functioning thyroid nodule. J Nucl Med 1991;32:30.

14. Wingo PA, Tong T, Bolden S. Cancer statistics,1995. CA J Clin 1995;45:8–30.

15. Clark OH, Quan-Yang D. Thyroid cancer. Med Clin North Am 1991;75:211–234.

16. Freitas JE, Freitas AE. Thyroid and parathyroid imaging. Semin Nucl Med 1994;24:234–245.

17. Tucker MA, Morris Jones PH, Boice JD Jr., et al. Therapeutic radiation at a young age is linked to secondary thyroid cancer. Cancer Res 1991;51:2885–2888.

18. Shore RE, Hildreth N, Dvoretsky P, et al. Thyroid cancer among persons given x-ray treatment in infancy for an enlarged thymus gland. Am J Epidemiol 1993;137:1068–1080.

19. Ron E, Modan B, Preston D, et al. Thyroid neoplasia following low-dose radiation in childhood. Radiat Res 1989;120:516–531.

20. Akslen LA, Haldorsen T, Thoresen SO, et al. Survival and causes of death in a thyroid cancer: a population-based study of 2478 cases from Norway. Cancer Res 1991;51:1234–1241.

21. Flynn MB, Tarter J, Lyons K, et al. Frequency and experience with carcinoma of the thyroid at a private, a Veterans Administration and a university hospital. J Surg Oncol 1991;48:164–170.

22. Som PM. Lymph nodes of the neck. Radiology 1987;165:593—600.

23. Hoefnagel CA, Delprat CC, Zanin D, et al. New radionuclide tracers for the diagnosis and therapy of medullary thyroid carcinoma. Clin Nucl Med 1988;13:159–165.

24. Dadparvar S, Krishna H, Brady LW, et al. The role of Iodine-131 and thallium-201 imaging and serum thyroglobulin in the management of differentiated thyroid carcinoma. Cancer 1993;71:3767–3773.

25. Miyamoto S, Kasagi K, Misaki T, et al. Evaluation of Technetium-99m MIBI scintigraphy in metastatic differentiated thyroid carcinoma. J Nucl Med 1997;38:352–356.

26. Lind P, Gallowitsch H, Langsteger W, et al. Technetium-99m Tetrofosmin whole-body scintigraphy in the follow-up of differentiated thyroid carcinoma. J Nucl Med 1997;38:348–352.

27. Title 10, Chapter 1, Code of Federal Regulation-Energy Part 35, Section 35.75(a)(2), November 30,1988.

28. Hall P, Holm LE, Lundell G, et al. Cancer risks in thyroid cancer patients. Br J Cancer 1991;64:159–163.

29. Hall P, Boice JD Jr, Berg G, et al. Leukaemia incidence after iodine-131 exposure. Lancet 1992;340:1–4.

30. McBiles M, Lambert AT, Cote MG, Kim SY. Sestamibi Parathyroid imaging. Sem Nucl Med 1995;25:221–234.

31. Thompson NW. Localization studies in patients with primary hyperparathyroidism. Br J Surg 1988;75:97–98.

32. Wilson NM, Gaunt J, Nunan TO, et al. Role of thallium-201/technetium 99m subtraction scanning in persistent or recurrent hypercalcaemia following parathyroidectomy. Br J Surg 1990;77:794–795.

33. Beierwaltes WH. Endocrine imaging: parathyroid, adrenal cortex and medulla, and other endocrine tumors. Part II. J Nucl Med 1991;32:1627–1639.

34. Fjeld JG, Erichsen K, Pfefer PF, et al. Technetium-99m-tetrofosmin for parathyroid scintigraphy: a comparison with sestamibi. J Nucl Med 1997; 38:831–834.

35. Reading CC. The parathyroid. In: Rumack CM, Wilson SR, Charboneau JW, eds. Diagnostic Ultrasound. St. Louis: Mosby Year Book, 1991:524–539.

36. Paltiel HJ, Gelfand MJ, Elgazzer A, et al. Neural crest tumors: 123I-MIBG imaging in children. Radiology 1994;190:117–121.

37. Krenning EP, Kwekkeboom DJ, Bakker WH, et al. Somatostatin receptor scintigraphy with 111-IN-DTPA-D-Phe) and 123-I-Try3-octreotide: the Rotterdam experience with more than 1000 patients. Eur J Nucl Med 1993; 20:716–731.

59

Gastrointestinal, Liver-Spleen, and Hepatobiliary Scintigraphy

Philip W. Wiest
Robert J. Telepak
Michael F. Hartshorne

GASTROINTESTINAL STUDIES

Nuclear medicine imaging studies can provide considerable information in the functional evaluation of the gastrointestinal system. Routine studies include hepatobiliary, gastrointestinal bleeding studies, and gastric emptying measurements. Other procedures that are less frequently ordered provide clinically valuable information.

Salivary Scanning

A quick look at the salivary glands of the mouth is frequently had in conjunction with the Tc-99m pertechnetate (Tc-99m-O$_4$) scan of the thyroid gland. One can scan the salivary glands intentionally with Tc-99m-O$_4$. A 5 to 10 mCi dose is injected intravenously (IV) with planar images performed immediately and after a delay during which lemon juice is washed around the mouth. In the past this study has been used to grade the severity of Sjögren's syndrome as inflammation degrades the secretory function of the glands. The salivary scan can be used as an adjunct to or replacement for sialography in some cases. Stimulation of the glands with lemon juice is important to document the drainage of saliva through the duct system to the mouth (Fig. 59.1).

Esophageal Imaging

The esophageal transit study, performed with swallowed solutions or solid boluses labeled with Tc-99m sulfur colloid, is an examination which can be done in lieu of esophageal manometry. It has been reported to detect esophageal dysmotility in 50% of symptomatic patients with an otherwise normal evaluation for dysphagia.

In the supine or upright position with a gamma camera imaging in the anterior projection, the patient swallows a radioactive bolus while dynamic data are obtained by a computer. The esophagus is divided into three regions of interest (ROI): upper, middle, and lower. Transit times are then calculated from time-activity curves representing the ROIs. The normal esophagus demonstrates sequential activity from proximal to distal with no visualized esophageal activity remaining after 10 seconds. Regional analysis may differentiate between achalasia and scleroderma. It is important to remember that esophageal scintigraphy is functional and does not provide detailed anatomic information. Barium or endoscopic study is necessary to exclude the possibility of neoplasm or infection as the cause of impaired esophageal function (Fig 59.2).

Gastroesophageal Reflux

The evaluation of heartburn and atypical chest pain in the adult commonly raises the clinical question of gastroesophageal reflux (GER) disease. In the pediatric population, failure to thrive and recurrent pneumonia often elicits the same question. A common diagnostic tool currently used in the diagnosis of GER disease is acid reflux monitoring. This examination unfortunately requires nasoesophageal intubation and 24 hour continuous recording. It is invasive and unwieldly, especially in the pediatric age group.

GER scintigraphy is performed with acidified orange juice mixed with Tc-99m-sulfur colloid. The acid decreases the lower esophageal sphincter pressure and also delays gastric emptying. Regions of interest are established via a computer to correspond to the stomach and segments (upper, middle, and lower) of the esophagus. In the pediatric population, ROIs over the lungs detect aspiration. Images may be recorded in adults with an abdominal binder that increases abdominal pressure sequentially in 10 mm Hg increments to a maximum of 100 mm Hg. Normal patients have no detectable GER activity. This examination is reported to have a 90% sensitivity in the detection of GER (Fig. 59.3).

Gastric Emptying

Gastric emptying is a complex physiologic process directed not only by neuroendocrine processes but also by

Figure 59.1. Warthin's tumor by salivary scan.
Immediate **(A)** and delayed **(B)** images after IV administration of Tc-99m pertechnetate show extra uptake in a palpable mass in the right parotid gland. Retention of the pertechnetate is prolonged in the mass (*arrows*) even after lemon juice stimulation of the salivary glands. This finding is characteristic of the functioning Warthin's tumor which is not drained by salivary ducts.

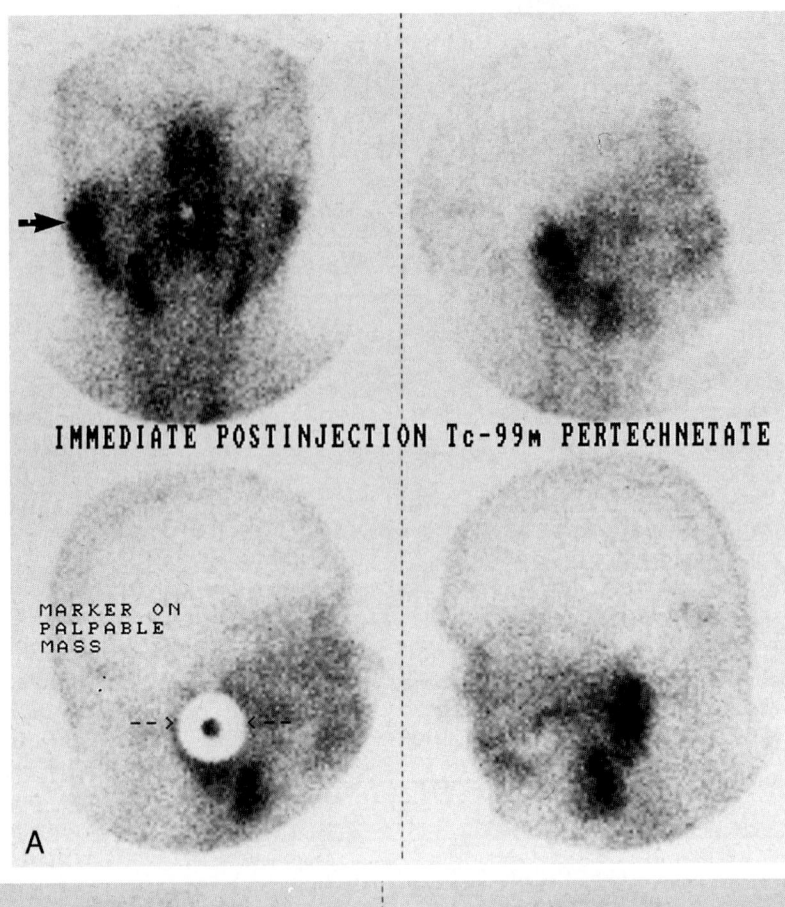

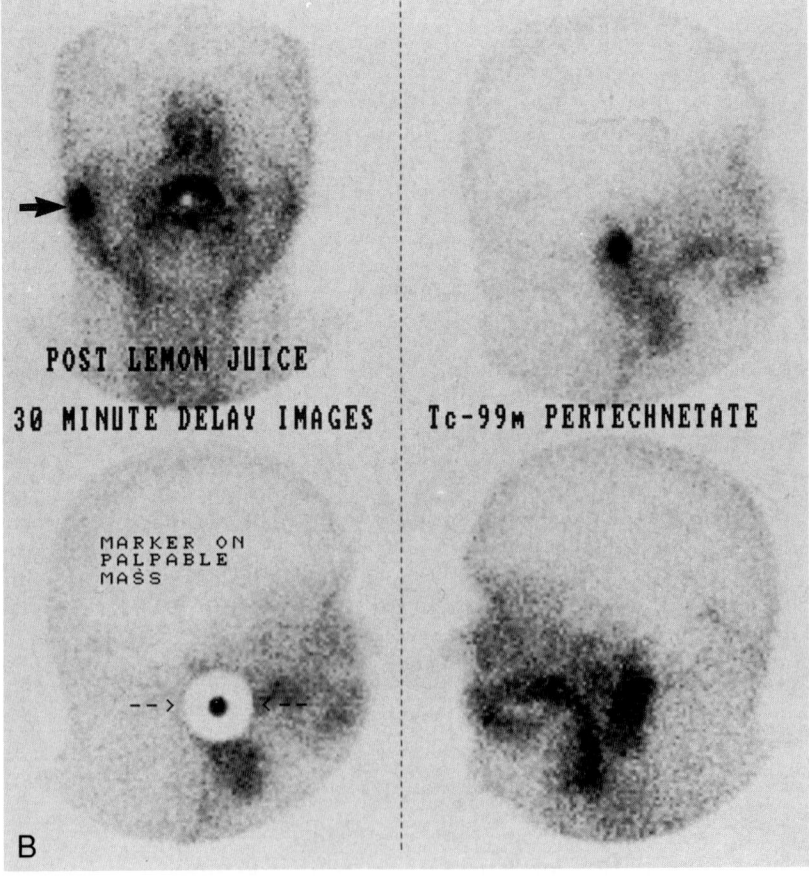

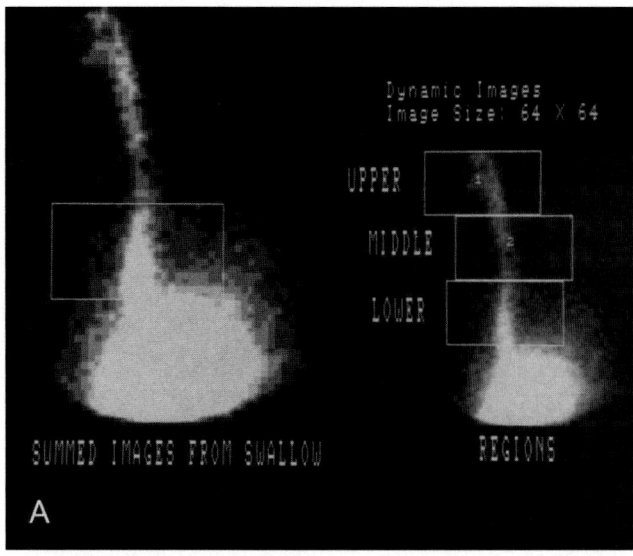

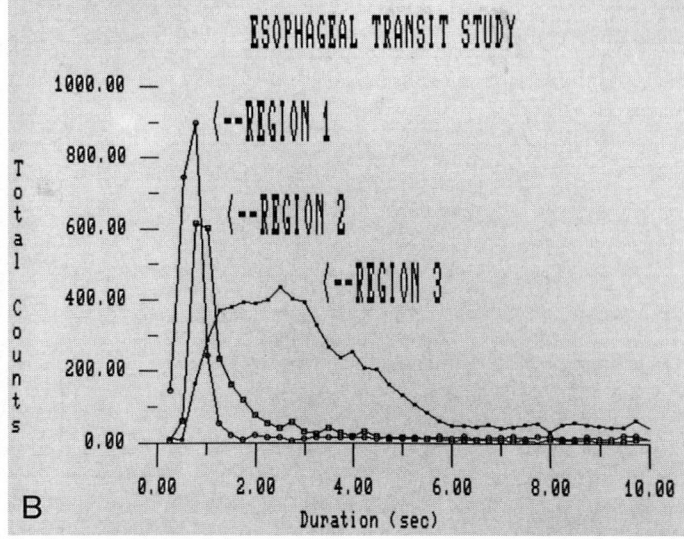

Figure 59.2. Normal Esophageal Transit Study. A. A composite image of the esophagus and stomach is used to generate ROIs around the upper, middle, and lower esophagus. **B.** Time-activity curves for each region are displayed for 10 seconds after the swallow. Inspection of the curves allows calculation of the transit time.

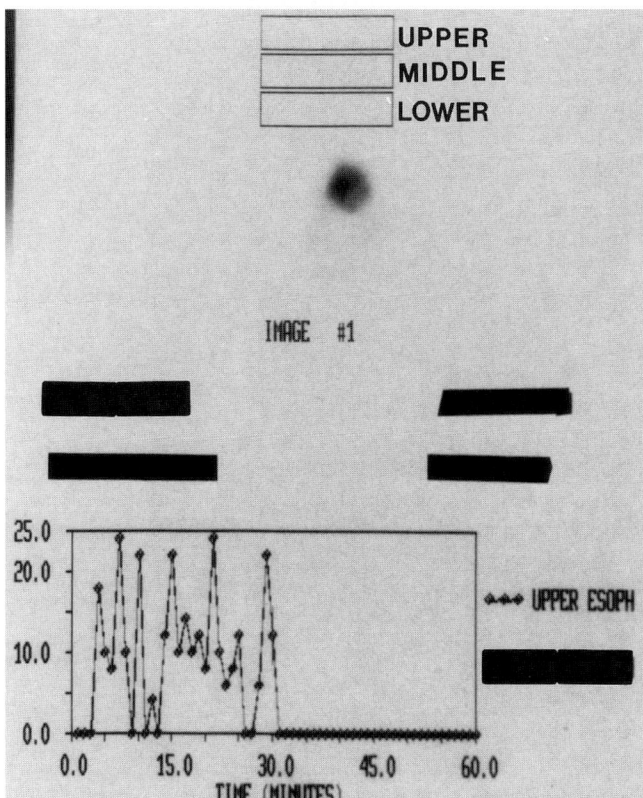

Figure 59.3. Abnormal GER Study. Three ROIs are established over the esophagus. A time-activity curve corresponding to the upper ROI for 60 minutes shows refluxed activity after 3 minutes, which continues for about 30 minutes.

a host of local factors. Food type and pH as well as food osmolality affect the rate of gastric emptying. Any process that interrupts this cycle can ultimately result in gastric stasis. Impaired gastric emptying can be caused by many disease states such as diabetes mellitus, electrolyte disturbances, postvagotomy syndromes, and some medications.

Excluding mechanical obstruction is important in diagnosing the cause of the patient's symptoms. Endoscopy or barium studies are superior in the detection of gastric ulcers, tumors, or bezoars. Gastric emptying scintigraphy has become the gold standard in the clinical evaluation of gastric motility. It is a simple test to perform, though interpretation is based upon complicated mathematical models. Solid food, liquids, or both are labeled with a radiotracer and consumed by the patient. Digital images of the stomach are acquired and a time-activity curve is generated for graphic analysis of the rate of emptying (Fig. 59.4).

The normal half emptying time (T1/2) of radioactive solids and liquids varies with the technique employed. In general, the normal T1/2 is less than 90 minutes for solids and less than 60 minutes for liquids. Each laboratory should establish its own normal T1/2 values. Visual interpretation of the stomach images is invaluable in understanding the "number" generated for T1/2. The gastric emptying technique can be extended to study and time the transit between stomach and colon to characterize disorders of the bowel's smooth muscle or enteric nervous system.

Gastrointestinal Bleeding Scintigraphy

Patients who present with clinically suspected upper gastrointestinal (GI) bleeding are usually evaluated and often treated by endoscopy. Scintigraphy is not usually needed. The patient with suspected lower gastrointesti-

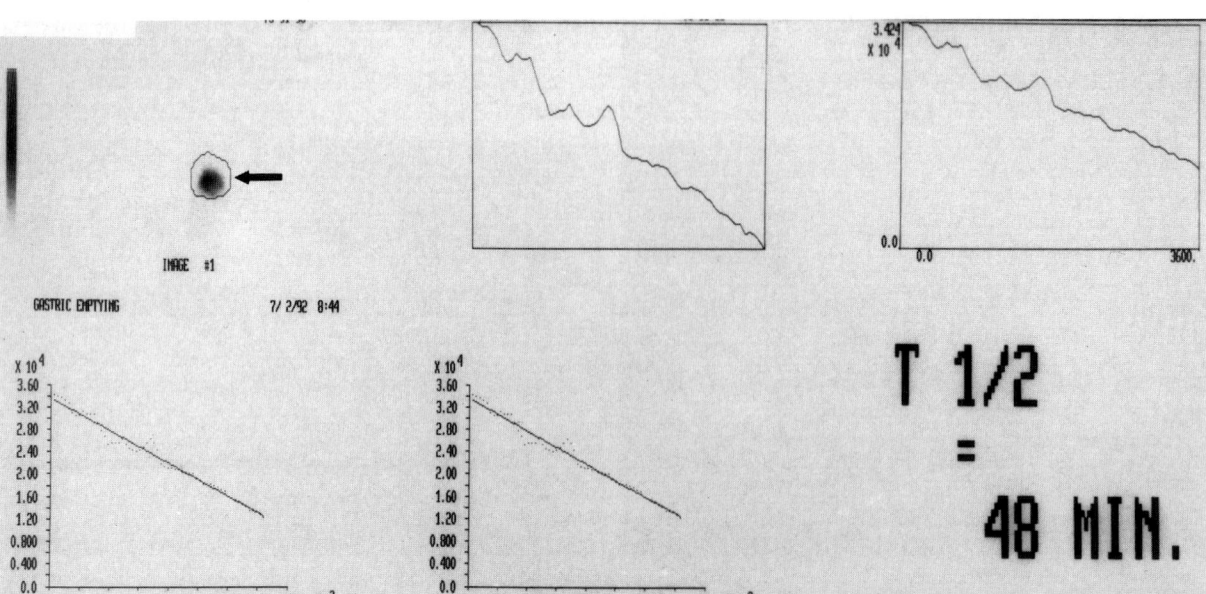

Figure 59.4. Normal Solid Gastric Emptying Study. In the *upper left-hand* image, an ROI (*arrow*) is established around the stomach. The next two graphics show the stomach's time-activity curve. The *bottom* two graphics show the linear best-fit to this data. The slope of the curve allows calculation of the T1/2 of 48 minutes.

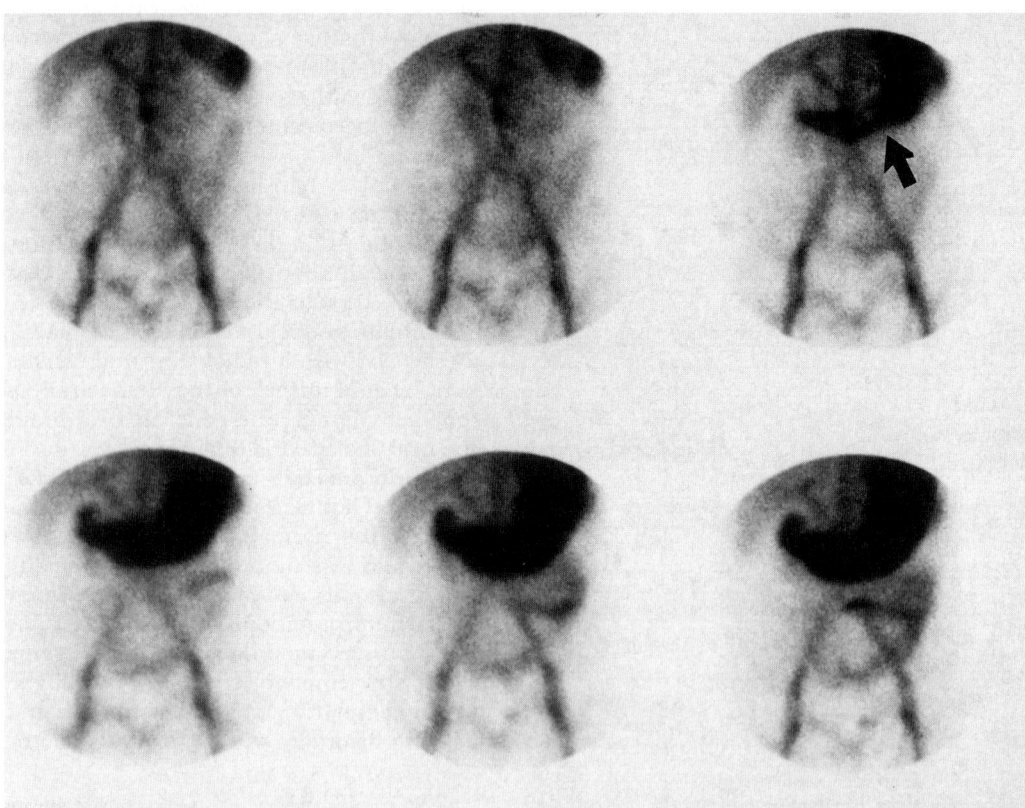

Figure 59.5. Upper Gastrointestinal Bleeding due to Gastric Varices. Sequential 5-minute images of the abdomen, in a patient with negative endoscopy, show tagged red cells filling the lumen of the stomach (*arrow*). This diagnosis cannot be made if there is free Tc-99m-O_4 mixed with the red cells; Tc-99m-O_4 is excreted physiologically in the stomach. The tagged red blood cells used had no free Tc-99m-O_4.

nal bleeding presents different problems in diagnosis and therapy. Proctosigmoidoscopy will exclude hemorrhoidal bleeding. Some GI physicians prefer emergent lower endoscopy. The authors prefer to proceed to an emergent gastrointestinal bleeding study with *in-vitro* Tc-99m-tagged red blood cells. Continuous 1 minute dynamic frames are acquired over the abdomen and pelvis in the anterior projection for at least 90 minutes or until the patient has bled enough to locate the source of hemorrhage. The study should be done emergently during the clinical period of maximal blood loss. The best chance of success in localizing the source of hemorrhage is had in orthostatic patients requiring a transfusion of at least two or more units of blood in the 24-hour period preceding scintigraphy. Repeated imaging can be done at any time up to 24 hours after red cell labeling.

Accurate hemorrhage localization is required for resection of a bleeding site. If angiographic therapy for a bleeding site is proposed, the more sensitive GI bleeding study is done first. The GI bleeding study will guide selection of appropriate vessels for embolization or infusion of vasoreactive drugs. Positive GI bleeding studies demonstrate three cardinal findings: *a)* an abnormal hot spot of radiotracer activity appears "out of no where" as it enters the bowel lumen; *b)* this activity persists and may increase with time; and *c)* the activity moves with peristalsis antegrade, retrograde, or in both directions (Fig. 59.5–59.7).

Meckel's Scan

A Meckel's diverticulum contains ectopic gastric mucosa which may ulcerate and bleed. Tc-99m-O$_4$ is given IV and the abdomen is imaged immediately and for one hour's worth of dynamic images. Tc-99m-O$_4$ localizes in gastric mucosa and can be used to detect the acid producing mucosa in the diverticulum. A focus of activity in the ectopic gastric mucosa in the middle or right lower quadrant of the abdomen, is detected as it accumulates the Tc-99m-O$_4$ in synchrony with the stomach. Detection may be enhanced by the use of pentagastrin to stimulate uptake or cimetidine to block the outflow of Tc-99m-O$_4$ from the diverticulum (Fig. 59.8).

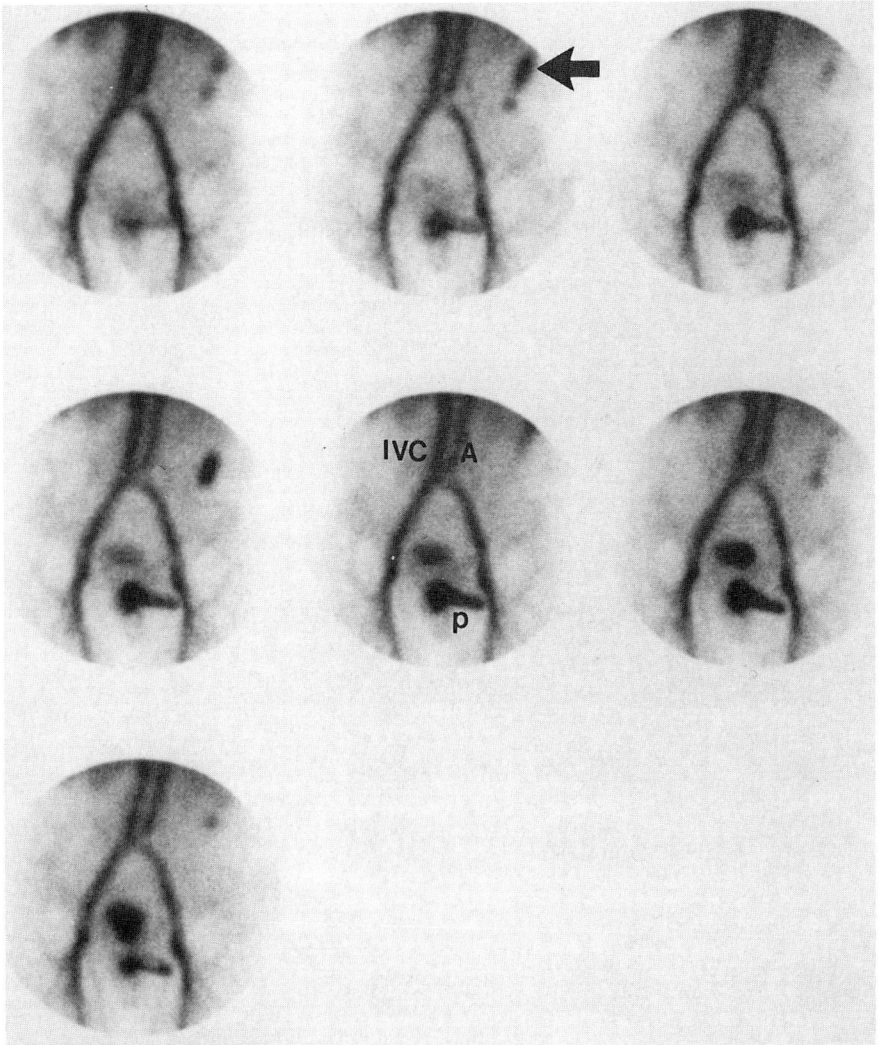

Figure 59.6. Splenic Flexure Bleeding in the Colon due to Diverticular Disease. Sequential 5-minute images show a small focus of bleeding (*arrow*) in the left upper quadrant that varies with intensity as it accumulates and moves through the colon. Note that the patient has a large, static blood pool in the penis. Unchanging blood pools such as the aorta (*A*), the inferior vena cava (*IVC*), and penis (*P*) should not be misinterpreted as hemorrhage.

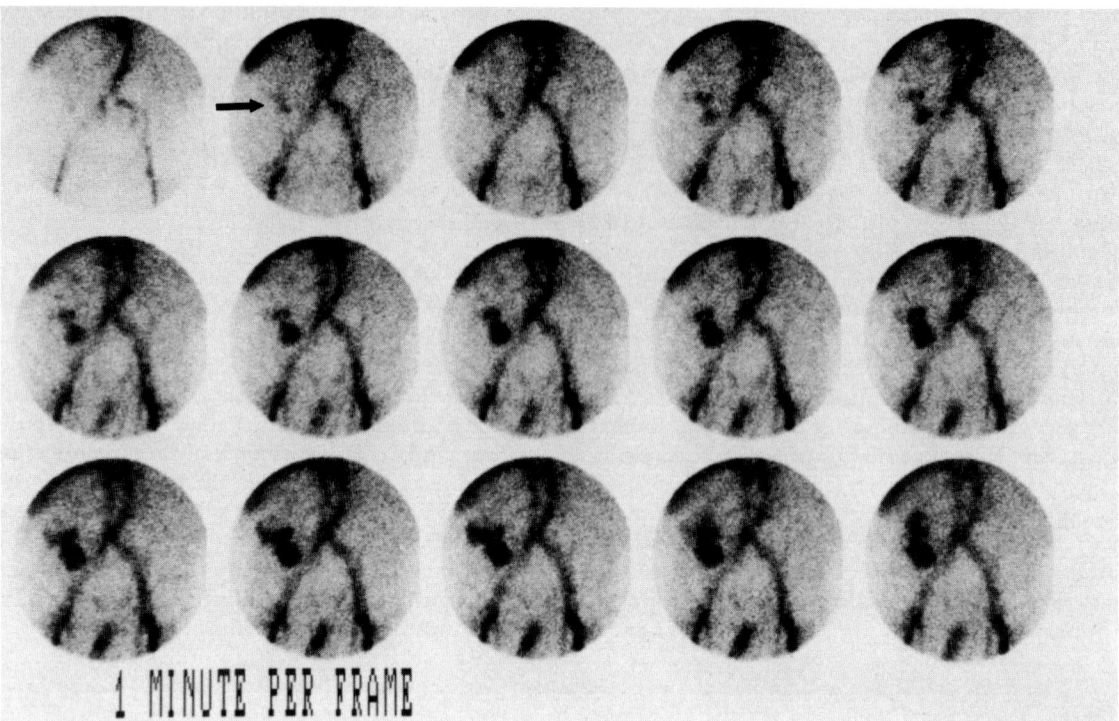

Figure 59.7. Cecal Bleeding due to Angiodysplasia. Images show a right lower quadrant hemorrhage (*arrow*).

Figure 59.8. Meckel's Diverticulum. A small focus (*arrow*) of Tc-99m-O$_4$ uptake gradually becomes visible in the ectopic gastric mucosa in a Meckel's diverticulum in the midabdomen.

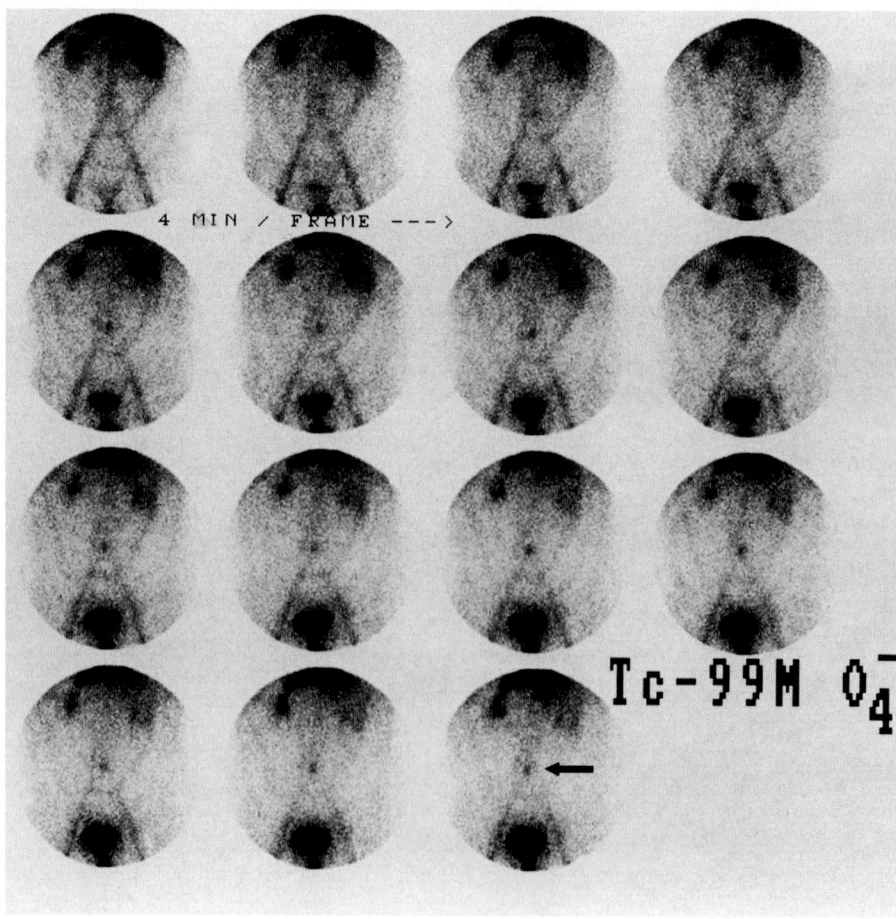

LIVER AND SPLEEN STUDIES

Liver Spleen Scan

Liver spleen scanning is performed by IV injection of Tc-99m-radiolabeled albumin or sulfur colloid. Colloid imaging provides information based upon organ perfusion and the distribution of reticuloendothelial cells which phagocytize the colloid particles. Kupffer cells in the liver and reticuloendothelial cells in the spleen are normally imaged. Reticuloendothelial cells in the bone marrow are minimally seen. The liver/spleen scan is an inexpensive and easy means to evaluate for focal or diffuse hepatic disease but it lacks disease specificity. Radiotracer uptake may be abnormal in a multitude of diseases. To make matters worse, hepatic lesions less than 1 cm in diameter are routinely missed even with SPECT. MR, CT and US have better resolution for hepatic masses. Liver spleen radionuclide imaging remains accurate and easy for evaluation of liver and spleen size, configuration, and position. This helps in the evaluation of suspected hepatomegaly in patients with obstructive lung disease causing diaphragmatic flattening or in patients with anatomic variants such as large left liver lobe or a Riedel's lobe on the right (Fig. 59.9).

Alterations in perfusion and reticuloendothelial system function caused by cirrhosis and hepatitis are seen as a "shift" of activity to the spleen, bone marrow, and lungs. The liver/spleen scan provides information that helps monitor the disease process and efficacy of therapy (Fig. 59.10).

Liver spleen scans can be "subtracted" from other nuclear medicine studies to provide spatial information about the liver or spleen in relation to a suspected abnormality. Indium-111 leukocyte scans (for infection), gallium-67 scans (for inflammation, lymphoma or hepatoma), In-111 Octreotide scans (for neuroendocrine tumors), and labeled antibody scans have physiologic uptake in the liver and/or spleen. Subtracting the liver/spleen scan from any these scans confirms "hot" abnormalities adjacent to the liver or spleen (Fig. 59.11).

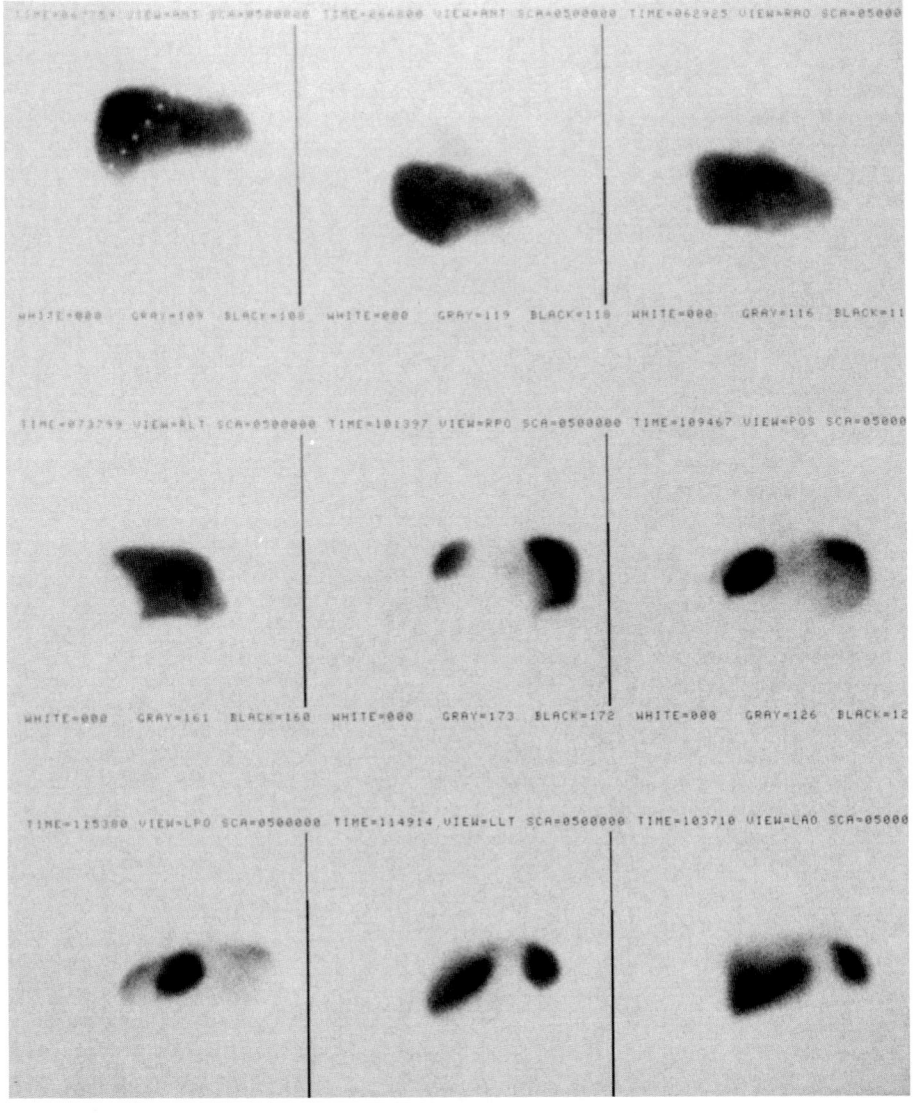

Figure 59.9. Normal Liver Spleen Scan. Sequential images begin with an anterior projection with a lead marker (row of cold dots) on the right costal margin. Subsequent images are anterior, right anterior oblique, right lateral, right posterior oblique, posterior, left posterior oblique, left lateral, and left anterior oblique from left to right, top to bottom. Note the homogeneous labeling of the liver and spleen and the relative size and position of these two organs in various projections.

Figure 59.10. Abnormal Liver/Spleen Scan in a Patient with Cirrhosis. The liver is small and labels poorly. The left lobe of the liver *(L)* is better seen than the right lobe *(R)*. Note the shift of the radiopharmaceutical to the bone marrow and spleen. Ascites separates the liver from the right ribs *(arrowheads)*. Compare this figure with Figure 59.9.

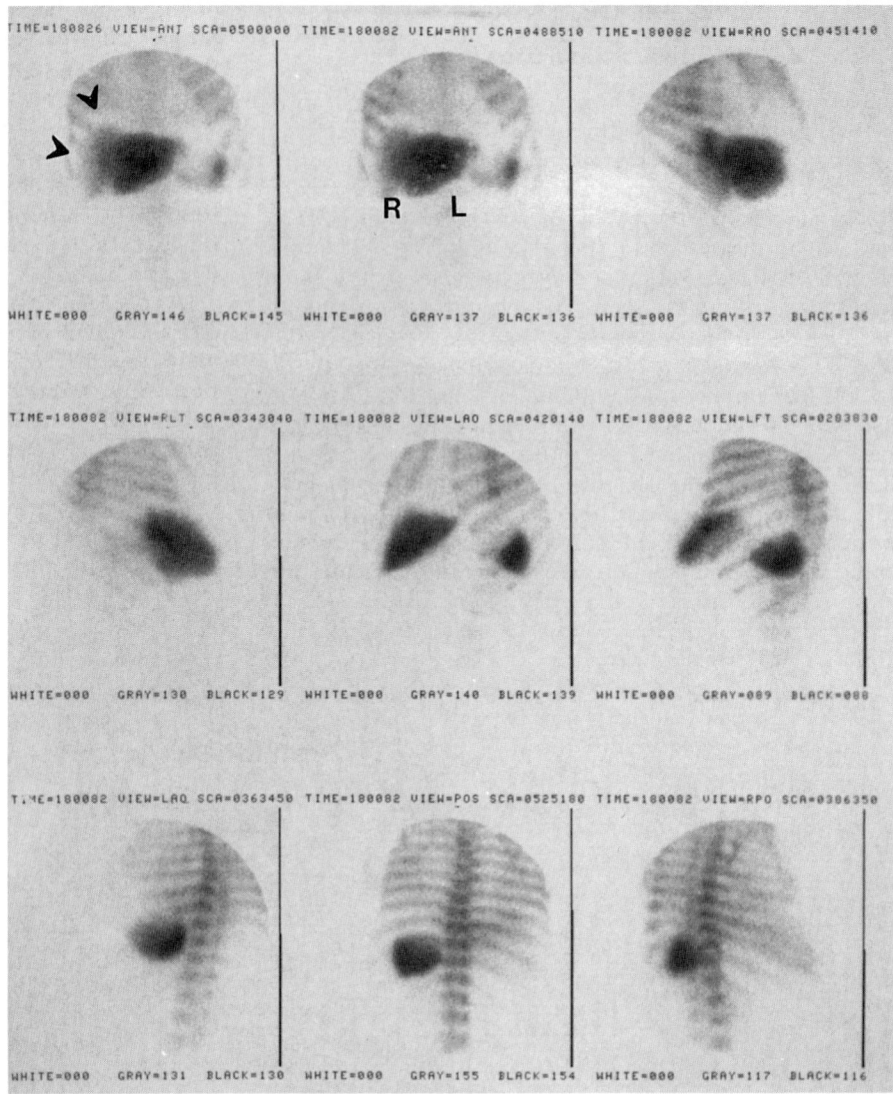

Figure 59.11. Liver/Spleen Subtraction from a Gallium-67 Scan in a Patient with a Hepatoma. A. Image of Ga-67 distribution in the anterior projection at 48 hours. **B.** Matched image of colloid distribution. Careful selection of the gamma camera energy windows allows simultaneous imaging of the two radiopharmaceuticals. The subtraction image **(C)** shows the gallium-avid hepatoma, which does not label with the colloid.

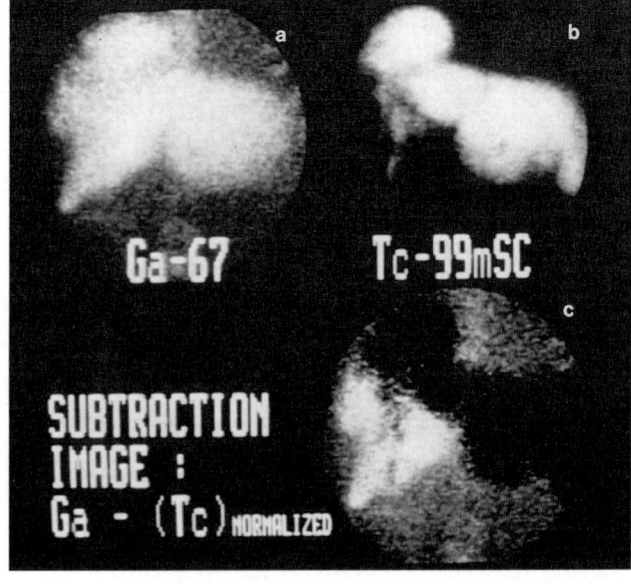

Heat-Damaged Red Blood Cell Scan for Splenic Tissue

Tc-99m-labeled red blood cells that have been damaged by heating are preferentially extracted from circulation by splenic tissue. Applications include diagnosis of polysplenia, splenosis, and confirmation of accessory splenic tissue.

HEPATOBILIARY IMAGING

Nuclear imaging of the gallbladder and biliary system is easily performed with Tc-99m-labeled iminodiacetic acid compounds. Several of the numerous iminodiacetic acid radiotracers that have been developed are commercially available. These radiopharmaceuticals are excreted unchanged into the biliary system and work even in the presence of elevated serum billirubin.

Acute Cholecystitis. Hepatobiliary scans are most commonly used to evaluate suspected acute cholecystitis. A minimum of 2 hours fasting is recommended in preparation for this scan. The anterior dynamic images of normal hepatobiliary scans show prompt and homogeneous uptake of the radiopharmaceutical by the liver. This activity decreases progressively as the radiotracer is excreted into the biliary system and drains into the small bowel. The activity should be seen in the major extrahepatic ducts, gallbladder, and small bowel within one hour (Fig. 59.12). Most patients with acute cholecystitis have a stone or stones obstructing the cystic duct. A small minority of patients, usually the chronically ill, have acalculous cholecystitis. The hallmark in the diagnosis of acute cholecystitis by cholescintigraphy is nonvisualization of the gallbladder at both one and four hour intervals after intravenous injection of the biliary agent.

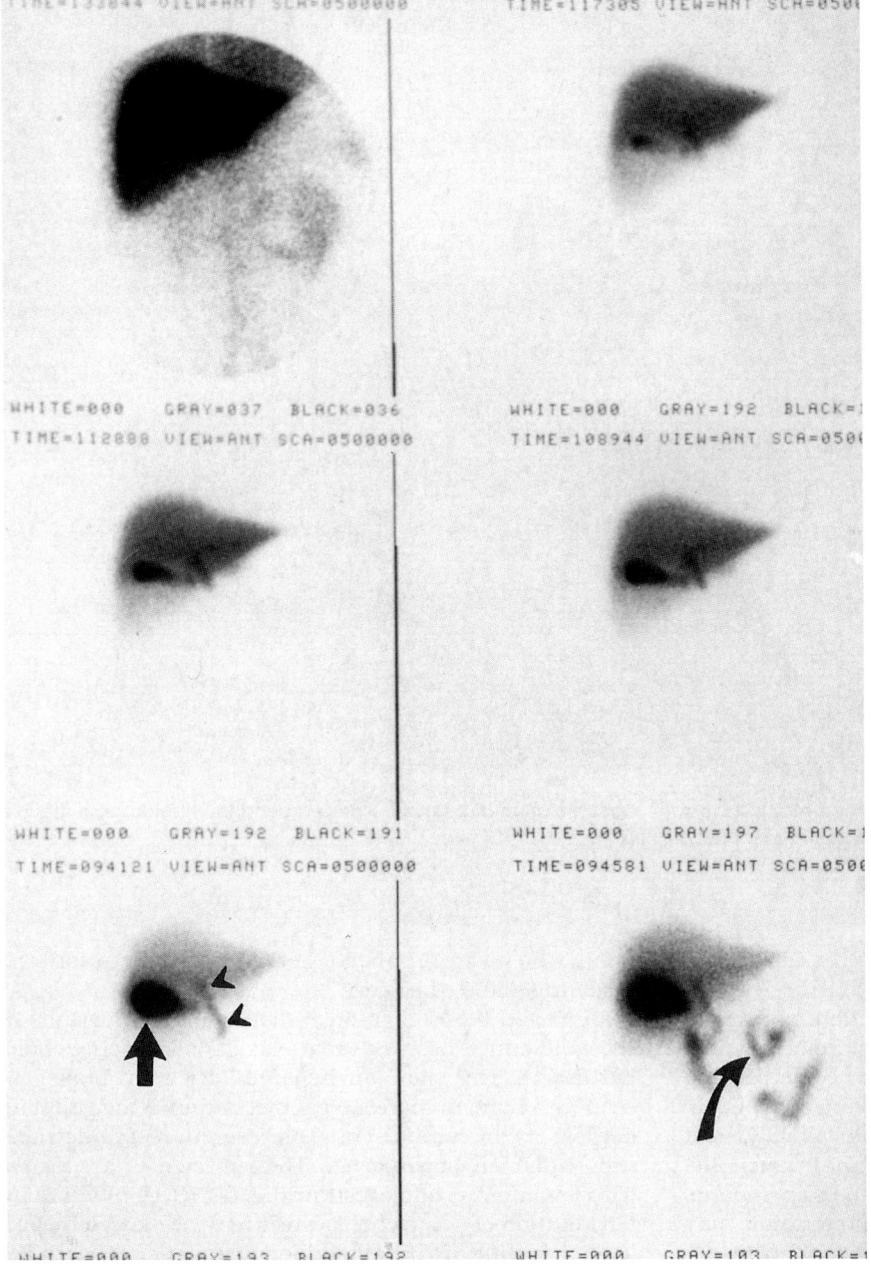

Figure 59.12. Normal Hepatobiliary Scan. Images of the liver immediately after injection and at subsequent 5-minute intervals show rapid clearance of the blood pool followed promptly by central biliary duct and gallbladder (*arrow*) activity. Activity continues to fill the common bile duct (*arrowheads*) at 20 minutes and the small bowel (*curved arrow*) at 25 minutes.

Figure 59.13. Acute Cholecystitis Diagnosed by Hepatobiliary Scan. The first hepatobiliary scan in this patient was positive for acute cholecystitis but the referring service did not believe the diagnosis. The scan was repeated on the next day. In it, the first image shows radioisotope left over from that first scan. A dim line of activity in the transverse colon is marked (*arrowheads*). CCK was used as a pre-treatment for the second scan. Starting with the second image the dose is rapidly concentrated and excreted by the liver into bile ducts and small bowel. The gallbladder never fills. As the liver clears a "hot rim" of activity is seen around the gallbladder fossa (*arrows*) which indicates inflammation caused by the severe acute cholecystitis.

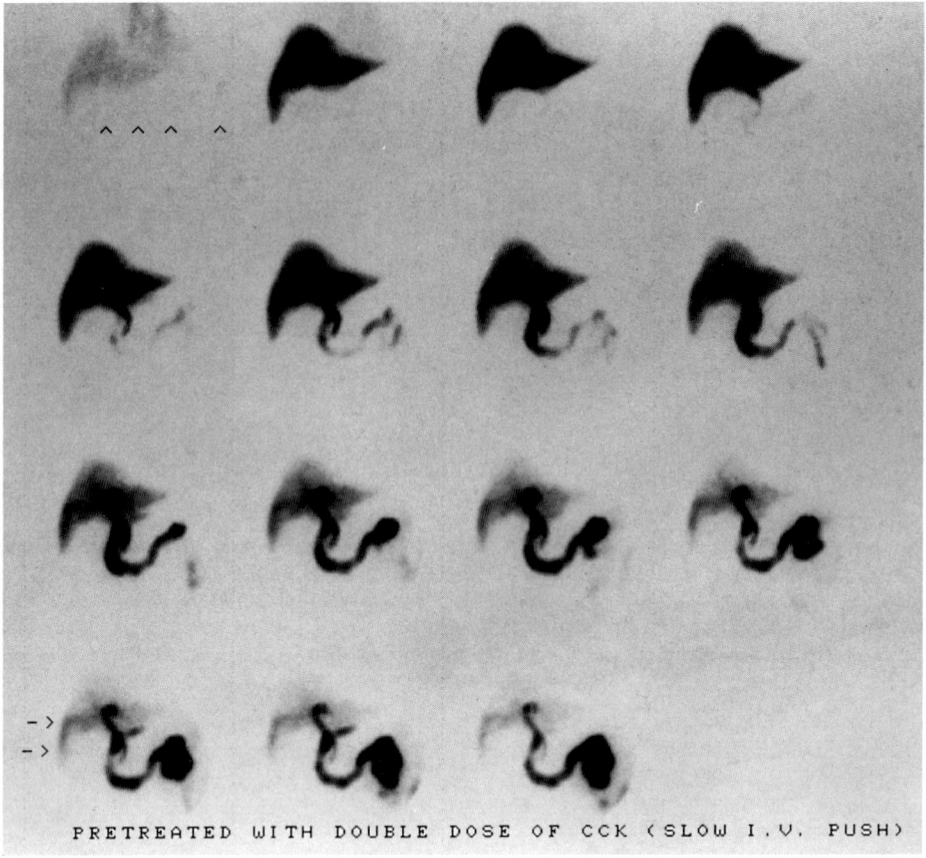

PRETREATED WITH DOUBLE DOSE OF CCK (SLOW I.V. PUSH)

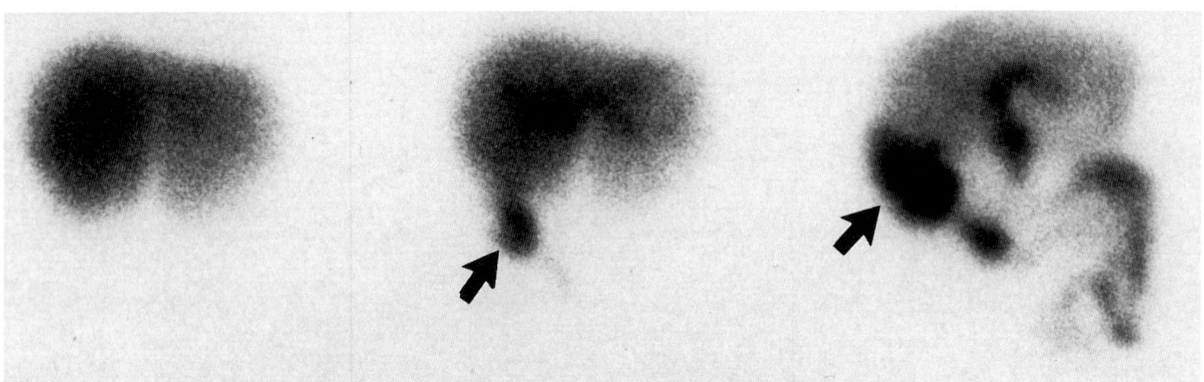

Figure 59.14. Biliary Leak after Cholecystectomy Detected by a Hepatobiliary Scan. Images (*left to right*) obtained immediately, 30 minutes, and 1 hour after administration of the biliary agent show accumulation of bile in the area around the right lobe of the liver (*arrows*).

Chronic cholecystitis is diagnosed when the nonvisualized gallbladder at one hour is seen at four hours. The nuclear medicine hepatobiliary examination has a 95% accuracy rate in the detection of acute cholecystitis. Small doses of IV morphine (1–2 mg) can be used during the scan to raise the pressure on the sphincter of Oddi. This helps push radiolabeled bile into the gallbladder. It is a handy way to speed up a "normal scan" because the diagnosis of acute cholecystitis is excluded as soon as the gallbladder is seen. Morphine administration may also allow true negative scans to be performed in pa-

tients who have stimulated their gallbladders to contract by eating before the scan.

Increased blood flow on radionuclide angiograms of the gallbladder fossa aids in the diagnosis of acute cholecystitis. A "rim sign" on hepatobiliary scan images is seen as a band of increased activity around the gallbladder fossa, which represents poor excretion of radiotracer from inflamed hepatocytes. The rim sign is associated with gangrenous cholecystitis (Fig. 59.13). A pitfall in interpretation of acute cholecystitis may be caused by prolonged fasting with gallbladder distension. The radiopharmaceutical will not enter the completely full gallbladder. This can be avoided by pretreating the patient with analogs of cholecystokinin (CCK). CCK is a short-acting, natural hormone that causes prompt gallbladder contraction. After emptying, the gallbladder refills, allowing entry of the biliary agent. A false-positive diagnosis of acute cholecystitis may also occur with previous cholecystectomy, tumor obstructing the cystic duct, and agenesis of the gallbladder.

Acalculous Biliary Disease includes chronic acalculous cholecystitis, cystic duct syndrome, and gallbladder dyskinesis. These patients present with similar complaints of right upper quadrant pain, fatty food intolerance, and epigastric distress. Cholescintigraphy and US may be normal. CCK-assisted cholescintigraphy in acalculous biliary disease demonstrates decreased gallbladder contraction. The normal gallbladder ejection fraction is greater than 35%.

Other uses for the hepatobiliary scan include the detection of postoperative complications and bile leaks in trauma (Fig. 59.14). The excretion phase of the scan is important in evaluating hepatic and common bile duct patency. A delay in visualization of the bile ducts of more than one hour suggests obstruction. Caution must be exercised to differentiate severe hepatocellular disease from obstruction, as both present with delays in biliary visualization. The hepatobiliary scan maintains a niche in differentiating neonatal hepatitis from biliary atresia. In the latter case radiolabeled bile will never enter the bowel. Unfortunately, if the hepatitis is bad enough the radiopharmaceutical may not leave the liver. When bowel activity is seen (and this may take 4–24 hours) the diagnosis of biliary atresia is excluded.

HEPATIC BLOOD POOL SCINTIGRAPHY

Cavernous Hemangiomas are the most common hepatic tumor. Frequently subcapsular in location, these tumors are often found incidentally by US, CT or MR. Although there are specific criteria for diagnosis of hepatic hemangioma by these techniques, no study is 100% specific. Because a significant risk of hemorrhage exists with biopsy, a noninvasive diagnostic approach is preferred. Scintigraphy with Tc-99m-labeled red blood cells using an in-vitro labeling technique has proved both sensitive and specific for cavernous hemangioma. A flow study should be performed initially and will demonstrate normal or decreased early uptake if the suspected lesion is a hemangioma. Tumors and inflammatory lesions tend to have increased arterial flow. Subsequent delayed SPECT imaging will reveal foci of activity within the liver that are hotter than surrounding parenchyma. Sensitivity decreases with lesions smaller than 1.5 cm, greater organ depth, and with single detector SPECT as opposed to multi-detector SPECT. Correlation with a second imaging technique is always advised as these lesions may be seen concomitant with malignancy. Specificity is generally high, although isolated cases of increased activity on delayed imaging with both colon and lung carcinoma metastases have been reported. In general, if two of the four imaging techniques demonstrate characteristic features of cavernous hemangioma, no further evaluation is warranted (Fig. 59.15).

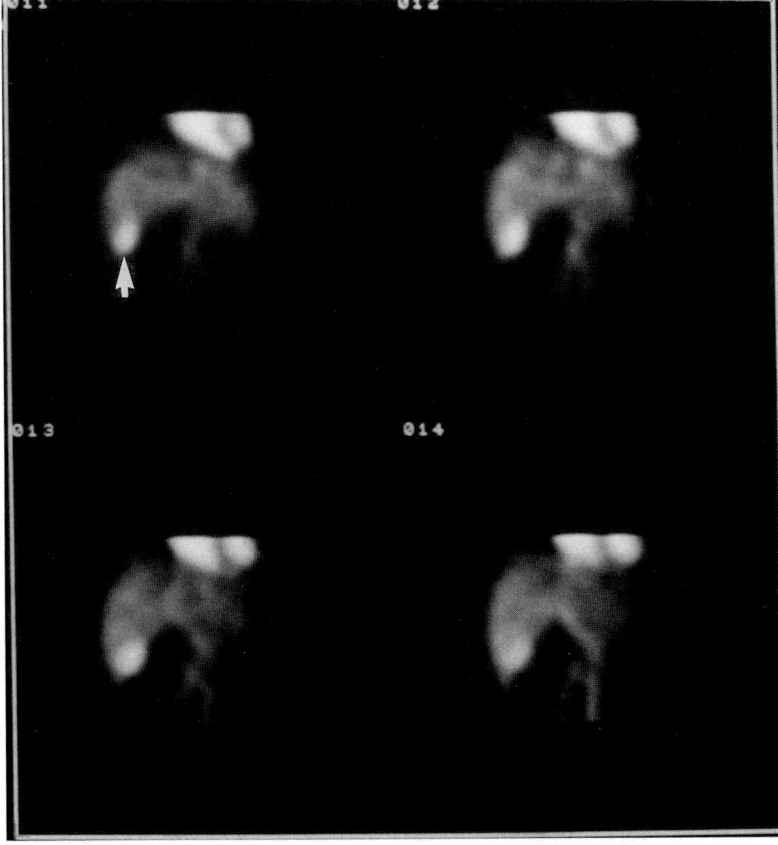

Figure 59.15. Hepatic Hemangioma. At first glance this study could be confused with a biliary scan. However note the vascular blood pool and that these are four coronal slices from a SPECT study of the liver performed 1 hour after the injection of 25 mCi of 99mTcO₄-red blood cells labeled with in-vitro technique. The area of increased activity (*arrow*) which simulates a gallbladder is actually a hemangioma in the liver of this hepatic transplant recipient.

Suggested Reading

Klein HA. Esophageal transit scintigraphy. Semin Nucl Med 1995;25:306–317.

Krishnamurthy S, Krishnamurthy GT. Cholecystokinin and morphine pharmacological intervention during ^{99m}Tc-HIDA cholescintigraphy: a rational approach. Semin Nucl Med 1996;26:16–24.

Mauree AH, Krevsky B. Whole-gut transit scintigraphy in the evaluation of small-bowel and colon transit disorders. Semin Nucl Med 1995;25:326–338.

Nadel HR. Hepatobiliary scintigraphy in children. Semin Nucl Med, 1996;26:25–42.

Royal HD, Drum DE. Liver-spleen scanning in benign disease. In: Mettler FA, ed. Radionuclide Imaging of the GI Tract. New York: Churchill-Livingstone, 1986:83–134.

Urbain J-L C, Charkes ND. Recent Advances in Gastric Emptying Scintigraphy. Semin Nucl Med 1995;25:318–325.

Wiest PW, Hartshorne MF. Atlas of gastrointestinal bleeding (RBC) scintigraphy. In: Ziessman HA, Van Nostrand, eds. Selected Atlases of Gastrointestinal Scintigraphy. New York: Springer-Verlag, 1992:35–74.

Ziessman HA. Atlas of cholescintigraphy: selective update. In: Ziessman HA, Van Nostrand D, eds. Selected Atlases of Gastrointestinal Scintigraphy. New York: Springer-Verlag. 1992:1–34.

60
Genitourinary System Scintigraphy

Mike McBiles
Peter W. Blue

RENAL IMAGING

Renal radionuclide imaging has always been an important part of the practice of nuclear medicine. As imaging modalities such as US, CT, and MR have replaced nuclear medicine anatomic imaging, there has been rapid development of the non-invasive functional nature of the radionuclide studies. Radionuclides are well suited for evaluating blood flow, nephron function and mass, and collecting system excretory function and drainage.

Radionuclide renal studies are safe, minimally invasive, and expose the patients to radiation doses comparable with competing radiologic procedures. They are used to study such disorders as renal collecting system obstruction, vesicoureteral reflux, renovascular hypertension, and pyelonephritis. Renal function parameters such as renal flow, differential function, glomerular filtration rate (GFR), and effective renal plasma flow (ERPF) are easily obtainable with radioisotopes. In patients with radiographic contrast sensitivity, radionuclide studies can frequently answer the clinical question, despite their limited spatial resolution.

This chapter highlights some of the areas that are best evaluated with radionuclides

Radiopharmaceuticals

Radionuclide renal imaging involves the assessment of the four major renal functions: blood flow; glomerular filtration; tubular function, which includes tubular reabsorption of filtered molecules (solutes and water) and active tubular secretion and; collecting system drainage. In order to assess these functions, the nuclear physician will choose a radiopharmaceutical tailored for the specific function or combination of functions to be studied. Only by understanding the sequential dynamic movement of the tracer from the blood to the bladder will accurate interpretation be possible.

Blood Flow. Renal perfusion can be assessed using any radioisotope that is given intravenously in sufficient dosage (>5 mCi) to acquire a usable series of 3–5 second images. Flow images are usually obtained using the commonly accepted doses of technetium-99m (Tc-99m) renal agents: diethylenetriamine pentaacetic acid (Tc-99m–DTPA) (10–20 mCi), mercaptoacetyltriglycine (Tc-99m–MAG3) (10–15 mCi), glucoheptonate(Tc-99m–GHA) (15–20 mCi), or even dimercaptosuccinic acid (Tc-99m–DMSA) (5 mCi).

Glomerular Filtration is a passive pumping of plasma components through the semipermeable glomerular membrane into Bowman's space. Plasma water and those molecules small enough to pass the membrane (e.g., electrolytes, creatinine, urea, etc.) are filtered and, if not fully reabsorbed, reach the renal collecting system. Proteins, in general, are too large to be filtered. Certain radioisotopes such as Tc-99m-DTPA are small enough and not significantly protein bound (5–10%) that they are almost fully filtered. Because there is no significant reabsorption of Tc-99m-DTPA, and since Tc-99m-DTPA does not reach the urine by any other mechanism than glomerular filtration, it traces this function well, and can be used to accurately measure the GFR. Although diffusion across the glomerulus is passive, the glomerular permeability must be maintained for filtration to continue. Disorders such as renal artery stenosis or cardiac pump failure decrease the preglomerular pressure. Renal obstruction and acute tubular necrosis may increase the postglomerular (Bowman's space) pressure. In either case, the net pressure drops, decreasing the GFR and the amount of tracer (Tc-99m-DTPA) passing through the kidney. Intrinsic diseases such as glomerulonephritis (chronic renal failure) disrupt glomerular membrane permeability, resulting in diminished filtration and tracer movement. Knowledge of how various pathologies affect renal tracer transfer is needed to fully interpret renal scintigraphy.

Two other radiotracers Tc-99m-GHA and Tc-99m-DMSA, are filtered by the glomerulus. Tc-99m-GHA is a glucose analog that is filtered and partially reabsorbed; 90% of the total dose reaches the urine while 10% is reabsorbed by the tubular cell, allowing for delayed cortical imaging. Tc-99m-DMSA has significantly greater tubular reabsorption and binding (40–50% of the total dose). Both agents may be used for cortical imaging, although many nuclear medicine physicians prefer Tc-99m-DMSA because collecting system activity is generally less of a problem and because image count statistics are slightly better using the usual clinical doses.

Tubular Secretion is an active process by which certain molecules are removed from the peri-tubular capillaries and secreted into the glomerularly filtered tubular urine that is passing by. For a radionuclide to effectively trace tubular function, most or all of the tracer must be removed in one pass by the tubule, that is, it must be secreted into the urine and not be reabsorbed. Until recently, I-131-orthoiodohippurate (I-131-OIH) has been the best of such agents with a 20% glomerular–60% tubular extraction efficiency. Its main limitations have been low spatial resolution and counting statistics using the requisite high energy collimated systems, and very high kidney dosimetry in situations of prolonged cortical retention. More recently, Tc-99m-MAG3 with a 5% glomerular–55% tubular extraction efficiency has become the agent of choice for tubular functional imaging because of its superiority in all of these areas. The Tc-99m-MAG3 clearance correlates very well with established renal plasma flow (ERPF) methods using I-131-OIH.

Because the clearance of Tc-99m-MAG3 (300–400 ml/min) (extraction efficiency = 60%) is so much greater than that of Tc-99m-DTPA (80–140 ml/min) (extraction efficiency = 20%), Tc-99m-MAG3 is the agent of choice for imaging kidneys in moderate to severe renal failure, immature kidneys, and in transplant kidneys where renal function is often in flux. It has replaced I-131-OIH for most purposes.

Collecting System. Isotopes for examining the collecting system include Tc-99m-DTPA, Tc-99m-GHA, and Tc-99m-MAG3. Because Tc-99m-MAG3 has the highest extraction of the Tc-99m agents and the greatest amount of tracer reaches the renal pelvis in the shortest time, it is the agent of choice for studies directed specifically at the collecting system, such as to rule out obstruction. Tc-99m-DTPA may be used when there is a need for a GFR determination. Any tracer not absorbed across urinary epithelium, including Tc-99m-DTPA, Tc-99m-O4, or even Tc-99m-sulfur colloid (1–3 mCi), may be instilled into the bladder to perform cystoureteral reflux studies.

Miscellaneous. Gallium-67 (Ga-67) citrate (6–10 mCi) is useful in evaluating infectious and neoplastic processes of the kidneys and perinephric spaces. Indium-111-labeled white blood cells (In-111-WBC) (0.5 mCi) are even more specific for the detection of focal inflammatory and acute infectious processes. Sodium pertechnetate (Tc-99m-O4) (5–10 mCi) is used in scrotal imaging. If possible, the thyroid should be blocked with oral potassium perchlorate prior to Tc-99m-O4 injection.

Image Acquisition

Recent advances in gamma camera technology and the increasing availability of SPECT allow for the quicker acquisition and processing of higher resolution and better quality images than have been previously available. Image acquisition matrix (64 × 64 or 128 × 128), and the computer or camera zoom should be chosen such that the resultant images include all desired structures and the pixel size is approximately one half the resolving capacity of the system at the distance of the organ of interest from the camera. Improved computer technology allows for the rapid processing of dynamic functional data and curve generation that is essential in the evaluation of renovascular hypertension and the assessment of collecting system obstruction. The availability of inexpensive high capacity digital image storage encourages rapid image retrieval for comparison studies, and allows for optimum image matrix sizes which correspond to the imaging system resolution.

Imaging Techniques. In all renal studies it is critical that the patient be immobilized during acquisition. The supine position is used routinely. The upright sitting position or semi upright position may be used, especially when ureteral drainage is evaluated or where renal pelvic activity might interfere with the study (e.g., evaluation for renovascular hypertension and the assessment of collecting system obstruction). The main drawback to nonsupine positions is that differential function determinations may be inaccurate because mobile kidneys may move from nearly the same depth when the patient is supine to different depths when not supine. Renal transplants and some renal variants (e.g., horseshoe kidney) and the urinary bladder are best imaged anteriorly.

Adequate hydration is mandatory in order to avoid false positive renovascular hypertension and collecting system obstruction studies, and to give reproducible results for quantitative washout parameters in follow-up studies. Many departments perform IV hydration and supplemental oral hydration routinely on all children and many adults because of the wide variability in the state of hydration upon presentation for the procedure.

For flow studies, an intravenous bolus of tracer is injected and a set of sequential images of 1–3 seconds are obtained. Tracer normally arrives at the kidney 1–2 seconds after the bolus has reached the adjacent aorta. Although flow studies are routinely performed for all dynamic renal studies in many clinics, some authors perform them only in acute renal failure, when there is a probability of rapidly changing renal function, such as transplantation, or in the evaluation of renal masses.

For the uptake and excretion phases of Tc-99m-GHA, Tc-99m-DTPA and Tc-99m-MAG3 imaging, a series of 15–60 second dynamic images are acquired over the following 20–30 minutes. In collecting system obstruction studies, an indwelling bladder catheter is often inserted to insure bladder decompression and to monitor urine output, and furosemide 20 mg IV is given at the end of the initial set of 20–30 minute images, and imaging continued for another 20–30 minutes.

For evaluation of renal vascular hypertension, an angiotensin converting enzyme inhibitor (ACEI) is given. This is accomplished either with enalaprilat 2.5 mg IV over 5 minutes beginning 15 minutes prior to radiopharmaceutical bolus, or with oral captopril 25–50 mg given one hour prior to the radiopharmaceutical. Blood pressures are recorded before ACEI administration, and at various times during the study. Many protocols require a baseline renal study without ACEI, which can be accomplished either on a separate day or on the same day with a smaller dose of radiopharmaceutical.

Static images using Tc-99m-DMSA are usually obtained with a pinhole collimator and/or a SPECT system 4 hours after injection to allow sufficient time for cortical localization, and background and collecting system washout.

Quantitative Analysis and Interpretation

Dynamic Imaging. The approach to interpreting dynamic renal studies can be divided into four phases, and sequential attention to each phase allows for a methodical evaluation of pertinent positive and negative findings so that a reasonable differential diagnosis can be reached (Fig. 60.1).

The *flow phase* lasts for the first minute after injection, when arterial flow to the kidney can be analyzed semi-quantitatively. Radiotracer is normally seen arriving at the kidneys within 1–2 seconds after appearance in the adjacent aorta, and appears at least as intense as the spleen. With Tc-99m-DTPA and Tc-99m-GHA, peak activity in the kidney is the reached six seconds later and declines, because of only 20% first pass extraction, until recirculation of the systemic bolus. With Tc-99m-MAG3 the intensity decline is less evident visually because of 60% first pass extraction. Areas of hyper- and hypo-perfusion are noted and correlated to delayed images.

The *uptake phase* continues until radiotracer begins to leave the parenchyma (3–4 minutes for Tc-99m-MAG3 and 4–5 minutes for Tc-99m-DTPA and Tc-99m-GHA). Time to collecting system appearance and areas of poor uptake should be noted. Differential function is computed by drawing regions of interest (ROI) and obtaining background subtracted 1–2 minute integrated unilateral whole kidney counts and expressing them as a percentage of total kidney counts. In many instances, this parameter is a crucial piece of information, and so careful examination of ROIs for proper position and artifacts is very important. Differential function can also be obtained on 4 hour delayed static images of Tc-99m-GHA and Tc-99m-DMSA, with excellent intra-patient and inter-radiopharmaceutical reproducibility of less than 5%.

The *cortical washout* and *excretory* phases begin after the uptake phase, and occur simultaneously but should be evaluated separately. Areas of prolonged or diminished cortical retention should be correlated with their uptake phase and their relation to the calyces. Although the calyces, renal pelvis and ureters may be seen in a

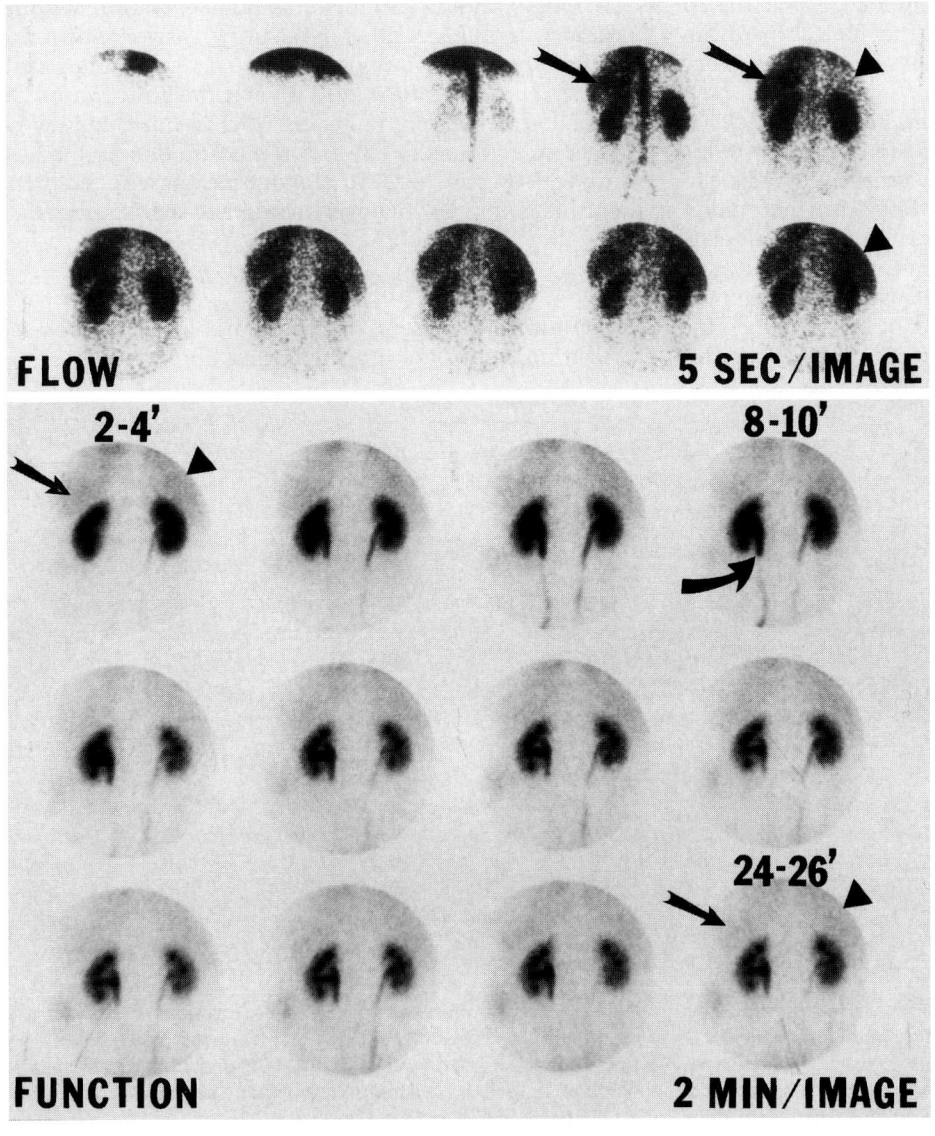

FLOW   **5 SEC/IMAGE**

2-4'   8-10'

24-26'

FUNCTION   **2 MIN/IMAGE**

Figure 60.1. Normal Tc-99m-DTPA Study. (Posterior Projection) **Renal Blood Flow** (*FLOW*-top): The bolus reaches the aorta (third image) and, within 2 seconds, the kidneys. The kidneys should be as hot or hotter than the spleen (*arrows*) on the image following the aorta bolus image. Hepatic activity (*arrowheads*) appears later than splenic activity because hepatic perfusion is predominantly from the portal vein. **Uptake** (*FUNCTION*-bottom): Tracer is rapidly cleared by the kidneys, resulting in peak cortical activity in the *2-4'* image. Intense cortical uptake in the *2-4'* image and rapid decrease of blood pool, liver (*arrowheads*) and spleen (*arrows*) activity is evidence of normal GFR. **Cortical Washput and Excretion**: This patient, allergic to iodinated contrast, was imaged after a renal stone had passed. Because tracer passes rapidly from an undilated collecting system to the bladder, there is no obstruction. The small column of tracer (*curved arrow*) represents ureteral spasm where the stone had probably impacted.

normal study, prolonged or intense accumulations, structural displacement or unusual contours should be noted. Background subtracted time activity curves for whole kidney, renal cortex, collecting system or renal pelvis (depending on the clinical question) are usually generated. Various parameters to quantitatively evaluate washout from these curves have been proposed, but the most common are the T1/2 and the 20 minute post injection to peak ratio. The T1/2 is defined as the time after either radiopharmaceutical injection or furosemide injection to half maximum activity. A normal value is less than 10 minutes, but in poor renal function or collecting system dilation, this parameter may not be determinable within the constraints of the usual 20-30 minute examination. The 20 minute post injection to peak ratio is the ratio of the 20 minute activity to the maximum activity. A normal value is less than 0.3.

Knowledge of the exact clinical question, results of other imaging modalities, laboratory results, and patient history markedly narrows the differential diagnosis, allows for selection of the appropriate radiopharmaceutical and imaging protocol, allows for the proper evaluation of artifacts, and increases the clinical usefulness of the scan. Every effort should be made, especially in transplant evaluations, to correlate the nuclear medicine images with available clinical, imaging, and laboratory data.

Absolute Function Quantitation. Renal tracer clearance (GFR with Tc-99m-DTPA or ERPF with Tc-99m-MAG3) can be visually estimated by assessing the rate of disappearance of tracer from the blood (cardiac blood pool and/or background), the rate of appearance of renal cortical activity, or the rate of appearance of urine (usually bladder) activity. Because of the well-recognized inadequacy of absolute functional quantitation using creatinine and blood urea nitrogen in patient with moderate to severe renal failure, radionuclide quantitative methods have been developed to accurately estimate the GFR and ERPF using more reliable methods. Radionuclide techniques for measurement of absolute renal function vary from counting of the radioactivity in the dose, plasma, and urine samples to pure imaging methods. Sometimes, a combination of imaging and serum and/or urine sample counting techniques are used. The most accurate methods, but most time-consuming and technically demanding, require well counter determination of either multiple (usually two) plasma sample collections, or urine and one plasma sample collection. These values are then used in empirically derived parametric equations to arrive at absolute function. The quickest but least accurate methods rely on initial renal cortical uptake, as determined by gamma camera images, expressed as a percentage of the dose administered. The choice of method depends on the clinical situation, the ability to perform the more complex methods, the need for a quick estimate of renal function during times of rapid change in critically ill patients, and the need for information that can only be determined by imaging, such as differential function.

In long-standing chronic renal failure, all radiographic and scintigraphic studies tend to be very sensitive but are not specific for any particular disease. Studies evaluating the GFR, ERPF, and differential function are of major use in helping to decide when a failed kidney no longer contributes to effective renal function and is best removed. Accurate GFR determinations can help the nephrologist in the dialysis decision-making process.

Clinical Applications

Anatomic Variants. Nuclear renal imaging is of use in evaluating anatomic variants when other imaging

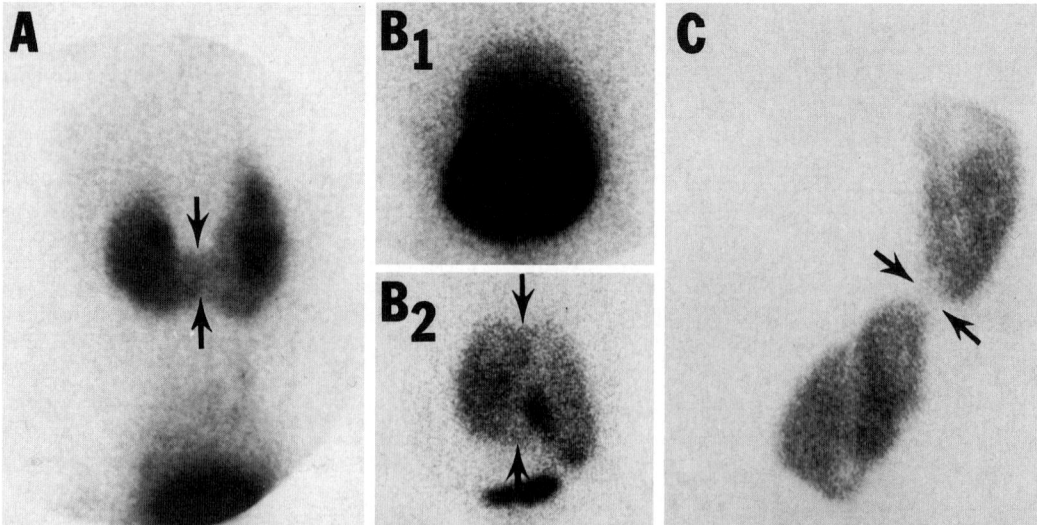

Figure 60.2. Congenital Renal Abnormalities. A. Horseshoe kidney (Tc-99m-DTPA). The medial angulation of the inferior renal poles and the connecting bridge characteristic of horseshoe kidney are best seen in this anterior view (*arrows*). Collecting system obstruction, a possible complication, is not seen. **B.** Lump or cake kidney (Tc-99m-DTPA). Anterior image of the bladder (*B1*) demonstrates no appreciable renal activity. After voiding (*B2*) the fused pelvic kidney was easily seen. The line of fusion (*arrows*) is apparent. **C.** Crossed-fused ectopia (Tc-99m-DMSA). The bridge of fusion (*arrows*) was best seen on this anterior Tc-99m-DMSA image.

modalities have not fully defined the abnormality. The ability to assess function makes scintigraphy even more valuable. A dromedary hump, a fetal lobulation, or a renal column of Bertin may appear as a mass on an US or CT. Tc-99m-DMSA or Tc-99m-GHA images (pinhole and/or SPECT) will demonstrate the questionable tissue to be normally functioning and rule out a pathologic lesion. Nuclear imaging is particularly useful in congenital abnormalities (Fig. 60.2) such as horseshoe kidney, lump or cake kidney, and crossed-fused ectopia when other modalities have not located or elucidated the nature of the abnormality.

Mass Lesions. Although radionuclide studies are not generally used to detect intra-renal masses, they may be of significant value in investigating hydronephrosis (HN) as a possible cause of a mass and in demonstrating functioning tissue associated with a mass (Fig. 60.3). In the neonate, multicystic dysplastic kidney and HN both present as fluid-filled masses. They can be differentiated by the presence (in HN) or the absence (in multicystic dysplastic kidney) of tracer in the fluid. On Tc-99m-DTPA or Tc-99m-MAG3 imaging, urine collections such as HN or urinoma increase tracer concentration with

time. Solid neoplasms, cysts, and abscesses may be difficult to differentiate on static imaging. However, renal tumors may be hypervascular on dynamic perfusion imaging, renal lymphoma generally demonstrates intense uptake on gallium imaging, and perinephric or intrarenal abscesses are hot on In-111-WBC imaging. In general, renal masses are investigated primarily with pyelography, US, CT, or MR, with scintigraphy providing additional supplemental information.

Acute Renal Failure. The differential diagnosis of acute renal failure includes acute vascular occlusion, acute collecting system or bladder outlet obstruction, and acute tubular necrosis. Unlike scintigraphic flow and function imaging, which can easily limit the diagnostic possibilities by distinguishing unilateral from bilateral processes, conventional anatomic imaging may be technically difficult or impossible. The renal perfusion (flow) study can demonstrate absent perfusion of one or both kidneys and may define the level of aortic cutoff from a dissecting aneurysm. In renal vein thrombosis (Fig. 60.4), decreased perfusion of an enlarged kidney with prolonged cortical retention of tracer is seen. Delayed images (Tc-99m-DTPA or Tc-99m-MAG3) demonstrating tracer in a dilated collecting system suggest a high-grade obstruction. In acute tubular necrosis

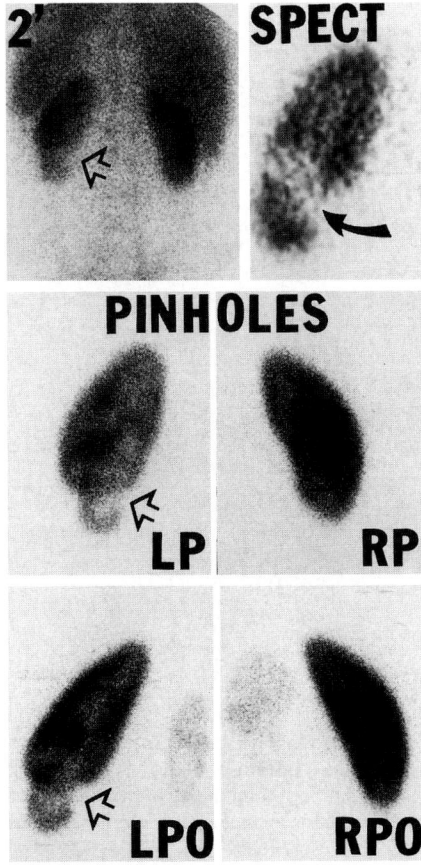

Figure 60.3. Renal Mass. Tc-99m-DTPA posterior image (*2'-upper left*) and Tc-99m-DMSA pinhole images (*middle and lower*) demonstrate a renal contour abnormality (*open arrows*) of the lower pole of the left kidney. The SPECT image (*upper right*) demonstrates the true cortical defect (*curved arrow*) that corresponds to a renal tumor. *LP*, left posterior; *RP*, right posterior; *LPO*, left posterior oblique; *RPO*, right posterior oblique.

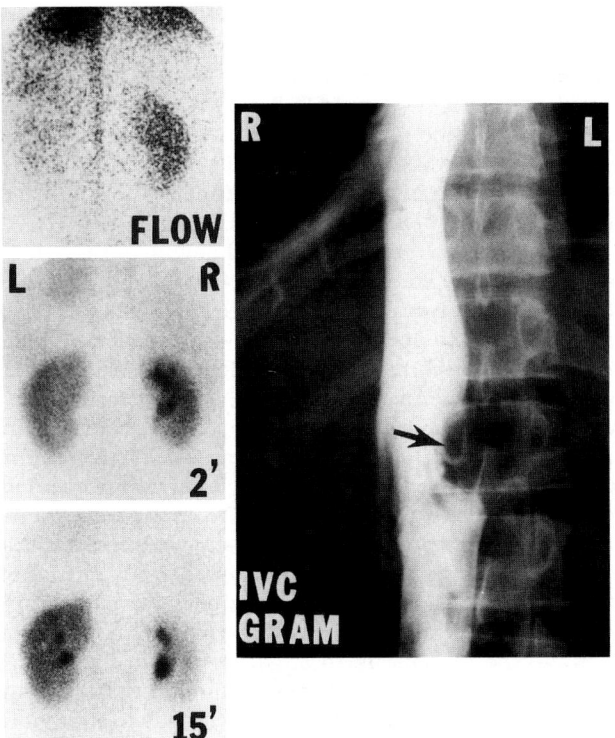

Figure 60.4. Renal Vein Thrombosis. Posterior scintigrams (*left*) demonstrate normal flow, cortical uptake, and excretion for the right kidney. The left kidney is enlarged with severely diminished flow and a progressive rise in cortical tracer through 15 minutes. The contrast inferior vena cavagram (*IVC GRAM*) (*right*) confirms thrombus in the left renal vein (*arrow*). Since 50% of patients with renal vein thrombosis develop pulmonary emboli, ventilation-perfusion scintigraphy should be considered.

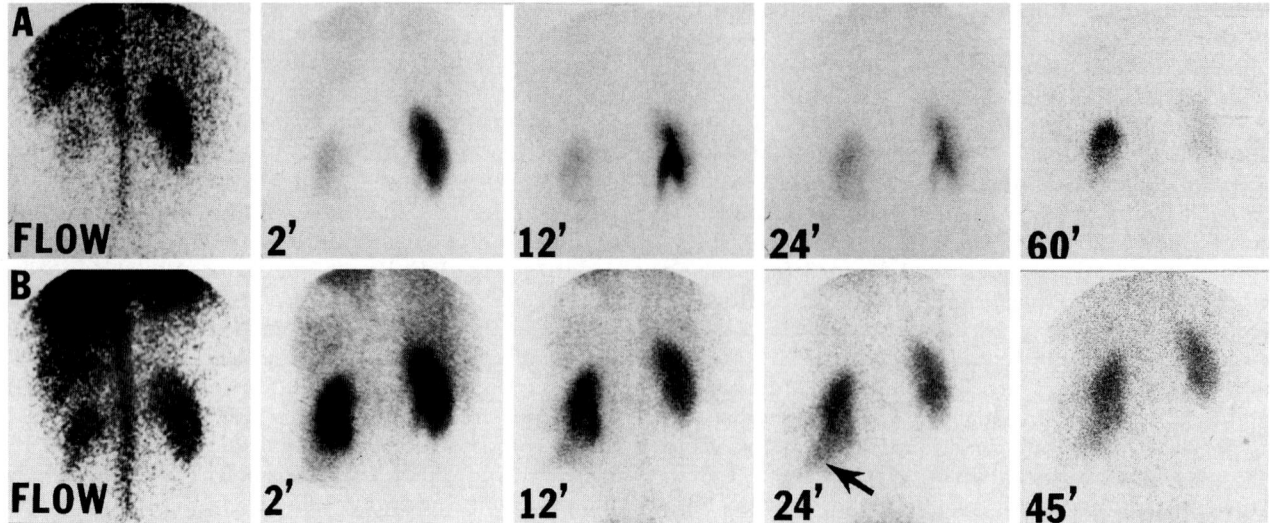

Figure 60.5. Acute Tubular Necrosis. A. Posterior Tc-99m-MAG3 renal scintigrams 48 hours after left renal ischemia during a surgical procedure reveals diminished left renal flow which is relatively well preserved compared to initial cortical uptake with slowly increasing cortical tracer retention through 60 minutes. GFR = 74 ml/min (left = 19 ml/min, right = 55 ml/min). **B.** A study performed 1 month later reveals almost full resolution of the unilateral ATN. GFR = 94 ml/min (left = 42 ml/min, right = 52 ml/min). Extrarenal tracer activity (*arrow*) indicates a urine leak along a postoperative nephrostomy tract.

(ATN) (Fig. 60.5), arterial flow is relatively well maintained in spite of almost absent transit of tracer to urine. In ATN, although glomerular filtration drops to near zero and Tc-99m-DTPA studies reveal no uptake, tubular cell uptake of Tc-99m-MAG3 continues as long as the cells are viable. The Tc-99m-MAG3 cortical activity can be used to gauge the prognosis of ATN. Progressive loss of cortical Tc-99m-MAG3 uptake is a poor sign for recovery, while the retention of accumulating ability, or the return of this function, is a favorable sign.

Renal Transplantation. Renal imaging of the anuric or oliguric transplanted kidney is performed to help distinguish acute tubular necrosis from transplant rejection as well as to detect other post-transplant complications. Differential diagnosis includes all of the diseases of concern in acute renal failure, with several others which are unique to transplantation. As a complementary modality to Doppler US, it can assist in situations where oliguric renal failure is a contraindication to nephrotoxic contrast agents. In ATN, renal perfusion is usually, but not invariably, relatively well preserved in comparison with the dramatic loss of renal function (GFR and cortical transit). Acute or chronic rejection results in a more balanced loss of perfusion and function because the damage is to small vessel perfusion with secondary and equivalent loss of function. The scintigraphic pattern of cyclosporine toxicity has been likened by some to that of ATN, and by others to that of rejection. A myriad of additional postoperative complications are seen following transplantation. Some that are well investigated scintigraphically include renal artery and renal vein thrombosis, renal infarction, renal infection, ureteral implant site obstruction or leakage, urinomas, and lymphoceles (Fig. 60.6).

As important as the patterns themselves may be, even more significant are the time after transplantation at

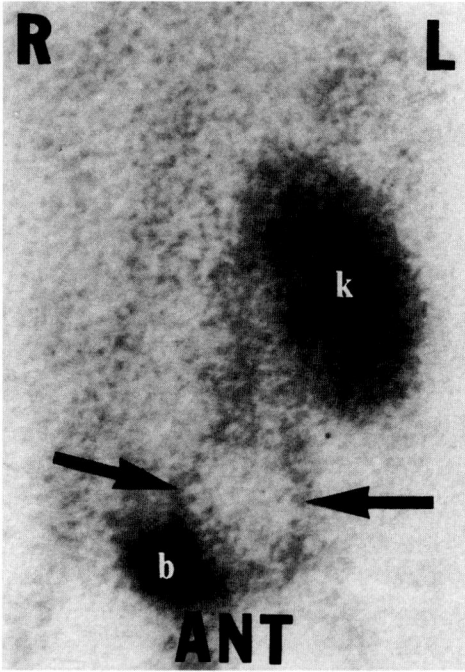

Figure 60.6. Lymphocele in a Renal Transplantation Patient. A lymphocele is seen as a photopenic area (*arrows*) adjacent to the bladder (*b*) on this anterior scintigram. Because it is not obstructing the transplant ureter, it is probably not clinically significant. *k*, transplant kidney.

which the patterns occur, the progression of sequential studies, and the correlation with clinical information. ATN usually occurs during the first week, and acute rejection from the first to the fourth week following transplantation. Cyclosporine toxicity occurs later and only in patients taking cyclosporine. Chronic rejection is a late sequela, which eventually occurs to some degree in all transplants. Urinomas tend to occur early, whereas lymphoceles usually occur several weeks after transplantation.

Renovascular Hypertension. Standard renal scintigraphy is neither sensitive nor specific in investigating hypertensive patients for renal artery stenosis (RAS) (Fig. 60.7). The value of scintigraphy is markedly enhanced by incorporating an ACEI (captopril or enalaprilat) into the study. Significant RAS decreases the blood pressure in the *afferent* glomerular arteriole, resulting in an increase in renin production by the juxtaglomerular apparatus. Renin stimulates the conversion of angiotensin I to angiotensin II. This local rise in angiotensin II causes con-

striction of the *efferent* arteriole, which maintains the glomerular perfusion pressure and thus the GFR. The ACEIs block the production of angiotensin II and, in compensated RAS, cause relaxation of the constricted efferent arteriole. The glomerular perfusion pressure and GFR drop and the transit of filtrate from glomerulus to renal pelvis is prolonged. In an unaffected kidney, the afferent arteriole is not constricted, so ACE inhibitors have little or no effect. Changes induced in the renogram curves are best documented by performing renography with Tc-99m-MAG3 before and after the administration of enalaprilat or captopril. Renogram changes are less apparent with Tc-99m-DTPA and Tc-99m-GHA, and differential function changes are more reliable indicators with these radiopharmaceuticals. Sensitivity and speci-

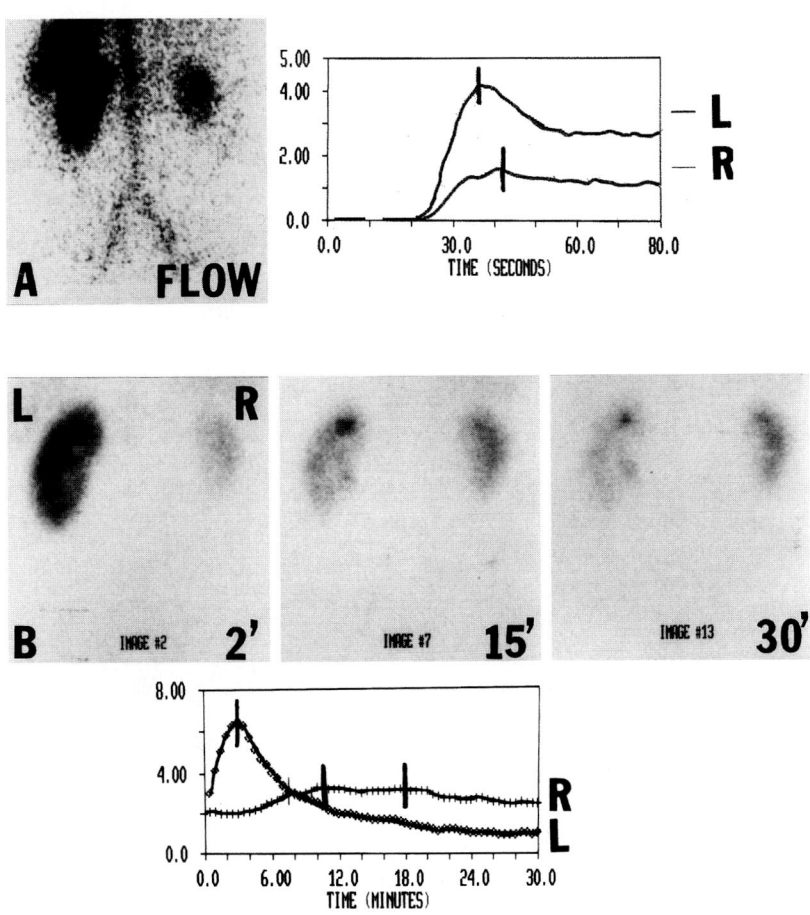

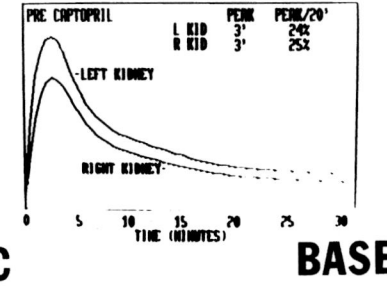

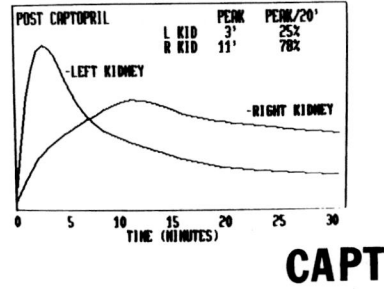

Figure 60.7. Renal Artery Stenosis. (Posterior scintograms). **A.** Flow to the small right kidney is decreased (*image*) and delayed (*curve*). **B.** Right cortical Tc-99m-DTPA activity (*top*) continues to rise during the first 12 minutes of the study. Orthoiodohippurate renography (*bottom*) (similar to Tc-99m-MAG3) reveals the characteristic of a severe RAS. **C.** Typical Tc-99m-MAG3 captopril curves of a patient with compensated right RAS. Both curves are normal in the baseline study. This is because of afferent arteriolar constriction that is maintaining glomerular perfusion pressure and GFR (see text). After captopril, the right GFR has dropped and the cortical glomerular to pelvis transit time has become prolonged. This is demonstrated by a prolonged time to peak, and a delayed washout on the stenotic side.

Figure 60.8. Furosemide Renography. (Posterior scintigrams). Furosemide (Lasix) administered at 15 minutes. A high-grade obstruction is seen on the left **(A,B,C)** with little tracer reaching the renal pelvis (*arrow*) and an absent furosemide response. On the right **(A,B,D)**, a dilated but unobstructed renal pelvis empties rapidly following furosemide administration. A follow-up study many months later **(E–H)** demonstrates that, following surgery, the left kidney has returned to normal. However, the right kidney has developed a high-grade obstruction with poor furosemide response.

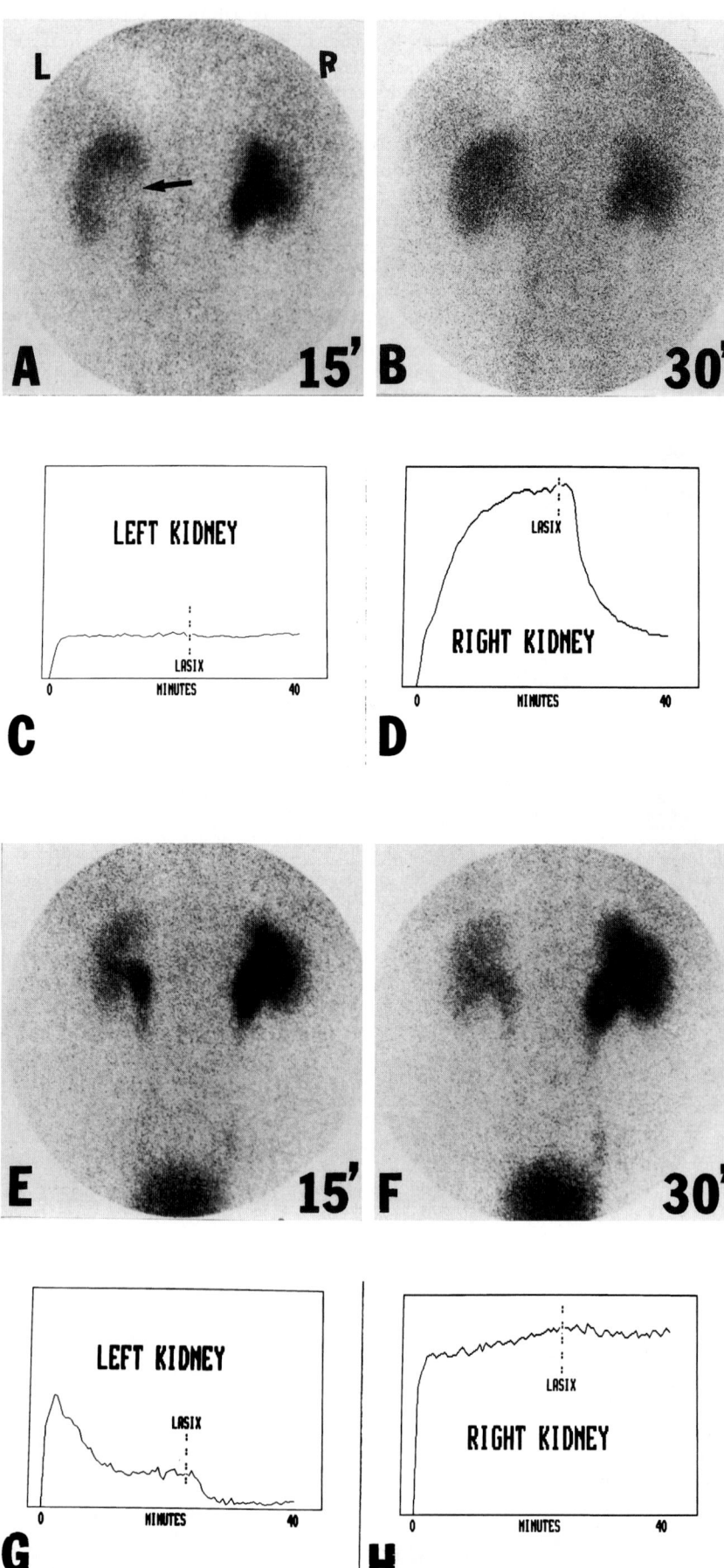

ficity for renovascular hypertension, as determined by response to lesion treatment, are both approximately 90%.

Urinary Tract Obstruction. Because radiopharmaceuticals such as Tc-99m-DTPA and Tc-99m-MAG3 are rapidly cleared through the kidneys, they are useful for the detection of both acute and chronic urinary tract ob-

struction (Figs 60.8, 60.9). These agents are also used to measure differential function in evaluation of stability and/or salvageability of obstructed kidneys.

When collecting system obstruction occurs, the postglomerular (Bowman's space) pressure rises and the GFR drops. Tubular damage occurs later than glomerular damage and takes significantly longer to reverse.

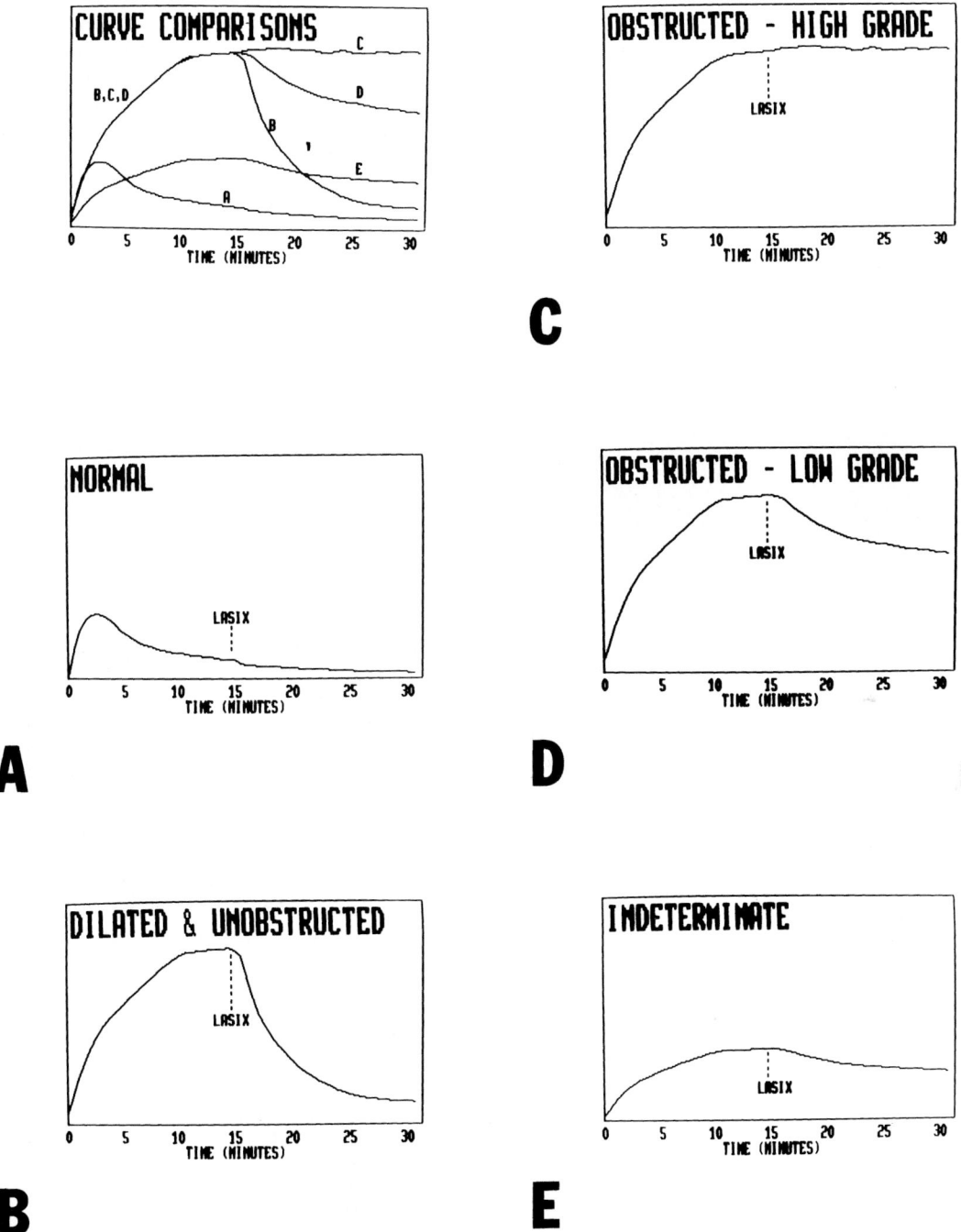

Figure 60.9. Furosemide Curve Patterns. Normal **(A)**, Dilated and unobstructed **(B)**, high-grade obstruction (no Lasix response) **(C)**. In a complete obstruction, no tracer would arrive at the renal pelvis. **D.** Low-grade obstruction. A partial response between that of curves **(B)** and **(C)** is seen. This pattern may be difficult to distinguish from an indeterminate study. If this pattern is seen with relatively good unilateral renal function, and if the collecting system is not markedly di-

lated, then low grade or partial obstruction can be confidently diagnosed. **E.** Indeterminate study. In a patient with a very large dilated collecting system or poor function in the kidney of interest, the furosemide dose may be insufficient to wash tracer from the collecting system. This curve represents a failed kidney that did not respond.

Renal imaging with Tc-99m-MAG3 or Tc-99m-DTPA reliably detects unilateral or bilateral urinary tract obstruction by demonstrating a dilated pelvocalyceal system and/or ureter with delayed drainage. However, since large but unobstructed collecting systems or decreased urine production in renal failure can mimic these obstructive patterns, the routine study is frequently augmented with furosemide. In the absence of renal failure, the post furosemide disappearance of tracer from the collecting system correlates with the severity of obstruction. In such cases in the adult, a T1/2 of 10 minutes or less is normal, and a T1/2 greater than 20 minutes confirms obstruction. However, positive obstructive renogram curves in the presence of compromised renal function should be interpreted with caution. The degree

of renal compromise at which renogram curves become unreliable is unknown and probably variable from patient to patient, but some authors use a unilateral GFR of less than 15 ml/minute (as estimated from the differential function and clinical or measured estimates of total renal function) as a point where positive curves are unreliable. Such curves should be interpreted as indeterminate, and not as partial obstruction. Also, in neonates and infants, obstructive curves are unreliable. It has been shown that, even in the presence of significantly decreased single kidney function, obstructive curves do not predict kidney deterioration, and that, in fact, these children may spontaneously improve in such cases. It is worth stressing, however, that at any age, level of renal function, or collecting system dilation, a non-obstructive curve effectively rules out obstruction, and more reliably than any other modality.

Infection. Imaging with Tc-99m-DMSA or Tc-99m-GHA is still the most sensitive modality for detecting pyelonephritis, despite recent advances in MR, US, and CT. Scintigraphy has the additional advantage that most neonates and infants do not require sedation. In acute pyelonephritis, decreased parenchymal uptake of Tc-99m-DMSA is seen either focally or diffusely within the normal renal contours (Fig. 60.10). In chronic pyelonephritis, scarring occurs and results in renal contour abnormalities with foci of diminished uptake. Renal or perinephric abscess and infected renal cysts may be imaged with Ga-67 or In-111-WBC.

Ureteral Reflux. Direct radionuclide cystography is the most sensitive imaging method for detecting ureteral reflux (Fig. 60.11). The radiation dose is significantly lower than with other radiographic techniques. The agent Tc-99m-O4 Tc-99m-DTPA, Tc-99m-MAG3 or Tc-99m-sulfur colloid is instilled into the bladder and is followed by a continuous computer acquisition during filling and voiding. Even the most transient reflux can be detected. The bladder volume is reported when reflux occurs. The low radiation dose, compared with contrast cystography, is especially desirable in pediatric screening or when multiple studies are needed to evaluate progression of disease and response to therapy.

Incidental Findings. Radiopharmaceuticals directed at other organ systems and accumulated by the

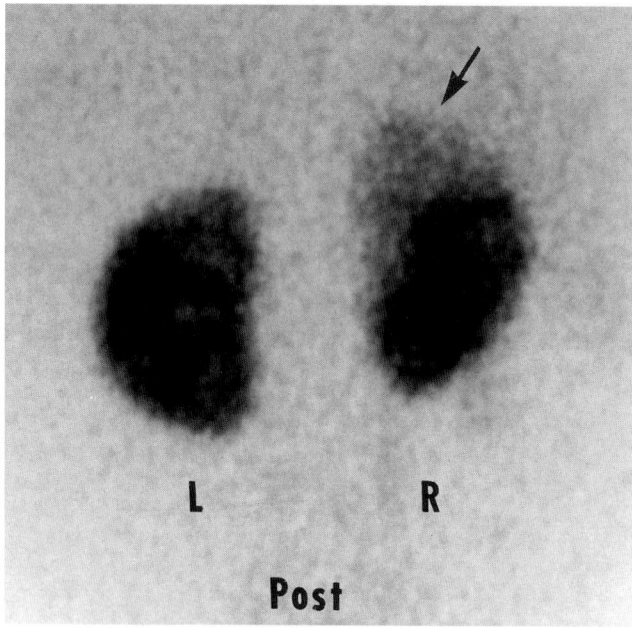

Figure 60.10. Acute Pyelonephritis. Posterior scintigrams show a photopenic area in the upper pole of the right kidney (*arrow*). Chronic pyelonephritis cannot be distinguished from acute pyelonephritis unless prior scans are available and show that the pattern is unchanged.

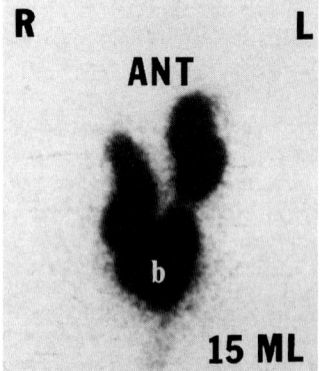 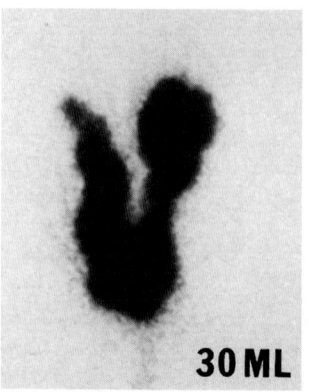 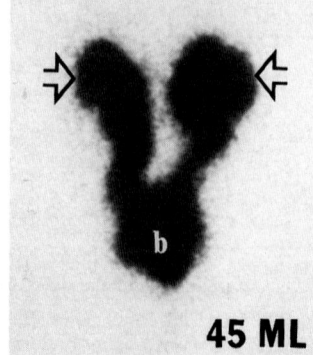 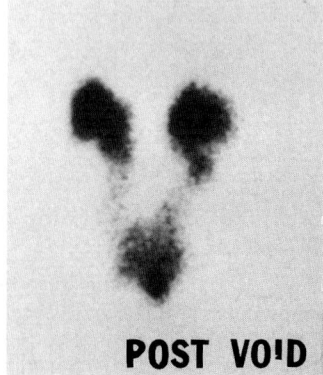

Figure 60.11. Ureteral Reflux. Anterior scintigrams demonstrate reflux of tracer to the renal pelvis (*arrows*) immediately on the left and at 45 ml bladder volume on the right. *b*, bladder.

kidneys may reveal unanticipated urinary tract abnormalities such as ureteral obstruction, urine leakage, abnormal renal position or shape, renal masses, and abnormal renal function. The kidneys are routinely demonstrated during skeletal imaging (Tc-99m-MDP) and may also be seen during thyroid imaging (Tc-99mO4), blood pool imaging of the heart and imaging for gastrointestinal bleeding (Tc-99m-RBC). The kidneys are the main excretory route for thallium-201 and, during the first 24 hours after injection, for Ga-67. Increased renal activity during lung perfusion imaging may be the result of a right-to-left intra-cardiac shunt.

TESTICULAR IMAGING

In many centers, radionuclide testicular imaging (Fig. 60.12) has been supplanted by Doppler US studies. Nevertheless, it remains a robust, non-operator dependent procedure with an extremely high sensitivity and specificity for acute torsion. Testicular torsion presents as a central hypovascular defect. As time passes, a hypervascular rim develops around the torsed testis and indicates loss of viability (delayed torsion). This rim may also be seen in abscess and hematoma. Epididymitis is hypervascular. Masses and other testicular lesions are best evaluated with other modalities.

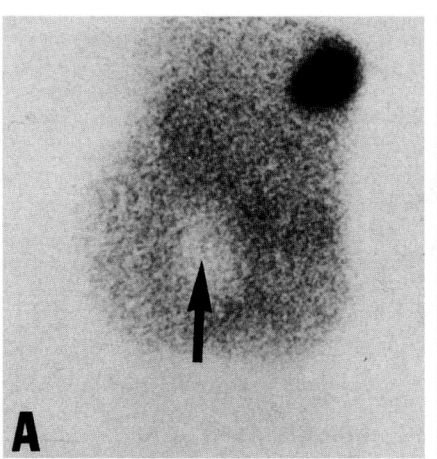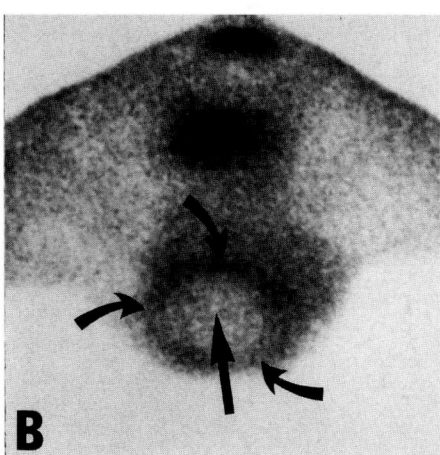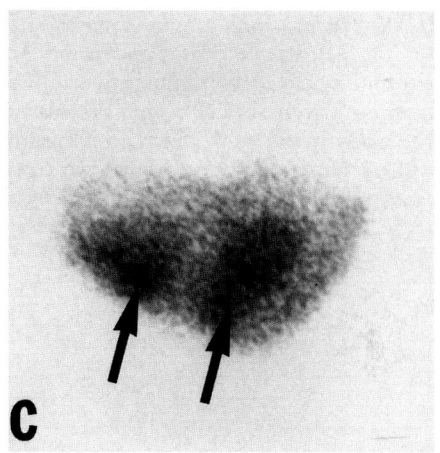

Figure 60.12. Imaging of the Painful Testis. (Anterior scintigrams). **A.** Testicular torsion is seen as a photon-deficient testis (*arrow*). **B.** The hyperemic rim (*curved arrows*) surrounding the photon-deficient testis (*straight arrow*) occurs when the diagnosis of torsion is delayed ("missed") and correlates well with loss of testicular viability. **C.** Hyperemic inflammation occurs with epididymitis resulting in increased radionuclide accumulation in the epididymis, in this case bilaterally (*arrows*).

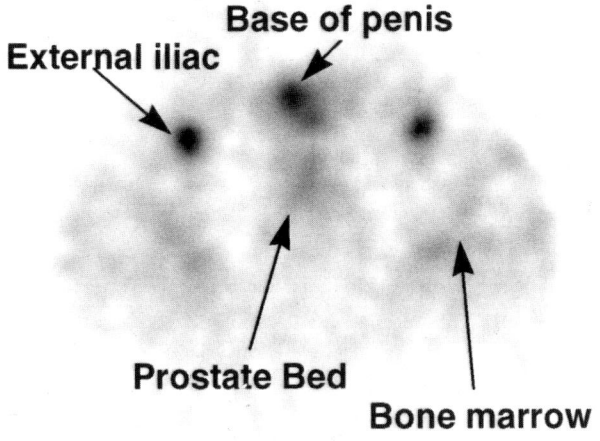

External iliac
Base of penis
Prostate Bed
Bone marrow

1 hour blood pool image, Transaxial pelvis

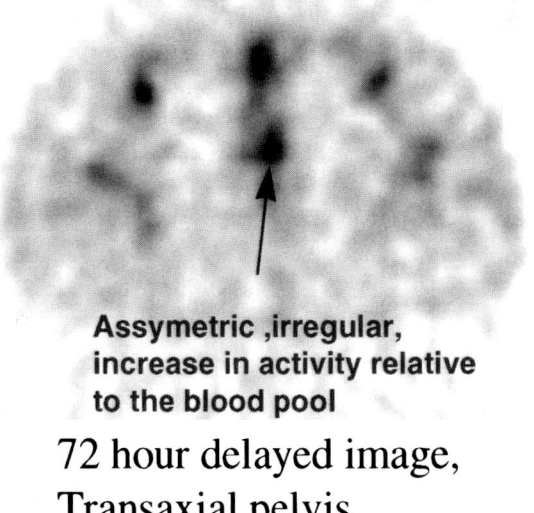

Assymetric ,irregular, increase in activity relative to the blood pool

72 hour delayed image, Transaxial pelvis

Figure 60.13. Prostate Cancer. (Transaxial scintigrams utilizing In-111 capromab pendetide). Early (*1 hour*) and late (*72 hour*) images through the prostate in a patient with rising PSA 3 years after radical prostatectomy. US-guided biopsy of the prostate bed nodules was negative for cancer. This study shows an unequivocal abnormality in the prostate bed on the late images. The patient was treated with external beam therapy to the prostate bed and the PSA fell to nondetectable. This implies that the prostate nodule biopsy was a false negative, a common scenario.

PROSTATE CANCER IMAGING

Prostate cancer spread is notoriously difficult to image, with all other imaging modalities demonstrating less than 50% sensitivity and specificity. Therapy depends on whether the patient has local disease versus distant metastasis. Indium-111 capromab pendetide (5mCi), a recently approved radiopharmaceutical, is a monoclonal antibody directed against cytoplasmic membrane antigens expressed only by prostate cancer. It has a sensitivity and specificity of 75% in detecting local disease and distant metastasis. It is helpful when positive for distant spread in patients with a reasonable pre-prostatectomy possibility of metastasis, and in patients with rising post-prostatectomy prostate specific antigen (PSA) to determine local recurrence or distant spread (Fig. 60.13). However, imaging with this agent requires exquisite attention to imaging protocol detail, knowledge of the normal scintigraphic distribution of the agent in the abdomen and pelvis, and a minimum of a dual head SPECT camera, preferably with multi-energy acquisition capabilities.

Suggested Readings

Blue PW, Manier SM, Chantelois AE, et al. Differential diagnosis of prolonged cortical retention of radiotracer in technetium-99m DTPA renal scintigraphy (nuclear medicine atlas). Clin Nucl Med 1987;12:77–84.

Fogelman I, Maisey M. Renal. In: An atlas of clinical nuclear medicine. St. Louis: Mosby, 1988:217–373.

Freeman LM, Blaufox MD, eds. Genitourinary imaging update. In: Seminars in nuclear medicine (entire issue). Philadelphia: WB Saunders 1992:59–137.

Sandler MP, et. al., eds. Diagnostic nuclear medicine. 3d ed. Baltimore: Williams & Wilkins, 1996:1177–1274,1331–1344.

Harbert JC, Eckelman WC, Neumann RD. Nuclear Medicine, Diagnosis and Therapy. Thieme, New York, 1996:713–744.

Mettler FA, Guiberteau MJ. Genitourinary system. In: Mettler FA, Guiberteau MJ, eds. Essentials of nuclear medicine imaging. 3d ed. Philadelphia: WB Saunders, 1991:237–251.

Thrall JH, Zeissman HA. Nuclear Medicine, The Requisites. St Louis: Mosey, 1995:283–320.

Treves ST. Pediatric Nuclear Medicine. New York. Springer-Verlag, 1994:339–429.

61
Scintigraphic Diagnosis of Inflammatory Processes

John M. Bauman

RADIOPHARMACEUTICALS
INFLAMMATORY PROCESSES
    Infection
    Noninfectious Inflammatory Processes
SUMMARY

The scintigraphic evaluation of inflammatory processes is extremely broad in scope and encompasses virtually all radiopharmaceuticals, imaging approaches, and inflammatory, benign and malignant diseases. Many of these topics have been discussed elsewhere and will not be further addressed. The focus of this discussion will be on the uses of Gallium-67 (Ga-67) and radiolabeled white blood cells (WBCs).

RADIOPHARMACEUTICALS

Gallium-67 (Ga-67) has been in use for more than 20 years to evaluate malignancy and inflammation after originally being introduced as a bone imaging agent. With principle photon energies of 93, 184, 296, and 388 keV and a poor photon yield per disintegration, Ga-67 is suboptimal as an imaging agent. Decay is by electron capture and the half-life is 78.1 hours. Typically, the three lower photopeaks are used for imaging and medium or high energy collimation is required.

Ga-67 is administered as the citrate and is rapidly bound to transferrin and lactoferrin in vivo. Five to 8 mCi doses are recommended when searching for infection; 10 mCi are recommended for tumor diagnosis. Higher doses are of particular help when SPECT imaging is planned.

The biodistribution is variable depending on age, sex, prior transfusions, chemotherapy, lactation status, underlying disease process, and time of imaging. Imaging is typically performed at several times during the 6–72 hours after injection. Earlier times are used for evaluation of infectious processes; later times for the evaluation of malignancy. During the first 24–48 hours, approximately 15% of the administered dose is excreted in the urine. Subsequently another 10–20% is excreted by the colon (1). The normal Ga-67 study shows uptake in the liver, spleen, skeleton, lacrimal glands, salivary glands, genitalia, and, the kidneys and colon at the appropriate times (Fig. 61.1). Laxative administration helps to clear unwanted colonic activity.

The exact mechanisms of Ga-67 localization in inflammatory lesions and tumors are unclear, but three principle components have been cited: blood flow and local capillary status, incorporation and transfer by leukocytes, and bacterial ingestion (1–4).

Indium-111 Labeled White Blood Cells (In-111-WBCs). Since the introduction of In-111-WBCs in 1976, a variety of labeling techniques have been reported. Typically, a WBC-rich, mixed cellular suspension from 60 ml of whole blood is incubated with In-111-oxine in a saline medium and injected. Autologous cells are usually used. However, in neutropenic patients and infants, ABO-compatible donor leukocytes may be used with appropriate type and cross-match precautions. Since HIV and hepatitis screening cannot be completed before injection of the donor cells, informed consent and careful donor selection are imperative. The labeling procedure requires approximately 2.5 hours to perform.

In-111 is superior to Ga-67 in its imaging characteristics, with peaks of 173 keV (89%) and 247 keV (92%). It decays by electron capture with a half-life of 67 hours. These energies require the use of a medium energy collimator but are easily imaged by the thinner crystals present in modern gamma cameras. The high target (abscess) to background ratios for In-111-WBC's provide excellent image contrast.

The spleen is the critical organ, receiving up to 20 rads per 0.5 mCi dose. There is no normal renal or intestinal excretion of In-111-WBCs, as is seen with Ga-67. Marrow activity is present because of normal cellular migration and marrow uptake of In-111. Moderate to marked lung activity is present on images obtained within 4 hours of injection. This activity represents margination of the cells in the lungs and is a physiologic response of the cells to contact with extracorporeal surfaces during labeling. Because of the low administered activity and the fact that a significant percentage of the cells are marginated early in the study, imaging is typically performed at 18–24 hours postinjection.

Technetium-99m Labeled White Blood Cells. Leukocytes labeled with Tc-99m-hexamethylpropylamine oxime (Tc-99m-HMPAO) are also used to image inflammation (5–8). With the higher doses possible with Tc-99m and its shorter half-life of 6 hours, imaging is performed much earlier, at 1–6 hours post injection. The biodistribution is similar to that of In-111-WBCs with some notable exceptions: renal, bladder, and intestinal activity may be seen because of excretion of the Tc-99m complex (Fig. 61.2). Hepatobiliary excretion with transit to gut is seen beginning approximately 3 hours after injection. Thus, gut and renal activity is less specific than with In-111-labeled cells. Although clinical experience with Tc-99m-HMPAO-WBCs is not as extensive as with In-111-WBCs, most reports are encouraging. Indium-

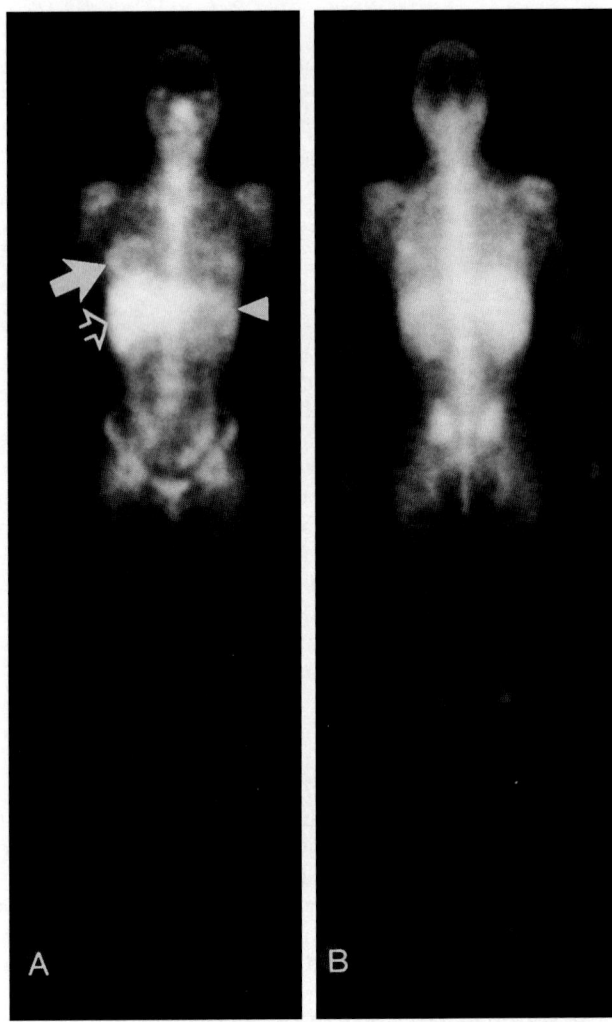

Figure 61.1. Normal Gallium Scan. A. Anterior view. **B.** Posterior view. The normal Ga-67 study has a variable appearance ranging from primarily soft-tissue localization to mostly skeletal uptake. Note the physiologic breast activity (*closed arrow*), which simulates the appearance of mildly abnormal pulmonary uptake in this middle-aged woman who was not lactating at the time of the study. The activity in the liver (*open arrow*) is much hotter than the activity in the spleen (*arrowhead*).

a complete history, physical examination and appropriate laboratory tests before an imaging evaluation is undertaken. Important questions to consider include the likely sites and sources of infection, the duration of the infection, and the physiologic response the most likely organism(s) elicit in the host.

For the purposes of this discussion, acute pyogenic infection is that which has been present for 3 weeks or less and is associated with fever, leukocytosis, and immature leukocytes on the peripheral smear. Also included are acute exacerbations of a chronic illness with similar acute manifestations. Illnesses of greater duration or lacking leukocytosis and sustained fever should be considered chronic.

If the initial evaluation suggests a likely source or site of infection, the appropriate anatomic study should be performed, e.g., sonographic evaluation of the right upper quadrant. If localizing signs are absent and the chest radiograph and urinalysis provide no clue, scintigraphy is indicated. For acute processes, the radiopharmaceutical of choice is radiolabeled autologous WBCs. The evaluation of chronic poorly localized infection is best performed using Ga-67 (9).

Acute Pyogenic Infections. Labeled leukocyte imaging has become the technique of choice in the evaluation of sepsis without localizing signs. Sensitivities and specificities of 85–95% have been reported, with some decline in specificity as the study has become more widely available (3,10). Abnormal activity is graded relative to splenic activity. Foci of activity with an intensity similar to that of the spleen are regarded as abscess or phlegmonous tissue until proven otherwise. Abnormal activity of lesser intensity than the spleen should not be discounted in a severely ill patient. Chronicity of infection, treatment, host defenses, and other factors affect the amount of inflammation present, and therefore the chemotactic ability of a lesion. When abnormal activity is identified an anatomic study (CT or US) may be of benefit in determining the need for percutaneous or surgical drainage.

In most patients, whole-body imaging should be performed since infectious foci will frequently be identified outside the area of clinical concern (Fig. 61.3). Upper abdominal infection may be difficult to diagnose because of normal hepatic and splenic activity. In such cases, concomitant imaging with Tc-99m sulfur colloid will help differentiate normal liver and spleen from adjacent or internal infection (Figs. 61.4,61.5). Similarly, other Tc-99m pharmaceuticals such as diethylene triaminepentaacetic acid (DTPA) and methylene diphosphonate (MDP) have been used successfully to localize infection to intrarenal or extrarenal sites and intraosseous or extraosseous sites, respectively. Such studies are optimally performed with the aid of computer subtraction techniques. Care should be taken, however, to use only the 247 keV peak of In-111 or to narrow the imaging window on the 173 keV peak when imaging after the injection of a Tc-99m agent. Otherwise the higher doses used with Tc-99m lead to acceptance of some Tc-99m counts into the lower window and may result in a false-positive diagnosis of infection.

111 is cyclotron-produced and therefore not always available. HMPAO, a lipophilic agent initially introduced as a brain blood flow imaging agent, is available in kit form for local compounding. HMPAO offers the ability to provide abscess imaging at any time, although the labeling procedure requires as much time as indium-111 labeling.

INFLAMMATORY PROCESSES

Infection

Infection represents the most common class of inflammatory processes with which we are concerned. The orderly evaluation of a potentially infected patient requires

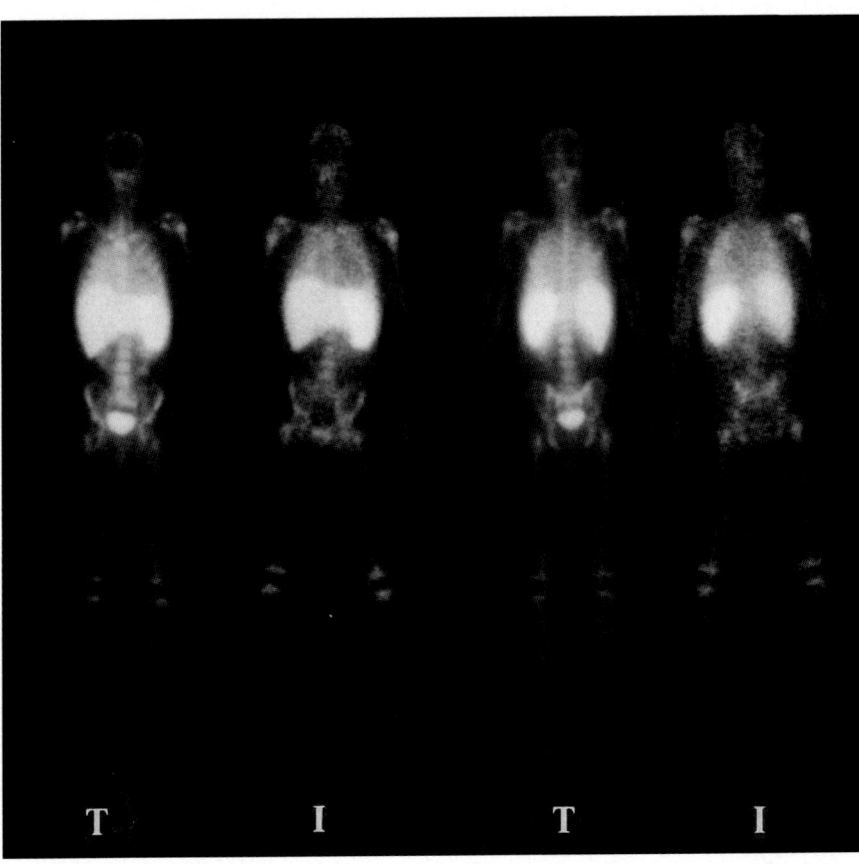

Figure 61.2. Normal Labeled Leukocyte Studies in the same adolescent male patient, approximately 2 weeks apart. Technetium-labeled study is captioned with *T*, and indium-labelled study is captioned with *I*. Anterior images on the left and posterior images on the right. Compare the biodistribution of Tc-99m-HMPAO labeled cells at 90 minutes post injection with that of In-111-WBC's at 18 hours post injection. Note the cardiac, femoral vessel, renal and bladder activity on the Tc-99m-HMPAO images which is not seen on the In-111-WBC images. Faint early intestinal activity is superimposed on the sacrum in the anterior Tc-99m-HMPAO image. Physeal plate activity is normal for age on both studies.

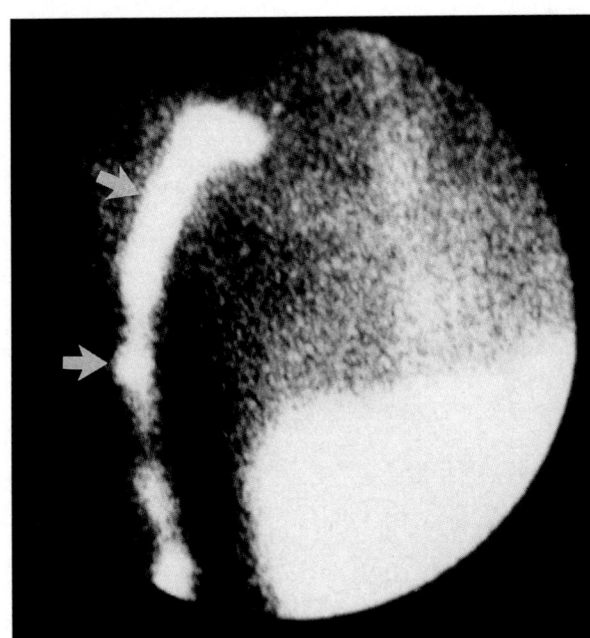

Figure 61.3. Septic Thrombophlebitis. In-111-WBC study demonstrates intense radionuclide activity in the right cephalic vein (*arrows*) in a patient with suspicion of intraabdominal sepsis. Septic thrombophlebitis was not suspected because the extremity was in a cast and the patient was taking narcotic analgesics.

Tc-99m-sulfur colloid may also be used to delineate the location of normal marrow or increased marrow activity in conjunction with In-111 leukocyte images in the evaluation of postoperative osteomyelitis (11,12). This is an excellent technique since post traumatic and postoperative bone recruits an increase in blood flow and therefore an increased delivery of labeled cells. The study may be misinterpreted as osteomyelitis unless the increased marrow activity is documented with the sulfur colloid study.

Lung activity on In-111-WBC images is nonspecific and may be seen in pneumonia, adult respiratory distress syndrome, congestive heart failure, endotoxemia, empyema, and other conditions. Abnormal lung activity should only be evaluated in light of clinical history and the chest radiograph, and then very carefully.

Liver and spleen activity mimics that of Tc-99m sulfur colloid. Incidental findings such as cold defects due to metastases, radiation therapy, or benign lesions may be seen (Fig. 61.6). The patchy pattern of diffuse liver disease is also demonstrated (Fig. 61.7).

Intestinal activity is never normal on an In-111-WBC study but may represent swallowed leukocyte activity from respiratory tract infection, dental abscess, or other inflammatory oropharyngeal lesion.

Figure 61.4. Abscess. In-111-WBC study, anterior projection **(A)** is superficially normal in a 40-year-old male who is 6 months status post Nissen fundoplication with recurrent fever and leukocytosis despite 2 courses of antibiotics. Multiple CT studies and endoscopy were negative. Note subtle activity in right colon (*short arrows*), not normally seen with In-111-WBCs. A simultaneously acquired liver-spleen scan with Tc-99m-sulfur colloid is shown in **(B)**. The image that results from subtraction of the sulfur colloid image from the In-111 image **(C)** reveals a left upper quadrant abscess (*long arrow*) at the surgical site. Internal drainage had spontaneously occurred resulting in the appearance of activity in the right colon on these images obtained 18 hours after injection.

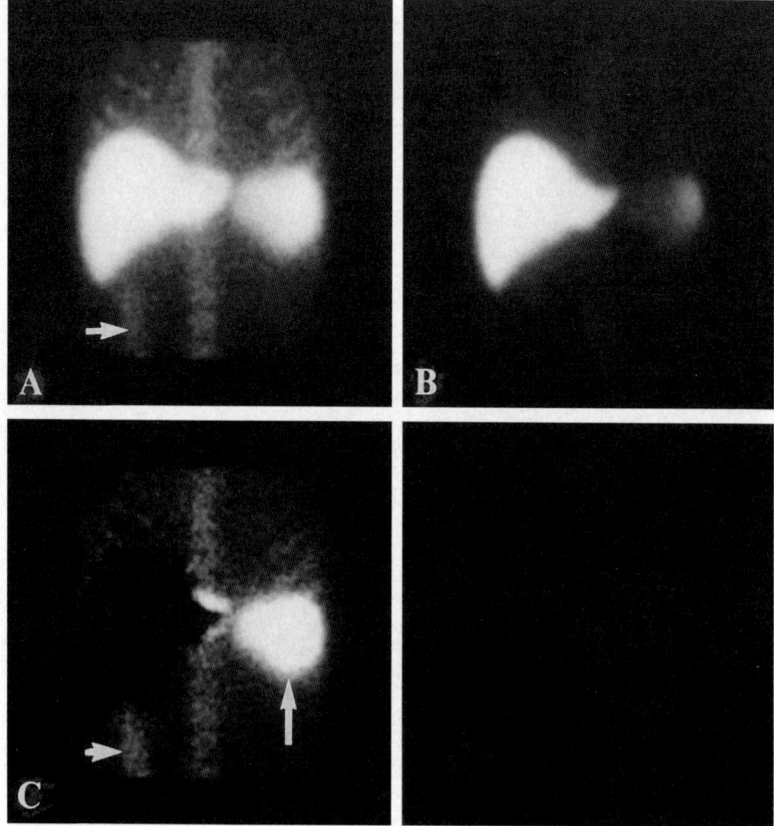

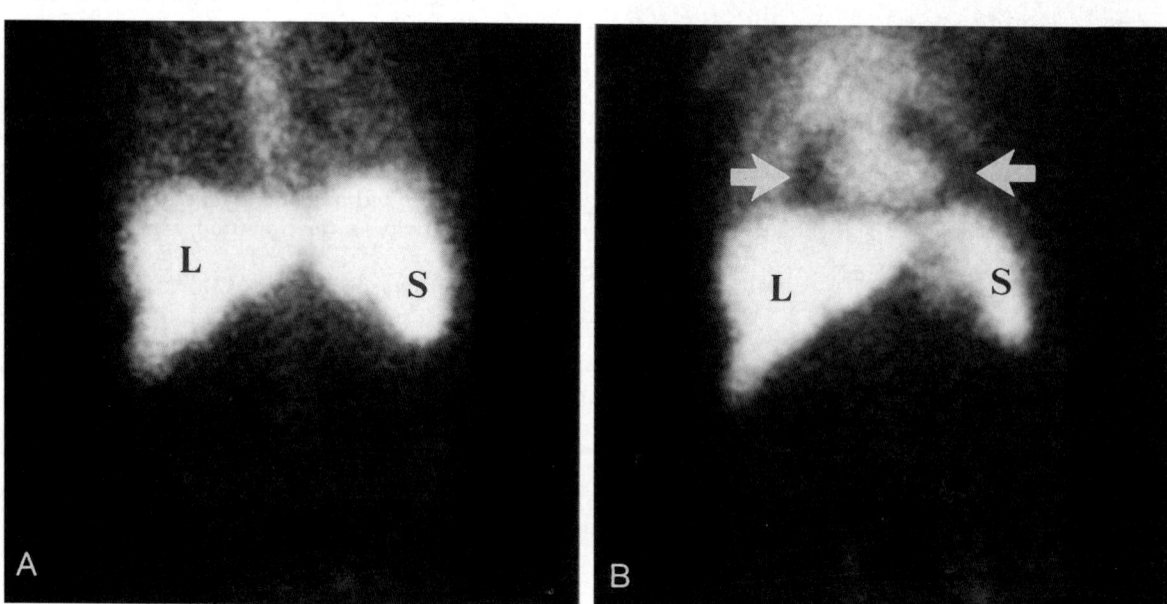

Figure 61.5. Unsuspected Pericardial Effusion. A. In-111-WBC study of the lower chest and upper abdomen was performed to evaluate fever and leukocytosis. **B.** Tc-99m-sulfur colloid image shortly after injection shows residual circulating colloid activity in the pulmonary and cardiac blood pool. The colloid study, performed to exclude perisplenic abscess, demonstrates a photopenic halo (*arrows*) surrounding the heart, indicative of pericardial effusion. *L*, liver; *S*, spleen.

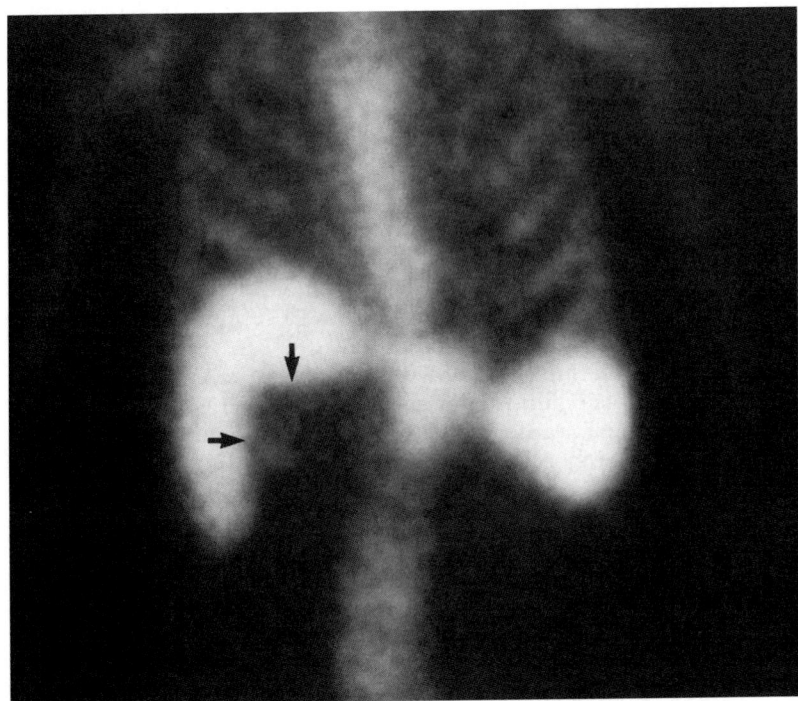

Figure 61.6. Radiation Therapy Portal. Anterior view from In-111-WBC study shows chest and upper abdomen of a patient being evaluated for fever and leukocytosis after surgery for carcinoma of the gallbladder. Note the rectangular "cut out" (*arrows*) from inferomedial aspect of the liver due to radiation therapy portal.

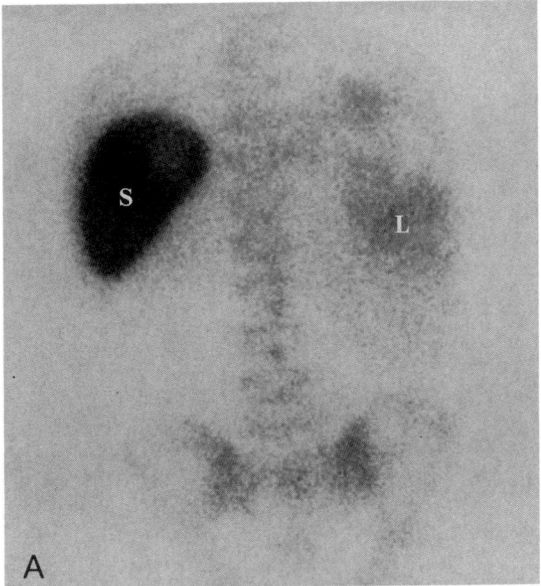

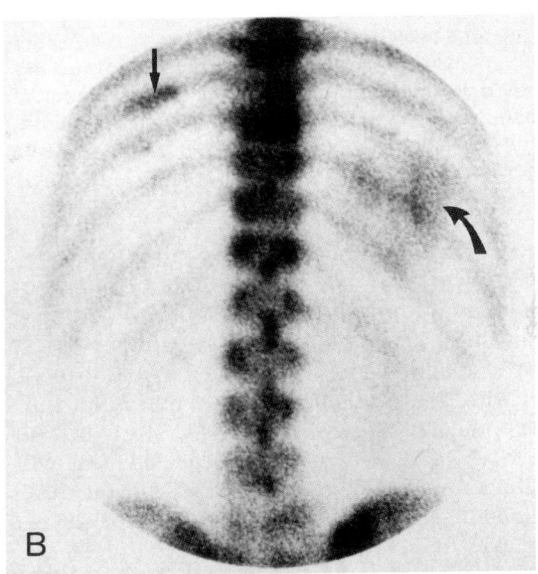

Figure 61.7. Metastatic Carcinoid Tumor. A. Posterior view of abdomen from In-111 study. The liver (*L*) is patchy, consistent with diffuse or multifocal disease. Photopenic defects are present in spleen (*S*) and bone marrow. **B.** Posterior bone scan image of the same area. Note the ill-defined soft-tissue activity (*curved arrow*) in the right upper quadrant corresponding to a photopenic defect in the liver, and focal areas of increased activity in the ribs (*straight arrow*) and spine. Metastatic carcinoid tumor involves the liver, spleen, and bone with calcification in the hepatic metastasis.

Most urinary tract infections are diagnosed clinically, but occasionally a patient fails to respond promptly to therapy and clinical concern leads to a search for other causes (Fig. 61.8). In-111-WBCs are also useful in defining which (if any) cysts are infected in patients with adult polycystic kidney disease and in confirming dialysis catheter infection.

The evaluation of osteomyelitis remains difficult and the literature is unclear as to the optimum imaging strategy (11–16). The three-phase bone scan remains

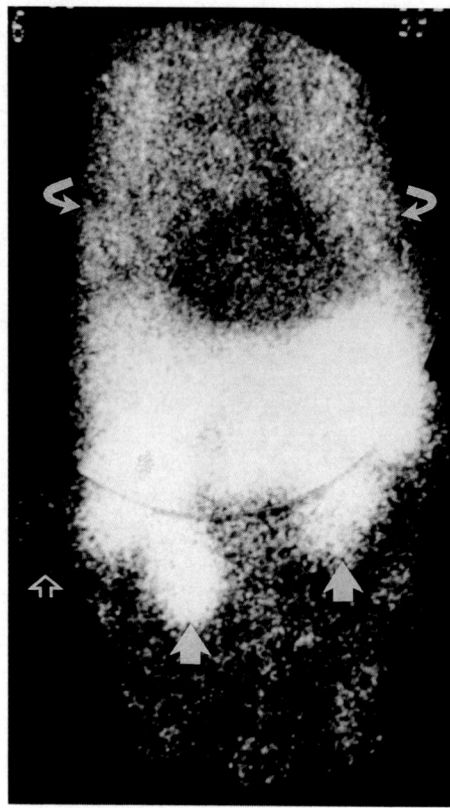

Figure 61.8. Bilateral Pyelonephritis. Composite image of anterior chest and abdomen demonstrates bilateral renal (*arrows*) and lung (*curved arrows*) activity due to pyelonephritis and adult respiratory distress syndrome secondary to sepsis. Activity adjacent to the patient's right side (*open arrow*) is located in an ostomy bag and was felt to be due to swallowed WBCs.

preeminent in excluding osteomyelitis, although rare, false-negatives are seen in the first 24–72 hours of infection and in infants. Some authors recommend adding a fourth phase at 24 hours in an effort to enhance specificity. For the diagnosis of acute osteomyelitis, most would start with the three-phase bone scan, and if that were positive, follow with an In-111-WBC study or less commonly, Ga-67 (Fig. 61.9). In most cases, Ga-67 will not add sufficient specificity to the bone scan for diagnosis, but may be of benefit in assessing therapeutic response (Fig. 61.10).

Cold defects may be seen in the skeleton on WBC imaging because of osteonecrosis, absent blood flow, or marrow packing with malignant cells (Fig. 61.11). Less commonly, osteomyelitis may present as a cold defect due to compromise of the vascular supply with elevated intraosseous pressure. It has been suggested that this mechanism may be one explanation for the reduced accuracy of In-111-WBC's in the diagnosis of vertebral osteomyelitis compared with other sites. Unlike Ga-67, normally healing wounds do not accumulate labeled leukocytes unless they are colonized (Fig. 61.4). Labeled WBCs are useful in evaluating vascular grafts for infection (Fig. 61.12,61.13). Caution is indicated in the first 6–8 weeks after graft placement because increased white cell activity is common with healing of tissues ad-

jacent to the graft. Recently several reports have appeared documenting the efficacy of Tc-99m-HMPAO WBC's in evaluating acute appendicitis in the outpatient setting.

Acute Nonpyogenic Infection. Ga-67 citrate remains the radiopharmaceutical of choice for the evaluation of all nonpyogenic inflammatory conditions. Although it can be used successfully in many of the acute pyogenic conditions just described, its suboptimal imaging characteristics and physiologic renal, intestinal, and wound accumulation have placed it in a second-string status for most acute infections.

The most notable exception is the evaluation of the febrile immunocompromised patient with a normal chest radiograph (2,4,17,18). *Pneumocystis carinii* pneumonia (PCP) is highly prevalent in this population and frequently presents with fever, dyspnea, and normal chest radiographs. The Ga-67 scan in PCP demonstrates diffuse bilateral pulmonary activity that may antedate radiographic findings by 2 weeks. The Ga-67 study has a sensitivity approaching 100% for PCP in the AIDS population. Unfortunately, lung uptake of Ga-67 is extremely nonspecific and may be due to cytomegalovirus pneumonia, cryptococcosis, lymphoma, atypical mycobacterial infection, bacterial pneumonia, or nonspecific pneumonitis, among many others. Factors that enhance the specificity for PCP in any immunocompromised patient include a normal chest radiograph and markedly intense heterogeneous bilateral pulmonary activity (Fig. 61.14).

In the AIDS population, both *Mycobacterium tuberculosis* (MTB) and *M. avium-intracellulare* (MAI) are prevalent. The former is more frequent among intravenous drug abusers. Ga-67 imaging reveals both pulmonary involvement and adenopathy. Again, however, the differential diagnosis is broad and includes lymphoma, cytomegalovirus, Cryptococcus, and bacterial lymphadenitis. It is important to note that neither the lymphadenopathy of the AIDS-related complex nor Kaposi's sarcoma are Ga-67 avid.

Despite the foregoing discussion, careful consideration should be given to the use of a labeled WBC study prior to Ga-67 administration in immunocompromised patients since they are also susceptible to bacterial infections, and Ga-67 administration will preclude the use of labeled WBCs for at least 1 week (19).

Chronic Infection. Ga-67 remains the radiopharmaceutical of choice for the investigation of low-grade chronic inflammatory processes. Such illnesses typically present as fever of unknown origin (FUO) in a relatively stable patient. Because a FUO by definition has been present for several weeks, labeled leukocyte scintigraphy would not be expected to be helpful. After history, physical examination, and routine laboratory data have been obtained, scintigraphy with Ga-67 is indicated. Although the results are often nonspecific, they may point toward additional diagnostic studies. The clinical differential diagnosis for FUO is extremely broad but includes chronic low-grade infections (e.g., fungus, tuberculosis, Epstein-Barr virus), malignancy (especially lymphoma and myeloproliferative disorders), vasculitides, collagen-vascular diseases, and endocrine disturbances.

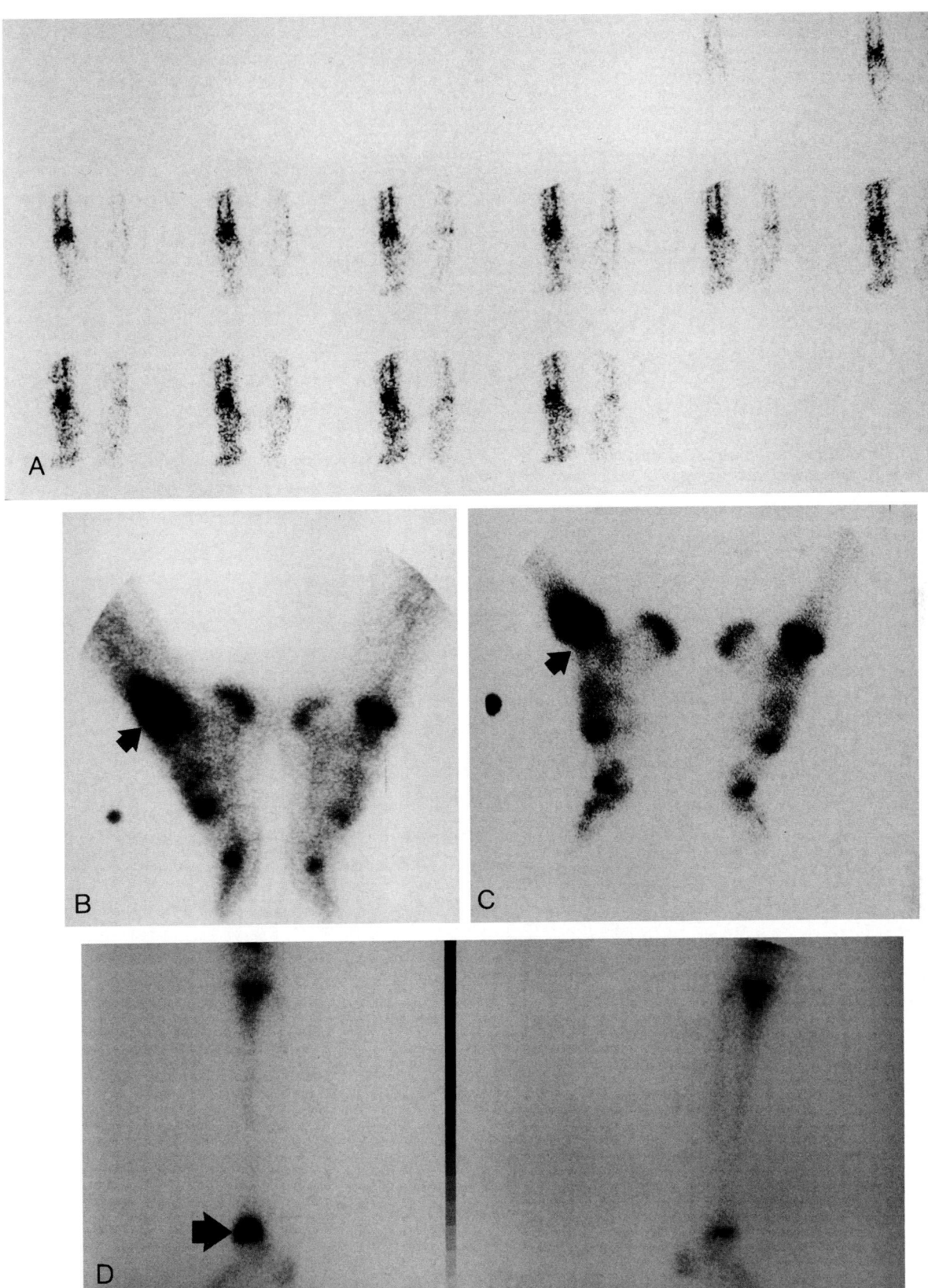

Figure 61.9. Acute Osteomyelitis. Three-phase bone scan **(A–C)** and Ga-67 scan **(D)** in a 13-year-old girl. Radiographs were normal. **A.** Anterior view of arterial flow study of the feet and ankles with Tc-99m-MDP, 2 seconds per frame. Note the early and increased flow to the right foot and ankle. **B.** Blood pool image, marker indicates the right side. Note the markedly increased activity in the distal tibia (*arrows* in **B** and **C**) extending to the physeal plate. **C.** Delayed static image in same view as **(B)**. **D.** Ga-67 study shows uptake (*arrow*) in same area of the distal right tibia.

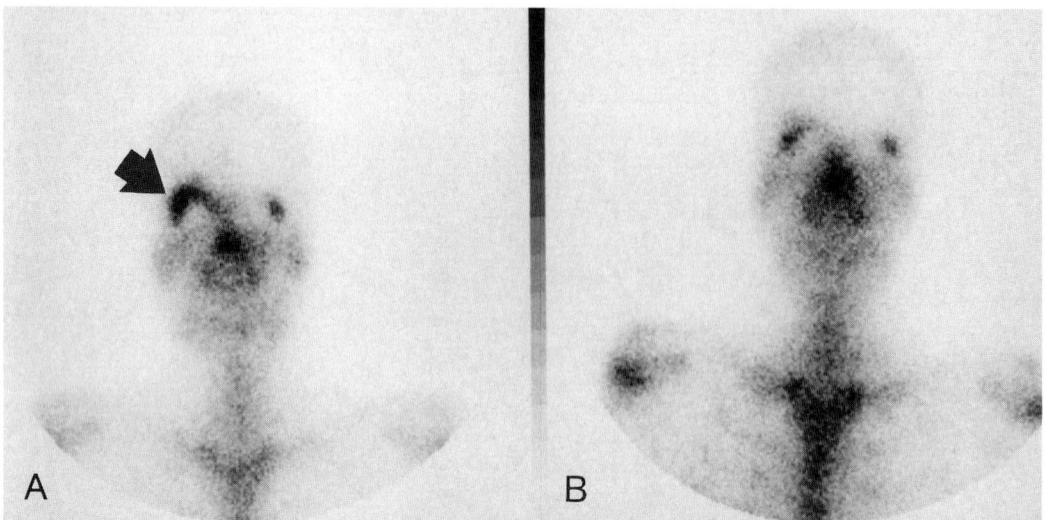

Figure 61.10. Osteomyelitis, Response to Therapy. A. Baseline Ga-67 scan in patient with proven right supraorbital rim osteomyelitis (*arrow*). **B.** Follow-up study demonstrates resolution after 6 weeks of therapy.

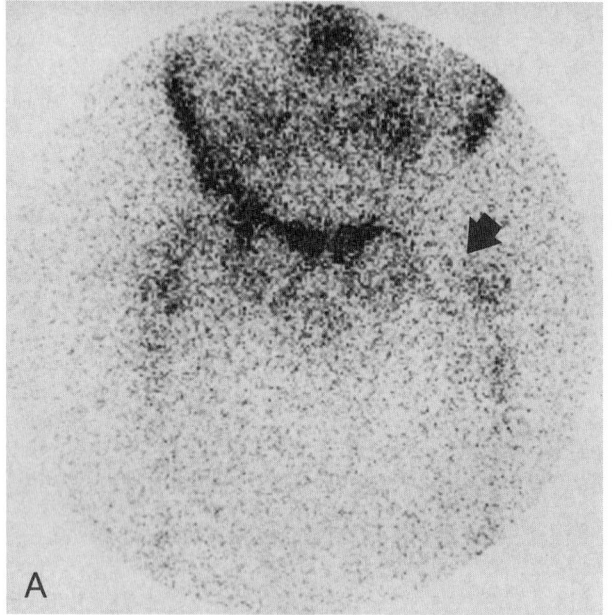
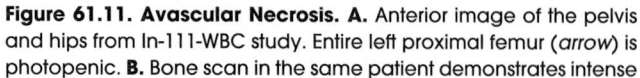
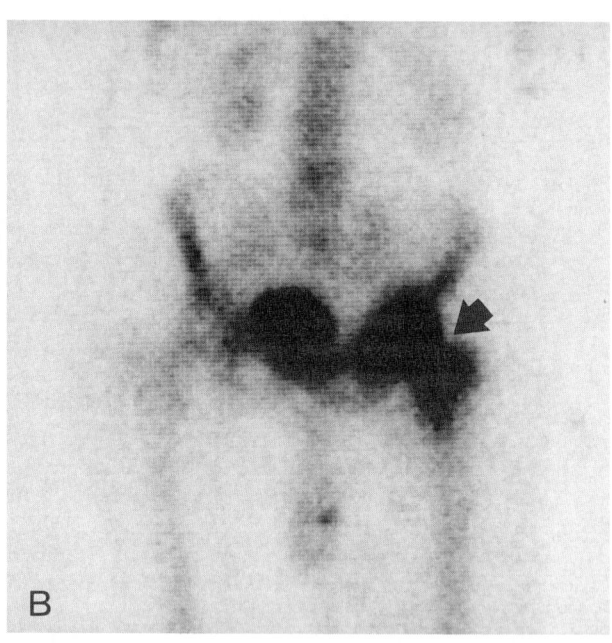

Figure 61.11. Avascular Necrosis. A. Anterior image of the pelvis and hips from In-111-WBC study. Entire left proximal femur (*arrow*) is photopenic. **B.** Bone scan in the same patient demonstrates intense radionuclide activity in proximal left femur (*arrow*). Avascular necrosis of the left femoral head and neck complicated a chronic femoral neck fracture.

Chronic osteomyelitis is a different cellular and clinical entity than acute osteomyelitis. As a result, the imaging approach is different, though still controversial. Most would begin with the three-phase bone scan, particularly in cases where the affected bone had been previously exposed to open trauma or surgical debridement. The bone study provides a better picture of the anatomy and physiology of the bone in the affected region. Subsequently, a Ga-67 study should be performed, with or without the aid of simultaneous Tc-99m bone imaging. Ga-67 activity at the suspicious site is as-sessed in comparison with the bone scan activity. Excess Ga-67 activity suggests the presence of continued infection. The imaging diagnosis of chronic osteomyelitis has a relatively low sensitivity and specificity. Although on theoretical grounds white blood cell imaging would not be expected to be helpful unless there were indications of acute recrudescence of the infection with recruitment of a polymorphonuclear leukocyte response, some authors have described results equal to or better than those obtained with combined Tc-99m-MDP and Ga-67 imaging.

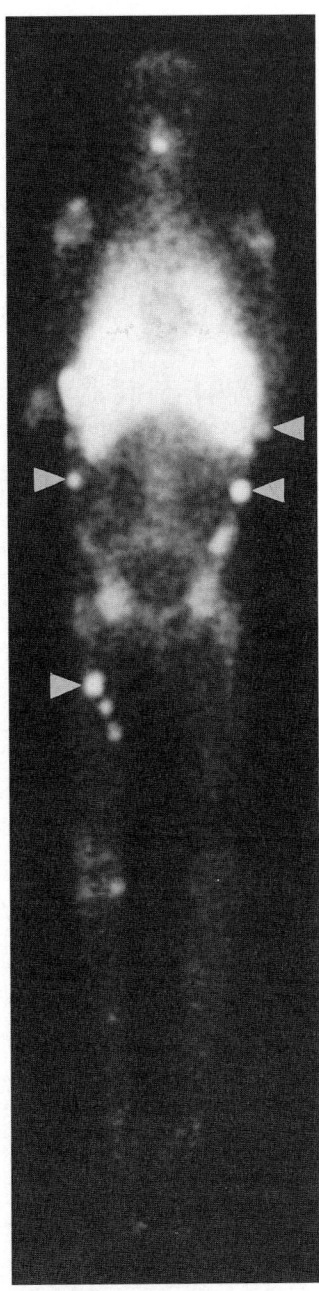

Figure 61.12. Vascular Graft Infection. Anterior whole-body In-111-WBC image demonstrates multiple foci of infection (*arrowheads*) involving both axillofemoral vascular grafts and the right femoropopliteal graft. Bilateral lung activity is related to sepsis. Increased nasopharyngeal activity is seen with nasotracheal and nasogastric intubation as well as sinusitis.

Noninfectious Inflammatory Processes

Inflammatory Bowel Disease. Both labeled WBCs and Ga-67 have been used to evaluate the extent and activity of inflammatory bowel disease (20). Since there is no physiologic intestinal or hepatobiliary excretion of In-111-WBCs, they are the radiopharmaceutical of choice although numerous reports document the efficacy of Tc-99m-HMPAO-WBC's as well. Excellent results have been obtained in the evaluation of the activity and extent of

disease in both ulcerative colitis and Crohn's disease, although discriminating between them is not possible. Pseudomembranous colitis also provokes a profound inflammatory response (Fig. 61.15).

Imaging should be performed within 30–90 minutes of injection of the labeled cells regardless of the isotope used for labeling. Serial imaging at 4 and up to 24 hours is recommended. The lesions of Crohn's disease and ulcerative colitis are intensely inflammatory and very early cell migration to the most involved areas is the rule. Subsequently, the cells are transported to the lumen of the intestine and migrate with peristalsis. Thus, if early imaging is not performed it will be impossible to differentiate inflammatory foci from intraluminal activity. Delayed imaging is important because patients with inflammatory bowel disease are at high risk for abscess, and very active inflammatory bowel disease may mask the presence of concomitant abscess.

Interstitial Lung Disease. Ga-67 imaging is an extremely sensitive indicator of inflammatory lung disease (2,21). Ga-67 uptake has been reported in sarcoidosis, interstitial pneumonitis in virtually all its forms and etiologies, drug reactions, collagen vascular disease, and pneumoconioses (Fig. 61.16). Unfortunately, a normal study does not exclude the possibility of low levels of inflammatory activity. Furthermore, the degree or pattern of activity is not diagnostic of specific illnesses. However, the degree of Ga-67 activity seems to reflect the severity of the underlying illness.

Ga-67 imaging is most useful in sarcoidosis where it has been shown to correlate with pulmonary disease activity and response to therapy (Fig. 61.17). Furthermore, Ga-67 scintigraphy has been reported to be up to 97% sensitive for detection of active sarcoidosis when considering both pulmonary and extrapulmonary sites. It has not been proven whether Ga-67 imaging can provide prognostic information or therapeutic insight for other inflammatory lung diseases.

Since determining the relative pulmonary Ga-67 activity may be helpful in assessing the level of inflammatory activity present, an objective index of Ga-67 activity has been sought. Some authors have chosen to compare pulmonary activity with sternal activity, others have compared pulmonary activity with hepatic activity, and still others have used semiquantitative techniques involving computer acquisitions, SPECT, and whole-body imaging to report activity ratios (2). As a result, no uniform method for quantifying Ga-67 pulmonary activity is available. Therefore, when reporting Ga-67 activity, the specific scale and reference standard should be stated. For clinical work we use a scale of 0 to 3 in which pulmonary activity is subjectively graded against liver activity. In this schema, 0 represents no pulmonary activity, 1 represents activity greater than normal but less than liver activity, 2 represents activity equal in intensity to liver activity, and 3 signifies activity greater than that seen in the liver (22). Obviously, quantitative techniques using other organs as reference points assume a normal healthy reference organ.

Figure 61.13. Infected Hematoma. A.
SPECT Tc-99m-HMPAO WBC study reveals an infected hematoma in the right lower quadrant that followed abdominal aortic graft placement. *a*, raw data frame; *b*, axial slice through the abscess, *c*, sagittal slice; *d*, coronal slice showing craniocaudad extent of the hematoma and the drain tract laterally. Note the drainage tract inflammation and ring of inflammation (*arrow*) around the relatively avascular hematoma. **B.** Axial CT slice. Compare with *b*. CT fails to reveal inflammatory changes at the graft site.

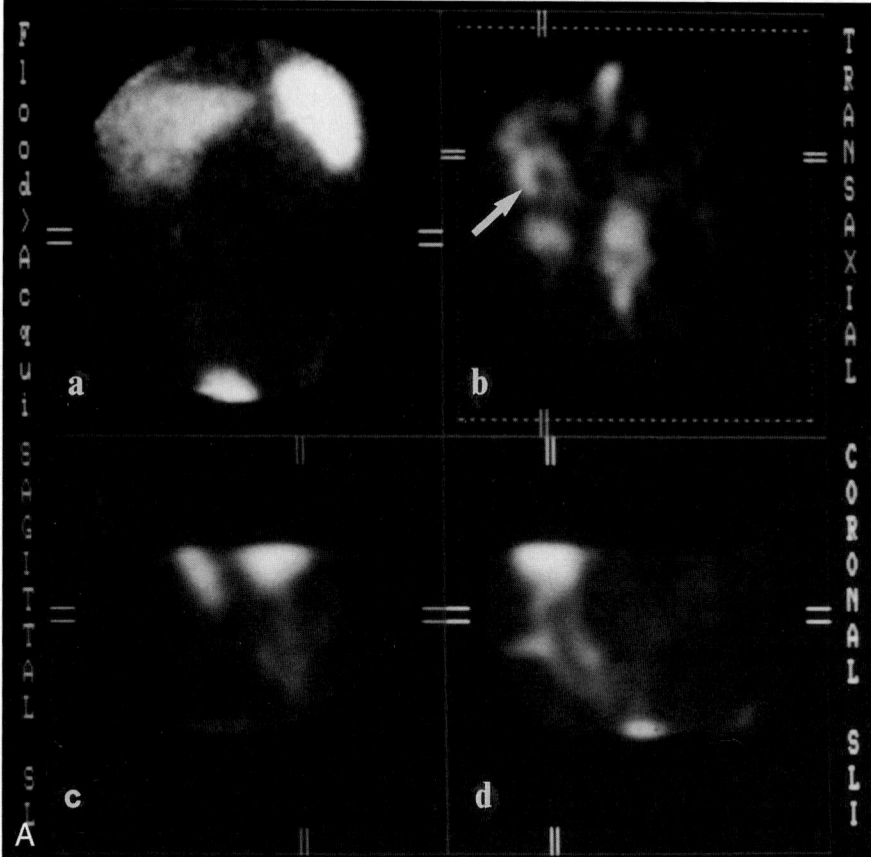

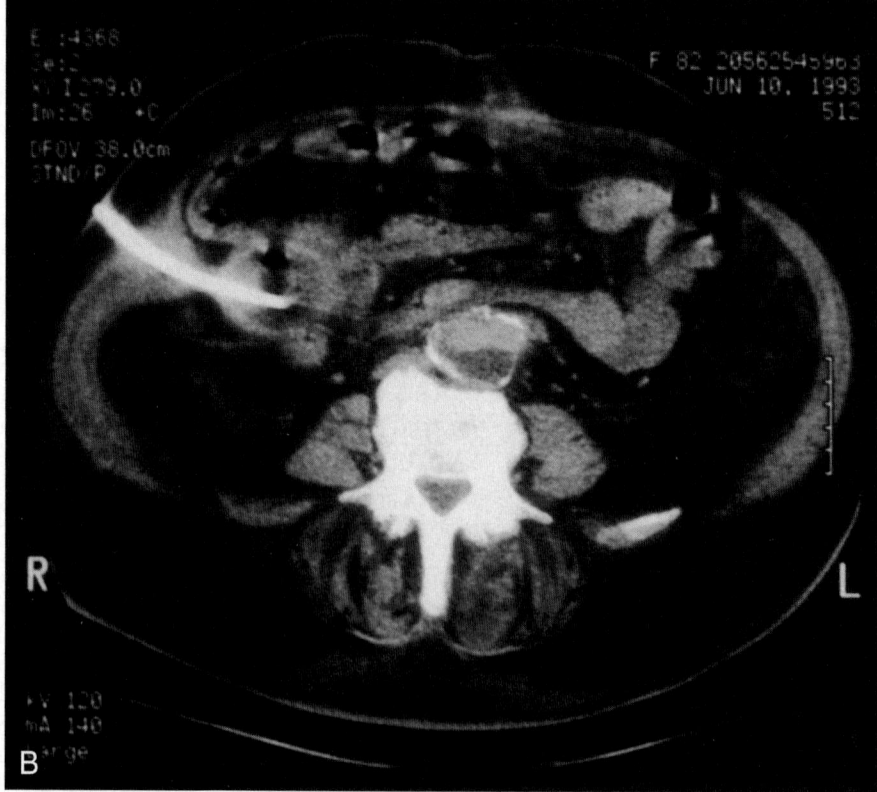

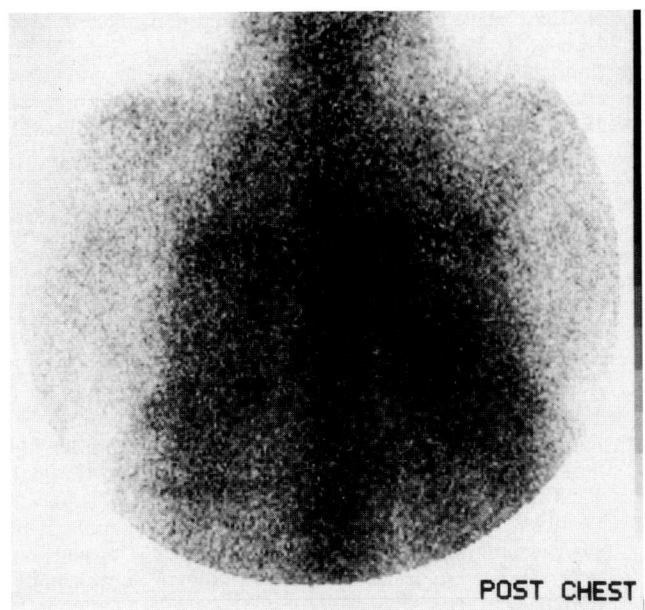

Figure 61.14. *Pneumocystis carinii* Pneumonia. Gallium study of the chest demonstrates markedly increased heterogeneous pulmonary activity in a pattern that, in an AIDS patient with a normal chest radiograph, strongly suggests *P. carinii* pneumonia.

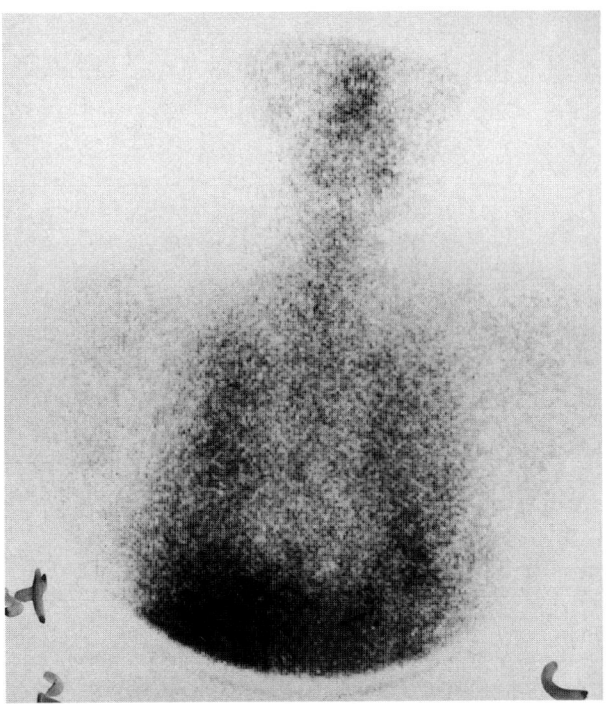

Figure 61.16. Inflammatory Lung Disease. Anterior Ga-67 scan of the chest demonstrates bilateral increased activity in the lung due to bleomycin toxicity in a patient treated for lymphoma.

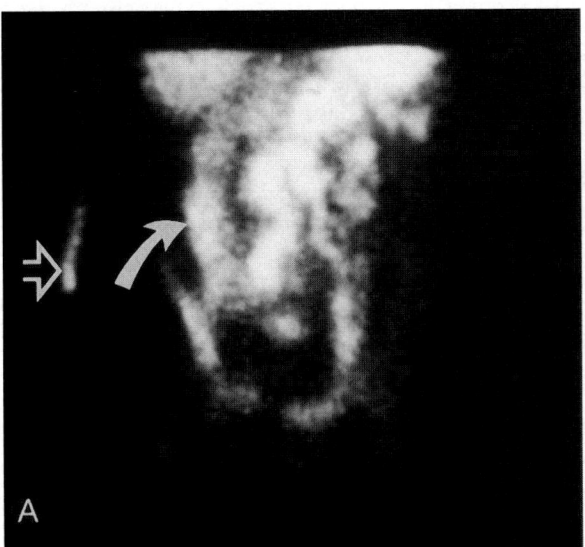

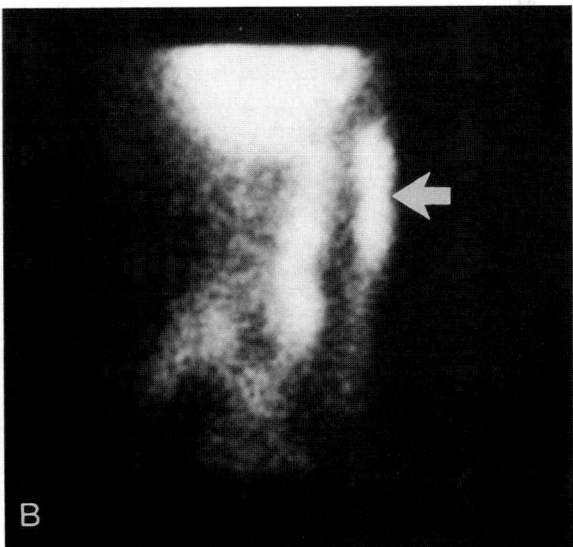

Figure 61.15. Pseudomembranous Colitis. Anterior **(A)** and right lateral **(B)** views of the abdomen and pelvis from In-111-WBC study. An anterior surgical wound infection is present in the midline (*arrow*). Septic thrombophlebitis is present in the right upper extremity on the anterior view (*open arrow*). Diffuse colonic activity (*curved arrow*), best seen in the right colon, is due to pseudomembranous colitis in this patient on multiple broad-spectrum antibiotics.

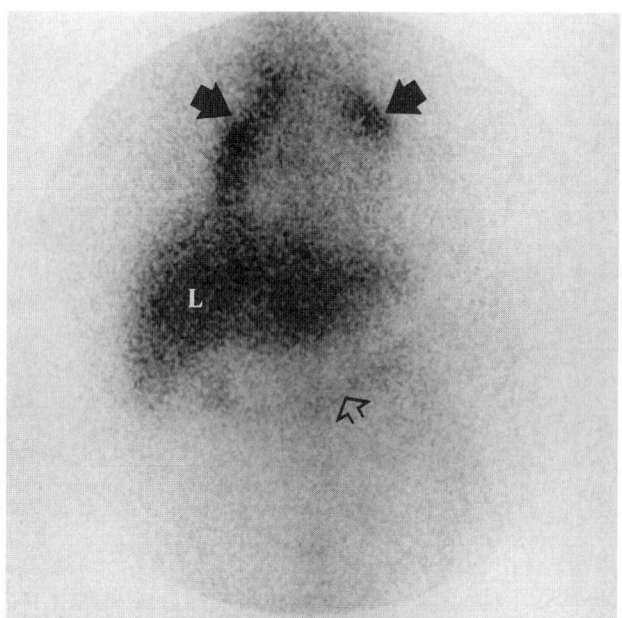

Figure 61.17. Sarcoidosis. Anterior chest and abdomen from a Ga-67 study shows bilateral hilar adenopathy (*closed arrows*), a pattern characteristic for sarcoidosis. Nonvisualization of the spleen is a normal variant and faint bowel activity (*open arrow*) is physiologic. *L*, liver.

SUMMARY

Scintigraphic imaging plays a pivotal role in the diagnosis of inflammatory conditions and will continue to do so in the foreseeable future. Optimal diagnosis requires careful consideration of the entire patient and the available imaging modalities. The scintigraphic techniques are best considered specific for inflammation rather than infection.

References

1. Halpern S, Hagan P. Gallium–67 citrate imaging in neoplastic and inflammatory disease. In: Freeman LM, Weissman HS, eds. Nuclear Medicine Annual 1980. New York: Raven Press, 1980:219–265.
2. Waxman AD. An update on the role of nuclear medicine in pulmonary disorders. In: Freeman LM, Weissman HS, eds. Nuclear Medicine Annual 1985. New York: Raven Press, 1985:199–231.
3. Froelich JW. Nuclear medicine in inflammatory diseases. In: Freeman LM, Weissman HS, eds. Nuclear Medicine Annual 1985. New York: Raven Press, 1985:23–71.
4. Bekerman C, Bitran J. Gallium-67 scanning in the clinical evaluation of human immunodeficiency virus infection: indications and limitations. Semin Nucl Med 1988;18:273–286.
5. Uno K, Yoshikawa K, Imazeki K, et al. Technetium-99m HMPAO labeled leukocytes in inflammation imaging. Ann Nucl Med 1991;5:77–81.
6. Lantto EH, Lantto TJ, Vorne M. Fast diagnosis of abdominal infections and inflammations with technetium-99m-HMPAO-labeled leukocytes. J Nucl Med 1991;32:2029–2034.
7. Mountford PJ, Kettle AG, O'Doherty MJ, Coakley AJ. Comparison of technetium-99m-HMPAO leukocytes with indium-111-oxine leukocytes for localizing intraabdominal sepsis. J Nucl Med 1990;31:311–315.
8. Roddie ME, Peters AM, Danpure HJ, et al. Inflammation: imaging with Tc-99m HMPAO-labeled leukocytes. Radiology 1988;166:767–772.
9. Froelich JW, Swanson D. Imaging of inflammatory processes with labeled cells. Semin Nucl Med 1984;14:128–140.
10. Lamki LM, Kasi LP, Haynie TP. Localization of indium-111 leukocytes in noninfected neoplasms. J Nucl Med 1988;29:1921–1926.
11. Seabold JE, Nepola JV, Marsh JL, et al. Postoperative bone marrow alterations: potential pitfalls in the diagnosis of osteomyelitis with In-111-labeled leukocyte scintigraphy. Radiology 1991;180:741–747.
12. Schauwecker DS. The scintigraphic diagnosis of osteomyelitis. AJR Am J Roentgenol 1992;158:9–18.
13. Devillers A, Bourguet P, Arvieux C, et al. Technetium-99m hexamethylpropylene amine oxime leucocyte scintigraphy for the diagnosis of bone and joint infections: a retrospective study in 116 patients. Eur J Nucl Med 1995; 22:302–307
14. Nepola JV, Seabold JE, Marsh JL, et al. Diagnosis of infection in ununited fractures. Combined imaging with indium-111-labeled leukocytes and technetium-99m methylene diphosphonate. Journal of Bone & Joint Surgery 1993;75:1816–22.
15. Johnson JE, Collier BD, Patel NC, et al. Prospective study of bone, indium-111-labeled white blood cell, and gallium-67 scanning for the evaluation of osteomyelitis in the diabetic foot. Foot Ankle Int 1996;17:10–16.
16. Kolindou A, Collier BD, Hellman RS, et al. In-111 WBC imaging of osteomyelitis in patients with underlying bone scan abnormalities. Clin Nucl Med 1996;21:183–191.
17. Kramer EL, Sanger JJ. Nuclear medicine in the management of the AIDS patient. In: Freeman LM, ed. Nuclear Medicine Annual 1990. New York: Raven Press, 1990:37–57.
18. Vanarthos WJ, Ganz WI, Vanarthos JC, et al. Diagnostic uses of nuclear medicine in AIDS. Radiographics 1992;12:731–752.
19. Fineman DS, Palestro CJ, Kim CK, et al. Detection of abnormalities in febrile AIDS patients with In-111-labeled leukocyte and Ga-67 scintigraphy. Radiology 1989;170:677–680.
20. Mansfield JC, Giaffer MH, Tindale WB, Holdsworth CD. Quantitative assessment of overall inflammatory bowel disease activity using labelled leucocytes: a direct comparison between indium-111 and technetium-99m HMPAO methods. Gut 1995; 37:679-83.
21. Kramer EL, Divgi CR. Pulmonary applications of nuclear medicine. Clin Chest Med 1991;12:55–75.
22. Niden AH, Mishkin FS, Khurana MM. Gallium-67 citrate lung scans in interstitial lung disease. Chest 1976;69:266–268.

62

Scintigraphic Tumor Imaging

James H. Timmons
John M. Bauman

There has been remarkable growth in the availability of scintigraphic methods for tumor imaging over the past few years. Many of these agents provide information which has not previously been available. Dramatic improvements in both sensitivity and specificity for detection and staging of tumors have been made. These agents are unique because they provide physiologic information concerning the imaged tumor, such as metabolic activity (and by extension viability), presence of specific cell surface receptors and presence of multidrug resistance apparatus. The development of these agents has depended heavily on the use of tracer techniques which do not significantly alter the physiologic activity of the substance being employed for imaging. Development has also been made possible by extensive "basic science" investigations into polypeptide chemistry and monoclonal antibodies and by "serendipitous" clinical observations. Significant recent advances in instrumentation and development of an industrial capacity for production and distribution of fluorine-18 based radiopharmaceuticals also seem likely to convert positron imaging from a research tool to a clinically relevant imaging approach. In a period of diminishing resources and managed care, agents are likely to be adopted only if they provide more cost effective detection and staging of tumors. Fortunately for the specialty of nuclear medicine, indications are that many of these agents will easily pass the "cost-effectiveness" test.

While this chapter is partially devoted to specific agents for imaging tumors, these should generally be considered only as examples. There are literally hundreds of agents currently under development for clinical use. It is much more important to understand the general principles behind imaging with the various classes of agents, and their potential benefits and limitations, than to understand the specific imaging appearances for any individual agent. By the time the next edition of this book is printed, it may be possible to be certain which agents will see the greatest clinical use.

CLASSES OF IMAGING ISOTOPES

Isotopes suitable for tumor imaging may be divided into positron emitters and isotopes which emit single gamma photons. The former are the basis for an imaging technology known as PET. The latter are employed in standard gamma camera imaging and in SPECT. Typical positron emitters are fluorine-18 (F-18), nitrogen-15 (N-15), oxygen-13 (O-13), and carbon (C-11). Typical gamma emitting isotopes are technetium-99m (Tc-99m) and iodine-123 (I-123).

PET has always been the "Cadillac" of nuclear medicine imaging studies. Positron imaging employs radioisotopes which decay to produce positrons (anti-matter electrons) which annihilate essentially immediately to form two 512 keV photons diverging at close to 180°. Because the photons strike detectors on opposite sides of the imaging device nearly simultaneously, the position of the emitting nucleus can be determined with fair accuracy from geometric considerations and time of flight. The radioisotopes which decay in this manner include the isotopes of the lighter elements which form the bulk of all biochemical substances, as well as other light elements such as F-18. Compounds made with these isotopes (except F-18) are chemically identical to the nonradioactive biochemicals upon which they are based. A neurotransmitter labeled with N-15 will have a biodistribution virtually identical to that of the unlabeled neurotransmitter. Even when F-18 is substituted for hydrogen, the chemical similarity to the original substrate is sufficient to assure similar biological behavior in most cases. PET radiopharmaceuticals are thus ideal for imaging biochemical processes in living systems.

The major disadvantage of positron emitting radiopharmaceuticals has been their short half-lives, ranging from a few minutes to two hours, and the relatively high energy of their photons. These disadvantages have required an on-site cyclotron for production of the isotopes, a skilled organic chemist for synthesis of appropriate imaging agents and a dedicated imaging apparatus with detectors optimized to the high energy photons produced. The high associated costs have severely limited clinical applications.

Gamma Emitting Isotopes are advantageous because they are available with a variety of half-lives, suitable to any purpose. There are several generator systems for convenient production of the desired isotope at the point of consumption, the most common being the molybdenum-99 (Mo-99)/Tc-99m generator system. The cost of the gamma camera and generator is significantly less than the cost of a PET scanner and cyclotron, and are similar to those for competing technologies such as CT and MR.

Gamma emitters are disadvantageous in that they are not easily incorporated into molecules without disrupting their biological function. The "atoms of life" generally do not have gamma emitting isotopes, although gamma isotopes are available for some less common biometallics, such as selenium-75. Incorporation of gamma emitters into biomolecules generally involves addition of significant bulk. It is difficult to produce a gamma labeled molecule which has biological behavior similar to that of the original molecule.

A recent development is the coincidence detection gamma camera (1). When equipped with collimators, this camera operates as a standard gamma camera for planar or SPECT imaging. When operated in coincidence mode without collimators, this instrument produces PET-like images with positron emitting radiopharmaceuticals. While these instruments have sensitivities inferior to those of true PET scanners, they are able to take advantage of the more physiologic imaging agents available through use of positron emitters, most importantly 18-fluorodeoxyglucose (F-18-DG). The development of gamma camera PET is likely to have a substantial effect on the availability of positron imaging.

RADIOIODINE: THE INDEX AGENT FOR TUMOR IMAGING

The first agent identified as having clear medical potential was radioiodine. The natural trapping of iodine by the thyroid made radioiodine a potentially ideal agent for imaging and therapy. We examine thyroid tumor imaging here briefly because it is paradigmatic of the choices involved in development and use of tumor imaging agents generally.

Iodine is trapped within the thyroid by conversion to thyroxine, which is stored within the colloid cells of thyroid tissue. Uptake is proportional to metabolic activity. Some thyroid tumors also trap iodine by the same mechanism. Since their metabolism is disordered however, they trap iodine at a much lower rate. This leads to an interesting phenomenon: thyroid tumors typically appear as cold spots in the thyroid gland on radioiodine imaging of the intact gland but as hot spots in the body when metastases are imaged after thyroid removal or ablation. Thyroid tumors arising from cells which do not trap and metabolize iodine, such as medullary carcinoma of the thyroid, will not take up radioiodine.

Multiple isotopes of iodine are available. Each is suitable for a particular purpose. Reactor produced iodine-131 (I-131) is relatively inexpensive. It has imageable photons but extensive beta-particle emission. It thus images and destroys thyroid tissue and can be used to ablate both malignant and benign thyroid tissue. The location of the tissues being ablated and the extent of uptake

within those tissues can be determined simultaneously. I-131 is suboptimal when imaging alone is desired however, as the significant beta radiation increases the risk of development of benign and malignant tumors. Cyclotron produced I-123 has no beta radiation and is safer for routine imaging. It also has a nearly ideal gamma energy of 159 keV. Cyclotron production means this agent is more expensive than I-131 and its relatively short half-life means the agent is limited to use at scheduled times.

Every imaging prescription involves issues of cost, likely tumor type, adequacy of the agent for the available equipment, availability of the agent, metabolic rate and route and their effect on timing of imaging, and patient radiation dose and safety. Every therapeutic dose must be planned to achieve adequate dose to the tissue to be ablated while minimizing whole-body and nontarget organ radiation. The choices involved are typical of those in other areas of oncologic scintigraphy.

THE IDEAL TUMOR IMAGING AGENT

What are the characteristics of an ideal tumor imaging agent? Foremost is specificity for the target tissue. This is never fully realized in practice. Radioiodine is secreted by the salivary glands and swallowed. Since bowel clearance is slow, whole body images for metastases may be problematic in the abdomen, where swallowed radioiodine in the bowel may mimic or obscure tumor. Similarly, F-18-DG localizes in metabolically active cardiac tissue, monoclonal antibodies are bound nonspecifically to liver tissue and gallium-67 (Ga-67) is bound to metabolically active bone and also taken up by normal liver. When uptake by normal tissue occurs, it is preferable that the tissue be one which is less frequently involved by the primary tumor or by metastatic disease. Since cardiac metastases and malignant pericardial effusion are much less common than liver metastases, the normal distribution of F-18-DG is preferable, in terms of imaging sensitivity, to that of a monoclonal antibody.

Rapid clearance of background activity is essential for short lived isotopes such as pertechnetate, which must be imaged within a few hours of administration. Clearance need not be as rapid for longer lived isotopes. For whole body I-131 scans, imaging of the abdomen may be delayed for a day to allow administration of a cathartic to purge nonspecific bowel radioactivity. Similarly, agents cleared rapidly, such as by renal excretion, are preferable to those cleared more slowly, such as by hepatic excretion. "Metabolic trapping" of an imaging agent within a tumor by any mechanism increases conspicuity and thus imaging sensitivity by increasing target activity over background. Trapping of radioiodine, for example, leads to increasing activity in tumor relative to background over time. An agent which is metabolically trapped, such as Tc-99m-Sestimibi (Tc-99m-MIBI), will generally be more sensitive than an agent which is easily washed out, such as thallium-201 (Tl-201). In general, the higher the target to background ratio at the time of imaging, the higher the sensitivity for detection of tumor.

BLOOD-FLOW AND CAPILLARY PERMEABILITY: A CAVEAT

Tumor imaging based on differential blood flow or capillary permeability is of incidental interest only, since these methods lack tissue specificity. Nevertheless, it is important to consider agents which localize in tumors by these mechanisms, because the potential for differential labeling on the basis of these mechanisms exists with any imaging tracer. Tc-99m-methylenediphosphonate (Tc-99m-MDP) is a typical example of a blood flow imaging agent and Tc-99m-glucoheptonate is a typical example of a capillary permeability agent.

During the flow and immediate static phases of a bone scan, it is occasionally possible to detect a hypervascular tumor because of increased blood flow to the tumor and a vascular blush within the tumor. On delayed static images, increased activity in bone usually results from increased osteoblast activity. However, the bone may have increased activity solely on the basis of increased blood flow to that bone, whatever the underlying cause. Similarly a cold defect on a bone scan can be the result of absence of osteoblast activity due to rapid tumor growth, or absence of blood flow due to tissue necrosis or vascular obstruction or compression. These findings based on alterations of blood flow may result in either unintentional or intentional detection of tumor, but are entirely nonspecific.

In the classic but obsolete brain scan, Tc-99m labeled glucoheptonate or diethylenetriamine pentaacetic acid (DTPA) were used to detect areas of increased capillary permeability. This break-down of the blood-brain barrier may be caused by a number of disease processes, including primary or metastatic tumors. When positive, these studies provided excellent "hot-spot" images which allowed detection of the tumor. The mechanism is again nonspecific, and diagnosis is limited to what can be determined through pattern recognition and clinical scenario.

It is important to realize that these mechanisms still apply when using modern imaging agents. A hypervascular structure may have activity which exceeds background due to high blood flow and nonspecific binding of the antibody. A tumor with high antibody affinity but poor blood flow can incidentally display activity similar or equal to background when imaged with a monoclonal antibody imaging agent. A tumor with high blood flow can appear to have high affinity for a radiolabeled antibody on the basis of preferential exposure to the imaging agent, without having specific affinity for that agent. If a brain tumor demonstrates increased activity after administration of Tc-99m-HMPAO, for example, it is difficult *a priori* to determine if the localization is due to increased blood flow, diffusion across a damaged blood brain barrier, or specific localization within the tumor. With all agents discussed in this review, the reader is urged to consider possible mechanisms for nonspecific localization when interpreting images.

CLASSES OF TUMOR IMAGING RADIOPHARMACEUTICALS

Markers of Metabolism

The rapid growth of tumors requires a rapid metabolic rate which provides a potential target for imaging agents. Early investigations into this type of imaging were performed with positron emitters and PET cameras. Agents were developed to image the DNA and protein synthesis required for cell division. Protein synthesis was assessed with C-11 methionine and C-11 tyrosine and DNA synthesis was assessed with F-18 deoxyuracil. Because of the limitations of early PET cameras, these agents were predominantly employed in imaging brain tumors.

With the exception of F-18, the positron emitters employed have such short half-lives that commercial distribution is prohibited. C-11, for example, has a half-life of 20 minutes. F-18, with a 110 minute half-life, is the preferred positron emitter. Agents based on amino acids and ribonucleic acids also present considerable difficulty in synthesis.

F-18-DG, an agent which targets glycolysis, has become the paradigmatic agent for metabolic imaging because it is relatively simple to synthesize. It is chemically stable and has reaction rates similar to those of glucose. There is also an extensive body of data on its clinical use, since it has been a standard agent for both brain and cardiac PET imaging for many years. Development of coincidence gamma cameras, the impending distribution system for the radiopharmaceutical, and strong evidence of cost-effectiveness and added value in staging lung tumors ensure that this agent will occupy a major niche in tumor imaging in coming years.

Like the agents previously mentioned, F-18-DG is metabolically trapped. Conversion to glucose-6-phosphate, the initial step in glycolysis, is the terminal metabolic step for F-18-DG. The agent accumulates at a rate proportional to the metabolic rate of the tissue being imaged. Since the protein and DNA synthesis required for cell division in the growing tumor require expenditure of energy and since most of this energy comes from glycolysis, F-18-DG activity parallels the activity of the protein and DNA synthesis agents in most cases. Since the mechanism of imaging is simple and well-understood, it is possible to predict quite accurately which tumors will localize the agent. Thus a rapidly growing tumor, such as non–small cell lung carcinoma, will usually localize the agent and a slow-growing tumor, such as an indolent lymphoma, is less likely to localize the agent. Since metastases tend to represent the most dedifferentiated and thus most metabolically active clones from the tumor, they are more likely than the primary to be imaged. The normal distribution is easy to predict from the known metabolic rates of various normal tissues. Brain tissue and cardiac tissue will have high activity and may tend to mask tumor in these locations.

Metabolic imaging agents complement the information available from anatomic imaging techniques such as CT or MR. In lung tumor imaging nodal staging by CT is based on size of the nodes. Because tumor may be present in very small nodes and very large inflammatory nodes may not contain tumor, this method is not simultaneously sensitive and specific for tumor. On the other hand cross sectional anatomic imaging techniques are more useful for direction of biopsy and for pre-surgical planning. By reducing the rate of unnecessary (meaning noncurative) surgery through improved staging, F-18-DG PET performed in addition to CT reduced the average cost per patient by over $1000 in a recent study (2). Fusion imaging, the accurate superimposition of metabolic images onto anatomic images through use of fiduciary markers, promises to further increase staging accuracy and provide anatomic localization of small metabolically active areas for biopsy.

Tc-99m Sestamibi (Tc-99m-MIBI) and Tc-99m Tetrofosmin (Tc-99m-TFos) are typical metabolic agents for gamma camera imaging. Both were developed for myocardial perfusion imaging. In oncology, they are of greatest potential interest for scintimammography. These agents were initially designed to substitute for Tl-201 in evaluating myocardial viability. Tl-201 had been serendipitously observed to localize within some tumors. Evaluation of Tc-99m-MIBI for tumor localization was a logical extension of this prior work. While the mechanism of localization is quite different, these agents fill a niche similar to that of F-18-DG. These agents are lipophilic, cationic materials whose uptake is dependent, in part, on cellular and mitochondrial membrane potentials (3). Malignant tumors have negative membrane potentials and high mitochondrial content to support their high metabolic rate. Thus, unlike F-18-DG, these agents are indirect markers of metabolic activity. Both agents also bind to P glycoprotein (P-gp), a mediator of multidrug resistance in breast cancer cells (4). When the multidrug resistance gene is present and active in a cell, P-gp is manufactured by the cell. P-gp traps cancer drugs by the same mechanism employed to trap these imaging pharmaceuticals: both are actively transported out of the cell. Thus, a breast cancer which localizes Tc-99m-MIBI or Tc-99m-TFos is likely to be responsive to chemotherapy. Alternatively, a breast cancer which does not localize these agents is likely to express multidrug resistance. Tl-201 apparently is not transported out of the cell by P-gp. This is reasonable, since Tl-201 is a simple ion, not representative of the types of large molecules (anthracyclines, vinca alkaloids, actinomycin D) usually transported by P-gp.

The greatest advantage of metabolic agents for staging is their ability to detect small or diffuse foci of primary or metastatic disease which are not detectable on anatomic images or are not pathologic by size criteria. They are also very useful for determining the presence or absence of recurrence in the bed of a treated tumor (5). The major disadvantage of these agents is that they are nonspecific. They image high metabolic activity rather than tumor *per se*. For example, F-18-DG may localize in an active tuberculous granuloma.

Monoclonal Antibodies

Polyclonal Antibodies are formed in response to an antigenic stimulus. The polyclonal antibody formed is really a set of chemically different substances which share the basic antibody structure, but have widely variant affinities for the intended target of the antigenic response. The variations occur because a large number of different cells respond with rapid division and antibody secretion when they are stimulated by an antigen. Each activated cell rapidly divides to form a clone of identical cells which produce one of the antibodies in the set. The set of antibodies produced by the many activated cell lines is thus termed polyclonal. Polyclonal antibodies have variable affinities for nontarget tissues. For an imaging agent, it is clearly desirable to have a single antibody of known and reliable affinity. A single antibody has the additional advantage of decreased nonspecific cross-reactivity with tissues other than the intended target. Such antibodies must be produced by a single clone, the descendants of a single cell. It is thus termed a monoclonal antibody.

Monoclonal Antibodies have three important advantages over polyclonal antibodies for imaging: maximum specificity, maximum sensitivity and predictable nontarget binding. By providing a high affinity, the monoclonal antibody reduces the dose of labeled antibody necessary to produce an acceptable target (tumor) to background ratio. By selecting a monoclonal antibody with high affinity, one simultaneously selects for greater specificity for that target. Nevertheless some cross reactivity may be inevitable, especially if the target tumor is very similar to a tissue normally present in the body. These cross reactions need to be constant so that the appearance of a normal scan may be determined with a high degree of certainty.

Basic Antibody Structure. A variety of antibody fragments and modified antibodies are employed for both imaging and therapy. Imaging agents to date have generally been based on the IgG antibody. This discussion will be limited to IgG for the sake of brevity, although there is no intrinsic reason that other antibody classes (IgA, IgE, IgD or IgM) could not be employed for imaging

Each IgG molecule has two binding regions for antigen (Fig. 62.1). An additional host binding region mediates effector functions such as blood clearance and nonspecific liver binding. When separated from the remainder of the antibody, the antigen-binding regions are termed Fab fragments and the effector mediator region is termed an Fc fragment. In the intact antibody, two Fab fragments are bound together by disulfide bonds. The Fc fragment is bound to each Fab fragment by covalent bonds. It is possible to remove the Fc region, while retaining the disulfide bonds between Fab regions. The resulting fragment is termed (Fab)$_2$. The antibody also consists of constant, variable and hypervariable regions. The constant regions are the same from antibody to antibody for a given antibody class and species of organism. The variable regions differ between antibodies within a class and contain the binding sites for antigen. The hypervariable regions have the greatest effect on antibody affinity and are those portions of the variable region which are most exposed at the antigen binding site.

The behavior of antibody fragments in biological systems is predictable in part on the basis of molecular weight alone. Smaller fragments partition more rapidly into various cellular and extracellular tissues because of

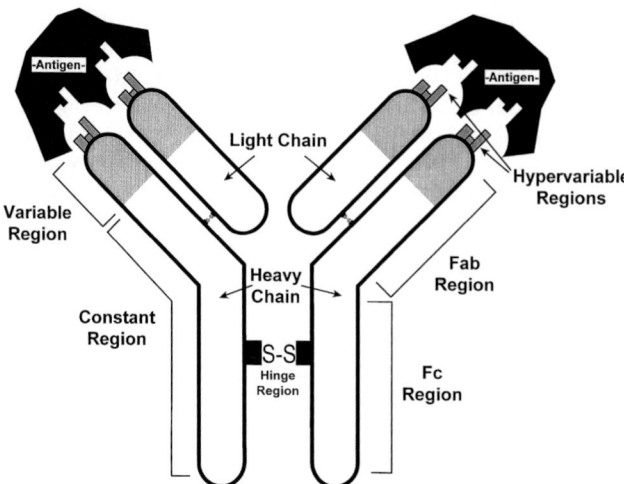

Figure 62.1. Monoclonal Antibody Structure. The basic antibody glycoprotein molecule consists of two identical heavy and light chains linked by a disulfide bridge. Each chain has a variable region responsible for antigenic binding, and a constant region involved in complement fixation and antibody-dependent cell toxicity. Each variable region, in turn, contains three hypervariable regions that form unique antigen-binding sites. The antibody can be fragmented into smaller units depending on the cleavage plane. Enzymatic digestion produces either an F(ab')2 fragment or two smaller Fab fragments and an Fc fragment. Fragment size dictates blood pool clearance rates, with the smaller ones clearing faster.

their smaller size. They are also metabolized and cleared from the blood stream more rapidly for the same reason. A small fragment is thus maximally exposed to the target tissue earlier, but for a shorter period of time. Smaller fragments will be favored for imaging when binding is rapid and strong, as this will result in rapid target labeling and rapid background clearance. Local recurrences, nodal metastases and peritoneal metastases may be better detected with fragments because their intact vasculature will insure that antigen will be exposed to the antibody (6). Smaller fragments will be advantageous, and often required, for isotopic labels having relatively short half-lives (7). The Tc-99m label, with a 6 hour half-life, requires rapid localization and background clearance so imaging can be performed within a day. Smaller fragments are also less immunogenic, and thus less likely to induce an undesirable immune response. Larger fragments or intact antibody may be preferable where a long reaction time is required, such as when binding is weak or slow, or for therapeutic applications where extended residence time in the target tissue is required to maximize radiation dose to the tumor. Since larger fragments and intact antibodies are cleared more slowly from the background, target to background ratios are lower. However, absolute uptake in tumor is higher with intact antibody (8). Slow background clearance increases whole body and nontarget dose in both imaging and therapeutic applications. Larger fragments allow, and may require, use of isotopes with longer half-lives.

Biochemical differences between fragments also affect biodistribution. The Fc region is of greatest interest, since it mediates nonspecific binding to the liver. For imaging agents, nonspecific liver binding significantly decreases sensitivity for detection of liver metastases. Metastases may even appear as photopenic rather than photoenhanced areas. High activity in the liver may also obscure activity in adjacent structures unless a lead shield is employed to cover the liver. Use of a shield however also carries the risk of obscuring an area of tumor activity. Dual isotope imaging with simultaneous acquisition of planar or SPECT data may allow digital subtraction of normal tissue or comparison of the biodistributions of an organ imaging agent (e.g., Tc-99m-sulfur colloid) with that of the labeled antibody to increase diagnostic accuracy. Finally, sequestration of an antibody or fragment in the liver reduces bioavailability of the agent for binding to the intended target. For a target outside the liver, rapid clearance of the background through nonspecific liver binding could improve imaging sensitivity. In practice, this advantage seldom outweighs the disadvantages listed. The use of antibody fragments for imaging began as an attempt to address the problem of nonspecific liver binding. Other techniques, such as pretreatment with Fc fragment to reduce nonspecific binding, have variable success.

The use of smaller fragments for imaging results in significantly increased renal activity. This can be addressed by administration of unlabeled leucine, which saturates the renal binding sites for the fragments and reduces their residence time in the kidneys. While pure pharmacologic grade leucine is not currently available, mixtures of amino acids, commercially available for total parenteral nutrition, appear to work just as well. Another approach to limiting renal activity is to use smaller fragments consisting only of the active binding site, or even of fragments of this active site.

It is important to recognize that monoclonal antibodies for imaging are usually produced from mouse hybridoma cells. These cells result from fusion of antibody-producing B lymphocytes with "immortal" myeloma cells. From the numerous fusion products which result, a single clone which produces high affinity antibody is selected. This cell line is then grown to produce the antibody. Since the mouse antibody is a foreign protein in the human bloodstream, it may incite an immune response. This results in production of human anti-mouse antibody (HAMA), which can cause mild to severe symptoms. Of greater concern, subsequent administrations of mouse antibody can result in mild to fatal (anaphylactic) reactions. This problem could limit the repeat use of monoclonal imaging or of therapeutic agents based on murine antibodies.

A variety of attempts have been made to reduce the antigenicity of the monoclonal imaging agents. Chimeric antibodies are formed from the variable regions of mouse antibodies and the constant regions of human antibodies. Humanized antibodies are formed by inserting the hypervariable region of the mouse antibody into a human antibody using recombinant DNA techniques. These modifications improve product safety at the cost of increased complexity and expense of production.

Clearly, monoclonal antibody imaging carries a significant risk of side effects. Before using these agents, physicians should thoroughly familiarize themselves with the side effect profile for the agent and be prepared to deal with any complications which arise. Prior to administration, the risk of HAMA reaction should be assessed in those patients who have previously undergone monoclonal antibody imaging or therapy.

It is likely that many of the future agents will be available with either a diagnostic or a therapeutic label, so that the likelihood of successful therapy can be assessed in advance of administration of the therapeutic agent. Beyond predicting response to radiotherapy with antibodies, imaging antibodies are most commonly used to assess equivocal findings at cross-sectional imaging (9). or to assess rising tumor markers in the absence of evident disease (10). Monoclonal antibody imaging agents currently approved for use are summarized in Table 62.1.

PEPTIDE RECEPTOR SCINTIGRAPHY

Regulatory peptides are a group of polypeptides which serve as internal messengers. They bind to targets on multiple tissues, most notably those of the brain and gastrointestinal system. They are expressed variably on the surfaces of a variety of human tumor cell lines. In cases where a stable radioactive label can be achieved without significantly decreasing the affinity of the receptors for the polypeptide, imaging and therapy are possible for specific tumor cells. The index compound and the only one commercially available at the time of this writing, is In-111-DTPA-D-Phe^1-octreotide (In-111-OCT). This protein binds with high affinity to the sst2 somatostatin receptor and with lesser affinity to two of the remaining five receptors for somatostatin.

Somatostatin Receptors are expressed by neuroendocrine tumors, some neural tumors (meningiomas, medulloblastomas, most astrocytomas and neuroblastomas), and small cell lung carcinomas. They are also highly expressed on the cell surfaces of carcinoid tumors and by cells in some nonmalignant conditions such as Wegener's granulomatosis, rheumatoid arthritis and tuberculosis (15). The sst2 receptor with the attached ligand is internalized by the cell, resulting in effective metabolic trapping of the radioligand within the tumor cell. In-111-OCT has >90% sensitivity for detection of carcinoid tumors. It can also be used to detect gastrinomas, insulinomas, glucagonomas and other (or unclassified) APUDomas (Fig. 62.2). It also has fair sensitivity for medullary thyroid carcinoma (65%). It detects primary small cell lung carcinoma with 90% sensitivity and nonliver metastases from small cell lung carcinoma with 70% sensitivity. It has successfully detected recurrent small cell lung carcinoma in patients who were in complete remission by standard criteria. The agent is rapidly cleared by renal excretion, with 90% excretion at 24 hours. It should be clear that the agent lacks specificity, but this is not significant in most tumor imaging applications. The agent will also image active granulomas, which are a potential source of false positive scans (16).

Other polypeptide imaging agents are under development and will likely find unique rolls in tumor imaging. These include a VIP receptor imaging agent for human epithelial tumors and adenocarcinomas; a substance-P receptor imaging agent for glial tumors, breast tumors and medullary thyroid carcinomas; and CCK-B/gastrin receptor imaging for medullary thyroid cancer and small cell lung cancer. Therapy has been attempted with Ytrium-90-somatostatin and VIP analogs and with the Auger and conversion electrons from In-111-somatostatin analogs used in high doses. Results are promising and further developments can be expected (17).

Mixed Mechanisms

The traditional gamma camera imaging agent Ga-67 depends on receptor binding but also falls within the category of metabolic marker agents. The metabolic activity imaged by gallium, at least in part, is the cellular competition for nutrient iron. Ga-67 ion, administered as the citrate salt, mimics free iron. It is rapidly bound to transferrin receptors on tumor cells, which are overexpressed in an attempt to maximize this scarce resource required for rapid growth. Limitation of free iron is a major defense mechanism of the body, although this is directed primarily at defense from pathogens. It is mediated by free transferrin protein in serum and by transferrin receptors on white cells. Pathogens also compete for free iron through production of soluble iron chelators termed siderophores. Gallium tumor activity thus depends both on the availability of transferrin receptors on the tumor and the metabolic activity of the tumor, which determines the extent to which these receptors will be expressed. For those tumors in which Ga-67 imaging is considered useful (predominantly lymphomas and hepatocellular carcinoma), it is generally recommended that a pretreatment baseline study be obtained before any therapy. If the baseline study is positive, Ga-67 will be more sensitive than any anatomic technique for detection of recurrence (Fig. 62.3). One problem is in children, where rebound thymic hyperplasia may result in significant Ga-67 uptake for several

Table 62.1. Monoclonal Antibody Imaging Agents

Name	Trade Name	Antigen	Ab Type	Label	Source
Satumomab (11)	OncoScint	TAG-72	Whole	In-111	Cytogen Corp.
Nofetumomab (12)	Verluma	40 kD Glycoprotein	Fab	Tc-99m	DuPont Pharma (13)
Arcitumomab (14)	CEA-Scan	CEA	Fab'	Tc-99m	Immunomedics, Inc.
Capromab Pendetide	ProstaScint	Prostate Specific Membrane Antigen	Whole	In-111	Cytogen Corp.

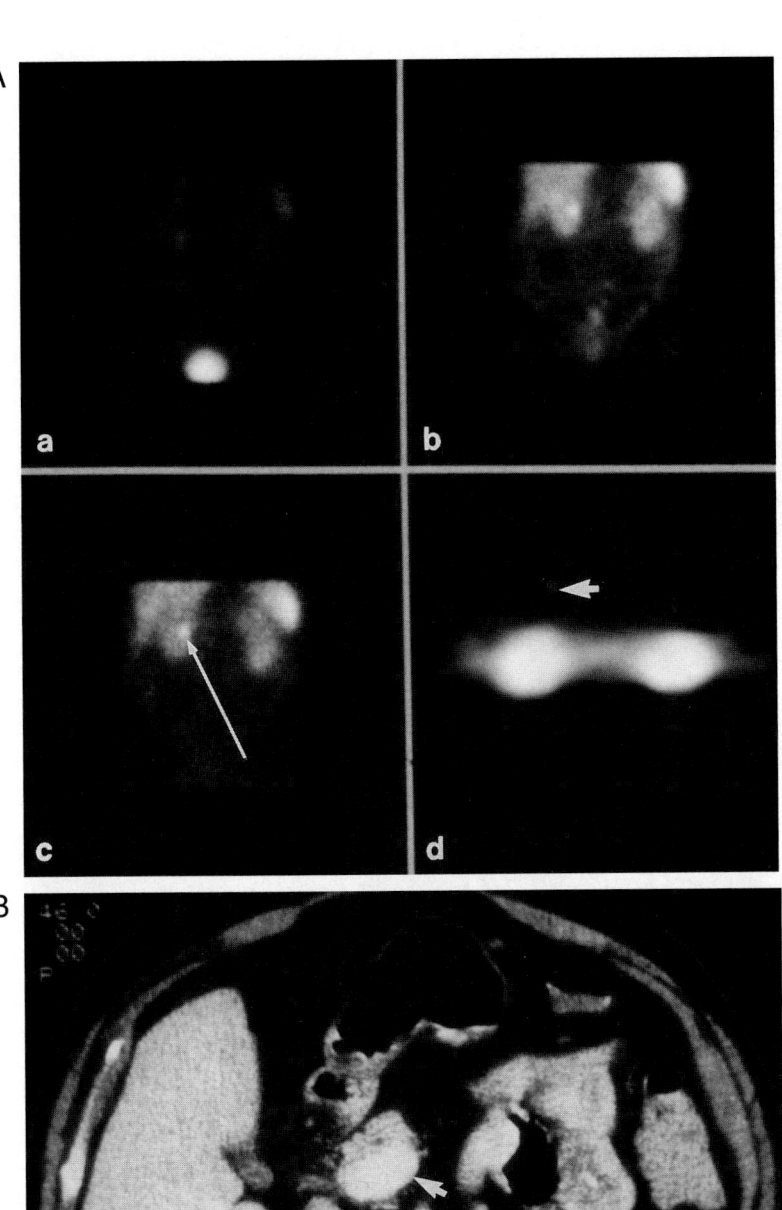

Figure 62.2. Gastrinoma. 52-year-old man with Zollinger-Ellison Syndrome. **A.** In-111-Octreotide images. **a.** 4-hour anterior abdomen. **b.** 24-hour anterior abdomen. **c.** 48 hour anterior abdomen. Note focus of increased activity (*arrow*) superimposed on upper pole of right kidney in all anterior planar images. **d.** Single axial slice through kidneys at 24 hours. The focus of activity representing the gastrinoma (*arrow*) is anterior to the right kidney. **B.** Corresponding CT slice. The enhancing soft tissue mass (*arrow*) immediately anterior to the inferior vena cava is the gastrinoma.

months post therapy and mimic or mask residual or recurrent tumor. If the baseline study is negative, no further Ga-67 imaging should be performed. An initially negative posttreatment study is not highly predictive of complete cure, at least for Hodgkin's disease (18).

Many early studies with Ga-67 were performed on rectilinear scanners and early generation gamma cameras with relatively low doses in the range of 1–4 mCi. As a result of using higher doses and SPECT, Ga-67 imaging has undergone a revival in recent years. SPECT provides much higher contrast resolution than planar imaging and therefore detects abnormalities that would otherwise have been missed. An increase in specificity with SPECT has also been reported. Whenever possible, SPECT imaging should be included in the evaluation of patients with malignancy.

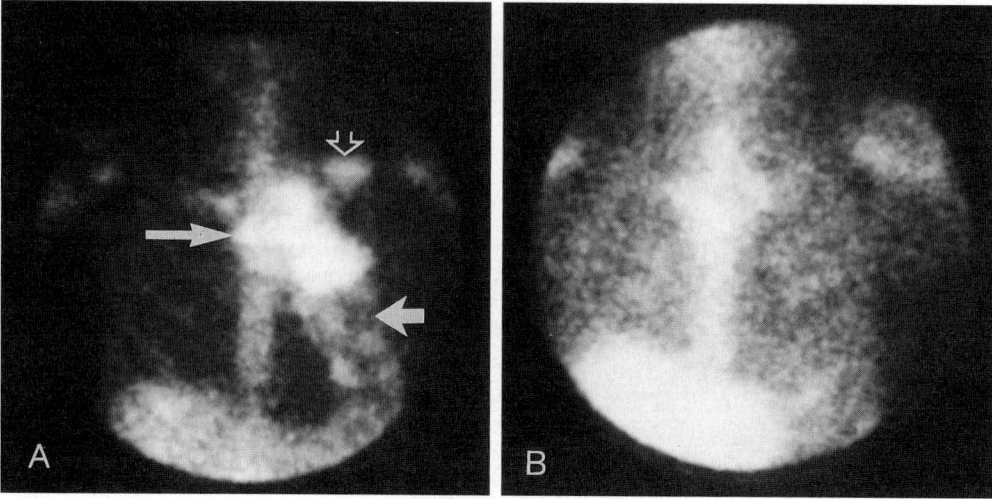

Figure 62.3. Lymphoma. Anterior chest images from Ga-67 studies pretreatment **(A)** and posttreatment **(B)** for lymphoma demonstrate the complete resolution of mediastinal (*long arrow*), parenchymal (*short arrow*), and left supraclavicular nodal (*open arrow*) disease.

Figure 62.4. Fibrolamellar Hepatocellular Carcinoma. Four anterior images of the liver. **A.** A Tc-99m sulfur colloid liver-spleen scan in a 22-year-old patient demonstrates a large photopenic mass (*arrow*) in the inferolateral aspect of the right lobe of the liver. **B.** A Ga-67 study demonstrates "fill in" of the mass (*arrow*). **C.** Hepatobiliary scan, 5 minutes after injection demonstrates limited patchy radionuclide activity in the mass (*arrow*) compared with the normal liver. **D.** Hepatobiliary scan, 70 minutes after the injection. Normal liver has washed out; mass (*arrow*) still retains activity; incidental finding of intrahepatic gallbladder (*open arrow*).

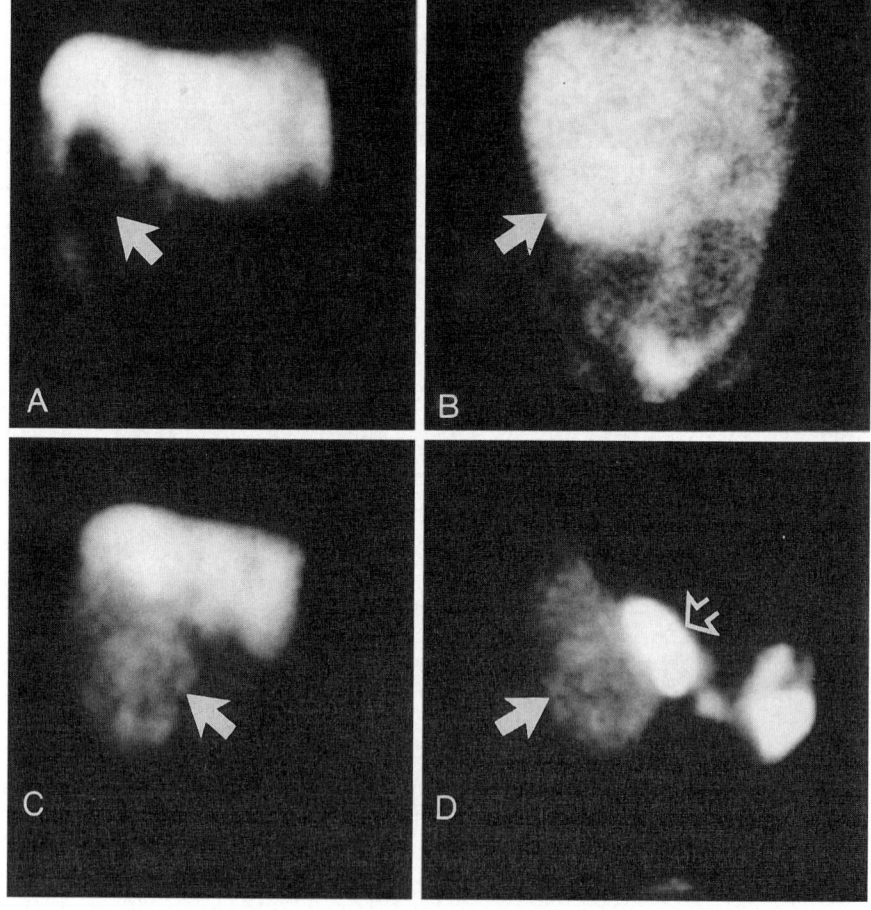

Ga-67 scintigraphy may be used to supplement Tc-99m-sulphur colloid (Tc-99m-SCOL) imaging.

Hepatocellular Carcinoma (HCC) is typically Ga-67 avid but contains no Kupffer cells, and so does not accumulate radiocolloid. The differential diagnosis for the pattern of cold defect on radiocolloid study with corresponding "fill-in" on the Ga-67 study includes abscess and metastasis. As a result, hepatobiliary imaging is sometimes performed. Well differentiated HCC may take up biliary agents albeit slower and to a lesser extent than surrounding normal liver, while poorly differentiated tumors will not. On delayed imaging, the HCC will be seen to retain the pharmaceutical because of the lack of connection to normal biliary radicles.

Hepatic Adenomas rarely contain Kupffer cells, and so usually appear cold on radiocolloid studies. The hepatobiliary scan pattern for hepatic adenoma is the same as that for well-differentiated HCC, although some appear cold because of central scarring and hemorrhage.

Focal Nodular Hyperplasia may have normal, increased, or most commonly, decreased activity compared with normal liver on radiocolloid imaging.

It should be emphasized that Ga-67 avidity of hepatic lesions may be manifest as a normal-appearing liver despite the presence of a space-occupying lesion documented by another imaging modality. Given the relative prevalences in the United States of the other lesions in the differential diagnosis, a Ga-67 avid hepatic lesion should be viewed as HCC until proved otherwise by tissue diagnosis.

A separate clinical and pathologic entity is the fibrolamellar subtype of HCC that is seen in younger patients and may have a better prognosis. In contrast to typical HCC, which occurs most commonly superimposed on underlying cirrhosis or chronic active hepatitis, fibrolamellar HCC occurs in otherwise normal livers. It is important to suggest the diagnosis of fibrolamellar HCC early so that potentially curative resection can be undertaken without delay (Fig. 62.4).

The localization of Ga-67 in foci of infection (due to transferrin receptors on macrophages and siderophores) and in foci of inflammation (due to transferrin receptors on macrophages) is potentially a major disadvantage in tumor imaging. This is especially true in patients where the tumor affinity for gallium is unknown and the patient has already undergone therapy resulting in inflammation and/or has a superimposed infection. Nevertheless, the 95% sensitivity of this agent for recurrent lymphoma insures it a continued place in the tumor imaging repertoire (19).

Lymphoscintigraphy

Lymphoscintigraphy has undergone a revival as the result of the sentinel node concept (20). Cutaneous melanoma tends to migrate to the nearest draining node without skip lesions in nodes further along the drainage chain. Since this tumor metastasizes almost exclusively by the lymphatic route, absence of tumor within the first draining lymph node makes presence of other metastatic disease highly unlikely. If this sentinel node can be located and demonstrated to be free of disease, more extensive lymph node dissection can be avoided. Any colloidal agent can in principle be employed for lymphoscintigraphy. Agents having particle sizes less than 50 nm are ideal. The most common agents employed are Tc-99m-SCOL and Tc-99m-human serum album (Tc-99m-HSA). Tc-99m-SCOL is somewhat suboptimal due to large particle size which results in significant retention at the injection site. This problem is partially overcome by filtration to obtain only the smaller particles. Tc-99m-HSA immediately enters the lymphatic system and allows rapid dynamic imaging of lymphatic channels with reduced overall imaging time. However retention in lymph nodes is significantly less than with Tc-99m-SCOL, which may make this agent less optimal for use of an intraoperative gamma probe to localize the sentinel node. In general HSA is probably preferable for imaging and SCOL for intraoperative use, but either can be used effectively.

Technical factors can significantly affect the outcome of the study. It is important to inject the agent intradermally, as subcutaneous injections may result in drainage to a different set of nodes. A transmission scan or other body image scan is required to allow effective interpretation of node location (Fig. 62.5). Head and neck lesions have especially short drainage chains. Since these lesions drain inferiorly, injection should occur above (cranial to) the level of the lesion to ensure the activity at the injection site does not obscure the sentinel node. Body wall lymphatics are highly variable. Both ipsilateral and contralateral imaging is required with body wall injections to insure all nodal groups draining the lesion are detected.

Lymphoscintigraphy is becoming accepted in some centers for evaluation of melanoma preoperatively. It can decrease the morbidity and cost of surgical therapy by reducing the extent of dissection required in a large number of cases. Lymphoscintigraphy has been investigated as a guide to radiation therapy in breast cancer and in evaluation of nodal metastases from prostate tumors. The predictive value of a sentinel node remains to be established in these tumors which also have significant hematogenous routes of spread.

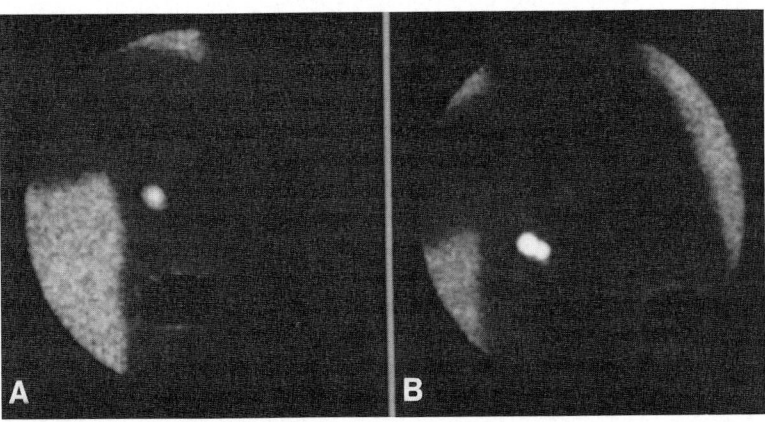

Figure 62.5. Malignant Melanoma. Lymphoscintigraphy with filtered Tc-99m sulfur colloid injected intradermally in four locations around the site of malignant melanoma located on the back at the inferior aspect of the left clavicle. Transmission imaging is performed with a Tc-99m flood source causing the patient to cast a "shadow" for positioning information. **A.** Image is slightly off-center, true posterior with left arm held out to the side. **B.** Image is a left lateral image. In both images the injection sites have been digitally subtracted ("halo" remains in the lower portion of each image) so that axillary nodal activity is more readily apparent. Imaging of the remainder of the trunk failed to demonstrate drainage elsewhere.

Other Tumor Imaging Agents

The use of MIBG for detection and therapy of neuro-blastoma and pheochromocytoma and iodinated cholesterol derivatives for adrenal cortical carcinoma are discussed in chapter 58. Bone imaging agents for both primary bone tumors and metastatic disease are discussed in chapter 55. In addition to localizing areas of increased or absent bone repair ("hot" and "cold" lesions respectively), these agents have a tendency to localize within malignant effusions and malignant ascites. The mechanism for this localization has yet to be fully explained.

A novel approach involves use of liposomes to image tumors (21). In addition to their intrinsic tendency to localize within tumor tissues, these agents are of special interest because they have the potential to be coated with antibodies or receptor targeting agents. If sufficient specificity for tumor can be achieved, these agents could be of great value for delivering large amounts of a therapeutic agent, such as a toxin or brachytherapy agent in a single package.

Pretreatment with agents designed to improve target to background ratios may become more common in the future. These agents may increase binding of the imaging agent to the intended target or they may decrease binding of the agent to nontarget tissues. Examples of the latter include use of amino acids to reduce renal activity after administration of monoclonal antibodies or pretreatment with cold octreotide to reduce nontarget accumulation of In-111-OCT.

DUAL AGENT SCINTIGRAPHY AND FUSION IMAGING

Dual Agent Imaging may improve sensitivity for detection of metastases from certain classes of tumors where the metastatic foci have variable receptor expression due to dedifferentiation or origin from different cell clones. F-18-DG and I-131 may be used in combination to simultaneously image differentiated (I-131) and dedifferentiated (F-18-DG) metastases from thyroid cancer. The combination of Tc-99m-MIBI and In-111-OCT has also been suggested as a means for determining multi-drug resistance in small cell lung carcinoma. Presumably, F-18-DG or Tl-201 in combination with any of the MIBI-like agents could achieve the same effect in tumors which do not have somatostatin receptors. Tc-99m-MIBI has been used in association with bone agent SPECT to exclude tumor spread suspected on the basis of the bone scan findings.

Fusion Imaging is the exact superimposition of the physiologic information from a nuclear medicine study with the anatomic information from CT or MR using fiduciary markers (22). This technology is already commercially available for brain imaging and will shortly be available commercially for SPECT and PET images of the whole body. This technique will allow the exact location of areas of physiologic activity to be determined for direction of biopsy, surgical intervention or refinement of radiation therapy fields.

Staging Lung Cancer. PET with F-18-DG is the most accurate method for imaging lung cancer. The sensitivity is over 95% for characterization of lung nodules, with specificity of 88% and overall accuracy of 94% (23). It also identifies and characterizes tumor spread in the mediastinum and elsewhere very accurately compared to CT. Sensitivity of PET F-18-DG imaging for this purpose is 88%, with specificity of 91% and overall accuracy of 91% (comparable numbers for CT are 80%, 58% and 70%)(24). The significance of the improved specificity of PET for lung cancer imaging is that it prevents unnecessary surgery by identifying patients who will not benefit from surgery. If PET is added to the staging of lung cancer, the average cost per patient is decreased by over $1000 by preventing unneeded surgery, and its morbidity and mortality.

Since cross-sectional anatomic imaging is well established for cancer imaging, nuclear medicine studies must gain a clinical foothold by establishing added value when used in addition to current imaging. The potential for wide application of F-18-DG imaging with coincidence gamma cameras means this technology could rapidly spread to all centers for staging of all lung cancers. This could have a major impact in decreasing the cost of care for these patients. In this respect, F-18-DG PET imaging for lung tumor is paradigmatic for the manner in which new oncologic imaging agents for nuclear medicine will have to be marketed. In most cases, it will be the specificity of the test which determines its added value. Fusion imaging may then be used to ensure identification of appropriate targets for resection in those patients who still merit surgical intervention.

Scintimammography. Radiographic mammography is the standard screening examination for breast cancer. Because of its relatively low cost, it is acceptable to have a poor specificity as long as sensitivity is high. Screening mammography misses 6–10% of breast carcinomas. Addition of physical examination significantly increases the value of screening. The relatively low specificity makes mammography less satisfactory for diagnostic evaluation. It nevertheless remains the gold standard for breast imaging. Specificity is obtained by addition of stereotactic or US directed biopsies. Most practices add US to detect benign causes of mammographic densities or palpable lesions (obviating biopsy of these lesions) and to evaluate for lesions hidden within dense portions of the breast. Some also advocate use of breast MR in diagnostically questionable cases.

Scintimammography can be performed with a variety of agents, including Tc-99m-MDP, Tl-201, Tc-99m-MIBI, Tc-99m-Tfos, F-18-DG and In-111-OCT. Of these, Tc-99m-MIBI currently offers the best compromise between cost and efficacy. Imaging can be performed with standard gamma cameras and requires little modification of equipment, although prone imaging is desirable (25). Reported sensitivities have been between 83 and 94% with reported specificities between 88 and 94% (26). Sensitivity for palpable lesions over 1.5 cm is high (90%) but specificity is lower (70%). Specificity for nonpalpable lesions is high (90%) but sensitivity is lower (approximately 60%)(27). Thus, while Tc-99m-MIBI scintigraphy can be performed at a reasonable cost, it is unlikely to compete with mammography for screening because it does not detect very small cancers with high sensitivity. F-18-DG PET imaging has better sensitivity and specificity (80-100%)(28). However, the cost of F-18-DG PET is prohibitive for a screening test. Both Tc-99m-MIBI and F-18-DG allow detection of axillary node metastases without additional administrations. Sensitivity for axillary node metastases with Tc-99m-MIBI has been variable but specificity exceeds 90%. Scintimammography with Tc-99m-MIBI appears to outperform MR in both sensitivity and specificity (29,30). As it is also simpler to perform and of lower or comparable cost, it is probably preferable as a confirmatory test for breast carcinoma.

Indications for scintimammography include search for a primary tumor in the patient with positive axillary nodes but no mammographically visible lesion, evaluation for multifocality in patients with extensive calcifications or densities on mammography and a positive biopsy, evaluation of chemotherapy response (especially in pre-surgical chemotherapy), obviating biopsy in the patient with an indeterminate or low-suspicion mammographic lesion, and assessing the patient with postsurgical scar after biopsy or lumpectomy. Scintimammography is often successful in patients with dense breasts and may be of value in patients with normal mammography and "lumpy" breasts (31).

The most interesting possibility for scintimammography is determination of multi-drug resistance prior to use of chemotherapy. Since P-gp actively transports Tc-99m-MIBI out of the cancer cell, the presence of multidrug resistance should, in principle, be detectable by use of this agent (32).

A scintimammogram is considered positive with focal breast uptake of any intensity. Where uncertainty exists, a false positive is preferable to a false negative; the former will be excluded by biopsy while the latter will result in delayed diagnosis of cancer and contribute to a poor outcome. As with any breast study, images should be read in correlation with clinical history, physical examination findings and mammography. Raw data as well as any masked images should be read to prevent unintentional masking of axillary or chest wall lesions. False negatives have been reported in patients with the multidrug resistance gene (33). Certain artifacts have been described. These include diffuse unilateral or bilateral uptake in 5-7%, for which the mechanism is not currently known. Other artifacts include Compton scattering from the imaging table or skin folds, shine through from the contralateral breast, nodal uptake related to infiltrated dose and secretion in sebaceous cysts.

TUMOR IMAGING

Brain Tumors may be imaged with a number of agents due to break down of the blood brain barrier. This usually occurs incidentally during bone scanning with Tc-99m-MDP. PET with F-18-DG, C-11-methionine, and other agents and SPECT with Tl-201 can be used to detect residual tumor after surgical ablation or radiation therapy. Tl-201 SPECT is significantly simpler and less expensive than F-18-DG PET and is also less expensive than coincidence gamma camera 18 FDG imaging. These

techniques are significantly more sensitive for residual tumor than anatomic cross-sectional imaging techniques. F-18-DG PET can also differentiate low-grade from high grade tumors of the CNS.

Thyroid Cancer. Both F-18-DG PET and In-111-OCT planar imaging and SPECT have been proposed for detection of dedifferentiated thyroid metastases which are no longer iodine avid. In-111-OCT can also be used to detect medullary thyroid carcinoma and its metastases. Sensitivity is only 65%, but receptor agents for other somatostatin receptors are under development and could improve on detection sensitivity. Tc-99mc-MIBI planar or SPECT imaging has been suggested for detection of thyroid metastases in patients while still on thyroid suppression drug regimens. The predictive value is high. This agent also has intense persistent uptake in Hurthle cell carcinoma, which may allow unique identification.

Head and Neck Tumors. Tc-99m-pertechnetate detects Warthin's tumor of the parotid gland with high specificity on planar imaging (chapter 59). Both F-18-DG PET and planar Tl-201 have been advocated for evaluation of nasopharyngeal carcinoma. Advantages include improved specificity for tumor (compared with CT or MR) and improved detection of residual or recurrent disease.

Lung Cancer. Use of F-18-DG in non–small cell lung carcinoma (NSCLC) has been discussed. Both Tl-201 and Tc-99m-MIBI have also been advocated for NSCLC imaging. In-111-OCT images the peptide receptors in small cell lung cancer. It also identified NSCLC, but did so by labeling adjacent lymphocytes or neuroendocrine cells rather than specific receptors. The Fab antibody fragment NR-LU-10 marketed as Verluma is also effective in detection and staging of both SCLC and NSCLC (Fig. 62.6)(34). Tl-201 has been used successfully to assess viability of lung cancer and thymic carcinoma after therapy. F-18-DG PET is also capable of detecting residual or recurrent lung carcinoma with high sensitivity (reported at 100%) but only moderate specificity (61%).

Colon Cancer. Monoclonal antibodies against carcinoembryonic antigen (CEA)(CEA scan, Fig.62.7) and against the TAG-72 antigen (Oncoscint, Fig. 62.8) are commercially available to evaluate colorectal metastases. These have the advantage of improved sensitivity and specificity over cross-sectional imaging. Both are indicated primarily in patients with rising serum CEA in whom no recurrent disease (or indeterminate post operative change) is detected by CT or MR (35). Liver imaging with Oncoscint is relatively insensitive due to high background activity in this organ and dual isotope imaging with Tc-99m-sulfur colloid and multi-detector SPECT are recommended to enhance sensitivity.

Pancreatic Adenocarcinoma may be detected by F-18-DG, with sensitivity of 96% compared with 64% for Tl-201 SPECT (36). In-111-OCT can be used to detect neuroendocrine tumors of the pancreas. This agent is especially useful for neuroendocrine tumors because it is very sensitive for follow-up and because positivity with the agent predicts response to octreotide therapy (Fig. 62.9). For neural crest derived neuroendocrine tumors, both In-111-OCT and I-131-metaiodobenzylguanidine (I-131-MIBG) may be employed. The latter agent is effective in detection of pheochromocytomas, especially those

Figure 62.6. Small Cell Lung Carcinoma. A. Anterior image with Tc-99m labeled antibody Nr-Lu-10 and corresponding Tc-99m-MDP bone scan **(B).** Note significant antibody localization in the primary tumor in the right upper lobe, the retromanubrial area, the right femoral neck and proximal left femur. All confirmed to represent tumor, and with little or no bony abnormality on the bone scan. **C.** Posterior labeled antibody images from the same patient. Note rib erosion by primary tumor and lumbar spine involvement which appears more extensive on the bone scan **(D)** but is also apparent on the antibody study.

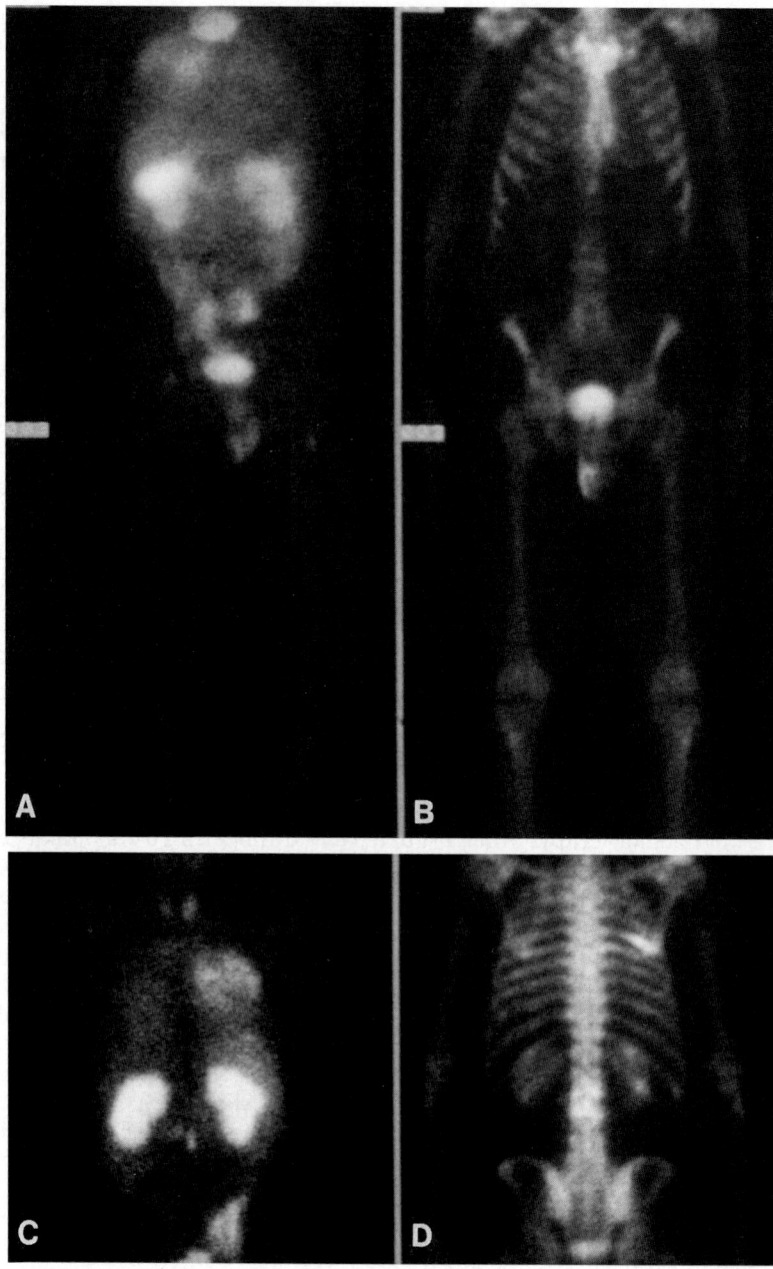

in extraadrenal locations (Fig. 62.10). It is also useful to detect metastatic disease sites in neuroblastoma. Another agent, I-131 labeled NP-59 (a norcholesterol derivative), is also available for adrenal cortical imaging. As this agent is not likely to be developed commercially it will continue to require institutional investigational new drug permits and is thus restricted to select centers.

Ovarian Carcinoma metastases may be imaged with Oncoscint. This radiopharmaceutical can demonstrate diffuse peritoneal tumor studding, which may be too small and diffuse to detect by cross-sectional imaging. F-18-DG has also been used to image ovarian cancer.

Prostate Cancer can be assessed with a monoclonal antibody to prostate specific antigen (PSA) released commercially as Prostascint (chapter 60). Prostascint is recommended for localization of lymph node metastases (sensitivity 62%, specificity 72%, accuracy 68%) and for recurrence detection in the patient with rising PSA in whom anatomic studies and bone scanning are negative. Neither of these agents is ideal as both have low target to background ratios, are expensive, and require considerable experience for correct interpretation.

Bone Tumors. Metabolic marker agents may be of value in assessing effectiveness of preoperative chemotherapy in limb sparing procedures (37). Strontium-89 is valuable for treatment of bone pain in metastatic prostate and breast cancer (38).

Summary. Oncologic nuclear medicine is an expanding field. The increasing number and type of radiopharmaceuticals effective for the detection and treatment of primary and metastatic cancer suggest that oncologic nuclear medicine holds promise not suspected even 5

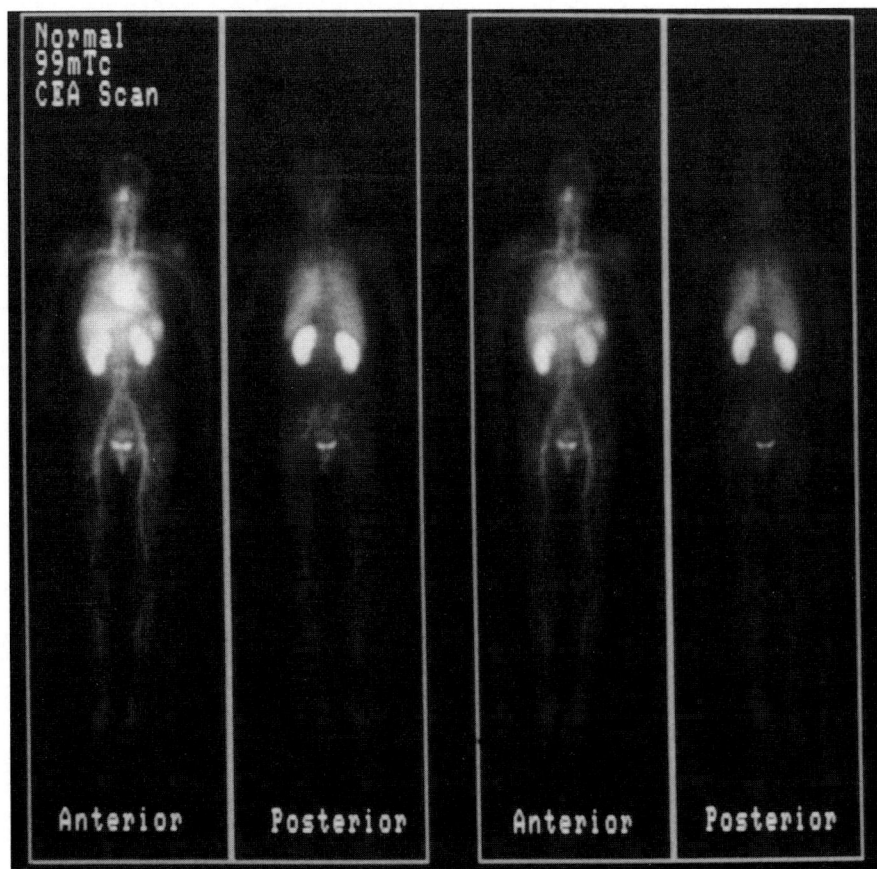

Figure 62.7. Normal CEA Scan. Whole-body anterior and posterior images.

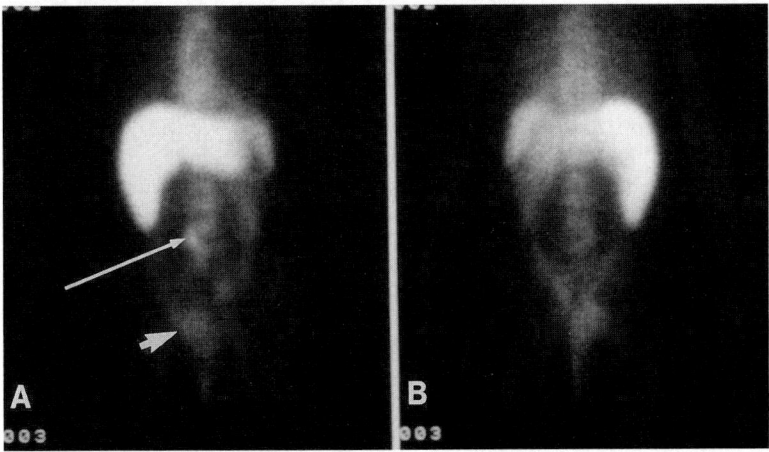

Figure 62.8. Metastatic Colon Carcinoma. In-111-Oncoscint study, **(A)** shows the anterior and **(B)** shows the posterior. Patient is status postresection of colon carcinoma with rising CEA. Study demonstrates paraspinous adenopathy (*long arrow*). Less obvious is the fixed uptake in the pelvis (*short arrow*) which remained unchanged over several days of imaging and was proven to be locally recurrent carcinoma.

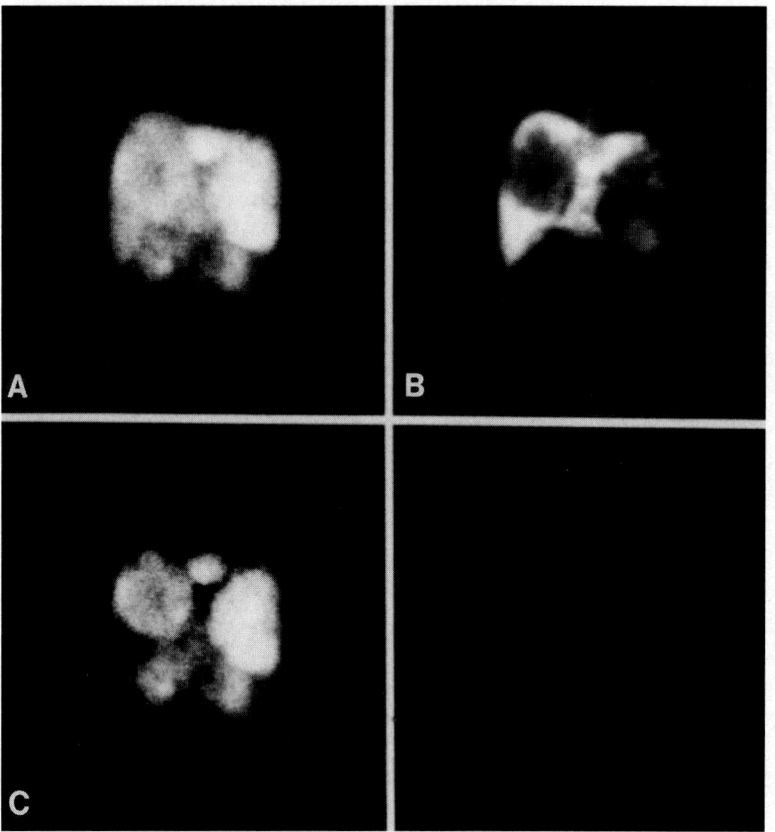

Figure 62.9. Metastatic Islet Cell Tumor. Patient with known metastatic islet cell tumor for evaluation of receptor status. **A.** Anterior liver and spleen with In-111-Octreotide. **B.** Tc-99m sulfur colloid liver spleen scan with multiple defects corresponding to the tumor. **C.** Subtraction study.

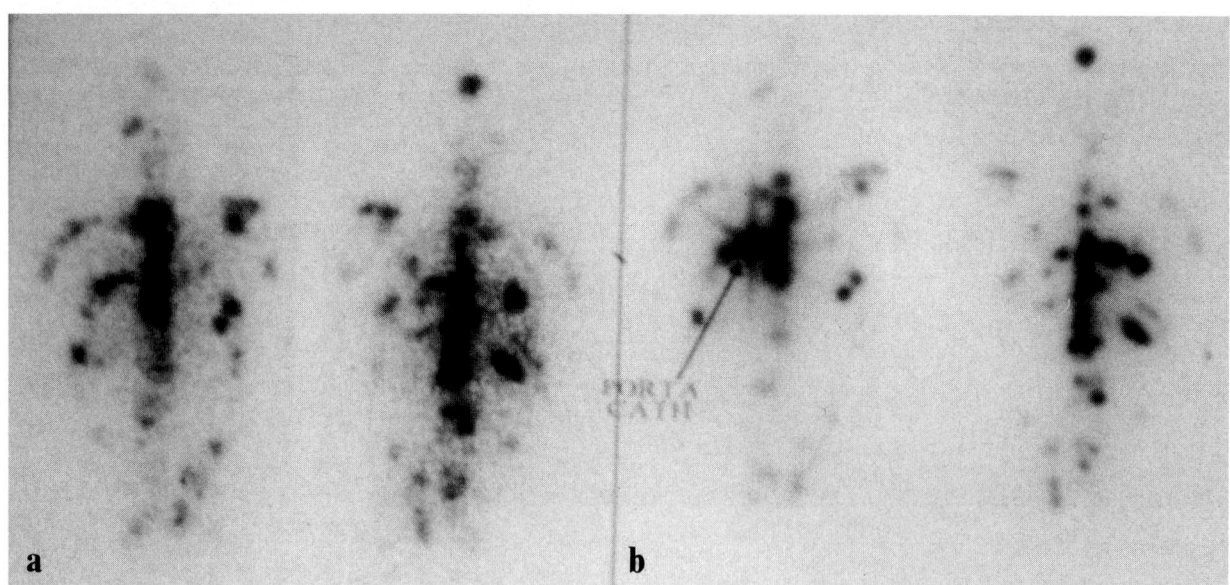

Figure 62.10. Metastatic Pheochromocytoma. Anterior and posterior whole body images with I-131-MIBG in a patient with widely metastatic pheochromocytoma. (Images courtesy of Dr. Peter Blue, Columbia, South Carolina.)

years ago. The advances in cost effective PET imaging technology with the availability of gamma camera PET from multiple vendors further strengthens the position of nuclear radiology in the managed care environment. Radiologists will need to understand not only the indications, contraindications and pitfalls of this new imaging technology, but also its position in the cost effective delivery of care.

References

1. Drane W, Abbott F, Nicole M, et al. Technology for FDG SPECT with a relatively inexpensive gamma camera. Radiology 1994;191:461–465.

2. Gambhir SS, Hoh CK, Phelps ME, et al. Decision tree sensitivity analysis for cost-effectiveness of FDG-PET in the staging and management of non–cell lung carcinoma. J Nucl Med 1996;37:1428–1436.

3. Arbab AS, Koizumi K, Toyama K, Araki T. Uptake of technetium-99m-tetrofosmin, technetium-99m-MIBI and thallium-201 in tumor cell lines. J Nucl Med 1996;37:1551–1556.

4. Ballinger JR, Bannerman J, Boxen I, et al. Technetium-99m-tetrofosmin as a substrate for P-glycoprotein: in vitro studies in multidrug-resistant breast tumor cells. J Nucl Med 1996;37:1578–1582.

5. Ojada J, Oonishi H, Yoshikawa K, et al. FDG-PET for the evaluation of tumor viability after anticancer therapy. Annals Nucl Med 1994;8:109–113.

6. Behr TM, Becker WS, Klein MW, et al. Diagnostic accuracy and tumor-targeting kinetics of complete versus fragmented 99mTc-labelled anti-carcinoembryonic antigen antibodies: an intraindividual comparison. Cancer Research 1995;55:5786s–5793s.

7. Behr T, Becker W, Hannappel E, et al. Targeting of liver metastases of colorectal cancer with IgG, F(ab')2, and Fab' anti-carcinoembryonic antigen antibodies labeled with 99mTc: the role of metabolism and kinetics. Cancer Research 1995;55:5777s–5785s.

8. Behr TM, Becker WS, Bair HJ, et al. Comparison of complete versus fragmented technetium-99m-labeled anti-CEA monoclonal antibodies immunoscintigraphy in colorectal cancer. J Nucl Med 1995;36:430–441.

9. Collier BD, Abdel-Nabi H, Doerr RJ, et al. Immunoscintigraphy performed with In-111-labeled CYT-103 in the management of colorectal cancer: Comparison with CT. Radiology 1992;185:179–186.

10. Patt YZ, Podoloff DA, Curley S, et al. Technetium 99m-labeled IMMU-4, a monoclonal antibody against carcinoembryonic antigen, for imaging of occult recurrent colorectal cancer in patients with rsing serum carcinoembryonic antigen levels. J Clin Oncol 1994;12:489–495.

11. Abdel-Nabi H, Doerr RJ, Chan H-W, et al. In-111-labeled monoclonal antibody immunoscintigraphy in colorectal carcinoma: safety, sensitivity, and preliminary clinical results. Radiology 1990;175:163–171.

12. Kasina S, Rao TN, Srinivasan A, et.al. Development and biologic evaluation of a kit for preformed chelate technetium-99m radiolabeling of an antibody Fab fragment using a diamide dimercaptide chelating agent. J Nucl Med 1991;32:1445–1451.

13. Developed by NeoRx Corp. Manufactured under license by Dr. Karl Thomas GmbH (Boehringer Ingelheim)

14. Moffat FL, Pinsky CM, Hammershaimb L, etal. Clinical utility of external immunoscintigraphy with the IMMU-4 99mTc-Fab' antibody fragment in patients undergoing surgery for carcinoma of the colon and rectum. Results of a pivotal Phase III trial. J Clin Oncol 1996;14:2295–2305.

15. Krenning EP, Kwekkeboom DJ, Pauwels S, et al. Somatostatin receptor scintigraphy. Nuclear Medicine Annual. New York: Raven Press, 1995;1–50 and references therein.

16. Krenning EP, KWekkeboom DJ, Bakker WH, et al. Somatostatin receptor scintigraphy with (111-In-DTPA-D-Phe1)- and (123I-Tyr3)-octreotide: the Rotterdam experience with more than 1000 patients. Eur J Nucl Med 1993;20:716–731.

17. Reubi JC. The molecular basis for peptide receptor scintigraphy. Continuing Education Course Manual 1997, Society of Nuclear Medicine, 294–297.

18. Salloum E, Brandt DS. Gallium scans in the management of patients with Hodgkin's disease: a study of 101 patients. J Clin Oncol 1997;15:518–527.

19. Front D, Israel O. The role of gallium-67 scintigraphy in evaluating the results of therapy of lymphoma patients. Sem Nucl Med 1995;25:60–71.

20. Morton DL et al. Intraoperative lymphatic mapping and selective cervical lymphadenectomy for early-stage melanomas of the head and neck. J Clin Oncol 1993;11:1751–1756.

21. Kubo A, Nakamura K, Sammiya T. et al. Indium-111-labeled liposomes: dosimetry and tumour detection in patients with cancer. Eur J Nucl Med 1993;20:107–113.

22. Wahl RL, Quint LE, Cieslak RD, et al. "Anatometabolic" tumor imaging: fusion of FDG PET with CT or MRI to localize foci of increased activity. J Nucl Med 1993;34:1190–1197.

23. Gupta NC, Maloof J, Gunel E. Probability of malignancy in solitary pulmonary nodules using fluorine-18-FDG and PET. J Nucl Med 1996;37:943–948.

24. Valk PE, Pounds TR, Hopkins DM, et al. Staging non–small cell lung cancer by whole-body positron emission tomographic imaging. Ann Thorac Surg 1995;60:1573–1581.

25. Khalkhali I, Mena I, Diggles L. Review of imaging techniques for the diagnosis of breast cancer: a new role of prone scintimammography using technetium-99m sestamibi. Eur J Nucl Med 1994;21:357–362.

26. Villanueva-Meyer J, Leonard MH Jr, Briscoe E, et al. Mammoscintigraphy with technetium-99m-sestamibi in suspected breast cancer. J Nucl Med 1996;37:926–930.

27. Preliminary results of multicenter trial as reported in Villanueva-Meyer J. Nuclear medicine breast imaging. Continuing Education Course Manual 1997, Society of Nuclear Medicine. 363–366.

28. Nieweg O, Kim E, Wong WH, et al. Positron emission tomography with fluorine-18-deoxyglucose in the detection and staging of breast cancer. Cancer 1996;71:3920–3925.

29. Tiling R, Sommer H, Pechmann M, et al. Comparison of technetium-99m-sestamibi scintimammography with contrast enhanced MRI for diagnosis of breast lesions. J Nucl Med 1997;38:58–62.

30. Helbich TH, Becerer A, Trattning S, et al. Differentiation of benign and malignant breast lesions: MR imgaing versus Tc99m sestamibi scintimammography. Radiology 1997;202:421–429.

31. Waxman AD. The role of Tc-99m-methoxyisobutylisonitrile in imaging breast cancer. Semin Nucl Med 1997;27:40–54.

32. Cordobes MD, Starzec A, Delmon-Moingeon L, et al. Technetium-99m-sestimibi uptake by human benign and malignant breast tumor cells: correlation with mdr gene expression. J Nucl Med 1996;37:286–289.

33. Moretti JL, Azaloux H, Boisseron D, et al. Primary breast cancer imaging with technetium-99m sestamibi and its relation with P-glycoprotein overexpression. Eur J Nucl Med 1996;23:980–986.

34. Breitz HB, Sullivan K, Nelp WB. Imaging lung cancer with radiolabeled antibodies. Sem Nucl Med 1993;23:127–132.

35. Poshyachinda M, Chaiwatanarat T, Saesow N, et al. Value of radioimmunoscintigraphy with technetium-99m labelled anti-CEA monoclonal antibody (BW431/26) in the detection of colorectal cancer. Eur J Nucl Med 1996;23: 624–630.

36. Inokuma T, Tamaki N, Torizuka T, et al. Value of fluorine-18-fluorodeoxyglucose and thallium-201 in the detection of pancreatic cancer. J Nucl Med 1995;36:229–235.

37. Rosen G., Loren GJ, Brien EW, et al. Serial thallium-201 scintigraphy in osteosarcoma. Correlation with tumor necrosis after preoperative chemotherapy. Clin Orthopedics Related Research 1993;293:302–306.

38. Robinson RG, Blake GM, Preston DF, et al. Strontium-89: Treatment results and kinetics in patients with painful matastatic prostate and breast cancer in bone. Radiographics 1989;9:271–281.

63

Central Nervous System Scintigraphy

James H. Timmons

TRADITIONAL BRAIN SCANS
CEREBROSPINAL FLUID STUDIES
FUNCTIONAL BRAIN IMAGING
    Positron Emission Tomography
    Single Photon Emission Computed Tomography

TRADITIONAL BRAIN SCANS

The traditional nuclear medicine brain scan detects a breakdown in the blood-brain barrier. The normal blood-brain barrier protects the CNS by preventing entry of harmful substances. Materials are excluded on the basis of molecular size and chemical characteristics. Active transport mechanisms are present for certain key materials.

Radiopharmaceuticals. Traditional brain scanning is typically performed with either Technetium-99m (Tc-99m) bound to diethylenetriaminepentaacetic acid (DTPA) or glucoheptonate (GH). Any agent that does not normally cross the blood-brain barrier can potentially be employed, although agents of cellular size (radiolabeled red blood cells, for example) will be excluded even by a damaged blood-brain barrier. Pertechnetate may be used but only if the patient is pretreated with 200–500 mg of potassium perchlorate. Perchlorate blocks the normal uptake of pertechnetate in the choroid plexus, which might otherwise be mistaken for an abnormality.

Technique. A dose of 15–20 mCi of Tc-99m-DTPA or GH is injected into an arm vein. Flow images are typically obtained at a rate of one image every 3 seconds for a total of 60 seconds, with the camera anterior to the head. Anterior, posterior, and lateral static images are subsequently obtained; vertex images are often useful. These are obtained by placing the camera at the vertex of the skull. A lead collar is employed to exclude radiation from radiopharmaceutical localized below the neck. Immediate static images are useful to evaluate blood pool abnormalities, while delayed static images after clearance of background activity are of greater value to detect breakdown of the blood-brain barrier.

Interpretation. Interpretation of static images depends primarily upon detecting or excluding radiopharmaceutical localization within the brain parenchyma. Some activity is invariably present from the radiopharmaceutical within the soft tissues of the scalp and within intracerebral blood vessels. Increased or asymmetric localization indicates breakdown of the blood-brain barrier. This finding is entirely nonspecific, being present in conditions as diverse as cerebral infarction, primary or metastatic tumor, and infectious processes. For this reason, clinical information is essential for interpretation. The presence of a lenticular photoenhanced (or occasionally photopenic) rim can be used to diagnose subdural hematoma.

The normal radionuclide angiogram is characterized by prompt symmetric perfusion. Asymmetric flow in the carotid arteries may indicate occlusive disease. The so-called flip-flop sign (decreased activity in the arterial phase, increased activity in the venous phase) may be seen in carotid occlusion. Vascular malformations, high-grade or vascular tumors, such as glioblastoma multiforme and meningioma, and inflammatory processes have increased flow. Low-grade or benign tumors, areas of porencephaly or edema, and occlusive processes have decreased flow. The complete absence of brain activity in the presence of prompt common carotid and scalp flow indicates brain death (1).

The traditional brain scan has largely been superseded by other techniques in current clinical practice, but still have a limited diagnostic role in the evaluation of brain death in potential organ transplant donors. There is little doubt that more modern brain radiopharmaceuticals such as Tc-99m-hexamethylpropylamine oxine (HMPAO) are capable of providing the same information. They are also much simpler to interpret although significantly more costly to perform.

CEREBROSPINAL FLUID STUDIES

Cerebrospinal fluid (CSF) is formed in the choroid plexus as an ultrafiltrate of plasma. It flows from the ventricles through the foramina of the fourth ventricle and ascends over the convexities of the brain to be absorbed predominantly by the arachnoid villa. Processes that impede flow over the convexities or absorption of the fluid by the villi result in communicating hydrocephalus. Tracer techniques are ideal for imaging of this process, because they are injected in small amounts and do not alter the CSF flow. Processes that obstruct the outflow from a ventricle are more difficult to assess by these techniques because injection must be made directly into the ventricle. Patency and flow in therapeutic shunts and reservoirs can easily be evaluated by injecting tracer directly into the device.

Radiopharmaceuticals and Technique. The standard cisternogram is performed by intrathecal injection of a sterile, pyrogen-free radiopharmaceutical. The only approved agent currently marketed for this purpose is indium-111 DTPA (half-life = 2.8 days). The injection of 0.5 mCi follows a spinal tap performed in the standard manner. Initial images may be obtained to ensure intrathecal injection. Subsequently, the radiopharmaceutical ascends to the basilar cisterns in approximately 4 hours and flows over the convexities within 24 hours in a normal individual. Images of the basilar cisterns are obtained at 4–6 hours. If images at 24 hours show ascent over the convexities with activity in the interhemispheric fissure and relative clearance of the basilar cisterns, imaging may be terminated. Otherwise, images should be obtained at 48 and 72 hours (2).

Shunt and reservoir studies are performed by direct injection of the device with 0.5 mCi In-111-DTPA in a small volume. Maintenance of sterile techniques during the injection is critical. It is also critical to understand the specific device being evaluated, as shunts often contain check valves and reservoir capacities are limited. A patient may also have several shunt tubes, some of which may be known to be occluded. In general, it is best to have direct input from the neurosurgeon involved in the case to ensure that the maximum amount of information is obtained (3).

Application to Hydrocephalus. Standard cisternography is performed primarily to evaluate for normal pressure hydrocephalus and for CSF leak. Normal pressure hydrocephalus is a form of communicating hydrocephalus classically associated with ataxia, dementia, and urinary incontinence. Cisternography demonstrates early localization of activity within the lateral ventricles, persisting beyond 24 hours, and delayed clearance over the convexities. While these findings indicate an increased likelihood of a clinical response to shunting, they neither definitively establish the diagnosis nor reliably predict the outcome of shunting (4). Other forms of communicating hydrocephalus (such as might result from radiation therapy or intrathecal chemotherapy) can also be evaluated with cisternography.

Application to CSF Leak. Cisternography has high sensitivity for CSF leak and remains the procedure of choice for this condition. The sensitivity results from the ability of tracer technique to detect very small amounts of activity. Imaging is performed between 1 and 3 hours after injection. Patient and camera position are chosen to maximize the likelihood of detection, with lateral views for CSF rhinorrhea and anterior views for CSF otorrhea. Cotton pledgets should be placed in the nostrils when evaluating CSF rhinorrhea. These are counted at 4–6 hours in a well counter. A serum sample from peripheral blood drawn concurrently is also counted. Pledget activity exceeding 1.5 times the serum concentration is evidence for CSF rhinorrhea (5).

Application to Shunts and Reservoirs. Shunts are evaluated primarily for patency. If the proximal portion is occluded manually (or contains a check valve), flow through the distal limb can be evaluated. The tracer should flow freely into the peritoneum (for ventriculoperitoneal shunts) or atrium (for ventriculoatrial shunts). Delayed flow or persistent activity at the shunt tip suggests malfunction. Diffusion will typically allow determination of the level of obstruction even when flow is absent. Reservoir injection tests for proper placement, patency, and proper functioning of the reservoir. If the reservoir empties directly into the ventricle (such as an Omaya shunt placed for intrathecal chemotherapy), noncommunicating hydrocephalus may be excluded by

normal progression of activity to the basilar cisterns and over the convexities. Ventriculospinal shunts may be evaluated only by direct injection of radiopharmaceutical into the ventricle.

FUNCTIONAL BRAIN IMAGING

Radiotracer techniques may be employed to evaluate blood flow in cerebral microvasculature. Agents suitable for this purpose include diffusable radiotracers such as xenon-133, tracers which are actively taken up by neural tissues, and tracers which effectively function as "ideal microspheres." True microspheres that lodge in and thus obstruct capillaries are contraindicated as they would create a stroke. Therefore, these agents must cross the blood-brain barrier and be permanently retained by some chemical process such as ionic trapping, nonspecific protein binding, or chemical breakdown. Glucose consumption and blood flow are linked in normally functioning brain tissues and in most pathologic processes. Therefore, the relative localization of these agents in various cortical tissues gives a reasonable qualitative indication of relative function.

Positron Emission Tomography Brain Imaging

Receptor Imaging. The paradigmatic technique for performance of in vivo biochemical and functional evaluation of the brain is positron emission tomography (PET). This technique allows qualitative or quantitative evaluation of receptor systems within the brain. Adrenergic, cholinergic, dopaminergic, serotonergic, benzodiazepine and opioid receptors have been extensively evaluated. PET allows true biochemical assessment of the properties of these receptor systems, such as affinity, saturation, and non-specific bindings, as well as more general information about distribution and uptake kinetics. These unique capabilities of the PET technique provide an extremely valuable research tool for evaluation of brain biochemistry and development of both imaging agents and pharmaceuticals. However, these studies are expensive, experimental and time-consuming. Experimental uses should be clearly differentiated from proven clinical indications; the associated ethical issues have been assessed and summarized by the Brain Imaging Council of the Society of Nuclear Medicine (6)

Metabolic Imaging with F-18-Fluorodeoxyglucose (F18-FDG). Clinical indications for PET almost exclusively involve F18-FDG, although a tailored examination with other agents may be warranted in evaluating the status of some brain tumors (7). The primary clinical indications are evaluation of epilepsy, dementia and glioma. PET use in epilepsy is predominantly in the presurgical evaluation of mesial temporal lesions resulting in partial complex seizures. Approximately 85% of these can be cured surgically if the focus of the abnormal brain is limited to a single temporal lobe. F18-FDG scanning must be performed interictally in seizure patients, as the 1.83 hour half-life of F-18 does not allow it to be held available for ictal scanning. Interictally, the seizure focus is hypometabolic. This is now thought to be due to interruption of connections with adjacent neurons which reduces neural activity and thus metabolism. Loss of neural connections can also result in decreased metabolism in more distant sites (diaschisis). Sites of temporal lobe epilepsy are identified as hypometabolic foci in 70% of interictal scans with a false positive rate of only 5% (8). Dementia evaluation is predominantly performed to separate dementia of the Alzheimer's type from other causes of dementia and from pseudodementia due to depression. While the only unequivocal test remains brain biopsy, detection of Alzheimer's disease is very reliable when applied to an appropriate population at risk. Patterns of activity with F18-FDG are similar to those described for SPECT agents subsequently in this review. The role of PET and SPECT scanning in evaluation of brain tumors has been discussed in the chapter on oncologic scintigraphy (chapter 62), and will not be repeated here. While PET is certainly a useful technique in each of these conditions, there are techniques available for SPECT imaging in each of these conditions which have similar sensitivity and specificity at decreased cost. Since both SPECT cameras and the appropriate imaging pharmaceuticals are more widely available than PET cameras and pharmaceuticals, SPECT is likely to occupy the predominant role in routine clinical application of functional brain imaging, with PET reserved for special circumstances. For this reason, the technique and interpretation of these studies is not discussed in detail. The interested reader is referred to one of the many excellent reviews available for PET brain imaging (9).

Single Photon Emission Computed Tomography

Radiopharmaceuticals. Much of the early work in this area was performed with xenon-133. This inhaled gas dissolves in blood to an extent adequate for imaging. The rapidity of perfusion and diffusion of this agent makes rapid imaging essential. Therefore, multiprobe-type cameras have predominantly been employed. This tracer is not well suited to rotating camera SPECT techniques. For this reason, and because of difficulties in handling and recovering a gaseous agent, this agent has largely been superseded by other radiopharmaceuticals.

Iodinated amphetamines tagged with iodine-123 replaced radioxenon for a time. These agents readily cross the blood-brain barrier. Both uptake and blood-brain barrier diffusion are reversible. This agent, therefore, will slowly redistribute over time. Iodoamphetamine (iofetamine) is also immediately sequestered by and slowly released from the lung. This effectively yields slow intraarterial injection over a period of hours. Because of these phenomena, iodoamphetamine images represent integration of all brain activity from the time of injection until completion of imaging. Because iodine-123 is cyclotron-produced and has a relatively short half-life (13.2 hours), availability proved problematic. This precluded use of these agents for ictal scanning of seizures. This agent also has been largely superseded. Agents currently in widespread use include Tc-99m labeled hexamethylproplyeneamine oxime (exametazine/HMPAO) and ethyl cisteinate dimer (bicisate/ECD).

Tc-99m-HMPAO is an agent of the "ideal microsphere" type. This agent crosses the blood-brain barrier and is trapped within the brain substance. The mechanisms proposed for trapping have included change in ionic state, binding to glutathione, and chemical decomposition (10). For purposes of scan interpretation, it is only necessary to understand that the agent essentially crosses the blood-brain barrier irreversibly. Unlike iodinated amphetamine, this agent provides a "snapshot" of brain activity for a short period after injection (approximately 10 minutes). The HMPAO is available as a kit that is combined with generator-produced pertechnetate prior to use. Availability is thus not problematic. The initial form of this agent was unstable in aqueous solution. It must be used immediately after preparation, which makes quality control procedures difficult. A stabilized form is now available which can be used for 4 hours after aqueous preparation.

Tc-99m-ECD is also an agent of the "ideal microsphere" type (11). This agent, unlike Tc-99m-HMPAO, does not localize in areas of luxury perfusion. While there are extensive subtle differences between this agent and HMPAO, the remaining differences are not of routine clinical relevance. Tc-99m-ECD is stable in aqueous solution for 6 hours and is therefore preferable when attempting ictal scanning of seizure disorders. This advantage is offset by higher pharmaceutical cost. Both agents have their proponents and are in common use (12).

Technique. Iofetamine and HMPAO scans are preferably performed with a triple-head rotating gamma camera. A dual head rotating camera can be employed, but single head cameras are not generally recommended at this time. Cameras limited to brain work are not generally necessary due to improvements in equipment since the first edition of this book, although they may be useful in practices with a large brain scanning referral base. High resolution collimators should be employed (13). The key issues are distance from the brain to the detector head and total counts acquired.

Prior to the procedure, the physician or an assistant should fill out a scanning worksheet consisting of history, brief neurologic physical examination and a mini mental status examination. Since the number of possible perfusion patterns is relatively small, it is important to be able to correlate these appropriately to the clinical situation. Historical data of importance include symptoms and duration, history of stroke, head injury or seizure, any medications (especially neurotropic or siezure medications), and whether CT or MR scans have been performed. Neurologic examination should include cognitive and motor examination and cranial nerve examination. Mental status examination should address orientation, registration, attention, recall and language functions.

The scanning agent is injected with the patient in a controlled stimulus state. This usually involves a supine, resting patient with closed eyes in a quiet room (or a room with white noise) and indirect lighting. The intravenous line should be established in advance and all instructions and questions should be dealt with prior to injection to avoid unintended stimulation of brain activity. The patient should remain in this controlled environment for at least 5 minutes after injection. 15–30 mCi of Tc-99m-HMPAO or Tc-99m-ECD should be employed (0.2–0.3 mCi/kg in pediatric patients). A delay after injection of no less than 60 minutes and preferably 90 minutes should be employed with Tc-99m-HMPAO, to allow for background clearance. No less than 30 minutes and preferably 60 minutes should elapse for Tc-99m-ECD. Quality control on the radiopharmaceutical should be performed prior to injection, according to the package insert. Careful patient monitoring is mandatory throughout the scan, since patients considered for the study by necessity have dementia, neurologic dysfunction, stroke, psychiatric disease, or another condition which would require monitoring.

If sedation is required, it should be given after injection of the radiopharmaceutical if at all possible. Attention to medications is critical, since both presence of and withdrawal from (prescription and illicit) drugs can affect biodistribution of the tracer within the brain. ECD or stabilized HMPAO should be prepared in advance if ictal scanning is to be attempted. The patient must be carefully and continuously monitored and injected very rapidly after seizure onset, since generalization of seizure foci can occur very rapidly. If acetazolamide (Diamox) is employed to assess vasodilatory reserve, this should be given as a slow IV push 15–20 minutes prior to radiotracer injection. The typical dosage is 1000 mg for adults and 14 mg/kg for children. This agent is *contraindicated* with known sulfa drug allergy, history of migraine headache, or within three days of acute stroke. It may cause postural hypotension, increasing the need for monitoring when arising from the scanning table. Dipyridamol has also been used to assess vascular reserve (14). All patients should void immediately prior to imaging to improve comfort. This is especially important when using acetazolamide, which is a diuretic.

Processing and Interpretation.
Filtering should be performed in all three dimensions. A low-pass filter is generally recommended, typically a Butterworth. Other filters can be used, but spatially varying filters may create artifacts. The whole brain should be reconstructed, taking care to include the vertex and cerebellum. Any summing of data should occur only after reconstruction at maximum resolution. Attenuation correction should always be performed and data should be evaluated in three orthogonal planes. It is also important to evaluate the raw data for acquisition errors. These should be evaluated on rotating display to check for patient motion during acquisition, which can also create serious artifacts. Rigorous quality control is required for these as well as other SPECT studies. A typical normal study is demonstrated in Figure 63.1.

In interpretation, it is important that background subtraction not be excessive and that a continuous color scale (or a continuous gray scale) be employed to avoid artifactual edges. The range of normal should be considered in rendering an opinion. Correlation with clinical data is required. Any regional perfusion defects should also be correlated with the positions of any CT or MR abnormalities. This is substantially easier if some type of fusion imaging (overlay of anatomic and functional images with or without the use of fiduciary markers) (15) is

employed, but can be performed visually. Extent and severity of defects should be reported.

The recommendations for image acquisition, processing and interpretation conform generally and specifically to the recommendations of the Brain Imaging Council of the Society of Nuclear Medicine current at the time this chapter was written. Readers are encouraged to check the current guidelines prior to initiating a brain imaging program.

Indications.
According to the American Academy of Neurology (AAN), the established indications for this technique are confirmation of Alzheimer's disease, presurgical ictal identification of seizure foci, and evaluation of acute brain ischemia (16). Use in brain death is considered promising but not established, apparently on the basis that the need for SPECT rather than planar imaging is not established. Most nuclear medicine physicians in clinical practice would consider brain death evaluation to be an established indication. Areas considered promising by the AAN are determination of stroke subtypes, assessment of vasospasm following subarachnoid hemorrhage, and (non-ictal) localization of seizure foci. The lack of viable therapeutic options in many of the conditions for which brain SPECT appears suited has certainly contributed to the lack of expansion of these indications. For this reason, the expansion of research into use of brain SPECT in psychiatric disorders (17), where therapeutic options are broad but objective evaluation of biologic aspects of the diseases is extremely weak, is especially promising. The remainder of the discussion will be limited primarily to the accepted indications, with brief discussion of other applications considered promising, applications to pre-surgical planning (balloon occlusion test and Wada test) and testing of vascular reserve.

APPLICATIONS

Stroke and Ischemia.
The extent of a stroke can be determined a short time after its occurrence with functional brain scanning (Figs. 63.2, 63.3, color plates). Sensitivities of 61–74% and specificities of 88–98% are reported in prospective blinded trials (18). This contrasts with several hours for MR (19) and days for CT (20), respectively. Molecular diffusion imaging may allow improved MR assessment of strokes acutely (21). Therapeutic administration of tissue plasminogen activator (TPA) is effective, but the time between initial onset and therapy is critical. The time of onset must be established and hemorrhagic stroke excluded prior to administration of TPA. CT is employed to radiply exclude hemorrhage and administration is begun as soon thereafter as possible (22). Functional imaging has not been widely employed on the theory it would delay therapy when stroke has already been confirmed clinically. Therapy of acute stroke has otherwise been limited to anticoagulation and supportive care. Anticoagulation requires only exclusion of hemorrhage, which is best accomplished with CT.

The use of functional imaging to confirm ischemia due to vasospasm after subarachnoid hemorrhage is very likely to see widespread use. Vasospasm of clinical significance occurs in 30% of patients after subarachnoid

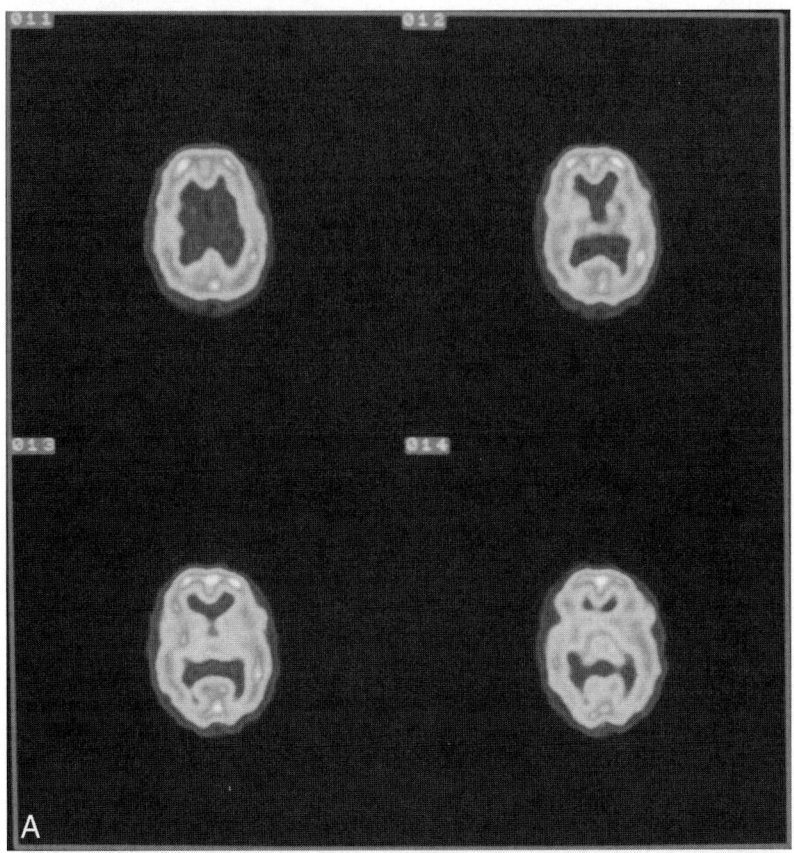

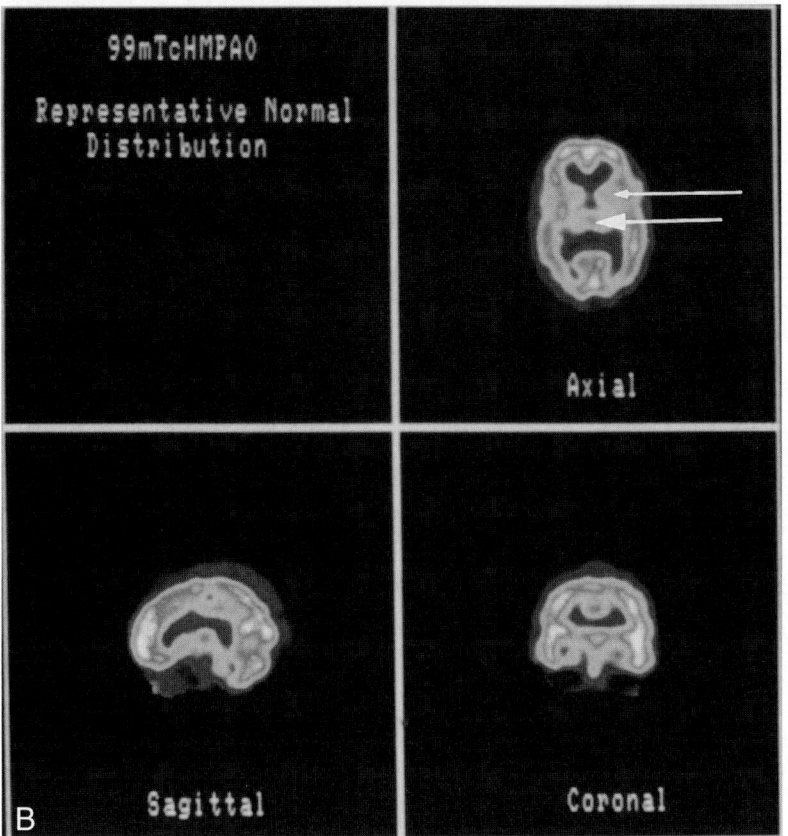

Figure 63.1. (Color Plates) Normal Study. Selected images from a normal Tc-99m-HMPAO study. **A.** Axial images. **B.** Representative central images in three standard planes (axial, sagittal, and coronal to long axis of brain). *Large arrow* indicates the brainstem; *small arrow* indicates the basal ganglia. With modern equipment, it should be possible to routinely obtain scans which resolve gyri, basal ganglia, and brainstem. Interpreters should consult an atlas to familiarize themselves with the normal distribution of radiotracer in the brain structures.

Figure 63.2. (Color Plates) Cerebral Infarction. Transaxial images reformatted into the plane of the orbitomeatal line (standard CT format) from a I-123-iofetamine scan show a large region of absent perfusion (*arrows*) in the distribution of the left middle cerebral artery after cerebral infarction. Note the decreased cerebellar activity on the side opposite the infarct (*arrow*), an example of crossed cerebellar diaschisis. This phenomenon results from decreased right cerebellar metabolism due to decreased neuronal communication between the right cerebellum and the infarcted portion of the left cerebral hemisphere. (All iofetamine images in this chapter were obtained during phase III trials of the agent under approved protocol. Modern equipment allows significant improvement in resolution.)

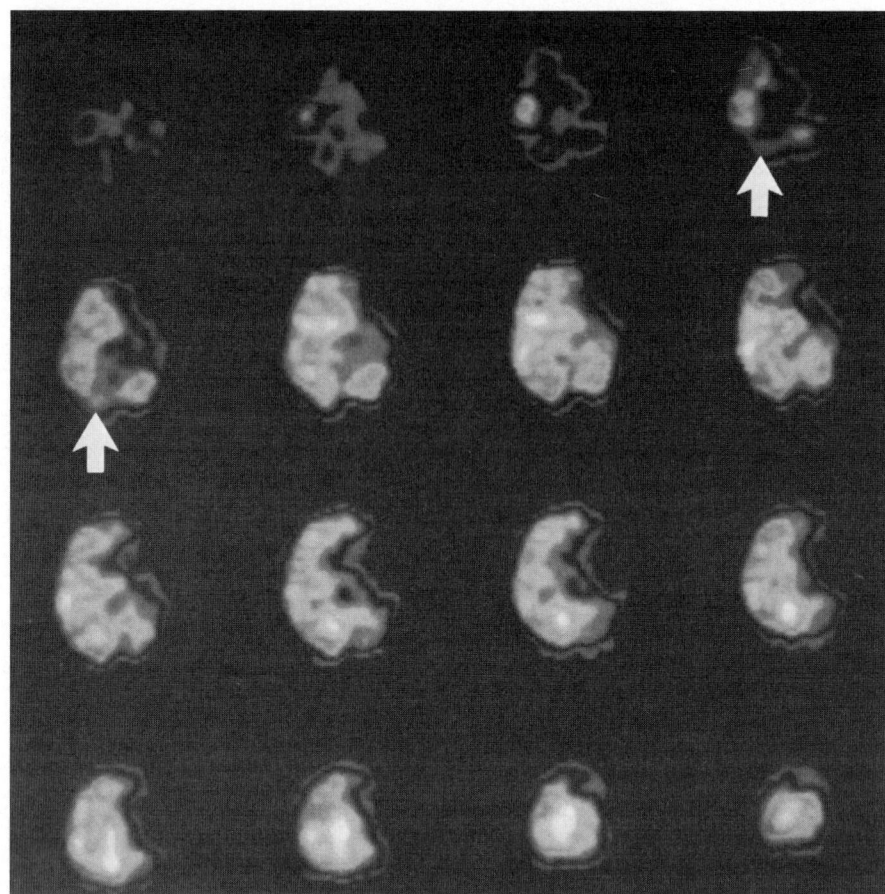

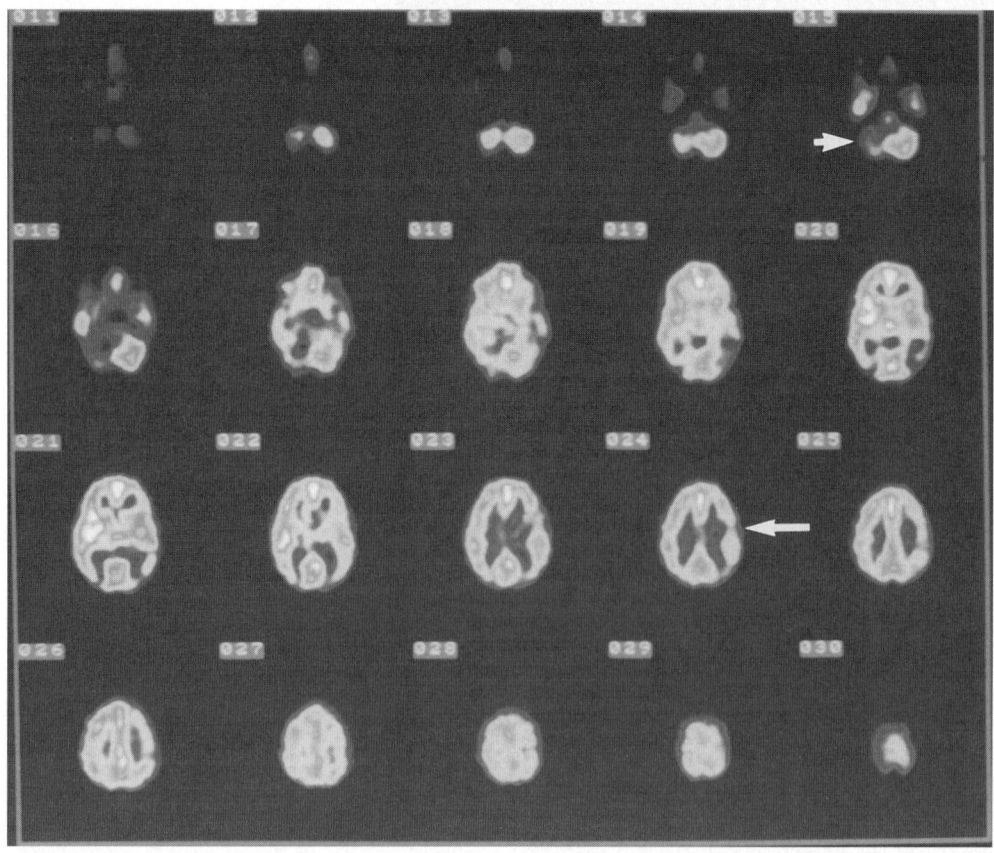

Figure 63.3. (Color Plates) Crossed Cerebral Diaschisis. After right cerebellar infarction (*arrowhead*), regional cerebral blood flow is reduced in left cerebrum (*arrow*). Radiopharmaceutical is 99m-Tc–HMPAO.

hemorrhage. SPECT brain imaging in association with neurologic examination and and transcranial doppler allows effective non-invasive monitoring and early intervention (23–25). As there are multiple potential therapies (hyperdynamic hypertension, hemodilution and hypervolemia, calcium channel blockers, micro-balloon cerebral angioplasty, intra-arterial papavarine) which require definitive diagnosis, this technique has significant clinical potential. In patients with hemispheric stroke, a normal brain SPECT study is an indication of lacunar infarction. Using this criterion, SPECT was 69% sensitive and 100% specific in identifying a lacunar stroke (26). Early differentiation is important, since embolic disease should prompt cardiac evaluation for a source and consideration of anticoagulant therapy. Prediction of prognosis after stroke or TIA is another area of likely application. Lesion volume correlates with early outcome in acute stroke (27) and large, severe perfusion defects are predictive of non-nutritive reperfusion (28). After transient ischemic attack (TIA), a prolonged deficit on functional scanning predicts high likelihood of ischemic stroke in the period following the TIA (29).

By judicious use of acetazolamide to test vasodilatory reserve of cerebral vessels it is possible to perform the equivalent of pharmacologic coronary stress imaging with thallium-210 for cerebral vessels. Studies with and without acetazolamide may provide information on the mechanism of ischemia (30). These studies may also be useful in presurgical planning when carotid surgery or intracranial/extracranial bypass surgery is contemplated because they can indicate the physiologic signifi-

cance of an anatomic vascular lesion. Interpretation of these studies depends on identification of a significant area of relatively decreased perfusion (actually indicating increased perfusion in the unaffected portions of the brain) after stimulation which was not present on the study without stimulation. This is exactly analogous to evaluation of coronary artery reserve with dipyridamol thallium-201 imaging as discussed in Chapter 57. The acetazolamide challenge study should be performed first, as a negative study with challenge precludes the need for the baseline study. As with coronary studies, evaluation of clinical data, accurate registration of images, and comparison to a normal database are important.

Injection during vascular occlusion of a carotid artery can test cross-circulation across the circle of Willis, demonstrating the precise areas of decreased perfusion during occlusion. This is the nuclear medicine version of the Matas test (31–33). (Figs. 63.4, 63.5, color plates). The distribution of amobarbital injected for localization of speech and memory functions (the Wada test) may also be assessed accurately using functional agents as tracers (34).

Dementia. Alzheimer's disease can be diagnosed with an accuracy of approximately 80% with functional brain scans (35). The typical pattern is decreased activity in parietal and posterior temporal regions bilaterally and symmetrically (Fig. 63.6, color plates). Logically, a positive diagnosis would be preferable to the tedious and low-yield procedures employed to exclude reversible causes of dementia. Unfortunately, the pattern of perfu-

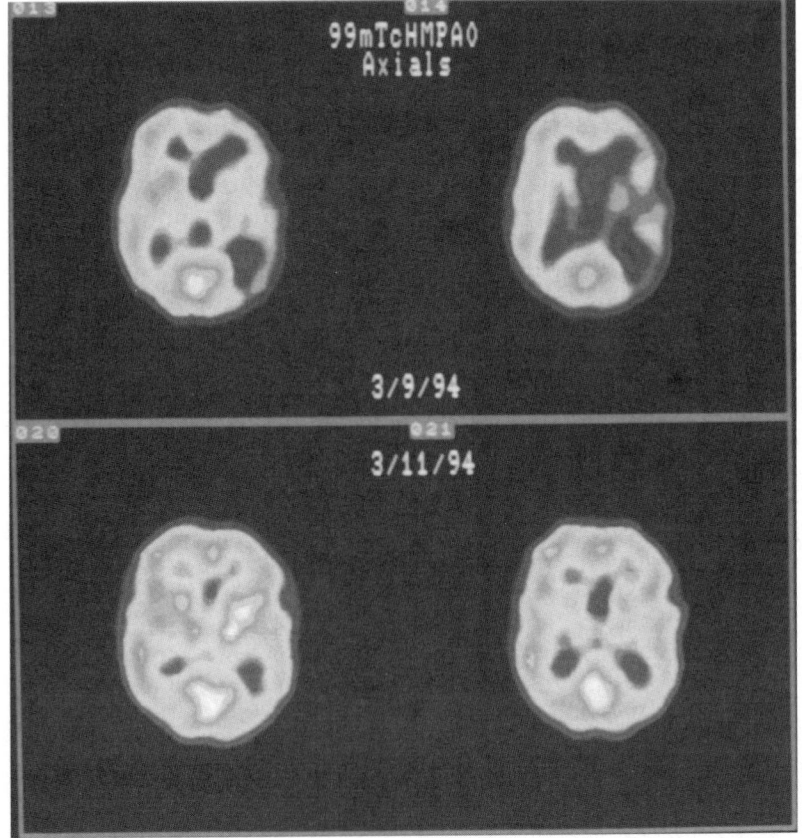

Figure 63.4. (Color Plates) Positive Balloon Occlusion Study. This patient was asymptomatic after inflation of the left carotid artery balloon, but images show decreased regional blood flow in the left middle cerebral artery distribution (*upper images*). Baseline study (*lower images*) shows normal tracer distribution. If occlusion study had been normal, the baseline images would be omitted. Radiopharmaceutical is Tc-99m–HMPAO.

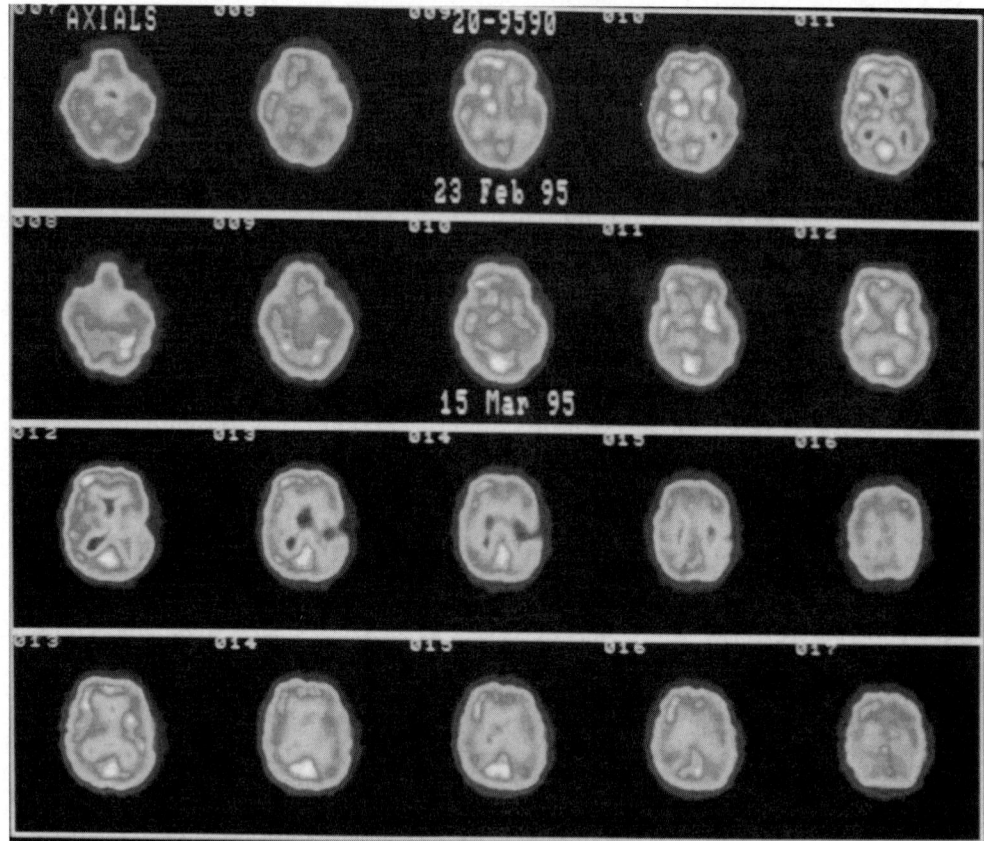

Figure 63.5. (Color Plates) Catheter-induced Resolving Ischemic Neurologic Deficit (RIND). This patient became aphasic with catheterization prior to balloon occlusion study of the left carotid artery (*first and third rows*). Images reveal marked decrease in left middle cerebral artery distribution regional blood flow. Images two weeks later, after resolution of aphasia, show normal distribution of tracer (*second and fourth rows*, matched with previous study). Radiopharmaceutical is Tc–99m–HMPAO.

sion defects in Alzheimer's disease is variable and nonspecific. The findings may be asymmetrical and may involve one or both frontal lobes. The classic bitemporoparietal defect of Alzheimer's can also be seen in other conditions including carbon monoxide poisoning, hypoglycemia, mitochondrial encephalomyelopathy, and other dementias. Functional brain SPECT therefore does not provide a pathognomonic diagnosis of the disease. Frontotemporal lobe degeneration (including the subtype Pick's disease) can generally be differentiated from Alzheimer's disease. Frontotemporal lobe degeneration is classically associated with frontotemporal perfusion defects on brain SPECT (36). Again, the pattern is not specific to this group of diseases. Vascular dementias can result in defects in any portion of the brain and can coexist with Alzheimer's disease in a large proportion of the elderly. Further complicating the picture is an increasing tendency for non-specific defects to occur in older patients, especially as a result of sulcal enlargement due to brain atrophy. The evaluation of dementia is therefore not straightfoward and may require anatomic as well as functional imaging.

With so many potential pitfalls and so few treatable causes of dementia, it might seem pointless to perform brain SPECT in the demented patient. However, there is a substantial clinical overlap between elderly patients with Alzheimer's disease, vascular dementia and pseudodementia due to depression. The functional scan may provide confirmation of the diagnosis of Alzheimer's disease. If the scan is unremarkable, a diagnosis of depression is much more likely and a trial of antidepressants may be indicated. Unfortunately, focal defects are more common in depressed, elderly patients. Vascular disease which is potentially reversible can be unmasked by administration of acetazolamide before scanning. The likelihood of development of etiologically specific therapies for at least some dementias remains high, making continued investigation of diagnostic techniques of utmost importance. Follow up scans improve sensitivity and specificity by demonstrating an appropriate pattern of progression in true dementias.

Seizure Disorders. Interictally, seizure foci tend to have a large aura or penumbra of decreased activity (Fig. 63.7,color plates). In simplistic terms, focal neuronal loss or damage result in a local phenomenon similar to diaschisis. (The actual situation is more complex and beyond the scope of this article.) Ictally, seizure foci have markedly increased blood flow and activity. Because of secondary activation and spread of the seizure foci, it is difficult to pinpoint the exact seizure focus unless injection can be made almost immediately after onset of the seizure. However, ictal SPECT may identify seizure foci

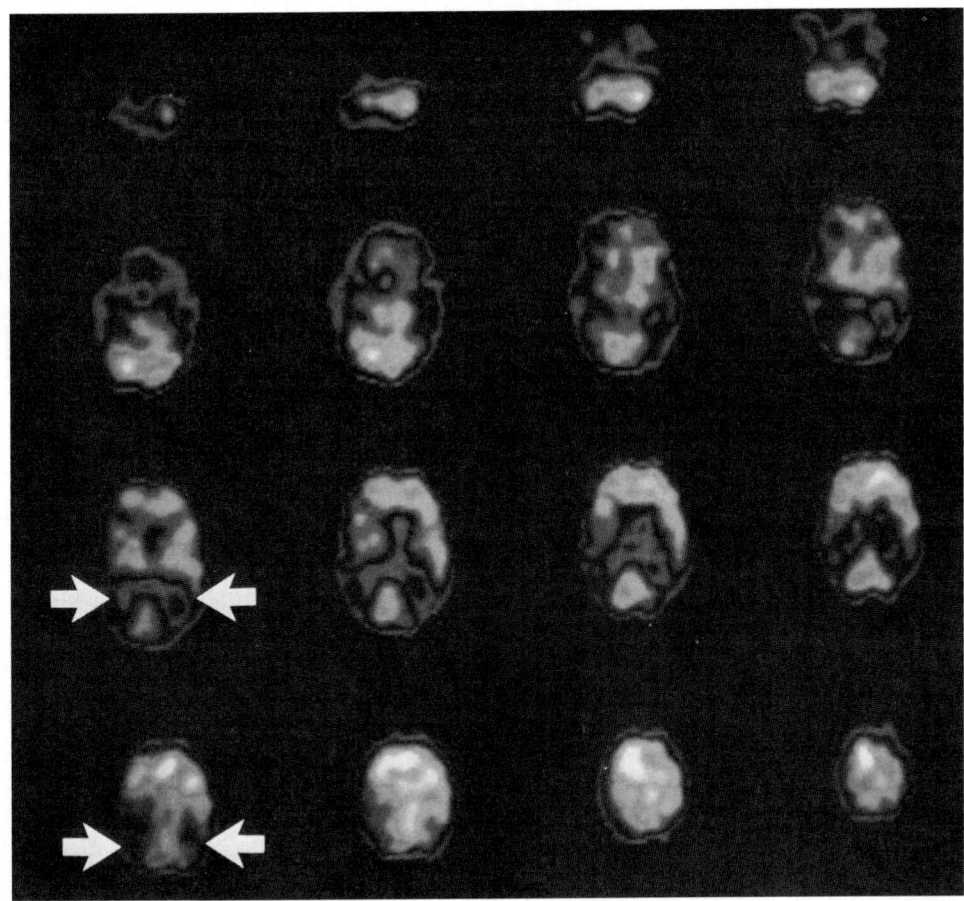

Figure 63.6. (Color Plates) Alzheimer's Dementia. An I–123–iofetamine scan in axial plane demonstrates bilateral decreased flow in the parietal and posterior temporal regions (*arrows*).

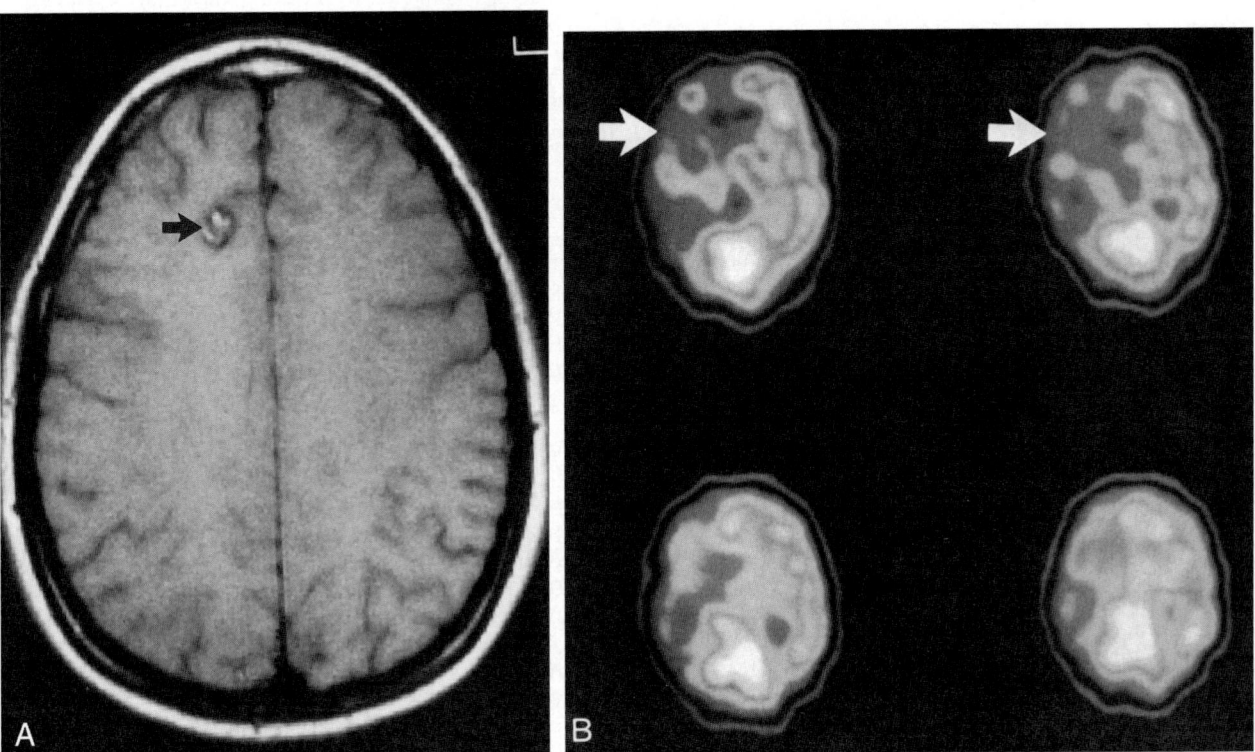

Figure 63.7. (Color Plates) Seizure Focus. A. Intermediate–weighted (proton density) MR image reveals prominent mixed signal right frontal lobe lesion (*arrow*), consistent with cavernous hemangioma. The patient suffers from a frontal lobe seizure disorder. **B.** Interictal I–123–iofetamine scan from the same patient shows an area of depressed flow/function (*arrows*) much larger than the underlying anatomic lesion.

which are not identified by MR and is especially useful in epileptogenic cortical developmental disorders (37), where electroencephalograms (EEG) often fail to identify the epileptogenic focus (38). An ictal SPECT study showing an area of increased regional blood flow which corresponds to an area of decreased regional blood flow on interictal SPECT is strong evidence for an epileptogenic lesion. If these findings also concur with the EEG findings and/or CT/MR evidence of a lesion, the need for more invasive depth electrocorticography or intraoperative electrocorticography may be obviated. For this indication, the technique will be applied mainly in larger referral centers that perform surgery for removal of seizure foci.

Brain Death criteria for Tc-99m-HMPAO scanning have been retrospectively validated (39). A flow study can be performed to give information equivalent to that obtained with DTPA. Additionally, the presence or absence of deposition of radiopharmaceutical in both supratentorial and infratentorial brain structures can be assessed.

SPECT imaging has been proposed to confirm the presence of an actual injury in patients with persistent symptoms after trauma but normal anatomic imaging studies. The increased sensitivity of functional SPECT relative to CT or MR favors this use, but this application is still considered investigational.

Readers interested in a more comprehensive discussion of functional brain imaging are referred to book length reviews cited below.

References

1. Bonetti MG, Ciritella P, Valle G, Perrone E. 99mTc HM–PAO brain perfusion SPECT in brain death. Neurology 1995;37:365–369.
2. Harbert JC. Radionuclide cisternography. Semin Nucl Med 1971;1:90–106
3. Harbert JC. Radionuclide techniques in the evaluation of cerebrospinal fluid shunts. CRC Crit Rev Diagn Imag 1977;9:207–228.
4. Hughes CP, Siegel BA, Coxe WS, et al. Adult idiopathic communicating hydrocephalus with and without shunting. J Neurology Neurosurg Psych 1978;41:961–971.
5. McKusick KA, Malmud LS, Kordela A, et al. Radionuclide cisternography: normal values for nasal secretion of intrathecally injected 111-In-DTPA. J Nucl Med 1973;14:933–934.
6. Society of Nuclear Medicine Brain Imaging Council. Ethical clinical practice of functional brain imaging. J Nucl Med 1996;37:1256–1259.
7. Conti PS. Introduction to imaging brain tumor metabolism with positron emission tomography (PET). Cancer Invest 1995;13:244–259.
8. Messa C, Fazio F, Costa DC, Ell PJ. Clinical brain radionuclide imaging studies. Sem Nucl Med 1995;15:111.
9. Hartshorne ME. Positron emission tomography. In Orrison WW, Lewine JD, Sanders JA, Hartshorne MF, eds. Functional Brain Imaging. St.Louis, MO: Mosby, 1995: pp.187–212.
10. Suess E, Malessa S, Ungersbock K, et al. Technetium-99m-d,l-hexamethylpropyleneamine oxime (HMPAO) uptake and glutathione content in brain tumors. J Nucl Med 1991;32:1675–1681.
11. Leveille J, Demonceau G, Walovitch RC. Intrasubject comparison between technetium–99m-ECD and technetium-99m-HMPAO in healthy human subjects. J Nucl Med1992;33:480–484 and references therein.
12. Moretti JL, Caglar M, Weinmann P. Cerebral perfusion imaging tracers for SPECT: which one to choose? J Nucl Med 1995;36:359–363.
13. Kim HJ, Karp JS, Mozley PD, et.al. Ann Nucl Med.1996;10:153–160.
14. Hwang TL, Saenz A, Farrell JJ, Brannon WL. Brain SPECT with dipyridamole stress to evaluate cerebral blood flow reserve in carotid artery disease. J Nucl Med 1996;37:1595–1599.
15. Pietrzyk U, Herholz K, Schuster A, et.al. Clinical applications of registration and fusion of multimodality brain images from PET, SPECT, CT, and MRI. Eur J Nucl Med 1996;21:174–182.
16. Assessment of brain SPECT: Report of the therapeutics and Technology Assessment Subcommittee of the American Academy of Neurology. Neurology 1996;46:278–285.
17. O'Connell RA. Psychiatric disorders. In Van Heertum RL, Tikofsky RS, eds. Cerebral SPECT Imaging. 2nd ed. Raven Press: New York, 1995.
18. Brass LM, Walovitch RC. Two prospective, blinded, controlled trials of Tc99m bicisate brain SPECT and standard neurological evaluation for identifying and localizing ischemic strokes. J Stroke Cerebrovasc Diseases 1992;1:S59.
19. Alberts MJ, Faulstich ME, Gray L. Stroke with negative brain magnetic resonance imaging. Stroke 1992;23:663–667.
20. Bose A, Pacia SV, Fayad P, et.al. Cerebral blood flow (CBF) imaging compared to CT during the initial 24 hours of cerebral infarction. Neurology 1990;40:190.
21. LeBihan D. Molecular diffusion nuclear magnetic resonance imaging. Mag Res Q 1991;7:1–30.
22. The National Institute of Neurological Disorders and Stroke rt–PA Stroke Study Group, Tissue plasminogen activator for acute ischemic stroke. N Engl J Med 1995; 33:1581–1587.
23. Soucy JP, McNamara D, Mohr G, et al. Evaluation of vasospasm secondary to subarachnoid hemorrhage with Technetium-99m-hexamethyl–propyleneamine oxime (HMPAO) tomoscintigraphy. J Nucl Med 1990;31:972–997.
24. Davis SM, Andrews JT, Lichtenstein M, et al. Correlations between cerebral arterial velocities, blood flow, and delayed ischemia after subarachnoid hemorrhage. Stroke 1992;23:492–497.
25. Lewis DH, Hsu S., Eskridge J, et al. Brain SPECT and transcranial Doppler ultrasound in vasospasm-induced delayed cerebral ischemia after subarachnoid hemorrhage. J Stroke Cerebrovasc Diseases 1992;2:12–21.
26. Brass LM, Walovich RC, Joseph JL, et al. The role of single photon emission computed tomography brain imaging with 99mTc-bicisate in the localization and definition of mechanism of ischemic stroke. J Cereb Blood Flow Metab 1994;14:S91–98.
27. Alexandrov AV, Black SE, Ehrlich LE, et al. Simple visual analysis of brain perfusion on HMPAO SPECT predicts early outcome in acute stroke. Stroke 1996;27:1537–1542.
28. Infield B, Davis SM, Donnan GA, et al. Streptokinase increases luxury perfusion after stroke. Stroke 1996;27:1524–1529.
29. Boboousslavsky J, Delaloye–Bischof A, Regli F, et al.

Prolonged hypoperfusion and early stroke after transient is-chemic attack. Stroke 1990:21:40–46.

30. Chollet F, Celsis P, Clanet M, et al. SPECT study of cere-bral:blood flow reactivity after acetazolamide in patients with transient ischemic attacks. Stroke 1989;20:458–464.

31. Matsuda H, Higashi S, Asli IN, et al. Evaluation of cerebral collateral circulation by technetium–99m HMPAO brain SPECT during Matas test: report of three cases. J Nucl Med 1988;29:1724–1729.

32. Monsein LH, Jeffery PJ, van Heerden BB, et al. Assessing adequacy of collateral circulation during balloon test occlu-sion of the internal carotid artery with 99mTc HMPAO SPECT. AJNR 1991;12:1045–1051.

33. Peterman SB, Taylor A Jr, Hoffman JC Jr. Improved detec-tion of cerebral hypoperfusion with internal carotid baloon occlusion and 99mTc–HMPAO cerebral perfusion SPECT imaging. AJNR 1991;12:1035–1041.

34. Jeffery PJ, Monsein LH, Szabo Z, et al. Mapping the distri-bution of amobarbital sodium in the intracarotid Wada test by use of Tc-99m HMPAO with SPECT. Radiology 1991; 178:847–850.

35. Holman BL, Johnson KA, Gerada B, et al. The scintigraphic appearance of Alzheimers's disease: a prospective study us-ing technetium-99m-HMPAO SPECT. J Nucl Med 1992;33: 181–185.

36. Brun A, Englung B, Gustafson L, et al. Clinical and neu-ropatholgical criteria for frontotemporal dementia. J Neurol Neurosurg Psychiatry 1994;57:416–418.

37. Kuniecky R, Mountz J, Wheatly G, Morawetz R. Ictal sin-gle–photon emission computed tomography demonstrates localized epileptogenesis in cortical dysplasia. Ann Neurol 1993;34:627–631.

38. Palmini A, Andermann F, Olivier A, et al. Focal neuronal migration disorders and intractable partial epilepsy: a study of 30 patients. Ann Neurol 1991;30:741–749.

39. Mrhac L, Zakko S, Parikh Y. Brain death: the evaluation of semi–quantitative parameters and other signs in HMPAO scintigraphy. Nuc Med Commun 1995;16:1016–1020.

Index

Page numbers followed by *t* and *f* indicate tables and figures, respectively.